Infections of the Gastrointestinal Tract

Infections of the Gastrointestinal Tract

Editors

Martin J. Blaser, M.D.
Addison B. Scoville Professor of Medicine
Director, Division of Infectious Diseases
Professor of Microbiology and Immunology
Vanderbilt University School of Medicine;
Nashville VA Medical Center
Nashville, Tennessee

Phillip D. Smith, M.D.
Professor of Medicine and Microbiology
Division of Gastroenterology;
Senior Scientist, Center for AIDS Research
University of Alabama School of Medicine
Birmingham, Alabama

Jonathan I. Ravdin, M.D.
Professor and Vice Chairman
Department of Internal Medicine
Case Western Reserve University;
Chief of Medicine
Cleveland VA Medical Center
Cleveland, Ohio

Harry B. Greenberg, M.D.
Professor of Medicine and Microbiology and
Immunology
Chief of Gastroenterology
Stanford University Medical Center;
Medical Investigator
Palo Alto VA Medical Center
Stanford, California

Richard L. Guerrant, M.D.
Chief, Division of Geographic and International Medicine
University of Virginia Health Sciences Center
Charlottesville, Virginia

Raven Press New York

Raven Press, 1185 Avenue of the Americas, New York, New York 10036

Made in the United States of America

Library of Congress Cataloging-in-Publication Data

Infections of the gastrointestinal tract / editors, Martin J. Blaser
 . . . [et al.].
       p.   cm.
   Includes bibliographical references and index.
   ISBN 0-7817-0226-7
   1. Gastrointestinal system—Infections.   I. Blaser, Martin J.
   [DNLM: 1. Gastrointestinal Diseases.   2. Communicable Diseases.
WI 140 I43 1995]
RC840.I53I54   1995
616.3'3—dc20
DNLM/DLC
for Library of Congress   95-2610
                                                            CIP

9 8 7 6 5 4 3 2 1

*To our families for their patience and
tolerance and to our colleagues, students,
and co-authors who continue to educate us*

Contents

Section 2: Viral Infections

Section 3: Parasitic Infections

Part VIII: Diagnostic Considerations in Gastrointestinal Infections

Part IX: Therapy for Gastrointestinal Infections

Part X: Prevention and Control

Contributors

Sharon L. Abbott
Supervisor in Enteric Bacteriology
Microbial Diseases Laboratory
California Department of Health Services
2151 Berkeley Way
Berkeley, California 94704-1011

David W. K. Acheson M.D.
Assistant Professor of Medicine
Division of Geographic Medicine and
* Infectious Diseases*
Tufts University School of Medicine
New England Medical Center
750 Washington Street
Boston, Massachusetts 02111

Karim A. Adal, M.D., M.Sc.
Fellow, Infectious Diseases
Department of Internal Medicine
University of Virginia Health Sciences
* Center*
Box 385
Charlottesville, Virginia 22908

Ban Mishu Allos, M.D.
Assistant Professor of Medicine and
* Preventive Medicine*
Departments of Medicine and Preventive
* Medicine*
Vanderbilt University School of Medicine
A3310 Medical Center North
Nashville, Tennessee 37232

Anne M. Anglim, M.D.
Fellow, Infectious Diseases
Department of Internal Medicine
University of Virginia Health Sciences
* Center*
Charlottesville, Virginia 22908

Donald Armstrong, M.D.
Professor of Medicine
Department of Medicine
Cornell University Medical College;
Memorial Sloan-Kettering Cancer Center
1275 York Avenue
New York, New York 10021

Stephen S. Arnon, M.D.
Senior Investigator and Chief
Infant Botulism Prevention Program
California Department of Health Services
2151 Berkeley Way
Berkeley, California 94704

John N. Aucott, M.D.
Assistant Professor of Medicine
Department of Medicine
Cleveland Veterans Affairs Medical Center
10701 East Boulevard
Cleveland, Ohio 44106

John G. Banwell, M.D.
Professor of Medicine
Department of Medicine
Case Western Reserve University;
University Hospital of Cleveland
2074 Abington Road
Cleveland, Ohio 44106

Michele Barry, M.D.
Professor of Medicine
Department of Medicine
Co-Director, International Health Program
Yale University School of Medicine
20 York Street
New Haven, Connecticut 06504

John G. Bartlett, M.D.
Professor of Medicine
Department of Medicine
The Johns Hopkins University School of
* Medicine*
Ross Research Building
720 Rutland Avenue
Baltimore, MD 21205

Dorsey M. Bass, M.D.
Assistant Professor
Department of Pediatrics
Stanford University School of Medicine
Stanford, California 94305-5119

A. Dean Befus, B.Sc. (Hon), M.Sc, Ph.D.
Professor of Medicine
Department of Medicine
University of Alberta
Edmonton, AB T6G 2S2
Canada

John E. Bennett, M.D.
Head, Clinical Mycology Section, LCI
National Institute of Allergy and Infectious
  Diseases
National Institutes of Health
9000 Rockville Pike
Bethesda, Maryland 20892

Michael L. Bennish, M.D.
Associate Professor
Departments of Pediatrics and Medicine
Division of Infectious Diseases
Tufts University School of Medicine-New
  England Medical Center
750 Washington Street
Boston, MA 02111

David G. Binion, M.D.
Gastroenterology Research Fellow
Department of Medicine
Case Western Reserve University;
University Hospital of Cleveland
2074 Abington Road
Cleveland, Ohio 44106

Robert Edward Black, M.D., M.P.H.
Professor and Chairman
Department of International Health
The Johns Hopkins University School of
  Hygiene and Public Health
615 North Wolfe Street
Baltimore, Maryland 21205

Neil R. Blacklow, M.D.
Richard M. Haidack Distinguished Professor
  of Medicine
Chairman, Department of Medicine
University of Massachusetts Medical School
55 Lake Avenue North
Worcester, Massachusetts 01655-0317

Martin J. Blaser, M.D.
Addison B. Scoville Professor of Medicine
Professor of Microbiology and Immunology
Vanderbilt University School of Medicine
A-3310 Medical Center North
Nashville, Tennessee 37232

William R. Brown, M.D.
Professor of Medicine
Department of Medicine
Gastroenterology Division
University of Colorado School of Medicine;
Denver Veterans Affairs Medical Center
1055 Clermont Street
Denver, Colorado 80220

Joan R. Butterton, M.Phil., M.D.,
  D.T.M.&H.
Clinical and Research Fellow
Infectious Disease Unit
Massachusetts General Hospital
Fruit Street
Boston, Massachusetts 02114

Steven B. Calderwood, M.D.
Associate Professor of Medicine
(Microbiology and Molecular Genetics)
Harvard Medical School;
Physician and Chief
Infectious Disease Unit
Massachusetts General Hospital
Fruit Street
Boston, Massachusetts 02181

Michael Cappello, M.D.
Postdoctoral Fellow
Department of Infectious Diseases
Yale University School of Medicine
20 York Street
New Haven, Connecticut 06504

John Cello, M.D.
Chief, Division of Gastroenterology
San Francisco General Hospital;
Professor of Medicine
University of California at San Francisco
500 Parnassus Avenue
San Francisco, California 94127

Mary F. Chan, M.D.
Assistant Professor of Medicine
Department of Medicine
Washington University School of Medicine
St. Louis, Missouri 63130

Eugene B. Chang, M.D.
Professor of Medicine and Cell Physiology
Department of Medicine
Gastroenterology Section
University of Chicago
5841 South Maryland Avenue
Chicago, Illinois 60637

Tien-lan Chang, M.D.
Department of Pediatric Gastroenterology
* and Nutrition*
Boston University School of Medicine;
Boston City Hospital
801 Albany Street
Boston, Massachusetts 02118

Judy H. Cho, M.D.
Fellow, Section of Gastroenterology
Department of Medicine
Gastroenterology Section
University of Chicago
5841 South Maryland Avenue
Chicago, Illinois 60637

H. Fred Clark, D.V.M., Ph.D.
Research Professor
Department of Pediatrics
University of Pennsylvania
Childrens Hospital Philadelphia
34th Street and Civic Center Boulevard
Philadelphia, Pennsylvania 19104

Mitchell B. Cohen, M.D.
Associate Professor of Pediatrics and
* Medicine*
Division of Pediatric Gastroenterology and
* Nutrition*
Children's Hospital Medical Center
3333 Burnet Avenue
Cincinnati, Ohio 45229

Mitchell L. Cohen, M.D.
Director, Division of Bacterial and Mycotic
* Diseases*
National Center for Infectious Diseases
Centers for Disease Control and Prevention
1600 Clifton Road
Atlanta, Georgia 30333

Timothy L. Cover, M.D.
Assistant Professor of Medicine
Division of Infectious Diseases
Vanderbilt University School of Medicine
Nashville Veterans Affairs Medical Center
A3310 Medical Center North
Nashville, Tennessee 37232

John K. Crane, M.D., Ph.D.
Assistant Professor of Medicine
Division of Infectious Diseases
BB103 SUNY Clinical Center
462 Grider Street
Buffalo, New York 14215

Sheila E. Crowe, M.D.
Assistant Professor of Medicine
Department of Internal Medicine
Division of Gastroenterology
University of Texas Medical Branch at
* Galveston*
4.111 John Sealy Hospital
301 University Boulevard
Galveston, Texas 77555-0564

Dickson D. Despommier, Ph.D.
Professor of Public Health and Microbiology
Department of Tropical Medicine
School of Public Health
Columbia University
630 West 168th Street
New York, New York 10032

Michael S. Donnenberg, M.D.
Assistant Professor of Medicine
Department of Medicine
Division of Infectious Diseases
University of Maryland School of Medicine;
Medical Services
Baltimore Veterans Affairs Medical Center
10 South Pine Street
Baltimore, Maryland 21201

J. Stephen Dummer, M.D.
Associate Professor of Medicine and
* Surgery*
Departments of Medicine and Surgery
Vanderbilt University Medical Center
911 Oxford House
Nashville, Tennessee 37232

Bruce E. Dunn, M.D., Ph.D.
Associate Professor and Vice Chairman
Department of Pathology
Medical College of Wisconsin;
Chief, Pathology and Laboratory Medicine
* Service (113)*
Clement J. Zablocki Veterans Affairs
* Medical Center*
5000 W. National Avenue
Milwaukee, Wisconsin 53295

Herbert L. DuPont, M.D.
Mary W. Kelsey Professor and Director
Center for Infectious Diseases
The University of Texas-Houston Medical
  School/School of Public Health
6431 Fannin
Houston, Texas 77030

Charles O. Elson, M.D.
Professor of Medicine
Department of Medicine
University of Alabama at Birmingham
845 19th Street South
Birmingham, Alabama 35294

Mary K. Estes, Ph.D.
Professor of Molecular Virology
Department of Molecular Virology
Baylor College of Medicine
1 Baylor Plaza
Houston, Texas 77030-3498

Stanley Falkow, M.D.
Professor of Microbiology and Immunology
Department of Microbiology and
  Immunology
Stanford University School of Medicine
300 Pasteur Drive
Stanford, California 94305-5402

Barry M. Farr, M.D., M.Sc.
William S. Jordan Associate Professor of
  Medicine
Department of Internal Medicine
University of Virginia Health Sciences
  Center
Charlottesville, Virginia 22908

Michael J. G. Farthing, BSc., M.D.
Professor of Gastroenterology
Division of Epidemiology
Digestive Diseases Research Centre
Medical College of St. Bartholomew's
  Hospital
Charterhouse Square
London EC1
United Kingdom

Roger A. Feldman, M.D., F.F.P.H.M.
Professor of Clinical Epidemiology
Department of Epidemiology and Medical
  Statistics
London Hospital Medical College
QMW Campus, Mile End Road
London, E1 4NS
United Kingdom

Sydney M. Finegold, M.D.
Professor of Medicine and Microbiology and
  Immunology
Departments of Medicine and Microbiology
  and Immunology
UCLA School of Medicine;
Staff Physician
Medical Service
West Los Angeles Veterans Affairs Medical
  Center
Wilshire and Sawtelle Boulevards
Los Angeles, California 90073

Janet F. Forstner, M.D., Ph.D.
The Research Institute
Division of Research Biochemistry
The Hospital for Sick Children
555 University Avenue
Toronto, Ontario, M5G 1X8
Canada

Scott L. Friedman, M.D.
Associate Professor of Medicine
Department of Medicine
Division of Gastroenterology
University of California at San Francisco
  School of Medicine;
San Francisco General Hospital
Liver Center Laboratory
San Francisco, California 94110

Glenn T. Furuta, M.D.
Instructor
Department of Pediatric Gastroenterology
Harvard Medical School
300 Longwood Avenue
Boston, Massachusetts 02116

Eugene J. Gangarosa, M.D., M.S.
Professor Emeritus
Emory University School of Public Health
Atlanta, Georgia 30322;
5305 Greencastle Way
Stone Mountain, Georgia 30087-1427

Gabriel Garcia, M.D.
Associate Professor of Medicine
Chief, Clinical Gastroenterology
Department of Medicine
Gastroenterology Division
Stanford University School of Medicine
300 Pasteur Drive
Stanford, California 94305-5202

Robert M. Genta, M.D.
Associate Professor of Pathology, Medicine,
  and Microbiology and Immunology
Baylor College of Medicine;
Associate Professor
Center for Infectious Diseases
University of Texas School of Public Health;
Pathology Service
Houston Veterans Affairs Medical Center
2002 Holcombe Boulevard
Houston, Texas 77030

Karen T. Giannasca, Ph.D.
Postdoctoral Research Fellow
Department of Pediatrics
Harvard Medical School
Children's Hospital
300 Longwood Avenue
Boston, Massachusetts 02115

Paul J. Giannasca, Ph.D.
Postdoctoral Research Fellow
Department of Pediatrics
Harvard Medical School
Children's Hospital
300 Longwood Avenue
Boston, Massachusetts 02115

Ralph A. Giannella, M.D.
Mark Brown Professor of Medicine
Department of Internal Medicine
Director, Division of Digestive Diseases
University of Cincinnati College of Medicine
231 Bethesda Avenue
Cincinnati, Ohio 45267-0595

Roger I. Glass, M.D., Ph.D.
Chief, Viral Gastroenteritis Unit
Centers for Disease Control and Prevention
1600 Clifton Road
Atlanta, Georgia 30333

Ramya Gopinath, M.B.
Fellow, Infectious Diseases
Division of Infectious Diseases
Department of Medicine
The Toronto Hospital;
University of Toronto
200 Elizabeth Street
Room EN G-214
Toronto, Canada M5G 2C4

Sherwood L. Gorbach, M.D.
Professor of Community Health and
  Medicine
Departments of Community Health and
  Medicine
Tufts University School of Medicine
136 Harrison Avenue
Boston, Massachusetts 02111

Gary M. Gray, M.D.
Professor of Medicine
Director, Digestive Disease Center
Department of Medicine
Gastroenterology Division
Stanford University School of Medicine
Stanford, California 94305-5487

Harry B. Greenberg, M.D.
Professor
Departments of Medicine and Microbiology
  and Immunology
Stanford University Medical Center
Palo Alto VA Medical Center
Stanford, California 94304

Patricia M. Griffin, M.D.
Acting Chief
Foodborne Diseases
Epidemiology Section
Foodborne and Diarrheal Diseases Branch
Division of Bacterial and Mycotic Diseases
National Center for Infectious Diseases
1600 Clifton Road
Atlanta, Georgia 30333

Richard L. Guerrant, M.D.
Chief, Division of Geographic and
  International Medicine
University of Virginia Health Sciences
  Center
Box 485
Charlottesville, Virginia 22908

Howard Hack, M.D.
Department of Medicine
Gastroenterology Division
Stanford University School of Medicine
300 Pasteur Drive
Stanford, California 94305

Michele E. Hardy, Ph.D.
Department of Molecular Virology
Baylor College of Medicine
1 Baylor Plaza
Houston, Texas 77030

Frederick P. Heinzel, M.D.
Department of Medicine
Case Western Reserve University;
Medical Service
Cleveland Veterans Affairs Medical Center
10701 East Boulevard
Cleveland, Ohio 44106

John E. Hermann, Ph.D.
Professor of Medicine, Molecular Genetics,
 and Microbiology
Division of Infectious Diseases and
 Immunology
University of Massachusetts Medical School
55 Lake Avenue North
Worcester, Massachusetts 01655

David R. Hill, M.D., D.T.M.&H.
Associate Professor of Medicine
International Traveler's Medical Service
University of Connecticut Health Center
Farmington, Connecticut 06030-3212

Elizabeth L. Hohmann, M.D.
Instructor of Medicine
Infectious Disease Unit
Harvard University;
Massachusetts General Hospital
Fruit Street
Boston, Massachusetts 02114

Gerald Holtmann, M.D.
Department of Gastroenterology
Division of Internal Medicine
University of Essen
Hufelandstr. 55
D-45122 Essen
Germany

Richard B. Hornick, M.D.
Department of Medical Education
Orlando Regional Medical Center
1414 S. Kuhl Avenue
Orlando, Florida 32806

C. Robert Horsburgh, Jr., M.D.
Associate Professor of Medicine
Emory University School of Medicine;
Grady Memorial Hospital
69 Butler Street
Atlanta, Georgia 30335

Peter J. Hotez, M.D., Ph.D.
Assistant Professor of Pediatrics
Department of Pediatrics
Yale University School of Medicine
333 Cedar Street
New Haven, Connecticut 06510

Alexander E. Hromockyj, Ph.D.
Postdoctoral Fellow
Department of Microbiology and
 Immunology
Stanford University School of Medicine
300 Pasteur Drive
Stanford, California 94305-5402

Stephen P. James, M.D.
Head, Division of Gastroenterology
Baltimore Veterans Affairs Medical Center;
Professor of Medicine, Immunology, and
 Microbiology
Department of Medicine
University of Maryland Hospital
22 S. Green Street
Baltimore, Maryland 21201

J. Michael Janda, Ph.D. (ABMM)
Chief, Enterics and Special Pathogens
 Section
Microbial Diseases Laboratory
California Department of Health Services
2151 Berkeley Way
Berkeley, California 94704-1011

Edward N. Janoff, M.D.
Associate Professor of Medicine
Department of Medicine
University of Minnesota;
Veterans Affairs Medical Center
One Veterans Drive
Minneapolis, Minnesota 55417

Caroline C. Johnson, M.D.
Associate Professor of Medicine
Department of Medicine
Medical College of Pennsylvania;
Staff Physician
Infectious Disease Section
Philadelphia Veterans Affairs Medical
 Center
Philadelphia, Pennsylvania 19104

Kevin C. Kain, M.D.
Assistant Professor
Department of Medicine
University of Toronto;
The Toronto Hospital
200 Elizabeth Street
Toronto, Ontario M5G 2C4
Canada

Allen B. Kaiser, M.D.
Professor of Medicine
Department of Medicine
Vanderbilt University Medical Center
D-3100 Medical Center North
Nashville, Tennessee 37232-2358

James B. Kaper, Ph.D.
Professor of Medicine, Microbiology, and
  Immunology
Departments of Medicine, Microbiology, and
  Immunology
Chief, Bacterial Genetics Section
Center for Vaccine Development
University of Maryland School of Medicine
22 South Greene Street
Baltimore, Maryland 21201

John E. Kellow, M.D.
Associate Professor of Medicine
Department of Gastroenterology
Royal North Shore Hospital of Sydney
St. Leonards
NSW 2065
Australia

Douglas S. Kernodle, M.D.
Assistant Professor of Medicine
Department of Medicine
Vanderbilt University School of Medicine
Chief, Infectious Diseases Section
Department Veterans Affairs Medical
  Center;
A-3300 Medical Center North
Nashville, Tennessee 37232-2605

Gerald T. Keusch, M.D.
Division of Infectious Disease
New England Medical Center
750 Washington Street
Boston, Massachusetts 02111

Jay S. Keystone, M.D., M.Sc. (CTM)
Professor of Medicine
University of Toronto;
Tropical Disease Unit
Division of Infectious Diseases
The Toronto Hospital
200 Elizabeth Street
Toronto, Ontario M5G 2C4
Canada

Christopher King, M.D.
Division of Geographic Medicine
Department of Medicine
Case Western Reserve University
University Hospitals of Cleveland
11100 Euclid Avenue
Cleveland, Ohio 44106

Robert E. Koehler, M.D.
Professor of Radiology
Department of Radiology
University of Alabama Hospital
619 South 19th Street
Birmingham, Alabama 35233-6830

Donald P. Kotler, M.D.
Associate Professor of Medicine
Columbia University College of Physicians
  and Surgeons;
Gastrointestinal Division
St. Luke's Roosevelt Hospital Center
421 West 113th Street
New York, New York 10025

Jean-Pierre Kraehenbuhl, M.D.
Professor of Biochemistry
Institute of Biochemistry
University of Lausanne
Membrane Biology Unit
ISREC
Ch. des Boveresses 155
CH-1066 Epalinges
Switzerland

Donald J. Krogstad, M.D.
Henderson Professor and Chair
Department of Tropical Medicine
Tulane School of Public Health and Tropical
  Medicine;
Professor and Chair
Department of Parasitology
Tulane University School of Graduate
  Studies;
Professor of Medicine
Tulane University School of Medicine
1501 Canal Street
New Orleans, Louisiana 70112

Jay A. Ladenheim, M.D.
Clinical Instructor/Staff Physician
Department of Gastroenterology
Sunnyvale Medical Clinic
401 Old San Francisco Road
Sunnyvale, California 94086

Michael E. Lamm, M.D.
Professor and Chairman
Department of Pathology
Case Western Reserve University;
University Hospitals of Cleveland
2085 Adelbert Road
Cleveland, Ohio 44106

Claudio F. Lanata, M.D., M.P.H.
Head, Nutrition and Infection Working
* Group*
Instituto de Investigacion Nutricional
A.P. 18-0191
Lima 18
Peru

Albert J. Lastovica, Ph.D.
Senior Specialist Scientist
Department of Medical Microbiology
Red Cross Children's Hospital
Rondebosch 7700
Cape Town, South Africa

Adrian Lee, B.Sc., Ph.D.
Professor of Medical Microbiology
School of Microbiology and Immunology
University of New South Wales
Sydney, New South Wales 2052
Australia

Myron M. Levine, M.D., D.T.P.H.
Professor of Medicine and Pediatrics
Department of Medicine and Pediatrics
Director, Center for Vaccine Development
University of Maryland Hospital
10 South Pine Street
Baltimore, Maryland 21201

Stuart B. Levy, M.D.
Professor of Molecular Biology and
* Microbiology*
Departments of Molecular/Microbiology and
* Medicine*
Tufts University School of Medicine-New
* England Medical School*
136 Harrison Avenue
Boston, Massachusetts 02111

Steven N. Lichtman, M.D.
Professor of Pediatrics
Division of Pediatric Gastroenterology
Department of Pediatrics
University of North Carolina School of
* Medicine*
Chapel Hill, North Carolina 27599

David M. Lyerly, Ph.D.
Research Scientist
Department of Biochemistry and Anaerobic
* Microbiology*
Virginia Polytechnic Institute and State
* University*
Blacksburg, Virginia 24061

Erich R. Mackow, Ph.D.
Assistant Professor
Departments of Medicine and Microbiology
State University of New York at Stony
* Brook*
Stony Brook, New York 11794;
Northport Veterans Affairs Medical Center
Middleville Road
Northport, New York 11768

Adel A. F. Mahmoud, M.D., Ph.D.
John H. Hord Professor and Chairman
Department of Medicine
Case Western Reserve University;
Physician-in-Chief
University Hospitals of Cleveland
11100 Euclid Avenue
Cleveland, Ohio 44106

Barbara J. Mann, Ph.D.
Assistant Professor
Department of Internal Medicine
University of Virginia School of Medicine
Charlottesville, Virginia 22908

David O. Matson, M.D., Ph.D.
Associate Professor
Department of Pediatrics and Microbiology
* and Immunology*
Eastern Virginia Medical School
855 West Brambleton Avenue
Norfolk, Virginia 23510

Suzanne M. Matsui, M.D.
Assistant Professor of Medicine
Department of Medicine
Stanford University School of Medicine
Stanford, California 94305-5487

Jiri F. Mestecky, M.D.
Professor of Microbiology and Medicine
Department of Microbiology
University of Alabama at Birmingham
845 19th Street South
Birmingham, Alabama 35294-2170

Patricia A. Mickelsen, Ph.D.
Clinical Associate Professor
Department of Medicine
Co-Director, Clinical Microbiology/Virology
Laboratory
Division of Infectious Diseases and
Geographic Medicine
Stanford University Medical Center
300 Pasteur Drive
Stanford, California 94305

Samuel I. Miller, M.D.
Associate Professor of Medicine
Infectious Disease Unit
Harvard University
Massachusetts General Hospital
Fruit Street
Boston, MA 02114

Desiree E. Morgan, M.D.
Instructor
Department of Diagnostic Radiology
University of Alabama Hospital
619 South 19th Street
Birmingham, Alabama 35233-6830

J. Glenn Morris, Jr. M.D., M.P.H.&T.M.
Professor of Medicine and of Epidemiology
and Preventive Medicine
Departments of Medicine and of
Epidemiology and Preventive Medicine
University of Maryland School of Medicine;
Veterans Affairs Medical Center
10 N. Greene Street
Baltimore, Maryland 21201

Jason D. Morrow, M.D.
Assistant Professor of Medicine and
Pharmacology
Department of Medicine and Pharmacology
Vanderbilt University School of Medicine
532 Medical Research Building
Nashville, Tennessee 37232-6602

James P. Nataro, M.D., Ph.D.
Assistant Professor of Pediatrics and
Medicine
Center for Vaccine Development
University of Maryland School of Medicine
10 S. Pine Street
Baltimore, Maryland 21201

Ann Marie Nelson, M.D.
Chief, Division of AIDS Pathology
Department of Infectious and Parasitic
Disease Pathology
Armed Forces Institute of Pathology
Washington, D.C. 20306-6000

Marian R. Neutra, Ph.D.
Professor of Pediatrics
Department of Pediatrics
Harvard Medical School
Children's Hospital
300 Longwood Avenue
Boston, Massachusetts 02115

Kathleen Maletic Neuzil, M.D.
Assistant Professor of Medicine
Department of Medicine
Vanderbilt University School of Medicine
Medical Research Building
Nashville, Tennessee 37232-6605

Richard A. Oberhelman, M.D.
Assistant Professor of Tropical Medicine
Department of Tropical Medicine
Tulane School of Public Health and Tropical
Medicine;
Assistant Professor of Pediatrics
Department of Pediatrics
Tulane University School of Medicine
1501 Canal Street
New Orleans, Louisiana 70112

Paul A. Offit, M.D.
Associate Professor
Department of Pediatrics
The University of Pennsylvania School of
Medicine
The Children's Hospital of Philadelphia
34th Street and Civic Center Boulevard
Philadelphia, Pennsylvania 19104

Mary G. Oliver, M.D.
Research Fellow
The Research Institute
The Hospital for Sick Children
555 University Avenue
Toronto, Ontario M5G 1X8
Canada

Jan M. Orenstein, M.D., Ph.D.
Professor
Department of Pathology
George Washington University School of
* Medicine*
2300 Eye Street, NW
Washington, D.C. 20037

Jani L. O'Rourke, B.Sc.
Project Scientist
School of Microbiology and Immunology
University of New South Wales
Sydney, New South Wales 2052
Australia

Julie Parsonnet, M.D.
Assistant Professor of Medicine and of
* Health Research and Policy*
Departments of Medicine and of Health
* Research and Policy*
Stanford University School of Medicine
Stanford, California 94305-5092

David A. Pegues, M.D.
Research Fellow in Medicine
Infectious Disease Unit
Harvard University
Massachusetts General Hospital
Fruit Street
Boston, Massachusetts 02214

Stephen I. Pelton, M.D.
Professor of Pediatrics
Department of Pediatric Infectious Disease
Boston University School of Medicine-
* Boston City Hospital*
818 Harrison Avenue, Finland 5
Boston, Massachusetts 02118

William A. Petri, Jr., M.D., Ph.D.
Associate Professor
Department of Medicine and Microbiology
University of Virginia
Charlottesville, Virginia 22908

Larry K. Pickering, M.D.
Professor of Pediatrics
Department of Pediatrics
Eastern Virginia Medical School;
Director, Center for Pediatric Research
Children's Hospital of The King's Daughters
855 West Brambleton Avenue
Norfolk, Virginia 23510-1001

Don W. Powell, M.D.
Edward Randall and Edward Randall, Jr.
* Professor and Chairman*
Department of Internal Medicine
Division of Gastroenterology
University of Texas Medical Branch at
* Galveston*
4.108 John Sealy Hospital
301 University Boulevard
Galveston, Texas 77555-0567

Thomas C. Quinn, M.D.
Professor of Medicine
Departments of Medicine and of Infectious
* Diseases*
The Johns Hopkins University School of
* Medicine*
720 Rutland Avenue
Baltimore, Maryland 21205-2196

Jonathan I. Ravdin, M.D.
Professor and Vice Chairman of Medicine
Department of Internal Medicine
Case Western Reserve University;
Chief of Medicine
Cleveland Veterans Affairs Medical Center
10701 East Boulevard
Cleveland, Ohio 44106

Sharon L. Reed, M.D.
Associate Professor of Pathology and
* Medicine*
Department of Pathology and Medicine,
Director of Microbiology Laboratory
University of California at San Diego
* Medical Center*
200 W. Arbor Drive
San Diego, California 92103-8416

David A. Relman, M.D.
Assistant Professor of Medicine and of
* Microbiology and Immunology*
Departments of Medicine (Infectious
* Diseases and Geographic Medicine) and*
* of Microbiology and Immunology*
Stanford University School of Medicine;
Palo Alto Veterans Affairs Medical Center
3801 Miranda Avenue
Palo Alto, California 94304

Susan J. Riegg, Ph.D.
Department of Pathology
Medical College of Wisconsin
8700 W. Wisconsin Avenue
Milwaukee, Wisconsin 53226

Lee W. Riley, M.D.
Associate Professor of Medicine
Department of Medicine
Cornell University Medical College
1300 York Avenue
New York, New York 10021

James K. Roche, M.D., Ph.D.
Associate Professor of Medicine
Department of Internal Medicine
University of Virginia Health Sciences
* Center*
Charlottesville, Virginia 22908

R. Balfour Sartor, M.D.
Professor of Medicine
Research Associate Professor of
* Microbiology and Immunology*
Departments of Medicine and of
* Microbiology and Immunology*
University of North Carolina
Division of Digestive Diseases
324 Burnett-Womack
Chapel Hill, North Carolina 27599-7080

William Schaffner, M.D.
Professor and Chairman
Department of Preventive Medicine
Professor of Medicine (Infectious Diseases)
Vanderbilt University School of Medicine
Nashville, Tennessee 37232-2637

Gary Schoolnick, M.D.
Associate Professor of Medicine
Howard Hughes Medical Institute
Beckman Center, MC 5428
Stanford University School of Medicine
Stanford, CA 94305

Cynthia L. Sears, M.D.
Associate Professor of Medicine
Divisions of Infectious Diseases and
* Gastroenterology*
The Johns Hopkins University School of
* Medicine*
Ross Building
720 Rutland Ave.
Baltimore, MD 21205-2196

Kent A. Sepkowitz, M.D.
Instructor
Department of Medicine
Cornell University Medical College;
Memorial Sloan-Kettering Cancer Center
1275 York Avenue
New York, New York 10021

Philip M. Sherman, M.D.
Professor of Pediatrics and Microbiology
Department of Gastroenterology
The Research Institute
The Hospital for Sick Children
University of Toronto
555 University Avenue
Toronto, Ontario M5G 1X8
Canada

Gary L. Simon, M.D.
Department of Medicine
The George Washington University
Washington, D.C. 20006

Daniel J. Skiest, M.D.
Assistant Professor of Medicine
Division of Infectious Diseases
University of Texas Southwestern Medical
* Center;*
Parkland Memorial Hospital
5323 Harry Hines Boulevard
Dallas, Texas 75235-9113

Martin B. Skirrow, M.B., Ph.D.,
** F.R.C.Path., D.T.M.&H.**
Honorary Emeritus Consultant
* Microbiologist*
Public Health Laboratory
Gloucestershire Royal Hospital
Great Western Road
Gloucester GL1 3NN
United Kingdom

Edward Slosberg, M.D.
Assistant Professor of Medicine
Division of Gastroenterology
Stanford University Medical Center
300 Pasteur Drive
Stanford, California 94305

Phillip D. Smith, M.D.
Professor of Medicine and Microbiology
Department of Medicine
Division of Gastroenterology;
Senior Scientist, Center for AIDS Research
University of Alabama School of Medicine
Birmingham, Alabama 35294

John D. Snyder, M.D.
Associate Professor of Pediatrics
Department of Pediatrics
University of California at San Francisco
500 Parnassus Avenue
San Francisco, California 94127

Charles R. Sterling, D.V.M.
Professor and Head
Department of Veterinary Science
University of Arizona
Tucson, Arizona 85721

Christina M. Surawicz, M.D.
Associate Professor of Medicine
Department of Medicine
Division of Gastroenterology
University of Washington;
Chief, Gastroenterology
Harborview Medical Center
325 9th Avenue
Seattle, Washington 98104

Kathryn Swanson, M.D.
Clinical Instructor
Division of Gastroenterology
Stanford University Medical Center
300 Pasteur Drive
Stanford, California 94305

Francisco A. Sylvester, M.D.
Research Fellow in Gastroenterology
The Research Institute
Division of Gastroenterology and Nutrition
The Hospital for Sick Children;
555 University Avenue
Toronto, Ontario M5G 1X8
Canada

Nicholas J. Talley, M.D., Ph.D.
Professor of Medicine
Division of Medicine
The Nepean Hospital
Clinical Sciences Building
Derby and Somerset Streets
Sydney, New South Wales 2570
Australia

Robert V. Tauxe, M.D.
Division of Bacterial and Mycotic Diseases
National Center for Infectious Diseases
Centers for Disease Control and Prevention
1600 Clifton Road
Atlanta, Georgia 30333

David N. Taylor, M.D.
Department of Clinical Trials
Walter Reed Army Institute of Research
14th and Dahlia Street, N.W.
Washington, DC 20307-5100

Nathan M. Thielman, M.D.
Department of Geographic and International
Medicine
University of Virginia School of Medicine
Charlottesville, Virginia 22908

Lucy S. Tompkins, M.D., Ph.D.
Associate Professor of Medicne
Director, Clinical Microbiology/Virology
Laboratory
Departments of Medicine (Infectious
Diseases and Geographic Medicine) and
of Microbiology and Immunology
Stanford University Medical Center
300 Pasteur Drive
Stanford, California 94305

Phillip P. Toskes, M.D.
Professor of Medicine
Director, Division of Gastroenterology,
Hepatology, and Nutrition
Associate Chairman for Clinical Affairs
University of Florida College of Medicine
1600 S.W. Archer Road
Gainesville, Florida 32610

Edmund C. Tramont, M.D.
Professor and Director
Medical Biotechnology Center
University of Maryland Biotechnology
Institute
University of Maryland
618 W. Lombard Street
Baltimore, Maryland 21201

Janice R. Verley, M.D.
Postdoctoral Fellow
Department of Medicine/Infectious Diseases
The Johns Hopkins University School of
Medicine
720 Rutland Avenue
Baltimore, Maryland 21205-2196

W. Allan Walker, M.D.
Conrad Taff Professor of Nutrition and
Pediatrics
Harvard Medical School;
Department of Medicine (Gastroenterology)
Children's Hospital
300 Longwood Avenue
Boston, Massachusetts 02115

Christine A. Wanke, M.D.
Division of Infectious Diseases
Harvard Medical School
New England
Deaconess Hospital
Boston, Massachusetts 02215

Ronald G. Washburn, M.D.
Associate Professor of Medicine
Division of Infectious Diseases
Bowman Gray School of Medicine of Wake
  Forest University
Medical Center Boulevard
Winston-Salem, North Carolina 27157

Tracy D. Wilkins, Ph.D.
Professor of Microbiology
Director of Biotechnology
Center for Biochemistry
Virginia Technical Institute and State
  University
Blacksburg, Virginia 24061

Harland S. Winter, M.D.
Department of Pediatric Gastroenterology
  and Nutrition
Boston University School of Medicine;
Boston City Hospital
801 Albany Street
Boston, Massachusetts 02118

Robert H. Yolken, M.D.
Professor of Pediatrics
Department of Pediatric Infectious Diseases
The Johns Hopkins University School of
  Medicine
600 N. Wolfe Street
Baltimore, Maryland 21287-4933

Harvey Young, M.D.
Assistant Professor of Medicine
Division of Gastroenterology
Stanford University Medical Center
300 Pasteur Drive H1121, MC 5202
Stanford, California 94305

Preface

Gastrointestinal infections are a major cause of disease and death, particularly in the developing world. New etiologic agents, including bacteria, viruses, and protozoans, have been identified; new diseases, such as AIDS, have appeared; and the pathophysiologic mechanisms of old diseases have been newly characterized. Widespread travel to developing countries has brought diseases associated with contaminated food and water to the immunologically naive populations of Main Street. The increased number of immunocompromised persons and the pandemic of HIV-infection have turned once-rare infections into everyday occurrences for the busy practitioner. New techniques permit quicker and more complete diagnosis of many infections.

These developments have increased the importance of understanding gastrointestinal infections not only by gastroenterologist and infectious diseases specialists, but by internists, pediatricians, pathologists, and surgeons as well. The goal of this book is to provide a comprehensive source that combines the scientific basis and the art of medicine, relevant to enteric infections. It is intended for the healthcare practitioner, the clinical investigator, and all who seek not only the latest clinical details but also an understanding of the breadth and limitations of our knowledge of enteric infections.

We recognize and reaffirm that medicine is both an art and a science; in this text we hope to emphasize both faces of this same coin. The clinician who understands the new technologies, be they preventive, diagnostic, or therapeutic, becomes their master, not their slave. Nevertheless, especially in this field, there are many opportunities for simple, low-technology, low-cost approaches for treating ill patients that must be considered as well.

This book is organized to permit readers to access information according to clinical presentation and by etiologic agent, as well as segregating information on infection in normal and immunocompromised hosts. This is a large text; to avoid dilution of interest and focus, we have not included the many infections that primarily involve the liver, which should be treated as a separate subject.

Part I provides an accounting of the importance of gastrointestinal infections in human history and reviews the major epidemiologic patterns of enteric infections today. Parts II and III cover the basic principles of gastrointestinal structure, physiology, and immunology, as they pertain to enteric infections. Parts IV, V, and VI consider the major clinical syndromes involving the gastrointestinal tract in normal and immunocompromised hosts. The pertinent features of each are described, emphasizing differential diagnosis and approach to therapy. Part VII describes the most important pathogens of the gastrointestinal tract. In this section, the emphasis is on microbiology of the agent, its epidemiology and pathophysiology, and the specific approaches to diagnosis and therapy. The final sections, Parts VIII, IX, and X provide information on special diagnostic and therapeutic considerations and prevention of gastrointestinal infections including new strategies in vaccine development.

Above all, we have tried to provide a volume that is both comprehensive and practical.

Martin J. Blaser
Phillip D. Smith
Jonathan I. Ravdin
Harry B. Greenberg
Richard L. Guerrant

Acknowledgments

The Editors wish to thank Proctor and Gamble
for their generous support of this book.

The Editors wish to thank Bayer Corporation, Pharmaceutical Division
for their generous support of this book.

Infections of the Gastrointestinal Tract

Infections of the Gastrointestinal Tract,
edited by M. J. Blaser, P. D. Smith, J. I. Ravdin,
H. B. Greenberg, and R. L. Guerrant
Raven Press, Ltd., New York © 1995.

CHAPTER 1

Cholera, Dysentery, and Diarrhea

Lessons of History

Edmund C. Tramont and Eugene J. Gangarosa

Probably because they are not glamorous and probably because they remind us of our vulnerabilities, the impact of infectious diseases on the history of humans is underappreciated (1). It is not our purpose here to catalog, examine, or discuss the long and well documented impact of gastrointestinal illnesses on the history of humans or their role in determining all military outcomes. Instead, we have focused on a few examples, namely, cholera and the epic battles at Gallipoli and El Alamein, since it can be argued that cholera served as the disease prototype that mobilized and focused public health officials to embrace the principles and practice of sanitation (the "sanitary revolution") and established the principles and practice of fluid replacement. It can also be argued that the outcome of the latter two historical military clashes had a significant impact on 20th century world events, which in turn influenced European and North American relationships, and hence our daily lives.

CHOLERA: OLD SCOURGE AND NEW CHALLENGES

When Vasco da Gama rounded the southernmost point of Africa, which he called the Cape of Good Hope, with all the flags of his gallant little ships flying, his officers and men clad in their gayest clothes and brightest armor, and his trumpets sounding, he little thought he was soon to meet with a new and dreadful pestilence at the courts of the great King of Calicut, low down on the southwestern or Malabar coast of India. He landed in 1498, and in 1503 Gaspar Correa, an officer of Vasco da Gama, says 20,000 men of Calicut died of

a disease which struck them suddenlike in the belly, so that some of them died in eight hours.

> J. C. Peters, 1885 (2)

Even as the seventh cholera pandemic sets new records for numbers of cases, deaths, and countries affected, cholera watchers are predicting the beginning of a new eighth pandemic. A resourceful new strain of *Vibrio cholerae* has appeared in Bangladesh and India. Cholerae watchers are predicting the beginning of the eighth pandemic (3). In the period of a few months, well over 100,000 cases and over 1000 deaths were attributed to this new strain following its extensive spread in South Asia. The fact that most cases occurred in adults in an area hyperendemic for cholera implies that the old strains induced little or no immunity against this new strain. Indeed cholera, a scourge of antiquity, remains a major public health problem today!

In the meantime, there is no end in sight to the seventh pandemic, which began in 1961 in Indonesia and Southeast Asia. The O1 El Tor strain of *V. cholerae* is responsible. It is thought to be the only pandemic caused by this strain. By June 1993, The World Health Organization (WHO) had reported three million cases and tens of thousands of deaths around the world since its beginning (WHO/47 Press Release, 22 June 1993).

Cholera is an acute and often deadly diarrheal disease (see chapter by Butterton and Calderwood). Cholera diarrhea, often referred to as *purging* to underscore its severity, may result in the loss of 10% or more of the body's vital fluids and electrolytes. The responsible pathogen, *V. cholerae*, causes the diarrhea by elaborating a toxin, known as cholera toxin, that poisons the upper small bowel through a cascade of chemical events resulting in a molecular derangement of the control of water and electrolytes. This results in a hypersecretion of chloride and a partial block of sodium absorption (4). The net result is an enormous outflow of fluid from the intestinal circula-

E. C. Tramont: Medical Biotechnology Center, University of Maryland, Baltimore, Maryland 21201.

E. J. Gangarosa: International Health Center, School of Public Health, Emory University, Atlanta, Georgia, 30329.

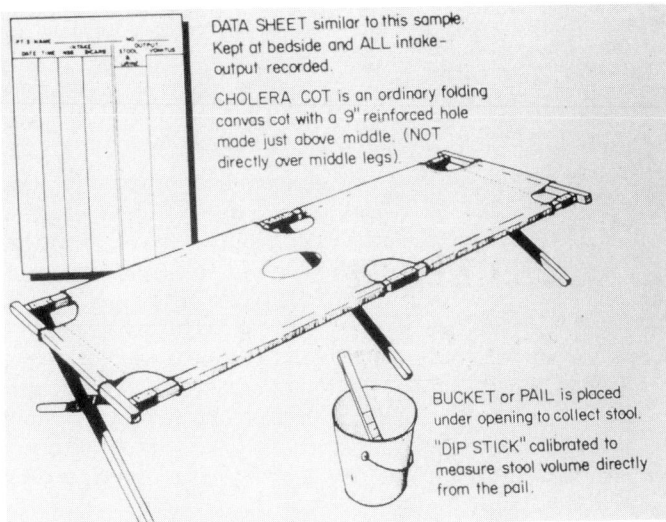 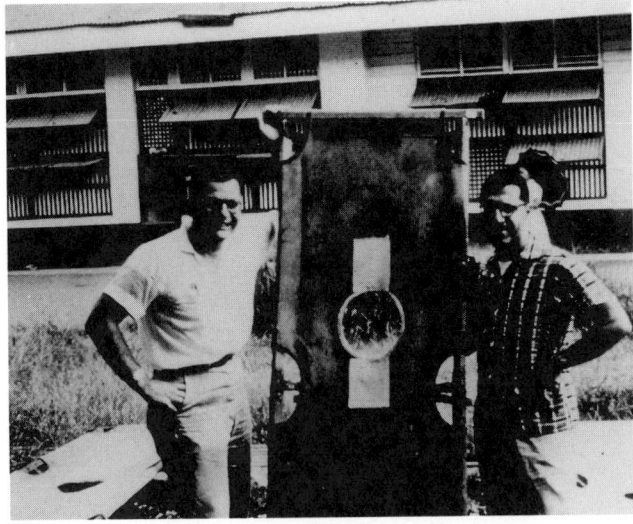

FIG. 1. The cholera cot was constructed to easily measure the volume of fluid loss as a guide for fluid replacement. One of the authors is shown holding such a cot.

tion into the lumen of the bowel (Fig. 1). Fluid mixed with mucus and containing large quantities of sodium, potassium, bicarbonate, and chloride gives the cholera stool its characteristic "rice-water" appearance. In severe cases, the result is shock, hypokalemia, hyponatremia, and metabolic acidosis. The process may be so fulminating as to cause death in a matter of hours, although for every severe case, there are many asymptomatic infections or cases with milder diarrhea indistinguishable from other forms of secretory diarrhea.

CHOLERA PANDEMICS

Before the current pandemic (outbreaks extended in time and crossing many national boundaries), historians described six pandemics, each originating on the Indian subcontinent. It is uncertain whether the disease was confined to Asia before 1817 but during the five decades following 1817, the disease spread in six pandemic waves out of India and across much of the world, including the Americas. Cholera receded after 1869, disappearing by the turn of the century from the Americas and most of Africa and Europe and by 1950 remained only on the Asian subcontinent. There is reason to believe that these six pandemics may, in fact, have been one single pandemic caused by the so-called classic strain (5). The seventh pandemic, caused by the El Tor biotype, was described early in the 20th century following its isolation at the El Tor quarantine station in Egypt from a pilgrim returning from Mecca. By 1960–1961, this strain had spread out of Indonesia, where an endemic focus had been described a quarter of a century earlier. In three decades, the pandemic moved rapidly to involve Southeast Asia, the Western Pacific, South Asia, the Middle East, Africa, South America, and most recently Latin America.

In January 1991, epidemic cholera appeared explosively in villages, towns, and cities along the Peruvian coast. In the ensuing months, it spread swiftly throughout Latin America, challenging the health care infrastructure of all the countries of that hemisphere. The intensity of the epidemic resembled the great urban epidemics of the past century in Europe and the United States, but what was conspicuous was the velocity of its spread—its transmission facilitated by modern air and land travel. In subsequent years, cholera assumed the characteristics of the pestilence of the past in terms of its persistence in foci that lacked safe water and good sanitation. At this writing, transmission has not been reported in the Caribbean countries although all adjacent Latin American countries have been affected and *V. cholerae* non-O1 has been isolated from the Gulf of Mexico (6). Cholera cases associated with travel and the ingestion of foods from infected countries have been reported in the United States (7). Despite the extraordinary numbers of patients needing emergency treatment straining medical resources, the mortality rates were surprisingly low. This has been attributed to the widespread use of fluid replacement therapy, especially the use of oral rehydration therapy (ORT).

UNIQUE CHARACTERISTICS OF THE CHOLERA ORGANISM AND ITS RESERVOIR

For years, traditional wisdom held that the only reservoir of this organism was in humans. Fecal–oral transmission was thought to be the exclusive means of spread. However, by 1977 evidence from the United States and Australia demonstrated a nonhuman reservoir.

Vibrio cholerae has unique survival mechanisms for persistence in aquatic environments. It is a halophilic organism, which enables it to find an ecological niche in estuarine waters, environments from which shellfish are commonly harvested. In these waters, the organism has a unique relationship with a wide range of aquatic plants including water hyacinths, duckweeds, and a variety of phytoplankton and zooplankton (8–11). From this niche, the organism persists and spreads periodically in a cycle involving seafood, especially shellfish, and humans.

This is also the nature of the endemic foci of cholera in the United States (6) and Australia and perhaps in other areas of the world as well. Thus humans still play the central role as a source of fecal–oral transmission, but the organism can persist in endemic foci and may spread when humans eat raw or undercooked seafoods. In parts of the world lacking water treatment and sanitation infrastructures, these two transmission mechanisms imperceptibly merge, causing food and waterborne outbreaks. Epstein (12) explained that "environmental conditions, e.g., sunlight, pH, temperature, salinity, and availability of nutrients, interact to affect both marine microflora and the physiological state, virulence, and survival of *V. cholerae*." He postulated that manipulation of the environment by humans may have contributed to the emergence of cholera in Peru. He surmised that the organism may have arrived in the bilge of a ship, and that it amplified in a permissive environment rich in abundant coastal sea life fertilized by increased atmospheric and coastal nitrate deposits as a result of a combination of global warming, the excessive use of agricultural fertilizers, discharge of industrial wastes and domestic sewage, and soil erosion. He also speculated that cholera may be only one example of the consequences of human "abuse of the environment" and speculated that humans may play a role through a "multiplicity of environmental changes," which collectively "may drastically alter disease reservoirs and vectors," setting the stage for "the emergence of new diseases" (12). Subsequently, at a landmark meeting on emerging pathogens in 1989, a widely held view was articulated that changing environments, not changing pathogens, were the main cause of emerging infectious diseases. Two of the meeting organizers, Nobel laureate Joshua Lederberg and virologist Stephen Morse, postulated that the so-called new viruses were in fact not "new" but may have existed for centuries in other hosts (13). Examples cited included human immunodeficiency virus (HIV), Ebola, Marburg, yellow fever, and Hanta viruses, which are normally monkey, mosquito, and rodent specified pathogens. Ways in which humans "abuse" the environment to bring about such changes were also noted by Gibbons (14), who stressed that some emerging pathogens may originate through ecologic imbalances created when forests are cleared for economic development (e.g., Lassa fever).

CHOLERA: A DIARRHEAL DISEASE PROTOTYPE AND THE TREATMENT BREAKTHROUGH

The seventh pandemic served as a powerful stimulus for researchers and health authorities. The rapid spread of the disease, its tendency to quickly kill previously healthy people, and its dramatic impact on affected communities energized scientists from many countries to address these issues.

At the beginning of the seventh pandemic, little was known about the pathogenesis of the disease and without

this understanding to guide therapy, mortality rates were high, often approaching 20% to 30% in hospitalized patients and higher in victims treated at home. In the early 1960s, studies conducted in Southeast Asia radically changed this situation.

During one of the first urban epidemics of cholera in modern times, an outbreak in Bangkok, Thailand, in 1959–1960, several landmark studies were conducted, which led to an understanding of the basic pathophysiology of the disease. One of these showed, contrary to contemporary views of the time, that the intestinal epithelium remained intact throughout the disease process and that intestinal epithelial cells continued their normal function (15). Another study defined the physiological deficits that occurred when cholera patients purge (16) and this subsequently provided the rationale for intravenous fluid and electrolyte replacement.

As the cholera pandemic moved quickly throughout Southeast Asia and across South Asia in the 1960s, the administration of intravenous fluids based on replacement of physiological losses resulted in a dramatic reduction of mortality in these patients to nearly zero. But this hospital-based therapy was expensive and out of the reach of most cholera victims. The development of a simpler, less costly regimen was therefore assigned a high research priority.

The success of the intravenous strategy stimulated research focused on oral rehydration. The subsequent discovery that glucose was necessary for the absorption of electrolytes that are administered orally was a landmark in the history of the treatment of cholera (17). Subsequent research demonstrated that cholera patients could be treated with oral fluids after cardiovascular collapse had been corrected with intravenous fluids. This advance in treatment greatly simplified the therapy of the disease. Patients survived using ORT that could easily be administered in remote settings and at a very low cost.

Soon after, investigators recognized that these discoveries were applicable to the treatment of all diarrheal diseases since the physiological losses differed only in degree. Thus cholera was recognized as the prototype of the so-called secretory diarrheas, which account for most of the diarrheal diseases, particularly those that kill untold numbers of infants each year.

Furthermore, in studies to demonstrate efficacy of this new oral rehydration strategy, and its applicability to other diarrheal diseases, investigators unexpectedly found that infants with diarrheal illnesses treated with ORT had a significant weight gain as compared to those treated by conventional regimens that did not include oral fluids. Thus it became evident that the vicious diarrhea/malnutrition and malnutrition/diarrhea cycle could at last be broken, at least for acute, watery diarrhea.

The impact of ORT on diarrheal disease mortality and morbidity has been dramatic. The number of lives saved each year by this inexpensive, easily administered therapy can be measured in the millions. Perhaps the most prophetic comments relative to this breakthrough were made in a *Lancet* editorial in 1978, which heralded ORT as perhaps the most significant medical breakthrough in this century (18). For the clinician the development of fluid replacement therapy means that cholera is no longer perceived as the dreaded disease it once was. This transformation from a highly malignant to an easily managed disease permits the clinician to shift focus from treating cholera as a single clinical entity to treating it as one of a generic group of acute secretory diarrheas that are all managed in essentially the same way. Anyone seen alive by a health care provider should survive!

But the implications of this relatively new treatment strategy go well beyond cholera, the other diarrheal diseases, or clinical medicine. ORT has provided the leverage and has proved to be the central point in the development of the multifaceted WHO-supported Diarrheal Diseases Control Programs now in place in most developing countries. This program has contributed substantially to the overall child-survival rates in these areas.

Challenge to the Clinician

The responsibility for treatment is not the only challenge for clinicians. They also have a responsibility to the patient and to the public to specifically diagnose these cases, allay unfounded fears, and give accurate advice on prevention. Patients who fit the high-risk criteria should be cultured to enable public health authorities to find and interrupt transmission. Clinicians should know that most clinical diagnostic laboratories do not routinely culture for *V. cholerae*. The clinical microbiology laboratory should be alerted when cholera is included in the differential diagnosis so that the appropriate culture media will be included. The clinician should also remember that rectal swabs or liquid stool are the specimens of choice when specimens have to be transported some distance. A variety of transport media such as Cary–Blair medium can be used.

One of us (EJG) has witnessed the anxiety, indeed sometimes panic, among clinicians called on to treat cholera patients for the first time. Clinicians need not fear for their own safety. Cholera is not transmitted by personal contact; the disease is spread only by ingestion of contaminated food or water. Measures such as the use of masks and gowns and patient isolation are inappropriate; only routine stool precautions are needed. Most patients will not need to be hospitalized unless there is evidence of cardiovascular deficiency.

Clinicians are frequently consulted by persons who seek travel advice. Although prevention strategies should encompass the full range of diseases a traveler may experience, clinicians should know that cholera is rare among Western travelers, that the risk of exposure in a cholera-affected area is no greater and probably considerably less than the risk of having an accident, and that cholera vaccines have limited value. In fact, most students of cholera, such as the authors, do not take the vaccine when they travel, even on cholera-related missions.

Clinicians practicing in the developed world usually do not think of cholera in the differential diagnosis of diarrhea. They should. Over 100 cases of cholera were documented in the United States in 1992 (6,7) and there has been a marked upward trend in documented cases over the past several years. Investigations of these cases revealed three groups. The largest number were cases exposed abroad who became ill after they returned to the United States. The second group were endemic cases occurring in persons who ingested contaminated shellfish. (As noted earlier, there are endemic foci in the United States and Australia and probably in other developed countries as well.) The third group were U.S. residents who consumed other contaminated imported foods. Thus far, the incriminated imported foods have been shellfish, usually hand-carried in personal luggage from affected countries of Latin America or other endemic areas, and coconut milk from Thailand (19). It is important to note that nearly all these cases have occurred in adults, in contrast to occurring in infants and children living in endemic areas.

With regard to treatment, the challenge to the clinician is to think "cholera." Cholera should be ruled out whenever a patient presents with watery diarrhea and a history of recent travel to a developing country or recent shellfish ingestion in this country or abroad. These patients should be seen and evaluated rather than being prescribed treatment over the telephone. Those who have evidence of shock should immediately be given intravenous solutions, usually lactated Ringer's solution. After circulatory stabilization is achieved (see chapter by Snyder), ORT should be given until the diarrhea has stopped. Commercial ORT solutions are readily available abroad and in the United States. Commonly available soft drinks and juices spiked with a heaping teaspoon of sucrose are acceptable substitutes (Tables 1 and 2).

Challenge to the Public Health Practitioner

Cholera represents only a small fraction of the morbidity and mortality due to diarrheal diseases worldwide but, given the large number of cases, represents a significant number. The magnitude of the global problem of the diarrheal diseases has been reported to be 3.3 million deaths each year, primarily in the developing world (21). In spite of the enormous advances made in our understanding of the pathogenesis and treatment of these diseases, they remain one of the most serious global health problems as we approach the 21st century. The great strides made in the primary care for the acute secretory diarrheas are overshadowed by the gaps in water and sanitation infrastructures, the root problems of all the diarrheal diseases.

One of us (EJG) has emphasized to his students that cholera should be seen as an opportunity for the public health practitioner. Few diseases provide such leverage to bring about constructive change. Those who lived through the polio era will recall how society was mobilized by the dread of that disease, particularly the bulbar form, which created respiratory emergencies, and the paralytic form, which left its victims crippled. In the same way, cholera has featured prominently as an energizer for public action.

In the early pandemics, moralism, interwoven with theology and piety, pervaded medical thinking. Leaders explained cholera in terms of divine displeasure. Rosenberg (22) noted the prevailing theme of the 19th century: "sin,

TABLE 1. *Comparison of electrolyte–glucose concentrations of solutions commonly administered at home*

Clear liquids	Na (mEq/L)	K (mEq/L)	HCO₃ (mEq/L)	Glucose (g/L)	Osmolarity (mM/L)
Cola	2	0.1	13	50–150 g glucose and fructose	550
Ginger ale	3	1	4	50–150 g glucose and fructose	540
Apple juice	3	20	0	100–150 g glucose and fructose	700
Chicken broth	250	5	0	0	450
Tea	0	0	0	0	5
Gatorade	20	3	3	45 g glucose and other sugars	330

From ref. 20.

in the scientific guise of predisposition, could still induce a case of cholera." Others explained epidemic diseases like cholera in terms of the miasmic theory, attributing environmental influences as the cause. Building on the lessons of the Civil War, a change occurred during the pandemic that reached the United States after that war. Despite clinging to religious and miasmic theories, some prominent medical leaders began to recognize the importance of sanitation in transmission. The work of John Snow, who demonstrated the role of contaminated water in the spread of cholera in the London outbreaks in the 1850s, influenced the thinking of enlightened leaders. For example, Rosenberg (22) quotes the health officer, William Clendenin, who wrote in the *Cincinnati Daily Gazette* of July 23, 1866 that "before erecting statues, building opera houses and art galleries, and buying expensive pictures, towns should be relieved of bad odors and fermenting pestilence. Good privies are far higher signs of civilization than grand palaces and fine art galleries." He was in the vanguard of a generation of public health workers who persuaded Americans of the need for *sanitary reform.*

Furthermore, the terror of cholera led to town meetings, which mobilized public support for change. Some actions taken, such as the implementation of fasting, played no role in control, but what was important is that communities recognized the need for standing committees to implement control. In a sense, these were desperate attempts to manage the unmanageable. From a historical point of view, however, many of these standing committees took on a life of their own and lasted well beyond the cholera crises when they evolved into boards of health and subsequently into municipal health departments. Thus the 1866 pandemic brought with it the beginnings of a scientific rationale for public health action and gave substance to these early health departments. Religious rhetoric was gradually replaced by rational actions; fast days were replaced by clean-up days, and eventually public health departments gained credibility as communities witnessed the success of their actions. Clearly, cholera provided considerable leverage in bringing about these changes and proved to be a powerful stimulus for the *sanitary revolution.*

The Sanitary "Revolution"

Documentation of waterborne transmission of cholera in the large urban outbreaks that occurred in London, England, in the 1850s and in Hamburg, Germany, in the 1890s, coincident with the urban outbreaks in the United States, set in motion the sanitary revolution. The essence of this revolution was the commitment of communities to long-term investments in the delivery of safe water by establishing water treatment plants coupled with sewage systems for the sanitary disposal of human wastes. Simultaneously, food handling practices were improved as the food-producing and the food-serving industries went

TABLE 2. *Comparison of electrolyte and carbohydrate concentrations of commercial oral rehydration solution (ORS) and solutions commonly administered at home*

Component of solution[a]	WHO[b]	Commercial ORS (manufacturer)		
		Pedialyte[c] (Ross)	Rehydralyte[c] (Ross)	Ricelyte[c] (Mead Johnson)
Sodium (mEq/L)	90	45	75	50
Potassium (mEq/L)	20	20	20	25
Chloride (mEq/L)	80	35	65	45
Citrate (mEq/L)	30	30	30	34
Glucose (g/L)	20	25	25	
Rice-syrup solids (g/L)				30

From ref. 20.
[a] Composition of solutions taken from package inserts.
[b] WHO-ORS is dispensed in packets. This product is considered the optimal. Manufactured and distributed in the United States by Jianas Brothers, Kansas City, MO.
[c] Pedialyte, Rehydralyte, and Ricelyte are dispensed in premixed liquid form.

through a slow process of improvement in food safety under the scrutiny of these newly formed public health departments.

The investments made in the sanitary revolution have had a profound impact on the industrialized nations. They eliminated cholera and other epidemic gastrointestinal diseases as a significant public health threat. As always, there are a few exceptions, such as the shellfish-related cholera outbreak in Naples, Italy, in 1973 (23) and the short-lived outbreak in Portugal in 1974 (24). There have also been imported cases into European and North American countries (19) but without subsequent transmission. These few exceptions serve to emphasize the rule that investments in community infrastructures that assure safe water, safe food, and effective sanitation have markedly reduced this threat. But, in addition to these benefits, these investments have resulted in an infrastructure that has profoundly improved all other aspects of health, quality of life, and economic development. The solution for those countries that still bear the burden of cholera and other diarrheal diseases lies in their own sanitary revolution.

The argument is often made that resources necessary to address these issues are simply not available. However, the priority given to health issues depends largely on the economic consequences of the disease. And economic policies that defer investments in a sanitary infrastructure because of the appeal of short-term gains from investments in vertical commercial programs need to be reconsidered. Tourism, for example, cannot flourish in countries where tourists frequently get sick from food and waterborne diseases. Quarantined and restricted imports are also an economic loss. The economic disasters created by cholera underscored how tenuous these investments can be when they are built on weak public health infra-

structures. In fact, the recent crisis has spurred some Latin American countries to accelerate their programs for water treatment and sewage system construction. The momentum of the seventh and the emergence of the eighth pandemic underscore the magnitude of the task that lies ahead.

THE IMPACT OF GASTROINTESTINAL ILLNESSES ON MILITARY CAMPAIGNS

> Soldiers have rarely won wars. They more often mop up after the barrage of epidemics. And typhus with its sisters, plague, cholera, typhoid and dysentery, have decided more campaigns than Caesar, Hannibal, Napoleon and all the inspector generals of history. The epidemics get the blame for defeat, the generals, the credit for victory. It ought to be the other way around.
> Hans Zinsser, 1935 (25)

Although the ravages of smallpox on Amerindians in the 16th and 17th centuries and the devastating effects of plague and tuberculosis in Europe have been duly recorded (26), the most conspicuous impact of infectious diseases has been on military campaigns. Simply stated, foodborne, waterborne, and vectorborne diseases have accounted for the outcome of more battles than the instruments of war (25,27) (Fig. 2). As noted above, whenever the normal lifestyle and sanitation of a community are disrupted, diarrheal illness becomes an important and critical determinant of human functionability; and war's legacy is just that!

Even if one argues that future conflicts will be conspicuous for the immensely destructive modern weaponry that may result in quick, decisive outcomes (as witnessed in military conflicts involving Western countries following

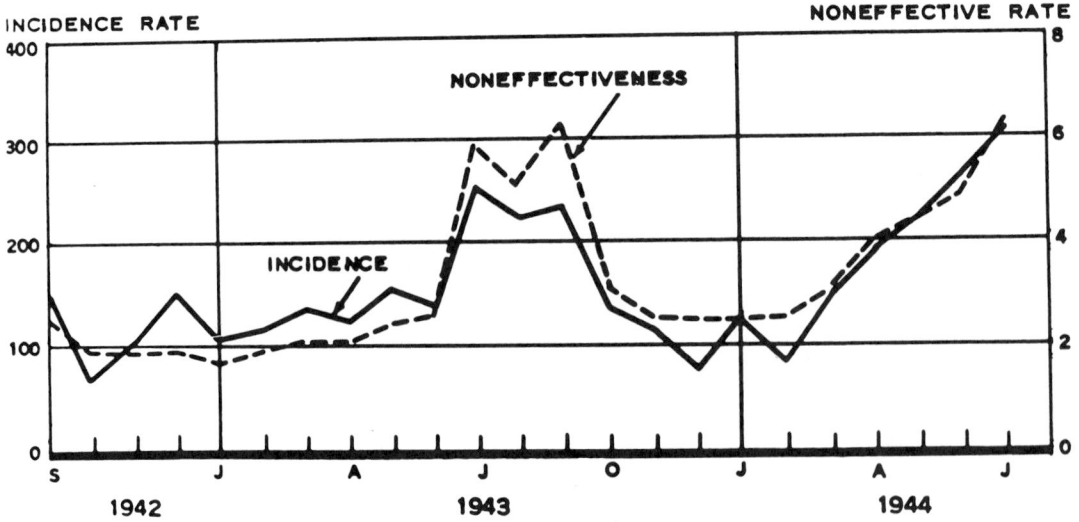

Source: Monthly Progress Report, Army Service Forces, War Department, 31 Aug. 1944, Section 7: Health.

FIG. 2. Impact of illnesses on troop effectiveness, Pacific Theater, World War II. In simple terms, troops cannot fight when they are sitting on their bottoms or weak from loss of fluid and electrolytes. The impact goes beyond the individual as it takes others to care for the ill and it fatigues those who have to fill in (31).

the Vietnam War), the aftermath of destruction and/or occupation will set the stage for an overwhelmingly increased incidence of gastrointestinal infections, and the least immunologically experienced (i.e., Americans, Canadians, and Western Europeans) and the most immunologically dysfunctional (i.e., the malnourished) will be the most vulnerable.

Gallipoli

From June onwards dysenteric diarrhoea spread through the Army and soon every man was infected by it. Many of the soldiers were able to endure it without reporting sick, but some soon became too weak even to drag themselves to the latrines, and by July, when over a thousand men were being evacuated every week, the disease had become far more destructive than the battle itself. Quite apart from the discomfort and the self-disgust, it created an overmastering lassitude. "It fills me," Hamilton wrote, "with a desperate

longing to lie down and do nothing but rest . . . and this, I think, must be the reason the Greeks were ten long years in taking Troy."

Alan Moorehead, 1956 (28)

It is always dangerous to describe a single episode in any protracted military conflict as the decisive event of that conflict; but there are major battles that mark a turning-of-the-tide in favor of the eventual "victor" (if there is such a thing in war). For example, the battles of Waterloo, Gettysburg, Midway, and the Tet offensive are considered from a historical perspective as the "turning points" of the Napoleonic War, the United States Civil War, the Pacific Theater in World War II, and the Vietnam War (29,30).

For World War I, the battle of Gallipoli is considered by many historians in the same vein. The Allied failure doomed any potential victory for Czarist Russia, thereby helping to set the stage for the Bolshevik Revolution and the eventual creation of the Communist Soviet Union and the subsequent Cold War. And Winston Churchill was

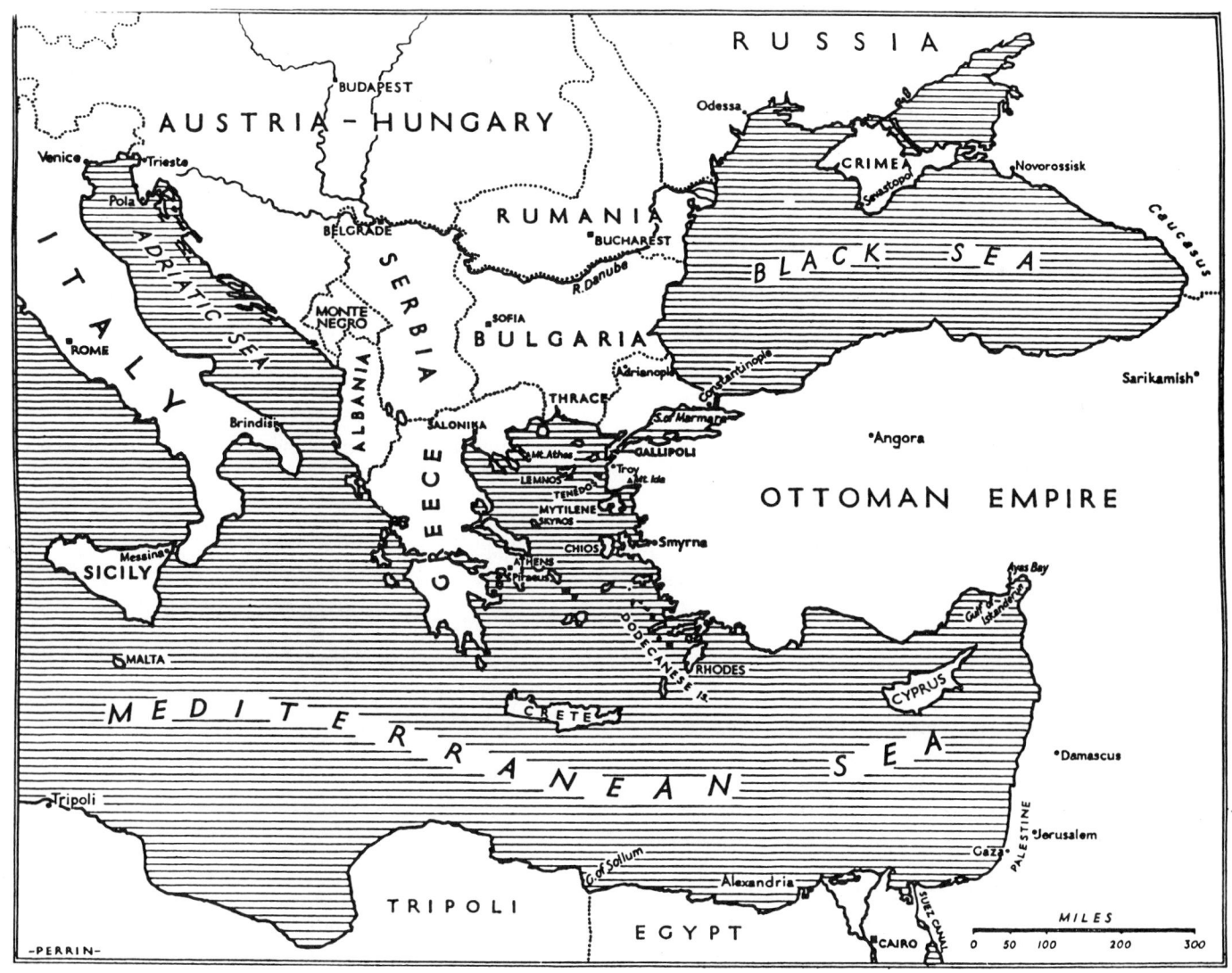

FIG. 3. Eastern Europe and the Middle East, 1912.

cast into the backwaters of political influence, which arguably made it easier for Hitler to ensconce Nazism (31,32).

Gallipoli is a peninsula (Fig. 3) that guards the Dardanelles, the entrance into the Black Sea, and hence a key supply route to Russia. During World War I, the Allied Forces, under a plan drawn up by Winston Churchill, then First Lord of the Admiralty of the British Navy, attempted to occupy Gallipoli and thus secure a logistic pipeline to Russia and maintain a second front against Germany. Gallipoli was defended by the Turks, then aligned with Germany. The Allied Forces, made up primarily of Australians, were defeated despite larger numbers of troops, superior battle equipment, and better training. The reason for the defeat was an epidemic of dysentery that disproportionately affected the relatively nonimmune Allied Forces in contrast to the local defenders (28).

El Alamein

> General Montgomery says the Eighth Army won, but Rommel claimed the victory for dysentery.
> Sir Sheldon F. Dudley (33).

Soon after the United States had entered into World War II, the brilliant German General Rommel was poised to gain control of the Suez Canal, thereby further blocking the transport of oil and other supplies to Great Britain and potentially starving the British out. But Rommel never accomplished his objective.

Perhaps because of the lessons learned at Gallipoli, or because of Great Britain's long-time occupation of the Middle East, the Allied forces employed superior preventive medicine measures; namely, they buried their excrement, thereby controlling the spread by flies of *Shigella* and other diarrheogenic microorganisms. The Axis Forces, on the other hand, relied on the sun to "bake" their excrement in the sand, allowing flies ample time to contaminate themselves and ultimately the human food chain.

Indeed, during the fateful and decisive battle at El Alamein, which preserved British control of the Suez Canal, Rommel was convalescing from dysentery in Germany. "But, as the Germans learned at El Alamein, dysentery can still win battles when hygienic discipline on one side is slack" (33).

Other Conflicts

> He who fails to learn from history is destined to repeat it.

A review of the major conflicts in which the U.S. military has participated (Table 3)—the Civil War (34), the Spanish–American War (35), World War I (36), World War II (37–40) (Fig. 2, Table 4), Korea (41–43), Lebanon (44–46), Vietnam (47–51) (Fig. 4) and Desert Storm (52)—reveals that diarrhea/dysentery has been monotonously recorded as a major problem of morbidity and troop dysfunction. In the Civil War, it was a major cause of mortality (32) (Table 5).

TABLE 3. *Hospital admissions for diarrhea/dysentery[a] (per 1000 troops/year)*

Conflict	Incidence	Death rate
Civil War	741	18
Spanish–American War	426	3.3
World War I	29	0.13
World War II	14	0.005
Korea	14	NA
Lebanon[b]	247	NA
Vietnam[c]	60	NA

[a] Includes all causes of diarrheal and dysenteric illnesses (infectious origin, gastroenteritis, ulcerative colitis, ileitis). Prior to the Spanish–American War, etiologic differences were not considered. Beginning with the Spanish–American War, typhoid fever was distinguished separately; amebiasis was considered separately during the Vietnam War.
[b] 13 August to 24 September 1958.
[c] January 1965 to March 1966.
NA, not available.

Control Of Gastrointestinal Illnesses by the Military

Every conflict leaves a legacy of improved medical care (27,53,54). The U.S. Civil War left us with, among other advances, the nascent principles and practice of public health that are still valid today (54,55). For example, by quarantining U.S. troops in fortified camps, and therefore foregoing local foodstuffs in favor of pre-prepared food rations (MREs), the U.S. military reduced gastrointestinal illnesses (and sexually transmitted diseases) in U.S. troops stationed in Somalia (1993) and maintained their occurrence at baseline levels. Mosquitoes, which obviously are not bound by such human-instituted policies, continued to spread malaria (56).

THE FUTURE

The importance of controlling gastrointestinal illnesses has often been forgotten. Unless we heed history's les-

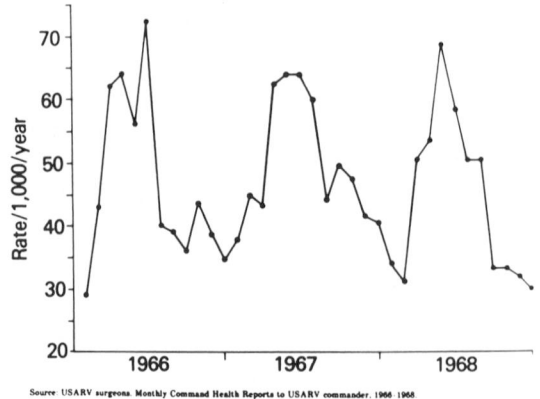

FIG. 4. Monthly diarrheal disease as documented by the U.S. Army during the Vietnam War (cases/1000 troops/year). The highest incidence occurred during the warmest months. Diarrhea due to *Escherichia coli* was demonstrated for the first time in a military setting (47).

TABLE 4. *Incidence of diarrhea and dysentery in the U.S. Army by area and year, 1940–1945,[a] parallels the availability of safe local water and sanitary disposal of fecal excrement*

Area	Number of cases/1000 troops/year						
	1940	1941	1942	1943	1944	1945	1942–1945
Continental United States	7	15	8	12	9	6	9
Overseas							
Europe[b]			17	12	13	14	14
Mediterranean			34	132	54	22	70
Africa–Middle East			196	170	115	79	128
Middle East			224	179	114	89	143
Persian Gulf Command			NA	NA	115	56	
China–Burma–India			123	146	181	93	131
China			NA	NA	68[c]	122	
India–Burma			NA		107[c]	86	
Southwest Pacific	27	28	59	70	55	74	67
Australian mainland			NA	NA	23	5[d]	
Philippine Islands	27	28			114	104	105
Other			NA	NA	54	32[d]	
Pacific Ocean	1	18	34	43	28	19	30
Central Pacific	1	18	15	11	21[e]	NA	
South Pacific			77	76	38[e]	NA	
North America		1	4	2	7	6	4
Latin America	8	13	21	21	17	16	19
Central America			104	86			
Alaska	f	f	5	8	3	1	5
Total overseas	9	17	30	66	38	33	40
Total Army	7	15	11	25	22	22	21

Adapted from ref. 31.

[a] Based on diagnoses reported on individual medical records, totals for 1940–1942 appear to be understated approximately as follows: one-half in 1940, one-quarter in 1941, and one-third in 1942. It is not known whether these proportions apply equally to each geographic area.

[b] United Kingdom and continental Europe.

[c] Data for November and December only.

[d] Data for first 8 months only.

[e] Data for first 7 months only.

[f] Included with continental United States.

NA, not available.

sons and intercede before the human gut is laid bear to the omnipresent and ever-changing horde of intestinal parasites, a weak link in the fortunes of all peoples and armies is the ever-present threat of gastrointestinal infections. The medical professionals practicing in all countries must know and understand cholera as the prototype disease: from clinical and laboratory diagnosis to treatment, from investigating and reporting cases, and most of all prevention.

The medical professional needs to recognize his/her special leadership role when deficiencies involve the water/food/sewage infrastructure and further recognize that careful investigation of an outbreak provides leverage to persuade decision-makers who control resources to address deficiencies, reorder priorities, and ensure the commitment needed to correct the root problems. Experiences in all countries ravaged by cholera underscore the importance of a multisectorial approach to prevention. The actors on this stage must come from ministries/departments responsible for health, agricultural development, transportation, and fisheries.

Countries that have already made the investments in the water/food/sewage infrastructure spawned during the sanitary revolutions of the past are generally protected. But this infrastructure cannot be taken for granted and must be nurtured, upgraded, and maintained. Obviously, countries where cholera and other diarrheal illnesses are actively transmitted must address the need for their own sanitary revolution if the long-term benefits of improved quality of life and enhanced economic development are to be realized.

Enforced public health measures offer the best protection for the masses; effective vaccines may someday offer

TABLE 5. *Death rate for diarrhea/dysentery per 1000 troops/year in the Civil War*

Year	Rate
1861–1862	4.2
1862–1863	16.0
1863–1864	26.7
1864–1865	28.8
1865–1866	21.5

Adapted from ref. 34.

a good chance of protection for the individual. But until more effective vaccines for *all* causes of gastrointestinal infections are developed, prevention through sanitation and public health intervention is our only tried and true weapon.

REFERENCES

1. McNeill WH. *Plagues and peoples*. Garden City, NY: Doubleday Publishing, 1976.
2. Peters JC. Early history of asiatic cholera in India as known to Europeans (AD 1503–1800). In: Wendt EC, ed. *Asiatic cholera*. New York: William Wood & Co, 1885.
3. Swerdlow DL, Ries AA. *Vibrio cholerae* non O1, the eighth pandemic. *Lancet* 1993;342:382–383.
4. Van Heyningen WE, Seal JR. *Cholera: the American scientific experience, 1947–1980*. Boulder, CO: Westview Press, 1983; chap. 9.
5. Blake PA. Epidemiology of cholera in the Americas. *Gastroenterol Clin North Am* 1993;3:639–660.
6. Levine WC, Griffin PM. *Vibrio* infections on the Gulf Coast: results of first year of regional surveillance. *J Infect Dis* 1993; 167:479–483.
7. Update: cholera—western hemisphere, 1992. *MMWR Morb Mortal Wkly Rep* 1993;42:89–91.
8. Colwell RR, Kaper J, Joseph SW. *Vibrio cholera, Vibrio parahaemolyticus* and other vibrios: occurrence and distribution in Chesapeake Bay. *Science* 1977;198:394–396.
9. Spira WM, Huq A, Ahmed QS, Sayeed A. Uptake of *Vibrio cholerae* biotype El Tor from contaminated water by water hyacinth (*Eichhoronia crassipes*). *Appl Environ Microbiol* 1981; 42:550–553.
10. Khan MU, Shahidullah M, Haque MS, Ahmed WU. Presence of vibrios in the surface water and their relation with cholera in the community. *Trop Geogr Med* 1984;36:335–340.
11. Islam MS, Drasar BS, Bradley DJ. Long-term persistence of toxigenic *Vibrio cholera* O1 in the mucilaginous sheath of a blue-green algae, *Anabaena variablis*. *J Trop Med Hyg* 1990;93:133–139.
12. Epstein PR. Cholera and the environment: an introduction to climate change. *PSR Q* 1992;2:146–160.
13. Culliton BJ. Emerging viruses, emerging threat. *Science* 1990; 247:279–280.
14. Gibbons A. Where are "new" diseases born? *Science* 1993;261: 680–681.
15. Gangarosa EJ, Beisel WR, Benyajati C, et al. The nature of the gastrointestinal lesion in Asiatic cholera and its relation to pathogenesis. *Am J Trop Med Hyg* 1960;9:125–135.
16. Watten RH, Morgan FM, Phillips RA, et al. Water and electrolyte studies in cholera. *J Clin Invest* 1959;38:1879–1891.
17. Nalin DR, Cash RA, Islam R, et al. Oral maintenance therapy for cholera in adults. *Lancet* 1968;2:370–374.
18. Water with sugar and salt. *Lancet* 1978;2:300–301.
19. Taylor JL, Tuttle J, Pramukul, T, et al. An outbreak of cholera in Maryland associated with imported commercial coconut milk. *J Infect Dis* 1993;167:1330–1335.
20. The management of acute diarrhea in children: oral rehydration, maintenance, and nutritional therapy *MMWR Morb Mortal Wkly Rep* 1992;41(RR-16).
21. Bern C, Martines J, de Zoysa I, and Glass RI. The magnitude of the global problem of diarrhoeal disease: a ten-year update. *Bull World Health Organ* 1992;70:705–714.
22. Rosenberg CE. *The cholera years: the United States in 1832, 1849, and 1866*. Chicago: The University of Chicago Press, 1987.
23. Baine WB, Zampiere A, Mazzotti M, et al. The epidemiology of cholera in Italy in 1973. *Lancet* 1974;2:1370–1374.
24. Blake PA, Rosenberg ML, Costa JB, et al. Cholera in Portugal, 1974. *Am J Epidemiol* 1977;105:344–348.
25. Zinsser H. *Rats, lice and history*. Boston: Little, Brown, 1935.
26. Cartwright FF. *Disease and history*. New York: Thomas Y Crowell, 1972.
27. Lacey SW. The arts of war and medicine; a study in symbiosis. *Am J Med Sci* 1993;305:407–420.
28. Moorehead A. *Gallipoli*. New York: Harper Brothers, 1956.
29. Summers HG. *On strategy, a critical analysis of the Viet Nam war*. Novato, CA: Presidio Press, 1982.
30. Karnow S. *Vietnam, a history*. New York: Viking Press, 1983.
31. Morgan T. *Churchill, young man in a hurry: 1874–1915*. New York: Simon & Shuster, 1982.
32. Manchester W. *The last lion, Winston Spenser Churchill, visions of glory 1874–1932*. Boston: Little, Brown, 1983.
33. Philbrook FR, Gordon JE. Diarrhea and dysentery. In: Hoff EB, ed. *Preventive medicine in World War II*, vol IV. Washington, DC: Office of the Surgeon General, Department of the Army, 1958;319–413.
34. Medical and surgical history of the War of the Rebellion (1861–1865). In: *Medical history, Parts II & III*. Washington, DC: US Government Printing Office, 1879.
35. Reed W, Vaughn C, Shakespeare EO. *Report on the origin and spread of typhoid fever in U.S. military camps during the Spanish War of 1898*. Washington, DC: US Government Printing Office, 1900.
36. Communicable and other diseases. In: *The medical department of the United States Army in the World War*, vol IX. Washington, DC: US Government Printing Office, 1928.
37. Bloom H. Dysentery in British prisoners of war. *Lancet* 1944; 2:558–560.
38. US War Department, Military Intelligence Division. *Merrill's Marauders (February–May 1944)*. American Forces in Action Series. Washington, DC: US Army Center of Military History, 1945.
39. Philbrook FR, Barnes LA, McGann WJ, Harrison RR. Prolonged laboratory observations on clinical cases and carriers of "*Shigella flexneri* III" following epidemic. *US Naval Med Bull* 1948;48:405–414.
40. Medical Department, United States Army. *Medical statistics in World War II*. Washington, DC: US Government Printing Office, 1975.
41. AR–TSG–*Medical statistics of the United States Army*. Annual Report of the Surgeon General. Calendar year 1953. Washington, DC: Office of the Surgeon General, 1955.
42. HOA–Office of the Surgeon General, United States Army. *Korea: A summary of medical experience, July 1950–Dec. 1952. Health of the Army*. Washington, DC: Office of the Surgeon General, 1953.
43. Crowdrey AE, ed. *The medic's war, United States Army in the Korean War*. Washington, DC: Center of Military History, US Army, 1987.
44. Hurewitz S. Military medical problems of the Lebanon crisis. *Mil Med* 1960;125:26–35.
45. Moore WS. Lessons learned from the Lebanon crisis. *Med Bull US Army Europe* 1959;16:61–65.
46. Long P. Office of the Surgeon General. *Preventive medicine lessons learned in Lebanon*. Disposition Form to Director, Historical Unit, 26 Jan 1960.
47. Gentry LO, Hedlund KW, Wells RF, Ognibene AJ. Bacterial diarrheal diseases. In: Ognibene AG, Barrett O, eds. *Internal medicine in Viet Nam*, vol II. Washington, DC: Office of the Surgeon General and Center of Military History, 1982.
48. Sheehy TW. Digestive disease as a national problem. VI. Enteric disease among United States troops in Vietnam. *Gastroenterology* 1968;55:105–112.
49. USARV surgeon. Monthly Command Health Reports to USARV commander, Jan. 1965–Apr. 1966. Washington, DC: US Army Center of Military History, 1966.
50. Stone GD. *Shigellosis in Saigon, Vietnam*. USARV Medical Bulletin (USARV Pam 40-7), Jan–Feb 1968. Washington, DC: Office of the Surgeon General, 1968.
51. Kalas P, Bearden H. Trip report to Vietnam, 18 February 1969 to 8 June 1969; to evaluate the problem of gastroenteritis in combat troops at the hospital, battalion aid station, and platoon (or company) level. Report to commander, US Army Medical Research and Development Command, Washington, DC, 25 July 1969.

52. Hyams KC, Bourgeois AL, Merrell BR, et al. Diarrheal disease during operation Desert Shield. *N Engl J Med* 1991;325: 1423–1428.

53. Bayne-Jones S. *The evolution of preventive medicines in the United States Army:* 1607–1939. Washington, DC: Office of the Surgeon General, Department of the Army, 1968.

54. Key JD. US Army Medical Department and Civil War medicine. *Mil Med* 1968;133:181–192.

55. Sartin JS. Infectious diseases during the Civil War: the triumph of the "Third Army." *Clin Infect Dis* 1993;16:580–584.

56. Walter Reed Army Institute Research Communicable Disease Report, vol 4, July 1993.

Infections of the Gastrointestinal Tract,
edited by M. J. Blaser, P. D. Smith, J. I. Ravdin,
H. B. Greenberg, and R. L. Guerrant
Raven Press, Ltd., New York © 1995.

CHAPTER 2

Epidemiology of Diarrheal Diseases in Developing Countries

Robert E. Black and Claudio F. Lanata

Diarrheal diseases are a serious public health problem in developing countries, especially in children who have high rates of diarrheal morbidity and related mortality (1,2). Under the conditions of poverty, poor environmental sanitation and hygiene, inadequate water supplies, and limited education prevalent in developing country settings, diarrheal diseases occur most frequently and have the most lethal consequences. When these conditions were present in the United States and Western Europe more than half a century ago, the problems with diarrheal diseases were similar (3,4). As these areas developed economically with provision of better water and sanitation, improved child feeding practices, and more education, the problems with diarrheal diseases were greatly diminished (3,4). Likewise, as developing countries undergo a similar economic and social improvement, the problems of infectious disease morbidity and mortality, including those of diarrheal diseases, are diminishing (5). Unfortunately, even countries undergoing rapid development, such as Brazil or Thailand, have sizable populations living in poverty and poor environmental conditions and suffering high rates of diarrheal disease morbidity and mortality (5). Furthermore, large areas of the developing world, such as South Asia and Sub-Saharan Africa, have had slow socioeconomic development and continuing high levels of morbidity and mortality, especially in children (6).

Substantial global efforts were directed at reduction of diarrheal disease mortality beginning in the 1980s (1). This effort was based on the recognition that acute dehydrating diarrheas played a substantial part in the fatal illnesses. Furthermore, it had been demonstrated in the preceding decade that this dehydration could be treated with oral fluid and electrolyte replacement, along with continued

feeding, rather than by expensive and difficult to administer intravenous fluids (7). This provided the possibility of making effective therapy much more widely available and resulted in the initiation of national diarrheal control programs in nearly all developing countries (1). These programs have led to greatly improved therapy for diarrhea in many settings and resulting reduction in diarrhea-related mortality (8,9). With reduction in diarrheal deaths related to dehydration, additional attention is being turned to the problems of dysentery and persistent diarrhea (often associated with malnutrition) that are also major causes of diarrhea-related mortality (10–13). These illnesses require additional therapeutic interventions (14–16). Furthermore, control program efforts are increasingly turning to preventive interventions (17). It is important to understand the etiology and epidemiology of the diarrheal diseases since this may provide the basis for specific therapeutic and preventive measures.

GENERAL EPIDEMIOLOGY

Definitions

Diarrhea is a symptom complex characterized by stools of decreased consistency and increased number. While on a clinical basis this can be thought of in relation to that individual's prior bowel habits, epidemiologic studies have commonly used a more precise definition for standardization (18). Although there is variability in the definitions used in the literature, most studies now consider diarrhea to be present when three or more liquid stools are passed during any 24-hr period. In the first 2 months of life, especially for breast-feeding infants, this may not be satisfactory and the definition is more commonly based on what the mother considers to be a decrease in stool consistency or an increase in stool frequency for that child. There is also variability in the definitions of diarrheal episodes in regard to the minimum number of

R. E. Black: Department of International Health, The Johns Hopkins University School of Hygiene and Public Health, Baltimore, Maryland 21205.

C. F. Lanata: Nutrition and Infection Working Group Instituto de Investigacion Nutricional, Lima 18, Peru.

healthy days that are necessary to determine the end of a diarrheal episode, but at least 2 days free of diarrhea are usually required to define an episode as terminated. Dysentery is a diarrheal disease defined by the presence of blood in liquid stools.

While most diarrheal episodes resolve during the first week, a small proportion continues for 2 weeks or more. Studies in children living in Bangladesh and Peru indicate that the distribution of episode durations is continuous, but skewed toward the longer durations (Fig. 1) (14,19–21). Similar findings have been reported from Brazil (22,23). Thus establishing a specific definition of persistent diarrhea as an illness of more than a given number of days is arbitrary. Nevertheless, doing so is useful for comparability in research studies and for implementing case management strategies. For these reasons, a World Health Organization (WHO) meeting recommended that persistent diarrhea be operationally defined as an episode of diarrhea that lasts for at least 14 days (24). Furthermore, this definition of persistent diarrhea operationally identifies children that tend to have heavy diarrheal burdens (22,23,29). The term persistent diarrhea is intended to encompass episodes that begin acutely and continue for longer than their expected duration, but not to include infrequent chronic diarrheal disorders, such as hereditary syndromes, gluten-sensitive enteropathy, granulomatous diseases, or tumors producing gastrointestinal hormones (24,25).

Incidence of Diarrhea

Diarrheal incidence has varied in the different settings in which it has been studied. This variation could be due to methodologic differences such as the definition of diarrhea and surveillance techniques used (18,26,27) or could be the result of actual differences in the study populations. A summary of prospective, community-based studies in developing countries found a median incidence of all diarrhea in children under 5 years of age of 2.6 episodes per child per year (2). Among these studies, the incidence was highest in those with a small number of children under surveillance and with frequent home visiting (e.g., two or three times per week), suggesting that larger studies with infrequent surveillance may have found lower rates because of underreporting of diarrhea. While it is likely that there are also differences in the incidence in different populations, the methodologic variations could account for a substantial part of the apparent differences.

The incidence of diarrhea varies with the age of the child within the first 5 years of life (Fig. 2) (21,23,28–32). Generally, children in the first 2 years of life have the highest incidence followed by a progressive fall with age. The peak incidence is often 6 to 11 months of age. The incidence in boys and girls as determined by community-based studies is similar; however, in some countries boys may be more commonly taken to health facilities, giving the appearance of higher rates of diarrhea.

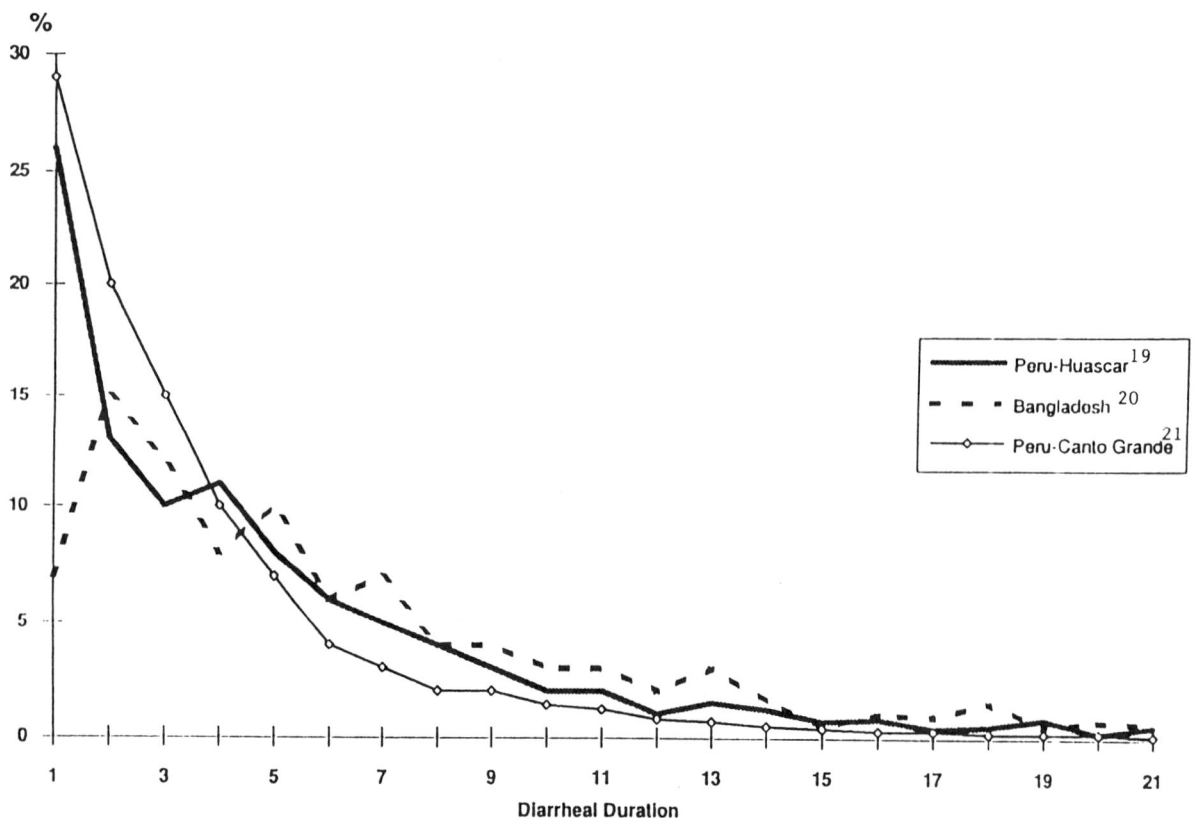

FIG. 1. Percentage distribution of diarrheal episode duration in days, ascertained from prospective community-based studies in Peru (19,21) and Bangladesh (20). (From ref. 14, with permission.)

Cases per 100 child-years

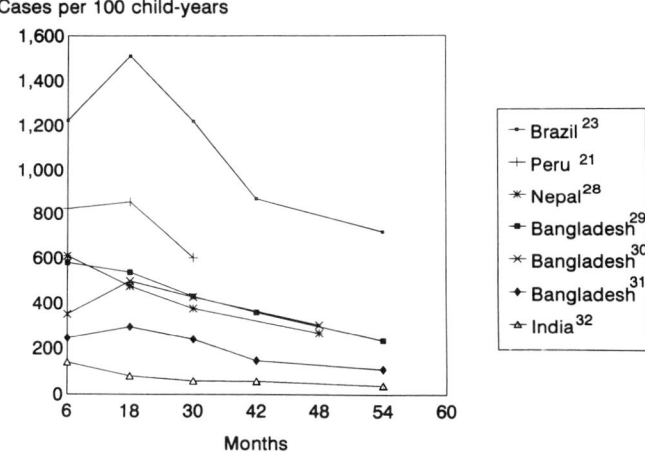

FIG. 2. Incidence of all diarrhea in selected developing countries by age.

Cases per 100 child-years

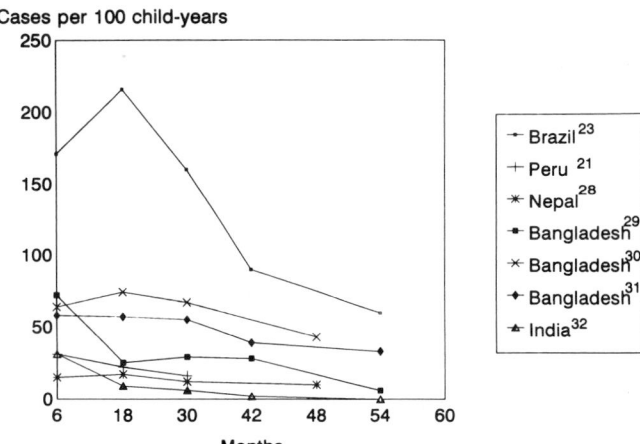

FIG. 3. Incidence of persistent diarrhea in selected developing countries.

Although high rates of diarrhea may occur throughout the year in developing country children, most settings have a peak during the hot and/or rainy months (33,34). The seasonality of all diarrhea is, in fact, a composite of the seasonality of individual agents causing diarrhea. Most of the bacterial causes of diarrhea appear to peak during the hot and/or wet months. Rotavirus may have little seasonality in tropical areas but often peaks in the cool and/or dry season in more temperate climates (35). The seasonality must be largely due to environmental influences on the transmission of the infectious agents, although seasonal shifts in the health of the children, such as seasonal deterioration in nutritional status, may also play a part.

Duration

In most settings a majority of diarrheal episodes are self-limited and resolve within 1 week (Table 1). A small fraction will take up to 2 weeks to resolve. Persistent diarrhea, illnesses of more than 2 weeks duration, rarely constitutes more than 20% of all episodes (Table 1). This proportion is also influenced by the study methodology but

is generally highest in the studies that find a high incidence of all diarrhea. The incidence of persistent diarrhea in children under 5 years of age has ranged up to 60 episodes per 100 child-years. The decline with age appears to be similar for persistent and all other diarrheas (Fig. 3).

Impact of Diarrhea

It has long been appreciated that diarrheal diseases are important causes of death in childhood. However, there is little direct information available on case fatality rates for diarrheal episodes at a community level. Case fatality rates in children under 5 years of age have been reported to be 0.1% in Bangui, Central African Republic (38), 0.3% in rural Egypt (39), 0.4% in rural North India (40), and 0.5% in rural Indonesia (41). The U.S. Institute of Medicine estimated that the diarrheal case fatality rate in children under 5 years of age in developing countries was 0.2% (42). The case fatality rate varies substantially with age, being highest in the youngest children. In a study from rural India, the case fatality rate was reported to be 0.7% for acute diarrhea but 14% for persistent diarrhea (13).

TABLE 1. *Duration of diarrheal episodes in children from community-based studies in developing countries*

Study (reference)	Age group (months)	Total episodes	Diarrheal incidence (per 100 child-years)	Diarrheal duration (days)		
				1–7	8–14	≥15
Indonesia (36)	0–11	618	311	83%	14%	4%
Guatemala (37)	0–11	262	334	53	27	19
Bangladesh (20)	0–59	941	557	66	21	14
Brazil (34)	0–71	519	600	82	15	3
Peru (19)	0–11	1299	984	79	14	7
India (32)	0–71	471	61	35	55	10
Brazil (23)	0–60	2896	1140	76	13	11
Peru (21)	0–35	5302	807	88	9	3
Bangladesh (29)	0–59	2609	455	71	22	7
Bangladesh (31)	0–71	1074	195	50	27	23

Recently, the World Bank reviewed the health problems of developing countries and concluded that diarrheal diseases were the second, after respiratory infections, most important cause of disability-adjusted life years lost (43). This is largely due to high childhood mortality from diarrheal diseases. It has been estimated that there are currently 3.2 to 3.5 million deaths from diarrhea in developing country children each year (2). The diarrheal mortality rate is highest in the first year of life at about 20 deaths per 1000 children. While the rate of about 5 deaths per 1000 children in the 1- to 4-year age group is lower, this age group still accounts for approximately half of the diarrheal deaths of childhood. Mortality rates appear to fall to very low levels after the first 5 years of life, although there may be a slight increase for older adults.

The infectious diseases of childhood have been found to have adverse effects on growth (44). Of all the infectious diseases, diarrhea seems to have the greatest adverse effect, possibly because of a reduction in appetite, altered feeding practices, and decreased nutrient absorption, along with the very high prevalence of diarrhea in young children (44,45). The magnitude of the effect of diarrheal diseases on growth in various studies has ranged from 10% to 80% of the growth retardation occurring in the first few years of life in comparison with an international reference population (44). The true estimate is probably closer to the lower end of this range. Furthermore, certain factors may moderate the effect of diarrheal illnesses on growth. Appropriate treatment of the illness may reduce the adverse effects of diarrhea; fluid replacement, continued breast-feeding, and a good diet during diarrhea can prevent weight faltering (44). In addition, children with an adequate regular diet will not only better withstand the illness but also have the potential to grow more rapidly after an illness, so-called catch-up growth, especially if they do not have subsequent episodes of diarrhea or other serious illness (46–48).

Diarrheal diseases are also an economic burden in developing countries because of the costs of medical care, medications, and lost work. While the illnesses can largely be managed by fluid and nutritional therapy, with selected use of antibiotics, pharmaceuticals are inappropriately widely used for managing diarrhea (49). Antibiotics and so-called antidiarrheal drugs are an unnecessary use of hundreds of millions of dollars in developing countries each year and, in addition to reducing the likelihood of appropriate therapy, must also contribute to antibiotic resistance among enteropathogens and other infectious agents (49).

MICROBIAL ETIOLOGIES

Relative Importance of Enteropathogens

A wide array of bacterial, viral, and parasitic agents have been associated with diarrhea in developing countries. Since the highest incidences of diarrhea and the most severe consequences are generally in young children, most studies have focused on this age group. Older children and adults may become ill from the same entero-

pathogens; however, the relative frequencies of these organisms may vary in different age groups because of immunity acquired from prior exposure.

Community-based studies are those in which household visits are made, usually at least once per week, to identify cases of diarrhea and to collect fecal specimens for culture. Results from these studies best represent the overall occurrence of diarrheal illnesses, regardless of severity or care-seeking. Based on 18 studies with comprehensive microbiology from nine countries (19,20,23,31,32,50–62), enterotoxigenic *Escherichia coli* (ETEC) has been found to constitute the largest proportion of episodes with a median of 14% (Table 2). The next most commonly found has been *Giardia lamblia,* but the proportion infected with this protozoan has been highly variable. *Campylobacter* species have been isolated from a median of 7%, rotaviruses from 5%, and *Shigella* species from 4%. *Cryptosporidium parvum* was found in 2% to 7% of episodes and *Entamoeba histolytica* was found in 2% or less in all but one study (median <1%).

Studies in health facilities, either outpatient clinics or hospital wards, evaluate a more selected group of patients for whom care was sought, often for an illness of greater severity. Based on 52 studies with comprehensive microbiology from 29 countries (33,63–108), rotavirus was the most frequent enteropathogen with a median of 20% (Table 3). However, these studies found that bacterial enteropathogens predominated overall. ETEC (median 12%), *Campylobacter* species (7%), and *Shigella* species (5%) have been most commonly identified. *Aeromonas, Salmonella* species, and vibrios, especially *Vibrio cholerae,* may be frequent in some settings. *Giardia lamblia* has been infrequently and *E. histolytica* rarely found in childhood diarrheas. *Cryptosporidium parvum* has been sought only more recently in etiology studies, but it has been found in each of nine studies seeking this agent, with a median identification rate of 5%.

Generally, the community-based studies have identified an enteropathogen in about half of the episodes and the facility-based studies in 60% to 70%. The tests employed to detect enteropathogens do not have optimal sensitivity and many other known enteropathogens exist than are evaluated in most studies. These other agents may each account for small proportions of the episodes without one of the more common enteropathogens identified.

The identification of an enteropathogen from feces during diarrhea does not necessarily mean that that agent is causing the illness. In fact, studies that have performed comprehensive microbiology frequently find two or more enteropathogens simultaneously and it is rarely possible to ascertain which is causing the illness or if they each are playing a role. These mixed infections could occur because the individual is exposed simultaneously to more than one agent through a common vehicle of transmission or is exposed to more than one vehicle of transmission. The individual may also have an asymptomatic infection with one enteropathogen when exposed to another.

Asymptomatic enteric infections are common in developing country populations. In community-based studies (19,20,23,31,50,52,53,55,58–61), the same children have been studied for enteropathogens on a routine basis (e.g.,

TABLE 2. *Percentage identification of selected enteropathogens from children with diarrhea in community-based studies in developing countries*

Characteristic	Aero-monas	Campylo-bacter	C. parvum	E. histolytica	ETEC	G. lamblia	Rota-virus	Sal-monella	Shigella	Vibrios
Number of studies	7	12	4	13	17	14	16	17	18	12
Median	2	7	2	<1	14	10	5	1	4	<1
Range	<1–13	2–24	2–7	0–9	5–37	<1–24	2–22	<1–16	1–27	0–3

TABLE 3. *Percentage identification of selected enteropathogens from children with diarrhea in health facilities in developing countries*

Characteristic	Aero-monas	Campylo-bacter	C. parvum	E. histolytica	ETEC	G. lamblia	Rota-virus	Sal-monella	Shigella	Vibrios
Number of studies	15	43	9	35	42	35	43	51	52	31
Median	4	7	5	1	12	2	20	4	5	2
Range	1–42	0–32	1–12	0–7	1–35	0–17	5–49	0–24	0–22	0–31

once per month), as well as when they had diarrhea. *Campylobacter* species were found as frequently when study children did not have diarrhea as when they did (Table 4). In most, but not all, studies, ETEC, *Shigella* species, and rotavirus were found more frequently during diarrhea, and the median values for percentage identification of these enteropathogens differed between diarrheal cases and controls.

In health-facility-based studies (63,65–67,70,75–77, 81–87,90,92–97,99,100,102,106), controls were usually children who came to the same facility for a reason other than diarrhea. Generally, the differences between diarrheal cases and controls were greater than in community-based studies. Most of the studies found *Campylobacter* species more frequently in diarrhea than in controls and nearly all did for ETEC and *Shigella* species (Table 4). The different rate of identification for rotavirus in cases and controls was quite striking. The rate in controls was 4% and all but one of the 27 studies found that less than 10% of controls were infected with rotavirus. In contrast, the median rate of identification in cases was 21% and more than one-quarter of studies found greater than 30% infected.

Some of the asymptomatic infections may represent convalescent carriage after an illness but could also reflect exposures to enteropathogens that were insufficient to cause illness, perhaps because of a low ingested number of organisms or immunity (109). The immunity could have been either passively transferred through breast milk or acquired from previous exposure to the organism (109–112). The high prevalence of these asymptomatic infections appears to be more indicative of frequent exposure to the agents, rather than of a long-term carrier state, which appears to be rare (19,20,111,112).

Few studies have focused specifically on enteropathogens associated with dysentery using recently developed microbiologic methods (20,113–115). However, older studies and more comprehensive recent studies have documented that *Shigella* species can be isolated in about half of dysenteric episodes (Table 5). Given the evidence that these organisms can be isolated from a single stool culture in only 60% to 70% of cases of shigellosis (116), the proportion of dysentery cases due to *Shigella* species is probably even higher. *Campylobacter* species may be the second-most frequent cause of dysentery, but its importance seems to vary by setting (113–115). Although enteroinvasive *E. coli* (EIEC) can cause dysentery, it has been isolated with very low frequency in the studies avail-

TABLE 4. *Percentage identification of* Campylobacter *species, enterotoxigenic* E. coli, *rotavirus, and* Shigella *species from cases of diarrhea (D) and children without diarrhea (C) in community-based and health facility-based studies in developing countries*

Type of study and characteristic	Campylobacter D	Campylobacter C	ETEC D	ETEC C	Rotavirus D	Rotavirus C	Shigella D	Shigella C
Community-based								
Number of studies	9		12		11		12	
Median	8	7	11	6	4	1	6	2
Range	3–22	1–48	2–34	1–22	2–22	0–21	2–27	0–19
Health facility-based								
Number of studies	24		23		27		30	
Median	8	2	13	4	21	4	4	<1
Range	0–20	0–14	3–26	0–17	6–49	0–28	0–22	0–3

TABLE 5. *Percentage identification of selected enteropathogens from children with dysentery in developing countries*

Country (reference)	Year	Age group (months)	Number of cases	*Camplylobacter*	EIEC	*Shigella*
Bangladesh (20)	1982	2–60	188	—	1	62
Thailand (113)	1986	12–120	200	12	4	44
Peru (115)	1986	3–60	170	18	—	26
Thailand (114)	1992	36–168	306	3	<1	49

able (Table 5). *Entamoeba histolytica* is capable of causing amebic colitis (117) but appears to be an infrequent cause of dysentery, especially in children (20,113,114). Other organisms such as *Salmonella* species, *V. parahaemolyticus,* and *Plesiomonas shigelloides* could be associated with dysentery in low frequency (113,114). Enterohemorrhagic (O157:H7) *E. coli* produces a hemorrhagic colitis (118). This organism has not yet been adequately studied in developing countries, but the distinctive clinical syndrome seen with this infection is uncommon. While a number of other enteropathogens such as ETEC, rotavirus, and *V. cholerae* have been isolated from feces of cases of dysentery, it is likely that these were part of a mixed infection and were not causing the invasive diarrhea.

Since persistent diarrheal episodes have particularly severe consequences for nutritional status and survival, a special effort has been focused on identifying enteropathogens associated with these episodes. To ascertain such an association it is necessary to determine the enteropathogens found in the first week of diarrhea for episodes that resolve in less than 2 weeks in comparison with episodes that persist longer, thus requiring a prospective study. Assessment of enteropathogens present during the third week of illness may also provide useful information if the organisms present in the initial stage of the same episode are known. Five studies using comprehensive microbiology provide data (31,32,61,62,119). Rotavirus was not found to be more frequent in persistent diarrhea; in fact, being more commonly found in acute diarrhea in two of four studies (31,61,62). *Aeromonas* species, *Campylobacter* species, and *G. lamblia* had similar rates of identification in acute and persistent diarrhea, and *E. histolytica* was rare in either. ETEC was frequently found in both acute and persistent episodes (Table 6). *Shigella* species have been associated with longer duration episodes (20), and their lack of association with persistent diarrhea in

these prospective studies may have been due to early antibiotic therapy.

Attention has been given recently to types of *E. coli,* demonstrating adherence properties in tissue culture assay that have been proposed as potentially important agents of acute and persistent diarrhea (120). These so-called enteroadherent *E. coli* (EAEC) are designated aggregative (AA), diffuse-adhering (DA), and localized-adhering (LA). EAEC-AA has been found to be more frequent in the initial days of persistent episodes in comparison with acute episodes in India (32), Bangladesh (31), and Mexico (119) (Table 6). On the other hand, it was found in similar frequency in acute and persistent episodes in Bangladesh (61), in Peru (62), and in Cambodian refugee children (64). EAEC-DA was found more frequently in persistent episodes only in Bangladesh (61). EAEC-LA has been the least frequently identified and was not associated with persistent diarrhea; rather, in Mexico it was associated with acute diarrhea (119).

Cultures of diarrheal episodes that have continued for more than 2 weeks have yielded enteropathogens in similar frequency to that found in the acute phase. However, examination of sequential cultures in the first and third weeks of the same episodes in Bangladesh and Peru indicates that persistent infection with the same organism during that episode is uncommon (61,62). A new enteropathogen is often found in the third week, suggesting that the prolonged episode duration in some cases is due to sequential infections with different pathogens.

In general, adults with diarrhea in developing countries seem to have predominantly bacterial infections (121,122). Enterotoxigenic *E. coli* infections are probably the most frequent (64). *Salmonella* species, *Shigella* species, and *Vibrio* species are commonly found (123–125). In areas, where *V. cholerae* O1 is endemic or where cholera epidemics are occurring, this organism may be frequent (64,126,127).

TABLE 6. *Percentage identification of selected enteropathogens during the first week of acute (A) or persistent (P) episodes of diarrhea in developing countries*

Country	*C. parvum*		EAEC-AA		EAEC-DA		EAEC-LA		ETEC		*Shigella*	
	A	P	A	P	A	P	A	P	A	P	A	P
India (32)	—	—	12	35	6	0	8	2	15	9	2	2
Bangladesh (31)	—	—	18	27	11	10	0	0	9	5	10	6
Bangladesh (61)	2	6	22	19	10	16	3	4	12	15	5	5
Peru (62)	4	1	11	12	12	13	3	4	25	24	6	8
Mexico (119)	—	—	8	51	28	33	19	4	—	—	—	—

In developing countries, diarrhea is a common complication of other infectious diseases, such as measles and the acquired immunodeficiency syndrome (AIDS). Measles-associated diarrhea has generally been linked to the same enteropathogens that cause childhood diarrhea in that setting (128,129). In one study *Campylobacter jejuni* was found more frequently in measles-associated diarrhea than in acute diarrheal controls (129). In adults with AIDS in developing countries a variety of pathogens, some uncommon causes of illness in normal hosts, have been associated with diarrhea. *Cryptosporidium parvum, Enterocytozoon bieneusi* (microsporidia), and *Isospora belli* may be especially important (130–132). However, in both adults and children common bacterial enteropathogens also play an important part in AIDS-associated diarrhea.

It appears that nosocomial diarrhea is common in developing country health facilities. Rotavirus may be especially common in nosocomial infections in pediatric wards (133), but many bacterial organisms, even *V. cholerae,* can be transmitted in treatment centers (134).

Bacterial Agents

Bacterial enteropathogens account for most of the diarrheal illnesses in both children and adults in developing countries. Most of the responsible agents were not detected until the development of appropriate conditions for their isolation and assays for identification of virulence properties in the last two decades.

Of the bacterial enteropathogens, diarrheogenic *E. coli* is clearly the predominant group causing illnesses in developing countries. Although *E. coli* organisms are an important part of the normal flora of the intestine, this organism can also cause diarrhea by a variety of mechanisms if it possesses the necessary virulence properties (135). The diarrheogenic potential of *E. coli* was recognized many years ago, with the so-called enteropathogenic *E. coli* (EPEC) (136). These organisms continued for many years to be identified by the serotypes of *E. coli* that were implicated in diarrheal outbreaks. *Escherichia coli* of these serotypes have commonly been identified in childhood diarrheas in developing countries, but this nomenclature has now been superceded. Diarrheogenic *E. coli* organisms are now designated based on the demonstration of virulence properties or laboratory characteristics felt to be associated with virulence properties (135). Some of the strains previously referred to as enteropathogenic have been found to produce attaching and effacing lesions in the intestine and localized adherence in the HEp-2 cell assay (135,137,138). The pathogenic role of EAEC-LA in acute diarrhea has been well documented (122,135); however, the importance of EAEC-DA or EAEC-AA in acute or persistent diarrhea is not yet clear (139–144).

Other strains of *E. coli* produce a heat-labile toxin (LT) or heat-stable toxin (ST) or both and a number of assays are now available to test for toxin production or the genetic capability of such production in *E. coli* (135). Although these assays are not optimally sensitive, the enterotoxigenic *E. coli* (ETEC) organisms are still the most commonly found enteropathogens. In addition, not all studies have sought both types of toxins, resulting in an underestimate of the frequency of ETEC in those studies. The relative frequencies of toxin production of each toxin by ETEC have varied from study to study, but either ST-only or LT-only strains usually predominate and strains producing both toxins are the least frequent. It has been demonstrated further that many ETEC organisms produce colonization factors that are important in pathogenesis, leaving open the possibility that not all toxin-producing strains may be capable of causing diarrhea (135). This may be a partial explanation for the high frequency of asymptomatic infections in developing country populations; however, it is also clear that acquired immunity may protect from illness but not colonization (145). Enteroinvasive and enterohemorrhagic *E. coli* do not appear to be common in developing countries, although epidemics of hemorrhagic colitis due to O157:H7 *E. coli* have occurred recently in South Africa and Swaziland.

Campylobacter jejuni or *C. coli* (often encompassed in epidemiologic studies as *C. jejuni*) appears to cause watery diarrhea and occasionally dysentery, especially in young children in developing countries (146). Immunity acquired from *C. jejuni* diarrhea is the likely explanation for the low rate of illness in adults and the high prevalence of asymptomatic infection (146). Other species of *Campylobacter* such as *C. hyointestinalis, C. lari,* or *C. upsaliensis* may cause diarrhea, but their importance is unknown (146).

Of the *Shigella* species found in diarrhea and dysentery in developing countries, *S. flexneri* is usually the most common, followed by *S. sonnei, S. boydii,* and *S. dysenteriae* (147,148). However, outbreaks of *S. dysenteriae* type 1 or Shiga bacillus have occurred in many countries (148–150). The resulting illnesses are often severe, resulting in high case fatality, and the organisms may be resistant to most commonly used antibiotics, rendering specific treatment ineffective (151).

Cholera occurs seasonally in endemic areas, such as the Ganges River delta of India and Bangladesh, as well as in global pandemics (152,153). In endemic areas cholera primarily affects children 2 to 15 years of age but may still cause a large proportion of severe watery diarrheal cases in adults during the season of transmission (152,153). Immunity develops after initial illness due to *V. cholerae,* although asymptomatic infections may still occur (154). In areas that have not had exposure to *V. cholerae* previously, the entire population is susceptible. Introduction of the organism in such a setting having poor sanitation and inadequately protected food and water can result in an explosive epidemic affecting the entire population (153,155). When the seventh pandemic of cholera, due to the El Tor biotype of *V. cholerae* O1, spread to Peru, hundreds of thousands of known cases and several thousand deaths were reported in that country (127,156). Within 1 year of introduction, 18 countries in the Western Hemisphere reported cholera, including most of South and Central America.

While El Tor *V. cholerae* O1 continues to spread, a new strain of vibrio recently caused a large epidemic of cholera-like watery diarrhea in Bangladesh and India (157). The involved *V. cholerae* non-O1 strain, assigned to serogroup O139, produces an enterotoxin apparently identical to cholera toxin. Since this epidemic has affected all age groups, similar to the pattern when *V. cholerae* O1 is newly introduced to an area, it is thought that previous experience with *V. cholerae* O1 does not provide immunologic protection from the new vibrio strain.

Aeromonas hydrophila is frequently and *Plesiomonas shigelloides* is less frequently found during diarrhea in developing countries (158). At least for *A. hydrophila,* the higher rate of isolation of the organism during diarrhea compared with controls in some studies suggests a causative role (159) (also see previously reported studies in Tables 2 and 3). However, their role as enteropathogens and the mechanisms by which they may cause diarrhea are still not resolved (160,161). *Yersinia enterocolitica* has been sought in a number of developing countries and appears to be found rarely in cases of diarrhea (162–164).

Clostridium difficile causes antibiotic-associated colitis and has been examined in this syndrome as well as in acute childhood diarrhea in a few developing countries (94,164). Limited evidence suggests that the organism may be found in acute diarrhea, but the causative relationship is not clear. The relationship of the organism to diarrhea associated with use of antibiotics has been better documented.

Viral Agents

Rotaviruses are clearly the most important cause of severe watery diarrhea in young children. The greater frequency of isolation of this agent in cases of diarrhea in health facilities than in the community undoubtedly reflects the greater severity of disease caused by rotavirus (165). This has also been documented in community-based studies where rotavirus has been associated with about 40% of the cases of diarrhea with dehydration, a potentially life-threatening complication (20).

Enteric adenoviruses of serotypes 40 and 41 may be the second most important cause of viral diarrhea (166–168). In 14 studies in developing countries (all but one of childhood diarrhea in health facilities), enteric adenoviruses were found in a median of 3% (range 0% to 6%) of episodes (57,85,89,90,92,97,107,108,169–171).

The Norwalk agent and related 27-nm caliciviruses (e.g., Hawaii and Snow Mountain agents) cause watery diarrhea and vomiting (172). Seroepidemiologic studies indicate that these agents occur worldwide (173,174). Several etiologic studies suggest that Norwalk agent alone may account for 2% to 5% of childhood diarrhea in developing countries (97,170,175). The importance of the other caliciviruses is unknown, but it is likely that they cause an additional small fraction of episodes (108).

Other viruses or virus-like particles have been proposed as causes of diarrhea. Coronaviruses (108,170) and astroviruses (176), as well as 25- to 30-mm round virus-like particles, have been found during diarrhea (108,112). Pestivirus has also been suggested as a pathogen (177). However, the causative role of these agents and their importance in developing countries are still uncertain.

Parasitic Agents

Giardia lamblia is an ubiquitous protozoan that has a very high carriage rate in many developing country populations, especially in children (178). While it could be a cause of diarrhea in specific cases, it is unlikely to be an important diarrheal pathogen in most settings (178–182). Likewise, amebiasis due to *E. histolytica* can be a serious disease with extraintestinal complications, such as liver abscess, but appears to be a very infrequent cause of childhood diarrhea or dysentery in developing countries (117,183–185) (also see Tables 2 and 3).

Cryptosporidium parvum, a small coccidian parasite, appears to be a cause of acute diarrhea and may have a particular association with persistent diarrhea or diarrhea in malnourished or immunocompromised hosts (186–188) (also see Tables 2, 3, and 6). It has a global distribution and may be the most important parasite causing childhood diarrhea in developing countries (186). Related organisms of the true coccidia, such as *I. belli,* may cause diarrhea but seem to be uncommon, except perhaps in association with AIDS (130–132). Diarrhea associated with microsporidia (*E. bieneusi*) also occurs with AIDS (189,190), but the role of this organism in immunocompetent individuals is unknown.

Cyclospora species, also referred to as "cyanobacterium-like bodies" and other names in the early literature, is a newly described protozoan enteropathogen (191–194). These coccidian parasites have been found in a number of developing countries. Infection is identified by the presence of spherical cyst-like organisms measuring 8 to 10 μm in diameter (larger than *C. parvum* oocysts, which are 3 to 5 μm) (194). Because the staining characteristics are similar to *C. parvum* and size discriminations have not been made in most previous studies, some of the cases attributed to *C. parvum* may have been due to *Cyclospora* species.

Other protozoan infections can be associated with diarrhea as well (195). *Balantidium coli* can cause diarrhea or dysentery, *Chilomastix mesnili* may result in mild diarrhea, and *Blastocystis hominis* is of uncertain pathogenicity.

Most intestinal helminthic infections are not associated with diarrhea, but dysentery and even rectal prolapse have been associated with severe *Trichuris trichiura* infections and diarrhea with other intestinal parasitic infections, such as with *Capillaria philippinensis, Trichostrongylus* species, *Strongyloides stercoralis, Necator americanus,* and *Ancylostoma duodenale* (196). Although diarrhea has been considered to occur as one of the clinical manifestations of other parasitic infections, such as malaria or schistosomiasis, a causative relationship is not clear; many of these diarrheal illnesses may be due to the highly prevalent bacterial and viral enteropathogens causing diarrhea in the same setting.

RISK FACTORS AND TRANSMISSION ROUTES

Diarrheal diseases are a consequence of two factors: exposure to a pathogenic organism and the susceptibility of the host to develop the disease. Nearly all diarrheal diseases are transmitted by direct contact with feces or indirectly through contact between feces and water, food, utensils, fingers, flies, or the ground. These routes of transmission usually coexist in a given community, although the intensity of each may vary and one or two of them may dominate (197). For an individual, one or more routes may be acting at a given time (198,199).

Socioeconomic Factors

Several studies have documented the role of socioeconomic status (SES) indicators associated with diarrheal diseases (34,200–209). Economic status and educational level may determine exposure to a particular transmission route. Even more basically, poverty and undereducation place families in poor environmental conditions, where they are exposed to multiple routes of transmission. In a prospective study in Brazil, the incidence of diarrhea was higher in poor rural and poor urban communities than in better SES urban areas (34). Family income (200–202), SES scales (202,203), ownership of valuable objects (202–207), and occupation of the household head (208) have been found associated with diarrheal diseases.

Other SES indicators have also been studied. Poorer household construction quality (204,207,210–213), crowding (200,208,214–217), larger family size (218), lower maternal education (204,208,219–221), lower maternal age (206), less access to improved water and sanitation (214,215,219,222,223), and the mother being absent from the home (224) have been found to be risk factors for diarrhea. Other studies, however, have found that lack of maternal education (203,206,207) and crowding (203, 206) were not associated with diarrhea.

SES factors affect diarrheal incidence through behavioral practices. In Lima, Peru (203), a SES scale was significantly associated with behavioral factors; such as children eating soil, adults using latrines, and children defecating outside the home. A multivariate analysis suggested that the SES scale was associated with diarrhea through the behavioral factors. A similar result was found in a study in rural Bangladesh (208).

Hygiene Practices

Hygiene practices are closely linked with person-to-person transmission of diarrhea, usually occurring indirectly through contaminated fingers. Of the hygiene practices, handwashing is probably the most widely studied. The risk of diarrhea with lack of handwashing, in particular of mothers after defecating or cleaning a child, has been documented (204,225–229). These findings have been confirmed by several studies that documented the efficacy of handwashing interventions in reducing the incidence of diarrhea (208,225,230–237).

Fecal contamination of mothers' hands has been documented to occur at the time of defecation or after cleaning their children's feces (221). The level of hand contamination with fecal coliforms was associated with diarrheal

incidence in Bangladesh (238). The association was stronger in communities with unimproved water and sanitation facilities, suggesting that the impact of handwashing might depend on the level of sanitary facilities and hygiene available in the community. This may be explained because the level of hand contamination with fecal coliforms is greater in communities without an adequate quantity of water and sanitation. Even the observation that a mother's hands were dirty (possibly correlated with fecal contamination) has been associated with more diarrhea in her child (229). Not only bacteria, but viruses, can adhere to the hands. Rotavirus was more frequently isolated from the hands of attendants of children with rotavirus diarrhea than from those attending children with nonrotavirus diarrhea in Bangladesh (239).

Handwashing with soap is effective in eliminating fecal contamination (221,225,240), even for viruses (241), and the absence of soap in the household has been found to be a risk factor for diarrhea (207). However, handwashing with ash, mud, or other agents that facilitate the removal of contaminants from the hands has also been found to be effective, but rinsing with water alone less so (204,242).

Another important hygiene behavior is the elimination of fecal material. All major enteropathogens are shed by infected persons via the feces, and therefore hygienic disposal of human excreta plays an important role in the control of diarrheal diseases (243,244).

Defecation of the child in the household area (205, 226,229,245) or in the yard or open areas (203,227), as well as nonhygienic methods of feces elimination (227,246) have been described as risk factors for diarrhea. Direct contact of the child with human feces (204) or the report of the child seen eating human feces (203) has been documented as a risk factor for diarrhea. Indirect contact of the child with feces by playing with toys or baby bottles contaminated on the ground (229) or the report of the child seen eating soil (203) has also been associated with increased risk of diarrhea. Another indirect route of exposure is the misuse of clothing, as demonstrated in a study in Bangladesh, where the mother's clothing (sari) was used for wiping the child's anus or dirty hands and then the same sari was used for cleaning eating utensils. This practice was found to be associated with an increased risk of diarrhea in children (247). Crawling infants, especially those who crawl further away or are more active, are at greater risk of fecal contamination, as demonstrated in a study in Bangladesh (204). Older children may also be at risk of increased diarrhea when exposed to dirty school toilets as shown in Cali, Colombia (248). An increased diarrheal risk has further been associated with the presence of rubbish in the house yard (207).

Other aspects related to the handling of feces may also be important. The use of paper after defecation has been shown to protect from the risk of fecal contamination of the fingers (221). Scraping the baby's feces off the ground for disposal was found to be protective for diarrhea in Bangladesh (204). The child defecating in the diaper or bucket was also found protective in Peru (203). In a structured observation study in Lima, it was found that households in which an infant's feces deposited in potties were discarded in a pit latrine had lower rates of diarrhea, while those that did not discard the feces in a latrine had higher rates (245). The use of pit latrines by adults may not be sufficient to reduce household diarrheal rates (203), although households without pit latrines have been found to have higher diarrheal rates (34) and populations moved to households with water and sanitation have reduced their diarrheal rates. Hygiene education may be an important component, as suggested by a study where the mother's failure to recognize the relationship between children feces and diarrhea was a risk factor for diarrhea and food contamination (249). Finally, interventions promoting hygienic disposal of feces may be more effective in the dry season, when water is scarce and sources more polluted, as suggested by a study in Nigeria (207).

Feeding Patterns

The increased incidence of diarrheal diseases at the age of introduction of weaning foods was recognized many years ago (250). An extensive review of the literature reported a median relative risk of diarrheal morbidity for infants not receiving breast milk, as compared to those receiving exclusive or partial breast-feeding, to be 3.0 for infants aged 0 to 2 months, 2.4 for those aged 3 to 5 months, 1.3 for those aged 6 to 8 months, and 1.5 for those aged 9 to 11 months (251). No protection was seen during the second year of life or after cessation of breast-feeding. In the first 6 months of life the relative risk was higher (3.5 to 5.9) for infants not receiving breast milk when compared with those who received breast milk and no other milks or solids. Breast-feeding was protective irrespective of the hygiene level of the study areas (251).

Several recent studies have provided further evidence of the benefits of breast-feeding (34,201,252–257). More importantly, several studies have clarified the risk of liquids and foods being added to breast milk. Two prospective studies have proved that in infants under 6 months of age, the simple addition of water or infusions to breast milk is associated with a 122% to 317% increase in diarrheal rates (252,253). The addition of other milks (128% to 235% increase) or solids (137% to 1330% increase) and the cessation of breast-feeding (280% to 1345% increase) were associated with higher rates of diarrhea, as compared with those in exclusively breast-fed infants (34,207,252–254). Not breast-feeding also has an increased risk of diarrhea when compared with partially breast-fed children and older infants. Interestingly, the protection of breast-feeding was greater in poor urban slums than in improved urban or rural areas (253,254), which had lower diarrheal incidence, suggesting that breast-feeding may be more protective in areas with a higher risk for diarrhea.

Breast-feeding may affect the duration of diarrhea (207,252). Non-breast-fed children in contrast to those at least partially breast-fed have a 25% to 200% increased diarrheal duration (14,29,258,259) or a 407% to 643% increased incidence of persistent diarrhea (258,260). Breast-feeding also reduces the severity of diarrhea. Several studies have documented the increased risk for hospitalization in children not breast-feeding as compared with

those who are breast-feeding (260–263). The protective effect has been shown for all diarrhea in children under 6 months of age (256) and for diarrhea due to *V. cholerae* or *Shigella* species in older children (256,261,262). However, the protection seems less clear for diarrhea due to rotavirus, *Campylobacter* species, and ETEC (256,264). This impact on severity may explain the documented reduced risk of death in breast-fed children (251,265–267). Bottle-fed children appeared to have higher case fatality rates for diarrhea, and in comparison with exclusively breast-fed children have a 25-fold increase in the relative risk for mortality in infants under 6 months of age (251). A Brazilian study has further documented the risk of death by feeding status, controlling for potential confounders (265–267); non-breast-fed infants were 14.2 times more likely to die of diarrhea than exclusive breast-fed infants. Partially breast-fed infants had an intermediate risk of death. Breast-feeding also protected from deaths due to persistent diarrhea, but not for dysenteric illness (267).

Food and Liquids

Bacterial contamination of weaning foods in developing countries has been documented extensively (19,224, 268–276). However, the relationship between contaminated weaning food and diarrhea has not been shown as clearly. In developed countries, food-related outbreaks of diarrheal diseases are frequent (277) but are not reliably reported in developing countries. The clear association between traveler's diarrhea and exposure to food from street vendors, restaurants, and even when prepared at home documents that food is able to transmit diarrheal diseases in developing countries (278–280). Adults in developing countries, however, do not commonly get ill when eating the same foods, most likely because of protection provided by acquired immunity. Nonimmune infants and young children are, however, at risk.

Food was suspected to be related to diarrheal diseases in children when the association between an increased incidence of diarrhea and the age of introduction of weaning foods was recognized many years ago (250). Children receiving much of their dietary intake from breast milk are at least partially protected from diarrhea (252–255,281), but the specific relationship with contaminated weaning foods has been somewhat more difficult to document. Studies in Bangladesh showed an association between ETEC infection in children and ETEC contaminated food and drinking water (145,269) but two other case–control studies in Thailand (272) and The Gambia (282) did not. Community-based longitudinal studies also have correlated the contamination of weaning foods with fecal coliforms and the incidence of diarrhea. Two studies have reported a positive association (249,269), while two other studies have not (273,283). Part of the variability in results may be due to the lack of sensitivity of the methods used in food microbiologic studies and sampling error (284).

Despite the lack of conclusive evidence, the wealth of data available indicates a very strong likelihood that weaning foods are an important route for the transmission of enteropathogens. Practically all major bacterial enteropathogens have been isolated from weaning food samples, in concentrations from 10^3 to 10^8 bacteria per gram or milliliter (19,268–276), a level that exceeds the known dose required to induce illness in a susceptible host (154). Moreover, food by itself reduces the need for a high inoculum to induce illness by the neutralization of gastric acid. For example, with cholera, instead of the 10^8 *V. cholerae* organisms required to induce illness in normal volunteers, only 10^3 organisms are needed when given with food (154).

The level and frequency of bacterial contamination vary by type of food. Foods that require cooking at high temperatures and are eaten hot (e.g., soups and stews) are less frequently contaminated than those that do not (19,268,269). Food seems to be more frequently contaminated and to have higher bacterial counts than drinking water (269). Among foods commonly given to young children, milk is more frequently contaminated and also has higher bacterial counts (tenfold higher) than other foods (19,269,270,285). One way of contaminating food is by poor hygienic practices in its manipulation, as suggested by the higher frequency of food contamination in households of low SES status (239). Dirty containers (285–287), contaminated water (19,269,285,288), and contaminated hands (19,272,285,288) are the most likely routes for entry of fecal organisms into the food.

The level of bacterial contamination is strongly influenced by the storage time between preparation and eating (19,249,268,269,282,286–289). Cooked foods cultured less than 1 hr after being prepared are often not contaminated or have low bacterial counts (19,269). The level of bacterial contamination rapidly increases in 4 to 6 hr, reaching a plateau at about 8 hr after preparation (19,249, 268,282,286–289). This bacterial proliferation is affected by ambient temperature, as demonstrated by a higher frequency of contaminated food and higher counts in samples studied during the warm compared with the cold season (268,269,272). Bacterial replication can be inhibited by keeping food at low temperature and the use of refrigerators for food storage has been found protective for diarrheal diseases (216,224). Only one study did not find any association between refrigerators and diarrhea (290), which could be explained by the use of the refrigerators for commercial or other purposes rather than storing weaning foods, as it has also been seen in Lima, Peru (C. Lanata, *unpublished data*). Inadequate cooking (268) or rewarming at temperatures up to 60°C (291) allows bacteria to survive, even in counts up to 10^3 bacteria/g (288). Cooking or rewarming food at high temperatures may destroy bacterial contaminants or reduce the content to a safe level (19,289). However, mothers in developing countries often do not warm foods to this level (i.e., >60°C) and this may not be a feasible intervention because of the need for extra time and fuel (292). Other alternatives could be the use of fermented foods (289,293) or yogurt (294) since these inhibit the growth of bacterial contaminants. Acid sauces (pH < 4) have been shown to reduce the risk of contamination in salads (295,296), but this may not be acceptable for weaning foods.

Food may also be contaminated before it reaches the home; 30% to 80% of uncooked fruits and vegetables have been reported to be contaminated with fecal coliforms and other enteropathogens, as well as a variety of other bacteria, viruses, and parasites (284,296–304). Vegetables growing close to the soil are more frequently contaminated than fruits and other vegetables grown in trees or above the ground (297,304). Fields irrigated with overhead sprinklers or with more contaminated water have a higher frequency of contamination (284,297,303,304) while vegetables grown in greenhouses irrigated with potable water are free from harmful bacteria (284,302). Polluted water has been found to contain a variety of bacteria, viruses, and parasites, which survive from 1 to 60 days (284). In the soil, fecal coliforms are more frequently isolated just after irrigation and in wet mud, while dry soil is sterile (284). Produce grown near cities that use irrigation water contaminated with sewage more frequently contains fecal bacteria than the same vegetables grown in fields away from big cities (301). Vegetables grown in contaminated water have been found to have pathogens contained in the water (284,305). Enteropathogens enter into vegetables either through the roots (284) or through the stem, as documented in experiments with healthy tomatoes exposed to test bacteria (303,304). For that reason, the elimination of irrigation with sewage-contaminated water should be considered as a high priority (306).

Irrigation is not the only source of contaminants. It is a common practice to wash vegetables at the time of harvesting to remove soil particles. Also, vegetables are kept moist with water spraying during transport and in markets. The water used for those practices is frequently of poor bacteriological quality (284). The bacterial content of vegetables has been shown to have a sixfold increase in the market as compared to the level found in the field before harvest (284).

The concentration of bacteria in vegetables and fruits has been reported to be between 10^3 and 10^8 bacteria per gram or milliliter (284,296,297,299,301–305). The concentration of bacteria is not uniform within the vegetable or fruit. In cucumbers, the highest concentration is close to the surface, suggesting that the bacteria got into the fruit through the external surface (302). In contrast, tomatoes do not allow the entrance of bacteria through their skin, but rather through the stem area (303,304). Lettuce seems to have a higher concentration of bacteria in the outer leaves (305).

Washing does reduce to some degree the level of contamination of fruits and vegetables, but not always to a safe level (297). In a laboratory experiment, the microbiologic content of lettuce, tomatoes, celery sticks, green peppers, and cucumbers did not change after a 1-min wash with plain or distilled water, a 0.01% bleach (chlorine) solution, and a 0.025% $KMnO_4$ solution (C. Lanata, *unpublished data*). Meats and dairy products can also carry enteropathogens (277,307). They may be inoculated in the abattoir by fingers of butchers contaminated after touching animal feces or internal organs, or by unhygienic surfaces or washing containers (308).

Finally, specific constituents of foods might contribute to diarrheal diseases. Lectins, present in some foods like beans and lentils, are hypothesized to facilitate the binding of bacteria with the intestinal mucosa, promoting the development of diarrhea or its prolongation (309–311). In Bangladesh, the consumption of lentils was associated with a 14% increase in the prevalence of diarrhea (14), but in Peru the consumption of beans was not associated with diarrhea (312).

Feeding Utensils

Baby bottles (19,260,313–316), baby bottle nipples (19,313,314,316,317), cups and spoons (19,314), and dirty food containers (285–287) have been found to be frequently contaminated with fecal bacteria, as well as specific diarrheogenic enteropathogens, *E. coli, Salmonella* species, *Shigella* species, *Staphylococcus aureus,* and others (19,316,317), even after being cleaned by the mother. Baby bottles have been found to be more frequently contaminated and to have higher bacterial counts than other food utensils. This is probably related to the difficulty to eliminate all food residuals and to the bottle's frequency of use, not allowing it to get completely dry. A small amount of liquid may permit bacteria to survive, and these bacteria replicate rapidly when milk or other liquids are added and kept at ambient temperature. A study in Peru has demonstrated that tea is practically sterile after its preparation (boiling water) and remains as such if served in cups to infants. However, if the same tea is served in a baby bottle, 35% of feedings had fecal coliforms (19).

The frequency of contamination of utensils and weaning foods with fecal coliforms has been associated with the hygiene level of the mother (316,317). The problem is accentuated by the fact that poor households may only own one or two feeding bottles and these will be in almost constant use (316,317). Although boiling or the use of sterilization solution for baby bottles and nipples is effective in eliminating contamination, the reported use of these methods has not been associated with a reduced occurrence frequency or level of contamination (263,313,314). This may be because the methods are infrequently or inadequately performed. Supporting this is one study that found that the same sterilization method was used more successfully by mothers of higher socioeconomic status and educational levels (317). The importance of the use of baby bottles as a risk factor for diarrhea has been difficult to document because it is closely linked to feeding patterns, that is, breast-feeding or the use of breast milk substitutes (202,203,252,253).

Water

Waterborne transmission has been documented for most enteropathogens (243), especially for *V. cholerae* (153,262,318–320), *S. typhi* (243), *G. lamblia* (243), and 27-nm Norwalk agent (321). The use of contaminated sources of water has been associated with an increased risk of diarrhea or poorer growth in several studies, probably related with its use for drinking, bathing, washing,

and cleaning feeding utensils (213,227,243,262,319,320, 322–325). The use of contaminated unboiled drinking water has been associated with diarrhea (145,207, 257,323,324). In some settings multiple water sources are frequently used for drinking and other purposes, obscuring the benefits of clean water from the primary source for drinking water (153,320). In areas without tap water, poor handling practices of water stored in the house, mainly by the introduction of contaminated hands (324) or contaminated buckets or jars (203,228), in uncovered water reservoirs (203,207) have been linked with an increased risk for diarrheal diseases. This contamination in water reservoirs at the home level is also indicated by greater levels of fecal coliforms found in the home container than at the water source (224,237). Finally, contaminated water may also introduce enteropathogens into food (285,288).

Several studies have now documented that water quantity is more important than water quality for diarrheal diseases (206,243,244,326), suggesting that the effect of water on diarrheal diseases is more through its use in hygiene behaviors than through ingestion. Nevertheless, water quality interventions have been effective in reducing diarrheal diseases (237,243,327), especially if combined with hygiene promotion (208). The use of adequate amounts of water has been found to prevent diarrheal deaths in a case–control study in Brazil, after controlling for SES and other confounding factors (326).

Flies

Many health professionals and lay personnel believe that flies transmit diarrhea. A variety of enteropathogens have been isolated from flies (328–330). These organisms can survive for some length of time: bacteria (3 to 30 days), parasites (1 day for *G. lamblia*), and viruses (12 to 17 days) (330). Survival appears longer for organisms ingested by the flies rather than carried on the surface (330). In one experiment, *S. typhimurium* could be picked up by flies from infected dog feces and inoculated into a beverage, which later infected human volunteers (330). Since flies feed once every 4 to 5 hr and deposit vomit and feces several times per hour, it is feasible that they could transmit diarrheal pathogens.

The evidence for flies as a route for transmission of enteropathogens is not conclusive. Initial studies tried to correlate fly density with diarrheal rates, providing conflicting results (330,331). Several studies have reported the isolation of enteropathogens, especially *Shigella* species, in flies captured in proximity of kitchens (328–331). In a case–control study, households with food left without fly covers were at twice the risk for having diarrhea, although the association was not significant (257). Initial fly control interventions provided unconvincing results, mostly because of the limitations in study design (330,331). An intervention in a military camp in Israel has recently shown that with a 60% fly reduction intervention, the outpatient attendance for diarrhea was reduced by 42% (85% for shigellosis) (328). Moreover, the fly intervention reduced seroconversion for ETEC by 56% and for shigella by 76% (328). These findings need to be confirmed in populations more typical of a developing country, without adequate water and sanitation and with poor hygiene habits, before fly control could be promoted as a public health intervention in developing countries. It is plausible that flies could contribute to transmission of diarrheal illnesses, especially those due to *Shigella* species, because of the low number of organisms required to cause shigellosis (332), but they may not be a predominant transmission route. Other insects, like cockroaches, could also play a minor role in the transmission of enteropathogens (333).

Animals

Animal feces have been reported to harbor a variety of enteropathogens, in particular, *Campylobacter jejuni*, *Salmonella* species, *C. parvum*, and ETEC (19,145, 334–337). The relationship varies by enteropathogen, since only a few cause diarrhea in both animals and humans. In a study in Bangladesh, the presence of ETEC in animal feces was not associated with ETEC diarrhea (145). On the other hand, *C. jejuni* may be very related to exposure to animal feces (146). Most chickens living in or around households in developing countries are positive for *C. jejuni* (19,334,336,337). In a case–control study in Peru, the strongest risk factor for *Campylobacter* species diarrhea was the presence of a chicken in the house (338). A similar association was found in a study done in Central Afican Republic (336). Using structured observation techniques, it was documented in a periurban community in Lima, Peru, that in a 12-hr period an infant crawling on the house floor had a mean of 2.9 contacts with chicken feces and that hands or objects contaminated by touching chicken feces were introduced into the child's mouth a mean of 3.9 times (337). *Campylobacter jejuni* was documented to survive up to 48 hr in the chicken's feces deposited on the household floor (337). In another study done in Lima, using a latex tracer given to chickens, it was possible to demonstrate recovery of the tracer from children's and mothers' hands and feces in all households studied (L. Roberts, *unpublished data*). Corraling the animals was 100% effective in preventing this contamination. However, an intervention study evaluating the effect of corraling free-living chickens in the household, done in Lima, failed to demonstrate any significant reduction of diarrheal rates or *C. jejuni* infections in children (C. Lanata, *unpublished data*). This may suggest other routes of transmission that are at least as important as the direct exposure to chicken feces.

Other Routes of Transmission

Other routes of transmission for diarrheal diseases could also exist. Air has been suggested as a vehicle for the transmission of rotavirus, but this has not been clearly shown (339,340).

HOST RISK FACTORS

Malnutrition

Malnutrition and diarrheal diseases have been found to be associated, in part because they both occur with high frequency in children living in poor socioeconomic and environmental conditions (341). However, malnutrition may be a more direct risk factor for diarrheal diseases through compromise of host immune and nonimmune defenses and regenerative capabilities.

Malnourished children, generally classified by low anthropometric status using a variety of indicators, have been found in some studies to have an increased incidence of diarrhea (an increase of 20% to 70%) (216,217,342–344). A number of other studies have found no increase in diarrheal incidence in malnourished children (345–347).

Malnourished children and adults have been shown to have diarrheal episodes of longer duration (217,345, 348,349). Health facility-based studies have found this relationship (348,349), but because they cannot ascertain if the malnutrition preceded or resulted from the diarrheal episode, the role of malnutrition as a risk factor needs to be established in prospective studies. Such prospective community-based studies in a number of countries have clearly documented that malnutrition is a risk factor for diarrheal episode duration, whether related to all episodes or those due to ETEC or *Shigella* species (345). The duration may increase 200% or more in malnourished children. As might then be expected, malnutrition is also a risk factor for persistent diarrhea, increasing incidence of persistent diarrhea in community-based studies by 200% to 300% (217,345,350,351).

Malnutrition may also be related to other measures of severity in diarrheal episodes. More malnourished children with rotavirus diarrhea were found to have more severe dehydration (352) and a higher rate of diarrheal stool output (353). Furthermore, malnourished children have a higher case fatality rate from diarrhea, especially persistent diarrhea (13), and an increased diarrheal mortality rate (12,354–356).

The mechanisms by which malnutrition may influence diarrhea and other infections have not been clearly established. Malnutrition is associated with decreased immune functions, as manifested in reduced production of secretory immunoglobulins (357,358) and depressed cell-mediated immunity (343,359), both of which could affect resistance to enteropathogens. It may also be related to nonimmune deficits in resistance, such as reduced gastric acid permitting entry of a greater infectious dose of enteropathogens (360,361). Furthermore, once infection and damage of intestinal mucosal cells have occurred, malnutrition may result in delayed epithelial regeneration (362).

Micronutrient Deficiencies

Specific micronutrient deficiencies may result in either a higher incidence or greater severity of diarrhea. Vitamin A deficiency is associated with a higher rate of severe diarrhea (363) and in a deficient population, vitamin A supplementation reduces diarrheal mortality (364–367). Zinc deficiency may also be related to diarrhea (368). Zinc supplementation has shortened the duration of diarrhea (369–371). Other micronutrients, such as folic acid, may be related to diarrhea as well. As with malnutrition in general, these specific deficiencies could have immune or nonimmune mechanisms to reduce resistance or delay recovery.

Previous Morbidity

A subset of the population of children in developing countries has a high prevalence of diarrhea (23,29,372). A strong predictor of an episode of diarrhea is a recent similar episode (342,344,350). This may again reflect high exposure to enteropathogens, reduced host resistance, or perhaps the prior episode actually contributed to the reduced resistance through mucosal damage, micronutrient losses, and/or immunosuppression. These possible mechanisms also apply to measles, which is known to increase the risk of diarrhea for a month or longer following an episode (373).

Gastric Acid

The acidic contents of the stomach form an important barrier to ingested enteropathogens, especially many of the bacterial agents. Hypochlorhydria may increase the likelihood of an illness-inducing level of the organism reaching the small intestine. Indeed, hypochlorhydria has been shown to be a risk factor for cholera and has been hypothesized for other diarrheal infections (374–377). It follows that medical conditions that reduce gastric acid or medications that neutralize acid might lead to a greater frequency or severity of diarrheal infections.

Helicobacter pylori infection of the stomach is common in children in developing countries (378). This infection may result in hypochlorhydria, perhaps leading to a greater risk of diarrhea (379).

Blood Group

Persons of blood group O have a greater risk of cholera, at least with *V. cholerae* El Tor infections, and of developing more severe illness (380–382). The mechanism has not been determined. Few studies have been done to examine such a relationship with other enteropathogens, but limited data suggest that a strong relationship does not exist for ETEC or for vibrios, other than *V. cholerae* O1 (383,384).

Immunity

The immune defenses clearly play an important role in susceptibility to enteropathogens. Maternal antibody passively acquired by the infant through breast milk pro-

tects against a variety of enteric infections and immunity is actively acquired by the child as a result of symptomatic and asymptomatic infections with enteropathogens.

Evidence is also accumulating that the competence of the immune system can be compromised, possibly reducing resistance to enteric infection and delaying recovery. Studies in Bangladesh and Peru have shown that children have depressed cell-mediated immunity, as assessed by delayed-type hypersensitivity to common antigens (343,344,350,385). Even controlling for anthropometric status or other variables, anergy was associated with a 100% increase in diarrhea and persistent diarrhea.

Immunocompetence of a child can be compromised by previous viral infections, such as measles (or measles vaccine) or influenza, or by other infections, such as tuberculosis or typhoid fever (386–390). The immune system can also be affected by a variety of micronutrient deficiencies, notably vitamin A and zinc (391,392). Thus these deficiencies could place children at greater risk of diarrhea or of severe illness through alterations in immune functions, as well as by a variety of other mechanisms.

STRATEGIES FOR CONTROL OF DIARRHEAL DISEASES

Reduction of mortality by prompt and appropriate treatment of diarrhea is the mainstay of diarrheal disease control programs (1). Prevention and correction of dehydration by oral rehydration therapy and maintenance of nutrition by continued feeding during illness are reducing mortality from dehydrating diarrheas (2). Antibiotic therapy of dysentery as presumed shigellosis will shorten the duration of illness and the dysentery case fatality rate (393). Finally, for persistent diarrhea, the most important diarrheal syndrome associated with mortality, dietary management can be effective to both treat the episode and improve the underlying nutritional deficits (14).

The remaining challenge for diarrheal disease control programs is prevention. A series of reviews of possible preventive interventions was completed in the 1980s (394). This effort identified a group of interventions for which there was evidence of high effectiveness and feasibility.

Promotion of breast-feeding and improved weaning practices are considered to be high priority. It has been estimated that successful breast-feeding promotion programs could reduce diarrhea prevalence by 40% in infants aged 0 to 2 months, 30% in those aged 3 to 5 months, and 10% in those aged 6 to 11 months (251). This might reduce diarrheal mortality rates in children under 5 years of age by 8% to 9%. Improving weaning practices could have the dual advantages of improving nutrient content and decreasing microbial contamination (395). It has been estimated that weaning education can improve nutritional status and thereby reduce diarrheal severity and case fatality. Between 2% and 12% reduction in childhood mortality could be expected by this indirect route (396). Reducing transmission of enteropathogens should be successful in reducing diarrheal incidence, based on the epidemiologic studies of diarrheal transmission to young children (397).

Since no intervention trials have been completed, it is not possible to estimate the magnitude of the reduction in incidence from an improvement in food safety.

Improved water supply, sanitation, and hygiene behaviors could also be expected to reduce diarrheal incidence. If both water supply and sanitation are improved, it has been estimated that diarrheal incidence and mortality could be reduced by about one-quarter (243). Improvements in water availability or in sanitation have been found to have greater impact on diarrheal diseases than improvement in water quality. Hygiene education may further enhance the impact. In fact, handwashing education programs have been found to reduce diarrheal incidence by 14% to 48% (225). It is expected then that well-designed projects combining water supply, sanitation, and hygiene education may reduce diarrheal morbidity by 35% to 50% (394).

Measles immunization as is currently being widely implemented in developing country health programs is likely having a substantial effect. It has been estimated that measles vaccination with 60% coverage may reduce diarrheal incidence by 2% and diarrheal mortality by 13% (398).

Improved cholera vaccines are in development and field testing. If successful, these vaccines may find public health use in related areas (399). An oral killed whole-cell vaccine with or without the B subunit of cholera toxin, given in three doses, has been shown to have 50% efficacy for at least 3 years (400). This vaccine might be useful for public health purposes in a cholera endemic area if given to young children or in an area where cholera was recently introduced if provided to the entire population. The long-term protection afforded by this vaccine enhances its potential for use. However, the lower level of protection shown in children (23% to 26% efficacy) may make the vaccine less useful in an endemic area or in an area not previously exposed, where the efficacy in the entire population may be similar to that of children in an endemic area. Other candidate cholera vaccines, including an attenuated live strain of *V. cholerae* O1, are in field trials (401,402). A potential drawback to all the cholera vaccines currently being developed is that they may not protect from the *V. cholerae* O139 currently causing epidemics in South Asia (157). Modified vaccines containing antigens of this new strain are being developed.

Rotavirus may be responsible for 5% of all diarrheal episodes and 20% of deaths in children under 5 years of age (399). The importance of rotavirus as a cause of mortality, the belief that there were only four rotavirus serotypes, and the ability to use animal rotavirus strains to construct animal–human rotavirus reassortants gave great impetus to rotavirus vaccine development. The most advanced vaccine, a tetravalent vaccine made with rhesus monkey rotavirus and three rhesus–human reassortant strains, has shown high-level protection, especially against severe rotavirus diarrhea (403,404). This or an improved vaccine may be useful for ultimate incorporation in the schedule of childhood immunizations.

It is still critical to ensure that all children in developing countries can receive effective case management for diarrhea. This will rightly remain the emphasis of diarrheal disease control programs in the next decade. However, there is also a pressing need to implement preventive interventions known to be efficacious, while continuing to seek even more effective and feasible technologies, such as vaccines, against the major enteropathogens.

REFERENCES

1. Claeson M, Merson MH. Global progress in the control of diarrheal diseases. *Pediatr Infect Dis J* 1990;9:345–355.
2. Bern C, Martines J, de Zoysa I, Glass RI. The magnitude of the global problem of diarrhoeal disease: a ten-year update. *Bull World Health Organ* 1992;70:705–714.
3. Stuart HC. Mortality among infants and children and progress in reduction in rates from certain causes. *J Pediatr* 1938;15:266–276.
4. Newsholme A. *Fifty years in public health.* London: George Allen and Unwin, 1939;321–360.
5. The World Bank. Households and health. In: World *development report 1993: investing in health.* Oxford: Oxford University Press, 1993;37–51.
6. Rutstein SO. Levels, trends and differentials in infant and child mortality in the less developed countries. In: *Child health priorities for the 1990s.* Baltimore: Johns Hopkins University Institute for International Programs, 1992;17–42.
7. Santosham M, Brown KH, Sack RB. Oral rehydration therapy and dietary therapy for acute childhood diarrhea. *Pediatr Rev* 1987;8:273–278.
8. Kielmann AA, Mobarek AB, Hammamy MT, et al. Control of deaths from diarrheal diseases in rural communities. 1. Design of an intervention study and effects on child mortality. *Trop Med Parasitol* 1985;36:191–198.
9. El-Rafie M, Hassouna WA, Hirschhorn N, et al. Effect of diarrhoeal disease control on infant and childhood mortality in Egypt. *Lancet* 1990;335:334–338.
10. Victora CH, Huttly SRA, Fuchs SC, et al. International differences in clinical patterns of diarrhoeal deaths: a comparison of children from Brazil, Senegal, Bangladesh, and India. *J. Diarrhoeal Dis Res* 1993;11:25–29.
11. Mølbak K, Aaby P, Ingholt L, et al. Persistent and acute diarrhea as the leading causes of child mortality in urban Guinea Bissau. *Trans R Soc Trop Med Hyg* 1992;86:216–220.
12. Fauveau V, Henry FJ, Briend A, et al. Persistent diarrhea as a cause of childhood mortality in rural Bangladesh. *Acta Paediatr* 1992;381(Suppl):15–21.
13. Bhan MK, Arora NH, Ghai KR, Khoshoo V, Bhandari N. Major factors in diarrhoea related mortality among rural children. *Indian J Med Res* 1986;83:9–12.
14. Black RE. Persistent diarrhea in children of developing countries. *Pediatr Infect Dis J* 1993;12:751–761.
15. Ashkenazi S, Cleary TG. Antibiotic treatment of bacterial gastroenteritis. *Pediatr Infect Dis J* 1991;10:140–148.
16. Richards L, Claeson M, Pierce N. Management of acute diarrhea in children: lessons learned. *Pediatr Infect Dis J* 1993;12:5–9.
17. The World Health Organization. Program for control of diarrheal diseases. *Interim programme report.* WHO/CDD/93.40, 1992.
18. Baqui AH, Black RE, Yunus MD, Hoque ARA, Chowdhury HR, Sack RB. Methodological issues in diarrhoeal diseases epidemiology: definition of diarrhoeal episodes. *Int J Epidemiol* 1991;20:1057–1063.
19. Black RE, Lopez de Romana G, Brown KH, Bravo N, Bazalar OG, Kanashiro HC. Incidence and etiology of infantile diarrhea and major routes of transmission in Huascar, Peru. *Am J Epidemiol* 1989;129:785–799.
20. Black RE, Brown KH, Becker S, Abdul Alim ARM, Huq I. Longitudinal studies of infectious diseases and physical growth of children in rural Bangladesh. II. Incidence of diarrhea and association with known pathogens. *Am J Epidemiol* 1982;115:315–324.
21. Lanata CF, Black RE, Gilman RH, Lazo F, Del Aquila R. Epidemiologic, clinical, and laboratory characteristics of acute

vs. persistent diarrhea in periurban Lima, Peru. *J Pediatr Gastroenterol Nutr* 1991;12:82–88.

22. McAuliffe JF, Shields DS, de Souza MA, Sakell J, Schorling J, Guerrant RL. Prolonged and recurring diarrhea in the northeast of Brazil: examination of cases from a community-based study. *J Pediatr Gastroenterol Nutr* 1986;5:902–906.

23. Schorling JB, Wanke CA, Schorling SK, McAuliffe JF, Aixiliadora de Souza M, Guerrant RL. A prospective study of persistent diarrhea among children in an urban Brazilian slum: patterns of occurrence and etiologic agents. *Am J Epidemiol* 1990; 132:144–156.

24. World Health Organization. Diarrhoeal diseases control. *Persistent diarrhoea in children*. CDD/DDM/85.1, 1985.

25. World Health Organization. Report of a WHO Meeting. *Persistent diarrhoea in children in developing countries*. WHO/CDD/88.27, 1988.

26. Martorell R, Habicht J-P, Yarbrough C, Lechtig A. Underreporting in fortnightly recall morbidity surveys. *Environ Child Health* 1976;June:129–134.

27. Alam N, Henry FJ, Rahaman MM. Reporting errors in one-week diarrhoea recall surveys: experience from a prospective study in rural Bangladesh. *Int J Epidemiol* 1989;18:697–700.

28. Laston S. *Risk factors for diarrheal disease in village children in Nepal* [Doctoral dissertation]. Cleveland: Case Western Reserve University, 1992.

29. Baqui AH, Black RE, Sack RB, Yunus MD, Siddique AK, Chowdhury HR. Epidemiological and clinical characteristics of acute and persistent diarrhea in rural Bangladeshi children. *Acta Paediatr* 1992;381(Suppl):15–21.

30. Huttly SRA, Hoque BA, Azia KMA, Hasan KZ, Patwary MY, Rahaman MM, Feachem RH. Persistent diarrhoea in a rural area of Bangladesh: a community-based longitudinal study. *Int J Epidemiol* 1989;18:964–969.

31. Henry FJ, Udoy AS, Wanke CA, Aziz K. Epidemiology of persistent diarrhea and etiologic agents in Mirzapur, Bangladesh. *Acta Paediatr* 1992;381(Suppl):27–31.

32. Bhan MK, Bhandari N, Sazawal S, et al. Descriptive epidemiology of persistent diarrhea among young children in rural northern India. *Bull World Health Organ* 1989;67:281–288.

33. Black RE, Merson MH, Rahman ASMM, et al. A two year study of bacterial, viral, and parasitic agents associated with diarrhea in rural Bangladesh. *J Infect Dis* 1980;142:660–664.

34. Guerrant RL, Kirchhoff LV, Shields DS, et al. Prospective study of diarrheal illnesses in northeastern Brazil: patterns of disease, nutritional impact, etiologies, and risk factors. *J Infect Dis* 1983;148:986–997.

35. Cook SM, Glass RI, LeBaron CW, Ho M-S. Global seasonality of rotavirus infections. *Bull World Health Organ* 1990;68:171–177.

36. Joe LK, Rukmono B, Oemijati S, et al. Diarrhoea among infants in a crowded area of Djakarta, Indonesia. A longitudinal study from birth to two years. *Bull World Health Organ* 1966;34:197–210.

37. Mata LJ, Urrutia JJ, Gordon JE. Diarrhoeal diseases in a cohort of Guatemalan village children observed from birth to age two years. *Trop Geogr Med* 1967;19:247–257.

38. Georges MC, Roure C, Tauxe RV, et al. Diarrhoeal morbidity and mortality in children in the Central African Republic. *Am J Trop Med Hyg* 1989;36:598–602.

39. El Alamy MA, Thacker SB, Arafat RR, et al. The incidence of diarrhoeal disease in a defined population in rural Egypt. *Am J Trop Med Hyg* 1986;35:1006–1012.

40. Kumar V, Kumar R, Dutta N. Oral rehydration therapy in reducing diarrhoea-related mortality in rural India. *J Diarrhoeal Dis Res* 1987;5:159–164.

41. Nazir M, Pardede N, Ismail R. The incidence of diarrhoeal diseases and diarrhoeal diseases related mortality in rural swampy low-land area of south Sumatra. *J Trop Pediatr* 1985; 31:268–272.

42. Institute of Medicine. Committee on Issues and Priorities for New Vaccine Development. *New vaccine development: establishing priorities, vol II. Diseases of importance in developing countries*. Washington, DC: National Academy Press, 1986.

43. The World Bank. Health and developing countries: successes and challenges. In: *World development report 1993: investing in health*. Oxford: Oxford University Press, 1993;17–36.

44. Black RE. Would control of childhood infectious diseases reduce malnutrition? *Acta Paediatr Scand Suppl* 1991;374:133–140.

45. Black RE, Brown KH, Becker S. Effects of diarrhea associated with specific enteropathogens on the growth of children in rural Bangladesh. *Pediatrics* 1984;73:799–805.

46. Black RE, Brown KH, Becker S. Influence of acute diarrhea on the growth parameters of children. In: Bellanti JA, ed. *Acute diarrhea: its nutritional consequences in children*, Nestle Nutrition Workshop Series, vol. 2. New York: Raven Press, 1983; 75–84.

47. Schorling JB, Guerrant RL. Diarrhea and catch-up growth. *Lancet* 1990;335:599–600.

48. Guerrant RL, Schorling JB, McAuliffe JF, de Souza MNA. Diarrhea as a cause and effect of malnutrition: diarrhea prevents catch-up growth and malnutrition increases diarrhea frequency and duration. *Am J Trop Med Hyg* 1992;47(1 Pt 2):28–35.

49. Harris S, Black RE. How useful are pharmaceuticals in managing diarrhoeal diseases in developing countries? *Health Policy Management* 1991;6:141–147.

50. Aye T, Nyien MM, Kanemasa Y, Hayashi Y. Etiological agents responsible for acute diarrhea in children in an urban community in Burma. *Microbiol Immunol* 1983;27:551–556.

51. Sircar BK, Deb BC, Sengupta PG, Mondal S, et al. A longitudinal study of diarrhoea among children in Calcutta communities. *Indian J Med Res* 1984;80:546–550.

52. Goh Rowland SGJ, Lloyd-Evans N, Williams K, Rowland MGM. The etiology of diarrhoea studied in the community in young urban Gambian children. *J Diarrhoeal Dis Res* 1985;3:7–13.

53. Mathur R, Reddy C, Naidu AN, Ravikumar, Krishnamachari KAVR. Nutritional status and diarrhoeal morbidity: a longitudinal study in rural Indian preschool children. *Human Nutr Clin Nutr* 1985;49C:447–454.

54. Guigliano LG, Bernardi MG, Vasconcelos JC, Costa CA, Giugliano R. Longitudinal study of diarrhoeal disease in a peri-urban community in Manaus (Amazon–Brazil). *Ann Trop Med Parasitol* 1986;80:443–450.

55. Cravioto A, Reyes RE, Ortego R, Fernandez G, Hernandez R, Lopez D. Prospective study of diarrhoeal disease in a cohort of rural Mexican children: incidence and isolated pathogens during the first two years of life. *Epidemiol Infect* 1988;101:123–134.

56. Tin-Aye, Mar-Mar-Nyein, Kyi-Kyi-Khin, et al. Epidemiology and aetiology of acute childhood diarrhoea in Burma: a rural community survey. *Trans R Soc Trop Med Hyg* 1989;83:827–830.

57. Linhares AC, Gabbay YB, Freitas RB, Travassos da Rosa ES, Mascarenhas JDP, Loureiro ECB. Longitudinal study of rotavirus infections among children from Belem, Brazil. *Epidemiol Infect* 1989;102:129–145.

58. Stanton B, Silimperi D, Khatun K, et al. Parasitic, bacterial and viral pathogens isolated from diarrhoeal and routine stool specimens of urban Bangladeshi children. *J Trop Med Hyg* 1989;92:46–55.

59. Loening WEK, Coovadia YM, Van Den Ende J. Aetiological factors of infantile diarrhoea: a community-based study. *Ann Trop Paediatr* 1989;9:248–255.

60. Nakano T, Binka FN, Afari EA, et al. Survey of enteropathogenic agents in children with and without diarrhoea in Ghana. *J Trop Med Hyg* 1990;93:408–412.

61. Baqui AH, Sack RB, Black RE, et al. Enteropathogens associated with acute and persistent diarrhea in Bangladeshi children <5 years of age. *J Infect Dis* 1992;166:792–796.

62. Lanata CF, Black RE, Máurtua D, et al. Etiologic agents in acute vs persistent diarrhea in children under three years of age in peri-urban Lima, Peru. *Acta Paediatr* 1992;381(Suppl):32–38.

63. Mutanda LN. Epidemiology of acute gastroenteritis in early childhood in Kenya: aetiological agents. *Trop Geogr Med* 1980; 32:138–143.

64. Stoll BJ, Glass RI, Huq MI, Khan MU, Holt JE, Banu H. Surveillance of patients attending a diarrhoeal disease hospital in Bangladesh. *Br Med J* 1982;285:1185–1188.

65. Thoren A, Stintzing G, Tufvesson B, Walder M, Habte D. Aetiology and clinical features of severe infantile diarrhoea in Addis Ababa, Ethiopia. *J Trop Paediatr* 1982;28:127–131.

66. Stintzing G, Möllby R, Habte D. Enterotoxigenic *Escherichia coli* and other enteropathogens in paediatric diarrhoea in Addis Ababa. *Acta Paediatr Scand* 1982;71:279–286.

67. Patel IU, Bhushan V, Chintu C, Bathirunathan N. Bacteriological study of diarrhoea in children at university teaching hospital, Lusaka, Zambia. *East Afr Med J* 1982;59:793–797.

68. Dosunmu-Ogunbi O, Coker AO, Agboniahor DE, Solanke SO, Uzoma KC. Local pattern of acute enteric bacterial infections in man—Lagos, Nigeria. International Symposium on Enteric Infections in Man and Animals: Standardization of Immunological Procedures, Dublin, Ireland, 1982. *Dev Biol Standard* 1983: 53;277–283.

69. DeMol P, Brasseur D, Hemelhof W, Kalala T, Butzler JP, Vis HL. Enteropathogenic agents in children with diarrhoea in rural Zaire. *Lancet* 1983;1:516–518.

70. Soenarto Y, Sebodo T, Suryantoro P, et al. Bacteria, parasitic agents and rotaviruses associated with acute diarrhoea in hospital in-patient Indonesian children. *Trans R Soc Trop Med Hyg* 1983;77:724–730.

71. Georges MC, Wachsmuth IK, Meunier DMV, et al. Parasitic, bacterial, and viral enteric pathogens associated with diarrhea in the Central African Republic. *J Clin Microbiol* 1984;19: 571–575.

72. Bogaerts J, Lepage P, Rouvry D, Vandepitte J. *Cryptosporidium* spp., a frequent cause of diarrhea in central Africa. *J Clin Microbiol* 1984;20:874–876.

73. Sen D, Saha MR, Balakrish Nair G, et al. Etiological spectrum of acute diarrhoea in hospitalised patients in Calcutta. *Indian J Med Res* 1985;82:286–291.

74. Echeverria P, Seriwatana J, Taylor DN, Yanggratoke S, Tirapat C. A comparative study of enterotoxigenic *Escherichia coli*, *Shigella*, *Aeromonas*, and *Vibrio* as etiologies of diarrhea in northeastern Thailand. *Am J Trop Med Hyg* 1985;34:547–554.

75. Trujillo H, Jaramillo C, Restrepo M, et al. Rotavirus y otros enteropatogenos en la etiologia de la diarrea aguda en Medellin, Colombia, 1982. *Bol Of Sanit Panam* 1985;98:251–260.

76. Bhat P, Macaden R, Unnyrishnan P, Rao HGV. Rotavirus and bacterial enteropathogens in acute diarrhoeas of young children in Bangalore. *Indian J Med Res* 1985;82:105–109.

77. Poocharoen L, Briun CW, Sirisanthana V, Vannareumol P, Leechanachai P, Sukhavat K. The relative importance of various enteropathogens as a cause of diarrhoea in hospitalized children in Chiang Mai, Thailand. *J Diarrhoeal Dis Res* 1986; 4:10–15.

78. Koornhof KH, Chaoub BD, Turnbull PCB, Miliotis MD, Richardson JL, Klugman KP, Khumalo Z. Bacterial enteritis of infancy and childhood in Soweto. *S Afr Med J* 1986 (Oct 11 suppl);51–54.

79. Shukry S, Zaki AM, DuPont HL, Shoukry I, El Tagi M, Hamed Z. Detection of enteropathogens in fatal and potentially fatal diarrhea in Cairo, Egypt. *J Clin Microbiol* 1986;24:959–962.

80. Mohandas V, Unni J, Mathew M, et al. Aetiology and clinical features of acute childhood diarrhoea in an outpatient clinic in Vellore, India. *Ann Trop Paediatr* 1987;7:167–172.

81. Moyenuddin M, Rahman KM, Sack DA. The aetiology of diarrhoea in children at an urban hospital in Bangladesh. *Trans R Soc Trop Med Hyg* 1987;81:299–302.

82. Bhan MK, Kumar R, Khoshoo V, et al. Etiologic role of enterotoxigenic *Escherichia coli* and rotavirus in acute diarrhoea in Delhi children. *Indian J Med Res* 1987;85:604–607.

83. Khan MMA, Khan A, Iqbal J, Ghafoor A, Burney M. Aetiologic agents of diarrhoeal diseases in hospitalised children in Rawalpindi, Pakistan. *J Diarrhoeal Dis Res* 1988;6:228–231.

84. Steele AD, Geyer A, Alexander JJ, Crewe-Brown HH, Fripp PJ. Enteropathogens isolated from children with gastro-enteritis at Ga-Rankuwa Hospital, South Africa. *Ann Trop Paediatr* 1988;8:262–267.

85. Al-Bwardy MAA, Ramia S, Al-Frayh AR, et al. Bacterial, parasitic, and viral enteropathogens associated with diarrhoea in Saudi children. *Ann Trop Paediatr* 1988;8:26–30.

86. Gueddana N, Saffen S, Ben Aissa, et al. Etudé etiologique des gastroenferites aigües de l'enfant en Tunisie. *Arch Fr Pediatr* 1988;45:207–211.

87. Casalino M, Yusuf MW, Nicoletti M, et al. A two-year study of enteric infections associated with diarrhoeal diseases in children in urban Somalia. *Trans R Soc Trop Med Hyg* 1988;82: 637–641.

88. Osisanya JOS, Daniel SO, Sehgal C, et al. Acute diarrhoeal disease in Nigeria: detection of enteropathogens in a rural Sub-Saharan population. *Trans R Soc Trop Med Hyg* 1988;82: 773–777.

89. Echeverria P, Taylor DN, Lexsomboon U, et al. Case–control study of endemic diarrheal disease in Thai children. *J Infect Dis* 1989;159:543–548.

90. Sethi S, Khuffash F. Bacterial and viral causes of acute diarrhoea in children in Kuwait. *J Diarrhoeal Dis Res* 1989;7: 85–88.

91. Mikhail IA, Hyams KC, Podgore JK, et al. Microbiologic and clinical study of acute diarrhea in children in Aswan, Egypt. *Scand J Infect Dis* 1989;21:59–65.

92. Sethi SK, Khuffash FA, Al-Nakib W. Microbial etiology of acute gastroenteritis in hospitalized children in Kuwait. *Pediatr Infect Dis J* 1989;8:593–597.

93. Gomes TAT, Blake PA, Trabulsi LR. Prevalence of *Escherichia coli* strains with localized, diffuse, and aggregative adherence to HeLa cells in infants with diarrhea and matched controls. *J Clin Microbiol* 1989;27:266–269.

94. Kim K-H, Suh I-S, Kim J-M, Kim C-W, Cho Y-J. Etiology of childhood diarrhea in Korea. *J Clin Microbiol* 1989;27(6): 1192–1196.

95. Mertens TE, Wijenayake R, Pinto MRM, et al. Microbiological agents associated with childhood diarrhoea in the dry zone of Sri Lanka. *Trop Med Parasitol* 1990;41:115–120.

96. Katouli M, Jaafari A, Farhoudi-Moghaddam AA, Ketabi GR. Aetiological studies of diarrhoeal diseases in infants and young children in Iran. *J Trop Med Hyg* 1990;93:22–27.

97. Huilan S, Zhen LG, Mathan MM, et al. Etiology of acute diarrhoea among children in developing countries: a multicentre study in five countries. *Bull World Health Organ* 1991;69: 549–555.

98. Ghosh AR, Nair GB, Dutta P, Pal SC, Sen D. Acute diarrhoeal diseases in infants aged below six months in hospital in Calcutta, India: an aetiological study. *Trans R Soc Trop Med Hyg* 1991;85:796–798.

99. Kain KC, Barteluk RL, Kelly MT, et al. Etiology of childhood diarrhea in Beijing, China. *J Clin Microbiol* 1991;29:90–95.

100. Pazzaglia G, Sack RB, Salazar E, et al. High frequency of coinfecting enteropathogens in *Aeromonas*-associated diarrhea of hospitalized Peruvian infants. *J Clin Microbiol* 1991;29: 1151–1156.

101. Na'was TE, Abo-Shehada MN. A study of the bacterial and parasitic causes of acute diarrhoea in northern Jordan. *J Diarrhoeal Dis Res* 1991;9(4):305–309.

102. Tardelli Gomes TA, Rassi V, MacDonald KL. Enteropathogens associated with acute diarrheal disease in urban infants in Sao Paulo, Brazil. *J Infect Dis* 1991;164:331–337.

103. Baqui AH, Zaman K, Yunus M, Mitra AK, Hossain KMB. Surveillance of patients attending a rural diarrhoea treatment centre in Bangladesh. *Trop Geogr Med* 1991;29:17–22.

104. Arthur JD, Bodhidatta L, Echeverria P, Phuphaisan S, Paul S. Diarrheal disease in Cambodian children at a camp in Thailand. *Am J Epidemiol* 1992;135(5):541–551.

105. Dutta P, Lahiri M, Sen D, Pal SC. Prospective hospital based study on persistent diarrhoea. *Gut* 1991;32:791–790.

106. Ming ZF, Xi ZD, Dong CS, et al. Diarrhoeal disease in children less than one year of age at a children's hospital in Guangzhou, People's Republic of China. *Trans R Soc Trop Med Hyg* 1991; 85:667–669.

107. San Pedro MC, Walz SE. A comprehensive survey of pediatric diarrhea at a private hospital in Metro Manila. *Southeast Asian J Trop Med Public Health* 1991;22:203–210.

108. Mathew M, Mathew MM, Mani K, et al. The relationship of

microbial pathogens to acute infectious diarrhoea of childhood. *J Trop Med Hyg* 1991;94:253–260.

109. Levine MM, Kaper JB, Black RE, Clements ML. New knowledge on pathogenesis of bacterial enteric infections as applied to vaccine development. *Microbiol Rev* 1983;47:510–550.

110. Glass RI, Svennerholm A-M, Stoll BJ, et al. Protection against cholera in breast-fed children by antibodies in breast milk. *N Engl J Med* 1983;308:1389–1392.

111. Ferreccio C, Prado V, Ojeda A, et al. Epidemiologic patterns of acute diarrhea and endemic *Shigella* infections in children in a poor periurban setting in Santiago, Chile. *Am J Epidemiol* 1991;134:614–627.

112. Cravioto A, Reyes RE, Trujillo F, et al. Risk of diarrhea during the first year of life associated with initial and subsequent colonization by specific enteropathogens. *Am J Epidemiol* 1990;131:886–904.

113. Taylor DN, Echeverria P, Pal Tibor T, et al. The role of *Shigella* spp., enteroinvasive *Escherichia coli* and other enteropathogens as causes of childhood dysentery in Thailand. *J Infect Dis* 1986;153:1132–1138.

114. Echeverria P, Sethabutr O, Serichantalergs O, Lexomboon U, Tamura K. *Shigella* and enteroinvasive *Escherichia coli* infections in households of children with dysentery in Bangkok. *J Infect Dis* 1992;165:144–147.

115. Salazar-Lindo E, Sack RB, Chea-Woo E, et al. Early treatment with erythromycin of *Campylobacter jejuni*-associated dysentery in children. *J Pediatr* 1986;109:355–360.

116. Harris JC, DuPont HL, Hornick RB. Fecal leukocytes in diarrheal illness. *Ann Intern Med* 1972;76:697–703.

117. Walsh JA. Problems of recognition and diagnosis of amebiasis: estimation of the global magnitude of morbidity and mortality. *Rev Infect Dis* 1986;8:228–272.

118. Riley LW, Remis RS, Helgerson SD, et al. Hemorrhagic colitis associated with a rare *Escherichia coli* serotype. *N Engl J Med* 1983;308:681–685.

119. Cravioto A, Tello A, Navarro A, et al. Association of *Escherichia coli* HEp-2 adherence patterns with type and duration of diarrhoea. *Lancet* 1991;337:262–264.

120. Mathewson JJ, Cravioto A. HEp-2 cell adherence as an assay for virulence among diarrheagenic *Escherichia coli*. *J Infect Dis* 1989;159:1057–1060.

121. Zaki AM, DuPont HL, El Alamy MA, et al. The detection of enteropathogens in acute diarrhea in a family cohort population in rural Egypt. *Am J Trop Med Hyg* 1986;35:1013–1022.

122. Korzeniowski OM, Dantas W, Trabulsi LR, Guerrant RL. A controlled study of endemic sporadic diarrhea among adult residents of southern Brazil. *Trans R Soc Trop Med Hyg* 1984;84:363–369.

123. Echeverria P, Pitarangsi C, Eampokalap B, Bivulbandhitkit S, Boonthai P, Rowe B. A longitudinal study of the prevalence of bacterial enteric pathogens among adults with diarrhea in Bangkok, Thailand. *Diagn Microbiol Infect Dis* 1983;1:193–204.

124. Choudari CP, Mathan M, Rajan DP, Raghavan R, Mathan VI. A correlative study of etiology, clinical features and rectal mucosal pathology in adults with acute infectious diarrhea in southern India. *Pathology* 1985;17:443–450.

125. Adkins HJ, Escamilla J, Santiago LT, Ranoa C, Echeverria PM, Cross JH. Two year survey of etiologic agents of diarrheal disease at San Lazaro Hospital, Manila, Republic of the Philippines. *J Clin Microbiol* 1987;25:1143–1147.

126. Sen D, Saha MR, Niyogi SK, et al. Aetiological studies on hospital in-patients with acute diarrhoea in Calcutta. *Trans R Soc Trop Med Hyg* 1983;77:212–214.

127. Ries AA, Vugia DJ, Beingolea L, et al. Cholera in Piura, Peru: a modern urban epidemic. *J Infect Dis* 1992;166:1429–1433.

128. Varavithya W, Aswasuwana S, Phuapradit P, Louisirirotchanakul S, Supavaj S, Nopchinda S. Etiology of diarrhea in measles. *J Med Assoc Thai* 1989;72(1):151–154.

129. Greenberg BL, Sack RB, Salazar-Lindo E, et al. Measles-associated diarrhea in hospitalized children in Lima, Peru: pathogenic agents and impact on growth. *J Infect Dis* 1991;163:495–502.

130. Colebunders R, Francis H, Mann JM, et al. Persistent diarrhea, strongly associated with HIV infection in Kinshasa, Zaire. *Am J Gastroenterol* 1987;82:859–864.

131. Guerrant RL, Bobak DA. Bacterial and protozoal gastroenteritis. *N Engl J Med* 1991;325(5):327–340.

132. Keusch GT, Thea DM, Kamenga M, Kakanda K, et al. Persistent diarrhea associated with AIDS. *Acta Pediatr* 1992;381(Suppl):45–48.

133. Lam BCC, Tam J, Ng MH, Yeung CY. Nosocomial gastroenteritis in paediatric patients. *J Hosp Infect* 1989;14:351–355.

134. Ryder RW, Rahman ASMM, Alim ARMA, Yunis MD, Houda BS. An outbreak of nosocomial cholera in a rural Bangladesh hospital. *J Hosp Infect* 1986;8:275–282.

135. Levine MM. *Escherichia coli* that cause diarrhea: enterotoxigenic, enteropathogenic, enteroinvasive, enterohemorrhagic, and enteroadherent. *J Infect Dis* 1987;155:377–388.

136. Robins-Browne RM. Traditional enteropathogenic *Escherichia coli* of infantile diarrhea. *Rev Infect Dis* 1987;9:28–53.

137. Clausen CR, Christie DL. Chronic diarrhea in infants caused by adherent enteropathogenic *Escherichia coli*. *J Pediatr* 1982;100:358–361.

138. Nataro JP, Baldini MM, Kaper JB, Black RE, Bravo N, Levine MM. Detection of an adherence factor of enteropathogenic *Escherichia coli* with a DNA probe. *J Infect Dis* 1985;152:560–565.

139. Scaletsky IC, Silva MLM, Trabulsi LR. Distinctive patterns of adherence of enteropathogenic *Escherichia coli* to HeLa cells. *Infect Immun* 1984;45:534–535.

140. Scaletsky ICA, Silva MLM, Toledo MRF, Davis BR, Blake PA, Trabulsi LR. Correlation between adherence to HeLa cells and serogroups, serotypes, and bioserotypes of *Escherichia coli*. *Infect Immun* 1985;49:528–532.

141. Mathewson JJ, Johnson PC, DuPont HL, Satterwhite TK, Winsor DK. Pathogenicity of enteroadherent *Escherichia coli* in adult volunteers. *J Infect Dis* 1986;154:524–527.

142. Tacket CO, Moseley SL, Kay B, Losonsky G, Levine MM. Challenge studies in volunteers using *Escherichia coli* strains with diffuse adherence in HEp-2 cells. *J Infect Dis* 1990;162:550–552.

143. Vial PA, Robins-Browne R, Lior H, et al. Characterization of enteroadherent-aggregative *Escherichia coli*, a putative agent of diarrheal disease. *J Infect Dis* 1988;158:70–79.

144. Yamamoto T, Koyama Y, Matsumoto M, et al. Localized, aggregative, and diffuse adherence to HeLa cells, plastic, and human small intestines by *Escherichia coli* isolated from patients with diarrhea. *J Infect Dis* 1992;166:1295–1310.

145. Black RE, Merson MH, Rowe B, et al. Enterotoxigenic *Escherichia coli* diarrhoea: acquired immunity and transmission in an endemic area. *Bull World Health Organ* 1981;59:263–268.

146. Nachamkin I, Blaser MJ, Tompkins LS, eds. *Campylobacter jejuni: current status and future trends.* Washington, DC: American Society for Microbiology, 1992.

147. Thisyakorn USA, Rienprayoon S, Shigellosis in Thai children: epidemiologic, clinical and laboratory features. *Pediatr Infect Dis J* 1992;11:213–215.

148. Khan MU, Roy NC, Islam R, Huq I, Stoll B. Fourteen years of shigellosis in Dhaka: an epidemiological analysis. *Int J Epidemiol* 1985;14:607–613.

149. Ebright JR, Moore EC, Sanborn WR, Schaeberg D, Kyle J, Ishida K. Epidemic Shiga bacillus dysentery in Central Africa. *Am J Trop Med Hyg* 1984;33:1192–1197.

150. Rahaman MM, Khan MM, Aziz KMS, Island MS, Golam Kibriya ARK. An outbreak of dysentery caused by *Shigella dysenteriae* type 1 on a coral island in the Bay of Bengal. *J Infect Dis* 1975;132:15–19.

151. Munshi MH, Sack DA, Haider K, Ahmed ZU, Rahaman MM, Morshed MG. Plasmid-mediated resistance to nalidixic acid in *Shigella dysenteriae* type 1. *Lancet* 1987;2:419–421.

152. Glass RI, Becker S, Huq MI, et al. Endemic cholera in rural Bangladesh, 1966–1980. *Am J Epidemiol* 1982;116:959–970.

153. Glass RI, Black RE. The epidemiology of cholera. In: Barua D, Greenough WB III, eds. *Cholera*. New York: Plenum Medical Book Company, 1992;129–154.

154. Levine MM, Black RR, Clements ML, Nalin DR, Cisneros L, Finkelstein RA. Volunteer studies in development of vaccines

against cholera and enterotoxigenic *Escherichia coli:* a review. In: Holme T, Holmgren J, Merson MH, Mollby R, eds. *Acute enteric infections in children: new prospects for treatment and prevention.* Amsterdam: Elsevier/North-Holland Biomedical Press, 1981;443–459.

155. Glass RI, Claeson M, Blake PA, Waldman RJ, Pierce NF. Cholera in Africa: lessons on transmission and control for Latin America. *Lancet* 1991;338:791–795.

156. Gangarosa EJ, Tauxe RV. Epilogue: the Latin American cholera epidemic. In: Barua D, Greenough WB III, eds. *Cholera.* New York: Plenum Medical Book Company, 1992;351–358.

157. Cholera Working Group, International Centre for Diarrhoeal Diseases Research, Bangladesh. Large epidemic of cholera-like disease in Bangladesh caused by *Vibrio cholerae* O139 synonym Bengal. *Lancet* 1993;342:387–390.

158. Rennels MB, Levine MM. Classical bacterial diarrhea: perspectives and update—*Salmonella, Shigella, Escherichia coli, Aeromonas,* and *Plesiomonas. Pediatr Infect Dis* 1986;5:S91–S100.

159. Gracey M, Burke V, Robinson J. *Aeromonas*-associated gastroenteritis. *Lancet* 1982;2:1304–1306.

160. Pitarangsi C, Echeverria P, Whitmire R, et al. Enteropathogenicity of *Aeromonas hydrophila* and *Plesiomonas shigelloides:* prevalence among individuals with and without diarrhea in Thailand. *Infect Immun* 1982;35:666–673.

161. Holmberg SD, Farmer JJ III. *Aeromonas hydrophila* and *Plesiomonas shigelloides* as causes of intestinal infections. *Rev Infect Dis* 1984;6:633–639.

162. Samadi AR Wachsmuth K, Huq MI, Mahbub M, Agbonlahor DE. An attempt to detect *Yersinia enterocolitica. Trop Geogr Med* 1982;34:151–154.

163. Agbonlahor DE, Odugbemi TO, Dosunmi-Ogunbi O. Isolation of species of *Yersinia* from patients with gastroenteritis in Nigeria. *J Med Microbiol* 1983;16:93–96.

164. Torres JF, Cedillo R, Sánchez J, Dillman C, Giono S, Múnoz O. Prevalence of *Clostridium difficile* and its cytotoxin in infants in Mexico. *J Clin Microbiol* 1984;20:274–275.

165. Black RE, Merson MH, Huq I, Alim ARMA, Yunus MD. Incidence and severity of rotavirus and *Escherichia coli* diarrhoea in rural Bangladesh. *Lancet* 1981;1:141–143.

166. Gary Jr GW, Hierholzer JC, Black RE. Characteristics of noncultivable adenoviruses associated with diarrhea in infants: a new subgroup of human adenoviruses. *J Clin Microbiol* 1979;10:96–103.

167. Kotloff KL, Losonsky GA, Morris JG, et al. Enteric adenovirus infection and childhood diarrhea: an epidemiologic study in three clinical settings. *Pediatrics* 1989;84:210–225.

168. Uhnoo I, Wadell G, Svensson L, Johansson ME. Importance of enteric adenoviruses 40 and 41 in acute gastroenteritis in infants and young children. *J Clin Microbiol* 1984;20:365–372.

169. Avery RM, Shelton AP, Beards GM, Omotade OO, Oyejide OC, Olaleye DO. Viral agents associated with infantile gastroenteritis in Nigeria: relative prevalence of adenovirus serotypes 40 and 41, astrovirus, and rotavirus serotypes 1 to 4. *J Diarrhoeal Dis Res* 1992;10:105–108.

170. Tiemessen CT, Wegerhoff FO, Erasmus MJ, Kidd AH. Infection by enteric adenoviruses, rotaviruses, and other agents in a rural African environment. *J Med Virol* 1989;28:176–182.

171. Herrmann JE, Blacklow NR, Perron-Henry DM, Clements E, Taylor DN, Echeverria P. Incidence of enteric adenoviruses among children in Thailand and the significance of these viruses in gastroenteritis. *J Clin Microbiol* 1988;26:1783–1786.

172. Dolin R, Treanor JJ, Madore HP. Novel agents of viral enteritis in humans. *J Infect Dis* 1987;155:365–376.

173. Greenberg HB, Valdesuso J, Kapikian AZ, et al. Prevalence of antibody to the Norwalk virus in various countries. *Infect Immun* 1979;26:270–273.

174. Ryder WR, Greenberg H, Singh N, et al. Seroepidemiology of heat-labile enterotoxigenic *Escherichia coli* and Norwalk virus infections in Panamanians, Canal Zone residents, Apache Indians, and United States Peace Corps Volunteers. *Infect Immun* 1982;37:903–906.

175. Black RE, Greenberg HB, Kapikian AZ, Brown KH, Becker S. Acquisition of serum antibody to Norwalk virus and rotavirus and relation to diarrhea in a longitudinal study of young children in rural Bangladesh. *J Infect Dis* 1982;145:483–489.

176. Kurtz JB, Lee TW, Pickering D. Astrovirus associated gastroenteritis in a children's ward. *J Clin Pathol* 1977;30:948–952.

177. Yolken R, Dubovi E, Leister F, Reid R, Almeido-Hill J, Santosham M. Infantile gastroenteritis associated with excretion of pestivirus antigens. *Lancet* 1989;1:517–520.

178. Stevens DP. Selective primary health care: strategies for control of disease in the developing world. XIX. Giardiasis. *Rev Infect Dis* 1985;7:530–535.

179. Gilman RH, Brown KH, Visvesvara GS. Epidemiology and serology of *Giardia lamblia* in a developing country: Bangladesh. *Trans R Soc Trop Med Hyg* 1985;79:469–473.

180. Mason PR, Patterson BA. Epidemiology of *Giardia lamblia* infection in children: cross-sectional and longitudinal studies in urban and rural communities of Zimbabwe. *Am J Trop Med Hyg* 1987;37:277–282.

181. Gilman RH, Marquis GS, Miranda E, Vestegui M, Martinez H. Rapid reinfection of *Giardia lamblia* after treatment in hyperendemic third world community. *Lancet* 1988;1:343–345.

182. Sullivan PS, DuPont HL, Arafat RR, et al. Illness and reservoirs associated with *Giardia lamblia* infection in rural Egypt: the case against treatment in developing world environments of high endemicity. *Am J Epidemiol* 1988;127:1272–1281.

183. Reed SL. Ambebiasis: an update. *Clin Infect Dis* 1992;14:385–393.

184. Wanke C, Butler T, Islam M. Epidemiologic and clinical features of invasive amebiasis in Bangladesh: a case control comparison with other diarrheal diseases and postmortem findings. *Am J Trop Med Hyg* 1988;38:335–341.

185. Nanda R, Bavaja U, Anand BS. *Entamoeba histolytica* cyst passers: clinical features and outcome in untreated subjects. *Lancet* 1984;2:301–303.

186. Current WL, Garcia LS. Cryptosporidiosis. *Clin Microbiol Rev* 1991;4:325–358.

187. Sarabia-Arce S, Salazar-Lindo E, Gilman RH, Naranjo J, Miranda E. Case–control study of *Cryptosporidium parvum* infection in Peruvian children hospitalized for diarrhea: possible association with malnutrition and nosocomial infection. *Pediatr Infect Dis J* 1990;9:627–631.

188. Petersen C. Cryptosporidiosis in patients infected with the human immunodeficiency virus. *Clin Infect Dis* 1992;15:903–909.

189. Shadduck JA. Human microsporidiosis and AIDS. *Rev Infect Dis* 11:1989;203–207.

190. Eeftinck Schattenkerk JKM, Van Gool T, Van Ketel RJ, et al. Clinical significance of small intestinal microsporidiosis in HIV-1-infected individuals. *Lancet* 1991;337:895–898.

191. Shlim DR, Cohen MT, Eaton M, et al. An alga-like organism associated with an outbreak of prolonged diarrhea among foreigners in Nepal. *Am J Trop Med Hyg* 1991;45:383–389.

192. Elder GH, Hunter PR, Codd GA. Hazardous freshwater cyanobacteria (blue-green algae). *Lancet* 1993;341:1519–1520.

193. Hoge CW, Shlim DR, Rajah R, et al. Epidemiology of diarrhoeal illness associated with coccidian-like organism among travellers and foreign residents in Nepal. *Lancet* 1993;341:1175–1180.

194. Ortega YR, Sterling CR, Gilman RH, Cama VA, Diaz F. *Cyclospora* species—a new protozoan pathogen of humans. *N Engl J Med* 1993;328:1308–1312.

195. Casemore DP. Foodborne protozoal infection. *Lancet* 1990;336:1427–1430.

196. Genta RM. Diarrhea in helminthic infections. *Clin Infect Dis* 1993;16(Suppl 2):S122–S129.

197. Briscoe J. Intervention studies and the definition of dominant transmission routes. *Am J Epidemiol* 1984;120:449–455.

198. Cairncross S. Ingested dose and diarrhea transmission routes. *Am J Epidemiol* 1987;125:921–922.

199. Briscoe J. Ingested dose and diarrhea transmission routes. *Am J Epidemiol* 1987;125:922–925.

200. Becker S, Black RE, Brown KH, Nahar S. Relations between socio-economic status and morbidity, food intake and growth in young children in two villages in Bangladesh. *Ecol Food Nutr* 1986;18:251–264.

201. Stanton BF, Clemens JD. Socioeconomic variables and rates of diarrhoeal disease in urban Bangladesh. *Trans R Soc Trop Med Hyg* 1987;81:278–282.

202. Winikoff B, Laukaran VH. The influence of infant feeding practices on morbidity and child growth. In: Winikoff B, Castle M, Lankaran V, eds. *Feeding infants in four societies. Causes and consequences of mother's choices*. Westport, CT: Greenwood Press, 1988;215–226.

203. Yeager BAC, Lanata CF, Lazo F, Verastegui H, Black RE. Transmission factors and socioeconomic status as determinants of diarrhoeal incidence in Lima, Peru. *J Diarrhoeal Dis Res* 1991;9:186–193.

204. Zeitlin MF, Guldan G, Klein RE, Ahmad N, Ahmad K. Sanitary conditions of crawling infants in rural Bangladesh. Report to the USAID Asia Bureau and to the HHS Office of International Health, Bangladesh.

205. Han AM, Moe K. Household faecal contamination and diarrhoea risk. *J Trop Med Hyg* 1990;93:333–336.

206. Esrey SA, Collett J, Miliotis MD, Koornhof HJ, Makhales P. The risk of infection from *Giardia lamblia* due to drinking water supply, use of water, and latrines among preschool children in rural Lesotho. *Int J Epidemiol* 1989;18:248–253.

207. Huttly SRA, Blum D, Kirkwood BR, Emeh RN, Feachem RG. The epidemiology of acute diarrhoea in a rural community in Imo State, Nigeria. *Trans R Soc Trop Med Hyg* 1987;81: 865–870.

208. Alam N, Wojtyniak B, Henry FJ, Rahaman MM. Mother's personal and domestic hygiene and diarrhoea incidence in young children in rural Bangladesh. *Int J Epidemiol* 1989;18:242–247.

209. Manderson L. Socioeconomic and cultural correlates of gastroenteritis amongst infants and small children in Malaysia. *J Trop Pediatr* 1981;27:166–176.

210. Stewart WH, McCabe LH, Hemphill EC, DeCagito T. Diarrhoeal disease control studies: the relationship of certain environmental factors to the prevalence of shigella infection. *Am J Trop Med Hyg* 1955;14:718–724.

211. Kournary M, Vasquez MA. Housing and certain socioenvironmental factors and prevalence of enteropathogenic bacteria among infants with diarrhoeal disease in Panama. *Am J Trop Med Hyg* 1969;18:936–941.

212. Freij L, Wall S. Quantity and variation in morbidity: THAID-analysis of the occurrence of gastroenteritis among Ethiopian children. *Int J Epidemiol* 1979;8:313–325.

213. Lenz R. Jakarta Kampung morbidity variations: some policy implications. *Soc Sci Med* 1988;26:641–649.

214. Moore HA, Cruz EDL, Vargas-Mendez O. Diarrheal disease studies in Costa Rica. *Am J Epidemiol* 1965;82:162–184.

215. Rahaman M, Rahaman MM, Wojtyniak B, Aziz KMS. Impact of environmental sanitation and crowding on infant mortality in rural Bangladesh. *Lancet* 1985;2:28–31.

216. Sepúlveda J, Willett W, Múnoz A. Malnutrition and diarrhea. A longitudinal study among urban Mexican children. *Am J Epidemiol* 1988;127:365–376.

217. Schorling JB, McAuliffe JF, de Souza MA, Guerrant RL. Malnutrition is associated with increased diarrhoea incidence and duration among children in an urban Brazilian slum. *Int J Epidemiol* 1990;19:728–735.

218. Khan AZ. Impact of family size on the morbidity pattern in school children. *Indian Pediatr* 1981;18:107–111.

219. Betrand WE, Walmus BF. Maternal knowledge, attitudes and practice as predictors of diarrhoeal disease in young children. *Int J Epidemiol* 1983;12:205–210.

220. Levine RJ, Khan MR, D'Souza S, Nalin DR. Failure of sanitary wells to protect against cholera and other diarrhoeas in Bangladesh. *Lancet* 1976;2:86–89.

221. Han AM, Nwe OO K, Aye T, Hlaing T. Personal toilet after defaecation and the degree of hand contamination according to different methods used. *J Trop Med Hyg* 1986;89:237–241.

222. Henry ES. Environmental sanitation, infection and nutritional status of infants in rural St. Lucia, West Indies. *Trans R Soc Trop Med Hyg* 1981;75:507–513.

223. Tomkins AM, Drasar BS, Bradley AK, Williamson WA. Water supply and nutritional status in rural northern Nigeria. *Trans R Soc Trop Med Hyg* 1978;72:239–243.

224. Molbak K, Hojlyng N, Jepsen S, Gaarslev K. Bacterial contamination of stored water and stored food: a potential source of diarrhoeal disease in West Africa. *Epidemiol Infect* 1989;102: 309–316.

225. Feachem RG. Interventions for the control of diarrhoeal diseases among young children: promotion of personal and domestic hygiene. *Bull World Health Organ* 1984;62:467–476.

226. Clemens JD, Stanton BF. An educational intervention for altering water-sanitation behaviours to reduce childhood diarrhea in urban Bangladesh. 1. Application of the case–control method for development of an intervention. *Am J Epidemiol* 1987;125: 284–291.

227. Alam N, Wai L. Importance of age in evaluating effects of maternal and domestic hygiene practices on diarrhoea in rural Bangladeshi children. *J Diarrhoeal Dis Res* 1991;9:104–110.

228. Saran M, Gaur SD. Epidemiologic correlates of diarrhea in a slum community in Varanasi. *Indian J Pediatr* 1981;48: 441–446.

229. Bartlett AV, Hurtado E, Schroeder DG, Mendez H. Association of indicators of hygiene behavior with persistent diarrhea of young children. *Acta Paediatr* 1992;381(Suppl):66–71.

230. Black RE, Dykes AC, Anderson KE, et al. Handwashing to prevent diarrhea in day-care centers. *Am J Epidemiol* 1981; 113:445–451.

231. Khan MU. Interruption of shigellosis by hand washing. *Trans R Soc Trop Med Hyg* 1982;76:164–168.

232. Torun B. Environmental and educational interventions against diarrhea in Guatemala. In: Chen LC, Scrimshaw NS, eds. *Diarrhea and malnutrition: interactions, mechanisms and interventions*. New York: Plenum Press, 1982;235–266.

233. Stanton BF, Clemens JD. An educational intervention for altering water-sanitation behaviours to reduce childhood diarrhea in urban Bangladesh. II. A randomized trial to assess the impact of the intervention on hygienic behaviours and rates of diarrhea. *Am J Epidemiol* 1987;125:292–301.

234. Stanton BF, Clemens JD, Khair T. Educational intervention for altering water-sanitation behavior to reduce childhood diarrhea in urban Bangladesh: impact on nutritional status. *Am J Clin Nutr* 1988;48:1166–1172.

235. Sircar BK, Sengupta PG, Mondal SK, et al. Effect of handwashing on the incidence of diarrhoea in a Calcutta slum. *J Diarrhoeal Dis Res* 1987;5:112–114.

236. Han AM, Hlaing T. Prevention of diarrhoea and dysentery by hand washing. *Trans R Soc Trop Med Hyg* 1989;83:128–131.

237. Pinfold JV. Faecal contamination of water and fingertip-rinses as a method for evaluating the effect of low-cost water supply and sanitation activities on faeco-oral disease transmission. II. A hygiene intervention study in rural north-east Thailand. *Epidemiol Infect* 1990;105:377–389.

238. Henry FJ, Rahim Z. Transmission of diarrhoea in two crowded areas with different sanitary facilities in Dhaka, Bangladesh. *J Trop Med Hyg* 1990;93:121–126.

239. Samadi AR, Huq MI, Ahmed QS. Detection of rotavirus in hand-washings of attendants of children with diarrhoea. *Br Med J* 1983;286:188.

240. Sprunt K, Redman W, Leidy G. Antibacterial effectiveness of routine hand washing. *Pediatrics* 1973;52:264–271.

241. Eggers HJ. Handwashing and horizontal spread of viruses. *Lancet* 1989;1:1452.

242. Hoque BA, Briend A. A comparison of local handwashing agents in Bangladesh. *J Trop Med Hyg* 1991;94:61–64.

243. Esrey SA, Feachem RG, Hughes JM. Interventions for the control of diarrhoeal diseases among young children: improving water supplies and excreta disposal facilities. *Bull World Health Organ* 1985;63:757–772.

244. Esrey SA, Habicht JP. Epidemiologic evidence for health benefits from improved water and sanitation in developing countries. *Epidemiol Rev* 1986;8:117–128.

245. Huttly SRA, Lanata CF, Gonzales H, et al. Structured observations of handwashing and defecation practices in a shanty town of Lima, Peru. *J Diarrhoeal Dis Res* (in press).

246. Baltazar JC, Solon FS. Disposal of faeces of children under two years old and diarrhoea incidence: a case–control study. *Int J Epidemiol* 1989;18(Suppl 2):S16–S19.

247. Stanton BF, Clemens JD. Soiled saris: a vector of disease trans- mission? *Trans R Soc Trop Med Hyg* 1986;80:485–488.
248. Koopman JS. Diarrhea and school toilet hygiene in Cali, Col- ombia. *Am J Epidemiol* 1978;107:412–420.
249. Bukenya GB, Nwokolo N. Transient risk factors for acute childhood diarrhoea in an urban community of Papua New Guinea. *Trans R Soc Trop Med Hyg* 1990;84:857–860.
250. Gordon JE, Chitkara ID, Wyon JB. Weanling diarrhea. *Am J Med Sci* 1963;130:345–377.
251. Feachem RG, Koblinsky MA. Interventions for the control of diarrhoeal disease among young children: promotion of breast- feeding. *Bull World Health Organ* 1984;62:271–291.
252. Brown KH, Black RE, Lopez de Romãna G, Creed de Kanash- iro H. Infant-feeding practices and their relationship with diar- rheal and other diseases in Huascar (Lima), Peru. *Pediatrics* 1989;83:31–40.
253. Popkin BM, Adair L, Akin JS, Black R, Briscoe J, Flieger W. Breast-feeding and diarrheal morbidity. *Pediatrics* 1990;86: 874–882.
254. Chakraborty AK, Das JC. Comparative study of incidence of diarrhea among children in two different environmental situa- tions in Calcutta. *Indian Pediatr* 1983;20:907–913.
255. Watkinson M. Delayed onset of weanling diarrhoea associated with high breast milk intake. *Trans R Soc Trop Med Hyg* 1981; 75:432–435.
256. Glass RI, Stoll BJ. The protective effect of human milk against diarrhea: a review of studies from Bangladesh. *Acta Paediatr Scand* 1989;351:131–136.
257. Knight SM, Toodayan W, Caique WJC, Kyi W, Barnes A, Desmarchelier P. Risk factors for the transmission of diarrhoea in children: a case–control study in rural Malaysia. *Int J Epide- miol* 1992;21:812–818.
258. Munir M. Infantile diarrhoea: breast and bottle feeding com- pared with special reference to their clinical role. *Paediatr In- donesia* 1985;25:100–106.
259. Khin-Maung U, Nyunt-Nyunt W, Myo K, Mu-Mu K, Tin U, Thane T. Effects on clinical outcome of breast feeding during acute diarrhoea. *Br Med J* 1985;290:587–589.
260. de Zoysa I, Rea M, Martines J. Why promote breastfeeding in diarrhoeal disease control programmes? *Health Policy Plan- ning* 1991;6:371–379.
261. Clemens JD, Stanton B, Stoll B, Shahid NS, Banu H, Chowd- hury AKMA. Breastfeeding as a determinant of severity in shigellosis. Evidence for protection throughout the first three years of life in Bangladeshi children. *Am J Epidemiol* 1986;123: 710–720.
262. Clemens JD, Sack DA, Harris JR, et al. Breastfeeding and the risk of severe cholera in rural Bangladeshi children. *Am J Epi- demiol* 1990;131:400–411.
263. Mahmood DA, Feachem RG, Huttly SRA. Infant feeding and risk of severe diarrhoea in Basrah City, Iraq. A case–control study. *Bull World Health Organ* 1989;67:701–706.
264. Dutta SR, Khalfan SA, Baig BH, Philipose L, Fulayfil R. Epi- demiology of rotavirus diarrhoea in children under five years in Bahrain. *Int J Epidemiol* 1990;19:722–727.
265. Victora CG, Smith PG, Vaughan JP, et al. Evidence for protec- tion by breast-feeding against infant deaths from infectious dis- eases in Brazil. *Lancet* 1987;2:319–322.
266. Victora CG, Smith PG, Vaughan JP, et al. Infant feeding and deaths due to diarrhea. A case–control study. *Am J Epidemiol* 1989;129:1032–1041.
267. Victora CG, Huttly SR, Fuchs SC, Nobre LC, Barros FC. Deaths due to dysentery, acute and persistent diarrhoea among Brazilian infants. *Acta Paediatr* 1992;381(Suppl):7–11.
268. Barrell RAE, Rowland MGM. Infant foods as a potential source of diarrhoeal illness in rural West Africa. *Trans R Soc Trop Med Hyg* 1979;73:85–90.
269. Black RE, Brown KH, Becker S, Abdul Alim ARM, Merson MH. Contamination of weaning foods and transmission of en- terotoxigenic *Escherichia coli* diarrhea in children in rural Bangladesh. *Trans R Soc Trop Med Hyg* 1982;76:259–264.
270. Agarwal DK, Chandra S, Bhatia BD, Sanyal SC, Agarawal KN. Bacteriology of weaning foods in some areas of Varanasi. *Indian Pediatr* 1982;19:131–134.
271. Echevarria P, Verhaert L, Basaca-Sevilla V, et al. Search for heat-labile enterotoxigenic *Escherichia coli* in humans, live- stock, food, and water in a community in the Philippines. *J Infect Dis* 1978;138:87–90.
272. Echevarria P, Taylor DN, Seriwatana J, et al. Potential sources of enterotoxigenic *Escherichia coli* in homes of children with diarrhoea in Thailand. *Bull World Health Organ* 1987;65: 207–215.
273. Han AM, Oo KN, Aye T, Hlaing T. Bacteriological studies of food and water consumed by children in Myanmar: 2. Lack of association between diarrhoea and contamination of food and water. *J Diarrhoeal Dis Res* 1991;9:91–93.
274. Henry FJ, Huttly SRA, Patwary Y, Aziz KMA. Bacterial con- tamination of weaning foods and drinking water in rural Bangla- desh. *Epidemiol Infect* 1990;104:79–85.
275. Bryan FL, Michanie S, Fernández NM, et al. Hazard analyses of foods prepared by migrants living in a new settlement at the outskirts of Lima, Peru. *J Food Protect* 1988;51:314–323.
276. Oo KN, Han AM, Hlaing T, Aye T. Bacteriologic studies of food and water consumed by children in Myanmar: 1. The na- ture of contamination. *J Diarrhoeal Dis Res* 1991;9:87–90.
277. Roberts D. Sources of infection: food. *Lancet* 1990;336: 859–861.
278. Merson MH, Morris GK, Sack DA, et al. Traveler's diarrhea in Mexico: a prospective study. *N Engl J Med* 1976;294: 1299–1305.
279. Tjoa WS, DuPont HL, Sullivan P, et al. Location of food con- sumption and traveler's diarrhea. *Am J Epidemiol* 1977;106: 61–66.
280. Wood LV, Ferguson LE, Hogan P, et al. Incidence of bacterial enteropathogens in foods from Mexico. *Appl Environ Microbiol* 1983;46:328–332.
281. Watkinson M. Delayed onset of weanling diarrhoea associated with high breast milk intake. *Trans R Soc Trop Med Hyg* 1981; 75:432–435.
282. Lloyd-Evans N, Pickering HA, Goh SGJ, Rowland MGM. Food and water hygiene and diarrhoea in young Gambian chil- dren: a limited case control study. *Trans R Soc Trop Med Hyg* 1984;78:209–211.
283. Henry FJ, Huttly SRA, Patwary Y, Aziz KMA. Environmental sanitation, food and water contamination and diarrhoea in rural Bangladesh. *Epidemiol Infect* 1990;104:253–259.
284. Geldreich EE, Bordner RH. Fecal contamination of fruits and vegetables during cultivation and processing for market. A re- view. *J Milk Food Technol* 1971;34:184–195.
285. Barrell RAE, Rowland MGM. Commercial milk products and indigenous weaning foods in a rural West African environment: a bacteriological perspective. *J Hyg (Camb)* 1980;84:191–202.
286. Rowland MGM, Barrell RAE, Whitehead RG. The weanling's dilemma: bacterial contamination in traditional Gambian wean- ing foods. *Lancet* 1978;1:136–138.
287. Barrell RA, Kolley SSMI. Cow's milk as a potential vehicle of diarrhoeal disease pathogens in a West African village. *J Trop Pediatr* 1982;28:48–52.
288. Capparelli E, Mata L. Microflora of maize prepared as tortillas. *Appl Microbiol* 1975;29:802–806.
289. Mensah PPA, Tomkins AM, Drasar BS, Harrison TJ. Fermen- tation of cereals for reduction of bacterial contamination of weaning foods in Ghana. *Lancet* 1990;336:140–143.
290. Barilaro MT, Rubeglio ED, Shugurensky AD, O'Donnell AM. Contaminacíon de alimentos a nivel domiciliario. *Rev Hosp Niños Bs As* 1982;26:132–139.
291. Makukutu CA, Guthrie RK. Behavior of *Vibrio cholerae* in hot foods. *Appl Environ Microbiol* 1986;52:824–831.
292. Gilman RH, Skillicorn P. Boiling of drinking water: can a fuel- scarce community afford it? *Bull World Health Organ* 1985;63: 157–163.
293. Mensah PPA, Tomkins AM, Drasar BS, Harrison TJ. Effect of fermentation of Ghanaian maize dough on the survival and proliferation of 4 strains of *Shigella flexneri*. *Trans R Soc Trop Med Hyg* 1989;82:635–636.
294. Ashworth A, Draper A. The potential of traditional technolo- gies for increasing the energy density of weaning foods. WHO/ CDD/EDP/92.4, 1992.

295. St Louis ME, Porter JD, Helal A, et al. Epidemic cholera in West Africa: the role of food handling and high-risk foods. *Am J Epidemiol* 1990;13:719–728.

296. Rodríguez-Rebollo M. Coliformes y *Escherichia coli* en frutas y verduras de mercado. *Microbiol Espãn* 1974;27:225–234.

297. Abdelnoor AM, Batshoun R, Roumani BM, et al. The bacterial flora of fruits and vegetables in Lebanon and the effect of washing on the bacterial content. *Zentralbl Bakteriol Mikrobiol Hyg* 1983;177:342–349.

298. Gerichter CB, Sechter I, Gavish A, Cahan D. Viability of *Vibrio cholerae* biotype El Tor and of cholera phage on vegetables. *Isr J Med Sci* 1975;11:889–895.

299. Jiwa SFH, Krovacek K, Wadstrom T. Enterotoxigenic bacteria in food and water from an Ethiopian community. *Appl Environ Microbiol* 1981;41:1010–1019.

300. Kolvin JL, Roberts D. Studies on the growth of *Vibrio cholerae* biotype El Tor and biotype classical in foods. *J Hyg (Camb)* 1982;89:243–52.

301. Lobos RH, García JM, Aguilar CA, et al. Estudio bacteriologico comparativo de lechugas (*Lactuca sativa*) provenientes de los alrededores de Santiago y región costera. *Bol Inst Bacteriol Chile* 1976;18:33–37.

302. Meneley JC, Stanghellini ME. Detection of enteric bacteria within locular tissue of healthy cucumbers. *J Food Sci* 1974;39:1267–1268.

303. Samish Z, Etinger-Tulczynska R. Distribution of bacteria within the tissue of healthy tomatoes. *Appl Microbiol* 1963;11:7–10.

304. Samish Z, Etinger-Tulkzynska R, Bick M. The microflora within the tissue of fruits and vegetables. *J Food Sci* 1963;28:259–266.

305. Ercolani GL. Bacteriological quality assessment of fresh marketed lettuce and fennel. *Appl Environ Microbiol* 1976;31:847–852.

306. Editorial. Use of sewage and sludge in agriculture. *Lancet* 1990;335:635–636.

307. Rasrinaul L, Suthienkul O, Echeverria P, et al. Foods as a source of enteropathogens causing childhood diarrhea in Thailand. *Am J Trop Med Hyg* 1988;39:97–102.

308. Pether JVS, Gilbert RJ. The survival of salmonellas on fingertips and transfer of the organisms to foods. *J Hyg (Camb)* 1971;69:673–681.

309. Banwell JG, Abramowsky CR, Weber F, Howard R, Boldt DH. Phytohemagglutinin-induced diarrheal disease. *Dig Dis Sci* 1984;29:921–929.

310. Pistole TG. Interaction of bacteria and fungi with lectins and lectin-like substances. *Annu Rev Microbiol* 1981;35:85–112.

311. Weiser MM. Dietary lectins and the possible mechanisms whereby they induce intestinal injury. In: Lebenthal E, ed. *Chronic diarrhea in children.* New York: Raven Press, 1984;279–287.

312. Lanata CF, Black RE, Creed-Kanashiro H, Lazo F, Gallardo ML, Verastegui H, Brown KH. Feeding during acute diarrhea as a risk factor for persistent diarrhea. *Acta Paediatr* 1992;381(suppl):32–38.

313. Hibbert JM, Golden MHN. What is the weanling's dilemma? Dietary faecal bacterial ingestion of normal children in Jamaica. *J Trop Pediatr* 1981;27:255–258.

314. Phillips I, Lwanga SK, Lore W, et al. Methods and hygiene of infant feeding in an urban area of Uganda. *J Trop Pediatr* 1969;15:167–171.

315. Surjono D, Ismadi SD, Suwardji, Rohde JE. Bacterial contamination and dilution of milk in infant feeding bottles. *J Trop Pediatr* 1980;26:58–61.

316. Cherian A, Lawande RV. Recovery of potential pathogens from feeding bottle contents and teats in Zaria, Nigeria. *Trans R Soc Trop Med Hyg* 1985;79:840–842.

317. Elegbe IA, Ojofeitimi EO, Elegbe I, Akinola MO. Pathogenic bacteria isolated from infant feeding teats: contamination of teats used by illiterate and educated nursing mothers in Ile-Ife, Nigeria. *Am J Dis Child* 1982;136:672–674.

318. Snow J. *Snow on cholera.* New York: Hafner Publications, 1962.

319. Tamplin ML, Parodi CC. Environmental spread of *Vibrio cholerae* in Peru. *Lancet* 1991;338:1216–1217.

320. Hughes JM, Boyce JM, Levine RJ, et al. Epidemiology of El Tor cholera in rural Bangladesh: importance of surface water in transmission. *Bull World Health Organ* 1982;60:395–404.

321. Taylor JW, Gary GW Jr, Greenberg HB. Norwalk-related viral gastroenteritis due to contaminated drinking water. *Am J Epidemiol* 1981;114:584–592.

322. Esrey SA, Habicht JP, Latham MC, Sisler DG, Casella G. Drinking water source, diarrheal morbidity and child growth in villages with both traditional and improved water supplies in rural Lesotho, Southern Africa. *Am J Public Health* 1988;78:1451–1455.

323. Mertens TE, Fernando MA, Cousens SN, Kirkwood BR, Marshall TF, Feachem RG. Childhood diarrhoea in Sri Lanka: a case–control study of the impact of improved water sources. *Trop Med Parasitol* 1990;41:98–104.

324. Swerdlow DL, Mintz ED, Rodriguez M, et al. Waterborne transmission of epidemic cholera in Trujillo, Peru: lessons for a continent at risk. *Lancet* 1992;340:28–33.

325. Moe CL, Sobsey MD, Samsa GP, Mesolo V. Bacterial indicators of risk of diarrhoeal disease from drinking-water in the Philippines. *Bull World Health Organ* 1991;69:305–317.

326. Victora CG, Smith PG, Vaughan JP, et al. Water supply, sanitation and housing in relation to the risk of infant mortality from diarrhoea. *Int J Epidemiol* 1988;17:651–654.

327. Deb BC, Sirca BK, Senegupta PG, et al. Studies on interventions to prevent El Tor cholera transmission in urban slums. *Bull World Health Organ* 1986;64:127–131.

328. Cohen D, Green M, Block C, Slepon R, Ambar R, Wasserman SS, Levine MM. Reduction of transmission of shigellosis by control of houseflies (*Musca domestica*). *Lancet* 1991;337:993–997.

329. Echeverria P, Harrison BA, Tirapat C, McFarland A. Flies as a source of enteric pathogens in a rural village in Thailand. *Appl Environ Microbiol* 1983;46:32–36.

330. Esrey SA. *Interventions for the control of diarrhoeal diseases among young children: fly control.* WHO/CDD/91.37. Geneva: World Health Organization, 1991.

331. Levine OS, Levine MM. Houseflies (*Musca domestica*) as mechanical vectors of shigellosis. *Rev Infect Dis* 1991;13:688–696.

332. Dupont HL, Levine MM, Hornick RB, Formal SB. Inoculum size, shigellosis and implications for expected mode of transmission. *J Infect Dis* 1989;159:1126–1128.

333. Agbodaze D, Owusu SB. Cockroaches (*Periplaneta americana*) as carriers of agents of bacterial diarrhoea in Accra, Ghana. *Cent Afr J Med* 1989;35:484–486.

334. Blaser MJ, LaForce FM, Wilson NA, Wang WL. Reservoirs for human campylobacteriosis. *J Infect Dis* 1980;141:665–669.

335. Cruz JR, Cano F, Caceres P, Chew F, Pareja G. Infection and diarrhea caused by *Cryptosporidium* sp among Guatemalan infants. *J Clin Microbiol* 1983;26:88–91.

336. Georges-Courbot MC, Cassel-Beraud AM, Gouandjika I, Monges J, Georges AJ. A cohort study of enteric campylobacter infection in children from birth to two years in Bangui (Central African Republic). *Trans R Soc Trop Med Hyg* 1990;84:122–125.

337. Marquis GS, Ventura G, Gilman RH, Porras E, Miranda E, Carbajal L, Pentafiel M. Fecal contamination of shanty town toddlers in households with non-corraled poultry, Lima, Peru. *Am J Public Health* 1990;80:146–149.

338. Grados O, Bravo N, Black RE, Butzler JP. Case–control study to identify risk factors for pediatric *Campylobacter* diarrhea in Lima, Peru. *Bull World Health Organ* 1988;66:369–374.

339. Santosham M, Yolken RH, Quiroz E, et al. Detection of rotavirus in respiratory secretions of children with pneumonia. *J Pediatr* 1983;103:583–585.

340. Ansari SA, Springthorpe VS, Sattar SA. Survival and vehicular spread of human rotaviruses: possible relation to seasonality of outbreaks. *Rev Infect Dis* 1991;13:448–461.

341. Gordon JE, Guzman MA, Ascoli W, et al. Acute diarrheal disease in less developed countries. I. An epidemiological basis for control. *Bull World Health Organ* 1964;31:1–7.

342. El Samani EFZ, Willett WC, Ware JH. Association of malnutrition and diarrhoea in children aged under five years. A prospective follow-up study in a rural Sudanese community. *Am J Epidemiol* 1988;128:93–105.

343. Black RE, Lanata CF, Lazo F. Delayed cutaneous hypersensitivity: epidemiologic factors affecting and usefulness in predicting diarrheal incidence in young Peruvian children. *Pediatr Infect Dis J* 1989;8:210–215.

344. Baqui AH, Black RE, Sack RB, Chowdhury HR, Yunus M, Siddique AK. Malnutrition, cell-mediated immune deficiency and diarrhea: a community-based longitudinal study in rural Bangladeshi children. *Am J Epidemiol* 1993;137:355–365.

345. Black RE, Brown KH, Becker S. Malnutrition is a determining factor in diarrheal duration, but not incidence, among young children in a longitudinal study in rural Bangladesh. *Am J Clin Nutr* 1984;37:87–94.

346. Bairagi R, Chowdhury MK, Kim YJ, Curlin GT, Gray RH. The association between malnutrition and diarrhoea in rural Bangladesh. *Int J Epidemiol* 1987;16:477–481.

347. Chen LC, Huq E, Huffman SL. A prospective study of the risk of diarrheal diseases according to the nutritional status of children. *Am J Epidemiol* 1981;114:284–292.

348. Palmer DL, Koster FT, Alam AKMJ, Islam MR. Nutritional status: a determinant of severity of diarrhea in patients with cholera. *J Infect Dis* 1976;134:8–14.

349. Karchmer AW, Curlin GT, Huq MI, Hirschhorn N. Furazolidone in paediatric cholera. *Bull World Health Organ* 1970;43:373–378.

350. Baqui AH, Sack RB, Black RE, Chowdhury HR, Yunus M, Siddique AK. Cell-mediated immune deficiency and malnutrition are independent risk factors for persistent diarrhea in Bangladeshi children. *Am J Clin Nutr* 1993;58:543–548.

351. Bhandari N, Bhan MK, Sazawal S, et al. Association of antecedent malnutrition with persistent diarrhoea: a case–control study. *Br Med J* 1989;298:1284–1287.

352. Black RE, Merson MH, Taylor PR, et al. Glucose vs sucrose in oral rehydration solutions for infants and young children with rotavirus-associated diarrhea. *Pediatrics* 1981;67:79.

353. Black RE, Merson MH, Eusof A, Huq I, Pollard R. Nutritional status, body size and severity of diarrhoea associated with rotavirus or enterotoxigenic *Escherichia coli. J Trop Med Hyg* 1984;87:83–89.

354. Bhandari N, Bhan MK, Sazawal S. Mortality associated with acute watery diarrhea, dysentery and persistent diarrhea in rural North India. *Acta Paediatr* 1992;381(Suppl):3–6.

355. Chen LC, Chowdhury AKMA, Huffman SA. Anthropometric assessment of energy-protein malnutrition and subsequent risk of mortality among preschool aged children. *Am J Clin Nutr* 1980;33:1836–1845.

356. Kielmann AA, McCord C. Weight-for-age as an index of risk of death in children. *Lancet* 1978;1:1247–1250.

357. Green F, Heyworth B. Immunoglobulin-containing cells in jejunal mucosa of children with protein-energy malnutrition and gastroenteritis. *Arch Dis Child* 1980;55:380–383.

358. Munson D, Franco D, Arbeter A, Velez H, Vitale JJ. Serum levels of immunoglobulins, cell-mediated immunity, and phagocytosis in protein-calorie malnutrition. *Am J Clin Nutr* 1974;27:625–628.

359. Schlesinger D, Steckel A. Impaired cellular immunity in marasmic infants. *Am J Clin Nutr* 1974;27:615–620.

360. Thomason H, Burke V, Gracey M. Impaired gastric function in experimental malnutrition. *Am J Clin Nutr* 1981;34:1278–1280.

361. Maffei HVL, Nobrega FJ. Gastric pH and microflora of normal and diarrhoeic infants. *Gut* 1975;16:719–726.

362. Brunser O, Reid A, Monckeberg F, Maccioni A, Contreras I. Jejunal mucosa in infant malnutrition. *Am J Clin Nutr* 1968;21:976–983.

363. Sommer A, Katz J, Tarwotjo I. Increased risk of respiratory disease and diarrhea in children with preexisting mild vitamin A deficiency. *Am J Clin Nutr* 1984;40:1090–1095.

364. Sommer A, Dijunaedi E, Tarwatjo I, et al. Impact of vitamin A supplementation on childhood mortality. *Lancet* 1986;327:1169–1173.

365. West KP, Pokhrel RP, Katz J, et al. Efficacy of vitamin A in reducing preschool child mortality in Nepal. *Lancet* 1991;338:67–71.

366. Daulaire NMP, Starbuck ES, Houstoni RM, Church MS, Stu-

kel TA, Pandey MR. Childhood mortality after a high dose of vitamin A in a high risk population. *Br Med J* 1992;304:207–210.

367. Ghana VAST Study Team. Vitamin A supplementation in northern Ghana: effects on clinic attendances, hospital admissions, and child mortality. *Lancet* 1993;342:7–12.

368. Hambidge KM. Zinc and diarrhea. *Acta Paediatr* 1992;381(Suppl):82–86.

369. Golden BE, Golden MHN. Zinc, sodium and potassium losses in the diarrhoeas of malnutrition and zinc deficiency. In: Mills CF, Bremmer I, Chesters JK, eds. *Trace elements in man and animals—TEMA 5.* Bucksburn, Aberdeen: Rowett Research Institute, 1985;228–232.

370. Sachdev HPS, Mittal NK, Mittal SK, Yadav HS. A controlled trial on utility of oral zinc supplementation in acute dehydrating diarrhea in infants. *J Pediatr Gastroenterol Nutr* 1988;7:877–881.

371. Sachdev HPS, Mittal NK, Yadav HS. Oral zinc supplementation in persistent diarrhoea in infants. *Ann Trop Paediatr* 1990;10:63–69.

372. Lima AAM, Fang G, Schorling JB, et al. Persistent diarrhea in northeast Brazil: etiologies and interactions with malnutrition. *Acta Paediatr* 1992;381(Suppl):39–44.

373. Feachem RG, Koblinsky MA. Interventions for the control of diarrhoeal diseases among young children: measles immunization. *Bull World Health Organ* 1983;61:641–652.

374. Cash RE, Music SI, Libonati JP, et al. Response of man to infection with *Vibrio cholerae.* I. Clinical, serologic, and bacteriologic responses to a known inoculum. *J Infect Dis* 1974;129:45–52.

375. Gitelson S. Gastrectomy, achlorhydria and cholera. *Isr J Med Sci* 1971;7:663–667.

376. Nalin DR, Levine RJ, Levine MM, et al. Cholera, non-vibrio cholera, and stomach acid. *Lancet* 1978;2:856–859.

377. Schiraldi O, Benvestito V, Di Bari C, et al. Gastric abnormalities in cholera: epidemiological and clinical considerations. *Bull World Health Organ* 1974;51:349–352.

378. Blaser MJ. *Helicobacter pylori:* its role in disease. *Clin Infect Dis* 1992;15:386–393.

379. Sullivan PB, Thomas JE, Wight DGD, et al. *Helicobacter pylori* in Gambian children with chronic diarrhoea and malnutrition. *Arch Dis Child* 1990;65:189–191.

380. Glass RI, Holmgren J, Haley CE, et al. Predisposition for cholera of individuals with O blood group. Possible evolutionary significance. *Am J Epidemiol* 1985;121:791–796.

381. Clemens JD, Sack DA, Harris JR, et al. ABO blood groups and cholera: new observations on specificity or risk and modification of vaccine efficacy. *J Infect Dis* 1989;159:770–773.

382. Levine MM, Nalin DR, Rennels MB, et al. Genetic susceptibility to cholera. *Ann Hum Biol* 1979;6:369–374.

383. Black RE, Levine MM, Clements ML, Hughes T, O'Donnell S. Association between O blood group and occurrence and severity of diarrhoea due to *Escherichia coli. Trans R Soc Trop Med Hyg* 1987;81:120–123.

384. van Loon FPL, Clemens JD, Sack DA, et al. ABO blood groups and the risk of diarrhea due to enterotoxigenic *Escherichia coli. J Infect Dis* 1991;163:1243–1246.

385. Koster FT, Palmer DL, Chakraborty J, Jackson T, Curlin GC. Cellular immune competence and diarrheal morbidity in malnourished Bangladeshi children: a prospective field study. *Am J Clin Nutr* 1987;46:115–120.

386. Mellman WJ, Wetton R. Depression of the tuberculin reaction by attenuated measles virus vaccine. *J Lab Clin Med* 1963;61:453–458.

387. Bloomfield AL, Mateer JG. Changes in skin sensitiveness to tuberculin during epidemic influenza. *Am Rev Tuberc Pulmonary Dis* 1919;3:166–168.

388. Starr S, Berkovich S. The depression of tuberculin reactivity during chickenpox. *Pediatrics* 1964;33:769–772.

389. Berkovich S, Starr S. Effects of live type 1 poliovirus vaccine and other viruses on the tuberculin test. *N Engl J Med* 1966;274:67–72.

390. Kauffman CA, Linnemann CC Jr, Schiff GM, Phair JP. Effect of viral and bacterial pneumonias on cell-mediated immunity in humans. *Infect Immun* 1976;13:78–83.

391. Beisel WR. Single nutrients and immunity. *Am J Clin Nutr* 1982;35:417–468.
392. Golden MHN, Golden BE. Zinc and delayed hypersensitivity responses. *Nutr Res* 1985;9(Suppl I):700–709.
393. Ronsmans C, Bennish ML, Weirzba T. Diagnosis and management of dysentery by community health workers. *Lancet* 1988; 2:552–555.
394. Feachem RG. Preventing diarrhoea: what are the policy options? *Health Policy Planning* 1986;1:109–117.
395. World Health Organization. Research on improving infant feeding practices to prevent diarrhoea or reduce its severity: memorandum from a JHU/WHO meeting. *Bull World Health Organ* 1989;67:27–33.
396. Ashworth A, Feachem RG. Interventions for the control of diarrhoeal diseases among young children: weaning education. *Bull World Health Organ* 1985;63(6);1115–1117.
397. Esrey SA, Feachem RG. Interventions for the control of diarrhoeal diseases among young children: promotion of food hygiene. WHO/CDD/89.30, 1989.
398. Feachem RG, Koblinsky MA. Interventions for the control of diarrhoeal diseases among young children: measles immunisation. *Bull World Health Organ* 1983;61:641–652.
399. de Zoysa I, Feachem RG. Interventions for the control of diarrhoeal diseases among young children: rotavirus and cholera immunization. *Bull World Health Organ* 1985;63: 569–583.
400. Clemens JD, Sack DA, Harris JR, et al. Field trial of oral cholera vaccines in Bangladesh: results from three-year follow-up. *Lancet* 1990;335:270–273.
401. Levine MM, Herrington D, Kaper J, et al. Safety, immunogenicity, and efficacy of recombinant live oral cholera vaccines, CVD 103 and CVD 103-HgR. *Lancet* 1988;2:467–470.
402. Suharyono, Simanjuntak C, Witham N, et al. Safety and immunogenicity of single-dose live oral cholera vaccine CVD 103-HgR in 5–9 year old Indonesian children. *Lancet* 1992;340: 689–694.
403. Kapikian AZ, Flores J, Hoshino Y, et al. Rotavirus: the major etiologic agent of severe infantile diarrhea may be controllable by a "Jennerian" approach to vaccination. *J Infect Dis* 1986; 153:815–822.
404. Flores J, Perea-Schael I, Marino G, et al. Protection against severe rotavirus diarrhoea by rhesus rotavirus vaccine in Venezuelan infants. *Lancet* 1987;1:882–884.

Infections of the Gastrointestinal Tract,
edited by M. J. Blaser, P. D. Smith, J. I. Ravdin,
H. B. Greenberg, and R. L. Guerrant
Raven Press, Ltd., New York © 1995.

CHAPTER 3

Epidemiology of Diarrheal Diseases in Developed Countries

|

Robert V. Tauxe and Mitchell L. Cohen

Although diarrheal disease is well recognized as a major cause of morbidity and mortality in the developing world, it is not often considered an important public health problem for the developed world. Diarrheal disease in these countries is often considered an inconvenience rather than an illness, and the morbidity and mortality are frequently underestimated or unknown. By the end of the 1980s, however, this attitude had begun to change. Particularly in the United States and Great Britain, public and media attention were drawn to problems such as *Salmonella enteritidis* in shell eggs, salmonellosis in poultry, *Escherichia coli* O157:H7 in hamburgers, and diarrheal disease in the day care setting. At the same time, new molecular biology techniques were applied to identify and study the organisms that caused diarrheal disease. Thus, in the last two decades, the epidemiology of diarrheal disease in the developed world has become much better understood. In this chapter, we examine the general epidemiology of diarrheal disease in the developed world, focusing on specific bacterial, viral, and parasitic etiologies, and conclude by examining potential strategies for prevention and control.

GENERAL EPIDEMIOLOGY

Definitions

The two most common approaches for studying diarrheal diseases are descriptive epidemiology and analytic epidemiology (1). Descriptive epidemiology typically involves collecting and analyzing data that describe the disease in the population. Analysis of these data generally

leads to the identification of trends and the development of hypotheses to explain the characteristics of a disease. Testing of these hypotheses involves analytic epidemiology. This is most frequently done by conducting case–control or cohort analyses to compare the characteristics or exposures of persons who are ill with those who are well. Outbreak investigations frequently use analytic epidemiology. Such analyses may lead to an association of disease with vehicles that transmit a specific disease, or host factors and behaviors that make individuals more susceptible to illness.

These two epidemiologic methods are often supplemented by laboratory methods that identify specific strains of microorganisms. They include traditional methods such as serotyping and, in recent years, molecular techniques such as deoxyribonucleic acid (DNA) fingerprinting or plasmid profile analysis. The use of newer methods has been referred to as molecular epidemiology. When used to subtype microorganisms associated with illness, molecular epidemiology allows better discrimination of strains that are associated with an outbreak and allows the epidemiologist to sort the "apples and oranges" of various microbial strains. In many instances, all three methods are used in combination to define the epidemiology of a particular diarrheal disease.

Sources and Limitations of Data

Data that define the epidemiology of diarrheal disease in the developed world come from three general sources: (a) surveillance, (b) outbreak investigations, and (c) prospective studies. Surveillance data are collected by either active or passive surveillance systems. Passive surveillance is a traditional approach in which health care workers report the occurrence of diseases to public health officials in local, state, or federal government. Active surveillance typically involves seeking out cases of a specific disease by outreach to physicians or clinical laboratories. Active surveillance requires more resources but gen-

R. V. Tauxe: Division of Bacterial and Mycotic Diseases, National Center for Infectious Diseases, Centers for Disease Control and Prevention, Atlanta, Georgia 30333.

M. L. Cohen: Division of Pediatric Gastroenterology and Nutrition, Children's Hospital Medical Center, Cincinnati, Ohio 45229.

erally yields more complete and timely data. Passive surveillance requires fewer resources and also may be more subject to underreporting and significant delays. Complete enumeration of all cases is usually impractical in either type of surveillance, so representative samples of cases are used to estimate and describe the total. Surveillance frequently supplies the data for descriptive epidemiology, such as the number of cases of a disease occurring in a given geographic area over a specific time period.

The other two sources of data are outbreak investigations and prospective studies of sporadic cases in a population. These frequently involve analytic and molecular techniques that identify mechanisms of transmission and risk factors for specific diarrheal diseases. When outbreaks of diarrheal illness occur, the microbial cause and the source of the illness are often unclear. Prompt epidemiologic investigation can determine the etiology, identify the groups affected, and implicate a source. These investigations provide a scientific base for emergency control measures to prevent further illness, such as closing restaurants, swimming beaches, or defective food processing plants. Careful tracing of the chain of events that produced the outbreak often leads to better understanding of how to prevent similar outbreaks in the future.

Prospective investigation of sporadic cases can also identify sources of infection, even in the absence of a recognized outbreak. Such investigations can be conducted over months to years, enrolling patients into the study as they occur, and comparing their pre-illness characteristics and exposures with those of healthy persons. For illnesses that can be acquired in a number of different ways, such studies can define the relative importance of the various sources. In general, prospective studies are more expensive and slower to conduct than outbreak investigations, are less driven by the pressure to respond to an emergency, and are less frequently performed.

There are various limitations to the epidemiologic data provided by each of these sources. Surveillance systems exist for only a limited number of diarrheal diseases or pathogens, and they vary greatly in what is reported and the completeness and speed of reporting. In the United States, only certain diseases are required by law to be reported, and the diseases that are legally reportable vary from state to state. The incidence of a disease identified through surveillance often underestimates the true occurrence of the disease.

Underreporting also occurs because of differences in the availability of laboratory tests. New methods are constantly being introduced to isolate and identify various pathogens. Some of these methods are identifying agents that were previously unrecognized, such as certain *Campylobacter* species, *E. coli* O157:H7, or a variety of viral agents. Other methods allow simpler and more rapid identification of well-recognized pathogens. However, because these methods are not uniformly applied in all clinical microbiologic laboratories, identification and subsequent reporting of disease will vary. A recent trend has been in the use of rapid methods that often do not require isolation of an organism in clinical laboratories or even physicians' offices. Such laboratory advances are likely to have considerable impact on the quantity and quality of epidemiologic data on diarrheal disease in the future. It is important to note that many microbiologic methods are more routinely available for bacterial agents than for certain viral and parasitic agents. This is likely to affect reporting as well as the estimates of the occurrence of disease. Because the degree of such underreporting varies substantially from one pathogen to another, surveillance data may be more useful in following trends for specific diseases over time rather than for comparing the number of cases of one infection with another.

Incidence

Data on the incidence of diarrheal disease in the developed world are limited. In 1982, it was estimated that one billion episodes of diarrheal diseases and almost five million deaths occurred annually in children under 5 years old (2). Most of this disease was thought to occur in the developing world, where children under the age of five had a median of three episodes of diarrheal disease per year, and adults less than one episode. In this analysis, the mortality rates in the developing world for children in the first year of life ranged from 8 to 50 per thousand live births. For the developed world, there are few similar analyses. One study conducted by the Centers for Disease Control and Prevention (CDC) estimated that over 25 million enteric infections, with over 10,000 deaths, occur each year in the United States (3). Others have estimated that foodborne disease alone accounts for over 80 million illnesses each year in the United States (4). A significant percentage of both these estimates would be diarrheal illness.

In the developed world, many studies focus on children less than 1 year or less than 5 years of age. In the National Health Interview Survey conducted by the National Center for Health Statistics the incidence of "intestinal virus" was ascertained (5). In this survey, the overall annual incidence was 3.4 per hundred persons, with the highest rates in children under 5 years of age (6.8 per hundred persons per year). Although the precise relationship of this category to diarrheal disease is unknown, these illnesses required medical attention one-third of the time, resulted in 4.1 days in bed, 7.0 school days lost, and 4.7 work days lost per 100 persons per year. A study of children visiting a group medical practice in Michigan identified annual rates of diarrhea per child as 0.82, 0.42, and 0.08 for the age groups of less than 1 year old, between 1 and 2 years old, and between 2 and 4 years old, respectively (6). Another study estimated that 16.5 million children under 5 years of age have between 21 and 37 million episodes of diarrhea each year in the United States (7). Approximately 10% of these episodes lead to a physician's visit, 220,000 children are hospitalized, and approximately 400 die. Several studies have suggested that the peak incidence of diarrheal disease in children is during the winter and that rotavirus is a primary cause (8). One Swedish study identified viral, bacterial, and parasitic agents in 58%, 14%, and 1% of diarrheal patients, respectively (9).

Diarrheal disease may also be an important public

health problem for another age group, the elderly. Using a hospital discharge diagnosis database, researchers estimated that adults accounted for 62% of hospitalizations for gastroenteritis, that 96% of diarrheal deaths occurred among adults, and that two-thirds of these deaths were among the elderly (10). Individuals older than 70 years of age had more than a 50-fold risk of dying from diarrheal disease compared with children under 5 years of age. A separate study associated a higher risk of dying of diarrhea with being white, female, and living in a long-term care facility (11).

In all these mortality studies, it is apparent that a significant proportion of these diarrheal deaths are preventable. It is likely that the occurrence of disease and the importance of specific etiologic agents vary according to the age, sex, geographic area, or specific exposure of the population involved (12,13). Certain populations have risk factors that increase their likely exposure to organisms spread by contaminated food, water, or other infected persons. Thus populations such as children in day care (14), homosexual men (15), or travelers (16) may be exposed to specific or different etiologic agents and have resulting differences in the frequency of disease.

Economic Cost

The economic cost of diarrheal disease in the developing world is unknown. In one hospital discharge data set, gastroenteritis was reported as a discharge diagnosis in approximately 2.5% of the total hospitalizations (10). Although the economic cost from these hospitalizations is large, additional economic costs are incurred through physicians' visits and medications, as well as indirectly through lost productivity. For one diarrheal disease, *Salmonella*, it has been estimated that the patient-related cost exceeds $1 billion per year. The cost for all foodborne disease in the United States has been estimated to be in excess of $28 billion (4). It is likely that diarrheal disease accounts for a significant proportion of foodborne disease cost and thus is a significant economic burden.

Reservoirs and Transmission Routes

Descriptive and analytic epidemiology are useful in identifying the reservoirs and the routes and specific mechanisms of transmission for diarrheal disease. For an organism to persist, it must have an ecologic niche or reservoir where it can replicate. Such reservoirs may exist either in the environment or in animal or human populations. Reservoirs for diarrheal pathogens can be in animal populations, such as *Salmonella* or *Campylobacter*, human populations, such as *Shigella*, or elsewhere in the environment, such as *Vibrio cholerae* 01. For an agent to cause diarrheal disease, it must be transmitted from the reservoir to a susceptible host in sufficient numbers and arrive at the site in the gastrointestinal tract where it can cause illness. Common routes of transmission for diarrheal pathogens include waterborne, foodborne, and person-to-person transmission by fecal–oral or respiratory

routes. The routes of transmission are often determined by characteristics of the organism and the host. Typically, *Salmonella*, which is usually foodborne, requires a relatively large infectious dose to cause severe illness in most individuals. Therefore severe salmonellosis is often related to mishandling of food that enables the *Salmonella* to grow to high numbers in the food and cause severe disease. On the other hand, *Shigella*, which requires only a low infectious dose to cause illness, is frequently transmitted person to person by fecal–oral contact, although this type of transmission does not provide special conditions that allow the growth of large numbers of organisms.

Tracing the precise mechanisms of transmission for many agents of diarrheal disease can be difficult, and more than one mechanism may be identified even in a single outbreak. In one outbreak of *Salmonella newport* infections, organisms that originated in a dairy herd in South Dakota were transmitted through the food chain by hamburger sold in a variety of supermarkets in multiple states (17). In addition, a nosocomial case occurred following person-to-person transmission by contaminated colonoscopy equipment.

Understanding the reservoirs and the required routes of transmission is important to defining potential prevention measures. As new agents are identified, and established agents appear in new food and water vehicles, investigations into transmission, often conducted in the outbreak setting, can clarify the utility of existing control measures and define the need and likely point of application of new ones.

Host-Specific Risk Factors

Exposure to a particular mode or vehicle of transmission is only one of the many risk factors that can be associated with diarrheal disease. Risk factors are frequently identified by case–control or cohort analyses that attempt to differentiate the associations in ill and well individuals. Studies have demonstrated large numbers of risk factors that may be associated with diarrheal disease. These include demographic factors such as age, sex, race, socioeconomic status, and area of residence, or other exposures such as food, medications, illicit drug use, travel, smoking, sexual activity, or day care attendance. Some factors may actually have a protective effect; for example, breast-feeding, washing hands with soap, or measles immunization may be associated with decreased risks for certain diarrheal diseases.

Global Trends

Several trends have been occurring in the spectrum of diarrheal diseases in recent years. Many of these trends are affecting the entire industrialized world. Changes in the epidemiology of specific infections in one country may herald changes soon to be observed in others.

New and Emerging Pathogens

A variety of new and emerging pathogens are being identified, making the challenge of diagnosis and treatment ever more complex (18). Examples include *E. coli* O157:H7, the growing variety of *Campylobacter* species, the 27-nm viral agents, and epidemic waterborne cryptosporidiosis. Many of these agents are transmitted through relatively low-dose infections, and many appear to have reservoirs in healthy food animals. Some of the newer agents were first identified as invasive pathogens in compromised hosts and were then found to affect the normal host as well, once methods for detecting them in stools were developed. Among the bacterial agents, there is a general increase in antimicrobial resistance. For some agents that have major food animal reservoirs, such as *Salmonella* and *Campylobacter*, this growing resistance appears to be the result of the widespread use of antimicrobial agents in animal husbandry (19). Among other agents that have human reservoirs, such as *Salmonella typhi* and *Shigella*, this resistance is related to the widespread use of over-the-counter antibiotics in the developing world (20).

Increasingly, the appearance of a new or reemerging pathogen in one part of the world is soon followed by international spread of that agent through rapid international travel and trade connections. Examples of this include the spread of *Yersinia enterocolitica* serotype O3 to all industrialized nations (21), the appearance of egg-associated *S. enteritidis* in epidemic form throughout North America, Europe, and parts of Asia (22), and the rapid spread of *Vibrio cholerae* O139 through Asia (23). Spread can occur from the developing world to the developed world. This was dramatically illustrated by the global epidemic of *Salmonella agona*, which followed the use of contaminated Peruvian anchovy fishmeal in chicken feed in North America and Europe, leading to the spread of this strain throughout the agricultural industry (24). Diseases can also spread from the industrialized world to the developing world. For example, in late 1992, *E. coli* O157 infections were recognized for the first time in Africa in refugee camps and ranches of Swaziland, where they were associated with devastating outbreaks of dysentery and hemolytic uremic syndrome (HUS) (25).

Another recent trend has been the recognition of a growing number of important postinfectious sequelae and chronic debility associated with diarrheal diseases. HUS and subsequent chronic renal failure have been linked definitively to infection with *E. coli* O157:H7 and other Shiga-like toxin-producing *E. coli* (26,27). Reiter's syndrome can follow infection with *Shigella* (28), *Salmonella* (29), *Y. enterocolitica* (30), and perhaps other enteric organisms. Most recently, a strong relationship between the presence of antibodies to *Campylobacter jejuni* and Guillain–Barŕe syndrome suggests that this paralytic illness may also be associated with enteric infection (31).

The Changing Population

Important changes have also occurred in the populations of the industrialized world themselves. The increase

in acquired immunodeficiency syndrome (AIDS) and the medical success stories of organ transplantation and cancer therapy mean that a growing proportion of the population is immunosuppressed. This high-risk subgroup is therefore susceptible to low doses of some pathogens that would be sufficient to produce only asymptomatic or mild infection in normal hosts. This brings increased concern to issues of food and water safety, and to the risk of nosocomial infections. The hospitalized immunosuppressed population may be the highest risk subgroup of all, and diarrheal illness may be a relatively common, though often overlooked, nosocomial infection. Although routine surveillance may rarely detect nosocomial gastroenteritis, intensive surveillance can identify rates as high as 8 cases per 100 admissions in a medical intensive care unit, and 2 cases per 100 admissions in a pediatric ward; *Salmonella, Clostridium difficile,* and rotavirus may be the most common pathogens involved (32).

The elderly are a second growing subgroup at higher risk. A substantial proportion of the population is now living in group homes and institutions for the elderly, providing a setting for common-source disease outbreaks among a very susceptible population. Child care is also becoming more institutionalized, and an increasing proportion of young children are being cared for in group settings such as day care centers. These settings greatly increase the number of children with whom a given child has contact, increasing the likelihood of person-to-person transmission of organisms, particularly those that infect at low doses. The disappearance of the traditional homemaker means that the impact of diarrheal illness on a family can go far beyond the cost of medical care itself to include the cost of missed work for whomever must stay home to care for the sick person or of an ill wage earner excluded from a sensitive occupation.

Another trend in recent years has been the explosive increase in international travel. Huge numbers of adventurous tourists, business travelers, international migrant labor pools, and immigrants revisiting their countries of origin cross national borders every year. In addition, large numbers of people travel involuntarily, fleeing war, famine, or poverty to surrounding nations. The public health impact of these population transfers is only beginning to be apparent, but these events intimately connect the developing and industrialized worlds. The array of pathogens from the developing world that cause traveler's diarrhea is only one manifestation of this trend; others include diseases brought by immigrants from refugee camps, nosocomial infections brought by orphanage children coming to the developed world for adoption, diseases of volunteer workers living in the developing world, and diseases of people in the developed nations whose vegetables are harvested, pigs are slaughtered, and oysters are shucked by recent immigrants from the developing world.

The Changing Food Supply

Changes in the nature of the global food supply are having an important effect on diarrheal illness in general. In industrialized nations, the small family farm is being replaced by large industrial-scale production units, which produce food more efficiently with less labor, coupled with large-scale centralized processing and distribution. As a result, a new ecology of large and crowded animal populations has been created. Substantial parts of the food supply are agricultural commodities, pooled anonymously in large central warehouses, processed in continuous fashion in giant plants, and distributed over large areas. As a result, just as a tankful of gasoline is a blend of the oil of an enormous number of individual oil wells, so a single hamburger, glass of milk, or fish stick may come from hundreds of different animals and farms; one bite can span continents. The same is true for animal feed, which is typically blended from a nonsterile menu of rendered offal, plant products, and fish protein from all corners of the earth. Large-scale production and broad distribution mean that when safety measures are carefully applied, they will protect large numbers of people. Conversely, when they fail and a food or fodder product is contaminated, huge numbers of people or animals can be affected virtually simultaneously.

SPECIFIC AGENTS

Bacterial Pathogens

Bacterial diseases are identified as the cause of illness in less than 15% of diarrheal disease cases in the developed world. In recent multicenter clinical studies in the United States, approximately 8% of all diarrheal stools yielded a bacterial pathogen, although 20% of specimens from patients with bloody diarrhea did so (33,34). Nevertheless, more data are available on these organisms than on the viral and parasitic pathogens.

The relative importance of the various bacterial agents has been estimated by a series of studies. The most important bacterial agents causing the highest incidence of disease are *Campylobacter, Salmonella, E. coli* O157:H7, and *Shigella*. A study conducted in Seattle, Washington, in the mid-1980s, identified frequencies of 47 per 100,000 population for *Campylobacter*, 22 per 100,000 for *Salmonella*, 8 per 100,000 for *E. coli* O157:H7, and 7 per 100,000 for *Shigella* (35). Other pathogens are identified less commonly but are important causes of morbidity and mortality. These include various enterotoxigenic, enteropathogenic, and enteroinvasive *E. coli, V. cholerae* and other *Vibrio* species, *Yersinia enterocolitica, Clostridium botulinum, Clostridium perfringens, Clostridium difficile, Bacillus cereus,* and *Staphylococcus aureus.*

Salmonella

Salmonella can be differentiated by a serotyping system that identifies both somatic (O) and flagellar (H) antigens. By this method, there are over 2000 serotypes of *Salmonella*. However, in the United States, three-fourths of cases of *Salmonella* infection are attributable to ten serotypes, and five, *S. typhimurium, S. enteritidis, S. heidel-*

berg, S. hadar, and *S. newport,* accounted for 58% of all isolates in 1991 (36). The approximately 40,000 isolates reported to CDC each year in the United States represent only a small proportion of the number of cases of salmonellosis that are thought to occur annually; an estimated 10 to 100 cases of *Salmonella* infection go unreported for every case that is reported (37). The highest attack rate is among infants, with a peak of 250 cases per 100,000 population per year occurring at 3 months of age (38). The elderly also appear to be at an increased risk for salmonellosis. The very young, the very old, and the immunosuppressed are particularly susceptible to severe or extraintestinal infections with *Salmonella*. Reported cases of salmonellosis have a marked summer–fall incidence, although this varies by serotype for reasons that remain unclear (39).

Salmonella species have become adapted to many different environments and hosts (39). Some are highly species specific: for example, *S. pullorum* and *S. gallinarum* have long been known to cause epidemic disease in their poultry hosts, and *S. choleraesuis* remains a major threat to swine health. These organisms rarely cause illness in humans. Other serotypes that commonly cause foodborne infections in humans have characteristic animal hosts, which are their primary reservoir but in which they do not cause disease. The healthy food animal reservoir for *S. heidelberg* and *S. infantis* is poultry, for *S. enteritidis* is egg-laying hens, and for *S. newport* and *S. dublin* is cattle. The marked geographic differences in distribution among the serotypes in the United States presumably reflect the underlying reservoirs; *S. enteritidis* predominates in the Northeast, *S. javiana* has been most common in the Southeast, and *S. weltevreden* is restricted to Hawaii.

In the developed world, salmonellosis is primarily a foodborne illness. Foodborne outbreaks of *Salmonella* infections are common; about 50 are reported annually (40). Over 90% are attributable to foods of animal origin, and the same sources are presumed to cause the large number of sporadic cases not associated with recognized outbreaks (41). Investigation of these outbreaks often identifies a two-step process, the initial introduction of bacterial contamination into a food, and subsequent foodhandling errors that allow the introduced bacteria to multiply. Common errors include undercooking foods of animal origin, such as meat or eggs, which have *Salmonella* in them when raw; cross-contamination that transfers *Salmonella* bacteria from raw meats to cooked foods, thus bypassing the protective effect of cooking; and holding food at temperatures that permit rapid bacterial multiplication, resulting in a large infectious dose. It is uncommon for foodhandlers themselves to be the source of *Salmonella* infection. In most instances, when infected foodhandlers are identified, it is apparent that they became infected by eating the contaminated food and are the victims of the outbreak themselves, rather than the cause (42).

In the last decade, several new aspects have complicated the epidemiology of *Salmonella* infection (43). A global pandemic of *S. enteritidis* infection has affected many countries of the developed world, with annual isolation rates as high as 80 to 100 per 100,000 population (22).

In the United States, between 1982 and 1991, the number of isolates of *S. enteritidis* increased almost fourfold (44). A variety of epidemiologic studies have implicated shell eggs or products containing inadequately cooked raw eggs as the vehicles of transmission (45). *Salmonella enteritidis* is able to silently colonize the ovaries of egg-laying hens and then pass to the contents of the egg in the oviduct of the chicken before the shell is formed (46).

A second growing challenge is increasing antimicrobial resistance of *Salmonella*, largely a result of the use of antibiotics in food animal reservoirs. In a series of three studies conducted by CDC from 1979 to 1989, the resistance of *Salmonella* to one or more antimicrobial agents increased from 16% to 32% (47). Although most cases of salmonellosis do not require antimicrobial treatment, it is often prescribed for the very young, the elderly, or people with underlying diseases. Increasing resistance will affect the efficacy of this treatment. Antimicrobial treatment of other infections may also be complicated by resistant salmonellosis. Because taking an antibiotic disrupts the protective effect of normal intestinal flora, even exposure to low doses of resistant *Salmonella* can be enough to cause illness in someone who is already taking an antibiotic for another reason (19). Antimicrobial agents are heavily used in animal husbandry as "growth promotants" and chemoprophylactic agents. Ironically, because these agents can suppress normal gut flora and reduce "colonization resistance," resistant strains can actually spread more easily in animals receiving such antibiotics than in those that do not.

The clinical spectrum of *Salmonella* infections has been expanding. *Salmonella* causes particularly severe and prolonged infections in AIDS patients. Some serotypes, such as *S. typhimurium*, *S. enteritidis,* and *S. dublin,* cause a typhoidal bacteremia in AIDS patients that can recur even after appropriate therapy; others, such as *S. heidelberg,* do not possess this property of opportunistic invasiveness (48). Reiter's syndrome, a chronic reactive arthropathy, has recently been reported to follow infection with *Salmonella* (29).

Campylobacter

Campylobacter species were first recognized as important human pathogens in the 1970s, after selective media for stool culture became available. Before this, *C. jejuni* was thought to be an uncommon cause of bacteremia in immunocompromised hosts; now it is recognized as the most common bacterial cause of diarrhea in the industrialized world. It is isolated from diarrheal patients' stools more frequently than *Salmonella* (49,50). Approximately 10,000 infections with *C. jejuni* are reported each year in the United States, a figure that represents only a tiny fraction of the estimated two to four million cases that actually occur each year (50). There is a marked summer–fall seasonality among reported *Campylobacter* isolates. *Campylobacter jejuni* can be serotyped using heat-stable and heat-labile (flagellar) antigens, but, unlike *Salmonella*, the various *Campylobacter* serotypes do not appear to have distinctive clinical, pathologic, or epidemiologic significance (51).

Although *C. jejuni* represents over 95% of cases reported to the national *Campylobacter* surveillance system, at least nine other *Campylobacter* species are potential human pathogens. Some, like *C. coli,* are common in other parts of the industrialized world but are relatively uncommon in the United States. Others, like *C. fetus* subspecies *fetus,* appear to be infrequent causes of bacteremia in immunocompromised hosts but are rarely isolated in stool culture. Most *Campylobacter* isolation media contain cephalothin, which inhibits the growth of a number of *Campylobacter* species including *C. fetus.* Thus these species, like *C. jejuni* before 1970, may be a more common cause of diarrheal illness than is currently recognized (52).

Campylobacter infections occur in all age groups, with the greatest incidence in children under 1 year of age, and a second peak in incidence in young adults. In young adults, *Campylobacter* is by far the most frequently diagnosed cause of diarrheal illness. This increased attack rate may be the result of food-handling errors made by young adults cooking for themselves for the first time with minimal culinary experience (53). In a survey of college students, *C. jejuni* was isolated ten times more often than *Salmonella* (54).

The principal animal reservoir for *C. jejuni* is the chicken. *Campylobacter* species have been isolated from many wild and domestic animals and appear to be particularly well adapted to the avian intestinal tract. Campylobacteriosis is primarily a sporadic foodborne illness, and poultry is the primary vehicle of transmission of *C. jejuni* to humans (55). Because the infectious dose is low, contact with raw poultry can cause illness even if the food is subsequently well cooked.

Outbreaks of *Campylobacter* infections are relatively infrequent and are typically traced to drinking raw milk or surface water. Waterborne disease typically follows consumption of untreated surface water that may be contaminated with bird feces (56). Surprisingly, for an organism with a low infectious dose, person-to-person transmission appears to be very rare, and outbreaks of campylobacteriosis in day care centers have not been reported in the United States (55).

Recently, a strong epidemiologic association has been reported between infection with *C. jejuni* and subsequent Guillain–Barré syndrome; this association may be restricted to a few serotypes of *C. jejuni* (31).

Shigella

The genus *Shigella* includes four serogroups, *S. dysenteriae, S. flexneri, S. boydii,* and *S. sonnei.* The first three serogroups can be further subdivided into multiple numbered serotypes; *S. sonnei* is a single serotype. *Shigella sonnei* is the most common cause of shigellosis in the United States, causing about 70% of reported infections, while *S. flexneri* accounts for about 25% (57). *Shigella dysenteriae* serotype 1 causes severe dysentery and HUS in the least developed parts of the world, where it has become highly resistant to many antimicrobial agents (58).

This serotype predominated in Europe until the 1920s, when it was replaced by various strains of *S. flexneri*. *Shigella flexneri* was in turn replaced by *S. sonnei* in the 1960s in both Europe and the United States (59,60). This also occurred in Japan, and in recent years, even *S. sonnei* has become rare in that country, appearing only in those returning from overseas and their contacts (61). This ecologic succession of serogroups is not easily explained, although it appears to be related in some fashion to improvements in sanitation and perhaps to differences in the transmissibility of the different species.

In the United States, approximately 20,000 isolates of *Shigella* are reported annually, an annual incidence of 8 per 100,000 population (57). Because of underreporting, the actual incidence of infection is likely to be 20 times greater (62). The highest incidence occurs in toddlers aged 1 to 4 years, among whom the national isolation rate was 27 per 100,000 in 1988 (57). *Shigella* is transmitted primarily from person to person via fecal–oral mechanisms, and the predominance among toddlers reflects the particular problem of shigellosis in child day care centers (63). Outbreaks of shigellosis in child day care centers can be especially difficult to control and are a persistent public health problem associated with the increased frequency of day care use. Other populations at risk for shigellosis include native Americans, homosexuals, and travelers to the developing world. Among these groups, *S. flexneri* is more frequently encountered (64). The disease has a marked summer–fall seasonal incidence. Foodborne outbreaks occasionally occur and are frequently attributed to infected foodhandlers. Waterborne outbreaks have occurred in association with swimming at crowded freshwater beaches (65).

Antimicrobial resistance has been a well-recognized feature of *Shigella* infections. In fact, shigellae were the first organisms identified to have multiple antimicrobial resistance that was plasmid mediated (66). Resistance is related to the use of antimicrobial agents used to treat shigellosis and other infections in humans. *Shigella* infections acquired during foreign travel are more likely to be resistant than those acquired in the United States; 76% of isolates acquired during foreign travel were resistant to multiple antibiotics in a recent study (64). The increasing frequency of antimicrobial resistance indicates the need for susceptibility testing of isolates from patients receiving antimicrobial therapy. Efforts to develop experimental vaccines have been hampered by the plasticity of the *Shigella* genome and the difficulty in achieving a reliably nonpathogenic live vaccine strain. However, transmission can be prevented even without a vaccine. Successful measures include providing safe water, promoting handwashing with soap, and fly control in selected settings (67–69). The increase in resistance of *Shigella* means that alternatives to antimicrobial therapy may be needed in the future and that attention to prevention is becoming more necessary than ever (70).

Enterohemorrhagic E. coli

In 1982, *E. coli* O157:H7 was first identified as the cause of hemorrhagic colitis, a distinctive dysentery (71). Since then, this organism has emerged as the most important cause of bloody diarrheal illness and the associated HUS on the North American continent and Europe (26). It produces two exotoxins, which resemble the Shiga toxin of *S. dysenteriae* type 1 in structure and biologic activity; they are known as Shiga-like toxins (SLT). These toxins are also called verotoxins because of their characteristic cytopathic effect on the Vero cell line. A group of SLT-producing *E. coli* serotypes have been identified; these are referred to collectively as enterohemorrhagic *E. coli* (EHEC). Although *E. coli* O157:H7 is by far the most frequently recognized, other members of the group can cause outbreaks, sporadic cases of hemorrhagic colitis, and HUS.

As of 1993, formal national surveillance for *E. coli* O157:H7 had not yet begun in the United States, although the infection was being made reportable in a growing number of states. Many laboratories did not routinely look for this organism in bloody stools. Limited local studies suggest that the incidence may be 20,000 cases per year, that persons of all age groups are affected, and that the infection has a summer–fall peak in frequency (35). In some parts of Canada, the incidence of diagnosed *E. coli* O157:H7 infections equals or exceeds that of *Salmonella*. Because the bloody diarrhea is typically not accompanied by fever or fecal leukocytes, noninfectious etiologies such as intussusception or ulcerative colitis are often suspected, and diagnostic stool cultures using sorbitol–MacConkey agar are not requested.

In the elderly, the infection is likely to be confused with ischemic colitis. Approximately 2% to 7% of infections with *E. coli* O157:H7 progress to HUS, the triad of microangiopathic hemolytic anemia, thrombocytopenia, and renal failure. In some cases, neurologic changes and fever occur, leading to the diagnosis of thrombotic thrombocytopenic purpura (TTP). HUS and TTP are more likely to occur in infected persons under 5 or over 55 years old, in infections caused by strains that produce SLT II, and possibly in persons whose initial diarrheal illness is treated with sulfa-containing antibiotics (72,73). In outbreaks, approximately 2% of patients with recognized O157 infection die (26). Of those who get HUS, 43% require dialysis, and 4% develop chronic renal failure (27).

Escherichia coli O157:H7 has emerged as a major public health threat in Canada, where it causes foodborne outbreaks and many sporadic cases in the general population and community-wide outbreaks among the native American population (26). In Europe, sporadic disease and occasional small outbreaks have been recognized. One outbreak that may have been caused by *E. coli* O111 has recently been reported from Italy (74).

The principal animal reservoir for *E. coli* O157:H7 is the cow. *Escherichia coli* O157:H7 has been isolated repeatedly from healthy beef and dairy herds on several continents (26). Transmission to humans typically follows consumption of undercooked ground beef or unpasteurized milk. The sources of other EHEC organisms have not been well demonstrated epidemiologically, although SLT-producing *E. coli* appear to be common in cattle herds. The infectious dose for *E. coli* O157:H7 has not been determined but it appears to be quite low, approximately several hundred organisms or less. Person-to-person transmission has been documented in day care centers and institutions for mental retardation (73,75). It is curious that, before 1993, *E. coli* O157:H7 had not been recognized as a cause of illness in the developing world. In that year, it was identified as the cause of a large outbreak of dysentery in southern Africa (25).

Vibrios

A variety of *Vibrio* species are pathogenic for humans. Most are halophilic or halotolerant, and infections are usually associated with consumption of raw seafood or contact with salt water (76). The species *V. cholerae* includes the O1 serogroup, which usually produces cholera toxin and can cause epidemic cholera, a variety of so-called non-O1 strains, which are associated with diarrheal and invasive infections but not with epidemic cholera, and the newly described serogroup O139, which also produces epidemic cholera (23). In North America, the non-O1 *V. cholerae* and *V. vulnificus* are the most common vibrios causing gastroenteritis and bacteremia (77). In Japan, *V. parahaemolyticus* is a frequent cause of diarrheal illness and outbreaks (78). In surveillance along the Gulf Coast of the United States, *Vibrio* infections were reported at a rate of 0.4 per 100,000 per year. They most commonly affected adults and occurred with a sharp summer seasonality, reflecting warm water temperatures conducive to the growth of vibrios in the environment (79).

The principal animal reservoir for vibrios is the marine invertebrate, particularly oysters, crabs, and shrimp. Vibrios are in a sense the coliforms of the sea, being well adapted to life in association with a variety of sea life. The appearance of vibrios in coastal waters and in shellfish harvested from those waters is a natural ecologic phenomenon, which can occur independent of human activity and sewage contamination. Toxigenic *V. cholerae* O1 has environmental reservoirs in the marshes of Louisiana and the rivers of northeast Australia, which appear to be independent of human contamination (77).

Vibrio infections most frequently follow consumption of raw oysters or other uncooked shellfish, leading to diarrheal illness and, in susceptible hosts, bacteremic invasion. Persons with underlying liver disease or iron overload states appear to be at higher risk for disseminated invasive disease. Bacteremia caused by *V. vulnificus* or non-O1 *V. cholerae* occurred in 28% of reported cases from the Gulf Coast, with a mortality of about 50% (79). Vibrios are also important causes of wound infections in wounds exposed to salt water, particularly in persons with underlying immunocompromising conditions (79).

Large outbreaks of seafood-associated *V. parahaemolyticus* infections occurred in the 1970s and early 1980s in the United States, but, since then, for reasons that are unclear, outbreaks have become rare. The appearance of epidemic *V. cholerae* O1 in Latin America beginning in 1991 and of epidemic *V. cholerae* O139 in Asia in 1993 has increased the chances of importation of these agents by travelers or imported foods into the industrialized world (23,77,80,81). *Vibrio cholerae* O1 strains character-

istic of the Latin American epidemic were found in the ballast water of freighters arriving in U.S. ports; routine transfer of millions of gallons of contaminated harbor water around the world in the ballast tanks of freighters is an efficient mechanism for rapid global spread of these and other harmful species (82).

Other Bacterial Enteric Pathogens

A variety of other bacterial agents are associated with diarrheal disease in the developed nations. Foodborne disease outbreaks and sporadic cases of gastrointestinal illness are frequently caused by other bacterial pathogens, such as *Staphylococcus aureus*, *Clostridium perfringens*, and *Bacillus cereus* (40). In the period 1973 to 1987, *Salmonella* caused 28% of outbreaks with known pathogen, and *S. aureus* (13%), *Clostridium botulinum* (8%), and *C. perfringens* (7%) were the second, third, and fourth most commonly reported causes of foodborne outbreaks in the United States. *Bacillus cereus* caused 58 outbreaks in this period, 2% of those for which the cause was known. It is most often associated with eating leftover cooked rice. *Clostridium perfringens* and *S. aureus* are commonly associated with foods of animal origin or foods high in protein, which may either be contaminated intrinsically by slaughtering or processing or be contaminated by food-handlers. The number of outbreaks caused by *C. perfringens* has decreased steadily in the last decade, for reasons that are unclear.

Another *Clostridium* species, *C. difficile*, can cause antibiotic-associated colitis and is a frequent cause of nosocomial diarrhea (83). The organism can also cause community-acquired diarrhea in normal adults whose protective natural flora are disrupted by antimicrobial use for other reasons. It is commonly found in the feces of infants and is presumed to be acquired by direct contact with other infected humans.

Yersinia enterocolitica is recognized as an important cause of disease in western Europe (30). The principal animal reservoir is the pig. In Belgium it has been as commonly identified as *Salmonella* and is related to the consumption of raw pork (84). Recent outbreaks in the United States occurred in infants who were cared for by persons preparing chitterlings, a dish made of pork intestines (85,86). This infection is more common in the cold months, when contamination of slaughtered pork is greatest (87–89).

Aside from EHEC, which was discussed earlier in greater detail, four other groups of pathogenic *E. coli* are currently recognized (90). These include enteropathogenic, enterotoxigenic, enteroinvasive, and enteroadherent *E. coli*. Acquisition of these types of *E. coli* in the developed world is uncommon and usually reflects travel to the developing world. Enterotoxigenic *E. coli* is a particularly common cause of traveler's diarrhea and also has caused recent outbreaks in the United States. Enteroinvasive strains of *E. coli* are very similar in pathogenesis and in microbial characteristics to *Shigella*; they have been associated with outbreaks caused by imported foods in the United States (91). Enteropathogenic *E. coli* is common in the developing world, where it can be multiply resistant and nosocomially acquired (92); it has been recognized as a rare cause of disease among children of migrant workers in day care.

The significance of two other pathogens, *Aeromonas hydrophila* and *Plesiomonas shigelloides,* is less clear. Some strains are likely to be diarrheal pathogens, but Koch's postulates have yet to be fulfilled (93). These organisms have been the subject of case–control studies that associated *Aeromonas* with drinking untreated water and *Plesiomonas* with eating raw shellfish and traveling abroad (94,95).

Viral Pathogens

The epidemiology of viral diseases has been hampered by the lack or difficulty of diagnostic tests. Thus there is little national surveillance for these diseases. Most data are from studies examining pediatric populations in specific geographic areas. Although most studies do not identify a causative agent in a large proportion of cases, the most commonly identified viral pathogens are rotavirus, the enteric adenoviruses, and the Norwalk-like viruses (96,97). A longitudinal hospital-based study identified rotavirus (34.5%), enteric adenoviruses (4.7%), and 27-nm (Norwalk-like) viruses (1.6%) as the causes of pediatric diarrhea (97). It is assumed that there are many, yet undefined, viral agents that are responsible for some of the diarrheal disease of unknown etiology. Potential candidates include caliciviruses, astroviruses, parvoviruses, non-group A rotaviruses, small round particles, and coronaviruses (98). For most of these viruses, their current role in diarrheal disease is unknown.

Rotavirus

Most studies suggest that rotavirus is the most common cause of pediatric diarrhea. In one study in the United States, most children had acquired antibody to rotavirus by 2 years of age (99). A Japanese study suggested that over 70% of winter diarrhea was associated with rotavirus (100). A study of hospital discharge diagnoses in the United States suggested that rotavirus might cause between 75 and 125 deaths and 65,000 to 70,000 hospitalizations each year in the United States (7). In one study of diarrheal disease among infants attending day care centers, rotavirus was the most commonly isolated pathogen (14). In another study of children seeking medical treatment for diarrhea in Michigan, 16% of episodes of diarrhea in children under 2 years of age was attributed to rotavirus (6). Rotavirus is also likely to be a cause of diarrheal disease in adults, potentially causing 5% to 10% of sporadic illness (101). Parents of ill children can become infected. Rotavirus has been associated with illness in travelers and may cause waterborne and nosocomial outbreaks. Disease appears to have a marked winter seasonality. The mechanism of transmission, although unknown, is thought to be person to person; this might include an airborne route.

Norwalk and Norwalk-like Viruses

The viruses in the Norwalk and Norwalk-like group are recognized through electron microscopy as 27-nm particles. It is likely that these viruses are a common cause of outbreaks of nonbacterial gastroenteritis (102). In one study, over a 4-year period, 42% of 74 outbreaks were attributed to the Norwalk virus (103). These viruses cause an illness that is often referred to as "winter vomiting disease." Its incubation period is between 24 and 48 hr, and secondary attack rates are high. The disease has been transmitted by foodborne, waterborne, and person-to-person spread. Although the illness generally has a winter seasonal incidence, outbreaks can occur throughout the year. The frequency of antibodies to Norwalk-like viruses increases with age, which suggests that these viruses may be a less important cause of diarrheal disease in children (104). One family of this type of virus contains many viruses named after the geographic areas in which they were first isolated; they include Cockle, Ditchling, Hawaii, Montgomery County, Norwalk, Snow Mountain, and Wollan (104).

Other Agents

Several studies suggest that other viral agents are important causes of diarrheal disease. A study in Canada suggested that enteric adenoviruses were the second most common viral pathogen in hospitalized patients (105). In a Swedish study, the enteric adenoviruses were identified in 13% of stool specimens from patients with acute gastroenteritis and from 1.5% of controls (106). Other viruses have been associated with specific outbreaks, such as astroviruses and caliciviruses with outbreaks in nurseries, pediatric wards, and schools, and parvoviruses with foodborne outbreaks associated with shellfish consumption (107).

Parasitic Pathogens

In the general population of the developed world, parasitic infections appear to be uncommon causes of diarrheal illness. However, these organisms do cause disease in certain populations such as day care attendees and employees, migrant workers and their families, and homosexual men. In the United States, the most frequent parasitic causes of diarrheal diseases are *Giardia lamblia, Cryptosporidium,* and the newly identified *Microsporidium.*

Giardia lamblia

Infection with *G. lamblia* (also known as *G. intestinalis*) is probably the most frequent parasitic cause of diarrheal disease in the developed world (108). Few reliable surveillance data are available because reporting is rarely mandated; in Vermont and in Wisconsin, symptomatic giardiasis had a reported annual incidence of 50 per 100,000;

incidence was highest among toddlers, with a second peak among young adults (109,110). A late summer peak in infections is typical though unexplained. Infections are passed person to person through the fecal–oral route by direct transfer of cysts or through contaminated water, and occasionally through food. *Giardia* frequently inhabits a variety of mammalian intestinal tracts, but because the organism is difficult to subtype, the importance of animal reservoirs in the epidemiology of this infection remains unclear (111).

Giardia infections are most commonly associated with attending child day care centers and with consuming untreated surface water (112). In the day care setting, carriage of *Giardia* may reach 50% or greater among pretoilet-trained children, and it may be the most frequently identified pathogen in toddlers in day care (113). The control of day care-related giardiasis remains a substantial challenge (114). Attempts to prevent transmission through aggressive detection and treatment of silent infection in children, family members, and even family pets have been generally unsuccessful in lowering infection rates.

Giardiasis is also a well-defined cause of outbreaks and sporadic cases of waterborne diarrhea (65). These typically follow consumption of untreated river or lake water contaminated with the feces of humans and of wild animals, such as beavers. Like other parasitic cysts, *Giardia* organisms are relatively resistant to the effects of chlorine treatment of water; water filtration is necessary to remove them. Outbreaks have followed the consumption of heavily contaminated water that was chlorinated but not filtered. Repeated outbreaks of giardiasis from partially treated water have led the Environmental Protection Agency to require filtration of surface water for all municipal water supplies in addition to chlorination (115). In recent years, several well-documented outbreaks of foodborne giardiasis have illustrated the potential for transmission via the foodborne route as well (116,117). In such outbreaks, the implicated food was contaminated by the hands of a food preparer who also changed the diapers of an infected toddler.

Cryptosporidium

Cryptosporidium has recently emerged as an important parasitic cause of diarrheal disease worldwide (118). It has been recognized as a diarrheal pathogen in patients with AIDS and also causes diarrheal illness in the normal host. In recent surveys in the state of Oregon and in Spain, cryptosporidia were identified in approximately 1% of the stools of diarrheal patients (119,120). Like *Giardia,* it has been identified as a cause of outbreaks in day care centers and as the cause of large waterborne outbreaks from municipal water systems. In a random survey of day care centers in Atlanta, cryptosporidia were identified in children at 12% of the centers and in 3% of children in affected centers (121). Recent waterborne outbreaks of cryptosporidial diarrheal illness have occurred in areas with large municipal water systems that were equipped with chlorination and filters and were functioning according to regulatory guidelines at the time the outbreak occurred

(122,123). Cryptosporidial cysts are even more resistant to chlorine then *Giardia* cysts, and apparently even minor fluctuations in the efficiency of filtration can permit outbreaks to occur if the incoming burden of cysts is sufficiently high. In a case–control study of sporadic cryptosporidiosis in Australia, illness was associated with consumption of surface water or municipal system water (124). An outbreak has also occurred after swimming in a chlorinated swimming pool (125). Better standard water treatment procedures are needed to prevent waterborne cryptosporidiosis (115). Cryptosporidia have been detected in a variety of animal species and appear to have an important bovine reservoir; the importance of this as a source of human illness remains to be established.

Other Agents

Other parasitic agents are occasional causes of intestinal disease in the developed world. *Microsporidium* was recognized as a cause of human illness in the 1980s, when it was detected in the intestines of AIDS patients with persistent diarrhea (126). The organism also causes disseminated disease in end-stage AIDS patients (127). Knowledge concerning the epidemiology of this pathogen is still evolving; it remains unclear whether it is a cause of illness in the normal host. The recently described pathogen *Cyclospora* (previously known as blue-green algae-like or cyanobacterium-like organism) has been recognized as a cause of diarrheal illness in AIDS patients and in travelers to the developing world, particularly Nepal (128,129). The nature of the organism has recently been clarified to be a new genus of protozoa (130).

Other well-recognized parasitic pathogens common in the developing world are occasionally identified in travelers. *Entamoeba histolytica* is uncommon in the United States, although infections are occasionally detected among foreign travelers and immigrants (131). Sustained person-to-person transmission of *E. histolytica* among homosexual men was reported in the 1970s (132). The agent has also been transmitted from patient to patient by colonic irrigation in a chiropractic clinic (133). *Anisakis* is an uncommon cause of hemorrhagic gastritis among persons eating raw infected salmon (40).

Chronic Diarrheas of Unknown Infectious Etiology

There are many noninfectious gastrointestinal diseases that cause chronic diarrhea in the developed world. A recently recognized syndrome, likely to be of an infectious etiology, deserves special comment. This syndrome, known as Brainerd diarrhea, was first described as the result of an outbreak in the small Minnesota town of Brainerd, associated with drinking raw milk (134). This disease begins with cramps, urgency, and frequent watery stools, suggesting acute gastroenteritis, but then resolves very slowly. Stool frequency among 122 patients averaged 30 motions per day and slowly decreased over the following year to 15 motions per day. The illnesses ultimately resolved, after a median duration of 16.5 months (135).

An outbreak of a similar illness followed consumption of untreated groundwater at a restaurant in rural Illinois (136). Extensive investigations have yet to identify an etiology, and the diagnosis is one of exclusion. Outside the outbreak setting, persons with abrupt onset of watery diarrhea that persists for more than 1 month, has no established etiology or alternate diagnosis, and does not respond to antimicrobial therapy may have the Brainerd syndrome. The relation of this illness to persistent diarrheas or chronic diarrheas of the developing world remains to be established, although a recent outbreak related to drinking contaminated water on a cruise ship off the coast of Ecuador suggests that there may be a connection (137).

STRATEGIES OF PREVENTION AND CONTROL

Preventing Exposure

Improvements in food and water sanitation in the last century have transformed the etiologic spectrum of diarrheal illness in the developed world, controlling or eliminating some of the most deadly infections. Nonetheless, diarrheal disease remains an important cause of morbidity in many developed nations and is a persistent challenge to clinicians, laboratory personnel, and public health officials. Surveillance of the various infectious causes of diarrhea is evolving as new agents are identified and their importance is established. Epidemiologic investigations of sporadic cases and outbreaks have greatly improved understanding of the mechanisms of transmission for well-established and for newly emerging pathogens. This understanding is important to guide diagnosis and to develop public health strategies to reduce the morbidity of diarrheal disease throughout the world. Many agents of diarrheal disease reach the patient at the end of a long chain of events. For these agents, understanding this chain of transmission often allows prevention measures to be targeted at a weak link.

Control at the Reservoir

For some diarrheal disease pathogens, prevention means preventing the pathogen from entering the chain of transmission in the first place. For example, large natural watershed areas are protected to prevent contamination of the reservoirs used for municipal water systems. The regulation of oyster beds is designed to prevent contamination of the harvest waters with sewage. For pathogens with large animal reservoirs, prevention may ultimately mean controlling the transmission of the pathogen among the animals. For example, *Campylobacter,* which is usually transmitted to humans by contact with undercooked poultry, may be controlled in the future by efforts to reduce infection among chickens in the hen house. These could include providing safe water for chickens to drink or vaccinating chickens against *Campylobacter* (138).

Prevention at the Processing Level: Controlling the Food or Water Vehicle

Contamination can also occur after a food has been harvested or drinking water collected, and so there are many possible points of intervention during processing and distribution to the consumer. Methods for disinfecting municipal water supplies have received enormous attention from public health engineers and officials over the last century. Nonetheless, identification of parasitic agents that are relatively resistant to current treatment procedures shows that further improvements are needed. Some food technologies have also advanced rapidly in the last century and are important bulwarks in the prevention of diarrheal illness. Pasteurization of milk and eggs and modern canning procedures are critical to the safety of the food supply. However, other technologies such as processing of meat and seafood have remained largely unchanged since industrial slaughterhouses and packing plants were invented; meat and fish inspection is a visual and olfactory process that was developed in the premicrobiologic era. Restaurant inspection is a useful tool that currently also depends largely on the visual inspection process (139). Introducing concepts of process control and microbial risk reduction into these processes is an important arena for future prevention. In the future, irradiation of certain high-risk foods is likely to be a useful addition to the control process; it is effective against a broad array of pathogens and can be used to sterilize some foods (140). The increasing centralization of food and water supplies of the industrialized world offers the opportunity to make these vehicles safer on a broad scale, but it also presents the specter of enormous outbreaks when a process is defective.

Consumer Self-Defense

For many pathogens, neither control at a distant reservoir nor prevention during processing is a current reality. For these, the main line of defense lies in the behavior of the consumers themselves. In the case of foodborne diseases, increasing public awareness about basic principles of food handling and the risks of consuming specific hazardous foods is becoming part of the practical reality of living in industrialized societies, as it already is in the developing world. Targeting specific education to groups at highest risk is needed as part of the preventive agenda. The protective benefit of breast-feeding in reducing infantile diarrhea may still be underappreciated. Other measures such as advising pregnant women of the risks of eating soft cheese and pâté appear to have decreased listeriosis in Europe and in the United States (141). Teaching AIDS patients to eat defensively may reduce their risks of diarrheal illness (142). Posting warnings in restaurants, which advise patients with liver disease not to eat raw oysters, is being attempted in several jurisdictions in the United States (143).

For many diarrheal diseases transmitted from person to person by contaminated hands, promotion of personal hygiene and handwashing may be the best preventive strategy. Promoting handwashing more aggressively in hospitals, in addition to reducing the indiscriminate use of antimicrobial drugs, may be needed to reduce nosocomial diarrheas. Because a growing proportion of toddlers are cared for in the day care setting, day care-based interventions can teach children good handwashing habits and prevent illness now and in the future in an entire generation.

Increasing Host Immunity

Another group of prevention and control strategies increase host resistance to infection following unavoidable exposure. The great strides made in vaccine development against some infectious diseases continue to spark hope for developing effective vaccines against a variety of diarrheal illnesses, including rotavirus, shigellosis, and cholera (144). Although no vaccine for a diarrheal illness has yet achieved practical public health utility, the availability of an inexpensive vaccine offering durable immunity against any of the major diarrheal pathogens after a single dose would be an important advance.

Host resistance can also be manipulated by increasing nonimmune resistance to colonization. In animal models, normal host flora form an important barrier to colonization with incoming pathogens. Transmission of *Salmonella* among chickens in Europe has been reduced by giving newly hatched chickens an extract of normal fecal flora, thereby conferring colonization resistance on them (145). In clinical settings, antimicrobial treatment that disrupts the host flora increases susceptibility to many enteric and respiratory pathogens, while treatments that do not affect gut flora preserve this important barrier to colonization (146). In an outbreak of Norwalk-like gastroenteritis in a nursing home, it was observed that persons already taking psyllium (Metamucil) were protected, suggesting that manipulations of gut ecology may also play a protective role in this infection (147). Other non-antimicrobial prophylactic strategies may be useful, including use of bismuth subsalicylate, or the simple addition of immunoglobulin to infant formula (148,149). In general, microbial manipulation that increases or restores resistance to colonization or infection remains a relatively unexplored but potentially fruitful arena for future research.

Eradication: A Distant Hope

Complexity of transmission, extensive environmental reservoirs, frequency of silent infections, and lack of vaccines make eradication extremely unlikely for most diarrheal pathogens in the developed world. For a few pathogens, eradication is theoretically possible. For example, both *Salmonella typhi* (the cause of typhoid fever) and *Shigella dysenteriae* type 1 (the cause of epidemic dysentery) are restricted to the human species without another animal reservoir; both may be preventable by vaccine and thus theoretically susceptible to eradication if all chains of transmission among humans can be broken. However,

difficulty in recognizing the disease and the carrier states makes this a remote possibility, even for these pathogens.

Anticipating the Unexpected

In recent years, a growing variety of bacterial, viral, and parasitic agents have been identified as important causes of enteric infections. Even for well-established pathogens, increases in antimicrobial resistance and in the immunosuppressed population make for new clinical challenges in diagnosis and appropriate therapy. Better understanding of the complex reservoirs and mechanisms of transmission has demonstrated the need for improvement in prevention strategies, which go far beyond the clinical setting. Many challenges recently identified in the developed world are likely to soon be recognized in the developing world, as accelerating contact between the developed and the developing world blends the problems of each area together. It is likely that changing human ecology will open up new evolutionary niches for known and currently unsuspected microbial pathogens, which will appear as new epidemics, new pathogens, and new vehicles of infection. This evolutionary context makes it likely that we will never know all the causes of diarrheal illness, nor how to prevent them. We can continue to expect the unexpected.

REFERENCES

1. Cohen ML. The epidemiology of community-acquired infections. In: Gorbach SL, Bartlett JG, Blacklow NR, eds. *Infectious diseases*. Philadelphia: Saunders, 1992;90–95.
2. Snyder JD, Merson MH. The magnitude of the global problem of acute diarrhoeal disease: a review of active surveillance data. *Bull World Health Organ* 1982;60:605.
3. Bennett JV, Holmberg SD, Rogers MF, et al. Infectious and parasitic diseases. *Am J Prev Med* 1987;3(Suppl):102.
4. Archer DL, Kvenberg JE. Incidence and cost of foodborne diarrheal disease in the United States. *J Food Protect* 1985;48:887–894.
5. National Center for Health Statistics, Ries PW. Current estimates from the National Health Interview Survey, United States—1984. DHHS publication no (PHS)86-1584. Washington, DC: Public Health Service, US Government Printing Office, 1986. (*Vital and health statistics;* series 10, no 156).
6. Koopman JS, Turkish VJ, Monto AS, et al. Patterns and etiology of diarrhea in three clinical settings. *Am J Epidemiol* 1984;119:114.
7. Glass RI, Lew JF, Gangarosa RE, LeBaron CW, Ho M. Estimates of morbidity and mortality rates for diarrheal disease in American children. *J Pediatr* 1991;118:27–33.
8. Ho M, Glass RI, Pinsky PF, Anderson LJ. Rotavirus as a cause of diarrheal morbidity and mortality in the United States. *J Infect Dis* 1988;158:1112–1116.
9. Uhnoo I, Wadell G, Svensson L, et al. Aetiology and epidemiology of acute gastroenteritis in Swedish children. *J Infect* 1986;13:73.
10. Gangarosa RE, Glass RI, Lew JF, Boring JR. Hospitalization involving gastroenteritis in the United States, 1985: the special burden of the disease among the elderly. *Am J Epidemiol* 1992;135:281–290.
11. Lew JF, Glass RI, Gangarosa RE, Cohen IP, Bern C, Moe CL. Diarrheal deaths in the United States, 1979 through 1987. *JAMA* 1991;265:3280–3284.
12. Guerrant RL, Lohr JA, Williams EK. Acute infectious diar-

rhea. I. Epidemiology, etiology and pathogenesis. *J Pediatr Dis* 1986;5:353.

13. Nelson JD. Etiology and epidemiology of diarrheal diseases in the United States. *Am J Med* 1985;78(Suppl 6B):76.
14. Bartlett AV, Moore M, Gary GW, et al. Diarrheal illness among infants and toddlers in day care centers. I. Epidemiology and pathogens. *J Pediatr* 1985;107:495.
15. Quinn TC, Stamm WE, Goodell SE, et al. The polymicrobial origin of intestinal infections in homosexual men. *N Engl J Med* 1983;309:576.
16. MacDonald KL, Cohen ML. Epidemiology of traveler's diarrhea: current perspectives. *Rev Infect Dis* 1986;8(Suppl 2):S117.
17. Holmberg SD, Osterholm MT, Senger KA, Cohen ML. Drug-resistant *Salmonella* from animals fed antimicrobials. *N Engl J Med* 1984;311:617–622.
18. Lederberg J, Shope RE, Oaks SC Jr, eds. *Emerging infections: microbial threats to health in the United States.* Washington, DC: National Academy Press, 1992.
19. Cohen ML, Tauxe RV. Drug-resistant *Salmonella* in the United States: an epidemiologic perspective. *Science* 1986;234:964.
20. Kunin CM, Lipton HL, Tupasi T, et al. Social, behavioral and practical factors affecting antibiotic use worldwide: report of Task Force 4. *Rev Infect Dis* 1987;9(Suppl 3):S270–S285.
21. World Health Organization. Worldwide spread of infections with *Yersinia enterocolitica*. *World Health Organ Chronicle* 1976;30:494–496.
22. Rodrigue DC, Tauxe RV, Rowe B. International increase in *Salmonella enteritidis:* a new pandemic? *Epidemiol Infect* 1990;105:21–27.
23. Centers for Disease Control and Prevention. Imported cholera associated with a newly described toxigenic *Vibrio cholerae* O139 strain—California, 1993. *MMWR Morb Mortal Wkly Rep* 1993;42:501–503.
24. Clark GM, Kaufmann AF, Gangarosa EJ, Thompson MA. Epidemiology of an international outbreak of *Salmonella agona*. *Lancet* 1973;2:1–10.
25. Isaacson M, Canter PH, Effler P, Arntzen L, Bomans P, Heenan R. Haemorrhagic colitis in Africa [Letter]. *Lancet* 1993;341:961.
26. Griffin PM, Tauxe RV. The epidemiology of infections caused by *Escherichia coli* O157:H7, other enterohemorrhagic *E. coli*, and the associated hemolytic uremic syndrome. *Epidemiol Rev* 1991;13:60–98.
27. Pavia AT, Siegler RL, Christofferson R, Milligan M. Predictors of severe disease and long term sequelae in post-diarrheal hemolytic uremic syndrome. Abstract 1456. *33rd Interscience Conference on Antimicrobial Agents and Chemotherapy,* New Orleans, Oct 17–20, 1993.
28. Finch M, Rodey G, Lawrence D, Blake P. Epidemic Reiter's syndrome following an outbreak of shigellosis. *Eur J Epidemiol* 1986;2:26–30.
29. Swerdlow DL, Lee LA, Tauxe RV, et al. Reactive arthropathy following a multistate outbreak of *Salmonella typhimurium* infections. Abstract 916. *30th Interscience Conference on Antimicrobial Agents and Chemotherapy,* Atlanta, Oct 21–24, 1990.
30. Ostroff SM, Kapperud G, Lassen J, Aasen S, Tauxe RV. Clinical features of sporadic *Yersinia enterocolitica* infections in Norway. *J Infect Dis* 1992;166:812–817.
31. Mishu B, Ilyas AA, Kosli CL, et al. Serologic evidence of previous *Campylobacter jejuni* infections in patients with the Guillain–Barfe syndrome. *Ann Intern Med* 1993;118:947–953.
32. Guerrant RL, Hughes JM, Lima NL, Crane J. Diarrhea in developed and developing countries: magnitude, special settings, and etiologies. *Rev Infect Dis* 1990;12(Suppl 1):S41–S50.
33. Ries AA, Griffin P, Greene K, *Escherichia coli* O157:H7 Study Group. *Escherichia coli* O157:H7 diarrhea in the United States: a 10 center surveillance study. Abstract 1454. *33rd Interscience Conference on Antimicrobial Agents and Chemotherapy,* New Orleans, Oct 17–20, 1993.
34. Blaser MJ, Wells JG, Feldman RA, et al. *Campylobacter* enteritis in the United States. A multicenter study. *Ann Intern Med* 1983;98:360.

35. MacDonald KL, O'Leary MJ, Cohen ML, et al. *Escherichia coli* O157:H7, an emerging gastrointestinal pathogen. *JAMA* 1988;259:3567–3570.
36. Centers for Disease Control. *Salmonella: annual summary, 1991.* Atlanta, GA: Centers for Disease Control, 1992.
37. Chalker RB, Blaser MJ. A review of human salmonellosis: III. Magnitude of *Salmonella* infections in the United States. *Rev Infect Dis* 1987;7:111–124.
38. Hargrett-Bean N, Pavia AT, Tauxe RV. *Salmonella* isolates from humans in the United States, 1984–1986. *MMWR CDC Surveill Summ* 1988;37(SS-2):25–31.
39. Martin SM, Hargrett-Bean N, Tauxe RV. An atlas of *Salmonella* in the United States: serotype-specific surveillance 1968–1986. Atlanta, GA: Centers for Disease Control, 1989; 179 pp.
40. Bean NH, Griffin PM. Foodborne disease outbreaks in the United States, 1973–1987: pathogens, vehicles and trends. *J Food Protect* 1990;53:804–817.
41. Cohen ML, Gangarosa EJ. Nontyphoid salmonellosis. *South Med J* 1978;71:1540.
42. Cruickshank JG, Humphrey TJ. The carrier food-handler and non-typhoid salmonellosis. *Epidemiol Infect* 1987;98:223–230.
43. Tauxe RV. *Salmonella:* a postmodern pathogen. *J Food Protect* 1991;54:563–568.
44. Centers for Disease Control. Outbreak of *Salmonella enteritidis* infection associated with consumption of raw shell eggs, 1991. *MMWR Morb Mortal Wkly Rep* 1992;41:369–372.
45. St Louis ME, Morse DL, Potter ME, DeMelfi TM, Guzewich JJ, Tauxe RV, Blake PA, the *Salmonella enteritidis* Working Group. The emergence of grade A eggs as a major source of *Salmonella enteritidis* infections: implications for the control of salmonellosis. *JAMA* 1988;259:2103–2107.
46. Gast RK, Beard CW. Production of *Salmonella enteritidis* contaminated eggs by experimentally infected hens. *Avian Dis* 1990;34:438–446.
47. Lee LA, Puhr ND, Maloney EK, Bean NH, Tauxe RV. Increase in antimicrobial resistant *Salmonella* infections in the United States, 1989–1990. *J Infect Dis [in press]*.
48. Levine WC, Buehler JW, Bean NH, Tauxe RV. Epidemiology of nontyphoidal *Salmonella* bacteremia during the human immunodeficiency virus epidemic. *J Infect Dis* 1991;164:81–87.
49. Blaser MJ, Taylor DN, Feldman RA. Epidemiology of *Campylobacter jejuni* infections. *Epidemiol Rev* 1983;5:157.
50. Tauxe RV. Epidemiology of *Campylobacter jejuni* infections in the United States and other industrialized nations. In: Nachamkin I, Blaser MJ, Tompkins L, eds. *Campylobacter jejuni: current status and future trends.* Washington, DC: American Society for Microbiology, 1992;9–19.
51. Patton CM, Wachsmuth IK. Typing schemes: are current methods useful? In: Nachamkin I, Blaser MJ, Tompkins L, eds. *Campylobacter jejuni: current status and future trends.* Washington, DC: American Society for Microbiology, 1992;110–128.
52. Mishu B, Patton CM, Tauxe RV. Clinical and epidemiologic features of non-jejuni, non-coli *Campylobacter* species. In: Nachamkin I, Blaser MJ, Tompkins L, eds. *Campylobacter jejuni: current status and future trends.* Washington, DC: American Society of Microbiology, 1992;31–41.
53. Deming MD, Tauxe RV, Blake PA, et al. *Campylobacter* enteritis at a university: transmission from eating chicken and from cats. *Am J Epidemiol* 1987;126:526–534.
54. Tauxe RV, Deming MS, Blake PA. *Campylobacter jejuni* infections on college campuses: a national survey. *Am J Public Health* 1985;75:659.
55. Tauxe RV, Hargrett-Bean N, Patton CM, Wachsmuth IK. *Campylobacter* isolates in the United States. 1982–1986. *MMWR CDC Surveill Summ* 1988;37(SS-2):1–13.
56. Taylor DN, McDermott KT, Little JR, Wells JG, Blaser MJ. *Campylobacter* enteritis from untreated water in the Rocky Mountains. *Ann Intern Med* 1983;99:38–40.
57. Lee LA, Shapiro CN, Hargrett-Bean N, Tauxe RV. Hyperendemic shigellosis in the United States: a review of surveillance data for 1967–1988. *J Infect Dis* 1991;164:894–900.
58. Ries AA, Wells JG, Olivola D, et al. Epidemic *Shigella dysent-*

eriae type 1 in Burundi: pan-resistance and the implications for prevention. *J Infect Dis* [*in press*].

59. Kostrzewski J, Stypulkowska-Misiurewicz H. Changes in the epidemiology of dysentery in Poland and the situation in Europe. *Arch Immunol Ther Exp* (*Warsz*) 1968;16:429–451.

60. Rosenberg ML, Weissman JB, Gangarosa EJ, Reller LB, Beasley RP. Shigellosis in the United States: ten-year review of nationwide surveillance, 1964–1973. *Am J Epidemiol* 1076;104:543–551.

61. Takeda Y. Shigellosis in Japan. In: Rahaman MM, Greenough WB, eds. *Proceedings of an international conference. Shigellosis: a continuing global problem* (Cox's Bazaar, Bangladesh). Dhaka, Bangladesh: International Center for Diarrheal Disease Research, 1983.

62. Rosenberg ML, Gangarosa EJ, Pollard RA, Wallace M, Bronitsky O, Marr JS. *Shigella* surveillance in the United States, 1975. *J Infect Dis* 1977;136:458–460.

63. Weissman JB, Gangarosa EJ, Schmerler A, et al. Shigellosis in day-care centers. *Lancet* 1975;1:88–90.

64. Tauxe RV, Puhr ND, Wells JG, Hargrett-Bean N, Blake PA. Antimicrobial resistance of *Shigella* isolates in the USA: the importance of international travelers. *J Infect Dis* 1990;162:1107–1111.

65. Herwaldt BL, Craun GF, Stokes SL, et al. Waterborne disease outbreaks, 1989–1990. *MMWR CDC Surveill Summ* 1991;40(SS-3):1–21.

66. Watanabe T. Infective heredity of multiple drug resistance in bacteria. *Bacteriol Rev* 1963;27:87–115.

67. Hollister AC, Beck D, Gittelsohn AM, Hemphill EC. Influence of water availability on *Shigella* prevalence in children of farm labor families. *Am J Public Health* 1955;45:354–362.

68. Khan MU. Interruption of shigellosis by handwashing. *Trans R Soc Trop Med Hyg* 1982;76:164–168.

69. Cohen D, Green M, Block C, et al. Reduction of transmission of shigellosis by control of house flies (*Musca domestica*). *Lancet* 1991;337:993–997.

70. Tuttle J, Tauxe RV. Antimicrobial-resistant *Shigella*: the growing need for prevention strategies. *Infect Dis Clin Pract* 1993;2:55–59.

71. Riley LW, Remis RS, Helgerson SD, et al. Hemorrhagic colitis associated with a rare *Escherichia coli* serotype. *N Engl J Med* 1983;308:681.

72. Ostroff SM, Tarr PI, Neill MA, Lewis JH, Hargrett-Bean N, Kobayashi JM. Toxin genotypes and plasmid profiles as determinants of systemic sequelae in *Escherichia coli* O157:H7 infections. *J Infect Dis* 1989;160:994–998.

73. Pavia AT, Nichols CR, Green DP, et al. Hemolytic-uremic syndrome during an outbreak of *Escherichia coli* O157:H7 infections in institutions for mentally retarded persons: clinical and epidemiologic observations. *J Pediatr* 1990;116:544–551.

74. Caprioli A, Luzzi I, Rosmini F, et al. Community-wide outbreak of hemolytic uremic syndrome associated with non O157, verocytotoxin-producing *Escherichia coli*. *J Infect Dis* 1994;169:208–211.

75. Spika JS, Parsons JE, Nordenberg D, Wells JG, Gunn RA, Blake PA. Hemolytic uremic syndrome and diarrhea associated with *Escherichia coli* O157:H7 in a day care center. *Pediatrics* 1986;109:287–291.

76. Blake PA, Weaver RE, Hollis DG. Diseases of humans (other than cholera) caused by vibrios. *Annu Rev Microbiol* 1980;34:341.

77. Blake PA. The epidemiology of cholera in the Americas. *Gastroenterol Clin North Am* 1993;22:639–660.

78. Fukami T, Saku K. Clinical epidemiology of infectious enteritis of outpatients at Tokyo Metropolitan Bokuto General Hospital. In: Saito M, Nakaya R, Matsubara Y, eds. *Infectious enteritis in Japan*. Tokyo: Saikon Publishing, 1986;211–220.

79. Levine WC, Griffin PM, the Gulf Coast Working Group. *Vibrio* infections on the Gulf Coast: results of first year of regional surveillance. *J Infect Dis* 1993;167:479–483.

80. Centers for Disease Control and Prevention. Cholera associated with international travel, 1992. *MMWR Morb Mortal Wkly Rep* 1992;41:664–667.

81. Taylor JL, Tuttle J, Pramukul T, et al. An outbreak of cholera in Maryland associated with imported commercial frozen fresh coconut milk. *J Infect Dis* 1993;167:1330–1335.

82. Centers for Disease Control and Prevention. Isolation of *Vibrio cholerae* O1 from oysters—Mobile Bay, 1991–1992. *MMWR Morb Mortal Wkly Rep* 1993;42:91–93.

83. Lyerly DM, Krwan HC, Wilkins TD. *Clostridium difficile* and its toxins. *Clin Microbiol Rev* 1988;1:1–18.

84. Tauxe RV, Vandepitte J, Wauters G, et al. *Yersinia enterocolitica* infections and pork: the missing link. *Lancet* 1987;1:1129–1132.

85. Lee LA, Gerber AR, Lonsway DR, et al. *Yersinia enterocolitica* O:3 infections in infants and children, associated with the household preparation of chitterlings. *N Engl J Med* 1990;322:984–987.

86. Lee LA, Taylor J, Carter GP, et al. *Yersinia enterocolitica* O:3: an emerging cause of pediatric gastroenteritis in the United States. *J Infect Dis* 1991;163:660–663.

87. Weber A, Knapp W. Nachweis von *Yersinia enterocolitica* und *Yersinia pseudotuberculosis* in Kotproben gesunder Slachtschweine in Abhaengigheit von der Jahrezeit. *Zentralbl Veterinarmed* [*B*] 1981;28:407–413.

88. Tsubokura M, Fukuda T, Otsuki K, et al. Studies on *Yersinia enterocolitica* 2. Relationship between detection from swine and seasonal incidence and regional distribution of the organism. *Jpn J Vet Sci* 1976;38:1–6.

89. Metchock B, Lonsway DR, Carter GP, Lee LA, McGowan JE. *Yersinia enterocolitica:* a frequent seasonal stool isolate from children at an urban hospital in the Southeast United States. *J Clin Microbiol* 1991;29:2868–2869.

90. Levine MM. *Escherichia coli* that cause diarrhea: enterotoxigenic, enteropathogenic, enteroinvasive, enterohemorrhagic, and enteroadherent. *J Infect Dis* 1987;155:377.

91. MacDonald KL, Eidson M, Stohmeyer C, et al. A multistate outbreak of gastrointestinal illness caused by enterotoxigenic *Escherichia coli* in imported semisoft cheese. *J Infect Dis* 1985;151:716.

92. Blake PA, Ramos S, MacDonald KL, et al. Pathogen-specific risk factors and protective factors for acute diarrheal disease in urban Brazilian infants. *J Infect Dis* 1993;167:627–632.

93. Holmberg SD, Farmer JJ III. *Aeromonas hydrophila* and *Plesiomonas shigelloides* as causes of intestinal infections. *Rev Infect Dis* 1984;6:633–639.

94. Holmberg SD, Schell WL, Fanning GR, et al. *Aeromonas* intestinal infections in the United States. *Ann Intern Med* 1986;105:683.

95. Holmberg SD, Wachsmuth IK, Hickman-Brenner FW, et al. *Plesiomonas* enteric infections in the United States. *Ann Intern Med* 1986;105:690.

96. Blacklow NR, Cukor G. Viral gastroenteritis. *N Engl J Med* 1981;304:397.

97. Brandt CD, Kim HW, Rodriguez NJ, et al. Pediatric viral gastroenteritis during eight years of study. *J Clin Microbiol* 1983;18:71.

98. Dolin R, Treanor JJ, Madore HP. Novel agents of viral enteritis in humans. *J Infect Dis* 1987;155:365.

99. Yolken RH, Wyatt RG, Zissis G, et al. Epidemiology of human rotavirus types 1 and 2 as studied by enzyme-linked immunosorbent assay. *N Engl J Med* 1978;299:1156.

100. Konno T, Suzuki H, Imai A, et al. A long-term survey of rotavirus infections in Japanese children with acute gastroenteritis. *J Infect Dis* 1978;138:569–576.

101. Hardy DB. Epidemiology of rotaviral infection in adults. *Rev Infect Dis* 1987;9:461.

102. Centers for Disease Control. Outbreak of viral gastroenteritis—Pennsylvania and Delaware. *MMWR Morb Mortal Wkly Rep* 1987;36:709.

103. Kaplan JE, Gary GW, Baron RC, et al. Epidemiology of Norwalk gastroenteritis and the role of Norwalk virus in outbreaks of acute nonbacterial gastroenteritis. *Ann Intern Med* 1982;96:756.

104. Kapikian AZ, Chanock RM. Norwalk group of viruses. In: Fields BN, Knipe DM, Chanock RM, et al., eds. *Virology*. Second Edition. New York: Raven Press, 1990;671–693.

105. Krajden M, Brown M, Petrasek A, et al. Adenovirus enteritis.

Clinical features of 131 cases with particular attention to the role of nosocomial illness (Abstract). *Twenty-Seventh Interscience Conference on Antimicrobial Agents and Chemotherapy,* New York, 1987.

106. Uhnoo I, Wadell G, Svensson L, et al. Two new serotypes of enteric adenovirus causing infantile diarrhoea. *Dev Biol Standard* 1983;53:311.

107. Appleton H. Small round viruses: classification and role in foodborne infections. *Ciba Found Symp* 1987;128:108.

108. Flanagan PA. *Giardia*—diagnosis, clinical course and epidemiology: a review. *Epidemiol Infect* 1992;109:1–22.

109. Birkhead G, Vogt RL. Epidemiologic surveillance for endemic *Giardia lamblia* infection in Vermont. The roles of waterborne and person-to-person transmission. *Am J Epidemiol* 1989;129:762–768.

110. Addiss DG, Davis JP, Roberts JM, Mast EE. Epidemiology of giardiasis in Wisconsin: increasing incidence of reported cases and unexplained seasonal trends. *Am J Trop Med Hyg* 1992;47:13–19.

111. Jakubowski W. Purple burps and the filtration of drinking water supplies. *Am J Public Health* 1988;78:123–125.

112. Dennis DT, Smith RP, Welch JJ, et al. Endemic giardiasis in New Hampshire: a case–control study of environmental risks. *J Infect Dis* 1993;167:1391–1395.

113. Black RE, Dykes AC, Sinclair SP, et al. Giardiasis in day-care centers: evidence of person-to-person transmission. *Pediatrics* 1977;60:486.

114. Steketee RW, Reid S, Cheng T, Stoebig JS, Harrington RG, Davis JP. Recurrent outbreaks of giardiasis in a child day care center, Wisconsin. *Am J Public Health* 1989;79:485–490.

115. Moore AC, Herwaldt BL, Craun GF, Calderon R, Highsmith A, Juranek DD. Waterborne disease outbreaks, 1991–1992. *MMWR CDC Surveill Summ* 1993;42:1–22.

116. Quick R, Paugh K, Addiss D, Kobayashi J, Baron R. Restaurant-associated outbreak of giardiasis. *J Infect Dis* 1992;166:673–676.

117. Mintz ED, Hudson-Wragg M, Mshar P, Cartter ML, Hadler JL. Foodborne giardiasis in a corporate office setting. *J Infect Dis* 1993;167:250–253.

118. Current WL, Garcia LS. Cryptosporidiosis. *Clin Microbiol Rev* 1991;4:325–358.

119. Skeels MR, Sokolow R, Hubbard CV, Andrus JK, Baisch J. *Cryptosporidium* infection in Oregon public health clinic patients 1985–1988: the value of statewide laboratory surveillance. *Am J Public Health* 1990;80:305–308.

120. Garcia-Rodriguez JA, Martin Sanchez AM, Canut Blasco A, Cedeno Montano J, Heras de Pedro MI. The incidence of cryptosporidiosis in children: a one-year prospective survey in a general hospital in Spain. *Eur J Epidemiol* 1989;5:70–73.

121. Addiss DG, Stewart JM, Finton RJ, et al. *Giardia lamblia* and *Cryptosporidium* infections in Fulton County, Georgia. *Pediatr Infect Dis J* 1991;10:907–911.

122. Hayes EB, Matte TD, O'Brien TR, et al. Large community outbreak of cryptosporidiosis due to contamination of a filtered public water supply. *N Engl J Med* 1989;320:1372–1376.

123. Richardson AJ, Frankenberg RA, Buck AC, et al. An outbreak of waterborne cryptosporidiosis in Swindon and Oxfordshire. *Epidemiol Infect* 1991;107:485–495.

124. Weinstein P, Macaitis M, Walker C, Cameron S. Cryptosporidial diarrhea in South Australia. An exploratory case–control study of risk factors for transmission. *Med J Aust* 1993;158:117–119.

125. Sorvillo FJ, Fujioka K, Nahlen B, Tormey MP, Kebabjian R, Mascola L. Swimming associated cryptosporidiosis. *Am J Public Health* 1992;82:742–744.

126. Weber R, Bryan RT, Owen RL, Wilcox CM, Gorelkin L, Visvesvara GS. Improved light-microscopical detection of *Microsporidia* spores in stool and duodenal aspirates. *N Engl J Med* 1992;326:161–166.

127. Orenstein JM, Dieterich DT, Kotler DP. Systemic dissemina-

tion by a newly recognized intestinal *Microsporidia* species in AIDS. *AIDS* 1992;6:1143–1150.

128. Long EG, White EH, Carmichael WW, et al. Morphologic and staining characteristics of a cyanobacterium-like organism associated with diarrhea. *J Infect Dis* 1991;164:199–202.

129. Shlim DR, Cohen MT, Eaton M, Rajah R, Long EG, Ungar BL. An alga-like organism associated with an outbreak of prolonged diarrhea among foreigners in Nepal. *Am J Trop Med Hyg* 1991;45:383–389.

130. Ortega YR, Sterling CR, Gilman RH, Cama VA, Diaz F. *Cyclospora* species—a new protozoan pathogen of humans. *N Engl J Med* 1993;328:1308–1312.

131. Krogstad DJ, Spencer HC, Healy GR, et al. Amebiasis: epidemiologic studies in the United States, 1971–1974. *Ann Intern Med* 1978;88:89.

132. Schmerin MJ, Gelston A, Jones TC. Amebiasis. An increasing problem among homosexuals in New York City. *JAMA* 1977;238:1386.

133. Istre GR, Kreiss K, Hopkins RS, et al. An outbreak of amebiasis spread by colonic irrigation at a chiropractic clinic. *N Engl J Med* 1982;307:339.

134. Osterholm MT, MacDonald KL, White KE, et al. An outbreak of a newly recognized chronic diarrhea syndrome associated with raw milk consumption. *JAMA* 1986;256:484.

135. Mintz ED, Parsonnet J, Osterholm MT. Chronic idiopathic diarrhea. *N Engl J Med* 1993;328:1713–1714.

136. Parsonnet J, Trock SC, Bopp CA, et al. Chronic diarrhea associated with drinking untreated water. *Ann Intern Med* 1989;110:985–991.

137. Mintz ED, Guris D, Wells JG, Tauxe RV. Darwin's revenge: an outbreak of chronic diarrhea among travelers to the Galapagos Islands. Abstract 1462. *33rd Interscience Conference on Antimicrobial Agents and Chemotherapy.* New Orleans, Oct 17–20, 1993.

138. Rollings DM. Potential for reduction in colonization of poultry by *Campylobacter* from environmental sources. In: Blankenship LC, ed. *Colonization control of human bacterial enteropathogens in poultry.* New York: Academic Press, 1991;47–56.

139. Irwin K, Ballard J, Grendon J, Kobayashi J. Results of routine restaurant inspections can predict outbreaks of foodborne illness: the Seattle–King County experience. *Am J Public Health* 1989;79:586–590.

140. Steele JH, Engel RE. Radiation processing of food. *J Am Vet Med Assoc* 1992;201:1522–1529.

141. Jackson LA, Wenger JD. Listeriosis: a foodborne disease. *Infect Med* 1993;10:61–66.

142. Griffin PG, Tauxe RV. Food counseling for patients with AIDS [Letter]. *J Infect Dis* 1988;158:668.

143. Centers for Disease Control and Prevention. *Vibrio vulnificus* infections associated with raw oyster consumption—Florida, 1981–1992. *MMWR Morb Mortal Wkly Rep* 1993;42:405–407.

144. Levine MM. Modern vaccines. Enteric vaccines. *Lancet* 1990;335:958–961.

145. Mulder RWAW, Bolder NM. Experience with competitive exclusion in the Netherlands. In: Blankenship LC, ed. *Colonization control of human bacterial enteropathogens in poultry.* New York: Academic Press, 1991;77–89.

146. Van der Waaij D, Verhoef J, eds. *New criteria for antimicrobial therapy: maintenance of digestive tract colonization resistance: Proceedings of a symposium,* Utrecht, Jan 1979. Oxford: Excerpta Medica, 1979.

147. Gustafson TL, Kobylik B, Hutcheson RH, Schaffner W. Protective effect of anticholinergic drugs and psyllium in a nosocomial outbreak of Norwalk gastroenteritis. *J Hosp Infect* 1983;4:367–374.

148. DuPont HL, Ericsson CD, Johnson PC, de la Cabada FJ. Use of bismuth subsalicylate for the prevention of traveler's diarrhea. *Rev Infect Dis* 1990;12(Suppl 1):S64–S67.

149. Tacket CO, Losonsky G, Link H, et al. Protection by milk immunoglobulin concentrate against oral challenge with enterotoxigenic *Escherichia coli*. *N Engl J Med* 1988;318:1240–1243.

Infections of the Gastrointestinal Tract,
edited by M. J. Blaser, P. D. Smith, J. I. Ravdin,
H. B. Greenberg, and R. L. Guerrant
Raven Press, Ltd., New York © 1995.

CHAPTER 4

Normal Alimentary Tract Microflora

Gary L. Simon and Sherwood L. Gorbach

The bacterial microflora of the human gastrointestinal tract is defined by the external environment, host physiology, and microbial interactions. Studies of the intestinal flora have shown that the microorganisms present within the gastrointestinal lumen are not merely passive inhabitants. The indigenous microflora play a profound role in normal human physiology as well as human disease.

COMPOSITION AND DISTRIBUTION OF THE FLORA

There are more than 400 different aerobic and anaerobic bacterial species (1–3) present in the human gastrointestinal tract. These organisms are not randomly distributed throughout the intestine, but rather reside in specific ecologic niches. The flora of the stomach and proximal small intestine differ significantly from that found in the terminal ileum and colon (Table 1).

Gastric acid and the normal propulsive peristaltic flow of the small bowel help to limit the bacterial populations of the proximal gastrointestinal tract. Most bacteria are destroyed by gastric acid. Individuals who produce normal amounts of gastric acid have few or none of the normal enteric flora present in gastric fluid (4). In those patients in whom bacteria are found the concentration is rather low, predominantly gram-positive and aerobic. The most frequently isolated species are streptococci, staphylococci, lactobacilli, and *Candida*.

A notable exception to the sparse bacterial population of the normal acid-producing stomach is *Helicobacter pylori*. These gram-negative bacteria are found in up to 25% of young asymptomatic patients and nearly 50% of those over the age of 60 (5). The presence of this organism is associated with histologic gastritis and duodenal ulcer disease (6,7) (see chapters by Riegg, Dunn, and Blaser and Taylor and Parsonnet).

G. L. Simon: Department of Medicine, The George Washington University, Washington, DC 20006.

S. L. Gorbach: Departments of Community Health and Medicine, Tufts University School of Medicine, Boston, Massachusetts 02111.

After eating, the bacterial population of the proximal bowel rises transiently to concentrations as high as 10^5/mL (8). These bacteria rapidly disappear as a result of the effects of both gastric acid and the rapid peristaltic flow present in the small bowel. In subjects with abnormal peristaltic flow, such as in a blind loop, the bacterial population of the small bowel is dramatically increased (9–11).

Within the small intestine there is a gradual transition from the sparse gram-positive microflora of the stomach to the more luxuriant gram-negative populations of the colon. It is in the distal ileum where gram-negative species begin to outnumber gram-positive organisms.

The bacterial population of the colon is both complex and large (1–3). Bacterial concentrations in excess of 10^{12}/mL are common. Anaerobic bacteria outnumber aerobic species by a factor of 10^2 to 10^4. The most frequently identified anaerobic microorganisms are Bacteroides, Bifidobacteria and Eubacteria, anaerobic gram-positive cocci, and *Clostridium* species. Aerobic isolates include species of Enterobacteriaceae, enterococci and other streptococci, staphylococci, and *Candida*.

EFFECT OF AGE ON THE FLORA

The gastrointestinal tract of newborn infants is colonized within a few days of birth (12–15). The first bacterial species to appear are facultative organisms such as *Escherichia coli* and streptococci, which are presumably acquired as a result of passage of the infant through the vaginal canal (15). In the colon, the concentration of these facultative microorganisms reaches 10^8 to 10^{10} within 2 weeks (16). One of the first metabolic effects of the microflora is to create a reducing environment by depleting the available oxygen. This leads to subsequent colonization of the colon by obligate anaerobic microorganisms.

The development of the intestinal microflora is affected by both the route of delivery and the microbiologic environment to which the infant is exposed. Among infants born by cesarean section Enterobacteriaceae other than *E. coli* are more frequently present and the colonization by anaerobes is delayed (14). For example, Long and

TABLE 1. *Principal microorganisms of the microflora at various sites*

Site	Log organisms/g
Stomach	
Total bacterial count	$0-10^8$
Aerobic bacteria	
H. pylori	$0-10^8$
Streptococci	$0-10^3$
Staphylococci	$0-10^2$
Lactobacilli	$0-10^3$
Enterobacteria	$0-10^2$
Fungi	$0-10^2$
Anaerobic bacteria	Rare
Upper small bowel	
Total bacterial count	$0-10^5$
Aerobic bacteria	
Streptococci	$0-10^4$
Staphylococci	$0-10^3$
Lactobacilli	$0-10^4$
Enterobacteria	$0-10^3$
Fungi	$0-10^2$
Anaerobic bacteria	
Bacteroides	$0-10^3$
Bifidobacteria	$0-10^4$
Streptococci	$0-10^3$
Clostridia	Rare
Eubacteria	Rare
Ileum	
Total bacterial count	10^3-10^9
Aerobic bacteria	
Streptococci	10^2-10^6
Staphylococci	10^2-10^5
Lactobacilli	10^2-10^5
Enterobacteria	10^2-10^7
Fungi	10^2-10^4
Anaerobic bacteria	
Bacteroides	10^3-10^7
Bifidobacteria	10^3-10^9
Streptococci	10^2-10^6
Clostridia	10^2-10^4
Eubacteria	Rare
Large bowel	
Total bacterial count	$10^{10}-10^{12}$
Aerobic bacteria	
Streptococci	10^5-10^{10}
Staphylococci	10^4-10^9
Lactobacilli	10^6-10^{10}
Enterobacteria	10^4-10^{10}
Fungi	10^4-10^6
Anaerobic bacteria	
Bacteroides	$10^{10}-10^{12}$
Bifidobacteria	10^8-10^{11}
Streptococci	$10^{10}-10^{12}$
Clostridia	10^6-10^{11}
Eubacteria	10^9-10^{12}

Swenson (13) found that by 4 to 6 days nearly all full-term, formula-fed, vaginally delivered infants were colonized with anaerobic bacteria and of these *Bacteroides fragilis* was found in 61%. On the other hand, anaerobes were noted in 59% and *B. fragilis* in only 9% of infants delivered by cesarean section. The flora of infants delivered by cesarean section are more closely akin to the hospital environment than to the microflora of the mother.

Colonization of the proximal and distal bowel occurs perorally. Studies in newborn infants with congenital intestinal obstruction distal to the ligament of Trietz revealed a fecal-type flora proximal to the obstruction, whereas the distal bowel remained sterile (17).

Differences in colonization are also noted when breast- and formula-fed babies are compared (16,18,19). Lactobacilli and bifidobacteria rapidly replace the initial bacterial flora in breast-fed infants. The concentration of *Bifidobacterium* exceeds that of Enterobacteriaceae by 100 to 1000-fold in the stools of normal breast-fed infants (16,18). *Clostridium* and *Bacteroides* species are also found in the feces of breast-fed infants. In contrast, Enterobacteriaceae predominate in the stools of infants who receive formula. In part, this may be due to the effect of iron that is often added to infant formulas (20). Breast milk is low in iron, which favors the development of a less complex flora in which lactobacilli and bifidobacteria predominate.

There is a shift in the predominant flora associated with weaning (21). The flora assume a more adult pattern with increasing numbers of anaerobic gram-positive cocci and *Bacteroides* species, while the concentrations of *Clostridium* and *E. coli* are reduced.

Although individual variations in the flora are common, there are relatively few changes associated with aging (22–25). There is a tendency for increased numbers of bacteria to be found in the stomach and proximal small bowel of elderly subjects, reflecting the greater incidence of hypochlorhydria and achlorhydria in this population (23). In general, studies of the fecal flora in the elderly revealed only modest changes (24). Elderly subjects tend to have a mild increase in aerobic gram-negative bacteria and fungi and a decrease in anaerobic organisms compared to younger subjects.

INFLUENCE OF HOST FACTORS ON THE MICROFLORA

The major host defense mechanisms that are active in the gastrointestinal tract are the cleansing action of normal peristaltic activity, the antibacterial activity of gastric acid, and the interactions that exist between the various microbial species that inhabit the tract (1,8,23,26–31). These properties not only help to prevent pathogenic organisms from gaining access to the host but also limit the population of bacteria within the intestinal lumen.

Gastric acid not only limits the bacterial population of the proximal gastrointestinal tract but also plays a major role in protection from colonization by exogenous pathogens. The high concentration of hydrochloric acid in the stomach is bactericidal to many microorganisms. Achlorhydria or reduced gastric acidity is associated with increased bacterial colonization of the stomach and small bowel as well as increased susceptibility to infection with enteric pathogens.

Decreased gastric acidity may occur as a result of aging, an underlying disease process, or from the use of pharmacologic agents. In such individuals there are higher concentrations of gastric and small bowel bacteria (1,23,29,30). The flora are qualitatively different as well.

Normally, gram-positive aerobic species predominate, whereas reduced acid is associated with colonization by coliforms and gram-negative anaerobic bacteria in the stomach and proximal small bowel.

Pharmacologic agents that cause hypochlorhydria such as H_2 antagonists or proton pump inhibitors may be associated with proliferation of bacteria within the stomach (32–35). In one study of 15 patients receiving cimetidine the median bacterial count increased from 0 to $10^{6.4}$ when the gastric pH was greater than 4.0 (32). Similar findings were noted with the proton pump inhibitor omeprazole (35).

The proliferation of aerobic gram-negative bacilli in the stomach of patients with decreased gastric acidity may have pathogenic significance. Driks and co-workers (36) followed patients in the intensive care units who were receiving antacids, sucralfate, or histamine antagonists. They noted an increased incidence of nosocomial gram-negative pneumonia among those patients with pharmacologically induced hypochlorhydria.

The role of gastric acid in preventing infection with enteric pathogens is well known (37). Patients who take antacids or histamine antagonists are at increased risk for developing infection. Furthermore, there is some evidence to suggest that patients with hypochlorhydria and salmonellosis tend to have more severe disease than do those with normal gastric secretory function.

Experimental studies with enteric pathogens have shown that the risk of infection increases dramatically with reduced gastric acidity (38,39). For example, in experimental *Vibrio cholerae* infection the mean infective dose is reduced from 10^{11} to 10^6 organisms following pretreatment with sodium bicarbonate (38). In another study volunteers were challenged with 10^8 viable *Campylobacter jejuni*. None of five volunteers given this inoculum with milk became ill, whereas diarrhea occurred in two of four given bacteria with sodium bicarbonate (39).

Normal peristalsis is the major host defense mechanism preventing bacteria from proliferating throughout the small intestine (26–28). A reduction in peristaltic activity, either from anatomic abnormalities, such as a blind loop or duodenal diverticula, or from physiologic disturbances such as diabetes mellitus or scleroderma, rapidly results in proliferation of bacteria within the small bowel (1,40–43). This may lead to a bacterial overgrowth syndrome with diarrhea and impaired intestinal absorption.

The ileocecal valve is an important barrier to prevention of retrograde colonization of the small bowel from the luxuriant bacterial populations of the colon. In patients with Crohn's disease or other syndromes in which the ileocecal valve is damaged or removed, there is spread of bacteria into the small bowel (1,41–44). This is most pronounced within the distal ileum. Malabsorption of both vitamin B_{12} and of bile acids via the enterohepatic circulation may occur since the ileum is the site at which these substances are normally absorbed (41,45–52).

The gastrointestinal microflora are most dense within the large bowel. Peristaltic flow is slower and, at this site, the major factors limiting the numbers of bacteria are microbial interactions. There are several mechanisms whereby the colonic flora collectively act to limit the bacterial population within the colon. These include the development of an acidic environment, production of inhibitory by-products such as short-chain fatty acids, and production of bacteriocins (1,28,53–58).

Ecologic forces are extremely important in defining the microbial flora of the gastrointestinal tract. At equilibrium each species occupies an assigned unique ecologic niche, which is remarkably stable over time. This is an extraordinarily complex ecosystem and its very complexity makes the system resistant to change. Studies in healthy individuals have shown that the flora are not easily altered (24,25). Ingested strains of *E. coli* are rapidly cleared from the intestinal tract. When the equilibrium is perturbed by alterations in host physiology, there may be transient changes in the flora. Alterations in the intestinal microflora frequently accompany systemic illness among hospitalized patients (59). Such patients are rapidly colonized by specific serogroups of *E. coli* as well as *Klebsiella*, *Pseudomonas*, and *Enterobacter*. Nevertheless, these changes are only transient and the combination of environmental pressures, host physiology, and microbial interactions allows the flora to rapidly assume a normal composition.

EFFECT OF DIET ON MICROBIAL FLORA

The effects of diet on the composition of the intestinal microflora have been studied by investigators for more than two decades with few consistent results. In general, alterations in diet are associated with very modest changes in the composition of the fecal flora.

An early study in the 1970s compared the Westernized diets of people living in Great Britain or the United States with the more vegetarian diets of individuals living in Uganda, Japan, and India (60). The most notable finding was the presence of greater concentrations of *Bacteroides* and fewer enterococci and other aerobic microorganisms in the fecal flora of Westerners.

These results have not been confirmed in subsequent studies. Finegold and co-workers (61) performed a very detailed study of diet and its effects on the microflora by examining stool samples from groups ingesting a Western diet or a Japanese diet. The Japanese diet was associated with modestly increased fecal concentrations of *Enterococcus faecalis*, *Eubacterium lentum*, and *E. contortum* and lower counts of *Bacteroides*. None of these differences were statistically significant. The same investigators examined the fecal flora of vegetarian and nonvegetarian Seventh Day Adventists in an effort to define high- and low-risk groups for developing colon cancer. Only minor changes in the fecal flora were noted in a comparison of the two groups. A similar study by Moore and Holdeman (2) failed to confirm the existence of a fecal flora that might represent a high-risk for development of colonic cancer.

Several studies have examined the flora of individuals who have been maintained on specific diets. Moore and Holdeman (2) detected no change in the fecal flora of individuals who were switched from an omnivorous to a vegetarian diet. Another study in which ten volunteers consumed a control diet, a meatless diet, and high beef diet revealed only a slight increase in anaerobes during the beef phase of the diet and a mild increase in coliforms during the meatless diet (62). Reddy and Wynder (63) examined the flora of volunteers who received a high meat diet, followed by 4 weeks of a nonmeat diet. The fecal flora during the nonmeat diet had lower concentrations of anaerobic bacteria, including decreased numbers of *Bacteroides,* bifidobacteria, and anaerobic gram-positive cocci.

Simple elemental diets are characterized by a decrease in total stool volume, but there are few changes in the actual microbial composition of the fecal flora (64–67). Analogously, adding fiber to diets may increase stool volume without significant changes in the concentrations of aerobic or anaerobic microorganisms (68).

These data suggest that low beef diets tend to be associated with higher fecal concentrations of aerobic bacteria and lower numbers of anaerobic microorganisms. However, there is little consistency between individual studies and the clinical significance of these differences is not readily apparent.

These studies were done utilizing classic bacteriologic techniques in which bacteria were identified by their morphology and ability to perform certain chemical reactions. The very complexity of the flora makes it difficult for any changes to be apparent using this approach. Studies examining the metabolic activity of the flora have shown that diet can alter the characteristics of the fecal flora (see below). These changes in bacterial metabolic activity may be of much greater significance to the host than are minor changes in the concentrations of individual constituents of the colonic bacterial population.

EFFECT OF ANTIBIOTICS ON THE MICROBIAL FLORA

Administration of antibiotics has a profound effect on the colonic and fecal flora depending on the specific antimicrobial activity of the agent involved, the route of administration, and the local luminal concentration of the drug (53,69–72). A marked reduction in the concentration of intestinal bacteria can be achieved with oral antibiotics, although this effect is usually short-lived. Nevertheless, this brief reduction in the colonic bacterial population can be beneficial. In patients undergoing colonic surgery, the administration of oral antibiotics, which decreases the number of bacteria, also reduces the incidence of postoperative wound infections (69,73,74) (see chapter by Kernodle and Kaiser). The preoperative administration of the combination of oral neomycin and erythromycin reduced the density of both aerobic and anaerobic bacteria within the colon. In a large Veterans Administration Cooperative Study there was a four- to fivefold reduction in the colonic aerobic and anaerobic bacterial populations (69). At the same time the incidence of postoperative wound infection was reduced from 35% in the placebo group to 9% receiving this regimen (73).

In another study, oral and intravenous metronidazole doses were combined with oral neomycin in patients who were undergoing elective colonic surgery (75). Both regimens were associated with a dramatic reduction in colonic bacterial concentrations. The mean reduction for *Bacteroides* species was $10^{-6.8}$ for oral metronidazole and $10^{-4.5}$ for intravenous drugs. There was rapid reconstitution of the normal flora following surgery after the antibiotics were discontinued. The concentration of *Bacteroides* species reached preantibiotic levels within 4 days for the group receiving intravenous therapy and within 6 days for those receiving oral drug.

A number of other prophylactic regimens have been examined and the results of these studies are quite similar (76–80). The administration of antibiotics that have activity against both the aerobic and anaerobic components of the colonic microflora is accompanied by a decrease in the colonic bacterial density and a decrease in the incidence of postoperative wound infections.

The administration of oral antibiotics in an effort to modify the fecal flora has been utilized in neutropenic patients in order to reduce the incidence of infectious complications (81–87). Surveillance studies have identified the gastrointestinal tract as a major reservoir from which infection arises. Intestinal colonization, especially with *Pseudomonas aeruginosa,* often precedes bacterial infection (88). The underlying hypothesis has been that through the use of selective antimicrobial regimens, intestinal colonization with potential pathogens can be prevented and the subsequent incidence of bacterial infection be reduced.

These studies have employed regimens consisting of either oral nonabsorbable antibiotics or selected systemic agents, which have activity against the aerobic gram-negative flora but leave the anaerobic bacterial populations intact (82,84,85,88). Colonization resistance, the ability of the flora to resist colonization by pathogenic species, is largely dependent on the anaerobic bacterial population. The use of selective regimens in which the antimicrobial agents employed have little activity against anaerobic bacteria helps to prevent overgrowth with pathogenic organisms (82,88–90). The results of these studies have suggested that the incidence of bacterial infections can be reduced in this population through the use of prophylactic antibiotics, although there appears to be no impact on overall mortality.

The effect of antibiotics in reducing the bacterial concentrations within the colon is not without hazards. By reducing the luminal bacterial density an ecologic vacuum is created, which may be filled with pathogenic bacteria. A dramatic example of this is pseudomembranous colitis in which toxin-producing anaerobic bacteria, *Clostridium difficile,* colonize the large bowel during treatment with antibiotics (90–92) (see chapter by Wilkins and Lyerly). Clindamycin and ampicillin are most frequently implicated, but virtually any antibiotic can cause this syndrome. The organism elaborates protein toxins, which cause ulceration and necrosis of the bowel mucosa.

EFFECT OF THE FLORA ON DEVELOPMENT OF THE IMMUNE SYSTEM

At the time of birth the immune system has not developed into a fully functional organ. Immunoglobulin (Ig) concentrations are reduced and even fall further within the first few months of life as a result of metabolism of maternal IgG. T cell numbers appear to be normal, but T cell effector activity is depressed. Studies in germ-free animals have shown that the physiologic development of the immune system is related directly to exposure to foreign antigens (53,89,93,94).

The single greatest site of immune system stimulation by antigenic challenge occurs in the gastrointestinal tract. The important role of the gut in immune function is evident by noting that nearly 25% of the gut mass is represented by lymphoid tissues (95). Histologic studies of the intestinal mucosa from germ-free and normal animals demonstrate that the presence of the microflora induces a state of "physiologic inflammation" (1,96,97). In the germ-free animal the intestinal wall is considerably thinner than normal (98). There is decreased cellularity within the lamina propria; lymphocytes and macrophages are sparse and plasma cells are noticeably absent. Peyer's patches are smaller and have fewer germinal centers.

Introduction of an intestinal microbial flora into germ-free animals induces an immune response involving T lymphocytes, B lymphocytes, plasma cells, macrophages, eosinophils, and mast cells (95,99). This population of cells, which provide immunologic competence to the host, is evident in the lamina propria of animals that have an intact microflora. Indeed, in situations where there is an increase in bacterial populations, such as in bacterial overgrowth syndromes or *H. pylori* infection, there is a further increase in the inflammatory response with a more pronounced cellular infiltrate demonstrated within the interstitium (1,41,42).

In the newborn infant, exposure of gut mucosa to bacterial antigens results in rapid production of large concentrations of secretory IgA (93). The critical role of IgA in protecting the host from infections originating at the mucosal surface is indicated by the fact that cells that synthesize IgA constitute more than 50% of the human lymphoid system and that more IgA is produced than any other immunoglobulin in the body. Immunofluorescent staining of plasma cells within the lamina propria reveals that 70% to 90% are IgA-producing cells (95).

IgM-producing cells are also relatively common in the lamina propria and there is significant synthesis of IgM antibodies as a result of gut stimulation within the first weeks of life (93). IgG-producing cells are less frequently encountered in gut-associated lymphoid tissue and synthesis of IgG antibodies is somewhat delayed in the neonate until the age of 6 months.

The role of the cellular immune system in the development of immunity in the gastrointestinal tract has not been well characterized. Population analyses indicate that the T lymphocyte population in the lamina propria is primarily CD4 helper/inducer cells (95). These cells play a major role in the development of the initial immunologic response to a new antigen, which is consistent with the concept that the gut represents a site of primary exposure of the host to many new antigens. Cytotoxic/suppressor (CD8) cells are less frequently seen.

It is clear that enteric encounters with microbial antigens result in stimulation of both a local intestinal immune response and a systemic immune response. The development of the immune system is highly dependent on this exposure. The normal intestinal flora play a major role in providing the antigenic stimulus for this process.

EFFECT OF THE FLORA ON ENTERIC PATHOGENS

The presence of an intact gastrointestinal microflora is an important factor in protecting the host from infection with exogenous pathogens (28,53,89). The effects of the normal intestinal bacterial population include depletion of essential nutrients, production of products that inhibit bacterial growth, suppression of bacterial adherence, and degradation of bacterial toxins (53).

It has been difficult to clearly define the effect of the normal flora on inhibiting *in vivo* growth of pathogens by limiting the availability of nutrients. Freter (100) demonstrated that in a highly reduced environment coliforms were able to inhibit the growth of *Shigella flexneri* in static and continuous flow cultures by successfully competing for carbon sources. The effect could be reversed by either adding glucose to the medium or increasing the oxidation–reduction potential through aeration.

Bacterial metabolism results in the production of various by-products, which may contribute to establishing an environment that is not conducive to growth of pathogens. These metabolic by-products include hydrogen ions, short-chain fatty acids, and alcohols (28).

Lactobacillus, Bifidobacterium, and streptococci produce lactic acid, which reduces the intracolonic pH and inhibits the growth of various facultative and anaerobic bacteria (101,102). An acidic environment is created by lactobacilli in the small intestine of newborn piglets, which inhibits the production of *E. coli* and *V. cholerae* enterotoxins (103,104). The low pH is also a factor in the inhibitory effects of short-chain fatty acids. These compounds, which are produced by anaerobic bacteria, can inhibit the growth of *S. flexneri* and *Salmonella typhimurium* providing that the environment is acidic (28,105–109).

Bacteriocins, high molecular weight protein antibiotics produced by streptococci (108–110) and gram-negative bacilli (111,112), suppress the growth of pathogens *in vitro*. The *in vivo* activity of bacteriocins is less well-defined. Kelstrup and Gibbons (113) suggested that these substances were inactivated within the intestinal lumen by bacterial proteolytic enzymes.

Mucosal attachment or adherence is one of the first steps in the pathogenesis of enteric infection. Adherence of pathogenic organisms to mucosal epithelial cells prevents the bacteria from being washed through the gastrointestinal tract by normal peristalsis. Recent studies have shown that the presence of an endogenous microflora competitively inhibits the adherence of pathogenic organisms to the epithelial surface (53,114). Adherence of *Candida albicans* to oral mouse epithelial cells of germ-free mice is increased twofold over that of conventional animals (115).

The mechanisms whereby the endogenous microflora

inhibit adherence by enteric pathogens are not well defined. However, at least in part, steric considerations appear to be a factor in this process; that is, the physical presence of high concentrations of endogenous bacteria prevents pathogens from gaining access to epithelial cell binding sites (53). This is suggested by studies in which the administration of antibiotics results in increased numbers of pathogenic bacteria adhering to mucosal cells. Pongpech and co-workers (116) found a 100-fold decrease in endogenous fusiform organisms in the mucous layer of the ceca of mice following streptomycin administration. Challenge of these mice with *Shigella sonnei* or enterotoxigenic *E. coli* led to increased numbers of these pathogenic bacteria compared to untreated animals.

METABOLIC ACTIVITY OF THE MICROFLORA

There is an enormous diversity of metabolic activity within the human gastrointestinal tract. Host enzymes from gastric mucosa, pancreas, and the brush border of intestinal cells break down complex molecules in order to facilitate absorption. At the same time, the luminal inhabitants, components of the intestinal microflora, produce enzymes that utilize ingested nutrients as well as products of human metabolism as substrate. The bacterially mediated transformation of compounds within the intestinal lumen is an important component of the normal and pathologic human condition.

There are three major types of chemical reaction that are mediated by the intestinal microflora (Table 2) (117–119). These include hydrolytic reactions, dehydroxylation reactions, and chemical reductions. Of these, the hydrolytic reactions are among the most well known and one of the best examples is hydrolysis of glycosidic bonds. A glycoside is a compound in which a carbohydrate compound is linked to a noncarbohydrate moiety, an aglycone. Common examples of glycosides include bilirubin glucuronide, digoxin, estriol-3-glucuronide, and conjugated bile acids. Within the lumen these compounds undergo bacterially mediated hydrolysis of the glycosidic linkage, leading to intraluminal release of the aglycone moiety.

One effect of intraluminal bacterially mediated hydrolysis of glycosidic bonds is the enterohepatic circulation of a variety of endogenous and exogenous compounds. Some examples of substances that undergo an enterohepatic circulation include endogenous compounds such as bilirubin, bile acids, estrogens, vitamin D, and cholesterol, as well as drugs such as digoxin, rifampin, morphine, and colchicine (118). Hepatic conjugation of these compounds with glucuronic acid, sulfate, glycine, taurine, or glutathione is followed by secretion into the bile. In the intestine, hydrolysis by β-glucuronidase, sulfatase, or other hydrolytic enzymes results in liberation of the unconjugated moiety (aglycone), which can be reabsorbed by the intestine. Loss of the hydrolytic enzymes results in less resorption of the aglycone and increased fecal excretion, which in turn leads to a reduced serum concentration of that specific compound.

Estrogen undergoes hepatic conjugation to form estrogen-3-sulfate-16-glucuronide, which is deconjugated within the lumen of the bowel by bacterial β-glucuronidase and sulfatase (120). The deconjugated estrogen is then reabsorbed by the intestinal cells and reconjugated to either estriol-16-glucuronide or estriol-3-glucuronide (121). The latter compound is resistant to further conjugation and thus does not undergo an enterohepatic circulation. The presence of estriol-3-glucuronide in the urine is an indicator of estrogen reabsorption in the lower gastrointestinal tract.

Exogenous factors can affect bacterial concentrations within the lumen and/or their metabolic activity. A number of investigators have examined the role of diet on the intestinal flora and its associated metabolic activity. As noted earlier, diet produces relatively little change in the actual composition of the flora. On the other hand, dietary alterations have a significant impact on the metabolic activity of the luminal bacteria. Dyer and co-workers (122) studied the effects of diet by examining the concentration of estrogen in the feces of vegetarian and omnivore American women. Vegetarian women excreted higher concentrations of estrogen in their feces than did omnivore women, indicating that there was less deconjugative activity in the bowel of vegetarian women.

Antibiotics also play a role in the enterohepatic circulation of estrogens. Oral antibiotics, which reduce the intestinal flora, also reduce the deconjugation reaction so that greater amounts of conjugated compounds are excreted in feces. Following the oral administration of ampicillin or neomycin, there is a marked reduction in urinary estrogen and a corresponding 60-fold increase in fecal excretion of conjugated estrogens and a threefold increase in unconjugated moieties (123–126). Ninety percent of the observed reduction in urinary estrogen is due to a de-

TABLE 2. *Metabolic reactions of microflora*

Reaction	Representative substrate
Hydrolysis	
Glucuronides	Bilirubin glucuronide
Glycosides	Cycasin
Sulfamates	Cyclamate
Amides	Methotrexate
Esters	Acetyldigoxin
Dehydroxylation	
C-hydroxyl groups	Bile acids
N-hydroxyl groups	*N*-hydroxyfluorenylacetamide
Decarboxylation	Amino acids
Deamination	Amino acids
Dehydrogenase	Cholesterol
Dehalogenation	DDT
Reduction	
Nitro groups	*p*-Nitrobenzoic acids
Double bonds	Unsaturated fatty acids
Azo groups	Food dyes
Aldehydes	Benzaldehydes
Alcohols	Benzyl alcohol
N-oxides	4-Nitroquinolone-1-oxide
Acetylation	Histamine
Nitrosamine formation	Demethylnitrosamine

crease in the urinary excretion of the 3-glucuronide. This confirms the gastrointestinal origin of this effect, since the synthesis of the 3-glucuronide moiety occurs only in the intestinal mucosal cells. These findings have important clinical implications. Administration of rifampin or ampicillin to women taking estrogens for birth control may result in lower serum concentrations of steroids, thereby reducing the effect of the birth control pill, resulting in "break-through" pregnancy (127–129).

Studies of individual bacterial species have shown that the enzymatic activity differs among species. The major bacterial glycosidase within the bowel lumen is β-glucuronidase. *Escherichia coli* and clostridia have the highest level of activity, whereas low levels of activity are found in bifidobacteria and lactobacilli (130). Conversely, *E. coli* had the lowest β-glucosidase activity whereas *E. faecalis* and *Bacteroides* species had the greatest activity of this enzyme.

Another major class of bacterially mediated enzymic activity is dehydroxylation. Dehydroxylation reactions include the removal of hydroxy groups from bile acids, decarboxylation and deamination of amino acids, and dehydrogenation of cholesterol and bile acids. Dehydroxylation of bile acids by bacterial 7α-steroid dehydrogenase is responsible for converting cholic and chenodeoxycholic acids into deoxycholic and lithocholic acids, respectively. Deoxycholic acid may be reabsorbed and then reexcreted in the bile; lithocholic acid is insoluble and is excreted in feces. Another bacterially mediated reaction of bile salts, nuclear dehydrogenation, results in chemical desaturation of steroid ring structure. These reactions may play a role in the etiology of colon cancer (131–133) (See below).

Both hydrolytic and reducing enzymes may be involved in the metabolism of digoxin. The pharmacologic activity of digoxin is dependent on bacterially mediated hydrolytic removal of a trisaccharide, which releases digoxigenin (134). However, in some individuals, there is a further reduction in the double bond of the lactone ring, which results in the formation of a pharmacologically inactive substance, dihydrodigoxigenin. This reaction is mediated by *Eubacterium lentum* (135).

Differences in diet appear to play a role in the frequency of digoxin inactivation (134). The reduction of digoxin occurs in 36% of New York City residents; 14% of a group of New Yorkers who were tested were found to excrete large amounts of digoxin metabolites. In contrast, this reaction occurs in only 13.7% of Indians living in southern India and only 1% excrete large amounts of metabolites.

Bacterial deamination is another important metabolic activity that is mediated by the bacterial flora. The breakdown of urea into carbon dioxide and ammonia is catalyzed by bacterial urease. Approximately 40% of the urea synthesized by the liver is broken down by a variety of bacteria including aerobic and anaerobic species (136).

Other reactions in which bacterial enzymes act on amines include esterification of primary amino groups, dealkylation of secondary and tertiary amines, and adding nitroso groups to secondary amines (117–119). The last reaction, N-nitrosation, is mediated by *E. faecalis,* clostridia, *Bacteroides,* and bifidobacteria (117).

SMALL BOWEL BACTERIAL OVERGROWTH

Anatomic and physiologic derangements of the gastrointestinal tract can lead to proliferation of bacteria in the proximal portion of the small intestine. Such "bacterial overgrowth" may be accompanied by a variety of metabolic disturbances including steatorrhea, vitamin deficiency, and fat, protein, and carbohydrate malabsorption.

Bacterial overgrowth in the small bowel may occur when there is reduced or absent gastric acid production. As noted earlier, gastric acid helps to limit the bacterial population of the proximal small bowel. Hypochlorhydria, which may result from atrophic gastritis, a surgical procedure, or drug therapy, is often accompanied by a substantial increase in the small bowel bacterial flora (1,23,31,34,137–139).

Disordered or ineffective peristalsis is a major etiologic factor in the development of small bowel bacterial overgrowth. Anatomic disorders such as small bowel diverticula, surgically created blind loops, or strictures with partial small bowel obstruction may lead to proliferation of bacteria within the small intestine (1,39,51,139). There have been several reports of bacterial overgrowth associated with a single duodenal diverticulum (1,139,140). In one patient, colonization was limited to the diverticulum and the small bowel just distal to it (43).

Physiologic derangements in which there is abnormal peristalsis may also be associated with small bowel bacterial overgrowth. Such disorders include diabetes mellitus, scleroderma, and intestinal pseudo-obstruction as well as a few systemic disorders such as cirrhosis, chronic malnutrition, and abdominal x-irradiation (1,141–145). Proliferation of enteric bacteria has also been seen in patients who have undergone extensive small bowel resection. Proliferation of bacteria was noted in both the remaining bowel segment and the bypassed loop of patients who underwent jejunoileal bypass for morbid obesity (146). Diarrhea with malabsorption and dense enteric bacterial growth has been seen in elderly patients who have no evidence of an underlying systemic illness or anatomic abnormality (147,148).

The bacterial flora present in the small bowel of patients with bacterial overgrowth syndrome are complex. Detailed microbiologic analysis has revealed more than 20 different species with bacterial counts ranging from 10^7 to 10^9 CFU/mL (1,49,149,150). Both aerobic and anaerobic species can be isolated, but it appears that the anaerobic flora are most frequently associated with physiologic disturbances (1,139,149,150). For example, aerobic coliforms and enterococci are often found in the small bowel of patients with acute diarrhea, cirrhosis, protein–calorie malnutrition, and hypochlorhydria without evidence of metabolic derangement (1,23,30,143,151). On the other hand, intestinal stasis with malabsorption is most often accompanied by colonization with anaerobic microorganisms.

The pathophysiologic role of the anaerobic microflora in intestinal overgrowth syndromes was illustrated in a patient with subtotal gastrectomy and a Billroth II anastomosis who had significant bacterial overgrowth, diarrhea, steatorrhea, and vitamin B_{12} malabsorption (149). Quantitative bacteriologic analysis of gastrojejunostomy fluid revealed bacterial counts of 10^{10} CFU/mL, of which 91% were *Bacteroides* and 8% coliform species. Treatment with oral neomycin reduced the coliform concentration but did not alter the patient's symptoms, whereas lincomycin, an antibiotic active against anaerobic bacteria but ineffective against coliforms, normalized both fat and vitamin B_{12} absorption.

Malabsorption of fat and fat-soluble vitamins accompanied by steatorrhea are the most frequently recognized clinical manifestations of small bowel bacterial overgrowth (1,41,45,48–52,152). The pathophysiologic mechanism of lipid malabsorption involves the deconjugation of bile salts within the small bowel lumen by the enteric bacteria. Under normal conditions, conjugated bile salts solubilize fatty acids through the formation of mixed micelles. Bacterially mediated hydrolysis within the small bowel lumen reduces the concentration of conjugated bile acids, which results in impaired micelle formation and fat malabsorption. This hydrolytic reaction is mediated primarily by anaerobic bacteria such as *Bacteroides, Bifidobacterium, Veillonella,* and *Clostridium* (153–159).

Small bowel bacterial overgrowth also is frequently associated with vitamin B_{12} deficiency and megaloblastic anemia (41,47,48,152). The malabsorption of vitamin B_{12} is due to binding of the vitamin to the bacteria present in the small bowel, thereby preventing absorption in the distal ileum. Virtually all the vitamin B_{12} ingested by patients with small bowel bacterial overgrowth is found in feces firmly bound to bacterial cell wall components (152,156).

The role of anaerobic bacteria in vitamin B_{12} malabsorption is suggested by studies performed in rats with surgically created blind loops. In these animals, administration of metronidazole, an antibiotic effective against anaerobic bacteria, corrected the malabsorption (157). Significant binding of the intrinsic factor–vitamin B_{12} complex by *Bacteroides* has been demonstrated *in vitro* (50,158). The irony of vitamin B_{12} deficiency in patients with small bowel bacterial overgrowth is that there is no vitamin available for absorption despite the fact that such patients actually have high intraluminal levels as a result of nonabsorbed dietary sources as well as from direct bacterial synthesis of the vitamin *in vivo*.

Amino acid and carbohydrate absorption also is impaired in patients with small bowel bacterial overgrowth. Fecal nitrogen content is increased, serum proteins are low, and, on occasion, a clinical picture of protein–calorie malnutrition is present (1,41,50,140). There also is reduced absorption of D-xylose as a result of intraluminal bacterial metabolism of this sugar (41,159,160). Elevated levels of fatty acids have been demonstrated in jejunal aspirates from patients with bacterial overgrowth, which indicates bacterial fermentation of carbohydrates within the small bowel (161,162).

TROPICAL SPRUE

Tropical sprue is a disorder of uncertain etiology with the clinical manifestations of chronic diarrhea, weight loss, and malabsorption of carbohydrates, fats, and vitamin B_{12}, which is present in a specific geographic distribution, predominantly the Caribbean area and the Indian subcontinent (163,164). The onset of illness is often traced to an episode of acute gastroenteritis, but the relationship between the acute episode and the development of the subsequent chronic illness is enigmatic (165–167). Although the pathogenesis of illness is not well defined, the pathophysiology appears to be related to an abnormal small intestinal microflora since treatment with antibiotics that are effective against the microbial species present within the small bowel is often curative (163,168).

Microbiologic studies of the proximal small intestine of patients with tropical sprue indicate that there is significant colonization with coliform bacteria. Studies of luminal fluid obtained from tropical sprue patients in Calcutta and Puerto Rico and from expatriates have confirmed that there are higher concentrations of aerobic gram-negative bacilli when compared with matched control populations who did not suffer from malabsorption (169–175). Aerobic enteric bacteria may be found in the small bowel of individuals who are suffering from malnutrition without evidence of tropical sprue, but the concentration of bacteria in this population is intermediate between normal controls and tropical sprue subjects (171,172).

Examination of both luminal fluid and mucosal biopsies from patients with tropical sprue indicates that the bacteria that are present are not merely transient colonizers but are directly associated with the surface of the intestinal epithelial cells. In one study of 16 Caucasians who acquired tropical sprue while traveling in endemic areas, there was increased enterobacterial concentrations adherent to mucosal tissues in 11 subjects (171). In 9 of the 11, the concentrations of mucosal bacteria actually exceeded the luminal concentrations. Those patients who had the most severe mucosal abnormalities tended to have higher bacterial counts.

These findings also are evident in the fecal flora of individuals with tropical sprue. In these patients, the concentration of aerobic microorganisms exceeds that of anaerobes (172). This is in sharp contrast to the findings in normal individuals where anaerobic bacteria outnumber aerobes by 1000-fold.

The pathophysiologic mechanisms of disease may be related to the production of enterotoxins (172–176). In a group of Puerto Rican patients with tropical sprue, jejunal aspirates revealed *Klebsiella pneumoniae, Enterobacter cloacae,* and *E. coli* capable of producing enterotoxin as measured by the rabbit ileal loop assay (174). This enterotoxin did not correlate with either the heat-labile or the heat-stable toxins that have previously been associated with enterotoxigenic *E. coli* (175). This enterotoxin induced fluid and electrolyte secretion in the small bowel of rodents, suggesting that some of the clinical manifestations of disease are related to persistent colonization with these enterotoxigenic organisms (167).

The bacterial colonization of the small bowel that is present in patients with tropical sprue is not merely an epiphenomenon (169,170,173). The response to antimicrobial agents, such as tetracycline, is dramatic with rapid improvement in clinical and physiologic parameters.

There is increased appetite, improved absorption of fat and vitamin B_{12}, and a decline in the bacterial population of the small bowel. Patients with tropical sprue have a net secretion of fluid and electrolytes into the small bowel lumen, which is rapidly reversed after the initiation of tetracycline therapy (177).

Tropical sprue is not analogous to the blind loop syndrome. In patients with small bowel bacterial overgrowth, the predominant bacterial organisms are anaerobic, unlike the predominantly aerobic flora of the tropical sprue subject. Not only are there bacteriologic differences, but examination of the mucosa from patients with tropical sprue reveals striking changes. The architecture of the small bowel of patients with tropical sprue includes marked blunting of the villi and inflammatory infiltration of the lamina propria (163,178,179). These changes are either absent or very mild in patients with small bowel bacterial overgrowth. Furthermore, in contrast to small bowel bacterial overgrowth in which bowel transit time is decreased, patients with tropical sprue have decreased motility and increased bowel transit time (180). This delay in small bowel transit time has been attributed to increased levels of enteroglucan as a result of mucosal cell injury. A consequence of delayed transit is increased bacterial stasis and further exposure of mucosal cells to bacteria and bacterial products.

The isolation of enterotoxigenic bacteria from tropical sprue patients suggests that these organisms play an important role in this disorder. This is reinforced by the salutary response seen with the administration of antibiotics. However, mucosal changes that are evident in tropical sprue cannot be reproduced in experimental germ-free animals that are challenged with the toxigenic organisms isolated from tropical sprue patients (171). This is the basic conundrum of tropical sprue and our understanding of the pathogenesis of this disorder is incomplete.

INTESTINAL FLORA AND CANCER

The role of the intestinal microflora in the pathogenesis of colon cancers has intrigued investigators for more than two decades. The incidence of colon cancer is higher among North Americans and Western Europeans than among Africans, Asians, and South Americans (181–185). Epidemiologic studies have suggested that the observed differences in incidence can be linked to the characteristic "Western" diet, which is high in beef fat and protein and low in dietary fiber. A positive correlation has been established between per capita consumption of beef, total fat, animal fat, and animal protein and the reported incidence of colon cancer (181,184).

The relationship between diet and colon cancer is even more apparent when examining migrant populations. Japanese living in Japan have a very low incidence of colon cancer, whereas among Japanese living in California the rate is increasing. The incidence of colon cancer among American-born Japanese approaches that of native Caucasian Americans (186). On the other hand, stomach cancer, which is common among Japanese living in Japan, is decreasing among Japanese living in California.

These findings were echoed by studies of Japanese migrants living in Hawaii. Those individuals who adopted a Western-style diet had a much higher incidence of colon cancer than did subjects who maintained a more traditional Japanese diet (187). In contrast to these findings, there was a lower than suspected incidence of colon cancer among Mormons living in Utah despite a rate of beef consumption that was very similar to the national average (188). Similarly, the incidence of colon cancer was not decreased among members of religious orders in England who abstained from meat (189).

Early studies attempted to correlate the epidemiologic findings and differences in diet with a "high-risk" flora. As noted earlier, the results of these studies failed to identify any consistent differences in the composition of the intestinal microflora of high-risk and low-risk populations. Classic taxonomic analysis of fecal samples from high- and low-risk populations does not appear to be worthwhile in identifying the link between the Western diet and colon cancer (2,61,133,190,191).

A more useful approach may be to examine the impact of diet on bacterial enzyme metabolism. Colon cancer can be induced in experimental animal models by metabolizing ingested procarcinogens into carcinogenic moieties (119,192). The site of this metabolic transformation is the colon and it is the bacterial enzymes that are present that mediate this mutagenic reaction (193,194). Many of these enzymes were described earlier and include β-glucosidase, β-glucuronidase, nitroreductase, azoreductase, 7α-dehydroxylase, and cholesterol dehydrogenase. These are inducible enzymes so that continued exposure of bacteria to an appropriate substrate leads to increased enzyme concentrations. If the substrate is a procarcinogen, there will be increased production of carcinogens.

Alteration of bacterial enzymes by diet has been demonstrated by several investigators. Rats fed a high beef diet developed significant increases in the activity of the fecal bacterial enzymes β-glucuronidase, azoreductase, and nitroreductase (192,195). A similar increase was noted in rats fed a grain diet supplemented only with 30% beef fat (196). A similar dietary induction of fecal bacterial enzymes in humans has also been demonstrated. β-Glucuronidase activity was monitored in a study in which volunteers were fed high meat diets followed by nonmeat diets (197). Higher fecal enzyme activity was noted in the subjects on a high meat diet.

The carcinogenic potential of these bacterial enzymes is illustrated by studies of cycasin-induced cancer in rats. Cycasin or methylazoxymethanol-β-D-glucoside is a naturally occurring glucoside that is found in the nut of tropical ferns. The aglycone of cycasin, methylazoxymethanol, is a carcinogen (198). When cycasin was fed to normal rats they subsequently developed hepatomas, renal sarcomas, squamous cell carcinomas of the ear duct, and, most frequently, intestinal adenocarcinoma (199). However, cycasin-induced cancer required intestinal bacteria since feeding cycasin to germ-free rats did not result in any tumor production (200).

Altering the route of administration and the age of the animal modified the results (198,200). Cycasin was inactive when given parenterally to adult conventional animals. On the other hand, tumors developed following subcutaneous or intraperitoneal administration in newborn conventional and newborn germ-free rats. Finally, administration of the aglycone, methylazoxymethanol, produced tumors in both germ-free and conventional animals regardless of the age of the animal or the route of administration (201).

The explanation for these findings is that the parent compound, cycasin, has no intrinsic carcinogenic activity. It must first be hydrolyzed to methylazoxymethanol, which is the active mutagen. This hydrolytic reaction is catalyzed by β-glucosidase. Within the intestine this reaction is mediated by bacterial β-glucosidase, which is absent in germ-free animals. The results of the experiments employing parenteral cycasin are due to high levels of tissue β-glucosidase, which is present in newborn, but not adult, animals.

Bacterial β-glucuronidase also plays an important role in colon carcinogenesis. This was noted by Weisburger et al. (202), who administered N-hydroxyfluorenylacetamide, a carcinogen, to germ-free and conventional rats. Germ-free rats excreted mostly the glucuronide conjugate in their feces, whereas the cecal and fecal metabolites were primarily free, unconjugated compounds in conventional animals.

The very low oxidation–reduction potential of the human colon strongly favors chemical reductions. The enzymes nitroreductase and azoreductase reduce nitro and azo compounds to aromatic amines, which are carcinogenic. Furthermore, this reaction involves highly reactive intermediate free radicals, which are also mutagenic (203). These enzymes are primarily associated with colonic bacteria.

Azo dyes are widely used in textiles, printing, and food-dye industries. Degradation of azo dyes within the colon results in liberation of toxic moieties, which may contribute to the high incidence of colon cancer in industrialized nations (204,205).

Aromatic nitro compounds are common chemical pollutants. These compounds are converted to aromatic amines by the enzyme nitroreductase. Intermediate compounds in this chemical reduction include highly reactive nitroso and N-hydroxy moieties (203). The role of bacterial nitroreductase in this conversion reaction was demonstrated by Wheeler and co-workers (206), who studied p-nitrobenzoic acid. When conventional animals were fed p-nitrobenzoic acid they rapidly converted it to p-aminobenzoic acid. In contrast, little reduction was noted when the compound was given to germ-free animals.

The effect of diet on the development of experimental colon cancer is illustrated in studies of dimethylhydrazine (DMH) and 3,2-dimethyl-4-aminophenyl (DMAB) (207–209). Both of these compounds are procarcinogens and require exposure to bacterial enzymes. Rats maintained on high beef diets (DMH) or high fat diets (DMAB) developed colon tumors more readily than did animals fed a low-fat or grain diet (210,211).

The impact of variations in diet on human fecal bacterial enzyme activity is similar to that noted in rats. Omnivores who ate a mixed Western diet had considerably higher levels of fecal β-glucuronidase, nitroreductase, and 7α-dehydroxylase than did lactovegetarians or strict vegetarians (212). Attempts to modify the fecal enzyme activity of the omnivore group by elimination of red meat and fiber supplementation revealed no significant changes except for a mild drop in 7α-dehydroxylase activity.

The enzymatic activity of the bacterial microflora can be modified by the administration of oral antibiotics. The incidence of DMH-induced tumors was strikingly reduced in rats given tetracycline or erythromycin (213). There was a corresponding reduction in fecal β-glucuronidase activity.

There is a structural similarity between bile acids and the carcinogenic polycyclic aromatic hydrocarbons. This has generated considerable interest in these compounds as potential carcinogens or cocarcinogens (60,63,131, 132,190,194,214,215). Epidemiologic studies have revealed that there is a correlation between the Western-style high beef diet and high fecal concentrations of secondary bile acids (60,63). Americans who consume a Western diet had higher levels of fecal bile acids, including deoxycholic acid and lithocholic acid, but not cholic acid, when compared with American vegetarians, Seventh Day Adventists, and Japanese or Chinese immigrants (63). In contrast, colon cancer patients living in Glasgow had decreased total fecal bile acids compared to control subjects (216).

The bacterial enzyme 7α-dehydroxylase converts primary bile acids to secondary bile acids. This enzyme is inducible and is affected by diet (193). The fecal microflora of North Americans or Western Europeans contain more bacterial strains capable of 7α-dehydroxylation than did those from Ugandans or Indians (60).

A similar enzyme, cholesterol dehydrogenase, is also higher in individuals who consume a Western diet. Such individuals have higher fecal concentrations of cholesterol degradation products, coprostanol and coprostanone. Mastromarino and co-workers (131) studied patients with colon cancer and found elevated fecal levels of both 7α-dehydroxylase and cholesterol dehydrogenase when compared with normal controls.

Bacteria may also play a protective role in this process by inactivating potential carcinogens. Escherichia coli, Bacteroides, Bifidobacterium, and Lactobacillus can degrade dimethylnitrosamine and diphenylnitrosamine to nitrite and the corresponding amine (217). In rats, cecal bacterial enzymes can dehydroxylate N-hydroxylacetamide, which reverses the process whereby amines are activated to proximal carcinogens (218).

The role of diet and bacterial enzymes in the pathogenesis of colon cancer is not fully elucidated. Nevertheless, the findings outlined above suggest that it is unlikely that these organisms are passive bystanders, but rather are contributors to the process through their metabolic activities.

PROBIOTIC EFFECTS OF THE MICROFLORA

The concept that some bacteria play a beneficial role in human health dates back to Metchnikoff, who suggested that the lactobacillus in yogurt was responsible for the longevity of the Balkan peasants. The beneficial effects of such bacteria have been termed the probiotic effect. Probiotic products include freeze-dried bacteria in tablets or capsules and fermented dairy products such as yogurts, fermented milks, and sweet acidophilus milks.

In order for a bacteria or a product to be considered as a probiotic it is necessary that there be clinically proven efficacy. Claims of benefit need to be supported by well-designed, randomized, double-blinded clinical trials. Few such studies exist and singular anecdotal claims of efficacy must be viewed with caution until further data are available.

Prerequisites for a bacterial species to exercise probiotic effects in humans are the capacity to adhere to human intestinal mucosal cells and the ability to grow in the intestinal lumen. Several species of lactobacilli as well as some strains of *Bifidobacterium* and *Saccharomyces* meet these criteria (218,220).

The claims for potential benefits of probiotics include a variety of disorders ranging from treatment of constipation to hepatic encephalopathy to hypercholesterolemia (221–225). The most notable effects are related to improved nutrition, relief of lactose intolerance, prevention of carcinogenesis, and treatment of intestinal infections (Table 3) (211,226–243).

There are several lines of evidence to suggest that yogurt provides a more nutritional benefit than does unfermented dairy products. Yogurt has a higher concentration of specific vitamins and minerals (244–246). In addition, protein and carbohydrate present in yogurt are found to be in a more digestible form (226,229). Finally, when fed to animals, cultured dairy products produce increased growth and feed efficiency compared to uncultured dairy products (226–228).

Lactase deficiency is a not uncommon disorder in people who consume lactose and is characterized by abdominal cramps and diarrhea. The clinical symptoms are caused by lack of the intestinal mucosal enzyme, β-galactosidase (lactase), which hydrolyses lactose to glucose and galactose. Lactobacilli produce lactase during fermentation and up to 50% of the lactose present in yogurt will be utilized by this enzyme during fermentation.

The presence of bacterial lactase in the intestines of patients consuming yogurt was evidenced by studies in which serum glucose was monitored in control subjects

and lactose-intolerant individuals given 500 mL of milk or yogurt (229). The lactose intolerant individuals had a much lower rise in serum glucose when given milk, indicating lactose utilization was impaired. On the other hand, when yogurt was given to lactose-intolerant subjects, the rate of increase in serum glucose was similar to that of control subjects given milk. In this and other studies, the consumption of yogurt by lactose-intolerant individuals is associated with improved glucose absorption and reduced diarrhea, flatulence, and abdominal distension when compared with a similar challenge with unfermented milk.

The potential beneficial role of fermented dairy products in the prevention of colon carcinogenesis has been shown in animal models in which the addition of these products reduces the incidence of experimentally induced colon tumors in rodents. Oral supplementation of an animal or human diet with *Lactobacillus acidophilus* results in a decline in fecal concentrations of the bacterial enzymes β-glucuronidase, azoreductase, and nitroreductase (210,212). As noted earlier, these enzymes are capable of catalyzing procarcinogens to carcinogenic moieties.

The carcinogen DMH is activated in the large intestine by β-glucuronidase. The addition of *L. acidophilus* to the diet of rats subsequently challenged with DMH reduced the incidence of colon tumors from 77% in control animals to 40% (211). This effect was seen after 20 weeks, but by 33 weeks there was little difference between the two groups, indicating that the impact of *L. acidophilus* was to delay tumor formation.

There have been several other studies that have shown that the addition of yogurt or milk and colostrum fermented with *L. acidophilus* resulted in a reduction in the incidence of experimentally induced tumors in animals (245,247–249). These studies suggest that under certain conditions these products may provide an inhibitory effect on tumor growth.

Fermented dairy products have been used in the treatment of intestinal infections with apparently beneficial results (235,238). *Lactobacillus acidophilus* exerts an antagonistic effect on the growth of *Salmonella typhimurium in vitro* (248). In one study, feeding yogurt to rats challenged with *Salmonella* resulted in less morbidity and improved weight gain compared with controls (236).

Studies in children with diarrhea have demonstrated a salutary effect with acidophilus milk. Among children with diarrhea due to salmonella or shigella, the administration of acidophilus milk led to resolution of symptoms in 43% of those with salmonella and 67% of those with shigella (238). No control group was included in this study.

In a controlled trial Isolauri and co-workers (250) studied three groups of infants with acute diarrhea. Group 1 received *Lactobacillus* GG fermented milk product, group 2 was given an equivalent number of organisms as a freeze-dried product, and group 3 received pasteurized yogurt containing no viable lactobacilli. The mean duration of diarrhea after beginning therapy with these additives was 1.4, 1.4, and 2.4 days, respectively ($P < 0.001$).

The beneficial effects of *L. caseii* GG were further demonstrated in another study in which it was shown that the intestinal immune response to rotavirus was augmented in

TABLE 3. *Beneficial (probiotic) effects of fermented dairy products*

Condition	References
Improved nutrition	223–225,243
Lactose intolerance	226–228
Chronic constipation	218
Enteric infections	232,233,235,237
Infantile diarrhea	236,239,240,247
Traveler's diarrhea	248–250
Antibiotic-associated diarrhea	217
Hypercholesterolemia	221,222
Hepatic encephalopathy	219,220
Experimental colon cancer	208,209,229

children who received this fermented milk product (242). Furthermore, in studies of rotavirus enteritis in suckling mice, administration of *Lactobacillus* GG counteracted the intestinal mucosal cell dysfunction induced by rotavirus (243).

Similar beneficial effects of fermented milk products have been noted by others. Niv et al. (239) treated two groups of children with diarrhea, one with neomycin/kaolin/pectin and the other with yogurt (239). Those receiving yogurt had a 50% shorter duration of disease compared to the other group. In another study that compared milk, yogurt, and diluted milk for the treatment of persistent diarrhea in young children, significant benefit was found for the group receiving yogurt compared to the other groups. Alm (241) administered 500 mL of acidophilus milk to individuals infected with salmonella and noted that this treatment shortened the carrier state.

Fermented milk products may also be of benefit in preventing traveler's diarrhea (251–253). A large group of Finnish travelers to southern Turkey were randomized to receive either *Lactobacillus* GG or placebo in a blinded study (251). Those who received *Lactobacillus* GG had a 40% reduction in diarrheal symptoms. In contrast to these findings, other studies have shown no clear-cut benefit of administering lactic acid bacteria to travelers.

Probiotic preparations also have been suggested as a possible therapeutic approach to antibiotic-associated diarrhea, which is often due to bacterial overgrowth (235,254,255). In some cases there appears to have been a beneficial effect. Bennett and colleagues (255) treated nine symptomatic patients with recurrent *C. difficile* diarrhea with high doses (10^9 CFU twice daily for 7 to 14 days) of *Lactobacillus* GG (255). All patients improved, but four patients had late recurrences from 60 to 180 days after initiation of therapy.

In summary, the microbial flora of the human gastrointestinal tract consist of a populous and extremely diverse group of organisms. These bacteria cannot be regarded as simply cohabitants, because they play a profound role in host physiology and pathophysiology.

REFERENCES

1. Simon G, Gorbach SL. Intestinal flora and gastrointestinal function. In: Christensen J, Jackson MJ, Jacobson ED, Walsh J, eds. *Physiology of the gastrointestinal tract.* New York: Raven Press, 1987;1729–1749.
2. Moore WEC, Holdeman LV. Discussion of current bacteriologic investigations of the relationships between intestinal flora, diet, and colon cancer. *Cancer Res* 1975;35:3418–3420.
3. Dunn D. Autochthonous microflora of the gastrointestinal tract. *Perspect Colon Rectal Surg* 1990;2:105.
4. Gorbach SL, Plaut AG, Hahas L, Weinstein L. Studies of intestinal microflora. II. Microorganisms of the small intestine and their relations to oral and fecal flora. *Gastroenterology* 1967;53:856–867.
5. Dooley CP, Cohen H, Fitzgibbons PL, et al. Prevalence of *Helicobacter pylori* infection and histologic gastritis in asymptomatic persons. *N Engl J Med* 1989;321:1562–1566.
6. Dooley CP, Cohen H. The clinical significance of *Campylobacter pylori. Ann Intern Med* 1988;108:70–79.
7. Blaser MJ. Gastric *Campylobacter*-like organisms, gastritis, and peptic ulcer disease. *Gastroenterology* 1987;93:371–383.
8. Hentges DJ. The anaerobic microflora of the human body. *Clin Infect Dis* 1993;16(Suppl 4):S175–S180.
9. Broido PW, Gorbach SL, Nyhus LM. Microflora of the gastrointestinal tract and the surgical malabsorption syndrome. *Surg Gynecol Obstet* 1972;135:449–460.
10. Drude RB Jr, Hines C Jr. The pathophysiology of intestinal bacterial overgrowth syndromes. *Arch Intern Med* 1980;140:1349–1352.
11. Dixon JMS. The fate of bacteria in the small intestine. *J Pathol Bacteriol* 1960;79:131–140.
12. Gareau FE, Mackel DC, Boring JR III, et al. The acquisition of fecal flora by infants from their mothers during birth. *J Pediatr* 1959;54:313–318.
13. Long SS, Swenson RM. Development of anaerobic fecal flora in healthy newborn infants. *J Pediatr* 1977;91:298–301.
14. Rotimi VO, Duerden B. The development of the bacterial flora in normal neonates. *J Med Microbiol* 1981;14:51–62.
15. Tannock GW, Fuller R, Smith SL, Hall MA. Plasmid profiling of members of the family Enterobacteriaceae, lactobacilli, and the bifidobacteria to study the transmission of bacteria from mother to infant. *J Clin Microbiol* 1990;28:1225–1228.
16. Copperstock MS, Zedd AJ. Intestinal flora of infants. In: Hentges DJ, ed. *Human intestinal microflora in health and disease.* New York: Academic Press, 1983;79–99.
17. Bishop RF, Anderson CM. The bacterial flora of the stomach and small intestine in children with intestinal obstruction. *Arch Dis Child* 1960;35:487.
18. Benno Y, Sawada K, Mitsuoka T. The intestinal microflora of infants: composition of fecal flora in breast-fed and bottle-fed infants. *Microbiol Immunol* 1984;28:975–986.
19. Lunderquist B, Nord CE, Winberg J. The composition of the faecal microflora in breast-fed and bottle-fed infants from birth to eight weeks. *Acta Paediatr Scand* 1985;74:45–51.
20. Mevissen-Verhage EA, Marcelis JH, de Vos MN, et al. *Bifidobacterium, Bacteroides,* and *Clostridium* spp. in fecal samples from breast-fed and bottle-fed infants with and without iron supplementation. *J Clin Microbiol* 1987;25:285–289.
21. Mata LV, Urrutia JJ. Intestinal colonization of breast-fed children in a rural area of low socio-economic level. *Ann NY Acad Sci* 1971;176:93–109.
22. Gorbach SL, Barza M, Guilano M, Jacobus NV. Colonization resistance of the human intestinal microflora: testing the hypothesis in normal volunteers. *Eur J Clin Microbiol Infect Dis* 1988;7:98–102.
23. Drasar BS, Shiner M, McLeod GM. Studies on the intestinal flora. I. The bacterial flora of the gastrointestinal tract in healthy and achlorhydric persons. *Gastroenterology* 1969;56:71–79.
24. Gorbach SL, Nahas L, Lerner PI, Weinstein L. Studies of intestinal microflora. I. Effects of diet, age, and periodic sampling on numbers of fecal microorganisms in man. *Gastroenterology* 1967;53:845–855.
25. Zubrycki L, Spaulding EH. Studies on the stability of the normal fecal flora. *J Bacteriol* 1962;83:968–974.
26. Dack GM, Petran E. Bacterial activity in different levels of the intestine and in isolated segments of small and large bowel in monkeys and dogs. *J Infect Dis* 1934;54:204–220.
27. Gorbach SL. Population control in the small bowel. *Gut* 1967;8:530–532.
28. Rolfe RD. Interactions among microorganisms of the indigenous intestinal flora and their influence on the host. *Rev Infect Dis* 1984;6:S59–S73.
29. Gray JDA, Shiner M. Influence of gastric pH on gastric and jejunal flora. *Gut* 1967;8:574–581.
30. Greenlee HB, Vivit R, Paez J, Dietz A. Bacterial flora of the jejunum following peptic ulcer surgery. *Arch Surg* 1971;102:260–265.
31. Muscroft TJ, Deane SA, Youngs D, Burdon DW, Keighley MRB. The microflora of the postoperative stomach. *Br J Surg* 1981;68:560–564.
32. Deane S, Youngs D, Poxon V, Keighley MRB, Alexander-Williams J, Burdon DW. Cimetidine and gastric microflora. *Br J Surg* 1980;67:371.
33. Muscroft TJ, Youngs D, Burdon DW, Keighley MRB. Cimeti-

dine and the potential risk of postoperative sepsis. *Br J Surg* 1981;68:557–559.

34. Ruddell WSJ, Axon ATR, Findlay JM, Bartholomew BA, Hill MJ. Effect of cimetidine on the gastric bacterial flora. *Lancet* 1980;1:672–674.

35. Sharma BK, Santana IA, Wood EC, et al. Intragastric bacterial activity and nitrosation before, during and after treatment with omeprazole. *Br Med J* 1984;289:717–719.

36. Driks MR, Craven DE, Celli BR, et al. Nosocomial pneumonia in intubated patients given sucralfate as compared with antacids or histamine type 2 blockers. *N Engl J Med* 1987;317:1376–1382.

37. Gianella RA, Broitman SA, Zamcheck N. Influence of gastric acidity on bacterial and parasitic enteric infections: a perspective. *Ann Intern Med* 1973;78:271–276.

38. Cash R, Music S, Libonati J, Snyder M, Wenzel R, Hornick R. Response of man to infection with *V. cholera*. I. Clinical, serologic and bacteriologic response to a known inoculum. *J Infect Dis* 1974;129:45–52.

39. Black RE, Levine MM, Clements ML, Hughes TP, Blaser MJ. Experimental *Campylobacter jejuni* infection in humans. *J Infect Dis* 1988;157:472–479.

40. Drude RB Jr, Hines C Jr. The pathophysiology of intestinal bacterial overgrowth syndromes. *Arch Intern Med* 1980;140:1349–1352.

41. King CE, Toskes PP. Small intestine bacterial overgrowth. *Gastroenterology* 1979;76:1035–1055.

42. Simon GL, Gorbach SL. Intestinal flora in health and disease. *Gastroenterology* 1984;86:174–193.

43. Tabaqchali S. The pathophysiological role of small intestinal bacterial flora. *Scand J Gastroenterol Suppl* 1970;6:139–163.

44. Prizont R, Hersh T, Floch MH. Jejunal bacterial flora in chronic small bowel disease. I. Celiac disease. II. regional enteritis. *Am J Clin Nutr* 1970;23:1602–1607.

45. Dawson AM, Isselbacher KJ. Studies of lipid metabolism in the small intestine with observation on the role of bile salts. *J Clin Invest* 1950;39:730–740.

46. Donaldson RM Jr. Studies on the pathogenesis of steatorrhea in the blind loop syndrome. *J Clin Invest* 1965;44:1815–1825.

47. Donaldson RM Jr. Malabsorption of ^{60}Co-labelled cyanocobalamin in rats with intestinal diverticula. I. Evolution of possible mechanisms. *Gastroenterology* 1962;43:271–281.

48. Gianella RA, Broitmen SA, Zamcheck N. Vitamin B$_{12}$ uptake by intestinal microorganisms: mechanism and relevance to syndromes of intestinal bacterial overgrowth. *J Clin Invest* 1971;50:1100–1107.

49. Gorbach SL, Tabachali S. Bacteria, bile and the small bowel. *Gut* 1969;10:963–972.

50. Gracey M. The contaminated small bowel syndrome: pathogenesis, diagnosis, and treatment. *Am J Clin Nutr* 1979;32:234–243.

51. Kim YS, Spritz N, Blum M, Terz J, Sherlock P. The role of altered bile acid metabolism in the steatorrhea of experimental blind loop. *J Clin Invest* 1966;45:956–962.

52. Tabaqchali S, Hatzioannou J, Boot CC. Bile-salt deconjugation and steatorrhea in patients with the stagnant loop syndrome. *Lancet* 1968;2:12–16.

53. Mackowiak PA. The normal microbial flora. *N Engl J Med* 1982;307:83–93.

54. Savage DC. Microbial ecology of the gastrointestinal tract. *Annu Rev Microbiol* 1977;31:107–133.

55. Simon GL, Gorbach SL. The human intestinal microflora. *Dig Dis Sci* 1986;1:147S–162S.

56. Byrne BM, Dankert J. Volatile fatty acids and aerobic flora in the gastrointestinal tract of mice under various conditions. *Infect Immun* 1979;23:559–563.

57. Freter R. In-vivo and in-vitro antagonism of intestinal bacteria against *Shigella flexneri*. II. The inhibitory mechanism. *J Infect Dis* 1962;110:38–46.

58. Hentges DJ, Maier BR. Inhibition of *Shigella flexneri* by the normal intestinal flora. III. Interactions with *Bacteroides fragilis* strains in vitro. *Infect Immun* 1970;2:364–370.

59. Cooke, EM, Ewins, SP, Shooter R. The changing fecal popula-

tion of *E. coli* in hospital medical patients. *Br Med J* 1969;4:593–595.

60. Hill MJ, Drasar BS, Aries V, Crowther JS, Hawksworth G, Williams REO. Bacterial and aetiology of cancer of large bowel. *Lancet* 1971;1:95–100.

61. Finegold S, Attebery HR, Sutter VL. Effect of diet on human fecal flora: comparison of Japanese and American diets. *Am J Clin Nutr* 1974;27:1456–1469.

62. Hentges DJ. Fecal flora of volunteers on controlled diets. *Am J Clin Nutr* 1978;31:S123–S124.

63. Reddy BS, Wynder EL. Large-bowel carcinogenesis: fecal constituents of populations with diverse incidence rates of colon cancer. *J Natl Cancer Inst* 1973;50:1437–1442.

64. Attebery HR, Sutter VL, Finegold SM. Effect of a partially chemically defined diet on normal human fecal flora. *Am J Clin Nutr* 1972;25:1391–1398.

65. Bornside GH, Cohn I Jr. Stability of normal human fecal flora during a chemically defined, low residue liquid diet. *Ann Surg* 1974;181:58–60.

66. Bounous G, Devroede GJ. Effects of an elemental diet on human fecal flora. *Gastroenterology* 1974;66:210–214.

67. Gorbach SL. The effect of diet on the intestinal microflora and its metabolic functions. In: Shills ME, ed. *Defined formula diets for medical purposes*. Chicago: American Medical Association, 1977.

68. Drasar BS, Jenkins DJA, Cummings JH. The influence of a diet rich in wheat fiber on the human fecal flora. *J Med Microbiol* 1976;9:423–431.

69. Bartlett JG, Condon RE, Gorbach SL, Clarke JS, Nichols RL, Ochi S. Veterans Administration cooperative study on bowel preparation for elective colorectal operations: impact of oral antibiotic regimen on colonic flora, wound irrigation cultures and bacteriology of septic complications. *Ann Surg* 1978;188:249–254.

70. Nichols RL, Condon RE, Gorbach SL, Nyhus LM. Efficacy of preoperative antimicrobial preparation of the bowel. *Ann Surg* 1972;176:227–232.

71. Nordenvall B, Hallberg D, Larsson L, Nord CE. The effect of clindamycin on the intestinal flora in patients with enteric hyperoxaluria. *Scand J Gastroenterol* 1983;18:177–181.

72. Giuliano M, Barza M, Jacobus NV, Gorbach SL. Effect of broad-spectrum parenteral antibiotics on composition of intestinal microflora of humans. *Antimicrob Agents Chemother* 1987;31:202–206.

73. Clarke JS, Condon RE, Bartlett JG, Gorbach SL, Nichols RL, Ochi S. Preoperative oral antibiotics reduce septic complications of colon operations: results of prospective, randomized, double-blind clinical study. *Ann Surg* 1977;186:251–259.

74. Nichols RL, Broido P, Condon RE, Gorbach SL, Nyhus LM. Effect of preoperative neomycin–erythromycin intestinal preparation on the incidence of infectious complications following colon cancer. *Ann Surg* 1973;178:453–462.

75. Dion YM, Richards GK, Prentis JJ, Hinchey EJ. The influence of oral versus parenteral preoperative metronidazole on sepsis following colon surgery. *Ann Surg* 1980;192:221–226.

76. Kager L, Ljungdahl I, Malmborg AS, Nord CE, Pieper R, Dahlgren P. Antibiotic prophylaxis with cefoxitin in colorectal surgery. *Ann Surg* 1981;193:277–282.

77. Washington JA II, Dearing WHH, Judd ES, et al. Effect of preoperative regimen on development of infection after intestinal surgery: prospective, randomized, double-blind study. *Ann Surg* 1974;180:567–572.

78. El-sefi Ta, El-awadi HM, Shehata MI, et al. The place of antibiotics in the prevention of post-appendicectomy sepsis: a prospective study of 400 cases. *Int Surg* 1986;71:18–21.

79. Busuttil RW, Davidson RK, Fine M, Tompkins R. Effect of prophylactic antibiotics in acute nonperforated appendicitis. *Ann Surg* 1981;194:502–509.

80. Gorbach SL. Antimicrobial prophylaxis for appendectomy and colorectal surgery. *Rev Infect Dis* 1991;13(Suppl 10):S815–S820.

81. Guiot HFL, van den Broek PJ, van der Meer JWM, van Furth R. Selective antimicrobial modulation of the intestinal flora of

patients with acute nonlymphocytic leukemia: a double-blind, placebo-controlled study. *J Infect Dis* 1983;147:615.

82. Guiot HFL, van der Meer JWM, van Furth R. Selective antimicrobial modulation of human microbial flora: infection prevention in patients with decreased host defense mechanisms by selective elimination of potentially pathogenic bacteria. *J Infect Dis* 1981;143:644–654.

83. Gurwith MJ, Brunton JL, Lank BA, Harding GKM, Ronald AR. A prospective controlled investigation of prophylactic trimethoprim/sulfamethoxazole in hospitalized granulocytopenic patients. *Am J Med* 1979;66:248–256.

84. Wade JC, Schimpff SC, Hargadon MS, Fortner CL, Young VM, Wiernik PH. A comparison of trimethoprim–sulfamethoxazole plus nystatin with gentamicin plus nystatin in the prevention of infections in acute leukemia. *N Engl J Med* 1981;304:1057–1062.

85. Sleijfer DT, Julder NH, de Bries-Hospers HG, Fidler V, Nieweg HO, van der Waaij D, van Saene HKF. Infection prevention in granulocytopenic patients by selective decontamination of the digestive tract. *Eur J Cancer* 1980;16:859–869.

86. Dekker A, Rozenberg-Arska M, Verhoef J. Infection prophylaxis in acute leukemia: a comparison of ciprofloxacin with trimethoprim–sulfamethoxazole and colistin. *Ann Intern Med* 1987;106:7–12.

87. GIMEMA. Prevention of bacterial infection in neutropenic patients with hematologic malignancies. A randomized multicenter trial compairing norfloxacin with ciprofloxacin. *Ann Intern Med* 1991;115:7–12.

88. Schimpff SC, Greene WH, Young VM, et al. Infection prevention in acute nonlymphocytic leukemia: laminar air flow room reverse isolation with oral, nonabsorbable antibiotic prophylaxis. *Ann Intern Med* 1975;82:351–358.

89. Van der Waaij D, De Vries JM, Ledderkerk JEC. Colonization resistance of the digestive tract in conventional and antibiotic treated mice. *J Hyg (Lond)* 1971;9:405.

90. van der Waaij D. The ecology of the human intestine and its consequences for overgrowth by pathogens such as *Clostridium difficile. Annu Rev Microbiol* 1989;43:69–87.

91. Bartlett JG, Chang TW, Gurwith M, Gorbach SL, Onderdonk AB. Antibiotic-associated pseudomembranous colitis due to toxin-producing clostridia. *N Engl J Med* 1978;198:531–534.

92. Bartlett JG. *Clostridium difficile:* clinical considerations. *Rev Infect Dis* 1990;12:S244.

93. Hanson LA, Ashraf R, Cruz JR, et al. Immunity related to exposition and bacterial colonization of the infant. *Acta Paediatr Scand* Suppl 1990;365:38–45.

94. Gordon HA, Pesti L. The gnotobiotic animal as a tool in the study of host microbial relationships. *Bact Rev* 1971;35:390–429.

95. Kagnoff MF. Immunology of the digestive system. In: Christensen J, Jackson MJ, Jacobson ED, Walsh J, eds. *Physiology of the gastrointestinal tract.* New York: Raven Press, 1987;1699–1728.

96. Abrams GD, Bauer H, Sprinz H. Influence of the normal flora on mucosal morphology and cellular renewal in the ileum. A comparison of germ-free and conventional mice. *Lab Invest* 1963;12:355–364.

97. Kenworthy R. Observations on the reaction of the intestinal mucosa to bacterial challenge. *J Clin Pathol* 1971;24:138–145.

98. Gordan HA, Bruchorer-Kardoss E. Effect of normal microbial flora on intestinal surface area. *Am J Physiol* 1961;201:175–182.

99. Bartnik W, ReMine SG, Chiba M, Thayer WR, Shorter RG. Isolation and characterization of colonic intraepithelial and lamina propria lymphocytes. *Gastroenterology* 1980;78:976–985.

100. Freter R. In vivo and in vitro antagonism of intestinal bacteria against *Shigella flexneri.* II. The inhibitory mechanism. *J Infect Dis* 1962;110:38–46.

101. Freter R. Interactions between mechanisms controlling the intestinal microflora. *Am J Clin Nutr* 1974;27:1409–1416.

102. Callahan LT III, Richardson SH. Biochemistry of vibrio cholera virulence. III. Nutritional requirements for toxin production and the effects of pH on toxin elaboration in chemically defined media. *Infect Immun* 1973;7:567–572.

103. Muralidhara KS, Sheggeby GG, Elliker PR, England DC, Sandine WE. Effect of feeding lactobacilli on the coliform and lactobacillus flora of intestinal tissue and feces from piglets. *J Food Protect* 1977;40:288–295.

104. Hentges DJ. Enteric pathogen-normal flora interactions. *Am J Clin Nutr* 1970;23:1451–1456.

105. Bohnhoff M, Miller CP, Martin JR. Resistance of the mouse's intestinal tract to experimental salmonella infection. 1. Factors which interfere with the initiation of infection by oral inoculation. *J Exp Med* 1964;120:805–816.

106. Hentges DJ, Maier BR. Inhibition of *Shigella flexneri* by the normal intestinal flora. III. Interactions with *Bacteroides fragilis* strains in vitro. *Infect Immun* 1970;2:364–370.

107. Meynell GG. Antibacterial mechanisms of the mouse gut. II. The role of Eh and volatile fatty acids in the normal gut. *Br J Exp Pathol* 1963;44:209–219.

108. Sanders E. Bacterial interference I. Its occurrence among the respiratory tract flora and characterization of inhibition of group A streptococci by viridans streptococci. *J Infect Dis* 1969;120:698–707.

109. Sanders CC, Sanders WE Jr, Harrowe DJ. Bacterial interference: effects of oral antibiotics on the normal throat flora and its ability to interfere with group a streptococci. *Infect Immun* 1976;13:808–812.

110. Crowe CC, Sanders WE Jr, Longley S. Bacterial interference. II. Role of the normal throat flora in prevention of colonization by group A streptococcus. *J Infect Dis* 1973;128:527–532.

111. Sprunt K, Redman W. Evidence suggesting importance of role of interbacterial inhibition in maintaining balance of normal flora. *Ann Intern Med* 1968;68:579–590.

112. Sprunt K, Leidy GA, Redman W. Prevention of bacterial overgrowth. *J Infect Dis* 1971;123:1–10.

113. Kelstrup J, Gibbons RJ. Inactivation of bacteriocin in the intestinal canal and oral cavity. *J Bacteriol* 1969;99:888–890.

114. Davidson JN, Hirsh DC. Bacterial competition as a means of preventing neonatal diarrhea in pigs. *Infect Immun* 1976;13:1773–1774.

115. Liljemark WF, Gibbons RJ. Suppression of *Candida albicans* by human oral streptococci in gnotobiotic mice. *Infect Immun* 1973;8:846–849.

116. Pongpech P, Hentges DJ, Marsh WW, Eberle ME. Effect of streptomycin administration on association of enteric pathogens with cecal tissue of mice. *Infect Immun* 1989;57:2092–2097.

117. Goldin BR, Lichtenstein AH, Gorbach SL. Nutritional and metabolic roles of intestinal flora. *Mod Nutr* 1994;8:569–582.

118. Plaa GL. The enterohepatic circulation. In: Gillete JR, ed. *Handbook of experimental pharmacology,* vol 28(3). New York: Springer-Verlag, 1975;130–149.

119. Scheline RR. Metabolism of foreign compounds by gastrointestinal microorganisms. *Pharmacol Rev* 1973;25:451–523.

120. Emerman S, Twombly GH, Levitz M. Biliary and urinary metabolites of estriol-15^{3}H-3-sulfate-^{35}S in women. *J Clin Endocrinol Metab* 1967;27:539–548.

121. Inoue N, Sandberg AA, Graham JB, Slaunwhite WR Jr. Studies on phenolic steroids in human subjects. IX. Role of the intestine in the conjugation of estriol. *J Clin Invest* 1969;48:390–396.

122. Dyer JT, Swenson L, Woods MN. Estrogen excretion patterns and plasma level in vegetarian and omnivorous women. *N Engl J Med* 1982;207:1542–1547.

123. Adlercreutz H, Martin F, Tikkanen MJ, Pulkkinen M. Effect of ampicillin administration on the excretion of twelve oestrogens in pregnancy urine. *Acta Endocrinol (Copenh)* 1975;80:551–557.

124. Adlercreutz H, Martin F, Pulkkinen M, Dencker H, Rimer U, Sjoberg NO, Tikkanen MJ. Intestinal metabolism of estrogens. *J Clin Endocrinol Metab* 1976;43:497–505.

125. Pulkkinen MO, Willman K. Reduction of maternal estrogen excretion by neomycin. *Am J Obstet Gynecol* 1973;115:1153.

126. Tikkanen MJ, Pulkkinen MO, Adlercreutz H. Effect of ampicillin treatment on the urinary excretion of estriol conjugation in pregnancy. *J Steroid Biochem* 1973;4:439–440.

127. Dossetar J. Drug interaction with oral contraceptives. *Fr Med J* 1975;4:467–468.

128. Reimer D. Rifampicin, ''pill'' do not go well together. *JAMA* 1974;227:608.

129. Sparros MJ. Pregnancies in reliable takers. *N Z Med J* 1989; 102:575–577.

130. Hawksworth G, Draser BS, Hill MJ. Intestinal bacteria and the hydrolysis of glycosidic bonds. *Med Microbiol* 1971;4:451–459.

131. Mastromarino A, Reddy BS, Wynder EL. Metabolic epidemiology of colon cancer: enzymic activity of fecal flora. *Am J Clin Nutr* 1976;29:1455–1450.

132. Salvioli G, Salata R, Bondi M, Fratalocchi A, Sala BM, Gibertini A. Bile acid transformation by the intestinal flora and cholesterol saturation in bile. *Digestion* 1981;23:80–81.

133. Hill MJ. Diet and the human intestinal bacterial flora. *Cancer Res* 1981;41:3778–3780.

134. Saha JR. Inactivation of digoxin by the gut flora: reversal by antibiotic therapy. *N Engl J Med* 1981;305:789–794.

135. Dobkin JF, Saha JR, Butler VP Jr, Neu HC, Lindenbaum J. Inactivation of digoxin by *Eubacterium lentum,* an anaerobe of the human gut flora. *Clin Res* 1982;30:551A.

136. Suzuksi K, Benno Y, Mitsuoka T, et al. Urease-producing species of intestinal anaerobes and their activities. *Appl Environ Microbiol* 1979;37:379–382.

137. Enanker LK, Nilsson F, Ryden AC, Schwan A. The aerobic and anaerobic microflora of the gastric remnant more than 15 years after Billroth II resection. *Scand J Gastroenterol* 1982; 17:715–720.

138. Bjorneklett A, Fuasa O, Midtvedt T. Small bowel bacterial overgrowth in the post gastrectomy syndrome. *Scand J Gastroenterol* 1983;18:277–287.

139. Drasar BS, Shiner M. Studies on the intestinal flora II. Bacterial flora of the small intestine in patients with gastrointestinal disorders. *Gut* 1969;10:812–819.

140. Goldstein F, Cozzolino HJ, Wirts CW. Diarrhea and steatorrhea due to a large solitary duodenal diverticulum. *Am J Diagn Dis* 1963;8:937.

141. Gracey M, Suharjono S, Stone DE. Microbial contamination of the gut. Another feature of malnutrition. *Am J Clin Nutr* 1973;26:1170–1174.

142. Goldstein F, Wirts CW, Kowlessar OD. Diabetic diarrhea and steatorrhea. Microbiologic and clinical observations. *Ann Intern Med* 1970;72:215–218.

143. Gorbach SL, Lal D, Levitan R. Intestinal micro-flora in Laennec's cirrhosis. *J Clin Invest* 1970;49:36A.

144. Kahn LJ, Jefferies GH, Sleisenger MH. Malabsorption in intestinal scleroderma: correction by antibiotics. *N Engl J Med* 1966;274:1339–1344.

145. Pearson AJ, Brezechwa-Ajdukiewicz A, McCarthy CF. Intestinal pseudo-obstruction with bacterial overgrowth in the small intestine. *Am J Dig Dis* 1969;14:200–205.

146. Corrodi P. Jejeunoileal bypass: change in the flora of the small intestine and its clinical impact. *Rev Infect Dis* 1984;6:S80–S84.

147. Robert SH, Jame O, Jarvis EH. Bacterial overgrowth syndrome without ''blind loop'': a cause for malnutrition in the elderly. *Lancet* 1977;2:1193–1195.

148. McEvoy A, Dutton J, James OFW. Bacterial contamination of the small intestine is an important cause of occult malabsorption in the elderly. *Br Med J* 1983;287:789–793.

149. Polter DE, Boyle JD, Miller LG, Finegold SM. Anaerobic bacteria as cause of the blind loop syndrome. A case report with observations on response to antibacterial agents. *Gastroenterology* 1968;54:1148–1154.

150. Tabaqchali S, Booth CC. Jejunal bacteriology and bile-salt metabolism in patients with intestinal malabsorption. *Lancet* 1966; 2:12–15.

151. Gorbach SL, Kean BH, Evans DG, Evans DJ Jr, Bessudo D. Traveler's diarrhea and toxigenic *Escherichia coli. N Engl J Med* 1975;292:933–936.

152. Donaldson RM Jr, Corrigon H, Natsios G. Malabsorption of ^{60}Co-labelled cyanocobalamin in rats with intestinal diverticula. II. Studies on contents of the diverticula. *Gastroenterology* 1962;43:282–290.

153. Aries V, Crowther JS, Drasar BS, Hill MJ. Degradation of bile salts by human intestinal bacteria. *Gut* 1969;10:575–576.

154. Lewis R, Gorbach S. Modification of bile acids by intestinal bacteria. *Arch Intern Med* 1972;130:545–548.

155. Drasar BS, Hill MJ, Shiner M. The deconjugation of bile salts by human intestinal bacteria. *Lancet* 1966;1:1237–1238.

156. Schjonsby H, Peters TJ, Hoffbrond AV, Tabaqchali S. The mechanism of vitamin B_{12} malabsorption in the blind loop syndrome (Abstr). *Gut* 1970;11:37.

157. Welkos S, Toskes P, Baer H. Importance of anaerobic bacteria in the cobalamin malabsorption of the experimental rat blind loop syndrome. *Gastroenterology* 1981;80:313–320.

158. Paulk EA Jr, Farrar WE Jr. Diverticulosis of the small intestine and megaloblastic anemia. Intestinal microflora and absorption before and after tetracycline administration. *Am J Med* 1964; 37:473–480.

159. Goldstein F, Karacadag S, Wirts CW, Kowlessar OD. Intraluminal small-intestinal utilization of D-xylose by bacteria. A limitation of the D-xylose absorption test. *Gastroenterology* 1970; 59:380–386.

160. Henegan JB. Influence of microbial flora on xylose absorption in rats and mice. *Am J Physiol* 1963;205:417–420.

161. Chernov AJ, Doe WF, Gompertz D. Intrajejunal volatile fatty acids in the stagnant loop syndrome. *Gut* 1972;13:103–106.

162. Prizont R, Whitehead JS, Kim YS. Short chain fatty acids in rats with jejunal blind loops. I. Analysis of SCFA in small intestine, cecum, feces, and plasma. *Gastroenterology* 1975;69: 1254–1264.

163. Klipstein FA. Tropical sprue. *Gastroenterology* 1968;54: 275–293.

164. Klipstein FA. Recent advances in tropical malabsorption. *Scand J Gastroenterol Suppl* 1970;6:93–114.

165. Cook GC. Tropical sprue: implications of Manson's concept. *J R Coll Physicians Lond* 1978;12:329–349.

166. Mathan VI, Baker SJ. Epidemic tropical sprue and other epidemics of diarrhea in south Indian villages. *Am J Clin Nutr* 1968;21:1077–1087.

167. Stefanni M. Clinical features and pathogenesis of tropical sprue. *Medicine (Baltimore)* 1948;27:379–427.

168. Maldonado N, Hortan E, Guerra R, Perez-Santiago E. Poorly absorbed sulfonamides in the treatment of tropical sprue. *Gastroenterology* 1969;57:559–568.

169. Gorbach SL, Banwell JG, Jacobi B, Chatterjee BD, Mitra R, Sen NN, Guha Mazumder DN. Tropical sprue and malnutrition in West Bengal. I. Intestinal micro-flora and absorption. *Am J Clin Nutr* 1970;23:1545–1558.

170. Gorbach SL, Mitra R, Jacobs B, Banwell JG, Chatterjee BD, Guha Mazumder DN. Bacterial contamination of the upper small bowel in tropical sprue. *Lancet* 1969;1:74–77.

171. Tomkins AM, Drasar BS, James WPT. Bacterial colonization of jejunal mucosa in acute tropical sprue. *Lancet* 1975;1:59–61.

172. Bhat P, Shantakumari S, Rajan D, Mathan VL, Kapadia CR, Swarnabai C, Baker SJ. Bacterial flora of the gastrointestinal tract in southern Indian control subjects and patients with tropical spure. *Gastroenterology* 1972;62:11–21.

173. Tomkins AM, Drasar BS, James WPT. Bacterial colonization of the upper intestine in mild tropical malabsorption. *Trop Med Hyg* 1980;74:752–755.

174. Klipstein FA, Holdeman LV, Corcino JJ, Moore WEC. Enterotoxigenic intestinal bacteria in tropical sprue. *Ann Intern Med* 1973;79:632–641.

175. Klipstein FA, Rowe B, Engert RF, Short HB, Gross RJ. Enterotoxigenicity of enteropathogenic serotypes of *Escherichia coli* isolated from infants with epidemic diarrhea. *Infect Immun* 1978;21:171–178.

176. Klipstein FA, Goetsch CA, Engert RF, Short HB, Schenk EA. Effect of monocontamination of germfree rats by enterotoxigenic coliform bacteria. *Gastroenterology* 1979;79:341–348.

177. Banwell JG, Gorbach SL, Mitra R, Cassells JS, Guha-Mazumder DN, Thomas J, Hardley JH. Tropical sprue and malnutrition in West Bengal. II. Fluid and electrolyte transport in the small intestine. *Am J Clin Nutr* 1970;21:1159–1168.

178. Banwell JG, Gorbach SL. Tropical sprue. *Gut* 1969;10:328.

179. Gerson CD, Kent TH, Saha JR, Siddiqi N, Lindenbaum J. Recovery of small-intestinal structure and function after residence

in the tropics. II. Studies in Indians and Pakistanis living in New York. *Ann Intern Med* 1971;75:41–48.

180. Cook GC. Aetiology and pathogenesis of postinfective tropical malabsorption (tropical sprue). *Lancet* 1984;1:721–723.

181. Armstrong B, Doll R. Environmental factors and cancer incidence and mortality in different countries, with special references to dietary practices. *Int J Cancer* 1975;15:617–631.

182. Burkitt DP. Epidemiology of cancer of the colon and rectum. *Cancer* 1971;28:3–13.

183. Doll R. The geographical distribution of cancer. *Br J Cancer* 1969;23:1–8.

184. Drasar BS, Irving D. Environmental factors and cancer of the colon and breast. *Br J Cancer* 1973;27:167–172.

185. Wynder EL. The epidemiology of large bowel cancer. *Cancer Res* 1975;35:3388–3394.

186. Dunn JE. Cancer epidemiology in the United States—with emphasis on Hawaii and California and Japan. *Cancer Res* 1975; 35:3240–3245.

187. Haenszel R, Berg JW, Segi M, Kurihara M, Locke FB. Large-bowel cancer in Hawaiian Japanese. *J Natl Cancer Inst* 1973; 51:1765–1779.

188. Lyon JL, Sorenson AW. Colon cancer in a low-risk population. *Am J Clin Nutr* 1978;31:S227–S230.

189. Kinlen LJ. Meat and fat consumption and cancer mortality: a study of strict religious orders in Britain. *Lancet* 1982;1: 946–949.

190. Mower HF, Ray RM, Shoff R, Stemmermann GN, Nokawa H. Fecal bile acids in two Japanese populations with different colon cancer risks. *Cancer Res* 1979;39:328–331.

191. Vargo D, Moskovita M, Floch MH. Faecal bacterial flora in cancer of the colon. *Gut* 1980;21:701–705.

192. Goldin BR, Gorbach SL. The relationship between diet and rat fecal bacterial enzymes implicated in colon cancer. *J Natl Cancer Inst* 1976;57:371–375.

193. Weisburger JH. Colon carcinogens: their metabolism and mode of action. *Cancer* 1971;28:60–70.

194. Hill MJ. The role of colon anaerobes in the metabolism of bile acids and steroids, and its relation to colon cancer. *Cancer* 1975;36:2387–2400.

195. Goldin B, Dwyer J, Gorbach SL, Gordon W, Swenson L. Influence of diet and age on fecal bacterial enzymes. *Am J Clin Nutr* 1978;31:S136–S140.

196. Goldin BR. The role of diet and the intestinal flora in the etiology of large bowel cancer (Abstr). International Symposium on Colorectal Cancer, New York.

197. Reddy BS, Weisburgher JH, Wynder EL. Fecal bacterial beta-glucuronidase: control by diet. *Science* 1974;183:416–417.

198. Laqueur GL. The induction of intestinal neoplasia with the glycoside of cycasin and its aglycone. *Virchows Arch Pathol Anat* 1965;340:151–163.

199. Laqueur GL, Mickelson O, Whiting MG, Kurland LT. Carcinogenic properties of nuts from *Cyclos circonilis*. *J Natl Cancer Inst* 1963;31:919–951.

200. Laqueur GL, Spatz M. Toxicology of cycasin. *Cancer Res* 1968;28:2262–2267.

201. Laqueur GL, McDaniel EG, Matsumoto H. Tumor induction in germfree rats with methylazoxymethanol (MAM) and synthetic MAM acetate. *J Natl Cancer Inst* 1967;39:355–371.

202. Weisburger JH, Grantham PM, Horton RE, Weisburger EK. Metabolism of the carcinogen *N*-hydroxy-*N*-2-fluorenylacetamide in germ free rats. *Biochem Pharmacol* 1970;19:151–162.

203. Gillette JR, Jamm JJ, Sasame HA. Mechanism of *p*-nitrobenzoate reduction in mice: the possible role of cytochrome P-450 in liver microsomes. *Mol Pharmacol* 1968;4:541–548.

204. Weisburgher JH, Weisburger EK. Biochemical formation and pharmacological, toxicological, and pathological properties of hydroxylamines and hydroxamic acid. *Pharmacol Rev* 1973; 25:1.

205. Morotomi M, Nanno M, Wantrobe T, et al. Mutagenic activation of biliary metabolites 1-nitropyrene by intestinal microflora. *Mutat Res* 1985;149:171–178.

206. Wheeler LA, Soderbert FB, Goldman P. The relationship between nitro group reduction and the intestinal microflora. *J Pharmacol Exp Ther* 1975;194:135–144.

207. Reddy BS, Narisawa T, Weisburger JH. Effect of a diet with high levels of protein and fat on colon carcinogenesis in F344 rats treated with 1,2-dimethylhydrazone. *J Natl Cancer Inst* 1976;57:567–569.

208. Reddy BS, Narisawa T, Wright P, Yukusich D, Weisburger JH, Wynder EL. Colon carcinogenesis with azoxymethane and dimethylhydrazine in germ-free rats. *Cancer Res* 1975;35: 287–290.

209. Reddy BS, Watanabe K. The effect of intestinal microflora on 3,2′-dimethyl-4-aminobiphenyl-induced carcinogenesis in F344 rats. *J Natl Cancer Inst* 1978;61:1269–1271.

210. Goldin BR, Gorbach SL. Diet and its effect on enzymes linked to colon cancer (Abstr). *Digestion* 1977;16:240–241.

211. Goldin BR, Gorbach SL. Effect of *Lactobacillus acidophilus* dietary supplements on 1,2-dimethylhydrazine dihydrochloride induced intestinal cancer in rats. *J Natl Cancer Inst* 1980;64: 263–265.

212. Goldin BR, Swenson L, Dwyer J, Sexton M, Gorbach SL. Effect of diet and *Lactobacillus* supplements on human fecal bacterial enzymes. *J Natl Cancer Inst* 1980;64:255–262.

213. Goldin BR, Gorbach SL. Effect of antibiotics on incidence of rat intestinal tumors induced by 1,2-dimethylhydrazine dihydrochloride. *J Natl Cancer Inst* 1981;67:877–880.

214. Hill MJ, Drasar BS, Williams REO. Faecal bile-acids and clostridia in patients with cancer of the large bowel. *Lancet* 1975; 1:535–538.

215. Kay RM. Effects of diet on the fecal excretion and bacterial modification of acidic and neutral steroids, and implications for colon carcinogenesis. *Cancer Res* 1981;42:3774–3777.

216. Murray WR, Blackwood A, Rotter JM, Calman KC, McKay C. Faecal bile acids and clostridia in the aetiology of colorectal cancer. *Br J Cancer* 1980;41:923–928.

217. Rowland LR, Grasso P. Degradation of *N*-nitrosamine by intestinal bacteria. *Appl Environ Microbiol* 1973;29:7–12.

218. Williams JR, Grantham PH, Marsh HH. Participation of liver fractions and of intestinal bacteria in the metabolism of *N*-hydroxy-*N*-2-fluorenylacetamide in the rat. *Biochem Pharmacol* 1970;19:173–188.

219. Elo S, Saxelin M, Salminen S. Attachment of *Lactobacillus casei* strain GG to human colon carcinoma cell line Caco-2: comparison with other dairy strains. *Lett Appl Microbiol* 1991; 13:154–156.

220. Surawicz CM, Elmer GW, Speelman P, et al. Prevention of antibiotic-associated diarrhea by *Saccharomyces boulardii*: a prospective study. *Gastroenterology* 1989;96:981–988.

221. Rajala SA, Salminen SJ, Seppänen JH, Vapaatalo H. Treatment of chronic constipation with lactitol sweetened yogurt supplemented with guar gum and wheat bran in elderly hospital in-patients. *Comp Gerontol* 1988;2:83–86.

222. Macbeth, WAAG, Kass EH, McDermott WV Jr. Treatment of hepatic encephalopathy by alteration of intestinal flora with *Lactobacillus acidophilus*. *Lancet* 1965;1:399–403.

223. Read AE, MCarthy CF, Heaton KW, Laidlow J. *Lactobacillus acidophilus* (ENPAC) in treatment of hepatic encephalopathy. *Br Med J* 1966;1:1267–1269.

224. Rao DM, Chawan CB, Pulusani SR. Influence of milk and thermophilic milk plasma cholesterol levels and hepatic cholesterogenesis in rats. *J Food Sci* 1981;46:1339–1341.

225. Hepner G, Fried R, St Jean S, et al. Hypocholesteremic effect of yogurt and milk. *Am J Clin Nutr* 1979;32:19–24.

226. Hargrove RE, Alford JA. Growth rate and feed efficiency of rats fed yogurt and other fermented milks. *J Dairy Sci* 1978; 61:11–19.

227. McDonough FE, Hitchins AD, Wong NP. Effect of yogurt and freeze dried yogurt on growth stimulation of rats. *J Food Sci* 1982;47:1463–1465.

228. Broussalian J, Westhoff D. Influence of lactose concentration on milk and yogurt growth of rats. *J Dairy Sci* 1983;66:438–443.

229. Alm L. Effect of fermentation on lactose, glucose and galactose content in milk and suitability of fermented milk products for lactose intolerant individuals. *J Dairy Sci* 1982;65:346–352.

230. Kim HS, Gilliland SE. *Lactobacillus acidophilus* as a dietary adjunct for milk to aid lactose digestion in humans. *J Dairy Sci* 1983;66:959–966.

231. DeWit O, Pochart P, Desjeux JF. Breath hydrogen concentration and plasma glucose, insulin and free fatty acid levels after lactose, milk, fresh or heated yogurt ingestion by healthy young adults with or without lactose malabsorption. *Nutrition* 1988; 4:131–135.

232. Goldin BR, Gorbach SL. Alterations in fecal microflora enzymes related to diet, age, *Lactobacillus* supplements, and dimethylhydrazine. *Cancer* 1977;40:2421–2426.

233. Goldin BR, Gorbach SL. Effect of milk and *Lactobacillus* feeding on human intestinal bacterial enzyme activity. *Am J Clin Nutr* 1984;39:756–761.

234. Goldin BR, Gorbach SL. Alterations of the intestinal microflora by diet, oral antibiotics and *Lactobacillus*. Decreased production of free amines from aromatic nitro compounds, azo dyes and glucuronides. *J Natl Cancer Inst* 1984b;73:689–695.

235. Gotz V, Romankiewicz JA, Moss J, Murray HW. Prophylaxis against ampicillin-associated diarrhea with a lactobacillus preparation. *Am J Hosp Pharmacol* 1979;36:754.

236. Hitchins AD, Wells P, McDonough FE, Wong NA. Amelioration of the adverse effect of a gastrointestinal challenge with *Salmonella enteritidis* on weanling rats by a yogurt diet. *Am J Clin Nutr* 1985;41:91–100.

237. Zychowicz C, Surazynmska A, Sietwierska B, Ciephinska T. Effect of *Lactobacillus acidophilus* cultures (acidophilus milk) on the carrier state of shigella and salmonella organisms in children. *Pediatr Polska* 1974;49:997–1003.

238. Zychowicz C, Kowalczyk S, Ciephinska T. Results of administration of *Lactobacillus acidophilus* cultures (acidophilus milk) in an endemic focus of dysentery. *Pediatr Polska* 1975;50: 429–435.

239. Niv M, Levy W, Greenstein NM. Yogurt in the treatment of infantile diarrhea. *Clin Pediatr* 1963;2:407–411.

240. Clements ML, Levine MM, Ristaino PA. Exogenous lactobacilli fed to man: their fate and ability to prevent diarrheal disease. *Prog Food Nutr Sci* 1983;7:29–37.

241. Alm L. The effect of *Lactobacillus acidophilus* administration upon the survival of *Salmonella* in randomly selected human carriers. *Prog Food Nutr Sci* 1983;7:13–17.

242. Kaila M, Isolauri E, Sopi E, Virtanen E, Laine S, Arvilommi H. Enhancement of the circulating antibody secreting cell response in human diarrhea by a human lactobacillus stain. *Pediatr Res* 1992;32(2):141–144.

243. Isolauri E, Kaila M, Arvola T, Majamaa H, Rantala I, Virtanen E, Arvilommi H. Diet during rotavirus enteritis affects jejunal permeability to macromolecule in suckling rats. *Pediatr Res* 1993;33(6):548–553.

244. Deeth HC, Tamine AY. Yogurt: nutritive and therapeutic aspects. *J Food Protect* 1981;44:78–86.

245. Shahani KM, Chandan RC. Nutritional and healthful aspects of cultured and culture-containing dairy foods. *J Dairy Sci* 1979;62:1685–1694.

246. Alm L. Effect of fermentation on B-vitamin content of milk in Sweden. *J Dairy Sci* 1982;65:353–359.

247. Reddy GV, Friend BA, Shahani KM, Farmer RE. Antitumor activity of yogurt components. *J Food Protect* 1983;46:8–11.

248. Friend BA, Farmer RE, Shahani KM. Effect of feeding and intraperitoneal implantation of yogurt culture cells on Ehrlich ascites tumor. *Milchwiss* 1982;37:708–710.

249. Gilliland SE, Speck ML. Antagonistic action of *Lactobacillus acidophilus* toward intestinal and foodborne pathogens in associative cultures. *J Food Protect* 1977;40:820–823.

250. Isolauri E, Juntunen M, Rautanen T. A human *Lactobacillus* strain (*Lactobacillus* GG) promotes recovery from acute diarrhoea in children. *Pediatrics* 1991;88:90–97.

251. Oksanen P, Salminen S, Saxelin M, et al. Prevention of travelers' diarrhoea by *Lactobacillus* GG. *Ann Med* 1990;22:53–56.

252. Clements ML, Levine MM, Black RE, et al. *Lactobacillus* prophylaxis for diarrhea due to enterotoxigenic *Escherichia coli*. *Antimicrob Agents Chemother* 1981;20:104–108.

253. Black FT, Anderson PL, Orskov F, et al. Prophylactic efficacy of lactobacilli on travelers' diarrhoea. *Travel Med* 1989;8: 333–335.

254. Lidbeck A, Edlund C, Gustafsson JA, et al. Impact of *Lactobacillus acidophilus* on the normal intestinal microflora after administration of two antimicrobial agents. *Infection* 1988;16: 329–336.

255. Bennett RG, Laghon B, Lindsay J, et al. *Lactobacillus* GG treatment of nosocomial infections (Abst). 3rd International Conference on Nosocomial Infections, Atlanta, 1990.

Infections of the Gastrointestinal Tract,
edited by M. J. Blaser, P. D. Smith, J. I. Ravdin,
H. B. Greenberg, and R. L. Guerrant
Raven Press, Ltd., New York © 1995.

CHAPTER 5

Production, Structure, and Biologic Relevance of Gastrointestinal Mucins

Janet F. Forstner, Mary G. Oliver, and Francisco A. Sylvester

GENERAL PROPERTIES OF MUCINS

Mucous glycoproteins, or mucins, are biopolymers responsible for the slimy gel-like consistency of mucous secretions. They consist of a family of heterogeneous, heavily glycosylated, high molecular weight glycoproteins illustrated schematically in Fig. 1. Most mucins contain sialic acid and sulfate attached to selected sugars and are therefore negatively charged under physiologic conditions. Mucins are often grouped into two classes: the secretory type and the membrane-associated type. The latter are expressed most strongly in certain tumor cell lines. Gastrointestinal mucins appear to be secretory-type mucins, arising from specialized mucus-producing cells of the salivary glands, stomach, pancreatic and bile ducts, gallbladder, and small and large intestine.

As listed in Table 1, mucins have many putative functional properties, most of which depend predominantly on their physical state as well-hydrated gels. These functions include lubrication, hydration of the mucosa, protection from harmful chemicals, and epithelial repair. Other mucin functions depend as well on specific chemical structures for recognition and binding processes. Membrane-associated mucins or mucin-like glycoproteins may function in the regulation of cellular morphology, growth, or differentiation and in enhancing local tumor metastases through interactions with the cellular cytoskeleton (chiefly actin), submucosal matrix proteins, cytotoxic T cells, and vascular selectins. Reviews of mucin classification, structure, and function can be found in ref. 1 to 21.

The relevance of mucins to intestinal infection and inflammation has begun to receive considerable attention. Under normal conditions, mucin gels form a layer over the contours of the mucosal surface. Interactions with the

mucin gel may determine whether an invading pathogen will establish residence in the intestine or be removed by fluid "flushing." In many cases pathogens secrete enzymes that weaken the mucous barrier and thereby gain access to mucosal cells. In other cases mucins provide a nutrient source for pathogens, which then have to compete with commensal bacteria for their survival. Mucin carbohydrates may serve as recognition targets for specific bacterial, viral, or parasitic adhesins, thereby setting the stage for early colonization of the mucous layer and release of toxins adjacent to mucosal cell receptors. Alternatively, mucin gels may physically entrap microorganisms and prevent their access to cells. In conditions of low flow rate of luminal fluid, as in obstruction and bacte-

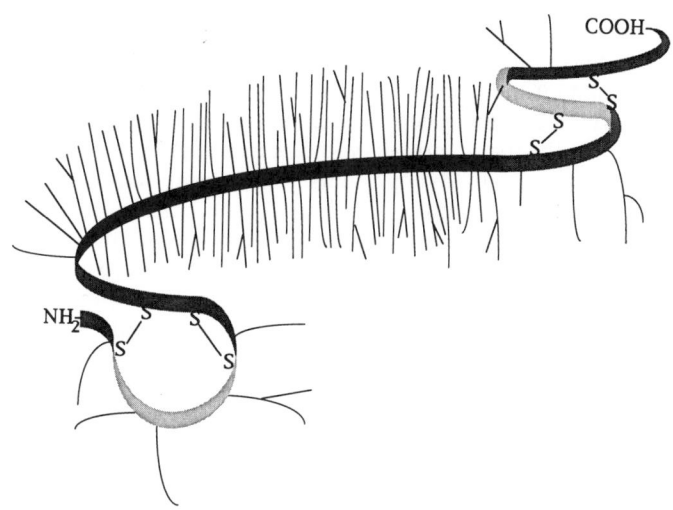

FIG. 1. Diagrammatic model of a mucin. The amino and carboxyl ends of the mucin peptide (*shaded*) are stabilized in a folded configuration by intramolecular S—S bonds and are less glycosylated than the extended (bottle-brush) central domain (*dark*).

J. F. Forstner, M. G. Oliver, and F. A. Sylvester: Divisions of Research Biochemistry and Gastroenterology and Nutrition, The Research Institute, The Hospital for Sick Children, Toronto, Ontario M5G 1X8, Canada.

TABLE 1. *Putative functional properties of mucins*

Lubrication
Hydration
Metal ion binding
Antioxidant
Mucus–bicarbonate barrier
Diffusion barrier for macromolecules, drugs, toxins, and
    other molecules
Interaction with surface immunoglobulins (secretory IgA)
    in host defense
Epithelial repair (reepithelialization)
Recognition sites for bacteria, parasites, and viruses
Nucleation site for bile stones
Membrane mucins—roles in tumor differentiation,
    growth, and metastases

rial overgrowth, stasis of mucus secretions favors bacterial colonization, and the bacteria may contribute further to stasis by stimulating mucus secretion (22). In conditions of rapid flow, as in the watery diarrhea of cholera infection, the bacteria, together with their toxins and surface mucins, are washed away (23). Therefore bacterial strategies for survival can be either thwarted or assisted by the dynamic state of the mucus gel layer. In obstruction of the biliary tree or gallbladder, mucins contribute significantly to the formation of bile stones (24–27), thus enhancing the tendency for secondary inflammation (cholecystitis).

MORPHOLOGY AND PHYSIOLOGY OF GOBLET CELLS

Goblet Cell Morphology

Production of mucins secreted along the length of the intestinal tract is delegated to a specific subset of epithelial cells: mucus cells in the stomach and goblet cells throughout the small and large intestine. Goblet cells are polarized columnar cells in the epithelium, optimally organized for the vectorial synthesis and secretion of high molecular weight glycoproteins in the apical (luminal) direction. In the mature cell (Fig. 2), the basal aspect of the cell forms the goblet's "stem" containing an ovoid nucleus surrounded by basophilic cytoplasm resulting from a concentration of rough endoplasmic reticulum (RER) (Fig. 3). Above the RER, in the supranuclear region, reside multiple Golgi stacks and numerous vesicles containing periodic acid–Schiff (PAS) positive material (Fig. 2). These condensing vacuoles represent mucin granules that have budded off the Golgi complex (Fig. 3). The upper region of the cell forms the "cup" of the goblet cell. It contains a tightly packed secretory granule mass and is delimited by the theca, a thin layer of cytoplasm containing a dense network of cytoskeletal elements that virtually excludes cellular organelles. This region is dedicated to the storage, movement, and secretion of mucin granules.

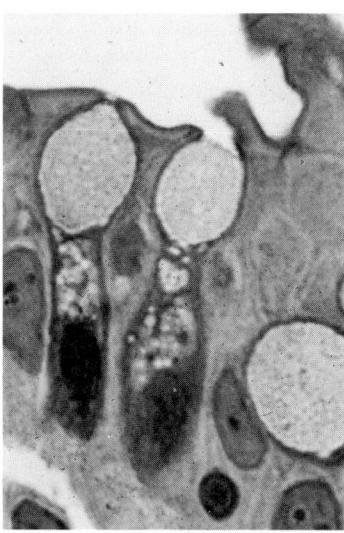

FIG. 2. Light micrography of a colonic goblet cell. The nucleus resides in the basal aspect of the cell and is surrounded by basophilic cytoplasm. The supranuclear region appears lighter stained due to the presence of numerous condensing vacuoles and nascent granules. The upper region of the cell contains a tightly packed mass of mucin granules.

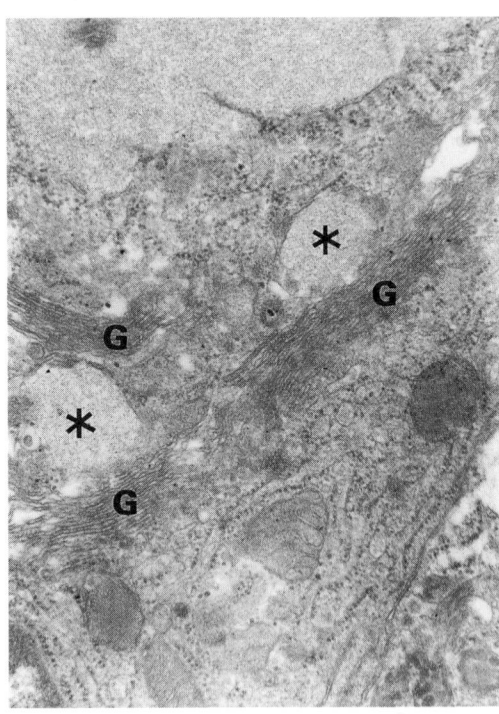

FIG. 3. Transmission electron micrograph of a colonic goblet cell. Abundant RER is present surrounding the cell nucleus and along the cell periphery. The supranuclear region contains numerous Golgi stacks (G) and condensing vacuoles (*).

Derivation, Maturation, and Life Span

Goblet cells arise by mitosis from either pluripotential stem cells located at the base of the crypts (28) or poorly differentiated oligomucus cells in the lower third of the crypt with characteristics of both absorptive and goblet cells (29). Studies using mouse aggregation chimeras have demonstrated that cells in individual crypts are derived from single progenitor cells; that is, crypts are monoclonal (30). Once propagated, these cells are short-lived. Kinetic analyses of goblet cell dynamics in mouse small intestine show that these cells migrate from the lower crypt to the villus tip in 2 to 3 days and then are sloughed into the lumen (31).

Morphometric studies on rabbit colonic goblet cells (32) have revealed that goblet cells, during migration to the epithelial surface, undergo a marked reorganization to attain the classic "goblet" shape (Fig. 4). After genesis, there is a vast proliferation of synthetic organelles, and the cells become very large, with an average volume of 1229 mm³. They are pyramidal in shape with a broad basal lamina contact and limited luminal contact (32). RER cisternae and Golgi stacks are spread throughout the cell and interspersed between mucin granules, which have not yet formed a definitive apical granule mass. Despite the emphasis on granule synthesis, mucin secretion has begun. As the cells migrate upwardly in the crypt, mean cell volume decreases; they become more columnar, and the polarization of cellular functions becomes evident. RER is more prominent at the base of the cell, and many of the Golgi stacks are relegated to their supranuclear location. Mucin granule density increases, and the apical granule mass coalesces (Fig. 4C). As cells move to the surface epithelium, the cell volume continues to decrease to an average of 542 mm³, less than 50% of its original volume, with a proportionate decrease in organelle components. The "stem" of the goblet cell becomes well defined and contact with the basal lamina continues to diminish (Fig. 4D). Upon reaching extrusion zones (33), the villus tips, or the colonic surface, the cell loses contact with the basal lamina and is exfoliated, releasing all cellular contents into the intestinal lumen.

The dramatic reorganization of the goblet cell from differentiation to death is accomplished in 3 to 4 days (29) by the baseline secretion of mucin granules (32). Throughout the cell life span, granules continually arise from the Golgi stacks and are transported to the cell apex, trapping cytoplasm and organelles between them. As granules are secreted and subjacent granules move apically, the trapped fragments are shed into the crypt lumen (32,34,35). This loss results in a profound remodeling of goblet cells.

Cytoarchitectural Organization

Mature goblet cells contain a pronounced cytoskeletal component. A dense network of intermediate filaments (IFs) is found from the cell base to the apex. This network, as in other epithelial cells, is comprised of keratin filaments and is presumed to be the structural component of the cytoskeleton; neither loss of secretory granules (36) nor elimination of other elements (37,38) perturbs goblet cell shape.

Microtubules (MTs) are also found in both the stem and cup, or theca, of the goblet cell. In the supranuclear region of the cell, MTs are seen to orient parallel, rather than perpendicular, to the longitudinal axis of the cell (38). Due to the density of organelles in this region, they maintain close proximity to the cell's synthetic machinery. MTs from the basal aspect of the cell course into the apical region and become part of the highly defined theca (39).

Actin filaments are sparsely present in the supranuclear region of goblet cells (40). Unlike enterocytes, goblet cells do not present an apical terminal web dense with actin-containing microvilli (40) but have few short microvilli (41). In addition, they have a cortical layer of actin filaments that forms a physical barrier between the granule mass and the apical plasma membrane (37,42).

Surrounding the apical granule mass is the theca, a highly defined cytoskeletal network (Fig. 5). The outermost layer is composed of bundles of IFs that encircle the cell like the hoops of a barrel. Immediately within this layer is a second layer of IFs that spiral around the apical granule mass and delimit the base of the theca, forming the cup-like shape. The innermost layer is comprised of 45 to 50 vertically oriented MTs that traverse the base of the theca. It is the MT component that directly contacts the peripheral mucin granules in the apical granule mass (39).

In mature cells, mucin granules are tightly apposed to each other, with very little intervening cytoplasm located in the angular spaces produced by multiple granule appositions. This very close packing of granules results in contact facets that are distinguished in freeze-fracture by the exclusion of intramembrane particles. The membranes of adjacent granules may appear as pentalaminar "prefusion" structures or as trilaminar, shared unit membrane structures. Groups of smaller granules are found just above the base of the theca. These granules, presumably newly formed, also form pentalaminar contacts and may coalesce here to form larger granules (43).

Secretion

Baseline Secretion

Under unstimulated conditions, goblet cells continually synthesize and secrete mucin granules into the external milieu. In the absence of added secretagogues, mucosal explants of both human and rat colon continually incorporate radiolabeled precursors into mucin glycoproteins, which are packaged into granules, transported to the cell surface, and secreted (37,38,44,45). Baseline granule turnover results from the preferential movement, as demonstrated by autoradiography (46), and secretion, as demonstrated by scanning electron microscopy (41), of mucin granules along the periphery of the apical granule mass.

Both MTs and actin filaments function in the maintenance of the baseline secretory pathway. MTs interact with Golgi elements in the supranuclear region and, as the innermost elements of the theca, contact peripheral

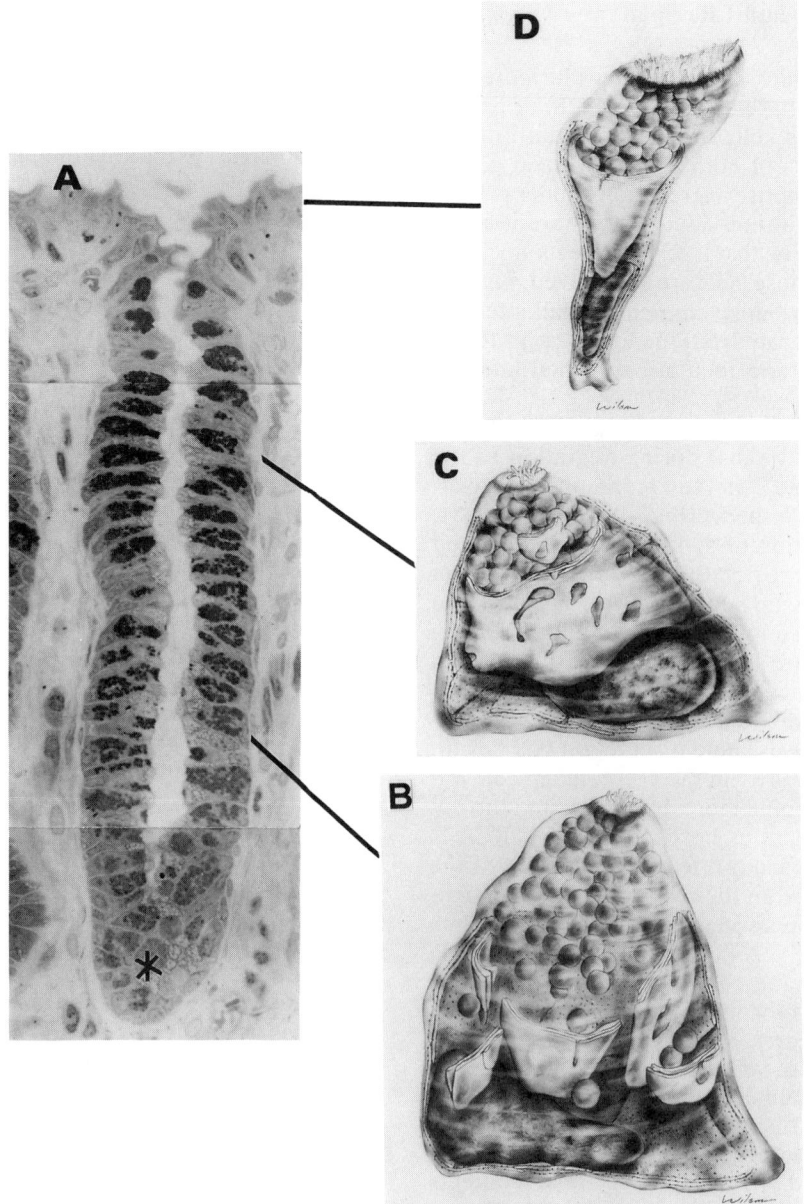

FIG. 4. Maturation of colonic goblet cells during migration to the epithelial surface. **A:** Light micrograph of rabbit colonic crypt. The colonic crypt contains two predominant cell types: dark-staining goblet cells and light-staining vacuolated cells. Progenitor cells reside in the crypt base(*), and the crypt lumen communicates with the intestinal lumen that contacts the surface cells. **B:** Schematic representation of colonic goblet cell in the lower one-third of the crypt. The cell demonstrates a pyramidal shape with little luminal contact. The RER is spread throughout the cell and numerous Golgi stacks are present. These elements intermingle with the mucin secretory granules filling the cytoplasm. **C:** Schematic representation of colonic goblet cell in the upper one-third of the crypt. The cell remains pyramidal but has reduced its cell volume. RER is concentrating along the basolateral aspects of the cell. The Golgi stacks are coalescing centrally in the cell, and the mucin granules are becoming more tightly packed. **D:** Schematic representation of colonic goblet cell on the epithelial surface. The basal region of the cell has narrowed, and luminal contact is greater than basal lamina contact. The organelles have become well ordered; the Golgi apparatus has coalesced in the supranuclear region, and RER surrounds the nucleus and Golgi along the periphery of the cell. The apical granule mass is tightly packed. (From ref. 32, with permission.)

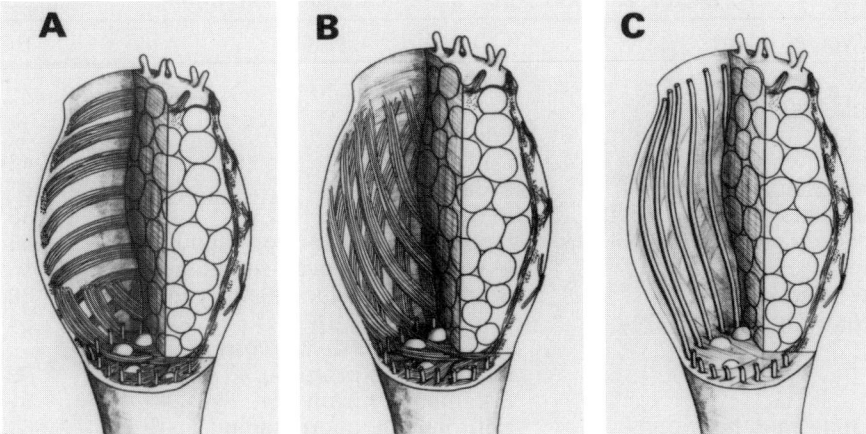

FIG. 5. Schematic representation of the theca of a colonic goblet cell. **A:** The outermost layer of the theca consists of intermediate filament bundles that girdle the apical granule mass. **B:** The middle layer is comprised of bundles of IFs that spiral around the apical granule mass like a basket and delimit the base of the theca. **C:** The inner layer consists of vertically oriented MTs immediately adjacent to the peripheral mucin granules. The MTs arise below the theca and cross the IF network at the base of the theca. (From ref. 39, with permission.)

granules in the apical granule mass (38,39) and spatially maintain the orderly baseline movement of mucin granules. MT depolymerization dramatically inhibits movement of mucin granules from the supranuclear region and along the apical granule mass. Disorganization of MTs in the supranuclear region by a tubulin polymerizing agent, taxol, impedes movement of mucin granules from the Golgi through the base of the theca. Normal MT density and orientation, however, are maintained in the theca; once granules enter the apical granule mass and contact these MTs, granule movement is unaffected.

Although actin is a minor component of the goblet cell cytoskeleton, it plays a substantial role in baseline secretion. For exocytosis to occur, the granule membrane must first contact the apical plasma membrane, requiring access to the plasma membrane across the cortical layer of actin filaments. Elimination of this layer by treatment with cytochalasins dramatically increases baseline movement of granules, but cavitation of the apical granule mass, suggesting secretion of centrally located granules, does not occur. These results suggest that baseline secretion of peripheral granules is solely dependent on access to the plasma membrane, and movement of granules through the apical granule mass is regulated by the rate of secretion. Central granules, even with elimination of the actin barrier, do not secrete and appear to require another signal for exocytosis to occur (37).

Accelerated Secretion

When exposed to a mucin secretagogue, goblet cells undergo an accelerated secretory event. In contrast to baseline secretion, it is initiated by the preferential exocytosis of centrally stored mucin granules. This is followed by compound exocytosis of granules that proceeds into the center of the apical granule mass, ultimately re-

cruiting peripheral granules until all granules stored within the theca have been secreted (36). This is a rapid event, the cell emptying its mucin granules in as little as 5 to 15 min.

Not all goblet cells respond equally to a secretory stimulus. When exposed to acetylcholine or cholinomimetic agents, crypt goblet cells respond more strongly than do those on the villi or surface (36,47–50). More than 75% of total mucin stored in crypt goblet cells is secreted, whereas only 25% to 30% of villus-stored mucin is secreted (48,50). It is remarkable that after removal of the stimulus, these cells rapidly resynthesize mucin granules and refill, returning to baseline stored mucin levels in less than 2 hr (50).

A wide variety of agents can alter mucin output by the epithelium (Table 2). For example, goblet cells respond to various luminal flora (21,51,52) and their toxins or other exoproducts (53,54) by increasing mucin secretion. Agents that are part of the natural defense system may also stimulate mucin secretion, including secretory products of macrophages and monocytes (55–59) and leukocytes (60). Inflammatory agents, such as prostaglandins (61), which are elaborated by a variety of cells, are also secretagogues. Agents that activate protein kinase C (61), increase intracellular calcium (61), or cyclic adenosine monophosphate (cAMP) (54) also stimulate mucin secretion. More extensive reviews of mucin secretagogues and their mechanisms are provided in refs. 14, 21, and 62.

Current research suggests that goblet cell responses to secretagogues may partially be inhibited. Treatment of mucin-producing colonic cell cultures with interferon-γ (63,64) or coincubation with *Helicobacter pylori* (65) decreases the secretory response of these cells to secretagogues such as cholera toxin or adenosine triphosphate (ATP). These agents, however, do not inhibit the baseline secretion of mucin. Indeed, no agents capable of abolishing baseline secretion have been reported to date.

TABLE 2. *Agents that stimulate/inhibit secretion*

Type of agent	Name	References
Stimulators		
Cholinergic agents	Acetylcholine	36, 58
	Pilocarpine	47, 50
	Carbachol	48, 49
Arachidonic acid metabolites	Prostaglandin E$_2$	61
Macrophage/monocyte products	Histamine	58
	Monocyte-derived secretagogue	56
	Macrophage-derived secretagogue	55, 57, 59
Leukocyte products	Neutrophil-derived secretagogue	60
Bacteria and exoproducts	Cholera toxin	54
	Pseudomonas aeruginosa	
	Elastase and protease	53
Parasites	*Entamoeba histolytica*	51
Neuropeptides and hormones	Neurotensin, neuromedin N	66
	Vasoactive intestinal peptide	61
Chemical irritants	Mustard oil	58
Inhibitors		
Bacteria and exoproducts	*Helicobacter pylori*	65
Cytokines	Interferon-γ	63, 64

Other Products of Goblet Cells

Although the major secretory products of goblet cells are mucins, other secreted proteins with potential bioregulatory activity have been described. These products may be copackaged into granules and released into the intestinal lumen during baseline or accelerated secretion. For example, goblet cells produce and secrete at least two serine proteases. One of these, termed ingobsin, has been localized in duodenal goblet cells in humans and rats, but little is present in secretory granules (67). Its secretion is, however, stimulated by infusion of acetylcholine, a mucin secretagogue (68). The second, kallikrein, is localized in the colonic goblet cells of humans and cats and is found within mucin granules and in the mucus overlying the epithelial surface (69). Although there is no reported function of these proteases, they probably either modulate the bioactivity of other luminal constituents or assist in removal of mucins by cleaving them into smaller fragments (see section on Susceptibility of Mucins to Damage).

Histochemical studies have demonstrated the presence of endogenous peroxidase activity in the RER, Golgi, and secretory granules of intestinal goblet cells (70,71). Preliminary investigations suggest that the peroxidase may be packaged and cosecreted with mucins into the intestinal lumen (72) and may function as the enzymatic component of a bactericidal system to protect the intestinal epithelium (73).

Immunocytochemical studies suggest that goblet cells may transport secretory IgA into the lumen (74). Antibodies to secretory component and IgA have been localized to the mucin granules of goblet cells in the epithelium overlying large populations of plasma cells. The conditions required for the appearance of secretory component expression in goblet cells are unknown.

Intestinal goblet cells may also produce bioactive peptides, which have been speculated to regulate mucosal growth, differentiation, and/or function. Intestinal trefoil factor (ITF), a 75 amino acid peptide and member of a cysteine-rich trefoil protein family (75), is synthesized and copackaged with mucins into secretory granules of both rat (76) and human (77,78) goblet cells. ITF has been immunolocalized in goblet cells, in the overlying mucus gel, and in columnar cells. Surprisingly, however, *in situ* hybridization revealed that messenger ribonucleic acid (mRNA) for ITF was present only within goblet cells, suggesting that the peptide may be secreted into the lumen by goblet cells and then internalized by columnar cells (77,78). Another trefoil protein, pancreatic spasmolytic polypeptide (PSP), demonstrates mitogenic activity *in vitro* (79) and the ability to regulate motility and to inhibit gastric acid secretion in rats (80), prompting speculation that ITF may have analogous feedback roles on intestinal cell function. PSP also shows resistance to digestion by luminal proteases (81), which is a distinct advantage for a putative regulatory protein in the luminal milieu. It is of interest that two frog skin mucins (FIM-A.1 and FIM-C.1) also contain multiple trefoil motifs (P domains) as integral parts of their C-terminal regions (82). Thus trefoil peptides (or domains) in mucus are likely to be important functionally and may herald a new dimension in goblet cell physiology.

PRIMARY STRUCTURE OF GASTROINTESTINAL MUCINS

Peptide Core

In purified mucins, the peptide component typically accounts for only about 20% of the dry weight, the rest consisting of carbohydrate and small amounts (2% to 3%) of sulfate. Partial complementary deoxyribonucleic acids (cDNAs) have been reported for two human intestinal mucins, MUC 2 (83–85) and MUC 3 (86), human gastric mucin, MUC 6 (87), and two rat intestinal mucins, MLP

(88–90) and M2 (RMUC 176) (91,92). Partial cDNAs are also available for two human tracheobronchial mucins, MUC 4 (93,94) and MUC 5 (95,96), and approximately six mucins of other species and organs (82,97–105). The cDNA for human MUC 1, a membrane-associated mucin of human breast, pancreas, and ovary (106,107), has been fully sequenced as has its mouse counterpart, Muc-1 (108).

Based on current information from cDNAs for human MUC 2 and MUC 3 and rat MLP and M2, intestinal apomucins are assumed to consist of three principal domains as illustrated in Fig. 1: a cysteine-rich unique N terminus of more than 800 amino acids (presumed on the basis of partial sequence information for human MUC 2); a long (but variable) extended central region arranged in the form of imperfect tandem repeats; and a folded cysteine-rich C-terminal domain of approximately 900 amino acids. In some of the membrane-associated mucins (ASGP-2, MUC 1, Muc-1), a putative transmembrane region of approximately 30 amino acids has been detected near the C terminus and a signal sequence near the N terminus. As more apomucin sequences become available, it is expected that a hydrophobic signal sequence will be recognized in all mucins and a transmembrane segment in all membrane-associated mucins.

Tandem Repeats: (TRs)

Tandem repeats are rich in proline, threonine, and/or serine (PST) and usually have a distinct consensus sequence. TRs of intestinal mucins (Fig. 6) vary from 6 (for M2) to 169 (for MUC 6) amino acids in length. Despite a similarity to MUC 2 in its C-terminal domain (85,88), rat MLP has not, as yet, been shown to possess a consensus TR motif in its central PST-rich region. The majority of serines and threonines in the TRs are probably glycosylated in all mature mucin molecules, since these residues provide attachment (acceptor) sites for N-acetyl-D-galactosamine (GalNAc), the first sugar added biosynthetically to initiate O-linked oligosaccharide branches. The six or seven flanking residues around the target hydroxy amino

acid, however, influence its acceptor function (109), particularly the presence of proline at position +3, which favors glycosylation of threonine (110).

In gastric mucin (MUC 6) the TRs are extraordinarily long (169 amino acids) (87), but they contain a lower proportion of serine plus threonine (49%) than the TRs of MUC 2 (61%), MUC 3 (71%), or M2 (66%). Since gastric mucins are as heavily glycosylated as the others, however, gastric mucins probably carry fewer but longer carbohydrate chains in each TR. Whether this influences the functional nature of the mucin gel or the susceptibility of the peptide core of gastric mucin to proteolytic enzymes has not been addressed.

Mature (glycosylated) mucins are normally not very reactive with antibodies generated against synthetic TR peptides, due to the "masking" of the latter by a "shield" of carbohydrate. However, in epithelial tumors with incomplete glycosylation, as in breast (111), ovarian (112), and colonic (113) tumor mucins, the TRs become more exposed and immunoreactive. This has both diagnostic and therapeutic implications (114).

Polymorphism

A common feature of mucin genes is that they exhibit genetic polymorphism, with allelic variations between individuals at the level of DNA and consequent protein isoforms (16,105). Variability probably arises from unequal chromosomal crossover events occurring within homologous TR regions of the genes, giving rise to a variable number of TRs (length polymorphisms), which are inherited in a stable fashion. Intestinal mucin MUC 2 is reported to contain from 40 to 115 TRs (83). If no alterations occur in the length of N- and C-terminal regions, mucin peptide isoforms are thus anticipated to vary from approximately 2600 to more than 5000 amino acids. Once glycosylated, the mucin size can be expected to range from about 1.4×10^6 to 2.5×10^6 daltons (assuming 80% carbohydrate by weight). These values correlate fairly closely with earlier biochemical determinations of the sizes of individual mucin "subunits" (115). One puzzle that has

MUCIN	LOCATION	CONSENSUS SEQUENCE
Human MUC2	Intestine, colon	PTTTPITTTTTVTPTPTPTGTQT (23 aa)
Human MUC3	Intestine, colon, gall bladder	HSTPSFTSSITTTETTS (17 aa)
Human MUC5	Stomach, lung	TTSTTSAP (8 aa)
Human MUC6	Stomach, gall bladder	169 aa per TR, rich in ser (18%), thr (31%), and pro (15%)
Rat MLP	Intestine, colon	Consensus TR not yet identified
Rat M2	Intestine, colon	TTTPDV (6 aa)

FIG. 6. TRs of the peptide core of secretory gastrointestinal mucins.

not been fully resolved is the extent of alternate splicing of mucin mRNAs. The mRNAs for human MUC 2 and rat M2, for example, exhibit significant size polydispersity in some Northern blot analyses (83,92) and very little size polydispersity in others (88,90,91). Possibly some of the apparent polydispersity can be attributed to degradation of the larger species of mucin mRNAs (>7 kb) on Northern blots.

Amino Terminal End

Sequence information is available for a region near, but not yet reaching, the N terminus of only one intestinal mucin, MUC 2 (85). This region of 775 amino acids is unique (nonrepetitive) and is much less glycosylated than the TRs. It also contains seven sites for N-linked oligosaccharides whose function is unknown. The N terminus is enriched in cysteine (10 mol %) and is therefore likely to be in a highly folded configuration. It is interesting that the N-terminal region exhibits many similarities in its sequence and cysteine distribution with the C-terminal end of the same mucin, suggesting that both ends may be suited for a common function, such as the generation of linear (end-to-end) disulfide-linked mucin polymers. As yet, no signal sequence has been reported for MUC 2.

Carboxyl Terminal End

Although the C-terminal sequence of MUC 3, MUC 6, and rat M2 are unknown, those of intestinal rat MLP and human MUC 2 have been sequenced and shown to have about 70% homology (85). They contain 869 and 845 amino acids, respectively, and are enriched in cysteine (10 mol %), with cysteine distribution patterns that are strikingly similar to those in the carboxy-terminal regions of two salivary mucins (PSM, BSM), a frog skin mucin (FIM-B.1), and the human blood clotting protein, von Willebrand factor (90). Thus a common structural motif appears to have been conserved at the C-terminal end of many mucins, in keeping with the notion that this structure subserves an important common function. Apart from a likely role in subunit polymerization (16), the S-S dependent folded regions are also required for the scavenging of oxygen radicals (see section on Susceptibility of Mucins to Damage).

In at least three membrane-associated mucins (MUC 1, Muc-1, and ASGP-2 of rat mammary ascites cell line 13762), there is a short (about 70 amino acids) cytoplasmic tail at the C terminus, which interacts with cellular cytoskeletal components, principally actin (99,116,117). Thus membrane-associated mucins may influence some aspects of cell morphology, growth, or differentiation.

In one cDNA clone (M2-798) for rat intestinal mucin M2, we have noted a sequence encoding an internal 82 amino acid hydrophobic domain (91). Since secretory mucins engage in many noncovalent hydrophobic interactions, this domain may constitute a hydrophobic "island." In another M2 clone (RMUC 176), a cysteine-rich segment of 92 amino acids has been identified (92). At

present it is unknown how the two unique segments are situated relative to each other near the C terminus of the mucin.

Expression of Mucin Genes

The genes for human mucins are not all present on the same chromosome, although human intestinal MUC 2, the lung (and gastric) mucin MUC 5, and gastric (and gallbladder) mucin MUC 6 are all clustered at the p terminus of chromosome 11 (p15.4-15.5) and thus may be members of a multigene family. Human intestinal MUC 3 is found on chromosome 7 (q22-24), and the mammary mucin gene, MUC 1, is found on chromosome 1 (q21-24). Very little is known about transcriptional regulation of mucin gene expression, although it is clear that each gene, including those that are clustered at 11 p15, has a different tissue-specific pattern of expression and is probably independently regulated (118). In normal conditions, MUC 2 is expressed predominantly in goblet cells of the intestine (jejunum and ileum) and right colon, whereas MUC 3, somewhat surprisingly, is expressed in columnar cells of the same regions (119). MUC 3 is also expressed in gallbladder. Rat MLP (120) and M2 (I. Khatri and J. Forstner, *unpublished data*) are both expressed in intestinal and colonic goblet cells, but not columnar cells. Thus the two rat genes are not strict expression homologues of human MUC 2 and MUC 3. MUC 6 is expressed in human stomach and gallbladder (87). Several colonic cancer cell lines show increased and ectopic expression of mucin genes (MUC 1, 2, 3, 4) (121,122), suggesting that some malignancy-associated factors, including connective tissue components (123), may upregulate mucin transcriptional processes. There is a growing interest in the possibility that enhanced or unusual mucin gene expression may also occur in intestinal infections (63).

Carbohydrate Structure

N-Linked Oligosaccharides

N-linked oligosaccharides are present in many mucins, but they comprise only a minor proportion of the total carbohydrate and appear to be confined mainly to the C- and N-terminal regions of the mucin molecule. In MUC 2 (85) and rat MLP (90), approximately 17 consensus sequences for N-glycosylation (asn-X-ser/thr) are present in the C-terminal region. It is not known whether all the target sequences become glycosylated during normal biosynthesis. Few compositional or structural details of the N-linked branches in mucins are known, although at least some of them in rat and human intestinal mucins must have exposed oligomannosyl residues, based on their recognition of *Escherichia coli* type 1 (mannose-sensitive) pili (124). Both hybrid and complex chains have been identified in a rodent salivary mucin (125). A physiologic function for mucin N-glycans has not been identified, although in one series of experiments, gastric mucin oligomerization was reduced by tunicamycin (126). The authors postulated that the biosynthetic addition of N-glycans to apomucins in the RER ensured the proper folding of the mucin for subsequent oligomerization and transport to the Golgi.

O-Linked Oligosaccharides

The majority of mucin oligosaccharides are of the O-glycan type, attached to the peptide TRs via an O-glycosidic linkage between the first carbon of GalNAc and the hydroxyl oxygen of threonine or serine. It is possible that this linkage is further stabilized, and the chains oriented with respect to the peptide, by a hydrogen bond between the amide group of GalNAc and the carbonyl oxygen of the threonine or serine (127) or an adjacent amino acid (128). The addition of GalNAc serves to "stiffen" the TR domain of the peptide core in an extended conformation (109,129,130). Although the O-glycans are closely packed side by side in the central TRs (Fig. 1), not all serines and threonines of each repeat are necessarily substituted, and thus the carbohydrate chains may exist in "clusters" rather than continually along the TRs (7), with intervening "naked" regions potentially vulnerable to physical or enzymatic rupture (18).

O-glycans contain GalNAc, N-acetylglucosamine (GlcNAc), fucose, galactose, and sialic acid. The chains vary in length (1 to 20 sugars), linkages (α or β), and degree of branching (131,132), all of which amplify their potential to generate different recognition sites for lectins, antibodies, and bacterial, viral, or parasite adhesins. The carbohydrate composition of mucins is heterogeneous and varies in different regions of the intestine, and even among different mucous cells of the same organ, such as the deep and superficial mucous cells of the stomach (133) or the crypt and surface goblet cells of the colon (134). A detailed review of mucin oligosaccharide structure is provided in ref. 17.

When GalNAc is transferred to serine or threonine of the nascent peptide, the Tn antigen structure is formed (Fig. 7) and other sugars are added sequentially through the concerted, interlocking actions of the multi-glycosyl transferase system of the Golgi network. Several genes for the transferases have now been cloned (135). Studies of regulatory factors governing their tissue-specific expression (136) will no doubt shed light on the normal diversity of mucin oligosaccharides and the changes in glycosylation of glycoproteins during normal development (137) and/or disease (138).

Typical core structures of mucin O-glycans consist of six different arrangements of Gal and GlcNAc bound to GalNAc (Fig. 7). The first four cores are common, particularly core 2 and core 3 in intestinal mucins. In addition to the typical cores, many mucins also express the sialosyl-Tn antigen [sialyl GalNAc], which is increased in tumor mucins (113) and mucins produced in some cases of ulcerative colitis (138). The core structures act as substrates for transferases, which add sugars one by one, and elongate the chains to produce backbone structures consisting of type 1 [Gal β1,3 GlcNAc] or type 2 [Gal

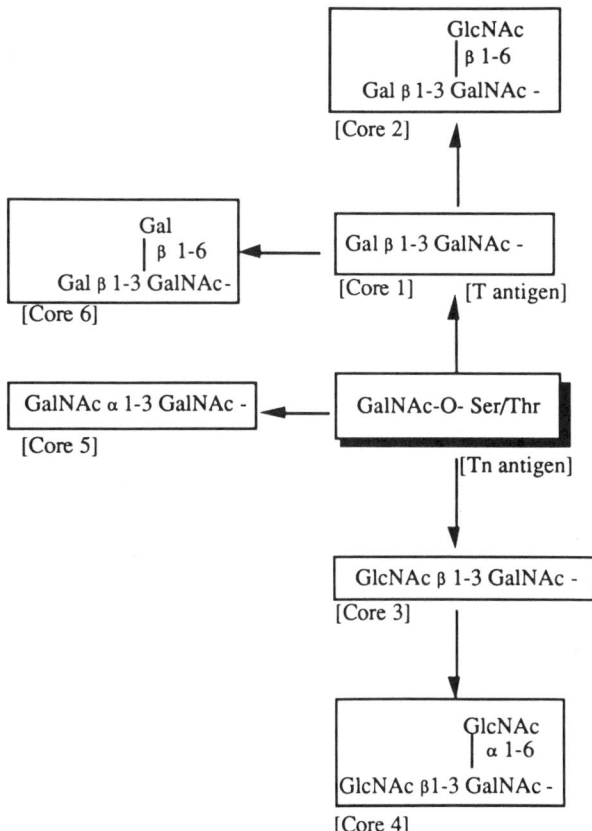

FIG. 7. O-glycan core structures. The cores are synthesized from the precursor Tn antigen by addition of galactose (Gal) and/or N-acetylglucosamine (GlcNAc). Cores 1 to 4 are most common in normal mucins.

β1,4 GlcNAc] units. The latter can be repeated or undergo branching at galactose residues by the addition of GlcNAc in β1,6 linkage. As oligosaccharide elongation proceeds, the more proximal core structures become "masked," and thus inaccessible to lectins, adhesins, or antibodies specific for them.

Peripheral sugars (fucose, galactose, GalNAc, and sialic acid) are transferred from their nucleotide sugar donors to terminal galactose residues of the backbones, as a final step in oligosaccharide synthesis. The peripheral sugars bond via α-glycosidic linkages, which stop further elongation, and give rise to the well-known ABH and Lewis blood group specificities of mucins (2). As shown several years ago (139,140), the A-, B-, or H-specific sugars can serve as nutrients for specific colonic commensals. To some extent the blood groups determine which species or strains will inhabit the human colon. Alterations of peripheral sugars occur in mucins of malignant tumors (113,138,141,142), in colonic mucins during immune responses to parasitic infestations (143), and in macrophage sialomucins as part of the response to inflammatory stimuli (144).

Peripheral sialylation is a relatively late Golgi-mediated event, and (together with sulfate) sialic acid imparts a negative charge to mucin chains. Sialic acid concentration of intestinal glycoproteins tends to be higher in the fetal and newborn period and to decrease with aging (137). Enhanced sialylation is one of the common abnormalities of tumor mucins (17).

Sulfation

Some of the peripheral or backbone residues (chiefly gal or GlcNAc) of mucin oligosaccharides acquire sulfate at the level of the Golgi membranes during biosynthesis (16). The longest or most branched chains are likely to carry the most sulfate (145). In respiratory mucins it has been shown that sulfate and sialic acid can be expressed on the same oligosaccharide, although usually on different branches (146). Most goblet cells of the gastrointestinal tract contain at least some sulfated mucin molecules, but sulfation increases from proximal to distal segments (147,148) and is highest in colonic areas that harbor high populations of fecal bacteria (149). Staining reactions with HID/alcian blue, pH 2.5, change from blue to brown-purple as the ratio of sulfate exceeds that of sialic acid in goblet cell granules (148). Mucin sulfation is decreased in ulcerative colitis (150) and increased in cystic fibrosis (151,152). To date there is no compelling evidence that bacteria, viruses, or parasites utilize sulfate residues as receptors for attachment. Indeed, the role of sulfate in mucins is thought to be one of protection against bacterial exoproducts (150,153). Gastric corpus and duodenal mucins are reported to be highly sulfated (154,155), with the suggestion that this confers protection against gastric pepsin and pancreatic proteases.

MUCIN OLIGOMERS AND GELS

Mucin Polymers

To attain viscoelastic and gel-forming properties, secretory mucin molecules must first link together to form polymers, presumably by end-to-end intermolecular disulfide bridges. Polymerization probably occurs in the RER prior to O-glycosylation (16). It is not known whether mucin polymers consist of more than one mucin peptide species (e.g., heteropolymers of MUC 2 and MUC 3) or in what orientation the subunits are assembled (head-to-head, head-to-tail, or tail-to-tail). The nature and configuration of the subunits in polymers, however, may be important determinants of the stability and quality of mucin gels. Once mucin polymers are assembled and fully glycosylated, they normally assume semiflexible "kinky" configurations, which, when extended by shearing stress and examined by electron microscopy, are seen to be extremely heterogeneous in length (156). Respiratory mucins have been particularly well studied and shown to range from 0.2 to as high as more than 10 µm in length. After reduction they decrease to 200 to 600 nm (157).

Gel Formation

Within goblet cell granules, mucin polymers are physically constrained in a highly condensed form, which tends to exclude water. Packing is enhanced by calcium ion neutralization of the fixed negative charges of sulfate and sialic acid. With secretion, polymers uncoil, Ca^{2+} diffuses outward, and the hydration volume increases explosively (158,159). The longer the polymer chain, the greater will be the radius of gyration and hydration sphere. With increasing mucin concentration, hydration spheres partially overlap, mucin "threads" intertangle, and mucin solutions become highly viscous. Strong noncovalent forces, probably hydrogen bonds (130), develop between the carbohydrates of the mucin threads, and a sol-to-gel phase transformation occurs when mucin reaches a concentration of 30 to 50 mg/mL (18). Cross-linkage of the gel structure provides considerable resistance to flow, which may explain why mucins are not completely cleared from the mucosal surface after a single fluid "flush."

Mucin gels flow slowly over the mucosal surface, creating a blanket that follows the undulations of the mucosal surface. If subjected to a strong shear stress, a mucin gel may rupture, but if left undisturbed, it will subsequently reanneal due to its intrinsic elasticity. Thus viscosity and elasticity are important properties for the continuity and stability *in vivo* of the surface mucous barrier. Gel thickness varies from about 50 to 450 µm (average 180 µm) in the human stomach and is thinner, possibly discontinuous, in the small intestine. The mucous layer is decreased by starvation (160) and increased in bacterial overgrowth (22). The gel does not cover the Peyer's patches, thus apparently does not impede the translocation of bacterial or other potentially antigenic luminal components across the bowel wall. In rat colon, the gel layer is approximately 150 µm. When epithelial tissues are injured, a thick mucoid coat (up to 1.5 µm thick in gastric lesions) develops over the site of injury. The coat is not simply a mucin gel; it is a gel-like "cap" comprised of mucin, fibrin, and necrotic cells, and it permits the rapid reepithelialization that constitutes repair of the underlying tissue (18).

Lubricant properties of mucin gels are important, but the physicochemical basis is not well understood. It can be assumed that to reduce frictional coefficients at mucosal surfaces, mucins, like other lubricants (161), have the ability to adhere to the mucosa as well as to spread over it. Hydrophobic interactions involving carbohydrates (162) may play a role in mucin adherence to the mucosa (or to particulate matter in the lumen), although the level of hydration of the mucin layer may be more critical to its functional adhesivity (158,163). The ability of mucin to spread over the mucosa probably depends on anionic charge repulsion (therefore sulfate and sialic acid) as well as repulsive hydration forces in the gel (161).

Nonmucin components that can be incorporated into the mucin gel include proteoglycans, lipids, electrolytes, DNA, and serum proteins [immunoglobulin A (IgA), lysozyme, albumin] (163,164). Some of these compounds may enhance the adhesivity of mucous secretions, but they also tend to produce weaker gels than those formed exclusively by mucin molecules. Thus mucous gels that form under inflammatory conditions or in regions of high cell sloughing may be "mixed" gels, which are more vulnerable to disruption by acid, detergents (bile), and denaturants (164).

SUSCEPTIBILITY OF MUCINS TO DAMAGE

Both the peptide core and the oligosaccharides of intestinal mucins are fragmented and then completely degraded by enzymes liberated into the lumen from normal host tissues and colonic bacteria (Fig. 8). Mucin degradation is thus a normal physiologic process. In addition, however, many pathogens, as well as host cells recruited for defense during inflammatory processes, elaborate enzymes that are mucolytic. An excess of these enzymes can alter the dynamic equilibrium between mucin production and degradation to cause a structural weakening of the protective mucous gel layer. Some of the sites on mucin molecules that have been recognized as particularly sensitive to damage are discussed below and are highlighted schematically in Fig. 8.

Peptide Cleavage

As deduced from cDNAs for human MUC 2 (85), rat MLP (90), and several other mucins, the C-terminal domains (but not the TRs) contain many lysine and arginine residues, as well as aromatic residues such as phenylalanine, tyrosine, and tryptophan. Thus these domains, and probably the N-terminal domains as well, are highly sensitive to proteolytic rupture by host and pathogen serine proteases. Experimental studies support this conclusion, since mucins are readily fragmented by digestion with serine proteases without any loss of carbohydrate (7,8,18,165–167). The enzymes cleave poorly glycosylated ("naked") peptide segments, and this disrupts the continuity of the linear polymers. There is a consequent dramatic reduction in molecular mass, viscoelasticity, and polymer length. Proteases capable of attacking mucins are produced in salivary, gastric, intestinal, and pancreatic tissues. Serine proteases detected in Paneth cells (168), duodenal goblet cells (67,68,169), and colonic enterocytes (69) might also be expected to act on mucins. Fecal bacteria elaborate a mixture of proteinases (167,170), although serine proteases cause the major damage to mucin structure.

In vivo, some protection of mucins against luminal proteases may be afforded by weak interactions of mucins with nonmucin components such as proteins, constituents of bile, anionic proteoglycans, lipids, and products of sloughed cells (2,16,18,164,171–173). It is also likely that

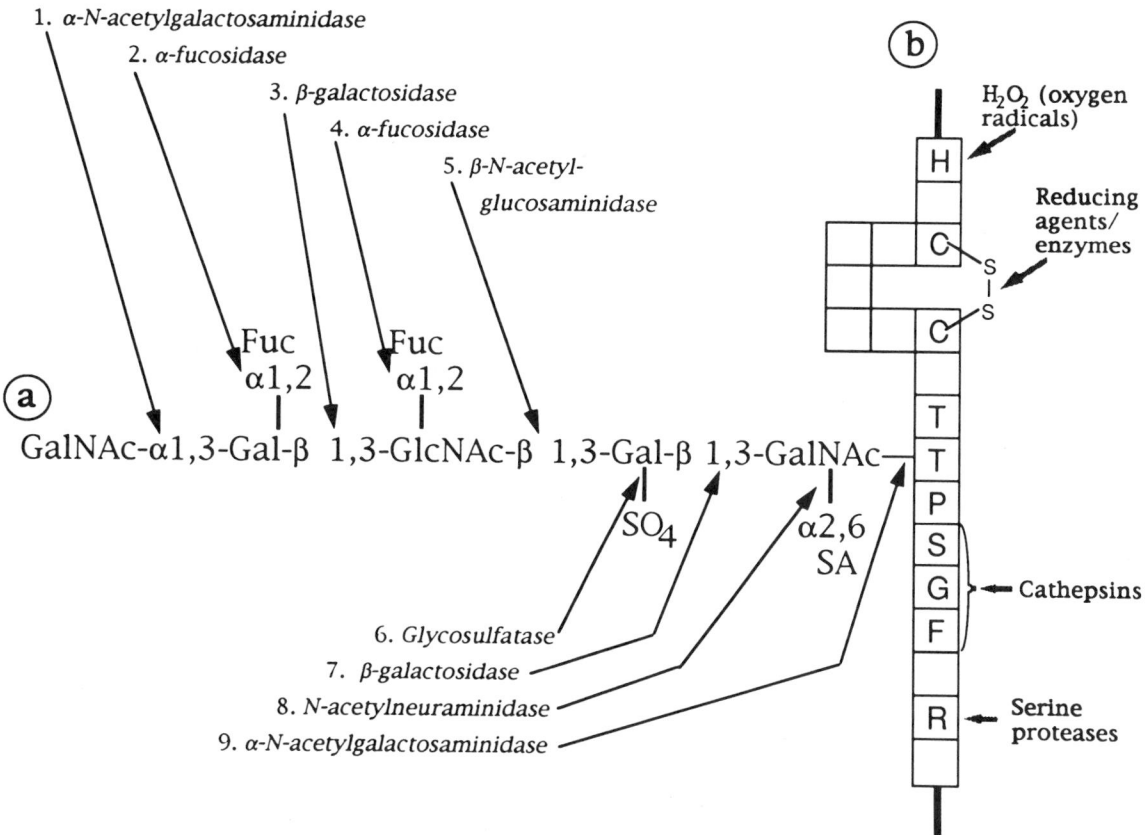

FIG. 8. Degradation of intestinal mucin. **a:** A hypothetical mucin oligosaccharide to show the sequential action of bacterial exoglycosidases and glycosulfatase. **b:** A portion of the polypeptide core to show amino acids (*squares*) vulnerable to chemical and enzymatic rupture. H, histidine; T, threonine; S, serine; P, proline; R, arginine; F, phenylalanine; G, glycine; C, cysteine. Many serine proteases of bacterial and host epithelial cells are mucolytic.

the normally folded state of the mucin peptide near the cysteine-rich termini "buries" some protease-sensitive regions, which only become vulnerable after disulfide bonds are ruptured (174).

During conventional purification procedures, mucins are exquisitely sensitive to the action of proteinases. For example, once the sequence of porcine submaxillary mucin was available from isolated cDNAs, it was realized that traditional purification procedures resulted in the loss of a long C-terminal domain of the mucin (98). Purification of human and rat intestinal mucins, even in the presence of three proteinase inhibitors, routinely allowed the "nicking" of a particular aspartyl–proline bond located in the C-terminal domain (92) and the liberation of a 118-kDa C-terminal glycopeptide previously called the "link" glycopeptide (175). Generally, aspartyl–proline bonds in proteins are sensitive to heating in the presence of acids (176), but since acidic conditions are not used during mucin purification, this is unlikely to be the cause of cleavage at these sites. A similar aspartyl–proline sequence, including many of the flanking residues, is also present in a rat ascites tumor sialomucin called pSMC-1. In this case the aspartyl–proline bond is cleaved enzymatically during the normal biosynthetic maturation of the mucin, allowing for the separation of the mucin into a 120-kDa membrane domain, ASGP-2, and a larger secreted component, ASGP-1 (99).

Various pathogens secrete proteases, some of which have been shown to affect mucins. For example, *H. pylori* secrete a mucin protease that is thought by some investigators (177,178), but debated by others (179), to increase the movement of the organism through the mucus gel to the gastric cells. *Vibrio cholerae* secrete a potent zinc-dependent metalloproteinase that lowers mucin viscosity and facilitates penetration of the enterotoxin to its GM1 ganglioside receptor on cell membranes (180). The mucus barrier may be damaged in inflammatory bowel disease by fecal proteinases, which are increased as a result of an alteration in the normal resident bacterial populations (181,182). Additionally, it is highly likely that inflammation itself contributes to mucin damage by the action of neutrophil proteases (183), mast cell proteases (184,185), and proteases of other inflammatory cells.

Reducing agents damage disulfide bonds that stabilize the tertiary structure of mucins, and these agents are widely recognized to be capable of destroying mucin polymers and collapsing mucin gels (8). Although specific bacterial reductases for these bonds have not been identified, reductases and glutathione are produced by colonic flora and host cells, and one might expect that they contribute to mucin depolymerization. Thiols in secretions also activate cathepsins, which can damage mucin peptide (186).

Mucins of stomach and bile have been shown to act as scavengers of oxygen radicals, thereby protecting the mucosa from damage by these agents (171,187,188). Mucin structure is compromised in the process, since a marked reduction in mucin viscosity occurs with oxygen radicals (171). The antioxidant function of mucin is probably associated with the rupture of histidine residues in the core peptide, since earlier studies revealed that hydrogen peroxide damages this amino acid (189,190). The effect depended on the presence of Cu^{2+} (or Fe^{2+}), suggesting that an oxidation–reduction reaction is involved. Since the C-terminal 850 (approximately) amino acid domain of two intestinal mucins (MUC 2 and MLP) contain at least ten histidine residues, it is likely that the C-terminal domain is involved in the antioxidant function. It is of interest, however, that the TRs of the gastric mucin MUC 6 also contain a rather high proportion (7.1 mol %) of histidine (87), leading to the speculation that they may also be damaged by hydrogen peroxide or its oxidation products.

Loss of Carbohydrate

Mucin oligosaccharides are degraded in a stepwise manner by the sequential removal of carbohydrates in a direction from the periphery to the internal core nearest the peptide linkage as shown schematically in Fig. 8. Specific subpopulations of normal colonic flora elaborate the required exoglycosidases (140,182,191–195). Host mucins can also induce or regulate the expression of at least some of the enzymes required for mucin deglycosylation (170,193,196,197). Mucolytic exoglycosidases, including neuraminidases (181,182) and blood-group-specific exoglycosidases (198), are increased in intestinal inflammation and/or infection. The importance of these enzymes as virulence determinants, however, is largely speculative. Antibiotics decrease mucin degradation and alter mucin composition to resemble that of mucins found in the germ-free state (192). A novel endoglycosidase has been described in a strain of *Streptomyces* and is expressed when the bacteria are grown in media containing mucin. The enzyme cleaves the O-glycosidic linkage between GalNAc and ser/thr to release the disaccharide Gal β1,3 GalNAc or a tetrasaccharide Gal β1-3 [Gal β1,4–GlcNAc β1,6] GalNAc (199). As mucin peptides become progressively deglycosylated, they are rendered more sensitive to rupture by proteolytic enzymes. Thus the alternating activities of bacterial (and host) glycosidases and proteases gradually degrade mucin macromolecules. Bacterial glycosulfatases (197) participate by removing sulfate from its attachment to galactose, GlcNAc, or GalNAc of the oligosaccharides. Since sulfate is thought to decrease the rate of mucin damage by glycosidases and proteases, those pathogens that elaborate sulfatases may accelerate mucin fragmentation. For example, a glycosulfatase purified from *H. pylori* (177,200) may play a role in degrading mucus, thus exposing the gastric mucosa to ulceration (201). In the same fashion, decreased mucin sulfate (150) and an increase in colonic sulfatases (198,202) by *Bacteroides* species may be important in perpetuating mucosal damage associated with chronic ulcerative colitis.

Mechanical Rupture

A heightened sensitivity to shear forces marks mucin gels as being different from the highly structured gels of alginate, agarose, gelatin, or other conventional gels. During purification and handling, mucin polymers are very easily broken (shortened) by shear forces (homogenization) (5). In a physiologic context mucin gel fragility is an asset, since *in vivo* mucin gels must be deformed and made to flow by the mild shearing forces of peristalsis and the waving motions of intestinal villi.

Mechanical fragility may be a factor in a recently described *in vitro* phenomenon termed "viscous fingering." In this process, hydrochloric acid injected through solutions of pig gastric mucin produced viscous fingering patterns dependent on pH, mucin concentration, and acid flow rate. HCl secreted by the gastric glands may thus penetrate the mucous gel layer (pH 5 to 7) through narrow fingers, whereas HCl in the lumen (pH 2) is prevented from diffusing back to the epithelium by the high viscosity of gastric mucous gel on the luminal side (203). Although acid-secreting channels have been observed *in vivo* in the adherent gastric mucous gel layer (204), it has been questioned (18) how the absence of viscous fingering in mucus below pH 4 *in vitro* is compatible with acid secretion through mucus *in vivo*.

MUCIN STRUCTURE–FUNCTION RELATIONSHIP

Consideration of the structural entities of mucin macromolecules in this chapter provides a basis for understanding the putative functions listed in Table 1. TRs or equivalent regions rich in serine and/or threonine serve as a scaffold for the attachment of numerous oligosaccharide chains. In turn, the abundant carbohydrates shield the long peptide cores and provide the necessary hygroscopic properties to permit formation of well-hydrated gels. The variable lengths of mucin core peptides and the heterogeneity of their oligosaccharide chains, however, probably serve to prevent the development of excessively rigid gel network structures and thus aid the spreading action of mucin gels over mucosal surfaces. Since most gastrointestinal mucins contain abundant sulfate and sialic acid within their oligosaccharide side chains, they offer appropriate sites for cation binding. Thus luminal mucins may help to screen ingested toxic heavy metals, drugs, and other cationic chemicals from gaining access to internal organs. The basis of the antioxidant role of mucins is not entirely clear but may involve the rupture of histidine residues in poorly glycosylated, folded regions at the termini of the peptide cores. Peroxidase activity associated with mucin granules in goblet cells may play an adjunctive role. In their disulfide-linked polymer forms, gastric mucins aggregate and form a continuous adherent gel over the gastric epithelium. As long as the gel structure remains intact, it provides a physical barrier and a stable unstirred layer largely resistant to luminal acid and hypertonic salt solutions. Bicarbonate secretions from underlying cells alkalinize the adherent gel layer and provide a further defense against potentially damaging hydrogen ion back-diffusion (the mucus–bicarbonate barrier). Mucins are also important as a first line of defense of the large intestine against a wide range of microorganisms. Many adhere by lectin-like adhesions to specific carbohydrate configurations within mucin oligosaccharides or are physically trapped in mucous gels. Provided mucous "flushing"

rates exceed bacterial colonization rates and mucin proteolytic degradation, the offending organisms are rapidly eliminated.

The present chapter has dealt mainly with secreted mucins, rather than membrane-attached mucins. The latter appear at present to be more important in tumor biology than in infections and are characterized by the possession of a short transmembrane segment near the C-terminal end of their core peptides. Examples include human MUC 1, mouse Muc-1, and mouse mammary sialomucin, ASGP-2. Through interactions of their short C-terminal cytoplasmic tails with cellular actin, the membrane mucins may have the potential to influence phosphorylation or other processes required for secretion, tumor cell adhesion, and/or growth. Mechanistic explanations for these functions are currently under investigation. No similar functions have as yet been ascribed to secreted mucins, but recent observations that cysteine-rich trefoil proteins are associated with mucins in goblet cells, or that trefoil motifs comprise an integral part of the mucin core peptide in some cases, raise the interesting (but unsubstantiated) possibility that secreted mucins might also participate in bioregulation, perhaps by a quasi-hormonal influence on cell mitogenesis or the response of epithelial cells to growth factors.

FUTURE DIRECTIONS

Extraordinary progress has been made during the last 6 years in elucidating the primary structure of mucus glycoproteins. Although many details are incomplete, the arrangement of the peptide domains within the basic mucin subunit makes clear, for the first time, how mucin molecules are constructed to facilitate polymer formation and sol-to-gel transformations. The existence of more than one mucin per organ is now firmly established, suggesting that the final secreted product of mucus cells is likely to consist of a heterogeneous mixture of mucin macromolecules. Equally impressive are demonstrations that mucins are not inert compounds but participate actively in the events of infection and inflammation. This is in part because they are recognition molecules and provide a diverse array of potential receptors for the attachment of microorganisms. A secretory response of goblet cells to a host of exogenous factors suggests that mucins may, in some circumstances, aggravate the infectious process, and in others create a more protective layer at the mucosal surface. The mechanisms involved in signal transduction and cytoskeletal changes, which regulate mucin granule movement through goblet cells, are important areas to pursue. It is safe to predict that the next few years will bring significant advances in this field.

Other pressing topics for future research include the structure and roles of cysteine-rich and hydrophobic subdomains of mucin polypeptides. With the tools of recombinant DNA and the ever-increasing knowledge of specific amino acid sequences in mucins, it should be possible to learn exactly how mucin subunits interact with each other during polymerization, with oxygen radicals during inflammation, and with bacterial exoenzymes and other mucolytic toxins. Interaction of mucins with lymphocytes is already an active area of research in tumor immunology and will no doubt shed increasing light on the way in which mucins participate in host defenses against infectious agents.

Knowledge is still rudimentary concerning the possible alterations of tissue-specific regulation of mucin gene expression and glycosylation by infectious agents and/or inflammatory cells. However, appropriate nucleotide probes for mucin mRNAs and the mRNAs encoding specific glycosyl transferases are now ready for application to animal and cell culture models of intestinal infections. The blueprint for approaching this field has, in some measure, already been provided by the strategies used to investigate mucin epitopes and altered gene expression during growth and differentiation of mucus-producing adenocarcinoma cells. It is anticipated that advances in the techniques for detailed carbohydrate analyses will allow correlations to be recognized between virulence determinants, mucin gene expression, and altered mucin receptors for microorganisms.

ACKNOWLEDGMENTS

The authors acknowledge financial support for this research from the Canadian Medical Research Council and the Canadian Cystic Fibrosis Foundation, and assistance in the photographic reproduction of figures by Dr. Robert Specian, Department of Cellular Biology and Anatomy, Louisiana State University Medical Center, Shreveport, Louisiana.

REFERENCES

1. Forstner GG, Forstner JF. Structure and function of gastrointestinal mucus. In: Desnuelle P, Sjöström H, Norén O, eds. *Molecular and cellular basis of digestion.* Amsterdam: Elsevier Science Publishers, 1986;125–143.
2. Neutra MR, Forstner JF. Gastrointestinal mucus synthesis, secretion and function. In: LR Johnson, ed. *Physiology of the gastrointestinal tract,* 2nd ed. New York: Raven Press, 1987; 975–1009.
3. Allen A, Hoskins LC. Colonic mucus in health and disease. In: Kisner R, Shorter RG, eds. *Diseases of the colon and rectum.* Baltimore: Williams & Wilkins, 1988;65–94.
4. Roussel P, Lamblin G, L'hermitte M, et al. The complexity of mucins. *Biochimie* 1988;70:1471–1482.
5. Carlstedt I, Sheehan K. Structure and macromolecular properties of mucus glycoproteins. *Monogr Allergy* 1988;24:16–24.
6. Harding SE. The macrostructure of mucus glycoproteins in solution. *Adv Carbohydr Chem Biochem* 1989;47:345–381.
7. Carlstedt I, Sheehan JK. Structure and macromolecular properties of cervical mucus glycoproteins. In: Chantler E, Ratcliffe NA, eds. *Mucus and related topics,* vol 43. Cambridge: Society for Experimental Biology, 1989;289–315.
8. Allen A, Hutton DA, Pearson JP, Sellers LA. The colonic mucus gel barrier: structure, gel formation and degradation. In: Peters TJ, ed. *The cell biology of inflammation in the gastrointestinal tract.* Hull, UK: Corners Publications, 1990;113–125.
9. Lundgren JD, Shelhamer JH. Pathogenesis of airway mucus hypersecretion. *J Allergy Clin Immunol* 1990;85:399–417.
10. Gendler SJ, Spicer AP, Lalani EN, et al. Structure and biology of a carcinoma-associated mucin, MUC 1. *Am Rev Respir Dis* 1991;144:S42–S47.
11. Bhavanandan VP. Cancer-associated mucins and mucin-type glycoproteins. *Glycobiology* 1991;1:493–503.
12. Hilkens J, Ligtenberg MJL, Vos HL, Litvinov SV. Cell membrane-associated mucins and their adhesion-modulating property. *Trends Biochem Sci* 1992;17:359–363.
13. Schachter H, Brockhausen I. The biosynthesis of serine (threonine)-N-acetylgalactosamine-linked carbohydrate moieties. In: Allen HJ, Kisailus EC, eds. *Glycoconjugates. composition, structure and function.* New York: Marcel Dekker, 1992; 263–332.
14. Rose MC. Mucins: structure, function and role in pulmonary diseases. *Am J Physiol* 1992;263:L413–L429.
15. Carraway KL, Hall SR. Cell surface mucin-type glycoproteins and mucin-like domains. *Glycobiology* 1991;1:131–138.
16. Strous GJ, Dekker J. Mucin-type glycoproteins. *Crit Rev Biochem Mol Biol* 1992;27:57–92.
17. Brockhausen I. Clinical aspects of glycoprotein synthesis. *Crit Rev Clin Sci* 1993;30:65–151.
18. Allen A, Pearson JP. Mucus glycoproteins of the normal gastrointestinal tract. *Eur J Gastroenterol Hepatol* 1993;5:193–199.
19. Allen A, Hutton DA, Leonard AJ, Pearson JP, Sellers LA. The role of mucin in the protection of the gastroduodenal mucosa. *Scand J Gastroenterol Suppl* 1986;21(125):71–77.
20. Cepinskas G, Specian RD, Kvietys PR. Adaptive cytoprotection in the small intestine—role of mucus. *Am J Physiol* 1993; 264:G921–G927.
21. Tse SK, Chadee K. The interaction between intestinal mucus glycoproteins and enteric infections. *Parasitol Today* 1991;7: 163–172.
22. Sherman P, Fleming N, Forstner J, Roomi N, Forstner G. Bacteria and the mucus blanket in experimental small bowel bacterial overgrowth. *Am J Pathol* 1987;126:527–534.
23. Sherr HP, Mertens BR, Broock R. Cholera toxin-induced glycoprotein secretion in rabbit small intestine. *Gastroenterology* 1979;77:18–25.
24. Sabinski F, Wosiewitz U, Leuschner U. Mucin-like high molecular mass protein fractions from total pig gallbladder bile mucus, pig gallbladder wall mucus, and total human gallbladder bile mucus. *Eur J Clin Chem Clin Biochem* 1992;30:753–759.
25. Yamasaki T, Nakayama F, Tamura S, Masahiko E. Characterization of mucin in the hepatic bile of patients with intrahepatic pigment stones. *J Gastroenterol Hepatol* 1992;7:36–41.
26. Smith BF. Gallbladder mucin as a pronucleating agent for cholesterol monohydrate crystals in bile. *Hepatology* 1990;11: 183S–188S.
27. Malet PF, Deng SQ, Soloway RD. Gallbladder mucin and cholesterol and pigment gallstone formation in hamsters. *Scand J Gastroenterol* 1989;24:1055–1060.
28. Cheng H, Leblond CP. Origin, differentiation and renewal of the four main epithelial cell types in the mouse small intestine. V. Unitarian theory of the origin of the four epithelial cell types. *Am J Anat* 1974;141:537–562.
29. Cheng H. Origin, differentiation and renewal of the four main epithelial cell types in the mouse small intestine II. Mucous cells. *Am J Anat* 1974;141:481–502.
30. Ponder BAJ, Schmidt GH, Wilkinson MM, Wood MJ, Monk M, Reid A. Derivation of mouse intestinal crypts from single progenitor cells. *Nature* 1985;313:689–691.
31. Merzel J, Leblond CP. Origin and renewal of goblet cells in the epithelium of the mouse small intestine. *Am J Anat* 1969; 124:281–306.
32. Radwin KA, Oliver MG, Specian RD. Cytoarchitectural reorganization of rabbit colonic goblet cells during baseline secretion. *Am J Anat* 1990;189:365–376.
33. Schmidt GH, Wilkinson MM, Ponder BAJ. Cell migration pathway in the intestinal epithelium: an *in situ* marker system using mouse aggregation chimeras. *Cell* 1985;40:425–429.
34. Trier JS. Studies on small intestinal crypt epithelium. I. The fine structure of the crypt epithelium of the proximal small intestine of fasting humans. *J Cell Biol* 1963;18:599–620.
35. Ichikawa M, Ichikawa A, Kidokoro S. Secretory process of mucus-secreting cells in mouse colonic mucosa studies by rapid freezing-substitution. *J Electron Microsc* 1987;36(3):117–127.
36. Specian RD, Neutra MR. Mechanism of rapid mucus secretion

in goblet cells stimulated by acetylcholine. *J Cell Biol* 1980;85: 626–640.

37. Oliver MG, Specian RD. Cytoskeleton of intestinal goblet cells: role of actin filaments in baseline secretion. *Am J Physiol* 1990; 259:G991–G997.

38. Oliver MG, Specian RD. Cytoskeleton of intestinal goblet cells: role of microtubules in baseline secretion. *Am J Physiol* 1991; 260:G850–G857.

39. Specian RD, Neutra MR. Cytoskeleton of intestinal goblet cells in rabbit and monkey. The theca. *Gastroenterology* 1984;87: 1313–1325.

40. Hagen SJ, Trier JS. Immunocytochemical localization of actin in epithelial cells of rat small intestine by light and electron microscopy. *J Histochem Cytochem* 1988;360:717–727.

41. Specian RD, Neutra MR. The surface topography of the colonic crypt in rabbit and monkey. *Am J Anat* 1981;160:461–472.

42. Sandoz D, Nicholas G, Laine MC. Two mucous cell types revisited after quick freezing and cryosubstitution. *Biol Cell* 1985; 54:79–88.

43. Neutra MR, Schaeffer SF. Membrane interactions between adjacent mucous secretion granules. *J Cell Biol* 1977;74:983–991.

44. Neutra MR, Leblond CP. Synthesis of the carbohydrate of mucus in the Golgi complex as shown by electron microscope radioautography of goblet cells from rats injected with glucose-H³. *J Cell Biol* 1966;30:119–136.

45. Neutra MR, Grand RJ, Trier JS. Glycoprotein synthesis, transport, and secretion by epithelial cells of the human rectal mucosa. *Lab Invest* 1977;36:535–546.

46. Oliver MG. *The baseline secretory pathway in rabbit colonic goblet cells* [Ph.D. dissertation]. Baton Rouge: Louisiana State University, 1990.

47. Specian RD, Neutra MR. Regulation of intestinal goblet cell secretion. I. Role of parasympathetic stimulation. *Am J Physiol* 1982;242:G370–G379.

48. Phillips TE. Both crypt and villus intestinal goblet cells secrete mucin in response to cholinergic stimulation. *Am J Physiol* 1992;262:G327–G331.

49. Phillips TE, Phillips TH, Neutra MR. Regulation of intestinal goblet cell secretion. III. Isolated intestinal epithelium. *Am J Physiol* 1984;247:G674–G681.

50. Kemper AC, Specian RD. Rat small intestinal mucins: a quantitative study. *Anat Rec* 1991;229:219–226.

51. Chadee K, Keller K. *Entamoeba histolytica* stimulates mucin secretion from colonic adenocarcinoma cells by a PK C-dependent mechanism. *Gastroenterology* 1992;102:A603.

52. Rothwell TL. Immune expulsion of parasitic nematodes from the alimentary tract. *Int J Parasitol* 1989;19:139–168.

53. Kapur R, Shriniwas. Effect of *Pseudomonas aeruginosa* protease and elastase on ligated rabbit ileal loops. *Indian J Med* 1987;86:295–297.

54. Roomi N, Laburthe M, Fleming N, Crowther R, Forstner J. Cholera-induced mucin secretion from rat intestine: lack of effect of cAMP, cycloheximide, VIP, and colchicine. *Am J Physiol* 1984;247:G140–G148.

55. Aisenberg J, Sperber K, Sylvester C, Itzkowitz S, Mayer L. Macrophage-derived mucus secretagogue, a product of lamina propria macrophages, induces mucus release from normal and inflammatory bowel disease epithelium. *Gastroenterology* 1992;102:A589.

56. Marom Z, Shelhamer JH, Kaliner M. Human monocyte-derived mucus secretagogue. *J Clin Invest* 1985;75:191–198.

57. Mehra M, Sperber K, Ogata S, Mayer L, Itzkowitz SH. Mucin secretion in inflammatory bowel disease (IBD): comparison of a macrophage-derived mucin secretagogue (MMS-68) with conventional secretagogues. *Gastroenterology* 1993;104:A1052.

58. Neutra MR, O'Malley LJ, Specian RD. Regulation of intestinal goblet cell secretion. II. A survey of potential secretagogues. *Am J Physiol* 1982;242:G380–G387.

59. Sperber K, Ogata S, Sylvester C, Aisenberg J, Chen A, Mayer L, Itzkowitz S. A novel human macrophage-derived intestinal mucin secretagogue: implications for the pathogenesis of inflammatory bowel disease. *Gastroenterology* 1993;104: 1302–1309.

60. Nash S, Parkos C, Nusrat A, Delp C, Madara JL. *In vitro*

model of intestinal crypt abscess. A novel neutrophil-derived secretagogue activity. *J Clin Invest* 1991;87:1474–1477.

61. McCool DJ, Marcon MA, Forstner JF, Forstner GG. The T84 human colonic adenocarcinoma cell line produces mucin in culture and releases it in response to various secretagogues. *Biochem J* 1990;267:491–500.

62. Lundgren JD. Mucus production in the lower airways. *Dan Med Bull* 1992;39:289–303.

63. Jarry A, Velcich A, Augenlicht L, Laboisse C. Effects of gamma-interferon on mucin biosynthesis in a human colonic goblet cell line. *Gastroenterology* 1993;104:A718.

64. Merlin D, Jarry A, Hopfer U, Laboisse CL. Gamma-interferon controls both chloride secretion and mucin exocytosis in a human intestinal goblet cell line. *Gastroenterology* 1993;104: A1052.

65. Micots I, Augeron C, Laboisse CL, Muzeau F, Megraud F. Mucin exocytosis: a major target for *Helicobacter pylori*. *J Clin Pathol* 1993;46:241–245.

66. Augeron C, Voisin T, Maoret JJ, Berthon B, Laburthe M, Laboisse CL. Neurotensin and neuromedin N stimulate mucin output from human goblet cells (C1.16E) via neurotensin receptors. *Am J Physiol* 1992;262:G470–G476.

67. Nexø E, Poulsen SS, Hansen SN, Kirkegaard P, Olsen PS. Characterisation of a novel proteolytic enzyme localised to goblet cells in rat and man. *Gut* 1984;25:656–664.

68. Kvist N, Olsen PS, Poulsen SS, Nexø E. Secretion of goblet cell serine proteinase, ingobsin, is stimulated by vasoactive intestinal polypeptide and acetylcholine. *Digestion* 1987;37: 223–227.

69. Schachter M, Peret MW, Billing AG, Wheeler GD. Immunolocalization of the protease kallikrein in the colon. *J Histochem Cytochem* 1983;31(11):1255–1260.

70. Venkatachalam MA, Soltani MH, Fahimi HD. Fine structural localization of peroxidase activity in the epithelium of large intestine of rat. *J Cell Biol* 1970;46:168–173.

71. Kataoka K, Nakai Y, Fujita H. The fine structural localization of peroxidase activity in digestive organs of rats and mice. *Histochemistry* 1974;38:5–18.

72. Childress RD, Sibley DA, Specian RD. Maturational distribution of intestinal peroxidase in rat small and large intestine: an immunochemical study. *Gastroenterology* 1992;102:A920.

73. Specian RD, Sibbley DA, Oliver MG. The intestinal mucus gel: a dynamic bactericidal and cytotoxic paradigm. *Anat Rec* 1991; 229:85A.

74. Oliver MG, Specian RD, Deitch E, Forstner JF, McCool D. Intragranular localization of secretory IgA in human intestinal goblet cells. *J Cell Biol* 1988;107:351a.

75. Wright NA. Trefoil peptides and the gut. *Gut* 1993;34:577–579.

76. Suemori S, Lynch-Devaney K, Podolsky DK. Identification and characterization of rat intestinal trefoil factor: tissue- and cell-specific member of the trefoil protein family. *Proc Natl Acad Sci USA* 1991;88:11017–11021.

77. Podolsky DK, Lynch-Devaney K, Stows JL, et al. Identification of human intestinal trefoil factor. *J Biol Chem* 1993;268(9): 6694–6702.

78. Wright NA, Poulsen R, Stamp G, et al. Trefoil peptide gene expression in gastrointestinal epithelial cells in inflammatory bowel disease. *Gastroenterology* 1993;104:12–20.

79. Hoosein NM, Thim L, Jorgensen KH, Brattain MG. Growth stimulatory effect of pancreatic spasmolytic polypeptide on cultured colon and breast tumor cells. *FEBS Lett* 1989;247: 303–306.

80. Frandsen ED, Jorgensen KH, Thim L. Receptor binding of pancreatic spasmolytic polypeptide (PSP) in rat intestinal mucosal cell membranes inhibits adenylate cyclase activity. *Regul Peptides* 1986;16:291–297.

81. Jorgensen KD, Diammand B, Jorgensen KH, Thim L. Pancreatic spasmolytic polypeptide (PSP) III: pharmacology of a new porcine pancreatic polypeptide with spasmolytic and gastric acid inhibitory effects. *Regul Peptides* 1982;3:231–243.

82. Hauser F, Hoffmann W. P-domain as shuffled cysteine-rich modules in integumentary mucin C.1 (FIM-C.1) from *Xenopus laevis*. *J Biol Chem* 1992;267:24620–24624.

83. Toribara NW, Gum JR Jr, Culhane PJ, et al. MUC-2 human

small intestinal mucin gene structure: repeated arrays and polymorphism. *J Clin Invest* 1991;88:1005–1013.

84. Gum JR, Byrd JC, Hicks JW, Toribara NW, Lamport DTA, Kim YS. Molecular cloning of human intestinal mucin cDNAs. *J Biol Chem* 1989;264:6480–6487.

85. Gum JR, Hicks JW, Toribara NW, Rothe EM, Lagace RE, Kim YS. The human MUC 2 intestinal mucin has cysteine-rich subdomains located both upstream and downstream of its central repetitive region. *J Biol Chem* 1992;267:21375–21383.

86. Gum JR, Hicks JW, Swallow DM, et al. Molecular-cloning of cDNAs derived from a novel human intestinal mucin gene. *Biochem Biophys Res Commun* 1990;171:407–415.

87. Toribara NW, Roberton AM, Ho SB, et al. Human gastric mucin. *J Biol Chem* 1993;268:5879–5885.

88. Xu G, Huan LJ, Khatri I, et al. Human intestinal mucin-like protein (MLP) is homologous with rat MLP in the C-terminal region, and is encoded by a gene on chromosome 11 p 15.5. *Biochem Biophys Res Commun* 1992;183:821–828.

89. Huan LJ, Xu G, Forstner G, Forstner J. A serine, threonine and proline-rich region near the carboxyl-terminus of a rat intestinal mucin peptide. *Biochim Biophys Acta* 1992;1132:79–82.

90. Xu G, Huan LJ, Khatri IA, et al. cDNA for the carboxyl-terminal region of a rat intestinal mucin-like peptide. *J Biol Chem* 1992;267:5401–5407.

91. Khatri IA, Forstner GG, Forstner JF. Suggestive evidence for two different mucin genes in rat intestine. *Biochem J* 1993;294:391–399.

92. Gum JR Jr, Hicks JW, Lagace RE, et al. Molecular cloning of rat intestinal mucin. *J Biol Chem* 1991;266:22733–22738.

93. Porchet N, Van Gong N, Dufosse J, et al. Molecular cloning and chromosomal localization of a novel human tracheo-bronchial mucin cDNA containing tandemly repeated sequences of 48 base pairs. *Biochem Biophys Res Commun* 1991;175:414–422.

94. Gross MS, Guyonnet-Duperat V, Porchet N, Bemheim A, Aubert JP, Nguyen VC. Mucin 4 (MUC4) gene: regional assignment (3q29) and RFLP analysis. *Ann Genet* 1992;35:21–26.

95. Van Cong N, Aubert JP, Gross MS, Porchet N, Degand P, Ffezal J. Assignment of human tracheobronchial mucin gene(s) to 11 p 15 and a tracheobronchial mucin-related sequence to chromosome 13. *Hum Genet* 1990;86:167–172.

96. Aubert JP, Porchet N, Crepin M, et al. Evidence for different human tracheobronchial mucin peptides deduced from nucleotide cDNA sequences. *Am J Respir Cell Mol Biol* 1991;5:178–185.

97. Timpte CS, Eckhardt AE, Abernethy JL, Hill RL. Porcine submaxillary gland apomucin contains tandemly repeated identical sequences of 81 residues. *J Biol Chem* 1988;263:1081–1088.

98. Eckhardt AE, Timpte CS, Abernethy JL, Zhao Y, Hill RL. Porcine submaxillary mucin contains a cysteine-rich, carboxyl-terminal domain in addition to a highly repetitive, glycosylated domain. *J Biol Chem* 1991;265:9678–9686.

99. Sheng Z, Wu K, Carraway KL, Fregien N. Molecular cloning of the transmembrane component of the 13762 mammary adenocarcinoma sialomucin complex: a new member of the epidermal growth factor superfamily. *J Biol Chem* 1992;267:16341–16346.

100. Bhargava AK, Woitach JT, Davidson EA, Bhavanandan VP. Cloning and cDNA sequence of a bovine submaxillary gland mucin-like protein containing two distinct domains. *Proc Natl Acad Sci USA* 1990;87:6798–6802.

101. Hoffman W. A new repetitive protein from *Xenopus laevis* skin highly homologous to pancreatic spasmolytic polypeptide. *J Biol Chem* 1988;263:7686–7690.

102. Hauser F, Gertzen EM, Hoffmann W. Expression of spasmolysin (FIM:A:1): an integumentary mucin from *Xenopus laevis*. *Exp Cell Res* 1990;189:157–162.

103. Probst JC, Gertzen EM, Hoffmann W. An integumentary mucin (FIM-B-1) from *Xenopus laevis* homologous with von Willebrand factor. *Biochemistry* 1990;29:6240–6244.

104. Probst JC, Hauser F, Joba W, Hoffmann W. The polymorphic integumentary mucin B.1 from *Xenopus laevis* contains the short consensus repeat. *J Biol Chem* 1992;267:6310–6316.

105. Sorimachi H, Emori Y, Kawasaki H, Kitajima K, Inoue S,

Suzuki K, Inoue Y. Molecular cloning and characterization of cDNAs coding for apo-polysialoglycoprotein of rainbow trout eggs. *J Biol Chem* 1988;263:17678–17684.

106. Gendler SJ, Burchell JM, Duhig T, Lamport D, White R, Parker M, Taylor-Papadimitriou J. Cloning of partial cDNAs encoding differentiation and tumor-associated mucin glycoproteins expressed by human mammary epithelium. *Proc Natl Acad Sci USA* 1987;84:6060–6064.

107. Gendler SJ, Lancaster CA, Taylor-Papadimitriou J, et al. Molecular cloning and expression of human tumor-associated polymorphic epithelial mucin. *J Biol Chem* 1990;265:15286–15293.

108. Spicer AP, Parry G, Patton S, Gendler SJ. Molecular cloning and analysis of the mouse homologue of the tumor-associated mucin, MUC1, reveals conservation of potential O-glycosylation sites, transmembrane, and cytoplasmic domains and a loss of minisatellite-like polymorphism. *J Biol Chem* 1991;266:15099–15109.

109. Tanpipat N, Mattice WL. Range of the influence of the carbohydrate moiety on the conformation of the poly(amino acid) backbone in glycosylated mucins. *Biopolymers* 1990;29:377–383.

110. O'Connell BC, Hagen FK, Tabak LA. The influence of flanking sequence on the O-glycosylation of threonine *in vitro*. *J Biol Chem* 1992;267:25010–25018.

111. Burchell J, Taylor-Papadimitriou J, Boshell M, Gendler S, Duhig T. A short sequence within the amino acid tandem repeat of a cancer-associated mucin, contains immunodominant epitopes. *Int J Cancer* 1989;44:691–696.

112. Layton GT, Devine PL, Warren JA, et al. Monoclonal antibodies reactive with the breast carcinoma-associated mucin core protein repeat sequence peptide also recognise the ovarian carcinoma-associated sebaceous gland antigen. *Tumor Biol* 1990;11:274–286.

113. Kim YS. Altered glycosylation of mucin glycoproteins in colonic neoplasia. *J Cell Biochem* 1992;16G:91–96.

114. Rughetti A, Turchi V, Ghetti CA, et al. Human B-cell immune response to the polymorphic epithelial mucin. *Cancer Res* 1993;53:2457–2459.

115. Carlstedt I, Sheehan JK, Corfield AP, Gallagher JT. Mucous glycoproteins: a gel of a problem. *Essays Biochem* 1985;20:40–76.

116. Parry G, Beck JC, Moss L, Bartley J, Ojakian GK. Determination of apical membrane polarity in mammary epithelial cell cultures: the role of cell–cell, cell–substream, and membrane–cytoskeleton interactions. *Exp Cell Res* 1990;188:302–315.

117. Sheng Z, Vanderpuye OA, Hull SR, et al. Topography and microfilament core association of a cell surface glycoprotein of ascites tumor cell microvilli. *J Cell Biochem* 1990;40:453–466.

118. Kovarik A, Peat N, Wilson D, Gendler SJ, Taylor-Papadimitrios J. Analysis of the tissue-specific promoter of the MUC 1 gene. *J Biol Chem* 1993;268:9917–9926.

119. Ho SB, Niehans GA, Lyftogt C, et al. Heterogeneity of mucin gene expression in normal and neoplastic tissues. *Cancer Res* 1993;53:641–651.

120. Xu G, Wang D, Huan LJ, Cutz E, Forstner G, Forstner J. Tissue-specific expression of a rat intestinal mucin-like peptide. *Biochem J* 1992;286:335–338.

121. Huet C, Sahuquillo-Merino C, Coudrier E, Louvard D. Absorptive and mucus-secreting subclones isolated from a multipotent intestinal cell line (HT-29) provide new models for cell polarity and terminal differentiation. *J Cell Biol* 1987;105:345–357.

122. Devine PL, Layton GT, Clark BA, et al. Production of MUC1 and MUC2 mucins by human tumor cell lines. *Biochem Biophys Res Commun* 1991;178:593–599.

123. Dohi DF, Sutton RC, Frazier ML, Nakamori S, McIsaac AM, Irimura T. Regulation of sialomucin production in colon carcinoma cells. *J Biol Chem* 1993;268:10133–10138.

124. Sajjan SU, Forstner JF. Role of the putative "link" glycopeptide of intestinal mucin in binding of piliated *Escherichia coli* serotype O157H7 strain CL-49. *Infect Immun* 1990;58:868–873.

125. Van Nieuw Amerongen A, Oderkerk CH, Roukema PA, Wolf

JH, Lisman JJW, Vliengenthart JFG. Primary structure of O- and N-glycosylic carbohydrate chains derived from murine submandibular mucin. *Carbohydr Res* 1987;164:43–49.

126. Dekker J, Strous GJ. Covalent oligomerization of rat gastric mucin occurs in the rough endoplasmic reticulum, is N-glycosylation dependent and precedes initial O-glycosylation. *J Biol Chem* 1990;265:18116–18122.

127. Mimura Y, Yamamoto Y, Inoue Y, Chûjô R. NMR study of interaction between sugar and peptide moieties in mucin-type model glycopeptides. *Int J Biol Macromol* 1992;14:242–248.

128. Butenhof KJ, Gerken TA. Structure and dynamics of mucin-like glycopeptides. Examination of peptide chain expansion and peptide–carbohydrate interactions by stochastic dynamics simulations. *Biochemistry* 1993;32:2650–2663.

129. Gerken TA, Butenhof KJ, Shogren R. Effects of glycosylation on the conformation and dynamics of O-linked glycoproteins, carbon-13 NMR studies of ovine submaxillary mucin. *Biochemistry* 1989;28:5536–5543.

130. Sterk H, Fabian W, Hayn E. Dynamic behaviour of mucus glycoproteins—a ^{13}C n.m.r. relaxation study. *Int J Biol Macromol* 1987;9:58–62.

131. Slomiany BL, Varahabhotla L, Murty N, Slomiany A. Isolation and characterization of oligosaccharides from rat colonic mucus glycoprotein. *J Biol Chem* 1980;255:9719–9723.

132. Slomiany BL, Zdebska E, Slomiany A. Structural characterization of neutral oligosaccharides of human H$^+$ Le^{b+} gastric mucin. *J Biol Chem* 1984;259:2863–2869.

133. Ishihara K, Hotta K. Comparison of the mucus glycoproteins present in the different layers of rat gastric mucosa. *Comp Biochem Physiol* 1993;104B:315–319.

134. Oliver MG, Specian RD. Intracellular variation of rat intestinal mucin granules localized by monoclonal antibodies. *Anat Rec* 1991;230:513–518.

135. Schachter H. Enzymes associated with glycosylation. *Curr Opin Structural Biol* 1991;1:755–765.

136. Jerome KR, Bu D, Olivera JF. Expression of tumor-associated epitopes on Epstein–Barr virus-immortalized B-cells and Burkitt's lymphomas transferred with epithelial mucin. *Cancer Res* 1992;52:5985–5990.

137. Shu-Heh WC, Walker WA. Bacterial toxin interaction with the developing intestine. *Gastroenterology* 1993;104:916–925.

138. Itzkowitz SH. Blood group-related carbohydrate antigen expression in malignant and premalignant colonic neoplasms. *J Cell Biochem Suppl* 1992;16:G97–G101.

139. Hoskins LC, Augustines M, McKee WB, Boulding ET, Kriaris M, Niedermayer G. Mucin degradation in human colon ecosystems. Isolation and properties of fecal strains that degrade ABH blood group antigens and oligosaccharides from mucin glycoproteins. *J Clin Invest* 1985;75:944–953.

140. Miller RS, Hoskins LC. Mucin degradation in human colon ecosystems. Estimation of fecal population densities by a "most probable number" method. *Gastroenterology* 1981;81:759–765.

141. Schoentag R, Primus FJ, Kuhns W. ABH and Lewis blood group expression in colorectal carcinoma. *Cancer Res* 1987;47:1695–1700.

142. Hirohashi S, Ino Y, Kodama T, Shimosato Y. Distribution of blood group antigens A, B, H, and 1 (Ma) in mucus-producing adenocarcinoma of human lung. *J Natl Canc Inst* 1981;72:1299–1305.

143. Ishikawa N, Horii Y, Nawa Y. Immune-mediated alteration of the terminal sugars of goblet cell mucins in the small intestine of *Nippostrongylus brasiliensis*-infected rats. *Immunology* 1993;78:303–307.

144. Rabinowitz SS, Gordon S. Macrosialin, a macrophage-restricted membrane sialoprotein differentially glycosylated in response to inflammatory stimuli. *J Exp Mol* 1991;174:827–836.

145. Wesley AW, Forstner J, Forstner G. Structure of intestinal mucus glycoprotein from human post-mortem or surgical tissue: inferences from correlation analyses of sugar and sulfate composition of individual mucins. *Carbohydr Res* 1983;115:151–163.

146. Mawhinney TP, Landrum DG, Gayer DA, Barbero GJ. Sulfated sialyl-oligosaccharides derived from tracheobronchial mucous glycoproteins of a patient suffering from cystic fibrosis. *Carbohydr Res* 1992;235:179–197.

147. Park CM, Reid PE, Owen DA, Sanker JM, Applegarth DA. Morphological and histochemical changes in intestinal mucin in the reserpine-treated rat model of cystic fibrosis. *Exp Mol Pathol* 1987;47:1–12.

148. Forstner J, Roomi N, Kharasani R, Kuhns W, Forstner G. Effect of reserpine on the histochemical and biochemical properties of rat intestinal mucin. *Exp Mol Pathol* 1991;54:129–143.

149. Filipe MI. Mucins in the human gastrointestinal epithelium: a review. *Invest Cell Pathol* 1979;2:195–216.

150. Raouf AH, Tsai HH, Parker N, Hoffman J, Walker RJ, Rhodes JM. Sulphation of colonic and rectal mucin in inflammatory bowel disease: reduced sulphation of rectal mucus in ulcerative colitis. *Clin Sci* 1992;83:623–626.

151. Morrisey SM, Tymvios MC. Acid mucins in human intestinal goblet cells. *J Pathol* 1978;126:197–208.

152. Cheng PW, Boat TF, Cranfill K, Yankaskas JR, Boucher RC. Increased sulfation of glycoconjugates by cultured nasal epithelial cells from patients with cystic fibrosis. *J Clin Invest* 1989;84:68–72.

153. Mian N, Anderson CE, Kent PW. Effect of O-sulfated groups in lactose and *N*-acetylneuraminyl-lactose on their enzymic hydrolysis. *Biochem J* 1979;181:387–389.

154. Goso Y, Hotta K. Types of oligosaccharide sulphation, depending on mucus glycoprotein source, corpus or antral, in rat stomach. *Biochem J* 1989;264:805–812.

155. Goso Y, Hotta K. Regional differences in sulfated oligosaccharides of rat gastrointestinal mucin as detected by two-dimensional chromatography. *Arch Biochem Biophys* 1993;302:212–217.

156. Sheehan JK, Oates K, Carlstedt I. Electron microscopy of cervical, gastric and bronchial mucus. *Biochem J* 1986;239:147–153.

157. Sheehan JK, Thornton J, Somerville M, Carlstedt I. The structure and heterogeneity of respiratory mucus glycoproteins. *Am J Respir Dis* 1991;144:S4–S9.

158. Verdugo P. Goblet cell secretion and mucogenesis. *Annu Rev Physiol* 1990;52:157–176.

159. Verdugo P. Mucin exocytosis. *Am J Respir Dis* 1991;144:S33–S37.

160. Sherman P, Forstner J, Roomi N, Khatri I, Forstner G. Mucin depletion in the intestine of malnourished rats. *Am J Physiol* 1984;248:G418–G423.

161. Jay GD. Characterization of a bovine synovial fluid lubricating factor. I. Chemical, surface activity and lubricating properties. *Connect Tissue Res* 1992;28:71–88.

162. Sundari CS, Raman B, Balasubramanian D. Hydrophobic surfaces in oligosaccharides: linear dextrins are amphiphilic chains. *Biochim Biophys Acta* 1991;1065:35–41.

163. Girod J, Zahm JM, Plotkowski C, Beck G, Purchelle E. Role of the physicochemical properties of mucus in the protection of the respiratory epithelium. *Eur Respir J* 1992;5:477–487.

164. Sellers LA, Allen A, Morris ER, Ross-Murphy SB. The rheology of pig small intestinal and colonic mucus: weakening of gel structure by non-mucin components. *Biochim Biophys Acta* 1991;1115:174–179.

165. Carlstedt I, Sheehan JK. Mucus glycoproteins—a short course. In: Glantz PO, Leach SA, Ericson T, eds. *Oral interfacial reactions of bone, soft tissue and saliva.* Oxford: IRL Press Limited, 1985;97–105.

166. Mantle M, Forstner G, Forstner J. Antigenic and structural features of goblet-cells mucin of human small intestine. *Biochem J* 1984;217:159–167.

167. Hutton DA, Pearson JP, Allen A, Fostern SNE. Mucolysis of the colonic mucus barrier by faecal proteinases: inhibition by interacting polyacrylate. *Clin Sci* 1990;78:265–271.

168. Bohe M, Borgstrom A, Lindstrom C, Ohlsson K. Trypsin-like immunoreactivity in human Paneth cells. *Digestion* 1984;30:271–275.

169. Poulsen SS, Nexø E, Olsen PS, Kirkegaard P. Localization of a new serine protease, ingobsin, in goblet cells in rat, pig and man. *Histochem J* 1985;17:487–492.

170. Macfarlane GT, Hay S, Gibson GR. Influence of mucin on gly-

cosidase, protease and arylamidase activities of human gut bacteria grown in a 3-stage continuous culture system. *J Appl Bacteriol* 1989;66:407–417.

171. Gong D, Turner B, Bhaskar KR, Lamont JT. Lipid binding to gastric mucin: protective effect against oxygen radicals. *Am J Physiol* 1990;259:G681–G686.

172. Magnusson KE, Stjernström I. Mucosal barrier mechanisms. Interplay between secretory IgA (SIgA), IgG and mucins on the surface properties and association of Salmonellae with intestine and granulocytes. *Immunology* 1982;45:239–248.

173. Murty VLN, Saarosiek J, Slomiany A, Slomiany BL. Effect of lipids and protein on the viscosity of gastric mucus glycoprotein. *Biochem Biophys Res Commun* 1984;121:521–529.

174. Sheehan JK, Carlstedt I. Electron microscopy of cervical mucus glycoproteins and fragments therefrom. The use of colloidal gold to make visible "naked" protein regions. *Biochem J* 1990;265:169–178.

175. Roberton AM, Mantle M, Fahim REF, et al. The putative "link" glycopeptide associated with mucus glycoproteins: composition and properties of preparations from the gastrointestinal tracts of several mammals. *Biochem J* 1989;261:637–647.

176. Marcus F. Preferential cleavage at aspartyl–prolyl peptide bonds in dilute acid. *Int J Peptide Protein Res* 1985;25:542–546.

177. Slomiany BL, Murty VLN, Piotrowski J, Liau YH, Sundaram P, Slomiany A. Glycosulfatase activity of *Helicobacter pylori* toward gastric mucin. *Biochem Biophys Res Commun* 1992;183:506–513.

178. Spychal RT, Goggin PM, Marrero JM, et al. Surface hydrophobicity of gastric mucosa in peptic ulcer disease. Relationship to gastritis and *Campylobacter pylori*. *Gastroenterology* 1990;98:1250–1254.

179. Sidebotham RL, Batten JJ, Karim QN, Spencer J, Baron JH. Breakdown of gastric mucus in presence of *Helicobacter pylori*. *J Clin Pathol* 1991;44:52–57.

180. Crowther RS, Roomi NW, Fahim REF, Forstner JF. *Vibrio cholera* metalloproteinase degrades intestinal mucin and facilitates enterotoxin-induced secretion from rat intestine. *Biochim Biophys Acta* 1987;924:393–402.

181. Corfield AP, Williams AJ, Clamp JR, Wagner SA, Mountford RD. Degradation by bacterial enzymes of colonic mucus from normal subjects and patients with inflammatory bowel disease: the role of sialic acid metabolism and the detection of a novel O-acetyl sialic acid esterase. *Clin Sci* 1988;74:71–78.

182. Corfield AP, Wagner SA, Clamp JR, Kriatis MS, Hoskins LC. Mucin degradation in the human colon: production of sialidase, sialate O-acetylesterase, N-acetylneuraminate lyase, arylesterase, and glycosulfatase activities by strains of fecal bacterial. *Infect Immun* 1992;60:3971–3978.

183. Takahashi H, Nukiwa T, Yoshimura K, et al. Structure of the human neutrophil elastase gene. *J Biol Chem* 1988;263:14739–14747.

184. Cole KR, Kumar S, Trong HL, Woodbury RG, Walsh KA, Neurath H. Rat mast cell carboxy peptidase: amino acid sequence and evidence of enzyme activity within mast cell granules. *Biochemistry* 1991;30:648–655.

185. Trong HL, Newlands GF, Miller HR, Charbonneau H, Neurath

186. Kooistra T, Millard PC, Lloyd JB. Role of thiols in degradation of proteins by cathepsins. *Biochem J* 1982;204:471–477.

187. Hiraishi H, Terano A, Ota S, et al. Role for mucous glycoprotein in protecting cultured rat gastric mucosal cells against toxic oxygen metabolites. *J Lab Clin Med* 1993;121:570–578.

188. Grisham MB, Von Ritter C, Smith BF, LaMont JT, Granger DN. Interaction between oxygen radicals and gastric mucin. *Am J Physiol* 1987;253:G93–G96.

189. Creeth JM, Cooper B, Donald ASR, Clamp JR. Mucus glycoproteins: scission at specific sites on the peptide backbone. *IRCS Med Sci* 1982;10:548–549.

190. Mantle M. Effects of hydrogen peroxide, mild trypsin digestion and partial reduction on rat intestinal mucin and its disulphide-bound 118 kDa glycoprotein. *Biochem J* 1991;274:679–685.

191. Variyam EP, Hoskins L. *In vitro* degradation of gastric mucin. Carbohydrate side chains protect polypeptide core from pancreatic proteases. *Gastroenterology* 1983;84:533–537.

192. Carlstedt-Duke B, Hoverstad T, Lingaas E, et al. Influence of antibiotics on intestinal mucin in healthy subjects. *Eur J Clin Microbiol* 1986;5:634–638.

193. Stanley RA, Ram SP, Wilkinson RK, Roberton AM. Degradation of pig gastric mucin and colonic mucins by bacteria isolated from pig colon. *Appl Environ Microbiol* 1986;51:1104–1109.

194. Nohle U, Schauer R. Metabolism of sialic acids from exogenously administered sialyllactose and mucin in mouse and rat. *Z Physiol Chem* 1984;365:1457–1467.

195. Macfarlane GT, Gibson GR. Formation of glycoprotein degrading enzymes by *Bacteroides fragilis*. *FEMS Microbiol Lett* 1991;61:289–293.

196. Barua RL, Tello R. Mucin: a probable substrate of intestinal fermentation. *Acta Gastroenterol Latinoam* 1984;14:279–283.

197. Rhodes JM, Black RR, Gallimore R, Savage A. Histochemical demonstration of desialylation and desulphation of normal and inflammatory bowel disease rectal mucus by faecal extracts. *Gut* 1985;26:1312–1318.

198. Prizont R. Degradation of intestinal glycoproteins by pathogenic *Shigella flexneri*. *Infect Immun* 1982;36:615–620.

199. Ishii-Karakasa I, Iwase H, Hotta K, Tanaka Y, Omura S. Partial purification and characterization of an endo-α-N-acetylgalactosaminidase from the culture medium of *Streptomyces* sp. OH-11242. *Biochem J* 1992;288:475–482.

200. Murty VL, Piotrowski J, Morita M, Slomiany A, Slomiany BL. Inhibition of *Helicobacter pylori* glycosulfatase activity toward gastric sulfomucin by nitecapone. *Biochem Int* 1992;26:1091–1099.

201. Slomiany A, Liau YH, Rosenthal WS, Slomiany BL. Sulfation of secretory and membrane glycolipids by human gastric mucosa in disease. *Gastroenterology* 1987;92:1644.

202. Tsai HH, Sunderland D, Gibson G, Hart CA, Rhodes JM. A novel mucin sulfatase from human feces: its identification, purification and characterisation. *Clin Sci* 1992;82:447–454.

203. Bhaskar KR, Garik P, Turner BS, et al. Viscous fingering of HCl through gastric mucin. *Nature* 1992;360:458–461.

204. Holm L, Flemstrom G. Microscopy of acid transport at the gastric surface *in vivo*. *J Int Med* 1990;228:91–95.

Infections of the Gastrointestinal Tract,
edited by M. J. Blaser, P. D. Smith, J. I. Ravdin,
H. B. Greenberg, and R. L. Guerrant
Raven Press, Ltd., New York © 1995.

CHAPTER 6

Nonimmune Defense Mechanisms of the Gastrointestinal Tract

G. T. Furuta and W. A. Walker

Despite a daily exposure to microbial particles, the gastrointestinal tract maintains a healthy state of "physiological inflammation." The oropharynx, stomach, esophagus, and small and large intestines utilize a complex and intricate system of defenses composed of both immune and nonimmune elements to protect the body from the deleterious effects of microbes. Typically the nonimmune elements lack the specificity of the immune defense but this is not always the case as seen by the antigen specificity of the enterocyte bacterial "receptors" or adherence factors. The nonimmune mechanisms often form the initial line of defense against microbes and participate as both chemical and mechanical barriers that decrease the ability of the microbial particles to attach to and invade the intestinal tract. This chapter will describe the major forms of nonimmune defense mechanisms (Table 1). A more detailed and specific discussion of these mechanisms as they pertain to certain microbial infections and a description of mucus will be covered in other chapters.

SALIVA

Three pairs of oral glands—the parotid, the submandibular, and the sublingual—contain mucous and serous cells that secrete saliva. Saliva is a complex mixture of water, ions, enzymes, glycoproteins, amylase, immunoglobulins, lysozyme, lactoperoxidase, and lactoferrin (1,2). The release of these substances is exclusively under neural control from the medulla and saliva is secreted at a rate of 0.3–0.5 mL/min (3). Stimuli include dryness of the oral mucosa, chewing, and certain food textures.

Saliva is the initial line of nonimmune defense of the intestinal tract. Several different components make saliva an effective chemical barrier. One is the peroxidase enzyme system. Peroxidase catalyzes the oxidation of thiocyanate (SCN−) to hypothiocyanous acid (HOSCN) and hypothiocyanate ion (OSCN−). The later two chemicals inhibit the growth and metabolism of bacteria, in particular *Lactobacillus* and *Streptococcus mutans,* and inhibit *S. mutans* glucose metabolism (4). In addition, lactoperoxidase from human milk inhibits growth of *Lactobacillus* and *S. mutans* (4,5).

Saliva contains antigen-specific glycoproteins and immunoglobulins. The glycoproteins bind to human epithelial cell receptors for *Streptococcus sanguis* and *salivarius,* thus inhibiting the attachment of these bacteria to epithelial cells and tooth enamel (6). They can facilitate the removal of these infective agents and desorb preattached bacteria. Although they constitute only a minority of total body immunoglobulin content, IgA, IgM, and IgG are secreted from the parotid gland (2).

Lactoferrin is present in saliva and human breast milk, and is released by epithelial cells and neutrophils. It has both bacteriostatic and bactericidal activities (1,7,8). By binding iron in areas of infection, lactoferrin decreases the pool of this nutrient necessary for bacterial growth. This bacterostatic effect is overcome if an excess of iron is given. Bactericidal effects of lactoferrin are secondary to their formation of hydroxyl radicals that are toxic to bacteria, direct effects which increase bacterial membrane permeability, inhibition of lipid peroxidation, and enhancement of the actions of lysozyme and sIgA (9–11). *In vitro* studies demonstrate lactoferrin's bactericidal effect on *Vibrio cholera, S. mutans, Pseudomonas aeruginosa, Escherichia coli,* and *Candida albicans* (12,13).

Lysozyme is a ubiquitous enzyme found in saliva, gastric juice, bile, and Paneth cells (8). The protein splits the muramic acid linkage in cell walls, producing bacterial lysis and phagocytosis (14,15). Its antibacterial action affects primarily gram-positive organisms, but it can act synergistically with lactoferrin to kill gram-negative organisms (10).

All of saliva's effect may not decrease oral bacteria. It

G. T. Furuta and W. A. Walker: Department of Pediatric Gastroenterology, Harvard Medical School and Boston Children's Hospital, Boston, Massachusetts 02116.

TABLE 1. *Nonimmune defense mechanisms of the gastrointestinal tract*

Oropharnx—saliva
    Blood group factors
    Adherence factors
Stomach—acid
    Lysozyme, lactoferrin
    Mast cells, eosinophils
    Nutrition
Intestinal tract—bile
    Cryptdins
    Lysozyme, lactoferrin
Peristalsis
    Adherence factos
Blood group factors
    Mast cells, eosinophils,
    Nutrition

contains binding proteins that attach to several organisms, including *C. albicans* (16,17) and *Streptococcus* sp. (18). These proteins bind the organism to the buccal mucosa and tooth enamel, thus creating a nidus for caries formation. Interestingly, *Helicobacter pylori* may acquire iron through the human lactoferrin system, thus enhancing this bacteria's virulence (19).

Permanent damage to the glands secondary to head and neck irradiation, Sjögren's syndrome, oral infections, and anticholinergic agents can disturb the flow of saliva. Any of these disorders can lead to xerostomia, increased dental caries, and potential infection. In fact, some elderly individuals with xerostomia have an increased incidence of aspiration pneumonia when compared to those with normal salivary flow (20).

GASTRIC ACIDITY

After passing through saliva, enteric pathogens encounter the gastric juices. This chemical barrier provides a major mechanism of defense against most bacteria and their products. Gastric secretions contain pepsin, lysozyme, and mucus but the main bactericidal component is acid (21). Hydrochloric acid is secreted from parietal cells following stimulation of histamine H_2, cholinergic, or gastrin receptors, and basal acid output is 7.0 mmol/hr (22).

In vitro, bacteria do not survive in aspirates of gastric juice with a pH less than 4.0 wheras bacteria exposed to achlorhydric juices can live for hours (23). Gastric acid is bactericidal for *Salmonella* sp., *Vibrio cholerae, Shigella* sp., *Serratia marcescens,* and *E. coli.* Bacterial counts of *E. coli, Salmonella* sp., and *S. marcescens* decrease by 99% after 15 min in gastric aspirates with a pH of 3.0 from normal subjects. In contrast, the gastric aspirates of patients with pernicious anemia have bacterial counts that are significantly higher (23). *Shigella sonnei* is killed within 10 min in gastric aspirates with a pH of 1.5–3.0 (24), but this finding is not confirmed in other *Shigella* species. Investigators have tried to simulate physiological gastric emptying conditions by incubating *Shigella* in media with a pH of 2.5 for 2 hr. *Shigella* survived this

environment but lost the ability to invade the epithelium (25).

Whether achlorhydria is secondary to surgery or medication, its association with an increased incidence of gastrointestinal infections is clear. After gastric resection, a higher incidence of *Salmonella* (26–28), *Giardia lamblia* (29), *V. cholerae* (30), and *Shigella* (31) infections is observed. Critically ill patients treated with antacid or acid-suppressing medication develop a higher incidence of gram-negative nosocomial pneumonia than those who maintain a gastric acid barrier. In these mechanically ventilated patients, gram-negative colonization of tracheal, pharyngeal, and gastric aspirates was more common in antacid or H_2 blocker-treated patients than in sucralfate-treated patients (32). Not only is there an increased incidence of gastrointestinal infection in patients with achlorhydria, but multiresistant salmonellosis has been observed in persons ingesting antacids (33). Studies examining the bacterial flora of the different anatomical compartments of the human gastrointestinal tract demonstrate that the acidic stomach is virtually void of bacteria. If achlorhydria develops, the gastric bacterial counts as well as bacterial counts distal to the stomach increase dramatically (34). The innoculating dose necessary to cause intestinal infection is higher in individuals with normal gastric acidity than in those with a higher pH. After the ingestion of 10^8 *V. cholerae* organisms by normal individuals, clinical symptoms of cholera develop. After neutralization of gastric pH, only 10^4 organisms were required to create a similar clinical syndrome (35).

Although acid is clearly effective in decreasing many bacterial infections, reports conflict as to whether an acidic environment is also effective in preventing parasitic infections such as *Diphyllobothrium latum, Strongyloides,* or *Giardia lamblia* (23). Acid's effect on *H. pylori* infection is not clear. This organism is found in stomachs with normal acid secretion, hyposecretion, or hypersecretion. It survives in a pH of 2.3 and can replicate at pH 4.3 (36).

ADHERENCE FACTORS

Adherence factors or bacterial receptors are expressed on the surface of epithelial cells and in the glycocalyx-covering enterocytes. These molecules are composed of carbohydrates (37), phospholipids, or glycoproteins (38). Each receptor has a hydrophobic end that is inserted into the epithelial lipid bilayer or glycocalyx and a hydrophilic end that is exposed to the intestinal lumen. The attachment of bacteria or their products by adhesins to these receptors is the initial event determining a microbe's capacity to colonize; if a host tissue does not express the receptor specific for the microbe or its products, the likelihood of infection is lessened. Binding can promote delivery of toxin or facilitate entry of the organism. The presence of these receptors is genetically determined, but they are also subject to later modification or induction (39).

A variety of carbohydrates and the protein fibronectin have been identified as bacterial receptors. Fibronectin binds gram-positive bacteria, including *Staphylococcus*

BACTERIAL ENTEROTOXIN INTERACTION
WITH THE **MATURE** ENTEROCYTE

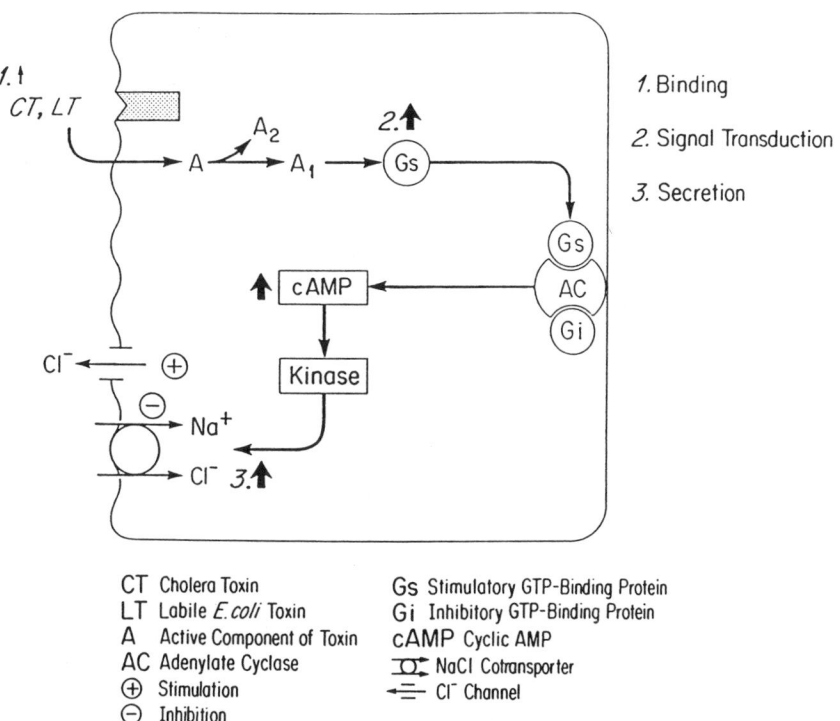

CT	Cholera Toxin
LT	Labile *E.coli* Toxin
A	Active Component of Toxin
AC	Adenylate Cyclase
⊕	Stimulation
⊖	Inhibition

Gs	Stimulatory GTP-Binding Protein
Gi	Inhibitory GTP-Binding Protein
cAMP	Cyclic AMP
	NaCl Cotransporter
	Cl⁻ Channel

FIG. 1. Mechanism of action of *Vibrio cholerae* enterotoxin.

aureus, Streptococcus pyogenes, mutans, salivarius, and *mitior,* but does not bind gram-negative bacteria as effectively (40). Three examples of bacteria or toxin with specific receptors are enteropathogenic *V. cholerae* toxin, *E. coli,* and *C. difficile* toxin. The receptor for the cholera toxin has been studied extensively. The human receptor has a terminal sugar on the glycolipid receptor, *N*-acetylgalactosamine, and a sialic acid residue. Three steps are involved in the series of events that produce clinical disease: toxin binding, signal transduction, and secretion. When the toxin binds to the intestinal surface receptor, it activates a cascade of transduction events that results in ribosylation of G proteins. These proteins stimulate adenylate cyclase, which produces an increase in intracellular levels of cAMP. The increase in cAMP stimulates fluid and electrolyte secretion into the intestinal lumen and decreases fluid and electrolyte absorption (41) (see Fig. 1).

To produce intestinal disease in the pig, enteropathogenic *E. coli* requires the production of enterotoxin and K88 antigen, a fimbrial adhesin. If the glycolipid receptor for the K88 antigen is not synthesized, clinical illness will not develop. For example, two porcine phenotypes differ in their susceptibility to the enteropathogenic diarrheal syndrome. The infection-resistant phenotype is K88 antigen receptor–negative and the infection-prone phenotype is receptor-positive. Cross-breeding follows Mendelian genetics and the receptor is coded by the autosomal domi-

nant gene. This describes a form of genetic immunity (39,42–44).

The glycoconjugate receptor for *Clostridium* toxin A has been identified in rat, rabbit, and human intestine (45,46) and its expression in the different species is age-dependent. For instance, in rabbits the receptors are present only in adulthood whereas in hamsters the receptors are present in both infancy and adulthood. The human receptor is present in adulthood but not infancy. This age-related difference in the human receptor may help explain the frequent detection of *C. difficile* toxin in the stools of healthy neonates.

BILE

After synthesis in the liver, the bile acids cholic and chendeoxycholic acid are conjugated with taurine or glycine. These bile salts are released into the duodenum from the gallbladder and after transit in the small intestine are deconjugated by bacteria to form deoxycholic and lithocholic acid. These are largely reabsorbed in the terminal ileum and returned to the liver. One liter of bile is produced each day and secretion is stimulated by cholecystokinin (47).

Authors suggest that bile acids participate in intestinal defense, but bile's exact role and mechanism of action is not clearly defined (48–52). *In vitro,* the unconjugated bile acids chenodeoxycholic, cholic, and deoxycholic inhibit the growth of stool isolates of *Clostridium, Bacteroides,* enterococcus sp, and *Lactobacillus,* but do not affect enteric aerobic organisms. Conjugated bile acids do not show this inhibitory effect. *In vitro* the unconjugated bile salt sodium cholate kills *Giardia.*

Conjugated bile acids from in diarrheal stools caused by *E. coli, Giardia,* and rotavirus infections are elevated. Unconjugated bile acids are increased in the stool specimens from these same recovered patients. This suggests that unconjugated bile acids may assist in controlling enteric pathogens (53). When *E. coli* endotoxin is pretreated with deoxycholate, clinical symptoms do not develop. The molecule is fragmented by the detergent action of the bile salt (54).

Although bile acids have been shown to have bactericidal effects, other studies are less suggestive. Bacterial cultures of the lumen of the human intestine performed in conjunction with intraluminal bile acid measurements do not correlate; specifically, gram-negative anaerobes are abundant in areas with a high intraluminal concentration of deoxycholic acid. This would not be predicted since *in vitro* anaerobic bacteria are killed by this bile salt (55). *Giardia lamblia* surface proteins and cell membrane antigens are modulated by bile, suggesting that bile may serve as a host factor for this organism (53,56). Also, conjugated bile salts assist in forming micelles thereby decreasing concentrations of oleic acid. Thus conjugated bile salts assist in protecting *Giardia* from the killing effects of oleic acid (52).

BLOOD GROUP FACTORS

The ABO blood group system is based on the expression of antigens on the surface of erythrocytes. These carbohydrate antigens are determined by the individual's genetic pattern and they can be released into saliva, mucus, and bile. People who release blood group antigens are secretors and those who do not are nonsecretors. The first association between blood groups and infectious diseases was made when similarities between blood group antigens and gram-negative bacteria, antigens were noted (57,58). Then epidemiological data showed an association between blood group type and frequency of gastrointestinal and urinary tract infections (59,60).

Blood group carbohydrates share cross-reactivity with antigens expressed by bacteria and their toxins. *Vibrio cholerae* O1 cell or toxin antigens share reactivity with blood type A or B carbohydrates. These blood group antigens can bind to intestinal receptors for this microbe, thus blocking the action of the bacteria or toxin, or they can bind to the bacterial adhesin to inhibit attachment to the gut (61). There is an increased frequency of nonsecretors among chronic *Salmonella typhi* carriers in Chile when compared to nonchronic carriers of *Salmonella* sp. This suggests that the lack of ABO carbohydrates in bile may allow the adherence of *S. typhi* to the biliary tract (62).

Nonsecretors have a higher incidence of clinical intestinal illness. Persons with group O blood type not only are at higher risk of developing cholera but also develop more severe disease than those with AB blood type (60,63). Epidemiological studies suggest that selective pressure of cholera may account for the low prevalence of blood group O in people living in the Gangetic delta, an endemic area for cholera (64). Nonsecretors also have a higher incidence of oral candidiasis (65,66).

In contrast to these benefits of secreting antigen, other studies find a different association. Epidemiological studies show that persons with blood group A have both a higher incidence and more severe illness with *G. lamblia* infection (29,67,68). ABO antigens on mucosal surfaces can function as receptors for *V. cholerae,* which can increase the likelihood of colonization and infection (65).

DEFENSINS/CRYPTDINS/CECROPINS

Defensins are a family of low molecular weight peptides isolated from human white blood cells. They possess antimicrobial activities against *E. coli, Listeria monocytogenes, Mycobacterium* sp., and *Candida albicans* (69–71). Cryptdins are a type of defensin whose name is derived from their anatomic location in the crypts of Lieberkuhn. Cryptdins are produced in Paneth cells and isolated from human and murine small intestine and the intestinal lumen (72). The regulation of cryptdin synthesis and release is not well understood, but a noticeable rise in the cryptdin mRNA occurs in the murine model at the time of gut closure (73). Cryptdins are released into the intestinal lumen from the Paneth cell by exocytosis. They are produced in the intestinal tract of germ-free mice, suggesting that bacteria are not needed to induce expression. They are also produced in mice who are void of T cells, suggesting independence from T-cell mediation (74). *In vitro,* cryptdins demonstrate antibacterial effects on the phoP mutant strain of *Salmonella typhimirum, L. monocytogenes,* and *E. coli,* ML-35p. Preliminary findings suggest that these peptides might provide an antimicrobial barrier in the intestinal tract (75–78), but their exact mechanism of action is unknown.

Mammals and insects possess another intestinal peptide with antibacterial properties. Initially cecoprins were found in the moth *Hyalophora cecropia* and recently they were isolated from the pig intestine. They kill gram-positive and gram-negative bacteria through lysis of the bacterial cell wall (79–84).

PERISTALSIS

Intestinal peristalsis provides a mechanical method for the removal of infectious particles. These sweeping actions occur as a result of migratory motor complexes (MMCs). MMCs are initiated by a variety of stimuli including cholinergic impulses; polypeptides such as histamine, motilin, somatastatin, gastrin, and cholecystokinin; and oxidative stress (85). When a motility response is initiated by an offending agent, it has been termed a "power propulsion." This peristaltic event is associated with diarrhea and abdominal distress in the animals. The small intestine is protected not only by peristalsis but by the ileocecal valve. In conjunction with peristalsis, this anatomic barrier helps prevent small intestinal bacterial overgrowth (86).

Animal models demonstrate that the cleansing action of peristalsis decreases the incidence of enteric pathology. In mice, rapid elimination of *V. cholerae* and *E. coli* occurs primarily as a result of intestinal peristaltic actions (87,88). After direct cecal inoculation with *Shigella flexneri,* adult guinea pigs, which are resistant to enteric dysentery, showed virtually normal ileal histology. Animals receiving opium to inhibit peristalsis developed ileal inflammation and significant mortality (89). Acute enteritis caused by *S. typhimurium* in opium-treated animals was histologically and clinically worse than that of the untreated controls (90). Humans receiving gastric inoculation of *Shigella* and treatment with Lomotil developed two to three times more systemic toxemia and prolonged carriage of the organism than untreated controls. Although this antiperistaltic medication decreased the amount of diarrhea these patients experienced, they were still systemically ill (91). These findings advise against the use of antimotility agents in the treatment of acute infectious diarrhea.

Peristalsis provides one of the main defenses against small-bowel bacterial overgrowth. Vantrappen et al. established the presence of a human intestinal motor complex and noted the association of small-bowel overgrowth with abnormal intestinal motility (92). When intestinal stasis develops, whether secondary to drugs, idiopathic pseudoobstruction, or systemic illness such as scleroderma or diabetes mellitus, the normal anatomic populations of bacteria are disrupted, promoting signs and symptoms of bacterial overgrowth. Usually the proximal small intestine contains $<10^5$ organisms/mL, primarily aerobic bacteria such as *Streptococcus* sp., the distal small intestine has $>10^8$ organisms/mL, primarily anaerobic bacteria such as *Bacteroides* and *E. coli,* and the colon contains 10^{10} organisms/mL, predominately anaerobes. When peristalsis is pharmacologically altered, bacterial populations begin to increase and change in hours. The proximal small intestine bacteria counts increase dramatically and the population of organisms assumes a character more like the lower small bowel (93,94). When the number of bacteria and the duration of contact time between bacteria and mucosa are increased, the likelihood of clinical illness increases (95). Morphine-induced peristaltic slowing results in increased bacterial translocation (96). The sequelae of increased bacterial counts and mucosal contact time include not only the possibility of increased bacterial translocation, but also nutrient malabsorption and anemia. Malabsorption occurs because of bile salt depletion and deconjugation, dissacharide loss, and disruption of enterocytes. Anemia is the result of vitamin B_{12} malabsorption and intestinal blood loss. The cleansing action of peristalsis is critical for intestinal health.

CELLULAR ELEMENTS

A variety of cells participate in the nonimmune defense of the intestinal tract. The epithelial layer, composed of four different cell types, provides a mechanical and chemical barrier against infection. Enterocytes form tight junctions with adjacent cells, and their apical surfaces are coated with mucus, sIgA, and cryptdins, all of which protect the immunologically potent lamina propria from antigenic exposure. Enteroendocrine cells produce acid and hormones. Goblet cells secrete mucus and Paneth cells release cryptdins, lysozyme, tumor necrosis factor-α, and other bioactive mediators. The lamina propria, depending on its degree of inflammation, contains a number of immunologically active cells such as white blood cells, eosinophils, and mast cells. After activation lymphocytes produce cytokines and immunoglobulins. Eosinophils produce cytokines and bioactive proteins. Two of these proteins, eosinophil major basic protein and eosinophil cationic protein, possess antibacterial properties (97). Mast cells in the lamina propria and submucosa can synthesize mediators that affect nerve, endocrine, and other intestinal cells. After sensitization to *Trichinella spiralis* and secondary exposure to this parasite, mast cells release chemical messengers including histamine, serotonin, prostaglandins, leukotrienes, platelet-activating factor, and cytokines. This massive release of mediators signals the enteric nervous system to generate a sequence of power propulsions and epithelial cell fluid secretions. This coordinated response of diarrhea and expulsion of infection demonstrates the synergy linking the immune and the nonimmune defenses of the bowel (98).

NUTRITION

The nutritional state of individuals can influence the development of infectious illnesses. Likewise infectious diseases can impact on the host's nutrition. Numerous clinical and laboratory studies suggest an intimate and complex relationship between nutrition, the immune system, and the development of infectious disease. Five hundred sixty million persons worldwide suffer from nutritional deficiencies (99). Twenty-four studies from third-world countries document almost 1 billion cases of diarrhea per year (100). The evidence suggesting that malnutrition predisposes to infectious illness is based on laboratory and clinical experiments in animals and humans, and on epidemiological observations. For several reasons, these studies are controversial and difficult to interpret. First, the term *malnutrition* is used in several ways. Some investigators include patients with marasmus (from the Greek *marasmos,* meaning "withering") or protein and calorie deprivation, others have included patients with kwashiorkor (from Ghana, meaning "displaced child") or protein-insufficient diets, and some include both (101). Next, it is difficult to examine nutritional deficiencies independently and separate confounding variables that may also predispose to infectious disease such as hygiene. Lastly, many epidemiological studies have an inadequate number of patients to demonstrate statistical significance or lack the data documenting specific nutritional deficiencies and infections. Despite these problems, clinical and laboratory information suggests that the malnourished patient is more predisposed to infectious disease. In a comprehensive review of clinical and laboratory studies, Scrimshaw et al. state that the relationship between nutrition and infection is synergistic; the morbidity and mortality of infectious illnesses are likely to be greater in those with malnutrition and infectious diseases can make the malnourished state worse (102).

When the immune and nonimmune defense mechanisms of normal individuals are compared to those of the malnourished, obvious differences are demonstrated. As starvation occurs, the epithelial layer atrophies, lymphoid tissue involutes, and antibody production decreases. Gross and histological samples of malnourished human thymus, lymph nodes, spleen, and gut-associated lymphoid aggregates weigh less and have fewer lymphocytes than normal (103). Protein-malnourished rats develop significant depletion of intraepithelial lymphocytes and decreased antibody formation when compared to their fed controls (104,105). Functional studies in humans demonstrate impaired cell-mediated immunity, decreased secretory antibody production and IgA producing plasma cells, altered intracellular killing, reduced complement activation, reduction in total number of intraepithelial lymphocytes, and lymphocyte responsiveness to interleukin 1 (106–108). Nonimmune mechanisms of defense are also affected. Gastric acidity and lysozyme secretion in individuals with marasmus or kwashiorkor are reduced (108).

Young, old, and immunocompromised malnourished individuals have more frequent and more severe gastrointestinal illness. The incidence and duration of diarrhea is increased twofold in children with protein calorie malnutrition. In large epidemiological studies, the highest morbidity and mortality from diarrheal illness is seen in children less than 1 year of age (100). Small-for-gestational-age infants have reduced sIgA response to poliovirus vaccine, fewer circulating lymphocytes, decreased opsonization, and decreased neutrophil oxidative metabolism (109). Protein-malnourished rodents and their offspring develop impaired qualitative and quantitative IgA responses that are reversed after refeeding (110–112). In some patients over the age of 60, cell-mediated immunity is impaired and this defect improves after nutritional supplementation (113–115). Although extensive prospective trials are incomplete, aggressive nutritional therapy may benefit AIDS patients, the newest population of malnourished individuals (103).

Not only is it important to receive sufficient protein and calories, but the route of intake of the calories seemingly is important. When rats are given the same quantities of nutrients either exclusively parenterally or enterally, intestinal atrophy develops in the group nourished parenterally (116). Functional studies in animals and human volunteers receiving all calories from parenteral nutrition show increased intestinal permeability when compared to their fed controls (116–118).

SUMMARY

The synergy between the nonimmune and immune elements protects the intestine from infectious disease. Microbial attachment is inhibited by glycoproteins and sIgA

and organisms are killed by the gastric acid. Those microbes or microbial products that survive passage through the stomach are swept into the small intestine and exposed to the antimicrobial actions of bile and cryptdins, and their attachment can be impeded by blood group factors or by peristalsis. If they penetrate the mucosa, microbes encounter the potent milieu of the lamina propria with its macrophages, T cells, eosinophils, and mast cells. These defenses are impaired when a part of the intestinal tract is excised or diseased or when protein/calorie deprivation ensues. When the continuity and integrity of the intestinal tract and mucosa are maintained, the individual elements of the gastrointestinal nonimmune defense mechanisms and the humoral and cellular elements of the immune system create an antagonistic environment for infectious diseases.

ACKNOWLEDGMENTS

This chapter was written with the support of NIH grants HD-121347, HD-31852, and DK-33506.

REFERENCES

1. Cole MF, Hsu SD, Baum BJ, et al. Specific and nonspecific immune factors in dental plaque fluid and saliva from young and old populations. *Infect Immun* 1981;31:998–1002.
2. Bowen WH. Defense mechanisms in the mouth and their possible role in the prevention of dental caries: a review. *J Oral Pathol* 1974;3:266–278.
3. Helm JF, Dodds WJ, Hogan WJ, Soergel KH, Egide MS, Wood CM. Acid neutralizing capacity of human saliva. *Gastroenterology* 1982;83:69.
4. Pruitt KM. The salivary peroxidase system: thermodynamic, kinetic and antibacterial properties. *J Oral Pathol* 1987;16:417–420.
5. Slowey RR, Eidelman S, Klebanoff SJ. Antibacterial activity of the purified peroxidase from human parotid saliva. *J Bacteriol* 1968;96:575–579.
6. Williams RC, Gibbons RJ. Inhibition of streptococcal attachment to receptors on human buccal epithelial cells by antigenically similar salivary glycoproteins. *Infect Immun* 1975;11:711–718.
7. Malamud D, Appelbaum B, Kline R, Golub EE. Bacterial aggregating activity in human saliva: comparisons of bacterial species and strains. *Infect Immun* 1981;31:1003–1006.
8. Florey H. The relative amounts of lysozyme present in the tissues of some mammals. *Br J Exp Pathol* 1930;251–261.
9. Weinberg ED. Iron witholding: a defense against infection and neoplasia. *Physiol Rev* 1984;64:65–103.
10. Ellison RT, Giehl TJ. Killing of gram negative bacteria by lactoferrin and lysozyme. *J Clin Invest* 1991;88:1080–1091.
11. Yamauchi K, Tomita M, Giehl TJ, Ellison RT. Antibacterial activity of lactoferrin and a pepsin derived lactoferrin peptide fragment. *Infect Immun* 1993;61:719–728.
12. Arnold RR, Cole MF, McGhee JR. A bactericidal effect for human lactoferrin. *Science* 1977;197:263–265.
13. Arnold RR, Brewer M, Gauthier JJ. Bactericidal activity of human lactoferrin: sensitivity of a variety of microorganisms. *Infect Immun* 1980;28:893–898.
14. Jolles P, Jolles J. What's new in lysozyme research? *Mol Cell Biochem* 1984;63:167–189.
15. Clamp JR, Creeth JM. Some non-mucin components of mucus and their possible roles. In: *Mucus and mucosa*. London: Pitman; 1984;121–136. Ciba Foundation symposium; vol 109.

16. Hoffman MP, Haidaris CG. Analysis of *Candida albicans* adhesion to salivary mucin. *Infect Immun* 1993;61:1940–1949.

17. Edgarton M, Scanapieco FA, Reddy MS, Levine MJ. Human submandibular-sublingual saliva promotes adhesion of *Candida albicans* to polymethylmethacrylate. *Infect Immun* 1993;61: 2644–2652.

18. Orstavik D, Kraus FW, Henshaw LC. In vitro attachment of streptococci to the tooth surface. *Infect Immun* 1974;9: 794–800.

19. Husson M, Legrand D, Spik G, Leclerc H. Iron acquisition by *Helicobacter pylori:* importance of human lactoferrin. *Infect Immun* 1993;61:2694–2697.

20. Terpenning M, Bretz W, Lopatin D, Langmore S, Dominguez B, Loesche W. Bacterial colonization of saliva and plaque in the elderly. *Clin Infect Dis* 1993;16(Suppl 4):314–316.

21. Giannella RA, Broitman SA, Zamcheck N. Gastric acid barrier to ingested microorganisms in man: studies in vivo and in vitro. *Gut* 1972;13:251–256.

22. Wise L, Ballinger WF. Gastric defense mechanisms. *Am J Surg* 1970;119:537–541.

23. Giannella R, Broitman SA, Zamcheck N. Influence of gastric acidity on bacterial and parasitic enteric infections. *Ann Intern Med* 1973;78:271–276.

24. Dare R, Magee JT, Mathison GE. In vitro studies on the bactericidal properties of natural and synthetic gastric juices. *J Med Microbiol* 1972;5:395–406.

25. Gorden J, Small PLC. Acid resistance in enteric bacteria. *Infect Immun* 1993;61:364–367.

26. Nordbring F. Contraction of salmonella gastroenteritis following previous operation on the stomach. *Acta Med Scand* 1956; 171:783–790.

27. Waddell WR, Kunz JJ. Association of salmonella enteritis with operation on the stomach. *N Engl J Med* 1956;255:555–559.

28. Gray JA, Trueman AM. Severe salmonella gastroenteritis associated with hypochlorhydria. *Scott Med J* 1971;16:255–258.

29. Roberts-Thomson IC. Genetic studies of human and murine giardiasis. *J Infect Dis* 1993;16(Suppl 2):S98–104.

30. Gitelson S. Gastrectomy, achlorhydria, and cholera. *Isr J Med Sci* 1971;7:663–667.

31. Dupont HL, Hornick RB, Snyder MJ, et al. Immunity in shigellosis. I. Response of man to attenuated strains of *Shigella. J Infect Dis* 1972;125:5–11.

32. Driks MR, Craven DE, Celli BR, et al. Nosocomial pneumonia in intubated patients given sucralfate as compared with antacids or histamine type 2 blockers. *N Engl J Med* 1987;317: 1376–1382.

33. Riley LW, Cohen ML, Seals JE, et al. Importance of host factors in human salmonellosis caused by multiresistant strains of *Salmonella. J Infect Dis* 1984;149:878–883.

34. Draser BS, Shiner M, McLeod GM. Studies on the intestinal flora I: The bacterial flora of the gastrointestinal tract in healthy and achlorhydric persons. *Gastroenterology* 1969;56:71–79.

35. Hornick RB, Music SI, Wenzel R, et al. The Broad Street pump revisited: response of volunteers to ingested cholera vibrios. *Bull NY Acad Med* 1971;47:1181–1191.

36. Hunt RH. pH and Hp − gastric acid secretion and helicobacter pylori: implications for ulcer healing and eradication of the organism. *Am J Gastroenterol* 1993;88:481–483.

37. Sharon N, Eshdat Y, Silverblatt FJ, Ofek I. Bacterial adherence to cell surface sugars. In: *Adhesion and microorganism pathogenicity.* Tunbridge Wells: Pitman; 1981:119–141. Ciba Foundation symposium; vol 80.

38. Elbein AD, Sanford BA, Ramsay MA, Pan YT. Effect of inhibitors on glycoprotein biosynthesis and bacterial adhesion. In: *Adhesion and microorganism pathogenicity.* Tunbridge Wells: Pitman; 1981:270–287. Ciba Foundation symposium; vol 80.

39. Warner L, Kim YS. Intestinal receptors for microbial attachment. In: Farthing MJG, Keusch GT, eds. *Enteric infection: mechanisms, manifestations and management.* New York: Raven Press; 1989:31–40.

40. Baddour LM, Christensen GD, Simpson WA, Beachey EH. Microbial adherence. In: Mandell GL, Douglas RG, Bennet JE, eds. *Principles and practice of infectious diseases.* 3rd ed. New York: Churchill Livingstone; 1990:9–22.

41. Chu SW, Walker WA. Bacterial toxin interaction with the developing intestine. *Gastroenterology* 1993;104:916–925.

42. Beachey EH. Bacterial adherence: adhesin-receptor interactions mediating the attachment of bacteria to mucosal surfaces. *J Infect Dis* 1981;143:325–345.

43. Sellwood R, Gibbon RA, Jones GW, Rutter JM. Adhesion of enteropathogenic *Escherichia coli* to pig intestinal brush borders: the existence of two pig phenotypes. *J Med Microbiol* 1975;8:405–411.

44. Schoolnik GK, Lark D, O'Hanley P. Bacterial adherence and anticolonization vaccines. In: Remington JS, Swartz MN, eds. *Current clinical topics in infectious diseases.* New York: McGraw-Hill; 1985:85–102. vol 6.

45. Rolfe RD, Song W. Purification of a functional receptor for *Clostridium difficile* toxin A from intestinal brush border membranes of infant hamsters. *Clin Infect Dis* 1993;16(Suppl 4): 219–227.

46. Pothoulakis C, Gao N, Dudeja P, Harig J, Brasitus TA, Lamont JT. The human colonic *Clostridium difficile* toxin A receptor is a trypsin sensitive glycoprotein. *Gastroenterology* 1992;102: A680.

47. Hoffman AF. Biliary secretions and excretions. In: West JB, ed. *Physiological basis of medical practice.* 12th ed. Baltimore: Williams and Wilkins; 1985:643.

48. Jackson SLO. Antibacterial action of bile. *Br Med J* 1972;(Nov 4):300.

49. Binder HJ, Filburn B, Floch M. Bile acid inhibition of intestinal anaerobic organisms. *Am J Clin Nutr* 1975;28:119–125.

50. Floch MH, Gershengoren W, Elliott S, Spiro HM. Bile acid inhibition of the intestinal microflora: a function for simple bile acids. *Gastroenterology* 1971;61:228–233.

51. Percy-Robb IW, Collee JG. Bile acids: a pH dependent antibacterial system in the gut. *Br Med J* 1972;3(September 30): 813–815.

52. Gillin FD, Das S, Reiner DS. Nonspecific defenses against human *Giardia.* In: Ruitenberg EJ, MacInnis AJ, eds. *Human parasitic diseases.* Amsterdam: Elsevier; 1990:199–213. vol 3.

53. Tazume S, Ozawa A, Yamamoto T, et al. Ecological study on the intestinal bacterial flora of patients with diarrhea. *Clin Infect Dis* 1993;16(Suppl 2):77–82.

54. Bertok L. Physico-chemical defense of vertebrate organisms: the role of bile acids in defense against bacterial endotoxins. *Persp Biol Med* 1977;21:70–76.

55. Mallory A, Kern F, Smith J, Savage D. Patterns of bile acids and microflora in the human small intestine. *Gastroenterology* 1973;64:26–42.

56. Kataelaris PH, Char S, Carnaby S, McHugh T, Naeem A, Farthing MJG. Bile modulates surface proteins and antigen expression of *Giardia lamblia. Gastroenterology* 1992;102:A644.

57. Muschel LH, Osawa E. Human blood group substance B and *Escherichia coli* 086. *Proc Soc Exp Biol Med* 1959;101:614–617.

58. Springer GF, Williamson P, Brandes WC. Blood group activity of gram-negative bacteria. *J Exp Med* 1961;113:1077–1093.

59. Sheinfeld J, Schaeffer AJ, Cordon-Cardo C, Rogatko AR, Fair WR. Association of the Lewis blood group phenotype with recurrent urinary tract infections in women. *N Engl J Med* 1989; 320:773–737.

60. Chaudhuri A, DasAdhikary CR. Possible role of blood group secretory substances in the aetiology of cholera. *Trans R Soc Trop Med Hyg* 1978;72:664–665.

61. Clemens JD, Sack DA, Harris JR, et al. ABO blood groups and cholera: new observations on specificity of risk and modification of vaccine efficacy. *J Infect Dis* 1989;159:770–773.

62. Hoffmann E, Chianale J, Rollan A, Pereira J, Ferrecio C, Sotomayor V. Blood group antigen secretion and gallstone disease in the *Salmonella typhi* chronic carrier state. *J Infect Dis* 1993; 167:993–994.

63. Barua D, Paguio AS. ABO blood groups and cholera. *Ann Hum Biol* 1977;4:489–493.

64. Glass RI, Holmgren J, Haley CE, et al. Predisposition for cholera of individuals with O blood group. *Am J Epidemiol* 1985; 121:791–796.

65. Burford-Mason A, Willoughby JMT, Weber JCP. Association between gastrointestinal tract carriage of *Candida,* blood group

O and nonsecretion of blood group antigens in patients with peptic ulcer. *Dig Dis Sci* 1993;38:1453–1458.

66. Lamey PJ, Darwazeh AMG, Muirhead J, Rennie JS, Samaranayake LP, MacFarlane TW. Chronic hyperplastic candidosis and secretor status. *J Oral Pathol Med* 1991;20:64–67.

67. Barnes GL, Kay R. Blood groups in giardiasis. *Lancet* 1976;2(April 9):808.

68. Zisman M. Blood group A and giardiasis. *Lancet* 1977;1(Dec. 17):1285.

69. Ogata K, Linzer TA, Zuberi RI, Ganz T, Lehrer RI, Catanzaro A. Activity of defensin from human neutrophilic granulocytes against *Mycobacterium avium–Mycobacterium intracellulare. Infect Immun* 1992;60:4720–4725.

70. Lehrer RI, Barton A, Daher KA, Harwig SSI, Ganz T, Selsted ME. Interaction of human defensins with *E. coli. J Clin Invest* 1989;84:553–561.

71. Lehrer RI, Ganz T, Szklarek D, Selsted ME. Modulation of the in vitro candidacidal activity of human neutrophil defensins by target cell metabolism and divalent cations. *J Clin Invest* 1988;81:1829–1835.

72. Lin MY, Munshi IA, Ouellette AJ. The defensin related murine CRS1C gene: expression in Paneth cells and linkage to Defcr, the cryptdin locus. *Genomics* 1992;14:363–368.

73. Eisenhauer PB, Harwig SSSL, Lehrer RI. Cryptdins:antimicrobial defensins of the murine small intestine. *Infect Immun* 1992;60:3556–3565.

74. Ouellette AJ, Greco RM, James M, Frederick D, Naftilan J, Fallon JT. Developmental regulation of cryptdin, a corticostatin/defensin precursor mRNA in mouse small intestinal crypt epithelium. *J Cell Biol* 1989;108:1687–1695.

75. Selsted ME, Miller SI, Henschen AH, Ouellette AJ. Enteric defensins: antibiotic peptide components of intestinal host defense. *J Cell Biol* 1992;118:929–936.

76. Miller SI, Pulkkien WS, Selsted ME, Mekalanos JJ. Characterization of defensin resistance phenotypes associated with mutations in the phoP virulence regulon of *Salmonella typhimurium. Infect Immun* 1990;58:3706–3710.

77. Jones DE, Bevins CL. Paneth cells of the human small intestine express an antimicrobial peptide gene. *J Biol Chem* 1992;267:23216–23225.

78. Jones DE, Bevins CL. Defensin 6 mRNA in human Paneth cells: Implications for antimicrobial peptides in host defense of the human bowel. *FEBS Lett* 1993;315:187–192.

79. Boman HG, Agerberth B, Boman A. Mechanisms of action on *Escherichia coli* of cecropin P1 and PR-39, two antibacterial peptides from pig intestine. *Infect Immun* 1993;61:2978–2984.

80. Boman HG, Faye I, Gudmundsson GH, Lee J, Lidholm D. Cell-free immunity in *Cepropia:* a model system for antibacterial proteins. *Eur J Biochem* 1991;201:23–31.

81. Agerberth B, Lee J, Bergman T, et al. Amino acid sequence PR-39: isolation from pig intestine of a new member of the family of proline-arginine rich antibacterial peptides. *Eur J Biochem* 1991;91:849–853.

82. Christensen B, Fink J, Merrifield RB, Mauzerall D. Channel forming properties of cecropins and related model compounds incorporated into planar lipid membranes. *Proc Natl Acad Sci USA* 1988;85:5072–5076.

83. Lee J, Boman A, Chuanxin S, et al. Antibacterial peptides from pig intestine: isolation of a mammalian cecropin. *Proc Natl Acad Sci USA* 1989;86:9159–9162.

84. Steiner S, Andreu D, Merrifield RB. Binding and action of cecoprin and cecoprin analogues: antibacterial peptides from insects. *Biochim Biophy Acta* 1988;939:260–266.

85. Vliet AVD, Tuinstra TJR, Bast A. Modulation of oxidative stress in the gastrointestinal tract and effect on rat intestinal motility. *Biochem Pharm* 1989;38:2807–2818.

86. Griffen WO, Richardson JD, Medley ES. Prevention of small bowel contamination by ileocecal valve. *South Med J* 1971;64:1056–1058.

87. Knop J, Rowley D. Antibacterial mechanism in the intestine: elimination of *V. cholerae* from the gastrointestinal tract of adult mice. *Austral J Exp Bio Med Sci* 1975;53:137–146.

88. Dixon JMS. The fate of bacteria in the small intestine. *J Pathol Bacteriol* 1960;79:131–140.

89. Formal SB, Abrams GD, Schneider H, Sprinz H. Experimental *Shigella* infections IV. Role of the small intestine in an experimental infection in guinea pigs. *J Bacteriol* 1963;85:119–125.

90. Kent TH, Formal SB, Labrec EH. Acute enteritis due to *Salmonella typhimurium* in opium treated guinea pigs. *Arch Pathol* 1966;81:501–508.

91. Dupont HL, Hornick RB. Adverse effect of lomotil therapy in shigellosis. *JAMA* 1973;226:1525–1528.

92. Vantrappen G, Janssens J, Hellemans J, Ghoos Y. The interdigestive motor complex of normal subjects and patients with bacterial overgrowth of the small intestine. *J Clin Invest* 1977;59:1158–1166.

93. Scott LD, Cahall DL. Influence of the interdigestive myoelectric complex on enteric flora in the rat digestive system. *Gastroenterology* 1982;82:737–745.

94. Hamilton I, Worsley BW, Cobden I, Cooke EM, Shoesmith JG, Axon AR. Simultaneous culture of salvia and jejunal aspirate in the investigation of small bowel bacterial overgrowth. *Gut* 1982;23:847–853.

95. Sprinz H. Pathogenesis of intestinal infection. *Arch Pathol* 1969;87:556.

96. Runkel NSF, Moody FG, Smith GS, et al. Alterations in rat intestinal transit by morphine promote bacterial translocation. *Dig Dis Sci* 1993;38:1530–1536.

97. Lehrer RI, Szklarek D, Barton A, Ganz T, Hamann KJ, Gleich GJ. Antibacterial properties of eosinophil major basic protein and eosinophil cationic protein. *J Immunol* 1989;142:4428–4434.

98. Boedeker EC, McQueen CE. Intestinal immunity to bacterial and parasitic infections. *Immunol Allergy Clin NA* 1988;8:393–421.

99. Chandra RK. Nutritional regulation of immunity and infection in the gastrointestinal tract. *J Pediatr Gastroenterol Nutr* 1983;(Suppl 1):181–187.

100. Snyder JD, Merson MH. The magnitude of the global problem of acute diarrhoeal disease: A review of active surveillance data. *Bull WHO* 1982;60:605–613.

101. Chandra RK. Nutritional deficiency and susceptibility to infection. *Bull WHO* 1979;57:167–177.

102. Scrimshaw NS, Taylor CE, Gordon JE. *Interactions of Nutrition and Infection.* Geneva: World Health Organization; 1968:329.; vol 57.

103. Hickey HS, Weaver KE. Nutritional management of patients with ARC or AIDS. *Gastroenterol Clin North Am* 1988;17:545–561.

104. Maffei HVL, Rodrigues MAM, Camarg JLVD, Campana AO. Intraepithelial lymphocytes in the jejunal mucosa of malnourished rats. *Gut* 1980;21:32–36.

105. Chandra RK. Antibody formation in first and second generation offspring of nutrionally deprived rats. *Science* 1975;190:288–289.

106. Chandra RK, Newberne PM. *Nutrition, Immunity, and Infection: Mechanisms of Interactions.* New York: Plenum Press; 1977:246.

107. Watson RR, McMurray DN, Martin P, Reyes MA. Effect of age, malnutrition and renutrition on free secretory component and IgA in secretions. *Am J Clin Nutr* 1985;42:281–288.

108. Ulijaszek SJ. Nutritional status and susceptibility to infectious disease. In: Harrison GA, Waterlow JC, eds. *Diet and Disease.* Cambridge: Cambridge University Press; 1990:137–154.

109. Chandra RK. Fetal malnutrition and postnatal immunocompetence. *Am J Dis Child* 1975;129:450–454.

110. Barry WS, Pierce NF. Protein deprivation causes reversible impairment of mucosal immune response to cholera toxoid/toxin in rat gut. *Nature* 1979;281:64–65.

111. Lim TS, Messiha N, Watson RR. Immune components of the intestinal mucosae of ageing and protein deficient mice. *Immunology* 1981;43:401–407.

112. McGee DW, McMurray DN. The effect of protein malnutrition on the IgA immune response in mice. *Immunology* 1988;63:25–29.

113. Chandra RK, Joshi P, Au B, Woodford G, Chandra S. Nutrition and immunocompetence of the elderly: effect of short term nu-

tritional supplementation on cell mediated immunity and lymphocyte subsets. *Nutr Res* 1982;2:223–232.

114. Chandra RK. Nutritional regulation of immunity and risk of infection in old age. *Immunology* 1989;67:141–147.

115. Sullivan DA, Vaerman JP, Soo C. Influence of severe protein malnutrition on rat lacrimal, salivary and gastrointestinal immune expression during development, adulthood and ageing. *Immunology* 1993;78:308–317.

116. Johnson LR, Copeland EM, Dudrick SJ, Lichtenberger LM, Castro GA. Structural and hormonal alteration in the gastrointestinal tract of parenterally fed rats. *Gastroenterology* 1975; 68:1177–1183.

117. McNeil LK, Hamilton JR. The effect of fasting on disaccharidase activity in the rat small intestine. *Pediatrics* 1971;47: 65–72.

118. Buchman AL, Moularzel AA, Ament ME, Hollander D. Intestinal permeability increases in normal volunteers receiving total parenteral nutrition. *Gut* 1993;34(Suppl):29.

Infections of the Gastrointestinal Tract,
edited by M. J. Blaser, P. D. Smith, J. I. Ravdin,
H. B. Greenberg, and R. L. Guerrant
Raven Press, Ltd., New York © 1995.

CHAPTER 7

The Role of Microbial Adherence Factors in Gastrointestinal Disease

Barbara J. Mann and William A. Petri, Jr.

The first step in the pathogenesis of many infectious diseases has been demonstrated to be adherence of the microorganism to the host. Adherence to the host is often paramount in establishing colonization and facilitating invasion, dissemination, toxin delivery, and host cell lysis. The harsh and dynamic environment found in the mammalian gastrointestinal (GI) tract presents a challenge to both pathogenic and commensal organisms that adhere to and colonize this site. Microbial adherence molecules (adhesins) must be protected against destruction by digestive enzymes and avoid recognition by the intestinal immune responses. Secretory IgA directed against adherence molecules may block colonization and therefore infection. Nonimmunological protective barriers, including a mucous lining, periodic sluffing of the lining, peristaltic movements, and cleansing actions, also may serve to block the establishment of infection by enteric pathogens. All of these factors necessitate that enteric microorganisms have specific means of attachment to the cells lining the GI tract in order to colonize and exert their pathogenic effects.

NATURE OF ADHESINS

An adhesin may be capable of interacting with more than one receptor and likewise a single receptor may be able to recognize multiple adhesins. This promiscuity allows organisms to adhere to different cell types and locations. The ability to recognize multiple receptors may facilitate colonization and invasion of organisms that invade through the intestinal epithelium and establish infection at extraintestinal sites. Type 1 fimbrial adhesins of *E. coli*, for example, recognize and bind to laminin, immobilized

fibronectin, and the CD11/CD18 leukocyte adhesion molecules (1–3).

The adhesin–receptor interaction plays a part in both tissue tropism and species specificity. Restricted expression of the receptor in a specific cell, tissue, or species can determine whether colonization and pathogenesis will occur. Glycosphingolipids have been identified as receptors for a number of adhesins (4). It may be directly relevant that specific glycolipids have been shown to have restricted expression in different species, cell, and tissue types (5–7). One of the best examples of tissue tropism due to adhesin–receptor interactions occurs in uropathogenic strains of *E. coli* where the expression of P fimbrial adhesins (which recognize globoseries glycolipids) promotes urinary tract colonization and invasion (8–10). In the case of swine coronavirus TGEV (transmissible gastroenteristis virus) the virus binds to an aminopeptidase N that is primarily expressed on the surface of intestinal mucosal cells (11).

Many strains of *E. coli* are known to cause disease in only certain animal species. In several cases the presence of a specific fimbrial type has been demonstrated to be required for infection. Strains of *E. coli* expressing K88 fimbria cause diarrheal illness only in certain strains of neonatal pigs. Studies comparing the epithelial brush border cells from genetically sensitive and resistant pigs suggest that resistance is due to the lack of a specific receptor for K88 fimbriae in the intestinal epithelial cells of resistant animals (12).

Poliovirus exhibits species restriction for primates. The receptor for poliovirus has been identified as a member of the immunoglobulin superfamily (13). Transgenic mice expressing the human poliovirus receptor are susceptible to poliovirus infection, indicating that the receptor is primarily responsible for species restriction (14). Poliovirus also exhibits a limited tissue tropism, replicating primarily in the lymphoid tissues of the pharynx and gut as well as and motor neurons. Somewhat paradoxically poliovirus receptor mRNA has been detected in a wide variety of

B. J. Mann and W. A. Petri, Jr: Department of Internal Medicine and Departments of Medicine and Microbiology, University of Virginia Health Sciences Center, Charlottesville, Virginia 22908.

TABLE 1. *Examples of host receptors and microbial adhesins*

Host cell ligand	Microbial adherin
Sugars	
Mannose	*Escherichia coli* type 1 fimbriae
Sialic acid	Influenza virus hemagglutinin
	Trypanosoma cruzi trans-sialidase
Galactose	*Entamoeba histolytica* lectin
	Escherichia coli P fimbriae
Galactosylcerebroside	HIV gp120/41
Immunoglobulin superfamily	
ICAM-1	Rhinovirus capsid (major group)
CD4	HIV gp120/41
Carcinoembryonic antigen	Mouse hepatitis virus
Growth factors/growth factor receptors	
EGF receptor	Vaccinia virus
Erhthropoietin receptor	Friend spleen focus-forming virus gp55
IL-6	Hepatitis B virus envelope glycoprotein
Integrins	
VLA-2	Echovirus 1
Poliovirus receptor	Poliovirus
β_1 integrins	*Yersinia* sp. Inv protein
CD11/CD18	*Escherichia coli* type 1 fimbriae
Extracellular matrix components	
Laminin	*Toxoplasma gondii*
	Escherichia coli type 1 fimbriae
Fibronectin	Streptococci
Transport proteins	
Basic amino acid	Ecotropic murine retrovirus
Phosphate transporter	Gibbon ape leukemia virus
Proteases	
Aminopeptidase N	Transmissible gastroenteritis virus
Complement receptors	
CR2	Epstein–Barr virus gp350/220
CR3	Leishmania
Glycosphingolipids	
GM_1	*E. coli* K88 fimbriae
Globoseries glycolipids	*E. coli* P fimbriae

tissue types, including kidney, which has been previously shown to lack poliovirus receptor sites (13). This suggests that expression of the receptor is necessary but not sufficient for poliovirus infection (14).

Host receptor molecules and microbial adhesins represent a diverse set of molecules. Microbial receptors identified to date consist of protein, lipid, or carbohydrate moieties. Tables 1 and 2 list some examples of the various types of receptor and adhesin molecules. The diversity of receptor types reflects the role that the adherence event can play in tissue tropism.

IDENTIFICATION OF ADHESINS

The identification of a molecule as an adhesin is not always straightforward. The development of a relevant adherence assay is key. An important consideration for an assay is the selection of an appropriate target cell that best represents the physiological situation. This would be especially true of organisms that exhibit cell, tissue, or species specificities for pathogenesis. One caveat in analyzing adherence properties of enteric organisms *in vitro*

TABLE 2. *Examples of different types of microbial adhesins*

Adhesin type	Organism
Fimbriae	
Type 1	*Escherichia coli*
P	*Escherichia coli*
K88	*Escherichia coli*
YadA	*Yersinia* sp.
Nonfimbrial bacteria	
Inv	*Yersinia* sp.
AIDA-I	*Escherichia coli*
Glycoproteins	
Galactose lectin	*Entamoeba histolytica*
gp120/41	HIV
gp350/220	Epstein Barr virus
Glycolipids	
Lipoteichoic acid	*Streptomyces pyogenes*
Lipophosphoglycan	*Leishmania* sp.
Enzymes	
trans-Sialidase	*Trypanosoma cruzi*
Toxins	*Bordetella pertussis*
Pertussis toxin	

is that it is not possible to recreate the microenvironment of the GI tract *in vitro* including the influences of the mucous lining, commensal microbial flora, and peristaltic movements on adherence. Another important aspect of a meaningful assay is that conditions should be designed to measure only adherence and limit other activities such as motility, invasion, and cell lysis.

The identification of an adhesin is often complicated by the fact that many organisms possess multiple adhesins that may be expressed simultaneously. Multiple adhesins may act independently or synergistically. The expression of some adhesins may be subject to specific regulatory controls that differ in microorganisms grown in cell culture vs. microorganisms infecting animals. In many bacterial species the study of individual putative adhesins can be accomplished by genetic manipulation including the ability to introduce and express a putative adhesin in a nonadherent strain of *E. coli*. For other organisms, such as protozoan parasites and viruses, the initial identification of an adhesin is usually accomplished by adherence inhibitory antibodies or by the carbohydrate recognition properties of the adhesin. Rigorous identification of a purified protein as an adhesin should include a demonstration that specific antibody inhibits adherence and that purified protein will competitively inhibit adherence. If a carbohydrate specificity is known, a demonstration that the carbohydrate is capable of blocking the adhesive activity of the protein should also be presented.

In bacteria the adhesin molecule is often a minor component of adherence organelles called *fimbriae* or *pili* (see Fig. 1). The most common type of fimbriae are the type 1 or mannose-sensitive fimbriae, which have been found on at least 70% of wild-type strains of *E. coli*. No direct association with disease has been demonstrated for type 1 fimbriae. Other examples of fimbriae include CFA1 (colonization factor antigen), CS1, and CS3, which are fimbriae found on strains of human enterotoxigenic *E. coli* (ETEC) and P fimbriae which have been isolated from pyelonephritis-associated strains of *E. coli*. Porcine and bovine examples of fimbriae are K88 and F41, respectively. *E. coli* fimbriae range of about 2–7 nm in diameter

and can only be seen by electron microscopy (15). They are easily distinguishable from flagella, which are about 20 nm in diameter (16). The various types of fimbriae exhibit distinct morphologies (17). Type 1, CFA1, CS1, and P pili represent a class of fimbriae that appear to be rigid rods of around 7 nm in diameter. K88, F41, and CS3 appear by electron microscopy to be thinner, about 2 nm in diameter, and more flexible. The adhesive subunit of type 1 fimbriae is a minor component of the fimbriae and has been localized to the tip as well as along the length of the fimbriae by immunolabeling (18). Some studies have suggested that only the adhesin located at the tip is a functional adhesin. Isolated fimbriae subjected to freeze fracture have an increased hemagglutinating activity over intact fimbriae, suggesting that the fracture process exposed cryptic binding sites located internally along the length of purified fimbriae (19). The location of the adhesive subunit in P fimbriae appears to be exclusively at the tip of morphologically distinct tip structures, termed *fibrillae* (20). The locations of PapG, the P fimbrial adhesin, and other major and minor subunits in the fimbrial organelle (Fig. 2) were determined by incubating fimbriae with subunit-specific antibodies and then visualizing bound antibody with gold-conjugated protein A in electron micrographs (21). In other types of fimbriae, which include K88 fimbriae, the adhesin appears to be a major subunit with adhesive activity located along the length of the fimbrial rod (22). Nonfimbrial types of bacterial adhesins such as AIDA-I (adhesin involved in diffuse adherence) have also been identified but they are not as well characterized (23).

CLASSIFICATION OF ADHESINS

Many microbial adhesins have been classified as lectins because they bind specific carbohydrate moieties. The complexity of carbohydrate structures and linkages has resulted in the creation of a large diversity of structures that could potentially be specifically recognized by microbial adhesins. The subtlety and specificity of adhesin–receptor interaction is illustrated by a study of the binding specificities of three allelic variants of P fimbrial–associated adhesins of *E. coli* that share antigenic cross-reactivity and sequence similarities (24). These three adhesin variants all recognized the same Gal (α1–4) Gal β–containing globoseries glycosphingolipids (GSLs) fixed to artificial surfaces. However, when tested in hemagglutination assays the adhesins differed in their ability to agglutinate erythrocytes with different GSLs in their membranes. Molecular modeling of the GSLs suggested that these GSLs have different saccharide orientations with respect to the membrane. Differential binding of the three P adhesins may result from differences in epitope presentation at the membrane by these GSLs (24).

EFFECTS OF ADHERENCE

The outcome of an adherence event may be colonization, invasion/internalization, toxicity, host cell lysis, or stimulation of specific cytokine production. The invasin

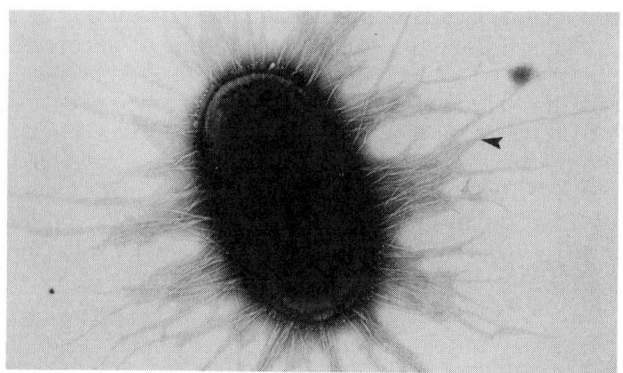

FIG. 1. Electron micrograph of *Escherichia coli* expressing P fimbriae. Bar = 0.25 µm. (From ref. 17, with permission).

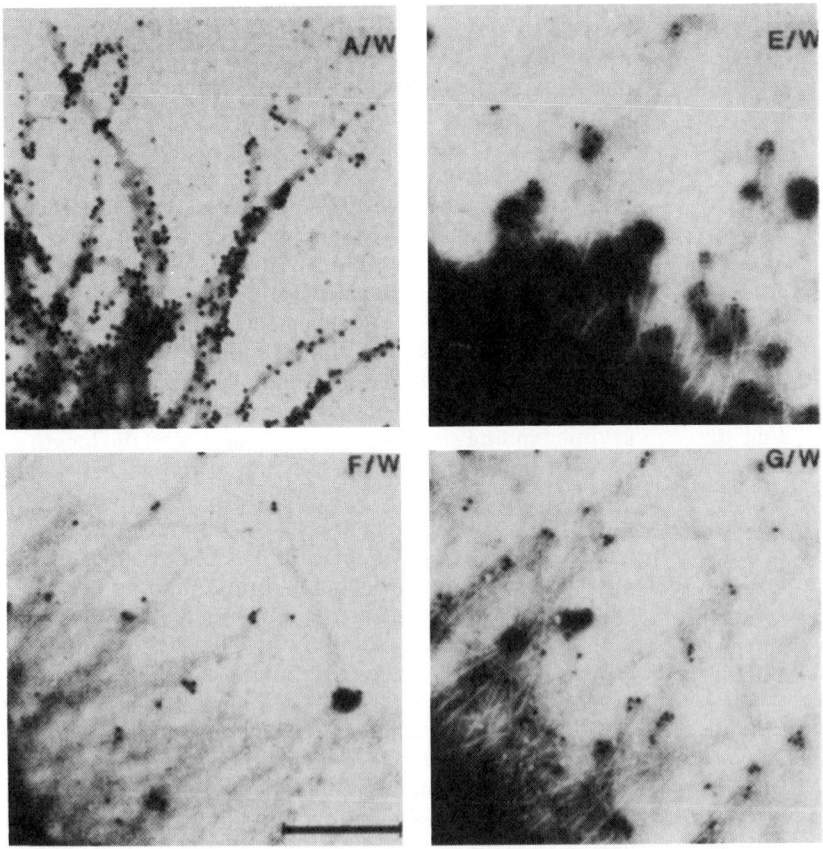

FIG. 2. Electron micrograph of P fimbriae reacted with sera specific for fimbrial subunits PapA in A/W, PapE in E/W, PapF in F/W, and PapG in G/W. Bound antibodies were visualized by the addition of colloidal gold-labeled protein A. Bar = 500 nm. (From ref. 21, with permission).

protein of *Yersinia* has been shown to mediate both adherence and invasion. Transfection of *E. coli* K12 with the invasin gene is able to confer an adherence and invasion phenotype to the normally noninvasive strain (25,26). Receptors for invasin have been identified as members of the β1 integrin family (27). Members of the integrin family are known to be transmembrane proteins associated with cytoskeleton proteins. *Yersinia* invasion can be inhibited by cytochalsin D suggesting that the invasion process involves cytoskeletal rearrangements facilitated by the interaction of the invasin protein with the β1 integrin (28).

Toxin activity and cytolysis can occur after adherence by virtue of the two membranes being in close contact and enabling a separate toxin or cytotoxic molecule to be efficiently delivered to its target. However, the pertussis toxin of *Bordetella pertussis* also mediates adherence to ciliated respiratory epithelium (29). Site-directed mutagenesis of the toxin subunits localized the adherence-mediating domains to the S2 and S3 subunits (30). A comparison of these regions revealed a significant amino sequence similarity with the carbohydrate recognition domains of calcium-dependent eukaryotic lectins.

The galactose-specific adhesin of *Entamoeba histolytica* has been shown to mediate amebic adherence and have a role in contact-dependent killing (Fig. 3). Inhibition of galactose adhesin activity by the addition of galactose or colonic mucins prevents contact-dependent lysis of host cells by amebic trophozoites *in vitro* (31–33). Inhibition of cytolysis is not merely due to a blocking of adherence since apposition of the plasma membranes of amebas and target cells, as can be achieved by centrifugation, does not result in target cell lysis in the presence of galactose (32,34). Galactose-specific adhesin monoclonal antibodies that apparently inhibit cytolysis but not adherence have been produced (35). The ability of the galactose adhesin-specific monoclonal antibody to block cytolysis after adherence suggests that the adhesin may be a cytolytic protein itself or that the adhesin plays a role in signaling the initiation of cytolysis (35).

Bacterial adherence can elicit inflammatory responses that include cytokine production. Elevated levels of interleukin 6 (IL-6) are found in the urine of mice within minutes after a mucosal challenge with P-fimbriated *E. coli* (36). The involvement of the adherence event was demonstrated by inoculating mice with purified preparations of the several fimbrial types via urethral catheterization (37). Only P fimbriae isolated from Adh⁺ bacteria (with a receptor binding domain) stimulated IL-6 production. No increase of IL-6 levels was observed when mice were inoculated with preparations of type 1, S or P fimbriae from Adh⁻ strains (without a receptor binding domain).

A few adhesins have been found to have additional biologic activities. Several adhesins, such as the invasin protein of *Yersinia,* mediate invasion as part of the adherence event (25,26). The galactose-specific adhesin of *E. histolytica* has been found to facilitate resistance to serum lysis by blocking assembly of the membrane attack complex

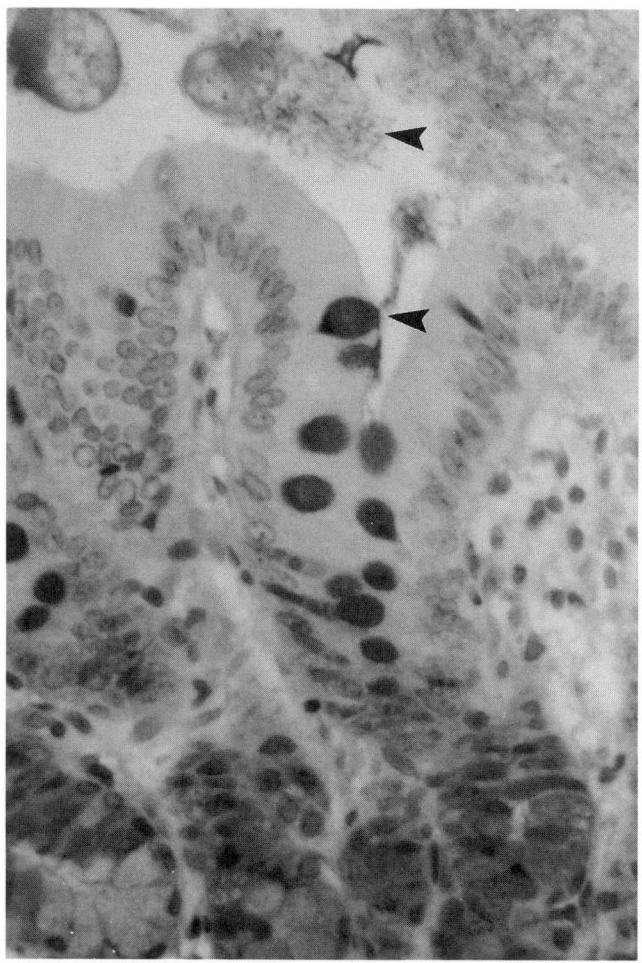

FIG. 3. *Entamoeba histolytica* trophozoites (*arrowhead*) adhering to colonic mucins in rat colon. Note the mucin-secreting goblet cell (*arrowhead*) in the interglandular epithelium. Scale bar is 0.06 mm. Hematoxylin-eosin, x312. (From ref. 52, with permission).

of complement (38). The adhesin YadA, encoded by the virulence plasmid of *Yersinia* sp., also appears to have a role in resistance to complement-mediated lysis (39). YadA appears to inhibit complement activation at early and late steps in the complement pathway, resulting in reduced amounts of C5b-9 complexes deposited on the surface of the bacteria.

REGULATION AND EXPRESSION OF ADHESINS

The expression of many bacterial adhesins is regulated. A number of strains of bacteria possess the ability to alternate between a state of expressing fimbriae on the surface to a state of nonexpression. This process, which has been called *phase variation,* may provide a mechanism for detaching from a substrate and/or may help the organism avoid detection by the host immune system. Phase variation for type 1 fimbriae occurs in about 1 of 1000 bacteria per generation (40,41). The expression of type 1 fimbriae is controlled by a 314-base-pair invertible element containing the promoter for expression of the *fim* genes that encode the type 1 fimbrial subunits. In one orientation of the element transcription of the *fim* genes occurs, in the opposite orientation the transcription of the *fim* genes is turned off. The inversion of this element is controlled by two gene products, *fimB* and *fimE*. The products of these two genes presumably encode site-specific recombinases. The mechanism for phase variation of type 1 fimbriae is similar to the mechanism that has been described for the switch of flagellar antigens in *S. typhimurium* (42). Other genes, unlinked to the *fim* gene cluster, have also been implicated in regulating phase variation, acting presumably as auxiliary factors or regulating the expression of *fimB* and *fimE* (43). Phase variation in P fimbriae is controlled by a distinctly different mechanism involving site-specific differential DNA methylation in the promoter region of the gene cluster encoding the P fimbrial subunits (44). The methylation state of this DNA influences the binding of different regulatory proteins which then either promote or prevent transcription.

The expression of many fimbriae is also under the influence of environmental factors such as temperature, catabolite repression, and osmolarity. Some of the genetic loci that have been shown to be involved in this type of regulation of fimbriae expression were first identified by their involvement in other biosynthetic or regulatory processes. Some examples are the Crp protein, which functions as a regulatory factor in catabolite repression (45), Lrp, a regulatory element of the leucine regulon (43), and *osmZ[pilG]* a loci involved in osmotic regulation (46).

Many adhesins require posttranslational processing, especially proteolytic fragmentation, to manifest full biological activity. The membrane fusion activity of the hemagglutinin (HA), which is required for viral infectivity, requires processing by a host protease of the intact hemagglutinin (HA_0) into HA_1 and HA_2. This proteolytic fragmentation exposes a highly conserved hydrophobic sequence at the amino terminus of HA_2 which, at acidic pH, is involved in viral entry into the cell by fusion of the viral membrane to the endocytic vacuole cell membrane (47). Similar processing events are required for the gp160 adhesin of human immunodeficiency virus (HIV) to have functional cell fusion activity (48). The requirement for host proteases to activate the fusion activity of adhesins may partly explain tropisms of microbial pathogens, since proteases required to activate the adhesins may only be present in certain tissues. This mechanism may help ensure that the virus will only infect the appropriate tissue type.

A microbial adhesin may also exist in active and inactive conformational states. Evidence for this is provided by the galactose-specific adhesin of *E. histolytica*. Monoclonal antibodies specific for different epitopes on the 170-kDa subunit of the galactose-specific adhesin can inhibit or enhance amebic adherence to target cells, presumably by altering the conformation of the protein to active or inactive conformations (49).

ADHESINS AS VACCINES

Adhesins are potential candidates for protective vaccines. Since many adhesins are critical for the establishment of colonization and/or the pathogenic process, antibodies or antimicrobial agents that block this interaction would have the potential to block infection. Vaccine trials in animals with purified fimbrial proteins have been shown to be effective vaccines. One of the first effective fimbrial vaccines was the case of K88 antigen to prevent diarrheal disease in newborn pigs (50). The galactose-specific adhesin of *E. histolytica* has also been shown to function as a protective antigen in a gerbil model of amebiasis (51). The potential to use DNA recombinant technology to alter or specifically express protective epitopes should help improve the effectiveness of these types of vaccines.

CONCLUSION

The adhesin molecules and corresponding receptors that mediate adherence have not been identified or well characterized for many pathogenic organisms. This should be an area of intensive research because it can provide practical information concerning targets for preventing or containing disease. The study of adhesin—receptor interactions can also contribute to our understanding of intermolecular interactions, cell–cell communication and signaling, which are important for many biological activities.

REFERENCES

1. Gbarah A, Gahmberg CG, Ofek I, Jacobi U, Sharon N. Identification of the leukocyte adhesion molecules CD11 and CD18 as receptors for type 1–fimbriated (mannose-specific) *Escherichia coli*. *Infect Immun* 1991;59:4524–4530.
2. Korhonen TK, Vaisanen-Rhen V, Rhen M, Pere A, Parkkinen J, Finne J. *Escherichia coli* fimbriae recognizing sialyl galactosides. *J Bacteriol* 1984;159:762–766.
3. Sokurenko EV, Courtney HS, Abraham SN, Klemm P, Hasty DL. Functional heterogeneity of type 1 fimbriae of *Escherichia coli*. *Infect Immun* 1992;60:4709–4719.
4. Warner L, Kim YS. Intestinal receptors for microbial attachment. In: Farthing MJG, Keusch GT, eds. *Enteric infections*. New York: Raven Press; 1988:31–40.
5. Karlsson K. Animal glycosphingolipids as membrane attachment sites for bacteria. *Annu Rev Biochem* 1989;58:309–350.
6. Breimer ME, Hansson GC, Karlsson K, Leffler H. Blood group type glycosphingolipids from small intestine of different animals analyzed by mass spectrometry and thin-layer chromatography. A note on species diversity. *J Biochem* 1981;90:589–609.
7. Breimer ME, Hansson GC, Karlsson K, Leffler H. Glycosphingolipids of rat tissues. Different composition of epithelial and nonepithelial cells of small intestine. *J Biol Chem* 1982;257: 557–568.
8. Kallenius G, Mollby R, Svensson SB, et al. The P^k antigen as receptor for the haemagglutinin of pyelonephritic *Escherichia coli* strains. *FEMS Microbiol Lett* 1980;7:297–302.
9. Kallenius G, Mollby R, Svensson S, et al. Occurrence of P-fimbriated *Escherichia coli* in urinary tract infections. *Lancet* 1981;2:1369–1372.
10. O'Hanley P, Low D, Romero I, et al. Gal–gal binding and hemolysin phenotypes and genotypes associated with uropathogenic *Escherichia coli*. *N Engl J Med* 1985;313:414–420.
11. Delmas B, Gelfi J, L'Haridon R, et al. Aminopeptidase N is a major receptor for the enteropathogenic coronavirus TGEV. *Nature* 1992;357:417–420.
12. Sellwood R, Gibbons RA, Jones GW, Rutter JM. Adhesion of enteropathogenic *Escherichia coli* to pig intestinal brush border: the existence of two pig phenotypes. *J Med Microbiol* 1975;4: 467–485.
13. Mendelsohn CL, Wimmer E, Racaniello VR. Cellular receptor for poliovirus: molecular cloning, nucleotide sequence and expression of a new member of the immunoglobulin superfamily. *Cell* 1989;56:855–865.
14. Ren R, Costantini F, Gorgacz EJ, Lee JJ, Racaniello VR. Transgenic mice expressing a human poliovirus receptor: a new model for poliomyelitis. *Cell* 1990;63:353–362.
15. Houwink AL, van Itersen W. Electron microscopic observations on bacterial cytology. II. A study on flagellation. *Biochim Biophys Acta* 1950;5:10–44.
16. Silverman M, Simon MI. Bacterial flagella. *Annu Rev Microbiol* 1977;31:397–419.
17. Klemm P. Fimbrial adhesins of *Escherichia coli*. *Rev Infect Dis* 1985;7:321–340.
18. Abraham SN, Goguen JD, Sun D, Klemm P, Beachey EH. Identification of two ancillary subunits of *Escherichia coli* type 1 fimbriae by using antibodies against synthetic oligopeptides of *fim* gene products. *J Bacteriol* 1987;169:5530–5536.
19. Ponniah S, Endres RO, Hasty DL, Abraham SN. Fragmentation of *Escherichia coli* type 1 fimbriae exposes cryptic D-mannose binding sites. *J Bacteriol* 1991;173:4195–4202.
20. Kuehn MJ, Heuser J, Normark S, Hultgren SJ. P pili in uropathogenic *E. coli* are composite fibres with distinct fibrillar adhesive tips. *Nature* 1992;356:252–255.
21. Lindberg F, Lund B, Johansson L, Normark S. Localization of the receptor-binding protein adhesin at the tip of the bacterial pilus. *Nature* 1987;328:84–87.
22. Jacobs AAC, Veneme J, Leeven R, van Pelt-Heerschap H, de Graaf FK. Inhibition of adhesive activity of K88 fibrillae by peptides derived from K88 adhesin. *J Bacteriol* 1987;169:735–741.
23. Benz I, Schmidt MA. Isolation and serologic characterization of AIDA-I, the adhesin mediating the diffuse adherence phenotype of the diarrhea-associated *Escherichia coli* strain 2787 (0126:27). *Infect Immun* 1992;60:13–18.
24. Stromberg N, Nyholm P, Pascher I, Normark S. Saccharide orientation at the cell surface affects glycolipid receptor function. *Proc Natl Acad Sci USA* 1991;88:9340–9344.
25. Young VB, Miller VH, Falkow S, Schoolnik GK. Sequence, localization and function of the invasin protein of *Yersinia enterocolitica*. *Mol Microbiol* 1990;4:1119–1128.
26. Isberg RR, Voorhis DL, Falkow S. Identification of invasin: a protein that allows enteric bacteria to penetrate cultured mammalian cells. *Cell* 1987;50:769–778.
27. Isberg RR, Leong JM. Multiple β$_1$ chain integrins are receptors for invasin, a protein that promotes bacterial penetration into mammalian cells. *Cell* 1990;60:861–871.
28. Young VB, Falkow S, Schoolnik GK. The invasin protein of *Yersinia enterocolitica*: internalization of invasin-bearing bacteria by eukaryotic cells is associated with reorganization of the cytoskeleton. *J Cell Biol* 1992;116:197–207.
29. Tuomanen E, Weiss A. Characterization of two adhesins of *Bordetella pertussis* for ciliated respiratory epithelial cells. *J Infect Dis* 1985;152:118–125.
30. Saukkonen K, Burnette WN, Mar V, Masure HR, Tuomanen E. Pertussis toxin has eukaryotic-like carbohydrate recognition domains. *Proc Natl Acad Sci USA* 1992;89:118–122.
31. Ravdin JI, Guerrant RL. Role of adherence in cytopathic mechanisms of *Entamoeba histolytica*. Study with mammalian tissue culture cells and human erythrocytes. *J Clin Invest* 1981;68: 1305–1313.
32. Guerrant RL, Brush JR JI, Sullivan JA, Mandell GL. Interaction between *Entamoeba histolytica* and human polymorphonuclear neutrophils. *J Infect Dis* 1981;143:83–93.
33. Chadee K, Petri WA Jr, Innes DJ, Ravdin JI. Rat and human colonic mucins bind to and inhibit the adherence lectin of *Entamoeba histolytica*. *J Clin Invest* 1987;80:1245–1254.
34. Ravdin JI, Croft BY, Guerrant RL. Cytopathogenic mechanisms of *Entamoeba histolytica*. *J Exp Med* 1980;152:377–390.

35. Saffer LD, Petri WA Jr. Role of the galactose lectin of *Entamoeba histolytica* in adherence-dependent killing of mammalian cells. *Infect Immun* 1991;59:4681–4683.

36. deMan P, van Kooten C, Aarden L, Engberg I, Linder H, Svanborg-Eden C. Bacterial attachment and inflammation in the urinary tract. *Infect Immun* 1989;57:3383–3388.

37. Linder H, Engberg I, Hoschuttzky H, Mattsby-Baltzer I, Svanborg C. Adhesion-dependent activation of mucosal interleukin-6 production. *Infect Immun* 1991;59:4357–4362.

38. Braga LL, Ninomiya H, McCoy JJ, et al. Inhibition of the complement membrane attack complex by the galactose-specific adhesin of *Entamoeba histolytica*. *J Clin Invest* 1992;90:1131–1137.

39. Pilz D, Vocke T, Heesemann J, Braade V. Mechanism of YadA-mediated serum resistance of *Yersinia enterocolitica* serotype 03. *Infect Immun* 1992;60:189–195.

40. Eisenstein BI. Phase variation of type 1 fimbriae in *Escherichia coli* is under transcriptional control. *Science* 1981;214:337–338.

41. Brinton CC Jr. Non-flagellar appendages of bacteria. *Nature* 1959;183:782–786.

42. Silverman M, Simon M. Phase variation and related systems. In: Shapiro J, ed. *Mobile genetic elements*. New York: Academic Press; 1983:537–557.

43. Blomfield IC, Calie PJ, Eberhardt KJ, McClain MS, Eisenstein BI. Lrp stimulates phase variation of type 1 fimbriation in *Escherichia coli* K-12. *J Bacteriol* 1993;175:27–36.

44. van der Woude MW, Braaten BA, Low DA. Evidence for global regulatory control of pilus expression in *Escherichia coli* by Lrp and DNA methylation: model building based on analysis of pap. *Mol Microbiol* 1992;6:2429–2435.

45. Goransson M, Forsman P, Nilsson P, Uhlin BE. Upstream activating sequences that are shared by two divergently transcribed operons mediated cAMP-CRP regulation of pilus-adhesin in *Escherichia coli*. *Mol Microbiol* 1989;3:1557–1565.

46. Kawula TH, Orndorff PE. Rapid site-specific DNA inversion in *Escherichia coli* mutants lacking the histone-like protein H-NS. *J Bacteriol* 1991;173:4116–4123.

47. Wiley DC, Skehel JJ. The structure and function of the hemagglutinin membrane glycoprotein of influenza virus. *Annu Rev Biochem* 1987;56:365–394.

48. Hallenberger S, Bosch V, Angliker H, et al. Inhibition of furin-mediated cleavage activation of HIV-1 glycoprotein gp160. *Nature* 1992;360:358–361.

49. Petri WA Jr., Snodgrass TL, Jackson TFHG, et al. Monoclonal antibodies directed against the galactose-binding lectin of *Entamoeba histolytica* enhance adherence. *J Immunol* 1990;144:4803–4809.

50. Rutter JM, Jones GW. Protection against enteric disease caused by *Escherichia coli*—a model for vaccination with a virulence determinant? *Nature* 1973;242:531–532.

51. Petri WAJ, Ravdin JI. Protection of gerbils from amebic liver abscess by immunization with the galactose-specific adherence lectin of *Entamoeba histolytica*. *Infect Immun* 1991;59:97–101.

52. Petri WA Jr. Invasive amebiasis and the galactose-specific lectin of *Entamoeba histolytica*. *ASM News* 1990;57:299–306.

Infections of the Gastrointestinal Tract,
edited by M. J. Blaser, P. D. Smith, J. I. Ravdin,
H. B. Greenberg, and R. L. Guerrant
Raven Press, Ltd., New York © 1995.

CHAPTER 8

Fluid and Electrolyte Transport During Enteric Infections

Sheila E. Crowe and Don W. Powell

Diarrhea is a cardinal manifestation of many gastrointestinal (GI) infections. Numerous pathophysiological mechanisms, including changes in gut muscle function, lead to this common symptom (1,2), but alterations of epithelial fluid and electrolyte transport are of particular importance (3–5). While toxins from infectious agents such as *Vibrio cholerae* are viewed as the sine que non of microbially induced perturbations of intestinal ion transport (6,7), microorganisms may alter electrolyte transport through other direct and indirect effects on enterocytes. For example, activation of the immune/inflammatory system by infectious agents may lead to changes in ion transport through products of immune and inflammatory cells which, analogous to neurohormonal factors (8,9), have proven to be important regulators of intestinal transport function (10,11). This chapter reviews the mechanisms involved in the normal homeostasis of fluid and electrolytes within the small and large intestine (12–16) and how these may be altered during enteric infections (17). Current and future applications of this knowledge are also discussed in the context of therapeutic strategies for the management of the diarrhea resulting from GI infection (18).

OVERVIEW OF INTESTINAL FLUID AND ELECTROLYTE BALANCE

The GI tract is uniquely designed to perform a variety of life-sustaining functions including the retrieval of nutrients, minerals, and water, as well as the exclusion or removal of microorganisms, toxins, and other potentially harmful macromolecules found within the contents of the gut lumen. During the course of a normal day, the GI tract must deal with a minimum of 8–9 L of fluid including

approximately 2000 mL of ingested material, 1500 mL of saliva, 2000 mL of gastric secretions, 2000 mL of pancreatic and biliary secretions, and at least 1000 mL of secretions from the intestine itself. Much of this volume is absorbed in the small intestine secondary to nutrient and electrolyte absorption leaving 1–2 L to enter the large intestine. Here, 90% of the remaining fluid is absorbed yielding an average daily stool volume of 100–200 mL (19). Even in situations where volumes several times greater than normal are presented to the colon, the large reserve absorptive capacity of the large bowel leads to relatively small amounts of stool water. However, in conditions such as cholera, the large volumes produced by the intestine [up to 10–20 L/day (20)] overwhelm the system. Colonic disease or dysfunction can give rise to increased stool volumes as well, even if relatively normal volumes of fluid are delivered to the large intestine. Although the consequence of abnormal fluid and electrolyte secretion and absorption is best illustrated by cholera, many other infectious diarrheas result from stimulation of secretion and/or inhibition of absorption. The fact that all segments of the intestine, from the proximal duodenum to the rectum, are able to secrete water and electrolytes underlies the immense secretory capacity of the intestinal tract.

The epithelial cells lining the GI tract are the key players in these absorptive and secretory events. Ions and solutes traverse the epithelium by passing through the cell (transcellular route) or between the cells (paracellular route) by mechanisms involving either active or passive transport. The gut epithelium is typical of other epithelia that are capable of vectorial fluid transport, being composed of polarized cells with distinct apical (luminal) and basolateral (antiluminal) membranes connected by tight junctions. These cells possess a sodium pump (Na^+,K^+-ATPase) on the basolateral membrane that exchanges intracellular sodium for extracellular potassium to maintain a low intracellular Na^+ concentration and a negative potential difference. Additional transporters are acquired and added to the basic epithelial cell with maturation and

S. E. Crowe, and D. W. Powell: Department of Internal Medicine, Division of Gastroenterology, University of Texas Medical Branch, Galveston, Texas 77555.

migration away from the stem cell zone located above the base of the crypt (21). This confers unique properties to certain cell populations and contributes to the variation of transcellular transport found along the crypt–villus axis, with secretion occurring largely in crypt (22) but also in villus cells (23) while absorption is largely regarded as a function of villus and surface cells. The significance of these differences is illustrated by situations in which injury to the villi results in a relatively selective loss of absorptive function (since Na^+-nutrient-coupled transporters are found primarily in the mature cells of the villus), while secretion may be unaffected. This is one of many mechanisms whereby enteric infections may give rise to diarrhea and malabsorption. Variation in the movement of ions and solutes through the paracellular route is also displayed within the intestinal tract. In general, the permeability of the intestine decreases distally through the tract so that the distal colon and rectum are the segments least permeable to the passive movement of fluids and electrolytes (24,25). Differences in permeability also occur along the crypt–villus axis with increased passive movement observed in the crypts (26). Net transport function differs within the various segments of the intestine. In health, the proximal small intestine is a source of net fluid secretion although significant absorption of nutrients and ions, including calcium and iron, takes place in this portion of the GI tract. The vast majority of nutrient absorption has occurred by the time the gut contents reach the distal third of the small bowel, although certain functions such as vitamin B_{12} uptake are unique to the ileum. The ileum has the potential to assume more proximal functions should disease or resection of the mid–small bowel necessitate this adaptation (27). For example, after 70% proximal small intestinal resection, ileal glucose-dependent Na^+ absorption increases 2.5-fold (28). Segmental variation in colonic transport has also been described with differential sensitivities to secretagogues, aldosterone, and Na^+ channel inhibitors found between the proximal and distal colon (29–31).

The adaptive nature of the GI epithelium is in part a consequence of rapidly proliferating and differentiating cells. Stem cells of the GI epithelium differentiate not only into the transporting cells discussed above, but also mucus-secreting goblet cells, specialized M cells overlying Peyer's patches, Paneth cells, and enteroendocrine cells (32). The lifespan of a mature differentiated intestinal epithelial cell is only 4–7 days (33,34). While the continual turnover of cells contributes to the sensitivity of the gut epithelium to certain injurious agents such as cytotoxic chemotherapeutic agents, this property also helps limit the disease manifestations of other agents to which epithelial cells are exposed for relatively short periods. For example, the diarrhea resulting from certain bacterial toxins (e.g., *V. cholerae*, *E. coli* STa toxin) and viruses (e.g., rotavirus) will resolve as a new population of epithelial cells replaces those altered during the initial infection. In these situations, the clinical outcome is good provided careful attention is paid to fluid and electrolyte replacement during the acute illness.

MECHANISMS OF INTESTINAL ION TRANSPORT

In order to comprehend how microbial infections may alter intestinal ion transport, some consideration of enterocyte transport mechanisms is in order. *In vivo* perfusion techniques have provided information about fluid and electrolyte transport in the intact organism, but knowledge of the mechanisms involved comes largely from *in vitro* experiments utilizing intestinal tissues or cultured epithelial cells. Studies of isolated intestinal segments, isolated enterocytes, and plasma membranes by everted gut sac, Ussing chamber, microelectrode, patch clamp, radionuclide efflux, or membrane vesicle techniques (15) have all contributed to our understanding of this area. The availability of human colonic epithelial cell lines that are capable of vectorial fluid transport has been particularly helpful (35,36). Of note is the T84 cell line, originally derived from a human colonic carcinoma, that is used extensively as a model of intestinal crypt cells (35,37). It should be noted that while certain differences exist between species and the various sites of the gut, an attempt is made to present an overview of the major processes and pathways identified to date.

Paracellular Pathway

Passive transport of ions and solutes between epithelial cells occurs in response to electrochemical gradients established across the epithelium and reflect the relative permeability or "tightness" of the epithelium. Tightness of a given epithelium correlates with the *in vitro* measurement of electrical resistance, and both are a function of the structure of the intercellular tight junction also referred to as the zona occludens. Ultrastructurally, the tight junction has been shown, using freeze-fracture techniques, to comprise interwoven strands (38,39). The number of these strands correlates with measurements of electrical resistance and passive ion flow and is connected to the cytoskeleton of epithelial cells (40,41). Increased intracellular Ca^{2+} and cAMP induce increased resistance of the tight junction whereas activation of protein kinase C has the opposite effect (42,43). Although the factors regulating the tight junctions have not been established to the extent that they have for transcellular mechanisms of fluid and electrolyte transport, it is clear that the tight junctions cannot be viewed as rigid structures (44).

The tight junction provides a route for the movement of water and charged ions to maintain electrical and osmotic balance across the epithelial layer (45). The osmotic gradient hypothesis of water transport maintains that increased osmolarity of the intercellular space, created by the active transport of ions and solutes, causes movement of water through and around cells (46). Solutes entrained in water are moved across the paracellular pathway by a process of solvent drag (47–49). Studies in animals suggest that carrier-mediated and passive absorption of D-glucose may be interrelated functionally, i.e., intracellular actomyosin filaments that are connected to the tight junctions contract in response to transcellular glucose absorption. This is accompanied by dilatations in tight junctions

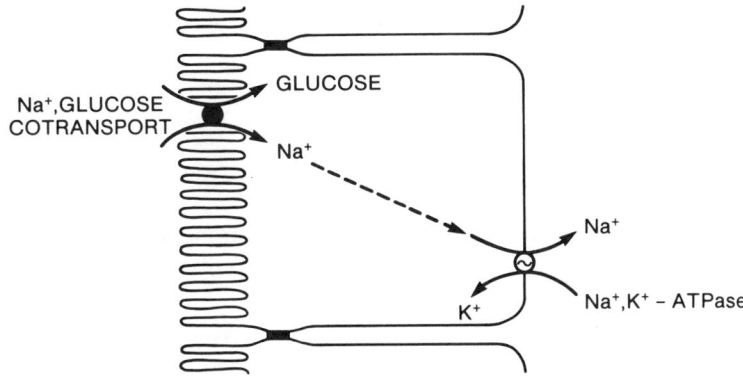

FIG. 1. Na$^+$-glucose cotransport. Glucose and Na$^+$ enter the cell via a Na$^+$-glucose cotransporter in the apical membrane. Na$^+$ is pumped out by active transport by the Na$^+$,K$^+$-ATPase and glucose is transported passively across the basolateral membrane by a specific carrier. Similar cotransport mechanisms exist for galactose, various classes of amino acids, peptides, vitamins, phosphates, and bile salts. (From ref. 15, with permission.)

between adjacent cells, which allows D-glucose present in the luminal fluid to move across the junctions during passive movement of fluid through this route (50). A recent *in vivo* study in humans did not support this concept that sodium-dependent nutrient transport increases tight junction permeability (51), but the validity of this study's conclusions have been questioned (52). Thus, the actual role of the paracellular route in the overall movements of sodium, glucose, and water remains ill defined.

Transcellular Mechanisms

Several key pathways facilitate the transfer of electrolytes in and out of the intestinal epithelial cell. These pathways take the form of pumps, carriers (cotransporters and exchangers), and channels. These are all membrane proteins that control the passage of specific molecules through what would be an otherwise impermeable lipid cell wall.

Pumps

Those membrane proteins that move a solute against an electrochemical gradient with a direct expenditure of energy are considered to be pumps. Foremost of the intestinal pumps is Na$^+$,K$^+$-ATPase, which harnesses the energy generated from the metabolism of ATP to drive sodium, against an electrochemical gradient, across the

basolateral membrane. This form of transport is called primary active transport. For every molecule of hydrolyzed ATP, three sodium ions are exchanged for two potassium ions rendering the cell interior electronegative (53). Thus, the pump creates an electrochemical gradient (low intracellular Na$^+$ concentration and electrical negativity) favoring sodium influx through Na$^+$ channels, Na$^+$-nutrient cotransporters, or Na$^+$ exchangers (Figs. 1–3). Inactivation of Na$^+$,K$^+$-ATPase by the cardiac glycoside, ouabain, inhibits all active transport mechanisms known to exist in intestinal epithelia, denoting the fundamental importance of this pump. Two subunits (α and β) of the Na$^+$,K$^+$-ATPase have been identified (54) and cloning studies indicate that the α subunit exists in three major isoforms, including α_1 found in the colon (55).

Other intestinal pumps include H$^+$,K$^+$-ATPase and Ca^{2+}- and Mg^{2+}-ATPases (56–60). A H$^+$,K$^+$-ATPase which has structural homology to the gastric form, as well as the three isoforms of Na$^+$,K$^+$-ATPase (61), has been localized to the apical membrane of crypt cells of the distal colon (62). However, unlike the related gastric pump, the colonic form does not generate high luminal hydrogen ion concentrations, perhaps reflecting neutralization by bicarbonate secretion by a Cl$^-$/HCO$_3^-$ exchanger present in the apical membrane of colonocytes (63).

Carriers

In contrast to pumps, carriers are facilitated transport pathways that allow ion movement in both directions ac-

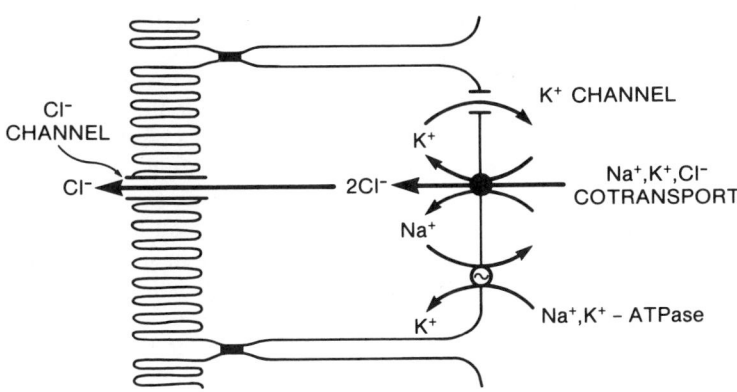

FIG. 2. Cl$^-$ secretion. Cl$^-$ is taken up by the Na$^+$,K$^+$,2Cl$^-$ cotransporter across the basolateral membrane. Na$^+$,K$^+$-ATPase provides the driving force and recycles Na$^+$. Excess K$^+$ is recycled via K$^+$ channels in the basolateral membrane. Cl$^-$ exits through a Cl$^-$ channel on the apical membrane. (From ref. 15, with permission.)

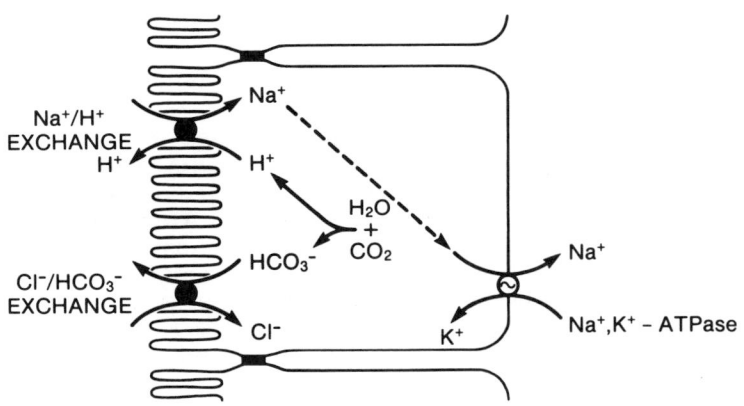

FIG. 3. Electroneutral NaCl transport. Na⁺ and Cl⁻ enter the cell across the apical membrane through a dual-exchange system consisting of an Na⁺/H⁺ exchanger and a Cl⁻/HCO₃⁻ exchanger. Na⁺ is extruded by Na⁺,K⁺-ATPase with Cl⁻ following to maintain electrical neutrality. (From ref. 15, with permission.)

cording to the prevailing electrochemical gradient. Those processes are coupled to an active transport pathway such as the Na⁺,K⁺-ATPase and are referred to as secondary transport pathways (e.g., Na⁺-nutrient and Na⁺,K⁺, 2Cl⁻ cotransporters, Na⁺/H⁺ exchanger). Tertiary transport pathways (e.g., Cl⁻/HCO₃⁻ exchanger) are driven by gradients produced by secondary active transport mechanisms (e.g., the intracellular alkalosis created by Na⁺/H⁺ exchange). Cotransport carriers or symports are major routes for intestinal absorption of various nutrients and electrolytes. The Na⁺-glucose cotransporter (64,65) (Fig. 1) is the best characterized of the nutrient cotransport carriers, but carriers for Na⁺-coupled amino acid, di- and tripeptide, and vitamin uptake also exist (66–69). The basolateral Na⁺,K⁺,2Cl⁻ cotransport carrier is an example of a cotransporter that deals with electrolytes only (70). This cotransporter, which has been purified, cloned, and sequenced (71), participates in transepithelial Cl⁻ transport (Fig. 2) as well as cell volume regulation (72). An Na⁺-Cl⁻ cotransporter was also recently cloned (73) and an electrogenic Na⁺-anion cotransporter mechanism identified in rat distal colon (74), but their roles in intestinal epithelial ion transport remain to be defined.

Exchange carriers or antiports move ions in one direction across the cell membrane in exchange for equivalently charged ions moving in the opposite direction. The two major exchangers found in the intestine, the Cl⁻/HCO₃⁻ and the Na⁺/H⁺ exchange carriers, when operating at identical stoichiometry constitute an electroneutral NaCl absorptive mechanism and are described in more detail below (Fig. 3). Another example is the Na⁺/Ca²⁺ exchanger, which maintains intracellular calcium lower than that of the surrounding extracellular environment (75).

Channels

Although channels also provide a facilitated route by which ions cross the cell membrane, there are several features that distinguish this type of pathway from carriers. First, membrane-spanning protein channels permit the rapid flow of ions when open but no movement occurs when they are closed. Second, flow through channels only occurs in a downhill fashion (passive transport) in contrast

to carriers that can move molecules against an electrochemical gradient. The rate at which ions are transported through the cell membrane differs between the two types of pathways; channels transport 10^8–10^9 ions per second whereas only 10^4–10^5 ions per second are moved via carriers. In addition, channels are highly selective allowing only specific ions to pass through the pore. The exact mechanisms that control this specificity are unclear. Opening and closing of channels is gated by different regulatory factors including voltage and intracellular messengers. Specific channels for Na⁺, K⁺, Cl⁻, Ca²⁺, and HCO₃⁻ (76–81) have been described and those transporting Na⁺, K⁺, and Cl⁻ are discussed in more detail below.

Absorptive Processes

Electrogenic Na⁺ Absorption

Sodium is actively absorbed throughout the intestine as a consequence of the sodium permeability of the apical membrane of all intestinal epithelial cells and because their basolateral membranes have Na⁺, K⁺-ATPase pumps. Utilizing the energy derived from ATP hydrolysis, sodium ions are pumped out in exchange for potassium. Extrusion of K⁺ through specific apical channels (76) permits the pump to maintain intracellular concentrations of sodium that are low relative to extracellular levels, thereby providing the driving force for the entry of sodium via Na⁺ channels or carriers. Movement of sodium into the cell by channels is referred to as "electrogenic" because it is not directly linked to the movement of other ions and there is a net transfer of charge across the epithelium. Electrogenic NaCl absorption predominates in the colon as a result of amiloride-sensitive, Na⁺-selective ion channels in apical membranes of absorptive cells in the distal colon (82,83). These Na⁺ channels are under the influence of aldosterone and are expressed in the more proximal colon and even the distal ileum in situations accompanied by increased aldosterone levels (e.g., sodium depletion, dehydration) (84–88). There is evidence for an additional Na⁺ channel in the colon that is much less sensitive to channel blockers including amiloride (89).

Electroneutral Na⁺ and Cl⁻ Transport

Electroneutral NaCl transport refers to the fact that there is no net transfer of charge involved in the process. The proposed mechanism whereby this occurs entails two separate carriers (90–92). One exchanges intracellular H^+ for extracellular Na^+, the other HCO_3^- for Cl^- (Fig. 3). The sodium gradient across the apical membrane facilitates sodium entry, which in turn drives apical H^+ exit. Sodium–hydrogen exchange is the principal mechanism for sodium absorption in the jejunum in the absence of luminal nutrients. Na^+/H^+ exchangers are also responsible for a "housekeeping" function in which excess hydrogen ions generated during intracellular metabolic processes are expelled to maintain intracellular pH. In villus cells of the ileum (93,94) and in colonocytes (63,95,96), sodium–hydrogen exchange is coupled to bicarbonate secretion and chloride entry. Assuming that these two exchangers operate at the same rate (stoichiometry of 1:1), the overall effect is to increase cell sodium and chloride, and to create water and CO_2 in the lumen while maintaining a constant intracellular pH (94). In the jejunum, the Na^+/H^+ exchanger is responsible for the acidification of jejunal luminal contents since there is no apparent Cl^-/HCO_3^- exchanger in this segment (90). A Cl^-/HCO_3^- exchanger is also present in the apical membrane of ileal crypt cells where neutral NaCl uptake does not take place (93).

Molecular cloning of the Na^+/H^+ exchanger has revealed that several forms exist in GI cells (97). A ubiquitous form (NHE-1) is found in all tissues examined (97) and is located in the basolateral membrane of gut epithelia (98). Of the epithelial types, NHE-2 is found in the stomach, liver, uterus, intestine, and kidney (97); NHE-3 in the kidney, small intestine, and colon; while NHE-4 is expressed in the stomach and, to a lesser extent, in the intestine (97). NHE-3 is located in the apical membrane of enterocytes and its distribution in jejunum, ileum, and proximal colon corresponds to the sites of electroneutral NaCl absorption (99). Recently a Cl^-/HCO_3^- exchanger that is expressed in the apical membrane of rabbit ileal crypt and villus cells was cloned (100), and functional studies suggest that two types of Cl^-/HCO_3^- exchanger may be present in rat small intestine (101).

Na⁺ Cotransporters

Sodium absorption in the small intestine occurs primarily through cotransport with nutrients. The intestinal Na^+-glucose cotransporter (SGLT1) was the first Na^+-cotransport carrier cloned (65,102) and is the best characterized of Na^+-nutrient cotransport mechanisms (64,103) (Fig. 1). Glucose is absorbed via an Na^+-glucose cotransporter located in the villus tip cells of the small intestine (104). The electrochemical gradient for sodium generated by the Na^+,K^+-ATPase provides the driving force for accumulation of intracellular nutrient against a concentration gradient. Glucose that accumulates within the cell exits across the basolateral membrane by passive diffusion, using the GLUT2 carrier. The charge of the ab-

sorbed Na^+ promotes Cl^- absorption via the paracellular pathway (the law of electroneutrality)[1] and water follows passively to maintain isotonicity of the intercellular space. Galactose coupling with sodium entry occurs through the Na^+-glucose carrier, while Na^+-coupled carriers for five separate amino acids, di- and tripeptides, phosphate, vitamins, and bile salts (66–69,105–107) are also present in the small intestine. The existence of Na^+-nutrient cotransporters and the fact that these remain operative during many diarrheal diseases provides the basis for the use of oral rehydration solutions that contain glucose, amino acids, or more complex sources of nutrients from which glucose, amino acids, or oligopeptides can be liberated by intraluminal and brush border digestive processes.

K⁺ Absorption

Until recently, it was assumed that K^+ leaked passively through the intercellular pathway in response to established gradients. It is now recognized that potassium is also absorbed and secreted by active transcellular mechanisms although the actual pathways are currently under investigation. It appears that H^+,K^+-ATPase in the apical membrane of epithelial cells of the distal colon is involved in electroneutral transepithelial potassium transport (56,57).

Secretory Processes

Electrogenic Cl⁻ Secretion

In the chloride secretory process, Cl^- is taken up across the basolateral membrane via the $Na^+,K^+,2Cl^-$ cotransporter. Na^+,K^+-ATPase provides the driving force for the entry of chloride by cotransport with sodium and also recycles Na^+. K^+ channels on the basolateral membrane (see below) allow for K^+ recycling (108,109). Chloride channels in the apical membrane permit the movement of chloride into the intestinal lumen. Since the cell interior is normally electronegative by 40–60 mV relative to the outside, the electrical gradient offsets the usual concentration gradient for chloride. Finally, since the epithelium cannot secrete chloride alone, the paracellular pathway permits the passive diffusion of sodium, potassium, and water in response to the transepithelial potential difference. The transcellular process is summarized in Fig. 2.

Several different chloride channels exist and are defined in part by their regulation by factors including intracellular levels of cyclic nucleotides or Ca^{2+} and cell volume (79,110–112). Cyclic nucleotide–activated low-conductance Cl^- channels are permeable to anions other than Cl^-. In cystic fibrosis, cAMP-activated Cl^- chan-

---

[1] The law of electroneutrality also applies to electrogenic Na^+ transport in the distal colon that occurs via amiloride-sensitive Na^+ channels. Thus, pure sodium is never absorbed alone but is accompanied by passive Cl^- absorption. The opposite is true for secretion: active Cl^- secretion is accompanied by passive Na^+ movement across tight junctions.

nels are defective (113). The CFTR (cystic fibrosis trans-membrane regulator) gene product is thought to be the Cl^- channel itself or a protein that regulates Cl^- channel function (114,115). Recent studies support the concept that CFTR can act as a low-conductance Cl^- channel gated by phosphokinase A (116). A Ca^{2+}-activated Cl^- channel, regulated by Ca^{2+}-calmodulin, was identified in airway epithelia and in colon carcinoma lines (117). This channel is not defective in cystic fibrosis. However, intestinal epithelia (unlike pulmonary epithelia) from patients with cystic fibrosis do not typically secrete Cl^- in response to Ca^{2+}-activating secretagogues (118–122). It was recently reported that Ca^{2+}-regulated Cl^- conductance is absent in intestinal epithelial cells (123), unlike pulmonary and pancreatic epithelial cells, in both (+/+) and (−/−) CFTR "knockout" mice (124). The absence of any alternative Cl^- (water) secretory process in the gut may explain the severity of disease expression in the intestine of cystic fibrosis "knockout" animals and patients (123,125). A third Cl^- channel regulated by cell volume (126–128) was identified as p-glycoprotein, the multidrug resistance gene product, which along with CFTR belongs to the ATP-binding cassette superfamily of membrane transport proteins (129). A novel G-protein-coupled Cl^- channel was also described in cultured human colonic cells (130).

K^+ Secretion

K^+ is secreted into the lumen of the mammalian colon under normal conditions using mechanisms similar to those implicated in Cl^- secretion (131,132). Although Na^+,K^+-ATPase and the $Na^+,K^+,2Cl^-$ cotransporter are involved in both Cl^- and K^+ secretion, it is the presence of barium-sensitive K^+ channels in the apical membrane that allows transepithelial potassium secretion (77). This process is electrogenic and can be stimulated by cAMP-acting secretagogues. These apical channels also facilitate ionic counterflow during electrogenic sodium absorption and are regulated by aldosterone (87,133,134). As discussed, potassium channels in the basolateral membrane allow potassium that enters via the sodium pump and the $Na^+/K^+/2Cl^-$ cotransporter to exit and prevent intracellular accumulation during electrogenic Cl^- secretion. Basolateral K^+ channels comprise at least two types, one localized to colonic surface cells and the other to crypt cells (135). In the crypt, two classes of basolateral K^+ channels have been identified, one regulated by cAMP (78) and the other through Ca^{2+} (136).

Bicarbonate Secretion

HCO_3^- is secreted by the duodenal epithelium where it contributes to the overlying mucus-bicarbonate layer. Although HCO_3^- is secreted elsewhere in the intestine, the mechanisms involved and physiologic role at these sites are less clear. Chloride–bicarbonate exchange in the human distal colon results in the alkalinization of the luminal contents due to the absence of an Na^+/H^+ exchanger

(137). The Cl^-/HCO_3^- exchanger is also present in the proximal colon and ileal brush border membrane, but at these sites, and in rat distal colon, it appears coupled to sodium–hydrogen exchange and is thus unlikely to account for alkalinization of the lumen in these segments (93–96). However, most bicarbonate secretion in the ileum is independent of chloride entry suggesting that additional mechanisms are involved. The ileum may secrete bicarbonate through either bicarbonate-selective channels in its brush border or electrogenic sodium-bicarbonate cotransporters (4). A recent study suggests that rabbit ileal HCO_3^- secretion is electrogenic and that at low intracellular Cl^- concentrations HCO_3^- can be secreted via anion channels activated by cAMP and cGMP (81). It is not clear if these HCO_3^- channels are the same or different from the Cl^- channel (or channels) that govern Cl^- secretion.

INTRACELLULAR MESSENGERS OF ION TRANSPORT

Regulation of intestinal electrolyte transport occurs via intracellular messengers that are modulated by various external stimuli and by other poorly understood factors such as acid–base balance (138), arterial and venous blood pressure, motility (139–141), and intraluminal pressure (142,143). Epithelial receptors for endogenous physiological stimuli are largely found on the basolateral membrane whereas receptors for bacterial enterotoxins are located in the apical membrane. Once receptor binding of the external stimulus occurs, a number of intracellular events mediate changes in various transport pathways to effect the observed stimulus-induced changes of ion transport. Cyclic nucleotides, both cAMP and cGMP, and ionized calcium (Ca^{2+}) are important players in these events and increased levels of these messengers within the epithelium act to stimulate Cl^- secretion by crypt epithelial cells and inhibit electroneutral NaCl absorption by surface or villus cells. These signal transduction pathways and the second messengers generated in response to external mediators are summarized here for the sake of completeness and are covered in more detail in the chapter by Chang and Cho.

Cyclic AMP

A variety of external stimuli act through cAMP (Tables 1 and 2). cAMP is generated from ATP through the activation of adenylate cyclase located in the basolateral membrane, a process regulated by stimulatory (G_s) and inhibitory (G_i) G proteins (144). Although a complete discussion of G proteins is beyond the scope of this chapter, over 17 types of α subunits, 4 types of β subunits, and 3 types of γ subunits have been reported (145). A number of external messengers including prostaglandins, histamine, vasoactive polypeptide, cholera toxin, adenosine (A_2), and β-agonists stimulate G_s and induce secretion. The α_2 agonists, somatostatin, enkephalin, (μ), and neuropeptide Y stimulate G_i and inhibit secretion (146). cAMP activates

TABLE 1. *Neuroendocrine modulators of intestinal ion transport*

Compound	ICM[a]	Enterocyte[b]	Neural[b]	Immune/mesenchymal[b,c]
Secretory				
Glucagon	cAMP	?	?	?
Histamine	cAMP	+	+	+ (P, L, F)
PHI	cAMP	+	−	?
Secretin	cAMP	?	?	?
VIP	cAMP	+	±	+ (L, M)
ANPs	cGMP	+	+	+ (F)
Guanylin	cGMP	+	?	?
Nitric oxide	cGMP	?	+	+ (P)
Acetylcholine	Ca^{2+}	+	+	+ (F?)
Bombesin	Ca^{2+}	+	?	?
Neurotensin	Ca^{2+}	?	+	?
Serotonin	Ca^{2+}	?	+	+
Substance P	Ca^{2+}	+	±	+ (L, M)
Calcitonin/CGRP	$?Ca^{2+}$	?	+	?
Cholecystokinin	$?Ca^{2+}$	?	?	?
Endothelin	$?Ca^{2+}$	?	−	?
Gastrin	?	?	?	?
GIP	?	?	?	?
Motilin	?	?	?	?
Vasopressin	?	?	?	?
Absorptive				
Aldosterone	?	+	−	?
α-adrenergic agents	G_i	+	+	?
Angiotensin	?	?	+	?
Dopamine	?	?	?	?
Enkephalins	?	±	?	?
Glucocorticoids	?	+	?	?
Neuropeptide Y	G_i	+	?	?
Opiates	?	±	+	?
Peptide YY	?	?	?	?
Prolactin	?	?	?	?
Somatostatin	G_i	+	?	?

ANPs, atrial natriuretic peptides; CGRP, calcitonin gene-related peptide; GIP, gastric inhibitory polypeptide; PHI, peptide histidine isoleucine; VIP, vasoactive intestinal polypeptide.

[a] ICM; intracellular mediator involved. Intracellular mediators for the absorptive stimuli of ion transport are largely unknown (?), although some act via inhibitory G proteins (G_i).

[b] Neurohumoral factors alter ion transport by acting directly on epithelial cells (enterocytes) and/or indirectly through regulatory systems (neural or immune/mesenchymal) to stimulate secretion or absorption. Involvement of these direct and indirect mechanisms for a given mediator is denoted as + (involved). − (not involved), ? (not tested or unclear), or ± (conflicting data).

[c] Various immune/mesenchymal cells include phagocytes (P), lymphocytes (L), mast cells (M), and fibroblasts (F). Their role is not well defined for absorptive stimuli.

TABLE 2. *Immune/inflammatory factors regulating intestinal ion transport*

Mediator	ICM[a]	Enterocyte[b]	Neural[b]	Immune/mesenchymal[b,c]
PAF	cAMP	+	+	+ (P)
Prostaglandins[d]	cAMP, Ca^{2+}	+	+	+ (L)
Nitric oxide	cGMP	?	+	+ (P)
Bradykinins	Ca^{2+}	+	+	+ (P)
Histamine	Ca^{2+}	+	+	+ (L)
ROS	Ca^{2+}	+	?	+ (P, F)
Serotonin	Ca^{2+}	−	+	+
Adenosine	?	+	+	+
Arachidonic acid	?	+	+	+
Cytokines	?	±	?	+ (L, M, F)
Leukotrienes	?	?	−	+ (P, F)

Note: The great majority of factors listed here stimulate secretion. PAF, platelet-activating factor; ROS, reactive oxygen species.

[a,b,c] See Table 1.

[d] Varying effects on transport and on the regulatory systems according to the class.

Cl⁻ channels (113,121) and inhibits coupled NaCl transporters (147). In T84 cells, cAMP-mediated Cl⁻ secretion is accompanied by cytoskeletal redistribution (148) with the $Na^+,K^+,2Cl^-$ cotransporter identified as the step functionally linked to the cytoskeleton (149). Receptor-mediated activation of adenylate cyclase and the subsequent secretory response are dependent on Ca^{2+}/calmodulin (147,150,151).

Cyclic GMP

Atrial natriuretic peptides (ANPs), *E. coli* STa, and nitric oxide all act to increase cGMP but the generation of cGMP from GTP involves the activation of three different forms of guanylate cyclase (soluble, particulate, and intestinal). The membrane-bound particulate form of guanylate cyclase, GCA, responds to ANPs and GCA mRNA is only found in lamina propria cells according to a recent *in situ* hybridization study (152). This supports previous studies suggesting that ANPs do not directly stimulate colonic epithelial cells (153,154). STa binds to receptor proteins in the brush border membrane that constitute forms of another membrane-bound type of guanylate cyclase, GCC (155), also classified as the intestinal or cytoskeletal-associated particulate form (156). In the *in situ* hybridization study, GCC mRNA was seen in epithelial cells throughout rat colonic crypts and to a lesser extent in the surface epithelial cells (152). In another study, mRNA for the STa receptor increased along the crypt–villus axis (157). mRNA expression for guanylin, an endogenous ligand for a guanylate cyclase similar to GCC, was strong in surface epithelial cells and the upper crypts of rat colon (152,158) as well as in villus cells in rat ileum (158). The ANP-stimulated guanylate cyclase (GCA) differs from the STa-stimulated form (GCC) in that protein kinase C inhibits only the latter type (159). Activation of the soluble guanylate cyclase occurs in response to nitric oxide.

cGMP has been shown to activate a unique isoform of cGMP-dependent protein kinase in the apical membrane of mammalian enterocytes, which, presumably through phosphorylation of specific brush border membrane proteins, triggers the opening of Cl⁻ channels and the inhibition of coupled Na^+, Cl⁻ transporters (160,161). As with cAMP-mediated secretion, cGMP-stimulated $Na^+,K^+,2Cl^-$ cotransport and Cl⁻ secretion is microfilament-dependent in T84 cells (162).

Calcium

Increases in the level of intracellular calcium constitute another primary signaling system known to regulate intestinal ion transport (163,164). To initiate this process, receptor-mediated activation of phospholipase C (PLC) stimulates the metabolism of membrane phosphatidylinositides to form inositol(1,4,5)triphosphate (IP₃) and 1,2-diacylglycerol (DAG). The latter activates protein kinase C (PKC), leading to phosphorylation reactions, or it is degraded by lipases to liberate arachidonic acid for eicosanoid production. The inositol phosphates, and especially

IP₃, elevate intracellular Ca^{2+} levels by mobilizing calcium from nonmitochondrial stores and also activate DAG/PKC. Increases of intracellular calcium due to calcium ionophores, muscarinic cholinergic agonists, and serotonin mediate their effects on ion transport through this mechanism (165,166). Recent evidence indicates that at least some forms of PLC are activated via G proteins; members of the novel G_q class of G proteins are coupled to the PLC stimulatory receptor for thromboxane A₂, bradykinin, angiotensin, histamine, vasopressin, and acetylcholine (167).

Intracellular calcium may also accumulate through an increased cell permeability to calcium (168). This mechanism appears responsible for the transport alterations due to neurotensin, bombesin, substance P, hydrogen peroxide, and carbachol. In avian systems cyclic nucleotides have been shown to stimulate release of calcium (147). In general, increases of intracellular Ca^{2+} activate anion secretion and inhibit NaCl absorption via the opening of basolateral K^+ channels (136,164). Cell calcium exerts its regulatory effects in several ways including direct effects on transport proteins and transport-related enzymes (163). Increased intracellular Ca^{2+} activates calmodulin, a 17-kDa calcium-binding regulatory protein, which in turn activates calmodulin-dependent protein kinases (169,170). Enterocyte receptor–mediated adenylate cyclase activity and cytoskeletal proteins are also regulated by calcium/calmodulin (151). As discussed, calcium acts to activate PKC and the effects of intracellular calcium can be modified by DAG/PKC (171) and by products of IP₃ metabolism (164,172).

Arachidonic Acid and Phospholipases

It has become apparent that certain stimuli of intestinal ion transport are not accompanied by increases in cAMP, cGMP, or cytosolic calcium, suggesting that additional second messenger pathways may exist. Recent studies indicate that arachidonic acid or its metabolites may be involved in the chloride secretion induced by adenosine and its precursor 5'-AMP (173,174). Other studies have implicated phospholipase A₂ pathways in the control of Cl⁻ secretion (175,176).

Kinases and Phosphatases

Specific enzymes that control phosphorylation of membrane proteins, referred to as protein kinases and phosphatases, mediate the effects of the primary second messengers, cyclic nucleotides, and calcium (177,178). The best defined enzyme of this type, protein kinase A, is involved in cAMP-dependent transport and has been shown to directly phosphorylate CFTR to open Cl⁻ channels (179,180). cGMP-dependent events may also be related to effects on protein kinase A (181) and this could explain why, in contrast to other systems, the two cyclic nucleotides mediate similar responses in intestinal epithelial cells. The protein kinase(s) modulating the secretory effects of calcium are not as well understood. Calcium/

calmodulin-dependent protein kinases are directly activated by increases in intracellular calcium. A brush border Ca^{2+}/calmodulin-dependent protein kinase II has been shown to inhibit rabbit ileal Na^{+}/H^{+} exchange, a process that participates in the regulation of basal NaCl absorption (182). Ca^{2+}/calmodulin-dependent protein kinases also modulate Cl^{-} secretion in cultured epithelial cells (183). Calcium acts with diacylglycerol to translocate PKC to the cell membrane and cause its activation (184). PKC appears to inhibit epithelial absorption (185) as well as stimulate secretion although the mechanisms of the latter process are complex (186).

REGULATORY SYSTEMS

Since absorptive and secretory epithelial cells are the effector cells of intestinal ion transport, it is important to understand their relationship with other cell populations within the gut wall (Fig. 4). In addition to transporting cells, the GI epithelium comprises mucus-secreting goblet cells, specialized M cells overlying Peyer's patches, as well as Paneth and other enteroendocrine cells. Together with intraepithelial lymphocytes, these epithelial and endocrine cells form a lining layer that separates the body from the contents of the gut lumen. Numerous other cell types including immune-inflammatory cells, mesenchymal cells, and nerves reside in the compartments below the basement membrane, the lamina propria, and the submucosa that are separated by the muscularis mucosae. By virtue of their close anatomic association, these cells have great potential to modify the epithelium. It is worth noting that some factors acutely regulate ion transport through the gating of ion channels and modulating carriers (187), whereas other mediators such as steroid hormones and cytokines have longer term effects by altering the expression of protein pumps, carriers, channels, or transport-related enzymes (85,188–190). It should be stated that the physiological significance of the regulatory sys-

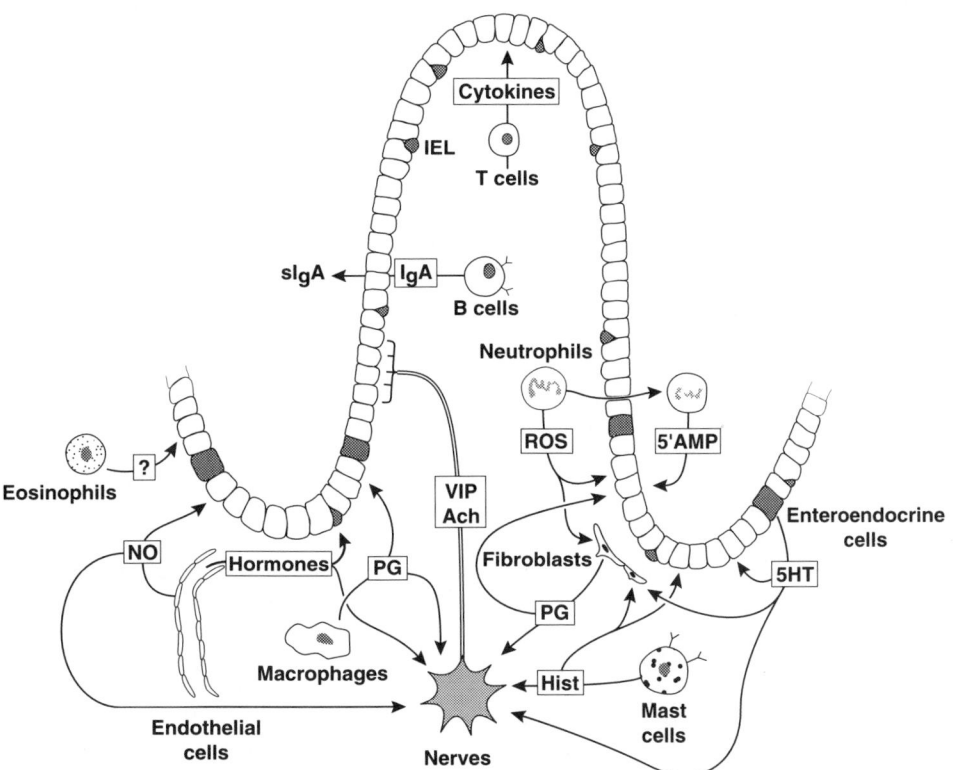

FIG. 4. Regulatory systems involved in intestinal ion transport. Enteroendocrine cells in the crypt release mediators, e.g., serotonin (5-HT) across the basolateral membrane to regulate adjacent epithelial cells (paracrine regulation). If released in large enough quantities in the bloodstream, these have endocrine actions (hormones). Peptides such as vasoactive intestinal peptide (VIP) or neurotransmitters such as acetylcholine (Ach) are released from the nerve endings of neurons to regulate epithelial cells (neurocrine regulation). Substances including reactive oxygen species (ROS), 5'-adenosine monophosphate (5'-AMP), prostaglandins (PG), and histamine (hist) released from activated immune cells such as phagocytes, mast cells, and lymphocytes can also regulate epithelial cells (immune regulation). Other mesenchymal cells, particularly fibroblasts, release mediators (e.g., PG) that alter epithelial ion transport. In addition to directly stimulating epithelial cells, immune/mesenchymal mediators may also act on nerves, other immune cells, and fibroblasts. Similarly, neuropeptides can affect immune cells, fibroblasts, and other nerves. Only key aspects of these complex interactions are depicted in this schematic diagram. IEL, intraepithelial lymphocytes; NO, nitric oxide; sIgA, secretory immunoglobulin A.

tems discussed briefly below is unknown since there are discrepancies between *in vivo* and *in vitro* studies, with many of the reported alterations of intestinal ion transport occurring only in response to concentrations of mediators that may be far higher than those likely to be released in disease situations. (For a more comprehensive discussion of this topic, see references 8, 10, and 11.)

Neurohumoral Control

Neurohormonal factors (Table 1) are recognized as a major controlling system for intestinal water and electrolyte transport (8,9). Neurohumoral regulation can be paracrine, neurocrine, or endocrine in nature with some overlap depending on the amount and cell source of the messenger produced. In certain pathological situations, messengers that would normally be classified as paracrine or neurotransmitter in nature are released into the blood in high enough concentrations to be considered as hormones. Examples of such conditions include endocrine cell tumors of the GI tract and pancreas (e.g., VIPomas, gastrinomas). Under normal circumstances, local release of chemical messengers from endocrine cells can influence the transport properties of the epithelium either by acting directly on the enterocytes (paracrine stimulation) or by modulating other regulatory elements of the mucosa such as nerves, leukocytes, or mesenchymal cells. Traditionally, hormones were viewed as agents that promoted absorption, but it is now apparent that hormonal as well as neural factors may stimulate either secretion or absorption (Table 1).

Intestinal ion transport is regulated by the autonomic nervous system, which consists of extrinsic sympathetic and parasympathetic nerves, and intrinsic enteric nerves. The enteric nervous system (ENS) is composed of the myenteric and submucosal plexuses and is an independent system that coordinates smooth muscle, epithelial and vascular functions of the gut. Submucosal neurons release a variety of neurotransmitters, including vasoactive intestinal polypeptide, enkephalins, acetylcholine, somatostatin, neuropeptide Y, and substance P. The central nervous system modulates ENS activity through parasympathetic and sympathetic pathways. Substance P is released from fibers that emanate from the dorsal root ganglia, whereas norepinephrine, somatostatin, and neuropeptide Y are released from neural fibers with cell bodies in prevertebral ganglia.

Traditionally, hormonal control of intestinal electrolyte transport was thought to be exerted mainly through the renin-angiotensin-aldosterone axis, an extraintestinal hormonal system that plays a major role in total body fluid and electrolyte balance. Angiotensin II stimulates the adrenal gland to release aldosterone, a hormone that regulates sodium transport in the distal colon and renal tubule. In the gut epithelium, aldosterone increases the number of Na^+ channels in the apical membrane, upregulates Na^+,K^+-ATPase activity, and alters K^+ and coupled NaCl transport in the colon (85,191). Angiotensin II itself stimulates absorption, an effect that may be mediated by sympathetic nerves and possibly due to direct actions on epithelial cells (192). Angiotensin II may function as a paracrine mediator in that it is formed locally within the gut. Glucocorticoids also have effects on ion transport to increase sodium absorption and sodium-coupled chloride absorption in the colon and small intestine (193,194). They stimulate rabbit ileal villus cell brush border Na^+/H^+ exchange with an increased mRNA for NHE-3 (195). Glucocorticoids also increase Na^+,K^+-ATPase in the basement membrane and induce the synthesis of lipocortin-1, a protein that inhibits phospholipase A_2, thereby inhibiting release of arachidonic acid from the plasma membrane (196).

ANPs are a group of peptides that are released from atrial myocytes into blood in response to atrial stretch or pressure. In addition to their role in overall body fluid homeostasis, ANPs have effects on intestinal transport. *In vivo* studies in rat small intestine suggest that these peptides inhibit absorption, whereas in Ussing chambered small intestine and in the colon, ANPs also stimulate chloride secretion (153,154,197,198). These effects appear to be mediated by cholinergic and noncholinergic nerves, and ANP receptors have been found on intestinal fibroblasts (199) suggesting that indirect mechanisms are involved. Vasopressin represents another hormone with secretory activity (200) but its mechanisms of action in the intestine are unclear.

Enteroendocrine cells constitute another component of the neurohormonal transport-regulating system. Amine-precursor uptake and decarboxylation (APUD) cells in both the large and small intestine contain serotonin (5-HT), glucagon, somatostatin, and substance P, while cells of the upper gut may also secrete GIP, secretin, neurotensin, cholecystokinin, motilin, gastrin, PYY, and enkephalins (8). Products from enteroendocrine cells operate in a paracrine or hormonal fashion, with epithelial ion transport affected by both direct or indirect mechanisms (Fig. 4, Table 1).

An understanding of how neuroendocrine factors alter intestinal ion transport (summarized in Table 1) has developed from a large numbers of studies in which exogenous neurohormonal substances were added *in vivo* or *in vitro* (70,201–214) or endogenous neurotransmitters were released by electrical field stimulation (215–219). As outlined in Table 1, these neuroendocrine substances have direct effects on intestinal epithelial cells but may also act on nonepithelial cells to affect ion transport. For example, certain mast cell populations possess receptors for substance P and may be activated by this peptide (220). The ENS is also subject to modulation by input from the immune and endocrine systems since submucosal neurons have receptors for eicosanoids, histamine, and platelet-activating factor and, possibly, acetylcholine, norepinephrine, 5-HT, enkephalins, and tachykinins (11). Thus, the potential for complex neuroimmune interactions in the regulation of intestinal ion transport is vast.

Immune/Inflammatory Cells

Knowledge of the normal intestinal immune-inflammatory system and how it may be activated during infection or other perturbations is essential to an understanding of how this system regulates intestinal ion transport in health and disease. A variety of immune and inflammatory cells are housed within the GI tract located predominantly below (lamina propria cells), but also within (intraepithelial cells), the epithelial layer. The immune cells of the intestinal lamina propria include approximately 60% T lymphocytes, 25% to 30% B cells or plasma cells (primarily IgA secreting), 8% to 10% macrophages, and 3% to 5% eosinophils and mast cells (221). Together with immune cells found in the lining surfaces of the respiratory, mammary, and urogenital tracts, these sites compose what is known as the common mucosal immune system or mucosa-associated lymphoid tissues (MALT). The corresponding term used to describe the GI immune system specifically is gut-associated lymphoid tissue (GALT). GALT consists of organized lymphoid follicles (Peyer's patches in the small intestine, lymphoid aggregates in the colon), the lymphoid and reticuloendothelial elements of the lamina propria, intraepithelial lymphocytes, and mesenteric lymph nodes. (For a comprehensive review of GI immune defense mechanisms, the reader is referred to Part III of this book.)

Phagocytes

The phagocytic immune-inflammatory cell system is composed of mononuclear phagocytes (monocytes and macrophages) and polymorphonuclear leukocytes (neutrophils and eosinophils). After leaving the bone marrow, monocytes circulate for ~24 hr before taking up residence in tissue sites, where they are referred to as macrophages. Neutrophils and eosinophils also circulate transiently before settling in various tissue sites. Significant numbers of eosinophils, macrophages, and neutrophils are found within the gut wall under normal conditions; increased numbers are seen with a variety of inflammatory and infectious states. Activation of these phagocytes, which exhibit chemotaxis and oxy radical–mediated killing of microorganisms, occurs in response to many stimuli including bacterial and immune cell products. Products of phagocyte secretion (Table 3) can have direct and/or

TABLE 3. *Secreted products of phagocytic leukocytes*

Enzymes and inhibitors
    Proteases and inhibitor, phospholipases and inhibitor, lysosomal hydrolases
Lipid metabolites
    PGE_2, $PGF_{2\alpha}$, PGI_2, TXA_2, LTB_4, C_4, D_4, E_4, HPETEs, HETEs, platelet-activating factor
Reactive oxygen metabolites
    O_2, H_2O_2, OH, HOCl
Hormones
    β-endorphins, ACTH, vitamin D_3
Complement components
Coagulation factors
    Kallikrein
Extracellular matrix
    Fibronectin, proteoglycans
Cytokines
    IL-1, IL-1RA, TNF-α, IFN-α, -γ, TGF-β, PDGF, IGFs

indirect effects on the epithelium to alter ion transport and also serve to amplify the inflammatory signal (Table 2). The bacterial chemotactic peptide, f-met-leu-phe (fMLF) (222), has been used to activate phagocytes (223) to induce a chloride secretory response in small intestinal and colonic tissues studied *in vitro* (224,225).

In vitro studies using T84 cell monolayers demonstrated that neutrophils can traverse the epithelium via tight junctions in response to chemotactic stimuli (226–228). The migration is mediated by the CD11b/CD18 adhesion molecule complex on neutrophils and is most efficient in the physiological direction (229). The epithelial ligand for CD11b/CD18 in this system has not yet been identified. This process is associated with a reduction in electrical resistance (226,230) and electrogenic chloride secretion is stimulated when luminal neutrophils are activated to release 5'-AMP [previously labeled as "neutrophil-derived secretagogue" (231)], which is cleaved to adenosine by an ecto-5'-nucleotidase located on the apical surface of intestinal epithelial cells (174). This may be an important mechanism contributing to the diarrhea occurring in diseases in which neutrophils are found within the gut lumen, particularly within crypts (crypt abscesses). Moreover, the biological relevance of apically located adenosine receptors (232) is now more apparent. *In vivo*, microbial inhabitants of the gut lumen may serve as stimuli that induce transepithelial migration and activation either by direct release of chemotactic peptides (e.g., fMLF) or via epithelial release of chemotactic factors that include IL-8 and other factors such as transmigration chemotactic factor (233,234). A recent communication suggests that activated eosinophils release a small molecular weight factor, possibly adenosine or its precursor, which stimulates T84 cells to secrete Cl^- (235).

Mast Cells

Intestinal mast cells arise from pluripotent hematopoietic stem cells and differentiate into two main phenotypes according to local environmental factors including the presence of certain cytokines and growth factors (220). Although mast cell heterogeneity has been best established in the rat (236), human intestinal mast cells also are also composed of two main populations (237–239). Mast cells release a variety of potential secretagogues including preformed mediators such as histamine and newly formed mediators generated by the metabolism of arachidonic acid (Table 4) (240). There is ample evidence that the activation of mast cells acutely stimulates intestinal secretion through both direct and indirect mechanisms (Table 2) (224,241–251). In addition, mast cell activation is accompanied by villus shortening and sloughing of villus tip cells (252,253), presumably through the action of mast cell proteases and oxy radicals. This damage to the villi could also impair absorptive processes allowing secretory mechanisms to predominate. A number of substances released during the inflammatory response to enteric infections (e.g., cytokines, neuropeptides, and other proinflammatory molecules) and certain microbial products, such as cholera toxin and *C. difficile* toxin A, are capable

TABLE 4. *Secreted products of mast cells*

Lysosomal enzymes
  Exoglycosidases, kininogenase, chymotrypsin/ trypsin, peroxidase, superoxide dismutase, aryl-sulfatases
Lipid metabolites
  PGD_2, LTB_4, C_4, D_4, E_4, HPETEs, HETEs, thromboxanes, platelet-activating factor
Reactive oxygen metabolites
Proteoglycans
  Heparin, chondroitin sulfate
Amines
  Histamine, serotonin
Cytokines
  IL-1-6, TNF-α, IFN-α, -γ, TGF-β, MIP-1 family, GM-CSF

of activating mast cells (254). A comprehensive discussion of the role of mast cells in intestinal immunity is presented in the chapter by Befus.

Lymphocytes

Although lymphocytes constitute a large proportion of the immune cells of the gut and they are clearly stimulated during the course of many GI infections, there is less evidence that this group of effector cells has direct effects on intestinal ion transport. Unlike phagocytes and mast cells, lymphocytes do not release a wide range of bioactive compounds that act as secretagogues. However, lymphocytes, by virtue of the production of cytokines, have great potential to modify the gut epithelium and the systems that regulate intestinal ion transport. While there is some evidence that a few cytokines have acute effects on ion transport (255,256), most studies demonstrated alterations of transport and other properties of the epithelium with more prolonged exposure to cytokines (257,258). Recent reports of experimental systems utilizing lymphocytes and T84 cells suggest that colonic epithelial cells cocultured with activated peripheral blood T cells (259) or juxtaposed with intraepithelial lymphocytes (IEL) (260) exhibit decreased electrical resistance and reduced secretory responses to agonists. In gut tissues, the net effect of lymphocyte activation is more complex and contributes to the development of villus atrophy and other manifestations of intestinal injury and repair. Work using human fetal intestinal explants demonstrates that mitogen-stimulated T cells and their cytokines induce villus atrophy and crypt hyperplasia (261–263). Similar mechanisms are involved in intestinal hypersensitivity reactions (264) and enteric parasitic infections (265). Thus, the classical morphological response to intestinal injury, villous atrophy, and crypt hyperplasia is a T-cell–driven process.

Epithelial Factors

Traditionally, the epithelium has been viewed as the target of gut inflammatory processes but current information suggests that the epithelium may also function as an active participant of the mucosal immune response. Epithelial cells interact with immune cells through the expression of adhesion and accessory molecules (266–268). The enterocyte produces a large number of cytokines and growth factors (269–277) although the biological relevance of their production is unknown since many have been detected only at the mRNA level and/or in cultured cells. Gut epithelial cells are a potential source of other inflammatory mediators including a variety of eicosanoids (278–281) and NO (282). Thus, it appears that the epithelium itself constitutes another source of immune-inflammatory mediators (Table 2), and as such the epithelium is capable of modulating the inflammatory response and may autoregulate intestinal ion transport.

Mesenchymal Cells

Although not readily classified as immune, neural, or hormonal control, there is recent evidence that nonimmune mesenchymal cells such as fibroblasts, and perhaps smooth muscle cells and endothelial cells, also play a role in regulating intestinal ion transport (11). This likely occurs through the release of factors acting in a paracrine fashion on epithelial cells and perhaps other elements of the intestinal mucosa. Intestinal smooth muscle also regulates the flow of intraluminal contents and thus regulates the contact time for absorption to occur (139). The importance of motility in the control of stool volume is illustrated by the effectiveness of many antidiarrheal drugs whose main action is control of motility. Additional intercellular transport-regulating interactions can be postulated since neural, endocrine, and immune factors may influence intestinal smooth muscle (283,284).

Specific Immune/Mesenchymal Factors and Their Effects on Ion Transport

Reactive Oxygen Species

Reactive oxygen species (ROS) including superoxide ($O_2^- \cdot$), hydroxyl radical (OH·), and hydrogen peroxide (H_2O_2), are generated during the respiratory burst in phagocytic cells through mitochondrial and microsomal electron transport chains and by various oxidant enzymes including xanthine oxidase, cyclooxygenase, and lipoxygenase. In the presence of myeloperoxidase, H_2O_2 combines with free chloride to form hypochlorous acid (HOCl), which in turn can combine with free primary amines to produce *N*-chloramines and monochloramine. H_2O_2 is the most stable of the ROS and its effects have been demonstrated to include stimulation of chloride secretion and inhibition of electroneutral sodium absorption in rat gut (285,286), and Ca^{2+}-mediated Cl^- secretion in T84 monolayers (287). The other ROS are capable of stimulating intestinal secretion as well (286,288,289).

Nitric Oxide

Mammalian cells synthesize inorganic oxides of nitrogen to form nitrites, nitrates, and NO. Although the production and role of NO is best established in neuronal and endothelial cells, NO is also produced by macrophages and neutrophils, as well as other cell types (290,291). NO appears to have direct effects on intestinal ion transport mediated through cGMP, but has indirect effects via the ENS and through metabolism of arachidonic acid (292,293). In one report, higher concentrations of NO stimulated net secretion while at lower concentrations absorptive processes were promoted.

Arachidonic Acid Metabolites

A major phospholipid component of all cell membranes is the unsaturated fatty acid arachidonic acid (AA), which is released by the action of phospholipases A_2 (PLA_2) or C (PLC). Metabolism by several different enzymatic pathways generates different groups of bioactive molecules. The major products of the cyclooxygenase pathway are prostaglandins (PGs) and thromboxanes while HPETEs, HETEs, and leukotrienes (LTs) are products of the lipoxygenase pathways. Eicosanoids are produced predominantly by subepithelial cell populations within the intestine (phagocytes, mast cells, and fibroblasts) and are metabolized by epithelial cells (11). They are released from the intestine in response to many factors including microbial products such as fMLF and LPS. Eicosanoids have multiple effects on gut function including fluid and electrolyte transport (11). In addition to direct epithelial effects, prostaglandins downregulate, whereas leukotrienes stimulate the immune cells known to regulate ion transport.

PGs, particularly PGE_2, induce cAMP-mediated Cl secretion and inhibit electroneutral NaCl and water absorption in both small and large intestines (109). K secretion is also stimulated in the colon. In contrast, PGD_2 has antisecretory effects (294,295). Although many nonprostaglandin eicosanoids (e.g., LTs) are reported to alter ion transport, most of these effects appear to be mediated through the release of cyclooxygenase products (296,297). There is recent evidence that AA itself may regulate the chloride secretory response to adenosine (173).

Platelet-Activating Factor (PAF)

The term *platelet-activating factor* (PAF) refers to a group of biologically active phosphoglyceride molecules which, like eicosanoids, are released upon activation of various cells including immune-inflammatory and mesenchymal elements. These compounds have multiple biological effects in addition to their ability to aggregate platelets. Studies in rat jejunum (298) and colon (224) demonstrate that PAF induces net ion transport due to electrogenic chloride secretion. While these studies showed that PAF had indirect effects on intestinal ion transport in native tissues, PAF-stimulated ion transport in T84 cells alone (299) implicates direct epithelial effects of PAF as well.

Purines

Until recently, adenosine-mediated alterations of intestinal ion transport were attributed to the activation of mast cells since adenosine is located within the secretory granules of these cells (240). However, it is now evident that neutrophils (174) and possibly eosinophils (235) may also act through adenosine to stimulate secretion. Adenosine has been shown to stimulate chloride secretion in rat intestine and in T84 cells (300). Although both studies demonstrated an increase in epithelial cAMP, a poor correlation between the magnitude of the secretory response and the increase in cyclic nucleotide levels to varying doses of adenosine was found in T84 cells. Subsequent studies by Barrett and coworkers suggest that arachidonic acid may function as an intracellular mediator coupling adenosine and chloride secretion (173). ATP also stimulates Cl^- secretion in T84 cells both directly and through the release of adenosine during conversion of ATP to ADP.

Histamine

Histamine synthesis occurs via enzymatic decarboxylation of the amino acid L-histidine (301). Mast cells constitute the major source of histamine in the intestine. Histamine stimulates anion secretion via histamine$_1$ receptors found on epithelial cells of the large and small intestine (302). The Isc response is short-lived and is mediated primarily by Cl^-. Histamine directly stimulates epithelial Cl^- secretion by increasing cytosolic free Ca^{2+} (303). Studies in intestinal tissues indicate that histamine acts via nerves as well, both directly on neural histamine receptors (302,304) and through PGs released from subepithelial cells (305). Histamine-induced PGs also stimulate epithelial cells to secrete Cl^- as described above.

Serotonin

Metabolism of the amino acid tryptophan results in the formation of serotonin, or 5-hydroxytryptamine (5-HT). 5-HT is present in specific populations of enteric neurons, in mucosal enterochromaffin cells, and in mast cells of certain species. 5-HT stimulates an increase in Isc in large and small intestine from rats, rabbits, guinea pigs, and humans (306–310), but the mechanisms for the increase (inhibition of electroneutral sodium absorption and/or stimulation of electrogenic Cl^- secretion) vary according to the species and gut segment involved. The use of 5-HT receptor antagonists to inhibit Isc changes suggests that different receptor subtypes are involved in the different species and intestinal sites. It is not clear at what level(s) this inhibition takes place since 5-HT receptors have been identified on various enteric cells including nerves and possibly enterocytes (310). 5-HT acts via nerves in the guinea pig intestine (310) and also appears to stimulate the release of PG from subepithelial cells (311).

Cytokines

Cytokines are important mediators of cell-to-cell communication and there is recent evidence to indicate that these proteins mediate acute and chronic effects on intestinal epithelial ion transport. Studies in avian (255) and rat small intestine (256) suggest that interleukins 1 and 3 (IL-1 and IL-3) act through mesenchymal and/or immune cells to indirectly stimulate epithelial ion transport. Preliminary communications indicate that tumor necrosis factor–α (TNF-α) and platelet-derived growth factor act in a similar fashion to induce alterations of ion transport (312,313). Cytokines do not appear to have an immediate effect on ion transport in cultured intestinal epithelial cells supporting the concept that acute cytokine-induced changes in intestinal tissues occur largely by indirect mechanisms. Epithelial growth factor (EGF) appears to be an exception to this general pattern of cytokine-activated ion transport since it is proabsorptive, effective on the mucosal surface and its actions are relatively acute and direct (314,315).

Epithelial exposure to cytokines for longer times appears to affect ion transport more directly since cultured epithelial cells exposed to interferon-γ (IFN-γ) for 24–48 hr exhibit reduced secretory responses to cAMP and Ca^{2+}-mediated agonists (257) and reduced Na^+-dependent brush border glutamine transport (316). Subtle changes in the T84 cell membrane protein composition led the authors in one study to speculate that ion channels regulating chloride secretion may have been affected (257). In another, the apical Cl^- channel, the basolateral $Na^+,K^+,2Cl^-$ cotransporter, the K^+ channel, and Na^+,K^+-ATPase were functionally downregulated by IFN-γ (258). In vitro experiments also indicate that certain cytokines [IFN-γ in T84 cells and TNF-α in HT-29 (317,318)] affect the tight junctions. Chronic cytokine exposure also impacts on other factors that regulate intestinal ion transport. Exposure of fibroblasts to IL-1β and/or TNF-α for 24–48 hr further augments (312,319) their ability to enhance, through the release of PGs, the secretory response of T84 cells to certain inflammatory mediators (299). While it is known that immune cells and nerves can also be modulated by cytokines, the consequence of such interactions has not been studied in the context of intestinal fluid and electrolyte transport. With continued investigation, it is likely that cytokines will be shown to influence all aspects regulating intestinal ion transport.

Another factor to consider in the intercellular regulation of intestinal ion transport is the potential for synergistic interactions between the mediators released from various regulatory cells (320,321). In a recent study, prior stimulation of T84 cells with the cAMP-acting neurohormonal secretagogue vasoactive intestinal peptide (VIP) was shown to augment the secretory response to the Ca^{2+}-mediated immune stimulus H_2O_2 (287). It should be clear that the regulation of fluid and electrolyte balance in both health and disease is a complex and partially understood process. Any discussion of how enteric infections alter intestinal ion transport must be considered with this limitation in mind.

MECHANISMS OF ALTERED ION TRANSPORT DURING INFECTION

Microbial pathogens can alter the movement of ions and water across the epithelium through various mechanisms, many of which may be operative in a single infection (Fig. 5). In order to cause disease, enteric pathogens entering the gut lumen must establish some form of communication with the epithelial cells lining the GI tract (322,323). This may occur by various mechanisms that include one or more of the following: toxin production; epithelial adherence; and epithelial invasion or translocation. Intestinal ion transport may be affected both acutely and directly by these interactions but the activation of various regulatory systems and the development of villous atrophy/crypt hyperplasia also play important roles in the alterations of fluid and electrolyte transport that accompany enteric infections (Fig. 6).

Toxin Production

Toxins are microbial proteins that may exhibit enterotoxicity (the ability to induce diarrhea), cytotoxicity (producing cytopathic effects), and/or neurotoxicity. Some enterotoxins such as cholera toxin as well as E. coli heat-labile (LT) and heat-stable enterotoxins (STa, STb) stimulate secretion without cytotoxicity. Other enterotoxins including Shiga toxin, C. difficile toxin A, and B. fragilis toxin have multiple effects on host cells. For some organisms, such as enterohemorrhagic E. coli (EHEC), which are noninvasive, cytotoxin production is important in disease pathogenesis whereas in others the role of the cytotoxin is less clear (see chapter by Sears, Guerrant, and Kaper).

Preformed Toxins

Certain bacterial pathogens elaborate toxins that cause disease without prior bacterial colonization of the GI tract. Foremost of these are staphylococcal enterotoxins A through E, which accumulate in S. aureus–contaminated foods that have been inadequately refrigerated. Their exact mechanism of action has not been determined but in animal models they cause net secretion of water and electrolytes from the gut (324) and they are thought to induce vomiting by stimulation of enteric autonomic sensory neurons (325). Bacillus cereus produces a preformed toxin that induces nausea, vomiting, and abdominal pain but B. cereus–associated diarrhea represents a different disease process in which sporulation of the organism takes place in vivo with the elaboration of a second, distinct enterotoxin (326).

A. Enterotoxins

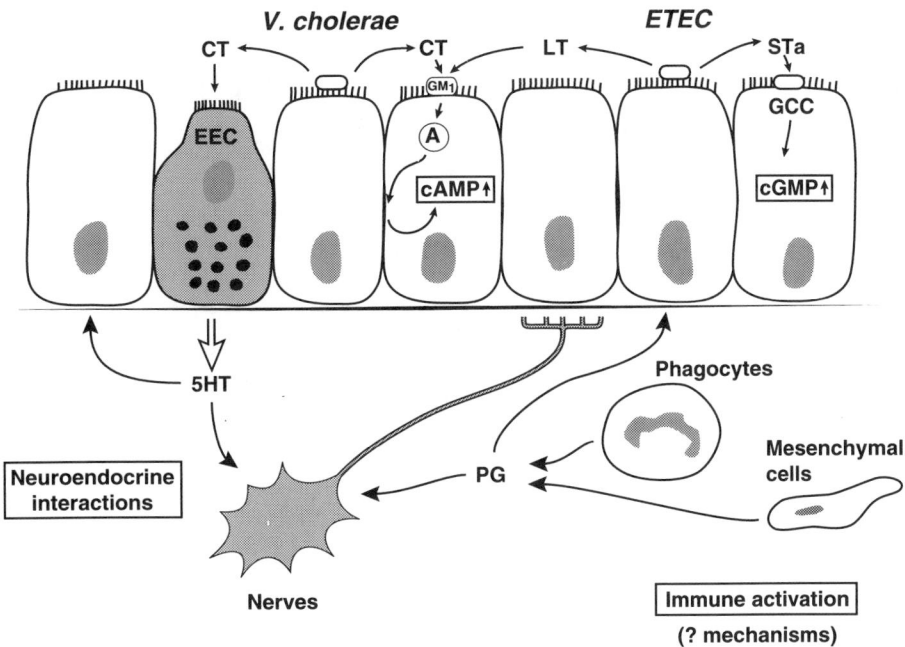

B. Cytotoxins

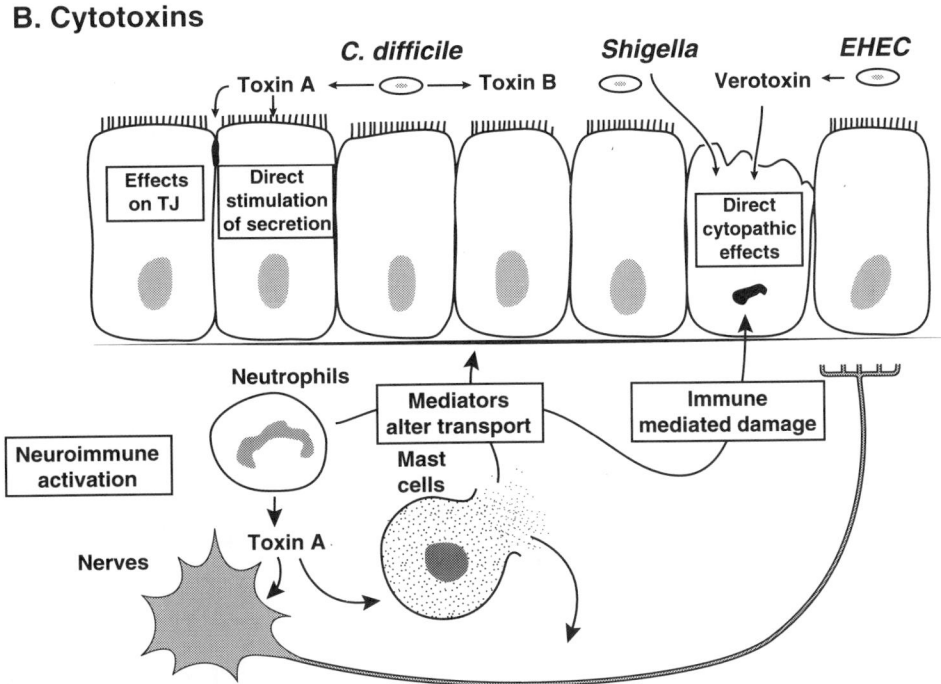

FIG. 5. Microbial–epithelial interactions. Schematic illustration of the major mechanisms leading to altered fluid and electrolyte secretion during enteric infections with representative microorganisms that (A) elaborate enterotoxins, (B) elaborate cytotoxins, (C) adhere only, and (D) invade or translocate. **A:** Enterotoxins such as *V. cholerae* cholera toxin (CT) or enterotoxigenic *E. coli* (ETEC) heat-labile (LT) and heat-stable (STa) toxins stimulate secretion and inhibit absorption by a receptor-mediated process in which cyclic nucleotide levels are increased. Preformed toxins, e.g., staphylococcal enterotoxin B (SEB), have similar actions but do not require prior microbial colonization. **B:** Cytotoxins elaborated by *C. difficile, Shigella,* and enterohemorrhagic *E. coli* (EHEC) have multiple effects on the epithelium including direct stimulation of secretion, increased epithelial permeability, and cell injury.

C. Enteroadherence

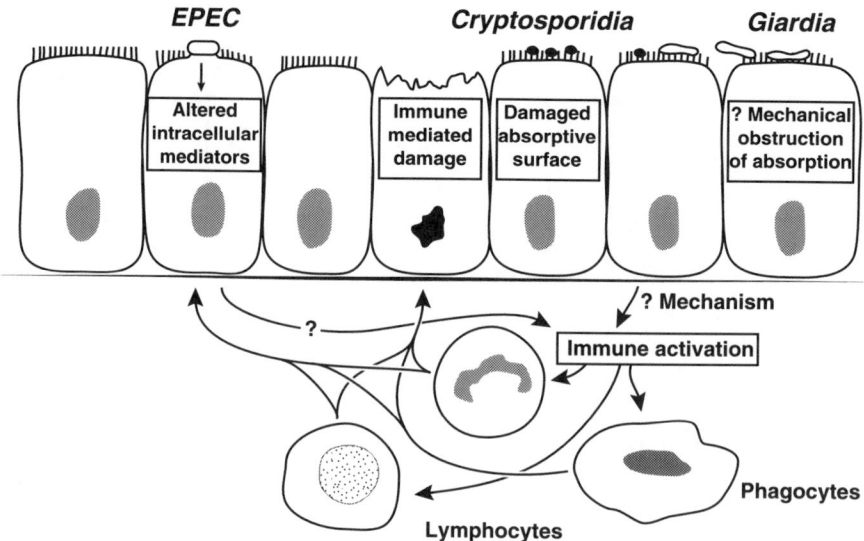

D. Invasion/ translocation

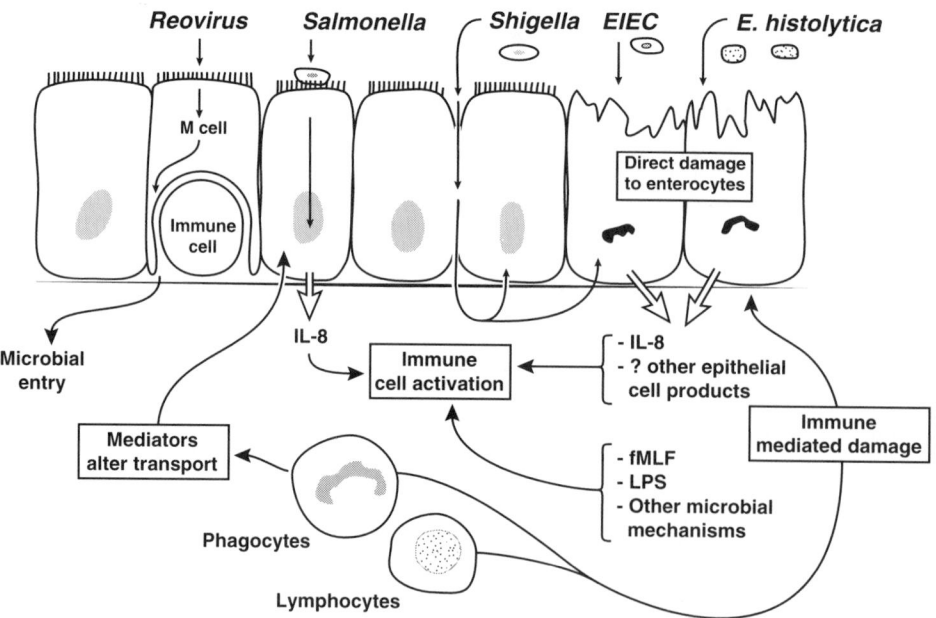

FIG. 5. *Continued.* **C:** Enteroadherent organisms such as enteropathogenic *E. coli* (EPEC), cryptosporidia, and *Giardia* stimulate secretion by unclear mechanisms that include altered intracellular messengers, and damaged or obstructed absorptive surfaces. **D:** Invasive organisms such as *Shigella,* enteroinvasive *E. coli* (EIEC), or *E. histolytica* produce marked epithelial injury while others, including reovirus, which translocates through M cells, and some *Salmonella* species, induce little direct epithelial damage.

Activation of immune/mesenchymal cells by bacterial, e.g., fMLF, lipopolysaccharide (LPS), or epithelial cell, e.g., IL-8, products (and often by unknown mechanisms) occurs in all of these categories of enteric infections. Products of these inflammatory cells may alter transport via receptor-mediated actions on enterocytes or by damaging the epithelium. Neuroendocrine involvement is best established for *V. cholerae* toxin in which 5-HT released from intestinal enteroendocrine cells (EEC) acts on nerves to stimulate alterations of ion transport but this regulatory system may mediate diarrhea associated with other infections.

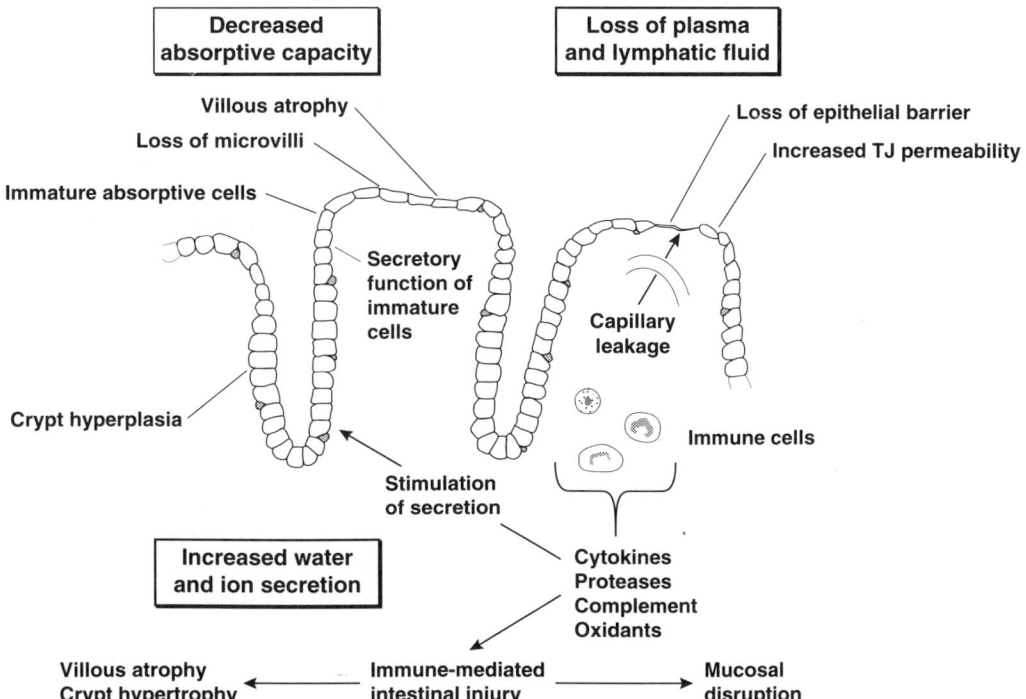

FIG. 6. Enteric infections and intestinal injury–repair processes. Stimulation of the immune system during many enteric infections can lead to a process of villous atrophy and crypt hyperplasia (*left*). This compounds any malabsorption or stimulated secretion associated with the initial infection. Villous atrophy, loss of microvilli, and immature absorptive cells contribute to a reduced absorptive capacity while secretion is enhanced by increased numbers of crypt cells (crypt hyperplasia) and, possibly, by the secretory effects of immune cell mediators.

Invasive or cytotoxin-producing microorganisms can impair the epithelial barrier directly by altering tight junctions or damaging enterocytes (*right*). Activation of inflammatory cells by these and other categories of enteric infections results in similar damage to the epithelium, in addition to endothelial injury, both of which lead to the loss of plasma and lymphatic fluid.

Enterotoxins

The products most studied for their ability to alter intestinal ion transport are those enterotoxins that stimulate secretion without cytotoxicity (Fig. 5A). Foremost of these is cholera toxin (choleragen) secreted by *Vibrio cholerae* and related species colonizing the upper small intestine. Following binding of cholera toxin β subunits to a specific glycolipid (G_{M1}) receptor, the active component (α subunit) in the plasma membrane is endocytosed and cleaved into A_1 peptide, which catalyzes the ADP ribosylation of the G protein, $G_{s\alpha}$. It is not clear as to whether the A_1 peptide itself or ADP-ribosylated $G_{s\alpha}$ moves to the basolateral membrane (327,328) where adenylate cyclase is activated to raise intracellular levels of cAMP (329), which stimulates electrogenic anion secretion in crypt cells and inhibits NaCl coupled transport in villus cells. *E. coli* heat-labile (LT) uses the same receptor and intracellular mediator mechanisms as cholera toxin. As will be discussed, cholera toxin has additional mechanisms by which it stimulates intestinal ion transport, including the activation of regulatory systems such as enteroendocrine cells, enteric nerves, and submucosal mesenchymal cells.

E. coli heat-stable enterotoxins (STa, STb) exert their effects on intestinal ion transport by different mechanisms. As discussed earlier, STa initiates intestinal secretion rapidly by stimulating intestinal brush border guanylate cyclase (GCC) and elevating intracellular levels of cGMP (161,181,330). STb stimulates cyclic nucleotide–independent intestinal secretion including bicarbonate secretion in weanling pig jejunum (331). *Salmonella typhimurium* enterotoxin-mediated fluid secretion involves PKC and AA metabolites (332). Enterotoxins elaborated by *Shigella* species and *Clostridium perfringens* also stimulate secretion (333–336).

Cytotoxins

Cytotoxic enterotoxins including Shiga toxin, (EHEC) verotoxins, *C. difficile* toxin A, and *B. fragilis* toxin induce fluid secretion through multiple and incompletely understood mechanisms (Fig. 5B). Shiga toxin selectively inhibits NaCl absorption without significantly altering anion secretion, which reflects a greater number of toxin receptors on villus vs. crypt cells (337,338). *E. coli* verotoxins produce mucosal and submucosal inflammation with necrosis and hemorrhage in association with alterations of colonic transport (339). Studies of *C. difficile* toxin A serve to illustrate the multiple mechanisms by which cytotoxins may cause disease since toxin A directly stimulates epithelial secretion, increases tight junction permeability (340,341), and activates regulatory systems entailing neutrophils (342,343), mast cells (254), and enteric nerves (344,345) (see below). *B. fragilis* enterotoxin displays similarly complex effects in the gut (346).

The observation that *C. difficile* toxin A alters the cytoskeletal structure of enterocytes and increases the permeability of tight junctions during chloride secretion (340,341) suggests that the paracellular route of ion transport can be altered during enteric infections. *V. cholerae* also elaborates a toxin, separate from cholera toxin, which affects the tight junctions (347). While disruption of the paracellular path would have some direct effect on intestinal epithelial ion transport, enhanced uptake of normally excluded and potentially inflammatory molecules from the gut lumen and increased migration of neutrophils through the tight junctions could have additional and indirect effects on intestinal transport.

Colonization/Adherence

An initial step in all pathogenic interactions between the microorganism and the gut epithelium is the process of microbial colonization or adherence. Microorganisms themselves elaborate colonization or adherence factors (reviewed in the chapter by Mann and Petri) and the epithelium possesses molecules that organisms utilize for binding and/or invasion. For many bacterial pathogens, a number of microbial as well as epithelial factors have been identified but the relationship of these factors to virulence is often unclear. Moreover, for some pathogens, the specific mechanisms by which the organism adheres to the intestinal epithelium are unknown.

The ability to colonize by means of adhesins is likely a prerequisite for virulence for most, if not all, infecting organisms, but adherence is the primary pathogenetic mechanism identified in certain bacterial and parasitic diarrheas (Fig. 5C). Enteropathogenic (or enteroadherent) *E. coli* (EPEC) are the best studied of this group of pathogens (348). Attachment of EPEC to the epithelium is accompanied by the formation of an enterocyte membrane pedestal, destruction of the microvilli, and localized condensation of actin microfilaments (349–351), a process referred to as "attaching and effacing" adherence (352). EPEC possess the *eae* gene, which encodes a 94-kDa membrane protein (353,354) and the EPEC adherence factor plasmid (355), both of which are necessary for the enteroadherent phenotype.

Pathogenic organisms that are categorized as enteroadherent (i.e., nontoxigenic and noninvasive *in vivo* and in most *in vitro* studies) are thought to cause diarrhea through brush border damage that interferes with epithelial absorption. Although the diarrhea associated with EPEC has been attributed to this mechanism, recent reports of altered concentrations of intracellular second messengers (356,357) that signal enterocyte cytoskeletal changes during EPEC infection imply a mechanism whereby cellular transport pathways can be modulated.

While a preliminary report suggests that transport is altered during EPEC infection of T84 cells, secretory responses were either unchanged (basal or Ca^{2+}-mediated stimulation) or reduced (to a cAMP-mediated agonist) (358). In experimental EPEC infection of rabbits, electroneutral NaCl and Na^+-coupled glutamine transport was reduced (359,360) and conductance, reflecting an effect on tight junctions, was increased in these and other studies (359–362). Together studies in T84 and animal intestine suggest that the secretory/antiabsorptive effects of EPEC infection may be mediated by indirect mechanisms such as immune cell activation, perhaps through signaling from the epithelium (Fig. 5C). Similar signaling mechanisms may be responsible for the altered intestinal motility that precedes diarrhea during experimental EPEC infection (363). In the case of *Giardia lamblia*, the mechanisms by which this noninvasive organism causes diarrhea are also not well established (364). Both mechanical obstruction of absorptive surfaces and damage to the brush border are postulated to produce malabsorption in giardiasis (365). Another explanation proposes that activated lymphocytes and macrophages induce enterocyte damage although the mechanisms by which *Giardia* activate these immune cells is not clear (366).

Adherence is also a requirement for the pathogenesis of toxin-producing microorganisms except for those infections in which preformed toxins cause disease. As an example, elaboration of diarrhea-inducing heat-stable and heat-labile toxins by enterotoxigenic *E. coli* (ETEC) requires prior bacterial colonization (17). Although several colonization factor antigens (CFAs) and putative colonization factors (PCFs) have been identified (367), the importance of these factors is not clear since these specific adhesins are only found in 50% to 70% of ETEC isolated from patients with diarrhea (368). In order for *V. cholerae* to produce diarrhea, microbial adherence to gut epithelial cells is necessary (322). This type of adherence is different from that found with enteropathogenic organisms since the microvilli are intact.

Colonization and attachment is also the initial step in the entry of invasive organisms into the epithelial cell (369,370). In the case of *E. histolytica*, surface carbohydrates on target cells can influence susceptibility to ameba-mediated cytotoxicity (371). Adhesion to intestinal mucin is also involved in infections with *Yersinia enterocolitica* and *E. histolytica* (369,372). For further details of how pathogens interact with the gut epithelium, the reader is referred to other chapters (see Part VII) that deal specifically with this subject.

Invasion/Translocation

The ability to enter the epithelial cell is characteristic of all enteric viruses, and many bacteria and parasites (Fig. 5D). Invasion of epithelial cells may result in cell damage leading to cell death in the case of some pathogens, such as rotavirus, *C. jejuni*, and *E. histolytica* (373), while for others, including reovirus and some *Salmonella* species (370,374), the organism translocates across the epithelium leaving the host cell relatively intact. Although almost all invasive bacteria can penetrate the epithelium, some, such as *Shigella* (375) and enteroinvasive *E. coli* (EIEC) (376), do not cross the epithelial layer. *Translocation* is a term that implies microbial passage from the GI tract to extraintestinal sites such as mesenteric lymph nodes, spleen, liver, peritoneal cavity, and bloodstream without specifying the mechanism of transfer (377). Increased translocation takes place when the epithelial barrier is damaged in association with extensive cutaneous thermal injury and during hypoxic, hypovolemic, endotoxic, and other forms of shock. Transcellular transport of endocytosed organisms are one potential mechanism of translocation (370,378,379). The tight junction has been proposed as another route of entry with studies confirming that bacteria can traverse tight junctions in cultured epithelial cells (380). Phagocytosis of organisms by intraepithelial leukocytes is, theoretically at least, an additional potential pathway for translocation. Viruses such as rotavirus enter enterocytes by direct cell membrane penetration (381). Entry via specialized epithelial cells overlying Peyers' patches (M cells) is a route of infection for reoviruses and other microorganisms (382).

Invasion of epithelial cells requires specific attachment followed by internalization, involving both microbial and host epithelial factors (383–386). In the case of EIEC and *Shigella* species, invasion and intracellular replication requires the 37-kb region of a large 180- to 210-kb plasmid (387,388). Flagellae and their function are factors determining the invasive nature of some pathogens including *C. jejuni* and *S. typhimurium* (389). Epithelial factors also mediate microbial invasion. Recently, stimulation of the EGF receptor was shown to be involved in the invasion of cultured intestinal epithelial cells by *S. typhimurium* (390). Rhinoviruses bind to the intercellular adhesion molecule, ICAM-1, which is expressed in a variety of cells including cultured intestinal epithelial cells (267,268). A particularly novel route of invasion has been proposed based on *in vitro* studies in which migration of neutrophils across T84 monolayers permitted passage of *S. flexnerii* through the tight junctions and entry into the epithelial cell via the basolateral membrane (380).

When invasive microorganisms damage the epithelium, cellular transport function is compromised along with disruption of barrier function. With frank loss of the epithelial barrier, fluid and electrolyte imbalances are compounded by the loss of plasma and lymphatic fluids. Selective loss of villus tip cells often occurs in small bowel infections with a loss of absorptive function but relative preservation of secretory capacity leading to malabsorption and net secretion (391). The mechanisms leading to altered ion transport during infections with invasive microorganisms are complex (Fig. 5D).

Activation of Regulatory Systems

As has been alluded to previously, the immune-inflammatory system plays a large role in the alterations of intestinal ion transport that occur during enteric infections. Microbial agents activate immune-inflammatory cells belonging to three main categories: mast cells, phagocytic cells, and lymphocytes.

Mast Cells

Both immune and nonimmune mechanisms are involved in the activation of mast cells and may play a role during various enteric infections. A number of substances released during the inflammatory response to enteric infections (e.g., cytokines, neuropeptides, and other proinflammatory molecules) can activate mast cells. In addition, certain microbial products such as cholera toxin and *C. difficile* toxin A are capable of directly activating mast cells with recent reports suggesting that mast cells play a role in the alterations of ion transport associated with *C. difficile* infection (254) and cholera toxin (Mary Perdue, personal communication).

Parasitic infestations are the most widely recognized to entail mast cell activation and are characterized by the stimulation of specific and nonspecific IgE antibodies which bind to high-affinity IgE receptors ($Fc_\epsilon R_I$) found on basophils and mast cells. Exposure to the specific parasite protein crosslinks IgE initiating the process of degranulation (intestinal anaphylaxis). Studies in nematode parasite infected animals have demonstrated that parasite antigens provoke intestinal secretory responses both *in vivo* and *in vitro* (245–247,250,392). It has been suggested that this process constitutes a mechanism of defense that aids in the expulsion of worms (10). Sloughing of the epithelium and intense intestinal muscle contractions are also part of this process. Thus, in intestinal anaphylaxis, the host sacrifices part of itself, the gut epithelium, in order to rid itself of the parasite. IgE binding to low-affinity receptors ($Fc_\epsilon R_{II}$) on eosinophils also occurs during parasitic infection and provides an additional mechanism whereby the infected host may clear the offending organism (393). However, alterations of intestinal ion transport resulting from the activation of eosinophils have not been well characterized.

Phagocytes

The idea that the inflammatory response to infections such as salmonellosis was important to the intestinal secretion associated with infection is not new. Indeed it was shown some time ago that animals rendered leukopenic did not respond to *Salmonella* infection with intestinal inflammation and secretion (394). However, it was relatively recently that the products of phagocytic white blood cells were shown to stimulate ion transport (395). Bacterial peptides such as fMLF are chemoattractant and activating for phagocytes and affect intestinal ion transport, presumably through the activation of neutrophils (223). A preliminary report suggests that fMLF can cross the epithelium through the paracellular pathway (396) providing a possible mechanism whereby noninvasive organisms may activate immune cells. Lipopolysaccharide (LPS), a component of the gram-negative bacterial cell wall, is a potent stimulus of immune-inflammatory effector cells and has been shown to alter colonic transport function (397). The strongest evidence that neutrophils are important in the alterations of fluid and electrolyte transport found during enteric infection is provided in a recent *in vivo* study demonstrating that anti-CD18 monoclonal antibodies inhibited the neutrophil infiltration, reduced NaCl absorption, and increased Cl⁻ secretion associated with rabbit EHEC infection (398,399). Other phagocytes such as macrophages may mediate enterocyte damage due to *Giardia* infection (366). Of the large number of inflammatory mediators known to modulate fluid and electrolyte transport, prostaglandins (PGs) have been most clearly identified to play a role in enteric infections. Cyclooxygenase inhibitors reduce the secretion associated with experimental *Salmonella* (400,401), cholera (402), ETEC (403), cryptosporidial (404), and amebic infections (405).

Lymphocytes

The evidence that lymphocytes are influential in the alterations of ion transport occurring during enteric infections is generally lacking. However, as T-cell activation causes villus atrophy and crypt hyperplasia (261–263), T cells may account for similar histopathological findings in various small intestinal infections including salmonellosis, shigellosis, protozoan, and rotavirus infections (see below). Staphylococcal enterotoxin B has been reported to activate mucosal T cells to induce this picture (406).

Neuroendocrine System

There is increasing information to implicate enteric nerves in the altered transport associated with certain intestinal infections. Animal studies suggest that enteric neural reflex pathways are activated by *E. coli* STa (407), *C. difficile* toxin A (344,345), cholera toxin (408–410), and *Salmonella typhimurium* infection (400). *In vitro* studies indicate that the enteric nervous system is also involved in the secretory response to the parasites, *Nippostrongylus brasiliensis* (245,392), *Trichinella spiralis* (247,250), and *Fasciolata hepatica* (411). It is not apparent as to how nerves are activated in all these instances. In the case of cholera toxin (Fig. 5A), stimulation of enterochromaffin cells to secrete 5-HT and neurotensin has been proposed as a potential mechanism whereby mucosal sensory nerves may be activated (407,412,413). Both mediators activate receptors on enteric neurons and evoke the release of secretory neurotransmitters, principally VIP, which act directly on enterocytes (414). Additionally, PGs released from leukocytes, fibroblasts, and perhaps the endothelium by 5-HT (415–417) may also alter neuronal excitability and have direct stimulatory transport effects on epithelial cells. *Entamoeba histolytica* lysates contain 5-HT, neurotensin, substance P, and acetylcholine (418), and *in vitro* studies have shown that amebic lysates produce alterations of intestinal ion transport through direct effects on the epithelium and/or indirectly through the release of prostaglandin E₂ (PGE₂) (405,419). Expansion and presumably activation of the phagocyte pool within the lamina propria is also a common response to infection with this and other parasites.

Epithelial Cells

Recently, it has become apparent that infection of epithelial cells stimulates the rapid release of the neutrophil chemoattracting and activating cytokine IL-8 (271,272). Although only invasive enteric pathogens stimulated IL-8 secretion from intestinal epithelial cell lines (420), studies in gastric, urinary, and pulmonary epithelial cells indicate that invasion is not necessary for bacterial stimulation of epithelial IL-8 secretion (421–423). Although LPSs can stimulate IL-8 in certain cells (233), LPSs did not appear responsible for *Helicobacter pylori*–induced IL-8 release from gastric epithelial cells (421) or in *Pseudomonas*-stimulated IL-8 production in pulmonary epithelial cells (423). This process constitutes a mechanism whereby immune cells can be recruited and activated by both invasive (Fig. 5D) and noninvasive (Fig. 5C) enteric pathogens. Microorganisms may also have effects on the production of other cytokines and proinflammatory molecules by epithelial cells. For example, phospholipase C elaborated by *C. perfringens* stimulated the production and release of PAF from cultured intestinal epithelial cells (424) and phospholipase A₂–dependent AA release (425). Recently, cholera toxin was shown to enhance IL-6 secretion by cultured intestinal epithelial cells (426).

Reparative Stages of Villus Atrophy/Crypt Hyperplasia

With sustained injury due to inflammation, both malabsorption and active secretion may be perpetuated with the development of villus atrophy and crypt hyperplasia (Fig. 6). While this is typically seen in immune-mediated conditions such as celiac disease (427,428) and experimental graft vs. host reactions (429), hyperplastic regenerative crypts are found in the repair process of most enteritides and some enterotoxigenic diseases involving immune activation. The immature "absorptive" cells (hyperplastic crypt cells) lack the full complement of transporting proteins and thus are relatively nonabsorptive. In addition, brush border damage results in malabsorption.

Transmissible gastroenteritis (TGE) virus infection is an experimental model of viral enteritis characterized by the development of villus atrophy and crypt hyperplasia (430), in which the following abnormalities have been shown to mediate diarrhea: impaired glucose and amino acid–coupled Na⁺ transport; defective NaCl absorption; diminished disaccharidase hydrolysis; and reduced mucosal absorptive surface (431–434). However, germane to the use of oral rehydration solutions in viral enteritides, rates for Na⁺-coupled glutamine and alanine transport are similar to those in uninfected control tissues and both amino acids were able to enhance jejunal Na⁺ absorption in the presence of glucose in the TGE model (435,436).

Although the organism is considered noninvasive, a similar pathophysiological and histological picture is seen

TABLE 5. *Categories of microbial–epithelial interactions leading to diarrhea*

Pathogenic process[a]	Microorganisms involved[b]
Preformed toxins	S. aureus, B. cereus
Enterotoxin production	V. cholerae, ETEC, Salmonella
Cytotoxin production	C. difficile, Shigella, EHEC, B. fragilis
Enteroadherence	EPEC, Giardia, cryptosporidia
Invasion/translocation	Salmonella, Shigella, EIEC, C. jejuni, Yersinia, E. histolytica, rotavirus
Immune activation	Salmonella, Shigella, EHEC, cryptosporidia, Giardia, E. histolytica, rotavirus
Neuroendocrine activation	V. cholerae, Salmonella, E. histolytica
Villous atrophy/crypt hyperplasia	Rotavirus, crytptosporidia, various bacterial enterides

[a] Multiple mechanisms are involved in some microbial infections.
[b] Only representative microbial agents are listed.

with cryptosporidial infections with loss of the villous absorptive surface, impaired Na$^+$-glucose absorption, crypt hypertrophy, and an inflammatory infiltrate of the lamina propria (437). An enterotoxigenic effect of stool supernatants from *Cryptosporidium*-infected calves has been reported (121) but the evidence that this "enterotoxin" is of microbial origin is lacking (438). Activation of various immune mechanisms during enteric infections may be responsible for the sequence of epithelial damage and repair, manifest as villus atrophy and crypt hyperplasia. Moreover, activated immune cells may also contribute to altered transport by elaborating factors with "enterotoxigenic" effects (121). The pathophysiological mechanisms leading to diarrhea are even more unclear in *Giardia* infection (364) where the pattern of villus atrophy and crypt hyperplasia is less pronounced (365). The mechanisms by which enteric infections alter intestinal fluid and electrolyte transport are complex (Table 5) and, as discussed, specific mechanisms are unclear in many instances.

Normal Gut Flora

The role of commensal gut flora (439–441) (see chapter by Simon and Gopbach) in the regulation of fluid and electrolyte transport is also unknown. The normal gut is considered to be in a state of chronic low-grade inflammation, due in part to the constant exposure to food antigens, ingested toxins, and luminal organisms. Germ-free animals have lower numbers of immune-inflammatory cells populating the GI tract (442) and presumably this modifies gut function although there are very few studies that have addressed this issue (441–444). The observation that secretory responses to stimuli such as electrical field stimulation, histamine, and substance P are altered in the small intestine of germ-free mice compared to conventionalized littermates (S. Crowe, unpublished data) suggests that the

normal intestinal flora participate in intestinal fluid and electrolyte homeostasis. However, further studies are needed to explore this hypothesis.

THERAPY TO CORRECT ALTERED TRANSPORT DURING INFECTION

Fluid and electrolyte imbalances during enteric infection are a consequence of altered intestinal secretion and absorption, often accompanied by a reduced intake of food and water. Such imbalances contribute to the morbidity and mortality of many enteric infections and necessitate corrective measures. Indeed, dehydration and not sepsis is what kills the vast majority of patients with enteric infections. Thus, the replacement and maintenance of fluid and electrolytes is the most important therapy of infectious diarrheas. Direct inhibition of the microbial agent or its products represents another treatment option that may ameliorate fluid and electrolyte imbalances (reviewed in the chapters by Morrow and Neuzil and Binion and Banwell). However, antimicrobial therapy has not proved to be useful in many diarrheal infections emphasizing the need for alternative effective therapies, e.g., targeting the systems that regulate ion transport that are activated during the infectious process. Finally, pharmacological attempts to repair altered epithelial transport mechanisms are being developed and may prove to be a clinically useful option (445,446). This section will focus on currently employed therapies that modulate the alterations of fluid and electrolyte transport associated with enteric infections.

Oral Rehydration Solutions

Oral rehydration solutions (ORS) are widely used in developing countries and to a lesser extent in developed nations for the replacement of fluid and electrolyte losses accompanying diarrheal diseases (447). The important and fundamental rationale for the inclusion of glucose and other nutrients in ORS is that Na$^+$-coupled nutrient absorptive processes remain unimpaired in secretory toxigenic diarrheas. Absorptive mechanisms are also sufficiently conserved to allow adequate uptake of these solutions in many invasive infections accompanied by injury to the absorptive surfaces of the intestine. Thus, replacement of secretory stool losses of Na$^+$, K$^+$, and HCO$_3^-$ can be achieved using specially formulated solutions containing glucose, amino acids, or polymeric compounds such as polysaccharides or polypeptides (18). The development of polymer-containing and cereal-based ORS provide superior replacement fluids that take advantage of the multiple Na$^+$-amino acid and -peptide carriers (compared to a single Na$^+$-glucose transporter) without the disadvantage of a high osmotic load, which stimulates additional fluid secretion into the gut lumen (448). A more comprehensive discussion of oral rehydration therapy is contained in the chapter by Snyder.

Modulation of Systems Regulating Ion Transport

Enteric infections can activate the regulatory systems that control intestinal ion transport and, as such, strategies to modulate the effect of these systems on the target epithelial cell have potential use in the treatment of infectious diarrhea. However, some of these strategies have not proved to be clinically effective whereas others remain untested in the setting of infectious diarrhea, leaving only a few agents of this general category to play a role in the management of altered fluid and electrolyte transport during enteric infections.

Immune/inflammatory System

Three hypothetical approaches to modulating immune system–altered intestinal ion transport include (a) inhibition of immune cell activation; (b) inhibition of specific mediator synthesis; and (c) inhibition of the action of the released secretory mediators. Mast cell stabilizers are one of the few drugs used in the treatment of diarrhea that can be classified in the first group. While sodium cromoglycate is used to treat the diarrhea associated with systemic mastocytosis (449), the role of mast cell stabilizers in infectious diarrhea is limited to experimental models of intestinal anaphylaxis involving parasitic infection (245).

Most drugs of the second type inhibit the metabolism of AA. Cyclooxygenase-inhibiting nonsteroidal antiinflammatory drugs (NSAIDs) such as aspirin, indomethacin, and bismuth subsalicylate have been tried in a variety of infectious diarrheal conditions with divergent results. There are studies in animal models to suggest that agents such as indomethacin reduce secretion in experimental *Salmonella* (400,401), cryptosporidial (404), amebic (405), ETEC (403), and cholera infections (402,450,451). Aspirin reduces acute diarrhea in pediatric populations (presumably mainly due to rotavirus infections) (452), but NSAIDs have not been consistently effective in cholera (453). In spite of the promising laboratory studies, NSAIDs are not accepted treatment for most infectious diarrheas. In contrast, bismuth subsalicylate does have a role in the prevention and management of traveler's diarrhea (454–456) and has beneficial effects in viral gastroenteritis (457). Recently, it was shown to reduce the duration of diarrhea and need for oral rehydration solutions in infants and children with acute watery diarrhea (458). Although the full spectrum of its mechanisms of action remain to be determined, its antisecretory effects on transport are unlikely to account for the reported improvements alone. Bismuth appears to inhibit bacterial attachment, growth, and toxin production (18).

Other agents that inhibit the generation of inflammatory mediators, including sulfasalazine, 5-aminosalicylic acid, and glucocorticoids, are effective treatment in various inflammatory gut conditions but there is no established role for these drugs in infectious diarrhea. Similarly, drugs that antagonize the effect of released mediators are not used in infectious diarrhea although receptor antagonists for histamine and 5-HT inhibit *in vitro* transport changes due to activation of intestinal mast cells sensitized during parasitic infections (245,247).

In general, pharmacological agents that modulate the immune-inflammatory system have not yet proved beneficial in infectious diarrhea. A recent report that monoclonal antibodies to neutrophil CD11/18 inhibit ion transport alterations associated with EHEC infection in rabbits (398) suggests that inhibition of immune cell recruitment and adhesion may offer a new and exciting approach to modulating the immune-inflammatory system (399). However, as this method also abrogates normal host defense mechanisms, such approaches may be more relevant to understanding disease pathogenesis than the treatment of disease.

Neuroendocrine System

Antidiarrheal drugs such as opiates, α_2-adrenergic receptor agonists, and anticholinergics act on receptors through which neurohumoral mediators exert their effects. Although these drugs may have activity at the level of the epithelium, most of their antidiarrheal action arises from effects on gut motility. For example, all anticholinergic drugs have antidiarrheal actions but their effects are largely mediated through muscarinic receptors on enteric nerves and intestinal smooth muscle. These agents are not recommended for the treatment of diarrhea although some anticholinergic drugs (hyoscyamine, dicyclomine) are used in antispasmodic therapy. Atropine is present in most preparations of the opiate diphenoxylate, but its main function is to diminish the potential for abuse since atropine has significant systemic anticholinergic side effects.

Opiates used to control diarrhea including natural substances such as paregoric and tincture of opium as well as the synthetic compounds codeine, diphenoxylate hydrochloride, and loperamide bind predominantly to μ-opiate receptors on muscle and decrease diarrhea by inhibiting small bowel motility (dilating the gut) and stimulating colonic nonperistaltic motility rather than through any effect on ion transport (459,460). Opiates may have indirect effects on epithelial transport through the modulation of neurotransmitter release. At high doses, opiates have been shown to have effects on electrolyte transport, presumably through δ receptors on epithelial cells, independent of their effects on motility (202,461). This suggests that opiates more specific for the δ receptor may be useful antidiarrheal therapy. Opiate drugs are generally avoided in most acute infectious diarrheas because their use predisposes to intestinal dilatation, strangulation, and perforation as well as reduced clearance of the infectious agent (462). Nonetheless, recent studies indicate that agents such as loperamide can be safely used to limit the symptoms associated with traveler's diarrhea (455,463,464).

Stimulation of α_2-adrenergic receptors on intestinal epithelial cells and secretory nerves of the ENS increases the basal absorption of fluid and electrolytes and inhibits stimulated secretion by a variety of agents. Clonidine is a specific α_2 agonist that has been used with some success in the treatment of diarrhea associated with diabetes (465) and with opiate withdrawal (466), but in cholera its antisecretory effects were minimal (467). The use of this class of drugs [including lidamidine, a structurally related drug (468)] is limited by significant centrally mediated side effects including hypotension, lightheadedness, sedation, and depression. The development of compounds with greater gut specificity may prove to be more useful for diarrheal diseases.

Somatostatin and its long-acting analog octreotide are proabsorptive hormones used in the management of secretory diarrhea due to endocrine tumors (469,470), short bowel syndrome (471), and the acquired immunodeficiency syndrome (AIDS) (472,473) with some success. Although native somatostatin inhibits stimulated electrolyte secretion via its action on G proteins, it is unclear as to what degree octreotide's antidiarrheal actions are due to modulation of epithelial ion transport since tumor hormone production and secretion as well as intestinal motility (474) are also inhibited. There is no proven role for somatostatin or octreotide in the management of infectious diarrhea, although they are used in certain refractory cases of AIDS-related diarrhea that may be of infectious origin (472,473).

Another agent that can be considered under the category of modulating regulatory pathways of intestinal ion transport is the natural plant product berberine. Although this alkaloid derivative from the root and bark of *Berberis arinstata* has been used for centuries in the treatment of diarrhea, its mechanisms of action are not completely known. Berberine has antimicrobial activity and effects on gut secretion and motility (475–477). There is evidence that berberine may be a muscarinic receptor antagonist and may also have α_2-adrenergic and opiate receptor agonist properties (476,477). This agent has been shown to be effective in certain toxigenic diarrheas (478).

Correction of Altered Transport Mechanisms

It is understandable why the previously discussed, specifically acting agents are generally unsuccessful in the management of infectious diarrhea since pathogens may alter transport via stimulation of the enteric nervous system and the intestinal immune system, in addition to direct epithelial effects. Therapeutic interventions directed toward final common intracellular events may provide a more rational basis for therapy and are reviewed here. Recently, the nonpathogenic yeast *Saccharomyces boulardii*, which has been used empirically in the treatment of acute infectious diarrhea and known to inhibit the secretion induced by cholera toxin and ETEC, was shown to inhibit cholera toxin and *E. coli* LT-mediated induction of cAMP implicating a receptor negatively coupled to adenylate cyclase (479).

Calmodulin Inhibitors

A number of drugs with calmodulin-inhibiting activity have been tried in the treatment of various secretory diarrheas (480). Chlorpromazine has been shown to reduce the diarrhea and the intravenous fluid requirements in *V. cholerae* infection (481) but the side effects of phenothiazines, particularly at the doses used in these studies, preclude the general use of such agents. Recently, a potent calmodulin inhibitor, zaldaride maleate, a pyrolobenzoxazepine derivative with GI antisecretory properties, was demonstrated to decrease the severity and duration of traveler's diarrhea due to ETEC or other bacterial agents as well as diarrhea without an identifiable bacterial cause (482).

Calcium Channel Blockers

Some drugs with antidiarrheal properties are known to have effects on intracellular calcium due to their effects on calcium channels. For example, although loperamide is commonly known to have opiate activity, it is also a calcium channel blocker (483). The calcium channel blocker verapamil stimulates water absorption and its use is often accompanied by the development of constipation. Experimentally verapamil has been shown to stimulate Na^+ and Cl^- absorption during viral (TGE) enteritis (484).

Chloride Channel Blockers

The idea that the final common pathway of chloride secretion could be blocked has provided an exciting alternative to the general approach of pharmacologically "repairing" altered transport. Three different classes of apical chloride channel blockers have been developed: anthranilic acid derivatives such as anthracene-9-carboxylic acid and 5-nitro-2-(3-phenylpropylamino)benzoic acid; indanyl alkanoic acids; and disulfonic stilbenes (485). These compounds have varying activity against the chloride channels of various types of epithelia (486) but these drugs have not proved to be effective *in vivo*. Although compounds that affect basolateral transport pathways involved in chloride secretion (i.e., the $Na^+,K^+,2Cl^-$ cotransporter) are also available, these agents (i.e., loop diuretics) are limited by their lack of specificity. Clearly, the development of effective agents to block apical chloride secretion continues to hold great promise in the treatment of secretory diarrhea.

CONCLUSIONS

It is clear that enteric infections can induce alterations of intestinal fluid and electrolyte transport by a number of different mechanisms. The enterocyte is the target of both direct and indirect processes that are initiated by microorganisms infecting the GI tract. Diarrhea results from the loss of absorptive surface, stimulation of secretory mechanisms, inhibition of absorptive pathways, or through plasma/lymph exudation. Often more than one of these processes is involved in a single infection. This is particularly true with invasive organisms that cause epithelial injury as well as activation of immune/inflammatory processes. Simpler transport-altering mechanisms are characteristic of bacteria that elaborate toxins such as *V. cholerae*. Even then, it is apparent that cholera toxin has effects on neuroendocrine and immune cells that provide indirect and more complex routes by which intestinal ion transport may be altered.

An understanding of the specific mechanisms involved in the altered intestinal ion transport induced by enteric pathogens is necessary for the effective treatment of these conditions. In situations where dehydration is a major feature, replacement of fluid and electrolytes is the cornerstone of any treatment regimen. In some circumstances antimicrobial therapy is appropriate. However, in many enteric infections, a specific organism is not readily identifiable or, if an agent is isolated, antibiotics have not necessarily been shown to be beneficial. Often the symptoms are sufficiently mild so as not to warrant potentially toxic therapy. Moreover, an already activated immune/inflammatory system may exert its pathophysiological influence even after the organism is eradicated. Thus, treatments directed against the final common pathways resulting in diarrhea may be the most appropriate strategy in many instances. The development of a successful pharmacological method to "repair" altered transport mechanisms will provide an important treatment option. Further investigation into the complex interactions involved in the alterations of ion transport during intestinal infections may lead to the development of novel therapies useful in infectious and other inflammatory diarrheas.

The authors gratefully acknowledge the assistance of Betty Jackson, Pat Ciano, and Eric Clemons as well as the financial support of National Institutes of Health Grant R37 DK-15350. S. E. Crowe is the recipient of an American Gastroenterological Association Foundation/ Industry Research Scholar Award.

REFERENCES

1. Powell DW. Approach to the patient with diarrhea. In: Yamada T, ed. *Textbook of gastroenterology.* Philadelphia: JB Lippincott; 1991:732–778.
2. Fine KD, Krejs GJ, Fordtran JS. Diarrhea. In: Sleisenger MH, Fordtran JS, eds. *Gastrointestinal disease. Pathophysiology/ diagnosis/management.* Philadelphia: WB Saunders; 1993: 1043–1072.
3. Fondacaro J. Intestinal ion transport, and diarrheal disease. *Am J Physiol* 1986;250:G1–G8.
4. Field M, Rao MC, Chang EB. Intestinal electrolyte transport and diarrheal disease (first of two parts). *N Engl J Med* 1989; 321:800–806.
5. Field M, Rao MC, Chang EB. Intestinal electrolyte transport and diarrheal disease. (Second of two parts). *N Engl J Med* 1989;321:879–883.
6. Grady GF, Madoff MA, Duhamel RC, Moore EW, Chalmers TC. Sodium transport by human ileum in vitro and its response to cholera toxin. *Gastroenterology* 1967;53:737–744.
7. Al-Awqati Q, Cameron JL, Greenough WB. Electrolyte transport in human ileum: effect of purified cholera exotoxin. *Am J Physiol* 1973;224:818–823.
8. Cooke HJ. Neural and humoral regulation of small intestinal electrolyte transport. In: Johnson LR, ed. *Physiology of the gastrointestinal tract.* New York: Raven Press; 1987: 1307–1350.
9. Lundgren O. Nervous control of intestinal fluid transport:
physiology and pathophysiology. *Comp Biochem Physiol* 1988; 90:603–609.
10. Castro G. Immunological regulation of epithelial function. *J Am Physiol Soc* 1982;G321–G329.
11. Powell DW. Immunophysiology of intestinal electrolyte transport. In: Schultz SG, ed. *Handbook of physiology. The gastrointestinal system.* Vol 4. Rockville, MD: The American Physiologic Society; 1991:591–641.
12. Powell DW. Intestinal water and electrolyte transport. In: Johnson LR, ed. *Physiology of the gastrointestinal tract.* New York: Raven Press; 1987:1267–1305.
13. Binder HJ, Sandle GI. Electrolyte absorption and secretion in the mammalian colon. In: Johnson LR, ed. *Physiology of the gastrointestinal tract.* New York: Raven Press; 1987: 1389–1418.
14. Donowitz M, Welsh MJ. Regulation of mammalian small intestinal electrolyte secretion. In: Johnson LR, ed. *Physiology of the gastrointestinal tract.* New York: Raven Press; 1987: 1351–1388.
15. Barrett KE, Dharmsathaphorn K. Secretion and absorption: small intestine and colon. In: Yamada T, ed. *Textbook of gastroenterology.* Philadelphia: JB Lippincott; 1991:265–294.
16. Sellin JH. Intestinal electrolyte absorption and secretion. In: Sleisenger MH, Fordtran JS, eds. *Gastrointestinal disease: pathophysiology/diagnosis/management.* Philadelphia: WB Saunders; 1993:954–976.
17. Guandalini S. Intestinal ion and nutrient transport in health and infectious diarrhoeal diseases. *Drugs* 1988;36 Suppl 4:26–38.
18. Powell DW, Szauter KE. Nonantibiotic therapy and pharmacotherapy of acute infectious diarrhea. *Gastroenterol Clin North Am* 1993;22:683–707.
19. Phillips SF, Giller J. The contribution of the colon to electrolyte and water conservation in man. *J Lab Clin Med* 1973;81: 733–746.
20. Phillips RA. Water and electrolyte losses in cholera. *Fed Proc* 1964;23:705.
21. Roth KA, Hermiston ML, Gordon JI. Use of transgenic mice to infer the biological properties of small intestinal stem cells and to examine the lineage relationships of their descendants. *Proc Natl Acad Sci USA* 1991;88:9407–9411.
22. Welsh MJ, Smith PL, Fromm M, Frizzell RA. Crypts are the site of intestinal fluid and electrolyte secretion. *Science* 1982; 218:1219–1221.
23. Stewart CP, Turnberg LA. A microelectrode study of responses to secretagogues by epithelial cells on villus and crypt of rat small intestine. *Am J Physiol* 1989;257:G334–G343.
24. Davis GR, Santa Ana CA, Morawski SG, Fordtran JS. Permeability characteristics of human jejunum, ileum, proximal colon and distal colon: results of potential difference measurements and unidirectional fluxes. *Gastroenterology* 1982;83:844.
25. Fordtran JS, Rector FC, Jr., Ewton MF, Soter N, Kinney J. Permeability characteristics of the human small intestine. *J Clin Invest* 1965;44:1935.
26. Marcial MA, Carlson SL, Madara JL. Partitioning of paracellular conductance along the ileal crypt-villus axis: a hypothesis based on structural analysis with detailed consideration of tight junction structure–function relationships. *J Membrane Biol* 1984;80:59.
27. Tilson MD, Wright HK. An adaptive change in ileal Na-K-ATPase activity after jejunectomy or jejunal transposition. *Surgery* 1971;70:421–424.
28. Schulzke JD, Fromm M, Bentzel CJ, Zeitz M, Menge H, Riecken EO. Ion transport in the experimental short bowel syndrome of the rat. *Gastroenterology* 1992;102:497.
29. Sandle GI, McGlone F. Segmental variability of membrane conductances in rat and human colonic epithelia. Implications for Na, K and Cl transport. *Pflugers Arch* 1987;410:173–180.
30. Sellin JH, De Soignie R. Ion transport in human colon in vitro. *Gastroenterology* 1987;93:441–448.
31. Schiller LR, Santa Ana CA, Morawski SG, Fordtran JS. Effect of amiloride on sodium transport in the proximal, distal, and entire human colon in vivo. *Dig Dis Sci* 1988;33:969–976.
32. Ponder BAJ, Schmidt GH, Wilinson MM, Monk M, Reid A.

Derivation of mouse intestinal crypts from single progenitor cells. *Nature* 1985;313:689–691.

33. Lipkin M, Sherlock P, Bell B. Cell renewal in stomach, ileum, colon and rectum. *Gastroenterology* 1963;45:721.

34. MacDonald WC, Trier JS, Everett NB. Cell proliferation and migration in the stomach, duodenum and rectum of man: radioautographic studies. *Gastroenterology* 1964;46:405.

35. Dharmsathaphorn K, Madara JL. Established intestinal cell lines as model systems for electrolyte transport studies. *Meth Enzymol* 1990;192:354–389.

36. Grasset E, Pinto M, Dussaulx E, Zweibaum A, Desjeux J. Epithelial properties of human colonic carcinoma cell line Caco-2: electrical parameters. *Am J Physiol* 1984;247:C260–C267.

37. Dharmsathaphorn K, McRoberts JA, Mandel KG, Tisdale LD, Masui H. A human colonic tumor cell line that maintains vectorial electrolyte transport. *Am J Physiol* 1984;246:G204–G208.

38. Claude P, Goodenough DA. Fracture faces of zonulae occludentes from "tight" and "leaky" epithelia. *J Cell Biol* 1973;58:390.

39. Madara J, Trier JR, Neutra MR. Structural changes in the plasma membrane accompany differentiation of epithelial cells in human and monkey small intestine. *Gastroenterology* 1980;78:970.

40. Madara JL, Moore R, Carlson S. Alteration of intestinal tight junction structure and permeability by cytoskeletal contraction. *Am J Physiol (Cell Physiol)* 1987;253:C854–C861.

41. Madara JL, Stafford J, Barenberg D, Carlson S. Functional coupling of tight junctions and microfilaments in T84 monolayers. *Am J Physiol* 1988;254:G416–G423.

42. Madara JL. Loosening tight junctions: lessons from the intestine. *J Clin Invest* 1989;83:1089–1094.

43. Stenson WF, Easom RA, Turk J, Riehl T. Regulation of paracellular permeability in Caco-2 cells by activation of protein kinase C. *Gastroenterology* 1992;102:A244 (abstr).

44. Madara JL. Tight junction dynamics: is paracellular transport regulated? *Cell* 1988;53:497–498.

45. Madara JL, Parkos C, Colgan S, Nusrat A, Atisook K, Kaoutzani P. The movement of solutes and cells across tight junctions. *Ann NY Acad Sci* 1992;664:47–60.

46. Diamond J. Twenty-First Bowditch Lecture. The epithelial junction: bridge, gate and fence. *Physiologist* 1977;20:10.

47. Fordtran JS, Rector FCJ, Carter NW. The mechanisms of sodium absorption in the human small intestine. *J Clin Invest* 1968;47:884–900.

48. Fordtran JS. Stimulation of active and passive sodium absorption by sugars in the human jejunum. *J Clin Invest* 1975;55:728–737.

49. Pappenheimer JR, Reiss KZ. Contribution of solvent drag through intercellular junctions to absorption of nutrients by the small intestine of the rat. *J Membrane Biol* 1987;100:123.

50. Madara JL, Pappenheimer JR. Structural basis for physiological regulation of paracellular pathways in intestinal epithelia. *J Membrane Biol* 1987;100:149–164.

51. Fine KD, Santa Ana CA, Porter JL, Fordtran JS. Effect of D-glucose on intestinal permeability and its passive absorption in human small intestine in vivo. *Gastroenterology* 1993;105:1117–1125.

52. Soergel KH. Showdown at the tight junction. *Gastroenterology* 1993;105:1247–1250.

53. Kirk KL, Halm DR, Dawson DC. Active sodium transport by turtle colon via an electrogenic Na-K exchange pump. *Nature* 1980;287:237–239.

54. Schneider JW, Mercer RW, Caplan M. Molecular cloning of rat brain Na,K-ATPase alpha-subunit cDNA. *Proc Natl Acad Sci USA* 1985;82:6357.

55. Fuller PJ, Verity K. Colonic sodium-potassium adenosine triphosphate subunit gene expression: ontogeny and regulation by adrenocortical steroids. *Endocrinology* 1990;127:32.

56. Suzuki Y, Kaneko K. Ouabain-sensitive H^+-K^+ exchange mechanism in the apical membrane of guinea pig colon. *Am J Physiol* 1989;256:G979–G988.

57. Castillo JR, Rajendran VM, Binder HJ. Apical membrane localization of ouabain-sensitive K^+-activated ATPase activities in rat distal colon. *Am J Physiol* 1991;261:G1005–G1011.

58. Carafoli E, Zurini M. The Ca^{2+}-pumping ATPase of plasma membranes: purification, reconstitution and properties. *Biochim Biophys Acta* 1982;683:279.

59. Haynes DH. Mechanism of Ca^{2+} transport by Ca^{2+}-Mg^{2+}-ATPase pump: analysis of major states and pathways. *Am J Physiol* 1983;244:G3.

60. Suzuki S, Ren LJ, Chen H. Further studies on the effect of aldosterone on Mg^{2+}-$HCO_3(-)$-ATPase and carbonic anhydrase from rat intestinal mucosa. *J Steroid Biochem* 1989;33:89.

61. Crowson MS, Shull GE. Isolation and characterization of a cDNA encoding the putative distal colon H^+,$K^+(+)$-ATPase. Similarity of deduced amino acid sequence to gastric H^+,$K^+(+)$-ATPase and Na^+,$K^+(+)$-ATPase and mRNA expression in distal colon, kidney, and uterus. *J Biol Chem* 1992;267:13740.

62. Takeguchi M, Asano S, Tabuchi Y, Takeguchi N. The presence of H^+,K^+-ATPase in the crypt of rabbit distal colon demonstrated with monoclonal antibodies against gastric H^+,K^+-ATPase. *Gastroenterology* 1990;99:1339.

63. Feldman GM, Stephenson RL. H^+ and HCO_3^- flux across apical surface of rat distal colon. *Am J Physiol* 1990;259:C35–C40.

64. Wright EM. The intestinal Na^+/glucose cotransporter. *Annu Rev Physiol* 1993;55:575.

65. Ikeda TS, Hwang E-S, Coady MJ, Hirayama BA, Hediger MA, Wright EM. Characterization of Na^+/glucose cotransporter cloned from rabbit small intestine. *J Membrane Biol* 1989;110:87.

66. Adibi SA, Morse EL, Masitamani SS, Amin PM. Evidence for two different modes of tripeptide disappearance in human intestine. *J Clin Invest* 1975;56:1355.

67. Adibi SA. Intestinal transport of dipeptides in man: relative importance of hydrolysis and intact absorption. *J Clin Invest* 1971;50:2266.

68. Alpers DH. Digestion and absorption of carbohydrates and protein. In: Johnson LR, ed. *Physiology of the gastrointestinal tract*. New York: Raven Press; 1987:1469.

69. Hopfer U. Membrane transport mechanisms for hexoses and amino acids in the small intestine. In: Johnson LR, ed. *Physiology of the gastrointestinal tract*. New York: Raven Press; 1987:1499–1526.

70. Dharmsathaphorn K, Mandel KG, Masui H, McRoberts JA. Vasoactive intestinal polypeptide-induced chloride secretion by a colonic epithelial cell line. Direct participation of a basolaterally localized Na^+,K^+,Cl-cotransport system. *J Clin Invest* 1985;75:462–471.

71. Lytle C, Xu JC, Biemesderfer D, Haas M, Forbush B. The Na-K-Cl cotransport protein of shark rectal gland. I. Development of monoclonal antibodies, immunoaffinity purification, and partial biochemical characterization. *J Biol Chem* 1992;267:25428.

72. Lytle C, Forbush B. The Na-K-Cl cotransport protein of shark rectal gland. II. Regulation by direct phosphorylation. *J Biol Chem* 1992;267:25438.

73. Gamba G, Salzberg SN, Lombardi M, et al. Primary structure, and functional expression of a cDNA encoding the thiazide-sensitive, electroneutral sodium-chloride cotransporter. *Proc Natl Acad Sci USA* 1993;90:2749.

74. Rajendran VM, Oesterlin M, Binder HJ. Sodium uptake across basolateral membrane of rat distal colon. Evidence for Na-H exchange and Na-anion cotransport. *J Clin Invest* 1991;88:1379–1385.

75. Eisner DA, Lederer WJ. Na-Ca exchange: stoichiometry and electrogenicity. *Am J Physiol* 1985;248:C189.

76. Smith PR, Benos DJ. Epithelial Na^- channels. *Annu Rev Physiol* 1991;53:509.

77. Wills NK. Apical membrane potassium and chloride permeabilities in surface cells of rabbit descending colon epithelium. *J Physiol (London)* 1985;358:433–445.

78. Kirk KL, Dawson DC. Basolateral potassium channel in turtle colon. *J Gen Physiol* 1983;82:297.

79. Hayslett JP, Gogelein H, Kunzelmann K, Greger R. Character-

istics of apical chloride channels in human colon cells (HT29). *Pflugers Arch* 1987;410:487–494.

80. Kunzelmann K, Gerlach L, Frobe U, Greger R. Bicarbonate permeability of epithelial chloride channels. *Pflugers Arch* 1991;417:616–621.

81. Minhas BS, Sullivan SK, Field M. Bicarbonate secretion in rabbit ileum: electrogenicity, ion dependence, and effects of cyclic nucleotides. *Gastroenterology* 1993;105:1617–1629.

82. Smith PR, Bradford AL, Dantzer V, Benos DJ, Skadhauge E. Immunocytochemical localization of amiloride-sensitive sodium channels in the lower intestine of the hen. *Cell Tissue Res* 1993;272:129–136.

83. Carey HV, Hayden UL, Spicer SS, Schulte BA, Benos DJ. Localization of amiloride-sensitive Na$^+$ channels in intestinal epithelia. *Am J Physiol* 1994;266:G504–G510.

84. Foster ES, Sandle GI, Hayslett JP, Binder HJ. Dietary potassium modulates active potassium absorption and secretion in rat distal colon. *Am J Physiol* 1986;251:G619–G626.

85. Will PC, DeLisle RC, Cortright RN, Hopfer U. Induction of amiloride-sensitive sodium transport in the intestines by adrenal steroids. *Ann N Y Acad Sci* 1981;372:64–78.

86. Turnheim K, Hudson RL, Schultz SG. Cell Na$^+$ activities and transcellular Na$^+$ absorption by descending colon from normal and Na$^+$-deprived rabbits. *Pflugers Arch* 1987;410:279–283.

87. Turnamian SG, Binder HJ. Regulation of active sodium and potassium transport in the distal colon of the rat. Role of the aldosterone and glucocorticoid receptors. *J Clin Invest* 1989;84:1924–1929.

88. Turnamian SG, Binder HJ. Aldosterone and glucocorticoid receptor-specific agonists regulate ion transport in rat proximal colon. *Am J Physiol* 1990;258:G492–G498.

89. Bridges RJ, Cragoe EJJ, Frizzell RA, Benos DJ. Inhibition of colonic Na$^+$ transport by amiloride analogues. *Am J Physiol* 1989;256:C67–C74.

90. Turnberg L, Fordtran JS, Carter N, Rector F. Mechanism of bicarbonate absorption and its relationship to sodium transport in human jejunum. *J Clin Invest* 1970;49:548–546.

91. Turnberg L, Bieberdorf F, Morawski S, Fordtran JS. Interrelationships of chloride, bicarbonate, sodium, and hydrogen transport in the human ileum. *J Clin Invest* 1970;49:557–567.

92. Knickelbein R, Aronson PS, Atherton W, Dobbins JW. Sodium and chloride transport across rabbit ileal brush border. I. Evidence for Na-H exchange. *Am J Physiol* 1983;245:G504–G510.

93. Knickelbein RG, Aronson PS, Dobbins JW. Membrane distribution of sodium-hydrogen and chloride-bicarbonate exchanges in crypt and villus cell membranes from rabbit ileum. *J Clin Invest* 1988;82:2158.

94. Sundaram U, Knickelbein RG, Dobbins JW. pH regulation in ileum: Na-H and Cl-HCO$_3$ exchange in isolated crypt and villus cells. *Am J Physiol* 1991;260:G440.

95. Foster ES, Dudeja PK, Brasitus TA. Contribution of Cl$^-$-OH$^-$ exchange to electroneutral NaCl absorption in rat distal colon. *Am J Physiol* 1990;258:G261–G267.

96. Foster ES, Dudeja PK, Brasitus TA. Na$^+$-H$^+$ exchange in rat colonic brush-border membrane vesicles. *Am J Physiol* 1986;250:G781–G787.

97. Orlowski J, Kandasamy RA, Shull GE. Molecular cloning of putative members of the Na/H exchanger gene family. cDNA cloning, deduced amino acid sequence, and mRNA tissue expression of the rat NaH exchanger NHE-1 and two structurally related proteins. *J Biol Chem* 1992;267:9331–9339.

98. Tse CM, Ma AL, Yang VW, et al. *EMBO J* 1991;10:1957–1067.

99. Tse C-M, Brant SR, Walker MS, Pouyssegur J, Donowitz M. Cloning and sequencing of a rabbit cDNA encoding an intestinal and kidney-specific Na$^+$/H$^+$ exchanger isoform (NHE-3). *J Biol Chem* 1992;267:9340–9346.

100. Chow A, Dobbins JW, Aronson PS, Igarashi P. cDNA cloning and localization of a band 3–related protein from ileum. *Am J Physiol* 1992;263:G345.

101. Vaandrager AB, De Jonge HR. A sensitive technique for the determination of anion exchange activities in brush-border membrane vesicles. Evidence for two exchangers with different affinities for HCO$_3^-$ and SITS in rat intestinal epithelium. *Biochim Biophys Acta* 1988;939:305.

102. Hediger MA, Coady MJ, Ikeda TS, Wright EM. Expression cloning and cDNA sequencing of the Na$^+$/glucose co-transporter. *Nature* 1987;330:379.

103. Wright EM, Turk E, Hager K, et al. The Na$^+$/glucose cotransporter (SGLT1). *Acta Physiol Scand (Suppl)* 1992;607:201–207.

104. Haase W, Heitmann K, Friese W, Ollig D, Koepsell H. Characterization and histochemical localization of the rat intestinal Na$^+$-D-glucose cotransporter by monoclonal antibodies. *Eur J Cell Biol* 1990;52:297–309.

105. Thwaites DT, McEwan GT, Cook MJ, Hirst BH, Simmons NL. H(+)-coupled (Na(+)-independent) proline transport in human intestinal (Caco-2) epithelial cell monolayers. *FEBS Lett* 1993;333:78–82.

106. Peerce BE. Identification of the intestinal Na-phosphate cotransporter. *Am J Physiol* 1989;256:G645–G652.

107. Rose RC. Intestinal absorption of water-soluble vitamins. In: Johnson LR, ed. *Physiology of the gastrointestinal tract*. New York: Raven Press; 1987:1581.

108. Mandel KG, McRoberts JA, Beuerlein G, Foster ES, Dharmsathaphorn K. Ba^{2+} inhibition of VIP- and A23187-stimulated Cl$^-$ secretion by T84 cell monolayers. *Am J Physiol* 1986;250:C486–C494.

109. Weymer A, Huott P, McRoberts JA, Dharmsathaphorn K. Chloride secretory mechanism induced by prostaglandin E1 in a colonic epithelial cell line. *J Clin Invest* 1985;76:1828–1836.

110. Halm DR, Rechkemmer GR, Schoumacher RA, Frizzell RA. Apical membrane chloride channels in a colonic cell line activated by secretory agonists. *Am J Physiol* 1988;254:C505–C511.

111. Tabcharani JA, Hanrahan JW. On the activation of outwardly rectifying anion channels in excised patches. *Am J Physiol* 1991;261:G992–G999.

112. Thiemann A, Gründer S, Pusch M, Jentsch TJ. A chloride channel widely expressed in epithelial and non-epithelial cells. *Nature* 1992;356:57–60.

113. Li M, McCann JD, Liedtke CM, Nairn AC, Greengard P, Welsh MJ. Cyclic AMP-dependent protein kinase opens chloride channels in normal but not cystic fibrosis airway epithelium. *Nature* 1988;331:358–360.

114. Chang EB, Bookstein C, Vaandrager A, DeJonge HR, Buse J, Musch MW. Cystic fibrosis transmembrane regulator mRNA expression relative to ion-nutrient transport in spontaneously differentiating human intestinal CaCo-2 epithelial cells. *J Lab Clin Med* 1991;118:377–381.

115. Bear CE, Li CH, Kartner N, et al. Purification and functional reconstitution of the cystic fibrosis transmembrane conductance regulator (CFTR). *Cell* 1992;68:809–818.

116. Bijman J, Dalemans W, Kansen M, et al. Low-conductance chloride channels in IEC-6 and CF nasal cells expressing CFTR. *Am J Physiol* 1993;264:L229–L235.

117. Vaandrager AB, Bajnath R, Groot JA, Bot AGM, De Jonge HR. Ca^{2+} and cAMP activate different chloride efflux pathways in HT-29.cl19A colonic epithelial cell line. *Am J Physiol* 1991;261:G958–G965.

118. Berschneider HM, Knowles MR, Azizkhan RG, et al. Altered intestinal chloride transport in cystic fibrosis. *FASEB J* 1988;2:2625–2629.

119. Taylor CJ, Baxter PS, Hardcastle J, Hardcastle PT. Failure to induce secretion in jejunal biopsies from children with cystic fibrosis. *Gut* 1988;29:957–962.

120. Veeze HJ, Sinaasappel M, Bijman J, Bouquet J, De Jonge HR. Ion transport abnormalities in rectal suction biopsies from children with cystic fibrosis. *Gastroenterology* 1991;101:398–403.

121. Anderson MP, Welsh MJ. Calcium and cAMP activate different chloride channels in the apical membrane of normal and cystic fibrosis epithelia. *Proc Natl Acad Sci USA* 1991;88:6003–6007.

122. O'Loughlin EV, Hunt DM, Gaskin KJ, et al. Abnormal epithelial transport in cystic fibrosis jejunum. *Am J Physiol Gastrointest Liver Physiol* 1991;260:G758–G763.

123. Clarke LL, Grubb BR, Yankaskas JR, Cotton CU, McKenzie A, Boucher RC. Relationship of a non-cystic fibrosis transmembrane conductance regulator-mediated chloride conductance to organ-level disease in Cftr(−/−) mice. *Proc Natl Acad Sci USA* 1994;91:479–483.

124. Clarke LL, Grubb BR, Gabriel SE, Smithies O, Koller BH, Boucher RC. Defective epithelial chloride transport in a gene-targeted mouse model of cystic fibrosis. *Science* 1992;257:1125–1128.

125. Veeze HJ, Halley DJJ, Bijman J, de Jongste JC, De Jonge HR, Sinaasappel M. Determinants of mild clinical symptoms in cystic fibrosis patients. Residual chloride secretion measured in rectal biopsies in relation to the genotype. *J Clin Invest* 1994; 93:461–466.

126. McEwan GT, Brown CD, Hirst BH, Simmons NL. Hypo-osmolar stimulation of transepithelial Cl⁻ secretion in cultured human T84 intestinal epithelial layers. *Biochim Biophys Acta* 1992;1135:180–183.

127. McEwan GT, Hunter J, Hirst BH, Simmons NL. Volume-activated Cl⁻ secretion and transepithelial vinblastine secretion mediated by P-glycoprotein are not correlated in cultured human T84 intestinal epithelial layers. *FEBS Lett* 1992;304: 233–236.

128. Worrell RT, Butt AG, Cliff WH, Frizzell RA. A volume sensitive chloride conductance in human colonic cell line T84. *Am J Physiol* 1989;256:C1111.

129. Valverde MA, Diaz M, Sepulveda FV, Gill DR, Hyde SC, Higgins CF. Volume-regulated chloride channels associated with the human multidrug-resistance P-glycoprotein. *Nature* 1992; 335:830–833.

130. Tilly BC, Kansen M, Van Gageldonk PGM, et al. G-proteins mediate intestinal chloride channel activation. *J Biol Chem* 1991;266:2036–2040.

131. McCabe RD, Smith PL, Sullivan SK. Ion transport by rabbit descending colon: mechanisms of transepithelial potassium transport. *Am J Physiol* 1984;246:G594.

132. Sullivan SK, Smith PL. Active potassium secretion by rabbit proximal colon. *Am J Physiol* 1986;250:G475.

133. Sweiry JH, Binder HJ. Characterization of aldosterone-induced potassium secretion in rat distal colon. *J Clin Invest* 1989;83:844–851.

134. Rechkemmer G, Halm DR. Aldosterone stimulates K⁺ secretion across mammalian colon independent of Na⁺ absorption. *Proc Natl Acad Sci USA* 1989;86:397.

135. Wills NK, Lewis SA, Eaton DC. Active and passive properties of rabbit descending colon: a microelectrode and nystatin study. *J Membrane Biol* 1979;45:81.

136. Loo DD, Kaunitz JD. Ca²⁺ and cAMP activate K⁺ channels in the basolateral membrane. *J Membr Biol* 1989;110:19–28.

137. Davis GR, Morawski SG, Santa Ana CA, Fordtran JS. Evaluation of chloride/bicarbonate exchange in the human colon *in vivo*. *J Clin Invest* 1983;71:201–207.

138. Feldman GM. Effect of chronic metabolic acidosis on net electrolyte transport in rate colon. *Am J Physiol* 1989;256: G1036–G1040.

139. See NA, Greenwood B, Bass P. Submucosal plexus alone integrates motor activity and epithelial transport in rate jejunum. *Am J Physiol* 1990;259:G593–G598.

140. Greenwood B, Davison JS. The relationship between gastrointestinal motility and secretion. *Am J Physiol* 1987;252: G91–G97.

141. Cooke HJ, Wang YZ, Rogers R. Coordination of Cl secretion and contraction by a histamine H₂-receptor agonist in guinea pig distal colon. *Am J Physiol* 1993;265:G973–G978.

142. Harris MS, Ramaswamy K, Kennedy JG. Induction of neurally mediated NaHCO₃ secretion by luminal distension in rat ileum. *Am J Physiol* 1989;257:G191–G197.

143. Schulzke J-D, Fromm M, Hegel U, Riecken E-O. Ion transport and enteric nervous system (ENS) in rat rectal colon: mechanical stretch causes electrogenic Cl-secretion via plexus Meissner and amiloride-sensitive electrogenic Na-absorption is not affected by intramural neurons. *Pflugers Arch* 1989;414:216–221.

144. Gilman AG. G proteins: transducers of receptor-generated signals. *Annu Rev Biochem* 1987;56:615–649.

145. Lewis DL, Lechleiter JD, Kim D, Nanavati C, Clapham DE. Intracellular regulation of ion channels in cell membranes. *Mayo Clin Proc* 1990;65:1127–1143.

146. Limbird LE. Receptors linked to inhibition of adenylate cy-

clase: additional signaling mechanisms. *FASEB J* 1988;2: 2686–2695.

147. Semrad CE, Change EB. Calcium mediated cyclic AMP inhibition of Na-H exchange in small intestine. *Am J Physiol* 1987; 252:C315–C322.

148. Shapiro M, Matthews J, Hecht G, Delp C, Madara JL. Stabilization of F-actin prevents cAMP-elicited Cl secretion in T84 cells. *J Clin Invest* 1991;87:1903–1909.

149. Matthews JB, Awtrey CS, Madara JL. Microfilament-dependent activation of Na⁺/K⁺/2Cl⁻ cotransport by cAMP,in intestinal epithelial monolayers. *J Clin Invest* 1992;90:1608–1613.

150. Chang EB, Semrad CE. Calcium mediated cyclic AMP inhibition of Na/H exchange in chicken small intestine. *Gastroenterology* 1985;88:1345.

151. Hardcastle J, Hardcastle PT, Ayton B, Chapman J, MacNeil S. Calcium-calmodulin-dependent activation of adenylate cyclase in prostaglandin-induced electrically-monitored intestinal secretion in the rat. *J Pharm Pharmacol* 1992;44:93.

152. Li Z, Goy MF. Peptide-regulated guanylate cyclase pathways in rat colon: in situ localization of GCA, GCC, and guanylin mRNA. *Am J Physiol* 1993;265:G394–G402.

153. Vaandrager AB, Bot AG, De Vente J, De Jonge HR. Atriopeptins and *Escherichia coli* enterotoxin STa have different sites of action in mammalian intestine. *Gastroenterology* 1992;102: 1161–1169.

154. Catto-Smith AG, Hardin JA, Patrick MK, O'Loughlin EV, Gall DG. The effect of atrial natriuretic peptide on intestinal electrolyte transport. *Reg Peptides* 1991;36:29–44.

155. Vaandrager AB, Schulz S, De Jonge HR, Garbers DL. Guanylyl cyclase C is an N-linked glycoprotein receptor that accounts for multiple heat-stable enterotoxin-binding proteins in the intestine. *J Biol Chem* 1993;268:2174–2179.

156. Hakki S, Crane M, Hugues M, OHanley P, Waldman SA. Solubilization and characterization of functionally coupled *Escherichia coli* heat-stable toxin receptors and particulate guanylate cyclase associated with the cytoskeleton compartment of intestinal membranes. *Int J Biochem* 1993;25:557–566.

157. Cohen MB, Mann EA, Lau C, Henning SJ, Giannella RA. A gradient in expression of the *Escherichia coli* heat-stable enterotoxin receptor exists along the villus-to-crypt axis of rat small intestine. *Biochem Biophys Res Commun* 1992;186: 483–490.

158. Lewis LG, Witte DP, Laney DW, Currie MG, Cohen MB. Guanylin mRNA is expressed in villous enterocytes of the rat small intestine and superficial epithelia of the rat colon. *Biochem Biophys Res Commun* 1993;196:553–560.

159. Crane JK, Wehner MS, Bolen EJ, et al. Regulation of intestinal guanylate cyclase by the heat-stable enterotoxin of *Escherichia coli* (STa) and protein kinase C. *Infect Immun* 1992;60: 5004–5012.

160. Lin M, Nairn AC, Guggino SE. cGMP-dependent protein kinase regulation of a chloride channel in T84 cells. *Am J Physiol* 1992;262:C1304–C1312.

161. Huott PA, Liu W, McRoberts JA, Giannella RA, Dharmsathaphorn K. Mechanism of action of *Escherichia coli* heat stable enterotoxin in a human colonic cell line. *J Clin Invest* 1988;82: 514–523.

162. Matthews JB, Awtrey CS, Thompson R, Hung T, Tally KJ. Na(+)-K(+)-2Cl⁻ cotransport and Cl⁻ secretion evoked by heat-stable enterotoxin is microfilament dependent in T84 cells. *Am J Physiol* 1993;265:G370–G378.

163. Dharmsathaphorn K, Cohn J, Beuerlein G. Multiple calcium-mediated effector mechanisms regulate chloride secretory responses in T₈₄-cells. *Am J Physiol* 1989;256:C1224–C1230.

164. Kachintorn U, Vajanaphanich M, Traynor-Kaplan AE, Dharmsathaphorn K, Barrett KE. Activation by calcium alone of chloride secretion in T84 epithelial cells. *Br J Pharmacol* 1993;109: 510–517.

165. Devor DC, Ahmed Z, Duffey ME. Cholinergic stimulation produces oscillations of cytosolic Ca²⁺ in a secretory epithelial cell line, T84. *Am J Physiol* 1991;260:C598–C608.

166. Donowitz M, Cohen ME, Gould M, Sharp GW. Elevated intracellular Ca²⁺ acts through protein kinase C to regulate rabbit ileal NaCl absorption. Evidence for sequential control by

Ca2+/calmodulin and protein kinase C. *J Clin Invest* 1989;83: 1953–1962.

167. Deckmyn H, Van Geet C, Vermylen J. Dual regulation of phospholipase C activity by G proteins. *News in Physiological Sciences* 1993;8:61–63.

168. Chang EB, Brown DR, Wang NS, Field M. Secretagogue-induced changes in membrane calcium permeability in chicken and chinchilla ileal mucosa. *J Clin Invest* 1986;78:281.

169. Stoclet JC, Gerard D, Kilhoffer MC, Lugnier C, Miller R, Schaeffer P. Calmodulin and its role in intracellular calcium regulation. *Prog Neurobiol* 1987;29:321–364.

170. Donowitz M, Wicks J, Madara JL, Sharp GW. Studies on role of calmodulin in Ca²⁺ regulation of rabbit ileal Na and Cl transport. *Am J Physiol* 1985;248:G726–G740.

171. Kachintorn U, Vongkovit P, Vajanaphanich M, Dinh S, Barrett KE, Dharmsathaphorn K. Dual effects of a phorbol ester on calcium-dependent chloride secretion by T84 epithelial cells. *Am J Physiol (Cell Physiol)* 1992;262:C15–C22.

172. Kachintorn U, Vajanaphanich M, Barrett KE, Traynor-Kaplan. Elevation of inositol tetrakisphosphate parallels inhibition of Ca(2+)-dependent Cl-secretion in T84 cells. *Am J Physiol* 1993;264:C671–C676.

173. Barrett KE, Bigby TD. Involvement of arachidonic acid in the chloride secretory response of intestinal epithelial cells. *Am J Physiol* 1993;264:C446–C452.

174. Madara JL, Patapoff TW, Gillece Castro B, Colgan SP, Parkos CA, Delp C, Mrsny RJ. 5′-Adenosine monophosphate is the neutrophil-derived paracrine factor that elicits chloride secretion from T84 intestinal epithelial cell monolayers (see comments). *J Clin Invest* 1993;91:2320–2325.

175. Plass H, Roden M, Wiener H, Turnheim K. Vanadium-induced Cl(−)-secretion in rabbit descending colon is mediated by prostaglandins. *Biochim Biophys Acta* 1992;1107:139.

176. Gustafson C, Franzen L, Tagesson C. Phospholipase activation and arachidonic acid release in isolated intestinal epithelial cells. *Scand J Gastroenterol* 1988;23:413.

177. Nishizuka Y. Studies and perspectives of protein kinase C. *Science* 1986;233:305–312.

178. Blackshear PJ, Nairn AC, Kuo JF. Protein kinases 1988: a current perspective. *FASEB J* 1988;2:2957–2969.

179. Anderson MP, Gregory RJ, Thompson S, et al. Demonstration that CFTR is a chloride channel by alteration of its anion selectivity. *Science* 1991;253:202.

180. Berger HA, Anderson MP, Gregory RJ, et al. Identification and regulation of the cystic fibrosis transmembrane conductance regulator-generated chloride channel. *J Clin Invest* 1991;88: 1422.

181. Forte LR, Thorne PK, Eber SL, et al. Stimulation of intestinal Cl⁻ transport by heat-stable enterotoxin: activation of cAMP-dependent protein kinase by cGMP. *Am J Physiol* 1992;263: C607–C615.

182. Cohen ME, Reinlib L, Watson AJM, et al. Rabbit ileal villus cell brush border Na⁺/H⁺ exchange is regulated by Ca²⁺/calmodulin-dependent protein kinase II, a brush border membrane protein. *Proc Natl Acad Sci USA* 1990;87:8990–8994.

183. Worrell RT, Frizzell RA. CaMKII mediates stimulation of chloride conductance by calcium in T84 cells. *Am J Physiol* 1991; 260:C877.

184. Cohen ME, Wesolek J, McCullen J, et al. Carbachol- and elevated Ca(2+)–induced translocation of functionally active protein kinase C to the brush border of rabbit ileal Na⁺ absorbing cells. *J Clin Invest* 1991;88:855–863.

185. Ahn J, Chang EB, Field M. Phorbol ester inhibition of Na-H exchange in rabbit proximal colon. *Am J Physiol* 1985;249: C527–C530.

186. Vaandrager AB, Vandenberghe N, Bot AGM, DeJonge HR. Phorbol esters stimulate and inhibit Cl⁻ secretion by different mechanisms in a colonic cell line. *Am J Physiol* 1992;262:P1, G249.

187. Helmle-Kolb C, Montrose MH, Stange G, Murer H. Regulation of *Na⁺/H⁺* exchange in opossum kidney cells by parathyroid hormone, cyclic AMP and phorbol esters. *Pflugers Arch* 1990; 415:461–470.

188. Tai YH, Decker RA, Marnane WG, Charney AN, Donowitz

189. Sardet C, Counillon A, Franchi J, Pouyssegur J. Growth factors induce phosphorylation of the Na⁺/H⁺ antiporter glycoprotein of 110 kD. *Science* 1990;247:723–726.

190. Watson AJM, Levine S, Donowitz M, Montrose MH. Serum regulates Na⁺/H⁺ exchange in Caco-2 cells by a mechanism which is dependent on F-actin. *J Biol Chem* 1992;267:956–962.

191. Sandle GI, Hayslett JP, Binder HJ. Effect of chronic hyperaldosteronism on the electrophysiology of rat distal colon. *Pflugers Arch* 1984;401:22–26.

192. Levens NR. Control of intestinal absorption by the renin-angiotensin system. *Am J Physiol* 1985;249:G3.

193. Sandle GI, Binder HJ. Corticosteroids and intestinal ion transport. *Gastroenterology* 1987;93:187–196.

194. Sellin JH, DeSoignie RC. Steroids alter ion transport and absorptive capacity in proximal and distal colon. *Am J Physiol* 1985;249:G113–G119.

195. Yun CH, Gurubhagavatula S, Levine SA, et al. Glucocorticoid stimulation of ileal Na⁺ absorptive cell brush border Na⁺/H⁺ exchange and association with an increase in message for NHE-3, an epithelial Na⁺/H⁺ exchanger isoform. *J Biol Chem* 1993; 268:206–211.

196. Lundgren JD, Hirata F, Marom Z. Dexamethasone inhibits respiratory glycoconjugate secretion from feline airways in vitro by the induction of lipocortin (lipomodulin) synthesis. *Am Rev Resp Dis* 1988;137:353–357.

197. Semrad CE, Cragoe EJ, Jr., Chang EB. Inhibition of Na/H exchange in avian intestine by atrial natriuretic factor. *J Clin Invest* 1990;86:585–591.

198. Argenzio RA, Armstrong M. ANP inhibits NaCl absorption and elicits Cl secretion in porcine colon: evidence for cGMP and Ca mediation. *Am J Physiol* 1993;265:R57–65.

199. Bianchi C, Thibault G, de Lean A, Genest J, Cantin M. Atrial natriuretic factor binding sites in the jejunum. *Am J Physiol Gastrointest Liver Physiol* 1989;256:G436–G441.

200. Soergel KH, Whalen GE, Harris JA, Geenen JE. Effect of ADH on human small intestinal water and solute transport. *J Clin Invest* 1968;47:1071.

201. Cooke HJ, Zafirova M, Carey HV, Walsh JH, Grider J. Vasoactive intestinal polypeptide actions on the guinea pig intestinal mucosa during neural stimulation. *Gastroenterology* 1987;92: 361–370.

202. Kachur JF, Miller RJ, Field M. Control of guinea pig intestinal electrolyte secretion by a δ-opiate receptor. *Proc Natl Acad Sci USA* 1980;77:2753–2756.

203. Isaacs PET, Corbett CL, Riley AK, Hawker PC, Turnberg LA. In vitro behavior of human intestinal mucosa. The influence of acetyl choline on ion transport. *J Clin Invest* 1976;58:535–542.

204. Dharmsathaphorn K, Pandol SJ. Mechanism of chloride secretion induced by carbachol in a colonic epithelial cell line. *J Clin Invest* 1986;77:348–354.

205. Roberts WG, Fedorak RN, Chang EB. In vitro effects of the long-acting somatostatin analogue SMS 201-995 on electrolyte transport by the rabbit ileum. *Gastroenterology* 1988;94: 1343–1350.

206. Brown DR, Overend MF, Treder BG. Neurohormonal regulation of ion transport in the porcine distal jejunum. Actions of somatostatin-14 and its natural and synthetic homologs. *J Pharmacol Exp Ther* 1990;252:126–134.

207. Hubel KA, Renquist KS. Effect of neuropeptide Y on ion transport by the rabbit ileum. *J Pharmacol Exp Ther* 1986;238: 167–169.

208. Greenwood B, Doolittle T, See NA, Koch TR, Dodds WJ, Davison JS. Effects of substance P and vasoactive intestinal polypeptide on contractile activity and epithelial transport in the ferret jejunum. *Gastroenterology* 1990;98:1509–1517.

209. Kuwahara A, Cooke HJ. Tachykinin-induced anion secretion in guinea pig distal colon: role of neural and inflammatory mediators. *J Pharmacol Exp Ther* 1990;252:1–7.

210. Hubel KA. Effects of pentagastrin and cholecystokinin on intestinal transport of ions and water in the rat. *Proc Soc Exp Biol Med* 1972;140:670–672.

211. Hubel KA. Effects of secretin and glucagon on intestinal transport of ions and water in the rat. *Proc Soc Exp Biol Med* 1972;139:656–658.

212. Donowitz M, Cusolito S, Battisti L, Fogel R, Sharp GW. Dopamine stimulation of active Na and Cl absorption in rabbit ileum: interaction with alpha 2-adrenergic and specific dopamine receptors. *J Clin Invest* 1982;69:1008–1016.

213. Chang EB, Field M, Miller RJ. Enterocyte alpha 2-adrenergic receptors: yohimbine and p-aminoclonidine binding relative to ion transport. *Am J Physiol* 1983;244:G76–G82.

214. Miller RJ, Kachur JF, Field M, Rivier J. Neurohumoral control of ileal electrolyte transport. *Ann N Y Acad Sci* 1981;372:571–593.

215. Cooke HJ, Shonnard K, Highison G, Wood JD. Effects of neurotransmitter release on mucosal transport in guinea pig ileum. *Am J Physiol* 1983;245:G745–G750.

216. Kuwahara A, Cooke HJ, Carey HV, Mekhjian H, Ellison EC, McGregor B. Effects of enteric neural stimulation on chloride transport in human left colon in vitro. *Dig Dis Sci* 1989;34:206–213.

217. Hubel KA, Renquist K, Shirazi S. Ion transport in human cecum, transverse colon, and sigmoid colon in vitro: baseline and response to electrical stimulation of intrinsic nerves. *Gastroenterology* 1987;92:501–507.

218. Hubel KA, Shirazi S. Human ileal ion transport in vitro: Changes with electrical field stimulation and tetrodotoxin. *Gastroenterology* 1982;83:63–68.

219. Hubel KA, Renquist KS. Ion transport in normal and inflamed human jejunum in vitro. Changes with electric field stimulation and theophylline. *Dig Dis Sci* 1990;35:815–820.

220. Galli SJ. New concepts about the mast cell. *Sem Med Beth Israel Hosp, Boston* 1994;328:257–265.

221. Sartor RB, Powell DW. Mechanisms of diarrhea in intestinal inflammation and hypersensitivity: immune system modulation of intestinal transport. In: Field M, ed. *Diarrheal diseases.* New York: Elsevier Science; 1991:75–114.

222. Schiffmann E, Corcoran BA, Wahl SM. N-Formylmethionyl peptides as chemoattractants for leucocytes. *Proc Natl Acad Sci USA* 1975;72:1059–1062.

223. Chadwick VS, Mellor DM, Myers DB, et al. Production of peptides inducing chemotaxis and lysosomal enzyme release in human neutrophils by intestinal bacteria in vitro and in vivo. *Scand J Gastroenterol* 1988;23:121–128.

224. Bern MJ, Sturbaum CW, Karaylacin SS, Berschneider HM, Wachsman JT, Powell DW. Immune system control of rat and rabbit colonic electrolyte transport: role of prostaglandins and enteric nervous system. *J Clin Invest* 1989;83:1810–1820.

225. Barrett TA, Musch MW, Chang EB. Chemotactic peptide effects on intestinal electrolyte transport. *Am J Physiol* 1990;259:G947–G954.

226. Nash S, Stafford J, Madara JL. Effects of polymorphonuclear leukocyte transmigration on the barrier function of cultured intestinal epithelial monlayers. *J Clin Invest* 1987;80:1104–1113.

227. Colgan SP, Parkos CA, Delp C, Arnaout MA, Madara JL. Neutrophil migration across cultured intestinal epithelial monolayers is modulated by epithelial exposure to IFN-gamma in a highly polarized fashion. *J Cell Biol* 1993;120:785–798.

228. Colgan SP, Serhan CN, Parkos CA, Delp-Archer C, Madara JL. Lipoxin A₄ modulates transmigration of human neutrophils across intestinal epithelial monolayers. *J Clin Invest* 1993;92:75–82.

229. Parkos CA, Delp C, Arnaout MA, Madara JL. Neutrophil migration across a cultured intestinal epithelium. Dependence on a CD11b/CD18-mediated event and enhanced efficiency in physiological direction. *J Clin Invest* 1991;88:1605–1612.

230. Parkos CA, Colgan SP, Delp C, Arnaout MA, Madara JL. Neutrophil migration across a cultured epithelial monolayer elicits a biphasic resistance response representing sequential effects on transcellular and paracellular pathways. *J Cell Biol* 1992;117:757–764.

231. Nash S, Parkos C, Nusrat A, Delp C, Madara JL. In vitro model of intestinal crypt abscess. A novel neutrophil-derived secretagogue activity. *J Clin Invest* 1991;87:1474–1477.

232. Barrett KE, Huott PA, Shah SS, Dharmsathaphorn K, Wasserman SI. Differing effects of apical and basolateral adenosine on colonic epithelial cell line T84. *Am J Physiol* 1989;256:C197–C203.

233. Schuerer-Maly C-C, Eckmann L, Kagnoff MF, Falco MT, Maly F-E. Colonic epithelial cell lines as a source of interleukin-8: stimulation by inflammatory cytokines and bacterial lipopolysaccharide. *Immunology* 1994;81:85–91.

234. McCormick BA, Colgan SP, Delp-Archer C, Miller SI, Madara JL. *Salmonella typhimurium* attachment to human intestinal epithelial monolayers: transcellular signalling to subepithelial neutrophils. *J Cell Biol* 1993;123:895–907.

235. Resnick MB, Colgan SP, Patapoff TW, et al. Activated eosinophils evoke chloride secretion in model intestinal epithelia primarily via regulated releast of 5′-AMP. *J Immunol* 1993;151:5716–5723.

236. Befus AD, Pierce FL, Gauldie J, Horsewood P, Bienenstock J. Mucosal mast cells I. Isolation and functional characteristics of rat intestinal mast cells. *J Immunol* 1982;128:2475–2480.

237. Befus AD, Dyck N, Goodacre R, Bienenstock J. Mast cells from the human intestinal lamina propria. Isolation, histochemical subtypes, and functional characterization. *J Immunol* 1987;138:2604–2610.

238. Befus AD, Goodacre R, Dyck N, Bienenstock J. Mast cell heterogeneity in man 1. Histological studies of the intestine. *Int Arch Allergy Appl Immunol* 1985;76:232–236.

239. Irani AM, Schecter NM, Craig SS, Deblois G, Schwartz LB. Two types of human mast cells that have distinct neutral protease compositions. *Proc Natl Acad Sci USA* 1986;83:4464–4469.

240. Serafin WE, Austen KF. Mediators of immediate hypersensitivity reactions. *N Engl J Med* 1987;317:30–34.

241. Cuthbert AW, McLaughlan P, Coombs RRA. Immediate hypersensitivity reaction to B-lactoglobulin in the epithelium lining the colon of guinea pigs fed cows' milk. *Int Arch Allergy Appl Immunol* 1983;72:34–40.

242. Baird AW, Coombs RR, McLaughlan P, Cuthbert AW. Immediate hypersensitivity reactions to cow milk proteins in isolated epithelium from ileum of milk-drinking guinea-pigs: comparisons with colonic epithelia. *Int Arch Allergy Appl Immunol* 1984;75:255–263.

243. Baird AW, Cuthbert AW, McVinish LJ. Type I hypersensitivity reactions in reconstructed tissues using syngeneic cell types. *Br J Pharmacol* 1987;91:857–869.

244. Perdue MH, Gall DG. Intestinal anaphylaxis in the rat: jejunal response to in vitro antigen exposure. *Am J Physiol* 1986;250:G427–G431.

245. Baird AW, Cuthbert AW, Pierce FL. Immediate hypersensitivity reactions in the epithelia from rats infected with *Nippostrongylus brasiliensis. Br J Pharmacol* 1985;85:787–795.

246. Russell DA. Mast cells in the regulation of intestinal electrolyte transport. *Am J Physiol* 1986;251:G253–G262.

247. Castro GA, Harari Y, Russell DA. Mediators of anaphylaxis-induced ion transport changes in small intestine. *Am J Physiol* 1987;253:G540–G548.

248. Crowe SE, Sestini P, Perdue MH. Allergic reactions of rat jejunal mucosa. Ion transport responses to luminal antigen and inflammatory mediators. *Gastroenterology* 1990;99:74–82.

249. Perdue MH, Masson S, Wershil BK, Galli SJ. Role of mast cells in ion transport abnormalities associated with intestinal anaphylaxis. Correction of the diminished secretory response in genetically mast cell-deficient W/Wv mice by bone marrow transplantation. *J Clin Invest* 1991;87:687–693.

250. Wang Y, Palmer JM, Cooke HJ. Neuroimmune regulation of colonic secretion in guinea pigs. *Am J Physiol* 1991;260:G307–G314.

251. Crowe SE, Perdue MH. Anti-immunoglobulin E–stimulated ion transport in human large and small intestine. *Gastroenterology* 1993;105:764–772.

252. D'Inca R, Ramage JK, Hunt RH, Perdue MH. Antigen-induced mucosal damage and restitution in the small intestine of the immunized rat. *Int Arch Allergy Appl Immunol* 1990;91:270–277.

253. Crowe SE, Soda K, Stanisz AM, Perdue MH. Intestinal perme-

ability in allergic rats. Nerve involvement in antigen-induced changes. *Am J Physiol Gastrointest Liver Physiol* 1994;27: G617–G623.

254. Pothoulakis C, Karmeli F, Kelly CP. Mast cell involvement in *Clostridium difficile* toxin A enteritis in rat. Studies with keotitfen. *Gastroenterology* 1993;105:701–707.

255. Chang EB, Musch MW, Mayer L. Interleukins 1 and 3 stimulate anion secretion in chicken intestine. *Gastroenterology* 1990;98:1518–1524.

256. Chiossone DC, Simon PL, Smith PL. Interleukin-1: effects on rabbit ileal mucosal ion transport in vitro. *Eur J Pharmacol* 1990;180:217–228.

257. Holmgren J, Fryklund J, Larsson H. Gamma-interferon–mediated down-regulation of electrolyte secretion by intestinal epithelial cells: a local immune mechanism. *Scand J Immunol* 1989;30:499–503.

258. Colgan SP, Parkos CA, Matthews JB, et al. Interferon-gamma induces a cell surface phenotype switch in intestinal epithelia: downregulation of ion transport function and upregulation of immune accessory ligands. *Am J Physiol* 1994;267:C402–C410.

259. McKay DM, Croitoru K, Perdue MH. Activation of T lymphocytes causes increased permeability of T84 epithelial monolayers and reduces responses to secretagogues. *Gastroenterology* 1993;104:A741 (abstr).

260. Kaoutzani P, Colgan SP, Cepek KL, et al. Reconstitution of cultured intestinal epithelial monolayers with intraepithelial lymphocytes (IEL): modulation of epithelial phenotype dependent on IEL-basolateral membrane apposition. *J Clin Invest* 1994;94:788–796.

261. Macdonald TT, Spencer J. Evidence that activated mucosal T cells play a role in the pathogenesis of enteropathy in human small intestine. *J Exp Med* 1988;167:1341–1349.

262. Ferreira RDC, Forsyth LE, Richman PI, Wells C, Spencer J, Macdonald TT. Changes in the rate of crypt epithelial cell proliferation and mucosal morphology induced by a T-cell–mediated response in human small intestine. *Gastroenterology* 1990; 98:1255–1263.

263. Evans CM, Phillips AD, Walker-Smith JA, Macdonald TT. Activation of lamina propria T cells induces crypt epithelial proliferation and goblet cell depletion in cultured human fetal colon. *Gut* 1992;33:230–235.

264. Ferguson A, Jarrett EEE. Hypersensitivity reactions in the small intestine. I. Thymus dependence of experimental "partial villous atrophy." *Gut* 1975;16:114–117.

265. D'Inca R, Ernst P, Hunt RH, Perdue MH. Role of T lymphocytes in intestinal mucosal injury. Inflammatory changes in athymic nude rats. *Dig Dis Sci* 1992;37:33–39.

266. Mayer L, Shlien R. Evidence for function of Ia molecules on gut epithelial cells in man. *J Exp Med* 1987;166:1471–1483.

267. Kvale D, Krajci P, Brandtzaeg P. Expression and regulation of adhesion molecules ICAM-1 (CD54) and LFA-3 (CD 58) in human intestinal epithelial cell lines. *Scand J Immunol* 1992; 35:669–676.

268. Kaiserlian D, Rigal D, Abello J, Revillard J-P. Expression, function and regulation of the intercellular adhesion molecule-1 (ICAM-1) on human intestinal epithelial cell lines. *Eur J Immunol* 1991;21:2415–2421.

269. Mayer L, Panja A, Li Y, et al. Unique features of antigen presentation in the intestine. *Ann N Y Acad Sci* 1992;664:39–46.

270. Lammers KM, Jansen J, Bijlsma PB, et al. Polarised interleukin 8 secretion by HT 29/19A cells. *Gut* 1994;35:338–342.

271. Eckmann L, Jung HC, Schurer-Maly C, Panja A, Morzycka-Wroblewska E, Kagnoff MF. Differential cytokine expression by human intestinal epithelial cell lines: regulated expression of interleukin 8. *Gastroenterology* 1993;105:1689–1697.

272. Shirota K, LeDuy L, Yuan S, Jothy S. Interleukin-6- and its receptor are expressed in human intestinal epithelial cells. *Virchows Arch B Cell Pathol* 1990;58:303–308.

273. Spriggs DR, Imamura K, Rodriguez C, Sariban E, Kufe DW. Tumor necrosis factor expression in human epithelial tumor cell lines. *J Clin Invest* 1988;81:455–460.

274. Koyama SY, Podolsky DK. Differential expression of transforming growth factors alpha and beta in rat intestinal epithelial cells. *J Clin Invest* 1989;83:1768–1773.

275. Barnard JA, Polk WH, Moses HL, Coffey RJ. Production of transforming growth factor-alpha by normal rat small intestine. *Am J Physiol* 1991;261:C994–1000.

276. Wright NA, Pike C, Elia G. Induction of a novel epidermal growth factor-secreting cell lineage by mucosal ulceration in human gastrointestinal stem cells. *Nature* 1990;343:82–85.

277. Fujiyama Y, Matsumoto T, Gutrion M, Strassmann G, Brown WR. Macrophage colony stimulating factor is present in gastrointestinal epithelial cells. *Gastroenterology* 1992;102:A625.

278. Gustafson C, Sjödahl R, Tagesson C. Phospholipase activation and arachidonic acid release in intestinal epithelial cells from patients with Crohn's disease. *Scand J Gastroenterol* 1990;25: 1151–1160.

279. Gustafson Svard C, Tagesson C, Boll RM, Kald B. Tumor necrosis factor-alpha potentiates phospholipase A2-stimulated release and metabolism of arachidonic acid in cultured intestinal epithelial cells (INT 407). *Scand J Gastroenterol* 1993;28: 323–330.

280. Gustafson C, Lindahl M, Tagesson C. Hydrogen peroxide stimulates phospholipase A_2-mediated arachidonic acid release in cultured intestinal epithelial cells (INT 407). *Scand J Gastroenterol* 1991;26:237–247.

281. Leduc LE, McRoberts JA, Vidrich A. Eicosanoid production by a differentiated canine colonic epithelial cell line, VNCC. *Gastroenterology* 1994;106:297–305.

282. Grisham MB. Nitric oxide production by intestinal epithelial cells. *Gastroenterology* 1993;104:A710 (abstr).

283. Muller MJ, Huizinga JD, Collins SM. Altered smooth muscle contraction and sodium pump activity in the inflamed rat intestine. *Am J Physiol* 1989;257:G570–G577.

284. Vermillion DL, Ernst PB, Scicchitano R, Collins SM. Antigen-induced contraction of jejunal smooth muscle in the sensitized rat. *Am J Physiol* 1989;255:G701–G708.

285. Karayalcin SS, Sturbaum CW, Wachsman JT, Cha JH, Powell DW. Hydrogen peroxide stimulates rat colonic prostaglandin production and alters electrolyte transport. *J Clin Invest* 1990; 86:60–68.

286. Grisham MB, Gaginella TS, von Ritter C, Tamai H, Be RM, Granger DN. Effects of neutrophil-derived oxidants on intestinal permeability, electrolyte transport, and epithelial cell viability. *Inflammation* 1990;14:531–542.

287. Nguyen TD, Canada AT. Modulation of human colonic T_{84} cell secretion by hydrogen peroxide. *Biochem Pharmacol* 1994;47: 403–410.

288. Tamai H, Kachur JF, Baron DA, Grisham MB, Gaginella TS. Monochloramine, a neutrophil-derived oxidant, stimulates rat colonic secretion. *J Pharmacol Exp Ther* 1991;257:887–894.

289. Tamai H, Gaginella TS, Kachur JF, Musch MW, Chang EB. Ca-mediated stimulation of Cl secretion by reactive oxygen metabolites in human colonic T84-cells. *J Clin Invest* 1992;89: 301–307.

290. Nathan C. Nitric oxide as a secretory product of mammalian cells. *FASEB J* 1992;6:3051–3064.

291. Stark ME, Szurszewski JH. Role of nitric oxide in gastrointestinal and hepatic function and disease. *Gastroenterology* 1992; 103:1928–1949.

292. MacNaughton WK. Nitric oxide-donating compounds stimulate electrolyte transport in the guinea pig intestine in vitro. *Life Sci* 1993;53:585–593.

293. Wilson KT, Xie Y, Musch MW, Chang EB. Sodium nitroprusside stimulates anion secretion and inhibits sodium chloride absorption in rat colon. *J Pharmacol Exp Ther* 1993;266: 224–230.

294. Keenan CM, Rangachari PK. Contrasting effects of PGE2 and PGD2: ion transport in the canine proximal colon. *Am J Physiol* 1991;260:G481–G488.

295. Georg K, Diener C, Diener M, Rummel W. Antisecretory effect of prostaglandin D2 in rat colon in vitro: action sites. *Am J Physiol* 1991;260:G904–G910.

296. Keenan CM, Rangachari PK. Eicosanoid interactions in the canine proximal colon. *Am J Physiol* 1989;256:G673–G679.

297. Smith PL, Chiossone DC, McCafferty GP. Characterization of LTC4 effects on rabbit ileal mucosa in vitro. *Naunyn Schmiedebergs Arch Pharmakol* 1990;341:94–100.

298. Hanglow AC, Bienenstock J, Perdue MH. Effects of platelet-activating factor on ion transport in isolated rat jejunum. *Am J Physiol* 1989;257:G845–G850.

299. Berschneider HM, Powell DW. Fibroblasts modulate intestinal secretory responses to inflammatory mediators. *J Clin Invest* 1992;89:484–489.

300. Barrett KE, Cohn JA, Huott PA, Wasserman SI, Dharmsathaphorn K. Immune-related intestinal chloride secretion. II. Effect of adenosine on T84 cell line. *Am J Physiol (Cell Physiol)* 1990;258:C902–C912.

301. Rangachari PK. Histamine: mercurial messenger in the gut. *Am J Physiol Gastrointest Liver Physiol* 1992;262:G1–G13.

302. Cooke HJ, Nameth PR, Wood JD. Histamine action on guinea pig ileal mucosa. *Am J Physiol* 1984;246:G372–G378.

303. Wasserman SI, Barrett KE, Huott PA, Beuerlein G, Kagnoff MF, Dharmsathaphorn K. Immune-related intestinal Cl secretion. I. Effect of histamine on the T84 cell line. *Am J Physiol* 1988;254:C53–C62.

304. Wang YZ, Cooke HJ. H2 receptors mediate cyclical chloride secretion in guinea pig distal colon. *Am J Physiol* 1990;258:G887–G893.

305. Wang Y-Z, Cooke HJ, Su H-C, Fertel R. Histamine augments colonic secretion in guinea pig distal colon. *Am J Physiol Gastrointest Liver Physiol* 1990;258:G432–G439.

306. Beesley A, Levin RJ. 5-Hydroxytryptamine induces electrogenic secretion and simultaneously activates a modulating inhibitory neural circuit in rat small intestine *in vitro*. *Exp Physiol* 1991;76:607–610.

307. Hardcastle J, Hardcastle PT, Redfern JS. Action of 5-hydroxytryptamine on intestinal ion transport in the rat. *J Physiol (London)* 1981;320:41–55.

308. Donowitz M, Tai YH, Asarkof N. Effect of serotonin on active electrolyte transport in rabbit ileum, gallbladder, and colon. *Am J Physiol* 1980;239:G463–G472.

309. Zimmerman TW, Binder HJ. Serotonin-induced alteration of colonic electrolyte transport in the rat. *Gastroenterology* 1984;86:310–317.

310. Cooke HJ, Wang YZ, Frieling T, Wood JD. Neural 5-hydroxytryptamine receptors regulate chloride secretion in guinea pig distal colon. *Am J Physiol* 1991;261:G833–G840.

311. Beubler E, Bukhave K, Rask-Madsen J. Significance of calcium for the prostaglandin-E2-mediated secretory response to 5-hydroxytryptamine in the small intestine of the rat in vivo. *Gastroenterology* 1986;90:1972–1977.

312. Kandil HM, Berschneider HM, Argenzio RA. Tumour necrosis factor alpha changes intestinal ion transport through a paracrine mechanism involving prostaglandins. *Gastroenterology* 1992;102:A217.

313. Wardle TD, Turnberg LA. Platelet derived growth factor stimulates chloride secretion in mammalian colon. *Gastroenterology* 1993;104:A289 (abstr).

314. Opleta-Madsen K, Hardin J, Gall DG. Epidermal growth factor upregulates intestinal electrolyte and nutrient transport. *Am J Physiol Gastrointest Liver Physiol* 1991;260:G807–G814.

315. Hardin JA, Gall DG. The effect of TGFα on intestinal solute transport. *Reg Peptides* 1992;39:169–176.

316. Souba WW, Copeland EM. Cytokine modulation of Na+-dependent glutamine transport across the brush border membrane of monolayers of human intestinal Caco-2 cells. *Ann Surg* 1992;215:536–545.

317. Madara JL, Stafford J. Interferon-g directly affects barrier function of cultured intestinal epithelial monolayers. *J Clin Invest* 1989;83:724–727.

318. Adams RB, Planchon SM, Roche JK. IFN-gamma modulation of epithelial barrier function. Time course, reversibility, and site of cytokine binding. *J Immunol* 1993;150:2356–2363.

319. Berschneider HM, Goralska M. Interleukin-1α (IL-1) and tumor necrosis factor–α (TNF) enhance the paracrine modulation of intestinal epithelial Cl⁻ secretion by fibroblasts. *Gastroenterology* 1992;102:A201.

320. Cartwright CA, McRoberts JA, Mandel KG, Dharmsathaphorn K. Synergistic action of cyclic adenosine monophosphate- and calcium-mediated chloride secretion in a colonic epithelial cell line. *J Clin Invest* 1985;76:1837–1842.

321. Warhurst G, Higgs NB, Tonge A, Turnberg LA. Stimulatory and inhibitory actions of carbachol on chloride secretory responses in human colonic cell line T84. *Am J Physiol* 1991;261:G220–G228.

322. Cantey JR. Infectious diarrhea. Pathogenesis and risk factors. *Am J Med* 1985;78:65–75.

323. Wick MJ, Madara JL, Fields BN, Normark SJ. Meeting review. Molecular cross talk between epithelial cells and pathogenic microorganisms. *Cell* 1991;67:651–659.

324. Liu CT, DuFault BR. Effects of intestinal infusion of staphylococcal enterotoxin B (SEB) on water and electrolyte fluxes: possible mechanisms of diarrhea. *Physiologist* 1977;20:57.

325. Elwell MR, Liu CT, Spertzel RO. Mechanisms of oral staphylococcal enterotoxin B–induced emesis in monkey. *Proc Soc Exp Biol Med* 1975;148:424.

326. Turnbull PCB, Kramer JM, Jorgensen K. Properties and production characteristics of vomiting, diarrheal, and necrotizing toxins of *Bacillus cereus*. *Am J Clin Nutr* 1979;32:219.

327. Lencer WI, Delp C, Neutra MR, Madara JL. Mechanism of cholera toxin action on a polarized human intestinal epithelial cell line: role of vesicular traffic. *J Cell Biol* 1992;117:1197–1209.

328. Lencer WI, de Almeida JB, Moe S, Stow JL, Ausiello DA, Madara JL. Entry of cholera toxin into polarized human intestinal epithelial cells. Identification of an early brefeldin A sensitive event required for A1-peptide generation. *J Clin Invest* 1993;92:2941–2951.

329. Hyun C, Kimmich GA. Effect of cholera toxin on cAMP levels and Na+ influx in isolated intestinal epithelial cells. *Am J Physiol* 1982;243:C107–C115.

330. Guandalini S, Rao MC, Smith PL, Field M. cGMP modulation of ileal ion transport: in vitro effects of *Escherichia coli* heat-stable enterotoxin. *Am J Physiol* 1982;243:G36–G41.

331. Weikel CS, Nellans HN, Guerrant RL. In vivo and in vitro effects of a novel enterotoxin, STb, produced by *Escherichia coli* [published erratum appears in *J Infect Dis* 1986 Dec; 154(6):1053]. *J Infect Dis* 1986;153:893–901.

332. Khurana S, Ganguly NK, Khullar M, Panigrahi D, Walia BN. Studies on the mechanism of *Salmonella typhimurium* enterotoxin-induced diarrhoea. *Biochim Biophys Acta* 1991;1097:171–176.

333. Donowitz M, Keusch GT, Binder HJ. Effect of *Shigella* enterotoxin on electrolyte transport in rabbit ileum. *Gastroenterology* 1975;69:1230–1237.

334. Donowitz M, Binder HJ. Effect of enterotoxins of *Vibrio cholerae*, *Escherichia coli*, and *Shigella dysenteriae* type 1 on fluid and electrolyte transport in the colon. *J Infect Dis* 1976;134:135–143.

335. McDonel JL. The molecular mode of action of *Clostridium perfringens* enterotoxin. *Am J Clin Nutr* 1979;32:210.

336. McDonel JL, Demers GW. In vivo effects of enterotoxin from *Clostridium perfringens* type A in the rabbit colon: binding vs. biologic activity. *J Infect Dis* 1982;145:490–494.

337. Keusch GT, Jacewicz M, Mobassaleh M, Donohue Rolfe A. Shiga toxin: intestinal cell receptors and pathophysiology of enterotoxic effects. *Rev Infect Dis* 1991;13 Suppl 4:S304–S310.

338. Kandel G, Donohue-Rolfe A, Donowitz M, Keusch GT. Pathogenesis of *Shigella* diarrhea. XVI. Selective targetting of Shiga toxin to villus cells of rabbit jejunum explains the effect of the toxin on intestinal electrolyte transport. *J Clin Invest* 1989;84:1509–1517.

339. Li Z, Bell C, Buret A, Robins-Browne R, Stiel D, O'Loughlin. The effect of enterohemorrhagic *Escherichia coli* O157:H7 on intestinal structure and solute transport in rabbits. *Gastroenterology* 1993;104:467–474.

340. Hecht G, Pothoulakis C, LaMont JT, Madara JL. *Clostridium difficile* toxin A perturbs cytoskeletal structure and tight junction permeability of cultured human intestinal epithelial monolayers. *J Clin Invest* 1988;82:1516–1524.

341. Moore R, Pothoulakis C, LaMont JT, Carlson S, Madara JL. *C. difficile* toxin A increases intestinal permeability and induces Cl⁻ secretion. *Am J Physiol Gastrointest Liver Physiol* 1990;259:G165–G172.

342. Pothoulakis C, Sullivan R, Melnick D. *Clostridium difficile* toxin A stimulates intracellular calcium release and chemotac-

tic response in human granulocytes. *J Clin Invest* 1988;81: 1741–1745.

343. Kelly CP, Becker SD, Linevsky J, et al. Neutrophil recruitment in *Clostridium difficile* toxin A enteritis in the rabbit. *J Clin Invest* 1994;93:1257–1265.

344. Pothoulakis C, Castagliuolo I, LaMont JT, O'Keane JC, Snider RM, Leeman SE. CP-96,345, a substance P antagonist, inhibits rat intestinal responses to *Clostridium difficile* toxin A but not cholera toxin. *Proc Natl Acad Sci USA* 1994;91:947–951.

345. Castagliuolo I, LaMont JT, Letourneau R. Neuronal involvement in the intestinal effects of *Clostridium difficile* toxin A and vibrio cholera enterotoxin in rat ileum. *Gastroenterology* 1994; in press.

346. Weikel CS, Grieco FD, Reuben J, Myers LL, Sack RB. Human colonic epithelial cells, HT29/C$_1$, treated with crude *Bacteroides fragilis* enterotoxin dramatically alter their morphology. *Infect Immun* 1992;60:321–327.

347. Fasano A, Baudry B, Pumplin DW, Wasserman SS, Tall BD, Ketley JM, Kaper JB. *Vibrio cholerae* produces a second enterotoxin, which affects intestinal tight junctions. *Proc Natl Acad Sci USA* 1991;88:5242–5246.

348. Hart CA, Batt RM, Fletcher J, Embaye H, Saunders JR. Interactions between enterocytes and enteropathogenic *Escherichia coli*. *Biochem Soc Trans* 1989;17:466–469.

349. Ulshen MH, Rollo JL. Pathogenesis of *Escherichia coli* gastroenteritis in man—another mechanism. *N Engl J Med* 1980; 302:99–101.

350. Rothbaum R, McAdams AJ, Giannella R, Partin JC. A clinicopathologic study of enterocyte-adherent *Escherichia coli:* a cause of protracted diarrhea in infants. *Gastroenterology* 1982; 83:441–454.

351. Tzipori S, Robins-Browne RM, Gonis G, Hayes J, Withers M, McCartney E. Enteropathogenic *Escherichia coli* enteritis: evaluation of the gnotobiotic piglet as a model of human infection. *Gut* 1985;26:570–578.

352. Moon HW, Whipp SC, Argenzio RA, Levine MM, Giannella RA. Attaching and effacing activities of rabbit and human enteropathogenic *Escherichia coli* in pig and rabbit intestines. *Infect Immun* 1983;41:1340–1351.

353. Jerse AE, Kaper JB. The *eae* gene of enteropathogenic *Escherichia coli* encodes a 94-kilodalton membrane protein, the expression of which is influenced by the EAF plasmid. *Infect Immun* 1991;59:4302–4309.

354. Jerse AE, Yu J, Tall BD, Kaper JB. A genetic locus of enteropathogenic *Escherichia coli* necessary for the production of attaching and effacing lesions on tissue culture cells. *Proc Natl Acad Sci USA* 1990;87:7839–7843.

355. Baldini MJ, Kaper JB, Levin MM, Candy DCA, Moon HW. Plasmid-mediated adhesion in enteropathogenic *Escherichia coli*. *J Pediatr Gastroenterol Nutr* 1983;2:534–538.

356. Baldwin TJ, Brooks SF, Knutton S, Hernandez HAM, Aitken A, Williams PH. Protein phosphorylation by protein kinase C in HEp-2 cells infected with enteropathogenic *Escherichia coli*. *Infect Immun* 1990;58:761–765.

357. Dytoc M, Fedorko L, Sherman M. Signal transduction in human epithelial cells infected with attaching and effacing *Escherichia coli* in vitro. *Gastroenterology* 1994;106: 1150–1161.

358. Perdue MH, Philpott DJ, McKay DM, Sherman PM. Enteropathogenic *Escherichia coli* infection alters T84 epithelial cell barrier and transport properties. *Gastroenterology* 1994;106: A751 (abstr).

359. Nath SK, Dechelotte P, Darmaun D, Gotteland M, Rongier M, Desjeux JF. [^{15}N]- and [^{14}C]glutamine fluxes across rabbit ileum in experimental bacterial diarrhea. *Am J Physiol* 1992; 262:G312–G318.

360. Tai YH, Gage TP, McQueen C, Formal SB, Boedeker EC. Electrolyte transport in rabbit cecum. I. Effect of RDEC-1 infection. *Am J Physiol* 1989;256:G721–G726.

361. Schlager TA, Wanke CA, Guerrant RL. Net fluid secretion and impaired villous function induced by colonization of the small intestine by nontoxigenic colonizing *Escherichia coli*. *Infect Immun* 1990;58:1337–1343.

362. Canil C, Rosenshine I, Ruschkowski S, Donnenberg MS,

Kaper JB, Finlay BB. Enteropathogenic *Escherichia coli* decreases transepithelial electrical resistance of polarized epithelial monolayers. *Infect Immun* 1993;61:2755–2762.

363. Sjogren RW, Sherman PM, Boedeker EC. Altered intestinal motility precedes diarrhea during *Escherichia coli* enteric infection. *Am J Physiol* 1989;257:G725–G731.

364. Cevallos AM, Katelaris PH, Farthing MJG. Pathogenesis of giardiasis (letter). *Gastroenterology* 1993;105:306–307.

365. Buret A, Hardin JA, Olson ME, Gall DG. Pathophysiology of small intestinal malabsorption in gerbils infected with *Giardia lamblia*. *Gastroenterology* 1992;103:506–513.

366. Goyal R, Mahajan RC, Ganguly NK, Sehgal R, Gorowara S, Singh K. Macrophage-mediated enterocyte damage in BALB/ c mice infected with different strains of *Giardia lamblia*. *Scand J Gastroenterol* 1993;28:845–848.

367. Viboud GI, Binsztein N, Svennerholm AM. A new fimbrial putative colonization factor, PCFO20, in human enterotoxigenic *Escherichia coli*. *Infect Immun* 1993;61:5190–5197.

368. Binsztein N, Jouve MJ, Viboud GI, et al. Colonization factors of enterotoxigenic *Escherichia coli* isolated from children with diarrhea in Argentina. *J Clin Microbiol* 1991;59:1290–1299.

369. Ravdin JI, Guerrant RL. Role of adherence in cytopathogenic mechanisms of *Entamoeba histolytica:* study with mammalian tissue culture cells and human erythrocytes. *J Clin Invest* 1981; 68:1305–1313.

370. Finlay BB, Falkow S. *Salmonella* interactions with polarized human intestinal Caco-2 epithelial cells. *J Infect Dis* 1990;162: 1096–1106.

371. Li E, Becker A, Stanley J. Chinese hamster ovary cells deficient in N-acetylglucosaminyltransferase I activity are resistant to *Entamoeba histolytica*–mediated cytotoxicity. *Infect Immun* 1989;57:8–12.

372. Mantle M, Husar SD. Adhesion of *Yersinia enterocolitica* to purified rabbit and human intestinal mucin. *Infect Immun* 1993; 61:2340–2346.

373. Duffy MC, Benson JB, Rubin SJ. Mucosal invasion in *Campylobacter* enteritis. *Am J Clin Pathol* 1980;73:706–708.

374. Montgomery LB, Kao C-YY, Verdin E, Cahill C, Maratos-Flier E. Infection of a polarized epithelial cell line with wild-type reovirus leads to virus persistence and altered cellular function. *J Gen Virol* 1991;72:2939–2946.

375. Rout WR, Formal SB, Dammin GJ, Giannella RA. Pathophysiology of *Salmonella* diarrhea in the Rhesus monkey: intestinal transport, morphological and bacteriological studies. *Gastroenterology* 1974;67:59–70.

376. DuPont HL, Formal SB. Pathogenesis of *Escherichia coli* diarrhea. *N Engl J Med* 1971;285:1–9.

377. Berg RD. Translocation of enteric bacteria in health and disease. *Curr Stud Hematol Blood Transfus* 1992;P 44–65.

378. Konkel ME, Hayes SF, Joens LA, Cieplak W, Jr. Characteristics of the internalization and intracellular survival of *Campylobacter jejuni* in human epithelial cell cultures. *Microb Pathog* 1992;13:357–370.

379. Oelschlaeger TA, Guerry P, Kopecko DJ. Unusual microtubule-dependent endocytosis mechanisms triggered by *Campylobacter jejuni* and *Citrobacter freundii*. *Proc Natl Acad Sci USA* 1993;90:6884–6888.

380. Perdomo JJ, Gounon P, Sansonetti J. Polymorphonuclear leukocyte transmigration promotes invasion of colonic epithelial monolayer by *Shigella flexneri*. *J Clin Invest* 1994;93:633–643.

381. Kaljot KT, Shaw RD, Rubin DH, Greenberg HB. Infectious rotavirus enters cell by direct cell membrane penetration, not by endocytosis. *J Virol* 1988;62:1136–1144.

382. Morrison LA, Sidman RL, Fields BN. Direct spread of reovirus from the intestinal lumen to the central nervous system through vagal autonomic nerve fibers. *Proc Natl Acad Sci USA* 1991; 88:3852–3856.

383. Finlay BB, Heffron F, Falkow S. Epithelial cell surfaces induce *Salmonella* proteins required for bacterial adherence and invasion. *Science* 1989;243:940–943.

384. Hale TL, Bonventre PF. *Shigella* infection of Henle intestinal epithelial cells: role of the bacterium. *Infect Immun* 1979;24: 879–886.

385. Hale TL, Morris RE, Bonventre PF. *Shigella* infection of Henle

intestinal epithelial cells: role of the host cell. *Infect Immun* 1979;24:887–894.

386. Miller VL, Falkow S. Evidence for two genetic loci in *Yersinia enterocolitica* that can promote invasion of epithelial cells. *Infect Immun* 1988;56:1242.

387. Small PLC, Falkow S. Identification of regions on a 230-kilobase plasmid from enteroinvasive *Escherichia coli* that are required for entry into HEp-2 cells. *Infect Immun* 1988;56:225–229.

388. Maurelli AT, Baudry B, deHauteville H, Hale TL, Sansonetti PJ. Cloning of plasmid DNA sequences involved in invasion of HeLa cells by *Shigella flexneri*. *Infect Immun* 1985;49:164–171.

389. Grant CC, Konkel ME, Cieplak W, Jr., Tompkins LS. Role of flagella in adherence, internalization, and translocation of *Campylobacter jejuni* in nonpolarized and polarized epithelial cell cultures. *Infect Immun* 1993;61:1764–1771.

390. Galan JE, Pace J, Hayman MJ. Involvement of the epidermal growth factor receptor in the invasion of cultured mammalian cells by *Salmonella typhimurium*. *Nature* 1992;357:588–589.

391. O'Loughlin EV, Pai CH, Gall DG. Effect of acute *Yersinia enterocolitica* infection on in vivo and in vitro small intestinal solute and fluid absorption in the rabbit. *Gastroenterology* 1988;94:664–672.

392. Perdue MH, Marshall J, Masson S. Ion transport abnormalities in inflamed rat jejunum. Involvement of mast cells and nerves. *Gastroenterology* 1990;98:561–567.

393. Capron A, Dessaint JP, Capron M, Joseph M, Ameisen JC, Tonnel AB. The second receptor for IgE (FceR2). *Immunol Today* 1986;7:15–18.

394. Giannella RA. Importance of the intestinal inflammatory reaction in *Salmonella*-mediated intestinal secretion. *Infect Immun* 1979;23:140–145.

395. Argenzio RA, Liacos JA. Endogenous prostanoids control ion transport across neonatal porcine ileum in vitro. *Am J Vet Res* 1990;51:747–751.

396. Riehl TE, Stenson WF. Mechanisms of transit of inflammatory mediators and bacterial peptides across intestinal epithelia. *Gastroenterology* 1993;104:A770 (abstr).

397. Ciancio MJ, Vitiritti L, Dhar A, Chang EB. Endotoxin-induced alterations in rat colonic water and electrolyte transport (see comments). *Gastroenterology* 1992;103:1437–1443.

398. Elliott E, Li Z, Bell C, et al. Modulation of host response to enterohemorrhagic *Escherichia coli* O157:H7 infection by anti-CD18 monoclonal antibody in rabbits. *Gastroenterology* 1994; (*in press*).

399. Powell DW. New paradigms for the pathophysiology of infectious diarrhea. *Gastroenterology* 1994;106:1705–1707.

400. Brunsson I. Enteric nerves mediate the fluid secretory response due to *Salmonella typhimurium* R5 infection in the rat small intestine. *Acta Physiol Scand* 1987;131:609–617.

401. Giannella RA, Rout WR, Formal SB. Effect of indomethacin on intestinal water transport in *Salmonella*-infected Rhesus monkeys. *Infect Immun* 1977;17:136–139.

402. Farris RK, Tapper EJ, Powell DW, Morris SM. Effect of aspirin on normal and cholera toxin-stimulated intestinal electrolyte transport. *J Clin Invest* 1976;57:916–924.

403. Madsen GL, Knoop FC. Inhibition of the secretory activity of *Escherichia coli* heat-stable enterotoxin by indomethacin. *Infect Immun* 1978;22:143–147.

404. Argenzio RA, Lecce J, Powell DW. Prostanoids inhibit intestinal NaCl absorption in experimental porcine cryptosporidiosis. *Gastroenterology* 1993;104:440–447.

405. McGowan K, Piver G, Stoff JS, Donowitz M. Role of prostaglandins and calcium in the effects of Entamoeba histolytica on colonic electrolyte transport (see comments). *Gastroenterology* 1990;98:873–880.

406. Lionetti P, Breese EJ, Murch SH, Taylor J, Walker-Smith JA, Macdonald TT. The superantigen staphylococcal enterotoxin B induces tissue damage in cultured human small intestine by T cell activation. *Gastroenterology* 1993;104:A732 (abstract).

407. Eklund S, Karlstrom L, Rokaeus A, Theodorsson E, Jodal M, Lundgren O. Effects of cholera toxin, *Escherichia coli* heat stable toxin and sodium deoxycholate on neurotensin release from the ileum in vivo. *Reg Peptides* 1989;26:241–252.

408. Cassuto J, Jodal M, Tuttle R, Lundgren O. On the role of intramural nerves in the pathogenesis of cholera toxin-induced intestinal secretion. *Scand J Gastroenterol* 1981;16:377–384.

409. Cassuto J, Siewert A, Jodal M, Lundgren O. The involvement of intramural nerves in cholera toxin induced intestinal secretion. *Acta Physiol Scand* 1983;117:195–202.

410. Jodal M, Holmgren S, Lundgren O, Sjoqvist A. Involvement of the myenteric plexus in the cholera toxin-induced net fluid secretion in the rat small intestine. *Gastroenterology* 1993;105:1286–1293.

411. O'Malley KE, Sloan T, Joyce P, Baird AW. Type I hypersensitivity reactions in intestinal mucosae from rats infected with *Fasciola hepatica*. *Parasite Immunol* 1993;15:449–453.

412. Cassuto J, Jodal M, Tuttle R, Lundgren O. 5-Hydroxytryptamine and cholera secretion. Physiological and pharmacological studies in cats and rats. *Scand J Gastroenterol* 1982;17:695–703.

413. Nilsson O, Cassuto J, Larson P-A, et al. 5-Hydroxytryptamine and cholera secretion: a histochemical and physiological study in cats. *Gut* 1983;24:542–548.

414. Cassuto J, Fahrenkrug J, Jodal M, Tuttle R, Lundgren O. Release of vasoactive intestinal polypeptide from the cat small intestine exposed to cholera toxin. *Gut* 1981;22:958–963.

415. Rask Madsen J, Bukhave K, Beubler E. Influence on intestinal secretion of eicosanoids. *J Intern Med (Suppl)* 1990;732:137–144.

416. Beubler E, Kollar G, Saria A, Bukhave K, Rask-Madsen J. Involvement of 5-hydroxytryptamine, prostaglandin-E_2, and cyclic adenosine monophosphate in cholera toxin-induced fluid secretion in the small intestine of the rat in vivo. *Gastroenterology* 1989;96:368–376.

417. Beubler E, Horina G. 5-HT_2 and 5-HT_3 receptor subtypes mediate cholera toxin-induced intestinal fluid secretion in the rat. *Gastroenterology* 1990;99:83–89.

418. McGowan K, Guerina V, Wicks J, Donowitz M. Secretory hormones of *Entamoeba histolytica*. In: Evered LD, Whelan J, eds. *Microbial toxins and diarrheal diseases*. London: Ciba Foundation Symposium II; 1985:139–150.

419. McGowan K, Kane A, Asarkof N, et al. *Entamoeba histolytica* causes intestinal secretion: role of serotonin. *Science* 1983;221:762–764.

420. Eckmann L, Kagnoff MF, Fierer J. Epithelial cells secrete the chemokine interleukin-8 in response to bacterial entry. *Infect Immun* 1993;61:4569–4574.

421. Crowe SE, Alvarez L, Dytoc M, et al. Expression of interleukin-8 and ICAM-1 by human gastric epithelium following *Helicobacter pylori* infection in vitro. *Gastroenterology* 1994; in press.

422. Agace W, Hedges S, Andersson U, Andersson J, Ceska M, Svanborg C. Selective cytokine production by epithelial cells following exposure to *Escherichia coli*. *Infect Immun* 1993;61:602–609.

423. Massion PP, Inoue H, Richman-Eisenstat J, et al. Novel *Pseudomonas* product stimulates interleukin-8 production in airway epithelial cells in vitro. *J Clin Invest* 1994;93:26–32.

424. Gustafson C, Kald B, Sjodahl R, Tagesson C. Phospholipase C from *Clostridium perfringens* stimulates formation and release of platelet-activating factor (PAF-acether) in cultured intestinal epithelial cells (INT 407). *Scand J Gastroenterol* 1991;26:1000–1006.

425. Gustafson C, Tagesson C. Phospholipase C from *Clostridium perfringens* stimulates phospholipase A2-mediated arachidonic acid release in cultured intestinal epithelial cells (INT 407). *Scand J Gastroenterol* 1990;25:363–371.

426. McGee DW, Elson CO, McGhee JR. Enhancing effect of cholera toxin on interleukin-6 secretion by IEC-6 intestinal epithelial cells: mode of action and augmenting effect of inflammatory cytokines. *Infect Immun* 1993;61:4637–4644.

427. Marsh MN. Grains of truth: evolutionary changes in small intestinal mucosa in response to environmental antigen challenge. *Gut* 1990;31:111–114.

428. Marsh MN. Gluten, major histocompatibility complex, and the small intestine—a molecular and immunobiologic approach to the spectrum of gluten sensitivity (celiac sprue). *Gastroenterology* 1992;102:330.

429. Mowat AM, Felstein MV, Borl A, Parrott DMV. Experimental studies of immunologically mediated enteropathy. Development of cell mediated immunity and intestinal pathology during a graft-versus-host reaction in irradiated mice. *Gut* 1988;29: 949–956.

430. Shepherd RW, Butler DG, Cutz E, Gall DG, Hamilton JR. The mucosal lesion in viral enteritis. Extent and dynamics of the epithelial response to virus invasion in transmissible gastroenteritis of piglets. *Gastroenterology* 1979;76:770–777.

431. Butler DG, Gall DG, Kelly MH, Hamilton JR. Transmissible gastroenteritis. Mechanisms responsible for diarrhea in an acute viral enteritis in piglets. *J Clin Invest* 1974;53:1335–1342.

432. McClung HJ, Butler DG, Kerzner B, Gall DH, Hamilton JR. Transmissible gastroenteritis. Mucosal ion transport in acute viral enteritis. *Gastroenterology* 1976;70:1091–1095.

433. Kerzner B, Kelly MH, Gall DG, Butler DG, Hamilton JR. Transmissible gastroenteritis: sodium transport and the intestinal epithelium during the course of viral enteritis. *Gastroenterology* 1977;72:457–461.

434. Rhoads JM, MacLeod RJ, Hamilton JR. Diminished brush border membrane Na-dependent L-alanine transport in acute viral enteritis in piglets. *J Pediatr Gastroenterol Nutr* 1989;9: 225–231.

435. Rhoads JM, MacLeod RJ, Hamilton JR. Alanine enhances jejunal sodium absorption in the presence of glucose: studies in piglet viral diarrhea. *Pediatr Res* 1986;20:879–883.

436. Rhoads JM, Keku EO, Quinn J, Woosely J, Lecce JG. L-Glutamine stimulates jejunal sodium and chloride absorption in pig rotavirus enteritis (see comments). *Gastroenterology* 1991;100: 683–691.

437. Argenzio RA, Liacos JA, Levy ML, Meuten DJ, Lecce JG, Powell DW. Villous atrophy, crypt hyperplasia, cellular infiltration, and impaired glucose-Na absorption in enteric cryptosporidiosis of pigs. *Gastroenterology* 1990;98:1129–1140.

438. Sears CL, Guerrant RL. Cryptosporidiosis: the complexity of intestinal pathophysiology. *Gastroenterology* 1994;106: 252–267.

439. Simon GL, Gorbach SL. Intestinal flora in health and disease. *Gastroenterology* 1984;86:174–193.

440. Carman RJ, Van Tassell RL, Wilkins TD. The normal intestinal microflora: ecology, variability and stability. *Vet Hum Toxicol* 1993;35 Suppl 1:11–14.

441. Boedeker EC. Adherent bacteria: breaching the mucosal barrier? *Gastroenterology* 1994;106:255–257.

442. Thompson GR, Trexler PC. Gastrointestinal structure and function in germ-free or gnotobiotic animals. *Gut* 1971;12: 230–235.

443. Caenepeel Ph, Janssens J, Vantrappen G, Eysson H, Coremans G. Interdigestive myoelectric complex in germ-free rats. *Dig Dis Sci* 1989;34:1180–1184.

444. Spitz J, Hecht G, Taveras M, Aoys E, Alverdy J. The effect of dexamethasone administration on rat intestinal permeability: the role of bacterial adherence. *Gastroenterology* 1994;106: 35–41.

445. Donowitz M, Wicks J, Sharp GWG. Drug therapy for diarrheal diseases: a look ahead. *Rev Infect Dis* 1986;8:S188–S201.

446. Barrett KE, Dharmsathaphorn K. Pharmacologic approaches to the therapy of diarrheal diseases. In: Field M, ed. *Diarrheal Diseases*. New York: Elsevier Science; 1991:501–516.

447. Hirschhorn N, Greenough I. Progress in oral rehydration therapy. *Sci Am* 1991;264:50–56.

448. *Cereal based oral rehydration therapy for diarrhoea: report of an international symposium, November 12–14, 1989*. Columbia, MD: Aga Khan Foundation; 1990.

449. Kirshenbaum AS, Metcalfe DD. The biology and therapy of mastocytosis. In: Galli SJ, Austen KF, eds. *Mast cell and basophil differentiation and function in health and disease*. New York: Raven Press; 1989:317–328.

450. Finck AD, Katz RL. Prevention of cholera-induced intestinal secretion in the cat by aspirin. *Nature* 1972;238:273–274.

451. Gots RE, Formal SB, Giannella RA. Indomethacin inhibition of *Salmonella typhimurium, Shigella flexneri,* and cholera-mediated rabbit ileal secretion. *J Infect Dis* 1974;130:280–284.

452. Burke V, Gracey M, Suharyono S. Reduction by aspirin of intestinal fluid loss in acute childhood gastroenteritis. *Lancet* 1980;1:1329.

453. Van Loon FP, Rabbani GH, Bukhave K, Rask Madsen J. Indomethacin decreases jejunal fluid secretion in addition to luminal release of prostaglandin E2 in patients with acute cholera. *Gut* 1992;33:643–645.

454. DuPont HL, Sullivan P, Pickering LK, Haynes G, Ackerman PB. Symptomatic treatment of diarrhea with bismuth subsalicylate among students attending a Mexican university. *Gastroenterology* 1977;73:715–718.

455. Johnson PC, Ericsson CD, DuPont HL, Morgan DR, Bitsura JA, Wood LV. Comparison of loperamide with bismuth subsalicylate for the treatment of acute travelers' diarrhea. *JAMA* 1986;225:757–760.

456. Graham DY, Estes MK, Gentry LO. Double-blind comparison of bismuth subsalicylate and placebo in the prevention and treatment of enterotoxigenic *Escherichia coli*–induced diarrhea in volunteers. *Gastroenterology* 1983;85:1017–1022.

457. Steinhoff MC, Douglas J, Greenberg HB, Callahan DR. Bismuth subsalicylate therapy of viral gastroenteritis. *Gastroenterology* 1980;786:1495–1499.

458. Figueroa-Quintanilla D, Salazar-Lindo E, Sack RB, et al. A controlled trial of bismuth subsalicylate in infants with acute watery diarrheal disease. *N Engl J Med* 1993;328:1653–1658.

459. Schiller LR, Santa Ana CA, Morawski SG. Mechanism of the antidiarrheal effect of loperamide. *Gastroenterology* 1984;86: 1475–1480.

460. Schiller LR, Davis GR, Santa Ana CA. Studies of the mechanism of the antidiarrheal effect of codeine. *J Clin Invest* 1982; 70:999–1008.

461. McKay JS, Linaker BD, Turnberg LA. Influence of opiates on ion transport across rabbit ileal mucosa. *Gastroenterology* 1981;80:279–284.

462. DuPont HL, Hornick RB. Adverse effect of lomotil therapy of shigellosis. *JAMA* 1973;93:284–285.

463. DuPont HL, Ericsson CD, DuPont MW, Luna AC, Mathewson JJ. A randomized, open-label comparison of nonprescription of loperamide and attipulgite in the symptomatic treatment of acute diarrhea. *Am J Med* 1990;88:20S–23S.

464. DuPont HL, Sanchez JF, Ericsson CD. Comparative efficacy of loperamide hydrochloride and bismuth subsalicylate in the management of acute diarrhea. *Am J Med* 1990;88:155.

465. Fedorak RN, Field M, Chang EB. Treatment of diabetic diarrhea with clonidine. *Ann Intern Med* 1985;102:197.

466. Sandgren JE, McPhee MS, Greenbergin NJ. Narcotic bowel syndrome treated with clonidine. *Ann Intern Med* 1984;101: 331.

467. Rabbani GH, Butler T, Patte D. Clinical trial of clonidine hydrochloride as an antisecretory agent in cholera. *Gastroenterology* 1989;97:321.

468. Edwards CA, Read NW. Effect of lidamidine, a proposed alpha 2-adrenoreceptor agonist, on salt and water transport in human jejunum. *Dig Dis Sci* 1986;31:817–821.

469. Kvols LK, Moertel CG, O'Connell MJ. Treatment of the malignant carcinoid syndrome: evaluation of a long-acting somatostatin analogue. *N Engl J Med* 1986;315:663–666.

470. Gorden P, Comi RJ, Maton PN. Somatostatin and somatostatin analogue (SMS 201-995) in treatment of hormone-secreting tumors of the pituitary and gastrointestinal tract and non-neoplastic disease of the gut. *Ann Intern Med* 1989;110:35.

471. Dharmsathaphorn K, Gorelick FS, Sherwin RS, Cataland S, Dobbins JW. Somatostatin decreases diarrhea in patients with the short-bowel syndrome. *J Clin Gastroenterol* 1982;4: 521–524.

472. Fanning M, Monte M, Sutherland LR. Pilot study of sandostatin (octreotide) therapy of refractory HIV-associated diarrhea. *Dig Dis Sci* 1991;36:476.

473. Girard P-M, Goldschmidt E, Vittecoq D. Vapreotide, a somatostatin analogue, in cryptosporidiosis and other AIDS-related diarrhoeal diseases. *AIDS J* 1992;6:715.

474. Dueno MI, Bai JC, Santangelo WC, Krejs GJ. Effect of somatostatin analog on water and electrolyte transport and transit time in human small bowel. *Dig Dis Sci* 1987;32:1092–1096.

475. Sack RB, Froehlich JL. Berberine inhibits intestinal secretory

response of *Vibrio cholerae* and *Escherichia coli* enterotoxin. *Infect Immun* 1982;35:471–475.

476. Tsai CS, Ochillo RF. Pharmacological effects of berberine on the longitudinal muscle of the guinea-pig isolated ileum. *Arch Int Pharmacodyn Ther* 1991;310:116.

477. Eaker EY, Sninsky CA. Effect of berberine on myoelectric activity and transit of the small intestine in rats. *Gastroenterology* 1989;96:1506.

478. Rabbani GH, Butler T, Knight J. Randomized controlled trial of berberine sulfate therapy due to enterotoxigenic *Escherichia coli* and *Vibrio cholerae*. *J Infect Dis* 1987;155:979.

479. Czerucka D, Roux I, Rampal P. *Saccharomyces boulardii* inhibits secretagogue-mediated adenosine 3′,5′-cyclic monophosphate induction in intestinal cells. *Gastroenterology* 1994; 106:65–72.

480. Shook JE, Burks TF, Wasley JW, Norman JA. Novel calmodulin antagonist CGS9343B inhibits secretory diarrhea. *J Pharmacol Exp Ther* 1989;251:247–252.

481. Rabbini GH, Greenough WB, Holmgren J, Lonnroth I. Chlor-promazine reduces fluid-loss in cholera. *Lancet* 1979;1: 410–412.

482. DuPont HL, Ericsson CD, Mathewson JJ, Marani S, Knellwolf-Cousin A-L, Martinez-Sandoval FG. Zaldaride maleate, an intestinal calmodulin inhibitor, in the therapy of travelers' diarrhea. *Gastroenterology* 1993;104:709–715.

483. Merritt JE, Brown BL, Tomlinson S. Loperamide and calmodulin (letter). *Lancet* 1982;1:283.

484. Homaidan FR, Torres A, Donowitz M, Sharp GW. Electrolyte transport in piglets infected with transmissible gastroenteritis virus. Stimulation by verapamil and clonidine. *Gastroenterology* 1991;101:895–901.

485. Wangemann P, Wittner M, DiStefano A, et al. Cl⁻-channel blockers in the thick ascending limb of the loop of Henle. Structure–activity relationship. *Pflugers Arch (Suppl)* 1986;2: S128–S141.

486. Singh AK, Afink GB, Venglarik CJ, Wang RP, Bridges RJ. Colonic Cl channel blockade by three classes of compounds. *Am J Physiol* 1991;261:C51–C63.

Infections of the Gastrointestinal Tract,
edited by M. J. Blaser, P. D. Smith, J. I. Ravdin,
H. B. Greenberg, and R. L. Guerrant
Raven Press, Ltd., New York © 1995.

CHAPTER 9

Pediatric Considerations Relevant to Enteric Infections

Philip M. Sherman and Steven N. Lichtman

Age-related variation in susceptibility to enteric infections is a well-known epidemiological finding. These differences frequently relate to infectious exposure and previous specific antigen challenge. Young children, who do not practice the handwashing precautions that prevent the fecal–oral transmission of enteric pathogens, are at increased risk of acquiring microbial pathogens. In addition, specific cellular and humoral immunity is poorly developed as a result of the lack of previous exposure to the offending microbial pathogens. These factors together result in the epidemiological observations of enteric infections being more frequent in children than in adults. For example, viral enteritides such as rotavirus and enteric adenovirus, bacterial infections caused by enteropathogenic *Escherichia coli* and enterohemorrhagic *E. coli,* and parasitic infections including *Giardia lamblia* occur more commonly among children than adults. Attendance at day care units is a risk factor for increased frequency of infection, including those affecting the gastrointestinal tract. Newborns and young infants are protected by transplacental transfer of maternal immunoglobulin G in the third trimester of gestation. Colostrum and breast milk also provide additional factors (discussed in more detail below) that provide protection to the immature host against microbial infections in the gut.

Certain infections produce different clinical manifestations in children than in adults. For example, cytomegalovirus infection in the stomach can produce a hypertrophic gastropathy in children that is acute and self-limited (1). In adults, cytomegalovirus has not been related to hypertrophic gastropathy (Menetrier's disease), which is a chronic, debilitating illness (2).

Acute enteric infections are also associated with an in-

creased frequency of complications in the young. During acute enteritis, for example, intravascular volume depletion, electrolyte disturbances (e.g., hyponatremia, hypernatremia), and metabolic derangements (e.g. hypoglycemia, acidosis) are more frequent in affected children. Associated protein calorie undernutrition is an additional risk factor promoting these complications in children. Systemic spread of the offending microbe is also more common among infants. For example, osteomyelitis, bacteremia, and meningitis can occasionally develop following *Salmonella, Shigella,* and *E. coli* infection in children under 1 year of age who have no other obvious feature of immunodeficiency.

Other gastrointestinal infections are less common among very young children than in adults. As discussed below, many asymptomatic infants harbor toxin-producing *Clostridium difficile* without adverse effects. Although rotavirus is a common cause of dehydrating acute diarrheal disease in infants and young children, the virus can be isolated from well newborn infants. These age-related differences may provide clues as to the pathogenesis of disease in older individuals and also provide considerations for novel strategies in the prevention and treatment of illness.

Helicobacter pylori infection of the stomach is uncommon in young children, and the frequency of this chronic gastric infection increases with advancing age (3). However, this epidemiological observation appears to be true only in developed countries. In developing nations, the frequency of infection is much higher in young children (3). Epidemiological parallels have been drawn to the varied prevalence of hepatitis A infection according to the socioeconomic status of different populations (4).

This chapter will consider selected aspects of gut development that impact on the susceptibility of the pediatric host to infection by gastrointestinal pathogens.

STRUCTURAL ABNORMALITIES

Congenital defects in embryogenesis and organogenesis occasionally result in structural abnormalities of the gas-

P. M. Sherman: Division of Gastroenterology, Research Institute, Hospital for Sick Children, Departments of Pediatrics and Microbiology, University of Toronto, Toronto, Ontario M5G 1X8 Canada.

S. N. Lichtman: Division of Pediatric Gastroenterology, Department of Pediatrics, University of North Carolina, Chapel Hill, North Carolina 27599.

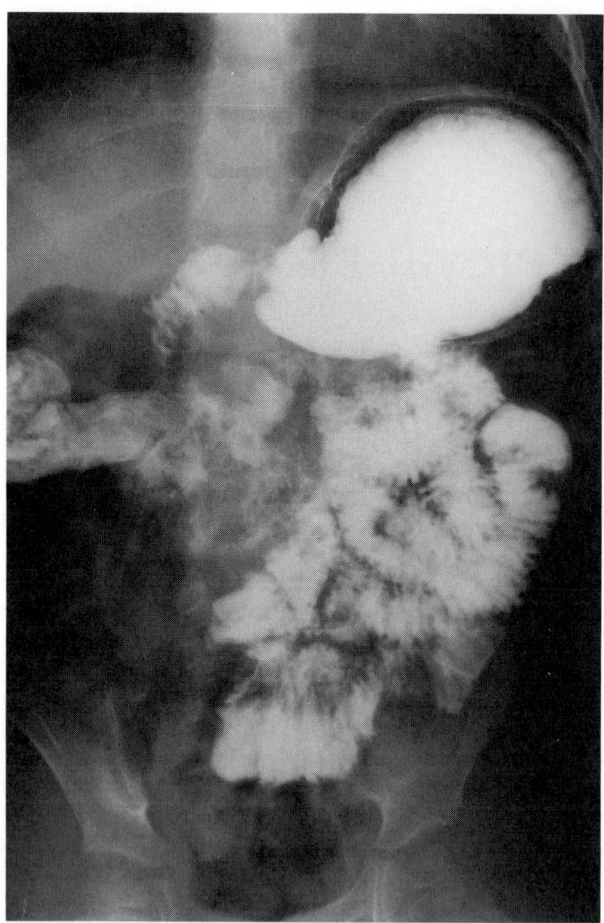

FIG. 1. Midjejunal diverticulum in a 10-month-old boy with chronic diarrhea, steatorrhea, and decreased growth. (From ref. 5, with permission.)

trointestinal tract that predispose affected individuals to enteric infections. For example, the in utero development of enteric duplications, diverticula (Fig. 1), webs, strictures, and stenoses (Fig. 2) predisposes to the development of small bowel bacterial overgrowth (5) (see Chapter by Toskes). These lesions provide an area of stasis that promotes the proliferation of a colonic-type microflora in the small intestine and results in the typical sequelae of the stagnant loop syndrome, including steatorrhea, cobalamin malabsorption, and chronic diarrhea (6–8). Short bowel syndrome also predisposes to small bowel bacterial overgrowth (9). This may result in an increased risk of both enteric and systemic infections, possibly related to increased bacterial translocation across the mucosal barrier (10).

HOST DEFENSES

Immune Defenses

In newborns, particularly premature newborns, the humoral and cellular immune responses may be less respon-

sive to microbial challenges than those of older subjects. Neutrophil and monocyte/macrophage responses to enteric infections, however, appear to be well developed in the human newborn, although, this may not apply to premature neonates and infants with protein calorie undernutrition (11). Because humoral and cellular immune responses in the newborn are less developed, breast milk and colostrum provide the newborn host an important source of protective factors. These factor's include specific sIgA antibodies (12), lymphocytes, granulocytes, and macrophages (13).

Nonimmune Defenses

As depicted in Fig. 3, the host has a number of complementary defense mechanisms to prevent microbial pathogens from entering, colonizing, and replicating in the gastrointestinal tract (14,15). Alterations in one or more of these host defenses, even in immunologically intact individuals, places the individual at increased risk for infection with enteric pathogens (16–18). Each of these host defenses may be poorly developed in the young infant, particularly those born prematurely and those suffering from protein calorie undernutrition (15,19). These nonimmune host defenses are discussed next.

Breast Milk

Colostrum and breast milk contain nonimmunological factors that assist the developing infant in resisting enteric microbial infections (Table 1). These may be broadly categorized as antiinflammatory, immunomodulatory, and antimicrobial factors. Antiinflammatory components of human milk include antioxidants such as tocopherols and β-carotenes as well as cytoprotective agents such as prostaglandins and epidermal growth factor (EGF) (20). Immunomodulatory agents present in breast milk include purines, inositol, and viable, activated neutrophils and macrophages (21). Nonimmune antimicrobial factors are also contained in human milk (22). For example, human breast milk, through the presence of bile salt–stimulated lipase (23), inhibits the growth of G. lamblia in vitro (24).

Other constituents of human milk that are reported to regulate the replication of enteric microbial pathogens in the gut include lactoferrin, lysozyme, lactoperoxidase (25), and whey protein (26). Membrane receptor analogs are also present in human milk (27). For example, the GM1 ganglioside receptor for choleragen, which inhibits toxin binding to membrane receptors in competitive inhibition assays, is excreted in breast milk in a functionally active form (28). A receptor that binds to the heat-stable enterotoxin of enterotoxigenic E. coli (ETEC) is also present in human milk (29). In addition, glycoprotein receptors for fimbrial adhesins of ETEC are contained in colostrum (30).

Gastric Acid and Pepsin

Gastric acid is an important nonimmune factor that protects the host against passage of orally ingested microbial

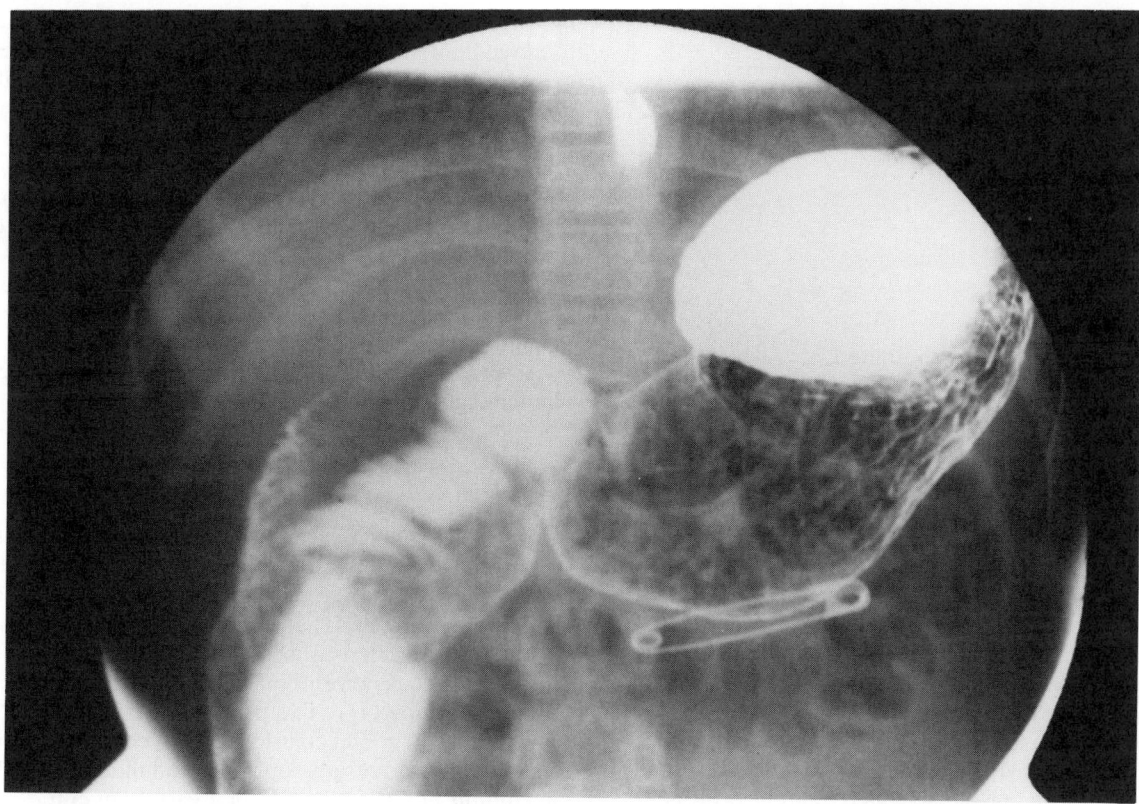

FIG. 2. Distention of duodenum and delayed transit of barium in a 6-year-old girl who presented during infancy with vomiting due to duodenal stenosis. (From ref. 5, with permission.)

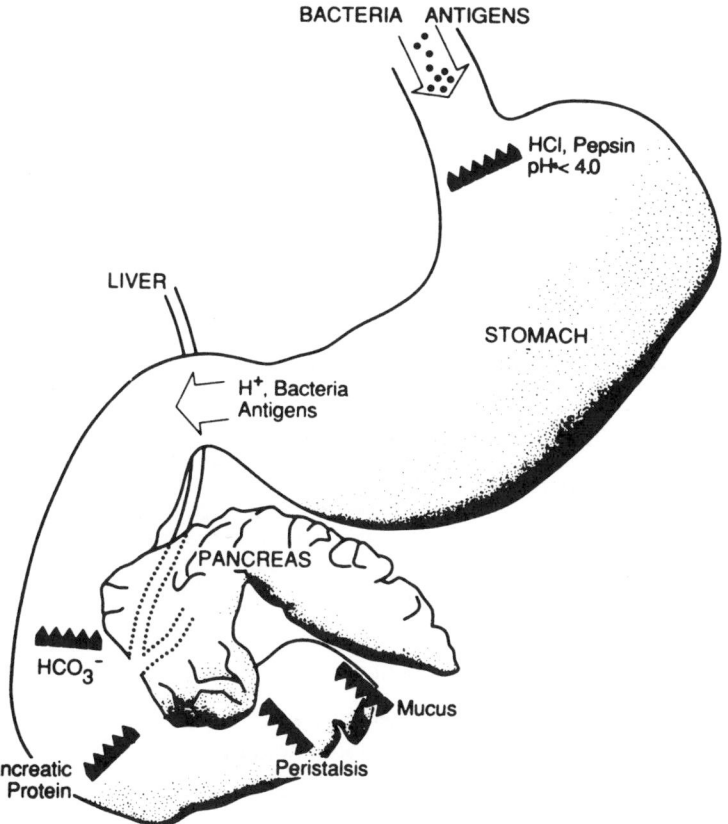

FIG. 3. Nonimmune defenses of the small intestine. These factors act in concert to protect the host from the adverse effects of ingested dietary antigens and microbial pathogens. (From ref. 15, with permission.)

TABLE 1. *Protective factors in human colostrum/breast milk*

Immunological
  Humoral antibodies
    sIgA
    sIgM, IgG
  Cellular immunity
    Macrophages
    Lymphocytes
    Neutrophils
  Complement
Nonimmunological
  Lipases, bile salt–stimulated
  Lysozome
  Lactoperoxidase
  Lactoferrin
  Receptor analogs
    Oligosaccharides
    Glycolipids

From ref. 15, with permission.

pathogens into the intestinal tract (16–18). Acid also activates pepsinogen to pepsin, which itself likely acts as a nonimmune defense factor against enteric pathogens. Inactivation of rotavirus, for example, is dependent on active pepsin activity (31). Acid production is developmentally regulated in rat pups, which secrete little acid and pepsin until the age of weaning (32). In contrast, newborn humans generally produce acid and pepsin normally in response to foods and hormonal stimuli (33). However, premature neonates, infants in intensive care settings, and undernourished children have reduced acid and pepsin synthesis by gastric parietal cells (34) and, as a result, a reduced gastric barrier to enteric infection.

Motility

Propulsive activity through the gastrointestinal tract is important not only for digestion but for maintaining the caudad flow of luminal contents. Interdigestive migratory motor complexes serve a housekeeper function that acts to move luminal contents distally and thereby prevent regions of intestinal stasis (35). Coordinated peristalsis is not fully developed until late in the third trimester of gestation (36,37). Premature infants, therefore, may be at increased risk for intestinal dysmotility, leading to regional stagnation and stasis of luminal contents that could promote microbial colonization and increase the risk of enteric infections (38).

Villus contractions may also play a role in reducing the access of microbial pathogens to receptors on host epithelial cell surfaces (39). Future studies should evaluate the possibility that villus contractility varies with both chronological age and nutritional status of the host.

Mucus

Mucus is the viscoelastic gel overlying the mucosal epithelial surface along the length of the gastrointestinal tract. Mucus in the large intestine serves as a reservoir for colonization (40,41) and as a probable nutrient source (42) for the commensal microflora. Mucus also acts as a barrier for access of enteric pathogens to the underlying mucosal surface (43). The principal constituent of intestinal mucus is a goblet cell–derived glycoprotein variously referred to as mucus glycoprotein and mucin (43,44). Mucins inhibit *in vitro* adhesion of a variety of enteric pathogens including ETEC, enteropathogenic *E. coli* (EPEC), and *Yersinia enterocolitica* (Table 2). Intestinal mucins also inhibit binding of parasites, such as *Entamoeba histolytica* (45), and viruses, such as rotavirus (46), to mucosal surfaces. Mucin-like glycoproteins present in human milk also inhibit adhesion of bacteria (47) and viral enteropathogens (48), which may provide another beneficial effect of mother's milk in reducing the risk of infectious enterocolitides in newborns and young infants.

Age-related changes in the terminal glycosylation of mucins in the small bowel (49) and colon (50,51) suggest that the functional properties of mucins in newborn animals and humans may differ from those in the adult. Reduced total carbohydrate and fucose levels and increased

TABLE 2. *Interactions between enteric bacteria and mucus*

Bacteria	Intestinal receptors	Effect of mucus on the bacteria
Shigella flexneri	60-kDa molecule; soluble agglutinin	Agglutination of serotype 1b, inhibits invasion of HeLa cells by 1b and 2a
Yersinia enterocolitica	Mucus; mucin; brush border membranes	Renders bacterial surface hydophilic, reduces virulence plasmid (pYV)–mediated adhesion to epithelial cell membrane
Campylobacter jejuni	Fucose/mannose residues on INT 407 cells; mucus (for lipopolysaccharide); sIgA in mucus	Adherence; bacterial aggregation
Escherichia coli, strain F-18	Mucus glycoprotein ($1.25–2.5 \times 10^5$) for lipopolysaccharide	Adherence/colonization
Escherichia coli, strain RDEC-1	Mucus; mucin	Adherence/colonization
Escherichia coli, strain CL-49	Mucin (membrane residues on N-linked oligosaccharide)	Bacterial aggregation

Adapted from ref. 45, with permission.

TABLE 3. *Chemical composition of purified mucus glycoproteins from rat small intestines*[a]

	Carbohydrate content (mol/1000 mol of total protein)	
	Newborn	Adult
Fucose	94.2 ± 16.3	265.8 ± 64.0
Mannose	6.4 ± 1.3	22.0 ± 2.0
Galactose	575.6 ± 78.9	617.9 ± 86.7
N-Acetylglucosamine	427.8 ± 13.3	435.4 ± 10.4
N-Acetylgalactosamine	376.8 ± 6.1	601.2 ± 3.5
N-Acetylneuraminic acid	245.5 ± 1.9	222.4 ± 26.2
Sulfate	262.4 ± 34.3	54.2 ± 2.0

Adapted from ref. 49, with permission.
[a] The neutral sugars and N-acetylneuraminic acid were measured by gas–liquid chromatography.

sulfate content (Table 3) correlate with changes in the physical properties of mucins derived from suckling rat small intestine (49). Whether these changes correspond to a reduced ability of the neonatal-derived mucins to block the adhesion of enteropathogenic parasites, viruses, and bacteria deserves experimental evaluation.

Cryptdins

Paneth cells are increasingly recognized as the cellular origin of antimicrobial factors present in the crypt lumen (52). These factors include peptides, referred to as cryptdins, which have a broad-spectrum of antimicrobial activity (53) (see chapter by Crowe and Powell). Whether cryptdins are subject to developmental regulation in humans is not known.

Pancreaticobiliary Secretions

Proteins of pancreatic origin inhibit bacterial colonization of the intestine (54). The exocrine pancreatic insufficiency of human infants (55) may reduce the production and excretion of these antibacterial proteins but this has not been confirmed experimentally. The role of biliary secretions in the inhibition of microbial replication and colonization in the gut has not been established. However, newborns and infants have a reduced choleretic response to bile acids and an immature enterohepatic circulation of bile acids (56).

Commensal Microflora

The indigenous bacterial flora provides a microenvironment that reduces replication and colonization of microbial pathogens (57). Following delivery from the sterile amniotic sac, the acquired colonic microflora varies considerably between exclusively breast-fed infants and those receiving nonhuman milk feedings (58). In addition,

infants hospitalized in an intensive care unit have an altered flora (59) that is characterized by reduced heterogeneity of culturable organisms (60). These changes may impair the ability of the immature host to resist colonization by microbial pathogens. These changes may also permit colonization by microorganisms that are more likely to result in intestinal complications. For example, one recent study showed that adult patients with pneumatosis cystoides intestinalis have a markedly reduced number of methanogenic and sulfate-reducing bacteria in the colon (61). Since necrotizing enterocolitis in premature infants is characterized by the presence of intramural air, it is of considerable interest to determine whether the composition of colonic microflora in such infants differs from that of unaffected infants of comparable age.

Cell Restitution

Surface epithelial cells in the gastrointestinal tract are replaced in rodents every 2–3 days and in humans every 5–7 days (62). In response to injury, accelerated cell proliferation and differentiation occurs in order to heal denuded or damaged epithelial surfaces. Whether premature infants and newborns can respond appropriately to required regenerative responses is not known. Malnourished infants in particular may have a reduced ability to repair local breaks in the intestinal epithelial cell barrier (63). Mucosal blood flow is an important factor in maintaining host epithelial cell integrity and function. Experimental findings (64) and clinical studies (65) indicate that the developing gut is especially susceptible to ischemia-reperfusion injury.

DEVELOPMENT OF HOST RECEPTORS

Age-related differences in the susceptibility to enteric infection may be due in part to the developmental regulation of receptor synthesis and expression in the gastrointestinal tract (66). Age-related differences to enteric infections could also be affected by the variability in effector responses following the binding of microbial attachment factors and microbial toxins to host receptors (66). This section will provide a summary of recent findings that support the hypothesis that developmental variation in the synthesis and expression of mucosal receptors promotes adhesion of microbes and their toxins (Table 4).

Toxin Receptors

Enterotoxigenic Escherichia coli

Enterotoxigenic *E. coli* are a common cause of both traveler's diarrhea (67) and infantile diarrhea in developing countries (68). Infants and young children are at increased risk of ETEC infection in whom it is a common cause of dehydrating illness (69). ETEC produces cytotonic enterotoxins that induce fluid accumulation in ligated intestinal loops in experimental animals. A heat-

TABLE 4. *Host susceptibility to toxigenic diarrhea in young children and animal models*

Pathogen	Host	Target tissue	Change with increasing age
V. cholerae	Children	Small intestine	↓
Enterotoxigenic *E. coli*	Children	Small intestine	↓
C. difficile	Children, rabbits	Large intestine, ileum	↑
Shigella dysenteriae type 1	Children, rabbits	Large intestine, ileum	↑

From ref. 66, with permission.

labile enterotoxin referred to as LT is structurally and functionally related to choleragen (70). Many ETEC isolates also produce heat-stable enterotoxins (ST), one of which is a small peptide rich in cysteine residues (71). ST binds to the guanylin cyclase C receptor on the apical aspect of enterocytes (72), thereby inducing an elevation in cGMP in the cytosol of enterocytes (73) and, ultimately, resulting in a diarrheal response. Sensitivity of young animals to the effects of ST is increased compared to that of adult animals (74,75). This is accompanied by an increase in both receptor-specific mRNA and receptor product present on the apical membrane of enterocytes. The affinities of binding of ST to the guanylin receptor in neonatal and adult intestinal membrane preparations are comparable (76). Cohen et al. (77) showed that the developing human intestine also contains increased levels of specific mRNA and the translated receptor product (Table 5). The same group has also shown that native ST is degraded to a product that does not bind to the guanylin receptor when placed into ligated loops in adult rats. In contrast, neonatal rat intestine lacks this proteolytic activity (78). The reduced degradation of ST, together with increased expression of the guanylin receptor, increases the responsiveness of the infant intestine to this bacterial enterotoxin.

Heat-Labile Enterotoxin of Vibrio cholera

Choleragen is a subunit toxin that binds to the GM1 ganglioside receptor and, through activation of the Gs protein, adenylate cyclase, and cAMP, results in chloride secretion from intestinal crypt cells and impaired sodium/chloride–coupled absorption in villus enterocytes (79). In neonatal animals, the affinity of toxin binding to the ganglioside receptor and the number of GM1 receptors are increased only slightly compared with adult intestine (80). However, there is a marked increase in the responsiveness of cAMP and Gs following exposure to cholera toxin (81). This suggests that there is an alteration in effector responsiveness to the toxin and therefore provides another mechanism whereby infants are at increased risk for enteric microbial infection (82).

Enterotoxins of Clostridium difficile

The etiological agent of antibiotic-associated colitis is *C. difficile,* a bacterial constituent of the normal colonic microflora in many infants up to 1 or 2 years of age (83). The reason that *C. difficile* colonization does not cause clinical symptoms in infants is not known but may relate to a developmental regulation in expression of the receptor that mediates toxin adhesion to the intestinal mucosa. *C. difficile,* including strains that colonize asymptomatic infants, elaborate both a cytotoxin (toxin B) and a 250-kDa polypeptide with enterotoxigenic properties (toxin A) (84). The enterotoxin binds to a brush border glycoprotein in rabbit ileum (85). As shown in Fig. 4, this toxin does not bind to brush border membranes in the intestine of newborn rabbits (86). This finding suggests that there is either an alteration in receptor numbers or a change in

TABLE 5. *Predicted heat-stable enterotoxin-receptor density as a function of age in human small intestine and colonic specimens*

Age (mo)	Predicted receptor number/μg protein (×10⁹)	
	Small intestine	Colon
1	1.82	2.03
2.7	1.43	1.54
7.4	1.12	1.13
20	0.89	0.80
54	0.74	0.55
150	0.67	0.38

From ref. 77, with permission.

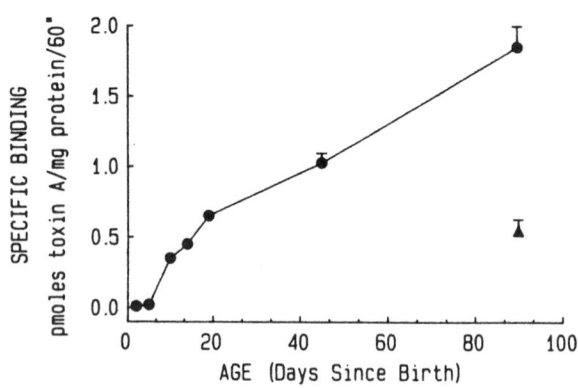

FIG. 4. Age-related increase in specific binding of *Clostridium difficile* toxin A to rabbit brush borders (BB). Vertical axis indicates tritiated toxin A specific binding to rabbit ileal brush borders. Closed triangle represents [³H]toxin A–specific binding to brush borders prepared from the ileum of a 3-month-old rabbit after preincubation of BB with the lectin BS-1. (From ref. 86, with permission.)

binding affinity of the toxin receptor. If receptor expression is developmentally regulated in the human gastrointestinal tract, it could potentially explain the observed lack of pathology and clinical symptoms in colonized infants. It should be noted, however, that developmental changes in toxin binding kinetics to the small intestine in hamsters are not evident (87).

Cytotoxins of Shigella dysenteriae *Type 1 and* Enterohemorrhagic *E. coli*

Shiga toxin of *S. dysenteriae* and the Shiga-like toxins of *E. coli*, which cause hemorrhagic colitis, are subunit toxins that bind to a specific glycolipid receptor (88). Following internalization of the A subunit of the toxin, which functions as a specific *N*-glycosidase to shut off ribosomal protein synthesis (89), the toxins induce a diarrheal response in ligated intestinal loops (90) and result in cytopathic effects in infected tissue culture cells. However, Shiga toxin has minimal effects on inducing fluid responses in infant rabbits compared to adult animals (91). As shown in Table 6, this age-related response correlates with the expression of the glycolipid globotriaosylceramide (Gb$_3$) receptor to which the B subunit of these toxins adheres (92). Specific transferase activities are reduced and α-galactoside activity is increased in the intestine of infant rabbits (93). The net effect is a reduced amount of functional Gb$_3$ receptor in the brush border membrane of infant rabbits. These findings suggest a mechanism for the reduced prevalence of *Shigella* infection in human infants (94) by virtue of reduced receptor binding sites for bacterial toxins. Whether the same glycolipid serves as a functional receptor in the human intestine and whether expression of the toxin-binding receptor is developmentally regulated in humans remain to be documented.

Receptors for Microbial Adhesins

Ontogeny changes also influence the development of receptor expression mediating the attachment of various

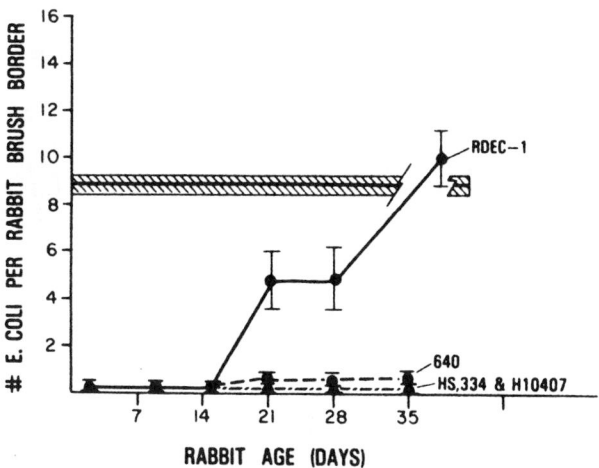

FIG. 5. Variation in the adherence of the *E. coli* enteropathogen strain RDEC-1 to intestinal brush borders from rabbits of varying age. Cross-hatched area represents the mean number of RDEC-1 adhered to adult rabbit brush borders (± 1 SE). *E. coli* strains 640 and HS are lapine and human fecal commensals, respectively. Strains 334 and H10407 are human ETEC strains. (From ref. 96, with permission.)

enteropathogens. For example, *E. coli* strain RDEC-1 (serotype O15:H$-$) is a lapine enteropathogen causing dehydrating diarrhea in postweanling rabbits. RDEC-1 adheres to a glycoprotein receptor that is present in ileal brush border membranes derived from weanling and adult rabbits (95) but, as shown in Fig. 5, not in suckling animals (96). Thus, susceptibility to RDEC-1 infection correlates with developmental expression of the glycoprotein receptor to which the fimbrial adhesin of the organism adheres (97).

Developmental changes in receptor expression also characterize the increased susceptibility of piglets to enterotoxigenic *E. coli* infection. For example, the K99 fimbrial adhesin binds to the ganglioside GM3 in porcine intestine (98). As shown in Fig. 6, GM3 content is greater in the intestine at birth compared to adult porcine intestine (99,100) and could account for the increased susceptibility of piglets to infection with strains of ETEC that elaborate K99 adhesins. Although this receptor is not present in human intestine (100), developmental regulation of the expression of receptors(s) mediating binding of human ETEC strains to the small bowel could similarly predispose young children to an increased risk of ETEC-induced infection. This issue, however, requires experimental confirmation. Although the exact receptor mediating intestinal binding of human ETEC strains has not been characterized, it appears that membrane glycoproteins (rather than lipid constituents of the plasma membrane) mediate binding of fimbrial adhesins (102).

The development of receptor expression in the overlying mucous layer with increasing age, rather than changes in receptor expression on the apical membrane of enterocytes, is reported to explain the resistance to infection of older pigs by ETEC expressing 987P fimbriae (103,104). Similar age-related changes in receptors present in por-

TABLE 6. Levels of major neutral glycolipid peaks from rabbit microvillus membrane at various ages[a]

Ages	Glycolipids (pmol/μg MVM protein)[a]		
	GlcCer	LacCer	Gb$_3$
<1 day	32.1 ± 6.2	95.3 ± 10.4	0.02 ± 0.02
16 days	21.8 ± 3.2	97.6 ± 16.0	0.2 ± 0.1
24 days	46.8 ± 4.1	46.7 ± 7.7	8.0 ± 0.5
34 days	30.2 ± 9.3	13.0 ± 2.2	10.4 ± 1.5
6 mo–1.5 yr	24.0 ± 10.8	3.6 ± 0.7	16.2 ± 5.0

From ref. 92, with permission.

Gb$_3$, globotriaosylceramide; GlcCer, glucosylceramide; LacCer, lactosylceramide; MVM, microvillus membrane.

[a] Measured by quantitative high-performance liquid chromatography.

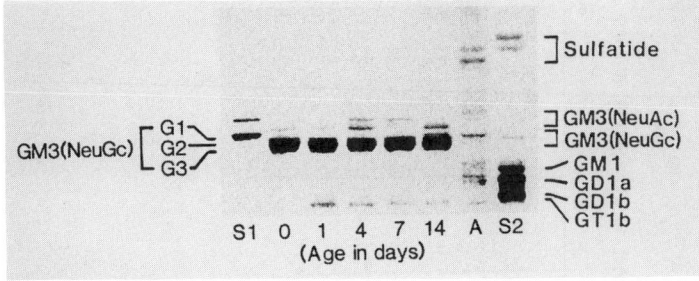

FIG. 6. Postnatal changes in pig intestinal ganglioside. Total intestinal gangliosides were assayed in 0- to 14-day-old piglets and adult pig (A) by thin-layer chromatography (TLC) and visualized with resorcinol. S1, GM3(NeuAc) isolated from dog erythrocytes (**upper band**) and GM3(NeuGc) isolated from horse erythrocytes (**lower band**). S2, Monkey brain gangliosides. GM3(NeuGc) of intestinal gangliosides was clearly separated into three bands (G1, G2, G3), when a smaller amount of gangliosides was applied to another TLC plate. (From ref. 99, with permission.)

cine mucus might also explain the increased susceptibility of piglets to infection with ETEC strains expressing K88 fimbrial adhesin (105,106). The possibility of developmental regulation of mucus-containing receptors for microbial enteropathogens in humans should be examined in future studies.

Whether there is developmental regulation of receptors mediating the adhesion of enteric parasites has not yet been examined in detail. For example, invasive *Entamoeba histolytica* isolates mediate binding via a galactose-binding lectin (107) to glycoconjugates (protein and lipids) present on eukaryotic cell surfaces (108,109). However, it is not known whether these are developmental changes in carbohydrate expression that are then reflected in age-related variations in the kinetics of parasite binding and subsequent invasion (Dr. K. Chadee, McGill University, personal communication).

Enteric viral pathogens also bind to specific host membrane receptors prior to cellular invasion (110). Whether receptor expression correlates with chronological age is not yet known. Recent evidence of age-related effects on rotavirus inactivation by gastric acid and pepsin (31) could also account for the increased risk of young children to viral enteritides.

The control mechanisms for these developmental changes in receptor expression should be defined since a variety of factors, such as drugs and hormones, could potentially be employed as novel strategies to either induce or downregulate the transcription and translation of microbial and toxin receptors by eukaryotic host cells and thereby reduce the susceptibility to enteric infection in high-risk individuals.

ACKNOWLEDGMENTS

Work in the authors' laboratories is supported by the Medical Research Council of Canada and the National Institutes of Health. P.S. is the recipient of a Career Scientist Award from the Ontario Ministry of Health.

REFERENCES

1. Qualman SJ, Hamoudi AB. Pediatric hypertrophic gastropathy (Menetrier's disease). *Pediatr Pathol* 1992;12:263–268.
2. Scharschmidt BF. The natural history of hypertrophic gastropathy (Menetrier's disease). Report of a case with 16 year follow-up and review of 120 cases from the literature. *Am J Med* 1977; 63:644–652.
3. Megraud F. Epidemiology of *Helicobacter pylori* infection. *Gastroenterol Clin North Am* 1993;22:73–88.
4. Perez-Perez GI, Taylor DN, Bodhidatta L, et al. Seroprevalence of *Helicobacter pylori* infections in Thailand. *J Infect Dis* 1990;161:1237–1241.
5. Sherman P. Bacterial overgrowth. In: Yamada T, Alpers DH, Owyang C, Powell DW, Silverstein FE, eds. *Atlas of gastroenterology.* Philadelphia: JB Lippincott; 1992:218–220.
6. Sherman PM. Bacterial overgrowth. In: Yamada T, Alpers DH, Owyang C, Powell DW, Silverstein FE, eds. *Textbook of gastroenterology.* Philadelphia: JB Lippincott; 1991:2:1530–1540.
7. Sherman P, Lichtman S. Small bowel bacterial overgrowth syndrome. *Surv Dig Dis* 1987;5:157–171.
8. Forstner G, Sherman P, Lichtman S. Bacterial overgrowth. In: Walker WA, Durie PR, Hamilton JR, Walker-Smith JA, Watkins JB, eds. *Pediatric gastrointestinal disease: pathophysiology, diagnosis, management.* Vol 1. Philadelphia: BC Decker; 1991:689–700.
9. Vanderhoof JA, Langnas AN, Pinch LW, Thompson JS, Kaufman SS. Short bowel syndrome. *J Pediatr Gastroentrerol Nutr* 1992;14:359–370.
10. Berg RD, Wommack E, Deitch EA. Immunosuppression and intestinal bacterial overgrowth synergistically promote bacterial translocation. *Arch Surg* 1988;123:1359–1364.
11. Chandra RK. Nutritional regulation of immunity and infection: from epidemiology to phenomenology to clinical practice. *J Pediatr Gastroenterol Nutr* 1986;5:844–852.
12. Hayani KC, Guerrero ML, Morrow AL, et al. Concentration of milk secretory immunoglobulin A against *Shigella* virulence plasmid-associated antigens as a predictor of symptom status in *Shigella*-infected breast-fed infants. *J Pediatr* 1992;121: 852–856.
13. Hanson LA, Cruz JR, Carlsson B. The immunology of human milk. *Immunol Infect Dis* 1991;1:303–306 (editorial).
14. Walker RI, Owen RL. Intestinal barriers to bacteria and their toxins. *Annu Rev Med* 1990;41:393–400.
15. Sherman PM, Forstner JF, Forstner GG. Mucosal barrier and its defense during the perinatal period. In: Lebenthal E, ed. *Human gastrointestinal development.* New York: Raven Press; 1989:687–698.
16. Giannella RA, Broitman SA, Zamcheck N. Influence of gastric acidity on bacterial and parasitic enteric infections. *Ann Intern Med* 1973;78:271–276.
17. Peterson WL, Mackowiak PA, Barnett CC, Marling-Cason M, Haley ML. The human gastric bactericidal barrier: mechanisms of action, relative antibacterial activity and dietary influences. *J Infect Dis* 1989;159:979–983.
18. Gorden J, Small PLC. Acid resistance in enteric bacteria. *Infect Immun* 1993;61:364–367.
19. Israel EJ, Walker AW. Host development in gut and related disorders. *Pediatr Clin North Am* 1988;35:1–14.
20. Goldman AS, Thorpe LW, Goldblum RM, Hanson LA. Anti-inflammatory properties of human milk. *Acta Pediatr Scand* 1985;75:689–695.

21. Holub BJ. The nutritional importance of inositol and the phosphoinositides. *N Engl J Med* 1992;326:1285–1287 (editorial).
22. May JT. Microbial contaminants and antimicrobial properties of human milk. *Microbiol Sci* 1988;5:42–46.
23. Gillin FD, Reiner DS, Gault MJ. Cholate-dependent killing of *Giardia lamblia* by human milk. *Infect Immun* 1985;47:619–622.
24. Gillin FD, Reiner DS, Wang C-S. Human milk kills parasitic intestinal protozoa. *Science* 1983;221:1290–1292.
25. Bullen JJ, Rogers HJ, Leigh J. Iron-binding proteins in milk and resistance to *Escherichia coli* infection in infants. *Br Med J* 1972;1:69–75.
26. Dolan SA, Boesman-Finkelstein M, Finkelstein RA. Inhibition of enteropathogenic bacteria by human milk whey in vitro. *Pediatr Infect Dis J* 1989;8:430–436.
27. Andersson B, Porras O, Hanson LA, Lagergard T, Svanborg-Eden C. Inhibition of attachment of *Streptococcus pneumoniae* and *Hemophilus influenzae* by human milk and receptor oligosaccharides. *J Infect Dis* 1986;153:232–237.
28. Laegreid A, Kolsto-Otnaess A-B. Trace amounts of ganglioside GM1 in human milk inhibit enterotoxins from *Vibrio cholerae* and *Escherichia coli*. *Life Sci* 1987;40:55–62.
29. Newburg DS, Pickering LK, McCluer RH, Cleary TG. Fucosylated oligosaccharides of human milk protect suckling mice from heat-stabile enterotoxin of *Escherichia coli*. *J Infect Dis* 1990;162:1075–1080.
30. Lindahl M. Binding of F41 and K99 fimbriae of enterotoxigenic *Escherichia coli* to glycoproteins from bovine and porcine colostrum. *Microbiol Immunol* 1989;33:373–379.
31. Bass DM, Baylor M, Broome R, Greenberg HB. Molecular basis of age-dependent gastric inactivation of Rhesus rotavirus in the mouse. *J Clin Invest* 1992;89:1741–1745.
32. Dial EJ, Lichtenberger LM. Development of the gastric barrier to acid. In: Lebenthal E, ed. *Human gastrointestinal development*. New York: Raven Press; 1989:353–363.
33. Weaver LT. Anatomy and embryology. In: Walker WA, Durie PR, Hamilton JR, Walker-Smith JA, Watkins JB, eds. *Pediatric gastrointestinal disease: pathophysiology, diagnosis, management*. Vol 1. Philadelphia: BC Decker, 1991:195–216.
34. Gilman RH, Partanen R, Brown KH, et al. Decreased gastric acid secretion and bacterial colonization of the stomach in severely malnourished Bangladeshi children. *Gastroenterology* 1988;94:1308–1314.
35. Quigley EMM. Small intestinal motor activity—its role in gut homeostasis and disease. *Q J Med* 1987;65:799–810.
36. Ruckebusch Y. Development of digestive motor patterns during perinatal life: mechanism and significance. *J Pediatr Gastroenterol Nutr* 1986;5:523–536.
37. Berseth CL. Gestational evolution of small intestine motility in preterm and term infants. *J Pediatr* 1989;115:646–651.
38. Ittmann PI, Amarnath R, Berseth CL. Maturation of antroduodenal motor activity in preterm and term infants. *Dig Dis Sci* 1992;37:14–19.
39. Erickson RA, Tarnawski A, Dines G, Stachura J. 16,16-Dimethyl prostaglandin E2 induces villus contraction in rats without affecting intestinal restitution. *Gastroenterology* 1990;99:708–716.
40. Bollard JE, Vanderwee MA, Smith GW, Tasman-Jones C, Gavin JB, Lee SP. Location of bacteria in the mid-colon of the rat. *Appl Environ Microbiol* 1986;51:604–608.
41. Rozee KR, Cooper D, Lam K, Costerton JW. Microbial flora of the mouse ileum mucous layer and epithelial surface. *Appl Environ Microbiol* 1982;43:1451–1463.
42. Corfield AP, Wagner SA, Clamp JR, Kriaris MS, Hoskins LC. Mucin degradation in the human colon: production of sialidase, sialate O-acetylesterase, *N*-acetylneuraminate lyase, arylesterase, and glycosulfatase activities by strains of fecal bacteria. *Infect Immun* 1992;60:3971–3978.
43. Neutra MR, Forstner JF. Gastrointestinal mucus: synthesis, secretion and function. In: Johnson LR, ed. *Physiology of the gastrointestinal tract*. New York: Raven Press; 1987:975–1008.
44. Specian RD, Oliver MG. Functional biology of intestinal goblet cells. *Am J Physiol* 1991;260:C183–C193.
45. Tse S-K, Chadee K. The interaction between intestinal mucus

glycoproteins and enteric infections. *Parasitol Today* 1991;7:163–172.
46. Chen CC, Baylor M, Bass DM. Murine intestinal mucins inhibit rotavirus infection. *Gastroenterology* 1993;105:84–92.
47. Schroten H, Lethen A, Hanisch FG, et al. Inhibition of adhesion of S-fimbriated *Escherichia coli* to epithelial cells by meconium and feces of breast-fed and formula-fed newborns: mucins are the major inhibitory component. *J Pediatr Gastroenterol Nutr* 1992;15:150–158.
48. Yolken RH, Peterson JA, Vonderfecht SL, Fouts ET, Midthun K, Newburg DS. Human milk mucin inhibits rotavirus replication and prevents experimental gastroenteritis. *J Clin Invest* 1992;29:1984–1991.
49. Shub MD, Pang KY, Swann DA, Walker WA. Age-related changes in chemical composition and physical properties of mucus glycoproteins from rat small intestine. *Biochem J* 1983;215:405–411.
50. Turck D, Feste AS, Lifschitz CH. Age and diet affect the composition of porcine colonic mucins. *Pediatr Res* 1993;33:564–567.
51. Colony PC, Steely J. Lectin binding patterns in developing rat colon. *Gastroenterology* 1987;92:1116–1126.
52. Jones DE, Bevins CL. Paneth cells of the human small intestine express an antimicrobial peptide gene. *J Biol Chem* 1992;267:23216–23225.
53. Eisenhauer PB, Harwig SSSL, Lehrer RI. Cryptdins: antimicrobial defensins of the murine small intestine. *Infect Immun* 1992;60:3556–3565.
54. Rubinstein E, Mark Z, Haspel J, et al. Antibacterial activity of the pancreatic fluid. *Gastroenterology* 1985;88:927–932.
55. Lebenthal E, Lee PC. The impact of intrauterine and postnatal malnutrition on the development of the exocrine pancreas and small intestine. *J Pediatr Gastroenterol Nutr* 1988;7:1–9 (editorial).
56. Balistreri WF. Neonatal cholestasis. *J Pediatr* 1985;106:171–184.
57. Mackowiak PA. The normal microbial flora. *N Engl J Med* 1982;307:83–93.
58. Yoshioka H, Iseki K, Fujita K. Development and differences of intestinal flora in the neonatal period in breast-fed and bottle-fed infants. *Pediatrics* 1983;72:317–321.
59. Bell MJ, Rudinsky M, Brotherton T, Schroeder K, Boxerman SB. Gastrointestinal microecology in the critically ill neonate. *J Pediatr Surg* 1984;19:745–751.
60. Lawrence G, Bates J, Gaul A. Pathogenesis of neonatal necrotising enterocolitis. *Lancet* 1982;1:137–139.
61. Christl SU, Gibson GR, Murgatroyd PR, Scheppach W, Cummings JH. Impaired hydrogen metabolism in pneumatosis cystoides intestinalis. *Gastroenterology* 1993;104:392–297.
62. Eastwood GL. Gastrointestinal epithelial renewal. *Gastroenterology* 1977;72:962–975.
63. Butzner JD, Butler DG, Miniats OP, Hamilton JR. Impact of chronic protein-calorie malnutrition on small intestinal repair after acute viral enteritis: a study in gnotobiotic piglets. *Pediatr Res* 1985;19:476–481.
64. Crissinger KD, Granger DN. Mucosal injury induced by ischemia and reperfusion in the piglet intestine: influences of age and feeding. *Gastroenterology* 1989;97:920–926.
65. Coombs RC, Morgan MEI, Durbin GM, Booth IW, McNeish AS. Abnormal gut blood flow velocities in neonates at risk of necrotising enterocolitis. *J Pediatr Gastroentrol Nutr* 1992;15:13–19.
66. Chu S-HW, Walker WA. Bacterial toxin interaction with the developing intestine. *Gastroenterology* 1993;104:916–925.
67. Black RE. Epidemiology of travelers' diarrhea and relative importance of various pathogens. *Rev Infect Dis* 1990;12(Suppl 1):S73–S79.
68. Echeverria P, Leksomboon U, Chaicumpa W, Seriwatana J, Tirapat C, Rowe B. Identification by DNA hybridisation of enterotoxigenic *Escherichia coli* in homes of children with diarrhoea. *Lancet* 1984;1:63–66.
69. Black RE, Brown KH, Becker S. Effects of diarrhea associated with specific enteropathogens on the growth of children in rural Bangladesh. *Pediatrics* 1984;73:799–805.

70. Sixma TK, Pronk SE, Kalk KH, et al. Crystal structure of a cholera toxin-related heat-labile enterotoxin from *E. coli*. *Nature* 1991;351:371–377.

71. Ozaki H, Sato T, Kubota H, Hata Y, Katsube Y, Shimonishi Y. Molecular structure of the toxic domain of heat-stable enterotoxin produced by a pathogenic strain of Escherichia coli. *J Biol Chem* 1991;266:5934–5941.

72. Shulz S, Green CK, Yuen PST, Garbers DL. Guanylyl cyclase is a heat-stable enterotoxin receptor. *Cell* 1990;63:941–948.

73. Dreyfus LA, Jaso-Friedmann L, Robertson DC. Characterization of the mechanisms of action of *Eschericha coli* heat-stable enterotoxin. *Infect Immun* 1984;44:493–501.

74. Cohen MB, Moyer MS, Luttrell M, Giannella RA. The immature rat small intestine exhibits an increased sensitivity and response to *Escherichia coli* heat-stable enterotoxin. *Pediatr Res* 1986;20:555–560.

75. Mezoff AG, Jensen NJ, Cohen MB. Mechanisms of increased susceptibility of immature and weaned pigs to *Escherichia coli* heat-stable enterotoxin. *Pediatr Res* 1991;29:424–428.

76. Katwa LC, Parker CD, White AA. Age-dependent changes in affinity-labeled receptors for *Escherichia coli* heat-stable enterotoxin in the swine intestine. *Infect Immun* 1991;59:4318–4323.

77. Cohen MB, Guarino A, Shukla R, Giannella RA. Age-related differences in receptors for *Escherichia coli* heat-stable enterotoxin in the small and large intestine of children. *Gastroenterology* 1988;94:367–373.

78. Cohen MB, Giannella RA. Jejunal toxin inactivation regulates susceptibility of the immature rat to STa. *Gastroenterology* 1992;102:1988–1996.

79. Spangler BD. Structure and function of cholera toxin and the related *Escherichia coli* heat-labile enterotoxin. *Microbiol Rev* 1992;56:622–647.

80. Lencer WI, Chu S-HW, Walker WA. Differential binding kinetics of cholera toxin to intestinal microvillus membranes during development. *Infect Immun* 1987;55:3126–3130.

81. Chu S-HW, Ely IG, Walker WA. Age and cortisone alter host responsiveness to cholera toxin in the developing gut. *Am J Physiol* 1989;256:G220–G225.

82. Seo JK, Chu S-HW, Walker WA. Development of intestinal host defense: an increased sensitivity in the adenylate cylase response to cholera toxin in suckling rats. *Pediatr Res* 1989;25:225–227.

83. Triadafilopoulos G, Lamont JT. Pseudomembranous colitis. In: Walker WA, Durie PR, Hamilton JR, Walker-Smith JA, Watkins JB, eds. *Pediatric gastrointestinal disease: pathophysiology, diagnosis, management.* Vol 1. Philadelphia: BC Decker, 1991:619–629.

84. Wilkins TD. Role of *Clostridium difficile* toxins in disease. *Gastroenterology* 1987;93:389–391 (editorial).

85. Pothoulakis C, LaMont JT, Eglow R, et al. Characterization of rabbit ileal receptors for *Clostridium difficile* toxin A: evidence for a receptor-coupled G protein. *J Clin Invest* 1991;88:119–125.

86. Eglow R, Pouthoulakis C, Itkowitz S, et al. Diminished *Clostridium difficile* toxin A sensitivity in newborn rabbit ileum is associated with decreased toxin A receptor. *J Clin Invest* 1992;90:822–829.

87. Rolfe RD. Binding kinetics of *Clostridium difficile* toxins A and B to intestinal brush border membranes from infant and adult hamsters. *Infect Immun* 1991;59:1223–1230.

88. Tesh V, O'Brien A. The pathogenic mechanisms of Shiga toxin and the Shiga-like toxins. *Mol Microbiol* 1991;5:1817–1822.

89. Saxena SK, O'Brien AD, Ackerman EJ. Shiga toxin, Shiga-like toxin II variant, and ricin are all single-site RNA *N*-glycosidases of 28S RNA when microinjected into *Xenopus* oocytes. *J Biol Chem* 1989;264:596–601.

90. Keenan KP, Sharpnack DD, Collins H, Formal SB, O'Brien AD. Morphologic evaluation of the effects of Shiga toxin and *E. coli* Shiga-like toxin on the rabbit intestine. *Am J Pathol* 1988;125:69–80.

91. Mobasseleh M, Donohue-Rolfe A, Jacewicz M, Grand RJ, Keusch GT. Pathogenesis of shigella diarrhea: evidence for a developmentally regulated glycolipid receptor for Shigella toxin involved in the fluid secretory response of rabbit small intestine. *J Infect Dis* 1988;157:1023–1031.

92. Mobassaleh M, Gross SK, McCluer RH, Donohue-Rolfe A, Keusch GT. Quantitation of the rabbit intestinal glycolipid receptor for Shiga toxin. Further evidence for the developmental regulation of globotriaosylceramide in microvillus membranes. *Gastroenterology* 1989;97:384–391.

93. Mobassaleh M, Koul O, Mishra K, McCluer R, Keusch G. The developmental pattern of the regulatory enzymes involved in the synthesis and breakdown of the Shiga toxin receptor in rabbit small intestine. *Gastroenterology* 1992;102:A567 (Abstract).

94. Haltalin KC. Neonatal shigellosis. Report of 16 cases and review of the literature. *Am J Dis Child* 1967;114:603–611.

95. Rafiee P, Leffler H, Byrd JC, Cassels FJ, Boedeker EC, Kim YS. A sialoglycoprotein complex linked to the microvillus cytoskeleton acts as a receptor for pilus (AF/R1) mediated adhesion of enteropathogenic *Escherichia coli* (RDEC-1) in rabbit small intestine. *J Cell Biol* 1991;115:1021–1029.

96. Cheney CP, Boedeker EC. Rabbit mucosal receptors for an enteropathogenic *Escherichia coli* strain: appearance of bacterial receptor activity at weaning. *Gastroenterology* 1984;87:821–826.

97. Berendson R, Cheney CP, Schad PA, Boedeker EC. Species-specific binding of purified pili (AF/R1) from the *Escherichia coli* RDEC-1 to rabbit intestinal mucosa. *Gastroenterology* 1983;85:837–845.

98. Ono E, Abe K, Nakazawa M, Naiki M. Ganglioside epitope recognized by K99 fimbriae from enterotoxigenic *Escherichia coli*. *Infect Immun* 1989;57:907–911.

99. Yuyama Y, Yoshimatsu K, Ono E, Saito M, Naiki M. Postnatal change of pig intestinal ganglioside bound by *Escherichia coli* with K99 fimbriae. *J Biochem* 1993;113:488–492.

100. Teneberg S, Willemsen P, deGraaf FK, Karlsson K-A. Receptor-active glycolipids of epithelial cells of the small intestine of young and adult pigs in relation to susceptibility to infection with *Escherichia coli* K99. *FEBS Lett* 1990;263:10–14.

101. Kyogashima M, Ginsburg V, Krivan HC. *Escherichia coli* K99 binds to N-glycosylsialoparagloboside and N-glycosyl-GM3 found in piglet small intestine. *Arch Biochem Biophys* 1989;270:391–397.

102. Wenneras C, Holmgren J, Svennerholm A-M. The binding of colonization factor antigens of enterotoxigenic *Escherichia coli* to intestinal cell membrane proteins. *FEMS Microbiol Lett* 1990;66:107–112.

103. Dean EA. Comparison of receptors for 987P pili of enterotoxigenic *Escherichia coli* in the small intestines of neonatal and older pigs. *Infect Immun* 1990;58:4030–4035.

104. Dean E, Whipp SC, Moon HW. Age-specific colonization of porcine intestinal epithelium by 987P-piliated enterotoxigenic *Escherichia coli*. *Infect Immun* 1989;57:82–87.

105. Willemsen PTJ, deGraaf FK. Age and serotype dependent binding of K88 fimbriae to porcine intestinal receptors. *Microb Pathogen* 1992;12:367–375.

106. Blomberg L, Krivan HC, Cohen PS, Conway PL. Piglet ileal mucus contains protein and glycolipid (galactosylceramide) receptors specific for *Escherichia coli* K88 fimbriae. *Infect Immun* 1993;61:2526–2531.

107. Adams SA, Robson SC, Gathiram V, et al. Immunological similarity between the 170 kD amoebic adherence glycoprotein and human β2 integrins. *Lancet* 1993;341:17–19.

108. Ravdin JI, Stanley P, Murphy CF, Petri WA Jr. Characterization of cell surface carbohydrate receptors for *Entamoeba histolytica* adherence lectin. *Infect Immun* 1989;57:2179–2186.

109. Bailey GB, Nudelman ED, Day DB, Harper CF, Gilmour JR. Specificity of glycosphingolipid recognition by *Entamoeba histolytica* trophozoites. *Infect Immun* 1990;58:43–47.

110. Bass DM, Mackow ER, Greenberg HB. Identification and partial characterization of a Rhesus rotavirus binding glycoprotein on murine enterocytes. *Virology* 1991;183:602–610.

Infections of the Gastrointestinal Tract,
edited by M. J. Blaser, P. D. Smith, J. I. Ravdin,
H. B. Greenberg, and R. L. Guerrant
Raven Press, Ltd., New York © 1995.

CHAPTER 10

The Mucosal Immune System

Charles O. Elson and Jiri F. Mestecky

Mucosal surfaces represent the major interface between the host and the environment. Thus, it is not surprising that most pathogens invade through or infect mucosal surfaces (1). The host has clearly evolved a number of defense mechanisms to deal with microbes in general and pathogens in particular. One of the most important of these is the mucosal immune system. This compartment of the immune system, quantitatively the largest, is marked by a number of distinguishing features that are unique to its specialized role. One of these features is the preferential production, transport, and secretion of IgA at all mucosal surfaces, a molecule that has been shown to limit the absorption of protein antigens, inhibit the attachment of bacteria, and neutralize a broad spectrum of viruses (2).

The precursors of mucosal IgA-producing plasma cells originate in organized lymphoepithelial structures that are present in the gastrointestinal tract (gut-associated lymphoreticular tissue, or GALT) and respiratory tract (bronchus-associated lymphoreticular tissue, or BALT). The discovery that antigen-stimulated GALT and BALT are the source of antigen-sensitized and IgA-committed plasma cell precursors that populate remote mucosal tissues and glands has led to the concept of a common mucosal immune system (3), in which an antigen exposure at one mucosal surface contributes cells to help protect remote mucosal sites as well (Fig. 1). For example, immunization of the gut through GALT can generate a mucosal response in the lung or in the vagina. This has led to a renewed interest in the development of oral vaccines to protect nonintestinal mucosal sites. Priming for a mucosal response via the intestine is convenient and effective, but an optimal immunity at distant mucosal sites seems to require local exposure of that mucosal surface to the antigen. In fact, the common mucosal immune system may contain certain subcompartments such that optimal vaginal immune responses occur after rectal immunization,

whereas optimal upper respiratory immune responses occur after nasopharyngeal or BALT immunization.

In regard to the intestine, lymphoid cells constitute approximately 25% of the cells present in the intestine; therefore the intestine is a major lymphoid organ (4,5). The mucosal immune system of the gut is organized into several interconnecting compartments representing either inductive or effector sites. Inductive sites consist of Peyer's patches and isolated lymphoid follicles, i.e., GALT; effector sites consist of the lamina propria and intraepithelial lymphocytes. The mesenteric lymph nodes, although outside the intestine proper, are frequently considered a fourth compartment. These different cell compartments are distinguished not only by differences in physical location and structure but by the types and functions of cells present within them.

The antigenic challenge to the intestinal immune system is enormous. It has been estimated that the number of microbial cells in the body, most of them in the intestine, exceeds the total number of cells in the body (6). One can add to these bacterial antigens the abundant antigens present in food and drink. Exactly how the intestinal mucosal system deals with this challenge is not yet known; however, it is apparent that the mucosal immune system is in a constant state of response, as witnessed by the large number of plasma cells present throughout the intestine and by studies on germ-free animals in which the mucosal lymphoid tissue is poorly developed (7–9). These observations have led to the concept of "physiological inflammation," in which the "normal" intestine is viewed as being in a state of mild inflammation (9) due to the massive antigenic challenge. Physiological inflammation may represent an important aspect of host defense against pathogens, many of which are likely to have antigens cross-reactive with those of the enteric flora. In this view, the "normal" stimulation of the intestinal immune system by the enteric flora "arms" or "primes" the system for accelerated and/or more effective immune responses to pathogenic microbes.

In the sections to follow, each compartment of the intestinal immune system will be considered separately, but

C. O. Elson, and J. F. Mestecky: Departments of Medicine and Microbiology, University of Alabama at Birmingham, Birmingham, Alabama 35294.

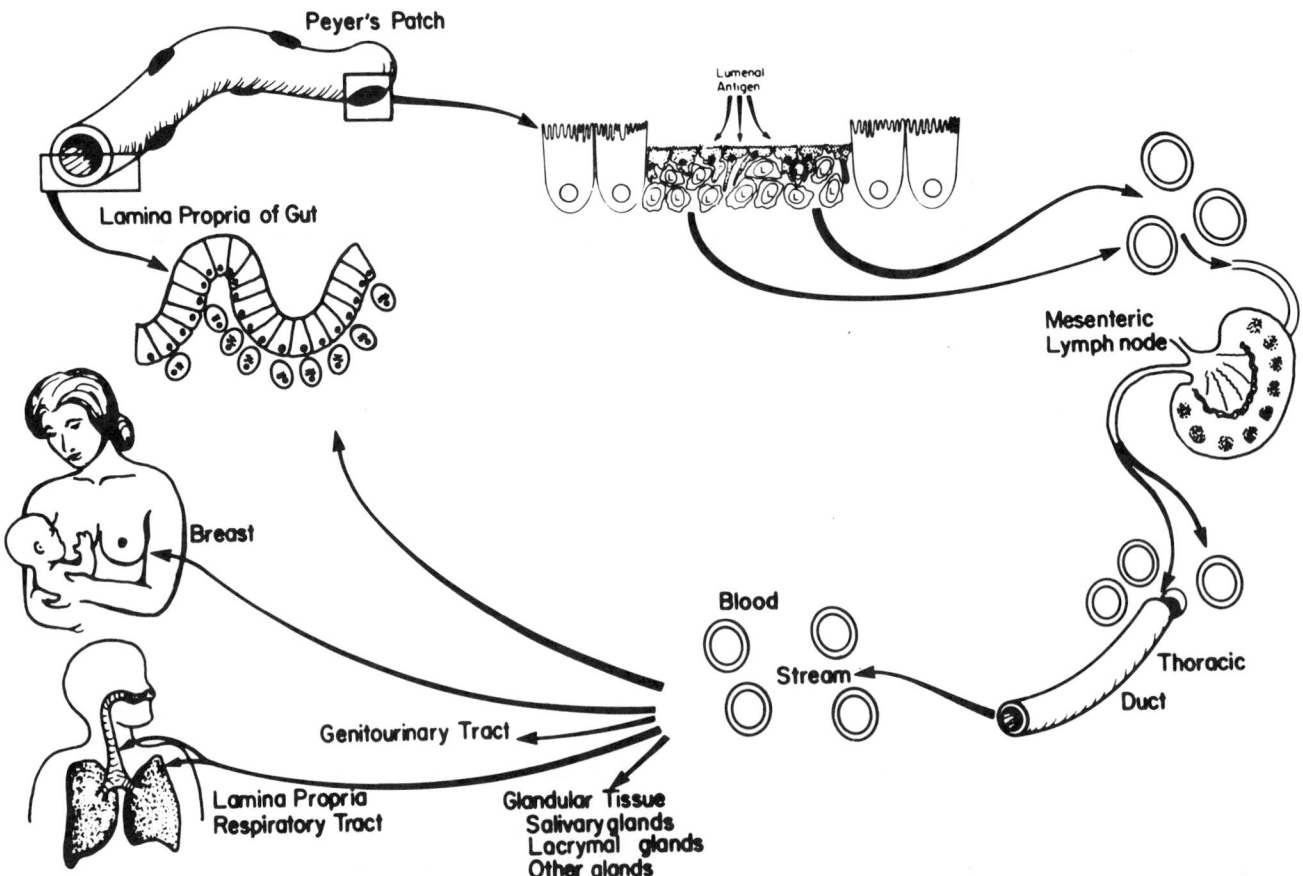

FIG. 1. Schematic diagram of the common mucosal immune system in humans. The intestine contains organized lymphoid structures known as Peyer's patches, as well as isolated lymphoid follicles. Luminal antigen enters these organized lymphoid tissues through a specialized epithelium containing pinocytotic and phagocytic M cells. Within the follicle, antigens interact with resident antigen-presenting cells, T cells, and B cells to generate IgA-committed and antigen-sensitized B cells and T cells. Once activated, cells leave the follicle and enter regional lymph nodes, then travel through the thoracic duct to the circulation, from which they populate various exocrine glands and mucosa-associated tissues in the salivary glands, respiratory tract, genitourinary tract, and lactating breast. Terminal differentiation into IgA-secreting plasma cells occurs in these mucosal tissues.

in reality those represent a dynamic and integrated system of host defense.

PEYER'S PATCHES AND LYMPHOID FOLLICLES

Peyer's patches (PPs) are organized lymphoid aggregates with one or more lymphoid follicles that extend from the epithelial layer into the lamina propria, and sometimes the submucosa. Although PPs are visible, macroscopic structures, clustered in certain regions such as the ileum in man, analogous small lymphoid follicles are dispersed abundantly throughout the intestine in humans and some other species (10,11). PPs and these small follicles together comprise GALT. PPs differ from other peripheral lymphoid tissues by their lack of afferent lymphatics, but they do have efferent lymphatics. Instead of afferent lymphatics, they have a specialized epithelium that actively

pinocytoses material present in the intestinal lumen and delivers it via trancytosis and exocytosis into the follicle (Fig. 1) (12). Distinguishing features of this specialized follicle-associated epithelium (FAE) include a relative lack of goblet cells and the presence of M, or membrane, cells that lack secretory component and alkaline phosphatase (5,13,14). The M cell serves as an important first step in the induction of intestinal immune responses, but relatively little is known about the factors determining its generation or function. At present, it is unclear that any selectivity except for the size of particles is exerted by the M cell in the material that it will pinocytose or phagocytose (Table 1). Soluble proteins, viruses, bacteria, protozoa, lysosomes, and microspheres have all been taken up by M cells (Table 1). Some organisms such as *Salmonella* exploit this feature, using M cells as a portal of entry into the body (15). M-cell uptake of *Salmonella* and particles such as microcapsules is being exploited to deliver vac-

TABLE 1. *Selected microbes and materials transported by M cells*

Macromolecules	Viruses	Bacteria	Parasites	Other
Ferritin	Reovirus 1,3	Mycobacteria	Cryptosporidia	Microcapsules < 10 μm size
Horseradish peroxidase	HIV-1 ?	Chlamydia		Liposomes
Ricin agglutinin I, II	Polio virus 1	*Vibrio cholerae*		Latex particles
Wheat germ agglutinin		*Salmonella* sp.		
Cholera-toxin		*E. coli* $O_{124}K_{72}$		
		Brucella abortus		
		Campylobacter jejuni		
		Yersinia enterocolitica		
		Shigella sp.		

cine antigens into GALT. Human M cells possess a lysosomal compartment and express HLA-DR molecules (5) and therefore have the potential to present antigen directly to the lymphocytes infiltrating the dome epithelium, but no direct evidence of antigen presentation by M cells exists (16).

Consistent with this active antigen uptake by the specialized dome epithelium, PP, and related lymphoid follicles serve as sites for the induction of mucosal immune responses. It is now recognized that the PPs contain all the cells needed for immune induction, i.e., B cells, T cells, and antigen-presenting cells (macrophages and dendritic cells). These cell types are structured in B-cell–dependent and T-cell–dependent areas similar to other peripheral lymphoid tissues. B cells predominate in the lymphoid follicles, whereas T cells predominate in the interfollicular areas and beneath the dome epithelium; macrophages appear to be scattered both beneath the dome epithelium and in the follicles (5,12,17). Quantitatively, B cells predominate in the PP of adult animals constituting some 60% to 70% of total cells, while T cells,

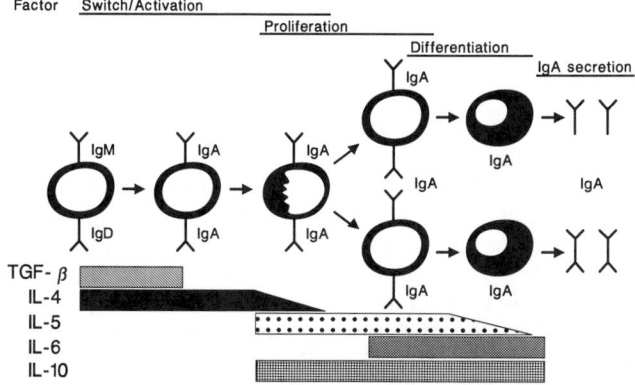

FIG. 2. Regulation of differentiation of IgA B cells by cytokines. Mature (sIgM⁺, sIgD⁺) B cells switch to sIgA⁺ cells under the influence of certain cytokines such as TGF-β. These cells can then be activated by antigen, mitogen, or IL-4. IL-5 induces activated B cells to proceed through the cell cycle, allowing for clonal expansion. IL-6 induces B cell differentiation into IgA-producing plasma cells. IL-10 affects both the proliferation and differentiation of B cells. Thus, as currently envisioned, a succession of cytokines drive B cells from the very earliest stages through plasma cell differentiation.

including both CD4+ and CD8+ cells, comprise about 20% of the total. Although T cells are present in smaller numbers, the rudimentary PP and the deficient IgA responses found in T-cell–deficient mice indicate that PP function is highly dependent on T cells (17). An important feature of PP cells is that they consist of precursor rather than effector cells. For example, although the PPs contain many B cells, few plasma cells are present, even after extensive immunization (18). The same appears to be true for cytotoxic T cells; the PPs contain precursors rather than effectors (19). One explanation is that differentiating B cells and T cells leave PPs and migrate to the gut and other lymphoid tissues (20,21). A second important feature of PPs is that the induction of immune responses there is highly dependent on the route of antigen exposure. PPs respond predominantly, if not exclusively, to antigen presented via the intestinal lumen, i.e., antigen transported via M cells (7–9).

GALT, BALT, and related tissues are sites in which there is preferential induction of IgA responses, an important function considering that IgA is the major immunoglobulin at mucosal surfaces. PP cells are enriched for IgA B-cell precursors relative to other lymphoid tissues (22,23), particularly for IgA B-cell precursors recognizing antigens present in the intestine (24). The mechanism for this preferential expression of IgA by PP B cells is not clear, but microenvironmental–B-cell interactions (25), the effects of an unusual switch T cell (26), the effects of a specialized dendritic cell (27), or the expression of cytokines such as tumor growth factor–β (TGF-β) in PPs (28) are possible explanations. Switch T cells, cloned from the murine PP, have been shown to cause B cells to change or switch from the production of IgM to the production of IgA. T cells regulate B-cell differentiation by secreting a variety of cytokines (Fig. 2); such T cells are present in the PP as well (29–31). These and other aspects of the T-cell regulation of IgA have been reviewed (32).

MUCOSAL LYMPHOCYTE TRAFFICKING

Lymphocytes induced in the GALT exit via efferent lymphatics and enter into mesenteric lymph nodes where they may undergo further division and differentiation (Fig. 1) (33). From there they travel via the thoracic duct into the circulation and are dispersed widely in the body (34). However, these cells selectively accumulate back (or "home") to the intestine and other mucosal sites such as the lactating breast, salivary and lacrimal gland, and perhaps genitourinary tissues (24,25), i.e., tissue of the common mucosal immune system (Fig. 1). The migration of IgA-producing cells from GALT to the lactating breast is an important mechanism that provides specific secretory IgA antibodies in mother's milk to protect the suckling newborn against the microbes with which it is most likely to be colonized (35). This dissemination of antigen-sensitized and IgA-committed cells from inductive sites to remote effector sites has important implications for the design of vaccines that would provide protective immunity at mucosal surfaces, the most frequent portals of entry of infectious agents. In order to populate the lamina propria of the intestine or remote secretory glands, such cells must exit the circulation. Numerous studies suggest that specific interactions between receptors on lymphocytes and those on the endothelial cells of specialized high endothelial venules (HEVs) regulate the selective distribution of lymphocytes to secondary lymphoid tissues (33). The molecular mechanisms of cell trafficking is an area of active research. A number of molecules important in cell migration into mucosae have been identified to date. These lymphocyte molecules and their respective endothelial cell ligands include LFA-1 (CD18/CD11a) binding to ICAM-1/ICAM-2, VLA-4 binding to VCAM-1, and CD44 binding to a 58- to 66-kDa molecule (36). Recent biochemical characterization of one mucosal vascular addressin that is selectively expressed on HEV of mucosal lymphoid organs and on lamina propria venules reveals that this receptor displays features common to members of the immunoglobulin supergene family (37). This receptor, designated the mucosal addressin cell-adhesion molecule (MAdCAM1) is composed of three immunoglobulin domains and a 37-amino-acid region localized between the second and third domains. This region is rich in serine and threonine, which are potential glycosylation sites for O-linked carbohydrates. Interestingly, the first and the second domains display sequences homologous to the human VCAM-1 molecule and the third domain to the CH2 domain of human IgA1; the intervening serine/threonine-rich region exhibits structural features characteristic of mucins. This unusual carbohydrate may play a role in lymphocyte binding and migration.

The entry of cells into a tissue such as the intestine is a critical component of mucosal immunity as well as of mucosal inflammation. In regard to the latter, inflammatory cytokines increase the expression of endothelial cell ICAM-1 and ELAM-1 during intestinal inflammation (38,39), thus facilitating entry of larger numbers of cells into inflammatory sites. The entry of nonspecific inflammatory cells into the intestine via these molecules is an important element of host defense against infectious pathogens, particularly during early infection before specific immunity has been triggered.

LAMINA PROPRIA LYMPHOCYTES

The intestinal lamina propria contains an abundance of B cells, plasma cells, T cells, and macrophages as well as a lesser number of other cell types such as eosinophils, mast cells, and dendritic cells (5). The intestinal lamina propria is the only site in the body where large numbers of plasma cells are present continuously. Approximately 70% to 90% of the plasma cells in the intestine produce IgA (40). The next most common isotype produced is IgM, representing 5% to 15%, followed by IgG, representing only 3% to 5%. IgE and IgD plasma cells are uncommon. Plasma cells are terminally differentiated, end-stage cells whose half-life is approximately 5 days (41), indicating that there must be a dynamic, continuous repopulation of lamina propria B cells. The proliferation and differentiation of B cells appears to be regulated by cytokines produced by a broad spectrum of resident cell types, particularly T cells, but also including macrophages and epithelial cells (32) (Fig. 2). With respect to differentiation of mucosal B cells into IgA plasma cells, interleukin-5 (IL-5), IL-6, IL-10, and TGF-β play prominent roles (42,43). Recent studies suggest that these cytokines are derived not only from T cells, but also from epithelial cells which can produce IL-6, IL-10, and TGF-β (44).

It is possible to isolate human lamina propria lymphocytes and study their functions in vitro (45). In such isolates B cells compose some 15% to 40% of the total cells with IgA-producing cells predominating (45). Considerable numbers of T cells are present also, ranging from 40% to 90% in different reports (46–48). Macrophages make up about 10% of lamina propria isolates (45), and mast cells form 1% to 3% (49). Interestingly, cells with neither B-cell or T-cell markers, i.e., null cells, and cells with natural killer (NK) cell markers seem to be deficient in the intestinal lamina propria (45,50,51), although cells capable of lymphokine-activated killer (LAK) activity are well represented (52).

The ability to isolate lamina propria cells from human and primate intestine has allowed lamina propria T cells to be characterized. Approximately two thirds of lamina propria T cells are CD4 + and one third are CD8 +, which is similar to their ratio in peripheral blood. However, lamina propria T cells differ in substantial ways from peripheral blood T cells. Most of the lamina propria T cells have the CD45RO + CD45RA − phenotype characteristic of memory cells, whereas the converse is true for peripheral blood T cells. Lamina propria T cells are in a higher state of activation based on expression of IL-2Rα chain, HLA-DR molecules, transferrin receptors, and CD98 (an activation molecule recognized by the monoclonal antibody 4F2). Upon activation lamina propria T cells produce greater amounts of cytokines such as IL-2, IL-4, IL-5, and interferon-γ (IFN-γ), which is consistent with their increased helper activity for B-cell responses (53). Perhaps reflecting this altered state of activation/differentiation, lamina propria T cells from lymphogranuloma venereum–infected nonhuman primates did not proliferate when stimulated by specific antigen, but instead produced high levels of cytokines (54). Human lamina propria T cells have diminished proliferative responses to stimulation via the CD3/T-cell receptor (TCR) complex but respond normally to stimulation via CD2 or CD28 (55). There appears to be a soluble mediator produced in the intestinal mucosa that downregulates the CD3/TCR pathway of T-cell activation (56). T cells with markers consistent with cytolytic T-cell function are present in the lamina propria, and functional cytolytic activity has been demonstrated in intestinal lymphocytes by redirected lysis assays (57). Whether such cytolytic activity is brought into play during normal intestinal immune responses is unclear, but such cells could be important in host defense against certain pathogens.

Intraepithelial Lymphocytes

Lymphocytes that are physically located within the epithelial layer, or intraepithelial lymphocytes (IELs), comprise one of every 6–10 cells in the epithelium (58–60). The cellular composition of this compartment is different from that in either the PP or the lamina propria. Plasma cells are not present, and B cells are absent or infrequent. The predominant cell type in small intestinal IEL is the CD8 + T cell, and in most mouse strains, about half bear γδ T-cell receptors and the other half αβ T-cell receptors. In mice IEL are quite heterogeneous based on expression of CD8 isoforms, Thy1, CD5, and on cell density (61). Whether similar heterogeneity exists in human IEL is unclear. Analysis of human IEL TCR gene expression shows evidence of oligoclonality (62); similar analysis of murine IEL TCR expression has not been done. In contrast to mice or chickens, Tγδ cells are a minor component in human IELs, most of which are TCRαβ +, CD8 +, CD45RO +. Most existing data on IEL come from studies done on small intestinal isolates. It is interesting, therefore, that mouse colon IELs have been found to consist mainly of CD4 +, TCRαβ + T cells, revealing previously unsuspected regional differences within the intestinal immune system (63). Whether similar regional differences exist for the lamina propria compartment is unknown. The environment in the small bowel and colon is dramatically different and so it should not be surprising that the mucosal immune system of these two sites is also different. It is quite possible that these regional differences in mucosal lymphoid populations are an important aspect of host defense against the enteric flora and against pathogens, but no direct evidence of this exists at present.

IEL Tαβ cells appear to originate in the PP and traffic to the epithelium via the lamina propria (64) but there is also evidence for a thymic-independent lineage of T cells in small intestinal IELs (61). The origin of these cells, which bear the CD8αα isoform and are CD5 –, remains unclear. In many species, a large proportion of the IELs contain granules that stain metachromatically and resemble mast cell granules, but contain little or no histamine (65).

The function of IELs in host defense remains unclear. First, IELs have full cytotoxic capabilities including NK, ADCC, and T-cell cytotoxicity. Because IELs increase in number after roundworm infestations, they might serve a cytotoxic function directed primarily at parasites. Second, IELs are increased in experimental graft versus host disease, prompting the suggestion that an increase in IELs may be a marker for cell-mediated immune responses in the intestine (66). Third, IELs might defend the epithelium

against viral infections by local secretion of IFN-γ (67) and perhaps by direct cytotoxicity. They may also produce other cytokines that may influence enterocyte functions. Although we know little about their precise function *in vivo*; IELs are situated in a site that would render them exposed to a variety of antigenic stimuli and thus they likely play an important role in mucosal host defense.

SECRETORY IgA AND ITS TRANSPORT SYSTEM

The appearance of large amounts of IgA in external secretions, and particularly in the intestinal tract, is the result of complex molecular and cellular interactions (Fig. 3) (for reviews, see Refs. 68–70) that have been studied in great detail. Most plasma cells at mucosal sites produce IgA in its polymeric (dimeric and tetrameric) form. Intracellular polymerization of monomers and the incorporation of an additional small glycoprotein J chain within the plasma cell results in the secretion of IgA molecules that can interact with a receptor specific for polymeric immunoglobulins of the IgA and IgM isotypes. This polyimmunoglobulin receptor, also called secretory component (SC), which is expressed on the surface of epithelial cells and, in some species, on hepatocytes, plays a key role in the selective epithelial transport of IgA. After SC is synthesized in the rough endoplasmic reticulum and heavily glycosylated in the Golgi complex, it reaches and is inserted into the basolateral membrane of the enterocyte, where it acts as a receptor. Biochemical studies reveal that SC belongs to the immunoglobulin superfamily and

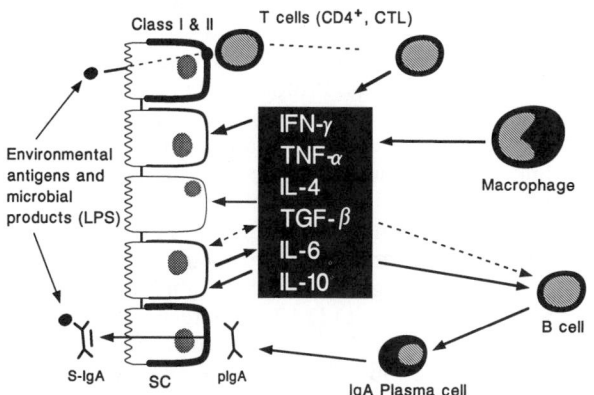

FIG. 3. Participation of epithelial cells in the mucosal immune system. Epithelial cells are in constant contact with antigen and bioactive products of microbes, which activate epithelial cells to produce a variety of cytokines that can interact with mucosal immune cells. Epithelial cells also can express class II MHC molecules and thus potentially act as antigen-presenting cells to induce either immunity or tolerance. In turn, mucosal immune cells produce local cytokines that act on epithelial cells. The physiological consequences for epithelial cell function are still being defined, but these cytokines can increase expression of certain molecules such as MHC class II molecules and secretory component, as well as to further enhance epithelial cell cytokine production.

consists of five immunoglobulin domains (71,72). After the initial interactions of polymeric IgA with SC on epithelial cells through noncovalent binding, the first domain of SC binds to the Cα3 domain, and the fifth SC domain binds covalently to the Cα2 domain. J chain is essential for polymeric IgA to interact with SC, probably by inducing conformational changes in IgA that permit SC binding. Following these molecular events, the membrane SC–polymeric IgA complex is internalized and transported in vesicles toward the apical surface of the epithelial cells. Once there, these vesicles fuse with the apical membrane. Proteolytic cleavage of SC releases the assembled molecule of secretory IgA (S-IgA) into external secretions. SC-mediated transport of polymeric IgA represents a unique system of interaction between a receptor and its ligand: SC is produced by epithelial cells regardless of the presence of its ligand and is not recycled. Instead, it remains permanently attached to polymeric IgA and confers an increased resistance of S-IgA to proteolytic enzymes in the intestinal tract. The magnitude of selective IgA transport is enormous, composing 3–5 g S-IgA produced and transported each day into the human intestine.

The synthesis and expression of both J chain and SC is regulated by cytokines and hormones (69): IL-5, IL-2, and possibly IL-6 upregulate J-chain synthesis while IL-4, IFN-γ, tumor necrosis factor–α (TNF-α), and TGF-β significantly enhance SC expression. Thus, the synthesis of all component chains of S-IgA is regulated by cytokines that are locally produced in the intestinal microenvironment.

In humans, IgA consists of two subclasses, IgA1 and IgA2. IgA1 composes about 80% to 90% of the IgA in serum, but only 40% to 50% of IgA in secretions. The expression of IgA1 appears to predominate in the proximal intestine, whereas IgA2 is expressed mainly in the distal intestine (73,74). Secretory and serum IgA antibodies display marked differences in IgA subclass usage to certain types of antigens. Protein antigens of microbial or food origin induce a predominantly IgA1 response, whereas endotoxins and polysaccharides induce both IgA1 and IgA2 responses, particularly in external secretions (75).

There are some functional differences in effector function between IgA1 and IgA2. In regard to host defense against enteric pathogens, the most significant is the susceptibility of IgA1 but not IgA2 to bacterial IgA proteases that cleave the Fc portion of IgA1, thus interfering with its biological functions. The predominant expression of IgA2 in the distal intestine and colon where bacteria are abundant thus can be viewed as an important adaptation of the IgA system for host defense. Once released into the lumen, secretory IgA has antiviral, antitoxin, and antibacterial functions, primarily by decreasing the ability of such cells or substances to bind to mucosa (76).

The liver can also transport IgA (77,78) as well as IgA immune complexes (79,80). This pathway is particularly important in certain rodents, such as rat, which transports 90% of its intestinal secretory IgA through the liver (78). In humans, this pathway appears to be of minor importance (81); moreover, IgA transport occurs in humans through bile ductular cells rather than through the hepatocyte (82,83).

EPITHELIAL AND NEURAL INTERACTIONS IN MUCOSAL IMMUNITY

The lymphocytes composing the intestinal immune system exist in a complex milieu in which they have close contact with other cell types. There is emerging realization that at least two of these cell types, the intestinal epithelial cell and the enteric neuron, may play a very significant role in mucosal immunity. Until recently, the epithelial cell was thought to be a passive partner whose functions were perhaps influenced or altered by products produced by immune cells. However, it is more likely that epithelial cells are active participants in the mucosal immune system (Fig. 3). Epithelial cells are able to produce cytokines such as TGF-β and IL-6 that are known to have profound effects on lymphocytes (84,85). Epithelial cells have receptors for certain cytokines as manifested by high-level IL-6 expression upon stimulation of epithelial IEC-6 cells with certain cytokines such as TGF-β or IL-1 (86). More recently, it was shown that epithelial cells produce IL-8 when invaded by various *Salmonella,* thus serving as an early response system to bacterial infection (87). In addition to cytokine production, some epithelial cells spontaneously express class II MHC molecules and this expression is increased by inflammation (88). A role for epithelial cells in antigen presentation has been proposed (89). However, because epithelial cells lack costimulatory molecules such as B7 (90), their main function may instead be tolerance of antigen-specific T cells. Lastly, the intestinal epithelium may act in an analogous fashion to thymic epithelium in supporting the thymic-independent lineage of T cells that is known to exist in the IELs (91).

Interactions between the nervous and immune systems are also likely to play an important role in mucosal immunity. The various compartments within the mucosal immune system differ in their innervation. The lamina propria in particular is richly innervated and it has been estimated that most lamina propria lymphocytes are within 1 cell diameter of a nerve fiber (92). Most of these nerves express the neuropeptides vasoactive intestinal peptide (VIP), substance P, or somatostatin. In addition, various subpopulations of mucosal T and B cells have receptors for these neuropeptides. Moreover, lymphocyte functions such as proliferation and immunoglobulin production are altered by *in vitro* exposure to these neuropeptides. The consequences of neurolymphoid interactions in the mucosa in the intact animal have yet to be defined and are likely to be very complex.

REGULATION OF THE INTESTINAL MUCOSAL IMMUNE SYSTEM

Immunity to antigens after intestinal exposure is well documented following natural infections in humans and oral immunization regimens in experimental animals (93). The large quantity of IgA produced in the intestine reflects a continuous and active mucosal immune response to antigens in the environment. The mechanisms by which this response is regulated are currently being defined. Mention has already been made of the helper function of the lamina propria CD4+ T cell. Murine CD4+ T cells in mice can be further subdivided into two types, based on the cytokines that they secrete and thus the functions that they serve (Fig. 4). Type 1 (Th1) CD4+ cells produce IL-2 and IFN-γ and mediate delayed hypersensitivity responses; type 2 (Th2) CD4+ T cells produce IL-4, IL-5, IL-6, and IL-10 and serve as helper cells for B-cell responses (94). Th1 and Th2 cells reciprocally regulate one another via the cytokines IL-10 and IFN-γ (Fig. 4). The balance between these two subsets may be very important in maintaining mucosal homeostasis and host defense because the Th1 vs. Th2 pattern of response in inbred mouse strains can mean death or survival of the host to various infectious agents (95). The factors that determine whether Th1 or Th2 cells will predominate in the response to a given pathogen are obviously important but as yet not understood. The current notion is that the initial encounter of the microbe with cells of the innate immune system (macrophages, granulocytes, mast cells, etc.) stimulates the production of certain cytokines, namely IL-12 or IL-4, which induce differentiation down the Th1 or Th2 pathway, respectively (Fig. 4).

The exact role of Th1 and Th2 cells in the regulation of mucosal immunity is not yet known; however, mucosal sites seem to have a propensity for Th2-type responses to antigens. For example, the same antigen (tetanus toxoid) when given parenterally induces predominantly Th1 responses in the spleen, but given orally induces predominantly Th2 responses in the lamina propria (96). The balance between Th1 and Th2 cells is likely to be an important factor in mucosal host defense toward microbial flora as well as microbial pathogens. The importance of this regulatory balance is illustrated by the development of chronic colitis in mice in whom IL-10 or IL-2,

cytokines important in maintaining such T-cell subset balance, have been genetically deleted (97,98). Much less is known about Th1 and Th2 cells in humans, but evidence is emerging that similar T-cell subsets are being found in humans with chronic parasitic and mycobacterial diseases (99).

The feeding of an antigen prior to parenteral immunization can induce a state of systemic unresponsiveness or "oral tolerance" (93) instead of immunity. The factors determining whether immunity or tolerance results from an antigen encounter in the gut are not well understood, but presumably the answer lies in complex regulatory cell interactions within GALT. Oral tolerance has been demonstrated in animals after the feeding of a variety of antigens including proteins, contact allergens, heterologous erythrocytes, and viral hemagglutinin (93). Some evidence exists that bacterial LPSs may sensitize the mucosal immune system in a manner that predisposes to development of oral tolerance (100) and to nonspecific suppression (101). Multiple mechanisms of tolerance have been demonstrated, but the most common one is the generation of suppressor CD8+ T cells in GALT. These CD8+ T cells may secrete TGF-β, an inhibitory cytokine, as a mechanism for their suppression (102). There seems to be differential cellular susceptibility to oral tolerance induction, with Th1 cells being most sensitive (103), followed by Th2 cells and then B cells. Feeding autoantigens has been used to abrogate or treat experimental autoimmune diseases, and recently trials have begun along a similar line in humans. A recent study showed that the feeding of a protein antigen to human volunteers did result in T-cell, but not B-cell, tolerance establishing for the first time that oral tolerance exists in humans (104). It is unclear as to whether protein antigens of bacterial origin can induce oral tolerance. Bacterial LPS given together with a nonbacterial antigen increased the degree of oral tolerance to

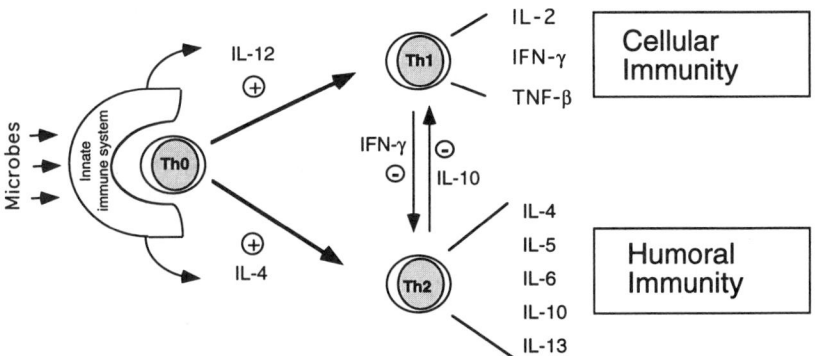

FIG. 4. T-Cell differentiation pathways induced by microbes. The initial encounter of microbes is with cells of the innate immune system (antigen-presenting cells, mast cells, granulocytes, stromal cells). This system provides a rapid but nonspecific response. Specific responses are generated by the presentation of microbial antigens by cells of the innate immune system to naive CD4+ T cells (Th0). Depending on the cytokine milieu in the microenvironment, CD4+ Th0 cells differentiate along either or both of two pathways, i.e., into Th1 cells that mediate cellular immune responses or into Th2 cells that mediate humoral immunity. Th1 and Th2 cells are distinguished by their production of certain cytokines as shown. They also produce many other cytokines in common. These two subsets regulate one another through interferon-γ (Th1) and IL-10 (Th2), which inhibit the reciprocal subset. For a given microbe, the predominant pathway stimulated can determine whether the infection results in disease or recovery.

the latter (105), so that the presence of highly stimulatory adjuvant molecules in microbes does not necessarily shift the mucosal response away from a tolerizing one. There have been a dearth of studies in which bacterial antigens have been tested for their ability to induce oral tolerance. The feeding of large amounts of *E. coli* alkaline phosphatase to mice did not result in oral tolerance (106), but whether this result can be extrapolated is unclear. The factors that determine whether tolerance or immunity occurs after a mucosal encounter with microbial antigens need to be defined. This is clearly an important consideration both for the outcome of any encounter with an intestinal pathogen, as well as for the possible development of oral vaccines against such infectious agents.

ACKNOWLEDGMENTS

This work was supported by NIH grants DK28623, DK44240, and AI35999.

REFERENCES

1. McGhee JR, Mestecky J. In defense of mucosal surfaces. Development of novel vaccines for IgA responses protective at portals of entry for microbial pathogens. *Infect Dis Clin North Am* 1990;4:315–341.
2. Kilian M, Mestecky J, Russell MW. Defense mechanisms involving Fc-dependent functions of immunoglobulin A (IgA) and their subversion by bacterial immunoglobulin A proteases. *Microbiol Rev* 1988;52:296–303.
3. Scicchitano R, Stanisz A, Ernst P, Bienenstock J. A common mucosal immune system revisited. In: Husband AJ, ed. *Migration and homing of lymphoid cells*. Vol 2. Boca Raton: CRC Press; 1988:1–35.
4. Strober W, Hanson LA, Sell KW (eds.). *Recent advances in mucosal immunity*. New York: Raven Press; 1982.
5. Brandtzaeg P. Research in gastrointestinal immunology. State of the art. *Scand J Gastroenterol* 1985;20:137–156.
6. Savage DC. Microbial ecology of the gastrointestinal tract. *Annu Rev Microbiol* 1977;31:107–133.
7. Crabbe PA, Bazin H, Eyssen H, Heremans JF. The normal microbial flora as a major stimulus for proliferation of plasma cells synthesizing IgA in the gut. The germ-free intestinal tract. *Int Arch Allergy* 1968;34:362–375.
8. Glaister JR. Factors affecting the lymphoid cells in the small intestinal epithelium of the mouse. *Int Arch Allergy* 1973;45:719–730.
9. Abrams GD, Bauer H, Sprinz H. Influence of the normal flora on mucosal morphology and cellular renewal in the ileum. *Lab Invest* 1963;12:355–364.
10. Keren DF, Holt PS, Collins HH, Gemski P, Formal SB. The role of Peyer's patches in the local immune response of rabbit ileum to live bacteria. *J Immunol* 1978;120:1892–1896.
11. Cornes JS. Number, size, and distribution of Peyer's patches in the human small intestine. I. The development of Peyer's patches. *Gut* 1965;6:225–233.
12. Bockman DE, Boydston WR, Beezhold DH. The role of epithelial cells in gut-associated immune reactivity. *Ann N Y Acad Sci* 1983;409:129–143.
13. Owen RL, Jones AL. Epithelial cell specialization within human Peyer's patches: and ultrastructural study of intestinal lymphoid follicles. *Gastroenterology* 1974;66:189–203.
14. Owen RL. Sequential uptake of horseradish peroxidase by lymphoid follicle epithelium of Peyer's patches in the normal unobstructed mouse intestine: and ultrastructural study. *Gastroenterology* 1977;72:440.
15. Owen RL. And now pathophysiology of M cells: good news

16. Trier JS. Structure and function of intestinal M cells. *Gastroenterol Clin North Am* 1992;20:531–548.
17. Guy-Grand D, Griscelli C, Vassalli P. Peyer's patches, gut IgA plasma cells and thymic function: study in nude mice bearing thymic grafts. *J Immunol* 1975;115:361–364.
18. Bienenstock J, Dolezel J. Peyer's patches: lack of specific antibody-containing cells after oral and parenteral immunization. *J Immunol* 1971;106:938–945.
19. Kagnoff MF. Effects of antigen feeding on intestinal and systemic immune responses. I. Priming of precursor cytotoxic T cells by antigen feeding. *J Immunol* 1978;120:395–399.
20. Kagnoff MF. Functional characteristics of Peyer's patch cells. IV. Effect of antigen feeding on the frequency of antigen-specific B cells. *J Immunol* 1977;118:992–997.
21. Guy-Grand D, Griscelli C, Vassalli P. The gut-associated lymphoid system: nature and properties of the large dividing cells. *Eur J Immunol* 1974;4:435–443.
22. Craig SW, Cebra JJ. Peyer's patches: an enriched source of precursors for IgA-producing immunocytes in the rabbit. *J Exp Med* 1971;134:188–200.
23. Tseng J. Transfer of lymphocytes of Peyer's patches between immunoglobulin allotype congenic mice: repopulation of the IgA plasma cells in the gut lamina propria. *J Immunol* 1981;127:2039.
24. Gearhart PJ, Cebra JJ. Differentiated B lymphocytes. Potential to express particular antibody variable and constant regions depends on site of lymphoid tissue and antigen load. *J Exp Med* 1979;149:216–227.
25. Cebra JJ, Komisar JL, Schweitzer PA. CH isotype switching during normal B-lymphocyte development. *Annu Rev Immunol* 1984;2:493–548.
26. Kawanishi H, Saltzman LE, Strober W. Mechanisms regulating IgA class-specific immunoglobulin production in murine gut-associated lymphoid tissues. I. T cells derived from Peyer's patches that switch sIgM B cells in vitro. *J Exp Med* 1983;157:433–449.
27. Spalding DM, Williamson SI, Koopman WJ, McGhee JR. Preferential induction of polyclonal IgA secretion by murine Peyer's patch dendritic cell-T cell mixtures. *J Exp Med* 1984;160:941–946.
28. Coffman RL, Lebman DA, Shrader B. Transforming growth factor beta specifically enhances IgA production by lipopolysaccharide-stimulated murine B lymphocytes. *J Exp Med* 1989;170:1039–1044.
29. Elson CO, Heck JA, Strober W. T-cell regulation of murine IgA synthesis. *J Exp Med* 1979;149:632–643.
30. Kiyono H, McGhee JR, Mostellar LM, et al. Murine Peyer's patch T cell clones. Characterization of antigen-specific helper T cells for immunoglobulin A responses. *J Exp Med* 1982;156:1115–1130.
31. Kiyono H, Mostellar-Barnum LM, Pitts AM, Williamson SI, Michalek SM, McGhee JR. Isotype-specific immunoregulation: IgA binding factors produced by Fcα receptor-positive T cell hybridomas regulate IgA responses. *J Exp Med* 1985;161:731–747.
32. McGhee JR, Mestecky J, Elson CO, Kiyono H. Regulation of IgA synthesis and immune response by T cells and interleukins. *J Clin Immunol* 1989;9:175–199.
33. Picker LJ, Butcher EC. Physiological and molecular mechanisms of lymphocyte homing. *Annu Rev Immunol* 1992;10:561–591.
34. Phillips-Quagliata JM, Lamm ME. Lymphocyte homing to mucosal effector sites. In: Ogra PL, Mestecky J, Lamm ME, Strober W, McGhee JR, Bienenstock J, eds. *Handbook of mucosal immunology*. San Diego: Academic Press; 1994:225–234.
35. Goldblum RM, Ahlstedt S, Carlsson B, et al. Antibody forming cells in human colostrum after oral immunization. *Nature* 1975;257:797–799.
36. Salmi M, Jalkanen S. Regulation of lymphocyte traffic to mucosa-associated lymphatic tissues. *Gastroenterol Clin North Am* 1991;20:495–510.
37. Brisken MJ, McEvoy LM, Butcher EC. MAdCAM-1 has ho-

and bad news from Peyer's patches. *Gastroenterology* 1983;85:468–470.

mology to immunoglobulin and mucin-like adhesion receptors and to IgA1. *Nature* 1993;363:461–464.

38. Koizumi M, King N, Lobb R, Benjamin C, Podolsky DK. Expression of vascular adhesion molecules in inflammatory bowel disease. *Gastroenterology* 1992;103:840–847.

39. Nakamura S, Ohtani H, Watanabe Y, et al. In situ expression of the cell adhesion molecules in inflammatory bowel disease. Evidence of immunologic activation of vascular endothelial cells. *Lab Invest* 1993;69:77–85.

40. Brandtzaeg P, Valnes K, Scott H, Rognum TO, Bjerke K, Baklein K. The human gastrointestinal secretory immune system in health and disease. *Scand J Gastroent* 1985;20:17–38.

41. Mattioli CA, Tomasi TBJ. The life span of IgA plasma cells from the mouse intestine. *J Exp Med* 1973;138:452–460.

42. Lebman DA, Lee FD, Coffman RL. Mechanism for transforming growth factor beta and IL-2 enhancement of IgA expression in lipopolysaccharide-stimulated B cell cultures. *J Immunol* 1990;144:952–959.

43. Banchereau J, de Paoli P, Valle A, Garcia E, Roussett F. Long-term human B cell lines dependent on interleukin-4 and antibody to CD40. *Science* 1991;251:70–72.

44. Beagley KW, Elson CO. Cells and cytokines in mucosal immunity and inflammation. *Gastroenterol Clin North Am* 1992;21:347–66.

45. Bull DM, Bookman MA. Isolation and functional characterization of human intestinal mucosal lymphoid cells. *J Clin Invest* 1979;59:966–974.

46. Goodacre R, Davidson R, Singal D, Bienenstock J. Morphologic and functional characteristics of human intestinal lymphoid cells isolated by a mechanical technique. *Gastroenterology* 1979;76:300–308.

47. Fiocchi C, Battisto JR, Farmer RG. Gut mucosal lymphocytes in inflammatory bowel disease: isolation and preliminary functional characterization. *Dig Dis Sci* 1979;24:705–717.

48. Eade OE, Andre-Ukens SS, Moulton C, MacPherson J, Beeken WL. Lymphocyte subpopulations of intestinal mucosa in inflammatory bowel disease. *Gut* 1980;21:675–682.

49. Fox CC, Dvorak AM, Peters SP, Kagey-Sobotka A, Lichtenstein LM. Isolation and characterization of human intestinal mucosal mast cells. *J Immunol* 1985;135:483–491.

50. MacDermott RP, Franklin GO, Jenkins KM, Kodner IJ, Nash GS, Weinrib IJ. Human intestinal mononuclear cells. I. Investigation of antibody-dependent, lectin-induced, and spontaneous cell-mediated cytotoxic capabilities. *Gastroenterology* 1980;78:47–56.

51. Targan S, Britvan L, Kendal R, Vimadalal S, Soll A. Isolation of spontaneous and interferon inducible natural killer like cells from human colonic mucosa: lysis of lymphoid and autologous epithelial target cells. *Clin Exp Immunol* 1983;54:14–22.

52. Hogan PG, Hapel AJ, Doe WF. Lymphokine-activated and natural killer cell activity in human intestinal mucosa. *J Immunol* 1985;135:1731–1738.

53. James SP. Mucosal T-cell function. *Gastroenterol Clin N Am* 1992;20:597–612.

54. Zeitz M, Quinn TC, Graeff AS, James SP. Mucosal T cells provide helper function but do not proliferate when stimulated by specific antigen in lymphogranuloma venereum proctitis in nonhuman primates. *Gastroenterology* 1988;94:353–366.

55. Qiao L, Schurmann G, Betzler M, Meuer SC. Activation and signaling status of human lamina propria T lymphocytes. *Gastroenterology* 1991;101:1529–1536.

56. Qiao L, Schurmann G, Autschbach F, Wallich R. Human intestinal mucosa alters T-cell reactivities. *Gastroenterology* 1993;105:814–819.

57. Shanahan F, Brogan M, Targan S. Human mucosal cytotoxic effector cells. *Gastroenterology* 1987;92:1951–7.

58. Ferguson A. Intraepithelial lymphocytes of the small intestine. *Gut* 1977;18:921–937.

59. Marsh MN. Functional and structural aspects of the epithelial lymphocyte, with implications for coeliac disease and tropical sprue. *Scand J Gastroenterol* 1985;20:55–75.

60. Ernst PB, Befus AD, Bienenstock J. Leukocytes in the intestinal epithelium: an unusual immunological compartment. *Immunol Today* 1985;6:50–55.

61. Cerf-Bensussan N, Guy-Grand D. Intestinal intraepithelial lymphocytes. *Gastroenterol Clin North Am* 1992;21:549–576.

62. Blumberg RS, Yockey C, Balk SP. Oligoclonal expansion of human intestinal alpha-beta T lymphocytes in epithelium and lamina propria. *Gastroenterology* 1992;102:A597.

63. Beagley KW, Fujihashi K, Lagoo AS, Elson CO. Regional differences in mucosal lymphoid cells of murine small vs. large bowel. *Gastroenterology* 1992;102:A593.

64. Guy-Grand D, Griscelli C, Vassalli P. The mouse gut T lymphocyte, a novel type of T cell. Nature, origin, and traffic in mice in normal and graft-versus-host conditions. *J Exp Med* 1978;148:1661–1667.

65. Cerf-Bensussan N, Guy-Grand D, Griscelli C. Intraepithelial lymphocytes of human gut: isolation, characterization and study of natural killer activity. *Gut* 1985;26:81–88.

66. Ferguson A. Why study T cell subsets in Crohn's disease? *Gut* 1983;24:687–691.

67. Cerf-Bensussan N, Quaroni A, Kurnick JT, Bhan AK. Intraepithelial lymphocytes modulate Ia expression by intestinal epithelial cells. *J Immunol* 1984;132:2244–2252.

68. Ahnen DJ, Brown WR, Kloppel TM. Secretory component: the polymeric immunoglobulin receptor. What's in it for the gastroenterologist and hepatologist? *Gastroenterology* 1985;89:667–682.

69. Mestecky J, Lue C, Russell MW. Selective transport of IgA. Cellular and molecular aspects. *Gastroenterol Clin North Am* 1991;20:441–471.

70. Brandtzaeg P, Krajci P, Lamm ME, Kaetzel CS. Epithelial and hepatobiliary transport of polymeric immunoglobulins. In: Ogra PL, Mestecky J, Lamm ME, Strober W, McGhee JR, Bienenstock J, ed. *Handbook of mucosal immunology.* San Diego: Academic Press; 1994:113–123.

71. Mostov KE, Friedlander M, Blobel G. The receptor for transepithelial transport of IgA and IgM contains multiple immunoglobulin-like domains. *Nature* 1984;308:37–43.

72. Eiffert H, Quentin E, Wiederhold M, et al. Determination of the molecular structure of the human free secretory component. *Hoppe-Seyler's Z. Biol Chem* 1991;372:119–128.

73. Crago SS, Kutteh WH, Moro I, et al. Distribution of IgA1-, IgA2-, and J chain-containing cells in human tissues. *J Immunol* 1984;132:16–18.

74. Kett K, Brandtzaeg P, Radl J, Haaijman JF. Different subclass distribution of IgA-producing cells in human lymphoid organs and various secretory tissues. *J Immunol* 1986;136:3631–3635.

75. Mestecky J, Lue C, Tarkowski A, et al. Comparative studies of the biological properties of human IgA subclasses. *Protides Biol Fluids* 1989;36:173–182.

76. Kilian M, Russell MW. Function of mucosal immunoglobulins. In: Ogra PL, Mestecky J, Lamm ME, Strober W, McGhee JR, Bienenstock J, ed. *Handbook of mucosal immunology.* San Diego: Academic Press, 1994;127–140.

77. Lemaitre-Coelho I, Jackson GDF, Vaerman JP. Relevance of biliary IgA antibodies in rat intestinal immunity. *Scand J Immunol* 1978;8:459–463.

78. Jackson GDF, Lemaitre Coelho I, Vaerman JP, Bazin H, Beckers A. Rapid disappearance from serum of intravenously injected rat myeloma IgA and its secretion into bile. *Eur J Immunol* 1978;8:123–130.

79. Peppard J, Orlans E, Payne AWR, Andrew E. The elimination of circulating complexes containing polymeric IgA by excretion into the bile. *Immunology* 1981;42:83–89.

80. Russell MW, Brown TA, Mestecky J. Role of serum IgA. Hepatobiliary transport of circulating antigens. *J Exp Med* 1981;153:968.

81. Delacroix DL, Hodgson HJF, McPherson A, Dive C, Vaerman J-P. Selective transport of polymeric immunoglobulin A in bile. *J Clin Invest* 1982;70:230.

82. Smith PD, Nagura H, Nakane PK, Brown WR. IgA in human hepatic bile and liver. *J Immunol* 1981;80:1476–1480.

83. Brown WR. Ultrastructural studies on the translocation of polymeric immunoglobulins by intestinal epithelium and liver. In: Strober W, Hanson LA, Sell KW, ed. *Recent advances in mucosal immunity.* New York: Raven Press; 1982:251–266.

84. Koyama SY, Podolsky DK. Differential expression of trans-

forming growth factors alpha and beta in rat intestinal epithelial cells. *J Clin Invest* 1989;83:1768–1773.

85. McGee DW, Beagley KW, Aicher WK, McGhee JR. Transforming growth factor-beta enhanced interleukin-6 secretion by intestinal epithelial cells. *Immunology* 1992;77:7–12.

86. McGee DW, Elson CO, McGhee JR. Enhancing effect of cholera toxin on interleukin-6 secretion by IEC-6 intestinal epithelial cells: mode of action and augmenting effect of inflammatory cytokines. *Infect Immun* 1993;61:4637–4644.

87. Eckmann L, Kagnoff MF, Fierer J. Epithelial cells secrete the chemokine interleukin-8 in response to bacterial entry. *Infect Immun* 1993;61:4569–4674.

88. Salomon P, Pizzimenti A, Panja A, Reisman A, Mayer L. The expression and regulation of class II antigens in normal and inflammatory bowel disease peripheral blood monocytes and intestinal epithelium. *Autoimmunity* 1991;9:141–149.

89. Bland PW, Kambarage DM. Antigen handling by the epithelium and lamina propria macrophages. *Gastroenterol Clin North Am* 1991;20:577–596.

90. Sanderson IR, Ouellette AJ, Carter EA, Walker WA, Harmatz PR. Differential regulation of B7 mRNA in enterocytes and lymphoid cells. *Immunology* 1993;79:434–438.

91. Mosley RL, Styre D, Klein JR. Differentiation and functional maturation of bone marrow-derived intestinal epithelial T cells expressing membrane T cell receptor in athymic radiation chimeras. *J Immunol* 1990;145:1369–1375.

92. Stead RH. Innervation of mucosal immune cells in the gastrointestinal tract. *Reg Immunol* 1992;4:91–99.

93. Elson CO. Induction and control of the gastrointestinal immune system. *Scand J Gastroenterol* 1985;Suppl.114:1–15.

94. Mosmann TR, Coffman RL. Th1 and Th2 cells: different patterns of lymphokine secretion lead to different functional properties. *Annu Rev Immunol* 1989;7:145–174.

95. Heinzel F, Sadick M, Holoday B, Coffman R, Locksley R. Reciprocal expression of interferon gamma or interleukin 4 during the resolution or progression of murine leischmaniasis. Evidence for expansion of distinct helper T cell subsets. *J Exp Med* 1989;169:59–72.

96. Xu-Amano J, Jackson RJ, Staats HF, et al. Helper T cell subsets for IgA responses. Oral immunization with tetanus toxoid and cholera toxin as adjuvant selectively induces Th2 cells in mucosa-associated tissues. *J Exp Med* 1993;178:1309–1320.

97. Kuhn R, Lohler J, Rennick D, Rajewsky K, Muller W. Interleukin-10–deficient mice develop chronic enterocolitis. *Cell* 1993; 75:263–274.

98. Sadlack B, Merz H, Schorle H, Schimpl A, Feller AC, Horak I. Ulcerative colitis-like disease in mice with a disrupted interleukin-2 gene. *Cell* 1993;75:253–261.

99. Romagnani S. Lymphokine production by human T cells in disease states. *Annu Rev Immunol* 1994;12:227–258.

100. Michalek SM, McGhee JR, Kiyono H, et al. The IgA response: inductive aspects, regulatory cells, and effector functions. *Ann N Y Acad Sci* 1983;409:48–69.

101. Mattingly JA, Eardley DD, Kemp JD, Gershon RK. Induction of suppressor cells in rat spleen: influence of microbial stimulation. *J Immunol* 1979;122:787–790.

102. Miller A, Lider O, Roberts AB, Sporn MB, Weiner HL. Suppressor T cells generated by oral tolerization to myelin basic protein suppress both in vitro and in vivo immune responses by the release of transforming growth factor beta after antigen-specific triggering. *Proc Natl Acad Sci USA* 1992;89:421–425.

103. Burstein HJ, Abbas AK. In vivo role of interleukin 4 in T cell tolerance induced by aqueous protein antigen. *J Exp Med* 1993; 177:457–463.

104. Husby S, Mestecky J, Moldoveanu Z, Holland S, Elson CO. Oral tolerance in humans. T cell but not B cell tolerance after antigen feeding. *J Immunol* 1994;152:4663–4670.

105. Khoury SJ, Lider O, Al-Sabbagh A, Weiner HL. Suppression of experimental autoimmune encephalomyelitis by oral administration of myelin basic protein. III. Synergistic effect of lipopolysaccharide. *Cell Immunol* 1990;131:302–10.

106. Dertzbaugh MT, Elson CO. Comparative effectiveness of the cholera toxin B subunit and alkaline phosphatase as carriers for oral vaccines. *Infect Immun* 1993;61:48–55.

Infections of the Gastrointestinal Tract,
edited by M. J. Blaser, P. D. Smith, J. I. Ravdin,
H. B. Greenberg, and R. L. Guerrant
Raven Press, Ltd., New York © 1995.

CHAPTER 11

M Cells and Microbial Pathogens

Marian R. Neutra, Paul J. Giannasca, Karen T. Giannasca,
and Jean-Pierre Kraehenbuhl

Over the immense surface area of the intestinal mucosa, luminal microorganisms are generally excluded from close contact with epithelial cell surfaces by the interplay of mucous and fluid secretions, secretory antibodies, peristaltic movements, and other defense mechanisms. The epithelial layer of the entire intestine is sealed by continuous tight junctions that permit charge-selective passage of certain ions, water, and some small organic molecules, but effectively exclude peptides, macromolecules, and microorganisms (1). The major cell type responsible for maintaining this crucial epithelial barrier, the absorptive cell or enterocyte, is well equipped to face the microorganism-rich environment of the lumen. Apical plasma membranes of enterocytes are highly differentiated structures that exclude most bacteria and viruses by means of rigid, closely packed microvilli (2) coated with an array of highly glycosylated, stalked glycoprotein enzymes (3) and a thick layer of membrane-associated glycoconjugates called the glycocalyx (4,5). This coat serves as a diffusion barrier that prevents contact of most microorganisms with integral components of the enterocyte plasma membrane and impedes access to the small intermicrovillus membrane domains involved in endocytosis (6).

For effective immune surveillance of potential pathogens and antigens in the intestinal lumen, antigens and microorganisms must be transported across the epithelial barrier of the intestine to cells of the mucosal immune system. Although such transport activity would seem to carry the risk of mucosal and systemic infection, the risk is apparently minimized by restriction of transport to specific sites in the mucosa that are organized for this purpose. Organized mucosal lymphoid tissues consist of cells equipped for phagocytosis, intracellular digestion, antigen

presentation, and induction of mucosal immune responses (7–9). Transepithelial transport of antigens and microorganisms into these "inductive" sites is accomplished by a distinct and relatively rare epithelial cell type, the M cell (10) (Fig. 1). The apical surfaces of M cells, unlike that of enterocytes, tend to allow close contact and adherence of particles and microorganisms while the basal surfaces of M cells interact in a unique fashion with cells of the mucosal immune system.

M CELLS: ROLE IN TRANSEPITHELIAL TRANSPORT OF ANTIGENS

Differentiation of M Cells

The cellular epithelial barrier lining the intestine is organized around crypts, the centers of cell proliferation. A small clonal group of stationary, undifferentiated cells located near the base of each crypt proliferates to produce daughter cells that give rise to several distinct cell phenotypes that migrate upward in orderly columns onto the surrounding villi (11). At sites of organized mucosal lymphoid tissue such as Peyer's patches, a ring of crypts surrounds each lymphoid follicle so that a typical crypt adjacent to a follicle contributes cells to a villus on one side and to the dome-shaped follicle-associated epithelium (FAE) on the other. Even deep in the crypt, the epithelium on the wall facing the follicle shows features that distinguish it from the common absorptive epithelium, such as a total lack of polymeric immunoglobulin receptors (12), and as these cells migrate up onto the dome epithelium, they differentiate to become M cells and follicle-associated absorptive cells (13). On the other wall of the same crypt, the conventional pattern of differentiation is seen with goblet cells and typical absorptive enterocytes bearing polymeric immunoglobulin receptors. Thymidine labeling studies indicate that M cells, like other intestinal epithelial cell types, arise from crypt stem cells,

M. R. Neutra, P. J. Giannasca, and K. T. Giannasca: Department of Pediatrics, Harvard Medical School and GI Cell Biology Laboratory, Children's Hospital, Boston, Massachusetts 02115.

J.-P. Kraehenbuhl: Swiss Institute for Experimental Cancer Research and Institute of Biochemistry, University of Lausanne, CH-1066 Epalinges, Switzerland.

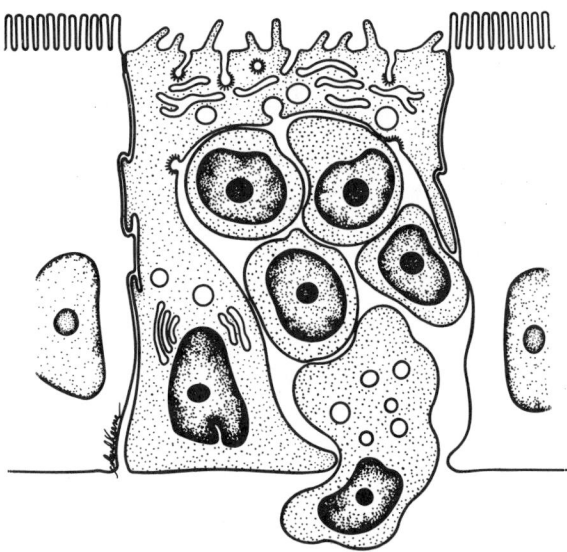

FIG. 1. Diagram of an M cell. The M-cell basolateral surface is modified to form an intraepithelial pocket into which lymphocytes and macrophages migrate. Antigens, microorganisms, and particles that adhere to the M-cell apical membrane are efficiently endocytosed and transported into the pocket, and hence to the underlying mucosal lymphoid tissue. (From ref. 55, with permission.)

migrate onto domes, and are sloughed into the lumen within a few days (13).

The distribution of M cells in the FAE varies. M cells are distributed over the entire dome in mouse and rabbit Peyer's patches (14–16) but are concentrated on the lateral dome margins in Peyer's patches of humans (17). The FAE shows other distinct features such as a relative lack of mucus-secreting goblet cells, and absorptive cells with atypical features (15,18). Lectin-binding studies in rabbits have revealed that M cells in the cecum (but not in Peyer's patches) have membrane glycoconjugates distinct from those of adjacent enterocytes (18). In some strains of mice, membranes of M cells in Peyer's patches are distinguished from enterocytes by specific lectin binding sites (19,20). We have observed that cell type–specific oligosaccharides appear on mouse M-cell apical and basolateral plasma membranes at an early stage of differentiation, deep in the follicle-associated crypts (21) (Fig. 2). This marker allows identification of cells committed to the M-cell phenotype prior to formation of the intraepithelial pocket or association with intraepithelial lymphocytes. Endocytosis is initiated as the immature M cells emerge from the crypts and shortly thereafter the lymphocyte-containing pocket appears (13).

The association of this unique epithelium with organized lymphoid tissue suggests that factors or cell contacts arising from the cells of the underlying lymphoid follicle induce the commitment of adjacent crypt cells to specific differentiation pathways. This hypothesis is consistent with the appearance of new FAE with M cells that accompanies the increase in mucosal lymphoid follicles observed after exposure of germ-free mice to a conventional environment (22) and after mucosal *Salmonella* infection

(23). This idea was recently supported by studies in immunodeficient (SCID) mice that apparently lack mucosal lymphoid follicles and have no detectable M cells. Injection of Peyer's patch cells from normal mice resulted in formation of new mucosal lymphoid follicles in the SCID mice, and this was accompanied by appearance of dome epithelia with M cells (T. Savidge, and M. Smith, *personal communication*). It is also possible, however, that local transport of antigens by a subpopulation of epithelial cells, perhaps reflecting local epithelial specializations or pre-M cells, determines the site of assembly of organized follicles in the mucosa. In humans, Peyer's patches appear before birth (24).

An important limitation in studies of M-cell biology is the lack of an *in vitro* culture system in which M-cell differentiation and function is maintained. Development of M-cell cultures may require a coculture system in which both appropriate epithelial precursors and lymphoid cells or their products are present.

The likelihood that a luminal microorganism will come into contact with an M-cell surface is determined in part by its motility and tropism, but also by intrinsic host factors such as the distribution and frequency of mucosal follicles, the microanatomy of the follicles, and the frequency of M cells in each FAE. All three parameters vary widely among species and in different intestinal regions. In mice, for example, patches of aggregated follicles are distributed throughout the small intestine and also occur in the cecum, colon, and rectum (15,25,26). In humans, large lymphoid follicle aggregates (Peyer's patches) are restricted to the ileum, but isolated lymphoid follicles occur throughout the large intestine with highest frequency in the rectum (27–30). In both mice and humans, small intestinal FAE is visible from the lumen as domes covering mucosal follicles (25) whereas the FAE in distal large intestine is sometimes sequestered at the base of a crypt-like epithelial invagination to form a "lymphoglandular complex" with a follicle deep in the mucosa (26,28,31). M cell numbers in the FAE vary widely: while they represent only about 10% of the FAE in mice, they comprise 50% of the FAE in rabbit Peyer's patch and appendix, often alternating with other cells (14) (Fig. 3). In humans, 10% or less of ileal FAE cells are M cells, and these tend to lie on the lateral margins of the dome epithelium (17). These characteristics influence the choice of species and mucosal site for studies of microbial–M-cell interactions. Many M-cell studies have used rabbit Peyer's patch or appendix, where M cells are relatively abundant. Extrapolation of such data to human M cells must be made with caution.

It should be emphasized that the proportion of the intestinal mucosa represented by FAE is extremely small, however, and M cells represent a tiny fraction of the epithelial surface area. The fact that microbial pathogens use M cells as entry points underscores the specificity of these microbial–host cell interactions.

Structural Organization of M Cells: Membrane Domains and Cytoskeleton

M cells form tight junctions with their epithelial neighbors that prevent paracellular passage of macromolecules

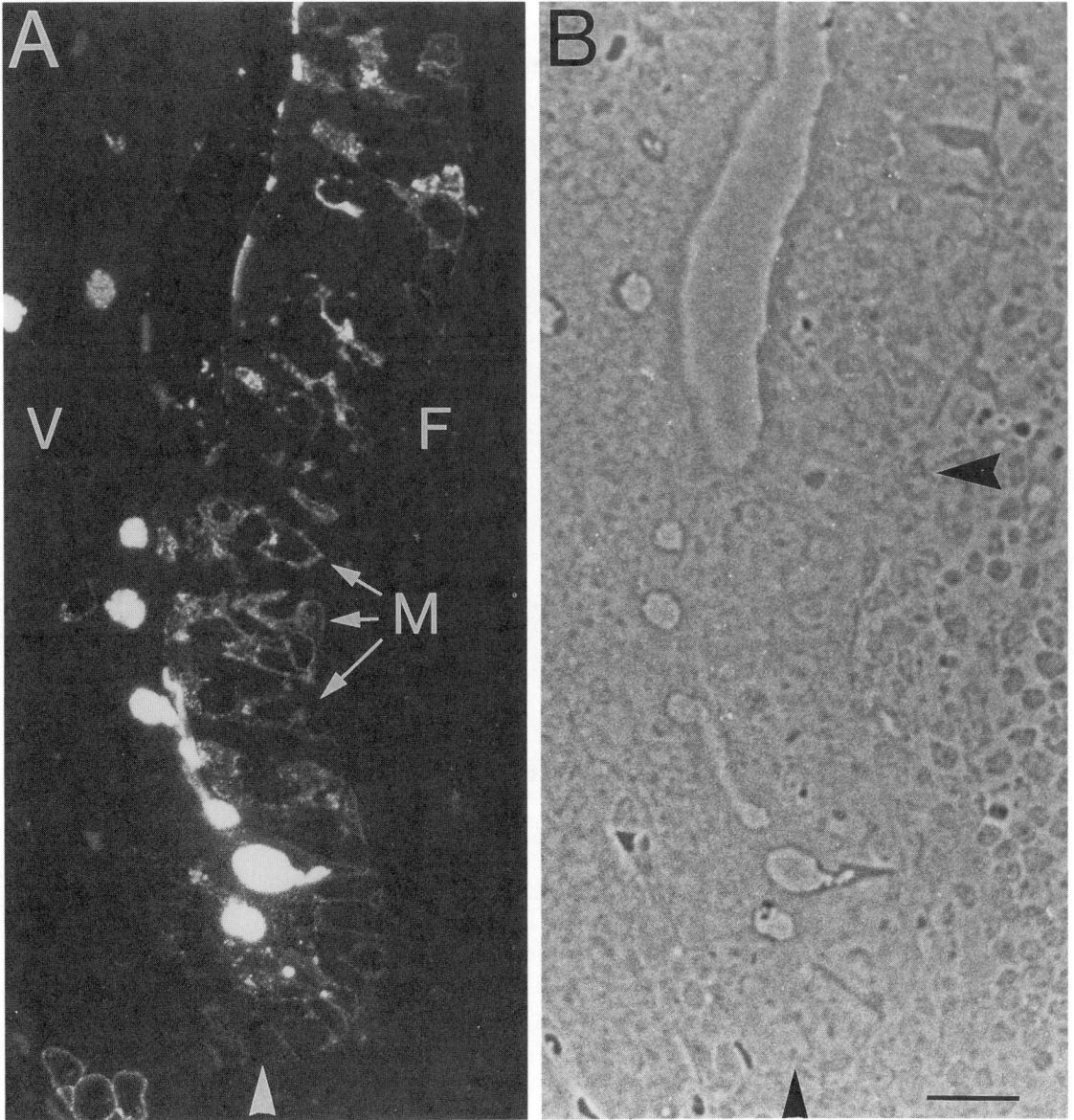

FIG. 2. Follicle-associated crypt epithelium from mouse Peyer's patch. Half-micrometer section stained with *Ulex europaeus* I lectin and visualized by fluorescence (**A**) and phase contrast microscopy (**B**). This crypt provides cells to the epithelium covering a villus (V, *on the left*) and a lymphoid follicle (F, *on the right*). Arrowheads mark the base of the crypt and the crypt–villus junction. Undifferentiated cells at the base of the crypt and cells committed to the M-cell phenotype (M) bind this lectin, but enterocytes destined for the villus do not. Goblet cells, enteroendocrine cells, and Paneth cells in adjacent crypts are also stained. Bar = 20 μm.

(32,33) but they have developed an unusual vesicular transport pathway (34,35). The basolateral cell surface is modified by a deep invagination that forms a large intraepithelial pocket lined by a distinct domain of the plasma membrane. The composition of this "pocket" domain has not been explored, but it clearly differs from either basal or lateral membrane domains in its relative lack of Na,K-ATPase (36) and in its ability to form close interaction sites with intraepithelial lymphocytes that migrate into the pocket. The unusual shape of the mature M cell appears to be supported by a dense network of intermediate fila-

ments (IFs) that surrounds the nucleus and courses through the cytoplasm around the pocket (36). In rabbits (but not in the other species examined so far) these filaments contain vimentin, an IF protein not found in other normal intestinal epithelial cell types, in addition to conventional epithelial cytokeratins (37,38). Although vimentin provides a convenient marker for normal rabbit M cells, it should be noted that epithelial cells can express vimentin in regenerating tissue, in neoplasia, and in culture (39,40).

Apical membranes of M cells in Peyer's patches show

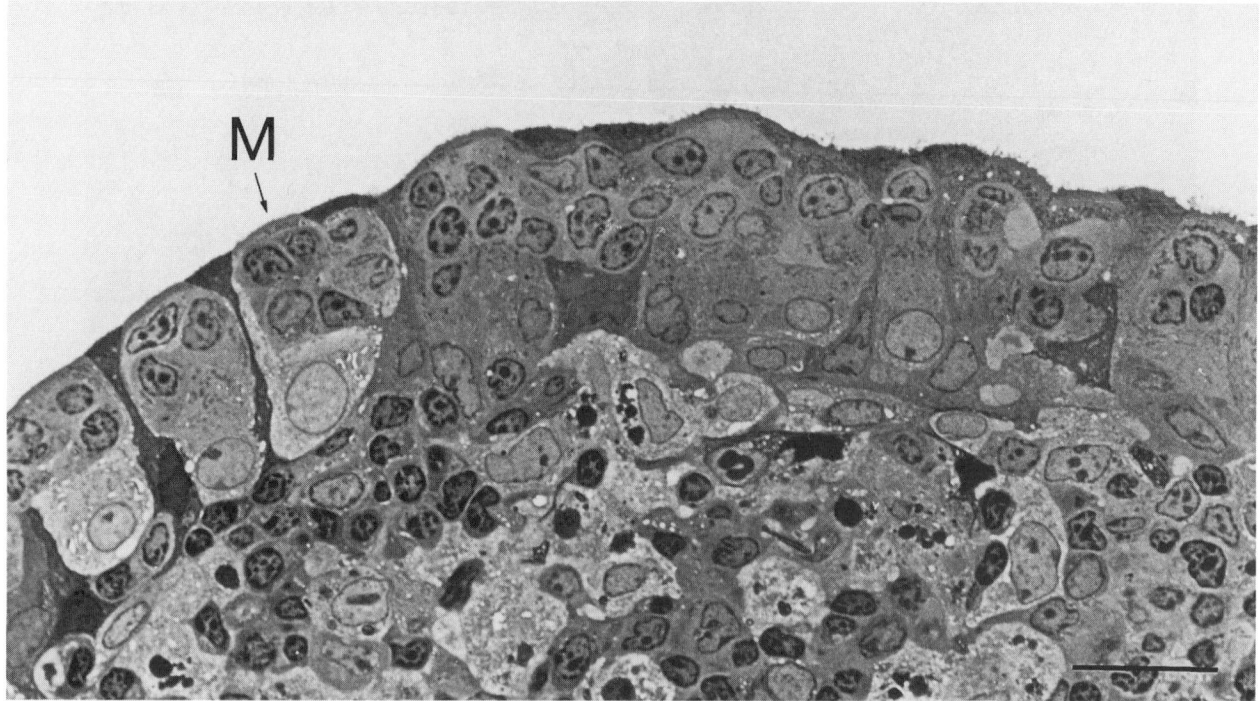

FIG. 3. Follicle-associated epithelium of rabbit appendix. The epithelium contains numerous M cells (M). Large, pale M-cell nuclei lie at the base of the cells, while densely staining lymphocyte nuclei are seen in the intraepithelial pockets. A variety of macrophages, lymphocytes, and other cells lie under the epithelium. Bar = 20 μm.

distinct features that have been used as identification markers. While enterocyte brush borders have abundant alkaline phosphatase, this enzyme is often reduced or absent on M cells (41,42). The apical cell surfaces of most M cells in Peyer's patches have fewer microvilli than absorptive cells, and may instead have branching microfolds (hence the name "M" cell; 43). M-cell apical surface features vary widely, however; short, closely packed microvilli may be present in Peyer's patch M cells (44) and rabbit cecal M cells have long, closely packed microvilli with high alkaline phosphatase activity (18). The cytoskeletal elements present in the M-cell apex are similar to those of absorptive cells in that microvilli and microfolds are supported by central actin bundles, and an actin ring is associated with the adherens junction that encircles the cell apex (32). Segmented bacteria that inhabit the rodent intestine can induce attachment sites on apical surfaces of either enterocytes or M cells, and in both cell types these sites are rimmed with submembrane assemblies of actin (45). However, the actin-associated proteins present in M cells are not yet fully defined. Such information will be useful for analyzing the intracellular events involved in the interactions of various microorganisms with M cells.

Adherence of Macromolecules, Antigens, and Particles to M-Cell Apical Membranes

M-cell transport may be a crucial first step in microbial infection as well as induction of secretory immune re-sponses. The factors that influence this transport are thus of great interest for understanding the mechanisms of microbial invasion and for design of mucosal immunization strategies (10). As in all cells, macromolecules or particles that can adhere to the apical plasma membranes of M cells are endocytosed or phagocytosed most efficiently. Double-tracer studies using rabbit Peyer's patches demonstrated that a lectin-ferritin conjugate that adhered to M cells was transcytosed at least 50 times more efficiently than a nonadherent bovine serum albumin (BSA) tracer (44). Thus identification of potential receptors for macromolecules and microorganisms on M cells is of great interest. However, there is very little information available concerning the molecular composition of M-cell surfaces. Early studies using nonadherent tracer proteins (native ferritin and horseradish peroxidase) demonstrated endocytosis, transcytosis, and delivery of soluble luminal material into the intraepithelial pocket (34,35). Later, cationized ferritin, a large (500-kDa) multivalent, positively charged protein, was shown to be endocytosed and transported very efficiently due to its ability to bind to anionic sites on M-cell surfaces (13,41,44). Polystyrene or latex beads also adhered to M cells and were transported into Peyer's patch mucosa (46,47). These observations suggested that particles or microorganisms with either hydrophobic or positively charged surfaces could interact with M-cell surfaces via relatively nonselective adherence mechanisms. The same particles would also interact with mucus and the glycocalyx of enterocytes on villi, however, and this would tend to reduce the efficiency of M-cell uptake.

Special fixation and lectin binding techniques have shown that M-cell apical membranes display abundant glycoconjugates that could potentially serve as binding sites for lectin-like microbial surface molecules (13,18,44). The use of lectins in studies of rabbit Peyer's patches failed to reveal carbohydrate sites unique to M-cell surfaces (18,44), but M-cell membrane glycoconjugates in other intestinal regions and other species do contain distinct lectin binding sites (19–21) and these may be important determinants in selective M-cell adherence of certain enteric pathogens. Despite evidence for the existence of unique components on M-cell surfaces, however, neither the microbial surface molecules that mediate adherence nor the M-cell surface molecules that serve as receptors have been identified.

The fact that particles and lectins that adhere either selectively or nonselectively to M-cell apical membranes are endocytosed and transcytosed with high efficiency may explain the observation that adherent immunogens tend to evoke strong secretory immune responses (48,49). For example, oral administration of lectins resulted in anti–lectin-specific secretory IgA whereas a comparable oral dose of a nonadherent immunogen, keyhole limpet hemocyanin, was ineffective (48). It has been suggested that inefficient M-cell transport of soluble luminal antigens and nonadherent particles prevents undesirable immune responses to food antigens and the normal intestinal flora (50). Small, repeated oral or inhaled doses of soluble immunogens result in immune tolerance (51), but the relationship between M-cell transport efficiency and either mucosal or systemic tolerance is not yet clear.

It should also be noted that selective adherence alone does not prove the existence of unique membrane receptors on M cells. The M-cell apical surface differs from that of intestinal absorptive cells in the increased accessibility of plasma membrane binding sites and apical membrane endocytic domains to large macromolecules and particulate ligands (44). For example, studies by us and others (52) showed that cholera toxin tagged with fluorescent rhodamine or visualized with immunoperoxidase histochemistry (52) adhered to both M-cell and enterocyte apical surfaces (presumably via the ubiquitous glycolipid receptor GM1), and that higher amounts adhered to the FAE than to villi. Uptake of toxin via M cells into sites of B-cell IgA switch and T-cell helper responses would explain in part the unique effectiveness of cholera toxin as mucosal antigen and adjuvant (52,53). Electron microscopic studies by us and by J. S. Trier and colleagues, however, showed that cholera toxin adsorbed to colloidal gold particles lost the ability to bind to enterocyte brush borders and adhered only to M cells. This observation suggests that large macromolecules and particulate ligands may be prevented by the thick enterocyte glycocalyx from contacting receptors on microvilli, while receptors and endocytic membrane domains are relatively accessible on M cells.

Although the FAE does not participate in receptor-mediated secretion of IgA, secretory IgA in the lumen can adhere selectively to the apical membranes of M cells. This was first observed in suckling rabbits as a local accumulation of milk sIgA on M cells of Peyer's patches and was suggested to play a role in maturation of the mucosal immune system (54). Subsequent studies in our laboratories showed that monoclonal mouse IgA, polyclonal rat sIgA, and polyclonal mouse IgG antibodies, either radiolabeled or coupled to colloidal gold, bound specifically to adult rabbit or mouse M cells and competed with each other for binding sites (55). Furthermore, IgA–antigen complexes adhered to M cells and were transported to the intraepithelial pocket. Binding of immunoglobulins appears not to be mediated by known Fc receptors, since antibodies against various epithelial and macrophage Fc receptors failed to recognize any M-cell component (55).

Regardless of the binding mechanism, it is clear that M cells can take up free sIgA and sIgA–antigen complexes (55) and this would result in repeated uptake of antigen into inductive sites. Antigens complexed with sIgA might be sampled by intraepithelial or subepithelial antigen-presenting cells to boost an existing secretory immune response to pathogens that have not been effectively cleared from the lumen. Reuptake of sIgA could also have other modulatory effects in the mucosal immune system (9). Fc α receptors are present on mucosal mononuclear cells (56) but their function in mucosal inductive sites is not established. The degree to which circulating IgA or IgG antibodies enter organized mucosal lymphoid tissues is not yet clear. An electron microscopic study showed that capillaries in the organized mucosal lymphoid tissue of Peyer's patches are nonfenestrated, and that diffusion of tracer proteins and circulating antibodies into Peyer's patch mucosa was impeded (57). Intravenous injection into adult mice of polyclonal or monoclonal anti–reovirus IgG antibodies failed to prevent entry and replication of virus in Peyer's patches (58). Thus mucosal Fc α receptors could be available for binding of IgA or immune complexes taken up from the lumen of the intestine.

Transepithelial Transport by M Cells

Between the short, irregular microvilli or microfolds on M-cell apical surfaces are many microdomains from which endocytosis occurs (6). M cells take up macromolecules, particles, and microorganisms by any or all of the endocytic mechanisms used by other cell types: adsorptive endocytosis via clathrin-coated pits and vesicles (36), fluid phase endocytosis in either coated (36) or uncoated vesicles (34,35), and phagocytosis involving extension of cellular processes and reorganization of submembrane actin assemblies. All of these uptake mechanisms result in transport of foreign material into a system of endosome-like tubules and vesicles located in the apical cytoplasmic layer above the intraepithelial pocket (36). There are also multivesicular bodies in this part of the cell (36,59). Like the multivesicular "transporting endosomes" or "late endosomes" characterized in many other cell types (60), this compartment in M cells contains the late endosome/lysosome membrane marker lgp 120 (59). Endosomes of most cells generate an acidic internal milieu (61), although specialized apical endosomes of some epithelial cells were recently found to be pH-neutral (62). M-cell apical vesicles accumulate weak bases, indicating that they are acidified, but their intravesicular pH is not determined (59). Some of these structures contain major histocompatibility complex (MHC) class II antigen, but this has been documented only in some species, and in a subpopulation of M cells (59). Endosomes of other cell types contain a subset of lysosomal enzymes (60,63). Immunocytochemical analysis has revealed the presence of an endosomal protease, cathepsin E, in human and rat M cells (64), but the possible presence of other endosomal hydrolases in M-cell transport vesicles has not yet been examined. Thus, it is not yet known as to what extent endocytosed materials are degraded during transepithelial transport or whether M cells participate in the processing and presentation of certain types of antigens. Most viruses and bacteria that are taken up by M cells appear ultrastructurally unaltered during transport but this does not rule out enzymatic processing of surface antigens. Typical dense lysosomes are infrequent in M cells and tend to lie deep in the cell, near the nucleus.

The M cell has shortened its transcytotic pathway by drawing its basolateral membrane up toward the apical surface, and by directing all vesicles derived from endocytosis or phagocytosis directly to the specialized basolateral "pocket" domain. The nature of the pocket subdomain and the mechanisms whereby endosomes are targeted directly to it are important areas for future study. The contents of M-cell vesicles are released by exocytosis at the invaginated pocket membrane as early as 10 min after apical endocytosis. Whether this final segment of the transepithelial transport pathway in M cells involves specialized transcytotic vesicles as in other cell types (65,66) or is accomplished by fusion of apical endosomes directly with the pocket membrane is unknown.

The capacity of an individual M cell for transcytosis is considerable, but its endocytic activity may vary over time. This was demonstrated by introducing nondegradable, fluorescent microspheres into ligated loops of rabbit ileum containing a Peyer's patch (47). The microspheres adhered to M cells and were rapidly and synchronously transcytosed into the intraepithelial pocket. During the following 90 min, however, additional luminal microspheres failed to adhere to M cells, suggesting that the M-cell apical surface had been temporarily depleted of the components necessary for particle adherence. Whether apical membrane molecules are replaced by de novo synthesis or by recycling of membrane from the pocket is not known. These aspects of M-cell biology have not been addressed because M cells have not been cultured as polarized monolayers. M-cell transcytotic activity is not dependent on the presence of lymphocytes in the intraepithelial pocket. Newly differentiated M cells that emerge from the crypts (13), as well as M cells in irradiated animals in which lymphocytes are depleted (67), conduct active endocytosis and transcytosis even though intraepithelial lymphocytes are not present.

M cells can transport immunogens across the epithelium in amounts sufficient to evoke mucosal immune responses. However, organized mucosal lymphoid tissues appear designed to retain macromolecules and microorganisms through efficient uptake by the numerous macrophages and dendritic cells in these sites (68). Thus, although antigens and particles that enter the Peyer's patches are subsequently found in mesenteric lymph nodes, they generally do not enter the circulation. There have been several attempts to measure and compare rates of transcytosis of proteins across Peyer's patch and nonpatch mucosa. While some investigators showed enhanced transport of protein into Peyer's patch (68,69), others did not (70). Such studies have been hampered by the use of tracer proteins of differing size, charge, and adherence properties, and by the complex architecture of the mucosa at these sampling sites. These methods have not been applied to microorganisms. New methods for quantitating the uptake of microorganisms and antigens by M cells and following their fates in the intestinal mucosa are sorely needed.

ROLE OF M CELLS IN SAMPLING ENTERIC MICROORGANISMS

In order to deliver a wide variety of microorganisms and particles to the mucosal immune system, M cells may use both selective and nonselective mechanisms for binding and uptake of luminal materials. It is tempting to think that common recognition mechanisms such as lectin–carbohydrate interactions allow the M cell to "sample" entire subclasses of potentially pathogenic luminal organisms. Such recognition could operate either by binding of a common set of bacterial protein lectins or adhesins to M-cell surface glycoconjugates or, conversely, M-cell surface lectins could recognize bacterial surface oligosaccharides. After transcytosis, bacteria are readily released from the membrane into the intraepithelial pocket. This suggests that initial binding occurs through multiple, low-affinity interaction sites and that the milieu of the transport vesicle or intraepithelial pocket allows rapid dissociation of the bacterium from the M-cell membrane receptors. Efficient transepithelial delivery and release of viruses and inert particles might also depend on multiple, low-affinity interactions with M-cell membrane components.

Due to the lack of stable M-cell culture systems, analysis of microbial–M-cell interactions has been limited to morphological studies. The ultrastructural appearance of various bacterial–M-cell interaction sites suggests that a variety of molecular mechanisms may be at play. Some bacteria form broad areas of very close interaction with M-cell apical membranes. In the case of *Vibrio cholerae*, for example, the bacterial outer membrane and the M-cell apical membrane are separated by a uniform 10- to 20-nm space consistent with participation of integral membrane components on both sides. This interaction induces recruitment and reorganization of M-cell submembrane actin filaments (Fig. 4) and results in an engulfment process that is morphologically similar to phagocytosis by macrophages. Studies of the interaction of *E. coli* with other cell types have shown that bacterial ligands bind to host cell receptors that in turn provide direct or indirect links to the host cell cytoskeleton and signaling machinery (71). In contrast, adherence of *Salmonella* to M-cell apical membranes initially occurs across a wider gap, implying

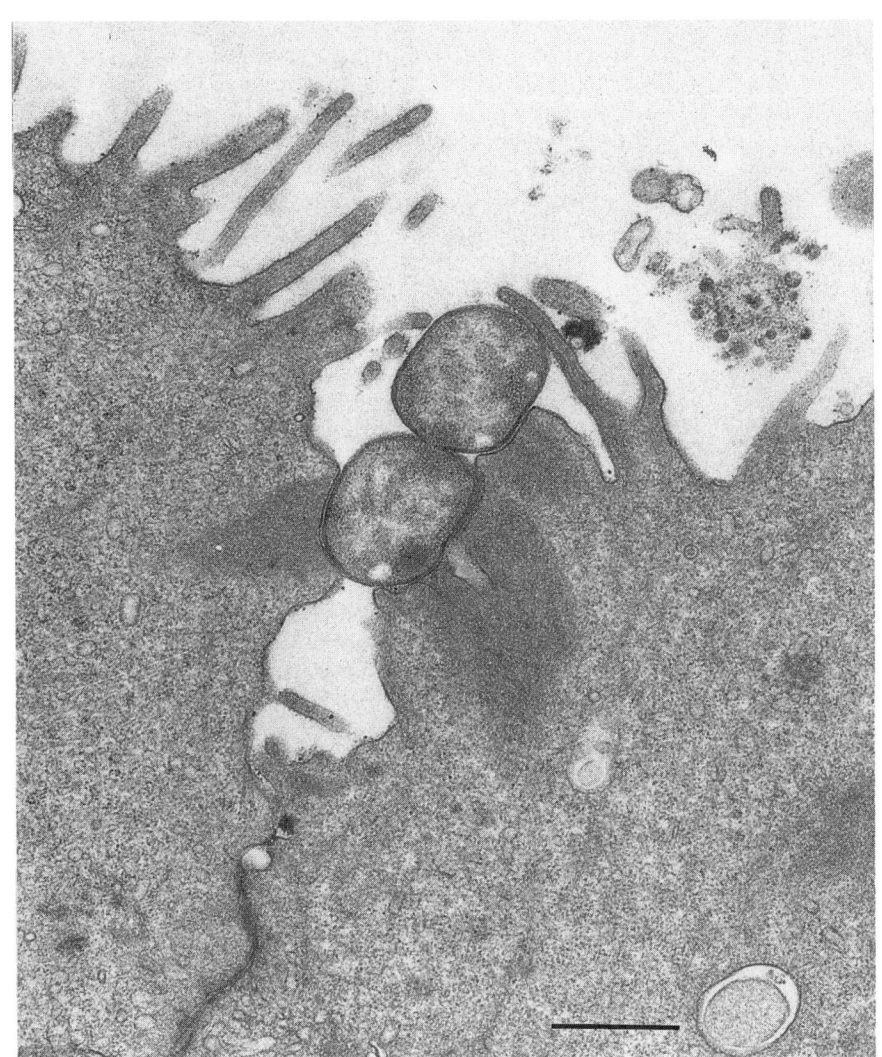

FIG. 4. Interaction of *Vibrio cholerae* with M cells in rabbit Peyer's patch epithelium. After injection into a ligated intestinal loop, *Vibrio cholerae* adhere to the apical surfaces of two adjacent M cells. At sites of bacterial–cell interaction, submembrane filaments (presumably actin) are associated with the M cell membrane. Electron micrograph by Dr. Julie Mack. Bar = 1 μm.

participation of relatively large structures on the bacterial surface and/or peripheral sites in the M-cell glycocalyx. The ensuing engulfment may be accompanied by severe disruption of apical cytoskeletal structures, which are described in more detail below. It is likely that M-cell adherence and uptake of any microorganism involves a sequence of molecular interactions including initial recognition (perhaps via a lectin–carbohydrate interaction) followed by more intimate associations that require recruitment of integral proteins of the M-cell membrane (72).

The role of M cells in mucosal defense is clearest for noninvasive microorganisms that cause disease by colonizing mucosal surfaces, such as *V. cholerae* and certain strains of *E. coli*. M-cell binding and uptake of these bacteria apparently results in efficient sampling by the mucosal immune system and secretion of antimicrobial sIgA antibodies that play a major role in limiting the duration of mucosal disease and preventing reinfection (7,73). However, M cells also bind and transport a wide variety of microorganisms that initiate mucosal and/or systemic disease by invading the intestinal mucosa. In these cases,

M-cell transport and induction of mucosal immunity carries the risk of infection and disease.

Vibrio cholerae

Vibrio cholerae are motile, uniflagellate, gram-negative bacteria that cause severe enterotoxin-induced secretory diarrhea. Within the small intestine, *V. cholerae* express a group of coregulated proteins including adhesins that allow them to adhere to epithelia of the proximal small intestine, pili that stabilize colonies on mucosal surfaces, and cholera toxin that induces secretion of chloride ions from intestinal epithelial cells (73–75). Colonization of the intestine by *V. cholerae* evokes a mucosal immune response in the host, including secretion of IgA antibodies (sIgA) directed against both cholera toxin and bacterial surface components including the outer membrane lipopolysaccharide (LPS) (76,77). Studies in various species, including humans, showed that secretion of IgA is associated with protection against subsequent oral challenge (76–78). Recent work in our laboratories has confirmed that sIgA alone can provide such protection and that M-cell transport plays a key role in the induction of specific IgA lymphoblasts (79–81).

When *V. cholerae* are inoculated into ligated intestinal loops containing Peyer's patches in rabbits or mice and the tissues are examined 30 min to 2 hr later, the bacteria are seen to selectively interact with M cells (79,82). M cells actively participate in the interaction of vibrios in both mice and rabbits, forming areas of close membrane apposition and assembly of local cytoskeletal specializations (Fig. 4). Owen et al. observed that after binding of *V. cholerae*, rabbit M cells formed pseudopod-like cell surface processes surrounding the organisms that were then transported in phagocytic vesicles and released, apparently unaltered, into the M-cell pocket below (82). The binding and uptake of vibrios in rabbits was shown to be dependent on bacterial viability, as M-cell adherence or uptake of *V. cholerae* killed by heat, fixation, acid treatment, or UV irradiation was not observed.

Subsequent studies confirmed that adherence requires live bacteria in the growth phase but does not require live host cells: binding of *V. cholerae* as well as *Vibrio parahemolyticus* to the surfaces of intestinal epithelial cells was demonstrated in formalin-fixed rabbit and human mucosal tissue (83–85). By eliminating the M-cell responses to bacterial binding such as reorganization of apical membrane and cytoskeleton, this approach allowed for identification of conditions required for initial recognition. This method showed that *V. cholerae* adhere to the surfaces of M cells with greater efficiency than to other epithelial cells, implying that M cells constitutively display surface receptors that are either unique or more accessible than those on enterocytes. It is not known whether the same *Vibrio* adhesins that mediate intestinal colonization are involved in M-cell adherence.

Cholera toxin also binds avidly (although not selectively) to M-cell surfaces and is efficiently transported into mucosa-associated lymphoid tissues (52). After mucosal immunization of mice with live, attenuated vibrios or subclinical doses of cholera toxin, colleagues in our laboratory isolated Peyer's patch lymphoblasts, fused them with myeloma cells, and recovered mucosa-derived hybridomas that secreted dimeric IgA antibodies directed against the surface LPS of the bacterial cells (79) and the B subunit of the toxin (80). This directly confirmed that M cell–mediated transport into Peyer's patch mucosa results in generation of antigen-specific IgA lymphoblasts at these local sites (55,86). Secretion of these monoclonal IgA antibodies from "backpack" hybridoma tumors showed that anti-LPS secretory IgA alone can protect against oral *V. cholerae* challenge but antitoxin IgA cannot (79,81). These results are consistent with the results of human cholera vaccine trials (77,78) and underscore the value of vaccines based on live, genetically engineered *V. cholerae* organisms that are capable of interacting with intestinal M cells and inducing anti-LPS IgA (87,88).

E. coli

The vast majority of the many types of *E. coli* found in the intestine do not selectively adhere to epithelial cell surfaces. Certain pathogenic strains do adhere and colonize and/or invade the mucosa, however, and these also interact with M cells. The interaction of two such strains with M cells has been analyzed ultrastructurally, and dramatic differences were observed. Within an hour of inoculation into ligated rabbit appendices, *E. coli* strain O:124 associated with the surfaces of rabbit M cells but did not induce close, organized adherence sites on M-cell surfaces (as seen in RDEC-1, described below). The bacteria were taken up into phagosome-like vesicles and later released into the intraepithelial pocket (89).

In contrast, the rabbit pathogen *E. coli* RDEC-1, which causes diarrheal disease analogous to enteropathogenic *E. coli* (EPEC) in humans, showed a complex interaction with M cells. When RDEC-1 was administered orally to rabbits, the bacteria initially bound preferentially to the surfaces of M cells (90). At early times RDEC-1 associated with peripheral components of the M-cell surface, but later M-cell microvilli/microfolds were effaced and the bacterium formed intimate adherence sites characterized by the presence of submembrane actin assemblies and formation of stable "pedestals" (90) similar to those observed at later times on absorptive enterocytes (91). Such adherence of RDEC-1 to M cells did not result in bacterial uptake. RDEC-1 is able to colonize the surface of the follicle-associated epithelium for up to 14 days postinfection (92). Thus, RDEC-1 appears to use a common mechanism to colonize enterocyte surfaces and to avoid being taken up by M cells. This strategy would avert a mucosal immune response and clearance by secretory antibodies, or an acute inflammatory response and eradication by other immune processes. The genes in EPEC that are involved in the induction of novel enterocyte apical surface structures have been extensively characterized (94,95) and analogous genes present in RDEC-1 are presumably relevant to the interaction of RDEC-1 with M cells.

Pili appear to play a role in initial adherence of RDEC-1 to M cells, since a nonadherent strain of *Shigella flexneri* engineered to express RDEC-1 pili adhered preferentially to M cells (93). These organisms did not induce pedestal formation but instead were phagocytosed and transported to the lamina propria. Thus, pilus-mediated adherence to M cells is not sufficient to induce new M-cell cytoskeletal structures but is sufficient to trigger phagocytosis and transepithelial transport.

Cryptosporidium

Cryptosporidium is a parasitic unicellular organism that causes diseases of the gastrointestinal, biliary, and respiratory epithelia in many hosts, including man (97). Although often believed to affect only immunocompromised patients such as those with AIDS, other studies suggest that *Cryptosporidium* may cause 1–10% of all cases of diarrhea in the normal population (98). Cryptosporidial organisms form a unique, intimate association with the apical surfaces of absorptive enterocytes that involves a complex series of events including deformation of microvilli and formation of a large, stable, phagosome-like compartment at the apical cell surface (99). Host cell cytoskeletal elements are recruited to form a dense "plate" under the parasite, which then uses host cell cytoplasmic nutrients to fuel its maturation and replication. *Cryptosporidium* apparently does not invade the mucosa beyond the apex of absorptive cells, but it is taken up by M cells. A spontaneous cryptosporidial infection in guinea pigs revealed organisms in the cytoplasm of M cells and within macrophages subjacent to M cells (99), but M cells did not form the specialized apical structures seen on absorptive cells. Thus, this organism mobilizes entirely different sets of intracellular machinery in the two epithelial cell types.

The role of M-cell uptake in the clearance of *Cryptosporidium* is not established, but the fact that cryptosporidiosis is self-limiting in immunocompetent humans suggests that uptake leads to a mucosal immune response that may prevent continued spread of organisms to new epithelial cells emerging from the crypts. To date, *Cryptosporidium* is the only protozoan for which M-cell transport has been directly documented, although *Giardia muris* was observed in phagocytic cells within Peyer's patches (100) and presumably entered via this route as well.

INVASION OF PATHOGENIC BACTERIA VIA M CELLS

Salmonella

Salmonella strains are responsible for both systemic and mucosal diseases in many host species. In humans, *S. typhi* causes typhoid fever while *S. typhimurium* is responsible for localized gastroenteritis commonly associated with food poisoning. However, infection of mice with *S. typhimurium* results in a lethal systemic typhoid-like disease that has provided researchers with a valuable animal model for human typhoid fever (101). The pathogenesis of *S. typhimurium* in mice following ingestion of bacteria involves development of initial foci of infection in small intestinal Peyer's patches (102,103). *Salmonella* can also invade directly through the absorptive villus epithelium (104). Subsequent infection of cells of the reticuloendothelial system leads to colonization of liver and spleen and general systemic dissemination.

Salmonella is an organism well equipped for invasion of many cell types. In the intestine it invades enterocytes through a mechanism that involves transient disassembly of microvilli and uptake in membrane-bound vesicles (104). Studies utilizing intestinal cell lines *in vitro* have shown that invasion is accompanied by local cytoplasmic Ca^{2+} spikes, cytoskeletal rearrangements, and membrane ruffling (105,106). The interaction of *Salmonella* with M cells has been studied in mice and rabbits by inoculating bacteria into ligated intestinal loops containing Peyer's patches. Mouse M cells show a dramatic response to *Salmonella* infection. Kohbata et al. (107) observed that within 30 min *S. typhi* selectively adhered to the surfaces of M cells and induced severe ballooning of the M-cell apical surface followed by degeneration and loss of M cells, which allowed the bacteria access to the underlying mucosa. *S. typhimurium* produced similar cytopathic ef-

fects in mice (108). In contrast, we have observed that exposure of rabbit Peyer's patches to *S. typhimurium* resulted in M-cell binding and transcytosis of bacteria without apparent cellular damage (Figs. 5 and 6). The differences in M-cell responses in mouse and rabbit could be due to virulence factors expressed specifically in the mouse gut environment (109) or to endogenous M-cell factors such as species differences in the membrane components used by *Salmonella* for adherence. We have observed in both mice and rabbits that invasion of enterocytes occurs after entry via M cells, perhaps because processing of brush border surface components is required.

The ability of *Salmonella* to adhere to M cells and to target themselves into Peyer's patches has been exploited in the use of attenuated strains as oral vaccines against typhoid fever (87). Genetically engineered *S. typhimurium* strains are currently being developed and tested in numerous laboratories as vectors for expression of foreign antigens in mucosal inductive sites (87,88). One of the challenges in this strategy has been achieving sufficient attenuation while still preserving M-cell adherence and proliferation in the mucosa (110). An additional complication is that secretory IgA directed against *Salmonella* surface components can prevent contact with M cells and entry into Peyer's patches (111) and this would reduce the effectiveness of repeated immunizations using this vector.

Yersinia

Certain *Yersinia* species are capable of invading the intestinal mucosa causing enteritis as well as mesenteric lymphadenitis in mammals. The pathogenic potential of *Yersinia* has been related to several virulence factors but little is known about the mechanism of adherence of *Yersinia* to the intestinal epithelium *in vivo*. Exposure of mouse Peyer's patch tissue in ligated loops to *Y. enterocolitica* resulted in nonselective binding of bacteria to M cells and enterocytes (112). While adherence to enterocytes did not result in invasion of these cells, binding to M cells was followed by uptake and transcytosis. Interestingly, both pathogenic and nonpathogenic strains adhered and were transported similarly. This finding suggests that, in the mouse, capacity to cause disease is related to the ability to survive and proliferate in the lamina propria and not the ability to bind to M cells. Similar studies examining *Y. pseudotuberculosis* interaction with rabbit M cells revealed selective binding of the organisms to M cells followed by their transcytosis (113).

Y. enterocolitica and *Y. pseudotuberculosis* express a protein, invasin, which has been shown to bind to $\beta 1$ integrins on cultured cells and to promote bacterial entry (114). Expression of invasin is also correlated with the ability of *Yersinia* to enter the Peyer's patch mucosa but not with subsequent steps in pathogenesis (115). On epithelial cells, however, $\beta 1$ integrins are present on basolateral and not apical membranes and basolateral localization has also been observed in human intestinal epithelium (116). Although the presence of low levels of integrins on M-cell apical surfaces has not been ruled out, whether

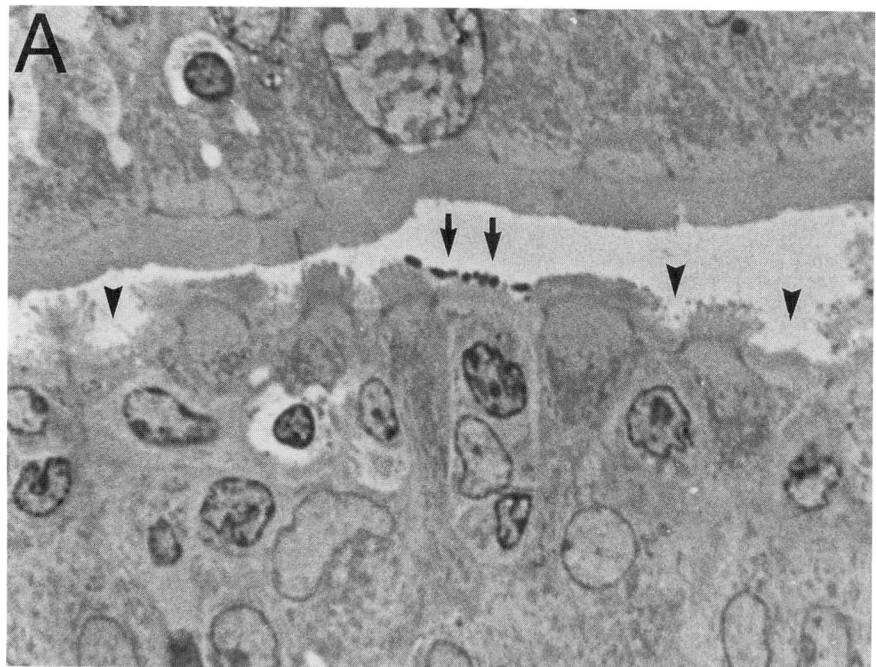

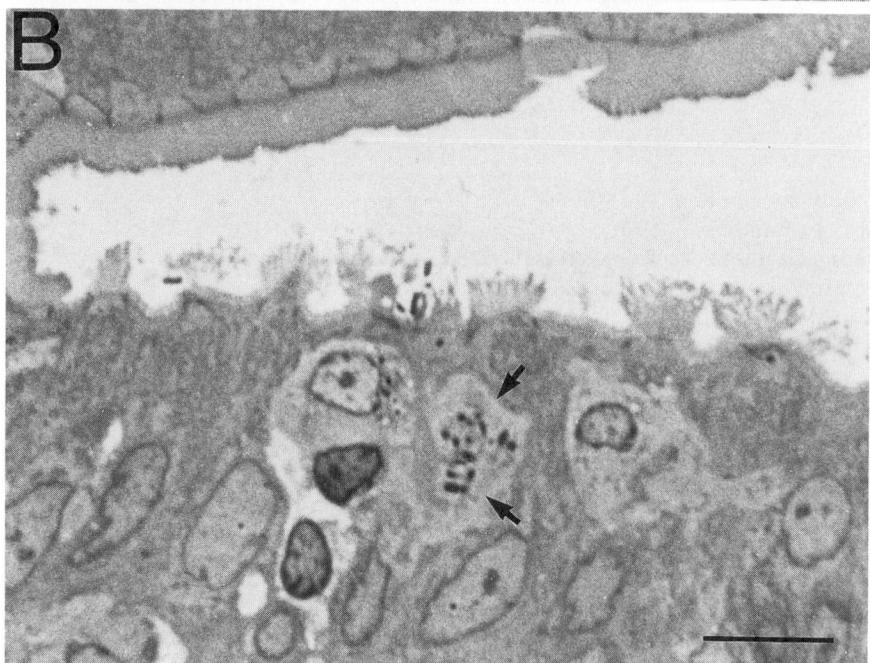

FIG. 5. Adherence and uptake of *Salmonella typhimurium* by rabbit M cells. *Salmonella* were injected into a ligated intestinal loop containing a Peyer's patch. **A:** Many bacteria (*arrows*) have adhered to the apical surface of a single M cell, while neighboring M cells (*arrowheads*) are free of bacteria. **B:** *Salmonella* have been taken up by an M cell and transported to the intraepithelial pocket (*arrows*). Bar = 10 μm.

invasin or other outer membrane components of *Yersinia* mediate M-cell adherence is not clear. The possibility remains that *Yersinia* invasin is a multifunctional molecule that can interact with M-cell surfaces via a domain not involved in integrin binding.

Shigella

Shigella are facultative intracellular pathogens that are responsible for bacillary dysentery or shigellosis. The organisms infect cells by adhering to the plasma membrane,

undergoing phagocytosis, and then disrupting the phagosome membrane to enter the cytoplasm. Once within the host cell cytoplasm, the bacteria proliferate, induce assembly of a "tail" of actin filaments, and are extruded in a cytoplasmic process that is phagocytosed by the neighboring cell, thus repeating the cycle of infection (117). Studies using polarized monolayers of intestinal enterocytes *in vitro* have shown that as long as epithelial tight junctions are intact, *Shigella flexneri* is unable to invade via the apical surfaces of enterocytes (118). General invasion of the intestinal epithelium *in vivo* may therefore require disruption of tight junctions, but entry via M cells

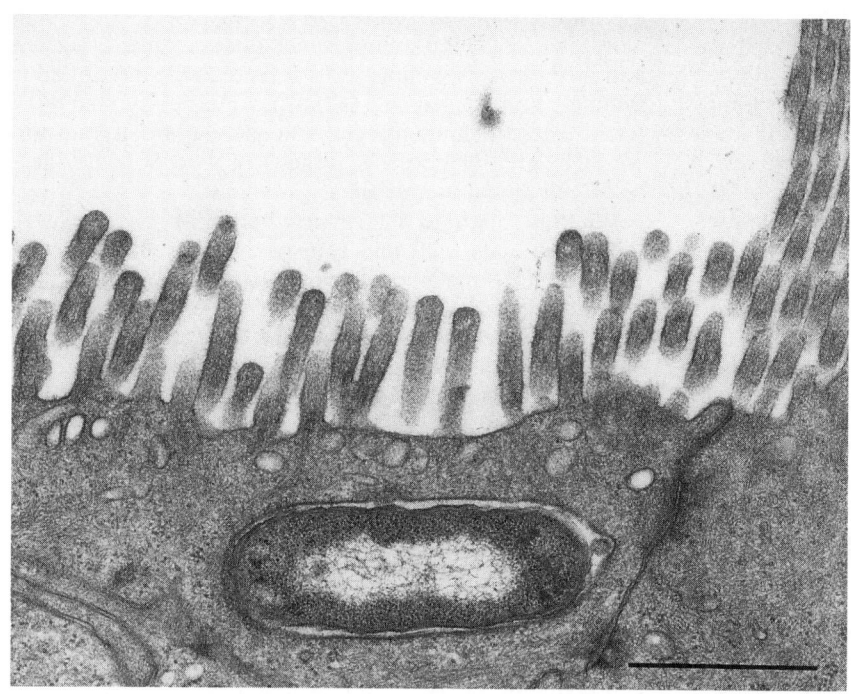

FIG. 6. A *Salmonella* within a phagocytic vacuole of a rabbit M cell. In the rabbit, uptake and transport of *Salmonella* does not cause M-cell damage. Bar = 1 μm.

occurs early, when junctions are intact. Inoculation of rabbit Peyer's patches with a pathogenic strain of *S. flexneri,* as well as selected nonpathogenic strains, resulted in selective binding and phagocytosis by M cells (119). Interestingly, heat-killed virulent bacteria were also taken up. Uptake of the virulent strain into Peyer's patches resulted in ulcerations in the FAE, whereas mucosal damage was not observed with any avirulent strains. How these experimental infections relate to the pathology of bacillary dysentery in humans is not known but it is intriguing that mucosal ulcerations typically found in *Shigella* infections are most frequent in the colon and ileum, sites where lymphoid follicles and M cells are relatively numerous.

M-Cell Transport of Other Pathogens

A growing number of pathogenic microorganisms have been shown to interact with M cells. *Campylobacter jejuni* was found to be transcytosed by rabbit M cells when incubated in intestinal loops (120). The authors suggested that the bacteremia that often follows oral administration of mice with *C. jejuni* could be a result of bacteria traversing the epithelium through M cells and gaining access to the circulation via the lymphatic drainage of the organized mucosal lymphoid tissue.

Mycobacteria also exhibit selective M-cell adherence and transcytosis. *Mycobacterium paratuberculosis,* inoculated into ligated ileal loops of calves, entered organized mucosal lymphoid tissues where they accumulated in macrophages (121). An electron microscopic study demonstrated that rabbit M cells efficiently transport BCG (bacillus Calmette-Guerin) into mucosal lymphoid tissue (122). The observed adherence and transport of BCG by

M cells lends support to the development of recombinant BCG as a vehicle for expression of foreign antigens in mucosal inductive sites (123,124).

INTERACTION OF INVASIVE VIRUSES WITH M CELLS

Relatively little is known about selective transport of viruses by M cells or the role of M cells in invasion of viral pathogens. To date, M-cell adherence and transport has been documented for only three viruses and in no case have the interacting viral and M-cell surface molecules responsible for these interactions been identified.

Reovirus

The best known example of M-cell–specific viral adherence is provided by the mouse pathogen, reovirus (125). Elegant studies have shown that processing of reovirus by proteases in the intestinal lumen increases viral infectivity through cleavage of the major outer capsid protein σ3 and through a conformational change in the σ1 protein that results in extension of the viral hemagglutinin (126,127). It was recently demonstrated in our laboratory that proteolytic processing of the outer capsid is also required for M-cell adherence: neither unprocessed virus (administered with protease inhibitors) nor capsidless cores can bind (128). Thus, the virus must use either the conserved, protease-resistant outer capsid protein μ1c or the extended σ1 protein to bind to M cells. The extended conformation and lectin-like nature of the σ1 protein would suggest that it mediates M-cell adherence. On the other hand, two distinct reovirus serotypes (type 1 Lang and type 3 Dearing) that show different target cell tropisms mediated by specific σ1 hemagglutinins both bind to M cells (129). If σ1 is involved in recognition of M cells, it must bind via a domain not involved in serotype-specific cell tropism. The reovirus adhesin, once identified, could potentially serve as an affinity ligand to target vaccines to M cells and to identify the M-cell receptors responsible for viral invasion.

The transepithelial transport pathway of M cells provides reovirus with multiple opportunities to infect both epithelial and lamina propria cells of the host. The virus may infect the M cell itself either by fusing directly with the membrane of the transport vesicle or by reentering the cell by endocytosis from the intraepithelial pocket, and this would explain the cytoplasmic viral factories observed in M cells within hours after M-cell uptake of virus *in vivo* (130). Bass et al. also observed that M cells infected by reovirus are selectively lost (130). This could lead to loss of epithelial barrier function and to impaired sampling of luminal antigens by the mucosal immune system. Perhaps the special vulnerability of M cells to damage by microorganisms explains the curious absence of M cells from the crest of the follicle-associated dome epithelium in human Peyer's patches (17).

Poliovirus

The pathogenesis of poliovirus in humans shows some intriguing parallels with reovirus in mice: poliovirus enters the body by the oral route and proliferates in Peyer's patches before spreading systemically (131). Although the efficacy of mucosal immunization with live, attenuated poliovirus was established decades ago (132) and the mucosal immune response to polio vaccine has been thoroughly documented (133), the mechanism of entry of virus into the mucosa was established only recently. Small explants of human Peyer's patches were exposed *in vitro* to wild poliovirus type 1 or to the attenuated Sabin strain, and were then examined by electron microscopy (134). Both viruses adhered to M cells and were endocytosed, whereas neither appeared to interact with enterocytes. The ability of poliovirus to exploit M-cell transport for penetration of the epithelial barrier makes it a candidate oral vaccine vector for delivery of foreign antigens either in recombinant viral particles (135) or as empty pseudovirus particles (136).

Human Immunodeficiency Virus

The majority of AIDS cases in the United States and the world are the result of sexual transmission of HIV, and infection through unprotected anal intercourse appears to be particularly efficient (137,138). It is now generally accepted that infection can occur without damage of the rectal epithelial lining. Although HIV uptake and infection in cultured epithelial cell lines has been documented (139,140), there is no clear evidence to date that normal absorptive enterocytes in adults become infected or serve as entry sites for the virus (141). The presence of M cells in human rectal epithelium is well documented, however, and free virus as well as virus-infected cells are found in infected human semen (142). The possibility that HIV could enter the human rectal mucosa via M-cell transport would be greatly increased if the virus were able to adhere to M-cell apical membranes.

We thus sought to determine whether M cells in experimental animals bind and transport HIV, as an indirect indication of such an uptake mechanism in humans (143). Live, infectious HIV-1 was applied to explants of rabbit and mouse Peyer's patch mucosa *in vitro* for 1 hr, and subsequent electron microscopic examination revealed that virus associated closely with M-cell apical membranes of both species. While some viral particles were seen on the glycocalyx of enterocytes, they did not make contact with enterocyte apical membranes and were not taken up by these cells. Endocytosis of HIV was seen only in M cells; in rabbit tissue, virus was observed in the intraepithelial pocket (143). Studies using explants of human rectal mucosa will be required to determine whether human M cells also bind and transport HIV. In the interim, however, it seems prudent to assume that M-cell transport of HIV does occur in human rectum and that delivery of virus to the intraepithelial pocket could be a rapid and efficient mechanism for infection of the CD4+ T cells and macrophages that lie within and beneath the epithelium (144,145). The fact that circulating antireovirus antibodies failed to protect mice against reovirus entry and proliferation in the Peyer's patch mucosa (58) suggests that systemic vaccines against HIV will fail to protect against rectal HIV infection. It is becoming increasingly clear that mucosal vaccine strategies that elicit secretory antibodies will be an important component of immune protection against sexual transmission of AIDS (146,147).

Future design of mucosal vaccines against HIV and other sexually transmitted diseases must take into account mounting evidence that the location in which M-cell transport and inductive events occur has a profound influence on the subsequent regional distribution of specific IgA plasma cells and IgA secretion. A secretory immune response against poliovirus, for example, was demonstrated in colon but not in nasopharynx following immunization of distal colon (133). Similarly, secretory immune responses to Sendai virus were concentrated in either the digestive tract or the airways, but not both, when administration of antigen was carefully restricted either to the stomach or to the trachea (148). The site of antigen exposure within the gastrointestinal tract is also important: immunization with cholera toxin into proximal intestine, distal intestine, or colon evoked highest levels of specific antitoxin secretory IgA in the segment of antigen exposure (149). We have used "wicks" made of an absorbent filter material for direct retrieval of secretions associated with mucosal surfaces of the gastrointestinal system and vagina of mice to show that immunization via the rectum is the only route that induces high levels of specific sIgA in the mucus coating the rectum and distal colon (150). Since inductive sites (lymphoid follicles with M cells) are particularly numerous in the distal colonic and rectal mucosa of humans (27–30), it is important to test the effectiveness of various types of mucosal vaccines by both oral and rectal immunization routes.

CONCLUSION

The importance of M cells in induction of mucosal immune responses, and in invasion of the intestinal mucosa by pathogenic microorganisms, is now widely recognized. However, we know almost nothing about the specific molecular recognition systems and nonspecific adherence mechanisms that underlie these phenomena. The same molecular mechanisms that allow M cells to selectively transport microorganisms to inductive sites of the mucosal immune system are presumably exploited by microbial pathogens to target themselves to these convenient invasion sites. In the absence of a cultured line of differentiated M cells, elucidation of these mechanisms remains an important but difficult challenge. A clearer understanding of the M cell will lead to design of more effective mucosal vaccines. Meanwhile, empirical information on the interactions of microorganisms with M cells, summarized in this chapter, is being used to target attenuated bacterial vaccine strains, live viral and bacterial vectors containing recombinant proteins or genes, and nonliving, particulate immunogens to the mucosal immune system.

ACKNOWLEDGMENTS

We are grateful to former members of our laboratory who contributed to the work summarized in this review: Richard Weltzin, Helen Amerongen, Julie Mack, and Felice Apter. We also acknowledge the collaboration of John Mekalanos and Bernard Fields of the Department of Microbiology and Molecular Genetics, Harvard Medical School. The authors are supported by NIH Research Grants HD17557, DK21505 and AI34757 and NIH Center Grant DK34854 to the Harvard Digestive Diseases Center (M.R.N.); and Swiss National Science Foundation Grant 31.246404.89 and Swiss League against Cancer Grant 373.89.2 (J.P.K.).

REFERENCES

1. Madara JL. Tight junction dynamics: Is paracellular transport regulated? *Cell* 1988;53:497–498.
2. Mooseker M. Organization, chemistry and assembly of the cytoskeletal apparatus of the intestinal brush border. *Annu Rev Cell Biol* 1985;1:209–241.
3. Semenza G. Anchoring and biosynthesis of stalked brush border membrane glycoproteins. *Annu Rev Cell Biol* 1986;2: 255–314.
4. Ito S. Form and function of the glycocalyx on free cell surfaces. *Phil Trans R Soc Lond (Biol)* 1974;268:55–66.
5. Bernadac A, Gorvel J-P, Feracci H, Maroux S. Human blood group A-like determinants as marker of the intracellular pools of glycoproteins in secretory and absorbing cells of A + rabbit jejunum. *Biol Cell* 1984;50:31–36.
6. Neutra MR, Wilson JM, Weltzin RA, Kraehenbuhl JP. Membrane domains and macromolecular transport in intestinal epithelial cells. *Am Rev Respir Dis* 1988;138:S10–S16.
7. Mestecky J, McGhee JR. Immunoglobulin A (IgA): molecular and cellular interactions involved in IgA biosynthesis and immune response. *Adv Immunol* 1987;40:153–245.
8. Brandtzaeg P, Sollid LM, Thrane PS, et al. Lymphoepithelial interactions in the mucosal immune system. *Gut* 1988;29: 1116–1130.
9. Kraehenbuhl JP, Neutra MN. Molecular and cellular basis of immune protection of mucosal surfaces. *Physiol Rev* 1992;72: 853–879.
10. Neutra MN, Kraehenbuhl JP. Transepithelial transport and mucosal defence I: the role of M cells. *Trends Cell Biol* 1992; 2:134–138.
11. Schmidt GH, Wilkinson MM, Ponder BAJ. Cell migration pathway in the intestinal epithelium: an in situ marker system using mouse aggregation chimeras. *Cell* 1985;40:425–429.
12. Pappo J, Owen RL. Absence of secretory component expression by epithelial cells overlying rabbit gut–associated lymphoid tissue. *Gastroenterology* 1988;95:1173–1177.
13. Bye WA, Allan CH, Trier JS. Structure, distribution and origin of M cells in Peyer's patches of mouse ileum. *Gastroenterology* 1984;86:789–801.
14. Pappo J, Steger HJ, Owen RL. Differential adherence of epithelium overlying gut-associated lymphoid tissue. An ultrastructural study. *Lab Invest* 1988;58:692–697.
15. Owen RL, Ermak TH. Structural specialization for antigen uptake and processing in the digestive tract. *Springer Semin Immunopathol* 1990;12:139–152.
16. Smith MW, Peacock MA. M cell distribution in the follicle-associated epithelium of mouse Peyer's patch. *Am J Anat* 1980; 159:167–175.
17. Fujimura Y, Kihara T, Ohtani K, et al. Distribution of microfold cells (M cells) in human follicle-associated epithelium. *Gastroenterol Jpn* 1990;25:130.
18. Gebert A, Hach G. Differential binding of lectins to M cells and enterocytes in the rabbit cecum. *Gastroenterology* 1993; 105:1350–1361.
19. Clark MA, Jepson MA, Simmons NL, Booth TA, Hirst BH. Differential expression of lectin-binding sites defines mouse intestinal M-cells. *J Histochem Cytochem* 1993;41:1679–1687.
20. Falk P, Roth KA, Gordon J. Lectins are sensitive tools for defining the differentiation programs of epithelial cell lineages in the developing and adult mouse gastrointestinal tract. *Am J Physiol (Gastroint Liver Physiol)* 1994;29:G987–G1003.
21. Giannasca PJ, Giannasca KT, Falk P, Gordon J, Neutra MR. Regional differences in glycoconjugates of mouse intestinal M cells: potential targets for mucosal vaccine delivery. *Am J Physiol (Gastroint Liver Physiol)* 1994; *(in press)*.
22. Smith MW, James PS, Tivey DR. M cell numbers increase after transfer of SPF mice to a normal animal house environment. *Am J Pathol* 1987;128:385–389.
23. Savidge TC, Smith MW, James PS, Aldred P. *Salmonella*-induced M-cell formation in germ-free mouse Peyer's patch tissue. *Am J Pathol* 1991;139:177–184.
24. Spencer J, MacDonald TT, Finn T, Isaacson PG. The development of gut-associated lymphoid tissue in the terminal ileum of fetal human intestine. *Clin Exp Immunol* 1986;64:536–543.
25. Owen RL, Nemanic P. Antigen processing structures of the mammalian intestinal tract: an SEM study of lymphoepithelial organs. *Scan Electron Microsc* 1978;2:367–378.
26. Owen RL, Piazza AJ, Ermak TH. Ultrastructural and cytoarchitectural features of lymphoreticular organs in the colon and rectum of adult BALB/c mice. *Am J Anat* 1991;190:10–18.
27. Langman JM, Rowland R. The number and distribution of lymphoid follicles in the human large intestine. *J Anat* 1986; 194:189–194.
28. O'Leary AD, Sweeney EC. Lymphoglandular complexes of the colon: structure and distribution. *Histopathology* 1986;10: 267–283.
29. Jacob E, Backer SJ, Swaminathan SP. M cells in the follicle-associated epithelium of the human colon. *Histopathology* 1987;11:941–952.
30. Fujimura Y, Hosobe M, Kihara T. Ultrastructural study of M cells from colonic lymphoid nodules obtained by colonoscopic biopsy. *Dig Dis Sci* 1992;37:1089–1098.

31. Kealy WF. Colonic lymphoid-glandular complex (microbursa): nature and morphology. *J Clin Pathol* 1976;29:241–244.

32. Madara JL, Bye WA, Trier JS. Structural features of and cholesterol distribution in M-cell membranes in guinea pig, rat and mouse Peyer's patches. *Gastroenterology* 1984;87:1091–1103.

33. Gebert A, Bartels H. Occluding junctions in the epithelia of the gut-associated lymphoid tissue (GALT) of the rabbit ileum and cecum. *Cell Tissue Res* 1991;266:301–314.

34. Bockman DE, Cooper MD. Pinocytosis by epithelium associated with lymphoid follicles in the bursa of Fabricius, appendix, and Peyer's patches. An electron microscopic study. *Am J Anat* 1973;136:455–478.

35. Owen RL. Sequential uptake of horseradish peroxidase by lymphoid follicle epithelium of Peyer's patches in the normal unobstructed mouse intestine: an ultrastructural study. *Gastroenterology* 1977;72:440–451.

36. Neutra MR, Phillips TL, Fishkind DJ, Mack JA. Membrane domains of the intestinal M cell. *J Cell Biol* 1986;103:466a.

37. Gebert A, Hach G, Bartels H. Co-localization of vimentin and cytokeratins in M-cells of rabbit gut-associated lymphoid tissue (GALT). *Cell Tissue Res* 1992;269:331–340.

38. Jepson MA, Mason CM, Bennett MK, Simmons NL, Hirst BH. Co-expression of vimentin and cytokeratins in M cells of rabbit intestinal follicle-associated epithelium. *Histochem J* 1992;24:33–39.

39. Grone HJ, Weber K, Grone E, Helmchen U, Osborn M. Coexpression of keratin and vimentin in damaged and regenerating tubular epithelium of the kidney. *Am J Pathol* 1987;129:1–8.

40. Franke WW, Mayer D, Schmid E, Denk H, Borenfreund E. Differences of expression of cytoskeletal proteins in cultured rat hepatocytes and hepatoma cells. *Exp Cell Res* 1981;134:345–365.

41. Owen RL, Bhalla DK. Cytochemical analysis of alkaline phosphatase and esterase activities and of lectin-binding and anionic sites in rat and mouse Peyer's patch M cells. *Am J Anat* 1983;168:199–212.

42. Smith MW, James PS, Tivey DR, Brown D. Automated histochemical analysis of cell populations in the intact follicle-associated epithelium of the mouse Peyer's patch. *Histochem J* 1988;20:443–448.

43. Owen RL, Jones AL. Epithelial cell specialization within human Peyer's patches: an ultrastructural study of intestinal lymphoid follicles. *Gastroenterology* 1974;66:189–203.

44. Neutra MR, Phillips TL, Mayer EL, Fishkind DJ. Transport of membrane-bound macromolecules by M cells in follicle-associated epithelium of rabbit Peyer's patch. *Cell Tiss Res* 1987;247:537–546.

45. Jepson MA, Clark MA, Simmons NL, Hirst BH. Actin accumulation at sites of attachment of indigenous apathogenic segmented filamentous bacteria to mouse ileal epithelial cells. *Infect Immun* 1993;61:4001–4004.

46. LeFevre ME, Olivo R, Joel DD. Accumulation of latex particles in Peyer's patches and their subsequent appearance in villi and mesenteric lymph node. *Proc Soc Exp Biol Med* 1978;159:298–302.

47. Pappo J, Ermak TH. Uptake and translocation of fluorescent latex particles by rabbit Peyer's patch follicle epithelium: a quantitative model for M cell uptake. *Clin Exp Immunol* 1989;76:144–148.

48. DeAizpurua HJ, Russell-Jones GJ. Oral vaccination: Identification of classes of proteins that provoke an immune response upon oral feeding. *J Exp Med* 1988;167:440–451.

49. Mayrhofer G. Physiology of the intestinal immune system. In: Newby TJ, Stokes CR, eds. *Local immune responses of the gut*. Boca Raton: CRC Press; 1984:1–96.

50. Stokes CR. Induction and control of intestinal immune responses. In: Newby TJ, Stokes CR, eds. *Local immune responses of the gut*. Boca Raton: CRC Press; 1984:97–142.

51. Mowat AM. The regulation of immune responses to dietary protein antigens. *Immunol Today* 1987;8:93–94.

52. Wilson AD, Robinson A, Iron L, Stokes CR. Adjuvant action of cholera toxin and pertussis toxin in the induction of IgA antibody response to orally-administered antigen. *Vaccine* 1993;11:113–118.

53. Nedrud JG, Lamm ME. Adjuvants and the mucosal immune system. In: Spriggs DR, Koff WC, eds. *Topics in vaccine adjuvant research*. Boca Raton: CRC Press, 1991:54–67.

54. Roy MJ, Varvayanis M. Development of dome epithelium in gut-associated lymphoid tissues: association of IgA with M cells. *Cell Tissue Res* 1987;248:645–651.

55. Weltzin RA, Lucia Jandris P, Michetti P, Fields BN, Kraehenbuhl JP, Neutra MR. Binding and transepithelial transport of immunoglobulins by intestinal M cells: demonstration using monoclonal IgA antibodies against enteric viral proteins. *J Cell Biol* 1989;108:1673–1685.

56. Fanger MW, Shen L, Pugh J, Bernier GM. Subpopulations of human peripheral granulocytes and monocytes express receptors for IgA. *Proc Natl Acad Sci USA* 1980;77:3640–3644.

57. Allan CH, Trier JS. Structure and permeability differ in subepithelial villus and Peyer's patch follicle capillaries. *Gastroenterology* 1991;100:1172–1179.

58. Tyler KL, Virgin DH, Bassel-Duby R, Fields BN. Antibody inhibits defined stages in the pathogenesis of reovirus serotype 3 infection of the nervous central system. *J Exp Med* 1989;170:887–895.

59. Allan CH, Mendrick DL, Trier JS. Rat intestinal M cells contain acidic endosomal-lysosomal compartments and express class II major histocompatibility complex determinants. *Gastroenterology* 1993;104:698–708.

60. Courtoy PJ. Dissection of endosomes. In: Steer CJ, Hanover JA, eds. *Intracellular trafficking of proteins*. Cambridge: Cambridge Univ. Press; 1991:103–156.

61. Maxfield FR, Yamashiro DJ. Acidification of organelles and the intracellular sorting of proteins during endocytosis. In: Steer CJ, Hanover JA, eds. *Intracellular trafficking of proteins*. Cambridge: Cambridge Univ. Press; 1991:157–182.

62. Lencer WI, Verkman AS, Arnaout A, Ausiello D, Brown D. Endocytic vesicles which retrieve the vasopressin-sensitive water channel do not contain a functional H^+ATPase. *J Cell Biol* 1990;111:379–389.

63. Diment S, Stahl P. Macrophage endosomes contain proteases which degrade endocytosed protein ligands. *J Biol Chem* 1985;260:15211–15317.

64. Finzi G, Cornaggia M, Capella C, et al. Cathepsin E in follicle associated epithelium of intestine and tonsils: localization to M cells and possible role in antigen processing. *Histochemistry* 1993;99:201–211.

65. Schaerer E, Neutra MR, Kraehenbuhl JP. Molecular and cellular mechanisms involved in transepithelial transport. *J Membr Biol* 1991;123:93–103.

66. Sztul E, Kaplin A, Saucan L, Palade G. Protein traffic between distinct plasma membrane domains: isolation and characterization of vesicular carriers involved in transcytosis. *Cell* 1991;64:81–89.

67. Ermak TH, Steger HJ, Strober S, Owen RL. M cells and granular mononuclear cells in Peyer's patch domes of mice depleted of their lymphocytes by total lymphoid irradiation. *Am J Pathol* 1989;134:529–537.

68. Ho NFH, Day JS, Barsuhn CL, Burton PS, Raub TJ. Biophysical model approaches to mechanistic transepithelial studies of peptides. *J Controlled Release* 1990;11:3–24.

69. Keljo DJ, Hamilton JR. Quantitative determination of macromolecular transport rate across intestinal Peyer's patches. *Am J Physiol* 1983;244:G637–G644.

70. Duroc R, Heyman M, Beaufrere B, Morgat JL, Desjeux JF. Horseradish peroxidase transport across rabbit jejunum and Peyer's patches in vitro. *Am J Physiol* 1983;245:G54–G58.

71. Rosenshine I, Donnenberg MS, Kaper JB, Finlay BB. Signal transduction between enteropathogenic *Escherichia coli* (EPEC) and epithelial cells: EPEC induces tyrosine phosphorylation of host cell proteins to initiate cytoskeletal rearrangement and bacterial uptake. *EMBO J* 1992;11:3551–3560.

72. Neutra MR. Ultrastructural studies of the interaction of bacteria with intestinal cell surfaces. In: Boedecker E, ed. *Attachment of organisms to the gut mucosa*. vol 1. Boca Raton: CRC Press; 1984:173–188.

73. Neutra MR, Kraehenbuhl JP. Secretory immunoglobulin A: structure, synthesis, and function. In: Johnson LR, ed. *Physiol-*

ogy of the gastrointestinal tract. 3rd ed. New York: Raven Press; 1994:975–1009.

74. Miller JF, Mekalanos JJ, Falkow S. Coordinate regulation and sensory transduction in the control of bacterial virulence. Science 1989;243:916–921.

75. Herrington DA, Hall RH, Losonsky G, Mekalanos JJ, Taylor RK, Levine MM. Toxin, toxin-coregulated pili, and the toxR regulon are essential for Vibrio cholerae pathogenesis in humans. J Exp Med 1988;168:1487–1492.

76. Jertborn M, Svennerholm AM, Holmgren J. Saliva, breast milk, and serum antibody responses as indirect measures of intestinal immunity after oral cholera vaccination or natural disease. J Clin Microbiol 1986;24:203–209.

77. Levine MM, Kaper JB, Black RE, Clements ML. New knowledge on pathogenesis of bacterial enteric infections as applied to vaccine development. Microbiol Rev 1983;47:510–550.

78. Levine MM, Nalin DR, Craig JP, et al. Immunity to cholera in man: relative role of antibacterial versus antitoxic immunity. Trans R Soc Trop Med Hyg 1988;73:3–9.

79. Winner LS III, Mack J, Weltzin RA, Mekalanos JJ, Kraehenbuhl JP, Neutra MR. New model for analysis of mucosal immunity: intestinal secretion of specific monoclonal immunoglobulin A from hybridoma tumors protects against Vibrio cholerae infection. Infect Immun 1991;59:977–982.

80. Apter FM, Lencer WI, Finkelstein RA, Mekalanos JJ, Neutra MR. Monoclonal immunoglobulin A antibodies directed against cholera toxin B subunit prevent the toxin-induced chloride secretory response and block toxin binding to epithelial cells in vitro. Infect Immun 1993;61:5271–5278.

81. Apter FM, Michetti P, Winner LS III, Mack JA, Mekalanos JJ, Neutra MR. Analysis of the roles of anti-lipopolysaccharide and anti-cholera toxin IgA antibodies in protection against Vibrio cholerae and cholera toxin using monoclonal IgA antibodies in vivo. Infect Immun 1993;61:5279–5285.

82. Owen RL, Pierce NF, Apple RT, Cray WCJ. M cell transport of Vibrio cholerae from the intestinal lumen into Peyer's patches: a mechanism for antigen sampling and for microbial transepithelial migration. J Infect Dis 1986;153:1108–1118.

83. Yamamoto T, Kamano T, Uchimura M, Iwanaga M, Yokota T. Vibrio cholerae O1 adherence to villi and lymphoid follicle epithelium: in vitro model using formalin-treated human small intestine and correlation between adherence and cell-associated hemagglutinin levels. Infect Immun 1988;56:3241–3250.

84. Yamamoto T, Yokota T. Adherence targets of Vibrio parahaemolyticus in human small intestines. Infect Immun 1989;57:2410–2419.

85. Yamamoto T, Yokota T. Vibrio cholerae O1 adherence to human small intestinal M cells in vitro. J Infect Dis 1989;160:168–169.

86. Cebra JJ, Gearheart PJ, Kamat R, Robertson SM, Tseng J. Origin and differentiation of lymphocytes involved in the secretory IgA response. Cold Spring Harbor Symp Quant Biol 1976;41:201–215.

87. Levine MM, Edelman R. Future vaccines against enteric pathogens. Infect Dis Clin North Am 1990;4:105–121.

88. Mekalanos JJ. Bacterial mucosal vaccines. In: Ciardi JE, McGhee JR, Kieth JM, eds. Genetically engineered vaccines. New York: Plenum Press; 1992;43–50. (Advances in Experimental Medicine and Biology; vol 327.)

89. Uchida J. An ultrastructural study on active uptake and transport of bacteria by microfold cells (M cells) to the lymphoid follicles in the rabbit appendix. J Clin Electron Microsc 1987;20:379–394.

90. Inman LR, Cantey JR. Specific adherence of Escherichia coli (strain RDEC-1) to membranous (M) cells of the Peyer's patch in Escherichia coli diarrhea in the rabbit. J Clin Invest 1983;71:1–8.

91. Knutton S, Lloyd DR, McNeish AS. Adhesion of enteropathogenic Escherichia coli to human intestinal enterocytes and cultured human intestinal mucosa. Infect Immun 1987;55:69–77.

92. Takeuchi A, Inman LR, O'Hanley PD, Cantey JR, Lushbaugh WB. Scanning and transmission electron microscopic study of Escherichia coli O15 (RDEC-1) enteric infection in rabbits. Infect Immun 1978;19:686–694.

93. Inman LR, Cantey JR. Peyer's patch lymphoid follicle epithelial adherence of a rabbit enteropathogenic Escherichia coli (strain RDEC-1). Role of plasmid-mediated pili in initial adherence. J Clin Invest 1984;74:90–95.

94. Jerse AE, Yu J, Tall BD, Kaper JB. A genetic locus of enteropathogenic Escherichia coli necessary for the production of attaching and effacing lesions on tissue culture cells. Proc Natl Acad Sci USA 1990;87:7839–7843.

95. Jerse AE, Kaper JB. The eae gene of enteropathogenic Escherichia coli encodes a 94-kilodalton membrane protein, the expression of which is influenced by the EAE plasmid. Infect Immun 1991;59:4302–4309.

96. Finlay BB, Rosenshine I, Donnenberg MS, Kaper JB. Cytoskeletal composition of attaching and effacing lesions associated with enteropathogenic Escherichia coli adherence to Hela cells. Infect Immun 1992;60:2541–2543.

97. Fayer R, Speer CA, Dubey JP. General biology of Cryptosporidium. In: Duley JP, Speers CA, Fayer R, eds. Cryptosporidiosis of man and animals. Boca Raton: CRC Press; 1990:1–30.

98. Flanigan TP, Soave R. Cryptosporidiosis. In: Sun T, ed. Progress in clinical parasitology. vol 3. New York: Springer-Verlag; 1993:1–20.

99. Marcial MA, Madara JL. Cryptosporidium: cellular localization, structural analysis of absorptive cell parasite membrane-membrane interactions in guinea pigs and suggestion of protozoan transport by M cells. Gastroenterology 1986;90:583–594.

100. Owen RL, Allen CL, Stevens DP. Phagocytosis of Giardia muris by macrophages in Peyer's patch epithelium in mice. Infect Immun 1981;33:591–601.

101. Hsu HS. Pathogenesis and immunity in murine salmonellosis. Microbiol Rev 1989;53:390–409.

102. Carter PB, Collins FM. The route of enteric infection in normal mice. J Exp Med 1974;139:1189–1203.

103. Hohmann AW, Schmidt G, Rowley D. Intestinal colonization and virulence of Salmonella in mice. Infect Immun 1978;22:763–770.

104. Takeuchi A. Electron microscope studies of experimental Salmonella infection. I. Penetration into the intestinal epithelium by Salmonella typhimurium. Am J Pathol 1967;50:109–136.

105. Rosenshine I, Finlay BB. Exploitation of host signal transduction pathways and cytoskeletal functions by invasive bacteria. BioEssays 1993;15:17–24.

106. Bliska JB, Galan JE, Falkow S. Signal transduction in the mammalian cell during bacterial attachment and entry. Cell 1993;73:903–920.

107. Kohbata S, Yokobata H, Yabuuchi E. Cytopathogenic effect of Salmonella typhi GIFU 10007 on M cells of murine ileal Peyer's patches in ligated ileal loops: an ultrastructural study. Microbiol Immunol 1986;30:1225–1237.

108. Jones BD, Ghori N, Falkow S. Salmonella typhimurium initiates murine infection by penetrating and destroying the specialized M cells of the Peyer's patches. J Exp Med 1994;180:15–23.

109. Mekalanos JJ. Environmental signals controlling expression of virulence determinants in bacteria. J Bacteriol 1992;174:1–7.

110. Curtiss R III, Goldschmidt RM, Kelly SM, Lyons M, Michalek SM, Pastian R, Stein S. Recombinant avirulent Salmonella for oral immunization to induce mucosal immunity to bacterial pathogens. In: Kohler H, LoVerde PT, eds. Vaccines: new concepts and developments. Essex, UK: Longman; 1987:261–271.

111. Michetti P, Mahan MJ, Slauch JM, Mekalanos JJ, Neutra MR. Monoclonal secretory IgA protects against oral challenge with the invasive pathogen Salmonella typhimurium. Infect Immun 1992;60:1786–1792.

112. Grutzkau A, Hanski C, Hahn H, Riecken EO. Involvement of M cells in the bacterial invasion of Peyer's patches: a common mechanism shared by Yersinia enterocolitica and other enteroinvasive bacteria. Gut 1990;31:1011–1015.

113. Fujimura Y, Kihara T, Mine K. Membranous cells as a portal of Yersinia pseudotuberculosis entry into rabbit ileum. J Clin Electron Microsc 1992;25:35–45.

114. Isberg RR. Pathways for the penetration of enteropathogenic Yersinia into mammalian cells. Mol Biol Med 1990;7:73–82.

115. Pepe JC, Miller VL. Yersinia enterocolitica invasin: a primary

role in the initiation of infection. *Proc Natl Acad Sci USA* 1993; 90:6473–6477.

116. Koretz K, Schlag P, Boumsell L, Moller P. Expression of VLA-α2, VLA-α6, and VLA-β1 chains in normal mucosa and adenomas of the colon, and in colon carcinomas and their liver metastases. *Am J Pathol* 1991;138:741–750.

117. Goldberg MB, Sansonetti PJ. *Shigella* subversion of the cellular cytoskeleton: a strategy for epithelial colonization. *Infect Immun* 1993;61:4941–4946.

118. Mounier J, Vasselon T, Hellio R, Lesourd M, Sansonetti PJ. *Shigella flexneri* enters human colonic Caco-2 cells through the basolateral pole. *Infect Immun* 1992;60:237–248.

119. Wassef JS, Keren DF, Mailloux JL. Role of M cells in initial antigen uptake and in ulcer formation in the rabbit intestinal loop model of shigellosis. *Infect Immun* 1989;57:858–863.

120. Walker RI, Schauder-Chock EA, Parker JL. Selective association and transport of *Campylobacter jejuni* through M cells of rabbit Peyer's patches. *Can J Microbiol* 1988;34:1142–1147.

121. Momotani E, Whipple DL, Thiermann AB, Cheville NF. Role of M cells and macrophages in the entrance of *Mycobacterium paratuberculosis* into domes of ileal Peyer's patches in calves. *Vet Pathol* 1988;25:131–137.

122. Fujimura Y. Functional morphology of microfold cells (M cells) in Peyer's patches. Phagocytosis and transport of BCG by M cells into rabbit Peyer's patches. *Gastroenterol Jpn* 1986;21:325–335.

123. Langermann S, Palaszynski S, Sadziene A, Stover CK, Koenig S. Induction of sustained systemic and mucosal immunity by a single intranasal immunization with recombinant BCG. *Proc Natl Acad Sci USA* 1994; in press.

124. Jacobs WR, Snapper SR, Tuckman M, Bloom BR. Mycobacteriophage vectors systems. *Rev Infect Dis* 1989;11:S404–S410.

125. Wolf JL, Rubin DH, Finberg RS, et al. Intestinal M cells: a pathway for entry of reovirus into the host. *Science* 1981;212:471–472.

126. Bass DM, Bodkin D, Dambrauskas R, Trier JS, Fields BN, Wolf JL. Intraluminal proteolytic activation plays an important role in replication of type 1 reovirus in the intestines of neonatal mice. *J Virol* 1990;64:1830–1833.

127. Nibert ML, Furlong DB, Fields BN. Mechanisms of viral pathogenesis. *J Clin Invest* 1991;88:727–734.

128. Amerongen HM, Wilson GAR, Fields BN, Neutra MR. Proteolytic processing of reovirus is required for adherence to intestinal M cells. *J Virol* 1994;68 (in press).

129. Wolf JL, Kaufman RS, Finberg R, Dambrauskas R, Fields BN, Trier JS. Determinants of reovirus interaction with the intestinal M cells and absorptive cells of murine intestine. *Gastroenterology* 1983;85:291–300.

130. Bass DM, Trier JS, Dambrauskas R, Wolf JL. Reovirus type 1 infection of small intestinal epithelium in suckling mice and its effect on M cells. *Lab Invest* 1988;55:226–235.

131. Bodian D. Emerging concept of poliovirus infection. *Science* 1955;122:105–108.

132. Koprowski H. Immunization of man against poliomyelitis with attenuated preparations of living virus. *Ann N Y Acad Sci* 1955; 61:1039–1049.

133. Ogra PL, Karzon DT. Distribution of poliovirus antibody in serum, nasopharynx and alimentary tract following segmental immunization of lower alimentary tract with poliovaccine. *J Immunol* 1969;102:1423–1430.

134. Sicinski P, Rowinski J, Warchol JB, et al. Poliovirus type 1 enters the human host through intestinal M cells. *Gastroenterology* 1990;98:56–58.

135. Choi WS, Pal-Ghosh R, Morrow CD. Expression of human immunodeficiency virus type 1 (HIV-1) gag, pol, and env proteins from chimeric HIV-1-poliovirus minireplicons. *J Virol* 1991;65:2875–2883.

136. Ansardi DC, Porter DC, Morrow CD. Coinfection with recombinant vaccinia viruses expressing poliovirus P1 and P3 proteins results in polyprotein processing and formation of empty capsid structures. *J Virol* 1991;65:2088–2092.

137. Friedland GH, Klein RS. Transmission of the human immunodeficiency virus. *N Engl J Med* 1987;317:1125–1135.

138. Quinn TC. The epidemiology of the acquired immune deficiency syndrome and the immunological responses to the human immunodeficiency virus. *Curr Opin Immunol* 1989;1:502–512.

139. Adachi A, Kownig S, Gendelman HE, et al. Productive, persistent infection of human colorectal cell lines with human immunodeficiency virus. *J Virol* 1987;61:209–213.

140. Bourinbaiar AS, Phillips DM. Transmission of human immunodeficiency virus from monocytes to epithelia. *J AIDS* 1991;4:56–63.

141. Fox CH, Kotler D, Tierney A, Wilson CS, Fauci AS. Detection of HIV-1 RNA in the lamina propria of patients with AIDS and gastrointestinal disease. *J Infect Dis* 1989;159:467–471.

142. Anderson DJ, O'Brien TR, Politch JA, et al. Effects of disease stage and zidovudine on the detection of human immunodeficiency virus type 1 in semen. *JAMA* 1992;267:2769–2774.

143. Amerongen HM, Weltzin RA, Farnet CM, Michetti P, Haseltine WA, Neutra MR. Transepithelial transport of HIV-1 by intestinal M cells: a mechanism for transmission of AIDS. *J AIDS* 1991;4:760–765.

144. Ermak TH, Steger HJ, Pappo J. Phenotypically distinct subpopulations of T cells in domes and M-cell pockets of rabbit gut-associated lymphoid tissues. *Immunology* 1990;71:530–537.

145. Bjerke K, Brandtzaeg P, Fausa O. T cell distribution is different in follicle-associated epithelium of human Peyer's patches and villous epithelium. *Clin Exp Immunol* 1988;74:270–275.

146. Forrest BD. The need for consideration of mucosal immunity in vaccine approaches to AIDS. *Vaccine Res* 1992;1:137–142.

147. McGhee JR, Mestecky J. The mucosal immune system in HIV infection and prospects for mucosal immunity to AIDS. *AIDS Res Rev* 1992;2:289–312.

148. Nedrud JG, Liang XP, Hague N, Lamm ME. Combined oral/nasal immunization protects mice from Sendai virus infection. *J Immunol* 1987;139:3484–3492.

149. Pierce FN, Cray WCJ. Determinants of the localization, magnitude, and duration of a specific mucosal IgA plasma cell response in enterically immunized rats. *J Immunol* 1982;128:1311–1315.

150. Haneberg B, Kendall D, Amerongen HM, et al. Induction of secretory immune responses in small intestine, colon-rectum, and vagina measured with a new method for collection of specific IgA from local mucosal surfaces. *Infect Immun* 1994;62:15–23.

Infections of the Gastrointestinal Tract,
edited by M. J. Blaser, P. D. Smith, J. I. Ravdin,
H. B. Greenberg, and R. L. Guerrant
Raven Press, Ltd., New York © 1995.

CHAPTER 12

Structure and Function of Mucosal IgA

Michael E. Lamm

Historically, the field of immunology, in particular the study of humoral immunity, developed in the context of resistance to infectious diseases. Since the early part of the century it has been recognized that the humoral immune system is compartmentalized in that antibodies in the mucosal secretions, as in the gastrointestinal tract, differ from those in the serum (1). Initially these differences were studied in terms of the kinetics of appearance of antibody and the time for peak responses after exposure to antigen. It was observed that after intestinal infection and immunization, specific antibodies appeared sooner in the intestinal secretions and peaked earlier than did antibodies in the serum (2,3). Furthermore, resistance to challenge by virulent organisms correlated better with the titer of antibodies in the intestinal secretions than with the titer of serum antibodies.

It was only much later that the various classes of antibody were defined, with subsequent investigation showing that the IgA isotype, while only a minor component of the immunoglobulins in serum, is the major class of antibody in the mucosal secretions throughout the body, including the intestinal tract (4). Moreover, mucosal IgA antibodies are synthesized locally by plasma cells situated in the lamina propria; in fact, the intestinal lamina propria contains the body's highest tissue density of plasma cells, and 90% of them make IgA (5). After secretion by these plasma cells, the IgA passes directly through the overlying epithelium to enter the mucosal fluids. In the course of its epithelial passage, IgA complexes with an epithelial cell receptor, part of which remains chemically bound to the IgA as it enters the luminal secretions (6); this extra polypeptide chain in secretory IgA is known as secretory component (SC).

Therefore the relatively small concentration of IgA present in serum does not reflect the amount of IgA actually being synthesized by the body. On a daily basis, the body synthesizes far more IgA, 66 mg/kg body weight, than all other immunoglobulin classes combined (7). Most of the body's IgA is produced in the mucous membranes, much of it in the intestines, where it acts as the body's first line of immunological defense, serving at the interface between the internal milieu and the external environment. Some 40 mg of secretory IgA per kg of body weight enters the intestinal secretions daily (8).

This chapter will consider the structure, transport, and function of mucosal IgA and will develop the thesis that it functions not only as a protective barrier in the luminal secretions but in two other locations as well, i.e., within the intestinal epithelium and in the mucosal lamina propria.

STRUCTURE OF IgA

The IgA in serum is synthesized to a great extent in the bone marrow and occurs mostly in monomeric form with a molecular weight of 160 kDa (9), i.e., the classical immunoglobulin structure of two H (α) and two L chains (either κ or λ in a given molecule) (Fig. 1). There are two subclasses of IgA—IgA1 and IgA2—defined by differences in the α chain, mostly due to a deletion in the hinge region at the midpoint of the α_2 chain (10). Within the α chains of the IgA2 subclass there are two allotypic variants, IgA2m(1) and IgA2m(2). As mediators of immune function, however, no major differences have been assigned to the two subclasses although their ratio can vary in the local population of plasma cells in different parts of the body, in different body fluids and secretions, in the antibody response to different kinds of antigens, and in certain diseases (11). The IgA1 subclass is uniquely susceptible to proteolysis by IgA proteases, a family of enzymes produced by certain pathogenic bacteria that manifest unusual substrate specificity for the hinge region of the α_1 chain, which is lacking in IgA2 (12,13). The IgA1 subclass thus appears to be at somewhat of a disadvantage in resisting infections caused by such pathogens.

In contrast to the IgA in serum, which is mostly monomeric IgA1, the IgA produced by mucosal plasma cells that enters the local secretions is relatively enriched in IgA2 (14), the extent of increase varying in different mu-

M. E. Lamm: Institute of Pathology, Case Western Reserve University, and Department of Pathology, University Hospitals of Cleveland, Cleveland, Ohio 44106.

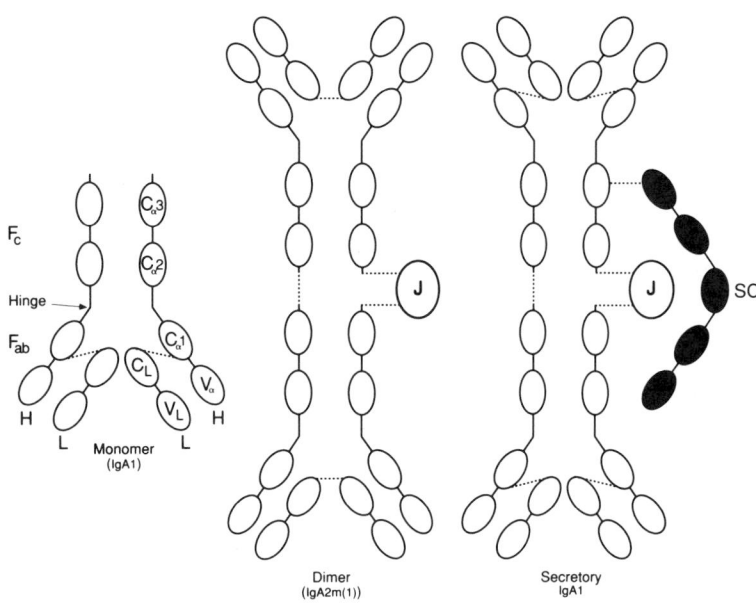

FIG. 1. Structure of IgA monomer, IgA dimer, and secretory IgA. The domains of the component polypeptide chains are indicated by ellipses, V for variable amino acid sequence domains and C for constant sequence domains. Selected interchain disulfide bonds are indicated by dashed lines. The monomer (*left*) is composed of two H (α) and two L chains. In the IgA1 subclass (*illustrated*) and the IgA2m(2) allotype of the IgA2 subclass, the H and L chains are conventionally covalently linked by disulfide bonds. The IgA1 subclass has an extended hinge region, which is susceptible to IgA proteases. Dimeric IgA is shown in the middle. In the IgA2m(1) allotypic variant (*shown*), but not the IgA2m(2) variant, the L chains are disulfide linked to each other instead of to the H chains. Dimeric IgA also contains a J chain, which is disulfide-bonded to C-terminal half-cystines in the two IgA monomer subunits. In secretory IgA (*right*), the dimer additionally contains a secretory component chain, whose C-terminal domain is disulfide bonded to the Cα2 domain of one of the IgA monomer subunits. The SC chain is formed during the release of secretory IgA from the epithelial cell when the external, IgA-binding portion of the pIgR is proteolytically cleaved from the membrane-spanning segment.

cous membranes. For example, the relative amount of IgA2 increases along the intestinal tract with the distance from the stomach (11). Mucosal IgA is also mostly dimeric, i.e., composed of two of the basic four-chain immunoglobulin subunits, so that the dimer possesses 4 α and 4 L polypeptide chains (Fig. 1). The two subunits of the dimer are joined covalently by disulfide bridges between the C termini of two of the α chains and by disulfide bridges from the other two α-chain C termini to a third type of polypeptide chain, the 17-kDa J chain (15–17). J chains, like immunoglobulin H and L chains, are synthesized by plasma cells and are present in all oligomeric immunoglobulins, i.e., all antibody molecules having more than one basic four-chain subunit, like dimeric IgA and pentameric IgM. The J chain is thought to play a role in initiating or stabilizing the oligomeric structure and in providing a conformation for IgA that enhances binding to the polymeric immunoglobulin receptor (pIgR), also known as transmembrane SC (18).

As mentioned, the externally secreted form of IgA contains a fourth kind of polypeptide chain, SC, derived by cleavage of a parent molecule, the pIgR, that is incorporated into dimeric IgA as it binds to and passes through the epithelial cell on its way to secretions. This SC, an 80-kDa subunit containing five domains, is a member of the immunoglobulin superfamily (19,20). It is disulfide-bonded to dimeric IgA because a labile intrachain disulfide bridge in the pIgR rearranges to enable bridging to an α chain of one of the two monomer subunits of the IgA dimer during epithelial transcytosis (21–23). Figure 1 shows the structure of the 420-kDa secretory IgA molecule.

The SC portion of secretory IgA serves two important functions. One, actually performed by its parent mole-

cule, the pIgR, is to promote binding of dimeric IgA to the mucosal epithelial cell and its transport through the cell into the secretions. The second function of SC, after secretion, is to stabilize and protect secretory IgA from proteolytic digestion by the enzymes present in the gastrointestinal fluids, both those secreted to aid in the digestion of food and those produced by the intestinal microflora (24–26).

BIOLOGICAL PROPERTIES OF IgA

The secretory form of IgA, containing an IgA dimer, has four combining sites for antigen. These multiple combining sites compared to the two in IgG, the principal immunoglobulin in serum, make secretory IgA a much more effective agglutinator of antigens (a property that is even more pronounced in IgM, which contains five four-chain immunoglobulin subunits and therefore ten antibody combining sites).

The term *biological properties of antibodies* is usually not used in the context of the combination of Fab portions with antigen, but rather to embrace those properties of antibodies that are mediated by their Fc regions, such as activation of complement and binding to receptors on phagocytic cells. The biological properties of IgA have been reviewed (11,13).

It is established that IgA can activate the alternative complement pathway that begins at the C3 step but is incapable of activating the classical pathway beginning with C1. Studies with mouse IgA antibody have suggested that its activation of the alternative pathway is inefficient, being largely confined to the fluid phase (27). There may be significant species variations in this regard, however, and rigorous studies with human IgA in antigen–antibody reactions have not been done. Furthermore, it is by no means clear that the intestinal secretions would have a fully functional complement system capable of activation by antibody or that if such activation were possible what significance it might have *in vivo*.

An analogous situation holds with respect to binding to leukocyte Fc receptors (Fc$_\alpha$ receptors), which either alone or in concert with cell surface complement receptors activate such functions as phagocytosis. Although Fc$_\alpha$ receptors have been described (28,29), it is again not clear as to what extent binding to such receptors in the milieu of the mucosal secretions is biologically significant.

It is noteworthy that in general the effector functions of antibodies that have been well characterized relate to the functions of immunoglobulins within the body proper, including serum, and not in the external secretions. In the author's view, even though IgA in internal body fluids may be capable of exerting some effector function, IgA is not particularly important within the body. It is clear, compared to IgG, IgE, and IgM, that IgA is certainly less effective (11,13,30). There is also no compelling evidence and perhaps no good reason to think that effector functions mediated by the Fc portion of antibodies are important in mucosal secretions. What is important for an exocrine immunoglobulin like dimeric IgA is that it be able to reach the secretions, which it does via a selective transepithelial pathway mediated by the pIgR, and that within the secretions it, like antibodies generically, can bind to antigen. As will be discussed later under "Function of IgA in Mucosal Defense," it should become evident that the usual effector functions of antibodies may not even be needed. Indeed, it is possible that during the course of evolution IgA has been selected not to mediate the typical effector functions of antibodies because it has to operate in parts of the body where foreign substances are ever present, the best example being the gastrointestinal tract with its content of food and microbial flora. Thus, the abundantly available IgA antibodies are constantly interacting with antigen, and if the resulting immune complexes were capable of activating inflammatory mediators, the intestine would be subject to a chronic state of immunologically mediated inflammation, clearly an undesirable situation. In fact, IgA antibodies may be able to dampen the proinflammatory properties of the other classes of immunoglobulins (13). Therefore it seems appropriate to consider that while the ability to bind antigens is important for IgA, the ability to trigger Fc effector functions may not be.

TRANSEPITHELIAL TRANSPORT OF IgA

Only dimers and higher polymers of IgA are actively transported across epithelia because monomeric IgA cannot effectively bind to pIgR. The transport of IgA and pIgR across epithelial cells has been studied mainly in intestinal epithelium and hepatocytes and in a model system employing transfected kidney epithelial cells (6,31–36). Initially, dimeric IgA secreted by plasma cells in the intestinal lamina propria diffuses across the epithe-

lial basement membrane to be able to bind noncovalently to pIgR on the basolateral surface of columnar epithelial cells, where it is especially prominent in intestinal crypts (Fig. 2). Following endocytosis, the complex enters a transcytotic vesicular system via which it reaches the apical (microvillous) surface (37–40). Close to the time of secretion from the epithelial cell the noncovalent binding between IgA and pIgR is stabilized by disulfide bond formation between the fifth domain of pIgR and the Cα2 domain of IgA (21,23,41). Finally, an enzyme thought to be present in the apical plasma membrane (42,43) cleaves the pIgR between its external and transmembrane portions so that the complex of dimeric IgA and the external segment of the pIgR, i.e., SC, is secreted into the lumen. Although IgA is very much the dominant secretory immunoglobulin, it should be kept in mind that IgM—also oligomeric, containing a J chain, and capable of binding to pIgR, but present in smaller amounts in the lamina propria—is transported across the epithelium by the same mechanism.

The possible role of the liver in transporting IgA into the intestinal contents should be considered. In rodents this is an important pathway because the hepatocyte expresses pIgR on its sinusoidal surface and their serum contains appreciable dimeric IgA, which can accordingly be transported into the bile (44–46). In humans, however, most of the IgA in serum is monomeric and hence incapable of binding to pIgR, and the hepatocyte does not express pIgR (32). The epithelium in the bile ducts and gallbladder in humans, on the other hand, does express pIgR and appears to be capable of transporting into bile small amounts of IgA, in part secreted by adjacent plasma cells.

FUNCTION OF IgA IN MUCOSAL DEFENSE

Initial concepts of local immunity in the early part of the century were based on observations that in response to immunization or challenge, the kinetics of intestinal antibody production did not mirror those in serum, and intestinal antibodies could not therefore be mere transudates from the serum. In the modern era of immunology, studies of the genesis of mucosal plasma cells and of the synthesis, structure, and transport of mucosal IgA have now clarified the origin of local humoral immunity. Throughout this period there has been general agreement that the role of mucosal IgA antibodies is to protect against infectious microorganisms (and other foreign matter), most of which either afflict mucous membranes or invade the body through a mucosal portal of entry. The concept that IgA offers such protection is supported by studies of oral (Sabin) vaccination against poliomyelitis, which induces intestinal IgA antibodies (47), as well as by studies of resistance to a variety of other mucosal infections, which have amply demonstrated that of various immunological parameters, resistance best correlates with the content of IgA antibodies in the local secretions (48–51). In addition, it is well established that patients with IgA deficiency manifest an increased incidence of mucosal infections as well as other disorders involving mucous membranes (52). This general background under-

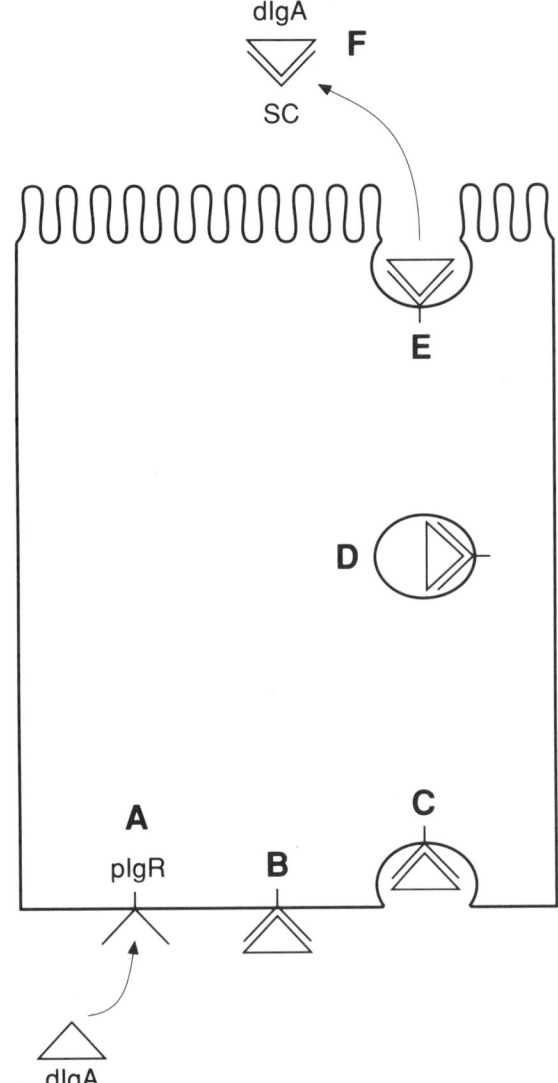

FIG. 2. Epithelial transcytosis of IgA. The cellular events associated with the transport of IgA across mucosal epithelia are illustrated. After synthesis in the rough endoplasmic reticulum, the pIgR passes through the Golgi apparatus, the trans-Golgi network, and vesicles that allow it to be inserted into the basolateral plasma membrane of the cell (**A**), with its IgA-binding portion on the outside and its cytoplasmic tail on the inside. A molecule of dimeric IgA, after secretion by a local plasma cell, binds noncovalently to the pIgR (**B**), and the complex is endocytosed (**C**). The complex enters a transcytotic system of vesicles (**D**) to reach the apical (microvillous) plasma membrane, where (**E**) a cell surface protease cleaves the external, IgA-binding portion of the pIgR (now termed SC) from the transmembrane segment, releasing the complex of dimeric IgA and secretory component (i.e., secretory IgA) into the lumen (**F**). Near the time of release the original noncovalent bonding of IgA to pIgR is stabilized by disulfide bonds.

lies modern efforts to develop oral immunization for intestinal pathogens like *Vibrio cholerae* (53,54).

In addition to clinical studies, there is also now good evidence from experiments in animals with monoclonal antibodies that IgA antibodies as the sole immunological effector are able to prevent viral and bacterial infections in the respiratory (55,56) and intestinal tracts (57–59). Thus, the immunological barrier/immune exclusion role for IgA, in which IgA antibodies in the luminal secretions defend against infection, is now well established. To mediate this protection, IgA antibodies bind to the surface of microorganisms and interfere with their motility and ability to bind to and penetrate the epithelial lining (60–63). In addition, IgA antibodies can neutralize bacterial toxins. As mentioned, IgA appears to be suited for this immune exclusion role more by virtue of having a selective mechanism to transport it into the secretions than by having any special abilities as an antibody per se.

It has long been believed that immune exclusion is the only major function of mucosal IgA and its *raison d'être*. Recently, however, experiments *in vitro* and *in vivo* have led to the proposal that IgA antibodies function importantly in host defense in two other locales, namely, within epithelial cells during the transport of IgA into the secretions and within the mucosal lamina propria prior to epithelial transport.

The original experiments underlying these two newly proposed functions were carried out with cultures of epithelial cell monolayers. In this system cells are polarized and attached to their neighbors by tight junctions, which prevent passive diffusion of macromolecules between cells and across the monolayer. The epithelial cells used express pIgR on their basolateral surface and are thus able to transport dimeric IgA (64). To test the hypothesis that during transepithelial cell transport specific IgA antibodies have the potential to neutralize intracellular pathogens, cell monolayers were infected at the apical surface with parainfluenza virus and exposed to monoclonal IgA antibody at the basal surface. In this model it was demonstrated by double immunofluorescence that IgA antibody colocalizes with viral protein within the epithelial cells and, even more significantly, can inhibit production of virus (65).

The second hypothesis to be tested in this polarized epithelial monolayer system was that immune complexes containing dimeric IgA antibodies would be transported by the same mechanism and route as free dimeric IgA. Accordingly, it was demonstrated that soluble immune complexes made in antigen excess with protein antigens and dimeric monoclonal IgA antibodies were transported from basal to apical surface and into the medium above the monolayer (66). Transport depended on cellular expression of the pIgR and on the IgA antibody being polymeric. Moreover, intact immune complexes were transported, with no evidence of intracellular degradation. It was also demonstrated that immune complexes containing IgG (or monomeric IgA) and dimeric IgA antibodies bound in the same molecular complex to multivalent antigen are transported in like manner (67). Therefore, in principle, any immune complex in the mucosal lamina propria that contains a molecule of dimeric IgA is capable of being transported across the mucosal epithelium into the luminal secretions. Such transport of IgA immune complexes is envisioned to function *in vivo* as an excretory immune system capable of excreting antigen from the mucosa, thereby ridding the body of potentially harmful immune complexes and minimizing the load of circulating immune complexes. However, there is also the untoward possibility that viruses in mucosal tissues could be complexed by IgA antibodies and thereby selectively introduced into epithelial cells (68).

These two newly proposed functions of IgA could be important in mucosal host defense. Certainly, mucous membranes are a common site of invasion by infectious agents, which can pass through or replicate in the lining epithelial cells. Therefore, the potential of IgA antibodies to encounter microbial pathogens within cells during their normal route of transport across the epithelium and to neutralize or excrete them is likely to be significant. However, even if the epithelial barrier should be breached by microorganisms, IgA antibodies secreted by local plasma cells would have the opportunity to bind and eliminate them and their products across the epithelium, either as intact microorganisms coated by IgA antibody or as soluble immune complexes.

Thus, mucosal IgA can now be envisioned as functioning in any of three tiers to protect the host (69) (Fig. 3). The innermost tier is the lamina propria, into which the abundant plasma cells secrete dimeric IgA. If IgA antibody binds antigen in the lamina propria, the complex can be directly excreted. The middle tier is the epithelial lining of the mucous membrane: if IgA antibody in transit to the secretions should meet an infectious pathogen inside an epithelial cell, it can neutralize or excrete it. The outermost tier, the traditional place where secretory IgA has been thought to function, is within the intestinal lumen, where IgA antibody can bind to microbes or their toxins and prevent attachment to and penetration through the mucosal epithelium.

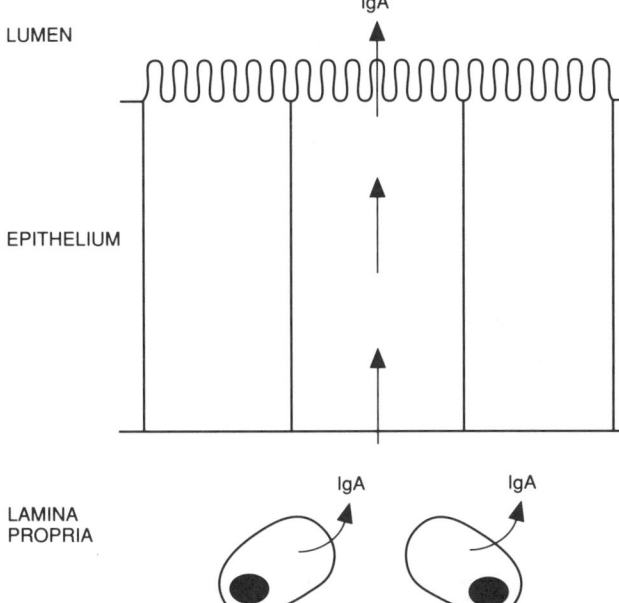

FIG. 3. Three tiers of mucosal IgA function in host defense. Intestinal IgA is thought to be capable of functioning at three different levels. First, dimeric IgA antibodies secreted from plasma cells in the lamina propria have an opportunity to combine with antigens, including infectious agents and their products, that may be present in the lamina propria. Such immune complexes can then bind to and be transported into the intestinal lumen by the plgR in the same manner as free dimeric IgA, an excretory function. Second, during their transepithelial transport, IgA antibodies have an opportunity to encounter intracellular microbes or their components within epithelial cells. In this way, they may be neutralized or excreted. Third, after epithelial transcytosis, secretory IgA antibodies may first encounter antigens within the intestinal lumen, where IgA can mediate its immune exclusion function.

REFERENCES

1. Besredka A. *Local immunization*. Baltimore: Williams and Wilkins; 1927.
2. Burrows W, Deupree NG, Moore DE. The effect of X-irradiation on experimental enteric cholera in the guinea pig. *J Infect Dis* 1950;87:158–168.
3. Burrows W, Deupree NG, Moore DE. The effect of X-irradiation on fecal and urinary antibody response. *J Infect Dis* 1950;87:169–183.
4. Tomasi TB. The discovery of secretory IgA and the mucosal immune system. *Immunol Today* 1992;13:416–418.
5. Lamm ME. Cellular aspects of immunoglobulin A. *Adv Immunol* 1976;22:223–290.
6. Brandtzaeg P. Role of J chain and secretory component in receptor-mediated glandular and hepatic transport of immunoglobulins in man. *Scand J Immunol* 1985;22:111–146.
7. Mestecky J, McGhee JR. Immunoglobulin A (IgA): Molecular and cellular interactions involved in IgA biosynthesis and immune response. *Adv Immunol* 1987;40:153–245.
8. Conley ME, Delacroix DL. Intravascular and mucosal immunoglobulin A: two separate but related systems of immune defense *Ann Intern Med* 1987;106:892–899.
9. Kutteh WH, Prince SJ, Mestecky J. Tissue origins of human polymeric and monomeric IgA. *J Immunol* 1982;128:990–995.
10. Kerr MA. The structure and function of human IgA. *Biochem J* 1990;271:285–296.
11. Mestecky J, Lue C, Tarkowski A, et al. Comparative studies of the biological properties of human IgA subclasses. *Protides Biol Fluids* 1989;36:173–182.
12. Plaut AG. The IgA1 proteases of pathogenic bacteria. *Annu Rev Microbiol* 1983;37:603–622.
13. Kilian M, Mestecky J, Russell MW. Defense mechanisms involving Fc-dependent functions of immunoglobulin A and their subversion by bacterial immunoglobulin A proteases *Microbiol Rev* 1988;52:296–303.
14. Kett K, Brandtzaeg P, Radl J, Haaijman JJ. Different subclass distribution of IgA-producing cells in human lymphoid organs and various secretory tissues. *J Immunol* 1986;136:3631–3635.
15. Mestecky J, Schrohenloher RE, Kulhavy R, Wright GP, Tomana M. Site of J chain attachment to human polymeric IgA. *Proc Natl Acad Sci USA* 1974;71:544–548.
16. Garcia-Pardo A, Lamm ME, Plaut AG, Frangione B. J chain is covalently bound to both monomer subunits in human secretory IgA. *J Biol Chem* 1981;256:11734–11738.
17. Bastian A, Kratzin H, Eckart K, Hilschmann N. Intra- and interchain disulfide bridges of the human J chain in secretory immunoglobulin A. *Biol Chem Hoppe-Seyler* 1992;373:1255–1263.
18. Brandtzaeg P, Prydz H. Direct evidence for an integrated function of J chain and secretory component in epithelial transport of immunoglobulins. *Nature* 1984;311:71–73.
19. Eiffert H, Quentin E, Wiederhold M, et al. Determination of the

molecular structure of the human free secretory component. *Biol Chem Hoppe-Seyler* 1991;372:119–128.

20. Krajci P, Kvale D, Tasken K, Brandtzaeg P. Molecular cloning and exon-intron mapping of the gene encoding human transmembrane secretory component (the poly-Ig receptor). *Eur J Immunol* 1992;22:2309–2315.

21. Cunningham-Rundles C, Lamm ME. Reactive half-cystine peptides of the secretory component of human exocrine immunoglobulin A. *J Biol Chem* 1975;250:1987–1991.

22. Garcia-Pardo A, Lamm ME, Plaut AG, Frangione B. Secretory component is covalently bound to a single sub-unit in human secretory IgA. *Molec Immunol* 1979;16:477–482.

23. Fallgreen-Gebauer E, Gebauer W, Bastian A, et al. The covalent linkage of secretory component to IgA. Strucure of sIgA. *Biol Chem Hoppe Seyler* 1993;374:1023–1028.

24. Brown WR, Newcomb RW, Ishizaka K. Proteolytic degradation of exocrine and serum immunoglobulins. *J Clin Invest* 1970;49:1374–1380.

25. Underdown BJ, Dorrington KJ. Studies of the structural and conformational basis for the relative resistance of serum and secretory immunoglobulin A to proteolysis. *J Immunol* 1974;112:949–959.

26. Lindh E. Increased resistance of immunoglobulin A dimers to proteolytic degradation after binding of secretory component. *J Immunol* 1975;114:284–286.

27. Pfaffenbach G, Lamm ME, Gigli I. Activation of the guinea pig alternative complement pathway by mouse IgA immune complexes. *J Exp Med* 1982;155:231–247.

28. Fanger MW, Goldstine SN, Shen L. Cytofluorographic analysis of receptors for IgA on human polymorphonuclear cells and monocytes and the correlation of receptor expression with phagocytosis. *Mol Immunol* 1983;20:1019–1027.

29. Monteiro RC, Kubagawa H, Cooper MD. Cellular distribution, regulation, and biochemical nature of an Fc_α receptor in humans. *J Exp Med* 1990;171:597–613.

30. Emancipator SE, Lamm ME. Pathways of tissue injury initiated by humoral immune mechanisms. *Lab Invest* 1986;54:475–478.

31. Solari R, Kraehenbuhl J-P. The biosynthesis of secretory component and its role in the transepithelial transport of IgA dimer. *Immunol Today* 1985;6:17–20.

32. Brown WR, Kloppel TM. The liver and IgA: immunological, cell biological and clinical implications. *Hepatology* 1989;9:763–784.

33. Underdown BJ. Transcytosis by the receptor for polymeric immunoglobulin. In: Metzger H, ed. *Fc receptors and the action of antibodies.* Washington, DC: American Society for Microbiology; 1990:74–93.

34. Mestecky J, Lue C, Russell MW. Selective transport of IgA. Cellular and molecular aspects. *Gastroenterol Clin North Am* 1991;20:441–471.

35. Apodaca G, Bomsel M, Arden J, et al. The polymeric immunoglobulin receptor. A model protein to study transcytosis. *J Clin Invest* 1991;87:1877–1882.

36. Mostov KE. Transepithelial transport of immunoglobulins. *Annu Rev Immunol;* 1994;12:63–84.

37. Renston RH, Jones AL, Christiansen WD, et al. Evidence for a vesicular transport mechanism in hepatocytes for biliary secretion of immunoglobulin A. *Science* 1980;208:1276–1278.

38. Takahashi I, Nakane PK, Brown WR. Ultrastructural events in the translocation of polymeric IgA by rat hepatocytes. *J Immunol* 1982;128:1181–1187.

39. Hoppe CA, Connolly TP, Hubbard AL. Transcellular transport of polymeric IgA in the rat hepatocyte: biochemical and morphological characterization of the transport pathway. *J Cell Biol* 1985;101:2113–2123.

40. Limet J, Quintart J, Schneider Y, Courtoy PJ. Receptor-mediated endocytosis of polymeric IgA and galactosylated serum albumin in the rat liver. Evidence for intracellular ligand sorting and identification of distinct endosomal compartments. *Eur J Biochem* 1985;146:539–548.

41. Chintalacharuvu KR, Tavill AS, Louis LN, Vaerman J-P, Lamm ME, Kaetzel CS. Disulfide bond formation between dimeric immunoglobulin A and the polymeric immunoglobulin receptor during hepatic transcytosis. *Hepatology,* 1994;19:162–173.

42. Musil LS, Baenziger JU. Proteolytic processing of rat liver membrane secretory component. Cleavage activity is localized to bile canalicular membranes. *J Biol Chem* 1988;263:15799–15808.

43. Solari R, Schaerer E, Tallichet C, Braiterman LT, Hubbard AL, Kraehenbuhl J-P. Cellular location of the cleavage event of the polymeric immunoglobulin receptor and fate of its anchoring domain in the rat hepatocyte. *Biochem J* 1989;257:759–768.

44. Jackson GDF, Lemaitre-Coelho I, Vaerman J-P, Bazin H, Beckers A. Rapid disappearance from serum of intravenously injected rat myeloma IgA and its secretion into bile. *Eur J Immunol* 1978;8:123–126.

45. Orlans E, Peppard J, Fry JF, Hinton RH, Mullock BM. Secretory component as the receptor for polymeric IgA on rat hepatocytes. *J Exp Med* 1979;150:1577–1581.

46. Fisher MM, Nagy B, Bazin H, Underdown BJ. Biliary transport of IgA: role of secretory component. *Proc Natl Acad Sci USA* 1979;76:2008–2012.

47. Ogra PL, Karzon DT. Formation and function of poliovirus antibody in different tissues. *Prog Med Virol* 1971;13:156–193.

48. Mills J, Van Kirk JE, Wright PF, Chanock RM. Experimental respiratory syncytial virus infection of adults. Possible mechanisms of resistance to infection and illness. *J Immunol* 1971;107:123–130.

49. Liew FY, Russell SM, Appleyard G, Brand CM, Beale J. Cross-protection in mice infected with influenza A virus by the respiratory route is correlated with local IgA antibody rather than serum antibody or cytotoxic T cell reactivity. *Eur J Immunol* 1984;14:350–356.

50. Offit PA, Clark HF. Protection against rotavirus-induced gastroenteritis in a murine model by passively acquired gastrointestinal but not circulating antibodies. *J Virol* 1985;54:58–64.

51. Gerber JD, Ingersoll JD, Gast AM, et al. Protection against feline infectious peritonitis by intranasal inoculation of a temperature-sensitive FIPV vaccine. *Vaccine* 1990;8:536–542.

52. Hanson LA, Björkander J, Oxelius VA. Selective IgA deficiency. In: Chandra RK, ed. *Primary and secondary immunodeficiency disorders.* New York: Churchill-Livingstone; 1983:62–84.

53. Clemens JD, Harris JR, Khan MR, et al. Field trial of oral cholera vaccines in Bangladesh. *Lancet* 1986;2:124–127.

54. Quiding M, Nordström I, Kilander A, et al. Intestinal immune responses in humans. Oral cholera vaccination induces strong intestinal antibody responses and interferon-γ production and evokes local immunological memory. *J Clin Invest* 1991;88:143–148.

55. Mazanec MB, Nedrud JG, Lamm ME. Immunoglobulin A monoclonal antibodies protect against Sendai virus. *J Virol* 1987;61:2624–2626.

56. Renegar KB, Small Jr PA. Passive transfer of local immunity to influenza virus infection by IgA antibody. *J Immunol* 1991;146:1972–1978.

57. Winner III L, Mack J, Weltzin R, Mekalanos JJ, Kraehenbuhl J-P, Neutra MR. New model for analysis of mucosal immunity: intestinal secretion of specific monoclonal immunoglobulin A from hybridoma tumors protects against *Vibrio cholerae* infection. *Infect Immun* 1991;59:977–982.

58. Michetti P, Mahan MJ, Slauch JM, Mekalanos JJ, Neutra MR. Monoclonal secretory immunoglobulin A protects mice against oral challenge with the invasive pathogen *Salmonella typhimurium. Infect Immun* 1992;60:1786–1792.

59. Czinn SJ, Cai A, Nedrud JG. Protection of germ-free mice from infection by *Helicobacter felis* after active oral or passive IgA immunization. *Vaccine* 1993;11:637–642.

60. Williams RC, Gibbons RJ. Inhibition of bacterial adherence by secretory immunoglobulin A: a mechanism of antigen disposal. *Science* 1972;177:697–699.

61. Fubara ES, Freter R. Protection against bacterial infection by secretory IgA antibodies. *J Immunol* 1973;111:395–403.

62. Svanborg-Eden C, Svennerholm A-M. Secretory immunoglobulin A and G antibodies prevent adhesion of *Escherichia coli* to human urinary tract epithelial cells. *Infect Immun* 1978;22:790–797.

63. Outlaw MC, Dimmock NJ. Mechanisms of neutralization of influenza virus on mouse tracheal epithelial cells by mouse mono-

clonal polymeric IgA and polyclonal IgM directed against the viral haemagglutinin. *J Gen Virol* 1990;71:69–76.

64. Mostov KE, Deitcher DL. Polymeric immunoglobulin receptor expressed in MDCK cells transcytoses IgA. *Cell* 1986;46: 613–621.

65. Mazanec MB, Kaetzel CS, Lamm ME, Fletcher D, Nedrud JG. Intracellular neutralization of virus by immunoglobulin A antibodies. *Proc Natl Acad Sci USA* 1992;89:6901–6905.

66. Kaetzel CS, Robinson JK, Chintalacharuvu KR, Vaerman J-P, Lamm ME. The polymeric immunoglobulin receptor (secretory component) mediates transport of immune complexes across ep-

ithelial cells: a local defense function for IgA. *Proc Natl Acad Sci USA* 1991;88:8796–8800.

67. Kaetzel CS, Robinson JK, Lamm ME. Epithelial transcytosis of monomeric IgA and IgG cross-linked through antigen to polymeric IgA. A role for monomeric antibodies in the mucosal immune system. *J Immunol* 1994;152:72–76.

68. Sixbey JW, Yao Q-Y. Immunoglobulin A-induced shift of Epstein–Barr virus tissue tropism. *Science* 1992;255:1578–1580.

69. Mazanec MB, Nedrud JG, Kaetzel CS, Lamm ME. A three-tiered view of the role of IgA in mucosal defense. *Immunol Today* 1993;14:430–435.

Infections of the Gastrointestinal Tract,
edited by M. J. Blaser, P. D. Smith, J. I. Ravdin,
H. B. Greenberg, and R. L. Guerrant
Raven Press, Ltd., New York © 1995.

CHAPTER 13

Secretory Antibody Responses to Enteric Pathogens

William R. Brown

One of the many complicated demands placed on the gastrointestinal immune system is that of existing peacefully with the indigenous intestinal microflora while, when called upon, responding vigorously to pathogenic microorganisms. The gut of germ-free animals (1) and the human neonate (2) contain few plasma cells, but after bacterial contamination the normal complement of the cells appears rapidly. The germ-free condition is associated with absence of immunoglobulin A (IgA) in the intestinal secretions, and the Ig appears as a response to colonization. Gastrointestinal secretions have antibody activity to a wide range of commensal organisms (3). Despite the presence of these "natural" antibodies, however, IgA antibodies, at least, probably have little influence on the composition of the flora. In support of this view is the observation that the normal flora of persons selectively deficient in IgA are not different from that of immunologically intact persons, and the IgA deficiency alone is not associated with overgrowth of bacteria in the upper intestine (4,5). In severe, generalized hypogammaglobulinemia, excess numbers of anaerobes have been cultured from upper intestinal fluids (4,5), a finding that may implicate antibodies of IgG or IgM isotype in limiting the growth of bacteria in the fluids, although the gastric hypochlorhydria resulting from chronic atrophic gastritis, or the associated T lymphocyte defects, which are common in such persons, also may aid the bacterial proliferation.

Despite the logical assumption that antibodies in gastrointestinal fluids play a major role in the protection against enteric pathogens, the evidence on the mechanisms by which the antibodies may be protective, and the importance of antibodies relative to nonimmunologic and other immunologic defense mechanisms of the gut, still is largely unclarified. The purpose of this chapter is to bring

together the existing data concerning this important issue. Although a serologic response to nearly all intestinal pathogens has been identified, a corresponding intestinal secretory antibody response often has not been sought, or information about the response is fragmentary. This state of ignorance is disappointing but understandable; collection of intestinal secretions and tissues is far more difficult than procurement of serum samples, and many technical difficulties confound the analysis of intestinal antibodies. Furthermore, the defenses against intestinal pathogens, just as in the regulation of the indigenous gut microflora, doubtless are complex and involve immunologic as well as nonimmunologic mechanisms. Thus assessing the importance of secretory antibodies amid numerous other defenses can be exceedingly difficult. Evidence favoring a limited role of antibodies in protection against intestinal pathogenic bacteria is that severe and frequent intestinal infections are not common in hypogammaglobulinemic patients (at least not in countries where hygiene is generally good), although infections with organisms such as salmonellae (4) and *Campylobacter jejuni* (6) do occur.

One area of great uncertainty is that of the mechanisms by which intestinal pathogens induce a secondary antibody response, in particular, IgA secretion. This is particularly true with respect to organisms that do not penetrate the epithelium. For example, how does an enterotoxin-secreting *Escherichia coli* organism induce an IgA response to the toxin, which binds to the epithelial surface and presumably is not in direct contact with the IgA-producing lymphoid cells? Some light may be shed on this complex and important issue by the recent observations that intestinal epithelial cells are sources of certain cytokines, for example, interleukin-1β (IL-1β) (7), IL-6 (8), and transforming growth factor-β (TGF-β) (9). IL-1 is known to induce IL-6 secretion by various cell types, and, in turn, IL-6, either alone or in combination with IL-5, is a potent inducer of IgA production by Peyer's patch B cells (10). Enhanced levels of IL-1 have been found in

W. R. Brown: Division of Gastroenterology, University of Colorado School of Medicine and Gastroenterology Section, Department of Veterans Affairs Medical Center, Denver, Colorado 80220.

mucosal tissues from rabbits infected with enteropathogenic *E. coli* (11), and *in situ* hybridization experiments have shown that the number of cells containing messenger ribonucleic acid (mRNA) for TGF-β were increased in both the lamina propria and epithelium of mice infected with *Trichinella spiralis* and in patients with chronic inflammatory bowel diseases (12). In addition, cholera toxin reportedly strongly promotes antigen presentation *in vivo* and *in vitro* by stimulating the production of IL-1 by antigen-presenting cells, including intestinal epithelial cells (13,14), and greatly promotes antigen priming of T cells (15). A less exotic mechanism by which some intestinal pathogens might stimulate antibody secretion is direct entry into the mucosa. Some intercellular passage of microorganisms and other particulate materials appears to occur through the villus tips of the small intestine, a phenomenon described as "persorption" (16).

The passive protection that can be conferred to the intestine through the ingestion of antibodies in breast fluids may be very important in the nursing infant. Quite appropriately, that topic also is reviewed in this chapter.

METHODS OF DEMONSTRATING ANTIBODY ACTIVITY IN THE INTESTINE

One of the difficulties in assessing the biologic significance of antibodies in gastrointestinal fluids lies in vexing technical problems. These problems include proteolytic degradation of the antibodies, especially those of IgM and IgG classes (17,18), in the fluids, which occurs *in vivo* or during storage; the interference from agglutination inhibitors; and the occurrence of various nonspecific reactions (19). Also, there is the issue of whether antibodies have immunologic activity, as opposed to merely being present, in the gut. For example, methods that demonstrate direct antibody–antigen interactions such as a radioimmunoassay, may indicate the presence of antibody, whereas a test of agglutination may be negative or reveal only low-titer antibody activity. Another factor that must be taken into account in evaluating the biologic significance of antimicrobial antibodies in the intestine is that many of the studies on this subject have been conducted in animals, and the relevance of the results to the situation in humans often is unclarified.

Recently, one advance seems to have been made at least in the methods for collecting intestinal fluids for the purpose of measuring antibodies—that is, intestinal lavage (20,21). The lavage is accomplished by having participants drink isotonic salt solution until 1000 mL or more of watery stool is passed, and antibodies are measured in concentrates of the fluid. Another useful approach to the study of mucosal immune responses is that of the enzyme-linked immunospot (ELISPOT) assay for measurement of functionally active antibody-secreting cells (22,23). This assay, which can be conducted either on circulating cells or on cells in intestinal biopsy specimens, may be a more accurate assessment of intestinal responses than measurement of antibodies in secretions.

ANTIBODIES TO BACTERIA

The presence of antibodies in intestinal secretions to intestinal pathogens has been known for over 70 years since Davies (24) found specific antibodies in the feces of patients suffering from dysentery. With resurgence of interest in intestinal immunity that occurred about 40 years later, intestinal antibody responses were demonstrated to infection with *Vibrio cholerae* (25,26), *E. coli* (27), and *Shigella* (28). These observations intensified interest in enteric immunization, and Freter (29) showed that a killed oral vaccine provided a more reliable stimulus of coproantibody then did parenteral vaccination.

The mechanisms by which antibodies may protect against enteric pathogenic bacteria are multiple and vary from one organism to another. The protective activities include inhibition of the attachment of bacteria to mucosal surfaces, inhibition of toxin production, and immobilization or lysis of organisms.

Vibrio cholerae

Vibrio cholerae is one organism that has been shown to induce a protective immune response that is partially if not entirely antibody mediated. Many years ago, Freter (30), using serum antibodies, showed that one effect of anti-cholera antibodies is to prevent the adherence of *V. cholerae* to intestinal mucosa. Later he showed that coproantibody and bacterial antagonism are protective factors in experimental cholera (31). In 1972, Fubara and Freter (32) showed that IgA antibodies obtained from the intestinal secretions of germ-free mice immunized with *V. cholerae* could protect against *V. cholerae* infection. The protection probably resulted from antibody agglutination and lysis of the organisms or, failing that, inhibition of bacterial attachment to epithelial cells.

There also is persuasive experimental evidence that IgA antibodies can neutralize the effect of cholera toxin. This neutralization appears to be accomplished by the antibodies preventing the binding of the toxin rather than interfering with the toxin's ability to activate adenylate cyclase (33). Direct evidence that IgA antibodies can prevent the secretory action of cholera toxin is our observation in rats that toxin, when mixed with bile from animals that had been immunized with the toxin, was virtually ineffective in inducing water secretion by ileal loops (34) (Fig. 1). This effect was shown to be due entirely to IgA antibodies in the bile, which is evidence not only of the specificity of the antibody action but also that IgA antibodies can be effective in the strong detergent environment of bile. Corroborative results have been reported by Vaerman's group (35).

In other work in animal models, a synergistic effect of antibodies to cholera toxin and whole vibrios or lipopolysaccharide has been observed (36,37). Also, both the secretory IgA (S-IgA) response and the plasma IgG anti-cholera toxin response after toxin feeding to mice have been found to be controlled by the I-A subregion of H-2 (38). There is debate in the literature over the issue of whether cholera toxin directly stimulates the secretion of

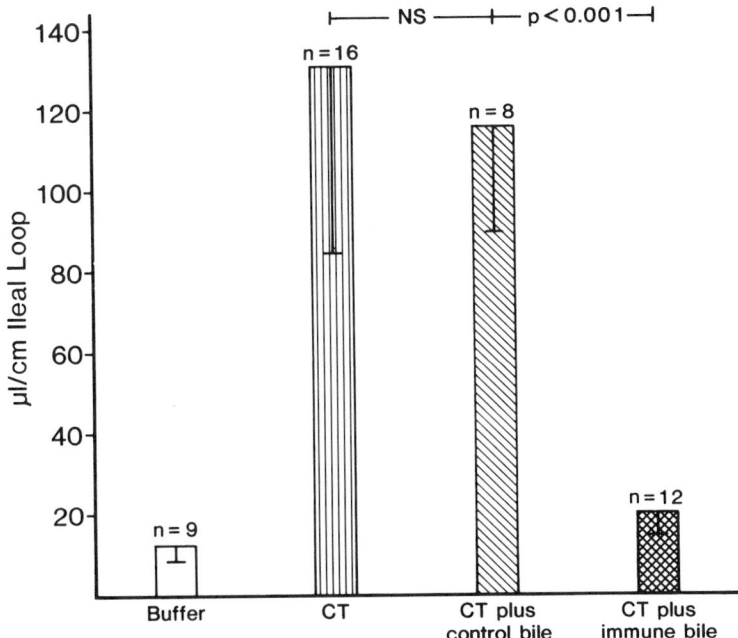

FIG. 1. The inhibiting effect of S-IgA antibodies on cholera toxin-stimulated water secretion by the intestine. The S-IgA antibodies in this work were present in bile of rats that had been immunized enterically with cholera toxin. The graph illustrates secretory response of *in situ* rat ileal loops after the instillation of buffer, cholera toxin (CT), or CT plus bile. Control bile was obtained either from uninoculated animals or from animals that had no anti-CT antibody response to inoculation. Immune bile contained IgA anti-CT antibodies but no anti-CT antibodies of other Ig isotypes. Whereas control bile had no effect on CT-induced secretion, immune bile almost completely inhibited CT-induced secretion. (From ref. 34, with permission.)

IgA into intestinal fluids, just as it stimulates water secretion. We (39) found that cholera toxin instilled into intestinal loops of rabbits did not induce IgA secretion even though an appropriate fluid response was obtained. On the other hand, cholera toxin has been used to enhance the collection of rabbit S-Igs (40), and enhanced secretion of IgA from intestinal crypt epithelium has been reported (41). The enhancement of IgA secretion, however, was modest and did not correspond kinetically or in magnitude with the secretion of fluid.

Human cholera and its prevention through various kinds of immunization have elicited much attention. Adult American volunteers experimentally infected with *V. cholerae* responded with high levels of specific antitoxin as well as antibacterial antibodies in jejunal fluids and serum (42,43). Clinical cholera has been shown to give rise to high levels of S-IgA antibodies not only against cholera toxin but also against the cell wall lipopolysaccharide locally in the intestine (36). Thus antibodies both to the toxin and the organisms may be important in the acquired immunity to cholera infection, but the relative importance of the two kinds of antibodies is not firmly established.

Considerable evidence indicates that natural infection with *V. cholerae* is highly effective in preventing recurrence of the disease, probably because of the production of high levels of specific S-IgA antibodies as well as immunologic memory for such antibody formation locally in the intestine (36,44). Recurrent symptomatic infections by *V. cholerae* appear to be uncommon, in contrast to the relatively poor protection conferred by standard vaccines. In Bangladesh, for example, a very low reinfection rate, suggesting approximately 90% protection against a second episode of cholera in endemic areas, has been reported (45). Human volunteers suffering from symptomatic cholera also were effectively protected against reinfection for several years after the initial cholera episode

(46). Thus Levine et al. (47) showed that four volunteers were immune to rechallenge with either homologous or heterologous serotypes of *V. cholerae* 33 to 36 months after initial infection: none developed diarrhea and only one was found to excrete the organisms after rechallenge. Prior to the rechallenge, S-IgA antibodies were not detectable in the jejunal fluids of the subjects who had been infected, but two of them had rises in S-IgA antibodies by day 8 postchallenge. This evidence of an intestinal IgA memory response to cholera antigen exposure has been corroborated by experiments in which oral administration of relatively low doses of cholera antigens to cholera convalescents resulted in considerably higher and earlier-appearing S-IgA antibody responses in intestinal secretions than observed in similarly immunized healthy controls (36). In mice, adoptive transfer of intestinal mucosal antitoxin memory by isolated B cells 1 year after oral immunization with cholera toxin has been reported (48).

Part of the explanation for the strong immunologic memory to cholera infection may be the potency of cholera toxin as an immunogen in the intestine (49). Indeed, the toxin actually can be an effective adjuvant for other enterically administered immunogens, a subject that is dealt with elsewhere (see chapter by Neutra). Moreover, unlike many other proteins, cholera toxin does not induce a state of systemic immunologic hyporesponsiveness (oral tolerance) when fed; it may in fact induce an IgG serum antibody response to itself and a heightened response (50).

Escherichia coli

The diarrhea-producing *E. coli* can conveniently be considered as three groups: enteropathogenic (EPEC), enterotoxigenic (ETEC), and enteroinvasive (EIEC). ETEC organisms are considerably more heterogeneous than *V. cholerae*, with numerous serotypes, colonization factors, and enterotoxins, although one of the enterotoxins, heat labile enterotoxin (LT), resembles cholera toxin in both structure and mechanism of action. Another *E. coli* enterotoxin (STa), which is heat stable, acts differently (via activation of guanylate cyclase), produces fluid accumulation in the suckling mouse assay but not in the rabbit ligated ileal loop assay, and is poorly immunogenic. Some strains of *E. coli,* previously known as enteropathogenic *E. coli,* may be more aptly termed enteroadherent organisms; although they can induce diarrhea, they lack the enteric pathogenic properties of other *E. coli* strains, such as LT or ST production, or the invasiveness of *Shigella.* In general, much less is known about immunologic protection against pathogenic *E. coli* than against *V. cholerae.*

With respect to *E. coli* enterotoxins, interestingly, there appears to be some cross-protection between antibodies to cholera toxin and *E. coli* enterotoxins. For example, cholera B subunit–whole cell cholera vaccine afforded substantial, though rather short-lasting, protection also against diarrhea caused by ETEC-producing LT enterotoxin (51), and, vice versa, anti-LT antibodies may be effective against experimental cholera, although immunity against the homologous toxin usually is somewhat better. Protection induced by *E. coli* enterotoxin may be less than that produced by cholera toxin, as shown by studies in Bangladesh and Mexico (52,53).

It is known also that the ability to produce enterotoxin is not sufficient to enable an *E. coli* strain to cause diarrhea; the organisms must also be able to colonize the mucosal surface of the small intestinal epithelial cells. This fact was first appreciated in studies of piglet diarrhea, where an adhesive factor (K88 antigen), controllable by a transferable plasmid, was found to be essential for the organism to cause diarrhea (54). Later it was learned that ETEC, which can cause diarrhea in humans, may require the presence of adhesive factors, known as colonization factor antigens (CFAs), for the induction of diarrhea (55). With respect to immunologic defense against certain pathogenic *E. coli,* these kinds of adhesive factors may be important because antibodies to the factors might prevent attachment of the bacteria to the mucosa and consequent interference with the production of enterotoxin. The plausibility of this concept is borne out in studies in both humans and animals.

In studies in humans, in which an intestinal lavage method was used to obtain intestinal secretions (20), an IgA response to CFA was found in 63% of CFA+ patients. A protective effect of such anti-CFA antibodies is suggested by the reports of the production of intestinal IgA antibodies to CFA/II in response to feeding CFA/II in biodegradable microspheres, with partial protection of the volunteers (56).

Details of immunologic protection against an enteroadherent *E. coli* have come from studies of the strain RDEC-1, which produces diarrhea in rabbits (57). RDEC-1 organisms adhere to the distal intestinal epithelium by means of fimbria. Considerable evidence indicates that antibodies to fimbrial proteins, for example, fimbrial adhesion AF/R1, can interfere with binding of the bacterium to the intestinal mucosa and prevent diarrheal illness in immunized rabbits. This evidence includes passive protection by milk IgA from infected rabbits (58), specific inhibition of RDEC-1 adherence to rabbit intestinal brush borders by milk S-IgA (59), and clearance of the organism from the guts of challenged animals in association with the appearance of antibody-forming cells in the intestinal mucosa and antibodies in bile and intestinal fluid to AF/R1 pilus antigens (60) (Figs. 2 and 3; Plate 1). Studies in the rabbit also have provided evidence that antibodies (in this case, monoclonal antibodies) to CFA/II could passively protect against infection with *E. coli* bearing these virulence factors, although the authors could not conclude whether the protection was due to interference with bacterial adherence or to agglutination of the organisms (61). The protective role of anti-pilus antibodies is supported also by the results of studies of protection by milk or colostral antibodies, as discussed later.

Another possible mechanism of immunologic protection against pathogenic *E. coli* is that of IgA-dependent bacterial killing, which has been demonstrated in pig ileal Thirty–Vella loops actively challenged with ETEC bearing a pilus adhesion, K88 (62).

Campylobacter Species

Campylobacter jejuni is one of the most commonly detected bacterial enteric pathogens, but thus far not much is known about immunologic defense against it, especially the possibility of secretory antibody defenses. Blaser et al. (63) found that specific serum IgA levels in Bangladeshi children rose with age while IgG antibody levels fell. The authors speculated that repeated exposure to the organism might cause the elevated serum IgA, and, intuitively, perhaps also S-IgA antibodies in the gut, which might prevent tissue invasion by the organism. Additional indirect evidence in favor of intestinal antibodies being important against *C. jejuni* infection is that *C. jejuni* diarrheal disease is self-limited in immunocompetent individuals but may cause chronic diarrhea in hypogammaglobulinemic persons, some of whom have documented deficiencies of secretory immunoglobulins (6,64). Also, Winsor et al. (65) demonstrated S-IgA to flagellar antigens and to the major outer membrane protein (43 kDa) of *C. jejuni* in stool extracts from patients with *C. jejuni* diarrhea. This antibody response may correlate with protection from infection with the organism. Experimentally, through the use of the removable intestinal tie adult rabbit diarrhea (RITARD) model, oral inoculation with *C. jejuni* stimulated primary intestinal and serum antibody responses (66). Anti-*Campylobacter* intestinal and serum IgA titers before the secondary challenge were the most reliable predictors of resistance to colonization and bacteremia.

Shigella

The role of antibodies in defense from *Shigella* infection is one of the best defined and most interesting of the intestinal antibacterial antibody responses. Many years ago,

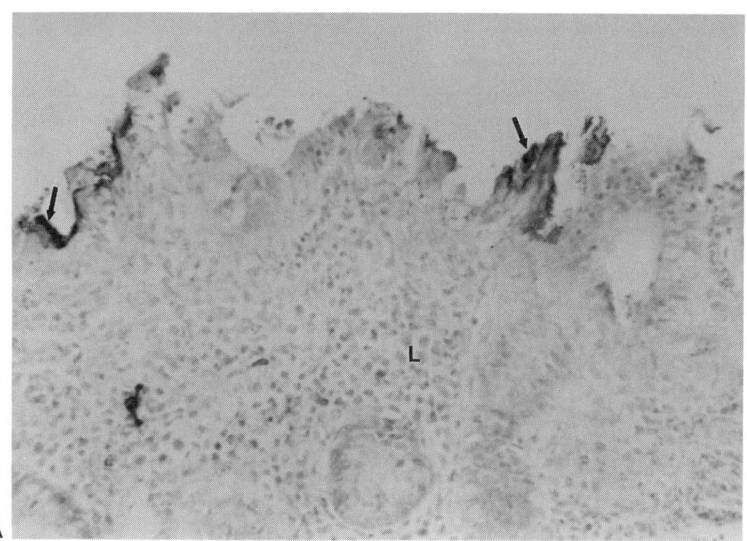

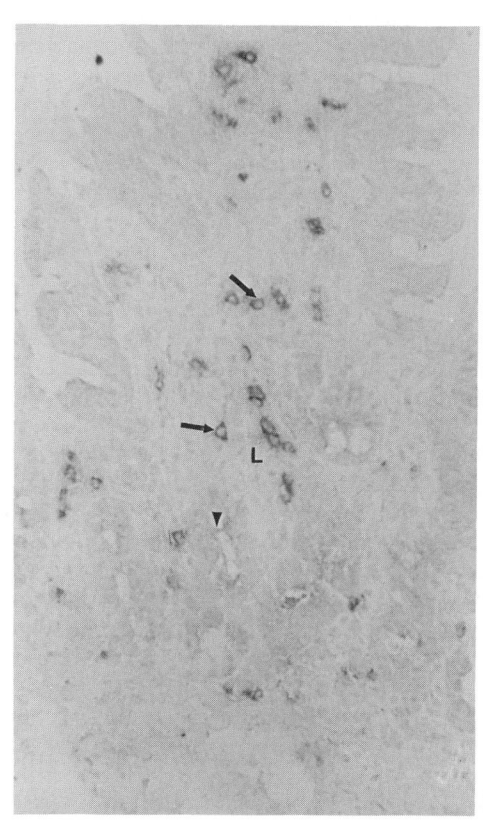

FIG. 2. Immunohistochemical studies in the rabbit diarrhea *E. coli* model, demonstrating anti-AF/R1 pilus-containing cells and adherent RDEC-1: (**A**) cecum and (**B**) jejunum. Animals were sacrificed 1 week after RDEC-1 infection. Tissue sections were reacted with pilus antigens, then with anti-RDEC-1 antibodies. In the cecum, a dense layer of RDEC-1 organisms is adherent to the epithelial surface (*arrows*), which is partially disrupted; anti-AF/R1 pilus antibody-containing cells are not present in the lamina propria (L). In the jejunum, numerous large plasma cells containing anti-AF/R1 pilus antibodies are present in the lamina propria (*arrows*); no RDEC-1 are adherent to the epithelium. (From ref. 60, with permission.) (See Plate 1.)

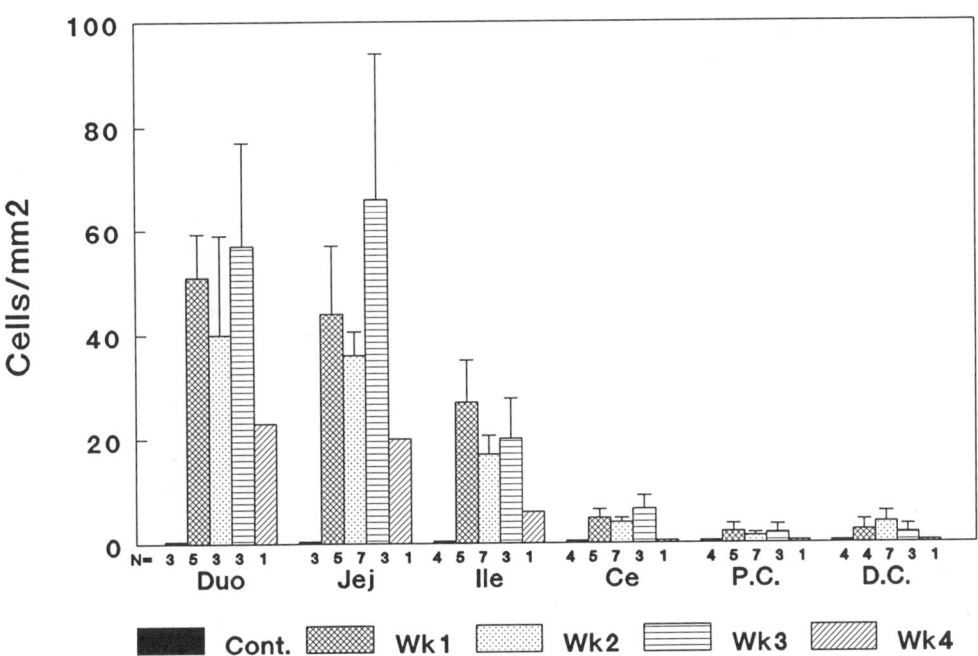

FIG. 3. Numbers of anti-AF/R1 pilus-containing cells in the lamina propria of RDEC-1-infected or control animals sacrificed at weekly intervals. Values are expressed as mean numbers of cells per square millimeter ± the standard error. N, numbers of animals used; Duo, duodenum; Jej, jejunum; Ile, ileum; Ce, cecum; P.C., proximal colon; D.C., distal colon; Cont., control.

Reed and Williams (28) found that fecal antibodies of the IgA, IgG, and IgM classes were increased after naturally acquired shigellosis, and the antibodies possessed anti-*Shigella* activity. Elucidation of mechanisms by which anti-*Shigella* antibodies might be produced and how they might exert a protective action has come from several studies. Thus *S. flexneri* organisms have been shown to preferentially colonize the follicle-associated epithelium of ligated rabbit intestinal loops, and virulent strains of shigellae can multiply within the M cells (67). The proclivity for the organisms to penetrate and proliferate within the follicle-associated epithelium has two consequences. On the one hand, it presumably facilitates the translocation of organisms to antigen-processing cells in the lymphoid follicle and the resultant production of antibodies, especially of IgA isotype. On the other hand, this easy entry of the organisms into the lymphoid tissue probably results in at least some of the mucosal lesions that characterize shigellosis. The antigenic stimulation of the gut-associated lymphoid tissue by *Shigella* no doubt results in the migration of antigen-specific B lymphocytes to the intestinal lamina propria and eventual secretion of IgA anti-*Shigella* antibodies into the intestinal lumen. In important studies with chronically isolated rabbit ileal loops, direct stimulation of the loops with either noninvasive or invasive strains of *Shigella* elicited strong local S-IgA responses against the somatic antigen of the challenge strain (68). A S-IgA memory response also has been demonstrated in rabbit ileal loops after peroral priming with *S. flexneri* (69,70).

The role of IgA antibodies in the protection from *Shigella* infection still requires clarification, however. S-IgA collected from ileal loops of rabbits immunized with invasive *E. coli–S. flexneri* 2a hybrid failed to inhibit the invasion of cultured mammalian cells by *S. flexneri* 2a (70). Antiserum elicited by parenteral immunization of rabbits with heat-killed *Shigella* also failed to inhibit the invasion of cultured cells (70). Thus the antibody recognizing the lipopolysaccharide somatic antigen may be ineffectual in inhibiting the initial uptake of shigellae to the intestinal epithelium. However, antibodies recognizing protein-aceous virulence determinants of *Shigella,* for example, plasmid-encoded invasion antigens and Shiga cytotoxin/enterotoxin, may be protective (68,71,72). In this regard, Keren et al. (68) have reported in rabbit ileal loop studies a strong correlation between the ability of loop fluids to neutralize the cytotoxicity of the toxin and IgA anti-Shiga toxin titers in the fluids.

In part, the mechanism of action of the secretory anti-*Shigella* antibodies seems to be through antibody-dependent cellular cytotoxicity (ADCC). Both intraepithelial lymphocytes and lamina proprial lymphocytes have shown ADCC against *S. flexneri,* and IgA recognizing the *Shigella* somatic antigen is more effective than IgG in arming the lymphocytes (73–75). In contrast, IgG and IgM are more effective than IgA in opsonizing shigellae for phagocytosis by polymorphonuclear neutrophils (76). Thus interstitial IgG and IgM recognizing the *Shigella* somatic antigens may be important in eliminating shigellae that are released from degenerating absorptive cells into the lamina propria.

Salmonella Species

Little direct experimental evidence bears on the possible role of antibodies in defense against salmonellae. However, the organism may penetrate the M cell (77), eventually leading to intestinal antibody production. Immunization studies have provided evidence that an anti-IgA antibody response to salmonellae can be elicited: immunization with strain *S. typhi* Ty21a evoked a specific S-IgA response to both lipopolysaccharide and flagellar antigens after oral administration (78), and IgA-driven T cell-mediated antibacterial immunity has been reported after giving live oral Ty21a vaccine to humans (79). These studies and similar immunization studies are discussed in more detail in the chapter by Miller and Pegues. Additional evidence that IgA-dependent cell-mediated activity may be important in defense against salmonellae comes from studies of *S. typhimurium* in mice, in which IgA-mediated killing of the organism by T cells isolated from Peyer's patches and spleens was observed (74). The systemically invasive *S. typhi,* which may rapidly be translocated to mesenteric lymph and may survive intracellularly in macrophages (80), can induce a systemic antibody response as well.

Helicobacter pylori

Helicobacter pylori is now recognized as causing gastroduodenal disease, but this bacterium is reviewed in the chapter by Taylor and Parsonnet.

ANTIBODIES TO VIRUSES

On the basis of information from patients with immunologic deficiencies, cell-mediated immune mechanisms appear to be more important than antibody-mediated mechanisms in defense against intestinal viral infections. For example, children who are recipients of bone marrow transplants or who have congenital T cell deficiencies have a high risk of developing chronic enteric adenovirus or rotavirus infections (81) and can develop severe and disseminated disease with high rates of mortality. In contrast, patients with Ig deficiencies do not seem to be especially prone to intestinal viral infections (4).

Nevertheless, intestinal antibody responses probably do have a role in prevention of enteric viral infections. S-IgA anti-viral antibodies as well as anti-viral antibodies of other immunoglobulin classes seem to prevent viral infections by similar mechanisms, that is, by inhibiting the penetration of viruses into susceptible cells (82); this is accomplished in the absence of any mediator substance such as complement.

Rotavirus

Rotavirus infection is the most common cause of severe diarrhea in infants and young children worldwide. Immune mechanisms of protection from rotavirus infection and clearance of established infection most likely depend on both humoral and cellular immune responses (83), and immunity to rotavirus gastroenteritis can be both homotypic (i.e., for the same serotype of virus) and heterotypic (i.e., for serotypes other than that of the primary infection) (83). Preexisting local neutralizing activity in intestinal fluid has been shown to be important in resistance to infection in calves and lambs (84).

In mice, rotavirus infection induces a very strong intestinal IgA response, as measured by an ELISPOT assay (22). In one study, after infection, about 50% of all antibody-secreting cells in the intestinal mucosa at the peak of the virus-specific response were rotavirus-specific cells. In a study of specific pathogen-free rabbits inoculated and challenged orally with rabbit Ala rotavirus, intestinal IgM was detected by 3 days postinoculation, and S-IgA was detected by 6 days postinoculation (85). Following challenge, rabbits were protected (no detectable virus shedding) from infection. All serologic and mucosal immune responses persisted at high levels until at least 175 days postchallenge.

Reovirus and Norwalk Agent

Although it seems likely that intestinal antibody responses to infection with these agents occur, apparently none has been described.

ANTIBODIES TO PARASITES

Giardiasis

Giardia lamblia is the causative organism in human giardiasis. Many experimental studies of immune protection from giardial infections have been conducted on mice, which can be infected with *G. muris*. The results of research in humans and mice suggest that there is a highly integrated and usually effective system of host defenses against giardiasis. Epidemiologic evidence indicates that a protective immunologic response to infection with *Giardia* probably occurs. Thus the prevalence of *G. lamblia* infection in Bangladesh is significantly higher in young children than in older persons (86), and in the Aspen, Colorado, outbreak there was a higher incidence of gastrointestinal infections in visitors to the community than in long-term residents (87). One piece of evidence favoring a role for antibody-mediated defense against the parasite is that patients with generalized hypogammaglobulinemia (e.g., common variable hypogammaglobulinemia) frequently are infected with *Giardia*, and the infection may be chronic (4). Persons selectively deficient in IgA, however, do not have an increased frequency of giardiasis (4,5), which raises doubt about the importance of IgA antibodies as opposed to those of other Ig classes in defense against *G. lamblia*. Nevertheless, other evidence that intestinal IgA antibody is involved in host defense against *Giardia* includes the observations that IgA antibodies in breast fluids may protect against giardiasis (discussed below) and that human volunteers experimentally inoculated with cultured trophozoites develop trophozoite-specific IgA in jejunal fluid (88).

The high frequency of giardiasis among Ig-deficient persons prompted us (89) to determine whether there is an unappreciated S-Ig deficiency among persons in the general population who acquire *G. lamblia* infection. However, we found that the levels of serum and intestinal fluid Igs were similar in patients recently infected with the parasite, except for an increased concentration of IgG in the patients' intestinal fluid.

Studies in mice, particularly by Heyworth and associates, have especially highlighted the likely role of IgA antibodies in clearance of murine *Giardia* infection. Heyworth has emphasized that T cell-deficient mice have difficulty in clearing *G. muris* and that the mice are deficient in helper T cells, not cytotoxic T cells (90,91). The helper T cell-depleted mice (and nude mice) do not generate a trophozoite-specific intestinal IgA response (91,92). Also, mice treated from birth onward with rabbit antiserum to mouse IgM to induce Ig deficiency lack the ability to clear *G. muris* infection or to develop an intestinal IgA response to the trophozoites (93).

Additional evidence favoring an important role for antibodies in anti-giardial defenses are the observations that acquired immunodeficiency syndrome (AIDS) patients who have reduced levels of anti-trophozoite antibodies frequently have symptomatic giardiasis, whereas AIDS patients with parasite-specific antibody do not have symptoms that can be attributed to *G. lamblia* infection (94).

The likely importance of monocyte-macrophages in defense against *Giardia* has been illustrated in several studies. Macrophages from various species were found capable of phagocytosing *Giardia* trophozoites (95). This activity could be important in the presentation of giardial antigens in immunologic reactions or in the killing of *Giardia*, by both spontaneous killing (96) and antibody-dependent killing (97).

Other Intestinal Parasites

Several other intestinal parasites such as *Cryptosporidia*, *Schistosoma*, and *Entamoeba histolytica* induce systemic antibody responses (97,98), but, regrettably, little or nothing is known about possible secretory antibody response to these organisms. This area urgently needs investigation.

COLOSTRAL AND MILK ANTIBODIES

The importance of colostrum in protecting the neonate has been recognized by owners of domestic animals for centuries. The protective value of breast fluids for human newborns has been less obvious. However, when resistance of breast-fed versus formula-fed infants is carefully evaluated, especially in underdeveloped countries, the immunologic value of colostrum for our own species becomes apparent (99).

The human breast is a major component of the S-IgA system, and breast fluids, especially colostrum during the

TABLE 1. *Specific antibody reactivity in human colostrum and milk*

Bacteria	Viruses	Fungi
Escherichia coli (O–K antigens and enterotoxin)	Rotavirus	*Candida albicans*
Salmonella	Poliovirus 1,2,3	
Shigella	Echovirus 6.9	
Vibrio cholerae	Coxsackievirus A9, B3	
Bacteroides fragilis	Respiratory syncytial virus	
Streptococcus pneumoniae	Cytomegalovirus	
Bordetella pertussis	Influenza A virus	
Corynebacterium diphtheriae	Herpes simplex virus	
Clostridium tetani	Arboviruses	
Streptococcus mutans	Semliki Forest	
Klebsiella pneumoniae	Ross River	
Chlamydia	Japanese B	

Adapted from ref. 100.

first 24 to 48 hr of lactation, are exceedingly rich in S-IgA (99). Human colostrum and milk differ from those fluids in many other mammals (e.g., rat, pig, and cow) in which IgG is a prominent or the predominant Ig; generally, the concentration of IgA in human breast secretions is at least ten times that of IgG or IgM. The numerous kinds of antibodies to bacteria, viruses, and fungi that have been identified in human colostrum and milk are listed in Table 1. Most of the antibodies of course are of the IgA class, and, not surprisingly, many of the antibacterial antibodies are directed toward intestinal bacteria. Ste-Marie et al. (101) found the amount of IgA antibodies to *E. coli* and *Bacteroides fragilis* in human breast fluids, measured by radioimmunoassay, to be about 0.5 µg per milligram of IgA, a value that remained fairly constant throughout lactation.

The true biologic role of breast fluid antibodies still is not fully clarified. Epidemiologic studies carried out in several rural and urban settings have demonstrated a striking resistance of breast-fed infants to *E. coli, Shigella, V. cholerae,* and protozoal infections (102). However, many medical, nutritional, and social behaviors that determine methods of feeding also are related to the acquisition of diarrheal disease, making a beneficial effect of breast-feeding difficult to assess.

A factor that confounds evaluation of the importance of antibodies in breast fluids is the presence of various immunologic cells. These include macrophages, neutrophils, regulatory T cells, effector T cells, and B lymphocytes (103). About 10^8 cells/day are delivered via milk to the nursing human newborn. A particularly interesting cell in breast fluids is that containing S-IgA (104). It has been proposed that these cells are transport vehicles for IgA to the newborn, although the amount of milk IgA transported by cells has been calculated to be trivial compared to the amount transported free (105). The cell-associated IgA may have a functional advantage, though, by releasing Ig during phagocytosis of colonizing microorganisms in the intestine (106).

Bacteria

One of the most persuasive pieces of evidence that milk IgA antibodies are effective in preventing diarrheal illness

is the observation that the frequency of diarrhea caused by *V. cholerae* was significantly lower in infants who ingested breast milk containing high titers of anti-cholera antibodies than in those ingesting low-antibody-titer milk (107). The protection was not associated with a decreased frequency of *V. cholerae* infection in infants' intestines, suggesting that the antibodies interfered with binding of the cholera enterotoxin to the mucosal surface.

Doubt has been raised about the importance of antibodies compared to other protective components of milk in defense against cholera in the newborn because of the reported presence of competing cholera toxin receptor-like glycocompounds (108) or other non-Ig components (109) present in milk. To try to help clarify this issue, we (110) evaluated the ability of milk from rabbits not immunized or immunized enterally during pregnancy with toxinogenic live *V. cholerae* to inhibit water secretion induced by *V. cholerae* in rat ileal loops. Nonimmune milk was not inhibitory, whereas immune milk was. The inhibitory component of the immune milk was Ig by virtue of its molecular weight and absorption by an anti-rat Ig immunosorbent. In addition, the inhibitory antibodies were principally antibodies to cholera toxin, because they could be removed from milk by a cholera toxin immunosorbent but were only partially removed by incubation with whole *V. cholerae*.

In animal studies, pigs and calves have been protected passively against an enterotoxigenic *E. coli* by luminal Ig directed against the organisms K88, K99, or 987 pilus adhesions received in the milk or colostrum from immunized sows or dams (111, 112). Passive protection of rabbits from infection with the rabbit diarrhea *E. coli* RDEC-1 also has been demonstrated (58).

Giardia Species

Giardia-specific IgA has been detected in human milk, and an inverse relationship between *Giardia*-specific IgA titer in maternal milk and prevalence of *G. lamblia* infection in suckling human infants has been reported (88, 113). In suckling mice, the ingestion of milk containing *Giardia*-specific IgA is temporarily protective against *G. muris* infection (114).

Viruses

From animal experiments, there is persuasive evidence for passive protection against rotavirus infection through the administration of breast fluids. Colostrum from cows vaccinated with rotavirus protected calves from experimentally induced rotavirus infection (115), and passive transfer of antibodies in milk or colostrum was protective when administered together with infective doses of viruses (115). In humans, however, the role of passive immunity in rotavirus infection is not established. Both breast-fed and bottle-fed children develop rotavirus infections and diarrhea. Totterdell et al. (117,118), however, found that the presence of rotavirus-specific antibody ingested in breast milk was associated with protection. Other reports have suggested a role for passive immune mechanisms in immunity to human rotavirus infection (119), as well as in reovirus-induced meningoencephalitis in neonatal mice (120).

In summary, antibodies, especially of IgA serotype, present in intestinal fluids probably are important in defense against enteric pathogens. Evidence of the protective effects of the antibodies is most convincing in the case of bacterial enterotoxins and certain enteroviruses. Intestinal antibodies also may be important deterrents to infection with *Shigella* and *Salmonella* species through the facilitation of cellular cytotoxicity reactions. In general, however, antibody-mediated defenses are probably a component of a very complex set of immunologic as well as nonimmunologic defenses that cooperate to protect the host from enteric infections.

REFERENCES

1. Thompson GR, Trexler PC. Gastrointestinal structure and function in germ-free or gnotobiotic animals. *Gut* 1971;12:230–235.
2. Crabbe PA, Heremans JF. The significance of local IgA in the physiology of the intestinal mucosa. *Folia Med Neerl* 1969;12:100–106.
3. McClelland DB, Samson RR, Parkin DM, Shearman DJC. Bacterial agglutination studies with secretory IgA prepared from human gastrointestinal secretions and colostrum. *Gut* 1972;13:450–458.
4. Brown WR, Butterfield D, Savage D, Tada T. Clinical, microbiological and immunological studies in patients with immunoglobulin deficiencies and gastrointestinal disorders. *Gut* 1972;13:441–449.
5. Brown WR, Savage DD, Dubois RB, Alp MH, Mallory A, Kern F Jr. The intestinal microflora of immunoglobulin-deficient and normal human subjects. *Gastroenterology* 1972;62:1143–1152.
6. Ahnen DJ, Brown WR. *Campylobacter* enteritis in immunedeficient patients. *Ann Intern Med* 1982;48:85–90.
7. Radema SA, Van Deventer SJH, Cerami A. Interleukin 1 beta is expressed predominantly by enterocytes in experimental colitis. *Gastroenterology* 1991;100:1180–1186.
8. McGee DW, Beagley KW, Aicher WK, McGhee JR. Transforming growth factor-β and IL-1β act in synergy to enhance IL-6 secretion by the intestinal epithelial cell line, IEC-6. *J Immunol* 1993;151:970–978.
9. Koyama S, Podolsky DK. Differential expression of transforming growth factors A and B in rat intestinal epithelial cells. *J Clin Invest* 1989;83:1768–1773.
10. Kunimoto DY, Harriman GR, Strober W. Regulation of IgA differentiation in CH12LX B cells by lymphokines. IL-4 induces membrane IgM-positive CH12LX cells to express membrane IgA and IL-5 induces membrane IgA-positive CH12LX cells to secrete IgA. *J Immunol* 1988;141:713–720.
11. Rachmilewitz D, Simon PL, Sjogren R, Fondacaro JD, Wasserman MA, Boedeker E. Interleukin-1: a sensitive marker of colonic inflammation. *Gastroenterology* 1988;9:A363.
12. Sinclair SB, Zettel LA, Lea R, Clark DA, Ernst BB. A role for transforming growth factor B in an antibody isotype regulation in inflamed bowel. *Gastroenterology* 1991;100:A616.
13. Bromander A, Holmgren J, Lycke N. Cholera toxin stimulates IL-1 production and enhances antigen presentation by macrophages in vitro. *J Immunol* 1991;146:2908–2914.
14. Bromander AK, Kjerrulf M, Holmgren J, Lycke N. Cholera toxin enhances alloantigen presentation by cultured intestinal epithelial cells. *Scand J Immunol* 1993;37:452–458.
15. Homqvist E, Lycke N. Cholera toxin adjuvant greatly promotes antigen-priming of T cells. *J Immunol* 1993;150:12A.
16. Raettig H. Mechanisms of oral immunization with inactivated microorganisms. *Prog Immunobiol Stand* 1970;4:337–346.
17. Brown WR, Newcomb RW, Ishizaka K. Proteolytic degradation of exocrine and serum immunoglobulins. *J Clin Invest* 1970;49:1374–1380.
18. Richman LK, Brown WR. Immunochemical characterization of IgM in human intestinal fluids. *J Immunol* 1977;119:1515–1519.
19. Shearman DJC, Parkin DM, McClelland DB. The demonstration and function of antibodies in the gastrointestinal tract. *Gut* 1972;13:483–499.
20. Stoll BJ, Svennerholm AM, Gothefors L, Barua D, Huda S, Holmgren J. Local and systemic antibody responses to naturally acquired enterotoxigenic *Escherichia coli* diarrhea in an endemic area. *J Infect Dis* 1986;153:527–534.
21. Slack DA, Islam A, Holmgren J, Svennerholm A-M. Development of methods for determining the intestinal immune response to V. cholerae antigens in humans. In: *Proceedings of the 15th Joint Conference on Cholera of the U.S.–Japan Cooperative Medical Science Program.* Publication no NIH-80-2003. Washington, DC: US Department of Health and Human Services, 1980;423–439.
22. Merchant AA, Groene WS, Cheng EH, Shaw RD. Murine intestinal antibody response to heterologous rotavirus infection. *J Clin Microbiol* 1991;29:1693–1701.
23. Czerkinsky CC, Nilsson L-A, Nygren H, Ouchterlong O, Tarkowski A. A solid-phase enzyme-linked immunospot (ELISPOT) assay for enumeration of specific antibody-secreting cells. *J Immunol Methods* 1983;65:109–121.
24. Davies A. An investigation into the serological properties of dysentery stools. *Lancet* 1922;2:1009–1012.
25. Freter R, De SP, Mondal A, Shrivastava DL, Sunderman FW Jr. Coproantibody and serum antibody in cholera patients. *J Infect Dis* 1965;115:83–87.
26. Northrup RS, Hussain SA. Immunoglobulins and antibody activity in the intestine and serum in cholera. II. Measurement of antibody activity in jejunal aspirates and sera of cholera patients by radioimmunodiffusion. *J Infect Dis* 1970;121(Suppl):142–146.
27. Lodinova R, Wagner V. Development of faecal immunoglobulins and coproantibodies in infants after artificial oral colonization with *E. coli* 083. *Experientia* 1970;26:188.
28. Reed WP, Williams RC Jr. Intestinal immunoglobulins in shigellosis. *Gastroenterology* 1971;61:35–45.
29. Freter R. Detection of coproantibody and its formation after parenteral and oral immunization of human volunteers. *J Infect Dis* 1962;111:37–48.
30. Freter R. Studies of the mechanism of action of intestinal antibody in experimental cholera. *Tex Rep Biol Med* 1969;27:299–316.
31. Freter R. Coproantibody and bacterial antagonism as protective factors in experimental enteric cholera. *J Exp Med* 1956;104:419–426.
32. Fubara ES, Freter R. Protection against enteric bacterial infection by secretory IgA antibodies. *J Immunol* 1973;111:395–403.
33. Svennerholm AM. The nature of protective immunity in chol-

era. In: Ouchterlony O, Holmgren J, eds. *Cholera and related diarrheal diseases.* Basel: Karger, 1980;171–184.

34. Tamaru T, Brown WR. IgA antibodies in rat bile inhibit cholera toxin-induced secretion in ileal loops in situ. *Immunology* 1985; 55:579–583.

35. Vaerman JP, Derijck-Langendries A, Rits M, et al. Neutralization of cholera toxin by rat bile secretory IgA antibodies. *Immunology* 1985;54:601–603.

36. Svennerholm A-M, Jertborn M, Gothefors L, Karim AMMM, Sack DA, Holmgren J. Mucosal antitoxic and antibacterial immunity after cholera disease and after immunization with a combined B subunit–whole cell vaccine. *J Infect Dis* 1984;149: 884–893.

37. Svennerholm A-M, Holmgren J. Synergistic protective effect in rabbits of immunization with *Vibrio cholerae* lipopolysaccharide and toxin/toxoid. *Infect Immun* 1976;13:735–740.

38. Elson CO, Ealding W. Ir gene control of the murine secretory IgA response to cholera toxin. *Eur J Immunol* 1987;17:425–428.

39. Borthistle BK, Isobe K, Brown WR. Studies on translocation of immunoglobulins across intestinal epithelium. III. Failure of cholera enterotoxin to stimulate secretion of IgA by rabbit intestine. *Am J Dig Dis* 1978;23:134–136.

40. Wood S, Clem SW. The use of cholera toxin for obtaining rabbit secretory immunoglobulins. *J Immunol Methods* 1974;4: 207–212.

41. Hamilton SR, Keren DF, Boitnott JK, Robertson SM, Yardley JH. Enhancement by cholera toxin of IgA secretion from intestinal crypt epithelium. *Gut* 1980;21:365–369.

42. Levine MM, Black RE, Clements ML, et al. Duration of infection derived immunity to cholera. *J Infect Dis* 1981;143: 818–820.

43. Levine MM. Vaccines against enterotoxigenic *Escherichia coli* infections. In: Woodrow GC, Levine MM, eds. *New generation vaccines.* Basel: Marcel Dekker, 1990;649–660.

44. Holmgren J, Svennerholm AM. Cholera and the immune response. *Prog Allergy* 1983;33:106–119.

45. Glass RI, Becker S, Huq MI, et al. Endemic cholera in rural Bangladesh, 1966–1980. *Am J Epidemiol* 1982;116:959–970.

46. Levine MM, Kaper JB, Black RE, Clements ML. New knowledge on pathogenesis of bacterial enteric infections as applied to vaccine development. *Microbiol Rev* 1983;47:510–550.

47. Levine MM, Black RE, Clements ML, et al. Duration of infection-derived immunity to cholera. *J Infect Dis* 1981;143: 818–820.

48. Lycke N, Holmgren J. Adoptive transfer of gut mucosal antitoxin memory by isolated B cells 1 year after oral immunization with cholera toxin. *Infect Immun* 1989;57:1137–1141.

49. Quiding M, Nordstrom I, Kilander A, Andersson G, Hanson L-A, Holmgren J, Czerkinsky C. Intestinal immune responses in humans. Oral cholera vaccination induces strong intestinal antibody responses, gamma-interferon production, and evokes local immunological memory. *J Clin Invest* 1991;88:143–148.

50. Elson CO, Ealding W. Cholera toxin feeding did not induce oral tolerance in mice and abrogated oral tolerance to an unrelated protein antigen. *J Immunol* 1984;133:2892–2897.

51. Clemens JD, Sack DA, Harris JR, et al. Field trial of oral cholera vaccines in Bangladesh: results from three-year follow-up. *Lancet* 1990;35:270–273.

52. Black RE. Overview of diarrheal diseases and strategies for their control. In: Sack DA, Freij L, eds. *Prospects for public health benefits in developing countries from new vaccines against enteric infections. SAREC Report.* Stockholm: SAREC, 1990;115–120.

53. Cravioto A, Reyes RE, Trujillo F, et al. Risk of diarrhea during the first year of life associated with initial and subsequent colonization by specific enteropathogens. *Am J Epidemiol* 1990; 131:886–904.

54. Smith HW, Linggood MA. Observations on the pathogenic properties of the K88, Hly and Ent plasmids of *Escherichia coli* with particular reference to porcine diarrhoea. *J Med Microbiol* 1971;4:467–485.

55. Evans DG, Evans DJ Jr. New surface-associated heat-labile colonization factor antigen (CFA/II) produced by enterotoxi-genic *Escherichia coli* of serogroups O6 and O8. *Infect Immun* 1978;21:638–647.

56. Boedeker E, Reid R, Bhagat H, et al. Safety, immunogenicity and efficacy in human volunteers of biodegradable, biocompatible microspheres containing colonization factor antigen/II (CFA/II) as an enteral vaccine against enterotoxigenic *E. coli* (ETEC). *Gastroenterology* 1993;104:A672.

57. Cantey JR, Hosterman DS. Characterization of colonization of the rabbit gastrointestinal tract by *Escherichia coli* RDEC-1. *Infect Immun* 1979;26:1099–1103.

58. Cantey JR. Prevention of bacterial infections of mucosal surfaces by immune secretory IgA. In: McGhee JR, Mestecky J, Babb JL, eds. *Secretory immunity and infection.* New York: Plenum Press, 1978;461–470.

59. Boedeker EC, Cheney CP, Cantey JR. Inhibition of enteropathogenic *Escherichia coli* (strain RDEC-1) adherence to rabbit intestinal brush borders by milk immune secretory immunoglobulin. *Adv Exp Med Biol* 1987;216B:919–930.

60. McQueen CE, Boedeker EC, Le M, Hamada Y, Brown WR. The mucosal immune response to RDEC-1 infection: study of lamina propria antibody-producing cells and biliary antibody. *Infect Immun* 1992;60:206–212.

61. Svennerholm A-M, Wenneras C, Holmgren J, McConnell MM, Rowe B. Roles of different coli surface antigens of colonization factor antigen II in colonization by and protective immunogenicity of enterotoxigenic *Escherichia coli* in rabbits. *Infect Immun* 1990;58:341–346.

62. Bhogal BS, Nagy LK, Walker PD. Neutrophil mediated and IgA independent antibacterial immunity against enteropathogenic *Escherichia coli* in the porcine intestinal mucosa. *Vet Immunol Immunopathol* 1987;14:23–44.

63. Blaser MJ, Black RE, Duncan DJ, et al. *Campylobacter jejuni*-specific serum antibodies are elevated in healthy Bangladeshi children. *J Clin Microbiol* 1985;21:164–167.

64. Dworkin B, Wormser GP, Abdoo RA, et al. Persistence of multiple antibiotic-resistant *Campylobacter jejuni* in a patient with the acquired immune deficiency syndrome. *Am J Med* 1986; 80:965–970.

65. Winsor DK Jr, Mathewson JJ, DuPont HC. Western blot analysis of intestinal secretory immunoglobulin. A response to *Campylobacter jejuni* antigens in patients with naturally acquired *Campylobacter* enteritis. *Gastroenterology* 1986;90: 1217–1222.

66. Burr DH, Caldwell MB, Bourgeois AL, Morgan HR, Wistar R Jr, Walker RI. Mucosal and systemic immunity to *Campylobacter jejuni* in rabbits after gastric inoculation. *Infect Immun* 1988;56:99–105.

67. Inman LR, Cantey JR, Formal SB. Colonization, virulence, and mucosal interaction of an enteropathogenic *Escherichia coli* (strain RDEC-1) expressing shigella somatic antigen in the rabbit intestine. *J Infect Dis* 1986;154:742–751.

68. Keren DF, Brown JE, McDonald RA, Wassef JS. Secretory immunoglobulin A response to Shiga toxin in rabbits: kinetics of the initial mucosal immune response and inhibition of toxicity in vitro and in vivo. *Infect Immun* 1989;57:1885–1889.

69. Keren DF, Scott PJ, McDonald RA, Kern SE. Local IgA memory response to bacterial antigens. *Ann NY Acad Sci* 1983;409: 734–744.

70. Hale TL, Keren DF. Pathogenesis and immunology in shigellosis: applications for vaccine development. *Curr Top Microbiol Immunol* 1992;180:117–137.

71. Oaks EV, Hale TL, Formal SB. Serum immune response to *Shigella* protein antigens in rhesus monkeys and humans infected with *Shigella* spp. *Infect Immun* 1986;53:57–63.

72. Dinari G, Hale TL, Austin SW, Formal SB. Local and systemic antibody responses to *Shigella* infection in rhesus monkeys. *J Infect Dis* 1987;155:1065–1069.

73. Tagliabue A, Boraschi D, Villa L, Keren DF, Lowell GH, Rappuoli R, Nencioni L. IgA-dependent cell-mediated activity against enteropathogenic bacteria: distribution, specificity, and characterization of the effector cells. *J Immunol* 1984;133: 988–992.

74. Tagliabue A, Villa L, Sestini P, et al. Antibody dependent cellular cytotoxicity against bacteria by intestinal and pulmonary

lymphocytes armed with IgA antibodies. In: Strober W, Lamm ME, McGhee R, James SP, eds. *Mucosal immunity and infections at mucosal surfaces.* New York: Oxford University Press, 1988;20–27.

75. Lowell GH, MacDermott RP, Summers PL, et al. Antibody-dependent cell-mediated antibacterial activity: K lymphocytes, monocytes, and granulocytes are effective against *Shigella. J Immunol* 1980;125:2778–2784.

76. Reed WP. Serum factors capable of opsonizing *Shigella* for phagocytosis by polymorphonuclear neutrophils. *Immunology* 1975;28:1051–1059.

77. Sneller MC, Strober W. M cells and host defense. *J Infect Dis* 1986;154:737–741.

78. Cancellieri V, Fara GM. Demonstration of specific IgA in human feces after immunization with live Ty21a *Salmonella typhi* vaccine. *J Infect Dis* 1985;151:482–484.

79. Tagliabue A, Villa L, DeMagistris MT, Romano M, Silvestri S, Boraschi D, Nencioni L. IgA-driven T cell-mediated antibacterial immunity in man after live oral Ty 21a vaccine. *J Immunol* 1986;137:1504–1510.

80. Gorbach SL. Infectious diarrhea. *Infect Dis Clin North Am* 1988;2:557–676.

81. Saulsbury FT, Winkelstein JA, Yolken RH. Chronic rotavirus infection in immunodeficiency. *J Pediatr* 1980;97:61–65.

82. Ganguly R, Waldman R. Development of local immunity. *Am J Clin Nutr* 1977;30:1843–1850.

83. Taterka JA, Cuff CF, Rubin DH. Viral gastrointestinal infections. *Gastroenterol Clin North Am* 1992;21:303–325.

84. Besser TE, Gay CC, McGuire TC, Evermann JF. Passive immunity to bovine rotavirus infection associated with transfer of serum antibody into the intestinal lumen. *J Virol* 1988;62:2238–2242.

85. Conner ME, Gilger MA, Estes MK, Graham DY. Serologic and mucosal immune response to rotavirus infection in the rabbit model. *J Virol* 1991;65:2562–2571.

86. Speelman P, Ljungstrom I. Protozoal enteric infections among expatriates in Bangladesh. *Am J Trop Med Hyg* 1986;35:1140–1145.

87. Istre GR, Dunlop TS, Gaspard GB, Hopkins RS. Waterborne giardiasis at a mountain resort: evidence for acquired immunity. *Am J Public Health* 1984;74:602–604.

88. Miotti PG, Gilman RH, Pickering LK, Ruiz-Palacios G, Park HS, Yolken RH. Prevalence of serum and milk antibodies to *Giardia lamblia* in different populations of lactating women. *J Infect Dis* 1985;152:1025–1031.

89. Jones EG, Brown WR. Serum and intestinal fluid immunoglobulins in patients with giardiasis. *Am J Dig Dis* 1974;19:791–796.

90. Heyworth MF, Carlson JR, Ermak TH. Clearance of *Giardia muris* infection requires helper/inducer T lymphocytes. *J Exp Med* 1987;165:1743–1748.

91. Heyworth MF. Intestinal IgA responses to *Giardia muris* in mice depleted of helper T lymphocytes and in immunocompetent mice. *J Parasitol* 1989;75:246–251.

92. Heyworth MF. Antibody response to *Giardia muris* trophozoites in mouse intestine. *Infect Immun* 1986;52:568–571.

93. Snider DP, Gordon J, McDermott MR, Underdown BJ. Chronic *Giardia muris* infection in anti-IgM-treated mice. I. Analysis of immunoglobulin and parasite-specific antibody in normal and immunoglobulin-deficient animals. *J Immunol* 1985;134:4153–4162.

94. Janoff EN, Smith PD, Blaser MJ. Acute antibody responses to *Giardia lamblia* are depressed in patients with AIDS. *J Infect Dis* 1988;157:798–804.

95. Saha TK, Gosh TK. Invasion of small intestinal mucosa by *Giardia lamblia* in man. *Gastroenterology* 1977;72:402–405.

96. Smith PD, Elson CO, Keister DB, et al. Human host response to *Giardia lamblia.* I. Spontaneous killing by mononuclear leukocytes in vitro. *J Immunol* 1982;128:1372–1376.

97. Smith PD. Parasitic infections. In: Targan SR, Shanahan F, eds. *Immunology and immunopathology of the liver and gastrointestinal tract.* New York: Igaku-Shoin, 1990;379–394.

98. Boedeker EC, McQueen CE. Intestinal immunity to bacterial and parasitic infections. *Immunol Allergy Clin North Am* 1988;8:393–421.

99. Strober W, Brown WR. The mucosal immune system. In: Samter M, Talmage DW, Frank MM, Austen NF, Claman HN, eds. *Immunological diseases,* 4th ed. Boston: Little, Brown, 1988;79–139.

100. Ogra PL, Losonsky GA, Fishaut M. Colustrum-derived immunity and maternal–neonatal interaction. *Ann NY Acad Sci* 1983;409:82.

101. Ste-Marie MT, Lee EM, Brown WR. Radioimmunologic measurements of naturally occurring antibodies. III. Antibodies reactive with *Escherichia coli* and *Bacteroides fragilis* in breast fluids and sera of mothers and newborn infants. *Pediatr Res* 1974;8:815–819.

102. Ogra PL, Greene HL. Human milk and breast feeding: an update on the state of the art. *Pediatr Res* 1982;16:266–271.

103. Losonsky GA, Ogra PL. Maternal–neonatal interactions and human breast milk. In: Gleicher N, ed. *Reproductive immunology.* New York: Liss, 1981;171–182.

104. Pittard WB III, Polmar SH, Fanaroff AA. The breast-milk macrophage: a potential vehicle for immunoglobulin transport. *J Reticuloendothel Soc* 1977;22:597–603.

105. Crago SS, Prince SJ, Pretlow TG, McGhee JR, Mestecky J. Human colostral cells. I. Separation and characterization. *Clin Exp Immunol* 1979;38:585–597.

106. Weaver EA, Rudloff HE, Goldblum RM, et al. Secretion of immunoglobulin A by human milk leukocytes initiated by surface membrane stimuli. *J Immunol* 1984;132:684–689.

107. Glass R, Svennerholm A-M, Stoll BJ, Khan MR, Hossain KMB, Huq MT, Holmgren J. Protection against cholera in breast-fed children by antibodies in breast milk. *N Engl J Med* 1983;308:1389–1392.

108. Laegreid A, Otnaess A-B, Fuglesang J. Human and bovine milk. Comparison of ganglioside composition and enterotoxin inhibitory activity. *Pediatr Res* 1986;20:416–421.

109. Lange S, Lonnroth I. Bile and milk from cholera toxin treated rats contain a hormone-like factor which inhibits diarrhoea induced by the toxin. *Int Arch Allergy Appl Immunol* 1986;79:270–275.

110. Yoshiyama Y, Brown WR. Specific antibodies to cholera toxin in rabbit milk are protective against *Vibrio cholerae*-induced intestinal secretion. *Immunology* 1987;61:543–547.

111. Acres SD, Isaacson RE, Babink Z, Zapitany RA. Immunization of calves against enterotoxigenic colibacillosis by vaccinating dams with purified K99 antigen and whole cell bacteria. *Infect Immun* 1975;2:121–122.

112. Rutter M, Jones W, Brown GTH, et al. Antibacterial activity in colostrum and milk associated with protection against enteric disease caused by K88 positive *Escherichia coli. Infect Immun* 1976;13:667–676.

113. Nayak N, Ganguly NK, Walia BNS, Wahi V, Kanwar SS, Mahajan RC. Specific secretory IgA in the milk of *Giardia lamblia*-infected and uninfected women. *J Infect Dis* 1987;155:724–727.

114. Andrews JS, Hewlett EL. Protection against infection with *Giardia muris* by milk containing antibody to *Giardia. J Infect Dis* 1981;143:242–246.

115. Castrucci G, Frigeri F, Ferrari M, et al. The efficacy of colostrum from cows vaccinated with rotavirus in protecting calves to experimentally induced rotavirus infection. *Comp Immunol Microbiol Infect* 1984;7:11–18.

116. Brussow H, Helperet H, Walther I, Sidoti J, Mietens C, Bachmann P. Bovine milk immunoglobulins for passive immunity to rotavirus gastroenteritis. *J Clin Microbiol* 1987;25:982–986.

117. Totterdell BM, Chrystie IL, Banatvala JE. Cord blood and breast milk antibodies in neonatal rotavirus infection. *Br Med J* 1980;280:828–830.

118. Totterdell BM, Nicholson KG, Macleod J, et al. Neonatal rotavirus infection: role of lacteal neutralizing alpha-anti-trypsin and non-immunoglobulin activity in protection. *J Med Virol* 1982;10:37–44.

119. McLean BS, Holmes IH. Effects of antibodies, trypsin, and trypsin inhibitors on susceptibility of neonates to rotavirus infection. *J Clin Microbiol* 1981;13:22–29.

120. Cuff CF, Lavi E, Cebra LK, et al. Passive immunity to fatal reovirus serotype 3-induced meningoencephalitis mediated by both secretory and transplacental factor in neonatal mice. *J Virol* 1990;64:1256–1263.

Infections of the Gastrointestinal Tract,
edited by M. J. Blaser, P. D. Smith, J. I. Ravdin,
H. B. Greenberg, and R. L. Guerrant
Published by Raven Press, Ltd., New York, 1995.

CHAPTER 14

Systemic Immune Response to Mucosal Pathogens

Edward N. Janoff

An elaborate array of host factors and pathogen-specific features affects whether an enteric pathogen causes acute or chronic infection and whether the infection is symptomatic. Certain enteric pathogens inhabit the bowel exclusively as superficial mucosal infections (e.g., *Giardia lamblia, Vibrio cholerae, Clostridium difficile,* and *Campylobacter jejuni*), whereas others also may produce a bacteremic phase (e.g., *Salmonella typhi* and *Campylobacter fetus*). Independent of the extent of anatomic invasion, most pathogens elicit a systemic immune response (1–13). This response is manifested by the presence of circulating antibodies to the organisms in serum and in mucosal secretions. The presence of enteric pathogen–specific antibodies in serum supports the diagnosis of acute enteric infections (6,11,12,14–17) and epidemiological investigations of outbreaks of enteric infections (18–23). Serological investigations also serve to define the ecological niche (e.g., age, race, sex, and geographic distribution) of newly described pathogens or routine pathogens in new populations (24–31). Finally, systemic antibody responses to mucosal infections have been examined as indirect markers of immunity to enteric infection and their associated symptoms (11,12,32–34). These data have been used to assess the risk of infection in a population and the efficacy of new vaccines (35–37). Moreover, analysis of the immunological reactivity of sera from patients with enteric infections allows characterization of the immunogenic epitopes, virulence factors, and potential antigens for protective vaccines (1,6,38).

The primary goal of mucosal immune defenses is "immune exclusion," i.e., keeping harmful elements out of the body (39). The intestine is constantly exposed to high concentrations of foreign antigens and bacteria and their proinflammatory components (e.g., polysaccharides and lipopolysaccharides). The mucosal immune system must minimize the local inflammatory response to these bacterial products and the damage they provoke (40–42), as well as recognize and respond to these antigens. A versatile system has evolved to serve these two potentially conflicting needs. This chapter will examine the relationship between mucosal infections and the systemic response that they elicit in order to understand the mechanisms, diagnostic value, and functional activities of these serum responses.

STIMULATION OF MUCOSAL AND SYSTEMIC IMMUNITY BY ENTERIC ANTIGENS

Induction of immune responses in the intestine involves a unique sequence of antigen sampling from the lumen, followed by processing and recognition by immune cells below the epithelial surface. Reactive immune cells disseminate to distant mucosal and systemic sites and return to the intestinal lamina propria (39,43–47). This sequence of events is relevant to generating systemic responses to enteric pathogens and is summarized below, using the nontoxic but highly immunogenic B subunit of cholera toxin (CTB) as a model antigen (Fig. 1) (48). Upon ingestion into the small bowel lumen, CTB avidly binds to ganglioside GM_1, a molecule abundantly present on mucosal epithelial cells (49,50). Antigens, such as CTB, are sampled from the lumen by modified membranous epithelial cells, M cells (or microfold cells), which transport antigens and organisms intact across the epithelial surface to organized mucosal lymphoid tissue below (51). These organized lymphoid follicles, or Peyer's patches, contain macrophages, T cells, and B cells, with germinal centers that generate the primary response to foreign antigens.

The induction of primary responses involves activation and proliferation of antigen-specific lymphocytes. However, in contrast to B cells in systemic sites, such as lymph nodes and the spleen, these activated cells do not differentiate into antibody-secreting plasma cells in this organized mucosal compartment. Rather, activated B and T lympho-

E. N. Janoff: Infectious Disease Section, Department of Medicine, Veterans Affairs Medical Center, and Department of Medicine, University of Minnesota School of Medicine, Minneapolis, Minnesota 55417.

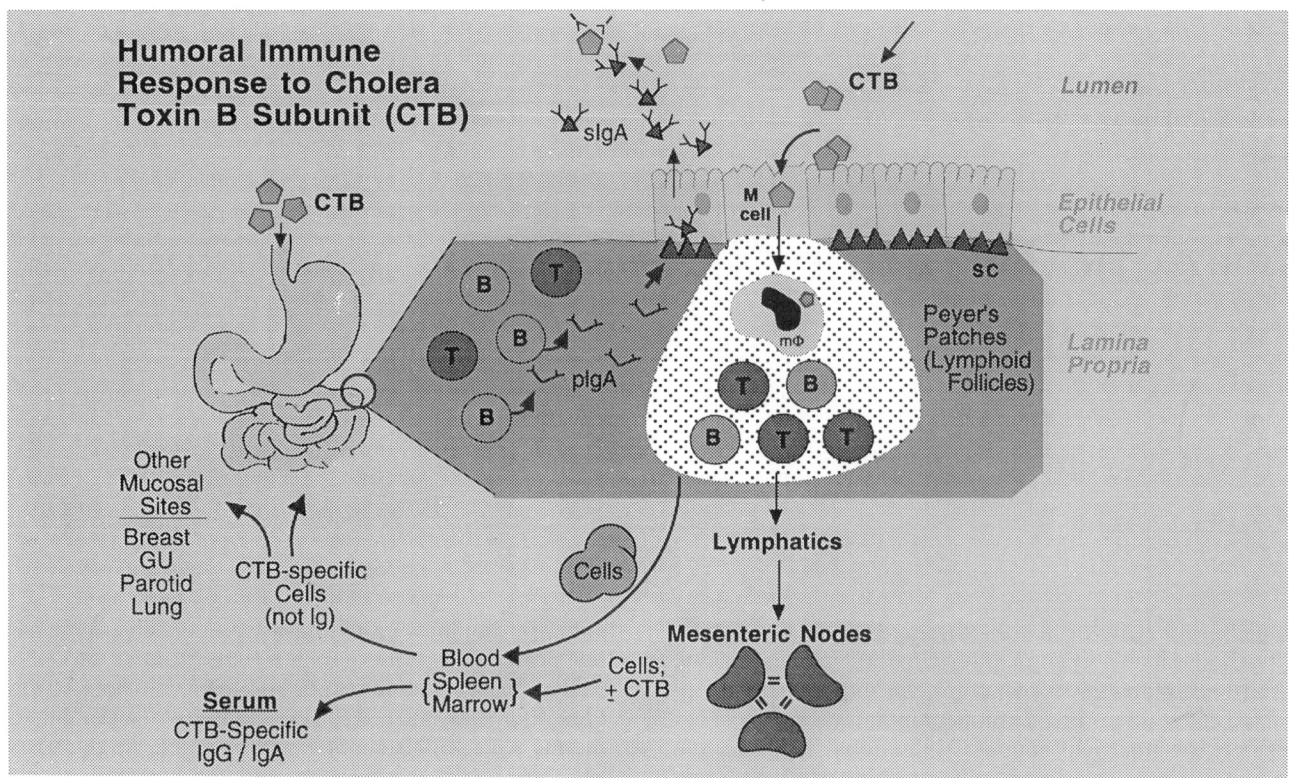

FIG. 1. Mucosal and systemic humoral immune response to cholera toxin B subunit.

cytes from mucosal lymphoid follicles are carried via lymphatics into the blood and migrate (or home) to the lamina propria of the intestine (43). In the lamina propria, in response to antigen, T cells, and cytokines (particularly interleukins 5 and 6), these antigen-stimulated B cells proliferate and differentiate into predominantly IgA-producing plasma cells. This IgA is produced in both its monomeric and polymeric forms (two or more molecules of IgA bound by a J chain) (52), but only polymeric IgA passes into the intestinal lumen.

The receptor for polymeric IgA is secretory component (SC), a protein distributed on the basolateral surface of mucosal epithelial cells (39). Whereas M cells transport antigens intact from the lumen to the lamina propria, SC binds to IgA and transports it intact in the opposite direction from the lamina propria to the lumen. SC also helps protect secretory IgA (sIgA) from enzymatic degradation in the bowel. As detailed in the chapter by Brown, specific sIgA may exhibit many protective roles in the intestinal lumen, which include prevention of binding of enteric pathogens or toxins (e.g., CTB) to the epithelial surface (immune exclusion), neutralization of toxins and viruses, or extrusion of antigens that have entered the lamina propria (53–59). sIgA may also inhibit complement activation and its associated inflammation (60,61). Thus, whereas the lymphoid follicles are considered the inductive sites of the mucosal immune system, the lamina propria is considered the functional or effector compartment (46). In addition to their migration to the lamina propria of the intestine, activated lymphocytes from intestinal lymphoid follicles also home to other mucosal sites (e.g., breast,

genitourinary tract, salivary glands, lungs) (39,54,62). The presence of antigen-specific B cells in blood within a week after mucosal exposure (47,63), the later appearance of these cells in distant mucosal sites (44), and the production at these sites of specific IgA are evidence for a common mucosal immune system (39,43,63). The clinical importance of this common mucosal system is exemplified by the protection afforded by breast milk to infants against intestinal infections (e.g., cholera, *Shigella* spp., *Giardia*, rotavirus) (64–67), particularly when infants are breastfed by mothers with prior enteric exposure to the organism and with pathogen-specific sIgA in their breast milk.

In addition to stimulation of *mucosal* IgA, antigens at mucosal surfaces also may induce *systemic* antibody responses. Once transported by M cells below the epithelial surface, CTB may be carried beyond the lymphoid follicles through lymphatics to regional mesenteric lymph nodes, where CTB-specific Ig (particularly IgA) may be produced and released into the serum (59,68). Residual antigen and activated cells from these nodes and from mucosal lymphoid follicles also may be carried by blood to spleen and bone marrow, where systemic (serum) Ig, particularly IgG, is produced (39).

ROLE OF SYSTEMIC ANTIBODY IN DIAGNOSIS OF MUCOSAL INFECTIONS

Microbiological tests complement immunological assays in the diagnosis of enteric infections. Microbiological tests are often sensitive and specific for determining the presence of the organism in stool, but they may require significant expertise and resources. Antigen detection methods may circumvent these obstacles but share with culture- and microscope-based methods the need to obtain stool samples at the time of interest (e.g., symptoms or survey). Serological tests may be useful in the acute setting or may allow diagnoses to be made retrospectively. With some infections (e.g., *Entamoeba histolytica*), serology also may help distinguish between invasive and asymptomatic infections, using small amounts of

TABLE 1. *Serum responses to enteric infections by antibody class*

Infection	n	IgG	IgM	IgA	Ref.
Bacteria					
• Acute *C. jejuni* enteritis	111			88[a]	4
Controls: 0–9 y.o.				4	
≥ 40 y.o.				54	
• Acute *C. jejuni* enteritis (ill for 21 days)	51	59	74	76	1
• Chronic *Helicobacter pylori* gastritis	59	97	Low	97	7
—Healthy adults	96	50		40–55	
• Enterotoxigenic *E. coli* diarrhea					
—Antigen: LT	10	70		80	13
CFA	10	70		100	
LPS	15	73		80	
• Children (Malaysia)					
—*S. typhi* (typhoid fever)	42	(95)[b]	(95)[b]		76
—Nontyphoid fever	49	(0)[b]	(0)[b]		
Protozoa					
• Acute *G. lamblia* diarrhea	27	67	41	78	6
—Healthy adults	66	6	2	2	
• Acute toxoplasmosis (seroconversion and/or lymphadonitis)	22	(100)[c]	100	100	73
—Chronic latent *T. gondii* infection	20	(100)[c]	0	0	
• *Entamoeba histolytica*					82
—Liver abscess (S. Africa)	83	99			
—Nonpathogenic strains (S. Africa)	69	25			
—Uninfected controls (S. Africa)	32	25			
—Healthy controls (U.S.)	40	0			
• *Cryptosporidium* diarrhea					163
—Acute—otherwise healthy adults	15	67[d]	80[d]		
—Chronic—patients with AIDS	26	100	15		
—Uninfected controls	42	5			
Viruses					
• Rotavirus gastroenteritis					70
—Infants >3 weeks old					
—Acute	44	7			
—One month	44	91	100	68[e]	
—Four months	43	100	14	93[e]	
• Rotavirus gastroenteritis					69
—Neonates (India)					
—Infected	37	8[f]	5	0	
—Uninfected	18	0	0	0	
• Rotavirus gastroenteritis					164
—Acute	8			0	
—Convalescent	8			75	

[a] Specific IgA was predominantly polymeric in patients compared with that in control subjects (median 90% vs. 17% polymeric, respectively).

[b] A positive test recorded if IgG and/or IgM positive. Either isotype alone was less sensitive, but percentages not noted.

[c] 100% positive by Sabin–Feldman dye test.

[d] IgG positive in 87% and IgM in 93% by 2 weeks after diagnosis.

[e] Specific serum secretory IgA was only rarely detected (14% and 0% in acute and convalescent sera, respectively).

[f] Rise in IgG level in three neonates; specific IgG detectable in all neonates in cord sera. Salivary IgA to rotavirus detectable in 62% of infected neonates and 5.5% of uninfected neonates.

more readily accessible and stable serum samples. A representative summary of reported assays is shown in Table 1.

The serological response to enteric infections is influenced by the timing of the sample relative to the infection, the age of the patient, and the extent of the host's previous exposure to the organism. In neonates with rotavirus who are less than 3 weeks of age, specific IgG, IgM, and IgA in serum was of no diagnostic value (69). During primary rotavirus infection in older infants, rotavirus-specific IgM was present within a week of the onset of symptoms in most infants, whereas IgA and IgG were not (70). By 1 and 4 months, however, the prevalence of IgM had decreased (only 14%), whereas specific IgG or IgA were detected in almost all children. Among adults, particularly those in endemic areas, specific IgM responses to most enteric pathogens are of considerably less diagnostic value than are IgG or IgA (e.g., *Shigella* sp. in Israel, *C. difficile* in elderly Americans, *G. lamblia* in Colorado residents) (5,6,71).

Enteric protozoan infections also often elicit circulating antibody responses. *Toxoplasma gondii* is transmitted through ingestion of infective cysts, which break down in the intestine and subsequently disseminate throughout the body. Whereas the presence of either anti–*T. gondii* IgG or a reactive Sabin–Feldman dye test is a reliable marker of either acute and chronic infection (72), detection of specific IgM and IgA, neither of which is present in chronic latent infection, suggests more recent infection (Table 1) (73–75). During acute symptomatic infections with *G. lamblia,* a noninvasive parasite of the upper small bowel, parasite-specific IgG and IgA were more sensitive indicators of infection than was IgM (6) (Fig. 2).

Antibody isotype also may be helpful as an adjunct to serological diagnosis of enteric infections. However, the usefulness is dependent on the organism, the assay, and the setting. Serological diagnosis of *Salmonella typhi* infections (typhoid fever) may be most sensitive and specific with immunoassays that detect either IgG or IgM (76). These assays compared favorably with the Widal test (bacterial agglutination), which depends primarily on IgM. Although widely used, the Widal test may lack specificity and reproducibility (11,77), problems that are most often improved with sensitive ELISA systems (10,14). IgG and particularly IgA were more sensitive as well as more specific markers of acute *Campylobacter jejuni* enteritis than was IgM (1,4). Following this acute infection, levels of specific IgA declined more rapidly than those of IgG or IgM. In an outbreak of *C. jejuni*–associated enteritis, specific IgG and IgM, but not IgA, rose in subjects exposed to the raw milk vector, whereas unexposed persons showed no rise. Baseline levels of IgG and IgM to *C. jejuni* were also increased in farm residents who chronically ingested raw milk. In contrast, during a waterborne outbreak of giardiasis, only parasite-specific IgA, not IgG or IgM, correlated with rates of exposure, infection, and symptoms (22).

In contrast to antibody responses to *S. typhi* and *C. jejuni,* specific IgG and IgA both were present at high levels in patients with chronic *Helicobacter pylori* infections, whereas IgM was not (7). The presence of circulating antibodies is a very sensitive indicator of ongoing *H. pylori* infection, but their presence does not reliably predict the presence of *H. pylori*–associated ulcer disease. Ongoing studies suggest, however, that a decrease in titers may accompany successful resolution of the infection following antimicrobial therapy. Detection of *H. pylori*–specific antibodies has also been used with banked sera to suggest a link between an increased incidence of both gastric adenocarcinoma and lymphoma and long-term *H. pylori* infection (78,79).

During certain bacterial infections, serological responses may accompany symptomatic but not asymptomatic infections (e.g., enterotoxigenic *E. coli* LT+ and *C. difficile*) (5,80). Similarly, serological responses are also clinically useful in differentiating invasive *Entamoeba histolytica* infections from asymptomatic colonization. IgG responses to the parasite are routinely reactive within 1–2 weeks of the onset of colitis and liver abscess (81–86). In contrast, persons asymptomatically infected with noninvasive strains do not typically develop antibodies in serum. Therefore, in areas of low endemicity of *E. histolytica,* a reactive serological test in a patient with appropriate symptoms is highly predictive of invasive infection. However, in highly endemic areas such as South Africa, Mexico, or India, positive tests are detected at high rates

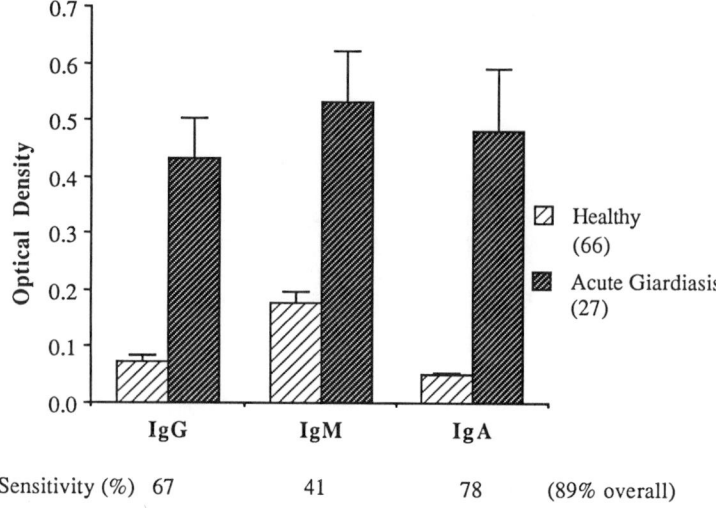

Sensitivity (%) 67   41   78   (89% overall)

FIG. 2. *Giardia lamblia*–specific antibodies in serum in 27 acutely infected immunocompetent adults and 66 healthy age-matched control subjects, Denver, Colorado. Adapted from Janoff et al. (6).

in the general population (82,86). These findings may result from persistence of IgG antibodies, which may last for years after acute invasive infection, or from asymptomatic infection with invasive strains (82). In the endemic setting, detection of *E. histolytica*–specific IgM may distinguish between active vs. previous infection in the symptomatic patient with detectable specific serum IgG (86).

Serological diagnosis of *E. histolytica* and other enteric pathogens is also useful in epidemiological studies in which microbiological specimens are not available or diagnostic facilities are inadequate. In a retrospective evaluation of an outbreak of amebic colitis in which six patients died, the use of "therapeutic" colonic irrigation was confirmed as the source of infection (87). Evidence of *E. histolytica* infection was more commonly confirmed in patients who received irrigation [20 of 54 persons (37%)] compared with only 1 of 42 (2%) who did not. Positive results of indirect hemagglutination tests of sera yielded the diagnosis in 19 of 20 cases, whereas the organism was detected in only 7 of these patients. Detection of IgG to *Cryptosporidium* in sera, but not IgM, helped establish the organism as a cause of large waterborne outbreaks of gastroenteritis (19,20) and alerted clinicians to the risk of person-to-person transmission in the hospital setting (21).

Thus, the presence and pattern of antibodies to enteric pathogens in serum may suggest prior exposure to a specific organism, acute or chronic infection, or infection with invasive vs. noninvasive strains. In epidemiological studies, serology is useful in establishing exposure rates in the community, risk factors for infection, and routes of transmission. These data are limited by differences in the sensitivity, specificity, and reproducibility of the assays. The use of international reference standards will help elucidate the effects of isotype, the age of the patient (80), the biology of the organism (3), the antigens being detected (1,6,38,88), the endemicity of the infection in the population studied, and the interaction of the organism with the mucosal immune system on determinations of seropositivity rates of specific antibodies.

RELATIONSHIP OF LOCAL AND CIRCULATING PATHOGEN-SPECIFIC ANTIBODIES

Detection of enteric pathogen-specific antibodies in serum often predicts their presence at mucosal sites. In studies of humoral responses to infection and immunization (*V. cholerae*, enterotoxigenic *E. coli*, *S. typhi*, rotavirus), the presence of specific IgG and IgA in serum shows a 70% to 80% correlation with organism-specific IgA in intestinal fluids; specific IgM correlates best during acute primary infection (3,13,33,70,89). Extraintestinal mucosal fluids, particularly breast milk, contain antibodies to many bacterial, viral, and parasitic enteric pathogens (31,90). The prevalence of *G. lamblia*–specific IgG in serum correlated with that of specific sIgA in breast milk among women in Texas and Mexico (31). Similarly, salivary antibodies often contain specific antibodies after mucosal antigenic exposure. However, these relationships are not consistent, and specific antibodies to different antigens (e.g., lipopolysaccharides, toxin, adherence factors) may be present in one site and not another, and they may vary in different patients. Overall, antibodies in serum and breast milk may be more predictive of intestinal responses than those in saliva, but none is consistently predictive of protection. Reliable and accessible indirect markers of protective immunity against enteric infections have remained elusive. Identification of these markers will facilitate testing of new vaccines in volunteers to limit the need for direct challenge studies. They will also help to determine what the protective mechanisms are when vaccines are successful. Novel methods for evaluating responses to mucosal challenge have been developed, such as detection of circulating antigen-specific antibody-secreting cells by ELISPOT, but correlations between results of these tests and protection against infection are uncertain (47,91,92). Appropriate markers of protection should allow accurate prediction of the degree of immunity in a population at risk to determine the need for large-scale vaccine delivery. Such success is typically determined by protection against illness rather than against infection (93).

Several general principles and caveats can be proposed about the interaction between mucosal and systemic immunity. First, oral immunization with non–pathogen-associated proteins, which elicit no intestinal damage or inflammation, are unlikely to provoke systemic immune responses (94,95). The immunogenicity of the nontoxic B subunit of cholera toxin given orally represents a striking exception to this principal. Second, parenteral immunization may not routinely elicit appreciable mucosal responses (94,96–99). Nevertheless parenteral immunization may be effective in preventing enteric disease (e.g., polio or *S. typhi*) (99–101). Third, parenteral immunization stimulates mucosal responses, e.g., sIgA, in subjects with prior mucosal exposure to the organism (2,99,102,103). This concept is consistent with the observation that parenteral killed cholera vaccines elicited intestinal secretory IgA responses in Pakistani women, among whom *V. cholerae* is endemic, but little local response among Swedish women, among whom these infections are absent (104). Thus, a positive correlation between the presence of specific antibodies in serum and intestinal fluids is dependent on initiation of the systemic immune response by mucosal stimulation.

Finally, the circulating antibody, particularly IgA, detected after mucosal infection or immunization does not originate in the mucosal lumen. Although levels of total secretory IgA in serum may be elevated in certain pathological conditions, such as during advanced human immunodeficiency virus (HIV) infection or liver disease (105,106), suggestions of a mucosal source for significant proportions of the specific IgA in serum are generally unfounded (107). However, analysis of pathogen-specific IgA in serum may reveal other clinically useful information about the character and kinetics of systemic responses to mucosal infections.

IgA SUBCLASSES AND MOLECULAR FORMS

In addition to pathogen-specific antibodies of the IgA class, investigators have sought more specific and predictive markers in serum that indicate a mucosal origin for these infections and antibodies. Such markers also may predict whether the serological response derives from stimulation of acute mucosal immunity or stimulation of systemic recall responses (108). Defining the origin of these antibodies in serum would also help define the physiological relationship and interaction of systemic and mucosal immune responses. Of greatest biological relevance is the predictive value of distinct antibodies in serum that reliably correlate with protection against pathogen-associated illness following previous infection or immunization.

One approach to determining a mucosal origin of infection has been to exploit anatomic differences in the subclass and molecular form of IgA. The IgA1 and IgA2 subclasses are distinguished by minor variations in the amino acid sequence of the heavy chain hinge region (109). As summarized in Table 2, the vast majority of IgA in serum is of the IgA1 subclass. The two subclasses, IgA1 and IgA2, are more equally distributed in mucosal fluids, although the moderate predominance of IgA1 in the upper intestinal tract is reversed in the colon (110–114). A more distinct anatomic disparity in IgA distribution is present in the molecular forms of the antibody: monomeric and polymeric. In serum, the predominance of monomeric IgA is similar to that of IgA1 (115). Thus, most IgA in serum is monomeric and of the IgA1 subclass.

In contrast to IgA in serum, virtually all IgA in mucosal fluids is polymeric (typically dimeric) (Table 2) (107, 111,114,115). Polymeric IgA is characterized by the presence of two complete IgA molecules joined by a J chain (111,116). The polymeric form shows no preference for IgA1 or IgA2 (4,114). The union of IgA (or IgM) with the J chain occurs intracellularly prior to secretion of the antibody (117–119). Both polymeric and monomeric IgA can be produced by the same cell and in both mucosal and systemic sites (120). However, polymeric IgA is the principal antibody found in secretions because the majority of plasma cells in mucosal tissues produce IgA, and J-chain–containing IgA (and IgM) requires facilitated transport across the epithelial cell to traverse from mucosa to lumen. This transfer is achieved by the binding of polymeric Ig to secretory component, a protein positioned at the basolateral portion of the epithelial cell that serves as the polymeric Ig receptor (121). Neither monomeric IgA nor IgG binds to secretory component, thereby precluding their routine access to luminal secretions. The complex of polymeric IgA with secretory component is called secretory IgA. Thus, polymeric IgA in serum may derive from systemic or mucosal sites, but secretory IgA in serum can only originate from the mucosal lumen.

Measurement of antigen-specific secretory IgA in serum had been limited in the past by technical factors, including the specificity of reagents available to most investigators. However, Gransfors and Toivanen reported that levels of *Yersinia enterocolitica*–specific IgA2, polymeric IgA, as well as secretory IgA in serum are increased in patients with postinfectious arthritis compared with values in patients without arthritis (122). These results may represent serological markers of the presence of persistent mucosal antigenic stimulation, but no chronic intestinal infection was documented. Other investigators have shown that although serum IgA is a sensitive indicator of rotavirus infection (Table 1), specific secretory IgA in serum is only rarely detected in serum (70).

PATHOGEN-SPECIFIC IgA1 AND IgA2

Following intestinal infection, IgA responses typically comprise both IgA1 and IgA2. However, similar to the distribution of total IgA in serum, pathogen-specific IgA in serum is most often of the IgA1 class (4,59). This predominance of antigen-specific IgA1 in serum following enteric infection or immunization is similar to the pattern of subclass responses following parenteral antigenic exposure. Although the anatomic source of antigenic stimulation may not influence the IgA subclass response, investigators have proposed that the composition of the antigen, whether protein or polysaccharide, may. Most subclass determinations are performed by solid phase radioimmunoassay or enzyme-linked immunosorbent assay (ELISA), which typically test for IgA to protein antigens (1,5,6,123–125) and show an IgA1 predominance (4,59). However, IgA2 may represent a larger proportion of the serum response to polysaccharide antigens, such as the capsular polysaccharides of *Streptococcus pneumoniae*, a mucosal respiratory pathogen (126).

A teleological explanation for the preferential IgA2 response to certain polysaccharides is that an enzyme (IgA1 protease) produced by several encapsulated mucosal pathogens (*S. pneumoniae*, *Haemophilus influenzae*, and *Neisseria meningitidis*) cleaves IgA1, but not IgA2, at the hinge sequence that distinguishes these subclasses. Adherence of the resultant antigen-binding F(ab')2 fragment to the surface polysaccharide without its associated Fc effector end may block binding by other antibodies as well as antibody-mediated clearance of the organism, thereby facilitating invasion across the mucosal barrier

TABLE 2. *Characterization of mucosal and systemic IgA by subclass and molecular form*

Subclass	Source of Ig	
	Intestine	Serum
	% Total Ig	
IgG	3–5	75–80
IgM	6–18	12–15
IgA	80–90	8–10
	% IgA	
IgA1	40–60	80–90
IgA2	40–60[a]	10–20
Monomeric	<10	80–95
Polymeric	>90	5–20[b]
Bound to secretory component[c]	>95	<5

[a] The proportion of IgA2 increases from the proximal small bowel to the colon.

[b] Polymeric IgA may be increased in patients with liver disease.

[c] Only the polymeric form of IgA may contain secretory component, to which it binds at the basolateral surface of mucosal epithelial cells.

(54). The prominance of polysaccharide-specific IgA2, as measured by ELISA in serum and by ELISPOT for circulating specific antibody-secreting cells, may reflect only the very early systemic response. Over time, polysaccharide-specific IgA may also evolve to comprise primarily IgA1 (127). Thus, measurement of IgA subclasses may not predict whether the infection or the antibodies detected are of mucosal or systemic origin, but may reflect in part the chemical composition of the antigen or, more likely, the timing of the response.

PATHOGEN-SPECIFIC MONOMERIC AND POLYMERIC IgA

The temporal sequence of humoral responses appears to more consistently influence the molecular form of specific IgA identified in serum following mucosal infection. Most studies have shown that the early acute IgA response to mucosal pathogens is primarily polymeric (Table 3); the predominant molecular form typically switches to monomeric IgA during convalescence (4,59) (Fig. 3). This switch in molecular form has been shown for several viruses acquired through the respiratory mucosa (rubella, mumps, and varicella) (125) and genital mucosa (herpes simplex) (128). Consistent with these findings, reactivations of both varicella (herpes zoster) and genital herpes more often elicited monomeric IgA, rather than the virus-specific polymeric IgA detected during acute primary infections.

In sera from patients with acute *C. jejuni* enteritis, polymeric IgA comprised the majority of specific IgA within 1–2 weeks of presentation (median 90%) (4). That these high molecular weight IgA molecules did not represent immune complexes or secretory IgA was excluded by their stability after acid treatment and lack of reactivity with antibodies directed to secretory component, respectively. The high proportion of polymeric IgA in acute sera decreased over time after resolution of infection, approaching that of specific IgA in healthy control subjects (median 17%). These data demonstrating the early but transient polymeric response to mucosal infections suggest that differentiating polymeric from monomeric IgA

TABLE 3. *Mucosal pathogens to which polymeric IgA responses have been demonstrated in acute sera[a]*

Bacteria:	*Campylobacter jejuni*
	Salmonella typhi
	Vibrio cholerae
	Clostridium difficile
	Streptococcus pneumoniae
Viruses:	Herpes simplex
	Measles
	Mumps
	Rubella
	Influenza

[a] Following infection or immunization.

reactive with mucosal pathogens may help to distinguish acute from previous infection, as well as primary from reactivated infection. However, the molecular form of IgA does not reliably predict the anatomic source of infection or antigenic exposure. Both mucosal and parenteral stimulation with either polysaccharide or protein antigens can elicit specific polymeric IgA in serum (3,59,98, 108,126,127,129).

Despite the consistency with which the transition from pathogen-specific polymeric to monomeric IgA has been shown, the immunological mechanism underlying this progression has not been demonstrated (3,129). These data do suggest, however, that the molecular form of specific IgA present in serum may be related to the extent and duration of prior exposure to the pathogen. That the evolving predominance of specific monomeric IgA reflects clonal maturation and, ultimately, memory responses is a reasonable hypothesis (3,130). It may also provide a useful approach to distinguish acute from reactivated infections.

FUNCTIONAL ACTIVITIES OF SERUM ANTIBODIES TO MUCOSAL PATHOGENS

Role of IgA

Recently, a functional correlate of this transition from specific polymeric to monomeric IgA was proposed. That

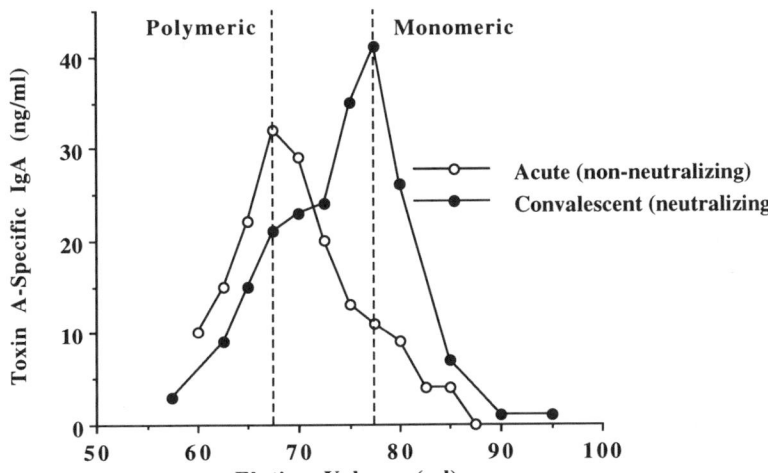

FIG. 3. Serum IgA response to toxin A of *Clostridium difficile* in association with antibiotic-associated colitis. As resolved on a Sephacryl S-300 HR molecular sieve column, the change in molecular form of specific IgA from polymeric in the acute sample to primarily monomeric in the convalescent sample was associated with the ability of IgA to neutralize the cytotoxic activity of toxin A (59).

the appearance of monomeric IgA accompanies the resolution of infection, often in the context of declining specific IgA levels in serum overall, suggests that an effective and potentially protective immune response has been generated (4). Among patients with *C. difficile* colitis, approximately a third develop antibodies in convalescent sera that neutralize the activity of the principal enterotoxin, toxin A (5,59,131). Although neutralizing activity correlated with levels of both toxin A–specific IgG and IgA, this functional activity resided almost exclusively in the IgA, not the IgG, fraction of convalescent sera. Thus, in this setting, a unique and selective relationship exists between the mucosal site of infection and the functional IgA response in serum.

Moreover, as with *C. jejuni, V. cholerae,* and *S. typhi* exposure, the IgA response to *C. difficile* toxin A also showed a transition in molecular form over time (59). However, the transition from polymeric to monomeric toxin A–specific IgA over time did not occur in all patients; only those patients who developed neutralizing activity produced predominantly monomeric IgA, whereas those who showed no neutralizing activity retained the polymeric form of specific IgA, which more typically accompanies acute or immature responses (Fig. 3). Therefore, the evolution in the molecular form of the IgA response from polymeric in acute sera to primarily monomeric in convalescent sera may correlate with distinct changes in the functional activity of these antibodies to limit damage to the host.

In addition to neutralization of toxins, antibodies in serum, including IgA, may also facilitate clearance of absorbed intestinal microbial antigens (116,132), which may limit further systemic immunogenicity and inflammation. Specific IgA may also serve a more active role in systemic defense. Although IgA binding is not typically associated with complement activation, deposition, and bacterial lysis, recent data confirm that two mucosal pathogens—*Neisseria meningitidis* and *Haemophilus influenzae*—are susceptible to IgA-driven complement-mediated lysis (133). The unique feature of these observations is that the lytic activity of IgA was only identifiable in the absence of IgG, which reacted with capsular polysaccharides; the IgA reacted with other surface proteins. Thus, circulating IgG and IgA may have distinct activities and antigen specificities.

In addition to its suggested role in complement-mediated lysis of gram-negative mucosal pathogens, circulating IgA may also facilitate non–complement-mediated cellular immune responses. IgA in adult sera that reacted with *S. typhi* showed antibody-dependent cell-mediated antibacterial activity. The IgA was obtained from adults immunized orally with the live *S. typhi* mutant strain Ty21A or normal sera (134–136). The effector cells in these assays were CD4+ lymphocytes, whereas IgA-driven complement-independent cellular activity against *N. meningitides* type C was monocyte-mediated (137). Thus, experimental evidence in humans suggests that circulating IgA has both complement-mediated and complement-independent cell-mediated activity against mucosal pathogens. These studies used high-titer specific IgA from patients convalescent from immunization of infection, but also circulating IgA from otherwise healthy subjects (136).

Role of Natural Antibodies, IgG and IgM

The ability of gram-negative enteric pathogens to evade the mucosal barrier and invade the systemic circulation is related to the bactericidal activity of normal human serum (138–141). Thus, *C. fetus* is relatively serum resistant and often causes invasive infections with bacteremia, whereas *C. jejuni* is typically serum sensitive and causes primarily mucosal infections and little bacteremia (140). The bactericidal activity of normal human serum involves both complement and antibody. Complement may bind to enteric gram-negative organisms without causing lysis; the specificity of the antibodies present may direct the location of complement deposition to lytic or nonlytic sites (142,143). The source of these "natural" antibodies in normal human serum is uncertain.

Natural antibodies are those present in serum in the absence of obvious prior infection or immunization. They may derive from subclinical infection or colonization, from cross-reactivity with other related antigens, or they may represent polyreactive antibodies (144). The first two sources may elicit IgG responses, whereas polyreactive antibodies are typically IgM. These antibodies react with low specificity and low affinity with many antigens; their ability to clear organisms from the circulation by complement-mediated or Fc-mediated mechanisms may serve as a first line of defense against systemic infection. Whether natural antibodies (especially IgM) or more specific antibodies found in convalescent serum (especially IgG and possibly IgA) represent the most important mechanism of systemic immunity against enteric infections is an area of active investigation (140,145).

Overall the clinically relevant contributions of serum antibodies to mucosal pathogens are poorly defined. The complement-mediated bactericidal activity of antibodies, particularly IgG and IgM, in serum to kill organisms such as *Salmonella* and *Campylobacter* species likely act to limit bacteremia and dissemination of these organisms beyond the intestine. That the *in vitro* activity of IgA to facilitate complement-mediated killing of mucosal gram-negative organisms occurs only in the absence of IgG (*N. meningitidis* and *H. influenzae*) (133) limits the relevance of these observations to systemic immunity. However, these observations do suggest mechanisms by which IgA may protect in an IgA-rich and IgG-poor environment such as intestinal and other mucosal tissues, where complement, CD4+ T cells, and macrophages are also present (133–137). Moreover, although the vast majority of mucosal antibodies are produced locally, low concentrations of both monomeric IgA and IgG are routinely detected in mucosal fluids (Table 2) (115,146). These low levels of monomeric antibodies may be passively transported from serum across the mucosal epithelium rather than originating in bile (115,116). Although levels of monomeric IgG and IgA from serum may increase following mucosal damage and inflammation, whether they are present in sufficient concentrations to have clinical antimicrobial effects in the intestinal lumen, where levels of complement are also low, remains to be determined.

PROTECTIVE ROLE OF SYSTEMIC ANTIBODY IN DEFENSE AGAINST ENTERIC PATHOGENS

Protection against acute symptomatic infections with specific enteric infections may be related to previous or recurrent exposure to the organism. Persons exposed to *G. lamblia* episodically, such as backpackers, travelers, and case contacts, experience high rates of symptomatic infection (147,148), whereas persons living in endemic areas and those with recurrent exposure to the organism, such as homosexual men and toddlers in day care centers, show low rates of symptomatic infection (25,149–151). Although differences in the virulence of individual *G. lamblia* strains may account for some of these clinical differences (152), these data suggest the development of acquired immunity following recurrent exposure. In this regard, during waterborne outbreaks of *G. lamblia* in Colorado mountain towns, recently arrived tourists and short-term residents showed significantly higher rates of illness than did long-term community residents (153,154). Similarly, 86% of infants in Bangladesh newly infected with *G. lamblia* showed symptoms compared with only 4% of infected mothers (155). The high rates of exposure and asymptomatic infections where *G. lamblia* is endemic are most often associated with high rates of seropositivity and increased levels of *G. lamblia*–specific antibodies in serum (6,25,156–158), particularly IgA (159).

These observations with *G. lamblia* infections are also consistent with those of other protozoan (e.g., *Cryptosporidium* sp.) (160), bacterial (e.g., enterotoxigenic *E. coli, Vibrio cholerae, C. jejuni*) (13,24,161), and viral pathogens (e.g., rotaviruses, calicivirus) (9,162). In each instance, lower rates of infection or increased rates of asymptomatic infection in specific populations correlate with increased levels of pathogen-specific antibodies in serum of these groups.

That increased levels of specific antibodies are associated with clinical protection does not confirm that these antibodies are the agents of this protection. In Bangladeshi children, higher titers of serum IgG to rotavirus by ELISA correlated with protection against both moderate and severe disease (9). However, further analyses of the neutralizing activity of antibodies to rotavirus in this population revealed that protection was not serotype-specific; protection against each of the four serotypes was more closely related to titers of heterotypic rather than homotypic neutralizing antibodies (8). Thus, in some settings, antibodies in serum to enteric pathogens may be markers of immunity rather than the direct mechanisms of protective immunity.

ACKNOWLEDGMENTS

This work was sponsored by the Veterans Affairs Research Service, Public Health Service/National Institutes of Health Grant AI-31373 and contract DE-42600. The author thanks Stuart Johnson and David N. Taylor for thoughtful discussions and Ann Emery for excellent secretarial support.

REFERENCES

1. Blaser MJ, Duncan DJ. Human serum antibody response to *Campylobacter jejuni* infection as measured in an enzyme-linked immunosorbent assay. *Infect Immun* 1984;44:292–298.
2. Svennerholm A-M, Holmgren J, Hanson LÅ, Lindblad BS, Quereshi F, Rahimtoola RJ. Boosting of secretory IgA antibody responses in man by parenteral cholera vaccination. *Scand J Immunol* 1977;6:1345–1349.
3. Mascart-Lemone F, Carlsson B, Jalil F, Hahn-Zoric M, Duchateau J, Hanson LÅ. Polymeric and monomeric IgA response in serum and milk after parenteral cholera and oral typhoid vaccination. *Scand J Immunol* 1988;28:443–448.
4. Mascart-Lemone FO, Duchateau JR, Oosterom J, Butzler J-P, Delacroix DL. Kinetics of anti-*Campylobacter jejuni* monomeric and polymeric immunoglobulin A1 and A2 responses in serum during acute enteritis. *J Clin Microbiol* 1987;25:1253–1257.
5. Johnson S, Gerding DN, Janoff EN. Systemic and mucosal antibody responses to toxin A in patients infected with *Clostridium difficile*. *J Infect Dis* 1992;166:1287–1294.
6. Janoff EN, Smith PD, Blaser MJ. Acute antibody responses to *Giardia lamblia* are depressed in patients with the acquired immunodeficiency syndrome. *J Infect Dis* 1988;157:798–804.
7. Perez-Perez GI, Dworkin BM, Chodos JE, Blaser MJ. *Campylobacter pylori* antibodies in humans. *Ann Intern Med* 1988;109:11–17.
8. Ward RL, Clemens JD, Knowlton DR, et al. Evidence that protection against rotavirus diarrhea after natural infection is not dependent on serotype-specific neutralizing antibody. *J Infect Dis* 1992;166:1251–1257.
9. Clemens JD, Ward RL, Rao MR, et al. Seroepidemiologic evaluation of antibodies to rotavirus as correlates of the risk of clinically significant rotavirus diarrhea in rural Bangladesh. *J Infect Dis* 1992;165:161–165.
10. Sarasombath S, Banchuin N, Sukosol T, Rungpitarangsi B, Manasatit S. Systemic and intestinal immunities after natural typhoid infection. *J Clin Microbiol* 1987;25:1088–1093.
11. Brodie J. Antibodies and the Aberdeen typhoid outbreak of 1964. *J Hyg* 1977;79:161–180.
12. Brodie J. Antibodies and the Aberdeen typhoid outbreak of 1964. II. *J Hyg* 1977;79:181–190.
13. Stoll BJ, Svennerholm A-M, Gothefors L, Barua D, Huda S, Holmgren J. Local and systemic antibody responses to naturally acquired enterotoxigenic *Escherichia coli* diarrhea in an endemic area. *J Infect Dis* 1986;153:527–534.
14. Beasley WJ, Joseph SW, Weiss E. Improved serodiagnosis of *Salmonella* enteric fevers by an enzyme-linked immunosorbent assay. *J Clin Microbiol* 1981;13:106–114.
15. Gary GW, Anderson LJ, Keswick BH, et al. Norwalk virus antigen and antibody response in an adult volunteer study. *J Clin Microbiol* 1987;25:2001–2003.
16. Christensen ML. Human viral gastroenteritis. *Clin Microbiol Rev* 1989;2:51–89.
17. Blacklow NR, Greenberg HB. Viral gastroenteritis. *N Engl J Med* 1991;325:252–264.
18. Kaplan JE, Gary GW, Baron RC, et al. Epidemiology of Norwalk gastroenteritis and the role of Norwalk virus in outbreaks of acute nonbacterial gastroenteritis. *Ann Intern Med* 1982;96:756–761.
19. Hayes EB, Matte TD, O'Brien TR, et al. Large community outbreak of cryptosporidiosis due to contamination of a filtered public water supply. *N Engl J Med* 1989;320:1372–1376.
20. D'Antonio RG, Winn RE, Taylor JP, et al. A waterborne outbreak of cryptosporidiosis in normal hosts. *Ann Intern Med* 1985;103:886–888.
21. Koch KL, Phillips DJ, Aber RC, Current WL. Cryptosporidiosis in hospital personnel. *Ann Intern Med* 1985;102:593–596.
22. Birkhead G, Janoff EN, Vogt RL, Smith PD. Elevated levels

of immunoglobulin A to *Giardia lamblia* during a waterborne outbreak of gastroenteritis. *J Clin Microbiol* 1989;27: 1707–1710.

23. Ungar BLP, Mulligan M, Nutman TB. Serologic evidence of *Cryptosporidium* infection in US volunteers before and during Peace Corps service in Africa. *Arch Intern Med* 1989;149: 894–897.

24. Echeverria P, Burke DS, Blacklow NR, Charoenkul C, Yanggratoke S. Age-specific prevalence of antibody to rotavirus, *Escherichia coli*, heat-labile enterotoxin, Norwalk virus, and hepatitis A virus in a rural community in Thailand. *J Clin Microbiol* 1983;17:923–925.

25. Gilman RH, Brown KH, Visvesvara GS, et al. Epidemiology and serology of *Giardia lamblia* in a developing country: Bangladesh. *Trans R Soc Trop Med Hyg* 1985;79:469–473.

26. Lengerich EJ, Addiss DG, Marx JJ, Ungar BLP, Juranek DD. Increased exposure to cryptosporidia among dairy farmers in Wisconsin. *J Infect Dis* 1993;167:1252–1255.

27. Ungar BLP, Gilman RH, Lanata CF, Perez-Schael L. Seroepidemiology of *Cryptosporidium* infection in two Latin American populations. *J Infect Dis* 1988;157:551–556.

28. Janoff EN, Reller LB. *Cryptosporidium* species, a protean protozoan. *J Clin Microbiol* 1987;25:967–975.

29. Current WL, Garcia LS. Cryptosporidiosis. *Clin Microbiol Rev* 1991;4:325–358.

30. Blaser MJ, Black RE, Duncan DJ, Amer J. *Campylobacter jejuni*–specific serum antibodies are elevated in healthy Bangladeshi children. *J Clin Microbiol* 1985;21:164–167.

31. Miotti PG, Gilman RH, Pickering LK, Ruiz-Palacios G, Park HS, Yolken RH. Prevalence of serum and milk antibodies to *Giardia lamblia* in different populations of lactating women. *J Infect Dis* 1985;152:1025–1031.

32. Kapikian AZ, Wyatt RG, Levine MM, et al. Oral administration of human rotavirus to volunteers: induction of illness and correlates of resistance. *J Infect Dis* 1983;147:95–106.

33. Jertborn M, Svennerholm A-M, Holmgren J. Saliva, breast milk, and serum antibody responses as indirect measures of intestinal immunity after oral cholera vaccination or natural disease. *J Clin Microbiol* 1986;24:203–209.

34. Parrino TA, Schreiber DS, Trier JS, Kapikian AZ, Blacklow NR. Clinical immunity in acute gastroenteritis caused by Norwalk agent. *N Engl J Med* 1977;2:86–89.

35. Clemens JD, Harris JR, Khan MR, et al. Field trial of oral cholera vaccines in Bangladesh. *Lancet* 1986;2:124–389.

36. Clemens JD, Sack DA, Harris JR, et al. Cross-protection by B subunit-whole cell cholera vaccine against diarrhea associated with heat-labile toxin-producing enterotoxigenic *Escherichia coli*: results of a large-scale field trial. *J Infect Dis* 1988;158: 372–377.

37. Simanjuntak CH, O'Hanley P, Punjabi NH, et al. Safety, immunogenicity, and transmissibility of single-dose live oral cholera vaccine strain CVD 103-HgR in 24- to 59-month-old Indonesian children. *J Infect Dis* 1993;168:1169–1176.

38. Osek J, Jonson G, Svennerholm A-M, Holmgren J. Role of antibodies against biotype-specific *Vibrio cholerae* pili in protection against experimental classical and El Tor cholera. *Infect Immun* 1994;62:2901–2907.

39. Mestecky J, McGhee J. Immunoglobulin A (IgA): molecular and cellular interactions involved in IgA biosynthesis and immune response. *Adv Immunol* 1987;40:153–245.

40. Ferretti M, Casini-Raggi V, Pizarro T, Eisenberg SP, Nast CC, Cominelli F. Neutralization of endogenous IL-1 receptor antagonist exacerbates and prolongs inflammation in rabbit immune colitis. *J Clin Invest* 1994;94:449–453.

41. Cominelli F, Nast CC, Clark BD, et al. Interleukin 1 (IL-1) gene expression, synthesis, and effect of specific IL-1 receptor blockade in rabbit immune complex colitis. *J Clin Invest* 1990; 86:972–980.

42. Kagnoff MF. A question of balance: ups and downs of mucosal inflammation. *J Clin Invest* 1994;94:1.

43. McDermott MR, Bienenstock J. Evidence for a common mucosal immunologic system. I. Migration of B immunoblasts into intestinal, respiratory, and genital tissues. *J Immunol* 1979;122: 1892–1898.

44. Weisz-Carrington P, Roux ME, McWilliams M, Phillips-Quagliata JM, Lamm ME. Organ and isotype distribution of plasma cells producing specific antibody after oral immunization: evidence for a generalized secretory immune system. *J Immunol* 1979;123:1705–1708.

45. McGhee JR, Mestecky J, Elson CO, Kiyono H. Regulation of IgA synthesis and immune response by T cells and interleukins. *J Clin Immunol* 1989;9:175.

46. McGhee JR, Mestecky J, Dertzbaugh MT, Eldridge JH, Hirasawa M, Kiyono H. The mucosal immune system: from fundamental concepts to vaccine development. *Vaccine* 1992;10: 75–88.

47. Quiding M, Nordström I, Kilander A, et al. Intestinal immune responses in humans. Oral cholera vaccination induces strong intestinal antibody responses and interferon-γ production and evokes local immunological memory. *J Clin Invest* 1991;88: 143–148.

48. Lycke N, Holmgren J. Strong adjuvant properties of cholera toxin on gut mucosal immune responses to orally presented antigens. *Immunol* 1986;59:301–308.

49. van Heyningen S. Cholera toxin: interaction of subunits with ganglioside G_{M1}. *Science* 1974;183:656–657.

50. Fishman PH, Atikkan EE. Mechanism of action of cholera toxin: effect of receptor density and multivalent binding on activation of adenylate cyclase. *J Membr Biol* 1980;54:51–60.

51. Wolf JL, Bye WA. The membranous epithelial (M) cell and the mucosal immune system. *Annu Rev Med* 1984;35:95–112.

52. Brandtzaeg P, Prydz H. Direct evidence for an integrated function of J chain and secretory component in epithelial transport of immunoglobulins. *Nature* 1984;311:71–73.

53. Stokes CR, Soothill JF, Turner MW. Immune exclusion is a function of IgA. *Nature* 1975;255:745–746.

54. Kilian M, Mestecky J, Russell MW. Defense mechanisms involving Fc-dependent functions of immunoglobulin A and their subversion by bacterial immunoglobulin A proteases. *Microbiol Rev* 1988;52:296–303.

55. Andre C, Lambert R, Bazin H, Vaerman J-P. Interference of oral immunization with the intestinal absorption of heterologous albumin. *Eur J Immunol* 1974;4:701.

56. Walker WA, Isselbacher KJ, Bloch KJ. Intestinal uptake of macromolecules: effect of oral immunization. *Science* 1972; 177:608.

57. Mazanec MB, Nedrud JG, Lamm ME. Immunoglobulin A monoclonal antibodies protect against Sendai virus. *J Virol* 1987;61:2624–2626.

58. Mazanec MB, Kaetzel CS, Lamm ME, Fletcher D, Nedrud JG. Intracellular neutralization of virus by immunoglobulin A antibodies. *Proc Natl Acad Sci USA* 1992;89:6901–6905.

59. Johnson S, Sypura WD, Gerding DN, Janoff EN. Neutralization of a bacterial enterotoxin by systemic IgA in response to mucosal infection (abstr). *J Immunol* 1993;150:117A.

60. Imai H, Chen A, Wyatt RJ, Rifai A. Lack of complement activation by human IgA immune complexes. *Clin Exp Immunol* 1988;73:479–483.

61. Russell MW, Mansa B. Complement-fixing properties of human IgA antibodies. Alternative pathway complement activation by plastic-bound, but not specific antigen-bound. *Scand J Immunol* 1989;30:175–183.

62. Roux ME, McWilliams M, Phillips-Quagliata J, Weisz-Carrington P, Lamm ME. Origin of IgA-secreting plasma cells in the mammary gland. *J Exp Med* 1977;146:1311.

63. Czerkinsky C, Prince SJ, Michalek SM, et al. IgA antibody-producing cells in peripheral blood after antigen ingestion: evidence for a common mucosal immune system in humans. *Proc Natl Acad Sci USA* 1987;84:2449–2453.

64. Glass RI, Svennerholm A-M, Stoll BJ, et al. Protection against cholera in breast-fed children by antibodies in breast milk. *N Engl J Med* 1983;308:1389–1392.

65. Nayak N, Ganguly NK, Walia BNS, Wahi V, Kanwar SS, Mahajan RC. Specific secretory IgA in the milk of *Giardia lamblia*–infected and uninfected women. *J Infect Dis* 1987;155: 724–727.

66. Hanson LA, Björkander J, Carlsson B, Robertson D, Söders-

tröm T. The heterogeneity of IgA deficiency. *J Clin Immunol* 1988;8:159–162.

67. Hayani KC, Guerrero ML, Ruiz-Palacios GM, Gomez HF, Cleary TG. Evidence for long-term memory of the mucosal immune system: milk secretory immunoglobulin A against *Shigella* lipopolysaccharides. *J Clin Microbiol* 1991;29:2599–2603.

68. Waldman RH, Benzic Z, Deb BC, et al. Cholera immunology. II. Serum and intestinal antibody response after naturally oc-curing cholera. *J Infect Dis* 1972;126:401–407.

69. Jayashree S, Bhan MK, Kumar R, Raj P, Glass R, Bhandari N. Serum and salivary antibodies as indicators of rotavirus in-fection in neonates. *J Infect Dis* 1988;158:1117–1120.

70. Grimwood K, Lund JCS, Coulson BS, Hudson IL, Bishop RF, Barnes GL. Comparison of serum and mucosal antibody re-sponses follow severe acute rotavirus gastroenteritis in young children. *J Clin Microbiol* 1988;26:732–738.

71. Cohen D, Block C, Green MS, Lowell G, Ofek I. Immunoglob-ulin M, A, and G antibody response to lipopolysaccharide O antigen in symptomatic and asymptomatic *Shigella* infections. *J Clin Microbiol* 1989;27:162–167.

72. Brooks RG, McCabe RE, Remington JS. Role of serology in the diagnosis of toxoplasmic lymphadenopathy. *Rev Infect Dis* 1987;9:1055–1062.

73. Stepick-Biek P, Thulliez P, Araujo FG, Remington JS. IgA anti-bodies for diagnosis of acute congenital and acquired toxoplas-mosis. *J Infect Dis* 1990;162:270–273.

74. Partanen P, Turunen HJ, Paasivuo RA, Leinikki PO. Immu-noblot analysis of *Toxoplasma gondii* antigens by human immu-noglobulins G, M, and A antibodies at different stages of infec-tion. *J Clin Microbiol* 1984;20:133–135.

75. Decoster A, Darcy F, Caron A, Capron A. IgA antibodies against P30 as markers of congenital and acute toxoplasmosis. *Lancet* 1988;2:1104–1107.

76. Choo KE, Oppenheimer SJ, Ismail AB, Ong KH. Rapid serodi-agnosis of typhoid fever by dot enzyme immunoassay in an endemic area. *Clin Infect Dis* 1994;19:172–176.

77. Schroeder SA. Interpretation of serologic tests for typhoid fever. *JAMA* 1968;206:839–840.

78. Parsonnet J, Friedman GD, Vandersteen DP, et al. *Helico-bacter pylori* infection and the risk of gastric carcinoma. *N Engl J Med* 1991;325:1127–1131.

79. Parsonnet J, Hansen S, Rodriguez L, et al. *Helicobacter pylori* infection and gastric lymphoma. *N Engl J Med* 1994;330:1267–1271.

80. Cushing AH, Smart J. Gastrointestinal carriage of toxigenic bacteria: relation to diarrhea and to serum immune response. *J Infect Dis* 1985;151:114–123.

81. Salata RA, Ravdin JI. Review of the human immune mecha-nisms directed against *Entamoeba histolytica*. *Rev Infect Dis* 1986;8:261–272.

82. Ravdin JI, Jackson TFHG, Petri Jr WA, et al. Association of serum antibodies to adherence lectin with invasive amebiasis and asymptomatic infection with pathogenic *Entamoeba histo-lytica*. *J Infect Dis* 1990;162:768–772.

83. Trissl D. Immunology of *Entamoeba histolytica* in human and animal hosts. *Rev Infect Dis* 1982;4:1154–1184.

84. Krupp IM. Antibody response in intestinal and extraintestinal amebiasis. *Am J Trop Med* 1970;19:57–62.

85. Katzenstein D, Rickerson V, Braude A. New concepts of ame-bic liver abscess derived from hepatic imaging, serodiagnosis, and hepatic enzymes in 67 consecutive cases in San Diego. *Medicine* 1982;61:237.

86. Jackson TFHG, Anderson CB, Simjee AE. Serological differ-entiation between past and present infection in hepatic amoebi-asis. *Trans R Soc Trop Med Hyg* 1984;78:342–345.

87. Istre GR, Kreiss K, Hopkins RS, et al. An outbreak of amebia-sis spread by colonic irrigation at a chiropractic clinic. *N Engl J Med* 1982;307:339–342.

88. Taylor GD, Wenman WM. Human immune responses to *Giar-dia lamblia* infection. *J Infect Dis* 1987;155:137–140.

89. Winsor DK, Jr, Mathewson JJ, DuPont HL. Western blot anal-ysis of intestinal secretory immunoglobulin A response to *Campylobacter jejuni* antigens in patients with naturally ac-quired *Campylobacter* enteritis. *Gastroenterology* 1986;90:1217–1222.

90. Yolken RH, Wyatt RG, Mata L, et al. Secretory antibody di-rected against rotavirus in human milk—measurement by means of enzyme-linked immunosorbent assay. *J Pediatr* 1978;93:916–921.

91. Kantele A, Arvilommi H, Jokinen I. Specific immunoglobulin-secreting human blood cells after peroral vaccination against *Salmonella typhi*. *J Infect Dis* 1986;153:1126–1131.

92. Forrest BD. Identification of an intestinal immune response using peripheral blood lymphocytes. *Lancet* 1988;1:81–83.

93. Clemens JD, Sack DA, Harris JR, et al. Field trial of oral chol-era vaccines in Bangladesh: results from three-year follow-up. *Lancet* 1990;335:270–273.

94. Kaplan ME, Zalusky R, Remington J, Herbert V. Immunologic studies with intrinsic factor in man. *J Clin Invest* 1963;42:368–382.

95. Husby S, Mestecky J, Moldoveanu Z, Holland S, Elson CO. Oral tolerance in humans. *J Immunol* 1994;152:4663–4670.

96. Ogra PL, Karzon DT, Righthand R, MacGillivray M. Immuno-globulin response in serum and secretions after immunization with live and inactivated poliovaccine and natural infection. *N Engl J Med* 1968;279:893–900.

97. Svennerholm A-M, Jertborn M, Gothefors L, Karim AMM, Sack DA, Holmgren J. Mucosal antitoxic and antibacterial im-munity after cholera disease and after immunization with a combined B subunit-whole cell vaccine. *J Infect Dis* 1984;149:884–893.

98. Bartholomeusz RCA, Forrest BD, Labrooy JT, et al. The serum polymeric IgA antibody response to typhoid vaccina-tion; its relationship to the intestinal IgA response. *Immunol-ogy* 1990;69:190–194.

99. Hone D, Hackett J. Vaccination against enteric bacterial dis-eases. *Rev Infect Dis* 1989;11:853–877.

100. Ashcroft MT, Ritchie JM, Nicholson CC. Controlled field trail in British Guiana school children of heat-killed phenolized and acetone-killed lyophilized typhoid vaccines. *Am J Hyg* 1964;79:196–206.

101. Robbins JB, Chu C, Schneerson R. Hypothesis for vaccine development: protective immunity to enteric diseases caused by nontyphoidal salmonellae and shigellae may be conferred by serum IgG antibodies to the O-specific polysaccharide of their lipopolysaccharides. *Clin Infect Dis* 1992;15:346–361.

102. Svennerholm A-M, Holmgren J, Sack DA, Bardhan PK. Intes-tinal antibody responses after immunisation with cholera B sub-unit. *Lancet* 1982;1:305–307.

103. Svennerholm A-M, Gothefors L, Sack DA, Bardhan PK, Holm-gren J. Local and systemic antibody responses and immunolog-ical memory in humans after immunization with cholera B sub-unit by different routes. *Bull WHO* 1984;62:909–918.

104. Svennerholm A-M, Hanson LÅ, Holmgren J, Lindblad BS, Nilsson B, Quireshi F. Different secretory immunoglobulin A antibody responses to cholera vaccination in Swedish and Paki-stani women. *Infect Immun* 1980;427–430.

105. Vincent C, Cozon G, Zittoun M, et al. Secretory immunoglobu-lins in serum from human immunodeficiency virus (HIV)–in-fected patients. *J Clin Immunol* 1992;12:381–388.

106. Delacroix DL, Elkon KB, Geubel AP, Hodgson HF, Dive C, Vaerman JP. Changes in size, subclass, and metabolic proper-ties of serum immunoglobulin A in liver diseases in other dis-eases with high serum immunoglobulin A. *J Clin Invest* 1983;71:358.

107. Conley ME, Delacroix DL. Intravascular and mucosal immu-noglobulin A: two separate but related systems of immune de-fense? *Ann Intern Med* 1987;106:892–901.

108. Layward L, Allen AC, Harper SJ, Hattersley JM, Feehally J. Increased and prolonged production of specific polymeric IgA after systemic immunization with tetanus toxoid in IgA ne-phropathy. *Clin Exp Immunol* 1992;88:394–398.

109. Mestecky J, Russell MW. IgA subclasses. *Monogr Allergy* 1986;19:277–301.

110. Delacroix DL, Dive C, Rambaud JC, Vaerman JP. IgA sub-classes in various secretions and in serum. *Immunology* 1982;47:383–385.

111. Brandtzaeg P. Humoral immune response patterns of human mucosae: induction and relation to bacterial respiratory tract infections. *J Infect Dis* 1992;165 (Suppl 1):S167–S176.

112. Brandtzaeg P, Kett K, Rognum TO, et al. Distribution of mucosal IgA and IgG subclass-producing immunocytes and alterations in various disorders. *Monogr Allergy* 1986;20:179–194.

113. Kett K, Brandtzaeg P, Radl J, Haaijman JE. Different subclass distribution of IgA-producing cells in human lymphoid organs and various secretory tissues. *J Immunol* 1986;136:3631–3635.

114. Crago SS, Kutteh WH, Moro I, et al. Distribution of IgA1-, IgA2-, and J chain-containing cells in human tissues. *J Immunol* 1984;132:16–18.

115. Jonard PP, Rambaud JC, Dive C, Vaerman JP, Galian A, Delacroix DL. Secretion of immunoglobulins and plasma proteins from the jejunal mucosa. *J Clin Invest* 1984;74:525–535.

116. Underdown BJ, Schiff JM. Immunoglobulin A: strategic defense initiative at the mucosal surface. *Annu Rev Immunol* 1986;4:389–417.

117. Brandtzaeg P. Immunohistochemical characterization of intracellular J-chain and binding site for secretory component (SC) in human immunoglobulin (Ig)-producing cells. *Mol Immunol* 1983;20:941–966.

118. Brandtzaeg P. Presence of J chain in human immunocytes containing various immunoglobulin classes. *Nature* 1974;252:418–420.

119. Moro I, Iwase T, Komiyama K, Moldoveanu Z, Mestecky J. Immunoglobulin A (IgA) polymerization sites in human immunocytes: immunoelectron microscopic study. *Cell Struct Funct* 1990;15:85–91.

120. Kutteh WH, Prince SJ, Mestecky J. Tissue origins of human polymeric and monomeric IgA. *J Immunol* 1982;128:990–995.

121. South MA, Cooper MD, Wollheim FA, Hong R, Good RA. The IgA system. I. Studies of the transport and immunochemistry of IgA in the saliva. *J Exp Med* 1966;123:615–627.

122. Granfors K, Toivanen A. IgA-anti-*Yersinia* antibodies in *Yersinia* triggered reactive arthritis. *Ann Rheum Dis* 1986;45:561–565.

123. Conley ME, Kearney JF, Lawton AR, Cooper MD. Differentiation of human B cells expressing the IgA subclass as demonstrated by monoclonal antibodies. *J Immunol* 1980;125:2311–2316.

124. Warny M, Vaerman J-P, Avesani V, Delmée M. Human antibody response to *Clostridium difficile* toxin A in relation to clinical course of infection. *Infect Immun* 1994;62:384–389.

125. Ponzi AN, Merlino C, Angerette A, Penna R. Virus-specific polymeric immunoglobulin A antibodies in serum from patients with rubella, measles, varicella, and herpes zoster virus infections. *J Clin Microbiol* 1985;22:505–509.

126. Tarkowski A, Lue C, Moldoveanu Z, Kiyono II, McGhee JR, Mestecky J. Immunization of humans with polysaccharide vaccines induces systemic predominantly polymeric IgA2-subclass antibody responses. *J Immunol* 1990;144:3770–3778.

127. Johnson S, Opstad N, Douglas Jr JM, Janoff EN. Selective production of polymeric IgA in response to *Streptococcus pneumoniae* capsular polysaccharides (abstract). Presented at the 34th Interscience Conference on Antimicrobial Agents and Chemotherapy, Orlando, FL, 1994.

128. Hashido M, Kawana T, Inouye S. Differentiation of primary from nonprimary genital herpesvirus infections by detection of polymeric immunoglobulin A activity. *J Clin Microbiol* 1989;27:2609–2611.

129. Mascart-Lemone F, Duchateau J, Conley ME, Delacroix DL. A polymeric IgA response in serum can be produced by parenteral immunization. *Immunology* 1987;61:409.

130. Moldoveanu Z, Egan ML, Mestecky J. Cellular origin of human polymeric and monomeric IgA: intracellular and secreted forms of IgA. *J Immunol* 1984;133:3156–3162.

131. Lyerly DM, Saum KE, Macdonald DK, Wilkins TD. Effects of *Clostridium difficile* toxins given intragastrically to animals. *Infect Immun* 1985;47:349–352.

132. Walker WA, Block KJ. Intestinal uptake of macromolecules: in vitro and in vivo studies. *Ann NY Acad Sci* 1983;409:593.

133. Jarvis GA, Griffiss JM. Human IgA1 initiates complement-me-diated killing of *Neisseria meningitidis*. *J Immunol* 1989;143:1703–1709.

134. Tagliabue A, Villa L, Boraschi D, Peri G, de Gori V, Nencioni L. Natural anti-bacterial activity against *Salmonella typhi* by human T4+ lymphocytes armed with IgA antibodies. *J Immunol* 1985;135:4178–4182.

135. Tagliabue A, Villa L, de Magistris MT, et al. IgA-driven T cell-mediated anti-bacterial immunity in man after live oral Ty 21a vaccine. *J Immunol* 1986;137:1504–1510.

136. Tagliabue A, Nencioni L, Mantovani A, et al. Impairment of in vitro natural antibacterial activity in HIV-infected patients. *J Immunol* 1988;141:2607–2611.

137. Lowell GH, Smith LF, Griffiss JM, Brandt BL. IgA-dependent, monocyte-mediated antibacterial activity. *J Exp Med* 1980;152:452–457.

138. Roantree RJ, Pappas NC. The survival of strains of enteric bacilli in the blood stream is related to their sensitivity to the bactericidal effect of serum. *J Clin Invest* 1960;39:82–88.

139. Schoolnik GK, Buchanan TM, Holmes KK. Gonococci causing disseminated gonococcal infection are resistant to the bactericidal action of normal human sera. *J Clin Invest* 1976;58:1163–1173.

140. Blaser MJ, Smith PF, Kohler PF. Susceptibility of *Campylobacter* isolates to the bactericidal acitivity of human serum. *J Infect Dis* 1985;151:227–235.

141. Blaser MJ, Smith PF, Repin JE, Joiner KA. Pathogenesis of *Campylobacter fetus* infections. II. Failure of encapsulated *Campylobacter fetus* to bind C3b explains serum and phagocytosis resistance. *J Clin Invest* 1988;81:1434–1444.

142. Joiner KA, Hammer CH, Brown EJ, Cole RJ, Frank MM. Studies on the mechanism of bacterial resistance to complement-mediated killing. I. Terminal complement components are deposited and released from *Salmonella minnesota* S218 without causing bacterial death. *J Exp Med* 1982;155:797–804.

143. Frank MM, Joiner K, Hammer C. The function of antibody and complement in the lysis of bacteria. *Rev Infect Dis* 1987;9:S537–S545.

144. Casali P, Notkins AL. Probing the human B cell repertoire with EBV: polyreactive antibodies and CD5+ B lymphocytes. *Annu Rev Immunol* 1989;7:513–535.

145. Pennie RA, Pearson RD, Barrett LJ, Lior H, Guerrant RL. Susceptibility of *Campylobacter jejuni* to strain-specific bactericidal activity in sera of infected patients. *Infect Immun* 1986;52:702–706.

146. Janoff EN, Jackson S, Wahl SM, Thomas K, Peterman JH, Smith PD. Intestinal mucosal immunoglobulins during HIV-1 infection. *J Infect Dis* 1994;170:299–307.

147. Steffen R, Rickenbach M, Wilhelm V, Helminger A, Shar M. Health problems after travel to developing countries. *J Infect Dis* 1987;156:84–91.

148. Barbour AG, Nichols CR, Fukushima T. An outbreak of giardiasis in a group of campers. *Am J Trop Med Hyg* 1976;25:384–389.

149. Phillips SC, Mildvan D, Williams DC, Gelb AM, White MC. Sexual transmission of enteric protozoa and helminths in a venereal-disease clinic population. *N Engl J Med* 1981;305:603–606.

150. Pickering LK, Woodward WE, DuPont HL, et al. Occurence of *Giardia lamblia* in children in day-care centers. *J Pediatr* 1984;104:522–526.

151. Zaki AM, DuPont HL, Elalmy MA, et al. The detection of enteropathogens in acute diarrhea in a family cohort population in rural Egypt. *Am J Trop Med Hyg* 1986;35:1013–1022.

152. Nash TE, Herrington DA, Losonsky GA, Levine MM. Experimental human infections with *Giardia lamblia*. *J Infect Dis* 1987;156:974–984.

153. Istre GR, Dunlop TS, Gaspard B, Hopkins RS. Waterborne giardiasis at a mountain resort: evidence for acquired immunity. *Am J Public Health* 1984;74:602–604.

154. Moore GT, Cross WM, McGuire D, et al. Epidemic giardiasis at a ski resort. *N Engl J Med* 1969;281:402–407.

155. Islam A, Stoll BJ, Ljungstrom I, Biswas J, Nazrul H, Huldt G. *Giardia lamblia* infections in a cohort of Bangladeshi moth-

ers and infants followed for one year. *J Pediatr* 1983;103: 996–1000.
156. Hossain MM, Ljungstrom I, Biswas J, Nazrul H, Huldt G. Amoebiasis and giardiasis in Bangladesh: parasitological and serological studies. *Trans R Soc Trop Med Hyg* 1983;77: 552–554.
157. Miotti PG, Gilman RN, Santosham M, Ryder RW, Yolken RH. Age-related rate of seropositivity of antibody to *Giardia lamblia* in four diverse populations. *J Clin Microbiol* 1986;24: 972–975.
158. Janoff EN, Smith PD. The role of immunity in *Giardia* infections. In: Meyer EA, eds. *Giardiasis*. Amsterdam: Elsevier, 1990:215–233.
159. Janoff EN, Taylor DN, Echeverria P, Glode M, Blaser MJ. Serum antibodies to *Giardia lamblia* by age in populations in Colorado and Thailand. *West G Med* 1990;152:253–256.

160. Janoff EN, Mead P, Mead J, et al. Clinical, nutritional, and immunologic response to *Giardia lamblia* and *Cryptosporidium* infection in Thai orphans. *Am J Trop Med Hyg* 1990;43: 248–256.
161. Blaser MJ, Sazie E, Williams Jr LP. The influence of immunity on raw milk-associated *Campylobacter* infection. *JAMA* 1987; 257:43–46.
162. Nakata S, Chiba S, Terashima H, Yokoyama T, Nakao T. Humoral immunity in infants with gastroenteritis caused by human calicivirus. *J Infect Dis* 1985;152:274–279.
163. Ungar BLP, Soave R, Fayer R, Nash TE. Enzyme immunoassay detection of immunoglobulin M and G antibodies to *Cryptosporidium* in immunocompetent and immunocompromised persons. *J Infect Dis* 1986;153:570–578.
164. Offit PA, Hoffenberg EJ, Santos N, Gouvea V. Rotavirus-specific humoral and cellular immune response after primary, symptomatic infection. *J Infect Dis* 1993;167:1436–1440.

Infections of the Gastrointestinal Tract,
edited by M. J. Blaser, P. D. Smith, J. I. Ravdin,
H. B. Greenberg, and R. L. Guerrant
Raven Press, Ltd., New York © 1995.

CHAPTER 15

Cellular Immune Mechanisms of Defense in the Gastrointestinal Tract

Stephen P. James

The mucosal immune system of the gastrointestinal (GI) tract is composed of specialized structures, including Peyer's patches, mesenteric lymph nodes, and the intestinal lamina propria. A complex mixture of cells within these structures undergoes continuous activation, migration and homing, terminal differentiation, and the expression of effector functions including release of antibodies and numerous mediators (1). This complicated system, the organization of which is reviewed in the previous chapters, provides the host with mechanisms to protect itself against invasion by potential pathogens and at the same time permits tolerance for potentially immunogenic products of digestion and normal intestinal flora. The balance between the mechanisms that control protective immune responses and inflammation and those that generate tolerance or nonresponsiveness determine the nature of the host response and the type of pathophysiology observed in response to different immunological stimuli. The aim of this chapter is to review the cellular immune mechanisms of the GI immune system. The major humoral immune function of the GI tract, IgA production, is reviewed in a separate chapter. While historically "cellular" and "humoral" immune function have been viewed as separate categories of immune function, this distinction is artificial because cellular and humoral function are closely intertwined.

MECHANISMS OF IMMUNITY AND INFLAMMATION

The immune system contains an array of specialized cells that interact with other nonimmune cells and mediators to generate complex, overlapping specific immune and nonspecific inflammatory responses. The coordinated effect of these responses is to generate immediate inflammatory responses to contain invading pathogens, generate specific cellular and antibody responses, and generate long-term immunological memory. The actions of the immune and inflammatory responses are also closely related to mechanisms of wound healing. Finally, the actions of immune and inflammatory mechanisms are also integrated with nonimmunological systems to produce physiological responses, such as secretion of water and electrolytes by the intestinal epithelium and neurologically controlled motor activity of the gut, which also are important in protecting the host from pathogens.

The effector mechanisms that are generated by immune and inflammatory mechanisms are classified into several categories. Specific antibodies can mediate *neutralization,* in which injurious effect of toxins and certain microorganisms are inhibited by binding to secretory antibodies. In the GI tract, the IgA promotes neutralization without generating potentially injurious inflammatory responses. Activated cells of the immune system also mediate *cytotoxicity,* to kill target cells and microorganisms by nonspecific or specific mechanisms. Many of the effects of the immune system are mediated by *cytokines,* which play numerous critical functions in cell proliferation, differentiation, effector functions, and wound healing. Finally, the combined functions of the immune system are critical in generating *inflammation,* characterized by a cascade of cellular responses by recruitment of macrophages, neutrophils, and lymphocytes; alteration of the vascular endothelium; release of inflammatory cytokines; and activation of different humoral factors (complement, kinin, coagulation). A unique feature of the GI tract is the continuous low-grade or "physiological" inflammation presumably due to the presence of food antigens and endogenous nonpathogenic microfora in the GI lumen. In contrast, pathological inflammation, such as that associated with GI pathogens, is characterized by an increased influx of inflammatory cells, lymphocytes, and cell activation with subsequent tissue injury.

S. P. James: Division of Gastroenterology, Department of Medicine, University of Maryland at Baltimore, and Baltimore VA Medical Center, Baltimore, Maryland 21201.

CELLS OF THE MUCOSAL IMMUNE SYSTEM

The cellular components of the mucosal immune system include cells of the so-called innate immune system that mediate host defense functions in the absence of antigen-specific recognition, and thus constitute the critical early warning system of the host defense system. These cells include cells of the myeloid lineage, such as monocytes, tissue macrophages, neutrophils, eosinophils, and mast cells, as well as lymphoid cells such as natural killer (NK) cells. Under some circumstances these cells can be "armed" to carry out antigen-specific immune functions by binding specific antibodies. The antigen-specific immune functions of the intestinal immune system are carried out by T cells, reviewed here, and IgA B cells, reviewed in a separate chapter.

PHAGOCYTIC CELLS

The GI mucosa is rich in tissue macrophages, many of which are activated even under normal physiological conditions. Macrophages in the mucosa are thought to carry out the functions of macrophages in other tissue sites: they are a first line of defense against invading pathogens, and serve the dual role of phagocytosing pathogens and activating lymphoid cells by presenting antigens and secreting cytokines to activate secondary specific immunological host defense mechanisms.

Neutrophils originate in the bone marrow and are the predominant circulating leukocyte. Mature neutrophils are very short-lived cells, having a circulation time of only about 10 hr before entering tissues or sites of inflammation. Although histologically inconspicuous in normal GI tissues, a large number of neutrophils normally traffic to the intestinal mucosa, where they are thought to traverse into the lumen. During intestinal inflammation, their influx into the mucosa and stool increases dramatically. Neutrophils are highly differentiated cells that exhibit stereotypical responses to specific stimuli. They are chemotactic in response to chemokines or bacterial products, a critical function for recruitment into areas of tissue injury. They also are phagocytic, allowing them to ingest opsonized microorganisms, and they generate an oxidative burst, the mechanism by which they kill microorganisms and mediate tissue injury. Neutrophils in the intestinal mucosa appear to have the same functions as neutrophils in other tissue sites.

Eosinophils, like neutrophils, are bone marrow–derived cells that are highly differentiated effector cells distinguished by their specific granules and morphological characteristics. Although normally infrequent in the circulation, they are present in large numbers in the mucosa. Eosinophils are less efficient *in vitro* in phagocytic activity than neutrophils. The major function of eosinophils appears to be release of granule contents and oxidants in response to certain types of tissue injury, such as parasitic infection. Eosinophils accumulate at sites of parasitism in response to chemotactic factors. Here they become activated by products from monocytes, mast cells, and T cells, including interleukin-3 (IL-3), IL-5, IL-1, and tumor necrosis factor (TNF), to differentiate into activated cells. Once activated they express cytotoxic activity toward the parasite by contact-mediated release of cytotoxic granules. Eosinophils are also prominent in many types of chronic inflammation and allergic responses.

Mast cells are numerous in the GI submucosa and they perform many functions that are reviewed in the following chapter.

GENERAL PROPERTIES OF T CELLS

T-cell precursors of the intestinal immune system originate in the bone marrow and then undergo a process of differentiation and T-cell selection (2). Selection of T cells may occur at sites other than the thymus, including mucosal epithelium (3). T-cell precursors that enter the thymus do not express CD4, CD8, or T-cell receptors (TCRs). During maturation in the thymus, these surface molecules are expressed and the immature T cells interact with the thymic epithelium, via major histocompatibility complex (MHC) class I and II molecules and self peptides. T cells that express high-affinity receptors for self MHC and peptides are eliminated through a process that signals the T cell to undergo apoptosis. Potentially autoreactive T cells that have very low affinity for self MHC are not activated and do not mature. T cells with intermediate affinity for self MHC undergo further maturation into mature CD4+ or CD8+ T cells.

TCRs do not bind soluble antigens with sufficient affinity to activate the cell. Rather, T cells must interact with antigens that are "presented" on the surface of another cell in which the antigen is displayed on an MHC class I or class II molecule (4). Antigens displayed on class I molecules represent endogenously synthesized peptides, including viral antigens (Fig. 1), whereas molecules displayed on class II molecules represent antigens that are

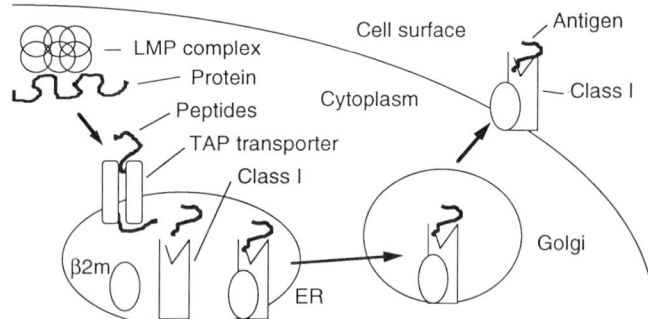

FIG. 1. Endogenously synthesized antigens are presented by HLA class I molecules on the cell surface. Normal cellular proteins and foreign proteins, from intracellular viruses or parasites, referred to as endogenous antigens, undergo degradation through interaction with proteins of the LMP complex and are transported by the TAP transporter across the endoplasmic reticulum (ER). Peptides associate with class I molecules and are transported via the Golgi to the cell surface. This is the primary mechanism for exposure of CD8 T cells to self- and foreign antigens.

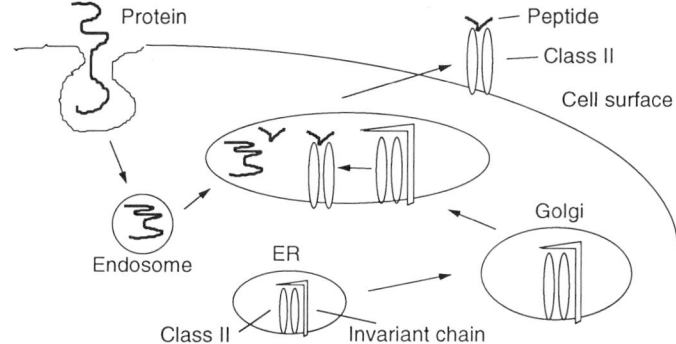

FIG. 2. Exogenous antigens are presented on the cell surface after uptake, intracellular processing, and re-expression on HLA class II molecules. Exogenous proteins are taken up into endosomes, degraded, and then associate with HLA class II molecules in fusion vesicles. HLA class II molecules are protected from taking up peptides in synthetic sites by the invariant chain. This is the primary mechanism for exposure of CD8 T-cell foreign antigens.

taken up, degraded ("processed"); and reexpressed on the surface of cells (5) (Fig. 2). The latter process occurs most efficiently in phagocytic cells such as macrophages, dendritic cells, Kupffer cells, and epidermal Langerhans cells, the so-called antigen presenting cells (APCs), although most cells that express class I or II molecules have the potential for presenting foreign antigens to T cells.

The majority of T cells mature from cells that initially expressed CD4 and CD8 into cells that express one or the other, but not both, molecules (Fig. 3). A small fraction of double-positive cells may escape into the circulation. CD4 molecules stabilize the interaction between foreign antigen on class II molecules and the CD4+ T cell whereas CD8 molecules stabilize the interaction expressed between endogenously processed antigens, such as viral peptides, on class I molecules and the CD8+ T cell. Although CD4 and CD8 T cells share many features, including the ability to produce lymphokines, the differences in the types of antigens that they recognize led originally to the concept that CD4 T cells are "helper" T cells and CD8 T cells are cytolytic T cells. Thus, the majority of T cells that provide "help" (through cognate interactions and lymphokine production) to B cells for antibody production in response to foreign exogenous antigens have the CD4 phenotype, and the majority of T cells that have cytolytic function directed against virally infected cells have the CD8 phenotype. In addition, the concept of CD4 T cells as helper cells and CD8 T cells as suppressor/cytolytic cells has been supplanted by the concept that these cell surface molecules contribute to antigen recognition by T cell (6,7).

The other set of molecules that are critical in determining specificity for antigens (or self peptides) is the TCR (8,9). There are two classes of heterodimers, one of which may be expressed on the surface of a mature T cell. Most T cells in humans have the α,β heterodimer, and only a minority have the γ,δ heterodimer. The latter receptors are of great interest in mucosal immunology because the most common site where they are found is the intestinal epithelium (so-called intraepithelial lymphocytes; see below) (10,11). Analogous to immunoglobulin molecules, each chain of the TCR is a product of a recombination process that links a variable region gene with a constant region gene for α, β, γ, or δ, along with additional intervening sequences. This recombination process generates a very large number (greater than 10^6) of different TCRs giving the individual a large "repertoire" of T cells capable of recognizing a large number of different antigens. Presumably, the driving genetic force for the evolution of this complex mechanism is the need for the host to defend itself against a myriad of pathogens. Analysis of differences in the frequency of T cells expressing different families of TCR genes, in addition to actually sequencing the individual TCR genes, has revealed important differences in the α,β and γ,δ classes of TCRs for different sites in the body. In addition, the distribution of specific receptors differs in sites such as skin, GI tract, and circulation, indicating that the T-cell repertoire varies in different sites. The γ,δ receptors on T cells have much less sequence diversity, suggesting that these receptors are more primordial in origin and may recognize more limited sets of antigens or self peptides.

CD4 T cell response to exogenous antigens

CD8 T cell response to endogenous antigens

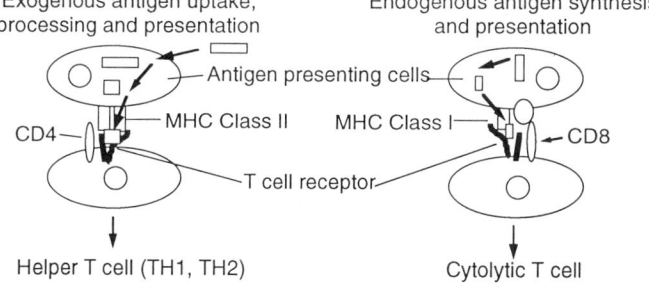

FIG. 3. CD4 and CD8 T cells are activated by different pathways of antigen presentation. CD4 T cells are activated by exogenous antigens presented on MHC class II molecules. The CD4 molecule stabilizes the interaction with the antigen-presenting cell. The activated CD4 T cell differentiates into cells with helper function, including TH1 and TH2 phenotypes. CD8 T cells recognize endogenously synthesized antigens expressed on class I molecules and differentiate into cytolytic T cells.

TCRs provide the specific recognition elements that confer antigen specificity, but activation of T cells occurs through a complex group of invariant molecules associated with the TCR, known as CD3, which transduce a cell signal when antigen binds to the receptor (12–14). The CD3 complex contains at least five different peptides (γ, δ, ϵ, ζ, η) that participate in cell activation through phosphorylation of other cellular proteins.

Many other surface molecules that are not unique to T cells participate in the interaction between T cells and other cells of the immune system, nonimmune cells, and the intercellular matrix (15). Such molecules include those that are important for cellular adhesion to counter receptors: CD2, the classical sheep erythrocyte receptor that binds to a cell surface ligand named LFA-2; CD11a (LFA-1 α chain) and CD54 (ICAM-1), CD29 (β chain of the VLA antigens), and CD44 (Pgp-1). Additional cell surface molecules are receptors for growth factors that are expressed during cell activation, such as CD25 (p55 chain of the IL-2 receptor) and CD71 (transferrin receptor). Other molecules, such as the CD45 series of isoforms, are associated with the level of cell maturation. Other cell surface molecules, such as CD28 (Tp44), may be additional ligands that are involved in signal transduction through alternative pathways (i.e., through the B-70 molecule on APCs). Finally, molecules such as HML-1 and the mucosal homing receptor are adhesion molecules that appear to be important in directing the trafficking of cells to mucosal sites.

When T cells are activated, they may undergo differentiation that alters their functional properties. Activated T cells may divide, providing many progeny cells with the same specificity, thus amplifying the immune response. T cells that have had prior antigen stimulation (memory cells) often have different, usually less stringent requirements for activation by the same antigen and they may recirculate for long periods. Some T cells differentiate into cells having high potential for cytokine production on subsequent stimulation, which causes the activation and function of both immune and nonimmunological cells. Yet another subpopulation of T cells differentiates into cells that have high potential for mediating cytolysis of target cells on subsequent contact through the release of various cytolytic mediators (see below).

INTESTINAL LAMINA PROPRIA T CELLS

The intestinal lamina propria is a unique immunological compartment (16). The effector functions mediated by lymphoid cells in this compartment are probably essential for effective host defense against pathogens. T cells in the diffuse compartment are located in the epithelial layer (intraepithelial lymphocytes; see below) and in the lamina propria. T cells normally constitute one third of the cells in the intestinal lamina propria and a significant number of these cells are activated (17). Due to the large size of the intestine, this represents the largest reservoir of T cells in the body.

The phenotypic distribution of CD4 and CD8 T cells is similar to that of peripheral blood (18). Human and primate lamina propria T cells are almost exclusively CD45RA-negative (19,20), whereas rodent T cells are CD45RB-negative, phenotypes that are typically found on "memory" lymphocytes. There are also phenotypic markers on CD8 cells that correlate with cytolytic and suppressor functions in the intestinal mucosa (19). In studies of a primate model of mucosal infection (lymphogranuloma venereum), T lymphocytes could be isolated from the intestinal mucosa that failed to proliferate in response to specific antigens but did release immunoregulatory factors (21,22), suggesting that they are short-term differentiated effector T cells (23–25). This correlates well with the observations described below that activation of lamina propria T cells can trigger high levels of lymphokine gene expression (26). The low proliferative rate of lamina propria lymphocytes under normal basal conditions has been confirmed by studies showing the presence of very rare Ki antigen (found in dividing cells)–positive cells in the normal intestinal mucosa. Most T cells in the human lamina propria express either CD4 or CD8 and α,β (TCRs), suggesting that they have arisen from the bone marrow and undergone prior thymic education. The TCR repertoire of lamina propria T cells is very diverse, and is not limited as it is in the epithelium and some other sites.

INTRAEPITHELIAL T CELLS

Interspersed among epithelial cells are specialized lymphocytes, referred to as intraepithelial lymphocytes (IELs). Although the major functions of these cells is still uncertain, a number of possibilities are under active study, including their role in host defense as cytolytic cells and their response to antigens presented on the surface of adjacent epithelial cells. It is possible that IELs and epithelial cells interact in ways that modify each other's functions through the production of cytokines. Human and murine IELs are phenotypically pleomorphic but are characterized by certain features. In humans, the majority of IELs are CD8+, CD3+ and have the morphology of large granular lymphocytes. In addition, while the majority in humans have α,β TCRs, an increased proportion of cells have γ,δ receptors, which are rarely expressed on peripheral blood T cells (10,11). In mice, many IELs are Thy-1–negative, and a substantially greater proportion of IELs have γ,δ TCRs, depending on environmental factors such as the presence or absence of enteric pathogens. In humans, an increased proportion of IELs express activation markers, such as CD25, compared to peripheral blood T cells, and a high proportion express the antigen HML-1, a late activation antigen (27). Interestingly, it is difficult to maximally activate IEL proliferation *in vitro* with mitogens or anti-CD3 alone. However, these cells can exhibit high levels of proliferation when triggered through the CD2 alternative pathway by using sheep erythrocytes or combinations of anti-CD2 monoclonal antibodies. These results clearly indicate that these IELs may require special types of cell–cell interactions for triggering.

Interest in IELs increased considerably when a significant proportion of these cells was shown to express γ,δ receptors. The diversity of TCRs expressed by this class of T cells is much greater in the intestine than in certain sites, such as skin. Although numerous characteristics of IELs have been described, their specific function *in vivo* is uncertain. They may recognize particular classes of highly conserved antigens, such as heat shock proteins. Furthermore, they may interact with classes of molecules expressed on epithelial cells besides typical HLA class I or II molecules, such as the CD1 molecules. Another recent insight concerning this class of T cells is that they localize to the intestinal epithelium in athymic animals (28,29). Furthermore, IELs are present in SCID mice, although these cells do not express mature TCRs (30). Finally, γ,δ IELs can be found in germ-free mice (31), indicating that bacterial antigens and mitogens are not necessary for development of these cells. These studies raise the intriguing possibility that the localization and maturation of IELs does not require "education" in the thymus, i.e., under certain circumstances, the intestinal epithelium may be a site of T-cell selection independent of the thymus.

CYTOLYTIC T-CELL FUNCTION

T cells of the CD8 phenotype that recognize endogenously synthesized foreign antigens, such as viral antigens, typically differentiate into cytolytic T lymphocytes (CTLs). These cells have the capacity to lyse "target" cells that express the foreign antigen. The recognition of the target cell is complex and involves multiple adhesion molecule interactions in addition to binding of the TCR. Activation of the T cell is followed by release of preformed cytolytic granule molecules, including perforin, onto the surface of the adjacent cell, which forms a pore in a fashion analogous to the membrane attack complex of the terminal complement cascade (32). Although formerly controversial, the role of perforin in CTL lysis is now generally accepted. This conclusion is confirmed by the observation that mice with an inactivated perforin gene have defective cytolysis and increased susceptibility to viral infections (33). In addition to release of perforins, it appears that other mechanisms may play a role in triggering apoptosis of target cells through non–perforin-mediated pathways (32). The intestinal lamina propria contains CD8 T cells that have the potential for mediating specific killing of virally infected target cells in murine model systems. However, the presence of cytolytic T cells in human intestinal mucosa has been technically more difficult to demonstrate. Using the "redirected lysis" assay in which CD8 T cells are triggered by anti-CD3 which crosslink target cells, human intestinal lamina propria has been shown to contain numerous T-cell precursors with cytolytic activity (34).

NATURAL KILLER LYMPHOCYTES

NK cells are specialized lymphocytes arising from bone marrow precursors (35) that populate the circulation (10% to 15% of circulating cells in adults), spleen, liver, and bone marrow but are generally infrequent in tissue sites such as the intestinal mucosa. NK cells are distinguished from mature T and B cells by the absence of CD3, TCRs, and immunoglobulin. In addition, NK cells typically express the surface glycoproteins CD16 and CD56. NK cells also have a distinctive morphology characterized by abundant cytoplasm and large azurophilic granules. This morphology is not specific, however, since activated CD8 lymphocytes may have the same appearance.

The first defined function of NK cells was tumor cell lysis. This function does not depend on antigen-specific recognition, since NK cells do not have TCRs, and does not require prior exposure to the tumor cells. Their ability to lyse tumor cells depends on the presence of specific glycoproteins on both the NK cell and the target cell, leading to release of preformed lytic factors by the NK cell. Whether tumor cell lysis by NK cells is important *in vivo* is uncertain, since for the most part NK cells have low lytic potential against freshly isolated tumor cells. The lytic activity of NK cells can be induced by cytokines, particularly IL-2. NK cells cultured in IL-2 are called lymphokine-activated killer cells (LAK cells), and these cells have much broader ability to lyse tumor cells, including freshly isolated tumor cells. NK cells have Fc receptors and can be "armed" with specific antibody to lyse target cells expressing the specific antigen. This form of cytotoxicity is called antibody-dependent cellular cytotoxicity (ADCC). While ADCC can be readily demonstrated *in vitro*, its significance *in vivo* is much less clear. A more important function of NK cells may be participation in the first line of defense against intracellular viral infections by lysis virus-infected target cells. Furthermore, IL-12 produced by activated macrophages is a potent stimulus for production of interferon-γ (IFN-γ) by NK cells, and in fact these cells may be a major source of this cytokine that is critical in triggering the early events of cellular immune responses.

IMMUNE CELLULAR COMMUNICATION: CELL CONTACT AND CYTOKINES

Cell Contact

Cells of the immune system communicate through the interaction of cell surface molecules, which require cellular contact, and through the release of soluble mediators such as cytokines, which mediate their effects through specific receptors on the responding cell. Many molecules on the surface of lymphocytes play a role in cell interactions. One classic example is the interaction of the TCR with MHC molecules on the surface of an APC. Other surface molecules that participate in cell interactions include CD2, CD11a (LFA-1 α chain), CD54 (ICAM-1), CD29 (β chain of the VLA antigens), CD44 (Pgp-1), and CD28 (Tp44) (36).

Cytokines

Cytokines are a diverse group of proteins secreted by cells of the immune system that are critical in controlling

Amplification	Differentiation
T-cell proliferation	Memory cells
B-cell proliferation	Cytolytic cells
Recruitment of cells	Antibody secreting cells

Inflammation	Tissue repair
Increased expression of adhesion molecules	Angiogenesis
	Epithelial growth
Induction of inflammatory cells	Fibroblast modulation
Chemotaxis	

FIG. 4. Cytokines are the soluble mediators by which cells of the immune system mediate their effects. Cytokines amplify the immune response by stimulating cell division and recruiting cells into sites of inflammation. Cytokines induce many differentiated functions of cells of the immune system and nonimmune cells. The process of inflammation is induced by soluble mediators that induce expression of adhesion molecules on vascular endothelial cells and by causing chemotaxis and differentiation of specialized functions of inflammatory cells. Cytokines also are important for repair of the damage induced by inflammation.

not only the growth, differentiation, and effector functions of cells of the immune system, but also in mediating a wide array of effects in nonimmune cells (37–39) (Fig. 4). The production of many of these secreted molecules is not unique to lymphoid cells, as they are produced by nonlymphoid cells as well.

Cytokines have a diverse array of overlapping functions. Cytokines and their receptors are expressed on many different types of cells. Therefore, one cytokine can have effects in different types of cells expressing the same receptor. Such receptors are often polymeric and their expression may be regulated by cell activation. Cytokines have a diverse array of physiological effects that often overlap. For some cytokines, this is due to cross-reactivity of the receptors for those cytokines. For other cytokines, it may be due to the fact that individual cytokines stimulate the production of another cytokine. Some cells respond to cytokines with a stereotypic response, i.e., different cytokines acting on the same cell elicit the same response. Finally, different types of cells can produce the same cytokine.

Cytokines are proteins that for the most part are secreted as newly synthesized molecules in response to different activation signals. They may have autocrine effects, i.e., they may affect the same cell type that secretes the cytokine. For example, IL-2 is secreted by T cells and is important for T-cell proliferation. Cytokines also may have effects on many other cell types in either nearby (paracrine effect) or distant sites (endocrine effect). Cytokines can have negative regulatory effects, as in the case of IL-10 discussed below.

It is helpful to classify cytokines according to their general class of effect (Fig. 5). Regulatory cytokines, such as IL-2, IL-4, IL-5, IL-10, IL-12, and IFN-γ, have important effects of the growth and differentiation of lymphoid cells. Proinflammatory cytokines, such as IL-1α and IL-1β, IL-6, IL-8, and TNF-α and β, are important in the recruit-

Inflammatory: Activation of myeloid cells
IL-1, IL-6, IL-8 family, TNF-α, TGF-β

Regulatory: Lymphocyte proliferation and differentiation
IL-2, IL-4, IL-5, IL-6, IL-10, IL-12, IL-13, IFN-γ, TGF-β

Hematopoietic: Growth of progenitor cells
IL-1, IL-6, IL-7, TNF-α, M-CSF, GM-CSF, Multi-CSF (IL-3)

FIG. 5. Cytokines are grouped in three broad classes of functions: inflammatory, regulatory, and hematopoietic. Cytokines have many overlapping functions and can act on many different cell types to mediate their effects.

ment and activation of inflammatory cells. Finally, some cytokines predominantly have effects on cell growth, and these include IL-3, IL-7, and GM-CSF.

PROPERTIES OF SELECTED CYTOKINES

Interleukin-1

IL-1 was first identified as a monokine produced by macrophages capable of augmenting T-cell responses to antigens and mitogens (40,41). IL-1 is not one but two distinct molecules (IL-1α and IL-1β) that are products of separate genes, both of which, in humans, are on chromosome 2. The two IL-1s are structurally dissimilar except for a region of homology that is likely to be the recognition site for the IL-1 receptor. IL-1β is the predominant secreted form and IL-1α is the main membrane-bound form of this molecule.

IL-1 is produced by macrophages and many other cells such as keratinocytes, astrocytes, and mesangial cells. In macrophages, IL-1 production is stimulated by a variety of agents such as lipopolysaccharides (LPS), phorbol esters, leukotrienes, immune complexes, UV irradiation, and agents that induce phagocytosis. In addition, T cells interacting with macrophages, via either cell contact or lymphokines, can induce IL-1 synthesis. Agents that suppress IL-1 secretion include those that downregulate immune responses generally such as cyclosporin A, corticosteroids, and prostaglandins. Finally, a naturally occurring inhibitor of IL-1, IL-1 receptor antagonist, has been identified; this molecule inhibits the action of IL-1 by competitive inhibition of binding to the IL-1 receptor.

The numerous functions of IL-1 reflect both direct effects of this interleukin and indirect effects due to mediators released in response to IL-1. Many of the effects of IL-1 are classified as inflammatory. In the central nervous system (CNS), IL-1 acts on the hypothalamic thermoregulatory center and other centers to cause fever and sleep, and acts in many areas of the CNS to increase secretion of various neuropeptides (including endorphins), corticotropin-releasing factor, and ACTH; the latter, in combination with direct effects of IL-1 on the adrenal gland, leads to increased circulating steroid levels. Similarly, IL-1 acts as an inflammatory mediator in the liver, where it increases synthesis of acute phase reactants and metallothioneines and decreases synthesis of albumin. In addition, it inhibits lipoprotein lipase synthesis and thus causes decreased lipid utilization and lactic acidosis.

Other inflammatory effects of IL-1 include its capacity to augment connective tissue cell growth and collagen formation, to increase bone resorption (osteoclast activity), and to induce prostaglandin synthesis. In addition, IL-1 augments the catabolic effects of TNF and is synergistic with the latter in the generation of hypertension and the capillary leak syndrome. Finally, IL-1 has notable inflammatory effects on the vascular system, including the enhancement of endothelial cell proliferation, the release of potent vasodilators, and the initiation of clot formation.

Interleukin-2

IL-2 is a 15.4-kDa protein that acts on activated T cells and (to a lesser extent) B cells, as well as on NK cells and thymocytes, causing these cells to proliferate and/or manifest differentiated cell function (e.g., cytotoxicity) (42). Lymphocytes have high-, intermediate-, and low-affinity receptors that are due to combinations of three different peptide receptor chains. The high-affinity receptor is a heterodimer composed of a p55 moiety (known as the "Tac" antigen) that binds IL-2 with low affinity and a p75 moiety that binds IL-2 with intermediate affinity (43,44). Activated lymphocytes express both high-affinity (p75/p55) and low-affinity (p55) receptors, whereas large granular lymphocytes (including NK cells) express receptors of intermediate affinity (p75). IL-2 receptors are also expressed on B cells and activated cells of the macrophage/monocyte lineage.

IL-2 is synthesized by both T cells and large granular lymphocytes. A variety of stimuli induce IL-2 synthesis, including specific antigens, antibodies reacting with cell surface molecules (CD3 and CD2 antigens) important in activation pathways, and nonspecific activating substances such as phorbol esters and mitogens. IL-2 synthesis is inhibited by immunosuppressive substances such as glucocorticoids, cyclosporin A, and prostaglandins.

IL-2 has been used for therapy of tumors. The basis of this therapy is the ability of IL-2 to induce LAK cells (see above), which have cytotoxic activity for various tumor cells (45).

Interleukin 3 and Other Colony-Stimulating Factors

IL-3 is representative of a family of cytokines involved in the growth and differentiation of hematopoietic and lymphoid precursor cells. This family consists of a group of molecules known as colony-stimulating factors (CSFs), which share the capacity to stimulate granulocyte and/or macrophage colony formation in bone marrow cultures (46,47). IL-3 (multi-CSF) is a glycoprotein derived from activated T cells that supports the growth of virtually all types of hematopoietic progenitor cells, usually at several stages of their development and in concert with other CSFs. Other members of this family include M-CSF (CSF-1), a glycoprotein that stimulates the growth of macrophage colonies and monocytic cell lines. GM-CSF,

a glycoprotein produced by various cells including fibroblasts, endothelial cells, and activated T cells, has growth-enhancing effects on granulocyte/macrophage/eosinophil colonies, and in combination with erythropoietin, on erythroid and multipotential colonies. In addition, GM-CSF has effects on mature cells, causing neutrophil and eosinophil activation and inducing neutrophil phagocytosis. G-CSF is a glycoprotein produced by macrophages and epithelial cells that stimulates predominantly granulocytes but may indirectly affect other precursors when present in high concentration. Erythropoietin is a 34- to 39-kDa glycoprotein produced in the kidney that predominantly stimulates erythroid precursor cells but also has effects on other precursors in association with other CSFs.

Interleukin-4

IL-4 was initially discovered as a factor that promotes B-cell proliferation. IL-4 can act on both resting and activated B cells (48,49). Other effects of IL-4 on B cells include the induction of class II MHC expression (50), the expression of CD23 (low-affinity IgE receptor) (51), and the upregulation of the IL-4 receptor itself (48); these effects allow the B cell to respond to other stimulatory lymphokines and to interact with other cells. IL-4 plays an important role in isotype differentiation of B cells: B cells stimulated with LPS in the presence of IL-4 preferentially express IgG1 (rather than IgG3) and IgE (52,53). Furthermore, IL-4 induction of IgG1 expression is inhibited by IFN-γ. Thus IL-4, as well as other lymphokines, have important effects on B-cell isotype differentiation. IL-4 also may stimulate resting T cells to undergo enhanced proliferation when exposed to other costimuli such as PMA. In addition, IL-4 acts to support proliferation and expansion of immature erythroid, myelomonocytic, and megakaryocytic precursors as well as macrophages and mast cells (in the mouse). These observations suggest that IL-4 is a broadly reactive growth and differentiation factor that is not limited to its effects on any one cell type.

Interleukin 5

IL-5 was initially identified as a factor present in supernatants of T-cell cultures that was capable of causing B cells to either differentiate into cells actively producing antibody or undergo proliferation. For this reason, IL-5 was initially called T-cell replacing factor (TRF) or B-cell growth factor II (BCGF-II) (55,56). A multimer of disulfide-linked subunits, IL-5 has isotype-specific effects: following LPS activation of murine B cells in the presence of IL-5, IgA but not IgG subclass production is increased (57). The effects of IL-5, like IL-4, are not restricted to B cells. In this regard, IL-5 has been shown to have colony-stimulating activity for eosinophils in liquid bone marrow culture (58) and to augment expression of T-cell cytotoxic capacity (59). The latter may relate to the ability of IL-5 to induce IL-2 receptors.

Interleukin-6

IL-6 induces terminal differentiation of B cells into plasma cells in the absence of proliferation. Although IL-6 does not augment normal B-cell proliferation, it has growth-enhancing effects on activated B cells. Thus, the effects of IL-6 on cells may depend somewhat on the preexisting state of cell activation. When the gene for IL-6 was discovered, it was found to be identical to IFN-β2. IL-6 is a protein with sequence and gene structure homology with G-CSF. Gene transcription of IL-6 is enhanced by IL-1 and, to a lesser extent, by other cytokines such as TNF, platelet-derived growth factor, and IFN-γ. In addition, LPS increases IL-6 mRNA synthesis in fibroblasts. Unlike the other type I interferon genes (IFN-α and IFN-β1 genes) that are located on chromosome 9, the human IL-6 (IFN-β2) gene is located on chromosome 7. In addition, the IL-6 gene has only a 20% homology with other type I interferons. IL-6 mediates its effects via the same receptor as other type I interferons and shares with the latter certain properties such as the ability to inhibit virus replication, to induce specific interferon-activated genes, and to have antimitogenic effects on fibroblasts. Thus, IL-6 is an interferon, but one that differs significantly from the other interferons.

In addition to its antiviral and B-cell effects, IL-6 also has important regulatory effects on the synthesis of acute phase reactants by hepatocytes. IL-6 is identical to monocyte-derived hepatocyte-stimulating factor (HSF) (62). The very diverse activities of IL-6 as well as the fact that IL-6 is produced by a variety of cell types indicates that IL-6 plays a central role during inflammation. Indeed, some of the inflammatory activities ascribed to IL-1 may be due to IL-6.

Tumor Necrosis Factors: TNF-α (Cachectin) and TNF-β (Lymphotoxin)

In 1975 Carswell et al. showed that the serum of BCG-primed, endotoxin-treated animals contains a macrophage-derived α factor, called tumor necrosis factor (TNF), which was capable of causing hemorrhagic necrosis of tumors (63). Independent of these studies, other investigators examined the mechanisms of cachexia associated with chronic inflammation. These studies led to the identification of a macrophage-derived factor that suppressed lipoprotein lipase synthesis and that, when ultimately purified and sequenced, was found to be identical to TNF. In other studies, a factor was isolated from activated lymphocytes which was able to lyse target cells, termed lymphotoxin (LT). LT and TNF share 26% identity and 51% homology (64). On the basis of this structural and functional similarity, a nomenclature was proposed: TNF-α for the macrophage factor and TNF-β for the lymphocyte factor.

In vivo administration of endotoxin to rabbits causes a rapid rise in TNF-α in plasma, followed by rapid clearance. The latter is thought to be caused by TNF-α membrane receptor-bearing cells present in the liver, skin, kidneys, lung, and gastrointestinal tract. It is now thought that many of the effects of administration of bacterial products and LPS are mediated directly by production of TNF-α (65). In addition, there is considerable evidence that TNF-α is the central mediator of the wasting that accompanies chronic disease (65). LPS is a potent inducer of TNF synthesis by macrophages, and large doses of TNF-α mimic the effects of endotoxic shock, suggesting that this protein is the major mediator of the deleterious effects of endotoxin.

TNF-α shares with IL-1 the capacity to act as a potent endogenous pyrogen; this is caused both by a direct effect on the hypothalamus and an indirect augmenting effect on IL-1 production. Other IL-1-like effects of TNF-α include the induction of prostaglandin E_2 and collagenase synthesis by human synovial cells and dermal fibroblasts and TNF-α–mediated bone resorption. TNF-β, on the other hand, has been shown to have a growth factor–like effect on human B cells and fibroblasts (66). The activities of both TNF-α and TNF-β may be due to their capacity to augment synthesis of other cytokines. In addition to the effect of TNF on IL-1 synthesis already mentioned, the TNFs cause production of GM-CSF and IFN-β2. In turn, other cytokines such as IFN-γ and LPS can cause increased TNF production. Finally, the antitumor effects of TNF are enhanced by INF-γ. TNF and, to a lesser extent, IL-1, are potent inducers of inflammation. TNF is chemotactic for neutrophils, and both induce endothelial cells to express adhesion molecules that are important in the initial steps of inflammation.

IL-8 Family

The IL-8 family of cytokines include two closely related groups of cytokines (chemokines α and chemokines β) that have proinflammatory activity (67). One of their important functions is chemotaxis for neutrophils and monocytes. These cytokines are produced by many types of cells, particularly activated monocytes. They are also produced by activated intestinal epithelial cell lines in response to potent stimuli or invasion by bacteria. These cytokines are thought to provide an important first step in host defense by triggering the influx of phagocytic cells to sites of tissue injury.

Interleukin 10

As indicated above, IL-10 was discovered as a cytokine produced by TH2 type T-cell clones (68). It has been shown to be produced by T cells, B cells, and macrophages. It has important negative immunoregulatory effects through its ability to inhibit macrophage expression of IL-1, IL-6, and IL-8 and TH1-type cell activation and IFN-γ production.

Interleukin 12

IL-12 appears to be produced primarily by macrophages and B cells, and is a potent stimulus for IFN-γ production by NK cells and, to a lesser extent, T cells (69). There is evidence both *in vitro* and *in vivo* that IL-12 is produced in response to intracellular infection of macrophages and is a powerful stimulus for TH1 cytokine production and granulomatous types of inflammatory responses. As indicated above, both IL-4 and IL-10 down-regulate production of IL-12 by macrophages, illustrating the complex interrelationship of cytokines during immune responses and inflammation.

Interferons

The interferons are proteins that were initially discovered because of their antiviral activity, i.e., they manifest "interference" with viral replication. The interferons are divided into two families: Type I interferons (IFN-α and IFN-β) are produced by many cell types and are encoded by numerous nonallelic genes (70). IFN-α is produced primarily by leukocytes, and IFN-β is the major interferon produced by nonleukocytes. Type II interferon, IFN-γ, is produced by T and NK cells in response to activation during immune responses.

The interferons have a large number of cellular effects, which vary depending on the type and dose of interferon and cell target. Interferons have antiviral activity against most types of viruses in virtually all cells through a complex series of intracellular events. In addition, interferons have numerous effects on the cells of the immune system by altering cell growth and differentiation. Interferons activate macrophages to increase their bactericidal and tumoricidal activity and enhance their antigen-presenting function. The effects of interferons on lymphocyte functions depend on the dose and timing of administration; these effects can be inhibitory or stimulatory. In general, as for other types of cells, the effects of interferons are antiproliferative and induce cellular differentiation. IFN-γ induces differentiation of precursors into cytolytic T cells and enhances the cytolytic function of NK cells.

Tumor Growth Factor

TGF-β was initially discovered as a cytokine that promotes proliferation of fibroblasts. There are at least three closely related forms of this cytokine. It is ubiquitous and is produced by many cell types and has a large number of known functions (71). Although TGF-β largely has a negative effect on the immune system, it also may induce specific differentiated cell functions such as the switch of B-cell precursors to IgA expressing cells. This cytokine is important in wound healing: it stimulates and mobilizes fibroblasts and stimulates collagen, fibronectin, and collagenase synthesis. TGF-β has antiproliferative effects on numerous types of cells, including epithelial cells, endothelial cells, smooth muscle cells, myeloid progenitors, and T and B cells. Despite its initial discovery as a growth factor, it primarily has antiproliferative effects and is important in inducing many differentiated functions of different types of cells.

PATTERNS OF LYMPHOKINE PRODUCTION IN THE REGULATION OF MUCOSAL IMMUNE RESPONSES

While the biological effects of individual cytokines have been described in considerable detail, more recently the complex and physiologically relevant issue has been the effect of combinations of cytokines in regulating immunological responses. The importance of this theme is best illustrated by numerous studies showing that IL-4 and IFN-γ have opposing effects in regulating IgE production (72). Furthermore, the pioneering studies of Mossman and colleagues demonstrated that individual clones of T cells in long-term culture differentiate in such a way that they tend to have a specialized pattern of lymphokine production, classified as type TH1 (including IL-2, IL-3, lymphotoxin, and IFN-γ) or type TH2 (including IL-4, IL-5, IL-6, IL-9, IL-10, and IL-13) (73–75) (Fig. 6). The cells of the former type were suggested to have helper activity for delayed-type hypersensitivity (DTH) responses and the latter for antibody synthesis. Since cells of these two types could differentially regulate murine immune responses, as in the case of IgE, it became important to determine whether cells with these properties exist *in vivo* and whether the same is true of human cells. In further studies of both murine and human clonal populations, it has become clear that individual cells can be identified that secrete patterns of lymphokines that do not fall into the TH1 and TH2 patterns. Furthermore, in humans IFN-γ and particularly IL-2, products of TH1 cells, may have important roles in B-cell differentiation. Nonetheless the original TH1–TH2 model has served as an important foundation for trying to understand the pathophysiology of certain types of diseases. The study of models of infectious diseases has been particularly revealing in this regard. It is noteworthy that from animals infected with *Brucella abortis*, it is possible to isolate T-cell clones primarily of the TH1 type, whereas animals colonized with *Nippostrongylus brasiliensis* have primarily TH2 cells *in vitro* (75). Some of the most convincing evidence for the importance of differences in the patterns of lymphokine production is that of murine leishmaniasis, an intracellular infection in which the cellular immune response is thought to be critical for recovery. Mouse strains that respond with a high "TH1-like" response have much lower mor-

Typical stimuli of TH1 responses
Intracellular pathogens: *Brucella*, mycobacteria, *Borrelia*, viruses, *Leishmania* (cutaneous)
Allografts
Encapsulated infectious agents

Typical stimuli for TH2 responses
Allergens
Parasites, schistosomes, *Leishmania* (visceral)

FIG. 6. TH1 and TH2 helper cell differentiation is induced by different types of stimuli. The TH1 response is typified by a granulomatous type of inflammatory response and production of IgG2 antibodies. The TH2 response is characterized by production of cytokines that induce production of IgG1 and IgE and differentiation of eosinophils.

bidity than animals having a "TH2-like" lymphokine response (76).

The ability of animals to resist parasite infection of the gastrointestinal tract with *Trichinella spiralis* is also genetically determined, and resistant strains have immune responses that are dominated by greater IFN-γ production and less IL-4 production by mesenteric lymph node cells (77). The implication of these important studies is that the genetic control of the immune response to infectious agents, including those that infect the gastrointestinal tract, is closely associated with the level of cytokines produced. The complex role of lymphokines in disease has also been demonstrated through studies in which the effects of cytokines are blocked by exogenously administered anticytokine antibodies. Animals parasitized with *N. brasiliensis* have marked eosinophilia that is likely dependent on IL-5, as confirmed by experiments in which the eosinophilia is blocked by infusion of anti-IL-5 (78). Indeed, eosinophils express IL-5 receptors, which can be upregulated by a T-cell lymphokine, GM-CSF (79). In murine schistosomiasis, anti-IL-5 blocks blood and tissue eosinophilia; however, antibody treatment does not block the granulomatous response (80). Thus, the regulation of immune responses *in vivo* in response to pathogens is complex and involves the production of multiple different cytokines. It is possible that the differentiation of T cells into TH1 or TH2 like cells is a process that is itself dependent on cytokines present in the microenvironment (81).

CYTOKINES AND THE MUCOSA

Important progress has been made in understanding the role of cytokines in the mucosal immune system. A discussion of this progress should be preceded by a reminder that the immunoglobulin response of the intestinal mucosa is highly skewed toward the production of IgA. Also, mucosal (lamina propria) are activated and T cells have primarily a "memory" phenotype. These fundamental observations would lead one to expect that the lymphokines and cytokines produced in the intestinal mucosa would differ from those produced in the systemic immune system. One important advance in identifying the lymphokines produced by individual cells in the mucosa has been the development of the ELISPOT assay. Applied to the study of gut-associated lymphoreticular tissue (GALT) in the mouse, the assay has revealed a number of interesting findings (82,83). First, the number of IFN-γ– and IL-5–producing cells is substantially higher in the Peyer's patch and intestinal lamina propria than in the systemic lymphoid sites such as the spleen. Furthermore, in the intestinal lamina propria, a site where large numbers of IgA plasma cells are normally present, significantly higher numbers of T cells produce IL-5 than IFN-γ.

An alternative approach has been used to study the potential for lymphokine production in normal primates. Following activation with mitogens, high levels of mRNA for IL-2, IFN-γ, IL-5, and, to a lesser extent, IL-4 are detected in mRNA prepared from intestinal lamina propria cells compared to cells obtained from other sites. These results indicate that the intestinal lamina propria may be a site of high lymphokine production by T cells under normal physiological conditions. Furthermore, it appears that intestinal lamina propria lymphocytes have the potential for both TH1 and TH2 types of cytokine production.

More recently, certain cytokines have been shown to play a key role in regulating the development of TH1 or TH2 responses (Fig. 7). IL-10 is a cytokine produced by TH2 murine T-cell clones that has the capacity not only to act as a B-cell growth factor but to inhibit the activation of TH1 clones of T cells (68). The inhibitory effect of IL-10 acts on macrophages, inhibiting the activation signals necessary for TH1 cell activation. IL-12 also appears to play a role in the development of TH1 responses, but in this case it has a positive effect on the development of cellular immune responses. IL-12 is produced primarily by macrophages and promotes cell-mediated immunity and granulomatous inflammation (69). One of its effects is to markedly stimulate IFN-γ production by NK cells. Importantly, recombinant IL-12 cures mice infected with *Leishmania major* (84). Conversely, anti-IFN-γ antibody can convert a *Leishmania*-resistant strain of mice to a susceptible strain. As indicated above, IFN-γ inhibits the IL-4–mediated induction of TH2 types of responses. Taken together, these observations suggest a certain symmetry in the regulation of TH1 or TH2 responses: IL-12 and IFN-γ promote cellular responses and inhibit TH2 types of responses, whereas IL-4 and IL-10 promote humoral immunity and inhibit cellular responses. The mechanisms that regulate TH1 vs. TH2 responses appear to influence the pathogenic outcome in certain disease conditions. The control may be initiated by interaction between the stimulus and target cell(s) of the immune system. Thus, intracellular infections localized in

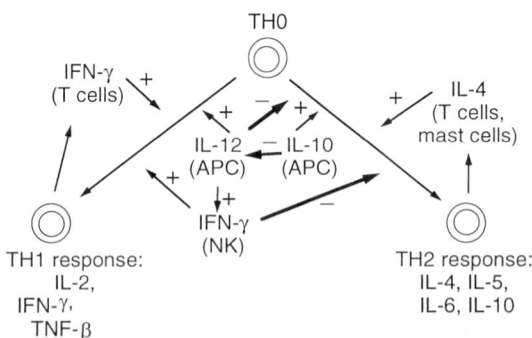

FIG. 7. The differentiation of undifferentiated TH0 T cells into specialized T-cell subsets is regulated by cytokines. IFN-γ, produced by T cells and NK cells, and IL-12, produced by antigen-presenting cells (APCs), promote differentiation of T cells into TH1 cells that secrete a pattern of cytokines associated with DTH and development of cytolytic T cells. The TH1 pathway is inhibited by IL-10 produced by APCs and T cells. Conversely, the TH2 pathway, which results in development of T cells that provide help for IgG1 and IgE responses, is promoted by IL-10 and IL-4, produced by T cells and mast cells. The TH2 pathway is inhibited by IL-12. Thus the balance of cytokines in the T-cell environment controls the development of specific T-cell phenotypes.

macrophages are potent inducers of cellular immune responses, probably due to the initial induction of IL-12 and IFN-γ production. In contrast, extracellular pathogens, such as intestinal parasites, appear to be strong inducers of cells that release IL-4 and IL-10.

CYTOKINE PRODUCTION IN HUMAN INFECTIOUS DISEASES

An extensive body of data indicates that specific patterns of T-lymphocyte cytokine production occur in response to different pathogens. Although some of the details differ from animal models in terms of specific cytokines, the overall concept remains the same: the immunopathology caused by different inciting agents is associated with specific patterns of cytokine production by cells responding to the agent (85).

The approaches to identifying the cytokines associated with human infectious diseases has included examining cytokine profiles of T-cell clones maintained *in vitro* and, more recently, analyzing the profiles of cytokines produced by cells from affected tissues or the tissues themselves using PCR-RT or *in situ* hybridization. As in animal models of granulomatous diseases, agents that induce strong granulomatous responses in humans are characterized generally by a TH1 pattern of cytokines. Purified protein derivative (PPD)–specific clones from patients with tuberculosis produce high levels of IFN-γ, whereas clones that do not react with PPD produce a TH0 pattern of cytokines (85). In studies of *Mycobacterium leprae* infection, patients with resistance have expression of predominantly TH1 cytokines in tissues, whereas patients with extensive disease have TH2 lymphokines (86). Furthermore, treatment of patients with *M. leprae* infection with IL-2 has been associated with restoration of delayed type hypersensitivity (DTH) and may aid in clearance of the organism (87). In Lyme disease, *Borrelia burgdorferi*–specific CD4 T-cell clones from peripheral blood or synovial fluid of infected patients also reveal a TH1 profile of lymphokines, whereas control (tetanus toxoid–specific) clones have a Th0 profile (88). A final example of the response to bacterial infections is that of *Yersinia enterocolitica*–induced reactive arthritis, in which, like Lyme disease, synovial fluid lymphocytes have a strong TH1 response (89).

Infection with viral pathogens in humans has also been shown to be associated with a TH1 type of cytokine profile. Interestingly, viruses tend to induce CD8 + CTL lymphocytes, which show a pattern of cytokine expression similar to that of CD4 + TH1 cells (90). In studies of responses to a variety of viruses, including infections with Epstein–Barr virus, HSV, and hepatitis B virus, a TH1 or Th0 pattern of response predominates (91–93). In contrast to the intracellular pathogens that lead to granulomatous and strong DTH responses with a TH1 profile of cytokines, infection with parasitic helminths is associated with eosinophilia, elevated IgE, and increased expression of TH2-type cytokines. The enlarging list of parasitic infections, including toxocariasis, loiasis, filariasis, strongyloidiasis, and onchocerciasis (94–96), that induce a TH2 response suggests that a TH2 pattern of cytokine production is the general rule in parasitic diseases. The roles that eosinophils and IgE play may be protective but, on the other hand, the TH2 response generated by helminths may also be one mechanism by which the parasites evade a protective TH1 type of response, since the TH2 cytokines IL-4 and IL-10 downregulate the TH1 response.

TRANSGENIC AND GENE-TARGETED MUTANT MICE: IMPLICATIONS FOR HOST DEFENSE IN THE GI IMMUNE SYSTEM

A number of important transgenic and gene disruption experiments in animal models convincingly demonstrate the critical role of specific cellular mechanisms in host defense in the gastrointestinal mucosa. Rats transgenic for human HLA-B27 and β2-microglobulin develop a spectrum of disease that closely resembles human spondyloarthropathies (97). Interestingly, these animals have a severe panintestinal inflammatory disease, and the susceptibility for this disease can be transferred to normal rats by bone marrow cells (98), indicating that susceptibility to the disease is dependent on expression of HLA B27 on cells of the immune system. Importantly, the disease is also dependent on the presence of a bacterial flora in the gut, since germ-free animals have little manifestation of disease. Thus, this model demonstrates that susceptibility to abnormal inflammation in the gastrointestinal tract can be triggered by the interaction of microbial products and specific HLA molecules on cells of the immune system.

Another approach to dissecting the role of specific immune mechanisms in host defense has been to disrupt specific genes in mice (99). In a series of experiments, Mombaerts et al. (100) produced murine strains deficient in certain T-cell–specific molecules, including TCR-α, TCR-β, TCR-δ, RAG-1 deficient, and CD4 (MHC class II–deficient). Surprisingly, animals deficient in TCR-α, TCR-β, or CD4 T cells developed an inflammatory disease of the colon characterized by wasting and bloody stools, reminiscent of human ulcerative colitis. As in the HLA-B27 transgenic model, these animals also expressed more severe disease when raised in a conventional, instead of a pathogen-free, environment, suggesting an important role for enteric flora in disease. Interestingly, TCR-δ–deficient mice had no apparent disease, raising questions concerning the significance of these cells in the IEL population for host defense. In addition, RAG-1–deficient mice that lacked mature T and B cells fared surprisingly well when kept in a pathogen-free environment; similar to immunodeficient humans, these animals were susceptible to opportunistic infections. These important observations suggest that specific populations of T cells are critical for maintaining the normal balance of immune response and tolerance in the gastrointestinal tract in the presence of a normal microbial flora.

Another series of highly informative experiments has involved the deletion of genes for specific cytokines. Animals having inactivation of the IL-2 gene develop an ulcerative colitis–like syndrome with autoantibodies when the gut contains bacterial flora (101). Interestingly, T cells of these animals demonstrated diminished T-cell proliferative responses and an increased tendency to a TH2 type of response (increased IgG1 and IgE). In contrast, animals with a disrupted IL-10 gene develop a panbowel inflammatory disease, again when housed in a conventional environment (102). These animals, as predicted, fail to mount a TH2 response to parasitic antigens but instead have an atypical TH1 type of response. Finally, an unexpected observation was that animals with disruption of the TGF-β gene also develop chronic inflammation of the bowel and wasting (103). These models have been highly instructive in demonstrating the crucial role of the presence of certain cellular mechanisms in the mucosal immune system and the importance of a balanced TH1 and TH2 response to main normal homeostasis in the gut. Studies of the responses of these animals to specific enteric pathogens should help elucidate the cellular factors critical for providing host protection against enteric infections.

REFERENCES

1. Strober W, Brown WR. The mucosal immune system. In: Samter M, ed. *Immunological diseases*. 4th Ed. Boston: Little, Brown; 1988.
2. Ramsdell F, Fowlkes BJ. Clonal deletion versus clonal anergy: the role of the thymus in inducing self tolerance. *Science* 1990; 248:1342–1348.
3. Lefrancois L, LeCorre R, Mayo J, Bluestone JA, Goodman T. Extrathymic selection of TCR γ,δ cells by class II major histocompatibility complex molecules. *Cell* 1990;63:333–340.
4. Schwartz, RH. T lymphocyte recognition of antigen in association with Gene products of the major histocompatibility complex. *Annu Rev Immunol* 1985;3:237–261.
5. Harding CV, Unanue ER. Cellular mechanisms of antigen processing and the function of class I and class II major histocompatibility complex molecules. *Cell* 1990;61:499.
6. Engleman EG, Benike CJ, Grumet FC, Evans RL. Activation of human T lymphocyte subsets: helper and suppressor/cytotoxic T cells recognize and respond to distinct histocompatibility antigens. *J Immunol* 1981;127:2124.
7. Meuer SC, Schlossman SF, Reinherz EL. Clonal analysis of human cytotoxic T lymphocytes: T4+ and T8+ effector cells recognize products of different major histocompatibility complex regions. *Proc Natl Acad Sci USA* 1982;79:4395.
8. Davis MM. T cell receptor gene diversity and selection. *Annu Rev Biochem* 1990;49:475.
9. Strominger JL. Developmental biology of T cell receptors. *Science* 1989;244:943.
10. Itohara S, Farr AG, Lafaille JJ, et al. Homing of a γδ thymocyte subset with homogeneous T cell receptors to mucosal epithelia. *Nature* 1990;343:754–757.
11. Haas W, Kaufman S, Martinez AC. The development and function of γδ T cells. *Immunol Today* 1990;11:340–343.
12. Baniyash M, Garcia-Morales P, Luong E, Samelson LE, Klausner RD. The T cell antigen receptor zeta chain is tyrosine phosphorylated upon activation. *J Biol Chem* 1988;263:18225.
13. Weissman AM, Baniyash S, Hou D, Samelson LE, Burgess WH, Klausner RD. Molecular cloning of the zeta chain of the T cell antigen receptor. *Science* 1988;239:1018.
14. Orloff DG, Frank SJ, Robey FA, Weissman AM, Klausner RD. Biochemical characterization of the eta chain of the T cell receptor. a unique subunit related to zeta. *J Biol Chem* 1989;264:14812.
15. Thomas M. The leukocyte common antigen family. *Annu Rev Immunol* 1989;7:339.

16. James SP. Mucosal T cell function. *Gastroenterology Clin North Am* 1991;20:597–612.
17. Zeitz M, Green WC, Peffer NJ, James SP. Lymphocytes isolated from the intestinal lamina propria of normal non-human primates have increased expression of genes associated with T cell activation. *Gastroenterology* 1988;94:647–655.
18. James SP, Fiocchi C, Graeff AS, Strober W. Immunoregulatory function of lamina propria T cells in Crohn's disease. *Gastroenterology* 1985;88:1143–1150.
19. James SP, Fiocchi C, Graeff AS, Strober W. Phenotypic analysis of lamina propria lymphocytes: predominance of helper-inducer and cytolytic T cell phenotypes and deficiency of suppressor-inducer phenotypes in Crohn's disease and control patients. *Gastroenterology* 1986;91:1483–1489.
20. James SP, Graeff AS, Zietz M. Predominance of helper-inducer T cells in mesenteric lymph nodes and intestinal lamina propria of normal non-human primates. *Cell Immunol* 1987;107:372–383.
21. James SP, Graeff AS, Zeitz M, Kappus E, Quinn TC. Cytotoxic and immunoregulatory function of intestinal lymphocytes in LGV proctitis of nonhuman primates. *Infect Immun* 1987;55:1137–1143.
22. Zeitz M, Quinn TC, Graeff AS, James SP. Mucosal T cells provide helper function but do not proliferate when stimulated by specific antigen in lymphogranuloma venereum proctitis in non-human primates. *Gastroenterology* 1988;94:353–366.
23. Swain SL, Weinberg AD, English M. CD4+ T cell subsets. Lymphokine secretion of memory cells and of effector cells that develop from precursors in vitro. *J Immunol* 1990;144:1788–1799.
24. Swain SL, Weinberg AD, Huston G. IL-4 and IFN-γ direct the development of distinct subsets of helper T cells. *Fed Proc* 1990;4:2020.
25. Weinberg AD, English M, Swain SL. Distinct regulation of lymphokine production is found in fresh versus in vitro primed murine helper T cells. *J Immunol* 1990;144:1800–1807.
26. James SP, Kwan WC, Sneller MC. T cells in inductive and effector compartment of the intestinal mucosal immune system of nonhuman primates differ in lymphokine mRNA expression, lymphokine utilization and regulatory function. *J Immunol* 1990;144:1251–1256.
27. Ullrich R, Schieferdecker HL, Ziegler K, Riecken EO, Zeitz M. Gamma delta T cells in the human intestine express surface markers of activation and are preferentially located in the epithelium. *Cell Immunol* 1990;128:619–627.
28. De Geus B, Van den Enden M, Coolen C, Nagelkerken L, Van der Heijden P, Rozing J. Phenotype of intraepithelial lymphocytes in euthymic and athymic mice: implications for differentiation of cells bearing a CD3− associated gamma delta T cell receptor. *Eur J Immunol* 1990;20:291–298.
29. Mosley RL, Styre D, Klein JR. Differentiation and functional maturation of bone marrow derived intestinal epithelial T cells expressing membrane T cell receptors in athymic radiation chimeras. *J Immunol* 1990;145:1369–75.
30. Croitoru K, Stead RH, Beinenstock J, et al. Presence of intestinal intraepithelial lymphocytes in mice with severe combined immunodeficiency disease. *Eur J Immunol* 1990;20:645–651.
31. Bandeira A, Mota-Santos T, Itohara S, et al. Localization of gamma/delta T cells to the intestinal epithelium is independent of normal microbial colonization. *J Exp Med* 1990;172:239–244.
32. Berke G. The binding and lysis of target cells by cytotoxic lymphocytes: molecular and cellular aspects. *Annu Rev Immunol* 1994;12:735–773.
33. Kägi D, Ledermann B, Bürki K, et al. Cytotoxicity mediated by T cells and natural killer cells is greatly impaired in perforin-deficient mice. Nature 1994;369:31–37.
34. Shanahan F, Deem R, Nayersina R, Leman B, Targan S. Human mucosal T cell cytotoxicity. *Gastroenterology* 1988;94:960–967.
35. Trinchieri G. Biology of natural killer cells. *Adv Immunol* 1989;47:187.
36. Springer TA. Adhesion receptors of the immune system. *Nature* 1990;346:425–434.

37. Balkwill FR, Burke F. The cytokine network. *Immunol Today* 1989;10:299.

38. Arai K, Lee F, Miyajima A, Miyatake S, Arai N, Yokota T. Cytokines: coordinators of immune and inflammatory responses. *Annu Rev Biochem* 1990;59:783.

39. Strober W, James SP. The interleukins. *Pediatr Res* 1988;24:549–557.

40. Durum SK, Schmidt JA, Oppenheim JJ. IL-1: an immunological prospective. *Annu Rev Immunol* 1985;3:263–287.

41. Dinarello CA. Biology of interleukin-1. *FASEB J* 1988;2:108–115.

42. Malkovsky M, Sondel PM. Interleukin 2 and its receptor: structure, function and therapeutic potential. *Blood Rev* 1987;1:1–12.

43. Robb RJ, Green WC, Rusk CM. Low and high affinity cellular receptors for interleukin 2: implications for the level of Tac antigen. *J Exp Med* 1984;160:1126–1146.

44. Waldmann TA. The structure, function and expression of interleukin 2 receptors on normal and malignant lymphocytes. *Science* 1986;232:727–732.

45. Grimm EA, Mazumder A, Zhang HZ, Rosenberg SA. The lymphokine activated killer cell phenomenon: lysis of NK resistant fresh solid tumor cells by IL-2 activated autologous human peripheral blood lymphocytes. *J Exp Med* 1982;155:1823–1841.

46. Nicola NA, Metcalf D. Specificity of action of colony-stimulating factors in the differentiation of granulocytes and macrophages. *Ciba Found Symp* 1986;118:7–28.

47. Sieff C. Hematopoietic growth factors. *J Clin Invest* 1987;79:1579–1557.

48. Paul WE, Ohara J. B cell stimulatory factor-1/interleukin-4. *Annu Rev Immunol* 1987;5:429–459.

49. Rabin EM, Mond JJ, Ohara J, Paul WE. B cell stimulatory factor (BSF)-1 prepares resting B cells to enter S phase in response to anti-IgM and to lipopolysaccharide. *J Exp Med* 1986;164:517–531.

50. Noelle R, Krammer PH, Ohara J, Uhr JW, Vitetta ES. Increased expression of Ia antigens on resting B cells: an additional role for B-cell growth factor. *Proc Natl Acad Sci USA* 1984;81:6149–6153.

51. DeFranco T, Aubry JP, Rousset F, et al. Human recombinant interleukin-4 induces Fcε receptors (CD23) on normal human B lymphocytes. *J Exp Med* 1984;165:11459–1467.

52. Vitetta ES, Ohara J, Myers C, Layton J, Krammer PH, Paul WE. Serological, biochemical, and functional identity of B cell-stimulatory factor 1 and B cell differentiation factor for IgG1. *J Exp Med* 1985;162:1726–1631.

53. Coffman RL, Ohara J, Bond MW, Carty J, Zlotnick E, Paul WE. B cell stimulatory factor-1 enhances the IgE response of lipopolysaccharide-activated B cells. *J Immunol* 1986;136:4538–4541.

54. Finkelman FD, Katona IM, Mosmann TR, Coffman RL. IFN-A regulates the isotypes of Ig secreted during in vivo humoral immune responses. *J Immunol* 1988;140:1022–1027.

55. Takatsu K, Tominaga A, Hamaoka T. Antigen-induced T cell-replacing factor (TRF). I. Functional characterization of a TRF-producing helper T cell subset and genetic studies on TRF production. *J Immunol* 1980;124:2414–2422.

56. Swain SL, Dennert G, Warner JF, Dutton RW. Culture supernatants of a stimulated T-cell line have helper activity that acts synergistically with interleukin-2 in the response of B cells to antigen. *Proc Natl Acad Sci USA* 1981;78:2517–2521.

57. Coffman RL, Shrader B, Carty J, Mosmann TR, Bond MW. A mouse T cell product that preferentially enhances IgA production. I. Biologic characterization. *J Immunol* 1987;139:3685–3690.

58. Sanderson CJ, O'Garra A, Warren DJ, Klaus GGB. Eosinophil differentiation factor also has B cell growth factor activity: proposed name interleukin 4. *Proc Natl Acad Sci USA* 1986;83:437–440.

59. Takatsu K, Kikuchi Y, Takahashi T, et al. Interleukin 5, a T cell-derived B cell differentiation factor also induces cytotoxic T lymphocytes. *Proc Natl Acad Sci USA* 1987;84:4234–4238.

60. Hirano T, Yasukawa K, Harada H, et al. Complementary DNA for a novel human interleukin (BSF-2) that induces B lymphocytes to produce immunoglobulin. *Nature* 1986;324:73–76.

61. Sehgal PB, May LT. Human β2-interferon. *J Interferon Res* 1987;7:521–527.

62. Gauldie J, Richards C, Harnish D, Lansdorp P, Baumann H. Interferon β2/B cell stimulatory factor type 2 shares identity with monocyte-derived hepatocyte stimulating factor and regulates the major acute phase protein response in liver cells. *Proc Natl Acad Sci USA* 1987;84:7251–7255.

63. Carswell EA, Old LJ, Kassel RL, Green S, Fiore N, Williamson B. An endotoxin-induced serum factor that causes necrosis of tumors. *Proc Natl Acad Sci USA* 1985;72:3666–3670.

64. Gray PW, Aggarwal BB, Benton CV, et al. Cloning and expression of cDNA for human lymphotoxin, a lymphokine with tumor necrosis activity. *Nature* 1984;312:721–724.

65. Dayer J-M, Beutler B, Cerami A. Cachectin/tumor necrosis factor stimulates collagenase and PGE2 production by human synovial cells and dermal fibroblasts. *J Exp Med* 1985;162:2163–2168.

66. Kehrl JH, Alvarez-Mon M, Delsing GA, Fauci AS. Lymphotoxin is an important T cell-derived growth factor for human B cells. *Science* 1987;238:1144–1146.

67. Oppenheim JJ, Zachariae CO, Mukaida N, Matsushima K. Properties of the novel proinflammatory supergene "intercrine" cytokine family. *Annu Rev Immunol* 1991;9:617–648.

68. Howard M, O'Garra A. Biological properties of interleukin-10. *Immunol Today* 1992;13:198.

69. Scott P. IL-12: initiation cytokine for cell-mediated immunity. *Science* 1993;260:496–497.

70. Pestka S, Langer JA, Zoon KC, Samuel CE. Interferons and their actions. *Annu Rev Biochem* 1987;56:727.

71. Massagué J. The transforming growth factor β family. *Annu Rev Cell Biol* 1990;6:597.

72. Chrétian I, Pène J, Brière F, De Waal Malefijt R, Rousset F, De Vries JE. Regulation of human IgE synthesis. I. Human IgE synthesis in vitro is determined by the reciprocal antagonistic effects of interleukin 4 and interferon-γ. *Eur J Immunol* 1990;20:243–251.

73. Cherwinski HM, Schumacher JH, Brown DK, Mosmann TR. Two types of mouse helper T cell revealed by RNA hybridization, functionally monospecific bioassays, and monoclonal antibodies. *J Exp Med* 1987;166:1229–1244.

74. Mosmann TR, Cherwinski H, Bond MW, Giedlin MA, Coffman RL. Two types of murine helper T cell clones. I. Definition according to profiles of lymphokine activities and secreted proteins. *J Immunol* 1987;136:2348–2357.

75. Street NE, TR Mosmann. Functional diversity of T lymphocytes due to secretion of different cytokine patterns. *FASEB J* 1991;5:171.

76. Scott P, Pearce E, Cheever AW, Coffman RL, Sher A. Role of cytokines and CD4 + T-cell subsets in the regulation of parasite immunity and disease. *Immunol Rev* 1989;112:161–182.

77. Pond L, Wassom DL, Hayes CE. Evidence for differential induction of helper T cell subsets during *Trichinella spiralis* infection. *J Immunol* 1989;143:4232–4237.

78. Rennick DM, Thompson-Snipes L, Coffman RL, Seymour BW, Jackson JD, Hudak S. In vivo administration of antibody to interleukin-5 inhibits increased generation of eosinophils and their progenitors in bone marrow of parasitized mice. *Blood* 1990;76:312–316.

79. Chihara J, Plumas J, Gruart V, et al. Characterization of a receptor for interleukin 5 on human eosinophils: variable expression and induction by granulocyte/macrophage colony-stimulating factor. *J Exp Med* 1990;172:1347–1351.

80. Sher A, Coffman RL, Hieny S, Scott P, Cheever AW. Interleukin 5 is required for the blood and tissue eosinophilia but not granuloma formation induced by infection with *Schistosoma mansoni*. *Proc Natl Acad Sci USA* 1990;87:61–65.

81. Seder RA, Paul WE. Acquisition of lymphokine-producing phenotype by CD4 + T cells. *Annu Rev Immunol* 1994;12:635–673.

82. Taguchi T, McGhee JR, Coffman RL, et al. Detection of individual mouse splenic T cells producing IFN-gamma and IL-5 using the enzyme-linked immunospot (ELISPOT) assay. *J Immunol Meth* 1990;128:65–73.

83. Taguchi T, McGhee JR, Coffman RL, et al. Analysis of Th1 and TH2 cells in murine gut-associated tissues. Frequencies of CD4+ and CD8+ T cells that secrete IFN-gamma and IL-5. *J Immunol* 1990;145:68–77.

84. Scott P, Pearce E, Cheever AW, Coffman RL, Sher A. Role of cytokines and CD4+ T cell subsets in the regulation of parasite immunity and disease. *Immunol Rev* 1989;112:161–182.

85. Romagnani S. Lymphokine production by human T cells in disease states. *Annu Rev Immunol* 1994;12:227–257.

86. Yamamura M, Uyemura K, Deans RJ, et al. Defining protective responses to pathogens: cytokine profiles in leprosy lesions. *Science* 1991;254:277–279.

87. Kaplan G, Britton WJ, Hancock GE, et al. The systemic influence of recombinant interleukin 2 on the mainfestion of lepromatous leprosy. *J Exp Med* 1991;173:993–1006.

88. Yssel H, Shanafelt MC, Soderberg C, Schneider PV, Anzola J, Peltz G. *Borrelia burgdorferi* activates a T helper type 1 like T cell subset in Lyme arthritis. *J Exp Med* 1991;174:593–601.

89. Schlaak J, Hermann E, Ringhoffer M, et al. Predominance of Th1-type T cells in synovial fluid of patients with *Yersinia* induced reactive arthritis. *Eur J Immunol* 1992;22:2771–2776.

90. Fong TAT, Mosmann TR. Alloreactive murine CD8+ T cell clones secrete the Th1 pattern of cytokines. *J Immunol* 1990;144:1744–52.

91. Andersson J, Andersson U. Characterization of cytokine production in infectious mononucleosis studied at a single-cell level in tonsil and peripheral blood. *Clin Exp Immunol* 1993;9:7–13.

92. Yasukawa M, Inatsuki A, Horiuchi T, Kobayashi Y. Functional heterogeneity among herpes simplex virus specific human CD4+ T cells. *J Immunol* 1991;146:1341–1347.

93. Ferrari C, Mondelli MU, Penna A, Fiaccadori F, Chisari FV. Functional characterization of cloned intrahepatic, hepatitis B virus nucleoprotein specific helper T cell lines. *J Immunol* 1987;139:539–544.

94. Mahanty S, Abrams JS, King CL, Limaye AP, Nutman TB. Parallel regulation of IL-4 and IL-5 in human helminth infections. *J Immunol* 1992;148:3567–3571.

95. Limaye AP, Abrams JS, Silver JE, Ottesen EA, Nutman TB. Regulation of parasite induced eosinophilia: selectively increased interleukin 5 production in helminth infected patients. *J Exp Med* 1990;172:399–402.

96. De Carli M, Romagnani S, Del Prete GF. Human T cell response to excretory secretory antigens of *Toxocara canis*. A model of preferential in vitro and in vivo activation of Th2 cells. In: Lewis JW, Maizels AM, eds. *Toxocara and toxocariasis: clinical, epidemiological, and molecular perspectives.* Birmingham: Birbeck; 141–148.

97. Hammer RE, Maika SD, Richardson JA, Tang J-P, Taurog JD. Spontaneous inflammatory disease in transgenic rats expressing HLA-B27 and human β2 m: an animal model of HLA-B27 associated human disorders. *Cell* 1990;63:1099.

98. Breban M, Hammer RE, Richardson JA, Taurog JD. Transfer of the inflammatory disease of HLA-B27 transgenic rats by bone marrow engraftment. *J Exp Med* 1993;178:1607–1616.

99. Pfeffer K, Mak TW. Lymphocyte ontogeny and activation in gene targeted mutant mice. *Annu Rev Immunol* 1994;12:367–411.

100. Mombaerts P, Mizoguchi E, Grusby MJ, Glimcher LH, Bhan AK, Tonegawa S. Spontaneous development of inflammatory bowel disease in T cell receptor mutant mice. *Cell* 1993;75:275–282.

101. Sadlack B, Merz H, Schorle H, Schimpl A, Feller AC, Horak I. Ulcerative colitis like disease in mice with a disrupted interleukin 2 gene. *Cell* 1993;75:253–261.

102. Kühn R, Löhler J, Rennick D, Rajewsky K, Müller W. Interleukin 10 deficient mice develop chronic enterocolitis. *Cell* 1993;75:263–274.

103. Shull MM, Ormsby I, Kier AB, et al. Targeted disruption of the mouse transforming growth factor beta 1 gene results in multifocal inflammatory disease. *Nature* 1992;359:693–699.

Infections of the Gastrointestinal Tract,
edited by M. J. Blaser, P. D. Smith, J. I. Ravdin,
H. B. Greenberg, and R. L. Guerrant
Raven Press, Ltd., New York © 1995.

CHAPTER 16

The Immunophysiology of Mast Cells in Intestinal Immunity and Symbiosis

A. Dean Befus

Fully differentiated mast cells are heavily granulated leukocytes that are widely distributed throughout the body (1). In association with acute allergic reactions, chronic inflammation, fibrosis, tissue repair, and host defenses, there are increases in mast cell numbers or in their activation. Mast cells are one of the few cell types that express high-affinity receptors for immunoglobulin E (IgE) antibodies (2). Sensitizing allergens interact with IgE molecules on these mast cell surface receptors and stimulate the release of several preformed and newly synthesized inflammatory mediators. In turn, a cascade of inflammatory events is generated, some of which are of short duration while others occur over longer periods of time (3). Although mast cells are best known for their role in IgE-mediated allergic reactions, they can be activated in several other ways and are involved in responses other than those with a known IgE association (4–6). Unfortunately, the biologic relevance of many of these activation pathways is largely unknown and much remains to be learned about the function of mast cells.

Despite the wide distribution of mast cells, only two phenotypes of mast cell are well known—one population scattered throughout tissues and known as the connective tissue mast cell (CTMC), and the other found at mucosal sites and known as the mucosal mast cell (MMC) (7–9). The most extensively studied MMCs are from the intestine (IMMCs). The lineage relationships of these two mast cell populations have been subject to much speculation and, at the present time, it is accepted that they are capable of phenotypic interchange under microenvironmental controls (10).

In this chapter, the characteristics of mast cells are reviewed and their functions are described. In the gastrointestinal tract, explosive anaphylactic degranulation of mast cells is central to the pathogenesis of allergic reactions and presumably to defenses against helminthic infec-

tions (9). However, there is also evidence that mast cells are involved in the maintenance of intestinal integrity and in adaptation to insult, albeit in a less dramatic fashion than anaphylactic degranulation (11). Physiologic levels of mediator release from IMMCs are likely to act on several targets in the intestinal microenvironment, including epithelial, endothelial, and mesenchymal cells, smooth muscle, and the immune and nervous systems.

There is a plethora of reviews on mast cells, their heterogeneity, and their roles in pathogenesis and host defenses in gastrointestinal helminthic infections (9–12). However, there are few reviews on the roles of mast cells in tissue repair (13,14) and immunophysiology (15–17). This chapter provides a brief review of mast cell ontogeny, heterogeneity, mediators, and activation; it then describes the regulation and functions of mast cells in the gastrointestinal microenvironment. This presents a broader overview of mast cell function than is generally presented and it is hoped that readers will be stimulated to integrate the potential functions of this cell more completely into models of gastrointestinal function, adaptation to injury, and normal homeostasis.

MAST CELL ONTOGENY

In our efforts to understand the development of mast cells and the factors that control their numbers, there have been descriptive studies of their pre- and postnatal development, their hyperplasia in response to stimuli, and their *in vitro* culture. Normally, mast cells begin to appear in most tissues before birth (18) and their numbers increase after birth to levels commonly found in adult tissues (18,19). Several stimuli influence the numbers of mast cells in tissues, including helminthic infections (20–22), acute or chronic inflammation (23), tumors (24), fibrosis and scarring (25,26), and tissue repair (13,14,27). Several growth and differentiation factors have been identified for mast cells, including the interleukins (ILs) IL-3, IL-4, IL-

A. D. Befus: Department of Medicine, University of Alberta, Edmonton, Alberta T6G 2S2, Canada.

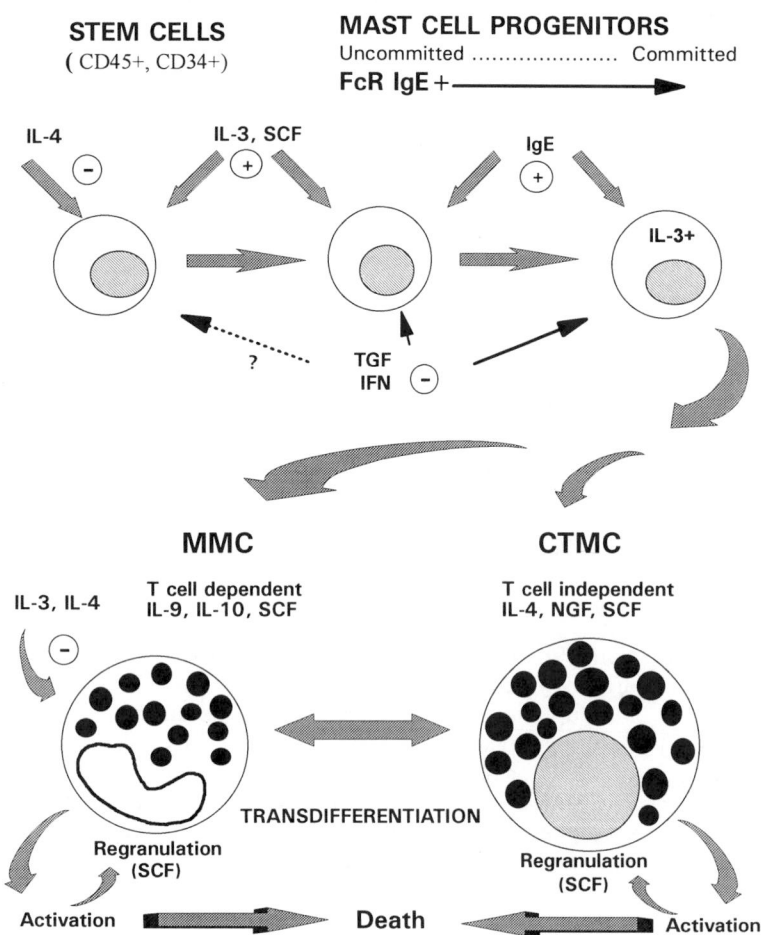

STEM CELLS
(CD45+, CD34+)

MAST CELL PROGENITORS
Uncommitted .... Committed
FcR IgE +————————————————▶

IL-4 (−)   IL-3, SCF (+)   IgE (+)   IL-3+

? ◀┈┈┈   TGF IFN (−)

MMC   CTMC

IL-3, IL-4 (−)   T cell dependent IL-9, IL-10, SCF   T cell independent IL-4, NGF, SCF

TRANSDIFFERENTIATION

Regranulation (SCF)   Regranulation (SCF)

Activation   Death   Activation

FIG. 1. The ontogeny of mast cells, factors that regulate their growth, differentiation, and survival. CTMC, connective tissue mast cell; FcR, Fc receptor; IFN, interferon; IL, interleukin; MMC, mucosal mast cell; NGF, nerve growth factor; SCF, stem cell factor; TGF, transforming growth factor.

9, and IL-10 and stem cell factor. Two strains of mice genetically deficient in mast cells, namely, W/Wᵛ and S1/S1ᵈ, have been powerful tools in clarifying many of these issues of mast cell ontogeny. The former are deficient in mast cell committed progenitors because of a deficiency in the stem cell factor receptor (c-kit), a tyrosine kinase based receptor, whereas S1/S1ᵈ mice are deficient in the production of stem cell factor (also called c-kit ligand or Steel factor) (10,28). Mast cells originate from pluripotent hematopoietic precursors that express CD34 (29) and CD45 (30) (Fig. 1). These precursors can be stimulated by stem cell factor and IL-3 and give rise to progenitors committed to mast cell development (31). Mast cell progenitors are responsive to IgE containing immune complexes (31) and ultimately become independent of exogenous IL-3 for their development, presumably because they begin to produce IL-3 themselves. Stem cell factor can be supplied by fibroblasts or fibroblast-derived conditioned medium (28). The progenitors become committed to the mast cell lineage and ultimately differentiate into mast cells with either the CTMC or MMC phenotype.

The development of mast cells from committed progenitors involves several factors that are incompletely understood at present, including IL-3, CD45, IgE immune complexes, IL-4, IL-9, IL-10, and stem cell factor (28,30–34). IL-4 and nerve growth factor facilitate development of mast cells with a CTMC-like phenotype (32,35), whereas

IL-10 induces the expression of some of the phenotypic characteristics of MMC, namely, MMC-specific proteinase expression (36). Several cytokines and growth factors may downregulate these pathways, including granulocyte–macrophage colony-stimulating factor (GM-CSF) (37), interferon-γ (IFN-γ) (38), transforming factor-β (TGF-β) (39), and histamine (40). Interestingly, IL-3 inhibits expression of MMC-specific proteinases (36). Work by Kitamura (10) has established that the commitment to a CTMC or IMMC phenotype is not irreversible, but that clonal populations of mast cells of one phenotype can change into mast cells of the other phenotype if subjected to the microenvironment normally associated with the other mast cell type. This process has been called transdifferentiation, but the extent to which it occurs *in vivo* remains to be determined.

It has been estimated that the half-life of a CTMC is approximately 180 days, whereas that of an IMMC is about 40 days (41). Unfortunately, the factors that influence mast cell survival in tissues have received little study. Recent emphasis on the role of programmed cell death (apoptosis) in the life history of many cell types, including inflammatory cells in tissue reactions (42), has lead to the discovery that stem cell factor can rescue mast cells from apoptosis induced by the withdrawal of IL-3 from IL-3-dependent cultures (43). This observation may be highly relevant *in vivo*, where there has been an increasing emphasis on connective tissue elements such as fibroblasts and processes of cell adhesion in the maintenance of normal homeostasis or in the pathogenesis of chronic inflammation. Apoptosis of mast cells may be the process that explains observations of glucocorticoid-induced disappearance of IMMCs (44) involving their phagocytosis by macrophages (45). Increased knowledge about mast cell survivorship in inflamed tissues may uncover novel therapeutic targets.

MAST CELL CHARACTERISTICS AND HETEROGENEITY

To study the characteristics and functions of mast cells, several mast cell lines have been developed from naturally occurring transformed cells or following transformation *in vitro* or *in vivo* using viral or chemical agents (46,47). Although cultures of *in vivo* derived mast cells or mast cell lines or clones have provided useful tools for study, it is widely recognized that they express only some of the characteristics of freshly isolated or *in situ* mast cells. Great care must be used in generalizations from studies of cultured mast cells. Thus mast cells have also been

studied shortly after their isolation by lavage from the peritoneal or pleural cavities, or following their isolation from solid tissues such as the gastrointestinal mucosa using enzymatic dispersion techniques (48–51).

With a focus on the role of CTMCs and IMMCs in IgE-mediated immediate hypersensitivity reactions, researchers have investigated the nature and extent of mast cell heterogeneity, including mediator content and biosynthetic potential, pathways of activation and downregulation, and function (Figs. 2 and 3). The repertoire of mast cell mediators and the diversity of pathways of activation or regulation suggest that mast cells have considerable potential for a broad involvement in acute and chronic inflammation, host defenses, and pathogenesis. Indeed, recent emphasis on their ability to produce a plethora of cytokines has led to the hypothesis that they may play a central role in decision making about the types of immune responses generated after initial exposure to an antigen or infectious agent (52). Two types of T helper cells have been identified, Th1 and Th2 cells (53). Th1 cells produce IL-2 and IFN-γ and induce many of the components of cellular immunity, whereas Th2 cells produce IL-4 and IL-5 and stimulate antibody responses, particularly IgE, and eosinophilia and mast cell hyperplasia. Romagnani

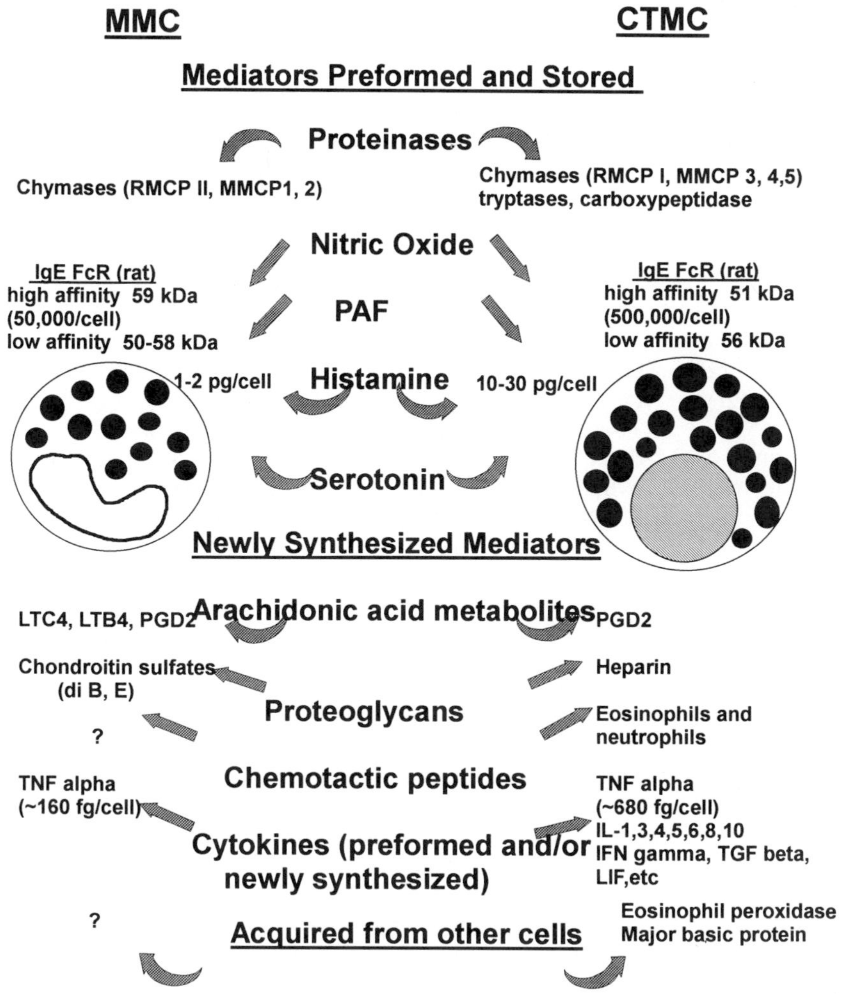

FIG. 2. Heterogeneity and mediators of mast cell populations. CTMC, connective tissue mast cell; IFN, interferon; FcR, Fc receptor; IL, interleukin; LIF, leukemia inhibitory factor; LT, leukotriene; MMC, mucosal mast cell; MMCP, mouse mast cell protease; PAF, platelet activating factor; PG, prostaglandin; RMCP, rat mast cell protease; TNF alpha, tumor necrosis factor alpha.

Activation

MMC   CTMC

Histamine releasing factors?

Cytokine priming   **Microbial factors**
IL-1, 4, 10, SCF

Cationic Moieties
48/80, neuropeptides (eg., substance P),
endorphins, defensins, peptide 401,
polylysine, polymyxin, mastoparan, C3a, et

substance P

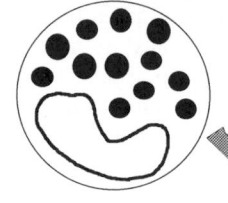

Antigen specific
IgE, IgG
T cell factors

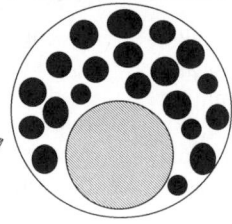

Inhibition

IFN alpha/beta, IFN gamma   IFN alpha/beta, IFN gamma
(TNF but not histamine)   (histamine and TNF)
PGE2   TGF beta, IL-1, PGE2,
                 Cytokines   lactoferrin, transferrin

Drugs

cromolyn and nedocromil   cromolyn and nedocromil
(TNF but not histamine)   (histamine and TNF),
sulfasalazine, steroids (apoptosis?)   cyclosporin A, FK506, sulfasalazine
                                   phosphodiesterase inhibitors,
                                   beta agonists, steroids (?)

?   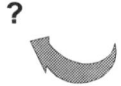   **Microbial Factors**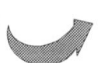

FIG. 3. The activation of mast cells and their regulation. CTMC, connective tissue mast cell; IFN, interferon; IL, interleukin; PG, prostaglandin; SCF, stem cell factor; TGF beta, transforming growth factor beta; TNF, tumor necrosis factor.

(52) postulated that IL-4 production by mast cells and basophils might be responsible for the IL-4-dependent amplification of Th2 cells and for their development during primary immune responses. It may be that CTMCs and IMMCs differ in this type of orchestration of immune responses in their local environments as a result of distinctive responsiveness to secretagogues or in their repertoire of stored and newly synthesized mediators.

Mast Cell Mediators

Mast cells produce a cornucopia of mediators, including histamine, serotonin, peptide chemotactic factors for neutrophils and eosinophils, prostaglandin D_2 (PGD_2) leukotrienes B_4, C_4, D_4, and E_4, heparin and chondroitin sulfate proteoglycans, proteinases and lysosomal enzymes, platelet activating factor (PAF), nitric oxide (NO), and several cytokines (Fig. 2). Given limitations of space, the reader is directed to current reviews for an extensive coverage of the field (7–9,54,55). Recently, studies of proteases, NO, and cytokines have dominated investigations of mast cell mediators and have raised fundamental ques-

tions about the role of mast cells in host defenses, pathogenesis, tissue integrity, and immunophysiology. NO and cytokines are not exclusively produced by mast cells. Therefore, when is the mast cell an important source of these mediators? Each of these mediators appears to be cytokine regulated and this regulation may be central to the control of mast cell phenotype and their role in the response of tissues to injury or antigen challenge.

Proteinases

Proteinases are surprisingly abundant in mast cells, perhaps representing more than 50% of total protein in some populations. Unfortunately, little is known about the functions of these proteinases. In the mouse, seven serine proteinases have been identified, five with chymase-like specificities [mouse mast cell protease (mMCP-1 to 5)] and two with tryptase-like specificities (mMCP-6,7) (56–58), all localized to mouse chromosome 14 with T cell granzymes (58). In addition, a metalloproteinase, MC carboxypeptidase A, has also been identified (59,60). MCP-1 and MCP-2 are preferentially expressed in mouse

IMMCs, whereas MCP-4,5,6 and MC carboxypeptidase A are preferentially expressed in CTMCs. mMCP-5,6 and mMC carboxypeptidase A are abundant in IL-3-cultured bone marrow-derived mast cells, whereas IL-9 and IL-10 induce messenger ribonucleic acid (mRNA) for mMCP-1 and mMCP-2, both of which are depressed by IL-3 and IL-4 (61). mMCP-4 is induced by stem cell factor (62).

In the rat, two chymases have been characterized, namely, RMCP-1 and RMCP-2. RMCP-1 is probably homologous to mMCP-4 and RMCP-2 is probably homologous to mMCP-1. RMCP-1 is expressed exclusively in CTMCs, whereas RMCP-2 is expressed solely in MMCs. RMCP-1 is insoluble and following mast cell activation it remains closely associated with the mast cell granules. By contrast, RMCP-2 is soluble and can be detected in the circulation following activation of IMMC (9,63). Rat peritoneal MC (PMCs) express three forms of MCP-5 and three forms of MC carboxypeptidase A. Rat PMCs also express tryptase, presumably equivalent to either mMCP-6 or mMCP-7, although it is of low abundance compared to tryptase in mouse or human mast cells (64).

Human mast cells also express chymase, tryptase, and MC carboxypeptidase A. A single chymase has been identified in human mast cells perhaps a homologue of m/RMCP-5 (65). Thus mast cell populations in several species exhibit differential expression of serine and metalloproteinases. Rat MCP-2 has been crystallized and its structure determined (66) and three-dimensional models of rat MCP-1, rat MC carboxypeptidase A, MC tryptase, and mMCP-1,2,4,5 have been prepared (67). Unfortunately, the substrate specificities and functions of these mast cell proteinases are incompletely known. Evidence suggests that they are involved in fibroblast activation (68), smooth muscle contraction (69), submucosal gland secretion (70), degradation of neuropeptides (71,72) and anaphylatoxins (73), protein processing (74,75), matrix degradation (76,77), and osteoblast attachment and spreading (77).

Nitric Oxide

NO, also known as endothelial-derived relaxing factor, stimulates relaxation of vascular smooth muscle and inhibits platelet aggregation and neutrophil activation (78). NO is produced by rat CTMCs and IMMCs and by many other cell types (79,80). It appears to have differential effects on mast cell mediators because it enhances mast cell-derived tumor necrosis factor-α (TNF-α) activity (80) but diminishes histamine and superoxide release (81). Recently, we established that inhibition of NO synthesis *in vivo* enhances mast cell-dependent intestinal permeability (11) and that IL-1β enhances the production of NO by mast cells and inhibits the production of PAF (82). Given the diversity of effects of NO, it is important to determine when mast cell-derived NO is the relevant source in the gastrointestinal tract or elsewhere and what its primary functions are.

Cytokines

Mast cells can produce several cytokines and, although the field is in its infancy, there is no evidence that there are major differences between mast cell populations in their ability to produce or secrete cytokines (83–88). In normal or inflamed tissues from humans or rodents, they may be a major source of IL-4, IL-5, IL-6, IL-8, and TNF-α (83–86). Several other cytokines have been identified in mast cells either as mRNA or as biologically active protein, including IFN-γ, IL-1, IL-3, GM-CSF, JE, MIP-1α, MIP-1β, TCA-3, and TGF-β (87,88). Some cytokines appear to be constitutively produced by some mast cell populations (e.g., TNF-α, TGF-β, and IL-4), whereas others can be induced by exposure of the mast cells to sensitizing antigens (83,85) or perhaps to other factors.

The immunosuppressive agent cyclosporin A (87), the anti-inflammatory drug sulfasalazine (89), and the anti-allergic agents nedocromil sodium and disodium cromoglycate (89) can depress the expression of some cytokines in mast cells. To determine the role played by mast cells in the cascades of cytokine production and networking, it will be essential to define the spectrum of cytokines produced by mast cells under different conditions and whether the patterns of expression are consistent with Th1/Th2 concepts. The nature of mast cell regulation in the gastrointestinal tract or elsewhere in response to infection or other stimuli needs further investigation.

Activation of Mast Cells

Although mast cell activation by allergens and IgE antibodies is well known, they can be activated in other ways, including by incompletely characterized antigen-specific T cell factors, cationic moieties, and several histamine-releasing factors (4,5,7). Many cationic moieties that activate histamine secretion from rat PMCs do not activate IMMCs. These cationic secretagogues appear to act by electrostatic and hydrophobic interactions with the cell membrane and then with the anionic C terminus of the G-protein α subunit (90), rather than by a classic surface receptor–ligand interaction. Many of these cationic moieties induce histamine secretion only at micromolar to millimolar concentrations and thus their *in vivo* role has been questioned.

Among the cationic moieties that activate rat CTMCs are the neuropeptides substance P, somatostatin, neurotensin, vasoactive intestinal polypeptide, and endorphins (5). Of these, only substance P induces histamine release from IMMCs. The *in vivo* role of mast cell activation by neuropeptides is poorly understood and is again questioned because of the high levels (micromolar to millimolar) needed to induce histamine secretion. However, data on the anatomic juxtaposition of mast cells and enteric nerves (91), on Pavlovian conditioning of release of rat mast cell proteinase II from IMMCs (92), and on the pathophysiology of intestinal epithelial transport (15,17, 93–95) and smooth muscle contraction (96,97) in acute allergic reactions provide strong evidence of mast cell–nervous system bidirectional communication (5).

Unfortunately, the nature and significance of this interaction is incompletely understood.

Several inflammatory cells produce histamine-releasing factors that activate basophils and/or mast cells (98), such as activated mononuclear cells producing histamine-releasing factors of 8 to 10, 15 to 17, and 35 to 41 kDa. The 8- to 10-kDa form has been identified as connective tissue-activating peptide and its cleavage product, neutrophil activating peptide. Neutrophil-derived histamine-releasing factor is different from these, because it is constitutively produced, heat stable, and less than 5 kDa. Given the role of cationic moieties in mast cell activation and the presence of highly cationic, cysteine-rich peptides in neutrophils, called defensins or corticostatins (99), it was postulated that defensins might be responsible for the neutrophil histamine-releasing factor activity. Indeed, defensins are potent histamine secretagogues from rat PMCs (100), but not from IMMCs (D. Befus, *unpublished data*). Whether they act like other cationic moieties or through classic ligand–receptor interactions remains to be determined. Five novel defensins, called cryptdins, have been identified from intestinal Paneth cells (101). Perhaps these intestinally derived cryptdins activate IMMCs, whereas neutrophil-derived defensins do not, thus providing a pathway for specific activation of IMMCs.

Other factors induce histamine secretion from CTMCs, but many have not been tested against IMMCs, or for their ability to induce secretion of other mediators. Stem cell factor is a potent secretagogue (102), a mast cell growth factor (103), and activates several early response genes in mast cells (104). Other cytokines have also been implicated in mast cell activation, although many of them have only been tested in basophils (98). Thus mast cells can be activated or primed by several stimuli, but only IgE-mediated ones have been well studied. The *in vivo* relevance of other pathways of mast cell activation and their actions on subpopulations of mast cells are unknown.

Regulation of Mast Cell Activation and Function

Anti-allergic and Anti-inflammatory Drugs

Many drugs that are widely used to treat allergic and other inflammatory conditions of the gastrointestinal tract or other tissues inhibit mast cell activation (105). Unfortunately, the mechanisms of drug action *in vivo* are unknown and no drug is specific for mast cells. Drugs may inhibit secretion of one mediator but are ineffective against others. Alternatively, some drugs inhibit mediator secretion from both IMMCs and CTMCs, whereas others, such as nedocromil sodium and disodium cromoglycate, inhibit histamine secretion from CTMCs, but not IMMCs. Interestingly, both drugs inhibit TNF-α activity of both PMCs and IMMCs (89), demonstrating that their actions are specific to certain mediators, as well as to mast cell populations.

Cytokines

There has been little emphasis on factors that regulate mast cell secretion *in vivo*. Corticosteroids inhibit development and activation of some mast cell populations (106) and induce macrophage engulfment of IMMCs (45), perhaps by a process involving apoptosis (43). Interestingly, IL-1β has differential effects on mast cell mediator secretion, potentiating the release of histamine, leukotriene C$_4$ (LTC$_4$), PGD$_2$, and NO but inhibiting PAF release (82). Recently, IL-4 has been shown to potentiate secretion of serotonin by murine mast cells (107) and to downregulate mRNA and immunoreactive protein for IL-1β (108). Pretreatment of rat CTMCs with TGF-β downregulates histamine and TNF-α secretion (85). Other endogenous factors that inhibit mast cell activation, such as lactoferrin, transferrin, and TGF-β, have been less well studied (105).

As a confirmation and extension of the Th1/Th2 model of regulation of immune and inflammatory responses (53), we have established that the Th1-associated cytokines IFN-α/β and IFN-γ inhibit synthesis and secretion of TNF-α from both CTMCs and IMMCs (109). However, IFN-α/β and IFN-γ inhibited histamine secretion from CTMCs but not from IMMCs (110). Thus IFNs have actions similar to some anti-allergic drugs; they are mast cell and mediator specific. Perhaps there are commonalities in the mechanisms of their actions.

MAST CELL FUNCTIONS

Defense Against Infections

It is well known that in response to many intestinal helminthic infections there is a marked hyperplasia of IMMCs (7,9,20) and synthesis of IgE antibodies. Similar mast cell hyperplasia is not found in bacterial, viral, and protozoan infections, although there is some evidence that bacterial products can modulate mast cell activity (111,112). For several years researchers have attempted to understand the significance of intestinal mastocytosis in helminthic infections, but the precise roles of this response remain unclear. Miller (9) and Rothwell (12) have extensively reviewed this field. Four major lines of investigation have been used (9), including:

1. Correlation of mast cell numbers and time course of parasite expulsion.
2. Analysis of parasite expulsion in mice genetically deficient in mast cells and their mast cell competent littermates.
3. Release of mast cell mediators in association with parasite expulsion and the role of exogenous mediators in induction of worm loss.
4. Effects of antagonists of mast cell activation or mediators on parasite expulsion.

Unfortunately, these approaches have not provided unequivocal evidence about the role of mast cells in defense against helminthic parasites. In some experimental systems there is good correlation between the time course of mast cell hyperplasia and parasite expulsion, whereas in other systems the correlation is poor (9,12). In several models mast cell activation and mediator secretion correlate with worm expulsion. Furthermore, the passive transfer of IgE antibodies can generate protective immunity in the intestinal milieu (113), perhaps as a result of mast cell activation, although other cell types bearing low-affinity receptors for IgE may also be involved.

Among the numerous studies of mast cell-deficient mice, there are data that suggest worm expulsion is either normal or delayed (9,12). In most cases the rejection of worms is delayed, rather than ablated. It has been proposed that in the absence of mast cells, other components of host defenses mediate worm expulsion. Studies of mast cell blocking agents or mediator antagonists have provided strong support for the role of monoamines (12) and arachidonic acid metabolites in some infections (114,115). From this spectrum of information Miller (9) concluded that "if mast cells serve a vital function it is probably not during primary nematode infection, since most data suggest that absence of enteric mast cells is associated with delayed rather than interrupted worm expulsion." Following challenge infections in sensitized hosts, mast cell activation occurs, but, as in primary infections, mast cells are not quintessential to worm expulsion. Given the experimental tools presently available the plethora and putative redundancy of defense mechanisms in the host prevent an unequivocal statement about intestinal mast cell function.

Mast Cells and the Immunophysiology of the Gastrointestinal Tract

Given the difficulties in identifying the broad functions of mast cells in host defense, it is not surprising that many investigators have taken reductionist approach to define the roles of mast cells in the physiology of the gastrointestinal tract. There is an abundance of studies on the actions of single mast cell mediators in the gut. For example, histamine, serotonin, and prostaglandins have several actions on the intestinal epithelium (15,17,93). Castro, Powell, Perdue, Gall, their colleagues, and many others have contributed to a large literature on the actions of antigen-induced secretion of inflammatory mediators on epithelial functions, particularly Cl secretion. Interestingly, inhibition of NO synthesis led to enhanced permeability of the intestinal epithelium, which appeared to be mast cell dependent. Other cells and tissues in the gastrointestinal tract, including smooth muscle, and the enteric nervous system have also been targets of similar investigations of the actions of mast cell mediators. For example, histamine has a complex series of actions in the regulation of enteric nervous function, at least in guinea pigs (16,116).

The actions of histamine are diverse and recent observations by Fujimoto and colleagues (117) have opened novel areas for investigation of intestinal mast cell functions. Interestingly, in a model of intestinal injury using ischemia-reperfusion, histamine and the enzyme responsible for its synthesis, histidine decarboxylase, increased in the jejunal mucosa following injury. Inhibition of these

increases with the suicide inhibitor of histidine decarboxylase, α-fluoromethylhistidine, was associated with a prolonged functional impairment in the intestine. Thus one function of mast cell activation in the intestine may be in restoration of normal function following injury.

Although mast cells produce several mediators that are pro-inflammatory and damage tissues, several of these mediators also appear to be involved in tissue repair and remodeling. Some of the mast cell proteinases can degrade components of the connective tissue matrix, while others activate some of the metalloproteinases involved in connective tissue turnover (76,77). Moreover, mast cell proteinases appear to be a component of the bidirectional communication between the cell and the nervous system, because many of the proteinases degrade neurotransmitters such as substance P and vasoactive intestinal polypeptide (71,72).

In summary, mast cell products play several roles in the induction and regulation of the functions of the epithelium, vasculature, smooth muscle, and nervous system in the gastrointestinal tract. Presumably, these mast cell functions are exaggerated during acute allergic reactions, such as those occurring in response to intestinal helminthic infections, but are ongoing at physiologic levels during normal gastrointestinal function, perhaps by mechanisms of mast cell activation that do not involve IgE antibodies.

A VIEW TO THE FUTURE

Although the questions posed by the study of mast cells in the gastrointestinal tract are challenging and many of them have frustrated investigators for years, we are in exciting times as new experimental tools are becoming widely available, which will help identify the roles of mast cells in normal gastrointestinal physiology and in the responses to infections. It will be critical to fully map the spectrum of cytokines produced by intestinal mast cells under different conditions of Th2- or Th1-dominated immune and inflammatory responses. Presumably, the microenvironment will dictate the selective expression of cytokines by mast cells. Similar questions apply to the mast cell as a source of NO. What are the pathways that induce and regulate the production of NO by mast cells and when is mast cell-derived NO important in the gastrointestinal tract, as opposed to NO derived from other cells? There is also much to be learned about mast cell proteinases, their regulation, substrates, and overall functions, alone and in concert with one another. These difficult questions will be addressed when specific inhibitors of the activation of mast cell subsets are developed, or when inhibitors of mast cell mediators, such as the proteinases, are available. It will also be essential to develop cellular and whole animal models in which mast cell numbers or functions can be manipulated by enhancing or ablating gene expression (transfections or knockouts). Knockouts will be particularly valuable when designed so that the animals are not totally deficient of mast cells, but selected for absence of expression of a specific gene critical to a specified mast cell function.

An important area for investigation is the microenvironmental control of intestinal mast cell function. What are the modes of activation and inhibition most relevant in the intestine, and are these unique to this microenvironment and to IMMCs? With such information, it will be possible to generate an integrative model of mast cell function in normal gastrointestinal physiology and in the pathophysiology of host responses to infection and injury. Such a model will be a critical tool in the rational design of therapeutic and preventative interventions.

REFERENCES

1. Selye H. *The mast cells*. Washington, DC: Butterworths, 1965.
2. Beaven MA, Metzger H. Signal transduction by Fc receptors: the fcεRI case. *Immunol Today* 1993;14:222–226.
3. Holgate ST. The mast cell and its function in allergic disease. *Clin Exp Allergy* 1991;3:11–16.
4. Befus D. Reciprocal interactions between mast cells and the endocrine system. In: Freier S, ed. *The neuroendocrine–immune network*. Boca Raton, FL: CRC Press, 1990;39–52.
5. Befus D. Reciprocity of mast cell–nervous system interactions. In: Tache Y, Wingate DL, Burks TF, eds. *Innervation of the gut. Pathophysiological implications*. Boca Raton, FL: CRC Press, 1994;315–330.
6. Askenase PW, Rosenstein RW, Ptak W. T cells produce an antigen-binding factor with in vivo activity analogous to IgE antibody. *J Exp Med* 1983;157:862–873.
7. Befus AD. Mast cells that are polymorphic. *Reg Immunol* 1989;2:176–187.
8. Galli SJ. New insights into "the riddle of the mast cells": microenvironmental regulation of mast cell development and phenotypic heterogeneity. *Lab Invest* 1989;62(1):5–33.
9. Miller HRP. Mast cells: their function and heterogeneity. In: Moqbel R, ed. *Allergy and immunity to helminths. Common mechanisms or divergent pathways?* London: Taylor and Francis, 1992;228–248.
10. Kitamura Y. Heterogeneity of mast cells and phenotypic change between subpopulations. *Annu Rev Immunol* 1989;7:59–76.
11. Kanwar S, Wallace JL, Befus D, Kubes P. Nitric oxide synthesis inhibition increases epithelial permeability via mast cells. *Am J Physiol* 1994;266:G222–G229.
12. Rothwell TLW. Immune expulsion of parasitic nematodes from the alimentary tract. *Int J Parasitol* 1989;19:139–168.
13. Whitting HW. The tissue mast cell and wound healing. *Int Rev Gen Exp Zoology* 1969;4:131–168.
14. Trabucchi E, Radaelli E, Marazai M, Foschi D, Musazzi M, Veronesi AM, Montorsi W. The role of mast cells in wound healing. *Int J Tissue React* 1988;10:367–372.
15. Powell DW. Immunophysiology of intestinal electrolyte transport. In: Schultz SG, ed. *Handbook of physiology. The gastrointestinal system*. Bethesda: American Physiological Society; 1990;591–641.
16. Cooke HJ, Wang Y-Z, Rogers RC. Neuro-immune interactions: histamine signals to the intestine. In: Tache Y, Wingate DL, Burks TF, eds. *Innervation of the gut. Pathophysiological implications*. Boca Raton, FL: CRC Press, 1994;307–314.
17. Crowe SE, Perdue MH. Gastrointestinal food hypersensitivity: basic mechanisms of pathophysiology. *Gastroenterology* 1992;103:1075–1095.
18. Watkins SG, Dearin JL, Yong LC, Wilhelm DL. Association of mastopoiesis with haemopoietic tissues in the neonatal rat. *Experientia* 1976;32:1339–1340.
19. Woodbury RG, Neurath H. Purification of an atypical mast cell protease and its levels in developing rats. *Biochemistry* 1978;7:4298–4304.
20. Miller HRP, Jarret WFH. Immune reactions to mucous membranes. 1. Intestinal mast cell response during helminth expulsion in the rat. *Immunology* 1971;20:277–288.

21. Chernin JH, Miller HRP, Newlands GFJ, McLaren DJ. Proteinase phenotypes and fixation properties of rat mast cells in parasitic lesions caused by *Mesocestoides corti*: selective and site-specific recruitment of mast cell subsets. *Parasite Immunol* 1988;10:433–442.
22. Weinstock JV, Boros DL. Modulation of granulomatous hypersensitivity. VI. T lymphocyte subsets influence mast cell density in liver granulomas of *Schistosoma mansoni*-infected mice. *J Immunol* 1983;131:959–961.
23. Bridges AJ, Malone DG, Jicinsky J, Chen M, Ory P, Engber W, Graziano FM. Human synovial mast cell involvement in rheumatoid arthritis and osteoarthritis: relationship to disease type, clinical activity, and antirheumatic therapy. *Arthritis Rheum* 1991;34:1116–1124.
24. Roche WR. The nature and significance of tumour-associated mast cells. *J Pathol* 1986;148:175–182.
25. Kischer CW, Bunce H III, Shetlar MR. Mast cell analyses in hypertrophic scars, hypertrophic scars treated with pressure and mature scars. *J Invest Dermatol* 1978;70:355–357.
26. Goto T, Befus D, Low R, Bienenstock J. Mast cell heterogeneity and hyperplasia in bleomycin-induced pulmonary fibrosis of rats. *Am Rev Respir Dis* 1984;130:797–802.
27. Severson AR. Mast cells in areas of experimental bone resorption and remodelling. *Br J Exp Pathol* 1969;50:17–21.
28. Galli SJ, Tsai M, Wershil BK. The c-kit receptor, stem cell factor, and mast cells. *Am J Pathol* 1993;142:965–974.
29. Kirshenbaum AS, Kessler SW, Goff JP, Metcalfe DD. Demonstration of the origin of human mast cells from CD34+ bone marrow progenitor cells. *J Immunol* 1991;146:1410–1415.
30. Broxmeyer HE, Lu L, Hangoc G, et al. CD45 cell surface antigens are linked to stimulation of early human myeloid progenitor cells by interleukin 3 (IL-3), a GM-CSF/IL-3 fusion protein, and mast cell growth factor (a c-kit ligand). *J Exp Med* 1991;174:447–458.
31. Ashman RI, Jarboe DJ, Conrad DH, Huff TF. The mast cell-committed progenitor. *In vitro* generation of committed progenitors from bone marrow. *J Immunol* 1991;146:211–216.
32. Hamaguchi Y, Kanakura Y, Fujita J, et al. Interleukin 4 as an essential factor for in vitro clonal growth of murine connective tissue type mast cells. *J Exp Med* 1987;165:268–273.
33. Hultner L, Druez C, Moeller J, et al. Mast cell growth-enhancing activity (MEA) is structurally related and functionally identical to the novel mouse T cell growth factor P40/TCGFIII (interleukin 9). *Eur J Immunol* 1990;20:1413–1416.
34. Thompson-Snipes L, Dhar V, Bond MW, Mosmann TR, Moore KW, Rennick D. Interleukin-10: a novel stimulatory factor for mast cells and their progenitors. *Agents Actions* 1991;20:10–16.
35. Matsuda H, Kannan Y, Ushio H, Kiso Y, Kanemoto T, Suzuki H, Kitamura Y. Nerve growth factor induces development of connective tissue-type mast cells in vitro from murine bone marrow cells. *J Exp Med* 1991;174:7–14.
36. Hamaguchi Y, Kanakura Y, Fujita J, et al. Interleukin 4 as an essential factor for in vitro clonal growth of murine connective tissue type mast cells. *J Exp Med* 1987;165:268–273.
37. Bressler RB, Thompson HL, Keefer JM, Metcalfe DD. Inhibition of the growth of IL-3-dependent mast cells from murine bone marrow by recombinant granulocyte-macrophage colony-stimulating factor. *J Immunol* 1989;143:135–139.
38. Takagi M, Koike K, Nakahata T. Antiproliferative effect of IFN-δ on proliferation of mouse connective tissue-type mast cells. *J Immunol* 1990;145:1880–1884.
39. Broide DH, Wasserman SI, Alvaro-Garcia J, Zvaifler NJ, Firestein GA. Transforming growth factor-β selectively inhibits IL-3 dependent mast cell proliferation without affecting mast cell function or differentiation. *J Immunol* 1989;143:1591–1597.
40. Schneider E, Piquet-Pellorce C, Dy M. New role for histamine in interleukin-3-induced proliferation of haematopoietic stem cells. *J Cell Physiol* 1990;143:337–343.
41. Enerback L. Mast cell heterogeneity: the evolution of the concept of a specific mucosal mast cell. In: Befus AD, Bienenstock J, Denburg JA, eds. *Mast cell differentiation and heterogeneity*. New York: Raven Press, 1986;1–26.
42. Cohen JJ. Apoptosis. *Immunol Today* 1993;14:126–130.
43. Mekori YA, Oh CK, Metcalfe DD. IL-3-dependent murine

mast cells undergo apoptosis on removal of IL-3. *J Immunol* 1993;151:3775–3784.

44. King SJ, Miller HRP, Newlands GFJ, Woodbury RG. Depletion of mucosal mast cell protease by corticosteroids: effect on intestinal anaphylaxis in the rat. *Proc Natl Acad Sci USA* 1985; 82:1214–1218.

45. Soda K, Kawabori S, Perdue MH, Bienenstock J. Macrophage engulfment of mucosal mast cells in rats treated with dexamethasone. *Gastroenterology* 1991;100:929–937.

46. Barsumian EL, Iserksy C, Petrino MG, Siraganian RP. IgE-induced histamine release from rat basophilic leukemia cell lines: isolation of releasing and nonreleasing clones. *Eur J Immunol* 1981;11:317–323.

47. Reynolds DS, Serafin WE, Faller DV, Dvorak AM, Austen KF, Stevens RL. Immortalization of murine connective tissue-type mast cells at multiple stages of their differentiation by coculture of splenocytes with fibroblasts that produce Kirsten sarcoma virus. *J Biol Chem* 1988;263:12783–12791.

48. Pearce FL, Behrendt H, Blum U, Poblete-Freundt G, Pult P, Stang-Voss CH, Schmutzler W. Isolation and study of functional mast cells from lung and mesentery of the guinea pig. *Agents Actions* 1977;7:45–56.

49. Befus AD, Pearce FL, Gauldie J, Horsewood P, Bienenstock J. Mucosal mast cells. I. Isolation and functional characteristics of rat intestinal mast cells. *J Immunol* 1982;128:2475–2480.

50. Schulman ES, MacGlashan DW, Peters SP, Schleimer RP, Newball HH, Lichtenstein LM. Human lung mast cells: purification and characterization. *J Immunol* 1982;129:2662–2667.

51. Benyon RC, Lowman LA, Church MK. Human skin mast cells: their dispersion, purification, and secretory characterization. *J Immunol* 1987;138:861–867.

52. Romagnani S. Induction of T$_H$1 and T$_H$2 responses: a key role for the "natural" immune response? *Immunol Today* 1992;13: 379–381.

53. Mosmann TR, Coffman RL. TH1 and TH2 cells: different patterns of lymphokine secretion lead to different functional properties. *Annu Rev Immunol* 1989;7:145–173.

54. Schwartz LB. Preformed mediators of human mast cells and basophils. In: Holgate ST, ed. *Mast cells, mediators and disease*. London: Kluwer Academic Publishers, 1988;129–147.

55. Robinson C. Mast cells and newly-generated lipid mediators. In: Holgate ST, ed. *Mast cells, mediators and disease*. London: Kluwer Academic Publishers, 1988;149–174.

56. Reynolds DS, Stevens RL, Lane WS, Carr MH, Austen KF, Serafin WE. Different mouse mast cell populations express various combinations of at least six distinct mast cell serine proteases. *Proc Natl Acad Sci USA* 1990;87:3230–3234.

57. Huang R, Blom T, Hellman L. Cloning and structural analysis of MMCP-1, MMCP-4 and MMCP-5, three mouse mast cell-specific serine proteases. *Eur J Immunol* 1991;21:1611–1621.

58. Gurish MF, Nadeau JH, Johnson KR, McNeil HP, Grattan KM, Austen KF, Stevens RL. A closely linked complex of mouse mast cell-specific chymase genes on chromosome 14. *J Biol Chem* 1993;268:11372–11379.

59. Reynolds DS, Stevens RL, Gurley DS, Lane WS, Austen KF, Serafin WE. Isolation and molecular cloning of mast cell carboxypeptidase A. A novel member of the carboxypeptidase gene family. *J Biol Chem* 1989;264:20094–20099.

60. Natsuaki M, Stewart C-B, Vanderslice P, Schwartz LB, Wintroub BU, Rutter WJ, Goldstein SM. Human skin mast cell carboxypeptidase: functional characterization, cDNA cloning, and genealogy. *J Invest Dermatol* 1992;99:138–145.

61. Eklund KK, Ghildyal N, Austen KF, Stevens RL. Induction by IL-9 and suppression by IL-3 and IL-4 of the levels of chromosome 14-derived transcripts that encode late-expressed mouse mast cell proteases. *J Immunol* 1993;151:4266–4273.

62. Gurish MF, Ghildyal N, McNeil HP, Austen KF, Gillis S, Stevens RL. Differential expression of secretory granule proteases in mouse mast cells exposed to interleukin 3 and c-*kit* ligand. *J Exp Med* 1992;175:1003–1012.

63. Miller HRP, Woodbury RG, Huntley JF, Newlands G. Systemic release of mucosal mast-cell protease in primed rats challenged with *Nippostrongylus brasiliensis*. *Immunology* 1983; 49:471–479.

64. Lagunoff D, Rickard A, Marquardt C. Rat mast cell tryptase. *Arch Biochem Biophys* 1991;291:52–58.

65. Caughey GH, Schaumberg TH, Zerweck EH, Butterfield JH, Hanson RD, Silverman GA, Ley TJ. The human mast cell chymase gene (CMA1): mapping to the cathepsin G/granzyme gene cluster and lineage-restricted expression. *Genomics* 1993;15: 614–620.

66. Remington SJ, Woodbury RG, Reynolds RS, Matthews BW, Neurath H. The structure of rat mast cell protease II at 1.9-Å resolution. *Biochemistry* 1988;27:8097–8105.

67. Sali A, Matsumoto R, McNeil HP, Karplus M, Stevens RL. Three-dimensional models of four mouse mast cell chymases. Identification of proteoglycan binding regions and protease-specific antigenic epitopes. *J Biol Chem* 1993;268:9023–9034.

68. Ruoss SJ, Hartmann T, Caughey GH. Mast cell tryptase is a mitogen for cultured fibroblasts. *J Clin Invest* 1991;88:493–499.

69. Sekizawa K, Caughey GH, Lazarus SC, Gold WM, Nadel JA. Mast cell tryptase causes airway smooth muscle hyperresponsiveness in dogs. *J Clin Invest* 1989;83:175–179.

70. Sommerhoff CP, Caughey GH, Finkbeiner WE, Lazarus SC, Basbaum CB, Nadel JA. Mast cell chymase. A potent secretagogue for airway gland serous cells. *J Immunol* 1989;142: 2450–2456.

71. Tam EK, Gaughey GH. Degradation of airway neuropeptides by human lung tryptase. *Am J Respir Cell Mol Biol* 1990;3: 27–32.

72. Bunnett NW, Goldstein SM, Nakazato P. Isolation of a neuropeptide-degrading carboxypeptidase from the human stomach. *Gastroenterology* 1992;102:76–87.

73. Kajita T, Hugli TE. Evidence for *in vivo* degradation of C3a anaphylatoxin by mast cell chymase: I. Nonspecific activation of rat peritoneal mast cells by C3a$_{des\ Arg}$. *Am J Pathol* 1991; 138:1359–1369.

74. Mizutani H, Schechter N, Lazarus G, Black RA, Kupper TS. Rapid and specific conversion of precursor interleukin 1β (IL-1β) to an active IL-1 species by human mast cell chymase. *J Exp Med* 1991;174:821–825.

75. Wypij DM, Nichols JS, Novak PJ, Stacy DL, Berman J, Wiseman JS. Role of mast cell chymase in the extracellular processing of big-endothelin-1 to endothelin-1 in the perfused rat lung. *Biochem Pharmacol* 1992;43:845–853.

76. Lohi J, Harvima I, Keski-Oja J. Pericellular substrates of human mast cell tryptase: 72,000 dalton gelatinase and fibronectin. *J Cell Biochem* 1992;50:337–349.

77. Banovac K, Banovac F, Yang J, Koren E. Interaction of osteoblasts with extracellular matrix: effect of mast cell chymase. *Proc Soc Exp Biol Med* 1993;203:221–235.

78. Moncada S. The L-arginine: nitric oxide pathway. *Acta Physiol Scand* 1992;145:201–227.

79. Salvemini DE, Masini E, Anggard E, Mannaioni PF, Vane J. Synthesis of a nitric-oxide like factor from L-arginine by rat serosal mast cells: stimulation of guanylate cyclase and inhibition of platelet aggregation. *Biochem Biophys Res Commun* 1990;169:596.

80. Bissonnette EY, Hogaboam CM, Wallace JL, Befus AD. Potentiation of tumor necrosis factor-α-mediated cytotoxicity of mast cells by their production of nitric oxide. *J Immunol* 1991; 147:3060–3065.

81. Salvemini D, Masini E, Pistelli A, Mannaioni PF, Vane J. Nitric oxide: a regulatory mediator of mast cell reactivity. *J Cardiovasc Pharmacol* 1991;17(Suppl 3):S258–S264.

82. Hogaboam CM, Befus AD, Wallace JL. Modulation of mast cell reactivity by interleukin-1 beta: divergent effects on nitric oxide and platelet-activiating factor release. *J Immunol* 1993; 151:3767–3774.

83. Bradding P, Feather IH, Howarth PH, et al. Interleukin 4 is localized to and release by human mast cells. *J Exp Med* 1992; 176:1381–1386.

84. Bradding P, Feather IH, Wilson S, Bardin PG, Heusser CH, Holgate ST, Howarth PH. Immunolocalization of cytokines in the nasal mucosa of normal and perennial rhinitic subjects. *J Immunol* 1993;151:3853–3865.

85. Gordon JR, Burd PR, Galli SJ. Mast cells as a source of multifunctional cytokines. *Immunol Today* 1990;11:458–464.

86. Moller A, Lippert U, Lessmann D, et al. Human mast cells produce IL-8. *J Immunol* 1993;151:3261–3266.
87. Burd PR, Rogers HW, Gordon JR, et al. Interleukin 3-dependent and -independent mast cells stimulated with IgE and antigen express multiple cytokines. *J Exp Med* 1989;170:245–257.
88. Pennington DW, Lopez AR, Thomas PS, Peck C, Gold WM. Dog mastocytoma cells produce transforming growth factor beta₁. *J Clin Invest* 1992;90:35–41.
89. Bissonnette EY, Befus AD. Modulation of mast cell function in the G.I. tract. In: Wallace JL, ed. *Immunopharmacology the gastrointestinal tract (handbook of immunopharmacology)*. London: Academic Press, 1993;95–101.
90. Mousli M, Bueb J-L, Bronner C, Rouot B, Landry Y. G protein activation: a receptor-independent mode of action for cationic amphiphilic neuropeptides and venom peptides. *Trends Pharmacol Sci* 1990;11:358–362.
91. Stead RH, Tomioka M, Quinonez G, Simon GT, Felten SY, Bienenstock J. Intestinal mucosal mast cells in normal and nematode-infected rat intestines are in intimate contact with peptidergic nerves. *Proc Natl Acad Sci USA* 1987;84:2975–2979.
92. MacQueen G, Marshall J, Perdue M, Siegel S, Bienenstock J. Pavlovian conditioning of rat mucosal mast cells to secrete rat mast cell protease II. *Science* 1989;243:83–85.
93. Castro GA. Immunophysiology of enteric parasitism. *Parasitol Today* 1989;5:11–19.
94. Crowe SE, Sestini P, Perdue MH. Allergic reactions of rat jejunal mucosa. Ion transport responses to luminal antigen and inflammatory mediators. *Gastroenterology* 1990;99:74–82.
95. Wang Y-Z, Palmer JM, Cooke HJ. Neuroimmune regulation of colonic secretion in guinea pigs. *Am J Physiol* 1991;260:G307–G314.
96. Scott RB, Diamant SC, Gall DG. Motility effects of intestinal anaphylaxis in the rat. *Am J Physiol* 1988;18:G505–G511.
97. Vermillion DL, Collins SM. Increased responsiveness of jejunal longitudinal muscle in *Trichinella*-infected rats. *Am J Physiol* 1988;17:G124–G129.
98. Kaplan AP, Reddigari S, Baeza M, Kuna P. Histamine releasing factors and cytokine-dependent activation of basophils and mast cells. *Adv Immunol* 1991;50:237–254.
99. Lehrer RI, Lichtenstein AK, Ganz T. Defensins' antimicrobial and cytotoxic peptides of mammalian cells. *Annu Rev Immunol* 1993;11:105–128.
100. Yamashita T, Saito K. Purification, primary structure, and biological activity of guinea pig neutrophil cationic peptides. *Infect Immun* 1989;57:2405–2409.
101. Selsted ME, Miller SI, Henschen AH, Ouellette AJ. Enteric defensins: antibiotic peptide components of intestinal host defense. *J Cell Biol* 1992;118:929–936.
102. Columbo M, Horowitz EM, Botana LM, et al. The human recombinant c-*kit* receptor ligand, rhSCF, induces mediator release from human cutaneous mast cells and enhances IgE-dependent mediator release from both skin mast cells and peripheral blood basophils. *J Immunol* 1992;149:599–608.
103. Tsai M, Takeishi T, Thompson H, et al. Induction of mast cell proliferation, maturation, and heparin synthesis by the rat c-kit ligand, stem cell factor. *Proc Natl Acad Sci USA* 1991;88:6382–6386.
104. Tsai M, Tam S-Y, Galli SJ. Distinct patterns of early response gene expression and proliferation in mouse mast cells stimulated by stem cell factor, interleukin-3, or IgE and antigen. *Eur J Immunol* 1993;23:867–872.
105. Benyon RC, Bissonnette EY, Befus D. Intestinal mast cells in IBD; pathogenesis and therapeutic implications. In: MacDermott RP, Stenson WF, eds. *Current topics in gastroenterology: inflammatory bowel disease*. New York: Elseiver Science Publishing, 1992;189–199.
106. Schleimer RP. Effects of glucocorticosteroids on inflammatory cells relevant to their therapeutic applications in asthma. *Am Rev Respir Dis* 1990;141:S59–S69.
107. Coleman JW, Holliday MR, Kimber I, Zsebo KM, Galli SJ. Regulation of mouse peritoneal mast cell secretory function by stem cell factor, IL-3 or IL-4. *J Immunol* 1993;150:556–562.
108. Sillaber C, Bevec D, Butterfield JH, et al. Tumor necrosis factor α and interleukin-1β mRNA expression in HMC-1 cells: differential regulation of gene product expression by recombinant interleukin-4. *Exp Hematol* 1993;21:1271–1275.
109. Bissonnette EY, Befus AD. Inhibition of mast cell-mediated cytotoxicity by IFN-α/β and -γ¹. *J Immunol* 1990;145:3385–3390.
110. Bissonnette EY, Chin B, Befus AD. IFN differentially regulates histamine and TNFα in rat intestinal mucosal mast cells. [*Submitted*].
111. Konig W, Konig B, Scheffer J, Hacker J, Goebel W. Role of cloned virulence factors (mannose-resistant haemagglutination, mannose-resistant adhesions) from uropathogenic *Escherichia coli* strains in the release of inflammatory mediators from neutrophils and mast cells. *Immunology* 1989;67:401–407.
112. Nakagomi K, Takeuchi M, Tanaka H, Tomizuka N. Studies of inhibitors of rat mast cell degranulation produced by microorganisms. I. Screening of microorganisms, and isolation and physico-chemical properties of eurocidins C, D and E. *J Antibiot* 1990;43:462–469.
113. Ahmad A, Wang CH, Bell RG. A role for IgE in intestinal immunity. Expression of rapid expulsion of *Trichinella spiralis* in rats transfused with IgE and thoracic duct lymphocytes. *J Immunol* 1991;146:3563–3570.
114. Moqbel R, King SJ, MacDonald AJ, Miller HR, Cromwell O, Shaw RJ, Kay AB. Enteral and systemic release of leukotrienes during anaphylaxis of *Nippostrongylus brasiliensis*-primed rats. *J Immunol* 1986;137:296–301.
115. Douch PGC, Harrison GBL, Buchanan LL, Greer KS. In vitro bioassay of sheep gastrointestinal mucus for nematode paralysing activity mediated by substances with some properties characteristic of SRS-A. *Int J Parasit* 1983;13:207–212.
116. Wood JD. Intestinal immuno-neuro physiology. In: Tache Y, Wingate DL, Burks TF, eds. *Innervation of the gut. Pathophysiological implications*. Boca Raton, FL: CRC Press, 1994;290–313.
117. Fujimoto K, Imamura I, Granger DN, Wada H, Sakata T, Tso P. Histamine and histidine decarboxylase are correlated with mucosal repair in rat small intestine after ischemia-reperfusion. *J Clin Invest* 1992;89:126–133.

Infections of the Gastrointestinal Tract,
edited by M. J. Blaser, P. D. Smith, J. I. Ravdin,
H. B. Greenberg, and R. L. Guerrant
Raven Press, Ltd., New York © 1995.

CHAPTER 17

Food Poisoning

John N. Aucott

Foodborne disease results from ingestion of either food or water contaminated with pathogenic microorganisms, microbial toxins, chemicals, or from consumption of naturally occurring plant and animal toxins. The diversity of microorganisms and toxins that can be involved in foodborne disease results in a wide spectrum of clinical syndromes. The focus of this chapter will be on foodborne disease with gastrointestinal symptoms occurring within 24 hr after ingestion. However, it is important to recognize that many serious foodborne illnesses such as hepatitis A (1,2), brucellosis (3), listeriosis (4,5), botulism (6), and diphylobrothium (7) do not have prominent gastrointestinal symptoms. In addition, foodborne illnesses may have prominent neurological symptoms in addition to gastrointestinal symptoms. This chapter will not directly discuss acute syndromes with neurological features such as fish-related toxins (see chapter by Morris) and botulism (see chapter by Arnon). Foodborne infections with longer incubation periods due to *Salmonella, Shigella* sp., *E. coli,* and *Campylobacter* sp. are discussed in depth elsewhere (Part VII).

The most important etiological factor for foodborne disease in the United States is bacterial agents, which cause 66% of the outbreaks and 92% of the individual cases in which a specific agent is eventually identified (Table 1). Chemical, parasitic, and viral agents are less common, accounting for 26%, 4%, and 5% of the identified outbreaks, respectively. An etiological agent cannot be determined in 62% of outbreaks (8), which are divided by the Centers for Disease Control (CDC) into four subgroups according to the incubation period: 1 hr, probable chemical poisoning; 1–7 hr, probable *Staphylococcus* food poisoning; 8–14 hr, probable *Clostridium perfringens* food poisoning; and more than 14 hr, probable other infectious or toxic agents (8).

RISK FACTORS FOR FOODBORNE ILLNESS

Risk factors for foodborne disease include the improper selection, preparation, or storage of food (Table 2). The

J. N. Aucott: Department of Medicine, Case Western Reserve University and Cleveland Veterans Affairs Medical Center, Cleveland, Ohio 44106.

most commonly reported food preparation practice that contributed to foodborne disease is improper storage or holding temperature, followed by poor personal hygiene of the food handler (8). Inadequate cooking and contaminated equipment ranked third or fourth in studies by the CDC in each year between 1983 and 1987. Food obtained from unsafe sources was the least common factor involved.

Chemical intoxication can be due to naturally occurring plant and animal toxins or by contamination of food with

TABLE 1. *Etiologies of foodborne disease outbreaks reported to the Centers for Disease Control, 1983–1987*

Etiologic agent	% of outbreaks with identified agent
Bacterial	
Salmonella	37.6
Clostridium botulinum	8.1
Staphylococcus aureus	5.2
Shigella	4.8
Campylobacter	3.1
Clostridium perfringens	2.6
Bacillus cereus	1.8
Escherichia coli	0.8
Streptococcus, group A	0.8
Vibrio parahemolyticus	0.4
Brucella	0.2
Other bacterial	0.5
Chemicals/Natural Toxins	
Ciguatoxin	9.6
Scombrotoxin	9.1
Mushrooms	1.5
Heavy metals	1.4
Monosodium glutamate	0.2
Shellfish poisoning	0.2
Other chemical	3.4
Parasitic	
Trichinella spiralis	3.6
Giardia	0.3
Viral	
Hepatitis A	3.1
Norwalk virus	1.1
Other viral	0.2

TABLE 2. *Risk factors for foodborne illness*

Risk factor	Examples
Food obtained from unsafe source	
Misidentification of unsafe foods	Mushrooms, ciguatera poisoning, shellfish
Chemical contamination of foods	Insecticides, heavy metals, MSG, toxic oil syndromes
Faulty food preparation practices	Botulism, brucellosis, listerosis
Food Handling Errors	
Poor personal hygiene of food handlers	*Staphylococcus*, viral, protozoal pathogens
	S. aureus, B. cereus
Inadequate storage of holding temperature	*C. perfringens,* most bacterial pathogens, scombroid
Improper storage containers	Heavy metal ingestion
Inadequate cooking of food	*E. coli* O157:H7, *Salmonella,* trichinosis
Consumption of uncooked foods	
Eggs	*Salmonella*
Shellfish	*Vibrio* species, hepatitis A,
Fish	anisakiasis, *Diphyllobothrium latum*
Beef	toxoplasmosis
Waterborne disease	Giardia lamblia, *Cryptosporidium, Shigella,* Norwalk virus,
	hepatitis A, chemicals

heavy metals, insecticides, or toxic oils. Fish and shellfish that are normally safe can accumulate toxins naturally present in the food chain (e.g., paralytic shellfish poisoning and ciguatera) or can be contaminated with bacteria that produce toxic levels compounds when the fish is improperly stored (scombroid or histamine fish poisoning) (9). Some "foods" are intrinsically toxic to humans with ingestion resulting from faulty identification of edible species, e.g., mushrooms (10) and ornamental and wild plants (11,12).

The variety of "foods" involved in foodborne disease includes food (8) and water (13), as well as substances added to food either intentionally or unintentionally. Important clues to the etiology of foodborne illness can be suggested by the implicated food. An obvious relationship may be suggested by the discovery of mushroom ingestion or may be more occult as in beverages stored in improper containers containing heavy metals. Bivalve molluscs such as oysters, clams, and mussels are particularly suspect because of their ability to transmit a variety of pathogens including hepatitis A (14), Norwalk agent (15,16), and *Vibrio* species (17–20), *Salmonella typhi,* and *Campylobacter* species (15). Fish and shellfish poisoning is often associated with prominent neurological and systemic symptoms such as ciguatera (21–23), scombroid (24–26), puffer fish poisoning (27), and paralytic shellfish poisoning (28,29). Ingestion of Chinese food may suggest monosodium glutamate (MSG) or *B. cereus*–contaminated fried rice (30,31). Raw meats present specific infectious risks. The increasing popularity of raw fish in sushi has increased the awareness of marine worm ingestions such as anisakis (32,33). Other associations include raw or undercooked beef with toxoplasmosis or *E. coli* (34) and undercooked pork or bear meat with trichinosis (35).

Waterborne diseases may include bacterial pathogens, especially *Escherichia coli, Shigella,* and viral pathogens such as hepatitis A, hepatitis E, or Norwalk, and parasitic disease due to *Giardia* or *Cryptosporidium* (13,36). Waterborne outbreaks may involve community water systems, well water, surface water, as well as bottled water. Recent

reports have documented the continued use of drinking water from wells after identification of chemical contamination by the CDC (37).

MAGNITUDE AND SIGNIFICANCE OF PROBLEM

Between 300 and 600 recognized outbreaks affecting 10,000–31,000 individuals are reported to the CDC each year (8). These figures include only the largest and most serious outbreaks and do not include sporadic foodborne disease. Therefore, this greatly underestimates the magnitude of the problem. The true incidence of foodborne disease in the United States has been estimated to be between 6.3 million and 81 million cases a year (38). The annual number of deaths in the USA from foodborne illness has been estimated between 523 and 7041 (38). Most foodborne illnesses are underdiagnosed because the majority are self-limited illnesses of short duration. As mentioned, no etiology is identified for 60% of outbreaks reported to the CDC (8). The inability to make a specific diagnosis results from the limited availability of assays for toxins, chemicals, viral agents, and certain disease-causing strains of bacteria, such as *E. coli* O157:H7.

Although symptoms of disease may often be mild, large outbreaks may have significant economic impact and result in closure of hospitals and schools (39). Cost estimates for all foodborne illness in the United States, including the medical expenses and lost productivity of those affected as well as lost revenues and legal fees incurred by the food supplier, range from $7.7 to $23 billion per year (38). Bacterial illness accounts for about 80% of this cost with salmonellosis accounting for 47% of the total (40).

ETIOLOGICAL AGENTS

Foodborne Viral Disease

Viral agents are increasingly recognized as important agents of water and foodborne disease. Unlike bacteria, viruses do not multiply or produce toxins in food. Food merely acts as a vehicle for their transfer. Most reported incidents of viral food- or waterborne illness are due to hepatitis A virus and Norwalk-like agents (13,39). Hepatitis A is an important source of waterborne outbreaks reported to the CDC. Hepatitis E should also be considered in any patient who has traveled abroad and is negative for serological markers for hepatitis A, B, and C (36).

Over 90% of foodborne viral gastroenteritis outbreaks in which the etiological agent is identified are due to Norwalk virus and related viruses (39). Norwalk virus is a single-stranded RNA virus that has many properties typical of caliciviruses but is difficult to study because of the inability to cultivate the virus in cell culture. Prevalence of antibodies to Norwalk agent is low in children and rises rapidly during adolescence and early adulthood. Immunity to reinfection is not complete after a single infection (42). Infection is spread by the fecal–oral route and possibly by airborne spread, with a 12- to 48-hr incubation period. Infectious virus may be excreted in the feces for at least 48 hr after clinical recovery resulting in spread by food handlers (43). Outbreaks occur throughout the year with large-scale family and community-wide epidemics due to secondary transmission of the virus. Common source outbreaks can afflict thousands of individuals as was seen in one example involving contaminated ice (44). Infection can result from ingestion of contaminated water, ice, and foods including poorly cooked clams and oysters, salads, cake frosting, and baked goods (45). Norwalk agent and Norwalk-like virus may also account for episodes of acute gastrointestinal disease where the etiological agent remains unclear (43).

Foodborne Bacterial Disease

Staphylococcal food poisoning is one of the most common types of foodborne disease in the United States, causing 5.2% of the recognized bacterial food poisoning outbreaks during 1983–1987 (8). *Staphylococcus* is capable of causing large outbreaks of illness involving over 1000 individuals. Staphylococcal food poisoning rarely results from commercially prepared food (46) and is due to contamination of foods by handlers in food service establishments or in the home (47). Humans are the usual source of such contamination of food, from an infected wound on the hands or occasionally from coughing or sneezing. It is estimated that 20% to 50% of healthy individuals carry *S. aureus,* most often in the nares, skin, or feces (47). Animals with mastitis can also transmit disease through infected milk (48). Over 99% of cases of staphylococcal food poisoning are due to *S. aureus.* Other coagulase-positive staphylococci including *S. hyicus* and *S. intermedius* produce small amounts of enterotoxin but have not been the cause of outbreaks of foodborne illness (47). Rarely are cases traced to coagulase-negative *Staphylococcus* sp. (49). Disease results from ingestion of one or more of the seven serologically distinct extracellular enterotoxins (A, B, C1, C2, C3, D, and E) (50,51). The majority of enterotoxigenic *Staphylococcus* involved in outbreaks of foodborne illness produce type A enterotoxin alone or in combination with type D toxin (52,53). Staphylococcal enterotoxins are resistant to heat, irradiation, pH extremes, and proteolysis (54–56) (Table 3). The purified toxins are small, 27–30 kDa, a single-chain polypeptide whose emetic activity may be related to a conserved histidine domain at the active site (57,58). As little as 100–200 ng will produce illness in humans. Assay for the presence of enterotoxin in food and its production *in vitro* provides an important epidemiological tool. Phage typing of species is useful for epidemiological investigations to trace the source of infection (59). Enterotoxigenic *Staphylococcus* of phage type III are most often associated with outbreaks of foodborne disease. Phage type I is less often involved in foodborne illness but can be found either alone or in combination with type III (47). Foods often implicated with outbreaks include dairy products, salads, and meats (especially ham). Food contaminated with *Staphylococcus* has a normal odor, taste, and appearance. High-protein foods favor the growth of *Staphylococcus* and present an especially high risk for food poisoning. Although a pH below 5.0 inhibits the growth of the bacteria, semipreserved products packaged with salt or sugar may still support growth of *Staphylococcus.*

Clostridium perfringens more commonly causes a mild form of foodborne illness but rarely can be severe (60). Approximately 3% of food poisoning reported to the CDC are due to the mild form of *Clostridium* food poisoning (8). *C. perfringens* type C causes rare cases of necrotic enteritis that are still reported from isolated regions of the world such as Papua New Guinea. This rare illness is due to production of the β toxin which is usually inactivated

TABLE 3. *Pathogenic mechanisms in bacterial foodborne illness*

Ingestion of preformed toxin	Toxin production *in vivo*	Tissue invasion

Staphylococcus
  27- to 30-kDa protein
  Stable to heat, protease, radiation, and pH extreme
	C. perfringens
	  35-kDa protein
	  Labile to heat, protease
		Salmonella
		  Cytotoxins
		  Heat-labile

Bacillus cereus
  5–10 kDa
  Stable to heat, protease, pH extreme
	Bacillus cereus
	  38- to 46-kDa
	  Labile to heat, protease
	Enterotoxigenic *E. coli,* LT, ST toxins
	Vibrio species, cholera toxin
		Shigella
		  Shiga cytotoxin

by proteolytic enzymes in the intestine. Susceptible individuals are either malnourished and lack these proteolytic enzymes, or have their enzymes inhibited by other substances in their diet (61). The vast majority of the typical cases of the mild diarrheal illness seen in developed countries are due to type A strains that are present in soil throughout the world and the intestinal tracts of virtually all vertebrate animals studied. Types B, C, D, E *Clostridium* are found only in animals and not soil. Spores are heat-resistant and survive cooking to germinate. The organism grows rapidly at temperatures of 15–50°C with a optimum growth temperature of 43–45°C. The organism can double in number in as little as 10 min (62). A 35-kDa protein enterotoxin is produced by type A *C. perfringens* during sporulation (Table 3). The enterotoxin alters the membrane ion permeability of intestinal epithelial cells and acts as a superantigen reactive with human T cells (63,64). The resultant illness only occurs after ingestion of heavily contaminated food with greater than 100 million bacteria per gram. Meats, meat products, and poultry are the foods most commonly implicated with outbreaks of food poisoning. High numbers of vegetative bacteria may be present while the food is palatable. Outbreaks are usually associated with food service establishments and domestic preparation. Commercially prepared processed food is rarely the cause of *Clostridium* foodborne disease (65).

Bacillus cereus is a less common source of foodborne illness in the United States, accounting for approximately 2% of outbreaks, with a confirmed etiology reported to the CDC during 1973–1987 (8). *B. cereus* is a ubiquitous, aerobic, spore-forming, gram-positive rod that causes two forms of toxin-mediated food poisoning: a short incubation emetic syndrome and a long incubation diarrheal syndrome (66,31). *B. cereus* is present in soil and water sources throughout the world and in most raw foods (61). In addition, 10% to 40% of humans are colonized with this bacteria. The spores of *Bacillus* are heat-resistant. The organism is capable of producing either the emetic or the diarrheal toxin depending on the food on which it grows (67,68). There is evidence that the emetic syndrome is caused by a preformed toxin with a molecular weight of 5000–10,000 kDa which is unaffected by heat, trypsin, pepsin, and pH extremes (Table 3). The emetic syndrome is associated with cooked rice in 95% of cases. In contrast, the diarrheal syndrome is associated with proteinaceous foods including vegetables, sauces, and puddings (61). The diarrheal enterotoxin is a heat-labile protein of molecular weight 38–46 kDa (69). There is no consistent relationship between the strain of *Bacillus* and the toxin produced. Outbreaks of foodborne illness due to *B. subtilis*, *B. licheniformis*, and *B. pumilus* have also been reported (61).

Foodborne Fungal Disease

Fungal mycotoxins are synthesized by numerous species of fungi including *Aspergillus flavus*, *Aspergillus parasiticus,* and *Fusariuma* species. Contamination of food, especially cereals and nuts, can occur in the field or during storage. Conditions of poor storage that favor growth of the fungi result in the production of these potent toxins. The toxins can contaminate meat, eggs, and milk when animals are fed contaminated grain. Historically, dramatic episodes of mycotoxin poisoning have included gangrenous ergotism and alimentary toxic aleukia resulting from *Fusarium*-contaminated cereals in postwar USSR (70). Aflatoxin from *A. flavus* is a potent carcinogen in certain animals but the relationship to human illness is unclear (71).

Food and Waterborne Parasitic Disease

Confirmed food- or waterborne parasitic infections are rare in developed countries but cases of trichinosis and giardiasis are reported to the CDC almost every year (8,13,43). Most parasites that are transmitted by contaminated food and water do not result in recognized outbreaks of acute foodborne illness (72). This may seem surprising given the wide prevalence of protozoans and helminths. Several factors may explain the lack of such outbreaks including the inability of parasites to multiply in food, the high rate of asymptomatic infection with these organisms, the difficulty with diagnosis, and the long delay (often years) before clinical presentation of many infections such as helminthic infections. Outbreaks of protozoal disease are more frequently associated with water than food in the United States. Waterborne outbreaks of *E. histolytica* have occurred in both the USA and UK, but are uncommon (72). Transmission of *Giardia* and *Cryptosporidium* by means of public water supplies in developed countries is being increasingly recognized. *Giardia lamblia* was implicated as the etiological agent in 7 of the 12 waterborne outbreaks between 1989 and 1990 in which an agent was identified. *Giardia* is commonly found in surface water throughout the world and is a hazard for outdoorsmen and campers. Because the cysts involved in the transmission of *Giardia* are relatively chlorine-resistant, public water supplies are a potential source of outbreaks as well. *Cryptosporidium* may contaminate water supplies that are exposed to livestock excreta. Waterborne outbreaks of cryptosporidiosis have been reported with increasing frequency in North America and may expose large numbers of individuals resulting in significant morbidity in immunocompromised hosts (73).

Foodborne parasitic disease can be due to food handlers or contaminated foods. Between 1983 and 1987, *Trichinella spiralis* and *G. lamblia* accounted for all the foodborne outbreaks where a parasitic cause was identified. Transmission of *Entamoeba histolytica* by food has been traced to contamination by food handlers in the past (72). There have been at least four foodborne outbreaks of *Giardia* in the USA (74,75). In all of these instances, the origin of *Giardia* was from food handlers who had contact with children who were excreting *Giardia* in their stool. *Cryptosporidium* infection has been epidemiologically linked to ingestion of raw sausage and raw milk, but contamination by food handlers excreting oocysts has not been documented (72). The increased popularity of sushi in North America has brought attention to foodborne illness due to anisakis, eustrongylides, and other fish tapeworms (32,33). These worms can be found in both fresh- and saltwater fish. Humans are exposed to these worms through the consumption of raw fish in sushi or occasionally through eating minnows or bait fish as a "stunt."

Foodborne Chemical Ingestions

Foodborne chemical ingestions may be the result of exogenous toxins contaminating foods or may result from naturally occurring toxins found in animals, plants, and fungi (76). Pesticides used in agriculture that contain potent cholinesterase inhibitors have resulted in foodborne outbreaks of serious illness (77). Addition of drugs to animal feed has been reported to result in β-agonist food poisoning from ingestion of contaminated beef liver (78). Heavy metal ingestion has accounted for one to four episodes reported to the CDC each year between 1983 and 1987. These episodes are often related to beverages that are stored in improper containers such as galvanized metal cans. The beverages are usually acidic and have included fruit punch, limeade, and tomato juice. Outbreaks have been reported from schools, restaurants, and homes. Other rare mechanisms of heavy metal ingestion have included cadmium from a refrigerator shell used as an improvised barbecue grill and copper from a corroded geyser (79,80).

Contamination of water with a wide variety of toxic chemicals can result in acute poisoning. Five of the 50 reported waterborne outbreaks between 1986 and 1988 were due to toxic chemicals. Chemicals can be introduced into public water systems through back-siphoning; one case involved concentrated sodium hydroxide (43). Faulty water treatment with water-softening agents can result in excessive alkalinity or acidity of water. Contact of copper pipes with acidic water will result in elevated copper levels and abdominal toxicity. Acute fluoride poisoning has been reported at least seven times in the United States. Fluoride and hydrogen ions in the stomach combine to form hydrofluoric acid, which is a gastric irritant. Outbreaks have affected hundreds of individuals and occasionally result in death, especially in patients with renal failure (81). Cross-connection of water systems with heating systems has resulted in the introduction of toxic levels of ethylene glycol into the water supply (43). In one episode well water was contaminated with nitrates resulting in fatal methemoglobinemia in an infant (43).

Food additives and substitutes can result in a variety of causes of food poisoning. Monosodium glutamate has been implicated in the Chinese restaurant syndrome in which patients experience a burning sensation or pressure in the chest, lacrimation, and diaphoresis. Wonton soup is frequently identified as the offending food, possibly because the effects of MSG are accentuated when it is consumed on an empty stomach. Large outbreaks of delayed neurological syndromes have been traced to the inadvertent ingestion of toxic oils. Examples have included industrial denatured rapeseed oil and a hydraulic fluid component, triorthocresyl phosphate. These industrial compounds have been used to adulterate olive oil, mus-

tard oil, Jamaican ginger, and cooking oil. The delayed neurological syndromes they produce are similar to that seen in eosinophilia-myalgia syndrome associated with L-tryptophan ingestion (82).

Animal toxins are primarily seen with ingestion of fish and shellfish (9,71,83). Fish and shellfish are associated with distinct food poisoning syndromes including ciguatera, scombroid, tetrodatoxin, paralytic, and neurotoxic shellfish poisoning, which are discussed in separate chapters.

Poisoning with plant toxins can be the result of ingestion of inedible plants as well as plants thought to be edible (71). Toxicity may result from improper preparation of the foods (cassava), misidentification of toxic species for edible species (mushrooms), or genetic susceptibility of the host to normally innocuous components of food (favism). Cyanide poisoning may result from ingestion of several foods including improperly prepared cassava, certain varieties of lima beans, apple seeds, bitter almonds, and laetrile produced from peach kernels. Unintentional overdoses of herbal remedies containing plant toxins may result in a variety of syndromes including neurological disease and hepatitis (84).

Edible plants may occasionally cause food poisoning under specific circumstances (71). Potato glycoalkaloids are produced under conditions of stress including exposure of potatoes to light, fungal, mechanical, or insect damage. Commercial blemish-free potato tubers will generally contain low levels of toxic glycoalkaloids that are further reduced by peeling the potatoes. However, poor quality or damaged potatoes can contain higher levels of the toxin. This results in acute potato poisoning, which presents with neurological symptoms including apathy, restlessness, drowsiness, and visual disturbance. Legumes contain a variety of biologically active compounds including estrogenic isoflavones and coumestans, hemagglutinins, tannins, and glycosides. Fava beans contain plant glycosides vicine and convicine, which are broken down to oxidants that cause favism in G6PD-deficient individuals of Mediterranean descent.

Ornamental and wild plants are common sources of potential food poisoning, especially in children (85). Fortunately, most ingestions involve house plants and ornamental plants with less than 0.04% of reported cases resulting in major toxicity (86). Highly toxic wild plants are occasionally mistaken for edible species and have resulted in at least 58 fatalities in the USA between 1979 and 1988. For example, water hemlock is a highly toxic species that may be mistaken for a wild edible plant and when ingested results in gastrointestinal symptoms, seizures, and respiratory distress with an overall mortality of 30% (11).

Mushroom poisoning is important because of the potential for lethal ingestion in addition to less severe but clinically varied syndromes. A large number of poisonous species grow abundantly and species identification can be exceedingly difficult even for expert mycologists. Mushrooms known to be edible in one location may be poisonous in a different geographic location. Poisonings occur more frequently in the fall when the reproductive part of the fungus is most easily harvested. Greater than 80% of reports of mushroom exposure to the American Association of Poison Control Centers were in children less than 6 years of age. Symptoms of mushroom poisoning vary from benign self-limited gastrointestinal symptoms to major systemic syndromes including liver and renal failure, hemolysis, disulfiram-like reactions, cholinergic symptoms, and psychoactive central nervous system (CNS) effects (87).

APPROACH TO FOOD POISONING SYNDROMES

The diagnosis of foodborne disease should be considered when an acute illness with gastrointestinal and/or neurological manifestations affects two or more persons who have previously shared a meal. The diagnostic approach to food poisoning should consider a combination of the specific symptoms including the presence of neurological or systemic symptoms, the incubation period, the duration of the illness, and the food associated with the illness (Table 4). This chapter will discuss illnesses occurring in the first 24 hr after exposure to a foodborne disease. However, many bacterial diseases that require replication in the host have incubation periods up to 3–5 days (see chapters on *Salmonella*, *E. coli*, etc.). Other foodborne illnesses have even longer incubation periods. Botulism may not present for 6 hr to 8 days after ingestion of toxin. The incubation period for trichinosis may range from 1 to 62 days, and *Giardia* has an incubation period of 1–4 weeks.

Searching for key historical clues and symptoms of food poisoning is essential to making the diagnosis and recognizing patients at risk for significant morbidity and mortality. The evaluation of gastrointestinal illness should focus on the presence or absence of vomiting and the differentiation of inflammatory from noninflammatory diarrhea. Diarrhea can be characterized as inflammatory by the presence of fecal leukocytes, heme-positive stool, fever, and leukocytosis. Such characterization of diarrheal illness may not always be clear-cut, as certain bacteria such as *Vibrio parahaemolyticus* may present with inflammatory or noninflammatory syndromes. Recognizing neurological symptoms of food poisoning is critical to diagnosing the rare life-threatening case of botulism and the unusual fish toxin–mediated syndromes such as ciguatera poisoning (see the chapters by Morris and Arnon). Other important systemic symptoms include signs of cholinergic excess in ingestion of a cholinesterase inhibitor insecticide or anticholinergic symptoms due to mushrooms containing ibotenic acid and muscimol. Symptoms of histamine excess occur in scombroid fish poisoning and the cutaneous burning and tightness seen with monosodium glutamate ingestion in the Chinese restaurant syndrome.

The specific pathogenic mechanism by which these agents produce disease helps explain the incubation period observed with different foodborne diseases. Foodborne bacterial disease is often toxin-mediated. Toxins may be preformed in the food before ingestion or produced *in vivo* as the result of replication of the bacteria in the gastrointestinal tract. Foodborne illness due to preformed toxins (*S. aureus* and *B. cereus*) results in a short-incubation illness with the rapid onset of toxin-mediated symptoms such as vomiting. In contrast, in *C. perfringens* and long-incubation *B. cereus* disease toxins are produced by bacteria in the gastrointestinal tract, resulting in a longer incubation period. These toxins typically result in noninflammatory, watery diarrhea without evidence of tissue invasion or fecal leukocytes. Organisms capable of tissue invasion include *Salmonella*, *Shigella* sp., invasive *E. coli*, and *Campylobacter*. Disease due to these agents exhibit even longer incubation periods and produce inflammatory colitis.

Acute Upper Gastrointestinal Symptoms, Nausea, Vomiting Within 0–6 Hr

The occurrence of acute gastrointestinal symptoms within 1–6 hr after the ingestion of food suggests the pres-

TABLE 4. *Clinical diagnosis of foodborne illness by incubation period and symptoms*

Predominant symptomatology	Incubation period			
	<2 hr	1–7 hr	8–14 hr	>14 hr
Upper intestinal, nausea/vomiting	Heavy metals, chemicals, mushrooms	*S. aureus*, *B. cereus*, Anisakis	Anisakis	Norwalk agent
Noninflammatory, diarrhea, no fecal leukocytes			*C. perfringens*, *B. cereus*	Enterotoxigenic *E. coli*, *V. cholerae, Giardia lamblia*, Norwalk agent
Inflammatory, ileocolitis				*Salmonella, Shigella, Campylobacter*, invasive, *E. coli*, *V. parahaemolyticus*, *E. histolytica*
Extragastrointestinal, neurological	Insecticides, mushroom and plant toxins, MSG, shellfish, scombroid	Shellfish, ciguatera		Botulism

ence of a preformed toxin or a chemical irritant. Both *S. aureus* and *B. cereus* produce toxin under conditions of improper food storage. The main noninfectious consideration is direct chemical irritation of the gastric mucosa by heavy metals or other direct toxins like fluoride ion. Rarely acute gastrointestinal symptoms are produced by direct invasion of the gastric mucosa by parasitic worms ingested in raw fish. The clinical features that these etiologies share in common include prominent nausea and vomiting. *S. aureus* and *B. cereus* syndromes can include headache, but should not include any motor or sensory neurological features.

Staphylococcal toxin-mediated disease is the prototype for preformed toxin-mediated acute gastrointestinal disease. Three conditions are necessary for staphylococcal food poisoning. First, food must be contaminated with an enterotoxin-producing strain of the bacteria. Second, suitable conditions for growth of the organism must be present. Finally, adequate time and suitable temperature for growth and toxin production must exist. Cooking food contaminated with *S. aureus* will kill the bacteria but will not destroy the heat-stable toxin that has been produced. The mechanism of action of staphylococcal enterotoxins is not completely understood but may include stimulation of interleukin-1, interferon, and tumor necrosis factor (88,89). Animal studies suggest that the enterotoxins produce the emetic response after stimulation of neural receptors and vagus and sympathetic nerves. These in turn activate the vomiting center in the CNS (90,91). Individuals have varied sensitivity to staphylococcal enterotoxin and in a given outbreak symptoms may be present in only a portion of the population exposed to the same dose of toxin. However, when concentration of the toxin is high, the attack rate approaches 100%. The diarrhea is not due to stimulation of adenylate cyclase activity and may be due to inhibition of water and sodium absorption in the small intestine by the enterotoxin (92,93).

Outbreaks of *S. aureus* toxin-mediated gastrointestinal disease have been characterized by potentially large numbers of affected individuals. Time to onset and severity of symptoms depend on the amount of toxin consumed. Symptoms begin with nausea. Severe abdominal cramps develop that are followed by forceful continuous vomiting at 5- to 20-min intervals. Emesis may occasionally be blood-streaked and blood may rarely be seen in the stool in severe cases. Diarrhea is seen in 77% of cases, is usually mild (94), and only rarely occurs in the absence of vomiting. Abdominal pain, if present, is moderate and diffuse and there is no tenesmus. Mild and transient headache and muscular cramps of the flexors of the legs as well as sweating are common. Fever is not characteristic but can occur in up to 23% of cases (94). Individuals may be quite disabled because of the extremely rapid onset of severe vomiting. Extreme vomiting has the potential to lead to severe metabolic alkalosis and rarely hypotension. Fortunately, acute symptoms are self-limited usually lasting 5–8 hr. Symptoms are almost completely resolved by 12 hr, though prostration may remain for up to 24–48 hr. Morbidity and mortality is limited to individuals at risk for severe dehydration and includes children, the elderly, and those with severe underlying medical conditions.

The diagnosis of staphylococcal food poisoning is made on the basis of the characteristic clinical syndrome. More than 10^5 colony-forming units of *Staphylococcus* per gram of food may be cultured. If *Staphylococcus* is cultured from the vomitus or feces of affected individuals or if food handlers are involved, the phage type should be the same as that in the food. Immunologically based assays, including enzyme-linked immunosorbent assay for enterotoxin, can detect as little as 0.1–1.0 ng of toxin per gram of food and may be useful for diagnosis in cases where the organisms have been killed by food processing (95–97). Antimicrobial therapy is not indicated since the illness is caused by a preformed toxin.

Bacillus cereus causes an emetic syndrome with a short 1- to 6-hr incubation period that is similar to that caused by *S. aureus*. In a small percentage of episodes, incubation periods that are shorter (15–30 min) or longer (6–12 hr) have been reported. Symptoms include vomiting (100%), abdominal cramps (100%), and often diarrhea (33% to 80%) (31,98–100). Fever is not associated with this syndrome. Recovery is usually rapid, taking from 6 to 24 hrs, though affected individuals often seek medical care in emergency rooms (101). Severe dehydration in infants, the elderly, or debilitated populations is a theoretical possibility, but rarely is hospitalization needed. No fatalities have been reported. The syndrome is probably due to a distinct enterotoxin different from that involved in the diarrheal form of *B. cereus* food poisoning. The toxin produces vomiting when fed to rhesus monkeys; however, the mechanism of action of the toxin is unknown (99,102). The diagnosis of outbreaks due to *B. cereus* can be documented by isolation of $>10^5$ organisms per gram of suspected food, but if the food was reheated prior to serving, the organism will be eliminated without decreasing the activity of the heat-stable toxin (101). Organisms may be cultured from the vomitus or stool specimens of affected individuals. Serotyping of *B. cereus*, if available, can be helpful in linking isolates to a common source as 14% of individuals may be transiently colonized in their gastrointestinal tract (102). Plasmid analysis may also play a role in epidemiological investigations (103). As in *S. aureus* foodborne disease, antimicrobial therapy is not indicated.

Bacillus subtilis has also been implicated in a short-incubation emetic syndrome. Vomiting is the major symptom followed by diarrhea occurring in 50% of cases. Additional symptoms include headaches (10%), flushing sensations, and sweating (61).

Heavy metals are a consideration in acute food poisoning especially when the incubation period is less than 1 hr (8). In a report of zinc ingestion due to storage of an acidic beverage in galvanized metal containers symptoms occurred from 5 min to 2 hr after ingestion (105). Zinc is a major constituent of galvanized metal and is converted to readily absorbable zinc salts on contact with acidic beverages. The emetic dose of zinc is 225–450 mg for adults, a level that can be achieved from storage in galvanized containers. Symptoms include nausea (83%), abdominal cramps (61%), metallic taste (33%), headache (33%), dizziness (22%), and chills (11%). Vomiting occurs in only 11% of individuals in contrast to bacterial toxin–mediated syndromes where vomiting is the characteristic feature.

Symptoms usually subside within 2–3 hr after emesis of the offending agent. In a recent outbreak of fluoride poisoning due to faulty fluoridation in a municipal water plant, the median interval between consumption and vomiting was 7 min and the median duration of symptoms was 24 hr. Ninety percent of patients had nausea, 80% vomiting, 52% abdominal pain, and 23% diarrhea. Fluoride ingestion resulted in profound hyperkalemia and hypocalcemia, which may result in cardiac dysrhythmias and death (81).

A major consideration in the differential diagnosis of these emetic syndromes is viral gastroenteritis. Viral gastroenteritis due to Norwalk agent shares many of the features of bacterial toxin–mediated disease. The sudden and widespread involvement in Norwalk virus outbreaks often suggests a common source outbreak that can be related to a foodborne source of infection, although many isolated cases occur as well (106). In addition, the onset of illness due to Norwalk virus is abrupt with explosive vomiting and/or watery diarrhea. Stools are loose and watery without blood, mucus, or fecal leukocytes. Associated symptoms include anorexia, nausea, abdominal cramping, malaise, headache, and myalgias. Fever may be present in as many as 40% of patients (106). There are important differences between Norwalk virus infection and bacterial toxin–mediated disease. The incubation period for Norwalk virus is longer, ranging from 10 to 51 hr, and the secondary attack rates are high resulting in recognition of an ongoing communitywide illness. The diagnosis of viral outbreaks is significantly limited by the current laboratory techniques for detecting these infections. Symptoms of Norwalk agent last 1–5 days, unlike the short duration of vomiting in staphylococcal disease. Carbohydrate and fat malabsorption may occur and last for 2–3 weeks after the initial onset of the illness. The diagnosis of viral gastroenteritis has depended on detection of viral particles in fecal specimens by electron microscopy. New polymerase chain reaction–based assays have been developed and have been used successfully to investigate outbreaks (106). Samples need to be collected within 48 hr after onset of symptoms and should be stored without freezing.

Gastrointestinal symptoms can occur after the ingestion of raw fish containing nematode larvae from the anisakis or eustrongylides family (32,33). Infection may localize acutely in the stomach or may be delayed with small intestine disease. In acute gastric anisakiasis, severe epigastric pain, nausea, and vomiting occur 1–12 hr after the ingestion of raw infected fish. Frequently the episode terminates when the worm is regurgitated. The worm can be visualized and removed during fiberoptic endoscopy. Occasionally invasion of the gastric mucosa occurs, which has been reported to cause perforation of the stomach or intestine. Invasion may also result in chronic gastrointestinal symptoms with a granulomatous response in the gastric mucosa.

Many types of mushrooms cause nonspecific gastrointestinal symptoms of nausea, vomiting, diarrhea, and abdominal cramping. In benign mushroom poisoning, the onset of symptoms ranges from a few minutes to 2–3 hr. The early onset distinguishes benign mushroom poisoning from the late-onset gastrointestinal symptoms that accompany the more serious mushroom poisoning syndromes. The onset of gastrointestinal symptoms is 6–12 hr in poisonings due to amitoxins or monomethylhydrazine containing mushrooms. These gastrointestinal symptoms subside before the onset of life-threatening hepatic and/or renal disease in the second phase of these syndromes. Unfortunately, ingestion of mushrooms often involves multiple species making the presence of early symptoms an unreliable indicator of a benign course.

Upper Small Bowel Symptoms, Noninflammatory Watery Diarrhea, Incubation Period 8–16 hr

The onset of abdominal cramps and diarrhea within 8–16 hr after food ingestion suggests toxin-mediated disease due to *C. perfringens* or *B. cereus*. The toxins produced by these organisms are heat-labile proteins that result in intestinal fluid secretion. The toxins are produced *in vivo*, accounting for the longer incubation period compared to that seen with preformed toxins due to *S. aureus* and the *B. cereus* emetic syndrome. Vomiting is not a prominent feature of these toxins and the presence of vomiting in more than one third of affected patients should suggest that these organisms are not involved. The diarrhea in this syndrome is typically noninflammatory and is usually accompanied by abdominal cramping and nausea. This is in contrast to the inflammatory diarrhea and fever that is often seen with invasive pathogens such as *Salmonella*, *Shigella*, and *Campylobacter*.

The usual symptoms of foodborne disease due to *C. perfringens* include severe abdominal cramps and diarrhea (60). Vomiting is unusual in these cases (61). The symptoms are due to toxin-mediated secretion of sodium and fluid and inhibition of chloride and glucose absorption throughout the small intestine (107,108). The enterotoxin is destroyed at 60°C after 10 min (109). The diagnosis of disease due to *C. perfringens* is difficult because the organism is found in the bowels 42% to 100% of normal individuals and antibody to the enterotoxin is found in 65% to 100% of individuals. In addition, serotyping of organisms, which is generally not available, implicates a specific serotype in only two thirds of outbreaks in the United Kingdom and 20% of outbreaks in the United States. Etiological confirmation is provided by finding 10^6 *C. perfringens* spores per gram of feces within 48 hr after the onset of illness or 10^5 organisms per gram of food (110). Demonstration of enterotoxin in the stool or a fourfold rise in antitoxin serum titers by reverse passive *Bacillus* hemagglutination may be helpful (111).

B. cereus causes a diarrheal syndrome distinct from the emetic syndrome described earlier. The duration of illness is usually less than 24 hr, but has been reported to last several days in at least one outbreak (101). *B. cereus* patients causes a diarrheal syndrome very similar to that of *C. perfringens*. Vomiting may be seen in up to 30% of cases. This syndrome is due to a 50,000-kDa heat-labile protein that activates intestinal adenylate cyclase and results in ileal fluid secretion (68). This toxin may also have cytotoxic activity in rabbit small intestine and guinea pig skin (68). The diagnosis of diarrheal illness due to *B. cereus* is based on culturing greater than 10^5 organisms from the implicated food. Isolation of the organism from the feces of affected individuals may include serotyping to confirm that the isolates were derived from a common source. There appears to be no consistent relationship between diarrheal and emetic toxin production by any given strain of *B. cereus*.

The differential diagnosis of noninflammatory diarrhea includes other infectious agents, mushrooms and other toxins, and primary gastrointestinal disorders. Many of these disorders, including infections with enterotoxigenic *E. coli* and viral agents, are difficult to diagnose without specialized laboratory facilities (112). Bacterial pathogens to consider include enterotoxigenic *E. coli*, *Vibrio parahaemolyticus,* and occasionally *Campylobacter jejuni, Salmonella,* and *Shigella.* These organisms typically have a median incubation period of 24–48 hr, which is longer than that seen with *B. cereus* and *C. perfringens.* Shorter incubation periods are seen though, presenting some potential for confusing these syndromes (112). The symptoms are similar with abdominal cramps and watery diarrhea and the absence of fever and vomiting. In contrast to infection with *B. cereus* and *C. perfringens,* patients with *E. coli* are often ill for 72–96 hr, which distinguishes these organisms. Viral gastroenteritis can mimic these syndromes, although vomiting is usually prominent and the occurrence of secondary cases not exposed to the suspected food is an important clue. Mushroom poisoning due to *Amanita* species presents with a biphasic disease that begins with self-limited abdominal cramps and diarrhea for less than 24 hours. This is followed by hepatic and renal failure 1–2 days later, which has a mortality rate of 30% to 50%.

Inflammatory Diarrhea with an Incubation Period Greater Than 16 hr

Organisms causing this syndrome are capable of tissue invasion and include *Salmonella, Shigella, C. jejuni, V. parahaemolyticus,* and invasive *E. coli.* Fever, abdominal cramps, and inflammatory diarrhea with fecal leukocytes and fecal blood are common with these organisms. The illnesses last 2–7 days and vomiting occurs in 35% to 80% of cases. *Yersinia enterocolitica* is a common cause of foodborne disease in northern Europe and Canada, and is notable for causing a syndrome of abdominal pain and fever resembling acute appendicitis. Hemorrhagic colitis complicated by hemolytic uremic syndrome has been traced to foodborne disease due to *E. coli* serotype O157: H7 (113).

Neurological or Systemic Symptoms With/Without Gastrointestinal Symptoms

The occurrence of neurological symptoms is critically important to recognize when evaluating possible food poisoning episodes. Important diseases that present with neurological symptoms include botulism, several distinct

fish- and shellfish-related syndromes, several types of mushroom poisoning, and chemical and pesticide poisoning. Muscular symptoms with eosinophilia should alert one to the possibility of trichinosis.

Mushroom syndromes include several defined syndromes with characteristic systemic features. Cyclopeptides found in *Amanita* mushrooms interfere with RNA metabolism and cause hepatic and renal necrosis, often requiring eventual transplantation. Mushrooms containing ibotenic acid and muscimol mimic alcohol intoxication. Species containing muscarine cause parasympathetic symptoms. Hallucinogenic mushrooms containing psilocibin and psilocin cause acute psychotic reactions with hallucinations and inappropriate behavior. Coprinus mushrooms contain a disulfiram-like substance that causes an antibuse-like reaction after ingestion of alcohol. *Gyromitra* species contain methyhydrazine, which may result in hepatic dysfunction, hemolysis, seizures, and coma. The treatment of mushroom poisoning is based on limited data and differs depending on the type of mushroom ingested (10).

The acute onset of abdominal pain, nausea, vomiting, and diarrhea in conjunction with peripheral and central nervous system symptoms and skeletal muscle symptoms should suggest the ingestion of a cholinesterase inhibitor (77). Symptoms of cholinergic excess can occur within 5 min of ingestion and include profuse sweating and salivation, blurred vision, pinpoint pupils, and excessive tearing. Muscle fasciculations and weakness, bradycardia and seizures, disorientation, and excitement also can occur. Both carbamate and organophosphate pesticides can cause this syndrome; however, because carbamates are reversible inhibitors of cholinesterases, poisoning with these compounds is less severe. Treatment is with atropine and supportive therapy.

The Chinese restaurant syndrome presents with a burning in the neck, chest, abdomen, or arms and a sense of tightness over the face and chest. Headache, flushing, diaphoresis, lacrimation, nausea, abdominal cramps, and thirst also frequently occur (114). Symptoms are probably due to ingestion of monosodium glutamate that is ingested on an empty stomach in wonton soup.

The differential diagnosis of foodborne illness with neurological symptoms includes several fish and shellfish toxin syndromes and botulism. A history of fish ingestion should suggest either histamine fish poisoning or ciguatera fish poisoning. Shellfish may be associated with either a paralytic syndrome including paralysis and respiratory insufficiency or a neurotoxic syndrome without paralysis.

DIAGNOSTIC MEASURES AND EPIDEMIOLOGICAL ASSESSMENT

The diagnosis of foodborne illness can be important in establishing an etiology and devising a therapeutic plan for a patient as well as for public health surveillance of an outbreak. The differing diagnostic tests available for each etiological agent is shown in Table 5. The diagnostic approach to an individual patient may consider both the importance of establishing a definitive diagnosis and the

TABLE 5. *Diagnosis of foodborne illness*

Source	Patient-based tests	Food
Bacterial		
Salmonella	Culture stool, blood	Culture
Clostridium botulinum	Culture stool, vomitus	Culture
	Toxin stool, vomitus, blood	Toxin[a]
Staphylococcus aureus	Culture stool, vomitus	>10^5 organisms/g food toxin[a]
Shigella	Culture stool	Culture
Campylobacter jejuni	Culture stool	Culture
Clostridium perfringens	Culture stool 10^6 org/gram stool, toxin stool[a]	>50^5 organisms/g food
Bacillus cereus	Culture stool, vomitus	>10^5 organisms/g food
Escherichia coli	Culture stool	
O157:H7	Sorbitol–MacConkey agar[a]	Culture
entertoxigenic	LT and ST toxin production[a]	
Vibrio parahaemolyticus	Culture stool	Culture
Vibrio cholerae	Culture stool	Culture
Chemicals/Toxins		
Ciguatoxin		Bioassay for toxin[a]
		RIA assay for toxin[a]
Scombrotoxin		Histamine concentration[a]
		>100 mg/100 g fish
Mushrooms	Hepatic transaminase levels	Toxin testing[a], identification by mycologist
Heavy metals	Clinical syndrome	Metal detection[a]
Monosodium glutamate		Toxin[a]
Shellfish poisoning		Toxin[a]
Parasitic		
Trichinella spiralis	Eosinophilia, serum antibody titer[a]	
Giardia	Stool exam, duodenal fluid exam	
Cryptosporidium	Stool acid-fast stain	
Anasakiasis	Gastroscopy	
Viral		
Hepatitis A	Serology anti-HAV IgM	
Norwalk virus	Stool PCR analysis[a], electron microscopy[a]	
	Acute/convalescent serum titers	

[a] Test may not be routinely available in some laboratories.

cost of the evaluation. For example, the cost of routine stool cultures in the evaluation of infectious gastroenteritis has been estimated to be about $950–$1200 per positive result (115). The cost of the evaluation can be reduced significantly by ordering stool cultures and stool ova and parasite exams only in selected patients, especially those with prolonged or inflammatory symptoms. When a specific diagnosis of foodborne illness is sought, the clinician must anticipate that some diagnostic tests will not be routinely available. Tests that must be specifically requested include identification of pathogenic *E. coli,* Norwalk virus identification, acid-fast staining for *Cryptosporidium,* and most assays for bacterial, plant, or animal toxins. Consultation with local experts in the hospital or health department may be helpful in facilitating the evaluation.

Foodborne disease surveillance addresses several objectives including timely disease prevention and control, knowledge of disease causation, and future guidance for food protection programs and public health programs (8). Surveillance may be complicated by transportation of foods over large areas with the potential for outbreaks to involve several states and countries from a single source of food (77,106). The meal responsible for an outbreak of food poisoning is identified through patient interviews. Food-specific attack rates can then be calculated for all the foods and beverages served at the meal. Controls should be found among those who ate at the meal but who did not become ill. The incriminated food should have a significantly higher attack rate for those who ingested the food than for those who did not, and most of those who became ill must have eaten the incriminated food. Laboratory diagnosis of outbreaks of foodborne illness is limited by the benign nature of many acute foodborne illnesses that results in a lack of reporting of most outbreaks. In addition, state laboratories may vary in the tests that they offer. For example, 20% of state laboratories do not offer *B. cereus* testing routinely (30). In addition, reporting requirements for important foodborne illnesses such as *E. coli* O15:H7 may vary significantly among states, with a majority of states not requiring reporting (13).

MANAGEMENT

Management of foodborne disease is based on recognizing that the majority of illness are self-limited and therapy

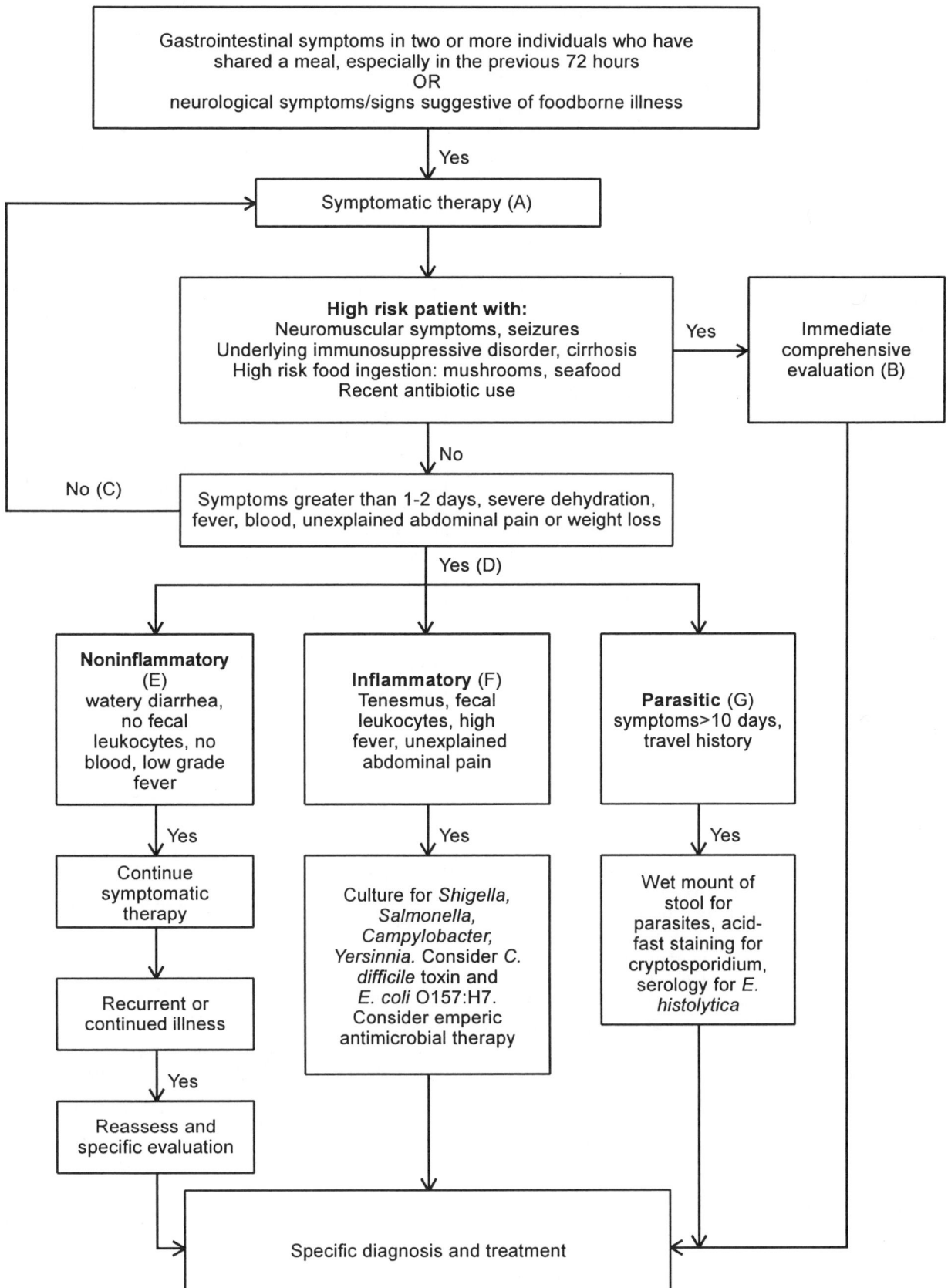

FIG. 1. Management of foodborne disease begins with symptomatic therapy (*A*) and the identification of high-risk patients requiring immediate comprehensive evaluation (*B*). Low-risk patients without prolonged symptoms or other risk factors are treated symptomatically (*C*). Patients with continued symptoms or suggestive signs (*D*) are differentiated into noninflammatory (*E*), inflammatory (*F*), and possible parasitic disease (*G*) for further management.

nonspecific and supportive (116). Initial management focuses on rehydration while identifying those cases requiring urgent diagnosis and intervention because of the potential for serious neurological or systemic involvement (Fig. 1). In low-risk patients with isolated gastrointestinal disease, management is based on the expectation of rapid recovery. Treatment is directed at replacing gastrointestinal fluid losses with oral or parenteral electrolyte solutions. Where toxin ingestion is recognized early, emesis may be induced if it has not occurred spontaneously. Antiemetics are contraindicated as they may allow further systemic absorption. Antiperistaltic agents should be avoided in patients with fever or fecal leukocytes, which suggest the presence of an invasive pathogen. The majority of the acute gastrointestinal illnesses discussed in this chapter resolve within 12–24 hr. The clinical course is not shortened by antibiotic therapy, and rarely do these illnesses result in significant morbidity or mortality. The diagnosis in these patients with self-limited illness can be inferred from the clinical presentation (Table 4). Identification of a specific etiology is usually not necessary for the management of individual patients. In contrast, diagnostic evaluation is indicated in patients who have either symptoms for more than 1–2 days duration, severe dehydration, fever, bloody diarrhea, or unexplained abdominal pain or weight loss. In these patients, further evaluation may identify a bacterial or parasitic agent that requires antimicrobial therapy. Despite this, most patients with prolonged symptoms have benign and self-limited viral or bacterial disease for which antimicrobial agents are not indicated. Emperic therapy for patients with febrile dysenteric illness may also be indicated (116).

PREVENTION

Foodborne diseases are largely preventable through the practice of proper food hygiene in combination with laws governing domestic and imported foods (117). In most outbreaks due to bacterial pathogens such as staphylococci, *B. cereus,* and *C. perfringens,* the disease occurred because food was stored at improper holding temperatures. Growth of pathogens can be prevented if cold food is rapidly cooled and kept adequately refrigerated (<40°F) and if hot food is held at temperatures above 140°Fahrenheit before serving (47). Poor personal hygiene of food handlers plays a role in bacterial as well as Norwalk agent outbreaks. Cooking of food before serving will eliminate the risk of disease for some agents, but not for staphylococcal toxins and disease due to other organisms capable of producing heat-stable toxins. Inadequate cooking is usually an important factor in outbreaks of trichinosis and shellfish-borne disease. Shellfish meat should be heated to a temperature of 85–90°C for 1.5 min in order to inactivate hepatitis A and other viruses (118). Contamination of food after cooking may result from poor food-handling practices. Chlorine-based compounds should be used to disinfect contaminated cooking surfaces.

Investigations of outbreaks suggest that food handlers may be unaware of even the most common hazards associated with foodborne disease such as fried rice (30). Outbreaks of potential hepatitis A need to be investigated rapidly to allow early administration of immunoglobulin to exposed individuals including other food handlers (2). High-risk patients, such as patients with liver cirrhosis and immunocompromised individuals, should be aware that foods such as raw oysters present a risk of fatal septicemia with *Vibrio vulnificus;* unfortunately, less than 15% of high-risk patients are aware of the risks associated with raw oyster consumption (17). These findings emphasize the need for education about basic practices for safe food handling and consumption.

Selection of foods plays an increasingly important role in preventing foodborne disease as food is transported worldwide and exotic foods are increasingly consumed. Raw or undercooked foods including milk, poultry, beef, pork, shellfish, fish, and eggs are important sources of foodborne pathogens. Application of polluted water or sewage sludge to fruit and vegetable crops can lead to transmission of bacterial, parasitic, and viral agents. Expertise in identification of safe food sources is necessary to prevent outbreaks of ciguatera and mushroom poisoning. Many chemical food poisonings result from use of defective storage containers, introduction of insecticides and other compounds into foods, or contamination of water supplies. Cysts of *Giardia* and *Cryptosporidium* are chlorine-resistant and require highly effective filtration to prevent their spread. Since suspected foodborne or waterborne illnesses may represent a threat to large numbers of people, these outbreaks should be recognized and promptly reported to the CDC and U.S. Department of Agriculture through local and state health departments.

REFERENCES

1. Ruddy S, Johnson R, Moseley J, Atwater J, Rossetti M, Hart J. An epidemic of clam-associated hepatitis. *JAMA* 1969;208: 649–655.
2. Skala M, Collier C, Hinkle CJ, et al. Foodborne Hepatitis S—Missouri, Wisconsin, and Alaska, 1990–1992. *MMWR* 1993;42:526–529.
3. Wise RI. Brucellosis in the United States—past, present, and future. *JAMA* 1980;244:2318–2322.
4. Schuchat A, Deaver K, Wenger JD, et al. Role of foods in sporadic listeriosis. I. Case-control study of dietary risk factors. *JAMA* 1992;267:2041–2045.
5. Linnan MJ, Mascola L, Lou XD, et al. Epidemic listeriosis associated with Mexican-style cheese. *N Engl J Med* 1988;319: 823–828.
6. St. Louis ME, Peck SHS, Bowering D, et al. Botulism from chopped garlic: delayed recognition of a major outbreak. *Ann Intern Med* 1988;108:363–368.
7. Ishizuka T, Ishizuka A. A case of diphyllobothriasis due to eating masousushi. *Med J Aust* 1986;145:114.
8. Bean NH, Griffin PM, Goulding JS, Ivey CB. Foodborne disease outbreaks, 5-year summary, 1983–1987. *MMWR* 1990; 39(SS-1):15–57.
9. Eastaugh J, Shepherd S. Infectious and toxic syndromes from fish and shellfish consumption. *Arch Intern Med* 1989;149: 1735–1740.
10. *The Medical Letter on Drugs and Therapeutics. Mushroom Poisoning* 1984;26:67–69.
11. Sweeney K, Gensheimer KF, Knowlton-Field J, et al. Water hemlock poisoning—Maine, 1992. *MMWR* 1994;43:229–231.
12. Litovitz TL. 1992 annual report of the American Association of Poison Control Centers Toxic Exposure Surveillance System. *Am J Emerg Med* 1993;11:494–555.

13. Herwaldt BL, Craun GF, Stokes SL, Juranek DD. Waterborne-disease outbreaks, 1989–1990. In: CDC *Surveillance Summaries,* December 1991. *MMWR* 1991;40(No. SS3):1–22.
14. O'Mahony MC, Gooch CD, Smyth DA, Thrussell AJ, Bartlett CLR, Noah ND. Epidemic hepatitis A from cockles. *Lancet.* 1983;1:518–520.
15. Morse DI, Guzewich JJ, Hanrahan JP, et al. Widespread outbreaks of clam- and oyster-associated gastroenteritis. Role of Norwalk virus. *N Engl J Med* 1986;314:678–681.
16. Appleton H, Pereira MS. A possible virus aetiology in outbreaks of food poisoning from cockles. *Lancet* 1977;1:780–781.
17. Hlady WG, Mullen RC, Hopkins RS. *Vibrio vulnificus* infections associated with raw oyster consumption—Florida, 1981–1992. *MMWR* 1993;42:405–407.
18. Wilson R, Lieb S, Roberts A, et al. Non-O group 1 *Vibrio cholerae* gastroenteritis associated with eating raw oysters. *Am J Epidemiol* 1981;114:293–298.
19. Blake P, Merson H, Weaver R, Hollis D, Heublein P. Disease caused by a marine vibrio. *N Engl J Med* 1979;300:1–4.
20. Eichold BH, Williamson JR, Woernle CH, et al. Isolation of *Vibrio cholerae* O1 from oysters—Mobile Bay, 1991–1992. *MMWR* 1993;42:91–93.
21. Engleberg N, Morris J, Lewis J, McMillan J, Pollard R. Ciguatera fish poisoning: a major common-source outbreak in the US Virgin Islands. *Ann Intern Med* 1983;98:336–337.
22. Frenette C, MacLean JD, Gyorkos TW. A large common-source outbreak of ciguatera fish poisoning. *J Infect Dis* 1988;158:1128–1131.
23. Chretien J, Fermaglich J, Garagusi V. Ciguatera poisoning presentation as a neurological disorder. *Arch Neurol* 1981;15:1225–1228.
24. Morrow JD, Margolies GR, Rowland J, Roberts LJ. Evidence that histamine is the causative toxin of scombroid-fish poisoning. *N Engl J Med* 1991;324:716–720.
25. Kim R. Flushing syndrome due to mahimahi (scombroid fish) poisoning. *Arch Dermatol* 1979;115:963–965.
26. Etkind P, Wilson M, Gallagher K, Cournoyer J. Bluefish-associated scombroid poisoning. *JAMA* 1987;258:3409–3410.
27. Sims J, Ostman D. Puffer fish poisoning: emergency diagnosis and management of mild human tetrodotoxication. *Ann Emerg Med* 1986;15:1094–1098.
28. Popkiss M, Horstman D, Harpur D. Paralytic shellfish poisoning: a report of 17 cases in Capetown. *South Afr Med J* 1979;55:1017–1022.
29. Acres J, Gray J. Paralytic shellfish poisoning. *Can Med Assoc J* 1978;119:1195–1197.
30. Khodr M, Hill S, Perkins L, et al. *Bacillus cereus* food poisoning associated with fried rice at two child day care centers—Virginia, 1993. *MMWR* 1994;43:177–178.
31. Mortimer PR, McCann G. Food-poisoning episodes associated with *Bacillus cereus* in fried rice. *Lancet* 1974;1:1043.
32. Wittner M, Turner JW, Jacquette G, Ash LR, Salgo MP, Tanowitz HB. Eustrongylidiasis—a parasitic infection acquired by eating sushi. *N Engl J Med* 1989;320:1124–1126.
33. Schantz PM. The dangers of eating raw fish. *N Engl J Med* 1989;320:1143–1145.
34. Turney C, Green-Smith M, Shipp M, et al. *Escherichia coli* O157:H7 outbreak linked to home-cooked hamburger—California, July 1993. *MMWR* 1994;43:213–215.
35. Bailey TM, Schantz PM. Trichinosis surveillance, 1985. *MMWR* 1986;36(SS-2):1–5.
36. Herrera JL, Hill S, Shaw J, et al. Hepatitis E among U.S. travelers, 1989–1992. *MMWR* 1993;42:1–4.
37. Crooke C. Continued use of drinking water wells contaminated with hazardous chemical substances—Virgin Islands and Minnesota, 1981–1993. *MMWR* 1994;43:89–91.
38. Todd E. Epidemiology of foodborne illness: North America. *Lancet* 1990;336:788–790.
39. Appleton H. Small round viruses: classification and role in foodborne infections. In: Bock J, Whelan J, eds. *Novel diarrhoea viruses (CIBA Foundation Symposium 128).* Chichester: Wiley; 1987:108–125.
40. Waites WM, Arbuthnott JP. Foodborne illness: an overview. *Lancet* 1990;336:722–725.
41. Bloch AB, Stramer SL, Smith JD, et al. Recovery of hepatitis A virus from a water supply responsible for a common source outbreak of hepatitis A. *Am J Public Health* 1990;80:428–430.
42. Blacklow NR, Greenberg HB. Viral gastroenteritis. *N Engl J Med* 1991;325:252–256.
43. Iverson AM, Gill M, Bartlett CL, Cubitt WD, McSwiggan DA. Two outbreaks of foodborne gastroenteritis caused by a small round structured virus: evidence of prolonged infectivity in a food handler. *Lancet* 1987;2:556–558.
44. Levine WC, Stephenson WT, Craun GF. Waterborne disease outbreaks, 1986–1988. *MMWR* 1990;39(SS-1):1–13.
45. Griffin MT, Surowiec JL, McCloskey DI, et al. Foodborne Norwalk virus. *Am J Epidemiol* 1982;115:178–184.
46. Collins RK, Henderson MN, Conwill DE, et al. Multiple outbreaks of staphylococcal food poisoning caused by canned mushrooms. *MMWR* 1989;38:417–418.
47. Tranter HS. Foodborne staphylococcal illness. *Lancet* 1990;336:1044–1046.
48. Santos EC dos, Genigeorgis C, Farver TB. Prevalence of Staphylococcus aureus in raw and pasteurized milk used for commercial manufacturing of Brazilian Minas cheese. *J Food Protect* 1981;44:172–176.
49. Breckinridge JC, Bergdoll MS. Outbreak of foodborne gastroenteritis due to a coagulase-negative enterotoxin-producing staphylococcus. *N Engl J Med* 1971;284:541.
50. Merson MH. The epidemiology of staphylococcal foodborne disease. *Proceedings of the Staphylococcus in Foods Conference.* University Park, PA: *Pennsylvania State University;* 1973:20.
51. Marrack P, Kappler J. The staphylococcal enterotoxins and their relatives. *Science* 1990;248:705–711.
52. Holmberg SD, Blake PA. Staphylococcal food poisoning in the United States: new facts and old misconceptions. *JAMA* 1984;251:487.
53. Bergdoll MS. *Staphylococcus aureus.* In: Doyle MP, ed. *Bacterial foodborne pathogens.* New York: Marcel Dekker; 1989:464–523.
54. Tatini Sr. Thermal stability of enterotoxins in food. *J Milk Food Technol* 1976;39:432–438.
55. Schwabe M, Notermans S, Boot R, Tatini SR, Kramer J. Inactivation of staphylococcal enterotoxins by heat and reactivation by high pH treatment. *Int Food Microbiol* 1990;10:33–42.
56. Spero L, Morlock BA. Biological activities of the peptides of staphylococcal enterotoxin C formed by limited tryptic hydrolysis. *J Biol Chem* 1978;253:8787–8791.
57. Stelma GN, Bergdoll MS. Inactivation of staphylococcal enterotoxin A by chemical modification. *Biochem Biophys Res Commun* 1982;105:121–126.
58. Scheuber PH, Golecki JR, Kickhofen F, Scheel D, Beck G, Hammer DK. Skin reactivity of unsensitized monkeys upon challenge with staphylococcal enterotoxin B: a new approach for investigating the site of toxic action. *Infect Immun* 1985;50:869–876.
59. De Saxe M, Coe AW, Wieneke AA. The use of phage typing in the investigation of food poisoning caused by *Staphylococcus aureus* enterotoxins. *Soc Appl Bacteriol Tech Ser* 1982;17:173–197.
60. Shandera WX, Tacket CO, Blake PA. Food poisoning due to *Clostridium perfringens* in the United States. *J Infect Dis* 1983;147:167.
61. Lund BM. Foodborne disease due to *Bacillus* and *Clostridium* species. *Lancet* 1990;336:982–986.
62. Labbe R. *Clostridium perfringens.* In: Doyle MP, ed. *Foodborne bacterial pathogens.* New York: Marcel Dekker; 1989:191–234.
63. McClane B, Hanna P, Wnek A. *Clostridium perfringens* enterotoxin. *Microb Pathog* 1988;4:317–323.
64. Bowness P, Moss PA, Tranter H, et al. *Clostridium perfringens* enterotoxin is a superantigen reactive with human T cell receptors V beta 6.9 and V beta 22. *J Exp Med* 1992;176:893–896.
65. Loewenstein MS. Epidemiology of *Clostridium perfringens* food poisoning. *N Engl J Med* 1972;286:1026.
66. Terranova W, Blake PA. *Bacillus cereus* food poisoning. *N Engl J Med* 1978;298:143.

67. Turnbull PCB, Kramer JM, Jorgensen K. Properties and production characteristics of vomiting, diarrheal, and necrotizing toxins of *Bacillus cereus*. *Am J Clin Nutr* 1979;32:219.

68. Melling J, Capel BJ, Turnbull PCB, et al. Identification of a novel enterotoxigenic activity associated with *Bacillus cereus*. *J Clin Pathol* 1976;29:938.

69. Spira WM, Goepfert JM. Biological characteristics of an enterotoxin produced by *Bacillus cereus*. *Can J Microbiol* 1975; 21:1236–1246.

70. Morgan MRA, Fenwick GR. Natural foodborne toxicants. *Lancet* 1990;336:1492–1495.

71. Stoloff L. Carcinogenicity of aflatoxins. *Science* 1987;237: 1283–1284.

72. Casemore DP. Foodborne protozoal infection. *Lancet* 1990; 336:1427–1432.

73. Smith JV, Rose JB. Waterborne cryptosporidiosis. *Parasitol Today* 1990;6:8–12.

74. Osterholm MT, Forfang JC, Ristinen TL, et al. An outbreak of foodborne giardiasis. *N Engl J Med* 1981;304:24.

75. Petersen LR, Cartter ML, Hadler JL. A foodborne outbreak of *Giardia lamblia*. *J Infect Dis* 1988;157:846–848.

76. Huxtable RJ. The toxicology of alkaloids in foods and herbs. In Tu AT (ed.), *Handbook of natural toxins. Vol 7. Food Poisoning*. Marcel Dekker: New York; 1992:238–262.

77. Jackson RJ, Stratton JW, Goldman LR, et al. Aldicarb food poisoning from contaminated melons—California. *MMWR* 1986;35:254–258.

78. Martinez-Navarro JF. Food poisoning related to consumption of illicit B-agonist in liver. *Lancet* 1989;336:1311.

79. Baker TD, Hafner WG. Cadmium poisoning from a refrigerator shelf used as an improvised barbecue grill. *Public Health Rep*. 1961;76:543.

80. Semple AB, Parry WH, Phillips DE. Acute copper poisoning: an outbreak traced to contaminated water from a corroded geyser. *Lancet* 1960;2:700.

81. Gessner BD, Beller M, Middaugh JP, Whitford GM. Acute fluoride poisoning from a public water system. *N Engl J Med* 1994;330:95–99.

82. Kibourne EM, Rigau-Perez JG, Heath CW Jr, et al. Clinical epidemiology of toxic-oil syndrome: manifestations of a new illness. *N Engl J Med* 1983;309:1408–1410.

83. Hughes J, Merson M. Fish and shellfish poisoning. *N Engl J Med* 1976;295:1117–1120.

84. Woolf GM, Rojter SE, Villamil FG, et al. Jin Bu Huan toxicity in adults—Los Angeles, 1993. *MMWR* 1993;42:920–922.

85. Kingsbury JM. Poisonous plants of the United States and Canada. Englewood Cliffs, NJ: Prentice-Hall; 1964.

86. Litovitz TL. 1992 annual report of the American Association of Poison Control Centers Toxic exposure surveillance system. *Am J Emerg Med* 1993;11:494–555.

87. Hall AH, Spoerke DG, Rumack BH. Mushroom poisoning: identification, diagnosis, and treatment. *Pediatrics in Review* 1987;8:291–298.

88. Marrack P, Kappler J. The staphylococcal enterotoxins and their relatives. *Science* 1990;248:705–711.

89. Yaqoob M, McClelland P, Murray AE, Mostafa SM, Ahmad R. Staphylococcal enterotoxins A and C causing toxic shock syndrome. *J Infect* 1990;20:176–177.

90. Sugiyama H, Hayama T. Abdominal viscera as site of emetic action for staphylococcal enterotoxin in the monkey. *J Infect Dis* 1965;115:330.

91. Clark WG, Vanderhooft GF, Borison HL. Emetic effect of purified staphylococcal enterotoxin in cats. *Proc Soc Exp Biol Med* 1962;111:205.

92. Elias J, Shields R. Influence of staphylococcal enterotoxin on water and electrolyte transport in the small intestine. *Gut* 1976; 17:527.

93. Beery JT, Taylor SL, Schlunz LR, Freed RC, Bergdoll MS. Effects of staphylococcal enterotoxin A on the rat gastrointestinal tract. *Infect Immun* 1984;44:234–240.

94. Feig M. Staphylococcal food poisoning. A report of two related outbreaks, and a discussion of the data presented. *Am J Public Health* 1950;40:279.

95. Tranter HS, Brehm RD. Production, purification and identification of the staphylococcal enterotoxins. *Soc Appl Bacteriol Symp Ser* 1990;19:109S–122S.

96. Fey H. Staphylococcal enterotoxins. In: Kohler RB, ed. *Antigen to diagnose bacterial infection*. Vol 2. Florida: CRC Press; 1986:211–238.

97. Berry PR, Rodhouse JC, Wieneke AA, Gilbert RJ. Use of commercial kits for the detection of *Clostridium perfringens* and *Staphylococcus aureus* enterotoxins. *Soc Appl Bacteriol Tech Ser* 1987;24:245–254.

98. Giannella RA, Brasile L. A hospital food-borne outbreak of diarrhea caused by *Bacillus cereus*. Clinical epidemiologic, and microbiologic studies. *J Infect Dis* 1979;139:366.

99. Terranova W, Blake PA. *Bacillus cereus* food poisoning. *N Engl J Med* 1978;298:143.

100. Midura T, Gerber M, Wood R, et al. Outbreak of food poisoning caused by *Bacillus cereus*. *Public Health Rep*. 1970;85:45.

101. Vandeloski J, Gensheimer KF. *Bacillus cereus*—Maine. *MMWR* 1986;35:408–410.

102. Turnbull PCB, Kramer JM, Jorgensen K. Properties and production characteristics of vomiting, diarrheal, and necrotizing toxins of *Bacillus cereus*. *Am J Clin Nutr* 1979;32:219.

103. Ghosh AC. Prevalence of *Bacillus cereus* in the faeces of healthy adults. *J Hyg* 1978;80:233.

104. DeBuono BA, Brondum J, Kramer JM, et al. Plasmid, serotypic, and enterotoxin analysis of *Bacillus cereus* in an outbreak setting. *J Clin Microbiol* 1988;26:1571–1574.

105. Lapham S, Vanderly R, Brackbill R, et al. Illness associated with elevated levels of zinc in fruit punch—New Mexico. *MMWR* 1983;32:257–258.

106. Conrad C, Hemphill K, Wilson S, et al. Multistate outbreak of viral gastroenteritis related to consumption of oysters—Louisiana, Maryland, Mississippi, and North Carolina, 1993. *MMWR* 1993;42:945–948.

107. McDonel JL, Duncan CL. Regional localization of activity of *Clostridium perfringens* type A enterotoxin in the rabbit ileum, jejunum and duodenum. *J Infect Dis* 1977;136:661.

108. McDonel JL, The molecular mode of action of *Clostridium perfringens* enterotoxin. *Am J Clin Nutr* 1979;32:210.

109. Stark RL, Duncan CL. Purification and biochemical properties of *Clostridium perfringens* type A enterotoxin. *Infect Immun* 1972;6:662.

110. Zimomra J, Wenderoth T, Snyder A, et al. *Clostridium perfringens* gastroenteritis associated with corned beef served at St. Patrick's Day meals—Ohio and Virginia, 1993. *MMWR* 1994;43:137–138,144.

111. Skjelkvale R, Uemura T. Detection of enterotoxin in faeces and anti-enterotoxin in serum after *Clostridium perfringens* food poisoning. *J Appl Bacteriol* 1977;42:355–358.

112. Benoit V, Raiche P, Smith MG, et al. Foodborne outbreaks of enterotoxigenic *Escherichia coli*—Rhode Island and New Hampshire, 1993. *MMWR* 1994;43:81,87–89.

113. Davis M, Osaki C, Gordon D, et al. Update: multistate outbreak of *Escherichia coli* O157:H7 infections from hamburgers—Western United States, 1992–1993. *MMWR* 1993;42: 258–263.

114. Schaumburg HH, Byck R, Gerstl R, et al. Monosodium L-glutamate: its pharmacology and role in the Chinese restaurant syndrome. *Science* 1969;163:826.

115. Guerrant RL, Shields DS, Thorson SM, et al. Evaluation and diagnosis of acute infectious diarrhea. *Am J Med* 1985;78: 91–98.

116. Guerrant RL, Bobak DA. Bacterial and protozoal gastroenteritis. *N Engl J Med* 1991;325:327–340.

117. Thompson P, Salsbury PA, Adams C, Archer DL. US Food legislation. *Lancet* 1990;336:1557–1559.

118. Millard J, Appleton H, Parry JV. Studies on heat inactivation of hepatitis A virus with special reference to shellfish. *Epidemiol Infect* 1987;98:397–414.

Infections of the Gastrointestinal Tract,
edited by M. J. Blaser, P. D. Smith, J. I. Ravdin,
H. B. Greenberg, and R. L. Guerrant
Raven Press, Ltd., New York © 1995.

CHAPTER 18

Natural Toxins Associated with Fish and Shellfish

J. Glenn Morris, Jr.

Fish and shellfish can sometimes carry natural toxins or toxic substances that cause human disease. Ciguatera fish poisoning is probably the most common of these intoxications, causing a unique clinical syndrome characterized by a combination of gastrointestinal and neurological symptoms (1–5). Paralytic shellfish poisoning is associated with neurologic symptoms, including, in severe cases, respiratory paralysis. Neurotoxic shellfish poisoning, diarrhetic shellfish poisoning, and amnesic shellfish poisoning occur with less frequency (1,2). In contrast to these entities, which are associated with toxins accumulated while fish or shellfish are alive, scombroid fish poisoning (1,2,6) results from mishandling of scombroid (tuna, mackerel, bonito) and related fish after capture: bacterial decomposition of the fish leads to release of histamine, which in turn causes "histamine poisoning." Each of these clinical syndromes will be considered in this chapter.

CIGUATERA FISH POISONING

Ciguatera fish poisoning is a clinical syndrome with characteristic gastrointestinal and neurological symptoms that occurs after the ingestion of tropical reef fish (3–5). The toxin or toxins that cause the syndrome originate in the dinoflagellate *Gambierdiscus toxicus* and other benthic algae that grow on reefs (7–10). Fish that eat the algae become toxic, and the effect is magnified through the food chain so that large predatory fish become the most toxic.

Pathogenesis

There appear to be multiple toxins responsible (either alone or in combination) for the clinical manifestations of

J. G. Morris, Jr.: Departments of Medicine and Epidemiology and Preventive Medicine, University of Maryland School of Medicine, and Department of Veterans Affairs Medical Center, Baltimore, Maryland 21201.

ciguatera. The toxins and toxin combinations that cause ciguatera may also vary among geographic areas, among fish species, and across time. One of the major contributors to toxic activity is "ciguatoxin," or CTX1. CTX1 is a small, lipid-soluble polyether with a molecular weight of 1112 and a molecular formula of $C_{60}H_{88}O_{19}$ (5,9,11,12). Two other distinct but closely related toxins, CTX2 and CTX3 (9,11,12), have also been identified in ciguatoxic fish, together with at least two minor toxins that may be further oxidized analogs of CTX1 and CTX2 (12). These toxins act primarily by opening voltage-dependent sodium channels in cell membranes (11,13,14). In mice, CTX1 is the most potent of the three (intraperitoneal 50% lethal dose = 0.25 μg/kg, vs. 2.3 and 0.9 μg/kg for CTX2 and CTX3, respectively); however, purified CTX2 and CTX3 induce mouse hindlimb paralysis, while CTX1 does not (11), suggesting that the structural differences in the toxins result in differences in *in vivo* activity.

Scaritoxin, another lipid-soluble neurotoxin, has also been associated with ciguatera by some investigators. This toxin has been shown to depress oxidative metabolic processes in rat brain and has a depolarizing action on excitable membranes. Generally, the pharmacological action is close to that of ciguatoxin, and indeed they may be related compounds. Maitotoxin is a water-soluble toxin that appears to interfere with or modify calcium movement or calcium conductance in tissues (15). Palytoxin, which can cause respiratory distress and severe muscle spasms, has also been isolated from some fish implicated as a cause of ciguatera (16).

While recognizing the diversity of toxins that may be present in ciguatoxic fish, there are certain general pathophysiological responses that have been associated with ciguatera toxins and toxic fish extracts. The gastrointestinal symptoms (diarrhea) seen in patients with ciguatera appear to result from direct stimulation of mucosal ion transport, without accompanying damage to the intestinal mucosa. Extracts from toxic fish cause a striking increase in transepithelial electrical potential difference and short-circuit current in Ussing chambers, with secretion apparently mediated by calcium (17). Neurological symptoms appear to be related to the direct effect of toxin on mammalian nerves, associated with prolongation of sodium channel activation. Electrophysiological studies on rats injected intraperitoneally with toxic fish extracts have demonstrated significant slowing of both mixed and motor nerve conduction velocities; in one study, motor and mixed nerve amplitudes were reduced, and absolute and supernormal periods prolonged (18). Comparable findings were reported in humans with acute ciguatera poisoning, with significant slowing of sensory conduction velocity and prolongation of the absolute refractory, relative refractory, and supernormal periods (19). Toxins and toxic extracts can also affect the cardiovascular system. In animal models, low doses of ciguatoxin cause mild hypotension and bradycardia. Higher doses give a biphasic response with an initial hypotension/bradycardia followed by hypertension/tachycardia; very high doses produce a phrenic nerve block with respiratory arrest (5).

Epidemiology

Ciguatera-associated toxins, produced by dinoflagellates and algae on tropical reefs, are concentrated as they are passed up the food chain. More than 400 fish species are said to have the potential for becoming toxic (20). However, the risk of toxicity is greatest for carnivorous, predatory fish, such as barracuda (over 70% of which may be toxic). Other fish that are commonly implicated in cases of ciguatera include amberjack (*Seriola* species), snappers (Lutjanidae), groupers (Serranidae), goatfish (Mullidae), and reef fish belonging to the Carrangidae (1). Toxicity is associated with fish size, with large fish within a species having a greater risk of toxicity; viscera also tend to have higher concentrations of toxin than fish flesh. The occurrence of toxic fish tends to be localized, but localization is not consistent and toxic fish may occur sporadically anywhere in a reef or island location (1,21,22). There are data suggesting that disruption of the reef environment by construction, military activities, storms, etc., can result in an increase in the incidence of ciguatoxic fish, due presumably to increases in toxic dinoflagellate and algal populations (23,24).

Ciguatera is a significant cause of morbidity in areas in which consumption of reef fish is common, including the Caribbean, southern Florida, Hawaii, the South Pacific, and Australia. The average incidence in the South Pacific from 1973 to 1983 was estimated to have been in the range of 500 cases per 100,000 population per year (25), with some island groups having rates many times higher [the average incidence for 1960–1984 for the Gambier Archipelago has been reported as 22,700 cases per 100,000 population per year (24)]. In a randomized, stratified community survey conducted in the U.S. Virgin Islands, the calculated incidence rate was 730 cases per 100,000 population per year (4). In Puerto Rico, 45 cases were reported to the Puerto Rico Poison Control Center in 1992. In an associated telephone survey, 7% of persons contacted reported that at least one family member had at one time had ciguatera (26). In Miami, on the edge of an endemic

area, 129 cases of ciguatera were reported to the Dade County Health Department between 1972 and 1976, for an annual incidence of 5 cases per 100,000 population; the actual incidence was estimated to be 10–100 times this figure (i.e., 50–500 cases per 100,000 population per year) (27).

Clinical Features

Ciguatera fish poisoning is a clinical diagnosis based on a characteristic sequence of gastrointestinal and neurological symptoms (3,5,21,27–29). As outlined in Table 1, gastrointestinal symptoms include diarrhea, vomiting, and abdominal pain and occur first, usually within 24 hr of eating an implicated fish. In severe cases, patients may also be hypotensive with a paradoxical bradycardia (21,28). These acute symptoms are accompanied or followed by neurological manifestations, which may persist for weeks or months. Neurological symptoms include pain and weakness in the lower extremities, a very characteristic symptom of patients in the Caribbean (21,28), and circumoral and peripheral paresthesias (Table 1). More bizarre symptoms such as temperature reversal (ice cream tastes hot, hot coffee seems cold) and "aching teeth" are frequently reported (3,27,28,30) and may prompt psychiatric referrals among physicians unacquainted with the disease. In very severe cases, particularly in the South Pacific, neurological symptoms may progress to coma and respiratory arrest within the first 24 hr of illness (31).

Toxicity can apparently be transmitted by breast milk (32) and by sexual intercourse (34). Maternal exposure at term may also result in symptoms in the newborn infant, although maternal intoxication during pregnancy does not appear to have a long-term effect on the fetus (35). Immunity does not occur after an initial intoxication; in contrast, intoxication may increase sensitivity to subsequent episodes of illness.

Within this general constellation of symptoms, the clinical syndrome may vary widely from patient to patient and from geographic area to geographic area. In one study of a cluster of ciguatera cases in the U.S. Virgin Islands, only 53% of affected persons had the typical combination of both gastrointestinal and neurological symptoms (21). In studies in the South Pacific, 89.1% of patients have been reported to experience circumoral paresthesias (3) compared with 54% of patients in Miami (27) and 36% of patients in St. Thomas, U.S. Virgin Islands (28). Variations in the symptom complex have also been associated with the type of fish eaten. In a Hawaiian study, circumoral paresthesias were reported in 75.7% of patients who had eaten *Ctenochaetus strigosus* (surgeon fish or kole), 68.4 of patients who had eaten *Seriola dumerili* (amberjack or kahala), and 28.4% of patients who had eaten *Caranx* spp. (ulua/papio or jack). Bradycardia, in contrast, was reported in 47.4% of patients who had eaten *S. dumerili*, but only 5.3% of patients who had eaten *Caranx* spp. and none of those who had consumed *S. dumerili* (36).

Although most patients recover completely within a few weeks, intermittent recrudescence of symptoms over a

TABLE 1. *Symptoms of 33 persons with ciguatera fish poisoning, St. Thomas, U.S. Virgin Islands, Jan. 1–April 10, 1990*

Symptom	No. (%) of patients with symptom	Median time between eating fish and onset, hr (range)	Median duration, days (range)
Gastrointestinal tract			
Diarrhea	30 (91)	6 (1–15)	1 (1–20)
Vomiting	23 (70)	5 (1–12)	1 (1–7)
Abdominal pain	13 (39)	3 (1–24)	2 (1–7)
Fatigue–malaise	23 (70)	6 (1–24)	7 (1–21)
Pruritus	19 (58)	12 (1–48)	3 (1–14)
Pain, weakness in lower extremities	19 (58)	8.5 (1–48)	10.5 (1–82)
Arthralgias	17 (52)	12 (1–36)	6 (1–30)
Circumoral paresthesia	12 (36)	6 (2–10)	21 (3–74)
Hot and cold reversal	12 (36)	12 (2–24)	14 (6–21)
Paresthesia in extremities	11 (33)	6 (2–10)	18 (3–28)
Headache	11 (33)	15.5 (1–30)	7.5 (1–14)
Myalgia	10 (30)	18 (4–24)	4.5 (1–21)
Bad taste—metallic taste	9 (27)	Insufficient data	Insufficient data
Chills	8 (24)	Insufficient data	Insufficient data
Tooth pain	8 (24)	Insufficient data	Insufficient data
Watery eyes	7 (21)	Insufficient data	Insufficient data
Dizziness	7 (21)	6 (1–12)	1 (1–7)
Sweating	6 (18)	12 (6–24)	1 (1–1)
Tremor	3 (9)	Insufficient data	Insufficient data
Rash	3 (9)	Insufficient data	Insufficient data

From Morris et al. *Arch Intern Med* 1982;142:1090–1092.

period of months to years can occur. These recrudescences can be triggered by a number of factors, including consumption of fish and alcohol (4). There is also a subset of patients who have long-term, chronic symptoms of fatigue and paresthesias that last for months or years. These symptoms can be quite severe, resulting in almost total disability. Development of chronicity is more likely in persons who had severe initial symptoms, a long interval to severe symptoms, or a long absolute duration of peak symptoms (29).

Diagnostic Measures

As noted above, ciguatera is a clinical diagnosis. There is no confirmatory test, such as a serologic assay (37), that will establish the diagnosis. Standard laboratory tests are usually within normal limits, although there is a report of elevated creatine phosphokinase (to 41,000 U/L) in one patient who ate fish containing palytoxin (16). As noted above, patients may have characteristic electrophysiological findings, including reduced sensory conduction velocity and prolongation of the absolute refractory, relative refractory, and supernormal periods (19).

Ciguatoxic fish have traditionally been identified by one of a number of bioassays, including, in endemic areas, feeding of suspect fish to the family cat (4). More recently, Hokama and colleagues in Hawaii developed a rapid "stick" immunoassay (38) and a solid phase immunobead assay (39) for toxic fish. The immunobead assay has excellent sensitivity; of 1037 fish tested, all illnesses occurred among persons eating fish identified as "positive" or

"borderline." However, specificity, as determined by occurrence of disease, is not as good; illness was reported in association with only 4 of 232 "borderline" fish and 5 of 17 "positive" fish.

Management

Intravenous infusion of mannitol (1 g/kg of 20% solution, infused over 45 min) may have a dramatic effect on acute symptoms of ciguatera fish poisoning, particularly in severe cases (30,40,41). Mannitol has the most pronounced effect on neurological symptoms and may be life saving in severe cases that progressed to coma (30). Whereas gastrointestinal and cardiac symptoms (bradycardia, hypotension) may show some response to mannitol infusion, they may also require symptomatic treatment, including administration of intravenous fluids and atropine (28). The mechanism of action of mannitol is not fully understood, although effects on axonal edema or a scavenger effect have been postulated (40). It should be noted that most of the data on mannitol have come from the South Pacific. Efficacy of therapy may be less in other geographic areas, such as the Caribbean, due to possible differences in the toxins responsible for the observed clinical syndromes.

Treatment of chronic manifestations is more difficult. In one small study (29), amitriptyline showed considerable benefit in two of nine cases and some benefit in an additional four cases. The mechanism of action of the drug is unclear but may be through sodium channel modification. In this same study, tocainide demonstrated some benefit in three of four cases; the fourth case reported worsening of symptoms. Benefit has also been reported with imipramine, nifedipine, and alprazolam (29). Mannitol outside of the acute setting does not appear to be of benefit, and there are no data to support the use of a variety of other proposed therapies, including vitamin B complex, ascorbic acid, and steroids (28,29). As is true for chronic pain syndromes, therapy in chronic cases needs to be individualized, with physician and patient working together to develop a rational, long-term plan of care.

Prevention

Ciguatoxic fish look and taste completely normal, and toxicity is not affected by cooking. In areas in which assays for toxic fish are available (i.e., Hawaii), the risk of toxicity can be reduced by screening all large, "high-risk" fish before their consumption; however, as noted above, the sensitivity of the current assays are not optimal, and their use would result in discarding a large number of borderline fish. In areas without access to laboratory assay systems, toxicity is best avoided by not eating large predacious reef fish; barracuda, in particular, should never be eaten. In such areas, a household cat may also be useful.

PARALYTIC SHELLFISH POISONING

Paralytic shellfish poisoning (PSP) results from eating bivalve molluscs (mussels, clams, oysters, scallops) that contain concentrated toxins produced by toxigenic dinoflagellates (1,2). Toxins associated with PSP are categorized as saxitoxins (42), of which at least 12 have been identified. Saxitoxins are thought to block the propagation of nerve and muscle action potentials by acting at the metal cation binding site in the sodium channels of the nerve membrane and interfering with changes in sodium permeability (2,43). In the United States, the dinoflagellates *Gonyaulax catenella* (West Coast) and *G. tamarenses* (East Coast) are responsible for most illnesses. Strains of these dinoflagellates develop characteristic toxin profiles that usually contain six to eight saxitoxins. Shellfish feeding on dinoflagellate blooms ingest all toxins but may selectively retain or biologically modify some derivatives, resulting in toxin profiles in the shellfish that differ from those of the dinoflagellate (44–46).

In the United States, PSP is primarily a problem in the New England states on the East Coast and in Alaska, California, and Washington on the West Coast (1,2,47). Blooms of the toxic dinoflagellates ("red tides") occur several times each year, primarily from April through October. It is currently not possible to predict occurrence of blooms. When blooms occur, shellfish become toxic and remain toxic for several weeks after the bloom subsides; some species remain toxic (i.e., butter clams in parts of Washington State and Alaska). Between 1976 and 1986, the Centers for Disease Control received reports of 12 PSP outbreaks in the United States involving 134 people, with one death (1). This relatively small number of cases is due, in large part, to aggressive surveillance of

shellfish by health departments in high-risk states, with toxicity identified by a standardized mouse bioassay. Identification of toxic shellfish results in closure of shellfish harvesting areas. When cases occur, they are often associated with noncommercial harvesting of shellfish in closed areas.

Symptoms of PSP are primarily neurological and usually appear within an hour of eating toxic shellfish (1,2,47,48). Symptoms include circumoral paresthesias and paresthesias of the extremities. In more severe cases, there may be ataxia, dysphagia, and mental status changes. In the most severe cases, respiratory paralysis occurs (generally within the first 24 hr of illness), leading to death if respiratory support is not available. The diagnosis is based on clinical presentation and a history of having eaten potentially toxic shellfish immediately before the onset of symptoms. Limited neurophysiological data suggest that patients have prolonged distal motor and sensory latencies, slowed conduction velocities, and moderately diminished amplitudes, compatible with incomplete sodium channel blockade (49).

Treatment of PSP is symptomatic. It has been suggested that treatment should include administration of a cathartic or enema in severe cases to remove unabsorbed toxin from the intestinal tract. Gastric lavage should also be considered if vomiting has not occurred (2). Recovery should be complete, with symptoms usually resolving within hours to days after shellfish ingestion.

Prevention is based on avoiding shellfish harvested from areas known to be toxic or to have had recent dinoflagellate blooms. However, it should be recognized that not all blooms are toxic, and toxicity can occur in the absence of a visible bloom. As noted above, surveillance of harvest areas in the United States is routinely conducted by state health departments. Areas are closed to harvesting when toxin levels in shellfish exceed 80 μg/100 g, with warnings about toxic conditions posted in the media and at harvest sites (47).

OTHER TYPES OF SHELLFISH POISONING

Neurotoxic Shellfish Poisoning

Neurotoxic shellfish poisoning is associated with blooms of *Gymnodinium breve*, which produce brevetoxin (1,2). Red tides caused by this organism occur sporadically in the Gulf of Mexico and off of the coast of Florida; one recent bloom with associated human illnesses was reported from North Carolina (50). Symptoms after eating toxic shellfish include circumoral paresthesias and paresthesias of the extremities, dizziness and ataxia, muscle aches, and gastrointestinal symptoms, including nausea, abdominal pain, vomiting, and diarrhea. Respiratory symptoms have also been reported, associated with aerosolization of the toxin by wind and wave action (51).

Diarrhetic Shellfish Poisoning

Diarrhetic shellfish poisoning is caused by eating mussels, scallops, or clams that have been feeding on *Dino-*

physis fortii or *D. acuminata* (1). In addition to diarrhea, symptoms of diarrhetic shellfish poisoning include nausea, vomiting, and abdominal pain. Okadaic acid and dinophysistoxin-1 have been implicated as the primary toxins responsible for the associated clinical syndrome (52,53). Cases are concentrated in Japan, with recent reports from Europe. No cases have been reported to date in the United States.

Amnesic Shellfish Poisoning

Amnesic shellfish poisoning has been proposed as a name for the clinical syndrome resulting from ingestion of shellfish containing domoic acid, which appears to originate in some varieties of the diatom *Nitzschia pungens* (54). A series of outbreaks due to this toxin were reported in the Atlantic provinces of Canada in 1987. Symptoms included vomiting, abdominal cramps, diarrhea, headache, and loss of short-term memory (54). On neuropsychological testing several months after the acute intoxication, patients were found to have severe anterograde memory deficits with relative preservation of other cognitive functions; patients also had clinical and electromyographic evidence of pure motor or sensorimotor neuropathy or axonopathy. Neuropathological studies in four patients who died demonstrated neuronal necrosis and loss, predominantly in the hippocampus and amygdala (55). Canadian authorities now analyze mussels and clams for domoic acid, and close shellfish beds to harvesting when levels exceed 20 µg/g (1).

SCOMBROID FISH POISONING

Scombroid fish poisoning results from the eating of fish containing high levels of free histamine. The syndrome was initially associated with fish in the families Scombridae and Scomberesocidae (tuna, mackerel, skipjack, and bonito). However, nonscombroid fish, such as mahimahi (dolphin), bluefish, and salmon, are commonly associated with illness (1,56–60).

In contrast to ciguatera and shellfish poisoning, which are caused by a preformed toxin derived from dinoflagellates or algae, scombroid is the result of bacterial decomposition of fish flesh after capture. Scombroid fish in particular contain substantial amounts of free histidine that can be decarboxylated to form histamine by enteric bacteria during spoilage (56,61). Illness may occur when free histamine levels exceed 20 mg/100 g of fish, levels that may be reached without overt evidence of spoilage. The U.S. Food and Drug Administration "action level" (i.e., the level at which further shipment or sale is prohibited) is 50 mg/100 g of fish. Symptoms in humans are associated with high urinary histamine excretion. A recent study demonstrated that this level is independent of mast cell activation (56). The number of reported outbreaks of scombroid fish poisoning in the United States approaches that of ciguatera (1,62). However, while ciguatera cases are concentrated in certain high-risk locations (i.e., areas

with high levels of consumption of reef fish), scombroid tends to occur at low levels throughout the country.

Symptoms of scombroid fish poisoning typically occur within a few hours of eating the implicated fish and can last for up to 12 hr. Typical symptoms include tingling and burning sensations around the mouth, facial flushing and sweating, nausea and vomiting, headache, palpitations, dizziness, rash, and occasionally, swelling of the face and tongue (2,56,57,63,64). Symptoms resolve spontaneously, but antihistamine drugs are effective and may be useful in more severe cases (56). There are no longterm sequelae. Although essentially a clinical diagnosis, the diagnosis can be confirmed by demonstrating high histamine levels in the fish that was eaten or in the patient's urine.

Prevention of scombroid fish poisoning is dependent on preventing spoilage of fish after capture. This is accomplished by rapid cool-down of large fish, such as tuna, and maintenance of a cold chain from the time of harvest until the fish is eaten. This is of particular concern for fish imported from tropical or semitropical areas, and for fish caught by recreational fishermen. For example, some outbreaks have resulted from eating recreationally caught tuna that had been left sitting on deck for several hours after capture. If suspected, toxicity can be confirmed by assaying fish for histamine, although it should be recognized that toxicity may vary from one part of a large fish to another. Toxic fish have been noted to have a "peppery" taste. Recognition of such a taste while eating suspect fish should be a warning not to proceed further with dinner.

REFERENCES

1. Institute of Medicine. *Seafood safety.* Washington, DC: National Academy Press; 1991.
2. Hughes JM, Merson MH. Fish and shellfish poisoning. *N Engl J Med* 1976;295:1117–1120.
3. Bagnis R, Kuberski T, Laugier S. Clinical observations on 3009 cases of ciguatera (fish poisoning) in the South Pacific. *Am J Trop Med Hyg* 1979;28:1067–1073.
4. Morris JG Jr, Lewin P, Smith CW, Blake PA, Schneider R. Ciguatera fish poisoning: epidemiology of the disease on St. Thomas, U.S. Virgin Islands. *Am J Trop Med Hyg* 1982;31:574–578.
5. Gillespie NC, Lewis RJ, Pearn JH, et al. Ciguatera in Australia: occurrence, clinical features, pathophysiology and management. *Med J Aust* 1986;145:584–590.
6. Morrow JD, Margolies GR, Rowland J, Roberts LJ II. Evidence that histamine is the causative toxin of scombroid-fish poisoning. *N Engl J Med* 1991;324:716–720.
7. Bagnis R, Chanteau S, Chungue E, Hurtel JM, Yasumoto T, Inoue A. Origins of ciguatera fish poisoning: a new dinoflagellate *Gambierdiscus toxicus* Adachi and Fukuyo definitely identified as a causal agent. *Toxicon* 1980;18:199–208.
8. Yasumoto T, Oshima Y, Murakami Y, Nakajima I, Bagnis R, Fukuyo Y. Toxicity of benthic dinoflagellates found in coral reef. *Bull Jap Soc Scientific Fisheries* 1980;46:327–331.
9. Hahn ST, Capra MF. The cyanobacterium *Oscillatoria erythraea*—a potential source of toxin in the ciguatera food chain. *Food Add Contam* 1992;9:351–355.
10. Holmes MJ, Lewis RJ, Poli MA, Gillespie NC. Strain dependent production of ciguatoxin precursors (gambiertoxins) by *Gambierdiscus toxicus* (*Dinophyceae*) in culture. Toxicon 1991;29:761–775.
11. Lewis RJ, Sellin M, Poli MA, Norton RS, MacLeod JK, Sheil MM. Purification and characterization of ciguatoxins from moray eel (*Lycodontis javanicus*, Muraenidae). Toxicon 1991;29:1115–1127.

12. Lewis RJ, Sellin M. Multiple ciguatoxins in the flesh of fish. *Toxicon* 1992;30:915–919.
13. Rayner MD. Mode of action of ciguatoxin. *Fed Proc* 1972;31:1139–1145.
14. Bidard J-N, Vijverberg HPM, Frelin C, et al. Ciguatoxin is a novel type of Na+ channel toxin. *J Biol Chem* 1984;259:8353–8357.
15. Takahashi M, Ohizumi Y, Yasumoto T. Maitotoxin, a Ca^{2+} channel activator candidate. *J Biol Chem* 1982;257:7287–7289.
16. Kodama AM, Hokama Y, Yasumoto T, Fukui M, Manea SJ, Sutherland N. Clinical and laboratory findings implicating palytoxin as cause of ciguatera poisoning due to *Decapterus macrosoma* (mackerel). *Toxicon* 1989;27:1051–1053.
17. Fasano A, Hokama Y, Russel R, Morris JG Jr. Diarrhea in ciguatera fish poisoning: preliminary evaluation of pathophysiological mechanisms. *Gastroenterology* 1991;100:471–476.
18. Cameron J, Flowers AE, Capra MF. Effects of ciguatoxin on nerve excitability in rats. I. *J Neurol Sci* 1991;101:87–92.
19. Cameron J, Flowers AE, Capra MF. Electrophysiological studies on ciguatera poisoning in man. II. *J Neurol Sci* 1991;101:93–97.
20. Representative list of fishes reported as ciguatoxic. In: Halstead BW. *Poisonous and venomous marine animals of the world.* Princeton, NJ: Darwin Press; 1978:326–348.
21. Engleberg NC, Moris JG Jr, Lewis J, McMillan JP, Pollard RA, Blake PA. Ciguatera fish poisoning: a major common source outbreak in the U.S. Virgin Islands. *Ann Intern Med* 1983;98:336–337.
22. Hokama Y, Asahina AY, Titus E, et al. A survey of ciguatera: assessment of Puako, Hawaii, associated with ciguatera toxin epidemics in humans. *J Clin Lab Anal* 1993;7:147–154.
23. Anderson BS, Sims JK, Wiebenga N, Sugi M. The epidemiology of ciguatera fish poisoning in Hawaii 1975–1982. *Haw Med J* 1983;42:326–334.
24. Ruff TA. Ciguatera in the pacific: a link with military activities. *Lancet* 1989;i:201–205.
25. Lewis ND. Disease and development: ciguatera fish poisoning. *Soc Sci Med* 1986;10:983–993.
26. Holt RJ, Miro G, Del Valle A. An analysis of poison control center reports of ciguatera toxicity in Puerto Rico for one year. *Clin Toxicol* 1984;22:177–185.
27. Lawrence DW, Enriquez MB, Lumish RM, Maceo A. Ciguatera fish poisoning in Miami. *JAMA* 1980;244:254–258.
28. Morris JG JR, Lewin P, Hargrett NT, Smith CW, Blake PA, Schneider R. Clinical features of ciguatera fish poisoning: a study of the disease in the US Virgin Islands. *Arch Intern Med* 1982;142:1090–1092.
29. Lange WR, Snyder FR, Fudala PJ. Travel and ciguatera fish poisoning. *Arch Intern Med* 1992;152:2049–2053.
30. Palafox NA, Jain LG, Pinano AZ, Gulick TM, Williams RK, Schatz IJ. Successful treatment of ciguatera fish poisoning with intravenous mannitol. *JAMA* 1988;259:2740–2742.
31. Deichmann WB, MacDonald WE, Cubit DA, Wunsch CE, Bartels JE, Merritt FR. Pain in jawbones and teeth in ciguatera intoxications. *Florida Scientist* 1977;40:227–237.
32. Blythe DG, deSylva DP. Mother's milk turns toxic following fish feast. *JAMA* 1990;264:2074.
34. Lange WR, Lipkin KM, Yang GC. Can ciguatera be a sexually transmitted disease? *J Toxicol Clin Toxicol* 1989;27:193–197.
35. Senecal PE, Osterloh JD. Normal fetal outcome after maternal ciguateria toxin exposure in the second trimester. *J Toxicol Clin Toxicol* 1991;29:473–478.
36. Kodama AM, Hokama Y. Variations in symptomatology of ciguatera poisoning. *Toxicon* 1989;27:593–595.
37. Emerson DL, Galbraith RM, McMillan JP, Higerd TB. Preliminary immunologic studies of ciguatera poisoning. *Arch Intern Med* 1983;143:1931–1933.
38. Hokama Y. A rapid, simplified enzyme immunoassay stick test for the detection of ciguatoxin and related polys/ethers from fish tissue. *Toxicon* 1985;23:939–946.
39. Hokama Y, Asahina AY, Shang ES, Hong TW, Shirai JL. Evaluation of the Hawaiian reef fishes with the solid phase immunobead assay. *J Clin Lab Anal* 1993;7:26–30.
40. Pearn JH, Lewis RJ, Ruff T, et al. Ciguatera and mannitol: experience with a new treatment regimen. *Med J Aust* 1989;151:77–80.
41. Stewart MP. Ciguatera fish poisoning: treatment with intravenous mannitol. *Trop Doctor* 1991;21:54–55.
42. Schantz E. Chemistry and biology of saxitoxins and related toxins. *Ann N Y Acad Sci* 1986;479:15–23.
43. Henderson R, Ritchie JM, Strichartz GR. Evidence that tetrodotoxin and szxitoxin act at a matal cation binding site in the sodium channels of nerve membranes. *Proc Natl Acad Sci USA* 1974;71:3936–3940.
44. Schantz EJ, Ghazarossia VK, Schnoes HK, et al. The structure of saxitoxin. *J Am Chem Soc* 1975;97:1238–1239.
45. Sullivan JJ, Iwaoka WT, Liston J. Enzymatic transformation of PSP toxins in the littleneck clam (*Protothacis staminea*). *Biochem Biophys Res Commun* 1983;114:465–472.
46. Anderson DM, Sullivan JJ, Reguera B. Paralytic shellfish poisoning in northwest Spain: the toxicity of the dinoflagellate *Gymnodinium catenatum*. *Toxicon* 1989;27:665–674.
47. Centers for Disease Control. Paralytic shellfish poisoning—Massachusetts and Alaska, 1990. *MMWP* 1991;40:157–161.
48. McCollum JPK, Pearson RCM, Ingham HR, Wood PC, Dewar HA. An epidemic of mussel poisoning in North-east England. *Lancet* 1968;2:767–770.
49. Long RR, Sargent JC, Hammer K. Paralytic shellfish poisoning: a case report and serial electrophysiologic observations. *Neurology* 1990;40:1310–1312.
50. Morris PD, Campbell DS, Taylor TH, Freeman JI. Clinical and epidemiological features of neurotoxic shellfish poisoning in North Carolina. *Am J Public Health* 1991;81:471–474.
51. Music SI, Howell JT, Brumback CL. Red tide: its public health implications. *J Fla Med Assoc* 1973;60:27–29.
52. Pleasance S, Quilliam MA, Marr JC. Ionspray mass spectrometry of marine toxins. IV. Determination of diarrhetic shellfish poisoning toxins in mussel tissue by liquid chromatography/mass spectroscopy. *Rapid Commun Mass Spectrosc* 1992;6:121–127.
53. Marr JC, Hu T, Pleasance S, Quilliam MA, Wright JL. Detection of new 7-O-acyl derivatives of diarrhetic shellfish poisoning toxins by liquid chromatography-mass spectrometry. *Toxicon* 1992;30:1621–1630.
54. Perl TM, Bedard L, Kosatsky T, Hockin JC, Todd ECD, Remis RS. An outbreak of toxic encephalopathy caused by eating mussels contaminated with domoic acid. *N Engl J Med* 1990;322:1775–1780.
55. Teitelbaum JS, Zatorre RJ, Carpenter S, et al. Neurologic sequelae of domoic acid intoxication due to injestion of contaminated mussels. *N Engl J Med* 1990;322:1781–1787.
56. Morrow JD, Margolies GR, Rowland J, Roberts LJ. Evidence that histamine is the causative toxin of scombroid-fish poisoning. *N Engl J Med* 1991;324:716–720.
57. Smart DR. Scombroid poisoning. A report of seven cases involving the Western Australian salmon, *Arripis truttaceus*. *Med J Aust* 1992;157:748–751.
58. Etkind P, Wilson ME, Gallagher K, Cournoyer J. Bluefish-associated scombroid poisoning: an example of the expanding spectrum of food poisoning from seafood. *JAMA* 1987;258:3409–3410.
59. Kim R. Flushing syndrome due to mahimahi (scombroid fish) poisoning. *Arch Dermatol* 1979;115:963–965.
60. Centers for Disease Control. Scombroid fish poisoning—New Mexico, 1987. *MMWP* 1988;37:451.
61. Taylor SL. Histamine food poisoning: toxicology and clinical aspects. *CRC Crit Rev Toxicol* 1986;17:91–128.
62. Hughes JM, Potter ME. Scombroid-fish poisoning: from pathogenesis to prevention. *N Engl J Med* 1991;324:766–768.
63. Kow-tong C, Malison MD. Outbreak of scombroid fish poisoning, Taiwan. *Am J Public Health* 1987;77:1335–1336.
64. Gilbert RJ, Hobbs G, Murray CK, Cruickshank JG, Young SEJ. Scombrotoxic fish poisoning: features of the first 50 incidents to be reported in Britain (1976–9). *Br Med J* 1980;281:71–72.

Infections of the Gastrointestinal Tract,
edited by M. J. Blaser, P. D. Smith, J. I. Ravdin,
H. B. Greenberg, and R. L. Guerrant
Published by Raven Press, Ltd., New York, 1995.

CHAPTER 19

Botulism as an Intestinal Toxemia

Stephen S. Arnon

Traditionally, botulism has been known as a foodborne disease and as such has always been of interest to gastroenterologists. Eighteen years ago the traditional view of botulism was revised and expanded following the recognition of a new form of the disease, i.e., infant botulism. Infant botulism is an infection of the intestinal tract in which ingested *Clostridium botulinum* spores germinate, multiply, and temporarily colonize the lumen of the large intestine and produce botulinum toxin in it. A minute fraction of the intraluminal toxin is then absorbed and carried by the bloodstream to peripheral cholinergic synapses, where it binds irreversibly. Clinically, the neuromuscular junction is the most important peripheral cholinergic synapse, and its poisoning by botulinum toxin results in hypotonia and flaccid paralysis. Botulinum neurotoxin is the most poisonous substance known. Its seven serologically distinguishable forms have arbitrarily been given the letters A–G. These seven toxin types serve as convenient clinical and epidemiological markers.

Recognition of infant botulism led to the discovery of two novel clostridial species that can make botulinumlike neurotoxins and colonize the human colon. Discovery of these additional neurotoxigenic clostridia necessitated a better descriptive term for the infectious form of botulism, now referred to as "the intestinal toxemias of infancy" or "intestinal toxemia botulism." The distinction from diseases caused by other toxin-producing intestinal bacteria (e.g., *Shigella dysenteriae* type 1, *Escherichia coli, Vibrio cholerae*) is that the intestinal toxemia clostridia neither invade the mucosa (like *Shigella* or some *E. coli*) nor produce a mucosally active toxin (like *V. cholerae* or other *E. coli*). Under exceptional circumstances (e.g., changes in normal anatomy and gut flora), adults can become ill with "infant-type" botulism. Intestinal toxemia botulism in infants and adults is the subject of this chapter.

S. S. Arnon, MD: Infant Botulism Prevention Program, California Department of Health Services, Berkeley, California 94704.

HISTORY

Reliable descriptions of foodborne botulism date to nineteenth century Germany, where Kerner described an illness known locally as "sausage poisoning." In 1895 in the small Belgian town of Ellezelles, an outbreak occurred among 34 musicians who had eaten from a raw ham preserved in salt brine. Twenty-three persons became sick, 13 severely, and 3 died. This episode of botulism became famous because Emile van Ermengem (1851–1922), Professor of Microbiology at the University of Ghent, carried out a now classical investigation that established the essential aspects of botulism. van Ermengem discovered the obligatorily anaerobic, spore-forming bacterium known today as *Clostridium botulinum* and its phenomenally potent heat-labile toxin, which caused a wide variety of vertebrate animals to die from flaccid muscle paralysis. Much subsequent work in the United States on the ecology of the bacterium and the eradication of its spores from canned foods was carried out in the early decades of the twentieth century by Meyer, Dack, and colleagues (1).

The second form of human botulism to be recognized, wound botulism, was first reported in 1951 (1). Wound botulism is an infectious disease and is the pathophysiological equivalent of tetanus. Wound botulism remains the rarest form of human botulism, with somewhat over 100 cases reported worldwide. An occasional case of wound botulism has occurred as a complication of intestinal surgery (2). Wound botulism was the subject of a recent review (3) and will not be discussed further here.

Infant botulism, the third form of human botulism, was recognized as a distinct clinical and epidemiological entity in 1976 (4,5), more than 50 years after Orr had first demonstrated the possibility experimentally (6). Shortly after modern recognition of the first cases and the naming of the entity, the novel pathogenesis of infant botulism was demonstrated (7,8). Discovery in the late 1970s of a laboratory-proven case of infant botulism that occurred in 1931, yet was misdiagnosed at the time, helped confirm that infant botulism was not a "new" disease but only a newly recognized one (9). The first case of infant botulism to be caused by type F botulinum toxin was recognized in New Mexico in 1979 (10); later the causative bacterium of this case was found to be a unique strain of *Clostridium baratii* that produced a type F–like botulinum toxin (11,12). The first and thus far only two cases of infant botulism caused by type E toxin were recognized in Rome, Italy in 1986 (13), which resulted in discovery of a unique strain of *Clostridium butyricum* that produced a type E–like botulinum toxin (12,14).

Once the intestinal toxemias of infancy had been recognized, it became apparent that intestinal toxemia botulism could occur in older children and adults under exceptional, nonphysiological circumstances. The first case report that provided impeccable evidence of infant-type botulism in an adult appeared in 1986 (15). To date, recognized intestinal toxemia botulism has resulted from any of the three neurotoxigenic clostridial species of *C. botulinum, C. baratii,* and *C. butyricum.* However, other systemic illnesses presently considered idiopathic may possibly find their explanation in the toxins of the various clostridial species that are capable of colonizing the large intestine, if a search for them is made.

Most recently, botulinum toxin has become celebrated as the first microbial toxin to be harnessed into service as a medicine for the treatment of human disease (16–18). The toxin is used to treat a variety of ophthalmological and neurological conditions characterized by overactivity or spasm of a particular muscle or muscle group (19).

INFECTIOUS AGENTS

Clostridia by definition are the obligatorily anaerobic, gram-positive, spore-forming rods. Clinical botulism from an intestinal toxemia may be caused by any of three clostridial species that produces either botulinum neurotoxin itself or a closely related botulinum-like neurotoxin. These three species are *C. botulinum* and one unique strain each within the species *C. baratii* and *C. butyricum* (11–14).

In general, each strain of *C. botulinum* produces a single toxin type. However, strains that produce predominantly one toxin type together with a lesser amount of a second toxin type are known and have been given the designations Ab (20), Af (21), Ba (22), and Bf (23). By use of the polymerase chain reaction, it was recently shown that 43/79 (54%) of type A strains examined also carried the gene for type B toxin (24). However, only 1 of these 43 type A strains expressed biologically active type B toxin, thus defining it as an Ab strain. A further remarkable finding was the discovery of the type B toxin gene in two strains of *Clostridium subterminale,* neither of which by bioassay expressed the toxin gene (24). The identification of the gene(s) for botulinum and botulinum-like toxins in an increasing variety of non–*C. botulinum* species suggests that these toxin-encoding genes may await discovery in other clostridial species not yet examined.

The fourth clostridial species known to produce a neurotoxin, *C. tetani,* is apparently unable to colonize the human infant intestinal tract, as least as judged by the absence of reported clinical cases. However, the almost universal immunization of women in the developed world with tetanus toxoid and the in utero transfer of maternal antibody to the fetus may prevent clinically evident cases of infant intestinal tetanus toxemia from occurring, while in the less developed world, tetanus in infancy is usually ascribed to "tetanus neonatorum." Perhaps tetanus neonatorum cases, especially those 2 months of age and older that lack an obvious wound source of toxin, should be evaluated for the possibility of intestinal colonization by *C. tetani.*

The bacterial species designated as *C. botulinum* is not a homogeneous collection of metabolically similar bacteria. Instead, the species was intentionally created as an aggregate of the strains that produce botulinum neurotoxin. This taxonomic decision preceded by several decades the discovery of the neurotoxigenic strains of *C. baratii, C. butyricum,* and *C. botulinum* type G. *Clostridium botulinum* is subdivided into four groups based on cultural and biochemical criteria. Group I consists of proteolytic strains that produce botulinum neurotoxin types A, B, and F; group II consists of nonproteolytic strains that produce neurotoxin types B, E, and F; group III consists of the strains that produce neurotoxin types C and D; and group IV consists of a single strain that produces neurotoxin type G (1). This latter group was recently proposed for inclusion in a new species, *C. argentinense* (25). In the next few years the nomenclature for all *C. botulinum* strains will probably be revised as ribosomal RNA and DNA hybridization techniques disclose the more correct taxonomic relationships between botulinum neurotoxin–producing strains and their nonneurotoxigenic clostridial counterparts (26, 26a, 26b).

Seven antigenic variations of botulinum neurotoxins exist and are distinguished from each other by the absence of cross-neutralization by monovalent antitoxins. These seven toxin types have been arbitrarily assigned the letters A–G (1). Because the neurotoxins produced by *C. butyricum* and *C. baratii* can be neutralized by either botulinum type E or type F antitoxin, respectively, these latter neurotoxins are referred to as "botulinum-like." The structural genes for the two botulinum-like toxins have been sequenced; the type E–like toxin has approximately 97% homology to classical botulinum type E toxin (27,28), while the type F–like toxin has approximately 70% homology to classical nonproteolytic type F botulinum toxin (29).

Botulinum toxin is the most poisonous poison known, and tetanus toxin is second only to botulinum toxin in potency (30). The extreme poisonousness of these two toxins derives from their specificity for synaptic neural cells and their enzymatic action that prevents synaptic transmission (see next section). The lethal (bloodstream) dose of botulinum toxin for a human has been estimated by extrapolation from primate and other animal studies to be less than, and perhaps substantially less than, 1 ng/kg (18,31); tetanus toxin is approximately one order of magnitude less potent (30,31).

PATHOGENESIS AND PATHOPHYSIOLOGY

As presently known, intestinal toxemia botulism results from ingestion of spores of any one of three neurotoxigenic clostridial species: *C. botulinum, C. butyricum,* and *C. baratii.* All three species produce either botulinum neurotoxin or botulinum-like neurotoxin in the lumen of the large intestine (32,33). The toxin is then absorbed from the colon and carried by the bloodstream to peripheral cholinergic synapses, the clinically most important of which is the neuromuscular junction. The toxin binds to unmyelinated terminal nerve endings and blocks their release of acetylcholine, thereby producing flaccid paralysis.

In its active form botulinum toxin consists of two peptide chains linked by at least one disulfide bond. The larger or "heavy" chain (~100,000 Da) contains the binding site by which the toxin attaches to the exterior surface of the nerve cell membrane. The different toxin serotypes apparently bind to different cell surface receptors (34). After the heavy chain attaches to the cell surface of the neuron, the "light" chain (~50,000 Da) and N terminal of the heavy chain are taken inside the cell by an endosome, the low internal pH of which apparently reduces the disulfide bond(s) and frees the light chain. The light chain then emerges into the cell cytoplasm and poisons acetylcholine release through its enzymatic action (35).

After centuries of curiosity and wonder, the basis of the extreme specificity and potency of the botulinum toxins was recently discovered (36). The light chain of the seven botulinum toxin serotypes and also of tetanus toxin was found to be zinc-containing endoproteases (37). Their substrates are various components of the "docking," or "togetherness," complex of proteins that enable the synaptic vesicle to fuse with the nerve cell terminal membrane and thereby release its acetylcholine into the synaptic cleft. These docking proteins have been given various names and acronyms, e.g., VAMP, SNAP-25, (38). Botulinum toxin type B and tetanus toxin were the first of the group to have their molecular mechanism understood (36). These two toxins as well as botulinum toxin types D, F, and G cleave the VAMP protein. Botulinum toxin types A and E cleave the SNAP-25 protein, and botulinum toxin type C cleaves the syntaxin protein (37,37a–c).

The central role of the normal intestinal microflora of adult animals in preventing *C. botulinum* spore germination and colonization of the large intestine has been elegantly shown in a mouse model system, in which the animals paradoxically remained asymptomatic (39–41). Administration of 10^6 type A spores failed to colonize the intestine of normal adult mice. However, after 2½ days treatment per os with a combination of erythromycin and kanamycin, half the mice could be colonized by just 2×10^4 spores, a 50-fold decrease in inoculum size. But when the antibiotic-treated mice were placed in cages with normal, untreated mice, they became resistant to intestinal colonization in 3 days (41). Because mice are coprophagic, the antibiotic-treated animals presumably had no difficulty in reacquiring a normal mouse intestinal flora from their cagemates. Additional work with germ-free animals emphasized the importance of normal flora as a protective barrier to colonization. Adult, germ-free mice could be colonized by just 10 *C. botulinum* type A spores, whereas after 3 days in a room that also housed conventional adult mice in different cages, the formerly germ-free animals

became resistant to colonization by 10^5 spores (40). Because this experimental design precluded coprophagy, the normal mouse intestinal flora must have been acquired by different means.

When infant mice rather than adult mice were used as the experimental animals, their intestines were found to be naturally susceptible to intestinal colonization by *C. botulinum* spores. Unlike the adult mice, pretreatment with antibiotics was not necessary to achieve colonization (39). However, like human infants, intestinal colonization of the normal flora infant mice occurred only within a restricted age interval (for mice, 7–13 days of age). Susceptibility of infant mice to intestinal colonization peaked between days 8 and 11 in a manner similar to the peaking of human infant susceptibility to intestinal *C. botulinum* colonization between 2 and 4 months of age (Fig. 1) (39,42). In addition, the infective dose of *C. botulinum* spores for infant mice was much smaller than that of their antibiotic-treated adult counterparts. For normal flora infant mice the 50% infective dose was only 700 spores. In one experiment, just 10 spores colonized an infant mouse (39). The minimum infective dose of *C. botulinum* spores for human infants is not known, but based on exposure to spore-containing honeys, it is estimated to be between 10 and 100 spores (43).

In the context of the pathophysiology of intestinal toxemia botulism, it should be emphasized that adults and older children regularly ingest small numbers of *C. botulinum* spores normally present in both cooked and fresh agricultural products (e.g., honey) without experiencing ill effects (44). The presumed explanation for this seeming paradox is that the fully developed and diversified intestinal microflora, present at a density of 10^{11}–10^{12} anaerobes per gram of feces, prevents germination and outgrowth by the few ingested *C. botulinum* spores.

Parenthetically, intestinal colonization with *C. tetani* could be achieved experimentally when adult germ-free rats were fed vegetative cells, but not spores, of *C. tetani,* yet the animals remained asymptomatic (45). Conventional flora adult mice fed *C. tetani* spores became colonized only when the inoculum contained 10^6 or more spores. Even at this inoculum size, no tetanus toxin was found in the intestinal lumen 24 hr after ingestion of the inoculum (46). Also, adult chickens (47) and infant and germ-free adult rats (48) have been studied as model systems for infant botulism, as have adult horses and foals (49). The illness produced in the foals after feeding *C. botulinum* spores may in actuality have been intestinal wound (necrotic ulcer) botulism (49).

Recognition of the central role of the host intestinal microflora in determining susceptibility or resistance to colonization by *C. botulinum* directed attention to factors that might influence the composition of the normal microflora. Diet is probably the most important of these factors in the infant. In comparison with the adult-type flora, the infant flora is simpler, with fewer genera and species. The dominant members vary, depending in part on whether the infant is fed only breast milk, only formula milk, or a mixture of the two (50,51). Also, the composition of intestinal flora is changed if solid food such as

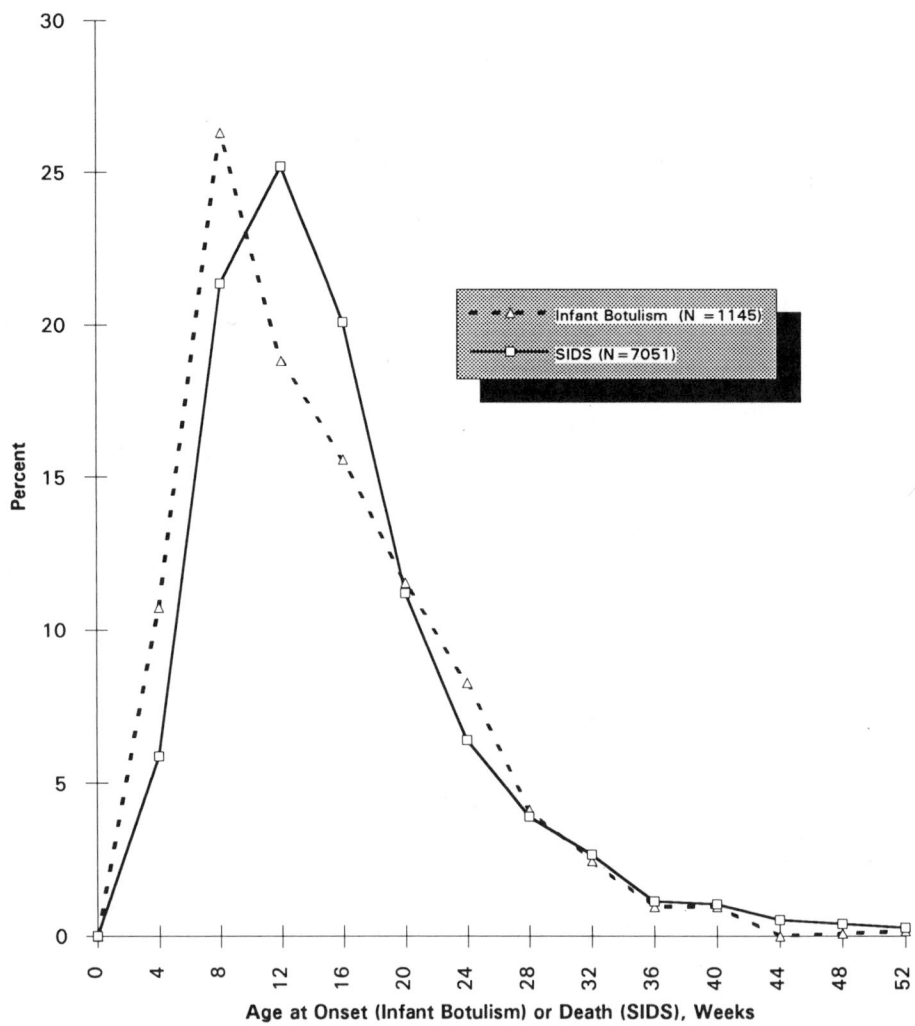

FIG. 1. Comparison of the age distribution of all hospitalized cases of infant botulism in the United States 1976–1992 (*N* = 1145) and all cases of sudden infant death syndrome (SIDS) in California (*N* = 7051). Age in days at onset (infant botulism) or at death (SIDS) converted to weeks.

cereals become part of the infant's diet (50,51). The normal human infant microflora contains several bacterial species, mainly *Bifidofacterium* and *Bacteroides,* that in vitro can inhibit the multiplication of *C. botulinum* (52).

Onset of infant botulism occurs at a significantly younger age in formula-fed infants (7.6 weeks) than in breast-fed infants (13.7 weeks) (53), perhaps reflecting the earlier availability in formula-fed infants of suitable ecological niches (50–53) and the formula-fed infant's lack of immune factors (e.g., SIgA, lactoferrin, lysozyme, etc.) contained in human milk (33,54,55). In addition, introduction of solid foods may "perturb" the intestinal microflora (50,51) and thereby aid in colonization by *C. botulinum* spores (33,42,56).

EPIDEMIOLOGY

The descriptive epidemiologies of intestinal toxemia botulism in infants and in adults are different. The adult

form will be discussed first, although generalizations are necessarily limited because less than a dozen cases of intestinal toxemia botulism in older children and adults are known (see end of section "Clinical Aspects" for specifics). Almost all adult intestinal toxemia botulism cases had either an underlying alteration of normal intestinal anatomy because of surgery or inflammatory bowel disease, or an alteration of the normal intestinal microflora from broad-spectrum antibiotic usage, or both. Adult intestinal toxemia botulism has affected both men and women in widely separated parts of the United States. No common source of ingested *C. botulinum* spores has been identified. Because the potentially at-risk population for adult intestinal toxemia botulism is so large, consisting of older persons who have had intestinal surgery, inflammatory bowel disease, and exposure to antibiotics, and because recognized cases are so few, either this illness occurs only rarely or it is often unrecognized.

The descriptive epidemiology of intestinal toxemia botulism in infants derives almost entirely from investigation of hospitalized cases, which represents only a portion of the clinical spectrum of illness (33,57–59). Present epidemiological generalizations may need to be revised as the outpatient and sudden death portions of the clinical spectrum become more clearly defined (42,60–63).

Notably, the infant is the only family member ill. Ninety-five percent of cases occur in children less than 6 months old. The age-at-onset distribution of infant botulism is matched only by one other condition, the sudden infant death syndrome (SIDS, crib death) (Fig. 1) (42,64). The youngest case showed symptoms at 6 days of age (65,66), while the oldest was 363 days old (67). The M/F ratio of cases is essentially 1:1. Cases have occurred in all major racial and ethnic groups. Infant botulism has now been reported from all inhabited continents except Africa.

Infant botulism has become the most common form of human botulism recognized in the United States (33). In the years 1976–1992, a total of 1145 cases of infant botulism were reported in the United States, where approximately 75–100 cases are recognized annually. Another 63 cases have been reported from 17 other countries. About half of the U.S. cases have been reported from California, which has the largest number of births of any U.S. state. However, California does not have the highest incidence of infant botulism once adjustment is made for differences in annual births (Table 1). Notably, only two of the ten highest incidence states are located east of the Rocky Mountains. However, the figures for absolute numbers of cases and for incidence should be viewed with caution because they depend on correct physician recognition and reporting of this uncommon illness. Only five U.S. cases have been outpatients, and all five were recognized by physicians with prior experience with the more classical hospitalized patient and who therefore requested the stool testing needed to document the mild part of the clinical spectrum. In the United States cases of infant botulism have occurred in all calendar months. When viewed nationally, seasonal fluctuation appears limited, with a slight surge in the three fall months August–October (30.4% of cases), and a slight trough in the three winter months December–February (22.2% of cases).

The geographic distribution of U.S. cases is uneven. Approximately two thirds of cases have been reported by the 13 states located in the Rocky Mountains and westward (including Hawaii and Alaska), while the remaining one third of cases was reported from the other 37 states (Table 1). In the 13 western states, *C. botulinum* type A was responsible for approximately two thirds of cases, whereas in the 37 easterly states, *C. botulinum* type B was responsible for approximately four fifths of cases. This asymmetrical distribution of case toxin types parallels the asymmetrical distribution of *C. botulinum* toxin types in American soils (68). Interesting geographic clusters of infant botulism have been recognized, such as in a small mountain town in Colorado (69) and in the "doughnut" distribution of cases around the core city of Philadelphia, Pennsylvania (56,57). All U.S. cases of infant botulism resulted from either type A or type B toxin except for one case with both toxin types (Hawaii), two cases with type Bf (both probably New Mexico), and one case caused by neurotoxigenic *C. baratii* type F (New Mexico).

Identified risk factors for illness include a slow intestinal transit time (less than one stool per day) (58,70) and ingestion of honey (42,43,58,70a,71,72). Honey from a variety of geographic origins is a known reservoir of *C. botulinum* spores (7,73–80), and all major pediatric and public health agencies in the United States have recommended that infants not be fed honey for the first 12 months of life (references in 42). Breastfeeding appears to provide protection against the fulminant, sudden death presentation of infant botulism (53).

IMMUNITY

No child who has recovered from infant botulism has experienced a second episode of the illness. Whether this outcome results from the development of immunity or from maturation of the intestinal microflora, or simply from the rarity of the disease, is unknown. Although "relapses" of infant botulism have been reported, a close reading of those reports suggests that the patients were just discharged too soon, i.e., before they had recovered adequate strength to feed and breathe on their own (81,82). However, patients may regain sufficient strength to permit hospital discharge even while still excreting *C. botulinum* toxin and organisms in their feces (7,83,84); in these circumstances, it is presumed that they have developed neutralizing antibody (serum or secretory or both) against the toxin. Such antibody, if present, can be demonstrated only with the mouse neutralization test. However, one study of three serum specimens from two patients with infant botulism that used only an enzyme-linked immunosorbent assay (ELISA) technique and crude botulinum toxoid as the capture antigen detected an antibody rise to this mixture of antigens of *C. botulinum* (85).

PATHOLOGY

Because botulinum toxin is not a cytotoxin, the acute illness does not result in observable histological or bio-

TABLE 1. *Cases and incidence of infant botulism, top ten incidence states, United States, 1977–1992*

State	Cases	Incidence[a]
Delaware	16	10.0
Hawaii	29	9.7
Utah	53	8.5
California	538	7.1
Pennsylvania	121	4.7
Washington	40	3.6
Oregon	24	3.6
New Mexico	15	3.5
Idaho	9	3.2
Arizona	24	2.6

[a] Per 100,000 live-births.

chemical pathology. With poisoning and loss of the trophic influence of acetylcholine, the synaptic cleft degenerates, and acetylcholinesterase activity spreads diffusely across the muscle cell membrane. Muscle atrophy also occurs. Recovery from botulinum toxin poisoning occurs through regeneration of the terminal unmyelinated nerve twigs. Once reformed, these twigs induce formation of new synaptic clefts, thereby restoring the neuromuscular junction. During recovery, new motor twigs emerge both terminally as well as preterminally from the distal nodes of Ranvier. With time the preterminal axonal sprouts atrophy, leaving the terminal neuromuscular junctions to initiate muscle contraction (86,87).

CLINICAL ASPECTS

Clinical Manifestations of Botulism

The classical triad of botulism consists of the acute to subacute onset of (a) a symmetrical, descending flaccid paralysis notably involving bulbar musculature, (b) a clear sensorium, and (c) the absence of fever. This triad may be useful in assessing adult cases, but it is less useful with infants because of their inability to describe symptoms. Infant botulism patients typically present with different complaints articulated by the parents.

Because toxemia is the pathophysiology common to all forms of botulism, and because blood flow to the head, face, throat, and neck musculature is relatively greater than blood flow to limb and trunk musculature, botulism always first manifests as weakness and paralysis of bulbar musculature. *It is not possible to have botulism without having at least some cranial nerve palsies.* However, careful and repetitive (i.e., sustained) examination may be required to identify bulbar palsies, particularly in mild cases. *Fatigability with any repetitive muscle activity is the clinical hallmark of botulism,* and this fact can be put to diagnostic use (Table 2). Botulism is a pure motor paralysis because only peripheral cholinergic synapses are affected; sensory nerves remain intact. Rarely, adult patients with botulism may complain of paresthesias; these paresthesias are thought to result from hyperventilation and anxiety as the patient perceives his or her muscles failing to work.

Like other infectious diseases, infant botulism displays a spectrum in its clinical severity (5,7,33,56,82,89). The onset ranges from the gradual to the abrupt. At one extreme are patients who returned to their physicians three or more times in a week as the signs of illness slowly became evident, while at the other extreme are patients who were nursing normally 6–8 hr before becoming so limp that acute meningitis was the diagnosis at presentation.

Because almost all patients recognized to date have been sufficiently paralyzed to need hospitalization, the present picture of infant botulism derives from the hospitalized patient. However, mildly weak and hypotonic cases managed as outpatients have been discerned by alert physicians familiar with the more "classical" manifestations. At the opposite end of the clinical spectrum are those few cases whose history and presentation are indistinguishable from typical cases of the SIDS (42,57, 58,60–63). There appears to be geographic variation in the proportion of SIDS cases that may be attributable to intestinal toxemia botulism (42,57,58,60–63). A recent autopsy study concluded that, like *C. botulinum*, *C. perfringens* and its toxin(s) may also play a role in SIDS via the intestinal toxemia pathway (90,91). Other bacterial toxins have also been proposed as causes of SIDS (92–97).

Parents typically notice constipation (defined as 3 or more days without a bowel movement in an infant previously defecating at least every other day), lethargy, listlessness, and poor feeding as the initial symptoms of infant botulism. A nursing mother may experience breast engorgement because of the child's weakened strength and duration of sucking. These early symptoms may be followed within hours to days by an expressionless face; a weak, moaning, or high-pitched cry; drooling (the inability to swallow); loss of head control ("head lag"); generalized weakness; hypotonicity; and, not infrequently, frank respiratory arrest. Iatrogenic respiratory arrest has occurred when positioning patients for lumbar puncture, thus compromising their already marginal airway and respiratory ability.

Mild cases or those with gradual onset often have been brought back repeatedly to office, clinic, or emergency room settings and been given alternative diagnoses (Table

TABLE 2. *Neurological signs helpful in the diagnosis of infant botulism*

Test	Findings
1. Take patient to dark room. Shine a bright light into the eye; note quickness of pupillary constriction. Remove the light when the constriction maximal; let pupil dilate again. Then immediately repeat the light, continuing thus for 1–3 min.	The initially brisk pupillary constriction may become sluggish and unable to constrict maximally. (Fatigability with repetitive muscle contraction is the clinical hallmark of botulism.)
2. Shine a bright light onto the fovea, keeping it there for 1–3 min, even if the infant tries to deviate his eyes.	Latent ophthalmoplegia may be elicited and/or purposeful efforts to avoid the light may diminish.
3. Place a clean fifth finger in the infant's mouth, taking care not to obstruct the airway. Note the strength and duration of the reflex sucking.	The suck is weak and poorly sustained.

Adapted from ref. 88, with permission.

TABLE 3. *Working differential diagnosis of infant botulism*

Admission diagnosis	Subsequent working diagnosis
r/o Sepsis	Amino acid metabolic disorder
Dehydration	Brainstem encephalitis
Viral	Drug ingestion
syndrome	Guillain–Barré syndrome
Pneumonia	Heavy metal poisoning (Pb, Mg, As)
Idiopathic	Hirschsprung disease
hypotonia	Hypothyroidism
Failure to	Medium-chain acetyl-CoA
thrive	dehydrogenase (MCAD) deficiency
	Metabolic encephalopathy
	Myasthenia gravis
	Poliomyelitis
	Viral polyneuritis
	Werdnig–Hoffmann disease

3). Consideration of any of these diagnoses should also call to mind the possibility of infant botulism. A history of having been fed honey is not necessary for making the diagnosis; at present less than 5% of confirmed cases (in California) have been fed honey before onset. The suspicion of infant botulism necessitates a careful cranial nerve examination, in which drooling and poor feeding are understood to represent dysphagia, a weak cry to represent dysphonia, and ptosis to represent oculomotor palsy rather than "sleepiness" or "systemic toxicity" (Fig. 2).

Laboratory findings in botulism are generally normal because botulinum toxin is not cytotoxic to any tissue. The normality of virtually all laboratory screening tests may also help suggest the possibility of infant botulism. However, a minimally elevated blood urea nitrogen (BUN), or a mild ketonemia and ketonuria from diminished intake of fluid and food, may be present at emergency room or admission evaluation. Dehydration occasionally results in a slightly elevated cerebrospinal fluid (CSF) protein concentration. Both serum and CSF abnormalities promptly reverse with feeding and hydration. Electromyography (EMG) is the one bedside diagnostic study that may be helpful in infant botulism (see below).

Differential Diagnosis and Diagnosis

The principal differential diagnostic considerations are Guillain–Barré syndrome and myasthenia gravis. The effects of various toxic substances (e.g., organophosphate poisoning, tick bite) and metabolic conditions (e.g., medium-chain acetyl dehydrogenase deficiency, hypocalcemia, etc.) can be mistaken for botulism but are identifiable by proper laboratory investigation. In adults, the Miller–Fisher variant of Guillain–Barré syndrome (ophthalmoplegia, ataxia, areflexia) (98) may cause confusion, particularly since the CSF may initially be normal. However, in this disorder the onset of paralysis may not be symmetrical or it may be ascending, with bulbar musculature affected later rather than earlier in the course of illness. Paresthesias, asymmetry of paralysis, and an abnor-

mal CSF or nerve conduction velocity help distinguish classical Guillain–Barré syndrome from botulism. Myasthenia gravis spares the pupillary light reflex and has available for it three relatively sensitive and specific diagnostic tests: the presence of antiacetylcholine receptor antibody, the edrophonium (Tensilon) test, and EMG. With repetitive stimulation at high (50-Hz) frequency the EMG in myasthenia shows a decremental pattern, in contrast to the incremental pattern ("facilitation") seen in botulism.

The differential diagnosis in infant botulism is straightforward, even though the variety of conditions initially considered may be lengthy (Table 3). Today, 18 years after its recognition, the most common admission diagnosis for infant botulism still remains "rule out sepsis." As with many conditions, often the most difficult step in diagnosis is considering the possibility (Table 3). A careful history and neurological examination are essential to prompt diagnosis; very few diseases in the first 6 months of life present like infant botulism. Clues to diagnosis may be found on radiographs done for other reasons. The chest roentgenogram may show an infiltrate in apical lung segments consistent with aspiration, while an abdominal roentgenogram may show dilated, gas-filled loops of large bowel.

In infants, myasthenia gravis in the first 6 months of life is usually congenital; a history of maternal myasthenia establishes the diagnosis. Guillain–Barré syndrome properly documented by an elevated CSF protein is almost

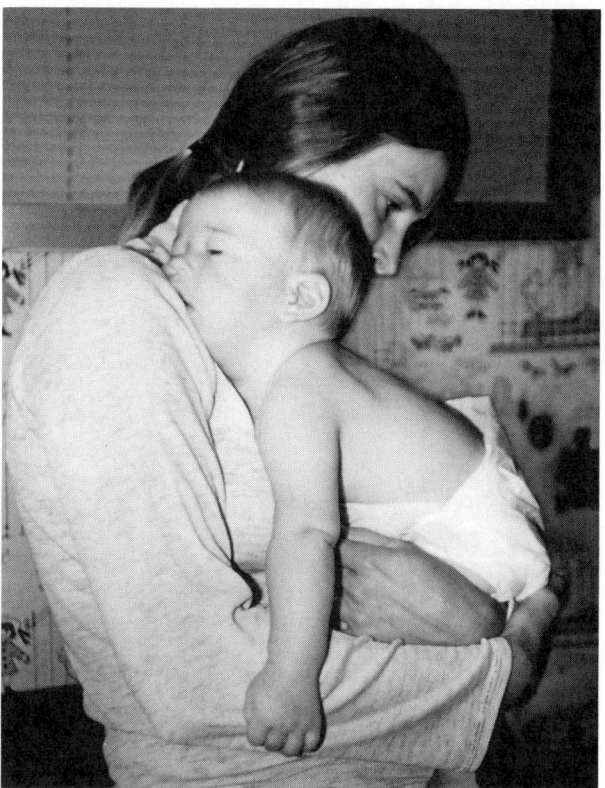

FIG. 2. Seven-week-old patient with mild infant botulism. Note ptosis, expressionless face, and lack of neck, arm, and truncal tone.

unknown in infancy. Metabolic disorders can be identified by appropriate testing of blood and urine. EMG is invasive, expensive, and painful, but can be helpful if the characteristic BSAP pattern is present (99,100). This pattern, seen in some but not all (101) patients with laboratory-confirmed infant botulism, has been given the acronym "BSAP" for "brief, small, abundant motor-unit potentials" (102). However, in a patient with a typical history and characteristic physical (especially neurological) examination, an EMG is usually not necessary if prompt testing of feces can be arranged through a state health department or Centers for Disease Control and Prevention (CDC) laboratory. The CDC's 24-hr notification telephone number is (404)639-2206 (Monday–Friday, 8:00 A.M.–5:00 P.M.) and (404)639-2888 (all other times). Other invasive and expensive diagnostic studies, such as MRI, CAT scan, EEG and muscle biopsy, yield normal or nonspecific results and are incapable of diagnosing infant botulism.

Definitive diagnosis of intestinal toxemia botulism is established by identification of neurotoxogenic *C. botulinum*, *C. baratii*, or *C. butyricum* organisms (with or without the concomitant presence of toxin) in the feces of a patient with an illness consisting of bulbar palsies, flaccid paralysis, and intact sensation and sensorium. Obtaining stool with which to carry out the necessary diagnostic studies may be difficult because of severe constipation; in this situation an enema with sterile, nonbacteriostatic water may be given. In suspect adult intestinal toxemia botulism cases, serum should also be examined for the possible presence of botulinum toxin. In the years ahead, molecular diagnostic (i.e., polymerase chain reaction) techniques may come to surpass the mouse bioassay in sensitivity and specificity (103–105).

Occasionally it is possible to identify small amounts (<5 mouse LD_{50}/mL) of botulinum toxin in the serum of infant patients if the specimen is collected early in the course of illness (13,83,106,107). In one report, almost one infant botulism patient in eight had toxin demonstrable in serum (106). Examination of feces by the mouse neutralization test remains the definitive diagnostic assay and should be done in all patients in whom the diagnosis is suspected. Clinically suspicious cases that lack an identified causative toxin type will not be included in official tallies of infant botulism (108). Physicians are also reminded that in most jurisdictions botulism or suspected botulism is an immediately reportable illness.

Clinical Course and Management

The course of infant botulism managed with meticulous supportive care has some generally predictable features. Following the acute to subacute onset of symptoms (hours to days), the progression of weakness eventually necessitates hospital admission. The nadir of hypotonicity and paralysis is generally reached about 1–2 weeks after admission. Patients may remain at this stage for as long as 2–3 weeks before showing improvement. Once improvement begins, it continues slowly over subsequent weeks (Fig. 3). Infant botulism does not have a relapsing course, and "regression" in a patient who has been improving should immediately launch a search for an occult complication (Table 4). The patient may be discharged once steady recovery is evident and gag reflex, sucking, and swallowing ability have returned, even though head lag and constipation may still be pronounced. Alternatively, the patient may be discharged somewhat earlier if the parents are able to feed the child by gavage at home.

Successful management of botulism is based on two

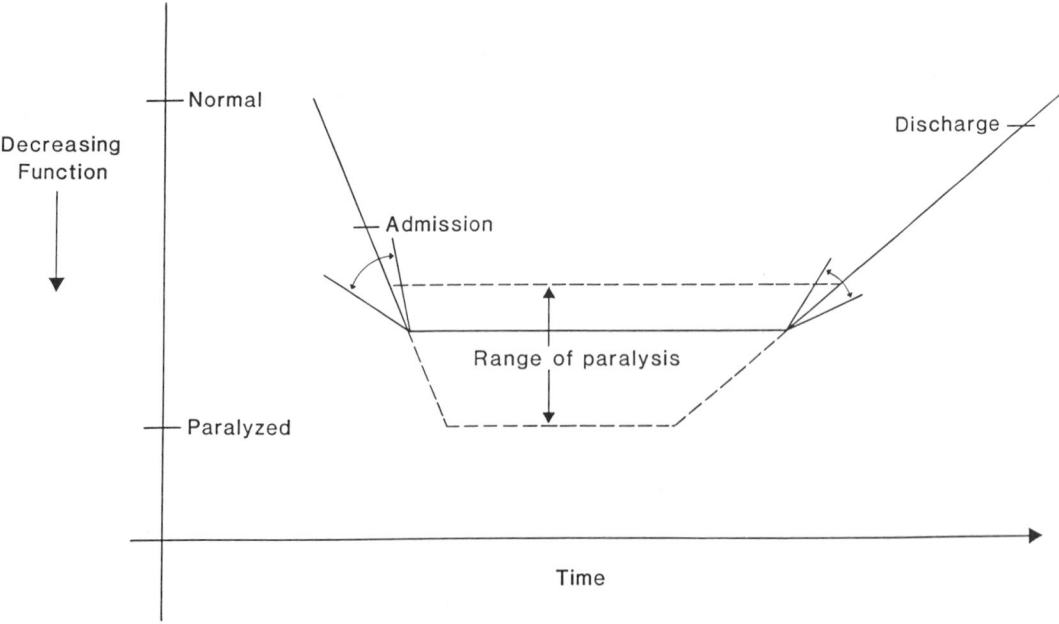

FIG. 3. Schematic course of infant botulism managed with meticulous supportive care. Time intervals intentionally omitted.

TABLE 4.—*Complications of infant botulism*

Adult respiratory distress syndrome
Aspiration
Fracture of the femur
Inappropriate antidiuretic hormone secretion
Misplaced or plugged endotracheal tube
Necrotizing enterocolitis
Otitis media
Pneumonia
Recurrent atelectasis
Seizures secondary to hyponatremia
Sepsis
Tension pneumothorax
Transfusion reaction
Urinary tract infection
Subglottic stenosis[a]
Tracheal granuloma[a]
Tracheitis[a]
Tracheomalacia[a]

[a] A single hospital's experience (82).

principles: (a) that fatigability with repetitive muscle activity is the clinical hallmark of the disease and (b) that complications can best be avoided by anticipating them. The first principle is most applicable to feeding and breathing. A simple positioning maneuver improves respiratory mechanics and ventilation (Fig. 4). The patient is placed face up on a rigid-bottomed crib, the entire floor of which is tilted head up at 30°. A small cloth roll is placed under the neck to support the cervical vertebrae and to tip the head back so that oral secretions will drain into the posterior pharynx, where they are most easily swallowed. Some support (e.g., a sandbag) is often needed under the pelvis to prevent the patient from gradually sliding downhill. Also as a consequence of this position, the abdominal viscera pull the diaphragm down and thereby expand the thorax, thus improving the respiratory mechanics. Also, any regurgitated stomach contents must travel uphill for aspiration to result. It is undesirable to elevate the patient's head by flexing the crib bed and patient so that a

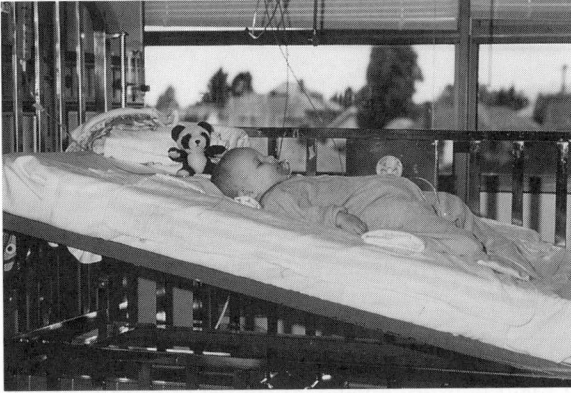

FIG. 4. Ideal positioning of an infant botulism patient. Note rigid mattress frame, 30° angle of entire body, small neck roll support. Brace under pelvis is to prevent downhill sliding.

bend occurs between thorax and abdomen. If this is done, the hypotonic thorax will settle onto the abdomen, making breathing difficult and tiring.

Intubation should be done prophylactically. Otherwise, fatigue of upper airway muscles will progress to pharyngeal musculature collapse, airway obstruction, and apnea. Transcutaneous carbon dioxide monitoring is useful in deciding when to intubate. A rising pCO_2 signals alveolar hypoventilation from fatigue and progressive paralysis of respiratory tract musculature. Approximately one third to one half of hospitalized patients will require intubation. Tracheostomy is almost never required because patients with global muscle paralysis and proper positioning can tolerate intubation for weeks or months without permanent sequelae (109,110).

Patients should be fed by nasogastric tube until it is certain that their strength of gag, suck, and swallow is sufficient to sustain them through an entire feeding by breast or bottle. Expressed breast milk is the nutritional fluid of choice, particularly because of the immune system components it contains (leukocytes, sIgA, lysozyme, lactoferrin, etc.). Tube feeding (nasogastric or nasojejunal) also assists in the resumption of peristalsis, a nonspecific but probably essential contributor to the eventual elimination of *C. botulinum* from the colonic microflora. Use of intravenous feeding (hyperalimentation) is discouraged both because of its potential for infection and because of the advantages of tube feeding.

Antibiotic administration is not part of the therapy of uncomplicated infant botulism. Botulinum toxin is primarily an intracellular molecule that is released by vegetative cell death and lysis. Consequently, clostridiocidal antibiotics may increase the amount of toxin available for absorption from a constipated large bowel and may actually worsen the patient's condition, a possibility apparently confirmed by recent clinical experience in California (California Department of Health Services, *unpublished data*). Antibiotic use in infant botulism should be reserved for the treatment of secondary infections. In these circumstances, a nonclostridiocidal antibiotic such as trimethoprim-sulfamethoxazole or nalidixic acid is preferred in order to minimize the release of additional toxin from *C. botulinum* vegetative cell death. Aminoglycoside antibiotics should be avoided because they may potentiate the blocking action of botulinum toxin at the neuromuscular junction (111).

Botulinum toxin does not cross the blood–brain barrier, but because the infant may appear comatose to the parents, they often need reassurance that brain damage has not occurred. Sensation remains intact, so patients are able to hear and feel normally. Accordingly, auditory, tactile, and visual stimuli should be provided, particularly in cases of prolonged hospital stay. Maintaining a strong central respiratory drive is essential in order to offset the peripheral blockade of neuromuscular transmission by botulinum toxin. For this reason, sedatives or other drugs that may cause central nervous system depression as a side effect, such as metoclopramide (Reglan), are contraindicated.

Constipation may be severe, so full hydration should be maintained. Stool softeners may be beneficial, but ca-

TABLE 5. *Adults or children with intestinal*

Patient age/sex (Ref.)	Location	Evidence for diagnosis
1. 37/F (15)	Maryland, USA	1. Type A botulinum toxin present in 2 serum specimens hospital days 11 and 13. Type A botulinum toxin present in 2 stool specimens hospital days 15 and 18. *C. botulinum* type A organisms present in 4 stool specimens hospital days 15–33. No evidence of wound or intraabdominal abscess by isotopic, computerized tomographic, endoscopic, or autopsy examination. *C. botulinum* type A organisms, but no toxin, found in the ingested creme of coconut. Husband who had also consumed the creme of coconut cocktails remained well.
2. 33/F (114, 116)	Oregon, USA	2. *C. botulinum* type A organisms present in feces hospital day 2.
3. 45/F (115)	Texas, USA	3. *C. botulinum* type B organisms present in feces at or after hospital admission.
4. ca. 70/M (116)	Kentucky, USA	4. Botulinum toxin type B present in serum on hospital day 30. Botulinum toxin type B present in feces hospital day 22. *C. botulinum* type B organisms present in feces hospital day 32.
5. 27/M (116)	Iceland	5. Onset of clinical botulism 40 days after eating home-made sausage. Type B botulinum toxin in serum 47 days after eating home-made sausage. *C. botulinum* type B organisms in feces 47 days after eating home-made sausage. No toxin in serum 19 days after eating home-made sausage. Type B botulinum toxin in enrichment culture of feces 19 days after eating home-made sausage, but organisms could not be isolated.
6. 54/M (117)	Georgia, USA	6. Botulinum toxin, probably type F, present in serum hospital day 4. *C. baratii* type F organisms present in stool specimens hospital days 4 and 14. *C. botulinum* type B organisms present in feces hospital day 4.
7. 3/F (118)	California, USA	7. *C. botulinum* type A toxin and organisms in two fecal specimens one month apart. Serum negative for toxin.
8. 67/M[c]	Oregon, USA	8. Type A botulinum toxin in serum at admission; *C. botulinum* type A organisms present in feces six months after onset.
9. 48/F[d]	Indiana, USA	9. *C. botulinum* type B in feces.
10. 51/F[e]	California, USA	10. *C. botulinum* type B in feces. Serum negative for toxin.

[a] French investigators reported type B botulinum toxin detectable in serum in 35.7% (10/28) of patients 2 or more weeks after they had eaten foods containing *C. botulinum* type B toxin and organisms. Fecal excretion of toxin and organisms was not studied. Three persons had type B toxin detectable in serum 87 or more days after eating a spoiled ham, two of whom inexplicably were reported to be asymptomatic (119).

[b] Swiss investigators reported a puzzling patient with Guillain–Barré syndrome in whom type F botulinum toxin was twice found in serum, once at days 10–28 and again at days 67–74 after onset, during which time the patient was continuously in the hospital. During these episodes, *C. botulinum* type F toxin and organisms were also present in feces. No food was suspected as a source of *C. botulinum* (120).

toxemia botulism (confirmed or possible)[a,b]

Possible predisposing circumstances	Comment
1. Onset 5 weeks s/p antrectomy, vagotomy, and Billroth type I anastomosis for peptic ulcer disease. Received broad-spectrum cephalosporin preoperatively. Five days before onset, patient consumed cocktails containing creme of coconut.	1. First case of adult intestinal toxemia botulism with impeccable supporting evidence. Probable source of *C. botulinum* spores identified, prior antibiotic exposure, no blind loop. Hospitalized continuously and died 8 months after onset.
2. Onset 3 years s/p ileojejunal bypass for obesity, with resultant shortened bowel and small bowel blind loop. Autopsy not obtained.	2. Blind loop; no prior antibiotic exposure. No wounds and no history suggestive of foodborne botulism. Died 17 days after onset.
3. Onset 10 years s/p cholecystectomy and 7 years s/p "gastric bypass" surgery for obesity, with resultant small bowel blind loop. Diarrhea, then constipation 1 month before admission.	3. Blind loop; possible prior antibiotic exposure, if any, unknown.
4. None known.	4. Evidence only suggestive. Wife became ill at same time and died before diagnostic studies done. *C. botulinum* type B organisms but no toxin found in three containers of unopened home-canned blackberries sufficiently acidic (pH $\leq$ 3.6) to prevent outgrowth of spores.
5. None known. To external appearances, intestinal tract apparently normal anatomically, physiologically, and microbiologically.	5. His 3 children developed type B foodborne botulism within 2 days after eating the home-made sausage. His wife developed type B botulism with toxin in her sum and type B organisms in her feces 12 days after eating the sausage. The sausage eaten by the husband may have contained only vegetative cells of *C. botulinum*, or a large number of spores, or both.
6. Onset 4 years s/p vagotomy, pyloroplasty, and cholecystectomy.	6. No prior antibiotics, no wounds, no history suggestive of foodborne botulism. Hospital stay of 31 days; chronic weakness and fatigue postdischarge.
7. Onset 7 weeks s/p radiation therapy, chemotherapy, and autologous bone marrow transplantation for neuroblastoma. Postoperative routine oral and occasional parenteral broad-spectrum antibiotic treatment. Ingestion of honey-coated dry cereal and vegetable-containing, microwave reheated frozen dinner prior to onset.	7. First case of nosocomially acquired intestinal toxemia botulism. Patient was treated with botulism immune globulin (IND-4283) under "compassionate use" provisions. Recovered from botulism, but died from recurrence of neuroblastoma.
8. Crohn's disease	8. Prior antibiotic exposure, if any, unknown.
9. Interval between colostomy for bowel cancer and onset not available.	9. Prior antibiotic and chemotherapy exposure, if any, unknown.
10. Onset 14 years s/p ileojejunal bypass for obesity. Began eating honey 2 weeks before onset, two aliquots of which were negative for *C. botulinum* spores.	10. Took an oral penicillin and an antacid for approximately one week before onset. First adult case with a history of honey exposure.

[c] Griffin PM et al., Centers for Disease Control and Prevention (CDC), *personal communication*.
[d] Hathaway CL et al., CDC, *personal communication*.
[e] California Department of Health Services and CDC, *unpublished data*.

thartics are not recommended. The majority of patients require no special measures beyond occasional rectal stimulation or a glycerin suppository. Infrequently, a small inspissated fecal plug can occupy the rectal vault and must be manually removed before regular defecation can resume. Enemas intended to remove *C. botulinum* and toxin are useless because the bacterium colonizes the entire length of the large bowel (32).

Patients with infant botulism excrete both *C. botulinum* toxin and organisms in the feces for periods ranging from weeks to months. Consequently, scrupulous handwashing should be practiced after changing the diapers, which should be autoclaved. Persons with open lesions on their hands should not handle soiled diapers. The potentially lengthy excretion of toxin and organisms (occasionally longer than 3 months) precludes close contact between recuperating patients and healthy infants during this time (e.g., sharing a crib or toys). The eventual exclusion of *C. botulinum* from the resident fecal flora, which occurs in all patients, further confirms that this bacterium is a pathogen when present in a symptomatic person.

Bladder atony may be present and increases the risk of urinary tract infection. Gentle manual pressure on the bladder (the Credé method) can be used to achieve emptying. Doing so is best done as a two-person maneuver, with one person sitting the infant up and supporting the head and airway, and the other using two hands (one behind the sacrum) to squeeze the bladder. Indwelling catheters or frequent intermittent catheterizations are not recommended because of their ability to initiate a urinary tract infection.

The second principle of management, the avoidance of complications, is aided by noting past experience (Table 4). Because daily change in an infant botulism patient may be almost imperceptible, there can be a deceptive dullness to its management that may lull the unwary physician into an erroneous complacency. All complications listed in Table 4 were nosocomially acquired, some iatrogenically. A few of these complications represent the irreducible minimum that accrues to critically ill, paralyzed infants who must reside in intensive care units for weeks or months while being entirely dependent on extracorporeal life support systems.

Efforts to improve the treatment of infant botulism continue. A human-derived botulinum antitoxin, known formally as botulism immune globulin, is undergoing investigational new drug evaluation for efficacy in California (112). The results of this randomized, placebo-controlled, double-blinded, phase II study, whose outcome measures are progression of paralysis, incidence of complications, and length and cost of hospital stay, are expected to become available by 1997.

Recovery and Prognosis

Recovery in botulism occurs through regeneration of terminal and subterminal unmyelinated nerve twigs. These sprouts then induce formation of new motor endplates, thereby restoring neuromuscular transmission. Clinically and in experimental animals, this process takes several weeks for completion (86,87). Once neuromuscular transmission is restored, movement resumes. No lasting neuromuscular effects of intestinal toxemia botulism have been observed in infants, but some adults with foodborne botulism have reported chronicity of weakness and fatigue (113). The reasons for this difference may include variation in the amount of toxin absorbed from the gut or variation in the regenerative capacity of adult and infantile motor nerve endings.

Infant botulism caused by type A toxin is potentially, but not invariably, more severe and expensive than that caused by type B toxin. In California, the mean hospital stay for 226 patients with type A illness was 5.6 weeks (median 4.6) at a mean (median) cost of $91,000 ($50,900) per case, whereas the mean hospital stay for 155 patients with type B illness was 3.7 weeks (median 3.4) at a mean (median) cost of $68,300 ($57,700) per case ($p < 10^{-4}$). Hospital costs for all patients from 1984 to 1993 averaged $2400 per day. One quarter of patient had hospital stays that cost $100,000 or more; the most expensive case was hospitalized for 10 months at a cost exceeding $890,000. (All dollar amounts are adjusted to 1993 constant dollars.)

Most patients recover fully from infant botulism. When death occurs, it is not a direct action of the botulinum toxin itself. Instead, death results from complications and the resulting need for intensive care. The case fatality ratio of infants hospitalized with intestinal toxemia botulism in the United States now stands at less than 1%. This remarkably low figure is a tribute to the high quality of intensive care available to these often critically ill, severely paralyzed infants. The experience in other parts of the world has not been so fortunate.

Clinical Circumstances of Adult and Toddler Intestinal Toxemia Botulism

Because botulism in older persons has traditionally been known as a foodborne intoxication, the special circumstances in which intestinal toxemia botulism has occurred in adults deserve description. Somewhat less than a dozen cases of intestinal toxemia botulism in adults and older children have been reported (15,114–118), a situation that is consistent with the presumed rarity of the condition and its current underrecognition.

The clinical circumstances, possible predisposing factors, and supporting diagnostic findings of the known cases of adult and childhood intestinal toxemia botulism are summarized in Table 5. The potentially predisposing features common to most—but not all—cases appear to consist of (a) an altered intestinal tract anatomy, either from surgery or inflammatory bowel disease, (b) an altered intestinal tract physiology (vagotomy, achlorhydria, parenteral nutrition, decreased motility), and (c) an altered intestinal microflora following broad-spectrum antibiotic treatment. The more puzzling circumstance is the Icelandic man who apparently had a normal intestinal tract and acquired intestinal toxemia botulism approximately 6 weeks after simply ingesting *C. botulinum* organisms, either as a large number of vegetative cells or spores, or both.

PREVENTION

Infant botulism and the intestinal toxemias of infancy result from ingestion of the spores of various neurotoxigenic clostridial species. Circumstantial evidence suggests that most infant patients inhale spores carried by microscopic (i.e., invisible) dust that then sticks to saliva and is swallowed. Such cases are presently unpreventable. The easy availability of dustborne botulinum spores in many parts of the world yet the rarity of clinical cases of infant botulism attests to the importance of host factors such as diet and microflora in determining whether or not a given child who swallows spores will develop clinical illness. Breastfeeding appears to slow the onset of illness and to diminish the risk of respiratory arrest in those infants in whom the disease develops (53).

The one identified, avoidable source of botulism spores for infants is honey (33,43). All major pediatric and public health agencies in the United States concur that honey should not be fed to any child less than 12 months of age [references in (42)]. Cases of infant botulism attributable to spore-containing honey have also been reported from Canada, Italy, and Japan (70a–72). Corn syrups were once considered a possible source of botulinum spores but on the basis of more recent evidence are no longer thought to be (121). Additional prevention measures may emerge from a better understanding of the composition and determinants of the infant intestinal microflora, the pathophysiological key to this unique infectious disease.

REFERENCES

1. Smith LDS, Sugiyama H. *Botulism: the Organism, its Toxins, the Disease*. 2nd Ed. Springfield, IL: Charles C. Thomas; 1988.
2. Isacsohn M, Cohen A, Steiner A, Rosenberg P, Rudensky B. Botulism intoxication after surgery in the gut. *Isr J Med Sci* 1985;21:150–153.
3. Weber JT, Goodpasture HC, Alexander H, Werner SB, Hatheway CL, Tauxe RV. Wound botulism in a patient with a tooth abscess: case report and review. *Clin Infect Dis* 1993;16: 635–639.
4. Pickett J, Berg B, Chaplin E, Brunstetter-Shafer M. Syndrome of botulism in infancy: clinical and electrophysiologic study. *N Engl J Med* 1976;295:770–772.
5. Midura TF, Arnon SS. Infant botulism: identification of *Clostridium botulinum* and its toxins in faeces. *Lancet* 1976;2: 934–936.
6. Orr PF. The pathogenicity of *Bacillus botulinus*. *J Infect Dis* 1922;30:118–127.
7. Arnon SS, Midura TF, Clay SA, Wood RM, Chin J. Infant botulism: epidemiological, clinical, and laboratory aspects. *JAMA* 1977;237:1946–1951.
8. Wilcke BW Jr, Midura TF, Arnon SS. Quantitative evidence of intestinal colonization by *Clostridium botulinum* in four cases of infant botulism. *J Infect Dis* 1980;141:419–423.
9. Arnon SS, Werner SB, Faber HK, Farr WH. Infant botulism in 1931: discovery of a misclassified case. *Am J Dis Child* 1979; 133:580–582.
10. Hoffman RE, Pincomb BJ, Skeels MR, Burkhart MJ. Type F infant botulism. *Am J Dis Child* 1982;136:270–271.
11. Hall JD, McCroskey LM, Pincomb BJ, Hatheway CL. Isolation of an organism resembling *Clostridium barati* which produces type F botulinal toxin from an infant with botulism. *J Clin Microbiol* 1985;21:654–655.
12. Suen JC, Hatheway CL, Steigerwalt AG, Brenner DJ. Genetic

13. Aureli P, Fenicia L, Pasolini B, Gianfranceschi M, McCroskey LM, Hatheway CL. Two cases of type E infant botulism in Italy caused by neurotoxigenic *Clostridium butyricum*. *J Infect Dis* 1986;54:207–211.
14. McCroskey LM, Hatheway CL, Fenicia L, Pasolini B, Aureli P. Characterization of an organism that produced type E botulinal toxin but which resembles *Clostridium butyricum* from the feces of an infant with type E botulism. *J Clin Microbiol* 1986; 23:201–202.
15. Chia JK, Clark JB, Ryan CA, Pollack M. Botulism in an adult associated with food-borne intestinal infection with *Clostridium botulinum*. *N Engl J Med* 1986;315:239–240.
16. Scott AB. Botulinum toxin injection into extraocular muscles as an alternative to strabismus surgery. *Ophthalmology* 1980; 87:1044–1049.
17. Jankovic J, Brin MF. Therapeutic uses of botulinum toxin. *N Engl J Med* 1991;324:1186–1194.
18. Schantz EJ, Johnson EA. Properties and use of botulinum toxin and other microbial neurotoxins in medicine. *Microbiol Rev* 1992;56:80–99.
19. Jankovic J, Hallet M (eds.). *Therapy with botulinum toxin*. New York: Marcel Dekker; 1994.
20. Poumeyrol M, Billon J, DeLille F, Hass C, Marmonier A, Sebald M. Intoxication botulique mortelle due a une souche de *Clostridium botulinum* de type AB. *Méd Mala Infect* 1983;13: 750–754.
21. Giménez DF, Ciccarelli AS. Studies on strain 84 of *Clostridium botulinum*. *Zbl Bakt I, Abt Orig A* 1970;84:215:212–220.
22. Giménez DF. *Clostridium botulinum* subtype Ba. *Zbl Bakt Hyg A* 1984;257:68–72.
23. Hatheway CL, McCroskey LM. Unusual neurotoxigenic clostridia recovered from human fecal specimens in the investigation of botulism. In: Hattori T, Ishida Y, Maruyama Y, Morita RY, Uchida A, eds. *Proceedings of the 5th International Symposium on Microbial Ecology: Recent Advances in Microbial Ecology*. Tokyo: Japan Scientific Societies Press; 1990: 477–481.
24. Franciosa G, Ferreira JL, Hatheway CL. Detection of types A, B, and E botulism neurotoxin genes in *Clostridium botulinum* and other *Clostridium* species by the polymerase chain reaction: evidence of unexpressed type B toxin genes in type A toxigenic organisms. *J Clin Microbiol* 1994;32:1911–1917.
25. Suen JC, Hatheway CL, Steigerwalt AG, Brenner DJ. *Clostridium argentinense* sp. nov.: a genetically homogeneous group composed of all strains of *Clostridium botulinum* toxin type G and some nontoxigenic strains previously identified as *Clostridium subterminale* or *Clostridium hastiforme*. *Int J System Bacteriol* 1988;38:375–381.
26. East AK, Thompson DE, Collins MD. Analysis of operons encoding 23S rRNA of *Clostridium botulinum* type A. *J Bacteriol* 1992;174:8158–8162.
26a. Hutson RA, Thompson DE, Collins MD. Genetic interrelationships of saccharolytic *Clostridium botulinum* types B, E, and F and related clostridia as revealed by small-subunit rRNA gene sequences. *FEMS Microbiol Lett* 1993;108;103–110.
26b. Hutson RA, Thompson DE, Lawson PA, Schocken-Itturino RP, Bottger EC, Collins MD. Genetic interrelationships of proteolytic *Clostridium botulinum* types A, B, and F and other members of the *Clostridium botulinum* complex as revealed by small-subunit rRNA gene sequences. *Antonie van Leeuwenhoek* 1993;64:273–283.
27. Poulet S, Hauser D, Quanz M, Niemann H, Popoff MR. Sequence of the botulinal neurotoxin E drived from *Clostridium botulinum* type E (strain Beluga) and *Clostridium butyricum* (strains ATCC 43181 and ATCC 43755). *Biochem Biophys Res Commun* 1992;183:107–113.
28. Fujii N, Kimura K, Yashiki T, et al. Cloning and whole nucleotide sequence of the gene for the light chain component of botulinum type E toxin from *Clostridium butyricum* strain BL6340 and *Clostridium botulinum* type E strain Mashike. *Microbiol Immunol* 1992;36:213–220.

29. Thompson DE, Hutson RA, East AK, Allaway D, Collins MD, Richardson PT. Nucleotide sequence of the gene coding for *Clostridium barati* type F neurotoxin: comparison with other clostridial neurotoxins. *FEMS Microbiol Lett* 1993;108: 175–182.

30. Gill DM. Bacterial toxins: a table of lethal amounts. *Microbiol Rev* 1982;46:86–94.

31. Morton HE. The toxicity of *Clostridium botulinum* type A toxin for various species of animals, including man. Philadelphia: University of Pennsylvania, Institute for Cooperative Research, 1961.

32. Mills DC, Arnon SS. The large intestine as the site of *Clostridium botulinum* colonization in human infant botulism. *J Infect Dis* 1987;156:997–998.

33. Arnon SS. Infant botulism: anticipating the second decade. *J Infect Dis* 1986;154:201–206.

34. Black JD, Dolly JO. Interacton of ^{125}I-labeled botulinum neurotoxins with nerve terminals. I. Ultrastructural autoradiographic localization and quantitation of distinct membrane acceptors for types A and B on motor nerves. *J Cell Biol* 1986;103: 521–534.

35. Simpson LL. Current concepts on the mechanism of action of clostridial neurotoxins. In: DasGupta BR, ed. *Botulinum and tetanus neurotoxins: neurotransmission and biomedical aspects.* New York: Plenum Press; 1993:5–15.

36. Schaivo G, Benfenati F, Poulain B, et al. Tetanus and botulinum-B neurotoxins block neurotransmitter release by proteolytic cleavage of synaptobrevin. *Nature* 1992;359:832–834.

37. Huttner WB. Snappy exocytoxins. *Nature* 1993;365:104–105.

37a. Blasi J, Chapman ER, Link E, et al. Botulinum neurotoxin A selectively cleaves the synaptic protein SNAP-25. *Nature* 1993; 365:160–163.

37b. Blasi J, Chapman ER, Yamasaki S, Binz T, Niemann H, Jahn R. Botulinum neurotoxin C1 blocks neurotransmitter release by means of cleaving HPC-1/syntaxin. *EMBO J* 1993;12: 4821–4828.

37c. Schiavo G, Rossetto O, Catsicas S, et al. Identification of the nerve terminal targets of botulinum neurotoxin serotypes A, D, and E. *J Biol Chem* 1993;268:23784–23787.

38. Barinaga M. Secrets of secretion revealed. *Science* 1993;260: 487–489.

39. Sugiyama H, Mills DC. Intraintestinal toxin in infant mice challenged intragastrically with *Clostridium botulinum* spores. *Infect Immun* 1978;21:59–63.

40. Moberg LJ, Sugiyama H. Microbial ecologic basis of infant botulism as studied with germfree mice. *Infect Immun* 1979; 25:653–657.

41. Burr DH, Sugiyama H. Susceptibility to enteric botulinum colonization of antibiotic-treated adult mice. *Infect Immun* 1982; 36:103–106.

42. Arnon SS, Damus K, Chin J. Infant botulism: epidemiology and relation to sudden infant death syndrome. *Epidemiol Rev* 1981;3:45–66.

43. Arnon SS, Midura TF, Damus K, Thompson B, Wood RM, Chin J. Honey and other environmental risk factors for infant botulism. *J Pediatr* 1979;94:331–336.

44. Easton EJ, Meyer KF. Occurrence of *Bacillus botulinus* in human and animal excreta. *J Infect Dis* 1924;35:207–212.

45. Wells CL, Balish E. *Clostridium tetani* growth and toxin production in the intestines of germfree rats. *Infect Immun* 1983; 41:826–828.

46. Ebisawa I, Kigawa M, Takayanagi M. Colonization of the intestinal tract of mice with *Clostridium tetani*. *Jpn J Exp Med* 1987; 57:315–320.

47. Miyazaki S, Sakaguchi G. Experimental botulism in chickens: the cecum as the site of production and absorption of botulinum toxin. *Jpn J Med Sci Biol* 1978;31:1–15.

48. Moberg LJ, Sugiyama H. The rat as an animal model for infant botulism. *Infect Immun* 1980;29:819–821.

49. Swerczek TW. Experimentally induced toxicoinfectious botulism in horses and foals. *Am J Vet Res* 1980;41:348–350.

50. Stark PL, Lee A. The microbial ecology of the large bowel of breast-fed and formula-fed infants during the first year of life. *J Med Microbiol* 1982;15:189–203.

51. Stark PL, Lee A. Clostridia isolated from the feces of infants during the first year of life. *J Pediatr* 1982;100:362–365.

52. Sullivan NM, Mills DC, Riemann HP, Arnon SS. Inhibition of growth of *Clostridium botulinum* by intestinal microflora isolated from healthy infants. *Microbiol Ecol Health Dis* 1988;1: 179–192.

53. Arnon SS, Damus K, Thompson B, Midura TF, Chin J. Protective role of human milk against sudden death from infant botulism. *J Pediatr* 1982;100:568–573.

54. Goldman AS, Goldblum RM. Immunologic system in human milk: characteristics and effects. In: Lebenthal E, ed. *Textbook of gastroenterology and nutrition in infancy.* 2nd Ed. New York: Raven Press; 1989:135–142.

55. Arnon SS. Breast feeding and toxigenic intestinal infections: missing links in crib death? *Rev Infect Dis* 1984;6:S193–S201.

56. Long SS, Gajeweski JL, Brown LW, Gilligan PH. Clinical, laboratory, and environmental features of infant botulism in southeastern Pennsylvania. *Pediatrics* 1985;75:935–941.

57. Long SS. Epidemiologic study of infant botulism in Pennsylvania: report of the infant botulism study group. *J Pediatr* 1985; 75:928–934.

58. Spika JS, Shaffer N, Hargrett-Bean N, Collin S, MacDonald KL, Blake PA. Risk factors for infant botulism in the United States. *Am J Dis Child* 1989;143:828–832.

59. Morris JG Jr, Snyder JD, Wilson R, Feldman RA. Infant botulism in the United States: an epidemiologic study of cases occurring outside of California. *Am J Public Health* 1983;73: 1385–1388.

60. Arnon SS, Midura TF, Damus K, Wood RM, Chin J. Intestinal infection and toxin production by *Clostridium botulinum* as one cause of sudden infant death syndrome. *Lancet* 1978;1: 1273–1277.

61. Peterson DR, Eklund MW, Chinn NM. The sudden infant death syndrome and infant botulism. *Rev Infect Dis* 1979;1:630–634.

62. Sonnabend OAR, Sonnabend WFF, Krech U, Molz G, Sigrist T. Continuous microbiological and pathological study of 70 sudden and unexpected deaths: toxigenic intestinal *Clostridium botulinum* infection in 9 cases of sudden infant death syndrome. *Lancet* 1985;1:237–240.

63. Byard RW, Moore L, Bourne AJ, Lawrence AJ, Goldwater PN. *Clostridium botulinum* and sudden infant death syndrome: a 10 year prospective study. *J Paediatr Child Health* 1992;28: 156–157.

64. Beckwith JB. The sudden infant death syndrome. *Curr Probl Pediatr* 1973;3:3–36.

65. Thilo EH, Townsend SF, Deacon J. Infant botulism at 1 week of age: report of two cases. *Pediatrics* 1993;92:151–153.

66. Hurst DL, Marsh WW. Early severe infantile botulism. *J Pediatr* 1993;122:909–911.

67. Hubert P, Roy C, Caille B. Un cas de botulisme chez un nourrisson de 11 mois. *Arch Fr Pediatr* 1987;44:129–130.

68. Smith LDS. The occurrence of *Clostridium botulinum* and *Clostridium tetani* in the soil of the United States. *Health Lab Sci* 1978;15:74–80.

69. Istre GR, Compton R, Novotny T, Young JE, Hatheway CL, Hopkins RS. Infant botulism: three cases in a small town. *Am J Dis Child* 1986;140:1013–1014.

70. Schwarz PJ, Arnon JM, Arnon SS. Epidemiologic aspects of infant botulism in California, 1976–91. In: DasGupta BR, ed. *Botulinum and tetanus neurotoxins: neurotransmission and biomedical aspects.* New York: Plenum Press; 1993:503–504.

70a. Hauschild AHW, Hilsheimer R, Weiss KF, Burke RB. *Clostridium botulinum* in honey, syrups, and dry infant cereals. *J Food Protect* 1988;51:892–894.

71. Tabita K, Sakaguchi S, Kozaki S, Sakaguchi G. Distinction between *Clostridium botulinum* type A strains associated with food-borne botulism and those with infant botulism in Japan and in the intraintestinal toxin production in infant mice and some other properties. *FEMS Microbiol Lett* 1991;79:251–256.

72. Fenicia L, Ferrini AM, Aureli P, Pocecco M. A case of infant botulism associated with honey feeding in Italy. *Eur J Epidemiol* 1993;9:671–673.

73. Sugiyama H, Mills DC, Kuo L-JC. Number of *Clostridium botulinum* spores in honey. *J Food Prot* 1978;41:848–850.

74. Midura TF, Snowden S, Wood RM, Arnon SS. Isolation of *Clostridium botulinum* from honey. *J Clin Microbiol* 1979;9:282–283.
75. Huhtanen CN, Knox D, Shimanuki H. Incidence and origin of *Clostridium botulinum* spores in honey. *J Food Prot* 1981;44:812–815.
76. Hauschild AHW, Hilsheimer R, Weiss KF, Burke RB. *Clostridium botulinum* in honey, syrups and dry infant cereals. *J Food Prot* 1988;51:892–894.
77. Nakano H, Okabe T, Hashimoto H, Sakaguchi G. Incidence of *Clostridium botulinum* in honey of various origins. *Jpn J Med Sci Biol* 1990;43:183–195.
78. Nakano H, Sakaguchi G. An unusually heavy contamination of honey products by *Clostridium botulinum* type F and *Bacillus alvei*. *FEMS Microbiol Lett* 1991;79:171–178.
79. Nakano H, Yoshikuni Y, Hashimoto H, Sakaguchi G. Detection of *Clostridium botulinum* in natural sweetening. *Int J Food Microbiol* 1992;16:117–121.
80. Berry PR, Gilbert RJ, Oliver RWA, Gibson AAM. Some preliminary studies on the low incidence of infant botulism in the United Kingdom (letter). *J Clin Pathol* 1987;40:121.
81. Glauser TA, Maguire HC, Sladky JT. Relapse of infant botulism. *Ann Neurol* 1990;28:187–189.
82. Schreiner MS, Field E, Ruddy R. Infant botulism: a review of 12 years' experience at the Children's Hospital of Philadelphia. *Pediatrics* 1991;87:159–165.
83. Paton JC, Lawrence AJ, Steven IM. Quantities of *Clostridium botulinum* organisms and toxin in feces and presence of *Clostridium botulinum* toxin in the serum of an infant with botulism. *J Clin Microbiol* 1983;17:13–15.
84. Paton JC, Lawrence AJ, Manson JI. Quantitation of *Clostridium botulinum* organisms and toxin in the feces of an infant with botulism. *J Clin Microbiol* 1982;15:1–4.
85. Rubin LG, Dezfulian M, Yolken RH. Serum antibody response to *Clostridium botulinum* toxin in infant botulism. *J Clin Microbiol* 1982;16:770–771.
86. Duchen LW. Motor nerve growth induced by botulinum toxin as a regenerative phenomenon. *Proc R Soc Med* 1972;65:196–197.
87. Angaut-Petit D, Molgo J, Comella JX, Faille L, Tabti N. Terminal sprouting in mouse neuromuscular junctions poisoned with botulinum type A toxin: morphological and electrophysiological features. *Neuroscience* 1990;37:799–808.
88. Arnon SS. Infant botulism. *Annu Rev Med* 1980;31:541–560.
89. Wilson R, Morris JG Jr, Snyder JD, Feldman RA. Clinical characteristics of infant botulism in the United States: a study of the non-California cases. *Pediatr Infect Dis* 1982;1:148–150.
90. Lindsay JA, Mach AS, Wilkinson MA, et al. *Clostridium perfringens* type A cytotoxic-enterotoxin(s) as triggers for death in the sudden infant death syndrome: development of a toxicoinfection hypothesis. *Curr Microbiol* 1993;27:51–59.
91. Mach AS, Lindsay JA. Activation of *Clostridium perfringens* cytotoxic enterotoxin(s) in vivo and in vitro: role in triggers for sudden infant death. *Curr Microbiol* 1994;28:261–267.
92. Telford DR, Morris JA, Hughes P, et al. The nasopharyngeal bacterial flora in the sudden infant death syndrome. *J Infect* 1989;18:125–130.
93. Bettelheim KA, Goldwater PN, Dwyer BW, Bourne AJ, Smith DL. Toxigenic *Escherichia coli* associated with sudden infant death syndrome. *Scand J Infect Dis* 1990;22:467–476.
94. McKendrick N, Drucker DB, Morris JA, et al. Bacterial toxins: a possible cause of cot death. *J Clin Pathol* 1992;45:49–53.
95. Malam JE, Carrick GF, Telford DR, Morris JA. Staphylococcal toxins and sudden infant death syndrome. *J Clin Pathol* 1992;45:716–721.
96. Drucker DB, Aluyi HS, Morris JA, Telford DR, Gibbs A. Lethal synergistic action of toxins of bacteria isolated from sudden infant death syndrome. *J Clin Pathol* 1992;45:799–801.
97. Murrell WG, Stewart BJ, O'Neill C, Siarakas S, Kariks S. Enterotoxigenic bacteria in the sudden infant death syndrome. *J Med Microbiol* 1993;39:114–127.
98. Berlit P, Rakicky J. The Miller Fisher syndrome: review of the literature. *J Clin Neuro-Ophthalmol* 1992;12:57–63.
99. Johnson RO, Clay SA, Arnon SS. Diagnosis and management of infant botulism. *Am J Dis Child* 1979;133:586–593.
100. Cornblath DR, Sladky JT, Sumner AJ. Clinical electrophysiology of infantile botulism. *Muscle and Nerve* 1983;6:448–452.
101. Graf WD, Hays RM, Astley SJ, Mendelman PM. Electrodiagnosis reliability in the diagnosis of infant botulism. *J Pediatr* 1992;120:747–749.
102. Engel WK. Brief, small, abundant motor-unit action potentials: a further critique of electromyographic interpretation. *Neurology* 1975;25:173–176.
103. Szabo EA, Pemberton JM, Desmarchelier PM. Specific detection of *Clostridium botulinum* type B by using the polymerase chain reaction. *Appl Environ Microbiol* 1992;58:418–420.
104. Szabo EA, Pemberton JM, Desmarchelier PM. Detection of the genes encoding botulinum neurotoxin types A to E by the polymerase chain reaction. *Appl Environ Microbiol* 1993;59:3011–3020.
105. Fach P, Hauser D, Guillou JP, Popoff MR. Polymerase chain reaction for the rapid identification of *Clostridium botulinum* type A strains and detection in food samples. *J Appl Bacteriol* 1993;75:234–239.
106. Hatheway CL, McCroskey LM. Examination of feces and serum for diagnosis of infant botulism in 336 patients. *J Clin Microbiol* 1987;25:2334–2338.
107. Takahashi M, Noda H, Takeshita S, et al. Attempts to quantify *Clostridium botulinum* type A toxin and antitoxin in serum of two cases of infant botulism in Japan. *Jpn J Med Sci Biol* 1990;43:233–237.
108. Centers for Disease Control. Case definitions for public health surveillance. *MMWR* 1990;39 (No. RR-13):6–7.
109. Arnon SS. Infant botulism. In: Feigen RD, Cherry JD, eds. *Textbook of pediatric infectious disease*. 3rd Ed. Philadelphia: WB Saunders; 1992:1095–1102.
110. Wohl DL, Tucker JA. Infant botulism: considerations for airway management. *Laryngoscope* 1992;102:1251–1254.
111. Santos JI, Swensen P, Glasgow LA. Potentiation of *Clostridium botulinum* toxin by aminoglycoside antibiotics: clinical and laboratory observations. *Pediatrics* 1981;68:50–54.
112. Arnon SS. Clinical trial of human botulism immune globulin. In: DasGupta BR, ed. *Botulinum and tetanus neurotoxins: neurotransmission and biomedical aspects*. New York: Plenum Press; 1993:477–483.
113. Mann JM, Martin S, Hoffman R, Marrazzo S. Patient recovery from type A botulism: morbidity assessment following a large outbreak. *Am J Public Health* 1981;71:266–269.
114. English WJ, Williams LP Jr, Bryant RE, Gillies MD. Case 48–1980: botulism (letter). *N Engl J Med* 1981;304:789–790.
115. Freedman M, Armstrong RM, Killian JM, Boland D. Botulism in a patient with jejunoileal bypass. *Ann Neurol* 1986;20:641–643.
116. McCroskey LM, Hatheway CL. Laboratory findings in four cases of adult botulism suggest colonization of the intestinal tract. *J Clin Microbiol* 1988;26:1052–1054.
117. McCroskey LM, Hatheway CL, Woodruff BA, Greenberg JA, Jurgenson P. Type F botulism due to neurotoxigenic *Clostridium botulinum* from an unknown source in an adult. *J Clin Microbiol* 1991;29:2618–2620.
118. Shen W-PV, Felsing N, Lang D, Goodman G, Cairo MS. Development of infant botulism in a 3-year-old female with neuroblastoma following autologous bone marrow transplantation: potential use of human botulism immune globulin. *Bone Marrow Transpl* 1994;13:345–347.
119. Sebald M, Saimot G. Toxémie botulique; intérêt de sa mise en évidence dans le diagnostic du botulisme humain de type B. *Ann Microbiol* 1973;124A:61–69.
120. Sonnabend WF, Sonnabend OA, Gründler P, Katz E. Intestinal toxicoinfection by *Clostridium botulinum* type F in an adult: case associated with Guillain–Barré syndrome. *Lancet* 1989;1:357–361.
121. Lilly T Jr., Rhodehamel EJ, Kautter DA, Solomon HM. *Clostridium botulinum* spores in corn syrup and other syrups. *J Food Protect* 1991;54:585–587.

Infections of the Gastrointestinal Tract,
edited by M. J. Blaser, P. D. Smith, J. I. Ravdin,
H. B. Greenberg, and R. L. Guerrant
Raven Press, Ltd., New York © 1995.

CHAPTER 20

Acute Watery Diarrhea

John K. Crane and Richard L. Guerrant

And so it was proven, by an insidious questioning, that the symptoms of love are the same as the symptoms of cholera.

GABRIEL GARCIA MARQUEZ,
Love in the Time of Cholera

The syndrome of acute watery diarrhea is so common, so much a part of the universal human experience, that all readers, unless they have spent their life in a sterile, protective bubble, have experienced it firsthand. Perhaps it was the lightheadedness and the rapid heart rate caused by dehydration that inspired Garcia Marquez's comparison of cholera and the emotion of love quoted above. Indeed, for intestinal pathogens that cause watery diarrhea without invading the gut mucosa, dehydration is the most life-threatening aspect of the illness.

Features of a diarrheal illness important in making a clinical assessment include the volume and frequency of the diarrhea, the character of the diarrhea (especially the presence or absence of blood or mucus in the stools), the presence of fever, and associated gastrointestinal symptoms such as vomiting and abdominal cramps. As opposed to watery diarrhea, *dysentery* consists of frequent but smaller stools, often with a gelatinous appearance containing blood and mucus, and frequently accompanied by fever and abdominal cramps. Acute inflammatory diarrheal illness such as dysentery is discussed in the next chapter. It should be noted, however, that even disease due to invasive pathogens (such as *Shigella* and *Entamoeba histolytica*) will usually begin with watery diarrhea and gradually evolve toward the more classic dysenteric features as the illness progresses. For example, Ericsson and DuPont report that, in their studies in Mexico where travelers had convenient access to medical care, about 90% of patients with *Shigella* infection initially presented with watery diarrhea (1). This illustrates the need for re-

J. K. Crane: Division of Infectious Diseases, SUNY Clinical Center, Buffalo, New York, 14215.

R. L. Guerrant: Division of Geographic Medicine, University of Virginia School of Medicine, Charlottesville, Virginia 22908.

evaluation of the patient with watery diarrhea if the patient worsens, if the character of the diarrhea changes, or if diarrhea persists for more than a few days.

MICROBIOLOGY

The causes of acute watery diarrhea are extremely varied and include toxic, noninfectious (Table 1) as well as infectious etiologies (Table 2; Fig. 1). Among travelers to developing countries, the most common causes of diarrhea are, in approximate descending order: *Escherichia coli* (primarily toxigenic, but also enteropathogenic strains), rotavirus, *Shigella, Campylobacter jejuni, Aeromonas* (especially in Thailand), *Salmonella* species, and noncholera *Vibrio.*

Among children in developing countries, the commonest causes of diarrhea include toxigenic *E. coli,* rotavirus, *Shigella,* and *Campylobacter.* Enteropathogenic *E. coli* may be important in children in large cities in the developing world (2). In studies of infants, a large proportion of cases (40–50%) may show no known pathogen.

Among outbreaks of diarrhea in children attending U.S. day care centers, the most common identified pathogens were rotavirus, enteric adenovirus, and *Giardia* (3). A high proportion of outbreaks (48% in this study) were of unknown etiology.

PATHOGENESIS

All of the causes of watery diarrhea have in common an imbalance between the amount of fluid secreted into the gastrointestinal tract (estimated to be at least 10 L/day in a normal adult) and the ability of the intestinal epithelium to reabsorb that fluid. Viral enteric pathogens such as rotavirus preferentially infect and kill villous tip enterocytes over large areas of the small intestine, markedly impairing absorptive capacity while allowing the spared, normal crypt cells to continue to secrete ions and fluid (Fig. 2). In these cases, the amount of fluid presented

TABLE 1. *Toxic and pharmacological causes of acute, watery diarrhea*

Type of poisoning	Associated symptoms	Ref.
Mushroom poisoning		
Amanita muscaria and *Chlorophyllum molybdites,* others	Salivation, lacrimation, constricted pupils	4,5
Poisoning from seafood		
Ciguatera	Numbness, tingling	6–9
Diarrhetic shellfish poisoning	Severe cramps	
Scombroid fish poisoning	Peppery taste, flushing	
Organophosphate pesticides		
Malathion	Salivation, lacrimation	10
Drugs		
Misoprostol		11,12
Laxatives		

to the colon may overwhelm its reabsorptive capacity, resulting in diarrhea.

Many cases of diarrhea may best be considered a pathological exaggeration of what is normally a host protective response to proliferation, attachment, or invasion by enteric microbes. Specialized crypt cells known as Paneth cells have been shown to contain antimicrobial peptides, termed cryptdins, which are related to the defensins of neutrophils (37). Although nothing is known about how the release of cryptdins is regulated, it is tempting to speculate that release may somehow be triggered by bacterial products within the crypts. Intestinal epithelial cells also

TABLE 2. *Common microbial causes of acute watery diarrhea*

Category	Common examples	Associated symptoms, comments	Settings	Ref.
Preformed bacterial toxins	Staphylococcal food poisoning, *Bacillus cereus* food poisoning	Nausea and vomiting predominate	Foodborne outbreaks	13,14
Viruses	Rotavirus	Fever common; 5- to 7-day duration	Increased incidence in winter in temperate climates	15–17
	Adenovirus	Fever and respiratory symptoms common; 10- to 12-day duration of vomiting and diarrhea; mustard yellow or tan watery stools	Children; AIDS	3,17–19
	Norwalk virus	Prominent vomiting; may have fever	Outbreaks; associated with raw shellfish	16,20
	Norwalk-like viruses	Illness similar to Norwalk virus		16,21
Bacteria	Enterotoxigenic *E. coli* (ETEC)	3- to 5- day duration; children often have fever	Travelers, infants in developing countries	22–25
	Enteropathogenic *E. coli* (EPEC)	May be associated with fever and vomiting; "fishy odor"; may have longer duration than ETEC	Infants, urban areas of developing countries	2,24
	Campylobacter jejuni	Fever and bloody stools common; propensity to relapse	Developed and developing countries; increased incidence in winter	1,26
	Vibrio cholerae (Fig. 1)	Massive watery diarrhea; "rice water stools," fishy odor	Epidemics	27–29
	Salmonella sp.	May also cause inflammatory diarrhea; fever common	Foodborne outbreaks	
	Many other enteric bacteria	*Aeromonas, Plesiomonas, Klebsiella, Citrobacter,* and others have been implicated		30,31
Parasites	*Giardia duodenalis*	Malabsorption syndrome; bloating; flatulence; foul-smelling stools; may produce persistent diarrhea	Travelers; backpackers; day care centers	32
	Cryptosporidium parvum	Watery diarrhea; persistent infections in immunocompromised patients	Travelers to St. Petersburg; outbreaks	33, 34
	Isospora belli	Malabsorption; eosinophilia	Developing countries; AIDS	32
	Cyclospora cayetenesis (formerly "CLOs; cyanobacteria-like organisms)	"Flu-like" onset with relapsing-remitting watery diarrhea lasting up to 2 months; stool exam shows nonrefractile spheres 8–10 μm in diameter	Travelers to Nepal; developing countries; waterborne outbreaks	35,36

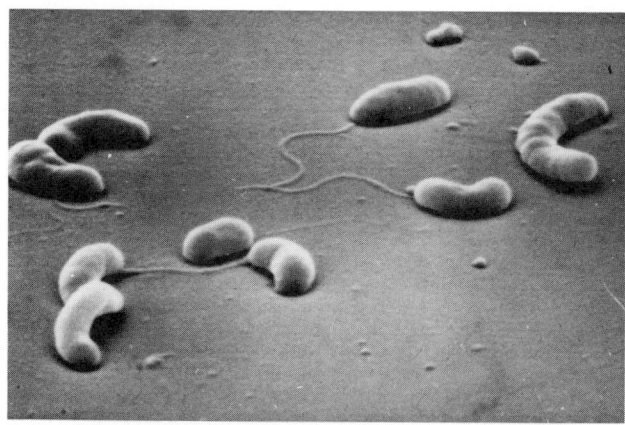

FIG. 1. Scanning electron micrograph of *Vibrio cholerae*. Note the presence of polar flagellae. (From ref. 76, with permission.)

produce guanylin, a peptide believed to be the endogenous ligand for the receptor for the heat-stable enterotoxin of *E. coli* (STa) (38–40). Guanylin probably serves as a local regulator of normal host secretion, but may also play a role in helping to purge crypts of proliferating or invading organisms.

Study of the secretory pathways stimulated by microbial toxins has enhanced our understanding of the regulation of the normal secretory and absorptive apparatus of the intestinal cell. Table 3 summarizes some of the microbial enterotoxins whose mechanism of action is known.

Activation of host cell protein kinases is a pathway by which several invasive bacteria (*Shigella*, *Salmonella*, *Yersinia*, *Listeria*) as well as other enteric pathogens classically considered as noninvasive (e.g., enteropathogenic *E. coli*, or EPEC) are hypothesized to invade cells or trigger diarrheal fluid secretion (41–43). At present the relative importance of different protein kinases in generating the intestinal fluid response is unclear, but tyrosine protein kinases, protein kinase C, and calmodulin-dependent protein kinase have all been reported to be stimulated by various organisms during different stages of adherence or invasion in cultured cells.

While the roles of various protein kinases are not yet well worked out in the pathogenesis of intestinal secretion in infection, evidence is stronger for the role of these kinases in the response to drugs and natural products, such as plant laxatives. For example, ricinoleic acid, considered the active ingredient in castor oil, stimulates protein kinase C (44). Similarly, the active compounds found in the oil of the purging croton (*Croton tiglii*), phorbol esters, are highly potent and specific stimulators of protein kinase C as well (45,46).

An important variable in the pathogenesis of diarrheal diseases is the infectious dose or the inoculum required to produce symptomatic disease in normal individuals. Table 4 lists the infectious dose for several enteric pathogens. The concept of the infectious dose has been criti-

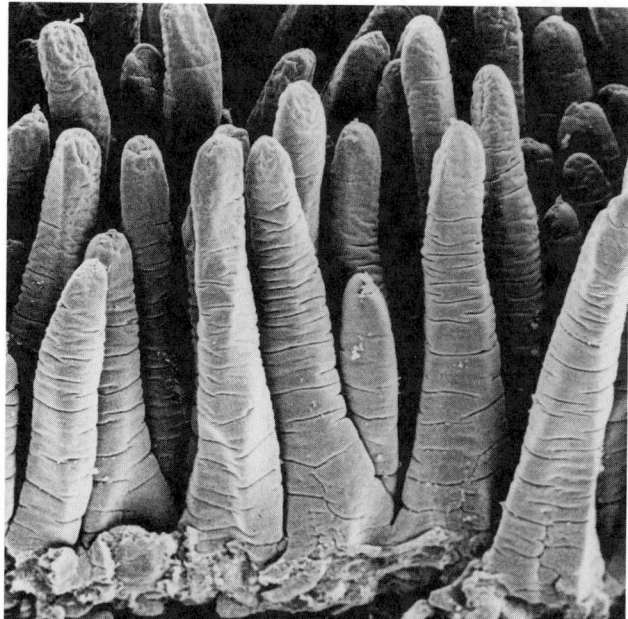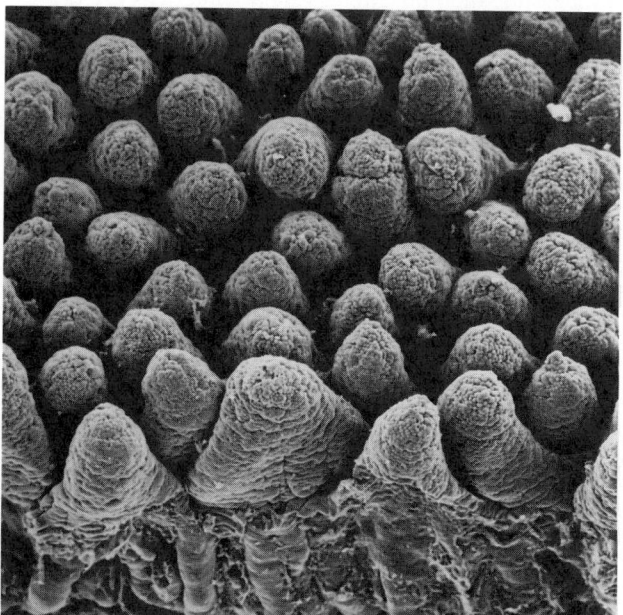

FIG. 2. Scanning electron micrograph of normal and rotavirus-damaged intestinal villi. Small intestinal mucosa is shown from normal, uninfected (**left**) and rotavirus-infected gnotobiotic calf (**right**), 6 days after infection. In the infected calf, the villi are markedly shortened, some villi are fused together, and the surface enterocytes are swollen and abnormally arranged. Depth of the crypts is markedly increased in the infected tissue due to compensatory hyperplasia at this stage of the infection. (Photographs courtesy of Dr. Graham A. Hall, Public Health Laboratory Service, Salisbury, Wiltshire, U.K.)

TABLE 3. *Activation of host secretory pathways by microbial enterotoxins and bacterial adhesion molecules*

Toxin or adhesion phenotype	Source	Second messenger or intracellular target	Ref.
Cholera toxin, heat-labile toxin, (LT)	*V. cholerae* *E. coli*, others	Bind to ganglioside GM$_1$; catalyzes ADP ribosylation of G$_{s-\alpha}$; elevate cyclic AMP	47
Heat-stable enterotoxins, (STa) (STp, STh, Y-ST); enteroaggregative heat-stable toxin (EAST1)	Toxigenic *E. coli* (STa), noncholera *Vibrio*, *Yersinia*, others; enteroaggregative *E. coli* (EAST1)	Bind to and activate membrane-bound guanylate cyclase; elevate cyclic GMP	48–50 51,52
Okadaic acid, microcystin	Produced by plankton or cyanobacteria such as *Microcyctis aeruginosa*; concentrated in sponges and shellfish (diarrhetic shellfish poisoning)	Inhibit protein phosphatases; unopposed protein kinase action may result in phosphorylation of and opening of membrane channels	8,9
STb	*E. coli*	Induces a rise in intracellular calcium from extracellular stores	52
Intimately adhering organisms	Enteropathogenic *E. coli* (EPEC)	Activation of host protein kinases, including tyrosine kinases, protein kinase C	41–43

cized because it emphasizes the virulent characteristics of the pathogenic organism without taking into account the wide variability of host defenses. Indeed, the infectious dose of many bacterial pathogens is lowered markedly in individuals with decreased gastric acidity, patients already receiving antibiotics, or patients with impaired intestinal motility or receiving antimotility drugs. In natural populations, behavioral factors such as food preferences, cooking methods, and hygienic practices are probably even more important than the above-mentioned "biological" factors in determining who becomes ill and who remains well after exposure to enteric pathogens. With these caveats in mind, the infectious dose can nevertheless be helpful in understanding the mode of transmission of disease and the approaches needed to interrupt

TABLE 4. *Infectious dose of various diarrheal pathogens*[a]

Pathogen	Infectious dose
"Low-inoculum" organisms	
Shigella[b]	10^1–10^2
Giardia lamblia	10^1–10^2 cysts
Entamoeba histolytica[b]	10^1–10^2 cysts
Rotavirus	10^1 plaque-forming units[c]
"Intermediate"-inoculum organisms	
Campylobacter jejuni[b]	10^2–10^6
"High-inoculum" organisms	
Vibrio cholerae	10^8
Salmonella	10^5
Escherichia coli	10^8

[a] Modified from ref. 53.
[b] Classically associated with inflammatory rather than watery diarrhea.
[c] From Ref. 54.

transmission. "Low-inoculum" agents such as *Giardia, Cryptosporidium,* rotavirus, and *Shigella* are easily spread from person to person, whereas "high-inoculum" agents such as *Vibrio cholerae, Salmonella,* and toxigenic *E. coli* are usually acquired by ingesting larger numbers of organisms via contaminated food or water.

EPIDEMIOLOGY

The modes of transmission and epidemiological features of the pathogens that cause acute watery diarrhea are quite varied, as emphasized by Tables 2 and 4. All of these infections are acquired by the inadvertent ingestion of organisms ultimately derived from feces ("fecal–oral route"). This statement, however, belies a great deal of ignorance in some cases about how enteric pathogens are actually spread.

Water

One of the most common adages heard by the traveler is, "Don't drink the water." The pioneering sleuthing that allowed Dr. John Snow to link the Broad Street water pump with the spread of cholera in London in 1854 remains a classic in medical history. The incidence of diarrheal disease is markedly increased in some areas in the rainy season (1,55), strongly suggesting contamination of water from runoff. Water has been implicated in the cholera outbreaks that began in Peru in 1991 and in Burundi in 1992 (27,28). Furthermore, evidence for direct acquisition of *Giardia* and *Cryptosporidium* from surface water or inadequately filtered municipal water supplies is well documented (33,34). However, solid evidence incriminating drinking water is lacking for many common pathogens such as toxigenic *E. coli* (1).

Food

For many pathogens, food is probably just as important, or more important, than water as a mode of transmission. Fish and shellfish have been incriminated in the spread of *Vibrio cholerae,* noncholera *Vibrio, Vibrio parahemolyticus,* and Norwalk virus (29). Eggs, including intact eggs, are a source of *Salmonella,* as are poultry and beef. Beef has also been the source of multistate outbreaks of enterohemorrhagic *E. coli,* including O157: H7, and other serotypes (56).

Vomitus and Other Modes of Transmission

Vomitus has been identified as the likely agent of transmission of Norwalk virus and other viral agents of gastroenteritis in outbreaks on cruise ships (57). Investigation of an outbreak of a Norwalk-like viral agent in a nursing home identified at least nine ill employees without any contact with patients or patients' body fluids, suggesting the possibility of airborne spread of virus (21).

Direct Person-to-Person Contact

Secondary spread among close household contacts is common for low-inoculum pathogens (see Table 4).

Insects

Flies and cockroaches have been blamed for contamination of food with enteric pathogens, but their role has not been conclusively proven. Cultures of microbes from the feet or digestive tracts of insects have been conducted and yielded pathogens such as *Salmonella* in a low percentage of individual insects (58). However, for a fair comparison, the rate of bacterial carriage in insects considered beneficial such as crickets, lady beetles, and praying mantises should be included as controls in future similar studies.

CLINICAL FEATURES AND DIFFERENTIAL DIAGNOSIS

The clinical setting of a diarrheal illness provides information as important to the clinician as that from the physical exam or inspection of the diarrheal fecal specimen. Is the patient an adult or a child? Has the patient traveled? What is known about the patient's immune system? Does the patient have a decrease in gastric acidity? Was the patient taking antibiotics before the onset of illness?

The history of the diarrheal illness itself is the next crucial part of the assessment. The character of the diarrhea (consistency, color, odor, volume, and frequency) is critical in determining subsequent management. Diarrhea associated with blood or mucus in the stools suggests an inflammatory cause (see previous chapter) and stool cul-

ture is usually indicated. Very high-volume diarrhea suggests rotavirus or, in the appropriate geographic setting, cholera or *Cryptosporidium.* Rotavirus and adenoviruses usually produce watery tan or yellowish stools. Cholera classically is associated with clear watery diarrhea containing light-colored flecks of mucus (''rice water'' stools). *Giardia*-induced diarrhea is often watery and greenish with bits of undigested food and associated with a foul odor. If the patient is unable to supply a fecal specimen at the time of the encounter, the appearance and odor of the stool must be elicited from the patient by direct questioning.

Prominent vomiting is often seen with rotavirus, adenovirus, enteropathogenic *E. coli,* Norwalk virus, and the Norwalk-like viruses.

Abdominal cramps are common in most diarrheal diseases and usually do not help distinguish one causative agent from another. Tenesmus, or painful rectal spasms, is an indication of proctitis and is an important clue toward invasive pathogens, such as *Shigella* or *Entamoeba histolytica.* High fever (>39°C) can be seen with these invasive pathogens but also with rotavirus and adenovirus (especially the classic, nonenteric serotypes) (18). Sexually transmitted causes of proctitis, including herpes simplex and cytomegalovirus, must be suspected if the patient has AIDS or is homosexually active. These patients may have rectal pain and mucoid rectal discharge but little actual diarrhea.

Physical examination of the patient with diarrhea is important to assess the patient's nutritional status, degree of dehydration (see Table 5), and signs of poisoning (cholinesterase inhibitors cause constricted pupils; botulism causes dilated pupils), and to rule out signs, such as splenomegaly, of multisystem disease. The degree of dehydration will usually have to be determined by physical examination, since it is difficult for the patient and physician to quantify the amount of diarrhea by history alone. In addition, the patient should be examined for physical signs of immune dysfunction, such as oral thrush, seborrheic dermatitis of the face, or lymphadenopathy, since the diagnostic approach will often be quite different in the patient immunocompromised by HIV or AIDS. A rectal examination is important in assessing proctitis and to determine if hemorrhoids are a confounding source of blood.

In this era where patients' body fluids are usually whisked to the laboratory in sealed biohazard bags, the importance to the clinician of actually inspecting the patient's diarrhea specimen for blood and mucus cannot be overemphasized. In many cases, this affords the opportunity to perform a wet mount of the fecal specimen for leukocytes immediately, before spontaneous lysis of neutrophils occurs due to prolonged standing at room temperature. Olfactory clues can be helpful in assessing diarrhea during inspection of the stool specimen. Frankly dysenteric stools due to *Shigella* are usually almost odorless. *Vibrio cholerae* and enteropathogenic *E. coli* have been said to impart a fishy odor to the diarrhea they produce. *Giardia* infections are associated with foul-smelling stools and flatulence. *Salmonella* infections have been reported anecdotally to give a hydrogen sulfide or ''rotten egg''

TABLE 5. *Assessment of dehydration*

Symptoms or signs	Mild or no dehydration (<5%)	Moderate dehydration (5–10%)	Severe dehydration (>10%)
General condition	Well, alert	Restless, irritable	Lethargic or unconscious; floppy
Eyes	Normal	Sunken	Very sunken and dry
Tears	Present	Absent	Absent
Mouth and tongue	Moist	Dry	Very dry
Thirst	Drinks normally, not thirsty	Thirsty, drinks eagerly	Drinks poorly or not able to drink
Skin	Pinch retracts immediately	Pinch retracts slowly (2 sec)	Pinch retracts very slowly (3–5 sec)
Estimated fluid deficit	<50 mL/kg	50–100 mL/kg	>100 mL/kg
Appropriate type of fluid therapy	Maintenance fluid with increased intake of home fluids such as fruit juice, soups, or ORS	Observed administration of ORS in the health facility; instruct caregivers on preparation	IV therapy initially; switch to oral when patient able to drink

Adapted from Refs. 59 and 60.
ORS, oral rehydration solution.

odor in the feces, correlating with the ability of nontyphoidal *Salmonella* to produce H_2S in vitro.

DIFFERENTIAL DIAGNOSIS

Recognition of acute diarrhea and suspicion of an infectious etiology will usually be performed by the patient before seeking medical attention. Occasionally, however, physicians will be confronted with patients whose illness is not due to an enteric pathogen but due to a toxic exposure (Table 1), a systemic illness, or noninfectious causes. Pernicious anemia may present with a preponderance of gastrointestinal symptoms, including diarrhea, fever, and malabsorption, which has been attributed to rapid turnover of intestinal epithelial cells due to megaloblastic changes. Pellagra due to niacin deficiency can also present with chronic diarrhea. Malaria in the returning traveler can present with a predominance of abdominal symptoms, including circulatory collapse and abdominal pain (the well-emphasized "algid malaria"). It is less appreciated that in a significant portion of malaria patients acute, watery diarrhea and fever may dominate the presentation. Harries et al. reported that acute watery diarrhea was the second most common symptom (in 23%) in a series of 150 consecutive adult patients with falciparum malaria in Malawi (61). A similar study in Uganda showed that acute diarrhea and/or vomiting was observed in 45% of HIV-negative children and 29% of HIV-negative adults with falciparum malaria (62). In typhoid fever, patients may be constipated early in their illness, but some may develop diarrhea. In both malaria and typhoid the presence of persistent high fever is a clue to ongoing systemic illness. Persistent diarrhea in a returning traveler occasionally leads to a gastroenterological evaluation and a diagnosis of inflammatory bowel disease or intestinal parasite. Even more commonly, patients with a history of inflammatory bowel disease may suffer a flare-up after an intercurrent bout of traveler's diarrhea due to the usual pathogens. In addition, patients may have their first episode of inflammatory bowel disease after foreign travel (63).

SPECIFIC DIAGNOSTIC MEASURES AND MANAGEMENT

Just as the usual impulse of the patient with diarrhea is to request antimotility medication to stop the diarrhea, the usual impulse of the physician is to send a stool culture. Although there are some situations in which these reflex actions are acceptable, in general the physician should resist them and instead apply critical thinking. Stool cultures obtained from otherwise healthy adults and children suffering from acute watery diarrhea in developed countries have such a low rate of positivity as to make them economically contraindicated, especially since most of the important therapeutic decisions will have to be made before the results of the cultures are known. Stool cultures in this setting may have a positivity rate as low as 2% or less and the cost per case detected may be $950–$1200, making the stool culture the "most expensive and least valuable microbiologic test in the hospital" (32,59,64,65). Stool exams for ova and parasites in the same population, or in patients hospitalized for other reasons who develop diarrhea while in the hospital, almost never yield a diagnosis relevant to the management of the diarrheal illness (a review of the patient's medication list and a test for *Clostridium difficile* or its toxin may be more helpful in the inpatient). Instead of a stool culture as the initial diagnostic test, a test for fecal leukocytes is preferred in those with more severe illness, a duration of diarrhea greater than 1 day, or those with fever or bloody diarrhea (Fig. 3). In the future, tests for a leukocyte marker such as fecal lactoferrin may be more sensitive

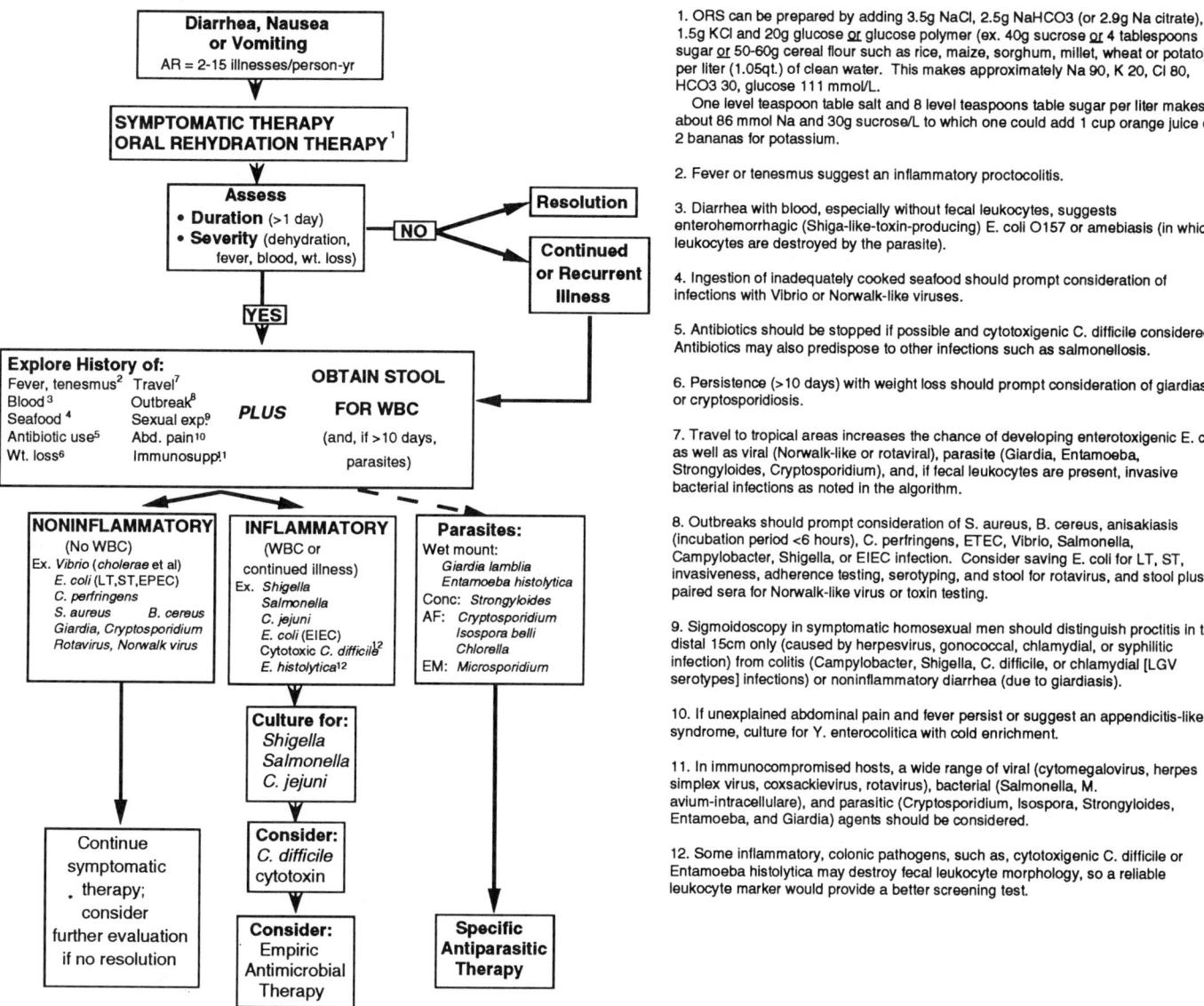

1. ORS can be prepared by adding 3.5g NaCl, 2.5g NaHCO3 (or 2.9g Na citrate), 1.5g KCl and 20g glucose or glucose polymer (ex. 40g sucrose or 4 tablespoons sugar or 50-60g cereal flour such as rice, maize, sorghum, millet, wheat or potato) per liter (1.05qt.) of clean water. This makes approximately Na 90, K 20, Cl 80, HCO3 30, glucose 111 mmol/L.
One level teaspoon table salt and 8 level teaspoons table sugar per liter makes about 86 mmol Na and 30g sucrose/L to which one could add 1 cup orange juice or 2 bananas for potassium.

2. Fever or tenesmus suggest an inflammatory proctocolitis.

3. Diarrhea with blood, especially without fecal leukocytes, suggests enterohemorrhagic (Shiga-like-toxin-producing) E. coli O157 or amebiasis (in which leukocytes are destroyed by the parasite).

4. Ingestion of inadequately cooked seafood should prompt consideration of infections with Vibrio or Norwalk-like viruses.

5. Antibiotics should be stopped if possible and cytotoxigenic C. difficile considered. Antibiotics may also predispose to other infections such as salmonellosis.

6. Persistence (>10 days) with weight loss should prompt consideration of giardiasis or cryptosporidiosis.

7. Travel to tropical areas increases the chance of developing enterotoxigenic E. coli, as well as viral (Norwalk-like or rotaviral), parasite (Giardia, Entamoeba, Strongyloides, Cryptosporidium), and, if fecal leukocytes are present, invasive bacterial infections as noted in the algorithm.

8. Outbreaks should prompt consideration of S. aureus, B. cereus, anisakiasis (incubation period <6 hours), C. perfringens, ETEC, Vibrio, Salmonella, Campylobacter, Shigella, or EIEC infection. Consider saving E. coli for LT, ST, invasiveness, adherence testing, serotyping, and stool for rotavirus, and stool plus paired sera for Norwalk-like virus or toxin testing.

9. Sigmoidoscopy in symptomatic homosexual men should distinguish proctitis in the distal 15cm only (caused by herpesvirus, gonococcal, chlamydial, or syphilitic infection) from colitis (Campylobacter, Shigella, C. difficile, or chlamydial [LGV serotypes] infections) or noninflammatory diarrhea (due to giardiasis).

10. If unexplained abdominal pain and fever persist or suggest an appendicitis-like syndrome, culture for Y. enterocolitica with cold enrichment.

11. In immunocompromised hosts, a wide range of viral (cytomegalovirus, herpes simplex virus, coxsackievirus, rotavirus), bacterial (Salmonella, M. avium-intracellulare), and parasitic (Cryptosporidium, Isospora, Strongyloides, Entamoeba, and Giardia) agents should be considered.

12. Some inflammatory, colonic pathogens, such as, cytotoxigenic C. difficile or Entamoeba histolytica may destroy fecal leukocyte morphology, so a reliable leukocyte marker would provide a better screening test.

FIG. 3. Approach to the diagnosis and management of infectious diarrhea. (From ref. 33, with permission.)

and less likely to give false-negative results if the analysis of the specimen is delayed (66,67). Figure 3 provides an algorithm for the approach to the patient with diarrhea in which the results of the fecal leukocyte test and the duration of the diarrhea are used as a "filter" to determine which patients should have a stool culture or an exam for parasites. Stool cultures may be indicated at the time of presentation or later if the patient has or develops symptoms suggestive of dysentery, is immunocompromised, is suspected of having cholera, or appears to be part of an outbreak. If cholera is suspected, cultures for *Vibrio* must be specifically requested. In situations where patients must be hospitalized for diarrhea the economic calculations change somewhat. For instance, although there is no specific therapy for rotavirus, a enzyme immunoassay (EIA) for rotavirus is probably indicated in the child hospitalized with diarrhea, since a confirmed diagnosis may

spare the patient more expensive and even invasive diagnostic tests.

REHYDRATION THERAPY

Rehydration of the dehydrated patient and maintenance of adequate hydration in the patient not yet dehydrated are the cornerstone of therapy for all patients with diarrhea. For adults and children without clinical signs of dehydration, maintenance of good hydration can be accomplished by increased intake of typical home fluids including water, fruit juices, sport beverages, and non–caffeine-containing carbonated beverages (60,68,69). Oral rehydrations solutions, such as Pedialyte and Rehydralyte, may also be used for maintenance hydration or mild dehydration. For the patient with moderate to severe dehydration, however, the common home fluids are not optimal (60,68). Fruit juices and soft drinks contain too much sugar (which results in too high an osmolarity) and too little salt to be useful in severe diarrhea. The osmolarity of Gatorade and similar sports/performance beverages, about 330 mmol/L, is close to physiological but the concentration of sodium (20 mmol/L) is still too low. The same criticism applies to Pedialyte, with a sodium concentration of 45 mmol/L, which is far below the value of 75–90 mmol/L recommended by the American Academy of Pediatrics and World Health Organization (WHO). Rehydralyte, with a sodium concentration of 75 mmol/L, is the only commercially available product in the United States with a sodium concentration optimal for oral treatment of severe dehydration. Packets of WHO rehydration salts, available in remote locations around the world, are paradoxically not readily available in the United States. However, hospitals and clinics in North America may purchase packets of WHO rehydration salts in lots of 125 or more (Jianas Brothers, Kansas City, MO 64108). The cost is less than 60 cents per packet, which may significantly increase compliance in low-income populations; by comparison, the cost of the commercially available premixed liquids is $6 to $7/L. A more detailed discussion of the theory and practice of oral rehydration therapy is found in the chapter by Snyder.

ANTIMICROBIAL THERAPY OF DIARRHEA

While oral rehydration is the cornerstone of antidiarrheal therapy, recent progress has shown that antimicrobial therapy may be a useful adjunct to oral rehydration. The best studied of these situations is that of traveler's diarrhea, where antibacterial agents such as the fluoroquinolones can markedly shorten the duration of illness (70). Details of the use of antibiotics for traveler's diarrhea will be found in the chapter by DuPont. A more controversial area is whether empiric antibiotic therapy (with quinolones or other antibiotics) has any role in the treatment of acute, nontraveler's diarrhea in adults (71). The high cost of the quinolones and the lower incidence of bacterial pathogens in developed countries in adults have prevented the widespread use of antibiotics for what is usually a short-lived illness.

The role of bismuth compounds, such as bismuth subsalicylate, in the treatment or prevention of acute diarrhea has attracted attention and investigation over the past decade. Bismuth subsalicylate is effective in both prophylaxis and treatment of traveler's diarrhea (72,73). In a study of children hospitalized with acute watery diarrhea in Peru, bismuth subsalicylate therapy resulted in a modest decrease in the severity and duration of illness that was evident by the third treatment day (74). It is unclear as to whether the modest benefits of bismuth subsalicylate warrant the trouble and cost of administering the drug to all of the potential recipients (75).

PREVENTION

Diarrheal disease due to "high-inoculum" pathogens such as *E. coli*, *Salmonella*, and *Vibrio cholerae* is theo-

retically easier to prevent than that attributable to "low-inoculum" organisms, since the former are usually spread through contamination of water distribution systems and violations of hygienic practices in the collection, storage, distribution, and preparation of food. In special situations such as child day care centers, measures to isolate diapering areas and personnel from food preparation, and to exclude children with diarrhea from attendance, can decrease but probably not eliminate transmission of enteric pathogens. Low-inoculum agents such as rotavirus and *Shigella* may spread easily among members of family and household; transmission may be decreased by personal hygiene measures such as handwashing.

REFERENCES

1. Ericsson C, DuPont H. Travelers' diarrhea: approaches to prevention and treatment. *Clin Infect Dis* 1993;16:616–626.
2. Tardelli Gomes TA, Rassi V, MacDonald KL, et al. Enteropathogens associated with acute diarrheal disease in urban infants in Sao Paulo, Brazil. *J Infect Dis* 1991;164:331–337.
3. Van R, Wun CC, O'Ryan M, Matson D, Jackson L, Pickering L. Outbreaks of human enteric adenovirus types 40 and 41 in Houston day care centers. *J Pediatr* 1992;120:516–521.
4. Hanrahan J, Gordon M. Mushroom poisoning: case reports and a review of therapy. *JAMA* 1984;251:1057–1061.
5. Lehmann P, Khazan U. Mushroom poisoning by *Chlorophyllum molybdites* in the midwestern United States. *Mycopathologia* 1992;118:3–13.
6. Hughes J, Merson M. Fish and shellfish poisoning. *N Engl J Med* 1976;295:1117–1120.
7. Eastaugh J, Shepherd S. infectious and toxic syndromes from fish and shellfish. *Arch Intern Med* 1989;149:1735–1740.
8. Yasumoto T, Muraa M, Oshima Y, Sano M, Matsumoto G, Clardy J. Diarrhetic shellfish toxins. *Tetrahedron* 1985;41: 1019–1025.
9. Cohen P, Holmes C, Tsukitani Y. Okadaic acid: a new probe for the study of cellular regulation. *Trends Biochem Sci* 1990; 15:98–102.
10. McGuigan M. Treatment of poisoning. *CIBA Clin Symp* 1984; 36:24–26.
11. Faich G, Frick M, Koffer H. Diarrhea after misoprostol in Crohn disease. *Ann Intern Med* 1991;114:342 (letter).
12. Kornbluth A, Gupta R, Gerson C. Life-threatening diarrhea after short-term misoprostol use in a patient with Crohn ileocolitis. *Ann Intern Med* 1990;113:474–475.
13. Terranova W, Blake P. *Bacillus cereus* food poisoning. *N Engl J Med* 1978;298:143–144.
14. Shandera W, Tacket C, Blake P. Food poisoning due to *Clostridium perfringens* in the United States. *J Infect Dis* 1983;147: 167–169.
15. Theil KW. Group A rotaviruses. In: Saif LJ, Theil KW, eds. *Viral diarrheas of man and animals*. Boca Raton: CRC Press; 1990:35–51.
16. Blacklow N, Cukor G. Viral gastroenteritis. *N Engl J Med* 1981; 304:397–406.
17. Uhnoo I, Olding-Stenkvist E, Kreuger A. Clinical features of acute gastroenteritis associated with rotavirus, enteric adenoviruses, and bacteria. *Arch Dis Child* 1986;61:732–738.
18. Svensson L, Uhnoo I, Wadell G. Enteric adenoviruses of man. In: Saif LJ, Theil KW, eds. *Viral diarrheas of man and animals*. Boca Raton: CRC Press; 1990:97–111.
19. Taterka J, Cuff C, Rubin D. Viral gastrointestinal infections. *Gastroenterol Clin North Am* 1992;21:303–330.
20. Eshali H, Breback K, Bennet R, Ehrnst A, Eriksson M, Hedlung K-O. Astroviruses as a cause of nosocomial outbreaks of infant diarrhea. *Pediatr Infect Dis J* 1991;10:511–515.
21. Gellert G, Waterman S, Ewert D, et al. An outbreak of acute gastroenteritis caused by a small round structured virus in a

geriatric convalescent facility. *Infect Control Hosp Epidemiol* 1990;11:459–464.

22. Guerrant RL, Kirchhoff LV, Shields DS, et al. Prospective study of diarrheal illnesses in northeastern Brazil: patterns of disease, nutritional impact, etiologies, and risk factors. *J Infect Dis* 1983;148:986–997.

23. Guerrant RL. Microbial toxins and diarrhoeal diseases: introduction and overview. In: Evered D, Whelan J, eds. *Microbial toxins and diarrhoeal disease*. London: Pitman; 1985:1–13. (Ciba Symposium 112.)

24. Cravioto A, Reyes RE, Trujillo F, et al. Risk of diarrhea during the first year of life associated with initial and subsequent colonization by specific enteropathogens. *Am J Epidemiol* 1990;131:886–904.

25. Huilan S, Zhen LG, Mathan MM, et al. Etiology of acute diarrhoea among children in developing countries: a multicentre study in five countries. *J WHO* 1991;69:549–555.

26. Blaser MJ, Reller LB. *Campylobacter* enteritis. *N Engl J Med* 1981;305:1444–1452.

27. Swerdlow D, Mintz E, Rodriguez M, et al. Waterborne transmission of cholera in Trujillo, Peru: lessons for a continent at risk. *Lancet* 1992;340:28–33.

28. Epidemic cholera—Burundi and Zimbabwe, 1992–1993. *MMWR* 1993;42:407–416.

29. Update: Cholera—Western hemisphere, 1992. *MMWR* 1992;41:667–668.

30. Holmberg S, Schell W, Fanning G, et al. *Aeromonas* intestinal infections in the United States. *Ann Intern Med* 1986;105:683–689.

31. Holmberg S, Wachsmuth I, Hickman-Brenner F, Blake P, Farmer J. *Plesiomonas* enteric infections in the United States. *Ann Intern Med* 1986;105:690–694.

32. Guerrant R, Bobak D. Bacterial and protozoal gastroenteritis. *N Engl J Med* 1991;325(5):327–340.

33. Herwaldt B, Craun G, Stokes S, Juranek D. Waterborne-disease outbreaks, 1989–1990. CDC Surveillance Summaries, Dec. 1991. *MMWR* 1991;40:SS1–SS22.

34. Hayes E, Matte T, O'Brien T, et al. Large community outbreak of cryptosporidiosis due to contamination of a filtered public water supply. *N Engl J Med* 1989;320:1372–1376.

35. Bendall RP, Lucas S, Moody A, Tovey G, Chiodini PL. Diarrhoea associated with cyanobacterium-like bodies: a new coccidian enteritis of man. *Lancet* 1993;341:590–592.

36. Ortega YR, Sterling CR, Gilman RH, Cama VA, Diaz F. Cyclospora species—a new protozoan pathogen of humans. *N Engl J Med* 1993;328:1308–1312.

37. Eisenhauer P, Harwig S, Lehrer R. Cryptdins: antimicrobial defensins of the murine small intestine. *Infect Immun* 1992;60:3556–3565.

38. Currie M, Fok K, Kato J, et al. Guanylin: an endogenous activator of intestinal guanylate cyclase. *Proc Natl Acad Sci USA* 1992;89:947–951.

39. de Sauvage FJ, Keshav S, Kuang WJ, Gillett N, Henzel W, Goeddel DV. Precursor structure, expression, and tissue distribution of human guanylin. *Proc Natl Acad Sci USA* 1992;89(19):9089–9093.

40. Schulz S, Chrisman TD, Garbers DL. Cloning and expression of guanylin. Its existence in various mammalian tissues. *J Biol Chem* 1992;267(23):16019–16021.

41. Rosenshine I, Donnenberg M, Kaper J, Finlay B. Signal transduction between enteropathogenic *Escherichia coli* (EPEC) and epithelial cells: EPEC induces tyrosine phosphorylation of host cell proteins to initiate cytoskeletal rearrangement and bacterial uptake. *EMBO J* 1992;11:3551–3560.

42. Baldwin T, Ward W, Aitken A, Knutton S, Williams P. Elevation of intracellular free calcium levels in HEp-2 cells infected with enteropathogenic *Escherichia coli*. *Infect Immun* 1991;59:1599–1604.

43. Manjarrez-Hernandez H, TJ B, Aitken A, Knutton S, Williams P. Intestinal epithelial cell protein phosphorylation in enteropathogenic *Escherichia coli* diarrhea. *Lancet* 1992;339:521–523.

44. Beubler E, Schirgi-Degen A. Stimulation of enterocyte protein kinase C by laxatives in vitro. *J Pharm Pharmacol* 1993;45:59–62.

45. Castagna M, Takai Y, Kaibuchi K, Sano K, Kikkawa UN Y. Direct activation of calcium-activated, phospholipid-dependent protein kinase by tumor-promoting phorbol esters. *J Biol Chem* 1982;257:7847–7851.

46. Weikel CS, Sando JJ, Guerrant RL. Stimulation of porcine jejunal ion secretion in vivo by protein kinase C activators. *J Clin Invest* 1985;76:2430–2435.

47. Gilman A. G proteins and dual control of adenylate cyclase. *Cell* 1984;36:577–579.

48. Thompson MR, Giannela RA. Revised amino acid sequence for a heat-stable enterotoxin produced by an *Escherichia coli* strain that is pathogenic for humans. *Infect Immun* 1985;47:834–836.

49. de Jonge HR. Mechanism of action of *Escherichia coli* heat-stable toxin. *Biochem Soc Trans* 1984;12:180–184.

50. Schulz S, Green CK, Yuen PST, Garbers DL. Guanylyl cyclase is a heat-stable enterotoxin receptor. *Cell* 1990;179:941–948.

51. Savarino S, Fasano A, Robertson D, Levine M. Enteroaggregative *Escherichia coli* elaborate a heat-stable enterotoxin demonstrable in an in vitro rabbit intestinal model. *J Clin Invest* 1991;87:1450–1455.

52. Dreyfus L, Harville B, Howard D, Shaban R, Beatty D, Morris S. Calcium influx mediated by the *Escherichia coli* heat-stable enterotoxin B (STb). *Proc Natl Acad Sci USA* 1993;90:3202–3206.

53. Guerrant R. Principles and syndromes of enteric infection. In: Mandel G, Douglas R, Bennett J, eds. *Principles and practice of infectious diseases*. 3rd ed. New York: Churchill Livingstone; 1990:839.

54. Ward RL, Bernstein DI, Young EC, Sherwood JR, Knowlton DR, Schiff GM. Human rotavirus studies in volunteers: determination of infectious dose and serological response to infection. *J Infect Dis* 1986;154:871–880.

55. Giron J, Jones T, Millan-Velasco F, et al. Diffuse-adhering *Escherichia coli* (DAEC) as a putative cause of diarrhea in Mayan children in Mexico. *J Infect Dis* 1991;163:507–513.

56. Update: multistate outbreak of *Escherichia coli* O157:H7 infections from hamburgers—Western United States, 1992–1993. *MMWR* 1993;42:258–263.

57. Ho M, Glass R, Monroe S, et al. Viral gastroenteritis aboard a cruise ship. *Lancet* 1989;2:961–964.

58. Devi S, Murray C. Cockroaches (*Blatta* and *Periplaneta* species) as reservoirs of drug-resistant salmonellas. *Epidemiol Infect* 1991;107:357–361.

59. Richards L, Claeson M, Pierce NF. Management of acute diarrhea in children: lessons learned. *Pediatr Infect Dis J* 1993;12:5–9.

60. Duggan C, Santosham M, Glass R. The management of acute diarrhea in children: oral rehydration, maintenance, and nutritional therapy. *MMWR* 1992;41:RR1–RR20.

61. Harries A, Speare R, Wirima J. Symptoms and responses to chemotherapy in adult Malawians admitted to hospital with *Plasmodium falciparum* malaria. *Ann Trop Med Parisitol* 1985;82:511–512.

62. Muller O, Moser R. The clinical and parasitological presentation of *Plasmodium falciparum* malaria in Uganda is unaffected by HIV-1 infection. *Trans R Soc Trop Med Hyg* 1990;84:336–338.

63. Schumacher G, Kollberg B, Ljungh A. Inflammatory bowel disease presenting as travellers' diarrhea. *Lancet* 1993;341:241–242.

64. Koplan J, Fineberg H, Ferraro M, Rosenberg M. Value of stool cultures. *Lancet* 1980;2:413–416.

65. Guerrant R, Shields D, Thorson S, Schorling J, Groschel D. Evaluation and diagnosis of acute infectious diarrhea. *Am J Med* 1985;78:91–98.

66. Guerrant R, Araujo V, Barrett L, Lee A, Cooper W, Groschel D. Measurement of fecal lactoferrin (LF) as a marker of inflammatory enteritis. *Clin Res* 1990;38:391A (abstract).

67. Guerrant R, Araujo V, Soares E, et al. Measurement of fecal lactoferrin as a marker of fecal leukocytes. *J Clin Microbiol* 1992;30:1238–1242.

68. Snyder J. Oral therapy for diarrhea. *Hosp Practice* 1991;26:86–88.

69. Avery M, Snyder J. Oral therapy for acute diarrhea. *N Engl J Med* 1990;323:891–894.
70. DuPont H, Ericsson C. Prevention and treatment of traveler's diarrhea. *N Engl J Med* 1993;328:1821–1827.
71. Quinolones in acute non-travellers' diarrhea. *Lancet* 1990;336:282 (editorial).
72. DuPont H, Sullivan P, Evans D, et al. Prevention of travelers' diarrhea (emporiatric enteritis). Prophylactic administration of subsalicylate bismuth. *JAMA* 1980;243:237–241.
73. DuPont H, Sullivan P, Pickering L, Haynes G, Ackerman P. Symptomatic treatment of diarrhea with bismuth subsalicylate among students attending a Mexican university. *Gastroenterology* 1977;73:715–718.
74. Figueroa-Quintanilla D, Salazar-Lindo E, Sack R, et al. A controlled trial of bismuth subsalicylate in infants with acute watery diarrheal disease. *N Engl J Med* 1993;328:1654–1658.
75. Snyder J. Can bismuth improve the simple solution for diarrhea? *N Engl J Med* 1993;328:1705–1706.
76. Banerjee DK. *Microbiology of Infectious Diseases*. London: Gower Medical Publishing; 19.

Infections of the Gastrointestinal Tract,
edited by M. J. Blaser, P. D. Smith, J. I. Ravdin,
H. B. Greenberg, and R. L. Guerrant
Raven Press, Ltd., New York © 1995.

CHAPTER 21

Acute Inflammatory Diarrhea (Dysentery)

Lee W. Riley

Oral rehydration therapy (ORT) is considered the cornerstone of global diarrheal disease control strategies. However, much of the life-saving benefits of ORT have applied to secretory and not to inflammatory diarrhea or dysentery. ORT has limited effect on mortality from inflammatory diarrhea, since deaths from inflammatory diarrhea are not caused by dehydration alone. In addition, inflammatory diarrhea is an important risk factor for persistent diarrhea—another manifestation of diarrhea associated with increased childhood mortality. The morbidity from inflammatory diarrhea, of course, is not limited to developing countries. In developed countries or highly industrialized sectors of middle-income countries, bacterial agents of inflammatory diarrhea have intimately established themselves into their complex food distribution network as well as to their highly specialized nosocomial practices. This chapter will highlight the pathogenesis, epidemiology, clinical features, and management of this syndrome.

DEFINITIONS

Inflammatory diarrhea is an acute enteric illness manifesting as diarrhea accompanied by fever and evidence in stool of an inflammatory process affecting the intestinal mucosa, such as pus, mucus, or blood. Dysentery is a severe manifestation of inflammatory diarrhea with blood or mucus in stool, accompanied by fever, crampy abdominal pain, and rectal tenesmus.

CLASSIFICATION

Syndromes that meet the above definition fall into two categories—those that are associated with recognized infectious agents, and those that have no clearly identified

infectious etiology (Table 1). Infectious agents that cause inflammatory diarrhea can be further divided into two subgroups—those organisms that elicit an inflammatory process by penetrating the intestinal mucosa, and those that elaborate cytotoxins without invading the cells.

MICROBIOLOGY

Worldwide, invasive bacterial agents constitute the most important subgroup of etiological agents of inflammatory diarrhea (1–13). Within the family Enterobacteriaceae, *Shigella* sp. (serogroups A–D: *dysenteriae, flexneri, sonnei,* and *boydii*), *Salmonella* sp. (*S. typhi* and nontyphoidal *Salmonella* sp.), enteroinvasive *Escherichia coli* (EIEC), and *Yersinia enterocolitica* cause inflammatory diarrhea. Among *Campylobacter* species, *Campylobacter jejuni* is the most common cause of inflammatory diarrhea. *Campylobacter coli* causes diarrhea in human hosts, but because most laboratories do not distinguish *C. coli* from *C. jejuni,* its true incidence is not known (14). Other species including *C. lari* (formerly *C. laridis*) and *C. hyointestinalis,* as well as *Helicobacter cindaedi* (formerly *C. cinaedi*) and *H. fenneliae* (formerly *C. fenneliae*), have been isolated from immunodeficient patients and homosexual men with enteritis and proctitis (15–17).

In patients with advanced acquired immunodeficiency syndrome (AIDS), one of the many causes of acute diarrhea may include *Mycobacterium avium* complex (MAC), which can invade the intestinal mucosa (18,19).

Noninvasive bacterial pathogens can elicit inflammatory response in the intestine. The most common cause, especially in nosocomial settings, is *Clostridium difficile,* a gram-positive, spore-forming, obligate anaerobe. Other agents include *Vibrio parahaemolyticus* and *Clostridium perfringens* (20,21). *Clostridium perfringens* type C is rarely associated with necrotizing enteritis in adults with poor nutrition or atypical dietary habits (22,23). A variety of bacterial agents have been implicated in necrotizing enterocolitis (NEC) in the newborn, including *Pseudomonas, Klebsiella, Clostridium butyricum, Salmonella,* and noninvasive *E. coli* strains (24–27).

L. W. Riley: Division of International Medicine, Cornell University Medical College, New York, New York 10021.

283

TABLE 1. *Classification of inflammatory diarrhea*

Diseases with recognized infectious etiology (pathogen) affecting all hosts:
  Invasive pathogen diseases:
  Amebic dysentery *(Entamoeba histolytica)*
  Bacillary dysentery, shigellosis *(Shigella* spp.*)*
  Balantidial dysentery *(Balantidium coli)*
  Bilharzial dysentery *(Schistosoma japonicum, mansoni)*
  Campylobacteriosis *(Campylobacter jejuni, coli)*
  Invasive *E. coli* diarrhea (enteroinvasive *E. coli*)
  Salmonellosis *(Salmonella* spp.*)*
  Typhoid fever *(Salmonella typhi)*
  Yersiniosis *(Yersinia enterocolitica)*

  Cytotoxin-producing pathogen diseases:
  Pseudomembranous colitis *(Clostridium difficile)*
  Vibriosis *(Vibrio parahaemolyticus)*

Diseases with recognized infectious etiology affecting predominantly hosts with underlying disease or immunodeficiency:
  Cytomegalovirus colitis (Cytomegalovirus)
  Herpes virus colitis *(Herpes simplex)*
  Intestinal mycobacteriosis *(Mycobacterium avium)*
  Isosporiasis *(Isospora belli)*
  Phycomycosis *(Mucor, Rhizopus, Absidia)*
  Strongylodiasis *(Strongyloides stercoralis)*

Diseases not recognized to be associated with specific infectious etiology:
  Ulcerative colitis
  Crohn's disease
  Ischemic colitis
  Neutropenic enterocolitis (typhlitis)
  Chemical or metal poisonings (thallium sulfate, barium carbonate, arsenic, lead)

Other inflammatory diarrhea syndromes (associated pathogens):
  Adult necrotizing entercolitis *(Clostridium perfringens* type C, others)
  Neonatal necrotizing enterocolitis (polymicrobial etiology)

E. coli strains belonging to the enterohemorrhagic *E. coli* (EHEC) group cause a distinct syndrome called hemorrhagic colitis (28–30). Although this syndrome includes bloody diarrhea, hemorrhagic colitis is not considered part of the syndromes of inflammatory diarrhea (see discussion below). The most common cause of hemorrhagic colitis and the only serotype associated with epidemics of this disease is *E. coli* O157:H7.

The most common parasitic cause of inflammatory diarrhea is *Entamoeba histolytica.* A ciliate protozoan *Balantidium coli* can penetrate with its rotary boring action the mucosa of the cecum and terminal ileum, and cause a dysenteric syndrome (balantidial dysentery) (31). The coccidian parasite *Isospora belli* can penetrate colonic mucosal cells in AIDS patients and elicit diarrhea (32,33). Eggs deposited by adult trematodes *Schistosoma mansoni* and *Schistosoma japonicum* in the intestinal venules can rupture the wall of the venules, thus eliciting focal inflammation, bleeding, and diarrhea (34). Heavy intestinal infestation by *Strongyloides stercoralis* can cause

dysentery, often associated with secondary bacterial infection (35).

Viral and fungal agents generally do not cause inflammatory diarrhea in immunocompetent hosts. Cytomegalovirus has been associated with colitis and bloody diarrhea in some patients with ulcerative colitis (36,37), AIDS (38,39), and other immunosuppressive disorders (40). A patient with AIDS often has several concurrent causes of diarrhea, and *Herpes simplex* and adenovirus have been attributed to some cases of colitis (41). Agents of phycomycosis have been rarely implicated in bloody diarrhea in diabetic patients (42,43).

Crohn's disease and ulcerative colitis are two major syndromes of chronic, relapsing inflammatory bowel disease for which infectious etiologies have not been demonstrated. Several recent studies have reported the possible association of *Mycobacterium paratuberculosis* in Crohn's disease (44,45). Using oligonucleotide primers based on *M. paratuberculosis* DNA sequences, several investigators have reported detecting *M. paratuberculosis* DNA sequences significantly more often from patients with than without Crohn's disease.

PATHOGENESIS

The ability of bacteria to produce dysentery is associated with their ability to elicit keratoconjunctivitis in guinea pigs (Sereny test) (46). The ability of the organism to enter cells, multiply, and spread from cell to cell is studied in vitro by infection of monolayers of cultured mammalian cells, such as HeLa, HEp-2, Henle, Caco-2 cells, and others. Cytotoxin elaboration is demonstrated by the detection of morphological changes and cytopathic effects elicited by organisms in cultured cells, such as Vero, HeLa, Chinese hamster ovary (CHO) cells, and human foreskin fibroblasts. These animal and tissue culture models have been used to identify a variety of virulence determinants that contribute to the pathogenesis of inflammatory diarrhea.

Invasive Pathogens

After attachment invasive organisms trigger a phagocytosis-like response in cultured cells that are not considered "professional phagocytes." It should be stressed that this capacity to invade cultured cells per se is neither sufficient nor a marker for an organism to elicit inflammatory diarrhea. For an invasive organism to produce a full spectrum of the dysenteric syndrome, it must be able to multiply intracellularly, spread intercellularly, and promote an inflammatory reaction by the host. The final characteristic diarrheal response is determined by the cell's specific signal transduction pathway elicited by products of an organism expressed during its entry into mammalian cells.

Yersinia pseudotuberculosis and *Yersinia enterocolitica* express a single 103-kDa chromosomally encoded protein product called invasin that mediates both attachment and invasion of the organism into cultured epithelial cells (47,48). Invasin interacts with the β_1 subunit of heterodimeric proteins belonging to an integrin subfamily (VLA proteins) of cell adhesion molecules (49). Integrins are transmembrane proteins that mediate cell attachment by linking extracellular matrix proteins with intracellular cytoskeletal elements. During entry, actin and actin-associated proteins, such as filamin and talin, accumulate around an invading bacillus (50). *Yersinia* organisms also express several virulence plasmid-encoded proteins called *Yersinia* outer membrane proteins (Yops) associated with phosphatase and kinase activities, microfilament disruption, and G-protein–linked receptor stimulation (51–53).

Shigella and enteroinvasive EIEC carry several genes (*ipa* genes) clustered on virulence plasmids of molecular mass between 180 and 230 kb that are associated with mammalian cell invasion (54,55). These genes are controlled by a complex regulatory system that includes chromosomal and plasmid-encoded products that respond to a variety of environmental stimuli. In contrast to other invasive enteric pathogens such as *Salmonella typhimurium* or *Yersinia enterocolitica,* once inside the cells, *Shigella* strains cause early lysis of the phogocytic membrane and escape into the cytoplasm, where they can proliferate. The lysis of the membrane is believed to be mediated by a hemolysin, encoded by *ipaB* (56). The spread of the bacteria to the lamina propria of the colonic mucosal cells triggers an inflammatory response that leads to the development of mucosal ulceration, a characteristic lesion seen in severe shigellosis.

The invasion of cells by *Salmonella* is believed to be mediated by several chromosomal genes located on a region called *inv* locus (57). *Salmonella typhimurium* strains enter cells by a pathway that is associated with activation of the epidermal growth factor receptor and a rapid increase in free cytosolic calcium levels (58,59). As with *Yersinia* and *Shigella,* the internalization of *Salmonella* is accompanied by accumulation of cytoskeleton-associated proteins, such as actin, α-actinin, talin, tubulin, and ezrin (60). The signal cascade elicited by *Salmonella* during entry into Henle cells also stimulates leukotrienes, which are known mediators of the inflammatory response (59).

Entamoeba histolytica causes amebic dysentery, and its pathogenesis is dependent on several organism and host factors. After excystation in the lumen of the intestines, *E. histolytica* trophozoites invade the colonic epithelium at the sites of their attachment mediated by a 260-kDa galactose-specific lectin (61,62). The lectin confers some protection against amebic liver abscess, a complication of amebic dysentery, in lectin-immunized gerbils, suggesting that this adhesin is an important virulence factor of the organism (63). The amebas characteristically produce cytolysis and tissue destruction at the site of attachment, and these effects are contact- and temperature- (37°C) dependent (64). Ravdin et al. reported that CHO cell lysis by *E. histolytica* trophozoites can be inhibited by antagonists of calcium-dependent phospholipase A activity (65). An antilectin monoclonal antibody that blocks the cytotoxic effect after adherence of the trophozoite has been identified, suggesting that the lectin itself may play a role in cytolysis (66). A number of other potential amebic

cytolethal substances have been identified, but their role in pathogenesis has not been defined. Trophozoites lyse infiltrating neutrophils at the site of infection, and the released neutrophil enzymes are believed to contribute to some of the tissue pathology (67).

The above observations reveal that mammalian cell entry of invasive pathogens is mediated by a variety of organism-specific protein or carbohydrate products that serve either as a ligand for a receptor component on the mammalian cell surface or as products that trigger cell signals that promote cytoskeletal rearrangement, free cytosolic calcium flux, other second-message response, or cell death. It should be noted, however, that most of these findings are based on observations made in vitro using cultured cells. Whether these cellular events actually occur during infection of intestinal cells in a patient with inflammatory diarrhea is not known. Furthermore, most of these studies have focused on cellular events that occur during internalization of invasive pathogens. How these events lead to the production of diarrhea (fluid output) in yersiniosis, shigellosis, salmonellosis, and amebiasis have not yet been satisfactorily answered.

Cytotoxin-Producing Pathogens

The invasive pathogen *Shigella dysenteriae* type 1, the cause of bacillary dysentery pandemics, produces a potent toxin called Shiga toxin that is cytotoxic to certain cultured cells and enterotoxic to ligated segments of rabbit ileum (68,69). It inhibits mammalian cell protein synthesis (70). After the recent discovery of related cytotoxins elaborated by *E. coli* strains associated with diarrhea, Shiga toxin has come to be considered a prototype of a family of toxins called Shiga-like toxins (SLTs) (71,72). The toxin consists of one A subunit linked to five B subunits. The B subunit is believed to bind the toxin to cellular neutral glycolipid Gb3 on the rabbit microvillus membrane, which is thought to inhibit the villus cell Na^+ absorption, and hence elicit net fluid secretion (73).

However, a *S. dysenteriae* 1 strain deleted in the toxin gene can produce cell death and diarrhea with pus in rhesus monkeys (74). Strains belonging to *Shigella* serogroups that elaborate only low levels of Shiga toxin can produce severe dysentery. Although direct cytotoxic effects of Shiga toxin on vascular endothelial cells have been demonstrated (75) and hence the toxin could conceivably produce the vascular damage that elicits bleeding, the above observations suggest that the inflammatory response may not be all related to the toxin effect.

Clostridium difficile, the etiological agent of pseudomembranous colitis, produces at least two toxins—an enterotoxin called toxin A and a cytotoxin called toxin B (76,77). Toxin A has been shown to be a potent chemoattractant of leukocytes and therefore probably contributes to the inflammatory response. It can elicit fluid accumulation in ligated rabbit ileal loops. The role of toxin B in diarrhea production has not been clearly demonstrated, but it is speculated that the toxin may require toxin A to express its full biological effect.

Most clinical isolates of *Vibrio parahaemolyticus* induce β-hemolysis (Kanagawa phenomenon, or KP) in Wagatsuma blood agar medium, whereas only 1–2% of environmental isolates exhibit this reaction (78,79). Hence, the KP is epidemiologically associated with diarrhea caused by *V. parahaemolyticus*. The KP is mediated by thermostable direct hemolysin (TDH), which has cytotoxic and enterotoxic activities. It can stimulate fluid accumulation in ligated rabbit ileal loop (80). Recently, a wild-type *V. parahaemolyticus* strain but not its isogenic TDH– mutant was shown to produce fluid accumulation in rabbit ileal loop (81). Invasion of the colonic mucosa by *V. parahaemolyticus* has also been reported (82).

Other Dysenteric Syndromes

Dysentery can be a component of syndromes in which infections result from a secondary complication of a primary disease process. These include necrotizing enterocolitis (NEC), ischemic colitis, and neutropenic enterocolitis.

A variety of infectious agents have been associated with neonatal NEC, including *Klebsiella, Salmonella, E. coli, Pseudomonas,* and *Clostridium butyricum* (24–27). The intestinal pathology of NEC resembles that observed in ischemic injury (see below), in which the areas of necrosis may become superinfected with intestinal flora. NEC in the newborn often follows episodes of asphyxia, apnea, respiratory distress syndrome, or hypothermia, which can contribute to the intestinal ischemia and devitalization. Others have suggested that the disease is promoted by a Shwartzman reaction following an infectious process (83). Neonatal NEC probably has a variety of causes, triggered by unknown factors that initially affect the gut mucosa, which is then secondarily infected with the gut flora; some of these organisms may produce gas and cause dissection through the friable bowel wall, and others may produce peritonitis or septicemia.

Neutropenic enterocolitis (typhlitis, ileocecal syndrome) has been described in patients treated for lymphoma and leukemia (84,85), transplant patients (86), and in patients with AIDS (87). Most of the cases were described before the association of *Clostridium difficile* with pseudomembranous colitis was recognized, and hence could represent antibiotic-associated or cancer chemotherapy–associated pseudomembranous colitis.

A patchy necrotizing small bowel disease progressing to segmental gangrene with pockets of gas occurs in adults in association with poor nutrition or certain dietary habits (22,23). *Clostridium perfringens* type C β toxin may play a role in its pathogenesis (88).

EPIDEMIOLOGY

Worldwide, the etiological agents of inflammatory diarrhea are isolated from 10% to over 50% of children with diarrhea less than 6 years of age, or from 22% to 66% of all diarrhea specimens in which a recognized enteric pathogen is identified (Table 2) (1–13). These differences, of course, result from variable study designs (geography, age, or socioeconomic groups examined, community vs. institution-based study, and the types of organisms sought).

The most common cause of diarrhea among travelers to Latin America, Africa, and Asia is enterotoxigenic *E. coli* (ETEC). However, *Shigella, Salmonella,* and *Campylobacter* organisms are important causes of traveler's diarrhea in Nepal, Morrocco, and Saudi Arabia (11–13), and may vary according to season of travel (13). Among American troops staying in Saudi Arabia during Operation Desert Shield in 1990, agents of inflammatory diarrhea composed 50% of all diarrhea cases in which a pathogen was identified (Table 2), and *Shigella* was isolated more frequently than any other pathogen except ETEC (11). *Yersinia enterocolitica* infections are rare in tropical countries.

According to the U.S. Public Health Service surveillance system, between the periods 1976–1980 and 1986–1990, the average annual reported incidence of salmonellosis increased from about 16/100,000 to 20/100,000, and the incidence of shigellosis increased by 20% from 9.2/100,000 to 10.1/100,000. The *Campylobacter* surveillance was initiated in 1983 (14). The annual reported incidence from the most recent reporting period (1989) was 3.8/100,000 (89). These reported isolation rates probably represent only 1–5% of the infections that actually occur each year in the United States (90).

In the United States, the peak isolation rates for *Salmonella* are observed in infants between 2 and 3 months of age, and for *Shigella,* 2 and 3 years of age. The isolation rate for *Campylobacter* remains constant through the first year of life and peaks in the young adult age group (20–40 years). With *Yersinia enterocolitica,* age-specific attack rates are highest for children between 1 and 3 years of age.

Globally, *E. histolytica* is estimated to infect about 500 million persons (excluding China) (91). Of these 8–10% develop diarrhea. In contrast to invasive bacterial pathogens, the rate of infection with *E. histolytica* increases with age. Disease manifestation also varies geographically. Invasive disease develops in one of every five infected persons in Mexico compared to one of every 100–1000 infections in the temperate areas (91).

Primates are the only reservoir of *Shigella* organisms, whereas *Salmonella* organisms have entrenched themselves into a variety of reservoirs, some of which are serotype-specific. For example, humans are the only reservoir for *Salmonella typhi.* Poultry has become a major reservoir for the serotype *Salmonella enteritidis* in the United States; between 1985 and 1992, this one serotype was responsible for 15,162 cases of salmonellosis, 1734 hospitalizations, and 53 deaths (92). *Salmonella* is the most commonly reported cause of foodborne gastroenteritis outbreaks in the United States. In industrialized countries, through their extensive food distribution network, a single contaminated food product can become a vehicle for infections in geographically widespread areas, and a single clone of *Salmonella* can be responsible for such epidemics (93,94).

TABLE 2. *Etiologic studies of acute diarrhea, 1984–1990*

Study site (Ref.)	Population	Period	Invasive bacteria			*Entamoeba histolytica* %
			No.	(%)[a]	(%)[b]	
Bangkok, Thailand[c] (1)	Children <5 yr	1988–89	119	(31)	(52)	<1
Hong Kong[c] (2)	All ages with diarrhea	1984–90	2004	(10)	(61)	NR
Sao Paulo, Brazil[c] (3)	Infants <12 mo	1985–86	87	(19)	(24)	NR
Western Australia[c] (4)	Aboriginal children <5 yr	1985–88	38	(NR)	(22)	0
Chiapas, Mexico[c] (5)	Children <6 yr	Summer '87	19	(36)	(66)	NR
Anapur-Palla, India (6)	Children <3 yr	1985–86	18	(10)	(25)	0
Djibouti, Djibouti (7)	All ages with diarrhea	Feb. 89	29	(14)	(30)	NR
Manila, Philippines[c] (8)	All ages with diarrhea	1984	466	(25)	(36)	0.1
Dhaka, Bangladesh[c] (9)	Children <6 yr	1984–86	29	(13)	(53)	<1
Aswan, Egypt[c] (10)	Children <5 yr	July 86	30	(20)	(22)	<1
Saudi Arabia (11)	U.S. troops in Desert Shield	Sept–Dec 1990	125	(29)	(50)	NR
Kathmandu, Nepal[c] (12)	Travelers and Peace Corp	1986–87	114	(35)	(75)	5
Morocco (13)	Travelers from Finland	1989	64	(37)	(63)	NR

NR, not reported.
[a] Proportion of all cases of acute diarrhea.
[b] Proportion of all cases of diarrhea with specific diagnosis; invasive bacterial pathogens sought for included *Shigella, Salmonella, Campylobacter,* enteroinvasive *E. coli,* and *Yersinia.*
[c] Studies in which rotavirus was sought.
NR, not reported.

Campylobacter jejuni is associated with the drinking of raw milk, but is also commonly found in poultry products. In Japan, *Vibrio parahaemolyticus* is the major cause of diarrhea in summer, and is associated with eating uncooked fish (sushi, sashimi) or shellfish (20). In northern Europe, the main reservoir for *Yersinia enterocolitica* is the swine (95), and in the United States yersiniosis outbreaks due to contaminated pasteurized milk (96), pig intestines (chitterlings) (97), and homemade tofu (98) have been reported.

Humans are the main reservoir of *E. histolytica,* but natural infections in macaque monkeys and pigs have been observed (99,100). Domesticated animals such as dogs and cattle may be secondarily infected from human feces. Pigs are the major reservoir of *Balantidium coli* (31).

Shigella infections are predominantly transmitted person-to-person and are a common cause of day care center outbreaks (101,102). However, large outbreaks of shigellosis due to contaminated foods are occasionally reported (103,104). As mentioned, animal food products are the major vehicles of *Salmonella* infections, but person-to-person transmission is also common. Often *Salmonella* is introduced into a household through a contaminated food product and the infection is sustained thereafter via person-to-person transmission (105). Now rare in the United States, nosocomial outbreaks of salmonellosis, particularly with drug-resistant strains, pose a serious problem in some middle-income countries (106). *Yersinia enterocolica,* which often causes bacteremia, can be enriched in phosphate buffer solution at 4–7°C. Hence, this organism may be transmitted by transfusion of contaminated blood (107,108). *E. histolytica* and *B. coli* are transmitted person-to-person. One form of necrotizing enterocolitis called "pig-bel," associated with *Clostridium perfringens*

type C β toxin, is associated with a large pork feast in the highlands of New Guinea (22).

Clostridium difficile is the most common cause of diarrhea in hospital settings, accounting for up to 45% of nosocomial diarrhea with a recognized cause (109). Widespread use of broad-spectrum antibiotics as well as antineoplastic agents contribute to its increasing incidence in hospitals.

Neonatal NEC is associated with low birthweight (24). Other reported associations include exchange transfusions, congenital deficiency of the bowel wall, trauma to the fetus in utero, use of umbilical catheters, the toxic effect of polyvinylchloride blood bags, and the infectious agents mentioned earlier (110–115).

CLINICAL FEATURES

As with all enteric pathogens, the agents of inflammatory diarrhea cause a wide spectrum of clinical manifestations, including asymptomatic carriage, explosive watery diarrhea, mucus- and blood-containing diarrhea, and extraintestinal or systemic complications. Disease manifestations and incubation periods are influenced by factors such as inoculum size, vehicles of infection, virulence properties of the organism, and host factors.

Factors That Influence Disease Manifestation

Information regarding minimum infective doses of organisms is usually derived from volunteer studies. One such study showed that approximately 10^5 *S. typhi* organisms caused symptoms in 28% of volunteers (116). These volunteer studies, however, are limited by the choice of strains used, the homogeneous age group of the volunteers (usually young males), and the choice of vehicle used to infect the volunteers (usually water). In natural settings, organisms can be introduced into the host via vehicles that buffer the organism from gastric acidity (fatty food items such as milk, cheese, chocolate). Thus, a lower inoculum dose can reach the intestines to cause symptomatic disease (117). In typhoid outbreaks traced to foods, the minimal infective dose of *S. typhi* was estimated to be less than 10^3 organisms (117). Organisms adapted to the human host, such as *Shigella* and *S. typhi*, are known to produce disease with lower infective doses. *Shigella* organisms can cause symptomatic disease with infective dose as low as ten organisms (118).

Virulence determinants of an organism affect disease expression. *S. typhi* organisms possessing the Vi antigen cause a higher attack rate and shorter incubation periods among volunteers (116). In general, *Shigella sonnei* causes milder disease than *Shigella flexneri* or *Shigella dysenteriae* 1. The isoenzyme patterns of *E. histolytica* strains that produce asymptomatic disease are distinct from those that produce symptomatic disease (119), although it is not known if these patterns represent differences in the organisms' virulence potentials.

Finally, it is well recognized that persons with underlying diseases such as malignancies, sickle cell anemia, schistosomiasis, gastrectomy, achlorhydria, AIDS, and persons taking antacids or antibiotics have increased susceptibility to symptomatic illness after *Salmonella* infection (120–127). Penicillins, in particular, increase the chance of symptomatic infection due to multidrug-resistant strains of *Salmonella* (128). The variable age-specific attack rates of shigellosis, salmonellosis, and campylobacteriosis suggest age-dependent susceptibility to symptomatic disease. Disease manifestation varies with age also. *Salmonella* bacteremia is more common in infants and the elderly (129). During a multistate outbreak in 1982, *Yersinia enterocolitica* was isolated from 14 persons with pharyngitis; all 14 were adults and enteritis occurred only in children (130). Host immunity influenced by the frequency of background exposures to pathogens affects disease manifestation. In two separate diarrhea outbreaks, the attack rate after *Campylobacter jejuni* infection was lower among farmers who regularly drank raw milk than among persons who were not previously exposed (131).

Asymptomatic Carriage

Asymptomatic chronic carriage (excretion of organism in stool for longer than a year) of *Shigella*, *Campylobacter*, or *Yersinia* is rare, is less than 1% with nontyphi *Salmonella*, and is 1–3% with *Salmonella typhi* (132). The median duration of excretion of nontyphi *Salmonella* after salmonellosis (convalescent carriage) has been estimated to be 5 weeks, and is longer in children. In Norway, 47% of the patients with *Y. enterocolitica* illness had prolonged shedding of the organism (mean 50.4 days) (133). Asymptomatic chronic carriage of *E. histolytica* varies geographically (80–99%) (91). About 40% of healthy neonates colonized with *Clostridium difficile* have high fecal toxin titers (134). High titers of fecal toxin are rarely detected in older children colonized with *C. difficile*, and although a few may develop diarrhea, they rarely develop pseudomembranous colitis (109).

Symptomatic Infections

It should be noted that although *Shigella dysenteriae* 1 usually produces a more severe dysenteric illness than other *Shigella* serotypes, in Bangladesh the highest mortality from shigellosis was associated with infection with *Shigella sonnei* (case fatality rate of 10.3%) (135). In developed countries, such as the United States, *S. sonnei* generally causes mild, self-limited illness. However, in the preantibiotic era, *S. sonnei* was associated with severe dysenteric syndrome with systemic complications such as seizures (136,137). These geographic or temporal differences in clinical manifestations may relate to the differences in background infectious inoculum size or pathogenicity of predominant clonal strains in the community.

S. typhi is associated with a clinical syndrome, distinct from typical salmonellosis, called typhoid or enteric fever in which enteritis is one component of a systemic illness. The incubation period is usually longer (7–14 days) than in nontyphoidal *Salmonella* infections (24–72 hr), and the first clinical manifestation is fever rather than gastrointestinal symptoms. Diarrhea is seen only in about half of the patients. Extraintestinal involvement such as splenomegaly and hepatomegaly occurs in about one third of patients, and erythematous maculopapular lesions (rose spots) on the abdomen is seen in about half. The systemic involvement results from bacteremia. The illness may last 2–3 weeks. In the preantibiotic era, 5–20% of the patients developed intestinal hemorrhage and 2–5% developed intestinal perforation. With appropriate antimicrobial therapy and supportive care, the mortality from typhoid fever is now less than 1%, and the complications of intestinal perforation and hemorrhage are rare (less than 1%) (138).

Nontyphoidal salmonellosis is characteristically accompanied by fever, nausea, anorexia, vomiting, crampy abdominal pain, and frequent loose bowel movements—manifestations clinically indistinguishable from the typical presentations of other invasive or cytotoxin-producing bacterial or invasive protozoal infections. Bloody diarrhea occurs with similar frequency (13–27%) as in *Campylobacter* enteritis, but with less frequency compared to shigellosis, and occurs more often in children (1–13).

Some cases of salmonellosis, especially during the early phase of the illness, can be mistaken for secretory diarrhea. They may present with explosive watery diarrhea, resembling cholera-like illness with mild fever, and develop profound dehydration. Such a presentation may depend on the serotype of the organism. A "choleriform syndrome" with *S. infantis* and *S. haardt* infections has been reported (139), and a possible role of an enterotoxin in some strains of *Salmonella* for this syndrome has been suggested (140).

Most patients with *Campylobacter jujuni* enteritis develop watery diarrhea initially, followed by blood-streaked stools, but severe dehydration is rare. In advanced disease, colitis or proctitis with crypt abscess formation resembling severe shigellosis, amebiasis, or ulcerative colitis can develop (141).

Bloody diarrhea with yersiniosis occurs mostly in children. In addition to enteritis, infected patients can develop mesenteric adenitis and terminal ileitis, which can be mistaken for appendicitis. However, suppuration of the appendix itself from *Y. enterocolitica* infection can occur (142,143).

Bloody diarrhea is seen in 5–10% of patients with *C. difficile*–associated diarrhea. Most patients have brown or clear watery diarrhea, but 85% of patients with pseudomembranous colitis will have mucus in the stool (144).

The characteristic symptomatic illness produced by *Entamoeba histolytica* is rectocolitis. Nearly all patients will have heme-positive stool, but, unlike shigellosis, stool leukocytes may not be abundant due to their lysis by the organism (145,146). Also in contrast to colitis from invasive bacterial pathogens, fever occurs in only about one third of the symptomatic patients.

Liver abscess caused by *E. histolytica* often is not preceded by any symptomatic intestinal disease (up to 50%), and develops within 2–5 months after exposure (145). It can present acutely with abdominal pain, fever, and diarrhea, or subacutely with vague abdominal pain without diarrhea accompanied only by weight loss. Hepatomegaly occurs in less than half, and jaundice is not a feature of this disease.

Cytomegalovirus (CMV) can cause severe gastrointestinal illness in patients receiving solid organ or bone marrow transplants, immunosuppressive drugs, or persons with AIDS or ulcerative colitis (36–40). The symptoms may include malaise, anorexia, nausea, vomiting, fever, abdominal pain, and diarrhea with blood. The disease can involve the entire gastrointestinal tract, which is quite distinct from dysenteric disease caused by other pathogens. Hence, a patient may have bright red blood per rectum or melena, depending on the site of involvement. Bleeding results from ulcerations of the gut mucosa. Colon appears to be more commonly involved in kidney transplant patients, as opposed to the esophagus in heart or heart–lung transplant patients (40).

Complications

In Bangladesh, during one year of active surveillance in 1984, 39% of 46,607 cases of diarrhea were found to be bloody, but deaths from bloody diarrhea accounted for 62% of all diarrhea deaths (147). Watery diarrhea was responsible for 41% of all diarrhea cases but 36% of all deaths. *Shigella* was identified from 64% of cultured bloody stool samples. Hence, in places like Bangladesh, bloody diarrhea and, in particular, shigellosis is a major cause of mortality. Worldwide *Shigella* is estimated to cause 200 million cases of diarrhea and 650,000 deaths each year (148).

Severe dehydration (>10% body weight) is not a prominent feature of most inflammatory diarrheal syndromes but can occur as a complication of these illnesses. In Bangladesh, patients with shigellosis rarely lost fluid of more than 30 mL/kg/day (149). In one study in Egypt, moderate to severe dehydration was most frequently seen with salmonellosis (91%), followed by *C. jejuni* diarrhea (10%), but not seen with shigellosis (10). A large study in Bangladesh showed that 12% of patients who died but only 1% of discharged patients had severe dehydration (135). However, a multivariate analysis showed that this association between dehydration and death was not apparent. Instead death was associated with younger age (<1 year), decreased serum protein, altered consciousness, and thrombocytopenia.

Other reported complications of shigellosis include seizures, ileus, intestinal perforation, toxic megacolon, rectal prolapse, hypoglycemia, hyponatremia, hemolytic-uremic syndrome, pneumonia, and bacteremia (150–153). Hypoglycemia is seen more often with *Shigella flexneri* than with *Shigella dysenteriae* type 1 dysentery (153). Toxic megacolon and bowel perforation are rare complications observed in many severe inflammatory conditions of the colon, including *C. difficile* pseudomembranous colitis, amebiasis, other invasive enteric bacterial infections, and ulcerative colitis.

Malnutrition and AIDS are risk factors for *Shigella* and *Salmonella* bacteremia (124,125,154,155). It should also be noted that shigellosis itself can provoke malnutrition in previously well-nourished children. In developing countries, invasive diarrhea can be a risk factor for persistent diarrhea (diarrhea lasting greater than 2 weeks), itself associated with high mortality and malnutrition (156).

In the United States, nontyphi *Salmonella* bacteremia occurs most commonly with *S. cholerasuis* (62%), *S. dublin* (40%), and *S. paratyphi* A (59%) intestinal infections (157). Other serotypes can cause bacteremia (0.8% with *S. newport* to 7.8% with *S. paratyphi* B), which is in contrast to *Shigella* or *C. jejuni* infections, which rarely cause bacteremia. The complications of salmonellosis, including rapid dehydration, convulsions, and septicemia, are more frequently seen in infants and elderly patients.

E. histolytica dysentery can be complicated by bowel perforation and peritonitis (1–4%). Pregnancy, malnutrition, and corticosteroid therapy are associated with fulminant colitis, which can be complicated by bowel necrosis, perforation, toxic megacolon, or liver abscess (158,159). An annular colonic mass, called ameboma, may develop in some patients. In addition to the hepatic abscess, other extraintestinal complications of amebiasis include direct or metastatic extension of the liver abscess into pleural or pericardial spaces, or, rarely, to the brain, kidneys, and lungs (145,146).

Patients with CMV enteritis may develop deep focal ulcerations extending to the submucosa into the muscularis. Such lesions may cause massive bleed, perforation, and shock. Gastrointestinal CMV disease is often a manifestation of systemic CMV infection and hence could be accompanied by CMV pneumonitis, hepatitis, or other organ involvement. CMV infection in patients with ulcerative colitis may develop as an infection superimposed on the inflamed mucosa or as a complication of the frequent use of immunosuppressive drugs. Mortality from CMV enteritis exceeded 80% before the availability of ganciclovir; nowadays death is relatively rare (40).

Complications of NEC include shock secondary to septicemia, fluid loss, or hemorrhage, and other features associated with the underlying illness. Many of the patients with NEC undergo surgery because of their signs of acute abdomen and may therefore develop intra- or postoperative complications.

Reactive arthritis and Reiter's syndrome may follow infections with *Shigella* (160), *Salmonella* (161), *Yersinia* (162,163), or *Campylobacter* (164). In a cohort involved in a common source *Shigella flexneri* outbreak, probable reactive arthritis developed in less than 3% of the infected persons (163). The susceptibility to reactive arthritis is associated with but not limited to persons belonging to the HLA-B27 histocompatibility group (163,165). Reactive arthritis following *Yersinia* infection is more common in northern Europe than in the United States, suggesting that there may be geographic differences in the prevalence of "arthrogenic" strains (162).

Differential Diagnosis

Except for some unusual but characteristic complications of inflammatory diarrhea, it is difficult to clinically distinguish among the different causes of inflammatory diarrhea. Patient history and epidemiological knowledge of the disease and pathogens help to narrow the possibilities. They can also be distinguished by their predilection to occur as sporadic illnesses only, as outbreaks, or as pandemics.

In North America or Europe, bloody diarrhea may be a manifestation of hemorrhagic colitis caused by a pathogen not considered to produce inflammatory diarrhea—*E. coli* O157:H7. The organism is not invasive and can produce an asymptomatic infection, watery diarrhea without blood, or grossly bloody diarrhea, with systemic complications that overlap the symptoms of inflammatory diarrhea (28–30). However, unlike dysentery, fever is either low grade or absent, even with profuse bloody diarrhea. However, fever may develop in more advanced disease, especially in the elderly (166), or in children who develop the complication of hemolytic uremic syndrome (HUS) (167). HUS is a major complication of hemorrhagic colitis, but it also occurs as a complication of shigellosis, especially after *Shigella dysenteriae* type 1 infection (168).

Only about a third of the patients with hemorrhagic colitis have fecal leukocytes. As mentioned, *E. histolytica* amebiasis can present with low-grade fever and dysenteric stool lacking fecal leukocytes. However, in North America or Europe, amebiasis is unusual among persons without a recent travel or homosexual history, and rarely occurs as outbreaks. On the other hand, like campylobacteriosis, yersiniosis, shigellosis, and salmonellosis, hemorrhagic colitis can occur sporadically or as part of an outbreak in community or institutional settings.

A distinct form of enterocolitis called ischemic colitis, characterized by an abrupt onset of abdominal pain followed by diarrhea and bloody discharge, was described by Wilson and Qualheim in 1954 (169), and further de-

tailed by others (170,171). At necropsy, the bowel is characteristically edematous with hemorrhage and scattered shallow ulcers affecting the entire intestinal tract in varying proportions. Leukocyte infiltration and necrosis of the mucosa accompany bacterial colonization and invasion. These lesions are believed to result from vascular insufficiency secondary to underlying cardiovascular disease, particularly following episodes of hypotension. Transient episodes as well as fulminant, gangrenous forms of ischemic colitis have been reported (172–174). Hemorrhagic colitis in the elderly can be mistaken for ischemic colitis, and a barium enema test in both may show a characteristic "thumbprinting" pattern, indicating submucosal edema or hemorrhage (28). A bloody diarrhea in the elderly that occurs as part of an outbreak is unlikely to be ischemic colitis.

Necrotizing enterocolitis (NEC) associated with neonates, neutropenic patients, or bowel ischemia presents with clinical manifestations that reflect their underlying disease. Symptoms include abdominal discomfort and severe pain with signs of acute abdomen (obstruction, perforation, or peritonitis) accompanied by fever and diarrhea that may be bloody. In patients with ileocecal involvement, abdominal pain localizes to the right lower quadrant, which may be mistaken for acute appendicitis or *Yersinia* enteritis. Features of the acute abdomen are more frequently observed in NEC than in diseases associated with invasive bacterial pathogens described above. Bacteremia with organisms normally associated with the gut flora in a patient with dysentery is highly suggestive of NEC.

Neonatal NEC can occur as a nosocomial outbreak (26,175), and adult forms of NEC have occurred as outbreaks in communities with atypical food habits, such as the pork feast in New Guinea (22), or in postwar Germany, where poor nutrition was shown to be associated with a form of enterocolitis called "Darmbrand" (23).

An acute exacerbation or the first manifestation of an inflammatory bowel disease may be difficult to distinguish from infectious inflammatory diarrhea. The possible role of an infectious agent, such as *Mycobacterium paratuberculosis,* which causes Johne's disease in ruminants, has been considered for Crohn's disease, but is not certain (44,45). Both Crohn's disease and ulcerative colitis produce diarrhea with blood accompanied by fever. Ulcerative colitis characteristically involves the entire colon, including the rectum, whereas Crohn's disease affects the colon and small intestine in a segmental fashion, sparing the rectum (176). The microabscesses in the superficial mucosa of the colon in ulcerative colitis may resemble those produced by severe amebiasis from *E. histolytica, Shigella,* or *Campylobacter.* However, in Crohn's disease, inflammation extends deeper into the bowel wall, and the macrophage predominance leads to the formation of noncaseating granulomas.

The arthritis of the spine and sacroiliac joints of inflammatory bowel disease resembles the reactive arthritis of shigellosis and yersiniosis, and is associated with the HLA-B27 histocompatibility type in all of these diseases. However, other manifestations such as uveitis and extraintestinal extension of fistulas may sway the diagnosis away from bacterial causes of inflammatory diarrhea. The chronic, relapsing pattern of the illness is also atypical for infectious inflammatory diarrhea, especially in adults.

Bloody diarrhea can be a manifestation of chemical or metal poisonings. Food items accidentally contaminated with the rodenticide thallium sulfate or barium carbonate produce acute watery or bloody diarrhea with nausea and vomiting, accompanied by neurological symptoms (177,178). Acute arsenic poisoning may produce bloody diarrhea, tenesmus, severe dehydration, and shock (179). Lead poisoning is associated with burning of the pharynx, abdominal pain, vomiting, and bloody diarrhea (179). All of these chemical poisonings can be distinguished from the infectious causes of bloody diarrhea by their extremely short incubation periods—minutes to 12 hr.

DIAGNOSTIC APPROACH

The initial approach to the diagnosis of inflammatory diarrhea involves careful history and physical examination, as well as familiarity with the epidemiology of the potential pathogens. These considerations influence the choice of laboratory tests.

Clinical and Epidemiological History

History and physical examination may help to distinguish inflammatory from secretory diarrhea, but the previous discussions show that the positive predictive values of symptoms and signs to distinguish specific causes of inflammatory diarrhea, especially in low-prevalence areas, would be unsatisfactorily low. The most discriminating features of the agents of inflammatory diarrhea, as described earlier, are their epidemiological and host characteristics.

Laboratory Tests

In developed countries, laboratory tests are usually performed to aid the clinical management of patients. However, in most parts of the world, such applications are not readily available or affordable. In such areas, diagnostic tests are instead used to characterize the epidemiology of an infectious agent, and it is this epidemiological information that is used to manage patients with diarrhea. In Bangladesh, the presence of bloody diarrhea in children had a positive predictive value of 50% for shigellosis (147). Hence, this single microbiological survey helped to establish a simple diarrhea management strategy that does not rely on stool culture from every patient: community health care workers are instructed to initiate antibiotics in all children who develop acute bloody diarrhea.

Some experts recommend microscopic examination of stool for leukocytes (180,181). The presence of fecal leukocytes indicates inflammatory process. A fresh fecal specimen is stained with methylene blue and examined for stained leukocytes. However, this method requires a microscope and a skilled microscopist. Leukocytes may be mistaken for amebas, such as E. histolytica. More recently, a latex agglutination method to detect lactoferrin, an iron-binding glycoprotein concentrated in secondary granules of leukocytes, was found to be a useful test to discriminate inflammatory from secretory diarrhea (182). The advantage of this test is that it does not require any trained personnel, and the test can be performed on specimens containing leukocytes that may have been lysed due to prolonged storage or transport. It should be pointed out that the absence of fecal leukocytes or their surrogates does not rule out agents of inflammatory diarrhea.

The microbiological diagnosis of inflammatory diarrhea pathogens is discussed in detail in the organism chapters. To assure detection of a pathogen, stool specimens should be plated within 2 hr of collection. Shigella is especially susceptible to acid pH that develops in unprocessed stool. If specimens cannot be processed immediately, such as in field situations, transport medium such as Cary–Blair or buffered glycerol saline should be used.

Agents belonging to the family Enterobacteriaceae are isolated by a combination of selective, differential, and enrichment media. Selective media (MacConkey, eosin–methylene blue agar [EMB]) are used to inhibit the growth of normal stool flora organisms, and differential media (xylose–lysine–deoxycholate [XLD], Salmonella–Shigella [SS], Hektoen enteric, Yersinia enteric agars) are used to allow isolation of colonies that can be further characterized for final identification. Enrichment broth media (gram-negative broth, selenite broth) are used to allow growth of organisms that may be present in low numbers (such as in specimens collected in later phase of an acute illness, or from convalescent or chronic carriers). Cold enrichment in phosphate-buffered saline is used to increase the recovery of Y. enterocolitica.

Campylobacter spp. require other differential media as well as selective growth temperatures and atmosphere (42°C at 4–6% oxygen, 6–10% carbon dioxide for C. jejuni). Patients residing at or traveling to the seacoast who develop dysentery should be cultured for Vibrio parahaemolyticus, which is isolated on thiosulfate citrate bile salt sucrose (TCBS) agar.

Suspected organisms isolated from the selective or differential media are further characterized morphologically, biochemically, serologically, genetically, or for their pathogenicity for final identification. Because of increased mortality, in endemic areas or during epidemics of Shigella dysenteriae type 1, it is important to rapidly examine suspected Shigella isolates with a slide agglutination test using antiserum against O antigens A–D. Although other serotypes of S. dysenteriae exist, an agglutination in A antiserum would be highly suspicious of the pandemic-prone type 1.

Absence in bloody stool samples of Shigella, Salmonella, Campylobacter, Yersinia, or Entamoeba histolytica from a patient with no known underlying disease in North America or Europe requires further examination of the E. coli for enterohemorrhagic strain, especially E. coli O157:H7. Most E. coli strains ferment sorbitol rapidly, whereas E. coli O157:H7 strains ferment sorbitol slowly or not at all (183,184). Therefore, MacConkey–sorbitol agar (available commercially) is used to select sorbitol-negative colonies, which are then tested for agglutination in O157 antiserum (184). Since *E. coli* O157 strains that have H antigens other than H7 are not associated with diarrhea, confirmatory diagnosis requires agglutination in H7 antiserum.

Blood cultures may be preferable to stool cultures in the diagnosis of typhoid fever. A variety of organisms may be detected in blood of patients with suspected NEC or ischemic colitis.

The diagnosis of *Salmonella*, *Shigella*, and *Campylobacter* spp., as well as *E. coli* O157:H7, should not end with their final isolation. They should be reported immediately to the local county or state public health laboratories. It is likely that an isolation of these pathogens represents occurrence of an unrecognized outbreak, and it is critical that outbreaks be "diagnosed" just as rapidly as the cause of dysentery in a patient.

Clostridium difficile can be isolated in differential and selective media, such as CCFA medium that contains cycloserine, cefoxitin, fructose, and egg yolk (185). Identification may be made with biochemical tests or gas–liquid chromatography (186). However, in hospitalized patients the asymptomatic carriage can be as high as 21%, and hence the isolation of the organism per se does not confirm an etiological diagnosis. Hence, cytotoxicity assays on filtered fecal specimen should be performed. Specificity of the cytotoxicity is confirmed by neutralization of the effect by *C. difficile* or *C. sordellii* antitoxin. Several kits for these assays are now commercially available.

In general, the serological diagnoses of bacterial inflammatory diarrhea are not helpful for acute management of the disease but may provide useful information for epidemiological studies, such as assessing asymptomatic carriage status or prevalence of infection in a community.

Pathogens identified at the genus or species level can be further subtyped. Subtyping information may help to distinguish pathogenic from nonpathogenic or other pathogenic variety of strains (e.g., enteroinvasive *E. coli* vs. other *E. coli* strains). *Salmonella*, *Shigella* spp., enteroinvasive *E. coli*, and *Yersinia enterocolitica*) are traditionally typed according to their O and flagellar antigens and their antibiotic susceptibility patterns. Molecular microbiological methods, such as plasmid profile analysis, restriction fragment length polymorphism analysis, and "ribotyping" provide additional subtyping information to assist epidemiological analyses (105,187–190).

The radiological diagnosis of inflammatory diarrhea is discussed elsewhere. The definitive diagnosis of inflammatory bowel disease involves endoscopy and mucosal biopsy histological examination. The mainstay of management of this syndrome is control of the inflammatory process, which requires antiinflammatory agents and immunosuppressive drugs—drugs that would not be indicated in infectious causes of inflammatory diarrhea. Hence, the definitive diagnosis is critical.

MANAGEMENT

Fluid and Electrolyte Balance

Oral glucose–electrolyte solutions were originally developed and evaluated in the treatment of cholera, and subsequently other secretory diarrheas due to organisms such as enterotoxigenic *E. coli* and rotavirus (191–193). Since the principal cause of death from secretory diarrhea is severe dehydration, the WHO advocates oral rehydration therapy (ORT) to prevent diarrhea mortality. The agents of dysentery can cause fluid loss but rarely produce the profound dehydration associated with agents of secretory diarrhea. However, electrolyte and glucose imbalance can be complications of dysentery associated with increased mortality (151). Hence, ORT may play a role in the prevention of such complications. Investigators in Thailand and Bangladesh have shown that ORT alone was effective for watery diarrhea from shigellosis manifesting predominantly as watery diarrhea instead of as dysentery (194,195).

Antimicrobial Therapy

WHO developed separate guidelines for the management of invasive diarrheas, emphasizing the use of specific antimicrobial agents (196). The choice of antibiotics depends on drug susceptibility data of the local agents of dysentery, cost, safety for children, and availability as an oral formulation. Resistance to amipicillin and trimethoprim-sulfamethoxazole, considered the drugs of choice for the treatment of shigellosis, has been observed with pandemic strains of *Shigella dysenteriae* 1 as well as other *Shigella* spp. in Asia and Africa (7,197,198). In the United States, 32% and 7% of the *Shigella* isolates were resistant to ampicillin and trimethoprim-sulfamethoxazole, respectively (199). Hence, in the United States, for shigellosis not associated with foreign travel, trimethoprim-sulfamethoxazole is considered the drug of choice. Fluoroquinolones are effective for shigellosis acquired abroad but are not approved for pediatric use.

In places like the United States, where diagnosis can be readily made, the empirical use of antimicrobial agents for inflammatory diarrhea must take clinical, host, and epidemiological factors into consideration. The use of ampicillin or ciprofloxacin in a patient with *Salmonella* gastroenteritis in an immunocompetent person may prolong the convalescent carriage state (200,201). On the other hand, treating mild diarrhea in a child with fever attending a day care center, where agents of inflammatory diarrhea have been implicated in outbreaks, may accelerate the clearance of organisms like *Shigella* and hence interrupt transmission.

The drug of choice for the treatment of *C. difficile* colitis is metronidazole. However, in severe or relapse cases, or in patients who cannot tolerate metronidazole, oral vancomycin is believed to be more effective (109). The choice, however, may also be influenced by the prevalence in the hospital of vancomycin-resistant gram-positive bacterial nosocomial infections, such as *Staphylococcus* or *Enterococcus* spp. infections. Intravenous vancomycin is not indicated in *C. difficile* colitis treatment since the drug may not be excreted into the intestinal lumen.

The therapy for amebiasis caused by *E. histolytica* is dependent on the sites of infection (lumen, bowel wall, or extraintestinal) and is reviewed in detail in the organism chapter. The management of diarrhea due to other parasitic causes is also discussed elsewhere in this book.

Antiperistaltic agents such as diphenoxylate hydrochloride with atropine sulfate should never be used in dysenteric syndromes.

In developing countries, and in inner cities and rural areas of developed countries, nutritional management of inflammatory diarrhea is important. As was mentioned earlier, hypoglycemia is a severe complication of dysentery associated with high mortality. Hypoglycemia may result from failure of gluconeogenesis secondary to deficiencies in protein or fat substrates for gluconeogenesis; hence, hypoglycemia is more likely to develop in malnourished children (151). Infants and small children should continue to be fed breast milk or weaning foods during their illness.

PREVENTION

The general approach to the prevention of dysentery is similar to that for prevention of all types of diarrhea—improving sanitation and hygiene. However, these improvements in hygiene can be focused if the local epidemiology of the pathogens of dysentery is known. Improved inspection and efficient regulation by the dairy, poultry, and meat industry in developed countries will contribute substantially to the control of salmonellosis, campylobacteriosis, and yersiniosis, as well as disease due to *E. coli* O157:H7. Proper food-handling practices, including cooking at the recommended temperature and time of meat products and eggs at restaurants (especially fast-food establishments) and at home, will significantly reduce the incidence of inflammatory diarrhea in the United States and Europe. Limiting the use of antimicrobial agents can prevent not only the emergence of drug-resistant *Salmonella,* especially in hospitals in middle-income countries, but *C. difficile* colitis in all hospitals. Chronic care facilities as well as day care centers should be aware of the potential for transmission of *C. difficile* and *Shigella* in their settings.

Handwashing with soap is an effective method to reduce shigellosis among inhabitants of developing countries (202), and *C. difficile* colitis in hospitals in all countries (109). During epidemics of *Shigella dysenteriae* 1, provision of large volumes of clean water can reduce the spread of disease. Availability of large volumes of water encourages handwashing. Water sources used for drinking should be separated from sources used for bathing and washing, and defecation should not be allowed or latrines located within 10 m of these water sources (196). The supply of chlorinated water or other chemicals for water treatment and of narrow-mouthed earthen jars with cov-

ers for storage will help to reduce transmission of enteric pathogens within families. Severe shigellosis occurs during or after measles in developing countries, and hence immunization against measles should be promoted. Bottle feeding is a recognized risk factor for death from shigellosis in infants, and early weaning in areas with poor sanitation is especially dangerous. Breastfeeding should be actively encouraged.

Travelers from developed countries to developing countries should avoid uncooked vegetables and untreated water. Data supporting the efficacy of antibiotic prophylaxis exist for causes of secretory diarrhea such as enterotoxigenic *E. coli,* but not for the agents of dysentery. Since dysentery is most likely to be treated with an antibiotic if a traveler develops it, the prophylactic use of antibiotics is discouraged; the potential emergence of drug-resistant infection will limit the choice of the drugs to use in such situations.

Vaccine Development

Cell-mediated mucosal immunity and systemic immunity (either humoral or cell-mediated) have been proposed to be important for protection against invasive pathogens such as *Shigella* and *Salmonella* (203). Therefore, antidysentery vaccine development efforts are directed at ways to promote these host responses. Currently, the only vaccines available for use against inflammatory diarrhea are typhoid vaccines. The parenteral, killed whole-cell vaccine offers 60–70% protection but is associated with many side effects. Multiple oral doses (three to four) of the enteric-coated, gal-epimerase–deficient, nonpathogenic strain of *Salmonella typhi* (Ty21a) have been shown to offer protection varying from 25% in a trial in Indonesian to 66% in Chilean children (204,205). Another injectable vaccine based on a single dose of purified Vi polysaccharide antigen has shown efficacy of about 65% over 18–21 months in trials in Nepal and South Africa (206,207).

Experimental parenteral killed *Shigella* whole-cell vaccine has not shown any protection and is associated with severe side effects (208). Therefore, efforts have been directed at developing attenuated oral vaccines. These approaches have included constructions of (a) nonpathogenic *E. coli* strains or attenuated *Salmonella* strains expressing *S. flexneri* invasion–protein antigens, as well as genes encoding *O*-polysaccharides (209,210), (b) deletion mutants, rendering *Shigella* auxotrophic for metabolites unavailable in mammalian cells (211,212), and (c) mutations in *Shigella* genes associated with virulence (213,214). Some of these constructs have shown protection in animal studies (212,215). Progress in vaccine development against nontyphoidal *Salmonella* and other agents of dysentery is still at preliminary stages.

In the developed world, despite their advanced technologies, diseases caused by agents of inflammatory diarrhea stubbornly remain unabated and may even be on the increase. In developing countries, dysentery is replacing secretory diarrhea as a major cause of diarrheal mortality. It is clear that control efforts for inflammatory diarrhea worldwide require a multifaceted approach, which includes increasing our understanding of their epidemiology and pathogenesis, and a commitment to basic public health intervention strategies.

REFERENCES

1. Varavithya W, Vathanophas K, Bodhidatta L, et al. Importance of salmonellae and *Campylobacter jejuni* in the etiology of diarrheal disease among children less than 5 years of age in a community in Bangkok, Thailand. *J Clin Microbiol* 1990;28:2507–2510.
2. Ling JM, Cheng AF. Infectious diarrhoea in Hong Kong. *J Trop Med Hyg* 1993;96:107–112.
3. Gomes TAT, Rassi V, MacDonald KL, et al. Enteropathogens associated with acute diarrheal disease in urban infants in Sao Paulo, Brazil. *J Infect Dis* 1991;164:331–337.
4. Gunzburg S, Gracey M, Burke V, Chang B. Epidemiology and microbiology of diarrhoea in young aboriginal children in the Kimberley region of Western Australia. *Epidemiol Infect* 1992;108:67–76.
5. Giron JA, Jones T, Millan-Velasco F, et al. Diffuse-adhering *Escherichia coli* (DAEC) as a putative cause of diarrhea in Mayan children in Mexico. *J Infect Dis* 1991;163:507–513.
6. Bhan MK, Raj P, Levine MM, et al. Enteroaggregative *Escherichia coli* associated with persistent diarrhea in a cohort of rural children in India. *J Infect Dis* 1989;159:1061–1064.
7. Mikail IA, Fox E, Habergerger Jr RL, Ahmed MH, Abbatte EA. Epidemiology of bacterial pathogens associated with infectious diarrhea in Djibouti. *J Clin Microbiol* 1990;956–961.
8. Adkins HJ, Escamilla J, Santiago LT, Ranoa C, Echeverria P, Cross JH. Two-year survey of etiologic agents of diarrhea disease at San Lazaro Hospital, Manila, Republic of the Philippines. *J Clin Microbiol* 1987;25:1143–1147.
9. Stanton B, Silimperi DR, Khatun K, et al. Parasitic, bacterial and viral pathogens isolated from diarrhoeal and routine stool specimens of urban Bangladesh children. *J Trop Med Hyg* 1989;92:46–55.
10. Mikhail IA, Hyams KC, Podgore JK, et al. Microbiologic and clinical study of acute diarrhea in children in Aswan, Egypt. *Scand J Infect Dis* 1989;21:59–65.
11. Hyams KC, Bourgeois AL, Merrell BR, et al. Diarrheal disease during operation Desert Shield. *N Engl J Med* 1991;325:1423–1428.
12. Taylor DN, Houston R, Shlim DR, Bhaibulaya M, Ungar BLP, Echeverria P. Etiology of diarrhea among travelers and foreign residents in Nepal. *JAMA* 1988;260:1245–1248.
13. Mattila L, Siitonen A, Kyronseppa H, et al. Seasonal variation in etiology of travelers' diarrhea. *J Infect Dis* 1992;165:385–388.
14. Riley LW, Finch MJ. Results of the first year of national surveillance of *Campylobacter* in the United States. *J Infect Dis* 1985;151:956–959.
15. Tauxe RV, Patton CM, Edmonds P, Barrett TJ, Brenner DJ, Blake PA. Illness associated with *Campylobacter laridis*, a newly recognized *Campylobacter* species. *J Clin Microbiol* 1985;21:222–225.
16. Fennell CL, Totten PA, Quinn TC, Patton DL, Holmes KK, Stamm WE. Characterization of *Campylobacter*-like organisms isolated from homosexual men. *J Infect Dis* 1984;149:58–66.
17. Edmonds P, Patton CM, Griffin PM, et al. *Campylobacter hyointestinalis* associated with human gastrointestinal disease in the United States. *J Clin Microbiol* 1987;25:685–691.
18. Hellyer TJ, Brown IN, Taylor NB, Allen BW, Easmon CSF. Gastrointestinal involvement in *Mycobacterium avium-intracellulare* infection of patients with HIV. *J Infect* 1993;26:55–66.
19. Horsburgh CR, Jr. *Mycobacterium avium* complex infection in the acquired immunodeficiency syndrome. *N Engl J Med* 1991;324:1332–1338.
20. Kudoh Y, Sakai S. Current status of bacterial diarrheal diseases in Japan. In: Takeda Y, Miwatani T, eds. *Bacterial diarrheal diseases*. Tokyo: KTK; 1985.
21. Blake PA, Weaver RE, Hollis DG. Disease of humans (other than cholera) caused by vibrios. *Annu Rev Microbiol* 1980;34:341–367.
22. Murrell TGC, Roth L, Egerton J, et al. Pig-bel: enteritis necroticans. *Lancet* 1966;1:217.
23. Hansen K, Jeckeln E, Jochims J, et al. *Dambrand-enteritis necroticanss*. Stuttgart: Georg Thiem Verlag; 1949.
24. Stein H, Beck J, Solomon, et al. Gastroenteritis with necrotizing enterocolitis in premature babies. *Br Med J* 1972;2:616–619.
25. Olarte J, Ferguson WW, Henderson NI, et al. *Klebsiella* strains isolated from diarrheal infants. *Am J Dis Child* 1961;101:763–770.
26. Howard FM, Flynn DM, Bradley JM, Noone P, Szawatkowski M. Outbreak of necrotising enterocolitis caused by *Clostridium butyricum*. *Lancet* 1977;2:1099–1102.
27. Santulli TY, Schullinger JN, Heird WC, et al. Acute necrotizing enterocolitis in infancy: a review of 64 cases. *Pediatrics* 1975;55:376–387.
28. Riley LW, Remis RS, Helgerson SD, et al. Hemorrhagic colitis associated with a rare *Escherichia coli* serotype. *N Engl J Med* 1983;308:681–685.
29. Griffin PM, Ostroff SM, Tauxe RV, et al. Illnesses associated with *Escherichia coli* O157:H7 infections: a broad clinical spectrum. *Ann Intern Med* 1988;109:705–712.
30. Griffin PM and Tauxe RV. The epidemiology of infections caused by *Escherichia coli* O157:H7, other enterohemorrhagic *E. coli*, and the associated hemolytic uremic syndrome. *Epidemiol Rev* 1991;13:60–98.
31. Brown HW, Neva FA, eds. *Basic clinical parasitology*. 5th ed. Norwalk: Appleton-Century-Crofts; 1983.
32. DeHovitz JA, Pape JW, Boncy M, Johnson WD Jr. clinical manifestations and therapy of *Isospora belli* infection in patients with acquired immunodeficiency syndrome. *N Engl J Med* 1986;315:87–90.
33. Forthal DN, Guest SS. *Isospora belli* enteritis in homosexual men. *Am J Trop Med Hyg* 1984;33:1060–1064.
34. Sanguino J, Peixe R, Guerra J, Rocha C, Quina M. Schistosomiasis and vascular alterations of the colonic mucosa. *Hepatogastroenterology* 1993;40:184–187.
35. Boyajian T. Strongyloidiasis on the Thai–Cambodian border. *Trans R Soc Trop Med Hyg* 1992;86:661–662.
36. Tamura H. Acute ulcerative colitis associated with cytomegalic inclusion virus. *Arch Pathol Lab Med* 1973;96:164–167.
37. Wolfe M, Cherry JD. Hemorrhage from cecal ulcers of cytomegalovirus infection: report of a case. *Ann Surg* 1971;177:490–494.
38. Jacobsen MA, Mills J. Serious cytomegalovirus disease in the acquired immunodeficiency syndrome (AIDS). *Ann Intern Med* 1988;108:585–594.
39. Frager HH, Frager JD, Wolf EL, et al. Cytomegalovirus colitis in acquired immunodeficiency syndrome: radiologic spectrum. *Gastroenterol Radiol* 1986;11:241–246.
40. Buckner FS and Pomeroy C. Cytomegalovirus disease of the gastrointestinal tract in patients without AIDS. *Clin Infect Dis* 1993;17:644–656.
41. Janoff EN, Orenstein JM, Manischewitz JF, Smith PD. Adenovirus colitis in the acquired immunodeficiency syndrome. *Gastroenterology* 1991;100:976–979.
42. Smith JMB. Mycoses of the alimentary tract. *Gut* 1969;10:1035–1040.
43. Centers for Disease Control. Diseases transmitted by foods. US Public Health Publication No. (CDC) 81-8237; 1979.
44. McFadden JJ, Butcher PD, Chiodini R, Hermon-Tayor J. Crohn's disease-isolated mycobacteria are identical to *Mycobacterium paratuberculosis*, as determined by DNA probes that distinguish between mycobacterial species. *J Clin Microbiol* 1987;25:796–801.
45. Sanderson JD, Moss MT, Tizard ML, Hermon-Taylor J. *Mycobacterium paratuberculosis* DNA in Crohn's disease tissue. *Gut* 1992;33:890–896.
46. Sereny B. Experimental *Shigella* keratoconjunctivitis. *Acta Microbiol Acad Sci Hung* 1955;2:293–295.
47. Isberg RR and Falkow R. A single genetic locus encoded by

Yersinia pseudotuberculosis permits invasion of cultured animal cells by *E. coli* K12. *Nature* 1985;317:262–264.

48. Isberg RR, Voorhis DL, Falkow S. Identification of invasin: a protein that allows enteric bacteria to penetrate cultured mammalian cells. *Cell* 1987;50:769–778.

49. Isberg RR, Leong JM. Multiple β₁ chain integrins are receptors for invasin, a protein that promotes bacterial penetration into mammalian cells. *Cell* 1990;60:861–871.

50. Young VB, Falkow S, Schoolnik GK. The invasin protein of *Yersinia enterocolitica*: internalization of invasin-bearing bacteria by eukaryotic cells is associated with reorganization of the cytoskeleton. *J Cell Biol* 1992;116:197–207.

51. Guan K and Dixon JE. Protein tyrosine phosphatase activity of an essential virulence determinant in *Yersinia*. *Science* 1990;249:553–556.

52. Leung KY, Straley SC. The *yopM* gene of *Yersinia pestis* encodes a released protein having homology with the human platelet surface protein GPIbα. *J Bacteriol* 1989;171:4623–4632.

53. Rosqvist R, Forsberg A, Wolf-Watz H. Intracellular targeting of the *Yersinia* YopE cytotoxin in mammalian cells induces actin microfilament disruption. *Infect Immun* 1992;59:4562–4569.

54. Goldberg MB, Sansonetti PJ. *Shigella* subversion of the cellular cytoskeleton: a strategy for epithelial colonization. *Infect Immun* 1993;61:4941–4946.

55. Hale TL, Oaks EV, Formal SB. Identification and antigenic characterization of virulence-associated, plasmid-coded proteins of *Shigella* spp. and enteroinvasive *Escherichia coli*. *Infect Immun* 1985;50:620–629.

56. Sansonetti PJ, Ryter A, Clerc P, Maurelli AT, Mournier J. Multiplication of *Shigella flexneri* within HeLa cells: lysis of the phagocytic vacuole and plasmid-mediated contact hemolysis. *Infect Immun* 1986;1:461–469.

57. Galan JE, Curtiss R III. Cloning and molecular characterization of genes whose products allow *Salmonella typhimurium* to penetrate tissue culture cells. *Proc Natl Acad Sci USA* 1989;86:6383–6387.

58. Galan JE, Pace J, Hayman MJ. Involvement of the epidermal growth factor receptor in the invasion of cultured mammalian cells by *Salmonella typhimurium*. *Nature* 1992;357:588–589.

59. Pace J, Hayman MJ, Galan JE. Signal transduction and invasion of epithelial cells by *S. typhimurium*. *Cell* 1993;72:505–514.

60. Finley BB, Gumbiner B, Falkow S. Cytoskeletal rearrangements accompanying *Salmonella* entry into epithelial cells. *J Cell Sci* 1991;99:383–394.

61. Ravdin JI. Pathogenesis of disease caused by *Entamoeba histolytica*: studies of adherence, secreted toxins, and contact-dependent cytolysis. *Rev Infect Dis* 1986;8:247–260.

62. Saffer LD, Petri WA Jr. *Entamoeba histolytica*: recognition of alpha- and beta-galactose by the 260-kDa adherence lectin. *Exp Parasitol* 1991;72:106–108.

63. Petri WA Jr, Ravdin JI. Protection of gerbils from amebic liver abscess by immunization with the galactose-specific adherence lectin of *Entamoeba histolytica*. *Infect Immun* 1991;59:97–101.

64. Ravdin JI, Guerrant RL. Role of adherence in cytopathogenic mechanisms of *Entamoeba histolytica*: study with mammalian tissue culture cells and human erythrocytes. *J Clin Invest* 1981;68:1305–1313.

65. Ravdin JI, Murphy CF, Guerrant RL, Long-Krug SA. Effect of calcium and phospholipase A antagonists in the cytopathogenicity of *Entamoeba histolytica*. *J Infect Dis* 1985;152:542–549.

66. Saffer LD, Petri WA Jr. Role of the galactose lectin of *Entamoeba histolytica* in adherence-dependent killing of mammalian cells. *Infect Immun* 1991;59:4681–4683.

67. Guerrant RL, Brush J, Ravdin JI, Sullivan JA, Mandell GL. Interaction between *Entamoeba histolytica* and human polymorphonuclear neutrophils. *J Infect Dis* 1981;143:83–93.

68. O'Brien AD and Holmes RK. Shiga and Shiga-like toxins. *Microbiol Rev* 1987;51:206–220.

69. Donohue-Rolfe A, Acheson DWK, Keusch GT. Shiga toxin: purification, structure, and function. *Rev Infect Dis* 1991;13(Suppl 4):S293–297.

70. Reisbig R, Olsnes S, Eiklid K. The cytotoxic activity of *Shigella* toxin. Evidence for catalytic inactivation of the 60 S ribosomal subunit. *J Biol Chem* 1981;256:8739–8744.

71. Knowalchuk J, Speirs JI, Stavric S. Vero response to a cytotoxin of *Escherichia coli*. *Infect Immun* 1977;18:775–779.

72. Karmali MA, Petric M, Lim C, Fleming PC, Arbus GS, Lior H. The association between idiopathic hemolytic uremic syndrome and infection by verotoxin-producing *Escherichia coli*. *J Infect Dis* 1985;151:775–782.

73. Jacewicz M, Clausen H, Nudelman E, Donohue-Rolfe A, Keusch GT. Pathogenesis of shigella diarrhea. XI. Isolation of a shigella toxin-binding glycolipid from rabbit jejunum and HeLa cells and its identification as globotriaosylceramide. *J Exp Med* 1986;163:1391–1404.

74. Fontaine A, Arondel J, Sansonetti PJ. Role of Shiga toxin in the pathogenesis of bacillary dysentery studied using Tox⁻ mutant of *Shigella dysenteriae* 1. *Infect Immun* 1988;56:3099–3109.

75. Obrig TG, DelVecchi PJ, Brown JE, et al. Direct cytotoxic action of Shiga toxin on human vascular endothelial cells. *Infect Immun* 1988;56:2373–2378.

76. Lyerly DM, Lockwood DE, Richardson SH, Wilkins TD. Biological activities of toxins A and B of *Clostridium difficile*. 1982;35:1147–1150.

77. Lyerly DM, Krivan HC, Wilkins TD. *Clostridium difficile*: its disease and toxins. *Clin Microbiol Rev* 1988;1:1–18.

78. Sakazaki R, Tamura K, Kato T, Obara Y, Yamai S, Hobo K. Studies on the enteropathogenic facultatively halophilic bacteria, *Vibrio parahaemolyticus*. III. Enteropathogenicity. *Jpn J Med Sci Biol* 1968;21:325–331.

79. Miyamoto Y, Kato T, Obara Y, Akiyama S, Takizawa K, Yamai S. In vitro hemolytic characteristics of *Vibrio parahaemolyticus*: its close correlation with human pathogenicity. *J Bacteriol* 1969;100:1147–1149.

80. Takeda Y. Thermostable direct hemolysin of *Vibrio parahaemolyticus*. *Pharmacol Ther* 1983;19:123–146.

81. Nishibuchi M, Fasano A. Russell RG, Kaper JB. Enterotoxigenicity of *Vibrio parahaemolyticus* with and without genes encoding thermostable direct hemolysin. *Infect Immun* 1992;60:3539–3545.

82. Chatterjee BD. Enteroinvasiveness model of *Vibrio parahaemolyticus*. *Indian J Med Res* 1984;79:151–158.

83. Hermann RE. Perforation of the colon from necrotizing colitis in the newborn: report of a survival and new etiological concept. *Surgery* 1965;58:436–441.

84. Steinberg D, Gold J, Brodin A. Necrotizing enterocolitis in leukemia. *Arch Intern Med* 1973;131:538–544.

85. Mower MJ, Hawkins JA, Nelson EW. Neutropenic enterocolitis in adults with acute leukemia. *Arch Surg* 1986;121:571–574.

86. Frankel AH, Barker F, Williams G, Benjamin IS, Lechler R, Rees AJ. Neutropenic enterocolitis in a renal transplant patient. *Transplantation* 1991;52:913–914.

87. Cutrona AF, Blinkhorn RJ, Crass J, Spagnuolo PJ. Probable neutropenic enterocolitis in patients with AIDS. *Rev Infect Dis* 1991;13:828–831.

88. Lawrence G, Shann F, Frestone DS, et al. Prevention of necrotizing enteritis in Papua New Guinea by active immunization. *Lancet* 1979;1:227–230.

89. Centers for Disease Control. *Campylobacter: annual tabulation 1987–89.* US Public Health Service; 1991.

90. Chalker RB, Blaser MJ. A review of human salmonellosis: III. Magnitude of *Salmonella* infection in the United States. *Rev Infect Dis* 1988;10:111–124.

91. Guerrant RL. The global problem of amebiasis: current status, research needs, and opportunities for progress. *Rev Infect Dis* 1986;8:218–227.

92. Centers for Disease Control and Prevention. Outbreaks of *Salmonella enteritidis* gastroenteritis—California, 1993. *MMWR* 1993;42:793–797.

93. Ryan CA, Nickels MK, Hargrett-Bean NT, et al. Massive outbreak of antimicrobial resistant salmonellosis traced to pasteurized milk. *JAMA* 1987;258:3268–3274.

94. Spika JS, Waterman SH, Soo Hoo G, et al. Chloramphenicol-resistant *Salmonella newport* traced through hamburger to

dairy farms: a major persisting source of human salmonellosis in California. *N Engl J Med* 1987;316:565–570.

95. Tauxe RV, Vandepitte J, Wauters G, et al. *Yersinia enterocolitica* infections and pork: the missing link. *Lancet* 1987;1: 1129–1132.

96. Tacket CO, Narain JP, Sattin R, et al. A multistate outbreak of infections caused by *Yersinia enterocolitica* transmitted by pasteurized milk. *JAMA* 1984;251:483–486.

97. Lee LA, Gerber AR, Lonsway DR et al. *Yersinia enterocolitica* O:3 infections in infants and children, associated with the household preparation of chitterlings. *N Engl J Med* 1990;322: 984–987.

98. Tacket CO, Ballard J, Harris N, et al. An outbreak of *Yersinia enterocolitica* infections caused by contaminated tofu (soybean curd). *Am J Epidemiol* 1985;121:705–711.

99. Hoare CA. Reservoir hosts and natural foci of human protozoal infection. *Acta Trop* 1962;19:281–317.

100. Dobell C. Researches on the intestinal protozoa of monkeys and man IV. An experimental study of the *histolytica*-like species of *Entamoeba* living naturally in macaques. *Parasitology* 1931;23:1–72.

101. Weissman JB, Schmerler A, Weiler P, et al. The role of preschool children and day-care centers in the spread of shigellosis in urban communities. *J Pediatr* 1974;84:797–802.

102. Black RE, Craun GF, Blake PA. Epidemiology of common-source outbreaks of shigellosis in the United States, 1961–1975. *Am J Epidemiol* 1978;108:47–52.

103. Lee LA, Ostroff SM, McGee HG, et al. An outbreak of shigellosis at an outdoor music festival. *Am J Epidemiol* 1991;133: 608–615.

104. Lew JF, Swerdlow DL, Dance ME, et al. An outbreak of shigellosis aboard a cruise ship caused by a multiple-antibiotic-resistant strain of *Shigella flexneri*. *Am J Epidemiol* 1991;134: 413–20.

105. Riley LW, DiFerdinando G, DeMelfi TM, Cohen ML. Evaluation of isolated cases of salmonellosis by plasmid profile analysis: introduction and transmission of a bacterial clone by precooked roast beef. *J Infect Dis* 1983;148:12–17.

106. Riley LW, Ceballos BSO, Trabulsi LR, Toledo MRF, Blake PA. The significance of hospitals as reservoirs for endemic multiresistant *Salmonella typhimurium* causing infection in urban Brazilian children. *J Infect Dis* 1984;150:236–241.

107. Tipple MA, Bland JJ, Murphy MJ, et al. Sepsis associated with transfusion of red cells contaminated with *Yersinia enterocolitica*. *Transfusion* 1990;30:207–213.

108. Jacobs J, Jamaer D, Vandeven J, Wouters M, Vermylen C, Vandepitte J. *Yersinia enterocolitica* in donor blood: a case report and review. *J Clin Microbiol* 1989;27:1119–1121.

109. Knoop FC, Owens M, Crocker IC. *Clostridium difficile*: clinical disease and diagnosis. *Clin Microbiol Rev* 1993;6:251–265.

110. Stein H, Kavin I, Faerber EN. Colonic strictures following nonoperative management of necrotizing enterocolitis. *J Pediatr Surg* 1975;10:943–947.

111. Touloukian RJ, Kadar A, Spencer RP. The gastrointestinal complications of neonatal umbilical venous exchange transfusions: a clinical and experimental study. *Pediatrics* 1973;52: 36–43.

112. Nienhuis L. Colon perforations in the newborn. *Am Surg* 1963; 29:835–840.

113. Stevenson JK, Graham CB, Oliver TK Jr, Goldenberg YE. Neonatal necrotizing enterocolitis. A report of 21 cases with 14 survivors. *Am J Surg* 1969;118:260–272.

114. Rogers AF, Dunn PM. Intestinal perforation, exchange transfusion and PVC. *Lancet* 1969;2:1203–1204.

115. Jaeger RJ, Rubin RJ. Migration of a phthalate ester plasticizer from polyvinyl chloride blood bags into stored human blood and its localization in human tissues. *N Engl J Med* 1972;287: 1114–1118.

116. Hornick RB, Greisman SE, Woodward TE, DuPont HL, Dawkins AT, Snyder MJ. Typhoid fever: pathogenesis and immunologic control. *N Engl J Med* 1970;283:686–691.

117. Blaser MJ, Newman LS. A review of human salmonellosis: I. Infective dose. *Rev Infect Dis* 1982;4:1096–1106.

118. DuPont HL, Levine MM, Hornick RB, et al. Inoculum size in shigellosis and implications for expected mode of transmission. *J Infect Dis* 1989;159:1126–1128.

119. Sargeaunt PG, Williamns JE. Electrophoretic isoenzyme patterns of the pathogenic and nonpathogenic intestinal amoebae of man. *Trans R Soc Trop Med Hyg* 1979;73:225–227.

120. Gianella RA, Broitman SA, Zamcheck N. Influence of gastric acidity on bacterial and parasitic enteric infections: a perspective. *Ann Intern Med* 1973;78:271–276.

121. Waddell WR, Kunz LJ. Association of salmonella enteritis with operation on the stomach. *N Engl J Med* 1956;255:555–559.

122. Han T, Sokal JE, Neter E. Salmonellosis in disseminated malignant diseases. *N Engl J Med* 1967;276:1045–1052.

123. Wolfe MS, Armstrong D, Louria DB, Blevins A. Salmonellosis in patients with neoplastic disease. A review of 100 episodes at Memorial Cancer Center over a 13-year period. *Arch Intern Med* 1971;128:546–554.

124. Celum CL, Chaisson RE, Rutherford GW, Barnhart JL, Echenberg DF. Incidence of salmonellosis in patients with AIDS. *J Infect Dis* 1987;156:998–1002.

125. Jacobs JL, Gold JW, Murray HW, Roberts RB, Armstrong D. *Salmonella* infections in patients with the acquired immunodeficiency syndrome. *Ann Intern Med* 1985;103:186–188.

126. Barret-Connor E. Bacterial infection and sickle cell anemia: an analysis of 250 infections in 166 patients and a review of the literature. *Medicine* 1971;50:97–112.

127. Black PH, Kunz LJ, Swartz MN. Salmonellosis—a review of some unusual aspects. *N Engl J Med* 1960;262:811–816, 846–870, 921–927.

128. Riley LW, Cohen ML, Seals JE, et al. Importance of host factors in human salmonellosis caused by multiresistant strains of *Salmonella*. *J Infect Dis* 1984;149:878–883.

129. Hook EW. Salmonellosis: certain factors influencing the interaction of *Salmonella* and the human host. *Bull NY Acad Med* 1961;37:499–512.

130. Tacket CO, Davis BR, Carter GP, et al. *Yersinia enterocolitica* pharyngitis. *Ann Intern Med* 1983;99:40–42.

131. Blaser MJ, Duncan DJ, Osterholm MT, Istre GR, Wang WL. Serologic study of two clusters of infection due to *Campylobacter jejuni*. *J Infect Dis* 1983;147:820–823.

132. Buchwald DS and Blaser MJ. A review of human salmonellosis: II. Duration of excretion following infection with nontyphi *Salmonella*. *Rev Infect Dis* 1984;6:345–356.

133. Ostroff SM, Kapperud G, Lassen J, Aasen S, Tauxe RV. Clinical features of sporadic *Yersinia enterocolitica* infections in Norway. *J Infect Dis* 1992;166:812–817.

134. Cooperstock M, Riegle L, Fabacher D, Woodruff CW. *Clostridium difficile* in formula-fed infants and sudden infant death syndrome. *Pediatrics* 1982;70:91–95.

135. Bennish ML, Harris JR, Wojtyniak BJ, Struelens M. Death in shigellosis: incidence and risk factors in hospitalized patients. *J Infect Dis* 1990;161:500–506.

136. Blatt ML, Shaw NG. Bacillary dysentery in children. A study of three hundred and fifty-six cases from the children's division in the Cook County Hospital, Chicago. *Arch Pathol Lab Med* 1938;26:216–239.

137. Dodd K, Buddingh GJ, Rapoport S. The etiology of ekiri, a highly fatal disease of Japanese children. *Pediatrics* 1949;3: 9–19.

138. Riley LW, Pape JW, Johnson WD Jr. Infections caused by *Salmonella* and *Shigella* species. In: Stein JH, ed. *Internal Medicine*. 4th ed. St. Louis: Mosby-Year Book; 1994: 2140–2147.

139. Aguero J, Faundez G, Nunez M et al. Choleriform syndrome and production of labile enterotoxin (CT/LT1)-like antigen by species of *Salmonella infantis* and *Salmonella haardt* isolated from the same patient. *Rev Infect Dis* 1991;13:420–423.

140. Giannella RA, Gots RE, Charney AN, Greenough WB, Formal SB. Pathogenesis of *Salmonella*-mediated intestinal fluid secretion. *Gastroenterology* 1975;69:1238–1245.

141. Blaser MJ, Parsons RB, Wang WL. Acute colitis caused by *Campylobacter fetus* ss jejuni. *Gastroenterology* 1980;78: 448–453.

142. Snyder JD, Christenson E, Feldman RA. Human *Yersinia enterocolitica* infections in Wisconsin. Clinical, laboratory, and epidemiologic features. *Am J Med* 1982;72:768–774.

143. Black RE, Jackson RJ, Tsai T, et al. Epidemic *Yersinia enterocolitica* infection due to contaminated chocolate milk. *N Engl J Med* 1978;298:76–79.
144. Tedesco F,J, Barton RW, Alpers DH. Clindamycin-associated colitis. A prospective study. *Ann Intern Med* 1974;81:429–433.
145. Adams EB, MacLeod IN. Invasive amebiasis. II. Amebic liver abscess and its complications. *Medicine* 1977;56:325–334.
146. Juniper K. Parasitic diseases of the intestinal tract. In: Paulson M, ed. *Gastroenterologic medicine.* Philadelphia: Lea & Febiger; 1969:172.
147. Ronsmans C, Bennish ML, Wierzba T. Diagnosis and management of dysentery by community health workers. *Lancet* 1988; 2:552–555.
148. World Health Organization. Research priorities for diarrhoeal disease vaccines: memorandum from a WHO meeting. *Bull WHO* 1991;69:667–676.
149. Rabbani GH, Gilman RH, Spira WM. Intestinal fluid loss in *Shigella* dysentery: role of oral rehydration therapy. *Lancet* 1983;1:654.
150. Bennish ML. Potentially lethal complications of shigellosis. *Rev Infect Dis* 1991;13(Suppl 4):S319–324.
151. Bennish ML, Azad AK, Rahman O, Phillips RE. Hypoglycemia during diarrhea in childhood. *N Engl J Med* 1990;322: 1357–1363.
152. Ashkenazi S, Dinari G, Zevulunov A, Nitzan M. Convulsions in childhood shigellosis. Clinical and laboratory features in 153 children. *Am J Dis Child* 1987;141:208–210.
153. Struelens MJ, Patte D, Kabir I, Salalm A, Nath SK, Butler T. *Shigella* septicemia: prevalence, presentation, risk factors, and outcome. *J Infect Dis* 1985;152:784–790.
154. Bhandari N, Bhan MK, Sazawal S. Mortality associated with acute watery diarrhea, dysentery and persistent diarrhea in rural north India. *Acta Paediatrica* (Suppl.) 1992;381:3–6.
155. Nelson MR, Shanson DC, Hawkins DA, Gazzard BG. *Salmonella, Campylobacter,* and *Shigella* in HIV-seropositive patients. *AIDS J* 1992;6:1495–1498.
156. Shahid NS, Sack DA, Rahman M, Alam AN, Rahman N. Risk factors for persistent diarrhea. *Br Med J* 1988;297:1036–1038.
157. Blaser MJ and Feldman RA. *Salmonella* bacteremia: reports to the Centers for Disease Control, 1968–1979. *J Infect Dis* 1981;143:743–746.
158. Wagner VP, Smale LE, Lischke JH. Amebic abscess of the liver and spleen in pregnancy and the puerperium. *Obstet Gynecol* 1975;45:562–565.
159. Kanani SR, Knight R. Relapsing amoebic colitis of 12 years' standing exacerbated by corticosteroids. *Br Med J* 1969;2: 613–614.
160. Simon DG, Kaslow RA, Rosenbaum J, Kaye RL, Calin A. Reiter's syndrome following epidemic shigellosis. *J Rheumatol* 1981;8:969–973.
161. Warren CPW. Arthritis associated with salmonella infections. *Ann Rheum Dis* 1970;29:483–487.
162. Olson DN, Finch WR. Reactive arthritis associated with *Yersinia enterocolitica* gastroenteritis. *Am J Gastroenterol* 1981; 76:524–546.
163. Finch M, Rodey G, Lawrence D, Blake P. Epidemic Reiter's syndrome following an outbreak of shigellosis. *Eur J Epidemiol* 1986;2:26–30.
164. Van de Putte LBA, Berden JHM, Boerbooms AMT, et al. Reactive arthritis after *Campylobacter jejuni* enteritis. *J Rheumatol* 1980;7:531–535.
165. Laitinen O, Leirisalo M, Skylv G. Relation between HLA-B27 and clinical features in patients with *Yersinia* arthritis. *Arthr Rheum* 1977;20:1121–1124.
166. Ryan CA, Tauxe RV, Hosek GW et al. *Escherichia coli* O157: H7 diarrhea in a nursing home: clinical, epidemiological, and pathological findings. *J Infect Dis* 1986;154:631–638.
167. Martin DL, MacDonald KL, White KE, Soler JT, Osterholm MT. Epidemiology and clinical aspects of the humolytic-uremic syndrome in Minnesota. *N Engl J Med* 1990;323:1161–1167.
168. Koster F, Levin J, Walker L, et al. Hemolytic-uremic syndrome after shigellosis. Relation to endotoxemia and circulating immune complexes. *N Engl J Med* 1978;298:927–933.
169. Wilson R, Qualheim RE. A form of acute hemorrhagic enterocolitis afflicting chronically ill individuals. *Gastroenterology* 1954;27:431–444.
170. Marston A, Pheils MT, Thomas ML, Morson BC. Ischemic colitis. *Gut* 1966;7:1–15.
171. McGovern VJ, Goulston JM. Ischaemic enterocolitis. *Gut* 1965;6:213–220.
172. Clark AW, Lloyd-Mostyn RH, Sadler MR de C. "Ischaemic" colitis in young adults. *Br Med J* 1972;4:70–72.
173. Miller WE, DePoto DW, Scholl HW, Raffensperger EC. Evanescent colitis in the young adult: a new entity? *Radiology* 1971;100:71–78.
174. Grossman H, Berdon WE, Baker DH. Reversible gastrointestinal signs of hemorrhage and edema in the pediatric age group. *Radiology* 1965;84:33–39.
175. Virnig NL, Reynolds JW. Epidemiological aspects of neonatal necrotizing enterocolitis. *Am J Dis Child* 1974;128:186–190.
176. Podolsky DK. Inflammatory bowel disease. 1 and 2. *N Engl J Med* 1991;325:928–937, 1008–1016.
177. Banks WJ, Pleasure DE, Suzuki K. Thallium poisoning. *Arch Neurol* 1972;26:456–464.
178. Ogen S, Rosenbluth S, Eisenberg A. Food poisoning due to barium carbonate in sausage. *Isr J Med Sci* 1967;3:565–568.
179. Hammond PR and Beliles RP. Metals. In: Doull J, Klaassen CD, Amdur MO, eds. *Casarett and Doulll's toxicology. The basic science of poisoning.* 2nd ed. New York: Macmillan; 1980.
180. Harris JC, DuPont HL, Hornick RB. Fecal leukocytes in diarrheal illness. *Ann Intern Med* 1972;76:697–703.
181. Korzeniowski OM, Barada FA, Rouse JD, Guerrant RL. Value of examination for fecal leukocytes in the early diagnosis of shigellosis. *Am J Trop Med Hyg* 1979;28:1031–1035.
182. Guerrant RL, Araujo V, Soares E, et al. Measurement of fecal lactoferrin as a marker of fecal leukocytes. *J Clin Microbiol* 1992;30:1238–1242.
183. Wells JG, Davis BR, Wachsmuth IK, et al. Laboratory investigation of hemorrhagic colitis outbreaks associated with a rare *Escherichia coli* serotype. *J Clin Microbiol* 1983;18:512–520.
184. Farmer JJ, Davis BR. H7 antiserum-sorbitol fermentation medium: a single tube screening medium for detecting *Escherichia coli* O157:H7 associated with hemorrhagic colitis. *J Clin Microbiol* 1985;22:620–625.
185. George WL, Sutter VL, Citron D, Finegold SM. Selective and differential medium for isolation of *Clostridium difficile*. *J Clin Microbiol* 1979;9:214–219.
186. Gopill S, Sims HV. Presumptive identification of *Clostridium difficile* by detection of p-cresol in prepared peptone yeast glucose broth supplemented with p-hydroxyphenylacetic acid. *J Clin Microbiol* 1990;28:1851–1853.
187. Litwin CM, Storm AL, Chipowsky S, Ryan KJ. Molecular epidemiology of *Shigella* infections: plasmid profiles, serotype correlation, and restriction endonuclease analysis. *J Clin Microbiol* 1991;29:104–108.
188. Wachsmuth IK. Molecular epidemiology of bacterial infections. Examples of methodology and investigations of outbreaks. *Rev Infect Dis* 1986;8:682–692.
189. Strockbine NA, Parsonnet J, Greene K, Kiehlbauch JA, Wachsmuth IK. Molecular epidemiologic techniques in analysis of epidemic and endemic *Shigella dysenteriae* type 1 strains. *J Infect Dis* 1991;163:406–409.
190. Faruque SM, Haider K, Rahman MM, et al. Differentiation of *Shigella flexneri* strains by rRNA gene restriction patterns. *J Clin Microbiol* 1992;30:2996–2999.
191. Pierce NF, Sack RB, Mitra RC, et al. Replacement of water and electrolyte losses in cholera by an oral glucose electrolyte solution. *Ann Intern Med* 1969;70:1173–81.
192. Nalin DR, Cash RA. Oral or nasogastric maintenance therapy for diarrhoea of unknown aetiology resembling cholera. *Trans R Soc Trop Med Hyg* 1970;64:769–771.
193. Black RE, Merson M, Taylor PR, et al. Glucose vs sucrose in oral rehydration solutions for infants and young children with rotavirus-associated diarrhea. *Pediatrics* 1981;67:79–83.
194. Nalin DR, Levine MM, Mata L, et al. Oral rehydration and maintenance of children with rotavirus and bacterial diarrhoeas. *Bull WHO* 1979;57:453–459.

195. Varavithya W, Sunthornkachit R, Eampokalap B. Oral rehydration therapy for invasive diarrhea. *Rev Infect Dis* 1991; 13(Suppl 4):S325–331.

196. World Health Organization. A manual for the treatment of acute diarrhoea. *WHO/CDD/SER* 80(2)Rev. 1; 1984.

197. Pal SC. Epidemic bacillary dysentery in West Bengal, India, 1984. *Lancet* 1984;1:1462 (letter).

198. Frost JA, Willshaw GA, Barclay EA, Rowe B. Plasmid characterization of drug-resistant *Shigella dysenteriae* 1 from an epidemic in Central Africa. *J Hyg* 1985;94:163–172.

199. Tauxe RV, Puhr ND, Wells JG, Hargrett-Bean N, Blake PA. Antimicrobial resistance of *Shigella* isolates in the USA: the importance of international travelers. *J Infect Dis* 1990;162: 1107–1111.

200. Aserkoff B, Bennett JV. Effect of antibiotic therapy in acute salmonellosis on the fecal excretion salmonellae. *N Engl J Med* 1969;281:636–640.

201. Neill MA, Opal SM, Heelan J, et al. Failure of Ciprofloxacin to eradicate convalescent fecal excretion after acute salmonellosis: experience during an outbreak in health care workers. *Ann Intern Med* 1991;114:195–199.

202. Aung MH, Thein H. Prevention of diarrhoea and dysentery by hand washing. *Trans R Soc Trop Med Hyg* 1989;83:128–131.

203. Tagliabue A, Boraschi D, Villa DF et al. Ig-A-dependent cell-mediated activity against enteropathogenic bacteria: distribution, specificity, and characterization of the effector cells. *J Immunol* 1984;133:988–992.

204. Levine MM. Development of vaccines against bacteria. In: Farthing MJG, Eeusch GT, eds. *Enteric infection: mechanisms, manifestations, and management*. London: Chapman and Hall; 1989:495.

205. World Health Organization. Annual report, Diarrheal Disease Control Programme. Geneva: 1988.

206. Acharya IL, Lowe CU, Thapa R, et al. Prevention of typhoid fever in Nepal with the Vi capsular polysaccharide of *Salmonella typhi*. A preliminary report. *N Engl J Med* 1987;317: 1101–1104.

207. Klugman KP, Gilbertson IT, Koornhof HJ, et al. Vaccination Advisory Committee. Protective efficacy of Vi capsular polysaccharide against typhoid fever. *Lancet* 1987;2:1165–1169.

208. Shaugnessey HJ, Olsson RC, Bass K, et al. Experimental human bacillary dysentery: polyvalent dysentery vaccine in its prevention. *JAMA* 1946;132:362–368.

209. Baron LS, Kopecko DJ, Formal SB, et al. Introduction of *Shigella flexneri* 2a type and group antigen genes into oral typhoid vaccine strain *Salmonella typhi* Ty21a. *Infect Immun* 1987;55: 2797–2801.

210. Formal SB, Hall TL, Kapfer C, et al. Oral vaccination of monkeys with an invasive *Escherichia coli* K12 hybrid expressing *Shigella flexneri* 2a somatic antigen. *Infect Immun* 1984;46: 465–469.

211. Lindberg A, Karnell A, Pal T et al. Construction of an auxotrophic *Shigella flexneri* strain for use as a live vaccine. *Microb Pathog* 1990;8:433–440.

212. Ahmed AU, Sarker MR, Sack DA. Protection of adult rabbits and monkeys from lethal shigellosis by oral immunization with a thymine-requiring and temperature-sensitive mutant of *Shigella flexneri* Y. *Vaccine* 1990;8:153–158.

213. Sansonetti PJ, Arondel J. Construction and evaluation of a double mutant of *Shigella flexneri* as a candidate for oral vaccination against shigellosis. *Vaccine* 1989;7:443–450.

214. Sansonetti PJ, Arondel J, Fontaine A, d'Hauteville H, Bernardini ML. OmpB (osmo-regulation) and icsA (cell-to-cell spread) mutants of *Shigella flexneri*: vaccine candidates and progress to study the pathogenesis of shigellosis. *Vaccine* 1991;9:416–422.

215. Karnell A, Stocker BAD, Katakura S, et al. An auxotrophic live oral *Shigella flexneri* vaccine: development and testing. *Rev Infect Dis* 1991;13(Suppl 4):S357–361.

Infections of the Gastrointestinal Tract,
edited by M. J. Blaser, P. D. Smith, J. I. Ravdin,
H. B. Greenberg, and R. L. Guerrant
Raven Press, Ltd., New York © 1995.

CHAPTER 22

Traveler's Diarrhea

Herbert L. DuPont

Traveler's diarrhea is most often narrowly defined as a clinically important illness (i.e., three or four unformed stools in 24 hr with an additional symptom of enteric infection such as abdominal pain and cramps) occurring in a person originating from a highly industrialized region during travel to a developing tropical region. More broadly defined, it may include an individual from any country who experiences diarrhea while away from his or her home region. The causes may differ when an individual from the United States visits Mexico from when a Mexican visits the United States; however, both usually result from the temporary relocation.

IMPORTANCE

Approximately 300 million persons cross international boundaries each year (1). Of these, 16 million or more venture into the developing regions where enteric pathogens are hyperendemic and diarrhea is an important threat. To the traveler, whether the travel is for business or pleasure, diarrhea is an important health matter. For the host country, the stakes may even be higher, however. Undoubtedly, many persons elect not to venture into high-risk areas for pleasure or to stimulate business opportunities because of a realistic fear of developing enteric disease with the uncertainty of prevention and adequate therapy. Considering that more than $100 billion is spent annually to support international travel and the fact that only 20% of this money finds its way into the developing regions (2), anything that can be done to promote additional tourism and business traffic will result in important economic benefit for the regions that need financial support the most.

While traveler's diarrhea represents an important factor in tourism and lost revenue to developing regions, the problem reflects inadequate general hygienic conditions, translating into high local rates of infant gastroenteritis

and enterocolitis and potentially preventable infant mortality. Thus, the health and economic burdens of low levels of hygiene and sanitation are enormous for the countries affected.

EPIDEMIOLOGY

Association of Travel with Diarrhea

Travel by its very nature will lead to diarrhea in a percentage of persons regardless of region of origin and destination. Persons leaving their own minienvironment must rely on food prepared and served by others that may contain microbes not found at home. Foods and beverages may contain nonmicrobial nonabsorbable materials that encourage passage of unformed stools. The travelers are under more stress, often keeping a chaotic schedule and consuming more alcohol than when at home. Not surprisingly, when persons from high-risk countries (e.g., Mexico) visit low-risk regions (e.g., United States), or when persons from one low-risk region (e.g., Switzerland) visit another low-risk region (e.g., United States, Caribbean), acute diarrhea occurs in approximately 2–4% of cases (3–5). This can be considered the background rate of illness attributed to travel independent of the special problem of travelers moving to developing tropical regions.

Host Factors

When persons go to a high-risk area from a highly industrialized country, the chance of developing diarrhea depends on their underlying health (6,7), whether they have previously visited or lived in another high-risk area (8), and where they elect to eat the majority of meals (9,10). The overall risk of illness among the persons from the industrialized world is about 40%. This was the rate of illness seen in U.S. students in Mexico by Kean nearly four decades ago (11). When persons from one developing tropical area visit another, they have reduced rates of

H. L. DuPont: Center for Infectious Diseases, University of Texas–Houston Medical School, School of Public Health, Houston, Texas 77030.

TABLE 1. *Occurrence of diarrhea among students, July 1975, Universidad de las Americas, Cholula, Puebla, Mexico*

Student group	No.	No. ill (5)
U.S. newly arrived	55	22 (40)
U.S. established[a]	142	28 (20)
Latin American	95	11 (12)

Adapted from ref. 8.
[a] Present at the school for at least one semester.

diarrhea compared to the group from the industrialized region; however, their rates of diarrhea are not negligible (8). In Table 1 the rates of illness among groups of students coming to a single school living in the same dormitories, student housing programs, or nearby apartments differ by region of origin and time in country. The newly arrived U.S. students showed a 40% rate for illness. It was reduced to 20% for the U.S. students who had been at the school for a semester or longer and 11% for Latin American students. For the Latin American students, it did not matter if they were from local Mexico or other region, or whether they were newly arrived or established students (8). While it is clear that natural immunity does occur through exposure, it is also clear that the immunity is not solid and a substantial risk remains even for those previously exposed.

Individuals differ importantly in their susceptibility to diarrhea when traveling to a high-risk area. Some of the factors that are known include gastric hypochlorhydria (7), apparent lack of intestinal receptors required for disease pathogenesis (12,13), age (rates of illness are higher in the young) (11), and immunological memory from previous exposure (14). Host genetics is an important area for future study. It is relevant that patients with blood group O have more severe cholera (15) and more frequently experience shigellosis (University of Texas, *unpublished data*) while infection by enterotoxigenic *Escherichia coli* does not appear to occur more commonly in individuals in certain blood groups (16).

Geographic Considerations

The world can be divided into three general regions in terms of risk of acquiring diarrhea: low, intermediate, and high. The low-risk areas include the United States, Canada, northwestern Europe, South Africa, Japan, New Zealand, and Australia. The intermediate areas consist of southern Europe and the northern Mediterranean countries, the Middle East, China, the Soviet Union, and parts of southern Africa (Zambia, Zimbabwe, and Botswana). The high-risk areas include most parts of Latin America, southern Asia, and Africa. As mentioned, the risk of acquiring diarrhea when nonimmune persons travel from low-risk to high-risk regions averages 40%. When the same individuals venture into intermediate risk areas, the chance of acquiring diarrhea is about 10% (3). As described above, when these people move from one low-risk area to another, even within the same country, the

chance of diarrhea occurrence probably is in the range of the 2–4% background rate. There are small regions within the larger areas that do not fit the expected risk pattern. Examples of this include Haiti and the Dominican Republic, which are high-risk countries within a low-risk region, while Singapore and Hong Kong are low-risk areas within high-risk settings.

Sources

Most travelers going to high-risk areas will tell you that the problem is in the water, possibly the food. There is little doubt, however, that food is the major source of diarrhea among persons going to larger cities of the developing world (9,10,17). For adventure travelers going to more remote rural areas, water may also be an important problem. Also, during rainy seasons even in urban areas of the developing world, water may become contaminated by fecal coliforms and pathogenic viruses (18) and become an important cause of diarrhea. In many tropical regions, crops are raised in soil fertilized with human excreta. This assures contamination with pathogenic microbes. Further errors occur. The foods frequently are not washed thoroughly when they reach the retail stores and restaurants; they are not properly refrigerated after preparation when not immediately consumed; and workers who may harbor enteric organisms without diarrhea (19) often do not use optimal standards of personal hygiene. The errors assure an exposure to enteric pathogens (10). Also, the food contains antibiotic-resistant coliforms (20) that may explain the common acquisition of antimicrobial-resistant flora during a stay in a region where traveler's diarrhea is prevalent (21).

CLINICAL FEATURES

Traveler's diarrhea characteristically begins within the week after arrival in the foreign locale. It may occur during the 7–10 days after returning home. The diarrheal illness characteristically consists of the passage of 3–10 unformed stools daily for 3–5 days without curative therapy (8,11). Most travelers experience abdominal pain or cramps, and for 10–20% of patients one or more of the following will result: fever, vomiting, and/or dysentery defined as the passage of small volume stools that contain gross blood and mucus (8,11,22). In 10% of affected persons the diarrhea will last more than a week and in 2% it will persist for a month or longer. During a bout of diarrhea, one fifth of patients are confined to bed for 1–2 days (1,3,22) Except for classical syndromes (i.e., febrile dysentery) it is not possible to determine the etiology of diarrhea based on clinical features (23).

ETIOLOGY

Bacterial agents cause approximately 85% of the cases of traveler's diarrhea (24,25). This explains the remarkable value of antibacterial drugs in both the prevention and

TABLE 2. *Epidemiology of traveler's diarrhea: approximate frequency of etiological agents*

Etiologic agent	Approximate percentage	Comment
Enterotoxigenic *E. coli* (ETEC)	5–40	The single most important agent, particularly in summertime, at least in semitropical areas
Enteroadherent *E. coli* (EAEC)	10	May explain one third of "culture-negative" traveler's diarrhea
Shigella and enteroinvasive *E. coli* (EIEC)	10–25	A major cause of fever and dysentery in travelers
Salmonella	5–10	Resembles *Shigella* and EIEC diarrhea
C. jejuni	3–15	More important in wintertime, at least in semitropical areas
Aeromonas	5	Particularly important in Thailand
Plesiomonas	5	Statistically related to travel to tropical areas and seafood consumption
Vibrio	0–10	Cholera is unusual in travelers, noncholera vibrios cause seafood-related diarrhea in travelers to coastal areas of southern Asia
Rotavirus and Norwalk virus	10	Rotavirus is particularly important in Mexico
G. lamblia	<2	Particularly common in travelers to mountainous regions and to St. Petersburg, Russia
Cryptosporidium	2	Particularly common in travelers to St. Petersburg, Russia
Unknown	20	Most of these patients have bacterial diarrhea; the illness will improve with antibacterial therapy

therapy of the illness (to be discussed later). The specific agents responsible show regional and seasonal variation. The accepted enteropathogenic agents in their order of occurrence include enterotoxigenic *E. coli* (ETEC); *Shigella* spp., *Campylobacter jejuni*, *Aeromonas* spp., *Plesiomonas shigelloides*, *Salmonella* spp., and noncholera vibrios (Table 2). Some pathogens appear to show a regional and seasonal increase in occurrence. ETEC is more common in summer months in Mexico and Morocco and in these areas during the autumn and winter *C. jejuni* becomes the most important agent identified (26,27). *Aeromonas* spp. occur more commonly in Thailand and may rival ETEC in importance (28). *Vibrio cholerae* infection will occur only very rarely in travelers to endemic areas (22), and then only if they consume heavily contaminated food, usually poorly cooked or inadequately handled seafood (29). Noncholera vibrios may occur in travelers to coastal areas of southeastern Asia (30).

We have been interested in determining the cause of diarrhea in the one fifth of persons with traveler's diarrhea in which an agent cannot be identified. One potentially important cause are *E. coli* that possess virulence properties other than conventional enterotoxin production. In studies carried out in Mexico, we have shown that in approximately 10% of patients with traveler's diarrhea and in one third of the pathogen-negative cases, HEp-2-adherent *E. coli* resembling enteropathogenic *E. coli* (EPEC) (31) can be detected in stool (32). In other studies carried out over two summers, we identified *Shigella*-like invasive *E. coli* in approximately 6% of cases (33).

In Mexico, rotavirus and Norwalk virus are important causes of enteric illness among travelers (34–37). When vomiting is the major clinical manifestation of enteric disease in travelers, viral gastroenteritis or foodborne intoxication due to preformed toxin of either *Staphylococcus aureus* or *Bacillus cereus* should be suspected. *Giardia lamblia* is an important cause of diarrhea among travelers to mountainous areas of North America (38) and of diarrhea in travelers to St. Petersburg, Russia (39). In the

latter setting, *Cryptosporidium* is also an important cause of traveler's diarrhea (39). *Entamoeba histolytica* infection is an unusual cause of illness among short-term travelers to developing regions (40). *Cyclospora* species, previously described as blue–green algae, or cyanobacteria-like organisms, have been shown to cause protracted diarrhea in immunocompetent travelers to developing countries including Nepal, Mexico, or Haiti and in patients with the acquired immune deficiency syndrome (AIDS) (41,42). *Cyclospora* are small spherical organisms resembling *Cryptosporidium*, yet in contrast to *C. parvum*, the organism shows variable staining when examined by light microscopy after acid-fast staining.

It is not possible to offer a complete list of pathogens and their relative importance in geographic areas given the lack of available data. However, the available studies suggest that there is a remarkable similarity of pathogens responsible regardless of the developing region to be visited (43,44). That most of the disease is bacterial in origin and the common pattern of agents regardless of specific geography justify the term "traveler's diarrhea" as a specific entity when considering approach to treatment and prevention despite the wide variation in potential etiological agents. The problems of traveler's diarrhea and pediatric diarrhea in the local country, with the possible exception of frequency of rotavirus infection, are similar in terms of incidence and etiology (45–48). Both represent highly susceptible nonimmune subjects who commonly become ill from infection by endemic enteropathogens.

As discussed under "Clinical Features," some of the patients with traveler's diarrhea will have protracted illness lasting weeks to months. The cause of this illness is highly variable, but the differential diagnosis includes infection by a protozoal pathogen, such as *G. lamblia*, *Cryptosporidium*, or *Cyclospora*, or in those with diarrhea lasting 1–3 weeks by an invasive bacterial pathogen including *Shigella*, *Salmonella*, *Campylobacter;* disaccharidase deficiency secondary to small bowel injury by an infecting organism; small bowel overgrowth syndrome caused by small bowel stasis (again, a result of small bowel infection); and a small bowel injury produced by repeated exposures to enteric pathogens or toxic substances resulting in a "tropical sprue"–like picture. There is a fairly well-characterized form of chronic diarrhea known as Brainerd diarrhea named after the initially reported outbreak that occurred in Brainerd, Minnesota (49). The disease consists of protracted diarrhea that may last years. It can usually be traced to consumption of raw (unpasteurized) milk or untreated surface water (49,50). The etiology is uncertain; however, it appears to be an as-yet-undiscovered infectious agent. It does not respond to antibacterial therapy and characteristically has a benign outcome as do most of the cases of prolonged diarrhea in travelers (51).

DIAGNOSIS

The history of travel is essential in making the diagnosis. Travel to specific region may suggest the cause (see "Etiology"). The clinical presentation often is important in leading to the proper diagnosis (see "Clinical Features" and "Etiology"). Since most patients with acute traveler's diarrhea will have a bacterial enteric infection, it is reasonable to initiate antibacterial therapy without microbiological evaluation. Laboratory study for parasites is largely reserved for those with protracted illness.

PREVENTION AND CONTROL

In attempting to prevent traveler's diarrhea, there are three general considerations: decreased exposure by modification and improvement of hygiene levels of the environment and education of the traveler designed to help the person consume the safest foods and beverages; chemoprophylaxis; and immunoprophylaxis.

Environmental and Educational Approaches

Unfortunately, physicians have not been effective in leading to a change in the way persons eat while in high-risk areas. More attention to effective education of the traveler is needed. Foods and beverages can be categorized as high-risk and low-risk based on a few basic principles. Table 3 lists the safe and unsafe foods. The most important principle is that heat kills microbes. The temperature of the food should be raised to approximately 59°C to assure killing of pathogens (52). A temperature that just reaches the point of being too hot to touch is 50°C. The careful traveler should warn the waitress/waiter at a restaurant that all cooked food must be brought to the table steaming hot or it will be returned to the kitchen. It would not be entirely unreasonable for the most cautious traveler to check the internal temperature of a served item with a clinical thermometer before consumption to be certain of its safety. Other safe foods include those that are dry (bread and crackers), those with high sugar content (i.e., jellies and syrups), citrus fruits with low pH, fruits and vegetables that have been peeled, peanut butter, self-prepared foods of all sorts that have been thoroughly washed with clean, previously boiled water prior to consumption, and bottled carbonated beverages. The foods that are often sources of enteric infection include moist items served at room temperature (often as part of a buffet), fruits and vegetables with intact skins (tomatoes, strawberries, and grapes), salads, milk (unless powdered milk is reconstituted with previously boiled water or boxed irradiated milk is used and refrigerated after preparation/opening), and tap water. Ice cubes should be considered contaminated since they are often made with tap water. It is not practical to attempt disinfection of ice cubes with alcoholic beverages (53). With attention to dietary and beverage restriction, it is possible to reduce the rate of diarrhea occurrence while in a high-risk area (54).

Chemoprophylaxis

It has been known for nearly four decades that antimicrobial drugs would decrease the threat of acquiring diarrhea during travels in high-risk regions (11). Contemporary data providing evidence of the value of chemoprophylaxis in preventing the disease can be dated back to the studies confirming enterotoxigenic *E. coli* as the major cause (24). Soon thereafter doxycycline (55) and trimethoprim-sulfamethoxazole (TMP-SMX) (56) were shown to prevent 80–90% of the disease that would occur without their use providing prevalent enteropathogenic bacteria were susceptible to the drugs (57). Because of the current frequent occurrence of doxycycline and TMP resistance, these drugs have limited value. Fortunately,

TABLE 3. *Safe and unsafe foods in developing tropical regions*

Low-risk foods and beverages	High-risk foods and beverages
1. Any item served steaming hot (>59°C) 2. Foods that are dry (i.e., bread and crackers) 3. Items with very high sugar content (syrups and jellies) 4. Fruits and vegetables that have been peeled 5. Peanut butter 6. Any fresh food item properly washed and prepared by the traveler 7. Bottled carbonated drinks including mineral water, soft drinks, and beer	1. Foods that are moist and served at room temperature, especially those at a buffet 2. Fruits and vegetables with skin intact—strawberries, tomatoes, grapes 3. Salads and other uncooked vegetables 4. Sauces and dressings in open containers on the table 5. Milk (other than powdered milk that is constituted with previously boiled water or irradiated milk kept refrigerated after preparing or opening) 6. Tap water or ice

TMP resistance is still unusual in the interior of Mexico and TMP-SMX continues to be of value (48). The most predictably active of the antibacterial drugs currently are the fluoroquinolones. Both norfloxacin (58,59) and ciprofloxacin (60) have been used for prophylaxis of traveler's diarrhea with protection rates near 90%. Amdinicillin, a drug with *in vitro* activity against the more resistant enteropathogens, was also shown to be an effective chemoprophylactic agent (61). With a protection rate of 90%, considering that 40% of untreated subjects will develop diarrhea during a period of risk, with antimicrobial prophylaxis illness will occur in 4% of persons.

Other approaches to chemoprophylaxis have been utilized. *Lactobacillus* preparations have been examined as prophylactic agents (62,63). The concept makes sense where the organism ferments intraluminal carbohydrates resulting in bactericidal organic acids. These agents have not been effective in preventing diarrhea, perhaps because of the intestinal location of the effects and their tendency to passively traverse the gut. Bismuth subsalicylate (BSS) has produced more impressive results (64–67). The prophylactic value of BSS probably relates to the antimicrobial property of the preparation as well as the intestinal reaction products produced after ingestion (68). BSS must be taken with meals when the challenge by bacterial agents occurs and at bedtime to be effective (65–67). The optimal dose is two 262-mg tablets chewed well four times a day with meals and at bedtime (65). When used in this dose, the protection rate will be about 65%. This translates into a rate of diarrhea of about 14% when the frequency of illness in untreated subjects is 40%.

In considering how prophylaxis might be used, the pros and cons of the approach must be thoroughly understood (1,6). Problems of prophylaxis include the side effects of the drugs, the false sense of security the traveler may have, and the difficulty in treating the diarrhea that results. Adverse experiences from the drugs may be considered minor (skin rash, insomnia, vaginitis in the case of the antimicrobials, and black tongue and stools and tinnitus in the case of BSS) and major (anaphylaxis, antibiotic-associated colitis, Stevens–Johnson syndrome). The minor reactions for the antibacterial drugs occur in about 3% of cases and major reactions in about 1 in 10,000 (69). For BSS in reasonably healthy persons, the minor reactions will occur commonly but severe reactions should

not occur. In patients taking excessive doses, especially with underlying medical impairment, bismuth encephalopathy may occur (70). A potential complication of antimicrobial chemoprophylaxis is development in antibiotic-resistant flora during the time the drug is taken (71).

The decision to recommend or approve the use of chemoprophylaxis is complex and revolves around a number of issues (6,72). Table 4 outlines one approach based on the underlying health of the future traveler, the importance of the trip and remaining disease-free, the willingness to follow dietary and beverage restrictions, and the orientation toward prophylaxis after understanding the limitations and risks of the approach. A majority of travelers should not use antibacterial chemoprophylaxis. The drugs used as well as their indications and doses are given in Table 5. The approach is used only for short-term travel. The longer the trip, the less valuable is chemoprophylaxis. When the time spent in the high-risk area exceeds 3 weeks, chemoprophylaxis should not be used. The drugs are begun the day of arrival in the high-risk area and continued for 2 days after the return home. Chemoprophylaxis is not appropriate for young infants or pregnant women. When the approach is desired for older children, BSS is recommended. Even for persons electing to take chemoprophylaxis, exercising care in what is eaten or drunk is required in order to have the lowest rates of illness (73).

Immunoprophylaxis

There is great interest in immunoprophylactic approaches to preventing acute infectious diarrhea. Considering the similarity of traveler's diarrhea and endemic diarrhea in children living in the developing world, a vaccine against one should have great utility in the other situation. Two approaches currently are being explored. The first is passive immunization using antibodies directed to enteropathogenic organisms or their purified virulence properties (74). The obvious limitation to this approach is that the preparation will need to be taken daily while in the period of risk, possibly with each meal. The protection will end when the preparation is discontinued. The advantage of passive immunoprophylaxis is that antibodies can be easily and cheaply produced in cows with purifi-

TABLE 4. *Factors used to determine the indication for chemoprophylaxis in travelers planning a trip to high-risk areas*

Host factor used in deciding about prophylaxis	Prophylaxis recommended
Important underlying disease: on omeprazole, diabetic on insulin, patient with heart disease, cancer, active inflammatory bowel disease, AIDS, those taking corticosteroids	Antibacterial agent is justified (see Table 5 for specific agent recommended and doses)
Importance of trip: mission could be ruined by illness rendered short term by effective therapy	Bismuth subsalicylate or an antibacterial drug is justified (see Table 5 for doses)
Restrictions on food and beverages: is not willing to exercise care in what is eaten or drunk	Bismuth subsalicylate is justified (see Table 5 for dose)
Interest in prophylaxis: traveler wishes prophylaxis after pros and cons are thoroughly explained and understood	Bismuth subsalicylate is appropriate (see Table 5 for dose)

Adapted from Refs. 6 and 72.

TABLE 5. *Drugs and dosages used in prophylaxis of traveler's diarrhea[a]*

Chemoprophylactic agent	Dose	Comment
Fluoroquinolones: norfloxacin (NF); ciprofloxacin (CF); ofloxacin (OF); fleroxacin (FO)	NF 400 mg; CF 500 mg; OF 300 mg; or FO 400 mg once daily	The most effective drugs available for adults for travel to all regions during all seasons
Trimethoprim (TMP) sulfamethoxazole (SMX)	160 mg TMP/800 mg SMX once daily	Remains effective for travel to the Mexican interior during summer
Doxycycline	100 mg once daily	Resistance is too common worldwide to recommend use without *in vitro* data confirming susceptibility
Bismuth subsalicyclate	Two 262-mg tablets chewed well four times a day (with meals and at bedtime)	Not as effective, but fewer side effects and probably effective in all regions and seasons

[a] All drugs are begun the day the destination is reached and continued for 2 days after returning home (not to be used for trips that exceed 3 weeks).

cation of multivalent antibody preparations that can be tailored to the region to be visited.

Probably of greater potential value is the development of active vaccines made up of the organisms or selected immunogenic properties that can be administered to subjects well in advance of their travels. A vaccine directed to enterotoxigenic *E. coli* and the prevalent types of *Shigella* could have great value in limiting illness. With time in the region, natural immunity to enterotoxigenic *E. coli* occurs (75,76). The immunity correlates with the occurrence of *E. coli* anti–heat-labile enterotoxin antibodies in the serum (77). An interesting preparation that is currently being evaluated as an anti-ETEC vaccine is a whole-cell *V. cholerae*/binding subunit of cholera or ETEC cholera-like toxin taken as two oral doses (78). The preparation should be effective in preventing cholera (78) and ETEC diarrhea (79) in view of the similarity of the two related heat-labile enterotoxins produced. Refinements of the immunizing agent will be taking place. Clearly, considering the multitude of etiological agents that cause traveler's diarrhea, immunoprophylaxis, despite having a valuable effect on reducing the frequency of illness, will not eliminate the problem.

MANAGEMENT

Regardless of approach, it will not be possible to prevent all illness among travelers. This plus the fact that by definition most cases of the diarrhea will occur while the individual is out of town and away from medical care underscores the need for empiric self-therapy of most cases of illness. All travelers to high-risk areas should be armed with therapeutic agents to treat the illness that might occur. As with other forms of diarrhea, there are three different types of therapy available: fluids and electrolytes, nonspecific symptomatic therapy, and antimicrobial therapy. They will be considered separately.

Fluids and Electrolytes

Fluids and electrolytes represent the standard and most fundamental form of treatment for all cases of diarrhea. In travelers with good underlying health, severe dehydration is unusual. For this reason, for most previously healthy older children and adults, it is recommended that they obtain flavored mineral water (hypotonic solutions containing glucose) to be consumed along with soups and broths augmented with saltine crackers to meet fluid and salt losses. For young infants and elderly persons, particularly when severe diarrhea and diarrhea and vomiting complicate the illness, more aggressive measures may rarely be needed. For infants under 2 years of age, parents are advised to take with them a supply of Pedialyte or Lytren should diarrhea occur. No therapy other than electrolyte solution should be given to young infants.

Nonspecific Therapy

There are three types of drugs that play a role in relieving symptoms associated with diarrhea. This approach is important among travelers where the symptomatically acting drugs may allow a person to function while out of town. The preparations used to treat symptoms of traveler's diarrhea include the antisecretory agents, the antimotility drugs, and the water-absorbing agents. Each can be shown to modify diarrheal illness. The symptomatic drugs have their major value in the treatment of mild forms of traveler's diarrhea. A number of travelers who pass only one or two unformed stools will have a nonprogressive course and antimicrobial agents may not be necessary. These patients may benefit from symptomatic therapy alone. Also, the antimotility drugs may be combined with the antimicrobial agents in patients with more intense illness providing there is no fever or dysentery. In Table 6 the drugs, their doses, and their indications for therapy of traveler's diarrhea are provided.

TABLE 6. *Therapy of traveler's diarrhea according to symptoms*

Clinical symptoms/signs	Suggested therapy
Passage of 1–2 unformed stools/24 hr without distressing enteric symptoms	Flavored mineral water and saltine crackers, no therapy
Passage of 1–2 unformed stools with distressing enteric symptoms	Symptomatic therapy in adults: BSS 30 mL or two tablets every 30 min for 8 doses; or, loperamide 4 mg initially followed by 2 mg after passage of each unformed stool not to exceed 8 tablets/day (prescription dose) or 4 caplets/day (OTC dose); drugs can be taken for 2 days
Vomiting without important diarrhea	BSS therapy (dose above)
Passage of >2 unformed stools in 24 hr, no fever, no dysentery or distressing abdominal pain/cramps with fewer stools	Antimicrobial drug (see Table 7) plus loperamide (dose above)
Diarrhea in a patient taking TMP-SMX or BSS prophylaxis	Fluoroquinolone therapy (see Table 7) plus loperamide (dose above) if no fever nor dysentery; antibacterial drug alone if fever/dysentery are present
Diarrhea in a patient taking fluoroquinolone prophylaxis	BSS therapy (dose above)
Diarrhea in a pregnant woman or an infant or young child	See text
Fever and or dysentery (diarrhea with passage of bloody stools)	Antimicrobial alone (see Table 7)

TMP-SMX, trimethoprim-sulfamethoxazole; BSS, bismuth subsalicylate.

Antisecretory Agents

The most useful antisecretory agent available currently is bismuth subsalicylate (BSS). For adults, BSS is taken in a dose of 524 mg (two tablets or 30 mL) every 30 min for 8 doses; it can be repeated in the same dose in 24 hr (80). When taken in this dose, it will reduce diarrhea (number of stools, duration of illness) by about 50% compared to a placebo preparation (80). BSS exerts antisecretory effects against bacterial enterotoxins (81,82). It apparently works though salicylate-dependent antisecretory mechanisms (83) other than prostaglandin inhibition and the preparation is entirely safe in terms of gastric effects. While aspirin is an effective antidiarrheal compound (84) the gastric toxicity is not acceptable to allow acetylsalicylic acid to be used routinely to treat diarrhea. Interestingly, BSS can be used to treat aspirin-induced gastritis in experimental animals (85). It is not known if the antimicrobial effects of the drug have any role in the antidiarrheal use of the drug. BSS is probably the treatment of choice for enteric illness of travelers where vomiting is the major clinical symptom (86).

With the available information to indicate that intestinal secretion is the most important pathophysiological mechanism leading to diarrheal disease, novel antisecretory agents are currently being developed. The enterotoxin-mediated diarrheal diseases such as ETEC diarrhea involves cyclic nucleotides, calmodulin, and intracellular calcium (87). A drug that inhibits intestinal calmodulin was shown to be an effective form of antisecretory therapy for traveler's diarrhea (88).

Antimotility Agents

The most effective of the symptomatic drugs are the antimotility agents, including paregoric, tincture of opium, codeine, diphenoxylate, and loperamide. The first of the useful synthetic opiates was diphenoxylate with atropine. While effective in treating diarrhea, this preparation has two problems. First, it possesses an important potential for central opiate effects in children who inadvertently take an overdose of their parents' medication. Second, atropine has been added to the drug to prevent overdose. Atropine, like other anticholinergic drugs, may produce additional objectionable symptoms such as dry mouth and blurred vision without antidiarrheal properties (89). The most useful preparation of the antimotility drugs is loperamide, which is as effective as diphenoxylate but with lessened central opiate effects and without the atropine. Loperamide will reduce diarrhea by 80% in terms of number of stools passed and duration of diarrhea during therapy (unpublished data) and it is more effective than BSS in treating traveler's diarrhea (90,91). The dose administered to adults is 4 mg (two capsules or two caplets) initially followed by 2 mg (one capsule or one caplet) after each unformed stool not to exceed eight capsules (16 mg) in 24 hr (prescription dose) or four caplets (8 mg) in 24 hr (over-the-counter dose), not to be used for more than 48 hr. Other antimotility drugs such as codeine, tincture of opium, or paregoric probably exert equivalent antidiarrheal effects as loperamide, although they do have greater potential for central toxicity.

The mechanism of action of this class of drugs is slowing of intestinal transit of the intraluminal column leading to increased reabsorption (92). Also, the drugs have an antisecretory effect that may play a role (93). There are three problems with loperamide use. Overdose is a potential problem in young children even though less than for diphenoxylate. Second, loperamide does not cure all cases of traveler's diarrhea and posttreatment clinical relapses are common (90). Finally, with the highly invasive bacterial enteropathogens, such as *Shigella, Salmonella,* and *Campylobacter*, intestinal invasion may be facilitated by a greater contact time between the infecting strain and the gut mucosa (94). For this reason, patients with fever and/or dysentery should be excluded from use of the drug.

Water-Absorbing Agents

The water-absorbing agents are the least effective in reducing diarrhea. However, they are the safest of the available drugs since the effects are strictly intraluminal. Attapulgite is the most important example in this group (95). It can be given to patients who cannot be given the other preparations since it remains unabsorbed. Young children and pregnant women with acute traveler's diarrhea should be able to be treated safely with attapulgite. The major result is passage of more formed stools with some relief of associated symptoms of enteric infection.

Antimicrobial Therapy

Since traveler's diarrhea is most often a bacterial infection, the antibacterials represent the most important drugs for therapy of the illness. The indications for antibacterial therapy are passage of three or more unformed stools in 24 hr, any diarrhea with distressing abdominal cramps or pain, presence of fever, and or passage of bloody stools (dysentery). Antimicrobial agents shorten the duration of posttreatment diarrhea from approximately 59–93 hr without therapy to 16–30 hr providing the prevalent organisms are susceptible to the drug employed (96–98). The standard and U.S. Food and Drug Administration approved antimicrobial for the treatment of traveler's diarrhea is TMP-SMX (96). It remains active in many regions of the developing world, including the noncoastal areas of Mexico (48,96–98). For areas of the world where susceptibility to TMP is not known and in other areas where *C. jejuni* is an important cause of traveler's diarrhea, the quinolones are preferred for empiric antimicrobial therapy (see Tables 6 and 7). The quinolones do not appear to differ in terms of therapeutic effect, and currently norfloxacin

(99), ciprofloxacin (97), ofloxacin (100), and fleroxacin (101) all appear to be equivalent. Unfortunately, children with traveler's diarrhea cannot be given one of the newer quinolones in view of the potential damage to growing articular cartilage (102). For children with diarrhea, optimal antimicrobial therapy for more severe disease includes either TMP-SMX plus erythromycin or furazolidone (see Table 7).

The antimicrobials will shorten the diarrhea associated with bacterial enteropathogens including ETEC and *Shigella* spp., the two major causes of illness. Also, the drugs will shorten the illness not associated with a definable pathogen providing further evidence that bacterial agents are responsible for this form of the disease (96,100,103).

The optimal duration of antimicrobial therapy for traveler's diarrhea has not been established. The approved duration of therapy is 5 days (96). Evidence would suggest that 3 days duration is sufficient for all cases (98,100) and single-dose treatment may be adequate for most (98). In all probability, treatment of this infection of the mucosal surface is similar to the situation seen in urinary tract infection. In both, drug concentrations at the site of infection reach very high levels (104,105). Until further definitive evidence is available, it might be reasonable to give single-dose therapy to those with milder forms of illness and give more prolonged treatment (3–5 days) for those with severe illness including those with febrile dysenteric diseases (106).

The importance of absorption of antibacterial drugs in traveler's diarrhea has not been established. In children with shigellosis, it was found that oral ampicillin (an absorbed drug) was more effective than oral neomycin (a poorly absorbed drug) (107). It was assumed that absorption of drug was important in treating the mucosal infection. An alternative possibility is that oral aminoglycosides are not effective in the treatment of shigellosis despite in vitro activity against strains of *Shigella* (108).

Evidence has been provided that the nonabsorbed drugs, bicozamycin and aztreonam, with in vitro activity against the prevalent bacterial agents, are effective in the treatment of traveler's diarrhea when taken orally

TABLE 7. *Antimicrobial therapy of traveler's diarrhea[a]*

Antimicrobial therapy	Indication
Travel to Mexican interior, summer	Adults: TMP-SMX 160 mg/800 mg bid Children: TMP-SMX 4 mg/20 mg/kg body weight/day in two daily doses; for 3 days
Travel to other high-risk areas, other seasons or Mexican interior during nonsummer months	Adults[b]: NF 400 mg bid, CF 500 mg bid, OF 300 mg bid, or FO 400 mg qd for 3 days Children[c]: TMP-SMX (above dose) plus erythromycin dose based on weight: <11 kg—250 mg/d; 11–18 kg—375 mg/day, 18.5–25 kg—500 mg/day, 25.5–36 kg—750 mg/day and >36 kg—1000 mg/day in four divided doses for 5 days
Diarrhea lasting 2 weeks or longer, unresponsive to antibacterial therapy (above) without presence of enteropathogen in examined stools	Adults: metronidazole 250 mg qid for 7 days Children: metronidazole 15 mg/kg in three divided doses for 7 days

[a] See Table 6 for indications.
[b] NF, norfloxacin; CF, ciprofloxacin; OF, ofloxacin; FO, fleroxacin.
[c] An alternative single agent that can be used is furazolidone 7.5 mg/kg/day in four divided doses for 5 days.

(103,109). Furthermore, bicozamycin was found to be effective in preventing the illness when employed as a prophylactic agent (110). Neither preparation is available currently. The search for nonabsorbed drugs with activity against enteric bacterial pathogens should continue in view of potential utility and safety of these preparations.

Combination Therapy

In studies conducted in U.S. and Swiss travelers, symptomatically acting drugs were shown to be more rapidly effective than antimicrobial drugs in improving diarrhea (111,112). Given the rapid response of the symptomatic agents and the curative effects of the antimicrobials, it was logical to attempt combined therapy (98,111, 113–115). The symptomatic drug selected for most of the trials has been loperamide based on the fact that BSS may bind to the antimicrobial preventing absorption (116). In a study carried out in Mexico with combined TMP-SMX and loperamide, the combination therapy led to more rapid resolution of symptoms than single-agent treatment (98). According to studies carried out in Egypt among U.S. military personnel where ciprofloxacin and loperamide were given together, combined therapy offered only minimal additions to the clinical response of the antimicrobial where after 24 hr the symptoms had improved or completely abated in 82% of patients receiving the combination compared to 67% for the group receiving the antimicrobial without loperamide ($P = 0.08$) (114). In the study carried out in Thailand among U.S. military personnel, once again only minimal additional benefits were seen when loperamide was combined with ciprofloxacin to treat diarrhea (115). In this trial subjects randomized to receive the combination of drugs reported passage of a lower cumulative number of unformed bowel movements at 48 and 72 hr after initiating therapy when compared to the subjects who were given only the antimicrobial. The most important pathogen in the Mexican and Egyptian trials was ETEC, while in the study carried out in Thailand *C. jejuni* was the most commonly identified enteropathogen. It is not known if TMP-SMX and the quinolones differ in terms of their interaction with loperamide. None of the studies showed a potentiation of illness or a failure of the antimicrobial to improve symptoms when the antimotility drug was administered.

EVALUATION OF PATIENTS WITH A HISTORY OF RECENT TRAVELS

Diarrheal illness in a person recently returning from a high-risk region is a common problem seen by physicians in practice. There are three common forms requiring evaluation: acute diarrhea, persistent or chronic diarrhea, and fever and toxicity. Each clinical presentation suggests special problems that should be approached in a different manner.

The Patient with Acute Diarrhea

When patients with diarrhea present for medical evaluation after undergoing travel in the recent past to a high or intermediate risk area, it is recommended to divide them into two groups: those with acute diarrhea and those with persistent diarrhea. For patients with acute diarrhea who have acquired diarrhea following travels to mountainous areas of North America or to Russia, it is recommended that stools be examined for protozoal pathogens including *Giardia* and *Cryptosporidium*. For others, it is appropriate to administer a course of antimicrobial therapy depending on region visited without laboratory evaluation (see Table 7).

The Patient with Prolonged Diarrhea

Most patients with persistent illness (>14 days duration) should have stool examined for routine enteric pathogens (see "Etiology" for discussion of causative agents). If a potential agent is identified, it should be treated specifically. Patients with negative etiological assessments should be given a short course of antibacterial therapy (see Table 7). For those who fail this treatment, a 7-day course of metronidazole can be given for empiric treatment of giardiasis or small bowel bacterial overgrowth. For those who fail the empiric treatment, a full workup is indicated by a gastroenterologist. It is not wise to continually treat these patients with prolonged diarrhea with antimicrobial drugs where the intestinal ecology will be severely disturbed leading to intermittent cycles of diarrhea and treatment often with temporary improvement in symptoms early in the course of treatment. Symptomatic treatment of these patients is warranted after evaluation if a cause is not identified. Fortunately, most of the patients who have protracted diarrhea following travel have a benign course and most eventually resolve (51).

The Febrile and Toxic Patient

When a previous traveler presents with fever and toxicity, an invasive bacterial infection should be considered. The list of possible etiologies includes *Shigella, Salmonella typhi, Salmonella enteritidis, C. jejuni, Brucella, Franciscella tularensis, Leptospira,* and *Yersinia enterocolitica*. Stool and blood cultures are indicated along with serological evaluation for brucellosis, tularemia, and leptospirosis. The patient is treated for the etiological agent identified. If diarrhea is a prevalent part of the picture, shigellosis or salmonellosis are the most likely diagnoses. If a diagnosis is not made rapidly, a 7-day course of fluoroquinolone is not unreasonable for empiric treatment of the more easily treated infections.

THE FUTURE

We need to improve our approach to educating travelers about the risks and means of minimizing exposures to enteric pathogens. Travelers should demand safe foods! For example, if most travelers required that all foods obtained in a public eating establishment be served steaming hot, the restaurants would soon learn that this is a minimum. Also, research should be continued in the attempt to reduce the threat of illness through strategies of chemoprophylaxis and immunoprophylaxis. Both of these approaches should play a role in dealing with the problem by reducing the threat of illness. However, they will not eliminate it.

The most feasible approach to reducing the threat of traveler's diarrhea is to do what is needed to make safer the environment into which the translocated individuals move. The requirements are easily understood and not impossible to achieve. There are two ways to accomplish the required improvements in hygiene. First is for the host countries to raise the importance of general health to a more important level in health planning and tackle the problem full scale by making improvements in water supply, sewage removal, general education, and monitoring and assuring food hygiene standards in public restaurants. While investigators in the industrialized regions have taken the lead in research in the area of traveler's diarrhea, the countries where the disease occurs should increasingly be involved. They have the most to gain. They should find it appalling that rates of traveler's diarrhea have not been reduced after four decades. They must realize not only that their economy depends on assuring the good health of their visitors, but that the real payoff of the changes would be the improved health of their own population.

If these countries are unwilling to do what is needed, then the second way to reduce the threat of traveler's diarrhea will be for the travel industry and research community to deal with hygienic improvements to assure a safer minienvironment for travelers. Club Med has attempted to do this. While data are unavailable to show how successful the approach has been, it is a wonderful idea. Presentation of genuinely safe water and food to persons temporarily living in a resort or hotel will go a long way toward stimulating travel and assuring good health and satisfaction with the experience. Regions of the developing world are among the most interesting and beautiful in the world, and should be made available to those who wish to visit.

REFERENCES

1. Gorbach SL, Edelman R, eds. Travelers' diarrhea: National Institutes of Health Consensus Development Conference. *Rev Infect Dis* 1986;8:Suppl 2:S109–S233.
2. International conference on the diarrhea of travelers—new directions in research: a summary. *J Infect Dis* 1978;137:355–369.
3. Steffen R, Rickenbach M, Wilhelm U, Helminger A, Schar M. Health problems after travel to developing countries. *J Infect Dis* 1987;156:84–91.
4. Dandoy S. The diarrhea of travelers: incidence in foreign students in the United States. *Calif Med* 1966;104;458–462.
5. Ryder RW, Wells JG, Gangarosa EJ. A study of travelers' diarrhea in foreign visitors to the United States. *J Infect Dis* 1977;136:605–607.
6. DuPont HL, Ericsson CD. Prevention and treatment of traveler's diarrhea. *N Engl J Med* 1993;328:1821–1827.
7. Wingate DL. Acid reduction and recurrent enteritis. *Lancet* 1990;335:222.
8. DuPont HL, Haynes GA, Pickering LK, Tjoa W, Sullivan P, Olarte J. Diarrhea of travelers in Mexico. Relative susceptibility of United States and Latin American students attending a Mexican university. *Am J Epidemiol* 1977;105:37–41.
9. Tjoa W, DuPont HL, Sullivan P, et al. Location of food consumption and travelers' diarrhea. *Am J Epidemiol* 1977;106:61–66.
10. Wood LV, Ferguson LE, Hogan P, Thurman D, DuPont HL, Ericsson CD. Incidence of bacterial enteropathogens in foods from Mexico. *Appl Environ Microbiol* 1983;46:328–332.
11. Kean BH. The diarrhea of travelers to Mexico: summary of five-year study. *Ann Intern Med* 1963;59:605–614.
12. Parrino TA, Schreiber DS, Trier JS, Kapikian AZ, Blacklow NR. Clinical immunity in acute gastroenteritis caused by the Norwalk agent. *N Engl J Med* 1977;297:86–89.
13. Rutter JM, Burrows MR, Sellwood R, Gibbons RA. A genetic basis for resistance to enteric disease caused by E. coli. *Nature* 1975;257:135–136.
14. DuPont HL, Olarte J, Evans DG, Pickering LK, Galindo E, Evans DJ Jr. Comparative susceptibility of Latin American and United States students to enteric pathogens. *N Engl J Med* 1976;295:1520–1521.
15. Glass RI, Holmgren J, Haley CE, et al. Predisposition for cholera of individuals with O blood group. Possible evolutionary significance. *Am J Epidemiol* 1985;121:791–796.
16. van Loon FPL, Clemens JD, Sack DA, et al. ABO blood groups and the risk of diarrhea due to enterotoxigenic *Escherichia coli*. *J Infect Dis* 1991;163:1243–1246.
17. Merson MH, Morris GK, Sack DA, et al. Travelers' diarrhea in Mexico: a prospective study of physicians and family members attending a congress. *N Engl J Med* 1976;294:1299–1305.
18. Deetz TR, Smith EM, Goyal SM, et al. Occurrence of rota- and enteroviruses in drinking and environmental water in a developing nation. *Water Res* 1984;18:567–571.
19. Pickering LK, DuPont HL, Evans DG, Evans DJ Jr, Olarte J. Isolation of enteric pathogens from asymptomatic students from the United States and Latin America. *J Infect Dis* 1977;135:1003–1005.
20. Wood LV, Jansen DM, DuPont HL. Antimicrobial resistance of gram-negative bacteria isolated from foods in Mexico. *J Infect Dis* 1983;148:766.
21. Murray BE, Mathewson JJ, DuPont HL, Ericsson CD, Reves RR. Emergence of resistant fecal *Escherichia coli* in travelers not taking prophylactic antimicrobial agents. *Antimicrob Agents Chemother* 1990;34:515–518.
22. Steffen R. Epidemiologic studies of travelers' diarrhea, severe gastrointestinal infections, and cholera. *Rev Infect Dis* 1986;8: Suppl 2:S122–S130.
23. Ericsson CD, Patterson TF, DuPont HL. Clinical presentation as a guide to therapy for travelers' diarrhea. *Am J Med Sci* 1987;294:91–96.
24. Gorbach SL, Kean BH, Evans DG, Evans DJ Jr, Bessudo D. Travelers' diarrhea and toxigenic *Escherichia coli*. *N Engl J Med* 1975;292:933–936.
25. DuPont HL, Ericsson CD, DuPont MW. Emporiatric enteritis: lessons learned from U.S. students in Mexico. *Trans Am Clin Climatol Assoc* 1985;97:32–42.
26. Mattila L, Siitonen A, Kyroseppa H, et al. Seasonal variation in etiology of travelers' diarrhea. *J Infect Dis* 1992;165:385–388.
27. Ericsson CD and DuPont HL. Travelers' diarrhea: approaches to prevention and treatment. *Clin Infect Dis* 1993;16:616–626.
28. Echeverria P, Sack RB, Blacklow NR, Bodhidatta P, Rowe B, McFarland A. Prophylactic doxycycline for travelers' diarrhea in Thailand: further supportive evidence of *Aeromonas hydrophila* as an enteric pathogen. *Am J Epidemiol* 1984;120:912–921.
29. Epidemiological Bulletin, Pan American Health Organization, Vol 12, No 1;1991:1–24.
30. Sriratanaban A, Reinprayoon S. *Vibrio parahaemolyticus*: a major cause of travelers' diarrhea in Bangkok. *Am J Trop Med Hyg* 1982;31:128–130.
31. Vial PA, Mathewson JJ, DuPont HL, Guers L, Levine MM: Comparison of two assay methods for patterns of adherence to HEp-2 cells of *Escherichia coli* from patients with diarrhea. *J Clin Microbiol* 1990;28:882–885.
32. Mathewson JJ, Johnson PC, DuPont HL, et al. A newly recog-

nized cause of travelers' diarrhea: enteroadherent *Escherichia coli. J Infect Dis* 1985;151:471–475.

33. Wanger AR, Murray BE, Echeverria P, Mathewson JJ, DuPont HL. Enteroinvasive *Escherichia coli* in travelers' diarrhea. *J Infect Dis* 1988;158:640–642.
34. Bolivar R, Conklin RH, Vollet JJ, et al. Rotavirus in travelers' diarrhea: study of an adult student population in Mexico. *J Infect Dis* 1978;137:324–327.
35. Vollet JJ, Ericsson CD, Gibson G, et al. Human rotavirus in an adult population with travelers' diarrhea and its relationship to location of food consumption. *J Med Virol* 1979;4:81–87.
36. Ryder RW, Oquist CA, Greenberg H. Traveler's diarrhea in Panamanian tourists in Mexico. *J Infect Dis* 1981;144:442–448.
37. Johnson PC, Hoy J, Mathewson JJ, Ericsson CD, DuPont HL. Occurrence of Norwalk virus infections among adults in Mexico. *J Infect Dis* 1990;162:389–393.
38. Wright RA, Spencer H, Brodsky RE, Vernon TM. Giardiasis in Colorado: an epidemiologic study. *Am J Epidemiol* 1977;105:330–336.
39. Jokipii L, Pohjola S, Jokipii AMM. Cryptosporidiosis associated with traveling and giardiasis. *Gastroenterology* 1985;89:838–842.
40. Frachtman RL, Ericsson CD, DuPont HL. Seroconversion to *Entamoeba histolytica* among short term travelers to Mexico. *Arch Intern Med* 1982;142:1299.
41. Shlim DR, Cohen MT, Eaton M, Rajah R, Long EG, Ungar BL. An algae-like organism associated with an outbreak of prolonged diarrhea among foreigners in Nepal. *Am J Trop Med Hyg* 1991;45:383–389.
42. Ortega YR, Sterling CR, Gilman RH, Cama VA, Díaz F. Cyclospora species—a new protozoan pathogen of humans. *N Engl J Med* 1993;328:1308–1312.
43. Taylor DN, Echeverria P. Etiology and epidemiology of travelers' diarrhea in Asia. *Rev Infect Dis* 1986;8:Suppl 2:S136–S141.
44. Steffen R, Mathewson JJ, Ericsson CD, et al. Travelers' diarrhea in West Africa and in Mexico: fecal transport systems and liquid bismuth subsalicylate for self-therapy. *J Infect Dis* 1988;157:1008–1013.
45. Evans DG, Olarte J, DuPont HL, et al. Enteropathogens associated with pediatric diarrhea in Mexico City. *J Pediatr* 1977;91:65–68.
46. Mathewson JJ, Oberhelman RA, DuPont HL, de la Cabada FJ, Garibay EV. Enteroadherent *Escherichia coli* as a cause of diarrhea among children in Mexico. *J Clin Microbiol* 1987;25:1917–1919.
47. Okhuysen PC, DuPont HL, Lopez JFF, Castell JP, Mathewson JJ. A comparative study of furazolidone and placebo in addition to oral rehydration in the treatment of acute infantile diarrhea. *Scand J Gastroenterol* 1989;24(Suppl 169):39–46.
48. Bandres JC, Mathewson JJ, Ericsson CD, DuPont HL. Trimethoprim/sulfamethoxazole remains active against enterotoxigenic *Escherichia coli* and *Shigella* spp in Guadalajara, Mexico. *Am J Med Sci* 1992;303:289–291.
49. Osterholm MT, MacDonald KL, White KE, et al. An outbreak of a newly recognized chronic diarrhea syndrome associated with raw milk consumption. *JAMA* 1986;256:484–490.
50. Parsonnet J, Trock SC, Bopp CA, et al. Chronic diarrhea associated with drinking untreated water. *Ann Intern Med* 1989;110:985–991.
51. Afzalpurkar RG, Schiller LR, Little KH, Santangelo WC, Fordtran JS. The self-limited nature of chronic idiopathic diarrhea. *N Engl J Med* 1992;327:1849–1852.
52. Bandres JC, Mathewson JJ, DuPont HL. Heat susceptibility of bacterial enteropathogens. Implications for the prevention of travelers' diarrhea. *Arch Intern Med* 1988;148:2261–2263.
53. Dickens DL, DuPont HL, Johnson PC. Survival of bacterial enteropathogens in the ice of popular drinks. *JAMA* 1985;253:3141–3143.
54. Kozicki M, Steffen R, Schär J. "Boil it, cook it, peel it or forget it"; does this rule prevent travellers' diarrhoea? *Int J Epidemiol* 1985;14:169–172.
55. Sack DA, Kaminsky DC, Sack RB, et al. Prophylactic doxycycline for travelers' diarrhea: results of a prospective double-

56. blind study of Peace Corps volunteers in Kenya. *N Engl J Med* 1978;298:758–763.
56. DuPont HL, Galindo E, Evans DG, Cabada FJ, Sullivan P, Evans DJ Jr. Prevention of travelers' diarrhea with trimethoprim/sulfamethoxazole and trimethoprim alone. *Gastroenterology* 1983;84:75–80.
57. Sack RB, Santosham M, Froehlich JL, Medina C, Ørskov F, Ørskov I. Doxycycline prophylaxis of travelers' diarrhea in Honduras, an area where resistance to doxycycline is common among enterotoxigenic *Escherichia coli. Am J Trop Med Hyg* 1984;33:460–466.
58. Johnson PC, Ericsson CD, Morgan DR, DuPont HL, Cabada FJ. Lack of emergence of resistant fecal flora during successful prophylaxis of travelers' diarrhea with norfloxacin. *Antimicrob Agents Chemother* 1986;30:671–674.
59. Wistrom J, Norrby SR, Burman LG, Lundholm R, Jellheden B, Englund G. Norfloxacin versus placebo for prophylaxis against travellers' diarrhoea. *J Antimicrob Chemother* 1987;20:563–574.
60. Rademaker CM, Hoepelman IM, Wolfhagen MJ, Beumer H, Rozenberg AM, Verhoef J. Results of a double-blind placebo-controlled study using ciprofloxacin for prevention of travelers' diarrhea. *Eur J Clin Microbiol Infect Dis* 1989;8:690–694.
61. Black FT, Gaarslev K, Ørskov F, et al. Mecillinam, a new prophylactic for travellers' diarrhoea: a prospective double-blind study in tourists traveling to Egypt and the Far East. *Scand J Infect Dis* 1983;15:189–1993.
62. de dios Pozo-Olano J, Warram JH Jr, Gomez RG, Cavazos MG. Effect of a lactobacilli preparation on traveler's diarrhea: a randomized, double blind clinical trial. *Gastroenterology* 1978;74:829–830.
63. Oksanen PJ, Salminen S, Saxelin M, et al. Prevention of travellers' diarrhoea by *Lactobacillus* GG. *Ann Intern Med* 1990;22:53–56.
64. DuPont HL, Sullivan P, Evans DG, et al. Prevention of travelers' diarrhea (emporiatric enteritis): prophylactic administration of subsalicylate bismuth. *JAMA* 1980;243:237–241.
65. DuPont HL, Ericsson CD, Johnson PC, Bitsura JM, DuPont MW, de la Cabada FJ. Prevention of travelers' diarrhea by the tablet formulation of bismuth subsalicylate. *JAMA* 1987;257:1347–1350.
66. Steffen R, DuPont HL, Heusser R, et al. Prevention of travelers' diarrhea by the tablet form of bismuth subsalicylate. *Antimicrob Agents Chemother* 1986;29:625–627.
67. Steffen R, Heusser R, DuPont HL. Prevention of travelers' diarrhea by non-antibiotic drugs. *Rev Infect Dis* 1986;8(Suppl):S151–S159.
68. Graham DY, Estes MK, Gentry LO. Double-blind comparison of bismuth subsalicylate and placebo in the prevention and treatment of enterotoxigenic *Escherichia coli. Gastroenterology* 1983;85:1017–1022.
69. Reves RR, Johnson PC, Ericsson CD, DuPont HL. A cost effectiveness comparison of the use of antimicrobial agents for treatment or prophylaxis of travelers' diarrhea. *Arch Intern Med* 1988;148:2421–2427.
70. Mendelowitz PC, Hoffman RS, Weber S. Bismuth absorption and myoclonic encephalopathy during bismuth subsalicylate therapy. *Ann Intern Med* 1990;112:140–141.
71. Murray BE, Rensimer ER, DuPont HL. Emergence of high-level trimethoprim resistance in fecal *Escherichia coli* during oral administration of trimethoprim or trimethoprim/sulfamethoxazole. *N Engl J Med* 1982;306:130–135.
72. Farthing MJG, DuPont HL, Guandalini S, Keusch GT, Steffen R. Treatment and prevention of travellers' diarrhoea. *Gastroenterol Int* 1992;5:162–175.
73. Ericsson CD, Pickering LK, Sullivan P, DuPont HL. The role of location of food consumption in the prevention of travelers' diarrhea in Mexico. *Gastroenterology* 1980;79:812–816.
74. Tacket CO, Losonsky G, Link H, et al. Protection by milk immunoglobulin concentrate against oral challenge with enterotoxigenic *Escherichia coli. N Engl J Med* 1988;318:1240–1243.
75. DuPont HL, Olarte J, Evans DG, Pickering LK, Galindo E, Evans DJ Jr. Comparative susceptibility of Latin American and

United States students to enteric pathogens. *N Engl J Med* 1976;295:1520–1521.

76. Brown MR, DuPont HL, Sullivan PS. Effect of duration of exposure on diarrhea due to enterotoxigenic *Escherichia coli* in travelers from the United States to Mexico. *J Infect Dis* 1982;145:582.

77. Evans DJ Jr, Ruiz-Palacios G, Evans DG, DuPont HL, Pickering LK, Olarte J. Humoral immune response to the heat-labile enterotoxin of *Escherichia coli* in naturally acquired diarrhea and antitoxin determination by passive immune hemolysis. *Infect Immun* 1977;16:781–788.

78. Clemens JD, Harris JR, Sack DA, et al. Field trial of oral cholera vaccines in Bangladesh: results of one year of follow-up. *J Infect Dis* 1988;158:60–69.

79. Peltola H, Siitonen A, Kyrönseppa H, et al. Prevention of travellers' diarrhoea by oral B-subunit/whole-cell cholera vaccine. *Lancet* 1991;338:1285–1289.

80. DuPont HL, Sullivan P, Pickering LK, Haynes G, Ackerman PB. Symptomatic treatment of diarrhea with bismuth subsalicylate among students attending a Mexican university. *Gastroenterology* 1977;73:715–718.

81. Ericsson CD, Evans DG, DuPont HL, Evans DJ Jr, Pickering LK. Bismuth subsalicylate inhibits activity of crude toxins of *Escherichia coli* and *Vibrio cholerae*. *J Infect Dis* 1977;136:693–696.

82. Gyles CL and Zigler M. The effect of adsorbent and anti-inflammatory drugs on secretion in ligated segments of pig intestine infected with *Escherichia coli*. *Can J Comp Med* 1978;42:260–268.

83. Powell DW, Tapper EJ, Morris SM. Aspirin-stimulated intestinal electrolyte transport in rabbit ileum in vitro. *Gastroenterology* 1979;76:1429–1437.

84. Burke V and Gracey M. Reduction by aspirin of intestinal fluid loss in acute childhood gastroenteritis. *Lancet* 1980;1:1329–1330.

85. Goldenberg MM, Honkomp LJ, Burrous SE, Castellion AW. Protective effect of pepto-bismol liquid on the gastric mucosa of rats. *Gastroenterology* 1975;69:636–640.

86. Steinhoff MC, Douglas RG Jr, Greenberg HB, Callahan DR. Bismuth subsalicylate therapy of viral gastroenteritis. *Gastroenterology* 1980;78:1495–1499.

87. Stoclet JC, Gerard D, Kilhoffer MC, Lugnier C, Miller R, Schaeffer P. Calmodulin and its role in intracellular calcium regulation. *Progr Neurobiol* 1987;29:321–364.

88. DuPont HL, Ericsson CD, Mathewson JJ, Marani S, Knellwolf-Cousin AL, Martinez-Sandoval FG. Zaldaride maleate (Zm), an intestinal calmodulin inhibitor in the therapy of travelers' diarrhea. *Gastroenterology* 1993;104:709–715.

89. Reves RR, Bass P, DuPont HL, Sullivan P, Mendiola J. Failure to demonstrate effectiveness of an anticholinergic drug in the symptomatic treatment of acute travelers' diarrhea. *J Clin Gastroenterol* 1983;5:223–227.

90. Johnson PC, Ericsson CD, DuPont HL, Morgan DR, Bitsura JA, Wood LV. Comparison of loperamide with bismuth subsalicylate for the treatment of acute travelers' diarrhea. *JAMA* 1986;225:757–760.

91. DuPont HL, Sanchez JF, Ericsson CD, et al. Comparative efficacy of loperamide hydrochloride and bismuth subsalicylate in the management of acute diarrhea. *Am J Med* 1990;88(Suppl 6a):15S–19S.

92. Schiller LR, Santa Ana CA, Morawski SG, Fordtran JS. Mechanism of the antidiarrheal effect of loperamide. *Gastroenterology* 1984;86:1475–1480.

93. Merritt JE, Brown BL, Tomlinson S. Loperamide and calmodulin. *Lancet* 1982;1:283.

94. DuPont HL, Hornick RB. Adverse effect of lomotil therapy in shigellosis. *JAMA* 1973;226:1525–1528.

95. DuPont HL, Ericsson CD, DuPont MW, Cruz Luna A, Mathewson JJ. A randomized, open-label comparison of nonprescription loperamide and attapulgite in the symptomatic treatment of acute diarrhea. *Am J Med* 1990;88(Suppl 6A):20S–23S.

96. DuPont HL, Reves RR, Galindo E, Sullivan PS, Wood LV, Mendiola JG. Treatment of travelers' diarrhea with trimethoprim/sulfamethoxazole and with trimethoprim alone. *N Engl J Med* 1982;307:841–844.

97. Ericsson CD, Johnson PC, DuPont HL, Morgan DR, Bitsura JM. Ciprofloxacin and trimethoprim/sulfamethoxazole as initial therapy for acute travelers' diarrhea. A placebo-controlled randomized trial. *Ann Intern Med* 1987;106:216–220.

98. Ericsson CD, DuPont HL, Mathewson JJ, West MS, Johnson PC, Bitsura JM. Treatment of travelers' diarrhea with sulfamethoxazole and trimethoprim and loperamide. *JAMA* 1990;263:257–261.

99. Wistrom J, Jertborn M, Hedstrom SA, et al. Short-term self-treatment of travellers' diarrhoea with norfloxacin: a placebo-controlled study. *J Antimicrob Chemother* 1989;23:905–913.

100. DuPont HL, Ericsson CD, Mathewson JJ, DuPont MW. Five versus three days of ofloxacin therapy for traveler's diarrhea: A placebo-controlled study. *Antimicrob Agents Chemother* 1992;36:87–91.

101. Steffen R, Jori R, DuPont HL, Mathewson JJ, Murray BE, Tschopp A. Fleroxacin, a long-acting fluoroquinolone, as effective therapy for travelers' diarrhea. *Rev Infect Dis* 1989;11(Suppl 5):S1154–S1155.

102. Gough A, Barsoum NJ, Mitchell L, McGuire EJ, de la Iglesia FA. Juvenile canine drug-induced arthropathy: clinicopathological studies on articular lesions caused by oxolonic acid and pipemidic acids. *Toxicol Appl Pharmacol* 1979;51:177–187.

103. DuPont HL, Ericsson CD, Mathewson JJ, de la Cabada FJ, Conrad DA. Oral aztreonam, a poorly absorbed yet effective therapy for bacterial diarrhea in US travelers to Mexico. *JAMA* 1992;267:1932–1935.

104. Cofsky RD, DeBouchet L, Landesman SH. Recovery of norfloxacin in feces after administration of a single oral dose to human volunteers. *Antimicrob Agents Chemother* 1984;26:110–111.

105. DuPont HL, Ericsson CD, Robinson A, Johnson PC. Current problems in antimicrobial therapy for bacterial enteric infection. *Am J Med* 1987;82(Suppl 4A):324–328.

106. Bennish ML, Abdus Salam M, Khan WA, Khan AM. Treatment of shigellosis: III. Comparison of one- or two-dose ciprofloxacin with standard 5-day therapy A randomized, blinded trial. *Ann Intern Med* 1992;117:727–734.

107. Haltalin KC, Nelson JD, Hinton LV, Kusmiesz HT, Sladoje M. Comparison of orally absorbable and nonabsorbable antibiotics in shigellosis: a double blind study with ampicillin and neomycin. *J Pediatr* 1968;72:708–720.

108. Nishida M, Mine Y, Nonoyama S, Kamimura T, Fukada S. Therapeutic efficacy of bicyclomycin for shigellosis experimentally induced in Rhesus monkeys. *J Antibiot* 1974;27:976–983.

109. Ericsson CD, DuPont HL, Sullivan P, Galindo E, Evans DG, Evans DJ Jr. Bicozamycin, a poorly absorbable antibiotic, effectively treats travelers' diarrhea. *Ann Intern Med* 1983;98:20–25.

110. Ericsson CD, DuPont HL, Galindo E, et al. Efficacy of bicozamycin in preventing travelers' diarrhea. *Gastroenterology* 1985;88:473–477.

111. Ericsson CD, Johnson PC, DuPont HL, Morgan DR. Role of a novel antidiarrheal agent, BW942C, alone or in combination with trimethoprim/sulfamethoxazole in the treatment of traveler's diarrhea. *Antimicrob Agents Chemother* 1986;29:1040–1046.

112. Steffen R, Heusser R, Tschopp A, DuPont HL. Efficacy and side-effects of six agents in the self-treatment of travellers' diarrhoea. *Trav Med Int* 1988;6:153–157.

113. Ericsson CD, Nicholls-Vasquez I, DuPont HL, Mathewson JJ. Optimal dosing of trimethoprim/sulfamethoxazole when used with loperamide to treat travelers' diarrhea. *Antimicrob Agents Chemother* 1992;36:2821–2824.

114. Taylor DN, Sanchez JL, Chandler W, Thornton S, McQueen C, Echeverria P. Treatment of travelers' diarrhea: ciprofloxacin plus loperamide compared with ciprofloxacin alone: a placebo-controlled, randomized trial. *Ann Intern Med* 1991;114:731–734.

115. Petruccelli BP, Murphy GS, Sanchez JL, et al. Treatment of traveler's diarrhea with ciprofloxacin and loperamide. *J Infect Dis* 1992;165:557–560.

116. Ericsson CD, Feldman S, Pickering LK, Cleary TG. Influence of subsalicylate bismuth on absorption of doxycycline. *JAMA* 1982;247:2266–2267.

Infections of the Gastrointestinal Tract,
edited by M. J. Blaser, P. D. Smith, J. I. Ravdin,
H. B. Greenberg, and R. L. Guerrant
Raven Press, Ltd., New York © 1995.

CHAPTER 23

Idiopathic Chronic Diarrhea

Julie Parsonnet, Christine A. Wanke, and Howard Hack

INTRODUCTION

Chronic diarrhea is commonly defined as three or more loose or watery stools daily for 30 days or longer (14 days for persistent diarrhea in children). Myriad illnesses may present with persistent loose stools as a primary or secondary manifestation of disease. Predominant in the differential diagnosis are noninfectious processes including inflammatory bowel diseases, endocrinopathies, malignancies, eating disorders, and somatoform illnesses (1). Only a small minority of chronic diarrheal illnesses are directly caused by infections. This is because infectious diarrheas typically are acute and self-limited and, when they do persist, are diagnosed and treated long before the 30 days that defines the chronic diarrhea syndrome. Despite these caveats, many organisms ranging from viruses to parasites have been reported to cause chronic diarrhea (Table 1). With few exceptions (most notably giardiasis), however, these infections either rarely progress to chronicity or are found only in immunocompromised hosts.

This chapter will not focus on the many microorganisms that can occasionally cause sustained illness. These are discussed extensively in chapters devoted to the specific infectious agents. While HIV-associated diarrheal illness may well become the most common persistent diarrheal illness syndrome seen in the United States and throughout the world, that syndrome is also covered elsewhere in this text. Instead, this chapter will focus on three chronic diarrhea syndromes that present diagnostic and treatment dilemmas to the gastroenterology and infectious disease specialist: Brainerd diarrhea, chronic sporadic diarrhea of adults, and chronic diarrhea of children in developing countries.

BRAINERD DIARRHEA

In 1983, an outbreak of a debilitating, chronic diarrheal illness occurred in rural Brainerd, Minnesota (2). One hundred twenty-two patients complained of sudden onset of watery diarrhea with up to 20 bowel movements per day. Extreme fecal urgency with fecal incontinence was common. Illness lasted for longer than one year in the majority of cases but no etiological agent was identified. Since the Minnesota outbreak, six other outbreaks of chronic diarrhea affecting 186 persons have been investigated (Table 2). The uniform clinical and epidemiological features of these outbreaks suggest a common underlying disease process. Thus, the syndrome has taken on the name "Brainerd diarrhea."

Clinical Features

Brainerd diarrhea is an impressive illness that causes marked disability and extensive medical costs. In the first weeks of illness, patients describe the sudden onset of frequent watery diarrhea accompanied by gas, borborygmi, and mild abdominal cramps (Table 3). Some patients describe up to 40 stools per day although 10–20 stools is more typical. Except for mild weight loss, there are usually no constitutional symptoms. Incontinence is the most debilitating feature; patients state that although they feel well, they try to be no more than one minute away from a bathroom. In the Henderson County, Illinois outbreak, affected truck drivers described wearing diapers to work and running into fields to defecate so they could complete their daily routes (3).

As Brainerd diarrhea persists, stools decrease in frequency and volume. Body weight stabilizes. Because stool frequency varies from day to day during the natural

J. Parsonnet: Division of Infectious Disease, Department of Medicine, and Division of Epidemiology, Department of Health Research and Policy, Stanford University School of Medicine, Stanford, California 94305.

C. A. Wanke: Division of Infectious Diseases, New England Deaconess Hospital, Harvard Medical School, Boston, Massachusetts 02215.

H. Hack: Division of Gastroenterology, Department of Medicine, Stanford University School of Medicine, Stanford, California 94305.

TABLE 1. *Infectious causes of chronic diarrhea in industrialized nations[a]*

Pathogen	Ref.
Viruses	
Rotavirus	68
Cytomegalovirus	69–71
Adenovirus	72
Astrovirus	73
Picobirnavirus	73
Bacteria	
Aeromonas hydrophila	74–76
Campylobacter jejuni	77–81
Clostridium difficile	82,83
Dysgonic fermenter-3	84
Enteropathogenic *E. coli*[b]	85–88
Mycobacterium tuberculosis	71,89
Atypical mycobacteria	90
Plesiomonas	91
Salmonella	92
Whipple's disease bacillus	93
Yersinia	94–97
Fungi	
Candida	98
Protozoa	
***Blastocystis hominis*[c]**	99,100
Cryptosporidium	71,101
Cyclospora	73,102–105
Entamoeba histolytica	106,107
Giardia lamblia	108,109
Isospora belli	110,112
Microsporidia	113–115
Helminths	
Strongyloides	108
Hookworm	108

[a] The organisms in bold represent infections that not uncommonly persist and cause chronic diarrhea in normal hosts. The remaining organisms either rarely result in chronic diarrhea in normal hosts (although they may commonly cause acute disease) or are exclusively pathogens in immunosuppressed patients.

[b] Reported as a cause of chronic diarrhea only in children.

[c] Remains a controversial cause of chronic diarrhea.

course of illness, treatment efficacy has been difficult to assess. No therapy (not antibiotics, steroids, antiinflammatory drugs, fiber, bismuth, or cholestyramine) is consistently effective, although opiate antimotility agents appear to provide temporary relief of symptoms in a subset of patients (2,4,5). Anecdotally, patients often claim to control their symptoms by adjusting their diets although no specific dietary changes are uniformly effective. Symptoms of loose stools persist for over a year in the majority of subjects. Eventually, however, symptoms subside. In the two studies with longest follow-up, all persons interviewed after 3 years were symptom-free (6).

Brainerd diarrhea is costly to the health care system. Approximately 80% of patients in the described outbreaks sought medical attention and 20% were hospitalized for extensive diagnostic tests and/or rehydration. Subjects with Brainerd diarrhea are as likely to be female as male although women have been more likely to seek medical

attention and be hospitalized (4). Brainerd diarrhea has been reported in relatively few children, and when it does occur, the duration of illness may be shorter than in adults (2,4).

Epidemiology

Of the seven outbreaks of Brainerd diarrhea, four have been reported in the medical literature (2,4,7,8); three smaller outbreaks investigated by state and federal public health departments remain unpublished (5,9) (Table 2). Six outbreaks occurred in the United States, five in rural settings. One outbreak occurred on a South American cruise ship.

Extensive epidemiological investigations were conducted in all outbreaks. In Brainerd, unpasteurized milk was identified as the vehicle for disease transmission. In a case-control study, the odds ratio for cases drinking milk from one particular dairy was 28.3. The investigators also reported the occurrence of similar milk-related outbreaks in other settings, although details of these outbreaks were not presented. Because of these findings, cases of chronic diarrhea were sought among raw milk drinkers in an outbreak in South Carolina. Although a relatively high attack rate was identified among raw milk drinkers [4 (15%) of 26 exposed], raw milk could not be named a risk factor for disease since no people without the exposure were interviewed (9).

Water has also been identified as a potential source for Brainerd diarrhea. In Henderson County, Illinois, illness was strongly linked to drinking untreated well water from a local restaurant (4). The restaurant's well had many construction deficiencies and contained unacceptable levels of fecal coliforms, a marker for contamination with human and/or animal waste. In Oklahoma, the outbreak was tentatively linked to a community water source (9). In this case, the water was not found to be contaminated despite many deficiencies in the system. Water was also identified as the likely vehicle for disease on a Galapagos Islands cruise ship (8). Again, there were marked deficiencies in the water system including intermittent lapses in chlorination but the water was not contaminated at the time of inspection. In all of these outbreaks, there were definitely no exposures to unpasteurized milk products (4,7,9).

As with transmissible diseases in general, exposure does not invariably cause illness. Only 8% of raw milk drinkers in Brainerd became ill (2). Although all Mountain View, Oklahoma residents were exposed to community water, only 1.6% became ill (5). In Henderson County, Illinois, three men who drank over 30 glasses of restaurant water during the outbreak period were among 15 (65%) of 23 exposed persons who did not get diarrhea (4). Common to each of these outbreaks, however, was a dose–response relationship between exposure and disease: the greater the exposure, the higher the risk. In all outbreaks, the attack rate was also consistently higher among the elderly than among the young. Persons age 65 years and older had a two- to threefold higher likelihood of acquiring disease than persons younger than 65 years (2,4,5,9).

There was one possible case of household transmission

TABLE 2. *Epidemiology of Brainerd diarrhea outbreaks*

Location	Year	N cases	Median age	% female	Source	Incubation period	Secondary transmission	Ref.
Baca County, CO	1977	20	54[a]	50	Unknown	Unknown	Not reported	(9)
Brainerd, MN	1983–84	122	41	49	Unpasteurized milk	15 days	Possibly two cases in one household	(2)
Iva, SC	1984	4	62	75	Unknown	Unknown	Not reported	(116)
San Antonio, TX	1984–85	10	NR	NR	Restaurant	20 to 30 days	Not reported	(7)
Henderson County, IL	1987	72	56	50	Untreated water, restaurant	10 days	None	(4)
Mountain View, OK	1988–89	22	60[b]	64	Probably water	NR	None	(5)
Cruise ship, Galapagos Islands	1992	58	66[c]	50	Probably water	12 days	None	(8)

[a] Estimated from reported data.
[b] Mean age.
[c] Based on 52 subjects.

described in the original Brainerd outbreak. Although person-to-person spread would corroborate an infectious etiology, no secondary cases were noted in any of the other six outbreaks.

Laboratory Investigations

Extensive clinical and laboratory studies have been conducted on selected patients. Hematological parameters and blood chemistries typically have been normal although hypokalemia has been reported with severe volume loss (4,5). The diarrhea causes moderate increases in stool volume (300 to 800 g/day). As with other secretory diarrheas, stool volume does not decrease with fasting (9–11). Serum levels of hormones that cause secretory diarrhea (i.e., gastrin, thyroxin, vasoactive intestinal polypeptide, pancreatic polypeptide, calcitonin) have also been within the normal range (11). There is no evidence of malabsorption. In a handful of subjects, however, small bowel motility was found to be abnormal with unusual,

prolonged, rapidly propagated, high-pressure waves in the jejunum (10).

Stool examinations have been unhelpful in identifying a cause for Brainerd diarrhea. A small number of fecal leukocytes may be observed in less than 20% of cases (2,4,5). Stool cultures, tests for bacterial toxins, and examinations for ova and parasites (including microsporidia) have revealed no consistent pathogen. In the first outbreak in Baca County, Colorado, *Klebsiella pneumoniae* was isolated from stool in 6 of 18 cases and in none of the controls (9). This finding has not been reproduced in other outbreaks. Other pathogens such as *Blastocystis hominis, Giardia lamblia, Campylobacter,* and *Salmonella* have each been isolated from one or two cases although eradication of these organisms did not ameliorate symptoms (2,4,8). Cultures of implicated milk and water have yielded no likely pathogens. No viral agents have been found by electron microscopy of stool or implicated water.

The only finding that may distinguish Brainerd diarrhea from other forms of chronic diarrhea has been found on

TABLE 3. *Clinical features of cases of Brainerd diarrhea from 5 outbreaks and from 17 cases of sporadic idiopathic chronic diarrhea*

Symptom or clinical finding	Brainerd diarrhea		Sporadic idiopathic chronic diarrhea	
	Number	Percent (range)	Number	Percent
Urgency	257/288	89 (75–100)	5/17	29
Weight loss	113/166	68 (55–76)	12/17	71
Incontinence	149/268	56 (51–81)	6/17	35
Cramps	150/289	52 (25–60)	5/17	29
Nausea	54/269	20 (14–28)	NA	NA
Fever or feverishness	14/289	5 (0–12)	2/17	12%
Vomiting	13/289	5 (0–18)	1/17	5.9%
Mean number of stools per day	10.5		10	
Median duration of illness	12 to 16.5 months		12 months	

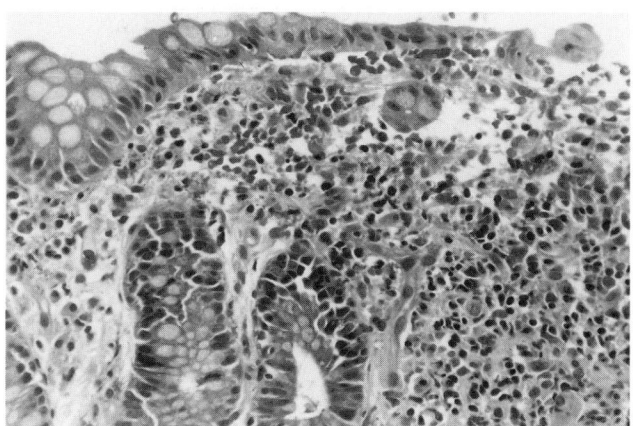

FIG. 1. A case of multifocal colitis from an outbreak of Brainerd diarrhea in Henderson County, IL. Focal areas of inflammation in the right colon are adjacent to mildly distorted crypts. Note the inflammation extending into the crypt and damge to surface epithelium. (H&E × 80.) (Courtesy Frank A. Mitros, MD, Department of Pathology, University of Iowa, Iowa City.)

colonoscopy (Fig. 1). Grossly, the bowel in Brainerd diarrhea looks either normal or mildly inflamed with nonspecific, patchy erythema and/or punctate hemorrhages (2,4,5,11). Histopathologically, however, Janda et al. identified an unusual inflammatory process that they termed *multifocal colitis* (Fig. 1). In four of five subjects, biopsy specimens showed patchy areas of acute inflammation in the lamina propria just beneath the surface epithelium (11). This inflammatory process included a predominance of lymphocytes but also a large number of neutrophils and eosinophils, the latter extending into a flattened surface epithelium. Crypt abscess were occasionally observed (11). Unfortunately, other pathologists evaluating Brainerd diarrhea specimens did not describe multifocal colitis but interpreted the biopsy findings as either mild, nonspecific inflammation (13 of 18 biopsies) or normal (4 of 18 biopsies) (2,4,5). Although the focality of multifocal colitis may hinder recognition of an inhomogeneous process, it remains to be confirmed that multifocal colitis is a characteristic feature of Brainerd diarrhea.

The cause of Brainerd diarrhea remains a matter of speculation. Minimal data (the one case of person-to-person transmission) supports an infectious etiology. On the other hand, antibiotics have had no effect on disease course suggesting against a bacterial etiology. Attempts have been made in the laboratory to develop an animal model for the disease. While Myers et al. reported transmitting severe diarrheal illness to rabbits after inoculating them with stools from three Brainerd outbreak cases, stools from two additional Brainerd cases did not cause disease (12). Furthermore, stools from other outbreaks did not yield similar results. Thus, few conclusions can yet be made from this work.

After all of the extensive investigations that have been conducted on Brainerd diarrhea, it is humbling to recognize that a pathogen has escaped detection. One reason the agent for Brainerd may be so elusive is that it may only

transiently exist in the gut. In the first stages of illness, the causative agent could permanently damage the gastrointestinal tract and then be eliminated. For instance, if stem cells or nonregenerative cells such as endocrine or neural cells were damaged, even a short-term insult could result in long-term disability. If the agent is only present in the initial stages of disease, it would be difficult to identify since by definition Brainerd diarrhea is diagnosed at a chronic stage. It also remains possible that Brainerd diarrhea is caused by a toxic rather than an infectious exposure. The hope for solving this disease rests in the expeditious investigation of chronic diarrhea outbreaks in which new, ongoing cases can be identified in the early stages of illness.

SPORADIC IDIOPATHIC CHRONIC DIARRHEA OF ADULTS

Chronic idiopathic diarrhea occurs not only in outbreaks but also sporadically throughout the country. The disease poses a frustrating problem to patients and clinicians alike. Chronic diarrhea is frequently debilitating, causing restriction of lifestyle and lost productivity at work. Before arriving at the specialist's office, patients with chronic diarrhea have often seen many doctors, undergone numerous diagnostic tests, and tried multiple home remedies and physician-prescribed therapies without success. For the majority of these patients, however, a cause for chronic diarrhea can eventually be identified. Usually this cause is not infectious (1). Among 27 intensively studied patients with chronic diarrhea reported in 1980, 9 were found to have surreptitiously used laxatives or diuretics, 8 had irritable bowel syndrome, 2 inflammatory bowel disease, 2 anal sphincter dysfunction, and 1 beef allergy. Only one subject had an infectious etiology of diarrhea: bacterial overgrowth of the small bowel. However, four subjects (three with secretory and one with osmotic diarrhea) remained undiagnosed. These cases that defied diagnosis despite extensive workup can be termed cases of sporadic idiopathic chronic diarrhea (SICD).

Clinical Disease and Investigation

Although data are extremely limited, the clinical features of SICD appear to be similar to those of Brainerd diarrhea (6) (Table 3). In the only systematic study done thus far, 17 SICD patients described sudden onset of watery diarrhea, accompanied rarely by nausea, vomiting, or feverishness (13). Bowel movements remained abnormal for months with patients not infrequently complaining of nocturnal or early morning bowel movements, fecal incontinence, and abdominal cramps. Seventy-one percent of patients lost weight with a median weight loss of 5 pounds.

As with Brainerd diarrhea, many therapies were tried to improve symptoms of SICD patients. Fifteen (88%) of 17 patients had been unsuccessfully treated with metronidazole before referral to the tertiary care center. Other antibiotics also provided no relief. Of subjects who received opiate antimotility agents, however, approximately 40% experienced some symptomatic improvement. The efficacy of loperamide in relieving SICD has similarly been observed in other studies (14). Other agents that were unsuccessfully tried in a few subjects included steroids, sulfasalazine, and cholestyramine. Despite the limited success of treatments, the chronic diarrheal illness eventually resolved in all patients with a mean duration of diarrhea was 15 months (range 7–31 months). In subsequent follow-up, patients had regained lost weight and described themselves as healthy.

Physical examination and routine blood tests on the Baylor patients were normal except for occasional hypokalemia (13). Stool cultures and tests for ova and parasites revealed no pathogens. No white cells were seen on Wright's stain of the stools. Diarrhea was secretory in nature with fecal fat increased in only one subject. Four subjects had excessive bacterial colonization of the jejunum but appropriate treatment with antibiotics did not ameliorate symptoms. Upper and lower gastrointestinal endoscopies and biopsies were generally normal. There was no evidence of multifocal colitis although one subject had colonic submucosal petechiae and erythema. In physiological studies of eight patients, there was evidence of bile acid malabsorption that did not correct with cholestyramine therapy (15). This suggested an ileal defect and was interpreted to indicate either an intestinal motility disorder or an underlying absorptive abnormality. The normal Shilling tests in these subjects, however, made the latter alternative somewhat less likely.

Epidemiology

The epidemiology of sporadic chronic diarrhea is largely undefined. To document disease prevalence, Mintz et al. surveyed 8000 members of the two largest professional gastroenterology societies in the United States (16). Members were asked to report chronic diarrhea cases (greater than 2 months of symptoms in a person older than 2 years) that had been seen in April 1991. HIV patients were excluded from the case definition. Although only 9% of gastroenterologists responded to the survey, a sampling of nonrespondents suggested that this group represented the overall population of specialists.

One hundred and sixty-five (28%) of the 589 respondents reported seeing 438 cases of chronic diarrhea in the preceding month. The median age of subjects was 47 years (range 9–88) and 58% were female. Despite the rural location of many Brainerd outbreaks, rural residence did not appear to increase risk for sporadic chronic diarrhea. Because many cases had not had extensive clinical evaluation (only one third had undergone colonoscopy), it is possible that a substantial proportion of reported cases do not represent true "idiopathic" disease. The epidemiological findings, however, do corroborate the observations of Afzalpurkar et al. The median age of their 17 SICD subjects was 54 with 41% of subjects being female; only one patient was from a rural location (13). Overall, Mintz et al. estimated that 5000–8000 patients with chronic diarrhea visit U.S. gastroenterologists on a monthly basis (16).

Chronic diarrhea is thought to be most common in travelers. Afzalpurkar et al. found that 59% of 17 patients had a history of recent travel before disease onset (13). This travel was usually local rather than international. Unfortunately, there is no information on the frequency of travel in a comparison control population and it is possible that local travel is equally common in both ill and well populations. In another study, Peace Corps volunteers who served in the late 1980s were found to have a very high incidence of chronic diarrhea (17). According to Peace Corps Medical Officers, 9 per 1000 volunteers experienced SICD. SICD appeared to be particularly likely in persons who were stationed in Haiti (one third of volunteers). Other areas of high risk included Nepal (31 per 1000 volunteers) and Tunisia (28 per 1000 volunteers). Illness was not thought to be related to rural residence or drinking of untreated water. The medical officers reported, however, that drinking of unpasteurized milk was a more common practice in countries with high risk for SICD.

While some of the cases of SICD in travelers may represent infection with now recognized diarrhea pathogens (i.e., cryptosporidia, microsporidia, or cyanobacteria), it is likely that a significant proportion would remain idiopathic if evaluated today. Some speculate that the increased incidence of chronic diarrhea among travelers may indicate replacement of the host's normal flora with alien "normal" flora. This remains unproved.

Comparison with Brainerd Diarrhea

It is unknown as to whether outbreak-related Brainerd diarrhea and SICD represent one or many diseases. During outbreak investigations of Brainerd diarrhea, cases of chronic diarrhea were identified that appeared to be unrelated to the outbreak (i.e., the date of onset was not during the outbreak period). These cases were clinically indistinguishable from Brainerd diarrhea (3,5). Upon extensive questioning of cases, it appeared possible that these sporadic cases were part of very small, unrecognized clusters of disease (5). Certainly the similarities between Brainerd and SICD are striking. Both begin with sudden onset of watery diarrhea and cause few constitutional symptoms except for mild weight loss. While outbreak-related cases described more urgency and incontinence, this may be due to the timing of the interview since outbreak cases tend to be evaluated earlier in the course of their illness when symptoms are most severe. Laboratory findings are minimal in both outbreak-related and sporadic disease. The finding of multifocal colitis, while unreported in sporadic chronic diarrhea, also needs substantiation in outbreak-related disease. Until the causative agent(s) are identified, however, the relationship of sporadic and outbreak-related diseases will remain uncertain (18).

PERSISTENT DIARRHEA IN CHILDREN IN DEVELOPING COUNTRIES

Diarrheal disease and malnutrition are widely accepted as two of the leading causes of morbidity and mortality in children in the developing world (19). It has become increasingly clear in the last decade that prolonged diarrheal illnesses and dysenteric diarrheal illnesses play a more prominent role in diarrheal morbidity and mortality than had been previously suspected (20). For the child in the developing world, prolonged or persistent diarrhea is defined as any diarrheal illness that lasts longer than 14 days. For the child with chronic, recurrent diarrheal illnesses, a 3-day diarrhea-free interval is generally required before a child can be said to have a new rather than a persistent diarrheal illness. Prolonged diarrhea is likely to become an increasingly important issue with the epidemic of AIDS advancing rapidly in children as well as adults in the developing world (21,22).

Significant progress has been made in the last 10 years in understanding the epidemiology, natural history, etiological agents, pathogenesis, and therapy of persistent diarrhea. As with acute diarrheal illness, it is difficult to generalize about persistent diarrhea. By definition, persistent diarrhea covers a spectrum of illnesses that extends from simple diarrheal illnesses that last 15 days to wasting diarrheal illnesses that persist for months; persistent diarrhea may be a watery or mucoid diarrheal illness or it may be a dysenteric illness. In this population of children, an intestinal injury inflicted by an infectious agent cannot be differentiated from an intestinal injury caused by malnutrition, food allergy, or the complications of systemic disease. The cumulative effect of all of these injuries is likely to be important in attempts to define the true etiology of persistent diarrheas (23). These physiological parameters are also likely complicated further by the socioeconomic and cultural environment in which the child lives. The complex interactions of intestinal physiology and social science have been difficult to study and have hindered the understanding of persistent diarrhea.

Epidemiology

Data from mostly retrospective studies suggest that between 3% and 27% of all childhood diarrhea is prolonged beyond 14 days in Indonesia, Bangladesh, and Guatemala (24–26). In recent prospective studies, 7.5% of all diarrheal illnesses were prolonged in children under the age of 5 years in rural Bangladesh although overall diarrheal incidence was particularly low in that population (27); 11% of all diarrheal episodes in children under the age of 5 years were prolonged beyond 14 days in a 2-year prospective study done in an urban slum in northeastern Brazil (28), the overall incidence of diarrhea was high in this population. Five percent of all the diarrheal episodes in this community lasted longer than 21 days, and 50% of the days that children spent with diarrheal disease were during episodes of persistent diarrhea. Eleven percent of all diarrheal illnesses were prolonged in a prospective study in Guatemala and 23% were prolonged in a study

in a rural community in Bangladesh (29,30). In Brazil, the peak incidence of persistent diarrhea was between the ages of 12 and 18 months. In the other studies, persistent diarrhea was seen most frequently in children under the age of 6 months in Guatemala and in the rural wetlands of Bangladesh, and between 6 and 12 months in the rural community in Bangladesh (27,29,30).

The disease burden in these populations is not evenly spread among all children, however. In rural Bangladesh, 16% of the children followed prospectively had eight or more episodes of diarrhea per year, and 11% of the children had diarrhea for more than 21% of the study days (27). In the Brazilian slum, children with one episode of persistent diarrhea spent an average of 135 days/year with diarrhea, whereas the children who did not have an episode of persistent diarrhea spent an average of 15 days/year with diarrhea (28).

Diarrheal disease mortality is also not evenly spread among these populations. Twelve percent of diarrheal deaths in northern India were associated with nondysenteric persistent diarrhea (31). Forty-nine percent of diarrheal deaths in Bangladesh were associated with persistent wasting diarrhea, and 62% of all diarrheal deaths were associated with persistent diarrhea in southern Brazil (32,33).

Natural History/Clinical Course

The spectrum of persistent diarrheal illness is so broad that it is extremely difficult to develop an understanding of the natural history of this syndrome or the ability to predict outcome. Few studies examine the total duration of diarrheal illnesses in these cases, and diarrheal illnesses are classified as either acute or persistent. However, some natural history data can be extracted from some of the studies. In the urban slums in northeastern Brazil, the average duration of the persistent diarrheal episodes was 26–27 days and diarrhea remitted spontaneously in all of these children without hospitalization and with no deaths (28). Twenty percent of these children had an infectious pathogen identified at day 14 of their illness. In rural Bangladesh, when 7.5% of all diarrheal illnesses were persistent, 5% of all diarrheal illnesses also lasted longer than 22 days; in these children disease was more severe as measured by dehydration, decreased activity, vomiting, and the need to bring the child to a health facility (27). The children with persistent diarrhea were also more likely to present with bloody or mucoid stool than with watery diarrhea. In many studies malnutrition and skin test anergy serve as markers that can identify children with prolonged diarrheal illness, but from the available literature it is difficult to predict which children will go on to spend 60–62% of days each year with prolonged diarrhea (Fig. 2).

Etiology

Bacteria

Small bowel overgrowth with aerobic and anaerobic bacteria has been postulated as a cause or a contributing

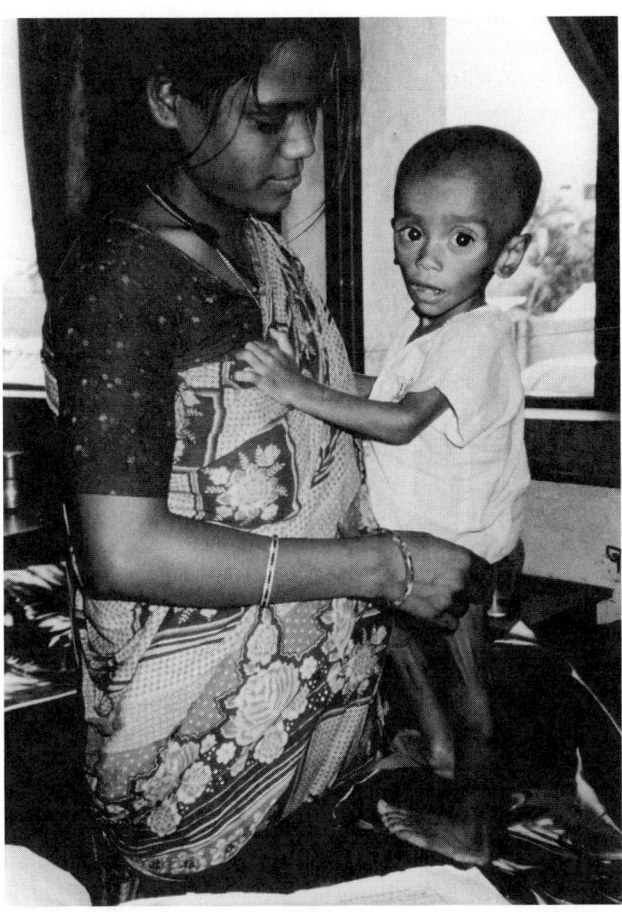

FIG. 2. An 18-month-old child hospitalized in Dhaka, Bangladesh for evaluation of chronic diarrhea. At admission at 18 months of age, this child weighed 6.2 kg and had suffered from diarrheal illness for longer than 10 months. No etiological agent was identified, although the child did have small bowel overgrowth with gram-negative rods. (Courtesy C. A. Wanke.)

factor of persistent diarrheal disease in children in the developing world for the last two decades (34–38). The studies that have attempted to examine this question have been problematic and difficult to compare either because of small numbers, lack of appropriate controls, or differences in intubation technique and microbiological evaluation. Most recently reviews and carefully done studies in Peru and India have suggested that nutritional status, age, and socioeconomic environment are more important in determining the number of bacteria within the small bowel than the clinical presence of acute or persistent diarrhea (39,40). While an animal model provides supporting data that small bowel overgrowth with nonvirulent E. coli can produce watery and persistent diarrheal illness, it has not been possible to confirm the association of overgrowth with persistent diarrhea in the absence of a recognized pathogen in studies in children in the developing world (41,42). Additionally, data that examine chronic diarrheal disease in HIV-positive patients have not shown an association between small bowel overgrowth and persistent diarrhea in this population (43,44).

E. coli are one of the most common causes of acute diarrheal disease in children in the developing world. While E. coli are more classically associated with acute, watery diarrheal disease, some of the E. coli have been associated with persistent diarrheal illness. Although the average duration of illness with the enterotoxigenic E. coli (ETEC) is 4–5 days, 7–8% of diarrheal illnesses in rural Bangladesh associated with ETEC lasted longer than 20 days (26). Twenty percent of children with persistent diarrhea in a northeastern Brazilian slum had ETEC when they were cultured after the fourteenth day of their illness (28). Forty-two percent of children with persistent diarrhea in Lima, Peru had ETEC isolated at during the first week of their illness; ETEC was isolated in 34% of a different group of children with persistent diarrhea in Lima during the second and third weeks of illness (45). ETEC was present in culture in 14% of children during the fourth week of illness. Whether children remain infected with organisms such as ETEC throughout the entire duration of a persistent diarrheal illness is more difficult to say; the study from Lima suggests that only 30% of the children with ETEC were infected throughout the first and second week of the diarrheal illness with the same ETEC and was not able to document any ETEC persisting in the same child for longer than 2 weeks.

In the developed world, the enteropathogenic E. coli (EPEC) have routinely been associated with chronic diarrhea of childhood, but in the developing world they are not common pathogens causing only 2–5% of childhood diarrheal illnesses. The burden of persistent diarrheal disease caused by the EPEC may therefore be less than that of the ETEC. The EPEC were associated with 8% of persistent diarrheal illnesses in Brazil and 4% in Lima, Peru and rural Bangladesh. In these studies the rates of occurrence of EPEC in persistent diarrhea were not significantly different from those seen in acute diarrheal disease. However, these studies did not examine the small bowel of the children with persistent diarrhea. It is possible that the tight attachment of EPEC to the effaced small bowel mucosa would have made small bowel aspirates more sensitive than stool cultures in identifying this organism (46). In a study from Brazil that did examine the small bowel fluid of children with persistent diarrhea, only 2 of 12 children studied had EPEC organisms identified, and then in small concentrations (47). Studies from India found that EPEC was more frequently cultured from the stool than from the small bowel fluid of children with persistent diarrhea (40).

The enteroaggregative E. coli (EAggEc) were recently identified as potential pathogens associated with diarrheal illness and in particular persistent diarrheal illness (48). To date these organisms have been identified more often in children with persistent diarrhea than in children with acute diarrhea or in children without diarrhea in Mexico, Brazil, India, and a rural community in Bangladesh (30,49–52). In these studies the EAggEc were associated with 19–53% of all episodes of persistent diarrhea, with 8–24% of episodes of acute diarrhea and were identified in 5–19% of stools from matched control children without diarrhea. Conversely, these organisms were not associated with persistent diarrhea in other studies done in Matlab, Bangladesh, in Peru, and in aboriginal children in Australia (45,53,54). Little is known about the clinical illness caused by the EAggEc, but the EAggEc were associated with bloody stool in the study done in Mexico (49). Studies to date have suggested that the EAggEc are a heterogeneous group of organisms with the same adherence phenotype and that strains from various geographic locales may harbor different virulence traits.

Another group of *E. coli*, those that adhere diffusely to cells in tissue culture rather than in the localized pattern of the EPEC or the stacked brick pattern of the EAggEc, has been less consistently associated with diarrheal disease. These diffusely adherent organisms were associated more frequently with persistent diarrhea in one study in Bangladesh and in older aboriginal children in Australia (53,54). The significance of these associations is not known.

The agents of dysenteric diarrheal illnesses have been associated with severe and complicated diarrheal illnesses but these have not been consistently documented to be prolonged illnesses. The incidence of shigellosis varies widely by geographic area, which has complicated studies of this pathogen in many parts of the developing world. The incidence of shigellosis is particularly high in Bangladesh; but in community studies of persistent diarrhea, *Shigella* was isolated in 5–9% of persistent diarrhea (30,53), rates that were not higher than those seen with acute diarrheal illness. Many diarrheal disease treatment regimens for children in the developing world suggest empiric antibiotics at presentation for bloody diarrheal disease, and this may explain the low incidence of *Shigella* in some studies of persistent diarrhea. As illnesses caused by *Shigella* may be more severe, studies of persistent diarrhea in patients requiring hospitalization might be of assistance in determining the role of *Shigella* in persistent diarrhea.

Other bacterial agents associated with dysentery include the nontyphoidal *Salmonella*, which were isolated more often from children with persistent diarrhea than from control children without diarrhea in a study done in northern India (52). *Campylobacter* has also been associated with persistent and relapsing diarrheal disease in both the developed and developing world. While these illnesses may be protracted in immunocompromised patients in the developed world, there are few data to establish a connection between severe malnutrition or cutaneous anergy and prolonged *Campylobacter* diarrhea in children in the developing world (55). Additionally, data regarding *Campylobacter* as a cause of persistent diarrhea is complicated by an extremely high asymptomatic carriage rate by children in parts of the developing world, with as many as 16% of children in South Africa, 25% of children in southern India, and 39% of 1-year-old children in Bangladesh found to harbor *Campylobacter* when free from diarrhea (56–58). In a study of persistent diarrhea done in a rural community in Bangladesh, *Campylobacter* was isolated from 8% of children with persistent diarrhea when they were cultured on day 14 of the persistent illness as opposed to 1–2% of children cultured at the onset of illness. *Campylobacter* was isolated at the same frequency of 8% in stools from nondiarrheal control children (30). A study done recently in Lima, Peru found *Campylobacter* to be isolated consistently from stools of children with persistent diarrhea over a 3-week period; however, the numbers of children with *Campylobacter* in this group was very small.

Viral Agents

Rotavirus is the only viral agent that has been included in routine studies of etiological agents in diarrheal illness in children in the developing world. While rotavirus has been documented as a cause of persistent diarrheal disease, its true role in causation of disease is as complicated as that discussed above for *Campylobacter*. Rotavirus has not been consistently identified more frequently from stools of children with prolonged diarrhea than from children with acute diarrhea although it can cause diarrhea that may persist for longer than 14 days. In diarrhea in the rural community in Bangladesh, it was identified more frequently on day 14 of the persistent illnesses than it was at the outset of the diarrheal illness. However, it was no more common in persistent than acute cases. In an earlier study from Bangladesh, 3% of all rotaviral illnesses were prolonged beyond 20 days (26).

Parasitic Agents

Giardia lamblia is one of the most commonly recognized intestinal protozoa and may routinely and asymptomatically colonize the intestines of up to 20% of children under the age of 5 years (59). As discussed with the *Campylobacter* and rotavirus above, it becomes extremely difficult to discern the true contribution of such highly endemic potential pathogens. There is a report of one child from Costa Rica who developed diarrhea at the age of 14 months that persisted for the following 2 years who was consistently found to carry and excrete *Giardia* during that period. *Giardia* was found in 18 of the 22 stools examined during that 2-year period (60). Two pieces of intriguing data that may be pertinent to understanding the role of *Giardia* in prolonged diarrheal illnesses were recently reported. Various clones of *Giardia* have been identified each of which has a distinctive phenotype. The clones varied in their response to serum cytotoxicity, ability to initiate infections in the intestine of an animal model, clinical severity of infection, and time to clear the intestine of the infection (61). Additionally, it has been reported that children in the Gambia with persistent diarrhea and giardiasis did not develop a *Giardia*-specific IgA antibody to a 57-kDa heat shock antigen, whereas those children who cleared giardia from their intestine had a clear response to the same heat shock antigen (62).

Chronic, nondysenteric amebiasis was originally described in West Pakistan as a syndrome of intermittent diarrhea with mucus, flatus, weight loss, food intolerance, and abdominal pain for months to years (63). A retrospective study of amebiasis in Bangladesh revealed that amebic dysentery was associated with a longer duration of symptoms and more severe malnutrition than the nonamebic diarrheal illnesses seen at the same hospital; this

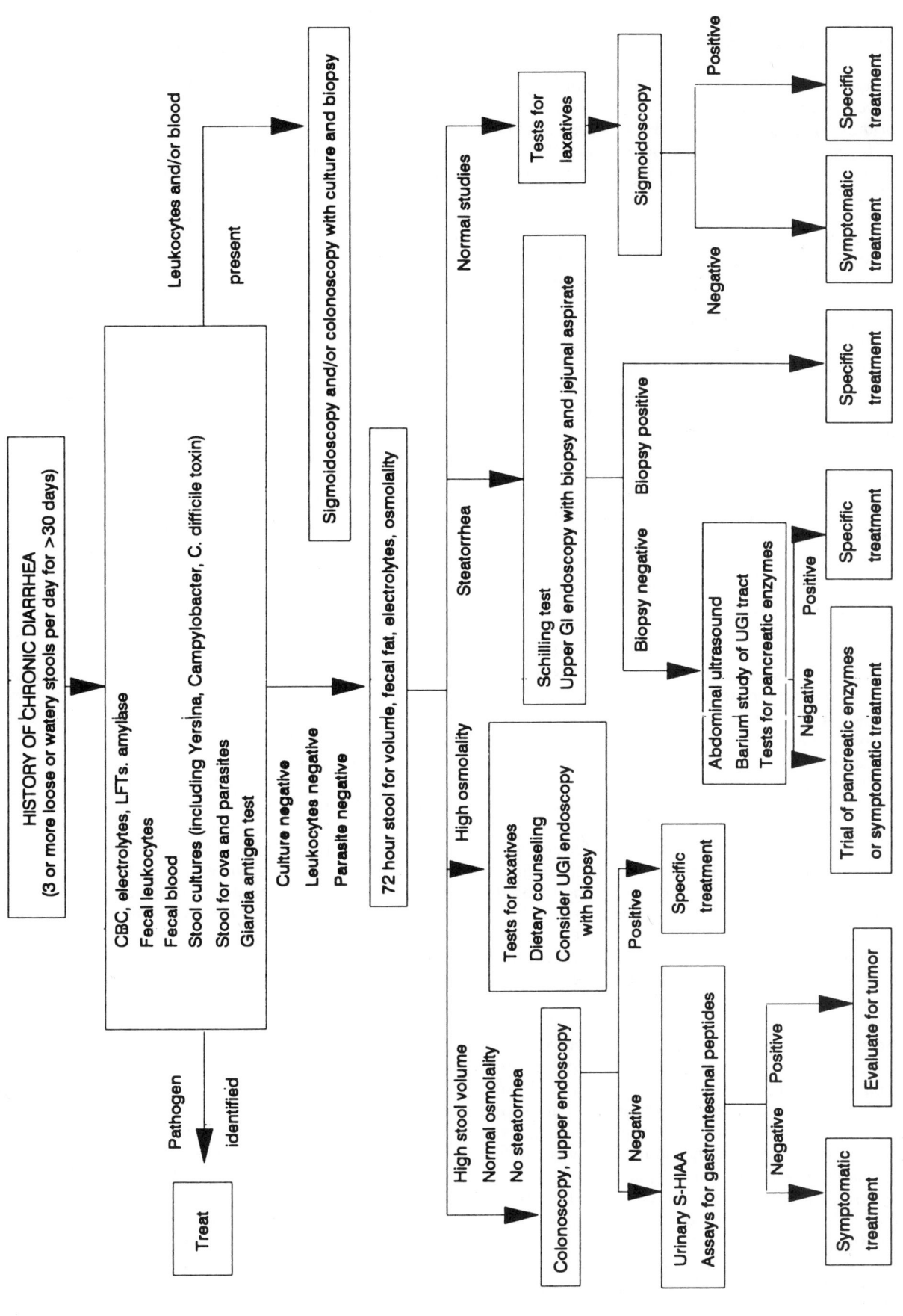

FIG. 3. Algorithm for the workup of chronic diarrhea.

syndrome occurred in persons of all ages including children, but was not seen in infants under the age of one year (64).

As techniques for identifying cryptosporidium in stool have improved, the ability to recognize the association of cryptosporidium with persistent diarrheal disease in children in the developing world has also increased. Although cryptosporidium had been recognized as a diarrheal pathogen since the turn of the century, it came to attention as a cause of severe watery diarrheal disease in HIV-positive patients early in the 1980s. Only recently has it been included in studies of etiological agents in persistent diarrhea in the developing world. It was recognized as a sole pathogen in 13% of stools from children with persistent diarrhea in an urban slum in northeastern Brazil and in 6% of stools from children with persistent diarrhea in rural Bangladesh (47,53). In this later study, cryptosporidium was the only recognized pathogen associated specifically with persistent diarrhea and not acute diarrhea, it was also present significantly less frequently in stools of children with acute diarrhea in the Brazilian study.

APPROACH TO A PATIENT WITH CHRONIC DIARRHEA

The differential diagnosis for chronic diarrhea in the immunocompetent host is substantial. As such, a careful history and physical examination are essential to direct the clinical investigation in a timely and cost-effective fashion. The clinician should obtain a detailed history of the diarrhea including appearance, consistency, and frequency of the stools and any associated weight loss or abdominal symptoms. A history of other medical problems, medications, allergies, recent travel, exposure to animals (including pets), well water use, and risk factors for HIV infection should also be elicited. It is especially useful to investigate the epidemiological context of the illness. This includes inquiring about other affected people in the patient's family, work environment, or community. The patient must be carefully questioned about symptoms of fecal incontinence that can occur secondary to anorectal sphincter disruption caused by diabetes mellitus, anorectal surgery, or epesiotomy (1); this is too commonly a missed diagnosis. An effort should be made to look at a stool sample.

Basic laboratory investigation should include a complete blood count, serum electrolytes, serum glucose, and liver function tests. Tests for fecal blood and fecal leukocytes and bacterial cultures of stools must be done. Physicians should be aware that many laboratories do not routinely culture for all bacterial diarrhea pathogens. Organisms that may be missed by routine culture include *Yersinia, Campylobacter, Aeromonas,* and pathogenic *E. coli* serotypes. If these are suspected, the laboratory must be informed. Three stools should be tested for ova and parasites with special stains requested for crytosporidia and cyanobacteria. Because *Giardia* is a common cause of chronic diarrhea, the stool should also be tested for *Giardia* antigens by ELISA. The sensitivity of these assays exceed those of routine ova and parasite examina-

tions (65,66). If there is a history of recent antibiotic use or hospitalization, stools should also be tested for *Clostridium difficile* toxin.

If the stool contains leukocytes and/or blood, the patient has an inflammatory diarrhea. In this case, the next step should be colonoscopy. In addition to gross inspection for pseudomembranes and ulcerative lesions, biopsies should be obtained and the mucosa should be swabbed for culture.

If the patient does not have inflammatory diarrhea, further laboratory investigations should be used to categorize chronic diarrhea into the different physiological categories: secretory, osmotic, or malabsoptive (Figure 3). A 3-day stool sample on a 100 g/day fat diet should be collected and measured for stool volume and fat content. A very high volume suggests a secretory process. This volume will remain high even during fasting. Elevated fecal fat, on the other hand, supports malabsorption. Testing fresh stool for electrolytes and osmolality can also be helpful. A high osmotic gap [osmolality $-2 \times$ (Na + K) > 160 mosmol] supports a diagnosis of osmotic diarrhea while a negative osmotic gap supports a secretory diarrhea (67). While some diarrheal diseases will have characteristics of more than one physiological category, categorizing chronic diarrhea by type may help direct the clinician to the most suitable follow-up tests studies. These studies are outlined in Figure 3.

Once a diagnosis is established, treatment should be directed at the specific etiology for diarrheal disease. If the studies outlined above are all negative and diarrhea persists, a diagnosis of SICD can be made. Unfortunately, treatment options are limited. The patient's diet can be investigated and potentially problematic items (i.e., caffeine, gluten, milk products) restricted. While success with dietary restriction may be limited, self-adjustment of diet often provides the patient with a sense of control over this disease. Opiate antimotility agents can also be expected to provide symptomatic relief in half of the cases. Most importantly, however, the patient should be reassured that although the disease is unpleasant, it is not life threatening. Furthermore, they can be heartened by the knowledge that the illness is virtually always self-limited.

REFERENCES

1. Read NW, Krejs GJ, Read MG, Santa Ana CA, Marawski S, Fordtran J. Chronic diarrhea of unknown origin. *Gastroenterology* 1980;78:264.
2. Osterholm MT, MacDonald KL, White KE, et al. An outbreak of a newly recognized chronic diarrhea syndrome associated with raw milk consumption. *JAMA* 1986;256:484–490.
3. Parsonnet J. Unpublished data.
4. Parsonnet J, Trock SC, Bopp CA, et al. Chronic diarrhea associated with drinking untreated water. *Ann Intern Med* 1989;110:985–991.
5. Harkess J and Oklahoma State Health Department. Unpublished data.
6. Mintz ED, Parsonnet J, Osterholm MT. Chronic idiopathic diarrhea (letter). *N Engl J Med* 1993;328:1713–714.
7. Martin DL, Hoberman LJ. A point source outbreak of chronic diarrhea in Texas: no known exposure to raw milk. *JAMA* 1986;256:469.

8. Mintz ED, Weber JT, Guris D, Tauxe RV. Outbreak of Brainerd type chronic diarrhea among travelers. *Gastroenterology* 1993;104:A747(Abstract).
9. Centers for Disease Control. Unpublished data.
10. Kellow J, Phillips S, Miller L, Osterholm MT, MacDonald KL. Abnormalities of motility and absorption in an outbreak of chronic diarrhea. *Gastroenterology* 1985;88:1442(Abstract).
11. Janda RC, Conklin JL, Mitros FA, Parsonnet J. Multifocal colitis associated with an epidemic of chronic diarrhea. *Gastroenterology* 1991;100:458–464.
12. Myers LL, Shoop DS, Potter ME, Wells JG. Enteric disease in rabbits inoculated with stool filtrates from persons with chronic diarrhea. *J Infect Dis* 1989;159:133–135.
13. Afzalpurkar RG, Schiller LR, Little KH, Santangelo WC, Fordtran JS. The self-limited nature of chronic idiopathic diarrhea. *N Engl J Med* 1992;327:1849–1852.
14. Palmer KR, Corbett CL, Holdsworth CD. Double-blind crossover study comparing loperamide codeine and diphenoxylate in the treatment of chronic diarrhea. *Gastroenterology* 1980; 79:1272–1275.
15. Schiller LR, Hogan RB, Morawski SG, et al. Studies of the prevalence and significance of radiolabeled bile acid malabsorption in a group of patients with idiopathic chronic diarrhea. *Gastroenterology* 1987;92:151–160.
16. Mintz ED, Mishu B, Guris D, Griffin PM. Prevalence of Brainerd type chronic diarrhea among patients of AGA and ACG members. *Gastroenterology* 1993;104:A747(Abstract).
17. Addiss DG, Tauxe RV, Bernard KW. Chronic diarrhoeal illness in US Peace Corps volunteers. *Int J Epidemiol* 1990;19: 217–218.
18. Afzalpurkar RG, Schiller LR, Fordtran JS. Chronic idiopathic diarrhea (letter). *N Engl J Med* 1993;328:1714.
19. Snyder JD, Merson MH. The magnitude of the global problem of acute diarrhoeal disease: a review of active surveillance data. *Bull WHO.* 1982;60:605–613.
20. McAuliffe JF, Shields DS, Auxiliadora de Sousa M, Sakell J, Schorling J, Guerrant RL. Prolonged and recurring diarrhea in the northeast of Brazil: examination of cases from a community-based study. *J Pediatr Gastroenterol Nutr* 1986;5: 902–906.
21. Prazuck T, Tall F, Nacro B, et al. HIV infection and severe malnutrition: a clinical and epidemiological study in Burkina Faso. *AIDS J* 1993;7:103–108.
22. Keusch GT, Thea DM, Kamenga M, et al. Persistent diarrhea associated with AIDS. *Acta Paediatr.* 1992;81 Suppl 381: 45–48.
23. Wanke CA. Infectious etiologies of prolonged diarrhea. In: Kalus G, ed. *Baillere's clinical Tropical medicine and communicable disease.* Vol 3. England: Balliere and Tindall; 1988: 567–590.
24. Joe LK, Rukmono B, Oemijati S, et al. Diarrhoea among infants in a crowded area of Djakarta, Indonesia. A longitudinal study from birth to two years. *Bull WHO* 1966;34:197–210.
25. Gordon JE, Ascoli W, Mata LJ, Guzman MA, Scrimshaw NS. Nutrition and infection field study in Guatemalan villages, 1959–1964. VI. Acute diarrheal disease and nutritional disorders in general disease incidence. *Arch Environ Health* 1968; 16:424–437.
26. Black RE, Merson MH, Rahman AS, et al. A two-year study of bacterial, viral, and parasitic agents associated with diarrhea in rural Bangladesh. *J Infect Dis* 1980;142:660–664.
27. Baqui AH, Black RE, Sack RB, Yunus MD, Siddique AK, Chowdhury HR. Epidemiological and clinical characteristics of acute and persistent diarrhoea in rural Bangladeshi children. *Acta Paediatr* 1992;81 Suppl 381:15–21.
28. Schorling JB, Wanke CA, Schorling SK, McAuliffe JF, de Souza MA, Guerrant RL. A prospective study of persistent diarrhea among children in an urban Brazilian slum. Patterns of occurrence and etiologic agents. *Am J Epidemiol* 1990;132: 144–56.
29. Cruz JR, Bartlett AV, Mendez H, Sibrian R. Epidemiology of persistent diarrhea among Guatemalan rural children. *Acta Paediatr* 1992;81 Suppl 381:22–26.
30. Henry FJ, Udoy AS, Wanke CA, Aziz KM. Epidemiology of

31. persistent diarrhea and etiologic agents in Mirzapur, Bangladesh. *Acta Paediatr* 1992;81 Suppl 381:27–31.
31. Bhandari N, Bhan MK, Sazawal S. Mortality associated with acute watery diarrhea, dysentery and persistent diarrhea in rural north India. *Acta Paediatr* 1992;81 Suppl 381:3–6.
32. Fauveau V, Henry FJ, Briend A, Yunus M, Chakraborty J. Persistent diarrhea as a cause of childhood mortality in rural Bangladesh. *Acta Paediatr* 1992;81 Suppl 381:12–14.
33. Victora CG, Huttly SR, Fuchs SC, Nobre LC, Barros FC. Deaths due to dysentery, acute and persistent diarrhoea among Brazilian infants. *Acta Paediatr* 1992;81 Suppl 381:7–11.
34. Gracey M, Stone DE. Small-intestinal microflora in Autralian aboriginal children with chronic diarrhoea. *Aust N Z J Med* 1972;2:215–219.
35. Coeelo-Ramirez P, Litshitz F. Enteric microflora and carbohydrate intolerance in infants with diarrhea. *Pediatrics* 1982;49: 233–238.
36. Challacombe DN, Richardson JM, Rowe B, Anderson CM. Bacterial microflora of the upper gastrointestinal tract in infants with protracted diarrhoea. *Arch Dis Child* 1974;49:270–277.
37. Heyworth B, Brown J. Jejunal microflora in malnourished Gambian children. *Arch Dis Child* 1975;50:27–33.
38. Rowland MG, Cole TJ, McCollum JP. Weanling diarrhoea in The Gambia: implications of a jejunal intubation study. *Trans R Soc Trop Med Hyg* 1981;75:215–218.
39. Penny ME. The role of the duodenal microflora as a determinant of persistent diarrhoea. *Acta Paediatr* 1992;81 Suppl 381: 114–120.
40. Bhatnagar S, Bhan MK, George C, et al. Is small bowel bacterial overgrowth of pathogenic significance in persistent diarrhea? *Acta Paediatr* 1992;81 Suppl 381:108–113.
41. Wanke CA, Guerrant RL. Small-bowel colonization alone is a cause of diarrhea. *Infect Immun* 1987;55:1924–1926.
42. Schlager TA, Wanke CA, Guerrant RL. Net fluid secretion and impaired villous function induced by colonization of the small intestine by nontoxigenic colonizing *Escherichia coli*. *Infect Immun* 1990;58:1337–1343.
43. Belitsos PC, Greenson JK, Yardley JH, Sisler JR, Bartlett JG. Association of gastric hypoacidity with opportunistic enteric infections in patients with AIDS. *J Infect Dis* 1992;166:277–284.
44. Wanke C. Unpublished data.
45. Lanata CF, Black RE, Maurtua D, et al. Etiologic agents in acute vs persistent diarrhea in children under three years of age in peri-urban Lima, Peru. *Acta Paediatr* 1992;81 Suppl 381: 32–38.
46. Ulshen MH, Rollo JL. Pathogenesis of escherichia coli gastroenteritis in man—another mechanism. *N Engl J Med* 1980; 302:99–101.
47. Lima AA, Fang G, Schorling JB, et al. Persistent diarrhea in northeast Brazil: etiologies and interactions with malnutrition. *Acta Paediatr* 1992;81 Suppl 381:39–44.
48. Vial PA, Robins-Browne R, Lior H, et al. Characterization of enteroadherent-aggregative Escherichia coli, a putative agent of diarrheal disease. *J Infect Dis* 1988;158:70–79.
49. Cravioto A, Tello A, Navarro A, et al. Association of *Escherichia coli* HEp-2 adherence patterns with type and duration of diarrhoea. *Lancet* 1991;337:262–264.
50. Wanke CA, Schorling JB, Barrett LJ, Desouza MA, Guerrant RL. Potential role of adherence traits of Escherichia coli in persistent diarrhea in an urban Brazilian slum. *Pediatr Infect Dis J* 1991;10:746–751.
51. Bhan MK, Raj P, Levine MM, et al. Enteroaggregative *Escherichia coli* associated with persistent diarrhea in a cohort of rural children in India. *J Infect Dis* 1989;159:1061–1064.
52. Bhan MK, Khoshoo V, Sommerfelt H, Raj P, Sazawal S, Srivastava R. Enteroaggregative *Escherichia coli* and *Salmonella* associated with nondysenteric persistent diarrhea. *Pediatr Infect Dis J* 1989;8:499–502.
53. Baqui AH, Sack RB, Black RE, et al. Enteropathogens associated with acute and persistent diarrhea in Bangladeshi children less than 5 years of age. *J Infect Dis* 1992;166:792–796.
54. Gunzburg ST, Chang BJ, Elliott SJ, Burke V, Gracey M. Diffuse and enteroaggregative patterns of adherence of enteric

Escherichia coli isolated from aboriginal children from the Kimberley region of Western Australia. *J Infect Dis* 1993;167: 755–758.

55. Lloyd-Evans N, Drasar BS, Tomkins AM. A comparison of the prevalence of campylobacter, Shigellae and Salmonellae in faeces of malnourished and well nourished children in the Gambia and Northern Nigeria. Trans R Soc Trop Med Hyg. 1983; 77:245–247.

56. Bokkenheuser VD, Richardson NJ, Bryner JH, et al. Detection of enteric campylobacteriosis in children. *J Clin Microbiol* 1979;9:227–232.

57. Mathan VI, Rajan DP, Klipstein FA, Engert RF. Enterotoxigenic *Campylobacter jejuni* among children in South India (letter). *Lancet* 1984;2:981.

58. Blaser MJ, Glass RI, Huq MI, Stoll B, Kibriya GM, Alim AR. Isolation of *Campylobacter* fetus subsp. *jejuni* from Bangladeshi children. *J Clin Microbiol* 1980;12:744–747.

59. WHO Scientific Working Group. Parasite-related diarrheas. *Bulletin WHO* 1980;53:819–830.

60. Mata L, Urrutia JJ, Simmon A. Infectious agents in acute and chronic diarrhea of childhood. In: Lebenthal E, ed. *Chronic diarrhea in children*. New York: Raven Press; 1984:237–257.

61. Udezulu IA, Visvesvara GS, Moss DM, Leitch GJ. Isolation of two *Giardia lamblia* (WB strain) clones with distinct surface protein and antigenic profiles and differing infectivity and virulence. *Infect Immun* 1992;60:2274–2280.

62. Char S, Cevallos AM, Yamson P, Sullivan PB, Neale G, Farthing MJ. Impaired IgA response to *Giardia* heat shock antigen in children with persistent diarrhoea and giardiasis. *Gut* 1993; 34:38–40.

63. Haider Z, Rasul A. Chronic nondysenteric intestinal amoebiasis: a review of 159 cases. *J Pakistan Med Assoc* 1975;75:78.

64. Wanke C, Butler T, Islam M. Epidemiologic and clinical features of invasive amebiasis in Bangladesh: a case-control comparison with other diarrheal diseases and postmortem findings. *Am J Trop Med Hyg* 1988;38:335–341.

65. Addiss DG, Mathews HM, Stewart JM, et al. Evaluation of a commercially available enzyme-linked immunosorbent assay for *Giardia lamblia* antigen in stool. *J Clin Microbiol* 1991;29: 1137–1142.

66. Janoff EN, Craft JC, Pickering LK, et al. Diagnosis of *Giardia lamblia* infections by detection of parasite-specific antigens. *J Clin Microbiol* 1989;27:431–435.

67. Shiau Y, Feldman GM, Resnick MA, Coff PM. Stool electrolyte and osmolality measurements in the evaluation of diarrheal disorders. *Ann Intern Med* 1985;102:773–775.

68. Oishi I, Kimura T, Murakami T, et al. Serial observations of chronic rotavirus infection in an immunodeficient child. *Microbiol Immunol* 1991;35:953–961.

69. Buckner FS, Pomeroy C. Cytomegalovirus disease of the gastrointestinal tract in patients without AIDS. *Clin Infect Dis* 1993;17:644–656.

70. Meiselman MS, Cello JP, Margaretten W. Cytomegalovirus colitis. Report of the clinical, endoscopic, and pathologic findings in two patients with the acquired immune deficiency syndrome. *Gastroenterology* 1985;88:171–175.

71. Simon D, Brandt LJ. Diarrhea in patients with the acquired immunodeficiency syndrome. *Gastroenterology* 1993;105: 1238–1242.

72. Janoff EN, Orenstein JM, Manischewitz JF, Smith PD. Adenovirus colitis in the acquired immunodeficiency syndrome. *Gastroenterology* 1991;100:976–979.

73. Grohmann GS, Glass RI, Pereira HG, et al. Enteric viruses and diarrhea in HIV-infected patients. Enteric Opportunistic Infections Working Group. *N Engl J Med* 1993;329:14–20.

74. King GE, Werner SB, Kizer KW. Epidemiology of *Aeromonas* infections in California. *Clin Infect Dis* 1992;15:449–452.

75. San Joaquin VH, Pickett DA. Aeromonas-associated gastroenteritis in children. *Pediatr Infect Dis J* 1988;7:53–57.

76. Holmberg SD, Schell WL, Fanning GR, et al. Aeromonas intestinal infections in the United States. *Ann Intern Med* 1986;105: 683–689.

77. Blaser MJ, Wells JG, Feldman RA, Pollard RA, Allen JR.

Campylobacter enteritis in the United States. A multicenter study. *Ann Intern Med* 1983;98:360–365.

78. Smalley JR, Klish WJ, Brown MR, Campbell MA. Chronic diarrhea associated with campylobacter. *Clin Pediatr (Phila)*. 1982;21:220.

79. Darbas H, Pelous C, Jean A, et al. [Chronic diarrhea caused by *Campylobacter jejuni* in a patient with AIDS] Diarrhee chronique due a *Campylobacter jejuni* chez un malade atteint de SIDA. *Pathol Biol (Paris)* 1988;36:888–890.

80. Perlman DM, Ampel NM, Schifman RB, et al. Persistent *Campylobacter jejuni* infections in patients infected with the human immunodeficiency virus (HIV). *Ann Intern Med* 1988; 108:540–546.

81. San Joaquin VH, Welch DF. *Campylobacter* enteritis. A 3-year experience. *Clin Pediatr (Phila)*. 1984;23:311–316.

82. Bartlett JG. Antibiotic-associated pseudomembranous colitis. *Rev Infect Dis* 1979;1:530–540.

83. Schwan A, Sjolin S, Trottestam U, Aronsson B. Relapsing Clostridium difficile enterocolitis cured by rectal infusion of normal faeces. *Scand J Infect Dis* 1984;16:211–215.

84. Heiner AM, DiSario JA, Carroll K, Cohen S, Evans TG, Shigeoka AO. Dysgonic fermenter-3: a bacterium associated with diarrhea in immunocompromised hosts. *Am J Gastroenterology* 1992;87:1629–1630.

85. Hill SM, Phillips AD, Walker-Smith JA. Enteropathogenic *Escherichia coli* and life threatening chronic diarrhoea. *Gut* 1991;32:154–158.

86. Clausen CR, Christie DL. Chronic diarrhea in infants caused by adherent enteropathogenic *Escherichia coli*. *J Pediatr* 1982; 100:358–361.

87. Lacroix J, Delage G, Gosselin F, Chicoine L. Severe protracted diarrhea due to multiresistant adherent *Escherichia coli*. *Am J Dis Child* 1984;138:693–696.

88. Rothbaum R, McAdams AJ, Giannella R, Partin JC. A clinicopathologic study of enterocyte-adherent *Escherichia coli:* a cause of protracted diarrhea in infants. *Gastroenterology* 1982; 83:441–454.

89. Klimach OE, Ormerod LP. Gastrointestinal tuberculosis: a retrospective review of 109 cases in a district general hospital. *Q J Med* 1985;56:569–578.

90. Gillin JS, Urmacher C, West R, Shike M. Disseminated *Mycobacterium avium-intracellulare* infection in acquired immunodeficiency syndrome mimicking Whipple's disease. *Gastroenterology* 1983;85:1187–1191.

91. Penn RG, Giger DK, Knoop FC, Preheim LC. *Plesiomonas shigelloides* overgrowth in the small intestine. *J Clin Microbiol* 1982;15:869–872.

92. Glynn JR, Palmer SR. Incubation period, severity of disease, and infecting dose: evidence from a Salmonella outbreak. *Am J Epidemiol* 1992;136:1369–1377.

93. Dobbins WO. Whipple's disease. In: Mandell GL, Douglas RG, Bennett JE, eds. *Principles and practice of infectious diseases*. 3rd ed. New York: Churchill Livingstone; 1990:909–911.

94. Ostroff SM, Kapperud G, Lassen J, Aasen S, Tauxe RV. Clinical features of sporadic *Yersinia enterocolitica* infections in Norway. *J Infect Dis* 1992;1166:812–817.

95. Mollee T, Tilse M. *Yersinia enterocolitica*. Isolation from faeces of adults and children in Queensland. *Med J Aust* 1985; 143:488–489.

96. Saebo A, Lassen J. Acute and chronic gastrointestinal manifestations associated with *Yersinia enterocolitica* infection. A Norwegian 10-year follow-up study on 458 hospitalized patients. *Ann Surg* 1992;215:250–255.

97. Saebo A, Lassen J. A survey of acute and chronic disease associated with *Yersinia enterocolitica* infection. A Norwegian 10-year follow-up study on 458 hospitalized patients. *Scand J Infect Dis* 1991;23:517–527.

98. Gupta TP, Ehrinpreis MN. *Candida*-associated diarrhea in hospitalized patients. *Gastroenterology* 1990;98:780–785.

99. Kain KC, Noble MA, Freeman HJ, Barteluk RL. Epidemiology and clinical features associated with *Blastocystis hominis* infection. *Diagn Microbiol Infect Dis* 1987;8:235–244.

100. Doyle PW, Helgason MM, Mathias RG, Proctor EM. Epide-

miology and pathogenicity of *Blastocystis hominis*. *J Clin Microbiol* 1990;28:116–121.

101. Wolfson JS, Richter JM, Waldron MA, Weber DJ, McCarthy DM, Hopkins CC. Cryptosporidiosis in immunocompetent patients. *N Engl J Med* 1985;312:1278–1282.

102. Smith PM. Traveller's diarrhoea associated with a cyanobacterium-like body (letter). *Med J Aust* 1993;158:724.

103. Anonymous. Outbreaks of diarrheal illness associated with cyanobacteria (blue-green algae)-like bodies—Chicago and Nepal, 1989 and 1990. *MMWR* 1991;40:325–327.

104. Long EG, Ebrahimzadeh A, White EH, Swisher B, Callaway CS. Alga associated with diarrhea in patients with acquired immunodeficiency syndrome and in travelers. *J Clin Microbiol* 1990;28:1101–1104.

105. Ortega YR, Sterling CR, Gilman RH, Cama VA, Diaz F. Cyclospora species—a new protozoan pathogen of humans. *N Engl J Med* 1993;328:1308–1312.

106. Matseshe JW, Phillips SF. Chronic diarrhea. A practical approach. *Med Clin North Am* 1978;62:141–154.

107. Adams EB, MacLeod IN. Invasive amebiasis. I. Amebic dysentery and its complications. *Medicine* 1977;56:315–323.

108. Butler T, Middleton FG, Earnest DL, Strickland GT. Chronic and recurrent diarrhea in American servicemen in Vietnam. An evaluation of etiology and small bowel structure and function. *Arch Intern Med* 1973;132:373–377.

109. Birkhead G, Vogt RL. Epidemiologic surveillance for endemic *Giardia lamblia* infection in Vermont: the roles of waterborne and person-to-person transmission. *Am J Epidemiol* 1989;129: 762–768.

110. Shaffer N, Moore L. Chronic travelers' diarrhea in a normal host due to *Isospora belli*. *J Infect Dis* 1989;159:596–597.

111. DeHovitz JA, Pape JW, Boncy M, Johnson WD. Clinical manifestations and therapy of Isospora belli infection in patients with the acquired immunodeficiency syndrome. *N Engl J Med* 1986;315:87–90.

112. Soave R, Johnson WD. *Cryptosporidium* and *Isospora belli* infection. *J Infect Dis* 1988;57:225–229.

113. Pol S, Roman CA, Richard S, et al. Microsporidia infection in patients with the human immunodeficiency virus and unexplained cholangitis. *N Engl J Med* 1993;328:95–99.

114. Eeftinck Schattenkerk JKM, Van Gool T, Van Ketel RJ, et al. Clinical significance of small-intestinal microsporidiosis in HIV-1-infected individuals. *Lancet* 1991;337:895–898.

115. Orenstein JM, Chiang J, Steinberg W, Smith PD, Rotterdam H, Kotler DP. Intestinal microsporidiosis as a cause of diarrhea in human immunodeficiency virus-infected patients: a report of 20 cases. *Hum Pathol* 1990;21:475–481.

116. Centers for Disease Control. Unpublished data.

Infections of the Gastrointestinal Tract, edited by M. J. Blaser, P. D. Smith, J. I. Ravdin, H. B. Greenberg, and R. L. Guerrant Raven Press, Ltd., New York © 1995.

CHAPTER 24

Enteric Fever

Richard B. Hornick

Enteric fever is a life-threatening infectious process that involves numerous organs and is manifested by prolonged fever, persistent bacteremia, and, as the name implies, significant inflammatory reaction in the intestines, especially the lymphoid tissue. In the early part of the nineteenth century, Bretonneau (1) in Paris described these latter lesions in patients with typhoid fever as "boil of the intestine" (dothoienenterite). Perforation through this severely compromised tissue usually resulted in the death of the diseased host. Appropriate antibiotic therapy prevents this catastrophe in most patients with typhoid fever, the classic example of enteric fever. *Salmonella* species are the bacteria that usually initiate this syndrome.

MICROBIOLOGY

Bacterial pathogens that can penetrate the epithelial lining and infect cells in Peyer's patches in the distal ileum have the potential to cause enteric fever. The most common etiological agent is *Salmonella typhi*. These organisms induce a wide spectrum of clinical manifestations from asymptomatic infections (2) to septic shock states and a unique chronic carrier condition. About 10–15% of patients are infected with other invasive bacterial species. What were formerly called the paratyphoid strains A, B, and C are the usual pathogens for most of this latter group. These strains are now known as *S. paratyphi, S. schott-mülleri,* and *S. hirschfeldii*. Other species of *Salmonella* may occasionally cause this infection, e.g., *S. sendai*. These species and the paratyphoid organisms usually induce a milder form of disease and rarely cause the chronic carrier state. *Yersinia enterocolitica* rarely may cause enteric fever. *Francisella tularensis* infection can produce typhoidal disease that is akin to enteric fever.

S. typhi are gram-negative bacilli that utilize glucose, maltose, and mannitol, but not sucrose or fructose in culture media. *S. typhi,* unlike other *Salmonella,* does not produce gas during fermentation of glucose in culture media. The virulence factors that enable salmonellae to produce enteric fever are only partially understood (see chapter by Miller, Pegues, and Hohmann). It is necessary to consider the importance of the cell wall as a virulence factor. Strains that are deficient in cell wall components, so-called "rough strains," are nonpathogenic and useful as oral vaccines (vide infra). The cell wall of *S. typhi* is a complex structure. The outer portion contains the potent, heat-stable, biologically active macromolecule endotoxin. Structurally, it is a lipopolysaccharide composed of three layers; the innermost is the lipid portion and it binds the other two layers to the remainder of the cell wall. The middle layer, or R core (R = rough strain), links the lipid with the outer section, the polysaccharide. The latter consists of repeating chains of sugars that determine the antigenic nature of the O antigen. When the polysaccharide side chains are removed or are not produced, exposing the middle or R core, the characteristic rough colonies on agar plates are produced. An "envelope," heat-labile antigen, Vi (for virulence), covers the O antigen and renders the strain nonagglutinable in the presence of "O"-specific antiserum (3). The Vi antigen interferes with phagocytosis by leukocytes, prevents binding by C3b, and slows the lysis of the salmonellae by hydrogen peroxide once ingested by the phagocytes (4). Strains lacking Vi antigen are rarely cultured from patients with enteric fever and are less virulent for healthy adults than are Vi-containing strains (5). The Vi antigen is almost always identified on *S. typhi* and *S. hirschfeldii* (paratyphoid C), and rarely on *Citrobacter freundii* strains. Phage typing of the Vi antigen has identified 80 distinct types. Antibodies to the Vi antigen may appear late in the course of typhoid fever, in low titer, and disappear during the convalescent stage. Such antibodies also are persistent in some patients who become chronic carriers. The motility of *Salmonella* is due to the flagellae, the H antigen. The virulence of strains lacking the H antigen is unknown; however, their conservation suggests a critical role in pathogenesis. The H and O antigens have been the two antigens used to classify *Salmonella* in the Kaufman–White (6) schema.

R. B. Hornick: Orlando Regional Healthcare System, Orlando, Florida 32806.

These identify the more than 2000 *Salmonella* serotypes. Among the many combinations of O and H antigens that distinguish these serotypes, *S. typhi* always has types 9 and 12, O antigens and dH, H antigen. At least 140 *Salmonella* have these and other O antigens as part of their cell wall. In addition, there are over 60 strains that have dH as part of their H antigen. The classic Widal reaction measures antibodies to the O and H antigens (7). This has been the most common serological test for diagnostic purposes. With many antigens shared with other *Salmonella,* the Widal is not a specific screening test for epidemiological purposes (see "Diagnostic Measures" below). A number of plasmids have been identified in typhoid bacilli. Most are associated with the ability to resist inhibitory activity of antibiotics. Study of these plasmids has not demonstrated any correlation with the clinical severity of disease (8). Other unknown factors must be involved. A variety of studies have indicated the clonal nature of *S. typhi* (8). In a comparison of strains isolated from Peru and Indonesia, including envelope protein profiles, chromosome restriction endonuclease digestion patterns, and immune responses to envelope antigens, genotypic and phenotypic differences were noted, but there was no correlation between strain characteristics and disease severity.

PATHOGENESIS

S. typhi are facultative intracellular organisms that resist intracellular destruction causing acute inflammatory illnesses. These bacteria are ingested with food or water, and do not invade the oropharyngeal mucosal linings. However, there are inflammatory changes, including granulomas seen in biopsy specimens from the upper small intestine taken during the incubation period of volunteers (9). These changes were not associated with any symptoms or signs of disease. Convalescent biopsies were normal. The primary focus of enteric fever is in the ileum and colon. In order for the etiological agents to be able to penetrate the epithelial cell lining of the lower intestinal tract, multiply in the lamina propria, and access the lymphatic and vascular circulations, they must survive the nonspecific and at times specific defense mechanisms of the gut. Volunteer studies have demonstrated that large numbers of one strain of *S. typhi* are necessary to initiate infection and disease in a high proportion of study subjects (5). Ingestion of 10^3 bacterial cells failed to produce disease, but evidence of infection was present; 10^5 organisms caused disease in 35% of healthy adult males; ingestion of 10^7 yielded an attack rate of 50%; and ingestion of 10^9 caused more than 90% to become ill. The organisms involved had had multiple *in vitro* passages since the original isolation; whether this has an effect in diminishing the virulence of the strain is unknown. The strain was from a carrier who had infected several family members. The relative degree of virulence of this strain for humans compared to others is also unknown. In some outbreak investigations it has been concluded that under actual field conditions fewer organisms ($<10^3$) may cause disease although with far lower attack rates (10). It is difficult under these circumstances to be certain about the virulence and size

of the inoculum once the epidemic has started, since these are retrospective analyses. It is apparent from the volunteer studies that small numbers of organisms can cause as severe an illness as large doses. The larger the inoculum, however, the shorter the incubation period. Thus, in the volunteer studies, the 10^5 dose was associated with an average incubation period of 13.2 days, and after the 10^9 dose the incubation period was 6 days. In many reported outbreaks of enteric fever, the incubation period averages 10–13 days. These inocula after ingestion were able to resist annihilation in the acid milieu of the stomach; withstand the pressures of host antibacterial substances, such as lysozymes and proteolytic enzymes, rapid transit, and commensal bacteria, to mention a few obvious obstacles; and penetrate the M cells of Peyer's patches and the lamina propria. The cell wall appears to be significant in the invasive process. Surface proteins produced by *Salmonella* can induce nonphagocytic cells to act as phagocytes and envelop the adherent bacteria (11); mutant strains that are avirulent for animals are unable to synthesize these proteins. The ingestion occurs through a ruffling of the cell wall that engulfs the organism. One essential element for growth of *S. typhi* is iron; in the gut lumen and in the lamina propria, as well as in some intracellular environments, little iron is available. These organisms, under these circumstances, also can express proteins such as enterochelin allowing capture of iron (12). Patients with typhoid fever produce antibodies to enterochelin. Other virulence factors are yet to be identified.

The increasing local concentration of bacteria in Peyer's patches induces a hyperplastic state of the lymphatic tissue, which may lead to abdominal pain in the patient. A high concentration of endotoxin in the Peyer's patch can lead to tissue necrosis, vascular thrombosis, and can act as a stimulus to initiate the process leading to a continuous febrile response (13). The entire ileum may be hyperemic because of the inflammatory process. The pathological changes occurring in the Peyer's patches can lead to perforation of the ileum or an intestinal hemorrhage, which are two of the significant complications of enteric fever. Peyer's patches extend from the mucosal surface to the serosal surface, facilitating the opportunity for perforation. In those patients who undergo laparotomy because of a perforation, the perforation usually is located in the antimesenteric surface of the ileum (14). Ulcerations without perforation also may be present in the ileum predominantly or in the colon.

These changes are the end results of unchecked multiplication of the pathogenic bacteria in the submucosal regions. Fortunately, with early and appropriate antibacterial therapy, such extreme life-threatening changes are rare. In the preantibiotic era the majority of patients were able to contain the inflammatory changes in the lamina propria or Peyer's patches; only about 3% developed perforations. Nevertheless, *S. typhi,* even though phagocytosized by monocytes and polymorphonuclear leukocytes, can remain viable and be transported to infect other elements of the reticuloendothelial system (RES). The bacteremia originates from lymphoid tissue in the RES and intestine. The liver reacts to invasion by the pathogens by producing granulomatous lesions and diffuse inflammatory changes with resulting hepatomegaly. Consistent with its generalized spread to organs with high RES concentrations, splenomegaly also occurs, and *S. typhi* can be isolated from bone marrow. *S. typhi* has been isolated from bone marrow as long as 1 year after successful treatment for typhoid fever. In addition, *S. typhi* and other enteric fever bacteria are discharged from the liver into the biliary tract, thereby infecting the gallbladder and distributing the pathogens back into the duodenum. Thus *S. typhi* can induce the acute febrile enteric fever syndrome in healthy persons and in a few patients, persist in the gallbladder producing the chronic carrier state. Other organ systems (e.g., lungs, central nervous system, skin) may develop significant pathological changes as a consequence of the bacteremia.

EPIDEMIOLOGY

The pathogens that cause enteric fever are acquired from contaminated food or water. *S. typhi* has no reservoir other than humans so the ultimate source of every infection is an infected person, usually a chronic carrier. As noted above, these organisms can persist intracellularly for a prolonged period. In carriers, they colonize diseased gallbladders. Most often they are contained inside gallstones; *S. typhi* and associated inflammatory debris may serve as a nidus for stone formation. *S. typhi* infects the epithelial lining of the gallbladder creating a chronically inflamed mucosa, which presumably interferes with normal emptying properties and aids in the formation of stones. This continuously inflamed environment is conducive to the development of adenocarcinoma of the gallbladder (15). Chronic carriers, especially those living in endemic areas, are more likely to develop this form of cancer than noncarriers with cholelithiasis. The previously healthy gallbladder is essentially resistant to induction of the carrier state. Chronic carriers may shed huge numbers of *S. typhi* in the stool, e.g., 10^6–10^{10} organisms per gram (16). However low-level or intermittent excretion is well documented (16). Despite the large number of virulent organisms in the lumen of the gut, chronic carriers do not develop enteric fever, presumably due to acquired immunity; the organisms remain confined in the lumen of the intestines. Those carriers who are food handlers and who do not wash their hands carefully can easily contaminate food; under proper environmental conditions, multiplication occurs and consumers are at risk. "Typhoid Mary," who served as a household cook, was the classic example (17). She worked for several families in and around New York City and was responsible for "at least 53 cases of typhoid fever and 3 deaths" (17). The investigation of the epidemics she started (1901–1915) cleared up the mystery that carriers—not bad air, food, or water—were the source of typhoid epidemics. The isolation of *S. typhi* from stool specimens was not available before 1901–1907 in the USA. As the technique became commonplace, the identification of carriers was finally achieved (17). Contaminated water is the most common source of organisms in developing countries. The World Health Organization (WHO) has been attempting to pro-

vide adequate water supplies and sewage systems for late-developing countries for the past 20 years. Civil unrest and wars as well as limited funds have disrupted these plans in some countries where typhoid is endemic. In the USA, the purification and chlorination of water supplies in the early twentieth century were the most significant public health measures instituted to control typhoid fever. Very dramatic declines in incidences occurred within months when such measures were initiated in particular localities (18). In Wheeling, West Virginia, the number of cases per year dropped from 91 to 23 after chlorination of the water supplied by the Ohio River. When filtration was added to the water processing, the number fell to 5. During this period, 1917 to 1928, the population increased from 41,587 to 60,816, further emphasizing the importance of water purification. The number of cases in the USA that were reported annually for the period 1982–1992 ranged from 360 to 500. Most of these cases occur in travelers to or immigrants from endemic countries. The majority of reported cases are from California and New York City. Currently, the number of deaths resulting from typhoid ranged from 0 to 3 per year. From 1980 to 1989, there were 4 years without any mortality. Occasional cases of typhoid fever occur in microbiology laboratory students and workers due to exposure to contaminated specimens, or "unknown" organisms as part of proficiency testing (19,20).

Small outbreaks of typhoid fever continue to occur in the USA, usually caused by a carrier who is involved in food preparation (21). Some of these carriers are recent immigrants from areas where enteric fever remains endemic. Since humans are the major reservoir for *S. typhi,* and it is spread by fecal–oral transmission, the use of toilet paper and careful handwashing serves to interdict this method of dispersal.

Carriers of paratyphoid strains are rare in the USA. These organisms also do not persist in the human host as long as *S. typhi*. The sources of these strains are the same as for *S. typhi,* but carriage is usually 4–6 months rather than for years postconvalescence.

Women are three times as likely to become typhoid carriers as men. They have a higher prevalence of gallbladder disease due to pregnancy and birth control pills. The incidence of carriers increases with age, so that women over age 40 developing typhoid fever (without specific therapy) had a 16% chance of developing chronic carriage (22). Younger women had a 2–4% chance. Many carriers give no history of having had a typhoid-like illness. (Typhoid Mary was such an example.) The incidence of carriers developing in patients recovering from typhoid fever and living in endemic areas is difficult to quantify because of lack of follow-up. However, some surveys estimate the number to be 1–3%, despite antibiotic therapy. Most carriers have high-titer serum antibodies to the Vi antigen (23), a useful survey tool, but difficult to utilize in developing countries. When identified, usually after an outbreak of enteric fever, carriers can be cured by cholecystectomy in order to remove the gallstones, and a few may be "cured" by prolonged antibiotic treatment. Many antibiotics have been tried without surgery and claimed to be effective only to have reappearance of positive stool cultures 4–5 years later (see chapter by Miller, Pegues, and Hohmann). *S. typhi* inside gallstones is shielded from the killing effect of antibiotics. The quinolone antibiotics were recently found to eliminate, perhaps permanently, the carrier state (24,25). Long-term follow-up is needed.

Urinary tract carriage of *S. typhi* occurs in countries where *Schistosoma haematobium* infections are endemic (26). These organisms have glycolipids on their surface that can serve as receptors for *S. typhi* type I pili (27). In addition, the worm may have the bacteria in its gut. This type of carrier has caused epidemics of typhoid fever in Egypt (26).

Direct person-to-person transmission of *S. typhi* had only been reported among homosexual persons (28). Once the AIDS epidemic was identified, typhoid fever was recognized as a very common infection in such persons living in endemic areas (29). The clinical presentation becomes atypical when the CD4 count is low. These patients are likely to have severe diarrhea and "ulcerative colitis" with enhanced relapse rates.

CLINICAL FEATURES

Enteric fever usually has an insidious onset. Low-grade fever appears first. The temperature recordings increase over the course of 48–72 hr and then remain constant at 39–40°C (102–104°F) for several weeks, unless modified by specific or nonspecific measures. Despite the fever, patients often do not have sweating or chills. A severe, generalized headache accompanies the fever. Anorexia, myalgia and fatigue are common complaints and dry cough also may be present. Abdominal pain, diffusely present, develops during this early period. Some patients will be constipated while others will have diarrhea. Examination of the abdomen will reveal tenderness to palpation and also the sensation of displacing air fluid contents in dilated loops of bowel. This indicates a paralytic ileus consistent with the pathological changes occurring in the ileum and colon. In contrast to the constipation associated with the ileus, some patients present with diarrhea. The diarrhea could result from the stimulation of secretory activity by prostaglandins released from the inflammatory cells or could also arise from enteropathogens ingested along with *S. typhi* (30). During the late stages of the first week of disease, in some patients with light-colored skin, a few rose spots may be detected after careful inspection. Rose spots are maculopapular, erythematous, small diameter, nontender lesions that will blanch with finger pressure. They are usually found in the skin of the abdominal wall and/or anterior thoracic wall. After a few days they no longer blanch but remain as a small hemorrhage into the skin. Biopsies of these lesions reveal a perivascular inflammatory exudate indicating a vasculitis induced by *S. typhi* and its endotoxin (31). Culture of these lesions will also yield *S. typhi*. These skin lesions indicate that similar changes are probably occurring in other organ systems. Splenomegaly and hepatomegaly often can be documented by physical examination. Encephalopathy (manifested as psychosis, mania, or marked apathy) is rare and

is indicative of progressive disease unaltered by specific therapy; however, even patients with appropriate antibacterial therapy frequently appear apathetic (32). Pneumonitis also is rare, but may be caused by *S. typhi* or secondary bacterial contaminants in a debilitated patient (33). One of the characteristic signs that is of diagnostic assistance is the presence of relative bradycardia in that the pulse is slower than expected with the high fever. This finding is unusual because of the widespread use of effective antibiotics. In the untreated patient, the fever remains constant at 39–40°C for weeks. For those patients who recover (the majority) without antibiotic therapy, there is a slow decline in the temperature curve over a 2-week period. Convalescence is prolonged in such patients in part because of the severe metabolic stresses associated with this chronic toxic infectious process. The use of effective antibiotics will control the disease and result in a period of defervescence of 2–5 days. This treatment has reduced mortality from 10–12% to less than 2% in some endemic countries. Children 1 year and younger and adults over 31 have the highest mortality in endemic regions (34). Death is associated with seizures, intestinal perforations, pneumonia, and delirium or coma (34).

The life-threatening complications of enteric fever have been briefly discussed in the "Pathogenesis" section. These primarily involve the intestinal wall, the site of multiplication of bacteria and therefore the accumulation of large concentrations of endotoxin. Perforation and intestinal hemorrhage occur when the disease processes have had an opportunity to progress. Thus, these events happen most often in the second week of disease. In untreated patients about 3% of patients develop perforation and for those the mortality rate approached 100% (14). In developing countries similar rates still exist due to late treatment, malnutrition, or immunocompromised patients. Even with surgical repair and antibiotics, the mortality rate ranges from 25% to 43%. Intestinal hemorrhage is less risky to the patient. The amount of bleeding is frequently physiologically tolerable and of short duration.

The pathogens that cause enteric fever are gram-negative rods. It is well known that gram-negative rod infections can cause septic shock with a mortality rate of 25–50%. What is unusual is that *S. typhi* has rarely been implicated in this condition. However, in southeastern Asia significant numbers of patients may develop septic shock caused by *S. typhi* (35). Such patients can be treated with large doses of steroids plus antibiotics, which appears to result in a lower mortality rate than antibiotics alone (35). In most cases of enteric fever, small numbers of the etiological agent are found in blood cultures. Furthermore, it has been difficult to demonstrate circulating endotoxin in these patients. However, those patients admitted with septic shock had circulating endotoxin and presumable large numbers of a virulent strain of *S. typhi*.

The intracellular habitat of *S. typhi* appears to promote relapse of disease. In the preantibiotic era, relapses occurred in 8–10% of patients. Subsequent to the utilization of antibiotics this incidence has increased to 15–20% of those treated with chloramphenicol, ampicillin, amoxicillin, and trimethoprim-sulfamethoxazole. Lower relapse rates (4–6%) have been noted in those patients treated with ceftriaxone and cefotaxime (36). These relapses are milder forms of the disease and occur about 2 weeks after cessation of treatment. In addition to relapses, second bouts of typhoid fever also may occur (37). Usually a different phage type has been involved in the subsequent disease. However, in the volunteer studies, rechallenge with the same dose, 10^5 organisms, induced a second illness in 5–15 men. These data indicate that the immunity acquired from a bout of typhoid is not total. Antibiotic treatment does not seem to prevent the development of solid resistance. Patients receiving no treatment also have developed second episodes (37). Carriers have solid intestinal immunity toward the resident strain. However, this level is not achieved after the usual episode of disease. Oral vaccines that interact with immune systems of the gut may induce excellent local immunity. This type of immunization appears to elicit a similar level of resistance as does the disease itself (see chapter by Levine). Patients recovering from typhoid fever have evidence of active cellular immune mechanisms, which are important in controlling the acute infection (38). However, this acquired resistance can be overcome, allowing the second bout of typhoid. Circulating antibodies to the O and H antigens have not been shown to predict resistance to later disease (5).

DIFFERENTIAL DIAGNOSIS

The clinical picture of fever, headache, abdominal pain, and myalgia suggests a number of infectious diseases. *F. tularensis* caused by the Jellison type A strain can cause a systemic disease without any cutaneous lesion. These patients have no rash and have a history of possible aerosol contact with or ingestion of meat from rabbits or other wild game animals. Infections with *Rickettsia rickettsii* in those patients with a faint rash, fever, severe headache, myalgia, and abdominal pain mimics the clinical picture of enteric fever. A search for a history of tick exposure or bite and even attached tick(s) and the peripheral location of the petechial rash (hands and feet) will lead to the correct diagnosis; Rocky Mountain spotted fever is a late spring to early fall disease, whereas typhoid may occur throughout the year. *Yersinia enterocolitica* has the propensity to produce mesenteric adenitis, which can cause abdominal pain and fever suggestive of typhoid fever. Stool and blood specimens properly cultured can reveal this pathogen. Similarly; primary septicemic forms of *Y. pseudotuberculosis* or *Y. pestis* infection may mimic the symptoms and signs of *S. typhi* disease. For persons living in endemic areas of the southwestern USA, plague should always be considered in community-acquired sepsis. In travelers returning from developing countries with acute febrile illnesses, malaria and hepatitis A also must be considered. Patients with various forms of lymphoma can present with fever, headache, and abdominal pain. Failure to isolate an infectious agent and the presence of generalized lymph node enlargement should suggest the possibility of a malignancy.

DIAGNOSTIC MEASURES

Enteric fever is usually diagnosed by isolating the pathogen in blood cultures (65–75% of patients with typhoid fever) during the first week of illness. Stool specimens yield *S. typhi* in about 70% of patients. Stool cultures often are negative during the first week of disease but become positive for varying periods, up to 4 months, even with antibiotic therapy. Culture of bone marrow aspirations gives the best yield, but this invasive procedure is not readily available in many endemic areas. Similarly, string cultures of duodenum secretions have yielded the diagnosis in 80% of patients (39); when one such culture, in addition to two blood cultures, was obtained in a series of 103 children, the yield was 92% (39). This was equal to two blood cultures plus a bone marrow culture. This procedure is acceptable to children and adults if appropriate devices are used. Measurement of the pH at the tip of the device when the string is withdrawn is important. When the pH value is greater than 6.0, the yield will be as stated above; a more acidic pH predicts that the culture will not be positive since the string has not reached the duodenum. This same device can be useful in detecting carriers (40). These patients often have erratic shedding of organisms in feces. The duodenal cultures can be a more reliable source of *S. typhi* in carriers.

Rose spots may be biopsied and cultured. However, this should not be necessary if the other more readily available specimens are obtained for culture. Liver biopsies are used in some countries as the source of cultures in patients suspected of having typhoid fever. While there is a high yield, this is the invasive procedure with a predictable potential for complications. It should be reserved for those situations when other sources for culture have failed and the patient is not responding to antibiotic therapy.

Serological studies have been employed for the diagnosis of typhoid fever since 1896 (7). The Widal test measures agglutinins to the O and H antigens. A fourfold increase in either or both titer(s) in paired serum samples obtained at least 2 weeks apart is significant and occurs in 50–75% of patients. It uses a poorly standardized test. The results are influenced by a number of factors that lower its sensitivity and specificity. There are numerous cross-reacting O and H antigens present in *Salmonella* species that cause the more common diarrheal diseases. Infections with cross-reacting organisms can produce false-positive results. The titer of agglutinins to the O and H antigens can increase rapidly in the first few days of disease and when the patient arrives at the hospital there already has been peak production of antibodies. The rise would have been missed because it occurred prior to initial testing. However, a single titer is diagnostic if the O ≥ 1:320 and/or the H ≥ 1:640. Chloramphenicol treatment has been shown to interfere with antibody production; this is an unpredictable effect because at least 65–70% of patients with typhoid fever who are treated with this antibiotic produce fourfold or greater rises in titer in specimens obtained 2–3 weeks apart. Not all patients without antibiotic therapy demonstrate significant titer rises. Patients with underlying diseases such as cirrhosis or AIDS may demonstrate variable serological results (41). The patient with cirrhosis may have false-positive results because of hypergammaglobulinemia, or cross-reacting antigens present in nosocomial, gram-negative organisms (41), while the immunosuppressed patient may not be able to develop antibodies.

The polymerase chain reaction (PCR) has been shown to rapidly (within 16 hr) detect *S. typhi* DNA in blood samples, providing an early diagnosis (42). It promises to be a much more sensitive and specific test.

MANAGEMENT

Patients with enteric fever require prompt antibiotic treatment in order to rapidly control the infectious process. Chloramphenicol, 2–4 g/day in divided doses for 14 days, had been the antibiotic of choice from 1948 to 1972 (43). The appearance of chloramphenicol-resistant strains of *S. typhi* in many endemic areas in the 1970s and their persistence has created therapeutic difficulties (44). This resistance pattern was first detected in 1950 in an isolated report, but did not cause any concern. Additional reports appeared in the mid-1960s (45). However, the large epidemic in Mexico City in 1972 was the major event that clearly indicated that chloramphenicol could no longer be assumed to be the drug of choice. This trend of *S. typhi* becoming resistant to other antibiotics continues. Ampicillin, amoxicillin, and trimethoprim-sulfamethoxazole have been used in place of chloramphenicol (46). These agents have provided effective and economic alternatives. However, resistance to these four antibacterial drugs is now fairly common (20–40%) in some endemic areas including the Indian subcontinent, Arabian Gulf, and northeastern Africa (47). The question of increased virulence associated with these multidrug-resistant strains has been raised (48). Several small series of patients suggests that this may be true, but prospective studies are needed to verify this suggestion. For patients with diagnosed typhoid fever returning from these areas of high prevalence of multidrug-resistant strains, treatment with ciprofloxacin or one of the cephalosporin antibiotics listed below should be started.

The newer cephalosporin antibiotics have been efficacious (e.g., cefoperazone, cefotaxime, and ceftriaxone), with cure rates ranging from 82% to 97% in small series (36). The dosage schedule for these drugs has been variable and the duration of treatment has ranged from 2 to 14 days. No standard regimen has been established. Reasonable therapy would be to maintain the antibiotic for at least 3 days after the patient has become afebrile.

The quinolone groups of antibacterial agents also have been shown to be effective (49). They have been used in children infected with multiresistant strains of *S. typhi* and no toxic effects on cartilage were noted. Ciprofloxacin, ofloxacin, and fleroxacin all have been used successfully to treat patients. In comparison trials, the clinical and bacteriological responses are as good as or better than those induced by chloramphenicol. The high concentrations of the quinolones achieved in the gallbladder and biliary tract have enabled these drugs to assist patients in clearing the acute disease, as well as those who are chronic carriers. The recommended dose has not been established. Of concern is the report of a strain of *S. typhi* isolated from a child who acquired the disease in India that was resistant to ciprofloxacin (50). The widespread use of the quinolones to treat diarrheal illnesses in areas of the world where these infections are common will lead to an increasing number of strains of *S. typhi* and other enteropathogens resistant to this useful group of therapeutic agents.

For those patients with enteric fever who present with or have signs and symptoms compatible with impending shock, the administration of high-dose dexamethasone can be life saving (35). Therefore, patients who are delirious, obtunded, stuporous, comatose, or in shock should receive 3 mg/kg initially over a 30-min period, then 1 mg/kg every 6 hr for 8 doses. An appropriate antibiotic should be given.

Patients with enteric fever receiving an effective antibiotic will become afebrile in 3–6 days. Rarely, a temperature elevation will persist beyond that time despite effective treatment. In these patients, careful search for unusual complications should be conducted. Those who develop perforation of the ileum or colon will have a resurgence of the fever, frequently a rise in the white blood cell count, and an increase in abdominal discomfort. They will be found to have rebound tenderness on palpation. These patients should have immediate laparotomy and surgical repair of the defect (14). Expanded antibiotic coverage is needed to counteract the aerobic and anaerobic flora that are contaminating the peritoneal cavity. The flushing of the abdomen with huge volumes of Ringer's lactate and saline solutions will help control the incipient infection. The addition of metronidazole and gentamicin and perhaps vancomycin will provide broad coverage. The high mortality associated with this complication requires the use of antibiotics and other supportive measures, e.g., fluid replacement and respiratory assistance.

Isolation of stools from patients with enteric fever should be done. Follow-up cultures are necessary to ensure that the chronic carrier state has not developed; three successive negative stool cultures are required. Convalescent carriage may persist for 3–4 months. Positive cultures after 1 year indicate that the patient is a carrier and will require an abdominal ultrasound or similar procedure to search for gallstones. Additional studies may be necessary to evaluate the functioning of the gallbladder if no stones are demonstrable. Obviously, carriers need to be prohibited from preparation of food.

PREVENTION

Control of enteric infections requires knowledge of the carriers, prohibiting their occupation as food handlers and adequate and safe disposal of their feces. The spread of the enteric fever pathogens is also blocked by providing safe water supplies. This measure has been the primary reason for the decline in the incidence of enteric fever in the developed countries. Sewage-contaminated rivers and streams have been sources of infection by direct and indirect routes. Water from these sources have been used to irrigate fields in which vegetables were grown (51). These vegetables served as a source of bacteria that spread from the lettuce, for example, or the fingers to the mouth. The huge investment required to provide clean water will be repaid many fold as the incidence of all enteric infections decline and the need for medical care decreases, as a result of these sanitation improvements.

There are several vaccines available to prevent typhoid fever (see chapter by Levine). The heat-killed, phenol-preserved vaccine has been shown to provide significant protection to those persons living in endemic areas (52). Presumably, the vaccine adds to the background-acquired immunity of this population. Its protective value is less in those persons who live in nonendemic areas (5). The vaccine-induced immunity will prevent disease in most individuals who are exposed to small size inocula (5). Larger numbers of bacteria overcome this protection (5). This vaccine is associated with pain and erythema and/or swelling at the site of injection, and headaches. The recommended second dose of vaccine can be administered in 4 weeks, even after those types of reactions. Reactions should be less likely with the second exposure. Because of significant neurological problems with this vaccine, several countries abandoned its use and championed the development of an oral vaccine. The two 0.5-mL doses of the killed vaccine are given subcutaneously at a 4-week interval. Booster doses should be given every 3 years if the need persists. Potential recipients of typhoid vaccines include travelers to endemic areas, especially, India, Pakistan, Chile, and Peru, and those technicians who may be exposed to S. typhi in a laboratory. Family members living with a carrier should also receive one of the vaccines.

An oral vaccine consisting of an attenuated, live strain of S. typhi (Ty21a) has been shown to provide better protection than the killed vaccine for adults living in a nonendemic area (53). In large-sized field trials in Egypt and Chile, children receiving the oral vaccine developed varied levels of immunity (54,55). Those in Egypt received a liquid formulation of the vaccine and these children had outstanding immunity. In Chile, the vaccine was administered in various formulations, e.g., enteric-coated capsules and liquid. The best results occurred in those who received the buffered liquid vaccine. The vaccine is now sold in enteric-coated capsule form (Vivotif, Berna-Swiss Serum and Vaccine Institute). The dose is four capsules, one every other day. The capsules need to be refrigerated and should be consumed at least a week prior to expected travel. These capsules contain strain Ty21a that has been attenuated by chemical mutagenesis (56). It is characterized by its inability to metabolize galactose and therefore in vivo it self-destructs as it attempts to multiply in the gut because the galactose block leads to an accumulation of carbohydrate precursors that eventually causes cell lysis. The protection induced by Ty21a is based on the development of cellular and humoral immunity. A previous dose of parenteral vaccine does not enhance or inhibit the local immunity induced by the oral vaccine (57). However, if several doses of killed vaccine are given after the

oral vaccine, an increase in specific IgA antibody has been measured. Very few reactions have been reported with the use of the live oral vaccine; some children had nausea and vomiting and a few people had complained of cramps and diarrhea. The live oral vaccine is contraindicated in immunocompromised hosts including persons with AIDS. This is a theoretical problem; there have not been reports of actual problems. Travelers to endemic areas are likely to receive other prophylactic measures in addition to typhoid vaccine. Those who receive antimalarial drugs, mefloquine, or chloroquine simultaneously with oral vaccine could manifest an antibacterial effect on the vaccine strain (58). Therefore, there should be a significant time interval between administration of the oral vaccine and the need to start malaria prophylaxis. Other antibiotics may also diminish the immunological response. The duration of efficacy of the oral vaccine is at least 3–4 years.

Another parenteral vaccine that has been shown to be highly effective consists of purified Vi polysaccharide (59). Like other polysaccharide vaccines, this has essentially no toxicity, and trials in South Africa and Nepal have shown efficacy rates comparable to or better than for the standard parental (phenol-extracted) vaccine (59,60). Its efficacy resides in the Vi antibodies induced. It is not commercially available in the United States but is available elsewhere.

REFERENCES

1. Bretonneau P. Notice sur le contagion de la dothinentérie. *Arch Gen Med* 1829;21:57.
2. Snyder MS, Hornick RB, McCrumb FR. Asymptomatic typhoidal bacteremia in volunteers. *Antimicrob Agents Chemother* 1963;3:604.
3. Felix A, Pitt RM. The pathogenic and immunogenic activities of *Salmonella typhi* in relation to its antigenic constituents. *J Hyg* 1951;49:92–110.
4. Looney RJ, Steigbigel RT. Role of the Vi antigen of *Salmonella typhi* in resistance to host defense in vitro. *J Lab Clin Med* 1986; 108:506–516.
5. Hornick RB, Greisman SE, Woodward TE, DuPont HL, Dawkins AT, Snyder MJ. Typhoid fever: pathogenesis and immunologic control. *N Engl J Med* 1970;283:686–691, 739–746.
6. Edwards PR, Ewing WH. *Identification of Entrobacteriaceae.* 3rd ed. Minneapolis: Burgess; 1972.
7. Widal F. Sérodiagnostic de la fièvre typhoide. *Sem Med* 1896; 16:259.
8. Franco A, Gonzalez C, Levine OS, et al. Further consideration of the clonal nature of *Salmonella typhi:* evaluation of molecular and clinical characteristics of strains from Indonesia and Peru. *J Clin Microbiol* 1992;30:2187–2190.
9. Sprinz H, Gangarrosa EJ, Williams M. Hornick RB, Woodward TE. Histopathology of the upper small intestine in typhoid fever. Biopsy study of experimental disease in man. *Am J Dig Dis* 1966;11:615–624.
10. Blaser MJ, Newman L. A review of human salmonellosis. I. Infective dose. *Rev Infect Dis* 1982;4(6):1096–1106.
11. Finlay BB, Heffron F, Falkow S. Epithelial cell surfaces induce *Salmonella* proteins required for bacterial adherence and invasion. *Science* 1989;243:940–943.
12. Fernandez-Beros ME, Gonzalez C, McIntosh MA, Cabello FC. Immune response to the iron-deprivation-induced proteins of *Salmonella typhi* in typhoid fever. *Infect Immun* 1989;57: 1271–1275.
13. Hornick RB, Greisman SE. On the pathogenesis of typhoid fever. *Arch Intern Med* 1978;138:357–359.

14. Butler T, Knight J, Nath SK, Speelman P, Roy SK, Azad MAK. Typhoid fever complicated by intestinal perforation: a persisting fatal disease requiring surgical management. *Rev Infect Dis* 1985;7:244–256.
15. Welton J, Man J, Friedman S. Association between hepatobiliary cancer and typhoid carrier state. *Lancet* 1979;1:791–794.
16. Merselis JG, Kage D, Connolly CS, Hook EW. Quantitative bacteriology of the typhoid carrier state. *Am J Trop Med Hyg* 1964;13:425–429.
17. Soper GA. The curious career of Typhoid Mary. *Bull NY Acad Med* 1939;15:698–712.
18. Veldee MV. An epidemiological study of typhoid fever in six Ohio River cities. *Public Health Rep* 1931;46:1460–1488.
19. Blaser MJ, Hickman FW, Farmer JJ, et al. The laboratory as a reservoir of infection. *J Infect Dis* 1980;142:934–938.
20. Blaser MJ, Lofgren JP. Fatal salmonellosis originating in a clinical microbiology laboratory. *J Clin Microbiol* 1981;13:855–858.
21. Birkhead GS, Morse DL, Levine WC, et al. Typhoid fever at a resort hotel in New York: a large outbreak with an unusual vehicle. *J Infect Dis* 1993;167:1228–1232.
22. Ames WR, Robins M. Age and sex as factors in the development of the typhoid carrier state and a method for estimating carrier prevalence. *Am J Public Health* 1943;33:221–230.
23. Lanata CF, Levine MM, Ristori C, Black RE, et al. Vi serology in detection of chronic *Salmonella typhi* carriers in an endemic area. *Lancet* 1983;2:441–443.
24. Gotuzzo E, Guerra JG, Benavente L, et al. Use of norfloxacin to treat chronic typhoid carriers. *J Infect Dis* 1988;157:1221–1225.
25. Ferreccio C, Morris JG Jr, Valdivieso C, Prenzel I, Sotomayor V, Drusano GL, Levine MM. Efficacy of ciprofloxacin in the treatment of chronic typhoid carriers. *J Infect Dis* 1988;157:1235–1238.
26. Hathont SE, El-Ghaffar YA, Awry AY, Hassan K. Relation between urinary schistosomiasis and chronic enteric urinary carrier state among Egyptians. *Am J Trop Med* 1966;15:156–161.
27. Melhem RF, LoVerde PT. Mechanism of interaction of *Salmonella* and *Schistosoma* species. *Infect Immun* 1984;44:274–281.
28. Dritz SK, Braff ED. Sexually transmitted typhoid fever (letter). *N Engl J Med* 1977;296:1359–1360.
29. Totuzzo E, Frisancho O, Sanchez J, Fiendo F, et al. Association between the acquired immunodeficiency syndrome and infections with *Salmonella typhi* and *Salmonella paratyphi* in an endemic typhoid area. *Arch Intern Med* 1991;151:381–382.
30. Roy SK, Speelman P, Butler T, Nath S, et al. Diarrhea associated with typhoid fever. *J Infect Dis* 1985;151:1138–1143.
31. Greisman SE, Hornick RB. Cellular inflammatory responses of man to bacterial endotoxin: a comparison with PPD and other bacterial antigens. *J Immunol* 1972;109:1210–1222.
32. Auntokun BO, Bademosi O, Ognenverni K, Wright SC. Neuropsychiatric manifestations of typhoid fever in 959 patients. *Arch Neurol* 1972;27:7–13.
33. Sharma AM, Sharma OP. Pulmonary manifestations of typhoid fever: two case reports and a review of the literature. *Chest* 1992;101:1144–1146.
34. Butler T, Islam A, Kabir I, Jones PK. Patterns of morbidity and mortality in typhoid fever dependent on age and gender: review of 552 hospitalized patients with diarrhea. *Rev Infect Dis* 1991;13:85–90.
35. Hoffman SL, Punjabi NH, Kumala S, et al. Reduction of mortality in chloramphenicol-treated severe typhoid fever by high-dose dexamethasone. *N Engl J Med* 1984;310:82–88.
36. Soe GB, Overturf GD. Treatment of typhoid fever and other systemic salmonelloses with cefotaxime, ceftriaxone, cefoperazone, and other newer cephalosporins. *Rev Infect Dis* 1987;9:719–735.
37. Marmion DE, Naylor GRE, Stewart IO. Second attacks of typhoid fever. *J Hygiene* 1953;52:260–267.
38. Murphy JR, Baqar S, Munoz C, Schlesinger L, et al. Characteristics of humoral and cellular immunity to *Salmonella typhi* in

residents of typhoid-endemic and typhoid-free regions. *J Infect Dis* 1987;156:1005–1009.
39. Avendano A, Herrera P, Horwitz I, et al. Duodenal string cultures: practicality and sensitivity for diagnosing enteric fever in children. *J Infect Dis* 1986;153:359–362.
40. Gilman RH, Islam S, Rabbani H, Ghosh H. Identification of gallbladder typhoid carriers by a string device. *Lancet* 1979;1:795–796.
41. Protell RL, Soloway RD, Martin WJ. Anti-salmonella agglutinins in chronic active liver disease. *Lancet* 1971;2:330–331.
42. Song J-H, Cho H, Park MY, et al. Detection of *Salmonella typhi* in the blood of patients with typhoid fever by polymerase chain reaction. *J Clin Microbiol* 1993;31:1439–1443.
43. Woodward RE, Smadel JE, Ley HL, Green R, Mankikar DS. Preliminary report on the beneficial effect of chloromycetin in the treatment of typhoid fever. *Ann Intern Med* 1948;49:131–134.
44. Vasquez V, Calderon E, Rodriquez RS. Chloramphenicol-resistant strains of *Salmonella typhosa* (letter). *N Engl J Med* 1972;286:1220.
45. Njoku-obi AN, Njoku-obi JC. Resistance of *Salmonella typhosa* to chloramphenicol. *J Bacteriol* 1965;90:552–553.
46. Gilman RH, Terminel M, Levine MM, Hernandea-Mendoza P, et al. Comparison of trimethoprim-sulfamethoxazole and amoxicillin in therapy of chloramphenicol-resistant and chloramphenicol-sensitive typhoid fever. *J Infect Dis* 1975;132:630–636.
47. Mourad AS, Metwally M, El Deen AN, et al. Multiple-drug-resistant *Salmonella typhi*. *Clin Infect Dis* 1993;17:135–136.
48. Bhutta ZA, Naqvi SH, Razzaq RA, Farooqui BJ. Multidrug-resistant typhoid in children: presentation and clinical features. *Rev Infect Dis* 1991;13:832–836.
49. Arnold K, Hong C-S, Nelwan R, et al. Randomized comparative study of fleroxacin and chloramphenicol in typhoid fever. *Am J Med* 1993;94(Suppl 3A):195S–200S.
50. Rowe B, Ward LR, Threlfall EJ. Ciprofloxacin and typhoid fever. *Lancet* 1992;339:740.
51. Sears SD, Ferreccio C, Levine MM, Cordano AM, et al. The use of Moore swabs for isolation of *Salmonella typhi* from irrigation water in Santiago, Chile. *J Infect Dis* 1984;149:640–642.
52. Cvjetanović B, Uemura K. The present status of field and laboratory studies of typhoid and paratyphoid vaccines: with special reference to studies sponsored by the world health organization. *Bull WHO* 1965;32:29–36.
53. Gilman RH, Hornick RB, Woodward WE, et al. Evaluation of a UDP-glucose-4-epimeraseless mutant of *Salmonella typhi* as a live oral vaccine. *J Infect Dis* 1977;136:717–723.
54. Wahdan MH, Serie C, Cerisier Y, Sallam S, Germanier R. A controlled field trial of live *Salmonella typhi* strain Ty21a oral vaccine against typhoid: three-year results. *J Infect Dis* 1982;145:292–295.
55. Levine MM, Ferreccio C, Cryz SC, Ortiz E. Comparison of enteric-coated capsules and liquid formulation of Ty21a typhoid vaccine in randomised controlled field trial. *Lancet* 1990;2:891–894.
56. Germanier R, Furer E. Isolation and characterization of gal E mutant Ty21a of *Salmonella typhi:* a candidate strain for a live oral typhoid vaccine. *J Infect Dis* 1975;131:553–558.
57. Forrest BD, LaBrooy JT, Dearlove CE, Shearman DJ. Effect of parenteral immunization on the intestinal immune response to *Salmonella typhi* Ty21a. *Infect Immun* 1992;60:465–471.
58. Horowitz H, Carbonaro CA. Inhibition of the *Salmonella typhi* oral vaccine strain, Ty21a, by mefloquine and chloroquine. *J Infect Dis* 1992;166:1462–1464.
59. Tachet CO, Ferreccio C, Robbins, et al. Safety and immunogenicity of two *Salmonella typhi* Vi capsular polysaccharide vaccines. *J Infect Dis* 1986;154:323–345.
60. Klugman KP, Gilbertson IT, Koornshof HJ, Robbins JB, et al. Protective activity of Vi capsular polysaccharide vaccine against typhoid fever. *Lancet* 1987;2:1165–1169.

Infections of the Gastrointestinal Tract,
edited by M. J. Blaser, P. D. Smith, J. I. Ravdin,
H. B. Greenberg, and R. L. Guerrant
Raven Press, Ltd., New York © 1995.

CHAPTER 25

Tropical Sprue

Chronic Intestinal Malabsorption in the Tropics

Gary M. Gray

Tropical sprue is a chronic malady of the small intestine manifested by the malabsorption of nutrients and vitamins that occurs in individuals residing in certain tropical locales. The essential features of the disease are an increased volume and number of stools, malabsorption of nutrients, and consequent weight loss in patients residing in a tropical region (1). It is uncertain as to when the disease was first recognized, but it may have been described as early as 600–1300 B.C. in Indian writings on the disorders of assimilation of food. Before 1800 in Barbados, Hillary (2) provided the typical clinical description of what is now thought to be tropical sprue. In 1880, Manson (3) adopted the Dutch term *Sprouw* that had been used to describe an illness involving buccal aphthous ulcers in children who developed what is now known to be nontropical sprue (synonyms: celiac sprue, gluten-sensitive enteropathy). Although tropical sprue involves primarily the small intestine (4–7), folic acid and vitamin B_{12} deficiency and megaloblastic anemia are commonly present at the outset of the disease and almost always occur when it becomes well established (8,9). Tropical sprue appears to compromise tissues that replicate rapidly and have a lifespan of only a few days. When patients with this tropical malabsorption respond dramatically to treatment with oral folic acid and broad-spectrum antibiotics, the diagnosis becomes secure.

EPIDEMIOLOGY

Tropical sprue is endemic in numerous locales in the tropics extending from the equator to both the north and the south slightly more than 30° latitude to include the Caribbean, India, and southern Africa (6). The disease is particularly prevalent in Cuba, the Dominican Republic, Haiti (10), and Puerto Rico (6), yet it has not been observed in Jamaica. It has also been well described in Columbia and Venezuela and probably occurs in Mexico (11). Perhaps the most extensive documentation of tropical sprue has been that in India (7,12). The disease has also been observed in Africa (13), Borneo, Burma, China, Hong Kong (14), Indonesia, Malaysia, Singapore, Vietnam, Sri Lanka (15), and the Philippines (16).

Besides occurring in indigenous populations, tropical sprue is contracted by those who visit the tropics for a month or longer. Typical tropical sprue developed in 10% of English military who were in the India–Burma region (17,18) during World War II, and in those stationed in Malaya (19,20) and Hong Kong (14). A similar proportion of the United States military serving in Puerto Rico developed tropical sprue (21) and, more recently, the disease was also found to be common in Vietnam among visitors from the United States, including both military personnel (22) and a medical professional team (11% after only 3 months exposure; 28% after a year) (23). The incubation period for North American expatriates traveling in these tropical lands may be a year or greater (21,24). Nearly half of Peace Corps volunteers from the United States residing in Pakistan developed malabsorption and abnormal intestinal morphology within 6 months (24). Subsequent recovery of absorptive function required 1–2 years after returning to the United States (25). Indians and Pakistanis who immigrate to the New York City area have a high prevalence of intestinal malabsorption, and the conversion to normal parameters usually requires a full year and sometimes as long as 2 or 3 years (26). The first symptoms of tropical sprue may emerge months or even years after expatriates have returned to their native temperate environments (27). It is rarely seen in short-term visitors to the tropics, probably because a prolonged exposure to a causative agent appears to be required and perhaps because antibiotics that may prevent intestinal infestations are now used extensively by travelers.

Although most cases of tropical sprue appear to arise sporadically in endemic form, a significant proportion of

Gary M. Gray: Digestive Disease Center, Stanford University Medical Center, Stanford, California 94305-5487.

individuals in the tropical region (5–10%) may contract the disease. Epidemics of tropical sprue have been reported, particularly from India (28,29). The maximal attack rate of tropical sprue in the slowly developing Indian epidemics is as high as 10–25 cases per 100 individuals per annum in adults. The frequency increases somewhat at about age 25 and may be even more common after age 40 (30–32). The attack rate in children is only about half that in adults, but the disease may be particularly severe and not infrequently lethal in young children (see below). Typically, the onset and spread among family members of a household occurs gradually, with new cases cropping up on a month-by-month basis over a period of a year or more. The incubation period within the household usually requires more than a month and, while initially affecting mainly adults, the disease is contracted by children as the epidemic evolves. Subsequent epidemics within the same community usually occur approximately every 5–6 years. The prevalence of symptomatic malabsorptive illness increases subsequently in children born after the first epidemic, suggesting that some immunity may be conferred in those who have contracted the disease (7). Perhaps because of the relatively slow evolution of such tropical sprue epidemics and the fact that there has been greater mobility of family members in recent years, the epidemic nature of the disease has not been established in tropical countries other than India. Furthermore, there are features of Indian epidemic tropical sprue that are not observed in sporadic endemic sprue. For instance, an acute enteritis, presumably infectious in nature and classically described as the first stage in Indian tropical sprue (32), is observed much less frequently in sprue elsewhere. Nevertheless, some experts consider an acute enteric episode to be an essential feature of the tropical sprue syndrome (33,34). Even though diarrheal syndromes, presumably caused by infectious organisms, occur commonly and recurrently in many of these tropical locales, they usually do not herald the onset of the chronic sprue condition. Also, the dramatic ameliorative response to antibiotic therapy usually reported for tropical sprue and used to support the putative bacterial etiology of the disease seems to be muted or absent in southern India (7,35). Hence, there is the lingering question as to whether tropical malabsorption observed in India may be a different disease than that seen in other tropical regions.

PATHOGENESIS

The Case for an Infectious Cause

Both because of the endemic nature and the fact that epidemics of tropical sprue have been repeatedly observed, an infectious agent has long been sought as the predominant or final eventual cause of chronic tropical sprue. Unfortunately, no unique organism has been identified and there is no animal model of the human tropical malabsorption syndrome. Nonetheless, numerous studies have demonstrated overgrowth of coliform organisms in the small intestine (36–39). In normal individuals, the upper jejunum harbors very few organisms and these are mainly gram-positive streptococci and lactobacilli. Higher titers of streptococci and fungi are present in the more distal bowel. Facultative anaerobic coliforms are present in the distal ileum in small numbers and are the normal inhabitants of the colon. Although recovery of small intestinal samples is fraught with error because of the contamination with nasopharyngeal organisms, studies of patients with tropical sprue have demonstrated facultative anaerobes in the upper small bowel, including *Klebsiella pneumoniae, E. coli,* and *Enterobacter cloacae* (37). A high proportion (~50 to >90%) of patients with untreated tropical sprue from southern India (38), Puerto Rico (39), and of Europeans traveling in Asia (33) were shown to harbor these coliform bacteria in small intestinal aspirates. In southern India, coliforms were demonstrated in the vast majority of patients with tropical sprue, but were also similarly frequent in healthy controls (38,40). Such enterobacteria have been shown to cause changes in mucosal structure in animals with intestinal stasis produced by experimental blind loops (41). Although toxins from these coliforms can produce a secretory diarrhea, they do not produce significant chronic intestinal histological changes like those seen in topical sprue.

Klipstein and colleagues (6) noted three features of the tropical sprue syndrome that led to the opinion that the disease is caused by a bacterium: (a) coliform overgrowth does not usually develop in other small intestine maladies such as celiac sprue; (b) enterotoxins of these coliforms produce intestinal structural and functional alterations in experimental animals; and (c) antibiotic therapy both eradicates the coliform overgrowth and improves the intestinal lesion. However, the overgrowth of coliforms may only be an epiphenomenon. Whereas these organisms are capable of emitting toxins and producing a secretory diarrhea, they have not been established to produce chronic pathological changes in the human small intestine or to cause chronic malabsorption. Furthermore, as estimated from the time required for orally ingested lactulose to be metabolized and expired as hydrogen, intestinal transit becomes prolonged in patients with tropical sprue (42); the long retention of nutrients and vitamins sets the stage for the bacterial overgrowth and consequent interference with nutrient assimilation. Admittedly, the organisms that overgrow in the small intestine in tropical sprue are facultative anaerobes rather than the anaerobes commonly seen in the classical stasis or small intestinal overgrowth syndrome. But factors other than stasis may allow overgrowth of the coliforms. Because of the higher ambient temperature in tropical regions, ingested food is likely to have a higher density of bacterial contamination. Control subjects in the tropics without malabsorption have often not been examined in parallel for possible bacterial overgrowth; but jejunal culture of coliforms has been observed in some control subjects from the same tropical environment who have no malabsorption (38,40). Although coliform overgrowth in the small intestine may set the stage for the chronic malabsorptive condition in the endemic tropical regions, the rapid elimination of the organism by antibiotics does not lead to the prompt reversal of the malabsorptive syndrome. Instead, the reversal of malabsorption and malnutrition induced by folic acid and antibiotics in tropical sprue often requires several weeks or even months (43,44). In essence, the case for a bacterial cause of tropical sprue is circumstantial, the coliform organisms that proliferate in the tropics having not been shown to produce a chronic malabsorptive condition. The isolation of a putative bacterial agent that is capable of producing the chronic tropical sprue syndrome remains elusive.

Viral infestations have been considered as a possible etiology for tropical sprue, but cultures of rectal swabs from patients have been negative (45). But culturing of excreted enteric viruses is commonly unsuccessful, and virus-like particles have been observed in stools of those affected by tropical sprue in Indian epidemics (46). Corona-like virus particles were reported to be chronically present in stools of a patient with tropical sprue (47), but the following features of the case make it less than compelling: (a) no antibodies against the virus were found in serum and (b) the patient also had undergone a vagotomy and a gastrojejunostomy for peptic disease, which may have permitted a chronic enteric viral infestation. Certainly, a more thorough analysis of possible role of infection with one or more viruses in chronic tropical sprue is indicated.

Other Causative Considerations

In addition to intestinal stasis and coliform overgrowth, alteration in plasma concentrations of gastrointestinal hormones including enteroglucagon, motilin, and peptide YY have been demonstrated in tropical sprue (33,48). While only moderately elevated in acute infectious diarrhea, peptide YY levels were tenfold higher than normal in tropical sprue patients (48). This dramatic finding deserves further study.

Although there has been the suggestion that poor hygiene and low socioeconomic status may predispose individuals in the tropics to develop the disease, there have been no comprehensive studies to document the role of altered nutrition or contaminated food in the etiology of tropical sprue.

The observations from India that the onset of tropical sprue is manifested by an acute enteritis that sets the stage for the chronic symptoms of the disease has prompted the hypothesis that tropical sprue is actually a postinfective tropical malabsorption (33,49). An enteritis produced by a variety of organisms is common in many tropical and subtropical regions and not infrequently produces a bloody colitis. In most instances of endemic tropical sprue, there is no discrete history of a preceding severe acute episode. Indeed, the acute episode itself, when it does occur, does not appear to be caused by a single or unique enteric pathogen. With the possible exception of Indian tropical sprue, it seems unlikely that an acute predisposing episode is an essential component of the chronic malabsorption syndrome typical of tropical sprue.

Whipple's Disease

Is there an analogy with Whipple's Disease? In many ways, the evolution of the illness in tropical sprue seems analogous to the chronic intestinal malabsorption seen in Whipple's disease where a specific bacterial cause was recently documented by the presence of a unique bacterial mRNA in intestinal tissues (50,51). Even though it is still not possible to cultivate the bacteria in Whipple's disease, the indolent onset, plodding but relentless progression to chronic weight loss and malnutrition, and the requirement for months of antibiotic therapy to ensure a complete remission are similar to those observed in tropical sprue. But certainly Whipple's is distinct from tropical sprue since a unique bacterium is found not only in the intestine but also in numerous lymph node groups, on heart valves (52), and in the brain (53). Whipple's disease is more common in temperate zones and the intestinal biopsy reveals the presence of periodic acid-Schiff (PAS)–positive macrophages in the intestinal tissue that contain bacterial bodies (54). Nevertheless, a comprehensive analysis of intestinal tissue from tropical sprue patients by the same approach used successfully to define the organism responsible for Whipple's disease may prove to be useful in determining whether a unique bacterium is present beneath the enterocyte layer in the intestinal mucosa of tropical sprue patients. Certainly the epidemiological features are most compatible with a permissive, chronic intestinal infection, primarily of the small intestine. Although the infectious agents remain to be identified, the dramatic, if somewhat delayed, response to antibiotic therapy strengthens this concept. It seems most likely that a fastidious organism, indigenous to the tropical climate, will be identified as the causative agent of chronic tropical sprue, just as the Whipple's bacillus appears to be ubiquitously present in the soils of temperate regions. In diseases such as these produced by the chronic harboring of fastidious bacteria, it remains to be established as to whether the putative organism itself produces the intestinal alteration by chronic infestation or whether there is a release of bioactive toxic products that produce the ultimate damage.

For the present, the primary etiology of the chronic malabsorption syndrome in the tropics must be said to be undiscovered. Certainly, tropical sprue is not an acute disease since an individual must reside in the tropics for a year or longer before contracting the chronic syndrome. Even in the studies of epidemics of tropical sprue in India (see above), the incubation period was one month or longer. Perhaps the stage must first be set in the tropics in those individuals who have a permissive constitution to develop the illness.

CLINICAL ILLNESS

Despite the report of acute diarrheal episodes preceding the onset of sprue in cases from southern India, in recent years the onset of tropical sprue in most locales within 30° north or south of the equator often has been very subtle. Although fatigue and malaise have not been emphasized as early symptoms, the author has observed a series of U.S. army recruits in Puerto Rico who developed midday fatigue, disinterest in work, and sleepiness that often prevented the accomplishment of even the most sedentary tasks. The symptoms of lassitude and weakness are often more disturbing than the increase in the number (to 3–10) and volume (1000 mL or greater) of stools per day. Understandably, some of these individuals are initially reprimanded by their superiors until evidence ensues that the patient is suffering from a systemic disease producing an obvious anemia or weight loss. The vitamin deficiencies are manifested by erythema and stinging pain of the tongue margins, and painful cracking at the corners of the mouth. Although it is generally believed that folate and vitamin B_{12} deficiency are late manifestations of the disease (6), a megaloblastic anemia is often the first abnormality noted by general physicians. The extent of fat malabsorption may be mild or moderate (15–25 g/day), probably because caloric intake is often reduced appreciably due to the severe anorexia and premature satiety associated with intestinal stasis and postprandial abdominal distention. But some patients excrete greater than 50 g/day. At least 90% of patients experience most of these abdominal symptoms and weight loss by the first month of the disease.

The disease may be particularly severe in childhood. Fevers, high-volume watery diarrhea (not infrequently bloody), and malnutrition are common (55,56). Death rates without medical intervention reach greater than 30% of patients. But mortality can be uniformly reduced to a negligible incidence with appropriate medical therapy (56).

Physical examination reveals apathy, evidence of appreciable weight loss, relatively retarded physical movement, loss of tongue papillae, cracking at the corners of the mouth, a paradoxically protuberant abdomen despite the loss of body weight, muscle wasting of the extremities, and an associated prominence of bowel sounds which often are audible without the aid of a stethoscope. About 25–30% of patients may have low-grade fevers at the beginning of the constitutional symptoms (57). After a few weeks of systemic manifestations, the patient usually shows a striking pallor, reflecting the associated anemia; an associated skin hyperpigmentation has been noted in the Indian studies (58). Systolic blood pressures of less than 100 and paradoxically slow pulse rates of less than 80 are common and may produce orthostasis. Pedal edema is usually present after a month of illness, and may be severe. In well-established disease, anasarca often develops.

Laboratory Findings

Megaloblastic anemia (Hct <30; MCV >105), much more severe than in nontropical enteropathies, often produces more dominant symptoms than the intestinal lesion and is a hallmark of tropical sprue (9,59). Hypoalbuminemia (<3 g/dL) can be expected in patients who have been ill for a month or longer due to the combination of malabsorption of dietary amino acids and peptides and to loss of serum proteins through the increased effective pore size in the diseased intestinal membrane (60). There is a marked reduction in capacity to absorb vitamin B_{12}, and bone marrow analysis almost always reveals severe

megaloblastosis. Steatorrhea (stool fat excretion, 15–50 g/day; normal = 6 g) and reduced xylose absorption (urine excretion of <4.0 g/5 hr after ingestion of the 25-g dose) are uniformly found. Brush border disaccharidases and hydrolysis of disaccharides at the intestinal surface are markedly impaired in tropical sprue (61). These tend to return to the normal range after treatment, but the depression of lactase may be more severe than the other disaccharidases and the recovery time may be delayed for months or years (62). Malabsorption of fat-soluble vitamins is common and vitamin D deficiency may produce hypocalcemia. In severe cases, secondary hyperparathyroidism can be manifested by an elevated serum parathyroid hormone level due to the chronic protracted calcium malabsorption. Although there is no evidence that the disease has an immunological basis, in the Puerto Rican population the presence of HLA types Aw-19 and especially Aw-31 appear to have a high association with tropical sprue (63).

Barium Contrast X-ray and Endoscopy

An upper small bowel X-ray series reveals prominent folds with an irregular contour from the jejunum through the distal ileum and retention of intraintestinal contents that dilute the barium contrast material. The radiologist may question whether the patient has failed to fast for the examination, but the findings are due to the substantial stasis related to altered motility (64,65). The important finding of ileal involvement is characteristic in tropical sprue and is rare in nontropical sprue, Whipple's disease, and other small intestinal enteropathies.

Upper gastrointestinal endoscopy frequently displays diminished prominence of the transverse duodenal folds, and close examination may demonstrate irregularities or scalloping when the view is parallel with the long axis of the folds (66). In addition, a patchy mosaic pattern of pale regions with prominent vessels, presumably representing atrophied areas of mucosa, may also be visualized. This finding may assist the operator in selecting the most seriously involved regions for endoscopic biopsy (66).

PATHOLOGY

Hematological Changes

Although the megaloblastic anemia seen in established tropical sprue is often said to be due to the chronic malabsorption and malnutrition, it is more severe than the anemias that develop in other small intestinal diseases that produce malabsorption. In part, this can be attributed to the involvement of the entire small intestine, including the ileum. But, not infrequently, severe megaloblastosis develops early in the course of the disease and the symptoms of anemia may be even more prominent than those of malabsorption (9,59). In addition, the prompt and often dramatic response to folic acid supplementation lends support to the fact that the vitamin B deficiencies may be pivotal in the pathogenesis of tropical sprue.

The Small Intestine

In the clinical setting of symptomatic small intestinal malabsorption with increased fat excretion and reduced D-xylose absorption occurring in the appropriate tropical locale, the definitive diagnosis can be made from the characteristic histological findings of the small intestinal biopsy. The hallmark of the disease is a generalized alteration in the small intestinal mucosa (67,68). In contrast to the normal small intestine, which displays tall villi with a scalloped or "sawtoothed" epithelial layer (Fig. 1), peroral biopsies from patients with tropical sprue reveal substantial blunting and broadening of the intestinal villi and deepening of the intestinal crypt epithelium (Fig. 2). Typical villus/crypt ratios decrease from a normal of 3–5:1 to 1:1 or less. The laminar propria is heavily infiltrated with chronic inflammatory cells, particularly lymphocytes, but an increase in plasma cells and histiocytes may also be seen. In severe disease, enterocytes become foreshortened from the normal, classic columnar shape to a cuboidal configuration, and there is a reduction of the height and numbers of luminal membrane microvilli when electron micrographs are examined. There is often a prominent infiltration of the single epithelial layer with migrating mononuclear cells from the underlying lamina propria. Although not generally realized, histological changes in untreated tropical sprue are distinctly characteristic and easily distinguishable from those of untreated celiac sprue (gluten-sensitive enteropathy, nontropical sprue), a disease that occurs more commonly in temperate zones. Even though the villi are markedly altered in tropical sprue, there is almost always preservation of identifiable villus and crypt units (12,67,68). In contrast, untreated celiac sprue is usually associated with the virtual absence of villi, marked elongation of crypts, and infiltration of plasma-type mononuclear cells rather than lymphocytes (69). In addition, the presence of fat accumulation at the basilar membrane underlying the enterocyte layer may be seen in tropical sprue but not in other enteropathies (70).

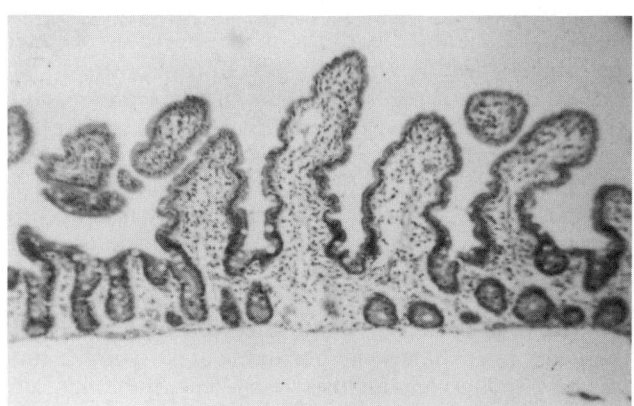

FIG. 1. Normal jejunal mucosa obtained by peroral biopsy. The tall, finger-like villi have a scalloped epithelial layer and display a ratio to the crypts of 3:1 or greater. There are moderate numbers of lymphocytes and plasma cells in the lamina propria, seen as small dots at this magnification (×100).

Interestingly enough, the reduction in villus height and the elongation of crypts producing an approximately one to one villus to crypt ratio is often seen in acquired immunodeficiency syndrome (AIDS) due to the HIV virus in patients who have watery diarrhea, even in the absence of intestinal malabsorption (71,72). Indeed, the intestinal histology in AIDS may be very similar to that in tropical sprue (Fig. 3), and in locales where it is an endemic disease, it is a more prevalent cause of intestinal injury than tropical sprue. Differentiation from Whipple's disease is relatively simple because of the PAS-positive macrophages and the presence of bacillary bodies on electron microscopy in that disease (54). In primary intestinal lymphoma (Mediterranean lymphoma), the paucity of intestinal crypts and dense infiltration with mononuclear cells, tightly packed in the lamina propria, serve to distinguish the disease from tropical sprue, even though malignant cells are uncommonly identified in primary lymphoma (73). Unlike the involvement with celiac sprue, which is most severe in the upper small intestine and usually spares the ileum, tropical sprue involves the entire small intestine, the ileal mucosa frequently being at least as damaged as the jejunum. The more severe malabsorption of vitamin B_{12} in tropical sprue as compared to celiac sprue can be explained by this.

DIFFERENTIAL DIAGNOSIS FROM OTHER ENTEROPATHIES

In temperate climates, the most common gastrointestinal enteropathy, *celiac sprue,* may present in a similar manner to tropical sprue, and it can be seen in the tropics (74). Besides the more severe histological abnormalities of the small intestine in celiac sprue, patients frequently know of family members who have had similar symptoms. Since the ileum is minimally involved, if at all, in celiac sprue, vitamin B_{12} absorption is likely to be normal and the dramatic response to the gluten-free diet clenches this diagnosis. The occasional response seen to gluten exclusion in tropical sprue is relatively muted by comparison. Diffuse *primary intestinal lymphoma* usually presents with chronic diarrhea often accompanied by bothersome abdominal pain, and malabsorption may not develop for months or even years. The paucity of crypts in the intestinal biopsy in primary lymphoma is also a tipoff (73). Extensive small intestinal *Crohn's disease* may produce severe malabsorption, but the intervening regions of normal mucosa and the development of strictures do not occur in tropical spure. *Intestinal tuberculosis* may be observed in some tropical countries and may mimic tropical sprue, but it is much less common, there being 100 patients with tropical sprue to every one identified with intestinal tuberculosis (7). *AIDS* is manifested by watery diarrhea with some malabsorption and alterations in the small intestinal histology that are very similar to that seen in tropical sprue (71,72) (cf. Figs. 2 and 3). Although an enteric infection can be identified in some AIDS patients, about half of these will have no detectable infectious cause. Hence in those individuals at risk for AIDS, appropriate diagnostic tests for AIDS are indicated. Small intes-

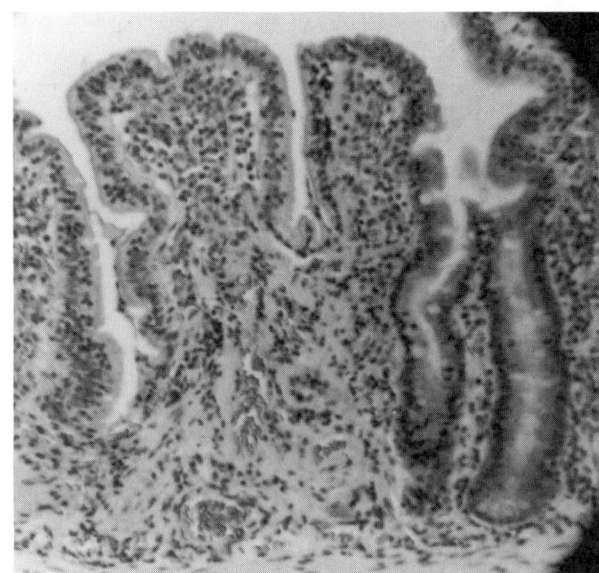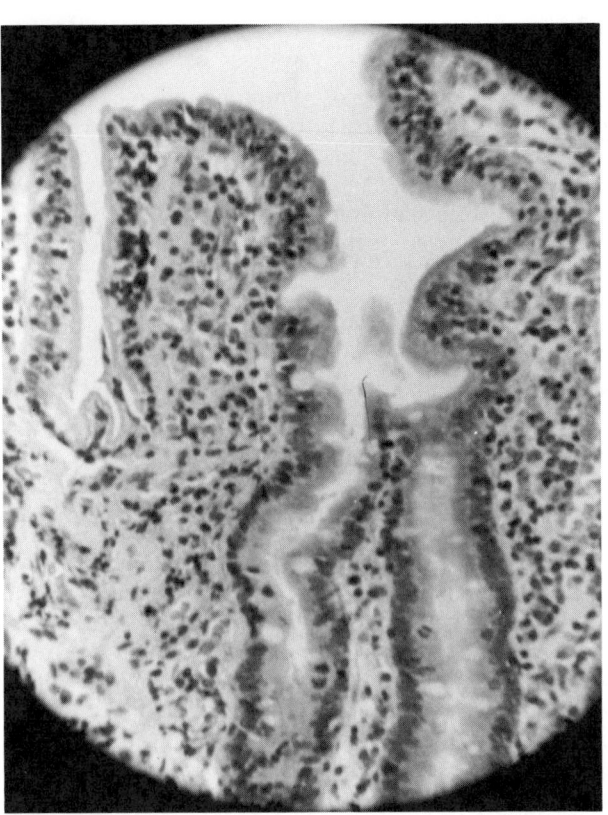

A   B

FIG. 2. Jejunal biopsy from a patient with tropical sprue. Villi are widened by increased infiltration of the lamina propria with inflammatory cells that also have migrated into the surface epithelial layer. **A:** ×100 magnification; **B:** ×400 magnification displaying the increased inflammatory cells, elongated crypts, and shortened villi, producing a villus/crypt ratio of 1:1.

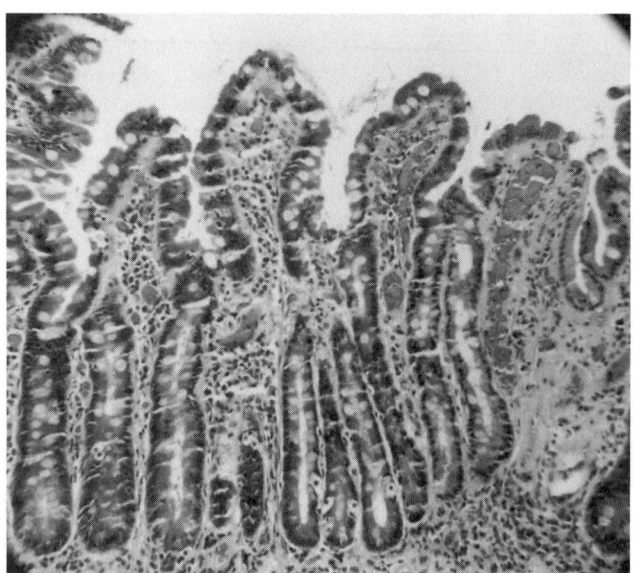

FIG. 3. Jejunal biopsy from a patient with AIDS. The widened lamina propria spaces, shortened villi, and elongated crypts are remarkably similar to the changes in tropical sprue. (Compare with Fig. 2.)

tinal *parasitic infestations* by *Cryptosporidium, Giardia,* and *Strongyloides* may cause diarrhea, and malabsorption may be intermittently manifested over many months or years. But the malabsorption secondary to parasitoses is usually mild and has little effect on the patient's nutrition and body weight. The diagnosis can be made by appropriate stool examination for ova and parasites. Notably, vitamin B_{12} deficiency due to the more severe involvement in tropical sprue is rarely observed in parasitoses. The *intestinal stasis syndrome* (*blind loop syndrome*) resulting in bacterial overgrowth caused by the slowed intestinal transit is usually due to the presence of numerous small intestinal diverticula or previous extensive gastric or intestinal surgery. Bacterial overgrowth may also occur in patients with achlorhydria, such as in pernicious anemia (75) or in the elderly (76,77), and may be associated with anorexia, diarrhea, mild malabsorption, and weight loss (78). This entity may also be produced by diseases that markedly alter the normal peristaltic activity in the small intestine such as amyloidosis, pseudoobstruction, scleroderma, and extensive injury of the small intestine. Bacterial overgrowth can usually be distinguished from tropical sprue by the minimal findings on the small intestinal X ray, by the presence of anaerobes rather than the coliforms seen in tropical sprue, and by the mild and nonspecific findings on the small intestinal biopsy (79). Severe histological lesions in the intestinal stasis syndrome are occasionally seen and a single biopsy may be indistinguishable from that seen in tropical sprue. But analysis of several biopsies from the same region will usually reveal minimal changes in most samples in the stasis syndrome (69,79). Finally, tropical sprue frequently develops in a community setting where there is a high prevalence of an entity frequently called tropical enteropathy (32,80). Such individuals are healthy and have no altered bowel habits, but intestinal biopsy may demonstrate nonspecific changes in the mucosal histology such as slight to moderate increase in the nuclear infiltration of the lamina propria below the epithelium. The normal villus-to-crypt ratio of 3–5:1 is maintained in tropical enteropathy, and persons with this subclinical condition do not appear to be at greater risk of developing tropical sprue than those with normal intestinal histology.

THERAPY

Because of the apparent vitamin deficiencies in tropical sprue, yeast and liver extracts were used in the 1930s to dramatically reverse the severe and often fatal anemia and malabsorption (81,82). Folic acid then became available in the late 1940s (83,84) and was very effective orally as the sole therapy, especially when given to patients who had the disease for only a few weeks or months. This vitamin improves the megaloblastic anemia within days (20,21) and, over the ensuing weeks, induces a dramatic reversal of anorexia and improvement in caloric intake and weight gain (43). The discrete response to therapy clinches the diagnosis of tropical sprue (6). A transient accentuation of pedal edema is common in the first week or so of therapy (43) but subsides as nutrition improves and the serum albumin levels increase. Although it is not necessary in the acute phase of treatment, vitamin B_{12} (1000 mg weekly) should be given also because its deficiency contributes to the malabsorption. But some intestinal malabsorption and altered histology often persists after vitamin therapy alone. When the disease has been well established over many months before the diagnosis is made, about 35–50% of patients may continue to have intestinal symptoms when treated only with folic acid, with or without vitamin B_{12} (20,21,43). For many of these patients, antibiotics are required to induce a complete remission. Antibacterial agents were first used in earnest during World War II when poorly absorbed oral sulfonamides were found successful as therapy of British military patients in the India–Burma region (18,85). Subsequently, both poorly absorbed sulfonamides (86) and particularly tetracycline have been given along with folic acid to achieve complete remission in the vast majority of patients with tropical sprue (44,87,88). Although the initial response may begin in only a few days, continual improvement and reversal of all aspects of the malabsorptive enteric syndrome and prevention of recurrence may require 6 months of therapy with oral folic acid, 5 mg and tetracycline, 250 mg q.i.d. (44,89). Even then, intestinal biopsies may still demonstrate crypt hyperplasia and mild villus shortening for many years, and relapses requiring additional courses of therapy will occur in 10–20% of patients who continue to reside in an endemic tropical region (90).

THE FUTURE

Despite the intense interest in tropical sprue for the latter half of this century, less has been written about the malady in the last few years. Certainly, it remains as a formidable chronic condition producing malnutrition in many countries near to the equator where general nutrition in the local seemingly healthy population is known to be frequently borderline. It seems paradoxical that there may be a waning interest in this disease even though several highly potent molecular techniques are now available for analysis of secretions and tissues. The time is ripe for a renewed examination of the microenvironmental factors in the intestinal cavity, the intestinal tissue, and the bone marrow where there seems certain to be a key to the etiology of tropical sprue.

ACKNOWLEDGMENTS

Work of the author related to this chapter is supported by a research grant (DK 11270) and a Digestive Disease Center grant (DK 38707) from the National Institutes of Health, National Institute of Diabetes, Digestive and Kidney Diseases.

REFERENCES

1. Klipstein FA, Baker SJ. Regarding the definition of tropical sprue. *Gastroenterology* 1970;58:717–721.
2. Hillary W. *Observations on the changes of the air and concomitant epidemical diseases in the Island of Barbados.* London: Hitch and Hawes; 1759:277.
3. Manson P. China maritime customs II—special series no. 2. Medical reports for the half year ended 31st March 1880. 19th issue. Shanghai: Statistical Department of the Inspectorate General; 1880:33.
4. Cook CG. Aetiology and pathogenesis of tropical sprue: do viruses play a role? *Trop Gastroenterol* 1985;6:1–3.
5. Klipstein FA, Short HB, Engert RF, Jean L, Weaver GA. Contamination of the small intestine by enterotoxigenic coliform bacteria among the rural population of Haiti. *Gastroenterology* 1976;70:1035–1041.
6. Klipstein FA. Tropical sprue in travelers and expatriates living abroad. *Gastroenterology* 1981;80:590–600.
7. Mathan VI. Tropical sprue in southern India. *Trans R Soc Trop Med Hyg* 1988;82:10–14.
8. Stefanini M. Clinical features and pathogenesis of tropical sprue: observations on a series of cases among Italian prisoners of war in India. *Medicine* 1948;27:379–427.
9. Gardner FH. A malabsorption syndrome in military personnel in Puerto Rico. *Arch Intern Med* 1956;98:44–60.
10. Klipstein FA, Samloff IM, Schenk EA. Tropical sprue in Haiti. *Ann Intern Med* 1966;64:575–593.
11. Garcia S. Malabsorption and malnutrition in Mexico. *Am J Clin Nutr* 1968;21:1066–1076.
12. Mathan M, Mathan VI, Baker SJ. An electron-microscopic study of jejunal mucosal morphology in control subjects and in patients with tropical sprue in southern India. *Gastroenterology* 1975;68:17–32.
13. Moshal MG. Tropical sprue in Africa. *Lancet* 1970;2:827.

14. Webb JF, Simpson F. Tropical sprue in Hong Kong. *Br Med J* 1966;2:1162–1166.
15. O'Brien W. Historical survey of tropical sprue affecting Europeans in southeast Asia. In: *Tropical sprue and megaloblastic anaemia: Wellcome Trust Collaborative Study 1961–1969.* London: Churchill Livingstone; 1971:13–24.
16. Sparberg M, Knudson KB, Frank S. Tropical sprue from the Philippines: report of three cases. *Milit Med* 1967;132:809–815.
17. Keele KD, Bound JP. Sprue in India: clinical survey of 600 cases. *Br Med J* 1946;1:77–81.
18. Ayrey F. Outbreaks of sprue during the Burma campaign. *Trans R Soc Trop Med Hyg* 1948;41:377–406.
19. O'Brien W, England NWJ. Military tropical sprue from southeast Asia. *Br Med J* 1966;2:1157–1162.
20. O'Brien W, England NWJ. Tropical sprue amongst British servicemen and their families in south-east Asia. In: *Tropical sprue and megaloblastic anaemia: Wellcome Trust Collaborative Study 1961–1969.* London: Churchill Livingstone; 1971:25–60.
21. Sheehy TW, Cohen WC, Wallace DK, et al. Tropical sprue in North Americans. *JAMA* 1965;194:1069–1076.
22. Pittman FE, Pittman JC. Tropical sprue in American servicemen following return from Vietnam. *Am J Dig Dis* 1976;21:393–398.
23. Catino D. Proctor RF, Colwell EJ, Legters LJ, Webb CR. Tropical sprue. Prospective studies on incidence, early manifestations, and association with abnormal bacterial flora and intestinal parasitemia, January 1967–March 1968. Annual Progress Report. U.S. Army Medical Research Team, (WRAIR), Vietnam and Institute Pasteur, Vietnam. 1 Sept 1967–30 June 1968.
24. Lindenbaum J, Kent TH, Sprinz H. Malabsorption and jejunitis in American Peace Corps volunteers in Pakistan. *Ann Intern Med* 1966;65:2101–1208.
25. Lindenbaum J, Gerson CD, Kent TH. Recovery of small-intestinal structure and function after residence in the tropics. *Ann Intern Med* 1971;74:218–222.
26. Gerson CD, Kent TH, Saha JR, Siddiqi N, Lindenbaum J. Recovery of small-intestinal structure and function after residence in the tropics. II. Studies in Indians and Pakistanis living in New York City. *Ann Intern Med* 1971;75:41–48.
27. Klipstein FA, Falaiye JM. Tropical sprue in expatriates form the tropics living in the continental United States. *Medicine* 1969;48:475–491.
28. Mathan VI, Baker SJ. Epidemic tropical sprue and other epidemics of diarrhea in South Indian villages. *Am J Clin Nutr* 1968;21:1077–1087.
29. Baker SJ, Mathan VI. An epidemic of tropical sprue in southern India. II Epidemiology. *Ann Trop Med Parasitol* 1970;64:453–467.
30. Mathan VI, Joseph S, Baker SJ. Tropical sprue in children. *Gastroenterology* 1969;56:556–569.
31. Santiago-Borrero PJ, Maldonado N, Horta E. Tropical sprue in children. *J Pediatr* 1970;76:470–479.
32. Baker SJ, Mathan VI. Tropical enteropathy and tropical sprue. *Am J Clin Nutr* 1972;25:1047–1055.
33. Cook GC. Aetiology and pathogenesis of postinfective tropical malabsorption (tropical sprue). *Lancet* 1984;1:721–723.
34. Glynn J. Tropical sprue—its aetiology and pathogenesis. *R Soc Med* 1986;79:599–606.
35. Baker SJ, Mathan VI. Tropical sprue in southern India. In: *Tropical sprue and megaloblastic anaemia: Wellcome Trust Collaborative Study 1961–1969.* London: Churchill Livingstone; 1971:189.
36. Tomkins AM, Drasar BS, James WPT. Bacterial colonization of jejunal mucosa in acute tropical sprue. *Lancet* 1975;1:59–62.
37. Gorbach SL, Banwell JG, Jacobs B, et al. Tropical sprue and malnutrition in West Bengal. I. Intestinal microflora and absorption. *Am J Clin Nutr* 1970;23:1545–1558.
38. Bhat P, Shantakumari S, Rajan D, et al. Bacterial flora of the gastrointestinal tract in southern Indian control subjects and patients with tropical sprue. *Gastroenterology* 1972;62:11–21.
39. Klipstein FA, Holdeman LV, Corcino JJ, Moore WE. Enterotoxigenic intestinal bacteria in tropical sprue. *Ann Intern Med* 1973;79:632–641.
40. Appelbaum PC, Moshal MG, Hift W, Chatterton SA. Intestinal bacteria in patients with tropical sprue. *South Afr Med J* 1980;57:1081–1083.
41. Toskes PP, Giannella RA, Jervis HR, Rout WR, Takeuchi A. Small intestinal mucosal injury in the experimental blind loop syndrome: light- and electron-microscopic and histochemical studies. *Gastroenterology* 1975;68:193–203.
42. Read NW. Small bowel transit time of food in man: measurement, regulation and possible importance. *Scand J Gastroenterol* 1984;96(Suppl):77–85.
43. Sheehy TW, Baggs B, Perez-Santiago E, Floch MH. Prognosis of tropical sprue. A study of the effect of folic acid on the intestinal aspects of acute and chronic sprue. *Ann Intern Med* 1962;57:892–908.
44. Guerra R, Wheby MS, Bayless TM. Long-term antibiotic therapy in tropical sprue. *Ann Intern Med* 1965;63:619–634.
45. Bayless TM, Guardiola-Rotger A, Wheby MS. Tropical sprue: viral cultures of rectal swabs. *Gastroenterology* 1966;51:32–35.
46. Mathan M, Mathan VI, Swaminathan SP, Yesudoss S, Baker SJ. Pleomorphic virus-like particles in human feces. *Lancet* 1975;1:1068–1069.
47. Baker SJ, Mathan M, Mathan VI, Jesudoss S, Swaminathan SP. Chronic enterocyte infection with coronavirus. One possible cause of the syndrome of tropical sprue? *Dig Dis Sci* 1982;27:1039–1043.
48. Adrian TE, Savage AP, Bacarese-Hamilton AJ, Wolfe K, Besterman HS, Bloom SR. Peptide YY abnormalities in gastrointestinal diseases. *Gastroenterology* 1986;90:379–384.
49. Baker SJ, Mathan VI. Syndrome of tropical sprue in south India. *Am J Clin Nutr* 1968;21:984–993.
50. Wilson KH, Blitchington R, Frothingham R, Wilson JA. Phylogeny of the Whipple's-disease-associated bacterium. *Lancet* 1991;338:474–475.
51. Relman DA, Schmidt TM, MacDermott RP, Falkow S. Identification of the uncultured bacillus of Whipple's disease. *N Engl J Med* 1992;327:293–301.
52. Ratliff NB, McMahon JT, Naab TJ, Cosgrove DM. Whipple's disease in the porcine leaflets of a Carpentier–Edwards prosthetic mitral valve. *N Engl J Med* 1984;311:902–903.
53. Bayless TM, Knox DL. Whipple's disease: a multisystem infection. *N Engl J Med* 1979;300:920–921.
54. Dobbins WO, Kawanishi H. Bacillary characteristics in Whipple's disease: an electron microsopic study. *Gastroenterology* 1981;80:1468–1475.
55. Santiago-Borrero PJ, Maldonado N, Horta E. Tropical sprue in children. *J Pediatr* 1970;76:470–479.
56. Mathan VI, Joseph S, Baker SJ. Tropical sprue in children. A syndrome of idiopathic malabsorption. *Gastroenterology* 1969;56:556–569.
57. Trier JS. Case 15-1990. Case Records of the Massachusetts General Hospital. Weekly clinicopathological exercises. *N Engl J Med* 1990;322:1067–1075.
58. Baker SJ. The recognition of vitamin B_{12} and folate deficiency. *N Z Med J* 1966;65:884–892.
59. Sparberg M, Knudson KB, Frank S. Tropical sprue from the Philippines: report of three cases. *Milit Med* 1967;809–815.
60. Vaish SK, Ignatius M, Baker SJ. Albumin metabolism in tropical sprue. *Q J Med* 1965;34:15–32.
61. Gray GM, Santiago NA. Disaccharide absorption in normal and diseased human intestine. *Gastroenterology* 1966;51:489–498.
62. Gray GM, Walter WM Jr, Colver EH. Persistent deficiency of intestinal lactase in apparently cured tropical sprue. *Gastroenterology* 1968;54:552–558.
63. Menendez-Corrada R, Nettleship E, Santiago-Delpin EA. HLA and tropical sprue. *Lancet* 1986;2:1183–1185.
64. Jayanthi V, Chacko A, Gani IK, Mathan VI. Intestinal transit in healthy southern Indian subjects in patients and tropical sprue. *Gut* 1989;30:35–38.
65. Cook GC. Delayed small-intestinal transit in tropical malabsorption. *Br Med J* 1978;2:238–240.
66. Tawil SC, Brandt LJ, Bernstein LH. Mosaic mucosa in tropical sprue. *Endoscopy* 1991;37:365–366.
67. Swanson VL, Thomassen RW. Pathology of the jejunal mucosa in tropical sprue. *Am J Pathol* 1965;46:511–551.
68. Swanson VL, Wheby MS, Bayless TM. Morphologic effects of

folic acid and vitamin B$_{12}$ on the jejunal lesion of tropical sprue. *Am J Pathol* 1966;49:167–197.

69. Perera DR, Weinstein WM, Rubin CE. Small intestinal biopsy. *Hum Pathol* 1975;6:157–217.

70. Schenk EA, Samloff IM, Klipstein FA. Morphologic characteristics of jejunal biopsy in celiac disease and tropical sprue. *Am J Pathol* 1965;47:765–781.

71. Kotler DP, Gaetz HP, Lange M, Klein EB, Holt PR. Enteropathy associated with the acquired immunodeficiency syndrome. *Ann Intern Med* 1984;101:421–428.

72. Madi K, Trajman A, da Silver CF, et al. Jejunal biopsy in HIV-infected patients. *J AIDS* 1991;4:930–937.

73. Gray GM, Rosenberg SA, Cooper AD, Gregory PB, Stein DT, Herzenberg H. Lymphomas involving the gastrointestinal tract. *Gastroenterology* 1982;82:143–152.

74. Misra RC, Kasthuri D, Chuttani HK. Adult coeliac disease in tropics. *Br Med J* 1966;2:1230–1232.

75. Lindenbaum J, Pezzimenti JF, Shea N. Small-intestinal function in vitamin B$_{12}$ deficiency. *Ann Intern Med* 1974;80:326–331.

76. Roberts SH, James O, Jarvis EH. Bacterial overgrowth syndrome without "blind loop": a cause for malnutrition in the elderly. *Lancet* 1977;2:1193–1195.

77. McEvoy A, Dutton J, James OFW. Bacterial contamination of the small intestine is an important cause of occult malabsorption in the elderly. *Br Med J* 1983;287:789–793.

78. King CE, Toskes PP. Small intestine bacterial overgrowth. *Gastroenterology* 1979;76:1035–1055.

79. Ament ME, Shimoda SS, Saunders DR, Rubin CE. Pathogenesis of steatorrhea in three cases of small intestinal stasis syndrome. *Gastroenterology* 1972;63:728–747.

80. Chaves FJZC, Veloso FT, Cruz I, et al. Subclinical tropical enteropathy in Angola: peroral jejunal biopsies and absorption studies in asymptomatic healthy men. *Mount Sinai J Med* 1981;48:47–52.

81. Wills L. Treatment of "pernicious anaemia of pregnancy" and "tropical anaemia" with special reference to yeast extract as a curative agent. *Br Med J* 1931;1:1059–1064.

82. Rhoads CP, Miller DK. Intensive liver extract therapy of sprue. *JAMA* 1934;103:387–391.

83. Spies TD, Milanes F, Menendez A, Koch MB, Minnich V. Observations on treatment of tropical sprue with folic acid. *J Lab Clin Med* 1946;31:227–241.

84. Suarez RM, Spies TD, Suarez RM Jr. Use of folic acid in sprue. *Ann Intern Med* 1947;26:643–677.

85. Keele KD, Bound JP. Sprue in India: a clinical survey of 600 cases. *Br Med J* 1946;1:77–81.

86. Maldonado N, Horta E, Guerra R, Perez-Santiago E. Poorly absorbed sulfonamides in the treatment of tropical sprue. *Gastroenterology* 1969;57:559–568.

87. French JM, Gaddie R, Smith NM. Tropical sprue: a study of seven cases and their response to combined chemotherapy. *Q J Med* 1956;25:333–351.

88. Sheehy TW, Perez-Santiago E. Antibiotic therapy in tropical sprue. *Gastroenterology* 1961;41:208–213.

89. Klipstein FA, Falaiye J. Tropical sprue in expatriates from the tropics living in the continental United States. *Medicine* (Baltimore) 1969;48:475–492.

90. Rickles FR, Klipstein FA, Tomasini J, Corcino JJ, Maldonado N. Long-term follow-up of antibiotic-treated tropical sprue. *Ann Intern Med* 1972;76:203–210.

Infections of the Gastrointestinal Tract,
edited by M. J. Blaser, P. D. Smith, J. I. Ravdin,
H. B. Greenberg, and R. L. Guerrant
Raven Press, Ltd., New York © 1995.

CHAPTER 26

Small Intestine Bacterial Overgrowth, Including Blind Loop Syndrome

Phillip P. Toskes

The development of malabsorption in a patient with overgrowth of bacteria within the small intestine is known as the blind loop, stagnant loop, stasis, or bacterial overgrowth syndrome. In this condition, the bacterial flora of the proximal small intestine resembles that of the normal colon. The qualitative and quantitative changes in flora that occur substantially alter the nutritional status of the human host. The overgrowth flora successfully compete with the human host for the ingested nutrients. What ensues is a complex array of clinical problems resulting from intraluminal bacterial catabolism of nutrients, often with production of toxic metabolites, and direct injury to the small intestine enterocyte (1,2).

In the past the most apparent conditions where bacterial overgrowth occurred were those related to intestinal blind loops. Thus this condition of antibiotic or surgically correctable malabsorption became known as the blind loop syndrome. Now it is appreciated that small intestine bacterial overgrowth may occur frequently with no definable blind loop.

DESCRIPTION OF NORMAL ENTERIC FLORA

The qualitative and quantitative aspects of the flora of the normal human gastrointestinal tract are described in Table 1. Normally the stomach and small intestine harbor relatively few bacteria. The bacteria found in the normal upper small intestine (the jejunum is the standard reference site for intestinal aspirates) consist of gram-positive aerobes or facultative anaerobes in concentrations of up to 10^4 organisms/mL of jejunal secretions. The jejunum of a healthy subject may contain coliforms transiently with concentrations rarely exceeding 10^3 bacteria/mL of secretions. The upper small intestine of healthy subjects does not contain anaerobic bacteroides.

P. P. Toskes: Division of Gastroenterology, Hepatology, and Nutrition, Department of Medicine, University of Florida, Gainesville, Florida 32610.

The ileum appears to represent a zone of transition from the sparse populations of aerobic flora present in the stomach and proximal bowel and the very dense bacterial populations of anaerobic microorganisms present in the colon. In the ileum the concentrations of microorganisms increase to levels of 10^5–10^9 organisms per gram of contents. Enterobacteria, including coliforms, occur only transiently and in small numbers in the proximal bowel, but are regularly found in substantial numbers in the ileum. Strict anaerobes, which normally cannot survive in the jejunum, frequently colonize the ileum.

The most dramatic change in the enteric flora occurs across the ileocecal valve. The total number of microorganisms increases up to 1 million fold and approximately 10^9–10^{12} microorganisms per gram of colonic contents. The large bowel flora is dominated by fastidious anaerobic organisms such as bacteroides, anaerobic lactobacilli, and clostridia. These microorganisms, although difficult to culture, actually outnumber aerobic and facultative organisms by as much as 10,000:1 within the lumen of the colon. When the ileocecal valve is resected, the populations of the most distal portions of the ileum tend to resemble those of the cecum.

TABLE 1. *Normal bacterial flora within the gastrointestinal tract*

	Stomach	Jejunum	Ileum	Cecum
Total bacterial counts[a]	0–3	0–4	5–8	10–12
Aerobes and facultative anaerobes	0–3	0–4	2–5	2–9
Anaerobes	0	0	3–7	9–12

[a] Log 10 of the number of viable microorganisms per gram of contents. Data compiled from Refs. 3–7. From ref. 2, with permission.

TABLE 2. *Endogenous defense mechanisms for preventing bacterial overgrowth*

Intestinal motility
Gastric acid secretion
Intact ileocecal sphincter
Immunoglobulins within intestinal secretions
Ill-defined mucosal factors
Bacteriostatic properties of pancreatic/biliary secretion

Table 2 lists in order of decreasing importance those factors normally preventing the development of bacterial overgrowth. Undoubtedly, the major factor responsible for limiting bacterial proliferation in the small bowel is the cleansing action of normal propulsive motility. In the relatively stagnant contents of the large bowel, bacterial growth is luxuriant, whereas microorganisms are rapidly cleared from the small intestine. Of particular importance in this regard is the interdigestive migrating motor complex. Mucus may aid in this mechanical process for removing bacteria, a possibility that is supported by the tendency for microorganisms to concentrate in the mucous layer that lines the gastrointestinal mucosa. The crucial importance of normal small bowel peristalsis is emphasized by the fact that whenever normal motility is slowed or interrupted, bacterial overgrowth (more than 10^4 microorganisms/mL of jejunal contents) rapidly ensues.

Bacterial interactions within the gut lumen represent an important, if still poorly understood, determinant of the bacterial populations inhabiting the alimentary canal. It is important to recognize, for example, that without the oxygen-utilizing aerobes such as coliforms and enterococci, the colon would not be sufficiently anaerobic to maintain the large populations of fastidious anaerobes such as the bacteroides. Anaerobes stabilize the enteric flora, thus preventing overgrowth with pathogens. In patients with bacterial overgrowth, the flora closely resembles that of the normal colon. Quantitative counts may reach 10^{10} viable bacteria/mL of secretions. Bacteroides and anaerobic lactobacilli usually predominate, but enterobacteria, enterococci, clostridia, and diphtheroids may also be present in high concentrations (1,2).

CLINICAL CONDITIONS ASSOCIATED WITH BACTERIAL OVERGROWTH

The recognized clinical conditions associated with bacterial overgrowth are listed in Table 3. In the past, when much more aggressive gastrointestinal surgery was performed on a more regular basis, anatomic abnormalities (e.g., Billroth II anastomosis, surgery for Crohn's disease) were the most common causes of clinically significant bacterial overgrowth. Blind pouches of the small intestine formed surgically by creation of an end-to-side enteroenteric anastomosis frequently produce bacterial overgrowth. Similarly, stagnant loops of intestine resulting from fistulae or surgical enterostomies allow for continuous recirculation of small intestinal contents and consequent bacterial overgrowth. Following partial gastrectomy and Billroth II anastomosis, dysfunction and stasis in the afferent loop may result in marked intraluminal proliferation of bacteria and consequent seeding of the remainder of the small intestine (8). Duodenal and jejunal diverticula may result in overgrowth, especially in the setting of hypo- or achlorhydria (Fig. 1) (9). Obstruction of the small intestine due to Crohn's disease (Fig. 2), adhesions, radiation damage, lymphoma, or tuberculosis may cause bacterial overgrowth (10–13). Patients with gastrocolic or gastrojejunocolic fistulae with colonic contents passing into the stomach and small intestine may develop a massive bacterial seeding of the small intestine and devastating malabsorption (14). Patients with Kock distal ileal pouches (continent ileostomy) may experience malabsorption secondary to bacterial overgrowth (15).

Abnormalities in intestinal motility often combined with decreased gastric acid secretion favor bacterial proliferation and subsequent malabsorption. Patients with scleroderma (16) (Fig. 3), intestinal pseudoobstruction (17), and diabetic autonomic neuropathy (18) are examples of such abnormalities. Patients with an absent or disordered migrating motor complex (MMC) may develop bacterial overgrowth and malabsorption (19). Such patients may have no radiographic abnormalities.

Elderly patients may develop malabsorption secondary to bacterial overgrowth. Indeed it has been suggested that bacterial overgrowth is the most common cause of clinically significant malabsorption in the elderly (20–23). The elderly often have motor disorders (often induced by prior gastrointestinal surgery) of the small intestine and decreased acid secretion. Some studies have demonstrated correction of the failure-to-thrive syndrome in elderly

TABLE 3. *Clinical conditions associated with bacterial overgrowth*

Gastric proliferation:
    Hypo- or achlorhydria, especially when combined with motor or anatomic disturbances
    Sustained hypochlorhydria induced by omeprazole
Small intestinal stagnation
Anatomic:
    Afferent loop of Billroth II partial gastrectomy
    Duodenal–jejunal diverticulosis
    Surgical blind loop (end-to-side anastomosis)
    Surgical recirculating loop (end-to-side anastomosis)
    Obstruction (stricture, adhesion, inflammation, neoplasm)
Motor:
    Scleroderma
    Idiopathic intestinal pseudoobstruction
    Absent or disordered migrating motor complex
    Diabetic autonomic neuropathy
Abnormal communication between proximal and distal gastrointestinal tract:
    Gastrocolic or jejunocolic fistula
    Resection of diseased ileocecal valve
Miscellaneous:
    Chronic pancreatitis
    Immunodeficiency syndromes
    Cirrhosis

Modified from ref. 2.

subjects following treatment with antibiotics. Other studies in healthy elderly subjects demonstrated a high frequency of bacterial overgrowth but it appeared to be of little clinical significance (24,25). The great majority of such individuals had normal absorption of nutrients despite significant overgrowth of the proximal small intestine. Such a condition has been called *simple colonization*. It may very well be a different situation if elderly subjects are ill or have associated hypomotility of the small intestine or anatomic abnormalities such as duodenal diverticula or previous gastrointestinal surgery (e.g., Billroth II anastomosis).

The importance of both normal intestinal motility and normal gastric acid secretion to prevent clinically significant bacterial overgrowth is underscored by recent clinical experiences wherein patients with scleroderma and reflux esophagitis who were doing relatively well on H2 receptor antagonist or antacid therapy developed marked malabsorption (diarrhea, steatorrhea) following institution of omeprazole. Omeprazole decreased markedly the remaining acid secretion in these patients, thus allowing

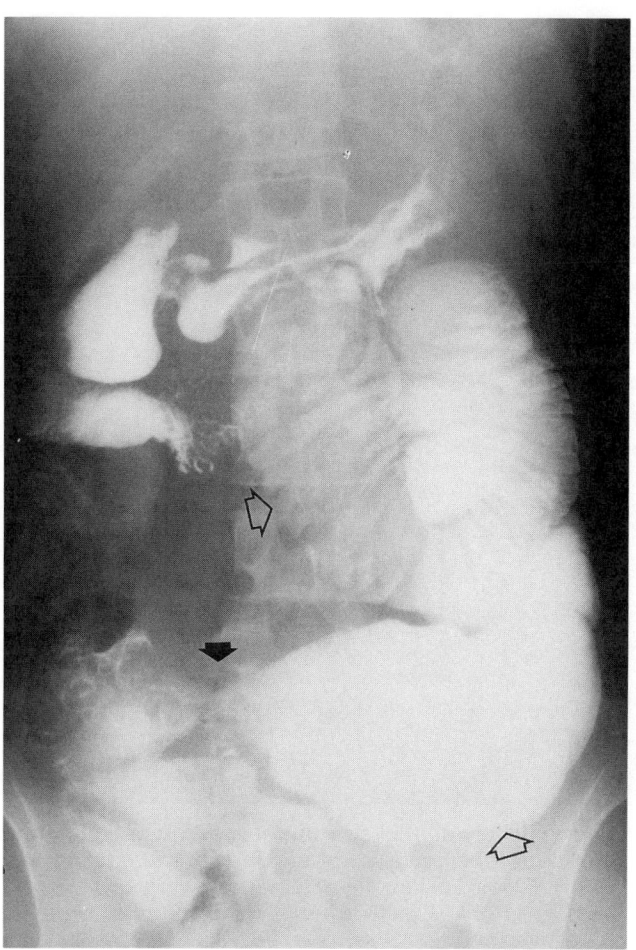

FIG. 2. Stricture in proximal ileum (*solid arrow*) with proximal dilated small bowel loops (*open arrows*) in a patient with Crohn's disease and clinically important malabsorption due to bacterial overgrowth. (From Toskes PP. Bacterial overgrowth syndromes. In: *Bockus gastroenterology* 5th ed. [*in press*], with permission.)

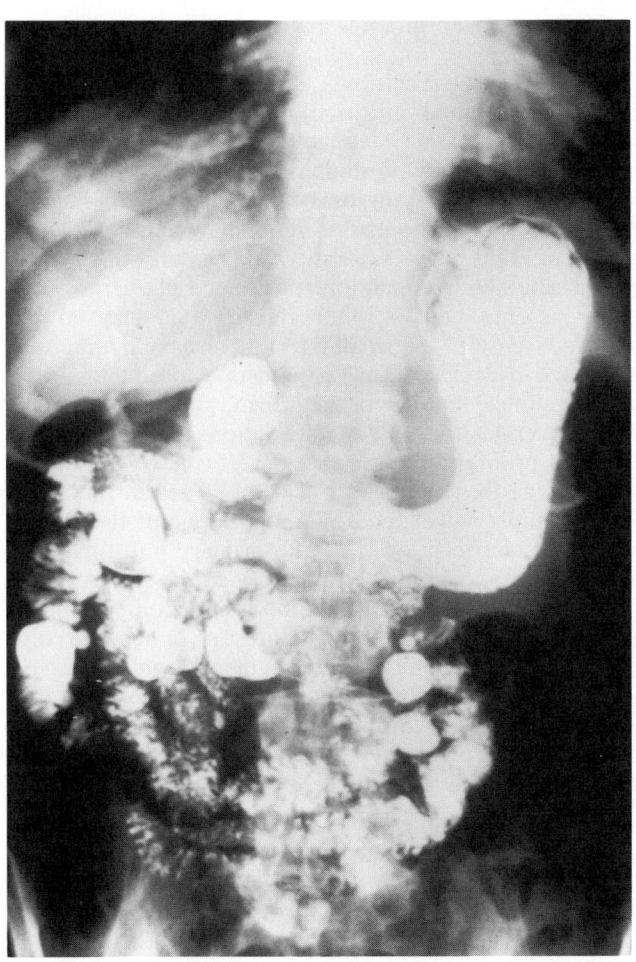

FIG. 1. Multiple duodenal and jejunal diverticula in a patient with malabsorption secondary to bacterial overgrowth. (From Toskes PP. Bacterial overgrowth of the gastrointestinal tract. *Adv Intern Med* 1993;38:387–407, with permission.)

bacterial overgrowth to occur. A recent preliminary report (26) documented bacterial overgrowth in 56% of 25 outpatients with reflux esophagitis and/or peptic ulcer disease who had received 40 mg of omeprazole for about 5 weeks. Whether this development of bacterial overgrowth in these types of ambulatory patients will have any clinical consequences remains to be determined. It appears that the bacterial overgrowth related to omeprazole treatment is similar to the "simple colonization" observed in the healthy elderly. Another study failed to show any effect of omeprazole therapy on fat or carbohydrate absorption despite the induction of bacterial overgrowth (25). It should be emphasized that in both of these studies the use of omeprazole was short term. Perhaps long-term use of omeprazole will lead to clinically significant overgrowth, especially if there is an associated abnormality (functional or structural) of the small intestine as discussed above.

Up to 40% of patients with chronic pancreatitis may have concomitant bacterial overgrowth (27). Bacterial

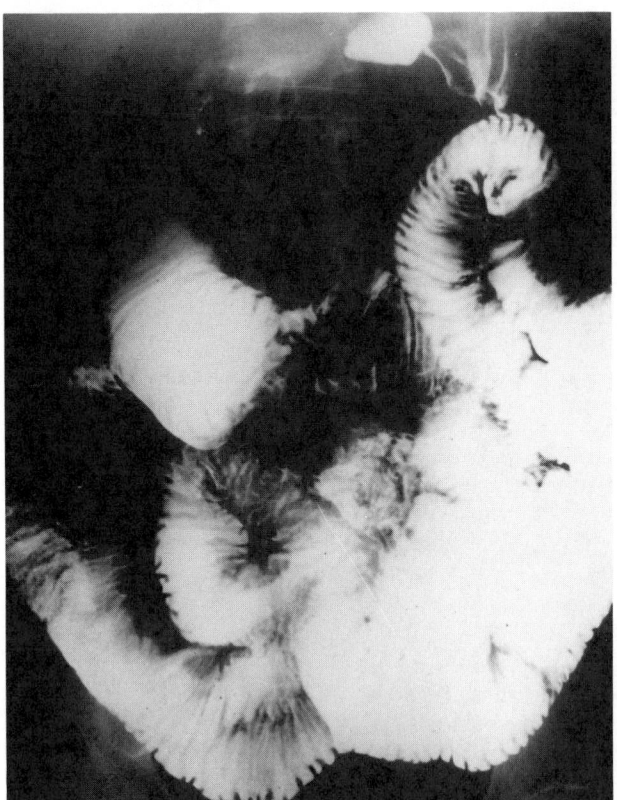

FIG. 3. Diffusely dilated small intestine in a patient with scleroderma and malabsorption due to bacterial overgrowth. (From Toskes PP. Bacterial overgrowth syndromes. In: *Bockus gastroenterology* 5th ed. [*in press*], with permission.)

overgrowth may occur in these patients because of a decrease in intestinal motility resulting from pain, fever, use of narcotics, and inflammatory changes or obstruction from the enlarged inflamed pancreas, or it may be due to previous pancreatic surgery. It is interesting to point out that canine pancreatic secretions have antibacterial activity (28). In addition, culture-proven bacterial overgrowth has been documented in dogs with pancreatic exocrine insufficiency (29). Appropriate therapy of steatorrhea in these patients may require both pancreatic extract and antimicrobial agents. The pathogenesis of the bacterial overgrowth in patients with immunodeficiency syndromes is poorly understood, but bacterial overgrowth is a common feature in these patients regardless of the immunological defect. These patients also have an increased intestinal permeability to macromolecules. A recent study in 17 children (30) demonstrated the presence of both bacterial overgrowth and abnormal intestinal permeability in 41% of the patients, suggesting a causal relation between the two. Several studies have documented the presence of small intestine bacterial overgrowth in patients with cirrhosis (31–33). The majority of these patients had alcohol-induced cirrhosis and may have had concomitant alcohol-induced pancreatic exocrine damage, perhaps contributing to the overgrowth (see above). The clinical relevance of the bacterial overgrowth in patients with cirrhosis has not been defined.

CLINICAL MANIFESTATIONS OF BACTERIAL OVERGROWTH

Although clinical manifestations vary greatly and depend, at least in part, on the nature of the small intestine abnormality causing the bacterial overgrowth, certain clinical features are hallmarks of the bacterial overgrowth syndrome. These features are pointed out in Table 4. Patients with bacterial overgrowth may demonstrate some or all of these features.

Patients with small intestinal diverticula are relatively asymptomatic until small intestinal bacterial populations are sufficiently established to cause steatorrhea with increased numbers of bowel movements, weight loss, and anemia. Because most patients with steatorrhea and anemia associated with small intestine diverticula are elderly, an interval of many years has been assumed between the development of the diverticula and the appearance of metabolic abnormalities. It seems likely that hypo- or achlorhydria, which is relatively common in the elderly, permits increased bacterial overgrowth in many cases. Although most symptomatic patients have multiple diverticula, development of the complications of bacterial overgrowth has been observed in some patients with a single large diverticulum.

Patients with strictures, surgically formed blind pouches of the small intestine, or functional dysmotility of the small intestine may note abdominal discomfort, bloating, and crampy periumbilical pain before diarrhea, steatorrhea, and the symptoms of anemia develop. In general, an interval of months or years may elapse between the time a blind pouch is formed and the onset of symptoms attributable to small intestine bacterial overgrowth. When patients have strictures or fistulae caused by Crohn's disease of the small intestine or have hypomotility caused by scleroderma or intestinal pseudoobstruction, the clinical features of the primary disease may completely overshadow any manifestations of intraluminal microbial proliferation. Furthermore, it may be difficult to determine in patients with Crohn's disease, radiation enteritis, short bowel syndrome, or lymphoma the extent to which malabsorption is due to primary intestinal disease or insufficiency or secondary bacterial overgrowth.

Whatever the cause of the abnormal proliferation of microorganisms within the small intestine lumen, the consequences for the patient are the same. Weight loss associated with clinically apparent steatorrhea has been observed in about one third of patients with small intestine bacterial overgrowth severe enough to cause cobalamin deficiency (34). Osteomalacia, vitamin K deficiency,

TABLE 4. *Clinical features of bacterial overgrowth*

Cobalamin (vitamin B_{12}) malabsorption and deficiency
Bloating
Abdominal pain
Steatorrhea
Diarrhea
Decreased urinary xylose excretion
Hypoalbuminemia

night blindness, and even hypocalcemic tetany have been known to develop as a consequence of lipid malabsorption in patients with this disorder. Appropriate therapy or surgical correction of the small intestine lesion conducive to stasis promptly reduced fecal fat excretion to normal or near-normal levels.

PATHOGENESIS OF NUTRIENT MALABSORPTION AND DEFICIENCY DUE TO BACTERIAL OVERGROWTH

Ample evidence indicates that the anemia that develops in patients with the blind loop syndrome is largely due to cobalamin deficiency. The anemia is usually megaloblastic and macrocytic, and serum cobalamin levels are low. Furthermore, neurological changes indistinguishable from those of pernicious anemia may develop, and the anemia can be corrected by physiological doses of the vitamin. Cobalamin (vitamin B_{12}) malabsorption that cannot be corrected by intrinsic factor is a hallmark of clinically significant small bowel bacterial overgrowth. Experiments performed three decades ago in rats with surgically induced bacterial overgrowth showed that bacterial uptake of cobalamin prevents the vitamin from being absorbed by enterocytes (35). This mechanism has now been confirmed in many experimental and clinical settings. Competitive uptake of the vitamin is particularly characteristic of gram-negative aerobes and various anaerobes that proliferate in the small bowel during stasis. Intrinsic factor effectively inhibits aerobic microbial uptake of cobalamin but has no effect on cobalamin uptake by gram-negative anaerobes (bacteroides) (36). Since *in vivo* intrinsic factor binds cobalamin before the vitamin comes in contact with intestinal bacteria, gram-negative anaerobes appear to be the bacteria responsible for the cobalamin malabsorption associated with bacterial overgrowth.

Enteric microorganisms synthesize cobalamin and thus become a rich source of this vitamin. Viable bacteria retain the vitamin, however, and it never becomes available to the host. In fact, these bacteria successfully compete with enterocytes for dietary cobalamin. Thus, patients with small bowel bacterial overgrowth face a paradoxical situation: they develop cobalamin deficiency even though they harbor large quantities of the vitamin in their small bowel.

In the experimental blind loop syndrome and in some patients with overgrowth, iron deficiency is secondary to blood lost through the gastrointestinal tract, perhaps secondary to ulcerated areas within stagnant loops (37). Under these circumstances, the patient may have guaiac-positive stools together with a microcytic and hypochromic anemia or in some instances anemia with two populations of red blood cells: microcytic and macrocytic. Folate deficiency is not a common occurrence in the blind loop syndrome. Unlike the situation with cobalamin, folate synthesized by microorganisms in the small intestine appears to be available for the host, and in patients with small intestine bacterial overgrowth, serum folate levels tend to be high rather than low (38).

Bloating and abdominal pain often result from an action of the overgrowth flora on fat and carbohydrate substrates within the lumen of the small intestine. Because of a decreased transport of nutrients across the damaged small intestine, more unabsorbed nutrients are presented to the distal intestine where further metabolism and production of toxic byproducts are produced leading to abdominal distention, pain, diarrhea, and/or steatorrhea.

Fat malabsorption associated with small bowel bacterial overgrowth results from bacterial alteration of bile salts (39). At the pH of intestinal contents conjugated bile salts normally exist as fully ionized, water-soluble bile salts capable of forming mixed micelles with the products of fat digestion. These conjugated bile salts are not readily reabsorbed from the proximal intestine and thus remain in the lumen to "solubilize" lipids. When bacteria proliferate in the small bowel, they deconjugate bile salts to form free bile acids that are present in small bowel contents as protonated bile acids and that are readily reabsorbed from the jejunum. If bacterial hydrolysis of conjugated bile salts is sufficiently rapid, bile salt micelle formation is impaired because of low bile acid concentration, and fat is poorly absorbed.

Deficiency of bile salt unquestionably limits intestinal transport of monoglyceride and fatty acids, but bile salt deficiency is probably not the only factor responsible for steatorrhea in bacterial overgrowth. Fat absorption is less impaired in rats with complete bile duct ligation, for example, than it is in rats with bacterial overgrowth (40). Accumulation of "toxic" concentrations of free bile acids may also contribute to steatorrhea in bacterial overgrowth (41), and the patchy intestinal mucosal lesion noted in the blind loop syndrome almost certainly plays a role in fat malabsorption.

Diarrhea may result from bacterial production of organic acids thereby increasing the osmolarity of small intestinal contents and decreasing intraluminal pH. Also, bacterial metabolites such as free bile acids, hydroxylated fatty acids, and organic acids stimulate secretion of water and electrolytes into the bowel lumen (39,41).

Experimental bacterial overgrowth in rats leads to small intestine motility disturbances that can be reversed with antibiotic therapy (42).

Decreased urinary xylose excretion is frequently seen in both the clinical and experimental blind loop syndrome. Although studies employing ^{14}C-xylose in the experimental blind loop syndrome have shown that the decreased urinary xylose excretion was due primarily to intraluminal catabolism of xylose to carbon dioxide, the decreased absorption of xylose in the setting of bacterial overgrowth may be secondary to both intraluminal catabolism of xylose by bacteria and diminished absorption due to small intestine mucosal dysfunction (43).

Hypoproteinemia is a frequent manifestation of the blind loop syndrome and is occasionally severe enough to cause edema. The etiology of the hypoproteinemia is multifactorial and may result from decreased uptake of amino acids by the damaged small intestine, intraluminal breakdown of protein and protein precursors by bacteria, and antibiotic-reversible protein-losing enteropathy (44–46).

In general, malabsorption can be attributed to intraluminal effects of proliferating bacteria combined with damage to the enterocyte itself. A patchy small bowel mucosal lesion of uncertain pathogenesis can be readily identified in experimental animals as well as in patients with bacterial overgrowth (44,46,47). Moderate blunting of villi, loss of structural integrity of some of the surface epithelial cells, and increased cellular infiltration of the lamina propria are characteristic.

DIAGNOSIS OF BACTERIAL OVERGROWTH

Overgrowth of bacteria within the small intestine should be considered in the differential diagnosis of any patient who presents with diarrhea, steatorrhea, weight loss, or macrocytic anemia, particularly if the patient is elderly or has had previous abdominal surgery. The development of diarrhea, weight loss, and macrocytic anemia months to years after gastric surgery suggests that the patient may have afferent loop dysfunction or a gastrojejunocolic fistula. A history of previous surgery for small intestinal obstruction should raise the question of whether the obstruction was bypassed by an end-to-side anastomosis, leaving a blind pouch, or a side-to-side anastomosis, resulting in recirculation of small intestine contents. On the other hand, a past history of recurrent bouts of intestinal obstruction may indicate stasis caused by a small intestinal stricture or adhesions. The presence of dysphagia should suggest the diagnosis of scleroderma, or repeated bouts of intestinal obstruction without obvious organic cause suggest intestinal pseudoobstruction.

When the clinical presentation suggests that proliferation of microorganisms in the small intestine lumen may cause or contribute to malabsorption, further evaluation is necessary for optimal management. The presence of steatorrhea should be documented. If the patient has clinically significant bacterial overgrowth, cobalamin absorption is frequently impaired, even though the patient may not yet have become cobalamin-deficient. Intrinsic factor will not improve cobalamin absorption in these patients. The urinary excretion of xylose may be decreased and the serum folate increased in some but not all patients with the blind loop syndrome.

A small intestinal biopsy is of value in excluding primary mucosal disease as the cause of the malabsorption. Although striking histological abnormalities of jejunal mucosa are not usually seen in patients with bacterial overgrowth, the biopsy is often abnormal. A patchy lesion of variable severity may be observed. Increased infiltration of the lamina propria with lymphocytes, plasma cells, and polymorphonuclear leukocytes, together with thickening and blunting of villi, may be seen. However, one does not find the diffuse alterations of the surface absorptive cells regularly present in celiac sprue. Although in some cases the biopsy specimen from a patient with the blind loop syndrome may show changes suggestive of tropical sprue, the history and intestinal culture should differentiate these two disorders.

The diagnosis of bacterial overgrowth requires a properly collected and appropriately cultured aspirate from the proximal small intestine. The specimen should be obtained under anaerobic conditions, serially diluted, and cultured on several selective media. In patients with clinically significant bacterial overgrowth, a number of different species are found, and the total concentration of bacteria generally exceeds 10^5 organisms/mL. Bacteroides, anaerobic lactobacilli, coliforms, and enterococci are all likely to be present in varying numbers. Although in most patients the intraluminal microbial proliferation can be documented in the proximal jejunum, it is important to recognize that pockets of overgrowth may be missed by a single culture and that bacterial overgrowth may occur only in the more distal portions of the small intestine. An intestinal culture requires intubation of the small intestine and time-consuming microbiological analyses.

A number of laboratory tests based on the metabolic actions of enteric bacteria have been proposed to assist in the diagnosis of the blind loop syndrome. Table 5 compares a number of these tests with the gold standard—the intestinal culture—with respect to ease of performance, sensitivity, specificity, and safety. The conclusions are based on a number of different studies from several laboratories throughout the world.

Quantitation of urinary excretion of indican, phenols, drug metabolites, and conjugated PABA does not adequately distinguish patients with bacterial overgrowth from those with other kinds of malabsorption. Analyses of intestinal aspirates for deconjugated bile acids or volatile fatty acids are difficult and suffer from many of the limitations previously stated for intestinal cultures (48,49). Increased free serum bile acids have been noted in several patients with the blind loop syndrome (50). Although of potential use as a diagnostic aid, this test depends on the presence of bacteria that have the capability of deconjugating bile salts (e.g., bacteroides).

Another approach to diagnosing bacterial overgrowth is the timed analysis of breath excretion of volatile metabolites produced by intraluminal bacteria. Both measurement of expired labeled CO_2 after oral administration of ^{14}C or ^{13}C-labeled substrates and breath hydrogen after administration of nonlabeled fermentable substrate have been employed.

The bile acid or ^{14}C-cholyglycine breath test was the first ^{14}C breath test used to diagnose bacterial overgrowth (51,52). Although frequently able to detect bacterial overgrowth, the bile acid breath test does not differentiate bacterial overgrowth from ileal damage or resection with excessive breath $^{14}CO_2$ production due to bacterial deconjugation within the colon of unabsorbed ^{14}C bile salt. This creates clinical difficulties because bacterial overgrowth may be superimposed on ileal damage in conditions such as Crohn's disease, lymphoma, and radiation enteritis. In addition, false-negative results have been described in 30% to 40% of patients with culture-proven overgrowth (53–55).

A 1-g ^{14}C-xylose breath test appears to be sensitive and specific enough to detect the presence of bacterial overgrowth (56). Elevated $^{14}CO_2$ levels appear within the breath in 85% of patients within the first 60 min of the test, with the 30-min breath sample being the most reliable. Xylose is attractive as a substrate because (a) xylose is catabolized by gram-negative aerobes, which are al-

TABLE 5. *Tests for bacterial overgrowth*

Test	Simplicity	Sensitivity	Specificity	Safety
Culture	Poor	Excellent	Excellent	Good
Urinary indican	Good	Poor	Poor	Excellent
Jejunal fatty acids	Poor	Fair	Excellent	Good
Jejunal bile acids	Poor	Fair	Excellent	Good
Fasting breath H_2	Excellent	Poor	Good	Excellent
^{14}C-bile acid BT	Excellent	Fair	Poor	Good
^{14}C-xylose BT	Excellent	Excellent	Excellent	Good
Lactulose-H_2 BT	Excellent	Fair	Fair-Good	Excellent
Glucose-H_2 BT	Excellent	Good	Fair-Good	Excellent

From ref. 2, with permission.

ways part of the overgrowth flora; (b) xylose is predominantly absorbed in the proximal small bowel as contrasted to the predominant ileal absorption of bile salts, leading to virtually no "dumping" of xylose into the colon; and (c) xylose is metabolized substantially less than other proximally absorbed substrates, such as glucose. Comparison with the bile acid breath test in a series of patients with culture-proven overgrowth demonstrated no false-negative results with the xylose breath test (54).

A number of laboratories throughout the world have evaluated the ^{14}C-xylose breath test and have documented its reliability in detecting small intestine bacterial overgrowth (57–59). In those studies that utilized the intestinal culture as the gold standard and evaluated shorter sampling intervals, particularly the 30-min time point, the sensitivity and specificity approximated 90%.

Breath hydrogen analysis allows a distinct separation of metabolic activity of the intestinal flora from that by the human host, for hydrogen production in mammalian tissue is unknown. Excessive breath hydrogen production has been noted in patients with bacterial overgrowth following the administration of 50–80 g of glucose or 10–12 g of lactulose (60–62). It should be pointed out that approximately one third of patients with culture-proven bacterial overgrowth will have elevated fasting levels of breath hydrogen (63).

Despite vigorous attention to methodological details such as avoiding foods (bread, pasta, fiber) that cause prolonged excretion of hydrogen the night before the test, preventing cigarette smoking, and avoiding physical exercise sufficient to produce hyperventilation for 2 hr before and during the test, breath hydrogen testing for bacterial overgrowth has been disappointing. Even performing a mouthwash before testing with 40 mL of chlorhexidine to eliminate the possibility of an early hydrogen peak due to interaction of the test sugar with oral bacteria, and adopting strict interpretation criteria such as requiring two consecutive hydrogen values more than 10 ppm above the baseline value, clearly distinguishable from the colonic peak (increase $\geq$20 ppm H_2 above baseline value) following lactulose administration, has not improved the sensitivity and specificity of breath hydrogen analysis for detecting small intestine bacterial overgrowth (64). A recent, well-carried-out study comparing the lactulose and glucose hydrogen breath tests to the intestinal culture found a sensitivity of 68% for lactulose and 62% for glucose and

a specificity of 44% and 83%, respectively (65). This same group of investigators found the fasting breath hydrogen level to be lacking not only in sensitivity but also in specificity.

Another recent study compared the 1-g ^{14}C-xylose breath test to a 10-g lactulose-H_2 test and an 80-g glucose-H_2 test in 20 subjects with culture-proven bacterial overgrowth and 10 control subjects (61). The ^{14}C-xylose breath test was positive (abnormal) in 19 of 20 subjects with overgrowth and 0 of 10 control subjects. In contrast, the H_2 breath tests demonstrated (a) uninterpretable results (absence of H_2-generating bacteria in 2 of 20 subjects with bacterial overgrowth and 1 of 10 control subjects, and (b) nondiagnostic increases in H_2 production in 3 of 18 80-g glucose-H_2 tests and 7 of 18 lactulose-H_2 tests in patients with culture-proven overgrowth.

It also must be emphasized that the factors that affect hydrogen production by intestinal bacteria require further attention. Recent studies demonstrate that up to 27% of normal subjects fail to show any rise in breath hydrogen following 12 g of lactulose (61,64,66). Also, the failure of abnormal H_2 expiration in patients with malabsorption may be due to production of organic acids or a "washout" effect of concomitant diarrhea (66).

The nonradioactive nature and ease of performance of H_2 breath tests make them attractive. Yet despite some views to the contrary, the preponderance of recent studies indicate that these tests have significant problems with both sensitivity and specificity. If one further considers that clinical laboratories do not pay attention to the methodological details listed above and the individual variation in the capacity of an individual's flora to produce H_2 from carbohydrate, then the hydrogen breath tests fare even worse than stated above.

The excellent sensitivity and specificity of the 1-g ^{14}C-xylose breath test makes it the test of choice to detect bacterial overgrowth. Although the ^{14}C-xylose test gives trivial radiation dosimetry, appreciably less than fluoroscopic placement of a jejunal culture tube, the test has not been recommended for children or fertile women. ^{13}C-xylose has been produced and the use of this stable isotope (no radiation to host) is under active investigation. Preliminary studies of a ^{13}C-labeled xylose breath test has demonstrated excellent distinction of subjects with culture-proven overgrowth from control subjects (67). Finally, the clinical efficacy committee of the American College of Physicians suggested that only two breath tests—the 1-g ^{14}C-xylose test for bacterial overgrowth and the 50-g lactose-H$_2$ test for lactose intolerance—are appropriate for routine clinical use.

TREATMENT OF BACTERIAL OVERGROWTH

The aim of therapy is the reduction of the bacterial overgrowth and consists of antibiotic administration or, when feasible, correction of the small intestine abnormality leading to stasis and microbial proliferation. Unfortunately, however, surgery is often impractical (e.g., scleroderma, multiple diverticula) or unacceptable to the patient. Thus, management of many patients with bacterial overgrowth is lifelong. It is important to emphasize again that bacterial overgrowth may be a treatable component of the malabsorption seen in patients with diseases such as Crohn's disease, intestinal lymphoma, or radiation enteritis. Deterioration in such patients may not be due to their primary disease process but to associated overgrowth. It also must be stressed that bacterial overgrowth may be present without causing any disease. An abnormal breath test or a pathological culture must be put in perspective by the clinician and appropriate decisions made.

Selection of an antimicrobial agent based on the sensitivity of the microorganisms present in the small bowel lumen is attractive in theory, but this approach is often difficult because there are usually many different bacterial species present, often with very different sensitivities. Under such circumstances, it may be extremely difficult to select what could be considered the most appropriate antibiotic on the basis of microbial sensitivity. Traditionally, treatment has been initiated with tetracycline. If the antibiotic is to be considered effective, diarrhea should subside and the absorption of fat and cobalamin should be distinctly improved within a week of beginning therapy. Unfortunately, up to 60% of patients with clinically significant malabsorption associated with bacterial overgrowth no longer respond to tetracycline, and treatment often must include other antimicrobial agents, some of which may have serious side effects. Thus it behooves the physician to establish the diagnosis rather than employ empirical therapy.

The most effective antimicrobial therapeutic program includes agents that are effective against both aerobic and anaerobic enteric bacteria. Although it is true that most patients with clinically significant malabsorption secondary to bacterial overgrowth have an intestinal flora that is largely overgrown with anaerobes, there are patients with malabsorption associated predominantly with an overgrowth of gram-negative aerobes such as *E. coli*, *Klebsiella*, or *Pseudomonas* (68).

The clavulonic acid derivative augmentin in a dose of 250–500 mg three times daily is effective in suppressing both the aerobic and anaerobic flora and correcting malabsorption. An alternative choice would be a cephalosporin (e.g., Keflex) 250 mg four times a day and metronidazole 250 mg three times a day. Tetracycline is another choice (250 mg four times a day) but the resistance problem, especially with bacteroides, must be appreciated. If these

agents are not effective, chloramphenicol (50 mg/kg in four divided doses) may be employed and is quite effective. Single anaerobic agents such as metronidazole or clindamycin do not appear to be as effective in clinical practice as agents effective against both aerobes and anaerobes.

There are agents that because of their known poor activity against anaerobes should not be used in treating bacterial overgrowth. Such antimicrobials to be avoided include penicillin, ampicillin, the oral aminoglycosides, kanamycin, and neomycin.

In many patients, a single course of therapy (e.g., 10 days) will suffice and the patient may remain symptom-free for months; in others, symptoms recur quickly and satisfactory results can be attained with cyclic therapy (one week out of every four); and in others continuous therapy may be needed for 1–2 months.

It should be recognized that there are no adequate controlled clinical trials in regard to choice of antimicrobial agent, duration of therapy, or appropriate management of recurrences.

Prolonged antibiotic therapy poses significant clinical problems including diarrhea, enterocolitis, patient intolerance, and bacterial resistance. A prokinetic agent that could help clear the small intestine of the overgrowth flora would be most welcome. Standard prokinetic agents have failed in this regard to date.

A recent provocative study in five patients with intestinal scleroderma and bacterial overgrowth is noteworthy (69). Octreotide stimulated motor activity in these patients, evoking phase 3 motor complexes that propagated at the same velocity as spontaneous complexes in normal subjects. Octreotide also decreased nausea, vomiting, bloating, and abdominal pain in these patients and cleared bacterial overgrowth as demonstrated by complete normalization of abnormal breath hydrogen tests. Such complete normalization of breath test results has rarely, if ever, been observed following antibiotic therapy. Doses of octreotide (100–500 µg three times daily) used clinically to treat acromegaly, the carcinoid syndrome, or vasoactive intestinal polypeptide–secreting tumors often induce hypomotility and would be predicted to lead to stasis and consequent overgrowth. However, in this study only a small dose of octreotide was used (50 µg) and only at bedtime so as to not impair the motor response to feeding. Although this is an exciting alternative to antimicrobial therapy, only a few patients were studied for just 3 weeks. The authors of this study have indicated that these good results have now been maintained for over 2 years. Whether this saluatory effect will be confirmed remains to be determined.

Nutritional support is an important part of the therapeutic program. Nutritional therapy may be needed despite maximally obtainable control of the bacterial overgrowth by antimicrobial agents. This is particularly true in the setting of incompletely reversible damage to the small intestine enterocyte. To reduce diarrhea and steatorrhea, a lactose-free diet and substitution of a large part of dietary fat by medium-chain triglycerides may be necessary. Patients with cobalamin malabsorption should receive monthly injections of this vitamin (100 µg). Deficiencies

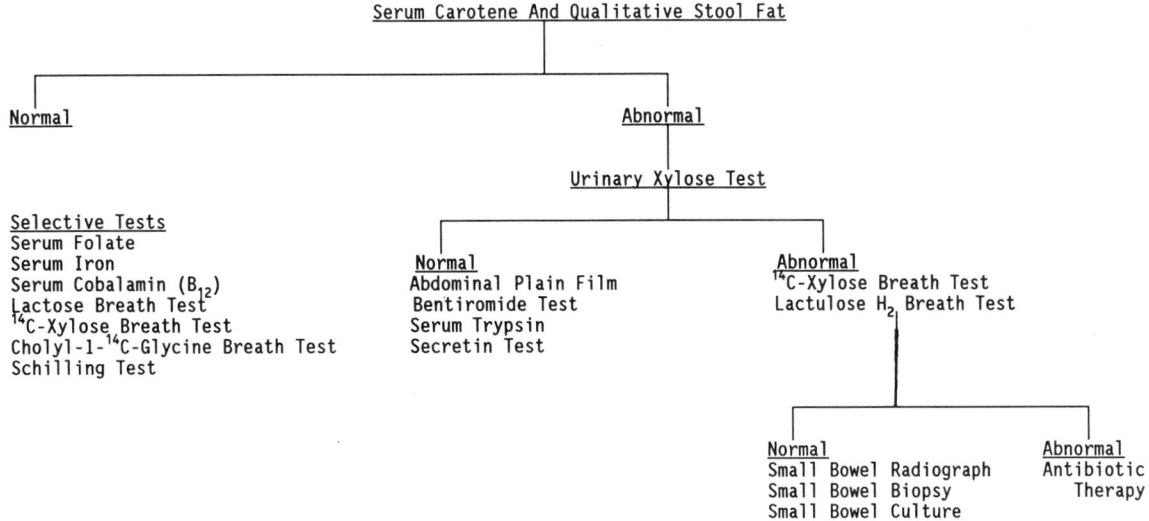

FIG. 4. Algorithm for evaluation of malabsorption. (From ref. 70, with permission.)

of other nutrients (i.e., calcium, vitamin K) should also be corrected.

Finally, it should be stressed that clinicians should have a low threshold for suspecting bacterial overgrowth as the cause of malabsorption in a given patient because the entity is rather common and readily treatable. Figure 4 presents a cost-effective, efficient algorithm for evaluating patients with malabsorption. The algorithm emphasizes the performance of noninvasive tests (breath tests for bacterial overgrowth, bentiromide and serum trypsin levels for pancreatic exocrine insufficiency) for the more common etiologies of malabsorption in contrast to an intestinal biopsy to document nontropical sprue, a somewhat rare cause of malabsorption in the United States.

It behooves the clinician to be aware of what normal and abnormal flora (both qualitative and quantitative) are within the gastrointestinal tract. The consequences of bacterial overgrowth within the small intestine can be serious malabsorption resulting in clinically important deficiencies of several nutrients. Alterations in gastric acid secretion and intestinal motility provide the setting for the development of bacterial overgrowth. The elderly in particular appear to be at risk for malabsorption secondary to bacterial overgrowth. Bacterial overgrowth can be easily diagnosed and readily treated if the clinician's index of suspicion for this entity is high.

REFERENCES

1. King CE, Toskes PP. Small intestine bacterial overgrowth. *Gastroenterology* 1979;76:1035–1055.
2. Toskes PP, Donaldson R. Enteric bacterial flora and bacterial overgrowth syndrome. In: Sleisenger MH, Fordtran JS, eds. *Gastrointestinal disease*. 5th ed. Philadelphia: WB Saunders; 1994:1106–1118.
3. Simon GL, Gorbach SL. The human intestinal microflora. *Dig Dis Sci* 1986;30(Suppl 9):147S.
4. Gorbach SL. Function of the normal human microflora. *Scand Infect Dis* 1986;(Suppl 49):17.
5. Simon GL, Gorbach SL. The intestinal flora in health and disease: a review. *Gastroenterology* 1984;86:174–193.
6. Donaldson RM. Role of indigenous enteric bacteria in intestinal function and disease. In: Code CF, ed. *Handbook of physiology*. Baltimore: Williams and Wilkins; 1968.
7. Savage DC. Gastrointestinal microflora in mammalian nutrition. *Annu Rev Nutr* 1986;6:1–55.
8. Goldstein F, Wirts CW, Kramer S. The relationship of afferent limb stasis and bacterial flora to the production of post-gastrectomy steatorrhea. *Gastroenterology* 1961;40:47–55.
9. Doig A, Girdwood RG. The absorption of folic acid and labeled cyanocobalamine in intestinal malabsorption with observations on the fecal excretion of fat and nitrogen and the absorption of glucose and xylose. *Q J Med* 1960;29:333–374.
10. Beeken WL, Kanish RE. Microbial flora of the upper small bowel in Crohn's disease. *Gastroenterology* 1973;65:390–397.
11. Bishop RF, Anderson CM. Bacterial flora of stomach and small intestine in children with intestinal obstruction. *Arch Dis Child* 1960;35:487–492.
12. Swan RW. Stagnant loop syndrome resulting from small bowel irradiation injury and intestinal bypass. *Gynecol Oncol* 1974;8:441–445.
13. Russell RM, Abadi P, Ismail-Beigi F. Role of bacterial overgrowth on the malabsorption syndrome of the primary small intestinal lymphoma. *Cancer* 1977;89:8579–8583.
14. Atwater JS, Butt HR, Priestley JT. Gastrojejunocolic fistulae with special reference to associated nutritional deficiencies and certain surgical aspects. *Ann Surg* 1943;117:414–419.
15. Kelly DG, Phillips SF, Kelly KA, et al. Dysfunction of the continent ileostomy: clinical features and bacteriology. *Gut* 1983;24:193–198.
16. Kahn I, Jeffries GH, Sleisenger MH. Malabsorption in intestinal scleroderma. Correction by antibiotics. *N Engl J Med* 1966;274:1339–1344.
17. Pearson AJ, Brzechwa-Adjukiewicz A, McCarthy CF. Intestinal pseudo-obstruction with bacterial overgrowth in the small intestine. *Am J Dig Dis* 1969;14:200–205.
18. Goldstein F, Wirts EC, Kowlessar OD. Diabetic diarrhea and steatorrhea. Microbiologic and clinical observations. *Ann Intern Med* 1970;72:215–218.
19. Vantrappen G, Janssens J, Hellemans J, et al. The interdigestive motor complex of normal subjects and patients with bacterial overgrowth of the small intestine. *J Clin Invest* 1977;59:1158–1166.
20. Roberts SH, James O, Jarvis EH. Bacterial overgrowth syndrome without "blind loop": a cause for malnutrition in the elderly. *Lancet* 1977;2:1193–1195.
21. McEvoy A, Dutton J, James OF. Bacterial contamination of the small intestine is an important cause of occult malabsorption in the elderly. *Br Med J* 1983;287:789–793.

22. Montgomery RD, Haboudi NY, Mike NH, et al. Causes of malabsorption in the elderly. *Age Ageing* 1986;15:235–240.
23. Haboudi N, Montgomery R. Small bowel bacterial overgrowth in elderly people: clinical significance and response to treatment. *Age Ageing* 1992;21:13–19.
24. Lipski P, Kelly P, James F. Bacterial comtamination of the small bowel in elderly people: is it necessarily pathological. *Age Ageing* 1992;21:13–19.
25. Saltzman J, Kowdley K, Pedrosa M, et al. Bacterial overgrowth without clinical malabsorption in elderly hypochlorhydric subjects. *Gastroenterology* 1994; 106:615–623.
26. Fried M, Slegrish H, Frei R, et al. Duodenal bacterial overgrowth during treatment with omeprazole in outpatients. *Gastroenterology* 1992;102:A71.
27. Lembeke B, Kraus B, Lankisch PG. Small intestinal function in chronic relapsing pancreatitis. *Hepatogastroenterology* 1985; 32:149–155.
28. Rubinstein E, Mark Z, Haspel J, et al. Antibacterial activity of the pancreatic fluid. *Gastroenterology* 1985;88:927–932.
29. Williams DA, Batt RM, McLean L. Bacterial overgrowth in the duodenum of dogs with exocrine pancreatic insufficiency. *J Am Vet Med Assoc* 1987;191:201–206.
30. Piqnata C, Budillon G, Monaco G, et al. Jejunal bacterial overgrowth and intestinal permeability in children with immunodeficiency syndromes. *Gut* 1990;31:879–882.
31. Martini GA, Phear EA, Ruebner E, et al. The bacterial content of the small intestine in normal and cirrhotic subjects: relation to the methionine toxicity. *Clin Sci* 1956;16:35–51.
32. Levitan R, Lai D, Borbach SL. Intestinal microflora in patients with alcoholic cirrhosis: urea-splitting bacteria and neomycin resistance. *Gastroenterology* 1972;62:275–279.
33. Correia JP, Garnel M, Monteiro E, et al. Bacteriology of the small intestine in cirrhotic subjects and its relation to malabsorption. *Am J Gastroenterol* 1971;56:428–435.
34. Tabaquchali S. The pathophysiological role of the small intestinal bacterial flora. *Scand J Gastroenterol* 1970;Suppl. 6: 139–163.
35. Donaldson RM Jr. Malabsorption of ^{60}Co-labelled cyanocobalamin in rats with intestinal diverticula. I. Evaluation of possible mechanisms. *Gastroenterology* 1962;43:271–281.
36. Welkos SA, Toskes PP, Baer H, et al. Importance of anaerobic bacteria in the cobalamin malabsorption of experimental rat blind loop syndrome. *Gastroenterology* 1981;80:313–320.
37. Giannella RA, Toskes PP. Gastrointestinal bleeding and iron absorption in the experimental blind loop syndrome. *Am J Clin Nutr* 1976;29:754–757.
38. Hoffbrand AV, Tabaquhali S, Moilin DL. High serum folate levels in intestinal blind loop syndrome. *Lancet* 1966;1: 1339–1342.
39. Kim YS, Spritz N, Blum M, et al. The role of altered bile acid metabolism in the steatorrhea of experimental blind loop syndrome. *J Clin Invest* 1966;45:956–962.
40. Donaldson RM Jr. Role of enteric microorganisms in malabsorption. *Fed Proc* 1967;26:1426–1431.
41. Wanitschke R, Ammon HV. Effects of dihydroxy bile acids and hydroxy fatty acids on the absorption of oleic acid in the human jejunum. *J Clin Invest* 1978;61:178–186.
42. Justus PG, Fernandez A, Martin JL, et al. Altered myoelectric activity in the experimental blind loop syndrome. *J Clin Invest* 1983;72:1064–1071.
43. Toskes PP, King CE, Spivey JC, et al. Xylose catabolism in experimental rat blind loop syndrome: studies including newly developed d-(^{14}C)xylose breath test. *Gastroenterology* 1978;74: 691–697.
44. Giannella RA, Rout WR, Toskes PP. Jejunal brush border injury and impaired sugar and amino acid uptake in the blind loop syndrome. *Gastroenterology* 1974;67:965–974.
45. Varcoe R, Holliday D, Tavill A. Utilization of urea nitrogen for albumin synthesis in the stagnant loop syndrome. *Gut* 1974;15: 898–902.
46. King CE, Toskes PP. Protein-losing enteropathy in the human and experimental rat blind loop syndrome. *Gastroenterology* 1981;80:504–509.

47. Toskes PP, Giannella RA, Jervis HR, et al. Small intestinal mucosal injury in the experimental blind loop syndrome. *Gastroenterology* 1975;68:1193–1203.
48. Setchell KD, Harrison DL, Gilbert JM, et al. Serum unconjugated bile acids: qualitative and quantitative profiles in ileal resection and bacterial overgrowth. *Clin Chim Acta* 1985;152: 297–302.
49. Hoverstad T, Bjorneklett A, Fausa O, et al. Short-chain fatty acids in the small bowel bacterial overgrowth syndrome. *Scand J Gastroenterol* 1985;20:492–496.
50. Tabaquchali S, Hatzionnou J, Booth CC. Bile salt deconjugation and steatorrhea in patients with the stagnant-loop syndrome. *Lancet* 1968;2:12–16.
51. Fromm H, Hofmann AF. Breath test for altered bile acid metabolism. *Lancet* 1971;2:621–625.
52. Sherr HP, Sasaki Y, Newman A, et al. Detection of bacterial deconjugation of bile salts by a convenient breath-analysis technique. *N Engl J Med* 1971;285:656–671.
53. Lauterburg BH, Newcomer AD, Hofmann AF. Clinical value of bile acid breath test. Evaluation of the Mayo Clinic experience. *Mayo Clin Proc* 1978;53:227–233.
54. King CE, Toskes PP, Guilarte TR, et al. Comparison of the one gram ^{14}C-xylose breath test to the ^{14}C-bile acid breath test in patients with small intestine bacterial overgrowth. *Dig Dis Sci* 1980;25:53–58.
55. Ferguson J, Walker K, and Thomson AB. Limitations in the use of ^{14}C-glycocholate breath and stool bile acid determinations in patients with chronic diarrhea. *J Clin Gastroenterol* 1986;8: 258–263.
56. King CE, Toskes PP, Spivey JC, et al. Detection of small intestine overgrowth by means of a ^{14}C-D-xylose breath test. *Gastroenterology* 1979;79:75–82.
57. Schneider A, Novis B, Chen V, et al. Value of the ^{14}C-D-xylose breath test in patients with intestinal bacterial overgrowth. *Digestion* 1985;32:86–91.
58. Rumessen JJ, Gudmand-Hoyer E, Bachmann E, et al. Diagnosis of bacterial overgrowth of the small intestine. *Scand J Gastroenterol* 1985;20:1267–1275.
59. Pruthi HS, Mehta SK, Pathak CM. Evaluation of ^{14}C-dxylose breath test in the diagnosis of small intestinal bacterial overgrowth. *Ind J Med Res* 1984;80:598–600.
60. Metz G, Cassull MA, Drasar BS, et al. Breath-hydrogen test for small intestinal bacterial colonization. *Lancet* 1976;1:688–689.
61. King CE, Toskes PP. Comparison of the 1-gram ^{14}C-xylose, 10-gram lactulose-H$_2$ and 80 gram glucose H$_2$ breath tests in patients with small intestine bacterial overgrowth. *Gastroenterology* 1986;91:1447–1451.
62. Rhodes JM, Middleton P, Jewell DP. The lactulose hydrogen breath test as a diagnostic test for small-bowel bacterial overgrowth. *Scand J Gastroenterol* 1979;4:333–336.
63. Perman JA, Modler S, Barr RG, et al. Fasting breath hydrogen concentration: normal values and clinical application. *Gastroenterology* 1984;87:1358–1363.
64. Strocchi A, Sorge M, Pranzo L, et al. Intraindividual variability in H$_2$ production capacity. *Gastroenterol Int* 1988;1(Suppl 1): 593.
65. Corazza GR, Menozzi MG, Strocchi A, et al. The diagnosis of small bowel bacterial overgrowth. *Gastroenterology* 1990;98: 302–305.
66. Gilat T, Ben Hur H, Gelman-Malachi E, et al. Alterations of the colonic flora and their effect on the hydrogen breath test. *Gut* 1978;19:602–605.
67. Lim H, Wagner DA, Toskes PP. A ^{13}C-Xylose breath test for bacterial overgrowth. *Gastroenterology* 1993;104:A259.
68. Kocoshis SA, Schletewitz K, Lovelace G, et al. Duodenal bile acids among children: keto derivatives and aerobic small bowel bacterial overgrowth. *J Pediatr Gastroenterol Nutr* 1987;6: 686–696.
69. Soudah HC, Hasler WL, Owyang C. Effect of octreotide on intestinal motility and bacterial overgrowth in scleroderma. *N Engl J Med* 1991;325:1461–1467.
70. Toskes P. Malabsorption. In Wyngaarden J, Smith L, Bennett J, eds. *Cecil's textbook of medicine.* 19th ed. Philadelphia: WB Saunders;1992:687–699.

Infections of the Gastrointestinal Tract,
edited by M. J. Blaser, P. D. Smith, J. I. Ravdin,
H. B. Greenberg, and R. L. Guerrant
Raven Press, Ltd., New York © 1995.

CHAPTER 27

Appendicitis

Christina M. Surawicz

Appendicitis is defined histopathologically as inflammation of the vermiform appendix. It is caused by obstruction of the appendix and associated with a characteristic clinical syndrome. The first report of appendicitis in 1886 remains a classic description of the clinical presentation (1). Occasionally, however, presentation may be atypical, making the diagnosis less obvious. When appendicitis is treated promptly by appendectomy, morbidity and mortality are low. However, missed diagnosis and improperly treated appendicitis may result in perforation with abscess formation.

MICROBIOLOGY

Most cases of appendicitis are idiopathic. Histopathology of appendixes removed from persons with idiopathic appendicitis show inflammation but usually no identifiable pathogen. Nevertheless, a variety of infections can cause appendicitis. In addition, inflammation of contiguous organs or tissue can mimic appendicitis.

Bacteria

Yersiniia enterocolitica has been reported to cause up to 6% of appendicitis in patients in northern European countries and Canada (2). Since 1981, additional strains have been reported to be associated with appendicitis, including the more invasive serotypes O3 and O9. In a prospective study of appendicitis in the United States, *Y. enterocolitica* was cultured from 9% (4/44) of inflamed appendixes and from none of 6 normal appendixes (2). In a retrospective study of nearly 3000 patients, *Y. enterocolitica* O3 and O9 were the most common pathogens (3.6%) isolated from resected appendixes (3) (Fig. 1; Plate 3).

Other bacteria that cause infections which can mimic appendicitis include *Escherichia coli* O157:H7, *Campylo-*

bacter spp., *Salmonella* spp., *Aspergillus,* and *Mycobacteria tuberculosis. E. coli* O157:H7 is an enterphemorrhagic *E. coli* that typically causes hemorrhagic colitis, resulting in bloody diarrhea. *Campylobacter* spp. can cause a pseudoappendicitis in which mesenteric lymph nodes are inflamed but the appendix is usually normal. *Salmonella enteritis* can be associated with abdominal pain that mimics appendicitis, but diarrhea eventually becomes the predominant symptom. Tuberculosis of the gastrointestinal tract has a predilection for the ileocecal area, causing a chronic pain syndrome that contrasts to the acute pain of appendicitis. *M. tuberculosis* may rarely cause appendicitis (5). An early report (1911) documented the presence of spirochetes in the feces of patients with acute appendicitis (6). In the 1930s, a study showed that 10% of appendixes from individuals with appendicitis-like symptoms had spirochetes (7). A large review of hundreds of appendectomy specimens found that spirochetosis was present in 12% of uninflamed appendixes compared to 0.7% from inflamed appendixes (8). The spirochetes, classified as *Brachyspira aalborgi,* are 2–4.8 μm long and 0.2 μm wide. Thus, the role of spirochetosis in the pathogenesis of appendicitis or pseudoappendicitis remains uncertain, but is not likely to be of major clinical significance.

Viruses

Viral causes of appendicitis and pseudoappendicitis are uncommon but include measles, adenovirus, and cytomegalovirus. Specimens from measles appendicitis have large multinucleate giant lymphoreticular cells. Adenovirus infection is characterized by intranuclear inclusions with viral particles identified by electron microscopy. Cytomegalovirus infection causes characteristic cytomegalic changes, typically in endothelial cells.

Parasites

Enterobius vermicularis, or pinworm, is the most common parasite found in appendectomy specimens, but the

C. M. Surawicz: Department of Medicine, Division of Gastroenterology, University of Washington School of Medicine and Harborview Medical Center, Seattle, Washington 98195.

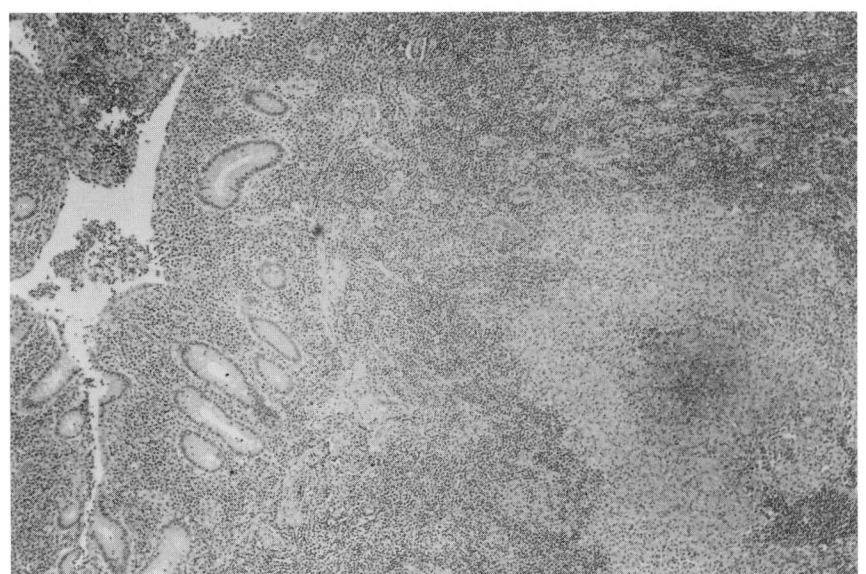

FIG. 1. Appendicitis due to *Yersina enterocolitica.* Diffuse inflammation and a submucosal granuloma with central necrosis are present in the veriform appendix (H & E). (Courtesy of Dr. Rodger Haggitt.) (See Plate 3.)

worms or eggs found in the lumen of the appendix are probably an incidental finding. Other parasites rarely associated with appendicitis include *Ascaris lumbricoides* (9), *Entamoeba histolytica, Schistosoma mansoni, Balantidium coli, Trichuris trichiura,* and *Strongyloides stercoralis* (Table 1). *Angiostrongylus costaricensis,* a nematode found in Central America, can also cause an appendicitis-like syndrome characterized by the presence of right lower quadrant mass with pain, fever, anorexia, and eosinophilia (10).

Fungi

Histoplasma capsulatum is the most common fungus associated with appendicitis, occurring in 9% of cases. Other fungi are rarely associated with appendicitis except in immunosuppressed persons. *Actinomyces* spp. have a predilection for the ileocecal area, causing a mass or sinus tracts. Actinomycosis should be considered in persons who develop a fistula following appendectomy. *Aspergillus* has been reported to cause appendicitis in patients with leukemia (11,12).

Granulomatous Appendicitis

Recent evidence suggests that granulomatous appendicitis, initially thought to be Crohn's disease of the appendix, is probably a distinct clinical entity due to an unknown infectious etiology (13) (Fig. 2; Plate 4). Other specific causes of appendiceal granulomas include Crohn's disease, sarcoidosis, tuberculosis, and yersiniosis.

Appendicitis in the Acquired Immunodeficiency Syndrome (AIDS)

Patients with AIDS infrequently develop appendicitis. A high index of suspicion is required in such patients since leukocytosis and fever may be absent in up to one third of cases. The differential diagnosis of appendicitis in such patients includes cytomegalovirus colitis, cryptosporidial and mycobacterial infections, as well as typhlitis and obstruction due to Kaposi's sarcoma. A recent case of cyto-

TABLE 1. *Infectious causes of appendicitis*

Bacteria
   Yersinia enterocolitica
   Campylobacter
   E. coli O157:H7
   Salmonella
   Shigella
   Mycobacterium tuberculosis
   non–*T. pallidum* spirochetes
Viruses
   Measles
   Adenovirus
   Cytomelagovirus
Parasites
   Enterobius vermicularis
   Ascaris lumbricoides
   Entamoeba histolytica
   Schistosoma mansoni
   Angiostrongylus
   Balantidium coli
   Trichuris trichiura, vulpis
   Strongyloides stercoralis
   Fascioa
   Toxocara
   Capillaria hepatica
Fungi
   Histoplasma
   Actinomycosis israelii
   Aspergillus

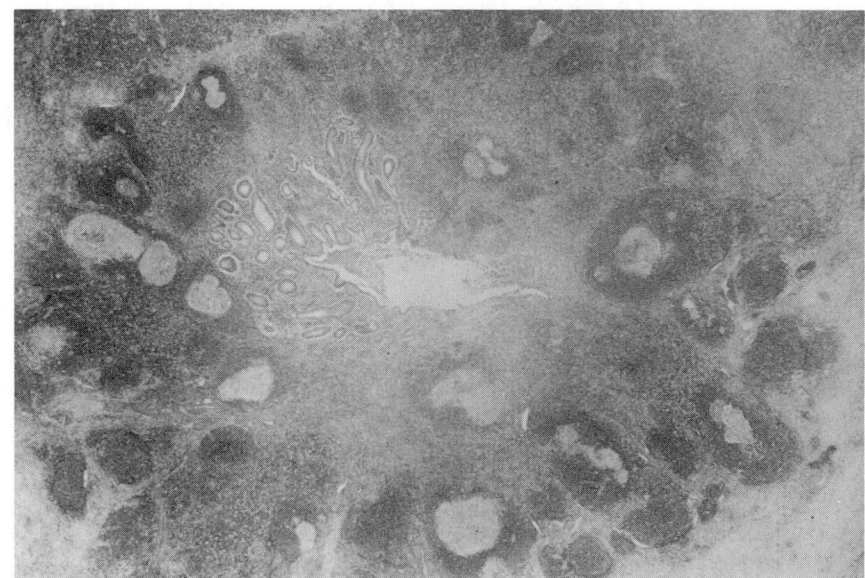

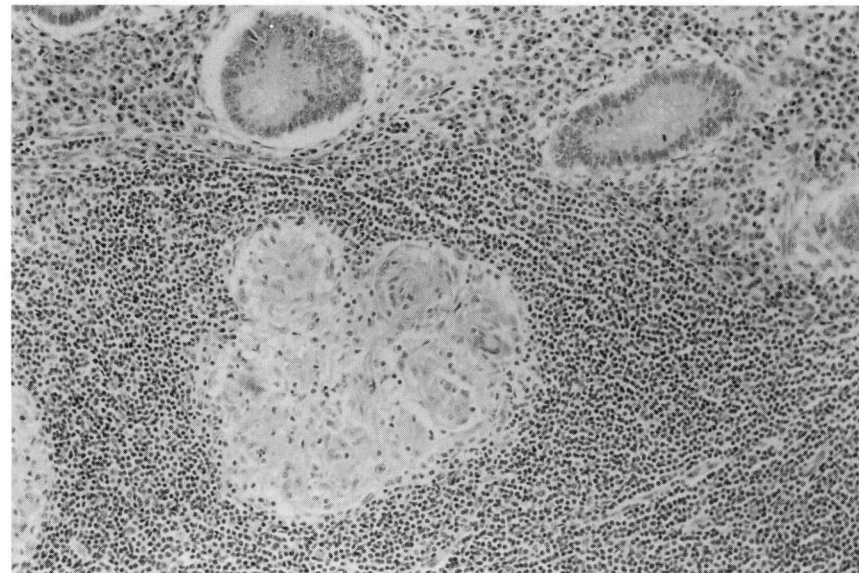

FIG. 2. Granulomatous appendicitis. **A:** The presence of multiple granulomas in the mucosa and submucosa of the appendix characterizes granulomatous appendicitis (H & E). **B:** The granuloma are discrete, noncaseating, and composed of epithelioid histiocytes with occasional multinucleated giant cells (H & E). (Courtesy of Dr. Rodger Haggitt.) (See Plate 4.)

megalovirus-associated ileal perforation in a patient with AIDS demonstrated the usefulness of in situ hybridization and immunohistochemical analysis for detecting cytomegalovirus nucleic acids and proteins in tissue specimens (14). Early use of diagnostic tests such as ultrasound and computed tomography scan may facilitate the diagnosis (15). Appendicitis does not appear to increase the morbidity in AIDS (16).

PATHOGENESIS

Appendicitis results when the lumen of the appendix becomes obstructed by objects such as a stone (fecalith) or parasite or by physical factors such as torsion. Less common causes of obstruction include tumor, foreign body, and lymphoid hyperplasia. Obstruction causes in-

creased pressure within the appendix as secretions accumulate; the resulting decrease in blood flow causes ischemia, which may progress to necrosis and perforation with peritonitis. A walled-off perforation results in a periappendiceal abscess.

Pseudoappendicitis occurs when an adjacent tissue or organ becomes inflamed, causing symptoms that simulate appendicitis, although the appendix is not involved. Periappendicitis is caused by inflammation of the serosa of the appendix. This results from intraabdominal inflammation of other causes, such as pelvic inflammatory disease or diverticulitis.

EPIDEMIOLOGY

While appendicitis can occur at any age, it is most common in children, although rare under 2 years of age. Appendicitis is more common in Western than Eastern countries, leading to speculation that a diet high in fiber is associated with a decreased incidence.

CLINICAL FEATURES

The most common presenting symptom of acute appendicitis is abdominal pain, which typically begins as a diffuse periumbilical pain that subsequently localizes to the right lower quadrant. The pain is constant and increases in severity. Such pain is present in 95% of patients with appendicitis. There is usually associated anorexia, nausea, vomiting, and low-grade fever.

On physical examination, right lower quadrant tenderness is present. Guarding and rebound tenderness at McBurney's point are present in 80% of cases. McBurney's point is 1.5–2 in. from the anterior superior iliac spine on a line from the spine to the umbilicus. Other findings on physical examination include the psoas, obturator, and Rovsing's signs, which are present in 80–90% of cases. A psoas sign is present if extending the thigh at the hip to stretch the peritoneum over the psoas muscle causes pain. The obturator sign, which is elicited when the obturator fascia is stretched by internal rotation of the thigh with the knee flexed, may be present in appendicitis, an inflamed retrocecal appendix, or a psoas muscle abscess. Rovsing's sign is elicited when pressing on the left iliac fossa causes referred right lower quadrant pain. Tenderness with digital examination of the rectum is elicited in over half (65%) of cases. In older patients, abdominal distention may be common.

Laboratory evaluation usually reveals an elevated white blood cell count ($>$10,000 cells/mm^3) with an increase in the percentage of polymorphonuclear neutrophils. Urinalysis can show the presence of red or white blood cells in the absence of urinary tract infection. A urine for serum βHCG should be considered in sexually active females of childbearing age.

A history, physical examination, evaluation of blood studies, and radiographic examination of the abdomen will be sufficient to make the diagnosis in most patients. Overall, clinical accuracy is 70–80%, falling to 30–50% in children and women of childbearing age. Missed diagnoses are more common in children due to the difficulty children have in communicating symptoms and in women, especially during pregnancy, due to confounding gynecological pathology. The rate of perforation is highest in preschool age children. The rate of appendectomy for an inflamed appendix (40%) is highest in young women with regular menses and right lower quadrant pain. Surgeons should be involved early in the evaluation of patients with suspected appendicitis. When the diagnosis is unclear, additional tests such as ultrasound may be helpful.

In a study of 150 children referred for possible appendicitis (17), half had immediate surgery. The most useful criteria to determine the need for immediate surgery were a history of epigastric pain localizing to the right lower quadrant, guarding, peritonitis, fever, and an elevated white blood cell count. When the diagnosis was unclear, close observation was the best approach to management.

Of the 76 children who were observed, one third ultimately had an appendectomy for histologically confirmed appendicitis, 3 of whom had already perforated. The other two thirds of the children improved and were discharged. These children were less likely to have had peritoneal signs, right lower quadrant tenderness, and guarding.

The diagnosis of appendicitis may be especially difficult in children with leukemia. In one recent study (18), the incidence of acute abdomen in this population was 4–5% and appendicitis 0.5%. Common symptoms were nausea, vomiting, and localized abdominal pain, but in children in whom diagnosis was delayed symptoms were vague abdominal pain, abdominal distention, fever, dehydration, and diarrhea; guarding was absent, even when the appendix had ruptured. A specific diagnosis in children with leukemia is typhlitis. This inflammation of the terminal ileum and cecum is related to chemotherapy, neutropenia, and bacterial overgrowth, and is present in 10% of leukemics at autopsy. Unlike appendicitis, it may improve with medical therapy (18).

The diagnosis of appendicitis in pregnancy is difficult, in part because the position of the appendix changes as the uterus enlarges. The loss of elasticity of the abdominal wall muscles may also change the presenting signs. In the fifth month of pregnancy, pain due to appendicitis may be present above the umbilicus. As the appendix becomes higher in location, signs and symptoms will be different. In addition, the appendix is less likely to be contained by the omentum, and perforation may more frequently lead to generalized peritonitis. Appendicitis is the most common cause of acute abdomen in the pregnant patient and, accordingly, is the most common surgical emergency in any trimester. It may be associated with premature labor and fetal distress (19). Prophylactic antibiotics and tocolytic drugs are often recommended.

The reliability of the classic symptoms of acute appendicitis was recently assessed (17). In the absence of nausea, vomiting, right iliac fossa tenderness, or the presence of symptoms for longer than 72 hr without evidence of perforation, the diagnosis is less likely. In women, pelvic inflammatory disease should be considered if symptoms occur near menses or if cervical or adnexal tenderness is present (17).

A specific scoring system with five clinical criteria has been developed to reduce the rate of appendectomy for inflamed appendixes (20). The criteria utilized by this system include abdominal pain, vomiting, right lower quadrant pain, low-grade fever, and either white blood cell count $>$10,000 cells/mm^3 or polymorphonuclear neutrophils $>$75%. The clinicians who developed the system recommend immediate laparotomy when four criteria are present and admission and observation when three criteria are present (20).

DIFFERENTIAL DIAGNOSIS

The most common differential diagnosis is infection or inflammation of adjacent tissues. Infections that involve the terminal ileum and cecum will cause right lower quadrant tenderness. Similarly, Crohn's ileocolitis usually causes right lower quadrant pain. The most common other diagnoses in a group of 150 children who were incorrectly suspected of having appendicitis were gastroenteritis, mesenteric adenitis, ovarian cyst, pneumonia, and constipation (21). *Y. enterocolitica* was the most common bacterial cause of appendicitis (see above). This bacterium may also cause right-sided colitis with terminal ileitis as well as acute mesenteric adenitis and/or terminal ileitis, which may be mistaken for appendicitis. *Y. pseudotuberculosis* also can cause a pseudoappendicitis syndrome as well as appendicitis (see Fig. 1). *Campylobacter* spp. and nontyphoidal *Salmonella* spp. are the second and third most common bacterial causes of appendicitis, after *Yersinia*. These infections involve the terminal ileum and cecum. When stool cultures are positive for one of these pathogens, acute appendicitis is less likely. Other bacterial, viral, fungal, and parasitic causes of appendicitis are described above.

In persons over 50 years of age, neoplasms should be considered among the differential diagnosis. Cecal tumor can present as appendicitis. Adenoma and adenocarcinoma occurring in the right colon occasionally mimics appendicitis or, when involving the appendix itself, can cause appendicitis (22,23). Ultrasound or computed tomography of the abdomen will facilitate differentiation between neoplasm and appendicitis. Right-sided diverticulitis should also be considered in older persons. The elderly may also have an atypical presentation without fever or leukocytosis, increasing their rate of complications. In women, pathology of the ovary, fallopian tubes, or uterus may cause right lower quadrant pain. This is most often due to pelvic inflammatory disease, but a ruptured ovarian cyst or ectopic pregnancy should also be considered. Rare causes of right lower quadrant pain include osteomyelitis of the iliac bones (24) and abscess of the psoas or gluteal muscles. Invagination of the appendix is unusual, but it also can cause symptoms such as recurrent right lower quadrant pain with nausea and vomiting (25).

DIAGNOSTIC MEASURES

As discussed above, appendicitis is easily diagnosed on the basis of history, physical examination, blood studies, and abdominal radiography. The abdominal X ray will be abnormal in only 10% of patients with an acute abdomen, a fecalith being the most common finding. A barium enema may be helpful when colonic disease is considered. Nonfilling of the appendix, which is suggestive of appendicitis, has a diagnostic accuracy of 80–98%. However, 10% of normal appendixes may not fill, and 20% of acutely inflamed appendixes may fill. Thus barium enema has a limited role as an ancillary diagnostic test. Upper gastrointestinal X-ray series may be helpful in the presence of ileal disease due to infection or Crohn's disease.

Abdominal ultrasound is useful when diagnosis is uncertain. In several series of patients in whom appendicitis was suspected but uncertain, ultrasound abnormalities were predictive of appendicitis in 80–90% of cases (26–28). When ultrasound is normal, the chance of appen-

dicitis is very low. Ultrasound in one series reduced the rate of negative laparotomies from 23% to 13% and was especially useful in evaluating in women of childbearing age (26). However, it altered clinical management in only 18%, confirming the importance of clinical evaluation and judgment.

Ultrasound also may indicate that perforation has occurred when loculated pericecal fluid, prominent pericecal fat, or circumferential loss of the submucosal layer of the appendix is present. The presence of periappendiceal fluid is specific for appendicitis (100%); however, because it is not always present the sensitivity is only 40% (29). In children, loculated fluid and the absence of the echogenic submucosal layer was highly predictive of perforation, but the presence of free fluid or appendicolith was not (30,31).

Ultrasound is especially useful in pregnant patients. However, it may be less helpful later in pregnancy (>35 weeks) when the appendix may not be visualized (32). In this circumstance, changes in patient positioning may be helpful.

Abdominal computed tomography (CT) scan also may be useful in evaluating certain patients with acute abdomen. In one prospective study of 40 patients with a nontraumatic acute abdomen, CT scan gave a correct diagnosis in 95% of cases compared to 50% based on clinical evaluation. In the same study, CT scan changed the clinical strategy in 12 patients (30%) and unnecessary laparotory was avoided in 7 patients (33). Overall, CT scan has a diagnostic accuracy of 93% and sensitivity of 98% (34). In summary, CT scan of the abdomen may be especially useful in patients with atypical presentations and in the elderly (34).

Technetium-99 scan to identify inflammation is rarely useful in the diagnosis of acute appendicitis because it has a high false-negative rate, is expensive, and is often not available (35).

Laparoscopy has been used as a diagnostic test, but it has an 18% technical failure rate, is invasive, and requires a general anesthetic. Moreover, the appendix may not always be visualized.

TREATMENT

When the diagnosis is obvious, acute appendicitis should be treated by immediate appendectomy. Although diagnostic accuracy increases with observation, the risk of perforation also increases with time. Perforation is associated with a 3-fold increase in wound infection, a 15-fold increase in intrabdominal abscess, a 50-fold increase in mortality, and, in women, tubal scarring that may contribute to infertility. Recently, appendectomy was performed by laparoscopic abdominal surgery. Although reported prior to laparoscopic cholecystectomy, laparoscopic appendectomy is performed less frequently because it takes longer and requires special training in laparoscopic techniques. Nevertheless, a randomized controlled trial of laparoscopic appendectomy compared to open appendectomy showed that laparoscopic surgery was associated with a more rapid recovery (36). Moreover, patients preferred the smaller scar (36).

The role of antibiotics in surgery for acute appendicitis has been debated, but when the appendix has perforated they are clearly indicated.

REFERENCES

1. McBurney C. Experience with early operative interference in cases of disease of the vermiform appendix. *NY Med J* 1989; 676–684.
2. Bennion RS, Thompson JE, Gil J, et al. The role of *Yersinia enterocolitica* in appendicitis in the southwestern United States. *Am Surgeon* 1991;57:766–768.
3. Van Noyen R, Selderslaghs R, Bekkaert J, et al. Causative role of *Yersinia* and other enteric pathogens in the appendicular syndrome. *Eur J Clin Microbiol Infect Dis* 1991;10:735–741.
4. Tarr PI, Weinberger E, Hatch EI Jr, Christie DL. Bacterial ileocecitis caused by Escherichia coli O157:H7. *J Pediatr Gastroenterol Nutr* 1992;14:261–263.
5. al-Hilaly MA, Abu-Zidan FM, Zayed FF, Suleiman JD, Farid LS. Tuberculous appendicitis with perforation. Department of Surgery, Al Adan Hospital, Ministry of Public Health Kuwait. *Br J Clin Prac* 1990 Dec;44(12):632–633.
6. Thiroloix J, Durand A. Spirochetemie au cours d'une appendicite aigue. Hemo et seroculture. Isolament et culture du parasite. Emploi du 606. Arreet de la septiciemie. *Bull Mem Soc Med Hosp III* 1911;31:653–662.
7. Mazza S. Espiroquetosis apendiculares. *Pren Med Argent* 1930; 17:464–468.
8. Henrik-Nielsen R, Lundbeck FA, Teglbjaerg PS, et al. Intestinal spirochetosis of the vermiform appendix. *Gastroenterology* 1985;88:971–977.
9. Chrungoo RK, Hangloo VK, Faroqui MM, Khan M. Surgical manifestations and management of ascariasis in Kasmir. Department of Surgery, Government Medical College, Srinagar. *J Indian Med Assoc* 1992 Jul;90(7):171–174.
10. Hulbert TV, Larsen RA, Chandrasoma PT. Abdominal angiostrongyliasis mimicking acute appendicitis and Meckel's diverticulum: report of a case in the United States and review. *Clin Infect Dis* 1992;14:836–840.
11. Rogers S, Potter MN, Slade RR. *Aspergillus* appendicitis in acute myeloid leukemia. Department of Haematology, Southmead Hospital, Westbury-on-Trym, Bristol. *Clin-Lab Haematol* 1990;12(4):471–476.
12. Bomelburg T, Roos N, von Lengerke HJ, Ritter J. Invasive aspergillosis complicating induction chemotherapy of childhood leukemia. Kinderklinik, University at Munster, Federal Republic of Germany. *Eur J Pediatr* 1992;July:151(7):485–487.
13. Dudley TH, Dean PJ. Idiopathic granulomatous appendicitis, or Crohn's disease of the appendix revisited. *Hum Pathol* 1993;24: 595–601.
14. Genta RM, Bleyzer I, Cate TR, Tandon AK, Yoffe B. In situ hybridization and immunohistochemical analysis of cytomegalovirus-associated ileal perforation. *Gastroenterology* 1993;104: 1822–1827.
15. Whitney TM, Macho JR, Russell TR, et al. Appendicitis in acquired immunodeficiency syndrome. *Am J Surg* 1992;164: 467–471.
16. Binderlow SR, Shaked AA. Acute appendicitis in patients with AIDS/HIV infection. Department of Surgery, Mount Sinai Medical Center, New York, NY 10029. *Am J Surg* 1991 July;162(1): 9–12.
17. Rasmussen OO, Hoffman J. Assessment of reliability of symptoms and signs of acute appendicitis. *J R Coll Surg Edinb* 1991; 36:372–377.
18. Angel CA, Rao BN, Wrenn E Jr, et al. Acute appendicitis in children with leukemia and other malignancies: still a diagnostic dilemma. *J Pediatr Surg* 1992;27:476–479.
19. Halvorsen AC, Brandt B, Andreasen JJ. Acute appendicitis in pregnancy: complications and subsequent management. *Eur J Surg* 1992;158:603–606.
20. Christian F, Christian GP. A simple scoring system to reduce the negative appendectomy rate. *Ann R Coll Surg Engl* 1992; 74:281–285.
21. Dolgin SE, Beck AR, Tartter PI. The risk of perforation when children with possible appendicitis are observed in the hospital. *Surg Gynecol Obstet* 1992;175:320–324.
22. Vander SA, Mandell GH. Villous adenoma of the appendix. Report of a case. *Arch Surg* 1968;97:562–564.
23. Munk JF. Villous adenoma causing acute appendicitis. *Br J Surg* 1977;64:593–595.
24. Ofiaeli O. Abnormal syndrome of iliac osteomyelitis presenting as acute appendicitis. Division of Orthopaedics and Traumatology, University Teaching Hospital, Anambra State, Nigeria. *Centr Afr J Med* 1992 Apr;38(4):171–173.
25. Lauwers GY, Prendergast NC, Wahl SJ, et al. Invagination of vermiform appendix. Case Report. *Dig Dis Sci* 1993;38:565–568.
26. Schwerk WB, Wichtrup B, Rothmund M, et al. Ultrasonography in the diagnosis of acute appendicitis: a prospective study. *Gastroenterology* 1989;97:630–639.
27. Larson JM, Pierce JC, Ellinger DM, et al. The validity and utility of sonography in the diagnosis of appendicitis in the community setting. *AJR* 1989;153:687–691.
28. Fa EM, Cronan JJ. Compression ultrasonography as an aid in the differential diagnosis of appendicitis. *Surg Gynecol Obstet* 1989;169:290–298.
29. Borushok KF, Jeffrey RB, Laing FC, et al. Sonographic diagnosis of perforation in patients with acute appendicitis. *AJR* 1990; 154:275–278.
30. Quillin SP, Siegel MJ, Coffin CM. Acute appendicitis in children: value of sonography in detecting perforation. *AJR* 1992; 159:1265–1268.
31. Sivit CJ, Newman KD, Boenning DA, et al. Appendicitis: usefulness of US in diagnosis in a pediatric population. *Radiology* 1992;185:549–552.
32. Lim HK, Bae SH, Seo GS. Diagnosis of acute appendicitis in pregnant women: value of sonography. *AJR* 1992;159:539–542.
33. Taourel P, Baron MP, Pradel J, et al. Acute abdomen of unknown origin: impact of CT on diagnosis and management. *Gastrointest Radiol* 1992;17:287–291.
34. Balthazar EJ, Megibow AJ, Siegel SE, et al. Appendicitis: prospective evaluation with high-resolution CT. *Radiology* 1991; 180:21–24.
35. Foley CR, Latimer RG, Rimkus DS. Detection of acute appendicitis by technetium 99 HMPAO scanning. *Am Surgeon* 1992;58: 761–765.
36. Attwood SEA, Hill ADK, Murphy PG, et al. A prospective randomized trial of laparoscopic versus open appendectomy. *Surgery* 1992;112:497–501.

Infections of the Gastrointestinal Tract,
edited by M. J. Blaser, P. D. Smith, J. I. Ravdin,
H. B. Greenberg, and R. L. Guerrant
Raven Press, Ltd., New York © 1995.

CHAPTER 28

Diverticulitis

Gabriel Garcia and Jay Ladenheim

Colonic diverticula are saccular outpouches that protrude through the wall of the colon. The diverticula can be any in number, can be variable in size (although generally smaller than 1 cm), and can occur anywhere along the length of the colon, but are most common in the sigmoid colon.

Diverticular disease is the general term that encompasses the wide variety of clinical conditions that arise from the presence of diverticula within the colon, a condition known as *diverticulosis*. About 70–80% of persons affected with diverticulosis are either completely asymptomatic or have uncomplicated courses characterized by pain and altered bowel habits. These latter symptoms can be similar in quality to those of irritable bowel syndrome (IBS). Complications can be seen in a sizable minority of those with diverticulosis and are most notable for (a) lower gastrointestinal bleeding that can range from a minor, self-limited process to one that is massive and life threatening, and (b) diverticulitis and its associated complications.

Diverticulitis is an inflammatory process that originates within a diverticulum and gives rise to a wide spectrum of clinical presentations. It is the most common significant complication of diverticular disease, affecting approximately 10–25% of those with colonic diverticula (1,2). This chapter will focus primarily on the pathogenesis, clinical syndromes, and approaches to the diagnosis and treatment of diverticulitis.

PATHOGENESIS OF DIVERTICULOSIS

Colonic diverticula are an acquired deformity that generally are not present at birth and increase in number with aging. Strictly speaking, they are pseudodiverticula because they lack the muscular layer of the colonic wall; the mucosa and submucosa herniate through the muscularis propia, acquire a serosal coat, and give rise to the forma-

tion of these diverticula (3,4). Histological sections reveal that the most likely sites of these herniations are at the point where the vasa recta, the colonic nutrient arteries, penetrate through the circular muscle bundles on either side of the mesenteric taenia and on the mesenteric side of the lateral taeniae (5,6). It is felt that these sites are areas of relative weakness and thus predispose to herniation (7,8).

What gives rise to the formation of diverticula? It is clear that multiple factors play a role. The key factors are the following:

1. A low-fiber diet
2. The aging process
3. Motility disorders
4. Connective tissue disorders, i.e., Marfan's and Ehlers–Danlos syndromes

Both epidemiological and clinical data help in our understanding of this process and support the etiological association with the factors listed above. First and foremost, this process has greatly different prevalences throughout the world (9–11). For example, in Africa and most of Asia, under 1% of adults have diverticula, while in most industrialized nations up to 50% of adults are affected. It has been postulated, but not proven, that low fiber content is the primary culprit in this disparity (11,12). By increasing stool volume and thus luminal radius (see below) and by decreasing intestinal transit time, fiber leads to a decreased intraluminal pressure (13). Milling of grains, which results in a refined, low-fiber product, became increasingly common in the Western world beginning in the late nineteenth century. At that time diverticula were an uncommon curiosity and the incidence of diverticulosis was only 5–7% in autopsy series published in the United States in the 1930s and 1940s (14,15). As the Western diet has become fiber-deficient, the prevalence of diverticulosis has greatly increased (12). Support for the dietary fiber hypothesis is found in the lower frequency of diverticulosis in vegetarians on higher fiber diets compared with case-matched controls (1,16). In the study by Gear, 12% of vegetarians (mean daily fiber intake of 41.5 g) compared

G. Garcia and J. Ladenheim: Department of Medicine, Division of Gastroenterology, Stanford University School of Medicine, Stanford, California 94305.

with 33% of nonvegetarians (mean fiber intake of 21 g) had diverticulosis by barium enema examination (17). Additional data arise from the observations that the prevalence of diverticulosis increases with time when people emigrate from low- to high-prevalence communities and when the diet changes from predominantly vegetarian to one that resembles a Western diet (18,19).

In Western industrialized countries the prevalence of diverticula clearly increases with age (2,14). Diverticula are rare before age 40, can be seen in 30–50% of those who are 50, and are found in up to 67% of people by age 80 (2). Increased elastin deposition, as opposed to decreased or abnormal collagen formation or muscular hypertrophy, occurs with aging, and is presently believed to be the underlying pathological process that gives rise to diverticula formation (20). Elastin deposition leads to foreshortening and contraction of the colonic wall, giving it a thickened and corrugated appearance that has been termed *mychosis*. Similarly, congenital abnormalities in connective tissue formation have been implicated in the frequent and early appearance of diverticulosis in patients with connective tissue disorders (21).

Motility disorders have been implicated as a cause of diverticulosis based primarily on extrapolations from limited human data and principles of physics (22). It appears that the sigmoid colon is the most common site for diverticula because it is the site of the highest pressure gradient between the colonic lumen and the peritoneal space. Intraluminal pressure is proportional to the wall tension and inversely proportional to the luminal diameter (22). This principle is derived from Laplace's law. Wall tension is greatest in areas of increased muscle activity and mass, such as the sigmoid colon, and luminal diameter is also the smallest in the mychotic sigmoid colon. In addition, Painter hypothesized that based on manometric and radiographic data, prominent contractions of the circular smooth muscles of the sigmoid colon can effectively close off afferent and efferent loops of colon within a short segment of sigmoid colon and thus lead to closed spaced compartments of focally high intraluminal pressure (23).

The location of colonic diverticula in the U.S. population is summarized as follows (24–26):

1. Ninety-six percent of patients with diverticula have sigmoid involvement.
2. Sixty percent have the diverticula confined to the sigmoid colon.
3. Eighty percent have the diverticula confined to the left colon.
4. Fifteen percent have the diverticula diffusely throughout the colon.
5. Four percent have the diverticula limited to the nonsigmoid colon, most commonly in the cecum.
6. Rectal involvement with diverticula is rare. This is probably because in part the taeniae coli fan out and form a completely circumferential muscle layer.

The incidence of diverticulitis parallels the distribution of colonic diverticula, and over 90% of all cases of diverticulitis involve the sigmoid colon (27). This distribution is not universal. In some Asian populations, diverticula are less common, tend to be right-sided, and appear to occur about 10 years earlier (28,29). The reasons for these differences are not fully understood.

PATHOGENESIS OF DIVERTICULITIS

Obstruction at the mouth of the diverticulum secondary to impaction of fecal material (i.e., fecolith) is felt to be the initial common pathway in diverticulitis (30,31). Obstruction leads to a compromised blood supply to the diverticulum, which subsequently becomes ischemic and more susceptible to bacterial invasion. What then takes place is a progressive series of developments whose course is determined by host systemic and local factors and by the timing of the initiation of medical treatment.

The earliest stage has been termed *pericolitis* or *peridiverticulitis*, which reflects the development of a focal area of inflammation at the apex of the diverticulum. This is felt to be secondary to a "microperforation" of the colonic wall with focal extravasation of luminal contents into the adjacent serosa. This subsequently leads to a localized inflammatory mass within the colonic wall, i.e., a pericolic phlegmon. Over a short period of time tissue necrosis occurs and a pericolic abscess, which is confined by the colonic mesentery, is formed. A pericolic abscess can enlarge and perforate and thus form a pelvic abscess (32). If this inflammatory process is not contained or walled off by host factors or by the early initiation of medical treatment, a pelvic abscess can rupture and lead to generalized peritonitis with possible fecal soilage. Although free perforation is considered the most dreaded consequence of diverticulitis, numerous other complications can arise, including (a) localized abscess formation, (b) obstruction of either the colon or small bowel secondary to mass effect, and (c) fistula formation. Frank bleeding, more commonly arising from a right-sided diverticulum, is an unusual manifestation of diverticulitis. Conversely, most patients with diverticular hemorrhage have a minimal or absent inflammatory reaction at the bleeding site (33).

NATURAL HISTORY

Most patients with diverticulosis are asymptomatic. The overall incidence of diverticulitis is ~25–30% in those patients with known diverticulosis (1,34,35). The mean age at presentation with diverticulitis is between 60 and 70 years (27,36). A number of studies have reported a gradual increase in the incidence of diverticulitis with known longer duration of diverticulosis. Horner et al. followed a group of 503 patients with radiological evidence of diverticulosis. The incidence of diverticulitis was 10% by 5 years, 25% by 10 years, and 37% by 20 years (24). Boles reported an incidence of ~30% in a group of 294 patients followed for a mean of 15 years (34). The true incidence of diverticulitis as a complication of diverticulosis, however, is unknown. Most studies likely overestimate the true percentage since many patients with diverticulosis are asymptomatic and are never identified or included in the published studies.

Recurrent attacks, 27–45%, are not uncommon in patients who experienced a prior bout of diverticulitis. In those patients whose first episode was managed solely medically, the likelihood of relapse is about 15–40% (2,34–36). For those who underwent operative resection, recurrence rates are on the order of 3–12% depending on the extent of colonic resection (34,37–39).

Certain groups of patients, however, need to be managed with specialized attention. The following sections will deal with the immunocompromised patient, the patient who uses nonsteroidal antiinflammatory drugs (NSAIDs), the patient with right-sided diverticulitis, and the patient under 40 years of age.

Immunocompromised patients, i.e., those who are on chronic steroids (40), have renal insufficiency (41), or have received a transplant (41–43), have an increased rate of morbidity and mortality with their attacks of diverticulitis. Current literature suggests that the incidence of diverticulitis in these populations is not increased, yet the impact of each event is magnified (44). This is felt to be secondary to a delay in the development of classic symptoms, the difficulty in sorting through the broadened differential diagnosis, and subsequent delay in definitive diagnosis and institution of medical treatment. Additionally, immunocompromised patients do not appear to "wall off" the inflammatory process as effectively. They more commonly have a free perforation, often with gross fecal soilage of the peritoneum, at first presentation. Tyau et al. retrospectively reviewed 209 cases of diverticulitis, 40 of which were considered to involve immunocompromised patients (45). During the index hospitalization course there was a 14% incidence of perforation in the immunocompetent group and a 43% incidence of perforation in the immunocompromised group. Surgical intervention was also more frequently required in the immunocompromised group. Mortality data from this study revealed significant differences with a death rate of 0.6% in the immunocompetent group and 25% in those who were immunocompromised.

Consensus favors an earlier consideration of definitive surgical intervention in the immunocompromised patient (40,42,44–46). Perkins et al. noted a 100% failure rate for medical management in a small cohort of immunocompromised patients (44). Surgical intervention was ultimately required for progressive sepsis, peritonitis, perforation, obstruction, or abscess formation. The role of percutaneous drainage of an abscess in immunocompromised patients has not been studied, yet those centers with the greatest published experience with these techniques generally avoid it in this setting and also recommend early surgical intervention (47,48).

Concurrent use of nonsteroidal antiinflammatory drugs has also been implicated in increased morbidity in patients with diverticular disease. A number of case reports and case-controlled studies have shown an increased rate of serious complications, including perforation and fistula formation, in patients presenting with diverticulitis who were on NSAIDs (49). A direct cause-and-effect relationship remains to be established.

Right-sided diverticulitis is an uncommon event in Western countries (50). In large part this is because di-

verticula are much less common in the right colon. Right-sided diverticulitis appears to have a predilection for younger patients (mean age is 41) (51,52). The average age is ~10–15 years lower than in patients with left-sided diverticula (38). The diagnosis is often confused with appendicitis, tubal or ovarian disorders, malignancy, Crohn's disease, or infectious processes secondary to tuberculosis, amebiasis, or actinomycosis (53). Clinically, a variety of reports reveal that patients with right-sided diverticulitis usually have less nausea and vomiting and a longer duration of symptoms at presentation than those with appendicitis (54). Imaging studies such as barium enema or computed tomography (CT) scanning can be helpful yet may not be diagnostic (55), and even intraoperatively malignancy can be difficult to exclude.

In an uncomplicated case in which the diagnosis of diverticulitis has been confidently made noninvasively, a trial of medical management, with or without a drainage procedure, has been shown to be effective (51,54,56). However, most authorities recommend surgical management in any patient with complications associated with right-sided diverticulitis with either a diverticulotomy, local excision, or partial right hemicolectomy (57). In addition, surgery needs to be considered when a right-sided inflammatory mass cannot be distinguished from a neoplasm or when there are recurrent episodes of diverticulitis (53,58). Although right-sided diverticulitis presents more commonly in younger patients, most young patients have the expected distribution of colonic diverticula (left-sided) and present with diverticulitis of the sigmoid colon. However, young patients, i.e., those less than 40 years of age, appear to have a different natural history than the older patient. In a number of large series, patients less than 40 account for 2–6% of the reported cases of diverticulosis (26,59–61). Although the prevalence of diverticula in young patients is quite low, less than 5–10% (2), the incidence of diverticulitis and its associated complications appears to be modestly increased (60–64).

Acosta looked at 285 patients admitted to a hospital for management of diverticular disease (diverticulosis and diverticulitis). Of the total cohort 6% were less than 40 years of age, whereas in the subgroup with diverticulitis 20% were less than 40. In the younger group there was a male-to-female ratio of 3:1, which was not seen when one looked at the group as a whole (59). Ouriel and Schwartz reported on 115 young patients who accounted for 2% of all the cases of diverticula disease seen at the University of Rochester Medical Center from 1961 through 1981 (61). In their series, 92 patients presented with diverticulitis; 17% needed urgent operations, 10% had elective surgery after a cooling-off period, and the rest were initially managed medically. Follow-up data over an average of 22 months showed that of the group initially managed successfully with medical therapy (67 patients), 55% required rehospitalization for diverticular disease, 23% had serious complications, and ultimately 45% required operative management. Freischlag et al. similarly reported that younger patients frequently presented with severe initial attacks and required surgery more frequently (63). In this series, 88% of young patients compared with 42% of patients over age 40 required urgent operations for complications of diverticulitis. All of these series reported a strong male predominance, and more than 80% of the episodes of diverticulitis involved the sigmoid colon. It would appear that either elective or (if needed) urgent operative resection should be considered in all young patients with an episode of diverticulitis at the time of their initial presentation.

CLINICAL FEATURES

Presenting signs and symptoms of diverticulitis are consistent with the underlying stage of illness. The earliest symptoms are acute onset of pain, most commonly in the left lower quadrant, followed by fever, anorexia, nausea, vomiting, and altered bowel habits, usually constipation. Physical examination at this time generally reveals a patient in moderate distress, with depressed bowel sounds and with localized tenderness and often a palpable fullness in the left lower quadrant. Digital rectal examination may reveal a tender mass. Laboratory evaluation is notable for an increased peripheral white blood cell count with a left shift, and frequently there is an abnormal urine analysis, especially if the colonic inflammatory process is adjacent to the genitourinary system. If the inflammatory process fails to be confined to the immediate pericolonic space, signs of diffuse peritoneal irritation (abdominal rigidity) or bacteremia (tachycardia, hypotension, and eventual circulatory collapse) will ensue.

DIAGNOSIS

The diagnosis of diverticulitis is generally made on history and physical examination. Symptoms of left lower quadrant pain, fever, and decreased frequency and caliber of stools are significant. A tender, left lower quadrant abdominal mass with signs of local peritoneal irritation should be sought. Radiographic and endoscopic confirmation may be required, yet generally play a more useful role in recognizing the complications that can be associated with diverticulitis. Plain films of the abdomen are generally nondiagnostic; they may be normal, or reveal an ileus or evidence of obstruction or pneumoperitoneum. Barium or water-soluble contrast enemas can be administered cautiously during the acute phase if the diagnosis is uncertain (3,65,66) yet are often deferred until later in the course. These studies may be diagnostic if contrast is seen outside the colonic lumen adjacent to a diverticulum. In addition, strictures, fistulas, or soft tissue inflammatory masses may be appreciated. Flexible sigmoidoscopy, like barium enemas, is also generally deferred during the acute setting because of the potential for converting a confined colonic perforation to a free peritoneal rupture and, as a consequence, causes fecal spoiling of the abdominal cavity. However, it can be employed if the diagnosis is uncertain and especially if one needs to rule out the possibility of malignancy, not diverticulitis, as the etiological factor of either stricture formation or colonic obstruction in a patient without localized signs of inflammation. The presence of pus exuding from a diverticular opening can be diagnostic but is rarely seen.

More recently, CT scanning has become the test of choice in the acute phase of diverticulitis, when barium enema and flexible sigmoidoscopy can lead to complications such as free perforation, increased severity of obstruction, and spillage of barium sulfate into the peritoneal cavity (67–70). CT is extremely sensitive in confirming the diagnosis of diverticulitis by visualizing both the colonic and pericolonic regions. This is logical since the most significant events in diverticulitis take place outside the colonic lumen. CT is also the ideal, noninvasive test for the critically ill patient when one is concerned about abscess or fistula formation or impending free perforation (68,71,72). CT effectively stratifies patients with diverticulitis according to severity of illness and helps to define subsequent treatment plans (73). The use of rectal contrast (500 cm^3 of water-soluble contrast medium) has been recommended to improve the sensitivity and specificity of CT images when evaluating a patient with clinically suspected diverticulitis (74). Certain groups, however, still favor the barium enema as the primary study with CT scanning reserved for further clarification (75). Ultrasound can also be used to help establish the diagnosis of diverticulitis (76–79). More importantly, ultrasound can be used to assess the abdomen for abscesses and screen for appendicitis or ovarian and tubal disorders, especially in a young patient with a clinical picture suggestive of right-sided diverticulitis.

DIFFERENTIAL DIAGNOSIS (Table 1)

1. *Irritable bowel syndrome (80)*. This syndrome is characterized by altered bowel habits associated with pain. The clinical presentation and management are similar to that of uncomplicated diverticulosis, except that diarrhea is frequent in irritable bowel syndrome.
2. *Appendicitis*. The most likely diagnosis in a young patient with right lower quadrant pain and fever is appendicitis. However, presentation can be identical to that of right-sided (cecal and ascending colon) diverticulitis.
3. *Colonic carcinoma*. Colorectal cancer has epidemiological features similar to those of diverticular disease and at times its presentation (e.g., obstructive symptoms) may overlap.
4. *Inflammatory bowel disease (81)*. Crohn's disease in particular may mimic diverticulitis, as both can present with fever, lower abdominal pain, abscess, etc.
5. *Ischemic, infectious, or radiation-induced colitis*.
6. *Pelvic lesions*. Pelvic pathology, especially ovarian, tuboovarian, and uterine lesions, needs to be considered in any woman presenting with abdominal complaints.

TREATMENT

For uncomplicated diverticulosis no specific treatment is required. For patients with uncomplicated diverticulo-

TABLE 1. *Diverticulitis: differential diagnosis*

Diagnosis	Prevalence	Clinical features	Diagnostic tests	Treatment
Diverticulosis	Female = male; increases with age	Often asymptomatic; can lead to pain, altered bowel habits, lack of systemic signs	Barium enema; colonoscopy	Fiber, fluids
Diverticulitis	Female = male; increases with age	Constellation of abdominal pain, altered bowel habits	CT scan; plain films; barium enema; colonoscopy	Hydration, antibiotics, may need surgery
Irritable bowel syndrome	Female > male; most present by age 50	Abdominal pain; altered bowel habits; lack of systemic signs. Lifelong condition with recurrent symptoms	Sigmoidoscopy; barium enema	Fiber, antidiarrheal agents, laxatives, antispasmodics; psychological support
Appendicitis	Male > female; peak incidence 2nd–3rd decade	Pain followed by anorexia, nausea, vomiting, and fever	Ultrasound; CT scan; surgery	Appendectomy
Colon cancer	Increases with age	Often asymptomatic; can lead to GI bleeding, pain, vomiting, and fever	Barium enema; colonoscopy; surgery	Colonoscopic polypectomy or surgical resection
Pelvic lesions (A) Acute salpingitis	Most common in sexually active young women	High fever; subacute onset of bilateral lower abdominal pain; variable vomiting	Ultrasound; pelvic exam	Hydration, antibiotics
(B) Ruptured ectopic pregnancy	Most common in sexually active young women	Acute onset of lower abdominal pain; can rapidly lead into shock	Ultrasound; pelvic exam	Hydration, antibiotics, emergent surgery
Ischemic colitis	Increases with age	Crampy abdominal pain; GI bleeding; low-grade fever; often with symptomatic coexisting vascular disease	Plain films; barium enema; colonoscopy	Generally medical. Hydration, antibiotics; surgical resection in selected cases of transmural disease
Inflammatory bowel disease	Any age yet usually by age 30 (bimodal age of onset)	Pain; fever; altered bowel habits common; lifelong condition with recurrent symptoms	Barium enema; colonoscopy; small bowel X-rays	Medical if possible: Steroids, asulfidine derivatives, immunosuppressives; selective surgical resection

sis who complain of chronic abdominal discomfort or altered bowel habits, current recommendations parallel those for irritable bowel, i.e., fiber (dietary or supplemental), fluids, antispasmodics such as dicyclomine, and, rarely, analgesics. The only therapy that has been validated by controlled trials is increased fiber intake, generally to 10–25 g daily (82,83). Fiber supplementation may lead initially to bloating or worsening of symptoms; thus beginning at a low dose and gradually increasing daily fiber intake is recommended.

Treatment for diverticulitis needs to be tailored to the medical condition at the time of presentation (31,32,70, 84,85). All patients with fever and leukocytosis in association with abdominal pain and evidence of local peritoneal irritation should be admitted to the hospital. Initial management includes bowel rest (with nasogastric decompression if nausea and vomiting are present), intravenous hydration, and parenteral antibiotics. Empiric antibiotic coverage is directed at the likely organisms predictably involved. The spectrum of bacteria that com-

plicates diverticulitis is the same as that found in the normal flora of the colon or feces. These include the enteric anaerobes (*Bacteroides fragilis*), the gram-negative aerobic bacilli (*E. coli*), and the gram-positive coliforms (*Streptococcus faecalis*).

Common choices for antibiotic coverage include "triple coverage" with ampicillin, gentamicin, and metronidazole. Recently, the use of broad-spectrum cephalosporins (cefoxitin or cefotetan) and extended spectrum penicillins (combined with a β-lactamase inhibitor) have been advocated. Duma and Kellum reviewed the efficacy of a wide variety of antibiotic regimens in patients with intraabdominal sepsis (86). They noted that aminoglycosides, broad-spectrum penicillins (87), cephalosporins (88,89), monobactams and carbapenems (90) are all effective drugs in treating patients with gram-negative bacilli. Although some of these drugs have anaerobic coverage, drugs such as clindamycin and metronidazole are often added for additional anerobic coverage (89). However, Kellum in a recently published, randomized, prospective study of 51 patients with diverticulitis compared the efficacy of cefoxitin to a combination of gentamicin and clindamicin. Both regimens had similar "cure rates" (greater than 85%) and were similarly well tolerated. On balance, these investigators favored the use of cefoxitin as a single agent given its reduced risk of nephrotoxicity in an elderly population and its narrower spectrum, thus avoiding the emergence of highly resistant organisms (88).

When diverticulitis is recognized and treated promptly, the course is often uncomplicated and successfully managed with medical therapy, as is true in 70–85% of patients (35,36,91). A favorable response is generally seen within 2–4 days with resolution of the signs and symptoms of the underlying illness. At this point one can return to an oral diet. Antibiotics should be continued for a total of 7–10 days. Radiographic or endoscopic evaluation of the colon and abdomen should be performed after the acute inflammatory process has subsided.

In those patients who fail to respond to medical management and remain with systemic or localized complaints, additional timely interventions are required. Workup may include the following:

1. Plain abdominal films—looking for free air or obstruction
2. Abdominal/pelvic CT scan—looking for abscess or fistula formation
3. "Gentle" lower GI series (barium or, more commonly, a water-soluble agent)—looking for fistula or stricture formation, localizing the site of inflammation
4. Colonoscopy—ruling out malignancy and evaluation of a stricture (92). Generally reserved for those patients in which radiographic studies are not helpful
5. Ultrasound—can be used to look for abscess, tuboovarian abscesses, ovarian cysts, or appendicitis (77,93,94)

CT scanning is becoming the primary diagnostic tool for evaluating patients in whom the diagnosis is uncertain or who are failing to respond to initial medical management. CT is regarded as a safe and highly sensitive tool. CT is useful in confirming the diagnosis as well as revealing the extent and nature of complications, including abscesses and fistulas (Fig. 1).

When a patient is failing medical therapy, a combination of the above tests is often required. The patient's clinical course as well as the physician's clinical judgment and local expertise are critical factors. The most likely interventions that may need to be considered are surgical intervention and percutaneous drainage of an abscess. Surgical treatment is generally divided into four categories: (a) emergent, (b) urgent, (c) abscess drainage, and (d) elective.

For the patient with frank peritoneal signs and free air on a plain film, indicative of free perforation into the abdominal cavity, attempts at stabilization should immediately be followed by operative intervention. In general, indications for immediate or urgent surgery include (a) progressive symptoms or sepsis despite antibiotics, (b) uncontained perforation, (c) large or small bowel obstruction not responsive to nasoenteral decompression, and (d) the persistence or progression of an abscess despite attempts at percutaneous drainage (27,95).

When a patient requires emergency surgery because of perforation or the inability to effectively stabilize with medical therapy, a two-stage operation is generally indicated. In this setting the surgeon is usually managing an unstable patient with an unprepped colon. The risks of performing a primary anastamosis at the time of colonic resection are quite high and include anastamotic breakdown, fistula formation, and increased patient operative mortality (27,95,96). Currently, a two-stage operation is

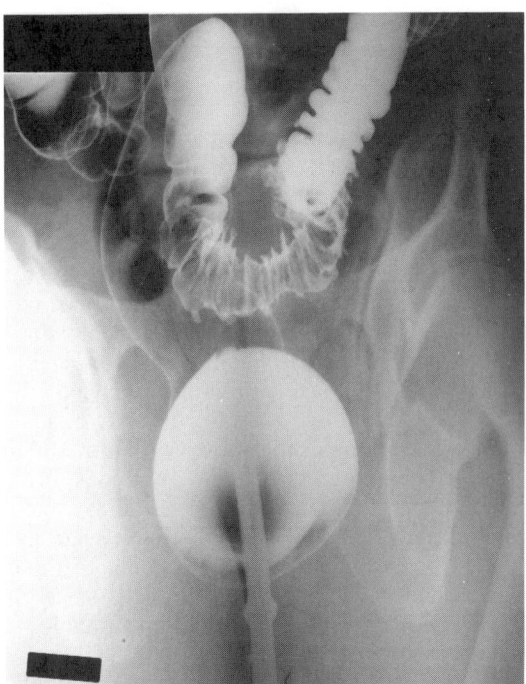
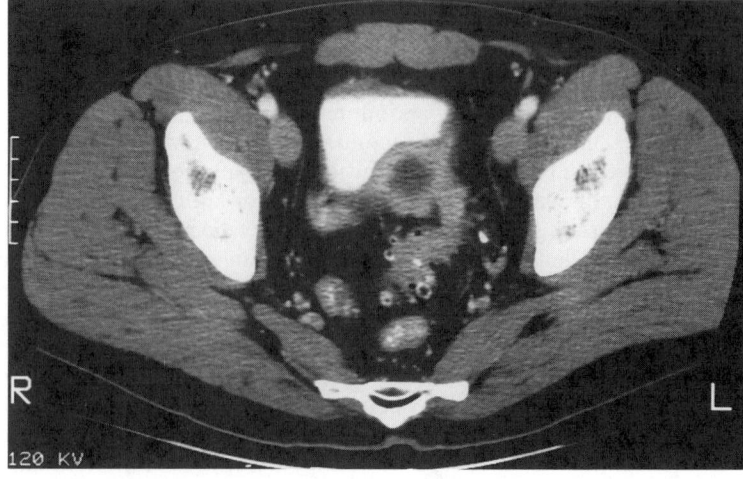

FIG. 1. A 47-year-old man presented with fever, left lower quadrant pain, and absence of stools for 4 days. A barium enema (*left*) showed diverticuli and narrowing of the sigmoid colon. A subsequent abdominal CT scan (*above*) showed a pericolonic abscess at the site of the diverticuli in the sigmoid colon.

recommended (27,38). During the first stage, the involved area of the colon is resected, the proximal loop is brought up as an end colostomy, the distal loop is either closed off (Hartmann pouch) or made into a mucous fistula, and the peritoneum is aggressively lavaged. At the time of the second stage, performed approximately 3 months later, restoration of colonic continuity can be accomplished.

For patients who can be stabilized with initial medical management yet go on to abscess formation, the surgical approach often can be done in a single stage. This is true for abscesses that are generally small and contiguous with the colonic mesentery (mesocolic abscess) as well as for pelvic abscesses. Small mesocolic abscesses have a better prognosis and often can be managed with a single-stage operative procedure with en bloc removal of the abscess cavity and the diseased segment of the colon (97). In fact, surgery is not always required in this setting, as a small mesocolic abscess can respond to medical treatment with antibiotics without a drainage procedure (98).

A number of recent reports have shown that the optimal treatment of a larger (>5 cm) pelvic or paracolic abscess generally includes preoperative percutaneous placement of a drainage catheter into the abscess cavity (48, 97,99–102). Percutaneous drainage is generally done under CT guidance and can be done in almost all patients with an abscess provided the abscess cavity is readily accessible and the patient is without signs of generalized peritonitis. Percutaneous drainage has been shown to effectively resolve the acute inflammatory process in the large majority of patients. Review of most series reveals an approximately 70% success rate in converting an anticipated multistage to a one-stage surgical procedure by preoperative percutaneous drainage (48,97). The one-stage operation includes a full bowel prep and subsequent resection of the involved area with primary colonic closure. In Stabile et al.'s series 14 of 17 patients, and in Mueller et al.'s series 13 of 21 patients, were successfully managed with preoperative percutaneous drainage followed by a one-stage procedure (48,97). Operative mortality is thus felt to be reduced in a patient who has been stabilized, hydrated, and prepped and requires only a one-stage surgical procedure.

In a small minority of patients with large abscesses who were successfully managed with percutaneous drainage, a definitive operative procedure was deferred for a variety of reasons including patient refusal. Despite initial success, however, preliminary data reveal a high incidence of recurrent abscess formation and signs and symptoms of diverticulitis over the ensuing months (48,97).

Fistula formation is also a well-recognized complication of diverticulitis and can occur in up to 20% of patients reported in surgical series, yet the true incidence is likely to be much lower if one includes all cases of diverticulitis (103–106). The fistula usually forms after an abscess extends and subsequently ruptures into a nearby structure. The signs and symptoms of fistula are often subacute and can present after the acute colonic inflammatory process has resolved. The most common site is a colovesical fistula, which accounts for approximately two thirds of all fistulas, yet others extend to the skin, vagina, uterus, or even other parts of the colon or small intestine. Treatment of a fistula tract is surgical with complete excision of the fistula tract.

Fistulas as well as strictures and partial obstructions can also frequently be dealt with in a one-stage procedure provided that bowel preparation can be done. In general, when surgical intervention is performed, the proximal line of resection should be at a site above the inflamed or involved area that is focally free of diverticula (more proximal segments that harbor diverticula may remain), and the distal line should be carried beyond the point of the most distal diverticulum, usually the proximal rectum (37).

CONCLUSION

Diverticulitis, which occurs in up to 30% of individuals with diverticulosis, is the most common complication of diverticular disease. Most patients with diverticulitis can be treated medically, yet a variety of diagnostic and therapeutic options are available for those with complicated courses. Although the classic scenario is left lower quadrant abdominal pain and fever in a middle-aged to elderly person, one must be aware of the different presentations of diverticulitis in other subgroups of patients, such as the immunocompromised.

REFERENCES

1. Almy TP, Howell DA. Medical progress. Diverticular disease of the colon. *N Engl J Med* 1980;302(6):324–331.
2. Parks TG. Natural history of diverticular disease of the colon. *Clin Gastroenterol* 1975;4(1):53–69.
3. Fleischner FG. Diverticular disease of the colon. New observations and revised concepts. *Gastroenterology* 1971;60(2):316–324.
4. Morson BC. Pathology of diverticular disease of the colon. *Clin Gastroenterol* 1975;4(1):37–52.
5. Drummond H. Sacculi of the large intestine, with special reference to their relations to the blood vessels of the bowel wall. *Br J Surg* 1916;4:407.
6. Meyers MA, Volberg F, Katzen B, Alonso D, Abbott G. The angioarchitecture of colonic diverticula. Significance in bleeding diverticulosis. *Radiology* 1973;108(2):249–261.
7. Noer RJ. Hemorrhage as a complication of diverticulitis. *Ann Surg* 1955;141:674–685.
8. Slack WW. The anatomy, pathology, and some clinical features of diverticulitis of the colon. *Br J Surg* 1962;50:185.
9. Kyle J, Adesola AO, Tinckler LF, de Beaux J. Incidence of diverticulitis. *Scand J Gastroenterol* 1967;2:77–80.
10. Mendeloff AI. Thoughts on the epidemiology of diverticular disease. *Clin Gastroenterol* 1986;15(4):855–877.
11. Painter NS, Burkitt DP. Diverticular disease of the colon: a deficiency disease of western civilization. *Br Med J* 1971;2(759):450–454.
12. Connell AM. Pathogenesis of diverticular disease of the colon. *Adv Intern Med* 1977;22(377):377–395.
13. Findlay JM, Smith AN, Mitchell WD, Anderson AJ, Eastwood MA. Effects of unprocessed bran on colon function in normal subjects and in diverticular disease. *Lancet* 1974;1(849):146–149.
14. Painter NS, Burkitt DP. Diverticular disease of the colon, a 20th century problem. *Clin Gastroenterol* 1975;4(1):3–21.
15. Rankin FW, Brown PW. Diverticulitis of the colon. *Surg Gynecol Obstet* 1930;50(5):836.
16. Brodribb AJ, Humphreys DM. Diverticular disease: three stud-

ies. Part I—Relation to other disorders and fibre intake. *Br Med J* 1976;1(6007):424–425.

17. Gear JS, Ware A, Fursdon P, et al. Symptomless diverticular disease and intake of dietary fibre. *Lancet* 1979;1(8115): 511–514.

18. Segal I, Solomon A, Hunt JA. Emergence of diverticular disease in the urban South African black. *Gastroenterology* 1977; 72(2):215–219.

19. Stemmermann GN, Yatani R. Diverticulosis and polyps of the large intestine. A necropsy study of Hawaii Japanese. *Cancer* 1973;31(5):1260–1270.

20. Whiteway J, Morson BC. Elastosis in diverticular disease of the sigmoid colon. *Gut* 1985;26(3):258–266.

21. Beighton PH, Murdoch JL, Votteler T. Gastrointestinal complications of the Ehlers-Danlos syndrome. *Gut* 1969;10(12): 1004–1008.

22. Eastwood MA, Watters DA, Smith AN. Diverticular disease—is it a motility disorder? *Clin Gastroenterol* 1982;11(3): 545–561.

23. Painter NS, Turelove SC, Ardran GM, Tuckey M. Segmentation and the localization of intraluminal pressures in the human colon, with special reference to the pathogenesis of colonic diverticula. *Gastroenterology* 1965;49(2):169.

24. Horner JL. Natural history of diverticulosis of the colon. *Am J Dig Dis* 1958;3(5):343.

25. Hughes LE. Postmortem survey of diverticular disease of the colon. I. Diverticulosis and diverticulitis. II. The muscular abnormality of the sigmoid colon. *Gut* 1969;10(5):336–351.

26. Parks TG. Natural history of diverticular disease of the colon: a review of 521 cases. *Br Med J* 1969;4(684):639–642.

27. Rodkey GV, Welch CE. Changing patterns in the surgical treatment of diverticular disease. *Ann Surg* 1984;200(4):466–478.

28. Sugihara K, Muto T, Morioka Y, Asano A, Yamamoto T. Diverticular disease of the colon in Japan. A review of 615 cases. *Dis Colon Rectum* 1984;27(8):531–537.

29. Vajrabukka T, Saksornchai K, Jimakorn P. Diverticular disease of the colon in a far-eastern community. *Dis Colon Rectum* 1980;23(3):151–154.

30. Ming S-C, Fleischner FG. Diverticulitis of the sigmoid colon: reappraisal of the pathology and pathogenesis. *Surgery* 1965; 58(4):627.

31. Morson BC. The muscle abnormality in diverticular disease of the sigmoid colon. *Br J Radiol* 1963;36(426):385.

32. Hinchey EJ, Schaal PG, Richards GK. Treatment of perforated diverticular disease of the colon. *Adv Surg* 1978;12(85):85–109.

33. Meyers MA, Alonso DR, Gray GF, Baer JW. Pathogenesis of bleeding colonic diverticulosis. *Gastroenterology* 1976;71(4): 577–583.

34. Boles RS, Jordan SM. The clinical significance of diverticulosis. *Gastroenterology* 1958;35(6):579.

35. Colcock BP. Surgical management of complicated diverticulitis. *N Engl J Med* 1958;259(12):570–573.

36. Larson DM, Masters SS, Spiro HM. Medical and surgical therapy in diverticular disease: a comparative study. *Gastroenterology* 1976;71(5):734–737.

37. Benn PL, Wolff BG, Ilstrup DM. Level of anastomosis and recurrent colonic diverticulitis. *Am J Surg* 1986;151(2): 269–271.

38. Chappuis CW, Cohn IJ. Acute colonic diverticulitis. *Surg Clin North Am* 1988;68(2):301–313.

39. Wolff BG, Ready RL, MacCarty RL, Dozois RR, Beart RJ. Influence of sigmoid resection on progression of diverticular disease of the colon. *Dis Colon Rectum* 1984;27(10):645–647.

40. ReMine SG, McIlrath DC. Bowel perforation in steroid-treated patients. *Ann Surg* 1980;192(4):581–586.

41. Starnes HJ, Lazarus JM, Vineyard G. Surgery for diverticulitis in renal failure. *Dis Colon Rectum* 1985;28(11):827–831.

42. Guice K, Rattazzi LC, Marchioro TL. Colon perforation in renal transplant patients. *Am J Surg* 1979;138(1):43–48.

43. Lao A, Bach D. Colonic complications in renal transplant recipients. *Dis Colon Rectum* 1988;31(2):130–133.

44. Perkins JD, Shield C, Chang FC, Farha GJ. Acute diverticulitis. Comparison of treatment in immunocompromised and non-

immunocompromised patients. *Am J Surg* 1984;148(6): 745–748.

45. Tyau ES, Prystowsky JB, Joehl RJ, Nahrwold DL. Acute diverticulitis. A complicated problem in the immunocompromised patient. *Arch Surg* 1991;126(7):855–859; discussion 858–859.

46. Alexander P, Schuman E, Vetto RM. Perforation of the colon in the immunocompromised patient. *Am J Surg* 1986;151(5): 557–561.

47. Rodkey GV. Letter. *Am J Surg* 1990;159:104.

48. Stabile BE, Puccio E, vanSonnenberg E, Neff CC. Preoperative percutaneous drainage of diverticular abscesses. *Am J Surg* 1990;159(1):99–104; discussion.

49. Bjarnason I, Hayllar J, MacPherson AJ, Russell AS. Side effects of nonsteroidal anti-inflammatory drugs on the small and large intestine in humans. *Gastroenterology* 1993;104: 1832–1847.

50. Williams KL. Acute solitary ulcers and acute diverticulitis of the caecum and ascending colon. *Br J Surg* 1960;47:351–358.

51. Bova JG, Hopens TA, Goldstein HM. Diverticulitis of the right colon. *Dig Dis Sci* 1984;29(2):150–156.

52. Wagner D, Zollinger R. Diverticulitis of the cecum and ascending colon. *Arch Surg* 1961;83:436–442.

53. Wyble EJ, Lee WC. Cecal diverticulitis: changing trends in management. *South Med J* 1988;81(3):313–316.

54. Fischer MG, Farkas AM. Diverticulitis of the cecum and ascending colon. *Dis Colon Rectum* 1984;27(7):454–458.

55. Balthazar EJ, Megibow AJ, Gordon RB, Hulnick D. Cecal diverticulitis: evaluation with CT. *Radiology* 1987;162:79–81.

56. Morris J, Stellato TA, Lieberman J, Haaga JR. The utility of computed tomography in colonic diverticulitis. *Ann Surg* 1986; 204(2):128–132.

57. Arrington P, Judd CJ. Cecal diverticulitis. *Am J Surg* 1981; 142(1):56–59.

58. Schmit PJ, Bennion RS, Thompson JJ. Cecal diverticulitis: a continuing diagnostic dilemma. *World J Surg* 1991;15(3): 367–371.

59. Acosta JA, Grebenc ML, Doberneck RC, McCarthy JD, Fry DE. Colonic diverticular disease in patients 40 years old or younger. *Am Surg* 1992;58(10):605–607.

60. Eusebio EB, Eisenberg MM. Natural history of diverticular disease of the colon in young patients. *Am J Surg* 1973;125(3): 308–311.

61. Ouriel K, Schwartz SI. Diverticular disease in the young patient. *Surg Gynecol Obstet* 1983;156(1):1–5.

62. Feczko PJ, Nish AD, Craig BM, Simms SM. Acute diverticulitis in patients under 40 years of age: radiologic diagnosis. *AJR* 1988;150(6):1311–1314.

63. Freischlag J, Bennion RS, Thompson JJ. Complications of diverticular disease of the colon in young people. *Dis Colon Rectum* 1986;29(10):639–643.

64. Hannan CE, Knightly JJ, Coffey RJ. Diverticular disease of the colon in the younger age group. *Dis Colon Rectum* 1961; 4:419–423.

65. Hiltunen JN, Kolehmainen H, Vuorinen T, Matikainen M. Early water-soluble contrast enema in the diagnosis of acute colonic diverticulitis. *Int J Colorect Dis* 1991;6:190–192.

66. Nicholas GG, Miller WT, Fitts WT, Tondreau RL. Diagnosis of diverticulitis of the colon: role of the barium enema in defining pericolic inflammation. *Ann Surg* 1972;176(2):205–209.

67. Ertan A. Colonic diverticulitis. Recognizing and managing its presentations and complications [see comments]. *Postgrad Med* 1990;88(3):67–72,77.

68. Hulnick DH, Megibow AJ, Balthazar EJ, Naidich DP, Bosniak MA. Computed tomography in the evaluation of diverticulitis. *Radiology* 1984;152(2):491–495.

69. Lieberman JM, Haaga JR. Computed tomography of diverticulitis. *J Comput Assist Tomogr* 1983;7(3):431–443.

70. Pohlman T. Diverticulitis. *Gastroenterol Clin North Am* 1988; 17(2):357–385.

71. Doringer E. Computerized tomography of colonic diverticulitis. *Crit Rev Diagn Imaging* 1992;33(5):421–435.

72. Pillari G, Greenspan B, Vernace FM, Rosenblum G. Computed

tomography of diverticulitis. *Gastrointest Radiol* 1984;9(3): 263–268.

73. Hachigian MP, Honickman S, Eisenstat TE, Rubin RJ, Salvati EP. Computed tomography in the initial management of acute left-sided diverticulitis. *Dis Colon Rectum* 1992;35(12): 1123–1129.

74. Raval B, Lamki N, St Ville E. Role of computed tomography in diverticulitis. *J Comput Tomogr* 1987;11(2):144–150.

75. Smith TR, Cho KC, Morehouse HT, Kratka PS. Comparison of computed tomography and contrast enema evaluation of diverticulitis. *Dis Colon Rectum* 1990;33(1):1–6.

76. Parulekar SG. Sonography of colonic diverticulitis. *J Ultrasound Med* 1985;4(12):659–666.

77. Schwerk WB, Schwarz S, Rothmund M. Sonography in acute colonic diverticulitis. A prospective study. *Dis Colon Rectum* 1992;35(11):1077–1084.

78. Wada M, Kikuchi Y, Doy M. Uncomplicated acute diverticulitis of the cecum and ascending colon: sonographic findings in 18 patients. AJR 1990;155(2):283–287.

79. Wilson SR, Toi A. The value of sonography in the diagnosis of acute diverticulitis of the colon. AJR 1990;154(6):1199–1202.

80. Otte JJ, Larsen L, Andersen JR. Irritable bowel syndrome and symptomatic diverticular disease—different diseases? *Am J Gastroenterol* 1986;81(7):529–531.

81. Schmidt GT, Lennard JJ, Morson BC, Young AC. Crohn's disease of the colon and its distinction from diverticulitis. *Gut* 1968;9(1):7–16.

82. Brodribb AJ. Treatment of symptomatic diverticular disease with a high-fibre diet. *Lancet* 1977;1(8013):664–666.

83. Weinreich J. Controlled studies with dietary fibre in the therapy of diverticular disease and irritable bowel syndrome. In: *Colon and nutrition. Proceedings of Falk Symposium #32.* Lancaster: MTP Press; 1981:239.

84. Hughes LE. Complications of diverticular disease: inflammation, obstruction and bleeding. *Clin Gastroenterol* 1975;4(1): 147–170.

85. Ulin AW, Pearce AE, Weinstein SF. Diverticular disease of the colon: surgical perspectives in the past decade. *Dis Colon Rectum* 1981;24(4):276–281.

86. Duma RJ, Kellum JM. Colonic diverticulitis: microbiologic, diagnostic, and therapeutic considerations. *Curr Clin Top Infect Dis* 1991;11(218):218–247.

87. Najem AZ, Kaminski ZC, Spillert CR, Lazaro EJ. Comparative study of parenteral piperacillin and cefoxitin in the treatment of surgical infections of the abdomen. *Surg Gynecol Obstet* 1983;157(5):423–425.

88. Kellum JM, Sugerman HJ, Coppa GF, et al. Randomized, prospective comparison of cefoxitin and gentamicin-clindamycin in the treatment of acute colonic diverticulitis. *Clin Ther* 1992; 14(3):376–384.

89. Tally FP, Ho JL. Management of patients with intraabdominal infection due to colonic perforation. *Curr Clin Top Infect Dis* 1987;8(266):266–295.

90. Jones RN. Review of the in vitro spectrum of activity of imipenem. *Am J Med* 1985;78(6A):22–32.

91. Konsten J, Gouma DJ, Obertop H, Soeters PB. Effect of preoperative risk factors on the outcome after surgery for complicated diverticular disease. *Neth J Surg* 1990;42(4):101–104.

92. Forde KA, Treat MR. Colonoscopy in the evaluation of strictures. *Dis Colon Rectum* 1985;28(10):699–701.

93. Jeffrey RJ, Laing FC, Townsend RR. Acute appendicitis: sonographic criteria based on 250 cases. *Radiology* 1988;167(2): 327–329.

94. Puylaert JB, Rutgers PH, Lalisang RI, et al. A prospective study of ultrasonography in the diagnosis of appendicitis. *N Engl J Med* 1987;317(11):666–669.

95. Lambert ME, Knox RA, Schofield PF, Hancock BD. Management of the septic complications of diverticular disease. *Br J Surg* 1986;73(7):576–579.

96. Colcock BP. Diverticular disease: proven surgical management. *Clin Gastroenterol* 1975;4(1):99–119.

97. Mueller PR, Saini S, Wittenburg J, et al. Sigmoid diverticular abscesses: percutaneous drainage as an adjunct to surgical resection in 24 cases. *Radiology* 1987;164(2):321–325.

98. Ambrosetti P, Robert J, Witzig JA, et al. Incidence, outcome, and proposed management of isolated abscesses complicating acute left-sided colonic diverticulitis. A prospective study of 140 patients. *Dis Colon Rectum* 1992;35(11):1072–1076.

99. Neff CC, vanSonnenberg E, Casola G, et al. Diverticular abscesses: percutaneous drainage. *Radiology* 1987;163(1):15–18.

100. Saini S, Mueller PR, Wittenberg J, Butch RJ, Rodkey GV, Welch CE. Percutaneous drainage of diverticular abscess. An adjunct to surgical therapy. *Arch Surg* 1986;121(4):475–478.

101. Sparks FC, Strauss EB, Corey JM. Percutaneous drainage of a diverticular abscess can make colostomy unnecessary in selected cases. *Conn Med* 1990;54(6):305–307.

102. vanSonnenberg E, Mueller PR, Ferrucci JJ. Percutaneous drainage of 250 abdominal abscesses and fluid collections. Part I., results, failures, and complications. *Radiology* 1984;151(2): 337–341.

103. McConnell DB, Sasaki TM, Vetto RM. Experience with colovesical fistula. *Am J Surg* 1980;140(1):80–84.

104. Small WP, Smith AN. Fistula and conditions associated with diverticular disease of the colon. *Clin Gastroenterol* 1975;4(1): 171–199.

105. Steele M, Deveney C, Burchell M. Diagnosis and management of colovesical fistulas. *Dis Colon Rectum* 1979;22(1):27–30.

106. Woods RJ, Lavery IC, Fazio VW, Jagelman DG, Weakley FL. Internal fistulas in diverticular disease. *Dis Colon Rectum* 1988; 31(8):591–596.

Infections of the Gastrointestinal Tract,
edited by M. J. Blaser, P. D. Smith, J. I. Ravdin,
H. B. Greenberg, and R. L. Guerrant
Raven Press, Ltd., New York © 1995.

CHAPTER **29**

Peritonitis and Intraabdominal Abscess

Sydney M. Finegold and Caroline C. Johnson

PERITONITIS

Peritonitis is inflammation of the serous lining of the peritoneal cavity. It represents a response to a variety of factors including microbial agents and chemical irritants. It is clearly much more of a problem than was appreciated by Stewardson (1), who wrote, in 1844, in Elliotson's *Practice of Medicine:*

> The treatment of peritonitis is easy enough, it consists of a general bleeding, followed by an abundance of local bleeding (by means of leeches), a rapid affection of the mouth by mercury and keeping the bowels well purged the whole time.

The surface area of the peritoneum approximates that of the skin. Normally, the peritoneal cavity is lubricated with about 20–50 mL of clear yellow fluid with characteristics of a transudate; there are fewer than 300 cells/mm^3 (mostly macrophages and lymphocytes), the specific gravity is low (<1.016), and the protein (chiefly albumin) content is low (<3 g/dL). In bacterial peritonitis, there may be inflow of 300–500 mL of fluid/hr into the peritoneal cavity (2).

Nonmicrobial peritonitis may follow the introduction into the peritoneal cavity of irritants such as blood, bile, pancreatic juice, other gastroduodenal juices, meconium, and starch or other foreign bodies. Peritonitis may occur in the course of sarcoidosis and familial Mediterranean fever (as part of familial paroxysmal polyserositis). Acute chylous peritonitis may have a sudden onset with crampy abdominal pain; the turbid ascitic fluid is typically sterile. On occasion chemical peritonitis may be related to intraperitoneal administration of antimicrobial agents, such as vancomycin (3).

S. M. Finegold: Medical Service, VA Medical Center, West Los Angeles, and Departments of Medicine, and Microbiology & Immunology, UCLA School of Medicine, Los Angeles, California.

C. C. Johnson: Infectious Disease Section, VA Medical Center, and Department of Medicine, Medical College of Pennsylvania, Philadelphia, Pennsylvania.

Infectious causes of peritonitis will be considered in the following categories: primary or spontaneous peritonitis, secondary peritonitis, peritonitis relating to peritoneal dialysis, and miscellaneous types of peritonitis (including actinomycotic, fungal, parasitic, tuberculous, and so forth).

Primary or Spontaneous Peritonitis

This syndrome, which is probably made up of several entities, is best defined as peritonitis without an evident gastrointestinal (GI) tract source (such as perforated viscus, etc.). For the most part, no local source is evident. It may, however, be related to female genital tract infection on occasion. There are variants to be kept in mind. Cases with positive ascitic fluid culture but no clinical findings of peritonitis have been designated as bacterascites. These cases may represent early colonization but their mortality is comparable to classic cases of spontaneous bacterial peritonitis. There are, conversely, patients with clinical evidence of peritonitis and increased white blood cell counts in ascitic fluid, but with negative cultures. These have been called culture-negative neutrocytic ascites.

Background Factors

Spontaneous bacterial peritonitis (SBP) in children is seen much less frequently than was true in the preantibiotic era; it presently accounts for only 1–2% of pediatric abdominal emergencies. In children, it is seen particularly in association with postnecrotic cirrhosis and with the nephrotic syndrome. There may be an association with urinary tract infection.

In adults, the major underlying factor is cirrhosis with ascites. The incidence of SBP in such patients has doubled to about 15% in the last decade (4), probably reflecting an increased awareness of the entity on the part of physicians and more frequent use of diagnostic paracenteses.

If culture-negative cases are included, the incidence of SBP in cirrhotics with ascites is 19%. Although alcoholic cirrhosis is the principal background illness, SBP has been seen in patients with ascites due to postnecrotic cirrhosis, chronic active hepatitis, acute viral hepatitis, congestive heart failure, malignancy, systemic lupus erythematosus, rheumatoid arthritis, lymphedema, nephrotic syndrome, gonococcal perihepatitis, and Budd–Chiari syndrome. Rarely, there is no apparent underlying disease.

Andreu et al. (5) prospectively studied 110 patients with cirrhosis and ascites and found an incidence of first-episode SBP of 25%. There were a number of risk factors that would predict the occurrence of SBP, but for clinical purposes the two that served well were ascitic fluid protein level (≤1 g/dL) and serum bilirubin level (>2.5 mg/dL).

Etiology

Prior to the availability of antimicrobial agents, *Streptococcus pneumoniae* and group A streptococci were important agents in SBP in children; these organisms are much less important now and have been replaced by gram-negative bacilli and, to a lesser extent, staphylococci. In adults, gram-negative bacilli also dominate, followed by streptococci and other gram-positive cocci. Garcia-Tsao (4) tabulated 806 organisms recovered from 746 cases of SBP in 27 reported series of cases; only 8% had a polymicrobial flora. Gram-negative bacilli were found in 72% of cases; included were *Escherichia coli* (in 47%), *Klebsiella* sp. (13%), and others. Roughly one fourth of cases had gram-positive cocci present; included were *Streptococcus pneumoniae*, other streptococci (primarily the viridans group), *Enterococcus,* and *Staphylococcus* (both *S. aureus* and catalase-negative forms). Anaerobes and microaerophiles were only seen in 5% of cases. A similar tabulation by Richardet and Beaugrand (6), involving 25 series published since 1978 and 532 patients, yielded similar results but with even fewer anaerobes. Targan et al. (7) found a 6% incidence of anaerobes or microaerophiles. It has been stated that anaerobes may be uncommon in SBP because of the relatively high oxygen content of ascitic fluid, which is comparable to that of venous blood (8); however, the redox potential may be relatively low as it can be in blood (9). It has also been noted that ascitic fluid may have antibacterial activity against *Bacteroides;* on the other hand, ascitic fluid was commonly used in the past as an excellent supplement for various media to facilitate growth of fastidious anaerobes. One must wonder about the suitability of media in common use for growth of very small numbers of such anaerobes. In any case, recovery of anaerobes from ascitic fluid, particularly in polymicrobial cases, should raise the possibility of secondary peritonitis. Specific organisms that have been reported in SBP are listed in Table 1.

Pathogenesis, Pathology

The frequency with which bowel organisms are found in SBP suggests that the gut is the major source of the

TABLE 1. *Organisms recovered from spontaneous bacterial peritonitis*

Gram-negative bacilli
  Enterobacteriaceae
    Citrobacter amalonaticus (10)
    Enterobacter aerogenes (11)
    Enterobacter cloacae
    Escherichia coli
    Klebsiella pneumoniae
    Proteus
    Providencia
    Salmonella
    Serratia
    Yersinia enterocolitica (12)
  Other
    Acinetobacter
    Aeromonas hydrophila
    Aeromonas sobria (13)
    Brucella melitensis (14)
    Campylobacter fetus
    Flavobacterium meningosepticum
    Haemophilus
    Moraxella
    Pasteurella multocida (15)
    Pseudomonas aeruginosa
Gram-negative cocci
  Neisseria meningitidis (16)
  Neisseria gonorrheae
Gram-positive cocci
  Enterococcus faecium (17)
  Enterococcus faecalis (18)
  Streptococcus, group A (19)
  Streptococcus, group B (20)
  Streptococcus, group D (non-enterococcal)
  Streptococcus (viridans group)
  Streptococcus, γ hemolytic
  Streptococcus pneumoniae
  Staphylococcus aureus
  Other staphylococci
Gram-positive bacilli
  Bacillus
  Corynebacterium (11)
  Listeria monocytogenes
Anaerobes
  Bacteroides fragilis (7)
  Bacteroides spp.
  Clostridium perfringens (7, 21)
  Clostridium cadaveris (22)
  Lactobacillus (23)
  Microaerophilic streptococci[a]
  Peptostreptococcus anaerobius
  Peptostreptococcus spp.
  Propionibacterium
Other
  Candida
  Chlamydia trachomatis
  Cytomegalovirus (24)
  ECHO virus, type 4 (25)
  Measles virus (26)
  Rubella virus (25)
  Mycobacterium tuberculosis
  Mycoplasma

[a] These organisms are not true anaerobes.

infection. However, other sources are evident as well. The urinary tract may be important as indicated by a study that found the same organism in urine and in ascitic fluid in 44% of patients with SBP (27). The genital tract may also be the source in women; transfallopian spread is probably particularly important (28). Seeding of ascitic fluid during bacteremia is often a common denominator for these various organisms. A major pathogenic mechanism is likely to be impaired clearance of bacteria from blood. The reticuloendothelial system, which normally removes a major portion of bloodborne organisms, exhibits decreased phagocytic activity in cirrhotics, probably due to shunting of blood via portosystemic shunts rather than because of inadequate intrinsic function (29). Peripheral destruction of microorganisms by neutrophils is impaired in patients with liver disease. In patients with cirrhosis, there has been demonstration of low serum complement (10,34), decreased serum opsonic activity (30), defective neutrophil chemotaxis (31), impaired IgM antibody activity (32), and decreased intracellular killing of phagocytized organisms (33). Both opsonic activity (10) and bactericidal activity of ascitic fluid (35) is reduced. Levels of interleukin-6 (IL-6) and tumor necrosis factor-α (TNF-α) are markedly increased in the ascitic fluid of patients with SBP (36). These cytokines have been implicated in the pathogenesis of septic shock and in the cytopathic effects noted in infections; their marked overproduction in ascitic fluid may be a factor in the severity of SBP and the poor prognosis related to liver decompensation.

Clinical Picture

The clinical features of spontaneous bacterial peritonitis are variable. In children, they may suggest acute appendicitis. There may be fever (often low-grade), abdominal pain, nausea, vomiting, diarrhea, diffuse abdominal tenderness, rebound tenderness, and hypoactive to absent bowel sounds. Adult patients with cirrhosis have preexisting ascites. Ten percent of cases will be totally asymptomatic; many patients will have fever, chills, abdominal tenderness and rebound, or decreased to absent bowel sounds. Patients most often have only one or two of the typical presenting symptoms and signs of peritonitis; fever and abdominal pain are the most common. Atypical manifestations such as hypothermia, hypotension, diarrhea, refractoriness to diuretics, or unexplained decrease in renal function may be clues to SBP. Unexplained encephalopathy, hepatorenal syndrome, variceal bleeding, or other deterioration in a cirrhotic patient should raise the suspicion of asymptomatic SBP. It should also be appreciated that the amount of ascites may be so small as to be clinically undetectable. Aside from complications noted above, the bacteremia that often accompanies SBP may be complicated by shock, renal failure, and disseminated intravascular coagulation. Spontaneous bacterial empyema may occur as a complication of SBP (37).

Diagnosis

The diagnosis of SBP requires ruling out the possibility of an intraabdominal source of infection. A high degree of suspicion is required. Examination of ascitic fluid is the only way to confirm the diagnosis or rule it out. Accordingly, paracentesis should be performed on any patient with new onset of ascites, any cirrhotic patient with ascites who develops any symptoms compatible with the diagnosis (including unexplained encephalopathy), and any cirrhotic patient who suddenly deteriorates. The principal indicator of SBP is the polymorphonuclear (PMN) count in ascitic fluid; counts $<250/mm^3$ rule out SBP and counts $>500/mm^3$ confirm it. PMN counts $>500/mm^3$ have a diagnostic sensitivity of 80%, a specificity of 97%, and a diagnostic accuracy of 92% (4). Counts between 250 and $500/mm^3$ indicate infection only in patients with a compatible clinical picture. In the asymptomatic patient, such a count probably means absence of infection, but a follow-up paracentesis should be performed in the next 12–24 hr. Measurements of ascitic fluid pH, lactate concentration, glucose, protein, and lactate dehydrogenase are not useful diagnostically. Bacteriological culture of ascitic fluid has had two problems—poor sensitivity and a relatively long delay for a result; both problems are decreased by culturing 10 mL of ascitic fluid in blood culture bottles at the patient's bedside (38,39). With this technique, cultures are positive in 63–93% of cases. Gram stains of ascitic fluid are often negative. The lysis-centrifugation blood culture technique was not as effective as direct inoculation of blood culture bottles (40). Blood cultures should always be obtained in SBP patients prior to therapy.

The culture-negative variety of SBP, also called culture-negative neutrocytic ascites and probable SBP, is characterized by a negative culture in the presence of increased PMN leukocytes and no local source of infection or inflammation. The incidence of culture-negative SBP in cirrhotics with ascites is 4%. Among patients with elevated PMN counts in ascitic fluid, the percentage who are culture-negative (with culture in blood culture bottles) is 7% (39). Patients with positive ascitic fluid culture but neutrophil counts of $<250/mm^3$ are seen with relative frequency; Runyon (20) calls these monomicrobial nonneutrocytic bacterascites. Two thirds of such patients were found to have resolved spontaneously (negative cultures of ascitic fluid on recheck, without treatment). However, the other third progress to spontaneous bacterial peritonitis—sometimes within a few hours.

The principle entity in the differential diagnosis of SBP is secondary peritonitis in which there is a local source of infection (usually perforation of the bowel or an abscess). Symptoms and physical findings are not adequate means for distinction between the two entities. Findings in the ascitic fluid that are indicative of secondary peritonitis are higher white blood cell count ($>10,000/mm^3$), protein >1 g/dL, glucose <50 mg/dL, and lactate dehydrogenase higher than the upper limits of normal for serum. After 48 hr of treatment, the number of ascitic fluid neutrophiles is typically back to the pretreatment level in all patients with spontaneous peritonitis, but this is true in only two thirds of patients with secondary peritonitis (41).

Therapy

Early institution of appropriate therapy is important for increased survival. Initial therapy will typically have to be empirical. Since over 90% of cases of SBP are caused by enteric gram-negative bacilli (chiefly *E. coli*) and gram-positive cocci (predominantly streptococci, including enterococci), empirical therapy should be directed against these organisms. Some clinicians feel that cefotaxime is the first drug of choice for initiating empirical therapy; this is based on a comparative study in which cefotaxime led to a cure rate of 85% whereas ampicillin plus tobramycin had a cure rate of only 56% (42). There were no side effects, no nephrotoxicity, and no superinfections noted in patients treated with cefotaxime. Other regimens that should be entirely satisfactory include ampicillin/sulbactam, ticarcillin/clavulanate, piperacillin/tazobactam, ticarcillin or piperacillin alone, ceftizoxime, cefoperazone, ceftriaxone, cefonicid (43), and carbapenems. Aminoglycosides are best avoided because of potential renal toxicity and because of unpredictable and relatively slow penetration into ascitic fluid. Drugs with relatively poor activity against gram-positive cocci, such as fluoroquinolones, ceftazidime, aztreonam, and trimethoprim-sulfamethoxazole, would not be as desirable as the others noted above. A randomized study comparing short- (5 days) and long- (10 days) duration therapy concluded that the shorter duration was as effective as the longer and no more likely to be complicated by recurrence of infection (44). It has been suggested (45) that measurements of TNF-α and IL-6 in ascitic fluid may be useful for monitoring response to therapy.

Prognosis

The prognosis in SBP is relatively poor. The mean mortality during hospitalization in series of cases of SBP reported in the literature, summarized by Garcia-Tsao (4), is 55%. Sepsis is the cause of death in one third of cases. Factors found to be associated with higher mortality in SBP patients are high bilirubin levels, decreased albumin levels, presence of encephalopathy, and development of renal insufficiency; this indicates that the severity of the underlying liver disease is a key element determining prognosis. Patients surviving an episode of SBP have a probability of survival of 38% at 1 year compared with a probability of 57% in cirrhotic patients with ascites but no history of SBP. Mortality is lower in patients with culture-negative neutrocytic ascites than in patients with culture-positive spontaneous bacterial peritonitis.

Prevention

Preventive measures must be concerned with both prevention of recurrences (which are common) and preven-

tion of the first episode of SBP. Parenteral therapy clearly is not a reasonable therapy because of the risk of development of resistant flora, potential for toxicity, and cost. Modification of the bowel flora, the source of the infecting organisms in SBP, is another approach that has received much attention. Long-term selective intestinal decontamination was achieved in a placebo-controlled, double-blind study with norfloxacin and this was effective in preventing recurrence of SBP due to gram-negative bacilli (46). Norfloxacin-treated patients had a 1-year probability of recurrence of SBP of 20%, compared with 68% in placebo-treated patients. However, the study failed to show any improvement in number of hospitalizations or in survival rate, and such prophylaxis would be quite expensive. The possibility of selection of a resistant (probably gram-positive) flora is also a concern. Until a prophylactic regimen can be shown to significantly decrease the hospitalization and mortality rates, antimicrobial prophylaxis should be limited to further controlled investigations and perhaps to patients anticipated to undergo liver transplantation in a relatively short time. Similarly, studies designed for primary prophylaxis (to prevent the first episode of SBP) failed to demonstrate improved survival even though there was a lower incidence of SBP and of bacteremia compared to patients receiving no treatment. Anticipation of SBP and early institution of therapy is the best approach at present.

Secondary Peritonitis

By definition, secondary peritonitis is associated with a predisposing GI lesion or event, and involves GI flora.

Background Factors

Numerous intraabdominal processes may give rise to peritonitis. Disease, trauma, or surgery involving any part of the GI tract or genitourinary tract may be responsible. The process may involve the stomach, small bowel, large bowel, gallbladder or biliary tract, liver, spleen, pancreas, urinary bladder, uterus, or vagina. A variety of disease processes may be implicated, including infection, inflammation due to other causes, vascular disease, low-flow states, malignancy, spontaneous perforation, and congenital disease. A foreign body may be responsible on occasion. Liver transplantation may be a background factor. Any type of microorganism may be responsible for underlying infections—bacterial, parasitic, viral, and fungal. Aside from the microbial agents, certain adjuvant substances such as bile, gastric juice, blood, and necrotic tissue play a role in the pathogenesis of peritonitis. An unusual background factor—endoscopic tattooing of the colon to provide an easily visible serosal stain for guidance of the surgeon—was reported by Park et al. (47); this resulted in an abscess in the colonic wall and focal peritonitis.

Etiology

The normal alimentary tract microflora is discussed elsewhere in this book. However, a brief summary here is in order as background for the discussion on etiology of secondary peritonitis. The stomach has a sparse flora, $<10^3$ organisms/mL, consisting chiefly of viridans group streptococci, anaerobic cocci, lactobacilli, and yeasts, which are transient flora from the oropharynx (48,49). Bacterial counts in the upper small intestine are $<10^5$ and the organisms recovered include streptococci, staphylococci, lactobacilli, and yeasts among the nonanaerobes and anaerobic streptococci and lactobacilli (50). In the distal ileum, however, counts are much higher (roughly 10^4–10^6) and the flora begins to resemble colonic flora, with coliforms, *Bacteroides,* and *Bifidobacterium.* Enterococci outnumber viridans streptococci in this location (50). Counts and diversity of the flora both increase as one traverses the large bowel; counts in the distal colon or feces are about 10^{12} per g of dry weight (51). Anaerobes outnumber nonanaerobes by a factor of about 1000:1. Predominant anaerobes are the *Bacteroides fragilis* group, *Peptostreptococcus, Eubacterium, Bifidobacterium,* and *Clostridium.* Both anaerobic and facultative lactobacilli are found in relatively large numbers. Among the facultative anaerobes, *Escherichia coli* predominates followed by various streptococci and *Enterococcus.*

Various factors may influence the bacteriology of the GI tract and thus of infections whose flora derives from it. There is a direct relationship between pH and quantity of gastric flora (52); the lower the pH, the lower the counts of microorganisms. In patients with bleeding or obstructing duodenal ulcer and those with gastric ulcer or malignancy, counts of gastric organisms are much higher than normal and many types are represented that are not seen normally (53). Patients receiving H_2 blockers or antacids have greater numbers of facultative gram-negative bacilli and other organisms in their stomachs. The most profound influence on GI flora is exerted by antimicrobial agents (54). Organisms typically associated with nosocomial infections (e.g., *Staphylococcus aureus, Staphylococcus epidermidis,* the *Klebsiella–Enterobacter–Serratia* group, *Pseudomonas aeruginosa, Enterococcus,* and *Candida*) may colonize the GI tract during hospitalization and by this means, or by direct introduction during surgery, become involved in postoperative infections following GI surgery. Marshall et al. (55) carried out a very important study in which they documented, by quantitative culture of gastric, duodenal, and proximal jejunal contents, that *Candida, Staphylococcus epidermidis,* and *Pseudomonas* were the most common isolates and that counts at times exceeded 10^8 organisms/mL. All but one of the patients demonstrating these organisms in the upper GI tract had invasive infection with the same organisms. It is important to note that the GI tract cultures were obtained via gastric or jejunal tubes that had been placed for therapeutic reasons; this may have facilitated entry of organisms into the upper GI tract from the external environment.

Anaerobes outnumber facultative bacteria by a ratio of 10:1 in the normal vaginal flora, anaerobic counts averaging 10^{8-9}/mL. The organisms most commonly encountered in relatively high counts are anaerobic and facultative lactobacilli, streptococci, *Peptostreptococcus, Prevotella bivia, P. disiens,* other *Prevotella,* pigmented anaerobic gram-negative bacilli, *Gardnerella,* diphtheroids, and *Staphylococcus epidermidis* (56–58). During menstruation, total bacterial counts decrease and the concentration of lactobacilli declines (59). Mårdh, in 1991 (60), found increased numbers of aciduric organisms such as lactobacilli and yeasts during pregnancy. By far the most comprehensive analysis of vaginal flora in pregnant women (with and without bacterial vaginosis) was performed by Hillier et al. (61). The most striking finding of this group was that hydrogen peroxide–producing lactobacilli were found in only 5% of women with bacterial vaginosis compared to 61% of women with a normal flora. The presence of a number of organisms was inversely related to vaginal colonization by H_2O_2-producing lactobacilli; included were *Gardnerella, Mycoplasma, Ureaplasma,* viridans streptococci, and seven different anaerobes. Other studies reveal that there are increased numbers of *Bacteroides* in the vaginal flora of women with trichomoniasis (58). Oral contraceptives have little effect on vaginal flora, but long-term use of intrauterine contraceptive devices increases the numbers of anaerobes isolated from the cervix (60,62). Antimicrobial agents certainly have an important impact on the normal vaginal flora, but there are relatively few studies of this. Finally, sexual exposure may lead to colonization or infection with *Neisseria gonorrheae* and *Chlamydia.*

Infections of the stomach per se are quite rare. An interesting recent report (63) discusses a fatal postoperative case with gastric necrosis, peritonitis, and bacteremia due to *Clostridium perfringens.* Shinagawa et al. (64) report on the bacteriology of 63 cases of perforated duodenal ulcer (44% positive cultures) and 13 cases of perforated gastric ulcer or carcinoma (11 cases of gastric ulcer) with 39% having positive cultures in comparison with perforations of the small bowel (72% positive), appendix (95% positive), colon (100% positive), and biliary tract (86% positive). Bacteria isolated, according to the site of perforation, are listed in Table 2. This is a unique and important study although it appears that anaerobic transport and/or culture techniques were not optimum. Mosdell et al. (65) describe 480 patients with peritonitis secondary to perforation of the appendix (281 cases); a diverticulum, 98; colon other than diverticulum, 32; peptic ulcer, 26; gallbladder, 13; and other sites, 30. Specimens were cultured from about two thirds of the patients and yielded an average of 2.6 isolates per culture. The most common isolates by far were *E. coli* and *B. fragilis.* Nonanaerobes also encountered relatively frequently included nonenterococcal streptococci, *Pseudomonas,* and *Klebsiella;* the other anaerobe encountered relatively often was *Peptostreptococcus* sp. Sirinek (66) summarized the bacteriology of secondary peritonitis from three studies in the literature. The predominant facultative bacteria recovered were *E. coli,* streptococci, staphylococci, *Klebsiella/Enterobacter,* and enterococci. The predominant anaerobes were *B. fragilis,* other *Bacteroides, Peptostreptococcus, Eubacterium,* and *Clostridium.* In a very detailed study of 71 patients with gangrenous or perforated appendicitis, Bennion et al. (67) found an average of 9.8 organisms per specimen in cases of gangrenous appendicitis and 12.7 per specimen in patients with perforated appendicitis; three

TABLE 2. *Isolated bacteria according to the site of perforation*

	Duodenum	Small intestine	Appendix	Colon	Others	Total
No. of cases	63	18	115	20	22	238
No. of positive cases	28	13	109	20	13	183
Gram-positive aerobes or facultatives						
S. aureus	3		5		2	10
Coagulase-negative Staph.	2	1	1	1	1	6
Streptococcus spp.	11		5	4	2	22
Enterococcus spp.	6	3	12	9	2	32
Subtotal	22	4	23	14	7	70
Gram-negative aerobes or facultatives						
E. coli	2	4	78	15	3	102
Klebsiella spp.	1	7	18	7	2	35
Enterobacter spp.	1	3	7	1		12
Citrobacter spp.		1	9	3		13
P. aeruginosa			10	2	1	13
Others			2	1	4	7
Subtotal	4	15	124	29	10	182
Gram-positive anaerobes						
Anaerobic streptococci	5		10	2	1	18
Peptostreptococcus spp.	4	5	16	7	3	35
Others	1	2	2	2		7
Subtotal	10	7	28	11	4	60
Gram-negative anaerobes						
B. fragilis group	2	5	64	13	6	90
Others		1	1	2	2	6
Subtotal	2	6	65	15	8	96
Total	38	32	240	69	29	408

Modified from ref. 64.

fourths of the isolates were anaerobes. Details of the bacteriological results of this study are given in Tables 3 and 4.

It has been noted that enterococci are seen more frequently in intraabdominal infection and in associated bacteremia when patients have been treated with cephalosporins (68). Nichols and Muzik (68) also noted that enterococci were isolated much more frequently postoperatively from patients with perforation of the GI tract (in 56% of postoperative infections in this group). Dougherty

TABLE 3. *Percentage of specimens yielding aerobic and facultative bacteria from patients with gangrenous and perforated appendicitis*

Bacteria	Gangrenous (n = 27)	Perforated (n = 44)	All (n = 71)
Escherichia coli	70.4	77.3	74.6
Viridans streptococci	18.5	43.2	33.8
Streptococcus, group D	7.4	27.3	19.7
Pseudomonas aeruginosa	11.1	18.2	15.5
Enterococcus sp.	18.5	9.1	12.7
Staphylococcus sp.	14.8	11.4	12.7
Pseudomonas sp.	7.4	9.1	8.5
Citrobacter freundii	3.7	6.8	5.6
β-Hemolytic Streptococcus, group F	7.4	4.5	5.6
β-Hemolytic Streptococcus, group C	3.7	4.5	4.2
Enterobacter sp.	7.4	2.3	4.2
Klebsiella sp.	3.7	4.5	4.2
β-Hemolytic Streptococcus, group G	0	4.5	2.8
Moraxella sp.	3.7	2.3	2.8
Corynebacterium sp.	0	2.3	1.4
Serratia marcescens	3.7	0	1.4
Eikenella corrodens	0	2.3	1.4
Hafnia alvei	3.7	0	1.4
Haemophilus influenzae	0	2.3	1.4

Modified from ref. 67.

TABLE 4. *Percentage of specimens yielding specific anaerobic bacteria from patients with gangrenous and perforated appendicitis*

Bacteria	Gangrenous (n = 27)	Perforated (n = 44)	All (n = 71)
Bacteroides fragilis	70.1	79.5	76.1
Bacteroides thetaiotaomicron	48.1	61.4	56.3
Bilophila wadsworthia	37.0	54.5	47.9
Peptostreptococcus micros	44.4	45.5	45.1
Eubacterium sp.	40.7	29.5	33.8
Bacteroides intermedius	33.3	27.3	29.6
Bacteroides vulgatus	18.5	34.1	28.2
Bacteroides splanchnicus	25.9	27.3	26.8
Fusobacterium sp.	22.2	27.3	25.4
Bacteroides ovatus	18.5	27.3	23.9
Microaerophilic streptococci[a]	29.6	20.5	23.9
Peptostreptococcus sp.	29.6	18.2	22.5
Lactobacillus sp.	22.2	20.5	21.1
Bacteroides uniformis	22.2	18.2	19.7
Bacteroides distasonis	14.8	20.5	18.3
Clostridium clostridioforme	18.5	18.2	18.3
Bacteroides gracilis	11.1	15.9	14.1
Actinomyces sp.	11.1	11.4	11.3
Clostridium ramosum	11.1	9.1	9.9
Porphyromonas sp.	18.5	2.3	8.5
Bacteroides buccae	3.7	6.8	5.6
Bacteroides caccae	7.4	4.5	5.6
Clostridium innocuum	7.4	4.5	5.6
Bacteroides stercoris	7.4	4.5	5.6
Clostridium sporogenes	3.7	6.8	5.6
Propionibacterium acnes	7.4	4.5	5.6
Clostridium leptum	11.1	0	4.2
Desulfomonas sp.	3.7	4.5	4.2
Bacteroides oralis	0	4.5	2.8
Bacteroides denticola	0	4.5	2.8
Bacteroides ureolyticus	3.7	2.3	2.8
Wolinelia sp.	3.7	2.3	2.8
Bacteroides oris	0	2.3	1.4
Mitsuokella multiacida	0	2.3	1.4
Veillonella sp.	0	2.3	1.4
Bacteroides eggerthii	0	2.3	1.4
Bacteroides capillosus	0	2.3	1.4
Desulfovibrio sp.	0	2.3	1.4
Unidentified gram-negative rod	37.0	36.4	36.6
Unidentified gram-positive rod	14.8	29.5	23.9
Unidentified pigmenting rod	18.5	18.2	18.3

[a] Not true anaerobes but placed here since good anaerobic transport and culture techniques are often required for their recovery.

Modified from ref. 67.

et al. (69) reported 19 cases of "breakthrough" enterococcal septicemia in surgical patients who are immunodepressed and/or receiving antimicrobial agents.

Patients in intensive care units with multiple organ failure may have a unique infecting flora. We previously cited the work of Marshall et al. (55); this study showed *Staphylococcus epidermidis*, *Candida*, and *Pseudomonas* to be the most common infecting organisms in such patients and correlated infection with these organisms with their presence in the upper GI tract. It is interesting to note that infections present at the time of admission to their surgical intensive care unit were most commonly due to *Escherichia coli*, *Bacteroides fragilis*, and enterococci in

contrast to the above data from patients who had been in the unit for some time and who had multiple organ failure. This latter entity has been termed "tertiary peritonitis" by Rotstein and Meakins (70). Mortality correlated highly with infection due to *S. epidermidis* or *Candida* and poorly with infection due to *Pseudomonas* or *E. coli*. It is noteworthy also that significant foci of invasive infection or of undrained abscesses were often absent at autopsy or exploration. These authors speculate on the importance of efforts to decrease gastric acidity in permitting the overgrowth of organisms demonstrated in the upper GI tract. They point out that translocation of organisms across the gut mucosal barrier might account for the invasive infection and that this proximal GI tract flora might alter normal systemic immune response, both antigen-specific and global immunity. In another study carried out in a surgical intensive care unit population, Rotstein et al. (71) documented a unique flora in peritoneal fluid collections and bacteremia. Twenty-five patients had undergone at least two surgical procedures for abdominal sepsis and 23 had at least three-system organ failure. The most common organisms from peritoneal cultures were *Staphylococcus epidermidis, Candida albicans, Pseudomonas aeruginosa, Enterobacter,* and *Enterococcus. E. coli* and *B. fragilis* were recovered relatively infrequently. In accompanying bacteremia, the most prevalent isolates were *S. epidermidis, Enterobacter, B. fragilis,* and *C. albicans.*

Neonatal peritonitis also has a unique infecting flora (72). *E. coli* was found in only 21% of such patients as compared with 69% of a control group of children with perforated appendicitis. In neonatal peritonitis, the most common gram-negative isolates were *Klebsiella* and *Enterobacter* and over half of the cultures yielded gram-positive cocci (most often coagulase-negative staphylococci and enterococci). Anaerobes were seldom recovered from neonatal peritonitis cases and from only 50% of appendicitis cases. *Candida* was found in 10% of neonatal peritonitis patients.

Patients with underlying immunosuppression, diabetes mellitus, or requiring prolonged antimicrobial therapy become at risk for superinfection with *Candida* (73), other fungi, cytomegalovirus (24), parasites such as *Strongyloides,* or other resistant organisms. On occasion, pseudomembranous colitis due to *Clostridium difficile* may be complicated by toxic megacolon with perforation and peritonitis (74). Miscellaneous other organisms may occasionally be involved in peritonitis, e.g., *Legionella* (75) or *Listeria* (76).

It is important to recognize that organisms that do not dominate the normal bowel (or vaginal) flora may still be very important in intraabdominal infection. Two examples of this are *Bacteroides fragilis* and *Bilophila wadsworthia* (Fig. 1). Because of their virulence, these organisms may be present in infection in disproportionately large numbers of cases considering their relatively low counts in normal flora. In the case of *Bilophila,* this may be readily overlooked because of the fastidious nature of this organism; it may require 7 days of incubation before growth is apparent.

The bacteriology of intraabdominal infection complicating female genital tract infection is very much like that seen in peritonitis due to a GI source. Differences include a higher incidence of *Peptostreptococcus* and of *Prevotella bivia* and *P. disiens* and a lower incidence of *Bacteroides fragilis.* In addition, the occurrence of gonococci, *Chlamydia trachomatis* (77), and actinomycosis related to intrauterine contraceptive devices (78) are unique. The latter infection may involve *Eubacterium nodatum* as well as various *Actinomyces* and *Propionibacterium propionicus.*

Bacteremia may be seen in 20–30% of patients with intraabdominal infection; organisms recovered have been chiefly *B. fragilis* and *E. coli* (79–82).

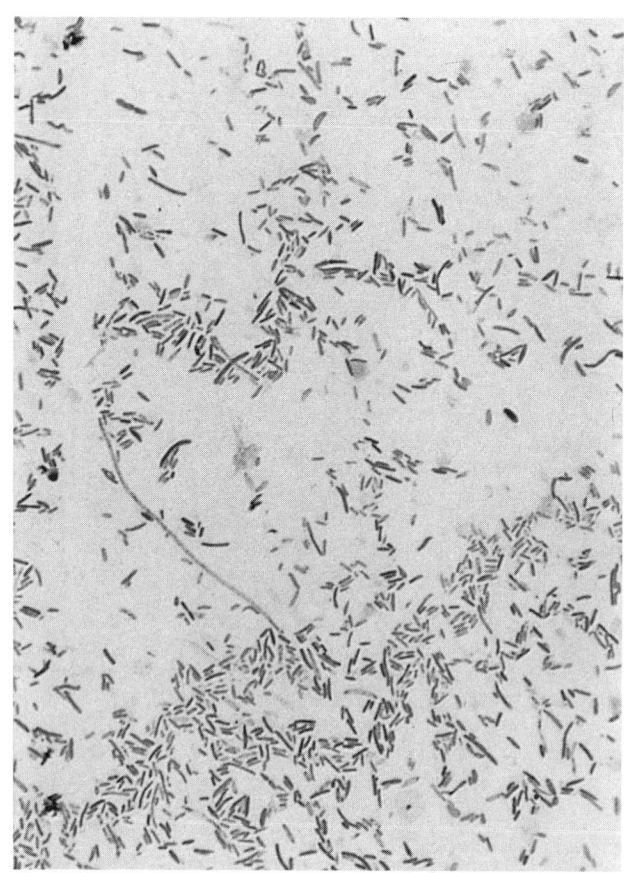

FIG. 1. *Bilophila wadsworthia.* Gram stain of pure culture. Organism is a large, gram-negative, anaerobic rod.

Pathogenesis, Pathology

Two major factors contribute to the establishment of peritonitis—a continuing source of infection and foreign material (such as intestinal contents, bile, gastric juice, or necrotic tissue) that protects bacteria from host defense mechanisms. Spillage of pancreatic enzymes results in enzymatic digestion and widespread necrosis. Bile in the peritoneal cavity is a serious problem and is associated with a poor prognosis. Free hemoglobin also facilitates peritonitis by enhancing bacterial virulence, perhaps by virtue of its iron content (83). Bacteria gain access to the peritoneal cavity through perforations in the GI tract or gallbladder or by translocation from an intact bowel in response to serosal inflammation.

Plaques of fibrinous material accumulate on the inflamed peritoneum and cause loops of bowel to adhere to one another and to the parietal peritoneum. There is an outpouring of leukocyte-containing serous fluid. The greater omentum tends to localize infection by adhering to areas of peritonitis; ileus also plays a role in localization of the process. The ratio of bacteria to leukocytes is an important factor determining the outcome of peritonitis. Ischemia, surgical or other trauma, malignancy, and other factors lead to devitalized tissue, which lowers the oxidation–reduction potential so that obligate anaerobes may grow well. Bacterial factors play an important role in peritonitis; included are such entities as endotoxin, collagenase, other proteolytic enzymes (84) deoxyribonuclease, heparinase, leukocidin, and urease (85). Various host factors such as removal and killing of bacteria by macrophages and PMN leukocytes (86), fibrin deposition to localize peritoneal infection (87), TNF, other interleukins, interferons, arachidonic acid metabolism and its products, platelet-activating factor, and coagulation abnormalities (88) play an important role in peritonitis and its complications. Synergy between various organisms appears to be a very important factor; this has been studied extensively with black-pigmented anaerobic gram-negative bacilli (89). The pigmenters with important pathogenic properties are *Prevotella intermedia, Porphyromonas gingivalis,* and *Porphyromonas endodontalis.*

Clinical Picture

The mode of onset of peritonitis varies according to the precipitating event. Perforated peptic ulcer with spillage of gastric contents may produce severe epigastric pain that spreads to involve the entire abdomen in minutes whereas pain from a perforated appendix is much more gradual. The usual findings are pain, abdominal distention, anorexia, nausea and vomiting, absence of abdominal respiratory movement, abdominal and rebound tenderness, diffuse muscle spasm and guarding, tenderness on rectal or vaginal examination, and fever. Patients characteristically lie quietly in bed with knees flexed; early in the course of the illness the patient is alert, restless, and irritable, but later the patient may be apathetic or delirious. There may be inability to pass feces or flatus and there may be more serious signs such as toxemia and shock. The very young or old, patients with lax abdominal musculature (postpartum patients or cirrhotics with ascites), patients in shock, and patients on corticosteroids may not manifest pain and muscle spasm. A high index of suspicion is necessary in such patients; early in the course of peritonitis there may be only an unexplained rise in pulse rate or hypotension; the most important physical finding is a completely silent abdomen on auscultation. The signs of peritonitis may be completely overshadowed by the manifestations of the underlying process.

Complications include bacteremia, shock, intraabdominal or retroperitoneal abscess, respiratory failure, adhesions, and GI fistulae, the latter sometimes associated with abdominal wall defects (90).

Diagnosis

The diagnosis of secondary peritonitis is primarily a clinical one. Specific information regarding the pain of peritonitis—the site of origin, the site of the most intense pain, and the character and radiation pattern of the pain—is crucial in differentiating peritonitis from myocardial infarction, sickle cell anemia, herpes zoster, tabetic crisis, lupus erythematosus, arachnidism, porphyria, diabetic ketoacidosis, plumbism, familial Mediterranean fever, pulmonary disease, and renal disease. Fever is common in peritonitis, but when it exceeds 39.4°C (103°F)

at the onset of the illness the causative process is not likely to be surgically reparable. The peripheral white blood cell (WBC) count is usually >12,000 but counts >20,000 cells/mm³ are rare in patients with an acute surgical abdomen. There is typically an increase in the percentage of PMN leukocytes and a moderate to marked shift to immature forms. Glycosuria and hyperglycemia may be seen in diabetic acidosis and in acute pancreatitis, but they are not typical in peritonitis. Hematuria and pyuria usually indicate primary involvement of the genitourinary tract, but they may reflect inflammatory disease such as appendicitis or diverticulitis adjacent to the ureter or bladder. Dehydration may lead to elevated hematocrit and blood urea nitrogen level. Very high levels of serum amylase are consistent with acute pancreatitis but lower levels may occur in peritonitis from any cause, intestinal obstruction, perforated viscus, uremia, and after injection of opiates. Both metabolic and respiratory acidosis are seen in severe or late peritonitis.

Supine, upright, or lateral decubitus radiographic films of the abdomen or computed tomography (CT) may reveal free gas in the peritoneal cavity, encapsulated gas in an abscess, features of ileus or obstruction, peritoneal fluid, volvulus, intussusception, vascular occlusion, calcification within the gallbladder or elsewhere, or obliteration of the psoas shadows or other peritoneal lines. Chest radiographs may also be helpful in detecting or ruling out pulmonary disease and in detecting free gas under the diaphragm. Ultrasound examination and radionuclide scanning may also aid in diagnosis.

Needle aspiration of peritoneal fluid is often helpful. The fluid may be purulent, bloody, turbid, or may contain fat globules (pathognomonic of fat digestion), bile, or fecal material. Negative findings are not useful diagnostically. If fluid cannot be obtained directly, peritoneal lavage with 1 L of saline may be considered; the presence of >500 WBC/mm³ correlates best with the presence of intraabdominal pathology (70). When pus or other fluid is obtained, Gram stain and aerobic and anaerobic cultures should be performed. Blood cultures should also always be done prior to initiating antimicrobial therapy. Peritoneoscopy or needle biopsy of the peritoneum may occasionally be useful.

Therapy

The principles of therapy are (a) to eliminate the primary source of infection by means of closure, excision, or isolation; (b) to aspirate as much of the infected peritoneal exudate as possible and to drain the site of the primary lesion; (c) to treat local or distant complications as needed; (d) to combat the effects of bacteria and their toxic metabolites; (e) to improve vascular perfusion by correcting fluid and electrolyte deficits; and (f) to reduce paralytic ileus (decompression of the gut by nasogastric tube, long intestinal tube, or enterostomy).

In most cases of secondary peritonitis, surgery is required for management of the underlying problem, for drainage of pus, and for excision of necrotic tissue. Surgery should be performed at the earliest possible time. Rotstein and Meakins (70) provide an excellent discussion of surgical principles and practices. For colonic pathology, surgery usually involves resecting the perforated segment of bowel and exteriorizing the proximal end as an end-colostomy; the distal end is either oversewn or a mucous fistula is created. A primary anastomosis in this setting creates a high risk of dehiscence and should be avoided. The risks associated with primary anastomosis of the small bowel are much lower; however, if there has been extensive peritoneal soiling or if there is concern about the viability of the intestine, resection with proximal and distal enterostomy may be indicated. Duodenal perforation related to peptic ulcer may be patched with a piece of omentum but perforated gastric ulcer requires local excision with primary closure or distal gastric resection with subsequent gastroduodenal or gastrojejunal anastomosis. Appendectomy is carried out for appendicitis. In the case of secondary infection of necrotic pancreas due to pancreatitis, laparotomy with finger debridement of the necrotic pancreas is important; laparostomy with repeated reexploration may be necessary (91).

At surgery, purulent exudates should be aspirated and loculations in the subphrenic spaces, paracolic gutters, and pelvis should be gently opened and debrided. Particulate debris such as feces or barium should be removed, but radical peritoneal debridement has not proven to be worthwhile and may lead to excessive bleeding. Intraoperative peritoneal lavage is standard practice during surgery for peritonitis but its efficacy is not well documented. However, there is no evidence that it is harmful and it reduces numbers of bacteria and removes substances such as blood, feces, and necrotic material. It is imperative to aspirate all fluid instilled and all collections of fluid prior to closure. The use of drains in patients with diffuse peritonitis is indicated only for postoperative lavage, drainage of abscess cavities, and to establish a controlled fistula. Drains left in place can be a hazard in that they may erode into bowel or blood vessels and may provide access to the peritoneal cavity for exogenous organisms.

Three other perioperative techniques have had their strong advocates, but properly designed prospective and well-controlled studies are needed to determine whether these procedures are truly effective and safe. They include (a) addition of antibiotics to peritoneal lavage solution (probably not needed when appropriate systemic antimicrobial therapy is used), (b) leaving the abdomen open following surgery, with or without scheduled relaparotomy, and (c) continuous postoperative peritoneal lavage.

Abdominal wall closure is effected with a single fascial layer of interrupted monofilament suture. In high-risk patients (elderly, malnourished, or immunocompromised), retention sutures through the full thickness of the abdominal wall may be used in addition. Delayed primary closure of the skin and subcutaneous tissues may be used. In such a case, if the wound appears clean and granulating on the third or fourth postoperative day, skin edges can be apposed with skin tapes or fine sutures. Primary wound closure over suction catheters that are irrigated with antimicrobials has not been shown to reduce wound infection. Some surgeons have used an absorbable mesh or a mesh-plus-zipper-technique as temporary closures in patients for whom primary closure is not considered desirable. Advocates of the mesh technique state that it reduces in-

traabdominal pressure, prevents evisceration, and allows for effective drainage; however, diffuse patchy necrosis of the bowel wall resulting in fistula formation has been described (92). The zipper offers easy access and prevents damage to the abdominal wall during relaparotomy but spontaneous drainage is prevented and a major reintervention is inevitably necessary. Various modifications of the zipper technique may represent improvements.

Detailed discussion of the management of appendicitis and diverticulitis and their complications will be given in other chapters in this book. In general, it appears that primary closure is essentially always reasonable in appendicitis. Laparoscopic appendectomy is utilized by some (93). For diverticulitis, medical therapy is adequate for about 75% of patients. Surgical intervention is reserved for those who fail medical management and those with recurrent acute attacks, diffuse peritonitis, abscess, persistent obstruction, or fistula formation. Abdominal CT scans allow guided percutaneous drainage of selected patients with large abscesses. With this approach, a single elective operation without a temporary colostomy is possible for most patients. For patients requiring emergency surgery, the two-stage approach with resection of the diseased colon at the initial operation is much preferred over the old three-stage approach (94).

Antimicrobial therapy is a second major approach to management of secondary peritonitis and its complications. Systemic antimicrobial therapy should be employed before and after surgical therapy. The choice of antimicrobial agents will depend on the microorganisms involved and the usual susceptibility patterns in the hospital being utilized. In complex bacterial mixtures, it is reasonable to target only pathogens known to be problems in terms of virulence and antimicrobial resistance as well as organisms present in large numbers, in blood cultures, and on repeated culture.

When *Staphylococcus aureus* is involved, one may use a penicillinase-resistant penicillin such as nafcillin or an antistaphylococcal cephalosporin such as cefazolin. In the case of methicillin-resistant *S. aureus* or *S. epidermidis,* vancomycin is the drug of choice. In the case of enterococci, many clinicians (95–97) feel that it is not necessary to provide antimicrobial coverage in non-ICU patients with the initial onset of secondary peritonitis unless these organisms are recovered from blood cultures. Patients who develop enterococcal infection later in the course of illness, following cephalosporin therapy, or in ICUs should have antimicrobial regimens that include coverage for enterococci. Ampicillin plus an aminoglycoside is often effective, but resistance is an increasingly serious problem with *Enterococcus.* Vancomycin plus an aminoglycoside is active against a number of strains resistant to ampicillin plus an aminoglycoside, but strains may be resistant to both of these agents as well. Agents that may be useful against these rare, highly resistant enterococci include teicoplanin, fluoroquinolones, and rifampin. Other streptococci (e.g., viridans streptococci, group A or B streptococci) are usually susceptible to penicillin or ampicillin.

For gram-negative nonanaerobic bacilli, many clinicians dealing with fairly sick patients use an aminoglycoside such as gentamicin or amikacin (at least initially, until the patient is improved) along with a β-lactam agent such as ticarcillin/clavulanic acid or piperacillin/tazobactam, or cefoxitin/cefoperazone/ceftazidime, or aztreonam or imipenem, depending on the particular gram-negative bacilli isolated, their likely susceptibility patterns, and how seriously ill the patient is. Some clinicians prefer to avoid aminoglycosides as initial empirical therapy because of their toxicity; in lieu of these agents, one may use combinations such as clindamycin plus aztreonam (98–100) or clindamycin plus ceftazidime (101). Trimethoprim-sulfamethoxazole, the fluoroquinolones (102), and chloramphenicol are other options that may be considered for gram-negative coverage. Gorbach (95) recommends reserving aminoglycosides for organisms resistant to other agents, for patients who have received other antibiotics within the past month, in association with reoperation or recurrence of infection, and for patients with prolonged hospitalization or nursing home residence preoperatively. Again, the usual susceptibility patterns of various gram-negative bacilli from the hospital in which the patient is being cared for and specific susceptibilities on the patient's isolates are important for consideration in devising initial regimens and revising them if necessary.

Among the anaerobes, the *Bacteroides fragilis* group is the most commonly encountered and is relatively resistant to antimicrobials. *Bacteroides thetaiotaomicron,* a member of the *B. fragilis* group, is encountered fairly often and is much more resistant to antimicrobials than *B. fragilis.* Other species in this group may also be quite resistant. Among the agents listed above, those with the greatest activity against the *B. fragilis* group and other anaerobes are the β-lactam/β-lactamase inhibitor combinations, imipenem and other penems, and chloramphenicol. The other drug with major activity against the anaerobes is metronidazole. Cefoxitin has moderately good activity against the *B. fragilis* group and many other anaerobes, as does clindamycin and broad-spectrum penicillins such as piperacillin or ticarcillin. Table 5 summarizes the activity of various antimicrobials against the anaerobes most commonly encountered in intraabdominal infection. Agents with poor or no activity against anaerobes include aminoglycosides, trimethoprim-sulfamethoxazole, quinolones, aztreonam, and some of the newer cephalosporins.

For *Candida,* amphotericin B is the drug of choice; flucytosine and fluconazole may also be useful.

In considering different empirical regimens with which to initiate therapy of secondary peritonitis, it should be appreciated that there are major problems of interpretation and comparability between various studies in the literature (104,105). The major problems in interpretation relate to variable diagnostic criteria, unmeasured severity of disease, wide differences in the quality of bacteriological studies, and unclear outcome measures. To address these deficiencies, a consistent system of definitions with minimum rules has been developed by a Joint Working Party of the Surgical Infection Societies of North America and Europe (106). Intraabdominal infection is defined as clinical peritonitis requiring both operative and microbiological confirmation of infection. The APACHE II system is proposed for grading severity of infection and for stratification of risk of mortality. The main outcome measures,

both independently and positively defined, are mortality and time until death on the one hand and recovery and time until recovery on the other.

It is generally agreed that it is important to have activity against both facultative gram-negative rods and anaerobes in initiating empirical therapy. Clindamycin plus gentamicin has been a popular initial regimen because clindamycin has given good coverage against anaerobes and most gram-positive organisms other than enterococci and the aminoglycoside covers most gram-negative nonanaerobic bacilli. This remains a much used regimen, but resistance of the *B. fragilis* group and other anaerobes such as some peptostreptococci in some centers has led some clinicians to seek other regimens. Clindamycin may be admixed with gentamicin and given every 8 hr without any loss of effectiveness and at least a 20% reduction in cost (107). Cefoxitin, with or without an aminoglycoside, has also been used widely (96,108–110). As noted above, a number of clinicians avoid the use of aminoglycosides, substituting various other agents with good activity against gram-negative nonanaerobic bacilli. Piperacillin (111,112) and ticarcillin have been used effectively in intraabdominal infection as have β-lactam/β-lactamase inhibitor combinations such as ampicillin/sulbactam (113) and ticarcillin/clavulanate (114–116). Regimens employing metronidazole for the anaerobic coverage along with one or more additional agents with activity against other categories of organisms that may be encountered have been very effective. Imipenem has also been used effectively as a single agent (97,117,118). For less severe peritonitis such as may be encountered with gangrenous or perforated appendicitis (localized rather than generalized peritonitis), ceftizoxime and cefotetan have been used as single agents to good effect (119).

The problem of antimicrobial therapy of persistent peritonitis in ICU patients is grim indeed. The organisms isolated (*S. epidermidis, Pseudomonas, Candida,* and enterococci) are relatively antimicrobial-resistant, but even when appropriate antimicrobial agents are administered these organisms tend to persist (71). This probably reflects impaired host defenses with multiple organ failure rather than failure of the antimicrobial agents. Mortality increases with increasing organ system failure (55).

Prognosis

The mortality rate in diffuse peritonitis has declined remarkably with the introduction of antimicrobials but there may still be significant mortality, depending on the underlying cause of the peritonitis and the presence of certain factors. The prognosis is poorer in the very old or very young; with prolonged contamination of the peritoneal cavity; with the presence of bile, pancreatic enzymes, or barium; with a serious underlying problem such as carcinoma; with significant associated problems (such as cardiovascular, respiratory, or renal disease); with certain organisms; and with associated bacteremia (120). The highest mortality, in terms of anatomic area involved, is associated with the pancreas and large bowel, with small intestine not far behind. Postoperative peritonitis carries a relatively high mortality. Septic shock and multisystem

TABLE 5. *Susceptibility of anaerobes*

Percent susceptible	B. fragilis	Other B. fragilis Group[a]	B. gracilis	Other Bacteroides spp.[b]
>95	Ampicillin + Sulbactam Cefoperazone + Sulbactam Piperacillin + Tazobactam Ticarcillin + Clavulanate Chloramphenicol Imipenem Metronidazole	Ampicillin + Sulbactam Cefoperazone + Sulbactam Piperacillin + Tazobactam Ticarcillin + Clavulanate Chloramphenicol Imipenem Metronidazole	Chloramphenicol Imipenem	Ampicillin + Sulbactam Cefoperazone + Sulbactam Ticarcillin + Clavulanate Cefoperazone Cefotaxime Cefoxitin Ceftizoxime Chloramphenicol Clindamycin Imipenem Piperacillin
85–95	Cefotetan Cefoxitin Clindamycin Piperacillin	Piperacillin	Metronidazole	Cefotetan Ceftazidime Ceftriaxone
70–84	Ceftozoxime Moxalactam	Cefoxitin Ceftizoxime Clindamycin	Ampicillin + Sulbactam Cefoperazone + Sulbactam Moxalactam Piperacillin	Moxalactam Penicillin G
50–69	Cefoperazone Cefotaxime Ceftazidime Ceftriaxone	Cefoperazone Cefotetan Moxalactam	Ticarcillan + Clavulanate Cefoperazone Cefotaxime Cefotetan Cefoxitin Ceftizoxime Clindamycin Penicillin G	
<50	Penicillin G	Cefotaxime Ceftazidime Ceftriaxone Penicillin G	Ceftazidime	

From ref. 103, with permission.
[a] Excluding *B. fragilis* species.
[b] Including organisms now in *Prevotella* and *Porphyromonas*
[c] Nonsporing gram-positive rods (e.g., *Actinomyces*, *Eubacterium*, etc.)

organ failure is a major factor in mortality; mortality is essentially 100% in tertiary peritonitis (121). The most frequent causes of death are respiratory, hepatic, and renal failure. The Apache II score cannot predict the outcome of peritonitis in individual patients but it is reliable for general risk stratification. Preliminary results suggest that IL-6 levels may serve as a predictor of outcome in peritonitis.

Prevention

Postoperative peritonitis may be avoided by preventing contamination of the peritoneal cavity with GI or vaginal secretions. Good surgical technique and antimicrobial prophylaxis are important. For surgery on the stomach or duodenum when the risk is relatively high because of decreased gastric acidity or motility (122), parenteral pro-

to antimicrobial agents

Fusobacterium	B. wadsworthia	Pepto-streptococcus	C. perfringens	Other Clostridium spp.	Nonsporing GPR[c]
Ampicillin + Sulbactam Piperacillin + Tazobactam Ceftizoxime Chloramphenicol Clindamycin Imipenem Metronidazole Penicillin G Piperacillin	Chloramphenicol Metronidazole Imipenem Ticarcillin Ticarcillin + Clavulanate Cefoxitin	Ampicillin + Sulbactam Cefoperazone + Sulbactam Ticarcillin + Clavulanate Cefoperazone Cefotetan Ceftazidime Ceftriaxone Chloramphenicol Imipenem Moxalactam Penicillin G Piperacillin	(All drugs are active at >95)	Ampicillin + Sulbactam Amoxicillin Ampicillin Carbenicillin Chloramphenicol Imipenem Metronidazole Penicillin G Piperacillin Ticarcillin	Ampicillin + Sulbactam Ticarcillan + Clavulanate Cefotaxime Ceftizoxime Chloramphenicol Imipenem Penicillin G Piperacillin
Cefoperazone + Sulbactam Ticarcillin + Clavulanate Cefoperazone Cefotaxime Cefotetan Cefoxitin Ceftriaxone	Clindamycin	Metronidazole			Cefoperazone + Sulbactam Cefotetan Cefoxitin Ceftazidime Ceftriaxone Clindamycin
Ceftazidime Moxalactam	Cefotaxime Cefotetan	Clindamycin		Cefoxitin Clindamycin Moxalactam	Cefoperazone Moxalactam
			Cefoperazone Cefotaxime Ceftozoxime Ceftriaxone	Metronidazole	
	Ceftizoxime Penicillin G			Ceftazidime	

phylactic antimicrobial therapy is clearly indicated. The *Medical Letter* (123) recommends cefazolin. Oral preoperative neomycin plus erythromycin "bowel prep" is clearly effective in reducing the amount of bowel flora and minimizing postoperative infection following colonic surgery (124). A short dosing period helps avoid colonization or overgrowth with resistant organisms. Whether parenteral therapy in addition would further improve results has not been determined definitively. A study by Schoetz et al. (125) showed that addition of parenteral cefoxitin significantly reduced the incidence of postoperative wound infection; however, it did not reduce the incidence of intraabdominal infection. Mechanical cleansing with a low-residue diet followed by a liquid diet, cathartics, and enemas is very important. For vaginal hysterectomy, cefazolin prophylaxis is recommended (123).

The early use of appropriate antimicrobials is efficacious in preventing infection following penetrating wounds of the abdomen that involve the bowel; cefoxitin would be a reasonable choice.

Systemic prophylactic antimicrobial usage should begin just prior to surgery so that adequate blood and tissue levels will be achieved and maintained during the operative procedure.

Peritonitis Complicating Peritoneal Dialysis

Background Factors

Since its development in the late 1970s, peritoneal dialysis has revolutionized the treatment of end-stage renal disease, providing a safe, cost-effective alternative to hemodialysis and transplantation (126,127). The number of patients receiving continuous ambulatory peritoneal dialysis (CAPD) worldwide has been estimated to be 65,000 (128). Despite extensive experience with this form of dialysis, peritonitis remains the most common complication and often limits its long-term utility. Peritonitis is the primary reason for discontinuing CAPD due to method failure (129).

The incidence of peritonitis complicating CAPD varies considerably among individual patients and centers. The rates tend to reflect the experience of the center, the specific technology used, and the participants' susceptibility to infection and ability to comply with procedures (130). Overall, however, the average incidence of peritonitis is 1.3–1.4 episodes per patient per year of dialysis (131). More than half of all episodes are experienced by only 25% of patients (133), and many CAPD patients remain free of peritonitis for years. In adults, men and women have equal risk of developing peritonitis, but persons of color and persons with less education and diabetics over 60 years of age are at increased risk (129,133,134). Children also seem to have a higher incidence of peritonitis (one episode per 7.7 months vs. one per 11.1 months) (135); however, in children whose parents perform the dialysate exchanges, the incidence of peritonitis approaches the rate seen in adults (136,137).

Etiology

In patients undergoing CAPD, peritonitis is usually caused by a single pathogen that originates from the normal flora of the skin or upper respiratory tract. Approximately 60–70% of cases are caused by gram-positive cocci, 20–30% by gram-negative bacilli, and the remainder by various anaerobic bacteria, fungi, and mycobacteria (Table 6) (138,139). Coagulase-negative *Staphylococcus* is the single most commonly encountered pathogen in most series, followed by *S. aureus* and species of streptococci. Among the gram-negative organisms, most Enterobacteriaceae have been associated with CAPD peritonitis but no single species predominates in all series. Nonfermentative gram-negative bacilli also occur sporadically, sometimes in association with environmental contamination (140). Although a rare pathogen in other types of peritonitis, *Pseudomonas aeruginosa* occurs

TABLE 6. *Common organisms associated with CAPD peritonitis*

Organism	%
Gram-Positive Bacteria	
Staphylococcus (coagulase-negative)	30–45
Staphylococcus aureus	10–20
Streptococcus	10–15
Enterococcus	3–5
Diphtheroids	1–2
Gram-Negative Bacteria	
Enterobacteriaceae	10–20
Pseudomonas aeruginosa	5–10
Other	2–3
Fungi	5–15
Mycobacteria	0–3
Anaerobes, polymicrobial	0–10

with relative frequency in CAPD peritonitis (5–10% of cases). It warrants special note because of its association with significant morbidity and late complications (141,142).

Fungi have become an important cause of CAPD-related peritonitis in recent years because of their increasing frequency and problematic management. Although many different fungi have been isolated, including *Aspergillus, Mucor, Rhizopus, Alternaria, Fusarium, Penicillium,* and *Drechslera, Candida albicans* accounts for 80–90% of cases (130,139,143). Risk factors for acquisition of fungal peritonitis are bacterial peritonitis within the preceding month, recent hospitalization, presence of extraperitoneal infection, use of immunosuppressive agents, and concomitant HIV infection; diabetes mellitus does not pose a special risk (143,144). *Mycobacterium* has been described as a pathogen in fewer than 3% of cases of CAPD-related peritonitis, but may also account for a portion of cases labeled as culture-negative (145). Overall, 86% of mycobacterial isolates reported in the literature are group IV (rapid growers), such as *M. fortuitum* and *M. chelonae* (146). One particularly large outbreak involved 17 patients who developed infection with *M. chelonae* following treatment with contaminated intermittent peritoneal dialysis machines (147). Other rare causes of peritonitis in patients undergoing CAPD are viruses (148), algae (149), and *M. tuberculosis* (150).

Pathogenesis

There are several potential routes of infection for development of peritonitis in CAPD patients. The two most important are (a) transluminal, resulting from a break in sterile technique during dialysate exchange, and (b) contiguous spread, in which microorganisms access the peritoneum along the tract of the dialysis catheter. In a review of factors leading to peritonitis at a single CAPD center, 36% of cases were due to suspected poor technique (transluminal contamination), 7% were attributed to known contamination, 20% to complicated exit site or tunnel infections, and 18% were of unknown origin (151). Less common portals of entry are hematogenous spread from a distant site of infection or direct contamination from the GI tract (138). Diverticular disease of the nonsigmoid colon appears to be a risk factor for acquisition of infection of intestinal origin, presumably through occult microperforations (152). However, isolation of multiple enteric pathogens from peritoneal fluid, especially anaerobic bacteria, suggests fecal contamination from gross colonic perforations (130).

Factors that may contribute to microbial pathogenicity include production of extracellular slime (biofilm) and ability to grow in dialysis fluids. It has been shown that both staphylococci and *C. albicans* can grow as microcolonies on polymeric surfaces (153,154). Surrounding biofilm serves to anchor the organisms and protect them from host defenses and antibiotic activity; thus it may play a role both in the initiation and relapse of CAPD-associated peritonitis (155). Once organisms gain access to the peritoneal cavity, further growth may depend on their survival in the presence of dialysis fluid. Fresh dialysate solutions are capable of supporting growth of *E. coli* but not staphylococci. However, after instillation into the peritoneal cavity, dialysis effluent supports growth of both organisms (156). Further studies have shown that the growth of *P. aeruginosa* and *E. coli* are enhanced 1000-fold in dialysis fluids from patients with peritonitis compared to uninfected controls (157). Accordingly, survival of bacteria contaminating the peritoneal cavity depends on timing of inoculation as well as the nature of the organism.

Another consideration in the pathogenesis of dialysis-associated peritonitis is the activity of host defenses (158). When used for dialysis, the peritoneal cavity does not provide a supportive milieu for operation of host defense mechanisms. The low pH (5.5–6.0), high osmolarity (300–400 mOsmol/kg), and dilution effects of the dialysate volume (2 L) act to diminish normal phagocytic function (158–160). Furthermore, dialysis has been shown to decrease the levels of immunoglobulin G (IgG) and complement (C3) in the peritoneum to approximately 1% of their normal levels (139). The significance of this observation is unclear since IgG levels in the dialysate do not correlate with occurrence of peritonitis (161). It is likely that the collective abnormalities in host defenses contribute to the pathogenesis of this infection.

Clinical Manifestations

Criteria for the diagnosis of CAPD-associated peritonitis are (a) signs and symptoms of peritoneal irritation, (b) cloudy dialysate effluent with a leukocyte count greater than $100/mm^3$, and (c) a positive culture of dialysate fluid. Any two of these criteria may be adequate to establish the diagnosis (154). Signs and symptoms of peritonitis vary from mild to severe, depending largely on the virulence of the pathogen and the time course of the infection (130). Infections due to coagulase-negative staphylococci tend to be indolent and mild, while those due to *S. aureus* and gram-negative bacilli are more fulminant in nature (162). Generally, turbid dialysate is the first and most common symptom to appear, followed shortly thereafter by abdominal pain and tenderness. Localized findings should suggest specific organ pathology such as cholecystitis or appendicitis. Other clinical manifestations of CAPD-related peritonitis are listed in Table 7.

TABLE 7. *Clinical manifestations of peritonitis in patients receiving continuous ambulatory peritoneal dialysis*

Manifestation	%
Cloudy dialysate	90–100
Abdominal pain	70–80
Fever	35–60
Nausea, vomiting	25–35
Diarrhea	<10
Abdominal tenderness	50–80
Drainage problems	15
Peripheral leukocytes	30–45

Diagnosis

Laboratory evaluation of dialysate effluent is critical to the diagnosis. Fluid should be sent for total cell count, differential leukocyte count, Gram stain, and culture. Although a leukocyte count of greater than $100/mm^3$ is a traditional cutoff for diagnosis, the value is not specific. In some cases of CAPD-associated peritonitis, WBC counts are less than $100/mm^3$; moreover, counts higher than that ($100–500/mm^3$) have been observed in the absence of infection (163,164). The differential cell count of dialysate may have a better predictive value. In one study, PMN leukocytes composed greater than 50% of the total count (mean = 85%) in infected patients while uninfected patients had less than 40% PMN leukocytes (mean = 12%) (165). On occasion, a preponderance of eosinophils may be noted in the fluid. This self-limited condition, eosinophilic peritonitis, often follows placement of the Tenckhoff catheter and may represent allergy to the tubing (166,167). Peritoneal eosinophilia also occurs with fungal peritonitis or recent intraperitoneal administration of antibiotics (139).

Gram stain of dialysis fluid is of low sensitivity, detecting only 20–30% of peritonitis episodes. Gram-positive organisms, especially *S. aureus,* are more likely to be detected than are gram-negative ones (163,168). Culture has a greater yield than Gram stain, although the precise method influences its sensitivity. Because there is a relatively small number of organisms contained in a large volume, optimal culturing techniques rely on some form of concentration, such as centrifugation, filtration, or lysis-centrifugation (169). Even with these specialized methods, 3–30% of peritonitis episodes are culture-negative. Presumably, most are due to fastidious, low-virulence organisms or coagulase-negative staphylococci that survive less well in dialysis fluid (130,157). Cases of culture-negative peritonitis that do not respond to empirical antibiotic treatment should be further investigated by obtaining dialysate fluid cultures for mycobacteria and fungi. Blood cultures are usually negative regardless of the etiological agent.

Therapy

Many patients with dialysis-related peritonitis can be managed on an ambulatory basis. Hospitalization is indicated for those patients who are severely ill or who are unable to manage administration of intraperitoneal antibiotics at home. A variety of antimicrobial agents have been used successfully for treatment, including penicillins, cephalosporins, aztreonam, imipenem, aminoglycosides, fluoroquinolones, and macrolide and glycopeptide antibiotics (170–177). Initial therapy is guided by results of the dialysis fluid Gram stain. If gram-positive bacteria are seen, a cephalosporin or vancomycin may be selected. Because of the high incidence of methicillin-resistant staphylococci in many centers, vancomycin is often preferred (178). For gram-negatives, an aminoglycoside is usually administered. In cases where no organisms are seen on the Gram stain, empirical treatment with a cephalosporin or vancomycin plus aminoglycoside is initiated. Alternatively, in relatively mild episodes of peritonitis, a single agent with antistaphylococcal activity may be suitable. Ultimately, empirical antibiotic selections are adjusted when the results of culture and sensitivity tests are known. A single specific agent is adequate treatment in the majority of cases of bacterial peritonitis. *P. aeruginosa*, however, has been associated with a high therapeutic failure rate and frequent relapses (179–181). A synergistic combination of antibiotics, such as an antipseudomonal β-lactam plus an aminoglycoside, has been recommended in addition to removal of the dialysis catheter. Intraperitoneal administration of antibiotics is the preferred method for drug delivery in CAPD-associated peritonitis because it achieves high local concentrations and permits self-treatment by the patient (182,183). Therapy is usually continued for 10–14 days but may need to be extended with unusually severe or slow to respond infections. Recommendations for specific drug doses and routes of administration have been published elsewhere (154,183,184).

Treatment of fungal peritonitis is controversial because of the lack of controlled studies and the small numbers of cases seen at any single center. Although there are reports of successful treatment with intraperitoneal and/or systemic antifungal agents alone (185–187), removal of the dialysis catheter is usually prudent to prevent relapse (130,188). A short course of systemic amphotericin B (250–500 mg) is often given following catheter removal. Some evidence has suggested that catheter removal alone may be curative in selected patients (188). Mycobacterial peritonitis also requires removal of the dialysis catheter for cure. Most of these organisms are resistant to conventional antituberculous agents, and susceptibilities vary greatly between the species. Antibiotic selections should be guided by either in vitro susceptibility tests or published recommendations (145–147).

Prognosis

CAPD-associated peritonitis is accompanied by reduction in ultrafiltration and protein loss in dialysis effluent. Rarely is it necessary to abandon use of the peritoneum for dialysis, but more frequent exchanges or hypertonic dialysate may be needed to prevent volume overload. The functional capacity of the peritoneal cavity returns to baseline in 7–10 days (189). After appropriate treatment of an episode of peritonitis, long-term resumption of CAPD is generally successful. Particularly severe or pro-

longed episodes of peritonitis may lead to formation of adhesions and an increased risk of peritoneal sclerosis but the same is not true of patients with repetitive bouts of infection (189). Mortality is 2–3% in younger patients (mean age = 45 years) but higher in elderly patients (7%) and those with fungal, mycobacterial, and polymicrobial infections (190,191). Required removal of the catheter is a major sequela of dialysis-related peritonitis. Relative indications for this are tunnel infection, catheter malfunction, relapse, bowel perforation, or fungal, mycobacterial, or *P. aeruginosa* infection. In general, catheters can be reinserted upon adequate resolution of the primary infection. Some evidence suggests that resumption of CAPD after a single episode of *Pseudomonas* peritonitis is often unsuccessful even with replacement of the catheter (180).

Prevention

Critical to prevention of peritonitis is careful patient selection with intensive education regarding aseptic technique and catheter care. Efforts to reduce the incidence of peritonitis by using oral or intraperitoneal antibiotics have largely been unsuccessful (192–195). Although a decrease in the number of random positive dialysate culture results has been observed in clinical studies, occurrence of clinical peritonitis was unaffected by prophylactic antibiotics. In cases of known contamination, such as documented breaks in asepsis or contaminated dialysate fluid or tubing, use of appropriate antibiotics for prophylaxis, or "early presumptive treatment," is probably judicious (196). More recent preventive measures have addressed specific reduction of *S. aureus* infections since evidence suggests that pre-CAPD nasal carriers are at high risk for subsequent exit site infection and peritonitis (197). Use of topical mupirocin eliminates colonization but has yet to be shown to significantly impact the incidence of peritonitis (198). Oral trimethoprim-sulfamethoxazole also decreases colonization and the number of episodes of staphylococcal peritonitis but not the overall incidence of peritonitis (199). Staphylococcal vaccines have also been used in CAPD patients, but studies show conflicting results as to efficacy (200,201).

The most significant advances in the prevention of dialysis-related peritonitis involve instrumentation changes. They fall into the following categories: (a) devices that facilitate connection of tubing, such as titanium adapters; (b) devices that help maintain field sterility during exchanges, such as UV light systems and in-line filters (202–204); and (c) devices that protect intraluminal sterility during exchanges, such as connector systems with disinfectant (Y connector, O set) (205,206). Most such devices have been shown to favorably impact the rate of peritonitis but add appreciably to the overall cost of CAPD.

Other Types of Peritonitis

Tuberculous Peritonitis (see chapter by Horsburgh and Nelson)

Although tuberculosis of the peritoneum is an uncommon disease, cases continue to occur in the USA, especially in the elderly, the urban poor, and those with HIV infection, cirrhosis, or debility (207). Currently, peritonitis is the sixth most common site of extrapulmonary tuberculosis (208). Most cases are thought to arise from reactivation of a latent focus of infection in the peritoneum or in an abdominal lymph node. Less commonly it arises from contiguous spread from the intestines or fallopian tubes (209). Concomitant active pulmonary tuberculosis occurs in 4–21% of patients, although abnormal chest radiographs are reported in nearly half of cases (210). The clinical manifestations of tuberculous peritonitis begin insidiously, with most patients having had symptoms for weeks to months prior to presentation (211). Fever, chills, weight loss, and abdominal pain are common complaints. Ascites is present in virtually all patients although it is not always detectable by clinical exam. The fluid is exudative (protein >2.5 g/dL) with a WBC count of 150–4000/mm^3 (211). Mononuclear cells predominate in most cases, but as many as 10% of patients will have an initial neutrophilic response (212). In cirrhotic patients the diagnosis of tuberculous peritonitis is often difficult because lymphocytes also do not predominate in all cases and the ascitic fluid may not be exudative due to low serum albumin levels (213).

Acid-fast smears of ascitic fluid are rarely positive in tuberculous peritonitis, and conventional cultures yield the pathogen in only 25% of cases. Concentrated ascitic fluid produces a higher yield on culture (66%), but requires large volumes of fluid and delays of 4–8 weeks before growth of the organism is recognized on solid media (214). At present laparoscopy with directed peritoneal biopsy is the best way to make a rapid specific diagnosis (210). Recently, determination of ascitic fluid adenosine deaminase activity was also proven to be a useful test in the diagnosis of peritoneal tuberculosis. Several studies have demonstrated that levels above 33 U/L are 100% sensitive and 95% specific to the diagnosis (215,216).

Drug regimens used for treatment of pulmonary tuberculosis are similarly efficacious in the treatment of peritoneal infection. Drugs with bactericidal activity, such as isoniazid and rifampin, are preferred first-line agents to be given for a period of 9 months. Addition of pyrazinamide may permit shortening of the duration of treatment to 6 months but requires careful monitoring. Because of the recent emergence of drug resistance in HIV-infected patients, therapy of suspected tuberculosis in these patients is usually initiated with a minimum of four agents. Therapy is readjusted in accordance with clinical response and results of susceptibility tests. Even with appropriate therapy, overall mortality is in the range of 7–13% (213,217). Early recognition is probably the key to improving survival.

Fungal Peritonitis (see chapter by Washburn, Gray, and Bennett)

With increasing numbers of immunosuppressed patients and advances in medical technology such as organ transplantation, opportunistic fungal infections of the peritoneum have emerged as a significant clinical problem. By far, *Candida* species are the most important of the fungal pathogens producing peritonitis. In non-CAPD patients, *Candida* peritonitis occurs as a complication of perforated abdominal organs or GI surgery (218). Recent antibiotic use is an important predisposing factor (219). Although *Candida* is the sole pathogen in some cases, most infections are polymicrobial, involving other endogenous flora of the GI tract.

The significance of *Candida* growing on culture of peritoneal fluid has been debated, even when it was found in the presence of gross peritoneal contamination. Many have argued that it is nonpathogenic and requires no specific antifungal therapy (220,221). However, development of intraperitoneal abscesses, systemic fungemia, and late mortality in some cases left untreated defines a definite pathogenic role (222,223). Therapy for *Candida* peritonitis usually consists of a specific antifungal antibiotic and surgical intervention to drain suppurative collections and repair perforations. Amphotericin B in low doses of 0.3 mg/kg/day for a total of 350–500 mg is recommended, provided there is no evidence of dissemination (218). In the case of polymicrobial infection, appropriate antibacterials are also administered. The role of fluconazole and other new azole antifungal agents in treatment of fungal peritonitis is uncertain. Mortality is low in adequately treated patients, but exceeds 50% in those in whom specific antifungal therapy is delayed or withheld (222) and in those acquiring disease as a complication of liver transplantation (224).

On rare occasions, fungi such as *Coccidioides, Histoplasma, Blastomyces,* and *Cryptococcus* may involve the peritoneum as part of a syndrome of dissemination. Clinical manifestations are similar to those produced by bacterial peritonitis. Therapy is as required for the disseminated infection.

INTRAABDOMINAL ABSCESS

Intraperitoneal Abscess

Abscesses are well-defined purulent collections walled off from the rest of the peritoneal cavity by inflammatory adhesions, loops of bowel and their mesentery, the greater omentum, and other abdominal viscera. Abscesses represent successful intervention by host defenses in the peritoneal cavity because the infection has been localized and prevented from entering the bloodstream. The chief anatomic sites of abscess within the abdomen are the subphrenic areas (including subhepatic and subdiaphragmatic abscesses), the pelvis, the lumbar gutters, and the intermesenteric folds. Subphrenic abscesses (Figs. 2 and 3) are divided into three groups: right and left subdiaphragmatic and subhepatic abscesses. The large spaces above and below the liver are typically subdivided about their midpoints by pyogenic membranes, leading to the designations of anterior and posterior spaces. Subdiaphragmatic abscesses remain a special problem. There are three subdiaphragmatic areas on each side: two intraperitoneal areas (anterior and posterior) and one extraperitoneal area which lies even further posteriorly. On the

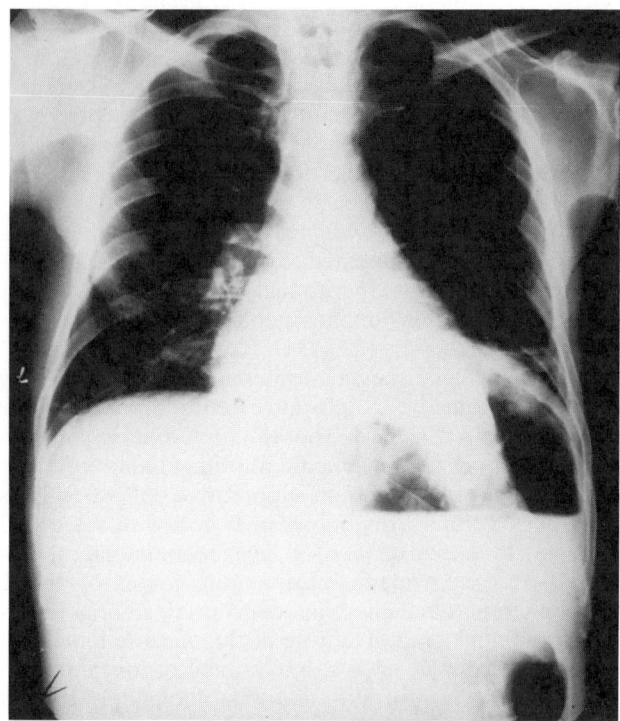

FIG. 2. Large left subphrenic abscess showing gas-fluid level in left upper quadrant (distinct from stomach air bubble), elevation of left hemidiaphragm, and slight atelectasis left lower lung field.

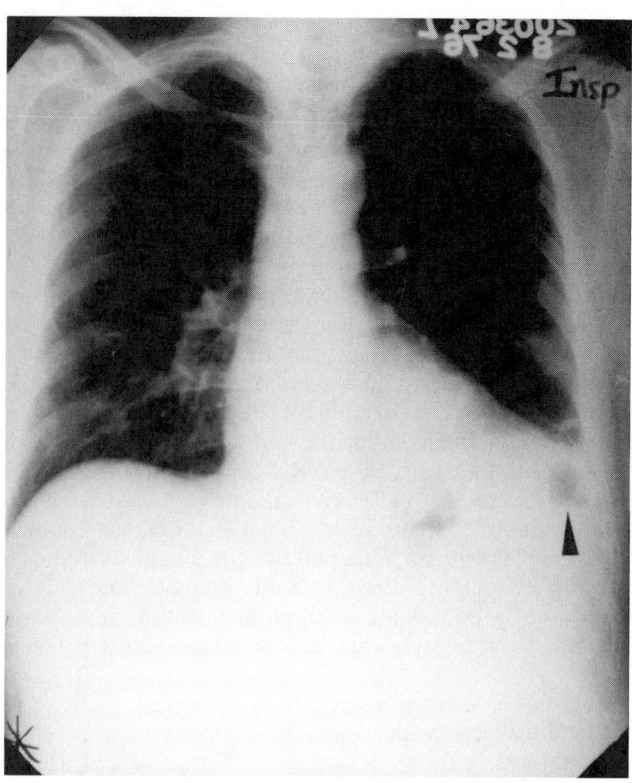

FIG. 3. Left subphrenic abscess. Arrow points to small gas-fluid level lateral to stomach bubble. Elevation of left hemidiaphragm and blunting of left costophrenic angle due to pleural effusion.

right, the extraperitoneal abscesses are in the layer of the crus of the diaphragm and coronary ligament; on the left, they arise above the superior pole of the left kidney. Abscesses may occur within abdominal viscera also, of course; these are usually due to hematogenous or lymphatic spread of microorganisms to the affected organ.

Etiology

The specific etiology relates to the underlying process and the flora of the GI, biliary, or female genital tract area that gave rise to the problem. Please refer to the extensive discussion of the normal flora of some of these areas in the section "Secondary Peritonitis." The major pathogens are ordinarily various Enterobacteriaceae, other gram-negative nonanaerobic bacilli, the *Bacteroides fragilis* group, other anaerobic gram-negative rods, clostridia, and anaerobic cocci. Many other organisms may become involved, as detailed in the earlier section. *Salmonella* may be involved in intraabdominal abscess in relation to prior gastroenteritis or biliary tract infection (225). Psoas abscess occurs primarily in children and typically is due to *Staphylococcus aureus,* but mycobacteria are also important causes and other organisms may be found (226,227).

Interestingly, *Clostridium septicum,* which is known for septicemia and a rapidly progressing course in association with colon malignancy, may also produce asymptomatic or minimally symptomatic abscesses in solid organs

such as the liver and in the retroperitoneum (228). These may also be associated with colonic carcinoma, leukemia involving the bowel, and neutropenia, and there may be accompanying asymptomatic bacteremia. Aggressive search for underlying pathology and aggressive treatment may prevent progression to fulminant toxemia.

Pathogenesis, Pathology

Again, the reader is referred to the earlier section on this topic, "Secondary Peritonitis." The underlying lesion in subphrenic abscess is almost always within the abdomen. Most recent cases have been related to the stomach or duodenum or the biliary tract, with relatively fewer cases of appendicitis than previously. A primary source in the lower intestinal tract or in the female genital tract is not uncommon. Abdominal surgery or trauma is also a relatively common cause of subphrenic abscess. The major route of infection is by direct extension or by way of lymphatic drainage. The suprahepatic space is much more likely to be infected than the infrahepatic space because the former is a closed space and has a negative pressure that is enhanced during inspiration. Left-sided subphrenic abscess is seen primarily after upper abdominal surgery or lesions of the stomach or duodenum.

The most common precursors of pelvic abscess are perforated appendix (Fig. 4) (usually the right lower quad-

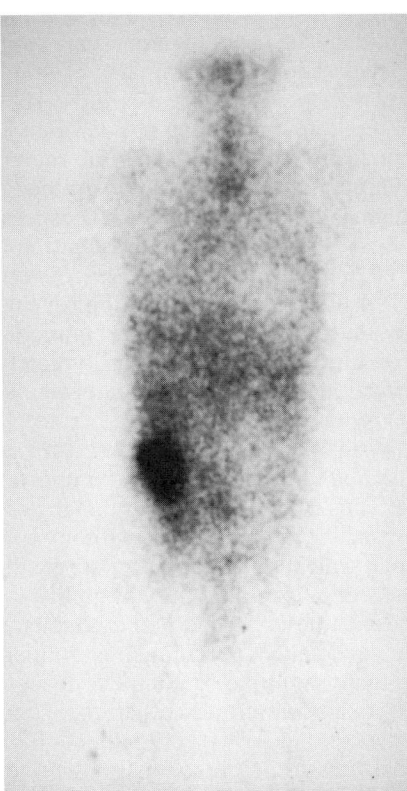

FIG. 4. Gallium scan showing right lower quadrant (appendiceal) abscess.

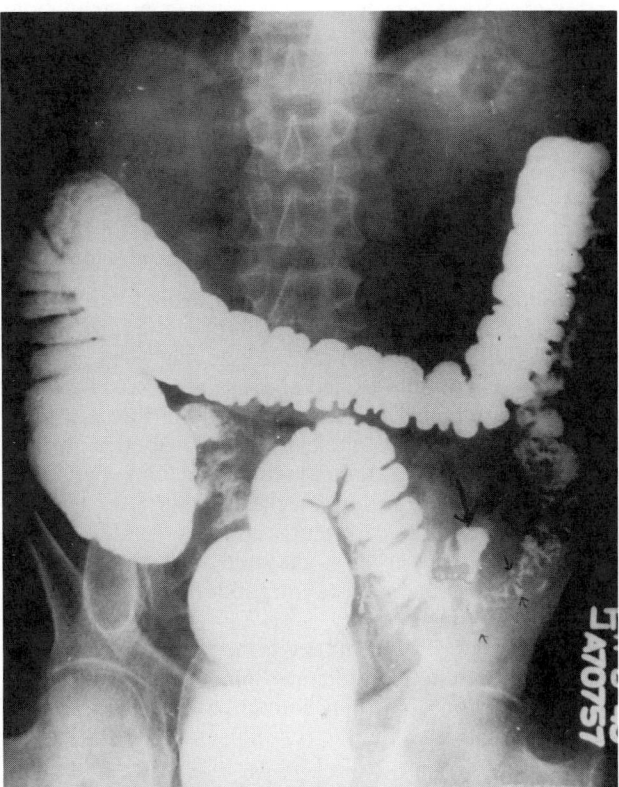

FIG. 5. Barium enema showing diverticulitis. Small arrows point to diverticula; large arrow points to abscess produced by rupture of an infected diverticulum.

rant), colonic diverticulitis (Fig. 5) (usually the left lower quadrant), and pelvic inflammatory disease. Pancreatitis is associated with lesser sac abscesses; perforation of the stomach or duodenum may also lead to lesser sac abscess. Acute diffuse peritonitis may also localize as a pelvic abscess. Paracolic abscess is more frequent on the right side.

Although host defenses may effectively localize infection by means of abscess formation, complete resolution of the abscess cannot usually be effected by host defense mechanisms because of local factors that impair these defense mechanisms or otherwise interfere with management (70,87). These include local hypoxia and low pH (which interfere with leukocyte migration and killing and with the antimicrobial activity of aminoglycosides), large numbers of stationary phase bacteria (interfering with antimicrobial efficacy), large concentrations of microbial byproducts and toxins (which impair phagocytic cell function, produce local tissue damage, and deplete complement), presence of necrotic debris (interferes with neutrophils and depletes complement), presence of hemoglobin (impairs phagocyte function), presence of fibrin (reduces access of host cells to bacteria), and sometimes the presence of barium sulfate (which impairs neutrophil function).

Clinical Picture

Many patients have an acute response with high intermittent fever, chills, abdominal pain, and tenderness.

However, intraabdominal abscess, especially subphrenic abscess, may be an insidious process; manifestations may be nonexistent, nonspecific, or misleading. Most patients have fever. The findings are not uncommonly those of an intrathoracic rather than an intraabdominal process. Pain, when present, is referred to the lower chest almost as often as to the upper abdomen. Hiccups may be present and persistent. Dyspnea, cough, chest or shoulder pain, and dullness or rales over the lung base may be noted. There may be tenderness and even local edema localized directly above the abscess, particularly at the costal margin. In subhepatic abscess, pain and tenderness are much less common. Prior therapy or prophylaxis may suppress the process sufficiently to further minimize findings and even contribute to a considerable delay between the time of the inciting event and the overt manifestations of intraabdominal abscess.

Pelvic abscess may be characterized by pain, deep tenderness in one or both lower quadrants, fever, urinary frequency, dysuria, and diarrhea. There may be mucus in the stools. There may be tenderness of the pelvic peritoneum and bulging of the anterior rectal wall on rectal or vaginal examination. Paracolic abscess results in fever and a tender, enlarging mass that may be difficult to palpate. Abscesses that have formed between or below the folds of the jejunoileal mesentery are characteristically small, multiple, and difficult to diagnose. They may result in fever, anorexia, vague pains, or partial small bowel obstruction.

Complications include bacteremia, fistulae (including external fistulae) (229), and mesenteric vein thrombosis (230).

Diagnosis

A high index of suspicion may be necessary in cases with minimal findings. Most patients exhibit leukocytosis with a left shift. Roentgenographic studies are usually quite helpful. As with the clinical findings, the roentgenographic signs of subphrenic abscess may be chiefly thoracic: elevation and decreased mobility of the diaphragm, lower lobe infiltrates, atelectasis, and obliteration of a costophrenic angle or larger pleural effusions. Obviously, in a postoperative patient, these findings may lead to a mistaken diagnosis of pneumonia. Gas under the diaphragm, gas bubbles or a gas-fluid level outside of the bowel, and displacement of intraabdominal organs are all important findings.

Ultrasonography, computed tomography (CT), and, occasionally, magnetic resonance imaging (MRI) are much more powerful tools than conventional radiography although the latter technique is still useful (231). CT is generally the most powerful of the available tools diagnostically; it is said to have sensitivity and specificity of 97% (66). One may see a low-density mass with a definable capsule that may be enhanced by intravenously administered contrast material. Contrast material is also administered orally and, at times, also rectally. With the bowel outlined in this manner, it is usually easy to determine that bubbles of gas or gas-fluid levels are extraluminal and therefore highly indicative of an abscess. CT can even detect the subtle thickening and edema of the colon wall and mesentery indicative of diverticulitis (94). Radionuclide scans (using technetium, gallium, or indium) may also be useful.

Blood cultures should always be obtained in cases of suspected intraabdominal abscess. The presence of a member of the *Bacteroides fragilis* group or two or more enteric nonanaerobes in a blood culture is indicative of intraabdominal infection. Obviously, if an abscess is drained surgically or percutaneously, both aerobic and anaerobic cultures and appropriate direct smears should be made.

Ultimately, laparoscopy (93) or even exploratory laparotomy may be required in very difficult cases, but nowadays this is rare due to the excellent diagnostic techniques available.

Therapy

Clearly, the principal approach to management of intraabdominal abscess is drainage. Most often this is best accomplished surgically although percutaneous drainage or laparascopic drainage (93) can be used successfully in many cases. The transperitoneal approach, rather than the posterior extraperitoneal approach, is now used almost exclusively because it permits the complete exploration and drainage of the subdiaphragmatic space while enabling visualization and drainage of the subhepatic space (many subphrenic abscesses have subhepatic extensions or separate collections of pus). Pelvic abscesses may be drained by incision through the rectum (232,233) or vagina. Paracolic abscesses can be drained retroperitoneally through an incision lateral to the abscess. Intermesenteric abscesses are drained by evacuation after gentle separation of the mesenteric folds.

When CT or ultrasound examination reveals a unilocular abscess that is accessible, percutaneous drainage under CT or ultrasound guidance is typically effective; usually, insertion of a drainage catheter is desirable. Haaga (231) reports an overall success rate of 80.8% in a number of series reported in the literature. Aside from accessibility and unilocular nature, important requirements for effective percutaneous drainage are an abscess that is not vascular and a patient without coagulopathy, concomitant surgical evaluation and surgical backup for complications or failure, and the possibility of dependent drainage via a catheter placed percutaneously. Actually, with further experience, percutaneous drainage has been effective in many multiple or complex abscesses; it may be necessary to insert multiple catheters, of course. Brolin et al. (234) report that 76% of 119 patients had successful drainage of abscesses percutaneously; the overall mortality rate was 16%, with a 75% mortality in the failure group. Failure with the percutaneous drainage procedure was greater in patients 60 years or older, patients with pancreatic abscess, and abscesses with large volumes (drainage persisting 3 days or longer). One should avoid traversing the pleural space for drainage of subphrenic abscesses (235) and it is best to avoid using a transhepatic or transplenic approach for drainage of lesser sac abscesses (231). Percutaneous drainage in properly selected patients will have lower morbidity and mortality than surgical drainage. Percutaneous drainage and surgical drainage should be considered complementary rather than competitive. Whatever technique is used, patients should be improved within 24–48 hr following drainage (236); if a patient is not improved following percutaneous drainage, he or she should be reevaluated with CT, and the surgeon and radiologist should review the case together to agree on an appropriate course of action. Patients with APACHE II scores of 15 or greater do not do as well with percutaneous drainage (8% survival) as with surgical drainage (30%), although the difference is not statistically significant (237); surgical treatment should not be avoided because the patient is considered to be "too ill." Intracavitary urokinase has been suggested to facilitate percutaneous drainage of multilocular abscesses (238).

Even patients with enteric fistulae may be managed successfully with the aid of percutaneous drainage of abdominal abscesses (239). Schuster et al. (239) found that 21 of 24 patients with various types of fistulae healed their fistulae without surgical intervention (over periods of up to 3 months). Percutaneous drainage has also been used successfully as the initial therapy of intraabdominal abscess associated with a perforated viscus, thus avoiding the first stage of the traditional two-stage surgical approach (240). Stabile et al. (241) found that percutaneous drainage obviated the need for colostomy and multiple-stage surgery in about 75% of patients with large diverticular abscesses. Percutaneous drainage has also been used in immunocompromised patients although the cure rate (53%) was lower than in nonimmunocompromised patients (73%) (242). Drainage of intraabdominal abscess with fistula formation has been effected via fistuloscopy in several patients in whom percutaneous drainage failed (243).

Antimicrobial agents are useful adjuncts to drainage procedures, but certainly are not a substitute. (See the section on therapy under "Secondary Peritonitis" for details on indications for various antimicrobial agents.) The low pH and low Eh environment in abscesses may impair the effectiveness of a number of antimicrobial agents (aminoglycosides as one example).

Serial imaging may be important for evaluating response to therapy.

Prognosis

Mortality with subphrenic abscess is still relatively high. Mortality is associated particularly with failure to detect and drain the abscess, delay in drainage, old age, and concominant serious underlying diseases.

The most frequent complications of subphrenic abscess are intrathoracic—serous effusion, empyema, necrotizing pneumonia, bronchial or bronchopleural fistula, pericarditis, and mediastinal abscess. Other complications include generalized peritonitis, and internal and external fistulae.

Prevention

Appropriate medical and surgical therapy of predisposing conditions should lower the incidence of intraabdominal abscess. Avoidance of postoperative drainage following splenectomy lowers the incidence of local complications, including abscess. Aseptic surgical technique is important in the prevention of postoperative infection.

The use of prophylactic antimicrobial agents in connection with abdominal surgery was discussed earlier in the section on prevention under "Secondary Peritonitis."

Pancreatic Abscess

Etiology

Pancreatic abscess develops primarily as a complication of pancreatitis of any origin (alcoholic, biliary, postoperative, or related to trauma). It occurs in 3–4% of cases of acute pancreatitis (244–247), frequently severe pancreatitis (248). Infected pancreatic necrosis develops in 3–6% of patients with acute pancreatitis (247). Less common causes are a complication of endoscopic retrograde cholangiopancreatography (249), a posterior penetrating peptic ulcer, or a secondary infection of a pseu-

docyst. Pancreatic abscess has also followed pancreatic and liver transplantation (250,251). Cytomegalovirus pancreatitis apparently may also predispose to pancreatic abscess (252). Males predominate over females in the incidence of pancreatic abscess by a ratio of about 2.5:1 and the peak incidence is in the 40- to 50-year age group (253).

Bacteriology

Enteric organisms are the organisms described most often from pancreatic abscess, with about half of cases showing a polymicrobial flora (245–247). E. coli is the organism found most often (35% of abscesses) with enterococci, viridans streptococci, and Klebsiella each found in about 20% of cases (247). S. aureus, Enterobacter, Pseudomonas, and Proteus are seen in less than 10% of cases (253,254). Candida is seen occasionally. The flora of infected pancreatic necrosis and of infected pancreatic pseudocyst is similar (247,255). The role of anaerobes is undoubtedly underestimated because optimal anaerobic techniques have often not been used, but a number of studies have documented the presence of anaerobes (244–247,253–266). The incidence of anaerobes in various studies has been listed as 6% (253), 9% (247), 14% (254), and 16% (256). "Bacteroides" were found in 4% of infected pancreatic pseudocysts, 9% of infected pancreatic necrosis cases, and 15% of pancreatic abscesses in one study (255). In the study by Shi et al. (245), 6 of 22 positive cultures from pancreatic abscesses yielded a mixed culture of aerobes and anaerobes. Anaerobes, including B. fragilis, have been recovered from bacteremia accompanying pancreatic abscess (264–266). Other anaerobes recovered from pancreatic abscesses include Clostridium difficile, C. cadaveris, "anaerobic streptococci," "Streptococcus milleri" (this group includes S. anginosus, S. constellatus, and S. intermedius), and S. anginosus. Eikenella corrodens and Haemophilus influenzae have been isolated from a pancreatic abscess (267) and Eikenella has been isolated from additional abscesses either in pure culture or together with other organisms (268). Mycobacterium tuberculosis has also been found.

Pathogenesis, Pathology

The bacteriology of the infected pancreas suggests an enteric origin. However, animal studies have shown that bacteria may reach the pancreas from many sources, including colon, gallbladder, and urinary tract. Bacteria may reach the pancreas by various routes including the circulation and the main pancreatic duct as well as transperitoneally. In animals, only those with inflamed glands develop infection and the rate of infection is proportional to the extent of the pancreatic necrosis. There is also some evidence for reduced host resistance to infection in patients with acute pancreatitis. Pancreatic abscesses consist of a collection of pus or necrotic material enclosed by a capsule or pseudocapsule. There may be adjacent areas of necrotic tissue, hemorrhage, and fat necrosis.

About two thirds of abscesses are multiple; they may be either unilocular or multilocular (247). About 25% involve the entire gland and the rest are relatively evenly distributed between the head, body, and tail of the pancreas although this varies in different reported series.

Clinical Picture

Persistence of fever, ileus, and tenderness or, more commonly, deterioration of the patient's condition 1–4 weeks after initial improvement in a patient with pancreatitis should raise the question of abscess. Most cases involve abdominal pain (usually epigastric in location and not uncommonly radiating to the back or flank), nausea and vomiting, and tenderness over the area of the abscess. There may also be guarding or rebound on examination. Low-grade fever to 40.6°C is common. About half the time either a mass or fullness is palpable. Leukocytosis (15,000–20,000/mm^3) is usual but elevation of the serum amylase and lipase are irregular and elevation of serum bilirubin uncommon. Hypoalbuminemia and elevated serum alkaline phosphatase are commonly seen. It must be appreciated that the clinical picture of pancreatic abscess is nonspecific; one cannot reliably distinguish between pancreatic abscess, sterile or infected pancreatic necrosis, and sterile or infected pancreatic pseudocysts.

Most cases are diagnosed 2–3 weeks after the onset of acute pancreatitis, but onset may be considerably later; it appears that the later the onset, the more favorable the prognosis.

Complications include perforation into the peritoneal cavity or into the stomach, bowel, biliary tree, or a bronchus; hemorrhage into the abscess cavity; GI bleeding; empyema; bacteremia; and diabetes mellitus.

Diagnosis

Chest roentgenograms may show abnormalities but findings are nonspecific. Abdominal films may show displacement of the gastric air bubble, retrogastric gas, or the classic "soap bubble" sign, all of which are suggestive of pancreatic infection. GI contrast studies may also show suggestive evidence (Fig. 6). Radionuclide studies are not particularly helpful diagnostically. Sonograms often detect phlegmon or pseudocyst but are rarely diagnostic of an abscess; however, CT scanning (Fig. 7) can detect secondary pancreatic infection in over 75% of patients (231,253). In addition, CT provides information on the site and size of the collection. High-dose intravenous contrast infusion in combination with CT scanning is said to be very helpful in predicting pancreatic necrosis.

Percutaneous CT-guided aspiration of material for Gram stain and culture is the most reliable method for differentiating secondary pancreatic infection from pancreatic inflammation. Several reports confirm the reliability and safety of this approach (253). Blood cultures should always be done both aerobically and anaerobically.

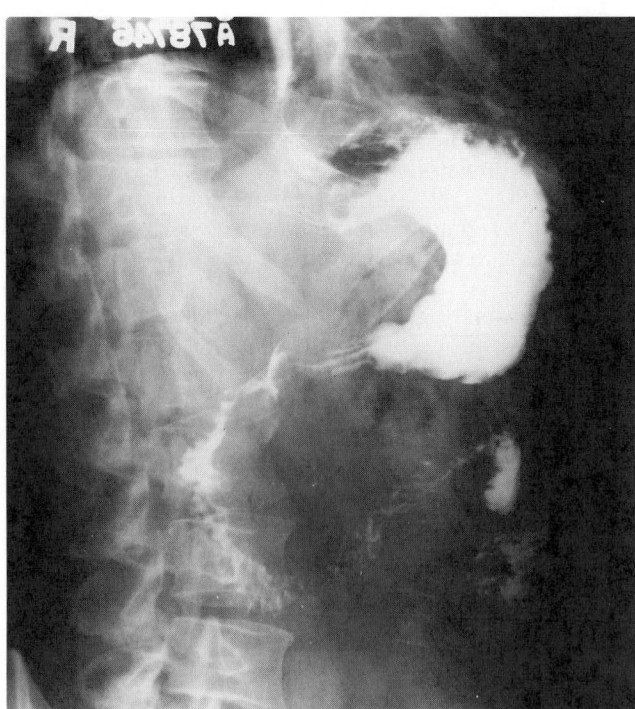

FIG. 6. Pancreatic abscess. Note widening of duodenal loop on upper GI series.

Therapy

The principal therapeutic approaches to pancreatic abscess are surgical debridement and drainage, percutaneous drainage, and antimicrobial therapy. Many feel that finding bacteria in material obtained by percutaneous CT-guided drainage mandates surgical intervention. Others would reserve surgery for patients with clinical evidence of sepsis together with demonstration on CT scan of a

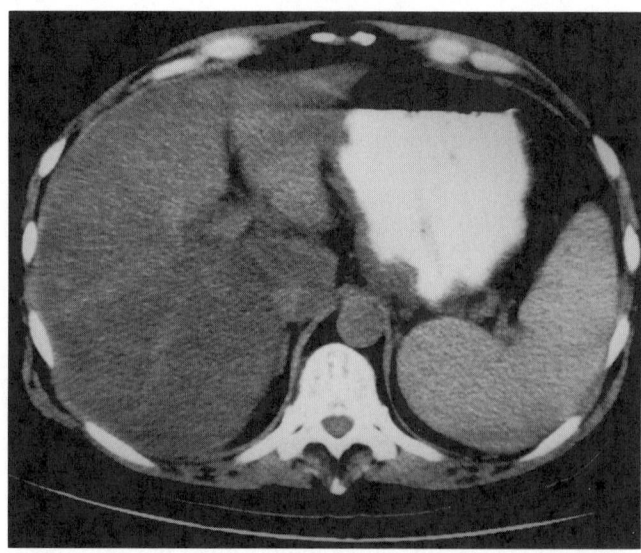

FIG. 7. CT scan showing large pancreatic abscess.

PERITONITIS AND INTRAABDOMINAL ABSCESS / 391

nonresolving pancreatic collection. The goals of surgical therapy are to remove devitalized pancreatic and peripancreatic tissue, to drain purulent collections, and to provide continuous drainage. Local debridement and drainage may have significantly higher mortality than retroperitoneal exploration; extensive unroofing of the superior retroperitoneum is needed because of the tendency of these infections to spread widely. Specific surgical approaches are discussed by Lumsden and Bradley (253). For infected pancreatic pseudocyst, operative or transcutaneous external drainage is done. For pancreatic abscess, surgical debridement and closed drainage are recommended (253); however, the success rate with percutaneous drainage is such that it is a reasonable alternative to surgery (231). The presence of gas bubbles, a gas-fluid level, or septations makes an abscess less amenable to percutaneous drainage (269). For more effective and safer surgery, intraoperative ultrasound has been recommended to localize fluid collections and the course of the pancreatic duct (270). For infected pancreatic necrosis, extensive surgical debridement and either closed or open drainage are performed. Reoperation is not uncommonly required. External drainage is effected by the use of multiple sumps and stuffed Penrose drains brought out through several separate sites. Sumps and drains should remain in the abscess cavity for at least a week. Evaluation of literature reports is rendered difficult by many authors failing to adequately distinguish between the above three types of pancreatic infection. Lumsden and Bradley (253) feel that for proven infected pancreatic necrosis, surgical intervention is necessary; particulate material in such patients would frequently occlude drainage tubes.

Antimicrobial therapy should always be used but plays only an adjunctive role. Ideally, information from Gram stain and culture should guide the choice of antimicrobial agents; empirical therapy follows the guidelines provided in the section on treatment of secondary peritonitis, since the flora of pancreatic abscess is typical of bowel flora. Antimicrobials that reach therapeutic levels in the pancreas include ceftazidime, cefotaxime, clindamycin, ciprofloxacin, rifampin, trimethoprim-sulfamethoxazole, and metronidazole (247,271). Buchler et al. (256) ranked drugs in three classes. Included in a class with low tissue levels were netilmicin and tobramycin; in a class with levels adequate to inhibit some, but not all, bacteria found in pancreatic infection were mezlocillin, piperacillin, ceftizoxime, and cefotaxime; and in a class with high pancreatic tissue levels and high bactericidal activity were ciprofloxacin, ofloxacin, and imipenem.

Prognosis

Stanten and Frey (260) summarized the mortality in 582 patients with pancreatic abscess from ten different series; mortality rates ranged from 9% to 38% with an average overall of 23%. Lumsden and Bradley (253) note that death is rare in infected pseudocyst of the pancreas but that mortality is 15–20% in pancreatic abscess and 20–50% in infected pancreatic necrosis. In addition to impressive mortality, there is a high incidence of serious complications; septicemia with multiple organ failure is a common event terminally. Respiratory failure occurs in 9–61%, renal failure 5–30%, hepatic failure 6–12%, GI tract hemorrhage 5–60%, peritonitis 12–17%, and intestinal obstruction 25–30%. Gastric outlet obstruction is also not uncommon.

Prevention

Early feeding after the onset of experimental pancreatitis results in an increased infection rate but there is no definite evidence that this occurs in humans. The value of early pancreatic resection or debridement requires further study; this may decrease or actually increase the incidence of subsequent infection. There is no evidence that early use of antimicrobials decreases the likelihood of infection. Fabian et al. (272) concluded from a randomized, prospective study that bacterial contamination via sump catheters was a problem in patients with pancreatic trauma and that septic complications were significantly reduced by use of closed suction drainage.

Pyogenic Liver Abscess

In the preantimicrobial era, *E. coli* and streptococci (particularly members of the viridans group and enterococci) predominated as etiological agents of liver abscess. Subsequently, other gram-negative bacilli such as *Klebsiella*, *Enterobacter*, *Proteus*, and *Pseudomonas* have been found with increasing frequency. Organisms encountered occasionally include *Listeria* (273), *Bartonella* (*Rochalimaea*) (274), *Aeromonas* (275), *Nocardia brasiliensis* (276), *Yersinia enterocolitica* (277), *Haemophilus* sp. (278), *Pediococcus* (279), *Chromobacterium* (280), *Edwardsiella* (281), *P. pseudomallei* (282), *Salmonella* (283), *Brucella* (284), *M. tuberculosis* (285), and *Aspergillus* (286). The exact incidence of anaerobes is uncertain because many studies have not utilized optimum anaerobic transport and culture techniques, and there has not been a proper prospective study. It appears, however, that if optimum techniques are used anaerobes would be found in at least 50% of liver abscesses, often in the absence of other organisms (287). A literature survey published in 1977 found 379 anaerobic isolates from liver abscess patients (288). Table 8 summarizes recent literature; 220 strains of anaerobes were found in this later survey, which was not intended to be complete. The most commonly encountered anaerobes currently are gram-negative rods (especially the *B. fragilis* group and other *Bacteroides* species, most of which would now be in *Prevotella* or *Porphyromonas*), and anaerobic and microaerophilic streptococci.

Hepatosplenic candidiasis is a localized but serious problem seen in immunocompromised patients. It is most often found in patients with myeloblastic leukemia, especially following cytosine arabinoside therapy, and in AIDS patients (315).

The incidence of liver abscess among hospital admissions or autopsies varies from 0.05% to 0.5%. There is a predominance of male patients. Multiple abscesses out-

TABLE 8. *Anaerobic and microaerophilic organisms isolated from liver abscesses*

Organism	No. isolates	Ref.
Gram-negative rods (GNR)		
Eikenella corrodens	2	286,289
Bacteroides ovatus	2	290,291
B. thetaiotaomicron	2	290,291
B. fragilis	45	286,288,292–299
B. uniformis	1	299
B. splanchnicus	1	300
Bacteroides spp.	34	259,275,286,288,295,296,301–303
Bilophila wadsworthia	3	299,300
Fusobacterium nucleatum	5	286,304–307
F. necrophorum	1	308
Fusobacterium spp.	14	288,293,298,309
Anaerobic GNR	3	288,303
Gram-negative cocci (GNC)		
Veillonella parvula	1	299
Anaerobic GNC	1	288
Gram-positive cocci (GPC)		
Microaerophilic *Strep.*	25	286,293,294,298,302,309
Streptococcus milleri	18	259,275,295,310,311
Peptostrep. anaerobius	8	288,298
Peptostreptococcus spp.	11	286,288,294,296
Anaerobic *Strep.*	10	301
Anaerobic GPC	2	288
Nonsporing gram-positive rods[a]		
Actinomyces israelii	1	242
A. meyeri	1	305
Actinomyces sp.	4	288,304,312,313
Lactobacillus sp.	1	314
Eubacterium sp.	2	286,294
Propionibacterium acnes	1	291
Propionibacterium sp.	1	288
Clostridia		
Clostridium septicum	1	228
C. perfringens	4	286,291,303,310
Clostridium sp.	5	259,288,303
Anaerobes, other	10	296–298

[a] See Section on actinomycosis (under "Intraabdominal Abscess") for additional data on *Actinomyces* sp.

number solitary abscesses; the right lobe is involved much more often than the left.

Most cases of liver abscess are secondary to pyleophlebitis but suppurative cholangitis is also a common background factor. Embolic abscesses may originate from anywhere in the body. Direct extension of infection, or extension by way of lymphatics, may follow a perforated gallbladder or duodenal ulcer, pancreatic abscess, perinephric or subdiaphragmatic abscess, or even lung abscess or thoracic empyema. Uncommon causes of liver abscess include retrograde infection via the hepatic vein and infection secondary to penetrating wounds or foreign bodies. It is not uncommon to be unable to find an underlying cause of liver abscess.

The most common clinical finding in liver abscess is fever, which may be accompanied by chills or sweats. The next most common finding is right upper quadrant pain. The pain is aching in character and tends to localize over the liver or the epigastrum; it may radiate to the right shoulder and be aggravated by inspiration. Percussion over the liver is painful. A mass may be localized beneath the costal margin or there may be fullness and tenderness of an intercostal space. Localized edema of the right lateral thoracic wall or the adjacent abdominal wall occurs at times. Nausea and vomiting are relatively uncommon. Upward enlargement of the liver may be detected in two thirds of cases. Abscesses high in the right lobe may lead to cough, splinting of the chest, dyspnea, pleural effusion, and atelectasis. Jaundice is uncommon. The course is most often indolent.

There is usually considerable leukocytosis ($>20,000/$mm^3) with a left shift. The serum alkaline phosphatase level is almost always elevated but liver function tests are usually normal. Blood cultures may be very helpful since they are positive in one third to one half of patients. Roentgenographic studies may show elevation of the diaphragm with reduced mobility and a change in contour; there may be pressure deformities or displacement of the stomach and duodenum. Occasionally there may be a gas-fluid level within the liver. CT, ultrasound (Fig. 8), and radionuclide studies are the most valuable procedures for diagnosing liver abscess and determining its location.

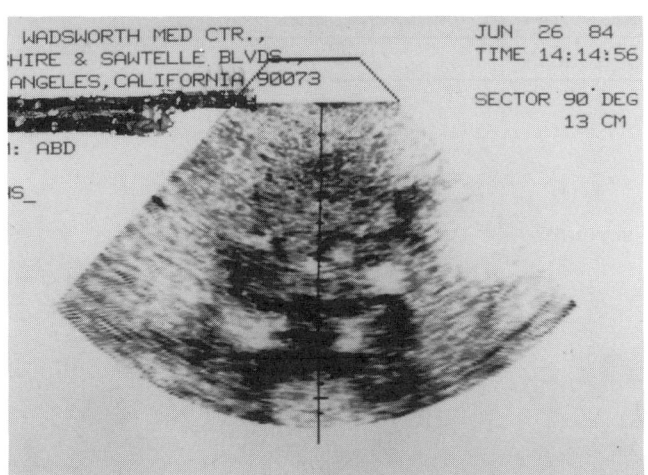

```
WADSWORTH MED CTR.,        JUN 26 84
HIRE & SAWTELLE BLVDS.,    TIME 14:14:56
ANGELES,CALIFORNIA/90073
                          SECTOR 90 DEG
I: ABD                            13 CM

IS_
```

FIG. 8. Ultrasonogram revealing multiple pyogenic liver abscesses.

Other types of studies are occasionally useful. Percutaneous aspiration may be undertaken for diagnostic purposes and to obtain material for Gram stain and aerobic and anaerobic culture. The principal entities to be considered in the differential diagnosis are amebic liver abscess (distinguished by epidemiologic factors, by the finding of amebae in the stools, or by serological testing) and subphrenic abscess.

Most patients can be managed with percutaneous drainage under ultrasound or CT guidance, augmented by antimicrobial therapy (236,242,293). A review of 252 patients treated with percutaneous drainage and antimicrobial therapy from 14 series in the literature showed an overall success rate of 77% (316). Surgical therapy will be required for some cases (317); some surgeons favor open drainage as the primary approach (309). Patients with multiple abscesses usually require an open drainage procedure (286). Ultrasound and CT are also important modalities for monitoring resolution of liver abscesses treated medically. Antimicrobial agents should be given for an extended period, depending on the speed of response as judged both clinically and by follow-up imaging procedures. The choice of agents depends on the specific infecting flora, as outlined in the treatment section under "Secondary Peritonitis." Metronidazole supplemented with ampicillin and at times other coverage for gram-negative bacilli is one good choice; metronidazole, of course, is also effective against amebic liver abscess.

The prognosis of liver abscess is relatively good, although patients with multiple liver abscesses still represent a serious problem. The prognosis depends primarily on the nature of the underlying disease. Complications of liver abscess include bacteremia, empyema, pneumonia, lung abscess, hepatobronchial fistula, rupture into the pericardium, peritonitis, subphrenic abscess, and metastatic abscesses in other organs.

Appropriate medical and surgical therapy of infections and other conditions that predispose to liver abscess will lower the incidence of this problem.

Splenic Abscess

Etiology

Splenic abscesses are uncommon. They usually are secondary to hematogenous dissemination of microorganisms. The original focus, of course, might be anywhere in the body. On occasion there may be direct inoculation related to surgery or trauma or spread of infection from nearby organs.

Bacteriology

Splenic abscesses secondary to endocarditis usually involve *Staphylococcus aureus* or various streptococci. Enterobacteriaceae, including *Salmonella*, have also been found. A polymicrobial flora is not unusual. Anaerobes have been recovered from a significant number of splenic abscesses; Table 9 is a summary of reports on splenic abscess involving anaerobes. Tuberculous splenic abscess is rare (285). Fungi, *Candida* species in particular, have been recovered from splenic abscesses in immunocompromised hosts; fungal splenic abscess is a part of the syndrome of hepatosplenic candidiasis. Blood cultures are positive in two thirds of patients with multiple splenic abscesses but in only a small percentage of those with solitary abscesses.

Pathogenesis

In addition to the background factors mentioned previously, splenic infarction is a relatively common underlying feature. The spleen may be seeded at the time of the infarction (e.g., with underlying endocarditis) or organisms may seed an area that had undergone infarction earlier. Patients with sickle cell disease may be predisposed on this basis. Hematoma may also predispose to splenic abscess. An enlarged spleen itself may develop subcapsular infarcts that may subsequently become infected and lead to abscess of the spleen.

Clinical Picture

Onset of illness associated with splenic abscess is often sudden, with chills and fever and left upper quadrant pain. When the upper pole of the spleen is involved, there is commonly left pleuritic pain radiating to the shoulder, elevation of the left diaphragm, and left pleural effusion. With lower pole abscess, there may be signs of peritoneal inflammation. In less than half of patients, the spleen is palpable and tender; rarely, a friction rub may be heard over the organ. Before the availability of modern imaging techniques, the diagnosis was frequently made late in the course of the illness or at autopsy. Because bacteremia is a common background for abscess of the spleen, many patients have abscesses in other organs such as the liver, kidneys, and brain. As noted earlier, endocarditis is a common underlying problem. Other complications in-

TABLE 9. *Splenic abscess involving anaerobes and microaerophiles*

Organism	No. isolates	Ref.
Gram-negative rods (GNR)		
Eikenella corrodens	1	318
Haemophilus aphrophilus	1	319
Actinobacillus	1	320
Bacteroides fragilis	8	219,321–327
Bacteroides sp.	several	328–330
Bacteroides melaninogenicus	3	324,331,332
Fusobacterium nucleatum	3	324,333,334
Fusobacterium necrophorum	3	329,334,335
Anaerobic GNR	2	324,336
Gram-positive cocci		
Microaerophilic *Strep.*	4	329,330,337
Streptococci milleri	2	327,338
Peptostrep. asaccharolyticus	1	339
Peptostreptococcus magnus	1	332
Peptostreptococcus sp.	6	324,329,332,338,340
Anaerobic *Strep.*	2	332
Nonsporing gram-positive rods		
Actinomyces israelii	1	341
Lactobacillus sp.	1	342
Eubacterium lentum	1	339
E. tenue	1	324
Eubacterium sp.	1	337
Propionibacterium acnes	1	343
P. avidum	1	344
Gram-positive *Coccobacillus*	1	324
Clostridia		
C. bifermentans	1	345
C. clostridioforme	1	345
C. perfringens	2	324,346
C. difficile	2	347,348
C. septicum	2	228,349
Clostridium sp.	4	327,346–348

clude thoracic empyema, subphrenic abscess, generalized peritonitis, and discharge of abscess contents into an adjacent viscus such as the colon or stomach.

Diagnosis

A high index of suspicion may be required. Splenic abscess should be considered in any patient with bacteremia and left upper quadrant symptoms or findings. Blood cultures, both aerobic and anaerobic, should be obtained; as noted earlier, bacteremia is relatively common. Leukocytosis is typically present but is not particularly helpful. Thrombocytosis is also commonly found (310), but this may be found in bacteremia and in various chronic bacterial infections. Roentgenograms may show compression of the gastric air shadow, displacement of other viscera, extraluminal gas or a gas-fluid level, elevation of the left diaphragm or left pleural effusion, left lower lung parenchymal infiltrates or atelectasis. Radionuclide scans (Fig. 9) and ultrasound are helpful diagnostically, but CT scan is the most useful diagnostic procedure.

Therapy

Surgery must be considered the procedure of choice presently (236) although increasing experience with per-

cutaneous drainage suggests that there is a role for this procedure (350), particularly for smaller solitary abscesses. Splenectomy is generally the surgical procedure of choice. Previously, when the spleen was grossly enlarged, surrounded by dense adhesions, and disrupted by extensive suppuration, patients were managed by spleno-

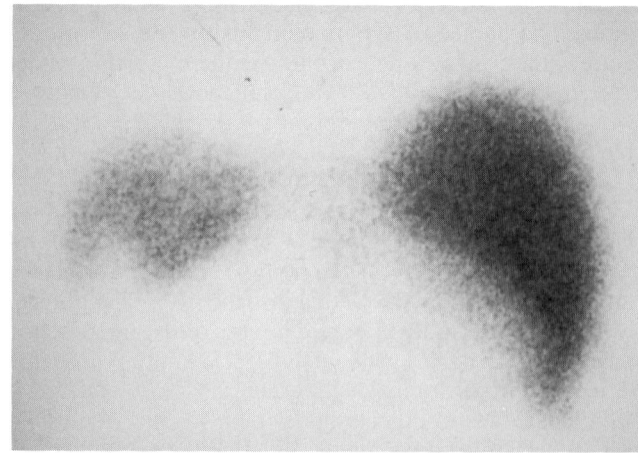

FIG. 9. Liver–spleen scan, posterior view. Note abscess in lower pole of spleen (*left*).

tomy and drainage of the abscess. With the early diagnosis that is now the rule with the available imaging techniques however, splenotomy is rarely necessary and presently splenectomy is the procedure of choice (328). Percutaneous drainage carries the potential risk of bleeding and of damage to neighboring organs. Adjunctive antimicrobial therapy plays an important role also. The specific agent(s) will depend on the nature of the organisms involved and their antimicrobial susceptibility. There is one report of successful treatment of a 5-cm solitary splenic abscess with antibiotics alone (339).

Prognosis

The ultimate prognosis of splenic abscess depends on the underlying process (324). Obviously, delay in diagnosis and definitive surgical therapy will lead to higher mortality. Higher mortality rates are also associated with the older age group, diabetes mellitus, alcoholism, and immunosuppressive disease or therapy (319). In two thirds of patients with abscess of the spleen, the infection is a terminal manifestation of uncontrolled disease of other organs, but often these patients have multiple small abscesses that produce no special clinical manifestations (328). Overall mortality rates may still be as high as 40% in unselected series (319).

Abdominal Actinomycosis

Etiology

The three major types of actinomycosis are cervicofacial, thoracic, and abdominal. Cervicofacial is clearly the most commonly encountered form; the other two varieties account for roughly 20% of cases each. The disease appears in a variety of forms from localized intraabdominal disease, to disease localized to the liver, to widespread involvement within the abdomen, and to widely disseminated disease. Hepatic involvement may be in the form of a small nodule (351), a pyogenic liver abscess (305), or multiple liver abscesses (304,312); involvement of the liver occurs in 15% of cases of abdominal actinomycosis. Miyamoto and Fang (305) present one case of pyogenic liver abscess and review 35 others from the literature. The ileocecal region of the intestine (and the appendix in particular) is the site most frequently involved in abdominal actinomycosis, but there are reports of involvement of the stomach, small bowel, rectum, sigmoid and transverse colon, liver, gallbladder, pancreas, pelvis (typically associated with intrauterine contraceptive devices) (352), and abdominal wall (353). Most often disease is limited to a single organ; disseminated infection is rare. It may be associated with an underlying disease such as neoplasm, appendicitis (354), or diverticulitis (355). The disease may originate in the thorax and extend through the diaphragm to involve the abdomen (356). A most unusual case of ruptured actinomycotic aneurysm of the splenic artery has been described (357).

Bacteriology

Any species of *Actinomyces* (*israelii, odontolyticus, naeslundii, viscosus, meyeri, georgiae,* or *gerencseriae*) may be involved as may *Propionibacterium propionicus* (formerly *Arachnia propionica*). Hill et al. (358) reported that *Eubacterium nodatum* may also be involved in pelvic infection in women using intrauterine contraceptive devices and that a clinical and pathological picture of actinomycosis may result. A variety of other anaerobic or microaerophilic bacteria may be found concurrently with the agents of actinomycosis, particularly pigmented anaerobic gram-negative bacilli and *Actinobacillus actinomycetemcomitans*.

Pathogenesis, Pathology

The causative agents of actinomycosis are part of the indigenous flora of the body. These agents may set up infection when some process such as surgery, trauma, or disease disrupts the mucosal barrier and lowers the oxidation–reduction potential so as to favor growth of anaerobic bacteria. In the case of abdominal actinomycosis, the Eh is normally quite low at the sites of normal carriage; furthermore, a number of *Actinomyces* are somewhat aerotolerant. Other predisposing factors are malignancy, the use of corticosteroids, and diabetes mellitus.

The disease typically spreads by direct extension, without regard for tissue planes, often producing sinus tracts or fistulae. The process classically involves suppuration, necrosis, acute and chronic inflammation, fibrosis, stricture formation, and obstruction.

Involvement of the liver in abdominal actinomycosis is usually due to spread via the portal vein from an intestinal source. However, it may occur by direct extension or via the hepatic artery during disseminated infection. It is not rare for no primary focus to be found (305).

Clinical Picture

The disease may be manifested by very firm, indurated masses or abscesses within the abdomen; sinus tracts and fistulae are relatively common. These classic findings may not be apparent, particularly early in the course of illness. The most common symptoms are pain, weight loss, and fever. Anorexia and chills may also be present, particularly with visceral involvement.

Hepatic actinomycosis has a nonspecific presentation and should be considered in the differential diagnosis of liver abscess and other space-occupying lesions of the liver.

Diagnosis

Diagnosis of abdominal actinomycosis is difficult and is usually not made without the aid of surgery or needle biopsy. Since this disease shows a predilection for the right iliac fossa, the diagnosis should be entertained in appropriate clinical settings. The classical findings of fibrotic induration, sinus tract and fistula formation, or abscess formation, when present, are very helpful in suggesting the possibility of actinomycosis although these findings are nonspecific. Among considerations in the differential diagnosis are carcinoma of the cecum, Crohn's disease, tuberculosis, and amebiasis. The presence of sulfur granules grossly visible in the pus from a draining sinus strongly enhances the possibility of actinomycosis.

Leukocytosis, elevated sedimentation rate, and elevated C-reactive protein are present but nonspecific. Elevation of the serum alkaline phosphotase is commonly present in liver abscess involving *Actinomyces* and related organisms but does not point to the specific etiology of the abscess. Conventional roentgenograms, ultrasound (359), and CT (360) are helpful in delineating masses, sinus tracts, and so forth, but definitive diagnosis depends on demonstrating the characteristic pathology and, specifically, sulfur granules on biopsy of appropriate materials (313,354). The sulfur granules are actually microcolonies of the organism with the eosinophilic, clubbed material at the edges of the granule in tissue sections representing the host response to the organism. On Gram stain, the organism is shown to be gram-positive with branching filaments. It is non–acid-fast, in contrast to *Nocardia* which is weakly acid-fast. The organisms of actinomycosis also show up well on Gomori methenamine-silver stain. Sulfur granules from pus should be cultured anaerobically and aerobically and crushed on a slide for Gram and acid-fast staining with a weak decolorizer. Cultures of pus or biopsy material for the agents of actinomycosis are positive in only 25–50% of cases that prove to be actinomycosis. The organisms are fastidious, even those that are relatively aerotolerant. Anaerobic blood cultures should be obtained.

Treatment

Most cases of intraabdominal actinomycosis require both surgical and antimicrobial therapy. The surgical approach depends on the exact nature and location of the disease process. The basic principles are incision and drainage of loculated pus, debridement, and excision of sinus tracts. Percutaneous drainage of abscesses may be adequate in selected cases (354), particularly in the case of isolated or even multiple liver abscesses (304,305). Intrauterine contraceptive devices should be removed in cases in which they served as the focus of the infection. Hyperbaric oxygen therapy failed in one patient on whom it was tried (353). Antimicrobial agents that are effective in actinomycosis include penicillin G, ampicillin, tetracycline, erythromycin, clindamycin, chloramphenicol, and imipenem. Penicillin G is the drug of choice for initiation of therapy and during periods of hospitalization. It should be given in high dosage—ordinarily 12–15 million units daily by the intravenous route in normal size adults with normal renal function. It must be kept in mind that certain of the agents may not be active against accompanying flora; for example, clindamycin is not active against *Actin-*

obacillus actinomycetemcomitans. Therapy, regardless of the agent employed, must be prolonged. The exact length of therapy will depend on the extent and location of disease and the speed of response, but ordinarily should not be for less than 6–9 months and often will need to be for a year or longer. CT is valuable for follow-up of patients on therapy (356).

Prognosis

Depending on the nature of any underlying disease (e.g., malignancy), most cases are amenable to cure but it is often necessary to do repeated surgeries or percutaneous drainage procedures and, as indicated above, antimicrobial therapy must be given for extended periods. Raz and Lev (353) describe a patient who had multiple relapses over a 7-year period despite long courses of several different antimicrobial agents, repeated surgical interventions, and even a course of hyperbaric oxygenation; this patient finally refused further therapy.

REFERENCES

1. Stewardson. Treatment of peritonitis. In: Elliotson J, ed. *Practice of medicine.* London: Carey & Hart; 1844:874.
2. Ahrenholz DH, Simmons RL. Peritonitis and other intraabdominal infections. In: Howard RJ, Simmons RL, eds. *Surgical infectious diseases.* 2nd ed. Norwalk: Appleton & Lange; 1988: 605–646.
3. Charney DI, Gouge SF. Chemical peritonitis secondary to intraperitoneal vancomycin. *Am J Kidney Dis* 1991;17:76–79.
4. Garcia-Tsao G. Spontaneous bacterial peritonitis. *Gastroenterol Clin North Am* 1992;21:257–275.
5. Andreu M, Sola R, Sitges-Serra A, et al. Risk factors for spontaneous bacterial peritonitis in cirrhotic patients with ascites. *Gastroenterology* 1993;104:1133–1138.
6. Richardet J-P, Beaugrand M. Infection péritonéale spontanée chez le cirrhotique. *Gastroenterol Clin Biol* 1991;15:239–249.
7. Targan SR, Chow AW, Guze LB. Role of anaerobic bacteria in spontaneous peritonitis of cirrhosis: report of two cases and review of the literature. *Am J Med* 1977;62:397–403.
8. Sheckman P, Onderdonk AB, Bartlett JG. Anaerobes in spontaneous peritonitis. *Lancet* 1977;2:1223.
9. Ziegler E. *The redox potential of the blood in vivo and in vitro, its measurement and significance.* Springfield, IL: Charles C Thomas; 1965:1–196.
10. Runyon BA, Morrissey RL, Hoefs JC, Wyle FA. Opsonic activity of human ascitic fluid: a potentially important protective mechanism against spontaneous bacterial peritonitis. *Hepatology* 1985;5:634–637.
11. McDougal WS, Izant RJ, Zollinger RM. Primary peritonitis in infancy and childhood. *Ann Surg* 1975;181:310–313.
12. Flament-Saillour M, de Truchis P, Risbourg M, Nordmann P. *Yersinia enterocolitica* peritonitis in an HIV-infected patient. *Clin Infect Dis;* in press.
13. Garcia M, Sanroman AL, Gisbert JP, Martin de Argila C, Moreira VF. Aeromonas sobria spontaneous bacterial peritonitis (letter). *Am J Gastroenterol* 1992;87:1890–1891.
14. Demirkan F, Akalin HE, Simsek H, Ozyilkan E, Telatar H. Spontaneous peritonitis due to *Brucella melitensis* in a patient with cirrhosis (letter). *Eur J Clin Microbiol Infect Dis* 1993;12: 66–67.
15. Gerding DN, Khan MY, Ewing JW, Hall WH. *Pasteurella multocida* peritonitis in hepatic cirrhosis with ascites. *Gastroenterology* 1976;70:413–415.
16. Leggiadro RJ, Lazar LF. Spontaneous bacterial peritonitis due

to *Neisseria meningitidis* serogroup Z in an infant with liver failure. *Clin Pediatr* 1991;30:350–352.

17. Pascual J, Sureda A, Lopez-San Roman A, et al. Spontaneous peritonitis caused by *Enterococcus faecium. J Clin Microbiol* 1990;28:1484–1486.

18. Toledo C, Salmeron JM, Rimola A, et al. Spontaneous bacterial peritonitis in cirrhosis: predictive factors of infection resolution and survival in patients. *Hepatology* 1993;17:251–257.

19. Christen RD, Moser R, Schlup P, Neftel KA. Fulminant group A streptococcal infections. Report of two cases. *Klin Wochenschr* 1990;68:427–430.

20. Runyon BA. Monomicrobial nonneutrocytic bacterascites: a variant of spontaneous bacterial peritonitis. *Hepatology* 1990; 12:710–715.

21. Tsurumi H, Tani K, Tajika K, et al. Spontaneous bacterial peritonitis due to *Clostridium perfringens* in a patient with liver cirrhosis and pure red cell aplasia. *Gastroenterol Jpn* 1992;27: 662–667.

22. Herman R, Goldman IS, Bronzo R, McKinley MJ. *Clostridium cadaveris:* an unusual cause of spontaneous bacterial peritonitis. *Am J Gastroenterol* 1992;87:140–142.

23. Propst T, Propst A, Schauer G, Judmaier G, Braunsteiner H, Vogel W. Spontane bakterielle peritonitis bei chronischer Lebererkrankung mit aszites. *Dtsch Med Wochenschr* 1993;118: 943–946.

24. Wilcox CM, Forsmark CE, Darragh TM, Yen TS, Cello JP. Cytomegalovirus peritonitis in a patient with the acquired immunodeficiency syndrome. *Dig Dis Sci* 1992;37:1288–1291.

25. Fowler R. Primary peritonitis: Changing aspects 1956–1970. *Aust Paediatr J* 1971;7:73–83.

26. Armitage TG, Williamson RCN. Primary peritonitis in children and adults. *Postgrad Med J* 1983;59:21–24.

27. Ho H, Guerra LG, Zuckerman MJ, Pere JF, Polly SM. Urinary tract infection: a predisposing factor for spontaneous bacterial peritonitis. *Gastroenterology* 1990;98:A593.

28. Bruyn GAW. Spontaneous pneumococcal peritonitis in young women. *Clin Infect Dis* 1993;16:728–729.

29. Rimola A, Soto R, Bory F, Arroyo V, Piera C, Rodes J. Reticuloendothelial system phagocytic activity in cirrhosis and its relation to bacterial infections and prognosis. *Hepatology* 1984; 4:53–58.

30. Wyke RJ, Rajkovic IA, Williams R. Impaired opsonization by serum from patients with chronic liver disease. *Clin Exp Immunol* 1983;51:91–98.

31. DeMeo AN, Anderson BR. Defective chemotaxis associated with a serum inhibitor in cirrhotic patients. *N Engl J Med* 1982; 286:635–640.

32. Fierer J, Finley F. Deficient serum bactericidal activity against *Escherichia coli* in patients with cirrhosis of the liver. *J Clin Invest* 1979;63:912–921.

33. Rajkovic IA, Williams R. Abnormalities of neutrophil phagocytosis, intracellular killing and metabolic activity in alcoholic cirrhosis and hepatitis. *Hepatology* 1986;6:252–262.

34. Bird G, Senaldi G, Panos M, et al. Activation of the classical complement pathway in spontaneous bacterial peritonitis. *Gut* 1992;33:307–311.

35. Fromkes JJ, Thomas FB, Mekhjam HS, et al. Antimicrobial activity of human ascitic fluid. *Gastroenterology* 1977;73: 668–672.

36. Deviere J, Content J, Crusiaux A, DuPont E. IL-6 and TNF alpha in ascitic fluid during spontaneous bacterial peritonitis. *Dig Dis Sci* 1991;36:123–124.

37. Xiol X, Castellote J, Baiellas C, et al. Spontaneous bacterial empyema in cirrhotic patients: analysis of eleven cases. *Hepatology* 1990;11:365–370.

38. Runyon BA, Canawati HN, Akriviadis EA. Optimization of ascitic fluid culture technique. *Gastroenterology* 1988;95: 1351–1355.

39. Runyon BA, Antillon MR, Akriviadis EA, McHutchison JG. Bedside inoculation of blood culture bottles with ascitic fluid is superior to delayed inoculation in the detection of spontaneous bacterial peritonitis. *J Clin Microbiol* 1990;28:2811–2812.

40. Siersema PD, de Marie S, van Zeijl JH, Bac D-J, Wilson JHP. Blood culture bottles are superior to lysis-centrifugation tubes

41. Akriviadis EA, Runyon BA. Utility of an algorithm in differentiating spontaneous from secondary bacterial peritonitis. *Gastroenterology* 1990;98:127–133.

42. Felisart J, Rimola A, Arroyo V, et al. Cefotaxime is more effective than is ampicillin-tobramycin in cirrhotics with severe infections. *Hepatology* 1985;5:457–462.

43. Gómez-Jiménez J, Ribera E, Gasser I, et al. Randomized trial comparing ceftriaxone with cefonicid for treatment of spontaneous bacterial peritonitis in cirrhotic patients. *Antimicrob Agents Chemother* 1993;37:1587–1592.

44. Runyon BA, McHutchison JG, Antillon MR, Akriviadis EA, Montano AA. Short-course versus long-course antibiotic treatment of spontaneous bacterial peritonitis. A randomized controlled study of 100 patients. *Gastroenterology* 1991;100: 1737–1742.

45. Zeni F, Tardy B, Vindimian M, et al. High levels of tumor necrosis factor-alpha and interleukin-6 in the ascitic fluid of cirrhotic patients with spontaneous bacterial peritonitis. *Clin Infect Dis* 1993;17:218–223.

46. Gines P, Rimola A, Planas R, et al. Norfloxacin prevents spontaneous bacterial peritonitis recurrence in cirrhosis: results of a double-blind, placebo-controlled trial. *Hepatology* 1990;12: 716–724.

47. Park SI, Genta RS, Romeo DP, Weesner RE. Colonic abscess and focal peritonitis secondary to India ink tattooing of the colon. *Gastrointest Endosc* 1991;37:68–71.

48. Giannella RA, Broitman SA, Zamcheck N. Gastric acid barrier to ingested microorganisms in man: studies in vivo and in vitro. *Gut* 1993;13:251–256.

49. Franklin MA, Skoryna SC. Studies on natural gastric flora. I. Bacterial flora of fasting human subjects. *Can Med Assoc J* 1966;95:1349–1355.

50. Gorbach SL, Nahas L, Lerner PI, Weinstein L. Studies of intestinal microflora. I. Effects of diet, age, and periodic sampling on numbers of fecal microorganisms in man. *Gastroenterology* 1967;53:845–855.

51. Finegold SM, Sutter VL, Mathisen GE. Normal indigenous intestinal flora. In: Hentges DJ, ed. *Human intestinal microflora in health and disease.* New York: Academic Press; 1983:3–31.

52. Drasar BS, Hill MJ. *Human intestinal flora.* New York: Academic Press; 1974:1–263.

53. Nichols RL, Smith JW. Intragastric microbial colonization in common disease states of the stomach and duodenum. *Ann Surg* 1975;182:557–561.

54. Finegold SM, Mathisen GE, George WL. Changes in human intestinal flora related to the administration of antimicrobial agents. In: Hentges DJ, ed. *Human intestinal microflora in health and disease.* New York: Academic Press; 1983:355–446.

55. Marshall JC, Christou NV, Horn R, Meakins JL. The microbiology of multiple organ failure. The proximal gastrointestinal tract as an occult reservoir of pathogens. *Arch Surg* 1988;123: 309–315.

56. Bartlett JG, Onderdonk AB, Drude E, et al. Quantitative bacteriology of the vaginal flora. *J Infect Dis* 1977;136:271–277.

57. Levison ME, Korman LC, Carrington ER, Kaye D. Quantitative microflora of the vagina. *Am J Obstet Gynecol* 1977;127: 80–85.

58. Levison ME, Trestman I, Quach R, Sladowski C, Floro CN. Quantitative bacteriology of the vaginal flora. *Am J Obstet Gynecol* 1979;133:139–144.

59. Onderdonk AB, Zamarchi GR, Walsh JA, Mellor RD, Muñoz A, Kass EH. Method for quantitative and qualitative evaluation of vaginal microflora during menstruation. *Appl Environ Microbiol* 1986;51:333–339.

60. Mårdh PA. The vaginal ecosystem. *Am J Obstet Gynecol* 1991; 165:1163–1168.

61. Hillier SL, Krohn MA, Rabe LK, Klebanoff SJ, Eschenbach DA. The normal vaginal flora, H_2O_2-producing lactobacilli, and bacterial vaginosis in pregnant women. *Clin Infect Dis* 1993; 16(Suppl 4):S273–S281.

62. Haukamaa M, Stranden P, Jousimies-Somer H, Siitonen A.

Bacterial flora of the cervix in women using different methods of contraception. *Am J Obstet Gynecol* 1986;154:520–524.

63. Holdsworth RJ. Fatal postoperative gastric necrosis caused by *Clostridium perfringens. Eur J Surg* 1992;158:447–449.

64. Shinagawa N, Muramoto M, Sakurai S, et al. A bacteriological study of perforated duodenal ulcers. *Jpn J Surg* 1991;21:1–7.

65. Mosdell DM, Morris DM, Voltura A, et al. Antibiotic treatment for surgical peritonitis. *Ann Surg* 1991;214:543–549.

66. Sirinek KR. Management of intraabdominal infections. *Pharmacotherapy* 1991;11:99S–104S.

67. Bennion RS, Thompson JE, Baron EJ, Finegold SM. Gangrenous and perforated appendicitis with peritonitis—treatment and bacteriology. *Clin Ther* 1990;12:31–44.

68. Nichols RL, Muzik AC. Enterococcal infections in surgical patients: the mystery continues. *Clin Infect Dis* 1992;15:72–76.

69. Dougherty SH, Flohr AB, Simmons RL. "Breakthrough" enterococcal septicemia in surgical patients. 19 cases and a review of the literature. *Arch Surg* 1983;118:232–238.

70. Rotstein OD, Meakins JL. Diagnostic and therapeutic challenges of intraabdominal infections. *World J Surg* 1990;14:159–166.

71. Rotstein OD, Pruett TL, Simmons RL. Microbiologic features and treatment of persistent peritonitis in patients in the intensive care unit. *Can J Surg* 1986;29:247–250.

72. Mollitt DL, Tepas JJI, Talbert JL. The microbiology of neonatal peritonitis. *Arch Surg* 1988;123:176–179.

73. Kujath P, Lerch K, Dammrich J. Fluconazole monitoring in *Candida* peritonitis based on histological control. *Mycoses* 1990;33:441–448.

74. Godet AS, Williams RD. Postoperative *Clostridium difficile* gastroenteritis. *J Urol* 1993;149:142–144.

75. Saura P, Vallés J, Jubert P, Ormaza J, Segura F. Spontaneous rupture of the spleen in a patient with legionellosis. *Clin Infect Dis* 1993;17:298.

76. Chetrit B, Lesur G, Bergemer AM, et al. [Listeria monocytogenes ascites infection in a patient with peritoneal carcinosis (letter)]. *Gastroenterol Clin Biol* 1991;15:861.

77. Yanagisawa N, Tomiyasu H, Hada T, et al. *Chlamydia trachomatis* peritonitis: report of a patient presenting spontaneous regression of ascites. *Intern Med* 1992;31:835–839.

78. Dawson JM, O'Riordan B, Chopra S. Ovarian actinomycosis presenting as acute peritonitis. *Aust N Z J Surg* 1992;62:161–163.

79. Chow AW, Guze LB. *Bacteroidaceae* bacteremia: clinical experience with 112 patients. *Medicine* (Baltimore) 1974;53:93–126.

80. Fry DE, Garrison RN, Polk HC Jr. Clinical implications in bacteroides bacteremia. *Surg Gynecol Obstet* 1979;149:189–192.

81. Bodner SJ, Koenig MG, Goodman JS. Bacteremic *Bacteroides* infections. *Ann Intern Med* 1970;73:537–544.

82. Gelb AF, Seligman SJ. Bacteroidaceae bacteremia. Effect of age and focus of clinical course. *JAMA* 1970;212:1038–1041.

83. Lee JT, Jr., Ahrenholz DN, Nelson RD, Simmons RL. Mechanisms of the adjuvant effect of hemoglobin in experimental peritonitis. V. The significance of the coordinated iron component. *Surgery* 1979;86:41–48.

84. Gharbia SE, Shah HN. Hydrolytic enzymes liberated by black-pigmented gram-negative anaerobes. *FEMS Immunol Med Microbiol* 1993;6:139–146.

85. Niederman R, Brunkhorst B, Smith S, Weinreb RN, Ryder MI. Ammonia as a potential mediator of adult human periodontal infection: inhibition of neutrophil function. *Arch Oral Biol* 1990;35:Suppl:205S–209S.

86. Dunn DL, Barke RA, Knight NB, Humphrey EW, Simmons RL. Role of resident macrophages, peripheral neutrophils, and translymphatic absorption in bacterial clearance from the peritoneal cavity. *Infect Immun* 1985;49:257–264.

87. Rotstein OD. Role of fibrin deposition in the pathogenesis of intraabdominal infection. *Eur J Clin Microbiol Infect Dis* 1992;11:1064–1068.

88. Hau T. Bacteria, toxins, and the peritoneum. *World J Surg* 1990;14:167–175.

89. Gharbia SE, Shah HN. Interactions between black-pigmented

90. Schein M, Decker GA. Gastrointestinal fistulas associated with large abdominal wall defects: experience with 43 patients. *Br J Surg* 1990;77:97–100.

91. Pollock AV. Nonoperative antiinfective treatment of intraabdominal infections. *World J Surg* 1990;14:227–230.

92. Farthmann EH, Schöffel U. Principles and limitations of operative management of intraabdominal infections. *World J Surg* 1990;14:210–217.

93. MacFayden BV Jr, Wolfe BM, McKernan JB. Laparoscopic management of the acute abdomen, appendix, and small and large bowel. *Surg Clin North Am* 1992;72:1169–1183.

94. Stabile BE. Therapeutic options in acute diverticulitis. *Compr Ther* 1991;17:26–33.

95. Gorbach SL. Treatment of intra-abdominal infections. *J Antimicrob Chemother* 1993;31(Suppl A):67–78.

96. Nichols RL, Smith JW, Klein DB, et al. Risk of infection after penetrating abdominal trauma. *N Engl J Med* 1984;311:1065–1070.

97. Solomkin JS, Dellinger EP, Christou NV, Busuttil RW. Results of a multicenter trial comparing imipenem/cilastatin to tobramycin/clindamycin for intra-abdominal infections. *Ann Surg* 1990;212:581–591.

98. Henry SA. Overall clinical experience with aztreonam in the treatment of intraabdominal infections. *Rev Infect Dis* 1985;7:729–733.

99. Berne TV, Yellin AE, Appleman MD, Gill MA, Chenella FC, Heseltine PN. Surgically treated gangrenous or perforated appendicitis. A comparison of aztreonam and clindamycin versus gentamicin and clindamycin. *Ann Surg* 1987;205:133–137.

100. Williams RR, Hotchkin D. Aztreonam plus clindamycin versus tobramycin plus clindamycin in the treatment of intraabdominal infections. *Rev Infect Dis* 1991;13(Suppl 7):S629–S633.

101. Bubrick MP, Heim-Duthoy KL, Yellin AE, et al. Ceftazidime/clindamycin in the treatment of intraabdominal infections. *Am Surg* 1990;56:613–617.

102. Smith JA. Treatment of intra-abdominal infections with quinolones. *Eur J Clin Microbiol Infect Dis* 1991;10:330–333.

103. Finegold SM, Jousimies-Somer HR, Wexler HM. Current perspectives on anaerobic infections: diagnostic approaches. *Infect Dis Clin North Am* 1993;7:257–275.

104. Solomkin JS, Meakins JL Jr, Allo MD, Dellinger EP, Simmons RL. Antibiotic trials in intra-abdominal infections. A critical evaluation of study design and outcome reporting. *Ann Surg* 1984;200:29–39.

105. Dellinger EP. Design and evaluation of clinical trials of antimicrobial agents in surgery. *Surg Gynecol Obstet* 1991;172(Suppl):65–72.

106. Nystrom PO, Bax R, Dellinger EP, et al. Proposed definitions for diagnosis, severity scoring, stratification, and outcome for trials on intraabdominal infection. *World J Surg* 1990;14:148–158.

107. Yellin AE, Berne TV, Heseltine PN, et al. Prospective randomized study of two different doses of clindamycin admixed with gentamicin in the management of perforated appendicitis. *Am Surg* 1993;59:248–255.

108. Corder AP, Prior JE, Bates T, Harrison M, Donaldson PJ. Metronidazole versus cefoxitin in severe appendicitis: a trial to compare a single intraoperative dose of two antibiotics given intravenously. *Postgrad Med J* 1983;59:720–723.

109. Oh SJ, Halsey JH Jr, Briggs DD Jr. Guanidine in type B botulism. *Arch Intern Med* 1975;135:726–728.

110. Wilson SE, Boswick JA Jr, Duma RJ, et al. Cephalosporin therapy in intraabdominal abscess. A multicenter randomized, comparative study of cefotetan, moxalactam, and cefoxitin. *Am J Surg* 1988;155:61–66.

111. Najem AZ, Kaminski ZC, Spillert CR, Lazaro EJ. Comparative study of parenteral piperacillin and cefoxitin in the treatment of surgical infections of the abdomen. *Surg Gynecol Obstet* 1983;157:423–425.

112. Paakkonen M, Alhava EM, Huttunen R, et al. Piperacillin com-

pared with cefuroxime plus metronidazole in diffuse peritonitis. *Eur J Surg* 1991;157:535–537.

113. Foster MC, Kapila L, Morris DL, Slack RC. A randomized comparative study of sulbactam plus ampicillin vs metronidazole plus cefotaxime in the management of acute appendicitis in children. *Rev Infect Dis* 1986;8:634–638.

114. Fink MP, Helsmoortel CM, Arous EJ, et al. Comparison of the safety and efficacy of parenteral ticarcillin/clavulanate and clindamycin/gentamicin in serious intra-abdominal infections. *J Antimicrob Chemother* 1989;24(Suppl B):147–156.

115. Pastorek JG Jr, Aldridge KE, Cunningham GL, et al. Comparison of ticarcillin plus clavulanic acid with cefoxitin in the treatment of female pelvic infection. *Am J Med* 1985;79:161–163.

116. Sirinek KR, Levine BA. A randomized trial of ticarcillin and clavulanate versus gentamicin and clindamycin in patients with complicated appendicitis. *Surg Gynecol Obstet* 1991;172(Suppl):30–35.

117. Solomkin JS, Fant WK, Rivera JO, Alexander JW. Randomized trial of imipenem/cilastatin versus gentamicin and clindamycin in mixed flora infections. *Am J Med* 1985;78:85–91.

118. Scandinavian Study Group. Imipenem/cilastatin versus gentamicin/clindamycin for treatment of serious bacterial infections. *Lancet* 1984;1:868–871.

119. Bennion RS, Thompson JE Jr, Baron EJ, Schmit PJ, Finegold SM. The use of single-agent antibacterial regimens in the treatment of advanced appendicitis with peritonitis. *Drug Invest* 1992;4(Suppl 1):7–12.

120. Pine RW, Wertz MJ, Lennard ES, Dellinger EP, Carrico CJ, Minshew BH. Determinants of organ malfunction or death in patients with intraabdominal sepsis. A discriminant analysis. *Arch Surg* 1983;118:242–249.

121. Meakins JL, Wicklund B, Forse RA. The surgical intensive care unit: Current concepts in infection. *Surg Clin North Am* 1980;60:117.

122. Gorbach SL. Antimicrobial prophylaxis for appendectomy and colorectal surgery. *Rev Infect Dis* 1991;13(Suppl 10):S815–S820.

123. Antimicrobial prophylaxis in surgery. *Med Lett* 1992;34:5–8.

124. Condon RE, Bartlett JG, Greenlee H, et al. Efficacy of oral and systemic antibiotic prophylaxis in colorectal operations. *Arch Surg* 1983;118:496–502.

125. Schoetz DJ Jr, Roberts PL, Murray JJ, Coller JA, Veidenheimer MC. Addition of parenteral cefoxitin to regimen of oral antibiotics for elective colorectal operations. *Ann Surg* 1990;212:209–212.

126. Popovich RP, Moncrief JW, Decherd JF, Bonner JB, Pyle WK. The definition of a novel portable-wearable equilibrium peritoneal technique (abst). *Abst Am Soc Artif Intern Organs* 1976;5:64.

127. Popovich RP, Moncrief JW, Nolph KD, et al. Continuous ambulatory peritoneal dialysis. *Ann Intern Med* 1978;88:449–456.

128. Nolph KD. Continuous ambulatory peritoneal dialysis as long-term treatment for end-stage renal disease. *Am J Kidney Dis* 1991;17:154–157.

129. Korbet SM, Vonesh EF, Firanek CA. A retrospective assessment of risk factors for peritonitis among an urban CAPD population. *Perit Dial Int* 1993;13:126–131.

130. Saklayen MG. CAPD peritonitis: incidence, pathogens, diagnosis, and management. *Med Clin North Am* 1990;74:997–1011.

131. Linblad AS, Novak JW, Nolph KD, Stablein DM, Cutler SJ. The 1987 USA National CAPD Registry report. *Trans Am Soc Artif Intern Organs* 1988;34:150–156.

132. Swartz RD. Chronic peritoneal dialysis: mechanical and infectious complications. *Nephron* 1987;40:29–37.

133. Rubin J, Ray R, Barnes T, Teal H, Hellems E, Bernheim J. Peritonitis in continuous ambulatory peritoneal dialysis patients. *Am J Kidney Dis* 1983;11:602–607.

134. Steinberg SM, Cutler SJ, Novak JK, Nolph KD. Report of the National CAPD Registry of the National Institutes of Health: characteristics of participants and selected outcome measures for the period January 1, 1981 through August 31, 1984. In: National CAPD Registry of the National Institute of Arthritis, Diabetes, and Digestive and Kidney Diseases. Washington DC: U.S. Public Health Service, 1985.

135. Howard RL, Millspaugh J, Teitelman I. Adult and pediatric peritonitis rates in a home dialysis program: comparison of continuous ambulatory and continuous cycling peritoneal dialysis. *Am J Kidney Dis* 1990;16:469–472.

136. Powell D, San Louis E, Calvin S, et al. Peritonitis in children undergoing continuous ambulatory peritoneal dialysis. *Am J Dis Child* 1985;139:29–32.

137. McClung MR. Peritonitis in children receiving continuous ambulatory peritoneal dialysis. *Pediatr Infect Dis* 1983;2:328–332.

138. Horton MW, Deeter RG, Sherman RA. Treatment of peritonitis in patients undergoing continuous ambulatory peritoneal dialysis. *Clin Pharm* 1990;9:102–118.

139. Von Graevenitz A, Amsterdam D. Microbiological aspects of peritonitis associated with continuous ambulatory peritoneal dialysis. *Clin Microbiol Rev* 1992;5:36–48.

140. Ashline V, Stevens A, Carter MJ. Nosocomial peritonitis related to contaminated dialysate warming water. *Am J Infect Control* 1981;9:50–52.

141. Krotrapelli R, Duffy WB, Lacke C, et al. *Pseudomonas* peritonitis and continuous ambulatory peritoneal dialysis. *Arch Intern Med* 1982;142:1862–1863.

142. Kaczmarski EB, Tooth JA, Anastassiades E, Manos J, Gokal R. *Pseudomonas* peritonitis with continuous ambulatory peritoneal dialysis: six year study. *Am J Kidney Dis* 1988;14:413–417.

143. Eisenberg ES, Leviton I, Soeiro R. Fungal peritonitis in patients receiving peritoneal dialysis: experience with eleven patients and review of the literature. *Rev Infect Dis* 1986;8:309–321.

144. Dressler R, Peters AT, Lynn RI. Pseudomonal and candidal peritonitis as a complication of continuous ambulatory peritoneal dialysis in human immunodeficiency virus-infected patients. *Am J Med* 1989;86:787–790.

145. Dunmire RB, Breyer JA. Nontuberculous mycobacterial peritonitis during continuous ambulatory peritoneal dialysis: case report and review of diagnostic and therapeutic strategies. *Am J Kidney Dis* 1991;18:126–130.

146. Hakim A, Hisam N, Reuman PD. Environmental mycobacterial peritonitis complicating peritoneal dialysis: three cases and review. *Clin Infect Dis* 1993;16:426–431.

147. Band JD, Ward JI, Fraser DW, et al. Peritonitis due to *Mycobacterium chelonae*–like organism associated with intermittent chronic peritoneal dialysis. *J Infect Dis* 1982;145:9–17.

148. Struijk DG, Van Ketel RJ, Krediet RT, et al. Viral peritonitis in a continuous ambulatory peritoneal dialysis patient. *Nephron* 1986;44:384.

149. Gibb AO, Aggarwal R, Sainson CO. Successful treatment of *Prototheca* peritonitis complicating continuous ambulatory peritoneal dialysis. *J Infect* 1991;22:183–185.

150. Ludlam H, Jayre D, Philips I. *Mycobacterium tuberculosis* as a cause of peritonitis in a patient undergoing continuous ambulatory peritoneal dialysis. *J Infect* 1986;12:75–77.

151. Prowant B, Nolph K, Ryan L, et al. Peritonitis in continuous ambulatory peritoneal dialysis: analysis of an 8-year experience. *Nephron* 1986;43:105–109.

152. Tranaeus A, Heimburger O, Granqvist S. Diverticular diseases of the colon: a risk factor for peritonitis in continuous ambulatory peritoneal dialysis. *Nephrol Dial Transplant* 1990;5:141–147.

153. Marrie TJ, Noble MA, Costerton JW. Examination of the morphology of bacteria adhering to peritoneal dialysis catheters by scanning and transmission electron microscopy. *J Clin Microbiol* 1983;18:1388–1398.

154. Peterson PK, Matzke G, Keane WK. Current concepts in the management of peritonitis in patients undergoing continuous ambulatory peritoneal dialysis. *Rev Infect Dis* 1987;9:604–612.

155. Holmes CJ, Evands R. Biofilm and foreign body infection—the significance to CAPD associated peritonitis. *Perit Dial Bull* 1986;6:168–177.

156. Verbrugh HA, Keane WF, Conroy WE, Peterson PK. Bacterial growth and killing in continuous ambulatory peritoneal dialysis fluids. *J Clin Microbiol* 1984;20:199–203.

157. Sheth NK, Bartell CA, Roth DA. In vitro study of bacterial

growth in continuous ambulatory peritoneal dialysis fluids. *J Clin Microbiol* 1986;23:1096–1098.

158. Lewis S, Holmes C. Host defense mechanisms in the peritoneal cavity of continuous ambulatory peritoneal dialysis patients. *Perit Dial Int* 1991;11:14–21.

159. Duwe AK, Vas SI, Weatherhead JW. Effects of the composition of peritoneal dialysis fluid on chemiluminescence, phagocytosis, and bactericidal activity in vitro. *Infect Immun* 1981;33:130–135.

160. Gordon DL, Rice JL, Avery VM. Surface phagocytosis and host defense in the peritoneal cavity during continuous ambulatory peritoneal dialysis. *Eur J Clin Microbiol* 1990;9:191–197.

161. De Vechi AF, Kopple JD, Young GA, et al. Plasma and dialysate immunoglobulin G in continuous ambulatory peritoneal dialysis patients: a multicenter study. *Am J Nephrol* 1990;10:451–456.

162. Tranaeus A, Heimburger O, Lindholm B. Peritonitis in continuous ambulatory peritoneal dialysis (CAPD): diagnostic findings, therapeutic outcome, and complications. *Perit Dial Int* 1989;9:179–190.

163. Males B, Walshe JJ, Amsterdam D. Laboratory indices of clinical peritonitis: total leukocyte count, microscopy, and microbiologic culture of peritoneal dialysis effluent. *J Clin Microbiol* 1987;25:2367–2371.

164. Korzets Z, Korzets A, Golan E, Zevin D, Bernheim J. CAPD peritonitis—initial presentation as an acute abdomen with a clear peritoneal effluent. *Clin Nephrol* 1992;37:155–157.

165. Flanigan MJ, Freeman RM, Lim VS. Cellular response to peritonitis among peritoneal dialysis patients. *Am J Kidney Dis* 1985;6:420–424.

166. Digenis GE, Khanna K, Panatlony D. Eosinophilia after implantation of the peritoneal catheter. *Perit Dial Bull* 1982;2:98–99.

167. Gokal R, Ramos JM, Ward MK, Kerr DNS. "Eosinophilic" peritonitis in continuous ambulatory peritoneal dialysis (CAPD). *Clin Nephrol* 1981;15:328–330.

168. Ludlam HA, Price TNC, Berry AJ, Phillips I. Laboratory diagnosis of peritonitis in patients on continuous ambulatory peritoneal dialysis. *J Clin Microbiol* 1988;26:1757–1762.

169. Bailie GR, Eisele G. Continuous ambulatory peritoneal dialysis: a review of its mechanics, advantages, complications, and areas of controversy. *Ann Pharmacother* 1992;26:1409–1420.

170. Krothapalli RK, Senekjian HO, Ayus JC. Efficacy of intravenous vancomycin in the treatment of gram-positive peritonitis in long-term peritoneal dialysis. *Am J Med* 1983;75:345–348.

171. Bailie GR, Morton R, Ganguli L, et al. Intravenous or intraperitoneal vancomycin for the treatment of continuous ambulatory peritoneal dialysis associated with gram-positive peritonitis? *Nephron* 1987;46:316–318.

172. Morse GD, Farolino DF, Apicella MA, et al. Comparative study of intraperitoneal and intravenous vancomycin pharmacokinetics during continuous ambulatory peritoneal dialysis. *Antimicrob Agents Chemother* 1987;31:173–177.

173. Merchant MR, Anwar N, Were A, et al. Imipenem versus netilmicin and vancomycin in the treatment of CAPD peritonitis. *Adv Perit Dial* 1992;8:234–237.

174. Cheng IK, Chan CY, Wong WT. A randomised prospective comparison of oral ofloxacin and intraperitoneal vancomycin in the treatment of bacterial peritonitis complicating continuous ambulatory peritoneal dialysis. *Perit Dial Int* 1991;11:27–30.

175. Nikolaidis P. Newer quinolones in the treatment of continuous ambulatory peritoneal dialysis (CAPD) related infections. *Perit Dial Int* 1990;10:127–133.

176. Dratwa M, Glupczynski Y, Lameire N, et al. Treatment of gram-negative peritonitis in patients undergoing continuous ambulatory peritoneal dialysis. *Rev Infect Dis* 1991;13(Suppl 7):S645–647.

177. Peterson J, Stewart RD, Catto GR, et al. Pharmacokinetics of intraperitoneal cefotaxime treatment of peritonitis in patients on continuous ambulatory peritoneal dialysis. *Nephron* 1985;40:79–82.

178. Flanigan MJ, Lim VS. Initial treatment of dialysis associated peritonitis: a controlled trial of vancomycin versus cefazolin. *Perit Dial Int* 1991;11:31–37.

179. Golper TA, Hartstein AI. Analysis of the causative pathogens in uncomplicated CAPD-associated peritonitis: duration of therapy, relapses, and prognosis. *Am J Kidney Dis* 1986;7:141–145.

180. Juergensen PH, Finklestein FO, Brennan R, et al. *Pseudomonas* peritonitis associated with continuous ambulatory peritoneal dialysis: a six year study. *Am J Kidney Dis* 1988;11:413–417.

181. Krothapalli R, Duff WB, Lack CH, et al. *Pseudomonas* peritonitis and continuous ambulatory peritoneal dialysis. *Arch Intern Med* 1982;142:1862–1863.

182. Bennet-Jones D, Wass V, Mawson P, et al. A comparison of intraperitoneal and intravenous/oral antibiotics in CAPD peritonitis. *Perit Dial Bull* 1987;7:31–33.

183. Keane WF, Everett ED, Fine RN, et al. CAPD related peritonitis management and antibiotic therapy recommendations: Travenol Peritonitis Management Advisory Committee. *Perit Dial Bull* 1987;7:55–62.

184. Keller E, Teetze P, Schollmeyer P. Drug therapy in patients undergoing continuous ambulatory peritoneal dialysis. Clinical pharmacokinetic considerations. *Clin Pharmacokinet* 1990;18:104–117.

185. Rubin J, Kirchner K, Walsh D, Green M, Bower J. Fungal peritonitis during continuous ambulatory peritoneal dialysis: a report of 17 cases. *Am J Kidney Dis* 1987;10:361–368.

186. Eisenberg ES. Intraperitoneal flucytosine in the management of fungal peritonitis in patients on continuous ambulatory peritoneal dialysis. *Am J Kidney Dis* 1988;11:465–467.

187. Venning MC, Ford M, Gould GK. Successful treatment of fungal peritonitis in CAPD using oral fluconazole. *Nephrol Dial Transplant* 1990;5:555.

188. Nagappan R, Collins JF, Lee WT. Fungal peritonitis in continuous ambulatory peritoneal dialysis—the Auckland experience. *Am J Kidney Dis* 1992;20:492–496.

189. Rubin J, Nolph K, Arfania D, et al. Follow-up of peritoneal clearances in patients undergoing continuous ambulatory peritoneal dialysis. *Kidney Int* 1979;16:619–623.

190. Smith JL, Flanigan MJ. Peritoneal dialysis catheter sepsis: a medical and surgical dilemma. *Am J Surg* 1987;154:602–607.

191. Valente J, Rappaport W. Continuous ambulatory peritoneal dialysis associated with peritonitis in older patients. *Am J Surg* 1990;159:579–581.

192. Sharma BK, Smith EC, Rodriquez H, et al. Trial of oral neomycin during peritoneal dialysis. *Am J Med Sci* 1971;262:175–178.

193. Axelrod J, Meyers BR, Hirschman SZ, et al. Prophylaxis with cephalothin in peritoneal dialysis. *Arch Intern Med* 1973;132:368–371.

194. Low DE, Vas SI, Oreopoulos DG, et al. Randomized clinical trial of prophylactic cephalexin in CAPD. *Lancet* 1980;2:753–754.

195. Churchill DN, Taylor DW, Vas SI, et al. Peritonitis in continuous ambulatory peritoneal dialysis patients: a randomized clinical trial of co-trimoxazole prophylaxis. *Perit Dial Bull* 1988;8:125–128.

196. Rubin J, McElroy R. Peritonitis secondary to dialysis tubing contamination among patients undergoing continuous ambulatory peritoneal dialysis. *Am J Kidney Dis* 1989;14:92–95.

197. Luzar MA. Peritonitis prevention in continuous ambulatory peritoneal dialysis. *Nephrologie* 1992;13:171–177.

198. Perez-Fontan M, Rosales M, Rodriguez-Carmona A, et al. Treatment of *Staphylococcus aureus* nasal carriers in CAPD with mupirocin. *Adv Perit Dial* 1992;8:242–245.

199. Swartz R, Messana J, Starmann B, Weber M, Reynolds J. Preventing *Staphylococcus aureus* infection during chronic peritoneal dialysis. *J Am Soc Nephrol* 1991;2:1085–1091.

200. Poole-Warren LA, Hallett MD, Hone PW, Burder SH, Farrell PC. Vaccination for prevention of CAPD associated staphylococcal infection: results of a prospective multicentre clinical trial. *Clin Nephrol* 1991;35:198–206.

201. Scatizzi A, Strippoli P. Prevention of *Staphylococcus aureus* peritonitis in continuous ambulatory peritoneal dialysis. In: Smeby LC, Jorstad S, Weideroe TE, eds. *Immune and meta-*

bolic aspects of therapeutic blood purification systems. Basel: Karger; 1986:191–196.

202. Ash SR, Hoswell R, Heefer EM, Bloch R. Effect of the Peridex filter on peritonitis in a CAPD population. *Perit Dial Bull* 1983; 3:89–93.

203. Nakamura Y, Hara Y, Ishida H, Moriwaki K, Shigemoto K. A randomized multicenter trial to evaluate the effects of UV-flash system on peritonitis rates in CAPD. *Adv Perit Dial* 1992; 8:313–315.

204. Stegmayr BG, Granbom L, Tranaeus A, Wikdahl AM. Reduced risk of peritonitis in CAPD with the use of a UV connector box. *Perit Dial Int* 1991;11:128–130.

205. Maiorca R, Cantaluppi A, Cancarini GC, et al. Prospective controlled trial of a Y-connector and disinfectant to prevent peritonitis in continuous ambulatory peritoneal dialysis. *Lancet* 1983; 1:642–644.

206. Dryden MS, McCann M, Wing AJ, Phillips I. Controlled trial of a Y-set dialysis delivery system to prevent peritonitis in patients receiving continuous ambulatory peritoneal dialysis. *J Hosp Infect* 1992;20:185–192.

207. Goth AA, Kim U. The reappearance of abdominal tuberculosis. *Surg Gynec Obstet* 1991;172:432–436.

208. Mehta JB, Dutt A, Harvill L, et al. Epidemiology of extrapulmonary tuberculosis: a comparative analysis with pre-AIDS era. *Chest* 1991;99:1134–1138.

209. Singh MM, Bhargava AN, Jain KP. Tuberculous peritonitis: an evaluation of pathogenetic mechanisms, diagnostic procedures, and therapeutic measures. *N Engl J Med* 1969;281:1091–1094.

210. Marshall JB. Tuberculosis of the gastrointestinal tract and peritoneum. *Am J Gastroenterol* 1993;88:989–999.

211. Sochocky S. Tuberculous peritonitis: a review of 100 cases. *Am Rev Respir Dis* 1967;95:398–401.

212. Karney WW, O'Donahue JM, Ostrow JH, et al. The spectrum of tuberculous peritonitis. *Chest* 1977;72:310–315.

213. Aguado JM, Pons F, Casafont F, San Miguel G, Valle R. Tuberculous peritonitis: a study comparing cirrhotic and noncirrhotic patients. *J Clin Gastroenterol* 1990;12:550–554.

214. Menzies RI, Fitzgerald JM, Mulpeter K. Laparoscopic diagnosis of ascites in Lesotho. *Br Med J* 1985;291:473–475.

215. Dwivedi M, Misra SP, Misra V, et al. Value of adenosine deaminase estimation in the diagnosis of tuberculous ascites. *Am J Gastroenterol* 1990;85:13–15.

216. Voigt MD, Kalvaria I, Trey C, et al. Diagnostic value of ascites adenosine deaminase in tuberculous peritonitis. *Lancet* 1989; 1:751–754.

217. Arend P, Valizadeh A, Dryjski J, Geens M. Tuberculous peritonitis. Description of 2 cases associated with another infection and literature review. *Acta Gastroenterol* 1990;53:307–314.

218. Sobel JD, Vasquez J. Candidemia and systemic candidiasis. *Semin Resp Infect* 1990;5:123–137.

219. Bayer AS, Blumenkrantz MJ, Montgomerie JZ, Galpin JE, Coburn JW, Guze LB. Candida peritonitis: report of 22 cases and review of the literature. *Am J Med* 1976;61:833–840.

220. Peoples JB. Candida and perforated peptic ulcers. *Surgery* 1986;100:758–762.

221. Rutledge R, Mandel SR, Wild RE. *Candida* species. Insignificant contaminant or pathogenic species. *Am Surg* 1986;52: 299–302.

222. Solomkin JS, Flohr AB, Quie PG, et al. The role of *Candida* in intra-peritoneal infections. *Surgery* 1980;88:524–530.

223. Marsh PK, Tally FP, Kellum J, et al. *Candida* infections in surgical patients. *Ann Surg* 1983;198:42–47.

224. Castaldo P, Stratta RJ, Wood RP, et al. Clinical spectrum of fungal infections after orthotopic liver transplantation. *Arch Surg* 1991;126:149–156.

225. Nathwani D, Morris AJ, Laing RB, Smith CC, Reid TM. *Salmonella virchow:* abscess former amongst the contemporary invasive salmonellae? *Scand J Infect Dis* 1991;23:467–471.

226. Gruenwald I, Abrahamson J, Cohen O. Psoas abscess: case report and review of the literature. *J Urol* 1992;147:1624–1626.

227. Ibanez Perez de la Blanca MA, Mediavilla Garcia JD, Martinez R, Mohamed-Balghata MO, Arrebola Nacle JP, Jimenez-Alonso J. Primary abscess of the psoas muscle caused by Streptococcus milleri (letter). *Clin Infect Dis* 1992;15:883–884.

228. Kolbeinsson ME, Holder WD Jr, Aziz S. Recognition, management, and prevention of *Clostridium septicum* abscess in immunosuppressed patients. *Arch Surg* 1991;126:642–645.

229. Prickett D, Montgomery R, Cheadle WG. External fistulas arising from the digestive tract. *South Med J* 1991;84:736–739.

230. Yu JS, Bennett WF, Bova JG. CT of superior mesenteric vein thrombosis complicating periappendiceal abscess. *J Comput Assist Tomogr* 1993;17:309–312.

231. Haaga JR. Imaging intraabdominal abscesses and nonoperative drainage procedures. *World J Surg* 1990;14:204–209.

232. Bennett JD, Kozak RI, Taylor BM, Jory TA. Deep pelvic abscesses: transrectal drainage with radiologic guidance. *Radiology* 1992;185:825–828.

233. Gazelle GS, Haaga JR, Stellato TA, Gauderer MWL, Plecha DT. Pelvic abscesses: CT-guided transrectal drainage. *Radiology* 1991;181:49–51.

234. Brolin RE, Flancbaum L, Ercoli FR, et al. Limitations of percutaneous catheter drainage of abdominal abscesses. *Surg Gynecol Obstet* 1991;173:203–210.

235. Samelson SL, Ferguson MK. Empyema following percutaneous catheter drainage of upper abdominal abscess. *Chest* 1992; 102:1612–1614.

236. Levison MA. Percutaneous versus open operative drainage of intraabdominal abscesses. *Infect Dis Clin North Am* 1992;6: 525–544.

237. Levison MA, Zeigler D. Correlation of APACHE II score, drainage technique and outcome in postoperative intra-abdominal abscess. *Surg Gynecol Obstet* 1991;172:89–94.

238. Lahorra JM, Haaga JR, Stellato T, Flanigan T, Graham R. Safety of intracavity urokinase with percutaneous abscess drainage. *Am J Roentgenol* 1993;160:171–174.

239. Schuster MR, Crummy AB, Wojtowycz MM, McDermott JC. Abdominal abscesses associated with enteric fistulas: percutaneous management. *J Vasc Interv Radiol* 1992;3:359–363.

240. Flancbaum L, Nosher JL, Brolin RE. Percutaneous catheter drainage of abdominal abscesses associated with perforated viscus. *Am Surg* 1990;56:52–56.

241. Stabile BE, Puccio E, vanSonnenberg E, Neff CC. Preoperative percutaneous drainage of diverticular abscesses. *Am J Surg* 1990;159:99–104.

242. Lambiase RE, Deyoe L, Cronan JJ, Dorfman GS. Percutaneous drainage of 335 consecutive abscesses: Results of primary drainage with 1-year follow-up. *Radiology* 1992;184:167–179.

243. Yamakawa T, Suzuki T, Kobayashi S, et al. Fistuloscopy for the management of postoperative intra-abdominal abscesses. *Endoscopy* 1992;24:218–221.

244. Becker JM, Pemberton JH, Diamgno EP, Ilstrup DM, McIlrath DC, Dozois RR. Prognostic factors in pancreatic abscess. *Surgery* 1984;96:455–460.

245. Shi EC, Yeo BW, Ham JM. Pancreatic abscesses. *Br J Surg* 1984;71:689–691.

246. Altemeier WA, Alexander JW. Pancreatic abscess. A study of 32 cases. *Arch Surg* 1963;87:80–89.

247. Widdison AL, Karanjia ND. Pancreatic infection complicating acute pancreatitis. *Br J Surg* 1993;80:148–154.

248. Ransom JHC, Balthazar E, Caccavale R, Cooper M. Computed tomography and the prediction of pancreatic abscess in acute pancreatitis. *Ann Surg* 1985;201:656–663.

249. Hurley JE, Vargish T. Early diagnosis and outcome of pancreatic abscesses in pancreatitis. *Am Surg* 1987;53:29–33.

250. Patel BK, Garvin PJ, Aridge DL, Chenoweth JL, Markivee CR. Fluid collections developing after pancreatic transplantation: radiologic evaluation and intervention. *Radiology* 1991;181: 215–220.

251. Dupuy D, Costello P, Lewis D, Jenkins R. Abdominal CT findings after liver transplantation in 66 patients. *AJR* 1991;156: 1167–1170.

252. Backman L, Brattstrom C, Reinholt FP, Andersson J, Tyden G. Development of intrapancreatic abscess—a consequence of CMV pancreatitis? *Transpl Int* 1991;4:116–121.

253. Lumsden A, Bradley ELI. Secondary pancreatic infections. *Surg Gynecol Obstet* 1990;170:459–467.

254. Bassi C, Vesentini S, Nifosi F, et al. Pancreatic abscess and

other pus-harboring collections related to pancreatitis: a review of 108 cases. *World J Surg* 1990;14:505–512.

255. Fedorak IJ, Ko TC, Djuricin G, McMahon M, Thompson K, Prinz RA. Secondary pancreatic infections: are they distinct clinical entities? *Surgery* 1992;112:824–831.

256. Büchler M, Malfertheiner P, Fries H, et al. Human pancreatic tissue concentration of bactericidal antibiotics. *Gastroenterology* 1992;103:1902–1908.

257. Aranha GU, Prinz RA, Greenlee HB. Pancreatic abscess: an unresolved surgical problem. *Am J Surg* 1982;144:534–538.

258. Bradley EL, Fulenwider JT. Open treatment of pancreatic abscess. *Surg Gynecol Obstet* 1984;159:509–513.

259. Ammann R, Münch R, Largiader F, Akovbiantz A, Marincek B. Pancreatic and hepatic abscesses: a late complication in 10 patients with chronic pancreatitis. *Gastroenterology* 1992;103:560–565.

260. Stanten R, Frey CF. Comprehensive management of acute necrotizing pancreatitis and pancreatic abscess. *Arch Surg* 1990;125:1269–1275.

261. Sofianou DC. Pancreatic abscess caused by *Clostridium difficile*. *Eur J Clin Microbiol Infect Dis* 1988;7:528–529.

262. Reuben AG, Musher DM, Hamill RJ, Broucke I. Polymicrobial bacteremia: clinical and microbiologic patterns. *Rev Infect Dis* 1989;11:161–183.

263. Rotman N, Mathieu D, Anglade M-C, Fagniez P-L. Failure of percutaneous drainage of pancreatic abscesses complicating severe acute pancreatitis. *Surg Gynecol Obstet* 1992;174:141–144.

264. Jones CE, Polk HC Jr., Fulton RL. Pancreatic abscess. *Am J Surg* 1975;129:44–47.

265. Molina F, Durán MT. Características microbiológicas y espectro de infecciones de '08 *Streptococcus anginosus* aislados. *Enf Infec Microbiol Clin* 1993;11:304–308.

266. Vazquez F, Mendez FJ, Pérez F, Mendoza MC. Anaerobic bacteremia in a general hospital: retrospective five-year analysis. *Rev Infect Dis* 1987;9:1038–1043.

267. Lutwick LI. Pancreatic abscess with Haemophilus influenzae and Eikenella corrodens. *JAMA* 1976;236:2091–2092.

268. Stein A, Teysseire N, Capobianco C, Bricot R, Raoult D. *Eikenella corrodens,* a rare cause of pancreatic abscess: two case reports and review. *Clin Infect Dis* 1993;17:273–275.

269. Mandel SR, Boyd D, Jaques PF, Mandell V, Staab EV. Drainage of hepatic, intraabdominal, and mediastinal abscesses guided by computerized axial tomography. Successful alternative to open drainage. *Am J Surg* 1983;145:120–125.

270. Printz H, Klotter H-J, Nies C, et al. Intraoperative ultrasonography in surgery for chronic pancreatitis. *Int J Pancreatol* 1993;12:233–237.

271. Drewelow B, Koch K, Otto C, Franke A, Riethling A-K. Penetration of ceftazidime into human pancreas. *Infection* 1993;21:229–234.

272. Fabian TC, Kudsk KA, Croce MA, et al. Superiority of closed suction drainage for pancreatic trauma. A randomized, prospective study. *Ann Surg* 1990;211:724–728.

273. Braun TI, Travis D, Dee RR, Nieman RE. Liver abscess due to *Listeria monocytogenes:* case report and review. *Clin Infect Dis* 1993;17:267–269.

274. Guerra LG, Neira CJ, Boman D, et al. Rapid response of AIDS-related bacillary angiomatosis to azithromycin. *Clin Infect Dis* 1993;17:264–266.

275. Karatassas A, Williams JA. Review of pyogenic liver abscess at the Royal Adelaide Hospital 1980–1987. *Aust N Z J Surg* 1990;60:893–897.

276. Ramseyer LT, Nguyen DL. Nocardia brasiliensis liver abscesses in an AIDS patient: imaging findings. *AJR* 1993;160:898–899.

277. Nemoto H, Murabayashi K, Kawamura Y, et al. Multiple liver abscesses secondary to *Yersinia enterocolitica*. *Intern Med* 1992;31:1125–1127.

278. O'Bryan TA, Whitener CJ, Katzman M, Appelbaum PC. Hepatobiliary infections caused by *Haemophilus* species. *Clin Infect Dis* 1992;15:716–719.

279. Sire JM, Donnio PY, Mesnard R, Pouedras P, Avril JL. Septicemia and hepatic abscess caused by *Pediococcus acidilactici. Eur J Clin Microbiol Infect Dis* 1992;11:623–625.

280. Martin J, Brimacombe J. *Chromobacterium violaceum* septicaemia: the intensive care management of two cases. *Anaesth Intensive Care* 1992;20:88–90.

281. Zighelboim J, Williams TW Jr, Bradshaw MW, Harris RL. Successful medical management of a patient with multiple hepatic abscesses due to *Edwardsiella tarda. Clin Infect Dis* 1992;14:117–120.

282. Vatcharapreechasakul T, Suputtamongkol Y, Dance DA, Chaowagul W, White NJ. *Pseudomonas pseudomallei* liver abscesses: a clinical, laboratory, and ultrasonographic study. *Clin Infect Dis* 1992;14:412–417.

283. Collazos J, Egurbide V, de Miguel J, Echevarria J, Usera MA. Liver abscess due to Salmonella enteritidis 19 months after an episode of gastroenteritis in a man who underwent a cholecystectomy. *Rev Infect Dis* 1991;13:1027–1028.

284. Vargas V, Comas P, Llatzer R, Esteban R, Guardia J. Brucellar hepatic abscess. *J Clin Gastroenterol* 1991;13:477–478.

285. Wilde CC, Kueh YK. Case report: tuberculous hepatic and splenic abscess. *Clin Radiol* 1991;43:215–216.

286. Swallow CJ, Rotstein OD. Management of pyogenic liver abscess in the era of computed tomography. *Can J Surg* 1990;33:355–362.

287. Sabbaj J, Sutter VL, Finegold SM. Anaerobic pyogenic liver abscess. *Ann Intern Med* 1972;77:629–638.

288. Finegold SM. *Anaerobic bacteria in human disease.* New York: Academic Press; 1977:1–710.

289. Branum GD, Tyson GS, Branum MA, Meyers WC. Hepatic abscess: changes in etiology, diagnosis, and management. *Ann Surg* 1990;212:655–662.

290. Wong E, Khardoir N, Carrasco CH, Wallace S, Patt Y, Bodey GP. Infectious complications of hepatic artery catheterization procedures in patients with cancer. *Rev Infect Dis* 1991;13:583–586.

291. Khardori N, Wong E, Carrasco CH, Wallace S, Patt Y, Bodey GP. Infections associated with biliary drainage procedures in patients with cancer. *Rev Infect Dis* 1991;13:587–591.

292. Lonardo A, Grisendi A, Pulvirenti M, et al. Right colon adenocarcinoma presenting as *Bacteroides fragilis* liver abscesses. *J Clin Gastroenterol* 1992;14:335–338.

293. Stain SC, Yellin AE, Donovan AJ, Brien HW. Pyogenic liver abscess: modern treatment. *Arch Surg* 1991;126:991–996.

294. Gupta U, Sharma MP. Etiology of liver abscess with special reference to anaerobic bacteria. *Ind J Med Res* 1990;91:21–23.

295. Shpitz B, Kaufman Z, Kantarovsky A, Freund U, Dinbar A. Pyogenic liver abscess. *Isr J Med Sci* 1990;26:564–567.

296. Cheng DL, Liu YC, Yen MY, et al. Pyogenic liver abscess: clinical manifestations and value of percutaneous catheter drainage treatment. *Taiwan I Hseuh Hui Tsa Chih* 1990;89:571–576.

297. Burt MJ, Chambers ST, Chapman BA. Pyogenic liver abscesses: a retrospective review of 24 cases. *N Z Med J* 1991;104:179–181.

298. Donovan AJ, Yellin AE, Ralls PW. Hepatic abscess. *World J Surg* 1991;15:162–169.

299. Kasten MJ, Rosenblatt JE, Gustafson DR. *Bilophila wadsworthia* bacteremia in two patients with hepatic abscess. *J Clin Microbiol* 1992;30:2502–2503.

300. Finegold S, Summanen P, Gerardo SH, Baron E. Clinical importance of *Bilophila wadsworthia. Eur J Clin Microbiol Infect Dis* 1992;11:1058–1063.

301. Bowers ED, Robison DJ, Doberneck RC. Pyogenic liver abscess. *World J Surg* 1990;14:128–132.

302. Steinhart AH, Simons M, Stone R, Heathcote J. Multiple hepatic abscesses: Cholangiographic changes simulating sclerosing cholangitis and resolution after percutaneous drainage. *Am J Gastroenterol* 1990;85:306–308.

303. Shimada H, Ohta S, Maehara M, Katayama K, Note M, Nakagawara G. Diagnostic and therapeutic strategies of pyogenic liver abscess. *Int Surg* 1993;78:40–45.

304. Bhatt BD, Zuckerman MJ, Ho H, Polly SM. Multiple actinomycotic abscesses of the liver. *Am J Gastroenterol* 1990;85:309–310.

305. Miyamoto MI, Fang FC. Pyogenic liver abscess involving *Actinomyces:* case report and review. *Clin Infect Dis* 1993;16:303–309.
306. Crippin JS, Wang KK. An unrecognized etiology for pyogenic hepatic abscesses in normal hosts: dental disease. *Am J Gastroenterol* 1992;87:1740–1743.
307. Scoular A, Corcoran GD, Malin A, Evans BA, Davies A, Miller RF. *Fusobacterium nucleatum* bacteraemia with multiple liver abscesses in an HIV-1 antibody positive man with IgG2 deficiency. *J Infect* 1992;24:321–325.
308. Zenon GJIII, Cadle RM, Hamill RJ. Ampicillin-sulbactam therapy for multiple pyogenic hepatic abscesses. *Clin Pharm* 1990;9:939–947.
309. Hansen N, Vargish T. Pyogenic hepatic abscess: a case for open drainage. *Am Surg* 1993;59:219–222.
310. Sridharan GV, Wilkinson SP, Primrose WR. Pyogenic liver abscess in the elderly. *Age Ageing* 1990;19:199–203.
311. Molina JM, Leport C, Bure A, Wolff M, Michon C, Vilde J-L. Clinical and bacterial features of infections caused by *Streptococcus milleri. Scand J Infect Dis* 1991;23:659–666.
312. Granger JK, Houn H-YD. Diagnosis of hepatic actinomycosis by fine-needle aspiration. *Diag Cytopathol* 1991;7:95–97.
313. Morrow JD, Neuzil KM. Primary hepatic actinomycosis—diagnosis by percutaneous transhepatic needle aspiration. *J Tenn Med Assoc* 1993;86:99–101.
314. Isobe H, Fukai T, Iwamoto H, et al. Liver abscess complicating intratumoral ethanol injection therapy for HCC. *Am J Gastroenterol* 1990;85:1646–1648.
315. Sobel JD, Vazquez J. Candidemia and systemic candidiasis. *Semin Resp Infect* 1990;5:123–137.
316. Dondelinger RF, Kurdziel JC, Gathy C. Percutaneous treatment of pyogenic liver abscess: a critical analysis of results. *Cardiovasc Intervent Radiol* 1990;13:174–182.
317. Pitt HA. Surgical management of hepatic abscesses. *World J Surg* 1990;14:498–504.
318. Pérez-Pomata MT, Domínguez J, Horcajo P, Santidrián F, Bisquert J. Spleen abscess caused by *Eikenella corrodens. Eur J Clin Microbiol Infect Dis* 1992;11:162–163.
319. Chun CH, Raff MJ, Contreras L, et al. Splenic abscess. *Medicine (Baltimore)* 1980;59:50–65.
320. Beaver DC, Thompson L. Actinobacillosis of man. Report of a fatal case. *Am J Pathol* 1933;9:603–622.
321. Chulay JD, Lankerani MR. Splenic abscess. Report of 10 cases and review of the literature. *Am J Med* 1976;61:513–522.
322. Galifer RB, Rodiere M, Peskine F, Ferran JL. [Splenic abscess caused by *Ristella fragilis:* a case report of a 2 year-old boy (author's transl)]. *Chir Pediatr* 1981;22:416–418.
323. Moraga Llop FA, Sarto Soliva J, Enriquez Civicos G, Sune Gracia J, Bertran Sangues JM. [Splenic abscess in an infant. Diagnostic value of echography]. *An Esp Pediatr* 1987;27:139–140.
324. Sarr MG, Zuidema GD. Splenic abscess—presentation, diagnosis, and treatment. *Surgery* 1982;92:480–485.
325. Drow DL, Mercer L, Peacock JB. Splenic abscess caused by *Shigella flexneri* and *Bacteroides fragilis. J Clin Microbiol* 1984;19:79–80.
326. Arazo P, Muñoz JR, Aguirre JM, et al. [Spleen abscess]. *An Med Interna* 1990;7:144–146.
327. Tikkakoski T, Siniluoto T, Päivänsalo M, et al. Splenic abscess. Imaging and intervention. *Acta Radiol* 1992;33:561–565.
328. Gadacz T, Way LW, Dunphy JE. Changing clinical spectrum of splenic abscess. *Am J Surg* 1974;128:182.
329. Westh H, Reines E, Skibsted L. Splenic abscesses: a review of 20 cases. *Scand J Infect Dis* 1990;22:569–573.
330. McSherry CK, Dineen P. The significance of splenic abscess. *Am J Surg* 1962;103:618–623.
331. Oehring H, Schulz H, Kramer B, Ehrhardt G. [*Bacteroides melaninogenicus* as the cause of multiple brain abscesses]. *Med Klin* 1967;62:1347–9 passim.
332. Linos DA, Nagorney DM, McIlrath DC. Splenic abscess—the importance of early diagnosis. *Mayo Clin Proc* 1983;58:261–264.
333. Haber SW, Perlino CA. Splenic abscess from *Fusobacterium nucleatum* (letter). *Ann Intern Med* 1989;110:948.
334. Kern W, Dolderer M, Krieger D, Büchler M, Kern P. Lemierresyndrom mit milzabszessen. *Dtsch Med Wochenschr* 1992;117:1513–1517.
335. Sastre J, Casas E, Sierra J, Puig JG, Gil A. Splenic abscess due to *Fusobacterium necrophorum. Rev Infect Dis* 1991;13:1249–1250.
336. Podgorny G. Splenic abscess causing obstruction of the large intestine: first reported case. *Am Surg* 1971;37:269–272.
337. Berkman WA, Harris SA Jr., Bernardino ME. Nonsurgical drainage of splenic abscess. *AJR* 1983;141:395–396.
338. Davis JM, Pober J, Kazam E, Dineen P. Diagnosis of splenic abscess: recent advances. *Infect Surg* 1983;2:90–96.
339. Dylewski J, Portnoy J, Mendelson J. Antibiotic treatment of splenic abscess (letter). *Ann Intern Med* 1979;91:493–494.
340. Conley TD, Vernino LA. Splenic abscess due to Peptostreptococcus spp. as a complication of cardiac catheterization. *Cathet Cardiovasc Diag* 1990;19:184–185.
341. Henry ML, Birken GA, Fabri PJ. Hyposplenism secondary to splenic actinomycosis. *Infect Surg* 1985;4:672–676.
342. Sherman ME, Albrecht M, DeGirolami PC, et al. An unusual case of splenic abscess and sepsis in an immunocompromised host. *Am J Clin Pathol* 1987;88:659–662.
343. Gekowski KM, Lopes R, LiCalzi L, Bia FJ. Splenic abscess caused by *Propionibacterium acnes. Yale J Biol Med* 1982;55:65–69.
344. Dunne WM Jr., Kurschenbaum HA, Deshur WR, et al. *Propionibacterium avidum* as the etiologic agent of splenic abscess. *Diag Microbiol Infect Dis* 1986;5:87–92.
345. Radulescu D. [Surgical infections with anaerobic bacteria (splenic abscess ruptured into the peritoneum)]. *Rev Chir* [Chir] 1979;28:129–136.
346. Gangahar DM, Delany HM. Intrasplenic abscess: two case reports and review of the literature. *Am Surg* 1981;47:488–491.
347. Saginur R, Fogel R, Begin L, Cohen B, Mendelson J. Splenic abscess due to *Clostridium difficile. J Infect Dis* 1983;147:1105.
348. Studemeister AE, Beilke MA, Kirmani N. Splenic abscess due to *Clostridium difficile* and *Pseudomonas paucimobilis. Am J Gastroenterol* 1987;82:389–390.
349. Kinnaird DW, Melo JC, McKeown JM. Splenic abscess due to *Clostridium septicum* in a patient with multiple myeloma. *South Med J* 1987;80:1318–1320.
350. Hadas-Halpern I, Hiller N, Dolberg M. Percutaneous drainage of splenic abscesses: an effective and safe procedure. *Br J Radiol* 1992;65:968–970.
351. Hisaoka M, Nakamura T, Haratake J, Horie A. Primary actinomycosis in the liver. *Sangyo Ika Daigaku Zasshi* 1991;13:29–34.
352. Muller-Holzner E, Gschwendtner A, Abfalter E, Solder E, Schrocksnadel H. Actinomycosis and long-term use of intrauterine devices. *Lancet* 1990;336:939.
353. Raz R, Lev A. Primary abdominal actinomycosis in a diabetic woman—an intractable disease. *J Infect* 1992;25:303–306.
354. Goldwag S, Abbitt PL, Watts B. Case report: percutaneous drainage of periappendiceal actinomycosis. *Clin Radiol* 1991;44:422–424.
355. Samuel I, Dixon MF, Benson EA. Actinomycosis complicating chronic diverticulitis of the sigmoid colon: a mixed association? *Postgrad Med J* 1992;68:57–58.
356. Lockhart GR, Williams GP, Gilbert-Barness E. Pathological case of the month. Thoracic and abdominal actinomycosis. *Am J Dis Child* 1993;147:317–318.
357. Kakkasseril J, Cabanas V, Saba K. Ruptured actinomycotic aneurysm of the splenic artery: a case report of successful resection. *Surgery* 1983;93:595–597.
358. Hill GB, Ayers OM, Kohan AP. Characteristics and sites of infection of *Eubacterium nodatum, Eubacterium timidum, Eubacterium brachy,* and other asaccharolytic eubacteria. *J Clin Microbiol* 1987;25:1540–1545.
359. Evans TN, Fitzgerald EJ. Abdominal actinomycosis. *Br J Clin Pract* 1990;44:499–500.
360. Manoussakis CA, Triantafillidis JK, Dadioti P, Papavasiliou E, Lissaios V. The role of computed tomography in the assessment of patients with abdominal actinomycosis. *Am J Gastroenterol* 1990;85:213–214.

Infections of the Gastrointestinal Tract,
edited by M. J. Blaser, P. D. Smith, J. I. Ravdin,
H. B. Greenberg, and R. L. Guerrant
Raven Press, Ltd., New York © 1995.

CHAPTER 30

Extraintestinal Manifestations of Enteric Infections

James K. Roche

In addition to the gastrointestinal manifestations of enteric infections, a variety of extraintestinal syndromes can occur either simultaneously or at a later time following detection of the enteric pathogen. These include nonseptic and septic arthritis, hemolytic uremic syndrome, Guillain–Barré syndrome, and symptoms of disseminated infection. Each will be described separately in this chapter, and evidence concerning mechanisms will be discussed where data exist.

NONSEPTIC ARTHRITIS

Nonseptic arthritis is seen in patients as two separate syndromes involving joints in association with enteric infection with several organisms, including *Salmonella, Shigella, Yersinia,* and *Campylobacter.* The first syndrome has been named *reactive arthritis* as well as *postinfectious arthritis* because it is usually seen after the onset of diarrhea but is present only in a minority of cases (1.9% of all cases of *Salmonella* colitis, for example) (1). Joint symptoms are usually asymmetric, migratory, with small-joint involvement predominating. Swelling, tenderness, and erythema of a joint may be associated with malaise, intermittent fever, and weight loss (2). After the onset of arthritis, joint fluid is usually serous, with cultures uniformly negative as are blood cultures (3). Anecdotal evidence indicates that neither antibiotics nor corticosteroids affect the natural history of the arthritis, although one report suggests that indomethacin in high doses is effective (4). A remarkable feature of this arthritis is its long duration, averaging 5 months in 2 reports and greater than 10 months in 9 of 13 cases reported in another series (1,3,5). In this syndrome, it should be noted that white blood cells in the joint fluid are present (average of 23,000/

mm³), but not in the septic range, and that there is eventual recovery in all cases for which long-term follow-up is available. Most patients (greater than 70%) are positive for the HLA B27 antigen (6). Carriage of the HLA B27 also strongly predisposes to spondylitis and acute anterior uveitis (7). Other features of reactive arthritis associated with *Salmonella, Campylobacter, Shigella,* or *Yersinia* are a male/female ratio approximately 1:1, a higher incidence of postinfectious arthritis after yersiniosis, and a recurrence one or more times in a substantial minority of patients (7).

A second syndrome occurring as a postinfective event to an intestinal pathogen is that of nonseptic arthritis associated with one or more other extraintestinal manifestations. This is most commonly an eye symptom (iritis or conjunctivitis), occurring in 88% of patients with arthritis and shigellosis, and in 2.3–26.5% of patients following *Salmonella, Campylobacter,* or *Yersinia* infections. The incidence of ocular lesions is said to vary with the location and stage of arthritis as well as its severity, and with the diligence with which lesions are sought. Uveitis is associated especially with severe or recurrent arthritis and, in particular, with sacroiliitis (8,9). Intraocular hemorrhage has been reported in severe cases, with corneal ulceration, keratitis, optic neuritis, and posterior uveitis being more rarely described (7). The second most common extraintestinal manifestation in addition to arthritis as a postinfectious syndrome is that of genital lesions, occurring in almost 70% of patients with arthritis following *Shigella* infection including circinate balanitis in 24%, and in 12.5–23.8% of arthritis patients with *Yersinia, Campylobacter,* or *Salmonella* (7). Other manifestations include circinate balanitis, occurring only in association with *Shigella* (23.7%), and erythema nodosum, occurring primarily in association with *Yersinia* (5.0%) (7). The term Reiter's syndrome is reserved for the classic triad, consisting of arthritis, urethritis, and conjunctivitis. *Shigella, Salmonella, Yersinia,* and *Campylobacter* species have all been implicated as enteric pathogens preceding Reiter's

J. K. Roche: Department of Internal Medicine, University of Virginia Health Sciences Center, Charlottesville, Virginia 22908.

syndrome (10). Of these, *Shigella flexneri* and *Salmonella typhimurium* are most closely associated with this clinical syndrome. Extraintestinal manifestations of *Yersinia, Salmonella,* and *Shigella* infections have all been linked to individuals with the HLA B27 antigen, and who tend to have a more chronic and aggressive course than B27–negative subjects, as well as a more frequent incidence of fever, weight loss, and eye involvement (11). For example, among 50 surviving patients with Reiter's syndrome from a 1944 *Shigella* epidemic, 39 were found to be B27-positive, compared with a frequency of 10% HLA B27 positivity in the general population (12). It has been calculated that a B27-positive person with dysentery has a 19–32% chance of developing Reiter's syndrome. The occasional occurrence of Reiter's syndrome in B27-negative persons indicates either that an environmental insult may be able to override genetic factors or that additional host susceptibility factors exist besides B27 (11). Studies of long-term follow-up indicate that morbidity may continue after the first episode of Reiter's syndrome. Disease persisted in 4 of 10 patients 13 years after symptom onset in one study (11) in which the recurrence rate for Reiter's syndrome was estimated to be 15% per patient per year. However, a prospective study in an unselected white adult population indicated that Reiter's syndrome complicates only 1–3% of infections due to *Shigella flexneri* (13), a number that would be expected if Reiter's syndrome complicated 19–32% of the 10% of the population with HLA-B27.

That spondylitis occurs in higher frequency in patient's with Reiter's syndrome is recognized and may relate to its association with the genetic marker HLA B27 (14). For patients with short-lived disease of the mild variety, symptoms are reported in about 9%, with sacroiliitis detected by X ray in 5–9% in retrospective studies. In patients with severe, chronic, or more recurrent Reiter's syndrome, an incidence of low back pain of 31–92% has been recorded, with an abnormal sacroiliac joint area by X ray in 73% of 33 patients with Reiter's syndrome (7).

Mechanism

The pathology of acute reactive arthritis may give some clue to etiology. Patchy, nonspecific changes are seen by microscopy of synovium, with infiltration by inflammatory cells, particularly polymorphonuclear leukocytes. While abnormalities of mitochondrial morphology of synovial lining cells have been reported, evidences of immunological abnormalities are few. Although serum levels of complement are normal, deposits of immunoglobulin and complement have been reported in synovium (15). This suggests that acute synovitis seen in Reiter's syndrome may be due to deposition of inflammatory immune complexes in the joint space. However, the involvement of microbial products, either as an antigen in the immune complex or as a substance that elicits immune complexes for deposition in tissue, has not been established. In contrast, arthritis that follows meningococcal infection as well as that associated with the prodromal phase of hepatitis B infection does show, in some instances, deposition of immune complexes containing microbial antigen in the

joint (16,17). These arthritides are different in their features in that they occur during or shortly after widespread antigen dissemination, are generally short lived, and rarely recur.

Evidence for mechanisms linking an enteric infectious agent with arthritis comes from three more recent studies. In one, Tsuchiua and coworkers (18) isolated a plasmid from erythrogenic *S. flexneri* strains, which was shown to encode an amino acid sequence analogous to HLA B27. They found elevated levels of antibodies to this peptide in 10.4% of 115 patients with ankylosing spondylitis and in 4.4% of 45 patients with Reiter's syndrome, suggesting that molecular mimicry, in which the peptide resembles B27 peptide, may be a mechanism for the pathogenesis of spondyloarthropathy. In a second study, more advanced techniques were used to look for microbial antigens in 15 patients with reactive arthritis after *Yersinia* infection whose synovial fluid was culture-negative. Synovial fluid cells, mostly polymorphonuclear leukocytes, from 10 of the 15 patients stained positively on immunofluorescence with a polyspecific as well as a monoclonal antibody elicited to *Yersinia* antigen. Only 1–10% of cells stained, but results in 6 of 10 patients were confirmed using Western blotting, with the same antibodies. None of ten cell deposits from control patients with rheumatoid arthritis showed *Yersinia* antigens (19). This, together with evidence that patients with *Yersinia* enteritis who develop reactive arthritis have a characteristically high and persisting IgA–anti-*Yersinia* antibody response (20), suggests that polysaccharides belonging to the *Yersinia* organism may be resistant to digestion and persist within phagocytic cells for long periods, providing a strong antigenic stimulus in patients destined to have arthritis. Organ localization may be due to antigen trapping in joint synovium, transported there by unknown means from the gastrointestinal tract. Further, chronic arthritis occurred in rats injected intravenously with live *Salmonella enteritidis,* most notably in adults and not in weanling animals, and was not found in joints that were directly injected with 10^3 viable organisms, suggesting that the syndrome is immunologically mediated. In comparison with adjuvant arthritis, which can be transferred to recipients with mononuclear cells from the infected host, repeated attempts to transfer *Salmonella*-associated arthritis in the rat model have failed for unknown reasons (18,20).

SEPTIC ARTHRITIS AT THE TIME OF ENTERIC INFECTION

Purulent synovitis occurring during enteric infection is relatively rare, with an incidence ranging from 0.2% to 2.5% after *Salmonella* infections, for example (21,22). As expected, most cases are monoarticular, generally involving large joints (knee, shoulder, and hip). Symptoms generally occur within 2 weeks, but as late as 7 weeks, after gastrointestinal symptoms begin, with peripheral leukocytosis, purulent joint fluid, and positive Gram stain in at least 50% of reported cases. Less than 30% of reported cases had a positive stool culture for an enteric pathogen at the time of septic arthritis despite the fact the arthritis was thought to represent hematogenous spread of organisms from the gastrointestinal tract (2). Relatively minor damage to the joints is reported in *Salmonella* and other enteric infections, and is generally of less than 3 months duration. Association with the HLA B27 antigen is not reported. Therapy with ampicillin, chloramphenicol, and trimethoprim-sulfamethoxazole in association with joint drainage has lead to successful outcomes (23,24).

HEMOLYTIC UREMIC SYNDROME

Although a large number of agents (drugs, chemicals, toxins, microbes) have been associated with individual cases of hemolytic uremic syndrome, the most common form occurs in infancy and childhood, characteristically a few days after an acute diarrheal illness. Many microbes have been associated with this condition including *Shigella dysenteria, Salmonella typhi, Campylobacter jejuni,* and *Yersinia pseudotuberculosis* (25). The triad of features characteristic of the syndrome are acute renal failure, thrombocytopenia, and microangiopathic hemolytic anemia. In a series of 40 pediatric patients reported with idiopathic hemolytic uremic syndrome, the most common clinical features were lethargy (34 patients), anuria (13 patients), oliguria (11 patients), disorientation or seizures (10 patients), peripheral edema (9 patients), temperature greater than 38°C (7 patients), and purpuric rash (6 patients). The mean white blood cell count was 20,200, and illness ranged in severity from mild to fulminant, culminating in fatal. Thirty-four patients fully recovered (85%), three (7.5%) had residual neurological deficits, two died, and one had chronic renal impairment (25). Strain O157:H7 has been the most frequently reported species of *Escherichia coli* to be associated with hemolytic uremic syndrome; both laparotomy and barium enema studies suggest that the right colon is the site of severest involvement for infection with this enteric organism; and culture of stool should be performed soon after presentation, since stool cultures have been found to be negative in the majority of cases when taken more than 5 days after the onset of illness (26,27).

Although the pathogenesis of hemolytic uremic syndrome is not well understood, it has been speculated that the primary event is injury to the endothelial cells of the glomerular capillaries, associated with local intravascular coagulation in the renal glomeruli, as well as thrombotic microangiopathy (28). Two factors have been suggested as the cause of endothelial cell damage. Because of their ability to damage vascular endothelium of renal glomeruli, as in the endotoxic shock syndrome (29), endotoxins have been implicated as an initiating mediator of injury. On the other hand, because immunoglobulin and complement have been detected in renal biopsy specimens of patients with hemolytic uremic syndrome (30), an immunological etiology has also been postulated. Direct support for both postulated mechanisms was reported by Coster and coworkers (31), where circulating immune complexes by the Raji cell immunoassay and the C1q solid phase assay were found in 10 of 20 patients with uncomplicated shigellosis and in 4 of 6 with severe hemolytic uremic syndrome, and the limulus assay for endotoxemia was positive in 9 of 18 patients with hemolysis and in 3 of 61 patients with uncomplicated shigellosis. These authors suggested that endotoxin is the mediator of renal cortical thrombosis and that intestinal pathogens may produce mucosal inflammation resulting in release of endotoxin and other mediators from the gastrointestinal tract into the circulation. Unanswered was why only certain patients develop the hemolytic uremic syndrome despite the presence of endotoxin and immune complexes in the circulation.

Karmali et al. (25) have gone on to identify a Shiga-like verocytotoxin (SLT) from *E. coli,* belonging to at least six different O sero groups that are now called "enterohemorrhagic *E. coli* because of the hemorrhagic colitis they characteristically cause (see Chapter by Griffin). Karmali detected SLT verotoxin in the stools of 24 of 40 (60%) of pediatric patients with idiopathic hemolytic uremic syndrome, with 75% of patients showing some evidence for renal involvement. The verotoxin was the only factor common to all strains associated with hemolytic uremic syndrome in their study, and detection of free fecal verotoxin was regarded as the most significant procedure for the early diagnosis of that infection (25).

OTHER EXTRAINTESTINAL MANIFESTATIONS

Involvement of skin and mucous membranes has been reported with some enteric pathogens. Pharyngitis, sometimes in association with cervical adenopathy, has been reported in adults with *Yersinia* enterocolitis as has erythema nodosum (32). Individual case reports of *Campylobacter* enteritis with erythema nodosum also exist (33). *Vibrio* infections of many species can cause direct cutaneous infections or severe hemorrhagic bullae as a part of sepsis, the latter characteristically seen with fulminant *V. vulnificus* infection, most often in patients with underlying liver disease who consume raw oysters.

NERVOUS SYSTEM INVOLVEMENT

A neurological syndrome reported in association with *Campylobacter jejuni* enteritis is that of Guillain–Barré syndrome. Speed and coworkers reported one case in association with stool culture positivity and three additional cases associated with an 8- to 64-fold increase in specific antibody to *Campylobacter* organism (34). Using similar means, Mishu and coworkers (35) detected a greater than twofold increase in immunoglobulin specific for *C. jejuni* in 43 (36%) of patients with Guillain–Barré syndrome and in 10 (10%) of controls ($p < 0.001$). Positive serological responses were greatest in the months of September through November, male patients predominated by a ratio of 3:1, and the association was more marked with increasing age. With regard to mechanism, host factors, particularly the immune response to *C. jejuni,* were speculated to predispose patients to the development of Guillain–Barré syndrome after intestinal infection. A link with the HLA B35 antigen was reported from Japan in 6 patients with the Guillain–Barré syndrome (36). Further definition of mechanism awaits data on the precise pathology involved with Guillain–Barré syndrome in association with enteritis and identification of a neurological target for immunological injury. Amako and coworkers showed that antibodies of one such patient reacted with a peripheral nerve myelin-specific protein, suggesting that infection elicits antibodies to some self-components (37). Other investigators have proposed that a myelin component, ganglioside, may be the ultimate target of antibodies elicited in response to enteric infection with *C. jejuni* (38).

EXTRAINTESTINAL MANIFESTATIONS ASSOCIATED WITH DISSEMINATED INFECTION

Of the organisms highlighted in this review of extraintestinal manifestations of enteric infections, the mucosa-invasive pathogens *Salmonella* and, rarely, *Shigella* are best recognized for their ability to be simultaneously present in blood, with the potential for infecting distant sites. *Yersinia*, *Vibrio*, or *Campylobacter* can cause a similar "sepsis" syndrome. For *Yersinia* septicemia, patients generally have one of two presentations. In acute septicemia, symptoms of pyrexia, headache, malaise, abdominal pain, and diarrhea predominate, similar to that found with systemic salmonellosis. Prognosis largely depends on early diagnosis as well as the natural history of the underlying diseases, discussed below. The second form, described as subacute, is found in patients who are chronically ill, in which a bacteremic episode may even go unnoticed. Localizing symptoms may be due to metastatic foci of infection, such as liver or splenic abscess. Prognosis in this case is much more guarded, with a mortality reported of up to 50% (39,40). The importance of the liver in resistance of the host to *Yersinia enterocolitica* infection, particularly septicemia, has been suggested by the frequency of cirrhosis and conditions of iron overload in the reported series (40). Two mechanisms have been proposed for this. Data in mice indicate that injection of ferric ammonium citrate increases the mortality of animals infected with *Y. enterocolitica,* and iron excess may be present in those with hemolytic anemia, hemochromatosis, and other chronic liver diseases. A second mechanism, suggested by Conn, proposes that cirrhotic livers may be less effective in reducing the number of bacteria in the portal bloodstream, since some blood flow bypasses the reticuloendothelial system of the liver through shunts, allowing the microorganism to spread to peripheral tissues (41). Other conditions apparently predisposing to bacteremia with *Yersinia* include transfusion-dependent blood dyscrasias, immunosuppressive therapy, diabetes mellitus, alcoholism, and malnutrition (42). A wide array of abnormalities in extraintestinal sites have been recorded after bacteremic spread of this organism. Besides hepatic and splenic abscesses noted above, endocarditis, mycotic aneurysm, meningitis, peritonitis, osteomyelitis, septic arthritis, pulmonary infiltrates, lung abscess, renal abscess, and cutaneous pustules have all been reported in association with *Y. enterocolitica* bacteremia (42).

With regard to *Campylobacter*, *C. fetus ss. fetus* is regarded as the most common etiological agent for septice-

mia, and pure septicemia without metastatic infectious foci is the most common presentation. Complications at a distance reported with septicemia due to this organism include carditis, phlebitis, meningitis, other pyogenic processes, and abortion (43,44). Because several series have shown septicemia with *Campylobacter* primarily limited to debilitated patients, it has been considered an opportunist by investigators who have studied it. Most commonly associated conditions are cirrhosis, carcinoma, Hodgkin's disease, agammaglobulinenemia, chronic leukemia, and lymphoma (43,44). Fetal loss is high with infected mothers, with fetal/neonatal mortality of 50%. Bacteremia is speculated to originate from the bowel, with seeding of organisms accounting for fetoplacental involvement. Mechanisms suggested to account for this latter phenomena include the finding that the organism localizes in the placenta *in vivo* following parenteral inoculation and grows preferentially in placental tissue extracts *in vitro* (44). Further, the known depression of cell-mediated immunity during pregnancy may also account for the occurrence of some cases (45). Another subspecies, *C. jejuni,* while commonly causing enteritis, relatively infrequently seeds the bloodstream, occurring predominantly in immunocompromised patients.

CONCLUSION

The extraintestinal manifestations of enteric infections reflect a wide range of infections and immunological consequences. While still poorly understood, the immunological mechanisms proposed raise intriguing hypotheses regarding microbial and/or host antigenicity and their roles in acute and chronic extraintestinal inflammatory processes. Knowledge of precise pathogenesis may shed light on important idiopathic intestinal diseases with manifestations outside the intestinal tract such as ulcerative colitis and Crohn's disease.

REFERENCES

1. Vertianinen J, Hurri L. Arthritis due to *Salmonella typhimurium*. *ACTA Med Scand* 1964;175:771.
2. Carroll WL, Balistreri WF, Brilli R, Parrish RA, Greenfield DJ. Spectrum of *Salmonella*-associated arthritis. *Pediatrics* 1981;68: 717–720.
3. Bergloff FE. Arthritis and intestinal infection. *ACTA Rheumatol Scand* 1963;9:141.
4. Stein HB, Abdullah A, Robinson HS, et al. *Salmonella* reactive arthritis in British Columbia. *Arthritis Rheum* 1980;22:206.
5. Warren CPW. Arthritis associated with *Salmonella* infections. *Ann Rheum Dis* 1970;29:483.
6. Hakensson U, Eitrem R, Low B, et al. HLA antigen B27 in cases with joint infection in an outbreak of Salmonellosis. *Scand J Infect Dis* 1976;8:245.
7. Keat A. Reiter's syndrome and reactive arthritis in perspective. *N Engl J Med* 1983;309:1606–1615.
8. Ford DK. Arthritis and venereal urethritis. *Br J Vener Dis* 1953; 29:123–133.
9. Oates JK, Young AC. Sacroiliitis and Reiter's disease. *Br Med J* 1959;1:1013–1015.
10. Leung F, Littlejohn GO, Bombardier C. *Arthritis Rheum* 1980; 23:948–950.

11. Calin A, Fries JF. An experimental epidemic of Reiter's syndrome revisited. *Ann Intern Med* 1976;84:564–566.
12. Sairanen E, Tilikainen A. HLA 27 in Reiter's disease following Shigellosis. *Scand J Rheumatol* 1975;4(Suppl. 8):30–41.
13. Zsonka GW. Recurrent attacks in Reiter's disease. *Arthritis Rheum* 1960;3:164–169.
14. Schlosstein L, Terasaki PI, Bluestone R, Pierson CM. High association of an HLA antigen, B27, with ankylosing spondylitis. *N Engl J Med* 1973;288:704–706.
15. Baldassare MR, Weiss TD, Tsai CC, Arthur RE, Moore TL, Zuckner J. Immunoprotein deposition in synovial tissue in Reiter's syndrome. *Ann Rheum Dis* 1981;40:281–285.
16. Herrick WW, Parkhurst GM. Meningococcal arthritis. *Am J Med Sci* 1919;158:473–481.
17. Scheumacher HR, Gall EP. Arthritis in acute hepatitis and chronic active hepatitis: pathology of the synovial membrane with evidence for the presence of Australia antigen in synovial membranes. *Am J Med Sci* 1974;57:655–664.
18. Tsuchiya N, Husby G, Williams RC Jr, Stieglitz H, Lipsky PE, Inman RD. Autoantibodies to the HLA-B27 sequence cross-react with the hypothetical peptide from the arthritis-associated *Shigella* plasmid. *J Clin Invest* 1990;86:1193–1203.
19. Granfors K, Jalkanen S, Essen R, et al. *Yersinia* antigens in synovial-fluid cells from patients with reactive arthritis. *N Engl J Med* 1989;320:216–221.
20. Granfors K, Toivanen A. IgA-anti-*Yersinia* antibodies in *Yersinia* triggered reactive arthritis. *Ann Rheum Dis* 1986;45:561–565.
21. Saphra I, Winter JW. Clinical manifestations in salmonellosis in man. *N Engl J Med* 1957;256:1128–1134.
22. Saphra I, Wussermann M. *Salmonella cholerae suis*. A clinical and epidemiological evaluation of 329 infections identified between 1940 and 1954 in the New York *Salmonella* Center. *Am J Med Sci* 1954;228:525–533.
23. Ortiz-Neu C, Marr JS, Cherubin CE, et al. Bone and joint infections due to *Salmonella*. *J Infect Dis* 1978;138:820–828.
24. Goldenberg DL, Cohen AS. Acute infectious arthritis. A review of patients with nongonococcal joint infections (with emphasis on therapy and prognosis). *Am J Med* 1976;60:369–377.
25. Karmali MA, Petric M, Lim C, Fleming PC, Arvus GS, Lior H. The association between idiopathic hemolytic uremic syndrome and infection by verotoxin-producing *Escherichia coli*. *J Infect Dis* 1985;151:775–782.
26. Spika JS, Parson JE, Nordenberg D, et al. Hemolytic uremic syndrome and diarrhea associated with *Escherichia coli* O157:H7 in a day care center. *J Pediatr* 1986;109:287–290.
27. Riley LW, Renis RS, Helgerson SD, et al. Hemorrhagic colitis associated with a rare *Escherichia coli* serotype. *N Engl J Med* 1983;308:681–685. Update. Sporadic hemorrhagic colitis. *MMWR* 1984;33:28–29.
28. Delans RJ, Biuso JE, Saba SR, Ramirez J. Hemolytic uremic syndrome after *Campylobacter*-induced diarrhea in an adult. *Arch Intern Med* 1984;144:1074–1076.
29. Thomas L, Goed RA. Studies on the generalized Shwartzman reactions: general observation concerning the phenomena. *J Exp Med* 1952;96:605–624.
30. McCoy RC, Abramowsky CR, Krueger R. The hemolytic uremic syndrome with positive immunofluorescence studies. *J Pediatr* 1974;85:170–174.
31. Coster F, Levin J, Walker L, et al. Hemolytic uremic syndrome after shigellosis. *N Engl J Med* 1978;298:927–933.
32. Cover TL, Aber RC. *Yersinia* enterocolitica—medical progress. *N Engl J Med* 1989;321:16–23.
33. Lambert M, Marion E, Coche E, Blutzler J-P. *Campylobacter* enteritis and erythema nodosum. *Lancet* 1982;1:1409.
34. Speed B, Kaldor J, Cavanaugh P. Guillain–Barré syndrome associated with campylobacter jejuni enteritis. Letter to the editor. *J Infect* 1984;8:85–86.
35. Mishu B, Amjad AI, Koski CL, et al. Serologic evidence of previous *Campylobacter jejuni* infection in patients with the Guillain–Barré syndrome. *Ann Intern Med* 1993;118:947–953.
36. Yuki M, Sato S, Itoh T, Miyatake T. HLA B35 and acute axonal polyneuropathy following *Campylobacter* infection. *Neurology* 1991;41:1561–1563.
37. Fujimoto S, Amako K. Guillain–Barré syndrome and *Campylobacter jejuni* infection (letter). *Lancet* 1990;335:1350.
38. Carpo M, Mobile-Orazio E, Meucci N, Scarlatto G. Anti-GM1 IgG antibodies in Guillain–Barré syndrome. *Clin Neuropathol* 1991;10:146.
39. Rabson AR, Hallett AF, Koornhof HJ. Generalized *Yersinia enterocolitica* infection. *J Infect Dis* 1975;131:447–451.
40. Bouza U, Dominguiz A, Meseguer M, et al. *Yersinia enterocolitica* septicemia. *Am J Clin Pathol* 1980;74:404–409.
41. Conn HO. Spontaneous peritonitis and bacteremia in lanexerosis caused by enteric organisms. *Ann Intern Med* 1964;60:568–580.
42. Cover TL, Aber RC. *Yersinia enterocolitica*. *N Engl J Med* 1989;321:16–23.
43. Walder M, Lindberg A, Schalen C, Ohman L. Five cases of *Campylobacter jejuni/coli* bacteremia. *Scand J Infect Dis* 1982;14:201–205.
44. Lowrie DP, Pearce JH. The placental localization of *Vibrio fetus*. *J Med Microbiol* 1970;3:607–614.
45. Weinberg ED. Pregnancy-associated depression of cell-mediated immunity. *Rev Infect Dis* 1984;6:814–831.

Infections of the Gastrointestinal Tract,
edited by M. J. Blaser, P. D. Smith, J. I. Ravdin,
H. B. Greenberg, and R. L. Guerrant
Raven Press, Ltd., New York © 1995.

CHAPTER 31

Sexually Transmitted Infections of the Anus and Rectum

Janice R. Verley and Thomas C. Quinn

Infections of the anus and rectum are frequently sexually transmitted, and occur primarily in homosexual men and heterosexual women who engage in anorectal intercourse. The most common anorectal infections observed in heterosexual women are caused by the classic venereal pathogens *Treponema pallidum, Neisseria gonorrhoeae,* and *Chlamydia trachomatis.* These pathogens also cause infections in homosexual men who are additionally at high risk for other bacterial, viral, and protozoan organisms, including herpes simplex virus (HSV), human papillomavirus (HPV), and *Entamoeba histolytica.* These infections are endemic in the homosexual male population and may cause perianal lesions, proctitis, or proctocolitis.

An epidemic of anorectal infections was first recognized in homosexual men in the 1970s (1,2). In the study by Sohn and Robilotti (2), infections with *N. gonorrhoeae, T. pallidum, E. histolytica,* and *C. trachomatis* accounted for less than 20% of the anorectal infections in their patients. The majority had condyloma acuminata infections and ''nonspecific proctitis'' that included hemorrhoids, fissures, and trauma from foreign bodies. However, in a later study, Quinn et al. (3) identified specific pathogens in more than 80% of symptomatic cases of proctitis and in 39% of asymptomatic homosexual men (Table 1). Multiple pathogens were found in 22% of symptomatic and 4% of asymptomatic cases. The high prevalence of anorectal infection in this population was related to high-risk behaviors, such as anogenital and oral–anal intercourse (anilingus), and oral–genital sex (fellatio) following anal intercourse, which allows pathogens to be ingested or inoculated onto the anorectal mucosa.

During the early 1980s, many of these sexually transmitted diseases (STDs) declined in homosexual men due to the adoption of safer sex practices because of the AIDS epidemic. Unfortunately, in the late 1980s the incidence

of anorectal gonorrhea in homosexual men started to increase again. This increase appeared to reflect a nationwide increase in STDs among both homosexual men and young heterosexuals, indicating decreased attention to safe sex practices in general (4–10).

Among heterosexual women, anorectal intercourse and cervical infections are associated with anorectal infections. In a study of women attending a gynecology clinic, anorectal infections were documented in a small proportion of women as they practiced anal receptive intercourse with a low number of infected partners (11). In women not practicing anal intercourse, anorectal infections are due to contamination of the anorectal area by cervicovaginal fluid from an infected cervix. Control of these infections has been complicated due to the practice of anonymous sex with large numbers of infected heterosexual or homosexual partners, an activity that enhances the spread of anorectal infections and impedes contact tracing. Additionally, the failure of physicians to recognize these infections and the delay of medical evaluation due to the asymptomatic nature of some infections perpetuates the human reservoir of these infections. This chapter reviews the common infections of the anorectal region of the gastrointestinal tract. Since the more traditional gastrointestinal pathogens will be discussed in detail in other chapters, this chapter will focus primarily on sexually transmitted pathogens.

ANATOMY AND CLINICAL SYMPTOMS

The epithelium of the skin and mucosa is an important barrier to infection of the perianal area, anus, and rectum (Fig. 1). Consequently, traumatic breaks in the epithelium due to anal intercourse or insertion of foreign bodies appear to promote local infections. The anal canal extends 2 cm internally from the anal verge to the anorectal (pectinate or dentate) line which separates the anal canal from the rectum. The cell lining, nervous supply, lymphatic

J. R. Verley and T. C. Quinn: Division of Infectious Diseases, Johns Hopkins University School of Medicine, Baltimore, Maryland 21205-2196.

TABLE 1. *Comparison of anatomic characteristics of the anus and rectum*

Characteristic	Anus	Rectum
Epithelium	Stratified squamous/cuboidal	Columnar
Nerve supply	Somatic sensory nerves	Autonomic nerves
Lymphatic drainage	Inguinal nodes	Pelvic nodes
Venous drainage	Inferior hemorrhoidal plexus/inferior vena cava	Superior hemorrhoidal plexus/portal vein
Common symptoms	Pruritus, discharge, pain	Hematochezia, discharge, tenesmus

and venous drainage are different for the anus and rectum (Table 2). Stretching of the rectum produces pain but the area is otherwise insensitive and infections of the rectum that spare the anus are relatively painless. Proctitis—inflammation of the anorectal mucosa—can lead to spasms of the underlying anal sphincter muscles, resulting in constipation and tenesmus (unproductive straining at stool), as well as pain, hematochezia, and mucopurulent rectal discharge (12). Visual inspection of the rectal mucosa in a patient with symptoms of proctitis may reveal normal mucosa or inflammation and ulcerations.

The spectrum of symptoms associated with anorectal infections ranges from asymptomatic to severe proctocolitis with rectal pain, constipation, tenesmus, hematochezia, mucoid rectal discharge, fever, and inguinal lymphadenopathy. The presence or absence as well as the severity of symptoms depends on the infecting organism, virulence of the strain, inoculum size, and immunity of the host. HSV infections are more often seen in symptom-

atic than asymptomatic patients, whereas *N. gonorrhoeae*, *T. pallidum*, and *E. histolytica* infections are more often asymptomatic. Nonlymphogranuloma venereum (LGV) strains of *C. trachomatis* often cause asymptomatic infection, whereas LGV strains may cause severe granulomatous proctitis simulating Crohn's disease.

HERPES SIMPLEX VIRUS

Microbiology

Anorectal herpetic infection is caused by herpes simplex virus type 2 (HSV-2) in 90% of cases and HSV-1 in 10% of cases. HSV is a member of the herpesvirus group that includes varicella zoster virus, cytomegalovirus, Epstein–Barr virus, and human herpesvirus type 6. These enveloped viruses are approximately 150–200 nm in size

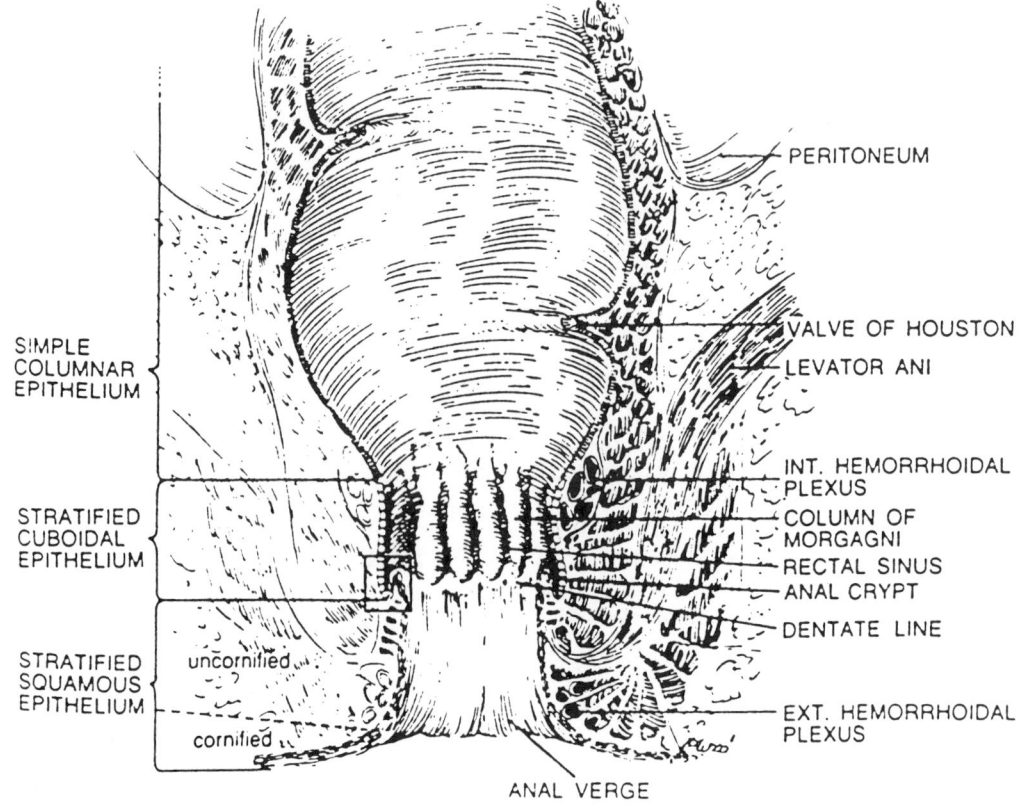

TABLE 2. *Etiologies of proctocolitis*

Infectious	Noninfectious
Chlamydia trachomatis	Ulcerative colitis
Treponema pallidum	Crohn's disease
Neisseria gonorrhoeae	Hemorrhoids
Haemophilus ducreyi	Polyps
Mycobacterium tuberculosis	Carcinoma
Campylobacter jejuni	Lymphoma
Salmonella sp.	Hydradenitis supprativa
Shigella sp.	Kaposi's sarcoma
Herpes simplex virus	
Human papilloma virus	
Cytomegalovirus	
Entamoeba histolytica	
Enterobius vermicularis	
Candida albicans	

with double-stranded DNA of 125,000–250,000 bp contained within an isocahedral capsid (14,15). There is approximately 50% base sequence homology between HSV-1 and HSV-2, and typing of isolates is generally performed using monoclonal antibodies (15). HSV attaches to the host cell surface via a cell surface receptor that has been identified as heparan sulfate (16). Three of the seven glycoproteins in the virus envelope, (gB, gD, and gH) are essential for infectivity (17). The virus can infect a wide range of cells, but infection in the immunocompetent human host is usually limited to mucocutaneous sites.

After entry into the cell, viral DNA is transcribed by host cell DNA polymerase under viral regulatory control. Viral proteins are synthesized in the cytoplasm that are then transported to the nucleus where the nucleocapsid is assembled. The viral envelope is acquired by budding through areas of the nuclear membrane that contain viral-specific glycoproteins. HSV infection ultimately kills cells by inhibiting cellular DNA replication, RNA processing, and protein synthesis. The neuron appears to be unique since production of the virion is not associated with cell lysis. Following replication in the dermis and epidermis, viral particles are transported to sensory neuronal ganglia where latency is established. Animal studies indicate that this occurs within 48 hr of infection (18). During latency the viral genome is maintained in an episomal state, and no viral genes that are necessary for lytic infection are expressed (19). The nondividing neuronal cells provide a sequestered environment for the virus from the host immune system. Reactivation of viral replication is associated with recurrent disease and the neuronal axon serves as a conduit for viral dissemination.

Pathogenesis and Immunity

Humoral immunity is important in controlling HSV infections (20,21). The major viral proteins that elicit antibody responses are surface glycoproteins (gC, gD, gAB), major capsid protein (VP5), and a group of low molecular weight proteins (20). Antibody-dependent cellular cytotoxicity is detectable within the first week of HSV infection. This mechanism of protection acts by destroying infected cells before release of progeny virus (21). In contrast, neutralizing antibody to HSV, which develops after 2 weeks of infection, appears to inhibit viral binding or penetration of target cells (20,22). The best evidence for protection by HSV-specific serum antibodies has been demonstrated in studies of neonatal exposure to HSV-2. Placental transfer of maternal antibodies appeared to protect newborns from HSV infection since infants born to seronegative mothers with primary genital HSV-2 infection at the time of delivery have a tenfold higher risk of infection than infants of seropositive mothers with recurrent HSV-2 infection (23,24). Both neutralizing and antibody-dependent cellular cytotoxicity (ADCC) antibodies were higher in the mothers of exposed infants without infection than mothers of infected infants. Local antibodies are also protective, as reflected in the inverse correlation between local HSV-specific IgA levels and isolation of HSV-2 from cervical samples (25). In addition, local antibody to HSV-1 appears to play a role in modulating HSV-2 infection in HSV-1–seropositive patients (20).

More severe HSV infections occur in immunosuppressed persons due to organ transplantation, cancer chemotherapy, human immunodeficiency virus (HIV) infection, and in neonates (26–30). In immunosuppressed persons, impaired cytotoxic lymphocyte activity and reduced levels of γ-interferon may contribute to the severity and recurrence of HSV infections (20,31–34).

Epidemiology

In the United States, approximately 500,000 persons acquire primary genital herpes each year, and an additional 10 million present with recurrent genital infection (19). HSV accounts for at least ten times more cases of genital ulcerative disease in the United States than syphilis. Between 1966 and 1989, the number of physician consultations for HSV increased 15-fold (Fig. 2) (35). Symptoms occur in only a small portion of cases as only one third of people with HSV-2 antibodies have a history of infection (36). Serological studies show that 30–50% of persons from higher socioeconomic groups and 80–100% from lower socioeconomic groups have been exposed to HSV (36–38). In addition to socioeconomic status, sexual activity is also a risk factor for acquisition of HSV. The seroprevalence of HSV-2 is 70% in prostitutes vs. 3% in nuns, and increases between the ages of 14 and 29 when there is increased sexual activity (38).

Humans are the only known reservoir of HSV. Transmission occurs by direct contact with a symptomatic or asymptomatic individual actively shedding virus. Transmission is more effective from male to female and the annual rate of viral acquisition is higher (31.8%) in susceptible female partners without antibody to HSV-1 or HSV-2 compared to females with antibody to HSV-1 (9.1%). Seventy percent of transmission appears to result from sexual contact during periods of asymptomatic viral shedding (39).

The proportion of cases of proctitis due to HSV has increased since the 1980s. Whereas safer sex practices have decreased the number of newly acquired herpetic

TABLE 3. *Diagnosis and treatment of infectious causes of proctocolitis*

Organism	Symptoms of proctitis	Histology	Diagnosis	Treatment	Anoscopy/ physical examination	Special considerations
C. trachomatis (non-LGV)	May be Asx	Follicles; neutrophil infiltrate of lamina propria/crypts	Culture; DFA	Doxycycline 100 mg PO bid × 7 d; or azithromycin 1 g	Normal or erythema; erosion or rectal discharge	
C. trachomatis (LGV)	Usually Sx	Diffuse inflammation; crypt abscesses; granulomas; giant cells	Culture; DFA; serology	Doxycyline 100 mg × 21 d	Purulent discharge; hematochezia; adenopathy; diffusely friable mucosa	Histology similar to Crohn's
Gonorrhea	May be Asx	Nonspecific cellular infiltrate	Culture; Gram stain	Ceftriaxone 125 mg/250 mg IM or Cefixime 400 mg/800 mg [quinolone/ spectinomycin]	Normal or purulent discharge; erythema/ erosion; able to express mucopus	Possible disseminated gonococcal infection
Syphilis	May be Asx	Nonspecific obliterative endarteritis; mononuclear cell infiltrate; granuloma crypt abscess	Dark field microscopy; immunohistochemical stain; serology	1°/2° PCN 2.4 million units IM; Latent— CN 2.4 million units q wk × 3	Chancre; polypoid mass; condyloma lata; irregular mucosa; adenopathy	Treatment may be inadequate with HIV
Herpes simplex virus	Often Sx; recurrence possible	Nonspecific inflamm; mononuclear infiltrate; intranuclear inclusions; multinucleated giant cells	Clin. syndr. (sacral radiculomyelopathy); viral culture; Tzank prep; serology; (WB; IgG immunoassay)	Acyclovir 400–800 mg 5×/d × 10 d; suppression: ACV 400 mg 2 ×/d. ACV resistance: Foscarnet	Discrete vesicles/ pustules; ulcers; erosion	
Human papillomavirus	May be Asx	Irregular epithelium; koilocytic cells; hyperkeratosis/ dyskeratosis; carcinoma	Clinical appearance; Papanicolau smear; biopsy; PCR/southern blot	Cryotherapy; TCA; surgical excision	Exophytic lesion erosion ulcer	Increased risk of anal carcinoma
E. histolytica	Often Asx	Nonspecific	Serology (invasive disease) stool exam for O&P (3–6 samples); erythrophagocytosis; zymodeme analysis	Metronidazole plus iodoquinol (invasive disease); or iodoquinol; or paromomycin; or diloxanide furoate (colonization)	May be normal	

LGV, lymphogranuloma venereum; Asx, asymptomatic; Sx, symptomatic; DFA, direct fluorescent antibody; WB, western blot; PCR, polymerase chain reaction; O&P, ova and parasites; PCN, penicillin; ACV, acyclovir; TCA, trichloroacetic acid.

infections, recurrent anorectal herpes infections have increased markedly in HIV-infected patients. Interestingly, several studies have shown an increased rate of acquisition of HIV-1 among persons with HSV infection (40–42). HSV disrupts the mucosa thereby facilitating cell-associated and cell-free transfer of HIV-1 between sexual partners (42). Activation of HIV-1 infection from latency by coinfection with HSV-2 has also been postulated to have a direct effect on viral replication of HIV and disease progression (43).

Clinical Illness

The spectrum of symptoms in HSV infection ranges from asymptomatic viral shedding to severe anal pain with ulcerative proctitis. Symptoms generally develop 4–21 days after exposure. The primary infection is self-limited and generally resolves within 3 weeks. Bacterial superinfection is more common for anorectal than for genital lesions and may prolong the course. Symptomatic recurrences tend to be less severe and of shorter duration than

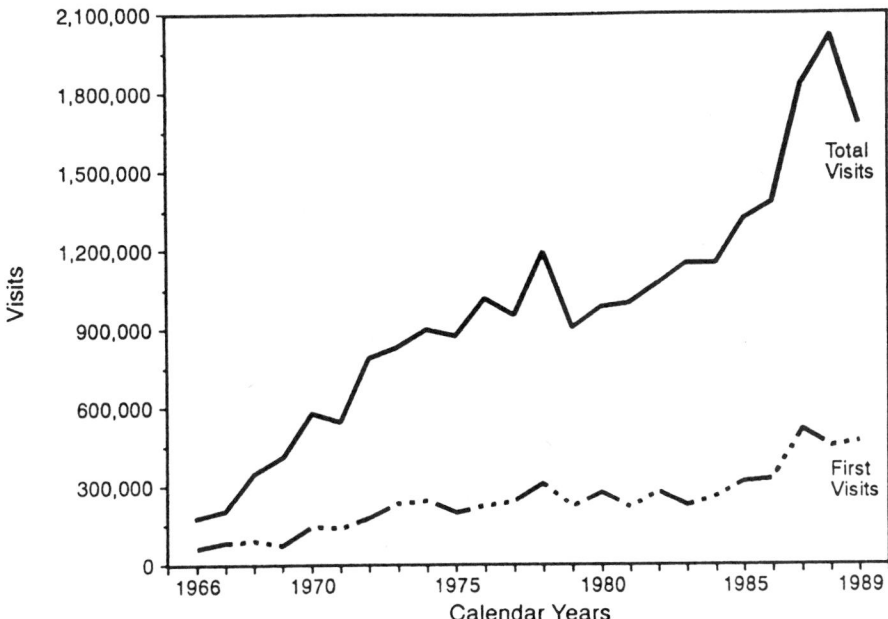

FIG. 2. Number of visits to private physicians' office in the United States between 1966 and 1989 for genital herpes simplex virus infections (35).

the primary infection. The frequency of recurrence is approximately four times greater with HSV-2 than HSV-1 (15,44,45).

Symptoms commonly associated with HSV proctitis include anorectal pain (100%), tenesmus (100%), constipation (78%), anal pruritus (80%), sacral paresthesia (26%), posterior thigh pain (26%), difficulty urinating (48%), perianal lesions (70%), inguinal adenopathy (57%), impotence (9%), and fever (48%) (46). The triad of constipation, anorectal pain, and urinary retention are strongly suggestive of herpetic proctitis. The constipation and urinary retention have been attributed to either a pain-induced reflex spasm of the anal and vesicular sphincters or a sacral radiculomyelopathy (47).

The presence of HIV-1 infection can adversely affect the clinical course of HSV proctitis. Unlike immunocompetent hosts who have spontaneous resolution of lesions within 2–3 weeks, HIV-1–infected patients tend to develop chronic progressive disease leading to large destructive perianal ulcers (48). Chronic mucocutaneous HSV in a person with a positive HIV serology is diagnostic of AIDS (49).

On physical examination, HSV proctitis is characterized by discrete vesicles, pustules, or shallow ulcers around the anus or in the anal canal and rectum. Anoscopic exam is often necessary to diagnose the lesions. In one study Quinn et al. (50) found that only 4 (27%) of 15 homosexual men with HSV anorectal infection had visible perirectal lesions. Koutsky et al. (51) found that 5 (19%) of 26 women with anorectal HSV-2 infection had perirectal lesions, and in 8 (31%) of 26 lesions were restricted to the anus or rectum. On anoscopic examination patients with HSV proctitis are likely to have diffuse friability of the distal 10 cm of the rectal mucosa.

Diagnosis

The diagnosis of HSV proctitis is based on the presence of the vesiculoulcerative lesions and characteristic symptoms. Viral culture of external lesions, a rectal swab, or a rectal biopsy specimen may be used to confirm the diagnosis. The sensitivity of culture for detection of HSV infection depends on the clinical stage of the lesion, the immune status of the host, and the site of infection. Immunofluorescent staining for HSV antigens in tissue biopsies may also be performed. A cytological scraping or Tzank prep for typical intranuclear inclusion bodies or multinucleated giant cells may be helpful.

Histological examination of rectal biopsy samples from patients with HSV proctitis usually shows acute nonspecific inflammation. The characteristic findings of perivascular mononuclear cell infiltrate, intranuclear inclusion bodies, and multinucleated giant cells may be present but are not unique to HSV infection. HSV serology can be used to confirm infection when paired serum samples demonstrate either seroconversion or a fourfold rise in titer (52). Commercially available enzyme immunoassays do not distinguish well between antibody subtypes (53). Recently, a type-specific glycoprotein, gG, was identified, and a serological assay using this protein to distinguish antibody to viral subtypes is highly specific (54). Additionally, western blot has been used to detect HSV-specific antibodies (55). Although isolation of HSV is the most specific means of confirming a primary episode of infection, detection of HSV-2–specific antibody is the most sensitive way to confirm symptomatic reactivation and to detect asymptomatic infection (51).

Polymerase chain reaction (PCR) is now being used for detection of HSV infection. In a study comparing PCR with culture, PCR detected HSV DNA from all culture-positive samples (56). In addition, PCR was able to detect HSV DNA in ulcerative lesions on 15 of 17 days compared with 3 of 17 days by viral isolation. PCR detection became negative only after the lesions reepithelialized. Although PCR does not differentiate between viable and nonviable HSV, it is more sensitive than culture for detection of infection.

Treatment

The decision to treat HSV proctitis depends on the severity of symptoms since the infection is usually self-limited in immunocompetent persons. Conservative therapy with sitz baths, stool softeners, and analgesics is used for mild proctitis. Antiviral therapy for initial infection consists of oral acyclovir 400–800 mg five times per day for 10 days, which decreases duration of symptoms and viral shedding (57,58). For severe mucocutaneous disease, such as that associated with immunosuppression, intravenous acyclovir, 5 mg/kg every 8 hr, should be used until the mucosal surface is healed (58–62). Since discontinuation of therapy is generally associated with recurrent disease, oral acyclovir 200 mg three to five times per day or 400 mg two times per day may be used to suppress clinical disease in immunosuppressed patients and in immunocompetent persons with more than four episodes of symptomatic HSV infection per year (58). Safety of daily dosing has been demonstrated in patients treated for up to 5 years; therapy should be stopped after 1 year to determine recurrence (58,63). Severity and duration of recurrences can be decreased if oral acyclovir 200 mg five times per day or 400 mg three times per day or 800 mg twice per day is initiated within 48 hr of onset of the lesion and continued for 5 days (58). Topical and intravenous vidarabine have proven to be ineffective for primary and recurrent genital herpes in immunocompetent patients (64,65).

HSV mutants resistant to acyclovir have been isolated from immunocompetent and immunocompromised patients after prolonged use of the drug (66–70). Deficiency of thymidine kinase, which prevents phosphorylation of acyclovir to its active form, is the most common mechanism of resistance (67,71); altered DNA polymerase occurs less frequently (68,72). Severe progressive mucocutaneous disease in HIV-infected patients can be associated with acyclovir-resistant HSV-2 (72). Foscarnet (phosphonoformic acid), 40–60 mg/kg every 8–12 hr, can produce clinical and microbiological cure in these patients (70,73). A randomized trial comparing foscarnet 40 mg/kg every 8 hr with vidarabine 15 mg/kg/day for HIV-infected patients with acyclovir-resistant ulcers demonstrated healing of all herpetic lesions after 10–14 days in the foscarnet group compared to complete failure of all six patients treated with vidarabine (74). HSV disease generally recurs after discontinuation of foscarnet, and these first recurrences are usually with an acyclovir-susceptible strain phenotypically similar to the one that established the initial infection (75). Foscarnet-resistant HSV strains have also been isolated from lesions that developed while patients were being treated with foscarnet. In several cases these isolates were sensitive to acyclovir and responded to therapy with either acyclovir alone or in combination with ganciclovir (76–78).

HUMAN PAPILLOMAVIRUS

Microbiology

The human papillomavirus is a member of the papovavirus family, which includes papillomaviruses, simian virus 40, and polyomaviruses (79). Human papillomaviruses are nonenveloped double-stranded DNA viruses of approximately 7900 base pairs encased in an icosahedral capsid. The genome is divided into early (E) and late (L) regions. The E regions code for eight regulatory gene products (E1–E8) and the L region codes for a 53-kDa protein that constitutes approximately 80% of the viral capsid proteins, and a 70-kDa minor capsid protein. Capsid proteins appear to mediate viral attachment to susceptible cells, host range, and neutralization (80,81). The E-region gene products are differentially expressed in different HPV strains; E6 and E7 regions code for proteins important in malignant transformation (82,83). Infection with HPV is initiated by entry and multiplication of the virus within the nucleus of cells of the basal germinal epithelium. Viral infection accelerates cell growth, leading to an irregularly thickened epithelium with foci of koilocytic cells containing perinuclear cavitation and nuclear atypia. Skin and mucosal lesions occur 3 weeks to 8 months following infection. Since only early gene products are expressed in the basal layers, viral particles and viral capsid proteins are absent in these cells but can be identified in the nondividing superficial cell layers. Transmission of the virus occurs by shedding of viral particles with the superficial epithelial cells (80).

Pathogenesis and Immunity

HPV infection leads to disruption of the normal skin morphology and excess proliferation of all epidermal layers except the basal layer. These changes lead to the development of acanthosis, parakeratosis, and sometimes hyperkeratosis (84). In some infected cells, koilocytic transformation occurs with characteristic shrinking of the nucleus. Certain HPVs are associated with exophytic and neoplastic lesions (85,86). The molecular basis for the difference in oncogenic potential of the HPVs is unclear, but duration of infection and cofactors such as sunlight and radiation may contribute to malignant transformation (87,88). In nonmalignant HPV lesions, viral DNA is located extrachromosomally, whereas in HPV-associated neoplasia it is generally integrated. This integration may occur at any site in the host cell chromosome but only at specific sites in the viral genome (80).

Humoral and cell-mediated immunity to HPV is poorly understood. The lack of an *in vitro* system to support replication of the virus has limited the ability to study responses to immunologically important antigens. However, observations of the natural history of HPV infection suggest that host immunity plays an important role in the pathogenesis of HPV infections. Warts are less common in adults than in children, presumably due to immunity acquired in childhood. Such lesions increase in size in conditions associated with impaired cell-mediated immunity, such as pregnancy (89), immunosuppressive therapy for organ transplantation (90), HIV infection and lymphoproliferative disorders (91).

Antibody to HPV-6b L1 fusion protein is reported to be present in 10% of children less than 5 years old and 60% of women attending a colposcopy clinic (92). Additional seroprevalence studies have shown that these antibodies are present in 44% of children, 39% of students from a university health service, and 56% of STD clinic patients, whereas 63% of patients with dysplasia, 67% of patients with vulvar carcinoma, and 66% patients with warts have such antibodies (92–94). Moreover, antibody reactivity to HPV-11 virions has been reported in 33% of patients with condyloma, but not in control subjects (95). Taken together, these studies indicate that antibodies to HPV proteins are common in the general population. HPV-specific antibodies are even more common in women with HPV-associated neoplasia (96–99). In particular, IgA antibodies to an E2 peptide of HPV-16 (peptide 245) may be up to threefold more common in women with carcinoma of the cervix than control subjects (96). Serum antibodies to HPV-16 and 18 E7 proteins also are more common in patients with invasive cervical cancer (98,99). Although antibodies to the E2 and E7 proteins have been suggested as markers for cervical or even anal cancer, their functional significance is still unknown.

Cell-mediated immunity also plays a role in the pathogenesis of HPV infection (90,91). Evidence indicates that natural killer cells from patients with anogenital tumors

have defective recognition of HPV-infected cells and are unresponsive to the stimulatory effects of cytokines such as IL-2 and IL-6 (100). There is also evidence for an important role for cytokines in mediating HPV expression in neoplastic cells (101). At least one mechanism appears to be suppression of transcription of mRNA for transforming proteins (E6/E7) by γ-interferon and leukoreglin (102). Another mechanism appears to be involved in HPV-associated neoplasia in patients with HIV, as suggested by the ability of the HIV-1 tat protein to increase transcription of E2-dependent HPV-16 (103).

Epidemiology

Anal papillomas are common in homosexual men and heterosexual women practicing anal intercourse. Between 46% and 90% of patients with anal warts have a history of engaging in anal sex. The lack of an accurate and reliable serological assay to test large numbers of people for HPV makes it impossible to determine the magnitude of HPV infection in the general population. However, genital warts probably represent only 10% of the total spectrum of genital HPV infection (104). The frequency of consultations for HPV increased ten-fold from 179,000 to 1.7 million between 1966 and 1987 (Fig. 3) and is nearly threefold that for HSV (35). HPV prevalence rates are estimated to vary between 9% in unselected women having cytological screening to 82% in repeatedly sampled prostitutes (105,106), and up to 51.5% in homosexual men (2).

Of the 60 HPVs identified, approximately 20% are detected in the anogenital tract, with HPV 6, 11, 16, 18, 31, 33, and 35 being the most common. HPV 6 and 11 are found in most exophytic anal condylomas and have little oncogenic potential (85). HPV 16 and 18 are found in 50%

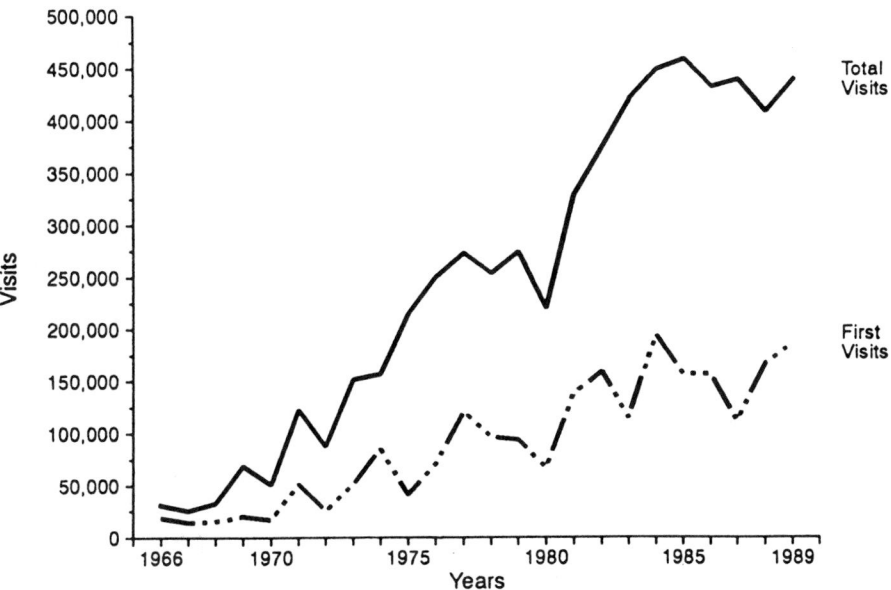

FIG. 3. Genital warts. Number of visits to private physicians' offices in the United States between 1966 and 1989 (35).

and 20%, respectively, of cervical cancers, and 56% and 5%, respectively, of anal cancers (85,86,107).

While the association of HPV and cervical cancer has long been recognized, there is now a growing body of evidence to support a role for HPV in anal cancer (108–111). Scholefield (109) prospectively followed 82 patients with anal HPV infection and found that 23 had evidence of anal intraepithelial neoplasm (AIN). The prevalence of HPV infection and AIN was higher in homosexual men than in heterosexual men. In patients without anal HPV infection no AIN was found. Several recent studies have examined the interaction of HPV and HIV, and reported an increased risk for HPV expression in anal intraepithelial lesions of HIV-infected individuals (111–114). In one study of 306 HIV-seropositive and 219-seronegative homosexual men, high-grade dysplasia was significantly more common in HIV-infected (4%) than HIV uninfected patients (0.5%) (111). The risk of having high-grade anal lesions in HIV-positive patients with CD4 counts less than 500 cells/mm^3 was 2.9-fold higher than for HIV-positive patients with CD4 counts greater than 500 cells/mm^3. The recognition of the association of HPV with anal cancer has led to recommendations for more aggressive diagnosis and therapy of these premalignant lesions.

Clinical Illness

Anal warts appear as white, pink, or grey flat or heaped-up lesions that vary in extent and number. They may be mistaken for condyloma lata, which are generally more moist and smooth in appearance. Anal warts can spontaneously resolve, likely due to an effective immune system (115). Patients with anorectal warts may be asymptomatic or complain of pruritus ani, rectal discharge, and bleeding. The warts are located in the perianal area or inside the anal canal (2). In cases where perianal lesions are detected, an anoscopic exam should be performed to rule out lesions within the canal.

Diagnosis

Diagnosis of anorectal HPV infection is based on clinical observation. Other lesions that may have a similar appearance include condylomata lata and squamous cell carcinoma. Distinction between benign and malignant lesions can only be made by histological examination of biopsy material, which should be performed for any lesion with an atypical appearance or a poor response to therapy. A Papanicolaou smear may reveal dyskeratosis and koilocytosis, classic signs of HPV infection, but this technique may be insensitive if only classic criteria are used, and DNA hybridization may be more likely to detect latent HPV infection without cellular abnormality (116,117). Southern blot analysis has been considered the gold standard for detection of HPV DNA. However, it is technically difficult to perform. Other DNA hybridization techniques such as dot-blot and filter *in situ* hybridization are simpler to perform, but less sensitive and specific (89).

PCR is now being developed for diagnosis of HPV (118–121). The amplified DNA can be subjected to hybridization using specific probes or restriction fragment length polymorphism (RFLP) for typing of the isolates (122).

Treatment

Effective curative therapy for HPV infection is not currently available. However, lesions can be treated with cryotherapy using a cryoprobe or liquid nitrogen. Such local treatment is effective in clearing 63–91% of lesions without scarring (123,124). In addition, a 20% podophyllin solution (<0.5 mL) in tincture of benzoin has been effective in removing up to 77% of lesions (125). The solution is applied to the warts and allowed to remain in place for up to 12 hr. Application can be repeated once or twice per week until all lesions are removed. Because the agent is caustic it cannot be used intranally, and because it has oncogenic and teratogenic potential it is contraindicated in pregnancy. Other side effects of podophyllin include blood dyscrasias, hepatotoxicity, and neuropathy. A less concentrated (0.5%) podophyllin solution has been effective and has the benefit of being able to be applied by the patient (126). Trichloroacetic acid (TCA) is another caustic agent that is effective in removing external lesions. A recent study comparing the efficacy of TCA with cryotherapy for external genital warts in 86 patients found an 86% rate of complete clearance with cryotherapy compared with 70% with TCA (127).

Electrocautery or electrodesiccation also can be used for removal of genital lesions, but such therapy is contraindicated for patients with pacemakers or for those with lesions proximal to the anal verge (58). CO$_2$ laser therapy and surgery are alternative treatment modalities, particularly for large lesions and those not amenable to other modes of treatment, but the requirement for local or general anesthesia limits their usefulness. In one study comparing podophyllin and surgery, surgery resulted in 93% clearance and 29% recurrence at 12 months compared with 77% clearance and 65% recurrence for podophyllin (128).

Several studies have examined the use of intramuscular and intralesional α- and β-interferon for genital warts (129–131). Intralesional α- and β-interferon appears more effective than placebo for the treatment of condyloma acuminata, and patients whose lesions contain detectable HPV nucleic acid or papillomavirus antigens or in whom koilocytes are observed seem more likely to respond to this treatment (132). The use of systemic interferon for genital warts is associated with variable results (129,132) and side effects, including fever, chills, headaches, and myalgia. The present Centers for Disease Control guidelines do not recommend its use for treatment of anogenital warts (58).

TREPONEMA PALLIDUM

Microbiology

Treponema pallidum, a member of the Spirochaetaceae family, is a unicellular, helical, tightly coiled organism approximately 6–15 μm long and 0.15 μm wide. The size of the organism is below the level of resolution by light microscopy, so dark field light microscopic examination is necessary for visualization. The spirochete is surrounded by an amorphous outer layer composed of mucopolysaccharides, an outer membrane, a mucopeptide layer or periplast, a peptidoglycan layer, and a cytoplasmic membrane. Three fibrils that arise from each end of the organism and insert in the opposite end contract to propel the organism in a characteristic rotary flexing motion. *T. pallidum* cannot be cultivated *in vitro* but can remain motile for up to 7 days if kept at 35°C in a highly enriched elevated CO_2 environment (133).

Pathogenesis and Immunity

T. pallidum is able to infect skin or mucosa in which there has been a break in the epithelial layer. The incubation period between exposure and development of a lesion depends on the size of the inoculum. In rabbits, 10^7 organisms will produce a lesion in 5–7 days, but as few as 4 organisms can establish infection. Since the organism divides slowly (30–33 hr per division), establishment of infection requires successful evasion of host immunity (133,134).

Although the clinical course of syphilis has been well described, the mechanisms of pathogenesis and immunity have not been fully elucidated. Early infection is associated with the development of a lesion (chancre) after an average of 21 days (range 10–90 days). After several weeks, the lesion heals spontaneously. The primary chancre contains spirochetes within a mucoid material consisting of hyaluronic acid and chondroitin sulfate which is rimmed by a cellular infiltrate composed primarily of neutrophils and macrophages known to phagocytose *T. pallidum* and lymphocytes (133–138). The origin of this mucoid material is uncertain, but it may contribute to the organisms evasion of host immune responses.

During secondary syphilis, *T. pallidum* disseminates to skin, mucosa, and organs despite the presence of *T. pallidum*–specific antibodies. The deposition of immune complexes in various tissues also occurs during secondary syphilis. Dissemination at this stage has been attributed to impaired cell-mediated immunity (139), as evidenced by the rapid and severe progression of disease in patients who are infected with HIV-1 or malnourished (140–142).

During the next stage of disease, referred to as latency, infection is effectively suppressed so that lesions are no longer apparent. It has been postulated that during latency the organism is "disguised" by concealing of *T. pallidum* antigens from host defense mechanisms, referred to as the "immunoprotective niche" (143,144). However, relapses with secondary syphilis, and subsequent development of neurosyphilis, indicate that viable organisms are still present.

Tertiary syphilis becomes clinically apparent 1–20 years after disseminated infection. Only one third of untreated patients will develop late manifestations of the disease. It has been postulated that failure to develop an effective delayed-type hypersensitivity response early in infection permits further disease progression. Cell-mediated immune responses likely contribute to host protection but may also play a pathological role since the development of large granulomatous lesions (gummas) during tertiary syphilis appear to represent a host-mediated hypersensitivity response to *T. pallidum* (145). These lesions often appear at sites prone to trauma (133).

Epidemiology

Between 1950 and 1978, the incidence of syphilis increased from 19,000 to 26,000 cases per year (146). The incidence continued to increase in the late 1970s and early 1980s, due largely to an increased number of cases in homosexual men (146,147). By the mid-1980s, however, the incidence of syphilis in homosexual men began to decrease in association with behavioral changes adopted in response to the HIV epidemic. In 1985, concurrent with the decreased rate in homosexual men, the incidence of syphilis in urban heterosexuals began to increase (148). Between 1985 and 1990, the rate of syphilis increased 126% in black men and 231% in black women (Fig. 4) (148,149), likely reflecting limited access to health care and promiscuous sexual activity related to the epidemic of illicit drug usage. Unfortunately, the same behavior patterns that place this population at risk for syphilis also enhance acquisition of HIV infection (146,150–152).

Although syphilis has decreased in homosexual men, anorectal syphilis still occurs primarily in homosexuals. In inner city STD clinics in the United Kingdom, 80% of cases of primary and secondary syphilis occur in homosexual men and 30% of these are anorectal (153). Indeed, among homosexual men attending one STD clinic, 12% had anorectal syphilis (50).

Clinical Illness

Gastrointestinal lesions due to syphilis occur most commonly in the primary and secondary stages of *T. pallidum* infection. The presence and type of symptoms depend on the form of the lesion. The primary lesion, which usually develops 2–6 weeks after exposure, has a variable appearance accounting for the high rate of misdiagnosis. The anal chancre is the most common presentation; it may be single and eccentrically placed or multiple with mirror images ("kissing chancres"). The chancres occur anywhere in the anus or rectum (154,155). Since chancres are often asymptomatic, painful lesions may be attributed to trauma or anal fissures. Superinfection of the chancre is often associated with the development of symptoms. Inguinal lymphadenopathy is often present with anorectal syphilis and helps to distinguish anorectal syphilis from fissures. Primary anorectal syphilis may also present as ulcerated masses that are typically located on the anterior wall of the rectum (156).

Secondary syphilis is associated with spirochetemia and typically develops 6 weeks to 6 months after the initial infection. Condyloma lata are the most common anorectal lesions associated with secondary syphilis. They are

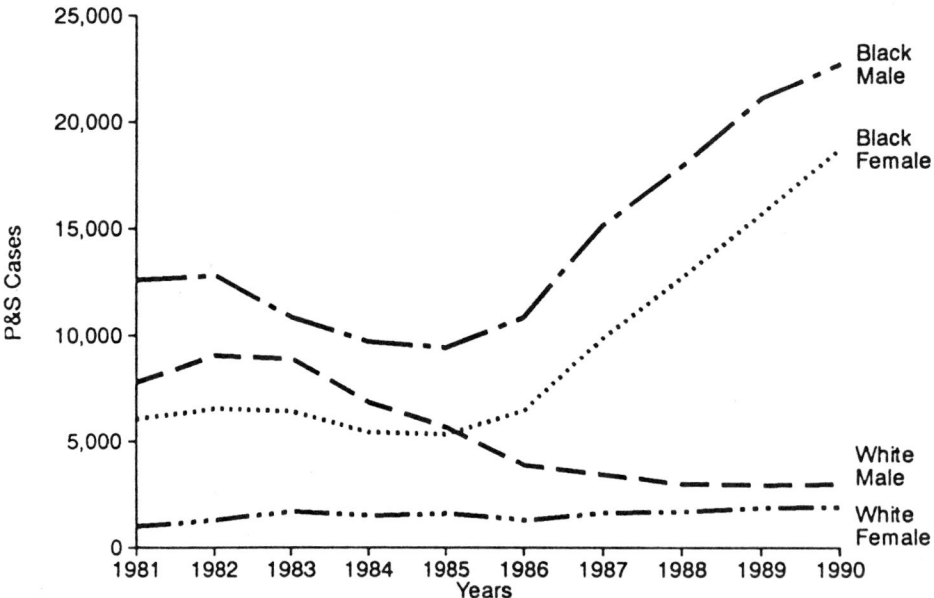

FIG. 4. Primary and secondary syphilis cases by gender and race in the United States between 1981 and 1990 (35).

smooth, warty masses in or near the rectum and must be differentiated from the more highly keratinized condyloma acuminata. Condyloma lata are often pruritic and produce a foul discharge that is highly infectious. Other presentations include proctitis without a clear ulcer, polypoid growth, pseudotumor, mucosal ulceration and erythema, or submucosal irregularities with rubbery nodes suggesting lymphoma. Constitutional symptoms, skin rashes, and mucous patches can also occur (157–159). Inflammation of the gastrointestinal tract from syphilis is usually limited to the distal 15 cm of the colon, but may reach the distal 20 cm with secondary syphilis. The anorectal lesions of primary and secondary syphilis may also coexist (157). Untreated, syphilitic proctitis will spontaneously resolve within 3–4 weeks. If the patient is not treated in the primary or secondary stage, a latent period ensues during which the patient is infected but asymptomatic. Some of these patients progress to develop tertiary syphilis. Although gastrointestinal lesions are unusual at this stage, rectal gummas may occur and can be mistaken for malignancy. During tertiary syphilis, anal sphincter paralysis and severe anal pain may develop in association with tabes dorsalis.

Although biopsies of syphilitic anal lesions are often nonspecific, histology may show an obliterative endarteritis with capillary proliferation; infiltration of the lamina propria by plasma cells, histiocytes, and lymphocytes; and occasionally granulomas (160,161).

Diagnosis

Diagnosis of primary or secondary syphilis is made by identification of the organisms in a lesion. Detection of typical organisms on dark field microscopy is useful for perianal lesions, but the presence of nonpathogenic treponemes makes the test less helpful for lesions in the rectum (162). Immunohistochemical stains of exudate from a lesion may be useful when the dark field examination is negative (163). However, silver-stained treponemes may be mistaken for tissue components, especially reticulin fibers (161). Routine histological examination is not useful as the findings are generally nonspecific and may be confused with other conditions such as inflammatory bowel disease. Newer diagnostic techniques that utilize PCR are being developed but are not yet available for clinical use.

Serological diagnosis of syphilis is based on the presence of antibodies to nontreponemal and treponemal antigens. Nontreponemal tests [Venereal Disease Research Lab (VDRL) and rapid plasma reagin (RPR)] are based on detection of antibodies to a cardiolipin antigen that is produced during infection. The VDRL generally becomes positive 2 weeks after development of a chancre. In untreated patients, titers will peak during secondary syphilis and subsequently decline. The sensitivity of the VDRL depends on the stage of infection. The test detects approximately 50–70% of cases of primary syphilis, 100% of cases of secondary syphilis, and 85–100% of cases of tertiary syphilis. A positive VDRL or RPR must be corroborated by a positive test specific for antibody to *T. pallidum* antigens such as the fluorescent treponemal antibody absorption (FTA-ABS) test or the microhemagglutination (MHATP) test. The specificity of the VDRL varies with the population tested and is higher in healthy than in sick persons (133,146). The FTA-ABS is the first serological test to become positive and is present in 70–90% of patients with a chancre. This test is generally 100% sensitive in secondary and tertiary syphilis. Treponemal antibody titers do not correlate with disease activity and usually remain positive after infection.

Concomitant infection with HIV-1 may impair antibody responses to *T. pallidum*. Delayed or absent serological test reactivity for syphilis occurs predominantly during the later stages of HIV infection (164–166). Higher RPR titers in HIV-1 seropositive patients with secondary syphilis than in HIV-1 seronegative patients (167). Serological false-positive tests, such as RPR-positive and FTA-ABS–negative tests, which occur in a wide variety of infectious and noninfectious conditions, have been associated with HIV infection (168,146). Because of the association between HIV and *T. pallidum* infections, HIV testing is recommended to all patients with syphilis.

Treatment

Penicillin is the treatment of choice for syphilis. Benzathine penicillin 2.4 million units IM is effective for primary, secondary, and early latent syphilis of less than 1 year. In latent syphilis of greater than 1 year and tertiary syphilis other than neurosyphilis, benzathine penicillin, 2.4 million units IM once per week for 3 weeks, is recommended (58). In patients intolerant of penicillin, doxycycline 100 mg orally twice per day, or tetracycline 500 mg four times per day, should be used for 2 weeks for early syphilis and for 4 weeks for latent or tertiary syphilis.

All patients with syphilis should be reexamined at 3 and 6 months since failure to eradicate syphilis can occur with any regimen. Nontreponemal antibody titers should decline fourfold by 3 months in primary and secondary syphilis, and by 6 months in early or latent syphilis. Lack of an appropriate decline in antibody titer, or persistence of clinical signs or symptoms suggests treatment failure or reinfection, in which case cerebrospinal fluid should be evaluated and retreatment started. Sexual contacts should be evaluated clinically and serologically. Since a partner may be infected yet be seronegative within 90 days of exposure, treatment is indicated during this period.

Several reports have documented poor responses to standard therapy for syphilis in patients with HIV infection (169–172). Syphilis may have a more aggressive course in these patients and single-dose therapy with benzathine penicillin for early syphilis has been associated with subsequent development of neurosyphilis. In addition, the serological titer may decrease more slowly after treatment in HIV-infected patients (172). Since patients with syphilis and HIV are at higher risk for failure of initial therapy, more frequent follow-up is recommended. HIV-infected patients with syphilis should be evaluated monthly for the first 3 months following treatment, and then at 6, 9, and 12 months to document lack of clinical or serological relapse (58).

NEISSERIA GONORRHOEAE

Microbiology

N. gonorrhoeae is a nonmotile, non–spore-forming, gram-negative diplococcus. The bacterium has a cyto-plasmic membrane, peptidoglycan layer, and outer membrane. Unlike meningococci, gonococci lack a polysaccharide capsule. *In vivo* the majority of *N. gonorrhoeae* have their outer cell surface covered by pili, which are individual fibrils or fibrillar aggregates involved in attachment and invasion of the organisms. Pili also serve as markers of pathogenicity, as piliated strains are more pathogenic than nonpiliated strains. Nonreciprocal recombinational events involving the pilus gene lead to antigenic variation of the pili as well as alternation between piliated and nonpiliated morphologies (173).

Several gonococcal plasmids have been identified, some of which mediate antibiotic resistance. For instance, derivatives of a 36-kDa plasmid confer tetracycline resistance (174) and several plasmids encode β-lactamases (175). Most gonococci also contain a cryptic 4.2-kilobase cryptic plasmid (176). The proportion of gonococcal infections due to β-lactamase–producing *N. gonorrhoeae* increased significantly during the 1980s. By 1989 over 5% of cases were due to strains with plasmid-mediated β-lactamases and over 17% had chromosomally mediated resistance to penicillin or tetracycline (177,178).

Pathogenesis and Immunity

N. gonorrhoeae most commonly infect columnar epithelial cells of the urethra and endocervix. However, other sites including the fallopian tubes, ovaries, rectum, and prostate also may be infected. After attachment to the epithelial cell, the organism is internalized by endocytosis and transported to the subepithelial space (179,180). Infection is associated with a vigorous neutrophil response, sloughing of epithelial cells, and development of submucosal microabscesses.

The lack of good animal models has limited study of the pathogenesis and immune response to this infection. Reinfection commonly occurs in both men and women, indicating that protective immunity does not occur following natural infection. However, partial protection against reinfection with the same serovar does occur. For example, Nairobi prostitutes generally have a two- to tenfold decreased risk of reinfection with the same serovar, and the risk of gonococcal infection is inversely related to the duration of prostitution (181). The ability of the organism to cause recurrent infections is due in part to antigenic variation and its ability mask relevant antigens. The relevant antigens include outer membrane components such as lipopolysaccharide (LPS), protein I, protein II (opa proteins), and protein III (182).

Protein I functions as a porin in the outer membrane and is used as an antigen for serotyping of gonococcal isolates (183). It is an important determinant of antibiotic susceptibility (184), serum resistance (185), and invasiveness (186). Gonococcal isolates that cause disseminated disease are typically IA and are resistant to the bactericidal effects of normal human serum, whereas isolates causing local disease are usually serum-sensitive (187,173). It appears that the bactericidal effect of normal human serum occurs primarily by binding IgM antibodies to complement and LPS (188,189). Protein III appears to contain epitopes for binding blocking antibodies and bactericidal antibodies (190).

Protein II, or the opa family of proteins, is important in the antigenic variation seen among gonococcal isolates. Gonococci undergo phase switching (on/off expression of opas), as well as switching from one opa to another (182). This antigenic variation likely contributes to bacterial evasion of host immune responses. Opas function as adhesins promoting adherence to epithelial cells (191) and neutrophils (192) and aggregation of organisms in a colony (193). They also stimulate production of bactericidal antibodies (194).

Delayed-type hypersensitivity responses to a variety of bacterial fractions and culture filtrates occurs in the majority of persons infected with *N. gonorrhoeae* (195). Additionally, lymphocytes from infected persons undergo transformation upon stimulation with gonococcal antigens. However, by 5 weeks after treatment, antigen-specific proliferation declines to undetectable levels (196,197), and the relationship between cellular immune responses and protection from gonococcal infection has not been elucidated.

Epidemiology

The incidence of *N. gonorrhoeae* infections decreased significantly between 1975 and 1987, with the greatest decline occurring in 25- to 44-year-old black males. By 1987, 15- to 24-year-old women had the highest incidence of gonorrhea (5). Since 1980, among homosexual men, the incidence of *N. gonorrhoeae* infections, particularly of the anorectal region, began a sharp decline; however, recent reports suggest that this trend may be changing (10,198–200).

N. gonorrhoeae is a common cause of anorectal infections in women as well as men. Between 1966 to 1977, 26–63% of women with gonorrhea had anorectal involvement, and in up to 20% the rectum was the only involved site (201). The role of rectal intercourse in the etiology of anorectal *N. gonorrhoeae* in women has been difficult to determine. Among homosexual men, *N. gonorrhoeae* is the most frequently identified sexually transmitted pathogen. Twenty-eight percent to 55% of homosexual men attending STD clinics have gonorrhea, and in 40% the anus is the only site of infection. The rectum is often more commonly involved than the urethra or pharynx (50,158,202). Homosexual men are more frequently infected with strains with the *mtr* mutation, which confers antibiotic susceptibility. This mutation is also associated with decreased membrane permeability, which is thought to enhance the ability of the strain to survive in the rectum (203). A study from the United Kingdom evaluated gonococcal isolates from 383 episodes of infections in women and found that one serovar, Bajk, was isolated with significantly higher frequency in rectal (27%) than genital (17%) infections (204). These studies suggest that different strains preferentially infect specific host sites.

Clinical Illness

Asymptomatic infections are common with anorectal gonorrhea and occur more frequently than urethral infections in homosexual men (50,205,206). When symptoms occur, they develop 5–7 days after exposure and include pruritus ani, bloody or mucopurulent discharge, tenesmus, and constipation. Anorectal gonorrhea may produce complications such as fistula, abscess, stricture, and disseminated infection. Disseminated gonococcal infection is typically associated with the AHU auxotype and host deficiency of complement components, particularly the terminal components (207,208).

On sigmoidoscopic examination the rectum may show normal mucosa or erythema, fissures, superficial erosion, and friability particularly at the anorectal junction (209,210). Mucus and pus also are commonly present (158,211). Histological findings are nonspecific and include patchy disorganization of the mucus-secreting cells, vascular engorgement, and infiltration of the lamina propria with neutrophils, lymphocytes, plasma cells, and monocytes (201).

Diagnosis

Diagnosis of anorectal gonorrhea is made by Gram stain or culture of the material obtained by swab of the rectum. In symptomatic patients, an anoscope should be used to perform the rectal swab as the diagnostic yield can be increased from 33% with a blind swab to 79% with a swab obtained under direct visualization (211). In asymptomatic patients, material from a blind swab is adequate since direct visualization does not increase the yield. Due to the relatively low sensitivity of Gram stain for rectal samples culture is the preferred method of diagnosis (50). A positive Gram stain should be confirmed by culture of the organism on selected media, such as Thayer–Martin which contains vancomycin, colistin, and trimethoprim to inhibit overgrowth of the gonorrhea by the endogenous intestinal bacteria.

Treatment

Ceftriaxone 250 mg IM is the recommended treatment for anorectal *N. gonorrhoeae* infection (58). This regimen has a cure rate of over 98% for genital and rectal infections. Ceftriaxone 125 mg IM is equally effective, less expensive, and easier to administer. To date, clinically relevant ceftriaxone resistance has not been reported with either dose of ceftriaxone (199,212). Due to the high rate of coinfection with chlamydia, all cases of *N. gonorrhoeae* should also receive a 7-day course of doxycycline 100 mg twice per day (58).

Recommended alternatives to ceftriaxone include spectinomycin 2 g IM, ciprofloxacin 500 mg orally, norfloxacin 800 mg orally, cefotaxime 1 g IM, ceftizoxime 500 mg IM, and cefuroxime axetil 1.0 g orally plus probenecid 1.0 g orally as single-dose regimens (58,213–216). Patients treated with an alternate regimen should have a follow-up culture (58). All patients with *N. gonorrhoeae* infection should also have a serological test for syphilis and be offered testing for HIV. In addition, sexual partners of infected patients exposed within the preceding 30 days should be treated presumptively.

CHLAMYDIA TRACHOMATIS

Microbiology

Chlamydiae are gram-negative obligate intracellular bacteria. They contain double-stranded DNA of approximately 600–850 kilobase pairs (660×10^6 Da). *C. trachomatis* also contain a plasmid (mol wt 4.4×10^6 Da) (217). The organisms have a biphasic growth cycle and exist as two discrete entities that differ in structure and function (218). They are unable to synthesize metabolic nutrients and high-energy compounds such as adenosine triphosphate (ATP) and are therefore dependent on host cells during the replicative phase of their growth cycle. *C. trachomatis* is divided into three biovars based in part on host susceptibility and DNA homology. Two of these biovars, the trachoma biovar and lymphogranuloma venerum (LGV) biovar, cause human infection; the third biovar does not. The trachoma biovar replicates only in columnar epithelial cells, and the LGV strains are also able to replicate in macrophages (219). The LGV and trachoma biovars have been serotyped into 15 serovars A–K, and L1, L2, and L3 based on differences in monoclonal antibody reactivity to the major outer membrane protein (MOMP), which is a cysteine-rich protein constituting 60% of the outer membrane of chlamydiae (220). Serovars A, B, Ba, and C are primarily associated with trachoma, serovars D–K with urogenital infections, and L1, L2, L3 with LGV.

The elementary body (EB) (diameter 300–400 nm) is the infectious form of chlamydiae. Although a specific host cell receptor has not been identified, inhibition of adherence of any *C. trachomatis* strain by a heterologous strain suggests that attachment involves a common host cell receptor that may be different for LGV and trachoma biovars (221). Following attachment the EB enters the host cell by active endocytosis (222). In polymorphonuclear leukocytes, lysosomes fuse with *C. trachomatis* leading to subsequent degradation of the organism. In infected epithelial cells phagolysosomal fusion does not occur until very late in infection; rather within 6–8 hr after entrance into the cell there is differentiation of the EB into a larger (800–1000 nm) reticulate body (RB). The RB, which is the metabolically active form of *Chlamydia*, differs structurally and morphologically from the EB. The RB multiplies by binary fission 8–24 hr after infection with expansion of the phagosome into the typical intracellular inclusion that displaces the cytoplasm. After 24 hr, progeny RBs condense into EBs which become evident in the phagosome. Subsequently phagolysosomal fusion occurs, and by 48–72 hr after infection, the cell ruptures, releasing infectious EBs that initiate new infection.

Pathogenesis and Immunity

Protective immunity to *C. trachomatis* is short-lived and appears to be serovar-specific. Seroepidemiological studies indicate that the presence of antichlamydial antibodies is associated with a reduced rate of isolation of *C. trachomatis*, suggesting that the antibodies are partially protective resulting in less severe infections (223,224). Previous infection is associated with a reduced likelihood of reinfection and less severe local disease. Additionally, serum antibodies may play a role in preventing the spread of infection. For example, postabortal salpingitis occurs more frequently in women infected with *Chlamydia* who have a lower serum antibody titer to *Chlamydia* before abortion (225). Neutralizing antibody directed against epitopes of the MOMP is the primary mechanism of protective humoral immunity (226–230). The mechanism of neutralization has been attributed to inhibition of attachment, as well as inhibition of infection following entry into the host cell (231,222).

Whereas humoral immunity appears to have a protective role in chlamydial infection, cellular immunity appears to play a dual role of contributing both to protection and to pathogenesis (232,233). In the monkey model of ocular *C. trachomatis* infection, a delayed-type hypersensitivity response is associated with trachoma, and in particular with recurrent exposure to a 57-kDa protein that is a member of the heat shock family of proteins (HSP) (234). Additionally, antibodies to the 57-kDa protein are more prevalent in women with *C. trachomatis* infection who develop the scarring sequelae of infection, tubal factor infertility, and ectopic pregnancy (235,236). In humans, lymphocytes proliferate *in vitro* in response to *C. trachomatis* antigens after initial infection (237), but such proliferation may be impaired in chronic infections (238). Cytokines, in particular γ-interferon, may be important in *C. trachomatis* infection. Several studies have shown *in vitro* inhibition of replication of *Chlamydia* by γ-interferon and in a mouse model depletion of γ-interferon results in exacerbation of infection (239–241). Although cellular cytotoxicity appears to play a protective role in *C. psittaci* infection, this has not been seen for cells infected with *C. trachomatis* (242).

Protection and pathogenesis in chlamydial infections are due to different types of immune responses to different antigens. Protection seems to be mediated in part by neutralizing antibody responses to MOMP and γ-interferon suppression of chlamydial replication. Atypical persistent infections may be produced in response to low levels of γ-interferon (243), and scarring and fibrosis appear due to recurrent infections, eliciting a delayed-type hypersensitivity reaction to the 57-kDa protein.

Epidemiology

C. trachomatis is the leading bacterial cause of STD in the United States. In 1986 *C. trachomatis* was estimated to cause over 4 million infections, 2.6 million among women and 1.8 million among men (244). In one STD population, 5% of homosexual men and 14% of heterosexual men had *C. trachomatis* infections. Prevalence decreased in both groups in individuals over 19 years of age (245). Since the first isolation of *C. trachomatis* from the rectum of a homosexual man (246), several studies have evaluated the rate of *C. trachomatis* infection of the urethra, cervix, and rectum in homosexual men and heterosexual women (3,13,247–250). Prevalence rates were higher for both men and women with symptoms of proctitis than asymptomatic patients. In women with anorectal *C. trachomatis* infection, rectal intercourse was associated with the presence of symptoms (248). Barnes et al. (251) compared serovars causing anorectal infection in homosexual and bisexual men with those causing cervical infections in heterosexual women in the same STD clinic. They demonstrated that 53% of rectal and 18% of cervical isolates were serovar D/D′, while serovar E was present in 32% of cervical and 6% of rectal isolates. The highly significant difference in serovar types from the two sites may be attributed to limited transmission between the two populations or to a decreased capability of certain serovars to survive at different mucosal sites.

Infections with the LGV biovar of *C. trachomatis* are endemic in eastern and western Africa, South America, and the Caribbean, but occur only sporadically in the United States and Europe. In the United States, LGV infections are more common in homosexual than heterosexual men. Anorectal LGV infections may occur as a primary anorectal infection in homosexual men and heterosexual women practicing receptive anal intercourse by spread from infected vaginal secretions in women or by lymphatic spread from genital infection.

Clinical Illness

The clinical presentation of anorectal *Chlamydia* infections ranges from asymptomatic to severe granulomatous proctitis, depending on the infecting immunotype, presence or absence of other rectal infection, quantity of the inoculum, and the patient's prior immunity to *C. trachomatis*. Infections with LGV serovars are more likely to cause severe disease than non-LGV serovars. Quinn et al. (13) found that all asymptomatic homosexual men infected with *C. trachomatis* had non-LGV serovars (D/E, D/G, C/J), whereas all three patients with LGV serovars were symptomatic. The less invasive non-LGV serovars were associated with asymptomatic infections or a less severe proctitis. On sigmoidoscopic examination of infection with non-LGV serovars, the mucosa may be normal or show focal areas of erythema, friability, and erosion. Corresponding histology shows neutrophil infiltration of the lamina propria and prominent follicles (13,252).

LGV often causes a severe proctocolitis with pruritus, purulent rectal discharge, diarrhea or constipation, hematochezia, fever, lymphadenopathy, and lower abdominal pain. The mucosa is usually friable or diffusely bloody with multiple ulcerations. Histology of this lesion shows diffuse inflammation with the presence of mononuclear cells, plasma cells, neutrophils, eosinophils, crypt abscesses, granulomas, and giant cells (13,247,253). The histopathology resembles that of Crohn's disease and misdiagnosis can occur.

If left untreated, anorectal LGV infection can progress to development of perirectal abscesses, with necrosis, fibrosis, strictures, stenosis, and fistula formation (254). The rectal strictures usually develop 2–5 cm above the anocutaneous margin, where there is a rich supply of lymphatics. Obstruction of lymphatic and venous drainage may cause perianal outgrowth of lymphatic tissue called lymphorrhoids or perianal condylomas (254).

Diagnosis

Rectal *Chlamydia* infection may be diagnosed by culture of rectal exudate in McCoy cells and identification of infected cells with a fluorescein-labeled monoclonal antibody to chlamydial antigens. Rompalo et al. (255) used the direct fluorescent antibody technique to evaluate rectal swab samples for *C. trachomatis* and found a 90% sensitivity and 100% specificity with this technique compared to culture. Immunoassays for chlamydial antigens give high false positivity rates and are not helpful for rectal samples (256,257).

The usefulness of serology for diagnosis of rectal *Chlamydia* infection depends on the duration, extent of disease, previous exposure, and infecting serotype. The high rate of antibodies to *C. trachomatis* in the adult population (80–90%) makes antibody detection in a single serum sample of little value in diagnosis of non-LGV infections (252). In addition, the most specific serological assay, the microimmunofluorescence test, is not widely available, is difficult to perform, and often detects cross-reactive antibodies with other chlamydial species (258–260). The complement fixation test is unable to distinguish *C. trachomatis* from other chlamydial infections (259), can cross-react with other gram-negative bacteria, and is nonsensitive, limiting its usefulness to systemic infections. Seroconversion or greater than a fourfold titer rise in acute and convalescent sera by microimmunofluorescence has been used as supportive evidence of infection.

Treatment

Tetracycline is the treatment of choice of chlamydial infections (261). Tetracycline 500 mg four times per day or doxycycline 100 mg twice per day for 21 days has been shown to eradicate anorectal infections including those with infections due to LGV biovar. Uncomplicated rectal infections due to non-LGV biovars may also be treated with doxycycline 100 mg bid for 7 to 10 days or oral azithromycin 1.0 g as a single dose. In patients unable to tolerate tetracycline or azithromycin, alternative regimens include ofloxacin 300 mg bid for 7 days, erythromycin base 500 mg qid for 7 days, erythromycin ethyl succinate 800 mg qid for 7 days, or sulfisoxazole 500 mg qid for 10 days. In pregnant women erythromycin base 500 mg qid for 7 days is recommended. In patients with stricture, antibiotics may reduce associated edema and inflammation, but surgical resection is usually necessary. If an alternate regimen is used, a test of cure should be performed.

ENTAMOEBA HISTOLYTICA

Microbiology

Entamoeba histolytica belongs to a family of amoeba that includes several nonpathogenic species such as *E. coli*, *E. hartmani*, and *E. gingivalis* (262). Infection is initiated by ingestion of the *E. histolytica* cyst by a susceptible host. Excystation occurs in the small bowel producing a metacystic ameba with four cystic nuclei from which eight metacystic trophozoites are produced by cytoplasmic division (263). Trophozoites multiply by binary fission in the colon and may either exist as commensals or cause invasive disease. Invasion of the colonic mucosa produces amebic dysentery whereas invasion of the portal vein and hepatic parenchyma produces hepatic abscesses. Trophozoites are classified as pathogenic or nonpathogenic based on their ability to cause invasive disease. Pathogenic trophozoites can be distinguished from nonpathogenic forms by trophozoite isoenzyme (hexokinase, glucophoshoisomerase, and phosphoglucomutase) mobility on starch gel electrophoresis, referred to as zymodeme analysis (264). Pathogenic forms can also be identified by the presence of erythrophagocytosis (ingestion of red blood cells), which is characteristic of pathogenic *E. histolytica* (263). Other techniques such as typing by monoclonal antibodies to surface antigens (265), ribosomal RNA sequence analysis (266), and RFLP also have been used to distinguish pathogenic and nonpathogenic forms (267).

Pathogenesis and Immunity

A protective role of humoral and cell-mediated immunity in *E. histolytica* infections has come from studies of natural infections. In addition, there is evidence that colonic mucus and host nutritional status are important in protection from invasive disease (268). Intestinal colonization does not induce protective immunity as serum antibodies to *E. histolytica* do not develop in the absence of tissue invasion (269,270). In contrast, invasive infection invariably induces *E. histolytica*–specific antibodies in the serum that are associated with resistance to subsequent invasive amebiasis (271). The mechanism of protective immunity appears to be inhibition of adherence of the trophozoites to host cells. Serum *E. histolytica*–specific antibodies from immune individuals primarily recognize a 170-kDa lectin that has been shown to mediate binding of the trophozoite to host cells (272). *In vitro* adherence of the trophozoite can be prevented by human immune sera (273). The ability of the trophozoite to adhere to host cells is one of the most important determinants of virulence. Adherence must be established in order for the trophozoite to lyse target cells (274,275). Petri et al (276) isolated a 170-kDa lectin galactose/*N*-acetyl-D-galactosamine (Gal/Gal NAc) that mediates binding of the trophozoite to host cells. Monoclonal antibodies that inhibit *E. histolytica* adherence bind this lectin and are able to competitively inhibit adherence of viable amebae to Chinese

hamster ovary cells (276). The purified lectin, when used to immunize gerbils, protected them from development of amebic liver abscess after infection with *E. histolytica* (277). Although this lectin plays a key role, other surface membrane lectins are also important for adherence (278). A role for complement in resolution of infection has been demonstrated by complement-mediated killing of trophozoite with serum from healthy controls and from patients infected with *E. histolytica* with high titers of antibody to *E. histolytica*. Trophozoites causing invasive disease, however, are resistant to complement-mediated lysis and can be selected *in vitro* by culture with normal human serum (279).

Regarding cellular responses, antigen-driven lymphocyte proliferation, and lymphokine production can be detected *in vitro* in invasive *E. histolytica* infection as evidenced by antigen-specific lymphocyte proliferation and lymphokine production (280,281). *In vitro* lymphokine production is associated with macrophage-induced killing of the organisms (282). In addition, *E. histolytica* induces cytotoxic T-cell activity in patients with invasive amebiasis (280). The benign course of *E. histolytica* infection in most patients who also have AIDS suggests that cellular responses do not play a significant role in the pathogenesis of invasive disease. Studies of *E. histolytica* infection in AIDS patients have shown that these patients are colonized with exclusively nonpathogenic trophozoites (283,284).

Epidemiology

Greater than 10% of the world's population is believed to be infected with *E. histolytica* (285). Transmission is primarily by waterborne route in areas of poverty and poor sanitation making the infection endemic in many developing countries. Humans are the only reservoir of infection. The majority of infections are asymptomatic and only 10% of those infected develop invasive intestinal disease or liver abscess (286). In the United States, where the overall prevalence of infection is estimated to be 4% (287), most infections occur in mentally retarded patients, persons in chronic care facilities with poor personal hygiene, immigrants from and travelers to endemic areas, and homosexual men.

E. histolytica infections in homosexual men without a history of foreign travel was first reported in 1968 (1). Subsequent studies in the mid-1970s to mid-1980s documented a 20–40% prevalence of amebiasis in homosexual men in New York and San Francisco (288–291). Quinn (3) detected *E. histolytica* in the stools of 28% of homosexual men in Seattle in the early 1980s whereas Sargeaunt (283) detected it in the stools of 11% of homosexual men in London. In the study by Quinn et al. (3), there was no significant difference in the prevalence of *E. histolytica* in homosexual men with (28.6%) and without (25%) gastrointestinal symptoms; 60% of symptomatic men with *E. histolytica* had coinfection with other pathogens. Asymptomatic infections in this population undoubtly facilitate transmission of the parasite.

Clinical Illness

Although the majority of persons infected with *E. histo-lytica* are asymptomatic, the organism causes a wide spectrum of intestinal disease, including mild colitis, fulminant colitis with toxic megacolon, and amebomas. Amebic co-litis in the homosexual population is characterized by the insidious onset of mild diarrhea, often accompanied by a bloody mucoid discharge alternating with constipation, as well as lower abdominal cramping, and tenesmus. Fulminant colitis with severe diarrhea and fever is much less common but occurs with increased frequency in patients

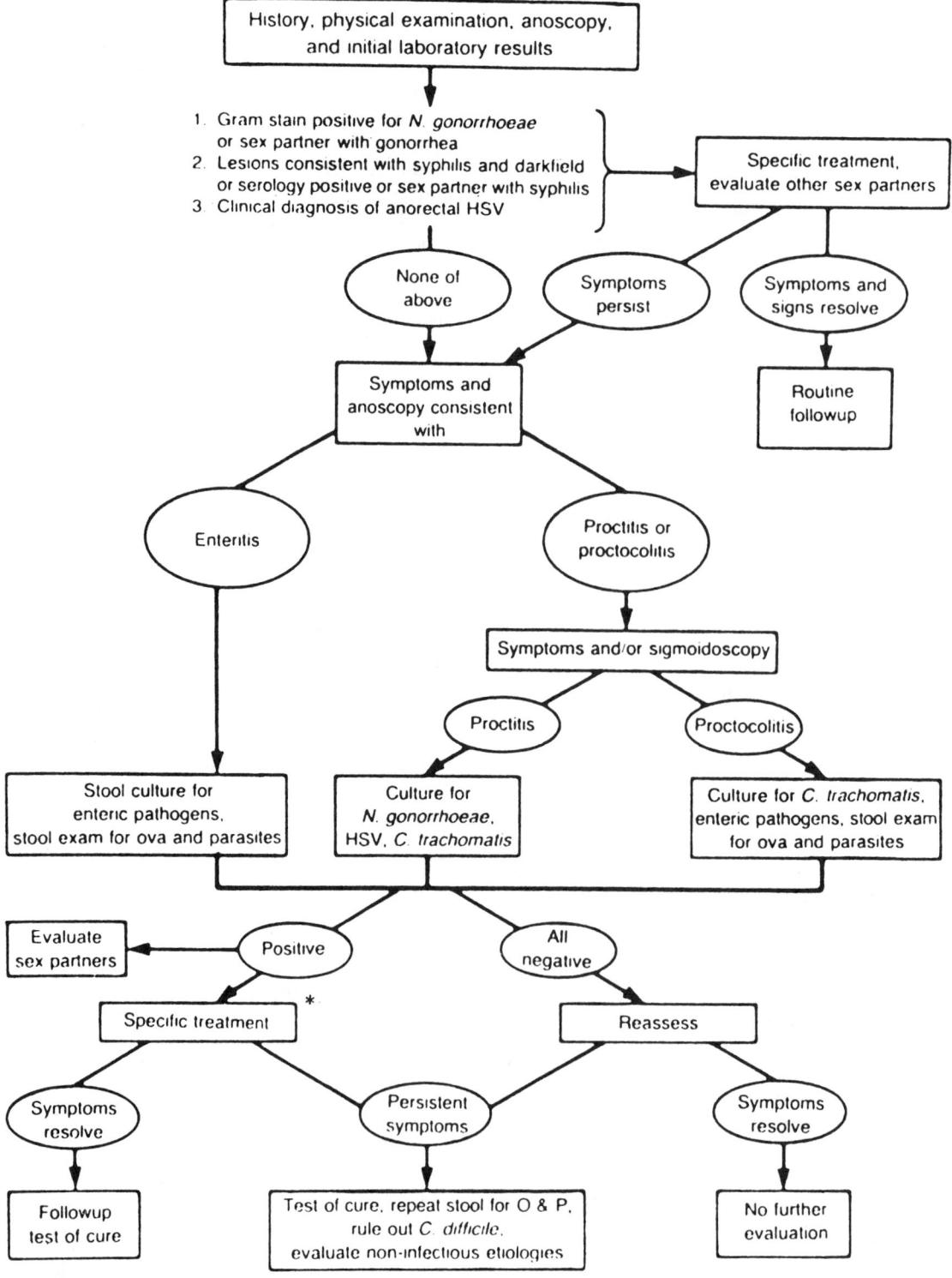

FIG. 5. Algorithm for the management of anorectal symptoms. (From ref. 3, with permission.)

receiving steroids (285). This form of amebic intestinal disease may progress to toxic megacolon and intestinal perforation. Concurrent liver abscess is not uncommon. *E. histolytica* can also cause granulomatous thickening of the bowel wall referred to as an ameboma (292). These masses occur in 1% of patients with *E. histolytica* infections and are generally found in the terminal colon. Amebic liver abscess is the most common extraintestinal infection of *E. histolytica*. Cerebral amebiasis is found in 1.2–2.5% of patients with amebiasis at autopsy though clinically it is seen in <0.1% of cases (285). These invasive infections rarely occur in homosexual men with *E. histolytica* infections.

Among homosexual men and patients with AIDS, infection with *E. histolytica* is usually asymptomatic, probably because the isolates in these patients are nonpathogenic (283,284). However, conversion from nonpathogenic to pathogenic zymodemes *in vitro* has been reported, but has never been seen in serial isolates from infected patients (293).

Diagnosis

Diagnosis of *E. histolytica* infection is generally made by microscopic examination of a wet mount of fresh stool or a rectal swab. Since cyst shedding is intermittent the diagnostic yield is increased by examining purged or multiple (three to six) samples of stool (294). It is important to distinguish *E. histolytica* cysts and trophozoites from those of the smaller, nonpathogenic *E. hartmani* and from neutrophils (295).

Serology is helpful for diagnosing disease due to invasive *E. histolytica*. The indirect hemagglutination test is the most widely used serological test and is positive in 81–98% of patients with proctocolitis. However, this test can remain positive for over 10 years after clinical and parasitological cure. The agar gel diffusion, counterimmunoelectrophoresis, and enzyme immunoassay techniques are quite sensitive (87–95% positive in patients with proctocolitis and 95–100% in patients with liver abscess) and offer the advantage of becoming negative 6–12 months after infection (296). Haque et al. recently developed an enzyme immunoassay to detect pathogen-specific epitopes of the galactose adhesin of *E. histolytica* in stool samples that is reportedly 100% sensitive and 97% specific compared to culture and zymodeme analysis (297). This new assay may become an important tool for more rapid determination of pathogenicity of *E. histolytica* infection.

Treatment

Treatment of *E. histolytica* depends on the type of infection. Asymptomatic carriage of the organisms should be treated to prevent continued infection with a possible pathogenic strain and to prevent continued transmission of the infection. The three luminal amebicides available to treat this type of infection include iodoquinol 650 mg orally three times per day for 20 days, which is the drug of choice (298). It is generally well tolerated but should not be used in patients allergic to iodine. A few case reports of optic atrophy, one leading to blindness, were noted in patients given doses higher than typically used for amebiasis (299,300). Paromomycin 25–30 mg/kg/day in three doses for 7 days is also active against asymptomatic infections and may be used for mild to moderate cases of symptomatic disease (301). Two cases of irreversible deafness with use of paromomycin with neomycin have been reported. Diloxanide furoate 500 mg three times per day for 10 days is widely used outside the United States for asymptomatic and mildly symptomatic infections (298) and in the United States is available from the Centers for Disease Control. Parasitological cure with this agent approaches 90%, similar to iodoquinol and paromomycin; side effects include flatulence, diarrhea, abdominal cramping, nausea, and headache (302). Diloxanide furoate is not effective for symptomatic dysentery.

Invasive intestinal disease should be treated with metronidazole 750 mg three times per day for 10 days (297). This drug is well absorbed and achieves good tissue levels but does not eradicate organisms in the lumen, so iodoquinol 650 mg three times per day for 20 days should be given subsequently (303). An alternate regimen for invasive disease is dihydroemitine 1.5 mg/kg/day (maximum 90 mg/day) IM for up to 5 days, or emetine 1 mg/kg/day IM for up to 5 days followed by iodoquinol (298).

CONCLUSION

Anorectal infections are common primarily in homosexual men and heterosexual women who practice receptive anal intercourse. The etiology is usually polymicrobial and the symptoms are variable depending on the pathogen and location of infection (anus vs. rectum). The asymptomatic nature of some of these infections promotes a high level of transmission and complications. Review of the patient's sexual history and an anoscopic examination should be considered in patients at risk for such infections as well as in patients with a relevant or suspicious perianal lesion. Appropriate management is outlined in Fig. 5 and should involve treatment of partners and follow-up evaluation for persistent infection. It is important to remember that patients presenting with anorectal infections are at risk for HIV and may have altered presentation and response to therapy, or develop associated conditions such as malignancy.

REFERENCES

1. Most H. Manhattan: "a tropic isle?" *Am J Trop Med Hyg* 1968; 217:333–354.
2. Sohn N, Robilotti JG Jr. The gay bowel syndrome. *Am J Gastroenterol* 1977;67:478–484.
3. Quinn TC, Stamm WE, Goodell SE. The polymicrobial origin of intestinal infections in homosexual men. *N Engl J Med* 1983; 309:576–582.
4. Booth RE, Watters JK, Chitwoud DD. HIV risk-related sex behaviors among injection drug users, crack smokers and injection drug users who smoke crack. *Am J Public Health* 1993; Aug 83(8):11448.

5. De Schryver A, Meheus A. Epidemiology of sexually transmitted diseases: the global picture. *Bull WHO* 1990;68(5):639–654.

6. Quinn TC, Cates W Jr. Epidemiology of sexually transmitted diseases in the 1990's. In: Quinn TC, ed. *Advances in host defense mechanisms*. vol. 8. *Sexually transmitted diseases*. New York: Raven Press; 1992:1–32.

7. Hook EW, III, Marra CM. Acquired syphilis in adults. *N Engl J Med* 1992;200:1060–1061.

8. Wald A, Corey L, Handsfield HH, Holmes KK. Influence of HIV infection on manifestations and natural history of other sexually transmitted diseases. *Annu Rev Public Health* 1993;14:19–42.

9. Finelli L, Budd J, Spitalny KC. Early syphilis: relationship to sex, drugs, and changes in high-risk behavior from 1987–1990. *Sex Trans Dis* 1993;20:89–95.

10. Handsfield HH, Schwebke J. Trends in sexually transmitted diseases in homosexually active men in King County, Washington, 1980–1990. *Sex Trans Dis* 1990;17(4):211–215.

11. Bolling DR Jr. Prevalence, goals and complications of heterosexual anal intercourse in a gynecologic population. *J Reprod Med* 1977;19:120–124.

12. Spiro HM. *Clinical gastroenterology*. 2nd ed. New York: Macmillan; 1977:881.

13. Quinn TC, Goodell SE, Mkritchian E. *Chlamydia trachomatis* proctitis. *N Engl J Med* 1981;305:195–200.

14. Spear GP. Biology of the herpesviruses. In: Holmes KK, ed. *Sexually transmitted diseases*. 2nd ed. New York: McGraw-Hill; 1990:379–389.

15. Mertz GJ. Genital herpes simplex virus infections. In: Martin DH, ed. *Medical Clin North Am* 1990;74(6):1433–1454.

16. WuDunn D, Spear PG. Initial interaction of herpes simplex virus with cells is binding to heparan sulfate. *J Virol* 1989;63:52–58.

17. Roizman BB, Batterson B. Herpes viruses and their replication. In: Fields BN, ed. *Virology*. New York: Raven Press; 1985:497.

18. Mirdel A, ed. *Herpes simplex virus*. New York: Springer-Verlag; 1989:15–18.

19. Roizman B. Introduction: objectives of herpes simplex virus vaccines seen from a historical perspective. *Rev Infect Dis* 1991;13(Suppl 11):S892–S894.

20. Ashley, R., Koelle DM. Immune responses to genital herpes infection. In: Quinn TC, ed. *Advances in host defense mechanisms*. vol 8. *Sexually transmitted diseases*. New York: Raven Press; 1992:201–331.

21. Shore SL, Cromeons TL, Romano JJ. Immune destruction of virus-infected cells early in the infection cycle. *Nature* 1976;262:695–696.

22. Highlander SL, Cai W, Person S, Levine M, Glorioso JC. Monoclonal antibodies define a domain on herpes simplex virus glycoprotein B involved in virus penetration. *J Virol* 1988;62:1881–1888.

23. Prober CG, Sullender WM, Yasukawa LL, Au DS, Yeager AS, Arvin AM. Low risk of herpes simplex virus infections in neonates exposed to the virus at the time of vaginal delivery to mothers with recurrent genital herpes simplex virus infections. *N Engl J Med* 1987;316:240–244.

24. Brown ZA, Benedetti J, Ashley R, et al. Neonatal herpes simplex virus infection in relation to asymptomatic maternal infection at the time of labor. *N Engl J Med* 1991;324:1247–1252.

25. Merriman H, Woods S, Winter C, Fahnlander A, Corey L. Secretory IgA antibody in cervicovaginal secretions in women with genital herpes simplex virus infection. *J Infect Dis* 1984;149:505–510.

26. Linnemann CC Jr, First MR, Alvira MM, Alexander JW, Schiff GM. Herpesvirus hominis type 2 meningoencephalitis following renal transplantation. *Am J Med* 1976;61:703–708.

27. Pollard RB, Arvin AM, Gamberg P, Rand KH, Gallagher JG, Merigan TC. Specific cell-mediated immunity and infections with herpes viruses in cardiac transplant recipients. *Am J Med* 1982;73:679–687.

28. Meyers JD, Fluornoy N, Thomas ED. Infection with herpes simplex virus and cell-mediated immunity after marrow transplant. *J Infect Dis* 1980;142:338–346.

29. Quinnan GV, Masur H, Rook AH, et al. Herpesvirus infections in the acquired immune deficiency syndrome. *JAMA* 1984;252:72–77.

30. Sullender WM, Miller JL, Yasukawa LL, et al. Humoral and cell-mediated immunity in neonates with herpes simplex virus infection. *J Infect Dis* 1987;155:28–37.

31. Mawle AC, Thieme ML, Ridgeway MR, McDonegal JS, Schmid DS. Inhibition of the in vitro generation of class II-restricted, HSV-1 specific, CD4+ CTL by HIV-1. *AIDS Res Hum Retrovir* 1990;6:229–41.

32. Toresth JW, Merigan TC. Significance of local gamma interferon in recurrent herpes simplex infection. *J Infect Dis* 1986;153:979–983.

33. Linnavuori KH. History of recurrent mucocutaneous herpes correlates with relatively low interferon production by herpes simplex virus-exposed cultured monocytes. *J Med Virol* 1988;25:61–68.

34. Cunningham AZ, Merigan TC. Gamma-interferon production appears to predict time of recurrence of herpes labialis. *J Immunol* 1983;130:2397–2400.

35. Centers for Disease Control. Division of STD/HIV prevention annual reports, 1990. Issued January 1991, Atlanta, Georgia.

36. Corey L. Genital herpes. In: Holmes KK, Mardh P, Sparling PF, Weisner PJ, eds. *Sexually transmitted diseases*. 2nd ed. New York: McGraw-Hill; 1990:391–414.

37. Guinan ME, Wolinsky SM, Reichman RC. Genital herpes simplex virus infection. *Epidemiol Rev* 1988;7:127.

38. Duenas A, Adam E, Melnick JZ, Rawls WE. Herpesvirus type 2 in a prostitute population. *Am J Epidemiol* 1972;95:483–489.

39. Mertz GJ, Benedetti J, Ashley R, Selke SA, Corey L. Risk factors for the sexual transmission of genital herpes. *Ann Intern Med* 1992;116:197–202.

40. Holmberg SD, Stewart JA, Gerber AR, et al. Prior herpes simplex virus type 2 infection as a risk factor for HIV. *JAMA* 1988;259:1048–1050.

41. Quinn TC. Epidemiology and serologic evidence for herpes simplex viruses in AIDS. In: Aurelian L, ed. *Herpes viruses, the immune system and AIDS*. Norwell, MA: Kluwer Academic Publishers; 1990:1–20.

42. Hook EW III, Cannon RO, Nahmias AJ, et al. Herpes simplex virus infection as a risk factor for human immunodeficiency virus infection in heterosexuals. *J Infect Dis* 1992;165:251–255.

43. Golden MP, Kim S, Hammer SM, et al. Activation of human immunodeficiency virus by herpes simplex virus. *J Infect Dis* 1992;166:494–499.

44. Corey L, Adams HG, Brown ZA, et al. Genital herpes simplex virus infection: clinical manifestations, course and complications. *Ann Intern Med* 1983;98:958–972.

45. Corey L, Spear PG. Infections with herpes simplex viruses. Parts 1 & 2. *N Engl J Med* 1986;314:686,749.

46. Goodell SE, Quinn TC, Mkrtichian E, Schuffler MD, Holmes KK, Corey L. Herpes simplex virus proctitis in homosexual men: clinical, sigmoidoscopic, and histopathological features. *N Engl J Med* 1983;308:868–871.

47. Samarasinghe RL, Oates JK, Maclennar IPD. Herpetic proctitis and sacral radiculomyelopathy: a hazard for homosexual men. *Br Med J* 1979;2:365–366.

48. Siegal FP, Lopez C, Hammer GS, et al. Severe acquired immunodeficiency in male homosexuals, manifested by chronic perianal ulcerative herpes simplex lesions. *N Engl J Med* 1981;305:1439–1444.

49. Centers for Disease Control. Revision of the CDC Surveillance Case Definition for Acquired Immunodeficiency Syndrome. *MMWR* 1987;36(Suppl):1–15.

50. Quinn TC, Corey L, Chaffee RG, Schuffler MD, Brancato FP, Holmes KK. The etiology of anorectal infections in homosexual men. *Am J Med* 1981;71:395–406.

51. Koutsky LA, Stevens CE, Holmes KK, et al. Underdiagnosis of genital herpes by current clinical and viral-isolation procedures. *N Engl J Med* 1992;326:1533–1539. *N Engl J Med* 1983;308:868–871.

52. Stalder H, Oxman MN, Herman K. Herpes simplex virus microneutralization: a simplification of the test. *J Infect Dis* 1975;131:423–430.

53. Ashley R, Cent A, Maggs V, Nahmias A, Corey L. Inability of enzyme immunoassays to discriminate between infections with herpes simplex virus types 1 and 2. *Ann Intern Med* 1991; 115:520–526.

54. Ashley RL, Mitoni J, Lee F, Nahmias A, Corey L. Comparison of western blot (immunoblot) and glycoprotein G-specific immunodot enzyme assay for detecting antibodies to herpes simplex virus types 1 and 2 in human sera. *J Clin Microbiol* 1988; 26:662–667.

55. Ashley RL et al. Comparison of western blot and IgG specific immunodot enzyme assay for detecting HSV-1 and HSV-2 antibodies in human sera. *J Clin Microbiol* 1988;26:662–667.

56. Cone RW, Hobson AC, Palmer J, Remington M, Corey L. Extended duration of herpes simplex virus DNA in genital lesions detected by the polymerase chain reaction. *J Infect Dis* 1991; 164:757–760.

57. Rompalo AM, Mertz GJ, Davis LG, et al. Oral acyclovir for treatment of first-episode herpes simplex virus proctitis. *JAMA* 1988;259:2879–2881.

58. Centers for Disease Control. 1993 Sexually transmitted diseases treatment guidelines. *MMWR* 1993;42:1–103.

59. Douglas JM, Critchlow C, Benedetti J, et al. A double-blind study of oral acyclovir for suppression of recurrences of genital herpes simplex virus infection. *N Engl J Med* 1984;310: 1551–1556.

60. Corey L, McCutchan JA, Ronald AR, Handsfield HH. Evaluation of new anti-infective drugs for the treatment of genital infections due to herpes simplex virus. Infectious Diseases Society of America and the Food and Drug Administration. *Clin Infect Dis* 1992;15(Suppl 1):S99–107.

61. Fletcher CV. Treatment of herpes virus infections in HIV-infected individuals. *Ann Pharmacother* 1992;26:955–962.

62. Drugs for sexually transmitted diseases. *Med Lett* 1991;33(860): 119–124.

63. Goldberg LH, Kaufman RH, Kurtz TO, et al. Continuous five-year treatment of patients with frequently recurring genital herpes simplex virus infection with acyclovir. *J Med Virol* 1993; Suppl 1:45–50.

64. Godman EL, Luby JP, Johnson MT. Prospective double-blind evaluation of topical adenine arabinoside in male herpes progenitalis. *Antimicrob Agents Chemother* 1975;8:693–697.

65. Whitley RJ, Spruance S, Hayden PG, et al. Vidarabin therapy for mucocutaneous herpes simplex virus infection in the immunocompromised host. *J Infect Dis* 1984;149:1–8.

66. Lehrman SN, Douglas JM, Corey L, Barry DW. Recurrent genital herpes and suppressive oral acyclovir therapy: relation between clinical outcome and in-vitro drug sensitivity. *Ann Intern Med* 1986;104:786–790.

67. Whitley RJ, Gnann JW Jr. Acyclovir: a decade later. *N Engl J Med* 1992;327(11):782–789.

68. Parker AC, Craig JIO, Collins P, Oliver N, Smith I. Acyclovir-resistant herpes simplex virus infection due to altered DNA polymerase. *Lancet* 1987;2:1461.

69. Wade JC, McLaren C, Meyers JD. Frequency and significance of acyclovir-resistant herpes simplex virus isolated from marrow transplant patients receiving multiple courses of treatment with acyclovir. *J Infect Dis* 1983;148:1077–1082.

70. Hardy WD. Foscarnet treatment of acyclovir-resistant herpes simplex virus infection in patients with acquired immunodeficiency syndrome: preliminary results of a controlled, randomized, regimen-comparative trial. *Am J Med* 1992;92(Suppl 2A): 30S–35S.

71. Oliver NM, Collins P, Van der Meer J, Van'T Wout JW. Biological and biochemical characterization of clinical isolates of herpes simplex virus type 2 resistant to acyclovir. *Antimicrob Agents Chemother* 1989;33:635–640.

72. Collins P, Larder BA, Oliver NM, Kemp S, Smith IW, Darby G. Characterization of a DNA polymerase mutant of herpes simplex virus from a severely immunocompromised patient receiving acyclovir. *J Gen Virol* 1989;70:375–382.

73. Safrin S. Treatment of acyclovir-resistant herpes simplex virus infections in patients with AIDS. *J AIDS* 1992;5(Suppl 1): S29–S32.

74. Safrin S, Crumpacker C, Chatis P, et al. A controlled trial comparing foscarnet with vidarabine for acyclovir-resistant mucocutaneous herpes simplex in the acquired immunodeficiency syndrome. *N Engl J Med* 1991;325:551–555.

75. Svennerholm B, Vahlne A, Lowhagen GB, Widell A, Lycke E. Sensitivity of HSV strains isolated before and after treatment with acyclovir. *Scand J Infect Dis* 1985;Suppl 47:149–154.

76. Safrin S, Berger TG, Gilson I, et al. Foscarnet therapy in five patients with AIDS and acyclovir-resistant varicella-zoster virus infection. *Ann Intern Med* 1991;115:19–21.

77. Safrin S, Kemmerly S, Plotkin B. Foscarnet-resistant herpes simplex virus infection in patients with AIDS. *J Infect Dis* 1994; 169:193–196.

78. Cotte L. Herpes simplex virus infection during foscarnet therapy. *J Infect Dis* 1992;166:447–448.

79. Shah KV. Howley PM. Papillomaviruses. In: BN Fields et al. eds. *Virology*. New York: Raven Press; 1990:1651.

80. Shah KV. Biology of human genital tract papillomaviruses. In: Holmes KK, ed. *Sexually transmitted diseases*. 2nd ed. New York: McGraw-Hill; 1990:425–431.

81. Viscidi RP, Shah KV. Immune response to genital tract infections with human papillomaviruses. In: Quinn TC, ed. *Advances in Host Defense Mechanisms*, vol 8. *Sexually transmitted diseases*. New York: Raven Press; 1982:239–260.

82. Androphy EJ, Hubbert NL, Schiller JT, Lowy DR. Identification of the HPV-16 E6 protein from transformed mouse cells and human cervical carcinoma cell lines. *EMBO J* 1987;6: 989–992.

83. Seedorf K, Oltersdorf T, Krammer G, Rowekamp W. Identification of early proteins of the human papilloma viruses type 16 (HPV 16) and type 18 (HPv 18) in cervical carcinoma cells. *EMBO J* 1987;6:139–144.

84. Reichman RC, Bonnez W. Papillomaviruses. In: Mandell G, Douglas RG Jr, Bennett JE, eds. *Principles and practice of infectious diseases*. 3rd ed. New York: Churchill-Livingstone; 1990:1191–1199.

85. Lorincz AT, Temple GF, Kurman RJ, Jenson AB, Lancaster WD. Oncogenic association of specific human papillomavirus types with cervical neoplasia. *JNCI* 1987;79:671–677.

86. Brown DR, Fife KH. Human papillomavirus infections of the genital tract. *Med. Clin. North Am. Sex Transm Dis* 1990;74(6): 1455–1485.

87. Rabbett WF. Juvenile laryngeal papillomatosis: the relation of irradiation to malignant degeneration in this disease. *Ann Otolog Rhinolog Laryngol* 1965;74:1149–1163.

88. Sandberg JP. Papillomavirus infections in animals. In: Syrjanen K, et al, eds. *Papillomaviruses and human diseases*. Berlin: Springer-Verlag; 1987:240.

89. Schneider A, Holtz M, Gissmann L. Increased prevalence of human papillomaviruses in the lower genital tract of pregnant women. *Int J Cancer* 1987;40:198–201.

90. Rudlinger RM, Smith JW, Bunney MH, et al. Human papillomavirus infections in a group of renal transplant patients. *Br J Dermatol* 1986;115:681–692.

91. Bernard C, Mougin C, Madoz L, et al. Viral co-infections in human papillomavirus-associated anogenital lesions according to the serostatus for the human immunodeficiency virus. *Int J Cancer* 1992;52:731–737.

92. Li C-CH, Shah KV, Seth A, Gilden RV. Identification of the human papillomavirus type 6b L1 open reading frame protein in condylomas and corresponding antibodies in human sera. *J Virol* 1987;61:2684–2690.

93. Jenison SA, Yu X-P, Valentine JM, et al. Evidence of prevalent genital type human papillomavirus infections in adults and children. *J Infect Dis* 1990;162:60–69.

94. Galloway DA, Jenison SA. Characterization of the humoral immune response to genital papillomaviruses. *Mol Biol Med* 1990;7:59–72.

95. Bonnez W, DaRin C, Rose RC, Reichman RC. Use of human papillomavirus type II virions in an ELISA to detect specific antibodies in humans with condylomata accuminata. *J Gen Virol* 1991;72:1343–1347.

96. Dillner J. Mapping of linear epitopes of human papillomavirus type 16: the E_1, E_2, E_3, E_4, E_5, E_6, & E_7 open reading frames. *Int J Cancer* 1990;46:703–711.

97. Mann VM, Loud de Lao, Brenes M, et al. Occurrence of IgA and IgG antibodies to select peptides representing human papillomavirus type 16 among cervical cancer cases and controls. *Cancer Res* 1990;50:7815–7819.

98. Bleul C, Muller M, Frank R, et al. Human papillomavirus (HPV) type 18 E6 and E7 antibodies in human sera: increased anti-E7 prevalence in cervical cancer patients. *J Clin Microbiol* 1991;29:1579–1588.

99. Jochmus-Kudielka J, Schneider A, Braun R, et al. Antibodies against the human papillomavirus type 16 early proteins in human sera correlation of anti-E7 reactivity with cervical cancer. *JNCI* 1989;81:1698–1704.

100. Malejczyk J, Malejczyk M, Majewski S, Orth G, Jablonska S. NK-cell activity in patients with HPV 16-associated anogenital tumors: defective recognition of HPV 16-harboring keratinocytes and restricted unresponsiveness to immunostimulatory cytokines. *Int J Cancer* 1993;53:917–921.

101. Evans CH, Flugelman AA, DiPaolo JA. Cytokine modulation of immune defenses in cervical cancer. *Oncology* 1993;50:245–251.

102. Woodworth CD, Lichti U, Simpson S, Evans CH, DiPaolo JA. Leukoregulin and gamma-interferon inhibit human papillomavirus type 16 gene transcription in human papillomavirus-immortalized human cervical cells. *Cancer Res* 1992;52:456–463.

103. Vernon SD, Hart CE, Reeves WC, Icenogle JP. The HIV-1 tat protein enhances E2-dependent human papillomavirus 16 transcription. *Virus Res* 1993;27:133–45.

104. Koutsky LA, Galloway DA, Holmes KK. Epidemiology of genital human papillomavirus infection. *Epidemiol Rev* 199;10:122–163.

105. de Villiers EM, Wagner D, Schneider A, et al. Human papilloma virus infections in women with and without abnormal cervical cytology. *Lancet* 1987;2:703–706.

106. Reeves WC, Arosemena JR, Garcia M, et al. Genital human papillomavirus infection in Panama City prostitutes. *J Infect Dis* 1989;160:599–603.

107. Lancaster WD and Jenson AB. Natural history of human papillomavirus infection of the anogenital tract. *Cancer Metas Rev* 1987;6:653–664.

108. Daling JR, Weiss NS, Klopfenstein LL, et al. Correlates of homosexual behavior and the incidence of anal cancer. *JAMA* 1982;247:1988–1990.

109. Scholefield JH, Sonnex C, Talbot IC, et al. Anal and cervical intraepithelial neoplasia: possible parallel. *Lancet* 1989;2:765–769.

110. Palmer JG, Scholefield JH, Coates PJ, et al. Anal cancer and human papillomaviruses. *Dis Col Rect* 1989;32:1016–1022.

111. Kiviat NB, Critchlow CW, Holmes KK, et al. Association of anal dysplasia and human papillomavirus with immunosuppression and HIV infection among homosexual men. *J AIDS* 1993;7:43–49.

112. Palefsky JM, Holly EA, Gonzales J, Lamborn K, Hollander H. Natural history of anal cytologic abnormalities and papillomavirus infection among homosexual men with group IV HIV disease. *J AIDS* 1992;5:1258–1265.

113. Kiviat N, Rompalo A, Bowden R, et al. Anal human papillomavirus infection among human immunodeficiency virus–seropositive and seronegative men. *J Infect Dis* 1990;163:358–361.

114. Caussy D, Goedert JJ, Palefsky J, et al. Interaction of human immunodeficiency and papilloma viruses: association with anal epithelial abnormality in homosexual men. *Int J Cancer* 1990;46:214–219.

115. Pyrohen S, Johansson E. Regression of warts: an immunological study. *Lancet* 1975;1:592–596.

116. Velasco J, Palacio V, Vazquez S, Mosquera C, Sampedro A. Diagnostic accuracy of the cytologic diagnosis of anal human papillomavirus infection compared with DNA hybridization studies. *Sex Trans Dis* 1993;20:147–151.

117. Law CLH, Qassim M, Thompson CH, et al. Factors associated with clinical and subclinical anal human papillomavirus infection in homosexual men. *Genitourin Med* 1991;67:92–98.

118. Snijders PJF, Meijer CJLM, Walboomers JMM. Degenerate primers based on highly conserved regions of amino acid sequence in papillomaviruses can be used in a generalized polymerase chain reaction to detect productive human papillomavirus infections. *J Gen Virol* 1991;72:2781–2786.

119. Evander M, Wadell G. A general primer pair for amplification and detection of genital human papillomavirus types. *J Virolog Meth* 1991;31:239–250.

120. Snijders PJF, Schulten EAJM, Mullink H. Detection of human papillomavirus and Epstein–Barr virus DNA sequences in oral mucosa of HIV-infected patients by the polymerase chain reaction. *Am J Pathol* 1990;137:659–666.

121. van den Brule AJC, Merjer CJLM, Bakeels V, Kenemans P, Walboomers JMM. Rapid detection of human papillomavirus in cervical scrapes by combined general primer-mediated and type-specific polymerase chain reaction. *J Clin Microbiol* 1990;28:2739–2743.

122. Pizzighella A, Rassu M, Piacentini I, Maschera B, Palú G. Polymerase chain reaction amplification and restriction enzyme typing as an accurate and simple way to detect and identify human papillomaviruses. *J Med Microbiol* 1993;39:33–38.

123. Bashi SA. Cryotherapy versus podophyllin in the treatment of genital warts. *Int J Dermatol* 1985;24:535–536.

124. Simmons PD, Langlet F, Thin RNT. Cryotherapy versus electrocautery in the treatment of genital warts. *Br J Vener Dis* 1981;57:273–274.

125. Simmons PD. Podophyllin 10% and 25% in the treatment of anogenital warts. *Br J Vener Dis* 1981;57:208–209.

126. Kinghorn GR, McMillan A, Mulcahy F, Drake S, Lacey C, Bingham JS. An open, comparative study of the efficacy of 0.5% podophyllotoxin lotion and 25% podophyllotoxin solution in the treatment of condylomata acuminata in males and females. *Int J STD AIDS* 1993;4:194–199.

127. Abdullah AN, Walzman M, Wade A. Treatment of external genital warts comparing cryotherapy (liquid nitrogen) and trichloracetic acid. *Sex Trans Dis* 1993;20:334.

128. Jensen SL. Comparison of podophyllin application with simple surgical excision in clearance and recurrence of perinatal condylomata acuminata. *Lancet* 1985;12:1146–1147.

129. Scholefield A, Schattner A, Crespi M, et al. Intramuscular human interferon-β injections in the treatment of condylomata acuminata. *Lancet* 1984;1:1038–1042.

130. Eron LJ, Judson F, Tucker S, et al. Interferon therapy for condylomata acuminata. *N Engl J Med* 1986;315:1059–1064.

131. Freidman-Kien A, Eron LJ, Conant M, et al. Natural interferon alpha for the treatment for the condylomata acuminata. *JAMA* 1988;259:533–538.

132. Reichman RC, Strike DG. Pathogenesis and treatment of human genital papillomavirus infections: a review. *Antiviral Res* 1989;11:109–118.

133. Musher DM. Biology of *Treponema pallidum*. In: Holmes KK, Mardh P, Sparling PF, Wiesner PJ, eds. *Sexually Transmitted Diseases*. 2nd ed. New York: McGraw-Hill; 1990:205–209.

134. Tramont EC. *Treponema pallidum*. In: Mandell GL, Douglas RG Jr, Bennett JE, eds. *Principles and practice of infectious diseases*. 3rd ed. New York: Churchill Livingstone; 1990:1794–1807.

135. Baker-Zander SA, Lukehart SA. Macrophage-mediated killing of opsonized *Treponema pallidum*. *J Infect Dis* 1992;165:69–74.

136. Sell S, Hsu P-L. Delayed hypersensitivity, immune deviation, antigen processing and T-cell subset selection in syphilis pathogenesis and vaccine design. *Immunol Today* 1993;14:576–582.

137. Fitzgerald TJ. Pathogenesis and immunology of *Treponema pallidum*. *Annu Rev Microbiol* 1981;35:29–54.

138. Lukehart SA. Immunology and pathogenesis of syphilis. In: Gallin J, Fauci AS, eds. Quinn TC, Shest ed. *Advances in host defense mechanisms*. New York: Raven Press; 1991:141–163.

139. Sell S, Norris SJ. The biology, pathology and immunology of syphilis. *Int Rev Exp Pathol* 1983;24:203–276.

140. Schell R, Marker D, eds. *Pathogenesis and immunology of treponemal infection*. New York: Marcel Dekker; 1983.

141. Shulkin D, Trippoli L, Abell E. *Lues maligna* in a patient with human immunodeficiency virus infection. *Am J Med* 1988;85:425–427.

142. Gregory N, Sanchez M, Buchness MR. The specrum of syphilis

in patients with human immunodeficiency virus infection. *J Am Acad Dermatol* 1990;22:1061–1067.

143. Goldmeier D, Hay P. A review and update on adult syphilis, with particular reference to its treatment. *Int J STD AIDS* 1993; 4:70–83.

144. Medici MA. The immunoprotective niche: a new pathogenic mechanism for syphilis, the systemic mycoses and other infectious diseases. *J Theor Biol* 1972;36:617–625.

145. Marshak LC, Rothman S. Skin testing with purified suspension of *Treponema pallidum*. *Am J Syph* 1951;35:35–41.

146. Hook EW III, Mara CM. Acquired syphilis in adults. *N Engl J Med* 1992;326:1060–1069.

147. Centers for Disease Control. Syphilis, United States. *MMWR* 1984;33:433–441.

148. Centers for Disease Control. Primary and secondary syphilis—United States, 1981–1990. *MMWR* 1991;40:314–323.

149. Rolfs RT, Nakashima AK. Epidemiology of primary and secondary syphilis in the United States, 1981 through 1989. *JAMA* 1990;264:1432–1437.

150. Stamm WE, Handsfield HH, Rompalo AM, et al. The association between genital ulcer disease and acquisition of HIV infection in homosexual men. *JAMA* 1988;260:1429–1433.

151. Quinn TC, Cannon RO, Glasser D, et al. The association of syphilis with risk of human immunodeficiency virus infection in patients attending STD clinics. *Arch Intern Med* 1990;150: 1297–1302.

152. Darrow WW, Echenberg DF, Jofee HW, et al. Risk factors for HIV infections in homosexual men. *Am J Public Health* 1987; 77:479–483.

153. British Cooperative Clinical Group. Homosexuality and venereal disease in the United Kingdom: a second study. *Br J Vener Dis* 1980;56:6–11.

154. Quinn TC, Stamm WE. Proctitis, proctocolitis, enteritis and esophagitis in homosexual men. In: Holmes KK, Mardh P, Sparling PF, Weisner PJ, eds. *Sexually transmitted diseases.* 2nd ed. New York: McGraw-Hill; 1990:663–684.

155. Mirdel A, Tovey SJ, Timmins DJ, Williams P. Primary and secondary syphilis, 20 years experience. Clinical features. *Genitourin Med* 1989;65:1–3.

156. Bassi O, Cosa G, Colavolpe A, Argentieri R. Primary syphilis of the rectum—endoscopic and clinical features: report of a case. *Dis Col Rect* 1991;34:1024–1026.

157. Akdamar K, Martin RJ, Ichinose H. Syphilitic proctitis. *Dig Dis Sci* 1977;22:701–704.

158. Wexner SD. Sexually transmitted diseases of the colon, rectum, and anus. The challenge of the nineties. *Dis Col Rect* 1990; 33:1048–1062.

159. Quinn TC, Lukehart SA, Goodell SE, Mkrtichian E, Schuffler MD, Holmes KK. Rectal mass caused by *Treponema pallidum:* confirmation by immunofluorescent staining. *Gastroenterology* 1982;82:135–139.

160. Hutchinson CM, Hook EW. Syphilis in adults. *Med Clin North Am* 1990;74(6):1389–1416.

161. Surawicz CM, Goodell SE, Quinn TC. Spectrum of rectal biopsy abnormalities in homosexual men with intestinal symptoms. *Gastroenterology* 1986;91:651–659.

162. Smibert RM. The spirochetes. In: Buchanan RE, Gibbons NE, eds. *Bergey's manual of determinative bacteriology.* 8th ed. Baltimore: Williams and Wilkins; 1974:167.

163. Hook EW III, Roddy RE, Lukehart SA, Horn J, Holmes KK, Tam MR. Detection of *Treponema pallidum* in lesion exudate with a pathogen-specific monoclonal antibody. *J Clin Microbiol* 1985;22:241–244.

164. Hicks CB, Benson PM, Cupton GR, Tramont EC. Seronegative secondary syphilis in a patient infected with the human immunodeficiency virus (HIV) with Kaposi sarcoma: a diagnostic dilemma. *Ann Intern Med* 1987;107:492–495 [Erratum: *Ann Intern Med* 1987;107:946].

165. Gregory N, Sanchez M, Brehness MR. The spectrum of syphilis in patients with human immunodeficiency virus infection. *J Am Acad Dermatol* 1990;22:1061–1067.

166. Tikjoh G, Russel M, Petersen CS, Gerstoft J, Kobayasi T. Seronegative secondary syphilis in a patient with AIDS: identifica-

tion of *Treponema pallidum* in a biopsy specimen. *J Am Acad Dermatol* 1991;24:506–508.

167. Hutchinson CM, Rompalo AM, Reichart CA, Hook EW III. Characteristics of patients with syphilis attending Baltimore STD clinics: multiple high-risk subgroups and interactions with human immunodeficiency virus infection. *Arch Intern Med* 1991;151:511–516.

168. Rompalo AM, Cannon RO, Quinn TC, Hook EW III. Association of biologic false-positive reactions for syphilis with human immunodeficiency virus infection. *J Infect Dis* 1992;165: 1124–1126.

169. Johns DR, Tierney M, Felsenstein D: Alteration in the natural history of neurosyphilis by concurrent infection with the human immunodeficiency virus. *N Engl J Med* 1987;316:1569–1572.

170. Berry CD, Hooten TM, Collier C, et al. Neurologic relapse after benzathine penicillin therapy for secondary syphilis in a patient with HIV infection. *N Engl J Med* 1987;316:1587–1589.

171. Musher DM, Hamill RJ, Baughn RE. Effect of human immunodeficiency virus (HIV) infection on the course of syphilis and the response to treatment. *Ann Intern Med* 1990;113:872–881.

172. Telzak EE, Greenberg MSZ, Harrison J, Stoneburner RL, Schutlz S. Syphilis treatment response in HIV-infected individuals. *AIDS* 1991;5:591–595.

173. Sparling PF. Biology of *Neisseria gonorrhoeae*. In: Holmes KK, Mardh P, Sparling PF, Weisner PJ, eds. *Sexually Transmitted Diseases.* 2nd ed. New York: McGraw-Hill; 1990: 131–147.

174. Morse SA, Johnson SR, Biddle JW, Roberts MC. High-level tetracycline resistance in *Neisseria gonorrhoeae* is the result of acquisition of streptococcal tetM determinant. *Antimicrob Agents Chemother* 1986;30:664–670.

175. Perine PL, Thornsberry C, Schalla W, et al. Evidence for two distinct types of penicillinase-producing *Neisseria gonorrhoeae*. *Lancet* 1977;2:993–995.

176. Robert M, Piot P, Falkow S. The etiology of gonococcal plasmids. *J Gen Microbiol* 1979;114:491–494.

177. Schwarcz SK, Zenilman JM, Schnell D, et al. National surveillance of antimicrobial resistance in *Neisseria gonorrhoeae*. *JAMA* 1990;264:1413–1417.

178. Centers for Disease Control. Plasmid-mediated antimicrobial resistance in *Neisseria gonorrhoeae,* United States, 1988 and 1989. *MMWR* 1990;39:284–287, 293.

179. Sparling PF. Biology of *Neisseria gonorrhoeae*. In: Holmes KK, Mardh P, Sparling PF, Weisner PJ, eds. *Sexually transmitted diseases.* 2nd ed. New York: McGraw-Hill; 1990:131–148.

180. Handsfield HH. *Neisseria gonorrhoeae*. In: Mandell G, Douglas RG Jr, Bennett JE, eds. *Principles and practice of infectious diseases.* 3rd ed. New York: Churchill Livingstone; 1990: 1613–1631.

181. Plummer FA, Simonsen JN, Chubb H, et al. Epidemiologic evidence for the development of serovar-specific immunity after gonococcal infection. *J Clin Invest* 1989;83:1472–1476.

182. Elkins C, Sparling PF. Immunobiology of *Neisseria gonorrhoeae*. In: Quinn TC, Cates W, eds. *Advances in host defense mechanisms.* vol 8. *Sexually transmitted diseases.* New York: Raven Press; 1992:113–139.

183. Knapp JS et al. Serological classification of *Neisseria gonorrhoeae* with use of monoclonal antibodies to gonococcal outer membrane protein I. *J Infect Dis* 1984;150:44–48.

184. Carbonetti NC, Simnand VS, Elkin C, Sparling PF. Construction of isogenic gonococci with variable porin structures: effect on susceptibility to human serum and antibiotics. *Mol Microbiol* 1990;4:1009–1018.

185. Hildebrandt JF, Mayer LW, Wang SP, Buchanan TM. *Neisseria gonorrhoeae* acquire a new principal outer membrane protein when transformed to resistance to serum bactericidal activity. *Infect Immun* 1978;20:267–272.

186. Virji M, Fletcher JN, Zak H, Heckels JE. The potential protective effect of monoclonal antibodies to gonococcal outer membrane protein IA. *J Gen Microbiol* 1987;133:2639–2646.

187. Eisenstein BI, Lee TJ, Sparling PF. Penicillin sensitivity and serum resistance of strains of *Neisseria gonorrhoeae* causing disseminated gonococcal infection. *Infect Immun* 1977;15: 834–841.

188. Apicella MA, Westerink MA, Morse SA, et al. Bactericidal antibody response of normal human serum to the lipooligosaccharide of *Neisseria gonorrhoeae*. *J Infect Dis* 1986;153:520–525.
189. Rice PA, Kasper DL. Characterization of serum resistance of *Neisseria gonorrhoeae* that disseminate: roles of blocking and outer membrane proteins. *J Clin Invest* 1982;70:157–167.
190. Virji M, Heckels JE. Location of a blocking epitope on outer-membrane protein III of *Neisseria gonorrhoeae* by synthetic peptide analysis. *J Gen Microbiol* 1989;135:1895–1899.
191. Sugasawara RJ, Cannon JG, Black WJ, et al. Inhibition of *Neisseria gonorrhoeae* attachment to HeLa cells with monoclonal antibody directed against protein II. *Infect Immun* 1983;42:980–985.
192. Fischer SH, Rest RF. Gonococci possessing only certain PII outer membrane proteins stimulate and adhere to neutrophils. *Infect Immun* 1988;56:1574–1579.
193. Blake MS. Functions of the outer membrane proteins of *Neisseria gonorrhoeae*. In: Jackson GG, Thomas H, eds. *The pathogenesis of bacterial infections*. Berlin: Springer-Verlag; 1985:51–66.
194. Black WJ, Schwalbe RS, Nachamkin I, Cannon JG. Characterization of *Neisseria gonorrhoeae* protein phase II phase variation by use of monoclonal antibodies. *Infect Immun* 1984;45:453–457.
195. Corbus BC, Corbus BC Jr. The cutaneous diagnosis of gonococcal infection. *JAMA* 1941;116:113–115.
196. Cooper MD, Moticka EJ. Cellular immune responses during gonococcal and meningococcal infections. *Clin Microbiol Rev* 1989;2(Suppl):S29–S34.
197. Wyle FA, Rowlett C, Blumenthal T. Cell-mediated immune response in gonococcal infections. *Br J Vener Dis* 1977;55:353–359.
198. Cates W. Epidemiology and control of STD: strategic evolution. *Infect Dis Clin North Am* 1987;1:1–23.
199. Judson FN. Gonorrhea. *Med Clin North Am Sex Transm Dis* 1990;74(6):1353–1366.
200. Centers for Disease Control. Declining rates of rectal and pharyngeal gonorrhea among men, New York City. *JAMA* 1984;252:327–331.
201. Klein EJ, Fisher LS, Chow AW, Guze LC. Anorectal gonococcal infection. *Ann Intern Med* 1977;86:340–346.
202. Judson FN, Miller KG, Schaffnet TM. Screening for gonorrhea and syphilis in the gay baths: Denver, Colorado. *Am J Public Health* 1977;67:740–742.
203. McFarland L, Mietzner TA, Knapp JS, Sandstrom E, Holmes KK, Morse SA. Gonococcal sensitivity to fecal lipids can be mediated by an MTR independent mechanism. *J Clin Microbiol* 1983;18:121–127.
204. Coghill DV, Young H. Genital gonorrhoea in women: a serovar correlation with concomitant rectal infection. *J Infect* 1989;18:131–141.
205. Quinn TC. Clinical approach to intestinal infections in homosexual men. *Med Clin North Am* 1986;70(3):611–634.
206. Pariser H, Marino AF. Gonorrhea: frequency of unrecognized reservoirs. *South Med J* 1970;63:198–202.
207. Eisenstein BI, Masi AT. Disseminated gonococcal infection (DGI) and gonococcal arthritis (GCA): I. Bacteriology, epidemiology, host factors, pathogen factors, and pathology. *Semin Arthritis Rheum* 1981;10(3):155–172.
208. McWhinney PHM, Langhorne P, Love WC, Whaley K. Disseminated gonococcal infection associated with deficiency of the second component of complement. *Postgrad Med J* 1991;67:297–298.
209. Harkness, A. The pathology of gonorrhea. *Br J Vener Dis* 1948;24:132.
210. Darcel DC, Felman YM, Riccardi NB. The utility of anoscopy in the rapid diagnosis of symptomatic anorectal gonorrhea in men. *Sex Trans Dis* 1981;8:16–17.
211. Deherogada P. Diagnosis of rectal gonorrhea by blind anorectal swabs compared with direct vision swabs taken via proctoscope. *Br J Vener Dis* 1977;53:311–313.
212. Handsfield HH, Hook EW III. Ceftriaxone for treatment of uncomplicated gonorrhea: routine use of a single 125 mg dose in a sexually transmitted disease clinic. *Sex Trans Dis* 1987;14:227–30.
213. Handsfield HH, McCormack WM, Hook EW III, et al. A comparison of single-dose cefixime with ceftriaxone as treatment for uncomplicated gonorrhea. *N Engl J Med* 1991;325:1337–41.
214. Verdon MS, Douglas JM Jr, Wiggins SD, Handsfield HH. Treatment of uncomplicated gonorrhea with single doses of 200 mg. cefixime. *Sex Trans Dis* 1993;20(5):290–293.
215. Tartaglione TA, Hooton TM. The role of fluoroquinolones in sexually transmitted diseases. *Rev Ther Pharmacother* 1993;13(3):189–201.
216. Veller-Fornasa C, Tarantello M, Cipriani R, Guerra L, Peserico A. Effect of ofloxacin on *Treponema pallidum* in incubating experimental syphilis. *Genitourin Med* 1987;63:214.
217. Bowie WR, Holmes KK. *Chlamydia trachomatis* (trachoma, perinatal infections, *Lymphogranuloma venereum* and other genital infections). In: Mandell GL, Douglas RG Jr, Bennett JE, eds. *Principles and practice of infectious disease*. 3rd ed. New York: Churchill Livingstone; 1990:1426–1440.
218. Ward ME. The chlamydial developmental cycle. In: Barron AL, ed. *Microbiology of Chlamydia*. Boca Raton: CRC Press; 1988:71–96.
219. Kuo CC. Cultures of *Chlamydia trachomatis* in mouse peritoneal macrophages: factors affecting organism growth. *Infect Immun* 1978;20:439.
220. Schachter J. Biology of *Chlamydia trachomatis*. In: Holmes KK, Mardh P, Sparling PF, Wiesner PJ, eds. *Sexually Transmitted Diseases*. 2nd ed. New York: McGraw-Hill; 1990:167–180.
221. Su H, Watkins NG, Zhang YX, Caldwell HD. *Chlamydia trachomatis* host cell interactions; role of the *Chlamydia* major outer membrane protein as an adhesin. *Infect Immun* 1990;58:1017–1025.
222. Lawn AM, Blyth WA, Tavern J. Interactions of TRIC agents with macrophages and BHK-21 cells observed by electron microscopy. *J Hyg* (London) 1973;72:515–528.
223. Brunham RC, Kuo CC, Cles L, Holmes KK, et al. Correlation of host immune response with quantitative recovery of *Chlamydia trachomatis* from the human endocervix. *Infect Immun* 1983;39:1491–1494.
224. Schachter J, Cles LD, Ray RM, Hesse FE. Is there immunity to chlamydial infections of the human genital tract? *Sex Trans Dis* 1983;10:123–125.
225. Brunham RC, Peeling R, Maclean I, McDowell J, Persson K, Osser S. Postabortal *Chlamydia trachomatis* salpingitis: correlating risk with antigen-specific serological responses and with neutralization. *J Infect Dis* 1987;155:749–755.
226. Caldwell HD, Perry LJ. Neutralization of *Chlamydia trachomatis* infectivity with antibodies to the major outer membrane protein. *Infect Immun* 1982;38:745–754.
227. Peeling R, Maclean IW, Brunham RC. In vitro neutralization of *Chlamydia trachomatis* with monoclonal antibody to an epitope on the major outer membrane protein. *Infect Immun* 1984;46:484–488.
228. Qu Z, Cheng X, de la Maza LM, Peterson EM. Characterization of a neutralizing monoclonal antibody directed at variable domain I of the major outer membrane protein of *Chlamydia trachomatis* C-complex serovars. *Infect Immun* 1993;61:1365–1370.
229. Stephens RS, Tam MR, Kuo CC, Nownski RC. Monoclonal antibodies to *Chlamydia trachomatis*: antibody specificities and antigen characterization. *J Immunol* 1982;128:1083–1089.
230. Zhang YX, Stewart SJ, Caldwell HD. Protective monoclonal antibodies to *Chlamydia trachomatis* serovar- and serogroup-specific major outer membrane protein determinants. *Infect Immun* 1989;57:636–638.
231. Su H, Caldwell HD. In vitro neutralization of *Chlamydia trachomatis* by monovalent fab antibody specific to the major outer membrane protein. *Infect Immun* 1991;59:2843–2845.
232. Morrison RP, Lyng K, Caldwell HD. Chlamydial disease pathogenesis. Ocular hypersensitivity elicited by a genus-specific 57 kd protein. *J Exp Med* 1989;169:663–675.
233. Morrison RP. Immune responses to chlamydia are protective and pathogenic. In: Bowie WR, Caldwell HD, Jones RP, Mardh

P, et al, eds. *Chlamydial infections*. Cambridge, UK: Cambridge University Press; 1990:164–172.

234. Morrison RP, Manning DS, Caldwell HD. Immunology of *Chlamydia trachomatis* infections. Immunoprotective and immunopathogenic responses. In: Gallin JJ, Fauci AS, eds. Quinn TC, guest ed. *Advances in host defense mechanisms*. New York: Raven Press; 1992:57–84.

235. Brunham RC, Peeling R, Maclean I, Kosseim ML, Paraskevas M. *Chlamydia trachomatis*–associated ectopic pregnancy: serologic and histologic correlates. *J Infect Dis* 1992;165: 1076–1081.

236. Brunham RC, Maclean IW, Binns B, Peeling RW. *Chlamydia trachomatis:* its role in tubal infertility. *J Infect Dis* 1985;152: 1275–1282.

237. Brunham RC, Martin DH, Kuo CC, et al. Cellular immune response during uncomplicated genital infection with *Chlamydia trachomatis* in humans. *Infect Immun* 1981;34:98–104.

238. Young E, Taylor HR. Immune mechanisms in chlamydial eye infection: cellular immune responses in chronic and acute disease. *J Infect Dis* 1984;150:745–751.

239. Rothermel CD, Byrne GI, Havell EA. Effect of interferon on the growth of *Chlamydia trachomatis* in mouse fibroblasts (L cells). *Infect Immun* 1983;39:362–370.

240. Byrne GI, Rothermel CD. Differential suceptibility of chlamydiae to exogenous fibroblast interferon. *Infect Immun* 1983;39: 1004–1005.

241. Williams DM, Grubbs BG, Schachter J, Magee DM. Gamma interferon levels during *Chlamydia trachomatis* pneumonia in mice. *Infect Immun* 1993;61:3556–3558.

242. Williams DM, Schachter J. Role of cell-mediated immunity in chlamydial infection: implications for ocular immunity. *Rev Infect Dis* 1985;7:754–759.

243. Beatty WL, Byrne GI, Morrison RP. Morphologic and antigenic characterization of interferon gamma-mediated persistent *Chlamydia trachomatis* infection in vitro. *Proc Natl Acad Sci USA* 1993;90:3998–4002.

244. Washington AE, Johnson RE, Sanders LL, et al. Incidence of *Chlamydia trachomatis* infections in the United States: using reported *Neisseria gonorrhoeae* as a surrogate. In: Oriel D, Ridgway G, Schachter J, et al, eds. Chlamydia infections. Cambridge, UK: Cambridge University Press; 1986:487.

245. Stamm WE, Koutsky LA, Benedetti JK, et al. *Chlamydia trachomatis* urethral infections in men. Prevalence, risk factors, and clinical manifestations. *Ann Intern Med* 1984;100:47–51.

246. Goldmeier D, Darougar S. Isolation of *Chlamydia trachomatis* from throat and rectum of homosexual men. *Br J Vener Dis* 1977;53:184–185.

247. Stamm WE, Quinn TC, Mkrtichian EE, Wang SP, Schuffler MD, Holmes KK. *Chlamydia trachomatis* proctitis. In: Mardh P-A, et al, eds. *Chlamydial infections*. London: Elsevier; 1982: 111–114.

248. Thompson CI, MacAulay AJ, Smith IW. *Chlamydia trachomatis* infections in the female rectum. *Genitourin Med* 1989;65: 269–273.

249. Sulaiman MZC, Foster J, Pugh SF. Prevalence of *Chlamydia trachomatis* infection in homosexual men. *Genitourin Med* 1987;63:179–181.

250. McMillan A, Sommerville RG, McKie PMK. Chlamydial infection in homosexual men. Frequency of isolation of *Chlamydia trachomatis* from the urethra, ano-rectum, and pharynx. *Br J Vener Dis* 1981;57:47–49.

251. Barnes RC, Rompalo AM, Stamm WE. Comparison of *Chlamydia trachomatis* serovars causing rectal and cervical infections. *J Infect Dis* 1987;156:953–958.

252. Mardh P, Paavonen J, Puolakkainen M. *Chlamydia*. New York: Plenum Press; 1989:15–55.

253. Levine JS, Smith PD, Bragge WR. Chronic proctitis in male homosexuals due to *Lymphogranuloma venereum*. *Gastroenterology* 1980;79:563–565.

254. Perine PL, Osoba AO. *Lymphogranuloma venereum*. In: Holmes KK, Mardh P, Sparling PF, Weisner PJ, eds. *Sexually transmitted diseases*. 2nd ed. New York: McGraw-Hill; 1990: 195–204.

255. Rompalo AM, Suchland RJ, Price CB, Stamm WE. Rapid diag-

nosis of *Chlamydia trachomatis* rectal infection by direct immunofluorescence staining. *J Infect Dis* 1987;155:1075–1076.

256. Pratt BC, Tait IA, Anyaegbunam WI. Rectal carriage of *Chlamydia trachomatis* in women. *J Clin Pathol* 1989;42:1309–1310.

257. Riordon T, Ellis DA, Mathews PI, Ratcliffe SF. False positive results with an ELISA for detection of chlamydial antigen. *J Clin Pathol* 1986;39:1276–1277.

258. Treharne JD, Forsey T, Thomas BJ. Chlamydial serology. *Br Med Bull* 1983;39(2):194–200.

259. Saikku P. Chlamydial serology. *Scand J Infect Dis* 1982(Suppl); 31:34–37.

260. Wang SP, Kuo CC, Grayston JT. Formalinized *Chlamydia trachomatis* organisms as antigen in the micro-immunofluorescence test. *J Clin Microbiol* 1979;10:259–261.

261. Centers for Disease Control. Recommendations for the prevention and management of *Chlamydia trachomatis* infections, 1993. *MMWR* 1993;42:1–38.

262. Ravdin JI, Petri WA. *Entamoeba histolytica* (amebiasis). In: Mandell GL, Douglas RG Jr, Bennett JE, eds. *Principles and practice of infectious diseases*. 3rd ed. New York: Churchill Livingstone; 1990:2036–2049.

263. Manson PEC, Bell DR. Medical protozoology (Appendix 1). *Manson's tropical diseases*. 19th ed. London: Bailliere-Tindall; 1987:1243–1249.

264. Sargeaunt PG, Williams JE, Greene JD. The differentiation of invasive and noninvasive *Entamoeba histolytica* by isoenzyme electrophoresis. *Trans R Soc Trop Med Hyg* 1978;72:519–521.

265. Petri WA Jr, Jackson TFHG, Gathiram V, et al. Pathogenic and nonpathogenic strains of *Entamoeba histolytica* can be differentiated by monoclonal antibodies to the galactose-specific adherence lecithin. *Infect Immun* 1990;58:1802–1806.

266. Clark CG, Diamond CS. Ribosomal RNA genes of pathogenic and nonpathogenic *Entamoeba histolytica* are distinct. *Mol Biochem Parasitol* 1991;49:297–302.

267. Zannich E, Horstmann RD, Knoblock J, Arnold HH. Genomic DNA differences between pathogenic and nonpathogenic *Entamoeba histolytica*. *Proc Natl Acad Sci USA* 1989;86: 5118–5122.

268. Chadee K, Petri WA Jr., Innes DJ, Ravdin JI. Rat colonic mucins bind to and inhibit the adherence of *Entamoeba histolytica*. *J Clin Invest* 1987;180:1245–1254.

269. Goldmeier D, Price AB, Billington O. Is entamoeba histolytica in homosexual men a pathogen? *Lancet* 1986;1:641–644.

270. Law C. Sexually transmitted diseases and enteric infections in the male homosexual population. *Semin Dermatol* 1990;9: 178–184.

271. Patterson M, Healy GR, Shabot JM. Serologic testing for amebiasis. *Gastroenterology* 1980;78:136–141.

272. Petri WA. Recognition of the galactose- or N-acetylgalactosamine-binding lectin of *Entamoeba histolytica* by human immune sera. *Infect Immun* 1987;55:2327–2331.

273. Petri WA, Ravdin JI. Cytopathogenicity of *Entamoeba histolytica*. *Eur J Epidemiol* 1987;3:123–126.

274. Ravdin JI, Guerrant RL. The role of adherence in cytopathogenic mechanisms of *Entamoeba histolytica*. Study with mammalian tissue culture cells and human erythrocytes. *J Clin Invest* 1981;68:1305–1313.

275. Ravdin JI, Croft BY, Guerrant RL. Cytopathogenic mechanisms of *Entamoeba histolytica*. *J Exp Med* 1980;152:377–390.

276. Petri WA et al. Isolation of the galactose-binding lectin which mediates the in vitro adherence of *Entamoeba histolytica*. *J Clin Invest* 1987;80:1238–1244.

277. Petri WA Jr, Ravdin JI. Protection of gerbils from amebic liver abscess by immunization with the galactose-specific adherence lectin of *Entamoeba histolytica*. *J Clin Invest* 1991;59:97–101.

278. Kobiler D, Mirelman D. Lectin activity in *Entamoeba histolytica* trophozoites. *Infect Immun* 1980;29:221–225.

279. Reed SL, Sargeaunt PG, Braude AI. Resistance to lysis by human immune serum of pathogenic *Entamoeba histolytica*. *Trans R Soc Trop Med Hyg* 1983;77:248–253.

280. Salata RA, Martinez-Palomo A, Murray HW, et al. Patients treated for amebic liver abscess develop a cell-mediated immune response effective in vitro against *Entamoeba histolytica*. *J Immunol* 1986;136:2633–2639.

281. Salata RA, Pearson RD, Ravdin JI. Interaction of human leukocytes with *Entamoeba histolytica*. Killing of virulent amebae by the activated macrophage. *J Clin Invest* 1985;76:491–499.
282. Salata RA, Martinez-Palomo A, Murray HW, et al. Patients treated for amebic liver abscess develop cell-mediated immune responses effective in vitro against *Entamoeba histolytica*. *J Immunol* 1986;136:2633–2639.
283. Sargeaunt PG, Oates JK, Mactennan I, et al. *Entamoeba histolytica* in male homosexuals. *Br J Vener Dis* 1983;59:193–195.
284. Reed SL, Wess DW. *Entamoeba histolytica* infection and AIDS. *Am J Med* 1991;90:269–270.
285. Reed SL. Amebiasis: an update. *Clin Infect Dis* 1992;14:385–393.
286. Walsh JA. Problems in recognition and diagnosis of amebiasis: estimation of the global magnitude of morbidity and mortality. *Rev Infect Dis* 1986;8:228–238.
287. Walsh JA. Prevalence of *Entamoeba histolytica* infection. In: Ravdin JI, ed. *Amebiasis: human infection by* Entamoeba histolytica. New York: Wiley; 1988:93–105.
288. Schmerin MJ, Gelston A, Jones TC. Amebiasis: an increasing problem among homosexuals in New York City. *JAMA* 1977;238:1387–1389.
289. Pomerantz BM, Marr JS, Goldman WD. Amebiasis in New York city 1958–1978: identification of the male homosexual high-risk population. *Bull NY Acad Med* 1980;56:232–244.
290. Dritz SK, Ainsworth TE, Back A, et al. Patterns of sexually transmitted enteric disease in a city. *Lancet* 1977;2:3–4.
291. Pearce RB. Intestinal protozoal infections and AIDS. *Lancet* 1983;2:51.
292. Higgs ES, Guerrant RL. Diagnosing intestinal parasites. In: Andriole VT, ed. *Mediguide to infectious diseases*. Vol 12. No 2. New York: Lawrence Dellaforte; 1992.
293. Mirelman D, Bracha R, Wexler A, Chayen A, et al. Changes in isoenzyme patterns of a cloned culture of nonpathogenic *Entamoeba histolytica* during axenization. *Infect Immun* 1986;54:827–832.
294. William DC. Amebiasis. In: Ostrow DG, Sandholzer TA, Felman YM, eds. *Sexually transmitted diseases in homosexual men: diagnosis, treatment and research*. New York: Plenum Press; 1983;:87–98.
295. Garcia LS. Parasitic infections in the compromised host. In: Isenberg HD, ed. *Clinical microbiology updates*. Vol 3. No. 1. Sommerville, NJ: Hoechst-Roussel; 1992.
296. Guerrant RL, Weikel CS, Ravdin JI. Intestinal protozoa: *Giardia lamblia, Entamoeba histolytica*, and *Cryptosporidium*. In: Holmes KK, ed. *Sexually transmitted diseases*. 2nd ed. New York: McGraw-Hill; 1990:493–514.
297. Haque R, Kress K, Wood S, et al. Diagnosis of pathogenic *Entamoeba histolytica* infection using a stool ELISA based on monoclonal antibodies to the galactose-specific adhesin. *J Infect Dis* 1993;167:347–349.
298. Drugs for parasitic infections. *Med Lett* 1988;30:15–22.
299. American Academy of Pediatrics Committee on Drugs. Blindness and neuropathy from diiodohydroxygenin-like drugs. *Pediatrics* 1974;54:378–379.
300. Behress MM. Optic atrophy in children after diiodohydroxygen therapy. *JAMA* 1974;228:693–694.
301. Sullam PM, Slutkin G, Gottlieb AB, Mills J. Paromamycin therapy of endemic amebiasis in homosexual men. *Sex Trans Dis* 1986;13:151–155.
302. McAuley JB, Herwaldt BL, Stokes SL, et al. Diloxanide furoate for treating asymptomatic *Entamoeba hisolytica* cyst passers: 14 years experience in the United States. *Clin Infect Dis* 1992;15:464–468.
303. Irusen EM, Jackson TFHG, Simjee AE. Asymptomatic intestinal colonization by pathogenic *Entamoeba hisolytica* in amebic liver abscess: prevalence, response to therapy, and pathogenic potential. *Clin Infect Dis* 1992;14:889–893.

Infections of the Gastrointestinal Tract,
edited by M. J. Blaser, P. D. Smith, J. I. Ravdin,
H. B. Greenberg, and R. L. Guerrant
Raven Press, Ltd., New York © 1995.

CHAPTER 32

Microbial Agents in the Pathogenesis, Differential Diagnosis, and Complications of Inflammatory Bowel Diseases

R. Balfour Sartor

Ulcerative colitis and Crohn's disease, collectively referred to as idiopathic inflammatory bowel disease (IBD), are chronic spontaneously relapsing disorders that affect between 500,000 and 1 million persons in the United States (1). Microbial agents appear to be intimately involved in the pathogenesis of these disorders and contribute to some of their most frequent complications (2–5). While it remains unclear whether specific infections initiate chronic, relapsing inflammation, it is apparent that common pathogens can reactivate underlying intestinal inflammation and produce disease in normal hosts that closely mimics idiopathic IBD. Moreover, ubiquitous intestinal bacteria seem to be essential in perpetuating chronic inflammation and in causing the frequent suppurative complications of Crohn's disease. This chapter discusses current evidence that IBD is caused by an infectious agent, examines the role of endogenous luminal bacteria in its pathogenesis, outlines ways to distinguish intestinal inflammation caused by pathogens from idiopathic IBD, identifies pathogens that can reactivate or suprainfect established ulcerative colitis and Crohn's disease, and discusses ways to recognize and treat the frequent septic complications of IBD.

ETIOLOGICAL CONSIDERATIONS: ARE CROHN'S DISEASE AND ULCERATIVE COLITIS CAUSED BY MICROBIAL AGENTS?

Ulcerative colitis and Crohn's disease are idiopathic disorders characterized by an unrestrained inflammatory response, but the factors initiating and perpetuating this

R. B. Sartor: Division of Digestive Diseases, University of North Carolina at Chapel Hill, Chapel Hill, North Carolina 27599-7080.

chronic immune reaction remain unclear (1). Genetic and environmental contributions are evident. Microbial influences in the pathogenesis of these disorders are strongly supported by observations that IBD occurs in the distal intestine (the area of highest luminal bacterial concentrations), that patients with Crohn's disease clinically improve when luminal bacterial concentrations are decreased, and that ulcerative colitis and Crohn's disease closely resemble enterocolonic infections (5). Chronic IBD could be either a predictable response to a specific pathogen or an inappropriate immunological response to ubiquitous microbial constituents. Clinical and experimental data support four etiological theories as outlined in Table 1.

Persistent Pathogen

Because Crohn's disease closely resembles ileocecal tuberculosis, *Yersinia,* and anorectal *Chlamydia* infections, and because ulcerative colitis mimics chronic *Campylobacter, Shigella,* and amebic colitis, investigators have diligently searched for specific pathogens in IBD. A number of organisms have been advanced as causes of ulcerative colitis and Crohn's disease (Table 2); most of these agents have not been confirmed by other investigators. Serum antibodies to a variety of conventional pathogens are increased in IBD, especially Crohn's disease (16,17), but may reflect an overly responsive immune reaction since antibody concentrations to a broad spectrum of commensal organisms are also increased (18–20). Sporadic reports of case clustering of Crohn's disease among family members (21) and close friends (22) support an infectious origin of this disorder. Two pathogens are under active investigation as possible causes of Crohn's disease: *Mycobacterium paratuberculosis* and *paramyxovirus* (measles). Although present data do not

TABLE 1. *Possible microbial etiologies of IBD*

1. Persistent pathogen
2. Induction of tissue injury by a transient pathogen, perpetuation by other mechanisms
3. Altered pathogenicity of endogenous enteric bacteria
4. Abnormal host response to ubiquitous bacteria or bacterial components

convincingly incriminate a single, persistent pathogen as a universal cause of Crohn's disease, this hypothesis must be considered in view of the possibility that this disorder may represent a heterogeneous group of diseases with similar phenotypes and with the knowledge that all gastrointestinal pathogens have not yet been discovered.

M. paratuberculosis

M. paratuberculosis is an extremely fastidious, slow-growing, mycobactin-dependent organism that causes Johne's disease (23,24). This disorder is a chronic, granulomatous enterocolitis in ruminants that does not respond to antimycobacterial therapy. In 1913, Dalziel noted the close similarity of the clinical and pathological features of human idiopathic granulomatous enteritis, ileocecal tuberculosis, and Johne's disease (25). Despite intense efforts by Crohn (26) and later investigators, mycobacteria were not linked with Crohn's disease until 1978 when Burnham and colleagues (13) cultured *M. kansasii* from a resected specimen. In 1984, Chiodini et al. (14) recovered slow-growing *M. paratuberculosis* from tissues of three patients with Crohn's disease, and subsequently ten apparently identical isolates of *M. paratuberculosis* were cultured from Crohn's disease tissues by five centers on three continents (24).

Recovery of *M. paratuberculosis* by culture is quite low (less than 15% of Crohn's cases) even in the most experienced hands. This organism, however, has not been cultured from ulcerative colitis or control tissues. Slow-growing spheroplasts have been recovered from 20% to 40% of Crohn's disease patients and a small number of controls (27–29). Recently, interest in this field has been stimulated by detection of *M. paratuberculosis* in the majority of Crohn's disease patients using polymerase chain

TABLE 2. *Infectious agents suggested to cause IBD*

Ulcerative colitis
    Diplostreptococcus (6)
    Bacteroides necrophorum (7)
    Shigella (8)
    RNA virus (9)
Crohn's disease
    Chlamydia (10)
    L forms of *Pseudomonas maltophilia* (11)
    Reovirus (12)
    Mycobacterium kansasii (13)
    Mycobacterium paratuberculosis (14)
    Paramyxovirus (measles) (15)

reaction (PCR) amplification based on a multicopy genomic DNA insertion element (IS-900) specific for *M. paratuberculosis* (30,31). Sanderson et al. (30) reported that 65% of Crohn's disease, 4% of ulcerative colitis, and 13% of control tissues had detectable IS-900 DNA. This observation has been confirmed by Dell'Isola and colleagues (31), who detected IS-900 sequences in intestinal tissues of 72% of children with Crohn's disease, 20% with ulcerative colitis, and 29% of disease controls. However, other groups have reported lower detection rates ranging from 0% to 8% (32,33). PCR technology has also been used to identify previously uncharacterized spheroplasts cultured from IBD patients. Results demonstrated that 33% to 38% of spheroplasts from Crohn's disease patients were *M. paratuberculosis* compared with 0% to 17% of spheroplasts from ulcerative colitis patients (28,29). *M. avium* subsp. *silvaticum* (wood pigeon bacillus, which can also cause Johne's disease) or uncharacterized mycobacterial strains were found in equal frequencies in Crohn's and control spheroplasts (29).

Additional evidence supporting *M. paratuberculosis* as a possible human pathogen is transmission of histological but not clinical inflammation to experimental animals by inoculating a human isolate (34,35) and identification of potential mechanisms of transmission. Viable *M. paratuberculosis* has been recovered in the milk of asymptomatic infected cows (36) and IS-900 has been detected in 7% of commercially distributed pasteurized milk samples, although no viable organisms have been recovered (37). Chiodini and Herman-Taylor (38) demonstrated that routine pasteurization does not kill *M. paratuberculosis* in milk. Furthermore, waterborne infections are suggested by high rates of Crohn's disease along rivers draining grazing lands inhabited by herds infected with Johne's disease (J. Herman-Taylor, unpublished data).

Although *M. paratuberculosis* as an etiological agent has several attractive features, it is probably not the cause of Crohn's disease in the majority of cases. There is no convincing epidemiological, immunological, histochemical, or clinical support for its etiological role. The incidence of Crohn's disease is not increased in spouses of patients, health care workers attending patients with Crohn's disease or animals with Johne's disease, or farm workers associated with *M. paratuberculosis* herds. While it is possible that infection with *M. paratuberculosis* may be limited to an early age, the absence of Crohn's disease in children living on farms with infected herds does not support this theory. Diligent searches for acid-fast bacilli and immunohistochemical evidence (39) of *M. paratuberculosis* antigen has been negative, although a preliminary report localized DNA of this organism to the lamina propria of one patient with Crohn's disease by *in situ* PCR (40). Although serum antibodies to *M. paratuberculosis* are elevated in some Crohn's disease patients (6,41), most investigators report nonspecific humoral or cellular immune responses to several mycobacterial species, indicating continuous environmental exposure to these organisms or defective immunoregulation of immunity to luminal antigens (41–46). Finally, antibiotic trials have not demonstrated convincingly an etiological role for mycobacteria in Crohn's disease (47–50). Swift and colleagues (49) showed no benefit from 12 months of therapy with rifampicin, isoniazid, and ethambutol. Prantera et al. (50) reported prevention of relapse with a 9-month course of ethambutol, clofazimine, and dapsone, with a one time dose of rifampicin on entry to the trial, but there was no endoscopic or radiological healing and clofazimine and dapsone have antiinflammatory activities. Controlled trials of clarithromycin, which has better *in vitro* activity against *M. paratuberculosis,* are in progress. At the present time, it is impossible to determine whether *M. paratuberculosis* causes Crohn's disease in a small subgroup of patients or whether the organism is an environmental contaminant that secondarily invades ulcerated tissue in Crohn's disease patients to a greater extent than in ulcerative colitis and inflammatory controls.

Measles

Wakefield and colleagues (15) suggest that persistent viral infection of vascular endothelial cells causes Crohn's disease by inducing focal granulomatous vasculitis. Paramyxovirus-like structures were visualized in the vascular endothelium of all nine Crohn's patients examined for the organism. Measles antigen and mRNA were localized to granulomas and endothelial cells by immunohistochemistry and *in situ* hybridization. Initially, antimeasles antibody was reported to be elevated, but a subsequent report indicated no difference in anti-measles IgG in Crohn's disease patients compared with ulcerative colitis and control patients (51). These authors postulate that measles infection induces focal vascular lesions that cause local ischemia and epithelial necrosis (52). Knibbs et al. (53) confirmed the presence of 18- to 200-nm-diameter structures in vascular endothelial cells and macrophages in Crohn's patients but were unable to demonstrate measles antigen by immunohistochemical staining. These provocative findings must be viewed with caution due to the inadequate number of controls, inconsistent localization of virus-like particles, lack of an immunological response, and discrepancies among the findings of different investigators.

Transient Pathogenic Infection

Infection with a conventional pathogen can precede the onset of typical idiopathic IBD. A small percentage of patients involved in epidemics of *Shigella, Salmonella,* or *Yersinia* develop classic ulcerative colitis or Crohn's disease with no evidence of persistent bacterial infection (54). Other patients with acute enteric infections acquired either sporadically or by traveling have been reported to progress to chronic, relapsing IBD despite clearance of the initial organism (55–59). Self-limited tissue injury caused by such agents could initiate inflammation subsequently perpetuated by separate mechanisms (Table 3), leading to chronic, spontaneously relapsing IBD (5). Many infections or environmental insults can break the mucosal barrier or induce acute inflammation; therefore, the initiating event may be nonspecific. Thus, the induc-

TABLE 3. *Mechanisms by which transient infections could induce chronic inflammation*

1. Disrupted mucosal barrier leading to stimulation of mucosal inflammatory cells
2. Induced inflammation perpetuated by alternative mechanisms
3. Modulation of host immune response
4. Autoimmune response

tion of IBD may be analogous to the initiation of juvenile onset diabetes mellitus by enteroviral coxackie and echo infections in HLA-DR3, DR4, and/or DQ3 hosts (60,61) and the induction of reactive arthritis by enteric bacteria (*Yersinia, Shigella, Salmonella, Chlamydia*) in HLA-B27 patients (62). Alternatively, delayed exposure to common enteric pathogens because of improved hygiene can have potentially detrimental consequences, analogous to polio (63).

Transient enteric infections could break the mucosal barrier by directly invading epithelial cells or by stimulating the release of enterotoxins, proinflammatory cytokines [tumor necrosis factor or interferon-γ (64)], or chemotactic peptides (64,65). The net result is epithelial necrosis or disruption of tight junctions that enhance uptake of proinflammatory luminal bacteria and bacterial components (5,66). In addition, transient inflammation could become self-sustaining due to defective downregulation of the immune response (5,67).

Alternatively, enteric infections could induce chronic intestinal inflammation by modulating the immune response. Enhanced immunoreactivity by adjuvant activity or induction of class II antigens on epithelial cells may initiate pathological responses to ubiquitous luminal epithelial antigens. Cell wall polymers such as peptidoglycan–polysaccharide complexes from ubiquitous luminal bacteria and pathogens, especially mycobacteria, have potent adjuvant activities (66,68) and a variety of infections can induce class II HLA antigens (69). Recent evidence shows that microbial agents can secrete molecules that modulate host immune responsiveness. For example, Epstein–Barr virus (EBV) protein (BCRF1) shares structural homology and immunosuppressive activity with IL-10 (70) and enteropathogenic *E. coli* secrete a partially characterized lymphokine inhibitory factor that inhibits expression of interleukin-2 (IL-2), IL-4, and IL-5 by mitogen-stimulated mononuclear cells and suppresses lymphocyte activation (71). Of interest, ulcerative colitis patients have increased mucosal concentrations of IL-10 (72), decreased concentrations of IL-2 (73), and a 76% detection rate of EBV infection (74). Spontaneous colitis that develops in IL-2 and IL-10 knockout mice clearly illustrate the detrimental consequences of dysregulation of mucosal lymphokines (75,76). Conversely, inflammatory mediators produced by activated immune cells can modulate bacterial function, as demonstrated by bacterial proliferation by IL-1 (77), and enhance production of formylated oligopeptides (f-met-leu-phe, or FMLP) in response to oxygen radicals (78).

A transient infection could induce chronic inflammation

by initiating an autoimmune response, either by exposing intracellular "hidden" antigens or by molecular mimicry, i.e., shared epitopes between microbial antigens and host proteins. Serum antibodies that react with both colonic epithelial cells and several Enterobacteriaceae have been demonstrated in ulcerative colitis (79,80). However, these antibodies are probably secondary responses to cellular damage since there is no compelling evidence that these antibodies cause epithelial cell injury. Das and colleagues (81) demonstrated that a 40-kDa colonic epithelial cell antigen, recently identified as the cytoskeletal protein tropomyosin, is specifically recognized by serum and mucosal-associated antibodies from ulcerative colitis patients. However, no homologous epitope has been found in microbial agents to suggest that molecular mimicry initiates production of this autoantibody. The close homology between bacterial (especially mycobacterial) and mammalian heat shock proteins (HSPs) raises the possibility that cross-reacting antibodies or cellular immune responses to these molecules could lead to chronic intestinal inflammation (82). Expression of these "stress proteins" is increased by a variety of stimuli, including inflammation and cytokines (83). These molecules protect the cell during stressful events and function as molecular chaperones for other cytoplasmic proteins. HSP60 expression is increased in epithelial cells from ulcerative colitis patients (84) and mononuclear cells within inflamed and histologically normal intestinal segments of ulcerative colitis and Crohn's disease patients, but not those with self-limited infectious colitis (85). Serum antibodies to HSP60 are increased in Crohn's disease and ulcerative colitis patients (86–88), although all patients do not show equal reactivity to human and mycobacterial HSPs (87). Similarly, circulating lymphocytes from IBD patients show selective responses to HSP60 (88,89). The ability of these molecules to mediate inflammation is illustrated by the induction or inhibition of experimental arthritis by T-lymphocyte clones reacting to HSP65 (90). Whether enhanced expression of mucosal HSP and immune responsiveness is a consequence of the inflammatory response or involved in its pathogenesis remains to be determined.

Altered Concentrations of Luminal Bacteria

Subtle alterations of the composition of the complex "normal" bacterial constituents ("dysbiosis") could lead to chronic stimulation of the mucosal immune system and result in chronic intestinal inflammation (2). These alterations could be a consequence of local environmental changes, such as exposure to antibiotics (91,92), genetic determinants (93), or anatomic changes such as loss of the ileocecal valve, partial obstruction, and enterocolonic fistulae. A number of investigators have described derangements of anaerobic bacterial constituents in Crohn's disease. Similar alterations have not been seen in ulcerative colitis, although nonspecific relative increases in aerobic bacteria and decreases in anaerobic flora occur in this disorder as well as in patients with diarrhea of many etiologies (2,93–95). Fecal concentrations of certain coccoid rods, such as *Eubacteria, Peptostreptococcus,* and

Coprococcus, are increased in patients with Crohn's disease (93,96) as are serum antibodies to these organisms (20,97). A provocative study by Van de Merwe et al. (93) of children of Crohn's disease patients suggests that profiles of fecal anaerobes are genetically determined and that abnormalities may precede clinical symptoms. One third of asymptomatic children had increased fecal concentrations of anaerobic coccobacilli; one third of these children with abnormal bacterial profiles developed intestinal symptoms during 5–7 years of prospective observation. Fecal concentrations of *Bacteroides vulgatus* are also increased in active Crohn's disease (96,98) and therapeutic efficacy of metronidazole correlates with decreased *Bacteroides* concentrations (96). Support for a role of anaerobic bacteria in the pathogenesis of Crohn's disease is provided by clinical responses to metronidazole (99), the requirement for *B. vulgatus* in carrageenan-induced colitis in guinea pigs (100,101), and the ability of cell wall polymers from certain *Eubacterial* species to induce chronic granulomatous inflammation in rats (66,102,103).

Abnormal Functional Properties

Emerging data implicate functional alterations in commensal bacteria in ulcerative colitis. Abnormal bacterial metabolites or altered virulence factors could have profound effects on epithelial cell function and lead to chronic mucosal injury. Such metabolites and factors may not be detected by conventional microbiological screening tests. Two groups have shown that *E. coli* from some patients with IBD adhere to epithelial cells by novel mechanisms (104,105), but findings are controversial (106). Bacterial adherence and/or invasion can directly or indirectly injure epithelial cells, as demonstrated by stimulated secretion of chemotactic peptides such as IL-8 by epithelial cell lines (65) and enhanced neutrophil transmigration across epithelial monolayers (107). Other functional abnormalities of *E. coli* from ulcerative colitis patients have been described, including production of verotoxin, Shiga-like toxin, necrotoxins, and hemolysins (108,109). More recently, Giaffer and colleagues (105) found no verotoxin production or hemolytic *E. coli* strains in IBD patients but did find cytotoxin production in 10% of Crohn's disease patients. Mucin-degrading enzymes are produced by *Bacteroides vulgatus* and group D streptococci (106,110), and enterococci from ulcerative colitis patients can secrete hyaluronidase (111). Production of superantigens and HSPs by luminal bacteria from IBD patients has not yet been investigated.

Recent data support the novel hypothesis by Roediger that ulcerative colitis is caused by defective metabolism of short-chain fatty acids (SCFAs) (112), leading to epithelial starvation. SCFAs are produced by anaerobic bacterial fermentation of nonabsorbed carbohydrates and proteins. Colonocytes preferentially use luminal SCFAs, especially butyrate, as fuel sources (113,114). Ulcerative colitis patients have decreased luminal concentrations of SCFAs and a selective defect in butyrate oxidation (112,114). Roediger recently demonstrated that hydrogen sulfide, which is produced by colonic bacteria, selectively inhibits epithelial cell butyrate metabolism, with the greatest effects in the distal colon (115). No blockade of glucose metabolism by butyrate was observed. In addition to inhibiting butyrate metabolism, hydrogen sulfide is toxic to colonic epithelial cells and mucus (116). Luminal hydrogen sulfide is increased in patients with ulcerative colitis (117) and sulfate-reducing bacteria are found in 96% of patients with ulcerative colitis compared with 50% of healthy controls (116). The majority of sulfate-reducing bacteria isolated from ulcerative colitis patients are *Desulfovibrio* sp., which are resistant to most antibiotics but sensitive to gentamicin (116). That altered production and metabolic blockade of SCFAs occurs in ulcerative colitis patients is supported by the therapeutic benefit of SCFA enemas (118,119) and aminoglycoside antibiotics (120).

Abnormal Host Response to Ubiquitous Luminal Bacterial Constituents

Based on observations in recent models, we believe that chronic, relapsing granulomatous intestinal and systemic inflammation is a genetically determined, abnormal host response to ubiquitous luminal bacterial constituents (4,5). In the normal host, detrimental responses to phlogistic luminal contents are prevented by several mechanisms including the epithelial barrier, mucus, and secretory antibodies that exclude toxic macromolecules, and downregulation of the inflammatory response by immunosuppressive mediators and T lymphocytes. Ineffective barrier function or defective immunosuppression in the genetically susceptible host results in continuous stimulation of the mucosal immune system and, consequently, chronic inflammation.

This hypothesis is supported by dramatic differences in the degree and chronicity of intestinal and systemic inflammation in rodents raised under conventional vs. sterile conditions. Lewis rats populated with specific pathogen-free conventional bacteria develop chronic mid–small bowel ulceration associated with intestinal fibrosis, hepatobiliary inflammation, anemia, and leukocytosis after subcutaneous injection of indomethacin. In contrast, littermates raised in a sterile (germ-free) environment have attenuated acute inflammation and no evidence of chronic intestinal or systemic inflammation (121). Human HLA B27/β_2-microglobulin transgenic rats raised in conventional rodent facilities develop colitis, gastritis, arthritis, dermatitis, and epididymitis by 3–4 months of age (122). However, under sterile conditions these rats do not develop arthritis, diarrhea, or biochemical evidence of colitis, although they manifest hair loss, nail changes, and epididymitis (123; R. B. Sartor, unpublished observations). Similarly, mice with embryonal stem cell deletion of IL-2 (IL-2 knockout mice) raised in a conventional environment develop aggressive pancolitis with bloody diarrhea. However, such mice kept under specific pathogen-free conditions have mild histological colitis but no clinical evidence of inflammation, and mice raised in a sterile environment have no clinical or histological colitis (75). Likewise, IL-10 knockout mice that develop enterocolitis in the conventional state exhibit only

colitis under specific pathogen-free conditions (76). Finally, germ-free hosts fail to develop cecal inflammation when challenged by ameba inoculation (124) or chronic oral administration of carrageenan (125). The latter model is of particular importance since *Bacteroides vulgatus* is uniquely capable of inducing injury (100), suggesting that all luminal bacterial constituents do not have equal inflammatory potential.

The importance of endogenous bacteria in the initiation and perpetuation of intestinal inflammation is also supported by changes in injury when concentrations of luminal bacteria are manipulated. Experimental jejunal bacterial overgrowth induces hepatobiliary inflammation that resembles sclerosing cholangitis (126) and reactivates quiescent arthritis (127). Indomethacin- and carrageenaninduced intestinal inflammation can be attenuated by antibiotics, particularly those with activity against anaerobic bacteria (128,129).

Patients with Crohn's disease improve when luminal bacterial concentrations are decreased by antibiotics, bowel rest, and lavage therapy (48). Metronidazole (10 mg/kg/day) is superior to placebo (99) and equal to sulfasalazine (130) as primary therapy of Crohn's colitis and enterocolitis. High-dose metronidazole (20 mg/kg/day) begun at the time of surgery and continued for 3 months decreased the recurrence rate of symptomatic Crohn's disease at 1 year but had no longlasting effects at 2 and 3 years postoperatively (131). Broad-spectrum antibiotics are routinely used by experienced investigators in primary treatment of Crohn's disease and are effective in uncontrolled trials (132,133), but have never been subjected to rigorously controlled trials. While most antibiotics only transiently alter bacterial concentrations due to emergence of resistant strains, metronidazole (98) and ciprofloxacin (120) have been reported to eliminate *Bacteroides* sp. and gram-negative coliforms, respectively, during 6 months of treatment.

Chronic antibiotic administration is not routinely advocated for primary treatment of ulcerative colitis, although several studies suggest an adjunctive role for agents active against gram-negative aerobes in addition to standard medical therapy. Turunen and colleagues (120) demonstrated clinical, endoscopic, and histological improvement following 6 months treatment with ciprofloxacin (500–750 mg bid) in a double-blind, placebo-controlled trial. Burke et al. (134,135) reported long-term benefits after brief tobramycin treatment and Danzi (136) found that 90% of ulcerative colitis patients improved with 8 months therapy with trimethoprim-sulfamethoxazole. In addition, Peppercorn (137) reports that patients with fulminant ulcerative colitis occasionally respond dramatically to broad-spectrum antibiotics. Most studies show that metronidazole has no effect in ulcerative colitis (48). These results suggest that aerobes are more important in the pathogenesis of ulcerative colitis and anaerobes in Crohn's disease.

We do not yet know whether luminal bacteria exert their effects by secondarily invading the ulcerated mucosa or by secreting toxic products. It is apparent that bacteria that normally inhabit the distal intestine produce proinflammatory molecules (5,66). Bacterial cell wall polymers, such as lipopolysaccharide (LPS, endotoxin) and peptidoglycan-polysaccharide (PG-PS), and formylated oligopeptide molecules, such as FMLP, can induce experimental intestinal inflammation (3,5,67,138–140). PG-PS derived from certain bacterial strains, including group D streptococci (enterococci), can induce chronic, spontaneously relapsing, granulomatous enterocolitis with associated arthritis, granulomatous hepatitis, anemia, and leukocytosis after intramural (subserosal) injection (67,141). Moreover, luminal PG-PS can potentiate acute indomethacin-induced enteritis (but not colitis) in germ-free rats (142) and has been implicated in the genesis of hepatobiliary inflammation accompanying jejunal bacterial overgrowth in rats (143,144). Increased serum antibodies to bacterial components (145) and circulating FMLP (76) and LPS (92,124) are found in patients with active Crohn's disease. Thus, it is possible that the continuous absorption of toxic products of luminal bacteria stimulate cells of the mucosal immune system, leading to sustained intestinal inflammation in the susceptible host.

Because most hosts do not develop intestinal inflammation despite continuous exposure to high concentrations of these proinflammatory bacteria, an essential component of this hypothesis is differential host susceptibility to chronic inflammation. In the normal state, inflammatory responses to luminal bacteria are prevented by exclusion of toxic molecules and downregulation of inflammation by carefully regulated immunosuppressive molecules and T lymphocytes. Thus, enhanced host susceptibility to luminal bacterial components could be due to defects in these defenses or an overly aggressive immune response to common stimuli. Moreover, defective barrier function or immunosuppression are likely genetically determined traits, reflected in increased familial incidence of IBD, higher concordance rate of Crohn's disease in monozygotic than dizygotic twins, familial patterns of disease, and differential susceptibility of inbred rodents to experimental enterocolitis (149,150).

Mucosal permeability appears to be increased in active Crohn's disease, but whether this abnormality is an intrinsic or acquired defect and whether it is a genetically determined susceptibility factor is unclear. Most studies demonstrate a correlation between disease activity and mucosal permeability, suggesting an acquired defect (1,151). Pooled results of a number of studies suggest that a subset of family members of Crohn's disease patients (approximately 10%) have a permeability defect (151). The observation that a subset of IBD family members responds inappropriately to challenge with nonsteroidal antiinflammatory drugs by exacerbating subtle permeability abnormalities (152) is potentially important for understanding genetic susceptibility to chronic inflammation. Podolsky's demonstration of specific alterations in colonic mucin glycoprotein profiles in ulcerative colitis patients, irrespective of disease activity (1), provides one explanation of defective barrier function. However, Pullan and colleagues (153) found that mucous gel thickness in the mildly inflamed ulcerative colitis patient is normal, but that the layer is denuded in moderately and severely active ulcerative colitis. Surprisingly, the mucous gel layer was intact in active Crohn's disease. The importance of an intact mucous gel layer to barrier function and exclusion of luminal bacterial products is illustrated by a 50-fold increased uptake of FMLP following dithiothreitol treatment, which removes surface mucus (154).

Host genetic susceptibility to luminal bacteria and bacterial components is demonstrated by differential progression of experimental inflammation in inbred rodent strains. Lewis rats, injected intramurally (subserosally) with PG-PS polymers, develop spontaneously relapsing granulomatous enterocolitis with fibrosis and extraintestinal inflammation. In contrast, Buffalo and Fischer F344 rats, the latter major histocompatibility complex matched with Lewis, exhibit self-limited intestinal inflammation, with no evidence of systemic manifestations (67). McCall and colleagues (67) reported a decreased ratio of IL-1 receptor antagonist (IL-1ra) relative to IL-1 in Lewis rats, suggesting that high-responding rats had a relative defect in immunosuppression. Likewise, Lewis rats injected subcutaneously with indomethacin develop chronic mid–small bowel ulcerations with granulomas, periportal hepatic inflammation, anemia, and fibrosis that persists for at least 77 days. Low-responding Fischer rats develop similar degrees of acute entercolitis, but inflammation resolves by 2 weeks, and there is no evidence of extraintestinal inflammation (155). In response to apparently identical luminal concentrations of anaerobic bacteria in the self-filling blind loop model, Lewis rats develop hepatobiliary inflammation within 2–4 weeks of jejunal bacterial overgrowth, Wistar rats display similar lesions after 8–12 weeks, but Fischer and Buffalo rats fail to develop any evidence of injury (126). Finally, C3H/HeJ mice infected with *Citrobacter freundii* develop chronic colitis whereas DBA/2J mice similarly inoculated exhibit only transient inflammation (156). These examples of dramatically different incidence, chronicity, and complications of experimental intestinal inflammation following identical exposure to bacteria and bacterial products in inbred rodent strains suggest the probability that humans with different genetic susceptibilities will respond differentially to noxious environmental stimuli. Indeed, recent data suggest that IBD patients display defective regulation of IL-1ra relative to IL-1 (157,158) as a possible mechanism of enhanced susceptibility to chronic inflammation.

CHRONIC ENTERIC INFECTIONS MIMICKING IBD

Ulcerative colitis and Crohn's disease strongly resemble several enteric infections (Table 4). Intestinal infections not only mimic the classic clinical features of ideopathic IBD, including diarrhea (with or without blood), abdominal pain, and weight loss (160,161), but can also present with identical extraintestinal manifestations and local complications. For example, a number of infectious agents can lead to toxic megacolon, perforation, abscesses, stricture, and fistula formation (161–165) as well as reactive arthritis, spondyloarthropathy, hepatobiliary inflammation, erythema nodosum, uveitis, and anemia of chronic disease (62).

TABLE 4. *Enteric pathogens that cause inflammation resembling IBD*

Resemble ulcerative colitis	Resemble Crohn's disease
Campylobacter jejuni	*Mycobacterium tuberculosis*
Salmonella sp.	*Yersinia enterocolitica*
Shigella sp.	Cytomegalovirus
Clostridium difficile	*Entamoeba histolytica*
Escherichia coli	*Chlamydia trachomatis*
O157:H7	*Histoplasma capsulatum*
Aeromonas sp.	*Actinomyces* sp.
Plesiomonas sp.	*Cryptococcus neoformans*
Vibrio noncholera sp.	*Mycobacterium avium*
Neisseria gonorrheal	complex
Legionella sp.	
Treponema pallidum	
Herpes simplex virus	
type II	
Blastocystis hominis	

Infectious Agents That Cause Intestinal Disease Resembling IBD

In developed countries, *Campylobacter jejuni, Salmonella* sp., *Aeromonas*, pathogenic *E. coli*, and *C. difficile* are the most common causes of acute enterocolitis (166–168). However, less common agents also must be considered because of their ability to induce chronic inflammation and because of exposure to more exotic organisms with today's more mobile society and international culinary practices. At least 40% of cases of probable infectious enterocolitis have no recoverable agent, either because of insensitive diagnostic methods or because many enteric pathogens remain to be discovered (169).

Campylobacter

In several clinical studies, *Campylobacter* is the most frequently isolated sporadic enteric infection, accounting for up to 31% of all pathogens recovered from patients with infectious diarrhea (166,167,170). Typically patients present with acute fever, malaise, and headache, followed by abdominal pain and diarrhea that resolves in 3–5 days, with the peak incidence occurring in the summer months (171). However, a more chronic presentation of invasive colitis manifested by bloody diarrhea and abdominal pain in a subset of patients may be confused with acute ulcerative colitis and Crohn's disease (170,172,173). Toxic megacolon (174), erythema nodosum (175), and relapses with abscess (176) may complicate the infection. Rarely, *C. jejuni* can cause acute ileocolitis, mimicking appendicitis (177). *Campylobacter* colitis is characterized by abdominal pain more severe than anticipated from the sigmoidoscopic findings (173). Endoscopic features of acute disease include mucosal edema, hyperemia, and shallow grey-based aphthous ulcers. In more chronic *Campylobacter* colitis (>1 week duration), the mucosa is granular and friable without ulceration, closely mimicking ulcera-

tive colitis. Histological changes also vary with the duration of infection (178). Acutely, predominant features include superficial ulceration, cryptitis, and mucus depletion; the lamina propria is edematous with neutrophilic and histiocytic infiltration. In latter stages, resolution is accompanied by regenerating epithelium, mononuclear cell infiltration, edema of the upper lamina propria, lymphoid hyperplasia, and no distortion of the crypt architecture.

Salmonella

Although *Salmonella typhimurium* or *enteriditis* is one of the most frequently isolated pathogens from patients with acute diarrhea, the vast majority of patients have transient gastroenteritis that resolves with a week. However, a minority of patients develop colitis with an average duration of 3 weeks, although symptoms may persist for 3 months. Patients with colitis exhibit bloody diarrhea with fecal leukocytes. Complications include sepsis, toxic megacolon, and perforation (163,179). Sigmoidoscopic features include nonspecific granularity, friability, and occasional ulceration; histology shows hemorrhage, mucosal ulceration, and crypt abscesses. Radiographic findings of granularity, fine ulceration, and loss of haustration are indistinguishable from ulcerative colitis, with the exception that rectal abnormalities may be absent (180). Segmental colitis with focal ulcers resembling Crohn's disease may rarely occur (181).

Shigella

In the United States, *Shigella sonnei* and *S. flexneri* account for 90% of reported cases of colitis. *S. sonnei* is more common in patients below the age of 15 years, whereas *S. flexneri* is more common in adolescents and adults. Mucosal invasion and enterotoxin production lead to colitis, which preferentially involves the distal colon, although the entire colon and terminal ileum may be inflamed (182). The most common clinical presentation is dysentery with bloody stools, mucus, and fever (183). Clinical symptoms usually persist for 5–7 days but may fluctuate over 2–3 weeks and rarely have a fulminant course leading to toxic megacolon and sepsis (165). *S. dysenteriae* type 1 has been reported to cause more virulent disease, possibly necessitating emergent colectomy (184). Histological features are nonspecific acute mucosal inflammation (see below).

E. coli

Enteroinvasive *E. coli,* enterohemorrhagic strains, and *E. coli* O157:H7 can produce acute colitis with bloody stools. *E. coli* O157:H7 is now recognized as a frequent cause of acute diarrhea (166,185). A broad spectrum of clinical presentations is described for *E. coli* O157:H7, ranging from nonbloody diarrhea to fulminant colitis complicated by the hemolytic-uremic syndrome and thrombotic thrombocytopenic purpura (186). Sporadic cases and outbreaks caused by the ingestion of unpasteurized milk and undercooked hamburger meat have been described (187). Bloody diarrhea is the most common symptom and severe abdominal cramps, fever, and fecal leukocytes are seen in about half of cases. A segmental distribution within the colon may suggest Crohn's disease, but rapid onset of symptoms more often resemble ischemic colitis or *C. difficile* toxin–induced colitis (188). Rarely, the distal ileum can be involved (189). Histological findings include focal necrosis with hemorrhage and acute inflammation in the superficial mucosa that resemble *C. difficile* toxin–mediated colitis (186,188). Of note, antibiotic therapy has not been shown to be beneficial.

Clostridium difficile

C. difficile is a frequent nosocomially acquired pathogen in patients treated with broad-spectrum antibiotics (188). The clinical spectrum of disease ranges from asymptomatic carriers to pseudomembranous colitis. Patients complain of diarrhea, tenesmus, lower abdominal cramps, nausea, and occasionally fever that begins 1–3 weeks after antibiotic exposure. Rectal bleeding is unusual, but occult blood and leukocytes in stool are common. Fulminant disease may result in toxic megacolon and perforation (190). Endoscopic examination reveals 2- to 5-mm diameter yellow–white, raised plaques that may become confluent. The diagnosis of *C. difficile*–associated colitis is more challenging when the rectum is spared (up to 30% of cases) and in early onset disease prior to the appearance of pseudomembranes (191). In longstanding, advanced cases, the correct diagnosis can usually be accomplished by toxin assays of stool and a flexible sigmoidoscopy in the setting of prior antibiotic exposure.

Aeromonas

Aeromonas hydrophilia and *A. sobria,* usually acquired from drinking untreated water, produce colitis in approximately 25% of infected patients. Symptoms usually resolve in a week, but 37% of children have symptoms for more than 2 weeks (192), and diarrhea persists for an average of 42 days in adults. Several cases have been described that have apparently progressed to typical ulcerative colitis (57,58).

Tuberculosis

Primary intestinal tuberculosis is extremely rare in developed countries, but ileocecal infections associated with active pulmonary tuberculosis may be anticipated to increase with the documented rise in pulmonary disease in recent years (194). Intestinal infections have been documented in up to 28% of patients with smear-positive, cavitating pulmonary tuberculosis (195). Conversely, two thirds of patients with ileocecal TB have evidence of pulmonary tuberculous lesions (196). Symptoms include ab-

dominal pain (90%), weight loss (74%), anorexia (60%), fever and diarrhea (56%) (197). An abdominal mass, usually tender and in the right lower quadrant, is present in over half of cases and ascites is detectable in 10%. Seventy-five percent of patients have ileocecal involvement (197); approximately 25% of patients have segmental colonic disease without cecal involvement. Isolated ileal disease is quite rare, but isolated duodenal involvement has been reported (198).

Pathological findings include transmural inflammation with large granulomas, frequent epithelioid cells, sharply defined mucosal ulcers with irregular margins, nodular mucosa, and serosal tubercles. Granulomas may be caseating, especially in mesenteric lymph nodes. Complications include stricture formation, fistulae, perforation, and bleeding (194).

Definitive diagnosis is difficult with noninvasive tests. A high index of suspicion can be based on the presence of pulmonary lesions, a positive skin test, or emigration from endemic areas. Ileocecal TB can closely mimic Crohn's disease on barium contrast studies and colonoscopy (Fig. 1). Features suggesting tuberculosis rather than Crohn's colitis include the absence of rectal and perianal involvement, transverse or circumferential ulcers rather than longitudinal ulcers, and a patulous ileocecal valve

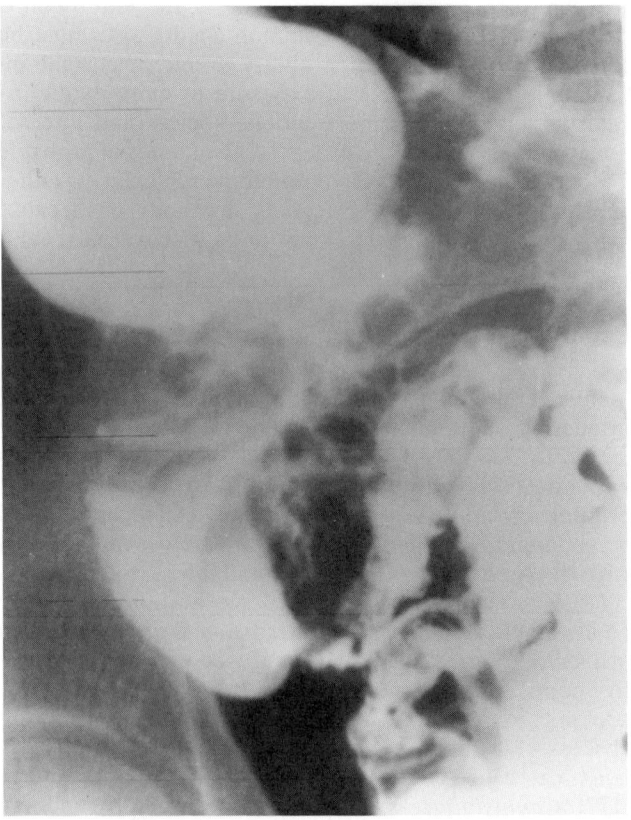

FIG. 1. Cecal tuberculosis. A barium enema shows concentric, focal narrowing and ulceration of the cecum, near the ileocecal valve. The terminal ileum is not well visualized, but proximal ileal loops are normal. Patient's chest x-ray showed bilateral apical infiltration with probable cavitation, consistent with TB.

(197). Small aphthous ulcers with normal surrounding mucosa, long strictures, and extraintestinal inflammation are more common in Crohn's disease. On biopsy, confluent or caseating granulomas suggest intestinal tuberculosis. Caseous necrosis of massively enlarged mesenteric lymph nodes may be detected by computed tomography (CT) scan (199). Serodiagnosis using enzyme-linked immunosorbent assay (ELISA) has been reported to have a diagnostic accuracy of 84% (200). Definitive diagnosis is made by identification of the organism on mucosal biopsies or resected tissue using acid-fast stains, immunohistochemistry, or culture. When suspicion is high, a therapeutic trial of triple antimycobacterial drugs is warranted while waiting for culture results. However, acid-fast stains of mucosal biopsies are positive in an extremely low percentage of cases. Clinical improvement should occur within 3–4 weeks of initiation of appropriate therapy.

Yersinia

Yersinia enterocolitica and *Y. pseudotuberculosis* generally affect persons less than 25 years of age, have a peak incidence during winter months, and are more common in Scandinavia that in the United States. Children <5 years of age usually develop acute gastroenteritis, whereas older persons more commonly have acute ileitis and mesenteric adenitis (201,202). Diarrhea and right lower quadrant abdominal pain are the most frequent symptoms; erythema nodosum, uveitis, and reactive arthritis may occur in HLA-B27 positive patients. Weight loss and vomiting are relatively rare whereas tenesmus, fever, fecal leukocytes, occult bleeding, and peripheral blood leukocytosis are frequently present.

Most patients have a self-limited course that resolves within 2 weeks, but 14% of patients in a long-term study were readmitted for abdominal pain or diarrhea (201). Rarely, patients have been reported to develop typical Crohn's disease after *Yersinia* infection (59). *Yersinia* bacteremia with focal abscesses is more common in patients with cirrhosis, hemolytic anemia, and diabetes.

Radiography and endoscopy of the ileum shows edema, ulceration, and lymphoid hyperplasia (Fig. 2). Aphthous ulcers may occur in the colon, but the rectum is usually spared (203,204). Fistulae, abscesses, stenosis, and skip lesions are uncommon. Because of the right lower quadrant pain, patients with *Yersinia* infections frequently undergo surgery, where acute ileitis and enlarged lymph nodes are found. Granulomas may be present in ileal biopsies and resected lymph nodes.

Amebiasis

Infection with *Entamoeba histolytica* is relatively unusual in developed countries. However, it should be considered in the differential diagnosis of IBD because of the risk of precipitating fulminant disease with corticosteroid therapy and complications such as hepatic abscess. High-risk groups include recent immigrants from endemic areas, male homosexuals, patients with AIDS, and institu-

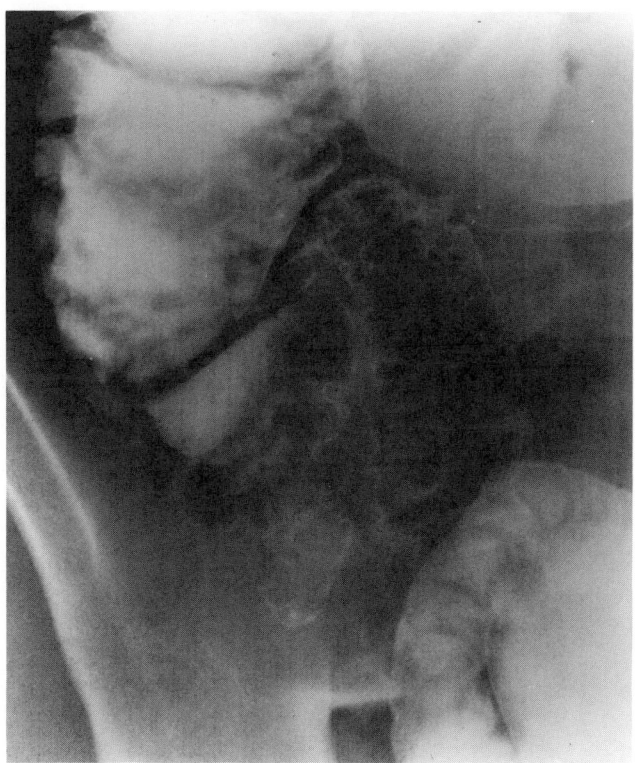

FIG. 2. *Yersinia* ileitis. A small bowel follow-through demonstrates nodularity of the distal ileum with no stenosis and minimal bowel wall thickening; stool grew *Yersinia enterocolitica.*

tionalized populations, especially the mentally retarded (205). Patients with invasive colonic infections present with bloody, mucoid diarrhea and abdominal pain. Fever, nausea, and vomiting are manifestations of fulminant disease (206). Radiographic and endoscopic features include flask-shaped ulcers that extend into the submucosa, lack of haustration, aphthoid ulcers, and marginal serration (207,208). Diagnosis is established by identification of trophozoites in stool samples, adherant mucus, or mucosal biopsies (207). Serology is a valuable adjunct to diagnosis of invasive amebiasis since detection of trophozoites in stool is relatively insensitive (209).

CMV

Cytomegalovirus (CMV) colitis is rare in immunocompetent hosts but is an important cause of mucosal ulceration in immunosuppressed patients. In nonimmunocompromised patients, the most common presentation is gastrointestinal bleeding secondary to ulceration in the colon and duodenum (210). Anal intercourse is a risk factor with an apparent incubation period of 1–2 weeks. In Cheung's (210) series, 10% presented with obstructive jaundice due to granulation tissue at the ampulla of Vater. CMV inclusion bodies were present in epithelial cells in areas of minimal inflammation and within endothelial cells in ulcerated areas (Fig. 3A), suggesting that ulceration is

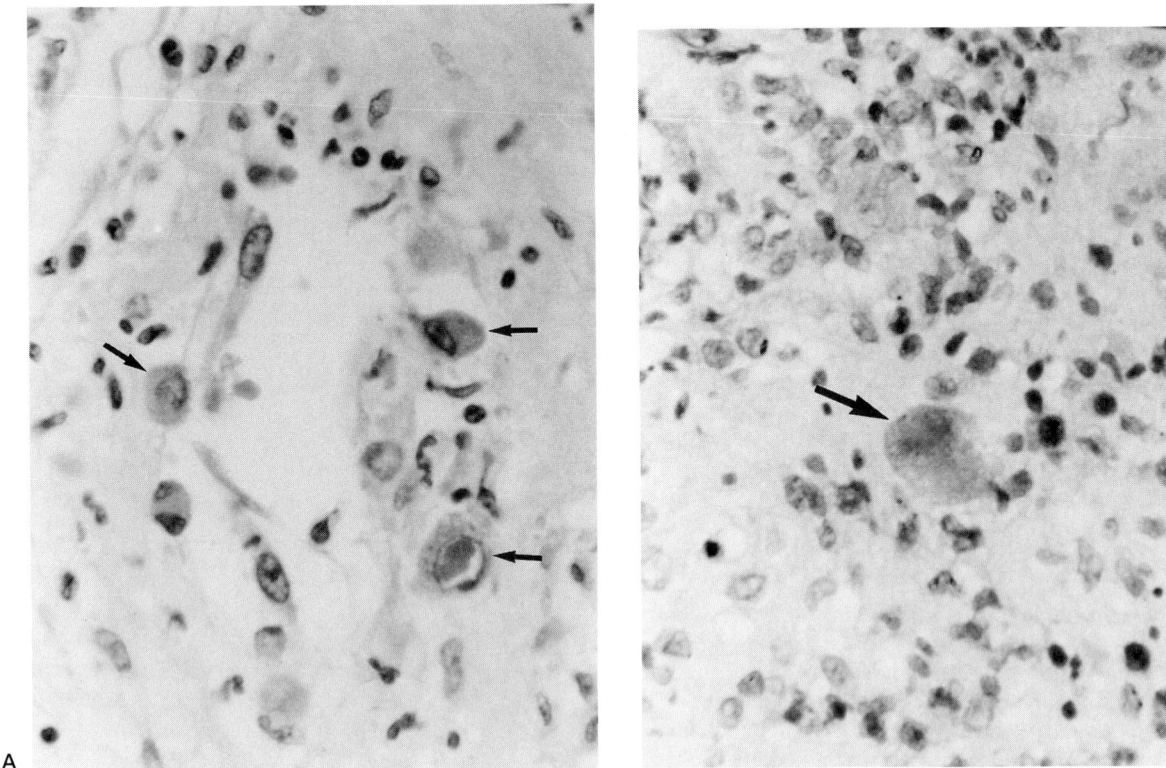

FIG. 3. A: CMV vasculitis. Viral inclusions are seen within the cytoplasm and nucleus of endothelial cells in the ulcerated intestine of an AIDS patient (*arrows*). **B:** CMV colitis. Cytoplasmic and intranuclear inclusions (*arrow*) in a mononuclear cell infiltrating the lamina propria of the colon. The overlying mucosa was ulcerated.

a result of ischemia caused by virally induced vasculitis (210). In immunocompromised patients, intestinal CMV infection can take a more fulminant, widespread course. CMV ileitis resembling Crohn's disease has been described as the sole opportunistic infection in an AIDS patient (211). Perforating ileocolitis, hemorrhagic proctocolitis, and toxic megacolon are causes of emergent surgery in immunocompromised patients with CMV intestinal inflammation (164,212).

Chlamydia

Chlamydia trachomatis, especially lymphogranuloma venereum (LGV) immunotypes, can cause chronic, granulomatous proctitis in homosexual men (213). Rectal disease can be complicated by strictures, fistulae, and abscesses (214). Non-LGV strains produce mild proctitis that mimics ulcerative colitis (213).

Clinical and Laboratory Criteria Distinguishing IBD from Infectious Enterocolitis

Crohn's disease and, to a lesser extent, ulcerative colitis typically have an indolent onset, with an average symptom duration of 3.2 years before correct diagnosis (215).

However, some IBD patients have an abrupt onset of symptoms similar to those of infectious enterocolitis, and some enteric infections have protracted courses. In all cases, infectious disorders must be excluded before the diagnosis of idiopathic ulcerative colitis or Crohn's disease can be established.

A careful history, physical examination, and routine laboratory screen can provide information to distinguish IBD from an infection (Table 5). An abrupt onset of symptoms in a previously healthy individual, particularly when associated with fever as one of the initial manifestations, favors an infectious origin. Between 15% and 25% of patients with IBD have a family history of these disorders (149), and up to 40% of patients with Crohn's disease will

TABLE 5. *Clinical criteria distinguishing IBD from infectious diarrhea*

Favoring IBD	Favoring infection
Chronic course (>4 weeks)	Acute course (<2 weeks)
Spontaneous relapses	No prior symptoms
Family history	Exposure history
Perianal complications	Antibiotics use
Growth retardation	Immunosuppression
Anemia	
Albumin <3.5 mg/dL	
Platelets >450,000/mL	

have associated perianal disease, particularly when there is colonic involvement (216). Exposure to untreated water, raw milk, undercooked ground beef, shellfish, other infected patients, travel, or oral or anal sex raises the possibility of an infectious etiology, as does suppression of the immune system by corticosteroids, immunosuppressive drugs, HIV infection, cirrhosis, and diabetes. Abdominal cramps, fever, rectal bleeding, fecal leukocytes, and occult blood are nonspecific findings. A right lower quadrant mass strongly suggests Crohn's disease, although ileocecal tuberculosis and periappendiceal abscess must be considered. A chronic, subclinical course is suggested by growth retardation in adolescents, unexplained weight loss, anemia, and hypoalbuminemia. In a retrospective study, approximately 60% of IBD patients had white blood cell counts >10,000/mL, hemoglobin <12 g/dL (females) or 14 g/dL (males), and serum albumin <3.5 g/dL, in contrast to 14% to 25% of patients with infectious diarrhea. Of note, the best discriminator between the patients was a platelet count of greater than 450,000/mL, which occurred in 59% of IBD patients but only 1.6% of patients with infections (168).

As mentioned above, endoscopic features of infectious colitis overlap considerably with those of idiopathic IBD. Patchy petechial hemorrhage, focal edema, and erythema in the rectosigmoid area are atypical findings for IBD and should alert the endoscopist to the possibility of an infectious etiology (217). Rectal sparing, discontinuous disease, and focal ulcers are not found in ulcerative colitis; and circumferential ulcers are more typical of intestinal tuberculosis than Crohn's disease (197).

Histological and immunohistological examination of rectal biopsies can be extremely helpful in distinguishing idiopathic IBD from infectious enterocolitis (Table 6). Surawicz and Belic (218) described seven histological features that have a predictive probability of 87% to 100% for ulcerative colitis and Crohn's disease. These include distorted crypt architecture, which was the most useful criterion and could appear within a month of onset of IBD symptoms, crypt atrophy, villous surface, mixed inflammatory cell populations in the lamina propria, granulomas, and basally located giant cells or lymphoid aggregates. Since this study examined self-limited infectious diseases of less than 1 month's duration, the discriminative value of these findings may be less for chronic infections. Granulomas are nonspecific and may be occur in

intestinal inflammation caused by *Mycobacterium, Chlamydia, Yersinia,* and syphilis, as well as in Crohn's disease Acid-fast and silver stains are helpful for identifying mycobacterial and fungal infections. Immunohistochemical staining and *in situ* hybridization are being used with increased frequency to sensitively detect a number of organisms. Van Spreeuwel et al. (167) demonstrated that IBD patients have a specific increase in IgG secreting plasma cells in the lamina propria.

Stool culture for bacteria, examination for enteric parasites, and immunoassay for *C. difficile* toxin are the most commonly used tests for identifying infectious etiologies of intestinal inflammation. Even in the best laboratories, stool cultures yield a diagnosis in only approximately 60% of cases of presumed infectious diarrhea cases. Serological tests for *E. histolytica, Yersinia,* and *Chlamydia* improve the chances of diagnosing agents with particularly poor recovery rates. Improved immunohistochemistry, molecular techniques, and discovery of new pathogens should improve this identification rate.

Management of Acute Colitis

Evaluation of patients with new onset diarrhea must be tailored to the aggressiveness of their symptoms. Healthy patients with recent onset of diarrhea without fever, abdominal tenderness, fecal leukocytes, rectal bleeding, or leukocytosis should be conservatively evaluated and treated symptomatically. Diarrhea that does not resolve within 7–10 days or that is associated with rectal bleeding, fever, fecal red blood cells or leukocytes, abdominal tenderness, or leukocytosis should be more aggressively evaluated with flexible sigmoidoscopy, stool culture, and an ova and parasite examination. A *C. difficile* toxin assay should be performed if patients have been exposed to antibiotics or recently hospitalized. Immunocompetent patients with symptoms greater than 4 weeks, anemia, thrombocytosis, hypoalbuminemia, and immunosuppressed patients with symptoms of shorter duration should be thoroughly evaluated by stool culture and microscopy, colonoscopy with biopsies, and small bowel follow-through x-ray. Patients with appropriate exposure histories and compatible clinical symptoms should be further evaluated with a TB skin test, chest x-ray, special stains of biopsies, and appropriate serologies. Prior to beginning corticosteroid therapy, all patients should have a skin test for TB and a serological assay for *E. histolytica*.

Once a diagnosis of infectious enterocolitis is established, specific therapy is indicated unless the symptoms are spontaneously resolving. Exceptions to this advice are *Salmonella* gastroenteritis, where antibiotic treatment of the uncomplicated infection may actually prolong the carrier state (219), and *E. coli* O157-H7, where antibiotics may not shorten the clinical course of enterocolitis and may increase the risk of the hemolytic-uremic syndrome (220,221). The decision to begin empirical therapy for IBD with immunosuppressive therapy must be weighed against the risk of potentiating CMV, tuberculosis, and amebiasis (222). When emergent coricosteroid therapy is essential, empirical coverage for TB or amebiasis should

TABLE 6. *Histologic features of IBD vs. infectious colitis*

IBD	Specific infectious diseases
Distorted crypt architecture	Pseudomembranes (*C. difficile, E. coli* O157:H7)
Basally located lymphoid aggregates	Viral inclusions (CMV, herpes simplex II)
	Caseating necrosis (*M. tuberculosis*)
Villous pattern of mucosa	Diagnostic organisms (*E. histolytica, Cryptosporidium*)
	Specific staining (*Mycobacterium, Histoplasma*)

be considered if there is a reasonable risk of infection. Sulfasalazine and other 5-aminosalicylic acid (5-ASA) compounds pose no risk of exacerbating infectious diseases, and metronidazole is effective for primary therapy of Crohn's colitis and certain infections, including amebiasis.

INFECTIONS EXACERBATING IBD

Abundant evidence inidicates that enteric infections are associated with relapses of established ulcerative colitis and Crohn's disease (Table 7) (5,223,224). Whether these infections have a primary or secondary role in the inflammation associated with relapse remains unresolved.

Epidemiology

Between 40% and 60% of relapses of IBD are associated with symptomatic respiratory infections (226,236). In a prospective study of children with IBD, Kangro et al. (226) showed an association between exacerbation of IBD and serologically diagnosed viral or mycoplasmic respiratory infections. This and other studies noted seasonal variations in exacerbations of IBD (236,237).

Between 4% and 32% of patients with acute relapse of IBD are infected with enteric bacterial or protozoal pathogens (224,230,232). C. difficile is the most common pathogen, followed by Salmonella, Shigella, Campylobacter, and Yersinia. Weber et al. (232) detected common enteric pathogens in 18% of patients with exacerbations of Crohn's disease and 13% of those with recurrent ulcerative colitis relapses. Gebhard et al. (225) demonstrated rotovirus or Norwalk agent in 8% of patients with relapses of either ulcerative colitis or Crohn's disease.

Microbiology

As listed in Table 7, a large number of pathogens have been associated with clinical relapses of IBD or recovered from tissues of patients with active disease. C. difficile has been the most thoroughly studied agent, but the relationship of this organism to relapses of IBD remains controversial. C. difficile or its cytotoxin is present in up to 32% of all patients with active IBD (228,238,239), and in 4% to 25% of patients with acutely relapsing disease (232,240). Trnka and LaMont (228) reported that 19% of IBD patients had detectable C. difficile toxin, including 60% of patients with severe flares. The suggestion that C. difficile infection is associated with severe exacerbations of IBD was confirmed by several groups, who found a particularly high rate of infection (20% to 50%) in hospitalized patients and those patients with fulminant or refractory colitis (28,141,242). However, in outpatients, C. difficile recovery did not correlate with disease activity (224,238,239,243). These studies suggest that the majority of IBD patients undergoing relapses do not have associated C. difficile infections and that it is not cost-effective to assay for C. difficile toxin in the outpatient experiencing a routine flare-up. However, the risk of C. difficile toxin–associated disease is substantially increased in hospitalized IBD patients, especially those with fulminant disease. Clinical responses to specific therapy for C. difficile illustrate the importance of establishing the correct diagnosis in flare-ups mediated by C. difficile toxin (228,241). The association between C. difficile infection and prior antibiotic use in IBD patients is controversial. Meyers et al. (239) found that all IBD patients with C. difficile infections had taken antibiotics within the previous 6 months, whereas fewer than 30% of infected patients had received antibiotics in studies by Trnka and LaMont (228) and McLauren (240).

In industrialized countries, 0% to 1.6% of patients with relapsing IBD prospectively evaluated were infected with Salmonella, Shigella, Campylobacter, or Yersinia (232). Even in developing countries, the detection rate of these organisms was only 4% (230). In retrospective studies of relapses of ulcerative colitis, the recovery of Salmonella was only 4.6% (245). These studies suggest that routine culture for "enteric pathogens" is not indicated in uncomplicated flare-ups of IBD.

CMV is a potential cause of exacerbation of IBD (223). Fifty to eighty percent of adults show serological evidence of infection, but gastrointestinal inflammation, which may be severe, is observed primarily in immunocompromised patients (211,222). Histological review of colonic resections in 46 patients with ulcerative colitis by Cooper et al. (246) revealed cytoplasmic and intranuclear inclusions characteristic of CMV in six patients (Fig. 3), all of whom were males with fulminant clinical courses. Five of these

TABLE 7. *Pathogens associated with IBD relapse*

Viral	Bacterial	Parasitic
Cytomegalovirus (55)	Clostridium difficile (228)	E. histolytica (230)
Rotavirus (225)	Salmonella sp. (229)	Giardia lamblia (234)
Norwalk agent (225)	Shigella sp. (230)	Blastocystis hominis (235)
Respiratory syncytial virus (226)	Campylobacter jejuni (176)	
Influenza A and B (226)	Yersinia sp. (231)	
Parainfluenza (226)	Enteropathogenic E. coli (232)	
Rubella (226)	Aeromonas sp. (233)	
Epstein–Barr virus (226)		
Herpes simplex virus (227)		
Adenovirus (226)		

six patients had toxic megacolon, and three had received corticosteroids before colonic dilatation occurred. A review of 16 published cases of CMV suprainfection of IBD (14 ulcerative colitis) described a severe clinical course with colectomy in 63% and a mortality rate of 43% (247). Bartlett et al. (224) described three patients (two with ulcerative colitis) who had exacerbation of their preexisting IBD while on steroid therapy. All had systemic symptoms of malaise, myalgias, fever, mild hepatitis, and atypical lymphocytes. Diagnosis was made by viral inclusion bodies (Fig. 3) and serology. Symptoms gradually improved when steroids were rapidly tapered. The frequent exposure of IBD patients to CMV is further documented by increased CMV antibody titers in ulcerative colitis patients compared with controls (248), and detection of CMV DNA in 81% of mucosal tissue from ulcerative colitis patients and 66% of Crohn's disease patients but only 29% of controls (249). The simultaneous presence of herpesvirus type 2 and CMV or EBV in 76% of ulcerative colitis patients but 29% of controls prompted the authors to postulate that synergistic viral infections play an important role in the activity of ulcerative colitis (249).

Pathogenesis

Improvement after metronidazole or vancomycin therapy (228,241,244) or steroid withdrawal (224,247) supports a causative role for C. difficile or CMV infection in relapses of IBD. In some patients, however, active inflammation persists after clearance of the infecting agent, raising the possibility that idiopathic, self-sustaining inflammation has been reactivated. Whether viral or bacterial suprainfection is a consequence of diminished resistance by an ulcerated mucosa, relative immunosuppression due to drug therapy or malnutrition, decreased colonization resistance caused by antibiotic therapy, or increased exposure to nosocomial infections is unclear.

Exacerbation of underlying IBD by upper respiratory infections (226) is more difficult to explain. It is possible that circulating cytokines liberated by inflammatory cells in the respiratory tract or viremia could preferentially activate intestinal lamina propria immune cells, which are in an enhanced state of responsiveness (primed state).

Clinical Features

Clinical or endoscopic features do not reliably indicate whether exacerbation of symptoms is due to microbial suprainfection or spontaneous reactivation of IBD. Of note, pseudomembranes are almost never found when C. difficile toxin is detected in active IBD. No studies have been performed to determine whether the histological features that distinguish IBD from self-limited colitis (218) are applicable to infectious exacerbations of IBD. CMV infections preferentially occur in patients receiving corticosteroids (224,246,247), and both CMV and C. difficile infections are associated with ulcerative colitis cases that pursue a fulminant course. A search for these infections must be aggressively undertaken in these clinical settings.

The presence of systemic symptoms, mildly elevated transaminases, and atypical circulating lymphocytes suggests CMV infection.

Diagnosis

The same strategies used to diagnose primary intestinal infections are used to detect microbial suprainfections causing clinical relapses of IBD. Outpatients with well-established IBD who display their typical pattern of recurrence should not be extensively evaluated for microbial pathogens unless they fail to respond appropriately to therapy directed toward active IBD. Outpatients who present with atypical flare-ups (e.g., nonbloody diarrhea in a patient with ulcerative colitis or bloody diarrhea in a patient with Crohn's ileitis) or with increased risk of infections, i.e., recent travel, antibiotic use, exposure to untreated water or hospitalization, merit appropriate evaluation. Patients with symptoms requiring hospitalization or patients unresponsive to conventional antiinflammatory therapy should also be evaluated. Fulminant intestinal inflammation dictates aggressive evaluation, with particular attention to C. difficile and CMV. The absence of pseudomembranes does not rule out C. difficile toxin–induced colitis, since this finding is extremely rare in IBD patients, even with severe exacerbations of inflammation (228).

Management

If a bacterial or parasitic pathogen is identified in a patient with an exacerbation of IBD, specific antibiotic therapy should be initiated. However, it should be noted that eradication of Salmonella may have no impact on the course of disease (245) and the majority of patients infected with B. hominis do not respond to metronidazole (235). The response of IBD patients with active colitis and C. difficile to vancomycin or metronidazole therapy is usually favorable, although some patients improve slowly (228,241,242,244). Metronidazole is effective in ulcerative colitis patients with toxic megacolon complicated by C. difficile infection (242). Most authorities advocate concurrent therapy of active IBD with 5-amino-salicylic acid (5-ASA) compounds while the evaluation for an enteric pathogen is in progress. Steroids should be used cautiously in patients with suspected microbial suprainfections but are frequently necessary for patients with fulminant inflammation. In such patients, empirical therapy for C. difficile may be warranted if this pathogen is suspected, since short-term therapy with metronidazole or vancomycin is relatively nontoxic and may be used as adjunctive therapy of IBD (48).

Management of patients with active IBD and CMV infections is not yet established. CMV is detected most frequently in IBD patients who are treated with steroids; such patients have a considerable mortality rate (247). In case reports, inflammation usually improves with rapid steroid tapering (224,247). Withdrawal of immunosuppressive therapy, which has not been prospectively evaluated, is potentially hazardous in the patient with fulminant colitis but merits consideration when a patient with CMV infection does not respond to appropriate management for the underlying IBD. Antiviral chemotherapy with gancyclovir or foscarnet has not been adequately evaluated in this setting. Timely tapering of antibiotics and immunosuppressive drugs should be a goal of all clinicians treating patients with IBD.

INFECTIOUS COMPLICATIONS OF IBD

Extraluminal spread of ubiquitous enteric bacteria accounts for some of the most frequent complications of IBD (250). These infectious complications are particularly prevalent in patients with Crohn's disease, in whom deep fissures, ulcers, increased luminal pressures due to stenoses, and chronic immunosuppressive therapy enhance translocation of luminal bacteria. The most common infectious complications (Table 8) are discussed below.

Intraabdominal Abscesses

Incidence

Abdominal abscess is one of the most common and dangerous complications of Crohn's disease but is extremely unusual in ulcerative colitis, where free perforations usually lead to peritonitis. Intraperitoneal abscesses complicate Crohn's disease in 10% to 20% of patients and retroperitoneal abscesses in 3% to 4% (251–255). Sex ratios appear to be equal in intraperitoneal abscesses, but males predominate by ninefold in retroperitoneal abscesses (252). A younger age of onset of IBD is characteristic of patients with abscesses (23 years) compared with those without abscesses (27 years). The distal ileum and sigmoid colon are the origin of most abscesses (216,251).

Pathogenesis and Microbiology

Abscesses can be spontaneous or postoperative. Spontaneous abscesses and abscesses presenting more than 6 months after surgery are probably a consequence of localized perforation of a mucosal ulcer (Fig. 4). Because of chronic transmural inflammation, the adjacent mesentery is thickened and local adhesions form, preventing

TABLE 8. Infectious complications of IBD

Abscess: intraabdominal, perianal, retroperitoneal abdominal wall, hepatic
Fistula: enteroenteric, enterovesical, enterocutaneous, perianal
Postoperative infection: intrabdominal abscesses, wound infections
Hematogenous infection: species, endocarditis
Opportunistic infection secondary to immunosuppressive therapy
Bacterial overgrowth: small bowel, pouchitis

free perforation in the vast majority of cases. Transmural extension of the ulcer leads to a localized abscess, which may drain spontaneously into adjacent bowel, bladder, psoas muscle, abdominal wall, or any adjacent structure. *E. coli, B. fragilis,* enterococci, and *Streptococcus viridans* are the principle bacteria isolated from intraabdominal abscess (251) and *E. coli* and streptococci invade tissue adjacent to fistulae (256). These organisms are similar to those reported in intraabdominal abscesses in patients without IBD (257).

Several factors may contribute to the high incidence of extramural extension of ulcers in Crohn's disease, including increased intramural pressures from obstruction, genetically determined host susceptibility, immunosuppression from medication(s) or malnutrition, and secondary invasion of ulcers by luminal bacteria (256). Sinus tracts and perforations in the small intestine are associated with strictures (258,259). In the colon, the length of the stenosis is a higher risk factor for abscesses and fistulae than wall thickness (259). Greenstein and colleagues (260) postulated that Crohn's disease can follow two distinct clinical courses, an aggressive form prone to abscesses and fistulae and a more indolent form that slowly strictures. The presence of these clinical patterns in families suggests a possible genetic predisposition to abscess formation (261).

Perioperative abscesses complicate 1% to 17% of operations for Crohn's disease and are related to anastomotic breakdown (262). In a series of 429 surgical procedures for Crohn's disease, the risk for serious complications was strongly correlated with surgery for intraabdominal abscesses and preoperative steroid use (262). The high risk of postoperative abscess in patients presenting with intraabdominal abscesses was confirmed by others who have described a 12% to 14% incidence (251,252). Experimental studies show that extremely high doses of corticosteroids are necessary to interfere with anastomotic healing in normal hosts (263) and other clinical studies have not demonstrated enhanced postoperative complications in patients receiving steroid therapy (264,265), suggesting that preoperative steroid use may be a marker of chronic aggressive disease rather than an actual risk for anastomotic dehiscence.

Clinical Presentation

Abdominal pain is the most common presenting symptom, manifesting as new onset, continuous, localized pain or as a change in character of existing symptoms (252). Two thirds of patients with retroperitoneal abscess have pain referred to the genitofemoral, lumbar, or other retroperitoneal nerve. Gastrointestinal bleeding occurs in 15% to 20% of patients (252). The most frequent physical findings include intraabdominal mass (occurring in two thirds of patients and in the right lower quadrant in 80%) and fever, which may be spiking in nature. Eighty percent of patients with retroperitoneal abscesses have a positive psoas sign, fixed flexion of the hip, or limitation of hip extension, indicating irritation of the psoas muscle. Laboratory values may be nonspecific, with leukocytosis, mild

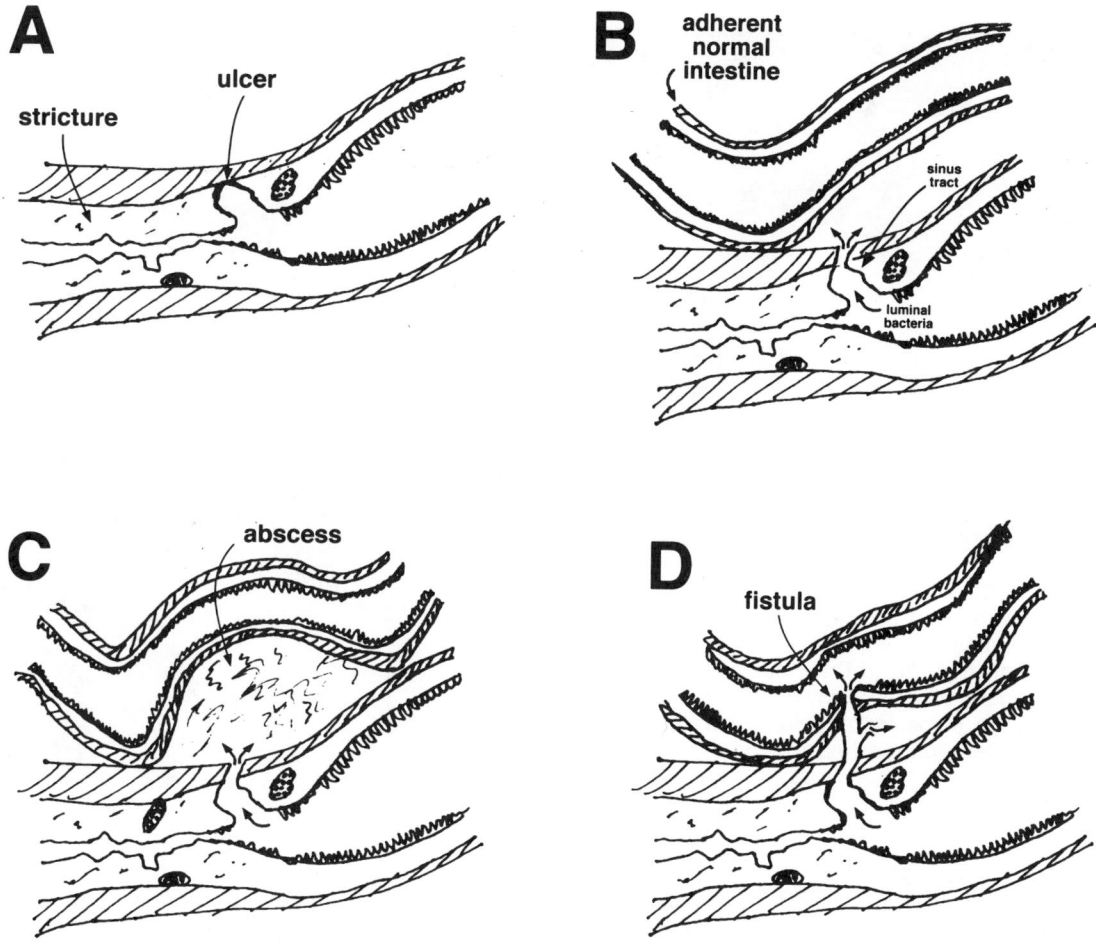

FIG. 4. Abscess and fistula formation in Crohn's disease. A fissure ulcer extending into the submucosa (**A**) and penetrating through the serosal surface leads to a sinus tract contained by an adherant loop of intestine (**B**). Extravasation of luminal bacteria into the contained space forms an intraabdominal abscess (**C**), which perforates into the adjacent normal bowel to form an enteroenteric fistula (**D**).

anemia, hypoalbuminemia, and elevated alkaline phosphatase. A normal white blood cell count does not rule out an abscess (252). Importantly, over half of grossly detectable abscesses at the time of surgery were clinically unsuspected (251).

Diagnosis

Distinguishing an intraabdominal abscess from active Crohn's disease with an associated mass of inflamed mesentery, enlarged lymph nodes, and adherent bowel can be difficult and is best accomplished by radiographic imaging studies. Plain films of the abdomen showing extraluminal air and ultrasound scans may be diagnostic but have a relatively low yield because of difficulty in distinguishing intra- and extraintestinal gas and fluid collections (266–268). Colonoscopy cannot visualize abscesses although opening of sinus tracts can be seen. Barium studies are relatively insensitive because the communication with the abscess may be intermittent; moreover, luminal barium has the disadvantage of delaying surgery and subse-

quent CT scans. Abdominal CT scan with luminal and intravenous contrast is a sensitive method of detecting abscesses and allows for the best anatomic correlation of abscesses with underlying intestinal inflammation (Fig. 5) (266–268). However, CT is relatively expensive and exposes the patient to relatively high levels of radiation. Indium-11 leukocyte scintigraphy has the advantage of being able to assess Crohn's disease activity and detect abscesses (268) but is relatively insensitive and lacks precise anatomic detail. Nuclear magnetic resonance imaging can precisely localize abscesses and assess disease activity when gadolinium chelates are injected (268), but has not been extensively evaluated in this setting and is the most expensive of all such modalities. Presently, CT scanning provides the best diagnostic approach and can be used to guide percutaneous drainage (see below).

Management

Intraabdominal abscesses require definitive therapy, which can be accomplished as a one- or two-stage proce-

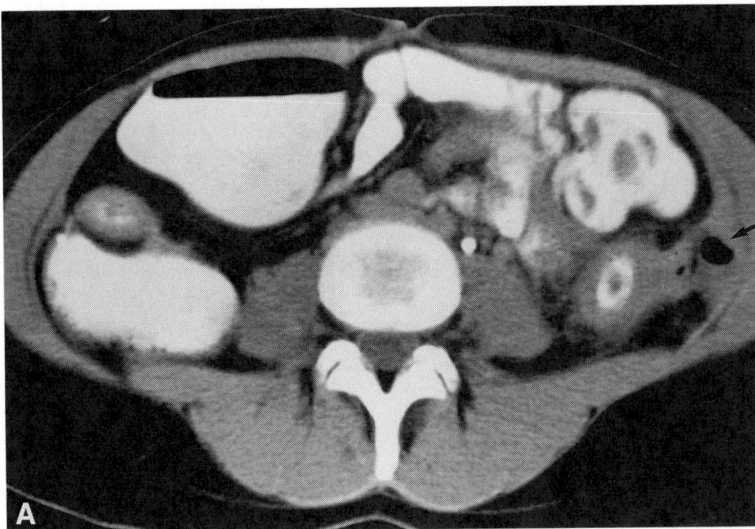
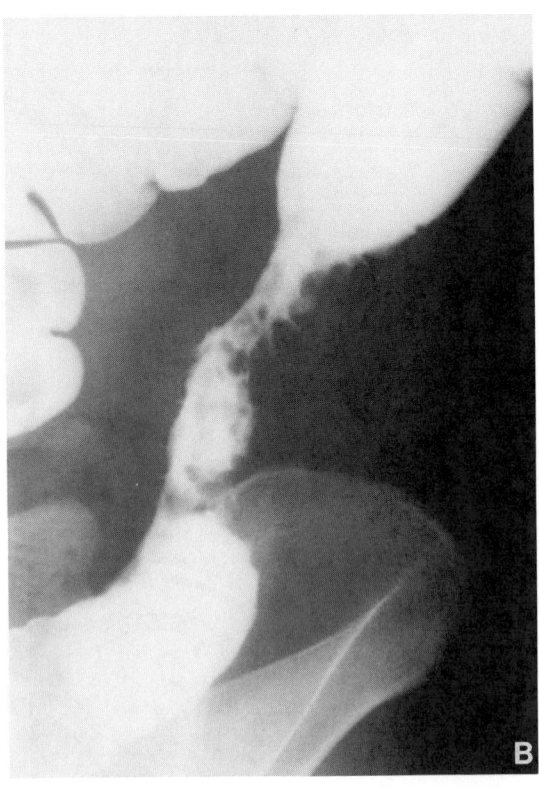

FIG. 5. A: Abdominal wall abscess. CT scan with oral contrast shows a left flank mass with air (*arrow*) adjacent to a thick-walled colon filled with contrast. Air in the mass connecting the abscess to the colon suggests a sinus tract. **B:** Active Crohn's disease. A barium enema in the same patient demonstrates segmental mucosal nodularity, ulceration, and narrowing.

dure. Abscesses large enough to be detected by CT scan will not respond to antibiotics. Definitive treatment includes resection of the disease bowel, since simple drainage of the abscess cavity usually leads to a chronic fistula. In Ribeiro's series, only 16% of patients were cured by surgical incision and drainage compared with 76% who underwent *en bloc* resection (252). Percutaneous drainage of the abscess under ultrasound or CT guidance followed by elective surgical resection is an alternative to the single-step surgical approach (270,271). This technique is advantageous for the extremely ill patient who can then undergo elective resection under optimal conditions after a period of antibiotic and nutritional support. Antibiotic coverage for aerobic and anaerobic organisms is used to prevent hematogenous spread of bacteria during drainage and to improve local healing.

Fistulae

As shown in Fig. 4, fistulae are a frequent complication of extramural perforation in Crohn's disease, due to a direct extension of an ulcer, spontaneous decompression of an abscess, or therapeutic drainage of an abscess. Although the microbiology of fistulae has not been fully evaluated, luminal flora secondarily invade tissues (256) and provide a rationale for antibiotic therapy (272–274). Enteric or colorectal fistulae occur (Fig. 6) in 20% to 40% of Crohn's disease patients but are rare in ulcerative colitis (250,254). In a recent analysis of 639 Crohn's patients who underwent abdominal surgery, 35% had at least one fistula: 69% within loops of intestine, 12% enterovesical,

16% enterocutaneous, 4% enterovaginal, and 95% from the ileum (275). Fistulous tracts in Crohn's disease can involve almost any organ, as documented by case reports of involving the epidural space (276), salpinx, ureter, and urethra (275). The clinical course and management of fistulae vary, depending on location (275,277–281). Symptomatic enterocutaneous, enterovesical, and rectovaginal

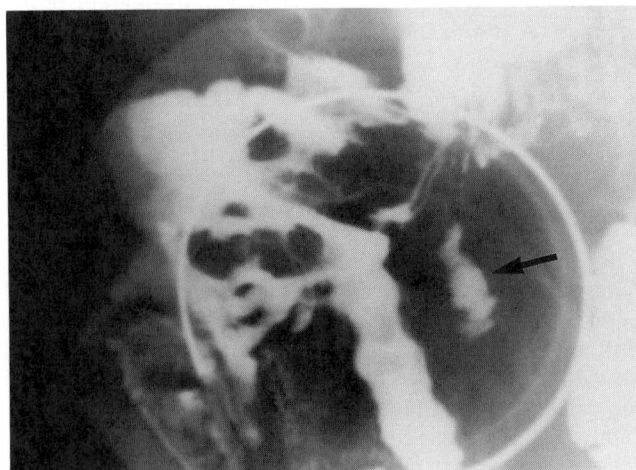

FIG. 6. Complex ileocecal fistula. A small bowel follow-through barium study demonstrates multiple fistulae between the distal ileum and cecum and a probable fistula from the distal ileum to proximal small bowel. Extravasated barium medial to the ileum denotes an abscess.

fistulae usually require surgical management, although immunosuppressive therapy may be effective (282–284). Perianal fistulae are particularly common in Crohn's disease and usually respond to long-term metronidazole therapy (272,273).

Postoperative Infections

Perioperative infectious complications of IBD range from wound infections to peritonitis with sepsis (285). As in most gastrointestinal surgical procedures, septic complications after surgery are more common in emergent procedures when bowel preparation is incomplete and when the indication for surgery is intraabdominal sepsis. In one prospective study (286), septicemia occurred in 7% of patients, anastomotic leakage in 4%, intraabdominal abscess in 4%, and wound infections in 12%. Complications were more common with colonic disease and when sepsis and intraabdominal abscess were present preoperatively. Emergent surgery and steroid therapy were not independent risk factors for infections. Increased incidence of postoperative infections following surgery for intraabdominal abscesses is a consistent feature in a number of studies (251–253,262), but only Post (262) found an increased risk of septic complications related to corticosteroid therapy.

Creation of internal ileal pouches with anastomosis to the anorectal verge is a complex procedure associated with a 7% risk of infection (287). A relatively common complication of total proctocolectomy for ulcerative colitis is a persistent perineal wound, which occurs in 7% to 40% of operations (285).

Hematogenous Spread of Enteric Bacteria in IBD

Although the incidence of bacteremia is unknown in active IBD, sporadic reports of sepsis (288), endocarditis (289–291), portal vein gas (292), and hepatic abscess (293) with enteric bacteria clearly demonstrate that heterogeneous distribution of luminal bacteria must occur. Bacteremia could occur more frequently in IBD patients because of enhanced translocation of luminal bacteria across the inflamed mucosa, overgrowth of luminal bacteria, immunosuppression due to medications or malnutrition, or increased frequency of colonoscopy with biopsy. There is universal agreement among investigators that mucosal permeability is increased in active Crohn's disease and, to a lesser degree, in active ulcerative colitis (1,5,151). Viable bacteria can secondarily invade inflamed mucosa and translocate to the lymphatic and portal circulations. Bacteria have been cultured from the serosa or mesenteric lymph nodes of 56% of resected tissues from patients with Crohn's disease, compared with 17% of controls (294); and up to 27% of ulcerative colitis patients have portal vein bacteremia (295). Translocation of viable luminal bacteria to mesenteric lymph nodes occurs in a variety of animal models of intestinal inflammation (296,297) and small bowel bacterial overgrowth (148). Mucosal translo-

cation of bacteria is potentiated by obstruction (298), antibiotic use (299), and immunosuppression (300,301).

Opportunistic Infections

Patients with IBD have increased susceptibility to infection with enteric pathogens, possibly due to impaired mucosal host defense mechanisms. In addition, the use of potent immunosuppressive drugs to treat IBD is associated with the acquisition of opportunistic infections and potentiation of local septic complications. Chronic steroid use is frequently complicated by mucosal and systemic candidiasis but rarely by bacterial and viral infections (302). In the National Cooperative Crohn's Disease study (303), steroid use was associated with a 27% risk of infection, including sepsis and liver abscess, compared with a 10% risk of infection in placebo-treated patients. In the European Crohn's study (304), no opportunistic infections were noted, but three of the five deaths occurred in steroid-treated patients with abdominal masses. In contrast, no risks were associated with steroid therapy of patients with abdominal masses in Felder's series (305). Azathioprine and 6-mercaptopurine at doses used in IBD are relatively safe, but surveys of large numbers of patients demonstrate a 7% incidence of infections, including disseminated CMV, herpes zoster encephalitis, and liver abscess in some cases (306). Use of cyclosporine is not yet widespread, but early reports indicate a substantial infectious risk, including *Pneumocystis* pneumonia, pulmonary abscess, mycotic aneurysm, and herpetic esophagitis (283,307,308). The infectious complications of combining high-dose corticosteroids, 6-mercaptopurine, and cyclosporine in critically ill patients with enhanced mucosal permeability and microscopic intestinal abscesses will probably prove to be substantial.

Bacterial Overgrowth

Approximately one third of patients with Crohn's disease have increased luminal concentrations of predominantly aerobic bacteria in jejunal fluid; most of these patients have had resection of their ileocecal valve (2). Intestinal strictures and fistulae, especially duodenal or jejunal fistulae to the colon, also predispose to proximal small bowel overgrowth by anaerobes.

The primary complication of the ileal pouch–anal anastomosis procedure performed after colectomy for ulcerative colitis is intermittent pouch inflammation (pouchitis), which appears to be caused by an overgrowth of bacteria. A clinical response to metronidazole in most patients with pouchitis (309) and increased concentrations of anaerobic bacteria in luminal contents of symptomatic patients (310) suggest that anaerobes induce pouch inflammation. However, other investigators have reported a relative increase of aerobic bacteria in pouchitis (311). *Bacteroides sp.* are present in low abundance (310), adhesive *E. coli* are increased but do not correlate with the degree of inflammation (312), and luminal pH is increased (311). Increased pH enhances proteolytic enzyme activity and increases mucin degradation (311), which could contribute to pouch mucosal injury. Of interest, clinical pouchitis occurs in 15% to 20% of patients with ulcerative colitis, but is extremely rare in patients undergoing colectomy for familial polyposis (313), suggesting differential host susceptibility or perhaps unique pathogenic flora in ulcerative colitis patients. Current data suggest that dysbiosis of luminal organisms contributes to pouch inflammation in a susceptible host.

CONCLUSION

The clinical and experimental data discussed in this chapter implicate microbial agents in the pathogenesis of chronic intestinal inflammation and its complications. Enteric pathogens induce inflammation that resembles the inflammatory responses of ulcerative colitis and Crohn's disease. It is possible that a specific transient pathogen, or a variety of pathogens, initiates IBD, which then is perpetuated by separate mechanisms involving ubiquitous luminal bacteria in genetically susceptible hosts, similar to that in susceptible inbred rodents. Endogenous bacteria are also responsible for abscesses and fistulae, which are among the most frequent complications of Crohn's disease. Careful attention to possible intestinal infections, judicious diagnostic evaluation, and appropriate treatment and prevention of suppurative complications of IBD should retard the progression of tissue damage in these disorders.

ACKNOWLEDGMENTS

The author gratefully acknowledges the expert secretarial and editorial assistance of Kelly Cannon and Brian Springer, and the careful editorial review by Dr. Phillip Smith. Original research described in this review was supported by NIH grants DK40249, DK47700, and DK34987, and the Crohn's and Colitis Foundation of America.

REFERENCES

1. Podolsky DK. Inflammatory bowel disease. *N Engl J Med* 1991;325:928–937, 1008–1016.
2. Gorbach, SL. Intestinal microflora in inflammatory bowel disease: Implications for etiology. In: Kirsner JB, Shorter RG, eds. *Inflammatory bowel disease.* 3rd ed. Philadelphia: Lea and Febiger; 1988:51–64.
3. Chadwick VS, Anderson RP. Microorganisms and their products in inflammatory bowel disease. In: MacDermott RP, Stenson WF, eds. *Inflammatory bowel disease.* New York: Elsevier; 1992:241–258.
4. Sartor RB. Role of the intestinal microflora in pathogenesis and complications. In: Scholmerich J, ed. *Inflammatory bowel disease: pathophysiology as basis of treatment.* Dordrecht: Kluwer; 1993:175–187.
5. Sartor RB. Microbial factors in the pathogenesis of Crohn's disease, ulcerative colitis and experimental intestinal inflammation. In: Kirsner JB, Shorter RJ, eds. *Inflammatory bowel disease.* 4th ed. Baltimore: Williams and Wilkins; in press.
6. Bargen JA. Experimental studies on etiology of chronic ulcerative colitis. *JAMA* 1924;83:332–336.
7. Dragsteadt IR, Dack GM, Kirsner JB. Chronic ulcerative coli-

tis: a summary of evidence implicating *Bacterium necrophorum* as an etiologic agent. *Ann Surg* 1941;114:653.
8. Macie TT. Ulcerative colitis due to chronic infection with Flexner-bacillus. *JAMA* 1932;98:1706.
9. Gitnick GL, Rosen VJ, Arthur MH, Hertweck SA. Evidence for the isolation of a new virus from ulcerative colitis patients. *Dig Dis Sci* 1979;24:609–619.
10. Munro J, Mayberry JF, Matthews N, Rhodes J. *Chlamydia* and Crohn's disease. *Lancet* 1979;2:45–46.
11. Parent K, and Mitchel P. Cell wall defective variants of *Pseudomonas* like (group Va) bacteria in Crohn's disease. *Gastroenterology* 1978;75:368–372.
12. Whorwell PJ, Phillips CA, Beeken WL, Little PK, Roessner KD. Isolation of reovirus-like agents from patients with Crohn's disease. *Lancet* 1977;1:1169–1171.
13. Burnham WR, Lennard-Jones JE, Stanford JL, Bird RG. Mycobacteria as a possible cause of inflammatory bowel disease. *Lancet* 1978;2:693–697.
14. Chiodini RJ, Van Kruiningen HJ, Thayer WR, Merkal RS, Coutu JA. Possible role of mycobacteria in inflammatory bowel disease. I. An unclassified mycobacterium species isolated from patients with Crohn's disease. *Dig Dis Sci* 1984;29:1073–1079.
15. Wakefield AJ, Pittilo RM, Sim R, et al. Evidence of persistent measles virus infection in Crohn's disease. *J Med Virol* 1993;39:345–353.
16. Stainsby KJ, Lowes JR, Allan RN, Ibbotson JP. Antibodies to *Mycobacterium paratuberculosis* and nine species of environmental mycobacteria in Crohn's disease and control subjects. *Gut* 1993;34:371–374.
17. Blaser MJ, Miller FA, Lacher J, Singleton JW. Patients with active Crohn's disease have elevated serum antibodies to antigens of seven enteric bacterial pathogens. *Gastroenterology* 1984;87:888–894.
18. Tabaqchali S, O'Donoghue DP, Bettelheim KA. *Escherichia coli* antibodies in patients with inflammatory bowel disease. *Gut* 1978;19:108–113.
19. Gump D, Caul E, Eade O, et al. Lymphocytotoxic and microbial antibodies in Crohn's disease and matched controls. *Antonie Van Leeuwenhoek* 1981;47:455–464.
20. Wensinck F, Van de Merwe JP, Mayberry JF. An international study of agglutinins to *Eubacterium, Peptostreptococcus* and *Coprococcus* species in Crohn's disease, ulcerative colitis and control subjects. *Digestion* 1983;27:63–69.
21. Van Kruiningen HJ, Colombel JF, Cartun RW, et al. An in-depth study of Crohn's disease in two French families. *Gastroenterology* 1993;104:351–360.
22. Aisenberg J, Janowitz HD. Cluster of inflammatory bowel disease in three close college friends. *J Clin Gastroenterol* 1993;17:18–20.
23. Chiodini RJ, Van Kruiningen HJ, Merkal RS. Ruminant paratuberculosis (Johne's disease): the current status and future prospects. *Cornell Vet* 1984;74:218–255.
24. Chiodini RJ. Crohn's disease and the mycobacterioses: a review and comparison of two disease entities. *Clin Microbiol Rev* 1989;2:90–117.
25. Dalzeil TK. Chronic intestinal enteritis. *Br Med J* 1913;2:1068–1069.
26. Crohn BB, Ginzbur L, Oppenheimer GD. Regional ileitis: a pathologic and clinical entity. *JAMA* 1932;99:1323–1329.
27. Graham DY, Markesich DC, Yoshimura HH. Mycobacteria and inflammatory bowel disease. Results of culture. *Gastroenterology* 1987;92:436–442.
28. Wall S, Kunze ZM, Saboor S, et al. Identification of spheroplast-like agents isolated from tissues of patients with Crohn's disease and control tissues by polymerase chain reaction. *J Clin Microbiol* 1993;31:1241–1245.
29. Moss MT, Sanderson JD, Tizard ML, et al. Polymerase chain reaction detection of *Mycobacterium paratuberculosis* and *Mycobacterium avium* subsp *silvaticum* in long term cultures from Crohn's disease and control tissues. *Gut* 1992;33:1209–1213.
30. Sanderson JD, Moss MT, Tizard ML, et al. *Mycobacterium paratuberculosis* DNA in Crohn's disease tissue. *Gut* 1992;33:890–896.

31. Dell'Isola B, Poyart C, Goulet O, Mougenot JF, et al. Detection of *Mycobacterium paratuberculosis* by polymerase chain reaction in children with Crohn's disease. *J Infect Dis* 1994;169:449–451.
32. Cellier C, De Benhouwer H, Faucheron JL, et al. *Mycobacterium paratuberculosis* and *Avium* subsp. *silvaticum* DNA cannot be detected in Crohn's disease tissues. *Gastroenterology* 1993;104:A678.
33. Fidler HM, Thurrell W, Johnson NM, Rook GA, McFadden JJ. Specific detection of *Mycobacterium paratuberculosis* DNA associated with granulomatous tissue in Crohn's disease. *Gut* 1994;35:506–510.
34. Van Kruiningen HJ, Chiodini RJ, Thayer WR, Coutu JA, Merkal RS, Runnels PL. Experimental disease in infant goats induced by a *Mycobacterium* isolated from a patient with Crohn's disease. A preliminary report. *Dig Dis Sci* 1986;31:1351–1360.
35. Van Kruiningen HJ, Ruiz B, Gumprecht L. Experimental disease in young chickens induced by a *Mycobacterium paratuberculosis* isolate from a patient with Crohn's disease. *Can J Vet Res* 1991;55:199–202.
36. Sweeney RW, Whitlock RH, Rosenberger AE. *Mycobacterium paratuberculosis* cultured from milk and supramammary lymph nodes of infected asymptomatic cows. *J Clin Microbiol* 1992;30:166–171.
37. Millar DS, Ford J, Sanderson JD, et al. IS900 PCR testing for *Mycobacterium paratuberculosis (Mptb)* in units of whole pasteurized cows milk widely obtained from retail outlets in England and Wales. In: Chiodini R, ed. *Proceedings of the 4th International Colloquium on Paratuberculosis*. Int Assoc Paratuberculosis, 1994; in press.
38. Chiodini RJ, Hermon-Taylor J. The thermal resistance of *Mycobacterium paratuberculosis* in raw milk under conditions simulating pasteurization. *J Vet Diag Invest* 1993;5:629–631.
39. Kobayashi K, Blaser MJ, Brown WR. Immunohistochemical examination for mycobacteria in intestinal tissues from patients with Crohn's disease (see comments). *Gastroenterology* 1989;96:1009–1015.
40. Fidler HM, Woolford A, Ray R, Wakefield A, McFadden J. Development of in situ polymerase chain reaction (PCR) to detect and localize *Mycobacterium paratuberculosis* within Crohn's disease tissue sections. *Gastroenterology* 1994;106:A680.
41. Elsaghier A, Prantera C, Moreno C, Ivanyi J. Antibodies to *Mycobacterium paratuberculosis*–specific protein antigens in Crohn's disease. *Clin Exp Immunol* 1992;90:503–508.
42. Dalton HR, Hoang P, Jewell DP. Antigen induced suppression in peripheral blood and lamina propria mononuclear cells in inflammatory bowel disease. *Gut* 1992;33:324–330.
43. Ibbotson JP, Lowes JR, Chahal H, et al. Mucosal cell-mediated immunity to mycobacterial, enterobacterial and other microbial antigens in inflammatory bowel disease. *Clin Exp Immunol* 1992;87:224–230.
44. Pirzer U, Schonhaar A, Fleischer B, Hermann E, Meyer zum Buschenfelde KH. Reactivity of infiltrating T lymphocytes with microbial antigens in Crohn's disease. *Lancet* 1991;338:1238–1239.
45. Stainsby KJ, Lowes JR, Allan RN, Ibbotson JP. Antibodies to *Mycobacterium paratuberculosis* and nine species of environmental mycobacteria in Crohn's disease and control subjects. *Gut* 1993;34:371–374.
46. Seldenrijk CA, Drexhage HA, Meuwissen SG, Meijer CJ. T-cellular immune reactions (in macrophage inhibition factor assay) against *Mycobacterium paratuberculosis, Mycobacterium kansasii, Mycobacterium tuberculosis, Mycobacterium avium* in patients with chronic inflammatory bowel disease. *Gut* 1990;31:529–535.
47. Rutgeerts P, Geboes K, Vantrappen G, et al. Rifabutin and ethambutol do not help recurrent Crohn's disease in the neoterminal ileum. *J Clin Gastroenterol* 1992;15:24–28.
48. Sartor RB. Antimicrobial therapy of inflammatory bowel disease: implications for pathogenesis and management. *Can J Gastroenterol* 1993;7:132–138.
49. Swift GL, Srivastava ED, Stone R, et al. Controlled trial of anti-tuberculosis chemotherapy for two years in Crohn's disease. *Gut* 1994;35:363–368.
50. Prantera C, Kohn A, Mangiarotti R, Andreoli A, Luzi C. Antimycobacterial therapy in Crohn's disease: results of a controlled, double-blind trial with a multiple antibiotic regimen. *Am J Gastroenterol* 1994;89:513–518.
51. Smith, MS, Khan K, Bradley NJ, et al. IgG antibodies to measles virus in children with inflammatory bowel disease. *Gastroenterology* 1994;106:A775.
52. Sankey EA, Dhillon AP, Anthony A, et al. Early mucosal changes in Crohn's disease. *Gut* 1993;34:375–381.
53. Knibbs DR, Van Kruiningen HJ, Colombe JF, Cortot A. Ultrastructural evidence of paramyxovirus in two french families with Crohn's disease. *Gastroenterology* 1993;104:A725.
54. Powell SJ, Wilmont AJ. Ulcerative post-dysenteric colitis. *Gut* 1966;7:438–443.
55. Diepersloot RJ, Kroes AC, Visser W, Jiwa NM, Rothbarth PH. Acute ulcerative proctocolitis associated with primary cytomegalovirus infection. *Arch Intern Med* 1990;150:1749–1751.
56. Orvar K, Murray J, Carmen G, Conklin J. Cytomegalovirus infection associated with onset of inflammatory bowel disease. *Dig Dis Sci* 1993;38:2307–2310.
57. Willoughby JM, Rahman AF, Gregory MM. Chronic colitis after *Aeromonas* infection. *Gut* 1989;30:686–690.
58. Leblanc M, Delage G, Rousseau E, Dobrescu O, Bernard-Bonnin AC. Prevalence of *Aeromonas spp.* pediatric gastroenteritis. *Can Med Assoc J* 1988;138:714–717.
59. Treacher DF, Jewell DP. *Yersinia* colitis associated with Crohn's disease. *Postgrad Med J* 1985;61:173–174.
60. Gill RG, Haskins K. Molecular mechanisms underlying diabetes and other autoimmune diseases. *Immunol Today* 1993;14:49–51.
61. Fohlman J, Göran F. Is juvenile diabetes a viral disease? *Ann Med* 1993;25:569–574.
62. Sartor RB, and Lichtman SN. Mechanisms of systemic inflammation associated with intestinal injury. In: Targan SR, Shanahan F, eds. *Inflammatory bowel disease: from bench to bedside*. Baltimore: Williams and Wilkins; 1993:210–229.
63. Gent AE, Hellier MD, Grace RH, Swarbrick ET, Coggon D. Inflammatory bowel disease and domestic hygiene in infancy. *Lancet* 1994;343:766–767.
64. Sartor RB. Cytokines in intestinal inflammation: pathophysiological and clinical considerations. *Gastroenterology* 1994;106:533–539.
65. Eckmann L, Kagnoff MF, Fierer J. Epithelial cells secrete the chemokine interleukin-8 in response to bacterial entry. *Infect Immun* 1993;61:4569–4574.
66. Schwab JH. Phlogistic properties of peptidoglycan-polysaccharide polymers from cell walls of pathogenic and normal-flora bacteria which colonize humans. *Infect Immun* 1993;61:4535–4539.
67. McCall RD, Haskill S, Zimmermann EM, Lund PK, Thompson RC, Sartor RB. Tissue Interleukin-1 and interleukin-1 receptor antagonist expression in enterocolitis in resistant and susceptible rats. *Gastroenterology* 1994;106:960–972.
68. Roediger WE. A new hypothesis for the aetiology of Crohn's disease: evidence from lipid metabolism and intestinal tuberculosis. *Postgrad Med J* 1991;67:666–671.
69. Hughes HP, Campos M, McDougall L, Beskorwayne TK, Potter AA, Babiuk LA. Regulation of major histocompatibility complex class II expression by *Pasteurella haemolytica* leukotoxin. *Infect Immun* 1994;62:1609–1615.
70. Hsu DH, de Waal Malefyt R, Fiorentino DF, et al. Expression of interleukin-10 activity by Epstein–Barr virus protein BCRF1. *Science* 1990;250:830–832.
71. Klapproth JM, Donnenberg MS, Abraham JM, Mobley HL, James SP. Lymphokine inhibitory products of enteric pathogens: a potential mechanism in UC. *Gastroenterology* 1994;106:A712.
72. Mullin GE, Vezza FR, Sampat A, et al. Abnormal IL-10 mRNA production in the intestinal mucosal lesions of inflammatory bowel disease. *Gastroenterology* 1993;104:A751.
73. Mullin GE, Lazenby AJ, Harris ML, Bayless TM, James SP. Increased interleukin-2 messenger RNA in the intestinal mu-

cosal lesions of Crohn's disease but not ulcerative colitis. *Gastroenterology* 1992;102:1620–1627.

74. Wakefield AJ, Fox JD, Sawyerr AM, et al. Detection of herpesvirus DNA in the large intestine of patients with ulcerative colitis and Crohn's disease using the nested polymerase chain reaction. *J Med Virol* 1992;38:183–190.

75. Sadlack B, Merz H, Schorle H, Schimpl A, Feller AC, Horak I. Ulcerative colitis-like disease in mice with a disrupted interleukin-2 gene. *Cell* 1993;75:253–261.

76. Kuhn R, Lohler J, Rennick D, Rajewsky K, Muller W. Interleukin-10-deficient mice develop chronic enterocolitis. *Cell* 1993;75:263–274.

77. Porat R, Clark BD, Wolff SM, Dinarello CA. Enhancement of growth of virulent strains of *Escherichia coli* by interleukin-1. *Science* 1991;254:430–432.

78. Broom MF, Sherriff RM, Ferry DM, Chadwick VS. Formylmethionyl-leucylphenylalanine and the SOS operon in *Escherichia coli*: a model of host-bacterial interactions. *Biochem J* 1993;291:895–900.

79. Lagercrantz RS, Hammerstrom S, Perlmann P, Gustafsson BE. Immunological studies in ulcerative colitis. IV. Origin of autoantibodies. *J Exp Med* 1968;128:1339–1352.

80. Thayer WR, Brown M, Sangree MH, Katz J, Hersh T. *Escherichia coli* 014 and colon hemagglutinating antibodies in inflammatory bowel disease. *Gastroenterology* 1969;57:311–318.

81. Vecchi M, Gionchetti P, Bianchi MB, et al. Circulating autoantibodies in ulcerative colitis (UC) against the MR 40K cytoskeleton protein tropomyosin provides a new clue in the pathogenesis of UC. *Gastroenterology* 1993;104:A796.

82. Kaufmann SH. Heat shock proteins and the immune response. *Immunol Today* 1990;11:129–136.

83. Yu RN, Barrett TA, Jurivich DA. Interferon and the heat shock response. *Gastroenterology* 1994;106:A1057.

84. Mojedhi G, Winrow VR, Blake DR, Rampton DS. Immunohistological localisation of stress proteins in rectal mucosa. *Gastroenterology* 1990;98:A464.

85. D'Haens G, Geboes K, Peetermans W, Rutgeerts P. Enhanced mucosal hsp60 expression in ulcerative colitis and Crohn's colitis but not in acute self-limited colitis. *Gastroenterology* 1994;106:A672.

86. Stevens TR, Winrow VR, Blake DR, Rampton DS. Circulating antibodies to heat-shock protein 60 in Crohn's disease and ulcerative colitis. *Clin Exp Immunol* 1992;90:271–274.

87. Elsaghier A, Prantera C, Bothamley G, Wilkins E, Jindal S, Ivanyi J. Disease association of antibodies to human and mycobacterial hsp70 and hsp60 stress proteins. *Clin Exp Immunol* 1992;89:305–309.

88. D'Haens G, Peetermans W, Hiele M, Ceuppens J, Geboes K, Rutgeerts P. Increased hsp65 antibody titers but decreased lymphocyte proliferative response to hsp65 in Crohn's disease. *Gastroenterology* 1994;106:A672.

89. Szewczuk MR, Depew WT. Evidence for T lymphocyte reactivity to the 65 kilodalton heat shock protein of mycobacterium in active Crohn's disease. *Clin Invest Med* 1992;15:494–505.

90. Van Eden W, Thole JE, Van der Zee R, et al. Cloning of the mycobacterial epitope recognized by T lymphocytes in adjuvant arthritis. *Nature* 1988;331:171–173.

91. Wurzelmann JI, Lyles CM, Sandler RS. Childhood infections and the risk of inflammatory bowel disease. *Dig Dis Sci* 1994;39:555–560.

92. Demling VL. Morbus Crohn durch antibiotika? *Fortschr Med* 1994;112:195–196.

93. Van de Merwe JP, Schroder AM, Wensinck F, Hazenberg MP. The obligate anaerobic faecal flora of patients with Crohn's disease and their first-degree relatives. *Scand J Gastroenterol* 1988;23:1125–1131.

94. Fabia R, Ar'Rajab A, Johansson M, et al. Impairment of bacterial flora in human ulcerative colitis and experimental colitis in the rat. *Digestion* 1993;54:248–255.

95. Hartley MG, Hudson MJ, Swarbrick ET, et al. The rectal mucosa-associated microflora in patients with ulcerative colitis. *J Med Microbiol* 1992;36:96–103.

96. Ruseler-van Embden JG, Both-Patoir HC. Anaerobic gram-negative faecal flora in patients with Crohn's disease and health subjects. *Antonie van Leeuwenhoek* 1983;49:125–132.

97. Auer IO, Roder A, Wensinck F, Van de Merwe JP, Schmidt H, et al. Selected bacterial antibodies in Crohn's disease and ulcerative colitis. *Scand J Gastroenterol* 1983;189:217–223.

98. Krook A, Lindstrom B, Kjellander J, Jarnerot G, Bodin L. Relation between concentrations of metronidazole and *Bacteroides spp.* in faeces of patients with Crohn's disease and healthy individuals. *J Clin Pathol* 1981;34:645–650.

99. Sutherland L, Singleton J, Sessions J, et al. Double-blind, placebo controlled trial of metronidazole in Crohn's disease. *Gut* 1991;32:1071–1075.

100. Onderdonk AB, Franklin ML, Cisneros RL. Production of experimental ulcerative colitis in gnotobiotic guinea pigs with simplified microflora. *Infect Immun* 1981;32:225–231.

101. Breeling JL, Onderdonk AB, Cisneros RL, Kasper DL. *Bacteroides vulgatus* outer membrane antigens associated with carrageenan-induced colitis in guinea pigs. *Infect Immun* 1988;56:1754–1759.

102. Severijnen AJ, Hazenberg MP, Van de Merwe JP. Induction of chronic arthritis in rats by cell wall fragments of anaerobic coccoid rods isolated from the faecal flora of patients with Crohn's disease. *Digestion* 1988;39:118–125.

103. Severijnen AJ, Van Kleef R, Hazenberg MP, Van de Merwe JP. Cell wall fragments from major residents of the human intestinal flora induce chronic arthritis in rats. *J Rheumatol* 1989;16:1061–1068.

104. Burke DA, Axon AT. Adhesive *Escherichia coli* in inflammatory bowel disease and infective diarrhea. *Br Med J* 1988;297:102–104.

105. Giaffer MH, Holdsworth CD, Duerden BI. Virulence properties of *Escherichia coli* strains isolated from patients with inflammatory bowel disease. *Gut* 1992;33:646–650.

106. Hartley MG, Hudson MJ, Swarbrick ET, Gent AE, Hellier MD, Grace RH. Adhesive and hydrophobic properties of *Escherichia coli* from the rectal mucosa of patients with ulcerative colitis. *Gut* 1993;34:63–67.

107. McCormick BA, Colgan SP, Miller SI, Madara JL. Apical binding of *Salmonella* to intestinal epithelia modulates neutrophil-epithelial interactions. *Gastroenterology* 1993;104:A740.

108. Cooke EM, Ewins SP, Hywel-Jones J, Lennard-Jones JE. Properties of strains of *Escherichia coli* carried in different phases of ulcerative colitis. *Gut* 1974;15:143–146.

109. Von Wulffen H, Russmann H, Karch H, et al. Verocytotoxin-producing *Escherichia coli* O2:H5 isolated from patients with ulcerative colitis (letter). *Lancet* 1989;1:1449–1450.

110. Ruseler Van Embden JG, Van der Helm R, Van Lieshout LM. Degradation of intestinal glycoproteins by *Bacteroides vulgatus*. *Fems Microbiol Lett* 1989;49:37–41.

111. Van der Wiel-Korstanje, JA, Winkler KC. The faecal flora in ulcerative colitis. *J Med Microbiol* 1975;8:491–501.

112. Roediger WE. The colonic epithelium in ulcerative colitis: an energy-deficiency disease? *Lancet* 1980;2:712–715.

113. Harig JM, Soergel KH, Komorowski RA, Wood CM. Treatment of diversion colitis with short-chain-fatty acid irrigation. *N Engl J Med* 1989;320:23–28.

114. Chapman MA, Grahn MF, Boyle MA, Hutton M, Rogers J, Williams NS. Butyrate oxidation is impaired in the colonic mucosa of sufferers of quiescent ulcerative colitis. *Gut* 1994;35:73–76.

115. Roediger WE, Duncan A, Kapaniris O, Millard S. Reducing sulfur compounds of the colon impair colonocyte nutrition: implications for ulcerative colitis. *Gastroenterology* 1993;104:802–809.

116. Pitcher MC, Gibson GR, Neale G, Cummings JH. Gentamicin kills multiple drug-resistant sulfate-reducing bacteria in patients with ulcerative colitis. *Gastroenterology* 1994;106:A753.

117. Gibson GR, Cummings JH, Macfarlane GT. Growth and activities of sulphate-reducing bacteria in gut contents of healthy subjects and patients with ulcerative colitis. *FEMS Microbiol Ecol* 1991;86:103–111.

118. Breuer RI, Buto SK, Christ ML, et al. Rectal irrigation with short-chain fatty acids for distal ulcerative colitis. Preliminary report. *Dig Dis Sci* 1991;36:185–187.

119. Scheppach W, Sommer H, Kirchner T, et al. Effect of butyrate enemas on the colonic mucosa in distal ulcerative colitis. *Gastroenterology* 1992;103:51–56.
120. Turunen U, Färkkilä M, Hakala K, et al. A double-blind, placebo controlled six-month ciprofloxacin treatment improves prognosis in ulcerative colitis. *Gastroenterology* 1994;106:A786.
121. Sartor RB, Bender DE, Grenther T, Holt LC. Absolute requirement for ubiquitous luminal bacteria in the pathogenesis of chronic intestinal inflammation. *Gastroenterology* 1994;106:A767.
122. Taurog JD, Maika SD, Simmons WA, Breban M, Hammer RE. Susceptibility to inflammatory disease in HLA-B27 transgenic rat lines correlates with the level of B27 expression. *J Immunol* 1993;150:4168–4178.
123. Taurog JD, Hammer RE, Montanez S, et al. Effect of the germ-free state on the inflammatory disease of HLA-B27 transgenic rats: a split result. *Arthritis Rheum* 1993;36:S46.
124. Phillips BP, Gorstein F. Effects of different species of bacteria on the pathology of enteric amebiasis in monocontaminated guinea pigs. *Am J Trop Med Hyg* 1966;15:863–868.
125. Onderdonk AB, Hermos JA, Bartlett JG. The role of the intestinal microflora in experimental colitis. *Am J Clin Nutr* 1977;30:1819–1825.
126. Lichtman SN, Sartor RB, Keku J, Schwab JH. Hepatic inflammation in rats with experimental small intestinal bacterial overgrowth. *Gastroenterology* 1990;98:414–423.
127. Lichtman SN, Holt LC, Keku J, Schwab JH, Sartor RB, et al. Small bowel bacterial overgrowth causes reactivation of arthritis in rats. *Gastroenterology* 1991;100:593A.
128. Onderdonk AB, Hermos JA, Dzink JL, Bartlett JG. Protective effect of metronidazole in experimental ulcerative colitis. *Gastroenterology* 1978;74:521–526.
129. Yamada T, Deitch E, Specian RD, Perry MA, Sartor RB, Grisham MB. Mechanisms of acute and chronic intestinal inflammation induced by indomethacin. *Inflammation* 1993;17:641–662.
130. Ursing B, Alm T, Barany F, et al. A comparative study of metronidazole and sulfasalazine for active Crohn's disease: the cooperative Crohn's disease study in Sweden. *Gastroenterology* 1982;83:550–562.
131. Rutgeerts P, Hiele M, Peeters M, Geboes K, Kerremans R. Prevention of clinical recurrence after ileal resection for Crohn's disease with metronidazole: a placebo controlled study. *Gastroenterology* 1994;106:A764.
132. Peppercorn MA. Is there a role for antibiotics as primary therapy in Crohn's ileitis? *J Clin Gastroenterol* 1993;17:235–237.
133. Moss AA, Carbone JV, Kressel HY. Radiologic and clinical assessment of broad-spectrum antibiotic therapy in Crohn's disease. *AJR* 1978;131:787–790.
134. Burke DA, Axon AT, Clayden SA, Dixon MF, Johnston D, Lacey RW. The efficacy of tobramycin in the treatment of ulcerative colitis. *Aliment Pharmacol Ther* 1990;4:123–129.
135. Burke DA, Clayden SA, Dixon MF, Axon AT, Johnston D, Lacey RW. A follow up study of adjunctive oral tobramycin therapy in acute ulcerative colitis. *Gastroenterology* 1988;94:A55.
136. Danzi JT. Trimethoprim-sulphamethoxazole therapy of inflammatory bowel disease. *Gastroenterology* 1989;96:A110.
137. Peppercorn MA. Are antibiotics useful in the management of nontoxic severe ulcerative colitis? *J Clin Gastroenterol* 1993;17:14–17.
138. Von Ritter C, Sekizuka E, Grisham MB, Granger DN. The chemotactic peptide N-formyl methionyl-leucyl-phenylalanine increases mucosal permeability in the distal ileum of the rat. *Gastroenterology* 1988;95:651–656.
139. Hsueh W, Gonzalez-Crussi F, Arroyave JL. Platelet-activating factor: an endogenous mediator for bowel necrosis in endotoxemia. *FASEB J* 1987;1:403–405.
140. Chester JF, Ross JS, Malt RA, Weitzman SA. Acute colitis produced by chemotactic peptides in rats and mice. *Am J Pathol* 1985;121:284–290.
141. Sartor RB, Cromartie WJ, Powell DW, Schwab JH. Granulomatous enterocolitis induced in rats by purified bacterial cell wall fragments. *Gastroenterology* 1985;89:587–595.
142. Davis SW, Holt LC, Sartor RB. Luminal bacterial and bacterial polymers potentiate indomethacin-induced intestinal injury in the rat. *Gastroenterology* 1990;98:444A.
143. Lichtman SN, Keku J, Schwab JH, Sartor RB. Evidence for peptidoglycan absorption in rats with experimental small bowel bacterial overgrowth. *Infect Immun* 1991;59:555–562.
144. Lichtman SN, Okoruwa EE, Keku J, Schwab JH, Sartor RB. Degradation of endogenous bacterial cell wall polymers by the muralytic enzyme mutanolysin prevents hepatobiliary injury in genetically susceptible rats with experimental intestinal bacterial overgrowth. *J Clin Invest* 1992;90:1313–1322.
145. Hazenberg MP, de Visser H, Bras MJ, Prins ME, Van de Merwe JP. Serum antibodies to peptidoglycan-polysaccharide complexes from the anaerobic intestinal flora in patients with Crohn's disease. *Digestion* 1990;47:172–180.
146. Anderson RP, Friend GM, Ferry DM, Chadwick VS. Formyl peptidemia in patients with inflammatory bowel disease and primary sclerosing cholangitis. *Gastroenterology* 1991;100:A557.
147. Wellmann W, Fink PC, Benner F, Schmidt FW. Endotoxaemia in active Crohn's disease. Treatment with whole gut irrigation and 5-aminosalicylic acid. *Gut* 1986;27:814–820.
148. Baldassano RN, Schreiber S, Johnston RBJ, Fu RD, Muraki T, MacDermott RP. Crohn's disease monocytes are primed for accentuated release of toxic oxygen metabolites. *Gastroenterology* 1993;105:60–66.
149. Yang H, Rotter JI. Genetics of inflammatory bowel disease. In: Targan SR, Shanahan F, eds. *Inflammatory bowel disease: from bench to bedside.* Baltimore: Williams and Wilkins; 1994:32–64.
150. Sartor RB. Genetic factors in animal models of intestinal inflammation. In: *Basic research and clinical implications of IBD.* Dordrecht: Kluwer Academic Press; in press.
151. May GR, Sutherland LR, Meddings JB. Is small intestinal permeability really increased in relatives of patients with Crohn's disease? *Gastroenterology* 1993;104:1627–1632.
152. Pironi L, Miglioli M, Ruggeri E, et al. Effect of non-steroidal anti-inflammatory drugs (NSAID) on intestinal permeability in first degree relatives of patients with Crohn's disease. *Gastroenterology* 1992;102:A679.
153. Pullan RD, Thomas GA, Rhodes M, et al. Thickness of adherent mucus gel on colonic mucosa in humans and its relevance to colitis. *Gut* 1994;35:353–359.
154. Hobson CH, Butt TJ, Ferry DM, et al. Enterohepatic circulation of bacterial chemotactic peptide in rats with experimental colitis. *Gastroenterology* 1988;94:1006–1013.
155. Sartor RB, Bender DE, Holt LC. Susceptibility of inbred rat strains to intestinal and extraintestinal inflammation induced by indomethacin. *Gastroenterology* 1992;102:A690.
156. Barthold SW, Osbaldiston GW, Jonas AM. Dietary, bacterial and host genetic interactions in the pathogenesis of transmissible murine colonic hyperplasia. *Lab Anim Sci* 1977;27:938–945.
157. Isaacs KL, Sartor RB, Haskill JS. Cytokine mRNA profiles in inflammatory bowel disease mucosa detected by PCR amplification. *Gastroenterology* 1992;103:1587–1595.
158. Isaacs KL, Sartor RB, Haskill JS. Relative expression of IL-1 and IL-1 receptor antagonist in IBD. *Gastroenterology* 1992;102:A279.
159. Farmer RG. Infectious causes of diarrhea in the differential diagnosis of inflammatory bowel disease. *Med Clin North Am* 1990;74:29–38.
160. Surawicz CM. Differential diagnosis of colitis. In: Targan SR, Shanahan F, eds. *Inflammatory bowel disease: from bench to bedside.* Baltimore: William and Wilkins; 1994:409–428.
161. Stuart RC, Leahy AL, Cafferkey MT, Stephens RB. *Yersinia enterocolitica* infection and toxic megacolon. *Br J Surg* 1986;73:590.
162. Moeller DD, Burger WE. Perforation of the ileum in *Yersinia enterocolitica* infection. *Am J Gastroenterol* 1985;80:19–20.
163. Raz R, Schonfeld S, Nassar F. Toxic megacolon in *Salmonella typhimurium* gastroenteritis. *Isr J Med Sci* 1988;24:719–720.
164. Orloff JJ, Saito R, Lasky S, Dave H. Toxic megacolon in cytomegalovirus colitis. *Am J Gastroenterol* 1989;84:794–797.

165. Christianson KA. Toxic megacolon complicating shigellosis. *J R Coll Surg Edinb* 1987;32:109–110.

166. Marshall WF, McLimans CA, Yu PK, Allerberger FJ, Van Scoy RE, Anhalt JP. Results of a 6-month survey of stool cultures for *Escherichia coli* O157:H7. *Mayo Clin Proc* 1990;65:787–792.

167. Van Spreeuwel JP, Lindeman J, Meijer CJ. A quantitative study of immunoglobulin containing cells in the differential diagnosis of acute colitis. *J Clin Pathol* 1985;38:774–777.

168. Harries AD, Beeching NJ, Rogerson SJ, Nye FJ. The platelet count as a simple measure to distinguish inflammatory bowel disease from infective diarrhoea. *J Infect* 1991;22:247–250.

169. Osterholm MT, MacDonald KL, White KE, et al. An outbreak of a newly recognized chronic diarrhea syndrome associated with raw milk consumption. *JAMA* 1986;265:484–490.

170. Blaser MJ, Reller LB. Campylobacter enteritis. *N Engl J Med* 1981;305:1444–1452.

171. Steingrimsson O, Thorsteinsson SB, Hjalmarsdottir M, Jonasdottir E, Kolbeinsson A. *Campylobacter ssp.* infections in Iceland during a 24-month period in 1980–1982. Clinical and epidemiological characteristics. *Scand J Infect Dis* 1985;17:285–290.

172. Blaser MJ, Parsons RB, Wang WL. Acute colitis caused by *Campylobacter fetus* ss. *jejuni*. *Gastroenterology* 1980;78:448–453.

173. Mee AS, Shield M, Burke M. *Campylobacter* colitis: differentiation from acute inflammatory bowel disease. *J R Soc Med* 1985;78:217–223.

174. Anderson JB, Tanner AH, Brodribb AJ. Toxic megacolon due to *Campylobacter* colitis. *Int J Colorectal Dis* 1986;1:58–59.

175. Frohli P, Hanselmann R, Koelz HR. Erythema nodosum in *Campylobacter jejuni* colitis. *Schweiz Med Wochenschr* 1990;120:946–947.

176. Simson JN, Ayling R, Stoker TA. *Campylobacter jejuni* associated with acute relapse and abscess formation in Crohn's disease. *J R Coll Surg Edinb* 1985;30:397.

177. Puylaert JB, Lalisan RI, Van der Werf SD, Doornbos L. *Campylobacter* ileocolitis mimicking acute appendicitis: differentiation with graded-compression US. *Radiology* 1988;166:737–740.

178. Van Spreeuwel JP, Duursma GC, Meijer CJ, Bax R, Rosekrans PC, Lindeman J. *Campylobacter* colitis: histological immunohistochemical and ultrastructural findings. *Gut* 1985;26:945–951.

179. Gill KP, Feeley TM, Keane FB. Toxic megacolon and perforation caused by *Salmonella*. *Br J Surg* 1989;76:796.

180. Nakamura S, Iida M, Tominaga M, Yao T, Hirata N, Fujishima M. *Salmonella* colitis: assessment with double-contrast barium enema examination in seven patients. *Radiology* 1992;184:537–540.

181. Vender RJ, Marignani P. *Salmonella* colitis presenting as a segmental colitis resembling Crohn's disease. *Dig Dis Sci* 1983;28:848–851.

182. Speelman P, Kabir I, Islam M. Distribution and spread of colonic lesions in shigellosis: a colonscopic study. *J Infect Dis* 1984;150:899–903.

183. Halpern Z, Dan M, Giladi M, Schwartz I, Sela O, Levo Y. Shigellosis in adults: epidemiologic, clinical, and laboratory features. *Medicine* 1989;68:210–217.

184. Caldwell GR, Reiss-Levy EA, De Carle DJ, Hunt DR. *Shigella dysenteriae* type 1 enterocolitis. *Aust N Z J Med* 1986;16:405–407.

185. Bokete TN, O'Callahan CM, Clausen CR, et al. Shiga-like toxin-producing *Escherichia coli* in Seattle children: a prospective study. *Gastroenterology* 1993;105:1724–1731.

186. Griffin PM, Olmstead LC, Petras RE. *Escherichia coli* O157:H7-associated colitis. A clinical and histological study of 11 cases. *Gastroenterology* 1990;99:142–149.

187. O'Brien AD, Melton AR, Schmitt CK, McKee ML, Batts ML, Griffin DE. Profile of *Escherichia coli* O157:H7 pathogen responsible for hamburger-borne outbreak of hemorrhagic colitis and hemolytic uremic syndrome in Washington. *J Clin Microbiol* 1993;31:2799–2801.

188. Gorbach SL, Graeme-Cook F, Smith RN. A 58-year-old woman with bloody diarrhea after chemotherapy for carcinoma of the tongue. *N Engl J Med* 1994;330:1811–1818.

189. Tarr PI, Weinberger E, Hatch EI, Christie DL. Bacterial ileocecitis caused by *Escherichia coli* O157:H7. *J Pediatr Gastroenterol Nutr* 1992;14:261–263.

190. Triadafilopoulos G, Hallstone AE. Acute abdomen as the first presentation of pseudomembranous colitis. *Gastroenterology* 199;101:685–691.

191. Tedesco FJ, Corless JK, Brownstein RE. Rectal sparing in antibiotic-associated pseudomembranous colitis: a prospective study. *Gastroenterology* 1982;83:1259–1260.

192. Gracey M, Burke V, Robinson J. *Aeromonas*-associated gastroenteritis. *Lancet* 1982;2:1304–1306.

193. Holmberg SD, Schell WL, Fanning GR, et al. Aeromonas intestinal infections in the United States. *Ann Intern Med* 1986;105:683–689.

194. Marshall JB. Tuberculosis of the gastrointestinal tract and peritoneum. *Am J Gastroenterol* 1993;88:989–999.

195. Pettengell KE, Larsen C, Garb M, Mayet FG, Simjee AE, Pirie D. Gastrointestinal tuberculosis in patients with pulmonary tuberculosis. *Q J Med* 1990;74:303–308.

196. Chen WS, Leu SY, Hsu H, Lin JK, Lin TC. Trend of large bowel tuberculosis and the relation with pulmonary tuberculosis. *Dis Colon Rectum* 1992;35:189–192.

197. Shah S, Thomas V, Mathan M, et al. Colonoscopic study of 50 patients with colonic tuberculosis. *Gut* 1992;33:347–351.

198. Vijayraghavan M, Aruna BH, Sarda AK, Sharma AK, Chatterjee TK. Duodenal tuberculosis: a review of the clinicopathologic features and management of twelve cases. *Jpn J Surg* 1990;20:526–529.

199. Balthazar EJ, Gordon R, Hulnick D. Ileocecal tuberculosis: CT and radiologic evaluation. *AJR* 1990;154:499–503.

200. Bhargava DK, Dasarathy S, Shriniwas MD, Kushwaha AK, Duphare H, Kapur BM. Evaluation of enzyme-linked immunosorbent assay using mycobacterial saline-extracted antigen for the serodiagnosis of abdominal tuberculosis. *Am J Gastroenterol* 1992;87:105–108.

201. Saebo A, Lassen J. Acute and chronic gastrointestinal manifestation associated with *Yersinia enterocolitica* infection. *Ann Surg* 1992;215:250–255.

202. Vantrappen G, Agg HO, Ponette E, Gegoes K, Bertrand PH. *Yersinia* enteritis and enterocolitis: gastrointestinal aspects. *Gastroenterology* 1977;72:220–227.

203. Matsumoto T, Mitsuo I, Matsui T, et al. Endoscopic findings in *Yersinia enterocolitica* enterocolitis. *Gastrointest Endosc* 1990;36:583–586.

204. Simmonds SD, Noble MA, Freeman HJ. Gastrointestinal features of culture-positive *Yersinia enterocolitica* infection. *Gastroenterology* 1987;92:112–117.

205. Ravdin JL. *Entamoeba histolytica*: from adherence to enteropathy. *J Infect Dis* 1989;159:420–429.

206. Aristizabal H, Acevedo J, Botero M. Fulminant amebic colitis. *World J Surg* 1991;15216–15221.

207. Matsui T, Iida M, Tada S, et al. The value of double-contrast barium enema in amebic colitis. *Gastrointest Radiol* 1989;14:73–78.

208. Radhakrishnan S, Al Nakib B, Shaikh H, Menon NK. The value of colonoscopy in schistosomal, tuberculous, and amebic colitis. Two-year experience. *Dis Col Rect* 1986;29:891–895.

209. Patel AS, DeRidder PH. Amebic colitis masquerading as acute inflammatory bowel disease. *J Clin Gastroenterol* 1989;11:407–410.

210. Cheung AN, Ng IO. Cytomegalovirus infection of the gastrointestinal tract in non-AIDS patients. *Am J Gastroenterol* 1993;88:1882–1886.

211. Wajsman R, Cappell MS, Biempica L, Cho KC. Terminal ileitis associated with cytomegalovirus and the acquired immune deficiency syndrome. *Am J Gastroenterology* 1989;84:790–793.

212. Wexner SD, Smithy WB, Trillo C, Hopkins BS, Dailey TH. Emergency colectomy for cytomegalovirus ileocolitis in patients with the acquired immune deficiency syndrome. *Dis Col Rect* 1988;31:755–761.

213. Quinn TC, Goodell SE, Mkrtichian E, et al. *Chlamydia trachomatis* proctitis. *N Engl J Med* 1981;305:195–200.

214. Mostafavi H, O'Donnell KF, Chong FK. Supralevator abscess due to chronic rectal lymphogranuloma venereum. *Am J Gastroenterol* 1990;85:602–606.
215. Sartor RB. Ulcerative colitis. *Consultant* 1983 (May);121–122.
216. Rankin GB, Watts HO, Melnyk CS, Kelley ML. National Cooperative Crohn's Disease Study: extraintestinal manifestations and perianal complications. *Gastroenterology* 1979;77:914–920.
217. Tedesco FJ, Hardin RD, Harper RN, Edward BH. Infectious colitis endoscopically simulating inflammatory bowel disease: a prospective evaluation. *Gastrointest Endosc* 1983;29:195–197.
218. Surawicz CM, Belic L. Rectal biopsy helps to distinguish acute self-limited colitis from idiopathic inflammatory bowel disease. *Gastroenterology* 1984;86:104–113.
219. Askerkoff B, Bennett JV. Effect of antibiotic therapy in acute salmonellosis on the fecal excretion of salmonellae. *N Engl J Med* 1969;281:636–640.
220. Riley LW, Remis RS, Helgerson SD, et al. Hemorrhagic colitis associated with a rare *Escherichia coli* serotype. *N Engl J Med* 1983;308:681–685.
221. Butler T, Islam MR, Azad MA, et al. Risk factors for the development of hemolytic uremic syndrome during shigellosis. *J Pediatr* 1987;110:894–897.
222. Aukrust P, Moum B, Farstad IN, Holter E, Bjorneklett A, Kremer D. Fatal cytomegalovirus (CMV) colitis in a patient receiving low dose prednisolone therapy. *Scand J Infect Dis* 1991;23:495–499.
223. Hermens DJ, Miner PB, Jr. Exacerbation of ulcerative colitis. *Gastroenterology* 1991;101:254–262.
224. Bartlett JG, Laughon BE, Bayless TM. Role of microbial agents in relapses of idiopathic inflammatory bowel disease. In: Bayless TM, ed. *Current management of inflammatory bowel disease.* Philadelphia: B. C. Decker; 1989:86–93.
225. Gebhard RL, Greenberg HB, Singh N, et al. Acute viral enteritis and exacerbations of inflammatory bowel disease. *Gastroenterology* 1982;83:1207–1209.
226. Kangro HO, Chong SK, Hardiman A, Heath RB, Walker-Smith JA. A prospective study of viral and mycoplasma infections in chronic inflammatory bowel disease. *Gastroenterology* 1990;98:549–553.
227. Ruther U, Nunnensiek C, Muller HA, et al. Herpes simplex-associated exacerbation of Crohn's disease. Successful treatment with acyclovir. *Dtsch Med Wochenschr* 1992;117:46–50.
228. Trnka YM, LaMont, JT. Association of *Clostridium difficile* toxin with symptomatic relapse of chronic inflammatory bowel disease. *Gastroenterology* 1981;80:693–696.
229. Szilagyi A, Gerson M, Mendelson J, Yusuf NA. *Salmonella* infections complicating inflammatory bowel disease. *J Clin Gastroenterol* 1985;7:251–255.
230. Kochhar R, Ayyagari A, Goenka MK, Dhali GK, Aggarwal R, Mehta SK. Role of infectious agents in exacerbations of ulcerative colitis in India. *J Clin Gastroenterol* 1993;16:26–30.
231. Payne M, Girdwood AH, Roost RW, Freson MJ, Kottler RE. *Yersinia enterocolitica* and Crohn's disease. A case report. *South Afr Med J* 1987;72:53–55.
232. Weber P, Koch M, Wolfgang RH, Scheurlen M, Jenss H, Hartmann F. Microbic superinfection in relapse of inflammatory bowel disease. *J Clin Gastroenterol* 1992;14:302–308.
233. Bayerdorffer E, Schwarzkopf-Steinhauser G, Ottenjann R. New unusual forms of colitis. Report of four cases with known and unknown etiology. *Hepatogastroenterology* 1986;33:187–190.
234. Scheurlen C, Kruis W, Spengler U, Weinzierl M, Baumgartner G, Lamina J. Crohn's disease is frequently complicated by giardiasis. *Scand J Gastroenterol* 1988;23:833–839.
235. Nagler J, Brown M, Soave R. *Blastocystis hominis* in inflammatory bowel disease. *J Clin Gastroenterol* 1993;16:109–112.
236. Mee AS, Jewell DP. Factors inducing relapse in inflammatory bowel disease. *Br Med J [Clin Res]* 1978;801–802.
237. Tysk C, Jarnerot G. Seasonal variation in exacerbations of ulcerative colitis. *Scand J Gastroenterol* 1993;28:95–96.
238. Greenfield C, Aguilar Ramirez JR, Pounder RE, et al. *Clostridium difficile* and inflammatory bowel disease. *Gut* 1983;24:713–717.
239. Meyers S, Mayer E, Buttone F, Desmond E, Janowitz HD, et al. Occurrence of *Clostridium difficile* toxin during the course of inflammatory bowel disease. *Gastroenterology* 1981;80:697–700.
240. McLaren L, Bartlett JG, Gitnick G. Infectious agents in inflammatory bowel disease: collaborative studies. *Gastroenterology* 1981;80:1228A.
241. Bolton RP, Sheriff RJ, Read AE. *Clostridium difficile* associated diarrhea: a role in inflammatory bowel disease? *Lancet* 1980;1:383–384.
242. Bolton RP, Read AE. *Clostridium difficile* in toxic megacolon complicating acute inflammatory bowel disease. *Br Med J* 1982;285:475–476.
243. Tremaine WJ, Bille J, Huizenga KA, Washington JA, Ilstrup DM. Factors which influence the occurrence of *Clostridium difficile* infections in inflammatory bowel disease. *Gastroenterology* 1983;84:A1337.
244. Keighley MR, Youngs D, Johnson M, Allan RN, Burdon DW. *Clostridium difficile* toxin in acute diarrhoea complicating inflammatory bowel disease. *Gut* 1983;23:410–414.
245. Lindeman RJ, Weinstein L, Levitan R, Patterson JF. Ulcerative colitis and intestinal salmonellosis. *Am J Med Sci* 1967;254:855–861.
246. Cooper HS, Raffensperger EC, Jonas L, Fitts WT Jr. Cytomegalovirus inclusions in patients with ulcerative colitis and toxic dilation requiring colonic resection. *Gastroenterology* 1977;72:1253–1256.
247. Berk T, Gordon SJ, Choi HY, Cooper HS. Cytomegalovirus infection of the colon: a possible in exacerbations of inflammatory bowel disease. *Am J Gastroenterol* 1985;80:355–360.
248. Farmer GW, Vincent MM, Fuccillo DA, et al. Viral investigations in ulcerative colitis and regional enteritis. *Gastroenterology* 1973;65:8–18.
249. Wakefield AJ, Fox JD, Sawyer AM, et al. Detection of herpesvirus DNA in the large intestine of patients with ulcerative colitis and Crohn's disease using the nested polymerase chain reaction. *J Med Virol* 1992;38:183–190.
250. Huizenga KA, Schroeder KW. Gastrointestinal complications of ulcerative colitis and Crohn's disease. In: Kirsner JB, Shorter RG, eds. *Inflammatory bowel disease.* 3rd ed. Philadelphia: Lea and Febiger; 1988:257–279.
251. Keighley MR, Eastwood D, Ambrose NS, Allan RN, Burdon DW. Incidence and microbiology of abdominal and pelvic abscess in Crohn's disease. *Gastroenterology* 1982;83:1271–1275.
252. Ribeiro MB, Greenstein AJ, Yamazaki Y, Aufses AH, Jr. Intraabdominal abscess in regional enteritis. *Ann Surg* 1991;213:32–26.
253. Greenstein AJ, Sachar DB, Greenstein RJ, Janowitz HD, Aufses AH Jr. Intraabdominal abscess in Crohn's (ileo) colitis. *Am J Gastroenterol* 1982;143:727–730.
254. Steinberg DM, Cooke WT, Alexander-Williams J. Abscess and fistulae in Crohn's disease. *Gut* 1973;14:865–869.
255. Kyle J. Psoas abscess in Crohn's disease. *Gastroenterology* 1971;61:149–155.
256. Cartun RW, Van Kruiningen HJ, Pedersen CA, Berman MM. An immunocytochemical search for infectious agents in Crohn's disease. *Mod Pathol* 1993;6:212–219.
257. Lorber B, Swenson RM. The bacteriology of intraabdominal infections. *Surg Clin North Am* 1975;55:1349–1354.
258. Kelly JK, Siu TO. The strictures, sinuses, and fissures of Crohn's disease. *J Clin Gastroenterol* 1986;8:594–598.
259. Tonelli F, Ficari F. Pathological features of Crohn's disease determining perforation. *J Clin Gastroenterol* 1991;13:226–230.
260. Greenstein AJ, Lachman P, Sachar DB, et al. Perforating and non-perforating indications for repeated operations in Crohn's disease: evidence for two clinical forms. *Gut* 1988;29:588–592.
261. Tokayer AZ, Reydel B, Bayless TM. Possible role of heredity in site and transmural aggressiveness of Crohn's disease. *Gastroenterology* 1992;102:A705.
262. Post S, Betzler M, Von Ditfurth B, Schurmann G, Kupper P, Herfarth C. Risks of intestinal anastomoses in Crohn's disease. *Ann Surg* 1991;213:37–42.
263. Aszodi A, Ponsky JL. Effects of corticosteroids on the healing bowel anastomosis. *Am Surg* 1984;50:546–548.

264. Allsop JR, Lee EC. Factors which influenced postoperative complications in patients with ulcerative colitis or Crohn's disease of the colon on corticosteroids. *Gut* 1978;19:729–734.

265. Knudsen L, Christansen L, Jarnum S. Early complications in patients previously treated with corticosteroids: a retrospective study of 250 operations on patients with Crohn's disease or ulcerative colitis. *Scand J Gastroenterol* 1976;37(Suppl): 123–128.

266. Knochel JQ, Koehler PR, Lee TG, Welch DM. Diagnosis of abdominal abscesses with computed tomography, ultrasound, and 111-In leukocyte scans. *Radiology* 1980;137:425–432.

267. Cybulsky IJ, Tam P. Intra-abdominal abscesses in Crohn's disease. *Am J Surg* 1990;56:678–682.

268. Wheeler JG, Slack NF, Duncan A, Whitehead PJ, Russell G, Harvey RF. The diagnosis of intraabdominal abscesses in patients with severe Crohn's disease. *Q J Med* 1992;n.s. 82: 159–167.

269. Shoenut JP, Semelka RC, Silverman R, Yaffe CS, Micflikier AB. Magnetic resonance imaging in inflammatory bowel disease. *J Clin Gastroenterol* 1993;17:73–78.

270. Gerzof SG, Robbins AH, Johnson WC, Birkett DH, Nabseth DC. Percutaneous catheter drainage of adominal abscesses. *N Engl Med* 1981;305:653–657.

271. Safrit HD, Mauro MA, Jaques PF. Percutaneous abscess drainage in Crohn's disease. *AJR* 1987;148:859–862.

272. Bernstein LH, Frank MS, Brandt LJ, Boley SJ. Healing of perineal Crohn's disease with metronidazole. *Gastroenterology* 1980;79:357–365.

273. Brandt LJ, Bernstein LH, Boley SJ, Frank MS. Metronidazole therapy for perineal Crohn's disease: a follow-up study. *Gastroenterology* 1982;83:383–387.

274. Wolf JL. Ciprofloxacin may be useful in Crohn's disease. *Gastroenterology* 1990;98:A212.

275. Michelassi F, Stella M, Balestracci T, Giuliante F, Marogna P, Block G. Incidence, diagnosis, and treatment of enteric and colorectal fistulae in patients with Crohn's disease. *Ann Surg* 1993;218:660–666.

276. Piontek M, Hengels K, Hefter H, Aulich A, Strohmeyer G. Spinal abscess and bacterial meningitis in Crohn's disease. *Dig Dis Sci* 1992;37:1131–1135.

277. Broe PJ, Bayless TM, Cameron JL. Crohn's disease: are enteroenteral fistulas an indication for surgery? *Surgery* 1982;91: 249–253.

278. McIntyre PB, Ritchie JK, Hawley PR, Bartram CI, Lennard-Jones JE. Management of enterocutaneous fistulas: a review of 132 cases. *Br J Surg* 1984;71:293–296.

279. Margolin ML, Korelitz BI. Management of bladder fistulas in Crohn's disease. *J Clin Gastroenterol* 1989;11:399–402.

280. Heyen F, Winslet MC, Andrew H, et al. Vaginal fistulas in Crohn's disease. *Dis Col Rect* 1989;32:379–383.

281. Williams DR, Coller JA, Corman ML, Nugent FW, Veidenheimer MC. Anal complications in Crohn's disease. *Dis Col Rect* 1981;24:22–24.

282. Korelitz BI, Present DH. Favorable effect of 6-mercaptopurine on fistulae of Crohn's disease. *Dig Dis Sci* 1985;30:58–64.

283. Hanauer SB, Smith MB. Rapid closure of Crohn's disease fistulas with continuous intravenous cyclosporin A. *Am J Gastroenterol* 1993;88:646–649.

284. Present DH, Lichtiger S. Efficacy of cyclosporine in treatment of fistula of Crohn's disease. *Dig Dis Sci* 1994;39:374–380.

285. Block GE, Schraut WH. Complications of the surgical treatment of ulcerative colitis and Crohn's disease. In: Kirsner JB, Shorter RG. *Inflammatory bowel disease.* 3rd ed. Philadelphia: Lea and Febiger; 1988:685–713.

286. Fasth S, Helleberg R, Hulten L, Magnusson O. Early complications after surgical treatment for Crohn's disease with particular reference to factors affecting their development. *Acta Chir Scand* 1980;146:519–526.

287. Becker JM. Surgical management of ulcerative colitis. In: MacDermott RP, Stenson WF, eds. *Inflammatory bowel disease.* New York: Elsevier; 1992:599–614.

288. Mellman RL, Spisak GM, Burakoff R. *Enterococcus avium bacteremia* in association with ulcerative colitis. *Am J Gastroenterol* 1992;87:375–378.

289. Kreuzpaintner G, Horstkotte D, Heyll A, Losse B, Stohmeyer G. Increased risk of bacterial endocarditis in inflammatory bowel disease. *Am J Med* 1992;92:391–395.

290. Moshkowitz M, Arber N, Wajsman R, Baratz M, Gilat T. *Streptococcus bovis* endocarditis as a presenting manifestation of idiopathic ulcerative colitis. *Postgrad Med J* 1992;68: 930–931.

291. Tomomasa T, Itoh K, Matsui A, et al. An infant with ulcerative colitis complicated by endocarditis and cerebral infarction. *J Pediatr Gastroenterol* 1993;17:323–325.

292. Al-Jahdali H, Pon C, Thompson WG, Matzinger FR. Non-fatal portal pyaemia complicating Crohn's disease of the terminal ileum. *Gut* 1994;35:560–561.

293. Kotanagi H, Sone S, Fukuoka T, et al. Liver abscess as the initial manifestation of colonic Crohn's disease: report of a case. *Jpn J Surg* 1991;21:348–351.

294. Ambrose NS, Johnson M, Burdon DW, Keighley MR. Incidence of pathogenic bacteria from mesenteric lymph nodes and ileal serosa during Crohn's disease. *Br J Surg* 1984;71:623–625.

295. Brooke BN, Dykes PW, Walker FC. A study of liver disorder in ulcerative colitis. *Postgrad Med J* 1961;37:245–251.

296. Yamada T, Deitch E, Specian RD, Perry MA, Sartor RB, Grisham MB. Mechanisms of acute and chronic inflammation induced by indomethacin. *Inflammation* 1993;17:641–642.

297. Gardiner KR, Erwin PJ, Anderson NH, Barr JG, Halliday MI, Rowland BJ. Colonic bacteria and bacterial translocation in experimental colitis. *Br J Surg* 1993;80:512–516.

298. Schoeffel U, Jaeger D, Pelz K, Salm R, Farthmann EH. Effect of human bowel wall distension on translocation of indigenous bacteria and endotoxins. *Dig Dis Sci* 1994;39:490–493.

299. Berg RD, Promotions of the translocation from the gastrointestinal tracts of mice by oral treatment with penicillin, clindamycin or metronidazole. *Infect Immun* 1981;33:854–861.

300. Berg RD. Bacterial translocation from the gastrointestinal tracts of mice receiving immunosuppressive chemotherapeutic agents. *Curr Microbiol* 1983;8:285–292.

301. Gautreaux MD, Deitch EA, Berg RD. T lymphocytes in host defense against bacterial translocation from the gastrointestinal tract. *Infect Immun* 1994;62:2874–2884.

302. Seale JP, Compton MR. Side-effects of corticosteroid agents. *Med J Aust* 1986;144:139–142.

303. Singleton JW, Law DH, Kelley ML, Jr., Mekhjian HS, Studevant RA. National Cooperative Crohn's Disease Study: adverse reactions to study drugs. *Gastroenterology* 1979;77: 870–882.

304. Malchow H, Ewe K, Brandes JW, et al. European Cooperative Crohn's Disease Study (ECCDS): results of drug treatment. *Gastroenterology* 1984;86:249–266.

305. Felder JB, Adler DJ, Korelitz BI. The safety of corticosteroid therapy in Crohn's disease with an abdominal mass. *Am J Gastroenterol* 1991;86:1450–1455.

306. Present DH, Meltzer SJ, Krumholz MP, Wolke A, Korelitz BI. 6-Mercaputopurine in the management of inflammatory bowel disease: short- and long-term toxicity. *Ann Intern Med* 1989; 111:641–649.

307. Baert F, Hanauer S. CYA in severe steroid-resistant UC: long-term results of therapy. *Gastroenterology* 1994;106(Suppl): A648.

308. Kozarek R, Bedard C, Patterson D, et al. Cyclosporin (Cy) use in the precolectomy chronic ulcerative colitis (CUC) pt in the Pacific northwest. *Gastroenterology* 1994;106(Suppl):A715.

309. Madden MV, McIntyre AS, Nicholls RJ. Double-blind cross-over trial of metronidazole versus placebo in chronic unremitting pouchitis *Dig Dis Sci* 1994;39:1193–1196.

310. Becker JM, Onderdonk AB. Bacterial dysbiosis in the pathogenesis of ileal pouchitis. *Gastroenterology* 1994;106:A650.

311. Ruseler-van Embden JH, Schoten WR, Lieshout LM. Pouchitis: result of microbial imbalance? *Gut* 1994;35:658–664.

312. Lobo AJ, Sagar PM, Rothwell J, et al. Carriage of adhesive *Escherichia coli* after restorative proctocolectomy and pouch anal anastomosis: relation with functional outcome and inflammation. *Gut* 1993;34:1379–1383.

313. Becker JM, Raymond JL. Ileal pouch–anal anastomosis. A single surgeon's experience with 100 consecutive cases. *Ann Surg* 1986;204:375–383.

Infections of the Gastrointestinal Tract,
edited by M. J. Blaser, P. D. Smith, J. I. Ravdin,
H. B. Greenberg, and R. L. Guerrant
Raven Press, Ltd., New York © 1995.

CHAPTER **33**

Esophageal Infections in HIV-1 Disease

Phillip D. Smith

The esophagus is a frequent site of infection by opportunistic pathogens in immunocompromised persons (1,2). Among patients with the acquired immunodeficiency syndrome (AIDS), such infections cause esophageal symptoms in 30–40% of cases (3–5) and represent the second most common gastrointestinal manifestation of AIDS. The esophageal symptoms caused by these infections include dysphagia (difficulty swallowing), odynophagia (painful swallowing), and, less frequently, substernal chest pain independent of deglutition. No one symptom or combination of symptoms is specifically associated with a particular infection. Consequently, the presence of exclusively dysphagia or odynophagia is an unreliable predictor of the etiology of the esophageal disease.

The infectious agents that cause esophageal disease in persons infected with human immunodeficiency virus type 1 (HIV-1), the causative agent of AIDS, include an array of fungal, viral, bacterial, and protozoal pathogens (Table 1). The majority of esophageal infections, however, are caused by three pathogens: *Candida albicans,* cytomegalovirus (CMV), and herpes simplex virus (HSV). These pathogens cause substantial morbidity in HIV-1–infected persons. The morbidity is due to the esophageal symptoms themselves as well as the secondary reduction in oral nutrition and the consequent decrease in caloric intake. Reduced caloric intake exacerbates the weight loss and cachexia that characterizes HIV-1 infection, particularly when diarrhea and malabsorption are present. In addition to infectious agents, non-infectious processes, including neoplasms, drugs, and acid peptic disease (Table 1), cause esophageal disease or injury in HIV-1–infected persons, although such manifestations are less common. This chapter reviews HIV-1–associated ulcerative disease of the esophagus and esophagitis caused by *C. albicans,* CMV, and herpes simplex virus in HIV-1–infected persons.

P. D. Smith: Department of Medicine and Microbiology, Division of Gastroenterology and Hepatology, Center for AIDS Research, University of Alabama School of Medicine, Birmingham, Alabama 35294.

HIV-1 ESOPHAGEAL ULCERATION

Description

The presence of esophageal ulcers without detectable opportunistic pathogens is now recognized as an important complication of HIV-1 infection (6). Aphthous ulcerations of the oral cavity and esophagus (7,8) likely represent a variation of HIV-1–associated ulcers. Histology of the lesions shows epithelial necrosis, accumulation of mononuclear and polymorphonuclear inflammatory cells, and collagen deposition. Histology and culture of biopsy specimens from the ulcer are negative for known pathogens, although *Candida* sp. may occasionally be present superficially, consistent with secondary infection. Electron microscopy (9), *in situ* hybridization (10,11), immunohistochemical staining (11), and coculture techniques (12) have revealed retrovirus-like particles or HIV-1 in association with the ulcers.

Pathogenesis

The pathogenesis of esophageal ulcerations in HIV-1–infected persons is likely multifactorial. During acute HIV-1 infection, high-titer viremia (13–15) presumably delivers high levels of virus to the tissues, including the esophagus. Since HIV-1 is capable of inducing inflammatory cytokines, such as interleukin-1 (16,17) and tumor necrosis factor–α (18–21), increased levels of these cytokines in esophageal mucosa would promote inflammation and its pathological sequelae. During late stage HIV-1 disease, however, the immunopathophysiology of alimentary tract mucosa is substantially altered, reflected in the suppression of local immune responses, dysregulation of cytokine production, and the presence of mild inflammation (22). These changes predispose the mucosa to increased numbers of HIV-1–infected mononuclear cells and likely account for our recent observation that HIV-1–expressing cells are 6- to 60-fold more prevalent in esophageal mucosa than in peripheral lymph nodes (23).

TABLE 1. *Reported causes of esophageal disease in HIV-1–infected persons*

Infectious agent	Neoplasm	Other
Fungal:	Kaposi's sarcoma	Zidovadine
Candida albicans	Lymphoma	Zalcitabine
Torulopsis glabrata	Squamous cell carcinoma	Reflux esophagitis
Histoplasma capsulatum		
Viral:		
Cytomegalovirus		
Herpes simplex virus		
Human immunodeficiency virus type 1		
Epstein–Barr virus		
Bacterial:		
Mycobacterium avium complex		
Mycobacterium tuberculosis		
Bacteriosis (unidentified)		
Protozoal:		
Cryptosporidium		
Pneumocystis carinii		
Leishmania sp.		

Adapted from ref. 68.

Thus, during late stage HIV-1 disease, the alimentary tract mucosa, including that of the esophagus, is a target for HIV-1–infected mononuclear cells and a site of increased levels of proinflammatory cytokines (24).

The association between the presence of HIV-1 in esophageal mucosa and esophageal ulceration, however, does not necessarily indicate that HIV-1 is the causative agent. We recently showed that in patients with AIDS the presence of HIV-1–infected mononuclear cells in esophageal lamina propria is not associated with localized accumulation of inflammatory cells, ulceration, or a specific esophageal symptom (25). Rather, the odynophagia and dysphagia were due to esophagitis caused by opportunistic agents or a pathological process such as Kaposi's sarcoma. Thus, alternative explanations for esophageal ulcerations in HIV-1–infected persons without detectable esophageal pathogens include missed diagnosis of known opportunistic microorganisms or infection by still undiscovered infectious agents. The ability to identify esophageal opportunistic pathogens or pathological processes in the vast majority of AIDS patients with esophageal symptoms (25) indicates that a vigorous diagnostic evaluation should be pursued before esophageal ulcerations are attributed to HIV-1.

Epidemiology

The epidemiology of HIV-1–associated ulcers has not been critically evaluated. Overall, they appear to be less common than CMV and HSV esophageal disease.

Clinical Features

Typically, patients with HIV-1–associated esophageal ulcers present with odynophagia and, less frequently, dysphagia, substernal chest pain, or a burning sensation independent of deglutition. Symptoms may be sufficiently se-

vere to limit the intake of food, thereby exacerbating the weight loss that accompanies HIV-1 infection. As shown in Fig. 1, the ulcers have well-demarcated edges, vary in size (usually 1–5 cm²), and occur throughout the esophagus as solitary or, more commonly, multiple lesions with normal intervening mucosa.

Differential Diagnosis

CMV is the most common cause of solitary esophageal ulcers in HIV-1–infected persons. In contrast to HIV-

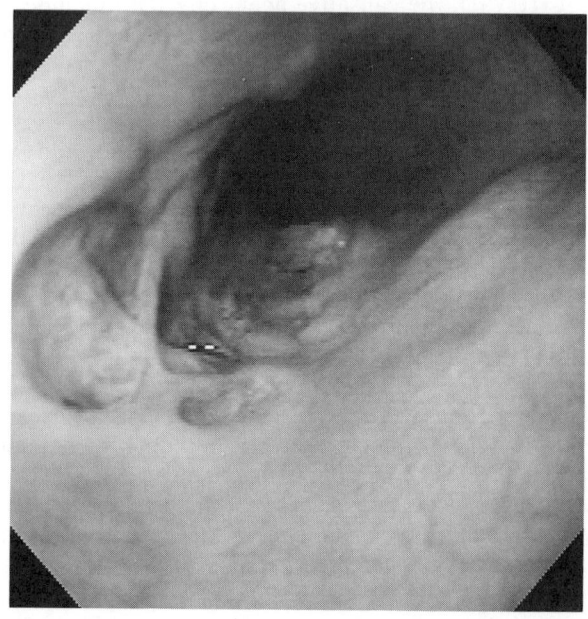

FIG. 1. Endoscopic photograph of two HIV-1–associated ulcers in which no other pathogens were identified. Note normal intervening mucosa. (Courtesy of C. M. Wilcox.) (See Plate 3.)

1–associated ulcers, however, CMV ulceration may be hemorrhagic and occasionally surrounded by inflamed mucosa. Esophageal ulcers caused by HSV are easily identified by the presence of multiple small vesicular erosions that coalesce into large superficial ulcerations. Rare causes of esophageal ulcers include Epstein–Barr virus (26), *Mycobacterium tuberculosis* (27,28), *Mycobacterium avium* complex (29), and *Torulopsis glabrata* (30). Mycobacterial ulcerations typically occur in the presence of severe eophagitis or an inflammatory mass. Finally, zidovudine (31) and zalcitabine (32) pill-induced injury may result in solitary midesophageal ulcers.

Diagnostic Measures

The definitive procedure for the evaluation of esophageal ulcers is esophagoscopy. This procedure allows both visual inspection and directed biopsy of abnormal mucosa. In a retrospective study of the role of endoscopy in the evaluation of gastrointestinal disease in HIV-1–infected persons, esophagoscopy yielded a diagnosis either by direct visualization of mucosa or histological evaluation of biopsied material in 94% of patients with esophageal symptoms and abnormal esophageal mucosa (33). The diagnosis of HIV-1–associated ulceration is usually based on the absence of known pathogens. The scientific rigor with which potential pathogens are excluded and the level of molecular techniques (*in situ* hybridization, DNA amplification) used to identify HIV-1 are important factors in establishing HIV-1 as the etiology of esophageal ulcers.

Management

Although the esophageal ulcerations associated with HIV-1 infection may heal spontaneously, the administration of high-dose steroids is effective therapy in many patients. Prednisone 40–60 mg/day given orally or methylprednisolone given intravenously when swallowing is impaired usually provides rapid clinical and endoscopic improvement (7,8,34,35). Steroid therapy should be administered with caution, however, because immunosuppression may be potentiated, leading to increased HIV-1 expression and the acquisition or exacerbation of opportunistic infections. Recently, aphthous ulcers of the oral cavity and esophagus in HIV-1–infected persons were shown to respond to thalidomide (5,36). A prospective trial of thalidimide for esophageal ulcers is currently underway.

Esophageal Ulceration and HIV-1 Progression

HIV-1–associated esophageal ulcers may signal HIV-1 disease progression in three settings. First, odynophagia due to esophageal ulcerations is occasionally the presenting symptom of initial HIV-1 infection (9,12) and the acute mononucleosis-like syndrome (37–39) that occurs in 30–70% of acutely infected persons (40,41). Second, a minority of persons with established acute HIV-1 syndrome may develop oral and esophageal ulceration (9–12,42–50) and candidiasis (14,43,48,50–57) as well as multisystemic complications (40,41). Such persons progress more rapidly to AIDS than those with mild or asymptomatic primary infection (39). In the majority of acutely infected persons the symptoms and high-titer viremia that accompany primary infection resolve shortly after seroconversion, and a period of prolonged clinical latency lasting 8–10 years ensues (58). Third, esophageal ulcerations (or candidiasis) can interrupt clinical latency, heralding rapid acquisition of life-threatening opportunistic infections and progression to AIDS. Thus, esophageal disease may be the presenting manifestation of acute HIV-1 syndrome, indicate rapid progression of acute HIV-1 syndrome to AIDS, or herald accelerated progression of clinical latency to AIDS.

CANDIDA ESOPHAGITIS

Description

C. albicans is a ubiquitous, dimorphic fungus that forms budding yeast, pseudohyphae, and occasionally true septate hyphae. The fungus is commonly present in the normal flora of the oral cavity and gastrointestinal tract of healthy adult humans. In immunocompetent persons, it does not cause esophageal disease and only rarely has been associated with diarrhea (59–61). In HIV-1–infected persons, however, this otherwise nonpathogenic commensal causes superficial mucosal disease of the oropharynx and esophagus. Indeed, the presence of oral candidiasis in persons at risk for AIDS is associated with the development of an AIDS-related infection or Kaposi's sarcoma in 60% of cases within 2 years (62).

Pathogenesis

The gastrointestinal tract is a reservoir for *Candida,* but the factors responsible for the change from asymptomatic commensal to esophageal pathogen are unclear. *Candida* overgrowth occurs throughout the esophagus, although more frequently in the distal region. Proliferation and overgrowth of the fungus in the superficial mucosa leads to keratinization and the raised "cheesy" white plaques that are pathognomonic of *Candida* esophagitis (Fig. 2). Histological examination of biopsy specimens from patients with esophageal candidiasis shows local invasion of the lamina propria but the absence of extension into the submucosa. The absence of penetration and disseminated candidiasis in HIV-1–infected persons is likely due to the relatively intact function of polymorphonuclear neutrophils in patients with even late stage HIV-1 disease.

The mechanism by which *Candida* causes mucosal inflammation is not known, but the mechanical shearing forces of the esophagus have been suggested to tear the mucosa underlying *Candida* microabscesses, leading to

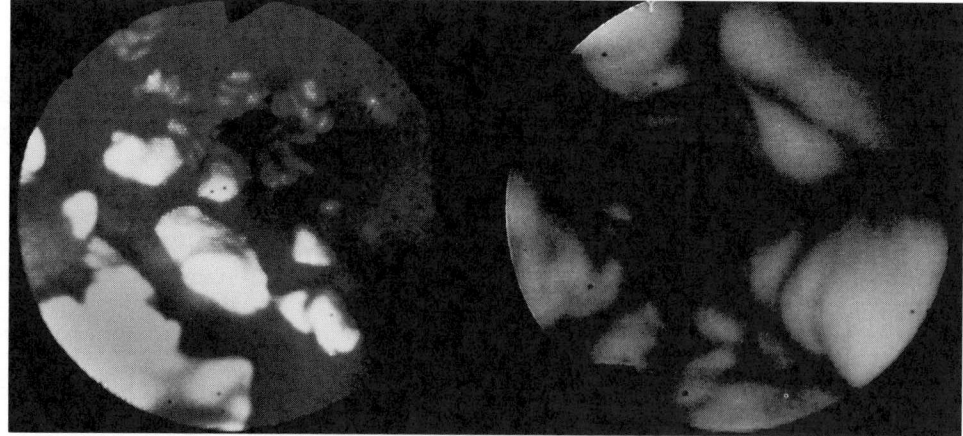

FIG. 2. Endoscopic appearance of *Candida* esophagitis. **Left:** Multiple exudative white plaques surrounded by inflamed erythematous mucosa. **Right:** Circumferential inflammatory membrane covering inflamed mucosa in a patient with severe *Candida* esophagitis.

ulceration (63). As summarized in Table 2, the similarity in phenotype and DNA characteristics among *C. albicans* isolated from AIDS patients and seronegative control subjects indicates that the candidiasis associated with AIDS is not caused by a virulent or unique strain of the organism (64). Rather, mucosal candidiasis in HIV-1–infected persons is likely the consequence of the proliferation of common isolates due to impaired local host defense mechanisms, in particular mononuclear cell antifungal activities.

Epidemiology

Although infection of the oropharynx and esophagus by *C. albicans* may occur independently, symptomatic candidiasis of both sites commonly occurs in the same patient. The frequency of infection in both locations has practical importance for the clinician and has been the subject of several studies. In an early study (65), 100% of ten AIDS patients with oral candidiasis (thrush) with or without esophageal symptoms had esophageal candidiasis. Subsequently, the sensitivity of thrush and esophageal symptoms as markers for esophageal candidiasis was reported to be 88% and 60%, respectively, and their specificity 81% and 100%, respectively (Table 3) (66). Combining both clinical parameters increased the sensitivity to 93% and specificity to 100%, and gave predictive values

of 100% for the presence of *Candida* esophagitis when both thrush and esophageal symptoms were present and 96% for the absence of *Candida* esophagitis when thrush and esophageal symptoms were absent (66).

Recently, larger studies of the predictive value of thrush and esophageal symptoms revealed that only 71–87% of AIDS patients with both clinical parameters have esophageal candidiasis (5,67). Moreover, approximately 40% of patients with esophageal symptoms reportedly have no thrush (67). Complicating the association between oral and esophageal candidiasis are observations that esophageal candidiasis may be asymptomatic (63,65). Thus, the presence of thrush and esophageal symptoms in an HIV-1–infected person, particularly after AIDS has developed, should alert the clinician to the possibility of concomitant esophageal candidiasis; however, the predictive value of thrush as a marker for esophageal candidiasis is less reliable than originally thought.

Clinical Features

Irrespective of the presence of oral infection, *C. albicans* is the most common cause of esophagitis in persons infected with HIV-1 (Table 4) (5,25,67). Esophageal candidiasis is associated with both odynophagia and dysphagia. Although odynophagia may occur more frequently

---

TABLE 2. *Similarities among isolates of* C. albicans *from AIDS patients and healthy subjects*

1. Resistance to 5-fluorocytosine
2. Induced synthesis of amino acids and nucleotides
3. Sugar utilization pattern
4. Enzyme (alkaline phosphatase, esterase, etc.) activity pattern
5. Restriction fragment length polymorphism of DNA
6. Frequency of the dimorphic DNA band encoding ribosomal RNA

Adapted from ref. 64.

TABLE 3. *Predictive value (%) of oral candidiasis and esophageal symptoms for* Candida *esophagitis in HIV-1–infected patients*

Condition	Sensitivity	Specificity	Predictive value	
			Positive	Negative
Oral candidiasis	88	81	81	88
Esophageal symptoms	60	100	100	73
Both	93	100	100	96

Adapted from ref. 66.

TABLE 4. *Esophageal disease in 25 AIDS patients with dysphagia and/or odynophagia*

Disease process	Number[a] n = 25(%)
C. albicans	15 (60%)
Cytomegalovirus	4 (16%)
Herpes simplex virus	4 (16%)
Kaposi's sarcoma	3 (12%)
Herpes zoster	1 (4%)
Mycobacterium avium complex	1 (4%)

Adapted from ref. 25.

[a] Three patients had two infections.

(65), neither symptom is predictive of *Candida* esophagitis. The symptoms occur with variable intensity, and the dysphagia may be associated with swallowing both solids and liquids. Occasionally, substernal chest pain is the primary symptom. Endoscopically, the pathognomonic lesion is a patchy or circumferential white plaque or membrane (containing exudate and fungal elements) overlying inflamed mucosa (Fig. 2).

Differential Diagnosis

As listed in Table 1, an array of infectious and noninfectious factors are responsible for symptomatic esophageal disease in HIV-1–infected persons. *C. albicans,* CMV, and HSV account for the majority of the causes and therefore must always be considered in the differential diagnosis. Moreover, approximately 20% of HIV-1–infected persons with symptomatic esophagitis have two of these opportunistic pathogens as the cause of their esophageal disease (25,63,67).

Diagnostic Measures

Esophageal symptoms in HIV-1–infected persons should be thoroughly evaluated with an appropriate diagnostic test for the following reasons. First, a particular esophageal symptom is not diagnostic of a specific pathogen. Second, oral thrush is not predictive of esophageal candidiasis. Third, *C. albicans* is the cause of the esophagitis in only about 50–60% of cases, and more than one pathogen may be present in 20% of cases. Fourth, therapy is available for the major causes of infectious esophageal disease in HIV-1–infected persons.

Barium esophagography and fiberoptic esophagoscopy are the two diagnostic modalities currently available for evaluating esophageal disease in HIV-1–infected patients. As reviewed by Wilcox (68), double-contrast barium esophagography is safe, noninvasive, and less expensive than barium esophagography. The characteristic radiographic feature of *Candida* esophagitis is multiple plaque-like lesions that give the esophagus a ragged or "shaggy" appearance. In contrast, esophagoscopy allows direct visualization and biopsy of the mucosa. In a comparison of the diagnostic accuracy of double-contrast barium eso-

phagography and esophagoscopy, Connolly et al. (69) showed that a correct and complete diagnosis was made radiographically in 30% of cases and endoscopically in 96%. Double-contrast barium radiography had a sensitivity of 25% and specificity of 100%, whereas endoscopy had a sensitivity of 98% and specificity of 100%. Thus, *Candida* esophagitis can be reliably diagnosed endoscopically by the presence of a white membrane or plaques overlying inflamed mucosa; histological identification of yeast and pseudohyphae in esophageal biopsies and cytological identification of these forms in brushing specimens confirm the endoscopic diagnosis but by themselves are not diagnostic since they may be present when the esophageal mucosa is endoscopically normal (67).

Management

C. albicans is one of the most readily treatable AIDS-defining opportunistic pathogens. A variety of topical agents, including nystatin, clotrimazole, and miconazole; oral agents, including ketoconazole, itraconazole, fluconazole, and 5-flucytosine; and the intravenous agent amphotericin B have been used to successfully treat *Candida* esophagitis (70–76). For oropharyngeal candidiasis, clotrimazole troches 10 mg five times daily or oral nystatin solution or tablets 500,000–1,000,000 units three to five times daily have been effective and relatively inexpensive (76–78). However, the inconvenience of multiple daily doses and treatment failures (79) have lead to the use of ketoconazole and fluconazole for oral candidiasis. Comparison of ketoconazole with fluconazole for oropharyngeal candidiasis in a randomized double-blind trial showed cure rates of 75% and 100% with ketoconazole (200 mg orally per day) and fluconazole (50 mg orally per day), respectively (80). Because of its higher cure rate and fewer side effects (see below), fluconzole is the oral agent of choice for oropharyngeal candidiasis and has been shown to be effective at preventing recurrences (78). Recently, a single oral dose of 150 mg of fluconazole was shown to be as effective as a daily oral dose of 50 mg for 7 days in curing oral candidiasis and preventing relapse during a 2-week follow-up (81).

For patients with esophageal candidiasis, topical agents are ineffective. Currently, fluconazole 100–200 mg orally once per day for 2–3 weeks is the drug of choice (78). In a multicenter, randomized, double-blind trial comparing fluconazole with ketoconazole therapy for *Candida* esophagitis, endoscopic cure occurred in 91% of patients with fluconzole and 52% with ketoconazole, and symptomatic cure occurred in 85% of patients with fluconazole and 65% with ketoconazole (82). Both drugs are generally safe and well tolerated (82,83). The major side effects of fluconazole are nausea, skin rash, and increases in hepatic aminotransferase levels; hepatic necrosis has occurred in a few patients. Also, fluconazole can be absorbed in the absence of gastric acid, which is a potentially important advantage since hypochlorhydria may be associated with AIDS (84). In contrast, ketoconazole absorption is dependent on the presence of acid. For fluconazole-resistant *C.*

albicans, amphotericin B 0.3 mg/kg intravenously daily for 7 days is the treatment of choice.

CYTOMEGALOVIRUS ESOPHAGEAL DISEASE

Description

CMV is one of the most common opportunistic pathogens in persons infected with HIV-1. Although serious gastrointestinal disease due to CMV occurs in only about 3% of cases (85), all organs of the gastrointestinal tract can be involved (86). In the esophagus, the principal manifestations of CMV disease are esophagitis, ulcerations, and, infrequently, pseudotumor.

Microbiology

CMV is a double-stranded DNA virus in the herpesviridae family. The naked virus is a spherical DNA–protein complex core surrounded by an icosahedral capsid with 162 capsomeres. It accumulates in nuclear and cytoplasmic inclusions of cells permissive to infection, such as endothelial and mononuclear cells, acquiring a single or double membrane upon budding from the nuclear and cytoplasmic membrane. The accumulation of viral particles in the nucleus and cytoplasm produces enlargement of the cell and the characteristic nuclear and cytoplasmic inclusions. After infection, the virus enters a latent phase during which CMV can be detected in certain cells, including circulating monocytes and lymphocytes, by molecular techniques but not cultured from these cells (87). This period of nonproductive latency can be interrupted when the host becomes immunosuppressed, such as during HIV-1 infection. As immunosuppression progresses, host antiviral mechanisms, including the natural killer (NK) and CMV-specific cytotoxic activities of lymphocytes, become depressed (88), and infection becomes productive. CMV can then be cultured from a variety of cells, including circulating mononuclear and polymorphonuclear cells; body fluids, such as semen and cervical secretions; and tissues, including the alimentary tract mucosa.

Pathogenesis

The reaction of latently infected cells and the wide dissemination of productively infected cells likely contribute to the expression of CMV in esophageal mucosa. The inflammation associated with CMV infection of esophageal mucosa is similar to that of other tissues and is characterized by the presence of cytomegalic inclusion cells, increased numbers of inflammatory cells, and frequently, although not invariably, vasculitis. The mechanism(s) by which the virus causes this inflammatory response is unclear, but investigations are currently underway to clarify this issue.

The intimate association between CMV and ulcerative lesions of the esophagus implicates the virus in pathogenesis of these lesions (89). This notion is supported by observations that the presence of increasing numbers of CMV inclusion cells in the mucosa of the esophagus, as well as other regions of the gastrointestinal tract, correlates directly with increasing grades of inflammation (90). Genta et al. (91) used *in situ* hybridization and immunohistochemistry to identify CMV in endothelial cells, enterocytes, fibroblasts, smooth muscle cells, and macrophages in the mucosa of the perforated ileum from an HIV-1–infected patient. Although previous reports suggested that CMV infection of endothelial cells and the associated vasculitis leads to vascular obstruction, ischemia, and tissue damage (92,93), the absence of vasculitis in the tissues studied by Genta (91) suggests that CMV causes local mucosal damage by a mechanism other than occlusive vasculitis. In this regard, we have shown that CMV-infected mucosal macrophages *in vivo* and peripheral blood monocytes *in vitro* express abundant levels of mRNA for tumor necrosis factor-α (TNF-α), a potent proinflammatory cytokine (94). Moreover, when the CMV-infected monocytes were stimulated with bacterial lipopolysaccharide, they produced levels of TNF-α peptide several fold greater than uninfected monocytes. Taken together, these data suggest that most cellular components of the mucosa are permissive to CMV infection and that CMV may prime some cells, such as lamina propria macrophages, causing increased transcription of cytokine mRNA. Secondary stimulation by bacterial products, which are abundant in the mucosa, activate the CMV-primed cells, leading to message translation and enhanced production of inflammatory cytokines. Other components of the mechanism(s) by which CMV induces mucosal inflammation are currently under investigation.

Epidemiology

In the largest study to date, CMV was the second most common cause of esophageal disease among 110 HIV-1–infected persons with esophageal symptoms (67). In smaller studies involving 20–48 patients (5,25,63), CMV and herpes simplex virus were equally common after *Candida* esophagitis as causes of esophageal disease. Among HIV-1–infected persons with esophageal symptoms, 10–20% have two and occasionally three opportunistic infections of the esophagus (5,25,67), and CMV is commonly a cause of one of these infections.

Clinical Features

The presenting symptoms associated with CMV esophageal disease are odynophagia and, less frequently, dysphagia. Wilcox et al. (94) reported that among 16 patients with CMV esophageal disease, odynophagia alone was present in 88% of cases and dysphagia alone in none. However, odynophagia is not predictive of CMV disease because it commonly accompanies other causes of esophagitis. Endoscopically, ulceration is the characteristic fea-

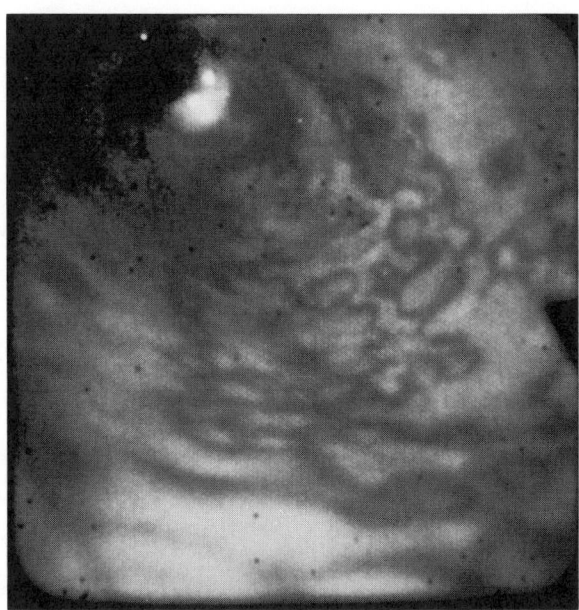

FIG. 3. Endoscopic photograph of a large solitary ulcer caused by CMV in the distal esophagus. (See Plate 4.)

ture of CMV esophagitis (Fig. 3). The ulcers are typically large (>5 cm²), solitary, often hemorrhagic, well demarcated at the edges, and located predominantly, but not exclusively, in the distal esophagus. Smaller ulcers occur and are more commonly located in the mid- and proximal regions of the esophagus. The mucosa between the ulcers usually appears normal.

Erosive inflammation with or without ulceration is the second most frequent manifestation of CMV infection of esophageal mucosa (96,97). In contrast to the normal intervening mucosa associated with CMV ulcers, the mucosa in this setting is diffusely erythematous and friable.

The least common manifestation of CMV esophageal disease is pseudotumor (97). This lesion resembles an exophytic mass, usually located in the distal esophagus, that radiographically and endoscopically may be mistaken for carcinoma.

Differential Diagnosis

The causes of esophageal symptoms that should be considered in the differential of CMV esophageal disease are listed in Table 1. Although odynophagia is more common than dysphagia in HIV-1–infected persons with CMV esophageal disease, the symptom is nonspecific. The differential for large, solitary esophageal ulcers is similar to that of HIV-1–associated ulcers and includes CMV, HIV-1, and Epstein–Barr virus (26). *M. tuberculosis* (27,28) and *Mycobacterium avium* complex (29) may cause ulcerations but usually when diffuse esophagitis or an inflammatory mass is present. The fungus *Torulopsis glabrata* is a rare cause of esophageal ulcers (29). Noninfectious causes of esophageal ulcers include the antiviral agents zidovudine (31) and zalcitabine (32), which can cause mid-esophageal pill-induced injury.

The diffuse esophagitis associated with CMV infection can also accompany infection by most of the other pathogens listed in Table 1. *C. albicans,* however, causes esophagitis that is easily distinguished from diffuse CMV esophagitis by a raised white membrane of fungal elements and exudate overlying the inflammation. The presence of *Candida* esophagitis, however, does not exclude the presence of underlying CMV esophagitis. Herpes simplex virus esophagitis begins with vesicular lesions, but after the lesions erode and coalesce an erosive esophagitis may be seen endoscopically. Novel causes of esophagitis include *Leishmania* sp. in endemic areas (98), cryptosporidiosis of the distal esophagus (99), and bacteriosis by unidentified bacteria (100).

The esophageal pseudotumor associated with CMV infection should be distinguished from processes with a potential for causing a mass-like effect, including Kaposi's sarcoma (25), lymphoma (101), squamous cell carcinoma (102), and *M. avium* complex (29). Although intestinal manifestations are more common, *Histoplasma capsulatum* has been reported to involve the esophagus in association with HIV-1 infection (103).

Diagnostic Measures

The diagnosis of CMV esophageal disease is firmly established by the presence of both endoscopic abnormality (ulcer and/or inflammation) and histological identification of cytomegalic inclusion cells with surrounding inflammation (104,105). Vasculitis may accompany the inflammation, but its presence is not required to diagnose CMV mucosal disease (89,91). Similarly, culture of CMV from a mucosal biopsy supports but is not required for the diagnosis.

Since the severity of inflammation correlates directly with the number of cells infected with CMV, it is reasonable to assume that the more severe the inflammation the greater the likelihood of identifying the pathognomonic inclusion cell. When endoscopic and histological evidence of inflammation is absent, the presence of CMV inclusion cells is consistent with the carrier state without CMV-associated disease. A problem arises, however, when ulcerative or inflammatory changes suggest CMV esophageal disease but CMV inclusion cells are not identified (89). Although the false-negative rate for detecting CMV inclusions in CMV-diseased tissue is not known, one explanation for the inability to detect inclusion cells in this setting is sampling error. The development of more sensitive diagnostic techniques should address this problem.

The newer diagnostic techniques being evaluated for the detection of CMV in gastrointestinal biopsies include immunocytochemical staining (106,107), *in situ* hybrization (107,108), and polymerase chain reaction (PCR) (109). The utility of immunocytochemistry was shown in a retrospective study in which inclusion cells were identified by staining in 92% of colon biopsies, whereas CMV was cultured in only 30% (105). Wu et al. (107) showed that *in situ* hybridization for CMV DNA was more sensitive than immunostaining and more sensitive than routine staining with hematoxylin and eosin for the detection of

CMV. The most promising and potentially sensitive and specific technique for detecting CMV gastrointestinal biopsies appears to be amplification of CMV DNA by PCR, which for enteric infection has a sensitivity of 92% and a specificity of 93–100% (109). These techniques may become more widely available after issues related to expense, the level of expertise required to perform the procedure, and the labor-intensive nature of performing the assays have been resolved.

Management

In response to the AIDS epidemic, substantial progress has been made toward the development of effective antiviral agents. The availability of agents such as ganciclovir and foscarnet offer reason for cautious optimism in the management of HIV-1–infected patients with CMV esophageal disease. Gancilovir [9-(1,3-cbdihydroxy-2-propoxymethyl)guanidine] is a nucleoside analog that inhibits replication of CMV DNA through its triphosphate derivative, which is a substrate and potent inhibitor of CMV DNA polymerase. In early uncontrolled studies in HIV-1–infected patients (110–115), ganciclovir reduced or stabilized the signs and symptoms of esophageal as well as enteric CMV disease in 63–100% of cases and lowered or cleared CMV from available culture sites in 68–100%. However, in the only randomized, double-blind, placebo–controlled study of ganciclovir therapy for CMV colitis, the drug reduced colonic inflammation, the number of colon cultures positive for CMV, and extracolonic disease, but did not significantly reduce the diarrhea, abdominal pain, or fever (116). The current recommended dose is 5 mg/kg intravenously twice daily for 14–21 days; side effects include neutropenia and thrombocytopenia, which are usually reversed after withdrawal, as well as confusion, rash, fever, nausea, vomiting, and diarrhea (114,115). Toxicity may be increased when the drug is used with zidovudine. In addition to side effects, the emergence of resistance and recurrence after termination of therapy are important clinical problems. Approximately 8% of patients treated with ganciclovir secrete resistant strains after 3 months of therapy (117). Because the drug is virustatic and not virucidal, recurrence will occur in the majority of patients after withdrawal of the drug. Thus, ganciclovir therapy should be individualized, with careful monitoring of patient improvement, potential side effects, and viral cultures.

Foscarnet (trisodium phosphonoformate) was developed in response to the emergence of ganciclovir-resistant CMV strains and refractory CMV disease. Shown to be effective for the treatment of CMV disease of other organs, foscarnet therapy was reported to induce remission of CMV esophageal ulceration within 2 weeks in 83% of patients (118). In this uncontrolled study, only 20% of 15 patients had a recurrence during 9 months of follow-up. The recommended dose of foscarnet is 60 mg/kg intravenously three times daily or 90 mg/kg intravenously twice daily for 14–21 days; side effects include renal dysfunction, seizures and other central nervous system disturbances, nausea, vomiting, and alterations in the levels of calcium, phosphate, potassium, and magnesium (119). Because recurrent disease is a potential problem, careful monitoring of the patient's clinical course is an important component of effective management.

HERPES SIMPLEX VIRUS

Description

Chronic HSV infection in homosexual men was one of the first infections to signal the emergence of AIDS (120). Since that initial description, HSV has remained one of the most prevalent opportunistic pathogens in persons infected with HIV-1.

Microbiology

HSV is a member of the herpesviridae family of viruses. Accordingly, its physical structure and replication cycle resemble that of other members of the group, such as that of CMV discussed above. Briefly, HSV is a double-stranded DNA virus composed of a DNA-protein core, an icosahedral capsid with 162 capsomeres, and a lipid-containing outer membrane. Key features of the life cycle include DNA replication in the host cell nucleus, assembly of the capsid in the cytoplasm, acquisition of the protein envelope upon budding from the nucleus, and lysis of the cell (except the neuron) with release of progeny virions. HSV establishes nonproductive latency in sensory nerve ganglia; reactivation of latent virus may occur in response to immunosuppression (HIV-1 infection), disruption of the skin (burns), and malnutrition (chronic hyperalimentation).

Pathogenesis

The pathogenesis of HSV disease of the esophageal mucosa likely follows the principles of infection of other mucocutaneous sites. As cell-mediated (NK and virus-specific cytotoxic lymphocyte) activity and humoral function deteriorates in response to HIV-1, HSV within sensory nerve ganglia is reactivated and the virus begins to spread peripherally along sensory nerve pathways. After reaching mucocutaneous sites, HSV spreads among epithelial cells by lysis and releases infectious virions that then infect and lyse adjacent cells. Small superficial vesicular lesions with an inflammatory base develop in response to the infection and lysis of epithelial cells. As infection spreads, the resulting small foci of necrotic epithelium become progressively more confluent, resulting in the development of superficial erosions and ulcerations.

Epidemiology

Since its initial description in the first patients with AIDS, HSV has remained a common problem in this population. The prevalence of HSV infections among AIDS patients has been reported to be 30% (121). In most studies (5,63,67), HSV is the third most frequent cause of esophagitis among HIV-1–infected persons, accounting for 4–14% of cases. As discussed above, approximately 25% of patients with esophagitis are coinfected with two, and sometime three, opportunistic pathogens, including HSV.

Clinical Features

The symptoms of HSV esophagitis are similar to those of *C. albicans* and CMV. Odynophagia and dysphagia occur, although odynophagia is the predominant symptom. Three progressive stages of mucosal abnormality have been observed endoscopically: first, discrete raised vesicles; second, coalescence of the vesicles into larger 0.5- to 2-cm^2 lesions with raised borders; and third, diffuse mucosal erosions and ulcerative esophagitis (122). The areas of erosion and ulceration may be hemorrhagic.

Differential Diagnosis

Because the symptoms of HSV are nonspecific, the differential diagnosis is similar to that of *C. albicans* and CMV esophageal disease. This differential includes the infectious agents listed in Table 1. The potential etiologies can be narrowed, however, when endoscopic visualization shows the characteristic mucosal changes described above (Fig. 4). Next to HSV, the most likely diagnosis is diffuse CMV esophagitis. Because advanced HSV lesions may have overlying plaques of exudate (122), *Candida* esophagitis is another, albeit less likely, consideration. Since large solitary ulcers and inflammatory mass are not

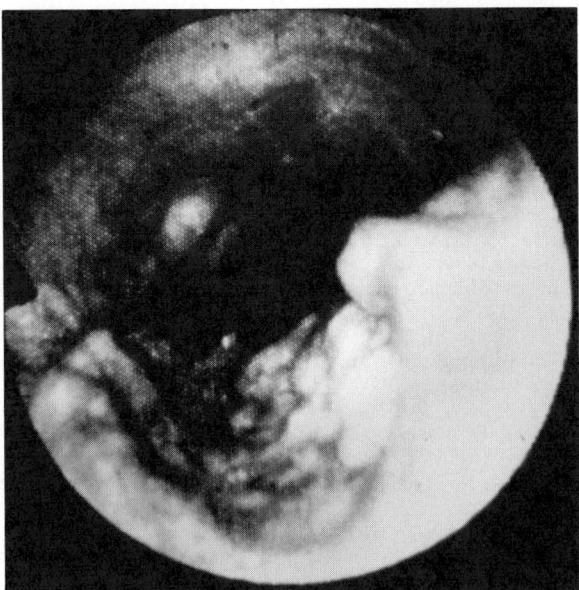

FIG. 4. Endoscopic appearance of multiple vesicular erosions, some of which have coalesced into small superficial ulcers, due to herpes simplex virus esophagitis.

a feature of HSV esophagitis, involvement by the pathogens that cause these manifestations is unlikely.

Diagnostic Measures

The diagnostic procedure of choice is esophagoscopy. Visual inspection may strongly suggest HSV, but the diagnosis is based on cytological identification of intranuclear (Cowdry type A) inclusions in multinucleated cells within a typical lesion and is confirmed by isolation of the virus.

Management

Acyclovir is the drug of choice for HSV esophagitis and is usually effective in reducing or clearing both symptoms and lesions. For primary or recurrent infection, acyclovir 200 mg orally five time per day for 14 days is recommended (119). Acyclovir is generally well tolerated, and the major side effects are nausea, vomiting, headaches, and reversible renal dysfunction with high doses.

Because recurrent HSV is common, long-term suppressive therapy with acyclovir 400 mg orally twice daily may be required (119). However, such therapy is associated with the emergence of resistant strains (123). Therefore, periodic monitoring of susceptibility to acyclovir is important for the early detection of resistance and individualization of therapy (124). Foscarnet 40 mg/kg intravenously three times daily for 21 days is effective for acyclovir-resistant mucocutaneous HSV (118,125). The side effects are discussed in the section on CMV.

In summary, esophageal infections remain a common and potentially debilitating problem for HIV-1–infected persons. Fortunately, effective diagnostic tools, improved therapeutic agents, and appropriate microbiological monitoring have enhanced our ability to meet this important clinical challenge.

ACKNOWLEDGMENTS

This work was supported in part by research grants DK47322 and AI35940 and contracts AI35163, AI45218, and AI45209 from the National Institutes of Health and the Department of Veterans Affairs.

REFERENCES

1. McDonald GB, Sharma P, Hackman RC, Meyers JD, Thomas ED. Esophageal infections in immunocompromised patients after marrow transplantation. *Gastroenterology* 1985;88: 111–117.
2. Wheeler RR, Peacock JE Jr, Cruz JM, Richter JE. Esophagitis in the immunocompromised host: role of esophagoscopy in diagnosis. *Rev Infect Dis* 1987;9:88–96.
3. Gelb A, Miller S. AIDS and gastroenterology. *Am J Gastroenterol* 1986;81:619–622.
4. Frager DH, Frager JD, Brandt LJ, et al. Gastrointestinal complications of AIDS: radiologic features. *Radiology* 1986;158: 597–603.
5. Connolly GM, Hawkins D, Harcourt-Webster JN, Parsons PA, Husain OAN, Gazzard BG. Oesophageal symptoms, their

causes, treatment, and prognosis in patients with acquired immunodeficiency syndrome. *Gut* 1989;30:1033–1039.

6. Wilcox CM, Schwartz DA. Endoscopic characterization of idiopathic esophageal ulceration associated with human immunodeficiency virus infection. *J Clin Gastroenterol* 1993;16:251–256.

7. Bach MC, Valenti AJ, Howell DA, Smith TJ. Odynophagia from aphthous ulcers of the pharynx and esophagus in the acquired immunodeficiency syndrome. *Ann Intern Med* 1988;109:338–339.

8. Bach MC, Howell DA, Valenti AJ, Smith TJ, Winslow DL. Aphthous ulceration of the gastrointestinal tract in patients with the acquired immunodeficiency syndrome. *Ann Intern Med* 1990;112:465–467.

9. Rabeneck L, Boyko WJ, McLean DM, McLeod WA, Wong KK. Unusual esophageal ulcers containing enveloped virus-like particles in homosexual men. *Gastroenterology* 1986;90:1882–1889.

10. Kotler DP, Wilson CS, Haroutiounian G, Fox CH. Detection of human immunodeficiency virus–1 by ^{35}S-RNA *in situ* hybridization in solitary esophageal ulcers in two patients with the acquired immune deficiency syndrome. *Am J Gastroenterol* 1989;84:313–317.

11. Frager D, Kotler DP, Baer J. Idiopathic esophageal ulceration in the acquired immunodeficiency syndrome: radiologic reappraisal in 10 patients. *Abdom Imag* 1994;19:2–5.

12. Rabeneck L, Popovic M, Gartner S, et al. Acute HIV infection presenting with painful swallowing and esophageal ulcers. *JAMA* 1990;263:2318–2322.

13. Daar ES, Moudgil T, Meyer RD, Ho DD. Transient high levels of viremia in patients with primary human immunodeficiency virus type 1 infection. *N Engl J Med* 1991;324:961–964.

14. Clark SJ, Saag MS, Decker WD, et al. High titers of cytopathic virus in plasma of patients with symptomatic primary HIV-1 infection. *N Engl J Med* 1991;326:954–960.

15. Piatak M, Saag MS, Yang LC, et al. High levels of cytopathic virus in plasma of patients with symptomatic primary HIV-1 infection determined by competitive PCR. *Science* 1993;259:1749–1754.

16. Wahl LM, Corcoran ML, Pyle SW, Arthur LO, Harel-Bellan A, Farrar WL. Human immunodeficiency virus glycoprotein (gp 120) induction of monocyte arachidonic acid metabolites and interleukin 1. *Proc Natl Acad Sci USA* 1989;86:621–625.

17. Clouse KA, Robbins PB, Fernie B, Ostrove JM, Fauci AS. Viral antigen stimulation of the production of human monokines capable of regulating HIV-1 expression. *J Immunol* 1989;143:470–475.

18. Wright SC, Jewett A, Mitsuyasu R, Bonvadia B. Spontaneous cytotoxicity and tumor necrosis factor production by peripheral blood monocytes from AIDS patients. *J Immunol* 1988;141:99–104.

19. Merrill JE, Koyanagi Y, Chen ISY. Interleukin-1 and tumor necrosis factor α can be induced from mononuclear phagocytes by human immunodeficiency virus type 1 binding to the CD4 receptor. *J Virol* 1989;63:4404–4408.

20. Molina J-M, Scadden DT, Byrn R, Dinarello C, Groopman JE. Production of tumor necrosis factor α and interleukin 1β by monocytic cells infected with human immunodeficiency virus. *J Clin Invest* 1989;84:733–737.

21. Voth R, Rossol S, Klein K, et al. Differential gene expression of INF-γ and tumor necrosis factor-α in peripheral blood mononuclear cells from patients with AIDS related complex and AIDS. *J Immunol* 1990;144:970–975.

22. Smith PD. Mucosal immunopathophysiology of HIV infection. In: Ogra PH, Mestecky JF, Lamm M, Strober W, McGhee JR, Bienenstock J, eds. *Handbook of mucosal immunology.* New York: Academic Press; 1994;719–728.

23. Smith PD, Fox CH, Masur H, Winter HS, Alling DW. Quantitative analysis of mononuclear cells expressing HIV-1 RNA in esophageal mucosa. *J Exp Med* 1994;180:1541–1546.

24. Kotler DP, Reka S, Clayton F. Intestinal mucosal inflammation associated with human immunodeficiency virus infection. *Dig Dis Sci* 1993;38:1119–1127.

25. Smith PD, Eisner MS, Manischewitz JF, Gill VJ, Masur H, Fox

26. Kitchen VS, Helbert M, Francis ND, et al. Epstein–Barr virus associated oesophageal ulcers in AIDS. *Gut* 1990;31:1223–1225.

27. Goodman P, Pinero SS, Rance RM, Mansell PWA. Mycobacterial esophagitis in AIDS. *Gastrointest Radiol* 1989;14:103–105.

28. Mokoena T, Shama DM, Ngakane H, Bryer JV. Oesophageal tuberculosis: a review of eleven cases. *Postgrad Med J* 1992;68:110–115.

29. Wall SD, Ominsky S, Altman DF, et al. Multifocal abnormalities of the gastrointestinal tract in AIDS. *Am J Radiol* 1986;146:1–5.

30. Tom W, Aaron JS. Esophageal ulcers caused by *Torulopsis glabrata* in a patient with acquired immune deficiency syndrome. *Am J Gastroenterol* 1987;82:766–768.

31. Edwards P, Turner J, Gold J, Cooper DA. Esophageal ulceration induced by zidovudine. *Ann Intern Med* 1990;112:65–66.

32. Indorf AS, Pegram PS. Esophageal ulceration related to zalcitabine (ddC). *Ann Intern Med* 1992;117:133–134.

33. Bonacini M, Skodras G. Gastrointestinal endoscopic pathology in patients seropositive for human immunodeficiency virus. *Missouri Med* 1993;90:85–89.

34. Wilcox CM, Schwartz DA. A pilot study of oral corticosteroid therapy for idiopathic esophageal ulcerations associated with human immunodeficiency virus infection. *Am J Med* 1992;98:131–134.

35. Kotler DP, Reka S, Orenstein JM, Fox CH. Chronic idiopathic esophageal ulceration in the acquired immunodeficiency syndrome. Characterization and treatment with steroids. *J Clin Gastroenterol* 1992;15:284–290.

36. Youle M, Clarbour J, Farthing C, et al. Treatment of resistant aphthous ulceration with thalidomide in patients positive for HIV antibody. *Br Med J* 1989;298:432.

37. Cooper DA, Gold J, Maclean P, Donovan B, et al. Acute AIDS retrovirus infection. Definition of a clinical illness associated with seroconversion. *Lancet* 1985;1:537–540.

38. Tindall B, Barker S, Donovan B, et al. Characterization of the acute clinical illness associated with human immunodeficiency virus infection. *Arch Intern Med* 1988;148:945–949.

39. Pederson C, Lindhardt BO, Jensen BL, et al. Clinical course of primary HIV infection: consequences for subsequent course of infection. *Br Med J* 1988;299:154–157.

40. Tindall B, Cooper DA. Primary HIV infection: host responses and intervention strategies. *AIDS* 1991;5:1–14.

41. Clark SJ, Shaw GM. The acute retroviral syndrome and the pathogenesis of HIV-1 infection. *Semin Immunol* 1993;15:149–155.

42. Bigger R, Johnson B, Musoke S, et al. Severe illness associated with appearance of antibody to human immunodeficiency virus in an African. *Br Med J* 1986;293:1210–1211.

43. Biggs B, Newton-John HF. Acute HTLV-III infection. A case from onset to seroconversion. *Med J Aust* 1986;144:545–547.

44. Lindskov R, Lindhart BO, Weismann K, et al. Acute HTLV-III infection with roseola-like rash. *Lancet* 1986;1:447.

45. Denning DW, Amos A, Wall RA. Oral and cutaneous features of acute human immunodeficiency virus infection. *Cutis* 1987;40:171–175.

46. von Sydow M, Gaines H, Sonnerborg A, Forsgren M, Pehrson PO, Strnnegard O. Antigen detection in primary infection. *Br Med J* 1988;296:238–240.

47. McMillan A, Bishop PE, Aw D, Peutherer JF. Immunohistology of the skin rash associated with acute HIV infection. *AIDS* 1989;3:309–312.

48. Hillman RJ, Tomlinson D, Taylor RD. Acute seroconversion to HIV in a male prostitute as a consequence of occupational exposure. *J AIDS* 1990;3:926–927.

49. Zeman A, Conaghy M. Acute infection with human immunodeficiency virus presenting with neurogenic urinary retention. *Genitourin Med* 1990;67:345–347.

50. Chawla SK, Ramani K, Chawla K, LoPresti P, Mahadevia P. Giant esophageal ulcers of AIDS: ultrastructural study. *Am J Gastroenterol* 1994;89:411–415.

51. Rustin M, Ridley C, Smith M, Kelsey M, Parker N. The acute exanthem associated with seroconversion to human T-cell lymphotropic virus III in a homosexual man. *J Infect* 1986;12:161–163.
52. Denning DW, Anderson J, Rudge P, Smith H. Acute myelopathy associated with primary infection with human immunodeficiency virus. *Br Med J* 1987;294:143–144.
53. Wiselka M, Nicholson K, Ward S, Flower A. Acute infection with human immunodeficiency virus associated with facial nerve palsy and neuralgia. *J Infect* 1987;15:189.
54. Cilla G, Perez TE, Furundarena JR, Cuadrado E, Iribarren JA, Neira F. Esophageal candidiasis and immunodeficiency associated with acute HIV infection. *AIDS* 1988;2:399–400.
55. Clotet B, Romeu J, Casals A, et al. Spontaneous resolution of candida esophagitis in a seroconverting patient for HIV antibodies. *Am J Gastroenterol* 1988;83:1433.
56. Dull JS, Sen P, Raffanti S, Middleton JR. Oral candidiasis as a marker for acute retroviral illness. *South Med J* 1991;84:733–735.
57. Pena JM, Martinez-Lopez MA, Arnalich F, Barbado FJ, Vasquez JJ. Esophageal candidiasis associated with acute infection due to human immunodeficiency virus. *Rev Infect Dis* 1991;13:872–875.
58. Schrage LK, Young JM, Fowler MG, Mathieson BJ, Vermund SH. Long-term survivors of HIV-1 infection: definitions and research challenges. *AIDS* 1994;8(suppl. 1):S95–S108.
59. Kane JG, Chretien JH, Garagusi VF. Diarrhea caused by Candida. *Lancet* 1976;1:335–336.
60. Talwar P, Chakrabarti A, Mehta S, Walia BNS, Kumar L, Chugh KS. Fungal diarrhea: association of different fungi and seasonal variation in their incidence. *Mycopathologia* 1990;110:101–105.
61. Gupta JP, Ehrinpreis MN. *Candida*-associated diarrhea in hospitalized patients. *Gastroenterology* 1990;98:780–785.
62. Klein RS, Harris CA, Small CB, Moll B, Lesser M, Friedland GH. Oral candidiasis in high-risk patients as the initial manifestation of the acquired immunodeficiency syndrome. *N Engl J Med* 1984;311:354–358.
63. Gould E, Kory WP, Raskin JB, Ibe MJ, Redlhammer DE. Esophageal biopsy findings in the acquired immunodeficiency syndrome: clinicopathologic correlation in 20 patients. *South Med J* 1988;81:1392–1395.
64. Whelan WL, Kirsch DR, Kwon-Chung KJ, Wahl SM, Smith PD. *Candida albicans* in patients with the acquired immunodeficiency syndrome: absence of a novel or hypervirulent strain. *J Infect Dis* 1990;162:513–518.
65. Tivitian A, Raufman JP, Rosenthal LE. Oral candidiasis as a marker for esophageal candidiasis in the acquired immunodeficiency syndrome. *Ann Intern Med* 1986;104:54–55.
66. Porro GB, Parente F, Cernuschi M. The diagnosis of esophageal candidiasis in patients with acquired immune deficiency syndrome: is endoscopy always necessary? *Am J Gastroenterol* 1989;84:143–146.
67. Bonacini M, Young T, Laine L. The causes of esophageal symptoms in human immunodeficiency virus infection. A prospective study of 110 patients. *Arch Intern Med* 1991;151:1567–1562.
68. Wilcox CM. Esophageal disease in the acquired immunodeficiency syndrome: Etiology, diagnosis, and management. *Am J Med* 1992;92:412–421.
69. Connolly GM, Forbes A, Gleeson JA, Gazzard BG. Investigation of upper gastrointestinal symptoms in patients with AIDS. *AIDS* 1989;3:453–456.
70. Kantrowitz PA, Fleischli DJ, Butler WT. Successful treatment of chronic esophageal moniliasis with a viscous suspension of nystatin. *Gastroenterology* 1969;57:424–430.
71. Medoff G, Dismukes WE, Meade RH III, Moses JM. A new therapeutic approach to *Candida* infections. A preliminary report. *Arch Intern Med* 1972;130:241–245.
72. Lalor E, Rabeneck L. Esophageal candidiasis in AIDS. Successful therapy with clotrimazole vaginal tablets taken by mouth. *Dig Dis Sci* 1991;36:279–281.
73. Deschamps MM, Pape JW, Verdier RI, DeHovitz J, Thomas F, Johnson WD Jr. Treatment of candida esophagitis in AIDS patients. *Am J Gastroenterol* 1988;83:20–21.
74. Fazio RA, Wickremesinghe PC, Arsura EL. Ketoconazole treatment of *Candida* esophagitis—a prospective study of 12 cases. *Am J Gastroenterol* 1983;78:261–264.
75. Smith DE, Midgley J, Allan M, Connolly GM, Gazzard BG. Itraconazole versus ketoconazole in the treatment of oral and oesophageal candidosis in patients infected with HIV. *AIDS* 1991;5:1367–1371.
76. Kirkpatrich CH, Alling DW. Treatment of chronic oral candidiasis with clotrimazole troches. A controlled clinical trial. *N Engl J Med* 1978;299:1201–1204.
77. Drugs for AIDS and associated infections. *Med Lett* 1993;35:79–86.
78. Systemic antifungal drugs. *Med Lett* 1994;36:16–18.
79. Lucatorio FM, Franker C, Hardy WD, Chafey S. Treatment of refractory oral candidiasis with fluconazole. A case report. *Oral Surg* 1991;71:42–44.
80. Dewit S, Weerts D, Goossens H, Clumeck N. Comparison of fluconazole and ketoconazole for oropharyngeal candidiasis in AIDS. *Lancet* 1989;1:746–748.
81. De Wit S, Goossens H, Clumeck N. Single-dose versus 7 days of fluconazole treatment for oral candidiasis in human immunodeficiency virus-infected patients: a prospective, randomized pilot study. *J Infect Dis* 1993;168:1332–1333.
82. Laine L, Dretler RH, Conteas CN, et al. Fluconazole compared with ketoconazole for the treatment of *Candida* esophagitis in AIDS. A randomized trial. *Ann Intern Med* 1992;117:655–660.
83. Gil A, Lavilla P, Valencia E, et al. Safety and efficacy of fluconazole treatment for Candida oesophagitis in AIDS. *Postgrad Med J* 1991;67:548–522.
84. Lake-Bakaar G, Tom W, Lake-Bakaar D, et al. Gastropathy and ketoconazole malabsorption in the acquired immunodeficiency syndrome (AIDS). *Ann Intern Med* 1988;109:471–473.
85. Jacobson MA, Mills J. Serious cytomegalovirus disease in acquired immunodeficiency syndrome (AIDS). Clinical findings, diagnosis, and treatment. *Ann Intern Med* 1988;108:585–594.
86. Smith PD, Quinn TC, Strober W, Janoff EN, Masur H. Gastrointestinal infections in AIDS. *Ann Intern Med* 1992;116:63–77.
87. Rice GPA, Schrier RD, Oldstone MBA. Cytomegalovirus infects human lymphocytes and monocytes: virus expression is restricted to immediate-early gene products. *Proc Natl Acad Sci USA* 1984;81:6134–6138.
88. Rook AH, Masur H, Lane HC, et al. Interleukin-2 enhances the depressed natural killer and cytomegalovirus-specific cytotoxic activities of lymphocytes from patients with acquired immune deficiency syndrome. *J Clin Invest* 1983;72:398–403.
89. Francis ND, Boylston AW, Roberts AHG, Parkin JM, Pinching AJ. Cytomegalovirus infection in gastrointestinal tracts of patients infected with HIV-1 or AIDS. *J Clin Pathol* 1989;42:1055–1064.
90. Hinnant KL, Rotterdam HZ, Bell ET, Tapper ML. Cytomegalovirus infection of the alimentary tract: a clinicopathological correlation. *Am J Gastroenterol* 1986;81:944–950.
91. Genta RM, Bleyzer I, Cate TR, Tandon AK, Yoffe B. In situ hybridization and immunohistochemical analysis of cytomegalovirus-associated ileal perforation. *Gastroenterology* 1993;104:1822–1827.
92. Kyriazis AP, Mitra SK. Multiple cytomegalovirus-related intestinal perforations in patients with acquired immunodeficiency syndrome. Report of two cases and review of the literature. *Arch Pathol Lab Med* 1992;116:495–499.
93. Tatum ET, Sun PCJ, Cohn DL. Cytomegalovirus vasculitis and colon perforation in a patient with the acquired immunodeficiency syndrome. *Pathology* 1989;21:235–238.
94. Smith PD, Saini SS, Raffeld M, Manischewitz JF, Wahl SM. Cytomegalovirus induction of tumor necrosis factor–α by human monocytes and mucosal macrophages. *J Clin Invest* 1992;90:1642–1648.
95. Wilcox CM, Diehl DL, Cello JP, Margaretten W, Jacobson MA. Cytomegalovirus esophagitis in patients with AIDS. A clinical, endoscopic and pathologic correlation. *Ann Intern Med* 1990;113:589–593.
96. Balthazar EJ, Megibow AJ, Hulnick DH. Cytomegalovirus

esophagitis and gastritis in AIDS. *Am J Radiol* 1985;144: 1201–1204.

97. Laguna F, Garcia-Samaniego J, Alonso MJ, Alvarez I, Gonzalez-Lahoz J. Pseudotumoral appearance of cytomegalovirus esophagitis and gastritis in AIDS patients. *Am J Gastroenterol* 1993;88:1108–1111.

98. Villanueva JL, Torre-Cisnoeros J, Jurado R, et al. Leishmania esophagitis in an AIDS patient: an unusual form of visceral leishmaniasis. *Am J Gastroenterol* 1994;89:273–275.

99. Kazlow PG, Shah K, Benkov KJ, Dische R, LeLeiko NS. Esophageal cryptosporidiosis in a child with acquired immune deficiency syndrome. *Gastroenterology* 1986;91:1301–1303.

100. Ezzell JH, Bremer J, Adamec TA. Bacterial esophagitis: an often forgotten cause of odynophagia. *Am J Gastroenterol* 1990;85:296–298.

101. Bernal Z, del Junco GW. Endoscopic and pathologic features of esophageal lymphoma: a report of four cases in patients with acquired immune deficiency syndrome. *Gastrointest Endosc* 1986;32:96–99.

102. Frager DH, Wolf EL, Competiello LS, Frager JD, Klein RS, Beneventano TC. Squamous cell carcinoma of the esophagus in patients with acquired immunodeficiency syndrome. *Gastrointest Radiol* 1988;358–360.

103. Forsmark CE, Wilcox CM, Darragh T, Cello JP. Disseminated histoplasmosis in AIDS: an unusual case of esophageal involvement and gastrointestinal bleeding. *Gastrointest Endosc* 1990; 36:604–605.

104. Smith PD, Lane HC, Gill VJ, et al. Intestinal infections in patients with the acquired immunodeficiency syndrome. *Ann Intern Med* 1988;108:328–333.

105. Smith PD. Infectious diarrheas in patients with AIDS. *Gastroenterol Clin North Am* 1993;22:535–548.

106. Culpepper-Morgan JA, Cutler DP, Scholes JV, Tierney AR. Evaluation of diagnostic criteria for mucosal cytomegalic inclusion disease in the acquired immune deficiency syndrome. *Am J Gastroenterol* 1987;82:1264–1270.

107. Wu G-D, Shintaku IP, Chien K, Geller SA. A comparison of routine light microscopy, immunohistochemistry, and in situ hybridization for the detection of cytomegalovirus in gastrointestinal biopsies. *Am J Gastroenterol* 1989;84:1517–1520.

108. Clayton F, Klein EB, Cutler DP. Correlation of in situ hybridization with histology and viral culture in patients with acquired immunodeficiency syndrome with cytomegalovirus colitis. *Arch Pathol Lab Med* 1989;113:1124–1126.

109. Cotte L, Drouet E, Bissuel F, Denoyel GA, Trepo C. Diagnostic value of amplification of human cytomegalovirus DNA from gastrointestinal biopsies from human immunodeficiency virus-infected patients. *J Clin Microbiol* 1993;31:2066–2069.

110. Collaborative DHPG Treatment Study Group. Treatment of serious cytomegalovirus infections with 9-(1,3-dihydroxy-2-propoxymethyl)guanine in patients with AIDS and other immunodeficiencies. *N Engl J Med* 1986;314:801–805.

111. Chachoua A, Dieterich D, Krasinski K, et al. 9-(1,3-Dihydroxy-2-propoxymethyl)guanine (ganciclovir) in the treatment of cytomegalovirus gastrointestinal disease with the acquired immunodeficiency syndrome. *Ann Intern Med* 1987;107:133–137.

112. Laskin OL, Stahl-Bayliss CM, Kalman CM, Rosecan LR. Use of ganciclovir to treat serious cytomegalovirus infections in patients with AIDS. *J Infect Dis* 1987;155:323–327.

113. Laskin OL, Cederberg DM, Mills J, Eron LJ, Mildvan D, Spector SA. Ganciclovir for the treatment and suppression of serious infections caused by cytomegalovirus. *Am J Med* 1987;83: 201–207.

114. Dieterich DT, Chachoua A, Lafleur F, et al. Ganciclovir treatment of gastrointestinal infections caused by cytomegalovirus in patients with AIDS. *Rev Infect Dis* 1988;10S:532–537.

115. Buhles WC, Mastre BJ, Tinker AJ, et al. Ganciclovir treatment of life- or sight-threatening cytomegalovirus infection: experience in 314 immunocompromised patients. *Rev Infect Dis* 1988; 10S:495–504.

116. Dieterich DT, Cutler DP, Busch DF, et al. Ganciclovir treatment of cytomegalovirus colitis in AIDS: a randomized, double-blind, placebo-controlled multicenter study. *J Infect Dis* 1993;167:278–282.

117. Drew WL, MKiner RC, Busch DF, et al. Prevalence of resistance in patients receiving ganciclovir for serious cytomegalovirus infection. *J Infect Dis* 1991;163:716–719.

118. Nelson MR, Connolly GM, Hawkins DA, Gazzard BG. Foscarnet in the treatment of cytomegalovirus infection of the esophagus and colon in patients with the acquired immune deficiency syndrome. *Am J Gastroenterol* 1991;86:876–881.

119. Drugs for non-HIV viral infections. *Med Lett* 1994;36:27–32.

120. Seigal FP, Lopez C, Hammer GS, et al. Severe acquired immunodeficiency in male homosexuals manifested by chronic herpes simplex lesions. *N Engl J Med* 1981;305:1439–1444.

121. Quinnan GV, Masur H, Rook AH, et al. Herpesvirus infections in the acquired immune deficiency syndrome. *JAMA* 1984;252: 72–77.

122. Agha FP, Lee HL, Nostrant TT. Herpetic esophagitis: a diagnostic challenge in immunocompromised patients. *Am J Gastroenterol* 1986;81:246–253.

123. Erlich DS, Mills J, Chatis P, et al. Acyclovir-resistant herpes simplex virus infections in patients with the acquired immunodeficiency syndrome. *N Engl J Med* 1989;320:293–296.

124. Englund JA, Zimmerman ME, Swierkosz EM, et al. Herpes simplex virus resistant to acyclovir. A study in a tertiary care center. *Ann Intern Med* 1990;112:416–422.

125. Safrin S, Crumpacker C, Chatis P, et al. A controlled trial comparing dfoscarnet with vidarabine for acycylovir-resistant mucocutaneous herpes simplex in the acquired immunodeficiency syndrome. *N Engl J Med* 1991;325:551–555.

Infections of the Gastrointestinal Tract,
edited by M. J. Blaser, P. D. Smith, J. I. Ravdin,
H. B. Greenberg, and R. L. Guerrant
Raven Press, Ltd., New York © 1995.

CHAPTER 34

Gastritis and Abdominal Pain in HIV-Infected Patients

Mary F. Chan and Scott L. Friedman

GASTRITIS

Description

Abdominal pain is a common gastrointestinal symptom in patients with human immunodeficiency virus (HIV) infection or the acquired immunodeficiency syndrome (AIDS). Understanding the clinical spectrum of abdominal pain in HIV disease is a significant challenge. Its frequency generally increases with progressive HIV disease due to the enlarging spectrum of infections and neoplasms as the illness progresses. Furthermore, the diagnosis and management of abdominal pain may be complicated by the use of medications, which themselves cause abdominal symptoms.

Gastritis is an important cause of abdominal pain in HIV-infected patients. The incidence of gastritic inflammation and infection in this setting is unknown, because gastritis is often asymptomatic. Although usually associated with endoscopic abnormalities, the diagnosis of gastritis usually requires endoscopy and histologic examination of biopsy specimens. However, even histologic abnormalities may be nonspecific. Gastritis in HIV disease can broadly be classified as infectious or noninfectious. Infectious gastritis may be further classified by the specific organism involved.

Microbiology and Pathogenesis

Infectious Gastritis

In HIV disease all classes of microorganism may involve the stomach and lead to gastritis. As with other

M. F. Chan: Department of Medicine, Washington University School of Medicine, St. Louis, Missouri 63130.

S. L. Friedman: Department of Medicine, University of California, San Francisco, and UCSF Liver Center Laboratory, San Francisco General Hospital, San Francisco, California 94110.

manifestations of HIV disease, however, the likelihood of infection with specific agents changes with progressive immunosuppression. For example, in the intermediate stage of HIV disease (i.e., CD4 lymphocyte count of 300 to 500 cells/mm^3), nonopportunistic bacteria including *Treponema pallidum* are more common, whereas in late stage disease (i.e., CD4 lymphocyte count below 200 cells/mm^3), cytomegalovirus (CMV), *Cryptosporidium*, and *Mycobacterium avium* complex (MAC) are typical. To date, HIV has been isolated from gastric mucosa (1) but not visualized by *in situ* hybridization, in contrast to its clear demonstration in other sites of the gastrointestinal tract (2,3). The specific features of organisms that cause infectious gastritis are reviewed in this section (Table 1).

Cytomegalovirus

Infection with CMV is a significant cause of morbidity and mortality in patients with HIV infection and CD4 lymphocyte counts less than 150 cells/mm^3. CMV may cause disease in any region of the gastrointestinal tract, including the stomach; gastrointestinal involvement is always part of systemic CMV infection (4,5). The high rate of CMV infection in homosexual men with late-stage HIV disease is related to the high prevalence of the infection in homosexual men (6).

In the stomach, CMV disease usually produces a single, large, shallow ulcer and occasionally diffuse ulceration (4). Alternatively, the mucosa may show thickened, nodular rugae or mass lesions (7–9). The virus can infect endothelial and epithelial cells, fibroblasts (10), mononuclear leukocytes (11), and muscle cells (12). One postulated mechanism of injury is the development of "endothelialitis," leading to mucosal ischemia (13,14) and, in severe disease, perforation, particularly in the small and large bowel, where the wall is thinner than in the stomach.

The diagnosis of gastric CMV is established by the presence of cells with typical intranuclear or cytoplasmic inclusion bodies (replicating virions) in endoscopic or surgi-

TABLE 1. *Infectious causes of gastritis in AIDS patients (see text for dosages)*

Infection	Endoscopic and pathologic findings	Treatment
Cytomegalovirus	Geographic ulcers; CMV inclusions	Ganciclovir, foscarnet
Mycobacterium avium complex	Nodules; acid-fast bacilli in foamy macrophages	Ethambutol, rifamprin, rifabutin amikacin, clarithromycin, clofazamine, ciprofloxacin
Cryptosporidium	Normal or erythema; oocysts on epithelial border	None proven effective
Helicobacter pylori	Normal or nodules and erythema; chronic active gastritis	Tetracycline, metronidazole, bismuth
Treponema pallidum	Ulcers, nodules; linitis plastica spirochetes	Penicillin
Bartonella henselae/ B. quintana	Red to purple macules or nodules; neovascularization	Erythromycin, cephalosporins, doxycycline
Phlegmonous gastritis	Necrotic ulcers	Broad-spectrum antibiotics, surgery

cal biopsy specimens (10) (Fig. 1; Plate 5). Inclusion cells are most easily identified at the edge of an ulcer rather than its base, where granulation and inflammatory tissue predominate. Demonstration of CMV inclusions is the gold standard for diagnosis, but it may be complemented by viral culture, immunohistochemical staining, or *in situ* hybridization (13,15,16). A positive culture in the absence of pathognomonic biopsy findings is not adequate to establish the diagnosis.

Mycobacterium avium Complex

(See chapter by Horsburgh and Nelson.) MAC is the most common systemic bacterial infection in HIV-in-

fected persons and is associated with gastrointestinal involvement in a significant percentage of patients with late-stage HIV disease (17–20). Infection of the stomach, which is always a manifestation of disseminated disease, is associated with abdominal pain, weight loss, and fever (18,21,22). When gastric involvement is accompanied by intestinal infection, diarrhea and malabsorption are common. Similar to CMV gastrointestinal disease, involvement of the small intestine and colon by MAC is more common than that of the stomach.

Endoscopic findings associated with gastrointestinal MAC are nonspecific and range from normal-appearing mucosa to erythema, edema, and friability. Small erosions and fine white nodules coating the small bowel mucosa

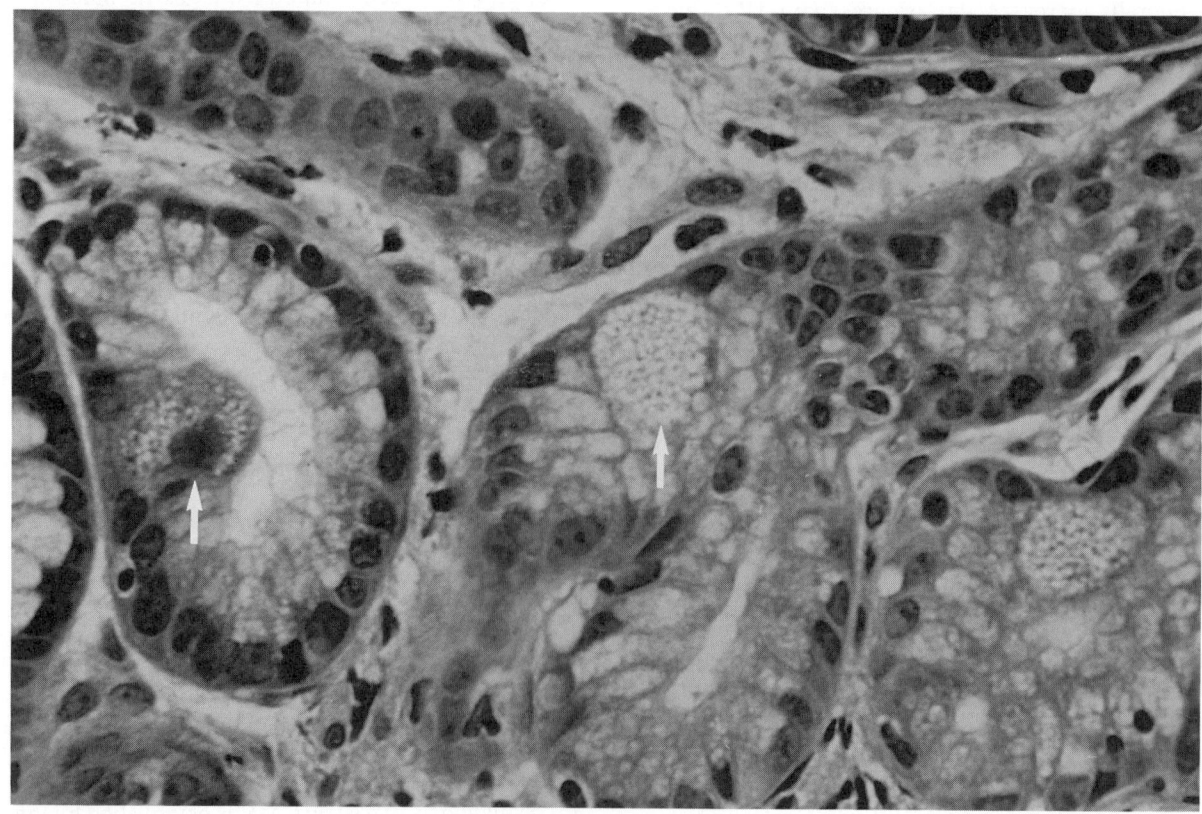

FIG. 1. Gastric mucosal biopsy from a patient with AIDS, demonstrating typical cytomegalic changes in epithelial cells (*arrows*). H&E stain. (See Plate 5.)

have also been described (23). Microscopic examination characteristically shows organisms within foamy, periodic acid–Schiff-positive lamina propria macrophages, mimicking Whipple's disease (18,24,25). However, in contrast to Whipple's organism, the MAC organism is acid-fast. Isolation and speciation are accomplished by culturing the organism (18,26–28).

Cryptosporidiosis

(See chapter by Adal et al.) Cryptosporidiosis also has been recognized as a cause of gastric infection (29–32). Pain is typically dull, nonradiating, and constant. Accompanying symptoms may include nausea and vomiting due to outlet obstruction (29–32). Gastritis, however, does not occur as an isolated finding, as all patients have concurrent small intestinal involvement. Endoscopic findings in cryptosporidiosis are subtle. Mild erythema and edema may be apparent, but the tissue often appears grossly normal. Diagnosis of gastric cryptosporidiosis requires histologic identification of the parasite either on the luminal surface of gastric epithelium by light microscopy or within an invagination of enterocyte plasma membrane by electron microscopy (33). The burden of organisms increases with progressive immunosuppression (34).

Identification of the organism in stool samples rather than biopsy establishes the presence of gastrointestinal cryptosporidiosis but does not localize the infection to the stomach. Radiologic studies of the gastrointestinal tract are not useful for establishing a specific diagnosis.

Helicobacter pylori

(See chapters by Riegg et al., Taylor and Parsonnet, and Holtman and Talley.) *Helicobacter pylori* has widely been recognized as a pathogen in the etiology of chronic gastritis and has closely been associated with peptic ulceration. The bacterium does not appear to be more prevalent or more symptomatic in patients with HIV infection (35–38). Indeed, its prevalence in this population may be lower than in the general population (13,39,40). In one study (41), *H. pylori* was identified in 28 (47%) of 59 control subjects and in only seven (14%) of 51 HIV seropositive patients ($p < 0.001$), and frequency of chronic active gastritis was similar in both groups, suggesting that cell-mediated immunodeficiency did not increase the risk of gastritis associated with *H. pylori*. In this and related studies (40), it has been speculated that the high prevalence of gastric achlorhydria in HIV disease might protect against *H. pylori* colonization.

Treponema pallidum

An increased incidence of syphilis has been reported in patients with HIV infection, often with atypical features and secondary and tertiary disease. Although true luetic gastritis is rare (less than 1% of patients with syphilis) (42), linitis plastica from syphilis was a well-described finding in late secondary and tertiary syphilis prior to the antibiotic era and has now been reported in patients with AIDS (43–45). Gastric syphilis has been documented in an illicit drug user with AIDS who previously had been treated with penicillin for a positive syphilis serology. Symptoms included abdominal pain, malaise, and weight loss. Endoscopic and radiographic studies raised the possibility of linitis plastica due to neoplasm because of the presence of a diffuse multinodular process with erosions and ulcerations extending from the distal stomach to the duodenal bulb. Warthin–Starry silver stain showed numerous spirochetes in the epithelium and lamina propria; the rapid plasma reagent test (RPR) and fluorescein treponemal antibody test (FTA) were positive. The symptoms resolved following retreatment with penicillin. This case illustrates that although the sensitivity of *T. pallidum* to penicillin is unchanged in HIV-infected patients, early syphilis may not be eradicated with standard courses of penicillin. The lack of a complete response to penicillin has been attributed to altered host defenses, underscoring the need for prolonged treatment, even in early infection (46).

Bartonella henselae/Bartonella quintana

Two newly identified organisms, *B. henselae* and *B. quintana* (previously called *Rochalimea* species), are the causative agents of a systemic opportunistic infection that can involve the stomach. The prevalence of these organisms is not established yet, but reports of the infections are likely to increase as clinicians and laboratories become aware of their role in HIV disease. Patients with gastric disease may complain of abdominal pain, nausea, and vomiting, in association with extragastric disease including fevers and bone, liver, and cutaneous lesions. Hepatic lesions (referred to as "bacillary peliosis" or "peliosis hepatitis") and cutaneous lesions ("bacillary angiomatosis") appear to be far more common than gastric disease.

Bartonella henselae and *B. quintana* are fastidious, gram-negative bacteria that can be recognized with a Warthin–Starry silver stain. The bacteria typically cause a pseudoneoplastic vascular proliferation resembling Kaposi's sarcoma, although the two lesions are not related etiologically. Like Kaposi's sarcoma, lesions of bacillary angiomatosis may involve the gastric mucosa and submucosa. In addition to a Warthin–Starry stain, other measures of diagnosis include polymerase chain reaction, culture on chocolate agar, and immunocytochemical techniques (47–50).

Phlegmonous Gastritis

Phlegmonous gastritis is another rare, but usually fatal, cause of infectious gastritis in patients with AIDS (51,52). Patients present with epigastric pain and tenderness, with or without fever. Peritonitis is rarely noted at presentation but may become evident within a few days. Radiographic findings are nonspecific. In 50% of cases the diagnosis is established at autopsy (51). The antemortem diagnosis has traditionally been made at laparotomy, which may reveal diffuse fibrinopurulent exudate in the peritoneal cavity and a thickened gastric wall. Tissue cultures are usually positive for oropharyngeal organisms. Endoscopy has been used to facilitate diagnosis of phlegmonous gastritis; findings include deep gastric ulcerations covered by a fibrinopurulent exudate. The histopathology typically demonstrates necrotic mucosa with intramural microabscesses. Aggressive surgical resection may be the most appropriate therapy, as an earlier study (53) reported a 100% mortality in patients treated with antibiotics alone compared to 18% mortality when gastric resection was combined with antibiotics (51).

Noninfectious Gastric Disease

In addition to infectious gastritis, AIDS patients may have noninfectious gastric lesions, including ulcerations associated with nonsteroidal anti-inflammatory drugs (NSAIDs), Kaposi's sarcoma, and lymphoma.

NSAID Injury

The clinical features and prevalence of gastric and duodenal ulcer disease are not appreciably altered in the setting of HIV infection. Gastric ulceration induced by NSAIDs is not an AIDS-associated lesion but should be considered in the differential diagnosis of patients with AIDS and abdominal pain, dyspepsia, or hemorrhage during NSAIDs therapy. NSAID-associated mucosal damage, which is thought to result from inhibition of prostaglandin E synthesis, will usually respond to treatment with H_2-receptor antagonists and removal of the offending agent. Prophylactic use of misoprostal, a prostaglandin E_1 analog, could be considered for the patient with a compelling indication for NSAID therapy and a known risk of ulceration, but the agent is expensive and may cause diarrhea. Its use in patients with HIV disease has not been reported.

Kaposi's Sarcoma

Kaposi's sarcoma (KS) is the most common tumor associated with HIV infection, occurring in 20% to 30% of all cases of AIDS, but almost exclusively in patients whose risk behavior is homosexual contact (54). KS is a multifocal tumor arising from lymphatic endothelial cells (55), which can involve the skin and/or viscera. Visceral involvement is detected in 10% of those with cutaneous disease. However, since most visceral KS lesions are asymptomatic, the actual incidence of KS may be higher (56).

KS lesions are common in the stomach, and involvement of the stomach and proximal small bowel is more common than that of the distal small bowel or colon. The lesions appear endoscopically as discrete, smoothly contoured red, purple, or blue polyps, with or without central umbilication, or erythematous macules that range from a

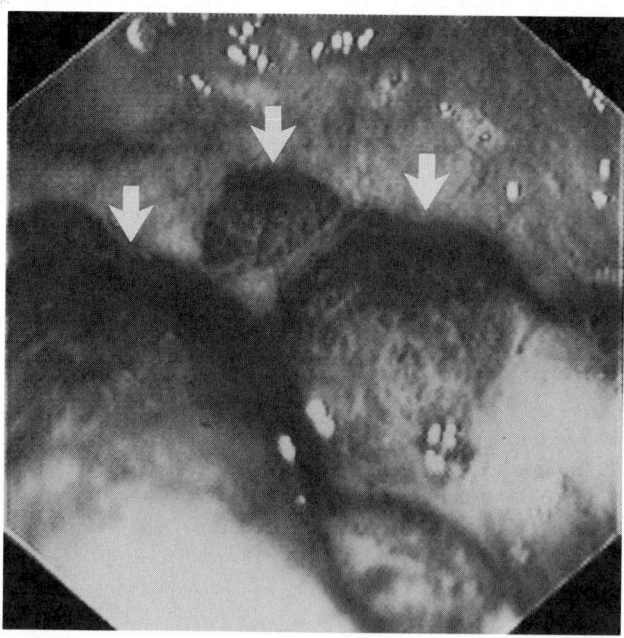

FIG. 2. Endoscopic view of the gastric antrum of a patient with KS appearing as erythematous nodules protruding into the lumen (*arrows*). (See Plate 6.)

few millimeters to several centimeters in size (Fig. 2; Plate 6). No region within the stomach is preferentially involved, and lesions may be single or multiple. Histologic examination confirms the diagnosis in only 25% of biopsied lesions, because KS is usually submucosal and beyond the reach of the standard biopsy forceps (57). KS is characterized histologically by the presence of spindle-shaped cells that produce a vascular structure with cleft-like spaces containing erythrocytes or hemosiderin (57). Although most KS lesions are clinically asymptomatic, advanced lesions may result in gastric bleeding or obstruction.

Non-Hodgkin's Lymphoma

Gastric involvement by non-Hodgkin's lymphoma (NHL) is relatively common in AIDS. NHL is 60 times more frequent in AIDS patients than in the general U.S. population (58), and the gastrointestinal tract is among the more common sites of extranodal disease (59). Abdominal pain, anorexia, nausea, and vomiting, although frequent presenting symptoms of gastric lymphoma, are nonspecific. Gastrointestinal bleeding, also nonspecific for malignancy, may occur in 10% to 30% of patients. On physical examination an abdominal mass is palpated in 20% of patients with gastric lymphoma. Radiographic contrast studies may demonstrate a mass, filling defect, ulceration, or thickened rugal folds. Because of the relative ease and safety of endoscopy, endoscopic biopsy is the preferred method of obtaining tissue for diagnosis. However, laparotomy and full thickness biopsy may be required to obtain sufficient tissue, as lymphoma may infiltrate only to the level of the submucosa. Endoscopic biopsies should be frozen so that immunoperoxidase studies can be performed to evaluate the infiltrate for immunoglobulin monoclonality.

Clinical Features

The clinical presentation of gastritis in HIV-infected patients depends on the extent and etiology of the gastric disease. Asymptomatic disease is not unusual, as gastritis is often diagnosed incidentally in patients undergoing endoscopy for other reasons. Symptomatic gastritis may be characterized by dyspepsia, epigastric pain, nausea, vomiting, fever, hematemesis, melena, or hematochezia. Although the presence of these symptoms does not establish a diagnosis, they may help narrow the diagnostic possibilities. For example, severe, continuous pain is more typical of CMV or phlegmonous gastritis (15), particularly when accompanied by fever, weight loss, and vomiting due to gastric outlet obstruction. Overt or subclinical bleeding also may be present (7,8,10,60). In contrast, dull pain more likely suggests neoplasm or infection with MAC, *Cryptosporidium, T. pallidum,* or *Bartonella.* Diarrhea may be present, indicating the possibility of an enteric pathogen with associated gastric involvement, such as cryptosporidiosis.

Diagnostic Measures

A specific diagnosis for symptomatic gastritis is best obtained with upper endoscopy and biopsy. Contrast radiography may reveal thickened gastric folds, nodules, or ulcerations, but these findings are nonspecific. Random endoscopic biopsies of the antrum and biopsies of lesions should be obtained with large biopsy forceps. Biopsies of macroscopically normal tissue are more likely to be of value in patients with low numbers of CD4 lymphocytes; biopsies are less useful in patients with early HIV disease (61). Biopsy sections should be stained with hematoxylin and eosin (H&E) and examined for histopathologic changes. Viral and bacterial cultures are not routinely indicated since histopathologic evaluation is the appropriate technique for the diagnosis of most gastric pathogens. Provided sampling is adequate, H&E stain sections are used to demonstrate lymphoma, CMV, *Cryptosporidium, H. pylori,* and foamy macrophages when MAC is present. If H&E stains are nondiagnostic, then the following special stains of either fresh or fixed tissue can be performed: Ziehl–Neelsen stain for acid-fast organisms; Warthin–Starry stain for *T. pallidum, H. pylori,* and *B. henselae;* and a modified Giemsa stain for *H. pylori.* Immunohistochemical stains for lymphocyte markers to establish the cell surface phenotype of the lymphomas can be performed on a fresh specimen.

Management

Cytomegalovirus

Tissue invasive CMV infection is treated with ganciclovir or foscarnet (5,62). Ganciclovir prevents viral replication by inhibiting DNA synthesis. The drug is inactive in its parenterally administered form and must be converted to the active triphosphate *in vivo.* An orally active form is not yet available. As a nucleoside analog, ganciclovir can be incorporated into host DNA, causing neutropenia (15). Concurrent therapy with granulocyte–macrophage colony-stimulating factor has been advocated to reduce the risk of neutropenia (63,64). Foscarnet, also an intravenous drug, is an effective alternative to ganciclovir in patients with marrow toxicity or progressive infection. Foscarnet (trisodium phosphonoformate) is a pyrophosphate analog that is a potent inhibitor *in vitro* of both the DNA polymerase of CMV and the reverse transcriptase of HIV. The drug is nephrotoxic and can lead to significant renal wasting of electrolytes, especially calcium; it must be given with 1 L of normal saline per day, with careful monitoring of serum electrolytes, calcium, and phosphorus (65).

We treat patients with gastrointestinal CMV disease and normal renal function with ganciclovir 5 mg/kg twice daily or 2.5 mg/kg every 8 hr for 14 to 21 days (63,64,66). Alternatively, foscarnet 60 mg/kg can be administered every 8 hr for 14 days. Foscarnet will induce remission in at least two-thirds of patients who fail to respond to ganciclovir (67). The role of chronic maintenance therapy for gastrointestinal CMV is not settled, unlike its role in CMV ocular disease for which maintenance is essential (69,70). In the absence of eye disease, we use maintenance ganciclovir (5 to 6 mg/kg once daily or five times per week) for patients who develop recurrent CMV disease after completing a 14- to 21-day course of therapy. Dosages must be reduced in patients with renal insufficiency, because the drug is excreted primarily via the kidneys (15).

Mycobacterium avium Complex

MAC is usually treated with multidrug antibiotic regimens, but these regimens are not curative (17,19,20,68–70). Thus the goal of treatment is to reduce symptoms, improve the quality of life, and prolong survival. Although the organism is generally resistant to standard antituberculous regimens, *in vitro* susceptibility has been demonstrated to ethambutol, rifampin, rifabutin, clofazimine, ciprofloxacin, cycloserine, imipenem, and amikacin (20,69). Treatment regimens consisting of amikacin, ethambutol, rifampin, and ciprofloxacin have shown promise in reducing both the mycobacterial burden and systemic symptoms in patients with MAC (69,71). Other regimens showing limited efficacy have included combinations of one or more of the aforementioned drugs and clarithromycin, azithromycin, and clofazimine (28,72). The U.S. Public Health Service Task Force in Prophylaxis and Therapy for *Mycobacterium avium* complex has recommended prophylactic rifabutin 300 mg po qd for patients with less than 100 CD4 cells/mm^3 and for disseminated MAC disease, a regimen consisting of either azithromycin or clarithromycin, and at least one additional agent from those listed above (73). More recent trials suggest that prophylaxis may be effective in patients with CD4 counts below 200 cells/mm³ (74).

Cryptosporidium

Specific therapy for *Cryptosporidium* is not currently available. However, clinical improvement has been reported anecdotally in patients treated with zidovudine (75), hyperalimentation (76), or somatostatin analogs to control diarrhea (77).

Helicobacter pylori

Although treatment recommendations are rapidly evolving, *H. pylori*-associated chronic active gastritis is usually eradicated by a regimen of tetracycline 500 mg qid, metronidazole 250 mg tid, and bismuth 300 mg qid for 2 weeks (78). Shorter two-drug regimens have been advocated (79,80) but have not been specifically used in patients with HIV infection.

Syphilis

Syphilitic gastritis is treated with penicillin G, 12 million units daily for 10 days (43). Early syphilis in an HIV-infected person may require a longer course of therapy to prevent secondary and tertiary disease (46).

Bartonella quintana/Bartonella henselae

Treatment for bacillary angiomatosis is erythromycin 250 to 500 mg qid for at least 1 month (81). Because the infection is multisystemic and involves deep tissues such as bone, longer courses of therapy or chronic prophylaxis may be necessary when resolution is slow or recurrences occur. In addition to erythromycin, case reports have documented efficacy with doxycycline, cephalosporins, and macrolide antibiotics (e.g., azithromycin and clarithromycin) (82).

Kaposi's Sarcoma

Hemorrhage from gastric KS can be controlled by endoscopic injection of lesions with epinephrine (1:10,000) or a sclerosant (e.g., ethanolamine oleate) in 1-cc increments to a total of 8 to 10 cc (83). Tumor size can be reduced by chemotherapy—the response generally paralleling that of cutaneous disease (84)—interferon-α in patients whose CD4 counts exceed 400 cells/mm³ (55,85–88), and radiation therapy for localized lesions (89). Bulky lesions associated with obstruction or refractory bleeding may require surgical resection.

Non-Hodgkin's Lymphoma

Protocols for the treatment of gastric lymphoma combine chemotherapy and/or surgical resection with or without postoperative radiation (90,91). There is no evidence that chemotherapy prolongs survival of AIDS patients with lymphoma (91).

ABDOMINAL PAIN

Description

Abdominal pain is a frequent symptom in patients with advanced HIV infection, occurring in up to 12% of patients (92,93). Its evaluation and therapy present many challenges. The clinician must consider not only the nature of the symptom but also the presence of associated complications and the degree of immunosuppression.

Clinical Features

Abdominal pain due to causes other than gastritis in the patient with AIDS usually falls into one of four "pain syndrome" categories (Table 2). Dull pain associated with diarrhea, nausea, and vomiting suggests infectious gastroenteritis. Acute, severe pain with peritonitis suggests perforation or transmural inflammation. Right upper quadrant pain and abnormal serum liver enzyme levels should alert the clinician to the possibility of cholecystitis, cholangitis, or infiltrative liver disease. Subacute pain with severe nausea and vomiting should lead the clinician to suspect bowel obstruction. Generalized upper abdominal pain is more frequently associated with pancreatic, gastric, and duodenal pathology; right upper quadrant abdominal pain with biliary and hepatic processes; and left lower quadrant pain with colitis (95).

Differential Diagnosis

The differential diagnosis of abdominal pain in the patient with AIDS includes biliary tract disorders, pancreatitis, and obstruction and perforation of the gastrointestinal tract (Table 3). The differential diagnosis includes not only the manifestations of opportunistic infection (95) and malignancy but also the more common causes of abdominal pain in the general population, such as peptic ulceration or calculous biliary disease. The lesions particularly common or unique to HIV disease are reviewed below.

Biliary Tract Disease

Diseases of the biliary tract commonly cause abdominal pain in patients with AIDS (95). The most common AIDS-related biliary tract disorders are idiopathic cholangiopathy and acalculous cholecystitis. In general, symptoms and signs of these diseases in HIV-infected patients are similar to those of uninfected persons and include right upper quadrant pain, fever, vomiting, and a cholestatic biochemical profile. Elevation of serum alkaline phosphatase levels is often dramatic with values as high as 20 times the upper limit of normal; jaundice is unusual, how-

TABLE 2. *Evaluation of abdominal pain: pain syndromes*

Symptoms	Suspect	Diagnostic method
Dull pain, diarrhea, nausea, vomiting	Infectious enteritis	Stool for C & S, ova and parasites; sigmoidoscopy
Acute, severe pain, peritonitis	Perforation	Abdominal films, surgical consult, liver function tests
Right upper quadrant pain, abnormal liver function tests	Cholecystitis, cholangitis, hepatic infiltates	Liver function tests, CT/ultrasound, possibly ERCP or liver biopsy
Subacute pain, severe nausea/vomiting	Obstruction	Contrast study

From ref. 94, with permission.

ever (96). Patients with symptoms and a biochemical profile suggesting AIDS-associated biliary tract disease should be evaluated initially with abdominal ultrasound or computed tomography (CT). These noninvasive tests will identify prominent or dilated intra- and extrahepatic bile ducts, thickened bile duct or gallbladder walls, and pericholecystic fluid. AIDS cholangiopathy is confirmed with endoscopic retrograde cholangiopancreatography (ERCP) (see below).

The spectrum of biliary tract disorders in HIV-infected patients includes the following: (a) papillary stenosis, (b) sclerosing cholangitis, (c) a combination of papillary stenosis and sclerosing cholangitis, and (d) long extrahepatic bile duct strictures (97) (Fig. 3). In one series (98), the most common pattern of biliary tract disease was the combination of papillary stenosis and sclerosing cholangitis (40%); intrahepatic ductal sclerotic changes were present in 17%, papillary stenosis alone in 8%, and high-grade bile

duct strictures in 11%. Twenty-three percent of patients had normal cholangiograms, suggesting that these patients' symptoms were not due to AIDS cholangiopathy (98).

The cholangiopathy is typically associated with CMV, *Cryptosporidium,* microsporidial species, and/or rarely atypical mycobacterial species (97–104). The primary site of local infection is uncertain in cases where organisms have been identified. In one series of 12 patients who underwent sphincterotomy for papillary stenosis, ampullary biopsies showed CMV in endothelial cells in four patients, one of whom had cryptosporidiosis; two other patients had only cryptosporidiosis; the remaining six patients had only acute and chronic inflammation (98).

Forty to 50% of patients with AIDS cholangiopathy have no organism identified by light microscopy. Recently, electron microscopy was used to detect *Enterocytozoon bieneusi* in the duodenum and bile of a patient with

TABLE 3. *Abdominal pain: AIDS-specific differential diagnosis*

Organ	Manifestation	Infections
Stomach	Gastritis	CMV, *Cryptosporidium*, MAC
	Ulcer	CMV, MAC, lymphoma
	Outlet obstruction	
Small intestine	Enteritis	*Cryptosporidium*, CMV, MAC, lymphoma, KS
		Cryptosporidium, CMV, MAC, microsporidium
	Obstruction	Lymphoma, KS, CMV
	Perforation	CMV, lymphoma
Colon/ appendix	Colitis	CMV
	Obstruction	Lymphoma, KS
	Perforation	CMV, lymphoma
	Appendicitis	KS, *Cryptosporidium*
Liver	Infiltration	MAC, KS, BA, CMV, lymphoma
Biliary tract	Cholecystitis	CMV, *Cryptosporidium*
	Cholangiopathy	CMV, *Cryptosporidium* microsporidium
Pancreas	Pancreatitis	CMV, pentamidine, DDI

From ref. 94, with permission.
CMV, cytomegalovirus; MAC, *Mycobacterium-avium* complex; KS, Kaposi's sarcoma; BA, bacillary angiomatosis; DDI, dideoxyinosine.

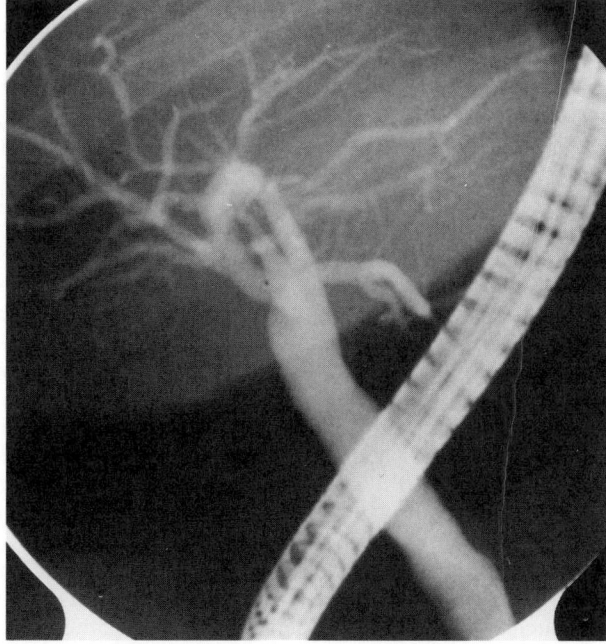

FIG. 3. Endoscopic retrograde cholangiogram demonstrating papillary stenosis with dilatation of the common hepatic and the common bile ducts in a patient with AIDS. The common duct is dilated to approximately 1 cm. The diameter of the endoscope, which is 1.1 cm, is used as a reference.

AIDS-associated diarrhea 3 months before he presented with sclerosing cholangitis, suggesting an etiologic role for microsporidiosis in AIDS cholangiopathy (102,103). Since electron microscopy is not routinely performed, the percentage of cases of AIDS cholangiopathy with no identifiable pathogen may be much lower than reported.

ERCP plays an important role in the therapy of AIDS cholangiopathy by facilitating internal drainage and decompression of the biliary system. AIDS-associated papillary stenosis is symptomatically responsive to common bile duct drainage by endoscopic sphincterotomy in at least half of affected patients (96,97). Despite pain relief in most patients, intrahepatic sclerosing cholangitis, if present, will progress, as manifested by continued rise in alkaline phosphatase (97). Acalculous cholecystitis is a late-stage consequence of HIV infection and is usually secondary to CMV infection or cryptosporidiosis. Its presentation is similar to cholecystitis and treatment often requires surgical intervention, including open or laparoscopic cholecystectomy or cholecystostomy in gravely ill patients.

Pancreatic Disease

Pancreatic disorders are less common than biliary tract disease in HIV-infected persons, although asymptomatic hyperamylasemia has frequently been noted (105).

Drugs

Drug-induced pancreatitis has been associated with pentamidine and trimethoprim-sulfamethoxazole, agents commonly used for the treatment of *Pneumocystis carinii* pneumonia (106). Pancreatitis also has been attributed to dideoxyinosine (DDI), an antiretroviral drug. DDI-associated pancreatitis is thought to reflect a hypersensitivity reaction and recurs after rechallenge with the drug (107).

Opportunistic pathogens, including CMV, *Cryptococcus neoformans,* and *Toxoplasma gondii,* have been associated with pancreatitis in HIV-infected patients (106,108). Antemortem diagnosis of infectious pancreatitis, however, is difficult to achieve, requiring a high index of suspicion by the clinician. CMV is probably the most common cause of infectious pancreatitis; symptoms are atypical and include anorexia, weight loss, and mild abdominal pain (108). Moreover, the diagnosis of CMV pancreatitis may be overlooked, because abdominal pain may be absent. Computed tomography and ultrasonography are used to detect pancreatic disease. Grossly, the pancreas is firm due to fibrosis and may show yellow-white discoloration. Microscopically, focal areas of necrosis with saponification of pancreatic parenchyma, chronic inflammatory cells, and nuclear debris may be present. The diagnosis is confirmed by the presence of cytoplasmic or intranuclear inclusions in ductal, acinar, endothelial, or islet cells.

Treatment

Treatment of pancreatitis of any cause is supportive. Medications known to cause pancreatitis should be dis-continued. Despite the lack of data showing efficacy, specific antimicrobial treatment should be considered if infectious pancreatitis is diagnosed. CMV pancreatitis may be treated with ganciclovir or foscarnet (see earlier discussion). Cryptococcosis responds to amphotericin B 0.5 to 0.8 mg/kg/day iv over 4 to 6 hr with or without 5-flucytosine 150 mg/kg po qd in divided doses for 6 weeks for a total dose of amphotericin 1.5 to 2 g, or amphotericin B with or without 5-flucytosine for 2 to 4 weeks followed by fluconazole 400 mg po qd (72). Toxoplasmosis is treated with sulfadiazine 1 g po q6h, pyrimethamine 75 to 100 mg po loading dose, then 25 to 75 mg po qd and leucovorin (folinic acid) 10 to 25 mg po qd. If the patient is allergic to sulfa, pyrimethamine 25 to 100 mg po qd and clindamycin 600 to 900 mg po or iv qid can be used (72).

Perforation and Obstruction: Incidence and Surgical Approach

Perforation and obstruction of the gastrointestinal tract are unusual in patients with AIDS (62,109) but can have devastating results. As in immunocompetent patients, presenting signs and symptoms include abdominal pain, nausea, vomiting, fever, leukocytosis, and signs of peritoneal irritation (e.g., rebound tenderness). There is no evidence that the signs or symptoms are diminished in patients with HIV disease.

Perforation commonly is a result of gastrointestinal ulceration due to CMV infection (109–114). The relatively high incidence of perforation in this infection may reflect the propensity of CMV to cause mucosal ischemia via endothelial cell infection. Obstruction may result from CMV, lymphoma, or KS, causing luminal encroachment or intussusception (62).

Complicated CMV enteritis is the most common AIDS-associated disease requiring emergency laparotomy (109–114). In one series of 35 patients undergoing 36 major abdominal operations, 11 patients had CMV enteritis, including 8 of 13 patients requiring emergency surgery for perforation or hemorrhage (114). In this same series NHL was the most common malignancy, presenting as an abdominal mass in four patients, bowel obstruction in three, and gastrointestinal bleeding in two (114).

Management

The management of intra-abdominal perforation or obstruction is surgical, as in the immunocompetent patient. However, high operative morbidity and mortality rates have been reported in AIDS patients undergoing laparotomy (112,113,115). Despite these high rates, patients with AIDS and surgical disease should not be denied an operation *a priori.* However, when planning patient management, the risks and benefits of treatment must be carefully considered. Healing rates and overall prognosis are directly related to the extent of immunosuppression and the indication for laparotomy; outcome in reported cases has not been affected by whether or not surgery was emergent. In a series of patients with late-stage HIV disease, surgical mortality was 20% (115). However, all deaths were considered to result from underlying disease and not from operative complications, suggesting that laparotomy does not jeopardize survival in patients with AIDS. These data contrast with another series (114) in which 1-month operative mortality rates of 9% for elective surgery and 46% for emergency surgery were reported in patients with AIDS. Thus poor surgical outcome in some patients may reflect late-stage disease.

Diagnostic Measures in the HIV-Infected Patient with Abdominal Pain

The evaluation of abdominal pain in the patient with HIV infection needs to be both expeditious and cost efficient; these requirements are particularly challenging given the broad differential diagnosis (Tables 2 and 3). In most cases, a diagnosis can be established using routine gastroenterological investigations and standard diagnostic criteria (95).

A thorough history is important in localizing the origin of the pain. The duration and severity of pain will dictate the urgency of evaluation. Associated signs and symptoms should suggest the particular organ(s) involved, and a diagnostic evaluation similar to that for a patient without AIDS should be undertaken. Abdominal ultrasound and/ or computed tomography are extremely useful and should be considered early in the evaluation (96,116,117). Stool cultures and examinations for ova and parasites and fecal leukocytes are indicated in the patient with suspected infectious enteritis. If these studies are nondiagnostic, then sigmoidoscopy with mucosal biopsy is appropriate (95). If there is evidence of peritoneal irritation, abdominal films to exclude perforation and a surgical consultation are necessary (see section on Perforation and Obstruction).

Management of Abdominal Pain in HIV-Infected Patients

The management of abdominal pain syndromes falls broadly into medical versus surgical therapy. The nonsurgical management of abdominal pain will be determined by the clinical evaluation. Treatable infections contributing to the symptoms should be managed with appropriate antimicrobial agents. Symptoms due to lymphoma or KS may respond to chemotherapy or radiation therapy. Symptomatic treatment with analgesics may be indicated as adjunctive therapy in patients undergoing disease-specific therapies or as primary treatment in patients without reversible or treatable disease. Indications for surgical intervention are considered in the preceding section.

REFERENCES

1. Gill MJ, Sutherland LR, Church DL. Gastrointestinal tissue cultures for HIV in HIV-infected AIDS patients. *AIDS* 1992; 6:553–556.
2. Kotler DP, Wilson CS, Haroutounian G, Fox CH. Detection of human immunodeficiency virus-1 by 35S-RNA in situ hybridization in solitary esophageal ulcers in two patients with the acquired immunodeficiency syndrome. *Am J Gastroenterol* 1989;84:313–317.
3. Fox CH, Kotler D, Tierney A, Wilson CS, Fauci AS. Detection of HIV-1 RNA in the lamina propria of patients with AIDS and gastrointestinal disease. *J Infect Dis* 1989;159:467–471.
4. Knapp AB, Horst DA, Eliopoulos G, et al. Widespread cytomegalovirus gastroenterocolitis in a patient with acquired immunodeficiency syndrome. *Gastroenterology* 1983;85: 1399–1402.
5. Smith PD, moderator. Gastrointestinal infections in AIDS. *Ann Intern Med* 1992;116(1):63–77.
6. Suttman U, Willers H, Gerdelmann R, Hopken W, Schedel I, Deicher H. Cytomegalovirus infection in HIV-1-infected individuals. *Infection* 1988;16:111–114.
7. Campbell DA, Piercey JRA, Shnitka TK, Goldsand G, Devine DO, Weinstein WM. Cytomegalovirus-associated gastric ulcer. *Gastroenterology* 1977;72(3):533–535.
8. Elta G, Turnage R, Eckhauser F, Agha F, Ross S. A submucosal antral mass caused by cytomegalovirus infection in a patient with acquired immunodeficiency syndrome. *Am J Gastroenterol* 1986;81(8):714–717.
9. Rich JD, Crawford JM, Kazanjian SN, Kazanjian PH. Discrete gastrointestinal mass lesions caused by cytomegalovirus in patients with AIDS: report of three cases and review. *Clin Infect Dis* 1992;15:609–614.
10. Culpepper-Morgan JA, Kotler DP, Scholes JV, Tierney AR. Evaluation of diagnostic criteria for mucosal cytomegalic inclusion disease in the acquired immune deficiency syndrome. *Am J Gastroenterol* 1987;82(12):1264–1270.
11. Smith PD, Saini SS, Raffeld M, Manischewitz JF, Wahl SM. Cytomegalovirus induction of tumor necrosis factor-alpha by human monocytes and mucosal macrophages. *J Clin Invest* 1992;90:1642–1648.
12. Lemstrom KB, Bruning JH, Bruggeman CA, Lautenschlager IT, Hayry PJ. Cytomegalovirus infection enhances smooth muscle cell proliferation and intimal thickening of rat aortic allografts. *J Clin Invest* 1993;92:549–558.
13. Francis ND, Boylston AW, Roberts AHG, Parkin JM, Pinching AJ. Cytomegalovirus infection in gastrointestinal tracts of patients infected with HIV-1 or AIDS. *J Clin Pathol* 1989;42: 1055–1064.
14. Meiselman MS, Cello JP, Margaretten W. Cytomegalovirus colitis: report of the clinical, endoscopic and pathologic findings in two patients with the acquired immunodeficiency syndrome. *Gastroenterology* 1985;88:171–175.
15. Drew WL. Cytomegalovirus infection in patients with AIDS. *J Infect Dis* 1988;158:449–456.
16. Wu G-D, Shintaku P, Chien K, Geller S. A comparison of routine light microscopy, immunohistochemistry, and in situ hybridization for the detection of cytomegalovirus in gastrointestinal biopsies. *Am J Gastroenterol* 1989;84(12):1517–1520.
17. Young LS, Inderlied CB, Berlin OG, Gottlieb MS. Mycobacterial infections in AIDS patients, with an emphasis on the *Mycobacterium avium* complex. *Rev Infect Dis* 1986;8:1024–1033.
18. Quinn TC. Bacterial infections in gastrointestinal infections in AIDS. *Ann Intern Med* 1990;116:67–68.
19. Hawkins CC, Gold JWM, Whimbey E, et al. *Mycobacterium avium* complex infections in patients with the acquired immunodeficiency syndrome. *Ann Intern Med* 1986;105:184–188.
20. Glatt AE, Chirgwin K, Landesman SH. Treatment of infections associated with human immunodeficiency virus. *N Engl J Med* 1988;318:1439–1448.
21. Gray JR, Rabeneck L. Atypical mycobacterial infection of the gastrointestinal tract in AIDS patients. *Am J Gastroenterol* 1989;84:1521–1524.
22. Horsburgh CRJ. *Mycobacterium avium* complex in the acquired immunodeficiency syndrome. *N Engl J Med* 1991;324: 1332–1338.
23. Monsour HP Jr, Quigley EMM, Markin RS, Dalke DD, Goldsmith JC, Harty RF. Endoscopy in the diagnosis of gastrointes-

tinal *Mycobacterium avium-intracellulare* infection. *J Clin Gastroenterol* 1991;13:20–24.

24. Gillin JS, Urmacher C, West R, Shike M. Disseminated *Mycobacterium avium-intracellulare* infection in acquired immunodeficiency syndrome mimicking Whipple's disease. *Gastroenterology* 1983;85:1187–1191.

25. Roth RI, Owen RL, Keren DF, Volberding PA. Intestinal infection with *Mycobacterium avium* in acquired immune deficiency syndrome (AIDS). *Dig Dis Sci* 1985;30:497–504.

26. Damsker B, Bottone EJ. *Mycobacterium avium—Mycobacterium intracellulare* from the intestinal tracts of patients with acquired immunodeficiency syndrome: concepts regarding acquisition and pathogenesis. *J Infect Dis* 1985;151:179–181.

27. Kiehn TE, Edwards FF, Brannon P, et al. Infections caused by *Mycobacterium avium* complex in immunocompromised patients: diagnosis by blood culture and fecal examination, antimicrobial and seroagglutination characteristics. *J Clin Microbiol* 1985;21:168–173.

28. Kerlikowske KM, Katz MH. *Mycobacterium avium* complex and *Mycobacterium tuberculosis* in patients infected with the human immunodeficiency virus. *West J Med* 1992;157:144–148.

29. Garone MA, Winston BJ, Lewis JH. Cryptosporidiosis of the stomach. *Am J Gastroenterol* 1986;81(6):465–470.

30. Guarda LA, Stein SA, Cleary KA, Ordonez NG. Human cryptosporidiosis in the acquired immune deficiency syndrome. *Arch Pathol Lab Med* 1983;107:562–566.

31. Navin TR, Juranek DD. Cryptosporidiosis: clinical, epidemiologic, and parasitologic review. *Rev Infect Dis* 1984;6(3):313–327.

32. Pitlik SD, Fainstein V, Garza D, et al. Human cryptosporidiosis: spectrum of disease. Report of six cases and review of the literature. *Arch Intern Med* 1983;143:2269–2275.

33. Marcial MA, Madara JL. *Cryptosporidium:* cellular localization, structural analysis of absorptive cell-parasite membrane–membrane interactions in guinea pigs, and suggestion of protozoan transport by M cells. *Gastroenterology* 1986;90:583–594.

34. Genta RM, Chappell CL, White AC Jr, Kimball KT, Goodgame RW. Duodenal morphology and intensity of infection in AIDS-related intestinal cryptosporidiosis. *Gastroenterology* 1993;105:1769–1775.

35. Harris M, Szabo J. *Helicobacter pylori* infection in an HIV-positive patient. *AIDS* 1992;6(11):1404–1405.

36. Meiseleman MS, Miller-Catchpole R, Christ M, Randall E. *Campylobacter pylori* in the acquired immunodeficiency syndrome. *Gastroenterology* 1988;95:209–212.

37. Rotterdam H, Dieterich DT. *Campylobacter pyloridis* in AIDS patients: a clinicopathological correlation. *Am J Gastroenterol* 1987;82:934.

38. Walker MM, Francis ND, Logan RPH, et al. *Campylobacter pylori* in the upper gastrointestinal tract of patients with HIV infection. In: Megraud FHL, ed. *Gastroduodenal pathology and Campylobacter pylori.* Amsterdam: Elsevier Science Publishers, 1989;553–556.

39. Battan R, Raviglione MC, Palagiano A, et al. *Helicobacter pylori* infection in patients with acquired immune deficiency syndrome. *Am J Gastroenterol* 1990;85(12):1576–1579.

40. Marano BJ Jr, Smith F, Bonanno CA. *Helicobacter pylori* prevalence in acquired immunodeficiency syndrome. *Am J Gastroenterol* 1993;88:687–690.

41. Francis ND, Logan RPH, Walker MM, et al. *Campylobacter pylori* in the upper gastrointestinal tract of patients with HIV-1 infection. *J Clin Pathol* 1990;43(1):60–62.

42. Cooley RN, Childers JH. Acquired syphilis of the stomach. *Gastroenterology* 1960;39:201–207.

43. Kasmin F, Reddy S, Mathur-Wagh U, et al. Syphilitic gastritis in an HIV-infected individual. *Am J Gastroenterol* 1992;87(12):1820–1822.

44. Patterson CO, Rouse MO. Description of gastroscopic appearance of luetic gastric lesions in late acquired syphilis. *Gastroenterology* 1948;10:474–485.

45. Raskin MM. Some specific radiological findings and considera-

46. Hook EW III. Syphilis and HIV infection. *J Infect Dis* 1989;160:530–534.

47. Relman D. The agent of bacillary angiomatosis—an approach to the identification of uncultured pathogens. *N Engl J Med* 1990;3233:1573.

48. Regnery R. Characterization of a novel *Rochalimaea* species, *R. henselae* sp. nov., isolated from blood of a febrile, human immunodeficiency virus-positive patient. *J Clin Microbiol* 1992;30:265.

49. Slater L. *Rochalimaea henselae* causes bacillary angiomatosis and peliosis hepatitis. *Arch Intern Med* 1992;152:602.

50. Welch D. *Rochalimaea henselae* sp. nov., a cause of septicemia, bacillary angiomatosis, and parenchymal bacillary peliosis. *J Clin Microbiol* 1992;30:275–280.

51. Zazzo J-F, Troche G, Millat B, Aubert A, Bedossa P, Keros L. Phlegmonous gastritis associated with HIV-1 seroconversion. Endoscopic and microscopic evolution. *Dig Dis Sci* 1992;37(9):1454–1459.

52. Mittleman RE, Suarez RV. Phlegmonous gastritis associated with the acquired immunodeficiency syndrome/pre-acquired immunodeficiency syndrome. *Arch Pathol Lab Med* 1985;109:765–767.

53. Miller AL, Smith B, Rogers AL. Phlegmonous gastritis. *Gastroenterology* 1975;68:231–238.

54. Gill PS, Rarick M, McCutchan JA, et al. Systemic treatment of AIDS-related Kaposi's sarcoma: results of a randomized trial. *Am J Med* 1991;90:427–433.

55. Scully PA, Steinman HK, Kennedy C, Trueblood K, Frisman DM, Voland JR. AIDS-related Kaposi's sarcoma displays differential expression of endothelial surface antigens. *Am J Pathol* 1988;130:244–251.

56. Rodgers VD, Kagnoff MF. Gastrointestinal manifestations of the acquired immunodeficiency syndrome. *West J Med* 1987;146:57–67.

57. Friedman SL, Wright TL, Altman DF. Gastrointestinal Kaposi's sarcoma in patients with acquired immunodeficiency syndrome—endoscopic and autopsy findings. *Gastroenterology* 1985;89:102–108.

58. Beral V, Peterman T, Berkelman R, Jaffe H. AIDS-associated non-Hodgkin lymphoma. *Lancet* 1991;337(8745):805–809.

59. Ziegler JL, Beckstead JA, Volberding PA, Abrams DI, Levine AM. Non-Hodgkin's lymphoma in 90 homosexual men; relationship to generalized lymphadenopathy and the acquired immunodeficiency syndrome. *N Engl J Med* 1984;311:565–570.

60. Victoria MS, Nangia BS, Jindrak K. Cytomegalovirus pyloric obstruction in a child with acquired immunodeficiency syndrome. *Pediatr Infect Dis* 1985;4(5):550–552.

61. Lim SG, Lipman MC, Squire S, et al. Audit of endoscopic surveillance biopsy specimens in HIV positive patients with gastrointestinal symptoms. *Gut* 1993;34:1429–1432.

62. Tanowitz HB, Simon D, Wittner M. Medical management of AIDS patients: gastrointestinal manifestations. *Med Clin North Am* 1992;76(1):45–62.

63. Jacobson MA, O'Donnell JJ, Porteous D, Brodie HR, Feigal D, Mills J. Retinal and gastrointestinal disease due to cytomegalovirus in patients with the acquired immuno-deficiency syndrome: prevalence, natural history and response to ganciclovir therapy. *Q J Med* 1988;67:473–486.

64. Jacobson MA, Mills J. Serious cytomegalovirus disease in the acquired immunodeficiency syndrome. *Ann Intern Med* 1988;108:585–594.

65. Dieterich DT, Poles MA, Dicker M, Tepper R, Lew E. Foscarnet treatment of cytomegalovirus gastrointestinal infections in acquired immunodeficiency syndrome patients who have failed ganciclovir induction. *Am J Gastroenterol* 1993;88:542–548.

66. Kotler DP, Culpepper-Morgan JA, Tierney AR, Klein EB. Treatment of disseminated cytomegalovirus infection with 9-(1,3-dihydroxy-2-propoxymethyl)guanine: evidence of prolonged survival in patients with the acquired immunodeficiency syndrome. *AIDS Res* 1986;2(4):299–307.

67. Dieterich DT, Poles MA, Dicker M, Tepper R, Lew E. Foscarnet treatment of cytomegalovirus gastrointestinal infections in

acquired immunodeficiency syndrome patients who have failed ganciclovir induction. *Am J Gastroenterol* 1993;88(4):524–548.

68. Baron EJ, Young LS. Amikacin, ethambutol, and rifampin for treatment of disseminated *Mycobacterium avium-intracellulare* infections in patients with acquired immune deficiency syndrome. *Diagn Microbiol Infect Dis* 1986;5:215–220.

69. Masur H, Tuazon C, Gill V, et al. Effect of combined clofazimine and ansamycin therapy of *Mycobacterium avium–Mycobacterium intracellulare* bacteremia in patients with AIDS. *J Infect Dis* 1987;155:127–129.

70. Wong B, Edwards FF, Kiehn TE, et al. Continuous high-grade *Mycobacterium avium-intracellulare* bacteremia in patients with the acquired immunodeficiency syndrome. *Am J Med* 1985;78:35–40.

71. Chiu J, Nussbaum J, Bozzette S, et al. Treatment of disseminated *Mycobacterium avium* complex infection in AIDS with amikacin, ethambutol, rifampin and ciprofloxacin. *Ann Intern Med* 1990;113:358–361.

72. Goldschmidt RH, Dong BJ. Treatment of AIDS and HIV-related conditions. *J Am Board Fam Pract* 1992;5:335–350.

73. US Public Health Service Task Force. Recommendations on prophylaxis and therapy for disseminated *Mycobacterium avium* complex for adults and adolescents infected with human immunodeficiency virus. *MMWR Morb Mortal Wkly Rep* 1993; 42:14–20.

74. Masur H. Recommendations on prophylaxis and therapy for disseminated *Mycobacterium avium* complex disease in patients infected with the human immunodeficiency virus. Public Health Service Task Force on Prophylaxis and Therapy for *Mycobacterium avium* Complex. *N Engl J Med* 1993;329: 898–904.

75. Flanigan T, Whalen C, Turner J, et al. *Cryptosporidium* infection and CD4 counts. *Ann Intern Med* 1992;116:840–841.

76. Tomlinson DR, Coker RJ, Waldron S, Harris JR. Early aggressive management of cryptosporidial infection in AIDS. *Int J STD AIDS* 1991;2(3):202–203.

77. Cello JP, Grendell J, Basuk P, et al. Prospective multicenter clinical trial of octreotide (Sandostatin) for refractory AIDS-associated diarrhea. *Ann Intern Med* 1991;115:705–710.

78. Graham DY, Lew GM, Klein PD, et al. Effect of treatment of *Helicobacter pylori* infection on the long-term recurrence of gastric or duodenal ulcer. *Ann Intern Med* 1992;116:705–708.

79. de Koster ED, Nyst JF, Deprez C, et al. *Helicobacter pylori* treatment: double vs. triple therapy: Who needs bismuth? *Gastroenterology* 1992;102:A58.

80. Bayerdorffer E, Mannes GA, Sommer A, et al. High dose omeprazole treatment combined with amoxicillin eradicates *H. pylori. Gastroenterology* 1992;102:A38.

81. Cockerell CJ, LeBoit PE. Bacillary angiomatosis: a newly characterized, pseudoneoplastic, infectious, cutaneous vascular disorder. *J Am Acad Dermatol* 1990;22(3):501–512.

82. Perkocha L, Geaghan S, Yen T, Nishimura S, Chan S, Garcia-Kennedy R. Clinical and pathological features of bacillary peliosis hepatitis in association with human immunodeficiency virus infection. *N Engl J Med* 1990;323(23):1581–1586.

83. Lew EA, Dieterich DT. Severe hemorrhage caused by gastrointestinal Kaposi's sarcoma in patients with the acquired immunodeficiency syndrome: treatment with endoscopic sclerotherapy. *Am J Gastroenterol* 1992;87:1471–1473.

84. Laine L, Amerian J, Rarick M, Harb M, Gill PS. The response of symptomatic gastrointestinal Kaposi's sarcoma to chemotherapy: a prospective evaluation using an endoscopic method of disease quantification. *Am J Gastroenterol* 1990;85:959–961.

85. Krown SE, Real FX, Cunningham-Rundles S, et al. Preliminary observations on the effect of recombinant leukocyte A interferon in homosexual men with Kaposi's sarcoma. *N Engl J Med* 1983;308:1071–1076.

86. Krown SE, Gold JWM, Niedzwiecki D, et al. Interferon-alpha with zidovudine: safety, tolerance and clinical and virologic effects in patients with Kaposi sarcoma associated with the acquired immunodeficiency syndrome (AIDS). *Ann Intern Med* 1990;112:812–821.

87. Lane HC, Feinberg J, Davey V. Anti-retroviral effects of interferon alpha in AIDS-associated Kaposi's sarcoma. *Lancet* 1988;2:1218–1222.

88. Volberding P. Therapy of Kaposi's sarcoma and AIDS. *Semin Oncol* 1984;11:60–67.

89. Nisce LZ, Safai B. Radiation therapy of Kaposi's sarcoma. *Front Radiat Ther Oncol* 1985;19:133–137.

90. Haber DA, Mayer RJ. Primary gastrointestinal lymphoma. *Semin Oncol* 1988;15(2):154–169.

91. Kaplan LD. HIV-associated lymphoma. *AIDS Clin Rev* 1993; :145–166.

92. Barone JE, Wolkomir AF, Muakkassa FF, Fares LG II. Abdominal pain and anorectal disease in AIDS. *Gastroenterol Clin North Am* 1988;17:631–638.

93. Penfold J, Clark AJM. Pain syndromes in HIV infection. *Can J Anaesth* 1992;39(7):724–730.

94. Friedman S. Gastrointestinal manifestations of AIDS and other sexually transmissible diseases. In: Sleisenger MH, Fordtran JS, Scharschmidt BF, Feldman M, eds. *Gastrointestinal disease,* 5th ed. Philadelphia: Saunders, 1993.

95. Thuluvath PJ, Connolly GM, Forbes A, Gazzard BG. Abdominal pain in HIV infection. *Q J Med* 1991;78(287):275–285.

96. Cello JP. AIDS and the gastroenterologist. *Scand J Gastroenterol* 1990;25:146–158.

97. Schneiderman DJ, Cello JP, Laing FC. Papillary stenosis and sclerosing cholangitis in the acquired immunodeficiency syndrome. *Ann Intern Med* 1987;106:546–549.

98. Cello JP. Acquired immunodeficiency syndrome cholangiopathy: spectrum of disease. *Am J Med* 1989;86:539–546.

99. Gremse DA, Bucuvalas JC, Bongiovanni GL. Papillary stenosis and sclerosing cholangitis in an immunodeficient child. *Gastroenterology* 1989;96:1600–1603.

100. Iannuzzi C, Belghiti J, Erlinger S, Menu Y, Fekete F. Cholangitis associated with cholecystitis in patients with acquired immunodeficiency syndrome. *Arch Surg* 1990;125:1211–1213.

101. Margulis S, Honig C, Soave R, Govoni A, Mouradian JA, Jacobson IM. Biliary tract obstruction in the acquired immunodeficiency syndrome. *Ann Intern Med* 1986;105:207–210.

102. Pol S, Romana C, Richard S, et al. *Enterocytozoon bieneusi* infection in acquired immunodeficiency syndrome-related sclerosing cholangitis. *Gastroenterology* 1992;102:1778–1781.

103. Pol S, Romana CA, Richard S, et al. Microsporidia infection in patients with the human immunodeficiency virus and unexplained cholangitis. *N Engl J Med* 1993;328(2):95–99.

104. Viteri AL, Greene JF Jr. Bile duct abnormalities in the acquired immune deficiency syndrome. *Gastroenterology* 1987;92: 2014–2018.

105. Zazzo JF, Pichon R, Regnier B. HIV and the pancreas. *Lancet* 1987;2:1212–1213.

106. Schwartz MS, Brandt LJ. The spectrum of pancreatic disease disorders in patients with the acquired immune deficiency syndrome. *Am J Gastroenterol* 1989;84:459–462.

107. Maxson E, Greenfield S, Turner J. Acute pancreatitis as a complication of ddI therapy in the acquired immune deficiency syndrome. *Am J Gastroenterol* 1990;85:1254.

108. Wilcox CM, Forsmark CE, Grendell JH, Darragh TM, Cello JP. Cytomegalovirus-associated acute pancreatic disease in patients with acquired immunodeficiency syndrome. *Gastroenterology* 1990;99:263–267.

109. Nugent P, O'Connell TX. The surgeon's role in treating acquired immunodeficiency syndrome. *Arch Surg* 1986;121: 1117–1120.

110. Ferguson CM. Surgical complications of human immunodeficiency virus infection. *Am Surg* 1988;54(1):4–9.

111. Kram HB, Hino ST, Cohen RE, et al. Spontaneous colonic perforation secondary to cytomegalovirus in a patient with acquired immune deficiency syndrome. *Crit Care Med* 1984;12: 469–471.

112. Robinson G, Wilson SE, Williams RA. Surgery in patients with acquired immunodeficiency syndrome. *Arch Surg* 1987;122: 170–175.

113. Wexner SD, Smithy WB, Trillo C, Hopkins BS, Dailey TH. Emergency colectomy for cytomegalovirus ileocolitis in patients with the acquired immune deficiency syndrome. *Dis Colon Rectum* 1988;31(10):755–761.

114. Wilson SE, Robinson G, Williams RA, et al. Acquired immune deficiency syndrome (AIDS): indications for abdominal surgery, pathology, and outcome. *Ann Surg* 1989;210(4):428–434.

115. Deziel DJ, Hyser MJ, Doolas A, Bines SD, Blaauw BB, Kessler HA. Major abdominal operations in acquired immunodeficiency syndrome. *Am Surg* 1990;56(7):445–450.

116. Lynch MA, Cho KC, Jeffrey J, Brooke R, Alterman DD, Federly MP. CT of peritoneal lymphomatosis. *AJR Am J Roentgenol* 1988;151:713–715.

117. Nyberg DA, Jeffrey J, Brooke R, Federle MP, Bottles K, Abrams DI. AIDS-related lymphoma: evaluation by abdominal CT. *Radiology* 1986;159(1):59–63.

Infections of the Gastrointestinal Tract,
edited by M. J. Blaser, P. D. Smith, J. I. Ravdin,
H. B. Greenberg, and R. L. Guerrant
Raven Press, Ltd., New York © 1995.

CHAPTER 35

Intestinal Infections in HIV-1 Disease

Phillip D. Smith

During the past 15 years, the world has witnessed the emergence of a new and devastating infectious disease—the acquired immunodeficiency syndrome (AIDS). The disease has now reached pandemic proportions and has been documented in virtually every country. Responding to this challenge, the medical and scientific communities of many countries have greatly advanced our knowledge of the clinical and immunopathophysiological features of this disease. As a result, it has become clear that the gastrointestinal tract plays several critical roles in the pathogenesis of AIDS. First, the gastrointestinal tract serves as an important portal of entry for human immunodeficiency virus type 1 (HIV-1), the causative agent of AIDS. Second, the entry of HIV-1 into the mucosa initiates a complex sequence of virological and immunological events that lead to local immunosuppression and altered intestinal physiology. Third, as a consequence of impaired immune and physiological function, the intestine is the target of infection by a diverse array of opportunistic pathogens. These pathogens cause diarrheal illnesses in a substantial proportion of HIV-1–infected persons in the developed world and in the majority of infected persons in the developing world.

This chapter summarizes the early, intermediate, and late virological and immunological events that occur in the mucosa during HIV-1 infection (Table 1) (1) and then reviews the corresponding diarrheal illnesses that are the consequence of those events. The chapter focuses in particular on the protozoal, viral, bacterial, and fungal intestinal infections that result from HIV-1–induced immunosuppression (Table 2).

PATHOGENESIS

Early Mucosal Events

The portal of entry for HIV-1 among homosexual men is the rectum. Trauma-induced (2) and infection-associated

P. D. Smith: Department of Medicine and Microbiology, Division of Gastroenterology and Hepatology, University of Alabama School of Medicine, and Center for AIDS Research, Birmingham, Alabama 35294.

(2,3) mucosal tears and erosions provide inoculated virus direct access to the underlying lymphoid cells and microcirculation. In the fetus and infants, the upper gastrointestinal tract likely serves as the portal of entry through the swallowing of HIV-1–infected fluids such as amniotic fluid *in utero,* cervical secretions and blood intrapartum, and breast milk during nursing. In the absence of disrupted mucosa, HIV-1 could be transported across the epithelium by M cells. These specialized epithelial cells bind macromolecules and microorganisms, such as poliovirus and reovirus (3,4), and transport them by a nondegradative process to the cell's basal surface where they are delivered to interdigitating mononuclear cells in the underlying lymphoid aggregate (5). The highest density of M cells is in the rectum (6), increasing the likelihood of contact between HIV-1 and M cells. Recent studies have shown that mouse M cells can take up and transport HIV-1 (7), but the role of human M cells in HIV-1 transport has not been elucidated. Finally, the detection of HIV-1 in or near the intestinal epithelium by some (8–10), but not all (11–15), investigators suggests that virus also might enter the mucosa through epithelial cells, but this remains controversial.

Once in the lamina propria, HIV-1 encounters an abundance of resident lymphocytes and macrophages. Infection of these cells likely occurs through the same CD4 receptor–mediated mechanism by which virus infects circulating cells (16,17). Subsequently, HIV-1–infected cells in the lymphoid aggregate could be distributed to mucosa throughout the body by the receptor-mediated homing mechanism that normally distributes antigen-stimulated lymphocytes from the lymphoid aggregate to distant mucosal sites (18). In addition, circulating cells that were infected as they passed through the mucosa could be distributed randomly to nonmucosal sites.

Several days to weeks after inoculation, virus reaches sufficient levels to trigger seroconversion and an acute mononucleosis-like illness, referred to as acute HIV-1 syndrome. The pathogenesis of this acute febrile illness, which may be accompanied by diarrhea, is unclear. However, the ability of HIV-1 to induce monocytes and macrophages *in vitro* to produce cytokines that mediate the fe-

TABLE 1. *Reported findings in the gastrointestinal tract mucosa of patients with HIV-1 infection*

1. HIV-1–infected cells present in rectal, colonic, ileal, duodenal, and esophageal mucosa
2. Prevalence of HIV-1 RNA-expressing mononuclear cells in mucosa 0.06%
3. Number of CD4+ cells and ratio of T4/T8 cells reduced
4. Proportion of plasma cells in mucosa producing IgA reduced
5. sIgA2 subclass reduced; HIV-1–specific sIgA predominantly against gp120 and gp160
6. Villus atrophy present; epithelial cell maturation impaired
7. Disaccharidase (lactase, sucrase) and enzyme (alkaline phosphatase) levels reduced
8. Cytokine (IL-1 and TNF-α) levels in mucosa increased
9. Gastric acid secretion reduced
10. Number of gastric and duodenal bacteria (anaerobes = aerobes) increased to >10^4 bacteria/mL

brile response, such as interleukin 1 (IL-1) (19–21) and tumor necrosis factor-α (TNF-α) (20–23), raises the possibility that HIV-1 induction of these cytokines *in vivo* is involved in the pathogenesis of acute HIV-1 syndrome. TNF-α also appears capable of influencing the transport of fluid and electrolytes by intestinal epithelial cells (24), raising the possibility that the diarrhea that may accompany acute HIV-1 syndrome is mediated by HIV-1–induced cytokines (25). Shortly after seroconversion, the immune response causes a rapid decline in viral burden, and the patient recovers symptomatically, albeit transiently.

Intermediate Mucosal Events

The intermediate stage of mucosal events corresponds to the period between HIV-1 infection and the develop-

ment of clinical AIDS with intestinal infections. This 8- to 10-year period (26) was previously thought to correspond to viral latency, but recent studies indicate that during this period systemic HIV-1 infection is active and progressive, leading to complete involution of lymph node germinal centers (27,28). Whether lymphoid structures in the mucosa also undergo progressive destruction during this stage of disease is not known.

As a consequence of the distribution of HIV-1–infected cells to distant mucosal sites, HIV-1–infected mononuclear cells have been identified in the mucosa of the rectum and colon (11), ileum (29), duodenum (12,30), and esophagus (15,31) (Fig. 1). Over time, infected and uninfected mucosal CD4+ cells are depleted by mechanisms that likely involve cell lysis (32), syncytia formation (33), and apoptosis (34). Since mucosal CD4+ helper cells play a central role in IgA B-cell differentiation, their selective depletion (35–37), together with a relative increase in the number of local suppressor CD8+ T cells (38) and a disturbance in mucosal regulatory cytokines (39,40), may contribute to the depletion of IgA-bearing B cells in the mucosa (31,41) and the secretory IgA2 subclass restriction reported in patients with advanced HIV-1 disease (42).

During the intermediate stage of mucosal HIV-1 infection, the mucosa undergoes villus atrophy and the numbers of crypt mitotic figures and levels of brush border enzymes decline, suggesting HIV-1–induced mucosal atrophy (12,43). In addition, intestinal dysmotility (44) and gastric acid secretory failure (45–47) occur in some patients with AIDS, contributing further to altered intestinal defense mechanisms and thereby predisposing the gastrointestinal tract to intestinal pathogens. Importantly, gastric acid and normal intestinal motility play critical roles in controlling the levels of intestinal bacteria, and the impairment of these mechanisms may promote an increase in number of bacteria (< 10^7 bacteria/mL) in the proximal small intestine in some HIV-1–infected persons

TABLE 2. *Diarrheal illnesses associated with the early, intermediate, and late stages of mucosal HIV-1 infection*

Early	Intermediate	Late
Acute HIV-1 syndrome	? AIDS enteropathy	Parasitic infections
	? Low-grade bacterial overgrowth	*Cryptosporidium*
		Microsporidians
		Isospora belli
		Viral infections
		Cytomegalovirus
		Herpes simplex virus
		Adenovirus
		Bacterial infections
		Mycobacterium avium complex
		Salmonella species
		Shigella flexneri
		Campylobacter jejuni
		Fungal infections
		Candida albicans
		Histoplasma capsulatum

Adapted from Smith PD. *Gastroenterol Clin North Am* 1993;22:535.

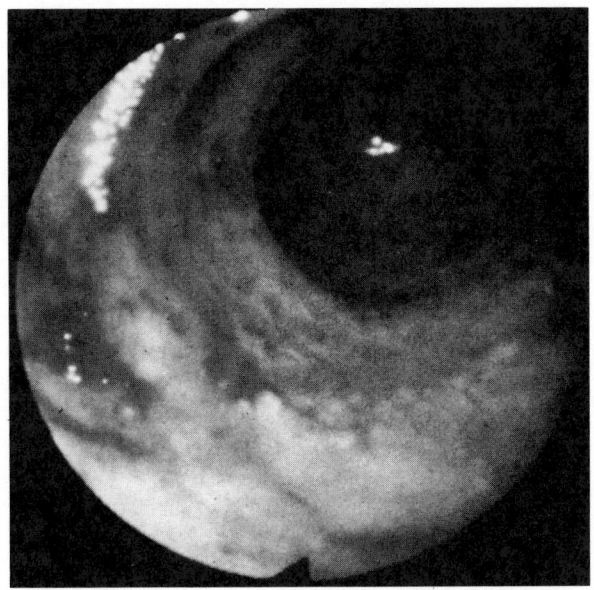 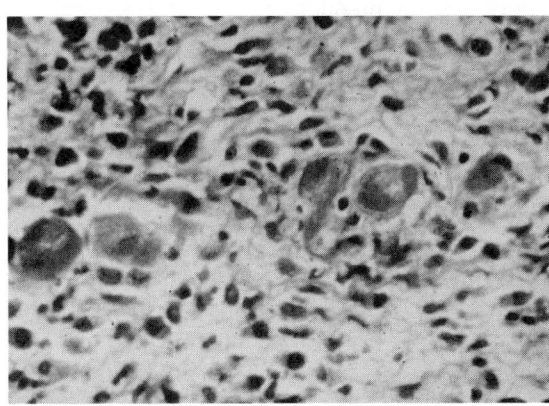

FIG. 1. Endoscopic and light microscopic appearance of cytomegalovirus colitis in an HIV-1–infected man. **A:** Direct visualization shows a diffusely ulcerated and bleeding mucosa with inflammation and exudate. **B:** Histology of the lesion in A shows numerous cytomegalic inclusion cells and inflammatory cells (×125). (From ref. 133, with permission.) (See Plate 6.)

(36,47,48). Although anaerobes are not predominant as in classic bacterial overgrowth syndrome, the increased number of bacteria may increase the local availability of bacterial products capable of stimulating cytokine and HIV-1 expression by mucosal macrophages.

As the largest lymphoid organ in the body, the lamina propria is not only a reservoir for HIV-1–infected cells but a site of HIV-1 expression. We recently determined the level of HIV-1 mRNA-expressing cells in the mucosa of AIDS patients with enteric infections to be 0.06% (31), which is approximately 6–60 times greater than the apparent frequency (0.001% to 0.01%) of cells reported to express viral RNA in lymph nodes from patients with AIDS (49). The prevalence of productively infected cells in the mucosa may reflect the local abundance of stimuli (bacterial endotoxin), certain cytokines (TNF-α, IL-6), and herpes group viruses (cytomegalovirus) capable of inducing viral transcription by HIV-1–infected mononuclear cells.

Late Mucosal Events

The reduction in the number of circulating CD4+ T cells and the decline in many of the functions of circulating T cells, B cells, and monocytes leads to the acquisition of systemic opportunistic infections. Since these cells populate the mucosa, the assumption that lymphoid function in the mucosa is also impaired seems reasonable. Impaired local immune function together with diminished nonspecific defense mechanisms as described above and summarized in Table 1 predispose the gastrointestinal tract to the diarrheal illnesses discussed next.

CLINICAL FEATURES, DIAGNOSTIC MEASURES, AND MANAGEMENT

Early Stage: Acute HIV-1 Infection

Clinical Illness

Several days to weeks after HIV-1 inoculation, 50% to 75% of patients experience an acute viral syndrome (Table 3) (50–52). This illness, acute HIV-1 syndrome is characterized by fever, headache, malaise, adenopathy, rash, pharyngitis, myalgias, and arthralgias. In addition, gastrointestinal symptoms occur in 33% to 67% of patients with acute HIV-1 syndrome and include anorexia, nausea, vomiting, and diarrhea (53–55). Rarely, acute HIV-1 syndrome is complicated by systemic manifestations, includ-

TABLE 3. Systemic and gastrointestinal features of acute HIV-1 syndrome

Systemic:	Fever
	Pharyngitis
	Headache/retrobulbar pain
	Malaise/lethargy
	Myalgias/arthralgias
	Lymphadenopathy
	Rash
Gastrointestinal:	Anorexia
	Nausea
	Vomiting
	Diarrhea
	Esophageal ulcers and candidiasis (rarely)

TABLE 4. *Differential diagnoses of acute HIV-1 syndrome*

Mononucleosis due to cytomegalovirus or Epstein–Barr virus infection
Viral hepatitis
Syphilis
Herpes simplex virus infection
Disseminated gonococcal infection
Rubella infection

ing aseptic meningoencephalitis, pneumonitis, acute renal failure, and esophageal ulcers and candidiasis (see preceding chapter). The presence of esophageal or systemic manifestations at this early stage of HIV-1 infection is associated with a more rapid progression to AIDS (56). Since acute HIV-1 syndrome, which lasts approximately 3 weeks, occurs prior to the acquisition of opportunistic intestinal infections but in the presence of high titer HIV-1 viremia (57,58), the cause of the symptoms is clearly HIV-1, possibly through the induction of cytokines as discussed above.

Diagnosis

The presence of symptoms consistent with acute HIV-1 syndrome in a person at risk for HIV-1 infection should alert the clinician to the possibility of initial HIV-1 infection. The presence of esophageal manifestations (ulcers, candidiasis) should strengthen that suspicion. Other etiologies that should be considered are listed in Table 4. The diagnosis of acute HIV-1 syndrome is established by the development of antibodies to HIV-1 as detected by enzyme-linked immunosorbent assay or immunoblotting. HIV-1-specific antibodies are usually detected shortly after onset of the syndrome (59,60). DNA amplification has been used to detect HIV-1 before antibodies are detectable in persons with long (window) periods between inoculation and seroconversion (61).

Treatment

The diarrhea associated with acute HIV-1 syndrome is transient and does not require treatment. Anecdotal reports indicate that esophageal ulcers can be successfully treated with steroids and thalidomide (see preceding chapter).

Intermediate Stage: Clinical Latency and Diarrhea without Detectable Pathogens

Clinical Illness

During the period between infection and clinical AIDS, which often lasts 8–10 years, the majority of HIV-1–infected persons do not have gastrointestinal manifestations. However, some patients develop diarrhea in the absence of detectable enteric pathogens. Previously referred to as "AIDS enteropathy" (43,62), this clinical condition is characterized by chronic, nonbloody, often watery diarrhea of variable severity and weight loss. In African patients, the diarrhea and weight loss may be extreme and life threatening (63). On physical examination, substantial reductions in both total body weight and muscle mass lead to cachexia (64); body cell mass at the time of death for many patients with AIDS approaches 50% of normal (65). Malabsorption of fat and carbohydrate is common (62,66). Histology of the small intestine shows partial villus atrophy with or without crypt hyperplasia (12,14,43,67,68). However, the reduction in surface area is only 17% (69) and villus atrophy and crypt hyperplasia occur as frequently in HIV-1–infected persons without diarrhea (67,68), suggesting that these changes alone are inadequate to account for the diarrhea. An alternative explanation is that occult infection with known pathogens or infection with yet-to-be-discovered pathogens is present.

Diagnosis

The strength of the diagnosis "AIDS enteropathy" rests on the scientific rigor with which other potential etiologies are excluded. To exclude other pathogens, important considerations include the epidemiology and microbiology of potential pathogens, the cost and feasibility of stool examination alone vs. stool examination plus an invasive diagnostic procedure, the ability of the patient to undergo an extensive endoscopic evaluation, and the therapeutic implication for identifying certain pathogens (70,71).

The three-phase diagnostic evaluation outlined in Table 5, which was used for 10 years at the National Institutes of Health, has yielded a specific pathogen in as many as 85% of patients with AIDS and diarrhea (48). Stool examination is the initial and most important diagnostic test. Based on only stool microbiological evaluation and culture, Laughon et al. (72) and Dryden et al. (73) identified enteric pathogens in 48% to 55% of HIV-1–infected patients with diarrhea. Steps 2 and 3 of the evaluation are performed successively when the previous step yields no identifiable pathogen or when the patient remains symptomatic despite therapy for an identified pathogen. These steps require the performance of an endoscopic procedure to obtain mucosal biopsy specimens. In this regard, Greenson et al. (68) showed that endoscopy (esophagoduodenoscopy and sigmoidoscopy) yielded a diagnosis in 50% of patients in whom no pathogen was detected by stool examination (68). Sigmoidoscopy is reportedly more sensitive than colonoscopy (97% vs. 62%, respectively) in providing a diagnosis of an enteric pathogen in HIV-1–infected persons (74). Until a prospective study has confirmed the presence of bacterial overgrowth and delineated its natural history in HIV-1–infected persons, small intestinal fluid is not routinely cultured for anaerobic and aerobic bacteria.

TABLE 5. *Diagnostic evaluation of diarrhea in HIV-1–infected persons*

Step 1:
Stool cultured for *Salmonella* species, *Shigella flexneri*, *Campylobacter jejuni*, and *Clostridium difficile* at least twice and assayed for *Clostridium difficile* toxin
Stool specimens (direct, concentrated, or both) examined for parasites using saline, iodine, trichrome, acid-fast preparations and for mycobacteria
Step 2:
Gastroduodenoscopy and colonoscopy performed to inspect tissue and obtain biopsy specimens and luminal material
Biopsy specimens stained with hematoxylin-eosin for protozoa and viral inclusion cells, with methenamine silver or Giemsa for fungi, and with Fite for mycobacteria
Duodenal biopsy specimens cultured for mycobacteria (if present in the stool)
Colonic biopsy specimens cultured for mycobacteria (if present in the stool) and for herpes simplex virus (rectal tissue)
Duodenal fluid specimens examined as above for parasites
Step 3:
Biopsy specimens examined by electron microscopy for microsporidians (duodenal tissue) and adenovirus (colonic tissue)

Adapted from Smith PD, et al. *Ann Intern Med* 1992; 116:63.

Treatment

A judicious approach to the therapeutic management of diarrheal illness in HIV-1–infected persons is outlined in Table 6. The importance of identifying the infectious etiology is underscored by observations that specific antimicrobial therapy can reduce the volume and frequency of diarrhea in 50% to 69% of HIV-1–infected patients with

TABLE 6. *Principles of therapy for infectious diarrhea in HIV-1–infected persons*

1. Supportive therapy with fluids, electrolytes, and antimotility drugs is important.
2. Specific therapy is preferable to empirical therapy because the differential diagnosis is extensive and because drug intolerance and drug interactions are common.
3. Etiology may be multifactorial; consequently, therapy may be partially but not completely beneficial.
4. Microorganisms may be resistant to currently used agents or may develop resistance.
5. Many infectious syndromes recur; consequently, long-term suppressive therapy is often necessary.
6. Role of total parenteral nutrition, anabolic steroids, and appetite enhancers is uncertain.
7. Specific antimicrobial therapy and supportive care can enhance the quality of life and duration of survival.

Adapted from Smith PD. *Gastroenterol Clin North Am* 1993;22:535.

diarrhea and an identifiable enteric pathogen (48,72). In the absence of detectable pathogens, supportive therapy with rehydration, electrolyte supplementation, and drugs that inhibit intestinal motility and secretion is associated with clinical improvement. Many patients may benefit symptomatically from therapy with loperamide, diphenoxylate, or paregoric. Some patients may also benefit from treatment with octreotide, a synthetic cyclic octapeptide analog of somatostatin, that has been shown to reduce stool frequency and volume in as many as 61% of AIDS patients with refractory diarrhea and no detectable pathogen (75). In addition, HIV-1–infected patients with intestinal symptoms but no identifiable pathogens who received zidovudine have been reported to have higher levels of intestinal brush border enzymes than comparable patients who did not receive the drug (43), but the effect of this antiviral agent on intestinal symptoms is unclear. To date, the mainstay of management of HIV-1–infected persons with diarrhea but no detectable enteric pathogens remains symptomatic therapy.

Late Stage: Opportunistic Pathogens

Protozoal Infections

Cryptosporidium

This protozoan parasite is present in approximately 20% of persons with AIDS and diarrhea in the United States (48,72,76,77) but as many as 55% of cases in developing countries such as Zaire and Haiti (78,79). *Cryptosporidium* is a relatively common cause of self-limited watery diarrhea in immunocompetent persons (76,80,81) but causes debilitating diarrhea in patients with AIDS. Typically, the diarrhea is relentless, voluminous, nonbloody, and watery; abdominal cramps and weight loss are also prominent symptoms (82). Asymptomatic carriage has been reported (83), but symptoms of dehydration and wasting are more common. Malabsorption of both fat and carbohydrate is associated with cryptosporidiosis. Rarely, *Cryptosporidium* may spread to the biliary tract, leading to biliary tract obstruction (84,85), or the esophagus, causing esophagitis (86). The parasite has been identified throughout the length of the gastrointestinal tract, developing within a parasitophorous vacuole beneath the epithelial cell membrane but outside the cytoplasm.

Diagnosis. Infection with *Cryptosporidium* is easily diagnosed by microscopic identification in stool with a modified acid-fast stain. Concentration of stool by zinc sulfate or Shether sucrose flotation enhances detection of rare or infrequent oocysts during intermittent shedding. Organisms may also be identified on small and large intestinal brush border by electron microscopy, but this technique is rarely necessary.

Treatment. Despite anecdotal reports of successful treatment of cryptosporidiosis in HIV-1–infected persons with spiramycin (87,88), paramomycin (89–91), bovine colostrum (92,93), transfer factor (94), somatostatin (75,95) and zidovudine (96), therapy with these agents has not been consistently effective and controlled clinical

TABLE 7. *Therapy for intestinal infections in HIV-1–infected adults*

Pathogen	Treatment	Alternative treatment
Protozoal:		
Cryptosporidium spp.	Paromomycin 500–750 mg PO qid	Azithromycin (being evaluated)
Microsporidium spp.	Albendazole 400 mg PO bid × 4 wks	
Isospora belli[a]	Trimethoprim-sulfamethoxazole 1 DS[b] tab PO qid × 10 d, then bid × 3 wks	
Giardia lamblia	Metronidazole 250 mg PO tid × 5 d	Quinacrine 100 mg PO tid × 5 d
Cyclospora[c]	NA[d]	
Viral:		
Cytomegalovirus[a,e,f]	Ganciclovir 5 mg/kg IV bid × 2–3 wk	Foscarnet 60 mg/kg IV tid or 90 mg IV bid × 2–3 wk
Herpes simplex[a,e,f]	Acyclovir 400 mg PO 5/d × 7–14 d	Foscarnet 40 mg/kg IV q 8 h × 3 wk
Adenovirus	NA	
Rotavirus[c]	NA	
Astrovirus[c]	NA	
Picobirnavirus[c]	NA	
Bacterial:		
Salmonella spp.[a,f]	Ceftriaxone 1–2 g PO qd × 7 d	Amoxicillin 1 g PO tid × 7–14 d
	Ciprofloxacin 500 mg PO bid × 7 d	Trimethoprim-sulfamethoxazole 1 DS tab bid × 10–14 d
Shigella flexneri[a,f]	Ciprofloxacin 500 mg PO bid × 7 d	Trimethoprim-sulfamethoxazole 1 DS tab bid × 10–14 d
	Ampicillin 500 mg PO qid × 5 d	Ceftriaxone 1–2 g PO qd × 7 d
Campylobacter jejuni[a,f]	Erythromycin 500 PO mg qid × 7 d	Tetracycline 500 mg PO qid × 7 d
	Ciprofloxacin 500 PO mg bid × 7 d	
Mycobacterium-avium complex[a,f]	Clarithromycin 500–1000 mg PO bid or Azithromycin 500 mg PO qd	Rifabutin 300 mg PO qd
	Ethambutol 15–25 mg/kg PO qd	Rifampin 600 mg PO qd
plus one or more:	Clofazamine 100–200 mg PO qd	Ethambutol 15 mg/kg PO qd
	Ciprofloxacin 750 mg PO bid	Cycloserine 250 mg PO bid
	Amikacin 7.5–15 mg/kg IV qd	Imipenum 500–750 mg IM bid
Clostridium difficile	Metronidazole 500 mg PO tid × 7–10 d	Vancomycin 15 mg PO qid × 7–10 d
Bacteriosis[c]	Ciprofloxacin 500 mg PO bid × 4 wk[g]	
Fungal:		
Histoplasma capsulatum[a]	Amphotericin B 0.5–0.6 mg/kg IV qd × 4–8 wks	Itraconazole 200 mg bid

[a] Chronic suppression at reduced dosage may be necessary.
[b] Double strength.
[c] Pathogenicity in HIV-1 infection not established.
[d] Not available.
[e] Reduce dosage for decreased creatinine clearance.
[f] Resistance may develop; susceptibility testing necessary.
[g] Based on ref. 197.

trials have not yet been performed. A course of paromomycin (see Table 7), a nonabsorbable aminoglycoside, is reasonable based on preliminary studies reporting symptomatic improvement and oocyst clearance in some patients (89–91). Somatostatin may reduce the frequency and volume of *Cryptosporidium*-associated diarrhea (75,95), but therapy is complicated by requirements that the drug be given chronically, several times daily and either intravenously or subcutaneously.

Microsporidium

Microsporidia are spore-forming, obligate intracellular protozoa that infect the small intestine *(Enterocytozoon*

bieneusi), small intestine with dissemination *(Septata intestinalis),* liver *(Encephalitozoon cuniculi),* and cornea *(Encephalitozoon hellem).* To date, microsporidia have been reported exclusively in HIV-1–infected persons. Infection with the parasite is associated with chronic, watery, nonbloody diarrhea of variable severity, frequently with substantial fluid and weight loss (97–99). Microsporidiosis has been reported to account for 40% to 50% of the cases of unexplained diarrhea among patients with HIV-1 infection (100,101). However, a recent report that *E. bieneusi* was as common in HIV-1–infected persons without diarrhea as in HIV-1–infected persons with diarrhea suggests that the parasite may not be as pathogenic as previous studies suggested (102); additional studies addressing this critical issue are indicated. The highest density of *E. bieneusi* is in the jejunum (103), where the parasite infects enterocytes and may cause villus atrophy (104). The organism is associated with and may cause AIDS-related cholangitis (105), presumably by ascending the proximal small intestine to infect the biliary tract. Ultrastructural features of the parasite are distinctive, and many organisms at different stages of development can be identified in the same enterocyte and cause cytopathic effect (106). *S. intestinalis,* which is ultrastructurally distinct from *E. bieneusi,* can penetrate into the lamina propria, infect macrophages and disseminate to other organs such as the kidney (107).

Diagnosis. Because of their small size, poor staining qualities, and minimal associated inflammation, microsporidia were formerly diagnosed exclusively by transmission electron microscopy. Today, trained observers can identify microsporidia by light microscopy in semithin plastic sections of small intestinal biopsies stained with methylene blue–azure II–basic fuchsin (98), touch preparations of mucosa stained with Giemsa (108,109) and stool specimens stained with a modified trichrome (chromotrope 2R) (110). Kotler et al. (111) compared these techniques and concluded that one light microscopic technique obviated the need for electron microscopy in over 50% of cases and a combination of any two techniques obviated the need in more than 75% of cases. A rapid fluorescence technique based on Uvitex 2B binding to chitin, a component of the spore wall, is reportedly effective for detecting microsporidia (106). However, since Uvitex 2B binds to any chitin-containing microorganism, morphological evaluation may be necessary to confirm the diagnosis. During endoscopy, biopsies should be taken at the most distal site, where the parasite burden is the highest.

Treatment. Curative therapy for microsporidiosis is not currently available. Albendazole, a benzimidazole derivative related to mebendazole, has been used to treat patients with both intestinal species of microsporidia (112). In open-label trials of albendazole (112,113), HIV-1–infected patients with microsporidia-associated diarrhea who received the drug experienced resolution or improvement in their diarrheal symptoms as well as weight gain or cessation of weight loss. While albendazole is being evaluated in a double-blind placebo-controlled trial, it is reasonable to treat patients with microsporidiosis with this agent (see Table 7).

Isospora belli

Intestinal infection with the protozoan *Isosopora belli* occurs in fewer than 3% of AIDS patients in the United States but as many as 15% of patients in developing nations such as Zambia and Haiti (114,115). Isosporosis is typically a chronic illness characterized by profuse, non-bloody, watery diarrhea that may be indistinguishable from the diarrheal illness associated with *Cryptosporidium* and *Microsporidium* infections. Weight loss of at least 10% may occur during the months prior to diagnosis (115,116). Nausea and abdominal cramps also typically accompany the illness; fever and vomiting are less fre-

quent. In Haitian patients, dehydration requiring hospitalization has been reported in nearly 50% of cases (115). Steatorrhea and eosinophilia may also be present. Histology usually shows inflammation associated with some degree of villus atrophy. Although concentrated in the small intestine, *I. belli* can be identified throughout the gastrointestinal tract. Rarely, the organism disseminates to extra-intestinal sites, including mesenteric and tracheobronchial lymph nodes (118).

Diagnosis. The diagnosis of *I. belli* is established by the identification of the typical highly refractile, spherical oocysts (containing two sporoblasts) in stool using the modified Kinyoun acid-fast stain (117). Stool concentration may be necessary to detect infrequent or rare oocysts.

Treatment. The most effective therapeutic agent for *I. belli* is trimethoprim-sulfamethoxazole. Because infection recurs in as many as 50% of cases following treatment, prolonged or repeat therapy with this agent may be required to suppress clinical illness.

Giardia lamblia and *Entamoeba histolytica*

These protozoan parasites are common enteric infections in seronegative homosexual men. In immunosuppressed HIV-1–infected persons, *G. lamblia* does not cause more frequent or severe infection than in seronegative persons and responds appropriately to antimicrobial therapy with metronidazole (119). In HIV-1–infected patients and in seronegative homosexual men, *E. histolytica* is a commensal belonging to non-pathogenic zymodemes (120–122).

Viral Infection

Cytomegalovirus

Cytomegalovirus (CMV) is one of the most common and potentially serious opportunistic pathogens of the gastrointestinal tract in HIV-1–infected persons. Among HIV-1–infected patients with a variety of gastrointestinal symptoms, CMV has been identified in intestinal biopsies in 8% of cases (123), whereas among AIDS patients with colitis or enteritis, it has identified in biopsies of as many as 45% of cases (48). Colitis appears to be the most common manifestation of gastrointestinal CMV disease (48,124), although firm epidemiological data to support this clinical impression are not available. CMV colitis is characterized by diarrhea, fever, and weight loss. Abdominal pain and hematochezia are frequently accompanying symptoms and help distinguish CMV colitis from the protozoan diarrheal illnesses described above. The colon appears to be particularly susceptible to progression to ischemic necrosis and perforation (125). Virtually all other organs of the alimentary tract are susceptible to CMV inflammatory disease, which manifests as esophagitis (126), gastritis (127), small intestinal enteritis (127), and, less frequently, as acalculous cholecystitis (128), papillary stenosis (129,130), sclerosing cholangitis (130), pancreatitis (131), and appendicitis (132). Regardless of whether or not diarrhea is present, CMV-associated disease of the biliary tract (usually without icterus or pruritus) should be included in the differential diagnosis of abdominal pain, nausea, and vomiting in patients with AIDS. Endoscopic findings that suggest CMV-induced disease range from localized hyperemia to hemorrhagic erythema to superficial or deep ulceration (Fig. 1A). The pathogenesis of CMV inflammation of the gastrointestinal tract mucosa and the potential role of CMV-induced inflammatory cytokines (133) are discussed in the section on CMV esophagitis in the preceding chapter.

Diagnosis. The endoscopic or colonoscopic visualization of discrete, often hemorrhagic, erosions or ulcerations with normal intervening mucosa in an HIV-1–infected person should suggest the possibility of CMV disease. Colitis may be patchy in as many as 41% of cases and involve only the right colon or cecum in 18% (134), indicating the potential importance of full colonoscopy in the evaluation of patients with suspected CMV colitis. The diagnosis of CMV gastrointestinal disease is established by the histopathological identification of large (cytomegalic) mononuclear, endothelial, epithelial, or smooth muscle cells containing intranuclear and/or cytoplasmic inclusions with surrounding inflammation (Fig. 1B) (48,135). The intranuclear inclusion (replicating virions) may be surrounded by a space, giving the appearance of an "owl's eye" halo. CMV can also be detected by culture, immunocytochemical staining, *in situ* hybridization, and DNA amplification (see previous chapter), but these sensitive techniques are difficult to perform, time-consuming, and expensive. Also, culture and DNA amplification may not differentiate between the presence of cytomegalovirus alone and cytomegalovirus with inflammation.

Treatment. The drugs of choice for CMV intestinal disease, ganciclovir and foscarnet (see Table 7), are the same as those used for CMV esophageal disease and are discussed in detail in the section on CMV esophagitis in the earlier chapter by Smith.

Herpes Simplex Virus

In contrast to the widespread involvement of the gastrointestinal tract by CMV, herpes simplex virus (HSV) disease is confined to the perianal region, rectum, and esophagus. The perianal lesions are typically chronic, cutaneous ulcers that cause localized pain but not diarrhea (136). Involvement of the rectum (proctitis) is often associated with perianal disease. Proctitis manifests as severe anorectal pain, tenesmus, constipation, inguinal lymphadenopathy, and less often, difficulty with urination and sacral paresthesias. Such symptoms may also be associated with proctitis in seronegative homosexual men (137). Diarrhea is not associated with typical proctitis, although the mucopurulent discharge may be misinterpreted as diarrhea. Proctocolitis, which occurs when the proctitis extends proximally into the distal sigmoid colon, can cause mild diarrhea associated with hematochezia, but the predominant symptoms are generally those of the proctitis. Overall, HSV proctocolitis is an infrequent cause of diarrhea in HIV-1–infected persons (48).

Diagnosis. Anoscopy and sigmoidoscopy are required to diagnose HSV proctitis and proctocolitis, respectively. Typical lesions begin as small vesicles and progress to erosions that often coalesce into diffuse ulcers. Diagnosis is predicated on the cytological identification of intranuclear (Cowdry type A) inclusions in cells within the lesion and is confirmed by virus isolation.

Treatment. The drugs of choice for HSV perianal disease and proctitis are acyclovir and foscarnet. These drugs are discussed in detail in the section on HSV esophagitis in the earlier chapter by Smith.

Adenovirus

Adenovirus is a recognized cause of diarrheal illness in healthy children and immunocompromised adults without HIV-1 infection (138). In immunosuppressed HIV-1–infected persons, the virus has been isolated from various body sites and may induce hepatic necrosis (139,140), but intestinal involvement is uncommon. In this regard, two reports indicate that among HIV-1–infected persons with diarrhea in the United States, adenovirus excretion is not more common than in patients without diarrhea (72,141). In contrast, 23% of Australian HIV-1–infected patients with diarrhea are reported to excrete adenovirus, whereas only 5.4% of asymptomatic HIV-1–infected patients excreted the virus (142). To date, only Janoff et al. (143) have examined intestinal tissue specimens from HIV-1–infected persons with diarrhea for the presence of adenovirus. Using culture and transmission electron microscopy, they identified adenovirus in inflamed colonic tissue of patients with AIDS who had chronic, watery, nonbloody, nonmucoid diarrhea. Weight loss was also a prominent symptom. Endoscopically, the colonic mucosa showed areas of discrete, often raised, erythematous lesions that were several millimeters in diameter. Light microscopy revealed chronic inflammation surrounding epithelial cells that contained large, amphophilic intranuclear inclusions. In contrast to the classic haloed appearance of CMV intranuclear inclusions, the inclusions in adenovirus-infected cells filled the nucleus, and cytoplasmic inclusions were not observed. Adenovirus appeared to infect only epithelial cells, especially goblet cells, sparing lamina propria cells, which are frequent targets of CMV. At the ultrastructural level, adenovirus was associated with degeneration, death, and focal necrosis of infected epithelial cells, some of which had been extruded into the lumen (Fig. 2). Although this study clearly showed that adenovirus can cause pathogenic changes in the colonic mucosa of HIV-1–infected persons with symptomatic colitis, a causal relationship between the pathological changes and the diarrhea has not been established.

Diagnosis. The diagnosis of adenovirus colitis is established by both the presence of mucosal inflammation and the identification of adenovirus by culture or transmission electron microscopy in a colonic biopsy specimen from a patient with diarrhea and no other detectable pathogens.

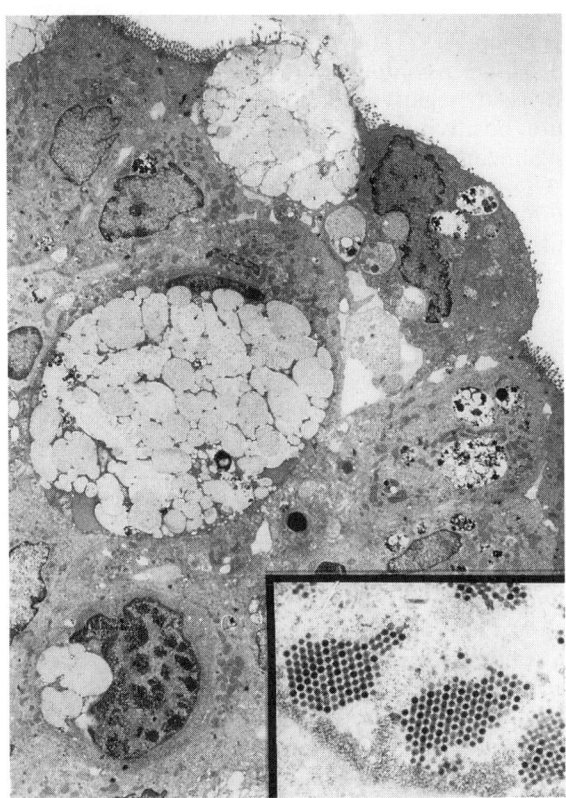

FIG. 2. Transmission electron micrograph of colonic epithelium from an HIV-1–infected person with adenovirus colitis. The degenerating goblet cell shows microvillus atrophy and a condensed nucleus containing a crystalline array of hexagonal nucleoids *(insert)* typical of adenovirus (×5390; insert ×33,600). (Courtesy of J. M. Orenstein.)

As pointed out by Janoff (144), when differences in the cytopathic effect of adenovirus vs. CMV in cell culture is not readily apparent, species- and type-specific antisera can be used to distinguish the two viruses. Although children are infected primarily with serotypes 40 and 41, HIV-1–infected patients excrete a range of serotypes (145).

Treatment. There is no known therapy for adenovirus colitis.

Bacterial Infections

Salmonella species, Shigella flexneri and Campylobacter jejuni

The diarrheal illnesses caused by *Salmonella* species (*S. typhimurium* and, less frequently, *S. enteriditis*) (145–152), *Shigella flexneri* (152–156) and *Campylobacter jejuni* (157,158) are clinically very similar and therefore are discussed together. In HIV-1–infected persons, these bacteria cause recurrent or chronic diarrhea commonly associated with fever and abdominal cramps. During symptomatic infection, the stool often contains fecal leukocytes and grossly visible or microscopic blood. Compared with salmonellosis, shigellosis, and *C. jejuni* infection in seronegative people, these infections in persons with AIDS occur substantially more frequently, cause a more prolonged or recurrent illness, and are more frequently associated with bacteremia and antibiotic resistance.

Diagnosis. These bacterial pathogens are diagnosed by culture of the organism in stool.

Treatment. Appropriate antimicrobial therapy for these organisms is listed in Table 7. Because recurrence is common and antimicrobial resistance may develop, repeat culture of stool and blood (when bacteremia is present) are required to monitor the response to antimicrobial therapy (see Table 6).

Mycobacterium-avium Complex

M. avium complex (MAC) is an acid-fast, obligate intracellular microorganism found throughout the world. The organism is the most common cause of systemic bacterial infection in HIV-1–infected persons in the United States, particularly those with AIDS. MAC is much less common in Africa and Haiti. End organ disease and bacteremia do not occur, however, until the number of CD4+ T cells declines to less than 100 cells/mm^3. Substantial gastrointestinal tract disease, which is usually a manifestation of disseminated infection, is associated with diarrhea, abdominal pain, malabsorption, weight loss, and fever, with or without night sweats (159,160). Concomitant hepatomegaly and/or splenomegaly due to MAC infection is often present. Evidence of numerous mycobacteria on histologic sections of biopsy or autopsy specimens suggests a causative or contributory role for MAC in the gastrointestinal manifestations. Endoscopic abnormalities are nonspecific and include erythema, friability, erosions, and fine white nodules. Occasionally, an inflammatory mass, which can be mistaken for a tumor, is the major gastrointestinal manifestation. The small intestine is reported to be involved more often than the colon (159), but this may reflect easier endoscopic access. Histological examination shows diffuse infiltration of the lamina propria by macrophages filled with bacilli (Fig. 3). These cells resemble the large, foamy macrophages containing periodic acid-Schiff bacilli in Whipple's disease, but electron microscopy and culture have confirmed the presence of MAC and the absence of *Tropheryma whippelii* (161,162). Granulomas are usually absent or poorly developed.

Diagnosis. The diagnosis of MAC is based on the visualization of typical acid-fast organisms in stool or mucosal biopsy specimens (fixed and touch preparations) (159,164). Retrospective analysis has suggested that culture of gastrointestinal tissue increases the positivity rate compared to acid fast staining alone (159), but this has not been evaluated in a controlled prospective study. Isolation and speciation is achieved by culture of organisms from stool and biopsy specimens (163,164). Although the incidence of *M. tuberculosis* pulmonary infections are increasing among HIV-1–infected persons, intestinal involvement is uncommon.

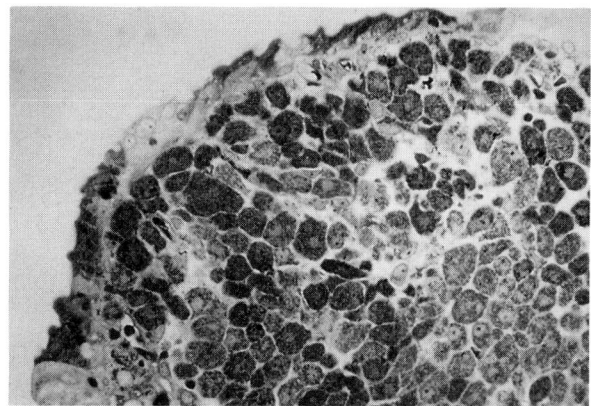

FIG. 3. Light micrograph of colonic mucosa infected with *M. avium* complex from a man with HIV-1 infection. Numerous lamina propria macrophages are filled with mycobacteria; stained with methylene blue-azure II, basic fuchsin (×100). (From ref. 179, with permission.)

Treatment. Although trials of antituberculous agents were initially disappointing (165–167), some combination regimens (i.e., rifampin, ethambutol, clofazimine, and ciprofloxacin) have produced rapid, albeit transient, clinical improvement and reduced bacteremia (168). More recently, there has been optimism for treating MAC with clarithromycin, azithromycin, and rifabutin (ansamycin), which have excellent *in vitro* activity. Ethambutol also appears to have activity against MAC. Clarithromycin monotherapy for disseminated disease can induce microbiological and clinical responses lasting 1–3 months. Combination regimens should produce more sustained benefit, but such regimens are expensive, toxic, difficult to tolerate and have not yet been proven to be more beneficial than clarithromycin alone. Nevertheless, the current recommended therapy is clarithromycin or azithromycin plus one or more of ethambutol, clofazimine, ciprofloxacin, and amikacin (169). For prophylaxis, rifabutin instituted when the CD4 count falls below 200 cells/mm^3 can reduce the frequency of disseminated MAC by 50% (170), although the duration of benefit has not been determined. There is also enthusiasm for clarithromycin or azithromycin for prophylaxis, but large clinical trials have not yet been completed. Rifabutin is a potent inducer of hepatic enzymes and, consequently, may alter the metabolism of other drugs. Clarithromycin inhibits hepatic metabolism and may have the opposite effect on drug levels.

Clostridium difficile

C. difficile, a gram-positive bacterium, is one of the most important causes of nosocomial intestinal infection. *C. difficile* infections appear not to be more common or more severe in HIV-1–infected persons than in seronegative persons (171,172). Nevertheless, because of the frequent use of antimicrobial agents, frequent hospitalizations, and immunosuppression, HIV-1–infected patients with diarrhea should be evaluated for infection with this organism with stool culture and toxin assay (173,174). Among non-HIV-1–infected persons with *C. difficile* culture-positive pseudomembranous colitis, 11% are cytotoxin assay-negative (174). In addition, rates of stool culture positivity (90% to 97%) have been shown to be significantly higher than stool toxin positivity (70% to 73%) for *C. difficile* among persons shown to have *C. difficile* infection (173), indicating that culture is more sensitive than toxin for detecting this organism. *C. difficile* in HIV-1–infected persons responds appropriately to metronidazole or vancomycin (see Table 7).

Fungal Infections

Histoplasma capsulatum

Disseminated *H. capsulatum* has emerged as an important opportunistic infection in HIV-1–infected persons who reside in endemic areas (175,176). Gastrointestinal involvement generally reflects disseminated disease, which is due primarily to reactivation of quiescent infection. Among persons with disseminated histoplasmosis, gastrointestinal involvement has been detected in approximately 70% of cases by evaluation of biopsy specimens, but gastrointestinal symptoms are present in only about 10% of patients (177). Symptoms include diarrhea, weight loss, fever, and abdominal pain. Similar to the infection with MAC, whether *H. capsulatum* itself causes these symptoms has not been proven. Most patients with gastrointestinal manifestations of *H. capsulatum* have colonic involvement. Colonoscopy in such patients may show inflammation, ulcerations, or fungating mass lesions.

Diagnosis. The histological examination of Giemsa-stained sections shows small intracellular yeast-like cells within macrophages or histiocytes. When infection is intense, the organism is not difficult to identify. However, the diagnosis of histoplasmosis is established by culture.

Treatment. Amphotericin B is the drug of choice for disseminated histoplasmosis (see Table 7). The recommended initial course of therapy in HIV-1–infected persons is amphotericin B 0.5–0.6 mg/kg intravenously daily for 4–8 weeks, or longer, depending on the clinical response (178). Long-term therapy with amphotericin B (50–80 mg intravenously every 2 weeks) is also highly effective in suppressing relapses after initial treatment (176).

Other Potential Enteric Pathogens

Recent investigations have identified other enteric microorganisms in HIV-1–infected persons with diarrhea. The association between the presence of these organisms and diarrheal illness suggests they have a pathogenic role in the illness, but proof of such a role awaits definitive epidemiological and clinical studies. These pathogens include Cyclospora species; the enteric viruses astrovirus, picobirnavirus and in some regions rotavirus; and an undefined enteroadherent bacteria.

Cyclospora

Cyclospora is a newly identified protozoan parasite with morphological and staining characteristics of a cyanobacterium-like organism (179,180). Microscopically, the spherical cyst-like organisms measure 8–10 μm in diameter and on modified acid-fast staining resemble *Cryptosporidium* (181). The cyclospora oocyst has two sporocysts, each containing two sporozoites, distinguishing the structure of this coccidian parasite from that of the larger *I. belli* whose oocysts have two sporocysts, each containing four sporozoites (181). The organism has been identified in persons with diarrhea from Latin America, the Caribbean, Southeast Asia, Eastern Europe, and the United States. In immunocompetent persons, the diarrhea is typically abrupt in onset, watery, and prolonged (lasting a mean of 6 weeks) but self-limited (182). The histopathology of the small intestine in patients with cyclospora-associated diarrhea shows acute and chronic inflammation, surface epithelial disarray, and varying degrees of villous atrophy and crypt hyperplasia (183). Cyclospora infection in persons with AIDS has been associated with prolonged (184) and self-limited (185) diarrhea, but the course of infection in immunosuppressed persons is to date unclear since too few of such patients have been studied.

Astrovirus, Picobirnavirus, and Rotavirus

Prospective evaluation of diarrhea in HIV-1–infected persons recently revealed an association between the presence of astrovirus and picobirnavirus and diarrhea in HIV-1–infected persons (186). Picobirnaviruses are small, bisegmented double-stranded RNA viruses that have been associated with diarrhea in animals, including pigs (187) and calves (188). Their identification in 10% of a cohort of HIV-1–infected persons with chronic diarrhea and prolonged viral shedding (186) suggests, but does not establish, a novel etiologic role in human diarrheal illness. Astroviruses are also small (28–30 nm in diameter) RNA viruses that have been identified in a variety of animal species. In humans, astroviruses are a recognized, although uncommon, cause of diarrhea in children (189–191). Astroviruses also were recently shown to be associated with diarrhea in 14% of cases in a cohort of HIV-1–infected persons (186). Further epidemiological and clinical studies are needed to define the etiologic role of these viruses in HIV-1 disease. In contrast to the preliminary study showing an increased prevalence of astroviruses and picobirnaviruses in HIV-1–infected persons with diarrhea (186), rotavirus appears not to be associated with diarrhea in HIV-1–infected persons in the United States (48,72,186,192) and Africa (Zaire) (193,194). However, in Australia rotavirus is the predominant virus detected in the stools of HIV-1–infected homosexual men with diarrhea (195), and in Germany the virus is associated with prolonged diarrhea in approximately 14% of adults with HIV-1–infection (196). These findings suggest geographic variation in the prevalence of rotavirus-associated diarrhea in HIV-1–infected persons.

Bacteriosis

Chronic intestinal infection with an enteroadherent coccobacillus has been reported in a few severely immunosuppressed (CD4+ T cells <100/mm^3) HIV-1–infected persons (197,198). The bacterium, which has not been isolated, appears to adhere to enterocytes predominantly in the right colon and ileum and to be associated with mild to moderate epithelial cell injury and nonspecific inflammation. HIV-1–infected patients with the infection typically have chronic diarrhea of variable severity, malabsorption, and weight loss. Studies are in progress to characterize this potentially important cause of diarrhea in HIV-1–infected persons.

In summary, the gastrointestinal tract plays a fundamental role in the pathogenesis of AIDS. As the largest lymphoid tissue in the body, the lamina propria of the intestinal mucosa is an important site of virological and immunological events that lead to local immunosuppression and the acquisition of the opportunistic infections discussed in this chapter. Increased knowledge regarding the natural history of these infections, better diagnostic modalities, and improved therapeutic options are the basis for a new optimism in caring for HIV-1–infected persons with gastrointestinal infections.

ACKNOWLEDGMENTS

This work was supported in part by research grants (DK-47322 and AI-35940) and contracts (AI-45218, AI-35163, and AI-45209) from the National Institutes of Health; a developmental grant from the Center for AIDS Research, University of Alabama; and the Department of Veterans Affairs.

REFERENCES

1. Smith PD. Mucosal immunopatholphysiology of HIV infection. In: Ogra PH, Mestecky JF, Lamm M, Strobe W, McGhee JR, Bienenstock J, eds. *Handbook of mucosal immunology.* San Diego: Academic Press; 1994:719–728.
2. Sohn N, Ribilotti JG. The gay bowel syndrome. A review of colonic and rectal conditions in 200 male homosexuals. *Am J Gastroenterol* 1977;67:478–484.
3. Surawicz CM, Goodell SE, Quinn TC, et al. Spectrum of rectal biopsy abnormalities in homosexual men with intestinal symptoms. *Gastroenterology* 1986;91:651–659.
4. Wolf JL, Rubin DH, Finberg BN, et al. Intestinal M cells: a pathway for entry of reovirus into the host. *Science* 1981;212:471–472.
5. Sicinski P, Rowinski J, Warchol JB, et al. Poliovirus type 1 enters the human host through intestinal M cells. *Gastroenterology* 1990;98:56–58.
6. O'Leary AD, Sweeney EC. Lymphoglandular complexes of the colon: structure and distribution. *Histopathology* 1986;10:267–283.
7. Amerongen HM, Weltzin R, Farnet CM, et al. Transepithelial transport of HIV-1 by intestinal M cells: a mechanism for transmission of AIDS. *J AIDS* 1991;4:760–765.
8. Nelson JA, Wiley CA, Reynolds-Kohler C, Reese CE, Margaretten W, Levey JA. Human immunodeficiency virus detected in bowel epithelium from patients with gastrointestinal symptoms. *Lancet* 1988;1:259–262.

9. Heise C, Dandekar S, Kumar P, Duplantier R, Donovan RM, Halsted CH. Human immunodeficiency virus infection of enterocytes and mononuclear cells in human jejunal mucosa. *Gastroenterology* 1991;100:1521–1527.

10. Clayton F, Reka S, Cronin WJ, Torlakovic E, Sigal SH, Kotler DP. Rectal mucosal pathology varies with human immunodeficiency virus antigen content and disease stage. *Gastroenterology* 1992;103:919–933.

11. Fox CH, Kotler DP, Tierney AR, Wilson CS, Fauci AS. Detection of HIV-1 RNA in the lamina propria of patients with AIDS and gastrointestinal disease. *J Infect Dis* 1989;159:467–471.

12. Ullrich R, Zeitz M, Heise W, L'age M, Hoffken G, Reiken EO. Small intestinal structure and function in patients infected with human immunodeficiency virus (HIV): Evidence for HIV-induced enteropathy. *Ann Intern Med* 1989;111:15–21.

13. Fleming SC, Kapembwa MS, MacDonald TT, Griffin GE. Direct in vitro infection of human gastrointestinal cells by HIV-1. *AIDS* 1992;6:1099–1104.

14. Ehrenprieis DD, Patterson BK, Brainer JA, et al. Histopathologic findings of duodenal biopsy specimens in HIV-infected patients with and without diarrhea and malabsorption. *Am J Clin Pathol* 1992;97:21–28.

15. Smith PD, Eisner MS, Manischewitz JF, Gill VJ, Masur H, Fox CH. Esophageal disease in AIDS is associated with pathologic processes rather than mucosal human immunodeficiency virus type 1. *J Infect Dis* 1993;159:547–552.

16. Dalgleish AG, Beverley PCL, Clapham PR, Crawford DH, Greaves MF, Weiss RA. The CD4 (T4) antigen is an essential component of the receptor for the AIDS retrovirus. *Nature* 1984;312:763–766.

17. Klatzman D, Champagne E, Chamaret S, et al. T lymphocyte T4 molecule behaves as the receptor for the human retrovirus LAV. *Nature* 1984;312:767–768.

18. Picker LJ, Butcher EC. Physiological and molecular mechanisms of lymphocyte homing. *Annu Rev Immunol* 1992: 561–591.

19. Wahl LM, Corcoran ML, Pyle SW, Arthur LO, HarelBellan A, Farrar WL. Human immunodeficiency virus glycoprotein (gp 120) induction of monocyte arachidonic acid metabolites and interleukin 1. *Proc Natl Acad Sci USA* 1989;86:621–625.

20. Merrill JE, Koyanagi Y, Chen ISY. Interleukin-1 and tumor necrosis factor-α can be induced from mononuclear phagocytes by human immunodeficiency virus type 1 binding to the CD4 receptor. *J Virol* 1989;63:4404–4408.

21. Molina J-M, Scadden DT, Byrn R, Dinarello C, Groopman JE. Production of tumor necrosis factor α by monocytic cells infected with human immunodeficiency virus. *J Clin Invest* 1990; 144:970–975.

22. Wright SC, Jewett A, Mitsuyasu R, Bonavida B. Spontaneous cytotoxicity and tumor necrosis factor production by peripheral blood monocytes from AIDS patients. *J Immunol* 1988;141: 99–104.

23. Voth R, Rossol S, Klein K, et al. Differential gene expression of IFN-α and tumor necrosis factor–α in peripheral blood mononuclear cells from patients with AIDS related complex and AIDS. *J Immunol* 1990;144:970–975.

24. Kandil HM, Berschneider HM, Argenzio RA. Tumour necrosis factor α changes porcine intestinal ion transport through a paracrine mechanism involving prostaglandins. *Gut* 1994;35: 934–940.

25. Fuller CM, Smith PD. Role of cytokines in AIDS diarrhea. *Reg Pept Lett* 1995; in press.

26. Schrager LK, Young JM, Fowler MG, Mathieson BJ, Vermund ST. Long-term survivors of HIV-1 infection: definitions and research challenges. *AIDS* 1994;8(Suppl. 1):S95–S108.

27. Pantaleo G, Graziosi C, Demarest JF, et al. HIV infection is active and progressive in lymphoid tissue during the clinically latent stage of disease. *Nature* 1993;362:355–358.

28. Embretson J, Zupancic M, Ribas JL, et al. Massive covert infection of helper T lymphocytes and macrophages by HIV during the incubation period of AIDS. *Nature* 1993;362:359–362.

29. Harriman GR, Smith PD, Horne MK, et al. Vitamin B12 malabsorption in patients with acquired immunodeficiency syndrome. *Arch Intern Med* 1989;149:2039–2041.

30. Jarry A, Cartez A, Rene E, Muzeau F, Brousse N. Infected and immune cells in the gastrointestinal tract of AIDS patients. An immunohistochemical study of 127 cases. *Histopathology* 1990;16:133–140.

31. Smith PD, Fox CH, Masur H, Winter HS, Alling DW. Quantitative analysis of mononuclear cells expressing HIV-1 RNA in esophageal mucosa. *J Exp Med* 1994;180:1541–1546.

32. Yolffe B, Lewis DE, Petrie BL, Noonan CA, Melnick JL, Hollinger FB. Fusion as a mediator of cytolysis in mixtures of uninfected CD4+ lymphocytes and cells infected by human immunodeficiency virus. *Proc Natl Acad Sci USA* 1987;84: 1429–1433.

33. Lifson J, Reyes GR, McGrath MS, Stein BS, Engleman EG. AIDS retrovirus induced cytopathology: giant cell formation and involvement of CD4 antigen. *Science* 1986;232:1123–1127.

34. Meyaard L, Otto SA, Jonker RR, Mijnster MJ, Keet RPM, Miedema F. Programmed death of T cells in HIV-1 infection. *Science* 1992;257:217–219.

35. Rodgers VD, Fassett R, Kagnoff MF. Abnormalities in intestinal mucosal T cells in homosexual populations including those with lymphadenopathy syndrome and acquired immunodeficiency syndrome. *Gastroenterology* 1986;90:552–558.

36. Budhraja M, Levendoglu H, Kocka F, Mangkornkanok M, Shere R. Duodenal mucosal T cell subpopulation and bacterial cultures in acquired immune deficiency syndrome. *Am J Gastroenterol* 1987;82:427–431.

37. Ellakany S, Whiteside TL, Schade RR, van Thiel DH. Analysis of intestinal lymphocyte subpopulations in patients with acquired immunodeficiency syndrome (AIDS) and AIDS-related complex. *Am J Clin Pathol* 1987;87:356–364.

38. Strober W. Mechanisms of mucosal immunity in relations to AIDS. In: Smith PD, moderator. Gastrointestinal infections in AIDS. *Ann Intern Med* 1992;116:63–77.

39. Steffen M, Reinecker HC, Petersen J, et al. Differences in cytokine secretion by intestinal mononuclear cells, peripheral blood monocytes and alveolar macrophages from HIV-infected patients. *Clin Exp Immunol* 1993;91:30–36.

40. Kotler DP, Reka S, Clayton F. Intestinal mucosal inflammation associated with human immunodeficiency virus infection. *Dig Dis Sci* 1993;38:1119–1127.

41. Kotler DP, Scholes JV, Tierney AR. Intestinal plasma cell alterations in acquired immunodeficiency syndrome. *Dig Dis Sci* 1987;32:129–138.

42. Janoff EN, Jackson S, Wahl SM, Thomas K, Peterman JF, Smith PD. Intestinal mucosal immunoglobulins during human immunodeficiency virus type 1 infection. *J Infect Dis* 1994;170: 299–307.

43. Ullrich R, Heise W, Bergs C, L'age M, Riecken EO, Zeitz M. Effects of zidovudine treatment on the small intestinal mucosa in patients infected with the human immunodeficiency virus. *Gastroenterology* 1992;102:1483–1492.

44. Reeves-Darby VG, Mathias JR, Clench MH. Abdominal gastrointestinal motility in patients with human immunodeficiency virus 1. *Gastroenterology* 1991;100:608A.

45. Lake-Bakaar G, Quadrox E, Beidas S, et al. Gastric secretory failure in patients with the acquired immunodeficiency syndrome (AIDS). *Ann Intern Med* 1988;109:502–504.

46. Lake-Bakaar G, Tom W, Lake-Bakaar D, et al. Gastropathy and ketoconazole malabsorption in the acquired immunodeficiency syndrome (AIDS). *Ann Intern Med* 1988;109:471–473.

47. Belitsos PC, Greenson JK, Yardley JH, Sisler JR, Bartlett JG. Association of gastric hypoacidity with opportunistic enteric infections in patient with AIDS. *J Infect Dis* 1992;166:277–284.

48. Smith PD, Lane HC, Gill VJ, et al. Intestinal infections in patients with the acquired immunodeficiency syndrome (AIDS). Etiology and response to therapy. *Ann Intern Med* 1988;108: 328–333.

49. Harper ME, Marselle LM, Gallo RC, Wong-Staal F. Detection of lymphocytes expressing human T-lymphocytes virus type III in lymph nodes and peripheral blood from infected individuals by in situ hybridization. *Proc Natl Acad Sci USA* 1986;83: 772–776.

50. Lange JMA, Parry JV, de Wolf F, Mortimer PP, Goutsmit J.

Diagnostic value of specific IgM antibodies in primary HIV infection. *Br Med J* 1986;293:1459–1462.

51. Fox R, Eldred LJ, Fuchs EJ, et al. Clinical manifestations of acute infection with human immunodeficiency virus in a cohort of gay men. *AIDS* 1987;1:35–38.

52. Pedersen C, Lindhardt BO, Jensen BL, et al. Clinical course of primary HIV infection: consequences for subsequent course of infection. *Br Med J* 1989;299:154–157.

53. Cooper DA, Gold J, Maclean P, et al. Acute AIDS retrovirus infection. Definition of a clinical illness associated with seroconversion. *Lancet* 1985;1:537–540.

54. Tindall B, Cooper DA. Primary HIV infection: host responses and intervention strategies. *AIDS* 1991;5:1–14.

55. Clark SJ, Shaw GM. The acute retroviral syndrome and the pathogenesis of HIV-1 infection. *Semin Immunol* 1993;5:149–155.

56. Pedersen C, Nielsen JO, Dickmeiss E, Jordal R. Early progression to AIDS following primary HIV infection. *AIDS* 1989;3:45–47.

57. Clark SJ, Saag MS, Decker WD, et al. High titers of cytopathic virus in plasma of patients with symptomatic primary HIV-1 infection. *N Engl J Med* 1991;324:954–960.

58. Daar ES, Moudgil T, Meyer RD, Ho DD. Transient high levels of viremia in patients with primary human immunodeficiency virus type 1 infection. *N Engl J Med* 1991;324:961–964.

59. Gaines H von Sydow M, Sonnenborg A, et al. Antibody response in primary human immunodeficiency virus infection. *Lancet* 1987;1:1249–1253.

60. Cooper DA, Imrie AA, Penny R. Antibody response to human immunodeficiency virus after primary infection. *J Infect Dis* 1987;155:1113–1118.

61. Wolinsky SM, Rinaldo CR, Kwok S, et al. Human immunodeficiency virus type 1 (HIV-1) infection a median of 18 months before a diagnostic Western blot. Evidence from a cohort of homosexual men. *Ann Intern Med* 1989;111:961–972.

62. Kotler DP, Gaetz HP, Lange M, et al. Enteropathy associated with the acquired immunodeficiency syndrome. *Ann Intern Med* 1984;101:421–428.

63. Serwadda D, Sewankambo NK, Carswell JW, et al. Slim disease: a new disease in Uganda and its association with HTLV-III infection. *Lancet* 1985;2:849–852.

64. Kotler DP, Wang J, Pierson RN. Body composition studies in patients with the acquired immunodeficiency syndrome. *Am J Clin Nutr* 1985;42:1255–1265.

65. Kotler DP, Tierney AR, Wang J, et al. Magnitude of body-cell-mass depletion and the timing of death from wasting in AIDS. *Am J Clin Nutr* 1989;50:444–447.

66. Gillin JS, Shike M, Alcock N, et al. Malabsorption and mucoal abnormalities of the small intestine in the acquired immunodeficiency syndrome. *Ann Intern Med* 1985;102:619–622.

67. Batman PA, Miller ARO, Forster SM, Harris JRW, Pinching AJ, Griffin GE. Jejunal enteropathy associated with human immunodeficiency virus infection: quantitative histology. *Am J Clin Pathol* 1989;42:275–281.

68. Greenson JK, Belitsos PC, Yardley JH, Bartlett JG. AIDS enteropathy: occult enteric infections and duodenal mucosal alterations in chronic diarrhea. *Ann Intern Med* 1991;114:366–372.

69. Ullrich R, Zeitz M, Heise W, et al. Mucosal atrophy is associated with loss of activated T cells in the duodenal mucosa of human immunodeficiency virus (HIV)-infected patients. *Digestion* 1990;46S:302–307.

70. Janoff EN, Smith PD. Perspectives on gastrointestinal infections in AIDS. *Gastroenterol Clin North Am* 1988;17:451–463.

71. Johanson JF, Sonnenber A. Efficient management of diarrhea in the acquired immunodeficiency syndrome (AIDS). *Ann Intern Med* 1990;112:942–948.

72. Laughon BE, Druckman DA, Vernon A, et al. Prevalence of enteric pathogens in homosexual men with and without acquired immunodeficiency syndrome. *Gastroenterology* 1988;94:984–993.

73. Dryden MS, Shanson DC. The microbial causes of diarrhoea in patients infected with the human immunodeficiency virus. *J Infect* 1988;17:107–114.

74. Connolly GM, Forbes A, Bleeson JA, Gazaard BG. The value of barium enema and colonoscopy in patients with infected with HIV. *AIDS* 1990;4:687–689.

75. Cello JP, Grendell JH, Basuk P, et al. Effect of octreotide on refractory AIDS-associated diarrhea. A prospective, multicenter clinical trial. *Ann Intern Med* 1991;115:705–710.

76. Janoff EN, Reller LB. *Cryptosporidium* species, a protean protozoan. *J Clin Microbiol* 1987;25:967–975.

77. Soave R, Armstrong D. *Cryptosporidium* and cryptosporidiosis in homosexual men. *Rev Infect Dis* 1986;8:1012–1023.

78. Colebunders R, Francis H, Mann JM, et al. Persistent diarrhea strongly associated with HIV infection in Kinshasa, Zaire. *Am J Gastroenterol* 1987;82:859–864.

79. Malebranche R, Arnoux E, Guerin JM, et al. Acquired immunodeficiency syndrome with severe gastrointestinal manifestations in Haiti. *Lancet* 1983;2:873–878.

80. Wolfson JS, Richter JM, Waldron MA, Weber DJ, McCarthy DM, Hopkins CC. Cryptosporidiosis in immunocompetent patients. *N Engl J Med* 1985;312:1278–1282.

81. MacKenzie WR, Hoxie NJ, Proctor ME, et al. A massive outbreak in Milwaukee of cryptosporidium infection transmitted through the public water supply. *N Engl J Med* 1994;331:161–167.

82. Soave R, Danner RL, Honig CL, et al. Cryptosporidiosis in homosexual men. *Ann Intern Med* 1984;110:504–511.

83. Janoff EN, Limas C, Gebhard RL, Penley KA. Cryptosporidial carriage without symptoms in the acquired immunodeficiency syndrome (AIDS). *Ann Intern Med* 1990;112:75–76.

84. Margulis SJ, Honig CL, Soave R, Govoni AF, Mouradian JA, Jacobson IM. Biliary tract obstruction in the acquired immunodeficiency syndrome. *Ann Intern Med* 1986;105:207–210.

85. Schneiderman DJ, Cello JP, Laing FC. Papillary stenosis and sclerosing cholangitis in the acquired immunodeficiency syndrome. *Ann Intern Med* 1987;106:546–549.

86. Kazlow PG, Shah K, Benkov KJ, Dische R, Leleiko NS. Esophageal cryptosporidiosis in a child with acquired immune deficiency syndrome. *Gastroenterology* 1986;91:1301–1303.

87. Portnoy D, Whiteside ME, Buckley E, McLeod CL. Treatment of intestinal cryptosporidiosis with spiramycin. *Ann Intern Med* 1984;101:202–204.

88. Moskovitz BL, Stanton TL, Kusmierek JJ. Spiramycin therapy for cryptosporidial diarrhea in immunocompromised patients. *J Antimicrob Chemother* 1988;22S:189–191.

89. Clezy K, Gold J, Blaze J, Jones P. Paromomycin for the treatment of cryptosporidial diarrhea in AIDS patients. *AIDS* 1991;5:12–13.

90. Armitage K, Flanigan T, Carey J, et al. Treatment of cryptosporidiosis with paromomycin. A report of five cases. *Arch Intern Med* 1992;152:2497–2499.

91. Danzinger LH, Kanyok TP, Novak RM. Treatment of cryptosporidial diarrhea in an AIDS patient with paromomycin. *Ann Pharmacother* 1993;27:1460–1462.

92. Ungar BP, Ward DJ, Fayer R, Quinn CA. Cessation of cryptosporidium-associated diarrhea in an acquired immunodeficiency syndrome patient after treatment with hyperimmune bovine colostrum. *Gastroenterology* 1990;98:486–489.

93. Shield J, Melville C, Novelli V, et al. Bovine colostrum immunoglobulin concentrate for cryptosporidiosis in AIDS. *Arch Dis Child* 1993;69:451–453.

94. Louie E, Borkowsky W, Klesius PH, et al. Treatment of *Cryptosporidium* with oral bovine transfer factor. *Clin Immunol Immunopathol* 1987;73:413–414.

95. Cook DJ, Kelton JG, Stanisz AM, Collins SM. Somatostatin treatment for cryptosporidial diarrhea in a patient with the acquired immunodeficiency syndrome (AIDS). *Ann Intern Med* 1988;108:708–709.

96. Greenberg RE, Mir R, Bank S, Siegal FP. Resolution of intestinal cryptosporidiosis after treatment of AIDS with AZT. *Gastroenterology* 1989;97:1327–1330.

97. Desportes I, Le Charpentier Y, Galian A, et al. Occurrence of a new microspoidian: *Enterocytozoon bieneusi* n. g., n. sp., in the enterocytes of a human patient with AIDS. *J Protozool* 1985;32:250–254.

98. Orenstein JM, Chang J, Steinberg W, Smith PD, Rotterdam H,

Kotler DP. Intestinal microsporidiosis as a cause of diarrhea in human immunodeficiency virus-infected patients: a report of 20 cases. *Hum Pathol* 1990;21:475–481.

99. Orenstein JM. Microsporidiosis in the acquired immunodeficiency syndrome. *J Parasitol* 1991;77:843–864.

100. Eeftinck Schattenkerk JKME, van Gool T, van Ketel RJ, et al. Clinical significance of small-intestinal microsporidiosis in HIV-1-infected individuals. *Lancet* 1991;1:895–898.

101. Molina J-M, Sarfati C, Beauvais B, et al. Intestinal microsporidiosis in human immunodeficiency virus-infected patients with chronic unexplained diarrhea: prevalence and clinical and biologic features. *J Infect Dis* 1993;167:217–221.

102. Rabeneck L, Gyorkey F, Genta R, et al. The role of microsporidia in the pathogenesis of HIV-related chronic diarrhea. *Ann Intern Med* 1993;119:895–899.

103. Orenstein JM, Tenner M, Kotler DP. Localization of infection by the microsporidian *Enterocytozoon bieneusi* in the gastrointestinal tract of AIDS patients with diarrhea. *AIDS* 1992;6:195–197.

104. Kotler DP, Rancisco A, Clayton F, Scholes JV, Orenstein JM. Small intestinal injury and parasitic diseases in AIDS. *Ann Intern Med* 1990;113:444–449.

105. Pol S, Romana CA, Richard S, et al. Microsporidia infection in patients with the human immunodeficiency virus and unexplained cholangitis. *N Engl J Med* 1993;328:95–99.

106. Cali A, Owen RL. Intracellular development of *Enterocytozoon*, a unique microsporidian found in the intestine of AIDS patients. *J Protozool* 1990;37:145–155.

107. Orenstein JM, Tenner M, Cali A, Kotler DP. A microsporidian previously undescribed in humans, infecting enterocytes and macrophages, and associated with diarrhea in an acquired immunodeficiency syndrome patient. *Hum Pathol* 1992;23:722–728.

108. Rijpstra AC, Canning EU, van Ketel, Eeftinck Schattenkerk JKM, Laarman JJ. Use of light microscopy to diagnose small-intestinal microsporidiosis in patients with AIDS. *J Infect Dis* 1988;157:827–831.

109. Simon D, Weiss LM, Tanowitz HB, Cali A, Jones J, Wittner M. Light microscopic diagnosis and variable response to octreotide. *Gastroenterology* 1991;100:271–273.

110. Weber R, Bryan R, Owen RL, et al. Improved light-microscopical detection of microsporidia spores in stool and duodenal aspirates. *N Engl J Med* 1992;326:161–166.

111. Kotler DP, Giang TT, Garro ML, Orenstein JM. Light microscopic diagnosis of microsporidiosis in patients with AIDS. *Am J Gastroenterol* 1994;89:540–544.

112. Dietrich D, Kotler D, Lew E, Poles M, Orenstein J. Albendazole treatment of two species of microsporidial enteritis. *Am J Gastroenterol* 1992;87:1312.

113. Banshard C, Ellis DS, Tovey DG, Dowell S, Gazzard BG. Treatment of intestinal microsporidiosis with albendazole in patients with AIDS. *AIDS* 1992;6:311–313.

114. Conlon CP, Pinching AJ, Perera CU, Moody A, Luo NP, Lucas SB. HIV-related enteropathy in Zambia: a clinical, microbiological and histological study. *Am J Trop Med Hyg* 1990;42:83–88.

115. DeHovitz J, Pape JW, Boncy M, Hohnson WD. Clinical manifestations and therapy of *Isospora belli* infection in patients with the acquired immunodeficiency syndrome. *N Engl J Med* 1986;315:87–90.

116. Ng E, Markell EK, Fleming RL, Freed M. Demonstration of *Isospora belli* by acid–fast stain in a patient with acquired immune deficiency syndrome. *J Clin Microbiol* 1984;20:384–386.

117. Whiteside ME, Barkin JS, May RG, Weiss SD, Fischl MA, MacLeod CL. Enteric coccidiosis among patients with the acquired immunodeficiency syndrome. *Am J Trop Med Hyg* 1984;33:1065–1072.

118. Restrepo C, Macher AM, Radany EH. Disseminated extraintestinal isosporiasis in a patient with acquired immune deficiency syndrome. *Am J Clin Pathol* 1987;87:536–542.

119. Janoff EN, Smith PD, Blaser MJ. Acute antibody responses to *Giardia lamblia* are depressed in patients with AIDS. *J Infect Dis* 1988;157:798–804.

120. Allason-Jones E, Mindel A, Sargeaunt P, Williams P. *Entamoeba histolytica* as a commensal intestinal parasite in homosexual men. *N Engl J Med* 1986;315:353–356.

121. Allason-Jones E, Mindel A, Sargeaunt P, Katz. Outcome of untreated infection with *Entamoeba histolytica* in homosexual men with and without HIV antibody. *Br Med J* 1988;297:654–657.

122. Aucott JN, Ravdin JI. Amegiasis and "nonpathogenic" intestinal protozoa. *Infect Dis Clin North Am* 1993;7:467–485.

123. Frances ND, Boylston AW, Roberts AH, Parkin JM, Pinching AJ. Cytomegalovirus infection in gastrointestinal tracts of patients infected with HIV-1 or AIDS. *J Clin Pathol* 1989;112:1055–1064.

124. Rene E, March C, Chevalier T, Rouzioux C, et al. Cytomegalovirus colitis in patients with acquired immunodeficiency syndrome. *Dig Dis Sci* 1988;33:171–175.

125. Meiselman MS, Cello JP, Margaretten W. Cytomegalovirus colitis. Report of the clinical, endoscopic, and pathologic findings in two patients with the acquired immune deficiency syndrome. *Gastroenterology* 1985;88:171–175.

126. Wilcox CM, Diehl DL, Cello JP, Margaretten W, Jacobson MA. Cytomegalovirus esophagitis in patients with AIDS. A clinical, endoscopic, and pathologic correlation. *Ann Intern Med* 1990;113:589–593.

127. Knapp AB, Horst DA, Eliopoulos G, et al. Widespread cytomegalovirus gastroenteritis in a patient with acquired immunodeficiency syndrome. *Gastroenterology* 1983;85:1399–1402.

128. Kavin Jones RB, Chowdhury L, Kabius S. Acalculous cholecystitis and cytomegalovirus infection in the acquired immunodeficiency syndrome. *Ann Intern Med* 1986;104:53–54.

129. Margulis SJ, Honig CL, Soave R, Govoni AF, Mouradian JA, Jacobson IM. Biliary tract obstruction in the acquired immunodeficiency syndrome. *Ann Intern Med* 1986;105:207–210.

130. Schneiderman DJ, Cello JP, Laing FC. Papillary stenosis and sclerosing cholangitis in the acquired immunodeficiency syndrome. *Ann Intern Med* 1987;106:546–549.

131. Wilcox CM, Forsmark CE, Grendell JH, Darragh TM, Cello JP. Cytomegalovirus-associated acute pancreatic disease in patients with the acquired immunodeficiency syndrome. Report of two patients. *Gastroenterology* 1990;99:263–267.

132. Valerdiz-Casasola S, Pardo-Mindan FJ. Cytomegalovirus infection of the appendix in a patient with the acquired immunodeficiency syndrome. *Gastroenterology* 1991;101:247–249.

133. Smith PD, Saini SS, Raffeld M, Manishewitz JF, Wahl SM. Cytomegalovirus induction of tumor necrosis factor-α by human monocytes and mucosal macrophages. *J Clin Invest* 1992;90:1642–1648.

134. Dieterich DT, Rahmin M. Cytomegalovirus colitis in AIDS: Presentation in 44 patients and a review of the literature. *J Acquir Immun Defic Syndr* 1991;4S:29–35.

135. Culpepper-Morgan JA, Kotler DP, Scholes JV, Tierney AR. Evolution of diagnostic criteria for mucosal cytomegalic inclusion disease in the acquired immune deficiency syndrome. *Am J Gastroenterol* 1987;82:1264–1270.

136. Siegal FP, Lopez C, Hammer GS, et al. Severe acquired immunodeficiency in male homosexuals manifested by chronic perianal ulcerative herpes simplex lesions. *N Engl J Med* 1981;305:1439–1444.

137. Goodell SE, Quinn TC, Mkrtichian E, Schuffler MD, Holmes KK, Corey L. Herpes simplex virus proctitis in homosexual men. Clinical, sigmoidoscopic, and histopathological features. *N Engl J Med* 1983;308:868–871.

138. Herrmann JE, Blacklow NR, Perron-Henry DM, et al. Incidence of enteric adenovirus among children in Thailand and the significance of these viruses in gastroenteritis. *J Clin Microbiol* 1988;26:1788–1796.

139. de Jong PJ, Valderrama G, Spigland I, Horwitz MS. Adenovirus isolates from urine of patients with acquired immunodeficiency syndrome. *Lancet* 1983;1:1293–1296.

140. Krilov LR, Rubin LG, Frogel M, et al. Disseminated adenovirus infection with hepatic necrosis in patients with human immunodeficiency virus infection and other immunodeficiency states. *J Infect Dis* 1990;12:303–307.

141. Kaljot KT, Ling JP, Gold JWM, et al. Prevalence of acute

entric viral pathogens in acquired immunodeficiency syndrome patients with diarrhea. *Gastroenterology* 1989;97:1031–1032.

142. Cunningham AL, Grohman GS, Harkness J, et al. Gastrointestinal viral infections in homosexual men who were symptomatic and seropositive for human immunodeficiency virus. *J Infect Dis* 1988;158:386–391.

143. Janoff EN, Orenstein JM, Manischewitz JF, Smith PD. Adenovirus colitis in the acquired immunodeficiency syndrome. *Gastroenterology* 1991;100:976–979.

144. Janoff EN. Diarrheal disease with viral enteric infections in immunocompromised patients. In: Owen R, Surawicz C, eds. *Gastrointestinal and hepatic infections.* Amsterdam: Elsevier; 1995; in press.

145. Bottone EJ, Wormser GP, Duncanson FP. Nontyphoidal *Salmonella* bacteremia as an early infection in acquired immunodeficiency syndrome. *Diag Microbiol Infect Dis* 1984;2:247–250.

146. Jacobs JL, Gold JWM, Murray HW, Roberts RB, Armstrong D. Salmonella infections in patients with the acquired immunodeficiency syndrome. *Ann Intern Med* 1985;102:186–188.

147. Glaser JB, Morton-Kute L, Berger SR, et al. Recurrent *Salmonella typhimurium* bacteremia associated with the acquired immunodeficiency syndrome. *Ann Intern Med* 1985;102:189–193.

148. Fischl MA, Dickinson GM, Sinave C, Pitchenik AE, Cleary TJ. *Salmonella* bacteremia as a manifestation of acquired immunodeficiency syndrome. *Arch Intern Med* 1986;146:113–115.

149. Smith PD, Macher AM, Bookman MA, et al. *Salmonella typhimurium* enteritis and bacteremia in the acquired immunodeficiency syndrome. *Ann Intern Med* 1985;102:207–209.

150. Sperber SJ, Schleupner CJ. Salmonella during infection with human immunodeficiency virus. *Rev Infect Dis* 1987;9:925–934.

151. Celum CL, Chaisson RE, Rutherford GW, Barnehart JL, Echenberg DF. Incidence of salmonellosis in patients with AIDS. *J Infect Dis* 1987;156:998–1002.

152. Pithie AD, Malin AS, Robertson VJ. Salmonella and shigella bacteraemia in Zimbabwe. *Cent Afr J Med* 1993;39:110–112.

153. Baskin DH, Lax JD, Barenberg D. Shigella bacteremia in patients with the acquired immune deficiency syndrome. *Am J Gastroenterol* 1987;82:338–341.

154. Gander RM, LaRocco MT. Multiple drug-resistance in *Shigella flexneri* isolated from a patient with human immunodeficiency virus. *Diag Microbiol Infect Dis* 1987;8:193–196.

155. Blaser MJ, Hale TL, Formal SB. Recurrent shigellosis complicating human immunodeficiency virus infection: failure of pre-existing antibodies to confer protection. *Am J Med* 1989;86:105–107.

156. Mandell W, Neu HC. Shigella bacteremia in adults. *JAMA* 1986;255:3116.

157. Dworkin B, Wormser GP, Abdoo RA, Cabello F, Aguero ME, Sivak SL. Persistence of multiply antibiotic-resistant *Campylobacter jejuni* in a patient with the acquired immune deficiency syndrome. *Am J Med* 1986;80:965–970.

158. Perlman DM, Ampel NM, Schifman RB, et al. Persistent *Campylobacter jejuni* infections in patients infected with human immunodeficiency virus (HIV). *Ann Intern Med* 1988;108:540–546.

159. Gray JR, Rabeneck L. Atypical mycobacterial infection of the gastrointestinal tract in AIDS patients. *Am J Gastroenterol* 1989;84:1521–1524.

160. Horsburgh CR Jr. *Mycobacterium avium* complex in the acquired immunodeficiency syndrome. *N Engl J Med* 1991;324:1332–1228.

161. Gillin JS, Urmacher C, West R, Shike M. Disseminated *Mycobacterium avium-intracellulare* infection in acquired immunodeficiency syndrome mimicking Whipple's disease. *Gastroenterology* 1983;84:1521–1524.

162. Roth RI, Owen RL, Keren DF, Volberding PA. Intestinal infection with *M. avium* in acquired immune deficiency syndrome (AIDS). Histological and clinical comparison with Whipple's disease. *Dig Dis Sci* 1985;30:497–504.

163. Kamsker B, Bottone EJ. *Mycobacterium avium–Mycobacterium intracellulare* from the intestinal tracts of patients with acquired immunodeficiency syndrome: concepts regarding acquisition and pathogenesis. *J Infect Dis* 1985;151:179–181.

164. Kiehn TE, Edwards FF, Brannon P, et al. Infections caused by *Mycobacterium avium* complex in immunocompromised patients: diagnosis by blood culture and fecal examination, antimicrobial susceptibility tests, and morphological and seroagglutination characteristics. *J Clin Microbiol* 1985;21:168–173.

165. Baron EJ, Young CS. Amikacin, ethambutol, and rifampin for treatment of disseminated *Mycobacterium avium-intracellulare* infections in patients with acquired immune deficiency syndrome. *Diag Microbiol Infect Dis* 1986;5:212–220.

166. Masur H, Tuazon C, Gill V, et al. Effect of combined clofazimine and ansamycin therapy on *Mycobacterium avium-intracellulare* bacteremia in patients with AIDS. *J Infect Dis* 1987;155:127–129.

167. Yajko DM, Nassos PD, Hadley WK. Therapeutic implications of inhibition versus killing of *Mycobacterium avium* complex by antimicrobial agents. *Antimicrob Agents Chemother* 1987;31:117–120.

168. Kemper CA, Meng T-C, Nussbaum J, et al. Treatment of *Mycobacterium avium* complex bacteremia in AIDS with a four-drug oral regimen. *Ann Intern Med* 1992;116:466–472.

169. The choice of antibacterial drugs. *Med Lett* 1994;36:53–60.

170. Nightingale SD, Cameron W, Gordin FM, et al. Two controlled trials of rifabutin prophylaxis against *Mycobacterium avium* complex infections in AIDS. *N Engl J Med* 1993;329:828–833.

171. Cozart JC, Kalangi SS, Clench MH, et al. *Clostridium difficile* diarrhea in patients with AIDS versus non-AIDS controls. *J Clin Gastroenterol* 1993;16:192–194.

172. Hutin Y, Molina J-M, Casin I, et al. Risk factors for *Clostridium difficile*–associated diarrhoea in HIV-infected patients. *AIDS* 1993;7:1441–1447.

173. Peterson LR, Olson MM, Shanholtzer CJ, Gerding DN. Results of a prospective, 18 month clinical evaluation of culture, cytotoxin testing, and culturette brand (CDT) latex testing in the diagnosis of *Clostridium difficile*–associated diarrhea. *Diagn Microbiol Infect Dis* 1988;10:85–91.

174. Gerding DN, Brazier JS. Optimal methods for identifying *Clostridium difficile* infections. *J Infect Dis* 1993;16S:439–442.

175. Wheat LJ, Connolly-Stringfield P, Kohler RB, Fram PT, Gupta MR. *Histoplasma capsulatum* polysaccharide antigen detection in diagnosis and management of disseminated histoplasmosis in patients with acquired immunodeficiency syndrome. *Am J Med* 1989;87:396–400.

176. McKinsey DS, Gupta MR, Riddler SA, Driks MR, Smith DL, Kurtin PJ. Long-term amphotericin B therapy for disseminated histoplasmosis in patients with the acquired immunodeficiency syndrome. *Ann Intern Med* 1989;111:655–659.

177. Driks MR, Gupta MR, McKinsey DS, Niehart RE, O'Connor MC. Gastrointestinal histoplasmosis in patients with the acquired immunodeficiency syndrome [Abstract]. Proceedings of the 30th Interscience Conference on Antimicrobial Agents and Chemotherapy. 1990;A1272.

178. Drugs for AIDS and associated infections. *Med Lett* 1993;35:7986.

179. Outbreaks of diarrheal illness associated with cyanobacteria (blue-green algae)-like bodies—Chicago and Nepal, 1989 and 1990. *MMWR Morb Mortal Wkly Rep* 1991;40:325–327.

180. Long EG, White EH, Carmichael WW, et al. Morphologic and staining characteristics of a cyanobacterium-like organism associated with diarrhea. *J Infect Dis* 1991;164:199–202.

181. Ortega YR, Sterling CR, Gilman RH, Cama VA, Diaz F. Cyclospora species—a new protozoan pathogen of humans. *N Engl J Med* 1993;328:1308–1312.

182. Shlim DR, Cohen MT, Eaton M, Rajah R, Long EG, Unger BLP. An alga-like organism associated with an outbreeak of prolonged diarrhea among foreigners in Nepal. *Am J Trop Med* 1991;45:383–389.

183. Connor BA, Shlim DR, Scholes JV, Rayburn JL, Reidy J, Rajah R. Pathologic changes in the small bowel in nine patients with diarrhea associated with a coccidia-like body. *Ann Intern Med* 1993;119:377–382.

184. Hart AS, Ridinger MT, Soundarajan R, Peters CS, Swiatlo AL,

Kocka FE. Novel organisms associated with chronic diarrhoea in AIDS. *Lancet* 1990;335:169–179.

185. Long EG, Ebrahimzadeh A, White EH, Swisher B, Callaway CS. Alga associated with diarrhea in patients with acquired immunodeficiency syndrome and in travelers. *J Clin Microbiol* 1990;28:1101–1104.

186. Grohmann GS, Blass RI, Pereira HG, et al. Enteric viruses and diarrhea in HIV-infected patients. *N Engl J Med* 1993;329:14–20.

187. Gatti MSV, de Castro AFP, Ferraz MMG, Fialho AM, Pereira HG. Viruses with bisegmented double-stranded RNA in pig faeces. *Res Vet Sci* 1989;47:397–398.

188. Vanopdenbosch E, Wellemans G. Birna-type virus in diarrhoeic calf faeces. *Vet Rec* 1989;125:610.

189. Kurtz JB, Lee TW, Pickering D. Astrovirus associated gastroenteritis in a children's ward. *J Clin Pathol* 1977;30:948–952.

190. Lew JF, Moe CL, Monroe SS, et al. Astrovirus and adenovirus associated with diarrhea in children in day care settings. *J Infect Dis* 1991;164:673–678.

191. Hermann JE, Taylor DN, Echeverria P, Blackow NR. Astroviruses as a cause of gastroenteritis in children. *N Engl J Med* 1991;324:1757–1760.

192. Kaljot KT, Ling JP, Gold JWM, et al. Prevalence of acute enteric viral pathogens in acquired immunodeficiency syndrome patients with diarrhea. *Gastroenterology* 1989;97:1031–1032.

193. Thea DM, Glass R, Grohmann GS, et al. Prevalence of enteric viruses among hospital patients with AIDS in Kinshasa, Zaire. *Trans R Soc Trop Med Hyg* 1993;87:263–266.

194. Oshitani H, Kasolo FC, Mpabalwani M, et al. Association of rotavirus and human immunodeficiency virus infection in children hospitalized with acute diarrhea, Lusaka, Zambia. *J Infect Dis* 1994;169:897–900.

195. Cunningham AL, Grohmann GS, Harkness J, et al. Gastrointestinal viral infections in homosexual men who were symptomatic and seropositive for human immunodeficiency virus. *J Infect Dis* 1988;158:386–391.

196. Albrecht H, Stellbrink HJ, Fenske S, Ermer M, Raedler A, Greten H. Rotavirus antigen detection in patients with HIV infection and diarrhea. *Scand J Infect Dis* 1993;28:307–310.

197. Kotler DP, Orenstein JM. Chronic diarrhea and malabsorption associated with enteropathogenic bacterial infection in a patient with AIDS. *Ann Intern Med* 1993;119:127–128.

198. Kotler DP, Giang TT, Orenstein JM. Chronic enteropathy in patients with AIDS. *Gastroenterology* 1994;106:A714.

Infections of the Gastrointestinal Tract,
edited by M. J. Blaser, P. D. Smith, J. I. Ravdin,
H. B. Greenberg, and R. L. Guerrant
Raven Press, Ltd., New York © 1995.

CHAPTER 36

Enteric Infections in HIV-Infected Children

Tien-lan Chang, Stephen I. Pelton, and Harland S. Winter

Infections of the gastrointestinal tract rank first among the worldwide causes of morbidity and mortality in children infected with human immunodeficiency virus (HIV) (1). In the United States, such infections result in malnutrition and disability in HIV-infected children but are less frequently a cause of death. Although the diagnostic approach to enteric infections is similar for pediatric and adult patients, the spectrum and management of enteric infections in the pediatric population infected with HIV differ from those in adult HIV-infected patients. This chapter will review the epidemiology of HIV infection in children; the risk factors for enteric infections; the clinical features common to HIV-infected children; and the diagnosis and management issues involved in the treatment of opportunistic infections in HIV-infected children.

EPIDEMIOLOGY OF HIV INFECTION IN CHILDREN

Modes of Infection

Children can acquire HIV infection either perinatally from their mother (vertical transmission) or from contaminated blood or blood products. Since the institution of stringent screening procedures for blood donors in 1983 and specific HIV testing of donated blood in 1985, the number of transfusion-acquired cases of acquired immunodeficiency syndrome (AIDS) in children in the United States has fallen dramatically. Only one case of HIV infection, transmitted via blood transfusion from a seronegative donor to an infant, has been reported since screening procedures began (2,3).

The risk of receiving a blood transfusion from an HIV-infected individual is estimated to be less than 1 in 40,000

(3,4). In the United States between 1981 and 1989, approximately 15% of pediatric patients with HIV infection acquired the infection from blood products and 85% from perinatal transmission (5). By 1992, however, greater than 95% of newly diagnosed cases of pediatric HIV infection were associated with vertical transmission. In developing countries, HIV transmission via blood transfusion remains a concern because many nations do not routinely screen donors for HIV (6).

The rate of perinatal vertical transmission of HIV-infected women to their infants ranges from 10% to 50% with a mean of 30% (7). Several factors may contribute to this variation in the transmission rate. First, transmission may occur more frequently in infants born to women who are symptomatic and consequently have more advanced AIDS (8). Data have shown that zidovudine given during pregnancy decreases the transmission rate to less than 10% (9). These observations suggest that viral replication and burden are important determinants of perinatal transmission. Second, the presence of maternal antibodies to specific epitopes of HIV gp120 may reduce the risk of transmission (10). Third, breastfeeding affects the rate of transmission since HIV may be present in the milk of HIV-infected women (11). In a prospective study of 16 breast-fed infants born to African women who seroconverted after delivery, the rate of postnatal transmission was estimated to be 36% to 53% (12). In Australia, the rate of perinatal transmission was 50% among breast-fed infants of HIV-infected women, 17% among the bottle-fed (13), and 27% for breast-fed infants of women who seroconverted postpartum (14). These and other studies suggest that breastfeeding is an additional risk for vertical transmission. Currently, because of the infant mortality associated with feeding formula in unsanitary living conditions, the World Health Organization (WHO) encourages the practice of breastfeeding regardless of the mother's HIV status (15). In countries in which infant mortality from enteric infection is low, HIV-infected mothers should not breast-feed their infants. This issue requires further examination as new data better assess the breastfeeding risk for HIV transmission.

T.-l. Chang, S. I. Pelton, and H. S. Winter: Department of Pediatric Gastroenterology and Nutrition, and Division of Infectious Disease, Department of Pediatrics, Boston City Hospital, Boston University School of Medicine, Boston, Massachusetts 02118.

Prevalence

Based on seroprevalence studies and mathematical models, the WHO estimates that 10 million persons have become infected with HIV in the past decade, including 3 million women, primarily of childbearing age, and 500,000 children (15). Approximately 80% of these women and children live in sub-Saharan Africa (6). In developed countries, approximately 2% of reported patients with AIDS are under the age of 13 years. However, in developing countries, the proportion of pediatric HIV-infected patients is higher, composing 15% to 20% of all AIDS cases (6). In the United States alone, 4249 cases of AIDS in children younger than 13 years of age had been reported by the end of 1992 (16). Significantly, the number of HIV-infected children approaches ten times the number of reported cases of AIDS in children.

Mortality and Morbidity

The mortality for children in the United States infected with HIV is related to the age of the child at diagnosis, the presence or absence of opportunistic infection, and the CD4 T-lymphocyte count or CD4/CD8 ratio. Children younger than 6 months with an AIDS-defining illness have a 1-year mortality rate of 45% to 55%, considerably higher than that of older children (15% to 28%) (17). Mortality is increased significantly for pediatric patients who develop certain opportunistic infections. For example, the median survival time is 4–10 months for pediatric patients with disseminated nontuberculous mycobacteria (18–20) and 9 months for those with *Pneumocystis carinii* pneumonia, compared to 63 months for those with pneumonia due to *Haemophilus influenzae* or gram-positive organisms (17). Among those pediatric patients who acquired opportunistic infections, 92% had an abnormal CD4/CD8 ratio or a low CD4 count; among those who died, 90% had a low CD4 count (21).

Gastrointestinal infections in the HIV-infected pediatric population is an important cause of morbidity. Diarrhea is present in 20% to 35% of children with AIDS, with malnutrition/growth failure present in 45% to 60% of cases (7,22–24). Gastrointestinal infections in children do not appear to shorten survival in HIV-infected children in developed countries (22). In contrast, in developing nations, diarrhea is the most common cause of death (1,25). The mortality attributed to diarrhea in Zairian infants followed from birth to the first 12 months of life was 132 per 1000 live births for HIV-infected infants and 12 per 1000 live births for uninfected infants (1). Persistent diarrhea lasting longer than 14 days occurred 4.8 times more often in HIV-infected Zairian children than in uninfected children (1). Moreover, 32% of all deaths in these HIV-infected children and 8% of deaths in HIV-uninfected children were attributed to persistent diarrhea (1).

In the United States and developed countries, morbidity and mortality from enteric infections may be more subtle (23–25). Diarrhea and malabsorption resulting from enteric infection may cause malnutrition, which in the growing child may impair T-cell function and increase the probability of opportunistic infection. Thus, rather than the rapid clinical deterioration observed in developing countries in HIV-infected children who develop diarrhea, in developed countries the clinical presentation often is chronic disease with malnutrition and growth failure.

PATHOBIOLOGY OF ENTERIC INFECTIONS IN HIV-INFECTED CHILDREN

The factors that may contribute to the pathobiology of enteric infections in HIV-infected children include gastrointestinal tract function, immunological alterations of the systemic and mucosal immune system, HIV infection of the intestinal mucosa, maternal health, and malnutrition.

Gastrointestinal Function

Gastrointestinal function of the newborn and infant may facilitate the translocation of pathogens, including HIV, across the mucosal barrier. Gastric acid secretion, an important barrier against enteric infection, is decreased in the first days of life and increases to adult levels by 1–3 months of age (26). Consequently, the neonate who swallows pathogenic organisms at birth may be at increased risk because of an ineffective gastric acid barrier. Secretion of enzymes such as enterokinase, chymotrypsin, and carboxypeptidase are decreased in the first year of life and in theory could contribute to impaired inactivation of enteric pathogens and toxins (27). The increased susceptibility to some enteric infections in infants may be explained by the higher number of receptor sites on the intestinal epithelial cell for rotavirus and *Escherichia coli* heat-stable enterotoxin (28–29). In addition to differences in epithelial cell membrane proteins, intestinal permeability for carbohydrates and proteins is increased in infants as compared to adults (30,31). Thus, multiple nonimmunological factors—secretion of gastric acid and proteolytic enzymes, binding of enteric pathogens to the mucosa, and intestinal permeability—may contribute to enhanced translocation of pathogens across the mucosal barrier of the child.

Immune Function

Newborn infants have reduced systemic immune responses to foreign antigens and infectious organisms (32,33) as well as reduced mucosal immune responses, reflected in reduced levels of fecal and salivary secretory IgA in the first month of life (34,35). Children with HIV infection, particularly those with opportunistic infections, have reduced absolute numbers of CD4 T cells, reduced CD4/CD8 ratios, impaired antibody response to immunizations, and abnormal lymphocyte proliferative responses to vaccine antigens (1,17,21,36,37). This alteration in systemic immune function is likely due to the consequences of HIV infection and/or the accompanying malnutrition. Little is known about the effects of HIV infection on the mucosal immune function of the HIV-infected child.

In the normal newborn, maternal IgG acquired transplacentally and breast milk IgA provide some mucosal immune function and reduce the severity and duration of intestinal symptoms during epidemics of enteric infections (38,39). Similarly, intravenous IgG (40) or breast milk (41) may protect the HIV-infected child from enteric infection, but transmission of HIV by breast milk negates its value when an alternate source of nutrition is available.

HIV Infection of the Intestinal Mucosa

HIV mRNA can be identified in the small intestinal mucosa of HIV-infected children (42) but, as in adults, HIV only infects lymphocytes or macrophages throughout the lamina propria. Unlike HIV-infected adults, the duodenal mucosa of HIV-infected children frequently has a nodular appearance (Fig. 1) caused by expansion of lymphoid elements of the lamina propria (Fig. 2). The cause of the proliferation of the cellular elements of the lamina propria is not known, but may be analogous to the lymphoid interstitial pneumonia commonly observed in HIV-infected children but rarely seen in HIV-infected adults.

There is no evidence in the adult or child that intestinal epithelial cells are infected with HIV (43). However, the observation that HIV-infected children develop lactose malabsorption earlier than would be predicted by normal genetic influences (42) supports the hypothesis that maturation of the enterocyte is altered. The mechanism for this epithelial cell dysfunction and any possible relationship to lymphoid proliferation is not known. However, there is a decrease in specific activity of the brush border enzyme lactase. This observation correlates with impaired lactose absorption in HIV-infected infants. In HIV-infected chil-

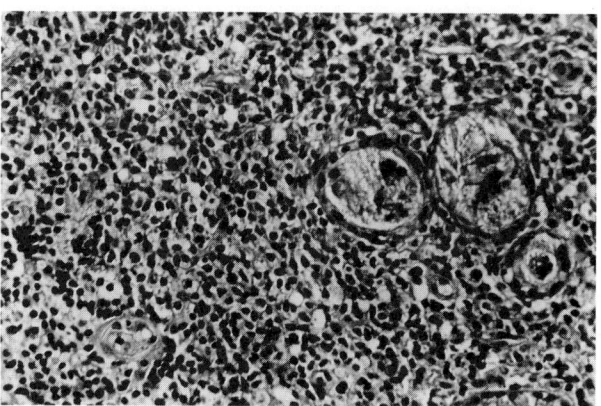

FIG. 2. Lymphoid proliferation of the small intestinal lamina propria in an HIV-infected child.

dren, lactase gene expression by *in situ* hybridization is decreased (Figs. 3 and 4) (42). A mosaic pattern recently reported in normal adults with alactasia (44) closely resembles the pattern of mRNA expression observed in HIV-infected children.

Maternal Health

An HIV-infected mother who becomes symptomatic with fever, weight loss, or diarrhea contributes to the illness of her child via at least two mechanisms. First, the mother may be a source of infectious agents for her child, either via placenta and breast milk (vertical transmission), or via the oral–fecal route (horizontal transmission). Second, a mother who is ill may be less able to care for an HIV-infected child for physical or psychological reasons. In HIV-uninfected infants, the incidence of persistent diarrhea is nearly double if the HIV-infected mother is symptomatic, and the risk is increased further if the

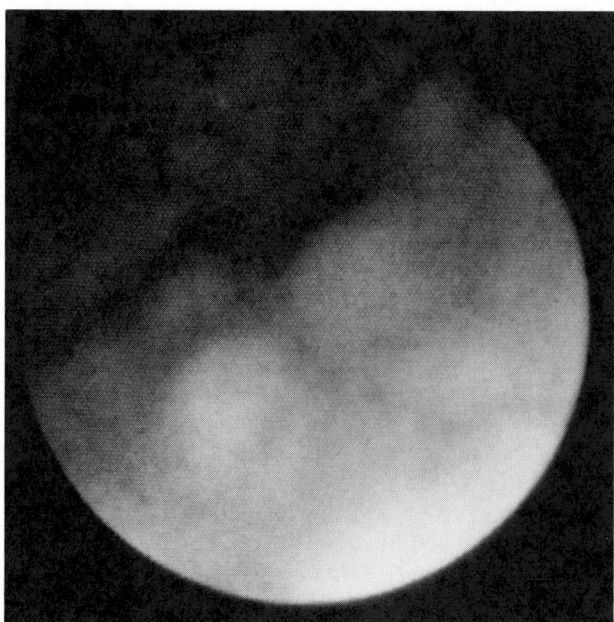

FIG. 1. Nodular duodenal mucosa in an HIV-infected child with an identifiable enteric pathogen.

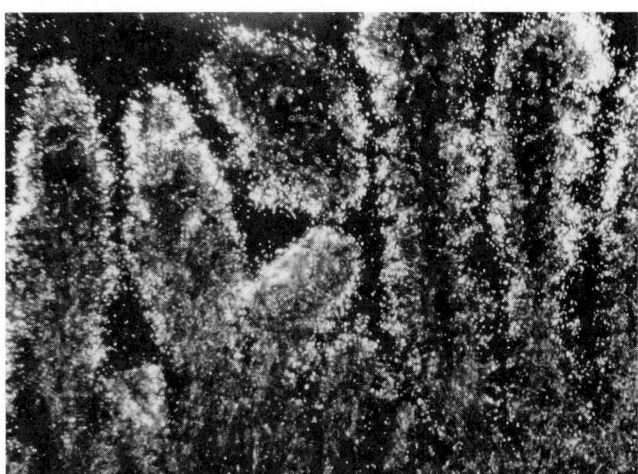

FIG. 3. Lactase mRNA expression as detected by *in situ* hybridization in the normal small intestine of a child. Detection of mRNA along the enteric villus.

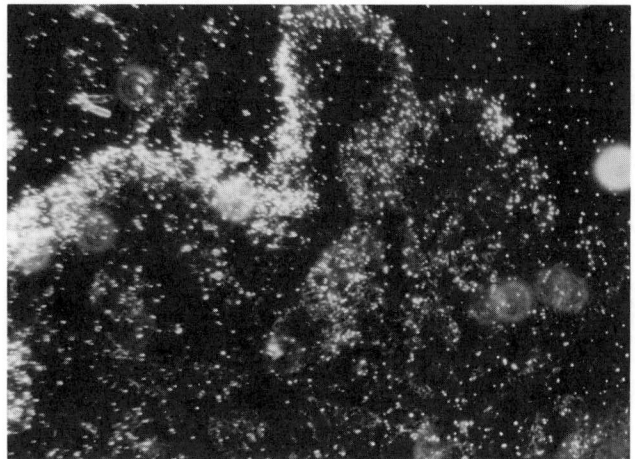

FIG. 4. Lactose mRNA is decreased along the villus an HIV-infected child.

mother dies (1). Regardless of the HIV status of the child, the early introduction of either milk formula or solid food into the infant's diet correlates with the occurrence of acute diarrhea (1). Thus, management of an HIV-infected child must consider maternal health status.

Malnutrition

In developing nations where chronic diarrhea, enteric infections, and malnutrition are prevalent, severe malnutrition is a recognized risk factor for malabsorption and chronic diarrhea (45). Because of altered gastrointestinal function, increased nutritional requirements, reduced nutrient reserves, and maternal health status, malnutrition is common in children infected with HIV. Protein-calorie malnutrition and deficiencies in micronutrients such as zinc and vitamin A are associated with defects in cellular immunity and absorptive function. The presence of these nutritional and immunological deficiencies is also a risk factor for diarrheal disease and enteric infection (46–48). Thus, a self-perpetuating cycle of malnutrition, malabsorption, immunodeficiency, and enteric infection occurs in HIV-infected children and is more severe in HIV-infected children than in adults.

CLINICAL ILLNESS

Viral Infections

Rotavirus usually causes diarrhea in children 3 months–3 years of age, whereas newborns and older children tend to be asymptomatic or have minimal symptoms (49). In outbreaks of gastroenteritis in day care centers in the United States, rotavirus accounts for approximately half of cases with an identifiable cause, followed in frequency by adenovirus (4% to 9%) (50,51) and astrovirus (2% to 7%) (51,52). However, in malnourished or immunocompromised children, including those infected with

HIV, rotavirus causes a protracted diarrhea (53), and in rare cases can disseminate beyond the intestinal tract and cause acute hepatitis (54). In contrast, rotavirus does not appear to be a significant pathogen in adult patients with HIV infection (55,56). Diagnosis of rotavirus infection is based on identification of the virus in the stool by an enzyme-linked immunoassay (57). Treatment of rotavirus-induced diarrhea consists of replacement of fluids and electrolytes. If the diarrhea persists for more than a week, nutritional support is necessary. Human serum immunoglobulin administered enterally may have a beneficial effect for children with intractable diarrhea (58,59), but its effectiveness in HIV-infected children remains unproven.

Adenoviruses are common pathogens of the respiratory and gastrointestinal tracts. Over 40 different serotypes have been identified but approximately 70% of adenovirus-associated enteric infections in normal children are attributable to serotypes 40 and 41 (60). The diarrhea in children caused by adenoviruses is related to injury of the small intestinal mucosa. In one fatal case of adenovirus gastroenteritis, in a non–HIV-infected individual, virus was identified by electron microscopy in the intestinal epithelial cell (61). In children with HIV infection and in other immunocompromised states, adenovirus can cause fulminant hepatitis as part of a disseminated infection that involves lungs, liver, bone marrow, heart, and brain (62,63). Gastrointestinal hemorrhage has been reported to occur in 30% of immunocompromised patients with disseminated adenovirus (63). Adenovirus can be identified in the stool by culture or an enzyme-linked immunoassay. It has been identified in colonic biopsies by electron microscopy in HIV-infected adult patients with adenovirus colitis (64) and in the stool from 15% of a group of adult men with HIV who had diarrhea (vs. 5% of patients without diarrhea). The serotypes that have been reported in HIV-infected patients have been serotypes other than types 40 and 41. Since adenovirus is also a common cause of pharyngitis and respiratory infections, a positive stool culture can be due to virus shed from the tonsils and airway secretions and does not necessarily indicate enteric infection. Other than supportive measures, there is no known specific treatment for adenovirus, although human serum globulin was used successfully in clearing adenovirus-induced pneumonia and hepatitis in a child with combined immunodeficiency (65). Ribavirin has potential as an experimental therapy.

The role of cytomegalovirus (CMV) as an enteric pathogen in immunocompetent children is unclear, except for its association with a protein-losing hypertrophic gastropathy (66). Children can acquire the infection vertically or horizontally. The risk of vertical transmission of CMV from a maternal carrier is approximately 1% in healthy infants. The majority of these infants are asymptomatic (67,68). In HIV-infected infants, however, the risk of infection is higher. In a group of children born to HIV-positive women and followed for 2–74 months, CMV was present in the urine in 46% of HIV-infected children and in 8% of children whose HIV status was indeterminate (69). In patients infected with HIV, CMV can cause inflammatory lesions anywhere in the gastrointestinal tract from the oral cavity to the rectum (70). Symptoms of

CMV-induced disease include dysphagia, abdominal pain, vomiting, diarrhea, and upper or lower gastrointestinal bleeding similar to adults, hemorrhagic gastritis, ileitis, and colitis have all been reported in HIV-infected children with CMV infection (71,72).

Establishing CMV as the cause of enteric disease poses a diagnostic challenge for the clinician. Positive CMV viral culture in the urine and serology as well as viral shedding in the gut can occur in children with or without active disease. Consequently, histopathological identification of CMV in the presence of inflammation is the best way presently to confirm its pathogenic role (73). *In situ* hybridization with DNA probes complimentary for CMV has been proposed as an alternative or supportive diagnostic tool (74); but its utility remains to be established.

Treatment of CMV-induced gastrointestinal disease in HIV-infected adults with ganciclovir is generally effective in ameliorating disease activity (67,75). In immunocompromised children (allograft recipients) with CMV disease involving different organs, a retrospective study showed that 54% of patients improved after receiving ganciclovir, 5–15 mg/kg/day for 1–5 weeks (78). Treatment with foscarnet is an alternative drug for patients who fail to respond to ganciclovir (76,77). Both ganciclovir and foscarnet are associated with significant marrow suppression. Human immunoglobulin may have a beneficial effect when used in conjunction with ganciclovir in the treatment of cytomegaloirus disease (79). The HIV-infected child with diarrhea, no focal or inflammatory enteric lesion, and cytomegalovirus in the stool should not be treated for cytomegalovirus-induced disease.

Other viruses have been detected by immunoassay or electron microscopy in the stools of HIV-infected adults with diarrhea. In HIV-infected children, astrovirus, picobirnavirus, and caliciviruses (80) have not been identified. Mucocutaneous herpes simplex virus infection has been reported in less than 1% of HIV-infected children (17).

Bacterial Infections

Bacterial infections, which include *Salmonella, Shigella, Campylobacter, Yersinia, Clostridium difficile,* and *E. coli,* account for only a minor proportion of enteric infections in the general population in most developed countries. The exact incidence of enteric bacterial infections in HIV-infected children is unknown, but some studies suggest an increased risk for *Salmonella* infection in HIV-infected patients (54,81,82) compared to the general population. In HIV-infected children, enteric organisms (including *Salmonella, Enterococcus, E. coli, Lactobacillus, Enterobacter* sp., and *Citrobacter*) accounted for almost half of the pathogens causing bacteremia (83). Because of the possibility for relapse and systemic dissemination, antimicrobial treatment of enteric pathogens in HIV-infected children may require a longer course than that recommended for the immunocompetent host.

Strains of *E. coli* may be important causes of diarrhea in children in developing nations (1,22). In a study of Zairian children with an identifiable cause of diarrhea, pathogenic

E. coli were isolated from the stool of 30% of HIV-negative children and 78% of HIV-infected children (22). These bacteria may be present in the colon or in the small intestine. *E. coli* and other bacteria, such as *Klebsiella,* have been found in high concentration in the small intestine of HIV-infected children with diarrhea (84,85). The frequency of bacterial overgrowth in HIV-infected children is not known, but should be suspected in a child with an elevated breath H_2 or an early rise in breath H_2 during a lactose breath test. The prevalence and importance of small bowel bacterial overgrowth to the development of diarrhea in HIV-infected children is unknown.

C. difficile is present in the stool of 29% of normal neonates and in 10% of children 4 months–2 years of age (86). Consequently, the significance of comparable levels of *C. difficile* in the stool of HIV-infected pediatric patients in these age groups with diarrhea is questionable. Certain serotypes of *C. difficile* appear to be associated with pathogenicity, even in infants (86). Although *C. difficile* colitis has been reported in infants and children (87,88), it has not been reported in HIV-infected children. Treatment of *C. difficile*–induced colitis with either vancomycin or metronidazole is effective in HIV-infected adults, but recurrence or treatment failure may occur (89).

Helicobacter pylori is recognized as an etiological agent for peptic ulcer and gastritis in both adults and children. Serological studies suggest a decreased incidence of *H. pylori* in both HIV-infected children and adults compared to the general population (90–92). Hypotheses to explain this decrease include increased antibiotic use and reduced acid production in HIV-infected patients (90).

Mycobacterial Infections

HIV-infected children infected with *Mycobacterium avium* complex (MAC) typically have multisystemic disease involving bone marrow, lungs, liver, mesenteric lymph nodes, and gastrointestinal tract (18–20). The prevalence rate of disseminated MAC in children infected with HIV is 11.4% (Pediatric Spectrum of Disease Project) (18). The gastrointestinal tract and respiratory systems are thought to be potential sites of entry for MAC (17) and a low CD4 cell count is the major risk factor for disseminated MAC. MAC is identified in 18% of children with a CD4 count less than 50/mm³ but only in 3% of children with a CD4 count greater than 100/mm³ (18). Abdominal pain and diarrhea are common in children with disseminated MAC and the organism can be grown from the stool. Although acid-fast bacilli-laden macrophages are found in the jejunal mucosa, gastrointestinal injury by MAC in HIV-infected children is rare. No effective treatment at present eradicates MAC from the gastrointestinal tract, but colony counts of MAC in blood cultures are decreased in response to single agents or combinations of drugs, such as azithromycin, clarithromycin, ethambutol, ciprofloxacin, amikacin, rifampin, and clofazamine (93). Clinical trials for the treatment of disseminated MAC in children are in progress.

In contrast to the high prevalence of MAC, few cases of *M. tuberculosis* and no cases of gastrointestinal tuberculosis have been reported in HIV-infected children in the United States (94). Two cases of intestinal perforation due to *M. tuberculosis* have been reported in HIV-infected adults (95). Since the populations at risk for tuberculosis and for HIV are similar in demographic characteristics, an increase in the number of HIV-infected children with tuberculosis is expected, and more cases with gastrointestinal tuberculosis likely will be identified.

Protozoan Infections

Giardia lamblia and *Cryptosporidium parvum* are the most common protozoan pathogens identified in HIV-infected children, but *Isospora belli* and *Microsporidium* have been found in immunodeficient adults. *Isospora* is a rare pathogen even in HIV-infected adults, but *Microsporidium* is identified in as many as 50% of HIV-infected adults with chronic diarrhea in whom no pathogen is identified by standard stool analysis (96–98). Although light microscopy on Giemsa-stained touch preparations or hematoxylin-eosin–stained paraffin-embedded sections of small intestine can detect *Microsporidium,* diagnosis is enhanced by electron microscopy (96–98). Because the jejunum is a preferential site for *Microsporidium* (96), difficulty in obtaining tissue samples from this area may explain the absence of reported *Microsporidium* in children with HIV.

Giardia usually causes watery diarrhea, bloating, and abdominal pain, but it can also be isolated from asymptomatic individuals. It occurs more frequently in children than in adults, although its prevalence is not increased in HIV-infected children compared to noninfected children with diarrhea (1,22,99). Giardiasis can be treated by metronidazole 10 mg/kg three times daily for 10–14 days or with furazolidone.

Cryptosporidium in HIV-infected children typically causes a chronic and debilitating secretory diarrhea. Only two cases have been reported out of 789 children with AIDS in New York from 1983 to 1990 (17). In contrast, in Tanzania *Cryptosporidium* is found in 13% of HIV-positive and 6% of HIV-negative children hospitalized for chronic diarrhea (99), and in Brazil in 7.1% of HIV-infected but only 0.4% of HIV-negative children (100). In addition to infection of the small and large intestine, *Cryptosporidium* can colonize gallbladder, bile duct, and pancreatic duct, and is implicated as a cause of cholangitis (101). Asymptomatic *Cryptosporidium* has been reported in HIV-infected adults (102), but its frequency is unknown. A retrospective study showed a 30% remission rate among 38 HIV-infected adults; those patients in clinical remission had a higher total lymphocyte count (102). Currently there is no proven effective treatment for eradicating *Cryptosporidium* in HIV-infected patients. Anecdotal reports suggest some clinical benefit (reduction of diarrhea) from octreotide in adults; human immunoglobulin administered enterally in a child with leukemia led to resolution of the infection (103,104). A clinical trial with bovine hyperimmune colostrum in HIV-infected children is currently underway, based on encouraging case reports (105).

Blastocystis hominis is a protozoan that is found in asymptomatic children and adults; its role as an enteric pathogen is still debated. In one study *B. hominis* was found more often in HIV-infected children (3 of 23) with diarrhea than in HIV-negative children (0 of 36) (99). In contrast, the incidence of *B. hominis* in HIV-infected adults may be lower than that in the HIV-negative population (56). The discrepancy in these observations could be due to the small sample size of reported studies or to the increased incidence of *Blastocystis* infection documented in children.

Fungal Infections

Fungal infections in HIV-infected children are mainly caused by *Candida* and *Histoplasma. Candida albicans* and other species can cause oral thrush in 15% to 40% of HIV-infected children (106), esophagitis in 13% (7), and disseminated candidiasis in 7% children (107). A retrospective review of 156 HIV-infected children in New York identified 11 cases of disseminated candidiasis over 7.5 years (107). Predisposing factors included central venous catheter placement, prolonged antibiotic use, oral thrush, and total parenteral nutrition. Neutropenia, defined as less than 200 cells/mm^3, was present in only two patients and therefore was not a risk factor. *Candida* was present in the esophagus in 45% of these 11 patients with candidiasis and in the gastrointestinal tract (location unspecified) in 18%. Other sites of *Candida* involvement included lungs, kidneys, brain, heart, liver, spleen, thyroid, skin, and bone. Coexistent enterococcal sepsis was present in 36% of patients and mycobacterial disease in 27%. The mortality rate in this series, reported by Leibovitz et al., was 90%. Four of the 11 cases were first diagnosed at postmortem, which suggests that the presentation of disseminated candiasis can be subtle (107). Treatment of *Candida* with fluconazole is effective for oral thrush and esophagitis (108), but for disseminated candidiasis amphotericin B remains the treatment of choice in the pediatric population.

Histoplasma capsulatum is endemic in the central United States. Disseminated histoplasmosis has been described in HIV-infected children and may be the AIDS-defining illness in as many as 8% of children and 25% of adults in the endemic region (109,110). Although gastrointestinal involvement in HIV-infected children has not been reported, 20% of other immunocompromised patients with systemic histoplasmosis have evidence of gastrointestinal involvement (111). Granuloma formation due to *Histoplasma* may mimic Crohn's disease radiologically, and intestinal obstruction and perforation are potential complications. Amphotericin B 1 mg/kg/day for 30 days is the recommended treatment for children with disseminated histoplasmosis (110).

DIAGNOSTIC EVALUATION

In evaluating a child with a putative enteric infection, the treating physician should consider the following:

First, diagnosis of some pathogens including cytomegalovirus, adenovirus, *Mycobacterium, Microsporidium,* and fungal infections requires histological examination of tissue biopsies. Second, despite thorough investigation, up to 50% to 60% of children will remain undiagnosed (1,23). Third, successful diagnosis of a pathogen(s) may not determine the cause of the patient's gastrointestinal symptoms. Many enteric pathogens can be found in the stool of asymptomatic individuals, and multiple pathogens can be present in a single patient. Finally, a definite diagnosis does not guarantee an effective specific treatment. The vigor of diagnostic investigation should be balanced by the severity of the child's symptoms. Some investigative procedures can be invasive and difficult for children. For adults a staged evaluation has been proposed (112). Figure 5 presents a similar diagnostic algorithm, based on the child's clinical status and ability to tolerate procedures that may help to make a diagnosis in the majority of patients (Fig. 2). According to this algorithm, initial evalua-

tion of a child with diarrhea should include stool cultures to test for bacterial pathogens, including *Salmonella, Shigella, Campylobacter, Yersinia,* and *C. difficile.* Culture for *E. coli* strain 0157:H7 is now routine for many clinical laboratories in the United States and should be done if there is blood in the stool. Parasites, including *Giardia lamblia, C. parvum,* and *Isospora belli,* can be identified in the stool by immunofluorescent techniques (e.g., *Giardia* antigen and *Cryptosporidium*) or by histological stains (e.g., Kinyoun stain for *Cryptosporidium* and *Isospora*) (113). Viruses such as rotavirus and adenovirus can be detected in the stool by enzyme-linked assays. These stool tests should be repeated at least once if no pathogen is isolated initially. Tests for enteroadherent factor–positive *E. coli* are not commonly available, but may be done at certain laboratories (e.g., Centers for Disease Control) if no other pathogens are isolated and there is a patient history of travel to regions where these bacteria are prevalent. Blood cultures should be obtained if there is fever

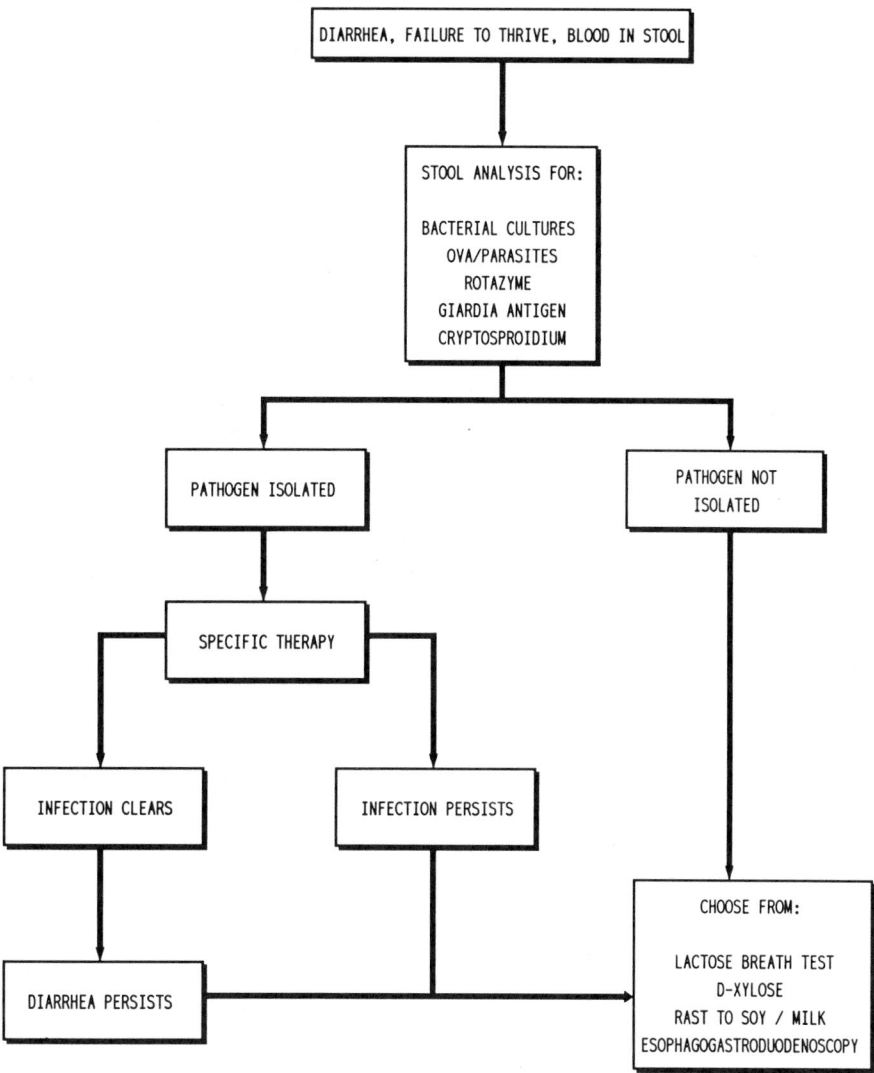

FIG. 5. Algorithm of diagnostic evaluation for the child suspected to have an enteric infection.

to identify disseminated fungal infection, mycobacterial infection, or a diagnosis of gastrointestinal bacterial infection, such as *Salmonella,* which has a propensity for bacteremia.

Endoscopy in HIV-infected children is indicated for evaluation of bleeding from the upper or lower gastrointestinal tract, dysphagia, and for persistent diarrhea causing significant wasting/malnutrition. Endoscopic biopsies should be obtained in saline for culture of fungi and *Mycobacteria,* viral culture medium for cytomegalovirus and adenovirus, formalin fixative for light microscopy, and glutaraldehyde fixative for electron microscopy to look for adenovirus, CMV, or *Microsporidium*. In addition, if clinically indicated, endoscopic aspirates of the small bowel fluid can be cultured quantitatively for aerobes and anaerobes to establish a diagnosis of bacterial overgrowth.

In addition to these specific tests for pathogens and stool tests for fat or reducing substances, tests that evaluate absorptive function may be helpful in the management of diarrhea in the pediatric patient. Malabsorption of specific sugars can be assessed by breath hydrogen tests and are of particular value in the pediatric population. In one study of 17 HIV-infected children, an abnormal lactose breath hydrogen test correlated significantly with the presence of diarrheal disease (114), but in another study no such correlation was found (115). Nevertheless, if the breath test is positive, management of a child with diarrhea may include a diet that avoids lactose. In addition, an early rise in the breath hydrogen concentration during a lactose breath test is an indication of small bowel bacterial overgrowth (116). Therefore, breath hydrogen tests may be used as diagnostic tools in children with diarrhea in whom a pathogen is not identified and for whom a modified formula must be selected.

Elevated serum levels of antibodies to food proteins are frequently present in children infected with HIV (117). The presence of these antibodies may only be an indication of increased mucosal permeability rather than true allergy; however, increased eosinophils in the stool (determined by Wright or Giemsa stain), blood, or intestinal/rectal biopsies provide additional evidence in support of an allergic cause.

MANAGEMENT OF PEDIATRIC HIV-RELATED ENTERIC INFECTION

If a specific treatable pathogen responsible for the HIV-related enteric infection is isolated, medications and their dosing schedules for children are listed in Table 1. In addition, since chronic carriage or prolonged fecal excretion is common for bacterial pathogens in the immunodeficient host, treatment may require an extended course. If no pathogen is found, an empiric course of antibiotic treatment may be considered for (a) a pathogen suspected to have been contracted by the child from travel to regions endemic for *E. coli* or (b) a positive breath hydrogen test that suggests small bowel bacterial overgrowth.

Beyond the acute phase of management, nutritional repletion has a key role in the overall medical care of children with HIV and enteric infection. Repletion should begin with an assessment of the nutritional status of the child and the establishment of the number of calories and quantity of protein necessary to achieve appropriate weight gain. A child's caloric needs should take into account the nutritional status (weight-for-age/weight-for-height percentiles, midarm circumference, and triceps skinfold thickness), activity level, and severity of infection, since fever and sepsis are known to increase energy demands. Serum total protein, albumin, prealbumin, and transferrin levels may help to assess the severity of protein deficiency. Deficiencies in micronutrients such as zinc, as previously mentioned, and selenium have been reported in children with HIV infection (118,119) and should be monitored in the malnourished child. Selection of a formula or nutritional supplement in the HIV-infected child with an enteric infection will depend on the severity

TABLE 1. *Antibiotics for enteric infections in children with HIV infection*

Pathogen	Antibiotic	Dose/duration
Salmonella	Ampicillin	100–200 mg/kg/d divided q6h × 10–14 days
	Ceftriaxone	100–150 mg/kg/d divided q21h × 10–14 days
	Chloramphenicol	80 mg/kg/d divided q6h × 10–14 days
	Ciprofloxacin	1000 mg/d divided q12h × 10–14 days
Campylobacter	Erythromycin	40 mg/kg/d divided q6h × 10 days
Shigella	TMP-SMX	10 mg TMP-SMX/kg/d divided q12h × 5 days
	Ampicillin	100 mg/kg/d divided q6h × 5 days
	Ciprofloxacin	1000 mg/d divided q12h × 5 days
C. difficile	Vancomycin	20 mg/kg/d divided q6h × 7 days
	Metronidazole	15–30 mg/kg/d divided q8h × 7 days
Giardia	Metronidazole	15–30 mg/kg/d divided q8h × 7 days
	Quinacrine HCl	6 mg/kg/d (max 300 mg/d) divided q8h × 7 days
	Furazolidone	6 mg/kg/d (max 400 mg/d) divided q6h × 7 days
Candida	Ketoconazole	5–10 mg/kg/d divided qd or q12h × 30 days
	Amphotericin B	0.5–1.5 mg/kg qd × 30 days
Histoplasma	Amphotericin B	0.5–1.5 mg/kg qd × 30 days

TMP/SMX, trimethoprim-sulfamethoxazole.

of intestinal injury. If the infection cannot be eradicated and the mucosa restored to normal, special care should be given to selecting a nutrient source that will sustain growth. Lactose-free formulas frequently are of benefit in HIV-infected children. In those children with severe injury to the mucosa, hydrolyzed preparations with medium chain triglyceride may be required. In children who are anorectic, a nasogastric catheter can be used temporarily (1 week to 1 month) for supplemental feedings in order to provide adequate nutrition. Because of a higher incidence of complications associated with a long-term indwelling nasogastric catheter (120,121), a gastrostomy may be preferable if supplemental feedings are required for more than a month. The supplemental feeding is best administered at night by a continuous drip, so that during the day the child can be orally stimulated with food. Daily monitoring of intake, output, and body weight will help to assess the adequacy of enteral feeding. Parenteral nutrition is indicated for chronic enteric infections, such as MAC, in children who are unable to maintain or gain weight on enteral feedings, and for those who cannot be fed enterally because of vomiting, gastrointestinal bleeding, or pancreatitis. The relative risks and benefits of a central venous catheter for parenteral nutrition vs. a gastrostomy should be considered carefully especially for those children who are neutropenic or thrombocytopenic. This group appears to be at risk for complications such as infection, bleeding, and poor wound healing.

SUMMARY

Enteric infections have a major global impact on the quality of life in children infected with HIV. Currently only 40% to 50% of enteric infections in children infected with HIV are attributable to specific pathogens. Identification of new enteric pathogens in HIV-infected children has not resulted in the development of effective therapies. Medical interventions for the treatment of these pathogens are therefore mostly supportive. Optimal nutritional support and provision of passive immunity may reduce the morbidity and frequency of enteric infection in HIV-infected children. However, to impact globally on the morbidity and mortality of infants infected with HIV, international public health efforts should be directed at providing appropriate nutrition for the HIV-infected child and his or her family.

REFERENCES

1. Thea DM, St. Louis ME, Atido U, et al. A prospective study of diarrhea and HIV-1 infection among 429 Zairian infants. *N Engl J Med* 1983;329:1696–1702.
2. MacCarthy VP, Charles DL, Unger JL. Transfusion-associated HIV infection in a neonate from a seronegative donor. *Am J Dis Child* 1987;2:84–87.
3. Ward JW, Holmberg SD, Allen JR, et al. Transmission of human immunodeficiency virus (HIV) by blood transfusions screened as negative for HIV antibody. *N Engl J Med* 1988;318:473–478.
4. Cohen ND, Munoz A, Reitz BA, et al. Transmission of retroviruses by transfusion of screened blood in patients undergoing cardiac surgery. *N Engl J Med* 1989;320:1172–1176.
5. Jones DS, Byers RH, Bush TJ, Oxtoby MJ, Rogers MF. Epidemiology of transfusion-associated acquired immunodeficiency syndrome in children in the United States, 1981 through 1989. *Pediatrics* 1992;89:123–127.
6. Quinn TC, Ruff A, Halsey N. Pediatric acquired immunodeficiency syndrome: special considerations for developing nations. *Pediatr Infect Dis J* 1992;11:558–568.
7. Oxtoby MJ. Perinatally acquired human immunodeficiency virus infection. *Pediatr Infect Dis J* 1990;9:609–619.
8. Ryder RW, Nsa E, Hassig SE, et al. Perinatal transmission of the human immunodeficiency virus type 1 to infants of seropositive women in Zaire. *N Engl J Med* 1989;320:1637–1642.
9. Centers for Disease Control. Zidovudine for the prevention of HIV transmission from mother to infant. *MMWR* 1994;43:285–287.
10. Rossi P, Moschese V, Broliden PA, et al. Presence of maternal antibodies to human immunodeficiency virus 1 envelope glycoprotein gp120 epitopes correlates with the uninfected status of children born to seropositive mother. *Proc Natl Acad Sci USA* 1989;86:8055–8058.
11. Ruff A, Coberly J, Farzadegan H, et al. Detection of HIV-1 by PCR in breast milk (Abst). Seventh International Conference on AIDS, Florence, Italy; 1991.
12. Van de Perre P, Simonon A, Msellati P, et al. Postnatal transmission of human immunodeficiency virus type 1 from mother to infant. A prospective cohort study in Kigali, Rwanda. *N Engl J Med* 1991;325:593–598.
13. Ziegler JB, Palasanthiran P, Cruickshank M, Langdon P. Pediatric HIV: Australian perspective. *J AIDS* 1993;6(Suppl 1):S20–S23.
14. Palasanthiran P, Ziegler JB, Stewart GJ, et al. Breastfeeding during primary maternal human immunodeficiency virus infection and risk of transmission from mother to infant. *J Infect Dis* 1983;167:441–444.
15. WHO/UNICEF. Statement on breast feeding and HIV. WHO/UNICEF consultative meeting of April 30–May 1. *Wkly Epidemiol Rec* 1992;67:177–184.
16. Centers for Disease Control. Statistics from CDC. AIDS 1993;7:601–603.
17. Turner BJ, Denison M, Eppes SC, et al. Survival experience of 789 children with acquired immunodeficiency syndrome. *Pediatr Infect Dis J* 1993;12:310–320.
18. Horsburgh CR Jr, Caldwell B, Simonds RJ. Epidemiology of disseminated nontuberculous mycobacterial disease in children with acquired immunodeficiency syndrome. *Pediatr Infect Dis J* 1993;12:219–222.
19. Rutstein RM, Cobb P, McGowan KL, Pinto-Martin J, Starr SE. *Mycobacterium avium intracellulare* complex infection in HIV-infected children. *J AIDS* 1993;7:507–512.
20. Hoyt L, Oleske J, Holland B, Connor E. Nontuberculous mycobacteria in children with acquired immunodeficiency syndrome. *Pediatr Infect Dis J* 1992;11:354–360.
21. Duliege AM, Messiah A, Blanche S, Tardieu M, Griscelli C, Spira A. Natural history of human immunodeficiency virus type 1 infection in children: prognostic value of laboratory tests on the bimodal progression of the disease. *Pediatr Infect Dis J* 1992;11:630–635.
22. Pavia AT, Long EG, Ryder RW, et al. Diarrhea among African children born to human immunodeficiency virus-infected mothers: clinical, microbiologic and epidemiologic features. *Pediatr Infect Dis J* 1992;11:996–1003.
23. Italian Multicenter Study. Epidemiology, clinical features, and prognostic factors of paediatric HIV infection. *Lancet* 1988;2:1043–1046.
24. Pratt RD, Hatch R, Dankner WM, Spector S. Pediatric human immunodeficiency virus infection in a low seroprevalence area. *Pediatr Infect Dis J* 1993;12:304–310.
25. Pahwa S, Kaplan M, Fikrig S, et al. Spectrum of human T-cell lymphotropic virus type III infection in children. *JAMA* 1986;255:2299–2305.
26. Grand RJ, Watkins JB, Torti FM. Development of the human gastrointestinal tract. *Gastroenterology* 1976;70:790–810.

27. Antonowicz I, Lebanthal E. Developmental pattern of small intestinal enterokinase and disaccharidase activities in the human fetus. *Gastroenterology* 1977;72:1299–1303.

28. Cohen MB, Guarino A, Shukla R, Giannella RA. Age-related differences in receptors for *Escherichia coli* heat-stable enterotoxin in the small and large intestine of children. *Gastroenterology* 1988;94:367–373.

29. Riepenhoff-Talty M, Lee PC, Carmody RJ, Barrett JH, Ogra PL. Age-dependent rotavirus-enterocyte interactions. *Proc Soc Exp Biol Med* 1982;170:146–154.

30. Bezzara J, Thompson S, Dos Santos B, Koldovsky O, Udall J. Urinary lactose excretion of infants and adults following ingestion of disaccharide. *J Am Coll Nutr* 1988;7:417.

31. Jakobsson I, Linberg T, Lothe L, Axelsson I, Benediktsson B. Human α-lactalbumin as a marker of macromolecular absorption. *Gut* 1986;27:1029–1034.

32. Kim KS, Wong VK, Adler R, Steinberg EA. Comparative immune responses to *Hemophilus influenzae* type b polysaccharide and a polysaccharide-protein conjugate vaccine. *Pediatrics* 1990;85:S648–S650.

33. Madore DV, Johnson C, Phipps DC, et al. Safety and immune response to *Haemophilus influenzae* type b oligosaccharide-CRM197 conjugate vaccine in 1- to 6-month-old infants. *Pediatrics* 1990;85:331–337.

34. Selner JC, Merrill DAK, Clamen HN. Salivary immunoglobulin and albumin: development during the newborn period. *Pediatrics* 1968;72:685–689.

35. Bradtzaeg P, Baklien K, Bjerke K, Rognum TO, Scott H, Valnes K. Nature and properties of the human gastrointestinal immune system. In: Miller K, Nicklin S, eds. *Immunology of the gastrointestinal tract.* vol 1. Boca Raton: CRC Press; 1987:1.

36. McKinney RE, Wilfert CM. Lymphocyte subsets in children younger than 2 years old: normal values in a population at risk for human immunodeficiency virus infection and diagnostic and prognostic application to infected children. *Pediatr Infect Dis J* 1992;11:639–644.

37. Borkowsky W, Rigaud M, Krasinski K, Moore T, Lawrence R, Pollack H. Cell-mediated and humoral immune responses in children infected with human immunodeficiency virus during the first four years of life. *J Pediatr* 1992;120:371–375.

38. Jason JM, Nieburg P, Marks JS. Mortality and infectious disease associated with infant-feeding practices in developing countries. *Pediatrics* 1984;74(Suppl):702–727.

39. Ruiz-Palacios GM, Calva JJ, Pickering LK, et al. Protection of breast-fed infants against Campylobacter diarrhea by antibodies in human milk. *J Pediatr* 1990;116:707–713.

40. Ochs HD. Intravenous immunoglobulin in the treatment and prevention of acute infections in pediatric acquired immunodeficiency syndrome patients. *Pediatr Infect Dis J* 1987;6:509–511.

41. Tozzi A, Pezzotti P, Greco D. Does breast-feeding delay progression to AIDS in HIV-infected children? *J AIDS* 1990;4:1293–1294.

42. Winter HS, Miller TL, Hobson CD, Naim HY. Enteropathy in congenital HIV infection: histological and molecular evaluation. *Gastroenterology* 1991;100:A626.

43. Fox CH, Cottler-Fox M. The pathobiology of HIV infection. *Immunol Today* 1992;13:353–356.

44. Maiuri L, Rossi M, Raia V, et al. Mosaic regulation of lactase in human adult-type hypolactasia. *Gastroenterology* 1994;107:54–60.

45. Berkowitz FE. Infections in children with severe protein-energy malnutrition. *Pediatr Infect Dis J* 1992;11:750–759.

46. Summer A, Katz J, Tarwotjo I. Increased risk of respiratory disease and diarrhea in children with pre-existing mild vitamin A deficiency. *Am J Clin Nutr* 1984;40:1090–1095.

47. El Bushra HE, Ash L, Coulson AH, Neumann CG. Interrelationship between diarrhea and vitamin A deficiency: is vitamin A deficiency a risk factor for diarrhea? *Pediatr Infect Dis J* 1992;11:380–384.

48. Keen CL, Gershwin ME. Zinc deficiency and immune function. *Annu Rev Nutr* 1990;10:415–431.

49. Bartlett AV III, Bednarz-Prashad J, DuPont HL, Pickering LK. Rotavirus gastroenteritis. *Annu Rev Med* 1987;38:399–415.

50. Van R, Wun CC, O'Ryan ML, Matson DO, Jackson L, Pickering LK. Outbreaks of human enteric adenovirus types 40 and 41 in Houston day care centers. *J Pediatr* 1992;120:516–521.

51. Mitchell DK, Van R, Morrow AL, Monroe SS, Glass RI, Pickering LK. Outbreaks of astrovirus gastroenteritis in day care centers. *J Pediatr* 1993;123:725–732.

52. Kotloff KL, Herrmann JE, Blacklow NR, et al. The frequency of astrovirus as a cause of diarrhea in Baltimore children. *Pediatr Infect Dis J* 1992;11:587–589.

53. Oshitani H, Kasolo FC, Mpabalwani M. Association of rotavirus and human immunodeficiency virus infection in children hospitalized with acute diarrhea, Lusaka, Zambia. *J Infect Dis* 1994;169:897–900.

54. Gilger MA, Matson DO, Conner ME, Rosenblatt HM, Finegold MJ, Estes MK. Extraintestinal rotavirus infections in children with immunodeficiency. *J Pediatr* 1992;120:912–917.

55. Smith PD, Lane HC, Gill VJ, et al. Intestinal infections in patients with the acquired immunodeficiency syndrome (AIDS). Etiology and response to therapy. *Ann Intern Med* 1988;108:328–333.

56. Laughon BE, Druckman DA, Vernon AA, et al. Prevalence of enteric pathogens in homosexual men with and without AIDS. *Gastroenterology* 1988;94:984–993.

57. Knisley CV, Bednarz-Prashad AJ, Pickering LK. Detection of rotavirus in stool specimens using monoclonal and polyclonal based assay systems. *J Clin Microbiol* 1986;23:897–900.

58. Guarino A, Guandalini S, Albano F, Mascia A, de Ritis G, Rubino A. Enteral immunoglobulins for treatment of protracted rotaviral diarrhea. *Pediatr Infect Dis J* 1991;10:612–614.

59. Melamed I, Griffiths AM, Roifman CM. Benefit of oral immune globulin therapy in patients with immunodeficiency and chronic diarrhea. *J Pediatr* 1991;119:486–488.

60. Brandt CD, Kim HW, Rodrigues WJ, et al. Adenoviruses and pediatric gastroenteritis. *J Infect Dis* 1985;151:437.

61. Whitlaw A, Davies H. Electron microscopy of fatal adenovirus gastroenteritis. *Lancet* 1977;1:361.

62. Janner D, Petro AM, Belchis D, Azimi PH. Fatal adenovirus infection in a child with acquired immunodeficiency syndrome. *Pediatr Infect Dis J* 1990;9:434–436.

63. Krilov LR, Rubin LG, Frogel M, et al. Disseminated adenovirus infection with hepatic necrosis in patients with human immunodeficiency virus infection and other immunodeficiency states. *Rev Infect Dis* 1990;12:303–307.

64. Janoff EN, Orenstein JM, Manischewitz JF, Smith PD. Adenovirus colitis in the acquired immunodeficiency syndrome. *Gastroenterology* 1991;100:976–979.

65. Dagan R, Schwartz RH, Insel RA, Menegus MA. Severe diffuse adenovirus 7a pneumonia in a child with combined immunodeficiency: possible therapeutic effect of human serum immunoglobulin containing a specific neutralizing antibody. *Pediatr Infect Dis J* 1984;3:246–251.

66. Cieslak TJ, Mullett CT, Puntel RA, Latimer JS. Menetrier's disease associated with cytomegalovirus infection in children: report of two cases and review of the literature. *Pediatr Infect Dis J* 1993;12:340–343.

67. Stagno S, Pass RF, Dworsky ME, Alford CA Jr. Maternal cytomegalovirus infection and perinatal transmission. *Clin Obstet Gynecol* 1982;25:563–576.

68. Yow MD, Williamson DW, Leeds LJ, et al. Epidemiologic characteristics of cytomegalovirus infection in mothers and their infants. *Am J Obstet Gynecol* 1988;158:1189–1195.

69. Frenkel LD, Gaur S, Tsolia M, Scudder R, Howell R, Kesarwala H. Cytomegalovirus infection in children with AIDS. *Rev Infect Dis* 1990;12:S820–S826.

70. Schooley RT. Cytomegalovirus in the setting of infection with human immunodeficiency virus. *Rev Infect Dis* 1990;12:S811–819.

71. Schwartz DL, So HB, Bungarz WR, et al. A case of life-threatening gastrointestinal hemorrhage in an infant with AIDS. *J Pediatr Surg* 1989;24:313–315.

72. Victoria MS, Nangia BS, Jindrak K. Cytomegalovirus pyloric

obstruction in a child with acquired immunodeficiency syndrome. *Pediatr Infect Dis J* 1985;4:550–552.

73. Strano A. Light microscopy of selected viral diseases (morphology of viral inclusion bodies). *Pathol Annu* 1976;11:53–75.

74. Schwartz DA, Wilcox CM. Atypical cytomegalovirus inclusions in gastrointestinal biopsy specimens from patients with the acquired immunodeficiency syndrome: diagnostic role of in situ nucleic acid hybridization. *Hum Pathol* 1992;23:1019–1026.

75. Dietrich DT, Kotler DP, Busch DF, et al. Ganciclovir treatment of cytomegalovirus colitis in AIDS: a randomized, double-blind, placebo-controlled multicenter study. *J Infect Dis* 1993;167:278–282.

76. Dietrich DT, Poles MA, Dicker M, Tepper R, Lew E. Foscarnet treatment of cytomegalovirus gastrointestinal infections in acquired immunodeficiency syndrome patients who have failed ganciclovir induction. *Am J Gastroenterol* 1993;88:542–548.

77. Nelson MR, Connolly GM, Francis N, et al. Foscarnet in the treatment of cytomegalovirus infection of the esophagus and colon in patients with the acquired immunodeficiency syndrome. *Am J Gastroenterol* 1991;86:876–881.

78. Gudnason T, Belani KK, Balfour HH. Ganciclovir treatment of cytomegalovirus disease in immunocompromised children. *Pediatr Infect Dis J* 1989;8:436–440.

79. Snydman DR. Cytomegalovirus immunoglobulins in the prevention and treatment of cytomegalovirus disease. *Rev Infect Dis* 1990;12(Suppl 7):S839–S848.

80. Grohman GS, Glass RI, Pereira HG, et al. Enteric viruses and diarrhea in HIV-infected patients. *N Engl J Med* 1993;329:14–20.

81. Sperber SJ, Schleupner CJ. Salmonellosis during infection with human immunodeficiency virus. *Rev Infect Dis* 1987;9:925–933.

82. Gotuzzo E, Frisancho O, Sanchez J, et al. Association between the acquired immunodeficiency syndrome and infection with *Salmonella typhi* or *Salmonella paratyphi* in an endemic typhoid area. *Arch Intern Med* 1991;151:381–382.

83. Bernstein LJ, Krieger BZ, Novick B, Sicklick MJ, Rubinstein A. Bacterial infection in the acquired immunodeficiency syndrome of children. *Pediatr Infect Dis J* 1985;4:472–475.

84. McLaughlin LC, Nord KS, Joshi VV, Oleske JM, Connor EM. Severe gastrointestinal involvement in children with the acquired immunodeficiency syndrome. *J Pediatr Gastroenterol Nutr* 1987;6:517–524.

85. Jain A, Reif S, O'Neil K, Gandhi A, Rossi T. Small intestinal bacterial overgrowth and protein-losing enteropathy in an infant with AIDS. *J Pediatr Gastroenterol Nutr* 1992;15:452–454.

86. Viscidi R, Willey S, Bartlett JG. Isolation rates and toxigenic potential of *Clostridium difficile* isolates from various patient populations. *Gastroenterology* 1981;81:5–9.

87. Buts JP, Corthier G, Delmee M. *Saccharomyces boulardii* for *Clostridium difficile*–associated enteropathies in infants. *J Pediatr Gastroenterol Nutr* 1993;16:419–425.

88. Sutphen JL, Grand RJ, Flores A, Chang TW, Bartlett JG. Chronic diarrhea associated with *Clostridium difficile* in children. *Am J Dis Child* 1983;137:275–278.

89. Cozart JC, Kalangi SS, Clench MH, et al. *Clostridium difficile* diarrhea in patients with AIDS versus non-AIDS controls. Methods of treatment and clinical response to treatment. *Am J Gastroenterol* 1993;16:192–194.

90. Marano BJ Jr, Smith F, Bonano CA. *Helicobacter pylori* prevalence in acquired immunodeficiency syndrome. *Am J Gastroenterol* 1993;88:687–690.

91. Edwards PD, Carrick J, Turner J, Lee A, Mitchell H, Cooper DA. *Helicobacter pylori*–associated gastritis is rare in AIDS: antibiotic effect or a consequence of immunodeficiency? *Am J Gastroenterol* 1991;86:1761–1764.

92. Blecker U, Keymolen K, Souayah H, Levy J, Vandenplas Y. *Helicobacter pylori* in children with acquired immunodeficiency syndrome. *Pediatrics* 1993;91:1217.

93. Masur H. Recommendations on prophylaxis and therapy for disseminated *Mycobacterium avium* complex disease in patients infected with the human immunodeficiency virus. *N Engl J Med* 1993;329:898–904.

94. Moss WJ, Dedyo T, Suarez M, Nicholas SW, Abrams E. Tuberculosis in children infected with human immunodeficiency virus: a report of five cases. *Pediatr Infect Dis J* 1992;11:114–120.

95. Friedenberg KA, Draguesku JO, Kiyabu M, Valenzuela JE. Intestinal perforation due to *Mycobacterium tuberculosis* in HIV-infected individuals: report of two cases. *Am J Gastroenterol* 1993;88:604–607.

96. Molina JM, Sarfati C, Beauvais B, et al. Intestinal microsporidiosis in human immunodeficiency virus-infected patients with chronic unexplained diarrhea: prevalence and clinical and biologic features. *J Infect Dis* 1993;167:217–221.

97. Kotler DP, Francisco A, Clayton F, Scholes JV, Orenstein JM. Small intestinal injury and parasitic diseases in AIDS. *Ann Intern Med* 1990;113:444–449.

98. Greenson J, Belitsos P, Yardley J, et al. AIDS enteropathy: occult enteric infection and duodenal alterations in chronic diarrhea. *Ann Intern Med* 1991;114:366–372.

99. Cegielski JP, Msengi AE, Dukes CS, et al. Intestinal parasites and HIV infection in Tanzanian children with chronic diarrhea. *J AIDS* 1993;7:213.

100. Santa Lucia MM, Ito HT, Castro M, DePaula MDN. Diarrheal illness: comparative study between AIDS patients and non-infected children. VII International Conference on AIDS, Florence, June 1991, Abstract WB2028.

101. Teixidor HS, Godwin TA, Ramirez EA. Cryptosporidiosis of the biliary tract in AIDS. *Radiology* 1991;180:51–56.

102. McGowan I, Hawkins AS, Weller IVD. The natural history of cryptosporidial diarrhea in HIV-infected patients. *J AIDS* 1993;7:349–354.

103. Romeu J, Miro JM, Sirera G, et al. Efficacy of octreotide in the management of chronic diarrhea in AIDS. *J AIDS* 1991;5:1495–1499.

104. Borowitz SM, Sausbury FT. Treatment of chronic cryptosporidial infection with orally administered human serum immune globulin. *J Pediatr* 1991;119:593–595.

105. Ungar BLP, Ward DJ, Fayer R, Quinn CA. Cessation of *Cryptosporidium*-associated diarrhea in an acquired immunodeficiency syndrome patient after treatment with hyperimmune bovine colostrum. *Gastroenterology* 1990;98:486–489.

106. Samaranayake LP, Holmstrup P. Oral candidiasis and human immunodeficiency virus infection. *J Oral Pathol Med* 1989;18:554–564.

107. Leibovitz E, Rigaud M, Chandwani S, et al. Disseminated fungal infections in children infected with human immunodeficiency virus. *Pediatr Infect Dis J* 1991;10:888–894.

108. Laine L, Dretler RH, Conteas CN, et al. Fluconazole compared to ketoconazole for the treatment of Candida esophagitis in AIDS. A randomized trial. *Ann Intern Med* 1992;117:655–660.

109. Schutze GE, Tucker NC, Jacobs RF. Histoplasmosis and perinatal human immunodeficiency virus. *Pediatr Infect Dis J* 1992;11:501.

110. Byers M, Feldman S, Edwards J. Disseminated histoplasmosis as the acquired immunodeficiency syndrome-defining illness in an infant. *Pediatr Infect Dis J* 1992;11:127–128.

111. Shull HJ. Human histoplasmosis: disease with protean manifestations often with digestive system involvement. *Gastroenterology* 1953;25:582.

112. Smith PD. Infectious diarrheas in patients with AIDS. *Gastroenterol Clin North Am* 1993;22:535–548.

113. Ma P, Soave R. Three-step stool examination for cryptosporidiosis in 10 homosexual men with protracted watery diarrhea. *J Infect Dis* 1983;147:824–828.

114. Yolken RH, Hart W, Oung I, Shiff C, Greenson J, Perman J. Gastrointestinal dysfunction and disaccharide intolerance in children infected with human immunodeficiency virus. *J Pediatr* 1991;118:359–363.

115. Miller TL, Orav EJ, Martin SR, Cooper ER, McIntosh K, Winter HS. Malnutrition and carbohydrate malabsorption in children with vertically transmitted human immunodeficiency virus 1 infection. *Gastroenterology* 1991;100:1296–1302.

116. Rhodes JM, Middleton P, Jewell DP. The lactulose hydrogen breath test as a diagnostic test for small-bowel bacterial overgrowth. *Scand J Gastroenterol* 1979;14:333–336.

117. Guarino A, Tarallo L, Guandalini S, Troncone R, Albano F, Rubino A. Impaired intestinal function in symptomatic HIV infection. *J Pediatr Gastroenterol Nutr* 1991;12:453–458.
118. Fabris N, Mocchigiani E, Galli M, et al. AIDS, zinc deficiency and thymic hormone failure. *JAMA* 1988;259:2850.
119. Kavanaugh-MacHugh A, Rowe S, Benjamin Y, et al. Selenium deficiency and cardiomyopathy in malnourished pediatric AIDS patients. Presented at the 5th International Conference on AIDS, Montreal; 1989.
120. Mobarhan S, Trumbore LS. Enteral tube feeding: a clinical perspective on recent advances. *Nutr Rev* 1991;49:129–140.
121. Bussy V, Marechal F, Nasca S. Microbial contamination of enteral feeding tubes occurring during nutritional treatment. *J Parent Ent Nutr* 1992;16:552–557.

Infections of the Gastrointestinal Tract,
edited by M. J. Blaser, P. D. Smith, J. I. Ravdin,
H. B. Greenberg, and R. L. Guerrant
Raven Press, Ltd., New York © 1995.

CHAPTER 37

Gastrointestinal Infections in Transplant Recipients

J. Stephen Dummer and Ban Mishu Allos

The outcomes for patients undergoing solid organ and bone marrow transplantations markedly improved during the 1980s, in part as a result of the development and use of the new immunosuppressive drug, cyclosporine. Transplantation is now an accepted form of therapy for patients with a variety of conditions previously considered untreatable and largely fatal. As a consequence, the number of transplants performed in the United States and in other parts of the world has dramatically increased since 1980. In the United States alone, there were 19,521 cadaveric kidney transplants performed between October 1987 and May 1991 (1). Between 1980 and 1990, there were 7.5 allogeneic bone marrow transplants performed per million population in the United States; more than 5500 were performed in 1990 alone (2). Worldwide, more than 2500 cardiac transplants are performed annually (3).

Infections of the gastrointestinal tract are frequent causes of morbidity and mortality among transplant patients. Among 131 emergency department visits by patients who had undergone heart or lung transplantation, 10% were due to gastrointestinal symptoms such as nausea, vomiting, or diarrhea (4). Gastrointestinal symptoms were the most common presenting complaint after fever and dyspnea. Among children undergoing bone marrow transplantation, 83% experienced diarrhea requiring a diagnostic workup within the first 21 months after transplantation (5). In a review of autopsy findings in 24 patients who had undergone bone marrow transplants, ten had serious infections of the gastrointestinal tract (6). Gastrointestinal infections were identified in autopsies of 11 (25%) of 44 cardiac transplant patients (7). Serious colonic infections occur in 1% to 4% of kidney transplant patients and the abdomen is the most frequent site of bacterial and

J. S. Dummer and B. Mishu Allos: Departments of Medicine and Surgery and Departments of Medicine and Preventive Medicine, Vanderbilt University Medical Center, Nashville, Tennessee 37232.

fungal infections among patients with liver transplants (8–12).

This chapter focuses on the general approach to gastrointestinal infections in transplant patients. A thorough discussion of the pathogenesis, clinical presentation, and treatment of specific pathogens is adequately covered in other chapters. Instead, we review the overall importance of enteric infections in transplant patients and try to place these in perspective with other pathologic processes of the gastrointestinal tract that are important in this population. The effects of immunosuppression on the gastrointestinal tract and discussion of the more relevant pathogens are also included.

MICROBIOLOGY

A broad range of organisms are capable of producing disease in transplant recipients. Table 1 illustrates the relative importance of pathogens causing infection in the gut or abdomen of transplant patients.

Bacterial Diseases

Listeria is one of the classic infections occurring in patients with defects in cell-mediated immunity (13). In experimental animal models, cytotoxic drugs, corticosteroids, and cyclosporine impair the development of immunity to this organism (14–16). Transplant patients account for 10% to 15% of cases of *Listeria* infections in large population-based surveys (17). These data suggest that the rate of *Listeria* infection in transplant patients is increased at least 1000-fold over normal populations. *Listeria* was identified in the stools of 5.6% of renal transplant recipients followed for 1 year (18). Both carriage of organisms and clinical disease in transplant patients are more common during summertime. Not surprisingly, the greatest risk of listeriosis occurs in the first year after

TABLE 1. *Relative importance of selected enteric pathogens in transplant patients compared with normal hosts*

Importance compared with normal hosts	Pathogen			
	Bacteria	Viruses	Fungi	Parasites
Much greater	*Listeria*	Cytomegalovirus Adenovirus Epstein–Barr virus Herpes simplex	*Candida* *Aspergillus*	
Greater	*Salmonella* *C. difficile*	Rotavirus	*Histoplasma*	*Strongyloides* *Cryptosporidium*
Equal	*Shigella* *Campylobacter* *Helicobacter*			*Giardia*
No data	*E. coli* *Aeromonas* *Yersinia*	Norwalk agent		

transplantation (18). *Listeria* organisms are highly susceptible to trimethoprim–sulfamethoxazole. The widespread use of this agent for *Pneumocystis* prophylaxis may have resulted in the decreased rate of *Listeria* infection in transplant recipients observed in recent years (19).

Infections with *Clostridium difficile* are most commonly reported after liver transplantation (3% to 6%) and bone marrow transplantation (14% to 15%), consistent with the greater use of antibiotics in these types of transplantation (5,8,9,20,21). They are less widely reported in renal and heart transplant populations. There is wide institutional variation in the incidence of *C. difficile* colitis (22). Furthermore, substantial evidence supports the nosocomial spread of *C. difficile* (22–25).

The frequency of *Salmonella* infections is increased in renal transplant patients. Of 592 renal transplant patients in Saudi Arabia, 20 developed *Salmonella* infection and of these 62.5% were bacteremic, 35% had focal abscesses outside the bowel, and 35% experienced relapse (26). High rates of salmonellosis in transplant patients have also been reported in a few European countries (27–29). Only sporadic cases of salmonellosis have been reported from transplant centers in the United States (30,31).

Reports of *Shigella* infections are infrequent among transplant patients (32–34). Indeed, the incidence and clinical severity may be similar to that in the general population. Although bacteremia was seen in three of four reported cases, the incidence of extra-intestinal *Shigella* infections in transplant patients is not known. *Campylobacter* infections are identified in human immunodeficiency virus (HIV)-infected persons 40 times more frequently than in the general population (35). *Campylobacter* infections are also more severe and difficult to eradicate in patients with HIV infection or hypogammaglobulinemia (35,36). Campylobacteriosis does not appear to be a frequent or important problem in transplant patients (37).

Ulcer disease and gastritis are frequently reported in some series of transplant recipients, but relatively little research has been done on *Helicobacter pylori* infection after transplantation. A single cross-sectional study of 202 renal transplant recipients showed that patients seropositive for *Helicobacter* described dyspeptic symptoms more frequently than seronegative transplant recipients (38). In another series of endoscopies of 33 renal transplant recipients, 48% had *Helicobacter* identified and its presence was associated with gastritis and symptomatic dyspepsia (39). By contrast, endoscopies of 276 patients before and after bone marrow transplantation revealed only one documented *Helicobacter* infection (40). In another study of 100 heart transplant recipients, 35% were seropositive and only one of 65 seronegative patients seroconverted during 3 years of follow-up (41). Forty percent of seropositive patients became seronegative during follow-up; these seroreversions were related to the use of oral and intravenous antibiotics. From these preliminary studies it appears that the importance of *Helicobacter* infection after transplantation may be variable and depend on factors such as the type of transplant, timing, and the use of antibiotics.

Viral Diseases

Cytomegalovirus (CMV) is likely the most important pathogen in transplant recipients. As defined by positive cultures, CMV infection occurs in 53% to 100% of solid organ transplant recipients and 32% to 52% of bone marrow recipients (42). The actual frequency with which CMV causes gastrointestinal disease is difficult to determine with certainty because definite diagnosis depends on endoscopy and involvement may be limited to areas of the bowel not accessible to endoscopy. Gastrointestinal complaints are common with CMV disease. In one series of heart and lung transplant patients with symptomatic CMV disease, 41% had abdominal pain without another explanation (43).

Other herpesviruses are also important in transplant patients. Enteric infection with herpes simplex virus is most often limited to the distal esophagus, but rare cases of herpes gastritis or herpes colitis are also seen and may be part of a picture of widely disseminated disease (44–46). Herpes zoster may rarely disseminate to the gut and prodromal shingles in an abdominal dermatome may also initially be confused with a severe intra-abdominal bacterial infection (47). Epstein–Barr virus (EBV) does not cause a gastroenteritis *per se* but EBV infection is linked to the development of B cell lymphoproliferative disease after transplantation, which often causes tumors in the bowel and may present with diarrhea, gastrointestinal hemorrhage, or abdominal pain (48).

Infections due to adenovirus occur only sporadically in adult solid organ transplant patients (49). They are more frequent (5% to 10%) after bone marrow transplantation and pediatric liver transplantation (50–53). The gut is frequently involved, often as part of a picture of disseminated disease involving the kidney, lung, and liver.

There are numerous descriptions of infection due to rotavirus in solid organ and bone marrow recipients. Infections occur most commonly in children but also occur in adults (54,55). Nosocomial transmission has been documented (56,57). The disease is generally self-limited, although prolonged illness has also been reported (58).

Enterovirus has caused sporadic and outbreak-related disease in bone marrow transplant recipients (21,59). In one reported outbreak of coxsackievirus A1 infection, six of seven infected bone marrow recipients died (59). Most patients experienced severe unrelenting diarrhea. Foamy vacuolization and sloughing of the mucosa were the predominant findings at autopsy.

Fungal Diseases

Candida species are ubiquitous in the normal gastrointestinal tract and may become invasive under conditions of immunosuppression, especially when the mucosa is injured by cytotoxic drugs or when high-dose corticosteroids are used (60,61). More than 60% of cancer patients developed thrush within 2 weeks of a course of chemotherapy, even in the absence of antibiotic therapy (62). Enteric involvement is usually limited to the throat and esophagus, but occasional cases of gastric or colonic candidiasis are described (63). The gut is thought to be the main portal of entry for disseminated candidiasis. Peritonitis and abscesses from *Candida* are reported in 3% to 19% of liver recipients and also may occur in other transplant patients after abdominal operations (64–67).

Although the gut is a common site for dissemination of *Aspergillus* infection, primary infection with *Aspergillus* in the bowel or abdominal cavity is rare (68). Wound and deep abdominal infection with *Aspergillus* has recently been described as a sequela to liver transplantation (69,70).

Disseminated histoplasmosis occurs in a small subset of transplant patients (71). Most patients with disseminated histoplasmosis have resided in or recently visited the endemic areas in the midwestern and southeastern United States. Involvement of the digestive tract is common with disseminated histoplasmosis; in some instances the digestive tract may be the only apparent site of disease (72). Gastrointestinal involvement may be asymptomatic or produce clinical manifestations such as diarrhea, abdominal pain, gastrointestinal bleeding, or malabsorption.

Parasites

Hyperinfection and disseminated infection with *Strongyloides* have been substantial problems in immunocompromised hosts including transplant recipients (73–76). Patients develop fever, abdominal pain, polymicrobial bacteremia, and pulmonary signs and symptoms. This entity was frequently described in transplant patients in the 1970s and early 1980s but seems to have virtually disappeared since the introduction of cyclosporine. This may be due to direct inhibition of the parasite by cyclosporine (77).

Infection with *Cryptosporidium* in transplant patients has been infrequently described. The range of disease has varied from asymptomatic carriage to intractable diarrhea (78,79). A nosocomial outbreak occurred in six patients in a bone marrow unit (79). This infection appears to be more frequent in transplant patients and also may be more morbid, leading to prolonged shedding of the organism. Three cases of *Giardia lamblia* infection have been reported in bone marrow recipients (5,80). Diarrhea was fulminant in one case but all patients responded to antibiotic therapy.

PATHOGENESIS

Microorganisms that are latent in the host and reactivate under immunosuppression are an important source of enteric infections in transplant recipients. CMV and other herpesviruses are the most important example of this type of organism. In addition to reactivation of latent infection, CMV may also be newly acquired from donated organs or blood transfusions (42). The exact site and molecular mechanism of CMV latency are not known. Herpes simplex virus is latent in dorsal root ganglia. Virus reaches the oral cavity by retrograde axonal spread from the trigeminal ganglion (81). Esophageal and gastric involvement by herpesvirus is thought to occur via aspiration of virus from the mouth. Most disease is due to reactivation of latent virus in seropositive individuals but rare cases of primary infection in seronegative transplant recipients have been described (82,83). EBV is also associated with enteric disease in transplant recipients. From 1% to 4% of transplant recipients develop B cell lymphoproliferative tumors related to EBV infection (84,85). The bowel is a common site for these tumors. They may occur in EBV-seropositive individuals but are more common in EBV-seronegative individuals who acquire the virus exogenously (86). The donor organ was shown to be the source of virus in two patients (87).

Some microorganisms are harmless commensals in normal hosts and become pathogenic during immunosuppression. Although all transplant recipients are at risk for mucocutaneous candidiasis, patients that receive extensive antibiotic treatment and also suffer injury to the bowel, either by surgical trauma (liver transplantation), radiation, cytotoxic drugs, or graft-versus-host disease (bone marrow transplantation), are at greatest risk for disseminated candidiasis. Patients normally at low risk for invasive candidiasis may have increased risk after abdominal surgery, long-term residence in the intensive care unit, or high-dose immunosuppressive therapy.

In contrast to CMV and *Candida,* common enteric infections that are exogenously acquired from food, water, animals, or other humans are not greatly increased in frequency in transplant populations. One exception is salmonella. Although salmonella infections are an uncommon problem at transplant centers in the United States, they are an important problem in less developed countries (33). Pathogens that are transmitted in the nosocomial setting (such as *C. difficile* or rotavirus) have also caused outbreaks in transplant recipients.

For some important pathogens the mode of acquisition is not clear. Adenovirus, like CMV, can latently infect cells and may reactivate under immunosuppression; however, nosocomial transmission may also occur (88,89). Because of their low incidence and the necessity of doing type-specific antibody studies to investigate protective immunity, adenovirus infections in transplant recipients have been less thoroughly investigated than CMV infections.

A major risk factor for infection in transplant patients is the mechanical trauma of surgery. Liver transplant surgery is lengthy and technically complicated. In 30% to 40% of cases the gut is entered via a Roux-en-Y loop to effect biliary drainage (90,91). Both ischemia and edema of the bowel can occur during transplant surgery; in one large liver transplant series 22% of 397 patients required a laparotomy for bleeding or infection and 17% required operative repair of biliary obstruction or leak (91). The rate of post-transplant bacterial and fungal infections in liver recipients is strongly associated with the duration of surgery (8,9,92). Abdominal abscesses and peritonitis are common in liver recipients during the first 4 to 6 months after transplantation. The organisms found in such infections are typical enteric flora (*Escherichia coli,* enterococcus, bacteroides) but also coagulase negative and positive staphylococcus. *Candida* is seen in approximately one-third of cases and *Aspergillus* infection occurs occasionally.

Procedure-related intra-abdominal infections are also a problem after pancreas transplantation (93–95). These infections are usually located near the allograft, which in North American transplant centers is most often placed superior to the bladder with drainage of the pancreatic exocrine secretions through a cuff of donor duodenum into the recipient's bladder.

Intra-abdominal infections in heart, kidney, and lung transplant recipients are less common and most often relate to preexisting pathology such as diverticulosis, cholelithiasis, or peptic ulcer disease. These infections occur both early and late after transplantation.

Immunosuppressive drugs are a risk factor for infection in the postoperative period. They may also produce symptoms that are confused with enteric or intra-abdominal infection. Corticosteroids are a mainstay of transplant immunosuppression. Pharmacologic actions of corticosteroids include reduction of vascular permeability, interference with neutrophil adherence, and blockage of the release of cytokines such as interleukin-1 from macrophages and other antigen-processing cells (96,97). The use of corticosteroids has been associated with the development of ulcers and pancreatitis (98,99). With long-term use, corticosteroids may cause thinning of the wall of the bowel and increase the risk for perforation from mural infections such as diverticulitis (100–102). Corticosteroids also remarkably decrease signs and symptoms of intra-abdominal inflammation, leading to delayed diagnosis of significant infections.

Azathioprine was introduced in the early 1960s for the prevention of allograft rejection (103). It is an antimetabolite and blocks replication of lymphocytes. It may cause nausea and vomiting at high doses or during initiation of therapy. Systemic signs such as fever, rash, or diffuse myalgias sometimes accompany these gastrointestinal symptoms. In long-term use and at low doses, azathioprine is usually well tolerated.

Cyclosporine has been used in transplant patients since its introduction in the early 1980s. Cyclosporine's main action is to block the antigen-stimulated release of interleukin-2 and interferon-γ from CD4 T cells (104). Mild gastrointestinal intolerance, consisting of bloating, anorexia, and nausea, is commonly seen with the use of cyclosporine, particularly on initiation and at higher doses. These symptoms almost always disappear with continued use (105). Cyclosporine has no known apparent chronic effects on the gastrointestinal tract (106).

A variety of anti-lymphocyte antibodies are used to prevent or treat organ rejection. These include the murine monoclonal antibody OKT3 (Muromonad-CD3) directed against the CD3 molecule on T cells and a variety of polyclonal anti-thymocyte or anti-lymphocyte antibody preparations produced by animal immunization (107,108). These preparations have no direct toxicity on the gastrointestinal tract, but they have been reported to increase the rate of serious infection with CMV, EBV, and fungi (9,109,110).

The pathogenesis of enteric and intra-abdominal infections in bone marrow recipients relates to two major factors: (a) the direct toxicity of radiation and cytotoxic drugs on the gastrointestinal tract and (b) graft-versus-host disease (GVHD), which occurs in up to 70% to 80% of individuals undergoing allogeneic marrow transplantation (111–114). Radiation and cytotoxic drugs cause direct injury to replicating cells in the gastrointestinal epithelium, which often leads to frank ulceration (111,114). There is extensive depletion of gut-associated lymphoid tissue with reduced T cell action and immunoglobulin production. Anorexia, odynophagia, nausea, vomiting, and diarrhea are common findings in the first 2 to 3 weeks after bone marrow transplantation. Although focal enteric and intra-abdominal infections are not common in this 2- to 3-week interval, bacteremias and fungemias that originate from bowel flora and reach the circulation through injured mucosa cause substantial morbidity (115,116). In autologous transplantation, the return of marrow function signals a marked improvement in immune function. Fatalities from infection are uncommon, once autologous engraftment has occurred. In allogeneic transplantation, however, acute GVHD supervenes in 70% to 80% of individuals and produces a secondary immunodeficiency. The gastrointestinal manifestations of acute GVHD include watery diarrhea, anorexia, nausea, and abdominal pain (114,116,117). Histology of the bowel shows dropout of crypts and foci of epithelial cell necrosis that can be visualized as edema, erythema, and ulceration of the epithelium on endoscopic examination. These changes can occur anywhere in the gastrointestinal tract but are most prominent in the distal small bowel and proximal large bowel. Concurrent with these structural changes in the bowel is the occurrence of pathological changes to multiple components of the immune system. Depression of specific B and T cell responses to new antigens appears to reverse more slowly in patients with GVHD. Local intestinal immunity is altered by the depletion of lymphocytes in the bowel wall and a decrease in secretory immunoglobulins (118–120). The immunosuppressive drugs used to treat GVHD add to the overall burden of immunosuppression. Consequently, the risk for serious local and systemic infection is clearly greater in patients with acute GVHD. If chronic GVHD follows acute GVHD, this state of immunosuppression may persist for years (114,121).

In contrast to GVHD, host-versus-graft disease is now described as a risk factor for infection in the emerging field of small bowel transplantation (122,123). Although this discipline is in its infancy, early reports identify acute bowel rejection as an important risk factor for bacterial translocation from the gut, producing spontaneous bacteremia. During episodes of rejection, disruption of the bowel mucosa can be visualized directly with an endoscope. Early studies also suggest that bowel recipients have a high rate of CMV enteritis (124). Future studies will be necessary to delineate the role of other enteric pathogens in this unique group of patients.

EPIDEMIOLOGY

The main predisposing factors and the usual temporal sequence for infectious complications after transplantation have been elucidated (125–127). The most useful insight for clinical management is that the risk for infection varies over time with the greatest risk occurring in the early post-transplant period. Thereafter, the risk declines but still remains higher than that of the general population. For example, the risk for infection late after liver transplantation is only about one-thirtieth of the risk during the first post-transplant month (9). The variety of pathogens encountered also decreases late after transplantation. This time course differs markedly from that observed in patients with AIDS, in whom the risk for infection rises inexorably over time and the array of infecting pathogens increases. In patients made neutropenic by chemotherapy, enhanced susceptibility to infection is usually brief (4 to 6 weeks), the array of infecting pathogens relatively narrow (fungi and nosocomial bacteria), and recovery of bone marrow brings a return of normal defense mechanisms.

The nature of the infectious complications changes as time elapses after transplantation. In the first 3 to 4 weeks, infections usually result from the transplant procedure or its direct complications. In bone marrow transplantation this is the period of profound marrow suppression; in solid organ transplantation the surgical procedure, intubation, anesthesia, and line and catheter placement are the main determinants of infection. Nosocomially acquired bacteria are the common pathogens. Fungal infections can also be seen in the more complex and invasive types of transplantation. Herpes simplex infections reactivate with a short incubation period and are also seen early after transplantation.

The second interval is from 1 to 6 months after transplantation. During this interval the predominant infectious risk is from opportunistic pathogens such as CMV, EBV, adenovirus, *Pneumocystis*, *Nocardia*, *Aspergillus*, and tuberculosis. Patients who receive augmented immunosuppression because of acute rejection or treatment of GVHD are at even greater risk during this interval (114,116). In bone marrow recipients with significant chronic GVHD, the enhanced risk for opportunistic pathogens may extend well beyond the 6-month period (114,121).

Finally, in the period beyond 6 months after transplantation, there is a chronic, but definitely increased, risk of infection. Many of these are common bacterial infections such as diverticulitis, sinusitis, or pneumonia, but some opportunistic pathogens such as *Cryptococcus*, *Listeria*, and *Nocardia* also may be seen. Community-acquired enteric pathogens are most often seen during this time.

CLINICAL FEATURES

The clinical presentation of enteric and intra-abdominal infection in transplant recipients may differ from those seen in immunocompetent patients. Abdominal symptoms and particularly abdominal pain are often milder in immunosuppressed patients; this is thought to be due to the anti-inflammatory effects of corticosteroids. Because both the immunologic control of disease and the patients' perception of disease are altered, presentation of infections at a relatively advanced stage is common. For example, a high proportion of salmonella infections are bacteremic and a high percentage of diverticulitis is perforated at presentation (10–12,26).

The most common infectious causes of gastrointestinal symptoms at various times after transplantation are shown in Table 2. Disease due to HSV is seldom a problem now because it can be effectively controlled with acyclovir prophylaxis (128,129). Pyogenic intra-abdominal infections are much more common in solid organ than in bone marrow transplant recipients. Peritonitis often occurs as a complication of abdominal surgery but also may be a result of bowel perforation from underlying conditions such as ulcer disease, CMV infection, diverticulitis, lymphoproliferative disease, and ischemia.

In the interval between 1 and 6 months after transplantation, CMV is the most important pathogen. Any abdominal symptom may be caused by CMV infection. In the late post-transplant period abdominal symptoms are most often noninfectious in origin or caused by common infectious conditions such as cholangitis or diverticulitis.

Fever accompanies most but not all enteric infections. Infections that may not produce febrile illness are (a) lo-

TABLE 2. *Common infectious causes of abdominal symptoms in transplant recipients according to time after transplantation*[a]

Symptom	Time after transplantation		
	0–30 days	1–6 months	>6 months
Esophageal symptoms	HSV *Candida* Bacterial	CMV *Candida* HSV	Mostly noninfectious
Nausea and vomiting	Sepsis Cholangitis Abscess *C. difficile*	CMV *C. difficile* Sepsis Abscess	Mostly noninfectious
Diarrhea	*C. difficile*	CMV *C. difficile* Adenovirus Other enteric pathogens	Common enteric pathogens
Upper abdominal pain	Cholangitis Abscess Peritonitis Wound infection HSV	CMV Cholangitis Abscess EBV lymphoma	Cholangitis Peritonitis
Lower abdominal pain	Typhlitis *C. difficile* Diverticulitis Wound infection	CMV *C. difficile* Diverticulitis Cystitis	Diverticulitis Peritonitis Appendiciitis Cystitis

[a] Cholangitis, abscess, peritonitis, and diverticulitis are seen primarily in solid organ transplant recipients. Typhlitis is restricted to bone marrow recipients. CMV, cytomegalovirus; HSV, herpes simplex virus.

calized mucocutaneous HSV infections, (b) peritonitis or abdominal abscesses due to relatively avirulent pathogens such as *Candida,* (c) mild cases of CMV gastritis or enteritis, (d) occasional cases of *C. difficile* colitis, and (e) diseases that do not cause fever in normal hosts such as giardiasis.

DIFFERENTIAL DIAGNOSIS

Many noninfectious conditions may mimic the infections listed in Table 2. The radiation and chemotherapeutic conditioning regimens given to bone marrow recipients cause severe mucositis that produces a wide variety of different symptoms during the first 2 to 3 weeks after transplantation. Common symptoms include diarrhea, which may be profuse and occasionally bloody, nausea, vomiting, and pain on swallowing (114,116,130). Abdominal pain may be caused by the conditioning regimens in two distinct ways. During profound neutropenia, a subset of patients will develop necrotizing enterocolitis, often called "typhlitis," because the primary site of involvement is in the cecum and right colon (131). Neutropenic colitis appears to be distinct from pseudomembranous colitis related to antibiotic use (131–133). In one study it occurred in 3 of 24 autopsied bone marrow patients (6). The cause of necrotizing colitis has not been firmly established. A major factor is thought to be toxic damage to the bowel from chemotherapy (114,133). This damage permits a necrotizing infection with bowel flora (usually gram-negative organisms or fungi) that causes transmural infection in the wall of the bowel. Typical symptoms are

fever, right lower quadrant pain, and abdominal distension.

Another important cause of abdominal pain occurring early after bone marrow transplantation is veno-occlusive disease (VOD) of the liver (134). The pathogenesis of this disease is unknown. It occurs most frequently in patients who receive intense conditioning regimens and have underlying hepatic disease. In one large series, 15% of bone marrow recipients developed severe VOD and 98% of these died. Histology of the liver shows occlusion of the hepatic venules by reticulum, collagen, or cell fragments associated with necrosis of hepatocytes around the central vein (135). The clinical manifestations are right upper quadrant pain and tenderness, hepatomegaly with weight gain, and ascites. Liver function tests, particularly bilirubin, also increase. Clinically, VOD can resemble cholecystitis, cholangitis, localized peritonitis, or intra-abdominal abscess but is more common than these other conditions.

After marrow engraftment, acute GVHD becomes a major source of gastrointestinal symptoms until 3 to 4 months after transplantation. Like CMV, GVHD may cause virtually any gastrointestinal symptom. The concurrence of skin and liver disease with gastrointestinal symptoms is helpful in establishing a clinical diagnosis of GVHD but is not an absolute criterion since skin rashes may be due to drug allergy, and liver injury may be due to residual VOD, drug toxicity, preexisting disease with hepatotrophic viruses, or new infection with CMV or adenovirus. GVHD can simulate CMV disease but is also a risk factor for CMV disease. Both CMV and GVHD also typically cause fever and leukopenia, but CMV does not usually cause a skin rash or significant hyperbilirubinemia.

Other noninfectious causes of abdominal symptoms occurring in marrow recipients from 1 to 6 months after transplantation include peptic disease in the esophagus or stomach, pancreatitis, and miscellaneous drug effects causing nausea, diarrhea, or abdominal pain.

In the late post-transplant period, chronic GVHD is the most common noninfectious cause of abdominal symptoms (114). Most patients with chronic GVHD have had acute GVHD, but in 20% to 30% it begins *de novo* 3 months or more after transplantation (113,114). Gut involvement with chronic GVHD is frequently restricted to the esophagus. Typical findings are fibrous bands or strictures and mucosal desquamation. Dysphagia, pain on swallowing, and weight loss are usual clinical manifestations. Some patients develop recurrent aspiration pneumonia from esophageal dysfunction. Occasionally, chronic GVHD involves the intestines and leads to obstruction or malabsorption.

The differential diagnosis of gastrointestinal symptoms is less complex in solid organ transplant recipients because of the absence of chemotherapy-related toxicity and the rarity of GVHD. Abdominal symptoms of gastritis or esophagitis are common in the early post-transplant period and have led some clinicians to use H$_2$ blocking medications routinely. In renal recipients who received peritoneal dialysis, catheters that are left in place postoperatively may cause pain. Thrombosis at the renal artery anastomosis can produce a clinical presentation similar to an abdominal abscess with fever, abdominal pain, and sepsis. If surgical removal of the kidney is delayed, bacterial superinfection of the ischemic allograft may occur. Leaks at the ureteral anastomosis can produce abdominal discomfort and graft dysfunction and also may lead to localized infection (136).

Heart transplant recipients do not routinely undergo abdominal surgery; therefore the differential diagnosis of abdominal complications is less extensive than after liver or renal transplantation. However, high rates of gastritis and esophagitis in the early post-transplant period have been reported from some centers (137–139).

An unusual cause of persistent vomiting in heart–lung recipients is gastric atony, possibly secondary to incidental vagotomy occurring during the transplant procedure. A pyloroplasty may be necessary to relieve the obstructive symptoms (140).

Noninfectious abdominal symptoms reported in liver recipients generally involve complications of surgery such as bile peritonitis or intra-abdominal hemorrhage. Superinfection with bacteria or fungi often occurs (9,66,141). Less severe complications such as drug-related nausea or diarrhea, noninfectious gastritis, or esophagitis also occur but have been overshadowed by more morbid complications.

DIAGNOSTIC APPROACH

Persistent gastrointestinal symptoms in transplant patients should lead to a prompt search for the causative agent, especially when the symptoms are accompanied by fever or other evidence of systemic involvement. Although the approach to diagnosis of gastrointestinal infections in transplant patients resembles in many ways the approach in immunocompetent hosts, there are some variations. Vague and nonspecific complaints may be the only presentation of serious gastrointestinal infections. Physical findings on abdominal examination, even in catastrophic conditions such as ischemic colitis, often are subtle (142). In a study of 23 heart and lung transplant patients with CMV disease, vague abdominal pain, gaseous distention, loss of appetite, or loose stools were frequently the only symptoms reported (137). It is often appropriate to move quickly to an aggressive, invasive diagnostic workup. Colonoscopic biopsy is the optimal method for early diagnosis of fungal colitis. In an autopsy series of renal transplant patients with colitis due to fungal pathogens, only 50% had documented fungemia (143). Wound drainage cultures growing *Aspergillus* or other fungi should not be ignored as these may indicate invasive disease (9). Endoscopy is also the only reliable way to diagnose CMV enteritis or colitis (144). Transplant patients undergoing endoscopy to evaluate chronic diarrheal symptoms should have a duodenal aspirate for microscopic examination for *Giardia* trophozoites as these may be difficult to detect on histologic sections in transplant patients (80).

Barium contrast studies may be an insensitive detector of gastrointestinal infections and mucosal lesions in transplant patients. In a study of 159 patients who had heart transplants between 1984 and 1990, 47 (30%) required procedures to evaluate the upper gastrointestinal tract; barium studies were frequently negative despite the fact that subsequent upper endoscopy revealed pathologic lesions (145). Despite the low sensitivity of barium studies in transplant patients, some controversy surrounds the use of upper endoscopy. In one series, 9 (19%) of 47 bone marrow transplant patients undergoing upper endoscopy during the first 100 days after transplantation developed hypotension, fever, and bacteremia within 24 hr of the procedure (146). Among patients who were receiving corticosteroids, the rate of bacteremia was greater than 50%. Other investigators, however, have not corroborated this finding. In a study of 27 endoscopies in 20 heart transplant patients, all of whom were taking steroids, no complications occurred (147). Similarly, of 53 endoscopies performed in bone marrow transplant patients (including 28 in patients not receiving broad spectrum antibiotics), no instance of bacteremia or hypotension occurred (148). Thirty-nine (74%) of these patients were taking corticosteroids.

Serologic testing to diagnose infections of the gastrointestinal tract is of limited usefulness in transplant patients. Seroconversions may occur late in the course of infection and some patients such as allogeneic bone marrow transplant patients do not mount a normal antibody response for up to 1 year post-transplant (149). Allogeneic bone marrow recipients also frequently receive intravenous immunoglobulin, which may result in false-positive serologic tests for CMV and other pathogens. Some tests for fungal antigens such as those for cryptococcal and histoplasma antigen are now well established (150). *Candida* antigen tests have suffered from poor sensitivity and specificity (151). A newer test for *Candida* enolase antigen has shown promising results in initial evaluation but further confirmation is necessary (152).

MANAGEMENT

The management of enteric infections in transplant patients is similar to the management in other hosts, both normal and compromised, and general guidelines can be sought from the chapters on individual infectious agents. A few important differences merit further discussion.

Cytomegalovirus

Before ganciclovir became available, there was no effective treatment for CMV infection. Ganciclovir is highly active against CMV (153); about 90% of infected individuals will develop negative viral cultures after 7 to 10 days of treatment. Ganciclovir entered clinical practice with few controlled studies having been done. Observational studies of transplant patients with CMV infection treated with ganciclovir have shown very variable results. The worst results were seen in bone marrow recipients with pneumonia, where only 10% to 15% survived (154,155); these results improved when intravenous immunoglobulin was administered with ganciclovir (156–158). Response rates in solid organ transplant patients with CMV infection varied from 37% to 100% (159–164). A small, randomized study of ganciclovir treatment of CMV enteritis after allogeneic bone marrow transplantation failed to show a definite benefit (165). Despite these disparate results, there is now a consensus that ganciclovir therapy is often beneficial (166,167). This belief is bolstered by the results of randomized studies of prophylaxis (168–171), the demonstrated antiviral effect, and retrospective analysis that shows less progression and dissemination of CMV after therapy (172).

After successful treatment of CMV disease, transplant recipients have a relapse about 15% to 25% of the time, usually within 3 or 4 weeks. Some of these relapses are mild and do not require retreatment.

Foscarnet (trisodium phosphonoformate) is also active against CMV but has been used less often than ganciclovir in transplantation because of its substantial renal toxicity (173,174). However, foscarnet is less toxic to the bone marrow than ganciclovir. This may be a significant advantage in bone marrow recipients with poor engraftment.

Antifungal Therapy

Azole drugs such as ketoconazole, fluconazole, and itraconazole are alternatives to amphotericin B for the treatment of susceptible fungi. However, experience with these agents is not extensive in transplant populations. Ketoconazole dramatically increases cyclosporine levels by interfering with its metabolism in the liver (175). Itraco-

nazole also appears to raise cyclosporine levels (176). Fluconazole's effect on cyclosporine metabolism is uncertain but appears to be much less than the other azoles (177). The intestinal absorption of ketoconazole and itraconazole may be erratic and dependent on the presence of acid and food in the stomach (178,179). Absorption is not a problem with fluconazole (177).

Amphotericin is still the mainstay of antifungal therapy in seriously ill patients, but other agents are assuming an increasing role in management (180,181). In neutropenic patients, amphotericin treatment is always continued until resolution of the neutropenia (181,182). Patients with significant invasive or fungal disease should receive amphotericin beyond neutrophil recovery but also should complete a course of amphotericin appropriate for the pathogen being treated (183). Empiric antifungal treatment of neutropenic patients who have fever that is unresponsive to broad spectrum antibacterial therapy and undetected by routine cultures is now a widely accepted practice; it is also supported by data from randomized trials (183,184). A similar approach may be reasonable in selected high-risk situations in solid organ transplantation such as a liver recipient who has recently undergone a difficult transplant operation and who has fever unresponsive to antibacterials.

Antibacterial Therapy

For the most part the treatment of bacterial enteric and intra-abdominal infections in transplant recipients follows guidelines for normal hosts. Neutropenic patients should always be treated at least until recovery of neutrophil counts and longer or more intense course of therapy may be advisable in allogeneic bone marrow recipients with significant GVHD. The use of longer courses of therapy for salmonella infections coupled with stool cultures to test for cure is a reasonable practice given the high rate of relapse in this population (26).

PREVENTION

Prevention of enteric and intra-abdominal infections in transplant patients is a complex topic. Inactivated vaccines are considered safe but may be less effective than in normal hosts (185). Live attenuated vaccines are usually avoided despite the absence of evidence that they represent a risk to transplant recipients. An attenuated vaccine made from the Towne strain of CMV was developed in the late 1970s and studied in renal transplant recipients but provided only minor clinical benefit (186). Environmental control to prevent infections has widely been practiced in bone marrow recipients as well as other neutropenic patients. When the use of laminar flow rooms is combined with other preventative measures such as the use of cooked food and nonabsorbable antibiotics, infectious morbidity is reduced in some studies (187,188). In solid organ transplantation, there is no evidence that any infection control measure beyond simple handwashing and the use of private rooms is beneficial (189).

The most common preventive effort in transplantation involves the use of prophylactic antibiotics to prevent infection. Intravenous antibiotics are used for wound prophylaxis for only a few days in the peritransplant period and are not discussed here. Oral nonabsorbable antibiotic regimens were the first type of prophylaxis to be investigated. Most studies were performed in the 1970s in neutropenic patients. The regimens were varied but combinations of neomycin, gentamicin, polymyxin B, or vancomycin were commonly used. Nystatin was often added to prevent *Candida* infections. The controlled studies show some benefit in terms of reduction of febrile days or infectious episodes but no consistent survival advantage was demonstrated (190–192). Most bone marrow centers have abandoned the use of these regimens, because they are unpalatable and difficult to administer to patients with severe mucositis (193). The use of oral nonabsorbable antibiotics has also been promoted in liver transplant recipients. Low rates of gram-negative infection have been reported in liver recipients taking a regimen of oral gentamicin, polymyxin B, and nystatin started before transplantation and continued until 21 days after transplantation (194). However, no controlled studies of nonabsorbable antibiotics have been done in solid organ transplantation and the use of these agents is not widely accepted.

Sulfamethoxazole–trimethoprim (SMX-TMP) was the next drug to receive extensive evaluation for the prevention of infection in neutropenic patients. Most studies of oral SMX-TMP prophylaxis showed an improvement in the rate of systemic infection without a definite impact on survival (195–204). The use of SMX-TMP was not without problems. In some studies a high rate of drug resistance developed in gram-negative rods (202,205,206). A few studies also demonstrated prolonged neutropenia in patients taking SMX-TMP and this has discouraged some bone marrow units from using this form of prophylaxis while patients are neutropenic (207,208).

Prevention of gram-negative infection during neutropenia is not the only indication for SMX-TMP. It is widely used for the prevention of *Pneumocystis* infection in all types of transplantation (209). The doses required for *Pneumocystis* prophylaxis are much lower than for neutropenic prophylaxis: doses of a single-strength tablet a day or three double-strength tablets a week appear to be adequate. When used for *Pneumocystis* prevention the drug is continued at least for the high-risk period of 6 to 12 months after transplantation and many centers continue SMX-TMP for the life of the patient. SMX-TMP is also effective for the prevention of urinary infection after renal transplantation (210).

Recently, fluoroquinolone antibiotics such as ciprofloxacin and norfloxacin have been employed to prevent bacterial infections in neutropenic patients. Gram-negative infections were reduced in the studies, but no definite improvement in survival was achieved (211–216). The incidence of gram-positive infections was not reduced. These agents have been well tolerated and ciprofloxacin can be given intravenously if necessary. An increase in a peculiar type of sepsis caused by *Streptococcus viridans* has been noted in some of the quinoline studies (217,218).

Development of drug resistance has not been a major problem in the published studies of quinolone prophylaxis in neutropenic patients but has occurred in other settings.

Antifungal therapy for prophylaxis against mucocutaneous *Candida* infection is a standard part of most transplant regimens. The most common regimen employed is oral nystatin solution 500,000 units qid. This regimen appears to be efficacious in preventing oral and esophageal candidiasis in solid organ and bone marrow recipients (219,220). It is uncertain whether it has any impact on systemic candidiasis. The regimen may be difficult to administer to intubated patients and patients with severe mucositis. Clotrimazole troches appear to work as well as nystatin and may be more palatable, but some *Candida* species are not susceptible to clotrimazole. Recently, interest has increased in regimens that can provide protection for systemic as well as mucosal fungal infection. Ketoconazole has provided superior protection against fungal mucositis but was poorly absorbed in some bone marrow recipients and led to increased colonization with *Torulopsis glabrata* in one study (221,222). Two large studies in neutropenic patients have shown that prophylactic fluconazole (400 mg/day) decreased systemic and superficial candidiasis (223,224). One of these studies also demonstrated decreased mortality in the fluconazole arm (224). A third controlled study did not show a definite benefit of fluconazole prophylaxis but did demonstrate trends in favor of fluconazole (225). *Candida* species such as *C. glabrata* and *C. krusei* are often resistant to azoles. For this reason, concerns have been voiced that widespread prophylactic use of azoles will encourage the development of resistance (226). Resistance of *C. albicans* to fluconazole has been reported in patients with AIDS but is not known to be a problem in transplant populations (227). A new recently released azole antibiotic, itraconazole, has more activity against *Aspergillus* than other azoles. However, the exclusively oral formulation may militate against its prophylactic use in the patients at highest risk for *Aspergillus* (176).

There is emerging interest in the use of low-dose intravenous (iv) amphotericin (0.1 to 0.2 mg/kg/day) as parenteral prophylaxis for fungal disease in high-risk patients. One randomized study of low-dose amphotericin B prophylaxis in autologous transplantation did not show a reduction in systemic fungal infections but did result in improved survival in the amphotericin arm (228). Low-dose iv amphotericin represents an interesting approach to prophylaxis against fungal infection, but it cannot be recommended for general use until further data are available.

Antiviral Prophylaxis

Acyclovir is the most effective form of prophylaxis for prevention of HSV infection. Relatively low doses (600 to 800 mg/day orally in divided doses) are able to prevent most oral, genital, and esophageal herpes infections in transplant patients (128,129). Apart from a small additional cost, there are no disadvantages to its routine prophylaxis in HSV-seropositive patients. Acyclovir prophylaxis should also prevent the occasional cases of tissue invasion or systemic disease due to HSV.

Prophylaxis of CMV infection has not been as successful. A large number of different regimens are being used, but none is ideal. Although acyclovir has no therapeutic efficacy in CMV disease, substantial evidence exists that high doses of oral acyclovir (800 mg qid) or iv acyclovir (500 mg/M^2 q8h) reduce the overall morbidity from CMV in kidney, heart, liver, and bone marrow transplant populations (229–232). Why the drug is effective prophylactically and not therapeutically is not clear but may relate to the intracellular accumulation of drug over time. Acyclovir's protection, however, is partial and breakthrough of CMV disease is not uncommon.

Numerous studies have investigated the efficacy of commercial iv immunoglobulins in the prevention of CMV disease, but no clear consensus has been reached about their efficacy (233). The best data exit for use of CMV hyperimmunoglobulin. CMV-seronegative kidney recipients receiving grafts from seropositive donors had a 65% reduction of CMV disease if they received infusions of CMV hyperimmunoglobulin in the first 16 weeks after transplantation (233,234).

Ganciclovir is the latest drug to be investigated for use in prophylaxis against CMV disease. A number of placebo-controlled studies in bone marrow transplant patients have demonstrated significant reductions in CMV disease when ganciclovir was administered after engraftment in asymptomatic patients at risk for CMV disease because of positive cultures or seropositivity (168–170). Neutropenia, however, is an important side effect, the consequences of which must be balanced against the risk of CMV disease (168). Another well-controlled study of ganciclovir showed a reduction of CMV disease in seropositive heart recipients who received the drug during the first month after transplantation (171). Unfortunately, the group with the highest risk for severe CMV disease—seronegative patients receiving organs from seropositive donors—did not benefit. Similar results have been noted in other studies of seronegative lung and liver recipients (235,236).

In conclusion, diagnosis and management of gastrointestinal infections in transplant patients require knowledge of the unique defects induced in nonimmune and immune host defense mechanisms, the epidemiology of these infections, and broad knowledge of the clinical syndromes and effective therapies for diverse viral, bacterial, and parasitic agents.

REFERENCES

1. Cecka JM, Cho YW, Terajaki PI. Analyses of the UNOS scientific renal transplant registry at three years—early events affecting transplant success. *Transplantation* 1992;53:59–64.
2. Bortin MM, Horowitz MM, Alfred AR. Increasing utilization of allogeneic bone marrow transplantation: results of the 1988–1990 survey. *Ann Intern Med* 1992;116:505–512.
3. Kniett JM, Kaye MP. The registry of the International Society for Heart Transplantation: seventh official report—1990. *J Heart Lung Transplant* 1990;9:323–330.
4. Sternbach GL, Varon J, Hunt SA. Emergency department pre-
sentation and care of heart and heart/lung transplant recipients. *Ann Emerg Med* 1992;21:1140–1144.
5. Blakey JL, Barnes GL, Bishop RF, et al. Infectious diarrhea in children undergoing bone-marrow transplantation. *Aust N Z J Med* 1989;19:31–36.
6. Bombi JA, Cardesa A, Llebaria C, et al. Main autopsy findings in bone marrow transplant patients. *Arch Pathol Lab Med* 1987; 111:125–129.
7. Graham AR. Autopsy findings in cardiac transplant patients: a ten year experience. *J Clin Pathol* 1992;97:369–375.
8. George DL, Arnow PM, Fox AS, et al. Bacterial infection as a complication of liver transplantation: epidemiology and risk factors. *Rev Infect Dis* 1991;13:387–396.
9. Kusne S, Dummer JS, Singh N, et al. Infections after liver transplantation: an analysis of 101 consecutive cases. *Medicine (Baltimore)* 1988;67:132–143.
10. Sawyerr OI, Garvin PJ, Codd JE, et al. Colorectal complications of renal allograft transplantation. *Arch Surg* 1978;113: 84–86.
11. Penn I, Brettschneider L, Simpson K, et al. Major colonic problems in human homotransplant recipients. *Arch Surg* 1970;100: 61–65.
12. Hadjiyannakis EJ, Evans DB, Smellie WAB, et al. Gastrointestinal complications after renal transplantation. *Lancet* 1971;2: 781–785.
13. Gellin BG, Broome CV. Listeroisis. *JAMA* 1989;261: 1313–1320.
14. Tripathy SP, Mackaness GB. The effect of cytotoxic agents on the primary immune response to *Listeria monocytogenes*. *J Exp Med* 1969;130:1–16.
15. Miller JK, Hedberg M. Effects of cortisone on susceptibility of mice to *Listeria monocytogenes*. *Am J Clin Pathol* 1965;43: 248–250.
16. Hugin AW, Cerny A, Wrann M, et al. Effect of cyclosporin A on immunity to *Listeria monocytogenes*. *Infect Immun* 1986; 52:12–17.
17. Schuchat A, Deaver KA, Wenger JD, et al. Role of foods in sporadic listeriosis: case–control study of dietary risk factors. *JAMA* 1992;267:2041–2045.
18. MacGowan AP, Marshall RJ, MacKay IM, et al. *Listeria* faecal carriage by renal transplant recipients, haemodialysis patients and patients in general practice; its relation to season, drug therapy, foreign travel, animal exposure and diet. *Epidemiol Infect* 1991;106:157–166.
19. Spitzer PG, Hammer SM, Karchmer AW. Treatment of *Listeria monocytogenes* infection with trimethoprim–sulfamethoxazole: case report and review of the literature. *Rev Infect Dis* 1986;8:427–430.
20. Gerding DN, Olson MM, Peterson LR, et al. *Clostridium difficile*—associated diarrhea and colitis in adults: a prospective case-controlled epidemiologic study. *Arch Intern Med* 1986; 146:95–100.
21. Yolken RH, Bishop CA, Townsend TR, et al. Infectious gastroenteritis in bone-marrow-transplant recipients. *N Engl J Med* 1982;306:1009–1012.
22. Fekety R, Kyung-Hee K, Brown D, et al. Epidemiology of antibiotic-associated colitis: isolation of *Clostridium difficile* from the hospital environment. *Am J Med* 1981;70:906–908.
23. McFarland LV, Mulligan ME, Kwok RYY, et al. Nosocomial acquisition of *Clostridium difficile* infection. *N Engl J Med* 1989;320:204–210.
24. Rampling A, Warren RE, Berry PJ, et al. Atypical *Clostridium difficile* colitis in neutropenic patients. *Lancet* 1982;2:162–163.
25. Wust J, Sullivan NM, Hardegger U, et al. Investigation of an outbreak of antibiotic-associated colitis by various typing methods. *J Clin Microbiol* 1982;16:1096–1101.
26. Dhar JM, Al-Khader AA, Al-Sulaiman M, et al. Non-typhoid *Salmonella* in renal transplant recipients: a report of twenty cases and review of the literature. *Q J Med* 1991;287:235–250.
27. Dupuis F, Vereerstraeten P, van Geertruyden J, et al. *Salmonella typhimurium* urinary infection after kidney transplantation: report of seven cases. *Clin Nephrol* 1974;2:131–135.
28. Ocharan-Corcuera J, Montejo-Baranda M, Lampreabe-Gaztelu

I, et al. Nontyphoid *Salmonella* infections after renal transplantation. *Transplantation* 1987;44:150–151.

29. Nielsen HE, Korsager B. Bacteremia after renal transplantation. *Scand J Infect Dis* 1977;9:111–117.

30. Anderson RJ, Schafer LA, Olin DB, et al. Septicemia in renal transplant recipients. *Arch Surg* 1973;106:692–694.

31. Smith EJ, Milligan SL, Filo RS. *Salmonella* mycotic aneurysm after renal transplantation. *South Med J* 1981;11:1399–1401.

32. Severn M, Michael J. *Shigella* septicaemia following renal transplantation. *Postgrad Med J* 1980;56:852–853.

33. Gueco I, Saniel M, Mendoza M, et al. Tropical infections after renal transplantation. *Transplant Proc* 1989;21:2105–2107.

34. Neter E, Merrin G, Surgalla MJ, et al. *Shigella sonnei* bacteremia. *Urology* 1974;4:198–200.

35. Perlman DM, Ampel NM, Schifman RB, et al. Persistent *Campylobacter jejuni* infections in patients infected with human immunodeficiency virus (HIV). *Ann Intern Med* 1988;108:540–546.

36. Ahnen DJ, Brown WR. *Campylobacter* enteritis in immune-deficient patients. *Ann Intern Med* 1982;96:187–188.

37. Blaser MJ, Wells JG, Feldman RA, et al. *Campylobacter* enteritis in the United States: a multicenter study. *Ann Intern Med* 1983;98:360–365.

38. Davenport A, Shallcross TM, Crabtree JE, et al. Prevalence of *Helicobacter pylori* in patients with end-stage renal failure and renal transplant recipients. *Nephron* 1991;59:597–601.

39. Teenan RP, Burgoyne M, Brown IL, et al. *Helicobacter pylori* in renal transplant recipients. *Transplantation* 1993;56:100–103.

40. Tobin A, Hackman RC, McDonald GB. *H. pylori* infection in the immunocompromised host: a prospective study of 276 patients. *Irish J Med Sci* 1992;161 (Suppl 10):64–65.

41. Dummer S, Perez-Perez G, Breinig MK, et al. Seroepidemiology of *H. pylori* infection in heart transplant (HTTX) recipients. Presented at 33rd ICAAC, Abstract 1291. New Orleans, LA, Oct 17–20, 1993.

42. Ho M. Human cytomegalovirus infections in immunosuppressed patients. In: Ho M, ed. *Cytomegalovirus: biology and infection*. New York: Plenum Press, 1991:249–300

43. Dummer JS, White LT, Ho M, et al. Morbidity of cytomegalovirus infection in recipients of heart or heart–lung transplants who received cyclosporine. *J Infect Dis* 1985;152:1182–1191.

44. Howiler W, Goldberg HI. Gastroesophageal involvement in herpes simplex. *Gastroenterology* 1976;70:775–778.

45. Adler M, Goldman M, Liesnard C, et al. Diffuse herpes simplex virus colitis in a kidney transplant recipient successfully treated with acyclovir. *Transplantation* 1987;43:919–921.

46. Buss DH, Scharyj M. Herpesvirus infection of the esophagus and other visceral organs in adults: incidence and clinical significance. *Am J Med* 1979;66:457–462.

47. Chang AE, Young NA, Reddick RL, et al. Small bowel obstruction as a complication of disseminated varicella-zoster infection. *Surgery* 1978;83:371–374.

48. Breinig MK, Zitelli B, Starzl TE, et al. Epstein–Barr virus, cytomegalovirus, and other viral infections in children after liver transplantation. *J Infect Dis* 1987;156:273–279.

49. Hierholzer JC. Adenoviruses in the immunocompromised host. *Clin Microbiol Rev* 1992;5:262–274.

50. Wasserman R, August CS, Plotkin SA. Viral infections in pediatric bone marrow transplant patients. *Pediatr Infect Dis* 1988;7:109–115.

51. Strickler JG, Singleton TP, Copenhaver CM, et al. Adenovirus in the gastrointestinal tracts of immunosuppressed patients. *Clin Microbiol Immunol* 1992;97:555–558.

52. Michaels MG, Green M, Wald ER, et al. Adenovirus infection in pediatric liver transplant recipients. *J Infect Dis* 1992;165:170–174.

53. Salt A, Sutehall G, Sargaison M, et al. Viral and *Toxoplasma gondii* infections in children after liver transplantation. *J Clin Pathol* 1989;43:63–67.

54. Willoughby RE, Wee SB, Yolken RH. Non-group A rotavirus infection associated with severe gastroenteritis in a bone marrow transplant patient. *Pediatr Infect Dis* 1988;7:133–135.

55. Peigue-Lafeuille H, Cluzel P, Deteix P, et al. Acute rotavirus gastroenteritis in an adult renal transplant recipient. *J Infect Dis* 1988;158:1400.

56. Kruger W, Stockschlader M, Zander AR. Transmission of rotavirus diarrhea in a bone marrow transplantation unit by a hospital worker. *Bone Marrow Transplant* 1991;8:507–508.

57. Peigue-Lafeuille H, Henquell C, Chambon M, et al. Nosocomial rotavirus infections in adult renal transplant recipients. *J Hosp Infect* 1991;18:67–70.

58. Saulsbury FT, Winkelstein JA, Yolken RH. Chronic rotavirus infection in immunodeficiency. *J Pediatr* 1980;97:61–65.

59. Townsend TR, Bolyard EA, Yolken RH, et al. Outbreak of coxsackie A1 gastroenteritis: a complication of bone-marrow transplantation. *Lancet* 1982;1:820–823.

60. Mathieson R, Dutta SK. *Candida* esophagitis. *Dig Dis Sci* 1983;28:365–370.

61. Cohen R, Roth FJ, Delgado E, et al. Fungal flora of the normal human small and large intestine. *N Engl J Med* 1969;280:638–641.

62. Samonis G, Rolston K, Karl C, et al. Prophylaxis of oropharyngeal candidiasis with fluconazole. *Rev Infect Dis* 1990;12:S369–S370.

63. Joshi SN, Garvin PJ, Sunwoo YC. Candidiasis of the duodenum and jejunum. *Gastroenterology* 1981;80:829–833.

64. Tollemar J, Ericzon BG, Barkholt L, et al. Risk factors for deep *Candida* infections in liver transplant recipients. *Transplant Proc* 1990;22:1826–1827.

65. Paya CV, Hermans PE, Washington JA II, et al. Incidence, distribution, and outcome of episodes of infection in 100 orthotopic liver transplantations. *Mayo Clin Proc* 1989;64:555–564.

66. Wajszczuk CP, Dummer JS, Ho M, et al. *Transplantation* 1985;40:347–353.

67. Hau T, Van Hook EJ, Simmons RL, et al. Prognostic factors of peritoneal infections in transplant patients. *Surgery* 1978;84:403–416.

68. Young RC, Bennett JE, Vogel CL, et al. Aspergillosis: the spectrum of the disease in 98 patients. *Medicine (Baltimore)* 1970;40:147–173.

69. Kusne S, Torre-Cisneros J, Manez R, et al. Factors associated with invasive lung aspergillosis and the significance of positive *Aspergillus* culture after liver transplantation. *J Infect Dis* 1992;166:1379–1383.

70. Durand F, Bernuau J, Dupont B, et al. *Aspergillus* intraabdominal abscess after liver transplantation successfully treated with itraconazole. *Transplantation* 1992;54:734–735.

71. Wheat LJ, Smith EJ, Sathapatayavongs G, et al. Histoplasmosis in renal allograft recipients. *Arch Intern Med* 1983;143:703–787.

72. Brett MT, Kwan JTC, Bending MR. Caecal perforation in a renal transplant patient with disseminated histoplasmosis. *J Clin Pathol* 1988;41:992–995.

73. White JV, Garvey G, Hardy MA. Fatal strongyloidiasis after renal transplantation: a complication of immunosuppression. *Am Surg* 1982;48:39–41.

74. Fagundes LA, Busato O, Brentano L. Strongyloidiasis: fatal complication of renal transplantation. *Lancet* 1971;2:439–440.

75. Stone WJ, Schaffner W. *Strongyloides* infections in transplant recipients. *Semin Respir Infect* 1990;5:58–64.

76. Morgan JS, Schaffner W, Stone WJ. Opportunistic strongyloidiasis in renal transplant recipients. *Transplantation* 1986;42:518–524.

77. Schad GA. Cyclosporine may eliminate the threat of overwhelming strongyloidiasis in immunosuppressed patients. *J Infect Dis* 1986;153:178.

78. Roncoroni AJ, Gomez MA, Mera J, et al. *Cryptosporidium* infection in renal transplant patients. *J Infect Dis* 1989;160:559.

79. Martino P, Gentile G, Caprioli A, et al. Hospital-acquired cryptosporidiosis in a bone marrow transplantation unit. *J Infect Dis* 1988;158:647–648.

80. Bromiker R, Korman SH, Or R, et al. Severe giardiasis in two patients undergoing bone marrow transplantation. *Bone Marrow Transplant* 1989;4:701–703.

81. Strauss SE, Rooney JF, Sever JL, et al. Herpes simplex virus

infection: biology, treatment, and prevention. *Ann Intern Med* 1985;103:404–419.

82. Kusne S, Schwartz M, Breinig MK, et al. Herpes simplex virus hepatitis after solid organ transplantation in adults. *J Infect Dis* 1991;163:1001–1007.

83. Dummer JS, Armstrong J, Somers J, et al. Transmission of infection with herpes simplex virus by renal transplantation. *J Infect Dis* 1987;155:202–206.

84. Nalesnik MA. Lymphoproliferative disease in organ transplant recipients. *Springer Semin Immunopathol* 1991;13:199–216.

85. Hanto DW, Frizzera G, Gajl-Peczalska KJ, et al. Epstein–Barr virus, immunodeficiency, and B cell lymphoproliferation. *Transplantation* 1985;39:461–471.

86. Ho M, Jaffe R, Miller G, et al. The frequency of Epstein–Barr virus infection and associated lymphoproliferative syndrome after transplantation and its manifestations in children. *Transplantation* 1988;45:719–727.

87. Cen H, Breinig MK, Atchison RW, et al. Epstein–Barr virus transmission via the donor organs in solid organ transplantation: polymerase chain reaction and restriction fragment length polymorphism analysis of IR2, IR3, and IR4. *J Virol* 1991;65:976–980.

88. Shields AF, Hackman RC, Fife KH, et al. Adenovirus infections in patients undergoing bone-marrow transplantation. *N Engl J Med* 1985;312:529–533.

89. Webb DH, Shields AF, Fife KH. Genomic variation of adenovirus type 5 isolates recovered from bone marrow transplant recipients. *J Clin Microbiol* 1987;25:305–308.

90. Starzl TE, Demetris AJ, Van Thiel D. Liver transplantation (first of two parts). *N Engl J Med* 1989;321:1014–1022.

91. Lebeau G, Yanaga K, Marsh JW, et al. Analysis of surgical complications after 397 transplantations. *Surg Gynecol Obstet* 1990;170:317–322.

92. Colonna JO, Winston DJ, Brill JE, et al. Infectious complications in liver transplantation. *Arch Surg* 1988;123:360–364.

93. Sutherland DER, Moudry KC, Fryd DS. Results of pancreas-transplant registry. *Diabetes* 1989;38 (Suppl 1):46–54.

94. Sollinger HW, Knechtle SJ, Reen A, et al. Experience with 100 consecutive simultaneous kidney–pancreas transplants with bladder drainage. *Ann Surg* 1991;214:703–711.

95. Ozaki CF, Stratta RJ, Taylor RJ, et al. Surgical complications in solitary pancreas and combined pancreas–kidney transplantations. *Am J Surg* 1992;164:546–551.

96. Swartz SL, Dluhy RG. Corticosteroids: clinical pharmacology and therapeutic use. *Drugs* 1978;16:238–255.

97. Wahl SM, Altman LC, Rosenstreich DL. Inhibition of in vitro lymphokine synthesis by glucocorticosteroids. *J Immunol* 1975;115:476–481.

98. Dayton MT, Kleckner SC, Brown DK. Peptic ulcer perforation associated with steroid use. *Arch Surg* 1987;122:376–380.

99. Fadul CE, Lemann W, Thaler HT, et al. Perforation of the gastrointestinal tract in patients receiving steroids for neurologic disease. *Neurology* 1988;38:348–352.

100. Alexander P, Schuman E, Vetto RM. Perforation of the colon in the immunocompromised patient. *Am J Surg* 1986;151:557–561.

101. Sautter RD, Ziffren SE. Adrenocortical steroid therapy resulting in unusual gastrointestinal complications. *Arch Surg* 1959;79:346–356.

102. Arsura EL. Corticosteroid-associated perforation of colonic diverticula. *Arch Intern Med* 1990;150:1337–1338.

103. Marsh JW, Vehe KL, White HM. Immunosuppressants. *Gastroenterol Clin North Am* 1992;21:679–693.

104. Bunjes D, Hardt C, Rollinghoff M, et al. Cyclosporin A mediates immunosuppression of primary cytotoxic T cell responses by impairing the release of interleukin 1 and interleukin 2. *Eur J Immunol* 1981;11:657–661.

105. Kahan BD. Cyclosporine. *N Engl J Med* 1989;321:1725–1738.

106. Drewe J, Beglinger C, Kissel T. The absorption site of cyclosporin in the human gastrointestinal tract. *Br J Clin Pharmacol* 1992;33:39–43.

107. Menkis AH, Powell AM, Novick RJ, et al. A prospective randomized controlled trial of initial immunosuppression with ALG versus OKT3 in recipients of cardiac allografts. *J Heart Lung Transplant* 1992;11:569–576.

108. Weir MR, Henry ML, Blackmore M, et al. Incidence and morbidity of cytomegalovirus disease associated with a seronegative recipient receiving seropositive donor-specific transfusion and living-related donor transplantation. *Transplantation* 1988;45:111–116.

109. Singh N, Dummer JS, Kusne S, et al. Infections with cytomegalovirus and other herpesviruses in 121 liver transplant recipients: transmission by donated organ and the effect of OKT3 antibodies. *J Infect Dis* 1988;158:124–131.

110. Swinnen LJ, Costanzo-Nordin MR, Fisher SG, et al. Increased incidence of lymphoproliferative disorder after immunosuppression with the monoclonal antibody OKT3 in cardiac-transplant recipients. *N Engl J Med* 1990;323:1723–1728.

111. Mitchell EP, Schein PS. Gastrointestinal toxicity of chemotherapeutic agents. *Semin Oncol* 1982;9:52–64.

112. Thomas ED, Storb R, Clift RA, et al. Bone-marrow transplantation (second of two parts). *N Engl J Med* 1975;292:895–902.

113. Ferrara JLM, Deeg HJ. Graft-versus-host disease. *N Engl J Med* 1991;324:667–673.

114. McDonald GB, Shulman HM, Sullivan KM, et al. Intestinal and hepatic complications of human bone marrow transplantation. *Gastroenterology* 1986;90:460–484.

115. Winston DJ, Ho WG, Champlin RE, et al. Infectious complications of bone marrow transplantation. *Exp Hematol* 1984;12:205–215.

116. Tutschka PJ. Infections and immunodeficiency in bone marrow transplantation. *Pediatr Infect Dis* 1988;7:S22–S29.

117. Jones B, Kramer SS, Saral R, et al. Gastrointestinal inflammation after bone marrow transplantation: graft-versus-host disease or opportunistic infection? *AJR Am J Roentgenol* 1988;150:277–281.

118. Tsoi MS, Storb R, Dobbs S, et al. Nonspecific suppressor cells in patients with chronic graft-vs-host disease after marrow grafting. *J Immunol* 1979;123:1970–1976.

119. Slavin RE, Santos GW. The graft versus host reaction in man after bone marrow transplantation: pathology, pathogenesis, clinical features, and implication. *Clin Immunol Immunopathol* 1973;1:472–498.

120. Beschorner WE, Yardley JH, Tutschka PJ, et al. Deficiency of intestinal immunity with graft-vs.-host disease in humans. *J Infect Dis* 1981;144:38–46.

121. Witherspoon RP, Storb R, Ochs HD, et al. Recovery of antibody production in human allogeneic marrow graft recipients: influence of time posttransplantation, the presence or absence of chronic graft-versus-host disease, and antithymocyte globulin treatment. *Blood* 1981;58:360–368.

122. Todo S, Tzakis AG, Abu-Elmagd K, et al. Cadaveric small bowel and small bowel–liver transplantation in humans. *Transplantation* 1992;53:369–376.

123. Grant D, Hurlbut D, Zhong R, et al. Intestinal permeability and bacterial translocation following small bowel transplantation in the rat. *Transplantation* 1991;52:221–224.

124. Kusne S, Manez R, Abu-Elmagd K, et al. Value of CMV DNA detection by polymerase chain reaction (PCR) in early diagnosis of CMV disease in small bowel allograft samples. Presented at the 12th Annual American Society of Transplant Physicians Meeting, Abstract P-1-46, Houston, TX, May 17–19, 1993.

125. Meyers JD. Infections in marrow transplant patients. In: Mandell GL, Douglas RG, Bennett JE, eds. *Principles and practice of infectious diseases*. New York: Churchill Livingstone, 1990;2291–2294.

126. Rubin RH. Infection in the renal and liver transplant patient. In: Rubin RH, Young LS, eds. *Clinical approach to infection in the compromised*. New York: Plenum Press, 1988;557–621.

127. Ho M, Dummer JS, Peterson PK, et al. Infections in solid organ transplant patients. In: Mandell GL, Douglas RG, Bennett JE, eds. *Principles and practice of infectious diseases*. New York: Churchill Livingstone, 1990;2294–2303.

128. Wade JC, Newton B, Flournoy N, et al. Oral acyclovir for prevention of herpes simplex virus reactivation after marrow transplantation. *Ann Intern Med* 1984;100:823–828.

129. Gluckman E, Lotsberg J, Devergie A, et al. Prophylaxis of

herpes infections after bone-marrow transplantation by oral acyclovir. *Lancet* 1983;2:706–708.

130. Jones B, Wall SD. Gastrointestinal disease in the immunocompromised host. *Radiol Clin North Am* 1992;30:555–577.

131. Dworkin B, Winawer SJ, Lightdale CJ. Typhlitis: report of a case with long-term survival and a review of the recent literature. *Dig Dis Sci* 1981;26:1032–1037.

132. Freeman HJ, Rabeneck L, Owen D. Survival after necrotizing enterocolitis of leukemia treated with oral vancomycin. *Gastroenterology* 1981;81:791–794.

133. Dosik GM, Luna M, Valdivieso M, et al. Necrotizing colitis in patients with cancer. *Am J Med* 1979;67:646–656.

134. McDonald GB, Hinds MS, Fisher LD, et al. Veno-occlusive disease of the liver and multiorgan failure after bone marrow transplantation: a cohort study of 355 patients. *Ann Intern Med* 1993;118:255–267.

135. Shulman HM, McDonald GB, Matthews D, et al. An analysis of hepatic venoocclusive disease and centrilobular hepatic degeneration following bone marrow transplantation. *Gastroenterology* 1980;79:1178–1191.

136. Fine RN, Terasaki PI, Ettenger RB, et al. Renal transplantation update. *Ann Intern Med* 1984;100:246–257.

137. Welch RW, Yokoyama Y, Cooper DKC, et al. The gastrointestinal management of patients undergoing heart transplantation. *J Okla State Med Assoc* 1991;84:557–562.

138. Villar HV, Neal DD, Levinson M, et al. Gastrointestinal complications after human transplantation and mechanical heart replacement. *Am J Surg* 1989;157:168–174.

139. Cates J, Chavez M, Laks H, et al. Gastrointestinal complications after cardiac transplantation: a spectrum of diseases. *Am J Gastroenterol* 1991;86:412–416.

140. Maurer JR. Therapeutic challenges following lung transplantation. *Clin Chest Med* 1990;11:279–290.

141. Castaldo P, Stratta RJ, Wood RP, et al. Clinical spectrum of fungal infections after orthotopic liver transplantation. *Arch Surg* 1991;126:149–156.

142. Flanigan RC, Reckard CR, Lucas BA. Colonic complications of renal transplantation. *J Urol* 1988;139:503–506.

143. Stylianos S, Forde KA, Benvenisty AI, et al. Low gastrointestinal hemorrhage in renal transplant recipients. *Arch Surg* 1988;123:739–744.

144. Lepinski SM, Hamilton JW. Isolated cytomegalovirus ileitis detected by colonoscopy. *Gastroenterology* 1990;98:1704–1706.

145. Steck TB, Durkin MG, Costanzo-Nordin MR, et al. Gastrointestinal complications and endoscopic findings in heart transplant patients. *J Heart Lung Transplant* 1993;12:244–251.

146. Bianco JA, Pepe MS, Higano C, et al. Prevalence of clinically relevant bacteremia after upper gastrointestinal endoscopy in bone marrow transplant recipients. *Am J Med* 1990;89:134–136.

147. Johnson R, Peitzman AB, Webster MW, et al. Upper gastrointestinal endoscopy after cardiac transplantation. *Surgery* 1988;103:300–304.

148. Kaw M, Przepiorka D, Sekas G. Infectious complications of endoscopic procedures in bone marrow transplant recipients. *Dig Dis Sci* 1993;38:71–74.

149. Lum LG. The kinetics of immune reconstitution after human marrow transplantation. *Blood* 1987;69:369–380.

150. Wheat LJ, Kohler RB, Tewari RP. Diagnosis of disseminated histoplasmosis by detection of *Histoplasma capsulatum* antigen in serum and urine specimens. *N Engl J Med* 1986;314:83–88.

151. Bennett JE. Rapid diagnosis of candidiasis and aspergillosis. *Rev Infect Dis* 1987;9:398–402.

152. Walsh TJ, Hathorn JW, Sobel JD, et al. Detection of circulating *Candida* enolase by immunoassay in patients with cancer and invasive candidiasis. *N Engl J Med* 1991;324:1026–1031.

153. Buhles WC Jr, Mastre BJ, Tinker AJ, et al. Ganciclovir treatment of life- or sight-threatening cytomegalovirus infection: experience in 314 immunocompromised patients. *Rev Infect Dis* 1988;10 (Suppl 3):S495–S506.

154. Reed EC, Dandliker PS, Meyers JD. Treatment of cytomegalovirus pneumonia with 9-[2-hydroxy-*I*-(hydroxymethyl)ethoxy-methyl]guanine and high-dose corticosteroids. *Ann Intern Med* 1986;105:214–215.

155. Shepp DH, Dandliker PS, de Miranda P, et al. Activity of 9-[2-hydroxy-*I*-(hydroxymethyl)ethoxymethyl]guanine in the treatment of cytomegalovirus pneumonia. *Ann Intern Med* 1985;103:368–373.

156. Reed EC, Bowden RA, Dandliker PS, et al. Treatment of cytomegalovirus pneumonia with ganciclovir and intravenous cytomegalovirus immunoglobulin in patients with bone marrow transplants. *Ann Intern Med* 1988;109:783–788.

157. Emanuel D, Cunningham I, Jules-Elysee K, et al. Cytomegalovirus pneumonia after bone marrow transplantation successfully treated with the combination of ganciclovir and high-dose intravenous immune globulin. *Ann Intern Med* 1988;109:777–782.

158. Schmidt GM, Kovacs A, Zaia JA, et al. Ganciclovir/immunoglobulin combination therapy for the treatment of human cytomegalovirus-associated interstitial pneumonia in bone marrow allograft recipients. *Transplantation* 1988;46:905–907.

159. Keay S, Petersen E, Icenogle T, et al. Ganciclovir treatment of serious cytomegalovirus infection in heart and heart–lung transplant recipients. *Rev Infect Dis* 1988;10(Suppl 3):S563–S572.

160. Paya CV, Hermans PE, Smith TF, et al. Efficacy of ganciclovir in liver and kidney transplant recipients with severe cytomegalovirus infection. *Transplantation* 1988;46:229–234.

161. Hrebinko R, Jordan ML, Dummer JS, et al. Ganciclovir for invasive cytomegalovirus infection in renal allograft recipients. *Transplant Proc* 1991;23:1346–1347.

162. Dunn DL, Mayoral JL, Gillingham KJ, et al. Treatment of invasive cytomegalovirus disease in solid organ transplant patients with ganciclovir. *Transplantation* 1991;51:98–106.

163. Snydman DR. Ganciclovir therapy for cytomegalovirus disease associated with renal transplants. *Rev Infect Dis* 1988;10 (Suppl 3):S554–S562.

164. Harbison MA, De Girolami PC, Jenkins RL, et al. Ganciclovir therapy of severe cytomegalovirus infections in solid-organ transplant recipients. *Transplantation* 1988;46:82–88.

165. Reed EC, Wolford JL, Kopecky KJ, et al. Ganciclovir for the treatment of cytomegalovirus gastroenteritis in bone marrow transplant patients: a randomized, placebo-controlled trial. *Ann Intern Med* 1990;112:505–510.

166. Erice A, Jordan MC, Chace BA, et al. Ganciclovir treatment of cytomegalovirus disease in transplant recipients and other immunocompromised hosts. *JAMA* 1987;257:3082–3087.

167. Paul S, Dummer JS. Topics in clinical pharmacology: ganciclovir. *Am J Med Sci* 1992;304:272–277.

168. Goodrich JM, Mori M, Gleaves CA, et al. Early treatment with ganciclovir to prevent cytomegalovirus disease after allogeneic bone marrow transplantation. *N Engl J Med* 1991;325:1601–1607.

169. Schmidt GM, Horak DA, Niland JC, et al. A randomized, controlled trial of prophylactic ganciclovir for cytomegalovirus pulmonary infection in recipients of allogeneic bone marrow transplants. *N Engl J Med* 1991;324:1005–1011.

170. Winston DJ, Ho WG, Bartoni K, et al. Ganciclovir prophylaxis of cytomegalovirus infection and disease in allogeneic bone marrow transplant recipients: results of a placebo-controlled, double-blind trial. *Ann Intern Med* 1993;118:179–184.

171. Merigan TC, Renlund DG, Keay S, et al. A controlled trial of ganciclovir to prevent cytomegalovirus disease after heart transplantation. *N Engl J Med* 1992;326:1182–1186.

172. Fletcher CV, Balfour HH Jr. Evaluation of ganciclovir for cytomegalovirus disease. *DICP* 1989;23:5–11.

173. Ringden O, Lonngvist B, Paulin T, et al. Pharmacokinetics, safety and preliminary clinical experiences using foscarnet in the treatment of cytomegalovirus infections in bone marrow and renal transplant recipients. *J Antimicrob Chemother* 1986;17:373–387.

174. Chrisp P, Clissold SP. Foscarnet: a review of its antiviral activity, pharmacokinetic properties and therapeutic use in immunocompromised patients with cytomegalovirus retinitis. *Drugs* 1991;41:104–129.

175. First MR, Schroeder TJ, Michael A, et al. Cyclosporine–keto-

conazole interaction: long-term follow-up and preliminary results of a randomized trial. *Transplantation* 1993;55:1000–1004.
176. Kramer MR, Marshall SE, Denning DW, et al. Cyclosporine and itraconazole interaction in heart and lung transplant recipients. *Ann Intern Med* 1990;113:327–329.
177. Grant SM, Clissold SP. Fluconazole: a review of its pharmacodynamic and pharmacokinetic properties, and therapeutic potential in superficial and systemic mycoses. *Drugs* 1990;39:877–916.
178. Brass C, Glagiani JN, Blaschke TF, et al. Disposition of ketoconazole, an oral antifungal, in humans. *Antimicrob Agents Chemother* 1982;21:151–158.
179. Grant SM, Clissold SP. Itraconazole: a review of its pharmacodynamic and pharmacokinetic properties, and therapeutic use in superficial and systemic mycoses. *Drugs* 1989;37:310–344.
180. Pizzo PA. Management of fever in patients with cancer and treatment-induced neutropenia. *N Engl J Med* 1993;328:1323–1332.
181. Meyer RD. Current role of therapy with amphotericin B. *Clin Infect Dis* 1992;14 (Suppl 1):S154–S160.
182. Walsh TJ, Lee J, Lecciones J, et al. Empiric therapy with amphotericin B in febrile granulocytopenic patients. *Rev Infect Dis* 1991;13:496–503.
183. EORTC International Antimicrobial Therapy Cooperative Group. Empiric antifungal therapy in febrile granulocytopenic patients. *Am J Med* 1989;86:668–672.
184. Pizzo PA, Robichaud RJ, Gill FA, et al. Empiric antibiotic and antifungal therapy for cancer patients with prolonged fever and granulocytopenia. *Am J Med* 1982;72:101–111.
185. Huang K, Armstrong JA, Ho M. Antibody response after influenza immunization in renal transplant patients receiving cyclosporine A or azathioprine. *Infect Immun* 1983;40:421–424.
186. Plotkin SA, Smiley ML, Friedman HM, et al. Towne-vaccine-induced prevention of cytomegalovirus disease after renal transplants. *Lancet* 1984;1:528–530.
187. Levine AS, Siegel SE, Schreiber AD, et al. Protected environments and prophylactic antibiotics: a prospective controlled study of their utility in the therapy of acute leukemia. *N Engl J Med* 1973;288:477–483.
188. Rodriguez V, Bodey GP, Freireich EJ, et al. Randomized trial of protected environment–prophylactic antibiotics in 145 adults with acute leukemia. *Medicine* (Baltimore) 1978;57:253–266.
189. Walsh TR, Guttenderf J, Dummer JS, et al. The value of isolation procedures in cardiac allograft recipients. *Ann Thorac Surg* 1989;47:1–5.
190. Storring RA, Jameson B, McElwain TJ, et al. Oral non-absorbed antibiotics prevent infection in acute non-lymphoblastic leukaemia. *Lancet* 1977;2:837–840.
191. Schimpff SC, Greene WH, Young VM, et al. Infection prevention in acute nonlymphocytic leukemia: laminar air flow room reverse isolation with oral, nonabsorbable antibiotic prophylaxis. *Ann Intern Med* 1975;82:351–358.
192. Dankert J, Gaus W, Gaya H, et al. Protective isolation and antimicrobial decontamination in patients with high susceptibility to infection: a prospective cooperative study of gnotobiotic care in acute leukaemia patients III: the quality of isolation and decontamination. *Infection* 1978;6:175–191.
193. Young LS. Antimicrobial prophylaxis against infection in neutropenic patients. *J Infect Dis* 1983;147:611–614.
194. Wiesner RH. The incidence of gram-negative bacterial and fungal infections in liver transplant patients treated with selective decontamination. *Infection* 1990;18(Suppl 1):S19–S21.
195. Starke ID, Donnelly P, Catovsky D, et al. Co-trimoxazole alone for prevention of bacterial infection in patients with acute leukaemia. *Lancet* 1982;1:5–6.
196. Enno A, Catovsky D, Darrell J, et al. Co-trimoxazole for prevention of infection in acute leukaemia. *Lancet* 1978;2:395–397.
197. Watson JG, Jameson B, Powles RL, et al. Co-trimoxazole versus non-absorbable antibiotics in acute leukaemia. *Lancet* 1982;1:6–9.
198. Wade JC, Schimpff SC, Hargadon MT, et al. A comparison of trimethoprim–sulfamethoxazole plus nystatin with gentamicin plus nystatin in the prevention of infections in acute leukemia. *N Engl J Med* 1981;304:1057–1062.
199. Gurwith MJ, Brunton JL, Lank BA, et al. A prospective controlled investigation of prophylactic trimethoprim/sulfamethoxazole in hospitalized granulocytopenic patients. *Am J Med* 1979;66:248–256.
200. Riben PD, Louie TJ, Lank BA, et al. Reduction in mortality from gram-negative sepsis in neutropenic patients receiving trimethoprim/sulfamethoxazole therapy. *Cancer* 1983;51:1587–1592.
201. Kramer BS, Carr DJ, Rand KH, et al. Prophylaxis of fever and infection in adult cancer patients: a placebo-controlled trial of oral trimethoprim–sulfamethoxazole plus erythromycin. *Cancer* 1984;53:329–335.
202. Gualtieri RJ, Donowitz GR, Kaiser DL, et al. Double-blind randomized study of prophylactic trimethoprim/sulfamethoxazole in granulocytopenic patients with hematologic malignancies. *Am J Med* 1983;74:934–940.
203. Weiser B, Lange M, Fialk MA, et al. Prophylactic trimethoprim–sulfamethoxazole during consolidation chemotherapy for acute leukemia: a controlled trial. *Ann Intern Med* 1981;95:436–438.
204. Pizzo PA, Robichaud KJ, Edwards BK, et al. Oral antibiotic prophylaxis in patients with cancer: a double-blind randomized placebo-controlled trial. *J Pediatr* 1983;102:125–133.
205. Goorin AM, Hershey BJ, Levin MJ, et al. Use of trimethoprim–sulfamethoxazole to prevent bacterial infections in children with acute lymphoblastic leukemia. *Pediatr Infect Dis* 1985;4:265–269.
206. Wilson JM, Guiney DG. Failure of oral trimethoprim–sulfamethoxazole prophylaxis in acute leukemia. *N Engl J Med* 1982;306:16–20.
207. Wade JC, de Jongh CA, Newman KA, et al. Selective antimicrobial modulation as prophylaxis against infection during granulocytopenia: trimethoprim–sulfamethoxazole vs. nalidixic acid. *J Infect Dis* 1983;147:624–634.
208. Dekker AW, Rozenberg-Arska M, Sixma JJ, et al. Prevention of infection by trimethoprim–sulfamethoxazole plus amphotericin B in patients with acute nonlymphocytic leukaemia. *Ann Intern Med* 1981;95:555–559.
209. Dummer JS. *Pneumocystis carinii* infections in transplant recipients. *Semin Respir Infect* 1990;5:50–57.
210. Fox BC, Sollinger HW, Belzer FO, et al. A prospective, randomized, double-blind study of trimethoprim–sulfamethoxazole for prophylaxis of infection in renal transplantation: clinical efficacy, absorption of trimethoprim–sulfamethoxazole, effects on the microflora, and the cost–benefit ratio. *Am J Med* 1990;89:255–274.
211. Karp JE, Merz WG, Hendricksen C, et al. Oral norfloxacin for prevention of gram-negative bacterial infections in patients with acute leukemia and granulocytopenia: a randomized, double-blind, placebo-controlled trial. *Ann Intern Med* 1987;106:1–6.
212. Karp JE, Dick JD, Merz WG. Systemic infection and colonization with and without prophylactic norfloxacin use over time in the granulocytopenic, acute leukemia patient. *Br J Cancer Clin Oncol* 1988;24(Suppl 1):S5–S13.
213. The Gimema Infection Program. Prevention of bacterial infection in neutropenic patients with hematologic malignancies: a randomized, multicenter trial comparing norfloxacin with ciprofloxacin. *Ann Intern Med* 1991;115:7–12.
214. Winston DJ, Ho WG, Nakao SL, et al. Norfloxacin versus vancomycin/polymyxin for prevention of infections in granulocytopenic patients. *Am J Med* 1986;80:884–890.
215. Dekker AW, Rozenberg-Arska M, Verhoef J. Infection prophylaxis in acute leukemia: a comparison of ciprofloxacin with trimethoprim–sulfamethoxazole and colistin. *Ann Intern Med* 1987;106:7–12.
216. Rozenberg-Arska M, Dekker AW, Verhoef J. Ciprofloxacin for selective decontamination of the alimentary tract in patients with acute leukemia during remission induction treatment: the effect on fecal flora. *J Infect Dis* 1985;152:104–107.
217. De Pauw BE, Donnelly JP, De Witte T, et al. Options and limitations of long-term oral ciprofloxacin as antibacterial pro-

phylaxis in allogeneic bone marrow transplant recipients. *Bone Marrow Transplant* 1990;5:179–182.

218. Elting LS, Bodey GP, Keefe BH. Septicemia and shock syndrome due to viridans streptococci: a case–control study of predisposing factors. *Clin Infect Dis* 1992;14:1201–1207.

219. Frick T, Fryd DS, Goodale RL, et al. Incidence and treatment of *Candida* esophagitis in patients undergoing renal transplantation: data from the Minnesota prospective randomized trial of cyclosporine versus antilymphocyte globulin–azathioprine. *Am J Surg* 1988;155:311–313.

220. Gombert ME, duBrucket L, Aulicino TM, et al. A comparative trial of clotrimazole troches and oral nystatin suspension in recipients of renal transplants. *JAMA* 1987;258:2553–2555.

221. Hann IM, Prentice HG, Corringham R, et al. Ketoconazole versus nystatin plus amphotericin B for fungal prophylaxis in severely immunocompromised patients. *Lancet* 1982;1: 826–829.

222. Shepp DH, Klosterman A, Siegel MS, et al. Comparative trial of ketoconazole and nystatin for prevention of fungal infection in neutropenic patients treated in a protective environment. *J Infect Dis* 1985;152:1257–1263.

223. Goodman JL, Winston DJ, Greenfield RA, et al. A controlled trial of fluconazole to prevent fungal infections in patients undergoing bone marrow transplantation. *N Engl J Med* 1992; 326:845–851.

224. Slavin M, Bowden R, Osborne B, et al. Fluconazole prophylaxis in marrow transplant recipients: a randomized placebo controlled double blind study. Presented at the 32nd International Conference on Antimicrobial Agents and Chemotherapy, Abstract 623, Anaheim, CA, Oct 11–14, 1992.

225. Winston DJ, Chandrasekar PH, Lazarus HM, et al. Fluconazole prophylaxis of fungal infections in patients with acute leukemia: results of a randomized placebo-controlled, double-blind, multicenter trial. *Ann Intern Med* 1993;118:495–503.

226. Wingard JR, Merz WG, Rinaldi MG, et al. Increase in *Candida krusei* infections among patients with bone marrow transplantation and neutropenia treated prophylactically with fluconazole. *N Engl J Med* 1991;325:1274–1277.

227. Troillet M, Durussel C, Bille J, et al. Fluconazole-resistant oral clindidiasis in HIV infected patients: in vitro–in vivo correlation. Presented at the 32nd International Conference on Antimicrobial Agents and Chemotherapy, Abstract 1202, Anaheim, CA, Oct 11–14, 1992.

228. Perfect JR, Klotman ME, Gilbert CC, et al. Prophylactic intravenous amphotericin B in neutropenic autologous bone marrow transplant recipients. *J Infect Dis* 1992;165:891–897.

229. Meyers JD, Reed EC, Shepp DH, et al. Acyclovir for prevention of cytomegalovirus infection and disease after allogeneic marrow transplantation. *N Engl J Med* 1988;318:70–75.

230. Balfour HH Jr, Chace BA, Stapleton JT, et al. A randomized, placebo-controlled trial of oral acyclovir for the prevention of cytomegalovirus disease in recipients of renal allografts. *N Engl J Med* 1989;320:1381–1384.

231. Mollison LC, Richards MJ, Johnson PDR, et al. High-dose oral acyclovir reduces the incidence of cytomegalovirus infection in liver transplant recipients. *J Infect Dis* 1993;168:721–724.

232. Elkins CC, Frist WH, Dummer JS, et al. Cytomegalovirus disease after heart transplantation: is acyclovir prophylaxis indicated? *Ann Thorac Surg* 1993;56:1267–1272.

233. Rubin RH, Tolkoff-Rubin NE. Antimicrobial strategies in the care of organ transplant recipients. *Antimicrob Agents Chemother* 1993;37:619–624.

234. Snydman DR, Werner BG, Heinze-Lacey B, et al. Use of cytomegalovirus immune globulin to prevent cytomegalovirus disease in renal transplant recipients. *N Engl J Med* 1987;317: 1049–1054.

235. Bailey TC, Trulock EP, Ettinger NA, et al. Failure of prophylactic ganciclovir to prevent cytomegalovirus disease in recipients of lung transplants. *J Infect Dis* 1992;165:548–552.

236. Martin M. Cytomegalovirus prophylaxis in solid organ transplantation. *Transplant Sci* 1992;2:83.

Infections of the Gastrointestinal Tract,
edited by M. J. Blaser, P. D. Smith, J. I. Ravdin,
H. B. Greenberg, and R. L. Guerrant
Raven Press, Ltd., New York © 1995.

CHAPTER 38

Gastrointestinal Infections in Neutropenic Patients

Kent A. Sepkowitz and Donald Armstrong

The gastrointestinal tract is the most common source of systemic infection in the neutropenic patient. The majority of documented bacteremias are due to bowel flora that enter the bloodstream in the setting of chemotherapy-induced neutropenia and thrombocytopenia. In addition, the neutropenic patient may develop fever and/or localized infection in several gastrointestinal sites, including the mouth, esophagus, intestine, cecum, and perianal area. This chapter reviews the clinical syndromes seen with infections of the gastrointestinal tract in the neutropenic patient. We consider an approach to the patient with neutropenia and abdominal pain and finally address the controversy surrounding gut decontamination for prevention of bacteremia in the patient receiving myelosuppressive chemotherapy.

MOUTH

Overview

Up to 40% of the one million new cancer patients diagnosed annually will develop oral complications that may be acute or chronic in nature (1). As the potency of treatment modalities intensifies, so too do the likelihood and the severity of oral complications. Periodontal or mucosal infection may be limited locally or serve as a site of entry into the bloodstream for viruses, bacteria, or fungi.

Pathogenesis

Several factors contribute to the high rate of oral complications. First, the normal flora of the mouth routinely

D. Armstrong and K. A. Sepkowitz: Infectious Disease Service, Memorial Sloan-Kettering Cancer Center, and Department of Medicine, Cornell University Medical College, New York, New York 10021.

enter the bloodstream with simple everyday acts such as chewing. Second, the likelihood of a significant inoculum of bacteria is greatly enhanced by local chemotherapy or radiation therapy-induced inflammation of the rapidly dividing mucosa. Many chemotherapeutic agents, including methotrexate, 5-fluorouracil, doxorubicin, and bleomycin, may cause mucositis. Third, control of the local infection is severely compromised by neutropenia, exemplified by the occurrence of symptoms in patients with cyclic neutropenia (2). Finally, the vast majority of the adult population has subclinical periodontal disease (3), which, in the setting of neutropenia, may flare and cause either local disease or bacteremia.

Several studies have defined attack rates by underlying cancer for development of oral complications. At M. D. Anderson, Dreizen et al. (4) found that 47% of 1500 leukemia patients had oral complications, including infection in 34%. A review at the same institution of patients with solid tumors found that oral infections occurred in 9.7% of 1000 patients (5), ranging from 8% among carcinoma patients to 18% among those with lymphoma. Peterson et al. (3) found that 24 (4.5%) of 534 patients with cancer were admitted with acute periodontal problems, including gingivitis and periodontitis. Most had an absolute neutrophil count less than 500. Sonis et al. (6) found that 39% of cancer patients admitted to several hospitals in Boston had oral complications.

Presentation

Patients with periodontal infection or mucositis (stomatitis) generally complain of pain on swallowing, talking, or chewing. Symptoms from other concurrent medical problems, such as pneumonia, may make mouth discomfort of secondary importance to the patient, or the oral discomfort may predominate and obscure other, more potentially life-threatening problems. Inability to eat or swallow may sufficiently compromise nutrition and hydration such that parenteral feedings are required.

The pathogens recovered locally include fungi, bacteria, and/or viruses. Attempts to define precisely which organism might be causing local oral infection are confounded by the presence of normal oral flora that overgrow many cultures. In most series, fungi, particularly *Candida albicans* (in the presence or absence of thrush), predominate. Among solid tumor patients, 67% of all oral infections were due to *C. albicans,* versus about 50% of all infections among leukemics (5). In all series, commonly recovered bacteria include *Pseudomonas aeruginosa, Klebsiella* species, and *Escherichia coli* (4). Gram-positive cocci were seen in 4% of leukemics (4). Streptococcal species are common in some series (7,8). Anaerobes also have been recovered (3).

Pseudomonas aeruginosa infection of the mouth may cause a specific clinical syndrome (5). *Pseudomonas aeruginosa* is angiophilic and may invade gingival blood vessels, causing ischemia and necrosis of local tissue. Bacteremia may ensue. If the infection is controlled with antibiotics and the neutropenia resolves, the necrotic core of tissue will slough and normal granulation will begin (5). If the infection is not well controlled locally, it may spread rapidly to involve face, neck, and mediastinum, with potentially catastrophic consequences (Fig. 1).

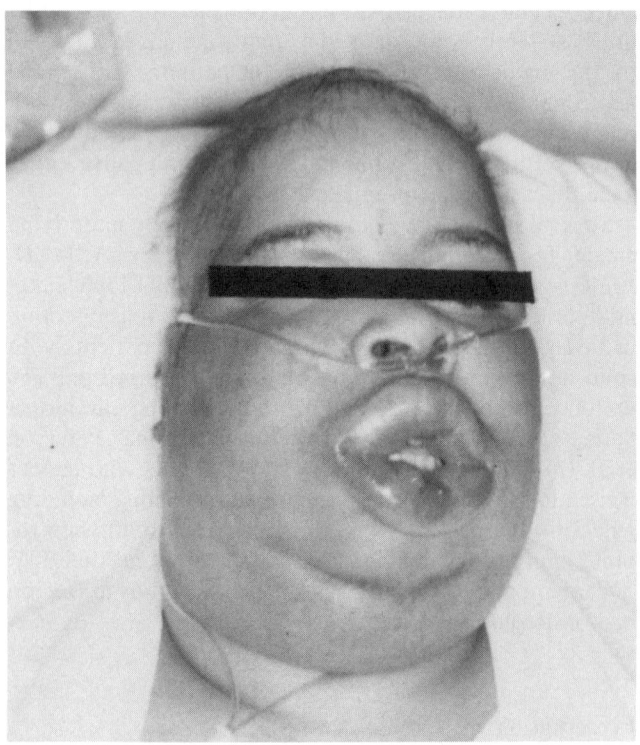

FIG. 1. Diffuse facial cellulitis due to *Pseudomonas aeroginosa* in a 22-year-old woman with aplastic anemia. Infection was introduced when patient pricked her gum with the tine of a fork while eating. The infection continued to spread despite antibiotics, and the patient died.

Herpes simplex is seen in about 10% of all patients with oral infection (4,5). Oral herpes simplex virus infection disrupts the integrity of the oral mucosa, thereby enhancing the opportunity for local bacterial flora to cause invasive and/or systemic disease. Identification and treatment of all oral herpes simplex infections are therefore crucial to control of bacterial infections in the neutropenic cancer patient.

Treatment

Empiric antibiotic therapy directed at the usual bacteria anticipated in the febrile neutropenic patient, such as ticarcillin–clavulanic acid with an aminoglycoside, is adequate to cover empirically the organisms likely to cause periodontal disease in many hospitals. The empiric therapy should be determined by the knowledge of the susceptibility patterns at each specific hospital. When an organism is recovered, treatment should be selected according to known susceptibilities. In patients with severe disease without a specific recovered organism and no response to standard antibiotics, metronidazole (500 mg q6–8h iv) may be added. Resistance of anaerobes is increasing, limiting the usefulness of metronidazole as an empiric agent for oral infection. In addition, control of pain with aggressive local care or systemically with narcotic analgesia is essential to allow the patient to eat, swallow, and speak.

ESOPHAGUS

Overview

Appreciation of the spectrum of infectious esophageal disease has increased in the wake of the acquired immunodeficiency syndrome (AIDS) epidemic. In cancer patients, esophageal infection due to fungal, bacterial, or viral pathogens can also be expected. Prompt institution of effective therapy is necessary to limit morbidity and prevent dissemination of an initially local infection.

In addition, the presence of esophagitis, specifically due to *C. albicans,* may be the presenting sign of underlying malignancy. In two prospective endoscopic series totaling over 3500 patients, an underlying cancer was found in 20 of 80 persons with *Candida* esophagitis (9).

Pathogenesis

Thoracic surgery, local radiation therapy, and chemotherapy all may predispose to esophageal disease by disrupting the integrity of the esophageal mucosa. In addition, chronic corticosteroid therapy, as might be given in patients with graft-versus-host disease (GVHD) or those with central nervous system cancer, also may provoke development of esophageal infection.

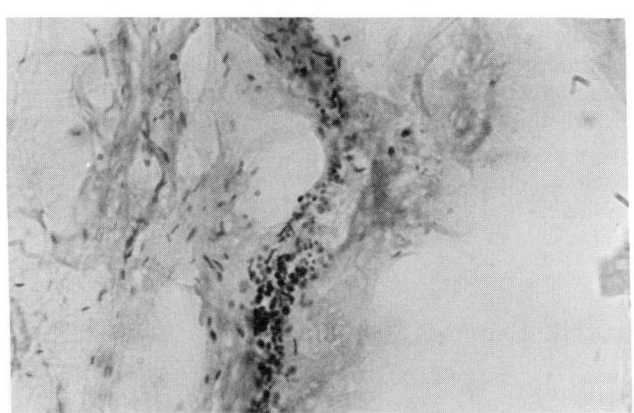

FIG. 2. Fungal esophagitis due to *Aspergillus flavus* in a bone marrow transplantation patient. *Aspergillus* is a rare cause of esophagitis in the absence of other signs of aspergillosis.

Presentation

Patients with esophagitis typically present with symptoms of dysphagia and/or odynophagia, or with a dull retrosternal ache. Three pathogens account for the majority of cases: *C. albicans,* herpes simplex, and cytomegalovirus (CMV). The pathogens do not each cause distinct clinical syndromes, although one series found that nausea and vomiting were particularly common features of herpes simplex esophagitis among bone marrow transplant patients (10). Additional etiologies include infection with *Aspergillus* species (Fig. 2) and gram-positive and -negative bacteria (Fig. 3) (11). One review of bacterial esophagitis found 20 cases among 5631 autopsies, and an additional 3 clinical cases of bacterial esophagitis (11). Cases were caused by *Staphylococcus* species, viridans strep, and *Bacillus* species.

Diagnosis is by endoscopic biopsy with culture. The practical algorithm developed for patients with human immunodeficiency virus (HIV) and esophagitis—initial treatment for fungal then herpetic disease, with endos-

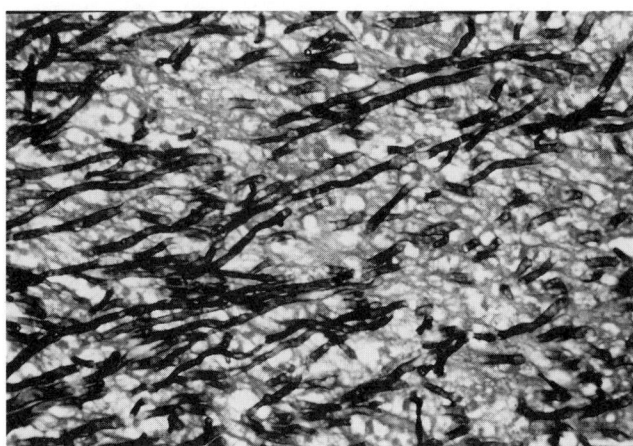

FIG. 3. Bacterial esophagitis. (See Plate 7.)

copy of nonresponders—may not be advisable for neutropenic patients who are already receiving antifungal and antiviral therapy. Biopsy, however, may be contraindicated by thrombocytopenia. Even with endoscopic biopsy, diagnosis of CMV may require an array of molecular diagnostic techniques (12).

Treatment

Treatment is directed at the recovered organism or empiricially, as noted.

CECUM: TYPHLITIS

Overview

Typhlitis is a necrotizing enterocolitis usually affecting the cecum that carries a mortality rate in some series that exceeds 50%. After early reports (13), Wagner et al. (14) described the syndrome, having reviewed autopsies of children dying of leukemia. They found an incidence of typhlitis of about 12% (14). Reviews have found children with acute leukemia to be the group at highest risk, although typhlitis has been diagnosed among children and adults with organ transplantation (15), drug-induced neutropenia (16), solid tumors (17), other hematologic neoplasms (17), sarcoma (17), aplastic anemia (18,19), cyclic neutropenia (20), AIDS (21), and other conditions. The disease is increasingly being diagnosed in adults (22–25).

The term "typhlitis" derives from *typhlon,* or blind pouch, referring to the cecum, where most cases are manifest. Other names for this syndrome have included neutropenic enterocolitis, necrotizing enterocolitis, and ileocecal syndrome.

Pathogenesis

The etiology of typhlitis is unknown. Anatomically, there are considered to be three types (18): confined to the cecum, involving the cecum as well as adjacent large and small bowel, and involving the cecum with scattered ulcers throughout the gastrointestinal tract.

Both chemotherapy and neutropenia appear to predispose patients to the development of typhlitis, but the occurrence of typhlitis in neutropenic patients who have not received chemotherapy, such as those with aplastic anemia or cyclic neutropenia, suggests that neutropenia is the more important risk factor. Cases, however, have occurred among patients with normal white blood cell counts (21). In most cases, disease occurs in the setting of chemotherapy-induced ulceration of intestinal mucosa, combined with neutropenia and thrombocytopenia. Under these conditions, bacteria and fungi appear to invade into the cecal wall.

Why the disease occurs predominantly in the cecum is also poorly understood. Peculiarities of the cecal blood supply, the motility, size, and distensibility of the cecum, or other factors may be pertinent.

Presentation

Most patients who develop typhlitis have received chemotherapeutic agents in the previous 30 days (17). Symptoms generally develop at the peak of neutropenia. The agents most commonly associated with development of typhlitis include vincristine (which can cause adynamic ileus), ara-C, and corticosteroids.

Common symptoms include fever, diarrhea, and right lower quadrant pain. Lower gastrointestinal bleeding is seen in up to 35% of patients. In one series (17), 62% of patients had a complaint of sore throat, reflecting diffuse chemotherapy-related mucositis, and suggesting the important contribution of such agents to development of bowel mucositis. Nausea and vomiting are also commonly seen. One study found that typhlitis seldom presented without symptoms (17). In severe cases, intestinal perforation often followed by shock may occur. Pseudomembranous colitis due to *Clostridium difficile* must be considered in the differential diagnosis.

Up to 70% of patients with typhlitis have positive blood cultures for bacteria (26). Often, multiple organisms may be recovered (17) (35% versus 8% in patients without typhlitis), reflecting a severely interrupted intestinal mucosa. Recovered organisms are predictable: aerobic intestinal flora including *E. coli, Klebsiella* species, and *P. aeruginosa. Staphylococcus aureus* has been noted in a pediatric series (18).

On gross examination of the cecum, bowel thickening and diffuse or discrete mucosal ulceration are seen. In addition, bowel wall edema, transmural hemorrhage, and necrosis occur. Microscopically, heavy invasion of bacteria into bowel wall with scant inflammatory response is noted. Fungi are also sometimes seen. Leukemia cells are seldom found in the bowel wall. These findings further emphasize the contribution of chemotherapy-induced mucositis and neutropenia/thrombocytopenia.

Radiologic evaluation can be very helpful (27–29). Abdominal plain films may reveal paralytic ileus, no gas in the large intestine, a distended, fluid-filled cecum, or intramural air (pneumatosis intestinalis). Computed tomography (CT) scan and sonography similarly may show typical features, including ascites in the area of the cecum, thickened bowel wall, and thickening of fascial planes. Barium enema and endoscopy are seldom performed given the relative contraindication of neutropenia and accompanying thrombocytopenia.

Treatment

There is no consensus regarding best therapy. Some experts recommend conservative management, including intravenous fluids, nasogastric suctioning, and broad spectrum antibacterial antibiotics. Antifungal antibiotics are added if no improvement is seen after 24 to 48 hr. Others favor surgery, including right hemicolectomy, with suggestions of improved survival in some series. Kunkel and Rosenthal (30) reviewed 22 cases of right hemicolectomy in the literature and found 16 survivors versus 6 fatalities. Alt et al. (24) found similar results.

Absolute indications for surgery include intractable gastrointestinal bleeding and cecal perforation.

Keiden et al. (25) suggested that, due to the high risk of recurrence of typhlitis in patients who survive the first episode but must undergo additional cycles of chemotherapy, elective right hemicolectomy should be recommended. This would be performed after the patient has stabilized and has normal white blood cell and platelet counts.

LARGE AND SMALL INTESTINE

Overview

Bowel flora are the source of most episodes of bacteremia in neutropenic patients. This is well demonstrated by the similar proportions of aerobic bacteria found in normal bowel flora and those causing bacteremia in neutropenic hosts: *E. coli, Klebsiella* species, and *P. aeruginosa* predominate (31). Thus, although never clinically evident, bowel flora are the most common source of infection in the neutropenic host.

Pathogenesis

Enteric organisms may enter the bloodstream through chemotherapy-induced mucosal ulcerations, many of which are microscopic. Neutropenia, aggravated by thrombocytopenia, contributes to poor healing of the ulcers, promoting further bacterial entry. Systemic illnesses that manifest in the gastrointestinal tract, including CMV infection or GVHD, may compromise the normal mucosal barrier. In addition, patients who have received radiation therapy to the abdomen or pelvis may develop radiation enteritis, wherein a friable mucosal surface is more likely to allow entry of bacteria from bowel into the bloodstream.

Many medical centers have published their experience with bacteremia and fungemia in neutropenic patients. The types and proportions of recovered organisms vary from one center to another, but at all medical centers, gram-negative enteric organisms, including *E. coli, Klebsiella* species, and *P. aeruginosa,* predominate. In recent years, with increasing use of central venous catheter devices, gram-positive organisms, including *Staphylococcus* species and *Streptococcus* species, have emerged. At Memorial Sloan-Kettering Cancer Center (MSKCC), reviews have confirmed the importance of enteric organisms. In 1982, gram-negative organisms, including *E. coli* (15%), *Klebsiella* species (15%), and *P. aeruginosa* (8%), predominated (31). Reviews of all episodes, including neutropenic and nonneutropenic, from the same institution from 1988 and 1993 demonstrate that these three gram-negative organisms continue to account for more than 20% of all episodes (T. E. Kiehn, *personal communication*).

Anaerobic bacteria are rarely recovered in the blood of febrile neutropenic patients, accounting for less than 3% of episodes in the 1982 MSKCC review, and continuing to account for about 3% of all recovered isolates in 1993. Anaerobes such as *Bacteroides* species or *Clostridium* species may be encountered, however, particularly when the bowel is necrotic and infiltrated with leukemia, lymphoma, or a solid tumor. *Clostridium difficile* is seen in neutropenic patients after the neutropenia resolves. The mechanism is the same as in nonneutropenic patients who receive multiple broad spectrum antibiotics. A *Clostridium* syndrome involving soft tissue may also occur: patients have a pulse–temperature dissociation and are alert despite hypotension. Cellulitis with crepitation is seen on physical examination. Aspiration of the crepitant tissue will demonstrate the organism.

Fungi, particularly *Candida* species, reside in normal bowel and may thrive as bacteria are suppressed by antibacterial therapy (32). Fungemia may ensue. *Trichosporon beigelii* is occurring more commonly as an opportunistic infection arising in the gastrointestinal tract of neutropenic patients. Molds, including *Aspergillus* species and the Mucorales, may rarely cause bowel infection and infarction, generally in the setting of overwhelming systemic infection. These organisms are almost never recovered in blood cultures.

Neutropenic patients who receive corticosteroids are at risk for the hyperinfection syndrome with *Strongyloides stercoralis*. This results in polymicrobic sepsis with bowel flora.

Adenovirus appears to disseminate from the gastrointestinal tract, causing skin lesions along with gastrointestinal symptoms resembling GVHD. Diagnosis requires a skin or gastrointestinal tract biopsy and culture. Adenovirus serotypes in the 30's are often responsible for this disease.

Presentation

The diagnosis must be made from the clinical presentation, namely, fever in a neutropenic patient without other explanation. The gastrointestinal source is usually not evident. Abdominal signs are often minimal since the inflammatory response is dampened by the cytotoxic therapy. Blood cultures are positive in only 10% to 20% of episodes (33).

Treatment

The treatment regimen should cover bowel flora anticipated in the patient and specific for the hospital. The susceptibility patterns will often vary so that the antibiotic regimen should be tailored for each hospital according to the blood culture isolates, which are reviewed on a monthly basis. Usually two or more antimicrobial agents are administered, including an antipseudomonal semisynthetic penicillin and an aminoglycoside (33). Antifungal therapy to treat *Candida* species is added in persistently febrile persons.

ANUS/RECTUM

Overview

Anorectal disease complicates 3% to 8% of patients hospitalized with malignant disease, and a higher proportion of those with hematologic neoplasm, ranging as high as 27% in nonlymphocytic leukemics and 8% in all leukemics (26,34). Grewal et al. (35) reviewed the MSKCC experience with anorectal disease in 2618 leukemia patients hospitalized from 1980 to 1990. Of these 151 (5.8%) had symptomatic anorectal disease, including infection, anal fissure or fistula, and hemorrhoids.

Pathogenesis

Patients with preexisting conditions, such as fissures or hemorrhoids, are more likely to develop complications (35). The normal local trauma of defecation interrupts the mucosal surface. Concurrent neutropenia and thrombocytopenia delay local healing and local infection may ensue.

Presentation

Common symptoms included fever, pain, and tenderness (26,35). Cellulitis and erythema are seen in less than half and purulence or fluctulance is seen in 13.5%. Bacteriologically, *P. aeruginosa* and *E. coli* predominate. Glenn et al. (36) demonstrated the importance of anaerobes and of enterococcus. In one series, *P. aeruginosa* alone predominated (34). In this series of 581 cancer patients, *P. aeruginosa* accounted for 15 of 22 abscesses and 12 episodes of resultant bacteremia. Several of these patients died.

Treatment

Treatment remains controversial although with the advent of potent broad spectrum antibiotics, more physicians are willing to try conservative measures. Glenn et al. (36) reviewed 57 episodes in 44 patients with cancer. Overall, antibiotic therapy alone was adequate for half of the episodes; proper selection of antibiotics to include both specific anaerobic coverage (metronidazole or clindamycin) and an aminoglycoside, as well as a broad spectrum beta-lactam antibiotic, resulted in an 88% response rate. In the review by Grewel et al. (35) 64% were treated conservatively and 36% operatively. Outcome was the same in the two groups and was more related to neutrophil count than to medical versus surgical management. This finding has been supported by others (36). In the series by Barnes et al. (37), surgical therapy resulted in high response rates with minimal surgical morbidity, leading the authors to recommend that early incision and drainage be considered in all patients.

Pseudomonas aeruginosa causing local cellulitis/is-

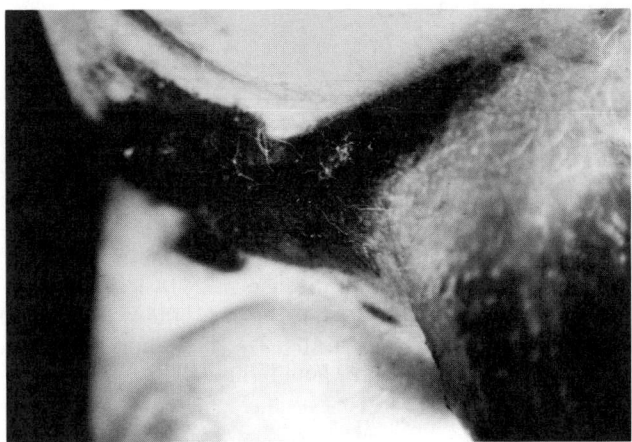

FIG. 4. Ischemia and necrosis of the perineum due to *Pseudomonas aeruginosa* infection in a woman with acute lymphoblastic leukemia who was neutropenic at the time.

TABLE 1. *Causes of abdominal pain in neutropenic patients*

Commonly seen in normal hosts (presentation may vary in neutropenic host)
    Perforation
    Appendicitis
    Peptic ulcer disease
    Pancreatitis
    Gallbladder disease
    Constipation
Unique to immunocompromised hosts
    Infiltration by malignant cells
    Hepatosplenic candidiasis
    Typhlitis
    Adynamic ileus
    Sweet's syndrome of bowel
    Graft-versus-host disease
    Cytomegalovirus
    Pneumocystis carinii of bowel

chemia is a dreaded complication (Fig. 4). In one series, these patients did well with conservative therapy (38). Discontinuation of taking rectal temperatures may have resulted in a decrease of this disease, at least among children (38).

OTHER SYNDROMES: *AEROMONAS*

Aeromonas hydrophila causes a mild, self-limited enteritis in healthy adults. Among the immunocompromised, it can cause a fulminant bloody diarrhea (26). In addition, *A. hydrophila* may cause a sepsis syndrome in neutropenic patients similar to that seen with *P. aeruginosa* (39), including development of ecthyma gangrenosum-like skin lesions. *Aeromonas hydrophila* may also cause recurrent disease (40).

APPROACH TO THE PATIENT WITH NEUTROPENIA AND ABDOMINAL PAIN

Abdominal pain is a common symptom in febrile, neutropenic patients. The list of potential causes, which is considerable in normal hosts, is even more extensive in the neutropenic patient. To further complicate matters, the physical examination may be less than dramatic, owing to the patient's poor inflammatory response. Because there is little margin for error in neutropenic patients, prompt diagnosis and institution of proper therapy are essential to limit morbidity and mortality. For those without an obvious source of fever, immediate empiric therapy must be considered.

Diseases that occur commonly in normal hosts, such as peptic ulcer disease, pancreatitis, and cholecystitis, are also seen in the neutropenic patient (Table 1). Peptic ulcer disease may be exacerbated by concurrent medicines, including corticosteroids. Gallbladder disease may be provoked by antibiotics, including ceftriaxone, and by admin-

istration of total parenteral nutrition. Pancreatitis too may be provoked by medications, such as L-asparaginase. Appendicitis may be particularly difficult to diagnose (41).

Diseases more specific to the immunocompromised host include typhlitis, a disease of the cecum, which was discussed earlier. Sweet's syndrome, also referred to as neutrophilic dermatosis, which generally causes one or several tender erythematous skin lesions, may also cause abdominal pain. GVHD, which occurs in some patients who have received allogeneic bone marrow transplantation, is a multisystem disease that particularly affects the skin, lung, and gastrointestinal tract. Patients may develop abdominal pain and bloody stool. Transplant patients are also at risk for CMV disease, which may affect the gastrointestinal tract, causing ulcers throughout. Pain and bleeding, as well as intestinal perforation, may be seen. With increasingly potent chemotherapeutic agents being used for a variety of cancers, other patients, besides those who have received bone marrow transplantation, may have sufficient immunosuppression to develop CMV disease. Intestinal *Pneumocystis carinii* has caused a similar syndrome and should be considered in cancer patients at risk for this infection. Also important to consider is infiltration by an aggressive tumor into visceral organs and lymph nodes. This may be seen in persons with either solid or hematologic neoplasm. Constipation/ileus should be considered, particularly in patients receiving large doses of narcotic analgesics for cancer-related pain. Vincristine commonly may cause an ileus. Hepatosplenic candidiasis may also present with abdominal pain, often after the white blood cell count has returned to normal.

A comprehensive evaluation should be conducted quickly. After a routine history is taken, a physical examination is conducted, and standard laboratory tests including amylase and lipase are drawn, abdominal radiographs should be performed to exclude intestinal perforation. Wade et al. (42) have suggested that patients be divided according to distribution of pain: those with localizing pain should receive an early radiographic study, such as sonogram or CT scan, while those with diffuse pain can be watched and treated conservatively. In all settings, surgical intervention is reserved for those with evidence of perforation, intra-abdominal hemorrhage, or clinical worsening.

GUT DECONTAMINATION: PROS AND CONS

The use of oral antibiotics to "sterilize" or decontaminate the gut and therefore lower the likelihood of neutropenia-associated bacteremia remains a controversial area (43–45). It has been a standard practice in many European medical centers, but less so in hospitals in the United States. Proponents point to fewer hospital days, less use of intravenous antibiotics, and lower morbidity with improved "quality of life." Those against routine use emphasize the failure of such decontaminating regimens to have an impact on mortality and on the rate of hospital admissions for febrile neutropenic episodes (44).

Perhaps the most compelling argument against routine use of gut sterilization is the inevitable emergence of resistant organisms, both within an individual and within the flora of a given hospital. A recent study from the European consortium, the EORTC, which has long advocated decontamination (Table 2), emphasizes how rapidly resistance can emerge (45). In our view, this argues strongly against use of gut decontamination in any setting. At MSKCC, a gut decontamination is not used in patients with neoplastic disease. As we have recently noted, the common gram-negative enteric organisms remain susceptible to most routinely used antibiotics, including gentamicin at our hospital, in contrast to reports from other centers (46). We believe that the policy not to use gut decontamination in our medical center has contributed greatly to the persistence of susceptibility of bacterial isolates to aminoglycosides. We therefore do not recommend use of prophylactic antimicrobial agents in neutropenic patients for eradication of organisms that might invade from the gastrointestinal tract, including fungi.

SUMMARY AND FUTURE CONCERNS

The use of empiric antimicrobial therapy in the febrile (or suspected infected) neutropenic patient has been the single most important advance in the management of such patients and has contributed greatly to the improved survival of cancer patients. The vast majority of bacteremic and fungemic episodes in the neutropenic patient have the gastrointestinal tract as their original nidus. Flora from the mouth, the esophagus, the intestines, or the perirectal area may enter the bloodstream under conditions of local perturbation by chemotherapy, surgery, or radiation therapy, particularly in the patient with chemotherapy-induced neutropenia. In addition, several specific syndromes, including esophagitis, typhlitis, and perirectal abscess, are seen commonly in the neutropenic patient. Improved survival rates depend on prompt diagnosis and institution of effective therapy, including broad spectrum antibiotics. Given growing concerns about the emergence of resistant organisms worldwide, we do not recommend selective gut decontamination in patients with chemotherapy-induced neutropenia.

In the future, as increasingly effective antibiotics, colony-stimulating factors, and lymphokines allow increasingly potent chemotherapeutic regimens to be administered, new and possibly unexpected syndromes will be seen, involving the gastrointestinal tract of cancer patients. Morbidity and mortality in such situations should be limited by an understanding of contributory host factors and by dogged persistence and vigilance in the care of the patient.

TABLE 2. *Emergence of resistance to quinolones given as part of gut decontamination regimen*

	1983–1985	1986–1990	1991–1993
Patients given prophylaxis/all patients (%)			
Prophylaxis	3/219 (1.4%)	228/694 (33%)	318/706 (45%)
Fluoroquinolone-resistant strains/strains tested (%)			
Escherichia coli	0/26	0/66	11/40 (28%)
Coagulase-negative Staphylococcus	0/22	44/172 (26%)	23/38 (61%)
Pseudomonas aeruginosa	1/25 (4%)	1/39 (3%)	1/13 (8%)
Klebsiella pneumoniae	0/3	1/17 (6%)	1/13 (8%)

From ref. 43, with permission.

REFERENCES

1. National Institutes of Health Consensus Panel. Consensus statement; oral complications of cancer therapies. In: *Oral complications of cancer therapy. NCI Monograph* 1990;9:3–8.
2. Kirstila V, Sewon L, Laine J. Periodontal disease in three siblings with familial neutropenia. *J Periodontol* 1993;64:566–570.
3. Peterson DE, Minah GE, Overholser D, et al. Microbiology of acute periodontal infection in myelosuppressed cancer patients. *J Clin Oncol* 1987;5:1461–1468.
4. Dreizen S, McCredie KB, Bodey GP, Keating MJ. Quantitative analysis of the oral complications of antileukemia chemotherapy. *Oral Surg Oral Med Oral Pathol* 1986;62:650–653.
5. Dreizen S, Bodey GP, Valdivieso M. Chemotherapy-associated oral infections in adults with solid tumors. *Oral Surg Oral Med Oral Pathol* 1983;55:113–120.
6. Sonis ST, Sonis AL, Lieberman A. Oral complications in patients receiving treatment for malignancies other than of head and neck. *J Am Dent Assoc* 1978;97:468–472.
7. Winegard JR. Infectious and noninfectious systemic consequences. In: *Oral complications of cancer therapy. NCI Monograph* 1990;9:21–26.
8. Cohen J, Worsley AM, Goldman JM, Donnelly JP, Catovsky D, Galton DAG. Septicaemia caused by viridans streptococci in neutropenic patients with leukaemia. *Lancet* 1983;2:1452–1454.
9. Baehr PH, McDonald GB. Esophageal infections: risk factors, presentation, diagnosis and treatment. *Gastroenterology* 1994;106:509–532.
10. Spencer GD, Hackman RC, McDonald GB, et al. A prospective study of unexplained nausea and vomiting after bone marrow transplantation. *Transplantation* 1986;42:602–607.
11. Walsh TJ, Belitsos NJ, Hamilton SR. Bacterial esophagitis in immunocompromised patients. *Arch Intern Med* 1986;146:1345–1348.

12. Hackman RC, Wolford JL, Cleaves CA, et al. Recognition and rapid diagnosis of upper gastrointestinal cytomegalovirus infection in marrow transplant recipients. *Transplant* 1994;57: 231–237.

13. Amromin GD, Salomon RD. Necrotizing enteropathy. A complication of treated leukemia or lymphoma patients. *JAMA* 1962; 182:133–139.

14. Wagner ML, Rosenberg HS, Fernbacj DJ, Singleton EB. Typhlitis: a complication of leukemia in childhood. *AJR Am J Roentgenol* 1970;109:341–350.

15. Nagler A, Pavel L, Naparstek E, Muggia-Sullam M, Slavin S. Typhlitis occurring in autologous bone marrow transplantation. *Bone Marrow Transplant* 1992;9:63–64.

16. Clary RM, Wyatt SB, Henley RW, et al. Fatal typhlitis secondary to procainamide-induced agranulocytosis. *Va Med Q* 1984; 3:697–698.

17. Dosik GM, Luna M, Valdivieso M, et al. Necrotizing colitis in patients with cancer. *Am J Med* 1979;67:646–656.

18. Katz JA, Wagner ML, Gresic MV, Mahoney DH, Fernbach DJ. Typhlitis: an 18-year experience and postmortem review. *Cancer* 1990;65:1041–1047.

19. Weinberger M, Hollingsworth H, Feuerstein IM, Young NS, Pizzo PA. Successful surgical management of neutropenic enterocolitis in two patients with severe aplastic anemia. *Arch Intern Med* 1994;153:107–113.

20. Geelhoed GW, Kane MA, Dale DC, Wells SA. Colon ulceration and perforation in cyclic neutropenia. *J Pediatr Surg* 1973;8: 379–382.

21. Till M, Lee N, Soper WD, Murphy RL. Typhlitis in patients with HIV-1 infection. *Ann Intern Med* 1992;116:998–1000.

22. Mower WJ, Hawkins JA, Nelson EW. Neutropenic enterocolitis in adults with acute leukemia. *Arch Surg* 1986;121:571–574.

23. Hiruki T, Fernandes B, Ramsay J, Rother I. Acute typhlitis in an immunocompromised host: a report of an unusual case and review of the literature. *Dig Dis Sci* 1992;37:1292–1296.

24. Alt B, Glass NR, Sollinger H. Neutropenic enterocolitis in adults: review of the literature and assessment of surgical intervention. *Am J Surg* 1985;149:405–408.

25. Keidan RD, Fanning J, Gatenby RA, Weese JL. Recurrent typhlitis: a disease resulting from aggressive chemotherapy. *Dis Colon Rectum* 1989;32:206–209.

26. Bodey GP, Fainstein V, Guerrant R. Infections of the gastrointestinal tract in the immunocompromised patient. *Annu Rev Med* 1986;37:271–281.

27. Merine DS, Fishman EK, Jones B, Nussbaum AR, Simmons T. Right lower quadrant pain in the immunocompromised: CT findings in 10 cases. *AJR Am J Roentgenol* 1987;149:1177–1179.

28. Jones B, Wall SD. Gastrointestinal disease in the immunocompromised host. *Radiol Clin North Am* 1992;30:555–577.

29. Wall SD, Jones B. Gastrointestinal tract in the immunocompromised host: opportunistic infections and other complications. *Radiology* 1992;185:327–335.

30. Kunkel JM, Rosenthal D. Management of the ileocecal syndrome: neutropenic enterocolitis. *Dis Colon Rectum* 1986;29: 196–199.

31. Whimbey E, Kiehn TE, Brannon P, Blevins A, Armstrong D. Bacteremia and fungemia in patients with neoplastic disease. *Am J Med* 1987;82:723–730.

32. Horn R, Wong B, Kiehn TE, Armstrong D. Fungemia in a cancer hospital: changing frequency, earlier onset, and results of therapy. *Rev Infect Dis* 1985;7:646–655.

33. Hughes W, Armstrong D, Bodey GP, et al. Guidelines for the use of antimicrobial agents in neutropenic patients with unexplained fever. *J Infect Dis* 1990;161:381–396.

34. Schimpff SC, Wiernik PH, Block JB. Rectal abscesses in cancer patients. *Lancet* 1972;2:844–847.

35. Grewel H, Guillem JG, Quan SHQ, Enker WE, Cohen AM. Anorectal disease in neutropenic leukemics: operative versus non-operative management. *Dis Colon Rectum* (*in press*).

36. Glenn J, Cotton D, Wesley R, Pizzo P. Anorectal infections in patients with malignant disease. *Rev Infect Dis* 1988;10:42–52.

37. Barnes SG, Sattler FR, Ballard JO. Perirectal infections in acute leukemia: improved survival after incision and drainage. *Ann Intern Med* 1984;100:515–518.

38. Angel C, Patrick CC, Lobe T, Rao B, Pui C-H. Management of anorectal/perineal infections caused by *Pseudomonas aeruginosa* in children with malignant disease. *J Pediatr Surg* 1991; 26:487–493.

39. Ketover BP, Young LS, Armstrong D. Septicemia due to *Aeromonas hydrophila:* clinical and immunologic aspects. *J Infect Dis* 1973;127:284–290.

40. Tapper ML, McCarthy LR, Mayo JB, Armstrong D. Recurrent *Aeromonas* sepsis in a patient with leukemia. *Am J Clin Pathol* 1075;64:525–530.

41. Angel CA, Rao BN, Wrenn E, Lobe TE, Kumar M. Acute appendicitis in children with leukemia and other malignancies: still a diagnostic dilemma. *J Pediatr Surg* 1992;27:476–479.

42. Wade DS, Douglass H, Nava HR, Piedmonte M. Abdominal pain in neutropenic patients. *Arch Surg* 1990;125:1119–1127.

43. Young LS. Antimicrobial prophylaxis in the neutropenic host: lessons on the past and perspective for the future. *Eur J Clin Microbiol Infect Dis* 1988;7:93–97.

44. Verhoef J. Prevention of infections in the neutropenic patient. *Clin Infect Dis* 1993;17(Suppl 2):S359–S367.

45. Cometta A, Calandra T, Bille J, Glauser MP. *Escherichia coli* resistant to fluoroquinolones in patients with cancer and neutropenia. *N Engl J Med* 1994;330:1240–1241.

46. Sepkowitz KA, Brown AE, Armstrong D. Empirical therapy for febrile, neutropenic patients: persistence of susceptibility of gram-negative bacilli to aminoglycoside antibiotics. [Correspondence]. *Clin Infect Dis* 1994;19:810–811.

Infections of the Gastrointestinal Tract,
edited by M. J. Blaser, P. D. Smith, J. I. Ravdin,
H. B. Greenberg, and R. L. Guerrant
Raven Press, Ltd., New York © 1995.

CHAPTER 39

Microbiology and Pathogenesis of *Helicobacter pylori*

Susan J. Riegg, Bruce E. Dunn, and Martin J. Blaser

The genus *Helicobacter,* created in 1989, originally contained two species: *H. pylori,* the human gastric pathogen, and *H. mustelae,* a similar bacterium found in the stomach of ferrets. As of 1994, it is anticipated that at least 12 *Helicobacter* species will have been named, based on 16S rRNA sequencing, DNA hybridization, and use of genus-specific probes (1). Distinguishing features of six of the species are compared in Table 1. *H. pylori, H. mustelae, H. memestrinae,* and *H. felis* are found in the stomachs of humans, ferrets, pigtail macaque monkeys, and cats and dogs, respectively. In contract, *H. fennelliae* and *H. cinaedi* reside in the intestines of humans or rodents.

MICROBIOLOGICAL CHARACTERISTICS

Morphology

H. pylori are curved or spiral-shaped gram-negative bacteria with bluntly rounded ends in gastric biopsy specimens. However, when cultured on solid medium, the bacterium assumes a rod shape; spiral forms may be few or absent. After prolonged culture, coccoid forms predominate. The organism measures 0.5–1.0 μm in width and 2.5–5.0 μm in length, and is unipolar with four to six sheathed flagella attached to one pole; each flagellum measures approximately 30 μm in length and 2.5 nm in thickness. Flagella characteristically exhibit a membra-

S. J. Riegg: Department of Pathology, Medical College of Wisconsin, Milwaukee, Wisconsin 53226.

B. E. Dunn: Department of Pathology, Medical College of Wisconsin, Milwaukee, Wisconsin 53226, and Pathology and Laboratory Medicine Service, Clement J. Zablocki Veterans Affairs Hospital, Milwaukee, Wisconsin 53295.

M. J. Blaser: Division of Infectious Diseases, Department of Medicine, and Department of Microbiology and Immunology, Vanderbilt University School of Medicine, Nashville, Tennessee 37232.

nous terminal bulb that is an extension of the flagellar sheath. The outer membrane is smooth and adheres closely to the cytoplasmic membrane (2,3). Ultrastructural studies using tannic acid as a mordant reveal that the organism has a distinctive surface glycocalyx-like structure up to 40 nm in thickness (3), which in biopsy specimens may be linked to the gastric epithelial microvilli by thread-like bridges (4). The surface of *H. pylori* grown on agar plates is studded with ring-like structures 12–15 nm in diameter that probably represent urease (5) and/or a heat shock protein homolog (see ref. 6). An afimbrial pilus-like structure approximately 2 nm in diameter has also been detected on the surface of the bacterium (7).

Genome and Plasmids

Beji et al. (8) studied the DNA composition of human isolates of *H. pylori* and found an average of 35.2 mol % G + C (range 34.1–37.5 mol %). Approximately 40% of *H. pylori* strains have been found to contain plasmids but none of the plasmids has been associated with a specific virulence factor (9). Taylor et al. (10) demonstrated that the genome sizes of 25 *H. pylori* isolates varied from 1.6 to 1.73 megabases, with an average size of 1.67 megabases. *H. pylori* contains at least two copies each of both 16S and 23S rRNA genes (11).

Several genes of *H. pylori* have been cloned and sequenced including urease structural and regulatory genes (12,13), a gene homologous to the groEL heat shock protein of *Escherichia coli* (14), the cytotoxin gene, a gene associated with expression of cytotoxin activity (15), a gene encoding a putative adhesin (16), and a gene encoding the recombinase (*recA*) protein. Placement of these genes in genomic maps (10,17) suggests that extensive rearrangement of the *H. pylori* chromosome has taken place.

TABLE 1. *Differential characteristics of* Helicobacter *species*

Characteristic	H. pylori	H. mustelae	H. nemestrinae	H. felis	H. fennelliae	H. cinaedi
Host	Human	Ferret	Pig-tailed macaque	Cat, dog	Human	Human, rodent
Primary site	Stomach	Stomach	Stomach	Stomach	Intestine	Intestine
Flagella	Multiple, unipolar	Multiple, bipolar, and lateral	Multiple, unipolar	Multiple, unipolar	Single, polar	Single, polar
Periplasmic fibers	−	−	−	+	−	−
Urease	+	+	+	+	−	−
Catalase	+	+	+	+	+	+
Nitrate reduction	−	+	−	+	−	+
Nalidixic acid (30 μg)	R	S	R	R	S	S
Cephalothin (30 μg)	S	R	S	S	S	PS
Microaerophilic growth at:						
42°C	V	V	V	V	−	−
30°C	+	+	+	+	+	+
25°C	−	−	−	−	−	−
Growth in:						
Air + 10% CO$_2$	V	−	V	−	−	−
Anaerobic	V	V	V	V	−	−
Growth in presence of:						
1% glycine	−	−	−	−	+	+
1% bile	−	−	−	−	+	+
G + C content (mol %)	34.1–37.5	35.1–42.2	24	42.5	37–38	37–38

+, positive; −, negative; R, resistant; S, sensitive; PS, partially sensitive; V, variable.

Antigens and Enzymes

To date, a variety of proteins and antigens of *H. pylori* have been characterized, as reviewed recently (18). These proteins include cytotoxin(s), urease, a homolog of the cpn60 heat shock protein family, two distinct flagellins, catalase, and several outer membrane proteins, among others. These antigens and enzymes will be discussed in detail below in the section dealing with pathogenesis.

Cellular Fatty Acid Composition

In 1985, Goodwin et al. (2) reported that the major fatty acids of *H. pylori* exhibited a unique profile including tetradecanoic (14:0), octadecanoic (18:0), and 19-carbon cyclopropane (19:0 cyc), with a small amount of hexadecanoic acid (16:0). In addition, Lambert et al. demonstrated that *H. pylori* is unique in producing 3-hydroxyoctadecanoic acid (3-OH-18:0) (19). The unusual fatty acid composition of *H. pylori* has been confirmed by Geis et al. (20). In contrast, *Campylobacter* species contain very small amounts of 14:0 and 18:0 fatty acid (2).

Nutritional Requirements

Defined media are not available for growing *H. pylori;* the organism requires complex basal media (either solid or liquid) with some form of supplementation, such as whole blood, heme, serum, charcoal, cornstarch, or egg yolk emulsion (4,21). While some of these supplements may serve as nutritional substrates, a key function is thought to be detoxification of the medium and protection of the organism (22). For instance, addition of exogenous catalase to basal media promotes growth of *H. pylori;* when bovine serum albumin also is added growth is similar to that on blood-supplemented medium, suggesting that protection from toxic peroxidated fatty acids is important (22). A recent report suggests that supplementation of solid and liquid media by cyclodextrins alone may be sufficient to support growth of *H. pylori* (23).

Fresh isolates of *H. pylori* grow best under microaerobic conditions. However, after laboratory passage, some strains become sufficiently aerotolerant to grow in 10% CO_2 in air. *H. pylori* grows poorly, if at all, under anaerobic conditions. Growth in most liquid media is enhanced by agitation and by incubation in a CO_2-rich atmosphere. Growth occurs at 30–37°C, but not at 25°C. Variable growth of *Helicobacter* sp. is observed at 42°C (4,21,23).

Metabolism

Using routine microbiological methods, *H. pylori* does not appear to utilize carbohydrates either fermentatively or oxidatively as a source of energy, but can use organic acids and amino acids via the Krebs cycle (24). However, Hazell and Mendz recently identified glucose kinase activity in *H. pylori* isolates (25). The substrate specificity, relatively high K_m, and absence of substrate inhibition suggested that the glucose phosphorylation observed was due to glucokinase rather than to hexokinase activity. Glucokinase activity appears to be associated with the bacterial cell membrane. In addition, enzyme activity characteristic of the pentose phosphate pathway has been identified in *H. pylori* isolates (26). Thus, *H. pylori* appears to be capable of catabolizing D-glucose. Additional studies are needed to fully understand carbohydrate utilization in this bacterium.

HISTOPATHOLOGY OF *H. PYLORI* INFECTION

The most common histological pattern of *H. pylori*-associated gastritis is chronic superficial gastritis. This pattern is usually characterized by mononuclear inflammatory cell infiltration associated with neutrophilic infiltration of the epithelium (27). It is not specifically associated with metaplastic change, granuloma formation, or fundic gland atrophy. The amount of inflammation may be highly variable, ranging from minimal inflammatory infiltration of the lamina propria with intact glandular architecture, to severe dense inflammation with microabscess formation, reactive epithelial atypia, and the presence of intraepithelial neutrophils.

In the earliest stages of *H. pylori*–associated gastritis, there is infiltration of neutrophils into the lamina propria (28). This association with neutrophils has been stressed because they are not normally present in the lamina propria. However, the number of mononuclear inflammatory cells, including immunocompetent B and T lymphocytes and plasma cells, is also increased (28). Concomitantly, there often are degenerative changes of the surface epithelial cells, including mucin depletion, cytoplasmic vacuolization, and irregularity and glandular disorganization. The epithelial mucin ranges from intact to markedly depleted, with mild depletion being the most common pattern. After eradication of *H. pylori* infection with antimicrobial agents, most of these features disappear rapidly (29); infiltration with mononuclear cells may persist for several months before disappearing.

Over the course of years or decades, there is extension of the inflammatory process into the deeper portions of the mucosa, partial loss of the pyloric glands and endocrine cells normally located in this region, and a progressive replacement of the mucosa by intestinal metaplasia (30). At endoscopy, the antral mucosa may show a slightly more granular appearance in advanced stages of infection, but this is not constant.

Most biopsy specimens with chronic superficial gastritis are associated with *H. pylori*. When present, the organisms tend to be sparse in areas of intense inflammation with reactive epithelial changes and loss of mucin, while they are easily identified in adjacent, less inflamed areas with a more normal mucus content. Bacteria are generally present in less than 5% of biopsy specimens that are histologically normal and, when present, are located most commonly in the gastric body (31,32). Since the distribution of bacteria may be patchy, occasional cases of chronic superficial gastritis with neutrophil activity may fail to show *H. pylori* organisms due to sampling error (33). Several investigators have demonstrated a positive correlation between number of *H. pylori* present and severity of inflammation (30,34). However, it is clear that bacterial load is not the only potential determinant of mucosal injury; other such variables include differences in host response and bacterial strain (30,34).

The epithelial abnormalities caused by *H. pylori* infection include mucin depletion, loss of nuclear polarity, and nuclear enlargement. These changes are more severe in the pit regions than in the surface epithelium. The presence of these changes should elicit a high index of suspicion for *H. pylori* infection, and a careful inspection of the biopsy slides including deeper levels and special stains is indicated.

The inflammatory response to *H. pylori* in children differs somewhat from that of adults. Endoscopy may reveal a finely granular or nodular mucosal surface. Microscopically, this nodularity corresponds to lymphonodular hyperplasia, especially in the antrum (35,36). Such lymphoid aggregates often contain activated germinal centers. In addition, the quantity of neutrophils may be less than that seen in adults.

Lymphoid hyperplasia with numerous lymphoid follicles is occasionally seen in adults (37) as well and has been referred to as follicular gastritis. In general, mild chronic gastric inflammation, including lymphoid follicle formation, is so common as to be considered a normal finding by many pathologists. However, recent studies have shown that lymphoid follicles represent a specific consequence of *H. pylori* infection (38,39). Genta and associates reported that lymphoid follicles are not present in gastric mucosa in the absence of a concurrent or past *H. pylori* infection (39) and suggested that *H. pylori* infection is a necessary precursor for the development of primary gastric lymphoma (40), by inducing lymphoid tissue in gastric mucosa.

Location of the Organism

The vast majority of *H. pylori* are located adjacent to surface and pit epithelial cells in the gastric mucosa. Bacteria can frequently be identified in hematoxylin and eosin (H&E)–stained sections, although special stains may be necessary to visualize bacteria by light microscopy. The organisms essentially are always found adjacent to gastric mucosal cells and are present in the small intestine only when there is gastric metaplasia. *H. pylori* does not overly areas of intestinal metaplasia in the stomach (41), an observation that may explain the low prevalence of *H. pylori* in patients with pernicious anemia (42). The absence of *H. pylori* overlying areas of intestinal metaplasia in severe atrophic gastritis does not rule out previous infection (43) or infection in other, less affected areas of the stomach.

Effects of Treatment

Several clinical trials have shown that gastritis improves after eradication of *H. pylori* (44,45); however, gastritis may recur or may become more severe with relapse of infection (44). Valle et al. reported that one year after eradication of *H. pylori* there was significant reduction in both acute and chronic inflammation (45). Acute inflammation was observed to resolve quickly after eradication. The decrease in chronic inflammation after eradication of *H. pylori* occurs more slowly; complete normalization of the mucosa typically requires months or even years (45).

EVIDENCE THAT *H. PYLORI* INFECTION CAUSES GASTRITIS

There is now extensive evidence implicating *H. pylori* in the pathogenesis of chronic superficial gastritis. For example, voluntary ingestion of the bacterium by two human investigators resulted in acute or chronic gastritis (46,47). Animal models of *H. pylori* infection have been developed. After experimental challenge with *H. pylori*, gnotobiotic piglets developed gastritis and a specific serological response (48). As noted above, treatment studies have shown that eradication of *H. pylori* by antimicrobial therapy clears gastritis (44,45). In addition, the titer of *H. pylori*-specific antibodies decreases after eradication. Further, *H. pylori* exhibits specificity of tissue involvement; it is exclusively associated with gastric mucosal cells and is not associated with intestinal epithelium either in the small intestine or intestinal metaplasia of the stomach. *H. pylori* is seen in the duodenal bulb only in association with gastric metaplasia. The organisms have been reported in cases of heterotopic gastric mucosa in Meckel's diverticula and in the rectum (49,50). In addition, *H. pylori* is associated with specific gastroduodenal pathology. Specifically, the bacterium is associated with chronic superficial and type B atrophic gastritis, but not with type A gastritis, bile reflux, or secondary gastritis. Nearly every individual infected with *H. pylori* shows evidence of a persistent immunological response to the bacterium. Finally, there have been several reported outbreaks of epidemic hypochlorhydria with gastritis. Based on clinical history, histopathological examination and serologic results, it appears that these cases were due to *H. pylori* infection (51).

DIAGNOSIS

A wide variety of tests is now available to diagnose *H. pylori* infection (Table 2). Histological examination of gastric tissue including use of DNA probes and polymerase chain reaction (PCR) analysis, culture, and rapid urease testing, when used to test gastric tissue all require endoscopy; therefore they incur expense and a risk, albeit slight, of complication due to the procedure. In contrast, breath tests, serology, gastric juice PCR, and urinary excretion of ^{15}N-ammonia are noninvasive tests that do not require endoscopy. The choice of test used for diagnosis of *H. pylori* infection will, in most cases, depend on the clinical information sought and the local availability and cost of individual tests. The microbiological basis for the tests used for detection of *H. pylori* will be discussed below.

The gold standard for detection of *H. pylori* has been defined as culture, histopathological examination of gastric biopsies, or serology, depending on the experience of various investigators (52). However, in many laboratories, cultures for *H. pylori* are positive less frequently than are histology or serology (52,53). This discrepancy is due in large part to the fastidious nature of the bacterium in culture.

At endoscopy, many adults with *H. pylori*-associated gastritis have normal-appearing gastric mucosa. The distribution of *H. pylori* and the associated inflammation is often patchy. The patchy nature of *H. pylori* infection can lead to endoscopic sampling error resulting in false-negative biopsy, culture, and rapid urease test results. At a minimum, two biopsies taken from within 5 cm of the pylorus should be obtained at endoscopy with multiple sections being examined histologically (54,55).

Histology

In most instances, *H. pylori* can be visualized at high magnification with conventional H&E-stained sections. Bacteria are located in the mucus adherent to the surface epithelium and are often found deep within the crypts. However, H&E staining may be unreliable when few bacteria are present. In addition, luminal debris on the surface of epithelium can be mistaken for *H. pylori* in H&E-stained sections. Histological identification of bacteria is facilitated with special stains such as the Warthin–Starry and modified Giemsa stains (56). The Warthin–Starry stain was recommended by Warren in his original report

TABLE 2. *Tests for detection of* Helicobacter pylori

Test	Sensitivity (%)	Specificity (%)	Endoscopy	Comments	Ref.
Histology	93–99	95–99	Yes	Multiple antral biopsies recommended	54,55
Culture	77–92	100	Yes	Variable results depending on experience of laboratory	4,21,52,83,84
Urease test (e.g., CLO)	89–98	93–98	Yes	Endoscopic method of choice for diagnosis of *H. pylori* infection	89–99
^{13}C breath test	90–100	98–100	No	Preferred when multiple tests required	100
^{14}C breath test	90–97	89–100	No	Small radiation exposure; well suited to follow-up of antimicrobial therapy	101–103
Serology	88–99	86–99	No	No appropriate for short-term follow-up of antimicrobial therapy	82,104–113
Gastric juice PCR	96	100	No	Technically very demanding	126,129

(57) and is quite reliable for visualizing *H. pylori*. However, it is labor-intensive, costly, and requires an experienced technician to perform reliably. The modified Giemsa stain is simpler and less labor-intensive.

Other stains that have been used for diagnosis of *H. pylori* include the modified Steiner stain (58), Brown–Hopps (59), acridine orange (60), cresyl–fast violet (61), histological half-Gram stain (62), Gimenez (63), carbol-fuchsin (64), modified Wright stain (65), Diff-Quik (66), Papanicolaou (67), and toluidine O (68). Practically speaking, the choice of stain is dependent on local availability and experience of the pathologist. If histological stains are negative, some investigators advocate examination of gastric biopsies by scanning electron microscopy (69). However, this approach is not practical outside of the research environment.

Immunologic techniques can also be used for the detection of *H. pylori* in formalin-fixed tissue (70), frozen sec-(71), and fresh biopsy material (72). A commercially vailable monoclonal antibody against a flagellar antigen resent in most *Campylobacter* species recognized *H. pyri* in formalin-fixed tissue (73). Using immunofluores-nt techniques, reported sensitivity is 93% to 96%, while ificity approaches 100% (74,75).

Phase contrast microscopy is another sensitive technique advocated for direct, rapid diagnosis. A fresh gastric biopsy specimen is placed on a glass slide, macerated, and suspended in a few drops of saline. After placement of a coverslip, the slide is examined using phase contrast microscopy. *H. pylori* is identified as dark, curved rods with characteristic motility (76).

Finally, Schneider et al. (77) developed a "nylon string test" for diagnosis of *H. pylori* infection, similar to that used for *Giardia* infection. After overnight fasting, a gelatin capsule is swallowed and recovered 4–5 hr later using the attached nylon string. Smears are prepared from mucus recovered on the distal 10 cm of the string and stained with Gram stain. This method was found to have a sensitivity of 95% and specificity of 100%.

Differential Diagnosis

Rarely, other tightly spiraled bacteria have been identified in the human gastric mucosa that measured up to 10 μm in length. They possess a corkscrew shape with four to nine tight, even spirals and lack periplasmic fibrils by electron microscopy. This bacterium was originally named "*Gastrospirillum hominis*" (78), but, based on rRNA sequencing and PCR analysis, the name "*H. heilmanii*" has been proposed (1). The importance of "*H. heilmanii*" in human gastritis is unknown. Monkeys often are infected with an organism of identical appearance.

In addition, chains of gram-negative cocci may occasionally be confused with the spiral shape of *H. pylori*. In some instances these cocci may represent degenerate forms of *H. pylori,* further confounding the problem of histological identification.

Culture

Culture is essential for identification, characterization, and antibiotic susceptibility testing, especially in cases of suspected antibiotic-resistant *H. pylori* infection. If the gastric biopsy cannot be directly inoculated onto culture medium in the endoscopy suite, then it must be placed into specialized medium for transport to the microbiology laboratory. The choice of transport media and avoidance of desiccation are vitally important to the subsequent success of culturing *H. pylori*. Useful transport media include nutrient, thioglycollate, *Brucella,* or brain–heart infusion broths, trypticase soy broth with 10% horse serum and 5 mM urea, 20% glucose, and physiological saline (4,79–81). Hazell et al. reported that viability of *H. pylori* decreases over several hours in saline, water, or 20% glucose but that viability is retained in brain–heart infusion broth supplemented with 0.5% neutral bovine serum albumin and 0.1% catalase (82). Current recommendations include placing the gastric biopsy immediately into transport medium maintained at 4–7°C until culture. Cultures should be set up as soon as possible after sampling due to the fastidious nature of *H. pylori*.

H. pylori can be grown on enriched, nonselective media such as sheep blood or chocolate agar. However, the organism requires a microaerobic (5% to 10% O_2) environment; primary cultures will not grow under standard aerobic or anaerobic conditions. A variety of primary culture media have been utilized including enriched, selective, and differential agars and broths. Some form of supplementation of basal media is necessary for growth of *H. pylori*; supplements have included starch, serum, charcoal, and hemin (4,21). In addition to one or more of the above primary enrichment media, a selective medium should be used for suppression of nasopharyngeal flora and other potential contaminants. Selective supplements include vancomycin, to inhibit gram-positive bacteria, and trimethoprim with polymyxin B or nalidixic acid or cefsulodin alone to inhibit gram-negative bacteria. Inhibition of fungi is accomplished by adding cycloheximide, nystatin, or amphotericin B. Since these selective supplements also may inhibit growth of *H. pylori,* Dent and McNulty (83) reported the use of a modified Skirrow's medium that improves the isolation of *H. pylori* and can be used without a nonselective medium. In most cases *H. pylori* can be isolated on nonselective media despite some contamination. Use of both nonselective fresh chocolate agar and a selective medium ensures optimal recovery of *H. pylori*.

Once inoculated, culture media are incubated under humid, microaerobic conditions with an optimal O_2 concentration of 5% to 10% at a temperature of 35–37°C for 5–7 days (84). The organism is slow-growing; therefore negative plates should be kept for 7–10 days. Colonies of *H. pylori* often are pinpoint in size, watery in consistency, translucent, and fail to produce hemolysis on blood agar. A hand-held magnifying glass can be used to detect very tiny colonies. Colonies also may be entire and easily visible.

Following isolation of colonies, confirmatory identification includes Gram stain, catalase, oxidase, and urease tests (84). By Gram stain, the organism is a curved or spiral-shaped gram-negative rod. Differentiation of *H. pylori* from *C. jejuni* can be easily accomplished by testing for urease (*C. jejuni* lacks urease activity) and nitrate reductase (positive in *C. jejuni*, negative in *H. pylori*). *H. pylori* is susceptible to cephalothin and resistant to nalidixic acid, while the opposite is true of *C. jejuni*. In addition, *C. jejuni* will hydrolyze hippurate whereas *H. pylori* will not (84).

There are numerous sources of error that create false-negative culture results. Successful culture of *H. pylori* can be confounded by endoscopic sampling error, recent antibiotic or bismuth compound use by the patient, use of antiseptic or other bacteriostatic agents during endoscopy, inappropriate handling or transport of the specimen, inadequate laboratory processing, ingestion of topical anesthetic or simethecone during endoscopy, and contamination of the biopsy forceps with other organisms or glutaraldehyde (4,21).

Growth of *H. pylori* in broth media is desirable for studies on physiology and metabolism. Broth culture is useful for determination of minimal inhibitory and bactericidal concentrations of antibiotics and potential antiulcer agents that may be used against *H. pylori* (4). Broth cultures are also convenient for production of large volumes of bacteria for antigen preparation or extraction of biologically active components.

Preservation of isolates for long-term storage is best achieved by storage in a cryopreservative in liquid nitrogen (85). Useful cryopreservatives include brucella broth supplemented with fetal bovine serum and 10% glycerol and 10% mucin solution (85–87). The organism also may be lyophilized by drying suspensions on cotton wool directly from the liquid state, since direct freeze-drying reduces viability of *H. pylori* (88).

Direct Urease Test on Endoscopic Biopsies

The early observation that *H. pylori* produced large amounts of urease activity led to the development of methods for the direct detection of the organism in gastric biopsy tissue. The direct urease test was the first rapid diagnostic test to be developed for *H. pylori* (89). This test is based on the ability of preformed urease to convert exogenous urea to ammonia, resulting in an increased pH of the medium, which is detected by a color change of an indicator. The urease protein produced by *H. pylori* has significantly higher activity than that of other urease-producing bacteria (90), thus contributing to the sensitivity of direct urease testing.

In the rapid urease tests, gastric tissue is placed in a broth medium containing a pH indicator, usually phenol red. The tissue should be crushed or macerated, resulting in a greater release of organisms and urease into the medium, giving a more rapidly positive result. A similar release of organisms can be achieved by vortexing the biopsy at high speed for 15 sec (91). Several broth media have been used, including 2% Christianson's urea broth, 6% urea broth, 10% urea broth, Stewart's broth, and urea

broth without glucose and peptone (91–95). Another modification is to absorb urea broth onto a piece of filter paper, place the fresh gastric tissue onto the urea-impregnated filter paper, then press between two glass slides (96). A positive color change appears within minutes.

In general, the sensitivity of broth tests is no more than 70%, with high specificity. Broth urease tests can be made very inexpensively; broth volume should not exceed 0.5 mL per test. Broth tests generally must be read within 1 hr to avoid false-positive reactions from urea hydrolysis by low numbers of contaminating urease–producing bacteria or autohydrolysis (97). The optimal temperature of *H. pylori* urease activity is 45°C (90). Rapid urease methods that involve incubation near or at this optimum have shown increased sensitivity and specificity compared to incubation at room temperature (97,98).

The CLO test, a gel containing phenol red as an indicator, is a commercially available modification of the broth urease test (99). The gastric biopsy specimen is placed directly on the gel, and the presence of preformed bacterial urease is detected by a color change to pink or magenta. If a significant quantity of urease is present, the color change occurs within minutes, but if only a small amount is present, then the reaction may require several hours. The advantage of the CLO test over the urea broth test is that the reaction is visible more rapidly, since the pH change is seen at the interface of the gel and the biopsy. In contrast, the pH change in broth tests is less intense since it is distributed uniformly throughout the medium. At 1 hr, the specificity of the test approaches 100%, but the sensitivity is only 60% to 70%. At 24 hr, these numbers reverse.

Urea Breath Tests

Urea breath tests are based on the principle that urea that has been labeled with a carbon isotope is administered orally and is hydrolyzed by urease produced by viable *H. pylori* in the stomach, if present. As a result, ammonia is produced and bicarbonate is excreted in the breath as CO_2. The amount of labeled CO_2 in the breath is indicative of the amount of urease activity (hence viable *H. pylori*) present. Urea breath tests are especially useful for assessing the eradication of *H. pylori* (100,101).

Two types of isotopically labeled urea are utilized: ^{13}C-urea and ^{14}C-urea. In both cases, the labeled urea is ingested by the patient, usually following a meal to delay gastric emptying, and labeled CO_2 in the breath is measured used either gas isotope mass spectrometry in the case of ^{13}C-urea or liquid scintillation counting in the case of ^{14}C-urea (67,68). Both tests measure active infection and are useful in making a primary diagnosis as well as monitoring response to therapy. The ^{13}C-urea breath test is more costly; however, the isotope is stable and nonradioactive, and therefore safer for use in children and pregnant women. On the other hand, the ^{14}C-urea test is less expensive and involves low exposure to a long-lived radioisotope (101–103). In the absence of prior therapy, the breath tests have a sensitivity and specificity approaching 97% and 100%, respectively (100–104). One month after therapy, a positive test indicates therapeutic failure with a specificity approaching 100%, but a negative test may be falsely negative (specificity about 80%).

Serology

H. pylori infection of the gastric mucosa results in a systemic as well as a local response that includes elevation of IgG and IgA in the serum, elevated secretory IgA, and low levels of gastric IgM (105), phenomena that have permitted development of a variety of serological tests for detection of *H. pylori*.

Serological methods are particularly useful in screening large numbers of individuals in epidemiological studies (106,107). Serological tests are noninvasive, relatively simple to perform, rapid, and cost-effective when compared to endoscopic biopsy. A variety of serological techniques have been utilized for detection of *H. pylori*–specific antibodies including complement fixation (108), hemagglutination (109), immunoblot (110), fluoroimmunoassay (82), and enzyme-linked immunosorbant assay (ELISA). Most studies have used ELISA assays (111). Recently, kits using enriched antigens for detecting *H. pylori*–specific IgG have become available commercially.

In untreated individuals with *H. pylori* infection, the antibody level is stably elevated. After successful bacterial eradication, the IgG levels tend to decrease, typically to approximately half of the pretreatment value within 6 months (112,113). Low levels of IgG may persist even after bacterial eradication; thus for optimal benefit, pre- and posttreatment samples should be compared. If *H. pylori* is suppressed but not eradicated, the IgG antibody level may decrease but then will eventually rise to the pretreatment value (114). Both saliva and urine have also been used to detect *H. pylori* antibodies; however, methodological problems currently preclude their use as diagnostic tests (115).

The utility of any serologic test for detecting *H. pylori*–specific antibodies is highly dependent on the antigen preparation used. In general, three types of antigen have been used for detection of *H. pylori*–specific antibodies. These preparations include crude antigens such as whole cells and whole-cell sonicates (116,117), cell fractions such as glycine extracts and heat-stable antigens (118), and enriched antigen fractions such as urease and a 120-kDa protein (119). The sensitivities and specificities using all three types of antigen preparation are generally greater than 95%. While analysis of whole-cell preparations of *H. pylori* by sodium dodecyl sulfate–polyacrylamide gel electrophoresis (SDS-PAGE) reveals a large number of protein bands, generally no more than 10 antigens are recognized by sera from infected individuals. Among the latter antigens are the 120-kDa antigen, the 62-kDa and 30-kDa subunits of urease, and the 54-kDa heat shock protein homolog (120).

Molecular Tests

Molecular tests, including DNA probes on gastric biopsies and PCR of biopsy material and gastric aspirates, offer the possibility of very precise diagnosis of *H. pylori* infection. DNA probes specific for *H. pylori* can be used on paraffin-embedded gastric biopsy specimens (121,122). The sensitivity of DNA probes is such that in some instances they may detect *H. pylori* when no bacteria are seen histologically. DNA probes are highly specific; contamination of specimens with DNA from other bacteria, including several species of *Campylobacter*, typically does not affect test results.

The method with the potential for greatest sensitivity is detection of *H. pylori*–specific DNA using PCR (123–125). Using gastric biopsy material, a variety of target DNA sequences have been used for PCR diagnosis including a portion of the 16S rRNA gene (123), a gene encoding for a urease subunit (124), and a portion of the gene encoding a species-specific 26-kDa protein (125). PCR has also been performed on gastric juice aspirates (126), which can be obtained using a nasogastric tube without the need for endoscopy. The reported sensitivity and specificity of all of these PCR tests have been high. In the study by Westblom et al. (126), clinical samples were collected at one institution and mailed to another where analysis was performed. Reverse transcriptase (RT) PCR also is highly accurate (127).

Urinary Excretion of ^{15}N-Ammonia

Wu et al. recently described a noninvasive test for *H. pylori* infection based on detection of ^{15}N-ammonia in urine (128). After oral ingestion, ^{15}N-urea is metabolized into CO_2 and ^{15}N-ammonia as a result of urease activity. The amount of ^{15}N-ammonia excreted in urine reflects urease activity; hence *H. pylori* load. In the initial report, sensitivity was 96% with 100% specificity (128).

In summary, many tests are available to diagnose *H. pylori* infection. If endoscopy is going to be performed, then histopathological examination and rapid urease testing should be performed at a minimum. Culture is especially important in suspected cases of antibiotic resistance. Serological testing methods are now very sensitive and specific, but antibody titers respond slowly to eradication of *H. pylori*. The major use of breath testing appears to be during follow-up of antimicrobial therapy, to assure that bacterial eradication has been achieved. Further studies are necessary to validate the ^{15}N-ammonia urinary excretion test. While molecular tests appear to be increasing in popularity, the lack of universal availability and labor-intensive nature of such tests may be restrictive. In addition, since molecular tests do not require viable bacteria for detection, such tests may prove problematic if used soon after therapeutic eradication of *H. pylori*, when residual DNA from nonviable bacteria might be present. Because PCR is extremely sensitive, minute amounts of contaminating nucleic acid within the laboratory may potentially result in a false-positive reaction; therefore the utmost effort must be made to prevent contamination. Laboratories wishing to perform PCR for diagnostic purposes must develop strict guidelines for the handling of clinical specimens (129).

PATHOGENESIS OF *H. PYLORI* INFECTION

Any model of *H. pylori* pathogenesis must take into account the fact that the bacterium is found associated only with gastric mucosal cells, either within the stomach or at sites of gastric metaplasia within the gastrointestinal tract. The bacterium induces chronic active inflammation, yet is able to persist in the gastric mucous gel despite inflammation and mucosal secretion of bacteria-specific immunoglobulins including sIgA.

Studies prior to the recognition of *H. pylori* determined that pathogenesis of peptic ulcer disease involves either increased acid production, decreased integrity of the gastric mucosal barrier, or both (130). Based on *in vitro* analyses, *H. pylori* isolates produce a variety of factors that might decrease gastric mucosal integrity directly and/or promote chronic active inflammation. In addition, *H. pylori* infection alters normal gastrin–hydrochloric acid homeostasis, which in many cases may result in increased secretion of acid and pepsin.

The success of *H. pylori* as a gastric pathogen appears to be dependent on maintenance factors and pathogenic mechanisms. Maintenance factors are those that are necessary to allow survival of *H. pylori* in the hostile environment of the gastric lumen; such factors presumably include spiral shape and motility, adaptive enzymes and proteins, and adherence to gastric mucosal cells and mucus (Table 3). Pathogenic mechanisms are those that lead directly to disruption of the gastric mucosal barrier, including toxins and mediators of inflammation, or increased gastric acid/peptic activity (Table 4). However, it must be recognized that this distinction may be arbitrary. *H. pylori* has successfully evolved to cause persistent infection of the human gastric mucosa. Inflammation may in fact be necessary for persistence (131,132); thus inflammatory mediators also may be maintenance factors.

The pathogenic roles of only two factors, bacterial motility and urease activity, have been demonstrated experimentally in animal models. The putative roles of inflammatory mediators and toxic products listed in Table 4 have been inferred from *in vitro* analyses and experiments. Studies of pathogenesis are limited by the suitability of animal models. For *H. pylori*, gnotobiotic piglets (48) or mice (133) have been useful, but each is limited by the cost and expertise necessary to maintain germ-free conditions. *H. mustelae,* which naturally infects ferrets (134), and *H. felis,* which can be used for experimental infection of mice (135), represent other possible options.

TABLE 3. *Putative maintenance factors of* Helicobacter pylori

Motility
    Spiral shape
    Flagella
Adaptive enzymes/proteins
    Urease
    Catalase
    Superoxide dismutase
    Protein inhibitor of gastric acid secretion
Bacterial adhesins

TABLE 4. *Putative pathogenic mechanisms of* Helicobacter pylori *inflammation*

Activation of inflammatory cells
Platelet-activating factor
    Autoimmune phenomena
    Lipopolysaccharide
Altered gastrin–hydrochloric acid homeostasis
    Decreased somatostatin release
    Hypergastrinemia
    Diminished responsiveness of parietal cells
Reduced mucosal integrity (toxic products)
    Cytotoxins
    Urease
    Mucinase
    Lipase
    Phospholipases (A and C)
    Hemolysin
    Alcohol dehydrogenase

Motility

The most convincing evidence that motility is a virulence factor for *H. pylori* comes from studies in gnotobiotic piglets (48). In the piglet model, the most motile strain of *H. pylori* also was the most virulent strain. The least virulent strain was the least motile. Active motility presumably promotes rapid passage of *H. pylori* through the acidic milieu of the gastric lumen, and penetration of the gastric mucous layer prior to reaching the neutral environment immediately overlying the gastric epithelium. Presumably, the key factors facilitating motility of *H. pylori* are its spiral shape and polar flagella. *H. pylori* strains possess two genes, *flaA* and *flaB,* located apart and encoding two distinct flagellar proteins; *flaA* is required for motility whereas *flaB* mutants have diminished motility (136).

Adaptive Enzymes and Proteins

Urease

There is abundant urease activity in *H. pylori.* The enzyme is a 550-kDa hexameric molecule composed of two subunits of 62–66 kDa and 29–31 kDa (137,138). With a K_m for urea of 0.3–0.8 mM, *H. pylori* urease is well adapted to the low urea concentrations present in the human stomach. Urease plays an essential role in infection and development of gastritis induced by *H. pylori* in gnotobiotic piglets (139). A mutant strain that exhibited essentially no urease activity was unable to infect piglets. In contrast, gastritis was induced in all piglets challenged with the same dose of the wild-type parental strain. *In vitro, H. pylori* in the absence of urea is not intrinsically resistant to the bactericidal effects of acid. However, addition of urea can protect *H. pylori,* although the exact mechanism is unknown (140,141). Functional urease activity is not essential for growth of *H. pylori* at neutral pH, since growth occurs in the presence of urease inhibitors, and in mutant strains lacking urease activity (13).

Regulation of urease activity is complex, and nine accessory genes that play roles in assembly of the macromolecule among other functions have been identified (142).

Catalase

Catalase protects bacteria against the toxic effects of reactive oxygen metabolites formed in neutrophils from hydrogen peroxide (H_2O_2) as a result of the well-characterized oxidative burst. The catalase molecule of *H. pylori* appears to be a 200-kDa tetrameric molecule with subunits of approximately 50 kDa (143). This basic protein has an isoelectric point of 9.0–9.3. All other known bacterial catalases have acidic isoelectric points. The enzyme is active over a broad pH range. By spectral analysis, catalase contains an iron porphyrin prosthetic group (143), similar to many other bacterial catalases.

Superoxide Dismutase

Superoxide dismutase catalyzes dismutation of the superoxide anion to form molecular oxygen; thus, like catalase, it protects bacteria against reactive oxygen metabolites. Superoxide dismutase activity has been detected in *H. pylori* isolates. The purified enzyme is a dimer composed of two identical subunits of approximately 20 kDa (Connors J, Parlow M, Dunn B, unpublished data). Presumably, superoxide dismutase along with catalase helps to protect *H. pylori* against reactive oxygen metabolites released by gastric neutrophils.

Protein Inhibitor of Gastric Acid Secretion

In an assay in which the weak base ^{14}C-aminopyrine is used to indirectly assess acid secretion from isolated rabbit parietal cells, most *Helicobacter* sp. produce a substance that is inhibitory (144). The inhibitor activity in *H. pylori* is partially heat-labile and is destroyed by pretreatment with pronase. Inhibition of gastric acid secretion may facilitate the early stages of *H. pylori* infection, since acid is deleterious to the bacterium. Direct inhibition of gastric secretion by *H. pylori* may help to explain the transient hypochlorhydria observed in individuals recently infected with *H. pylori*. Alternatively, induction of inflammation may be responsible for inhibition of acid secretion.

Bacterial Adhesins

In vivo, *H. pylori* is associated primarily with gastric mucus-secreting cells including foci of gastric metaplasia. By electron microscopy, adherence of *H. pylori* to human gastric mucus cells in some cases involves formation of "attachment pedestals." At such sites there is effacement of microvilli and disruption of cytoskeletal elements (5). In experimentally infected animals, *H. pylori* is found only in the stomach and not in other regions of the gastrointestinal tract. Taken together these observations suggest that *H. pylori* associates specifically with gastric mucus-secreting cells.

Specificity of bacterial adherence implies interaction between bacterial adhesins and mucosal cell receptors. A variety of putative *H. pylori* adhesins have been identified including a fibrillar hemagglutinin (145), a protein that co-purifies with urease by size exclusion chromatography (146), a 31-kDa adhesin (16), a 19.6-kDa pilus-like protein (7), and a molecule antigenically similar to exoenzyme S, a potent virulence factor produced by *Pseudomonas aeruginosa* (147). The potential ligands for these adhesins include sialic acid (145), fucosylated glycoconjugates (148), and other glycolipids (149).

H. pylori induces gastric inflammation. A variety of putative mediators of inflammation produced by *H. pylori* have been identified.

Activation of Inflammatory Cells

H. pylori products are capable of stimulating neutrophils (150), monocytes, and macrophages *in vitro*. Soluble *H. pylori* surface proteins, known to be enriched for urease activity, can induce expression of the monocyte surface antigen HLA-DR and interleukin-2 receptor, synthesis of the inflammatory cytokines interleukin-1 and tumor necrosis factor (TNF), and secretion of the reactive oxygen metabolite superoxide anion (151). This activation is independent of the presence of lipopolysaccharide (LPS). By immunoperoxidase staining, urease, but not intact bacteria, can be detected within the macrophages of the lamina propria of infected individuals (152). Gastric mucosal biopsies cultured from *H. pylori*–infected individuals release significantly greater amounts of TNF-2 into culture supernatants than do biopsies from uninfected individuals (153). *In vivo*, mucosal resorption of secreted *H. pylori* proteins may activate macrophages residing in the lamina propria or mucosal monocytes by mechanisms similar to those described above (151).

Phospholipase A

H. pylori express phospholipase A (PLA) activity in vitro (154). PLA-induced degradation of membrane phospholipids results in formation of arachidonic acid, which can be converted into leukotrienes, prostaglandins, or thromboxanes. These compounds are known to be chemotactic and can alter cell membrane permeability (155). Phospholiase C activity also is present (156).

Platelet-Activating Factor

Paf-acether, first described as platelet-activating factor, is a potent inflammatory mediator produced by both prokaryotic and eukaryotic cells. Paf can produce severe pathological changes including gastric ulceration. Paf has been detected in *H. pylori* grown on blood agar plates. However, Paf was synthesized by *H. pylori* grown in broth medium only if specific metabolic precursors were added (157). Paf precursors, but not Paf itself, have been detected in gastric biopsy material from *H. pylori*–infected individuals with duodenal ulcers. Thus, *H. pylori* may add to local production of Paf in the gastric mucosa (157) promoting mucosal injury.

Autoimmune Phenomena

Heat shock proteins (HSPs) are a group of highly conserved proteins found in all prokaryotic and eukaryotic cells studied (158), and bacterial HSPs also are potent immunogens. T cells with the γ/δ receptor are specialized to recognize the mycobacterial 65-kDa HSP (158). *H. pylori* infection stimulates formation of antibodies that cross-react with human antral gastric antigens (159). In addition, there is induced expression of major histocompatibility complex (MHC) class II antigens on gastric cells in individuals with *H. pylori*–associated gastritis (160) and an increased number of γ/δ T cells within the epithelium (161). Furthermore, a monoclonal antibody against the 65-kDa mycobacterial heat shock protein cross-reacts with gastric epithelial cells in *H. pylori*–infected, but not *H. pylori*–uninfected, tissue biopsies and with *H. pylori* directly (161). A major *H. pylori* antigen has been purified (162), cloned, and sequenced (14), showing extensive homology with the cpn60 family of HSPs.

Taken together, these observations suggest that γ/δ T cells play a role in host defense against *H. pylori* infection and that *H. pylori* may trigger an autoimmune response to HSPs expressed by gastric epithelial cells.

Lipopolysaccharide

In general, LPS from a variety of gram-negative bacteria has been shown to function as a mediator of inflammation. The LPS molecules of *H. pylori* strains are structurally heterogeneous and may have variable degrees of endotoxicity (163). Interestingly, the LPS of *H. pylori* shows very low biological activity (164), similar to that of *Bacteroides,* another organism that persists in the gastrointestinal tract (132).

Altered Gastrin–Hydrochloric Acid Homeostasis

Gastrin is a peptide secreted by antral G cells that stimulates parietal cells to secrete acid and, to a lesser extent, chief cells to secrete pepsin. Gastrin secretion is at least as important as is vagal stimulation in control of gastric secretion (165). A variety of observations indicate that *H. pylori* infection perturbs gastrin–hydrochloric acid homeostasis in infected individuals. For example, *H. pylori* is known to be preferentially localized within gastric antral crypts, the site of greatest concentration of G cells. Inflammation of antral crypts is generally more severe than is inflammation of superficial gastric mucosa. In *H. pylori* infection, the absolute number of G cells is preserved; G cells in infected individuals contain higher levels of immunoreactive gastrin per cell than do G cells of uninfected

individuals (166). Further, G-cell gastrin levels appear to be inversely correlated with the magnitude of bacterial colonization (166). Compared with uninfected persons, *H. pylori*–infected individuals demonstrate fasting and meal-induced hypergastrinemia; eradication of infection eliminates hypergastrinemia (167,168). Thus, hypergastrinemia, which was thought to predispose to duodenal ulceration, is a consequence of *H. pylori* infection (167). Low pH inhibits gastrin release to the same extent in infected and uninfected individuals. As noted above, *H. pylori* supernatants contain a protein capable of inhibiting gastric acid secretion by parietal cells (144).

Two key aspects of gastrin–hydrochloric acid homeostasis are altered in individuals infected with *H. pylori* (169). First, normal acid levels do not reduce gastrin secretion. Possible explanations include ammonia production by *H. pylori* urease resulting in neutralization of the environment in the vicinity of G cells or somatostatin-secreting (D) cells, which monitor luminal acidity. Another possibility is that chronic antral inflammation may upregulate gastrin production (131). The second important physiological alteration is that hydrochloric acid appears not to be increased in the face of elevated gastrin levels in most individuals. This apparent alteration may be due to the inability of parietal cells to respond to gastrin either due to inflammation or to the direct effects of an inhibitor of gastric acid secretion. Many studies have demonstrated that basal and meal-stimulated gastrin levels are elevated in *H. pylori*–infected individuals with DU. However, significant differences between *H. pylori*–infected and uninfected persons in basal and peak acid output have not been demonstrated consistently. Eradication of *H. pylori* characteristically decreases basal and meal-stimulated gastrin secretion; whether or not basal or peak acid output is affected is not clear (168,170). Augmenting *H. pylori* ammonia production by infusing urea into the stomach of *H. pylori*–infected individuals with DU significantly increases intragastric ammonia levels without affecting the plasma gastrin concentration (171,172). Thus, access of H^+ ion to the pH-sensitive sites governing gastrin release by mucosal ammonia produced by *H. pylori* urease does not appear to be a critical factor involved in acute regulation of gastrin levels (168). Whatever the mechanism, the effect of *H. pylori* infection on gastrin release is more profound than the effect on acid (170). However, prolonged hypergastrinemia associated with *H. pylori* infection may contribute to the increased parietal cell mass characteristically present in DU patients.

Decreased Mucosal Integrity

The two major mechanisms whereby *H. pylori* infection might lead to decreased mucosal integrity include elaboration of toxic bacterial products and induction of mucosal inflammation.

Cytotoxins

Broth culture supernatants from approximately 50% of *H. pylori* isolates tested produce a toxin that induces vacuolization of a variety of cell lines. The purified 87-kDa toxin shows limited sequence homology with various ion channel transport proteins and human gastric H$^+$, K$^+$-ATPase (173). Intact activity of the vacuolar ATPase of eukaryotic cells appears to be essential in the pathogenesis of vacuolization induced by the cytotoxin (174). Genetic studies indicate that the gene encoding this toxin, *vacA*, is present in nearly all *H. pylori* strains, regardless of whether they express toxin activity *in vitro* (175–178). The *vacA* sequences of tox + and tox − strains are dissimilar and other heterogeneities of *vacA* structure have been observed (175).

In naturally infected humans, vacuolizing cytotoxin may be an important virulence factor. Cytotoxic activity is more prevalent in isolates of *H. pylori* from individuals with peptic ulcer disease than with gastritis only (179). A gene (*cagA*) associated with expression of cytotoxin activity has been identified (15), but mutation of *cagA* indicates that it is not necessary for cytotoxin activity (180).

Bacterial lysates from *H. pylori* strains also express a protein that is cytotoxic for Chinese hamster ovary cells and appears to be distinct from the vacuolizing cytotoxin (181).

Urease

Besides its role as a maintenance factor, urease activity may have direct toxic effects on gastric cells and mucus *in vivo*. *In vitro*, ammonia produced by urease is toxic to gastric carcinoma and other cell types (182). Triebling et al. observed a significant correlation between severity of gastric inflammation and concentration of gastric juice ammonia in *H. pylori*–positive patients with chronic renal failure (183). In rats, ammonia infused in concentrations present in uremic humans disrupts the mucosal barrier (184). Accumulation of ammonia produced by hydrolysis of urea may disturb the ionic integrity of gastric mucus and may allow back-diffusion of H$^+$ toward the gastric mucosa, resulting in tissue injury.

Mucinase

Chronic *H. pylori* infection is associated with depletion of the mucous layer overlying gastric cells. This depletion of mucus may be due either to inhibition of mucus secretion or to degradation of mucus after its secretion. Mucus depletion also may represent increased mucin turnover (185). *In vitro, H. pylori* secretes a protease capable of degrading porcine gastric mucus (186). In contrast, Sidebotham et al. (187) failed to detect mucinase activity in cell infiltrates of *H. pylori*. Mucinase-associated degradation of gastric mucus would likely disrupt the normal barrier function facilitating back diffusion of H$^+$ ions leading to injury of gastric epithelial cells. Reduction of gastric mucus viscosity might also facilitate penetration of *H. pylori* toward the gastric mucosa and release essential nutrients for *H. pylori* survival and growth.

Lipase and Phospholipases

H. pylori filtrates exhibit lipase activity based on their ability to convert glycerol trioleate into free oleic acid, mono- and dioleates; expression of phospholipase A (PLA) and phospholipase C (PLC) activity also occur (154,156). These enzymes may contribute to the degradation of rat gastric mucus observed *in vitro* in the presence of *H. pylori* filtrates. Thus, *H. pylori*–induced formation of lysophospholipids could impair the protective function of the gastric mucus gel (154,188).

Hemolysin

Some strains of *H. pylori* grown in broth, but not on solid medium, secrete a factor that induces weak hemolysis in a variety of erythrocytes, including those from human, horse, guinea pig, rabbit, and sheep (188). Hemolysins produced by other bacteria are known to be cytotoxic and can mediate inflammation. By analogy, *H. pylori* hemolysin may have a deleterious effect on the gastric mucosal barrier.

Alcohol dehydrogenase

Alcohol dehydrogenase activity has been identified in isolates of *H. pylori*. It has been suggested that conversion of ethanol to the toxic metabolite acetaldehyde by alcohol dehydrogenase may promote gastric mucosal injury (189). To date, there is no report regarding characteristics of the purified enzyme.

Inflammation and Pathogenesis

A model was previously developed describing the relationship between *H. pylori* infection and gastroduodenal pathology (131,132). According to this model, *H. pylori* releases products that result in tissue inflammation; inflammation in turn leads to release of host factors into the mucous layer, in which the bacterium resides, that *H. pylori* can use for nutrition. Chronic inflammation has effects on both gastrin secretion and parietal cell function, but host immunological suppressor activity downregulates this process. In addition, to maintain its ecological niche, *H. pylori* also downregulates the inflammatory process to the level necessary for persistent survival (132). Possible outcomes of infection include chronic superficial gastritis, duodenal ulceration, gastrin ulceration, and gastric atrophy, a precursor lesion for gastric carcinoma. According to this model, the outcome of infection is based on the interaction of bacteria-induced inflammation and host immune suppression of inflammation on gastric secretory physiology.

While not directly addressed by this model, gastric and duodenal ulceration may result from direct injury to the gastric mucosal barrier induced by toxic bacterial products, such as ammonia, LPS, urease, toxins, acetaldehyde, and others, in addition to the deleterious effects provided by chronic inflammation. The factors that determine the consequences of disordered regulation of inflammation, acid production, and mucosal injury induced by *H. pylori* infection are not presently known. Differences in bacterial strain characteristics, host genetic factors, and environmental cofactors are likely to be involved.

REFERENCES

1. Goodwin CS, Worsley BW. The *Helicobacter* genus: the current history of *H. pylori* and taxonomy of current species. In: Goodwin CS, Worsley BW, eds. *Helicobacter pylori biology and clinical practice.* Boca Raton: CRC Press; 1993:1–13.
2. Goodwin CS, McCulloch RK, Armstrong JA, Wee SH. Unusual cellular fatty acids and distinctive ultrastructure in a new spiral bacterium (*Campylobacter pyloridis*) from the human gastric mucosa. *J Med Microbiol* 1985;19:257–267.
3. Goodwin CS, Armstrong JA, Chilvers T, et al. Transfer of *Campylobacter pylori* and *Campylobacter mustelae* to *Helicobacter* gen. nov. as *Helicobacter pylori* comb. nov. and *Helicobacter mustelae* comb. nov., respectively. *Int J Syst Bacteriol* 1989;39:397.
4. Goodwin CS, Armstrong JA. Microbiological aspects of *Helicobacter pylori* (*Campylobacter pylori*). *Eur J Clin Microbiol Infect Dis* 1990;9:1–13.
5. Lee A, O'Rourke J. Ultrastructure of *Helicobacter* organisms and possible relevance for pathogenesis. In: Goodwin CS, Worsley BW, eds. *Helicobacter pylori biology and clinical practice.* Boca Raton: CRC Press; 1993:15–35.
6. Austin JW, Doig P, Stewart M, Trust TJ. Structural comparison of urease and a GroEL analog from *Helicobacter pylori. J Bacteriol* 1992;174:7470–7473.
7. Doig P, Austin JW, Kostrzynska M, Trust TJ. Production of a conserved adhesin by the human gastroduodenal pathogen *Helicobacter pylori. J Bacteriol* 1992;174:2539–2547.
8. Beji A, Megraud F, Vincent P, Gavini F, Izard D, Leclerc H. GC content of DNA of *Campylobacter pylori* and other species belonging or related to the genus *Campylobacter. Ann Inst Pasteur Microbiol* 1988;139:527–534.
9. Kleanthous H, Clayton CL, Tabaqchali S. Characterization of a plasmid from *Helicobacter pylori* encoding a replication protein common to plasmids in gram-positive bacteria. *Mol Microbiol* 1991;5:2377–2389.
10. Taylor DE, Simons M, Chang N, Salama S. Differentiation of *Helicobacter pylori* isolates by pulsed-field gel electrophoresis of genome DNA. *Microbiol Ecology in Health and Disease* 1991;4:S172.
11. Taylor DE, Eaton M, Chang N, Salama SM. Construction of a *Helicobacter pylori* genome map and demonstration of diversity at the genome level. *J Bacteriol* 1992;174:6800–6806.
12. Clayton CL, Pallen MJ, Kleanthous H, Wren BW, Tabaqchali S. Nucleotide sequence of two genes from *Helicobacter pylori* encoding for urease subunits. *Nucleic Acids Res* 1990;18:362.
13. Labigne A, Cussac V, Courcoux P. Shuttle cloning and nucleotide sequences of *Helicobacter pylori* genes responsible for urease activity. *J Bacteriol* 1991;173:1920–1931.
14. Macchia G, Massone A, Burroni D, Covacci A, Censini S, Rappuoli R. The Hsp60 protein of *Helicobacter pylori*: structure and immune response in patients with gastroduodenal disease. *Mol Microbiol* 1993;9:645–652.
15. Tummuru MKR, Cover TL, Blaser MJ. Cloning and expression of a high molecular weight major antigen of *Helicobacter pylori*: evidence of linkage to cytotoxin production. *Infect Immun* 1993;61:1799–1809.
16. Evans DG, Karjalainen T, Evans DJ, Graham D, Lee C. Cloning of the adhesin subunit gene of *Helicobacter pylori. Ital J Gastroenterol* 1991;23:30.
17. Bukanov NO, Berg DE. Ordered cosmid library and high-resolution physical-genetic map of *Helicobacter pylori* strain NCTC 11638. *Mol Microbiol* 1994;11:509–523.
18. Dunn BE. Proteins, antigens, and typing methods for *Helicobacter pylori.* In: Goodwin CS, Worsley BW, eds. *Helicobacter pylori biology and clinical practice.* Boca Raton: CRC Press; 1993:191–208.
19. Lambert MA, Patton CM, Barrett TJ, Moss CW. Differentiation of *Campylobacter* and *Campylobacter*-like organisms by cellular fatty acid composition. *J Clin Microbiol* 1987;25:706–713.
20. Geis G, Leying H, Suerbaum S, Opferkuch W. Unusual fatty acid substitution in lipids and lipopolysaccharides of *Helicobacter pylori. J Clin Microbiol* 1990;28:930–932.
21. Hazell SL, Markesich DC, Evans DJ, Evans DG, Graham DY. Influence of media supplements on growth and survival of *Campylobacter pylori. Eur J Clin Microbiol Infect Dis* 1989;8:597–602.
22. Hazell SL, Graham DY. Unsaturated fatty acids and viability of *Helicobacter* (*Campylobacter*) *pylori. J Clin Microbiol* 1990;28:1060–1061.
23. Olivieri R, Bugnoli M, Armellini D, et al. Growth of *Helicobacter pylori* in media containing cyclodextrins. *J Clin Microbiol* 1993;31:160–162.
24. Megraud F. Microbiological characteristics of *Campylobacter pylori. Eur J Gastroenterol Hepatatol* 1989;1:5–12.
25. Hazell SL, Mendz GL. The metabolism and enzymes of *Helicobacter pylori*: function and potential virulence effects. In: Goodwin CS, Worsley BW, eds. *Helicobacter pylori biology and clinical practice.* Boca Raton: CRC Press; 1993:115–142.
26. Mendz GL, Hazell SL. Evidence for a pentose phosphate pathway in *Helicobacter pylori. FEMS Microbiol Lett* 1991;84:331–336.
27. Robert ME, Weinstein WM. *Helicobacter pylori*–associated gastric pathology. *Gastroenterol Clin North Am* 1993;22:59–72.
28. Sipponen P, Kekki M, Siurala M. The Sydney system: epidemiology and natural history of chronic gastritis. *J Gastroenterol Hepatol* 1991;6:244–248.
29. Rauws EA, Langenberg W, Houthoff HJ, et al. *Campylobacter pyloridis*–associated chronic active antral gastritis: a prospective study of its prevalence and the effects of antibacterial and antiulcer treatment. *Gastroenterology* 1988;94:33–39.
30. Karttunen T, Niemela S, Lehtola J. *Helicobacter pylori* in dyspeptic patients: quantitative association with severity of gastritis, intragastric pH, and serum gastrin concentration. *Scand J Gastroenterol* (Suppl) 1991;186:124–134.
31. Collins JS, Hamilton PW, Watt PC, Sloan JM, Love AH. Superficial gastritis and *Campylobacter pylori* in dyspeptic patients—a quantitative study using computer-linked image analysis. *J Pathol* 1989;158:303–310.
32. Siurala M, Sipponen P, Kekki M. *Campylobacter pylori* in a sample of Finnish population: relations to morphology and functions of the gastric mucosa. *Gut* 1988;29:909–915.
33. Bayerdorffer E, Oertel H, Lehn N, et al. Topographic association between active gastritis and *Campylobacter pylori* colonization. *J Clin Pathol* 1989;42:834–839.
34. Satoh K, Kimura K, Yoshida Y, Kasano T, Kihira K, Taniguchi Y. A topographical relationship between *Helicobacter pylori* and gastritis: quantitative assessment of *Helicobacter pylori* in the gastric mucosa. *Am J Gastroenterol* 1991;86:285–291.
35. Bujanover Y, Konikoff F, Baratz M. Nodular gastritis and *Helicobacter pylori. J Pediatr Gastroenterol Nutr* 1990;11:41–44.
36. Hassall E, Dimmick JE. Unique features of *Helicobacter pylori* disease in children. *Dig Dis Sci* 1991;36:417–423.
37. Stolte M, Eidt S. Lymphoid follicles in antral mucosa: immune response to *Campylobacter pylori? J Clin Pathol* 1989;42:1269–1271.
38. Isaacson PG, Spencer J. Is gastric lymphoma an infectious disease? *Hum Pathol* 1993;24:569–570.
39. Genta RM, Hamner HW, Graham DY. Gastric lymphoid follicles in *Helicobacter pylori* infection: frequency, distribution, and response to triple therapy. *Hum Pathol* 1993;24:577–583.
40. Parsonnet J, Hansen S, Rodriguez L, et al. *Helicobacter pylori* infection and gastric lymphoma. *N Engl J Med* 1994;330:1267–1271.
41. Wyatt JI, Rathbone BJ. Immune response of the gastric mucosa

to *Campylobacter pylori*. *Scand J Gastroenterol (Suppl)* 1988; 142:44–49.

42. Fong T-L, Dooley CP, Dehesa M, et al. *Helicobacter pylori* infection in pernicious anemia. A prospective controlled study. *Gastroenterology* 1991;100:328–332.

43. Karnes WEJ, Samloff IM, Siurala M, et al. Positive serum antibody and negative tissue staining for *Helicobacter pylori* in subjects with atrophic body gastritis. *Gastroenterology* 1991; 101:167–174.

44. Patchett S, Beattie S, Leen E, Keane C, O'Morain C. *Helicobacter pylori* and duodenal ulcer recurrence. *Am J Gastroenterol* 1992;87:24–27.

45. Valle J, Seppala K, Sipponen P, Kosunen T. Disappearance of gastritis after eradication of *Helicobacter pylori*. A morphometric study. *Scand J Gastroenterol* 1991;26:1057–1065.

46. Marshall BJ, Armstrong JA, McGechie DB, Glancy RJ. Attempt to fulfill Koch's postulates for pyloric *Campylobacter*. *Med J Aus* 1985;142:436–439.

47. Morris A, Nicholson G. Ingestion of *Campylobacter pyloridis* causes gastritis and raised fasting gastric pH. *Am J Gastroenterol* 1987;82:192–199.

48. Eaton KA, Morgan DR, Krakowka S. *Campylobacter pylori* virulence factors in gnotobiotic piglets. *Infect Immun* 1989;57: 1119–1125.

49. Morris A, Nicholson G, Zwi J, Vanderwee M. *Campylobacter pylori* infection in Meckel's diverticula containing gastric mucosa. *Gut* 1989;30:1233–1235.

50. de Cothi GA, Newbold KM, O'Connor HJ. *Campylobacter*-like organisms and heterotopic gastric mucosa in Meckel's diverticula. *J Clin Pathol* 1989;42:132–134.

51. Peterson WL. *Helicobacter pylori* and peptic ulcer disease. *N Engl J Med* 1991;324:1043–1048.

52. Barthel JS, Everett ED. Diagnosis of *Campylobacter pylori* infections: the "gold standard" and the alternatives. *Rev Infect Dis* 1990;12(Suppl 1):S107–S114.

53. Dooley CP, Fitzgibbons PL, Cohen H, Appleman MD, Pérez-Pérez GI, Blaser MJ. Prevalence of *Helicobacter pylori* infection and histologic gastritis in asymptomatic persons. *N Engl J Med* 1989;321:1562–1566.

54. Morris A, Ali MR, Brown P, Lane M, Patton K. *Campylobacter pylori* infection in biopsy specimens of gastric antrum: laboratory diagnosis and estimation of sampling error. *J Clin Pathol* 1989;42:727–732.

55. Wyatt JI, Primrose J, Dixon MF. Distribution of *Campylobacter pylori* in gastric biopsies. *J Pathol* 1988;155:350A.

56. Madan E, Kemp J, Westblom TU, Subik M, Sexton S, Cook J. Evaluation of staining methods for identifying *Campylobacter pylori*. *Am J Clin Pathol* 1988;90:450–453.

57. Warren JR. Unidentified curved bacilli on gastric epithelium in chronic active gastritis. *Lancet* 1983;2:1273.

58. Garvey W, Fathi A, Bigelow F. Modified Steiner stain for the demonstration of spirochetes. *J Histotech* 1985;8:15–18.

59. Westblom TU, Madan E, Kemp J, Subik MA, Tseng J. Improved visualisation of mucus penetration by *Campylobacter pylori* using a Brown–Hopps stain. *J Clin Pathol* 1988;41:232.

60. Simor AE, Cooter NB, Low DE. Comparison of four stains and a urease test for rapid detection of *Helicobacter pylori* in gastric biopsies. *Eur J Clin Microbiol Infect Dis* 1990;9: 350–352.

61. Burnett RA, Brown IL, Findlay J. Cresyl fast violet staining method of *Campylobacter* like organisms. *J Clin Pathol* 1987; 40:353–355.

62. Britt DP, Painchaud SM, Tungekar MF, et al. Detection of *Helicobacter pylori* in gastric brushings. *Trans R Soc Trop Med Hyg* 1990;84:581–582.

63. McMullen L, Walker MM, Bain LA, Karim QN, Baron JH. Histological identification of *Campylobacter* using Gimenez technique in gastric antral mucosa. *J Clin Pathol* 1987;40: 464–467.

64. Rocha GA, Queiroz DM, Mendes EN, Lage AP, Barbosa AJ. Simple carbolfuchsin staining for showing *C. pylori* and other spiral bacteria in gastric mucosa. *J Clin Pathol* 1989;42: 1004–1008.

65. Butler GA. Butler modified Wright stain for demonstration of *Campylobacter pylori*. *J Histotech* 1990;13:109–113.

66. Skipper R, DeStephano DB. A rapid stain for *Campylobacter pylori* in gastrointestinal tissue sections using Diff-Quik. *J Histotech* 1989;12:303–305.

67. Pinto MM, Meriano FV, Afridi S, Taubin HL. Cytodiagnosis of *Campylobacter pylori* in Papanicolaou-stained imprints of gastric biopsy specimens. *Acta Cytol* 1991;35:204–206.

68. Slater B. Superior stain for *Helicobacter pylori* using toluidine O. *J Clin Pathol* 1990;43:961.

69. Bonvicini F, Versura P, Pretolani S, Gasbarrini G, Laschi R. Scanning electron microscopy in the study of *Campylobacter pylori* associated gastritis. *Scann Electron Microsc* 1989;3: 355–360.

70. Rivera E, Lopez Vidal Y, Lugueno V, Ruiz Palacios GM. Indirect immunofluorescence assay for detection of *Helicobacter pylori* in human gastric mucosal biopsies. *J Clin Microbiol* 1991; 29:1748–1751.

71. Steer HW, Newell DG. Immunological identification of *Campylobacter pyloridis* in gastric biopsy tissue. *Lancet* 1985; 2:38–39.

72. Husson MO, Leclerc H. Detection of *Helicobacter-pylori* in stomach tissue by use of a monoclonal antibody. *J Clin Microbiol* 1991;29:2831–2834.

73. Cartun RW, Kryzmowski GA, Pedersen CA, Morin SG, Van Kruiningen HJ, Berman MM. Immunocytochemical identification of *Helicobacter pylori* in formalin-fixed gastric biopsies. *Mod Pathol* 1991;4:498–502.

74. Schaber E, Umlauft F, Stoffler G, Aigner F, Paulweber B, Sandhofer F. Indirect immunofluorescence test and enzyme-linked immunosorbent assay for detection of *Campylobacter pylori*. *J Clin Microbiol* 1989;27:327–330.

75. Parsonnet J, Welch K, Compton C, et al. Simple microbiologic detection of *Campylobacter pylori*. *J Clin Microbiol* 1988;26: 948–949.

76. Pinkard KJ, Jarrison B, Capstick JA, Medley G, Lambert JR. Detection of *Campylobacter pyloridis* in gastric mucosa by phase contrast microscopy. *J Clin Pathol* 1986;39:112–116.

77. Schneider RE, Torres M, Solis C, Passarelli L, Schneider FE, Vettorazzi M. A simple method to detect *Helicobacter pylori* in gastric specimens. *Br Med J* 1990;300:1559.

78. McNulty CA, Dent JC, Curry A, et al. New spiral bacterium in gastric mucosa. *J Clin Pathol* 1989;42:585–591.

79. Taylor DE, Hargreaves JA, Laiking NG, Sherbaniuk RW, Jewell LD. Isolation and characterization of *Campylobacter pyloridis* from gastric biopsies. *Am J Clin Pathol* 1987;87:49–54.

80. Owen RJ, On SL, Costas M. Potential transport medium for *Campylobacter pylori*. *J Clin Pathol* 1988;41:1337–1338.

81. Coudron PE, Kirby DF. Comparison of rapid urease tests, staining techniques, and growth on different solid media for detection of *Campylobacter pylori*. *J Clin Microbiol* 1989;27: 1527–1530.

82. Aceti A, Pennica A, Leri O, et al. Time-resolved fluoroimmunoassay for *Campylobacter pylori* antibodies. *Lancet* 1989;2: 505.

83. Dent JC, McNulty CA. Evaluation of a new selective medium for *Campylobacter pylori*. *Eur J Clin Microbiol Infect Dis* 1988; 7:555–558.

84. Penner JL. *Campylobacter, Helicobacter,* and related spiral bacteria. In: Balows A, Hausler WJ Jr, Herrmann KL, Isenberg HD, eds. *Manual of clinical microbiology*. Washington, DC: Am Soc Microbiol; 1991:402–409.

85. Ribeiro CD, Gray SJ. Long-term freeze storage of *Campylobacter pyloridis*. *J Clin Pathol* 1987;40:1265–1267.

86. Drumm B, Sherman P. Long-term storage of *Campylobacter pylori*. *J Clin Microbiol* 1989;27:1655–1656.

87. Ansorg R, von Recklinghausen G, Pomarius R, Schmid EN. Evaluation of techniques for isolation, subcultivation, and preservation of *Helicobacter pylori*. *J Clin Microbiol* 1991;29: 51–53.

88. Goodwin CS, McCullough C, Boehm J. Successful lyophilization of *Campylobacter pylori* and spiral organisms from the stomachs of animals. *Pathology* 1989;21:227–229.

89. McNulty CAM, Wise R. Rapid diagnosis of *Campylobacter*-associated gastritis. *Lancet* 1985;1:1443–1444.

90. Mobley HL, Cortesia MJ, Rosenthal LE, Jones BD. Characterization of urease from *Campylobacter pylori*. *J Clin Microbiol* 1988;26:831–836.

91. Hazell SL, Borody TJ, Lee A. *Campylobacter pyloridis* gastritis I: detection of urease as a marker of bacterial colonization and gastritis. *Am J Gastroenterol* 1987;82:292–298.

92. Vaira D, Holton J, Cairns S, et al. Urease tests for *Campylobacter pylori*: care in interpretation. *J Clin Pathol* 1988;41:812–813.

93. Yeung CK, Yuen KY, Fu KH, Tsang TM, Seto WH, Saing H. Rapid endoscopy room diagnosis of *Campylobacter pylori*-associated gastritis in children. *J Pediatr Gastroenterol Nutr* 1990;10:357–360.

94. Czinn SJ, Carr H. Rapid diagnosis of *Campylobacter pyloridis*-associated gastritis. *J Pediatr* 1987;100:569–572.

95. Khanna MU, Kochar N, Nair NG, Bhatia SJ, Abraham P. Evaluation of a modified medium for the one hour urease test for *Helicobacter pylori* infection. *Indian J Gastroenterol* 1990;9:219–220.

96. Zhong Y, Xiancun Z, Hong Y, Shengyi J. Rapid diagnosis of *Campylobacter pylori* by urea test paper. *J Gastroenterol Hepatol* 1990;5:514–516.

97. Westblom TU, Madan E, Kemp J, Subik MA. Evaluation of a rapid urease test to detect *Campylobacter pylori* infection. *J Clin Microbiol* 1988;26:1393–1394.

98. Abdalla S, Marco F, Perez RM, et al. Rapid detection of gastric *Campylobacter pylori* colonization by a simple biochemical test. *J Clin Microbiol* 1989;27:2604–2605.

99. Marshall BJ, Warren JR, Francis GJ, Langton SR, Goodwin CS, Blincow ED. Rapid urease test in the management of *Campylobacter pyloridis*-associated gastritis. *Am J Gastroenterol* 1987;82:200–207.

100. Graham DY, Klein PD, Evans DJJ, et al. *Campylobacter pylori* detected noninvasively by the ^{13}C-urea breath test. *Lancet* 1987;1:1174–1177.

101. Marshall BJ, Surveyor I. Carbon-14 urea breath test for the diagnosis of *Campylobacter pylori* associated gastritis. *J Nucl Med* 1988;29:11–16.

102. Rauws EA, Royen EA, Langenberg W, Woensel JV, Vrij AA, Tytgat GN. ^{14}C-urea breath test in *C. pylori* gastritis. *Gut* 1989;30:798–803.

103. Debongnie JC, Pauwels S, Raat A, et al. Quantification of *Helicobacter pylori* infection in gastritis and ulcer disease using a simple and rapid carbon-14-urea breath test. *J Nucl Med* 1991;32:1192–1198.

104. Marshall BJ, Plankey MW, Hoffman SR, et al. A 20-minute breath test for *Helicobacter pylori*. *Am J Gastroenterol* 1991;86:438–445.

105. Rathbone BJ, Wyatt JI, Worsley BW, et al. Systemic and local antibody responses to gastric *Campylobacter pyloridis* in non-ulcer dyspepsia. *Gut* 1986;27:642–647.

106. Megraud F, Brassens Rabbe MP, Denis F, Belbouri A, Hoa DQ. Seroepidemiology of *Campylobacter pylori* infection in various populations. *J Clin Microbiol* 1989;27:1870–1873.

107. Reiff A, Jacobs E, Kist M. Seroepidemiological study of the immune response to *Campylobacter pylori* in potential risk groups. *Eur J Clin Microbiol Infect Dis* 1989;8:592–596.

108. von Wulffen H, Heisemann J, Butzow GH, Loning T, Laufs R. Detection of *Campylobacter pylori* in patients with antrum gastritis and peptic ulcers by culture, complement fixation tests and immunoblot. *J Clin Microbiol* 1986;24:716–722.

109. Marshall BJ, McGechie DB, Francis GJ, Utley PJ. Pyloric *Campylobacter* serology. *Lancet* 1984;2:281–283.

110. Kaldor J, Tee W, Nicolacopolous C, Demirtzoglon K, Noonan D, Dwyer B. Immunoblot confirmation of immune response to *Campylobacter pyloridis* in patients with duodenal ulcers. *Med J Aust* 1986;145:133–135.

111. Pérez-Pérez GI, Dunn BE. Diagnosis of *C. pylori* infection by serologic methods. In: Blaser MJ, ed. *Campylobacter pylori in gastritis and peptic ulcer disease*. New York: Igaku-Shoin; 1989:163–174.

112. Vaira D, Holton J, Cairns SR, et al. Antibody titers to *Campylobacter pylori* after treatment for gastritis. *Br Med J* 1988;297:397.

113. van Bohemen CG, Langenberg ML, Rauws EA, Oudbier J, Weterings E, Zanen HC. Rapidly decreased serum IgG to *Campylobacter pylori* following elimination of *Campylobacter* in histological chronic biopsy *Campylobacter*-positive gastritis. *Immunol Lett* 1989;20:59–61.

114. Kosunen TU, Seppala K, Sarna S, Sipponen P. Diagnostic value of decreasing IgG, IgA, and IgM antibody titres after eradication of *Helicobacter pylori*. *Lancet* 1992;339:893–895.

115. Smith MT, Dobek AS, Maydonovitch CL, et al. Salivary antibody response to *Helicobacter pylori*: a pilot study. *Gastroenterology* 1990;98:A127.

116. Pérez-Pérez GI, Dworkin BM, Chodos JE, Blaser MJ. *Campylobacter pylori* antibodies in humans. *Ann Intern Med* 1988;109:11–17.

117. Hirschl AM, Pletschette M, Hirschl MH, Berger J, Stanek G, Rotter ML. Comparison of different antigen preparations in an evaluation of the immune response to *Campylobacter pylori*. *Eur J Clin Microbiol Infect Dis* 1988;7:570–575.

118. Newell DG, Stacey A. Antigens for the serodiagnosis of *Campylobacter pylori* infections. *Gastroenterol Clin Biol* 1989;13:37B–41B.

119. Hirschl AM, Rathbone BJ, Wyatt JI, Berger J, Rotter ML. Comparison of ELISA antigen preparations alone or in combination for serodiagnosing *Helicobacter pylori* infections. *J Clin Pathol* 1990;43:511–513.

120. Andersen LP, Espersen F. Immunoglobulin G antibodies to *Helicobacter pylori* in patients with dyspeptic symptoms investigated by the western immunoblot technique. *J Clin Microbiol* 1992;30:1743–1751.

121. Van den Berg FM, Zijlmans H, Langenberg W, Rauws E, Schipper M. Detection of *Campylobacter pylori* in stomach tissue by DNA in situ hybridisation. *J Clin Pathol* 1989;42:995–1000.

122. Morotomi M, Hoshina S, Green P, et al. Oligonucleotide probe for detection and identification of *Campylobacter pylori*. *J Clin Microbiol* 1989;27:2652–2655.

123. Hoshina S, Kahn SM, Jiang W, et al. Direct detection and amplification of *Helicobacter pylori* ribosomal 16S gene segments from gastric endoscopic biopsies. *Diag Microbiol Infect Dis* 1990;13:473–479.

124. Valentine JL, Arthur RR, Mobley HL, Dick JD. Detection of *Helicobacter pylori* by using the polymerase chain reaction. *J Clin Microbiol* 1991;29:689–695.

125. Hammar M, Tyszkiewicz T, Wadstrom T, O'Toole PW. Rapid detection of *Helicobacter pylori* in gastric biopsy material by polymerase chain reaction. *J Clin Microbiol* 1992;30:54–58.

126. Westblom TU, Phadnis S, Yang P, Czinn SJ. Diagnosis of *Helicobacter pylori* infection by means of a polymerase chain reaction assay for gastric juice aspirates. *Clin Infect Dis* 1993;16:367–371.

127. Peek RM Jr, Miller GG, Tham KT, et al. Reverse transcription and polymerase chain reaction detection of *Helicobacter pylori* in gastric biopsies and in vivo expression of *H. pylori* genes. *Gastroenterology* 1994; (in press).

128. Wu JC, Liu GL, Zhang ZH, Mou YL, Chen QA, Yang SL. 15NH4+ excretion test: a new method for detection of Helicobacter pylori infection. *J Clin Microbiol* 1992;30:181–184.

129. Westblom TU. The comparative value of different diagnostic tests for *Helicobacter pylori*. In: Goodwin CS, Worsley BW, eds. *Helicobacter pylori biology and clinical practice*. Boca Raton: CRC Press; 1993:329–342.

130. Peterson WL. Pathogenesis and therapy of peptic ulcer disease. *J Clin Gastroenterol* 1990;12:S1–S6.

131. Blaser MJ. Hypotheses on the pathogenesis and natural history of *Helicobacter pylori*–induced inflammation. *Gastroenterology* 1992;102:720–727.

132. Blaser MJ, Parsonnet J. Parasitism by the "slow" bacterium *Helicobacter pylori* leads to altered gastric homeostasis and neoplasia. *J Clin Invest* 1994;94:4–8.

133. Karita M, Kouchiyama T, Okita K, Nakazawa T. New small animal model for human gastric *Helicobacter pylori* infection:

success in both nude and euthymic mice. *Am J Gastroenterol* 1991;86:1596–1603.

134. Fox JG, Paster BJ, Dewhirst FE, et al. Helicobacter mustelae isolation from feces of ferrets: evidence to support fecal-oral transmission of a gastric *Helicobacter*. *Infect Immun* 1992;60: 606–611.

135. Chen M, Lee A, Hazell S. Immunisation against gastric helicobacter infection in a mouse/Helicobacter felis model. *Lancet* 1992;339:1120–1121.

136. Suerbaum S, Josenhans C, Labigne A. Cloning and genetic characterization of the Helicobacter pylori and Helicobacter mustelae flaB flagellin genes and construction of H. pylori flaA- and flaB-negative mutants by electroporation-mediated allelic exchange. *J Bacteriol* 1993;175:3278–3288.

137. Dunn BE, Campbell GP, Pérez-Pérez GI, Blaser MJ. Purification and characterization of *Helicobacter pylori* urease. *J Biol Chem* 1990;265:9464–9469.

138. Hu LT, Mobley HL. Purification and N-terminal analysis of urease from *Helicobacter pylori*. *Infect Immun* 1990;58: 992–998.

139. Eaton KA, Brooks CL, Morgan DR, Krakowka S. Essential role of urease in pathogenesis of gastritis induced by *Helicobacter pylori* in gnotobiotic piglets. *Infect Immun* 1991;59: 2470–2475.

140. Marshall BJ, Barrett LJ, Prakash C, McCallum RW, Guerrant RL. Urea protects Helicobacter (*Campylobacter*) *pylori* from the bactericidal effect of acid. *Gastroenterology* 1990;99: 697–702.

141. McGowan CC, Cover TL, Blaser MJ. The proton pump inhibitor, omeprazole, inhibits survival of *Helicobacter pylori* at low pH by a urease-independent mechanism. *Gastroenterology* 1994; (*in press*).

142. Cussac V, Ferrero RL, Labigne A. Expression of *Helicobacter pylori* urease genes in *Escherichia coli* grown under nitrogen-limiting conditions. *J Bacteriol* 1992;174:2466–2473.

143. Hazell SL, Evans DJJ, Graham DY. *Helicobacter pylori* catalase. *J Gen Microbiol* 1991;137:57–61.

144. Vargas M, Lee A, Fox JG, Cave DR. Inhibition of acid secretion from parietal cells by non-human-infecting *Helicobacter* species—a factor in colonization of gastric mucosa. *Infect Immun* 1991;59:3694–3699.

145. Evans DG, Evans DJJ, Moulds JJ, Graham DY. N-Acetylneuraminyllactose-binding fibrillar hemagglutinin of *Campylobacter pylori*: a putative colonization factor antigen. *Infect Immun* 1988;56:2896–2906.

146. Fauchere J-L, Blaser MJ. Adherence of *Helicobacter pylori* cells and superficial components to HeLa cell membranes. *Microb Pathog* 1990;9:427–439.

147. Lingwood CA, Cheng M, Krivan HC, Woods D. Glycolipid receptor binding specificity of exoenzyme S from *Pseudomonas aeruginosa*. *Biochem Biophys Res Commun* 1991;175: 1076–1081.

148. Boren T, Falk P, Roth KA, Larson G, Normark S. Attachment of *Helicobacter pylori* to human gastric epithelium mediated by blood group antigens. *Science* 1993;262:1892–1895.

149. Lingwood CA, Huesca M, Kuksis A. The glycerolipid receptor for Helicobacter pylori (and exoenzyme S) is phosphatidylethanolamine. *Infect Immun* 1992;60:2470–2474.

150. Mooney C, Keenan J, Munster D, et al. Neutrophil activation by *Helicobacter pylori*. *Gut* 1991;32:853–857.

151. Mai UEH, Pérez-Pérez GI, Wahl LM, Wahl SM, Blaser MJ, Smith PD. Soluble surface proteins from *Helicobacter pylori* activate monocytes/macrophages by lipopolysaccharide-independent mechanism. *J Clin Invest* 1991;87:894–900.

152. Mai UE, Pérez-Pérez GI, Allen JB, Wahl SM, Blaser MJ, Smith PD. Surface proteins from *Helicobacter pylori* exhibit chemotactic activity for human leukocytes and are present in gastric mucosa. *J Exp Med* 1992;175:517–525.

153. Crabtree JE, Shallcross TM, Heatley RV, Wyatt JI. Mucosal tumour necrosis factor alpha and interleukin-6 in patients with *Helicobacter pylori* associated gastritis. *Gut* 1991;32: 1473–1477.

154. Slomiany BL, Nishikawa H, Piotrowski J, Okazaki K, Slomi-

any A. Lipolytic activity of *Campylobacter pylori*: effect of sofalcone. *Digestion* 1989;43:33–40.

155. Lewis RA, Austin KF, Soberman RJ. Leukotrienes and other products of the 5-lipoxygenase pathway. *N Engl J Med* 1990; 323:645–651.

156. Weitkamp JH, Pérez-Pérez GI, Bode G, Malfertheiner P, Blaser MJ. Identification and characterization of *Helicobacter pylori* phospholipase C activity. *Zent Bacteriol* 1993;280:11–27.

157. Denizot Y, Sobhani I, Rambaud JC, Lewin M, Thomas Y, Benveniste J. Paf-acether synthesis by *Helicobacter pylori*. *Gut* 1990;31:1242–1245.

158. Born W, Happ MP, Dallas A, et al. Recognition of heat shock proteins and gamma-delta cell function. *Immunol Today* 1990; 11:40–46.

159. Negrini R, Lisato L, Zanella I, et al. *Helicobacter pylori* infection induces antibodies cross-reacting with human gastric mucosa. *Gastroenterology* 1991;101:437–445.

160. Scheynius A, Engstrand L. Gastric epithelial cells in *Helicobacter pylori*–associated gastritis express HLA-DR but not ICAM-1. *Scand J Immunol* 1991;33:237–241.

161. Engstrand L, Scheynius A, Pahlson C. An increased number of gamma/delta T-cells and gastric epithelial cell expression of the groEL stress-protein homologue in *Helicobacter pylori*–associated chronic gastritis of the antrum. *Am J Gastroenterol* 1991;86:976–980.

162. Dunn BE, Roop RM, Sung C-C, Sharma SA, Pérez-Pérez GI, Blaser MJ. Identification and purification of a cpn 60 heat shock protein homolog from *Helicobacter pylori*. *Infect Immun* 1992; 60:1946–1951.

163. Pérez-Pérez GI, Blaser MJ. Conservation and diversity of *Campylobacter pyloridis* major antigens. *Infect Immun* 1987; 55:1256–1263.

164. Muotiala A, Helander IM, Pyhala L, Kosunen TU, Moran AP. Low biological activity of *Helicobacter pylori* lipopolysaccharide. *Infect Immun* 1992;60:1714–1716.

165. Wolfe MM, Soll AH. The physiology of gastric acid secretion. *N Engl J Med* 1988;319:1707–1714.

166. Sankey EA, Helliwell, Dhillon AP. Immunostaining of antral gastrin cells is quantitatively increased in *Helicobacter pylori* gastritis. *Histopathology* 1990;16:151–156.

167. Graham DY, Opekun A, Lew GM, Evans DJJ, Klein PD, Evans DG. Ablation of exaggerated meal-stimulated gastrin release in duodenal ulcer patients after clearance of Helicobacter (*Campylobacter*) *pylori* infection. *Am J Gastroenterol* 1990;85: 394–398.

168. Levi S, Beardshall K, Swift I, et al. Antral *Helicobacter pylori*, hypergastrinaemia, and duodenal ulcers: effect of eradicating the organism. *Br Med J* 1989;299:1504–1505.

169. Strauss RM, Wang TC, Kelsey PB, et al. Association of *Helicobacter pylori* infection with dyspeptic symptoms in patients undergoing gastroduodenoscopy. *Am J Med* 1990;89:464–469.

170. el-Omar E, Penman I, Dorrian CA, Ardill JES, Mccoll KEL. Eradicating *Helicobacter pylori* infection lowers gastrin mediated acid secretion by two thirds in patients with duodenal ulcer. *Gut* 1994;34:1060–1065.

171. Chittajallu RS, Neithercut WD, Macdonald AM, McColl KE. Effect of increasing *Helicobacter pylori* ammonia production by urea infusion on plasma gastrin concentrations. *Gut* 1991; 32:21–24.

172. Graham DY, Opekun A, Lew GM, Klein PD, Walsh JH. *Helicobacter pylori*–associated exaggerated gastrin release in duodenal ulcer patients. The effect of bombesin infusion and urea ingestion. *Gastroenterology* 1991;100:1571–1575.

173. Cover TL, Reddy LY, Blaser MJ. Effects of ATPase inhibitors on the response of HeLa cells to *Helicobacter pylori* vacuolating toxin. *Infect Immun J* 1993;61:1427–1431.

174. Cover TL, Blaser MJ. Purification and characterization of the vacuolating toxin from *Helicobacter pylori*. *J Biol Chem* 1992; 267:10570–10575.

175. Cover TL, Tummuru MKR, Cao P, Thompson SA, Blaser MJ. Divergence of genetic sequences for the vacuolating cytotoxin among *Helicobacter pylori* strains. *J Biol Chem* 1994;269: 10566–10573.

176. Phadnis SH, Ilver D, Janzon L, Normark S, Westblom TU.

Pathological significance and molecular characterization of the vacuolating toxin gene of *Helicobacter pylori*. *Infect Immun* 1994;62:1557–1565.

177. Schmitt W, Haas R. Genetic analysis of the *Helicobacter pylori* vacuolating cytotoxin: structural similarities with the IgA protease type of exported protein. *Mol Microbiol* 1994;12:307–319.

178. Telford JL, Ghiara P, Dell'Orco M, et al. Gene structure of the *Helicobacter pylori* cytotoxin and evidence of its key role in gastric disease. *J Exp Med* 1994;179:1653–1658.

179. Figura N, Guglielmetti P, Rossolini A, et al. Cytotoxin production by *Campylobacter pylori* strains isolated from patients with peptic ulcers and from patients with chronic gastritis only. *J Clin Microbiol* 1989;27:225–226.

180. Tummuru MKR, Cover TL, Blaser MJ. Mutation of the cytotoxin-associated *cagA* gene does not affect the vacuolating cytotoxin activity of *Helicobacter pylori*. *Infect Immun* 1994;62:2609–2613.

181. Hupertz V, Czinn S. Demonstration of a cytotoxin from *Campylobacter pylori*. *Eur J Clin Microbiol Infect Dis* 1988;7:576–578.

182. Smoot DT, Mobley HL, Chippendale GR, Lewison JF, Resau JH. *Helicobacter pylori* urease activity is toxic to human gastric epithelial cells. *Infect Immun* 1990;58:1992–1994.

183. Triebling AT, Korsten MA, Dlugosz JW, Paronetto F, Lieber CS. Severity of *Helicobacter*-induced gastric injury correlates with gastric juice ammonia. *Dig Dis Sci* 1991;36:1089–1096.

184. Tsujii M, Kawano S, Tsuji S, et al. Cell kinetics of mucosal atrophy in rat stomach induced by long-term administration of ammonia. *Gastroenterology* 1993;104:796–801.

185. Lee A, Fox J, Hazell S. The pathogenicity of *Helicobacter pylori*: a perspective. *Infect Immun J* 1993;661:1601–1610.

186. Sarosiek J, Bilski J, Murty VL, Slomiany A, Slomiany BL. Colloidal bismuth subcitrate (De-Nol) inhibits degradation of gastric mucus by *Campylobacter pylori* protease. *Am J Gastroenterol* 1989;84:506–510.

187. Sidebotham RL, Batten JJ, Karim QN, Spencer J, Baron JH. Breakdown of gastric mucus in presence of *Helicobacter pylori*. *J Clin Pathol* 1991;44:52–57.

188. Goggin PM, Northfield TC, Spychal RT. Factors affecting gastric mucosal hydrophobicity in man. *Scand J Gastroenterol (Suppl)* 1991;181:65–73.

189. Roine RP, Salmela KS, Hook Nikanne J, Kosunen TU, Salaspuro M. Alcohol dehydrogenase mediated acetaldehyde production by *Helicobacter pylori*—a possible mechanism behind gastric injury. *Life Sci* 1992;51:1333–1337.

Infections of the Gastrointestinal Tract,
edited by M. J. Blaser, P. D. Smith, J. I. Ravdin,
H. B. Greenberg, and R. L. Guerrant
Raven Press, Ltd., New York © 1995.

CHAPTER **40**

Epidemiology and Natural History of *Helicobacter pylori* Infection

David N. Taylor and Julie Parsonnet

Since *Helicobacter pylori* was first isolated 10 years ago, this organism has aroused widespread interest. *Helicobacter pylori* is the only organism known to live in the human stomach and has changed our understanding of the stomach as a barrier to bacteria. Epidemiologic studies have defined *Helicobacter* infection as having a worldwide distribution and it rivals *Streptococcus mutans,* the cause of tooth decay, as one of the most common human pathogens. Although much has been learned about the risk factors for acquisition of infection, relatively little is known about transmission. *Helicobacter pylori* infection is usually acquired silently without knowledge of the time of exposure, the source, or the magnitude of the infecting dose. Little is known about the role of host factors in preventing infection or the possibility of spontaneously clearing the infection.

Helicobacter pylori infection causes superficial gastritis that persists for years, leading to chronic inflammation. The response to *H. pylori* infection is highly variable. Infection may involve the entire stomach or be restricted to either antrum or corpus. Antral gastritis caused by *H. pylori* is associated with gastric ulcers. The duodenum, which is normally resistant to infection because of its small intestinal mucosa, may become infected when gastric metaplasia occurs, greatly increasing risk for duodenal ulceration. Most importantly, eradication of infection in either the antrum or duodenum prevents ulcer relapse. Inflammation may progress and result in loss of glandular structures in the stomach (atrophic gastritis) and/or reactive growth of intestinal-type tissue within the stomach (intestinal metaplasia). Atrophic gastritis appears to be an important predisposing factor in gastric cancer. The factors that determine the diverse responses

are not known but may include age at acquisition of infection, host immune response, characteristics of the infecting organism, or environmental exposures. The site of infection within the stomach and its progression over time may determine the outcomes of *H. pylori* infection (i.e., gastritis, cancer, or ulcer). Perhaps the most perplexing aspect of *H. pylori* epidemiology is the high infection/disease ratio. Only a small percentage of infections are associated with peptic ulcer disease or gastric cancer, suggesting that other factors must be involved to manifest these diseases. Understanding the interplay of *H. pylori* infection with other factors is the greatest challenge.

DESCRIPTIVE EPIDEMIOLOGY

Prevalence by Age and Sex

Helicobacter pylori has been detected in nearly every population in the world by direct isolation of the organism from the stomach or by indirect measurements such as serum antibody or urea breath tests. *Helicobacter pylori* infection can be acquired at any age from infant to adult. Seroepidemiologic studies indicate that the prevalence of infection increases with age. The magnitude of the immunoglobulin (Ig) G serologic response to infection is remarkably constant over time. Among a U.S. adult population who were tested 8 years apart, the serum antibody titers among those who were seropositive both times were similar, indicating that the serologic response to infection is chronic and constant (1). Since *H. pylori* infection lasts years to decades and can be lifelong, the age-specific seroprevalence curves reflect the cumulative infection rate. Studies from the developed world, including North America, Europe, Australia, and Japan, demonstrate an increase in prevalence with increasing age (2). The continuous increase suggests that infection occurs in all age groups. In most developed countries the rate of increase

D. N. Taylor: Department of Clinical Trials, Walter Reed Army Institute of Research, Washington, DC 20307-5100.
J. Parsonnet: Departments of Medicine and of Health Research and Policy, Stanford University Medical School, Stanford, California 94305.

551

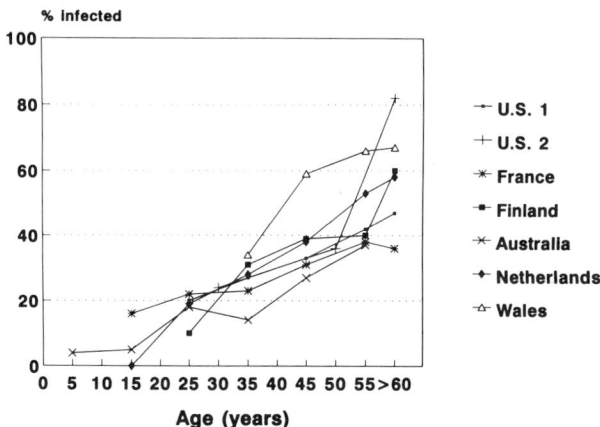

FIG. 1. Relationship between age and prevalence of *Helicobacter pylori* infection among healthy persons in developed countries. U.S. 1 (*n* = 113), U.S. 2 (*n* = 53), France (*n* = 1199), Finland (*n* = 500), Australia (*n* = 785), Netherlands (*n* = 401), Wales (*n* = 1175).

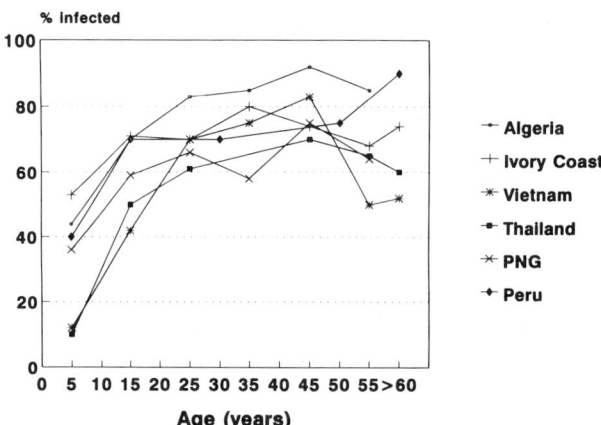

FIG. 2. Relationship between age and prevalence of *Helicobacter pylori* among healthy persons in developing countries. Algeria (*n* = 277), Ivory Coast (*n* = 374), Vietnam (*n* = 365), Thailand (*n* = 161), Papua–New Guinea (PNG) (*n* = 157), Peru (*n* = 361).

is about 1% per year (Fig. 1). The prevalence at age 20 is about 20% and 50% of the population is infected at age 55 or 60 years. However, there is considerable variation between population groups even within the United States. For example, among 366 public health officers studied from age 30 to 50, the annual seroconversion rate was 0.49% (1). In this high socioeconomic group the rate of new infections was low in adults. In contrast, the calculated infection rate among 1000 U.S. army recruits 17 to 26 years old was 2.5% per year (3). Follow-up studies after treatment in developed countries suggest that the rate of reinfection is 2% or less per year (4–7). Thus, among adults in developed countries, the prevalence of the infection increases with age and the incidence is low (0% to 5% per year). *Helicobacter pylori* prevalence is especially high among persons at an institution for the mentally retarded, where annual incidence was determined as 5% per year in an Australian study (8). In this regard the seroepidemiology of *H. pylori* resembles hepatitis A with a higher incidence in institutionalized populations.

Helicobacter pylori infection rates are considerably higher among populations in developing countries. The seroprevalence curves depicting infection rates from developing world populations indicate that, at age 20, at least 60% are infected and, in some areas, 50% of persons are infected by age 5 (9,10). Unlike the steady rise in seroprevalence seen in the developed world, infection occurs early in childhood in the developing world (11). After childhood there is little correlation of *H. pylori* prevalence with age in the developing world because such a large part of the population is already infected (Fig. 2). Indicative of the high rate of childhood infection in developing countries, immigrants to developed countries have a high rate of infection, which they retain for their lifetimes (12,13). Within the developing world institutionalized populations have high infection rates. For example, in a Thai urban orphanage, 74% of children 1 to 4 years old were seropositive compared to 18% of children 5 to 9 years old living

in villages (10). Thus, in developing countries, *H. pylori* infection is acquired earlier in life and more frequently than in developed countries.

A decrease in infection rate has become evident in countries that have undergone rapid socioeconomic development. This apparent change in infection rate by birth cohort has been described in Japan, where persons born after 1950 have a rate of rise of about 1% per year while Japanese born before 1950 have a rate two to three times higher (14). Declining rates of infection have also been observed in the United States and in Europe (1,15). For example, *H. pylori* prevalence declined from 22% among professionals in the U.S. Public Health Service born from 1940 to 1944 to 12% among those born from 1955 to 1959 (1) (Fig. 3). Since age at the time of infection may be a risk factor for gastric cancer, a delay in acquisition of infection may be associated with a decrease in cancer rate.

In a number of studies in both developed and developing countries, the age-specific prevalence of infection in men and women was nearly equal (2,9). Among U.S. military recruits, women had higher seroprevalence rates than men (32% versus 22%) (3). Women had higher rates in all race–ethnic groups, but the gender difference was especially prominent among Hispanics and blacks. Similarly, in a study of children in Arkansas, black girls had higher infection rates than black boys (16). Chilean women were more likely to be infected than Chilean men (39% versus 28%) (17). However, no differences were observed among Peruvians (18). Mothers of children who were infected with *H. pylori* were more likely to be infected than their fathers, suggesting that women may be important in transmitting *H. pylori* to children (19). Other data suggest that a female predominance may not be correct.

Race–Ethnic Differences

Helicobacter pylori infection is highly associated with race or ethnic group. In the United States among adults,

Percent infected

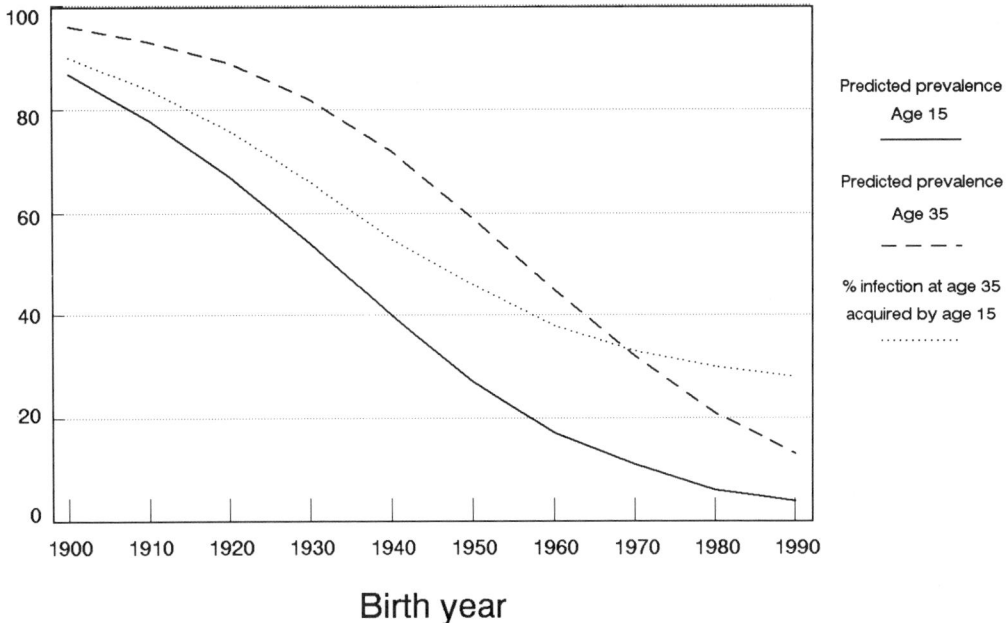

FIG. 3. Modeling of the birth year cohort effect of *Helicobacter pylori* infection. In a study done using sera collected from 341 people between 1969 and 1987, the prevalence of *H. pylori* infection by age and year of birth was modeled using logistic regression. The model indicates that persons born early in the century are more likely to have infection than persons born later. Persons born early in the century are also more likely to have acquired their infection in childhood (before age 15 years). (Data from ref. 1.)

healthy Hispanic and black populations have seropositivity rates several-fold higher than non-Hispanic white populations (2,3,20). In a Maryland study, the overall seropositivity rate among blacks was 57% compared with 26% for whites (21) and was independent of age, gender, dietary practice, and geographic location (urban versus rural). The frequency of *H. pylori* infection was higher in blacks (70%) than whites (34%) in a study of 485 asymptomatic adults in Houston, Texas (22), which also remained significant after adjustments for age, gender, educational level, current income, and use of tobacco or alcohol. In a Denver study of men attending a clinic for sexually transmitted diseases, 42% of healthy Hispanic and black men were seropositive compared to 12% among non-Hispanic, white men (23). The reasons for these highly significant differences in seroprevalence rates among race–ethnic groups are not well understood, but socioeconomic conditions during childhood such as crowding, poor sanitation, and close contact with infected persons appear to be important risk factors.

Among military recruits aged 17 to 18 years, the prevalence of *H. pylori* infection was 41% for blacks, 26% for Hispanics, and 14% for whites (3). To achieve these rates requires a constant annual infection rate from birth of 3% for blacks, 1.7% for Hispanics, and 0.7% for whites. However, from age 17 to 26 years, the rate of increase was about 2.5% per year for nonwhite and white populations. These data suggest that there is constant high incidence

of infection in nonwhite populations so that 60% are infected by age 25. In contrast, among white populations the incidence increases from less than 1% per year below the age of 20 to 2.5% per year during young adulthood. This conclusion is also compatible with the age-associated prevalence data from Houston and suggests that at least in white populations risk of infection actually increases during young adulthood (22).

Studies from outside the United States suggest that the race–ethnic differences are more a reflection of poor socioeconomic conditions and crowding, rather than related to genetic factors. In New Zealand, infection rates among adults were high in native populations (39% to 70%) and low in white New Zealanders (15%) (24). The exception is Australian aborigines who have *H. pylori* infection rates of only 0.5% compared to 15% of Caucasian Australians (25). That duodenal ulcers are also rare in this group of aborigines lends support to the hypothesis that *H. pylori* may be a necessary factor for the development of duodenal ulcers. In Singapore, ethnic Chinese have a rate of peptic ulcer disease that is seven times higher than that of Malaysians (26). Similarly, antral gastritis and *H. pylori* infection are twice as common in Singapore Chinese. Whether these differences reflect an increase in susceptibility among certain ethnic groups, or differences in type of and extent of exposure to *H. pylori* remains to be determined.

Socioeconomic Differences

Helicobacter pylori infection is more prevalent in low socioeconomic groups. In the United States low socioeconomic groups may be defined in terms of income or years of education. *Helicobacter pylori* infection was more common in low-income than in high-income families in an Arkansas study of 247 healthy children and in a Texas study of 485 adults living in Houston (16,22). Since infection is often acquired during childhood, particularly in nonwhite populations in the developed world, socioeconomic factors of the parents may better reflect seropositivity rates. Similarly, in Wales, age-adjusted *H. pylori* infection rates were highest in the lowest social classes (62%), less in the middle class (57%), and least in the higher classes (49%) (27).

Similar trends were observed in developing world populations. In Saudi Arabia, *H. pylori* infections were found in 77% of non-college graduates and 54% of college graduates (28). In Peru, among persons less than 30 years old, *H. pylori* seropositivity rates were 88% and 82% in men and women in public clinics, respectively, and 66% and 43% in men and women in private clinics, respectively (18).

Geographic Differences

The geographic distribution of gastric and duodenal ulcers is not uniform and thus the risk factors for these illnesses may not be uniform (29). Differences in seropositivity rates were observed among the various geographic regions of the United States (3). In general, seroprevalence rates in young adults are higher in the South (31%). However, when racial distribution patterns were taken into account, the geographic differences were not significant. Minor geographic differences have also been noted in a study from Peru that found higher rates of infection among inhabitants of the mostly rural interior of Peru (30).

MECHANISMS AND ROUTES OF TRANSMISSION

The natural host for *H. pylori* is humans. Person-to-person spread is likely the dominant mode of transmission although controversy exists over whether fecal–oral or oral–oral spread predominates. The high infection rates among persons in developing countries, institutionalized populations, and low socioeconomic groups suggest fecal–oral transmission similar to the epidemiology observed with hepatitis A.

By maintaining specimens under microaerobic conditions, *H. pylori* was isolated from the feces of 9 of 23 children from The Gambia, an area that is hyperendemic for *H. pylori* where more than 90% of children under 5 years old are infected (31). This study was the first to demonstrate that *H. pylori* could pass from the stomach through the entire gut. Although special care was used in handling specimens, isolation was also aided by extremely rapid intestinal transit times in these children. *Helico-*

bacter pylori was most recently isolated from the feces of adult dyspeptic patients in England using the same methods (32). Studies from the ferret animal model suggest that hypochlorhydria might also aid in the transmission of viable organisms in the feces (33).

Oral–oral transmission is also a possibility. *Helicobacter pylori* has been isolated directly from dental plaque (34) and saliva (35), and, by the polymerase chain reaction, the *H. pylori* genome has been detected in dental plaque and saliva (36–38). An *H. pylori* strain isolated from saliva was identical to the strain colonizing the stomach (35). However, rates of infection among dental workers were not elevated compared to age-matched control groups (39).

Whether by oral–oral or fecal–oral transmission, intrafamilial spread appears to occur in North American and European populations (19,40–42). When a parent is infected, the other family members are also likely to be infected. Crowded or unsanitary conditions may be risk factors for adults. German submarine crews had higher seroprevalence rates than other military personnel, suggesting that crowding on board a submarine may be a risk factor for *Helicobacter* infection (43). Among 206 U.S. soldiers deployed to the Persian Gulf, there were five seroconversions to *H. pylori*. In this group of 107 soldiers who were susceptible, five seroconverted during the 7.5-month deployment for a 4.6% rate during that time. The seroconversion rate per year during deployment was 7.6% or three times higher than if the soldiers had stayed at home (3).

Traveler's diarrhea is usually acquired through ingestion of contaminated food and water. So if *Helicobacter* infection was found to be travel related, food and water would be likely sources. In Lima, Peru, persons who drank from the municipal water system had a much higher risk of *H. pylori* infection than did persons who drank from private wells (44). This association was significant across socioeconomic groups. Nonculturable *H. pylori* organisms were detected in river water, suggesting that *H. pylori* can remain dormant in water for months (45). In Chile consumption of uncooked vegetables was associated with higher rates of *H. pylori* infection (46). While these studies from Latin America are suggestive, numerous confounding variables make these data difficult to interpret. In developed countries there is no epidemiologic evidence to suggest foodborne or waterborne transmission. Vegetarians, for example, were at equal risk for infection as meat-eaters in England (47). A study of Seventh Day Adventists in Maryland, another vegetarian group, also showed no significant differences in *H. pylori* infection rates compared with meat-eating controls (21). In another survey, Canadian farmers had higher seroprevalence rates at younger ages than did other Canadians without animal exposure (48). Whether these data indicate higher rates of infection with human strains of *H. pylori* is not yet known; and if so, socioeconomic differences might be important. Seropositivity rates were found to be higher in Italian abattoir workers than clerks who had no exposure to animal parts (49), although there were numerous confounding factors.

Person-to-Person Transmission

Transmission in Institutionalized Populations

Helicobacter pylori seropositivity rates are higher in persons living in institutions. For example, at a Bangkok orphanage H. pylori seropositivity was 74% in children 2 to 4 years old, well above the rates in children living in rural Thailand (10). In Australia inmates of a mental institution were much more frequently H. pylori seropositive than were healthy blood donors (50). Similarly, in Germany, persons living in closed communities such as psychiatric centers and orphanages had higher seropositivity rates than did control groups (51).

Sexual Transmission

There is little evidence for transmission between couples (12). Nor is there a correlation with sexual preference, number of sexual partners, history of sexually transmitted diseases, or human immunodeficiency virus (HIV) status among those infected with H. pylori compared with those who were not infected (23). There is no evidence to suggest sexual transmission of H. pylori.

Iatrogenic Transmission

Transmission of H. pylori in the endoscopy suite can occur. Patient-to-patient transmission by an endoscope was proved by isolation of the identical strain of H. pylori from patients undergoing procedures in the same endoscopy suite (52). The endoscope had been mechanically cleaned between patients using a detergent and treated with 70% ethanol. The frequency of endoscopic transmission of H. pylori infection was 3 for every 1000 gastroduodenoscopies (52). Contact with secretions from infected patients may also subject endoscopists to risk of infection. The prevalence of H. pylori infection in a group of gastroenterologists was 52%, compared with 21% in an age-matched group of blood donors ($p < 0.01$) (53).

NATURAL HISTORY OF HELICOBACTER PYLORI INFECTION

Helicobacter pylori infection, once acquired, persists as evidenced by the isolation of strains with identical restriction endonuclease profiles from infected persons taken on multiple occasions over several years (54). Follow-up over 1 to 2 years indicates that the infection is stable, with little change in histologic grading of gastritis or fluctuation of antibody titer (4). Prolonged elevation of serum antibody titers also suggests that infection persists for years, decades, or possibly for life. Spontaneous eradication of infection with gastric healing may occur but is probably uncommon (55). Eradication of H. pylori usually results in a healing, or at least a pronounced improvement, of gastritis in adults and children (7,56). Chronic

superficial gastritis caused by H. pylori may be either symptomatic or asymptomatic. Early in the course of infection there may be changes in acid secretion. Later in the course, infection may be associated with non-ulcer dyspepsia, peptic ulcer disease, type B atrophic gastritis, or gastric carcinoma. The progression of H. pylori infection chronic superficial gastritis to one of these syndromes may require cofactors, including genetic predisposition, smoking, alcohol, and diet (57–59). Finally, differences in the virulence properties of H. pylori strains may have an impact on disease progression.

Acute Symptomatic Gastritis

The acute infection and incubation periods associated with H. pylori infection were best observed in two self-inoculation experiments (60,61). Each experimenter had a normal gastric biopsy prior to ingestion of H. pylori. Seven days after swallowing 10^9 H. pylori organisms after inhibition of gastric acidity, an Australian experimenter developed epigastric distress and general irritability (60). Gastroscopy showed antral gastritis associated with H. pylori. He began treatment with tinidazole, had no further symptoms, and did not develop an antibody response to the organism. This infection induced an acute self-limited gastritis.

A New Zealand investigator ingested 3×10^5 H. pylori organisms after first neutralizing stomach acidity (61). He developed severe epigastric pain, stomach cramping, nausea, vomiting, and insomnia after 3 days. He continued to have mild abdominal symptoms until day 11 when his symptoms ceased. On day 5, biopsies showed intense inflammation of the antrum, normal histologic appearance of the gastric fundus, and a gastric pH of 1.2. By day 8, fasting gastric pH was 7.6. Following infection, he had an early, transient IgM seroconversion, and later he had seroconversion in both IgA and IgG. After a 4-week course of bismuth, organisms and pathology cleared (61). However, re-biopsy a year later showed the recurrence of both H. pylori and chronic inflammation (62). The infection, pathology, and specific immune response persisted for more than 3 years until combination antimicrobial therapy was successful (62).

Hypochlorhydria with Acute Gastritis

As evidenced by the second volunteer's case, hypochlorhydria may accompany the gastritis in the earliest phase of H. pylori infection. Several outbreaks of acute onset hypochlorhydria with marked gastritis have been reported following gastric secretion studies (63,64). Four of six persons developed an acute upper gastrointestinal illness after undergoing gastric secretion studies in England in which gastric juice was extracted and assessed with a common pH electrode and then reinfused (63). They became markedly hypochlorhydric, with severe gastritis, and retrospective examination showed organisms with the same appearance as H. pylori in the biopsies (65). In another outbreak that occurred in Texas, 46% of 37 healthy volunteers who underwent gastric secretion studies developed hypochlorhydria (64). About 1 week after intubation occurred, subjects became ill, with epigastric pain, nausea, and vomiting lasting 1 to 4 days. An increased pH was detected 7 to 49 days (mean 25 days) after the illness began and occurred in some subjects who did not develop symptoms. The duration of hypochlorhydria was 2 to 8 months (mean 4 months). During periods of hypochlorhydria all patients had severe fundal and antral gastritis. A retrospective analysis of the biopsy and serum specimens suggested that this outbreak was caused by *H. pylori,* apparently introduced into the stomachs of volunteers by a contaminated pH electrode (64). Serologic response to *H. pylori* antigens was also demonstrated in most of these patients. Intraluminal acid levels are normal in dyspeptic patients with and without *H. pylori* despite increases in gastrin level in the *H. pylori*-infected patients (66).

Asymptomatic Infection

Most infected persons do not have symptoms despite histologic evidence of inflammation at the site of *H. pylori* infection. Histologic gastritis is a relatively common finding in asymptomatic populations. In a study conducted in Los Angeles, California, inflammation was detected in gastric biopsies in 37% of 113 adult volunteers who had no upper gastrointestinal symptoms (67).

Chronic Gastritis

The characteristic pathologic lesion caused by *H. pylori* is chronic superficial gastritis (also called chronic active gastritis), an acute and chronic inflammatory process of the gastric submucosa. Superficial gastritis is very rarely found in the absence of *H. pylori* (68). In longitudinal studies in Finland, Estonia, and Colombia, chronic superficial gastritis has been found to be a lifelong disease (69–72). Furthermore, the extent and degree of gastritis are fairly stable. In a 6-year, population-based, follow-up study, little change in superficial gastritis occurred over time in adults although antral gastritis occasionally healed in young children (73). In the longest follow-up study, gastritis in 377 subjects largely remained unchanged or slowly progressed over 30 to 34 years (71).

Because superficial gastritis is chronic and unremitting, it has been presumed that *H. pylori* behaves similarly. There is little reason to doubt this is the case. Despite a decade of *H. pylori* research, there has yet to be one documented spontaneous cure of naturally acquired infection. Serologic data also cast doubt on spontaneous eradication of infection. In subjects tested for *H. pylori* antibodies twice (with a mean of 8 years between serum samples), titers remained remarkably stable over time (1). Fifty-seven (90%) of 63 subjects who initially had positive titers for *H. pylori* IgG remained positive years later. Of the six subjects whose sera reverted to negative, only two had the 50% drop in titer one might expect with elimination of infection (74). While the titer drop in these two

subjects could have represented spontaneous cure, a laboratory error or acquired hypoglobulinemia could also explain the finding. It remains possible, however, that a scattered handful of persons can naturally eradicate *H. pylori*.

In approximately 3% to 5% of persons per year, chronic superficial gastritis progresses to chronic atrophic gastritis (72,75,76). In gastric atrophy, there is destruction of gastric glands resulting in hypochlorhydria and loss of digestive proenzymes, particularly pepsinogens (77). While atrophic gastritis of the antrum tends to heal with aging, atrophic gastritis of the body tends to be progressive (71). As corpus atrophy worsens, patches of intestinal metaplasia arise and the gastric epithelium transforms to either small or large bowel morphology. The abnormal mucosa of atrophic gastritis and intestinal metaplasia are inhospitable to *H. pylori* and biopsies taken from these areas yield no organisms (78–80). In patients with these lesions, however, *H. pylori* will very often continue to be identified in nonatrophic locations of the stomach (81). Some elderly subjects with extensive atrophic gastritis and/or intestinal metaplasia may have no *H. pylori* in any of multiple gastric biopsies. In the majority of these subjects, anti-*H. pylori* IgG will be found in serologic assays, suggesting smoldering, low-grade infection (78,81–83). Some investigators maintain, however, that *H. pylori* can be completely lost and antibody responses disappear when gastric epithelium is entirely replaced by atrophic or metaplastic tissue. This theory has been invoked to explain the drop in *H. pylori* seroprevalence seen in the oldest age groups (14).

While gastric atrophy and intestinal metaplasia rarely occur in the absence of *H. pylori*-related superficial gastritis (one exception being pernicious anemia), it is not known whether *H. pylori* directly plays a part in destruction of glands and epithelial transformation. In support of a causal role, one study has suggested that cytotoxin-producing strains of *H. pylori* are more common in persons with chronic atrophic gastritis than in persons with only chronic superficial gastritis (84). In the ferret model, gastric atrophy develops after prolonged infection with a related *Helicobacter, H. mustalae* (85). An important hypothesis, however, is that dietary factors—in particular, low intake of dietary antioxidants such as beta-carotene and ascorbic acid—are responsible for progressive transformation of the gastric mucosa (86).

Gastric Cancer

Gastric cancer is second only to lung cancer as a cause of cancer death worldwide (87). In many countries of Latin America and Asia, gastric cancer is the most common malignancy among men and the second most common among women with incidence rates up to 80 per 100,000 per year (88,89). In the United States, where socioeconomic and hygienic factors have improved dramatically over the last century, the incidence of gastric cancer has plummeted from being the most common form of cancer in the 1930s, to the ninth most common in the 1980s; it now afflicts less than 10 per 100,000 persons per year

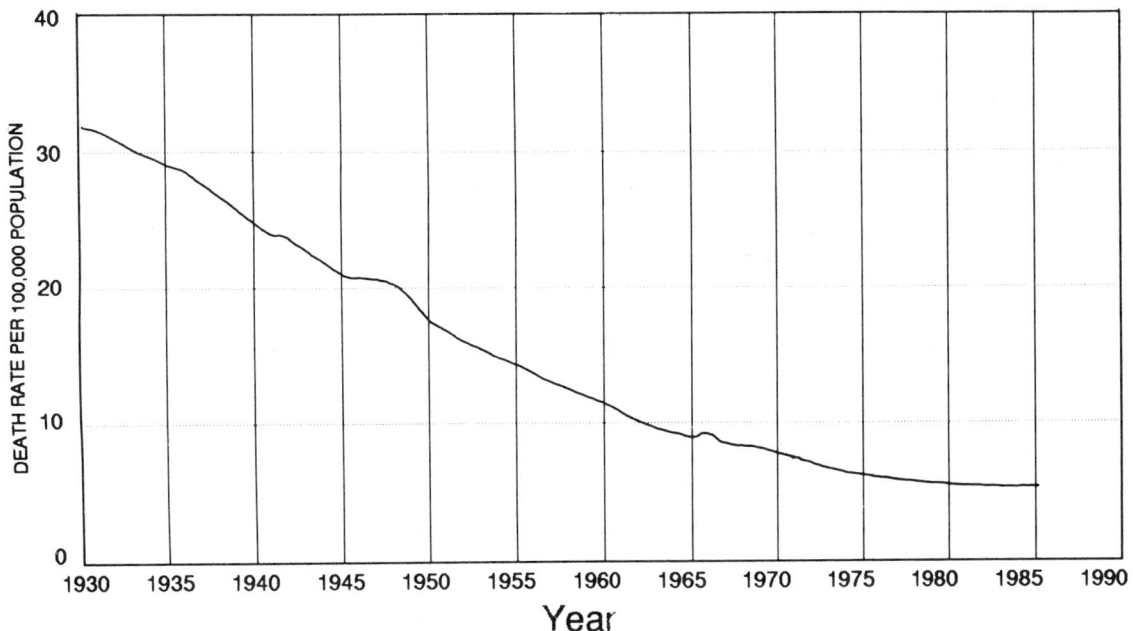

FIG. 4. Decline in gastric cancer mortality from 1930 to 1985 in the United States. (Adapted from ref. 90, with permission.)

(Fig. 4) (91). This decline has been restricted to the more common cancers of the gastric body and/or antrum (distal cancers); cancers located more proximally in the stomach (in the gastroesophageal junction and/or cardia) have slowly increased in incidence (92,93). Certain ethnic groups within the United States, however, retain an increased risk for distal cancer. For example, the incidence of gastric cancer among African-Americans, Asian-Americans, and Hispanics is almost double that among whites (91).

Clues to the events leading to the decline in gastric cancer incidence derive from studies of persons who moved from regions of high gastric cancer risk to regions of low risk. For instance, persons who moved from Japan, a high-risk country, to regions of lower risk in the United States only moderately lessened their cancer risk even if they immigrated at a young age (94,95). Children of immigrants, however, adopted a gastric cancer risk much closer to that of their new country. Similar results have been found in European immigrants to Australia and Puerto Rican immigrants to New York (96,97). These studies suggest that an environmental factor is critical in causing cancer and that this factor exerts its influence in childhood and is somehow related to socioeconomic conditions (98,99).

While dietary factors undoubtedly play an important role in gastric carcinogenesis, *H. pylori* infection is now considered to be the most important single risk factor in gastric carcinogenesis (100). Support for this hypothesis comes from two types of data: (a) studies of the natural history of gastric cancer and (b) epidemiologic studies evaluating the association of *H. pylori* with cancer.

Long before *H. pylori* was first isolated, it was known that the stomach undergoes a sequence of histopathologic changes before distal cancer occurs. In chronological progression, these "preoplastic" conditions are superficial gastritis, atrophic gastritis, intestinal metaplasia, dysplasia, and finally cancer (72,75,99,100). By virtue of its strong causal association with superficial gastritis, it seemed likely that *H. pylori* would be associated with the other lesions as well. Numerous biopsy-based studies have shown that *H. pylori* is commonly found in normal gastric tissue of persons with preoplastic lesions (72,81,101). It has also been found in 50% to 100% of persons with gastric cancer (72,81,101). *Helicobacter pylori* is common in all populations, however, and these biopsy-based studies have not confirmed that infection is more common in malignancy and premalignancy than in normal hosts. Atrophic gastritis involving the body of the stomach appears to be particularly critical for carcinogenesis (100), although it is controversial whether atrophy is a marker for the long-term effects of superficial gastritis or whether atrophy itself leads to malignancy by virtue of hypochlorhydria or loss of digestive enzymes (102–106).

The most compelling data linking *H. pylori* with cancer come from serologic investigations (Table 1). These include ecologic studies that correlate prevalence of *H. pylori* infection and incidence of gastric cancer in multiple regions (83,107–113), case–control studies of cancer patients (114–119), and nested case–control studies within large cohort populations followed for cancer (113,120–122). The combination of studies provides convincing evidence that gastric cancer occurs in regions of high *H. pylori* prevalence, that *H. pylori* is more common in cancer patients than in controls, and that *H. pylori* infection precedes the onset of cancer by many years. Approximately half of gastric cancers might not occur if *H. pylori* did not exist (121,122).

TABLE 1. *Seroepidemiologic studies that evaluate the association of* Helicobacter pylori *with noncardia gastric cancer*

Study design and population	Significant association?	Comment	References
Ecologic, cross-sectional studies			
China	Yes	46 Chinese counties	107,108
Colombia and Louisiana	Yes	Two regions each in Colombia and New Orleans; socioeconomic factors found to be important in determining risk for *H. pylori*	109
Costa Rica	No	Children in one high-risk and one low-risk region	110
Italy	No	Adults in two high-risk and two low-risk regions	111
Japan	No	Five counties	83
Multinational	Yes	17 Adult populations in 13 countries	112
Taiwan	Yes	Three townships; strongest correlation found in persons younger than 20 years	113
Case–control studies			
Finland	Yes	OR = 2.3[a]; controls with nongastric malignancies	114
Greece	No	Small sample size	115
Minnesota	Yes	OR = 2.7; cancer-free controls	116
Netherlands	Yes	OR = 4.2[a]; blood donor controls	117
Netherlands	No	OR = 0.9[a]; controls with clinical indication for endoscopy (but without ulcers, gastric atrophy, or metaplasia)	118
Sweden	Yes	OR = 2.7; hospital controls	119
Nested case–control studies			
California	Yes	OR = 3.6; peptic ulcer disease found to be protective	120
Japanese–American men in Hawaii	Yes	OR = 12.0; increasing OR found with increasing antibody titer	121
Taiwan	No	OR = 1.6; few cases and short follow-up period	113
United Kingdom	Yes	OR = 2.8[b]	122

[a] Calculated from age-adjusted data presented in the manuscript.
[b] Gastric cancers occurring in the cardia and/or gastroesophageal junction included in case group.

Of the few studies that do not support an association between *H. pylori* and cancer, many can be faulted for inadequate sample size (Table 1). In particular, ecologic studies cannot show a correlation between exposure and outcome unless many sites are evaluated. Despite this, the negative studies indicate that infection is common in all populations and that the overwhelming majority of infections will not result in cancer. The age at which infection begins (infected children at worse risk), the site of infection within the stomach (corpus involvement worse than antral infection only), and the host response to infection all appear to determine the degree of risk (100,123). In most people, infection alone does not appear to be sufficient to cause cancer.

Peptic Ulcer Disease

The peak incidence for peptic ulcer disease in North America, Europe, and Japan occurred in the 1950s. Since then, hospitalizations and mortality from peptic ulcer disease, like gastric cancer, have been declining steadily (Fig. 5) (124–132). While some of the decline represents changes in clinical practice (i.e., widespread use of histamine-blockers for dyspepsia reducing diagnosis, hospitalization, and complications of ulcers), it is not clear that this can entirely explain the remarkable downward trend (126,129). Part of the decrease, which pertains to both gastric and duodenal ulcers, appears to be accounted for by a birth year (cohort) phenomenon (125–127,131). Persons born toward the end of the 19th century are at higher risk for ulcer disease than those born either later or earlier (125–127,131). Because the turn of the century appears to be the period of maximal risk, aspects of modern industrialization (i.e., urbanization, stress engendered by World War I, dietary changes, cigarette use) have been thought responsible for causing disease (127). Yet no single environmental factor could satisfactorily explain the 20th century rise and fall in disease incidence (125).

Over the last 10 years, it has become clear that *H. pylori* is the major cause of ulceration of both gastric and duodenal mucosas. The critical experiments showing that eradication of infection prevents recurrent ulceration confirm unequivocally the importance of *H. pylori* in these diseases (6,7). Unless a subject uses nonsteroidal antiinflammatory agents or has a predisposing condition (i.e., Zollinger–Ellison syndrome), an ulcer can be assumed to be *H. pylori* related (68,133,134).

Unfortunately, the natural history of infection that leads to ulceration has not been well defined. With duodenal ulcers, diffuse superficial gastritis of the antrum appears to precede and be coincident with ulcer develop-

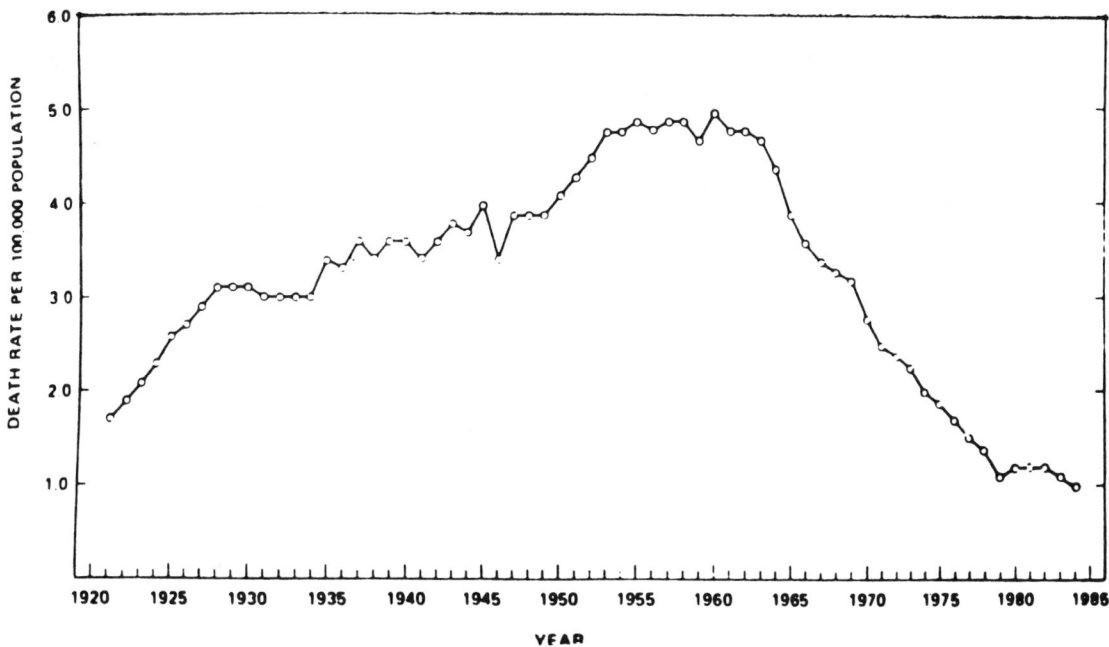

FIG. 5. Duodenal ulcer mortality rates for U.S. men, 1920 to 1985. (Adapted from ref. 126, with permission.)

ment. Longitudinal studies show that approximately 20% of people with *H. pylori*-related antral gastritis or pangastritis will develop duodenal ulcer within 10 years (68). *Helicobacter pylori,* however, cannot normally colonize small intestinal epithelium. For *H. pylori* to attach and survive in the duodenum, inflammation with gastric metaplasia is necessary (135). Thus *H. pylori*-infected persons at highest risk for duodenal ulceration are those in the subset with superficial antral gastritis, duodenitis, and gastric metaplasia of the duodenal mucosa (134). Since acid is typically necessary for the development of duodenal ulcers, duodenal ulcer patients rarely have significant atrophy of the acid-producing corpus (100). In contrast, gastric cancer subjects usually have extensive corpus atrophy. It thus appears that the natural history of *H. pylori* infection in persons with duodenal ulcer is distinct and dissimilar from those with gastric cancer. This may explain both the low incidence of gastric cancer in subjects with a history of duodenal ulcers (2) and the low incidence of peptic ulcers in regions with high cancer incidence (136).

The natural history of gastric ulcers is even less well established than duodenal ulcers. It has been suggested, however, that antral gastritis with antral atrophy but no corpus atrophy is the histologic lesion that engenders the greatest risk for gastric ulceration (68). Until animal models for *H. pylori* infection satisfactorily reproduce human disease, however, ulcer natural history will remain difficult to dissect.

Gastric Lymphoma

Non-Hodgkin's lymphoma (NHL) primary to the stomach, or gastric lymphoma, is a rare malignancy. It ac-
counts for only 10% of lymphomas and 3% of gastric neoplasms (137). According to national cancer registry data from 1985, there were only 7.1 cases of gastric lymphoma per million population per year (138). Gastric lymphoma remains, however, the most common extranodal form of NHL, accounting for 20% of primary extranodal disease (139). Almost all gastric lymphomas are of B cell lineage.

The stomach, unlike the intestine, is not a lymphoid organ (140). In infancy and early childhood, lymphocytes and plasma cells are not found in the stomach. With acquisition of *H. pylori* infection, however, chronic inflammation develops and lymphocytes accumulate in the submucosa, gradually increasing their depth of penetration and forming lymphoid follicles (141). When persons are treated for *H. pylori* infection, lymphoid follicles diminish in size and may regress entirely (141,142). It is from areas of chronic inflammation, often in the form of lymphoid follicles, that the majority of gastric lymphomas arise (143).

Epidemiologically, a few studies link *H. pylori* to gastric lymphoma. One small study found *H. pylori* to be more common in a region with high primary gastric lymphoma incidence than in a low incidence area (144). A much larger ecologic study also identified a potential link between *H. pylori* and lymphoma although in this study the primary site of lymphoma was not specified and the association was weak (107). Two groups have demonstrated high coincident rates of *H. pylori* infection in patients with gastric lymphoma (116,145); one of these studies linked infection to a specific type of gastric lymphoma derived from mucosa-associated lymphoid tissue (MALT lymphomas) (145). The strongest epidemiologic support for an association, however, comes from a nested case–control study in Norway and the United States (146). In this study, persons with *H. pylori* infection were found to have a sixfold higher rate of later developing gastric lymphoma than controls. *Helicobacter pylori* infection did not increase risk of developing lymphoma in other sites.

Although data from epidemiologic studies cannot definitively determine cause, clinical data from one study strongly support a role for *H. pylori* in low-grade MALT lymphomas (147). Infection was eradicated in six patients with this tumor and the lymphoma remitted completely in five. Lymphocytes obtained from the stomach before and after treatment changed from monoclonal to polyclonal. In the laboratory, B lymphocytes from MALT tissue proliferated when T cells in the culture were exposed to *H. pylori* (148). Without T cells in the system, no proliferation occurred, suggesting a T-cell-mediated proliferative response. While it is not clear that the pathogenesis of low-grade MALT lymphomas and that of the more common high-grade, diffuse large-cell lymphomas of the stomach are the same, these results mandate investigations of antigenic stimulation by *H. pylori* as a local factor in lymphomagenesis.

REFERENCES

1. Parsonnet J, Blaser MJ, Perez-Perez GI, Hargrett-Bean N, Tauxe R. Symptoms and risk factors of *Helicobacter pylori* infection in a cohort of epidemiologists. *Gastroenterology* 1992; 102:41–46.
2. Taylor DN, Blaser MJ. Epidemiology of *Helicobacter pylori* infection. *Epidemiol Rev* 1991;13:42–59.
3. Smoak B, Kelley P, Taylor DN. Seroprevalence of *Helicobacter pylori* infections in a cohort of U.S. Army recruits. *Am J Epidemiol* 1994;139:513–519.
4. Langenberg W, Rauws EA, Houthoff HJ, Oudbier JH, van Bohemen CG, Tytgat GN, Rietra PJ. Follow-up study of individuals with untreated *Campylobacter pylori*-associated gastritis and of noninfected persons with non-ulcer dyspepsia. *J Infect Dis* 1988;157:1245–1249.
5. Marshall BJ, Goodwin CS, Warren JR, et al. Prospective double-blind trial of duodenal ulcer relapse after eradication of *Campylobacter pylori*. *Lancet* 1988;2:1437–1442.
6. Grahan DY, Lew GM, Klein PD, Evans DG, Evans DJ, Saeed Z, Malaty HM. Effect of treatment of *Helicobacter pylori* infection on the long-term recurrence of gastric or duodenal ulcer: a randomized, controlled study. *Ann Intern Med* 1992;116: 705–708.
7. Hentschel E, Brandstatter G, Dragosics B, et al. Effect of ranitidine and amoxicillin plus metronidazole on the eradication of *Helicobacter pylori* and the recurrence of duodenal ulcer. *N Engl J Med* 1993;328:308–312.
8. Lambert JR, Lin SK, Nicholson L, et al. Seroepidemiological study of *Helicobacter pylori* antibodies in institutionalized adults [Abstract]. *Rev Esp Enferm Dig* 1990;78:S41–S42.
9. Megraud F, Brassens-Rabbe M-P, Denis F, Belbouri A, Hoa DQ. Seroepidemiology of *Campylobacter pylori* infection in various populations. *J Clin Microbiol* 1989;27:1870–1873.
10. Perez-Perez GI, Taylor DN, Bodhidatta L, et al. Seroprevalence of *Helicobacter pylori* infections in Thailand. *J Infect Dis* 1990;161:1237–1241.
11. Mitchell HM, Li YY, Hu PJ, et al. Epidemiology of *Helicobacter pylori* in southern China: identification of early childhood as the critical period for acquisition. *J Infect Dis* 1992; 166:149–153.
12. Perez-Perez GI, Witkin SS, Decker MD, Blaser MJ. Seroprevalence of *Helicobacter pylori* infection in couples. *J Clin Microbiol* 1991;29:642–644.
13. Dwyer B, Kaldor J, Tee W, Marakowski E, Raios K. Antibody

response to *Campylobacter pylori* in diverse ethnic groups. *Scand J Infect Dis* 1988;20:349–350.
14. Asaka M, Kimura T, Kudo M, et al. Relationship of *Helicobacter pylori* to serum pepsinogens in an asymptomatic Japanese population. *Gastroenterology* 1992;102:760–766.
15. Banatvala N, Mayo K, Megraud F, Jennings R, Deeks JJ, Feldman RA. The cohort effect and *Helicobacter pylori*. *J Infect Dis* 1993;168:219–221.
16. Fiedorek SC, Malaty HM, Evans DL, et al. Factors influencing the epidemiology of *Helicobacter pylori* infection in children. *Pediatrie* 1991;88:578–582.
17. Hopkins RJ, Vial PA, Ferreccio C, et al. Seroprevalence of *Helicobacter pylori* in Chile: vegetables may serve as one route of transmission. *J Infect Dis* 1993;168:222–226.
18. Ramirez-Ramos A, Leon-Barua R, Gilman RH, Gastrointestinal Physiology Working Group. *Helicobacter pylori* and gastritis in Peruvian patients: relationship to socioeconomic level, age, and sex. *Am J Gastroenterol* 1990;85:819–823.
19. Drumm B, Perez-Perez GI, Blaser MJ, Sherman PM. Intrafamilial clustering of *Helicobacter pylori* infection. *N Engl J Med* 1990;322:359–363.
20. Dehesa M, Dooley CP, Cohen H, Fitzgibbons P, Perez-Perez GI, Blaser MJ. High prevalence of *Helicobacter pylori* infection and histologic gastritis in an asymptomatic Hispanic population. *J Clin Microbiol* 1991;29:1128–1131.
21. Hopkins RJ, Russell RG, O'Donnoghue JM, Wasserman SS, Lefkowitz A, Morris JG Jr. Seroprevalence of *Helicobacter pylori* in Seventh-Day Adventists and other groups in Maryland. Lack of association with diet. *Arch Intern Med* 1990;150: 2347–2348.
22. Graham DY, Malaty HM, Evans DG, Evans DJ, Klein PD, Adam E. Epidemiology of *Helicobacter pylori* in an asymptomatic population in the United States: effect of age, race and socioeconomic status. *Gastroenterology* 1991;100:1495–1501.
23. Polish LB, Douglas JM, Davidson AJ, Le YK, Perez-Perez GI, Blaser MJ. Characterization of risk factors for *Helicobacter pylori* infection among men attending a sexually transmitted disease clinic: lack of evidence for sexual transmission. *J Clin Microbiol* 1991;29:2139–2143.
24. Morris A, Nicholson G, Lloyd G, Haines D, Rogers A, Taylor D. Seroepidemiology of *Campylobacter pyloridis*. *N Z Med J* 1986;99:657–659.
25. Dwyer B, Sun NX, Kaldor J, Tee W, Lambert J, Luppino M, Flannery G. Antibody response to *Campylobacter pylori* in an ethnic group lacking peptic ulceration. *Scand J Infect Dis* 1988; 20:63–68.
26. Kang JY, Wee A, Math MV, Guan R, Tay HH, Yap I, Sutherland IH. *Helicobacter pylori* and gastritis in patients with peptic ulcer and non-ulcer dyspepsia: ethnic differences in Singapore. *Gut* 1990;31:850–853.
27. Sitas F, Forman D, Yarnell JWG, Burr ML, Elwood PC, Pedley S, Marks KJ. *Helicobacter pylori* infection rates in relation to age and social class in a population of Welsh men. *Gut* 1991; 32:25–28.
28. Al-Moagel MA, Evans DG, Abdulghani ME, Adam E, Evans DJ Jr, Malaty HM, Graham DY. Prevalence of *Helicobacter* (formerly *Campylobacter*) *pylori* infection in Saudi Arabia, and comparison of those with and without upper gastrointestinal symptoms. *Am J Gastroenterol* 1990;85:944–948.
29. Sonnenberg A. The US temporal and geographic variations of diseases related to *Helicobacter pylori*. *Am J Public Health* 1993;83:1006–1010.
30. The Gastrointestinal Physiology Working Group of the Cayetano Heredia and the Johns Hopkins University. Ecology of *Helicobacter pylori* in Peru: infection rates in coastal, high altitude, and jungle communities. *Gut* 1992;33:604–605.
31. Thomas JE, Gibson GR, Darboe MK, Dale A, Weaver LT. Isolation of *Helicobacter pylori* from human feces. *Lancet* 1992;340:1194–1195.
32. Kelly SM, Cummings JH, MacFarlane GT, Grimes V, MacFarlane S, Gibson GR. Occurrence of *Helicobacter pylori* in fecal specimens from patients with dyspepsia in the UK [Abstract]. *Gastroenterology* 1993;104:A116.
33. Fox JG, Blanco MC, Yan L, Shames B, Polidoro D, Dewhirst

FE, Paster BJ. Role of gastric pH in isolation of *Helicobacter mustelae* from the feces of ferrets. *Gastroenterology* 1993;104: 86–92.

34. Desai HG, Gill HH, Shankaran K, Mehta PR, Prabhu SR. Dental plaque: a permanent reservoir of *Helicobacter pylori*. *Scand J Gasteroenterol* 1991;26:1205–1208.

35. Ferguson DA, Chuanfu L, Patel N, Mayberry WR, Chi DS, Thomas E. Isolation of *Helicobacter pylori* from saliva. *J Clin Microbiol* 1993;31:2802–2804.

36. Krajden S, Fuksa M, Anderson J, et al. Examination of human stomach biopsies, saliva, and dental plaque for *Campylobacter pylori*. *J Clin Microbiol* 1989;27:1397–1398.

37. Nguyen AM, Engstrand L, Genta RM, Graham DY, el-Zaatari FA. Detection of *Helicobacter pylori* in dental plaque by reverse transcription–polymerase chain reaction. *J Clin Microbiol* 1993;31:783–787.

38. Mapstone NP, Lynch DA, Lewis FA, Axon AT, Tompkins DS, Dixon MF, Quirke P. Identification of *Helicobacter pylori* DNA in the mouths and stomachs of patients with gastritis using PCR. *J Clin Pathol* 1993;46:540–543.

39. Malaty HM, Evans DJ Jr, Abramovitch K, Evans DG, Graham DY. *Helicobacter pylori* infection in dental workers: a seroepidemiology study. *Am J Gastroenterol* 1992;87:1728–1731.

40. Malaty HM, Graham DY, Klein PD, Evans DG, Adam E, Evans DJ. Transmission of *Helicobacter pylori* infection: studies in families of healthy individuals. *Scand J Gastroenterol* 1991;26:927–932.

41. Mendall MA, Goggin PM, Molineaux N, Levy J, Toosy T, Strachan D, Northfield TC. Childhood living conditions and *Helicobacter pylori* seropositivity in adult life. *Lancet* 1992;339: 896–897.

42. Mitchell JD, Mitchell HM, Tobias V. Acute *Helicobacter pylori* infection in an infant associated with gastric ulceration and serological evidence of intra-familial transmission. *Am J Gastroenterol* 1992;87:382–386.

43. Hammermeister I, Janus G, Schamarowski F, Rudolf M, Jacobs E, Kist M. Elevated risk of *Helicobacter pylori* infection in submarine crews. *Eur J Clin Microbiol Infect Dis* 1992;11: 9–14.

44. Klein PD, Graham DY, Gaillour A, Opekun AR, Smith EO. Water source as risk factor for *Helicobacter pylori* infection in Peruvian children. *Lancet* 1991;337:1503–1506.

45. Shahamat M, Mai U, Paszko-Kolva C, Kessel M, Colwell RR. Use of autoradiography to assess viability of *Helicobacter pylori* in water. *Appl Environ Microbiol* 1993;59:1231–1235.

46. Hopkins RJ, Vial PA, Ferreccio C, et al. Seroprevalence of *Helicobacter pylori* in Chile: vegetables may serve as one route of transmission. *J Infect Dis* 1993;168:222–226.

47. Webberley MJ, Webberley JM, Newell D, Lowe P, Melikian V. Seroepidemiology of *Helicobacter pylori* infection in vegans and meat eaters. *Epidemiol Infect* 1992;108:457–462.

48. Perez-Perez GI, Marrie T, Meiklejohn G, Shimoyama T, Inouye H, Marshall G, Blaser MJ. The effect of age on seroprevalence of *Campylobacter pylori* infection. *Can J Infect Dis* 1992; 3:134–138.

49. Vaira D, D'Anastasio C, Holton J, Grauenfels P, Salmon PR, Gondolfi L. *Campylobacter pylori* in abattoir workers: is it a zoonosis? *Lancet* 1988;2:725–6.

50. Berkowicz J, Lee A. Person-to-person transmission of *Campylobacter pylori* [Letter]. *Lancet* 1987;2:680–681.

51. Reiff A, Jacobs E, Kist M. Seroepidemiological study of the immune response to *Campylobacter pylori* in potential risk groups. *Eur J Clin Microbiol Infect Dis* 1989;8:592–596.

52. Langenberg W, Rauws EA, Oudbier JH, Tytgat GN. Patient-to-patient transmission of *Campylobacter pylori* infection by fiberoptic gastroduodenoscopy and biopsy. *J Infect Dis* 1990; 161:507–511.

53. Mitchell HM, Lee A, Carrick JTI. Increased incidence of *Campylobacter pylori* infection in gastroenterologists: further evidence to support person-to-person transmission of *C. pylori*. *Scand J Gastroenterol* 1989;24:396–400.

54. Langenberg W, Rauws E, Widjojkusumo A, Tygat G, Zanen H. Identification of *Campylobacter pyloridis* isolates by restriction endonuclease DNA analysis. *J Clin Microbiol* 1986;24: 414–417.

55. Kuipers EJ, Pena AS, van Kamp G, et al. Seroconversion of *Helicobacter pylori*. *Lancet* 1993;342:328–331.

56. Drumm B, Sherman P, Chiasson D, Karmali M, Cutz E. Treatment of *Campylobacter pylori*-associated gastritis in children with bismuth subsalicylate and ampicillin. *J Pediatr* 1988;113: 908–912.

57. Mentis A, Blackwell CC, Weir DM, Spiliadis C, Dailianas A, Skandalis N. ABO blood group, secretor status and detection of *Helicobacter pylori* among patients with gastric and duodenal ulcers. *Epidemiol Infect* 1991;106:221–229.

58. Martin DF, Montgomery E, Dobek AS, Patrissi GA, Peura DA. *Campylobacter pylori*, NSAIDS, and smoking: risk factors for peptic ulcer disease. *Am J Gastroenterol* 1989;84:1268–1272.

59. Hook-Nikanne J. Effect of alcohol consumption on the risk of *Helicobacter pylori* infection. *Digestion* 1991;50:92–98.

60. Marshall BJ, Armstrong JA, McGechie DB, Glancy RJ. Attempt to fulfill Koch's postulates for pyloric *Campylobacter*. *Med J Aust* 1985;142:436–439.

61. Morris A, Nicholson G. Ingestion of *Campylobacter pyloridis* causes gastritis and raised fasting gastric pH. *Am J Gastroenterol* 1987;82:192–199.

62. Morris AJ, Ali MR, Nicholson GI, Perez-Perez GI, Blaser MJ. Long term follow-up of voluntary ingestion of *Helicobacter pylori*. *Ann Intern Med* 1991;114:662–663.

63. Gledhill T, Leicester RJ, Addis B, et al. Epidemic hypochlorhydria. *Br Med J* 1985;290:1383–1386.

64. Ramsey EJ, Carey KV, Peterson WL, et al. Epidemic gastritis with hypochlorhydria. *Gastroenterology* 1979;76:1449–1457.

65. Graham DY, Klein PD. *Campylobacter pyloridis* gastritis: the past, the present, and speculations about the future. *Am J Gastroenterol* 1987;82:283–286.

66. Barthel JS, Westblom TU, Havey AD, Gonzalez F, Everett D. Gastritis and *Campylobacter pylori* in healthy, asymptomatic volunteers. *Arch Intern Med* 1988;148:1149–1151.

67. Dooley CP, Cohen H, Fitzgibbons PL, Bauer M, Appleman MD, Perez-Perez GI, Blaser MJ. Prevalence of *Helicobacter pylori* infection and histologic gastritis in asymptomatic persons. *N Engl J Med* 1989;321:1562–1566.

68. Sipponen P. Natural history of gastritis and its relationship to peptic ulcer disease. *Digestion* 1992;5:70–75.

69. Sipponen P, Kekki M, Siurala M. The Sydney system: epidemiology and natural history of chronic gastritis. *J Gastroenterol Hepatol* 1991;6:244–251.

70. Kekki M, Ihamaki T, Kaukkonen M, Varis K, Siurala M. Progression of gastritis at a population level: comparison of long-term follow-up with stochastic analysis of cross-sectional data. *Scand J Gastroenterol* 1980;15:651–655.

71. Ihamaki T, Kekki M, Sipponen P, Siurala M. The sequelae and course of chronic gastritis during a 30- to 34-bioptic follow-up study. *Scand J Gastroenterol* 1985;20:485–491.

72. Correa P, Haenszel W, Cuello C, et al. Gastric precancerous process in a high risk population: cohort follow-up. *Cancer Res* 1990;50:4737–4740.

73. Kekki M, Maaroos HI, Sipponen P, et al. Grade of *Helicobacter pylori* colonisation in relation to gastritis: a six-year population-based follow-up study. *Scand J Gastroenterol Suppl* 1991;186:142–150.

74. Kosunen TU, Seppala K, Sarna S, Sipponen P. Diagnostic value of decreasing IgG, IgA, and IgM antibody titres after eradication of *Helicobacter pylori*. *Lancet* 1992;339:893–895.

75. Siurala M, Varis K, Kekki M. New aspects on epidemiology, genetics and dynamics of chronic gastritis. *Front Gastroenterol Res* 1980;6:148–166.

76. Varis K. Epidemiology of gastritis. *Scand J Gastroenterol Suppl* 1982;79:44–51.

77. Massarrat S, Schmitz-Moorman P, Fritsch W, Hausamen T, Kappert J. Morphological findings of different areas of gastric mucosa in patients with achlorhydria, normochlorhydria and their relationship to serum gastrin level: evidence for two different types of gastritis. *Klin Wochenschr* 1977;55:1095–1102.

78. Karnes WE, Samloff IM, Siurala M, et al. Postive serum antibody and negative tissue staining for *Helicobacter pylori* in

subjects with atrophic gastritis. *Gastroenterology* 1991;101:167–174.

79. Siurala M, Sipponen P, Kekki M. *Campylobacter pylori* in a sample of Finnish population: relations to morphology and functions of the gastric mucosa. *Gut* 1988;19:909–915.

80. Faisal MA, Russell RM, Samloff IM, Holt PR. *Helicobacter pylori* and atrophic gastritis in the elderly. *Gastroenterology* 1990;99:1543–1544.

81. Guarner J, Mohar A, Parsonnet J, Halperin D. The association of *Helicobacter pylori* with gastric cancer and other preneoplastic gastric lesions in Chiapas, Mexico. *Cancer* 1993;71:297–301.

82. Fukao A, Komatsu S, Tsubono Y, et al. *Helicobacter pylori* infection and chronic atrophic gastritis among Japanese blood donors: a cross-sectional study. *Cancer Causes Control* 1993;4:307–312.

83. Tsugane S, Kabuto M, Imai H, et al. *Helicobacter pylori*, dietary factors, and atrophic gastritis in five Japanese populations with different gastric cancer mortality. *Cancer Causes Control* 1993;4:297–305.

84. Fox JG, Correa P, Taylor NS, et al. High prevalence and persistence of cytotoxin-positive *Helicobacter pylori* strains in a population with high prevalence of atrophic gastritis. *Am J Gastroenterol* 1992;87:1554–1560.

85. Fox JG, Otto G, Murphy JC, Taylor NS, Lee A. Gastric colonization of the ferret with *Helicobacter* species: natural and experimental infections. *Rev Infect Dis* 1991;13(Suppl 8):S671–S680.

86. Correa P. Human gastric carcinogenesis: a multistep and multifactorial process—First American Cancer Society Award lecture on cancer epidemiology and prevention. *Cancer Res* 1992;52:6735–6740.

87. Parkin DM, Laara E, Muir CS. Estimates of the worldwide frequency of sixteen major cancers in 1980. *Int J Cancer* 1988;41:184–197.

88. Parkin DM, ed. *Cancer occurrence in developing countries.* Lyon, France: International Agency for Research on Cancer, 1986.

89. Waterhouse J, Muir CS, Shanmugaratnam K, Powell J, eds. *Cancer incidence in five continents.* Lyon, France: International Agency for Research on Cancer, 1986.

90. Thomas DB. Cancer. In: Last JM, Wallace RB, eds. *Public health and preventive medicine.* Norwalk, CT: Appleton and Lange, 1992;814.

91. Young JL, ed. *Surveillance, epidemiology and end results: incidence and mortality data, 1973–1977.* Bethesda: Department of Health and Human Services, 1981.

92. Zheng T, Mayne ST, Holford TR, et al. The time trend and age–period–cohort effects on incidence of adenocarcinoma of the stomach in Connecticut from 1955–1989. *Cancer* 1993;72:330–340.

93. Rios-Castellanos E, Sitas F, Shepard NA, Jewell DP. Changing pattern of gastric cancer in Oxfordshire. *Gut* 1992;33:1312–1317.

94. Haenszel W, Kurihara M, Segi M, Lee RK. Stomach cancer among Japanese men in Hawaii. *J Natl Cancer Inst* 1972;49:969–988.

95. Kmet J. The role of migrant population in studies of selected cancer sites: a review. *J Chronic Dis* 1970;23:305–324.

96. McMichael AJ, McCall MG, Hartshorne JM, Woodings TL. Patterns of gastro-intestinal cancer in European migrants to Australia: the role of dietary change. *Int J Cancer* 1980;25:431–437.

97. Rosenwaike I. Cancer mortality amoung Puerto Rican-born residents in New York City. *Am J Epidemiol* 1984;2:177–185.

98. Armijo R, Gonzalez A, Orellana M, et al. Epidemiology of gastric cancer in Chile. I. Case–control study. *Int J Epidemiol* 1981;10:53–56.

99. Correa P, Cuello C, Duque E. Carcinoma and intestinal metaplasia of the stomach in Columbian migrants. *J Natl Cancer Inst* 1970;44:297.

100. Sipponen P, Seppala K. Gastric carcinoma: failed adaptation to *Helicobacter pylori*. *Scand J Gastroenterol Suppl* 1992;27:33–38.

101. Wee A, Kang JY, Teh M. *Helicobacter pylori* and gastric can-

cer: correlation with gastritis, intestinal metaplasia, and tumour histology. *Gut* 1992;33:1029–1032.

102. Correa P, Cuello C, Duque E, et al. Gastric cancer in Colombia. III. Natural history of precursor lesions. *J Natl Cancer Inst* 1976;57:1027–1035.

103. Parsonnet J, Samloff IM, Nelson LM, Orentreich N, Vogelman JH, Friedman GD. *Helicobacter pylori*, pepsinogen and risk for gastric adenocarcinoma. *Cancer Epidemiol Biomarkers Prev* 1993;2:1–7.

104. Moller H, Nissen A, Mosbech J. Use of cimetidine and other peptic ulcer drugs in Denmark 1977–1990 with analysis of the risk of gastric cancer among cimetidine users. *Gut* 1992;33:1166–1169.

105. Colin-Jones DG, Langman MJ, Lawson DH, Logan RF, Paterson KR, Vessey MP. Postmarketing surveillance of the safety of cimetidine: 10 year mortality report. *Gut* 1992;33:1280–1284.

106. La Vecchia C, Negri E, Franceschi S, D'Avanzo B. Histamine-2-receptor antagonists and gastric cancer: update and note on latency and covariates. *Nutrition* 1992;8:177–181.

107. Forman D, Sitas F, Newell DG, et al. Geographic association of *Helicobacter pylori* antibody prevalence and gastric cancer mortality in rural China. *Int J Cancer* 1990;46:608–611.

108. Kneller RW, Guo WD, Hsing AW, et al. Risk factors for stomach cancer in sixty-five Chinese counties. *Cancer Epidemiol Biomarkers Prev* 1992;1:113–118.

109. Correa P, Fox JG, Fontham E, et al. *Helicobacter pylori* and gastric carcinoma: serum antibody prevalence in populations with contrasting cancer risks. *Cancer* 1990;66:2569–2574.

110. Sierra R, Munoz N, Pena AS, et al. Antibodies to *Helicobacter pylori* and pepsinogen levels in children from Costa Rica: comparison of two areas with different risks for stomach cancer. *Cancer Epidemiol Biomarkers Prev* 1992;1:449–454.

111. Palli D, Decarli A, Cipriani F, et al. *Helicobacter pylori* antibodies in areas of Italy at varying gastric cancer risk. *Cancer Epidemiol Biomarkers Prev* 1993;2:37–40.

112. Eurogast Study Group. An international association between *Helicobacter pylori* infection and gastric cancer. *Lancet* 1993;341:1359–1362.

113. Lin JT, Wang LY, Wang JT, Wang TH, Yang CS, Chen CJ. Weak association between *Helicobacter pylori* infection and gastric cancer risk: epidemiologic evidence from Taiwan. *Gastroenterology* 1993;104(Suppl):A421.

114. Sipponen P, Kosunen TU, Valle J, Riihela M, Seppala K. *Helicobacter pylori* infection and chronic gastritis in gastric cancer. *J Clin Pathol* 1992;45:319–323.

115. Archimandritis A, Bitsikas J, Tjivras M, et al. Gastric adenocarcinoma and *Helicobacter pylori* infection. *Gastroenterology* 1993;104(Suppl):A384(abst).

116. Talley NJ, Zinmeister AR, Weaver A, et al. Gastric adenocarcinoma and *Helicobacter pylori* infection. *J Natl Cancer Inst* 1991;83:1734–1739.

117. Loffeld RJLF, Willems I, Flendrig JA, Arends JW. *Helicobacter pylori* and gastric carcinoma. *Histology* 1990;17:537–541.

118. Kuipers EJ, Garcia-Casanova M, Flendrig JA, Arends JW. *Helicobacter pylori* serology in patients with gastric cancer. *Scand J Gastroenterol* 1993;28:433–437.

119. Hansson L-E, Engstrand L, Evans DJ, Nyren O. *Helicobacter pylori* seropositivity is a risk factor for gastric adenocarcinoma. *Gastroenterology* 1992;102(Suppl):A361(abst).

120. Parsonnet J, Friedman GD, Vandersteen DP, et al. *Helicobacter pylori* infection and the risk of gastric carcinoma. *N Engl J Med* 1991;325:1127–1131.

121. Nomura A, Stemmerman GN, Chyou P, Kato I, Perez-Perez GI, Blaser MJ. *Helicobacter pylori* infection and gastric carcinoma in a population of Japanese-Americans in Hawaii. *N Engl J Med* 1991;325:1132–1136.

122. Forman D, Newell DG, Fullerton F, et al. Association between infection with *Helicobacter pylori* and risk of gastric cancer: evidence from a prospective investigation. *Br Med J* 1991;302:1302–1305.

123. Mitchell HM, Bohane TD, Tobias V, et al. *Helicobacter pylori* infection in children: potential clues to pathogenesis. *J Pediatr Gastroenterol Nutr* 1993;16:120–125.

124. Kawai K, Shirakawa K, Misaki F, Hayashi K, Watanabe Y. Natural history and epidemiologic studies of peptic ulcer disease in Japan. *Gastroenterology* 1989;96:581–585.
125. Sonnenberg A. Occurrence of a cohort phenomenon in peptic ulcer mortality from Switzerland. *Gastroenterology* 1984;86: 398–401.
126. Kurata JH. Ulcer epidemiology: an overview and proposed research framework. *Gastroenterology* 1989;96:569–580.
127. Susser M. Period effects, generation effects and age effects in peptic ulcer mortality. *J Chronic Dis* 1982;35:29–40.
128. Kurata JH, Haile BM. Epidemiology of peptic ulcer disease. *Clin Gastroenterol* 1984;13:289–307.
129. Kurata JH, Elashoff JD, Haile BM, Honda GD. A reappraisal of time trends in ulcer disease and factors related to changes in ulcer hospitalization and mortality rates. *Am J Public Health* 1983;73:1066–1072.
130. Tilvis RS, Vuoristo M, Varis K. Changed profile of peptic ulcer disease in hospital patients during 1969–1984. *Scand J Gastroenterol* 1987;22:1238–1244.
131. Sonnenberg A, Fritsch A. Changing mortality of peptic ulcer disease in Germany. *Gastroenterology* 1983;84:1553–1557.
132. Kurata JH, Honda GD, Frankl H. Hospitalization and mortality rates for peptic ulcers: a comparison of large health maintenance organization and United States data. *Gastroenterology* 1982;83:1008–1016.
133. Graham DY. Treatment of peptic ulcers caused by *Helicobacter pylori* [Editorial]. *N Engl J Med* 1993;328:349–350.
134. Wyatt JI, Rathbone BJ. Gastric metaplasia in the duodenum and *Campylobacter pylori*. *Gastroenterol Clin Biol* 1989;13: 78B–82B.
135. Malfertheiner P, Bode G, Stanescu A, Ditschuneit H. Gastric metaplasia and *Campylobacter pylori* in duodenal ulcer disease: an ultrastructural analysis. *Gastroenterol Clin Biol* 1989; 13:71B–74B.
136. Burstein M, Monroe E, Leon-Barua R, Lozano R, Berendson R, Gilman RH. Low peptic ulcer and high gastric cancer prevalence in a developing country with a high prevalence of infection by *Helicobacter pylori*. *J Clin Gastroenterol* 1991;13: 154–156.
137. Spiro HM. Lymphoma of the stomach. In: *Clinical gastroenterology*. New York: Macmillan, 1983;292–297.
138. Severson RK, Davis S. Increasing incidence of primary gastric lymphoma. *Cancer* 1990;66:1283–1287.
139. Rubin E, Farber JL. The gastrointestinal tract. In: Rubin E, Farber JL, eds. *Essential pathology*. Philadelphia: Lippincott, 1988;352–393.
140. Ming S. Adenocarcinoma and other malignant epithelial tumors of the stomach. In: Ming S, Goldman H, eds. *Pathology of the gastrointestinal tract*. Philadelphia: Saunders, 1992;584–618.
141. Genta RM, Hamner HW, Graham DY. Gastric lymphoid follicles in *Helicobacter pylori* infection: frequency, distribution, and response to triple therapy. *Hum Pathol* 1993;24:577–583.
142. Stolte M. *Helicobacter pylori* gastritis and gastric MALT-lymphoma [Letter]. *Lancet* 1992;339:745–746.
143. Boland CR, Scheiman JM. Tumors of the stomach. In: Yamada T, Alpers DH, Owyang C, eds. *Textbook of gastroenterology*. Philadelphia: Lippincott, 1991;1353–1379.
144. Doglioni C, Wotherspoon AC, Moschini A, De Boni M, Isaacson PG. High incidence of primary gastric lymphoma in northeastern Italy. *Lancet* 1992;339:834–835.
145. Wotherspoon AC, Ortiz-Hidalgo C, Falzon MR, Isaacson PG. *Helicobacter pylori*-associated gastritis and primary B-cell gastric lymphomaa. *Lancet* 1991;338:1175–1176.
146. Parsonnet J, Hansen S, Rodriguez L, et al. *Helicobacter pylori* and primary gastric lymphoma. *N Engl J Med* 1994;330: 1267–1271.
147. Wotherspoon AC, Doglioni C, Diss TC, Pan L, Moschini A, De Boni M, Isaacson PG. Regression of primary low-grade B-cell gastric lymphoma of mucosa-associated lymphoid tissue type after eradication of *Helicobacter pylori*. *Lancet* 1993;342: 575–577.
148. Hussell T, Isaacson PG, Crabtree JE, Spencer J. The response of cells from low-grade B-cell lymphomas of mucosa-associated lymphoid tissue to *Helicobacter pylori*. *Lancet* 1993;342: 571–574.

Infections of the Gastrointestinal Tract,
edited by M. J. Blaser, P. D. Smith, J. I. Ravdin,
H. B. Greenberg, and R. L. Guerrant
Raven Press, Ltd., New York © 1995.

CHAPTER 41

Clinical Approach to the *Helicobacter*-Infected Patient

Gerald Holtmann and Nicholas J. Talley

In 1982, *Helicobacter pylori* (initially called *Campylobacter pyloridis* and then *Campylobacter pylori*) was first successfully cultured and identified (1). The development of sensitive and specific diagnostic methods, including serology and breath testing, and the application of therapies that can eliminate the infection have resulted in an appreciation of the clinical relevance of *H. pylori* in gastroduodenal diseases. It is now accepted that *H. pylori* is the most important cause of chronic histological gastritis in humans. However, most infected persons have no symptoms (2–4). In developed countries, the prevalence rates of infection range from 30% to 50% (5–24); infection is related to advancing age (11), lower socioeconomic status (10,11,25), certain ethnic groups (26), sanitary conditions (27), and country of origin (7,21,28). The reported prevalence rates in developing countries are considerably higher than in developed countries (29–31). The high prevalence is clinically very important because *H. pylori* is now recognized to play a key role in the pathogenesis of chronic peptic ulcer and probably gastric cancer.

DIAGNOSTIC TESTS

A number of tests have been developed for the diagnosis of *H. pylori* infection. These tests can be categorized into those that are based on direct assessment of gastric biopsies and indirect tests that detect an immunological response (i.e., antibodies against *H. pylori*) or metabolic products of *H. pylori* (i.e., urease activity) (Table 1).

Biopsy Methods

Histology

At upper gastrointestinal endoscopy, gastric biopsies can safely be obtained for diagnostic purposes in most

G. Holtmann: Department of Gastroenterology, University of Essen, H5122 Essen, Germany.
N. J. Talley: Division of Medicine, The Nepean Hospital, Sydney NSW 2750, Australia.

patients. The conventional hematoxylin–eosin (HE) stain at high power is able to detect most cases of *H. pylori* infection unless there is a very low number of organisms (32). The organisms are best seen in or near adherent mucus on the luminal side of the gastric surface and pit epithelial cells. There are more sensitive staining methods for the diagnosis of *H. pylori,* including the modified Giemsa or Warthin–Starry silver stain (33–37) (Fig. 1). *Helicobacter pylori* is a gram-negative organism that can also be detected by Gram staining if there is dense infection but this is a less useful diagnostic test. Overall, the sensitivity and specificity of histology for the diagnosis of *H. pylori* are over 95% *in experienced hands,* although there is some interobserver variation (38,39).

Helicobacter pylori can colonize the mucosa of the antrum and corpus, but colonization is patchy and may be antral predominant (38,40–42); as fundic gland mucosa can extend into the antrum, antral gland mucosa is most reliably sampled by taking biopsies within 2 cm of the pylorus. Sampling error may often explain why histology is negative when other tests indicate *H. pylori* infection. A single gastric biopsy does not yield optimal sensitivity; it is therefore recommended that two biopsies be taken from the antrum and two from the gastric body to assess for *H. pylori* and accompanying gastritis.

Culture

The most specific method to diagnose infection is culture of *H. pylori* from tissue biopsies. Unfortunately, relying on culture of *H. pylori* alone can miss a substantial proportion of infected cases for technical reasons including overgrowth of other bacteria or small bacterial loads (4). Thus the "gold standard" for the detection of *H. pylori* remains a combination of histological staining and culture. Attention to transport of the biopsy material is particularly crucial for an adequate diagnostic yield. *Helicobacter pylori* suspended in distilled water or physi-

TABLE 1. *Diagnostic tests for* Helicobacter pylori *infection*

Test	Advantages	Disadvantages	Approximate sensitivity and specificity
Histology	Allows evaluation of the degree of inflammation	Requires upper endoscopy, depends on the experience of the pathologist	Sensitivity >95% Specificity >95%
Microbiology	Allows identification of antibiotic-resistant strains	Requires upper endoscopy, difficult to culture, considerable risk of false-negative results	Sensitivity >75% Specificity 100%
Biopsy urease testing (24 h)	Rapid, inexpensive, can be performed in the endoscopy room	Requires upper endoscopy, may be falsely negative immediately after antibiotic treatment or during treatment with omeprazole	Sensitivity >95% Specificity >80%
Serology	Noninvasive, inexpensive	Less useful to verify the outcome of eradication therapy since a long time is required for seroreversion	Sensitivity >90% Specificity >90%
^{13}C and ^{14}C breath testing	Respond rapidly to changes in *H. pylori* colonization, noninvasive, inexpensive	Needs expensive equipment, exposure to radiation (^{14}C only)	Sensitivity >95% Specificity >95%

ologic saline may be successfully cultured after days if stored at 7°C, but the organism rapidly loses viability at room temperature (43,44). One way to improve the sensitivity of culture is to use specific transport media (e.g., blood agars) (32). Nevertheless, the sensitivity of culture ranges from 77% to 98% even in expert hands (45–48). Currently, the main value of culture outside research protocols is not for diagnosis of *H. pylori* infection but for determination of antibiotic resistance, which is becoming an increasing problem (49–52).

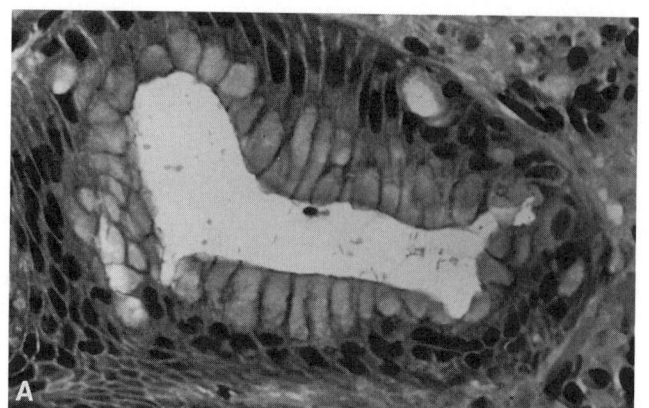
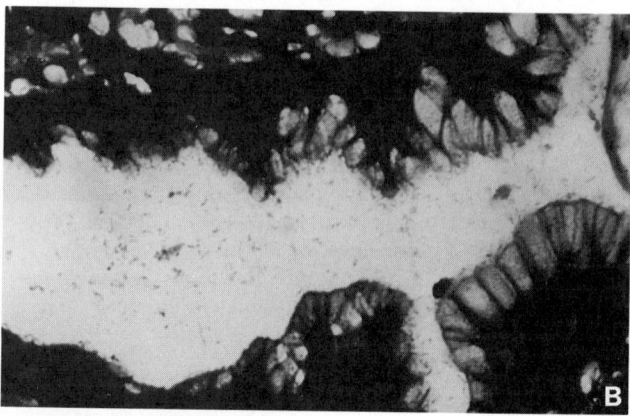
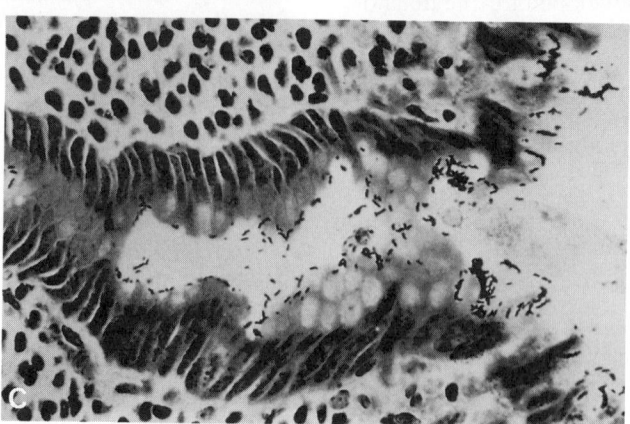

FIG. 1. *Helicobacter pylori* identified by hematoxylin–eosin (**A**), Giemsa (**B**), and Warthin–Starry silver stains (**C**). (From ref. 278, with permission.) (See Plate 8.)

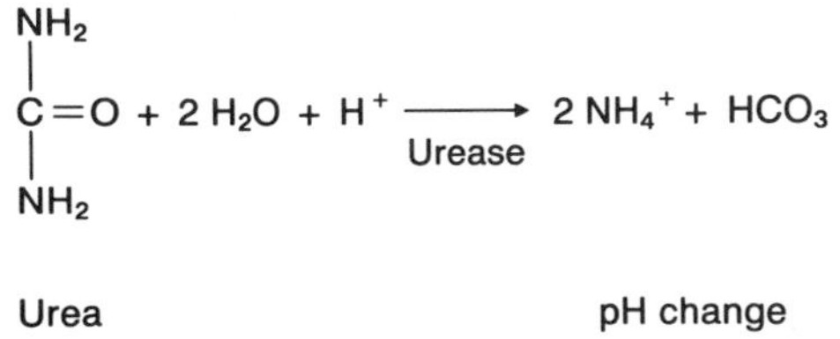

$$\begin{array}{c} NH_2 \\ | \\ C=O + 2\,H_2O + H^+ \xrightarrow{\text{Urease}} 2\,NH_4^+ + HCO_3 \\ | \\ NH_2 \end{array}$$

Urea   pH change

FIG. 2. Hydrolysis of urea by *Helicobacter pylori* urease.

Biopsy Urease Tests

Helicobacter pylori is a potent producer of the enzyme urease that hydrolyzes urea to ammonia and bicarbonate (Fig. 2). This metabolic characteristic can be used to verify the presence of *H. pylori* in gastric biopsies (34,53–57). In patients undergoing upper gastrointestinal endoscopy, urease testing is performed by obtaining a biopsy and placing it into a vial containing urea broth and a color indicator (e.g., phenol red). A change of pH following liberation of bicarbonate by urease will lead to a color change (Fig. 2). The commercially available *Campylobacter*-like organism (CLO) test uses a pellet of modified Christensen's urea agar and an indicator; a color reaction can be visualized in 75% of infected cases within 60 min, but a negative result can only be assumed if the color reaction is not visible within 24 hr. Since the color reaction is directly related to the amount of urease activity in the sample obtained, a rapid color reaction generally indicates dense colonization by *H. pylori*. However, false-negative results occur if only small numbers of organisms are present and false-positive results occasionally are found because of bacterial overgrowth by other urease-producing bacteria. Rapid urease tests (e.g., the modified rapid urease test, MRU) have been developed with liquid urea broth containing phenol red or bromothymol blue as indicators; they yield a result within a few minutes with a sensitivity and specificity similar to that of the CLO test (46,55,57–59). In clinical practice, biopsy urease testing has the advantage of diagnosing *H. pylori* status in most cases soon after endoscopy, which is helpful for the clinician planning therapeutic interventions. This test also is less expensive than histology or culture of gastric biopsies.

Immunohistochemical/Fluorescence

Immunohistochemical or fluorescence techniques have been developed with the aim of increasing the diagnostic yield of histology (60). These tests are more difficult to perform and require a fluorescent microscope (61). Moreover, these methods have not been shown to be more sensitive or specific than routine histology (62,63).

Molecular Testing

Molecular biology techniques may become more relevant in the future for the diagnosis of *H. pylori* infection.

Recently, polymerase chain reaction (PCR) methods for the detection of the structural gene encoding urease production have been developed, and initial results have yielded promising sensitivities and specificities (64). Such methods can accurately identify *H. pylori* in gastric biopsies and in gastric juice. Gel electrophoresis and restriction endonuclease techniques have begun to identify various *H. pylori* strains. Molecular biological approaches may eventually allow clinicians to determine whether a particular *H. pylori* strain is of high or low virulence, although the issue of strain virulence remains unresolved at present (65–68).

Noninvasive

Serology

Standard

Infection with *H. pylori* is chronic and results in histological gastritis. This is associated with a local and systemic immune response characterized by induction of circulating specific immunoglobulin G (IgG), IgA, and, acutely, IgM antibodies (69,70). Moreover, spontaneous eradication of *H. pylori* infection seldom occurs. The presence of *H. pylori* antibodies is therefore an indirect indicator of infection with *H. pylori*.

Enzyme-linked immunoadsorbent assays (ELISAs) are currently considered the optimal method for testing for *H. pylori* antibodies. It is noteworthy that assays testing for IgG antibodies have yielded the highest sensitivities while IgM levels cannot discriminate between infected and uninfected cases (71). Pooled whole-cell antigens may cross-react with sera containing other bacterial antibodies (e.g., *Campylobacter jejuni*) and so various methods have been employed to extract more specific *H. pylori* antigenic material. However, the commercially available ELISA tests generally all yield sensitivities and specificities between 90% and 100% compared to histology and/or urease testing (39,71–75). The high sensitivity and specificity of most of the tests are remarkable since there is considerable antigenic variation between different strains of *H. pylori* (76) (Fig. 3). Serology is therefore a very useful test for identification of *H. pylori* infection in the patient care setting (77) as well as in epidemiological studies (12,73,78–83).

Other investigators have utilized a flow cytometric immunofluorescence assay (FMIA) to diagnose *H. pylori*. In this assay, polystyrene microspheres coated with a multicomponent antigen are incubated with the serum sample. Thereafter, fluorescein-labeled goat anti-human immunoglobulin is added and fluorescence quantitated. This method, however, has yielded similar sensitivities and specificities to standard ELISAs (74). Salivary antibody levels have also been used to diagnose infection but it is difficult to collect noncontaminated fluid.

The possibility of false-negative results has to be considered in any patient with an impaired immune response (e.g., the elderly, patients on hemodialysis, or patients

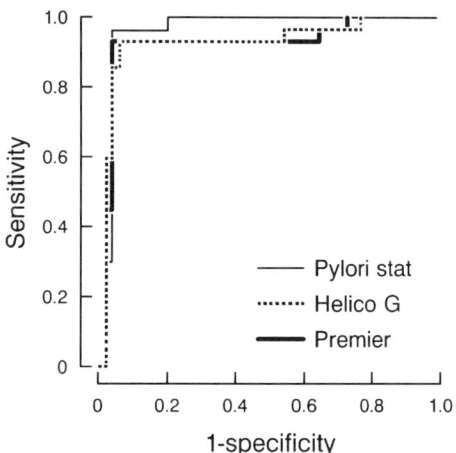

FIG. 3. Receiver operator characteristic curves for three commercially available ELISA tests for IgG to *Helicobacter pylori*. (From ref. 71, with permission.)

treated with immunosuppressants after organ transplantation) (84). In addition, chronic nonsteroidal anti-inflammatory drug (NSAID) treatment may suppress infection and decrease the sensitivity of some serological tests (85,86). False-negative results may occur during the first few weeks of infection.

In the future, determination of *H. pylori* antibody status may be useful to follow up the success of eradication therapy. After 3 to 6 months, *H. pylori* titers decrease in subjects who have had their infection successfully eradicated (70,87,88), but 50% of these patients do not become seronegative even after prolonged follow-up. Thus, if the baseline antibody titer is known, a change of titer during follow-up may provide useful information. However, other indirect methods such as breath testing, which is discussed later, are more suitable for judging if treatment has eliminated the infection.

Rapid Serological Tests

There have been efforts made to speed up laboratory determination of *H. pylori* antibody status to allow more rapid diagnosis of infection in clinical practice (89,90). To date, these tests have yielded similar sensitivities to conventional ELISAs and therefore may eventually become widely used in the office-based care of patients.

Breath Testing

Helicobacter pylori hydrolyzes urea, which is metabolized to ammonia and bicarbonate; the bicarbonate is absorbed and excreted as carbon dioxide (CO_2) by the lungs. If urea is labeled with a radioactive carbon isotope and the labeled urea is metabolized, it can be detected in the breath as labeled carbon dioxide. The exhalation of labeled carbon dioxide can be measured and used as a

marker for *H. pylori* infection (91,92) (Fig. 4). Initially, this method was developed with the stable (nonradioactive) ^{13}C isotope, but to measure ^{13}C excretion requires a gas isotope ratio mass spectrometer. Although the availability of this equipment is increasing and it is becoming less expensive, these factors have limited the use of the ^{13}C test in clinical practice. However, the method has been adapted for use with the radioactive isotope ^{14}C that can easily be detected by the widely available scintillation counters (93–98). The sensitivity and specificity of breath testing to detect *H. pylori* infection is over 95%. Moreover, this test essentially samples the entire stomach for the presence of infection and can be repeated after treatment to accurately document infection status. Although many protocols have been proposed, a single breath sample obtained 20 min after ingestion of labeled urea in water has been reported to be sufficient to diagnose an infected case.

Although the radiation exposure from ^{14}C is extremely low (97,99), nonradioactive testing using ^{13}C is preferred in children and pregnant women (29,49,100–114).

Blood Bicarbonate

Based on the principles of the urea breath test, an increase of ^{13}C-bicarbonate after ingestion of a meal with ^{13}C-labeled urea can be measured in the serum in *H. pylori*-infected patients (105). However, the breath test is simpler and even less invasive.

Overview of Diagnostic Testing in Clinical Practice

A number of good tests are available to document infection status. However, diagnostic testing should only be performed if treatment is a consideration. The choice of which test depends on the clinical circumstances. For example, if there is a clinical indication for endoscopy, endoscopic biopsy with histology and biopsy urease testing is the method of choice to optimize sensitivity and specificity. Breath testing is useful to document current infection in patients in whom endoscopy is not planned and to follow up treatment success. Serology is most useful to screen dyspeptic patients for evidence of infection if this will alter management (e.g., determine who should be endoscoped or not).

CONSEQUENCES OF *H. PYLORI* INFECTION

Helicobacter pylori infection is associated with a number of clinical conditions summarized in Table 2. These will each be discussed in turn.

Acute Infection

Acute infection with *H. pylori* may result in as many as 60% of infected subjects developing short-lived symptoms associated with acute gastritis, characterized by a neutro-

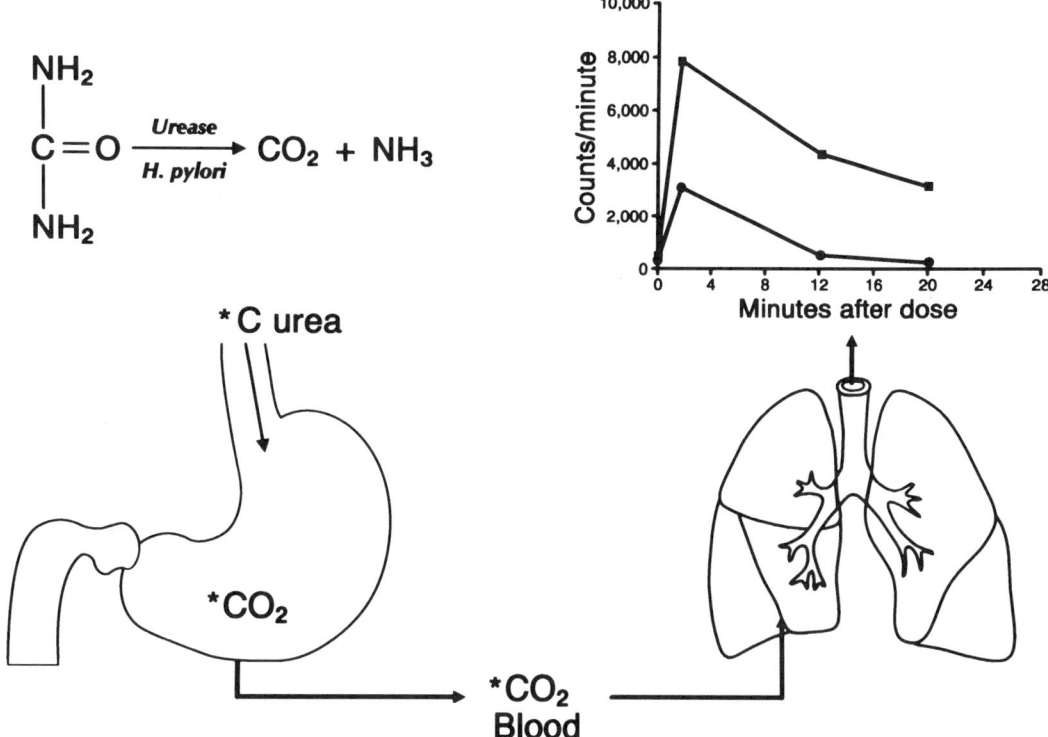

FIG. 4. Schematic representation of the ^{14}C and ^{13}C breath test. After ingestion of labeled urea, urea is metabolized by urease into ammonia and bicarbonate. Bicarbonate is exhaled as CO_2 via the lungs and the concentration of labeled carbon atoms can be determined in the exhaled air. More than 1000 counts/min at 20 min defines a positive ^{14}C urea breath test (*upper curve*). An early peak can occur in both *Helicobacter pylori*-positive and -negative cases from hydrolysis of urea by mouth flora.

philic and mononuclear cell infiltrate, and later in many cases transient hypochlorhydria (115–120). In Marshall's experiment (117), symptoms of fullness and a sensation of early morning hunger developed on the seventh day after self-inoculation, but these resolved spontaneously. In another experiment, Morris ingested *H. pylori* but had symptoms for only 10 days (118) even though the infection persisted for years and eradication therapy was initially unsuccessful (119). Similarly, there are reports of patients or normal volunteers who became infected after participation in research protocols involving gastric intubation for measurement of gastric acid secretion (115–117,120). In a study from Dallas, 17 of 37 volunteers experienced a considerable decrease in acid output (hypochlorhydria) associated with histological gastritis that was later attributed to *H. pylori* probably transmitted by a contaminated pH electrode (120). The hypochlorhydria occurred a mean of 25 days after the illness began, but acid secretion did not return to normal in most subjects until a mean of 125 days. The mechanisms explaining the reversible hypochlorhydria are uncertain; parietal cell morphology and numbers are not affected by infection, but *H. pylori* can produce a toxin *in vitro* that reduces acid secretion by isolated guinea pig parietal cells. *Helicobacter pylori* survives some of the clinically used disinfection procedures (121), and thus the infection also can be transmitted iatrogenically by endoscopic procedures.

The exact sequence of events after first ingestion of the organisms remain to be fully defined, but the following sequence is thought to occur. After ingestion, the bacteria penetrates into the mucous layer of the antrum and corpus, where they colonize the mucosa below the mucous layer. Hypochlorhydria may help the organisms to become established. Urease activity helps to protect the bacteria from acid attack. *Helicobacter pylori* is highly motile because of its flagella. The penetration into the mucous layer may be facilitated by motility and enzymatic products (e.g., phospholipase A, lipase, mucinase) (122–124). Bacterial multiplication then occurs within the mucous layer. The adhesion of *H. pylori* to gastric epithelial cells is also probably important (123,125,126). Release of hemagglutinin and the presence of receptors for specific mucosal surface antigens may facilitate the adhesion of the microorganism (127,128). A few organisms may be able to invade between mucocytes. Most often the infection is not cleared by the host inflammatory and humoral response, but the host response is usually able to control the infection and there is downregulation of the immune response to a chronic disease pattern.

Symptoms in acutely infected subjects usually resolve within a few days and chronic complaints have not been reported in any of these cases to date (115–120). Thus acute *H. pylori* infection is rarely identified as such and often is misdiagnosed as viral gastroenteritis.

TABLE 2. *Clinical features of gastroduodenal diseases associated with* Helicobacter pylori *infection*

1. Acute infection
   Symptoms
       Incubation period: 3–7 days
       Duration of illness: 2–7 days
   Hypochlorhydria
       Prevalence: >50% of those acutely infected
       Incubation period: 25 days (range, 7–49 days)
       Duration: 4 months (range, 2–8 months)
2. Chronic gastritis (histologic)
       Incubation period: 3–7 days
       Duration: years, probably lifelong
       Risk factors for symptoms: uncertain association
       Incidence (new cases): <1 per 100 population per
           year in developed countries
       Prevalence: varies by race and age in developed
           countries
       Higher rates in persons from developing countries
3. Chronic peptic ulcer
       Incubation period: variable
       Duration: years, eradication of organism essen-
           tially abolishes ulcer relapse
       Incidence: 1–3 per 1000 population per year in de-
           veloped countries
       Risk factors predisposing persons with asymp-
           tomatic *H. pylori* gastritis to duodenal ulcer:
           unknown
4. Gastric cancer
       Incubation period: probably decades
       Atrophic gastritis and intestinal metaplasia are
           precursor lesions for gastric adenocarcinoma
       H. pylori infection often seen in adjacent gastric
           tissue

Adapted from ref. 279.

Chronic Infection

Chronic Gastritis

Most frequently, chronic infection with *H. pylori* results in an asymptomatic superficial gastritis. The evidence that *H. pylori* is causally linked to gastritis is presented in Table 3. At endoscopy in adults, there is a very poor correlation between the presence or severity of *H. pylori* gastritis and endoscopic appearance, and therefore biopsies are essential to document the presence of gastritis.

The inflammatory cell infiltrate usually comprises a combination of neutrophils and mononuclear cells (commonly referred to as active chronic gastritis). In the majority of cases inflammatory cells are concentrated in the superficial part of the lamina propria. Epithelial damage can often be identified on light microscopy, but the organisms are less often found in areas with intense epithelial damage and mucus depletion. The inflammatory response tends to differ in children; in these cases there may be fine nodularity of the mucosa macroscopically associated with lymphoid hyperplasia, predominantly in the antrum. Unless *H. pylori* gastritis progresses to gastric atrophy or metaplasia (129,130), the infection persists for life in most untreated patients.

TABLE 3. *Evidence implicating* Helicobacter pylori *in the pathogenesis of chronic gastritis*

Direct evidence
1. Voluntary ingestion of *H. pylori* results in gastritis.
2. Experimental animal challenge simulates human infection with resulting chronic gastritis.
3. Antimicrobial therapy that eradicates infection heals gastritis.

Indirect evidence
1. *Helicobacter pylori* only overlies gastric or gastric-type epithelium.
2. *Helicobacter pylori* infection is associated with only certain types of gastroduodenal inflammation, not all types.
3. There is a universal systemic immune response to *H. pylori*.
4. Levels of *H. pylori*-specific antibodies decrease with therapy, concomitant with diminution in inflammation.
5. *Helicobacter pylori* is associated with epidemic gastritis and hypochlorhydria.

* Adapted from ref. 280.

The pathogenesis of the gastritis linked to *H. pylori* infection remains inadequately understood. It is unclear how much is directly due to the bacteria, and how much is due to the host inflammatory and immune response. There has been intense interest in a number of putative virulence factors of the bacteria in the pathogenesis of gastritis, but whether the factors identified represent cause and effect is unknown. *Helicobacter pylori* theoretically may produce mucosal damage by production of toxins or release of destructive enzymes (122,130). A vacuolizing cytotoxin has been found in approximately 50% of *H. pylori* strains (130). Another potential virulence factor may be urease, which hydrolyzes urea into ammonia; ammonia and the formation of monochloramines have been postulated to be directly toxic to mucosal cells, but recent evidence suggests that this is not a key factor (122,131). *Helicobacter pylori* produces mucinase, which is able to disrupt the protective mucous layer (123). Other enzymes that may disrupt gastric mucosal integrity include lipopolysaccharide, lipase, phospholipase A, and hemolysin. Other putative mediators of gastric inflammation by the organism include mucosal invasion, activation of inflammatory cells by *H. pylori* proteins, synthesis of platelet-activating factor, and induction of eosinophil degranulation. On the other hand, how much of gastritis is an immunologically related "innocent bystander" effect because of failure of the immune response to eliminate the infection is unknown. Local and systemic antibodies to a 120- 140-kDa molecular weight protein (*cagA* product) also has been linked to more severe gastritis (130).

Peptic Ulcer Disease

Duodenal Ulcer

A chronic peptic ulcer is defined as a break in the gastrointestinal mucosa that extends through the muscularis mucosae. A chronic ulcer usually has a diameter of 0.5 cm or greater and is characterized by depth and the presence of fibrous tissue in the ulcer base. The lifetime prevalence of peptic ulcer is approximately 10% and the annual incidence is 0.3% (132).

In duodenal ulcer disease, the prevalence of *H. pylori* infection is over 95%, strongly suggesting a cause and effect relationship (133,134). During the last four decades the incidence of duodenal ulcers has decreased (132), and this decrease in ulcer incidence has paralleled a decrease in the acquisition of *H. pylori* infection in persons born in more recent decades in Western countries (135). The most convincing evidence for a pathogenetic role of *H. pylori* in duodenal ulcers comes from experimental studies on the effects of treating the infection. Traditionally, antisecretory therapy (e.g., with a H_2-receptor blocker or an acid pump inhibitor) or sucralfate have been used to heal peptic ulceration. In patients healed with conventional therapy who are not given maintenance treatment, however, 80% of duodenal ulcers will relapse in 1 year. Eradication of *H. pylori,* on the other hand, alters the natural history of duodenal ulcer disease; it reduces the ulcer relapse rate over 1 year by more than 90% (Table 4, Fig. 5) (110,136–147).

Pathophysiology of H. pylori-*Induced Duodenal Ulcer.* The gastritis induced by *H. pylori* infection probably directly results in a number of changes of structure and function in gastric and duodenal mucosa that can result in ulcer disease. Some findings that were originally considered to be genetic markers of duodenal ulcer disease (e.g., elevated hyperpepsinogenemia I levels) are now known to be the result of the infection.

Effects of Gastric H. pylori *Colonization in Duodenal Ulcer Disease.* Gastrin from the antrum stimulates the parietal cells in the gastric body to secrete acid, and this hormone is as important as the vagus nerve in controlling gastric acid secretion. The basal and meal-stimulated release of gastrin is increased in duodenal ulcer patients and in patients with *H. pylori* infection who do not have an ulcer, but this rapidly reverts to normal with eradication of the infection (124,148–157). Recent studies suggest that the increase of gastrin is mainly due to G17 rather than G34; G17 is released from the antral mucosa where *H. pylori* is predominant while G34 is released from the duodenum (158).

How *H. pylori* alters gastrin release continues to be a subject of intense study. It was initially postulated that the bacterial urease would lead to production of an alkaline

TABLE 4. *Published studies of the effect of eradication of* H. pylori *on the relapse rate of duodenal ulcers*

Authors (reference)	Study design	Treatment	*H. pylori* eradication rate	DU relapse rate in *H. pylori* eradicated	DU relapse rate in *H. pylori* noneradicated	Duration of follow-up (months)
Bianchi Porro et al., 1993 (269)	Crossover, randomized	CBS, amoxicillin, tinidazole	83%	12%	100%	12
Sepalla et al., 1992 (138)	Open trial	CBS, amoxicillin, metronidazole	84%	1%	30%	12
Rauws and Tytgat, 1990 (144)	Prospective, randomized, controlled trial	CBS, amoxicillin metronidazole	62%	0%	89%	
Marshall et al., 1988 (136)	Prospective, double-blind, randomized	Cimetidine, CBS, tinidazole, placebo	Unknown	21%	84%	12
Graham et al., 1992 (141)	Randomized, controlled	Ranitidine, tetracycline, metronidazole, bismuth subsalicylate	89%	0%	95%	≤24
Hentschel et al., 1993 (147)	Prospective, parallel groups	Amoxicillin, metronidazole, ranitidine	89%	2%	85%	12
Coghlan et al., 1987 (146)	Randomized, single blind, clinical trial	CBS	52% (but no data on *H. pylori* status or prior treatment given)	27%	79%	12
Borody et al., 1989 (273)	Prospective, unblinded	CBS, tetracycline, metronidazole	94% (also patients with nonulcer dyspepsia included)	7%	Not available	12–37
George et al., 1990 (262)	Follow-up	Ranitidine, CBS, tetracycline, metronidazole	96%	0%	Not available	12
O'Riordan et al., 1990 (274)	Parallel groups	CBS, metronidazole, amoxicillin	74%	Data not available	Not available	None

CBS, colloidal bismuth subcitrate; DU, duodenol ulcer.

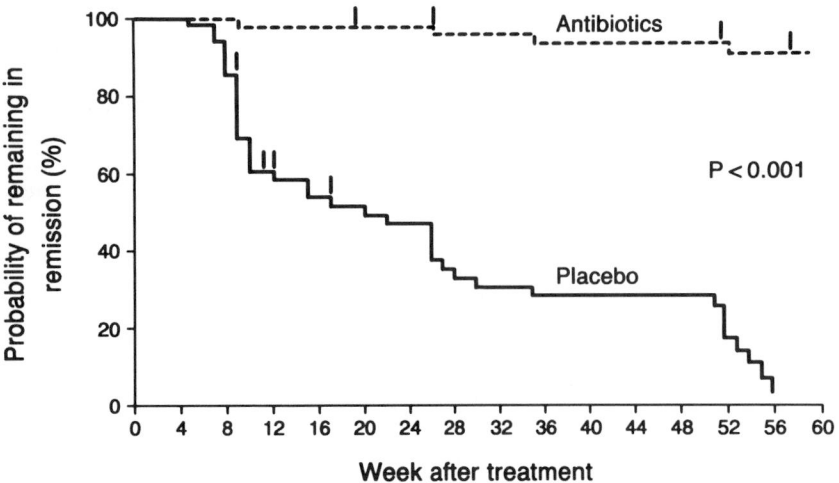

FIG. 5. Influence of eradication therapy with ranitidine, metronidazole, and amoxicillin ($n = 50$) compared with ranitidine alone ($n = 49$) on duodenal ulcer relapse. Note that bismuth was not included in the treatment regimen, indicating that the mucosal protective effects of bismuth are unlikely to explain the significantly lowered duodenal ulcer relapse rates identified by previous investigators. (From ref. 147, with permission.)

environment in the antrum that would in turn prevent the physiological suppression of gastrin release by acid. However, experiments that increased *H. pylori* ammonia production by intragastric infusion of urea have failed to alter gastrin levels, indicating that hypergastrinemia is not secondary to urease. It has been postulated that antral inflammation interferes with the normal somatostatin-mediated inhibition of gastrin release. *Helicobacter pylori* gastritis is associated with a decrease in the number of antral D cells (which produce the inhibitory hormone somatostatin) and G cells (which produce gastrin). However, the ratio of D to G cells is probably unchanged (159), and the rapid normalization of gastrin release after eradication therapy suggests that chemical mediators are most likely responsible for the increased gastrin release. Increased gastrin release may be mediated by increased release of luminal gastrin releasing peptide (GRP) secondary to the bacteria–host inflammatory interaction (152).

The increased gastrin induced by *H. pylori* appears to have limited effects on gastric acid secretion in subjects without ulcer disease; although some studies have found an increased gastric acid secretion in infected subjects (160), others suggest that basal and peak gastric acid outputs are similar in infected and noninfected subjects (161–163). Moreover, eradication of *H. pylori* only reduces acid output in a subset of duodenal ulcer patients. However, it is conceivable that prolonged hypergastrinemia associated with *H. pylori* infection leads to a more permanent increase in parietal cell mass that is known to characterize duodenal ulcer disease, and that this is not reversible in the short term with elimination of the infection.

Effects of H. pylori *on Duodenal Mucosa.* Since *H. pylori* colonizes only gastric mucosa, it was initially difficult to explain how *H. pylori* could be involved in the pathogenesis of duodenal ulceration. However, foci of gastric metaplasia in the duodenum are found in many healthy subjects and in the majority of patients with chronic duodenal ulcers (164,165). This gastric metaplasia is believed to be a response of pluripotential epithelial stem cells that differentiate into gastric-type rather than absorptive-type intestinal epithelium in response to acid

injury of the duodenum. This morphological change allows colonization by *H. pylori* in the duodenum that in turn leads to focal inflammation and mucosal damage, facilitating further tissue damage by gastric acid or pepsin (7,164–169). With eradication of *H. pylori*, there is normalization (disappearance of metaplasia) of the duodenal mucosa. In contrast, suppression of acid secretion can lead to resolution of gastric metaplasia (169).

Integrated Concept of H. pylori-*Induced Mucosal Damage.* The "leaking roof" hypothesis proposed by Goodwin (170) provides one model for duodenal ulcer disease; it is assumed that an intact mucosal barrier (roof) is essential to protect the underlying tissue from gastric acid (rain). Decreased mucosal integrity ("leaking roof") from *H. pylori*-induced impairment of the protective mucous layer and focal inflammation in the duodenum predispose to backdiffusion of H^+ ions that in turn results in focal tissue damage and ulcer formation (Fig. 6). However, the pathology of duodenitis and ulceration suggests that bacteria-induced inflammation is the primary defect, and hyperacidity may only add to the tissue injury.

It is unclear why some patients with *H. pylori* infection develop a duodenal ulcer, while most do not. Both host

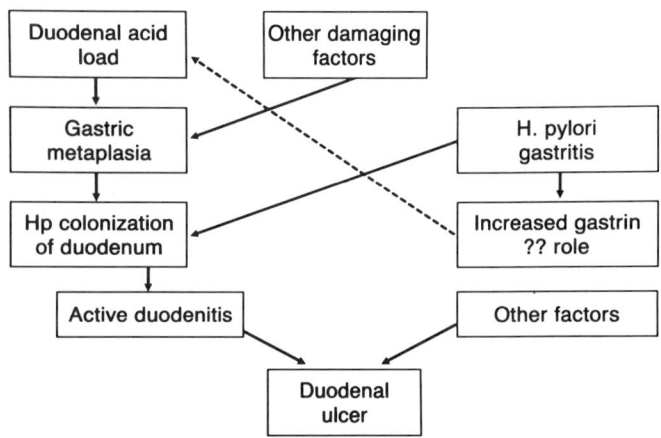

FIG. 6. Possible pathogenesis of chronic duodenal ulcer.

and bacterial factors may be relevant. Thus patients predisposed to duodenal ulcer may be those who naturally are in the upper normal range for gastric acid secretory capacity; such patients are predisposed to develop gastric metaplasia in the duodenum because of their higher acid load, and if these areas become infected the sequence to duodenal ulcer has begun. In addition, some *H. pylori* strains may have specific virulence factors that produce more severe inflammation and damage in the duodenum (125,171). For example, utilizing DNA–DNA hybridization, differences have been found between *H. pylori* strains from patients with duodenal ulcers and asymptomatic gastritis (68). These results, however, do not prove that genetic differences identified in *H. pylori* strains are of pathogenic importance; they may simply reflect divergent evolution. A vacuolizing cytotoxin has been found more often in *H. pylori* isolates from patients with duodenal ulceration (130), and the *cagA* product also has been associated with more severe gastric inflammation and peptic ulceration (130). Thus despite the central importance of *H. pylori* infection, duodenal ulcer may be the result of a multifactorial process involving both the host response and the bacteria.

Gastric Ulcer

While chronic gastric ulcers may occur in the absence of infection (172), gastric ulcers also are strongly associated with *H. pylori* infection. The proportion of subjects with chronic gastric ulcer and *H. pylori* infection approaches 80% to 90% (38,105,173,174). Moreover, gastric ulcer relapse is very substantially reduced by eradication of *H. pylori* infection (141,175) (Fig. 7). Nevertheless, the prevalence of *H. pylori* infection in patients with gastric ulcers is significantly lower than the prevalence rate in patients with duodenal ulcer, probably due in part to the relatively larger contribution of aspirin and NSAIDs to gastric ulcers.

Acid secretion tends to be normal or low in gastric ulcer patients perhaps because of more extensive gastritis in-

volving the acid-secreting corpus mucosa. Gastric ulcers tend to occur in antral type, non-acid-secreting mucosa usually adjacent to acid-secreting areas where the acid load is likely to be higher. It is yet unknown how *H. pylori* infection can result in a gastric ulcer, which is a focal lesion, when *H. pylori* gastritis is known to be a diffuse gastric process. Ormand and Talley have suggested that the gastric mucous layer is markedly degraded in the areas where *H. pylori* colonization is densest and acid secretion highest, which then allows hydrogen ion backdiffusion to occur (176). The subsequent change in mucosal pH stimulates the bacteria to migrate elsewhere, leading to a reduction in the density of *H. pylori* colonization that may allow healing to occur. The balance between healing and other noxious factors at the injured site determines if focal ulceration occurs.

The consumption of NSAIDs is recognized also to be an important risk factor for the development of gastric ulcers, and it is likely that *H. pylori* and NSAIDs induce gastric ulcers by independent mechanisms. Less certain is whether *H. pylori* has the potential to cause ulceration more often in the presence of NSAID intake. Supporting the concept of a synergistic action, Heresbach et al. (177) found more severe acute gastropathy in NSAID-treated patients with *H. pylori* colonization compared to patients without *H. pylori*. However, other studies have failed to confirm this finding (178).

Nonulcer Dyspepsia

Symptoms of upper gastrointestinal distress in the absence of peptic ulcer disease or any identifiable structural abnormality are among the most frequent complaints in Western countries, with a prevalence of 25% (179). The pathophysiology of nonulcer (also called functional) dyspepsia is very poorly understood (180), but one potential explanation in a subset of patients may be *H. pylori* infection (73,179,181–184).

If *H. pylori* plays a pathogenic role in nonulcer dyspepsia, then the infection should be more common in nonulcer

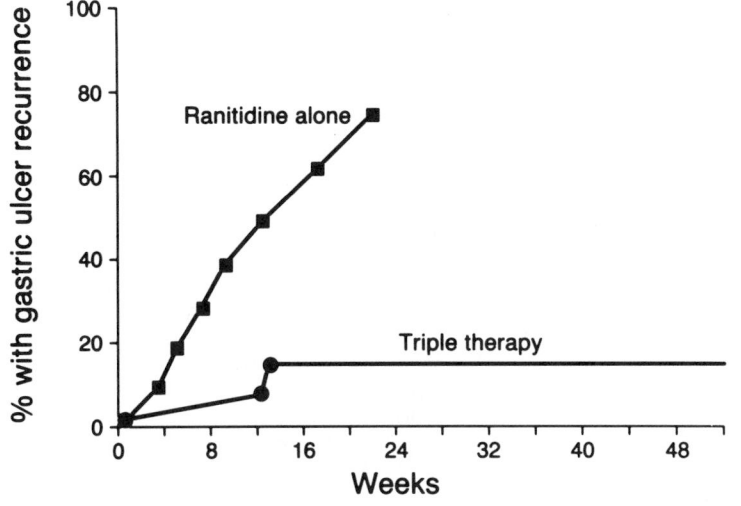

FIG. 7. Gastric ulcer recurrence (life table) for the year after successful ulcer healing with triple therapy (bismuth subsalicylate, metronidazole, and tetracycline) plus ranitidine compared with ranitidine alone. The recurrence rate of gastric ulcer was significantly greater in the ranitidine alone group. (From ref. 141, with permission.)

TABLE 5. *Symptoms associated with* Helicobacter pylori—*positive nonulcer dyspepsia*

Author (reference)	Number of subjects	H. pylori positive (%)	Individual symptom(s) associated with H. pylori
Marshall and Warren (4)	65	58	Burping
Rokkas et al. (190)	55	45	Postprandial bloating
Rathbone et al. (191)	193	54	Regurgitation (not esophagitis), previous dyspepsia
Andersen et al. (192)	33	39	None except symptom duration
Deltenre et al. (193)	200	64	Ulcer-like symptoms
Tucci et al. (189)	45	60	Epigastric pain or burning
Loffeld et al. (184)	109	56	None
Börsch et al. (194)	69	52	Flatulence a negative predictor
Jeena et al. (195)	69	78	None
Sobala et al. (196)	186	41	None
Collins et al. (182)	18	50	None
Guerre et al. (197)	96	40	None
Strauss et al. (73)	32	63	None
Vaira et al. (198)	107	58	Postprandial bloating
Goh et al. (199)	71	56	None
Schubert et al. (181)	474	36	None
Holtmann et al. (24)	44	26	None

dyspepsia than in healthy persons and specific symptoms should be associated with the infection. The prevalence rate of infection with *H. pylori* in outpatients with nonulcer dyspepsia approaches 50% (185–187) although infection is also common in asymptomatic persons (9,11). Thus in a careful population-based study, the prevalence of *H. pylori* in patients with nonulcer dyspepsia was 48% while the prevalence in age- and gender-matched controls was 36%, a significant difference (188). On the other hand, in a recent study in healthy blood donors without evidence of organic disease, no difference was found in the prevalence of *H. pylori* in subjects with and without dyspepsia. Furthermore, no differences were detected in subjects with specific patterns of dyspeptic symptoms (i.e., dysmotility-like, ulcer-like, or reflux-like dyspepsia) (24). Data on the relationship between specific upper abdominal symptoms and *H. pylori* also remain conflicting, with some studies reporting a positive association and most failing to confirm any link (4,73,182,184,189–199) (Table 5).

Only equivocal evidence for a role of *H. pylori* in nonulcer dyspepsia has come from treatment studies (199–207) (Table 6). Several studies have observed improvement of symptoms in patients in whom infection was suppressed, but other studies have failed to detect a significant benefit. However, these investigators used treatments that rarely eradicated infection, and long-term follow-up was usually not undertaken. The effects of eradicating *H. pylori* have similarly produced conflicting evidence but few reports have been published in full (208).

Gastric Malignancy

Adenocarcinoma

The incidence of gastric adenocarcinoma varies widely among different populations, ranging from fewer than 10 per 100,000 in Western Europe and the United States to 80 per 100,000 in Colombia and Japan (209). There is also

TABLE 6. *Anti-*Helicobacter pylori *therapy in nonulcer dyspepsia*

Author (reference)	n	Drug regiment (duration of treatment, weeks)	H. pylori suppression (%)	Response
McNulty et al. (200)	50	BSS (4 wk)	78	Improvement just short of significant.
		Erythromycin (2 wk)	7	No improvement.
Rokkas et al. (202)	52	CBS (8 wk)	83	Pain and bloating improved.
Lambert et al. (203)	82	CBS (4 wk)	59	Pain during the day and night improved.
Loffeld et al. (204)	50	CBS (4 wk)	30	No significant improvement.
Kang et al. (205)	51	CBS (8 wk)	89	More likely to become asymptomatic and lower use of antacids in cleared group.
Goh et al. (199)	71	CBS (4 wk)	81	Mean symptom score improved.
Marshall et al. (275)	50	BSS (3 wk)	70	No significant improvement.
Glupczynski et al. (206)	45	Amoxicillin (8 days)	91	No significant improvement.
Gastroenterology Physiology Working Group (207)	69	Nitrofurantoin (2 wk)	58	No significant improvement.
		Furazolidone (2 wk)	86	No significant improvement.

BSS, bismuth subsalicylate; CBS, colloidal bismuth subcitrate.

TABLE 7. Helicobacter pylori *and gastric adenocarcinoma*

Author (reference)	Odds ratio	95% Confidence interval
Forman et al. (212)	2.8	1.04–7.97
Nomura et al. (211)	6.0	2.1–17.3
Parsonnet et al. (213)	3.6	1.8–7.3
Talley et al. (214)	2.7	1.2–5.1
Guarner et al. (78)	4.0	1.1–14.9
Lin et al. (276)	1.0	0.6–1.8
Eurogast Study Group (215)	Sixfold[a]	—

[a] Increase of the gastric cancer risk in populations with a 100% *H. pylori* prevalence.

considerable variability of cancer incidence in different ethnic groups (209). Furthermore, the gastric cancer risk is altered by changes in geographical location. For example, the descendants of Japanese moving from their high-risk home country to a low-risk area have the same risk of gastric cancer as other people living in the low-risk area after several generations. Thus it has been speculated that an environmental factor must be associated with gastric carcinogenesis (210).

More recently, infection with *H. pylori* has been identified as an important risk factor in gastric adenocarcinoma (78,211–215) (Table 7). Striking parallels between the prevalence of *H. pylori* and gastric cancer have been found. In areas with high incidence rates of gastric cancer such as Peru (216–218) or Mexico (78), the prevalence rate of *H. pylori* approaches 90% in adults. In contrast, in countries with a low *H. pylori* prevalence, the incidence of gastric cancer is also low. Of particular note, noncardia gastric adenocarcinoma and *H. pylori* share a number of similar epidemiological patterns (Table 8). In Western countries there has been a considerable decrease of gastric cancer incidence during the last decades (210) and this decrease has been paralleled by a decrease of *H. pylori* infection in younger persons over recent decades (219,220). Case–control studies have evaluated whether an association between *H. pylori* infection and gastric cancer exists. Most studies have detected a significantly increased gastric cancer risk in *H. pylori*-infected subjects (78,211–215,276). Furthermore, the studies generally suggest that the risk is confined to noncardia gastric cancer.

Helicobacter pylori gastritis can progress to chronic atrophic gastritis, which is widely accepted as a precursor of gastric carcinoma (221). Studies from Scandinavia on the natural history of gastritis suggest that it usually takes decades for superficial gastritis to progress to atrophy (222–224). It is unknown if this is a reversible process; although one case of gastric mucosal atrophy apparently reversing to normal after successful eradication therapy of *H. pylori* has been reported, the findings were not confirmed by histology (225). How many subjects with *H. pylori* will finally progress to atrophic mucosa has been evaluated in Finnish studies, which suggest that 30% to 40% of infected individuals will do so. It is unknown whether or not specific bacterial virulence factors contribute to this progression, but the prevalence of a pH-dependent vacuolating cytotoxin was increased in patients with chronic atrophic gastritis compared to subjects with gastritis alone (226).

Gastric cancer develops only in a small proportion of infected subjects and may occur in subjects without evidence of past *H. pylori* infection. Thus *H. pylori* may be neither necessary nor sufficient to explain gastric adenocarcinoma; other variables such as nutritional intake (e.g., the ingestion of vitamin C) or genetic factors may be important (Fig. 8). The mechanisms by which *H. pylori* may result in malignant transformation are yet to be clearly identified. The production of superoxide and hydroxyl radicals in inflamed gastric mucosa may be able to induce mutations and malignant transformation in the gastric epithelium in predisposed individuals. Furthermore, the rapid turnover of cells with gastritis may favor growth of transformed malignant cells. It is unknown whether some strains of *H. pylori* are particularly carcinogenic.

In summary, current data strongly suggest that chronic *H. pylori* infection is associated with the development of chronic atrophic gastritis, which in a minority of otherwise predisposed individuals can result in the development of gastric adenocarcinoma.

Lymphoma

There is now evidence that *H. pylori* plays a key role in the development of mucosa associated lymphoid tissue (MALT) lymphoma. Lymphoid tissue is absent in normal gastric mucosa, but lymphoid tissue aggregates typically

TABLE 8. *Features of gastric adenocarcinoma and* Helicobacter pylori *in industrialized nations*

Features	Noncardia gastric cancer	H. pylori
Prevalence	Increases with age	Increases with age
Male/female	2:1	1:1
Ethnic groups	Incidence higher in blacks and Hispanics than Caucasians in U.S.	Prevalence higher in blacks and Hispanics than Caucasians in U.S.
Socioeconomic status	Disease of the poor	Higher prevalence in lower socioeconomic groups
Time trends	Mortality rate decreasing over past 50 years	Incidence diminishing with time (cohort effect)
Family history	Relatives of cases have two to three times greater risk of cancer	Parents and siblings of infected children more often infected

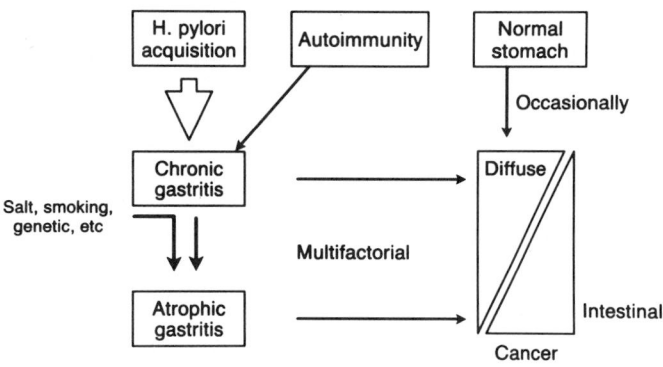

FIG. 8. A scheme for the pathogenesis of gastric adenocarcinoma. (From ref. 277, with permission.)

occur as a local response to infection with *H. pylori*. In one study (227), 125 out of 450 patients infected with *H. pylori* showed mucosal lymphoid follicles. In eight patients, the lymphoid infiltrates had features of MALT lymphoma. In a separate group of patients, 92% with MALT lymphoma were infected with *H. pylori* (227). Five patients with MALT lymphoma who tested positive for *H. pylori* were followed; four of them had complete remission after successful *H. pylori* eradication therapy, without undergoing additional therapeutic interventions (228). It has thus been speculated that infection with *H. pylori* may play a role in the multifactorial genesis of MALT lymphoma (229).

The observation that eradication of *H. pylori* can result in "retransformation" of malignant cells is most spectacular (230). The findings, however, remain to be confirmed in larger studies. Indeed, the MALT lymphomas may represent a continuum, and perhaps only the truly premalignant stages are reversible with eradication of the infection. Until more data are available, it remains essential to closely follow up patients by endoscopic surveillance who have only been treated by eradication of the infection. Histologic changes and endosonographic assessment of the thickness of the gastric wall may both be of value during follow-up. An association between *H. pylori* and non-Hodgkin's lymphoma of the stomach has also been reported (230).

Other Sites

Barrett's Esophagus

Barrett's esophagus is characterized by columnar metaplasia of the esophagus that is believed to be induced by chronic reflux of gastric acid or bile (231). While there is no convincing evidence that *H. pylori* is associated with gastroesophageal reflux disease or duodenogastric reflux (232), *H. pylori* has been found in esophageal tissue in patients with Barrett's esophagus and gastric-type epithelium in 20% to 50% of cases (233–235). However, patients with *H. pylori* do not have more esophageal inflammatory change than those without the infection (233,236,237), and

thus *H. pylori* in Barrett's esophagus is most likely an epiphenomenon of no clinical importance.

Meckel's Diverticulum

Ectopic gastric mucosa is found in a Meckel's diverticulum in 25% of cases. While it has been speculated that *H. pylori* might increase the risk of inflammation and ulceration in the diverticulum, *H. pylori* has been found in less than 2% of resected Meckel's diverticula and ulceration has not been associated with the infection (238,239).

TREATMENT REGIMENS

In the past 10 years, the pathophysiologic role of *H. pylori* in gastritis and chronic peptic ulceration has been established beyond doubt. However, optimal therapy has yet to be defined. *In vitro*, *H. pylori* is susceptible to bismuth and various antibiotics, but these findings have not translated into success *in vivo*. If antimicrobial therapy has been unsuccessful, most patients will have a recrudescence of infection within 1 month of stopping treatment. Testing for the organism may be misleading if done soon after stopping treatment. Therefore, eradication of *H. pylori* is currently defined as the absence of infection at least 4 weeks after stopping treatment.

Initially, bismuth alone was prescribed to eliminate *H. pylori* from the gastric mucosa, but it was soon discovered that bismuth only temporarily suppressed *H. pylori* in most cases and usually was unable to achieve permanent eradication. As a consequence, many combinations of bismuth and antibiotics were tested empirically. Even though some of these combinations have proved to be highly effective, concerns about side effects have tended to limit their widespread use. More recently, a combination of a single antibiotic with an acid pump inhibitor has been tested successfully. A summary of the efficacy of eradication therapy is presented in Table 9.

Bismuth Compounds

Bismuth preparations have been used for decades for the treatment of upper gastrointestinal symptoms. Several

TABLE 9. *Effects of different treatment regimens on eradication of* Helicobacter pylori

Therapy (reference)	Eradication rate
Monotherapy (244)	
Colloidal bismuth subcitrate	21%
Bismuth subsalicylate	10%
Amoxicillin	23%
Dual therapy (244)	
Bismuth/metronidazole	55%
Bismuth/amoxicillin	44%
Triple therapy (244)	
Bismuth/metronidazole	
plus amoxicillin	73%
or	
plus tetracycline	94%
Acid suppression plus antibiotics	
Acid pump inhibitor	
(omeprazole)	82%
plus amoxicillin (250)	

studies have shown that bismuth preparations alone promote duodenal ulcer healing and reduce ulcer relapse rates (133,200,240–243). However, at best only about 20% of patients have *H. pylori* eradicated using bismuth alone (244). No direct comparisons between bismuth subsalicylate and bismuth subcitrate taken four times a day are available, but the latter may be more effective in eradicating *H. pylori*.

Antibiotics

Monotherapy with single agents yield eradication rates from nil to at best 30%. The low pH of the stomach and the ecological niche of the organism in the mucous layer probably help to protect it. A recent meta-analysis of empiric therapy reported a 23% eradication rate for amoxicillin monotherapy compared with only 8% for other antibiotics (244). Moreover, rapid induction of bacterial resistance with single antibiotic use has been reported to occur, especially with metronidazole, erythromycin, clarithromycin, and ciprofloxacin. On the other hand, bismuth, amoxicillin, tetracycline, furazolidone, and nitrofurantoin do not induce antibiotic resistance if used alone. Thus treatment with a single antibiotic does not achieve reliable eradication of *H. pylori*.

Combinations

Double Therapy

The efficacy of bismuth compounds is increased if they are combined with an antibiotic. Thus a combination of bismuth plus amoxicillin yields eradication rates from 28% to 60%, with a mean of 44% (244). Combinations of bismuth and metronidazole yield higher eradication rates, ranging from 32% to 79%, with a mean of 55%. In patients with metronidazole-resistant strains, clarithromycin is an alternative that has produced similar results to amoxicillin in double therapy. In one study, amoxicillin and metroni-

dazole in combination with ranitidine eradicated *H. pylori* in 89% of patients with a duodenal ulcer (147).

Triple Therapy

Triple therapy refers to the combination of a bismuth preparation, metronidazole, and either amoxicillin or tetracycline. Cumulated data yield a mean eradication rate with such a regimen of 94% (244). Amoxicillin has a slightly lower eradication rate than tetracycline in triple therapy. Even though triple therapy is highly effective, compliance with this therapy is relatively poor because of the numbers of tablets required. It has been shown that most patients taking triple therapy will be successful in eradicating the infection if more than 60% of the prescribed medications are taken (111). Moreover, side effects including nausea, diarrhea, sore mouth, and rash occur in up to 20% of cases. *Clostridium difficile* colitis and candidiasis occur rarely. The optimal duration of therapy is also not defined, but generally a 2-week course is recommended. One-week therapeutic regimens are being tested but may be less effective. For example, colloidal bismuth 120 mg, amoxicillin 500 mg four times a day for 7 days, and metronidazole 400 mg five times daily on days 5, 6, and 7 eradicated 72% of cases (93% were eradicated who had metronidazole-sensitive isolates) (245).

Acid Inhibition and Antibiotics

The H_2-receptor blockers (cimetidine, ranitidine, famotidine, and nizatidine) lack any significant anti-*H. pylori* effect *in vitro* and *in vivo,* but the acid pump inhibitors (omeprazole, lansoprazole, and pantoprazole) have *in vitro* antimicrobial activity against *H. pylori* (246,247). The acid pump inhibitors can temporarily suppress infection in up to 60% of patients (248), although eradication is rare (248–253). In contrast, several studies have shown that the combination of an acid pump inhibitor and a single antibiotic results in eradication rates of 60% to 80% although some centers have had poorer results (250,254–256). The most widely used combination has been omeprazole plus amoxicillin, although combinations with other antibiotics (e.g., clarithromycin) have yielded similar results (147,257). Further work to optimize and simplify the eradication protocols is currently underway but it appears that an acid pump inhibitor and antibiotic taken twice daily for 2 weeks is best (244). Addition of a third agent (e.g., metronidazole, or clarithromycin) for several days may improve efficacy.

Time Course

With successful antimicrobial treatment, the polymorphonuclear cells and surface cell damage disappear within 48 hr of starting treatment, while the mononuclear cells markedly decrease within 2 weeks. However, complete disappearance of the chronic inflammatory reaction may take 6 months or more following successful eradication (124,258).

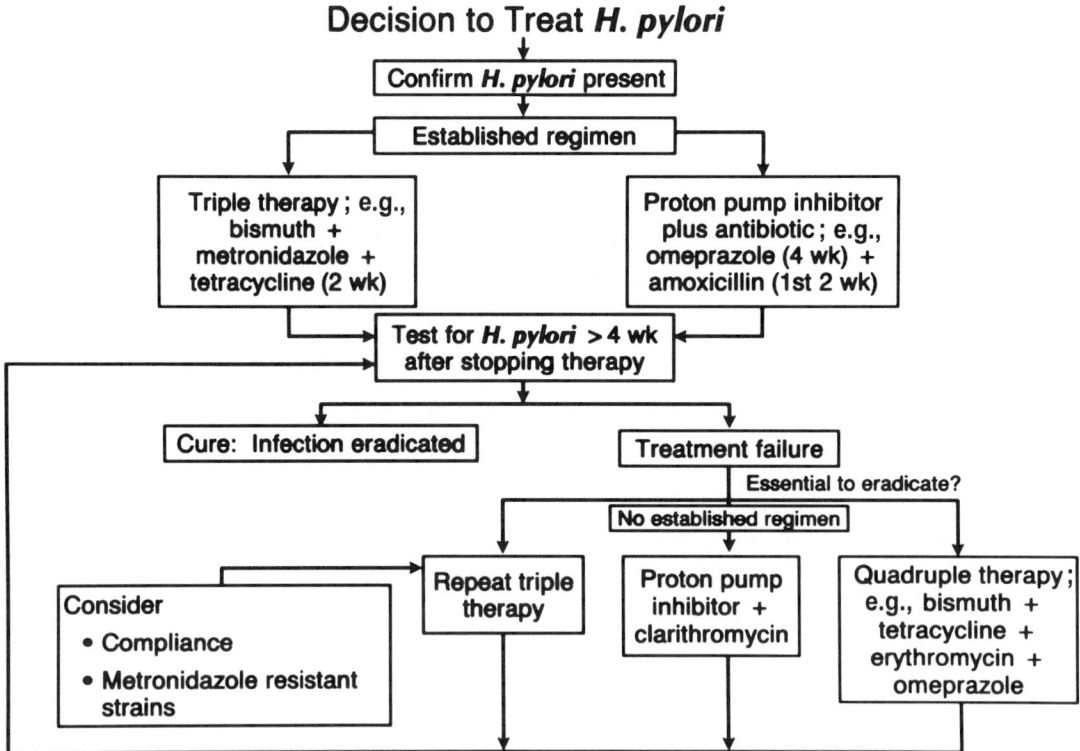

FIG. 9. Strategy for the treatment of *Helicobacter pylori* infection.

Eradication Therapy: Current Recommendations

The combination of either bismuth subsalicylate (two tablets four times a day) or bismuth subcitrate (two tablets twice a day) plus metronidazole (250 to 500 mg three times a day) and tetracycline (500 mg four times a day) or, if this cannot be used, amoxicillin (500 mg four times a day) for 2 weeks is the practical first choice for eradication therapy. Bismuth should be taken before meals and should be taken 30 min apart from the antibiotics. Alternatively, a combination of omeprazole (20 mg twice a day for 2 weeks) and amoxicillin (1 g twice a day for 2 weeks) is a reasonable but more expensive alternative. Note that addition of an antibiotic after a period of treatment with an acid pump inhibitor may produce poorer results. If infection fails to be eradicated by these alternatives, no well-defined options exist; however, retreatment with triple therapy frequently is successful. Other combinations that may be effective include two weeks of omeprazole and clarithromycin or a one-week triple therapy with an acid pump inhibitor, clarithromycin, and tinidazole. A strategy for treating *H. pylori* is summarized in Fig. 9.

INDICATIONS FOR DIAGNOSTIC TESTING AND THERAPY

Acute *H. pylori* Infection

Acute infection with *H. pylori* may result in dyspeptic symptoms, but because symptoms are self-limited, specific testing and treatment are not required.

Peptic Ulcer Disease

Duodenal Ulcer (Uncomplicated)

Virtually all patients with duodenal ulcer test positive for *H. pylori;* the absence of *H. pylori* most often suggests intake of NSAIDs or the presence of Zollinger–Ellison syndrome as the cause of ulceration. Very rare causes of *H. pylori*-negative duodenal ulcers include Crohn's disease, tuberculosis, malignancy, and viral infections (172,259). Successful eradication of *H. pylori* essentially abolishes relapse of duodenal ulcer disease (110,136–138,141,142,144–147,253,260–262). While smoking has been identified as an important risk factor for duodenal ulcer recurrence (263), after successful eradication of *H. pylori* smoking does not increase the risk of ulcer recurrence (140). Whether eradication of *H. pylori* leads to faster ulcer healing than acid suppression alone is not yet well-established (264,265). In general, patients treated with acid suppression plus antibiotics have had higher healing rates than patients treated with acid suppression alone (Fig. 10), but the healing rates in these trials have been lower than expected (266,267).

An attempt should be made to eradicate *H. pylori* in all duodenal ulcer patients who have documented infection (Fig. 11). Similarly, patients currently being treated with maintenance antisecretory therapy for ulcer disease who are infected should be offered therapy for *H. pylori* if this has not been tried. In the United States, bismuth subsalicylate is the only currently available bismuth compound and its efficacy in healing ulcers is unknown. Therefore,

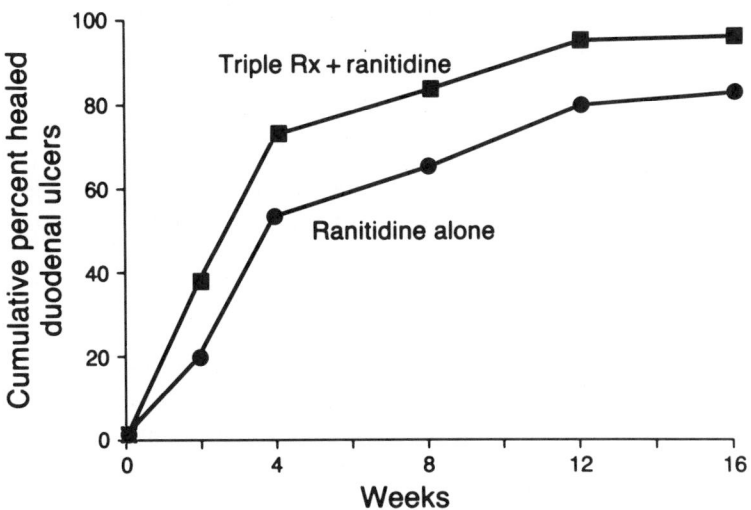

FIG. 10. Healing of duodenal ulcer was significantly more rapid in patients assigned to receive triple therapy (bismuth subsalicylate, metronidazole, and tetracycline) plus ranitidine (*n* = 53) compared to those assigned to receive ranitidine alone (*n* = 52). (From ref. 265, with permission.)

if triple therapy is given to a patient with an active ulcer, an ulcer healing agent such as an H_2 blocker or an acid pump inhibitor must be added. For this reason, an acid pump inhibitor plus amoxicillin may be the preferred first-line treatment for active duodenal ulcer disease.

It must be remembered that the currently available eradication regimens are not successful in approximately 20% of patients. Ideally, the physician should therefore confirm that *H. pylori* has been eradicated after treatment as this helps in planning future management. In patients with multiple ulcer recurrences who fail to have their infection successfully eradicated despite repeated courses

of treatment, conventional long-term acid suppression remains the major treatment option.

Gastric Ulcer (Uncomplicated)

Intake of NSAIDs always should be curtailed whether or not *H. pylori* infection is present. Otherwise, the treatment principles discussed earlier for duodenal ulcer disease similarly apply in gastric ulcer. In contrast to duodenal ulcers, however, the risk of an ulcer relapse is higher in successfully eradicated patients since other fac-

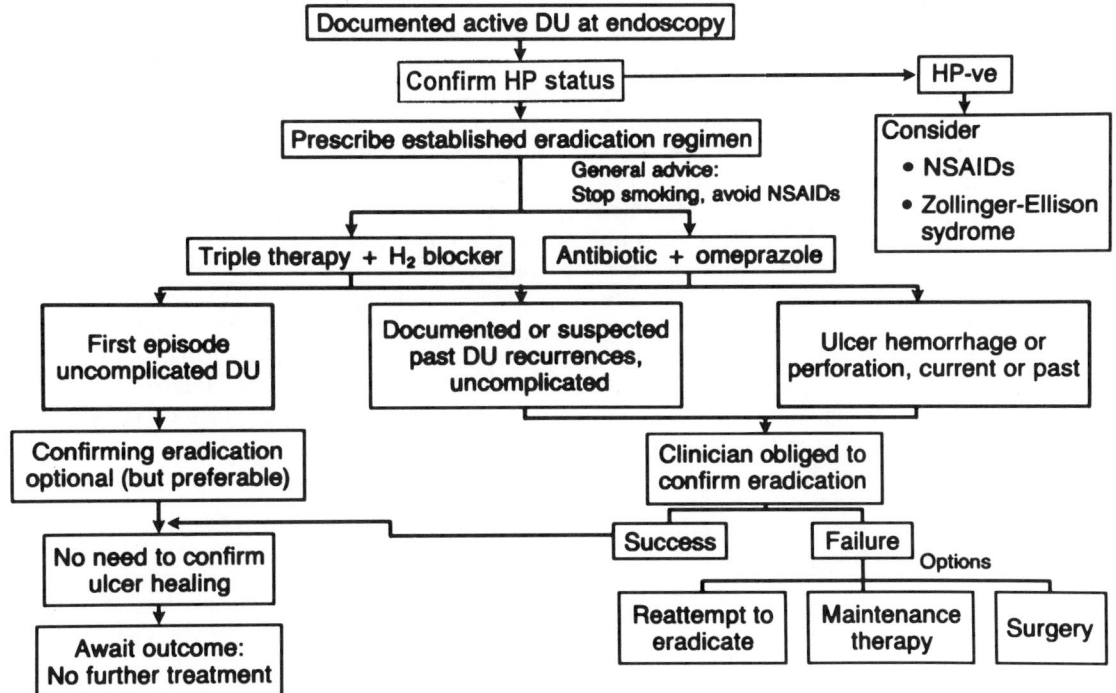

FIG. 11. Strategy for the treatment of duodenal ulcer disease.

tors such as NSAIDs also cause gastric ulcers. Moreover, it is recommended that ulcer healing be confirmed at a follow-up endoscopy 8 to 12 weeks later and gastric malignancy be excluded by taking multiple gastric biopsies at the ulcer site.

Refractory Disease

More than 80% of chronic peptic ulcers are healed within 8 weeks by conventional acid suppression using H$_2$ blockers (266–268). The small group of patients who do not heal within this time interval are considered to have refractory disease. Clinically, it is sometimes difficult to distinguish between an early ulcer relapse after weeks of treatment or a real nonresponder to treatment. Refractory ulcers necessitate further diagnostic workup to exclude Zollinger–Ellison syndrome and consumption of nonsteroidals as a cause of delayed healing. In gastric ulcer disease, exclusion of malignancy is essential. In the absence of another cause, therapy to eradicate H. pylori is the treatment of choice in patients with refractory disease who have not been so treated; the prevalence of refractory ulcer disease is probably very low in patients in whom H. pylori has been successfully eradicated. One study in patients with refractory duodenal ulcers demonstrated an 88% four-week healing rate after eradication therapy with colloidal bismuth subcitrate, amoxicillin, and tinidazole, but this study did not include any appropriate control group (269). In patients who fail to have the infection eradicated, more substantial acid suppression (e.g., by the use of an acid pump inhibitor) will heal the majority of ulcers (270).

Patients with Increased Risk of Ulcer Complications

Little data are available on whether eradication of H. pylori in patients who have had non-NSAID ulcer bleeding or perforation abolishes the risk of recurrent complications, although this makes perfect sense based on current knowledge. In a small randomized controlled trial of 31 patients presenting after a major ulcer bleed, Graham et al. (271) found that hemorrhage occurred significantly more often in those treated with ranitidine alone (and no maintenance antisecretory therapy) compared with those given triple therapy. Although larger and better trials are needed, anti-H. pylori therapy therefore remains the treatment of choice in these patients. However, it is absolutely essential to confirm that the organism has been eradicated in patients who have had ulcer complications before maintenance antisecretory treatment is stopped, and to ensure that NSAIDs are not being taken. If eradication fails, other treatment options for the prevention of ulcer complications such as long-term maintenance therapy with acid-suppressing agents has to be considered (272).

Nonulcer Dyspepsia

There is as yet no convincing evidence that H. pylori causes nonulcer dyspepsia. Thus it is not justifiable to routinely eradicate the infection in patients with nonulcer dyspepsia. The present data, however, do not exclude the possibility that there is a small subgroup of patients that will profit from eradication therapy. In practice, patients with severe symptoms that have not responded to conventional therapy, such as use of prokinetics or acid-reducing drugs, may be candidates for anti-H. pylori therapy if infected, but the benefit in such cases is not established.

Patients at Risk of Developing Gastric Cancer

Helicobacter pylori gastritis is associated with an increased risk of gastric cancer. It is likely, however, that the infection must be prolonged and associated with the development of atrophic gastritis and intestinal metaplasia for gastric cancer to occur. Little is known about the effects of eradication therapy on precursor lesions.

Until further studies are available, it seems reasonable to consider offering anti-H. pylori treatment to infected patients with a strong family history of gastric cancer or histologically documented intestinal metaplasia. However, the benefit of such treatment, if any, is unknown. Primary prevention of infection in childhood may be the most effective way to eliminate gastric cancer in high-risk populations, but this must await the development of a vaccine.

OUTLOOK

Much progress has been made in the last decade, and the clinical role of H. pylori infection is becoming unraveled. However, many key clinical questions remain to be answered. Exactly how does H. pylori produce such diverse clinical endpoints, from ulcer to possibly cancer? Is H. pylori a cause of nonulcer dyspepsia? Can the gastric cancer sequence be interrupted by treating the infection? Who among those with asymptomatic gastritis should we target for therapy, or should everyone be treated? What is the best strategy for those who fail current regimens to eradicate infection?

The public health implications of a policy of treating all or even most infected persons are enormous. Still, in the near future, physicians will be able to identify H. pylori infection in their offices using rapid, highly accurate, noninvasive diagnostic procedures, and it is then likely that eradication therapies will be more widely applied. The rapid developments in this field have changed medical practice, and we are likely to see even more change over the next decade.

REFERENCES

1. Marshall B, Warren JR. Unidentified curved bacillus on gastric epithelium in active chronic gastritis. *Lancet* 1983;1: 1273–1275.
2. Heatley RV. *Helicobacter pylori* infection and inflammation. *Scand J Gastroenterol Suppl* 1991;187:23–30.
3. Johnston BJ, Reed PI, Ali MH. Prevalence of *Campylobacter*

pylori in duodenal and gastric mucosa—relationship to inflammation. *Scand J Gastroenterol Suppl* 1988;142:69–75.

4. Marshall BJ, Warren JR. Unidentified curved bacilli in the stomach of patients with gastritis and peptic ulceration. *Lancet* 1984;1:1311–1315.

5. Blecker U, Hauser B, Lanciers S, Peeters S, Suys B, Vandenplas Y. The prevalence of *Helicobacter pylori*-positive serology in asymptomatic children. *J Pediatr Gastroenterol Nutr* 1993;16:252–256.

6. Megraud F. Epidemiology of *Helicobacter pylori* infection. *Gastroenterol Clin North Am* 1993;22:73–88.

7. Asaka M, Kimura T, Kudo M, et al. Relationship of *Helicobacter pylori* to serum pepsinogens in an asymptomatic Japanese population. *Gastroenterology* 1992;102:760–766.

8. Parsonnet J, Blaser MJ, Perez Perez GI, Hargrett Bean N, Tauxe RV. Symptoms and risk factors of *Helicobacter pylori* infection in a cohort of epidemiologists. *Gastroenterology* 1992;102:41–46.

9. Dehesa M, Dooley CP, Cohen H, Fitzgibbons PL, Perez Perez GI, Blaser MJ. High prevalence of *Helicobacter pylori* infection and histologic gastritis in asymptomatic Hispanics. *J Clin Microbiol* 1991;29:1128–1131.

10. Graham DY, Adam E, Reddy GT, et al. Seroepidemiology of *Helicobacter pylori* infection in India. Comparison of developing and developed countries. *Dig Dis Sci* 1991;36:1084–1088.

11. Graham DY, Malaty HM, Evans DG, Evans DJ Jr, Klein PD, Adam E. Epidemiology of *Helicobacter pylori* in an asymptomatic population in the United States. Effect of age, race, and socioeconomic status. *Gastroenterology* 1991;100:1495–1501.

12. Sitas F, Forman D, Yarnell JW, et al. *Helicobacter pylori* infection rates in relation to age and social class in a population of Welsh men. *Gut* 1991;32:25–28.

13. Pateraki E, Mentis A, Spiliadis C, et al. Seroepidemiology of *Helicobacter pylori* infection in Greece. *FEMS Microbiol Immunol* 1990;2:129–136.

14. Hirschl AM. Frequency of occurrence of *Campylobacter pylori* and analysis of the systemic and local immune response. *Zentralbl Bakteriol Mikrobiol Hyg A* 1987;266:526–542.

15. Jones DM, Eldridge J, Fox AJ, et al. Antibody to the gastric *Campylobacter*-like organism—clinical correlations and distribution in the normal population. *J Med Microbiol* 1986;22:57.

16. Newell DG, Caygill CPJ, Stacey AR, et al. The distribution of anti-*C. pylori* antibodies in patients undergoing endoscopy and in the normal population relative to age and geographical distribution. In: Takemoto T, Kawai K, Shimoyama T, eds. Campylobacter pylori *and gastroduodenal diseases*, 2nd ed. Tokyo: Taisho, 1990;54.

17. Kosunen TU, Hook J, Rautelin HI, et al. Age dependent increase of *Campylobacter pylori* antibodies in blood donors. *Scand J Gastroenterol* 1989;24:110.

18. Mégraud F, Bonnet F, Garnier M, et al. Characterization of *Campylobacter pyloridis* by culture, enzymatic profile, and protein content. *J Clin Microbiol* 1985;22:1007.

19. Basso L, Clune J, Beattie S, et al. Epidemiology of *Helicobacter pylori* infestion. *Rev Esp Enferm Dig* 1990;78(suppl I):40.

20. Fich A, Carel R, Keret D, et al. Seroepidemiology of *Helicobacter pylori* in the Israeli population. *Gastroenterology* 1992;102:A68.

21. Dwyer B, Kaldor J, Tee W, Marakowski E, Raios K. Antibody response to *Campylobacter pylori* in diverse ethnic groups. *Scand J Infect Dis* 1988;20:349–350.

22. Morris A, Nicholson G, Lloyd G, et al. Seroepidemiology of *Campylobacter pyloridis*. *N Z Med J* 1986;99:657.

23. Perez Perez GI, Dworkin BM, Chodos JE, Blaser MJ. *Campylobacter pylori* antibodies in humans. *Ann Intern Med* 1988;109:11–17.

24. Holtmann G, Goebell H, Holtmann M, Talley NJ. Dyspepsia in healthy blood donors: pattern of symptoms and association with *Helicobacter pylori*. *Dig Dis Sci* 1994;39:1090–1098.

25. Malaty HM, Evans DG, Evans DJ Jr, Graham DY. *Helicobacter pylori* in Hispanics: comparison with blacks and whites of similar age and socioeconomic class. *Gastroenterology* 1992;103:813–816.

26. Graham DY, Klein PD, Opekun AR, et al. Epidemiology of *Campylobacter pylori* infection: ethnic considerations. *Scand J Gastroenterol Suppl* 1988;142:9–13.

27. Hammermeister I, Janus G, Schamarowski F, Rudolf M, Jacobs E, Kist M. Elevated risk of *Helicobacter pylori* infection in submarine crews. *Eur J Clin Microbiol Infect Dis* 1992;11:9–14.

28. Nomura A, Stemmermann GN, Chyou P, et al. *Helicobacter pylori* infection and gastric carcinoma in a population of Japanese–Americans in Hawaii. *N Engl J Med* 1991;325:1132.

29. Glupczynski Y, Bourdeaux L, Verhas M, DePrez C, DeVos D, Devreker T. Use of a urea breath test versus invasive methods to determine the prevalence of *Helicobacter pylori* in Zaire. *Eur J Clin Microbiol Infect Dis* 1992;11:322–327.

30. Holcombe C, Omotara BA, Eldridge J, Jones DM. *H. pylori,* the most common bacterial infection in Africa: a random serological study. *Am J Gastroenterol* 1992;87:28–30.

31. Diomande MI, Flejou JF, Potet F, et al. Chronic gastritis and *Helicobacter pylori* infection on the Ivory Coast. A series of 277 symptomatic patients. *Gastroenterol Clin Biol* 1991;15:711–716.

32. Barthel JS, Everett ED. Diagnosis of *Campylobacter pylori* infections: the "gold standard" and the alternatives. *Rev Infect Dis* 1990;12(Suppl):S107–S114.

33. Brown KE, Peura DA. Diagnosis of *Helicobacter pylori* infection. *Gastroenterol Clin North Am* 1993;22:105–115.

34. Gray SF, Wyatt JI, Rathbone BJ. Simplified techniques for identifying *Campylobacter pyloridis*. *J Clin Pathol* 1986;39:1279.

35. Gustavsson S, Phillips SF, Malagelada JR, et al. Assessment of *Campylobacter*-like organisms in the postoperative stomach, iatrogenic gastritis, and chronic gastroduodenal diseases: preliminary observations. *Mayo Clin Proc* 1987;62:265–268.

36. Montgomery EA, Martin DF, Peura DA. Rapid diagnosis of *Campylobacter pylori* by Gram's stain. *Am J Clin Pathol* 1988;90:606–609.

37. Madan E, Kemp J, Westblom TU, Subik M, Sexton S, Cook J. Evaluation of staining methods for identifying *Campylobacter pylori*. *Am J Clin Pathol* 1988;90:450–453.

38. Haruma K, Okamoto S, Sumii K, et al. *Helicobacter pylori* infection and gastroduodenal disease: a comparison of endoscopic findings, histology, and urease test data. *Hiroshima J Med Sci* 1992;41:65–70.

39. Lin SK, Lambert JR, Schembri M, et al. A comparison of diagnostic tests to determine *Helicobacter pylori* infection. *J Gastroenterol Hepatol* 1992;7:203–209.

40. Hedenbro JL, Benoni C, Schalen C, et al. *Helicobacter pylori* and atrophic gastritis. *Tokai J Exp Clin Med* 1992;17:1–4.

41. Rocha GA, Queiroz DM, Mendes EN, Barbosa AJ, Lima GF Jr, Oliveira CA. *Helicobacter pylori* acute gastritis: histological, endoscopical, clinical, and therapeutic features. *Am J Gastroenterol* 1991;86:1592–1595.

42. Petross CW, Appleman MD, Cohen H, et al. Prevalence of *Campylobacter pylori* and association with antral mucosal histology in subjects with and without upper gastrointestinal symptoms. *Dig Dis Sci* 1988;33:649.

43. West AP, Millar MR, Tompkins DS. Effect of physical environment on survival of *Helicobacter pylori*. *J Clin Pathol* 1992;45:228–231.

44. Hartmann D, von Graevenitz A. A note on name, viability and urease tests of *Campylobacter pylori*. *Eur J Clin Microbiol* 1987;6:82–83.

45. Morris A, Ali MR, Brown P, et al. *Campylobacter pylori* infection in biopsy specimens of gastric antrum: laboratory diagnosis and estimation of sampling error. *J Clin Pathol* 1989;42:727–732.

46. Nysaeter G, Berstad K, Weberg R, Berstad A, Hardardottir H. Diagnosis of *Helicobacter pylori* infection. Rapid urease test, microscopy of smears and culture from ventricular biopsy compared with the ^{14}C-urea breath test. *Tidsskr Nor Laegeforen* 1992;112:2356–2358.

47. Carvalho AS, Queiroz DM, Mendes EN, Rocha GA, Penna FJ. Diagnosis and distribution of *Helicobacter pylori* in the gastric

mucosa of symptomatic children. *Braz J Med Biol Res* 1991; 24:163–166.

48. Hernandez F, Rivera P, Sigaran M, Miranda J. Diagnosis of *Helicobacter pylori:* comparison of an urease test, histological visualization of curved bacteria and culture. *Rev Inst Med Trop Sao Paulo* 1991;33:80–82.

49. Bell GD, Powell KU, Burridge SM, et al. Short report: omeprazole plus antibiotic combinations for the eradication of metronidazole-resistant *Helicobacter pylori. Aliment Pharmacol Ther* 1992;6:751–758.

50. Loo VG, Sherman P, Matlow AG. *Helicobacter pylori* infection in a pediatric population: in vitro susceptibilities to omeprazole and eight antimicrobial agents. *Antimicrob Agents Chemother* 1992;36:1133–1135.

51. Rautelin H, Seppala K, Renkonen OV, Vainio U, Kosunen TU. Role of metronidazole resistance in therapy of *Helicobacter pylori* infections. *Antimicrob Agents Chemother* 1992; 36:163–166.

52. European Study Group on Antibiotic Susceptibility of *Helicobacter pylori.* Results of a multicentre European survey in 1991 of metronidazole resistance in *Helicobacter pylori. Eur J Clin Microbiol Infect Dis* 1992;11:777–781.

53. Kolts BE, Joseph B, Achem SR, Bianchi T, Monteiro C. *Helicobacter pylori* detection: a quality and cost analysis. *Am J Gastroenterol* 1993;88:650–655.

54. Qureshi H, Ahmed W, Zuberi SJ, Kazi J. Use of CLO test in the detection of *Helicobacter pylori* infection and its correlation with histologic gastritis. *J Pak Med Assoc* 1992;42:292–293.

55. Ng TM, Fock KM, Ho J, et al. CLOtest (rapid urease test) in the diagnosis of *Helicobacter pylori* infection. *Singapore Med J* 1992;33:568–569.

56. Guelrud M, Mendoza S, Gelrud D, Essenfeld E. Comparison of urease test (CLOtest) and histology in the diagnosis of *Campylobacter pylori. G E N* 1989;43:279–282.

57. Oderda G, Dell'Olio D, Morra I, Ansaldi N. Rapid urease test (CLO-test) for early detection of *Campylobacter pylori* infection in children. *Am J Gastroenterol* 1988;83:792.

58. Katelaris PH, Lowe DG, Norbu P, Farthing MJ. Field evaluation of a rapid, simple and inexpensive urease test for the detection of *Helicobacter pylori. J Gastroenterol Hepatol* 1992;7: 569–571.

59. Thillainayagam AV, Arvind AS, Cook RS, Harrison IG, Tabaqchali S, Farthing MJ. Diagnostic efficiency of an ultrarapid endoscopy room test for *Helicobacter pylori. Gut* 1991;32: 467–469.

60. Engstrand L, Gustavsson S, Jorgensen A, Schwan A, Scheynius A. Inoculation of barrier-born pigs with *Helicobacter pylori:* a useful animal model for gastritis type B. *Infect Immun* 1990;58:1763–1768.

61. Chodos JE, Dworkin BM, Smith F, Van Horn K, Weiss L, Rosenthal WS. *Campylobacter pylori* and gastroduodenal disease: a prospective endoscopic study and comparison of diagnostic tests. *Am J Gastroenterol* 1988;83:1226–1230.

62. Rivera E, Lopez Vidal Y, Luqueno V, Ruiz Palacios GM. Indirect immunofluorescence assay for detection of *Helicobacter pylori* in human gastric mucosal biopsies. *J Clin Microbiol* 1991; 29:1748–1751.

63. Engstrand L, Pahlson C, Gustavsson S, et al. Monoclonal antibodies for rapid identification of *Campylobacter pyloridis. Lancet* 1986;2:1402–1403.

64. Westblom TU, Phadnis S, Yang P, Czinn SJ. Diagnosis of *Helicobacter pylori* infection by means of a polymerase chain reaction assay for gastric juice aspirates. *Clin Infect Dis* 1993;16: 367–371.

65. Owen RJ, Bell GD, Desai M, et al. Biotype and molecular fingerprints of metronidazole-resistant strains of *Helicobacter pylori* from antral gastric mucosa. *J Med Microbiol* 1993;38:6–12.

66. Labigne A, Cussac V, Courcoux P. Development of genetic and molecular approaches for the diagnosis and the study of the pathogenic power of *Helicobacter pylori,* agent of inflammatory gastric diseases. *Ann Gastroenterol Hepatol (Paris)* 1992;28:93–97.

67. Engstrand L, Nguyen AM, Graham DY, el Zaatari FA. Reverse transcription and polymerase chain reaction amplification of rRNA for detection of *Helicobacter* species. *J Clin Microbiol* 1992;30:2295–2301.

68. Yoshimura HH, Evans DG, Graham DY. DNA–DNA hybridization demonstrates apparent genetic differences between *Helicobacter pylori* from patients with duodenal ulcer and asymptomatic gastritis. *Dig Dis Sci* 1993;38:1128–1131.

69. Collins JS. Role of *Helicobacter pylori* in gastritis and duodenitis in man. *Agents Actions* 1992;Spec No:C47–C49.

70. Glupczynski Y, Burette A, Goossens H, DePrez C, Butzler JP. Effect of antimicrobial therapy on the specific serological response to *Helicobacter pylori* infection. *Eur J Clin Microbiol Infect Dis* 1992;11:583–588.

71. Talley NJ, Kost L, Haddad A, Zinsmeister AR. Comparison of commercial serological tests for detection of *Helicobacter pylori* antibodies. *J Clin Microbiol* 1992;30:3146–3150.

72. Crabtree JE, Shallcross TM, Heatley RV, Wyatt JI. Evaluation of a commercial ELISA for serodiagnosis of *Helicobacter pylori* infection. *J Clin Pathol* 1991;44:326–328.

73. Strauss RM, Wang TC, Kelsey PB, et al. Association of *Helicobacter pylori* infection with dyspeptic symptoms in patients undergoing gastroduodenoscopy. *Am J Med* 1990;89:464–469.

74. Best LM, Veldhuyzen van Zanten SJ, Bezanson GS, Haldane DJ, Malatjalian DA. Serological detection of *Helicobacter pylori* by a flow microsphere immunofluorescence assay. *J Clin Microbiol* 1992;30:2311–2317.

75. Talley NJ, Newell DG, Ormand JE, et al. Serodiagnosis of *Helicobacter pylori:* comparison of enzyme-linked immunosorbent assays. *J Clin Microbiol* 1991;29:1635–1639.

76. Lelwala Guruge J, Nilsson I, Ljungh A, Wadstrom T. Cell surface proteins of *Helicobacter pylori* as antigens in an ELISA and a comparison with three commercial ELISA. *Scand J Infect Dis* 1992;24:457–465.

77. Sobala GM, Crabtree JE, Pentith JA, et al. Screening dyspepsia by serology to *Helicobacter pylori. Lancet* 1991;338:94–96.

78. Guarner J, Mohar A, Parsonnet J, Halperin D. The association of *Helicobacter pylori* with gastric cancer and preneoplastic gastric lesions in Chiapas, Mexico. *Cancer* 1993;71:297–301.

79. Gubbins GP, Schubert TT, Attanasio F, Lubetsky M, Perez Perez GI, Blaser MJ. *Helicobacter pylori* seroprevalence in patients with rheumatoid arthritis: effect of nonsteroidal anti-inflammatory drugs and gold compounds. *Am J Med* 1992;93: 412–418.

80. Mitchell HM, Li YY, Hu PJ, et al. Epidemiology of *Helicobacter pylori* in southern China: identification of early childhood as the critical period for acquisition. *J Infect Dis* 1992; 166:149–153.

81. Polish LB, Douglas JM Jr, Davidson AJ, Perez Perez GI, Blaser MJ. Characterization of risk factors for *Helicobacter pylori* infection among men attending a sexually transmitted disease clinic: lack of evidence for sexual transmission. *J Clin Microbiol* 1991;29:2139–2143.

82. Perez Perez GI, Witkin SS, Decker MD, Blaser MJ. Seroprevalence of *Helicobacter pylori* infection in couples. *J Clin Microbiol* 1991;29:642–644.

83. Hopkins RJ, Russell RG, O'Donnoghue JM, Wasserman SS, Lefkowitz A, Morris JGJ. Seroprevalence of *Helicobacter pylori* in Seventh-Day Adventists and other groups in Maryland. Lack of association with diet. *Arch Intern Med* 1990;150: 2347–2348.

84. von Wulffen H, Grote HJ, Kramer Hansen H. Serological screening for *Campylobacter pylori* in candidates for renal transplantation. *Lancet* 1987;1:1140–1141.

85. Taha AS, Boothman P, Nakshabendi I, et al. Diagnostic tests for *Helicobacter pylori:* comparison and influence of non-steroidal anti-inflammatory drugs. *J Clin Pathol* 1992;45:709–712.

86. Taha AS, Reid J, Boothmann P, et al. Serological diagnosis of *Helicobacter pylori*—evaluation of four tests in the presence or absence of non-steroidal anti-inflammatory drugs. *Gut* 1993; 34:461–465.

87. Kosunen TU, Seppala K, Sarna S, Sipponen P. Diagnostic value of decreasing IgG, IgA, and IgM antibody titres after eradication of *Helicobacter pylori. Lancet* 1992;339:893–895.

88. Goossens H, Glupczynski Y, Burette A, et al. Evaluation of a commercially available complement fixation test for diagnosis

of *Helicobacter pylori* infection and for follow-up after antimicrobial therapy. *J Clin Microbiol* 1992;30:3230–3233.

89. Westblom TU, Lagging LM, Midkiff BR, Czinn SJ. Evaluation of QuickVue, a rapid enzyme immunoassay test for the detection of serum antibodies to *Helicobacter pylori*. *Diagn Microbiol Infect Dis* 1993;16:317–320.

90. Westblom TU, Madan E, Gudipati S, Midkiff BR, Czinn SJ. Diagnosis of *Helicobacter pylori* infection in adult and pediatric patients by using Pyloriset, a rapid latex agglutination test. *J Clin Microbiol* 1992;30:96–98.

91. Graham DY, Klein PD, Evans DJ, et al. *Campylobacter pylori* detected noninvasively by the 13-C-urea breath test. *Lancet* 1987;1:1174–1177.

92. Lotterer E, Ramaker J, Ludtke FE, Tegeler R, Geletneky JV, Bauer FE. The simplified ^{13}C-urea breath test—one point analysis for detection of *Helicobacter pylori* infection. *Z Gastroenterol* 1991;29:590–594.

93. Moshkowitz M, Peled Y, Baratz M, Halpern Z, Tiomny E, Gilat T. ^{14}C-urea breath test—a simple, noninvasive method for the detection of *Helicobacter pylori* infection. *Isr J Med Sci* 1993;29:94–97.

94. Novis BH, Gabay G, Leichtmann G, Peri M, Bernheim J, Pomeranz IS. Two point analysis 15-minute ^{14}C-urea breath test for diagnosing *Helicobacter pylori* infection. *Digestion* 1991;50:16–21.

95. Debongnie JC, Pauwels S, Raat A, de Meeus Y, Haot J, Mainguet P. Quantification of *Helicobacter pylori* infection in gastritis and ulcer disease using a simple and rapid carbon-14-urea breath test. *J Nucl Med* 1991;32:1192–1198.

96. Newell DG, Hawtin PR, Stacey AR, MacDougall MH, Ruddle AC. Estimation of prevalence of *Helicobacter pylori* infection in an asymptomatic elderly population comparing [^{14}C] urea breath test and serology. *J Clin Pathol* 1991;44:385–387.

97. Marshall BJ, Plankey MW, Hoffman SR, et al. A 20-minute breath test for *Helicobacter pylori*. *Am J Gastroenterol* 1991;86:438–445.

98. Coelho LG, Chausson Y, Passos MC, et al. ^{14}C-urea breath test to diagnose gastric *Helicobacter pylori* colonization. *Gastroenterol Clin Biol* 1990;14:801–805.

99. Stubbs JB, Marshall BJ. Radiation dose estimates for the carbon-14-labeled urea breath test. *J Nucl Med* 1993;34:821–825.

100. Logan RP, Gummett PA, Misiewicz JJ, Karim QN, Walker MM, Baron JH. Two-week eradication regimen for metronidazole-resistant *Helicobacter pylori*. *Aliment Pharmacol Ther* 1993;7:149–153.

101. Fraser AG, Lam WM, Luk YW, et al. Effect of ranitidine bismuth citrate on postprandial plasma gastrin and pepsinogens. *Gut* 1993;34:338–342.

102. Cutler AF, Schubert TT. Patient factors affecting *Helicobacter pylori* eradication with triple therapy. *Am J Gastroenterol* 1993;88:505–509.

103. Drumm B. *Helicobacter pylori* in the pediatric patient. *Gastroenterol Clin North Am* 1993;22:169–182.

104. Graham DY, Lew GM, Ramirez FC, Genta RM, Klein PD, Malaty HM. Short report: a non-metronidazole triple therapy for eradication of *Helicobacter pylori* infection—tetracycline, amoxicillin, bismuth. *Aliment Pharmacol Ther* 1993;7:111–113.

105. Moulton Barrett R, Triadafilopoulos G, Michener R, Gologorsky D. Serum ^{13}C-bicarbonate in the assessment of gastric *Helicobacter pylori* urease activity. *Am J Gastroenterol* 1993;88:369–374.

106. Lotterer E, Ludtke FE, Tegeler R, Bauer FE. The ^{13}C-urea breath test, *Helicobacter pylori* infection, and the operated stomach. *J Clin Gastroenterol* 1993;16:82–84.

107. Rowe PA, el Nujumi AM, Williams C, Dahill S, Briggs JD, McColl KE. The diagnosis of *Helicobacter pylori* infection in uremic patients. *Am J Kidney Dis* 1992;20:574–579.

108. Malaty H, Klein PD, Graham DY. Short report: cefprozil for the eradication of *Helicobacter pylori* infection. *Aliment Pharmacol Ther* 1992;6:503–506.

109. Vandenplas Y, Blecker U, Devreker T, et al. Contribution of the ^{13}C-urea breath test to the detection of *Helicobacter pylori* gastritis in children. *Pediatrics* 1992;90:608–611.

110. Coelho LG, Passos MC, Chausson Y, et al. Duodenal ulcer

and eradication of *Helicobacter pylori* in a developing country. An 18-month follow-up study. *Scand J Gastroenterol* 1992;27:362–366.

111. Graham DY, Lew GM, Malaty HM, et al. Factors influencing the eradication of *Helicobacter pylori* with triple therapy. *Gastroenterology* 1992;102:493–496.

112. Weil J, Bell GD, Powell K, et al. *Helicobacter pylori:* treatment with combinations of pivampicillin and tripotassium dicitrato bismuthate. *Aliment Pharmacol Ther* 1991;5:543–547.

113. Bell GD, Powell K, Weil J, Harrison G, Brookes S, Prosser S. ^{13}C-urea breath test for *Helicobacter pylori* infection. *Gut* 1991;32:551–552.

114. Cooreman M, Hengels KJ, Krausgrill P, Strohmeyer G. ^{13}C-Harnstoff-Atemtest als nicht-invasive Methode zum Nachweis von *Helicobacter (Campylobacter) pylori*. *Dtsch Med Wochenschr* 1990;115:367–371.

115. Frommer DJ, Carrick J, Lee A, et al. Acute presentation of *Campylobacter pylori* gastritis. *Am J Gastroenterol* 1988;83:1168–1171.

116. Graham DY, Alpert LC, Smith JL, et al. Iatrogenic *Campylobacter pylori* infection is a cause of epidemic achlorhydria. *Am J Gastroenterol* 1988;83:974–980.

117. Marshall BJ, Armstrong JA, McGechie DB, et al. Attempt to fulfill Koch's postulates for pyloric *Campylobacter*. *Med J Aust* 1985;142:436–439.

118. Morris A, Nicholson G. Ingestion of *Campylobacter pyloridis* causing gastritis and raised fasting pH. *Am J Gastroenterol* 1987;82:192–199.

119. Morris AJ, Ali MR, Nicholson GI, Perez Perez GI, Blaser MJ. Long-term follow-up of voluntary ingestion of *Helicobacter pylori*. *Ann Intern Med* 1991;114:662–663.

120. Ramsey EJ, Carey KV, Peterson WL, et al. Epidemic gastritis with hypochlorhydria. *Gastroenterology* 1979;76:1449–1457.

121. Katoh M, Saito D, Noda T, et al. *Helicobacter pylori* may be transmitted through gastrofiberscope even after manual Hyamine washing. *Jpn J Cancer Res* 1993;84:117–119.

122. Marshall BJ. Virulence and pathogenicity of *Helicobacter pylori*. *J Gastroenterol Hepatol* 1991;6:121–124.

123. Sarosiek J, Peura DA, Guerrant RL, et al. Mucolytic effects of *Helicobacter pylori*. *Scand J Gastroenterol Suppl* 1991;187:47–55.

124. Jaskiewicz K, Louw JA, Marks IN. Local cellular and immune response by antral mucosa in patients undergoing treatment for eradication of *Helicobacter pylori*. *Dig Dis Sci* 1993;38:937–943.

125. Newell DG. Virulence factors of *Helicobacter pylori*. *Scand J Gastroenterol Suppl* 1991;187:31–38.

126. Rathbone BJ, Wyatt JI, Heatley RV. Possible pathogenetic pathways of *Campylobacter pylori* in gastro-duodenal disease. *Scand J Gastroenterol Suppl* 1988;142:40–43.

127. Evans DG, Evans DJ Jr, Moulds JJ, Graham DY. *N*-acetyl-neuraminyllactose-binding fibrillar hemagglutinin of *Campylobacter pylori:* a putative colonization factor antigen. *Infect Immun* 1988;56:2896–2906.

128. Neman Simha V, Megraud F. In vitro model for *Campylobacter pylori* adherence properties. *Infect Immun* 1988;56:3329–3333.

129. Sipponen P. Natural history of gastritis and its relationship to peptic ulcer disease. *Digestion* 1992;51(Suppl 1):70–75.

130. Blaser MJ. Hypotheses on the pathogenesis and natural history of *Helicobacter pylori*-induced inflammation. *Gastroenterology* 1992;102:720–727.

131. Mobley HL, Cortesia MJ, Rosenthal LE, Jones BD. Characterization of urease from *Campylobacter pylori*. *J Clin Microbiol* 1988;26:831–836.

132. Kurata JJ. Ulcer epidemiology: an overview and research framework. *Gastroenterology* 1989;96:569–580.

133. Dooley CP, McKenna D, Humphreys H, et al. Histological gastritis in duodenal ulcer: relationship to *Campylobacter pylori* and effect of ulcer therapy. *Am J Gastroenterol* 1988;83:278–282.

134. Graham DY, Klein PD, Opekun AR, Boutton TW. Effect of age on the frequency of active *Campylobacter pylori* infection diagnosed by the [^{13}C]urea breath test in normal subjects and

patients with peptic ulcer disease. *J Infect Dis* 1988;157: 777–780.

135. Banatvala N, Mayo K, Megraud F, Jennings R, Deeks JJ, Feldman RA. The cohort effect and *Helicobacter pylori*. *J Infect Dis* 1993;168:219–221.

136. Marshall BJ, Goodwin CS, Warren JR, et al. Prospective double-blind trial of duodenal ulcer relapse after eradication of *Campylobacter pylori*. *Lancet* 1988;2:1437–1442.

137. Marshall BJ, Warren JR, Goodwin CS. Duodenal ulcer relapse after eradication of *Campylobacter pylori*. *Lancet* 1989;1: 836–837.

138. Seppala K, Farkkila M, Nuutinen H, et al. Triple therapy of *Helicobacter pylori* infection in peptic ulcer. A 12-month follow-up study of 93 patients. *Scand J Gastroenterol* 1992;27: 973–976.

139. Oderda G, Vaira D, Ainley C, et al. Eighteen month follow-up of *Helicobacter pylori* positive children treated with amoxycillin and tinidazole. *Gut* 1992;33:1328–1330.

140. Borody TJ, George LL, Brandl S, Andrews P, Jankiewicz E, Ostapowicz N. Smoking does not contribute to duodenal ulcer relapse after *Helicobacter pylori* eradication. *Am J Gastroenterol* 1992;87:1390–1393.

141. Graham DY, Lew GM, Klein PD, et al. Effect of treatment of *Helicobacter pylori* infection on the long-term recurrence of gastric or duodenal ulcer. A randomized, controlled study. *Ann Intern Med* 1992;116:705–708.

142. Patchett S, Beattie S, Leen E, Keane C, O'Morain C. *Helicobacter pylori* and duodenal ulcer recurrence. *Am J Gastroenterol* 1992;87:24–27.

143. Fiocca R, Solcia E, Santoro B. Duodenal ulcer relapse after eradication of *Helicobacter pylori*. *Lancet* 1991;337:1614.

144. Rauws EA, Tytgat GN. Cure of duodenal ulcer associated with eradication of *Helicobacter pylori*. *Lancet* 1990;335:1233–1235.

145. Lam SK. Duodenal ulcer relapse after eradication of *Campylobacter pylori*. *Lancet* 1989;1:384.

146. Coghlan JG, Gilligan D, Humphries H, et al. *Campylobacter pylori* and recurrence of duodenal ulcers—a 12-month follow-up study. *Lancet* 1987;2:1109–1111.

147. Hentschel E, Brandstatter G, Dragosics B, et al. Effect of ranitidine and amoxicillin plus metronidazole on the eradication of *Helicobacter pylori* and the recurrence of duodenal ulcer. *N Engl J Med* 1993;328:308–312.

148. Nakanishi T, Shinomura Y, Kanayama S, Matsuzawa Y. Eradication of *Helicobacter pylori* normalizes serum gastrin concentration and antral gastrin cell number in a patient with primary gastrin cell hyperplasia. *Am J Gastroenterol* 1993;88:440–442.

149. Moss SF, Playford RJ, Ayesu K, Li SK, Calam J. pH-dependent secretion of gastrin in duodenal ulcer disease: effect of suppressing *Helicobacter pylori*. *Digestion* 1992;52:173–178.

150. Archimandritis A, Tjivras M, Kapsalas D, et al. Preliminary observations in the fasting serum gastrin in patients with duodenal ulcer; further evidence of the "clearing" effect of omeprazole on *H. pylori*? *Ital J Gastroenterol* 1992;24:378–379.

151. Chittajallu RS, Neithercut WD, Ardill JE, McColl KE. *Helicobacter pylori*-related hypergastrinaemia is not due to elevated antral surface pH. Studies with antral alkalinisation. *Scand J Gastroenterol* 1992;27:218–222.

152. Beardshall K, Moss S, Gill J, et al. Suppression of *Helicobacter pylori* reduces gastrin releasing peptide stimulated gastrin release in duodenal ulcer patients. *Gut* 1992;33:601–603.

153. Rangachari PK. *Helicobacter* and hypergastrinemia: the Quisling option. *Scand J Gastroenterol Suppl* 1991;187:85–90.

154. Prewett EJ, Smith JT, Nwokolo CU, Hudson M, Sawyerr AM, Pounder RE. Eradication of *Helicobacter pylori* abolishes 24-hour hypergastrinaemia: a prospective study in healthy subjects. *Aliment Pharmacol Ther* 1991;5:283–290.

155. Graham DY, Opekun A, Lew GM, Klein PD, Walsh JH. *Helicobacter pylori*-associated exaggerated gastrin release in duodenal ulcer patients. The effect of bombesin infusion and urea ingestion. *Gastroenterology* 1991;100:1571–1575.

156. Levi S, Beardshall K, Swift I, et al. Antral *Helicobacter pylori*, hypergastrinaemia, and duodenal ulcers: effect of eradicating the organism. *BMJ* 1989;299:1504–1505.

157. Peterson WL, Barnett Cora C, Evans DJ, et al. Acid secretion

and serum gastrin in normal subjects and patients with duodenal ulcer: the role of *Helicobacter pylori*. *Am J Gastroenterol* 1993;88:2038–2043.

158. Mulholland G, Ardill JEDS, Fillmore D, Chittajallu RS, Fullarton GM, McColl KEL. *Helicobacter pylori* related hypergastrinaemia is the result of a selective increase in gastrin 17. *Gut* 1993;34:757–761.

159. Murthy UK, Linscheer R, Cho C. The hypergastrinemia in *Helicobacter pylori* (HP-)gastritis is due to a decrease in antral D cell density and D:G cell ratio. *Gastroenterology* 1992;102: A130.

160. Kang JY, Wee A. *Helicobacter pylori* and gastric acid output in peptic ulcer disease. *Dig Dis Sci* 1991;36:5–9.

161. Montbriand JR, Appelman HD, Cotner EK, Nostrant TT, Elta GH. Treatment of *Campylobacter pylori* does not alter gastric acid secretion. *Am J Gastroenterol* 1989;84:1513–1516.

162. McColl KE, Fullarton GM, Chittajalu R, et al. Plasma gastrin, daytime intragastric pH, and nocturnal acid output before and at 1 and 7 months after eradication of *Helicobacter pylori* in duodenal ulcer subjects. *Scand J Gastroenterol* 1991;26: 339–346.

163. Graham DY, Opekun A, Lew GM, Evans DJ Jr, Klein PD, Evans DG. Ablation of exaggerated meal-stimulated gastrin release in duodenal ulcer patients after clearance of *Helicobacter* (*Campylobacter*) *pylori* infection. *Am J Gastroenterol* 1990;85: 394–398.

164. Fitzgibbons PL, Dooley CP, Cohen H, Appleman MD. Prevalence of gastric metaplasia, inflammation, and *Campylobacter pylori* in the duodenum of members of a normal population. *Am J Clin Pathol* 1988;90:711–714.

165. Carrick J, Lee A, Hazell S, et al. *Campylobacter pylori*, duodenal ulcer, and gastric metaplasia: possible role of functional heterotopic tissue. *Gut* 1989;30:790–797.

166. Fraser AG, Prewett EJ, Pounder RE, Samloff IM. Short report: twenty-four-hour hyperpepsinogenaemia in *Helicobacter pylori*-positive subjects is abolished by eradication of the infection. *Aliment Pharmacol Ther* 1992;6:389–394.

167. Crabtree JE, Shallcross TM, Wyatt JI, et al. Mucosal humoral immune response to *Helicobacter pylori* in patients with duodenitis. *Dig Dis Sci* 1991;36:1266–1273.

168. Price AB. Histological aspects of *Campylobacter pylori* colonisation and infection of gastric and duodenal mucosa. *Scand J Gastroenterol Suppl* 1988;142:21–24.

169. Noach LA, Rolf TM, Bosma NB, et al. Gastric metaplasia and *Helicobacter pylori* infection. *Gut* 1993;34:1510–1514.

170. Goodwin CS. Duodenal ulcer, *Campylobacter pylori*, and the "leaking roof" concept. *Lancet* 1988;2:1467–1469.

171. Dunn BE. Pathogenic mechanisms of *Helicobacter pylori*. *Gastroenterol Clin North Am* 1993;22:43–57.

172. Borody TJ, Brandl S, Andrews P, Jankiewicz E, Ostapowicz N. *Helicobacter pylori*-negative gastric ulcer. *Am J Gastroenterol* 1992;87:1403–1406.

173. Kachintorn U, Luengrojanakul P, Atisook K, et al. *Helicobacter pylori* and peptic ulcer diseases: prevalence and association with antral gastritis in 210 patients. *J Med Assoc Thai* 1992; 75:386–392.

174. Sobala GM, Axon ATR. *Helicobacter pylori*, gastric ulceration and the postoperative stomach. In: Rathbone BJ, Heatley RV, eds. Helicobacter pylori *and gastroduodenal disease*, 2nd ed. Oxford: Blackwell Scientific, 1992;150–157.

175. Tatsuta M, Ishikawa H, Iishi H, Okuda S, Yokota Y. Reduction of gastric ulcer recurrence after suppression of *Helicobacter pylori* by cefixime. *Gut* 1990;31:973–976.

176. Rademaker JW, Hunt RH. Acid and barriers. Current research and future developments for peptic ulcer therapy. *Scand J Gastroenterol Suppl* 1990;175:19–26.

177. Heresbach D, Raoul JL, Bretagne JF, et al. *Helicobacter pylori*: a risk and severity factor of non-steroidal anti-inflammatory drug induced gastropathy. *Gut* 1992;33:1608–1611.

178. Loeb D, Talley NJ, Ahlquist DA, Carpenter HA, Zinsmeister AR. Long-term nonsteroidal anti-inflammatory drug use and gastroduodenal injury: the role of *Helicobacter pylori*. *Gastroenterology* 1992;102:1899–1905.

179. Jones RH, Lydeard S. Prevalence of symptoms of dyspepsia in the community. *BMJ* 1989;298:30–32.
180. Talley NJ, Phillips SF. Non-ulcer dyspepsia: potential causes and pathophysiology. *Ann Intern Med* 1988;108:865–879.
181. Schubert TT, Schubert AB, Ma CK. Symptoms, gastritis, and *Helicobacter pylori* in patients referred for endoscopy. *Gastrointest Endosc* 1992;38:357–360.
182. Collins JS, Knill Jones RP, Sloan JM, et al. A comparison of symptoms between non-ulcer dyspepsia patients positive and negative for *Helicobacter pylori*. *Ulster Med J* 1991;60:21–27.
183. Uppal R, Lateef SK, Korsten MA, Paronetto F, Lieber CS. Chronic alcoholic gastritis. Roles of alcohol and *Helicobacter pylori*. *Arch Intern Med* 1991;151:760–764.
184. Loffeld RJ, Potters HV, Arends JW, Stobberingh E, Flendrig JA, Van Spreeuwel JP. Campylobacter associated gastritis in patients with non-ulcer dyspepsia. *J Clin Pathol* 1988;41:85–88.
185. Takayasu H, Harasawa S, Miwa T, Yamada Y. Investigation of gastric function and prevalence of *Helicobacter pylori* in non-ulcer dyspepsia. *Nippon Shokakibyo Gakkai Zasshi* 1993;90:743–754.
186. Greenberg RE, Bank S. The prevalence of *Helicobacter pylori* in nonulcer dyspepsia. Importance of stratification according to age. *Arch Intern Med* 1990;150:2053–2055.
187. Loffeld RJ, Stobberingh E, Flendrig JA, Arends JW. Presence of *Helicobacter pylori* in patients with non-ulcer dyspepsia revealing normal antral histological characteristics. *Digestion* 1990;47:29–34.
188. Bernersen B, Johnsen R, Bostad L, Straume B, Sommer AI, Burhol PG. Is *Helicobacter pylori* the cause of dyspepsia? *BMJ* 1992;304:1276–1279.
189. Tucci A, Corinaldesi R, Stanghellini V, et al. *Helicobacter pylori* infection and gastric function in patients with chronic idiopathic dyspepsia. *Gastroenterology* 1992;103:768–774.
190. Rokkas T, Pursey C, Uzoechina E, et al. Campylobacter pylori and non-ulcer dyspepsia. *Am J Gastroenterol* 1987;82:1149–1152.
191. Rathbone BJ, Wyatt J, Heatley RV. Symptomatology in *C. pylori* positive and negative dyspepsia. *Gut* 1988;29:A1473.
192. Andersen LP, Elsborg L, Justesen T. Campylobacter pylori in peptic ulcer disease. III. Symptoms and paraclinical and epidemiologic findings. *Scand J Gastroenterol* 1988;23:347–350.
193. Deltenre M, Nyst JF, Jonas C, et al. Données cliniques, endoscopiques et histologiques chez 1100 patients dont 574 colonisés pas *Campylobacter pylori*. *Gastroenterol Clin Biol* 1989;13:89B–95B.
194. Börsch G, Schmidt G, Wegener M, et al. *Campylobacter pylori*: prospective analysis of clinical and histological factors associated with colonization of the upper gastrointestinal tract. *Eur J Clin Invest* 1988;18:133–138.
195. Jeena CP, Simjee AE, Pettengell KE, et al. Comparison of symptoms in *Campylobacter pylori* positive and negative patients presenting with dyspepsia for upper gastrointestinal endoscopy. *S Afr Med J* 1988;73:659.
196. Sobala GM, Dixon MF, Axon ATR. Symptomatology of *Helicobacter pylori* associated dyspepsia. *Eur J Gastroenterol Hepatol* 1990;2:445–449.
197. Guerre J, Berthe Y, Chaussade S, et al. Has *Campylobacter pylori* gastritis a specific clinical symptomatology. *Klin Wochenschr* 1989;67 (Suppl 18):25–26.
198. Vaira D, Holton J, Osborn J, et al. Endoscopy in dyspeptic patients: is gastric mucosal biopsy useful? *Am J Gastroenterol* 1990;85:701–704.
199. Goh KL, Parasakthi N, Peh SC, Wong NW, Lo YL, Puthucheary SD. *Helicobacter pylori* infection and non-ulcer dyspepsia: the effect of treatment with colloidal bismuth subcitrate. *Scand J Gastroenterol* 1991;26:1123–1131.
200. McNulty CAM, Gearty JC, Crump B, et al. Campylobacter pyloridis and associated gastritis: investigator blind placebo-controlled trial of bismuth salicylate and erythromycin ethylsuccinate. *BMJ* 1986;293:645–649.
201. Borody T, Hennessy W, Daskalopoulos G, et al. Double-blind trials of De-Nol in non-ulcer dyspepsia associated with *Campylobacter pylori* gastritis. *Gastroenterology* 1987;92:1324.
202. Rokkas T, Pursey C, Uzoechina E, et al. Non-ulcer dyspepsia and short term De-Nol therapy: a placebo controlled trial with particular reference to the role of *Campylobacter pylori*. *Gut* 1988;29:1386–1391.
203. Lambert RJ, Dunn K, Borromeo M, et al. *Campylobacter pylori*—a role in non-ulcer dyspepsia. *Scand J Gastroenterol Suppl* 1989;160:7–13.
204. Loffeld RJLF, Potters HVJP, Stobberingh E, et al. *Campylobacter* associated gastritis in patients with non-ulcer dyspepsia: a double-blind placebo controlled trial with colloidal bismuth subcitrate. *Gut* 1989;30:1206–1212.
205. Kang JY, Tay HH, Wee A, et al. Effect of colloidal bismuth subcitrate on symptoms and gastric histology in non-ulcer dyspepsia: a double-blind placebo controlled study. *Gut* 1990;31:476–489.
206. Glupczynski Y, Burette A, Labbe M, DePrez C, De Reuck M, Deltenre M. *Campylobacter pylori*-associated gastritis: a double-blind placebo-controlled trial with amoxycillin. *Am J Gastroenterol* 1988;83:365–372.
207. Gastrointestinal Physiology Working Group of Cayetano Heredia and the Johns Hopkins Universities. Nitrofurans in the treatment of gastritis associated with *Campylobacter pylori*. *Gastroenterology* 1988;95:1178–1184.
208. Patchett S, Beattie S, Leen E, Keane C, O'Morain C. Eradicating *Helicobacter pylori* and symptoms of non-ulcer dyspepsia. *BMJ* 1991;303:1238–1240.
209. Young JL. *Surveillance, epidemiology, and end results: incidence and mortality data, 1973–1977*. Bethesda, MD: National Cancer Institute Monograph, US Department of Health and Human Services, 1981.
210. Haenszel W, Kurihara M, Mitsuo S, et al. Stomach cancer among Japanese in Hawaii. *J Natl Cancer Inst* 1972;49:969.
211. Nomura A, Stemmermann GN, Chyou PH, Kato I, Perez Perez GI, Blaser MJ. *Helicobacter pylori* infection and gastric carcinoma among Japanese Americans in Hawaii. *N Engl J Med* 1991;325:1132–1136.
212. Forman D, Newell DG, Fullerton F, et al. Association between infection with *Helicobacter pylori* and risk of gastric cancer: evidence from a prospective investigation. *BMJ* 1991;302:1302–1305.
213. Parsonnet J, Friedman GD, Vandersteen DP, et al. *Helicobacter pylori* infection and risk for gastric cancer. *N Engl J Med* 1991;325:1127.
214. Talley NJ, Zinsmeister AR, Weaver A, et al. Gastric adenocarcinoma and *Helicobacter pylori* infection. *J Natl Cancer Inst* 1991;83:1734–1739.
215. EUROGAST Study Group. An international association between *Helicobacter pylori* infection and gastric cancer. *Lancet* 1993;341:1359–1362.
216. Klein PD, Graham DY, Gaillour A, Opekun AR, Smith EO. Water source as risk factor for *Helicobacter pylori* infection in Peruvian children. Gastrointestinal Physiology Working Group. *Lancet* 1991;337:1503–1506.
217. Ubilluz Dhaga del Castillo R. Uncomplicated peptic ulcer disease. The therapeutic prospects and practice. *Rev Gastroenterol Peru* 1991;11:40–48.
218. The Gastrointestinal Physiology Working Group of the Cayetano Heredia and the Johns Hopkins University. Ecology of *Helicobacter pylori* in Peru: infection rates in coastal, high altitude, and jungle communities. *Gut* 1992;33:604–605.
219. Oderda G, Forni M, Tavassoli K, Ansaldi N. Campylobacter pylori and gastroduodenal pathology in children. *Pediatr Med Chir* 1988;10:19–23.
220. Mégraud F, Brassens-Rabbe MP, Denis F, et al. Seroepidemiology of *Campylobacter pylori* infection in various populations. *J Clin Microbiol* 1989;27:1870.
221. Caselli M, Pazzi P, La Corte R, Trevisani L, Osnato R, Stabellini G. Do nonsteroidal anti-inflammatory drugs have a protective effect against *Campylobacter pylori*? *Presse Med* 1988;17:1762.
222. Siurala M, Varis K, Wiljasalo M. Studies of patients with atrophic gastritis: a 10–15 year follow-up. *Scand J Gastroenterol* 1966;1:40–48.
223. Faisal MA, Russell RM, Samloff IM, Holt PR. *Helicobacter*

pylori infection and atrophic gastritis in the elderly. *Gastroenterology* 1990;99:1543–1544.

224. Dooley CP, Cohen H, Fitzgibbons P, et al. Prevalence of *Helicobacter pylori* and histologic gastritis in asymptomatic persons. *N Engl J Med* 1989;321:1562–1566.

225. Borody TJ, Andrews P, Jankiewicz E, Ferch N, Caroll M. Apparent reversal of early gastric atrophy after triple therapy for *Helicobacter pylori*. *Am J Gastroenterol* 1993;88:1266–1268.

226. Fox JG, Correa P, Taylor NS, et al. High prevalence and persistence of cytotoxin-positive *Helicobacter pylori* strains in a population with high prevalence of atrophic gastritis. *Am J Gastroenterol* 1992;87:1554–1560.

227. Wotherspoon AC, Ortiz-Hidalgo C, Falzon MR, Isaacson PG. *Helicobacter pylori*-associated gastritis and primary B-cell gastric lymphoma. *Lancet* 1991;338:1175–1176.

228. Wotherspoon AC, Doglioni C, Diss TC, et al. Regression of primary low-grade B-cell gastric lymphoma of mucosa-associated lymphoid tissue type after eradication of *Helicobacter pylori*. *Lancet* 1993;342:575–577.

229. Isaacson PG. Is gastric lymphoma an infectious disease? *Hum Pathol* 1993;24:569–579.

230. Parsonnet J, Hansen S, Rodriguez L, et al. *Helicobacter pylori* infection and gastric lymphoma. *N Engl J Med* 1994;330:1267–1271.

231. Meyer W, Vollmar F, Barr W. Barrett-esophagus following total gastrectomy. *Endoscopy* 1979;2:121–126.

232. Karttunen T, Niemela S. *Campylobacter pylori* and duodenogastric reflux in peptic ulcer disease and gastritis. *Lancet* 1988;1:118.

233. Loffeld RJ, Ten Tije BJ, Arends JW. Prevalence and significance of *Helicobacter pylori* in patients with Barrett's esophagus. *Am J Gastroenterol* 1992;87:1598–1600.

234. Queiroz DM, Barbosa AJ, Mendes EN, et al. Distribution of *Campylobacter pylori* and gastritis in the stomach of patients with and without duodenal ulcer. *Am J Gastroenterol* 1988;83:1368–1370.

235. Feng YY, Wang Y. *Campylobacter pylori* in patients with gastritis, peptic ulcer, and carcinoma of the stomach in Lanzhou, China. *Lancet* 1988;1:1055.

236. Talley NJ, Cameron AJ, Shorter RG, Zinsmeister AR, Phillips SF. *Campylobacter pylori* and Barrett's esophagus. *Mayo Clin Proc* 1988;63:1176–1180.

237. Paull G, Yardley JH. Gastric and esophageal *Campylobacter pylori* in patients with Barrett's esophagus. *Gastroenterology* 1988;95:216–218.

238. Fich A, Talley NJ, Shorter RG, Phillips SF. Does *Helicobacter pylori* colonize the gastric mucosa of Meckel's diverticulum? *Mayo Clin Proc* 1990;65:187–191.

239. Kumar S, Small P, Nawroz I, Mohammed R. *Helicobacter pylori* and Meckel's diverticulum. *J R Coll Surg Edinb* 1991;36:225–226.

240. Miller JP. Colloidal bismuth in the treatment of duodenal ulceration: the benefit for the patient. *Scand J Gastroenterol Suppl* 1989;157:16–20.

241. Eberhardt R, Kasper G, Dettmer A, Hochter W, Hagena D. Effect of bismuth subsalicylate versus cimetidine on *Campylobacter pylori*, ulcer healing and rate of recurrence. *Med Klin* 1988;83:402–405.

242. Humphreys H, Bourke S, Dooley C, et al. Effect of treatment on *Campylobacter pylori* in peptic disease: a randomised prospective trial. *Gut* 1988;29:279–283.

243. Rokkas T, Sladen GE. Bismuth: effects on gastritis and peptic ulcer. *Scand J Gastroenterol Suppl* 1988;142:82–86.

244. Chiba N, Rao BV, Rademaker JW, Hunt RH. Meta-analysis of the efficacy of antibiotic therapy in eradicating *Helicobacter pylori*. *Am J Gastroenterol* 1992;87:1716–1727.

245. Logan RP, Gummett PA, Misiewicz JJ, Karim QN, Walker MM, Baron JH. One week eradication regimen for *Helicobacter pylori*. *Lancet* 1991;338:1249–1252.

246. Suerbaum S, Leying H, Klemm K, Opferkuch W. Antibacterial activity of pantoprazole and omeprazole against *Helicobacter pylori*. *Eur J Clin Microbiol Infect Dis* 1991;10:92–93.

247. Iwahi T, Satoh H, Nakao M, et al. Lansoprazole, a novel benzimidazole proton pump inhibitor, and its related compounds

248. Sherman P, Shames B, Loo V, Matlow A, Drumm B, Penner J. Omeprazole therapy for *Helicobacter pylori* infection. *Scand J Gastroenterol* 1992;27:1018–1022.

249. Daw MA, Deegan P, Leen E, O'Morain C. Short report: the effect of omeprazole on *Helicobacter pylori* and associated gastritis. *Aliment Pharmacol Ther* 1991;5:435–439.

250. Labenz J, Gyenes E, Ruhl GH, Börsch G. Omeprazole plus amoxicillin: efficacy of various treatment regimens to eradicate *Helicobacter pylori*. *Am J Gastroenterol* 1993;88:491–495.

251. Wagner S, Varrentrapp M, Haruma K, et al. The role of omeprazole (40 mg) in the treatment of gastric *Helicobacter pylori* infection. *Z Gastroenterol* 1991;29:595–598.

252. Weil J, Bell GD, Powell K, et al. Omeprazole and *Helicobacter pylori*: temporary suppression rather than true eradication. *Aliment Pharmacol Ther* 1991;5:309–313.

253. Hosking SW, Ling TK, Yung MY, et al. Randomised controlled trial of short term treatment to eradicate *Helicobacter pylori* in patients with duodenal ulcer. *BMJ* 1992;305:502–504.

254. Labenz J, Gyenes E, Ruhl GH, Börsch G. Two weeks treatment with amoxicillin/omeprazole for eradication of *Helicobacter pylori*. *Z Gastroenterol* 1992;30:776–778.

255. Labenz J, Gyenes E, Ruhl GH, Börsch G. Short-term therapy with high dosage omeprazole and amoxicillin for *Helicobacter pylori* eradication. A pilot study. *Med Klin* 1992;87:118–119.

256. Adamek RJ, Wegener M, Birkholz S, Opferkuch W, Ruhl GH, Ricken D. Modified combined omeprazole/amoxicillin therapy for *Helicobacter pylori* eradication: a pilot study. *Leber Magen Darm* 1992;22:222–224.

257. Cellini L, Marzio L, Di Girolamo A, Allocati N, Grossi L, Dainelli B. Enhanced clearing of *Helicobacter pylori* after omeprazole plus roxithromycin treatment. *FEMS Microbiol Lett* 1991;68:255–257.

258. Sorf M, Krislo V, Gogora M, Masek O. Morphologic changes in chronic active superficial *Campylobacter pylori*-positive antrum gastritis after treatment with bismuth. *Vnitr Lek* 1990;36:759–762.

259. Laine L, Marin Sorensen M, Weinstein WM. Nonsteroidal antiinflammatory drug-associated gastric ulcers do not require *Helicobacter pylori* for their development. *Am J Gastroenterol* 1992;87:1398–1402.

260. Nanivadekar SA, Sawant PD, Patel HD, Shroff CP, Popat UR, Bhatt PP. Relapse of *Helicobacter pylori* infection after different treatment regimens. A 3-month follow-up study. *J Assoc Physicians India* 1990;38(Suppl 1):712–715.

261. Morris A, Lane M, Hamilton I, et al. Duodenal ulcer relapse after eradication of *Helicobacter pylori*. *N Z Med J* 1991;104:329–331.

262. George LL, Borody TJ, Andrews P, et al. Cure of duodenal ulcer after eradication of *Helicobacter pylori*. *Med J Aust* 1990;153:145–149.

263. Armstrong D, Blum AL, Arnold R, et al. RUDER: a 2-year prospective study of risk factors for recurrent duodenal ulceration (DU) in 1899 patients. *Gastroenterology* 1991;100:A27.

264. Bayerdorffer E, Kasper G, Pirlet T, Sommer A, Ottenjann R. Ofloxacin in the therapy of *Campylobacter pylori*-positive duodenal ulcer. A prospective controlled randomized study. *Dtsch Med Wochenschr* 1987;112:1407–1411.

265. Graham DY, Lew GM, Evans DG, Evans DJ Jr, Klein PD. Effect of triple therapy (antibiotics plus bismuth) on duodenal ulcer healing. A randomized controlled trial. *Ann Intern Med* 1991;115:266–269.

266. Holtmann G, Armstrong D, Pöppel E, et al. Influence of stress on the healing and relapse of duodenal ulcers. A prospective, multicenter trial of 2109 patients with recurrent duodenal ulceration treated with ranitidine. *Scand J Gastroenterol* 1992;27:917–923.

267. Holtmann G, Armstrong D, Goebell H, et al. Does long-term maintenance therapy with ranitidine affect the natural course of duodenal ulcer disease. *Eur J Gastroenterol Hepatol* 1993;5:311–317.

268. Deakin M, Williams JG. Histamine H2-receptor antagonists in peptic ulcer disease. Efficacy in healing peptic ulcers. *Drugs* 1992;44:709–719.

269. Bianchi Porro G, Parente F, Lazzaroni M. Short and long term outcome of *Helicobacter pylori* positive resistant duodenal ulcers treated with colloidal bismuth subcitrate plus antibiotics or sucralfate alone. *Gut* 1993;34:466–469.

270. Hixson LJ, Kelley CL, Jones WN, Tuohy CD. Current trends in the pharmacotherapy for peptic ulcer disease. *Arch Intern Med* 1992;152:726–732.

271. Graham DY, Hepps KS, Ramirez FC, Lew GM, Screed ZA. Treatment of *Helicobacter pylori* reduces the rate of rebleeding in peptic ulcer disease. *Scand J Gastroenterol* 1993;28:939–942.

272. Holtmann G, Armstrong D, Blum AL, et al. Effects of 2-year maintenance therapy with ranitidine on the natural course of duodenal ulcer (DU) disease. *Gastroenterology* 1992;102:A84.

273. Borody TJ, Cole P, Noonan S, et al. Recurrence of duodenal ulcer and *Campylobacter pylori* infection after eradication. *Med J Aust* 1989;151:431–435.

274. O'Riordan T, Mathai E, Tobin E, et al. Adjuvant antibiotic therapy in duodenal ulcers treated with colloidal bismuth subcitrate. *Gut* 1990;31:999–1002.

275. Marshall BJ, Valenzuela JE, McCallum RW, et al. Bismuth subsalicylate suppression of *Helicobacter pylori* in nonulcer dyspepsia: a double-blind placebo-controlled trial. *Dig Dis Sci* 1993;38:1674–1680.

276. Lin JT, Wang JT, Wang TH, Wu MS, Lee TK, Chen CJ. *Helicobacter pylori* infection in a randomly selected population, healthy volunteers, and patients with gastric ulcer and gastric adenocarcinoma. A seroprevalence study in Taiwan. *Scand J Gastroenterol* 1993;28:1067–1072.

277. Sipponen P, Seppala K. A scheme for the pathogenesis of gastric adenocarcinoma. *Scand J Gastroenterol* 1992;27(Suppl 193):33–38.

278. Peterson WL, Lee E, Feldman M. Relationship between *Campylobacter pylori* and gastritis in healthy humans after administration of placebo or indomethacin. *Gastroenterology* 1988;95:1185–1197.

279. Taylor DN, Blaser MJ. The epidemiology of *Helicobacter pylori* infection. *Epidemiol Rev* 1991;13:42–59.

280. Blaser MJ. *Helicobacter pylori* and the pathogenesis of gastroduodenal inflammation. *J Infect Dis* 1990;161:626–633.

Infections of the Gastrointestinal Tract,
edited by M. J. Blaser, P. D. Smith, J. I. Ravdin,
H. B. Greenberg, and R. L. Guerrant
Raven Press, Ltd., New York © 1995.

CHAPTER 42

Gastrospirillum hominis (*Helicobacter heilmannii*) and Other Gastric Infections of Humans

Adrian Lee, Jani L. O'Rourke, and John E. Kellow

Bacterial infections of the stomach have, until recently, been considered to be rare in humans, most commonly manifesting as secondary infections associated with other disease states such as syphilis and tuberculosis (1). Our concepts of the stomach as an inhospitable environment for bacterial colonization, however, have been altered by the discovery that the bacterium *Helicobacter pylori* (2,3) commonly colonizes the human stomach (4).

The observation of colonization of the gastric mucosa by large numbers of spiral-shaped bacteria is not new, as for over 100 years these organisms have been reported in almost every one of the many studies on the stomach of a wide range of animals (5–7). The data were much less definitive for humans. Scattered reports of spiral bacteria in human gastric samples appeared early this century (8,9) with the most systematic and accurate description of human gastric spiral-shaped bacteria coming from Doenges in 1939 (10). Doenges described four different types of bacteria in human gastric samples obtained at autopsy. The most prevalent organism, a "thick spirochaete with 2–3 turns" is now accepted to have been *H. pylori*. Moreover, in two cases he described a "spirochaete which showed sharp angulation, with 6–8 turns," which he had seen regularly in monkeys and corresponded to earlier descriptions of the bacteria commonly seen in several other animal species (7).

The importance of Doenges' work became apparent with the discovery and acceptance of *H. pylori* as a human pathogen. But of more relevance to this chapter was his finding of a second morphological type of bacterium, one that was commonly encountered in animal studies, in

human gastric mucosa. Confirmation of his findings came in 1987 when Dent and colleagues (11) described three cases of gastritis in humans associated with such an organism. *Helicobacter pylori* was not observed in any of these patients. The unofficial name *Gastrospirillum hominis* was assigned to this organism (12). The possibility arose that this represented another bacterium that could be associated with gastric disease in humans. This initial report alerted histopathologists to the existence of this organism and since then many other cases have appeared in the literature of the association of *G. hominis* with a variety of disease states (13–24). Two recent reports describe large surveys in Belgium and the Peoples Republic of China in which a total of 64 patients (34/~15,000 and 30/1931, respectively) were found to be colonized with *G. hominis* (25,26). The diagnoses in these patients ranged from acute and chronic gastritis to duodenal ulceration, gastric ulceration, and gastric cancer.

A third spiral bacterium has now been associated with human gastric disease. It is another *Helicobacter* species, *H. felis*, which was originally isolated from cats and dogs (27,28). It has now been found associated with two cases of gastritis in humans (18,29). Electron microscopic analysis of gastric biopsies from these patients allowed direct visualization of bacteria with the characteristic morphology of *H. felis*.

While the prevalence rates of human infection with *G. hominis* and *H. felis* are low (less than 1% to 1.5%), studies of these bacteria in their natural and experimental animal hosts have provided useful information with respect to the disease processes of both these organisms and *H. pylori* in humans. To date, animal studies with these bacteria have been utilized in screening trials for anti-*H. pylori* chemotherapeutic agents (30), studies of pathogenic mechanisms (31–35), and in the development of possible immunization strategies (36–38).

A. Lee and J. L. O'Rourke: School of Microbiology and Immunology, University of New South Wales, Sydney, New South Wales, Australia 2052.

J. E. Kellow: Department of Medicine, Royal North Shore Hospital, St. Leonards, New South Wales, Australia 2065.

This chapter draws attention to the rare group of non-*H. pylori* gastric infections that includes the newly discovered organisms *G. hominis* and *H. felis* together with syphilis, tuberculosis, anthrax, and various mycotic infections. In addition to resulting in serious illness in some instances, these infections can also complicate diagnosis of more serious illnesses (e.g., gastric carcinoma) because they may mimic the symptoms of these diseases. Also discussed is the potential deleterious effects of bacterial overgrowth in the stomach, which accompanies the continual use of antimicrobial, immunosuppressive, and acid-suppressive therapies.

GASTROSPIRILLUM HOMINIS (HELICOBACTER HEILMANNII)

Description

Gastrospirillum hominis is a gram-negative, tightly spiraled/helical shaped organism with between 4 and 20 turns (12,16,24). These organisms are 4 to 10 μm in length, 0.5 to 1 μm in width, and they possess at least 12 sheathed flagella, 28 nm in diameter (Fig. 1A). Electron microscopic analysis has shown these bacteria to have truncated ends, an electron lucent area in the terminal region of the organism, and a "polar membrane," similar to that found in other *Helicobacter* species and spiral-shaped bacteria (39).

Helicobacter felis is indistinguishable from *G. hominis* by light microscopy, with the morphological trait that dif-

ferentiates between these two organisms, the presence or absence of periplasmic fibers, only observed by electron microscopy (Fig. 1B). *Helicobacter felis* is entwined by such periplasmic fibers; although the fibers usually are in pairs, their number can vary from one to three (27).

Microbiology

Gastrospirillum hominis

In addition to the standard methods used for the cultivation of other *Helicobacter* species a variety of different types of enriched media and atmospheric conditions have been employed in attempts to culture *G. hominis* from human gastric biopsies. However, to date, none have been successful (12,22). By applying methods used by Salomon (7), we have been able to maintain human isolates of this bacterium *in vivo* (21,30). Specific pathogen-free (SPF) mice were inoculated orally with gastric biopsies obtained from human patients known to harbor *G. hominis*. The gastric mucosa of the mice is rapidly colonized with the helical organisms and can be kept alive by passage from mouse to mouse via oral administration of infected gastric homogenates. The original isolate from an Indonesian male (21) has now been kept alive via animal passage for 5 years.

Recently, by utilizing this mouse model and molecular techniques, Solnick et al. (40) have sequenced the 16s ribosomal ribonucleic acid (rRNA) gene of *G. hominis*. The 16s rRNA gene has been a highly conserved gene over

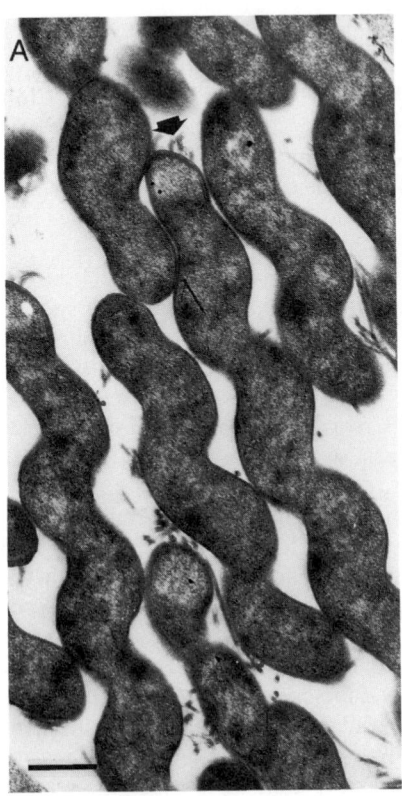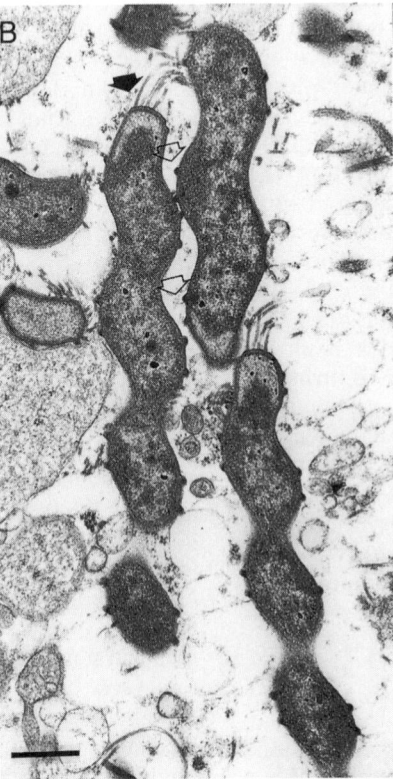

FIG. 1. Transmission electron micrograph of *G. hominis* (**A**) and *H. felis* (**B**), showing the characteristic spiral/helical morphology of the bacteria and the tufts of flagella (*closed arrow*). The periplasmic fibers, characteristic of *H. felis,* are also indicated (*open arrow*). (Bars = 0.5 μm).

the course of bacterial evolution and is used to determine evolutionary differences among bacteria (41). Indeed, *H. felis* and *H. mustelae,* originally isolated from cat and ferret stomachs, respectively, while both very different bacteria morphologically, were assigned to the genus *Helicobacter* due to the similarity of their 16s rRNA to that of *H. pylori* (28). Gastric material was obtained from mice that had been colonized with biopsies from two individual patients infected with *G. hominis.* Deoxyribonucleic acid (DNA) was extracted and the 16s rRNA gene was amplified by polymerase chain reaction (PCR) and cloned into *Escherichia coli* and sequenced. The sequences obtained from the two samples were distinct (96.5% similarity) with both of them showing high degrees of homology with *H. felis* and *H. pylori* (97% to 98% and 95%, respectively). These data confirm that *G. hominis* is a new member of the *Helicobacter* genus. There appears to be several distinct types of this organism, which may have arisen from a variety of animal sources. The new name proposed for these bacteria is *Helicobacter heilmannii* (in honor of the German histopathologist Konrad Heilmann) (42).

The only biochemical trait that has been described for *G. hominis* is the presence of the enzyme urease. Urease has been detected in approximately two-thirds of biopsies of infected persons by the urease biopsy test (12,15, 16,18,20,22,24,43,44). Monoclonal antibodies directed against the urease of *H. pylori* have been shown to cross-react with *G. hominis* and similar *G. hominis*-like organisms (GHLOs) from monkeys and baboons (45). Sequence analysis of the urease gene of *G. hominis* has also shown a high degree of homology with the urease genes of *H. pylori* and *H. felis* (46).

Helicobacter felis

Helicobacter felis was first cultured from the gastric mucosa of a cat, and, like *H. pylori,* it can be cultivated on blood agar plates containing Skirrow's selective supplement (Oxoid, Basingstoke, U.K.) with microaerobic conditions and a high percentage of humidity (27). This organism shares many phenotypic traits with *H. pylori* that is, it is urease, catalase, and oxidase positive and does not readily utilize carbohydrates (28).

As stated previously, confirmation of the identity of this organism is by visualization of the presence of periplasmic fibers. It is recognition of these characteristic fibers in electron micrographs of two human patients that is the only evidence that this organism can infect humans. Human infection could be more common than is thought, as many of the reported *G. hominis* cases have been diagnosed by light microscopy, which does not allow distinction between *G. hominis* and *H. felis. Helicobacter felis* has never been cultured from a human patient but much more work has to be done on the feline and canine isolates.

Epidemiology

Although the number of cases of human gastric colonization with either *G. hominis* or *H. felis* is expanding due to the increased awareness of these bacteria, the prevalence of gastric infection with these bacteria is still low, that is, 0.25% to 1.5%. There is no apparent predisposition in patients relating to either sex or age, the bacteria being found in either sex and in patients ranging from 2 to 79 years of age (12,16,47,48).

The epidemiology of these infections is not completely understood. However, it is clear that human infections are likely to be zoonoses with patients becoming infected due to close contact with animals, most likely cats and dogs. *Gastrospirillum hominis* and GHLOs and, to a lesser extent, *H. felis* are widespread in the animal kingdom with hosts ranging from domestic pets, such as cats and dogs, farm animals, such as pigs, and even more exotic species including several nonhuman primates, "big cats," and even the Tasmanian devil. In a few instances in these hosts, the bacteria have been associated with a mild form of gastritis (34,49–54). An association with animals has been found in some (but not all) of the reported cases of human infection with *G. hominis* and *H. felis.* One patient was known to have kept 14 cats (22), another to have eaten dog meat (55), and others to work with animals (12,23,24,29,56).

Given the ubiquity of *G. hominis* and *H. felis* infected animals, it is surprising that more humans are not infected with these bacteria. The bacteria must be relatively difficult to transmit, an observation that has been made in discussions of the epidemiology of human *H. pylori* infection. It is unlikely that fecal–oral spread is involved, otherwise the infection rate in developing countries would be very high given the contamination of food and drinking water with animal excreta. Current evidence would suggest an oral–oral route of transmission. There are experimental data in laboratory animals that support this hypothesis. The gastric helicobacters *G. hominis* and *H. felis* were shown not to transfer to noninfected germ-free and SPF rodents from infected animals when they were housed in the same cage even though these animals are known to be coprophagic. By contrast, *H. pylori* and *H. felis* were transferred to uninfected beagle puppies from their infected litter mates. During play puppies are known to come into very close contact with each other especially via licking and biting (57). Thus humans most probably become infected when they are licked by their overenthusiastic and affectionate domestic pets.

Pathogenesis and Immunity

The contribution of these non-*H. pylori* organisms to gastric disease is at present unproven. To date, approximately 170 cases of infection with this organism have been reported in the world literature. Most are associated with mild gastritis; however, there have been reports of duodenal ulceration (eight cases), gastric ulceration (eight cases), and two cases of gastric carcinoma (the latter in association with *H. pylori*). The presence of these organisms is usually associated with an active chronic gastritis that tends to be less aggressive than *H. pylori* infections in humans (Fig. 2). This is characterized by an infiltrate of polymorphonuclear leukocytes, lymphocytes, and plasma

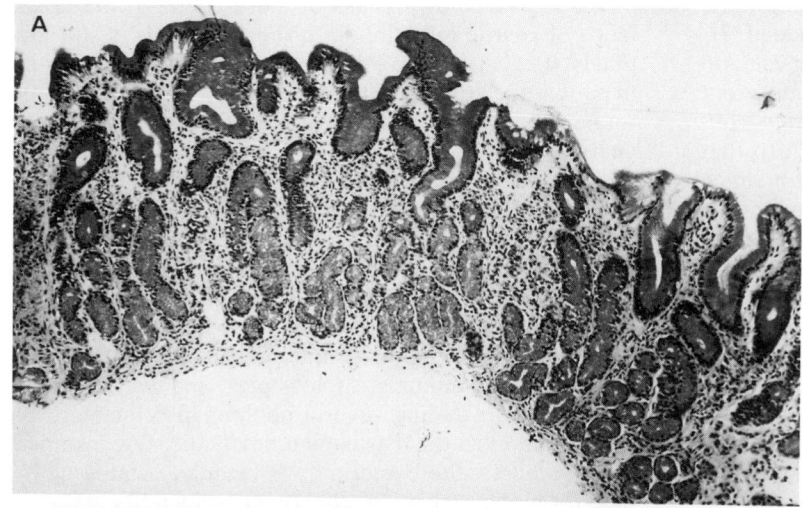

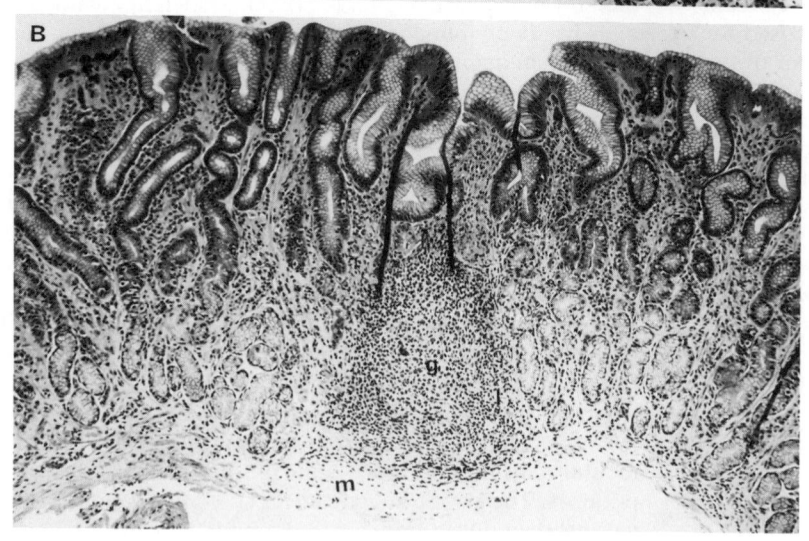

FIG. 2. Gastric biopsies of patients colonized with *G. hominis*, revealing mild chronic gastritis as indicated by (**A**) diffuse infiltrate of lymphoid cells as well as scattered eosinophils in the lamina propria of the mucosae (×450) and (**B**) as above, with a distinct lymphoid follicle abutting the muscularis mucosa (m). The germinal center (g) and a marginal zone of small lymphocytes (l) are also apparent (×450). (Biopsy specimens courtesy of Dr. F. Bonar and Dr. G. Daskalopoulos, respectively.)

cells in the lamina propria. In some cases superficial chronic gastritis, gastric neoplasia, or infiltration into the foveolar epithelium also has been present. One acute infection has been associated with *G. hominis* in which the antral mucosa histologically showed acute erosions, congestion, and edema with a severe infiltrate of polymorphonuclear neutrophil leukocytes in the lamina propria, intraepithelially and in the glands (55).

Gastrospirillum hominis has been found to localize in the surface gastric mucosa and in the necks of and deep within the gastric glands (Fig. 3) (24). There does not appear to be evidence of direct attachment of the bacteria to the gastric epithelial cells, unlike *H. pylori* (58). A higher proportion of antral biopsies compared to the body biopsies show these organisms; they were found in all antral biopsies from 39 patients of one study versus only 20% of the body biopsies (16). This finding is in accordance with reports of a predominant antral localization of *H. pylori* however, this issue remains controversial (59,60).

Intracellular localization has only been observed on two occasions; however, this may not be an accurate representation of localization due to the small number of cases in which biopsies were examined using electron micros-

copy (16,22). In these cases the bacteria were seen in the cytoplasm and canniculi of parietal cells, associated with mitochondrial swelling and more severe degenerative changes in cytoplasmic organelles. Heilmann suggested that a possible cytopathic effect may be indicated by the presence of lysozymes and vacuoles (Fig. 4).

In their natural hosts the presence of *G. hominis* organisms is associated with primary infiltration of mononuclear cells and lymphoid aggregates with little active inflammation with neutrophils. However, the mononuclear infiltration can be very extensive and tissue damage does appear in some cases (50,51,54,61). In a foreign host, these animal helicobacters can induce significant pathology, and this has been the basis of many small animal model studies. *Helicobacter felis* will induce a very aggressive active/chronic gastritis in germ-free mice (62). It is of interest that in the one well-documented case of human *H. felis* associated gastritis, a significant neutrophil infiltration was observed (18). This can be seen in Fig. 5, which shows a gastric biopsy from a 61-year-old woman who presented with severe, diffuse, acute gastritis. Very long-term infection (more than 18 months) of conventional Swiss mice with these same organisms re-

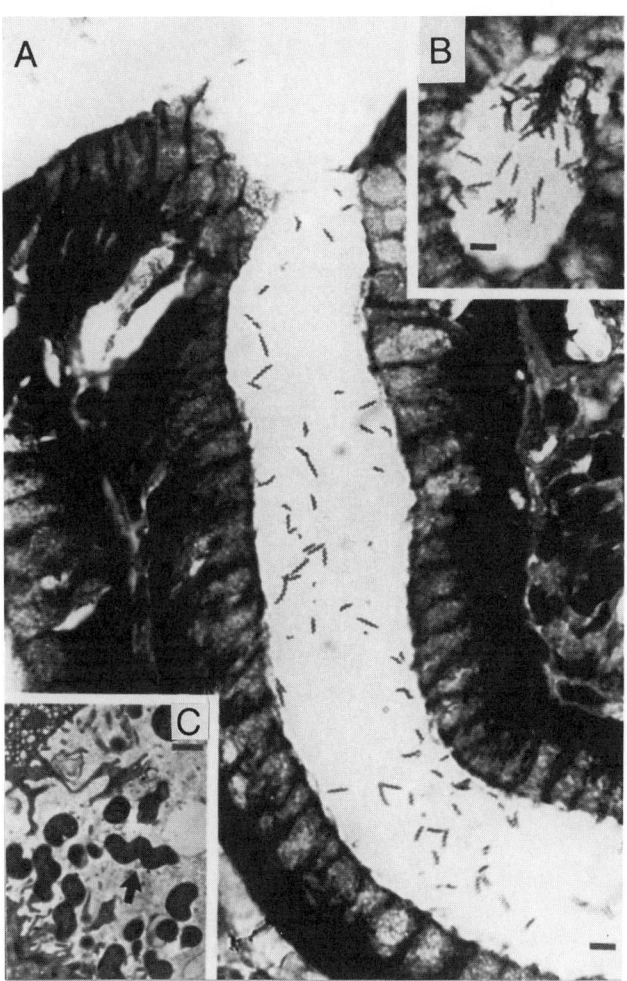

FIG. 3. Gastric biopsy of a patient colonized with *G. hominis*, showing the localization of the bacteria in the gastric lumen and deep into gastric glands (**A,B**) (bars = 5 μm) with higher magnification revealing the close association with microvilli (**C**) (bar = 1 μm). (From ref. 30, with permission.)

sults in a progressively destructive atrophic gastritis (63) that is very similar to that seen in some patients with *H. pylori* infection.

Long-term infection (18 to 26 months) of SPF BALB/c mice with *G. hominis* or *H. felis* has been shown to induce large lymphoid aggregates with lymphoepithelial lesions indicative of MALToma (M. Dixon and A. Jack, *personal communication*). The lesions were largely centered on the corpus mucosa immediately distal to the squamoepithelial junction of the esophagus. Lymphoid aggregates were detected in 73.8% of infected animals (8% of control animals) with lymphoepithelial lesions developing in 22.6% of the infected animals. No lymphoepithelial lesions were observed in the control, uninfected animals (*unpublished data*). These lesions are similar to those now being proposed to be induced by *H. pylori* in humans (64,65).

In summary, the pathology associated with *G. hominis* (*H. heilmannii*) and *H. felis* in humans is likely to be simi-

lar to that induced by *H. pylori*. Only when more cases are reported will compelling evidence accumulate. The eradication trials that aided in the proof that *H. pylori* is a pathogen are more difficult with these organisms due to the small numbers of infected persons. We know *G. hominis* presence is associated with inflammation of varying severity; ulcers have been seen and long-term infection (i.e., 4 and 10 years) is possible (16). Thus in a clinical situation it is probably best to deal with a *G. hominis* infection in the same manner as one would a *H. pylori* infection.

Clinical Features

In the majority of published reports of infection with *G. hominis* the usual complaints of patients are epigastric pain or discomfort. The prevalence of other symptoms appears to be variable, although nausea and, to a lesser extent, vomiting, anorexia, weight loss, and diarrhea have also been features in a number of cases. Occasional patients have presented with gastrointestinal bleeding due to gastric or duodenal ulceration (D. Querioz *personal communication*). According to the classification of functional dyspepsia proposed by Drossman et al. (66), most patients appear to fit the category of "ulcer-like" dyspepsia. In those cases in which the organism has been documented in the absence of concomitant *H. pylori* infection, there are no apparent differences from the symptom clusters reported in association with the latter organism (12,16,21–24). However, there is no evidence at present that *G. hominis* causes these symptoms.

Diagnosis

Upper gastrointestinal panendoscopy, in approximately half of the *G. hominis* cases reported to date, has demonstrated macroscopically normal gastroduodenal mucosa (12,16,21,56,67). In the other half, findings have ranged from antral erythema to more severe antral gastritis, including erosions and gastric ulceration (15,22–26). Lymphoid follicles have also been observed in one adult case and in two cases of chronic gastritis in 4- and 10-year-old children (T. Bohane, J. Mitchell, and D. Queiroz, *personal communication*). Duodenal erosions were present in three cases (14,44). In nearly all cases, histology has revealed moderate to severe active chronic gastritis. There have been two cases of acute infection—one associated with *G. hominis* (55) and the other with *H. felis* (18).

The bacteria can be identified in gastric biopsies by observation of their distinct morphology. While they can be seen in hematoxylin and eosin stained sections, they are more obvious when a Giemsa or Warthin–Starry silver stain is used. As more histopathologists become aware of the existence of these bacteria, the detection rate is increasing; however, as yet there is no way to distinguish between *G. hominis* or *H. felis* unless electron microscopy is performed.

As *H. pylori* is thought to be responsible for the major-

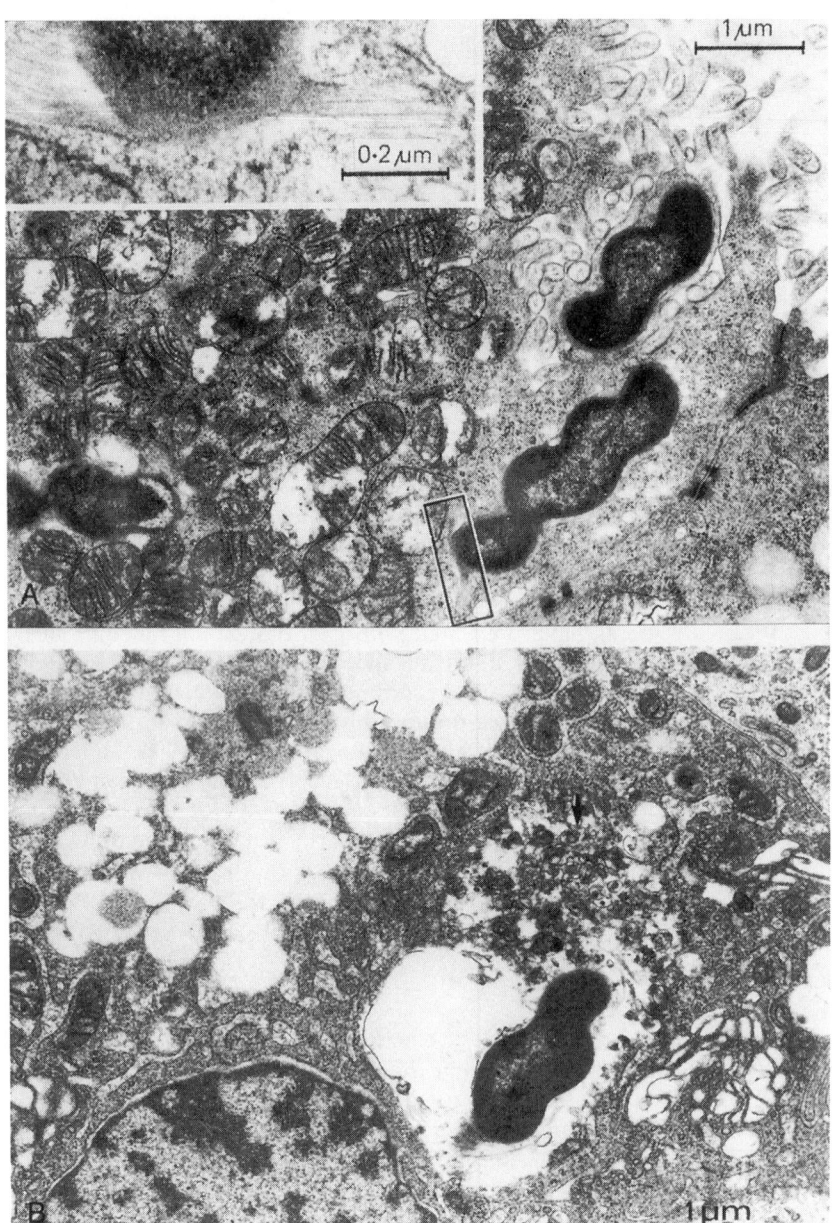

FIG. 4. Transmission electron micrographs of gastric biopsies, showing intracellular location of *G. hominis* bacteria. **A:** Bacteria within a parietal cell causing degeneration-like mitochondrial swelling with the **inset** showing twisting bacterial filaments (bar = 1 μm). (From ref. 16, with permission.) **B:** Formation of a large vacuole with microvesicular disintegration of organelles (*arrow*) in an antral mucopeptic cell next to the organism (bar = 1 μm). (From ref. 51, with permission.)

ity of gastric infections, urease biopsy tests and serology have in some instances been used to aid diagnosis. The rate of detected urease positivity (approximately 66%) appears to be lower than that for *H. pylori*. This may be misleading as in many cases a much slower change in the urease reaction than that commonly seen for *H. pylori* infections has been reported (24). This is probably due not to the presence of urease-negative helicobacters but to the lower numbers of *G. hominis* that appear to colonize the gastric mucosa compared to *H. pylori*. Serology results in which *H. pylori* is used as the antigen are controversial, with positive results in 8 of 13 patients (12,21,26) and negative results in another five patients (24,43,56). Our own studies, utilizing either *H. pylori* or *H. felis* as the antigen, show a much higher rate of seropositivity,

$^{12}/_{15}$ (80%) with *H. felis* as the antigen compared to 60% when *H. pylori* is used as the antigen (*unpublished data*).

Mixed infection with both *H. pylori* and *G. hominis* is possible (17 cases to date), although monoinfection appears the norm (15,16,19,20,23,26,68).

Treatment

Treatment with bismuth, amoxicillin, and metronidazole in various combinations has been undertaken in a number of reported cases. Complete or near complete resolution of symptoms has occurred in the majority of patients to date (12,16,19,20,22,23,24,44). In the absence of placebo-controlled studies, however, it is difficult to

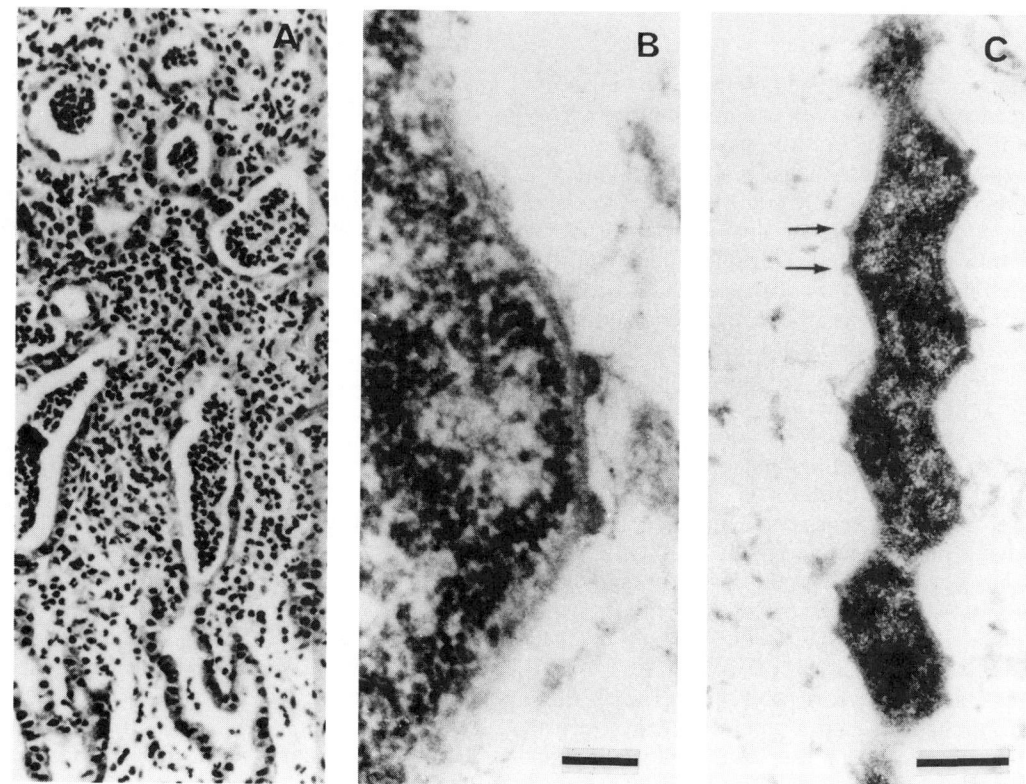

FIG. 5. Micrographs of a patient colonized with *H. felis*, revealing (**A**) acute diffuse gastritis (×200) and (**B,C**) the bacteria with the characteristic morphology and presence of periplasmic fibers (*arrows*) (bar = 0.1 μm and 0.5 μm, respectively). (From ref. 18, with permission.)

gauge the significance of symptomatic improvement in functional dyspepsia. Clearance of the organism has usually been obtained with such "triple therapy" regimens. Follow-up biopsies, taken 1 to 5 months after treatment, have been obtained in a number of cases in which the characteristic bacteria could not be detected and the histological appearance of the gastric tissue had improved or returned to normal (19,22,24). At the present time it is not clear whether eradication is easier to obtain than in the case of *H. pylori*. Several reports describe the disappearance of the bacterium and resolution of symptoms without any treatment being undertaken.

It is possible that diagnosis of *G. hominis* infection should be treated exactly the same as though *H. pylori* infection had been diagnosed. Demonstration of endoscopic or histological gastritis and/or association with dyspeptic symptoms should not be an indication for treatment. However, in the rare case when an ulcer is diagnosed, antimicrobial therapy should be instituted together with an appropriate acid-inhibiting agent (68). Current anti-*H. pylori* regimens are likely to be more than adequate for *G. hominis* and *H. felis* infections.

TREPONEMA PALLIDUM

Description

Even though gastric lesions associated with syphilitic infections are uncommonly detected (less than 1%) the relationship between gastric infection and syphilis has been known for over 100 years. A history of untreated or inadequately treated syphilis (primary, secondary, tertiary, latent, or congenital) usually has been regarded as a necessary criterion to establish a clinical diagnosis of gastric syphilis (69). It has been suggested that stomach involvement is a normal part of the pathophysiology of syphilis (70). The causative organism, *T. pallidum*, is a long slender spirochaete (8 to 15 μm × 0.2 μm), which is best visualized by dark-field microscopy or by the Warthin–Starry stain, as it is not readily stained by conventional techniques.

Clinical Features

Symptoms of gastric syphilis are nonspecific and depend on the stage of the illness (particularly for tertiary syphilis), the site of the gastric lesion (body or antrum), and the degree of associated deformity. In the early secondary stage, ulcer-like abdominal pain and vomiting may occur and, rarely, gastrointestinal bleeding. In some patients, however, there may be no gastrointestinal symptoms. In the late secondary or tertiary stage, characteristic symptoms include weight loss, nausea, vomiting, early satiety, and abdominal pain, usually occurring postprandially (71). Physical examination may demonstrate other clinical features of syphilis.

Diagnosis

In its secondary or tertiary stage, syphilis can cause a wide range of gastric lesions, which can mimic other entities such as benign gastric ulceration, gastric carcinoma, or lymphoma. In the early secondary stage, radiological findings are nonspecific, with diffusely hypertrophied or thickened folds, or a nodular appearance, with or without mucosal ulceration (72,73). In the tertiary stage, antral narrowing, which produces a funnel-shaped deformity or even a "linitis plastica" appearance, is the most frequent anatomical deformity. An hourglass stomach may be produced if the predominant reaction has occurred in the fundus. Antral ulceration also may be observed, as can a gumma within the gastric wall. An association has been suggested between gastric syphilis and the development of squamous cell carcinoma of the stomach (74).

At upper gastrointestinal endoscopy, in early secondary syphilis, edematous erythematous mucosa with scattered erosions has been documented (75,76). In late secondary syphilis an erosive gastritis, particularly an edematous, friable, ulcerated antral mucosa, can be observed (77,78). In tertiary syphilis the inflammatory response produces a fibrotic narrowing of the antrum of the body. In addition, shallow gastric ulceration may occur with a characteristic violaceous hue on the edges of the ulcers (79). Histologically, biopsies demonstrate a nonspecific chronic gastritis with an infiltrate of lymphocytes and plasma cells. A submucosal mononuclear inflammatory reaction is often noted around arteries and veins (80). There has also been a case report of mixed infection of gastric tissue with both *T. pallidum* and *H. pylori* in association with chronic active gastritis (81).

Diagnosis of gastric syphilis can be confirmed by visualization of *T. pallidum* during examination of fresh biopsy material by dark-field microscopy or by positive staining of fixed tissue by specific fluorescent antibodies or by Warthin–Starry silver stain (77,78). Antibodies induced by *T. pallidum* infection also can be detected in patients' sera, the most commonly used technique is the VDRL (Venereal Disease Research Laboratory) slide flocculation test. The VDRL test also is useful for follow-up studies to determine whether treatment has been successful in eradicating the bacterium. This is indicated by a falling titer during the year following treatment.

Treatment

Penicillin (e.g., benzathine penicillin G) remains the treatment of choice for gastric syphilis. The specific regimen depends on the stage and duration of the illness. The Centers for Disease Control and Prevention (CDC) have outlined a recommended therapy. For early syphilis (primary, secondary, or latent infections of less than 1 year), 2.4 million units of penicillin G are given intramuscularly at a single session; the dosage is increased to three successive weekly intramuscular injections of 2.4 million units for syphilis of more than 1-year duration (1). Higher doses have been given for neurosyphilis. Alternative treatments utilizing tetracycline have also been described for patients allergic to penicillin.

Symptomatic improvement occurs after a variable period. Gain in weight is a characteristic feature of improvement after commencement of therapy. Healing of lesions can be detected radiologically and endoscopically, although the length of time required to influence the specific defects depends on the type of lesion and the degree of fibrosis. Gastric mucosal changes have been shown to revert to a macroscopically normal appearance approximately 1 month after therapy (82).

MYCOBACTERIUM TUBERCULOSIS

Description

Gastric tuberculosis is rarely encountered, although persons with primary pulmonary tuberculosis are at a higher risk of gastric infection. Older studies have shown prevalence levels ranging from 0.2% in normal necropsy specimens to 2.3% in necroscopy specimens obtained from patients with pulmonary tuberculosis (69). The causative organism, *M. tuberculosis,* is a slender curved rod (2 to 4 μm × 0.2 to 0.5 μm) that exhibits properties of a intracellular parasite, primarily infecting macrophages. The organism is very slow growing but it can be cultured on specialized media. As it is resistant to conventional staining methods, the bacteria are most easily visualized by a Ziehl–Neelsen stain due to their acid-fast properties.

The bacteria can directly invade the gastric mucosa, enter via the bloodstream or lymphatic system, or invade by direct extension from adjacent structures. In patients with pulmonary tuberculosis, a gastric infection with *M. tuberculosis* can readily be superimposed on a preexisting, nonspecific lesion in the stomach (69). There also appears to be an association of gastric tuberculosis with gastric carcinoma.

Clinical Features

As with the other chronic gastric infections, the symptoms of gastric tuberculosis are nonspecific and include ulcer-like dyspepsia, weight loss, vomiting, and gastric bleeding. The lesion, however, may be asymptomatic, while gastrointestinal symptoms may occur in patients with pulmonary tuberculosis in the absence of gastric involvement (83). The majority of patients have symptoms and signs of tuberculosis at other sites in the body, including the intestine; clinical features of gastric outlet obstruction may be present. The duration of symptoms, when present, can extend from weeks to years. A palpable abdominal mass occurs in about 50% of cases (84).

Diagnosis

The presence of advanced pulmonary tuberculosis raises the possibility of associated gastric involvement. However, a negative chest radiograph does not always exclude the presence of gastric tuberculosis (85), and a strongly positive tuberculin reaction in the absence of demonstrable tuberculosis elsewhere strengthens the diagnosis (83). Radiological findings in the stomach are nonspecific. Thus single or multiple gastric ulcerations are frequently present and may simulate benign gastric ulceration, gastric carcinoma, lymphoma, or Crohn's disease. There is often a continuity of ulceration from the duodenum into the antrum of the stomach. A hypertrophic response in the submucosa can produce gastric wall thickening and annular constriction of the lumen (86). Pyloric stenosis, or even fistula formation, also may occur (83,87).

Endoscopically, the lesions are typically small, often multiple, shallow ulcerations that are more prominent in the distal stomach. Biopsies may demonstrate gastritis only; definitive diagnosis depends on the demonstration of tubercle bacilli or a caseating granuloma. Mycobacteria, however, can be demonstrated in tissue in only one-third of cases (88).

Treatment

Usually, treatment with three antituberculosis drugs is the appropriate management. The drugs of choice are isoniazid (300 mg/day), rifampicin (600 mg/day), and pyrazinamide (2 g/day) with ethambutol (1.2 g/day) and streptomycin (1 g/day) being used in some instances. Response to such chemotherapy is usually relatively rapid and effective, although treatment for periods in excess of 9 months is recommended. In the hypertrophic form of the disease, however, chemotherapy may not be as effective, necessitating surgical resection or bypass.

MYCOTIC INFECTIONS

Description

A number of systemic mycotic infections can involve the stomach in an invasive fashion, but these are exceedingly rare. Examples are species of *Candida, Mucor,* and *Rhizophus, Histoplasma capsulatum* (89,90), *Torulopsis glabrata, Actinomyces israelii* (91,92), and *Aspergillus fumigatus* (93). *Candida albicans* has been the most frequently reported. Predisposing factors that result in increased frequency of gastric infection include diabetes, malignancies, burns, trauma, pregnancy, and immunodeficiency syndromes.

Clinical Features

Symptoms such as epigastric pain, anorexia, nausea, vomiting, and weight loss have been reported (94). However, symptoms are usually more pronounced if candidiasis is present in other areas of the gastrointestinal tract. Gastric candidiasis may be more prevalent in patients with previous partial gastrectomy (94). Yeast bezoars also are a complication of gastric surgery, especially vagotomy with antrectomy or a drainage procedure (95,96); when the bezoars are present, cultures of gastric aspirates usually grow *Candida* or *Torulopsis* species.

Diagnosis

Stool culture is usually not of value in the diagnosis of gastric candidiasis, as yeasts are found in a significant proportion of healthy people (97). The radiological appearance of gastric candidiasis reflects mucosal ulceration and submucosal invasion. Gastric sponge-like semifluid masses appear to be typical of severe cases, in addition to filling defects, superficial ulceration, enlarged gastric folds, and a lack of gastric distensibility (98,99). Gastric fistulas have also been reported in mycotic infections (100).

At endoscopy the presence of single or multiple whitish plaques, which are confluent and may form white or grey membranes, are characteristic of gastric candidiasis (101). Mucosal brushings of the lesions have a greater yield than biopsies. Mycotic membranes dislodged with the biopsy forceps and retrieved can be stained to allow visualization of the organisms (102). Mucosal biopsies often demonstrate acute or chronic inflammation with absence of fungi. For definitive diagnosis of most lesions of gastric candidiasis, histological evidence of mycelial invasion of the mucosa or ulcer slough should be present, but this depends on the endoscopic findings and clinical situation.

Gastric infection with *Histoplasma capsulatum* can result in polypoid nodules that, by microscopy, are found to be submucosal focal aggregates of macrophages heavily infected with the fungi. Other mycotic infections manifest as necrotic lesions in which the causative organism often can be detected (89).

Treatment

Culture is required to determine the species and susceptibility to antifungal agents. For *Candida albicans,* oral nystatin therapy is simple and often effective in cases that appear superficial as visualized by endoscopy. Amphotericin B or ketoconazole is useful in deeply invasive disease states. Yeast bezoars can usually be treated satisfactorily by mechanical disruption and oral nystatin.

OTHER GASTRIC INFECTIONS

The stomach has been shown to be susceptible to infection by other microorganisms including *Bacillus anthracis,* the causative organism of anthrax, protozoans, especially *Giardia lamblia,* and parasites such as *Strongyloides stercoralis* and *Anisakis* species.

Primary anthrax may develop in the stomach through the ingestion of contaminated foodstuffs. Infection can result in the invasion of the gastric mucosa and secondary ulceration, which then may disseminate to the bloodstream, possibly resulting in meningitis. Patients present with nonspecific symptoms; however, bleeding with hematemesis and/or melena may occur. The characteristic gram-positive spore-forming rod can be detected by culture or in biopsies. Penicillin G remains the drug of choice for treatment (1).

Giardia lamblia has been reported in 0.3% of patients with upper gastrointestinal symptoms, usually in the presence of intestinal metaplasia and/or *H. pylori* infection (103). The protozoa can be found in the foveolar pits and in the overlying epithelium. Affected persons usually are found to have moderate or severe chronic atrophic gastritis. The infection has been associated with a decrease in gastric acidity as some patients only become colonized with the protozoa after treatment with H_2 antagonists.

There also has been a recent case report of a *S. stercoralis* infection of the stomach. A 70-year-old man presented with symptoms of high fever, diarrhea, and weight loss. Endoscopy revealed a large prepyloric ulcer with evidence of recent bleeding. The lumen and mucosal crypts were found to be infiltrated by helminthic eggs and larvae. The patient was treated with thiabendazole. The gastric ulcer had healed when the patient was reexamined 3 weeks later (104).

Two cases of stomach granuloma have been associated with *Anisakis*-like nematodes (105). The worms were found to penetrate into the stomach wall, causing severe diffuse inflammatory reactions, and had been detected in submucosal granulomata associated with necrosis, extensive eosinophilic infiltration, and ulcerative lesions.

BACTERIAL OVERGROWTH IN THE STOMACH

Introduction

Gastric acidity is of benefit to the human host in two major ways—as an aid to digestion and as a barrier to the entry of pathogens into the intestinal tract. It is this latter property of gastric acidity that will be considered here. If the acidity of the stomach is lowered, the gastric lumen may become colonized with large numbers of bacteria, including coliform bacteria, staphylococci, streptococci, and other bacteria originating from the oral cavity. This overgrowth may be associated with a number of clinical consequences.

Predisposing Factors to Bacterial Overgrowth in the Stomach

Acid-Suppressive Therapy

There is a clear inverse relationship between the number of bacteria in gastric and duodenal secretions and the level of gastric acid. Drasar et al. (106) showed that normal subjects with gastric pH < 4 have fewer than 10^4 bacteria/mL in their fasting gastric juice. For a short time (2 hr) after a meal, this number may increase due to the transient presence of oral bacteria. In contrast, patients on acid-suppressive therapy show a significant rise in the numbers of gastric bacteria (107,108); gastric colonization may occur after only 12 hr of acid suppression.

Age

There is extensive literature on the relationship between gastric acid secretion and advancing age (109). Many claim that gastric acid output declines with age. In a Norwegian study of 15 healthy old persons with a mean age of 84 years, 12 (80%) were hypochlorhydric with a pH of 6.6 and a mean bacterial count of 10^8 colony forming units (CFU) per milliliter (range 10^5 to 10^{10}) in their fasting gastric aspirate (110). In contrast, Wormsley and Grossman (111) studied 75 control subjects including 14 subjects over 60 years of age and found no significant difference in acid secretion. The reason for these differences could probably be due to differences in rates of *H. pylori* infection and/or the degree of atrophic gastritis, the latter known to impair acid secretion due to ablation of parietal cell function. Given that more than half of the world is infected with *H. pylori* and, in certain countries, have been infected for decades, it is likely that there are currently many elderly hypochlorhydrics in the world with significant bacterial overgrowth.

Another similar but unrelated cause of hypochlorhydria, which is not a consequence of aging but with which it would correlate, is pernicious anemia. Of relevance is that classic pernicious anemia is associated with severe atrophic gastritis involving the fundus with destruction of parietal cells and, as with *H. pylori*-associated atrophy, bacterial overgrowth results. The inflammation also inhibits intrinsic factor production, leading to cobolamine malabsorption and thus to megablastic anemia.

Origin of Overgrowing Bacteria

There is controversy with respect to the contribution of overgrowing bacteria to disease. In part, this probably reflects an uncertainty as to the origin of these organisms. In the group of healthy elderly persons with fasting hypochlorhydria described above, the microbial flora were dominated by viridans streptococci, coagulase-negative staphylococci, and *Hemophilus* species (110), indicating that the normal site of contamination is from the oral cavity. In another study of 108 patients, the majority were shown to have bacteria in the duodenum with a predominance of *E. coli* and *Enterococcus faecalis* (112). Thus, when duodenogastric reflux occurs, these fecal-type bacteria could seed the stomach. There are groups in which this phenomenon occurs with increased frequency (e.g., the severe atrophic gastritis associated with gastric cancer) (113), explaining why patients with gastric carcinoma have a high rate of colonization with bacteria typical of the lower gastrointestinal tract (114,115). The other group of patients with very significant increase in reflux are those nursed in intensive care units (ICUs). Compared to a control group of healthy persons, patients in ICUs were found to have three to four times higher concentrations of bile in gastric juice, indicating significant duodenogastric reflux (116). Thus the organisms overgrowing in a hypochlorhydric person could originate from the intestinal tract.

To compound the difficulties in determining the sources

of organisms present in the stomach, it should be remembered that the oral flora can change, particularly in response to antimicrobial therapy, and intestinal bacteria such as *E. coli* can predominate.

Bacterial Growth as a Predisposition to Nosocomial Pneumonia

There is no unified opinion supporting the hypothesis that gastric bacteria are a source of bronchopulmonary infection. However, it has been claimed that acid suppression employed in intensive care patients, to prevent the development of stress ulcers, predisposes to nosocomial pneumonia. This controversy has been excellently reviewed by Tryba (117), who concludes that drugs that increase the frequency of patients with gastric pH > 4 significantly increase the risk of pulmonary infection, at least among ventilated patients in the ICU (117). This phenomenon will vary depending on the type of patient. In neurosurgical patients, gastric reflux is reduced and the stomach is not considered to be an important source for nosocomial infection or endotoxemia. In contrast, Craven et al. (118) have shown that the pneumonia rate in patients without stress-bleeding prophylaxis was 8% while patients receiving cimetidine alone or cimetidine with an antacid showed a pneumonia rate of 37% to 38%. Based on these observations, it has been suggested that stress ulcers should be prevented by administration of agents, such as sucralfate, that are mucosal protectants and do not affect gastric pH (119). However, the evidence is too uncertain to be able to make firm recommendations. For example, another source of nosocomial infection in critically ill patients may be translocation of intestinal bacteria across ischemic gastrointestinal epithelium (120).

CONCLUSION

Helicobacter pylori is the major pathogen infecting the human stomach. However, this chapter draws attention to a miscellany of other organisms that can in certain circumstances proliferate in the gastric mucosa with potentially deleterious effects to the host. These uncommon conditions should be considered when managing the small subsets of patients for whom a pathogen is suspected and *H. pylori* is not isolated or detected.

ACKNOWLEDGMENTS

This work is supported by the National Health and Medical Research Council of Australia. We would also like to thank the following for providing us with unpublished data relating to patients colonized with *G. hominis*: Dr. T. Bohane, Dr. J. Mitchell, Dr. T. Borody, Dr. C. Meredith, Dr. L. Hillman, Dr. W. Davies, Dr. G. Daskalopoulos, Dr. F. Bonar, Dr. R. Fischer, Dr. N. Figura, Prof. W. Wegmann, Dr. D. Queiroz, Dr. B. Marshall, Dr. A. Morris, Dr. H. Yang, and Dr. E. Ierardi.

REFERENCES

1. Manten HD, Harary AM. Chronic infections of the stomach. In: Berk JE, ed. *Bockus gastroenterology,* 4th ed. Philadelphia: Saunders, 1985;1328–1342.
2. Marshall BJ. Unidentified curved bacillus on gastric epithelium in active chronic gastritis. *Lancet* 1983;1:1273–1275.
3. Warren JR. Unidentified curved bacilli on gastric epithelium in active chronic gastritis. *Lancet* 1983;1:1273.
4. Mitchell HM. The epidemiology of *Helicobacter pylori* infection and its relation to gastric cancer. In: Goodwin CS, Wormsley BW, eds. *Helicobacter pylori: biology and clinical practice.* Boca Raton, FL: CRC Press, 1993;95–114.
5. Bizzozero G. Ueber die schlauchfoermigen drusen des magendarmkanals und die beziehungen ihres epithels zu dem oberfachenepithel der schleimhaut. *Arch Mikrosk Anat* 1892;42:82–152.
6. Rappin JP. Contr a l'etude de bacterium de la bouche a l'etat normal. Quoted by Breed RS, Murray EGD, Hitchens AP, eds. In: *Bergey's manual of determinative bacteriology,* 6th ed. Baltimore: Williams & Wilkins, 1981;68.
7. Salomon H. Spirillum of the mammalian stomach and its behaviour with respect to parietal cells. *Zentralbl Bakt* 1896;19:433–441.
8. Kreinitz W. Ueber das auftreten von spirochaeten verschiedener form im magenihalt bei carcinoma ventriculi. *Deutsch Med Wochenschr* 1906;32:872.
9. Luger A, Neuberger H. Uber spirochatenbefunde im magensaft und dev diagnostische bedeutung fur das carcinoma ventriculi. *Z Klin Med* 1921;92:54–75.
10. Doenges JL. Spirochaetes in the gastric glands of *Macaca rhesus* and humans without definite history of related disease. *Arch Pathol* 1939;27:469–477.
11. Dent JC, McNulty CAM, Uff JC, Wilkinson SP, Gear MWL. Spiral organisms in the gastric antrum. *Lancet* 1987;2:96.
12. McNulty CAM, Dent JC, Curry A, et al. New spiral bacterium in gastric mucosa. *J Clin Pathol* 1989;42:585–591.
13. Flejou JF, Diomande I, Molas G, et al. Human chronic gastritis associated with non-*Helicobacter pylori* spiral organisms (*Gastrospirillum hominis*). Four cases and review of the literature. *Gastroenterol Clin Biol* 1990;14:806–810.
14. Borody TJ, George LL, Brandl S, et al. *Helicobacter pylori*-negative duodenal ulcer. *Am J Gastroenterol* 1991;86:1154–1157.
15. Fischer R, Samisch W, Schwenke E. "*Gastrospirillum hominis*": another four cases. *Lancet* 1990;335:59.
16. Heilmann KL, Borchard F. Gastritis due to spiral shaped bacteria other than *Helicobacter pylori*: clinical, histological, and ultrastructural findings. *Gut* 1991;32:137–140.
17. Logan RP, Karim QN, Polson RJ, Walker MM, Baron JH. "*Gastrospirillum hominis*" infection of the stomach. *Lancet* 1989;2:672.
18. Wegmann W, Aschwanden M, Schaub N, Aenishanslin W, Gyr K. Gastritis associated with *Gastrospirillum hominis*—a zoonosis? *Schweiz Med Wochenschr* 1991;121:245–254.
19. Kubonova K, Trupl J, Jancula L, Polak E, Viablik V. Presence of spiral bacteria (*Gastrospirillum hominis*) in the gastric mucosa. *Eur J Clin Microbiol Infect Dis* 1991;10:459–460.
20. Ierardi E, Monno R, Mongelli A, et al. *Gastrospirillum hominis* associated chronic active gastritis: the first report from Italy. *Ital J Gastroenterol* 1991;23:86–87.
21. Lee A, Eckstein RP, Fevre DI, Dick E, Kellow JE. Non-*Campylobacter pylori* spiral organisms in the gastric antrum. *Aust N Z J Med* 1989;19:156–158.
22. Dye KR, Marshall BJ, Frierson HFJ, Guerrant RL, McCallum RW. Ultrastructure of another spiral organism associated with human gastritis. *Dig Dis Sci* 1989;34:1787–1791.
23. Kern SE, Yardley JH, Kafonek DR, et al. Three cases of gastric spirochetelike organisms. *Gastroenterology* 1989;96:266–267.
24. Morris A, Ali MR, Thomsen L, Hollis B. Tightly spiral shaped bacteria in the human stomach: another cause of active chronic gastritis? *Gut* 1990;31:139–143.
25. Debongnie JC, Donnay M, Jouret A, Deprez C, Burette A.

Gastrospirillum hominis in Belgium. *Acta Gastroenterol Belg* 1993;56 (Suppl):88.

26. Zhou Y, Yang HT, Xu ZM. Gastritis due to "*Helicobacter heilmannii.*" *Acta Gastroenterol Belg* 1993;56(Suppl):49.

27. Lee A, Hazell SL, O'Rourke J, Kouprach S. Isolation of a spiral-shaped bacterium from the cat stomach. *Infect Immun* 1988;56:2843–2850.

28. Paster BJ, Lee A, Fox JG, et al. Phylogeny of *Helicobacter felis* sp. nov., *Helicobacter mustelae,* and related bacteria. *Int J Syst Bacteriol* 1991;41:31–38.

29. Lavelle J, Conklin F, Mitros S, Landas S. Transmission of "*Gastrospirillum hominis*" from cat to man. *Gastroenterology* 1992;104:306.

30. Dick E, Lee A, Watson G, O'Rourke J. Use of the mouse for the isolation and investigation of stomach-associated, spiral-helical shaped bacteria from man and other animals. *J Med Microbiol* 1989;29:55–62.

31. Krakowka S, Morgan DR, Eaton KA, Radin MJ. Animal models of *Helicobacter pylori* gastritis. In: Menge H, Gregor M, Tytgat GNJ, Marshall BJ, McNulty CAM, eds. *Helicobacter pylori 1990.* Berlin: Springer-Verlag, 1991;74–80.

32. Fox JG, Lee A. Gastric *Campylobacter*-like organisms: their role in gastric disease of laboratory animals. *Lab Anim Sci* 1989;39:543–553.

33. Eaton KA, Radin MJ, Krakowka S. Animal models of bacterial gastritis—the role of host, bacterial species and duration of infection on severity of gastritis. *Zentralbl Bakt (Int J Med Microbiol)* 1993;280:28–37.

34. Dubois A, Tarnawski A, Fiala N, et al. Direct evidence for parietal cell invasion and injury by *Campylobacter pylori*-like (CPLO) organisms in rhesus monkeys. An animal model for gastritis. *Gastroenterology* 1988;94:A105.

35. Fox JG, Lee A. Gastric *Helicobacter* infection in animals: natural and experimental infections. In: Goodwin CS, Worsley BW, eds. *Helicobacter pylori: biology and clinical practice.* Boca Raton, FL: CRC Press, 1993;407–430.

36. Chen M, Lee A, Hazell SL. Immunisation against *Helicobacter* infection in a mouse/*Helicobacter felis* model. *Lancet* 1992;1:1120–1121.

37. Chen MH, Lee A, Hazell S, Hu PJ, Li YY. Immunisation against gastric infection with *Helicobacter* species—first step in the prophylaxis of gastric cancer? *Zentralbl Bakt (Int J Med Microbiol)* 1993;280:155–165.

38. Czinn SJ, Cai A, Nedrud JG. Protection of germ-free mice from infection by *Helicobacter felis* after active oral or passive IgA immunisation. *Vaccine* 1993;11:637–642.

39. Lee A, O'Rourke JL. Ultrastructure of *Helicobacter* organisms and possible relevance for pathogenesis. In: Goodwin CS, Worsley BW, eds. *Helicobacter pylori: biology and clinical practice.* Boca Raton, FL: CRC Press, 1993;15–35.

40. Solnick JV, O'Rourke J, Lee A, Paster BJ, Dewhirst FE, Tompkins LS. An uncultured gastric spiral organism is a newly identified helicobacter in humans. *J Infect Dis* 1993;168:379–385.

41. Woese CR. Bacterial evolution. *Microbiol Rev* 1987;51:221–271.

42. O'Rourke JL, Solnick J, Lee A, Tompkins LS. "*Helicobacter heilmannii*" (previously *Gastrospirillum*), a new species of *Helicobacter* in humans and animals. *Irish J Med Sci* 1992;161(Suppl 10):31.

43. Figura N, Guglielmetti P, Quaranta S. Spiral shaped bacteria in gastric mucosa. *J Clin Pathol* 1990;43:173.

44. Nakshabendi IM, Peebles SE, Lee FD, Russell RI. Spiral shaped microorganisms in the human duodenal mucosa. *Postgrad Med J* 1991;67:846–847.

45. Newell DG, Lee A, Hawtin PR, Hudson MJ, Stacey AR, Fox J. Antigenic conservation of the ureases of spiral- and helical-shaped bacteria colonising the stomachs of man and animals. *FEMS Microbiol Lett* 1989;65:183–186.

46. Solnick J, O'Rourke J, Lee A, Tompkins LS. Cloning, sequencing, and expression of urease genes from "*Helicobacter heilmannii*" (formerly "*Gastrospirillum hominis*"). *Acta Gastroenterol Belg* 1993;56 (Suppl):50.

47. Lee A. *Helicobacter pylori* and helicobacter-like organisms in animals: overview of mucus-colonising organisms. In: Rathbone BJ, Heatley RV, eds. *Helicobacter pylori and gastroduodenal disease,* 2nd ed. Oxford: Blackwell Scientific Publications, 1992;259–275.

48. Lee A. Human gastric spirilla other than *Campylobacter pylori*. In: Blaser M, ed. *Campylobacter in gastritis and peptic ulcer diseases.* New York: Igaku-Shoin Medical Publishers, 1989; 225–240.

49. Curry A, Jones DM, Skelton-Stroud P. Novel ultrastructure in a helical bacterium found in the baboon (*Papio anubis*) stomach. *J Gen Microbiol* 1989;135:2223–2231.

50. Eaton KA, Radin MJ, Kramer L, et al. Gastric spiral bacilli in captive cheetahs. *Scand J Gastroenterol* 1991;26:38–42.

51. Heilmann KL, Borchard F. Further observations on human spirobacteria. In: Menge H, Gregor M, Tytgat GNJ, Marshall BJ, McNulty CAM, eds. *Helicobacter pylori 1990.* Berlin: Springer-Verlag, 1991;63–70.

52. O'Rourke JL, Lee A. The diversity of gastric microbiota from a wide range of mammals including the human. *Acta Gastroenterol Belg* 1993;56(Suppl):53.

53. Queiroz DM, Rocha GA, Mendes EN, Lage AP, Carvalho AC, Barbosa AJ. A spiral microorganism in the stomach of pigs. *Vet Microbiol* 1990;24:199–204.

54. Geyer C, Colbatzky F, Lechner J, Hermanns W. Occurrence of spiral-shaped bacteria in gastric biopsies of dogs and cats. *Vet Record* 1993;133:18–19.

55. Yang HT, Zhou DY, Blum AL. "*Helicobacter heilmannii*" associated acute gastritis. *Acta Gastroenterol Belg* 1993;56(Suppl):75.

56. Waring PM, Shilkin KB. "Corkscrew-like" bacteria associated with gastritis. *Histopathology* 1989;15:647–649.

57. Lee A, Fox JG, Otto G, Dick EH, Krakowka S. Transmission of *Helicobacter* spp.: a challenge to the dogma of faecal–oral spread. *Epidemiol Infect* 1991;107:99–109.

58. O'Rourke JL, Lee A, Fox JG. *Helicobacter* infection in animals: a clue to the role of adhesion in the pathogenesis of gastroduodenal disease. *Eur J Gastroenterol Hepatol* 1992;4:S31–S37.

59. Genta RM, Graham DY. The gastric cardia in *Helicobacter pylori* infection. *Gastroenterology* 1993;104:A86.

60. Lynch DAF, Mapstone NP, Clarke AMT, et al. Correlation between cell proliferation in *H. pylori* associated gastritis and histological scoring using the Sydney system. *Acta Gastroenterol Belg* 1993;56(Suppl):54.

61. Henry GA, Long PH, Burns JL, Charbonneau DL. Gastric spirillosis in beagles. *Am J Vet Res* 1987;48:831–836.

62. Lee A, Fox JG, Otto G, Murphy J. A small animal model of human *Helicobacter pylori* active chronic gastritis. *Gastroenterology* 1990;99:1315–1323.

63. Lee A, Chen MH, Coltro N, et al. Long term infection of the gastric mucosa with *Helicobacter* species does induce atrophic gastritis in an animal model of *Helicobacter pylori* infection. *Zentralbl Bakt (Int J Med Microbiol)* 1993;280:38–50.

64. Isaacson PG, Spencer J. Is gastric lymphoma an infectious disease? *Hum Pathol* 1993;24:569–570.

65. Wotherspoon AC, Ortiz-Hidalgo C, Falzon MR, Isaacson PG. *Helicobacter pylori*-associated gastritis and primary B-cell gastric lymphocytes. *Lancet* 1991;338:1175–1176.

66. Drossman DA, Thompson WG, Talley NJ, Funch-Jensen P, et al. Identification of subgroups of functional gastrointestinal disorders. *Gastroenterol Int* 1990;3:159–172.

67. Lord MG, Taylor CJ, Nour S. "*Gastrospirillum hominis*" infection of the stomach. *Lancet* 1989;2:672.

68. Queiroz DM, Cabral MM, Nogueira AM, Barbosa AJ, Rocha GA, Mendes EN. Mixed gastric infection by "*Gastrospirillum hominis*" and *Helicobacter pylori*. *Lancet* 1990;2:507–508.

69. Bockus HL. Syphilis and the stomach. In: Bockus HL, ed. *Gastroenterology,* 3rd ed. Philadelphia: Saunders, 1974; 1041–1059.

70. Palmer ED. *Clinical gastroenterology.* New York: Harper & Row, 1963.

71. Eusterman GB. Gastric syphilis. Observations based on 93 cases. *JAMA* 1931;96:173–179.

72. Jones BV, Lichtenstein JE. Gastric syphilis: radiological findings. *AJR Am J Roentgenol* 1993;160:59–61.
73. Morin ME, Tan A. Diffuse enlargement of gastric folds as a manifestation of secondary syphilis. *Am J Gastroenterol* 1980; 74:170–172.
74. Vaughan WP, Straus FH, Paloyan D. Squamous carcinoma of the stomach after luetic linitis plastica. *Gastroenterology* 1977; 72:945–948.
75. Schwartz I. Gastroscopic observations in secondary syphilis. *Gastroenterology* 1948;10:227–230.
76. Mitchell R, Bralow S. Acute erosive gastritis due to early syphilis. *Ann Intern Med* 1964;61:933–938.
77. Sacha D, Klein R, Swerdlow F, et al. Erosive syphilitic gastritis: dark-field and immunofluorescent diagnosis from biopsy specimen. *Ann Intern Med* 1974;80:512–515.
78. Reisman T, Leverett F, Hudson J, Kalser M. Syphilitic gastropathy. *Am J Dig Dis* 1975;20:588–593.
79. Patterson C, Rouse M. Description of gastroscopic appearance of luetic gastric lesions in late acquired syphilis. *Gastroenterology* 1948;10:474–485.
80. Singer HA, Dyas FG. Syphilis of the stomach with special reference to certain diagnostic criteria. *Arch Intern Med* 1928;42: 718–734.
81. Rank EL, Goldenberg SA, Hasson J, Cartun RW, Grey N. *Treponema pallidum* and *Helicobacter pylori* recovered in a case of chronic active gastritis. *Am J Clin Pathol* 1992;97: 116–120.
82. Fanche PS. Syphilis of the stomach. *Ann Intern Med* 1951;35: 240–248.
83. Gaines W, Steinbach HL, Lowenhaupt E. Tuberculosis of the stomach. *Radiology* 1952;58:808–819.
84. Walters W, Kirklin BR, Clagett OT. Tuberculosis of the stomach. *Proc Staff Meet Mayo Clin* 1936;11:83–85.
85. Pinto RS, Zausner J, Beranbaum ER. Gastric tuberculosis: report of a case with discussion of angiographic findings. *AJR Am J Roentgenol* 1970;110:808–812.
86. Abrams JS, Holden WD. Tuberculosis of the gastrointestinal tract. *Arch Surg* 1964;89:282–293.
87. Ackermann AJ. Roentgenological study of gastric tuberculosis. *AJR Am J Roentgenol* 1940;44:59.
88. Chazan B, Aitchison J. Gastric tuberculosis. *Br Med J* 1960; 2:1288–1290.
89. Goodwin RA, Shapira JL, Thurman GH, et al. Disseminated histoplasmosis: clinical and pathologic correlations. *Medicine (Baltimore)* 1980;59:1–33.
90. Nudelman HL, Radatansky H. Gastric histoplasmosis: a case report. *JAMA* 1966;195:134–136.
91. Fuller CC, Wood H. Actinomycotic granuloma of the stomach. *JAMA* 1945;129:1163.
92. Behring I. The occurrence of actinomycosis of the stomach and the duodenum. *Acta Pathol Microbiol Scand* 1933;16(Suppl): 18–30.
93. Landau JW, Newcomer VD, Schulz J. Aspergillosis: report of the pertinent literature. *Mycopathologia* 1963;20:177–224.
94. Ahnlund HO, Pallin B, Peterhoff R, Schonebeck J. Mycosis of the stomach. *Acta Chir Scand* 1967;133:555–562.
95. Borg I, Heijkenskjold F, Nilehn B, Wehlin L. Massive growth of yeasts in resected stomach. *Gut* 1966;1:244–249.
96. Konok G, Haddad H, Strom B. Postoperative gastric mycosis. *Surg Gynecol Obstet* 1980;150:337–341.
97. Kozinn PJ, Taschdjian CL. Enteric candidiasis: diagnosis and clinical considerations. *Pediatrics* 1962;30:71–85.
98. Pugh TF, Fitch SJ. Invasive gastric candidiasis. *Pediatr Radiol* 1986;16:67–68.
99. Shanks SC, Kerley P. *A text book of x-ray diagnosis*. London: HK Lewis & Co, 1958.
100. Bearse C. Mycotic infections of the stomach. *Am J Dig Dis* 1938;5:674.
101. Minoli G, Terruzi V, Butti G, Frigerio G, Rossini A. Gastric candidiasis: an endoscopic histology study in 26 patients. *Gastrointest Endosc* 1982;28:59–61.
102. Knoke M, Bernhardt H. Endoscopic aspects of mycosis in the upper digestive tract. *Endoscopy* 1980;12:295–298.
103. Doglioni C, De Boni M, Cielo R, et al. Gastric giardiasis. *J Clin Pathol* 1992;45:964–967.
104. Dees A, Batenburg PL, Umar HM, Menon RS, Verweij J. *Strongyloides stercoralis* associated with a bleeding gastric ulcer. *Gut* 1990;31:1414–1415.
105. Asami K, Watanuki T, Sakai H, Imano H, Okamoto R. Two cases of stomach granuloma caused by *Anisakis*-like larval nematodes in Japan. *Am J Trop Med Hyg* 1965;14:119–123.
106. Drasar BS, Shiner M, McLeod GM. Studies on the intestinal flora. I. The bacterial flora of the gastric tract in healthy and achlorhydric persons. *Gastroenterology* 1969;56:71–79.
107. Ruddell WSJ, Axon ATR, Findlay JM, Bartholomew BA, Hill MJ. Effect of cimetidine on the gastric bacterial flora. *Lancet* 1980;1:672–674.
108. Snepar R, Poporad GA, Romano JM, Kobasa WD, Kaye D. Effect of cimetidine and antacid on gastric microbial flora. *Infect Immun* 1982;36:518–524.
109. Goldschmiedt M, Feldman M. Age-related changes in gastric acid secretion. In: Holt PR, Russell RM, eds. *Chronic gastritis and hypochlorhydria in the elderly*. Boca Raton, FL: CRC Press, 1993;13–30.
110. Husebye E, Skar V, Hoverstad T, Melby K. Fasting hypochlorhydria with gram positive gastric flora is highly prevalent in healthy old people. *Gut* 1992;33:1331–1337.
111. Wormsley KG, Grossman MI. Maximal histalog test in control subjects and patients with peptic ulcer. *Gut* 1965;6:427–435.
112. Bach-Nielsen P, Amdrup E. Preoperative bacteriologic examination of the stomach and duodenum. *Acta Chir Scand* 1965; 129:521–529.
113. Houghton PWJ, Mortensen NJ, Cooper MJ, Morgan AP, Burton P. Intragastric bile acids and histological changes in gastric mucosa. *Br J Surg* 1986;73:354–356.
114. Sjostedt S, Kager L, Heimdahl A, Nord CE. Microbial colonisation of tumours in relation to the upper gastrointestinal tract in patients with gastric carcinoma. *Ann Surg* 1988;207:341–346.
115. Sjostedt S, Heimdahl A, Kager L, Nord CE. Microbial colonisation of the oropharynx, esophagus and stomach in patients with gastric disease. *Eur J Clin Microbiol* 1985;4:49–51.
116. Schindlbeck NE, Lippert M, Heinrich C, Muller-Lissner SA. Intragastric bile acid concentrations in critically ill, artificially ventilated patients. *Am J Gastroenterol* 1989;84:624–628.
117. Tryba M. The gastropulmonary route of infection—fact or fiction. *Am J Med* 1991;91(Suppl 2A):135S–146S.
118. Craven DE, Kunches LM, Kilinsky V, Lichtenberg DA, Make BJ, McCabe WR. Risk factors for pneumonia and fatality in patients receiving continuous mechanical ventilation. *Am Rev Respir Dis* 1986;133:792–796.
119. Driks MR, Craven DE, Celli BR, et al. Nosocomial pneumonia in intubated patients given sucralfate as compared with antacids or histamine type 2 blockers. *N Engl J Med* 1987;317: 1376–1382.
120. Fiddian-Green RG, Baker S. Nosocomial pneumonia in the critically ill: product of aspiration or translocation. *Crit Care Med* 1991;119:763–769.

Infections of the Gastrointestinal Tract,
edited by M. J. Blaser, P. D. Smith, J. I. Ravdin,
H. B. Greenberg, and R. L. Guerrant
Raven Press, Ltd., New York © 1995.

CHAPTER 43

Interactions of Bacteria with the Gut Epithelium

Alexander E. Hromockyj and Stanley Falkow

Certain bacterial pathogens are adapted uniquely for survival and persistence in the human intestine. Ingested by their hosts in contaminated food or water, these organisms encounter a series of host defenses against infection, such as the acid pH in the stomach, digestive enzymes, bile, the mucus overlying the intestinal epithelium, and competition with the host's normal gut flora for nutrients. Adaptation of these microbes to these hostile host factors is associated with their capacity to express specific pathogenic determinants that promote survival within the host. In parallel, these pathogenic bacteria have evolved cellular receptors to detect environmental stimuli and coordinately regulate virulence gene expression in response to these cues.

Enteric bacterial pathogens can broadly be categorized into three groups: *enteroadherent,* which adhere to and colonize the surface of the intestinal epithelium where they remain for the duration of the infection; *enterotoxigenic,* which, in addition to adherence and colonization of the intestinal epithelium, produce potent toxins; and *enteroinvasive,* which are capable of actively crossing the intestinal epithelium. The enteroinvasive group can be further divided into organisms that remain localized to the mucosal epithelial layers and organisms that penetrate into deeper tissue and cause systemic infection.

Because bacterial enterotoxins and the cellular effects they elicit have been reviewed comprehensively elsewhere in this volume (see chapters by Crowe and Powell, Crane and Guerrant, DuPont, Chang, Butterton and Calderwood, and Cohen and Gianella), we will focus here on the enteroadherent and enteroinvasive groups of enteropathogens, specifically the enteropathogenic derivative of *Escherichia coli,* EPEC (enteropathogenic *E. coli*), the enteropathogenic *Yersinia* and *Salmonella* species, and *Shigella* species. For all enteric pathogens, attachment of the enteropathogen to the gut epithelium is the critical first step in establishing a niche within the host. However, for the enteroinvasive species, the hallmark of infection after attachment is entry into the intestinal mucosa and subsequent spread to the lamina propria. The initial bacteria–host cell events and changes that occur in the host cell will be emphasized in this chapter.

GENETIC BASIS AND CELL BIOLOGY OF BACTERIA–HOST CELL INTERACTIONS

Our current understanding of enteric bacterial infections is based on histopathological observations from human and animal infection. Moreover, *in vitro* studies of bacterial interactions with cultured mammalian cells have been valuable in dissecting the genetic basis of enteric bacterial virulence and the host cellular mechanisms exploited by these organisms. Bacterial invasion of epithelial cells is often referred to as "parasite directed phagocytosis." As implied by this term, invasive enteropathogens trigger specific host cell signaling events to facilitate their uptake by normally nonphagocytic cells, while the morphological, cytoskeletal, and cytochemical events that occur in the target mammalian cell during invasion resemble phagocytosis.

The ability of enteropathogenic bacteria to adhere to and enter mammalian cells is a multigenic virulence trait. Classic genetic techniques and recombinant DNA technology have provided considerable information about the genetic organization and structure–function of these virulence determinants. It is clear that seemingly diverse pathogenic enteric bacteria share a number of analogous and even related virulence themes. For example, virulence genes of EPEC, *Shigella, Salmonella,* and *Yersinia* species are encoded both on the bacterial chromosome and on large virulence plasmids characteristic of each group of organisms. Ranging in size from 70 kb for the *Yersinia* species (1) up to 220 kb for the *Shigella* species (2), genes

A. E. Hromockyj: Department of Microbiology and Immunology, Stanford University School of Medicine, Stanford, California 94305-5402.

S. Falkow: Department of Microbiology and Immunology, Stanford University School of Medicine, Stanford, California 94305-5402; and Microscopy Branch, Rocky Mountain Laboratories, National Institutes of Health, Hamilton, Montana 59840.

604 / Chapter 43

on these virulence plasmids encode gene products essential for adherence and invasion of host cells. Another emerging theme among these enteric organisms is that expression of virulence determinants on the bacterial surface or their extracellular export involves accessory proteins that comprise a distinct, specialized secretory mechanism. Meanwhile, superimposed on this network of virulence genes is a hierarchy of regulatory factors, which for enteric pathogens, as for all pathogenic bacteria, consist of transcriptional activators and repressors that respond to various environmental stimuli, including temperature, osmolarity, oxygen tension, and calcium ion and phosphate concentrations (3,4).

Phagocytosis by macrophages and neutrophils is characterized by a number of cellular changes that occur during ingestion of foreign particles. Primary among these changes is the rearrangement of cytoskeletal proteins localized underneath the plasma membrane and in contact with the particle being internalized. Not surprisingly, studies of bacterial invasion have focused on these same proteins and their association with bacteria attaching to and invading epithelial cells. The involvement of cytoskeletal contractile proteins, actin and myosin, as well as the actin-associated proteins α-actinin, vinculin, paxillin, talin, and ezrin, have all been investigated. The actin-associated proteins are of particular interest due to their putative role of linking the actin cytoskeletal network to transmembrane proteins that are involved in receptor recognition of various ligands (5,6). Evaluation of bacterial invasion has also focused on the variations in host cell cytosolic calcium concentrations, which are thought to regulate microfilamentous actin assembly and serve as a signal for phagocytosis (7). In addition, the study of host cell signal transduction pathways affected by bacterial invasion has been directed toward protein phosphorylation. Protein phosphorylation within a cell is a mechanism used in cellular regulation of growth, cell cycle, and cytoskeletal integrity, which is dependent on the opposing activities of protein kinases (PK) and protein phosphatases (PT) (8). The following sections will therefore highlight the morphological, cytoskeletal, and cytochemical events that occur during bacterial attachment to and invasion of epithelial cells with reference to the genetic determinants involved in the bacteria–host cell interactions.

Yersinia: A Paradigm of Bacterial Pathogenicity

The genus Yersinia is made up of a number of species that cause zoonotic infections in birds, pigs, and rodents. Humans are not the normal reservoir of yersiniae in nature. Disease in humans, caused by the pathogenic strains Y. pestis, Y. enterocolitica, and Y. pseudotuberculosis, usually results from accidental infection. Yersinia pestis, the causative agent of bubonic plague, is transmitted to humans by the bite of an infected flea, while Y. enterocolitica and Y. pseudotuberculosis cause gastroenteritis as a result of the ingestion of contaminated food. For the enteropathogenic strains of Yersinia, the primary sites of infection are the Peyer's patch lymphoid follicles located in the small intestine (9). Evidence from the murine model of yersiniosis indicates that following transcytosis of the

lymphoid follicle-associated epithelium, yersiniae that colonize the Peyer's patches are exclusively extracellular (10). It is from this site that yersiniae are capable of spreading and causing systemic infection (Fig. 1).

All enteropathogenic yersiniae have a number of chromosomal and virulence plasmid-encoded proteins that facilitate a direct interaction with target cells and alter host cell signaling pathways. The 103-kDa invasin (Inv) protein, encoded by the chromosomal inv gene, is the best characterized yersiniae virulence protein that mediates adherence to and entry into cultured mammalian cells (11). Inv facilitates a high-affinity binding of yersiniae to several of the mammalian cell heterodimeric $\alpha\beta_1$ integrin proteins and subsequent entry of the bacteria into the target cell (12). Integrins are a family of eukaryotic cell surface receptors that mediate both cell–cell and cell–extracellular matrix (ECM) protein interactions possibly through linkage with the eukaryotic cell cytoskeleton (5,6). A cascade of intracellular events result from ligands binding cellular integrin receptors, which suggest that these proteins transmit signals into the mammalian cell perhaps through the association of integrin cytoplasmic domains with cytoskeletal proteins like talin and α-actinin. As such, the binding of Inv to a β_1 integrin can be received as a specific signal to the bound cell that results in internalization of the bacterium. Bacteria binding mammalian cells via Inv cause a clustering of the β_1 integrin receptors, which is accompanied by alterations in the target cell cytoskeleton (13). Polymerized actin and the actin-associated proteins, filamin and talin, also accumulate around the invading bacterium (13). Evidence from studies with fibroblasts and blood platelets indicates that ligand binding of integrin receptors on these cells triggers several intracellular events. Included among these signals are the activation of phospholipases, the elevation of cytoplasmic pH and Ca^{2+}, as well as the activation of protein kinases (6). Whether or not similar cytochemical events occur during the interaction of Inv with a β_1 integrin receptor has yet to be determined. Inv-mediated invasion of epithelial cells is inhibited by pretreatment of the eukaryotic cells with tyrosine-protein kinase inhibitors, which suggests that protein phosphorylation may be an important cellular event triggered by interaction of yersiniae with β_1 integrin receptors (14).

Two other proteins that mediate yersinia–mammalian cell interactions in vitro are Ail and YadA. The 17-kDa Ail protein, encoded by a chromosomal gene in Y. enterocolitica, promotes binding to a variety of cultured cells while mediating efficient entry into a limited number of these cells (15). As yet, the host cell surface receptor for Ail is unknown. YadA, a 45-kDa fimbrillar protein encoded by the yersiniae virulence plasmid yadA gene (16), also mediates attachment to and invasion of epithelial cells via a β_1 integrin receptor (17,18). However, based on YadA binding of the ECM proteins, collagen, fibronectin, and laminin (19–21), which are also β_1 integrin receptor ligands, it is unclear whether YadA mediates invasion directly by binding the β_1 integrin receptor or indirectly via ECM proteins. Both Ail and YadA also facilitate bacterial resistance to human serum complement (22–24), which may reflect their major function in yersiniae pathogenesis as opposed to epithelial cell invasion. Expression of Inv,

Yersiniae

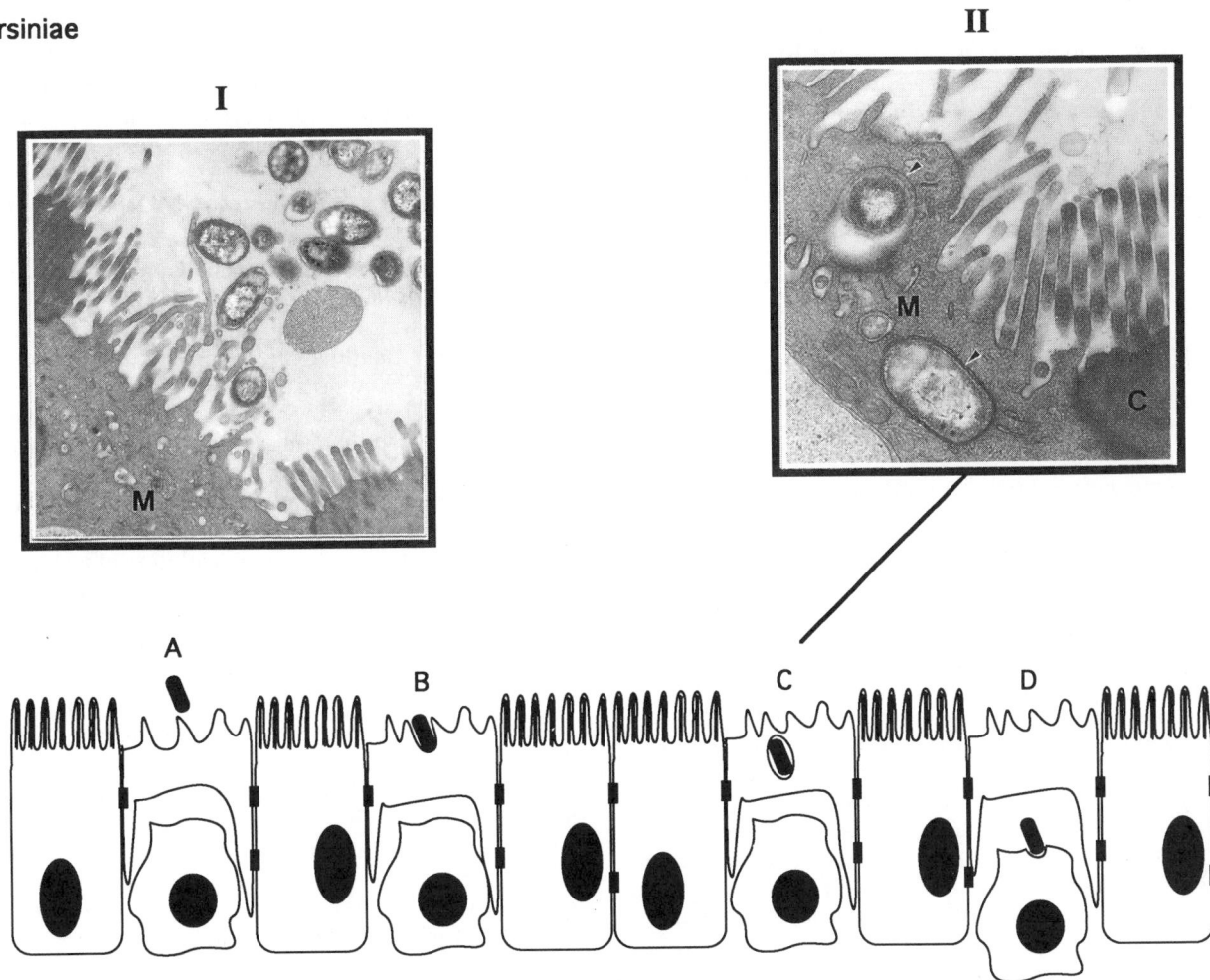

FIG. 1. Interaction of enteropathogenic *Yersinia* species with the intestinal epithelium. Diagrammed is the interaction of yersiniae with M cells overlying the Peyer's patch (PP) follicle-associated epithelium. **A,B:** Adherence to and intimate association of yersiniae with an M cell. **C:** Bacterium localized within an intracellular vacuole. **D:** Bacterium having trancytosed M cell and interacting with Peyer's patch macrophage where the bacterium inhibits phagocytosis. **I,II:** Transmission electron micrographs (TEMs) of *Y. pseudotuberculosis* attachment to and internalization by rabbit intestinal M cells (111). M and C denote M cells and absorptive epithelial cells, respectively. *Arrowheads* indicate location of yersiniae bacteria.

Ail, and YadA is regulated by temperature. Inv is optimally expressed by yersiniae cultured at 28°C (25), whereas Ail and YadA are maximally expressed by bacteria cultured at 37°C (23,26). While the regulatory mechanisms for YadA expression have been elucidated, the molecular mechanisms that regulate Inv and Ail expression remain undefined. All virulent strains of enteropathogenic yersiniae tested harbor a functional *inv* gene (27), homologous nucleotide sequences for *ail* (28), and the 70-kb virulence plasmid (1), which suggests that three distinct adherence and entry pathways are potentially involved in *Yersinia* species virulence.

In addition to the invasion proteins described above, the *Yersinia* outer membrane proteins, Yops, are potent putative effector molecules of the host reticuloendothelial system. Like YadA, the genes that code for the Yops are located on the *Yersinia* species virulence plasmid. Under conditions of low calcium concentrations (<100 μM) at 37°C, Yop expression is maximal (29). The synthesis of Yops in response to these environmental signals is tightly controlled by two independent regulatory loops. A positive regulatory loop requires the activity of the temperature-regulated VirF protein, a transcriptional activator of the *yadA* (30) and *yop* genes (31), which itself is regulated by the chromosomally encoded YmoA protein (32). In addition to VirF, the LcrV protein is also thought to be involved in the positive regulatory loop of Yop expression (33). The *lcr* (low calcium response) genes constitute the negative regulatory loop, which in conditions of high Ca^{2+} concentration are activated to repress Yop expression (33). Following initial Yop synthesis within the bacterial cytoplasm, subsequent Yop extracellular secretion requires the specialized function of the Ysc (*Yersinia* secretion) proteins encoded by the *ysc* operon (33,34). Expression of the *ysc* operon is also regulated by the positive and negative regulatory loops in response to temperature and Ca^{2+}. Several of these Lcr and Ysc regulatory proteins (33,34) share homology with the *mxi/spa* gene clusters in *Shigella* species (35–37) and the *spa/inv* genes of *Salmonella* species (38), which are involved in the expression of virulence proteins on the surfaces of these organisms. Exported out of the bacterial cytoplasm into the extracellular environment, the Yops are then capable of acting on target cells. The function of the Yops has been deduced from their shared sequence homologies with previously identified proteins. YopH, YopM, and YpkA, while sharing no significant homology with other bacterial proteins, exhibit striking homology with eukaryotic proteins. YopM is homologous with the platelet receptor for von Willebrand factor (39) and has been shown to inhibit platelet aggregation through an interaction with thrombin (40). YpkA shares protein sequence homology with serine/threonine kinases and expresses kinase activity *in vitro* (41). YopH has protein tyrosine phosphatase activity and contains a catalytic site, which is identical to that of eukaryotic phosphatases (42). Another of the Yops, YopE, mediates a contact-dependent cytotoxicity, which results in host cell actin depolymerization (43). Through the concerted effects of the tyrosine phosphatase activity of YopH and the depolymerization of actin mediated by YopE, yersiniae inhibit macrophage and neutrophil phagocytosis (43). While the actual eukaryotic cell targets of YopE activity have yet to be identified, two proteins of 120 kDa and 55 kDa in size have been identified as targets of YopH (44). The identity and function of these proteins are unknown, although preliminary evidence suggests that they are protein tyrosine kinases (45). In addition, the more recently discovered YpkA serine/threonine kinase activity points to a possible function for this protein in altering host cell signal transduction pathways. In order to elicit their effects on the target cell, three additional Yops—YopD, YopN, and YopB—have been described as essential for YopH and YopE delivery into the host cell cytoplasm. The mechanism of this delivery has not yet been determined. What is clear, however, is that the specific interaction of yersiniae with the target phagocyte via the adherence and invasion proteins Inv and YadA is the requisite first step in mediating the antiphagocytic properties of YopH and YopE (17,43; A. E. Hromockyj and S. Falkow, *personal observations*).

Therefore the primary pathogenic strategy of the *Yersinia* species following transcytosis of the intestinal epithelium is to inhibit macrophage and neutrophil phagocytosis, and perhaps cytokine signaling, thereby negating the functions of the host cellular immune response. This is in contrast to the salmonellae that enter and survive within phagocytic cells populating the Peyer's patches. Whereas the salmonellae and shigellae utilize specialized secretory processes to express invasion proteins on their surface, the yersiniae use an analogous system to secrete the antiphagocytic Yops, YopH and YopE. Furthermore, enteropathogenic yersiniae utilize the adherence and invasion protein Inv not only to cross the intestinal epithelium (46) but also to subvert host phagocytes. It is interesting that the antiphagocytic mechanism employed by yersiniae to avoid phagocytosis is a similar strategy to the intimate epithelial cell attachment exhibited by enteropathogenic *E. coli*. While EPEC colonize the epithelial cell surface and remain sequestered from the host immune system, yersiniae attack the immune system and, in a sense, seem to colonize the surface of macrophages.

Enteropathogenic *Escherichia* (EPEC)

The EPEC are recognized as a distinct group of *E. coli* serotypes that cause significant outbreaks of neonatal diarrhea primarily in developing countries. In contrast to the other enteropathogenic organisms discussed in this chapter, EPEC strains appear to elicit their pathogenic effects primarily by attachment and surface colonization of the intestinal epithelium as opposed to invasion of these cells. EPEC pathogenesis is characterized by a distinct histopathological feature referred to as an "attaching and effacing" lesion in which EPEC organisms intimately adhere to enterocytes and cause dissolution of microvilli and cupping of the enterocyte membrane around the bacteria (47). Presumably loss of the microvilli leads to host malabsorption and in turn the diarrheal symptoms exhibited during EPEC infection. Similar histopathology has been described for the rabbit diarrheogenic *E. coli* (RDEC-1) (48) and *Citrobacter freundii*, which causes murine colonic hyperplasia (49).

EPEC virulence is dependent on the presence of the approximately 95-kb EAF (EPEC adherence factor) virulence plasmid and at least nine distinct chromosomal loci (48). The best characterized of the EPEC virulence genes is *eaeA*, which is part of the chromosomal *eae* gene cluster and codes for the 94-kDa outer membrane protein, intimin (48,50). Intimin plays a crucial role in the ability of EPEC to adhere closely to cultured mammalian cells *in vitro*. Intimin-defective EPEC mutants fail to cause diarrhea in human volunteers (50). The predicted amino acid sequences of intimin and the enteropathogenic yersiniae invasin protein display a high degree of homology in domains associated with their export. An EAF plasmid-encoded gene designated *per* has been identified as a regulatory protein involved in *eaeA* expression (48). Another gene mapped to the EAF plasmid, *bfpA*, appears to code for the bundle forming pilis (BFP), which cause EPEC to aggregate and are thought to mediate the initial adherence of EPEC to epithelial cells (51). Additional EPEC chromosomal virulence loci have been identified as genetic mutants altered in phenotypes characteristic of EPEC pathogenesis. Although EPEC is not classically defined as an invasive organism, several of these chromosomal loci, designated *cfm*, mediate EPEC entry into cultured epithelial cells (52). Although identification of these invasion loci has challenged the traditional notion of EPEC as a noninvasive organism, the clinical significance of EPEC invasion remains unclear. Earlier studies have shown that EPEC can disseminate later in infection (53). Further characterization of these various mutants may lead to the identification of additional genes and a role for invasion in EPEC virulence.

Based on detailed *in vitro* studies of the genetic basis of EPEC interactions with mammalian cells described earlier, a three-stage model of EPEC pathogenesis has been

I

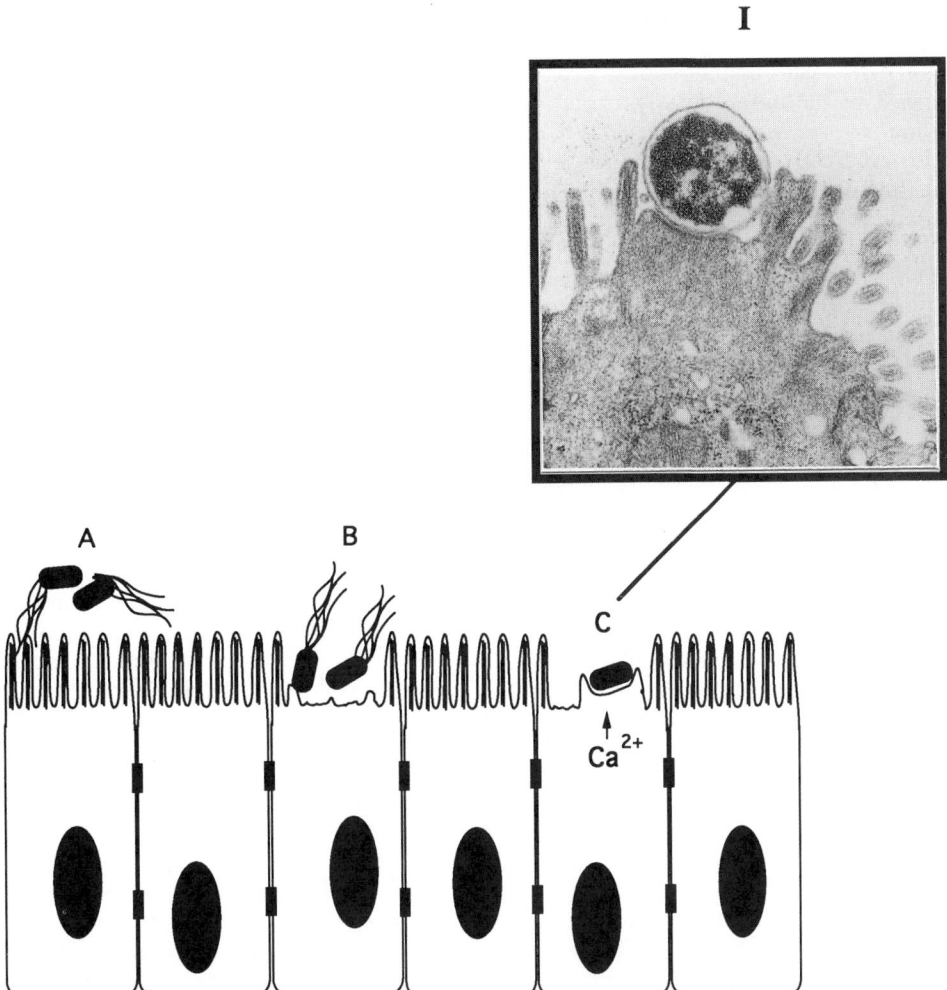

FIG. 2. Interaction of EPEC with the intestinal epithelium. Diagrammed are the proposed steps of EPEC interaction with the gut epithelium. **A:** BFP-mediated adherence to brush border of epithelium. **B,C:** Intimin protein mediated "localized adherence" to and dissolution of epithelial microvilli, followed by the formation of an "attaching and effacing" lesion and associated with a release of intracellular calcium. **I:** TEM of attaching and effacing lesion caused by *Citrobacter freundii* in mouse small intestine (124), a histopathological lesion resembling those observed in human EPEC infection.

proposed (48) (Fig. 2). Following an initial BFP-mediated interaction of the bacteria with the epithelial microvilli, the EPEC form a distinct pattern of microcolonies on the epithelial cell surface referred to as "localized adherence," which is associated with effacement of microvilli and fluid secretion. As the infection progresses the intimin protein is thought to be expressed and is known to mediate the "attaching and effacing" lesion. The morphological changes exhibited by epithelial cells following EPEC adherence are accompanied by both cytoskeletal and cytochemical events thought to be essential in the intimate adherence of the bacteria to the host cell. High concentrations of the host cell cytoskeletal protein actin are found to be associated with the characteristic "pedestal" formed beneath attached EPEC (54). Other cytoskeletal microfilament-associated proteins such as α-actinin, talin, and ezrin are also localized to EPEC attaching and effacing lesions (55).

Target cell cytochemical responses to EPEC infection *in vitro* include elevations of free intracellular calcium ($[Ca^{2+}]_i$) and the phosphorylation of several host cell proteins. The calcium release is thought to originate from intracellular stores since the inhibition of increased $[Ca^{2+}]_i$ prevents the formation of attaching and effacing lesions (48,56). Five proteins with apparent molecular masses of 21, 27, 90, 100, and 130 kDa are known to be phosphorylated during EPEC attachment and invasion. Of the two smallest proteins, the 21-kDa protein has been identified as the myosin light chain. Both the 21- and 27-kDa proteins appear to be phosphorylated by protein kinase C activity induced by EPEC invasion (57,58). The two largest proteins have been identified as α-actinin and vinculin, respectively (48). The 27- and 90-kDa proteins have yet to be identified. The importance of host cell protein phosphorylation in EPEC invasion is further supported by evidence that protein kinase inhibitors, specifically protein tyrosine kinase (TPK) inhibitors, inhibit EPEC invasion (52).

The interaction of EPEC with epithelial cells provides an interesting contrast to the enteroinvasive organisms discussed in this chapter. Whereas *Yersinia, Salmonella,* and *Shigella* species efficiently invade epithelial cells *in vitro* and this invasion correlates with their ability to invade the intestinal epithelium, EPEC elicits many of the same cytoskeletal and cytochemical changes in host cells but remains on the host cell surface. As mentioned earlier, the cell surface colonization by EPEC is similar to the antiphagocytic phenotype expressed by enteropathogenic *Yersinia* species. It may be that the interaction of intimin with a host cell surface receptor, as is the case with yersiniae invasin, serves to inhibit EPEC internalization by mammalian cells. Therefore intimin binding of a host cell surface receptor may act as a signal that alters host cell signaling activities.

Salmonella

Human disease caused by salmonellae range from a self-limiting gastroenteritis to a severe systemic infection, typhoid fever. The *Salmonella* species are a diverse group of pathogenic organisms that have been isolated from birds, mammals, and reptiles. Infections in animals constitute the principal reservoir of nontyphoidal infection in humans. Person-to-person transmission, while possible, is less likely. As is the case with infections caused by both the *Shigella* and the enteropathogenic *Yersinia* species, the ability of *Salmonella* to cause disease requires that these organisms penetrate the intestinal epithelial barrier. The primary site of *Salmonella* infection, based on the murine model of salmonellosis, appears to be the Peyer's patches of the distal ileum.

Among the *Salmonella* species, several genetic loci have been identified that mediate mammalian cell invasion. Genetic loci associated with invasion have been mapped to several chromosomal positions that include genes required for LPS expression and chemotaxis (59,60). In *S. typhimurium,* a chromosomal region spanning approximately 100 kb appears to contain the key genes for mediating salmonellae invasion. At least 15 different genes—*invA–D* and *H* (61,62), *spaM–T* (38), *orgA* (B. D. Jones and S. Falkow, *personal communication*), *prgH* (63), and *hil* (64)—have been mapped to this region. The specific function of many of these loci in invasion is not entirely clear. The predicted protein sequence homologies of InvA and InvE with shigellae, Mxi/Spa (35,37) and yersiniae, Lcr/Ysc proteins (33,34), together with the ability of the *Shigella flexneri spa47* gene to complement a *S. typhimurium spaP* mutation (38), suggest that these *S. typhimurium* genes encode for proteins that are involved in the surface expression of proteins with a direct role in the invasion process. Additional loci that are distinct from these have been identified in both *S. typhi* (65) and *S. choleraesuis* (59). In the human pathogenic species *S. typhi* a group of invasion associated genes, also designated *invA–D, H,* have been identified (65). Although this region of deoxyribonucleic acid (DNA) is present in *S.*

typhimurium, it appears to serve a different function from that of *S. typhi.* (65). Environmental growth conditions of low oxygen tension and high osmolarity have been shown to enhance epithelial cell invasion by *S. typhimurium* (66) and *S. typhi* (67), respectively. Transcription of several *S. typhimurium* invasion-associated genetic loci and specifically *org* are enhanced by low-oxygen growth conditions (B. D. Jones and S. Falkow, *personal communication*).

Electron microscopic studies of the events that lead to salmonellae penetration of the intestinal epithelium in animal models and *in vitro* studies with cultured mammalian cells present a picture of dynamic interaction between salmonellae and target epithelial cells (68–70) (Fig. 3). Characteristic of the dramatic morphological changes that occur during *Salmonella* species invasion are destruction of the brush border microvilli on the apical surface of epithelium and an increase in permeability of the epithelial cell tight junctions, followed by entry of the bacterium within a membrane-bound vacuole (68,71). These gross morphological changes occur rapidly, and entry begins within a few minutes of the salmonella–host cell interaction (70). There is a profound rearrangement of the host cell cytoskeletal protein actin at the site of bacterial entry, along with an accumulation of the actin-associated proteins talin, ezrin, α-actinin, tropomysin, and tubulin (69). The rearrangement of these proteins accompanying entry of the bacterium is transient, and they rapidly dissociate and return to their normal distribution following salmonellae entry into the host cells (69). The morphological and cytoskeletal alterations of the host cell plasma membrane induced by salmonellae closely resemble normal eukaryotic cell ruffling. Ruffles are specialized plasma membrane ultrastructures of mammalian cells composed in part by rearranged filamentous actin and temporally associated with increased pinocytosis (72). They are considered to be an integral part of mammalian cell growth, development, and locomotion and are triggered by signaling events such as growth factors, mitogens, and oncogene expression (72–75). Ruffles induced in the presence of invasive salmonellae or by other stimuli facilitate epithelial cell internalization of noninvasive bacteria, which indicates that salmonella invasion may represent an exploitation of the host cell machinery that mediates pinocytosis (76).

In addition to profound morphological and cytoskeletal changes, salmonella invasion also triggers a cascade of target cell cytochemical events. *Salmonella typhimurium* epithelial cell invasion causes a rapid increase in intracellular $[Ca^{2+}]_i$ that is required for salmonella entry and a transient increase in inositol 1,4,5-triphosphate (IP$_3$) concentrations (77,78). IP$_3$ is a product of phospholipase C, and its primary role is mobilization of Ca^{2+} from intracellular stores (77). These data have been interpreted as an indication of the possible activation of phospholipase C during salmonella invasion, which results in the observed release of $[Ca^{2+}]_i$ (77). Phosphorylation of the epidermal growth factor receptor (EGFR) has also been observed when *S. typhimurium* invades epithelial cells expressing this receptor (79). Therefore it has been suggested that salmonellae mediate invasion via EGFR (79). Based on

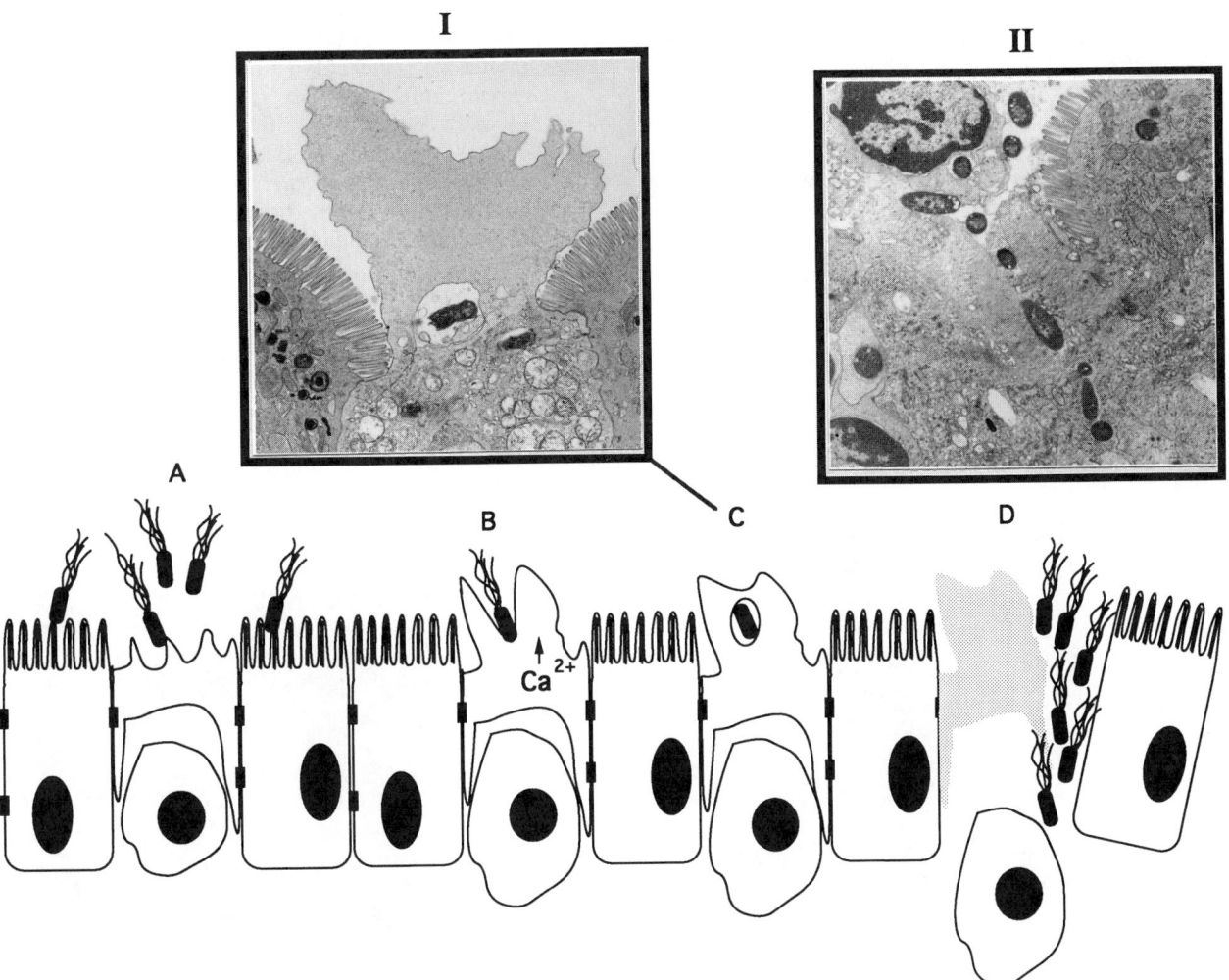

FIG. 3. Interaction of enteropathogenic *Salmonella* species with the intestinal epithelium. Diagrammed are the interaction and invasion of salmonellae with an M cell and an absorptive epithelial cell overlying the PP follicle. Salmonella invasion is shown for an M cell. **A:** Adherence of salmonellae to an M cell followed by a salmonella invasion-induced membrane ruffle. **C:** Bacterium localized within an intracellular vacuole. **D:** Destruction of the invaded M cell followed by an influx of bacteria into the epithelial cell breach and entry into PP. **I:** TEM of *S. typhimurium* following invasion of a murine intestinal M cell (124). **II:** TEM of bacteria entering a murine PP. (Courtesy B. Jones.)

the observed increase in phospholipase A_2 and 5-lipooxygenase activity following stimulation of the EGFR, the role of these proteins in *S. typhimurium* infection of epithelial cells has also been investigated (78). The activity of both of these enzymes is required for *S. typhimurium* invasion and a product of the 5-lipoxygenase, leukotriene A4, induces epithelial cell entry of noninvasive *S. typhimurium* (78). However, the increased activity of these enzymes may not be the direct result of *S. typhimurium* invasion. Other studies have demonstrated that cells that do not express the EGFR are still permissive for salmonella invasion (76,80). Alternatively, salmonellae may utilize several pathways for entry into various cell types. Attempts to determine the signaling events that lead to the induction of *Salmonella* invasion have focused on the role of the small GTPases *rac* and *rho,* proteins that are

involved in the regulation of growth factor-induced membrane ruffling and stress fiber formation (75,81). However, these studies demonstrated that *Salmonella* invasion is a *rac-* and *rho*-independent mechanism (80).

Salmonella invasion has been characterized extensively from several perspectives. However, unlike the yersiniae, shigellae, and EPEC, the identity and nature of the salmonella protein(s) directly involved in promoting bacterial entry remain elusive. It seems likely that the distinct membrane ruffles induced by invading salmonellae represent the secretion of bacterial products that stimulate host cell macropynocytic machinery. Therefore salmonellae invading epithelial cells induce more global effects in contrast to *Yersinia* and *Shigella* invasion, which resembles classic phagocytosis, that is, the binding and clustering of a host cell surface receptor followed by internalization of the invading organism. Once having penetrated the intestinal epithelial barrier, salmonellae may utilize the same invasion mechanisms to invade host macrophages (D. Monack and S. Falkow, *personal communication*). Thus the pathogenic strategy of the *Salmonella* species, like that of the *Shigella* species, is intracellular parasitism whereby these organisms enter a privileged site to elude the host immune system.

Shigella

Shigellosis of bacillary dysentery is exclusively a disease of humans and higher primates caused by one of four shigella serotypes: *S. flexneri*, *S. sonnei*, *S. boydii*, and *S. dysenteriae*. In contrast to the other groups of organisms described in this chapter, the primary site of *Shigella* species infection is the colon (82). Also, while *Salmonella* and *Yersinia* infections may spread systemically, *Shigella* infections are generally confined to the superficial layers of the intestinal mucosa. Based on the events observed in animal models and *in vitro* cell culture, *Shigella* invasion can be divided into three steps; entry, intracellular spread, and intercellular invasion (Fig. 4). *Shigella* invasion of epithelial cells, like EPEC adherence and *Salmonella* invasion, is characterized by destruction of the brush border of the intestinal epithelium followed by epithelial cell invasion (83). Once inside the eukaryotic cell, the shigellae reside only temporarily within a cytoplasmic vacuole from which they escape and multiply rapidly in

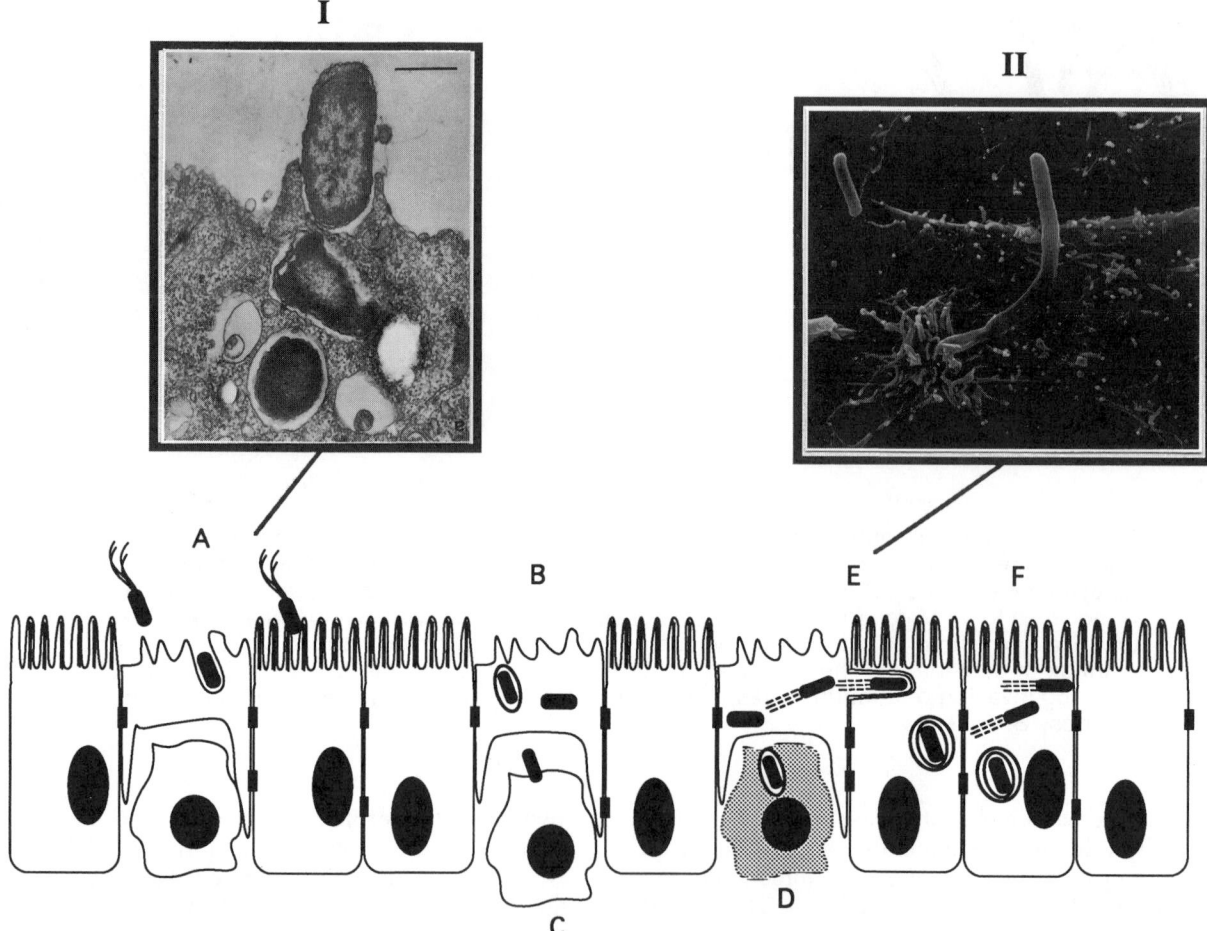

FIG. 4. Interaction of *Shigella* species with the gut epithelium. Diagrammed is the putative interaction of shigellae with M cells overlying PP follicles as well as absorptive epithelial cells. Invasion is diagrammed for an M cell. **A,B:** Adherence to and intimate association of yersiniae with an M cell followed by localization of the invading organism within an intracellular cytoplasmic vacuole. **D,E:** Bacteria, having trancytosed the M cell, may interact with Peyer's patch macrophages and induce macrophage apoptosis. Bacteria free within the target cell cytoplasm also move within the host cell via an actin-associated tail. **F:** Shigella intercellular invasion through a host cell membrane protrusion, followed by residence of the invading organism within a double-membraned intracellular cytoplasmic vacuole and escape from that vacuole. **I:** TEM of *S. flexneri* attachment to and invasion of a cultured mammalian epithelial cell (84). **II:** Scanning EM of *S. flexneri*-induced membrane protrusion in a HeLa cell as it passes out of the cell (107). Bar = 0.5 μm.

the cytoplasm (84). Bacteria free in the cytoplasm move to the periphery of the cell cytoplasm and spread laterally from the initially infected cell to adjacent cells through membrane-bound protrusions (85,86). Subsequently, the bacteria are located in a cytoplasmic vacuole in the newly invaded cell from which they escape and repeat the intercellular invasion process. Repeated rounds of rapid intracellular multiplication and intercellular spread lead to death of the infected cells.

Shigella invasion requires a 30-kb region of the 220-kb virulence plasmid (87). To date, 20 invasion-associated genes have been identified within this region. The *ipa* operon, which maps to this region of the virulence plasmid, consists of four genes that encode for the invasion plasmid antigen proteins IpaB (62 kDa), C (43 kDa), D (37 kDa), and A (78 kDa) (88,89). These proteins were first recognized as the major immunogenic peptides in convalescent sera of patients recovering from *S. flexneri* infections (90). The IpaB, C, and D proteins are expressed on the bacterial surface and direct shigella invasion of cultured mammalian cells (88,91). The role that each Ipa protein plays in mediating invasion and the identity of a specific eukaryotic cell surface receptor to which they may bind have yet to be determined. A second distinct set of genes that map upstream of the *ipa* operon, referred to as the *mxi* (membrane expression of Ipa) or *spa* (surface presentation of Ipa antigens), code for proteins indirectly involved in shigella invasion (35,37,92). The Mxi and Spa proteins are required for proper surface expression of the IpaB, C, and D proteins.

Transcription of the *ipa* operon and the *mxi/spa* genes is tightly temperature regulated and is dependent on a network of two transcriptional activators, VirF and VirB, and the transcriptional repressor, VirR (93). VirR, a histone-like protein, encoded by the chromosomal *virR* gene, is the central regulatory protein in the shigella temperature-dependent regulatory network (93,94). VirR is believed to repress virulence gene expression at 30°C either by downregulation of *virF* and *virB* expression or by directly repressing *ipa* and *mxi/spa* gene transcription (93). At 37°C, the VirR protein is inactive and the VirF and VirB proteins can function to activate *ipa* and *mxi* gene expression. Homologs of *virR* have been identified in *E. coli* (95,96) and *S. typhimurium* (97,98) and the presence of the histone-like protein YmoA in *Yersinia* (32) suggests that a common thermoregulatory pathway may exist in all these organisms. Two other genes, *icsA (virG)* and *icsB,* which map to the 30-kb invasion region of the shigella virulence plasmid, are essential for intracellular movement and intercellular invasion mediated by shigellae during infection of epithelial cells (99–101).

The initial entry step of shigellae into epithelial cells is an energy-requiring endocytic process characterized by the accumulation of polymerized actin and myosin at the site of bacterial entry (102,103). The association of these proteins with the invading bacterium is transient. In contrast with EPEC adherence and salmonella invasion, *S. flexneri* invasion occurs without an increase in cytosolic $[Ca^{2+}]_i$ (104). Although the eukaryotic receptor for shigellae is unknown, invasion appears to occur at cellular focal adhesion plaques (105,106). These structures are defined as regions where converging filaments of intracellular actin and actin-associated cytoskeletal proteins adhere to components of the ECM and suggest a possible role for integrins in the shigella entry process (107). Within 15 min of entry into an epithelial cell, shigellae break out of their membrane-enclosed vacuoles through the activity of the IpaB protein and enter the host cell cytoplasm (84). Short filaments of cytoplasmic actin immediately accumulate around the shigellae and are bundled to form an actin tail behind the organism as it moves through the cytoplasm (100). Several other cytoskeletal proteins are localized to the actin tail, and they include the actin binding protein, plastin, an actin gelation protein, filamin, and vinculin (100). The role that these proteins play in the cytoplasmic movement of these organisms is still unclear. The virulence plasmid encoded IcsA protein is also associated with the actin tail. IcsA binds to and hydrolyzes adenosine triphosphate (ATP) and as a result of this activity is thought to provide the energy required for shigella intracellular movement (108).

Intercellular invasion is characterized by a hollow membrane protrusion containing a single bacterium (85,86). The shigellae within the protrusion continue to associate with the actin tail and the actin-associated cytoplasmic proteins (86). Formation of the protrusion is followed by phagocytosis of this structure and the bacterium it contains by the adjoining cell. This phagocytic mechanism requires the cellular cadherin protein, L-CAM, and the association of α- and β-catenin, vinculin, and α-actinin, all cellular components that comprise the intermediate junctions (107). Thus the shigellae are never exposed to the extracellular environment when invading adjacent cells. The newly invaded cell then contains an organism in a double-bound vacuole and it has been demonstrated that the shigella IcsB protein is required for lysis of the double membrane (101).

Shigella species display yet another variation of enterobacterial invasion. In contrast to *Salmonella* and *Yersinia,* once *Shigella* organisms have invaded an epithelial cell, they pass from one cell to another without ever being exposed to the extracellular environment. Therefore *Shigella* organisms are capable of subverting the host cell signaling and cytoskeletal systems on two levels. First, these organisms trigger their own entry into the host cells. Second, they recruit cytoskeletal proteins within the host cell cytoplasm to facilitate movement within the cell, followed by entry into adjoining cells. Whereas *Salmonella* and *Yersinia* have developed mechanisms for subverting the host immune system by directly interacting with immune cell populations, the shigellae appear to use their intercellular invasion mechanism as a strategy to avoid direct contact with the host immune system.

PERSPECTIVE

Bacterial attachment and invasion of the intestinal epithelium consist of a series of many subcellular events. Proteins expressed by the enteropathogen incite a series of complex responses in the target enterocyte that ultimately result in sufficient bacterial growth to colonize the human intestine or to ensure transmission to a new susceptible host. The pathogenic strategies of the organisms we have described share a number of common mechanisms, but each organism clearly has a unique "pathogenic signature." Yet, with all that we understand about the early events in enterobacterial infections, questions remain. Numerous virulence proteins have been identified in *Yersinia, Shigella,* EPEC, and *Salmonella* species with putative roles in attachment and invasion. Therein lie the limitations in information that is obtainable from *in vitro* mammalian cell culture systems. The next step will be to understand the actual role of these various proteins in infection. Based on animal model experiments, there is increasing evidence that the interaction of enteropathogenic bacteria with the gut epithelium involves a specific interaction with the host antigen sampling system. Enteroinvasive shigellae, yersiniae, and salmonellae exploit the host antigen sampling system to penetrate the intestinal mucosa as opposed to direct invasion of the absorptive epithelial cells. Found in the epithelium overlying Peyer's patches, M cells are specialized epithelioid cells that sample the luminal contents, thereby delivering antigens to the immune cells that populate the lymphoid follicle (109,110). Whether or not enteropathogenic bacteria target M cells for entry into Peyer's patches is an area of intense investigation. All the enteroinvasive species discussed here have been shown adherent to the surface of or within M cells in various animal models (111–115). It has been demonstrated that *S. typhi* preferentially adheres to murine M cells, which suggests a similar event in humans (113). *Salmonella typhimurium,* which is invasive for mammalian cells *in vitro,* causes membrane ruffles in murine M cells, while a noninvasive mutant is rarely found within M cells (114). Evidence for the correlation between epithelial cell invasion mediated by the *Yersinia* invasin protein and the ability of yersiniae to penetrate the intestinal epithelium has also been described (46). Therefore it would appear that the cytoskeletal and cytochemical changes observed for bacterial invasion of mammalian cells *in vitro* may reflect M cell events occurring during infection. Once these pathogens transcytose the M cells, they then employ various strategies to avoid the host cellular immune response. While the *Salmonella* species survive within macrophages, *Yersinia* species inhibit macrophage phagocytosis. Meanwhile, *Shigella* species escape macrophage killing by inducing programmed cell death or apoptosis in the macrophages (116). The RDEC-1 model of EPEC infection in rabbits reveals that these organisms are also localized to the Peyer's patch follicle-associated epithelium early in infection (117). However, although these organisms adhere to the M cell surface, they are rarely found within these same cells. It is therefore possible that the pedestal formation observed may serve as a mechanism to actually prevent the internalization of these organisms by M cells. As such, EPEC could avoid the host immune system altogether.

Interaction with the immune system is therefore another field that is drawing greater attention in the study of enterobacterial pathogens. Moreover, studies have shown that enterocytes themselves may play a key role in mediating the host intestinal immune response. Whereas M cells are thought only to transport antigens into the Peyer's patches, human and murine intestinal epithelial cells express both class II major histocompatibility markers on their surfaces (118–120) and present antigen *in vitro* (121). In addition, bacterial invasion of epithelial cells *in vitro* induces proinflammatory cytokine secretion by the infected cells (122,123). Thus interaction of bacteria with the intestinal epithelium may involve another dimension of the host–parasite interaction. As the current mysteries concerning each unique host–parasite relationship become clarified, we can expect to learn new ways to think about the prevention and treatment of bacterial enteric infection.

ACKNOWLEDGMENTS

We thank S. Fisher for editing and critical review of the manuscript and N. Ghori for electron microscopy images of *S. typhimurium* invasion of M cells. Research in the laboratory of S.F. was funded by the National Institutes of Health (Grants AI26195, DK38707, and DK07056-19 for A.E.H.).

REFERENCES

1. Portnoy DA, Falkow S. Virulence associated plasmids from *Yersinia enterocolitica* and *Yersinia pestis. J Bacteriol* 1981; 148:877–883.
2. Sansonetti PJ, Kopeko DJ, Formal SB. Involvement of a plasmid in the invasive ability of *Shigella flexneri. Infect Immun* 1982;35:852–860.
3. DiRita JV, Mekalanos JJ. Genetic regulation of bacterial virulence. *Annu Rev Genet* 1989;23:455–482.
4. Miller JF, Mekalanos JJ, Falkow SF. Coordinate regulation and sensory transduction in the control of bacterial virulence. *Science* 1989;243:916–922.
5. Schwartz MA. Transmembrane signaling by integrins. *Trends Cell Biol* 1992;2:304–307.
6. Hynes RO. Integrins: versatility, modulation and signaling in cell adhesion. *Cell* 1992;69:11–25.
7. Pollard TD, Cooper JA. Actin and actin-binding proteins. A critical evaluation of mechanisms and functions. *Annu Rev Biochem* 1986;55:987–1035.
8. Guan K-L, Dixon JE. Bacterial and viral protein tyrosine phosphatases. *Semin Cell Biol* 1993;4:389–396.
9. Carter PB. Pathogenicity of *Yersinia enterocolitica* for mice. *Infect Immun* 1975;11:164–170.
10. Hanski C, Kutschka U, Schmoranzer HP, et al. Immunohistochemical and electron microscopic study of interaction of *Yersinia enterocolitica* serotype O8 with intestinal mucosa during experimental enteritis. *Infect Immun* 1989;57:673–678.
11. Isberg RR, Voorhis DL, Falkow S. Identification of invasin: a protein that allows enteric bacteria to penetrate cultured mammalian cells. *Cell* 1987;50:769–778.
12. Isberg RR, Leong JM. Multiple b1 chain integrins are receptors for invasin, a protein that promotes bacterial penetration into mammalian cells. *Cell* 1990;60:861–871.
13. Young VB, Falkow S, Schoolnik GK. The invasin protein of *Yersinia enterocolitica:* internalization of invasin-bearing bacteria by eukaryotic cells is associated with reorganization of the cytoskeleton. *J Exp Med* 1992;116:197–207.
14. Rosenshine I, Duronio V, Finlay BB. Tyrosine protein kinase inhibitors block invasin-promoted bacterial uptake by epithelial cells. *Infect Immun* 1992;60:2211–2217.
15. Miller VL, Falkow S. Evidence for two genetic loci in *Yersinia*

enterocolitica that can promote invasion of epithelial cells. *Infect Immun* 1988;56:56:1242–1248.

16. Skurnik M, Wolf-Watz H. Analysis of the *yopA* gene encoding the Yop1 virulence determinant *Yersinia* spp. *Mol Microbiol* 1989;3:517–529.

17. Bliska JB, Copass MC, Falkow S. The *Yersinia pseudotuberculosis* adhesin YadA mediates intimate bacterial attachment to and entry into HEp-2 cells. *Infect Immun* 1993;61:3914–3921.

18. Yang Y, Isberg RR. Cellular internalization in the absence of invasin expression is promoted by the *Yersinia pseudotuberculosis yadA* product. *Infect Immun* 1993;61:3907–3913.

19. Tertti R, Skurnik M, Vartio T, Kuusela P. Adhesion protein YadA of *Yersinia* species mediates binding of bacteria to fibronectin. *Infect Immun* 1992;60:3021–3024.

20. Schulze-Koops H, Burkhardt H, Heesemann J, von der Mark K, Emmrich F. Plasmid-encoded outer membrane protein YadA mediates specific binding of enteropathogenic yersiniae to various types of collagen. *Infect Immun* 1992;60:2153–2159.

21. Schulze-Koops H, Burkhardt H, Heesemann J, et al. Outer membrane protein YadA of enteropathogenic yersiniae mediates specific binding to cellular but not plasma fibronectin. *Infect Immun* 1993;61:2513–2519.

22. China B, Sory M-P, N'guyen BT, De Bruyere M, Cornelis GR. Role of the YadA protein in prevention of opsonization of *Yersinia enterocolitica* by C3b molecules. *Infect Immun* 1993;61:3907–3913.

23. Bliska JB, Falkow S. Bacterial resistance to complement killing mediated by the Ail protein of *Yersinia enterocolitica*. *Proc Natl Acad Sci USA* 1992;89:3561–3565.

24. Pierson DE, Falkow S. The *ail* gene of *Yersinia enterocolitica* has a role in the ability of the organism to survive serum killing. *Infect Immun* 1993;61:1846–1852.

25. Isberg RR, Swain A, Falkow S. Analysis of expression and thermoregulation of the *Yersinia pseudotuberculosis inv* gene with hybrid proteins. *Infect Immun* 1988;56:2133–2138.

26. Martinez RJ. Thermoregulation-dependent expression of *Yersinia enterocolitica* protein 1 imparts serum resistance to *Escherichia coli* K-12. *Infect Immun* 1989;61:3732–3739.

27. Pierson DE, Falkow S. Nonpathogenic isolates of *Yersinia enterocolitica* do not contain functional *inv*-homologous sequences. *Infect Immun* 1990;58:1059–1064.

28. Miller VL, Farmer J, Hill WE, Falkow S. The *ail* locus is found uniquely in *Yersinia enterocolitica* serotypes commonly associated with disease. *Infect Immun* 1989;57:121–131.

29. Pollack C, Straley SC, Klempner MS. Probing the phagolysosomal environment of human macrophages with a Ca²⁺-responsive operon fusion in *Yersinia pestis*. *Nature* 1986;322:834–837.

30. Skurnik M, Toivanen P. LcrF is the temperature-regulated activator of the *yadA* gene of *Yersinia enterocolitica* and *Yersinia pseudotuberculosis*. *J Bacteriol* 1992;174:2047–2051.

31. Lambert de Rouvroit C, Sluiters C, Cornelis GR. Role of the transcriptional activator, VirF, and temperature in the expression of the pYV plasmid genes of *Yersinia enterocolitica*. *Mol Microbiol* 1992;6:395–409.

32. Cornelis GR, Sluiters C, Delor I, et al. *ymoA*, a *Yersinia enterocolitica* chromosomal gene modulating the expression of virulence functions. *Mol Microbiol* 1991;5:1023–1034.

33. Straley SC, Plano GV, Skrzypek E, Haddix PL, Fields KA. Regulation by Ca²⁺ in the Yersinia low-Ca²⁺ response. *Mol Microbiol* 1993;8:1005–1010.

34. Forsberg A, Rosqvist R, Wolf-Watz H. Regulation and polarized transfer of the *Yersinia* outer proteins (Yops) involved in antiphagocytosis. *Trends Mirobiol* 1994;2:14–19.

35. Andrews GP, Hromockyj AE, Coker C, Maurelli AT. Two novel virulence loci, *mxiA* and *mxiB*, in *Shigella flexneri* 2a, facilitate excretion of invasion plasmid antigens. *Infect Immun* 1991;59:1997–2005.

36. Andrews GP, Maurelli AT. *mxiA* of *Shigella flexneri* 2a, which facilitates export of invasion plasmid antigens, encodes a homolog of the low-calcium-response protein, LcrD, of *Yersinia pestis*. *Infect Immun* 1992;60:3287–3295.

37. Venkatesan MM, Buysse JM, Oaks EV. Surface presentation of *Shigella flexneri* invasion plasmid antigens requires the products of the *spa* locus. *J Bacteriol* 1992;174:1990–2001.

38. Groisman EA, Ochman H. Cognate gene clusters govern invasion of host epithelial cells by *Salmonella typhimurium* and *Shigella flexneri*. *EMBO J* 1993;12(10):3779–3787.

39. Leung KY, Straley SC. The *yopM* gene of *Yersinia pestis* encodes a released protein having homology with the human platelet surface protein GPIba. *J Bacteriol* 1989;171:4623–4632.

40. Reisner BS, Straley SC. *Yersinia pestis* YopM: thrombin binding and overexpression. *Infect Immun* 1992;60:5242–5252.

41. Gaylov EE, Hakansson S, Forsberg A, Wolf-Watz H. A secreted protein kinase of *Yersinia pseudotuberculosis* is an indispensable virulence determinant. *Nature* 1993;361:730–732.

42. Guan K, Dixon JE. Protein tyrosine phosphatase activity of an essential virulence determinant in *Yersinia*. *Science* 1990;249:553–556.

43. Rosqvist R, Forsberg A, Rimpilainen M, Bergman T, Wolf WH. The cytotoxic protein YopE of *Yersinia* obstructs the primary host defence. *Mol Microbiol* 1990;4:657–667.

44. Bliska JB, Guan K, Dixon JE, Falkow S. Tyrosine phosphate hydrolysis of host proteins by an essential *Yersinia* virulence determinant. *Proc Natl Acad Sci USA* 1991;88:1187–1191.

45. Bliska JB, Clemens JC, Dixon JE, Falkow S. The *Yersinia* tyrosine phosphatase: specificity of a bacterial virulence determinant for phosphoproteins in the J774A.1 macrophage. *J Exp Med* 1992;176:1625–1630.

46. Pepe JC, Miller VL. *Yersinia enterocolitica* invasin: a primary role in the initiation of infection. *Proc Natl Acad Sci USA* 1993;90:6473–6477.

47. Moon HW, Whipp SC, Argenzio RA, Levine MM, Gianella RA. Attaching and effacing activities of rabbit and human enteropathogenic *Escherichia coli* in pig and rabbit intestines. *Infect Immun* 1983;41:1340–1351.

48. Donnenberg MS, Kaper JB. Enteropathogenic *Escherichia coli*. *Infect Immun* 1992;60:3953–3961.

49. Schauer DB, Falkow S. The *eae* gene of *Citrobacter freundii* biotype 4280 is necessary for colonization in transmissible murine colonic hyperplasia. *Infect Immun* 1993;61:4654–4661.

50. Jerse AE, Kaper JB. The *eae* gene of enteropathogenic *Escherichia coli* encodes a 94-kilodalton membrane protein, the expression of which is influenced by the EAF plasmid. *Infect Immun* 1991;59:4302–4309.

51. Giron JA, Ho ASY, Schoolnik GK. An inducible bundle forming pilus of enteropathogenic *Escherichia coli*. *Science* 1991;254:710–713.

52. Rosenshine I, Donnenberg MS, Kaper JB, Finlay BB. Signal transduction between enteropathogenic *Escherichia coli* (EPEC) and epithelial cells: EPEC induces tyrosine phosphorylation of host cell proteins to initiate cytoskeletal rearrangement and bacterial uptake. *EMBO J* 1992;11:3551–3560.

53. Drucker MM, Polliack A, Yeivin R, Sacks TG. Immunofluorescent demonstration of enteropathogenic *Escherichia coli* in tissues of infants dying with enteritis. *Pediatrics* 1970;46:855–864.

54. Knutton S, Baldwin T, Williams PH, McNeish AS. Actin accumulation at sites of bacterial adhesion to tissue culture cells: basis of a new diagnostic test for enteropathogenic and enterohemorrhagic *Escherichia coli*. *Infect Immun* 1989;57:1290–1298.

55. Finlay BB, Rosenshine I, Donnenberg MS, Kaper JB. Cytoskeletal composition of attaching and effacing lesions associated with enteropathogenic *Escherichia coli* adherence to HeLa cells. *Infect Immun* 1992;60:2541–2543.

56. Baldwin TJ, Ward W, Aitken A, Knutton S, Williams PH. Elevation of intracellular free calcium levels in HEp-2 cells with enteropathogenic *Escherichia coli*. *Infect Immun* 1991;59:1599–1604.

57. Manjarrez-Hernandez HA, Amess B, Sellers L, et al. Purification of a 20 kDa phosphoprotein from epithelial cells and identification as a myosin light chain. Phosphorylation induced by enteropathogenic *Escherichia coli* and phorbol ester. *FEBS Lett* 1991;292:121–127.

58. Baldwin TJ, Brooks SF, Knutton S, Manjarrez-Hernandez HA, Aitken A, Williams PH. Protein phosphorylation by protein kinase C in HEp-2 cells infected with enteropathogenic *Esche-*

richia coli. Infect Immun 1990;58:761–765 [Erratum. *Infect Immun* 1990;58:2024.]

59. Finlay BB, Starnbach MN, Francis CL, et al. Identification and characterization of Tn*phoA* mutants of *Salmonella* that are unable to pass through a polarized MDCK epithelial cell monolayer. *Mol Microbiol* 1988;2:757–766.

60. Jones BD, Lee CA, Falkow S. Invasion by *Salmonella typhimurium* is affected by the direction of flagellar rotation. *Infect Immun* 1992;60:2475–2480.

61. Galan JE, Curtiss R III. Cloning and molecular characterization of genes whose products allow *Salmonella typhimurium* to penetrate tissue culture cells. *Proc Natl Acad Sci USA* 1989;86: 6383–6387.

62. Ginocchio C, Pace J, Galan JE. Identification and molecular characterization of a *Salmonella typhimurium* gene involved in triggering the internalization of salmonellae into cultured epithelial cells. *Proc Natl Acad Sci USA* 1992;89:5976–5980.

63. Behlau I, Miller S. A phoP-repressed gene promotes *Salmonella typhimurium* invasion of epithelial cells. *J Bacteriol* 1993; 175:4475–4484.

64. Lee CA, Jones BD, Falkow S. Identification of a *Salmonella typhimurium* invasion locus by selection of hyperinvasive mutants. *Proc Natl Acad Sci USA* 1992;89:1847–1851.

65. Elsinghorst EA, Baron LS, Kopeko DJ. Penetration of human intestinal epithelial cells by *Salmonella*: molecular cloning and expression of *Salmonella typhi* invasion determinants in *Escherichia coli. Proc Natl Acad Sci USA* 1989;86:5173–5177.

66. Lee CA, Falkow S. The ability of *Salmonella* to enter mammalian cells is affected by bacterial growth state. *Proc Natl Acad Sci USA* 1990;87:4304–4308.

67. Tartera C, Metcalf ES. Osmolarity and growth phase overlap in regulation of *Salmonella typhi* adherence to and invasion of human intestinal cells. *Infect Immun* 1993;61:3084–3089.

68. Takeuchi A. Electron microscope studies of experimental *Salmonella* infection. I. Penetration into the intestinal epithelium by *Salmonella typhimurium. Am J Pathol* 1967;50:109–136.

69. Finlay BB, Ruschkowski S, Dedhar S. Cytoskeletal rearrangements accompanying *Salmonella* entry into epithelial cells. *J Cell Sci* 1991;99:283–296.

70. Francis CL, Starnbach MN, Falkow S. Morphological and cytoskeletal changes in epithelial cells occur immediately upon interaction with *Salmonella typhimurium* grown under low-oxygen conditions. *Mol Microbiol* 1992;6:3077–3087.

71. Finlay BB, Gumbiner B, Falkow S. Penetration of *Salmonella* through a polarized Madin–Darby canine kidney epithelial cell monolayer. *J Cell Biol* 1988;107:221–230.

72. Kadowaki T, Kayasu S, Nishida E, et al. Insulin-like growth factors, insulin, and epidermal growth factor cause rapid cytoskeletal reorganization in KB cells. *J Biol Chem* 1986;261: 16141–16147.

73. Miyata Y, Nishida E, Sakai H. Regulation of the intracellular Ca^{2+} and cyclic AMP of the growth factor-induced ruffling membrane formation and stimulation of fluid-phase endocytosis. *Exp Cell Res* 1989;175:286–297.

74. Bar-Sagi D, Feramisco JR. Induction of membrane ruffling and fluid phase pinocytosis in quiescent fibroblasts by *ras* proteins. *Science* 1986;233:1061–1068.

75. Ridley AJ, Paterson HF, Johnston CL, Diekmann D, Hall A. The small GTP-binding protein rac regulates growth factor-induced membrane ruffling. *Cell* 1992;70:401–410.

76. Francis CL, Ryan TA, Jones BD, Smith SJ, Falkow S. Ruffles induced by *Salmonella* and other stimuli direct macropinocytosis of bacteria. *Nature* 1993;364:639–642.

77. Ruschkowski S, Rosenshine I, Finlay BB. *Salmonella typhimurium* induces an inositol phosphate flux in infected epithelial cells. *FEMS Microbiol Lett* 1992;95:121–126.

78. Pace J, Hayman MJ, Galan JE. Signal transduction and invasion of epithelial cells by *S. typhimurium. Cell* 1993;72: 505–514.

79. Galen JE, Pace J, Hayman MJ. Involvement of the epidermal growth factor receptor in the invasion of cultured mammalian cells by *Salmonella typhimurium. Nature* 1992;357:588–589.

80. Jones BD, Paterson HF, Hall A, Falkow S. *Salmonella typhimurium* induces membrane ruffling by a growth factor-recep-

tor-independent mechanism. *Proc Natl Acad Sci USA* 1993; 90:10390–10394.

81. Ridley AJ, Hall A. The small GTP-binding protein rho regulates the assembly of focal adhesions and actin stress fibers in response growth factors. *Cell* 1992;70:389–399.

82. LaBrec EH, Schneider H, Magnani TJ, Formal SB. Epithelial cell penetration as an essential step in the pathogenesis of bacillary dysentery. *J Bacteriol* 1964;88:1503–1518.

83. Takeuchi A, Formal SB, Sprinz H. Experimental acute colitis in the rhesus monkey following peroral infection with *Shigella flexneri*. An electron microscope study. *Am J Pathol* 1968;52: 503–509.

84. Sansonetti PJ, Ryter A, Clerc P, Maurelli AT, Mounier J. Multiplication of *Shigella flexneri* within HeLa cells: lysis of the phagocytic vacuole and plasmid-mediated contact hemolysis. *Infect Immun* 1986;1:461–469.

85. Kadurugamuwa JL, Rohde M, Wehland J, Timmis KN. Intercellular spread of *Shigella flexneri* through a monolayer mediated by membranous protrusions and associated with reorganization of the cytoskeletal protein vinculin. *Infect Immun* 1991;59:3463–3471.

86. Prevost MC, Lesourd M, Arpin M, et al. Unipolar reorganization of F-actin layer at bacterial cell division and bundling of actin filaments by plastin correlate with movement of *Shigella flexneri* within HeLa cells. *Infect Immun* 1992;34:75–83.

87. Maurelli AT, Baudry B, d'Hauteville H, Hale TL, Sansonetti PJ. Cloning of plasmid DNA sequence involved in invasion of HeLa cells by *Shigella flexneri. Infect Immun* 1985;49:164–171.

88. Baudry B, Maurelli AT, Clerc P, Sadoff JC, Sansonetti PJ. Localization of plasmid loci necessary for the entry of *Shigella flexneri* into HeLa cells and characterization of one locus encoding four immunogenic polypeptides. *J Gen Microbiol* 1987; 133:3403–3413.

89. Venkatesan MM, Buysse JM, Kopeko DJ. Characterization of invasion plasmid antigen genes *(ipaBCD)* from *Shigella flexneri. Proc Natl Acad Sci USA* 1988;85:9317–9321.

90. Hale TL, Oaks EV, Formal SB. Identification and antigenic characterization of virulence-associated, plasmid-coded proteins of *Shigella* spp. and enteroinvasive *Escherichia coli. Infect Immun* 1985;50:620–629.

91. High NJ, Mournier M, Prevost C, Sansonetti PJ. IpaB of *Shigella flexneri* causes entry into epithelial cells and escape from the phagocytic vacuole. *EMBO J* 1992;11:1991–1999.

92. Hromockyj AE, Maurelli AT. Identification of *Shigella* invasion genes by isolation of temperature-regulated *inv::lacZ* operon fusions. *Infect Immun* 1989;57:2963–2970.

93. Maurelli AT, Hromockyj AE, Bernardini ML. Environmental regulation of *Shigella* virulence. In: Sansonetti PJ, ed. *Current topics in microbiology and immunology*. Berlin: Springer-Verlag, 1992;95–115.

94. Hromockyj AE, Tucker SC, Maurelli AT. Temperature regulation of *Shigella* virulence: identification of the repressor gene *virR*, an analogue of *hns*, and partial complementation by tyrosyl transfer RNA (tRNA1^{Tyr}). *Mol Microbiol* 1992;6: 2113–2124.

95. Hromockyj AE, Maurelli AT. Identification of an *Escherichia coli* gene homologous to *virR*, a regulator of *Shigella* virulence. *J Bacteriol* 1989;171:2879–2881.

96. Goransson M, Sonden B, Nilsson P, et al. Transcriptional silencing and thermoregulation of gene expression in *Escherichia coli. Nature* 1990;344:682–685.

97. Hulton CSJ, Seirafi A, Hinton JCD, et al. Histone-like protein H1 (H-NS), DNA supercoiling, and gene expression in bacteria. *Cell* 1990;63:631–642.

98. Marsh M, Hillyard DR. Nucleotide sequence of *hns* encoding the DNA-binding protein H-NS of *Salmonella typhimurium. Nucleic Acids Res* 1990;18:3397.

99. Makino S, Sasakawa C, Kamata K, Kurata T, Yoshikawa M. A genetic determinant required for continuous reinfection of adjacent cells on large plasmid in *S. flexneri* 2a. *Cell* 1986;46: 551–555.

100. Bernardini ML, Mounier J, d'Hauteville H, CoquisRondon M, Sansonetti PJ. Identification of *icsA*, a plasmid locus of *Shigella flexneri* that governs bacterial intra- and intercellular spread

through interaction with F-actin. *Proc Natl Acad Sci USA* 1989;86:3867–3871.

101. Allaoui A, Mounier J, Prevost C, Sansonetti PJ, Parsot C. *icsB:* a *Shigella flexneri* virulence gene necessary for the lysis of protrusions during intercellular spread. *Mol Microbiol* 1992;6: 1605–1616.

102. Clerc P, Sansonetti PJ. Entry of *Shigella flexneri* into HeLa cells: evidence for directed phagocytosis involving actin polymerization and myosin accumulation. *Infect Immun* 1987;55: 2681–2688.

103. Hale TL, Bonventre PF. *Shigella* infection of Henle intestinal epithelial cells: role of the bacterium. *Infect Immun* 1979;24: 879–886.

104. Clerc PL, Berthon B, Claret M, Sansonetti PJ. Internalization of *Shigella flexneri* into HeLa cells occurs without an increase in cytosolic Ca2+ concentration. *Infect Immun* 1989; 2919–2922.

105. Mounier J, Vasselon T, Hellio R, Lesourd M, Sansonetti PJ. *Shigella flexneri* enters human colonic Caco-2 epithelial cells through the basolateral pole. *Infect Immun* 1992;60:237–248.

106. Vasselon T, Mounier J, Hellio R, Sansonetti PJ. Movement along actin filaments of perijunctional area and do novo polymerization of cellular actin are required for *Shigella flexneri* colonization of epithelial Caco-2 cell monolayers. *Infect Immun* 1992;60:1031–1040.

107. Goldberg MB, Sansonetti PJ. *Shigella* subversion of the cellular cytoskeleton: a strategy for epithelial colonization. *Infect Immun* 1993;12:4941–4946.

108. Goldberg MB, Parsot C, Barzu O, Sansonetti PJ. Unipolar localization and ATPase activity of IcsA, a *Shigella flexneri* protein involved in intracellular movement. *J Bacteriol* 1993;175: 2189–2196.

109. Owen TL, Jones AL. Epithelial cells specialization within human Peyer's patches: an ultrastructural study of intestinal lymphoid follicles. *Gastroenterology* 1974;66:189–203.

110. Owen RL, Ermak TH. Structural specializations for antigen uptake and processing in the digestive tract. *Can J Microbiol* 1988;34:1142–7.

111. Fujimora Y, Kihara T, Mine H. Membranous cells as a portal of *Yersinia pseudotuberculosis* entry into rabbit ileum. *J Clin Electron Microscopy* 1992;25:35–45.

112. Grutzkau A, Hanski C, Hahn H, Riecken EO. Involvement of M cells in the bacterial invasion of Peyer's patches: a common mechanism shared by *Yersinia enterocolitica* and other enteroinvasive bacteria. *Gut* 1990;31:1011–1015.

113. Kohbata S, Yokoyama H, Yabuuchi E. Cytopathogenic effect of *Salmonella typhi* GIFU 10007 on M cells of murine ileal Peyer's Patches in ligated ileal loops: an ultrastructural study. *Microbiol Immunol* 1986;30:1225–1237.

114. Jones BD, Ghori N, Falkow S. Salmonella typhimurium initiates murine infection by penetrating and destroying the specialized epithelial M cells of the Peyer's patches. *J Exp Med* 1994; 180:15–23.

115. Wassef JS, Keren DF, Mailloux JL. Role of M cells in initial bacterial uptake and in ulcer formation in the rabbit intestinal loop model in shigellosis. *Infect Immun* 1989;57:858–863.

116. Zychlinsky A, Prevost MC, Sansonetti PJ. *Shigella flexneri* induces apoptosis in infected macrophages. *Nature* 1992;358: 167–169.

117. Inman LR, Cantey JR, Formal SB. Colonization, virulence, and mucosal interaction of an enteropathogenic *Escherichia coli* (strain RDEC-1) expressing *Shigella* somatic antigen in the rabbit intestine. *J Infect Dis* 1986;154:742–751.

118. Matsumoto S, Setoyama H, Umesaki Y. Differential induction of major histocompatibility complex molecules on mouse intestine by bacterial colonization. *Gastroenterology* 1992;103: 1777–1782.

119. Bland PW, Kambarage DM. Antigen handling by the epithelium and lamina propria macrophages. *Gastroenterology Clinics of North America* 1991;20:577–96.

120. Brandtzaeg P, Bjerke K. Immunomorphological characteristics of human Peyer's patches. *Digestion* 1990;2:262–273.

121. Mayer L, Shlien R. Evidence for function of Ia molecules on gut epithelial cells in man. *J Exp Med* 1987;166:1471–1483.

122. Arnold R, Scheffer J, Konig B, Konig W. Effects of *Listeria monocytogenes* and *Yersinia enterocolitica* on cytokine gene expression and release from human polymorphonuclear granulocytes and epithelial (HEp-2) cells. *Infect Immun* 1993;61: 2545–2552.

123. Agace W, Hedges S, Andersson U, Andersson J, Ceska M, Svanborg C. Selective cytokine production by epithelial cells following exposure to *Escherichia coli*. *Infect Immun* 1993;61: 602–609.

124. Bliska JB, Galan JE, Falkow S. Signal transduction in the mammalian cell during bacterial attachment and entry. *Cell* 1993; 73:903–920.

Infections of the Gastrointestinal Tract,
edited by M. J. Blaser, P. D. Smith, J. I. Ravdin,
H. B. Greenberg, and R. L. Guerrant
Raven Press, Ltd., New York © 1995.

CHAPTER 44

Enteric Bacterial Toxins

Cynthia L. Sears, Richard L. Guerrant, and James B. Kaper

Bacteria that colonize the intestine and produce one or more toxins are important etiological agents of diarrheal disease in both industrialized and developing countries. The focus of this chapter will be to provide an overview of the toxins produced by enteric pathogens and to delineate their linkage to human disease. To accomplish these goals, the range of criteria utilized to demonstrate pathogenicity of an enteric bacterial toxin will be reviewed followed by a discussion of the criteria used to classify a given bacterial enteric toxin. Using these definitions, Table 1 classifies the enteric bacterial toxins into their identified general mode of action(s) as well as by genus and species. In classifying the toxins, emphasis has been given to data derived from studies of toxins in potentially relevant models of disease, namely, intestinal mucosa *in vivo* and/or intestinal epithelial cells *in vitro* (Table 2). More detailed information on each of these toxins is available in other chapters in this volume. Lastly, the potential mechanisms by which enteric bacterial toxins contribute to intestinal secretion will be discussed (Table 4). The most striking observation from these latter data are that despite the elegance of the mechanistic data available for a few enteric bacterial toxins, the knowledge of the secretory mechanisms of most toxins are only crudely understood.

CRITERIA FOR ESTABLISHING THE PATHOGENICITY OF AN ENTERIC BACTERIAL TOXIN

The most convincing criterion to determine if an enteric toxin contributes to the pathogenicity of an organism is to demonstrate that the purified toxin causes diarrhea when ingested by human volunteers. This stringent criterion is met for only one enteric bacterial toxin, i.e., cholera. Ingestion of as little as 5 μg of cholera toxin resulted in diarrhea in four of five subjects with a mean stool volume of 2.5 L and ingestion of 25 μg resulted in diarrhea in two of two subjects with a mean stool output of 21.9 L (1). These data unequivocally establish the potent secretory activity of cholera toxin in the human intestine but do not identify the mechanism(s) resulting in the secretory response.

An alternative strategy for establishing the significance of a toxin in volunteer trials is to feed subjects isogenic bacterial strains specifically engineered so that the only difference between the strains is expression of an active toxin. Studies with strains of *Vibrio cholerae* specifically mutated in genes encoding cholera toxin (*ctx*) demonstrated that volunteers ingesting the wild-type strain expressing cholera toxin experienced the severe diarrhea characteristic of cholera while individuals ingesting the same strain mutated in the *ctx* genes did not experience clinical cholera (2). However, ~50% of the volunteers in the latter group did experience mild to moderate diarrhea of low volumes indicating that although cholera toxin is responsible for the severe diarrhea that is cholera, there are additional secretogenic factors produced by *V. cholerae* that can cause mild diarrhea.

Short of volunteer trials, there are other criteria for associating an enteric toxin with human disease. Supporting evidence for such an association could include (a) detection of a toxin directly in a clinical specimen; (b) measurement of an intestinal or serum antibody response to the toxin; or (c) epidemiological association of bacteria producing the toxin with clinical disease. Fulfillment of the first two criteria indicates *in vivo* production of the toxin. However, because enteric bacteria most often produce numerous virulence proteins in addition to an enteric toxin such as attachment and/or invasion factors, the detection of toxin in a clinical specimen, the demonstration of an antitoxin response, or an epidemiological association is only supportive and not definitive in determining

C. L. Sears: Department of Medicine, Divisions of Infectious Diseases and Gastroenterology, Johns Hopkins University School of Medicine, Baltimore, Maryland 21205.

R. L. Guerrant: Department of Medicine, University of Virginia School of Medicine, Charlottesville, Virginia 22908.

J. B. Kaper: Departments of Medicine, Microbiology and Immunology, and Bacterial Genetics Section of the Center for Vaccine Development, University of Maryland School of Medicine, Baltimore, Maryland 21201.

that the toxin contributes to the intestinal secretion observed in the infection.

Examples of toxins that have been detected directly in stools from infected patients include *C. difficile* toxin A [reviewed in (3)], Shiga toxin (4), cholera toxin [reviewed in (5)], and heat-labile toxin (LT) and heat-stable toxin (ST) from enterotoxigenic *E. coli* (6). However, failure to detect toxins in stools may be due to the insensitivity of the detection assay, the toxin-binding effects of free gangliosides present in mucin found in stools, proteolytic degradation of the toxin in the intestinal tract, or other reasons.

The production of an immune response against a toxin can also be taken as evidence of *in vivo* toxin production but failure to detect an immune response does not rule out *in vivo* toxin production. While serum and intestinal antibody responses against cholera toxin and LT are seen, an antibody response against ST has not been demonstrated [reviewed in (1)]. The lack of an immune response to ST is probably due to the fact that ST is nonimmunogenic, due to its small size, unless it is experimentally conjugated to a larger carrier protein. The poor immune response against Shiga toxin in patients infected with *S. dysenteriae* 1 occurs for quite different reasons. In the early 1970s, Keusch et al. (7) reported that volunteers ingesting this pathogen developed no serum IgG responses against Shiga toxin but did develop low levels of IgM antibodies. It is now recognized that the globotriosylceramide (Gb3) receptor for Shiga toxin is a B-cell differentiation antigen known as CD77. Shiga toxin selectively kills IgG- and IgA-committed lymphocytes whereas most IgM-producing cells are resistant to Shiga toxin (8).

Many examples of an epidemiological association of toxin production with human disease can be cited but such studies have been particularly useful for establishing the significance of LT I and STa-producing ETEC and enterotoxigenic *Bacteroides fragilis* (ETBF). *E. coli* and *B. fragilis* are both members of normal intestinal flora but the strains isolated from healthy individuals usually do not produce enterotoxins. Epidemiological studies have demonstrated that *E. coli* producing LT I or STa (9,10) or ETBF (11–13) are found significantly more often in individuals with diarrheal disease than in healthy individuals.

Additional approaches to studying the pathogenicity of enteric bacterial toxins utilize one or more nonhuman experimental approaches including animal models, Ussing chambers, and *in vitro* assays. Most data on the pathogenicity of bacterial enteric toxins are based on these approaches and then, by analogy, the toxin is proposed as important in human diarrheal disease. Although only gross intestinal secretion is typically measured, a classic approach to determining whether an enteric toxin stimulates secretion is ligated intestinal segments or loops as originally described by De using sterile culture filtrates of *V. cholerae* inoculated into rabbit ileal loops (14). For this experimental approach, small intestinal (jejunal or ileal) ligated intestinal segments are inoculated with toxin preparations or bacterial cultures and the subsequent presence or absence of secretion is assessed at time points up to 18 hr. For the reservations discussed above, inoculation of whole bacterial cultures is less definitive in estab-

lishing the importance of the toxin to disease pathogenesis unless the experiments are conducted using isogenic mutant strains of bacteria. Isogenic strains of enteric bacteria differing only in the presence or absence of a toxin gene are a potent tool for establishing the pathogenicity of a toxin in the animal model. For example, isogenic strains of *Yersinia enterocolitica* have been utilized to establish that the heat-stable enterotoxin produced by most pathogenic strains contributes to the severity of disease in a rabbit animal model (15). Similarly, isogenic strains of *Vibrio parahaemolyticus* differing only in production of the thermostable direct hemolysin (TDH) were tested in ligated rabbit ileal loops to demonstrate the contribution of TDH in causing the secretion (16). An alternative approach to establishing the relevance to secretion of an enteric bacterial toxin is oral inoculation of an animal with the toxin and demonstration of either diarrhea or intestinal fluid accumulation. Examples of animal models where this approach has proved valuable are suckling mice in which oral inoculation of the *E. coli* heat-stable enterotoxin (STa) stimulates intestinal secretion (17) and the sealed adult mouse model (SAM) that has been used, for example, to study host genetics modulating the secretory response to cholera toxin (18).

A valuable *in vitro* experimental approach used to identify secretory responses to enteric bacterial toxins is the Ussing chamber. For this technique, either native intestinal epithelium or monolayers of cultured intestinal epithelial cells are mounted between Lucite chambers under conditions of ionic, osmotic, and electrical ("voltage-clamped") equilibrium. The ability of an enteric toxin to stimulate anion (usually chloride) secretion and/or to inhibit NaCl absorption, both potentially contributing to net intestinal secretion, can be measured under these conditions. Three measurements related by Ohm's law ($V = IR$) are made in Ussing chambers: (a) short circuit current (I_{sc} or I); (b) potential difference (PD or V); and (c) resistance (R). Increases in I_{sc} and PD in monolayers of intestinal epithelial cells indicate the secretion of chloride. In native intestinal tissue, increases in I_{sc} and PD in combination with secretion in a ligated intestinal segment also is consistent with net intestinal anionic secretion. This technique has been used extensively to identify the secretory potential of numerous enteric bacterial toxins including cholera toxin (19), the *E. coli* heat-stable enterotoxins (STa, STb) (20–22), the enteroaggregative *E. coli* heat-stable enterotoxin (EAST-1) (23,24), Shiga toxin (25), and the recently identified enterotoxins of enteroinvasive *E. coli* (26,27) and *Shigella flexneri* (28) to name a few.

A third experimental approach to identify activities of enteric bacterial toxins is the use of a wide variety of nonintestinal cell lines. Most often the activity of a particular toxin is identified due to a change in the shape of the cells or due to cytotoxicity in response to treatment with the enteric toxin. For example, Chinese hamster ovary (CHO) and Y-1 adrenal cells have proven useful for identifying toxins that increase intracellular cyclic AMP such as cholera toxin [reviewed in (29,30)], the *Salmonella* toxin (31,32), and the heat-labile enterotoxins of *E. coli* [reviewed in (33)]. In response to an increase in intracellular cyclic AMP, CHO cells stretch (34) and Y-1 adrenal cells become round (35). Another example is the use of HeLa or Vero cells for identification of the cytotoxicity due to inhibition of protein synthesis by Shiga and Shiga-like toxins (36). Although the use of these cell lines has been very valuable in identifying one or more activities of enteric toxins, these experimental data do not aid in determining the secretory activity of enteric toxins, and thus must be interpreted with caution in discussions of the importance of the results to pathogenicity.

CLASSIFICATION OF ENTERIC BACTERIAL TOXINS

Classification of enteric bacterial toxins is most often based on an identified general mode of action. However, a strict classification of enteric bacterial toxins is often problematic. In some instances, this is due to the fact that the available data are incomplete; in other cases, it is due to the complexity of the mode of action. For the purposes of this chapter, four classes of toxins will be defined: (a) enterotoxins; (b) cytoskeleton-altering toxins; (c) cytotoxins; and (d) toxins with neural activity. To be included within a particular toxin class, only one of the listed criteria (see below) must be fulfilled. Several of the toxins can be placed in more than one category.

A toxin is classified as an *enterotoxin* if (a) the toxin stimulates net secretion in ligated intestinal segments without either histological evidence of intestinal damage by light microscopy (if data are available) or evidence from *in vitro* assays of injury to nonerythrocytic cells; or (b) the toxin stimulates secretion as measured in Ussing chambers.

The second class of enteric toxins are the *cytoskeleton-altering* toxins. This group of toxins, including *Clostridium difficile* toxin A or the toxin produced by ETBF, produce an alteration in cell shape without inducing significant cell injury. When studies are available, toxin-induced changes in cell shape have most often been demonstrated to be due to rearrangement of F or filamentous actin in the affected cells.

The third class of enteric toxins are *cytotoxins*. These toxins produce cellular damage documented either by gross findings (e.g., intestinal hemorrhage), evidence of light microscopic intestinal damage, or by studies identifying toxicity to cells (e.g., inhibition of protein synthesis, release of lactic dehydrogenase from cells). As delineated in Tables 1 and 2, the activity of enteric cytotoxins may or may not be associated with secretion in *in vivo* or *in vitro* intestinal models of disease.

Lastly, enteric bacterial toxins may have *neural activity*. A toxin is classified in this group if available data suggest that at least part of the secretory activity of the toxin is attributable to the release of one or more neurotransmitters from the enteric nervous system or that the toxin alters smooth muscle activity in the intestine. At present, no enteric toxin is clearly identified as stimulating secretion solely through these potential mechanisms.

ENTERIC BACTERIAL TOXINS CATEGORIZED BY GENUS AND SPECIES

Table 1 is a compendium of the enteric bacteria and the toxins they produce. These bacteria have been linked to human illnesses predominantly through epidemiological studies and, in many cases, volunteer trials (see below). The clinical expression of disease associated with infection with the vast majority of these bacteria is diarrhea which is watery or, uncommonly, dysenteric. Exceptions are (a) infection with *Bacillus cereus,* which produces two clinical syndromes, one dominated by emesis and the second by diarrhea (37); and (b) ingestion of food containing toxin(s) produced by *Staphylococcus aureus* that result in a prominent emetic response sometimes accompanied by diarrhea (38). This latter food poisoning syndrome is an intoxication and not an infection. Each bacterium listed in Table 1 has been identified to produce one or more toxins with biological activity either on native intestinal mucosa, intestinal epithelial cell lines, or nonintestinal cell lines. These enteric bacterial toxins are categorized by the definitions described in the text above and emphasis has been given to data on the toxin's mode of action derived from intestinal models of disease. Question marks indicate toxins for which the data are too limited to confidently classify the general activity of the toxin. In limited instances, toxin-producing bacteria are listed in Table 1 that are not known to play a significant role in human disease or have only a weak association with disease. A pertinent example is the C2 toxin produced by *Clostridium botulinum,* which is secretory in mouse intestinal loops but is not a neurotoxin like other *C. botulinum* toxins (39,40). The role of the C2 toxin in human disease is unknown. Similarly, *Vibrio metschnikovii* and strains of *E. coli* producing the cytolethal distending toxins (CLDT) and the cytoxic necrotizing factors 1 and 2 are associated with human disease only by limited anecdotal reports at present (41–46). Table 2 (which is abstracted from Table 1) specifically lists toxins by bacterial genus and species for which experimental data are available indicating activity in intestinal models of disease and indicates which toxins have been identified to stimulate an intestinal secretory response.

As shown in Table 3, human volunteer data have established the pathogenicity of most of the important enteric bacterial pathogens. In some instances, such as the toxin-producing *Aeromonas hydrophila* and *Plesiomonas shigelloides,* pathogenicity could not be demonstrated in adults despite inocula as large as 10^9–10^{10} organisms administered with 2g of sodium bicarbonate to neutralize gastric acid and enhance the likelihood of survival of the inoculum through the stomach. To provide a complete listing of enteric pathogens studied in human volunteers, Table 3 also lists enteropathogenic *E. coli* (EPEC), diffusely adherent *E. coli* (DAEC), and *Salmonella typhi.* To date, none of these bacteria have been identified to produce toxins stimulating an intestinal secretory response. In fact, although EPEC, a pathogen primarily in children less than 1 year of age, yielded diarrhea in adult volunteers, DAEC, which have also been associated with diarrheal illnesses in children in some but not all epidemiological

TABLE 1. *Enteric bacterial toxins: functional classification by genus and species[a]*

Genus and species	Enterotoxin	Cytoskeleton-altering	Cytotoxin	Neural activity	Ref.
Aeromonas hydrophilia[b]					
Aerolysin[c]			+(s)[d]		119,121,122
Other toxins[5]	+	+			120,138–140
Bacillus cereus					
"Emetic toxin"				+(?)	109,141
"Diarrheal toxin"			+(s)		109,110
Bacteroides fragilis (ETBF)					
Toxin		+(i,s)[f,g]			112,142,143 (Sears, Koshy, Chambers, unpublished data)
Campylobacter jejuni[b]					
LT-like	+	+			144,145
Cytotoxin			+		146–148
CLDT		+[h]	+		149
Clostridium botulinum					
C2 toxin		+[h]	+(s)		39,124,150,151
Clostridium difficile					
Toxin A		+(i,s)	+(s)[i]	+	90,94,99,100,152
Toxin B		+(i)	+		129,152,153
Clostridium perfringens type A					
CPE			+(s)		113,114,117,154,155
Clostridium perfringens type C					
β toxin			+		156,157
α toxin			+		158,159
"Enterotoxin" (CPE)			+(s)		160,161
Enteroaggregative *E. coli* (EAggEC)[b]					
EAST	+				23,24
Heat-labile toxin	+(?)[j]		+(?)[j]		162
Enterohemorrhagic *E. coli* (EHEC)					
Shiga-like toxin			+(s)		25,36,130,163,164
Enteroinvasive *E. coli* (EIEC)[b]					
EIET	+				26,27,165
Cytotoxin			+		26
TieA	+				27,165
Enterotoxigenic *E. coli* (ETEC)[b]					
STa	+	+		+	17,20,21,84,85,88,89,166
STb	+[k]				22,167–171
LT I	+	+			33
LT II	+	+			172–175
Other *E. coli* toxins					
CLDT		+[h]			42,176
CNF 1 and 2		+			45,126–128
Plesiomonas shigelloides[b]					
Heat-labile enterotoxin	+	+			133,177
Heat-stable enterotoxin	+				177,178
Salmonella sp. (non-*typhi*)[b]					
Enterotoxin (Stn)	+	+			179,180
Shigella dysenteriae[b]					
Shiga toxin			+(s)		25,36,130,163,181
Other *Shigella* sp.[b]					
ShET 1 and 2	+				28
Shiga-like toxin			+		36
Staphylococcus aureus					
Enterotoxins A-E	+			+	38,182–185
δ toxin	+		+[l]		186–189

TABLE 1. *Continued.*

Genus and species	Enterotoxin	Cytoskeleton-altering	Cytotoxin	Neural activity	Ref.
Vibrio cholerae O1/O139[b,m]					
CT	+	+		+	19,29,33,64
Zot		+			52,53
Ace	+				54
Hemolysin			+(s)		190–192
Vibrio cholerae non-O1, non-O139[b]					
ST-like	+				75
Vibrio metschnikovii					
Cytolysin			+(s)		41
Vibrio parahaemolyticus[b,n]					
TDH hemolysin[o]	+				16,118
Yersinia enterocolitica					
Heat-stable enterotoxins I and II	+				15,76,193

[a] Ace, accessory cholera enterotoxin; CLDT, cytolethal distending toxin; CNF, cytotoxic necrotizing factor; CPE, *Clostridium perfringens* enterotoxin; EAST, enteroaggregative *E. coli* heat-stable enterotoxin; EIET, enteroinvasive *E. coli* enterotoxin; ETBF, Enterotoxigenic *Bacteroides fragilis*; LT, enterotoxigenic *E. coli* heat-labile enterotoxin; ShET, *Shigella* enterotoxin; ST, enterotoxigenic *E. coli* heat-stable enterotoxin; Stn, *Salmonella* enterotoxin; TDH, thermostable direct hemolysin; TieA, toxin of enteroinvasive *E. coli*, type A.

[b] Indicates that organism has been tested in volunteers (see Table 3).

[c] Other names for the β-hemolysin of *A. hydrophila* are aerolysin, cytotoxic enterotoxin, or CT cross-reactive cytolytic enterotoxin (CTC-cytolysin).

[d] (s) = cytotoxin that is secretory in animal intestine and/or Ussing chambers *in vitro*.

[e] At least four other nonhemolytic toxins have been described for *Aeromonas* sp. All either cause elongation of CHO cells or rounding of Y-1 adrenal cells; one is cross-reactive with CT antisera; and three have been demonstrated to stimulate secretion in suckling mice or ligated intestinal segments in rats or rabbits.

[f] The ETBF toxin stimulates secretion in lamb and calf ligated intestinal segments. Histopathology of lamb intestine after 18 hr of exposure to ETBF reveals intestinal epithelial cell rounding and detachment from the lamina propria (Sears CL, Chambers F, Myers L, unpublished observations). However, the time course of secretion versus changes in epithelial cell morphology is unknown.

[g] (i) = Alteration of the cytoskeleton or change in cell morphology has been shown in intestinal cells *in vivo* or *in vitro*. (i,s) = alteration of the cytoskeleton as above plus evidence for secretion in an intestinal model such as ligated intestinal segments or Ussing chambers *in vitro* using native intestinal tissue of monolayers of intestinal epithelial cells.

[h] Cells display altered morphology for up to 3 days with lethality (cytotoxicity) occurring later.

[i] *In vivo* studies with *C. difficile* toxin A demonstrates that secretion is consistently associated with inflammation and damage to the intestinal epithelium. However, *in vitro* studies with intestinal epithelial cells and nonintestinal cell lines have not revealed cytotoxicity activity with *C. difficile* toxin A. Thus it seems likely that this toxin stimulates a striking inflammatory response by as yet unknown mechanisms that is cytotoxic to the intestinal epithelium.

[j] Based on data in HEp-2 cells, the heat-labile toxin of EAggEC is postulated to act as an enterotoxin by increasing intracellular calcium and/or to act as a cytotoxin based on its cross-reactivity with *E. coli* hemolysin antisera.

[k] In detailed studies, alterations in villous cell morphology has been identified in rat intestine after treatment with *E. coli* STb.

[l] Delayed histologic damage is seen *in vivo* after treatment of the intestine with δ toxin. However, δ toxin rapidly (within minutes) alters intestinal transport by increasing potential difference and decreasing resistance in guinea pig ileum studied in Ussing chambers.

[m] O1/O139 refers to the O1 and O139 serogroups of *V. cholerae*. These serogroups comprise the epidemic strains of *V. cholerae* that produce cholera toxin and produce clinical cholera. Although some strains of *V. cholerae* belonging to serogroups other than O1 or O139 may express cholera toxin, the majority of strains in these serogroups are either nonpathogenic or express virulence factors other than cholera toxin.

[n] *V. parahaemolyticus* produces other potential toxins, but data are very limited.

[o] Other species of *Vibrio* implicated in diarrheal disease, namely, *V. mimicus* and *V. hollisae* have also been reported to produce TDH and possess the *tdh* gene (194).

TABLE 2. *Enteric bacterial toxins with demonstrated activity on native intestine or intestinal epithelial cell lines*

Genus	Native intestinal activity	Activity in intestinal epithelial cell lines	Secretion
A. hydrophilia			
Aerolysin	Enterotoxin[a]		+
Other toxins	+[a]		+
B. cereus			
"Emetic toxin"	+[b]		
"Diarrheal toxin"	Cytotoxin		+
B. fragilis			
Toxin	+[c]	Cytoskeleton-altering	+
C. jejuni			
Heat-labile	+[d]		+
Heat-labile cytotoxin		Cytotoxin	
CLDT	Cytotoxin		+
C. botulinum	+[e]		+
C. difficile			
Toxin A	Cytotoxin	Cytoskeleton-altering	+
Toxin B		Cytoskeleton-altering	
C. perfringens type A			
CPE	Cytotoxin		+
C. perfringens type C			
β toxin	Cytotoxin		
α toxin	+[f]		
CPE	Cytotoxin		+
EAgg *E. coli*			
EAST	Enterotoxin		+
EHEC			
Shiga toxin	Cytotoxin		+
EIEC			
EIET	Enterotoxin		+
TieA	+[e]		+
ETEC			
STa	Enterotoxin, neural activity	Enterotoxin Cytoskeleton-altering	+
STb	Enterotoxin[g]		+
LT I	Enterotoxin	Cytoskeleton-altering[h]	+
LT II	+[i]	Cytoskeleton-altering[h]	+
E. coli			
CLDT	−[j]		
CNF1	−[j]		−
CNF2	+[e]		+
P. shigelloides			
Heat-labile	+[k]		+
Heat-stable	+[k]		+
Salmonella sp.			
Enterotoxin	Enterotoxin[g]	Cytoskeleton-altering	+
S. dysenteriae			
Shiga toxin	Cytotoxin		+
Other *Shigella* sp.			
ShET 1 and 2	+		+
S. aureus			
Enterotoxins A–E	+[b]		
	Enterotoxin[l]		+
δ toxin	Cytotoxin		
V. cholerae			
CT	Enterotoxin	Cytoskeleton-altering[h]	+
Ace	Enterotoxin		+
Zot	Cytoskeleton-altering	Cytoskeleton-altering	
Hemolysin	Cytotoxin		+
V. cholerae non-O1, non-0139			
ST-like	+[e]		+
V. metschnikovii			
Cytolysin	+[e]		+

TABLE 2. *Continued.*

Genus	Native intestinal activity	Activity in intestinal epithelial cell lines	Secretion
V. parahaemolyticus			
TDH	Enterotoxin		+
Y. enterocolitica			
Heat-stable enterotoxin I	+ [e]		+
Heat-stable enterotoxin II	+ [e]		+

[a] The aerolysin of *A. hydrophila* is cytotoxic to nonintestinal cells but caused secretion without histological changes in perfused rat jejunum (122). Data on intestinal secretory activity exist for three of the four other toxins of *A. hydrophila,* but no intestinal histology is available.

[b] Toxins elicited vomiting in monkeys.

[c] Histological examination of lamb intestine exposed to 18 hr of ETBF organisms revealed rounded intestinal epithelial cells with detachment of some cells.

[d] Culture supernatants of *C. jejuni* have elicited hemorrhagic fluid in rat ileal loops that was neutralized with cholera antitoxin (145). Rabbit ileal loop and suckling mice assays were negative. It is unclear as to whether the secretory activity observed was due to the heat-labile enterotoxin or the heat-labile cytotoxin potentially produced by *C. jejuni* strains.

[e] Results of histological examination of intestinal tissue have not been reported.

[f] The α toxin of *C. perfringens* type C has been reported to increase Isc in Ussing chambers only when added to the serosal side of rat colonic mucosa. Histological results are not available.

[g] Mild histological changes have been reported.

[h] Intestinal epithelial cell chloride secretion stimulated by increases in intracellular cyclic AMP has been shown to be dependent in part on rearrangement of F actin (57,58). Thus, by analogy, it is postulated that enteric bacterial toxins that increase cyclic AMP may also be cytoskeleton-altering toxins in intestinal epithelial cells.

[i] *E. coli* heat-labile enterotoxin (LT) II, unlike *E. coli* LT I, does not stimulate secretion in rabbit ileal segments. However, *E. coli* LT II does stimulate secretion in the sealed adult mouse (SAM) model. Histological studies of intestinal tissue are not available.

[j] These toxins did not yield secretion when tested in rabbit ileal segments.

[k] Culture filtrates of *P. shigelloides* may contain heat-labile or heat-stable secretory factors detectable in rabbit ileal loops that do not alter the histology of the intestine (177,178).

[l] δ toxin stimulates a rapid PD change in intestinal tissue with delayed damage by histopathology.

investigations (47–51), did not cause diarrhea in adult volunteers. Similarly, infection with *S. typhi,* the etiological agent of typhoid fever, predominantly causes a systemic illness.

Three general observations are apparent from the data in Tables 1 and 2, each of which will be discussed separately below. First, although most enteric toxins have been reported to have one identified activity to date, recent data available for the best studied toxins, in particular cholera toxin, *E. coli* STa, and *C. difficile* toxin A, highlight the potential complexity of toxin action in stimulating intestinal secretion. For example, *E. coli* STa and most likely cholera toxin can be classified as enterotoxins, cytoskeleton-altering toxins, and toxins with neural activity. Similarly, the complexity of the action of *C. difficile* toxin A is clear from a comparison of *in vivo* and *in vitro* studies, as will be discussed below. Second, certain enteric toxins have been "misnamed," commonly referred to as enterotoxins when in fact the data indicate that an alternative classification may be more appropriate. Third, several toxins produced by enteric bacteria can be classified as hemolysins based on the ability of the toxin to lyse erythrocytes of one or more species but only in limited instances has this activity been correlated with the pathogenesis of intestinal secretion.

The Potential Complexity of Enteric Bacterial Toxin Action: Cholera Toxin, *E. coli* STa, and *C. difficile* Toxin A

The disease cholera is characterized by rapidly dehydrating noninflammatory diarrhea caused by *Vibrio cholerae*. Although recent data have identified other toxins produced by *V. cholerae* (52–54), the secretion observed in cholera is largely ascribed to its ability to produce cholera toxin (CT). CT is a classic enterotoxin and does not injure intestinal epithelial cells. The first recognized and most ubiquitous activity of CT is to stimulate intracellular production of cyclic AMP via activation of adenylate cyclase [reviewed in (29,30,33)]. *In vitro* studies indicate that cyclic AMP stimulates chloride secretion and inhibits the absorption of NaCl (19,55). The chloride secretion is most likely mediated by activation of A kinase with phosphorylation of the cystic fibrosis transmembrane regulator (CFTR), a major chloride channel present in intestinal epithelia (56). However, a combination of *in vivo* and *in vitro* observations also suggest that the pathogenesis of secretion in response to CT may be more complex. Most likely, the additional mechanisms described below by which CT may stimulate intestinal secretion aug-

TABLE 3. *Enteric bacteria and toxins studied in volunteers*

Bacteria	Inoculum[a]	Outcome	Reference
Vibrio cholerae[b]			
O1 (CT+)	10^{3*} (10^3)	Diarrhea	195
O139	10^{4*} (10^4)	Diarrhea	196
Non-O1/non-O139 (ST+)	10^6 (10^6)	Diarrhea	197
Non-O1/non-O139 (ST−)	10^9	No diarrhea	197
Shigella sp.			
dysenteriae	10^{1*} (2×10^2)	Diarrhea/dysentery	198
flexneri	10^{2*} (10^4)	Diarrhea/dysentery	198
sonnei	$5 \times 10^{2*}$ (5×10^2)	Diarrhea/dysentery	198
Escherichia coli			
enterotoxigenic	10^{6*} (10^6)	Diarrhea	199
enteropathogenic	10^{6*} (10^{10})	Diarrhea	200
enteroinvasive	10^8 (10^8)	Diarrhea/dysentery	201
enteroaggregative	7×10^8 (−)	Diarrhea	202
diffusely-adherent	10^{10}	No diarrhea	203
Salmonella typhimurium	2×10^9	Diarrhea	204
Salmonella typhi	10^5 (10^7)	Typhoid fever	205
Campylobacter jejuni	$8 \times 10^{2*}$ (10^8)	Diarrhea	206
Vibrio parahaemolyticus	3×10^7 (10^8)	Diarrhea	207
Aeromonas hydrophila	10^{10}	No diarrhea	208
Plesiomonas shigelloides	4×10^9	No diarrhea	209

[a] Lowest inoculum giving diarrhea in one or more subjects is shown; * indicates that this inoculum was the lowest one studied. The inoculum in parenthesis is the lowest-causing diarrhea in 50% or more of subjects receiving that inoculum; (−) indicates that no inoculum tested gave diarrhea in 50% or more of subjects. Most but not all studies have administered sodium bicarbonate prior to ingestion of the inoculum to neutralize stomach acidity.

[b] *V. cholerae* O1 lacking both cholera toxin (CT) and the TCP intestinal colonization factor have been fed to volunteers and did not cause diarrhea at inocula of 10^8 (210). Genetically engineered *V. cholerae* O1 strains deleted of cholera toxin have caused diarrhea in volunteers at inocula of 10^4 (2). *V. cholerae* non-O1/O139 indicate those strains belonging to serogroups other than O1 or O139; one such strain expressed a toxin similar to the *E. coli* heat-stable enterotoxin (ST).

ment and/or supplement (but do not supplant) cyclic AMP–mediated intestinal secretion.

First, CT may utilize the intestinal epithelial cell cytoskeleton to yield secretion. Immobilization of F actin in intestinal epithelial monolayers inhibits the chloride secretory response to agonists known to increase intracellular cyclic AMP, suggesting that modulation of intestinal epithelial cell F actin may be necessary for CT to stimulate maximal epithelial cell chloride secretion (57). Subsequent data have indicated that the Na/K/2Cl cotransporter, which is key to the transepithelial secretion of chloride, is functionally linked to the cytoskeleton (58). These data suggest that toxins that increase intracellular cyclic AMP may also be classified as cytoskeleton-altering toxins. Second, *in vitro* and *in vivo* data implicate prostaglandins of the E series (PGE_1 and PGE_2) (59,60) and, recently, platelet-activating factor (PAF) (61–63) in the pathogenesis of intestinal secretion stimulated by CT. However, the mechanisms for these responses are not known. Third, part of the secretory response to CT may be due to an effect on the enteric nervous system, possibly by stimulating peptide hormone release by intestinal enterochromaffin cells and/or by increasing the smooth muscle activity of the small bowel (64–66). Serotonin and vasoactive intestinal peptide (VIP), both intestinal secretory agonists, are released into the human small bowel *in vivo*

after treatment with CT and release of VIP can be blocked by the ganglionic blocker, tetrodotoxin, suggesting a neuronal source for the VIP (67). Additional *in vivo* data showing that CT-induced secretion is inhibited by several neurotransmitter and ganglionic blockers also support a role for the enteric nervous system in the intestinal secretion stimulated by CT (68–70) and indicate that CT can be classified as a toxin with neural activity.

E. coli producing an 18- or 19-amino-acid peptide with a molecular weight of ~2 kDa (71,72) are important causes of traveler's diarrhea and dehydrating diarrheal illnesses in children of the developing world. In most but not all studies (73), STa amino acid residues 5–17 or 6–18 confer full binding and enterotoxic activities and it is this region that shares a striking identity with heat-stable enterotoxins secreted by other enteric pathogens including *Yersinia enterocolitica* and *Vibrio cholerae* non-O1 (74–76). *E. coli* STa appears to act by binding to guanylate cyclase type C (GC-C) (77). STa binding activates particulate intestinal guanylate cyclase or GC-C, thereby producing elevated cellular levels of cyclic GMP that stimulate chloride secretion and inhibit NaCl absorption resulting in net intestinal fluid secretion (17,20,21). The endogenous agonist for GC-C is a 15-amino-acid hormone guanylin that contains four cysteines and is less potent than STa in activating GC-C and in stimulating chloride secretion (78–80). Guanylin presumably plays a role in basal gut homeostasis and STa opportunistically utilizes GC-C to alter ion transport in the gut. *In vitro* data using human intestinal epithelial cell lines indicate that cyclic GMP via activation of a kinase stimulates CFTR (81–83). Although STa is a classic enterotoxin without *in vivo* or *in vitro* evidence of histological damage, the secretory response to STa *in vitro* in T84 cells (human intestinal epithelial cells) was recently reported to involve microfilament (F actin) rearrangement only at the basal pole of these polarized cells (84), revealing that this toxin may also be classified as a cytoskeleton-altering toxin. Whether cyclic GMP alone accounts for the full secretory response to STa is controversial. In rat jejunum, the secretory response to STa has been completely abrogated by 5-hydroxytryptamine (5-HT, or serotonin) receptor antagonists without altering the cyclic GMP response to STa (85). These results suggest that serotonin mediates STa secretion possibly through an effect on prostaglandin synthesis (HT-2 receptors) and/or neurons (HT-3 receptors). Although *in vitro* studies using isolated rat intestinal epithelial cells suggest that STa may increase intracellular calcium and activate protein kinase C, correlation of these data with a secretory response is not yet available (80,86,87). Lastly, a role for the enteric nervous system in STa-stimulated secretion has been suggested by studies of myoelectric activity in STa-treated rabbit small intestine and by studies employing neuronal inhibitors that diminished the STa secretory response *in vivo* (88,89). These data suggest that *E. coli* STa may also be regarded as a toxin with neural activity.

Strains of *C. difficile* associated with antibiotic-associated diarrhea or, in its most severe clinical expression, pseudomembranous colitis produce two toxins, the "enterotoxin" (toxin A) and cytotoxin (toxin B). The bulk of data from *in vivo* intestinal disease models indicates that toxin A is of primary importance in disease pathogenesis. Although often described as an enterotoxin, toxin A causes rounding of many nonintestinal cell types that usually precedes evidence of cell membrane injury (90,91). In addition, *in vivo* studies indicate that toxin A induces hemorrhagic fluid secretion and markedly damages ileal and colonic epithelium (92–98). In guinea pig and/or rabbit ileal tissues mounted in Ussing chambers, toxin A stimulates chloride secretion, increases intestinal epithelial permeability, and alters epithelial cell structure (94,99). In contrast, in monolayers of human colonic epithelial cells (T84 cells) studied *in vitro*, toxin A markedly diminishes monolayer resistance over time without evidence of cellular damage (100). Staining of F actin is strikingly diminished in T84 cells at the tight junctional ring by toxin A without cellular damage or disruption of the tight junctions evident by transmission electron microscopy (100). The mechanism by which toxin A disrupts F actin has not been identified. The contrast between the *in vivo* and *in vitro* intestinal epithelial responses to toxin A are probably due to three sets of observations. First, toxin A may stimulate, by a yet undefined mechanism, neutrophil recruitment, possibly through a G protein–linked neutrophil toxin A receptor (101). Second, treatment of the intestinal epithelium with toxin A stimulates release of numerous inflammatory mediators (e.g., leukotrienes, prostaglandin

E$_2$, PAF, histamine) that are potentially secretory and/or may modify intestinal permeability (98,102–107). Third, the inflammatory and secretory effects of toxin A are reduced by an antagonist of the peptide substance P in rats (108). Substance P is a transmitter of submucosal primary sensory neurons known to participate in inflammatory responses. Together these data indicate that toxin A stimulates secretion and inflammation most likely by direct effects on intestinal epithelial cells and indirect effects via activation of submucosal immune effector cells and the enteric nervous system. Thus, *C. difficile* toxin A is best classified as a cytotoxin with neural activity based on the *in vivo* data and as a cytoskeleton-altering toxin based on its effects on intestinal epithelial cells *in vitro*.

"Misnamed" Enteric Bacterial Toxins

The experimental, but not the clinical, data available on four enteric bacterial toxins suggest that these toxins are "misnamed." These toxins are the *Bacillus cereus* "diarrheal toxin," the *Bacteroides fragilis* enterotoxin, *Clostridium difficile* toxin A, and the *Clostridium perfringens* enterotoxin (CPE). The clinical illnesses associated with infection with each of these bacteria are most often characterized by watery diarrhea, not dysentery. One exception is the occurrence of pseudomembranous enterocolitis, which is the extreme of the clinical expression of infection with strains of *C. difficile* producing toxin A. It is important to note that the histopathology of human intestinal tissue in these infections is generally not known nor are detailed clinical evaluations examining for an intestinal inflammatory response typically available. Thus, a ready explanation for the discrepancy between the clinical presentation of these infections and the experimental data on the activity of these toxins as delineated below is not obvious at present.

The diarrheal toxin of *B. cereus,* frequently referred to as an enterotoxin in the literature, consists of a two- to three-component protein complex with possible hemolytic activity (109–111). Individual components of this toxin complex are biologically inactive until added together. This toxin stimulates secretion and necrosis in rabbit ligated ileal segments and is cytotoxic for Vero cells indicating that it is a secretory cytotoxin not an enterotoxin. The *B. fragilis* enterotoxin stimulates secretion in lamb- and calf-ligated intestinal segments (112). However, recent data examining the histopathology of intestinal epithelial cells treated with purified toxin and lamb intestine treated with ETBF indicate that intestinal epithelial cells develop dramatic morphological changes such as rounding and loss of intestinal microvilli after exposure (C. Sears, F. Chambers, S. Koshy, L. Myers, unpublished observations). These morphological changes in intestinal epithelial cells *in vitro* occur without evidence of significant cytotoxicity suggesting that this toxin is best classified at present as a secretory cytoskeleton-altering toxin. *C. difficile* toxin A is commonly referred to as an enterotoxin. However, as delineated in the data discussed above, there is no evidence of secretion stimulated by this toxin in the absence of histological damage and, in addition, no secretion in response to this toxin has been identified in the studies examining the action of this toxin specifically on an intestinal epithelial cell line (T84). These data suggest that *C. difficile* toxin A is best classified as a cytotoxin with neural activity based on the *in vivo* data and as a cytoskeleton-altering toxin based on its effects on T84 cells *in vitro*. Lastly, CPE stimulates secretion that is associated with histologic damage in, for example, rat- and rabbit-ligated ileal segments (113,114). In addition, detailed studies of the mode of action of CPE using rabbit brush border membranes and lipid bilayers suggest that this toxin binds irreversibly to cells creating an ion-permeable channel by direct membrane insertion (113,115–117). The resulting membrane permeability changes are lethal for eukaryotic cells. Thus, CPE is most likely a cytotoxin, not an enterotoxin.

Relationship of Enteric Bacterial Hemolysins to Intestinal Secretion

Much of the historic literature on bacterial toxins has focused on toxins capable of lysing erythrocytes. Hemolytic toxins have been studied not only for extraintestinal diseases, but also for diarrheal diseases, where the linkage between lysis of erythrocytes and a secretory response in intestinal epithelial cells is not intuitive. There are many examples of hemolysins that play no role in intestinal disease but there are also several examples of toxins that are linked to secretory diarrhea and were first discovered on the basis of hemolytic activity.

One such toxin is the thermostable direct hemolysin (TDH) or Kanagawa phenomenon hemolysin of *V. parahaemolyticus*. This toxin was first discovered and characterized on the basis of lysis of erythrocytes. Despite the lack of a mechanistic linkage between hemolysis and secretion, there was a striking epidemiological linkage with diarrheal disease wherein TDH + strains were isolated almost exclusively from diarrheal stools while TDH – strains were isolated almost exclusively from nonclinical specimens. An isogenic mutant of *V. parahaemolyticus* was constructed in which the genes encoding TDH were specifically mutated (16). The TDH + strain caused fluid accumulation in ligated rabbit loops whereas the TDH – strain did not. Furthermore, culture supernatants from the TDH + strain increased I_{sc} in Ussing chambers whereas supernatants from the TDH – strain did not increase I_{sc}. Histological examination of rabbit intestine exposed to TDH in these experiments showed no evidence of cell damage (16). Further work using purified TDH in Ussing chambers suggests that TDH stimulates chloride secretion and that calcium may be the intracellular mediator of secretion since the Ussing chamber response is blocked by preincubation with the calcium-buffering compound BAPTA/AM (118).

Another example of a hemolytic toxin for which a linkage to secretion has been established is the aerolysin of *Aeromonas hydrophila* and *A. sobria*. This toxin, also known as β-hemolysin, or "cholera toxin cross-reactive cytolytic enterotoxin," lyses rabbit erythrocytes as well as a wide variety of nonintestinal cells such as CHO cells

(119–121). The purified hemolysin causes fluid accumulation in rabbit ileal loops and infant mouse intestines (119,121). Furthermore, culture filtrates of *A. sobria* produce enterotoxic activity in a rat jejunal perfusion system that is neutralized by monoclonal antibody against the aerolysin (122). In the rat perfusion system, the culture filtrates induced net water, potassium, and sodium loss with a rapid onset (less than 5 min) without changes in intestinal histology.

These examples illustrate that cytotoxic activity on erythrocytes should not be a contraindication to intestinal secretory relevance. However, use of hemolytic assays in studying such toxins should be limited to toxin purification studies or similar applications and mechanistic studies should be conducted on relevant intestinal cells and tissues.

MECHANISMS BY WHICH ENTERIC BACTERIAL TOXINS STIMULATE INTESTINAL SECRETION

Two approaches will be used to analyze how enteric bacterial toxins act to stimulate intestinal secretion. First, the relationship between how the toxins have been classified using the general mode of action (e.g., enterotoxin, cytotoxin, etc.) and their mechanisms of action will be discussed. Second, as detailed in Table 4, the enteric bacterial toxins will be classified by how clearly their mechanism of action is established. Of note, most of these toxins have one or more activities for which a mechanism is incompletely established (possible or postulated mechanism of action) or not known at all.

Relationship Between the General Mode of Activity of the Enteric Bacterial Toxins and Mechanisms of Secretion

The primary mechanism of action documented for unequivocal enterotoxins such as cholera toxin, the heat-labile and heat-stable enterotoxins of *E. coli* (*STa*, LT I, LT II), and EAST 1 is activation of either adenylate cyclase or GC-C with subsequent elevation of intracellular cyclic nucleotide levels (cyclic AMP, cyclic GMP). As already discussed earlier in this chapter, one note of caution is that, for example, cholera toxin and *E. coli* STa may also employ alternative mechanisms that contribute to the secretory response to these toxins. Elevation of intracellular calcium by, for example, *E. coli* STb (123) or *V. parahaemolyticus* TDH (118) may be an alternative mechanism by which enterotoxins may stimulate intestinal secretion. However, as discussed below, an increase in intracellular calcium has not yet been established as a mechanism of action for an enteric bacterial toxin.

For most of the cytoskeleton-altering toxins, the cytoskeletal protein(s) involved in a cellular morphological change in response to toxin treatment is unknown. Of the three major cytoskeletal proteins—actin, tubulin, and keratin—only F actin has repeatedly been shown to be altered by enteric bacterial toxins (e.g., ETBF toxin, *E.*

coli STa, *C. difficile* toxins A and B, C2 toxin of *C. botulinum*, *E. coli* CNFs 1 and 2) that alter cell shape without usually causing cellular damage. In general, how these toxins modulate the microfilament (or F-actin) structure of cells is unknown. However, two mechanisms have been identified. First, the C2 toxin of *C. botulinum* ADP-ribosylates arginine-177 of G (monomeric) actin preventing polymerization of G to F actin (124,125). Second, recent data have suggested that three enteric bacterial toxins, *E. coli* CNFs 1 and 2 and *C. difficile* toxin B, alter the GTP-binding protein Rho that modulates microfilament structure in eukaryotic cells (126–129). The molecular basis by which Rho is altered has not been identified for any of these toxins. Neither of these mechanisms altering F-actin structure have been linked to secretion. However, the relationship between the ability of a toxin to alter the cellular cytoskeleton and secretion is an active area of study. Recent data suggest that the regulation of Na/K/2Cl cotransporter, a key protein in transepithelial chloride transport, is functionally linked to the cytoskeleton (58). Moreover, chloride secretion stimulated by *E. coli* STa (84) and cyclic AMP–dependent agonists (57) are reduced when F actin is immobilized in monolayers of intestinal epithelial cells studied in Ussing chambers.

The best established mechanism of action for any of the enteric bacterial cytotoxins is inhibition of protein synthesis. This has only been studied in detail for the Shiga and Shiga-like toxins that possess *N*-glycosidase activity, which cleaves adenine 4324 from the 3′ end of the 28S rRNA component of the eukaryotic ribosomal complex, inhibiting peptide elongation and terminating protein synthesis (36,130,131). The Gb3 receptor for Shiga toxin is present in greater concentrations in the absorptive villous cells compared to the secretory crypt cells and the preferential killing of the villous cells leads to decreased fluid absorption (25). In addition, CPE is lethal to eukaryotic cells presumably by creating an ion-permeable membrane pore that leads to irreversible inhibition of vital cell functions such as protein and nucleotide synthesis through leakage of intracellular potassium (113,115,116). The C2 toxin of *C. botulinum* is also ultimately lethal to eukaryotic cells (124). How ADP ribosylation of G actin by the C2 toxin of *C. botulinum* results in cell lethality is unknown.

Precise mechanisms for how enteric bacterial toxins such as cholera toxin or *E. coli* STa stimulate secretion through their neural activity are not available. The most precise data available on this category of activity is the demonstration that the secretion and inflammation stimulated by *C. difficile* toxin A is inhibited by an antagonist of peptide substance P release, a transmitter of submucosal primary sensory neurons involved in inflammatory responses (108).

Enteric Bacterial Toxins with Established, Possible/Postulated, or Unknown Mechanisms of Action

Table 4 lists the enteric bacterial toxins by degree of certainty regarding their mechanism of action. Toxins are considered to have an established mechanism of action if

the molecular mechanism of action has been identified and the activity of the toxin has been linked to intestinal secretion. However, except for the documented ability of cyclic nucleotides to stimulate the chloride channel CFTR by activating protein kinases in the intestinal epithelial cell, direct data indicating that these molecular mechanisms of action can activate one or more intestinal epithelial cell ion transporters or even lead to secretion by an intestinal epithelial cell (e.g., by pore formation) are lacking.

Within the established mechanisms of action, there are three general categories: (a) toxins that bind to a receptor stimulating the release of a second messenger (e.g., cyclic nucleotides); (b) toxins with an A/B structure where the B subunit mediates cell binding and the enzymatically active A subunit is translocated across the eukaryotic cell membrane to its cytosolic substrate; and (c) toxins that insert directly into the cell membrane creating an ion-permeable pore (132). Conspicuously absent from the list of established mechanisms of enteric bacterial toxin action are toxins known to stimulate secretion by calcium/protein kinase C–dependent, calcium/calmodulin–dependent, or tyrosine kinase–dependent mechanisms. Preliminary data on several toxins (particularly the *E. coli* STb toxin and the *V. parahaemolyticus* TDH toxin) are very suggestive of a calcium-dependent mechanism, but the mechanism is not definitively established because either direct measurements of intracellular calcium and/or protein kinase C activity are missing or else the detection of the potential intracellular mediator has not been correlated with a secretory response (see discussion below). Among the established mechanisms of action, the best understood mechanisms at the molecular level are the ADP-ribosyltransferase activity of CT and the *E. coli* LTs (29,30,33), the *N*-glycosidase activity of Shiga and Shiga-like toxins (130), and the ADP-ribosyltransferase activity of the *C. botulinum* C2 toxin (125). In each of these examples, the specific residue modified by the enzymatic activity of the toxin has been identified.

Toxins with possible or postulated mechanisms of action have been included in this category based on one of several criteria. First, the mechanism of action of the toxin has been inferred by identification of a biological activity specific for another toxin with a known mechanism of action. For example, similar to CT, the LT of *P. shigelloides* causes CHO cell elongation neutralizable by antisera against CT, suggesting that this toxin elevates intracellular cyclic AMP (133). Second, the possible mechanism of action has been demonstrated only in nonintestinal cells. For example, in addition to its ability to form an ion-permeable channel in lipid bilayers (134), the δ toxin of *S. aureus* has been reported to stimulate a eukaryotic cell phospholipase A2 suggesting that stimulation of arachidonic acid metabolism may contribute to the secretory response to this toxin (135). Third, the toxin has been shown to elevate a second messenger in intestinal epithelial cells but the relevance to secretion has not yet been demonstrated. This criterion applies to the increases in intracellular calcium reported for the *E. coli* STa and STb toxins. *E. coli* STa has been reported to elevate intracellular calcium and to stimulate the release of diacylglyc-

TABLE 4. *Enteric bacterial toxins: mechanistic classification*

I. *Toxins with Established Mechanisms of Action[a]*
   A. *Cyclic Nucleotides*
      1. *Cyclic AMP* Cholera toxin (29,30)
          Escherichia coli LT I and II[b] (33)
      2. *Cyclic GMP Escherichia coli* STa[b] (17,20)
          Enteroaggregative *Escherichia coli* heat-stable enterotoxin (EAST 1) (23,24)
          Yersinia enterocolitica heat-stable enterotoxin I (211)
   B. *ADP-ribosylation*
      Cholera toxin (29,30)
      Escherichia coli LT I and II (33)
      Clostridium botulinum C2 toxin (125)
   C. *Inhibition of Protein Synthesis*
      Shiga toxin (36)
      Shiga-like toxins I and II (36)
   D. *Pore Formation*
      Staphylococcus aureus δ toxin (134)
      Clostridium perfringens enterotoxin (CPE) (117)
II. *Toxins with Possible or Postulated Mechanisms of Action*
   A. *Cyclic AMP*
      Plesiomonas shigelloides heat-labile toxin (177)
      Campylobacter jejuni heat-labile enterotoxin (145)
      Salmonella typhimurium heat-labile enterotoxin (31,32,137)
   B. *Arachidonic Acid Cascade*
      Cholera toxin (59–61)
      Clostridium difficile toxin A (98,102,105–107)
      Escherichia coli STb (136)
      Staphylococcus aureus δ toxin (135)
      Salmonella typhimurium enterotoxin (31,137)
   C. *Calcium/Protein Kinase C*
      Escherichia coli STb (123)
      Enteroaggregative *Escherichia coli* heat-labile toxin (162)
      Escherichia coli STa (80,86,87)
      Vibrio parahaemolyticus thermostable direct hemolysin (TDH) (118)
   D. *Pore Formation*
      Vibrio cholerae O1 accessory cholera enterotoxin (Ace) (54)
      Enteroaggregative *Escherichia coli* heat-labile toxin (162)
   E. *Alteration of the GTP-Binding Protein, Rho*
      Escherichia coli cytotoxic necrotizing factors 1 and 2 (126,128)
      Clostridium difficile toxin B (129)
III. *Toxins with Unknown Mechanism of Action*
   A. *Enterotoxins*
      Clostridium perfringens α toxin (phospholipase C) (159)
      Enteroinvasive *Escherichia coli* enterotoxin (26)
      Plesiomonas shigelloides heat-stable enterotoxin (178)
      Staphylococcus aureus enterotoxins A–E (182–184)
      Yersinia enterocolitica heat-stable enterotoxin II (Yst-II) (193)
   B. *Cytotoxins*
      Bacillus cereus "diarrheal toxin" (109,110)
      Clostridium difficile toxin A (92–98)
      Campylobacter jejuni cytotoxin (146,147)
      Campylobacter jejuni cytolethal distending toxin (CLDT) (149)
      Clostridium perfringens β toxin (157)
      Enteroinvasive *Escherichia coli* cytotoxin (26)
      Escherichia coli cytolethal distending toxin (CLDT) (42,176)
      Vibrio metschnikovii cytolysin (41)

TABLE 4. *Continued.*

C. *Cytoskeleton-Altering Toxins*
    Campylobacter jejuni cytolethal distending toxin (CLDT) (149)
    Cholera toxin[c] (57,58)
    Clostridium difficile toxin A (100)
    Enterotoxigenic *Bacteroides fragilis* toxin (Sears CL, Koshy S, Van Tassel R, Chambers F, unpublished observations)
    Escherichia coli cytolethal distending toxin (CLDT) (42,176)
    Escherichia coli STa[d] (84)
    Escherichia coli LT I and II[c] (57,58)
    Salmonella typhimurium enterotoxin[c] (57,58)
    Vibrio cholerae 01 zonula occludens toxin (Zot) (52)
D. *Neural Activity*
    Bacillus cereus "emetic toxin" (109,141)
    Cholera toxin (64–70)
    Clostridium difficile toxin A (108)
    Escherichia coli STa (88,89)
    Staphylococcus aureus enterotoxins A–E (38,212)

[a] A toxin is considered to have an "established" mechanism of action if the molecular mechanism of action has been identified and the toxin stimulates intestinal secretion.

[b] LT, heat-labile enterotoxin; ST, heat-stable enterotoxin.

[c] Chloride secretion in intestinal epithelial monolayers stimulated by agonists such as vasoactive intestinal peptide that increase cyclic AMP is regulated by F actin, most likely through the Na/K/2Cl cotransporter that plays a key role in transepithelial Cl⁻ secretion. By analogy, a similar response to cholera toxin, *E. coli* LT I and II the *Salmonella typhimurium* enterotoxin is hypothesized.

[d] *E. coli* STa has been shown to alter the appearance of F actin in the basal portion of T_{84} cells, a human intestinal epithelial cell line, but the mechanism of this effect is unknown.

erol in isolated rat intestinal epithelial cells (80,86,87). However, the relevance of these observations to secretion has not been demonstrated. The *E. coli* STb toxin has also been shown to elevate intracellular calcium in several cell types including human intestinal epithelial cells, HT29/C1 (123). This appears to occur through activation of a calcium channel regulated by a GTP-binding protein. Similar to the data on *E. coli* STa, experiments to demonstrate a secretory response correlating with the increase in intracellular calcium stimulated by *E. coli* STb have not yet been done. Fourth, the mechanism of action of the toxin has been suggested by experiments using inhibitors or chelators of, for example, protein kinases or calcium, respectively, but direct data demonstrating kinase activation or increases in intracellular calcium are lacking. For example, secretion stimulated by the *V. parahaemolyticus* TDH is abrogated by chelation of intracellular calcium using BAPTA/AM (118). These data suggest, but do not prove, a role for calcium in the secretory activity of this toxin. Fifth, the mechanism of action of the toxin is based on computer modeling of the toxin's structure deduced from the DNA sequence for the toxin. For example, the potential pore-forming toxin, *V. cholerae* O1 Ace toxin, is predicted to be amphipathic suggesting that multimers of these toxin molecules could insert in the intestinal epithelial cell membrane to create an ion-permeable channel (54). Sixth, as already discussed, recent data have suggested that three enteric bacterial toxins, *E. coli* CNFs 1 and 2 and *C. difficile* toxin B, alter the GTP-binding protein Rho, which modulates microfilament structure in eukaryotic cells (126–128). However, the molecular basis for this activity has not been identified for any of these

toxins and, except for *E. coli* CNF2, these toxins have not been linked to intestinal secretion. Thus this is a potential mechanism of action that requires further study. Lastly, several toxins including cholera toxin (59–61), *C. difficile* toxin A (98,102,105–107), *E. coli* STb (136), and the *S. typhimurium* heat-labile enterotoxin (31,137) stimulate the release of arachidonic acid metabolites in the intestine. Furthermore, each of these toxins has been linked to secretion in one or more experimental intestinal models. However, the mechanistic steps between binding of the toxin to its intestinal epithelial cell receptor and the ultimate release of arachidonic acid metabolites are likely to be multiple and have not been delineated for any of these toxins.

The last category of enteric bacterial toxins are those with unknown mechanisms of action. Most enteric bacterial toxins have been classified by demonstrating various biological activities in one or more experimental systems. However, many biological activities have been identified for which precise mechanistic explanations do not exist at present. Even among the best-studied toxins, there are examples of biological activities for which the mechanism(s) are unknown. For example, the mechanism by which *E. coli* STa alters the appearance of F actin in intestinal epithelial cells *in vitro* is unknown (84).

CONCLUSIONS

Despite the many years of research into bacterial enteric toxins, there are many gaps in our knowledge of the mechanisms by which these toxins cause diarrhea. The accumulated knowledge on these toxins spans a wide spectrum from recently discovered and unpurified toxins to toxins for which exquisite molecular detail is known. Even for those toxins that have been studied for years and whose mechanism of action was believed to be known, there are recent data indicating that our previous mechanistic schemes were too simplistic. The power of recombinant DNA technology to study structure–function relationships and the accelerating accumulation of information about eukaryotic signal transduction pathways provide unprecedented opportunities for great improvements in our understanding of how these toxins cause disease.

REFERENCES

1. Levine MM, Kaper JB, Black RE, Clements ML. New knowledge on pathogenesis of bacterial enteric infections as applied to vaccine development. *Microbiol Rev* 1983;47:510–550.
2. Levine MM, Kaper JB, Herrington D, et al. Volunteer studies of deletion mutants of *Vibrio cholerae* O1 prepared by recombinant techniques. *Infect Immun* 1988;56:161–167.
3. Kelly CP, Pothoulakis C, LaMont JT. *Clostridium difficile* colitis. *N Engl J Med* 1994;330:257–262.
4. Lopez EL, Diaz M, Grinstein S, et al. Hemolytic uremic syndrome and diarrhea in Argentine children: the role of Shiga-like toxins. *J Infect Dis* 1989;160:469–475.
5. Nair GB, Takeda Y. Detection of toxins of *Vibrio cholerae* O1 and non-O1. In: Wachsmuth IK, Blake PA, Olsvik Ø, eds. *Vibrio cholerae and cholera: molecular to global perspectives.* Washington, DC: Am Soc Microbiol, 1994;53–67.
6. Merson MH, Yolken RH, Sack RB, et al. Detection of *Escherichia coli* enterotoxins in stools. *Infect Immun* 1980;29:108–113.
7. Keusch GT, Jacewicz M, Levine MM, Hornick RB, Kochwa S. Pathogenesis of *Shigella* diarrhea. Serum anticytotoxin antibody response produced by toxigenic and nontoxigenic *Shigella dysenteriae* 1. *J Clin Invest* 1976;57:194–202.
8. Cohen A, Madrid Marina V, Estrov Z, Freedman MH, Lingwood CA, Dosch HM. Expression of glycolipid receptors to Shiga-like toxin on human B lymphocytes: a mechanism for the failure of long-lived antibody response to dysenteric disease. *Int Immunol* 1990;2:1–8.
9. Merson MH, Morris GK, Sack DA, et al. Travelers' diarrhea in Mexico: a prospective study of physicians and family members attending a congress. *N Engl J Med* 1976;294:1299–1305.
10. Guerrant RL, Moore RA, Kirschenfeld PM, Sande MA. Role of toxigenic and invasive bacteria in acute diarrhea of childhood. *N Engl J Med* 1975;293:567–573.
11. Sack RB, Myers LL, Almeido-Hill J, et al. Enterotoxigenic *Bacteroides fragilis*: epidemiologic studies of its role as a human diarrhoeal pathogen. *J Diarrh Dis Res* 1992;5:4–9.
12. Sack RB, Albert MJ, Alam K, Neogi PKB, Akbar MS. Isolation of enterotoxigenic *Bacteroides fragilis* from Bangladeshi children with diarrhea: a case-control study. *J Clin Microbiol* 1994;32:960–963.
13. San Joaquin VH, Griffis JC, Lee C, Sears CL. Association of *Bacteroides fragilis* with childhood diarrhea. *J Clin Microbiol* 1994; submitted.
14. De SN. Enterotoxicity of bacteria-free culture filtrate of *Vibrio cholerae. Nature* 1959;183:1533–1534.
15. Delor I, Cornelis GR. Role of *Yersinia enterocolitica* Yst toxin in experimental infection in young rabbits. *Infect Immun* 1992;60:4269–4277.
16. Nishibuchi M, Fasano A, Russell RG, Kaper JB. Enterotoxigenicity of *Vibrio parahaemolyticus* with and without genes encoding thermostable direct hemolysin. *Infect Immun* 1992;60:3539–3545.
17. Hughes JM, Murad F, Chang B, Guerrant RL. Role of cyclic GMP in the action of heat-stable enterotoxin of *Escherichia coli. Nature* 1978;2;71:755–756.
18. Richardson SH, Giles JC, Kruger KS. Sealed adult mice: new model for enterotoxin evaluation. *Infect Immun* 1984;43:482–486.
19. Field M, Fromm D, Al-Awqati Q, Greenough WB III. Effect of cholera enterotoxin on ion transport across isolated ileal mucosa. *J Clin Invest* 1972;51:796–804.
20. Field M, Graf LH, Laird WJ, Smith PL. Heat-stable enterotoxin of *Escherichia coli: in vitro* effects on guanylate cyclase activity, cyclic GMP concentration, and ion transport in small intestine. *Proc Natl Acad Sci USA* 1978;75:2800–2804.
21. Guandalini S, Rao MC, Smith PL, Field M. cGMP modulation of ileal ion transport: in vitro effects of *Escherichia coli* heat-stable enterotoxin. *Am J Physiol* 1982;243:G36–G41.
22. Weikel CS, Nellans HN, Guerrant RL. In vivo and in vitro effects of a novel enterotoxin, STb, produced by *Escherichia coli. J Infect Dis* 1986;153:893–901.
23. Savarino SJ, Fasano A, Watson J, et al. Enteroaggregative *Escherichia coli* heat-stable enterotoxin 1 represents another subfamily of *E. coli* heat-stable toxin. *Proc Natl Acad Sci USA* 1993;90:3093–3097.
24. Savarino SJ, Fasano A, Robertson DC, Levine MM. Enteroaggregative *Escherichia coli* elaborate a heat-stable enterotoxin demonstrable in an in vitro rabbit intestinal model. *J Clin Invest* 1991;87:1450–1455.
25. Kandel G, Donohue-Rolfe A, Donowitz M, Keusch GT. Pathogenesis of *Shigella* diarrhea. 16. Selective targeting of shiga toxin to villus cells of rabbit jejunum explains the effect of the toxin on intestinal electrolyte transport. *J Clin Invest* 1989;84:1509–1517.
26. Fasano A, Kay BA, Russell RG, Maneval DR, Levine MM. Enterotoxin and cytotoxin production by enteroinvasive *Escherichia coli. Infect Immun* 1990;58:3717–3723.
27.
28. Fasano A, Maneval DR Jr, Noriega F, Nataro JP, Levine MM. Enterotoxic factors elaborated by *Shigella flexneri* 2a. *Abstr 29th Joint Conference on Cholera and Related Diarrheal Diseases* 1993;158–162.
29. Kaper JB, Fasano A, Trucksis M. Toxins of *Vibrio cholerae.* In: Wachsmuth IK, Blake P, Ølsvik O, eds. Vibrio cholerae and cholera. Washington, DC: Am Soc Microbiol; 1993:145–176.
30. Kaper JB, Morris JG Jr, Levine MM. Cholera. *Clin Microbiol Rev* 1994 [*in press*].
31. Peterson JW. Salmonella toxin. *Pharmacol Ther* 1980;11:719–724.
32. Peterson JW, Molina NC, Houston CW, Fader RC. Elevated cAMP in intestinal epithelial cells during experimental cholera and salmonellosis. *Toxicon* 1983;21:761–775.
33. Spangler BD. Structure and function of cholera toxin and the related *Escherichia coli* heat-labile enterotoxin. *Microbiol Rev* 1992;56:622–647.
34. Guerrant RL, Brunton LL, Schnaitman TC, Rebhun LI, Gilman AG. Cyclic adenosine monophosphate and alteration of Chinese hamster ovary cell morphology: a rapid, sensitive in vitro assay for the enterotoxins of *Vibrio cholerae* and *Escherichia coli. Infect Immun* 1974;10:320–327.
35. Donta ST, Moon HW, Whipp SC. Detection of heat-labile *Escherichia coli* enterotoxin with the use of adrenal cells in tissue culture. *Science* 1974;183:334–336.
36. O'Brien AD, Holmes RK. Shiga and Shiga-like toxins. *Microbiol Rev* 1987;51:206–220.
37. Terranova W, Blake PA. *Bacillus cereus* food poisoning. *N Engl J Med* 1978;298:143–144.
38. Tranter HS. Foodborne staphylococcal illness. *Lancet* 1990;336:1044–1046.
39. Ohishi I. Response of mouse intestinal loop to botulinum C_2 toxin: enterotoxic activity induced by cooperation of nonlinked protein components. *Infect Immun* 1983;40:691–695.
40. Ohishi I, Iwasaki M, Sakaguchi G. Purification and characterization of two components of botulinum C_2 toxin. *Infect Immun* 1980;30:668–673.
41. Miyake M, Honda T, Miwatani T. Purification and characterization of *Vibrio metschnikovii* cytolysin. *Infect Immun* 1988;56:954–960.
42. Johnson WM, Lior H. Response of Chinese hamster ovary cells to a cytolethal distending toxin (CDT) of *Escherichia coli* and

possible misinterpretation as heat-labile (LT) enterotoxin. *FEMS Microbiol Lett* 1987;43:19–23.

43. Bouzari S, Varghese A. Cytolethal distending toxin (CLDT) production by enteropathogenic *Escherichia coli*. *FEMS Microbiol Lett* 1990;71:193–198.

44. Caprioli A, Falbo V, Roda LG, Ruggeri FM, Zona C. Partial purification and characterization of an *Escherichia coli* toxic factor that induces morphological cell alterations. *Infect Immun* 1983;39:1300–1306.

45. De Rycke J, Gonzalez EA, Blanco J, Oswald E, Blanco M, Boivin R. Evidence for two types of cytotoxic necrotizing factor in human and animal clinical isolates of *Escherichia coli*. *J Clin Microbiol* 1990;28:694–699.

46. Blanco J, Blanco M, Alonso MP, Blanco JE, Garabal JI, Gonzalez EA. Serogroups of *Escherichia coli* strains producing cytotoxic necrotizing factors CNF1 and CNF2. *FEMS Microbiol Lett* 1992;96:155–160.

47. Gunzburg ST, Chang BJ, Elliott SJ, Burke V, Gracey M. Diffuse and enteroaggregative patterns of adherence of enteric *Escherichia coli* isolated from aboriginal children from the Kimberley region of western Australia. *J Infect Dis* 1993;167:755–758.

48. Jallat C, Livrelli V, Darfeuille-Michaud A, Rich C, Joly B. *Echerichia coli* strains involved in diarrhea in France: high prevalence and heterogeneity of diffusely adhering strains. *J Clin Microbiol* 1993;31:2031–2037.

49. Levine MM, Prado V, Robins-Browne R, et al. Use of DNA probes and HEp-2 cell adherence assay to detect diarrheagenic *Escherichia coli*. *J Infect Dis* 1988;158:224–228.

50. Cravioto A, Tello A, Navarro A, et al. Association of *Escherichia coli* HEp-2 adherence patterns with type and duration of diarrhoea. *Lancet* 1991;337:262–264.

51. Giron JA, Jones T, Millanvelasco F, et al. Diffuse-adhering *Escherichia coli* (DAEC) as a putative cause of diarrhea in Mayan children in Mexico. *J Infect Dis* 1991;163:507–513.

52. Fasano A, Baudry B, Pumplin DW, et al. *Vibrio cholerae* produces a second enterotoxin, which affects intestinal tight junctions. *Proc Natl Acad Sci USA* 1991;88:5242–5246.

53. Scaletsky ICA, Silva MLM, Trabulsi LR. Distinctive patterns of adherence of enteropathogenic *Escherichia coli* to HeLa cells. *Infect Immun* 1984;45:534–536.

54. Trucksis M, Galen JE, Michalski J, Fasano A, Kaper JB. Accessory cholera enterotoxin (Ace), the third toxin of a *Vibrio cholerae* virulence cassette. *Proc Natl Acad Sci USA* 1993;90:5267–5271.

55. Field M. Ion transport in rabbit ileal mucosa. II. Effects of cyclic 3′,5′-AMP. *Am J Physiol* 1971;221:992–997.

56. Kartner N, Hanrahan JW, Jensen TJ, et al. Expression of the cystic fibrosis gene in non-epithelial invertebrate cells produces a regulated anion conductance. *Cell* 1991;64:681–691.

57. Shapiro M, Matthews J, Hecht G, Delp C, Madara JL. Stabilization of F-actin prevents cAMP-elicited Cl⁻ secretion in T84 cells. *J Clin Invest* 1991;87:1903–1909.

58. Matthew JB, Awtrey CS, Madara JL. Microfilament-dependent activation of Na⁺/K⁺/2Cl⁻ cotransport by cAMP in intestinal epithelial monolayers. *J Clin Invest* 1992;90:1608–1613.

59. Peterson JW, Ochoa LG. Role of prostaglandins and cAMP in the secretory effects of cholera toxin. *Science* 1989;245:857–859.

60. de Jonge HR. Intracellular mechanisms regulating intestinal secretion. In: Wadström T, Mäkelä PH, Svennerholm A-M, Wolf-Watz H, eds. *Molecular pathogenesis of gastrointestinal infections*. New York: Plenum Press; 1991:107–114.

61. Guerrant RL, Fang GD, Thielman NM, Fonteles MC. Role of platelet activating factor (PAF) in the intestinal epithelial secretory and Chinese hamster ovary (CHO) cell cytoskeletal responses to cholera toxin. *Proc Natl Acad Sci USA* 1994;91:9655–9658.

62. Thielman NM, Fang GD, Barrett LJ, Fonteles MC, Guerrant RL. Inhibition of cholera toxin effects on intestinal secretion and Chinese hamster ovary cell elongation by platelet activating factor antagonists. *Abstr 29th Joint Conference on Cholera and Related Diarrheal Diseases,* Monterey, CA 1993:172–176.

63. Fang GD, Fonteles MC, Barrett LJ, Guerrant RL. Inhibition by platelet activating factor (PAF) antagonists of the effects of

choleratoxin on intestinal secretion and cytoskeleton of Chinese hamster ovary (CHO) cells. *Clin Res* 1993;41:222A.

64. Cassuto J, Jodal M, Tuttle R, Lundgren O. On the role of intramural nerves in the pathogenesis of cholera toxin-induced intestinal secretion. *Scand J Gastroenterol* 1981;16:377–384.

65. Mathias JR, Carlson GM, DiMarino AJ, Bertiger G, Morton HE, Cohen S. Intestinal myoelectric activity in response to live *Vibrio cholerae* and cholera enterotoxin. *J Clin Invest* 1976;58:91–96.

66. Lind CD, Davis RH, Guerrant RL, Kaper JB, Mathias JR. Effects of *Vibrio cholerae* recombinant strains on rabbit ileum in vivo. Enterotoxin production and myoelectric activity. *Gastroenterology* 1991;101:319–324.

67. Nilsson O, Cassuto J, Larsson P-A, et al. 5-Hydroxytryptamine and cholera secretion: a histochemical and physiological study in cats. *Gut* 1983;24:542–548.

68. Cassuto J, Fahrenkrug J, Jodal M, Tuttle R, Lundgren O. The release of vasoactive intestinal polypeptide from the cat small intestine exposed to cholera toxin. *Gut* 1981;22:958–963.

69. Cassuto J, Jodal M, Lundgren O. The effect of nicotinic and muscarinic receptor blockade on cholera toxin induced intestinal secretion in rats and cats. *Acta Physiol Scand* 1982;114:573–577.

70. Cassuto J, Siewert A, Jodal M, Lundgren O. The involvement of intramural nerves in cholera toxin induced intestinal secretion. *Acta Physiol Scand* 1983;117:195–202.

71. Thompson MR, Giannella RA. Revised amino acid sequence for a heat-stable enterotoxin produced by an *Escherichia coli* strain (18D) that is pathogenic for humans. *Infect Immun* 1985;47:834–836.

72. Dreyfus LA, Frantz JC, Robertson DC. Chemical properties of heat-stable enterotoxins produced by enterotoxigenic *Escherichia coli* of different host origins. *Infect Immun* 1983;42:539–548.

73. Waldman SA, O'Hanley P. Influence of a glycine or proline substitution on the functional properties of a 14-amino-acid analog of *Escherichia coli* heat-stable enterotoxin. *Infect Immun* 1989;57:2420–2424.

74. Yoshimura S, Ikemura H, Watanabe H, et al. Essential structure for full enterotoxigenic activity of heat-stable enterotoxin produced by enterotoxigenic *Escherichia coli*. *FEBS Lett* 1985;181:138–141.

75. Arita M, Honda T, Miwatani T, Ohmori K, Takao T, Shimonishi Y. Purification and characterization of a new heat-stable enterotoxin produced by *Vibrio cholerae* non-O1 serogroup Hakata. *Infect Immun* 1991;59:2186–2188.

76. Delor I, Kaeckenbeeck A, Wauters G, Cornelis GR. Nucleotide sequence of *yst*, the *Yersinia enterocolitica* gene encoding the heat-stable enterotoxin, and prevalence of the gene among pathogenic and nonpathogenic Yersiniae. *Infect Immun* 1990;58:2983–2988.

77. Schulz S, Green CK, Yuen PST, Garbers DL. Guanylyl cyclase is a heat-stable enterotoxin receptor. *Cell* 1990;63:941–948.

78. Currie MG, Fok KF, Kato J, et al. Guanylin: an endogenous activator of intestinal guanylate cyclase. *Proc Natl Acad Sci USA* 1992;89:947–951.

79. Forte LR, Eber SL, Turner JT, Freeman RH, Fok KF, Currie MG. Guanylin stimulation of Cl⁻ secretion in human intestinal T₈₄ cells via cyclic guanosine monophosphate. *J Clin Invest* 1993;91:2423–2428.

80. Knoop FC, Owens M, Marcus JN, Murphy B. Elevation of calcium in rat enterocytes by *Escherichia coli* heat-stable (STa) enterotoxin. *Curr Microbiol* 1991;23:291–296.

81. Lin M, Nairn AC, Guggino SE. cGMP-dependent protein kinase regulation of a chloride channel in T84 cells. *Am J Physiol (Cell Physiol)* 1992;262:C1304–C1312.

82. Forte LR, Thorne PK, Eber SL, et al. Stimulation of intestinal Cl⁻ transport by heat-stable enterotoxin: activation of cAMP-dependent protein kinase by cGMP. *Am J Physiol (Cell Physiol)* 1992;263:C607–C615.

83. Tien X-Y, Brasitus TA, Kaetzel MA, Dedman JR, Nelson DJ. Activation of the cystic fibrosis transmembrane conductance regulator by cGMP in the human colonic cancer cell line, Caco-2. *J Biol Chem* 1994;269:51–54.

84. Matthews JB, Awtrey CS, Thompson R, Hung T, Tally KJ, Madara JL. Na⁺-K⁺-2Cl⁻ cotransport and Cl⁻ secretion

evoked by heat-stable enterotoxin is microfilament dependent in T84 cells. *Am J Physiol* 1993;265:G370–G378.

85. Beubler E, Badhri P, Schirgi-Degen A. 5-HT receptor antagonists and heat-stable *Escherichia coli* enterotoxin-induced effects in the rat. *Eur J Pharmacol* 1992;219:445–450.

86. Banik ND, Ganguly U. Diacylglycerol breakdown in plasma membrane of rat intestinal epithelial cells. *FEBS Lett* 1989;250: 201–204.

87. Banik N, Ganguly U. Stimulation of phosphoinosites breakdown by the heat stable *E. coli* enterotoxin in rat intestinal epithelial cells. *FEBS Lett* 1988;236:489–492.

88. Eklund S, Jodal M, Lundgren O. The enteric nervous system participates in the secretory response to the heat stable enterotoxins of *Escherichia coli* in rats and cats. *Neuroscience* 1985; 14:673–681.

89. Mathias JR, Nogueira J, Martin JL, Carlson GM, Giannella RA. *Escherichia coli* heat-stable toxin: its effect on motility of the small intestine. *Am J Physiol* 1982;242:G360–G363.

90. Fiorentini C, Thelestam M. *Clostridium difficile* toxin A and its effects on cells. *Toxicon* 1991;29:543–567.

91. Tucker KD, Carrig PE, Wilkins TD. Toxin A of *Clostridium difficile* is a potent cytotoxin. *J Clin Microbiol* 1990;28: 869–871.

92. Lyerly DM, Lockwood DW, Richardson SH, Wilkins TD. Biological activities of toxins A and B of *Clostridium difficile*. *Infect Immun* 1982;35:1147–1150.

93. Lyerly DM, Saum KE, MacDonald DK, Wilkins TD. Effects of *Clostridium difficile* toxins given intragastrically to animals. *Infect Immun* 1985;47:349–352.

94. Mitchell TJ, Ketley JM, Burdon DW, Candy DCA, Stephen J. The effects of *Clostridium difficile* crude toxins and purified toxin A on stripped rabbit ileal mucosa in Ussing chambers. *J Med Microbiol* 1987;23:199–204.

95. Triadafilopoulos G, Pothoulakis C, O'Brien MJ, LaMont JT. Differential effects of *Clostridium difficile* toxins A and B on rabbit ileum. *Gastroenterology* 1987;93:273–279.

96. Lima AAM, Lyerly DM, Wilkins TD, Innes DJ, Guerrant RL. Effects of *Clostridium difficile* toxins A and B in rabbit small and large intestine in vivo and on cultured cells in vitro. *Infect Immun* 1988;56:582–588.

97. Lima AAM, Innes DJ, Jr., Chadee K, Lyerly DM, Wilkins TD, Guerrant RL. *Clostridium difficile* toxin A: interactions with mucus and early sequential histopathologic effects in rabbit small intestine. *Lab Invest* 1989;61:419–425.

98. Triadafilopoulos G, Pothoulakis C, Weiss R, Giampaolo C, LaMont JT. Comparative study of *Clostridium difficile* toxin A and cholera toxin in rabbit ileum. *Gastroenterology* 1989;97: 1186–1192.

99. Moore R, Pothoulakis C, LaMont JT, Carlson S, Madara J. *C. difficile* toxin A increases intestinal permeability and induces Cl⁻ secretion. *Am J Physiol* 1990;259:G165–G172.

100. Hecht G, Pothoulakis C, LaMont JT, Madara JL. *Clostridium difficile* toxin A perturbs cytoskeletal structure and tight junction permeability of the cultured human intestinal epithelial monolayers. *J Clin Invest* 1988;82:1516–1524.

101. Kelly CP, Becker S, Linevsky JK, et al. Neutrophil recruitment in *Clostridium difficile* toxin A enteritis in the rabbit. *J Clin Invest* 1994;93:1257–1265.

102. Pothoulakis C, Karmeli F, Kelly CP, et al. Ketofifen inhibits *Clostridium difficile* toxin A–induced enteritis in rat ileum. *Gastroenterol* 1993;105:701–707.

103. Fang GD, Lima AM, Adams R, Lyerly DM, Guerrant RL. Inhibition by quinacrine of the effects of *C. difficile* toxin A on intestinal secretion, and on T84 cell tissue resistance and F-actin. *Clin Res* 1991;39(2):185A.

104. Fang GD, Fonteles MC, Lima AAM, Lyerly DM, Guerrant RL. Inhibitors of phospholipase A₂ cyclooxygenase, and platelet activating factor (PAF) block the secretory and cytoskeletal effects of *C. difficile* toxin A. *IDSA Ann Mtg, Anaheim, CA, October 1992; #37* 1992.

105. Fang GD, Lima AAM, Thielman NM, et al. Role of phospholipase A₂ in the histologic, epithelial and secretory responses to *Clostridium difficile* toxin A. *Mol Medicine* 1994; [in press].

106. Fonteles MC, Fang GD, Thielman NM, Yotseff PS, Guerrant RL. Role of platelet activating factor in the inflammatory and secretory effects of *Clostridium difficile* toxin A. *J Lipid Mediators* 1994; [in press].

107. Guerrant RL. Lessons from diarrheal diseases: demography to molecular pharmacology. *J Infect Dis* 1994;169:1206–1218.

108. Pothoulakis C, Castagliuolo I, LaMont JT, et al. CP-96,345, a substance P antagonist, inhibits rat intestinal responses to *Clostridium difficile* toxin A but not cholera toxin. *Proc Natl Acad Sci USA* 1994;91:947–951.

109. Turnbull PCB. *Bacillus cereus* toxins. *Pharmacol Ther* 1981; 13:453–505.

110. Thompson NE, Ketterhagen MJ, Bergdoll MS, Schantz EJ. Isolation and some properties of an enterotoxin produced by *Bacillus cereus*. *Infect Immun* 1984;43:887–894.

111. Beecher DJ, Macmillan JD. A novel biocomponent hemolysin from *Bacillus cereus*. *Infect Immun* 1990;58:2220–2227.

112. Myers LL, Shoop DS, Firehammer BD, Border MM. Association of enterotoxigenic *Bacteroides fragilis* with diarrheal disease in calves. *J Infect Dis* 1985;152:1344–1347.

113. McClane BA, Hanna PC, Wnek AP. *Clostridium perfringens* enterotoxin. *Microb Pathog* 1988;4:317–323.

114. McDonel JL. In vivo effects of *Clostridium perfringens* enteropathogenic factors on the rat ileum. *Infect Immun* 1974;10: 1156–1162.

115. McClane BA, Wnek AP, Hulkower KI, Hanna PC. Divalent cation involvement in the action of *Clostridium perfringens* type A enterotoxin. *J Biol Chem* 1988;263:2423–2435.

116. McClane BA, McDonel JL. The effects of *Clostridium perfringens* enterotoxin on morphology, viability, and macromolecular synthesis in Vero cells. *J Cell Physiol* 1979;99:191–200.

117. Sugimoto N, Takagi M, Ozutsumi K, Harada S, Matsuda M. Enterotoxin of *Clostridium perfringens* type A forms ion-permeable channels in a lipid bilayer membrane. *Biochem Biophys Res Commun* 1988;156:551–556.

118. Raimondi F, Kaper JB, Kao JPY, Guandalini S, Fasano A. Calcium-dependent intestinal chloride secretion induced by the thermostable direct hemolysin of *Vibrio parahaemolyticus* in rabbit ileum; [submitted].

119. Asao T, Kinoshita Y, Kozaki S, Uemura T, Sakaguchi G. Purification and some properties of *Aeromonas hydrophila* hemolysin. *Infect Immun* 1984;46:122–127.

120. Houston CW, Chopra AK, Rose JM, Kurosky A. Review of *Aeromonas* enterotoxins. *Experientia* 1991;47:424–426.

121. Rose JM, Houston CW, Kurosky A. Bioactivity and immunological characterization of a cholera toxin-cross-reactive cytolytic enterotoxin from *Aeromonas hydrophila*. *Infect Immun* 1989;57:1170–1176.

122. Millership SE, Barer MR, Mulla RJ, Maneck S. Enterotoxic effects of *Aeromonas sobria* haemolysin in a rat jejunal perfusion system identified by specific neutralization with a monoclonal antibody. *J Gen Microbiol* 1992;138:261–267.

123. Dreyfus LA, Harville B, Howard DE, Shaban R, Beatty DM, Morris SJ. Calcium influx mediated by the *Escherichia coli* heat-stable enterotoxin B (ST$_B$). *Proc Natl Acad Sci USA* 1993; 90:3202–3206.

124. Aktories K, Wegner A. Mechanisms of the cytopathic action of actin-ADP-ribosylating toxins. *Mol Microbiol* 1992;6: 2905–2908.

125. Vandekerckhove J, Schering B, Bärmann M, Aktories K. Botulinum C₂ toxin ADP-ribosylates cytoplasmic beta/gamma-actin in arginine 177. *J Biol Chem* 1988;263:696–700.

126. Oswald E, Sugai M, Labigne A, et al. Cytotoxic necrotizing factor type 2 produced by virulent *Escherichia coli* modifies the small GTP-binding proteins Rho involved in assembly of actin stress fibers. *Proc Natl Acad Sci USA* 1994;91: 3814–3818.

127. Fiorentini C, Arancia G, Caprioli A, Falbo V, Ruggeri FM, Donelli G. Cytoskeletal changes induced in HEp-2 cells by the cytotoxic necrotizing factor of *Escherichia coli*. *Toxicon* 1988; 26:1047–1056.

128. Fiorentini C, Falzano L, Donelli G, Oswald E, Popoff MR, Boquet P. *E. coli* cytotoxic necrotizing factor I (CNF1) and its effects on cells. *Toxicon* 1993;31:501.

129. Just I, Fritz G, Aktories K, et al. *Clostridium difficile* toxin B acts on the GTP-binding protein Rho. *J Biol Chem* 1994;269: 10706–10712.

130. Tesh VL, O'Brien AD. The pathogenic mechanisms of Shiga

toxin and the Shiga-like toxins. *Mol Microbiol* 1991;5: 1817–1822.

131. Endo Y, Tsurugi K, Yutsudo T, Takeda Y, Ogasawara K, Igarashi K. The site of action of a verotoxin (VT2) from *Escherichia coli* O157:H7 and of Shiga toxin on eukaryotic ribosomes: RNA *N*-glycosidase activity of the toxins. *Eur J Biochem* 1988;171:45–50.

132. Wren BW. Bacterial enterotoxin interactions. In: Hormaeche CE, Penn CW, Smyth CJ, eds. *Molecular biology of bacterial infection: current status and future perspectives.* Cambridge: Cambridge University Press; 1992:127–147.

133. Gardner SE, Fowlston SE, George WL. Effect of iron on production of a possible virulence factor by *Plesiomonas shigelloides. J Clin Microbiol* 1990;28:811–813.

134. Mellor IR, Thomas DH, Sansom MSP. Properties of ion channels formed by *Staphylococcus aureus. Biochim Biophys Acta* 1988;942:280–294.

135. Bernheimer AW, Rudy B. Interactions between membranes and cytolytic peptides. *Biochim Biophys Acta* 1986;864:123–141.

136. Harville BA, Dreyfus LA. Involvement of 5-hydroxytryptamine and prostaglandin E2 in the intestinal secretory action of *Escherichia coli* heat-stable enterotoxin B (STb); [submitted].

137. Giannella RA, Gots RE, Charney AN, Greenough WB, Formal SB. Pathogenesis of *Salmonella*-mediated intestinal fluid secretion: activation of adenylate cyclase and inhibition by indomethacin. *Gastroenterology* 1975;69:1238–1245.

138. Chopra AK, Vo TN, Houston CW. Mechanism of action of a cytotonic enterotoxin produced by *Aeromonas hydrophila. FEMS Microbiol Lett* 1992;70:15–19.

139. Ljungh Å, Eneroth P, Wadström T. Cytotonic enterotoxin from *Aeromonas hydrophila. Toxicon* 1982;20:787–794.

140. Potomski J, Burke V, Robinson J, Fumarola D, Miragliotta G. *Aeromonas* cytotonic enterotoxin cross reactive with cholera toxin. *J Med Microbiol* 1987;23:179–186.

141. Turnbull PCB, Kramer JM, Jorgensen K, Gilbert RJ, Melling J. Properties and production characteristics of vomiting, diarrheal, and necrotizing toxins of *Bacillus cereus. Am J Clin Nutr* 1979;32:219–228.

142. Weikel CS, Grieco FD, Reuben J, Myers LL, Sack RB. Human colonic epithelial cells, HT29/C1, treated with crude *Bacteroides fragilis* enterotoxin dramatically alter their morphology. *Infect Immun* 1992;60:321–327.

143. Van Tassell RL, Lyerly DM, Wilkins TD. Purification and characterization of an enterotoxin from *Bacteroides fragilis. Infect Immun* 1992;60:1343–1350.

144. Walker RI, Caldwell MB, Lee EC, Guerry P, Trust T, Ruiz-Palacios GM. Pathophysiology of *Campylobacter* enteritis. *Microbiol Rev* 1986;50:81–94.

145. Ruiz-Palacios GM, Torres J, Torres NI, Escamilla E, Ruiz-Palacios BR, Tamayo J. Cholera-like enterotoxin produced by *Campylobacter jejuni. Lancet* 1983;2:250–252.

146. Guerrant RL, Wanke CA, Pennie RA, Barrett LJ, Lima AAM, O'Brien AD. Production of a unique cytotoxin by *Campylobacter jejuni. Infect Immun* 1987;55:2526–2530.

147. Mahajan S, Rodgers FG. Isolation, characterization, and host-cell-binding properties of a cytotoxin from *Campylobacter jejuni. J Clin Microbiol* 1990;28:1314–1320.

148. Perez-Perez GI, Cohn DL, Guerrant RL, Patton CM, Reller LB, Blaser MJ. Clinical and immunologic significance of cholera-like toxin and cytotoxin production by *Campylobacter* species in patients with acute inflammatory diarrhea in the USA. *J Infect Dis* 1989;160:460–467.

149. Johnson WM, Lior H. A new heat-labile cytolethal distending toxin (CLDT) produced by *Campylobacter* spp. *Microb Pathog* 1988;4:115–126.

150. Ohishi I, Miyake M, Ogura H, Nakamura S. Cytopathic effect of botulinum C_2 toxin on tissue-culture cells. *FEMS Microbiol Lett* 1984;23:281–284.

151. Just I, Wille M, Chaponnier C, Aktories K. Gelsolin-actin complex is target for ADP-ribosylation by *Clostridium botulinum* C2 toxin in intact human neutrophils. *Eur J Pharm* 1994;246:293–297.

152. Lyerly DM, Krivan HC, Wilkins TD. *Clostridium difficile:* its disease and toxins. *Clin Microbiol Rev* 1988;1:1–18.

153. Pothoulakis C, Barone LM, Ely R, et al. Purification and properties of *Clostridium difficile* cytotoxin B. *J Biol Chem* 1986; 261:1316–1321.

154. Bartholomew BA, Stringer MF. *Clostridium perfringens* enterotoxin: a brief review. *Biochem Soc Trans* 1984;12:195–197.

155. McDonel JL. The molecular mode of action of *Clostridium perfringens* enterotoxin. *Am J Clin Nutr* 1979;32:210–218.

156. Lawrence G, Cooke R. Experimental pigbel: the production and pathology of necrotizing enteritis due to *Clostridium welchii* type C in the guinea pig. *Br J Exp Pathol* 1980;61:261–271.

157. Hunter SE, Brown JE, Oyston PCF, Sakurai J, Titball RW. Molecular genetic analysis of beta-toxin of *Clostridium perfringens* reveals sequence homology with alpha-toxin, gamma-toxin, and leukocidin of *Staphylococcus aureus. Infect Immun* 1993;61:3958–3965.

158. Titball RW, Leslie DL, Harvey S, Kelly D. Hemolytic and sphingomyelinase activities of *Clostridium perfringens* alpha-toxin are dependent on a domain homologous to that of an enzyme from the human arachidonic acid pathway. *Infect Immun* 1991;59:1872–1874.

159. Diener M, Eglème C, Rummel W. Phospholipase C-induced anion secretion and its interaction with carbachol in the rat colonic mucosa. *Eur J Pharmacol* 1991;299:267–276.

160. Skjelkvåle R, Duncan CL. Characterization of enterotoxin purified from *Clostridium perfringens* type C. *Infect Immun* 1975; 11:1061–1068.

161. Skjelkvåle R, Duncan CL. Enterotoxin formation by different toxigenic types of *Clostridium perfringens. Infect Immun* 1975; 11:563–575.

162. Baldwin TJ, Knutton S, Sellers L, Hernandez HAM, Aitken A, Williams PH. Enteroaggregative *Escherichia coli* strains secrete a heat-labile toxin antigenically related to *E. coli* hemolysin. *Infect Immun* 1992;60:2092–2095.

163. Moyer MP, Dixon PS, Rothman SW, Brown JE. Cytotoxicity of Shiga toxin for primary cultures of human colonic and ileal epithelial cells. *Infect Immun* 1987;55:1533–1535.

164. Sjogren R, Neill R, Rachmilewitz D, et al. Role of Shiga-like toxin I in bacterial enteritis: Comparison between isogenic *Escherichia coli* strains induced in rabbits. *Gastroenterology* 1994;106:306–317.

165. Nataro JP, Seriwatana J, Fasano A, Noriega F, Guers L, Morris JG Jr. Cloning and sequencing of a new plasmid-encoded enterotoxin in enteroinvasive *E. coli* and *Shigella. Abstr 28th Joint Conference on Cholera and Related Diarrheal Diseases* Monterey 1993;144–147.

166. Huott PA, Liu W, McRoberts JA, Giannella RA, Dharmsathaphorn K. Mechanism of action of *Escherichia coli* heat stable enterotoxin in a human colonic cell line. *J Clin Invest* 1988;82:514–523.

167. Whipp SC. Protease degradation of *Escherichia coli* heat-stable mouse-negative pig-positive enterotoxin. *Infect Immun* 1987; 55:2057–2060.

168. Whipp SC. Assay for enterotoxigenic *Escherichia coli* heat-stable toxin b in rats and mice. *Infect Immun* 1990;58:930–934.

169. Weikel CS, Tiemens K, Moseley S, Guerrant RL. Species specificity and lack of production of STb enterotoxin by *Escherichia coli* strains isolated from humans with diarrheal illness. *Infect Immun* 1986;52:323–325.

170. Whipp SC, Moseley SL, Moon HW. Microscopic alterations in jejunal epithelium of 3-week-old pigs induced by pig-specific, mouse-negative, heat-stable *Escherichia coli* enterotoxin. *Am J Vet Res* 1986;47:615–618.

171. Whipp SC, Kokue E, Morgan RW, Rose R, Moon HW. Functional significance of histologic alterations induced by *Escherichia coli* pig-specific, mouse-negative, heat-stable enterotoxin (ST$_b$). *Vet Res Commun* 1987;11:41–55.

172. Chang PP, Moss J, Twiddy EM, Holmes RK. Type II heat-labile enterotoxin of *Escherichia coli* activates adenylate cyclase in human fibroblasts by ADP ribosylation. *Infect Immun* 1987;55:1854–1858.

173. Donta ST, Tomicic T, Holmes RK. Binding of class II *Escherichia coli* enterotoxins to mouse Y1 and intestinal cells. *Infect Immun* 1992;60:2870–2873.

174. Lee CM, Chang PP, Tsai SC, et al. Activation of *Escherichia coli* heat-labile enterotoxins by native and recombinant adeno-

sine diphosphate-ribosylation factors, 20-kD guanine nucleo-tide-binding proteins. *J Clin Invest* 1991;87:1780–1786.

175. Holmes RK, Twiddy EM, Pickett CL. Purification and characterization of type II heat-labile enterotoxin of *Escherichia coli*. *Infect Immun* 1986;53:464–473.

176. Scott DA, Kaper JB. Cloning and sequencing of the genes encoding *Escherichia coli* cytolethal distending toxin. *Infect Immun* 1994;62:244–251.

177. Saraswathi B, Agarwal RK, Sanyal SC. Further studies on enteropathogenicity of *Plesiomonas shigelloides*. *Ind J Med Res* 1983;78:12–18.

178. Matthews BG, Douglas H, Guiney DG. Production of a heat stable enterotoxin by *Plesiomonas shigelloides*. *Microb Pathog* 1988;5:207–213.

179. Chopra AK, Peterson JW, Chary P, Prasad R. Molecular characterization of an enterotoxin from *Salmonella typhimurium*. *Microb Pathog* 1994;16:85–98.

180. Khurana S, Ganguly NK, Khullar M, Panigrahi D, Walia BNS. Studies on the mechanism of *Salmonella typhimurium* enterotoxin-induced diarrhoea. *Biochim Biophys Acta* 1991;1097:171–176.

181. Fontaine A, Arondel J, Sansonetti PJ. Role of Shiga toxin in the pathogenesis of bacillary dysentery, studied by using a Tox⁻ mutant of *Shigella dysenteriae* 1. *Infect Immun* 1988;56:3099–3109.

182. Sullivan R, Asano T. Effects of staphylococcal enterotoxin B on intestinal transport in the rat. *Am J Physiol* 1971;220:1793–1797.

183. Huang KC, Chen TST, Rout WR. Effect of staphylococcal enterotoxins A,B, and C, on ion transport and permeability across the flounder intestine. *Proc Soc Exp Biol Med* 1974;147:250–254.

184. Elias J, Shields R. Influence of staphylococcal enterotoxin on water and electrolyte transport in the small intestine. *Gut* 1976;17:527–535.

185. Johnson HM, Russell JK, Pontzer CH. Staphylococcal enterotoxin microbial superantigens. *FASEB J* 1991;5:2706–2712.

186. Kapral FA. *Staphylococcus aureus* delta toxin as an enterotoxin. In: Evered D, Whelan J, eds. *Microbial toxins and diarrhoeal disease*. London: Pitman; 1985:215–229.

187. Kapral FA, O'Brien AD, Ruff PD, Drugan WJ Jr. Inhibition of water absorption in the intestine by *Staphylococcus aureus* delta-toxin. *Infect Immun* 1976;13:140–145.

188. O'Brien AD, McClung HJ, Kapral FA. Increased tissue conductance and ion transport in guinea pig ileum after exposure to *Staphylococcus aureus* delta-toxin in vitro. *Infect Immun* 1978;21:102–113.

189. O'Brien AD, Kapral FA. Increased cyclic adenosine 3′,5′-monophosphate content in guinea pig ileum after exposure to *Staphylococcus aureus* delta-toxin. *Infect Immun* 1976;13:152–162.

190. Ichinose Y, Yamamoto K, Nakasone N, et al. Enterotoxicity of El Tor-like hemolysin of non-O1 *Vibrio cholerae*. *Infect Immun* 1987;55:1090–1093.

191. Krasilnikov OV, Muratkhodjaev JN, Zitzer AO. The mode of action of *Vibrio cholerae* cytolysin. The influences on both erythrocytes and planar lipid bilayers. *Biochim Biophys Acta* 1992;1111:7–16.

192. Honda T, Finkelstein RA. Purification and characterization of a hemolysin produced by *Vibrio cholerae* biotype El Tor: another toxic substance produced by cholera vibrios. *Infect Immun* 1979;26:1020–1027.

193. Robins-Browne RM, Takeda T, Fasano A, et al. Assessment of enterotoxin production by *Yersinia enterocolitica* and identification of a novel heat-stable enterotoxin produced by a noninvasive *Y. enterocolitica* strain isolated from clinical material. *Infect Immun* 1993;61:764–767.

194. Nishibuchi M, Khaeomanee-iam V, Honda T, Kaper JB, Miwa-

tani T. Comparative analysis of the hemolysin genes of *Vibrio cholerae* non-01, *V. mimicus*, and *V. hollisae* that are similar to the *tdh* gene of *V. parahaemolyticus*. *FEMS Microbiol Lett* 1990;55:251–256.

195. Levine MM, Black RE, Clements ML, Nalin DR, Cisneros L, Finkelstein RA. Volunteer studies in development of vaccines against cholera and enterotoxigenic *Escherichia coli*: a review. In: Holme T, Holmgren J, Merson MH, Mollby R, eds. *Acute enteric infections in children. New prospects for treatment and prevention.* Amsterdam: Elsevier; 1981:443–459.

196. Beubler E, Hinterleitner T, Horina G. Protein kinase C and intestinal fluid secretion: involvement of prostaglandin E2 but not of 5-hydroxytryptamine. *Eur J Pharmacol* 1990;182:543–548.

197. Morris JG Jr, Takeda T, Tall BD, et al. Experimental non-0 group 1 *Vibrio cholerae* gastroenteritis in humans. *J Clin Invest* 1990;85:697–705.

198. DuPont HL, Levine MM, Hornick RB, Formal SB. Inoculum size in shigellosis and implications for expected mode of transmission. *J Infect Dis* 1989;159:1126–1128.

199. Levine MM, Nalin DR, Hoover DL, Bergquist EJ, Hornick RB, Young CR. Immunity to enterotoxigenic *Escherichia coli*. *Infect Immun* 1979;23:729–736.

200. Levine MM, Bergquist EJ, Nalin DR, et al. *Escherichia coli* strains that cause diarrhoea but do not produce heat-labile or heat-stable enterotoxins and are non-invasive. *Lancet* 1978;1:1119–1122.

201. DuPont HL, Formal SB, Hornick RB, et al. Pathogenesis of *Escherichia coli* diarrhea. *N Engl J Med* 1971;285:1–9.

202. Mathewson JJ, Johnson PC, DuPont HL, Satterwhite TK, Winsor DK. Pathogenicity of enteroadherent *Escherichia coli* in adult volunteers. *J Infect Dis* 1986;154:524–527.

203. Tacket CO, Moseley SL, Kay B, Losonsky G, Levine MM. Challenge studies in volunteers using *Escherichia coli* strains with diffuse adherence to HEp-2 cells. *J Infect Dis* 1990;162:550–552.

204. Hormache E, Peluffo C-A, Aleppo P-L. Nueva contribucion al estudio etiologica de las "Diarrheas infantiles de Verano." *Arch Urug Med* 1936;9:113–162.

205. Hornick RB, Greisman SE, Woodward TE, DuPont HL, Dawkins AT, Snyder MJ. Typhoid fever: pathogenesis and immunological control. *N Engl J Med* 1970;283:686–691.

206. Black RE, Levine MM, Clements ML, Hughes TP, Blaser MJ. Experimental *Campylobacter jejuni* infection in humans. *J Infect Dis* 1988;157:472–479.

207. Sanyal SC, Sen PC. Human volunteer study on the pathogenicity of *Vibrio parahaemolyticus*. In: Fujino T, Sakaguchi G, Sakazaki R, Takeda Y, eds. *International symposium on Vibrio parahaemolyticus*. Tokyo: Saikon; 1974:227–230.

208. Morgan DR, Johnson PC, DuPont HL, Satterwhite TK, Wood LV. Lack of correlation between known virulence properties of *Aeromonas hydrophila* and enteropathogenicity for humans. *Infect Immun* 1985;50:62–65.

209. Svennerholm AM, Gothefors L, Sack DA, Bardhan PK, Holmgren J. Local and systemic antibody responses and immunological memory in humans after immunization with cholera B subunit by different routes. *Bull WHO* 1984;62:909–918.

210. Levine MM, Black RE, Clements ML, et al. The pathogenicity of nonenterotoxigenic *Vibrio cholerae* serogroup O1 biotype El Tor isolated from sewage water in Brazil. *J Infect Dis* 1982;145:296–299.

211. Inoue R, Okamoto K, Moriyama T, Takahashi T, Shimizu K, Miyama A. Effect of *Yersinia enterocolitica* ST on cyclic guanosine 3′,5′-monophosphate levels in mouse intestines and cultured cells. *Microbiol Immunol* 1983;27:159–166.

212. Elwell MR, Liu CT, Spertzel RO, Beisel WR. Mechanisms of oral staphylococcal enterotoxin B-induced emesis in the monkey. *Proc Soc Exp Biol Med* 1975;148:424–427.

Infections of the Gastrointestinal Tract,
edited by M. J. Blaser, P. D. Smith, J. I. Ravdin,
H. B. Greenberg, and R. L. Guerrant
Raven Press, Ltd., New York © 1995.

CHAPTER 45

Intracellular Mediators and Mechanisms of Pathogen-Induced Alterations in Intestinal Electrolyte Transport

Judy H. Cho and Eugene B. Chang

Pathogen-induced diarrheal diseases result when the balance that normally exists between intestinal absorption and secretion is lost and excessive net secretion of fluid and electrolytes occurs. Although the intracellular mechanisms that mediate these events are complex and only partially understood, we will highlight signal transduction and cellular events known to be initiated by diarrhea-associated pathogens and review how intracellular mediators might cause excessive net secretion. In addition, we will describe potential molecular mechanisms that may affect the expression of specific ion transport proteins and discuss recently described cellular mechanisms that may mediate the diarrheal actions of certain pathogens.

GENERAL MECHANISMS OF PATHOGEN-INDUCED DIARRHEAL DISEASES

Gastrointestinal infections cause diarrhea through a number of different mechanisms depending on the specific pathogen involved. Some of these processes are summarized in Table 1. In the classic toxin-mediated diarrheas induced by noninvasive pathogens such as *Vibrios cholerae,* binding of the bacterial toxin to intestinal epithelial cell receptors has no effect on mucosal histology, but results in a severe functional derangement of water and electrolyte transport, mediated via an increase in the concentration of cAMP (1). Other toxins such as the Shiga toxin have cytotoxic properties that result in significant compromise of intestinal barrier function (2). Barrier and absorptive functions can also be compromised by noncytotoxic toxins from organisms such as *Clostridium difficile,*

J. H. Cho and E. B. Chang: Department of Medicine, Gastroenterology Section, University of Chicago, Chicago, Illinois 60637.

which secretes toxin A which appears to alter epithelial cytoskeletal elements essential for microvillar and tight junction integrity (3). It is important to note, however, that some diarrheal processes resulting from gastrointestinal infections are in fact not mediated by bacterial enterotoxins. For example, following penetration across the mucosal barrier, pathogens frequently evoke an inflammatory response that produces a wide array of immune and inflammatory mediators within the bowel wall, which are capable of directly and indirectly stimulating net intestinal secretion. Alternatively, some lysates of the pathogens themselves contain neurohumoral mediators known to stimulate net secretion. Details of these pathogenic processes are described below.

ABSORPTION AND SECRETION IN THE NORMAL INTESTINE

Most infectious pathogens that cause diarrhea target normal processes involved in intestinal water and electrolyte transport. Although patients and physicians consider the development of diarrhea undesirable, the stimulation of net secretions and the resulting diarrhea are important host defenses that purge the gut of harmful pathogens and provide the aqueous vehicle for luminal delivery of secreted IgA antibodies. Equally important, however, the presence of endogenous counterregulatory mechanisms is essential, as the perturbations caused by the pathogens have to be bridled to prevent life-threatening volume and metabolic disturbances, and, during the recovery period, normal salt and water homeostasis must be restored (4). Thus, it is important that the normal physiological events and regulation of fluid and electrolyte transport by the gut be briefly reviewed.

The average daily fluid load to the gastrointestinal tract

TABLE 1. *Mechanism by which gastrointestinal infections cause diarrhea*

Agent in process	Mechanism	Consequences
(1) Enterotoxins	Increased net secretion Increased mucosal permeability	Luminal accumulation of fluid Decreased absorptive capability, "leaky bowel"
(2) Cytotoxin	Mucosal destruction and destruction and inflammation	Loss of absorptive area Transudation
(3) Inflammation	Elaboration of inflammatory mediator secretagogues Stimulation of enteric secretomotor neurons Alteration of blood flow	Increased net secretion Loss of surface area Decreased transit time

is 9 L, which comes from approximately 2 L of ingested fluids and 7 L of endogenous secretions originating from salivary, intestinal, pancreatic, and biliary sources. The intestinal tract must absorb most of the fluid load and excrete less than 200 mL of stool volume per day (assuming a Western culture diet), or diarrhea, defined as greater than 200 g/day, would be a regular and unconscionable event. In addition, the absorptive and secretory functions of the gut must be adaptable so that rapid compensations to potentially large fluctuations in fluid and dietary loads can be made. Fortunately, this is possible because absorptive and secretory functions of the gut are tightly regulated by complex neural and hormonal mechanisms that can adjust regional fluid and electrolyte transport processes in response to variations in luminal load and metabolic or volume requirements of the body.

Several neurohumoral agents present in the intestine have been identified that can stimulate net absorption (proabsorptive agents) or net secretion (secretagogues). Secretagogues stimulate net secretion by inhibiting active absorption of NaCl and/or stimulating active secretion of anions such as chloride. Conversely, proabsorptive agents stimulate net absorption by stimulating active absorption of NaCl and/or inhibiting anion secretion. They can affect intestinal transport by directly binding to epithelial cell receptors of the intestine that increase concentrations of intracellular mediators such as cAMP, calcium, and cGMP, resulting in net secretion. In contrast, norepinephrine, released from sympathetic neurons within the intestinal wall, is a proabsorptive agent that binds to α_2-adrenergic receptors of intestinal epithelia to enhance Na absorption and inhibit active anion secretion. Although the precise cellular mechanisms mediating its effects are incompletely understood, norepinephrine may in part act

by decreasing stimulated levels of intracellular cAMP (5,6). Table 2 lists several known neurohumoral agents and their corresponding second messengers that appear to have direct epithelial effects on intestinal water and electrolyte transport.

Neural, paracrine, and humoral agents also indirectly affect intestinal water and electrolyte transport. Some are known to affect secretomotor neurons of the gut, which can augment and amplify the actions of the original agent. As an example, prostaglandins secreted by lamina propria cells such as resident macrophages and subepithelial fibroblasts (7) stimulate secretomotor neurons and directly activate epithelial receptors to cause net secretion (8–10). The former results in the release of several neural secretagogues (e.g., acetylcholine and serotonin), which further stimulates net intestinal secretion and initiates propulsive motor contractions. In addition, these agents may affect blood flow, which may play an important part in the secretory process (11,12). Table 3 lists several agents that can cause net secretion through a variety of pathways.

CELLULAR MECHANISMS OF PATHOGEN-INDUCED NET INTESTINAL SECRETION

Direct Effects of Pathogens on Intestinal Epithelial Cell Ion Transport Function

Enterotoxin-Stimulated Increases in cAMP of Intestinal Epithelial Cells

Vibrio cholerae is the classic noninvasive pathogen that produces profuse watery diarrhea via an enterotoxin-me-

TABLE 2. *Hormones and neurotransmitters that directly stimulate secretion or inhibit absorption in intestine*

Vasoactive intestinal	Calcium	Cyclic GMP
Vasoactive intestinal peptide	Acetylcholine	Guanylin
Bradykinin	Serotonin	Acetylcholine (?)
Histamine	Bradykinin	
Prostaglandins		

TABLE 3. *Secretagogues and their sites of action*

Secretagogue	Epithelial cells	Enteric neurons	Lamina propria cells
Prostaglandins	X	X	X
Bradykinin	X	—	X
Adenosine	X	?	?
Histamine	X	X	—
ROMs	X	X	X
PAF	X	X	X
Serotonin	X	X	—
Acetylcholine	X	X	—
Nitric oxide	X	X	X

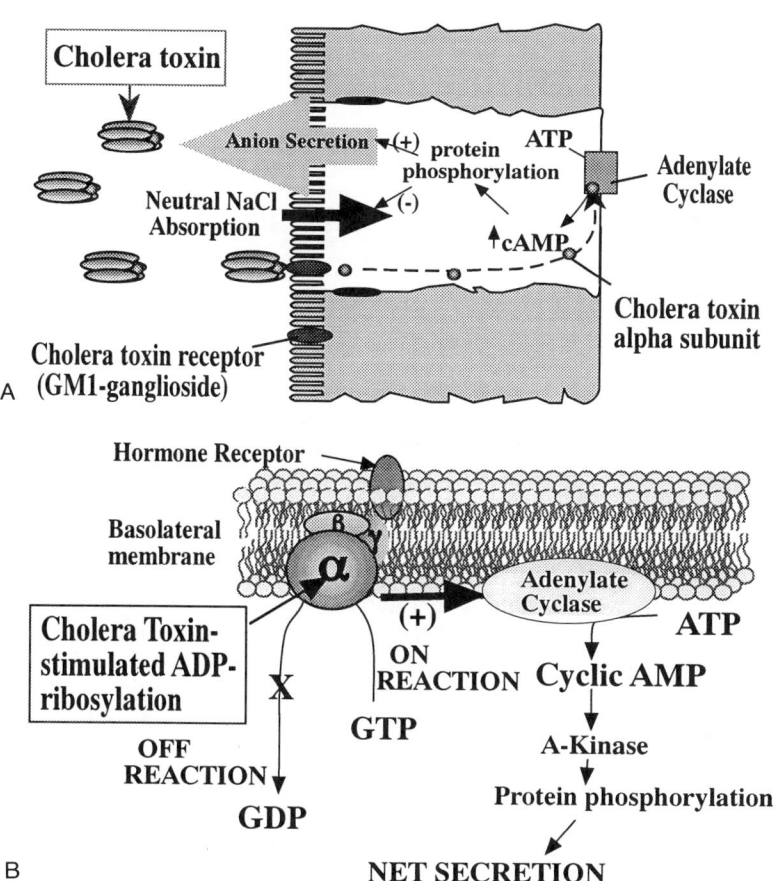

FIG. 1. Mechanism of action of cholera toxin. **A:** Binding of cholera toxin increases cAMP production by adenylate cyclase, resulting in phosphorylation of transport proteins that stimulates anion secretion and inhibits neutral NaCl absorption. **B:** Regulation of adenylate cyclase is under the dual control of stimulatory and inhibitory, G_s and G_i, subunits of membrane-transducing heterotrimeric G proteins.

diated increase in intracellular cAMP. The cholera toxin consists of α and β subunits, their properties described in greater depth by other chapters of this book. As shown in Fig. 1A, the β subunits bind to a specific receptor, GM1 ganglioside, on the apical surface of the intestinal enterocyte, but it is the α subunit that eventually enters the cell, probably through an endocytic pathway. Then it irreversibly stimulates ADP ribosylation of an arginine residue on G_s, the stimulatory subunit of a heterotrimeric G protein, located in the basolateral membrane of enterocytes. G proteins are membrane-associated heterotrimers that normally act to transduce extracellular signals from neurohumoral agents across the plasma membrane into the cell, resulting in an alteration in the concentrations of intracellular second messengers. As shown in Fig. 1B, adenylate cyclase is under the dual regulatory control of stimulatory, G_s, and inhibitory, G_i, subunits. Binding of the cholera toxin causes irreversible activation of G_s and thus adenylate cyclase, resulting in significant increases in cytosolic cAMP (1,13–15).

A significant part of cAMP effects are mediated via activation of cAMP-dependent protein kinases (A kinases). Protein kinases catalyze the transfer of the terminal phosphate of ATP to the hydroxyl group on a serine, threonine, or tyrosine residue of target proteins to form a phosphomonoester bond. This adds two negative charges to the substrate protein, resulting in a conformational change that affects the protein's activity (16,17). Although most of the substrates that are relevant to the processes of acti-

vated anion secretion and inhibited NaCl absorption are not known, it is speculated that these proteins are either involved in the regulation of ion transport or are themselves transport proteins. Examples of the latter may be the cystic fibrosis transmembrane regulator (CFTR) protein and luminal membrane Na/H exchangers (NHE). As will be discussed later, CFTR is involved in Cl secretion and appears to be phosphorylated by cAMP-dependent protein kinase, resulting in increased Cl^- conductance (18–20). On the other hand, the luminal NHE isoforms, NHE-2 and NHE-3, have consensus regions in their c-terminal domains for phosphorylation by cAMP-dependent protein kinase (21–24). Whether these are actual sites of phosphorylation and whether they lead to altered Na transport activity is not known. A greater discussion of these mechanisms is provided later.

Enterotoxin-Induced Alterations in Intracellular cGMP

Infections with *E. coli* producing heat-stable enterotoxin, ST_a, result in the stimulation of net intestinal secretion caused by an increase in the concentration of the intracellular mediator cyclic GMP (cGMP) (25–27). ST_a does not appear to stimulate concomitant increases in intracellular cAMP or calcium. In contrast to cholera toxin where activation of adenylate cyclase follows several intermediate events, the ST_a receptor itself appears to have intrinsic guanylyl cyclase activity. The binding of the

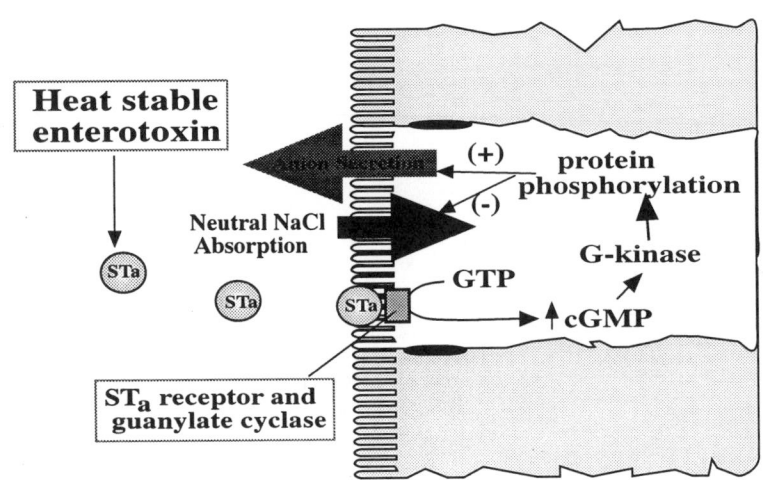

FIG. 2. Mechanism of action of *E. coli*–associated heat-stable enterotoxin, ST_a. Binding of ST_a to its receptor directly results in activation of guanylate cyclase and an increase in intracellular cGMP.

toxin to this receptor activates the enzyme, which then hydrolyzes GTP, resulting in increases in intracellular concentrations of cGMP (Fig. 2). It is not known at the present time whether the activation of guanylate cyclase activity involves a GTP-binding protein. In addition, the ST_a receptor guanyl cyclase is a particulate form of guanylyl cyclase (28), as opposed to the soluble forms, which are stimulated by agents such as nitric oxide.

Much insight has been gained in the past several years into the nature of the ST_a receptor. For years, the conundrum of why the gut would have a specific ST_a receptor or why physiological activators of enterocyte guanyl cyclase activity could not be identified remained unsolved. However, in 1992 Currie et al. (29) identified a unique gut peptide called guanylin that specifically bound and activated the ST_a receptor. Because this subject is extensively discussed in other chapters of this book, its review here will be brief and aspects only relevant to ion transport will be discussed. Guanylin appears to be made by intestinal epithelial cells, albeit its expression is greater in intestinal crypt cells. In contrast, the expression of the guanylin and putative ST_a receptor (30) appears to be highest in the midvillus regions of the small intestine and upper crypt areas of the colon. Although ST_a and guanylin bind to the guanylin receptor, ST_a appears to have greater affinity. This has led some to suspect that other guanylin-like receptors may exist (31). Indeed, this may be true, as other binding sites and molecular forms of the guanylin receptor have now been identified.

The activation of guanylyl cyclase by binding of exogenous agents such as heat-stable enterotoxin, ST_a, or endogenous agents such as guanylin results in an increase in the hydrolysis of GTP to form cGMP. Two groups of cGMP-dependent kinases (G kinases) have been identified, and G kinase II is localized to intestinal brush border (32). In addition, gradients of expression of G kinase II have been demonstrated with higher levels of expression being noted in the absorptive villus regions than in the crypt regions. This correlates with the pattern of expression observed with guanylyl cyclase, with definite levels of transcript being observed at the crypt–villus junction, and increasing levels of expression observed at the villus

tip (33). Of note is that activation of G kinases results in less stimulation of secretion compared to activation by A kinases, whereas the inhibition of NaCl absorption induced by the two types of kinases is comparable (34).

While stimulation of net intestinal secretion with ST_a is unassociated with increases in intracellular cAMP or calcium, addition of ST_a to either carbachol or phorbol esters (which activate protein kinase C, similar to the effects of endogenously produced diacylglycerol) results in a synergistic effect on net secretion. This effect has been attributed to protein kinase C (PKC)–stimulated phosphorylation of guanylyl cyclase, resulting in its activation (35).

Pathogen-Induced Intestinal Secretion Mediated by Increases in Cytosolic Calcium

Besides enterotoxins, gastrointestinal pathogens are known to produce a variety of neurohumoral agents that may directly increase net intestinal secretion. This has been best defined with *Entamoeba histolytica* lysates, which have been shown to contain serotonin, neurotensin, substance P, and acetylcholine, i.e., secretagogues that appear able to increase intestinal epithelial cytosolic calcium (36). Because the receptors for these agents are believed to be located in the basolateral membrane of epithelial cells, it is likely that the pathogens must breach the mucosal barrier to be able to stimulate net secretion by such a mechanism. Stimulation of cholinergic muscarinic and serotonin receptors results in the activation of phospholipase C, which hydrolyzes the membrane phospholipid, phosphatidylinositol 4,5-bisphosphate (PIP2), to yield diacylglycerol (DAG) and inositol 1,4,5-trisphosphate (IP_3) (37) (Fig. 3). These G-protein–linked receptors are characterized by having seven transmembrane spanning domains. Following binding of the agonist to the receptor, a conformational change in the second and third cytoplasmic loops causes the membrane-associated G protein to dissociate into α and βγ subunits. Both subunits are then able to activate different phospholipase C isoenzymes (38).

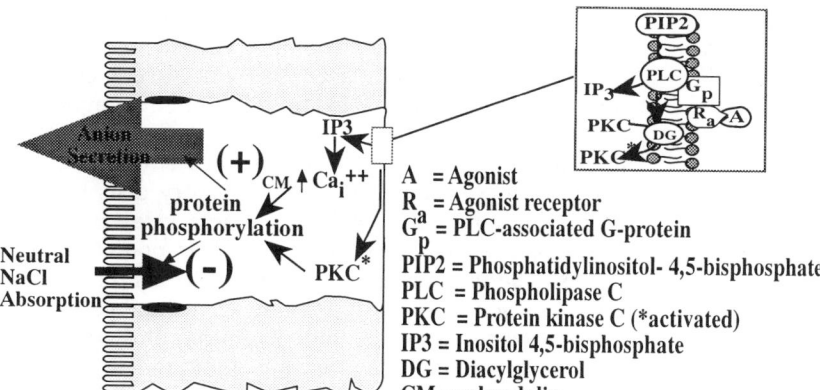

A = Agonist
R_a = Agonist receptor
G_p^a = PLC-associated G-protein
PIP2 = Phosphatidylinositol- 4,5-bisphosphate
PLC = Phospholipase C
PKC = Protein kinase C (*activated)
IP3 = Inositol 4,5-bisphosphate
DG = Diacylglycerol
CM = calmodulin

FIG. 3. Net intestinal secretion can be mediated by increases in cytosolic calcium and activation of protein kinase C.

As will be discussed below, the formation of DAG activates PKC, which may stimulate intestinal secretion directly and indirectly through the activation of arachidonic acid metabolism. IP_3, on the other hand, increases cytosolic calcium by binding to specific receptors primarily located on organelles such as endoplasmic reticulum (39). This binding results in a conformational change in the tetrameric intracellular calcium channel, thereby releasing calcium into the cytosol, increasing cytosolic calcium concentrations. IP_3 may also regulate calcium influx across the plasma membrane of cells. There is some evidence that IP_3 may have direct effects on calcium channels in the plasma membranes. In addition, influx of calcium across plasma membranes is linked to intracellular stores of calcium via a capacitance mechanism (40,41). For example, when calcium stores within the endoplasmic reticulum are depleted by agents such as thapsigargin, calcium entry across the plasma membrane of some cells is stimulated. The resulting cytoplasmic concentrations of calcium stimulated by agonists are tightly regulated by the complex interplay of pumps to sequester calcium into disparate intracellular stores, binding proteins such as calsequestrin and calreticulum, and calcium channels through which calcium is released from intracellular stores into the cytoplasm (38). Increases in IP_3 levels are observed as early as 5 sec after exposure to the muscarinic agonist carbachol. However, the addition of carbachol also results in the production of other phospholipid metabolites, such as inositol tetrakisphosphate, IP_4, in a time course consistent with cessation of muscarinic agonist-induced stimulation of secretion. This inhibition of intestinal secretion occurs in the presence of increased intracellular concentrations of calcium, suggesting that IP_4 inhibits intestinal secretion induced by increased intracellular concentrations of calcium (42).

A second mechanism whereby increases in pathogens may increase intracellular calcium is via elaborated enterotoxins. A noncyclic GMP-associated heat-stable enterotoxin, ST_b, produced in *E. coli* infection has also been associated with stimulating intestinal secretion by increasing intracellular concentrations of calcium. This effect is dependent on external calcium concentrations and is inhibited by pertussis toxin, suggesting that ST_b binds to a receptor linked to a GTP-binding regulatory G protein that acts directly to open calcium channels on the plasma

membrane. This G-protein gating of ion channels has also been described in association with K^+ channels as well.

Toxin A produced by *C. difficile* also appears to stimulate increases in cytosolic calcium in neutrophils, resulting in their activation. Because this toxin also stimulates intestinal anion secretion (43), it is not unreasonable to speculate that this may occur through a Ca-dependent mechanism. However, this remains to be proven. Enterotoxins such as cholera toxin or the heat-labile toxin made by *E. coli* may also stimulate increases in cytosolic calcium by increasing cyclic nucleotide concentrations in enterocytes. Stimulated increases in both cAMP and cGMP appear to increase cytosolic calcium, which may be important in potentiating the secretory response. However, this effect is highly species-specific and has been best shown in isolated avian enterocytes (44,45).

More recently, a third mechanism has been described by which pathogens increase intestinal epithelial cytosolic calcium. Organisms such as *Salmonella typhimurium* appear to stimulate increases in cytosolic calcium coinciding with their invasion of cultured epithelial cells (46,47). These events are apparently interdependent because invasion-defective mutants did not increase cytosolic calcium, and inhibition of the induced increases in cytosolic calcium caused by wild-type *S. typhimurium* blocked bacterial entry. The cellular mechanisms mediating these events turn out to quite unique. *S. typhimurium* appears to bind to the epidermal growth factor receptor (EGFR), which results in the activation of phospholipase A2 (PLA2), presumably mediated by EGF tyrosine kinase stimulation of distal serine/threonine kinases and MAP kinases (see Figure 7). PLA2 in turn hydrolyzes membrane phospholipids to release arachidonic acid (AA), which is metabolized by 5-lipoxygenase (5-LO) to form leukotrienes. In the cell system in which these experiments were performed, the major leukotriene metabolite that was formed was LTD4, which may cause increased membrane permeability to Ca influx directly or indirectly through the activation of other intermediary processes.

Unfortunately, far less is known about the events distal to the stimulated increases in cytosolic calcium that are involved in regulating intestinal epithelial ion transport. As will be discussed later, increased cytosolic calcium may directly alter membrane conductance of Cl and K, by mechanisms that are still not well understood. Alternatively, it appears that some transport processes are affected following calcium binding to calcium regulatory protein calmodulin. The resulting activated calcium–calmodulin complex may activate essential protein kinases that ultimately cause phosphorylation of specific transport proteins, affecting their activity.

Activation of Protein Kinase C

Agents that increase intracellular calcium, such as serotonin and acetylcholine, in part exert their effects on electrolyte transport by increasing the activity of PKC, a calcium-dependent protein kinase (48). Calcium induces activation of PKC by stimulating the translocation of the enzyme from an inactive cytosolic fraction to the membrane fraction where it exerts its effects, presumably by causing phosphorylation of specific membrane proteins (49). A characteristic feature of muscarinic agonist-induced effects on electrolyte transport *in vitro* is that its onset is rapid, with maximal effects present by 90 sec, and that the duration of effect is short-lived, lasting only several minutes. Part of the short-lived duration can be attributed to the fact that regulation of intestinal secretion can occur at different sites, a fact that will be discussed in more detail in the next section. Specifically, PKC-α acutely stimulates intestinal secretion by its effects on the chloride channel; however, over the course of several minutes, it chronically inhibits electrolyte secretion by inhibiting the efflux of potassium through K^+ channels located on the basolateral membrane (50). Diacylglycerol activates PKC while IP_3 regulates intracellular concentrations of calcium, primarily by mobilizing calcium from intracellular stores such as the endoplasmic reticulum (38).

Other Mechanisms of Pathogen-Induced Net Intestinal Secretion and Diarrhea

This section will outline other mechanisms of pathogen-induced secretion occuring via secretagogues elaborated during the inflammatory response as well as the amplification and modulation of this response by the intestinal nervous system and the local production of prostaglandins.

Acute Inflammatory Effects of Gastrointestinal Infections

The range of histological responses seen in the intestine varies widely depending on the specific pathogen involved. Toxin-mediated diarrheas resulting from noninvasive pathogens such as *Vibrio cholerae* are noninvasive and result in a minimal inflammatory response. In contrast, invasive infections resulting in the disruption of the mucosal barrier can produce diarrhea by exudative processes. In addition, some gastrointestinal infections cause a form of secretory diarrhea associated with submucosal and lamina propria inflammation, but structurally intact intestinal mucosa. Infiltration of the lamina propria occurs

by a host of inflammatory cells including phagocytes [polymorphonuclear neutrophils (PMNs), eosinophils, and macrophages] and mast cells, with the cell composition varying with the specific infection. For example, *Salmonella* infections are associated with a significant PMN infiltration, while rejection of parasites is dependent on increased mast cells. These inflammatory cells result in the production of a broad but variable array of soluble inflammatory mediators that can act as potent secretagogues. The inflammatory response thus serves the purpose of purging the gut of noxious agents and pathogens, but also exacerbates the acute symptom of diarrhea.

Of the known inflammatory mediators that are capable of stimulating net intestinal secretion, those resulting from the metabolism of AA have been best studied (Fig. 4). Local production of AA metabolites, or prostaglandins, has been demonstrated in a number of gastrointestinal infections. While enterocytes themselves have been shown to produce some prostaglandins (51,52), it is believed that the most significant production of prostaglandins associated with infections results from inflammatory cells in the lamina propria as well as the subepithelial mesenchymal compartment (53). This compartment consists of fibroblasts and myofibroblasts that form a sheath directly beneath the epithelial layer basement membrane. During inflammation, the fibroblasts are stimulated by mediators such as histamine, bradykinin, interleukins, and cytokines. Fibroblast activation results in the stimulation of prostaglandin release and production. By virtue of its location immediately beneath the epithelial layer, it has been postulated that prostaglandin release by the subepithelial mesenchymal compartment represents a final amplification mechanism for secretory stimuli.

Receptors for PGE_2, one of the major prostaglandins that induce intestinal secretion, have been demonstrated on the basolateral membrane of enterocytes. PGE_2 has been shown to stimulate anion secretion and inhibit NaCl absorption via both cAMP- and calcium-mediated pathways (54–56). While PGE_2 effects on intestinal secretion can be direct (8–10), via binding to its receptor on the enterocyte, other prostaglandins, such as PGI_2, PGD_2,

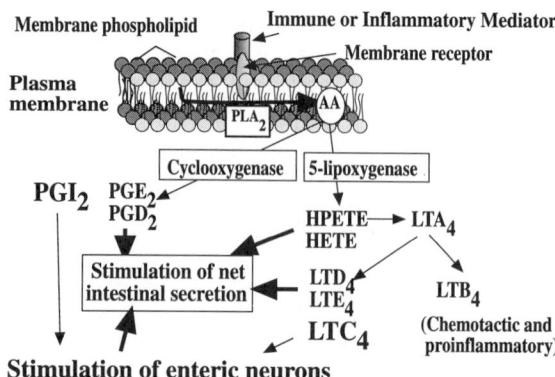

FIG. 4. Stimulation of net intestinal secretion in acute inflammatory states. A number of secretagogues are elaborated by subepithelial inflammatory cells. In addition, modulation of secretory stimuli occurs via enteric neurons and the subepithelial myofibroblast layer.

and the peptidoleukotriene LTC$_4$, are believed to act primarily via enteric neurons (see below) (57–59). Specifically, PGI$_2$ induces intestinal secretion by stimulating acetylcholine and inhibiting norepinephrine release.

In addition to the prostaglandins, many 5-lipoxygenase metabolites released by phagocytic cells are capable of stimulating net secretion; these include 5-hydroperoxy- and 5-hydroxyeicosatetraenoic acid (5-HPETE and 5-HETE) and leukotrienes C$_4$, D$_4$, and E$_4$ (60,61). Although direct stimulation of epithelial cells by these mediators has been demonstrated in animal models, little is known about their significance in humans.

Inflammatory Mediators of Intestinal Secretion

Central to the understanding of inflammation-induced intestinal secretion is the concept that a given secretagogue may act to induce secretion through multiple mechanisms, reflecting the complex regulatory network controlling intestinal secretion and absorption. For example, infection with parasites can result in mast cell infiltration and activation within the lamina propria. Mast cell degranulation results in the production of multiple soluble mediators, including histamine. Histamine is capable of directly inducing intestinal secretion via the presence of H1 receptors on enterocytes. However, neurotoxins and prostaglandin synthetase inhibitors are capable of decreasing but not abolishing the secretory response to histamine (62–64). The net inflammatory response within the intestine then consists of (a) soluble mediators produced by inflammatory cells within the lamina propria that can directly stimulate enterocyte secretion, (b) amplification by local prostaglandin production; and (c) modulation of secretory stimuli by the intestinal nervous system. A brief discussion of some inflammatory mediators is presented below (Fig. 5).

Reactive Oxygen Metabolites

Reactive oxygen metabolites (ROMs) are oxygen-centered free radicals that are released from the respiratory burst by activated phagocytic cells. Examples include H$_2$O$_2$, superoxide, hydroxyl radical, and monochloramine. They have a small direct effect on inducing enterocyte secretion though calcium-mediated mechanisms and have a more profound stimulatory effect on secretion via release of prostaglandins from the lamina propria (65,66).

Platelet-Activating Factor

Platelet-activating factor (PAF) is formed by phospholipase A$_2$ hydrolysis of AA. Its major sources in the intestine are activated phagocytes, mast cells, platelets, and vascular endothelium. Like ROMs, PAFs have a small direct effect on enterocyte secretion via calcium-mediated pathways, but the majority of their effects are mediated via release of prostaglandins (53,67).

Histamine

Histamine is released from activated mast cells and is known to contribute to the diarrhea associated with parasite rejection. Histamine can directly increase enterocyte calcium levels, initiating phosphoinositol and PKC activity via H$_1$ receptors on the enterocyte. However, a significant amount of histamine's effects are mediated by local prostaglandin production and enteric neurons (62–64).

Serotonin

Serotonin is present in mast cells, platelets, mucosal enterochromaffin cells, and a subset of myenteric neurons. Serotonin has been shown to inhibit NaCl absorption and stimulate anion secretion. Its effects are mediated directly via calcium-mediated events and indirectly via enteric neurons and subepithelial prostaglandin release (68–70).

Bradykinin

Activation of kallikrein to produce bradykinin occurs in activated phagocyte- and mast cell–mediated inflam-

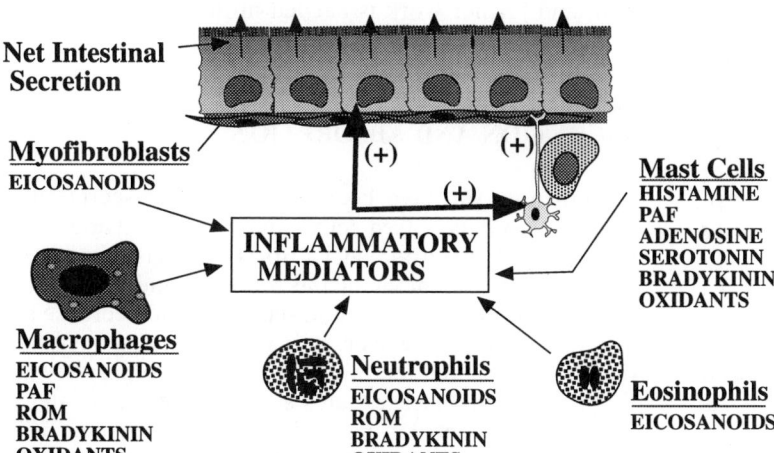

FIG. 5. Immune or inflammatory mediators of inflammation. Many prostaglandins and 5-lipoxygenase inhibitors are capable of stimulating net secretion.

mation. Bradykinin is a potent anion secretagogue. Its receptors have been demonstrated on enterocytes and its direct effects occur through calcium-mediated effects. A significant amount of its secretagogue activity is mediated via subepithelial prostaglandin production (51,52,71).

Nitric Oxide

The gaseous free radical nitric oxide is produced by the action of nitric oxide synthetase on L-arginine in a wide variety of cells such as endothelial cells and neurons. Nitric oxide inhibits NaCl exchange and stimulates anion secretion. The mechanisms of these actions are numerous and include an increase in soluble cGMP in the lamina propria as well as effects mediated via enteric neurons and local prostaglandin production (72–74).

Amplification by Local Prostaglandin Production: Neuronal Innervation of the Intestine

The intestine is extrinsically innervated by postganglionic sympathetic neurons and preganglionic parasympathetic neurons. In addition, the intestine is unique among organ systems in that it is also richly innervated by an intrinsic enteric neuronal system. The intrinsic enteric reflex arc consists of (a) sensory neurons with nerve endings terminating in the mucosa, (b) interneurons contained within the intestinal wall which coordinate local neuronal networks, and (c) motor neurons that act as the final effector cells. One type of motor neuron is the secretomotor neuron whose cell bodies are located within the submucosal plexus (Meissner's plexus). The net effect of the intrinsic reflex arc is that it provides the intestine with a mechanism to modulate intestinal secretion and absorption in response to luminal concentrations of nutrients (such as glucose) as well as local production of mediators produced by the inflammatory response (4).

The effector secretomotor neurons release neurotransmitters in proximity to enterocytes to induce secretion and inhibit absorption during neural stimulation (75). Secretomotor neurons can be divided into cholinergic and noncholinergic types. Cholinergic neurons release acetylcholine, which acts at muscarinic receptors located on enterocytes. Acetylcholine acts via calcium mobilized from intracellular stores by phosphoinositide metabolites. Putative noncholinergic neurotransmitters operational in the enteric nervous system include vasoactive intestinal peptide (VIP) (76) and substance P (75). VIP receptors have been demonstrated on enterocytes and VIP in vitro stimulates chloride secretion and inhibits NaCl absorption. Substance P, a neuropeptide, has been shown to stimulate anion secretion and inhibit apical Na-H exchange, one of the steps involved in electroneutral NaCl absorption. Substance P receptors, NK-1, have been demonstrated on neurons and epithelial cells. A number of other putative secretory neurotransmitters have been identified within the intestine, but significance *in vivo* has not yet been established.

That enteric neurons contribute to intestinal secretion induced by a secretagogue can be demonstrated by studies of neurotoxins such as tetrodotoxin. For example, histamine-induced increases in intestinal short-circuit current, I_{sc}, a measure of anion secretion, is decreased but not abolished by the addition of tetrodotoxin. This suggests that histamine induces secretion in part via stimulation of neurons innervating the intestine, but that other pathways exist. It has been estimated that as much as 50% of inflammation-induced intestinal secretion is mediated through enteric neurons.

Neutrophil-Derived Secretagogue (5'-AMP), Adenosine, and Novel Intracellular Mediators of Intestinal Electrolyte Transport

A novel mechanism of intestinal secretion, not operating via previously discussed intracellular mediators, was recently described (77,78). One of the histological hallmarks of active intestinal inflammation is the formation of crypt abscesses. Activation of intestinal neutrophils results in their transmigration from the lamina propria, across the epithelial layer, into intestinal crypts. Madara and coworkers recently identified a product of neutrophils, 5'-AMP, which, when applied to the apical surface of epithelial cells, results in active anion secretion. 5'-AMP is metabolized by an apical ectoenzyme to adenosine, a well-known intestinal secretagogue.

Activation of intestinal secretion by adenosine has many of the characteristics of cAMP-induced secretion. Addition of adenosine to supramaximal doses of cAMP does not result in any additional stimulation of secretion. Furthermore, when combined with calcium-mediated secretagogues such as muscarinic agonists and serotonin, adenosine has a synergistic effect on secretion. Finally, in large doses, adenosine does increase cAMP levels. However, adenosine at low doses stimulates secretion not associated with increases in cAMP. These results suggest that at low doses adenosine increases secretion by an intracellular mediator other than cAMP, cGMP, or calcium, and that this mediator may function through a common path with cAMP-mediated secretion, but at a point distal to cAMP production. AA has been forwarded as a putative intracellular mediator of adenosine-induced secretion, and further work is needed in this area (79).

MOLECULAR BASIS OF INTESTINAL SECRETION AND ABSORPTION

Until now we have been discussing net secretion as resulting from increased active anion secretion and/or decreased electroneutral NaCl absorption. In isolated intestinal studies, a number of the secretagogues previously discussed both increase anion secretion and decrease salt absorption (80). However, it is important to understand that absorption and secretion are regulated separately and that in different disease states each may play a greater or lesser role in contributing to the resulting diarrhea. With the cloning of specific transporters, greater understanding of the molecular basis of the regulation of intestinal transport is possible. The major effect of cAMP, calcium, and cGMP on intestinal transport is believed to occur via activation of respective kinases and phosphorylation of transport proteins, resulting in their activation or inhibition. In the not-too-distant future, a complete understanding of the specific sites of phosphorylation on transport proteins resulting from regulation by intracellular mediators will be possible.

Regulation of Active Anion Secretion

Figure 6A outlines the present model of active anion secretion (82–84). The Na^+, K^+-ATPase pump provides the energy for the active chloride secretion by creating the necessary ion gradients for favorable vectorial transport. The Na-K-2Cl cotransporter and K channel are located on the basolateral surface and the chloride channel is located on the apical membrane. These basolateral membrane processes result in the accumulation of intracellular Cl^-. Activation of chloride channels results in the active secretion of chloride across the apical membrane, down its electrochemical gradient. Na ions passively accompany the secretion of Cl and the secretion of water results. While regulation of anion secretion has been demonstrated at several of these steps, it is believed that a crucial step in the regulation of active anion secretion occurs at the level of apical chloride channels, which will be discussed first.

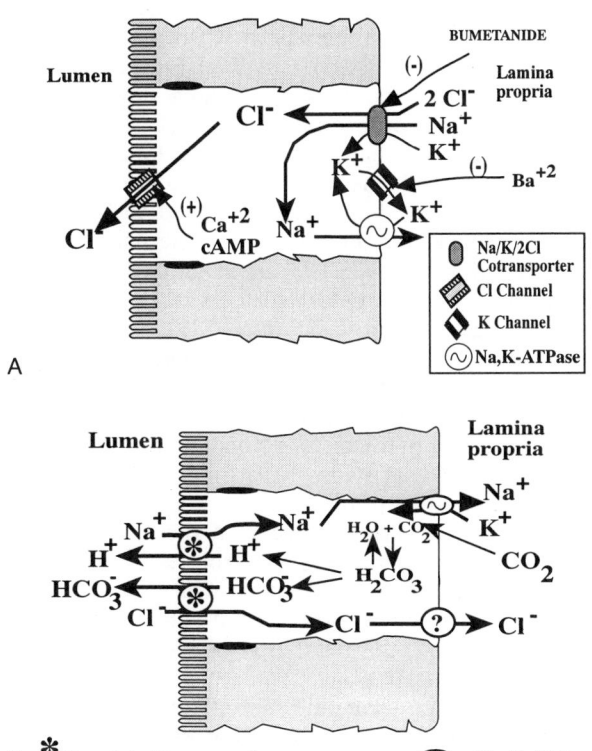

FIG. 6. Models of intestinal absorption and secretion. A: Active chloride secretion. B: Electroneutral NaCl absorption.

Regulation of the Apical Chloride Channel

The gene responsible for the genetic defect resulting in cystic fibrosis was cloned by the technique now known as positional cloning (18). The corresponding protein, the cystic fibrosis transmembrane regulator (CFTR), functions as a chloride channel. The mutations associated with cystic fibrosis result in malfunction and aberrant membrane trafficking of CFTR, resulting in the clinical syndrome of defective chloride secretion apparent in multiple organs including intestine, lung, and pancreas.

Multiple lines of evidence have been forwarded to suggest that CFTR represents a major chloride channel in the apical domain of intestine (18). In contrast to the situation in cystic fibrosis, where too little chloride secretion occurs, activation of the wild-type CFTR by cAMP has been demonstrated (19,20), resulting in activation of chloride secretion and the production of diarrhea. The CFTR protein consists of five separate domains: two transmembrane spanning domains, two nucleotide binding domains, and a regulatory R domain, which contains several consensus phosphorylation sequences (85). It is known that PKA phosphorylates four serine residues of the CFTR on the R domain. Simultaneous mutations of these four serine residues to alanines prevented cAMP-stimulated activation. These results suggest that a major mechanism of the cAMP-induced chloride secretion occurs via A-kinase activation of the CFTR. In addition, the presence of consensus domains for PKC and other protein kinases suggests that CFTR may also be regulated by alternative pathways.

Other regulatory mechanisms are involved in cAMP-stimulated chloride secretion. Under conditions of enterocyte shrinkage, activation of the channel by cAMP does not occur, suggesting the presence of a protective mechanism against excessive secretion under conditions of volume depletion. This sensitivity of cAMP-induced secretion to cell volume changes suggests an association of the secretory response with cytoskeletal components, a possibility that will be discussed later (86).

Multiple chloride channels exist (87) and the transport characteristics of calcium-stimulated chloride channel efflux differ from those of cAMP-mediated transport, suggesting that multiple chloride channels may be operative in epithelial mucosa. For example, in studies on airway epithelia, the effects of cAMP and calcium on net chloride secretion are additive. In addition, DIDS, an inhibitor of multiple chloride channels, inhibits calcium-stimulated chloride currents but not cAMP-stimulated currents (18). Finally, anion selectivity studies demonstrate differences between calcium and cAMP-mediated chloride currents, suggesting that different chloride channels (with different conductances to various anions) are operational. Taken together, these studies suggest that disparate chloride channels function on the apical domain of epithelia. While poorly defined at present, calcium-stimulated chloride secretion may function in part through activation of apical chloride channels, but regulation at other sites in the secretory pathway, such as regulation of K^+ efflux, may play an equal if not more important role (88).

Regulation of K⁺ Efflux

In several intestinal cultured cell lines that serve as models of chloride secretion, such as T84 and HT-29 clone 19A (both derived from human colon adenocarcinomas), Ca^{2+}-activated chloride channels have not been demonstrated in apical membrane preparations (87,88). In these cells, it is believed that most of the apical chloride conductance occurs via the cAMP-responsive CFTR. These results would indicate that calcium does not directly activate CFTR. However, calcium-stimulated chloride secretion in intestinal epithelia of patients with cystic fibrosis is defective. Taken together, these results would indicate that calcium regulation at sites other than the apical chloride channels, such as regulation of potassium efflux, are functionally important.

In T84 colonic epithelial cells that do not contain Ca^{2+}-activated chloride channels, calcium-mediated secretion is believed to be driven by activation of basolateral K^+ efflux via potassium channels. The resulting decrease in intracellular potassium provides the driving force for chloride uptake by the basolateral Na-K-2Cl cotransporter and subsequent exit across constitutively open apical chloride (CFTR) channels. In cystic fibrosis patients, this final step of passive exit across the CFTR is impaired, explaining how calcium-stimulated chloride secretion can be impaired in cystic fibrosis patients even though calcium has no known direct effects on the CFTR (88).

Regulation of the Na-K-2Cl Cotransporter

Stimulation of chloride secretion by intracellular mediators is decreased under conditions of enterocyte shrinkage, presumably serving as a protective mechanism against excessive secretion in conditions of volume depletion. While described with calcium-induced secretion, this effect is observed most strikingly with cAMP-induced secretion. It is believed that coordination of cell volume status with transport activity is mediated by the cytoskeletal architecture. The molecular mechanisms underlying this coordination have recently been defined with respect to the Na-K-2Cl cotransporter.

One of the differences observed between cAMP and calcium-mediated secretagogues is that only cAMP-mediated secretagogues induce profound changes in the cytoskeletal architecture of the enterocyte. If this rearrangement is inhibited by cytoskeletal poisons such as NBD-phalloidin, cAMP-induced (and not calcium-mediated) secretion is significantly inhibited. Activity of the Na-K-2Cl cotransporter (as measured by the bumetanide-sensitive rubidium-86 uptake) was found to be inhibited in the presence of NBD-phalloidin, but the activities of the chloride channel, the K channel, and the Na^+, K^+-ATPase pump were not affected (89). A number of bacterial enterotoxins (e.g., *C. difficile* toxin A) (3) have been shown to produce profound cytoskeletal rearrangements and the present data suggest that at least one mechanism of the toxin-induced secretion is via activation of the Na-K-2Cl cotransporter. Cytoskeletal rearrangements are increasingly being recognized as playing a major role in a number of

infection-induced intestinal responses and will be discussed separately.

In summary, the secretory response results from the coordinated function of multiple membrane transport proteins located on the apical and basolateral domains. Functionally significant regulation has been defined at a number of these sites, including cAMP-induced activation of the apical chloride channel, which is crucial in *V. cholerae* infection, calcium-induced inhibition of the K channel, and cytoskeletal regulation of the Na-K-2Cl cotransporter. Regulation of these membrane proteins can occur through multiple mechanisms as well. For example, phosphorylation at specific sites has been defined for the CFTR. In contrast, the observed activation of basolateral Na-K-2Cl cotransport activity associated with cAMP-induced cytoskeletal rearrangements is believed to result from recruitment of additional protein molecules to the membrane surface.

Regulation of Electrolyte Absorption

The model of electroneutral absorption of NaCl is diagrammed in Fig. 6B. Active absorption of NaCl is driven by a Na^+, K^+-ATPase pump on the basolateral membrane. The Na^+, K^+-ATPase pump is located on the basolateral domain and extrudes Na from the cell, maintaining intracellular Na concentrations low relative to the extracellular concentration. This electrochemical gradient provides the driving force for the absorption of sodium into intestinal epithelial cells by an Na-H exchanger on the apical domain. The absorption of NaCl across the apical domain occurs via the paired activity of Na-H and $Cl-HCO_3$ exchangers (90,91) (see Fig. 6B). The apical membrane process is the rate-limiting step and regulation of intestinal absorption occurs at this site. Multiple isoforms of the Na-H exchanger have been cloned (21–24), and localization of at least one isoform to the apical domain has been established (92). The apical $Cl-HCO_3$ exchanger has not been cloned thus far. The nature of the coupling reaction between the Na-H and $Cl-HCO_3$ exchangers as well as regulatory aspects of the apical $Cl-HCO_3$ exchanger remain to be defined (91,92).

In addition to electroneutral NaCl absorption, absorption of sodium in the intestine occurs via Na-glucose, Na-amino acid, and other sodium–nutrient cotransporters in the small intestine. In the distal colon, sodium absorption via sodium channels provides for a final, highly efficient phase of sodium absorption.

Secretion and absorption occur in distinct locations within the intestinal epithelium; electrolyte absorption occurs in villi and surface enterocytes while secretion has been postulated to occur primarily in subsurface crypts (81). Concomitantly, the regulation of secretion and absorption in the intestine are separate processes. While many secretagogues have the dual effect of stimulating secretion and inhibiting absorption, correlation of the two processes does not always occur. An important example of this is that in many infectious diarrheas, such as cholera, stimulation of chloride secretion and inhibition of electroneutral NaCl absorption are seen. However, sodium absorption by nutrient cotransporters such as Na-glucose transporters is unaffected and provides the basis for glucose-based oral rehydration formulas used in the treatment of infectious diarrheas.

The following section will discuss the regulation of electroneutral NaCl absorption, with emphasis on apical Na-H exchange. This process is impaired in many infectious diarrheas and, as will be discussed, its regulation often mirrors that of chloride secretion.

Regulation of the Apical Na-H Exchanger

It is known that both cAMP- and calcium-mediated secretagogues can decrease electroneutral NaCl absorption and multiple lines of evidence suggest that these secretagogues may act by decreasing the activity of apical Na-H exchange (45). At least two isoforms of Na-H exchange are functionally important in mediating apical sodium transport, NHE-2 and NHE-3, both of which have multiple putative phosphorylation sites for kinase activity (21,23,24). Phorbol esters (which increase PKC activity) decrease brush border Na-H exchange in chicken enterocytes (93). In addition, translocation of PKC from cytosolic to membrane fractions occurs in a time course consistent with PKC activation, causing a decrease in apical Na-H exchange (94). Finally, NHE-3 (an apical Na-H exchanger) transfectants when exposed to phorbol esters demonstrate decreased apical Na-H exchange (95).

Regulation of the Apical Cl-HCO₃ Exchanger

The electroneutral absorption of NaCl occurs via the paired activity of Na-H and Cl-HCO₃ exchangers on the apical membrane (see Fig. 6B) (96). Much is known regarding the regulation of apical Na-H exchange. However, studies in rabbit ileum suggest that regulation of apical Cl-HCO₃ may also occur. In isolated villus cells, serotonin appears to inhibit NaCl vectorial transport by an HCO₃-dependent, Na-independent process, suggesting that inhibition is being mediated primarily via the Cl-HCO₃ exchanger and not Na-H exchange. In contrast, in crypt cells, serotonin-induced alkalinization is HCO₃-independent, Na-dependent, and amiloride-sensitive, suggesting primary mediation occurring by stimulation of basolateral membrane Na-H exchange (97).

Thus regulation of NaCl absorption by second-messenger systems may be mediated at Na-H or Cl-HCO₃ exchange, or both. In addition, the cellular pathways affecting these exchangers may be dependent on the state of epithelial cell differentiation or possibly by differential expression of exchanger isoforms during cell development.

OTHER CELLULAR MECHANISMS THAT MAY MEDIATE PATHOGEN-INDUCED DIARRHEAL DISEASE: EFFECTS OF CYTOSKELETAL ELEMENTS

Fundamental alteration of the actin cytoskeleton appears to be a major effect of several enterotoxins, such as *C. difficile* toxin (4) and the zonula occludens toxin (ZOT) associated with cholera infection (98). Remodeling of the cytoskeletal architecture has been reported to result in the effacement of microvilli causing loss of absorptive surface area, which in turn decreases brush border membrane hydrolase activity and thus malabsorption of nutrients and electrolytes. In addition, alterations in mucosal permeability may result from disruption of tight junction integrity as the actin microfilament skeleton inserts into the zonula adherens and zonula occludens components of the tight junctions. Recent studies of ZOT have suggested that this effect may be mediated by activated PKC (99).

Recent studies elucidated the membrane transduction events associated with bacterial adherence and entry into enterocytes (47,48). An important virulence factor common to all *Salmonella* is their ability to cross the intestinal epithelial barrier, which involves entry into enterocytes. Studies with *S. typhimurium* demonstrated that binding to the EGFR sets into motion a host of responses (Fig. 7), including profound cytoskeletal rearrangements at the point of the bacterial–host cell contact as well as increases in intracellular calcium concentrations. Binding of the EGFR activates the membrane-bound phospholipase A₂, which results in the production of AA, which is ultimately converted to leukotriene D₄ (LTD₄). LTD₄ activates a Ca^{2+} channel, causing an influx of calcium across the plasma membrane, increasing the intracellular concentration of calcium (47,48). While these studies do not directly address the effects of increases in intracellular calcium

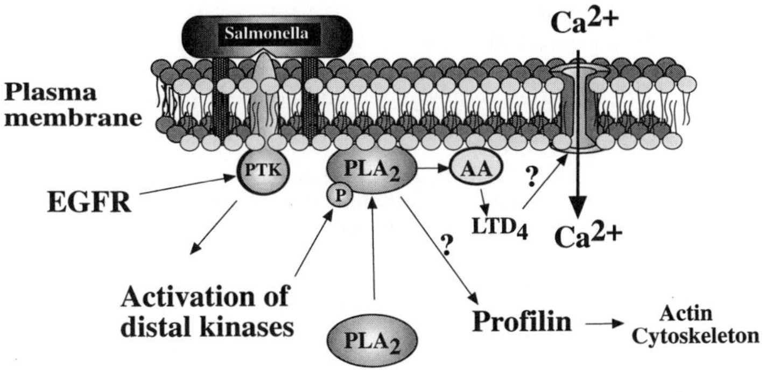

FIG. 7. Signal transduction events in *Salmonella typhimurium* infection. Cytoskeletal rearrangements as well as increases in cytosolic calcium levels have been demonstrated. EGFR, epidermal growth factor receptor; PLA₂, phospholipase A₂; AA, arachidonic acid; PTK, protein kinases; LTD₄, leukotriene D₄.

concentrations on electrolyte transport, they do open up an entirely new mechanism of pathogen-induced alterations in electrolyte transport. Increases in intracellular mediators of electrolyte transport may result not only from elaborated toxins and inflammatory secretagogues produced by the epithelial defense response, but also directly from membrane processes involved in pathogen adherence and entry into the intestinal epithelia.

REFERENCES

1. Field M, Semrad CE. Toxigenic diarrheas, congenital diarrheas, and cystic fibrosis: disorders of intestinal ion transport. *Annu Rev Physiol* 1993;55:631–655.
2. Keusch GT, Donohue-Rolfe A, Jacewizc M. *Shigella* toxin and the pathogenesis of shigellosis. *Ciba Found Symp* 1985;112:193–214.
3. Hecht G, Koutsouris A, Pothoulakis C, LaMont JT, Madara JL. *Clostridum difficile* toxin B disrupts the barrier function of T84 monolaters. *Gastroenterology* 1992;102:416–423.
4. Chang EB, Rao MC. Intestinal water and electrolyte transport. *Physiology of the gastrointestinal tract.* New York: Raven Press; 1994:2027–2081.
5. Chang EB, Field M, Miller RJ. Alpha-2 adrenergic receptor regulation of ion transport in rabbit ileum. *Am J Physiol* 1982;242:G237–G242.
6. Chang EB, Field M, Miller RJ. Enterocyte alpha-2-adrenergic receptors: Yohimbine and p-aminoclonidine binding relative to ion transport. *Am J Physiol* 1983;244:G76–G82.
7. Berschneider HM, Powell DW. Fibroblasts modulate intestinal secretory responses to inflammatory mediators. *J Clin Invest* 1992;89:484–489.
8. Al-aqwati Q, Greenough WB. Prostaglandins inhibit intestinal sodium transport. *Nature* 1972;238:26–27.
9. Racusen L, Binder HJ. Effect of prostaglandins on ion transport across isolated colonic mucosa. *Dig Dis Sci* 1980;25:900–904.
10. Musch MW, Field M, Miller RJ, Stoff JS. Homologous desensitization to prostaglandins in rabbit ileum. *Am J Physiol* 1987;252:G120–G127.
11. Granger DN. Intestinal microcirculation and transmural fluid transport. *Am J Physiol* 1981;240:G343–349.
12. Granger DN, Perry MA, Kvietys PR, Taylor AE. Interstitium-to-blood movement of macromolecules in the absorbing small intestine. *Am J Physiol* 1981;241:G31–G36.
13. Dominguez P, Barros F, Lazo PS. The activation of adenylate cyclase from small intestinal epithelium by cholera toxin. *Eur J Biochem* 1985;146:533–538.
14. Dominguez P, Velasco G, Barros F, Lazo PS. Intestinal brush border membranes contain regulatory subunits of adenylyl cyclase. *Proc Natl Acad Sci USA* 1987;84:6965–6969.
15. Lynch CJ, Morbach L, Blackmore PF, Exton JH. a-Subunits of N_s are released from the plasma membrane following cholera toxin activation. *FEBS Lett* 1986;200:333–336.
16. Shenolikar S. Protein phosphorylation: hormones, drugs and bioregulation. *FASEB J* 1988;2:2753–2764.
17. Taskulkao C, Nash NT, Leach K, Rao MC. Second messenger-specific protein kinases in a salt absorbing intestinal epithelia. *Am J Physiol* 1990;258:C879–C888.
18. Anderson MP, Sheppard DN, Berger HA, Welsh MJ. Chloride channels in the apical membrane of normal and cystic fibrosis airway and intestinal epithelia. *Am J Physiol* 1992;263:L1–L14.
19. Anderson MP, Gregory RJ, Thompson S, et al. Demonstration that CFTR is a chloride channel by alteration of its anion selectivity. *Science* 1991;253:202–207.
20. Berger HA, Anderson MP, Gregory RJ, Smith SAE, Welsh MJ. Identification and regulation of the cystic fibrosis transmembrane conductance regulator-generated chloride channel. *J Clin Invest* 1991;88:1422–1431.
21. Orlowski J, Kandasamy RA, Shull GE. Molecular cloning of putative members of the Na/H exchanger gene family. *J Biol Chem* 1992;267:9331–9339.
22. Sardet CA, Franchi A, Pouyssegur J. Molecular cloning, primary structure, and expression of the human growth factor-activatable Na$^+$/H$^+$ antiporter. *Cell* 1989;56:271–280.
23. Tse CM, Brant SR, Waler S, Pouyssegur J, Donowitz M. Cloning and sequencing of a rabbit cDNA encoding an intestinal and kidney-specific Na$^+$/H$^+$ exchanger isoform (NHE-3). *J Biol Chem* 1992;267:9340–9346.
24. Wang Z, Orlowski J, Shull GE. Primary structure and functional expression of a novel gastrointestinal isoform of the rat Na/H exchanger. *J Biol Chem* 1993;268:11925–11928.
25. Hughes JM, Murad F, Chang B, Guerrant RL. Role of cyclic GMP in the action of heat stable enterotoxin of *Escherichia coli*. *Nature* 1978;271:755–756.
26. Field J, Graff LH Jr, Laird WJ, Smith PL. Heat stable enterotoxin of *Escherichia coli:* in vitro effects on guanylate cyclase activity, cyclic GMP concentration and ion transport in small intestine. *Proc Natl Acad Sci USA* 1978;75:2800–2804.
27. Huott PA, Liu W, McRoberts GA, Giannella RA, Dharmsathaphorn K. The mechanism of *E. coli* heat stable enterotoxin in a human colonic cell. *J Clin Invest* 1988;82:514–523.
28. Mittal CK, Murad F. Guanylate cyclase: regulation of cyclic GMP metabolism. In: Nathanson JA, Kebabian JW, eds. *Handbook of experimental pharmacology.* Berlin: Springer-Verlag; 1982:225–260.
29. Currie MG, Fok KF, Kato J, et al. Guanylin: an endogenous activator of intestinal guanylate cyclase. *Proc Natl Acad Sci USA* 1992;89:947–951.
30. Schulz S, Green CK, Yuen PST, Garbers DL. Guanylyl cyclase is a heat-stable enterotoxin receptor. *Cell* 1990;63:941–948.
31. Krause WJ, Forter LR, Eber SL, Freeman RH, Cullingford GL. Localization and distribution of guanylin/heat-stable enterotoxin receptors in the intestinal mucosa of man and other vertebrates. *Gastroenterology* 1993;104:A835.
32. Edelman AM, Blumenthal DK, Krebs EG. Protein serine/threonine kinases. *Annu Rev Biochem* 1987;56:567–613.
33. Cohen MB, Mann EA, Lau C, Henning SJ, Giannella RA. A gradient in expression of the *Escherichia coli* heat-stable enterotoxin receptor exists along the villus-to-crypt axis of rat small intestine. *Biochem Biophys Res Commun* 1992;186:483–490.
34. Field MJ, Rao MC, Chang EB. Intestinal electrolyte transport and diarrheal disease (2 part article). *N Engl J Med* 1989;321:800–806, 879–883.
35. Khare S, Wilson D, Tien XY, Bissonnette M, Brasitus TA. Calcium activates rat colonic membrane guanylate cyclase via protein kinase C (PKC). *Gastroenterology* 1993;104:A256.
36. McGowan K, Piver G, Stoff JS, Donowitz M. Role of prostaglandins and calcium in the effects of *Entamoeba histolytica* on colonic electrolyte transport. *Gastroenterology* 1990;98:873–880.
37. Matozaki T, Sakamoto C, Nagao M, Nishizaki H, Baba S. G protein in stimulation of PI hydrolysis by CCK in isolated rat pancreatic acinar cells. *Am J Physiol* 1988;255:E652–E659.
38. Berridge MJ. Inositol trisphosphate and calcium signaling. *Nature* 1993;361:315–325.
39. Meldolesi J, Villa A, Volpe P, Pozzan T. Cellular sites of IP$_3$ action. In: Putney JW, Jr, ed. *Advances in second messenger and phosphoprotein research: inositol phosphates and calcium signaling.* Vol 26. New York: Raven Press; 1993:187–208.
40. Putney JW Jr. A model for receptor-regulated calcium entry. *Cell Calcium* 1986;7:1–12.
41. Putney JW. Capacitative Ca^{2+}-entry revisited. *Cell Calcium* 1991;11:611–624.
42. Kachintorn U, Vajanaphanich M, Barrett KE, Traynor-Kaplan AE. Elevation of inositol tetrakisphosphate parallels inhibition of Ca^{2+}-dependent Cl$^-$-secretion in T84 cells. *Am J Physiol* 1993;264:C671–C676.
43. Pothoulakis C, Sullivan R, Melnick DA. *Clostridium difficile* toxin A stimulates intracellular calcium release and chemotactic response in human granulocytes. *J Clin Invest* 1988;81:1741–1715.
44. Semrad C, Chang EB. Inhibition of Na/H exchange in avian intestine by atrial natriuretic factor. *J Clin Invest* 1990;86585–591.
45. Semrad CE, Chang EB. Calcium-mediated cyclic AMP inhibi-

tion of Na/H exchange in the small intestine. *Am J Physiol* 1987; C315–C322.

46. Pace J, Hayman MJ, Galan JE. Signal transduction and invasion of epithelial cells by *S. typhimurium*. *Cell* 1993;72:505–514.

47. Bliska JB, Galan JE, Falkow S. Signal transduction in the mammalian cell during bacterial attachment and entry. *Cell* 1993;73: 903–920.

48. Nishizuka Y. Intracellular signaling by hydrolysis of phospholipids and activation of protein kinase C. *Science* 1992;258: 607–614.

49. Hyun CS, Karl PI, Martello LA. Protein kinase C isoforms in rabbit ileal enterocytes. *Gastroenterology* 1993;104:A255.

50. vandenBerghe N, Vaandrager AB, Bot AG, Parker PJ, deJonge HR. Dual role for protein kinase C alpha as a regulator of ion secretion in the HT29c1.19A human colonic cell line. *Biochem J* 1992;285:673–679.

51. Lawson LD, Powell DW. Bradykinin-stimulated eicosanoid synthesis and secretion by rabbit ileal components. *Am J Physiol* 1987;252:G783–G790.

52. Craven PA, DeRubertis FR. Profiles of eicosanoid production by superficial and proliferative colonic epithelial cells and subepithelial colonic tissue. *Prostaglandins* 1986;32:387–399.

53. Hinterleitner TA, Powell DW. Immune system control of intestinal ion transport. *Proc Soc Exp Biol Med* 1991;197:249–260.

54. Kimberg DV, Field M, Johnson J, Henderson, Gershon E. Stimulation of intestinal mucosal adenylate cyclase by cholera toxin and prostaglandins. *J Clin Invest* 1971;50:1218–1230.

55. Calderaro V, Giovane A, DeSimone B. Arachidonic acid metabolites and chloride secretion in rabbit distal colonic mucosa. *Am J Physiol* 1991;261:G443–G450.

56. Beubler E, Bukhave K, Rask-Madsen J. Significance of calcium for the prostaglandin-E2-mediated secretory response to 5-hydroxytryptamine in the small intestine of the rat *in vivo*. *Gastroenterology* 1986;90:1972–1977.

57. Gaion RM, Trento M. The role of prostacyclin in modulating cholinergic neurotransmission in guinea-pig ileum. *Br J Pharmacol* 1983;80:279–286.

58. Yagasaki O, Takai M, Yanagiya I. Acetylcholine release from the myenteric plexus of guinea-pig ileum by prostaglandin E1. *J Pharm Pharmacol* 1981;33:521–525.

59. Traynor T, Brown DR, O'Grady SM. Neuroregulation of Na and Cl transport across the porcine distal colon. *Gastroenterology* 1990;98:A558.

60. Musch MW, Kachur JF, Miller RJ, et al. Bradykinin stimulated electrolyte secretion in rabbit and guinea pig intestine: involvement of arachidonic acid metabolites. *J Clin Invest* 71: 1073–1083.

61. Musch MW, Miller RJ, Field M, Siegel MI. Stimulation of colonic secretion by lipoxygenase metabolites of arachidonic acid. *Science* 1982;217:1255–1256.

62. Wasserman SI, Barrett KE, Huott PA. Immune-related intestinal Cl-secretion. I. Effect of histamine on the T84 cell line. *Am J Physiol* 1988;254:C53–C62.

63. Hardcastle J, Hardcastle PT. The secretory actions of histamine in rat small intestine. *J Physiol* 1987;388:521–532.

64. Cooke HJ, Nemeth PR, Wood JD. Histamine action on guinea pig ileal mucosa. *Am J Physiol* 1984;246:G372–G377.

65. Tamai H, Gaginella TS, Kachur JF, Musch MW, Chang EB. Ca-mediated stimulation of Cl secretion by reactive oxygen metabolites in human colonic T84 cells. *J Clin Invest* 1992;89: 301–307.

66. Karayalcin SS, Sturbaum CW, Wachsman JT, Cha JH, Powell DW. Hydrogen peroxide stimulates rat colonic prostaglandin production and alters electrolyte transport. *J Clin Invest* 1990; 86:60–68.

67. Hanglow AC, Bienenstock J, Perdue MH. Effects of platelet-activating factor on ion transport in isolated rat jejunum. *Am J Physiol* 1989;257:G845–G850.

68. Donowitz M, Asarkof N, Pike G. Calcium dependence of serotonin-induced change in rabbit ileal electrolyte transport. *J Clin Invest* 1980;66:341–352.

69. Hirose R, Chang EB. Effects of serotonin on Na/H exchange and intracellular calcium in isolated chicken enterocytes. *Am J Physiol* 1988;254:G891–G897.

70. Bern MJ, Sturbaum CW, Darayalcin SS, Berschneider HM, Wachsman JT, Powell DW. Immune system control of rat and rabbit colonic electrolyte transport: role of prostaglandins and enteric nervous system. *J Clin Invest* 1989;83:1810–1820.

71. Gaginella TS, Kachur JF. Kinins as mediators of intestinal secretion. *Am J Physiol* 1989;:G1–G15.

72. Wilson KT, Vaandrager AB, De Venter J, et al. Second messenger pathways involved in sodium nitroprusside-stimulated colonic electrolyte transport: localization of cyclic nucleotide and PGE2 production to the subepithelium. *Gastroenterology* 1993; 104:A290.

73. Wilson KT, Xie Y, Musch MWM, Chang EB. Nitric oxide stimulates anion secretion and inhibits NaCl absorption in rat distal colon. *Gastroenterology* 1992;102:A253.

74. Stark ME, Szurszewski JH. Role of nitric oxide in gastrointestinal and hepatic function and disease. *Gastroenterology* 1992; 103:1928–1949.

75. Lundgren O. Nervous control of intestinal transport. *Balliere's Clin Gastroenterol* 1988;2:85–106.

76. Schwartz CJ, Kimberg DV, Sheerine HE, Field M, Said SI. Vasoactive intestinal peptide stimulation of adenylate cyclase and active electrolyte secretion in intestinal mucosa. *J Clin Invest* 1974;54:536–544.

77. Madara JL, Parkos C, Colgan S, et al. Cl-secretion in a model intestinal epithelium induced by a neutrophil derived secretagogue. *J Clin Invest* 1992;89:1938–1944.

78. Madara JL, Patapoff RW, Gillece-Castro B, et al. 5'-AMP is the neutrophil derived paracrine factor that elicits chloride secretion from T84 intestinal epithelial cell monolayers. *J Clin Invest* 1993; 91:2320–2325.

79. Barrett KE, Bigby TD. Involvement of arachidonic acid in the chloride secretory response of intestinal epithelial cells. *Am J Physiol* 1993;264:C446–452.

80. Sullivan SK, Field M. Ion transport in mammalian small intestine. In: Field M, Frizzell RA, eds. *Handbook of physiology, Sect 6, The gastrointestinal system, Vol 4. Intestinal absorption and secretion.* Bethesda: Am Physiol Soc; 1991:287–302.

81. Welsh MJ, Smith PL, Fromm M, Frizzell RA. Crypts are the site of intestinal fluid and electrolyte secretion. *Science* 1982; 218:1219–1221.

82. Dharmasathaphorn K, Mandel KG, Masui H, McRoberts JA. Vasoactive intestinal polypeptide-induced chloride secretion by a colonic epithelial cell line: direct participation of a basolaterally localized Na$^+$, K$^+$, Cl$^-$ cotransport system. *J Clin Invest* 1985;75:462–471.

83. Mandel KG, Dharmsathaphorn K, McRoberts JA. Characterization of a cyclic AMP-activated Cl-transport pathway in the apical membrane of a human colonic epithelial cell line. *J Biol Chem* 1986;261:704–712.

84. Barrett KE. Positive and negative regulation of chloride secretion in T84 cells. *Am J Physiol* 1993;265:C859–C868.

85. Riordan JR, Rommens JM, Kerem B, et al. Identification of the cystic fibrosis gene: cloning and characterization of complementary DNA. *Science* 1989;245:1066–1073.

86. Fine DM, Blackmon DL, Montrose MH. Cell chloride and volume homeostasis in HT29-Cl cells: asymmetric cyclic AMP stimulation of chloride efflux versus chloride uptake. *Gastroenterology* 1993;104:A248.

87. Anderson MP, Welsh MJ. Calcium and cAMP activate different chloride channels in the apical membrane of normal and cystic fibrosis epithelia. *Proc Natl Acad Sci USA* 1991;88:6003–6007.

88. Dharmsathaphorn K, Pandol SJ. Mechanisms of chloride secretion induced by carbachol in a colonic epithelial cell line. *J Clin Invest* 1986;77:348–354.

89. Matthews JB, Awtrey CS, Madara JL. Microfilament-dependent activation of Na$^+$/K$^+$/2Cl$^-$ cotransport by cAMP in intestinal epithelial monolayers. *J Clin Invest* 1992;90:1608–1613.

90. Knickelbein RG, Aronson PS, Dobbins JW. Membrane distribution of sodium-hydrogen and chloride-bicarbonate exchangers in crypt and villus cell membranes from rabbit ileum. *J Clin Invest* 1988;82:2158–2163.

91. Knickelbein R, Aronson PS, Schron CM, Seifter J, Dobbins JW. Sodium and chloride transport across rabbit ileal brush border.

II. Evidence for Cl-HCO₃ exchange and mechanism of coupling. *Am J Physiol* 1985;249:G236–G245.

92. Bookstein CM, DePaoli AM, Xie Y, Niu P, Musch MW, Rao MC, Chang EB. Na⁺/H⁺ exchangers, NHE-1 and NHE-3, of rat intestine: expression and localization. *J Clin Invest* 1994;93: 106–113.

93. Chang EB, Musch MW, Drabik-Arvans D, Rao MC. Phorbol ester inhibition of chicken intestinal brush-border sodium-proton exchange. *Am J Physiol* 1991;260:C1264–C1272.

94. Musch MW, Drabik-Arvans D, Rao MC, Chang EB. Bethanechol inhibition of chicken intestinal brush border Na/H exchange: role of protein kinase C and other calcium-dependent processes. *J Cell Physiol* 1992;152:362–371.

95. Tse CM, Levine SA, Yun CHC, et al. Functional characteristics of a cloned epithelial Na⁺/H⁺ exchanger (NHE3): resistance to amiloride and inhibition by protein kinase C. *Proc Natl Acad Sci USA* 1993;90:9110–9114.

96. Sundaram U, Knickelbein RG, Dobbins JW. pH regulation in ileum: Na⁺-H⁺ and Cl⁻-HCO3⁻ exchange in isolated crypt and villus cells. *Am J Physiol* 1991;260:G440–G449.

97. Sundaram U, Knickelbein RG, Dobbins JW. Mechanism of intestinal secretion: effect of serotonin on rabbit ileal crypt and villus cells. *J Clin Invest* 1991;87:743–746.

98. Fassano A, Baudry B, Pumplin DW, et al. *Vibrio cholerae* produces a second enterotoxin, which affects tight junctions. *Proc Natl Acad Sci USA* 1991;88:5242–5246.

99. Fassano A, Margaretten K, Ding X, Goldblum S, Kaper JB. Mechanisms of action of zonula occludens toxin (ZOT) elaborated by *Vibrio cholerae* (abstract). AGA fall symposium, 1993.

Infections of the Gastrointestinal Tract,
edited by M. J. Blaser, P. D. Smith, J. I. Ravdin,
H. B. Greenberg, and R. L. Guerrant
Raven Press, Ltd., New York © 1995.

CHAPTER 46

Vibrio cholerae O1

Joan R. Butterton and Stephen B. Calderwood

Vibrio cholerae O1 is a gram-negative bacterium that causes a severe, dehydrating, and occasionally fatal diarrhea in humans. There are an estimated 5.5 million cases worldwide of cholera each year, with more than 100,000 deaths (1). Over the last several decades, cholera has been considered to occur primarily in developing countries of Asia and Africa, but over the past several years it has reached epidemic proportions in regions of South and Central America as well (2,3).

TAXONOMY

The genus *Vibrio* is a member of the family Vibrionaceae and is closely related to members of the Enterobacteriaceae. Although vibrios were originally distinguished from the Enterobacteriaceae by biochemical characteristics, more recent studies of the amino acid sequence divergence of enzymes (4) and ribosomal RNA homologies (5) have confirmed the ancestral relationship between the genus *Vibrio* and the family Enterobacteriaceae. At present, 34 *Vibrio* species are recognized, a third of which are known to be pathogenic in humans (6).

Vibrio cholerae is divided into 139 serotypes on the basis of the O antigen of the cell surface lipopolysaccharide (7). The dominant part of the O1 antigen is a homopolymer containing the amino sugar D-perosamine substituted with 3-deoxy-L-glycerotetronic acid (8,9). Until 1993, only *V. cholerae* of the O1 serotype was believed to be responsible for epidemic cholera in humans; all other serotypes are referred to as non-O1. The non-O1 group has been associated with occasional cases of gastroenteritis and extraintestinal infections (as discussed in the chapter by Morris), but has not been believed to cause large epidemics (10). However, a strain of *V. cholerae* non-O1 associated with epidemic cholera appeared in southern

J. R. Butterton: Infectious Disease Unit, Massachusetts General Hospital, Boston, Massachusetts 02114.

S. B. Calderwood: Department of Microbiology and Molecular Genetics, Harvard Medical School, Boston, Massachusetts 02115.

and eastern India in October 1992 (11) and in Bangladesh in January 1993 (12). This novel non-O1 serotype will be discussed in detail below.

BIOTYPES

V. cholerae O1 is divided into two biotypes: classical and El Tor. The El Tor strains were first isolated in 1905 from returning Mecca pilgrims at the quarantine camp of El Tor in the Sinai Peninsula of Egypt (13). These strains agglutinated in O1 typing antiserum and produced typical cases of cholera, but differed from previously isolated strains by producing hemolysins. Characteristics used to differentiate the classical and El Tor biotypes are shown in Table 1.

SEROTYPES

Both classical and El Tor biotypes can be further divided according to the antigenic subspecificity of the O1 antigen into Ogawa, Inaba, and Hikojima serotypes. The O1 antigen can be fractionated into A, B, and C antigens (14–16). Ogawa strains express the A and B antigens and a small amount of C antigen; Inaba strains express the A and C antigens; and Hikojima strains, which are rare, express all three antigens. *V. cholerae* O1 strains can interconvert between the Ogawa and Inaba serotypes (17,18). The *V. cholerae* O1 antigen is synthesized by genes in the *rfb* gene cluster; these have been cloned and sequenced, and the differences between the Ogawa and Inaba serotypes determined (19). The product of the *rfbT* gene is required for determining the Ogawa serotype specificity; Inaba strains are *rfbT* mutants. A variety of changes in *rfbT* may produce an Inaba strain, but correction of such mutations will be rare, explaining observations that conversion from Ogawa to Inaba is more frequent than that from Inaba to Ogawa (19). Inaba strains may arise as a result of selection of *rfbT* mutants due to anti-Ogawa antibodies produced by the immune response

TABLE 1. *Differentiation of the classical and El Tor biotypes of* Vibrio cholerae 01

Characteristics	Classical	El Tor
Hemolysis	−	+
Agglutination of chicken red cells	−	+
Susceptibility to polymyxin B (50 IU)	+	−
Voges–Proskauer reaction	−	+
Susceptibility to bacteriophages:		
IV	+	−
V	−	+

during an infection (17–19). Since Inaba strains are likely independent *rfbT* mutants, the serotype of a strain is not necessarily a suitable marker for epidemiological studies (19).

MICROBIOLOGY

Cell Morphology

V. cholerae cells are single, short (1.5–3.0 by 0.5 μm), slightly curved gram-negative rods; *vibrio* is Greek for *comma*. Many variants may appear in culture. Cells may rarely appear straight, spherical, or as spirilla, or S- or C-shaped if joined (20). Bacilli may lie parallel to each other in smears from mucus in rice water stool. Although essentially nonencapsulated, cells may occasionally look encapsulated (20). Cells have a single, long, polar flagellum (see Fig. 1) and show a characteristic rapid linear motility. This motility forms the basis for identification by an immobilization test (21).

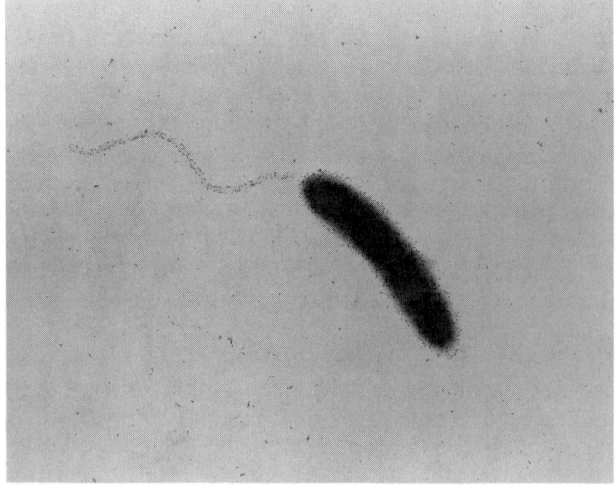

FIG. 1. Electron micrograph of *Vibrio cholerae,* stained with immunogold antilipopolysaccharide antibodies. Courtesy of Dr. John J. Mekalanos and Dr. Marian R. Neutra.

Colonial Morphology and Pigmentation

After primary isolation in bile salt agar (BSA) or lactose teepol agar (LTA), *V. cholerae* form clear, translucent colonies with a sharp, round margin and a flat top, which are easily distinguished from the opaque, convex, grayish white colonies of enteric bacteria (20). The bile salts inhibit the growth of aerobic gram-positive bacilli and add to the translucency of the colonies. *V. cholerae* colonies on BSA show greenish to red–bronze iridescence under stereoplate microscopy (20). After one week, minute secondary colonies appear over the initial growth, while needle-shaped crystals develop underneath. Colony morphology may undergo variations, appearing opaque, rugose, or dwarf (20).

Thiosulfate citrate bile salts–sucrose (TCBS) agar is the most extensively used selective medium for the isolation of *V. cholerae;* the growth of most enteric bacteria is inhibited (22). The sucrose-fermenting colonies of *V. cholerae* on TCBS appear large, yellow, smooth, and opaque. On sucrose teepol tellurite (STT) agar, *V. cholerae* appears translucent yellow; on TCBS lauryl sulfate agar (*Vibrio* agar), colonies are translucent bluish gray; and on lauryl sulfate tellurite agar (cholera medium), they are grayish translucent (20). Colonies cultured on TCBS and *Vibrio* agar are sticky and cannot be used for direct slide agglutination, but must first be subcultured on nutrient agar.

A selective and differential agar medium, polymyxin–mannose–tellurite (PMT) agar, has been developed to differentiate *V. cholerae* O1 from non-O1 strains (23). All strains of *V. cholerae* O1 but only 20% of non-O1 strains ferment mannose in 24 hr. Colonies of *V. cholerae* O1 are yellow with a brown center and are easily agglutinated with O1 antiserum; non-O1 strains are smaller and violet in color.

Biochemical Characteristics

Cholera vibrios are facultative anaerobes that are characterized by their positive oxidase, catalase, and nitrate reduction tests. The positive oxidase reaction differentiates them from the oxidase-negative Enterobacteriaceae; their fermentative metabolism distinguishes them from the oxidase-positive *Pseudomonas* spp. *Aeromonas* spp. are resistant to the vibriostatic compound O/129, to which most *V. cholerae* are susceptible (24). *V. cholerae* is lysine decarboxylase–positive and arginine dihydrolase–negative, grows in nutrient broth without added NaCl, and ferments sucrose (25).

Typing Systems

Species identification is rapidly confirmed by slide agglutination tests with polyvalent O1 antiserum and type-specific Inaba and Ogawa antisera. Biotyping is performed as described above.

Many phage typing schemes for classifying *V. cholerae*

O1 have been developed (26). The most widely used are those of Basu and Mukerjee (27), Lee and Furniss (28), and Drozhevkina and Arutyunov (29). Each contains only a small number of El Tor–specific phages, thus limiting the number of phage types defined; in addition, only a few phage types account for the majority of the strains examined. To address these limitations, five newly isolated phages have been incorporated into the conventional Basu and Mukerjee phage typing scheme, greatly increasing the ability to classify strains of *V. cholerae* O1 biotype El Tor (30). Given the difficulties of quality control, phage typing has been limited to reference laboratories.

EPIDEMIOLOGY

Pandemics

Ancient medical texts from India, Asia, and Europe contain descriptions of severe diarrheal diseases with vomiting that resemble cholera caused by *V. cholerae* O1 (31,32). The enormous impact that cholera has had throughout history contributed to the sanitary revolutions of North America and Europe, to the evolution of health care systems, and to many scientific discoveries. The history of cholera is discussed in detail in the chapter by Tramont and Gangarosa.

In the nineteenth century, six pandemics of cholera spread throughout the world, beginning in Asia, spreading to Europe, and then to the Americas (31). Three waves of cholera entered the United States in 1832, 1849, and 1866, causing heavy casualties (33,34). During the epidemic in London in 1849 John Snow demonstrated that transmission was linked to fecal contamination of water at the infamous Broad Street pump (35). Curved organisms were isolated from cholera victims in 1854 by Filippo Pacini and again by Robert Koch in 1883, who demonstrated the etiological relationship of the comma-shaped organisms with the disease (36).

Throughout the early part of the twentieth century, cholera was a seasonal endemic disease in Asia. The current seventh pandemic began in 1961, spreading from an endemic focus in Sulawesi (Celebes), Indonesia (37) to the Pacific Islands, southeast Asia, and the Middle East. In 1970 cholera reached Africa (38) and Europe (39,40). Although the classical biotype of *V. cholerae* O1 caused the fifth and sixth pandemics, the seventh pandemic has been caused by the El Tor biotype. Biological factors allowing the El Tor strain to replace the classical strain are discussed below. However, 6 years after the El Tor strain replaced classical cholera in Bangladesh, the classical strain reappeared in 1979 (41–44). Reasons for its reappearance and current coexistence with El Tor strains are poorly understood (45).

In late January 1991, *V. cholerae* O1, serotype Inaba, biotype El Tor, appeared with explosive intensity in several coastal Peruvian cities (46), making its first appearance in South America since 1895. The epidemic spread rapidly to other urban areas and then to neighboring countries, jumping southward to Santiago, Chile, and northward to Central America within months (2,47). The same

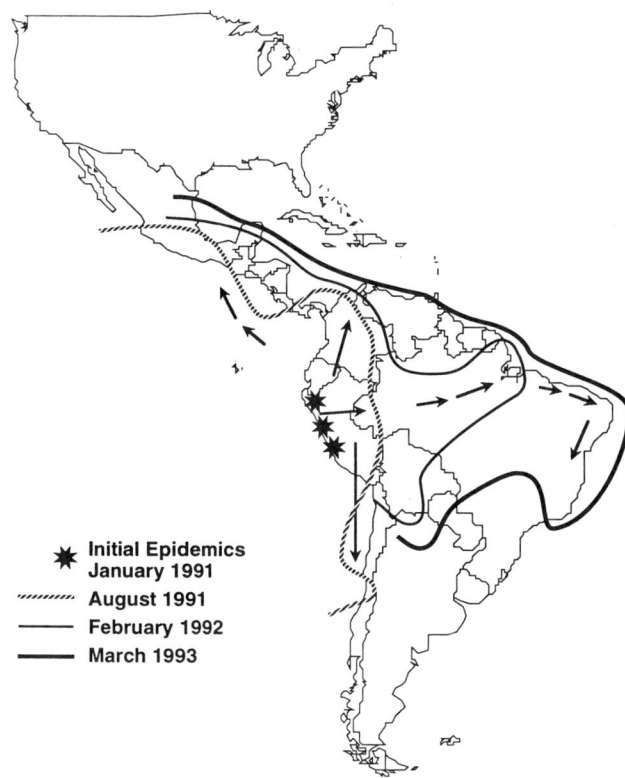

FIG. 2. Spread of cholera through the Americas, 1991–1993. Courtesy of Dr. Robert V. Tauxe, Centers for Disease Control and Prevention.

strain was isolated from all of the affected countries, suggesting a single introduction (48). The strain is related to the seventh pandemic *V. cholerae* O1 strains present in Africa and Asia, but can be clearly distinguished by microbiological and genetic markers (48,49). It is distinct from the endemic strain of *V. cholerae* O1 present along the Gulf of Mexico since 1973 (48–50).

The spread of cholera through the Americas is shown in Fig. 2 (51). Cumulative cholera case totals reported to the Pan American Health Organization as of June 1993 are listed in Table 2.

In the United States from 1961 to 1990, 41 cases of cholera were imported by travelers returning from countries with cholera (3), representing an estimated rate of less than 1 per 500,000 travelers to affected areas (52). In addition, in 1973 an endemic focus was identified in the Gulf of Mexico (53). Through 1992, 65 cases associated with this focus have been reported (53–55). No secondary transmission has been documented. Most of the cases associated with the endemic focus followed consumption of raw shellfish; in 1988 raw oysters from the Gulf of Mexico caused single cases in six states (56). Cholera has spread on a Gulf Coast oil rig, when food was contaminated by a cross-connection in water lines (57).

From 1991 through March 1993, 30 cases of cholera were reported in U.S. residents who had traveled to South America (58–60). Another 11 cases occurred in U.S. residents who ate crabs brought back from Ecuador by other

TABLE 2. *Cumulative cholera case totals reported to the Pan American Health Organization as of June 1993*

Country	1991[a] Cases	1992 Cases	1992 Deaths	1993 Cases	1993 Deaths
Peru	322,562	206,565	709	58,565	295
Ecuador	46,320	31,870	208	3,291	29
Brazil	2,101	24,039	312	5,103	81
Bolivia	206	21,324	383	7,652	192
Guatemala	3,674	15,178	207	1,237	19
Colombia	11,979	15,129	23[a]	182	4
El Salvador	947	8,109	45	3,191	8
Mexico	2,690	7,814	99	1,415	25
Nicaragua	1	3,067	46	701	34
Venezuela	13	2,456	62	63	3
Panama	1,178	2,416	49	42	4
Argentina	0	553	15	1,515	24
Honduras	11	384	17	22	2
Guyana	0	290	4	58	2
Belize	0	154	4	14	0
United States	26 (8[b])	102 (11[b])	1	14 (1[b])	0
Chile	41	71	1	28	0
French Guyana	1	16	0	2	0
Surinam	0	12	1	0	0
Costa Rica	0	12	0	4	0
Paraguay	0	0	0	3	0
Canada	1[b]	0	0	0	0

[a] Incomplete reporting.
[b] Not associated with the Latin American epidemic (these are included in country total).

Hemisphere total:

	1993 cumulative	1992	1991
Cases =	83,102	339,561	391,751
Deaths =	722	2,163	4,002
Death/case ratio =	0.87%	0.64%	1.02%

Centers for Disease Control and Prevention, unpublished data.

travelers (58,59), and 75 cases were associated with food served aboard a 1992 airline flight from Peru (61). Although the South American *V. cholerae* O1 strain has been cultured from oysters in Mobile Bay, Alabama and from the ballast water of ships returning from Latin America, no disease has originated in the United States (62,63). During this same period, 10 U.S. cases occurred in travelers to regions of the world other than South America, and 3 cases were traced to imported frozen coconut milk from Asia (64).

An epidemic outbreak of cholera began in southern and eastern India in October 1992 (11) and in Bangladesh in January 1993 (12), and rapidly spread (65–69). The strains isolated during this outbreak did not agglutinate with O1 antiserum or with monoclonal antibodies against the A, B, and C antigens of *V. cholerae* O1, and were thus identified as non-O1 strains. These strains did not react with a panel of the 137 known non-O1 antisera and have been designated as a new serogroup, O139, with the suggested name of "Bengal" (70). Genetic analysis suggests that *V. cholerae* O139 Bengal is an O-antigen mutant of an El Tor strain rather than a non-O1 strain that has acquired virulence genes (71). *V. cholerae* O139 Bengal contains the cholera toxin gene, the zonula occludens toxin (ZOT) gene, and the gene for the toxin coregulated pilus, but not the gene for the heat-stable enterotoxin of *V. cholerae*

non-O1 (11,12,71). The strain produces cholera toxin, which is neutralized by antitoxin antibodies (11,12,68,71). Initial isolates have been resistant to cotrimoxazole, streptomycin, and furazolidone, but sensitive to tetracycline (11).

The recent spread of *V. cholerae* O139 Bengal is the first time a non-O1 strain has been responsible for epidemic cholera. Many of the cases are in adults, suggesting that immunity to *V. cholerae* O1 does not protect against the O139 serotype (68). *V. cholerae* O139 has displaced *V. cholerae* O1 from the environment in areas in which it is causing disease, suggesting that *V. cholerae* O139 may have an intrinsic survival advantage over *V. cholerae* O1 (72,73), or that the lack of immunity to *V. cholerae* O139 allows its niche to expand from infected persons into the environment through sewage contamination. *V. cholerae* O139 is spreading faster than the *V. cholerae* O1 El Tor strain responsible for the seventh pandemic, appearing in Thailand in April 1993 (69); a case was imported into the United States from India in February 1993 (66). These observations have raised concern that the appearance of *V. cholerae* O139 may mark the beginning of the eighth cholera pandemic (74). A specific diagnostic antiserum for *V. cholerae* O139 is available (67); all cases of illness caused by *V. cholerae* O139 should be reported to the World Health Organization (WHO) as cholera (67).

Natural Reservoirs

V. cholerae O1 is a freeliving inhabitant of brackish water and estuarine systems (75). Many studies have investigated the ability of *V. cholerae* O1 to be cultured from stool, sewage, water, and other environments (76,77). Survival is prolonged in cold, saline conditions (77). *V. cholerae* O1 is sensitive to desiccation; cells only survive several hours on dry surfaces (78).

The presence of *V. cholerae* O1 in the environment, perhaps serving as a reservoir between epidemics of human disease, was questioned because organisms could not be cultured from water sources uncontaminated by active cholera cases (79). However, *V. cholerae* O1 can change from a viable, culturable form to a nonculturable form under certain environmental conditions. Nonculturable forms do not grow on routine laboratory media but can be detected by fluorescent antibody staining or gene probes; they remain responsive to nalidixic acid and continue to take up radiolabeled substrate (80–84). Under starvation conditions, *V. cholerae* O1 cells become small and ovoid; such cells can survive, perhaps for years, in the culturable state in the environment (75). When starved cells are placed in a cold, saline environment, such as seawater, they become nonculturable, but viability can be demonstrated when they are introduced into rabbit ileal loops (80). *V. cholerae* O1 therefore appear able to survive through cold seasons in a dormant state but remain potentially pathogenic.

Plankton and shellfish may serve as reservoirs of *V. cholerae* O1 in the environment. At least 10^4–10^5 organisms may attach to a single copepod. During a copepod bloom, the number of *V. cholerae* O1 may rise to the number needed to cause human disease (85). *V. cholerae* O1 may also adhere to water plants (86) and algae (87). Raw bivalves (clams, oysters, and mussels) and undercooked shellfish (shrimp, crabs) have been documented as important vehicles of transmission (39,54,56,88,89).

Transmission

V. cholerae O1 is transmitted by the fecal–oral route and is spread primarily through contaminated food and water. Since the classic observations by John Snow during the cholera epidemic in London in 1854 (35), water has been considered a major vehicle for cholera transmission. During the recent outbreak in Peru, fecal contamination of the municipal water supplies of large urban areas was associated with the majority of cases (90,91). Factors leading to contamination were clandestine taps into water lines, low water pressure, frequent cutoffs, and lack of chlorination (90,91). Storage of water has also been associated with transmission of *V. cholerae* O1. In Peru, illness was strongly associated with drinking water into which others had introduced their hands (90). Contamination of water in household storage containers was also demonstrated in Calcutta (92); when narrow-necked water containers were used to prevent hands from entering, cholera attack rates were reduced (93). Contaminated noncarbonated bottled water (94) and contaminated ice

(91,95) have been implicated in other outbreaks. Use of contaminated surface water for cooking, bathing, and washing also may lead to illness (96).

Foodborne transmission plays an important role in many cholera outbreaks (76,77). The duration of survival of *V. cholerae* O1 in various foods is influenced by the pH, humidity, temperature, and inoculum size (77,97–100). Organisms can survive on vegetables for 1–2 days at room temperature, or longer if moist or cooler (98); survival is also enhanced in alkaline foods (99). Cases of cholera have been associated with crops irrigated with sewage (101), with lettuce (90), millet gruel (102), rice (99), raw and cooked seafood (39,40,54–56, 88,89,103), pickled or dried fish (103), and frozen coconut milk (64).

During active cholera outbreaks, human carriers provide a large reservoir of infection. Although asymptomatic carriers can be an important source of transmission during outbreaks (45), chronic carriage appears rare (104). Excretion of organisms rarely lasts longer than 2 weeks (77), although a few patients have been documented to excrete vibrios for months (105,106) or, in the case of "Cholera Dolores," for years (107). Direct person-to-person spread, rather than through contamination of food or water, is not usually an important route of transmission. Direct spread has been implicated in outbreaks in hospitals (108,109), during burial ceremonies in which intestinal contents are removed from the dead body (110), through sweat (111), and from ill children to their mothers (112), but in some of these cases contamination of food or water may have occurred.

Flies can carry vibrios (45,113) but have not been documented to transmit disease. Similarly, fomites may become contaminated, but since *V. cholerae* O1 survives only a short time on dry surfaces, fomites are an unlikely source for disease transmission. Fecally contaminated wet cloth should, however, be washed in ways that prevent further environmental contamination (45).

Risk Factors

The previous exposure of a population is an important factor in the risk of contracting cholera. Patients who recover from *V. cholerae* O1 infection have longlasting, perhaps lifelong, immunity to reinfection (114). In endemic areas such as eastern India and Bangladesh, cholera primarily affects nonimmune children 2–15 years of age (112), while in areas with little preexisting immunity, such as in Latin America or in regions affected by *V. cholerae* O139 Bengal, cholera is a disease affecting persons of all ages (68,90,91).

Persons with low gastric acidity, due to malnutrition, gastritis, surgery, or drugs such as antacids, H_2 receptor antagonists, and marijuana, are at increased risk for cholera infection (115–120). *V. cholerae* O1 are killed rapidly in gastric acid of pH <2.4 (115). Ingesting organisms with sodium bicarbonate or food reduces the infectious dose from 10^{11} organisms to 10^4–10^6 organisms (121,122). Infection with *Helicobacter pylori,* common in Latin American countries, has been proposed as a factor increasing the risk of *V. cholerae* O1 infection during the recent Latin American epidemic (2).

Blood group O is associated with an increased risk of severe cholera, although the reasons for this association are unknown (123–127). The population of the Ganges Delta has the lowest prevalence of O blood group genes in the world. Only 30% of Bangladeshis but at least 75% of Peruvians are of blood group O, suggesting not only that cholera has selected against persons of the O blood group in the Ganges Delta (126) but also that Latin American populations may be predisposed to particularly severe clinical infection (2).

Bottle feeding of infants is associated with a greater risk of cholera, while breast feeding appears protective (128–130). Breast milk antibodies against cholera do not appear to protect children from colonization with *V. cholerae* O1 but do protect against disease in those who are colonized (130). Maternal vaccination may provide protection to their nonvaccinated breast-fed children (129). The reduced risk of cholera in breast-fed children could be a result of decreased ingestion of contaminated food or water, the antibacterial effect of lactoferrin in breast milk, a protective effect of breast milk antibodies, or improved nutrition. However, children with chronic malnutrition have not been demonstrated to have an increased risk of infection or disease with *V. cholerae* O1 (131).

The biotype of the infecting *V. cholerae* O1 strain may have an influence on the risk of infection. The El Tor biotype may be less immunogenic than the classical biotype (132) and produces higher rates of asymptomatic or mildly symptomatic infections (1 clinical case per 30–100 infections with the El Tor biotype vs. 1 case for each 2–4 infections with classical strains) (133–135). Duration of carriage following infection is longer with the El Tor biotype (136). The El Tor biotype may also survive longer in the environment (such as in water, feces, and sewage) and on food than the classical biotype (97,100,137).

PATHOGENESIS AND IMMUNITY

Pathogenesis

Colonization

After ingestion, *V. cholerae* O1 must pass through the gastric acid barrier of the stomach to colonize the small intestine. There the organism penetrates the mucus gel, adheres to the brush border of intestinal epithelial cells via specific adhesins, and produces a number of extracellular secreted proteins, including cholera toxin, neuraminidase, and hemolysin. Full virulence of *V. cholerae* depends on the coordinate regulation of many of these virulence factors.

The importance of the gastric acid barrier in preventing organisms from reaching the small bowel has been discussed above (115–119,121,122). Vibrios that survive passage through the stomach—due to a large inoculum size, a hypochlorhydric host, protection within a bolus of food, or a rapid gastric emptying time—must colonize the small

intestine in order to produce disease. Adherence to the brush border of the intestinal epithelium is the initial step in colonization. *V. cholerae* O1 adheres to the mucous coat of the human small intestine more than to the epithelial surface of the villi, suggesting that the mucous coat is a primary adherence target in human infection (138). Adherence to the sugar residues in the mucous coat may be mediated by cell-associated hemagglutinins (discussed below) (138). After attaching to the mucous gel, vibrios move by unknown mechanisms to their final adherence sites on the absorptive cell microvilli (139–142).

Pili are important factors in the adherence of vibrios to the small intestine. The classical biotype of *V. cholerae* O1 produces a pilus, the toxin-coregulated pilus (TCP), which is necessary for human colonization (143,144). Antibodies to the 20.5-kDa major subunit of the pilus, TcpA, inhibit attachment of bacteria to epithelial cells in vitro, and are protective in an animal model (145–147). In volunteer studies, mutant strains lacking pili fail to colonize the intestine or produce an immune response (144). Although both classical and El Tor biotypes possess the *tcpA* gene (146,148), TCPs are poorly expressed on El Tor vibrios (149,150) and have not been demonstrated to be virulence factors in the El Tor biotype.

Two additional types of fimbriae, types B and C, have been identified as morphologically distinct from TCP (149); the role of these fimbrial types in virulence remains to be determined. Other pili have been demonstrated to have hemagglutinating activity but play no role in colonization (151).

Other factors have been demonstrated to be important for the colonization of the small intestine by *V. cholerae* O1. Protease production may allow degradation of the mucous gel (152). An accessory colonization factor (ACF) is encoded by the clustered *acfA, B, C,* and *D* genes. Mutations in any of these genes reduce the ability of vibrios to colonize the intestine of suckling mice (153–155).

A number of hemagglutinins (HA) are produced by *V. cholerae* and may function as adherence factors (156–159; for reviews, see 160–162). Both cholera biotypes produce a soluble HA protease (156), encoded by the *hap* gene (163), which is a zinc-dependent metalloprotease (164,165) that cleaves mucin, fibronectin, and lactoferrin (166), and nicks and activates the A subunit of cholera toxin (167). The HA protease appears not to play a primary role in virulence (168); studies on cultured human intestinal cells suggest that the HA protease is a "detachase," responsible for detachment of the vibrios from the intestinal epithelium, perhaps by destroying host cell receptors for several adhesins (168). Besides the soluble HA protease, several cell-associated HAs have been described (157), including the D-mannose–D-fructose–sensitive HA (MSHA) expressed by El Tor strains, the L-fucose–sensitive HA expressed by classical strains, and the D-mannose–, L-fucose–resistant HA (MFRHA) expressed by both biotypes. Both the MSHA and the MFRHA appear to be important colonization factors in animal models (169–171).

Motility appears to be an important factor in colonization by *V. cholerae* (172–174). Although flagellar antigens may play a role (175), they are less important (174). Motility combined with chemotaxis (176) may allow organisms to avoid clearance by peristalsis.

Cholera toxin itself may contribute to *V. cholerae* virulence by enhancing mucosal colonization. Mutant nontoxinogenic organisms show decreased colonization of rabbit intestinal mucosa compared to parent toxinogenic strains; when purified toxin is added to the nontoxinogenic strain, colonization increases to the level of the parent strain (177). Other investigators, however, have not detected a colonization defect in toxin-negative strains (169).

A variety of outer membrane proteins have been characterized that appear to play a role in the intestinal colonization of vibrios. Antibodies to several porin-like outer membrane proteins have been demonstrated to protect against infection by inhibiting intestinal colonization (178,179).

Cholera Toxin

The major virulence factor for *V. cholerae* O1 is cholera toxin. The structure, mechanism of action, and genetic regulation of cholera toxin have been the focus of intense scientific activity over the past several decades. The history of research in these areas was recently extensively reviewed (180).

Cholera toxin (CT) is a multimeric protein composed of one A subunit (molecular weight 27,215) noncovalently attached to five B subunits (molecular weight 11,677) (181). The A subunit undergoes proteolytic nicking to produce A1 and A2 fragments linked by a disulfide bond (182). The A1 fragment (approximate molecular weight 22,500) contains the enzymatic activity of the toxin (183). The A2 fragment (approximate molecular weight 5500) attaches the A subunit to the B-subunit pentamer (181). The proteolytic cleavage of the A subunit is necessary for expression of the enzymatic activity of the toxin (184).

The B subunit pentamer binds holotoxin to the enterocyte surface receptor, the ganglioside GM1 (185,186). *V. cholerae* produces a neuraminidase (NANase), encoded by the *nanH* gene (187), which catalyzes conversion of gangliosides to GM1 (188). The role of NANase in cholera pathogenesis is still unclear; it has been postulated that NANase may produce locally high concentrations of GM1 receptor for cholera toxin, thereby increasing the binding and uptake of CT by enterocytes (189).

Following binding of holotoxin, the A1 fragment catalyzes the ADP ribosylation of a GTP-binding protein and causes persistent activation of adenylate cyclase (190,191). The end result is an increase of cAMP within the intestinal mucosa, stimulating chloride secretion and decreasing sodium absorption, leading to loss of fluid and electrolytes and the production of diarrhea (Fig. 3) (for reviews, see 192–196).

The heat-labile enterotoxin (LT) produced by some enterotoxigenic strains of *Escherichia coli* shares an identical mode of action with cholera toxin. CT and LT have structural, antigenic, and DNA sequence homology (197–200), suggesting a common evolutionary origin (201).

cAMP may not be the sole mediator of intestinal water

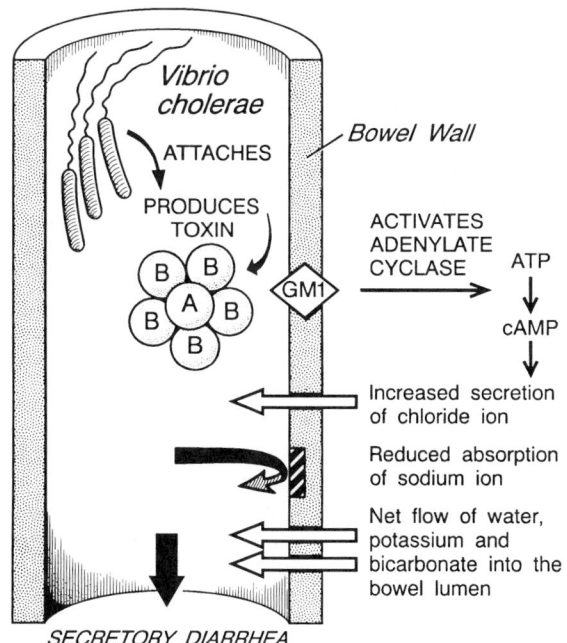

FIG. 3. Pathophysiology of *V. cholerae* infection. See text for details.

and electrolyte transport in cholera. Cholera toxin may lead to increased production of prostaglandins, which may independently contribute to the massive loss of water and electrolytes in cholera. Such a role for prostaglandins is suggested by the observations that drugs that inhibit prostaglandin synthesis reduce the effects of cholera toxin on fluid secretion in experimental animals (202,203), while patients with active disease have elevated prostaglandin E_2 concentrations in jejunal aspirates (204). In a rabbit model, treatment with cholera toxin caused a dose-dependent synthesis and release of PGE that correlated better than cAMP levels with fluid accumulation in the intestinal lumen (205).

The factors influencing cholera toxin production in vivo are not known. In vitro conditions that enhance production are low temperature (25–30°C), osmolarity (NaCl concentration of 50–60 mM), rich media, high aeration, a slightly acidic pH (6.5), and the presence of certain amino acids (asparagine, serine, glutamate, and arginine), phosphate, and trace elements (143,206–209). Different strains also show differing levels of toxin production. The fact that cholera toxin expression is regulated by environmental conditions has led to the identification of other similarly regulated *V. cholerae* virulence factors (143,153) that will be discussed below.

The cholera toxin structural genes (*ctxAB*) were cloned with the use of homologous *E. coli* LT gene probes (210–212). Cholera toxin genes are poorly expressed in *E. coli* (211,213); the A subunit is not proteolytically nicked and the assembled holotoxin remains in the periplasm and is not secreted extracellularly (211). The DNA sequence of *ctxAB* has been determined for both El Tor

(201,214–216) and classical (201,217) strains. Minor differences in the amino acid sequences of the various strains exist. *ctxB* lies immediately downstream of *ctxA*, overlapping by four nucleotides. The predicted length of CtxA is 258 amino acids, with the first 18 residues serving as a likely signal sequence; CtxB is 124 amino acids in length, with a 21-residue signal sequence. *ctxA* and *ctxB* are transcribed as an operon; consistent with the 5:1 ratio of B subunit to A subunit in holotoxin, the B subunit is more highly expressed, likely due to translational control (201).

V. cholerae strains of the classical biotype contain two identical, nontandem copies of the *ctxAB* operon (218); both express active cholera toxin (201). In contrast, about 70% of El Tor strains have a single copy of *ctxAB*, with the rest having two or more tandemly repeated copies (218). The presence of multiple copies loosely correlates with increased toxin production (218). *ctxAB* lies within a larger transposon-like cholera toxin genetic element (219), composed of a 4.5–kilobase pair (kbp) "core region," flanked by one or more copies of a 2.7- or 2.4-kbp directly repeated region called, respectively, RS1 or RS2 (Fig. 4) (218,220). The RS sequences allow tandem duplication and amplification of the core region through *recA*–dependent recombination (219). All classical strains, as well as some El Tor strains, lack a downstream RS copy; in these strains no gene amplification is seen (218,221). Amplification of the core region in El Tor strains has been demonstrated to occur during intestinal passage in animals, associated with the selection of hypertoxinogenic variants (218). The importance of such amplification in human disease remains to be defined.

Nontoxinogenic *V. cholerae* O1 strains are naturally occurring (222,223), perhaps through loss of the core region by rearrangements through the RS regions (213,224). A 17-bp "end-repeat" (ER) sequence is arranged in direct repeats at the ends of RS1. The ER element shares 17 of 18 bp with a sequence on the *V. cholerae* chromosome called *attRS1* (220). This element therefore can act as a site-specific recombination system, providing a mechanism for conversion between toxigenic and nontoxigenic strains (220,225).

Investigations into the molecular regulation of cholera toxin production have led to the realization that many *V. cholerae* virulence genes are coordinately regulated by a single regulator (for reviews, see Refs. 226 and 227). As described above, cloned *ctxAB* genes are poorly expressed in *E. coli* (211,213). A *ctx–lacZ* fusion was created on the chromosome of an *E. coli* strain; then a genomic library of *V. cholerae* was introduced. A plasmid that increased *lacZ* expression carried a gene, *toxR*, that en-

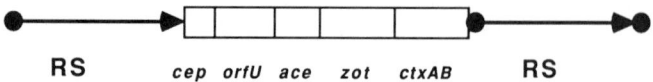

FIG. 4. Schematic of the cholera toxin genetic element, with the 4.5-kbp "core region" flanked by 2.7-kbp direct repeats (RS elements). End-repeat sequences are indicated by dots. Open reading frames in the core region: *cep*, core-encoded pilin; *orfU*, open reading frame of unknown function; *ace*, accessory cholera enterotoxin; *zot*, zonula occludens toxin; *ctxAB*, cholera toxin operon.

codes a positive regulator of *ctxAB* (213). Introducing *toxR* with the cloned *ctxAB* genes in *E. coli* increased toxin expression dramatically (213).

toxR appears to be present in all *V. cholerae* O1 strains, both toxinogenic and nontoxinogenic (228). The gene product, ToxR, is a 32.5-kDa protein that activates transcription of *ctxAB* following binding to a 7-bp repetitive region in the *ctxAB* promoter (208); levels of cholera toxin production are related to the number of tandem repeats present (201). ToxR is a transmembrane protein (208); the amino terminus is a DNA binding region that is similar to the activator class of proteins in the family of prokaryotic two-component regulators (229). The periplasmic carboxy terminus of ToxR senses environmental changes, leading to conformational changes in the DNA-binding amino terminus and altered gene transcription (229).

toxR expression is modulated by the *V. cholerae* heat shock gene, *htpG* (230). The *htpG* gene lies directly upstream of and in the opposite orientation from *toxR*. At low temperatures (22°C), σ70 RNA polymerase binds to the *toxR* promoter and transcribes *toxR;* at high temperatures (37°C), more σ32 RNA polymerase is made, which binds to the *htpG* promoter and represses *toxR* transcription. Although temperature, osmolarity, pH, and amino acid concentration all regulate the function of ToxR, the latter three parameters do not appear to act at the level of *toxR* expression (208).

A second gene in the *toxR* operon is *toxS*, which lies immediately downstream of *toxR* and is part of the same transcriptional unit (231,232). *toxS* encodes for a 19-kDa protein that is located in the periplasm (232). ToxS is necessary for ToxR activation, perhaps by facilitating dimerization (232).

In addition to directly activating the *ctxAB* promoter, ToxR activates transcription of another gene, *toxT* (233). ToxT is a 32-kDa member of the AraC family of transcriptional control proteins (234). ToxT can independently activate *ctxAB* expression, suggesting that the *ctxAB* promoter contains regulatory sites for two different activators. *toxT* lies within the *tcp* cluster of genes responsible for production of the toxin-coregulated pilus (143,153); it was initially sequenced as *tcpN* (235).

ctxAB is the only operon directly activated by ToxR; all other defined ToxR-activated genes (*tag* genes) are activated by ToxT (233). These include the *tcp* genes encoding the TCP (143,153), the *acf* genes encoding the accessory colonization factor (153), the genes encoding the two major outer membrane proteins OmpU and OmpT (209), the *aldA* gene encoding the enzyme aldehyde dehydrogenase (236), and other still undefined *tag* genes (153). The regulatory cascade controlling many virulence genes in *V. cholerae* is shown in Fig. 5. Such regulatory cascades controlling virulence factors have likely evolved to allow pathogens to control precisely when virulence genes will be expressed, thus conferring a survival advantage by allowing organisms to adapt to varying environmental conditions (227).

Other Toxins

Several other enterotoxins, besides cholera toxin, have been described in *V. cholerae* O1. The genes encoding

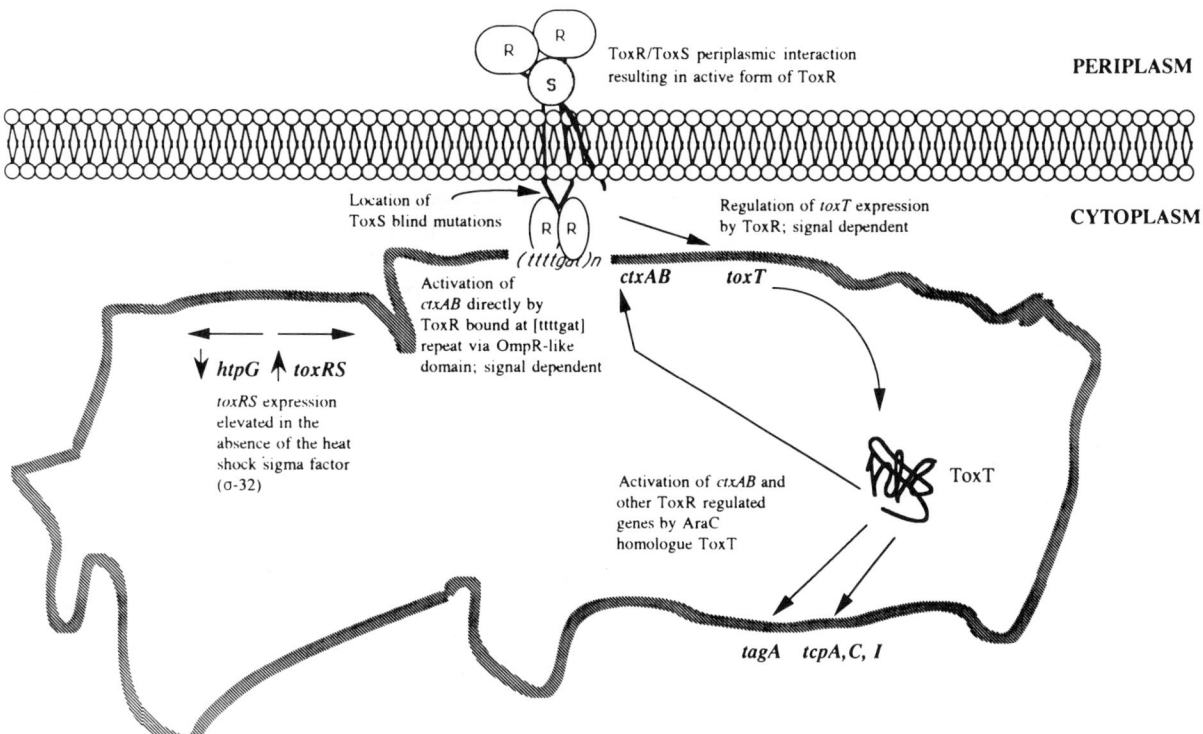

FIG. 5. Model for the ToxR regulatory system of *V. cholerae*. See text for details. (From ref. 227, with permission.)

two of these, *zot* and *ace*, lie upstream of *ctxAB* within the 4.5-kbp core region of the cholera toxin genetic element. Zot (zonula occludens toxin) increases the permeability of the small intestinal mucosa by affecting the structure of the intercellular tight junctions (237). *zot* lies immediately upstream of *ctxAB*, with the end of *zot* overlapping the *ctxAB* promoter (238). Expression of *zot* does not require ToxR (238). The third toxin of the core region, Ace (accessory cholera enterotoxin), is encoded by a gene that lies immediately upstream of *zot*; the termination codon of *ace* overlaps with the initiation codon of *zot* (239). Ace increases ion transport across rabbit ileal mucosa and causes fluid secretion in ligated rabbit ileal loops. The mechanism of action of Ace is unknown, but its predicted protein sequence is similar to eukaryotic ion-transporting ATPases, including the product of the cystic fibrosis gene (239). An open reading frame of unknown function, *orfU*, lies immediately upstream of *ace* (239); the gene for a colonization factor, *cep* (core-encoded pilin), lies upstream of *orfU* (220). The genes in the core region of the cholera toxin genetic element are depicted in Fig. 4.

Additional toxins are encoded outside of the cholera toxin genetic element. *V. cholerae* O1 produces four molecular species of heat-stable enterotoxins, all homologous to the heat-stable enterotoxin of some *V. cholerae* non-O1 strains (240). At the protein level, these toxins are homologous to the ST enterotoxin of enterotoxigenic *E. coli*, although the genes encoding these proteins lack nucleotide similarity. The relevance of these enterotoxins to human disease is not yet known. In addition, *V. chol-*

erae may produce a Shiga-like toxin, analogous to the Shiga-like toxins found in a variety of strains of enterohemorrhagic *E. coli* (241). However, cloned fragments from one *V. cholerae* strain, which showed homology to *E. coli* *slt-I* probes at low stringency, showed no significant homology to the *slt-I* open reading frame when sequenced (225).

Other Virulence Factors

Other virulence factors, distinct from the ToxR regulon, have also been described. Iron is an important signal for the regulation of many bacterial virulence factors, and *in vivo*–grown *V. cholerae* O1 express proteins that are similar to those seen following *in vitro* growth in low-iron conditions, suggesting that the organism senses low-iron conditions *in vivo* in the intestine (242). The major 77-kDa iron-regulated outer membrane protein of *V. cholerae* O1 has been shown to be a virulence factor for this organism and is encoded by the gene *irgA* (243). A mutation in *irgA* produces a 100-fold defect in the virulence of *V. cholerae* O1 in a suckling mouse model and a 10-fold defect in colonization compared to the wild-type parent strain (243). Expression of *irgA* depends on a second iron-regulated gene, *irgB*, whose protein product acts as a transcriptional activator for *irgA* (244,245). The mechanism by which IrgA and IrgB affect the pathogenesis of *V. cholerae* O1 infection, however, remains undefined (246).

The *V. cholerae* O1 hemolysin used to distinguish the usually hemolytic El Tor biotype from the nonhemolytic classical biotype has been the subject of intensive investigations. Hemolysin genes have been cloned from both biotypes (247–251). All examined classical strains have an 11-bp deletion in the structural gene, *hlyA*, of the El Tor biotype (252,253). However, both hemolytic and nonhemolytic variants of one El Tor strain have identical *hlyA* sequences, suggesting that other genes may affect hemolysis (254). Another gene, *hlyB*, may contribute to expression of the hemolytic phenotype (249,255). Two potential regulatory loci, *hlyR* (256) and *hlyU* (257), have also been described. Hemolytic activity is negatively regulated by iron concentration (258), perhaps by affecting *hlyU* transcription (257). The *V. cholerae* O1 hemolysin also has enterotoxic and cytotoxic activity (259–262). Volunteer studies, however, have not revealed a difference in the ability of hemolytic and nonhemolytic strains to cause diarrhea (263), leaving unresolved the question of the role of hemolysin in the pathogenesis of cholera.

Immunity

Naturally Occurring Immunity

Patients who recover from cholera infection are believed to have longlasting immunity to reinfection (114). In volunteer challenge studies, clinical infection with *V. cholerae* of the classical biotype provides complete protection against illness after rechallenge with classical Ogawa or Inaba strains; organisms cannot be recovered from stool after rechallenge (114,121,122,264,265). Protection lasts for at least 3 years (114). In contrast, infection with El Tor strains provides only 90% protection against rechallenge with El Tor Ogawa or Inaba strains (114,122) and organisms can be recovered from the stools of 30% of the rechallenged volunteers (122,265). Population studies in endemic areas give conflicting estimates of the protection provided by natural infection, ranging from none (266) to 90% (267). The protection conferred by an initial episode of cholera may be influenced by the biotype of the initial infection (132). In a large field study in Bangladesh, the overall incidence of cholera was 61% lower in persons who had been previously ill with cholera than in persons who had not had a known prior infection. In this study, initial episodes of classical cholera provided complete protection against subsequent cholera, while initial episodes of El Tor cholera were associated with negligible protection (132).

Mucosal Immunity

As a mucosal pathogen, *V. cholerae* adheres selectively to the M cells of the gastrointestinal tract (268) and is a strong stimulus to the common mucosal immune system (269); oral cholera vaccination in humans produces a strong secretory immune response, as judged by salivary IgA directed against cholera toxin B subunit (270). Secretory IgA by itself is sufficient to protect against subsequent intestinal disease from *V. cholerae* (271). Animal studies have demonstrated that prior colonization with *V. cholerae* produces substantial resistance to recolonization, suggesting that mucosal colonization is essential for immunizing efficiency (272). The observation that prior oral immunization with nontoxigenic strains interferes with stimulation of a mucosal antitoxin response by toxigenic strains also points to the importance of colonization in the induction of a mucosal immune response (273). However, cholera toxin clearly plays a role in enhancing mucosal colonization, as discussed above; in addition, cholera toxin is a strong adjuvant, enhancing mucosal secretory antibody responses to a variety of oral antigens (274–276).

Systemic Immunity

Intestinal antibodies are felt to provide the primary protection against disease caused by *V. cholerae;* serum antibodies are likely not protective but are used as markers for the presence of secretory IgA directed against the same antigens. Both antibacterial and antitoxic immunity are important in the host response to infection with *V. cholerae*. Parenteral immunization of animals with cholera toxin, toxoids, or B subunit alone provides only brief protection as serum antitoxin antibodies fall rapidly (277–280); field trials of parenteral toxoid vaccines have not shown evidence of protection (281,282). Oral B subunit alone, however, given with oral killed whole-cell vaccine, produces both serum and intestinal antitoxin antibody responses and leads to a greater protective effect than with whole-cell vaccine alone (283). Serum IgG antitoxic antibodies rise after clinical cholera and can persist for several years (284–287). However, epidemiological studies have not demonstrated a correlation between the presence of serum antitoxic antibodies and protection against infection (284,288). The presence of secretory IgA antitoxic antibodies in breast milk, however, is correlated with protection of breast-fed children, suggesting that serum antitoxic antibody levels may not fully reflect intestinal secretory IgA protection (130).

Antibacterial immunity is an essential component to protection against cholera. Both parenteral and oral killed whole-cell vaccines, which produce no antitoxin response, can lead to protection against clinical disease (for a review, see Ref. 289). Live oral vaccines that lack the genes for cholera toxin also provide protection against disease (290). The presence of serum vibriocidal antibodies, which are measured by their ability to kill bacteria in the presence of complement, clearly correlates with protection against disease; epidemiological studies have shown a clear relationship between the vibriocidal antibody titer and protection against cholera (291–293). Most vibriocidal antibodies appear to be antilipopolysaccharide antibodies, though other components of the cell surface may play a role (265,294–296). Vibriocidal antibody titers are also used in cholera diagnosis. Titers peak 10–21 days after infection; a fourfold rise between acute (days 1–5) and early convalescent (days 10–21) sera, or a fourfold fall in antibody titers between early and late (>2 months) convalescent sera, is considered diagnostic (297).

Other antigens that may play a role in protection, such

as the toxin-coregulated pilus, the accessory colonization factor, cell-associated hemagglutinins, flagellar antigens, and other outer membrane proteins, have been discussed above.

CLINICAL ILLNESS

Incubation Period

The incubation period of cholera is usually 1–3 days, with a range of a few hours to 5 days (121,298,299). Human volunteer studies have demonstrated an inverse relationship between the incubation period and the ingested dose of organisms (121,298), as well as with the gastric pH (45).

Asymptomatic and Mild Disease

As discussed earlier, the majority of persons infected with *V. cholerae* O1 remain asymptomatic, with the El Tor biotype producing higher rates of asymptomatic or mildly symptomatic infections than the classical biotype (30–100:1 for El Tor vs. 2–4:1 for classical) (133–135). Similarly, the ratio of persons with severe disease to those with mild disease varies with biotype, from 1:7 for El Tor to 1:1 for classical strains (135). Mild disease is indistinguishable from many other forms of infectious diarrhea, with no prodromal symptoms, a few episodes of watery stools without mucus or blood, rare nausea and vomiting, and no significant fluid loss (300). In areas experiencing an epidemic outbreak, however, the majority of cases of diarrhea are likely to be a result of *V. cholerae* infection; during the recent outbreak in Peru, *V. cholerae* O1 was recovered from 79% of patients presenting with diarrhea (90).

Cholera Gravis

Severe disease, called cholera gravis, is characterized by severe watery diarrhea, vomiting, and dehydration (300). Clinical findings are due to rapid and massive fluid and electrolyte loss. Diarrhea may begin slowly or abruptly and is painless; stools quickly become watery and clear with flecks of mucus. Cholera stools are classically described as "rice water" stools, for their similarity to water in which uncooked rice has been washed. Stools characteristically have a mild "fishy" odor. Vomiting is common, often beginning after the onset of diarrhea but sometimes before (121). There is no abdominal pain or fever.

Severe cholera is distinguished by how rapidly a healthy person can become dramatically ill. Patients may present after only a few hours of illness and may look cadaveric in appearance (Fig. 6). Fluid loss due to diarrhea and vomiting may be massive, between 500 mL and 1 L of fluid per hour, and can lead to the rapid loss of more than 10% of body weight (300). Diarrhea is most severe during the first 48 hr, then slows, ending after 4–6 days in patients treated with appropriate rehydration (301–303). Total vol-

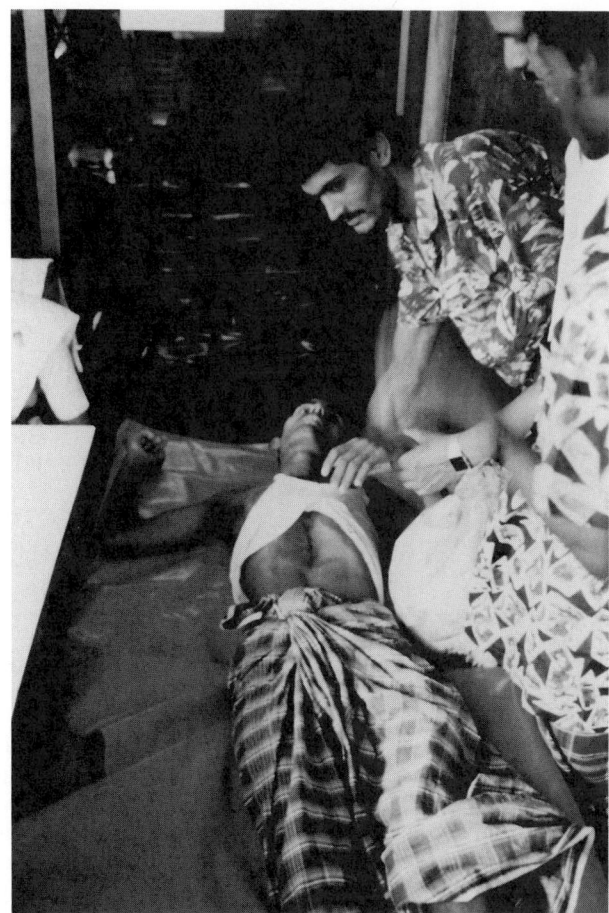

FIG. 6. Cholera patient with severe dehydration. Courtesy of Dr. John J. Mekalanos.

ume loss during illness may reach 100% of body weight (302). Along with rapid fluid losses come large electrolyte losses; cholera stools contain high concentrations of sodium, potassium, chloride, and bicarbonate (Table 3).

Patients with severe cholera present with signs of volume and electrolyte loss. Mild dehydration is indicated by thirst, dry mouth, decreased axillary sweat, and slight weight loss. Signs of moderate dehydration include tachycardia, an orthostatic fall in blood pressure, skin tenting, and sunken eyes or fontanelle. Signs of severe dehydration are hypotension, anuria, and mental status changes. Rapid assessment of the degree of dehydration is essential for optimal rehydration therapy of patients with cholera (see Table 4).

Complications of severe cholera are the result of sus-

TABLE 3. *Electrolyte composition of cholera stool (mEq/L)*

	Sodium	Potassium	Chloride	Bicarbonate
Adults	135	15	100	45
Children	105	25	90	30

Adapted from ref. 313, with permission.

TABLE 4. *Signs and symptoms of dehydration among patients with diarrhea*

Examination	Outcome		
	No signs of dehydration	Some dehydration	Severe dehydration
Look at			
Mental status	Well, alert	Restless, irritable[a]	Lethargic or unconscious; floppy infant[a]
Eyes	Normal	Sunken	Very sunken and dry
Tears	Present	Absent	Absent
Mouth/tongue	Moist	Dry	Very dry
Thirst	Drinks normally, not thirsty	Thirsty, drinks eagerly[a]	Drinks poorly or not able to drink[a]
Feel			
Skin pinch	Goes back rapidly	Goes back slowly[a]	Goes back very slowly[a]
Pulse	Normal	Faster than normal[a]	Very fast, weak or nonpalpable[a]
Fontanelle	Normal	Sunken	Very sunken
Decide degree of dehydration	*No* signs of dehydration, <2.5% of body weight	If two or more of these signs exist, including at least one important sign, then there is *some* dehydration, from 2.5% to 10% of body weight	If two or more of these signs exist, including at least one important sign, then there is *severe* dehydration, >10% of body weight

From ref. 3, with permission.
[a] Important signs and symptoms for assessment of dehydration.

tained volume loss or electrolyte imbalances. Severe acidosis is the result of loss of bicarbonate in the stool, along with lactic acidemia from shock, hyperphosphatemia from renal failure, and hyperproteinemia from dehydration (304). Acidosis may be manifested as tachypnea, Kussmaul breathing, or, in end-stage cases, pulmonary edema (305). Loss of potassium in the stool may lead to hypokalemia, which can cause cardiac arrhythmias, paralytic ileus, and painful leg cramps. Renal failure follows acute tubular necrosis from hypovolemia (306). Hypoglycemia may be a severe complication of cholera, especially in children (307), and is a poor prognostic sign (308,309). Hypoglycemia is caused by defects in gluconeogenesis (310). Hypoglycemia has been implicated in mental status changes and seizures seen in severe cholera, particularly in children (301,311). Cholera in pregnancy carries a high mortality, with a 50% risk of fetal death during the third trimester (312).

Mortality

The large, rapid volume losses in cholera gravis can lead to hypovolemic shock and death within 2–3 hr. More commonly, untreated patients progress to shock in 4–12 hr and death in 18 hr to several days (313). Mortality in untreated patients may be as high as 50–70% (314). In endemic areas, children have a ten times greater case fatality rate than adults (315).

DIAGNOSIS

Clinical Diagnosis

Although cholera cannot be definitively distinguished clinically from other causes of severe watery diarrhea and

vomiting, cholera should be considered in all such cases, particularly those with rapid progression and severe dehydration (3). Many infectious diseases cause severe diarrhea in children, but dehydrating diarrhea in an adult is uncommon and raises the suspicion of cholera (316). Clinical suspicion should be increased for travelers to areas with cholera who develop diarrhea within 5 days of leaving the area, or in persons who recently ingested raw or undercooked shellfish (3,47,316).

Laboratory Diagnosis

To confirm a case of cholera requires laboratory identification of toxinogenic *V. cholerae* O1 or *V. cholerae* O139 Bengal from a person with diarrhea (316). It is essential, however, not to wait for laboratory confirmation before treating patients who are suspected of having cholera since death by dehydration can occur quickly.

Stool specimens or rectal swabs should be collected soon after the start of illness and before antibiotic treatment, if possible. If specimens must be held or transported, they should be placed in transport medium; semisolid Cary–Blair medium is the one most extensively used (317–319). Swabs in holding medium can be kept at room temperature, whereas liquid stool should be refrigerated (320). Vibrios can survive for up to 5 weeks in stools placed on blotting paper and kept in sealed plastic bags (321). Several practical methods have been developed to isolate *V. cholerae* from water (322) or sewage (323) for use in surveillance.

The stools of patients with acute, untreated cholera contain extremely large numbers of vibrios (10^6–10^8 per mL) (324), so Gram's stain of such stools revealing sheets of vibrio forms may suggest the diagnosis. Direct plating of acute stool specimens on selective media, such as TCBS agar, is usually sufficient for the isolation of organisms. Enrichment in alkaline peptone water for 6–8 hr, which selects for vibrios because of their tolerance to high pH, increases the recovery of *V. cholerae* when bacterial numbers are low, as in convalescent carriers (320). The appearance of *V. cholerae* on a variety of selective media has been discussed above.

Yellow colonies on TCBS are subcultured and biochemically confirmed as *V. cholerae*. Non-O1 strains are differentiated from *V. cholerae* O1 by slide agglutination tests with polyvalent O1 antiserum and type-specific Inaba and Ogawa antisera, which are available commercially (25). Biotyping has been described above. The recent spread of an epidemic strain of toxinogenic non-O1 *V. cholerae*, O139 Bengal, has highlighted the need to test strains for the production of cholera toxin. A specific diagnostic antiserum for *V. cholerae* O139 is available (67). Enzyme-linked immunosorbent assays, a latex agglutination assay, and the polymerase chain reaction have all been used to detect toxinogenic strains (325–327).

Several methods have been developed for the rapid laboratory diagnosis of *V. cholerae* from stool (320). These include agglutination of organisms in stool with cholera antiserum (328), coagglutination with *Staphylococcus aureus* and specific *V. cholerae* antiserum (329), observation of typical colonies on nutrient agar with oblique light illumination (330), and fluorescent antibody techniques (331). A rapid and effective method involves detection of vibrios in stool by dark field or phase contrast microscopy. Both *Vibrio* and *Campylobacter* demonstrate a characteristic motility, called "shooting stars." Motility of vibrios is inhibited when specific antisera is added (21).

Vibriocidal and antitoxin antibody titers can be used retrospectively to confirm *V. cholerae* O1 infection. A rise in antitoxic antibody titers, which increases 2–4 weeks after the onset of disease and remains elevated, may be diagnostic. Specific reagents must be used to avoid cross-reaction with antibodies against *E. coli* heat-labile toxin (332). The use of vibriocidal antibody titers in diagnosis has been discussed above.

Because epidemic strains of *V. cholerae* O1 can acquire plasmids carrying antibiotic resistance, it is important to determine the antimicrobial susceptibility of strains isolated in the laboratory. This can be done using disk diffusion methods or other standard techniques.

TREATMENT

Degree of Dehydration

The prime consideration in treatment of clinical cholera is rapid, appropriate volume replacement. Physicians should be aware that fluid losses may be greater than for most diarrheas usually seen and that aggressive rehydration with large volumes of fluid may be necessary (3). The rapid assessment of the degree of dehydration of an individual patient should guide the course of treatment. WHO guidelines for deciding if patients have *no* (<2.5%

body weight), *some* (2.5–10% body weight), or *severe* (>10% body weight) dehydration are shown in Table 4.

Oral Rehydration

The treatment of cholera was revolutionized by the promotion of oral rehydration solutions, which depends on the fact that glucose-facilitated sodium and water absorption in the small intestine remains intact in the presence of cholera toxin. The availability of oral rehydration solutions has reduced mortality from cholera from over 50% to less than 1% (90,99,102). The WHO recommends a solution containing 3.5 g of sodium chloride, 2.5 g of sodium bicarbonate, 1.5 g of potassium chloride, and 20 g of glucose (or 40 g of sucrose) per liter of water (333). Guidelines for rehydration and maintenance therapy with oral rehydration solutions are reviewed in detail in the chapter by Snyder.

Intravenous Rehydration

Patients who are severely dehydrated (>10% of body weight) or in whom mental status changes or vomiting preclude the use of oral therapy should be treated with intravenous solutions such as Ringer's lactate, which is the only generally available solution with the appropriate electrolyte composition (334). Normal or half-normal saline solutions can be used if Ringer's lactate is not available, but do not contain needed bicarbonate or potassium. Plain glucose in water is ineffective in replacing intravascular fluid and electrolyte losses in cholera (334). Oral rehydration solution should be given as soon as a patient can drink. Severely dehydrated patients will need to have large volumes of fluid given rapidly. Patients must be monitored for complications of fluid overload, but if oral rehydration therapy is begun when initial rehydration is complete, this should be unusual; insufficient hydration is much more common than overhydration. Volumes of intravenous fluids to be given and rates of administration are shown in Table 5.

Antimicrobial Therapy

Rehydration therapy is the only treatment necessary for cholera patients. Use of antibiotics, however, can reduce the duration and thus the expense of treatment, an

TABLE 5. *Guidelines for intravenous treatment of patients with severe dehydration*

Age	First give 30 mL/kg	Then give 70 mL/kg
Infants (under 12 mo)	1 h[a]	5 hr
Children and adults	30 min[a]	2.5 hr

From ref. 3, with permission.
[a] Repeat if radial pulse is still very weak or not detectable.

TABLE 6. *Antibiotics for treatment of cholera*

	Antibiotics	Administration	Dose Children	Dose Adults
First choices	Tetracycline	Four times per day for 3 d	12.5 mg/kg	500 mg
	Doxycycline	One single dose	6 mg/kg	300 mg
Alternatives (tetracycline-resistant strains)	Erythromycin	Adults: four times per day for 3 d Children: three times per day for 3 d	10 mg/kg	250 mg
	TMP-SMX[a]	Two times per day for 3 d	5 mg/kg TMP, 25 mg/kg SMX	160 mg TMP, 800 mg SMX
	Furazolidone	Four times per day for 3 d	1.25 mg/kg	100 mg

From ref. 3, with permission.
[a] TMP indicates trimethoprim; and SMX, sulfamethoxazole.

important consideration for cholera control. Antibiotics have been demonstrated to reduce the volume and duration of diarrhea by about half and reduce the duration of *Vibrio* excretion to an average of one day (301,335). Oral antibiotics can be given when vomiting stops, usually about the time that initial rehydration is completed. Injectable antibiotics are unnecessary (334).

Antibiotics used in the treatment of cholera are shown in Table 6. Tetracycline is the drug most commonly used; doxycycline is preferable as only a single dose is needed. Alternative drugs that may be used if strains are tetracycline-resistant are furazolidone, trimethoprim-sulfamethoxazole, erythromycin, chloramphenicol, or one of the fluoroquinolones (334,336).

V. cholerae O1 was originally found to be universally sensitive to tetracycline (335), but large outbreaks of multiple antibiotic-resistant organisms have since been documented in Tanzania and Bangladesh (337–339); antibiotic-resistant *V. cholerae* is present in South America as well (3). Resistances are carried on plasmids belonging to incompatibility group Inc6-C (339). Antibiotic-resistant organisms are likely selected for by the use of tetracycline for prophylaxis; in areas where prophylaxis is not common, such as Bangladesh, resistance plasmids are rapidly lost (338). Clinicians should determine the antibiotic susceptibility pattern in their area to guide therapy.

Tetracycline treatment of family contacts of patients with cholera has been demonstrated to be effective in preventing illness (340,341). Because of the difficulties in determining who is a close contact (and limiting treatment to such persons), in treating before infection can spread, in isolating treated contacts to prevent reinfection, and in the cost of surveillance and treatment programs, the WHO only recommends the use of selective chemoprophylaxis if surveillance shows that an average of one household member in a family of five becomes ill after the first case (334). None of the cholera cases imported by the United States since 1961 have resulted in secondary transmission (52); chemoprophylaxis of family contacts in the United States is therefore not recommended (342). Families should be instructed in proper handwashing and in cleaning contaminated clothes and bedding with soap and chlorine bleach. Homes should be inspected to confirm that sewage treatment is sufficient to decontaminate feces (342). Mass chemoprophylaxis of an entire community has not been successful in limiting the spread of cholera (334,343). Such treatment gives a false sense of security, may lead to the emergence of drug-resistant strains, may cause adverse drug reactions, and draws resources from effective control measures (334,343).

Other Therapies

Many antisecretory drugs have been tested in cholera patients; none have proven to be of benefit (344). The WHO recommends against the use of antidiarrheal, antiemetic, antispasmodic, cardiotonic, or corticosteroid medications in the treatment of cholera (334).

PREVENTION

Hygiene

Prevention of the spread of epidemic cholera requires interruption of fecal–oral transmission. Ensuring the safety of food and water depends on the availability of adequate sewage collection and disposal, the protection of clean water sources, and effective water treatment (345). Many developing countries do not possess the infrastructure to provide clean water and sewage treatment to their populations.

Measures that can be taken on a local level include the construction of latrines, education concerning the importance of handwashing after defecation, and education on how to make food and water safe at home (334). Water can be disinfected with chlorine or iodine, by filtration, or by bringing water to a rolling boil for 30 sec at sea level or for 3 min at higher altitudes (345). Carbonated bottled water may be safe, as *V. cholerae* will not survive in an acidic environment for more than a day (40). In emergencies, two drops of household bleach (5.25% chlorine) may be mixed well in a quart of water and allowed to stand for 10 min before consumption; such water should not be used for more than short periods (345). Food should be cooked until hot and eaten while hot. Utensils should be washed and thoroughly dried after use and hands should be washed before preparing and eating food (334).

Surveillance

Cholera is an internationally notifiable disease. In the United States, physicians must report cases of cholera to local and state health departments; isolates from presumed cases should be sent to state health departments and to the Centers for Disease Control (CDC) for laboratory confirmation. The CDC will test strains for the production of cholera toxin. The CDC investigates outbreaks, assisted by the U.S. Environmental Protection Agency if transmission appears to be by water (345). Confirmed cases are reported to the WHO, which is responsible for global surveillance.

Vaccines

The currently licensed parenteral killed whole-cell vaccine preparation provides less than 50% protection from disease, for a duration of only 3–6 months. The vaccine does not reduce the rate of asymptomatic infections and so does not prevent transmission of disease (346). The vaccine is no longer recommended for international travelers and should not be used in contacts of patients with cholera (346). Because of these limitations, the 26th World Health Assembly abolished the requirement in the International Health Regulations for a certificate of vaccination against cholera (334).

The development of improved vaccines is an area of intense research activity. These include oral, killed, whole-cell vaccines that are administered both with and without the B subunit of cholera toxin; live, oral vaccine strains constructed with the use of molecular genetic techniques to delete cholera toxin and other virulence genes; and the use of attenuated strains of *V. cholerae* to deliver heterologous antigens to the mucosal immune system. These vaccines are discussed in the chapter by Levine.

ACKNOWLEDGEMENTS

This work was supported by Public Health Service Grants AI27329 and AI34968 (to S.B.C.) from the National Institute of Allergy and Infectious Diseases and by a grant from the WHO/UNDP Programme for Vaccine Development. J.R.B. is a Howard Hughes Medical Institute Physician Research Fellow.

REFERENCES

1. Development of vaccines against cholera and diarrhoea due to enterotoxigenic *Escherichia coli*: memorandum from a WHO meeting. *Bull WHO* 1990;68:303–312.
2. Tauxe RV, Blake PA. Epidemic cholera in Latin America. *JAMA* 1992;267:1388–1390.
3. Swerdlow DL, Ries AA. Cholera in the Americas. *JAMA* 1992; 267:1495–1499.
4. Baumann L, Bang SS, Baumann P. Study of relationship among species of *Vibrio*, *Photobacterium*, and terrestrial enterobacteria by an immunological comparison of glutamine synthetase and superoxide dismutase. *Curr Microbiol* 1980;4:133–138.
5. MacDonell MT, Swartz DG, Ortiz-Conde BA, Last GA, Colwell RR. Ribosomal RNA phylogenies for the *Vibrio*-enteric group of eubacteria. *Microbiol Sci* 1986;3:172–178.
6. Janda JM, Powers C, Bryant RG, Abbott SL. Current perspectives on the epidemiology and pathogenesis of clinically significant *Vibrio* spp. *Clin Microbiol Rev* 1988;1:245–267.
7. Sakazaki R, Donovan TJ. Serology and epidemiology of *Vibrio cholerae* and *Vibrio mimicus*. In: Bergen T, ed. *Methods in microbiology*. vol 16. London: Academic Press; 1984:271–289.
8. Kenne L, Lindberg B, Unger P, Gustafsson B, Holme T. Structural studies of the *Vibrio cholerae* O-antigen. *Carbohydr Res* 1982;100:341–349.
9. Redmond JW. The structure of the O-antigenic side chain of the lipopolysaccharide of *Vibrio cholerae* 569B (Inaba). *Biochim Biophys Acta* 1979;584:346–352.
10. Morris JG. Non-O group 1 *Vibrio cholerae:* a look at the epidemiology of an occasional pathogen. *Epidemiol Rev* 1990;12: 179–191.
11. Ramamurthy T, Garg S, Sharma R, et al. Emergence of novel strain of *Vibrio cholerae* with epidemic potential in southern and eastern India. *Lancet* 1993;341:703–704.
12. Albert MJ, Siddique AK, Islam MS, et al. Large outbreak of clinical cholera due to *Vibrio cholerae* non-O1 in Bangladesh. *Lancet* 1993;341:704.
13. Gotschlich T. Vibrios Choleriques isoles au compement de Tor. Retour du pelerinage de l'annee, 1905. Report adresse au President du Conseil quarante naine d'Egypt, Alexandria. *Bull Inst Louis Pasteur* 1905;3:726.
14. Sugiyama J, Gondaira F, Matsuda J, Soga M, Terada Y. New method for serological typing of *Vibrio cholerae* O:1 using a monoclonal antibody-sensitized latex agglutination test. *Microbiol Immunol* 1987;31:387–391.
15. Sakazaki R, Tamura K. Somatic antigen variation in *Vibrio cholerae*. *Jpn J Med Sci Biol* 1971;24:93–100.
16. Redmond JW, Korsch MJ, Jackson GD. Immunochemical studies of the O-antigens of *Vibrio cholerae*. Partial characterization of an acid-labile antigenic determinant. *Aust J Exp Biol Med Sci* 1973;51:229–235.
17. Sack RB, Miller CE. Progressive changes of Vibrio serotypes in germ-free mice infected with *Vibrio cholerae*. *J Bacteriol* 1969;99:688–695.
18. Sheehy TW, Sprinz H, Augerson WS, Formal SB. Laboratory *Vibrio cholerae* infection in the United States. *JAMA* 1966;197: 321–326.
19. Stroeher UH, Karageorgos LE, Morona R, Manning PA. Serotype conversion in *Vibrio cholerae* O1. *Proc Natl Acad Sci USA* 1992;89:2566–2570.
20. Chatterjee BD. Vibrios and campylobacters. In: Braude AI, Davis CE, Fierer J, eds. *Infectious diseases and medical microbiology*. 2nd ed. Philadelphia: WB Saunders; 1986:303–314.
21. Benenson AS, Islam MR, Greenough WB III. Rapid identification of *Vibrio cholerae* by darkfield microscopy. *Bull World Health Organ* 1964;30:827.
22. Kobayashi T, Enomoto S, Sakazaki R. A new selective isolation medium for the vibrio group on a modified Nakanishi's medium (TCBS agar medium). *Jpn J Bacteriol* 1963;18: 387–392.
23. Shimada T, Sakazaki R, Fujimara S, et al. A new selective differential agar medium for isolation of *Vibrio cholerae* O1:PMT (polymyxin mannose–tellurite agar). *Jpn J Med Sci Biol* 1990;43:37–41.
24. Baumann P, Furniss AL, Lee JV. Genus I. *Vibrio* Pacini 1854, 411. In: Kreig NR, Holt JG, eds. *Bergey's manual of systematic bacteriology*. vol 1. Baltimore: Williams & Wilkins; 1984: 518–538.
25. Kelly MT, Hickman-Brenner FW, Farmer JJ III. *Vibrio*. In: Balows A, Hausler WJ, Herrmann KL, Isenberg HD, Shadomy HJ, eds. *Manual of clinical microbiology*. 5th ed. Washington, DC: American Society for Microbiology; 1991:384–395.
26. Rowe B, Frost JA. Vibrio phages and phage-typing. In: Barua D, Greenough WB III, eds. *Cholera*. New York: Plenum Press; 1992:95–105.
27. Basu S, Mukerjee S. Bacteriophage typing of *Vibrio eltor*. *Experientia* 1968;24:299–300.
28. Lee JV, Furniss AL. The phage typing of *Vibrio cholerae* sero-

var O1. In: Holme T, Holmgren J, Merson MH, Mollby R, eds. *Acute enteric infections in children: new prospects for treatment and prevention.* Amsterdam: Elsevier; 1981:119–122.

29. Drozhevkina MS, Arutyunov YI. Phage-typing of *Vibrio cholerae* using a new collection of phages. *J Hyg Epidemiol Microbiol Immunol* 1971;23:340–347.

30. Chattopadhyay DJ, Sarkar BL, Ansari MQ, et al. New phage typing scheme for *Vibrio cholerae* O1 biotype El Tor strains. *J Clin Microbiol* 1993;31:1579–1585.

31. Barua D. History of cholera. In: Barua D, Greenough WB III, eds. *Cholera.* New York: Plenum Press; 1992:1–36.

32. MacPherson J. *Annals of cholera from the earliest periods to the year 1817.* 2nd ed. London: HK Lewis; 1884.

33. Duffy J. The history of Asiatic cholera in the United States. *Bull NY Acad Med* 1971;47:1152–1168.

34. Rosenberg CE. *The cholera years.* Chicago: University of Chicago Press; 1962.

35. Snow J. *On the mode of communication of cholera.* London: John Churchill; 1849.

36. Koch R. An address on cholera and its bacillus. *Br Med J* 1884; 2:403–407, 453–459.

37. Barua D. The global epidemiology of cholera in recent years. *Proc R Soc Med* 1972;65:423–428.

38. Goodgame RW, Greenough WBG III. Cholera in Africa: a message for the West. *Ann Intern Med* 1975;82:101–106.

39. Baine WB, Zampieri A, Mazzotti M, et al. Epidemiology of cholera in Italy in 1973. *Lancet* 1974;2:1370–1376.

40. Blake PA, Rosenberg ML, Bandeira Costa J, et al. Cholera in Portugal, 1974. I. Modes of transmission. *Am J Epidemiol* 1977; 105:337–343.

41. Huq MI, Glass RI, Stoll BJ. Epidemiology of cholera. *N Engl J Med* 1980;303:643–644.

42. Shahid NS, Samadi AR, Khan MU, et al. Classical vs. El Tor cholera. A prospective family study of a concurrent outbreak. *J Diarrh Dis Res* 1984;2:73.

43. Samadi AR, Huq MI, Shahid NS, et al. Classical *Vibrio cholerae* biotype displaced El Tor in Bangladesh. *Lancet* 1983;1: 805–807.

44. Hugo MI, Sanyal SC, Samadi AR, et al. Comparative behaviour of classical and El Tor biotypes of *Vibrio cholerae* O1 isolated in Bangladesh during 1982. *J Diarrh Dis Res* 1983;1: 5–9.

45. Glass RI, Black RE. The epidemiology of cholera. In: Barua D, Greenough WB III, eds. *Cholera.* New York: Plenum Press; 1992:129–154.

46. Centers for Disease Control. Cholera—Peru, 1991. *MMWR* 1991;40:108–109.

47. Centers for Disease Control. Update: Cholera—Western Hemisphere. *MMWR* 1991;40:860.

48. Wachsmuth IK, Bopp CA, Fields PI. Difference between toxigenic *Vibrio cholerae* O1 from South America and US Gulf Coast. *Lancet* 1991;337:1097–1098.

49. Wachsmuth IK, Evins GM, Fields PI, et al. The molecular epidemiology of cholera in Latin America. *J Infect Dis* 1993; 167:621–626.

50. Almeida RJ, Cameron DN, Cook WL, Wachsmuth IK. Vibriophage VcA-3 as an epidemic strain marker for the U.S. Gulf Coast *Vibrio cholerae* O1 clone. *J Clin Microbiol* 1991;30: 300–304.

51. Centers for Disease Control. Update: cholera—western hemisphere, 1992. *MMWR* 1993;42:89–91.

52. Snyder JD, Blake PA. Is cholera a problem for US travelers? *JAMA* 1982;247:2268–2269.

53. Weissman JB, De Witt WE, Thompson J, et al. A case of cholera in Texas, 1973. *Am J Epidemiol* 1974;100:487–498.

54. Blake PA, Allegra DT, Snyder JD, et al. Cholera: a possible endemic focus in the United States. *N Engl J Med* 1980;302: 305–309.

55. Lowry PW, Pavia AT, McFarland LM, et al. Cholera in Louisiana: widening spectrum of seafood vehicles. *Arch Intern Med* 1989;149:2079–2084.

56. Pavia AT, Campbell JF, Blake PA, Smith JD, Martin DL. Cholera from raw oysters shipped interstate. *JAMA* 1987;258:2374.

57. Johnston JM, Martin DL, Perdue J, et al. Cholera on a Gulf Coast oil rig. *N Engl J Med* 1983;309:523–526.

58. Centers for Disease Control. Cholera—New Jersey and Florida. *MMWR* 1991;40:287–289.

59. Centers for Disease Control. Cholera—New York, 1991. *MMWR* 1991;40:516–518.

60. Centers for Disease Control. Importation of cholera from Peru. *MMWR* 1991;40:258–259.

61. Centers for Disease Control. Cholera associated with an international airline flight, 1992. *MMWR* 1992;41:134–135.

62. DePaola A, Capers GM, Motes ML, et al. Isolation of Latin American epidemic strain of *Vibrio cholerae* O1 from US Gulf Coast. *Lancet* 1992;339:624.

63. McCarthy SA, McPhearson RM, Guarino AM, Gaines JL. Toxigenic *Vibrio cholerae* O1 and cargo ships entering Gulf of Mexico. *Lancet* 1992;339:624–625.

64. Centers for Disease Control. Cholera associated with imported frozen coconut milk—Maryland, 1991. *MMWR* 1991;40: 844–845.

65. Bhattacharya MK, Bhattacharya SK, Garg S, et al. Outbreak of *Vibrio cholerae* non-O1 in India and Bangladesh. *Lancet* 1993;341:1346–1347.

66. Centers for Disease Control. Imported cholera associated with a newly described toxigenic *Vibrio cholerae* O139 strain—California, 1993. *MMWR* 1993;42:501–503.

67. World Health Organization. Epidemic diarrhea due to *Vibrio cholerae* non-O1. *Week Epidemiol Rec* 1993;68:141–2.

68. Cholera Working Group, International Centre for Diarrhoeal Diseases Research, Bangladesh. Large epidemic of cholera-like disease in Bangladesh caused by *Vibrio cholerae* O139 synonym Bengal. *Lancet* 1993;342:387–390.

69. Chongsa-nguan M, Chaicumpa W, Moolasart P, et al. *Vibrio cholerae* O139 Bengal in Bangkok. *Lancet* 1993;342:430–431.

70. Shimada T, Nair GB, Deb BC, Albert MJ, Sack RB, Takeda Y. Outbreak of *Vibrio cholerae* non-O1 in India and Bangladesh. *Lancet* 1993;341:1346.

71. Hall RH, Khambaty FM, Kothary M, Keasler SP. Non-O1 *Vibrio cholerae.* *Lancet* 1993;342:430.

72. Islam MS, Hasan MK, Miah MA, et al. Isolation of *Vibrio cholerae* O139 Bengal from water in Bangladesh. *Lancet* 1933; 342:430.

73. Jesudason MV, John TJ. Major shift in prevalence of non-O1 *Vibrio cholerae.* *Lancet* 1993;341:1090–1091.

74. Swerdlow DL, Ries AA. *Vibrio cholerae* non-O1—the eighth pandemic? *Lancet* 1993;342:382–383.

75. Colwell RR, Spira WM. The ecology of *Vibrio cholerae.* In: Barua D, Greenough WB III, eds. *Cholera.* New York: Plenum Press; 1992:107–128.

76. Pollitzer R. *Cholera.* Geneva: WHO; 1959.

77. Feachem R, Miller C, Drasar B. Environmental aspects of cholera epidemiology. II. Occurrence and survival of *Vibrio cholerae* in the environment. *Trop Dis Bull* 1981;78:865–880.

78. Pesigan TP, Plantilla J, Rolda M. Applied studies on the viability of El Tor vibrios. *Bull WHO* 1967;37:779–786.

79. McCormack WM, Islam MS, Fahimuddin M, Mosley WH. Endemic cholera in rural East Pakistan. *Am J Epidemiol* 1969;89: 393–404.

80. Colwell RR, Brayton PR, Grimes DJ, Roszak DR, Huq SA, Palmer LM. Viable but nonculturable *Vibrio cholerae* and related pathogens in the environment: implications for release of genetically engineered microorganisms. *Biotechnology* 1985;3: 817–820.

81. Huq A, Colwell RR, Rahman R, et al. Detection of *Vibrio cholerae* O1 in the aquatic environment by fluorescent-monoclonal antibody and culture methods. *Appl Environ Microbiol* 1990; 56:2370–2373.

82. Roszak DB, Grimes DJ, Colwell RR. Viable but nonrecoverable stage of *Salmonella enteritidis* in aquatic systems. *Can J Microbiol* 1984;30:334–338.

83. Xu H-S, Roberts N, Singleton FL, Attwell RW, Grimes DJ, Colwell RR. Survival and viability of non-culturable *Escherichia coli* and *Vibrio cholerae* in the estuarine and marine environment. *Microb Ecol* 1982;8:313–323.

84. Brayton PR, Colwell RR. Fluorescent antibody staining

method for enumeration of viable environmental *Vibrio cholerae* O1. *J Microbiol Meth* 1987;6:309–314.

85. Tamplin ML, Gauzens AL, Huq A, Sack DA, Colwell RR. Attachment of *Vibrio cholerae* serogroup O1 to zooplankton and phytoplankton of Bangladesh waters. *Appl Environ Microbiol* 1990;56:1977–1980.

86. Spira WM, Huq A, Ahmed QS, Saeed YA. Uptake of *Vibrio cholerae* biotype El Tor from contaminated water by water hyacinth (*Eichornia crassipes*). *Appl Environ Microbiol* 1981; 42:550–553.

87. Islam MS, Drasar BS, Bradley DJ. Long-term persistence of toxigenic *Vibrio cholerae* O1 in the mucilaginous sheath of a blue–green alga, *Anabaena variabilis*. *J Trop Med Hyg* 1990; 193:133–139.

88. Salamaso S, Freco D, Bonfiglio B, et al. Recurrence of pelecypos-associated cholera in Sardinia. *Lancet* 1980;2: 1124–1128.

89. Joseph PR, Tamayo JF, Mosley WH, et al. Studies of cholera El Tor in the Philippines. 2. A retrospective investigation of an explosive outbreak in Bacalod City and Talisay, November 1961. *Bull WHO* 1965;33:637–643.

90. Swerdlow DL, Mintz ED, Rodriguez M, et al. Waterborne transmission of epidemic cholera in Trujillo, Peru: lessons for a continent at risk. *Lancet* 1992;340:28–33.

91. Ries AA, Vugia DJ, Beingolea L, et al. Cholera in Piura, Peru: a modern urban epidemic. *J Infect Dis* 1992;166:1429–1433.

92. Deb BC, Sircar BK, Sengupta PG, et al. Intra-familial transmission of *Vibrio cholerae* biotype El Tor in Calcutta slums. *Ind J Med Res* 1982;76:814–819.

93. Deb BC, Sircar BK, Genegupta PG, et al. Studies on interventions to prevent eltor cholera transmission in urban slums. *Bull WHO* 1986;64:127–131.

94. Blake PA, Rosenberg ML, Florencia J, et al. Cholera in Portugal, 1974. II. Transmission in bottled mineral water. *Am J Epidemiol* 1977;105:344–348.

95. Glass RI, Alim ARMA, Eusof A, et al. Cholera in Indonesia: epidemiologic studies of transmission in Aceh Province. *Am J Trop Med Hyg* 1984;33:933–939.

96. Hughes JM, Boyce JM, Levine RJ, et al. Epidemiology of El Tor cholera in rural Bangladesh: importance of surface water in transmission. *Bull WHO* 1982;60:395–404.

97. Kolvin JL, Roberts D. Studies on the growth of *Vibrio cholerae* biotype eltor and biotype classical in foods. *J Hyg* 1982;89: 243–252.

98. Gerichter ChB, Sechter I, Gavish A, Cahan D. Viability of *Vibrio cholerae* biotype El Tor and of cholera phage on vegetables. *Isr J Med Sci* 1975;11:889–895.

99. St. Louis ME, Porter JD, Helal A, et al. Epidemic cholera in West Africa: the role of food handling and high-risk foods. *Am J Epidemiol* 1990;131:719–728.

100. Felsenfeld O. Notes on food, beverages and fomites contaminated with *Vibrio cholerae*. *Bull WHO* 1965;33:725–734.

101. Cohen J, Klasmer R, Ghalayini H, Schwartz T, Pridan D, Davies AM. Epidemiological aspects of cholera El Tor outbreak in a non-endemic area. *Lancet* 1971;2:86–89.

102. Tauxe RV, Holmberg SD, Dodin A, Wells JG, Blake PA. Epidemic cholera in Mali: high mortality and multiple routes of transmission in a famine area. *Epidemiol Infect* 1988;100: 279–289.

103. McIntyre RC, Tira T, Flood T, Blake PA. Modes of transmission of cholera in a newly infected population on an atoll: implications for control measures. *Lancet* 1979;1:311–314.

104. McCormick WM, Isam MS, Fahimuddin M, et al. A community study of inapparent cholera infections. *Am J Epidemiol* 1969; 89:658–664.

105. Dizon JJ. Cholera carriers. In: Barua D, Burrows W, eds. *Cholera*. Philadelphia: WB Saunders; 1974:367–380.

106. Pierce NF, Banwell JG, Sack RB, et al. Convalescent carriers of *Vibrio cholerae*: detection and detailed investigation. *Ann Intern Med* 1970;72:357–364.

107. Azurin JC, Kobari K, Barua D, et al. A long-term carrier of cholera: cholera Dolores. *Bull WHO* 1967;37:745–749.

108. Mhalu FS, Mtango FDE, Msengi AE. Hospital outbreaks of cholera transmitted through close person-to-person contact. *Lancet* 1984;2:82–84.

109. Ryder RW, Mizanur Rahman ASM, Alim ARMA. An outbreak of nosocomial cholera in a rural Bangladesh hospital. *J Hosp Infect* 1986;8:275–282.

110. Mandar MP, Mhalu FS. Cholera control in an inaccessible district in Tanzania: importance of temporary rural centers. *Med J Zambia* 1980;15:10–13.

111. Isaacson M, Clarke KR, Ellacombe GH, et al. The recent cholera outbreak in the South African gold mining industry: a preliminary report. *S Afr Med J* 1974;48:2557–2560.

112. Glass RI, Becker S, Huq MI, et al. Endemic cholera in rural Bangladesh. *Am J Epidemiol* 1982;116:959–970.

113. Wolff HL, van Zijl WJ. Houseflies, the availability of water, and diarrhoeal diseases. *Bull WHO* 1969;41:952–959.

114. Levine MM, Black RE, Clements ML, Cisneros L, Nalin DR, Young CR. Duration of infection-derived immunity to cholera. *J Infect Dis* 1981;143:818–820.

115. Nalin DR, Levine RJ, Levine MM, et al. Cholera, non-vibrio cholera, and stomach acid. *Lancet* 1978;2:856–859.

116. Abdou S. Susceptibility to cholera. *Lancet* 1948;1:903–904.

117. Gitelson S. Gastrectomy, achlorhydria and cholera. *Isr J Med Sci* 1971;7:663–667.

118. Sack GH, Pierce NF, Hennessey KN, et al. Gastric acidity in cholera and noncholera diarrhoea. *Bull WHO* 1972;47:31–36.

119. Schiraldi O, Benvestito V, Di Bari C, et al. Gastric abnormalities in cholera: epidemiological and clinical considerations. *Bull WHO* 1974;51:349–352.

120. Nalin DR, Levine MM, Rhead J, et al. Cannabis, hypochlorhydria, and cholera. *Lancet* 1978;2:859–861.

121. Cash RA, Music SI, Libonati JP, et al. Response of man to infection with *Vibrio cholerae*. I. Clinical, serologic, and bacteriologic responses to a known inoculum. *J Infect Dis* 1974;129: 45–52.

122. Levine MM, Black RE, Clements ML, et al. Volunteer studies in development of vaccines against cholera and enterotoxigenic *Escherichia coli*: a review. In: Holme T, Holmgren J, Merson MH, Mollby R, eds. *Acute enteric infections in children: new prospects for treatment and prevention*. Amsterdam: Elsevier; 1981:443–459.

123. Barua D, Paguio AS. ABO blood groups and cholera. *Ann Hum Biol* 1977;4:489–492.

124. Chandhuri A. Cholera and blood-group. *Lancet* 1977;2: 404–405.

125. Levine MM, Nalin DR, Rennels MB, et al. Genetic susceptibility to cholera. *Ann Hum Biol* 1979;6:369–374.

126. Glass RI, Holmgren J, Haley CE, et al. Predisposition for cholera of individuals with O blood group: possible evolutionary significance. *Am J Epidemiol* 1985;121:791–796.

127. Clemens JD, Sack DA, Harris JR, et al. ABO blood groups and cholera: new observations on specificity of risk and modification of vaccine efficacy. *J Infect Dis* 1989;159:770–773.

128. Gunn RA, Kimball AM, Pollard RA, et al. Bottle feeding as a risk factor for cholera in infants. *Lancet* 1979;2:730–732.

129. Clemens JD, Sack DA, Harris JR, et al. Breast feeding and the risk of severe cholera in rural Bangladeshi children. *Am J Epidemiol* 1990;131:400–411.

130. Glass RI, Svennerholm A-M, Stoll BJ, et al. Protection against cholera in breast-fed children by antibodies in breast milk. *N Engl J Med* 1983;308:1389–1392.

131. Glass RI, Svennerholm A-M, Stoll BJ, et al. Effects of undernutrition on infection with *Vibrio cholerae* O1 and on response to oral cholera vaccine. *Pediatr Infect Dis J* 1989;8:105–109.

132. Clemens JD, Van Loon F, Sack DA, et al. Biotype as determinant of natural immunising effect of cholera. *Lancet* 1991;337: 883–884.

133. Woodward WE, Mosley WH. The spectrum of cholera in rural Bangladesh. II. Comparison of El Tor, Ogawa and classical Inaba infection. *Am J Epidemiol* 1972;96:342–351.

134. Gerichter CB, Sechter I, Cohen J, Davies AM. A serological survey for cholera antibodies in the population of Jerusalem and surroundings. *Isr J Med Sci* 1973;9:980–985.

135. Bart KJ, Huq Z, Khan M, Mosley WH. Seroepidemiologic studies during a simultaneous epidemic of infection with El Tor

Ogawa and classical Inaba *Vibrio cholerae*. *J Infect Dis* 1970; 121(Suppl):S17–S24.

136. Dizon JJ, Alvero MG, Joseph PR, et al. Studies on El Tor in the Philippines: 1. Characteristics of cholera El Tor in Negros Occidental Province, November 1961 to September 1962. *Bull WHO* 1965;33:627.

137. Neogy KN. Viability of *V. cholerae* and *V. eltor* in food and water. *Bull Calcutta School Trop Med* 1965;13:10–11.

138. Yamamoto T, Yokota T. Electron microscopic study of *Vibrio cholerae* O1 adherence to the mucus coat and villus surface in the human small intestine. *Infect Immun* 1988;56:2753–2759.

139. Jones GW, Abrams GD, Freter R. Adhesive properties of *Vibrio cholerae*: adhesion to isolated rabbit brush border membranes and hemagglutinating activity. *Infect Immun* 1976;14: 232–239.

140. Jones GW, Freter R. Adhesive properties of *Vibrio cholerae*: nature of the interaction with isolated rabbit brush border membranes and human erythrocytes. *Infect Immun* 1976;14: 240–245.

141. Nakasone N, Iwanaga M. Quantitative evaluation of colonizing ability of *Vibrio cholerae* O1. *Microbiol Immunol* 1987;31: 753–761.

142. Nelson ET, Clements JD, Finkelstein RA. *Vibrio cholerae* adherence and colonization in experimental cholera: electron microscopic studies. *Infect Immun* 1976;14:527–547.

143. Taylor RK, Miller VL, Furlong DB, Mekalanos JJ. Use of *phoA* gene fusions to identify a pilus colonization factor coordinately regulated with cholera toxin. *Proc Natl Acad Sci USA* 1987; 84:2833–2837.

144. Herrington DA, Hall RH, Losnosky GA, Mekalanos JJ, Taylor RK, Levine MM. Toxin, toxin-coregulated pili, and the *toxR* regulon are essential for *Vibrio cholerae* pathogenesis in humans. *J Exp Med* 1988;168:1487–1492.

145. Sun D, Mekalanos JJ, Taylor RK. Antibodies directed against the toxin-coregulated pilus isolated from *Vibrio cholerae* provide protection in the infant mouse experimental cholera model. *J Infect Dis* 1990;161:1231–1236.

146. Sharma DP, Stroeher UH, Thomas CJ, Manning PA, Attridge SR. The toxin-coregulated pilus (TCP) of *Vibrio cholerae*: molecular cloning of genes involved in pilus biosynthesis and evaluation of TCP as a protective antigen in the infant mouse model. *Microb Pathog* 1989;7:437–448.

147. Sharma DP, Thomas C, Hall RH, Levine MM, Attridge SR. Significance of toxin-coregulated pili as protective antigens of *Vibrio cholerae* in the infant mouse model. *Vaccine* 1989;7: 451–456.

148. Taylor R, Shaw C, Peterson K, Spears P, Mekalanos JJ. Safe, live *Vibrio cholerae* vaccines? *Vaccine* 1988;6:151–154.

149. Hall RH, Vial PA, Kaper JB, Mekalanos JJ, Levine MM. Morphological studies on fimbriae expressed by *Vibrio cholerae* O1. *Microb Pathog* 1988;4:257–265.

150. Jonson G, Holmgren J, Svennerholm A-M. Analysis of expression of toxin-coregulated pili in classical and El Tor *Vibrio cholerae* O1 in vitro and in vivo. *Infect Immun* 1992;60:4278–4284.

151. Iwanaga M, Nakasone N, Ehara M. Pili of *Vibrio cholerae* O1 biotype El Tor: a comparative study of adhesive and non-adhesive strains. *Microbiol Immunol* 1989;33:1–9.

152. Schneider DR, Parker CD. Isolation and characterization of protease-deficient mutants of *Vibrio cholerae*. *J Infect Dis* 1978;138:143–151.

153. Peterson KM, Mekalanos JJ. Characterization of the *Vibrio cholerae* ToxR regulon: identification of novel genes involved in intestinal colonization. *Infect Immun* 1988;56:2822–2829.

154. Parsot C, Taxman E, Mekalanos JJ. ToxR regulates the production of lipoproteins and the expression of serum resistance in *Vibrio cholerae*. *Proc Natl Acad Sci USA* 1991;88:1641–1645.

155. Parsot C, Mekalanos JJ. Structural analysis of the *acfA* and *acfD* genes of *Vibrio cholerae*: effects of DNA topology and transcriptional activators on expression. *J Bacteriol* 1992;174: 5211–5218.

156. Finkelstein RA, Hanne LF. Purification and characterization of the soluble hemagglutinin (cholera lectin) produced by *Vibrio cholerae*. *Infect Immun* 1982;36:1199–1208.

157. Hanne LF, Finkelstein RA. Characterization and distribution

158. Booth BA, Finkelstein RA. Presence of hemagglutinin/protease and other potential virulence factors in O1 and non-O1 *Vibrio cholerae*. *J Infect Dis* 1986;154:183–186.

159. Honda T, Booth BA, Boesman-Finkelstein M, Finkelstein RA. Comparative study of *Vibrio cholerae* non-O1 protease and soluble hemagglutinin with those of *Vibrio cholerae* O1. *Infect Immun* 1987;55:451–454.

160. Booth BA, Sciortino CV, Finkelstein RA. Adhesins of *Vibrio cholerae*. In: Mirelman D, ed. *Microbial lectins and agglutinins: properties and biological activity*. New York: John Wiley and Sons; 1986:169–182.

161. Booth BA, Sciortino CV, Finkelstein RA. On the trail of adherence mechanisms in *Vibrio cholerae*: many scents but not much sense. In: Robbins JB, ed. *Bacterial vaccines*. New York: Praeger; 1987:220–241.

162. Booth BA, Dyer TJ, Finkelstein RA. Adhesion of *Vibrio cholerae* to cultured human cells. In: Sack RB, Zinnaka Y, eds. *Advances in research on cholera and related diarrheas*. Tokyo: KTK; 1990:19–35.

163. Hase CC, Finkelstein RA. Cloning and nucleotide sequence of the *Vibrio cholerae* hemagglutinin/protease (HA/protease) gene and construction of an HA/protease-negative strain. *J Bacteriol* 1991;173:3311–3317.

164. Booth BA, Boesman-Finkelstein M, Finkelstein R. *Vibrio cholerae* soluble hemagglutinin/protease is a metalloenzyme. *Infect Immun* 1983;42:558–560.

165. Hase CC, Finkelstein RA. Comparison of the *Vibrio cholerae* hemagglutinin/protease and the *Pseudomonas aeruginosa* elastase. *Infect Immun* 1990;58:4011–4015.

166. Finkelstein RA, Boesman-Finkelstein M, Holt P. *Vibrio cholerae* hemagglutinin/lectin/protease hydrolyzes fibronectin and ovomucin: F. M. Burnet revisited. *Proc Natl Acad Sci USA* 1983;80:1092–1095.

167. Booth BA, Boesman-Finkelstein M, Finkelstein R. *Vibrio cholerae* hemagglutinin/protease nicks cholera enterotoxin. *Infect Immun* 1984;45:558–560.

168. Finkelstein RA, Boesman-Finkelstein M, Chang Y, Hase CC. *Vibrio cholerae* hemagglutinin/protease, colonial variation, virulence, and detachment. *Infect Immun* 1992;60:472–478.

169. Finn TM, Reiser J, Germanier R, Cryz SJ. Cell-associated hemagglutinin-deficient mutant of *Vibrio cholerae*. *Infect Immun* 1987;55:942–946.

170. Osek J, Svennerholm A-M, Holmgren J. Protection against *Vibrio cholerae* El Tor infection by specific antibodies against mannose-binding hemagglutinin pili. *Infect Immun* 1992;60: 4961–4964.

171. Franzon VL, Barker A, Manning PA. Nucleotide sequence encoding the mannose-fucose-resistant hemagglutinin of *Vibrio cholerae* O1 and construction of a mutant. *Infect Immun* 1993; 61:3031–3037.

172. Guentzel MN, Berry LJ. Motility as a virulence factor for *Vibrio cholerae*. *Infect Immun* 1975;11:890–897.

173. Yancey RJ, Willis DL, Berry LJ. Role of motility in experimental cholera in adult rabbits. *Infect Immun* 1978;22:387–392.

174. Richardson K. Roles of motility and flagellar structure in pathogenicity of *Vibrio cholerae*: analysis of motility mutants in three animal models. *Infect Immun* 1991;59:2727–2736.

175. Attridge SR, Rowley D. The role of the flagellum in the adherence of *Vibrio cholerae*. *J Infect Dis* 1983;147:864–872.

176. Freter R, Allweiss B, O'Brien PCM, Halstead SA, Macsai MS. Role of chemotaxis in the association of motile bacteria with intestinal mucosa: in vitro studies. *Infect Immun* 1981;34: 241–249.

177. Pierce NF, Kaper JB, Mekalanos JJ, Cray WC. Role of cholera toxin in enteric colonization by *Vibrio cholerae* O1 in rabbits. *Infect Immun* 1985;50:813–816.

178. Sengupta DK, Sengupta TK, Ghose AC. Antibodies to outer membrane proteins of *Vibrio cholerae* induce protection by inhibition of intestinal colonization of vibrios. *FEMS Microbiol Immunol* 1992;89:261–266.

179. Sengupta DK, Sengupta TK, Ghose AC. Major outer membrane proteins of *Vibrio cholerae* and their role in induction of

protective immunity through inhibition of intestinal colonization. *Infect Immun* 1992;60:4848–4855.

180. Finkelstein RA. Cholera enterotoxin (choleragen): a historical perspective. In: Barua D, Greenough WB III, eds. *Cholera.* New York: Plenum Press; 1992:155–188.

181. Gill DM. The arrangement of subunits in cholera toxin. *Biochemistry* 1976;15:1242–1248.

182. Gill DM, Rappaport RS. The origin of A1. In: *Proceedings of the 12th joint conference on cholera.* US–Japan Cooperative Medical Science Program, Japan. Bethesda: National Institutes of Health; 1977.

183. Gill DM, King CA. The mechanism of action of cholera toxin in pigeon erythrocyte lysates. *J Biol Chem* 1975;250:6224–6432.

184. Mekalanos JJ, Collier RJ, Romig WR. The enzymatic activity of cholera toxin. II. Relationships to proteolytic processing, disulfide bond reduction, and subunit composition. *J Biol Chem* 1979;254:5855–5861.

185. van Heyningen WE, Carpenter CC, Pierce NF, Greenough WB 3d. Deactivation of cholera toxin by ganglioside. *J Infect Dis* 1971;124:415–418.

186. Cuatrecasas P. *Vibrio cholerae* choleragenoid: mechanism of inhibition of cholera toxin action. *Biochemistry* 1973;2:3577–3581.

187. Vimr ER, Lawrisuk L, Galen J, Kaper JB. Cloning and expression of the *Vibrio cholerae* neuraminidase gene *nanH* in *Escherichia coli. J Bacteriol* 1988;170:1495–1504.

188. Holmgren J, Lonnroth I, Mansson J.-E, Svennerholm L. Interaction of cholera toxin and membrane G_{M1} ganglioside of small intestine. *Proc Natl Acad Sci USA* 1975;72:2520–2524.

189. Galen JE, Ketley JM, Fasano A, Richardson SH, Wasserman SS, Kaper JB. Role of *Vibrio cholerae* neuraminidase in the function of cholera toxin. *Infect Immun* 1992;60:406–415.

190. Cassel D, Pfeuffer T. Mechanism of cholera toxin action: covalent modification of the guanyl-binding protein of the adenylate cyclase system. *Proc Natl Acad Sci USA* 1978;75:2669–2673.

191. Gill DM, Meren R. ADP-ribosylation of membrane proteins catalyzed by cholera toxin: basis of the activation of adenylate cyclase. *Proc Natl Acad Sci USA* 1978;75:3050–3054.

192. Field M. Regulation of small intestine ion transport by cyclic nucleotides and calcium. In: Field M, Fordtran JS, Schultz SG, eds. *Secretory diarrhea.* Bethesda: American Physiology Society; 1980:21.

193. Holmgren J. Actions of cholera toxin and the prevention and treatment of cholera. *Nature* 1981;292:413–417.

194. Lai C-Y. The chemistry and biology of cholera toxin. *CRC Crit Rev Biochem* 1980;9:171–206.

195. Moss J, Vaughan M. Activation of adenylate cyclase by choleragen. *Annu Rev Biochem* 1979;48:581–600.

196. Gilman AG. G proteins and dual control of adenylate cyclase. *Cell* 1984;36:577–579.

197. Gyles CL. Relationships among heat-labile enterotoxins of *Escherichia coli* and *Vibrio cholerae. J Infect Dis* 1974;129:277–283.

198. Clements JD, Finkelstein RA. Isolation and characterization of homogeneous heat-labile enterotoxins(s) (LT(s)) with high specific activity from *Escherichia coli* cultures. *Infect Immun* 1979;24:760–769.

199. Dallas WS, Falkow S. Amino acid sequence homology between cholera toxin and *Escherichia coli* heat-labile toxin. *Nature* 1980;288:499–501.

200. Gilligan PH, Brown JC, Robertson DC. Immunological relationships between cholera toxin and *Escherichia coli* heat-labile enterotoxin. *Infect Immun* 1983;42:683–691.

201. Mekalanos JJ, Swartz DJ, Pearson GDN, Harford N, Groyne F, de Wilde M. Cholera toxin genes: nucleotide sequence, deletion analysis, and vaccine development. *Nature* 1983;306:551–557.

202. Wald A, Gotterer GS, Rajendra GR, Turjjman NA, Hendrix TR. Effect of indomethacin on cholera-induced fluid movement, unidirectional sodium fluxes, and intestinal cAMP. *Gastroenterology* 1977;72:106–110.

203. Jacoby HI, Marshall CH. Antagonism of cholera enterotoxin by antiinflammatory agents in the rat. *Nature* 1972;235:163–165.

204. Speelman P, Rabbani GH, Bukhave K, Rask-Madesn K. Increased jejunal prostaglandin E2 concentrations in patients with acute cholera. *Gut* 1985;26:188–193.

205. Peterson JW, Ochoa LG. Role of prostaglandins and cAMP in the secretory effects of cholera toxin. *Science* 1989;245:857–859.

206. Evans DJ, Richardson SH. In vitro production of choleragen and vascular permeability factor by *Vibrio cholerae. J Bacteriol* 1968;96:126–130.

207. Richardson SH. Factors influencing in vivo skin permeability factor production by *Vibrio cholerae. J Bacteriol* 1969;100:27–34.

208. Miller VL, Taylor RK, Mekalanos JJ. Cholera toxin transcriptional activator ToxR is a transmembrane DNA binding protein. *Cell* 1987;48:271–279.

209. Miller VL, Mekalanos JJ. A novel suicide vector and its use in construction of insertion mutations: osmoregulation of outer membrane proteins and virulence determinants in *Vibrio cholerae* requires *toxR. J Bacteriol* 1988;170:2575–2583.

210. Kaper JB, Levine MM. Cloned cholera enterotoxin genes in study and prevention of cholera. *Lancet* 1981;2:1162–1163.

211. Pearson GDN, Mekalanos JJ. Molecular cloning of *Vibrio cholerae* enterotoxin genes in *Escherichia coli* K-12. *Proc Natl Acad Sci USA* 1982;79:2976–2980.

212. Gennaro ML, Greenaway PJ, Broadbent DA. The expression of biologically active cholera toxin in *Escherichia coli. Nucleic Acids Res* 1982;10:4883–4890.

213. Miller VL, Mekalanos JJ. Synthesis of cholera toxin is positively regulated at the transcriptional level by *toxR. Proc Natl Acad Sci USA* 1984;81:3471–3475.

214. Lockman HA, Galen JE, Kaper JB. *Vibrio cholerae* enterotoxin genes: Nucleotide sequence analysis of DNA encoding ADP-ribosyltransferase. *J Bacteriol* 1984;159:1086–1089.

215. Lockman H, Kaper JB. Nucleotide sequence analysis of the A2 and B subunits of *Vibrio cholerae* enterotoxin. *J Biol Chem* 1983;258:13722–13726.

216. Gennaro ML, Greenaway PJ. Nucleotide sequences within the cholera toxin operon. *Nucleic Acids Res* 1983;11:3855–3861.

217. Sanchez J, Holmgren J. Recombinant system for overexpression of cholera toxin B subunit in *Vibrio cholerae* as a basis for vaccine development. *Proc Natl Acad Sci USA* 1989;86:481–485.

218. Mekalanos J. Duplication and amplification of toxin genes in *Vibrio cholerae. Cell* 1983;35:253–263.

219. Goldberg I, Mekalanos JJ. Effect of a *recA* mutation on cholera toxin gene amplification and deletion events. *J Bacteriol* 1986;165:723–731.

220. Pearson GDN, Woods A, Chiang SL, Mekalanos JJ. CTX genetic element encodes a site-specific recombination system and an intestinal colonization factor. *Proc Natl Acad Sci USA* 1993;90:3750–3754; Correction *Proc Natl Acad Sci USA* 1993;90:8302.

221. Mekalanos JJ. Cholera toxin: genetic analysis, regulation, and role in pathogenesis. *Curr Top Microbiol Immunol* 1985;118:97–118.

222. Morris JG Jr, Picardi JL, Lieb S, et al. Isolation of nontoxigenic *Vibrio cholerae* O group 1 from a patient with severe gastrointestinal disease. *J Clin Microbiol* 1984;19:296–297.

223. Goldberg S, Murphy JR. Molecular epidemiological studies of United States Gulf Coast *Vibrio cholerae* strains: integration site of mutator vibriophage VcA-3. *Infect Immun* 1983;42:224–230.

224. Kaper JB, Moseley SL, Falkow S. Molecular characterization of environmental and nontoxigenic strains of *Vibrio cholerae. Infect Immun* 1981;32:661–667.

225. Pearson GDN, DiRita VJ, Goldberg MB, Boyko SA, Calderwood SB and Mekalanos JJ. New attenuated derivatives of *Vibrio cholerae. Res Microbiol* 1990;141:893–899.

226. Mekalanos JJ, DiRita VJ. Signal transduction in the control of cholera toxin expression. In: Moss J, Vaughan M, eds. *ADP-ribosylating toxins and G proteins: insights into signal transduction.* Washington, DC: American Society for Microbiology; 1990.

227. DiRita VJ. Co-ordinate expression of virulence genes by ToxR in *Vibrio cholerae*. *Mol Microbiol* 1992;6:451–458.

228. Miller VL, Mekalanos JJ. Genetic analysis of the cholera toxin positive regulatory gene *toxR*. *J Bacteriol* 1985;163:580–585.

229. Miller JF, Mekalanos JJ, Falkow S. Coordinate regulation and sensory transduction in the control of bacterial virulence. *Science* 1989;243:916–922.

230. Parsot C, Mekalanos JJ. Expression of ToxR, the transcriptional activator of the virulence factors in *Vibrio cholerae*, is modulated by the heat shock response. *Proc Natl Acad Sci USA* 1990;87:9898–9902.

231. Miller VL, DiRita VJ, Mekalanos JJ. Identification of *toxS*, a regulatory gene whose product enhances ToxR-mediated activation of the cholera toxin promoter. *J Bacteriol* 1989;171:1288–1293.

232. DiRita VJ, Mekalanos JJ. Periplasmic interaction between two membrane regulatory proteins, ToxR and ToxS, results in signal transduction and transcriptional activation. *Cell* 1991;64:29–37.

233. DiRita VJ, Parsot C, Jander G, Mekalanos JJ. Regulatory cascade controls virulence in *Vibrio cholerae*. *Proc Natl Acad Sci USA* 1991;88:5403–5407.

234. Higgins DE, Nazareno E, DiRita V. The virulence gene activator ToxT from *Vibrio cholerae* is a member of the AraC family of transcriptional activators. *J Bacteriol* 1992;174:6974–6980.

235. Ogierman MA, Manning PA. Homology of TcpN, a putative regulatory protein of *Vibrio cholerae*, to the AraC family of transcriptional activators. *Gene* 1992;116:93–97.

236. Parsot C, Mekalanos JJ. Expression of the *Vibrio cholerae* gene encoding aldehyde dehydrogenase is under the control of ToxR, the cholera toxin transcriptional activator. *J Bacteriol* 1991;173:2842–2851.

237. Fasano A, Baudry B, Pumplin DW, et al. *Vibrio cholerae* produces a second enterotoxin, which affects intestinal tight junctions. *Proc Natl Acad Sci USA* 1991;88:5242–5246.

238. Baudry B, Fasano A, Ketley J, Kaper JB. Cloning of a gene (*zot*) encoding a new toxin produced by *Vibrio cholerae*. *Infect Immun* 1992;60:428–434.

239. Trucksis M, Galen JE, Michalski J, Fasano A, Kaper JB. Accessory cholera enterotoxin (Ace), the third toxin of a *Vibrio cholerae* virulence cassette. *Proc Natl Acad Sci USA* 1993;90:5267–5271.

240. Yoshino K-I, Miyachi M, Takao T, et al. Purification and sequence determination of heat-stable enterotoxin elaborated by a cholera toxin-producing strain of *Vibrio cholerae* O1. *FEBS Lett* 1993;326:83–86.

241. O'Brien AD, Chen ME, Holmes RK, Kaper JB. Environmental and human isolates of *Vibrio cholerae* and *Vibrio parahaemolyticus* produce a *Shigella dysenteriae* 1 (Shiga)-like cytotoxin. *Lancet* 1985;1:77–78.

242. Sciortino CV, Finkelstein RA. *Vibrio cholerae* expresses iron-regulated outer membrane proteins in vivo. *Infect Immun* 1983;42:990–996.

243. Goldberg MB, DiRita VJ, Calderwood SB. Identification of an iron-regulated virulence determinant in *Vibrio cholere*, using Tn*phoA* mutagenesis. *Infect Immun* 1990;58:55–60.

244. Goldberg MB, Boyko SA, Calderwood SB. Transcriptional regulation by iron of a *Vibrio cholerae* virulence gene and homology of the gene to the *Escherichia coli* Fur system. *J Bacteriol* 1990;172:6863–6870.

245. Goldberg MB, Boyko SA, Calderwood SB. Positive transcriptional regulation of an iron-regulated virulence gene in *Vibrio cholerae*. *Proc Natl Acad Sci USA* 1991;88:1125–1129.

246. Goldberg MB, Boyko SA, Butterton JR, Stoebner JA, Payne SM, Calderwood SB. Characterization of a *Vibrio cholerae* virulence factor homologous to the family of TonB-dependent proteins. *Mol Microbiol* 1992;6:2407–2418.

247. Goldberg SL, Murphy JR. Molecular cloning of the hemolysin determinant from *Vibrio cholerae* El Tor. *J Bacteriol* 1984;160:239–244.

248. Goldberg SL, Murphy JR. Cloning and characterization of the hemolysin determinants from *Vibrio cholerae* RV79 (Hly +), RV79 (Hly −), and 569B. *J Bacteriol* 1985;162:35–41.

249. Manning PA, Brown MH, Heuzenroeder MW. Cloning of the structural gene (hly) for the haemolysin of *Vibrio cholerae* El Tor strain O17. *Gene* 1984;31:225–231.

250. Richardson K, Michalski J, Kaper JB. Hemolysin production and cloning of two hemolysin determinants from classical *Vibrio cholerae*. *Infect Immun* 1986;54:415–420.

251. Yamamoto K, Ichinose Y, Shinagawa H, et al. Two-step processing for activation of the cytolysin/hemolysin of *Vibrio cholerae* O1 biotype El Tor: Nucleotide sequence of the structural gene (hlyA) and characterization of the processed products. *Infect Immun* 1990;58:4106–4116.

252. Alm RA, Stroeher UH, Manning PA. Extracellular proteins of *Vibrio cholerae*: nucleotide sequence of the structural gene (hlyA) for the haemolysin of the haemolytic El Tor strain O17 and characterization of the *hlyA* mutation in the non-haemolytic classical strain 569B. *Mol Microbiol* 1988;2:481–488.

253. Alm RA, Manning PA. Biotype-specific probe for *Vibrio cholerae* serogroup O1. *J Clin Microbiol* 1990;28:823–824.

254. Rader AE, Murphy JR. Nucleotide sequences and comparison of the hemolysin determinants of *Vibrio cholerae* El Tor RV79 (Hly +) and RV79 (Hly −) and classical 569B (Hly −). *Infect Immun* 1988;56:1414–1419.

255. Alm RA, Manning PA. Characterization of the *hlyB* gene and its role in the production of the El Tor haemolysin of *Vibrio cholerae* O1. *Mol Microbiol* 1990;4:413–425.

256. von Mechow S, Vaidya AB, Bramucci MG. Mapping of a gene that regulates haemolysin production in *Vibrio cholerae*. *J Bacteriol* 1985;163:799–802.

257. Williams SG, Manning PA. Transcription of the *Vibrio cholerae* haemolysin gene, hlyA, and cloning of a positive regulatory locus, hlyU. *Mol Microbiol* 1991;5:2031–2038.

258. Stoebner JA, Payne SM. Iron-regulated hemolysin production and utilization of heme and hemoglobin by *Vibrio cholerae*. *Infect Immun* 1988;56:2891–2895.

259. Alm RA, Mayrhofer G, Kotlarski I, Manning PA. Amino-terminal domain of the El Tor haemolysin of *Vibrio cholerae* O1 is expressed in classical strains and is cytotoxic. *Vaccine* 1991;9:588–594.

260. Hall RH, Drasar BS. *Vibrio cholerae* HlyA hemolysin is processed by proteolysis. *Infect Immun* 1990;58:3375–3379.

261. Honda T, Finkelstein RA. Purification and characterization of a hemolysin produced by *Vibrio cholerae* biotype El Tor: another toxic substance produced by cholera vibrios. *Infect Immun* 1979;26:1020–1027.

262. Ichinose Y, Yamamoto K, Nakasone N, et al. Enterotoxicity of El Tor-like hemolysin of non-O1 *Vibrio cholerae*. *Infect Immun* 1987;55:1090–1093.

263. Levine MM, Kaper JB, Herrington D, et al. Volunteer studies of deletion mutants of *Vibrio cholerae* O1 prepared by recombinant techniques. *Infect Immun* 1988;56:161–167.

264. Levine MM, Nalin DR, Craig JP, et al. Immunity to cholera in man: relative role of antibacterial versus antitoxic immunity. *Trans R Soc Trop Med Hyg* 1979;73:3–9.

265. Levine MM, Kaper JB, Black RE, et al. New knowledge on pathogenesis of bacterial enteric infections as applied to vaccine development. *Microbiol Rev* 1983;47:510–550.

266. Woodward W. Cholera reinfection in man. *J Infect Dis* 1971;123:61–66.

267. Glass R, Becker S, Huq M, et al. Endemic cholera in rural Bangladesh, 1966–1980. *Am J Epidemiol* 1982;116:959–70.

268. Owen RL, Pierce NF, Apple RT, Cray WC. M cell transport of *Vibrio cholerae* from the intestinal lumen into Peyer's patches: a mechanism for antigen sampling and for microbial transepithelial migration. *J Infect Dis* 1986;153:1108–1118.

269. Svennerholm A-M, Sack DA, Holmgren J, Bardhan PK. Intestinal antibody responses after immunisation with cholera B subunit. *Lancet* 1982;1:305–308.

270. Czerkinsky C, Svennerholm A-M, Quiding M, Jonsson R, Holmgren J. Antibody-producing cells in peripheral blood and salivary glands after oral cholera vaccination of humans. *Infect Immun* 1991;59:996–1001.

271. Winner L III, Mack J, Weltzin KR, Mekalanos JJ, Kraehenbuhl J-P, Neutra MR. New model for analysis of mucosal immunity: intestinal secretion of specific monoclonal immunoglobulin A

from hybridoma tumors protects against *Vibrio cholerae* infection. *Infect Immun* 1991;59:977–982.

272. Cray WC, Tokunaga E, Pierce NF. Successful colonization and immunization of adult rabbits by oral inoculation with *Vibrio cholerae* O1. *Infect Immun* 1983;41:735–741.

273. Pierce NF, Kaper JB, Mekalanos JJ, Cray WC, Richardson K. Determinants of the immunogenicity of live virulent and mutant *Vibrio cholerae* O1 in rabbit intestine. *Infect Immun* 1987;55: 477–481.

274. Lycke N, Holmgren J. Strong adjuvant properties of cholera toxin on gut mucosal immune responses to orally presented antigens. *Immunology* 1986;59:301–308.

275. Black RE, Levine MM, Clements ML, Young CR, Svennerholm AM, Holmgren J. Protective efficacy in humans of killed whole-vibrio oral cholera vaccine with and without the B subunit of cholera toxin. *Infect Immun* 1987;55:1116–1120.

276. Czerkinsky C, Russell MW, Lycke N, Lindblad M, Holmgren J. Oral administration of a streptococcal antigen coupled to cholera toxin B subunit evokes strong antibody responses in salivary glands and extramucosal tissues. *Infect Immun* 1989; 57:1072–1077.

277. Fujita K, Finkelstein RA. Antitoxic immunity in experimental cholera: comparison of immunity induced perorally and parenterally in mice. *J Infect Dis* 1972;125:647–655.

278. Holmgren J, Svennerholm A-M, Ouchterlony O, et al. Antitoxic immunity in experimental cholera: protection and serum and local antibody responses in rabbits after enteric and parenteral immunization. *Infect Immun* 1975;12:463–470.

279. Pierce NF, Sack RB, Sircar BK. Immunity to experimental cholera. III. Enhanced duration of protection after sequential parenteral-oral toxoid administration to dogs. *J Infect Dis* 1977; 135:888–896.

280. Pierce NF, Reynolds HY. Immunity to experimental cholera. I. Protective effect of humoral IgG antitoxin demonstrated by passive immunization. *J Immunol* 1974;113:1017–1023.

281. Curlin G, Levine R, Aziz KMS, et al. Field trial of cholera toxoid. In: *Proceedings of the 11th Joint Conference on Cholera*. U.S.–Japan Cooperative Medical Science Program, Bethesda: National Institutes of Health; 1975:314–329.

282. Norili H. Evaluation of toxic field trial on the Philippines. In: Fukumi H, Zinnaka Y, eds. *Proceedings of the 12th Joint Conference on Cholera*. Tokyo: U.S.–Japan Cooperative Medical Science Program. Sapporo, 1976:302–310.

283. Clemens JD, Sack DA, Harris JR, et al. Field trial of oral cholera vaccines in Bangladesh. *Lancet* 1986;2:124–127.

284. Benenson AS, Saad A, Mosley WH, et al. Serological studies in cholera. 3. Serum toxin neutralization—Rise in titre in response to infection with *Vibrio cholerae*, and the level in the "normal" population of East Pakistan. *Bull WHO* 1968;38: 287–295.

285. Levine MM, Young CR, Hughes TP, et al. Duration of serum antitoxin response following *Vibrio cholerae* infection in North Americans: relevance for seroepidemiology. *Am J Epidemiol* 1981;114:348–354.

286. Levine MM, Young JCR, Black RE, et al. Enzyme-linked immunosorbent assay to measure antibodies to purified heat-labile enterotoxins from human and porcine strains of *Escherichia coli* and to cholera toxin: application in serodiagnosis and seroepidemiology. *J Clin Microbiol* 1985;21:174–179.

287. Svennerholm A-M, Jertborn M, Gothefors L, et al. Mucosal antitoxic and antibacterial immunity after cholera disease and after immunization with a combined B subunit whole cell vaccine. *J Infect Dis* 1984;149:884–893.

288. Glass RI, Svennerholm A-M, Khan RN, et al. Seroepidemiological studies of El Tor cholera in Bangladesh: association of serum antibody levels with protection. *J Infect Dis* 1985;151: 236–242.

289. Levine MM, Pierce NF. Immunity and vaccine development. In: Barua D, Greenough WB III, eds. *Cholera*. New York: Plenum Press; 1992:285–328.

290. Levine MM, Kaper JB, Herrington D, et al. Volunteer studies of deletion mutants of *Vibrio cholerae* O1 prepared by recombinant techniques. *Infect Immun* 1988;56:161–167.

291. Mosley WH, McCormack WM, Ahmed A, et al. Report of the

1966–67 cholera field trial in rural East Pakistan. 2. Results of the serological surveys in the study population—the relationship of case rate to antibody titre and an estimate of the inapparent infection rate with *Vibrio cholerae*. *Bull WHO* 1969;40: 187–197.

292. Mosley WH. The role of immunity in cholera. A review of epidemiological and serological studies. *Texas Rep Biol Med* 1969;27:227–244.

293. Mosley WH, Woodward WE, Aziz KMS, et al. The 1968–1969 cholera vaccine field trial in rural East Pakistan. Effectiveness of monovalent Ogawa and Inaba vaccines and a purified Inaba antigen, with comparative results of serological and animal protection tests. *J Infect Dis* 1970;121:S1–S9.

294. Neoh SH, Rowley D. Protection of infant mice against cholera by antibodies to three *Vibrio cholerae* antigens. *J Infect Dis* 1972;126:41–47.

295. Neoh SE, Rowley D. The antigens of *Vibrio cholerae* involved in the vibriocidal action of antibody and complement. *J Infect Dis* 1970;121:505–513.

296. Attridge SR, Rowley D. Prophylactic significance of the non-polysaccharide antigens of *Vibrio cholerae*. *J Infect Dis* 1983; 148:931–939.

297. Young CR, Wachsmuth IK, Olsvik O, Feeley JC. Immune response to *Vibrio cholerae*. In: Rose NR, Friedman H, Fahey JL, eds. *Manual of clinical immunology*. Washington, DC: American Society for Microbiology; 1986:363–370.

298. Hornick RB, Music SI, Wenzel R, et al. The Broad Street pump revisited: response of volunteers to ingested cholera vibrios. *Bull NY Acad Med* 1971;47:1181–1191.

299. Oseasohn R, Ahmad S, Islam MA, Rahaman ASMM. Clinical and bacteriological findings among families of cholera patients. *Lancet* 1966;1:340–342.

300. Rabbani GH, Greenough WB III. Pathophysiology and clinical aspects of cholera. In: Barua D, Greenough WB III, eds. *Cholera*. New York: Plenum Press; 1992:209–228.

301. Carpenter CCJ, Barua D, Wallace CK, et al. Clinical studies in Asiatic cholera. IV. Antibiotic therapy in cholera. *Bull Johns Hopkins Hosp* 1966;118:216–229.

302. Hirschhorn N, Kinzie JL, Sachar DB, et al. Decrease in net stool output in children during intestinal perfusion with glucose-containing solution. *N Engl J Med* 1968;279:176–181.

303. Pierce NF, Banwell JG, Mitra RC, et al. A controlled comparison of tetracycline and furazolidone in cholera. *Br Med J* 1968; 3:277–280.

304. Wang F, Butler T, Rabbani GH, Jones PK. The acidosis of cholera: contributions of hyperproteinemia, lactic acidemia, and hyperphosphatemia to an increased serum anion gap. *N Engl J Med* 1986;315:1591–1595.

305. Greenough WB III, Hirschhorn N, Gordon RS Jr, Lindenbaum J, Ally KKM. Pulmonary edema associated with acidosis in patients with cholera. *Trop Geogr Med* 1976;28:86–90.

306. Benyajati C, Keoplug M, Beisel WR, Gangarosa EJ, Sprinz H, Sitprija V. Acute renal failure in Asiatic cholera: clinicopathologic correlations with acute tubular necrosis and hypokalemic nephropathy. *Ann Intern Med* 1960;52:960–975.

307. Hirschhorn N, Lindenbaum J, Greenough III WB, Alam SM. Hypoglycemia in children with acute diarrhea. *Lancet* 1966;2: 128–132.

308. Molla AM, Hossain M, Islam R, Bardhan PK, Sarkar SA. Hypoglycemia: a complication of diarrhea in childhood. *Ind Pediatr* 1981;18:181–185.

309. Jones RG. Hypoglycemia in children with acute diarrhea. *Lancet* 1966;2:643.

310. Bennish ML, Azad AK, Rahman O, Phillips RE. Hypoglycemia during diarrhea in childhood: Prevalence, pathophysiology, and outcome. *N Engl J Med* 1990;322:1357–1363.

311. Mahalanabis D, Brayton JB, Mondal A, Pierce NF. The use of Ringer's lactate in the treatment of children with cholera and acute noncholera diarrhea. *Bull WHO* 1972;46:311–319.

312. Hirschhorn N, Chaudhury AKMA, Lindenbaum J. Cholera in pregnant women. *Lancet* 1969;1:1230–1232.

313. Greenough WB. *Vibrio cholerae*. In: Mandell GL, Douglas GR, Bennett JE, eds. *Principles and practice of infectious diseases*. 3rd ed. New York: Churchill Livingstone; 1990:1636–1646.

314. Lindenbaum J, Greenough WB III, Islam MR. Antibiotic therapy of cholera. *Bull WHO* 1967;36:871–833.
315. Mosley WH, Benenson AS, Barui KR. A serological survey of cholera antibodies in rural East Pakistan. I. The distribution of area and the relation of antibody titer to the pattern of endemic cholera. *Bull WHO* 1968;38:327–334.
316. Centers for Disease Control. Surveillance for epidemic cholera in the Americas: an assessment. In: CDC surveillance summaries, March 1992. *MMWR* 1992;41(No. SS-1):27–34.
317. Zafari Y, Zarifi A, Zomorodi F. A comparative study of sea water and Cary–Blair media for transportation of stool specimens. *J Trop Med Hyg* 1968;71:178–179.
318. Cary SG, Blair EB. New transport medium for shipment of clinical specimens. 1. Faecal specimens. *J Bacteriol* 1964;88:96–98.
319. Gaines S, Haque SU, Paniom W, et al. A field trial of a new transport medium for collection of faeces for bacteriological examination. *Am J Trop Med Hyg* 1965;14:136–140.
320. Pal SC. Laboratory diagnosis. In: Barua D, Greenough WB III, eds. *Cholera*. New York: Plenum Press; 1992:229–252.
321. Barua D, Gomez CZ. Blotting-paper strips for transportation of cholera stools. *Bull WHO* 1967;37:798.
322. Spira WM, Ahmed QS. Gauze filtration and enrichment procedures for recovery of *Vibrio cholerae* from contaminated waters. *Appl Environ Microbiol* 1981;42:730–733.
323. Barrett TJ, Blake PA, Morris GK, Puhr ND, Bradford HB, Wells JG. Use of Moore swabs for isolating *Vibrio cholerae* from sewage. *J Clin Microbiol* 1980;11:385–388.
324. Gorbach SI, Banwell JG, Jacob B, et al. Intestinal microflora in Asiatic cholera. I. Rice-water stool. *J Infect Dis* 1970;121:32–37.
325. Almeida RJ, Hickman-Brenner FW, Sowers EG, Puhr ND, Farmer JJ III, Wachsmuth IK. Comparison of a latex agglutination assay and an enzyme-linked immunosorbent assay for detecting cholera toxin. *J Clin Microbiol* 1990;28:128–130.
326. Fields PI, Popovic T, Wachsmuth K, Olsvik O. Use of polymerase chain reaction for detection of toxigenic *Vibrio cholerae* O1 strains from the Latin American cholera epidemic. *J Clin Microbiol* 1992;30:2118–2121.
327. Keasler SP, Hall RH. Detecting and biotyping *Vibrio cholerae* O1 with multiplex polymerase chain reaction. *Lancet* 1993;341:1661.
328. Lam SYS. A rapid test for the identification of *Vibrio cholerae* in stool. *J Diarrh Dis Res* 1983;2:87–89.
329. Rahman M, Sack DA, Wadood A, et al. A low cost and rapid slide agglutination test for diagnosis of cholera using faecal samples. In: *Proceedings of the 23rd joint conference on cholera*. US–Japan Cooperative Medical Science Program, Bethesda: National Institutes of Health; 1987:88.
330. Barua D. Laboratory diagnosis of cholera cases and carriers. In: *Principles and practices of cholera control*, Public Health Paper No. 40. Geneva: WHO; 1970:47–52.
331. Zinnaka Y, Shimodori S, Takeya K. Application of fluorescent antibody technique to the detection of cholera vibrio. *Jpn J Infect Dis* 1965;39:51–58.
332. Centers for Disease Control. Case definitions for public health surveillance. *MMWR* 1990;39:9–10.
333. World Health Organization. *A manual for the treatment of diarrhea*. Geneva, Programme for Control of Diarrhoeal Diseases. Publication WHO/CDD/SER/80.2 rev 2, 1990.
334. World Health Organization. *Guidelines for cholera control*. Geneva: Programme for Control of Diarrhoeal Disease. Publication WHO/CDD/SER/80.4 rev 2, 1991.
335. Greenough WB III, Rosenberg IS, Gordon RS, et al. Tetracycline in the treatment of cholera. *Lancet* 1964;1:355–357.
336. Bhattacharya SK, Bhattacharya MK, Dutta P, et al. Double-blind, randomized, controlled clinical trial of norfloxacin for cholera. *Antimicrob Agents Chemother* 1990;34:939–940.
337. Mhalu FS, Mmari PW, Ijumba J. Rapid emergence of El Tor *Vibrio cholerae* resistant to antimicrobial agents during first six months of fourth cholera epidemic in Tanzania. *Lancet* 1979;1:345–347.
338. Glass RI, Huq I, Alim ARMA, Yunus M. Emergence of multiply antibiotic-resistant *Vibrio cholerae* in Bangladesh. *J Infect Dis* 1980;142:939–942.
339. Ouellette M, Gerbaud G, Courvalin P. Genetic, biochemical and molecular characterization of strains of *Vibrio cholerae* multiresistant to antibiotics. *Ann Inst Pasteur Microbiol* 1988;139:105–113.
340. McCormack WM, Chowdhury AM, Jahangir N, Fariduddin Ahmed AB, Mosley WH. Tetracycline prophylaxis in families of cholera patients. *Bull WHO* 1968;38:787–792.
341. Gupta PGS, Sircar BK, Mondal S, et al. Effect of doxycycline on transmission of *Vibrio cholerae* infection among family contacts of cholera patients in Calcutta. *Bull WHO* 1978;56:323–326.
342. Centers for Disease Control. Update: Cholera—Western hemisphere, and recommendations for treatment of cholera. *MMWR* 1991;40:562–565.
343. Gangarosa EJ, Saghari H, Emile J, Sanati A, Siadat H, Watanabe Y. Search for a mass chemotherapeutic drug for cholera control. *Bull WHO* 1966;35:669–674.
344. Mahalanabis D, Molla AM, Sack D. Clinical management of cholera. In: Barua D, Greenough WB III, eds. *Cholera*. New York: Plenum Press; 1992:253–284.
345. Craun G, Swerdlow D, Tauxe R, et al. Prevention of waterborne cholera in the United States. *J Am Waterworks Assoc* 1991;83:40–46.
346. Centers for Disease Control. ACIP: cholera vaccine. *MMWR* 1988;37:617–624.

Infections of the Gastrointestinal Tract,
edited by M. J. Blaser, P. D. Smith, J. I. Ravdin,
H. B. Greenberg, and R. L. Guerrant
Raven Press, Ltd., New York © 1995.

CHAPTER 47

"Noncholera" *Vibrio* Species

J. Glenn Morris, Jr.

A major concern of early cholera investigators was the differentiation of epidemic-associated strains of *Vibrio cholerae* from other, "atypical" *Vibrio* strains. Work by Gardner and Venkatraman and others in the 1930s (1,2) led to the concept that *V. cholerae* strains could be divided into two groups: those in O group 1, which agglutinated with antisera directed against antigens present on strains isolated from cholera patients, and other "nonagglutinating" or "noncholera" *Vibrio* strains, which were regarded primarily as nonpathogenic, environmental isolates. Some early writers discussed the possibility that nonagglutinating isolates were responsible for "paracholera" or similar clinical syndromes (2). However, it was not until the 1950s and 1960s that investigators began to identify outbreaks of disease directly attributable to these strains (3–7).

As more attention was paid to nonagglutinating vibrios, it became increasingly obvious that these isolates were a heterogeneous group, including species besides *V. cholerae*. These observations have led, since the late 1970s, to the designation of a number of new *Vibrio* species. As shown in Table 1, there are now 11 *Vibrio* species other than *V. cholerae* that have been associated with human illness (8,9). At the same time, there has been increasing recognition that *V. cholerae* strains in O groups other than 1 (non-O1 *V. cholerae*) can cause both epidemic and endemic disease (10–17). *V. cholerae* in O group 1 and in O group 139 [a newly recognized serovar associated with rapidly spreading epidemic disease in Asia (10–13)] cause epidemic cholera; they are described separately, in the chapter on cholera. Infections with *V. cholerae* in other O groups, as well as other *Vibrio* species, which are acquired through the gastrointestinal tract (*V. parahaemolyticus, V. fluvialis, V. mimicus, V. hollisae, V. furnissii,* and *V. vulnificus*) will be dealt with in this chapter. *V. alginolyticus* and *V. damsela* (18) are generally acquired by exposure of wounds to seawater. Descriptions of infections with *V. cincinnatiensis* (19), *V. carchariae* (20), and

J. G. Morris, Jr: Departments of Medicine and Epidemiology and Preventive Medicine, University of Maryland School of Medicine, and Veterans Affairs Medical Center, Baltimore, Maryland 21201.

V. metschnikovii (21,22) have been restricted to case reports, and the significance of their isolation from humans remains to be determined.

Vibrios are free-living, naturally occurring (autochthonous) bacteria in estuarine or marine environments. Aside from the 12 species cited above, there are at least another 23 *Vibrio* species that have been isolated from environmental sources (8). Based on numerical taxonomy studies (23), it is likely that the actual number of *Vibrio* species is much greater, with isolates obtained during environmental surveys often belonging to as yet unidentified or unnamed *Vibrio* species. Even within species that have been identified as human pathogens, there may be only a minority of strains that have the necessary virulence characteristics to cause illness; however, differentiation of potentially pathogenic from nonpathogenic strains within these species is not always possible.

VIBRIO CHOLERAE IN O GROUPS OTHER THAN 1 (NON-O1 *VIBRIO CHOLERAE*)

As noted above, it has traditionally been assumed that epidemic cholera is caused only by *V. cholerae* strains in O group 1. This assumption has been challenged by the emergence of *V. cholerae* O139 Bengal, a non-O1 *V. cholerae* strain that has now spread in epidemic form across much of Asia (10–13). These observations indicate that the presence or absence of the O1 antigen is an inadequate marker for epidemic potential. However, with the exception of the O139 isolates [and some non-O1 strains that have been isolated during the course of cholera epidemics caused by *V. cholerae* O1 (4,15)], it is still true that non-O1 strains are primarily a cause of sporadic illness, probably reflecting occasional introduction of environmental isolates into human populations (24). It is the strains responsible for this sporadic disease that will be discussed in this section.

Microbiology

All *V. cholerae* share essentially identical microbiological and biochemical characteristics (25). Like other *Vibrio*

TABLE 1. Vibrio *species implicated as a cause of human disease*

Species	Clinical presentations[a]		
	GI	Wound/ear	Septicemia
V. cholerae			
O1	+ +	(+)	
non-O1	+ +	+	+
V. mimicus	+ +	+	
V. parahaemolyticus	+ +	+	(+)
V. fluvialis	+ +		
V. furnissii	+ +		
V. hollisae	+ +		(+)
V. vulnificus	+	+ +	+ +
V. alginolyticus		+ +	
V. damsela		+ +	
V. cincinnatiensis			+
V. carchariae		+	
V. metschnikovii	?		?

[a] + + denotes most common presentation, + other clinical presentations, and (+) very rare presentation

species, *V. cholerae* is a facultatively anaerobic, asporogenous, gram-negative rod. *V. cholerae* is oxidase-positive, reduces nitrate, and is motile by a single polar, sheathed flagellum. Growth is stimulated by the addition of 1% NaCl; however, in contrast to other *Vibrio* species, *V. cholerae* will grow in the absence of NaCl. Biochemical characteristics are summarized in Table 2.

Differentiation of O group 1 and non-O1 *V. cholerae* is based on expression of the O1 antigen and agglutination with O1 antisera. The O1 biosynthetic gene cluster in *V. cholerae* (VcRfb) contains 20 kb of DNA (26). Probes to

internal gene sequences within the Vcrfbr and Vcrfbs genes do not hybridize with non-O1 strains, indicating that some or all of the genes in this gene complex are absent in non-O1 *V. cholerae* (27). Non-O1 strains have been subdivided by several investigators into a series of O groups; the two most commonly used schemes have been developed by Smith and Sakazaki, respectively (28,29).

V. cholerae strains can also be classified based on enzyme electrophoretic patterns (zymovar analysis). In the system developed by Salles and colleagues (30,31), virtually all epidemic-associated *V. cholerae* strains fall into one of two closely related zymovars: zymovar 13 (O1 classical strains) or zymovar 14 [O1 El Tor and O139 Bengal strains (27)]. In contrast, nonepidemic *V. cholerae* strains (O1 and non-O1) can be classified into close to 100 zymovars, with a degree of genetic diversity that approaches that of *E. coli*. These observations emphasize the heterogeneity of *V. cholerae* strains; as is true for *E. coli*, this diversity should prompt caution in making generalizations about nonepidemic *V. cholerae* isolates.

Approximately 70% of non-O1 *V. cholerae* strains are able to produce a polysaccharide capsule (32). Strains undergo phase variation, shifting at a rate of $\sim10^{-5}$ between encapsulated forms having an opaque colonial morphology and unencapsulated or minimally encapsulated forms having a translucent morphology. Preliminary studies suggest that there are multiple capsular types.

Epidemiology

The most common clinical manifestation of "sporadic" non-O1 *V. cholerae* infections is gastroenteritis (Table 3).

TABLE 2. *Tests for differentiation of selected* Vibrio *species[a]*

Test	*V. cholerae* O1 and non-O1	*V. mimicus*	*V. parahaemolyticus*	*V. fluvialis*	*V. furnissili*	*V. hollisae*	*V. vulnificus*
Oxidase	+	+	+	+	+	+	+
NO₃-NO₂ + 1% NaCl	+	+	+	+	+	+	+
Indole + 1% NaCl	+	+	+	−	−	+/−	+
Voges–Proskauer + 1% NaCl	+/−	−	−	−	−	−	−
Urease	−	−	−/+	−	−	−	−
Lysine decarboxylase + 1% NaCl	+	+	+	−	−	−	+
Ornithine decarboxylase + 1% NaCl	+	+	+	−	−	−	+/−
Arginine dihydrolase + 1% NaCl	−	−	−	+	+	−	−
Fermentation of							
Sucrose	+	−	−	+	+	−	−/+
Lactose	(+)/−	+/−	−	−	−	−	+
L-Arabinose	−	−	+	+	+	+	−
Gas from glucose	−	−	−	−	+	−	−
Growth in nutrient broth							
0% NaCl	+	+	−	−	−	−	−
3% NaCl	+	+	+	+	+	+	+
6% NaCl	+/−	+/−	+	+/−	+/−	+/−	+/−
8% NaCl	−	−	+	−	−	−	−
10% NaCl	−	−	−	−	−	−	−
Susceptibility to O/129							
10 μg	S	S	R	R	R	R	S
150 μg	S	S	S	S	S	S	S
Growth on TCBS	Y	G	G	Y	Y	G/−	G/Y

Data from ref. 8.

[a] +, Most strains positive; −, most strains negative; +/− or −/+, variable reaction (predominant reaction shown as the numerator); ( ) = delayed reaction; S, susceptible; R, resistant; Y, yellow colonies; G, green colonies. TCBS, thiocitrate sulfate bile salts.

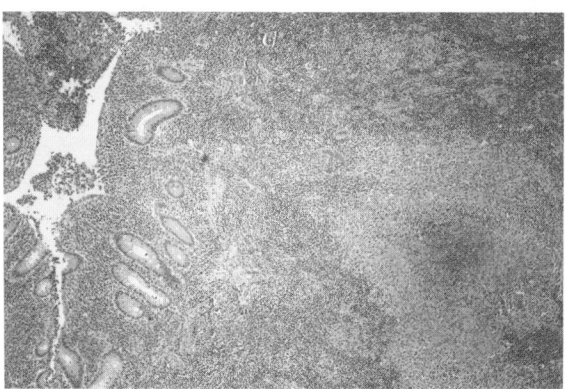

PLATE 1. Appendicitis due to *Yersina enterocolitica*. Diffuse inflammation and a submucosal granuloma with central necrosis are present in the veriform appendix (H & E). (Courtesy of Dr. Rodger Haggitt.)

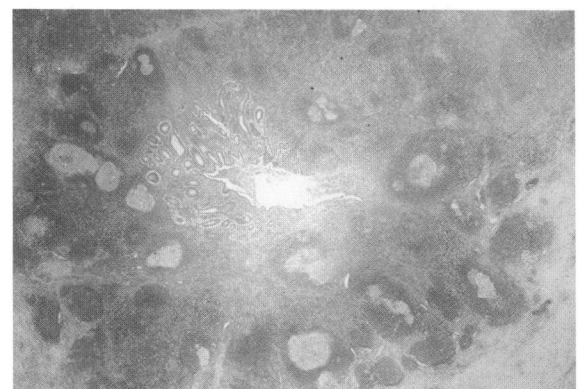

A

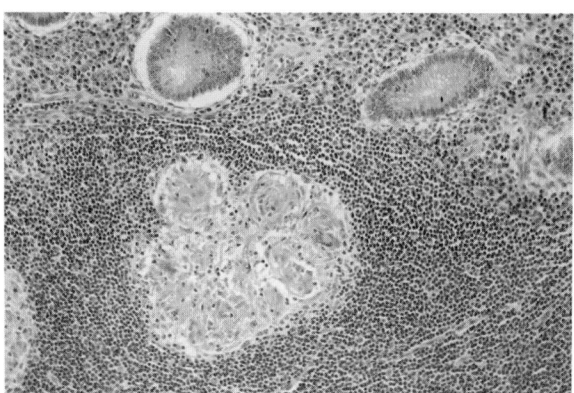

B

PLATE 2. Granulomatous appendicitis. **A:** The presence of multiple granulomas in the mucosa and submucosa of the appendix characterizes granulomatous appendicitis (H & E). **B:** The granuloma are discrete, noncaseating, and composed of epithelioid histiocytes with occasional multinucleated giant cells (H & E). (Courtesy of Dr. Rodger Haggitt.)

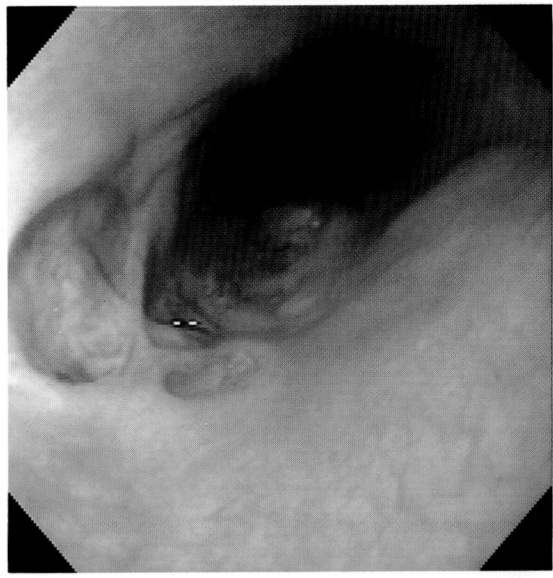

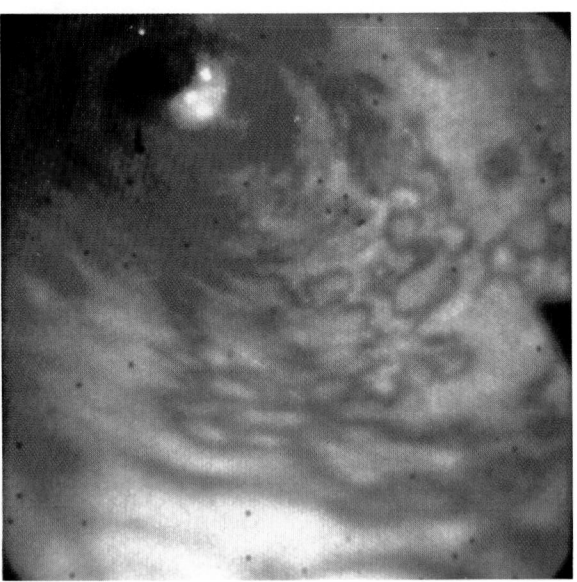

PLATE 3. Endoscopic photograph of two HIV-1–associated ulcers in which no other pathogens were identified. Note normal intervening mucosa. (Courtesy of C. M. Wilcox.)

PLATE 4. Endoscopic photograph of a large solitary ulcer caused by CMV in the distal esophagus.

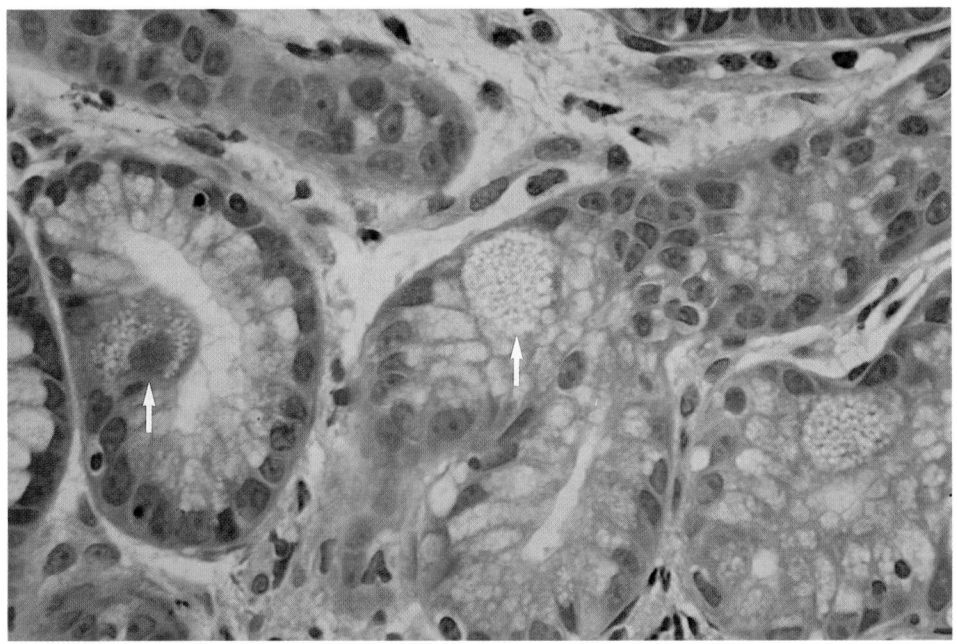

PLATE 5. Gastric mucosal biopsy from a patient with AIDS, demonstrating typical cytomegalic changes in epithelial cells (*arrows*). H&E stain.

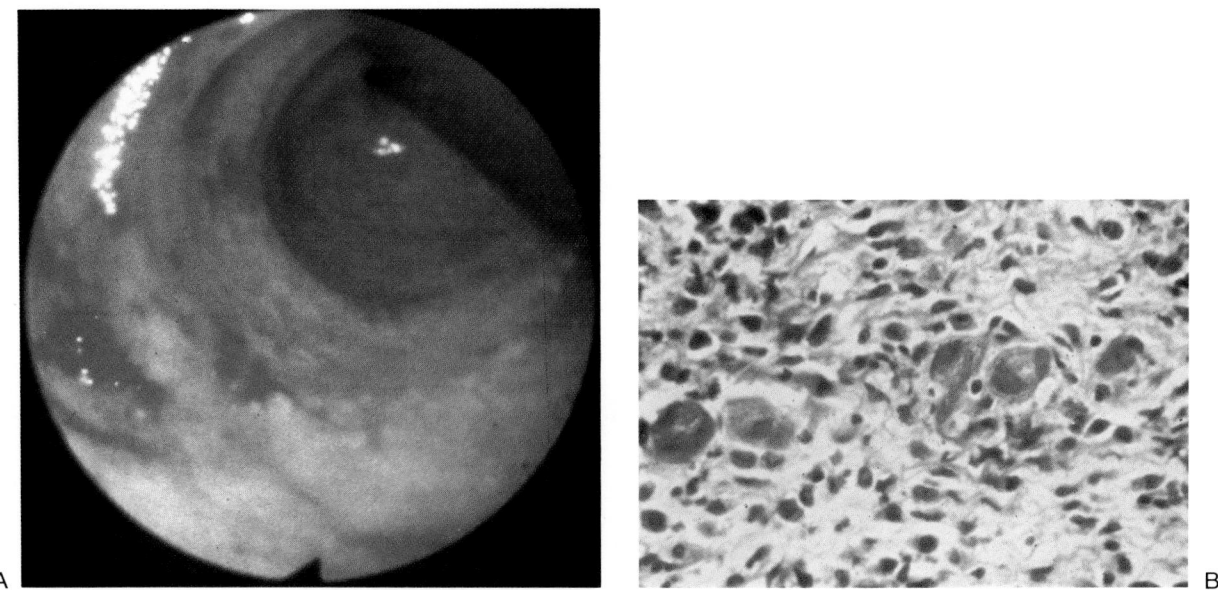

A   B

PLATE 6. Endoscopic and light microscopic appearance of cytomegalovirus colitis in an HIV-1–infected man. **A:** Direct visualization shows a diffusely ulcerated and bleeding mucosa with inflammation and exudate. **B:** Histology of the lesion in A shows numerous cytomegalic inclusion cells and inflammatory cells (×125). (From ref. 133, with permission.)

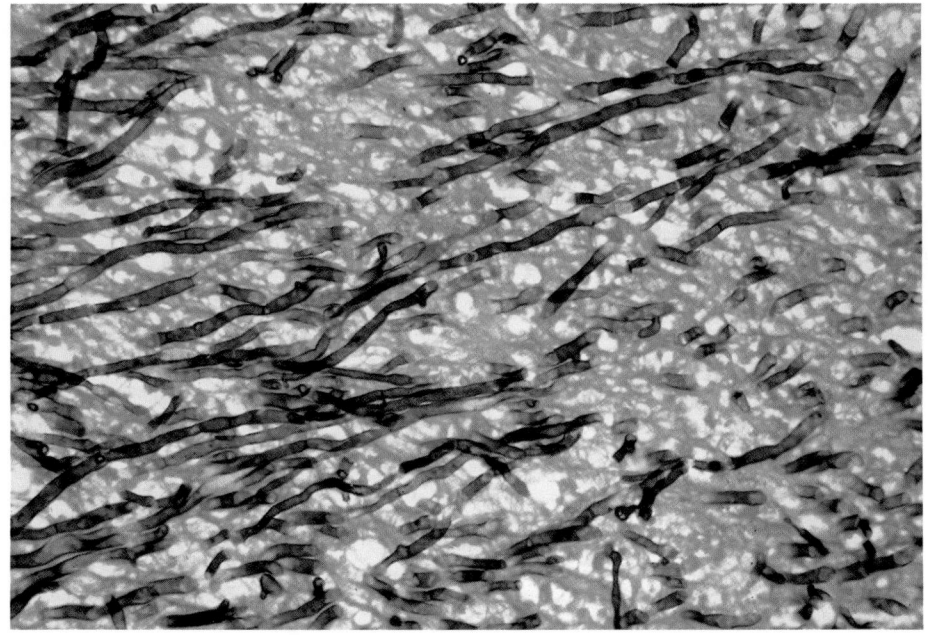

PLATE 7. Bacterial esophagitis.

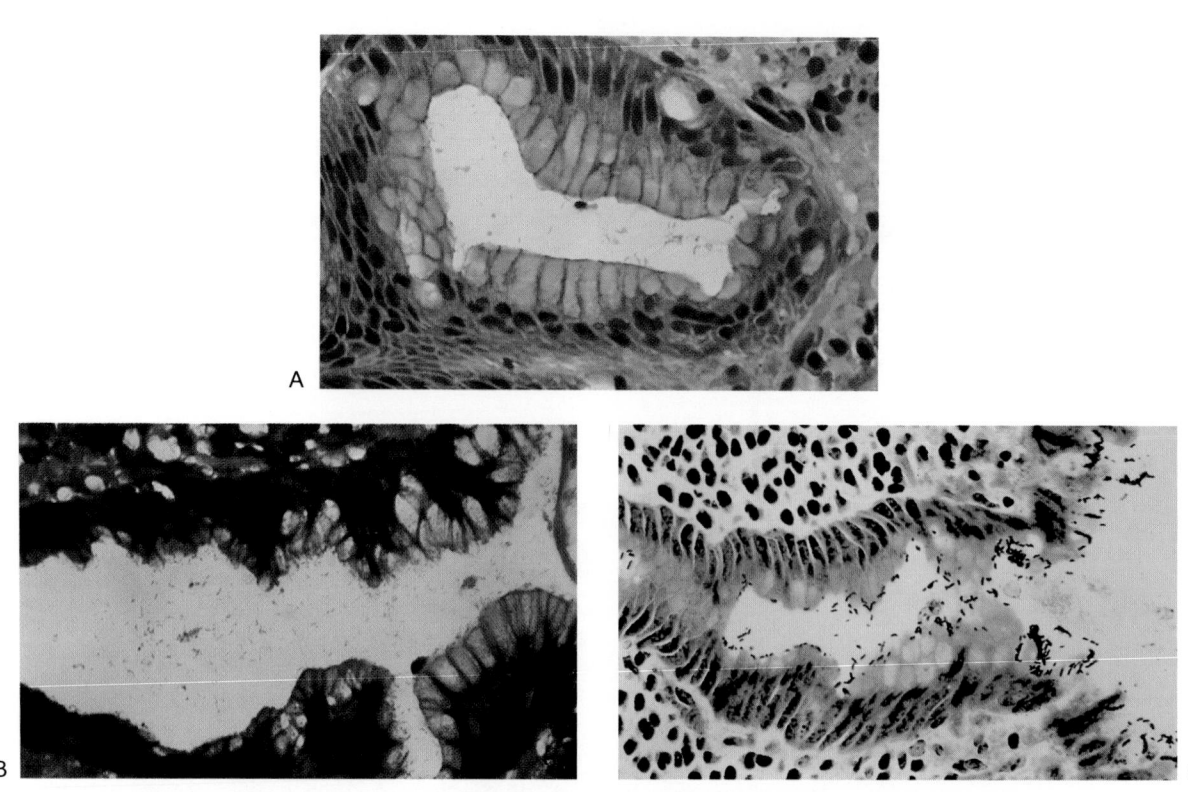

PLATE 8. *Helicobacter pylori* identified by hematoxylin–eosin (**A**), Giemsa (**B**), and Warthin–Starry silver stains (**C**). (From ref. 278, with permission.)

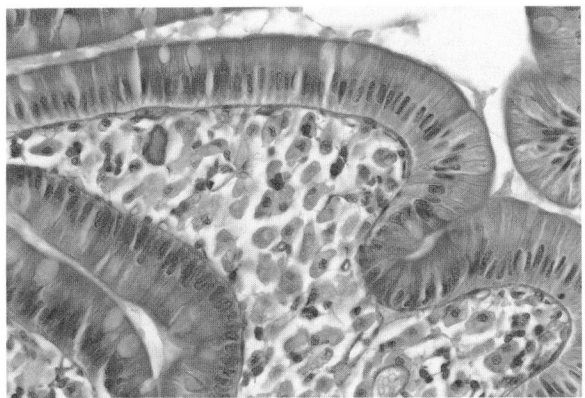

PLATE 9. Typical histology of the duodenal mucosa in a patient with Whipple's disease. Numerous vacuolated macrophages crowd the lamina propria. (H&E, ×300.) (Courtesy of Dr. Donald Regula.) (From ref. 2, with permission.)

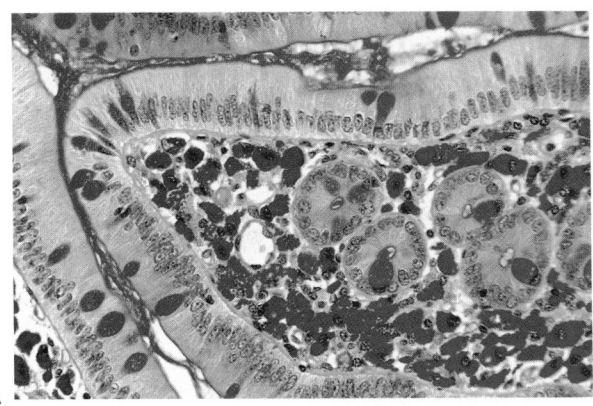
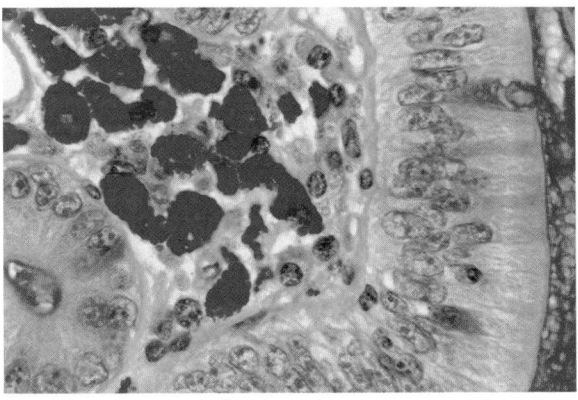

A

B

PLATE 10. **A:** Duodenal mucosa of same patient as mentioned in Fig. 2, Chapter 41, stained with periodic acid–Schiff (PAS) reagent. Vacuoles of the macrophages within the lamina propria react intensely and appear purple, indicating the presence of glycoprotein (in this case, bacterial cell wall). Epithelial goblet cells are also PAS-positive. (×300). (From ref. 2, with permission.) **B:** Same tissue, higher magnification. ×750. (Courtesy of Dr. Donald Regula.)

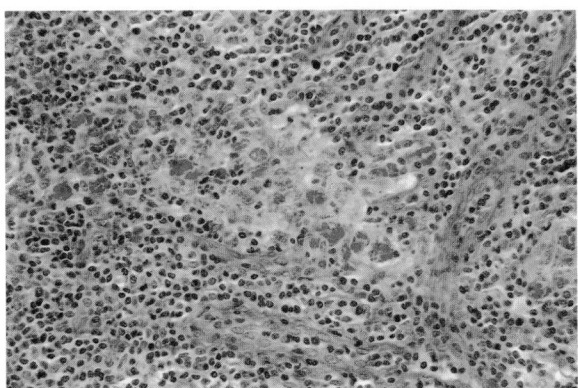

PLATE 11. Lymph node from a patient with Whipple's disease. Dark, PAS-positive clumps correspond to macrophage vacuoles. There is also a pronounced fibrotic reaction that stains less intensely, in a streak-like pattern. ×250. Periodic acid–Schiff reaction. (Courtesy of Dr. Donald Regula and Dr. Mark Feldman.)

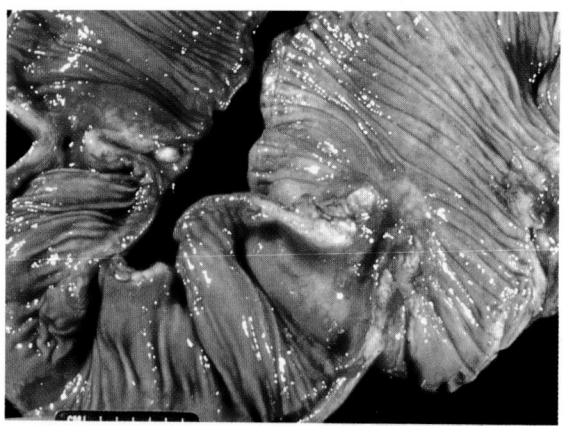

PLATE 12. Tuberculous enteritis, ulcerative, ileocolostomy specimen. Multiple ulcerations are present with focal thickening, especially at the ileocecal junction. (Courtesy of Mount Sinai Hospital, Miami.)

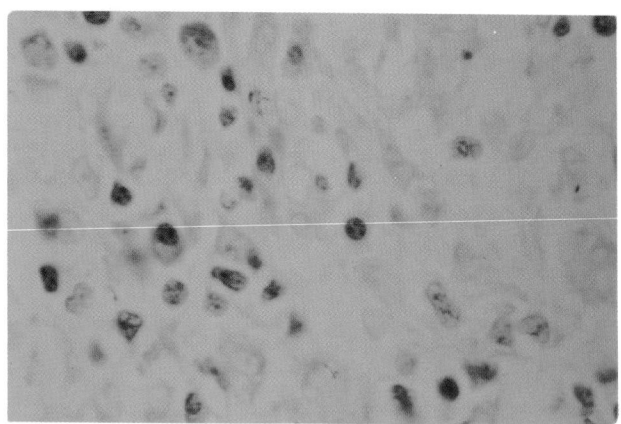

PLATE 13. Tuberculous enteritis, acute (×600). Ziehl–Neelsen–stained section of intestinal wall (see Fig. 1) reveals a loosely formed granuloma with numerous acid-fast bacilli. (Courtesy of Mount Sinai Hospital, Miami.)

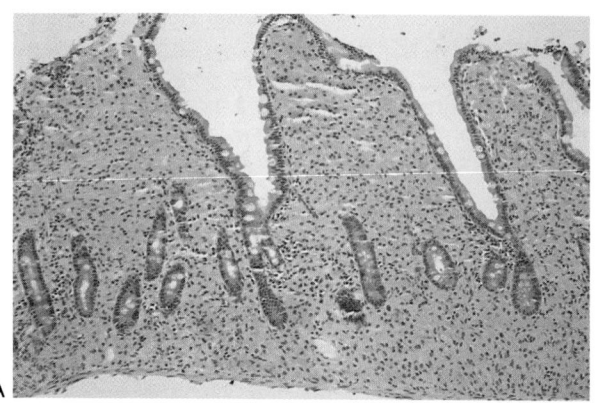

A

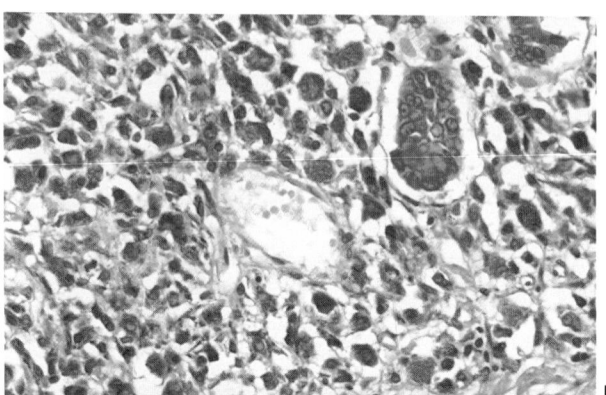

B

PLATE 14. *Mycobacterium avium* complex (MAC) disease. **A:** Histological section of intestine with marked expansion of villi and submucosa by a diffuse infiltrate of foamy histiocytes (H&E stain) (×100). (Courtesy of Dr. Charles M. Wilcox.) **B:** Ziehl–Neelsen stained section shows histiocytes stuffed with acid-fast bacilli (×300).

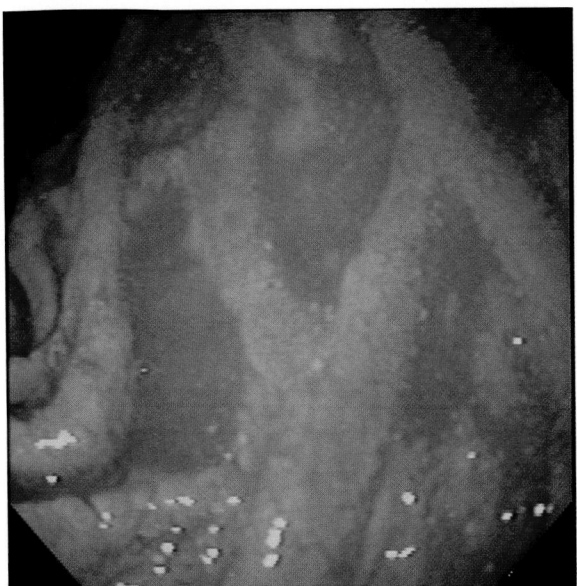

PLATE 15. Endoscopic appearance of the duodenal mucosa of a patient with disseminated *Mycobacterium avium* complex (MAC) disease. There are markedly thickened intestinal folds and multiple/plaques yellow. (Courtesy of Dr. Charles M. Wilcox.)

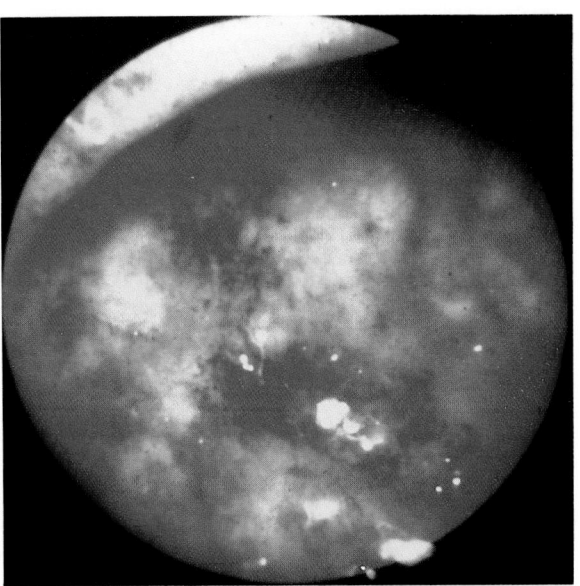

PLATE 16. Patient with amebic colitis at colonoscopy. Note punctate hemorrhagic ulcers with normal appearing mucosa. (Courtesy of H. Jinich, UCSD Medical Center.)

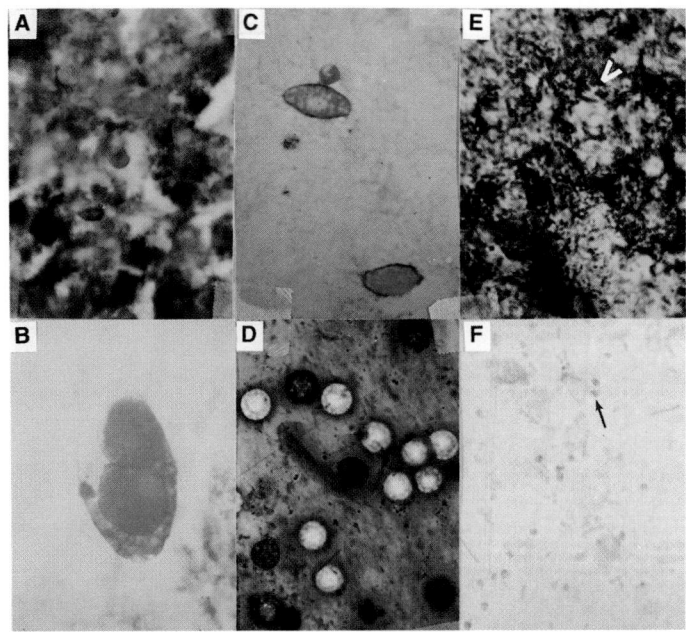

PLATE 17. Causes of diarrhea in AIDS patients. **A:** *Cryptosporidium* oocysts in fecal specimen. **B:** *Isospora belli* oocyst with bilobed nuclei. **C:** *I. belli* and *Cryptosporidium* together in the stool of a patient with AIDS **D:** *Cyclospora* (formerly called "cyanobacterium-like organism") in the stool of a patient with AIDS and diarrhea. **E:** *M. avium* complex organisms (arrow) in the stool of a patient with AIDS and protracted fever and diarrhea. **F:** *Microsporidia.* A–E, acid-fast stain; F, chromotrope stain. (Courtesy of Rosemary Soave, Cynthia Sears, Earl Long, Madeline Boucy, and Ralph Bryan.)

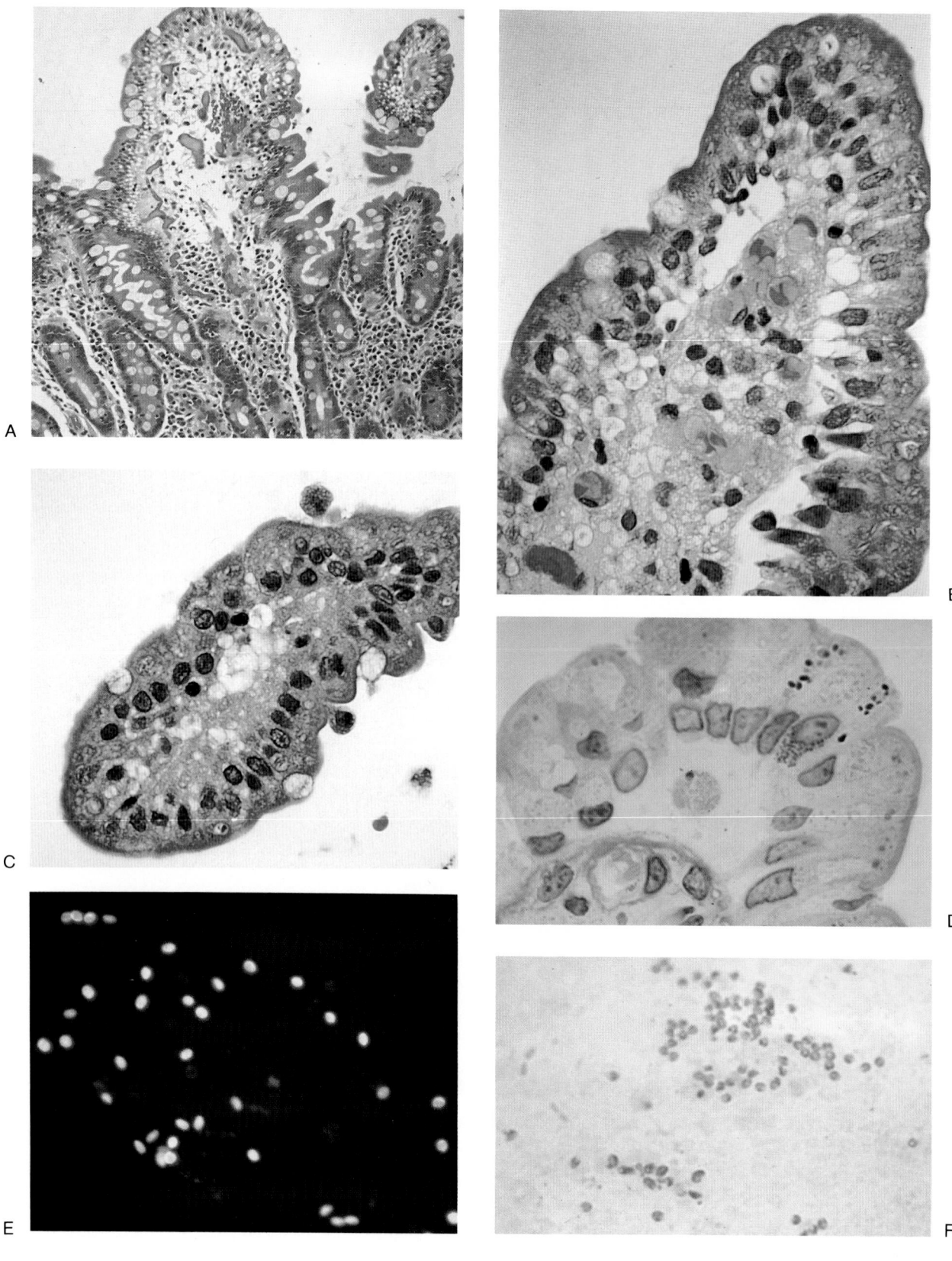

A

B

C

D

E

F

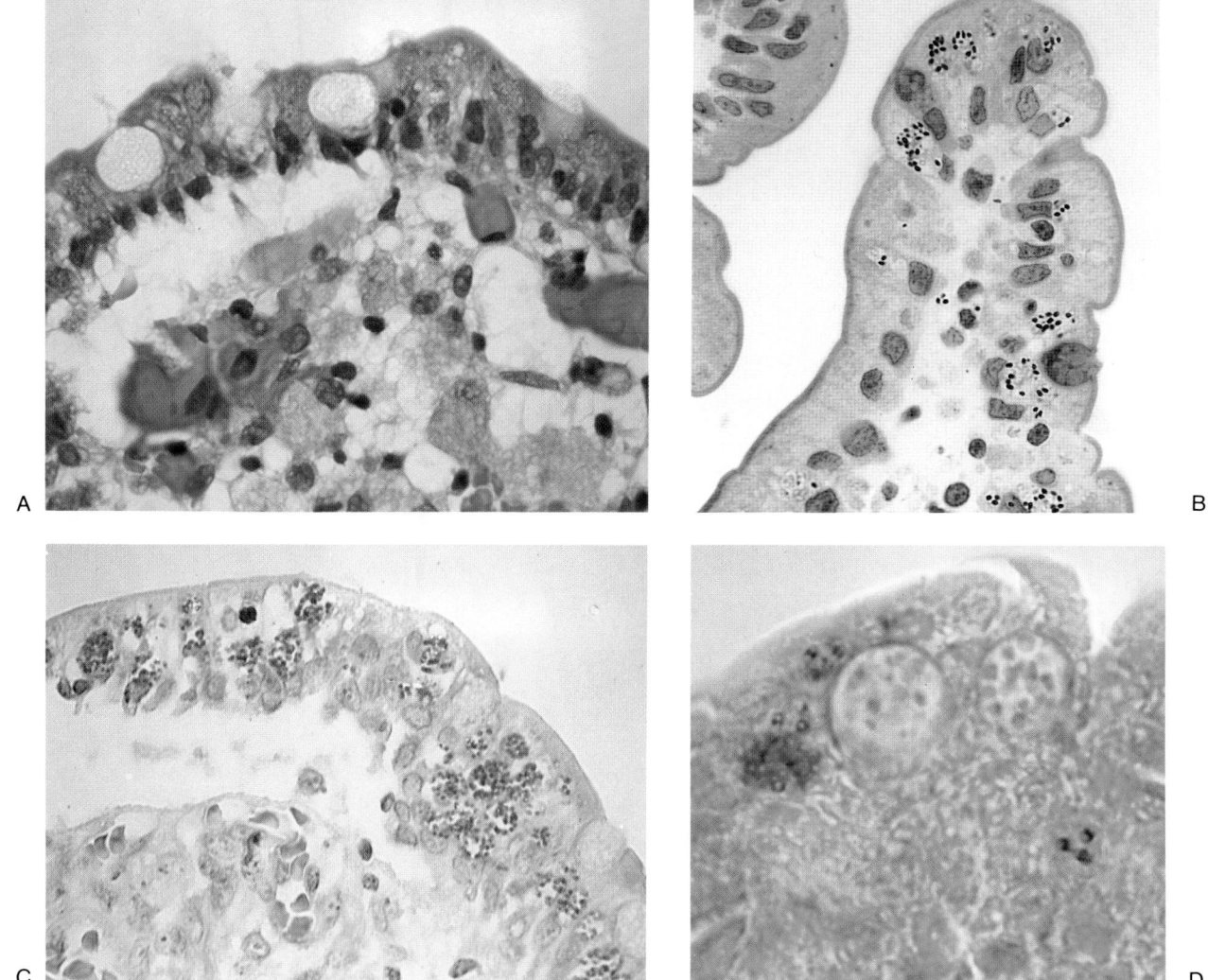

PLATE 19. Light microscopy of *S. intestinalis*. **A:** In H&E-stained sections the spores appear as supranuclear collections of refractile bluish bodies. Strips of enterocytes are frequently seen shedding. Some of the prominent lamina propria macrophages contain spores. (×576). **B:** In plastic sections the spores stain dark blue. (×576). **C:** A partially polarized Brown–Brenn, Gram stain showing the pink birefringence of some of the dark red-staining spores. (×576). **D:** A characteristic dark-staining central band is visible in some of the spores. Brown–Brenn-stained paraffin section. (×1080).

PLATE 18. Light microscopy of *E. bieneusi*. **A:** A distorted villus and elongated crypts typical of microsporidia infection. Several shed enterocytes are visible. (×152, H&E). **B:** Clear clefts are visible in some of the many bluish supranuclear plasmodia at the tip of a villus. Note the characteristic vacuolization and separation of enterocytes at the basement membrane. (×608, H&E). **C:** The spores in one (**upper**) of the two shedding enterocytes are slightly refractile. Many bluish supranuclear plasmodia are visible. (×608, H&E). **D:** The spores stain dark blue while the plasmodia stain lighter than the cytoplasm in semithin plastic sections. The darker "dots" within the plasmodia are nuclei. There is a spore in a shed cell within the space created by the sloughing enterocytes. ×950; methylene-blue, basic fuchsin, azure II). **E:** The spores fluoresce white to pink using the Calcifluor whitening agent. (Courtesy of Dr. Elizabeth Didier.) (Duodenal fluid, ×1520). **F:** The spores stain pink and the background light blue in the modified trichrome, chromotrope 2R stain (61). The polar vacuole and a central band can be seen in several of the spores. (×1425).

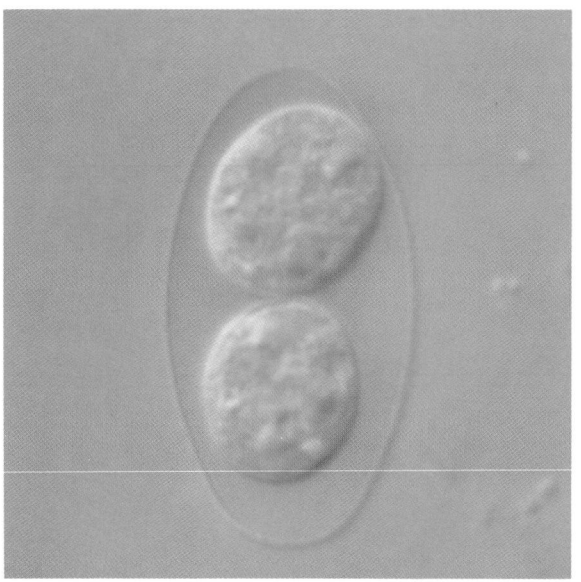

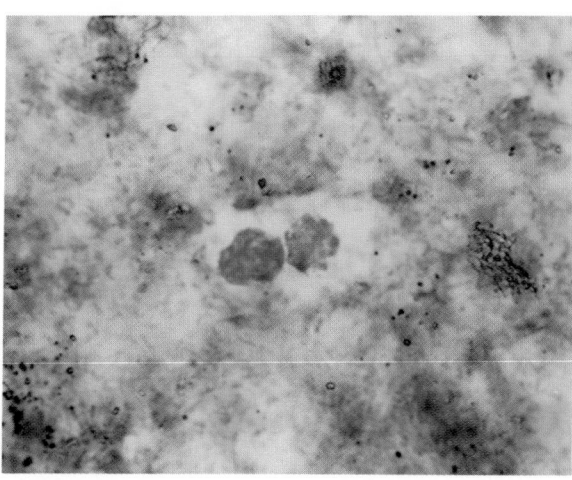

PLATE 20. Oocyst of *Isospora belli*. A mature sporulated oocyst containing two sporocysts, using Nomarski optics (×1250). (Courtesy of Dr. Murray Wittner.)

PLATE 21. Direct smear of stool sample from a patient with isosporiasis (modified acid-fast stain, ×600). (Courtesy of Dr. Jim Yang.)

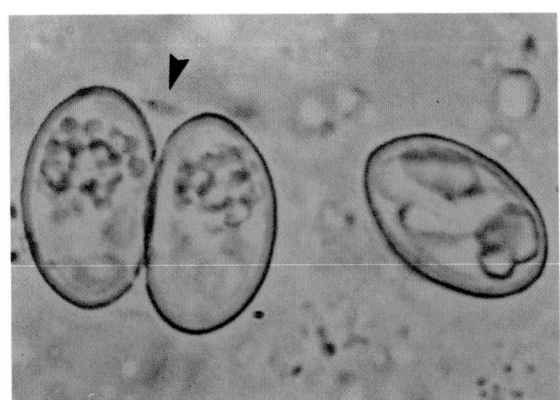

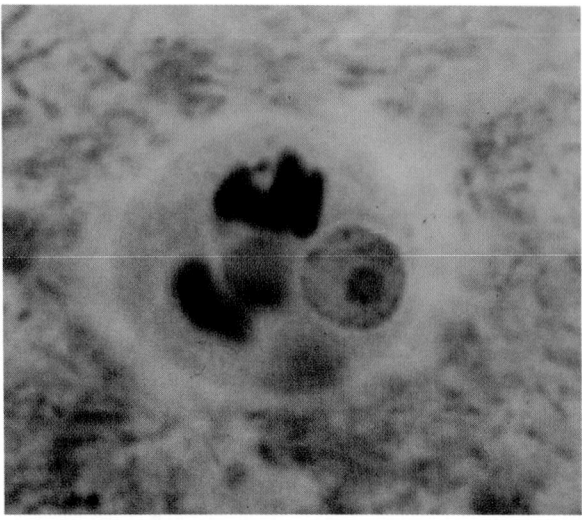

PLATE 22. Oocyst and free sporocyst of *Sarcocystis* species. The thin-walled (*arrow*) oocyst usually ruptures so that individual sporocysts are more commonly seen. In the oocyst, residual bodies are seen in each sporocyst overlying the individual sporozoites (formalin-fixed wet preparation, ×800). (From ref. 23, with permission.)

PLATE 23. Cyst of *Entamoeba polecki*. This photograph illustrates some of the morphologic features that distinguish *E. polecki* from other intestinal ameba. Uninucleate cysts that have large numbers of chromatoid bodies of varied morphology strongly suggest *E. polecki* infection (iron hematoxylin stain). (From ref. 23, with permission.)

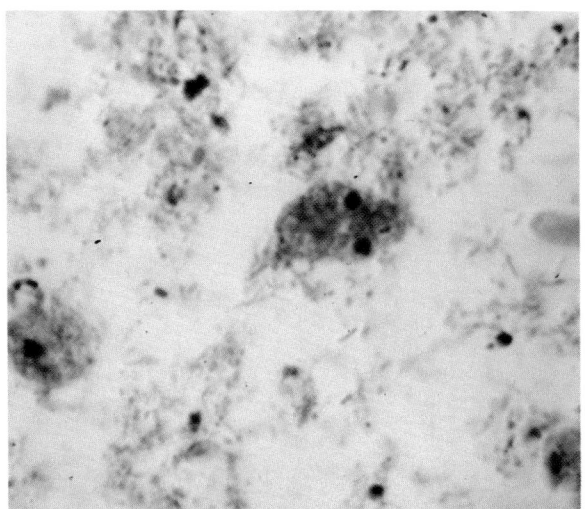

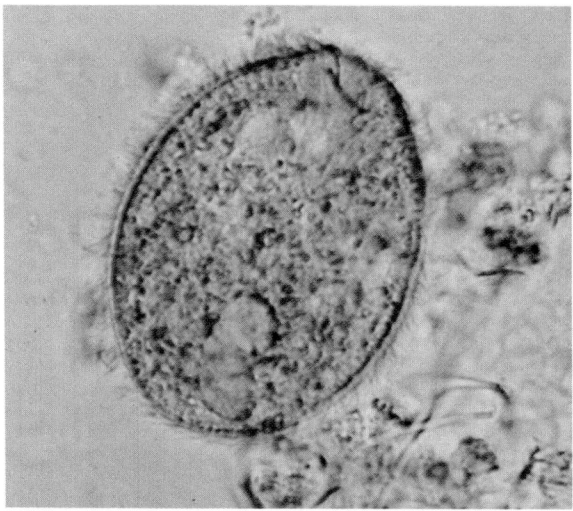

PLATE 24. Trophozoites of *Dientamoeba fragilis.* Uninucleate and more typical binucleate trophozoites of *D. fragilis.* A typical nucleus with a karyosome in the form of a tetrad is observed in the binucleate organism (iron hematoxylin stain, ×600).

PLATE 25. *Balantidium coli* trophozoite in stool. These organisms can be recognized by their large size, ciliated surface, prominent cytosome, and large kidney bean-shaped macronucleus (formalin-preserved wet mount). (From ref. 23, with permission.)

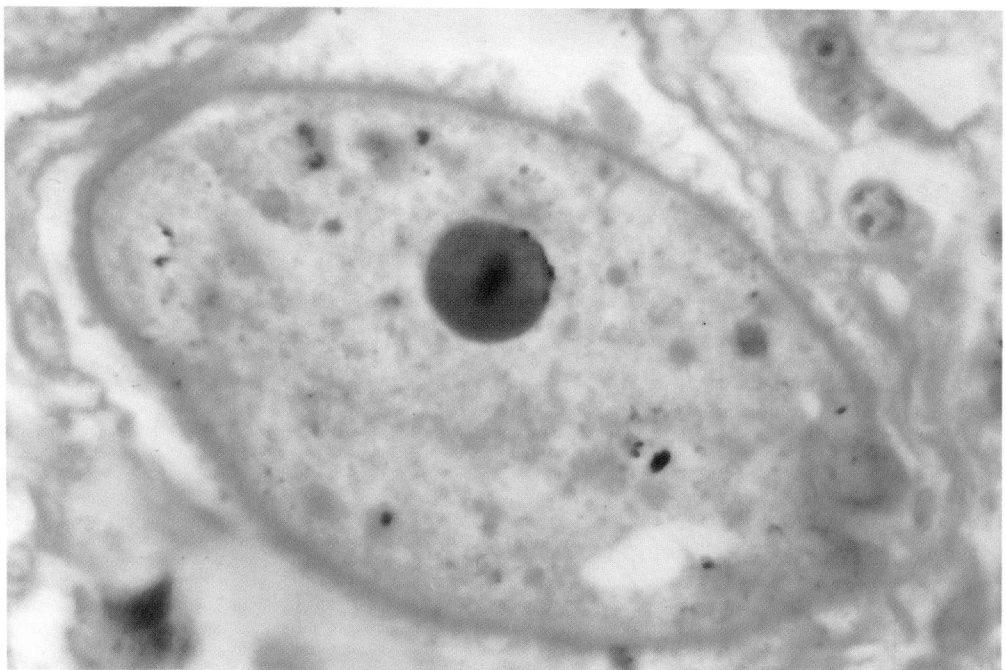

PLATE 26. Colonic biopsy showing trophozoite of *Balantidium coli.* Trichrome stain shows the prominent cytosome and the usual kidney bean-shaped macronucleus that has been bisected in this tissue section. (Courtesy of Dr. Jim Yang.)

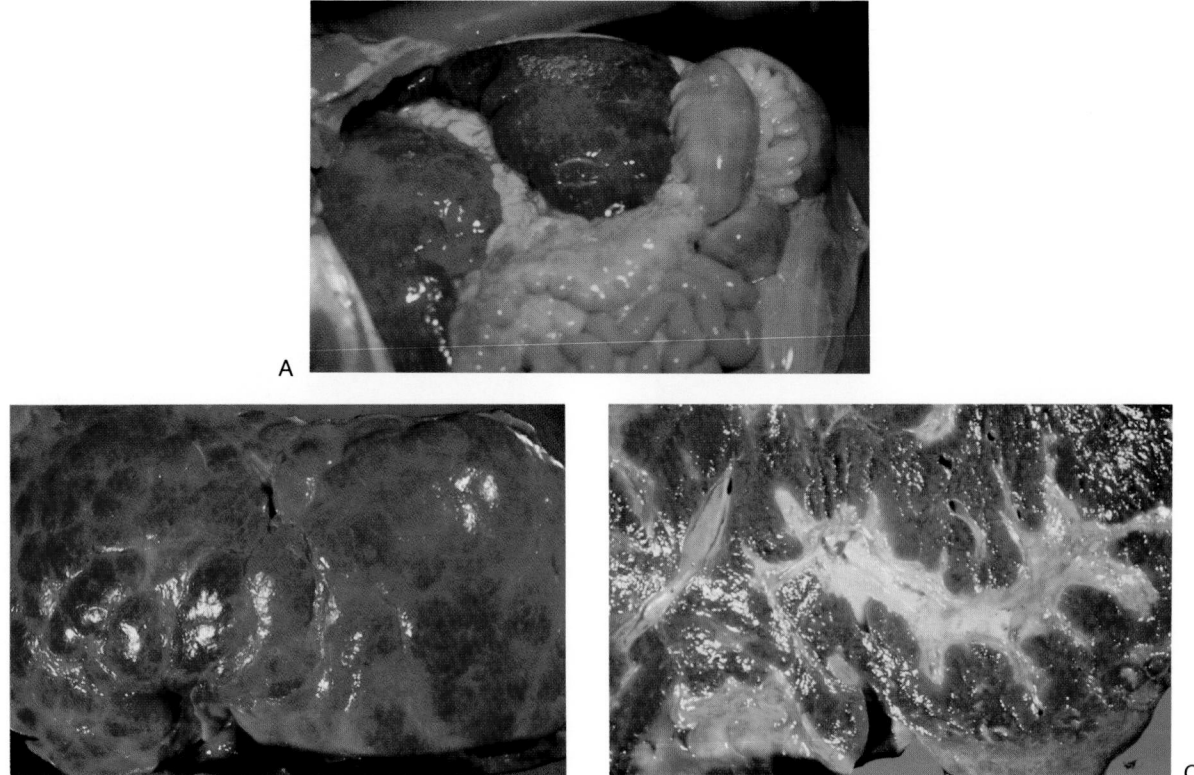

PLATE 27. Hepatosplenomegaly (liver, *red;* spleen, *purple*) at autopsy in patient with *Schistosoma mansoni* **(A).** Nodular changes on the surface of the liver **(B)** and the presinusoidal (Symmers' pipe-stem) fibrosis of the liver in cross section **(C)** (Courtesy of M. Mittermeyer.)

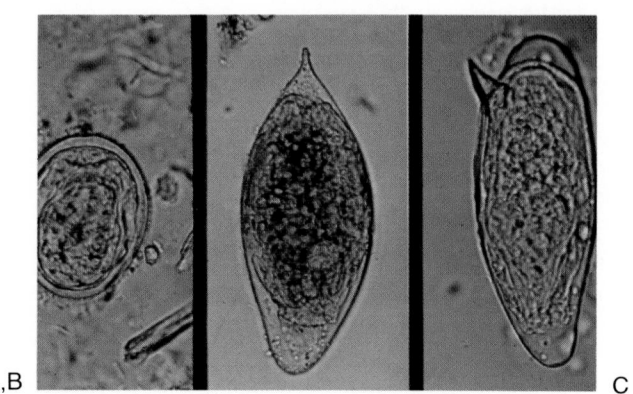

PLATE 28. *Schistosoma japonicum* **(A),** *S. haematobium* **(B),** and *S. mansoni* **(C)** ova in the stool or urine.

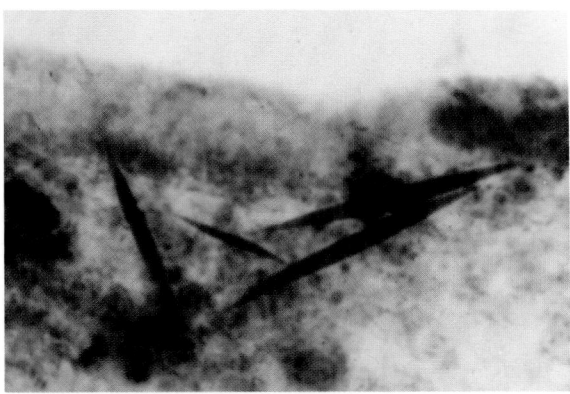

PLATE 29. Charcot–Leyden crystals (trichrome stain, oil immersion). Note the characterisitic shape; various sizes will be present in a single specimen. The presence of these crystals indicates the presence of eosinophils in the contents of the intestinal lumen. (Courtesy of L. Garcia and D. Bruckner.)

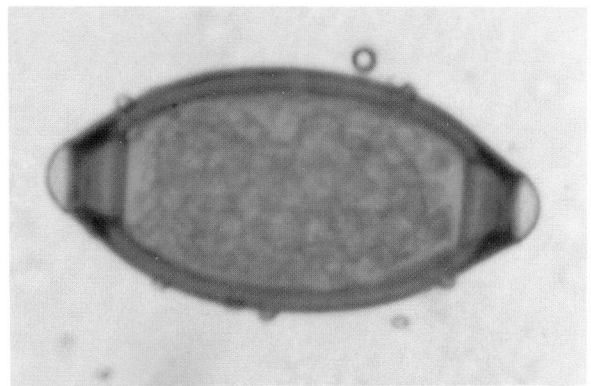

PLATE 30. *Trichuris trichiura* egg; iodine stain, wet mount. (Courtesy of L. Garcia and D. Bruckner.)

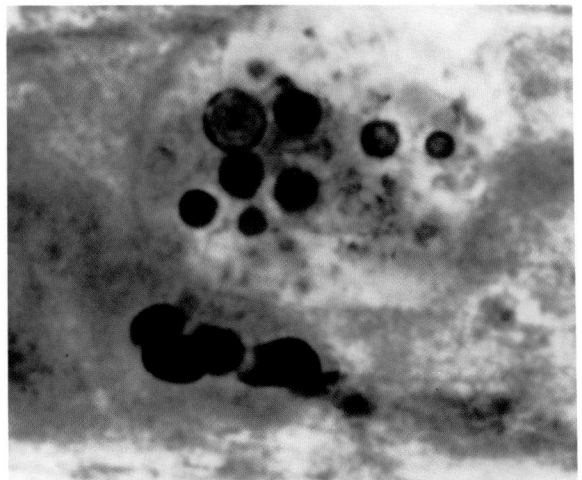

PLATE 31. *Entamoeba histolytica* trophozoite; trichrome stain. Note the presence of ingested red blood cells in the cytoplasm, which stain red with trichrome stain. (Courtesy of L. Garcia and D. Bruckner.)

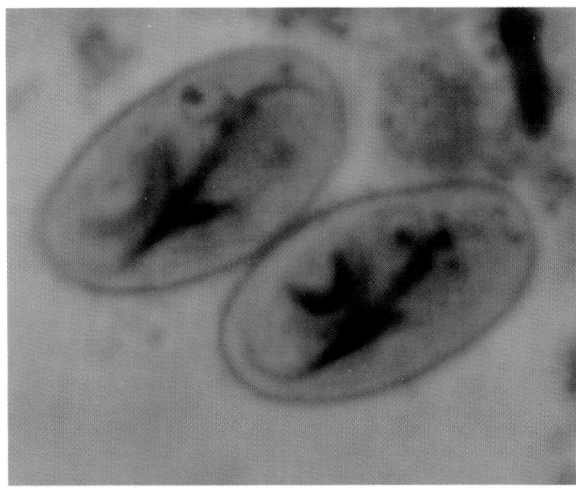

PLATE 32. *Giardia lamblia* cysts; iron and hematoxylin stain. (Courtesy of L. Garcia and D. Bruckner.)

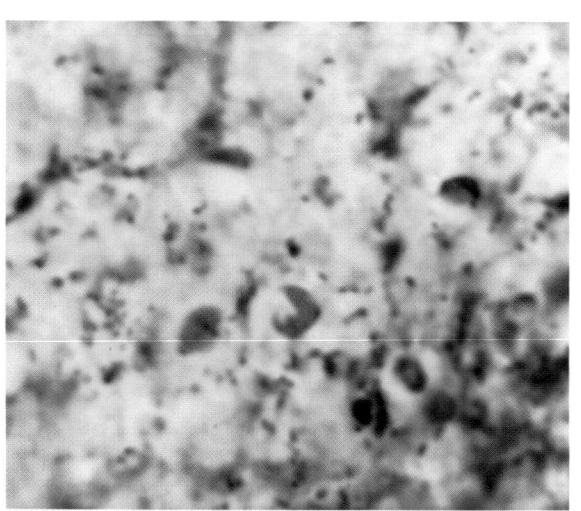

PLATE 33. *Cryptosporidium parvum* oocyts, modified acid-fast stain. (Courtesy of L. Garcia and D. Bruckner.)

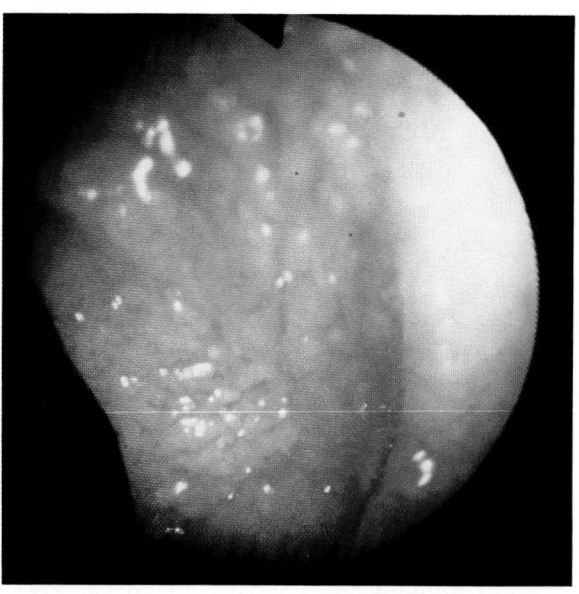

PLATE 34. Whipple's disease. Note characteristic coarsening of the villous pattern and pale, yellow, shaggy mucosa. (From ref. 14a, with permission.)

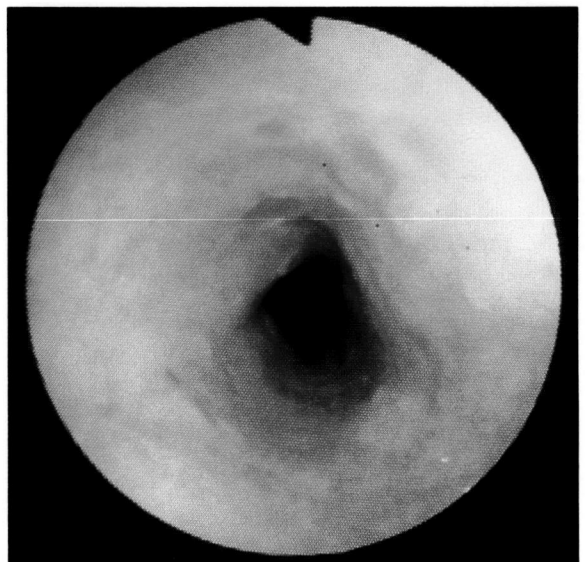

PLATE 35. HSV esophageal ulcer, early. Discrete punched-out ulcerations with normal intervening mucosa. (From ref. 14a, with permission.)

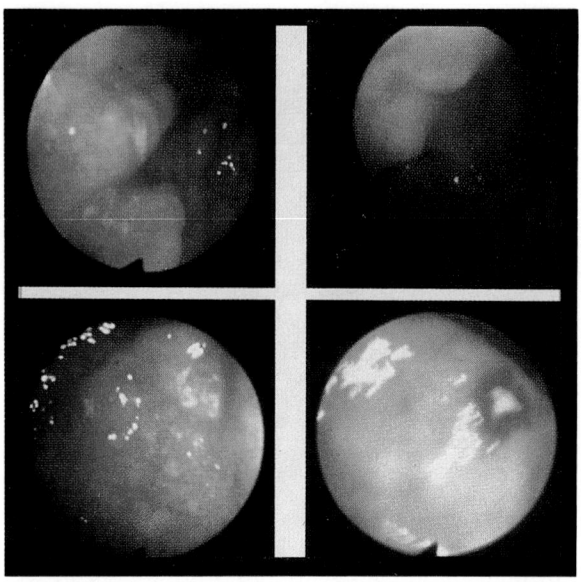

PLATE 36. Varied endoscopic appearance of CMV gastric lesions. Top left: Nodular gastritis with erosions. Top right: Nodular gastritis with minimal inflammation. Bottom left: Erosive gastritis. Bottom right: Gastric ulcerations. (From ref. 37, with permission.)

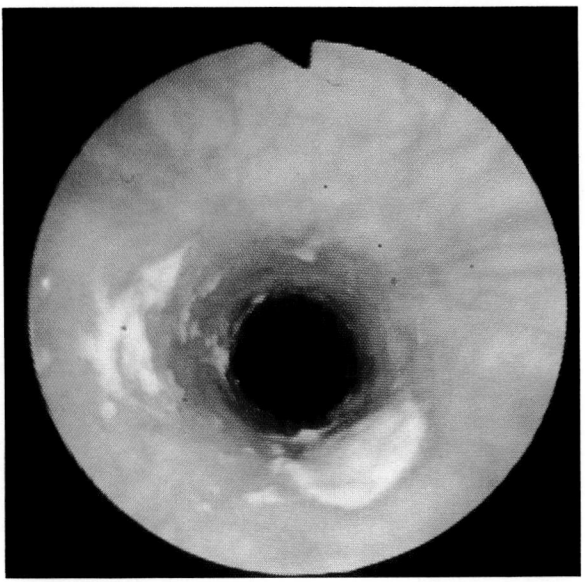

PLATE 37. *Candida* esophagitis. Discrete ulcer with white exudate and normal surrounding mucosa. (From ref. 14a, with permission.)

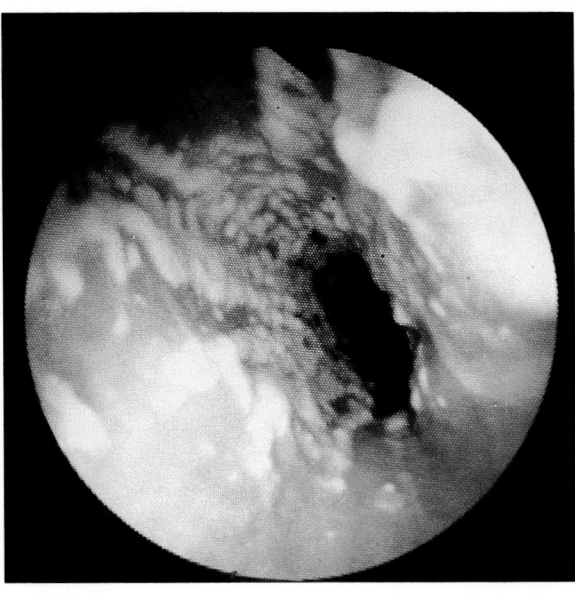

PLATE 38. *Candida* esophagitis. Severe, with extensive exudate and erythema. (From ref. 14a, with permission.)

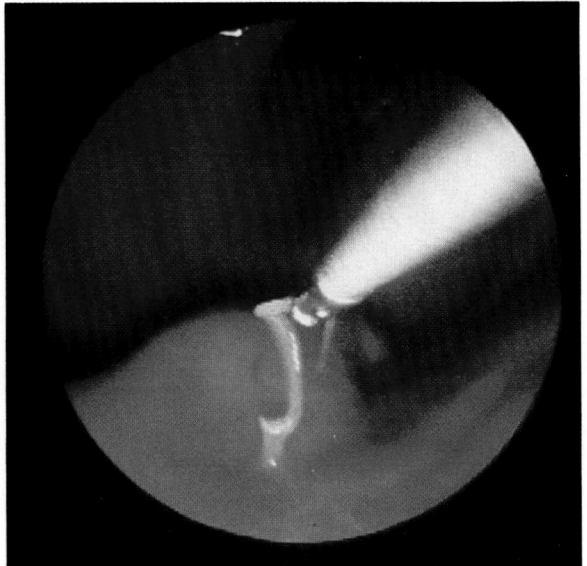

PLATE 39. Gastric anisakiasis. Anisakis larva being removed from the top of the inflammatory nodule. (From ref. 66, with permission.)

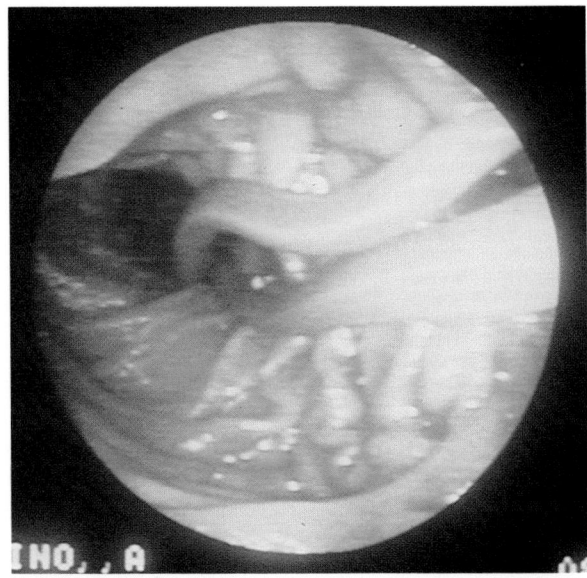

PLATE 40. *Ascaris* in duodenum. (Courtesy Dr. C. Michael Knauer.)

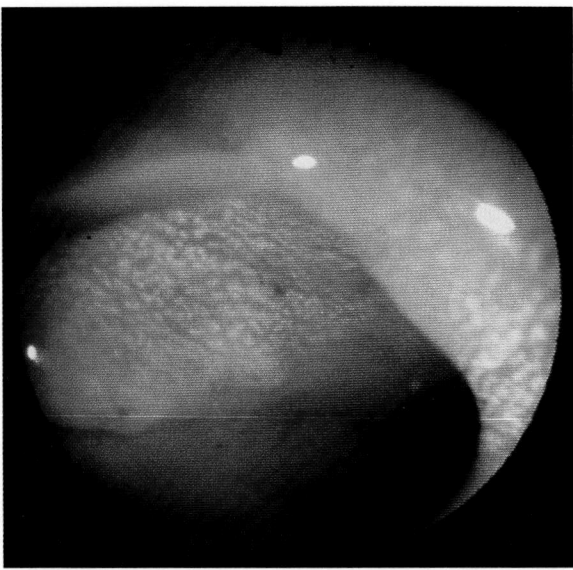

PLATE 41. MAI of the duodenum. Coarse, pale whitish-yellow, granular mucosa resembling Whipple's disease. (From ref. 116a, with permission.)

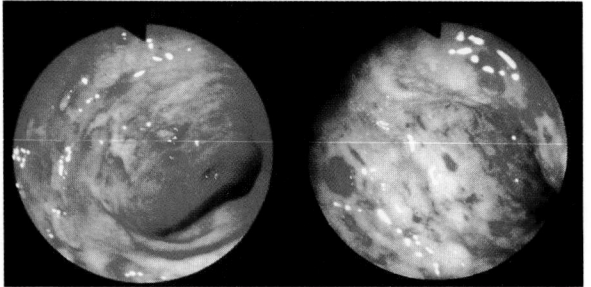

PLATE 42. Left: Severe *Shigalla flexineri* colitis with extensive coalescent superficial ulceration involving nearly the entire bowel circumference. Right: Improved appearance after two weeks of antibiotic therapy. (From ref. 14a, with permission.)

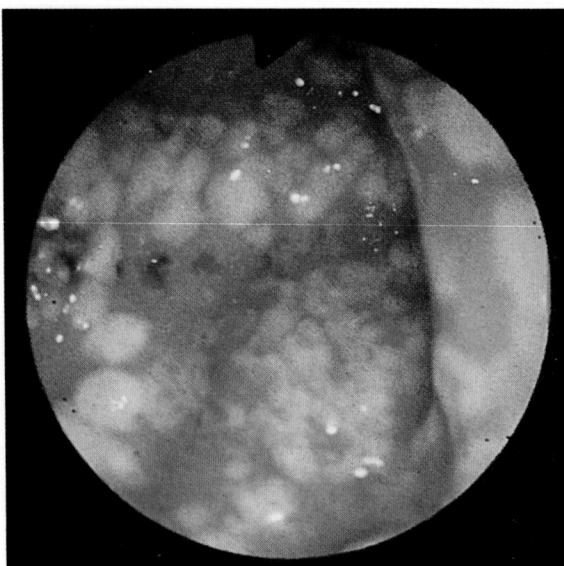

PLATE 43. Pseudomembranous colitis. Confluent colonic inflammation with pseudomembrane formation. This colonoscopic view illustrates the greenish pseudomembrane overlying the inflamed mucosal surface. (From ref. 133a, with permission.)

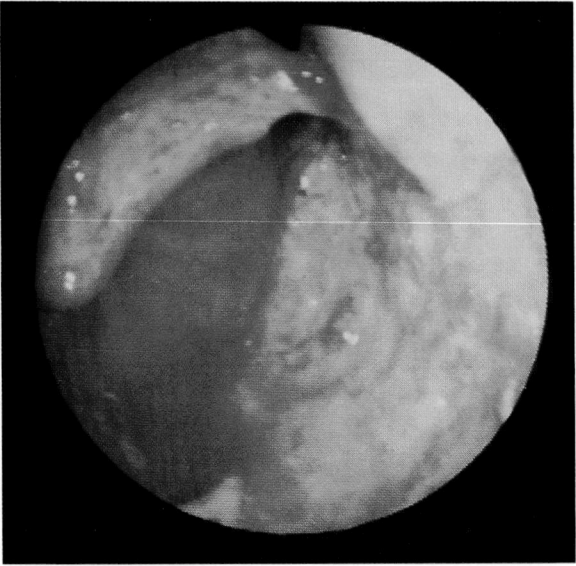

PLATE 44. HSV proctitis. Confluent, nearly circumferential ulceration of the anal canal and distal rectum. (From ref. 14a, with permission.)

TABLE 3. *Sources of non-O1* V. cholerae *submitted for species confirmation to the Centers for Disease Control, through 1985*

Source	Number of isolates submitted (%)
Feces or intestinal	94 (46.5%)
Spinal fluid	1 (0.5%)
Blood	42 (20.8%)
Wound	
hand or arm	2 (1.0%)
foot or leg	9 (4.5%)
other or unknown	3 (1.5%)
Ear	24 (11.9%)
Gallbladder	1 (0.5%)
Urine	4 (2.0%)
Respiratory tract	10 (5.0%)
Other or unknown	12 (5.9%)
Total	202 (100%)

Data from ref. 25.

However, non-O1 *V. cholerae* strains have also been isolated from blood [~20% of isolates submitted to Centers for Disease Control (CDC) for species confirmation (25)], wound and ear infections (~20% of isolates), and other clinical sites.

Reservoirs

Non-O1 *V. cholerae* organisms have been isolated from surface water in multiple sites in North America, Europe, Asia, and Australia, and it is likely that they are present in coastal and estuarine areas throughout the world (23). As would be expected with a free-living estuarine organism, environmental studies have generally shown no correlation between isolation of non-O1 *V. cholerae* and the presence of fecal coliforms (33–36). Isolation rates are influenced by salinity (isolation generally occurs in water with a salinity of 2–20 ppt) and water temperature (optimally >17°C)(21,34,37). However, isolation has been reported from freshwater (38), and infections have occurred after exposure to freshwater inland lakes (39,40).

Non-O1 *V. cholerae* are a common isolate from shellfish, particularly from filter feeders such as oysters. In one study conducted by the U.S. Food and Drug Administration, non-O1 *V. cholerae* were isolated from 111 (14%) of 790 samples of freshly harvested oyster shellstock (41). Isolation rates were highest during warm, summer months, when counts of the organism would be expected to be highest in harvesting waters. Non-O1 *V. cholerae* have also been isolated from a variety of wild and domestic animals (35,42–45). It is unclear as to what role animal carriage plays in maintaining the organism in the environment. Asymptomatic carriage of non-O1 *V. cholerae* by humans also is known to occur (46,47).

Transmission

Virtually all cases of non-O1 *V. cholerae* gastroenteritis acquired in the United States are associated with eating raw or undercooked shellfish (particularly raw oysters) (16). While the linkage is less strong, there is also a suggestion that septicemia can result from ingestion of the organism in seafood (48,49).

Seafood remains an important vehicle of infection for sporadic non-O1 disease outside of the United States. However, it is clear that transmission can also occur through other routes (3,16,24,50), including water (5) and a variety of other foods (51,52).

Frequency of Isolation

There is wide variability in the reported frequency of isolation of non-O1 *V. cholerae* from stool cultures of persons with diarrhea (24). The highest reported isolation rate has been 16%, among 134 children and adults with diarrhea in Cancun, Mexico, seen during a single 2-month period in July and August 1983 (51). While matched controls were not examined, no non-O1 *V. cholerae* were isolated from a group of 22 well children in this same study. In a comparable study conducted in Mexico City (at a high altitude and at some distance from the coast), no non-O1 strains were identified from patients with diarrhea (53). In Bangladesh, isolation rates of nonepidemic non-O1 strains from persons with diarrhea at the Cholera Research Laboratory in Dhaka (6) and the Matlab Treatment Center (54) have been reported to be 3% and 7%, respectively.

Rates of isolation in the United States appear to be much lower. In passive, laboratory-based studies in the United States, non-O1 *V. cholerae* have rarely been isolated. Seven coastal area hospitals in four southern states isolated only seven specimens of non-O1 *V. cholerae* (including five isolates from a single outbreak) from approximately 11,000 stool cultures performed with use of thiocitrate sulfate bile salts (TCBS) media (9). Comparable data were obtained during a 14-year period in a single hospital in Annapolis, Maryland (55). In 1989, the first year of coordinated *Vibrio* surveillance in four Gulf Coast states (Alabama, Florida, Louisiana, and Texas), 28 non-O1 *V. cholerae* isolates were reported (56) (Table 4). Non-O1 strains were isolated from 13 (2.7%) of 479 persons in a cohort of physicians attending a convention in New Orleans in late September (46). Despite this relatively high colonization rate, only 2 (15%) of the 13 culture-positive persons were symptomatic, comparable to the overall 14% rate of diarrhea reported in the entire cohort.

Pathophysiology

From the time they were first identified, questions have arisen about the pathogenicity of non-O1 *V. cholerae* strains. There is now compelling evidence from volunteer studies that nonepidemic non-O1 strains can indeed cause human disease (17). At the same time, the relatively low rates of disease occurrence (and the corresponding high rate of isolation of the organism from the environment and from seafood) suggest that only a minority of strains carry the necessary virulence factors to cause human ill-

674 / CHAPTER 47

TABLE 4. *Patients with clinical syndromes associated with* Vibrio *species reported from Alabama, Florida, Louisiana, and Texas in 1989*

Vibrio species	No.	Primary septicemia	Syndromes Gastroenteritis	Wound infection	Complications Hospitalization	Death
Patients with one species isolated						
V. alginolyticus[a]	0	0	0	5 (17)	3 (5)	0
V. cholerae						3 (33)
Non-O1	28	6 (43)	18 (25)	4 (14)	20 (30)	0
O1 nontoxigenic	1	0	1 (1)	0	0	0
V. damsela	1	0	0	1 (3)	0	0
V. fluvialis	7	0	7 (10)	0	3 (5)	
V. hollisae	9	0	8 (11)	1 (3)	2 (3)	0
V. mimicus	4	0	4 (6)	0	2 (3)	0
V. parahaemolyticus	33	1 (7)	26 (37)	6 (21)	20 (30)	2 (22)
V. vulnificus	18	7 (50)	3 (3)	8 (28)	15 (23)	4 (44)
Not speciated	2	0	0	2 (7)	0	0
Patients with two species isolated[b]	6	0	4 (6)	2 (7)	1 (2)	0
Total	116	14 (100)	71 (100)	29 (100)	66 (100)	9 (100)

Data from ref. 56.

Note: Data are number (%) and do not include five from whom isolates were reported without sufficient clinical data to characterize by syndrome: 2 with *V. mimicus,* 2 with *V. cholerae* non-O1, and 1 with *V. parahaemolyticus.*

[a] Two patients had syndromes other than wound infections. *V. alginolyticus* was isolated from ear infection drainage and from a gangrenous gallbladder, 1 each.

[b] Six patients had 2 *Vibrio* species isolated: *V. alginolyticus* and *V. cholerae* non-O1 from 1 with a wound infection, *V. cholerae* non-O1 and *V. mimicus* from 2 with primary septicemia, *V. damsela* and *V. parahaemolyticus* from 1 with a wound infection, and *V. parahaemolyticus* and *V. vulnificus* from 2 with gastroenteritis. Only the patient with *V. parahaemolyticus* and *V. vulnificus* was hospitalized; none died.

ness. At this point no single virulence factor has been identified that can account for all reported cases. Analogous to our current understanding of diarrheagenic *E. coli* (and in keeping with the genetic diversity seen among non-O1 strains), there may be several subgroups of non-O1 *V. cholerae* that are able to cause disease, each through a different pathogenic mechanism. Possible mechanisms are summarized below.

Extracellular Toxins

Cholera Toxin

Some non-O1 strains can produce cholera toxin (CT) or cholera-like toxins (57–61). In one study in Bangladesh, CT-producing strains were isolated from 29% of cases of sporadic non-O1 *V. cholerae* gastroenteritis; patients infected with these strains had more severe illness, with greater weight loss, a significantly higher admission specific gravity, and more prolonged and profuse diarrhea (58). Cholera toxin-producing strains of non-O1 *V. cholerae* have always been found at relatively high rates in Bangladesh and India, with one Indian study finding CT activity in 9 (26%) of 34 clinical isolates from sporadic cases as compared with 1 of 10 environmental isolates (57). However, the frequency of isolation of CT-positive strains has been much lower outside the Indian subcontinent (60,61).

NAG-ST

Some non-O1 strains produce a 17-amino-acid, heat-stable enterotoxin (designated NAG-ST) that closely resembles the heat-stable toxin produced by enterotoxigenic strains of *E. coli* and *Yersinia enterocolitica* (62,63). In volunteer studies, a colonizing, NAG-ST–producing strain of non-O1 *V. cholerae* caused diarrhea in healthy North American adults (17). In epidemiological studies it has been possible to identify a subgroup of non-O1 strains that are closely related genetically (based on zymovar analysis), are characterized by a common capsular type and production of NAG-ST, and are significantly more likely to be isolated from patients with diarrhea than from the environment (64). Again, however, the strains within this group account for only a small minority of all clinical non-O1 *V. cholerae* isolates (65,66).

El Tor Hemolysin

All non-O1 *V. cholerae* strains are hemolytic and all appear to carry the gene for the El Tor hemolysin. The El Tor hemolysin has been shown to have enterotoxic activity, and it has been postulated that the enterotoxigenicity of non-O1 strains is due to this toxin (66–69). A similar role for the El Tor hemolysin has been proposed in explaining the virulence of CT-negative strains of *V. cholerae* O1. However, at this point there is not a clear consensus on the importance of the hemolysin in either O1 (70,71) or non-O1 disease (24,72).

Other Putative Toxins

A variety of other possible toxins have been identified, including a hemolysin that is very closely related to the thermostable direct hemolysin (or Kanagawa hemolysin) of *V. parahaemolyticus* (see section on *V. parahaemolyticus* below) (63,66), a Shiga-like toxin (66,73), the zonula occludens toxin (ZOT) recently described in *V. cholerae* O1 [which, however, appears to be almost always linked to CT (74)], and various cell-associated hemagglutinins (59,75). Further studies, including volunteer studies and studies with isogeneic mutants, are needed to define the importance of these and other factors in the pathogenesis of non-O1 *V. cholerae*–associated disease.

Colonization Factors

Non-O1 strains differ in their ability to colonize and cause disease in rabbits (76): isolates from patients with diarrhea are significantly more likely to colonize and cause disease than are environmental isolates. Differences in colonizing ability have been confirmed in volunteer studies (17), and it appears reasonable to hypothesize that colonization is a necessary prerequisite for occurrence of disease. However, colonization alone is not sufficient to cause human illness; in volunteer studies, one strain that was an excellent colonizer failed to cause diarrhea even after administration of 10^9 colony-forming units (CFU) (17). While some non-O1 strains are fimbriated, colonization can occur in the absence of fimbriae (17,77).

Encapsulation

Non-O1 strains are able to produce a polysaccharide capsule that confers resistance to serum bactericidal activity and that is associated with increased virulence in mice (32). Heavily encapsulated strains are significantly more likely to be isolated from patients with septicemia than strains with minimal or no capsular polysaccharide (78). Strains of *V. cholerae* O1 are not encapsulated; with one or two possible exceptions, *V. cholerae* O1 has not been isolated from blood.

Clinical Syndromes

Gastroenteritis

The gastroenteritis associated with non-O1 *V. cholerae* can range from mild illness to profuse, watery diarrhea comparable to that seen in epidemic cholera. In a group of 19 sporadic cases of non-O1 *V. cholerae* gastroenteritis in Dhaka, Bangladesh (6), illness ranged from mild diarrhea, requiring no therapy, to heavy, cholera-like purges. The maximum stool volume among these 19 patients was

8 L (recorded during hospitalization), and the longest duration of diarrhea was 2.5 days; however, the median stool volume during hospitalization was less than 1 L, and diarrhea lasted for less than 24 hr in half of the cases. In a group of 14 U.S. cases identified retrospectively on the basis of positive stool cultures (16), symptoms included diarrhea (100% of patients), abdominal cramps (93%), and fever (71%), with nausea and vomiting occurring less frequently (21%). A quarter of the U.S. patients reported bloody diarrhea. Median duration of illness was 6.4 days, with 8 of the 14 requiring hospitalization; however, as these patients were identified on the basis of positive cultures, hospitalized patients and patients with more severe, prolonged diarrhea may have been overrepresented.

While the above data provide a general picture of the gastroenteritis which can be seen in association with non-O1 *V. cholerae*, it should be recognized that they probably reflect symptoms from a heterogeneous group of non-O1 strains (with a heterogeneous group of virulence mechanisms). A more accurate assessment of symptoms associated with a single strain or subset of strains can be obtained from volunteer studies and from outbreak reports.

Three non-O1 strains have been administered to volunteers in doses as high as 10^9 CFU (17). Two of the strains colonized volunteers. However, only one of these strains (an O31 strain isolated from a patient with traveler's diarrhea at Narita Airport, Tokyo) caused diarrhea; this strain produced NAG-ST. The median incubation period before onset of gastroenteritis for volunteers receiving NRT-36S was 10 hr (range 5.5–96 hr). Diarrheal stool volumes ranged from 140 to 5397 mL (Table 5). The diarrheal illness tended to be short-lived, with a median duration of 21 hr (range 3.5–48 hr). Abdominal cramps were prominent, with one volunteer (who received 10^6 CFU) having only abdominal cramps and no diarrhea.

Two foodborne outbreaks attributable to non-O1 *V. cholerae* have been reported. In one, on an airplane flight to Australia (50), the mean incubation period was 11.5 hr (range 5.25–37.5 hr); in an outbreak at a technical school in Czechoslovakia (3) the incubation period was estimated to be 20–30 hr. Attack rates in both outbreaks exceeded 60%, emphasizing that a virulent non-O1 strain, at a high enough inoculum, can consistently cause illness in healthy adults. In both outbreaks diarrhea was generally mild and resolved in the majority of cases in less than 24 hr. However, it was also noted that some patients had severe diarrhea (12 or more bowel movements in 24 hr, up to 6 bowel movements in a half-hour), and that illness was often accompanied by abdominal cramps and vomiting.

Septicemia

Non-O1 *V. cholerae* also has been isolated from blood (49). The majority of these cases have involved immunocompromised patients, particularly those with hematological malignancies or cirrhosis, suggesting that host susceptibility is a critical factor in determining whether septicemia will occur. The case fatality rate among reported cases is 61.5% (49). As noted above, strains re-

TABLE 5. *Symptoms of volunteers ingesting non-O1* V. cholerae *strains NRT-36S*

Inoculum size	No. of volunteers	No. of volunteers with:			Stool volumes (mL)
		Diarrhea	Fever	Abd. pain	
10^5	2	0	0	0	—
10^6	3	2	0	2	5397;140
10^7	2	1	0	0	589
10^9	3	3	0	3	2091;276;273

Data from ref. 17.

sponsible for septicemia have uniformly been found to be heavily encapsulated (78).

Infections at Other Sites

Non-O1 *V. cholerae* has been isolated from a variety of other sites, including wounds, ears, sputum, urine, and cerebrospinal fluid (25,55,56,79,80). The clinical significance of the wound, ear, and sputum isolates is unclear. In many such cases non-O1 *V. cholerae* has been isolated together with a variety of other potential pathogens (55). In the absence of subsequent bacteremia, it is difficult to determine whether the isolate reflected significant non-O1 *V. cholerae* infection, or was simply a commensal or colonizing strain.

Diagnosis

Methodology for isolation of non-O1 strains is identical to that for *V. cholerae* O1. For isolation from stool, a selective media such as TCBS is generally necessary (Table 2). Non-O1 strains grow well on blood agar and other nonselective media that may be used for wound cultures; they also grow well in standard blood culture media.

Therapy

As with *V. cholerae* O1, the mainstay of therapy of diarrheal disease is oral rehydration (81,82). There have been no controlled trials of antimicrobial therapy in persons infected with non-O1 *V. cholerae* strains. Gastroenteritis due to non-O1 *V. cholerae* is generally self-limited and does not require therapy. For patients with a more prolonged course (>5 days of diarrhea) administration of tetracycline would appear to be reasonable, based on data from studies with *V. cholerae* O1 (81–83). Non-O1 *V. cholerae* are susceptible *in vitro* to a number of antibiotics, including tetracycline, chloramphenicol, trimethoprim-sulfamethoxazole, and ciprofloxacin (8,84). Strains show variable resistance to ampicillin, and there are data suggesting that ampicillin has reduced efficacy in the treatment of cholera (85); ampicillin is not recommended for therapy. In instances in which tetracycline cannot be used, ciprofloxacin would be a reasonable alternative.

In cases of septicemia, supportive care and correction of shock is essential. Optimal antimicrobial agents would again include tetracycline and ciprofloxacin. If broader coverage is desired (or for empiric therapy before culture results are available), a third-generation cephalosporin may be added to the antimicrobial regimen.

Prevention

In countries such as the United States, non-O1 infections can be prevented by not eating raw or undercooked seafood, particularly during warm months in the late summer and early fall. For healthy adults, the risk of infection is low, and if it occurs, the resultant gastroenteritis is generally mild. Persons who have underlying liver disease or who are immunosuppressed also are at risk for septicemia. Given the high fatality rates associated with septicemia, persons in these groups should not consume raw oysters. In third-world countries, transmission of non-O1 *V. cholerae* appears to parallel that of other enteric pathogens, with the risk of illness minimized by making certain that food and water come from clean sources.

VIBRIO MIMICUS

Prior to 1981, *V. mimicus* was identified as encompassing sucrose-negative strains of *V. cholerae*. DNA–DNA homology studies at that time demonstrated that these strains constituted a separate species (86); the name *mimicus* was proposed because of the similarity of these strains to *V. cholerae*. Clinical isolates of *V. mimicus* received by the CDC primarily have come from stool (83%) and ear (13%) cultures (25). *V. mimicus* also has been isolated from a number of environmental sources, including oysters (86,87); gastroenteritis is significantly associated with raw oyster consumption (88). The total number of human *V. mimicus* isolates submitted to the CDC for identification is approximately 25% of that of non-O1 *V. cholerae* (25). In the 1989 surveillance in four Gulf Coast states (Alabama, Florida, Louisiana, and Texas) four cases of *V. mimicus* gastroenteritis were identified (Table 4) (56).

Between 10% and 16% of isolates (including environmental isolates) produce a heat-labile toxin that appears to be identical to cholera toxin (86,89–91). Some *V. mimicus* strains produce a heat-stable enterotoxin (Vm-ST) that is closely related to NAG-ST produced by non-O1 *V. cholerae* (90,92). Strains also can produce a thermostable direct hemolysin-like hemolysin (Vm-TDH) that is virtually identical to the thermostable direct hemolysin of *V. parahaemolyticus* (93,94).

In a study of 19 cases identified retrospectively based on isolation of *V. mimicus* from stool (88), symptoms included diarrhea (94%), nausea, vomiting, and abdominal cramps (67%), fever (44%), and headache (39%). Three patients had bloody diarrhea. Diarrhea lasted a median of 6 days. Diagnosis is based on isolation of the organism from stool. As with other *Vibrio* species, isolation is facilitated by use of a selective media such as TCBS.

No data are available on therapy. As in other diarrheal diseases, the mainstay of therapy should be correction of dehydration. Isolates are sensitive *in vitro* to tetracycline, trimethoprim-sulfamethoxazole, chloramphenicol, and ciprofloxacin (25,84). Based on experience with other *Vibrio* species, it would be reasonable to administer tetracycline in more severe cases (>5 days diarrhea).

VIBRIO PARAHAEMOLYTICUS

In the fall of 1950 there was an outbreak of food poisoning in Osaka, Japan; of 272 patients with acute gastroenteritis, 20 died. These deaths led to an intensive investigation of the outbreak and, ultimately, to the identification of an etiological agent that was first named *Pasteurella parahaemolyticus,* with subsequent reclassification as *Vibrio parahaemolyticus* (95). *V. parahaemolyticus* is now recognized worldwide as a cause of diarrheal disease and is generally reported as the most common cause of foodborne illness in Japan (8,96–99).

Microbiology

Typical biochemical characteristics of *V. parahaemolyticus* are summarized in Table 2. The bacterium is halophilic, or salt loving, and requires NaCl for growth. As outlined below, clinical isolates tend to be hemolytic for human erythrocytes when grown on special media (Wagatsuma agar) (95,100,101); this is termed the Kanagawa reaction, named for the Japanese prefecture where the original study was done.

Prior to the 1980s, most *V. parahaemolyticus* isolated were urease-negative (102,103). However, since that time urease-positive isolates have been seen with increasing frequency, particularly along the Pacific Coast of North America (8,104–108). Seventy percent of *V. parahaemolyticus* isolates submitted to the California state health department laboratory for identification since 1980 have been urease-positive (8); in one survey, 58% of environmental *V. parahaemolyticus* isolates from Washington State were urease-positive (108). In contrast to the traditional experience with urease-negative strains, urease-positive strains isolated from patients with gastroenteritis are often Kanagawa-negative (105,107,108).

Epidemiology

As with *V. cholerae,* *V. parahaemolyticus* is part of the normal, free-living bacterial flora in estuarine areas throughout the world. As halophilic (salt-loving) bacteria, *V. parahaemolyticus* are a very common isolate from estuarine and marine water, sediment, suspended particulates, plankton, fish, and shellfish (95,108,110,111); counts in oysters may exceed those in water by 100-fold (110). In temperate climates, isolation is seasonal, with *V. parahaemolyticus* apparently passing the winter in sediments and then proliferating as water temperatures rise (95,110).

In Japan, *V. parahaemolyticus* has been implicated as the etiological agent in 24% of reported cases of foodborne disease (96). In the United States it has been associated with a number of major foodborne disease outbreaks, often involving mishandling of shellfish after cooking (97–99). In the 1989 four-state survey of rates of isolation of *Vibrio* species (Table 4), *V. parahaemolyticus* was the most common *Vibrio* species isolated, and the most common isolate from cases of *Vibrio*-associated gastroenteritis (56).

Pathogenesis

The virulence of *V. parahaemolyticus* for humans has traditionally been correlated with hemolytic activity: >95% of strains isolated from patients with gastroenteritis in Japan are Kanagawa-positive, in contrast to ≤2% of environmental isolates (95,100,101,112). The association of a positive Kanagawa reaction with clinical disease has been confirmed in volunteer studies. Volunteers fed up to 10^{10} CFU of *V. parahaemolyticus* strain 255/72 (a Kanagawa-negative strain) remained asymptomatic. In contrast, diarrheal illness was seen in two of four volunteers who ingested 3×10^7 CFU of *V. parahaemolyticus* strain 129/71 (a Kanagawa-positive strain), with one of four volunteers receiving 2×10^5 CFU of this strain reporting abdominal cramps (but no diarrhea) (113).

Hemolytic activity in Kanagawa-positive strains appears to be due to the production of thermostable direct hemolysin (Vp-TDH) (114–117). While the actual role of this hemolysin in the pathogenic process has been the subject of some controversy (116), recent studies with isogeneic mutants have demonstrated that deletion of the Vp-TDH gene results in loss of enterotoxic activity in Ussing chamber and rabbit ileal loop models (117).

At the same time, there are other thermostable direct hemolysin-related hemolysins (Vp-TRH) that appear to have phenotypic activity similar to that of Vp-TDH and that share sequence homology with Vp-TDH (118–121). These genes have been found almost exclusively in clinical isolates and may be present in more than half of disease-associated Kanagawa-negative strains (including urease-positive strains). Finally, there are clinical urease-positive, Kanagawa-negative *V. parahaemolyticus* strains that carry neither Vp-TDH or Vp-TRH but that can elicit fluid accumulation in ligated rabbit ileal loops (i.e., have enterotoxic activity) (109). The virulence factors responsible for this enterotoxigenicity remain to be determined.

V. parahaemolyticus can cause a dysentery-like syndrome (122,123), suggesting that some strains have invasive capabilities. In limited studies, isolates have not given a positive reaction in the Sereny test (which tests for invasiveness in the guinea pig or rabbit eye) (122); however, it has been shown that Kanagawa-positive strains are able to penetrate the intestinal epithelium of infant rabbits (124).

Clinical Manifestations

V. parahaemolyticus most commonly causes gastroenteritis. In a summary of eight culture-confirmed outbreaks in the United States (97), manifestations included diarrhea (98%), abdominal cramps (82%), nausea (71%), vomiting (52%), headache (42%), fever [rarely >38.9°C (102°F), 27%], and chills (24%). The incubation period ranged from 4 to 96 hr. The illness was usually self-limited, with a median duration of 3 days. A dysentery-like syndrome associated with *V. parahaemolyticus* has been reported in India and Bangladesh (122); although it is apparently not as common in the United States, there is one report of a U.S. patient with blood and leukocytes in her stool, and superficial colonic ulcerations noted on sigmoidoscopy (123). There are anecdotal reports of cardiac arrhythmias and sudden death in persons infected with *V. parahaemolyticus*.

V. parahaemolyticus also is a cause of infection in seawater-associated wounds (55,56). Wound infections may progress to septicemia, particularly in persons with reduced host defenses. While occasional cases of primary septicemia have been reported (i.e., septicemia without an obvious focus of infection), rates are much lower than those reported for non-O1 *V. cholerae* or *V. vulnificus* (Table 4).

Diagnosis

Blood agar and other nonselective media support the growth of *V. parahaemolyticus,* but isolation from feces generally requires the use of a selective medium such as TCBS. The colonies of *V. parahaemolyticus* on TCBS are blue–green (sucrose-negative). Species identification is based on standard biochemical tests (Table 2). Unlike *V. cholerae, V. parahaemolyticus* will not grow in 0% sodium chloride but will grow in the relatively high concentrations of 6–8% NaCl. A positive Kanagawa reaction [as identified by hemolytic activity on Wagatsuma agar or hybridization with DNA probes for Vp-TDH (125,126)] may be useful in differentiating potentially pathogenic from nonpathogenic strains; as noted above, this distinction is not useful for isolates from along the Pacific coast of North America, where recent *V. parahaemolyticus* isolates from patients with gastroenteritis have been urease-positive and Kanagawa-negative (105,106).

Therapy

As in other diarrheal diseases (81), the key to management of patients with *V. parahaemolyticus* gastroenteritis is provision of adequate rehydration. *V. parahaemolyti-*

cus is susceptible *in vitro* to tetracycline, chloramphenicol, trimethoprim/sulfamethoxazole, and the quinolones; the minimum inhibitory concentration 90% for gentamicin is 4 μg/mL and that of ampicillin >128 μg/mL (25,84). Although there are no data regarding antimicrobic efficacy, patients with persistent diarrhea (>5 days) may benefit from treatment with tetracycline or a quinolone.

VIBRIO FLUVIALIS

Vibrio fluvialis includes strains previously designated as enteric group EF-6 or group F *Vibrio. Fluvialis* is from the Latin for "river," reflecting the early isolation of the organism from river and estuarine waters; the name was proposed in 1981 (127). Biochemically, *V. fluvialis* is very similar to *Aeromonas* species; when the British Public Health Laboratories reviewed all their old anaerogenic, lysine decarboxylase-negative *Aeromonas* strains, they found that one third were actually *V. fluvialis* (127). Identification systems in common use in hospital microbiology laboratories in the United States will often identify *V. fluvialis* as *Aeromonas hydrophilia* (128); isolates should be screened for salt requirements to try to differentiate the two species [*V. fluvialis* grows in 6–7% NaCl, while *Aeromonas* does not (8,95,127,128)].

V. fluvialis has been isolated from estuarine environments (127,128). There are anecdotal data suggesting that infections in the United States are associated with the eating of seafood (129,130). Although there is known to have been at least one major outbreak of *V. fluvialis*–associated gastroenteritis in Bangladesh (131), reported isolations are rare, generally occurring at a rate less than one tenth of that of non-O1 *V. cholerae* (25).

V. fluvialis (whole cells) has been shown to stimulate fluid accumulation in rabbit ileal loops (129). The organism has been reported to produce a variety of cell-free and cell-associated products, including factors that cause cell elongation and cell death in tissue culture assays using Chinese hamster ovary (CHO) cells. Oral challenge of infant mice results in intestinal fluid accumulation, diarrhea, and death (132).

Symptoms that occurred in an outbreak in Bangladesh in 1976–1977 (131) included diarrhea (100%), vomiting (97%), abdominal pain (75%), moderate to severe dehydration (67%), and fever (35%). Seventy-five percent of the patients were reported to have leukocytes and blood cells in their stools. There are anecdotal reports of the organism being associated with intestinal ulceration. There has been at least one reported death associated with the organism in the United States (133).

Diagnosis is based on stool culture results. No data are available on therapy, although based on antimicrobial susceptibility patterns and experience with other *Vibrio* species, treatment with tetracycline would appear to be reasonable in cases in which diarrhea has persisted for >5 days or in cases with bloody diarrhea.

VIBRIO FURNISSII

The species *V. furnissii* includes aerogenic strains (strains that produce gas from glucose) previously classified as biovar II of *V. fluvialis* (127,134). The name *furnissii*, honoring A. L. Furniss, a researcher at the British Public Health Laboratories at Maidstone, was proposed in 1983. The organism is present in the marine environment (127). Binding of *V. furnissii* to chitin is facilitated by chemotaxis to chitin hydrolysis products (135). There is a suggestion that gastroenteritis is associated with eating seafood. Reported isolation rates in the United States have been roughly comparable to those of *V. fluvialis* (25).

An outbreak of gastroenteritis associated with an organism retrospectively identified as *V. furnissii* occurred in 1969 on a flight from Tokyo to Seattle (136,137). Patients' symptoms included diarrhea (91%), abdominal cramps (79%), nausea (65%), and vomiting (39%). One of 23 sick passengers died, and two others required hospitalization.

VIBRIO HOLLISAE

DNA hybridization studies conducted in 1982 determined that *Vibrio* strains previously designated as belonging to enteric group EF-13 constituted a separate species, which was subsequently designated *Vibrio hollisae,* honoring Dannie Hollis, an investigator at the CDC (138). Illness in the United States has been associated with eating raw seafood (18). The number of isolates that have been reported to CDC is approximately 15% of that of non-O1 *V. cholerae* (25). *V. hollisae* can produce an enterotoxin that causes fluid accumulation in infant mice and elongation of CHO cells (139); some strains produce a hemolysin that is homologous with the thermostable direct hemolysin of *V. parahaemolyticus* (140).

In a retrospective study of U.S. cases identified on the basis of stool isolates (18), symptoms associated with *V. hollisae* included diarrhea, vomiting (five of nine patients), and fever (five of nine patients). Septicemia may occur in patients with underlying liver disease (141,142). The diagnosis of *V. hollisae* infections is complicated by the organism's tendency to grow poorly on TCBS medium, which is normally used to screen for *Vibrio* species; isolation may require the identification of colonies on blood agar plates.

VIBRIO VULNIFICUS

V. vulnificus, initially identified simply as a halophilic lactose-positive marine *Vibrio,* received its present name in 1979 (143,144). The organism can cause severe wound infections, septicemia, and possibly gastroenteritis (143,145–148). Because *V. vulnificus* is biochemically very similar to *V. parahaemolyticus,* it is possible that some severe infections previously attributed to *V. parahaemolyticus* were actually caused by *V. vulnificus.*

Microbiology

Biochemical characteristics of *V. vulnificus* are summarized in Table 2. While *V. vulnificus* was initially classified based on its ability to ferment lactose, 10–15% of isolates may be lactose-negative (25). Definitive identification of the organism can be difficult based on biochemical reactions alone; confirmation of species identity may require use of DNA probes (149,150) or numerical taxonomy techniques.

As reported for non-O1 *V. cholerae, V. vulnificus* strains produce a polysaccharide capsule (151–154). Strains are able to undergo phase variation, shifting between encapsulated forms having an opaque colony morphology and unencapsulated forms having a translucent colony morphology. There are numerous capsular types: in one study, 15 different capsular types were identified among 19 *V. vulnificus* isolates from clinical and environmental sources (155).

Epidemiology

V. vulnificus is a free-living estuarine organism, and is frequently isolated from water and shellfish, particularly oysters. In the United States, it is present in estuarine areas along the Atlantic, Gulf, and Pacific coasts (149,156–159). The density of *V. vulnificus* is a function of the temperature of the estuarine water, with isolations most frequent at temperatures >20°C (149,158,159). Counts of *V. vulnificus* in oysters are generally 100-fold higher than those found in the surrounding water (149). During warm, summer months virtually 100% of oysters carry the organism.

Bacteremia without an obvious focus of infection ("primary septicemia") occurs in persons who are alcoholic or who have chronic underlying illnesses, such as liver disease, cirrhosis, or hemochromatosis (Table 6) (143, 145–148); in one study, an increased risk of infection was associated with consumption of as little as one ounce of alcohol per day (147). Infection is thought to be acquired by eating oysters containing the organism. Wound infections occur after exposure to estuarine water: typical exposures include wounds acquired while opening an oyster or in a boating accident. Wounds may become infected in normal hosts. However, the most severe manifestations are seen in persons with underlying defects in host defense mechanisms.

V. vulnificus is the most common cause of serious *Vibrio* infections in the United States. The incidence of infections caused by *V. vulnificus* in coastal regions approximates 0.5/100,000 population/year (55,146,147), with primary septicemia accounting for two thirds of the cases. Based on the number of cases reported to the Florida Health Department between 1981 and 1992, the annual rate of illness from *V. vulnificus* infection for adults with self-reported liver disease in Florida who ate raw oysters was 7.2 per 100,000 adults, 80 times the rate for adults without known liver disease who ate raw oysters (0.09 cases per 100,000 population) (160). Large series of cases have been reported from Korea (148), and it is likely that *V. vulnificus* is distributed worldwide.

Pathogenesis

As noted above, *V. vulnificus* undergoes phase variation, shifting between an unencapsulated form with a

TABLE 6. *Epidemiologic features and clinical manifestations of patients with primary septicemia caused by* Vibrio vulnificus

Feature	USA/CDC $(n = 42)^a$	Korea $(n = 70)^b$
Risk factors		
Liver disease	74%	67%
Alcoholic cirrhosis	31%	43%
Hemochromatosis	12%	—
Chronic hepatitis, cirrhosis (unspecified etiology), other	31%	24%
Alcohol abuse without documented liver disease	12%	27%
Other chronic illnesses^c	8%	7%
Mean age (years)	56^d	51
Symptoms		
Fever	93%	54%
Chills	86%	33%
Hypotension	36%	54%
Diarrhea	26%	33%
Vomiting	31%	20%
Skin lesions	71%	91%
Mortality	52%	79%

^{a} Data from ref. 143 and 145.

^{b} Data from ref. 148.

^{c} Includes diabetes mellitus, thalassemia major, chronic renal failure, "preleukemia," lymphoma, tuberculosis, rheumatoid arthritis.

^{d} Mean ages not available for patients in ref. 143.

translucent colonial morphology and an encapsulated form that produces opaque colonies (151–153). Encapsulated strains are resistant to the bactericidal activity of normal human serum and to phagocytosis, and are highly virulent in animal models. Loss of the capsule correlates with loss of virulence (153). All clinical isolates are able to produce a capsule, as are the majority of environmental isolates. There is a suggestion that certain capsular types are more common among clinical than environmental isolates (155). However, no one capsular type predominates among clinical isolates, and at this point it is not possible to differentiate clinical from environmental isolates on the basis of capsule structure or type.

V. vulnificus is also very sensitive to the degree of binding of iron by transferrin in the host (161,162); *V. vulnificus* grows rapidly in serum with transferrin 70% saturated with iron, while growth is severely restricted at <70% (in normal adults, transferrin is around 30% saturated). These observations may explain the increased risk of disease in persons with hemochromatosis, or in malnourished alcoholics with low concentrations of transferrin and correspondingly high saturation of transferrin (161). The ability to grow under iron-limited conditions in the presence of saturated transferrin is coregulated with capsule expression: when strains shift to an unencapsulated phase, they also lose the ability to use transferrin-bound iron for growth. However, factors responsible for iron utilization are distinct from encapsulation. Transposon mutants have been identified that have lost the ability to express a cap-

sule but that retain the ability to grow under iron-limited conditions in the presence of saturated transferrin (153).

V. vulnificus produces a variety of extracellular products, including a cytolysin, proteases, collagenase, and phospholipases (163–166), which have been implicated as possible virulence factors. These products have clear biological activity (167,168) and may contribute to specific manifestations observed in patients infected with the organism; for example, the purified cytolysin has been shown to cause skin damage/skin lesions similar to those seen in patients with septicemia (167). At the same time, these products do not appear to be essential to the disease process. In studies with genetically engineered isogenic mutants, deletion or inactivation of the gene encoding the cytolysin or the protease had a minimal effect on virulence of the organism in animals (169,170).

Given the frequency of isolation of *V. vulnificus* from oysters, the incidence of disease is still much less than might be expected, even taking into account the need for an appropriate host (160). This may reflect the need for a high infectious dose (although no data are currently available to support this hypothesis). Alternatively, strains of *V. vulnificus* may differ in their ability to cause illness. While this latter hypothesis is attractive, there currently is no way to clearly differentiate strains with increased potential for causing human disease (if such strains exist) from less virulent environmental isolates.

Clinical Manifestations

One third of patients with primary bacteremia have shock when first seen or become hypotensive within 12 hr of hospitalization (Table 6). Three fourths of patients have distinctive bullous skin lesions (Fig. 1). Thrombocytopenia is common, and there is often evidence of disseminated intravascular coagulation; gastrointestinal bleeding is not infrequent. Over 50% of patients with primary bacteremia die; the mortality rate exceeds 90% for those who are hypotensive. Persons with bacteremia often have

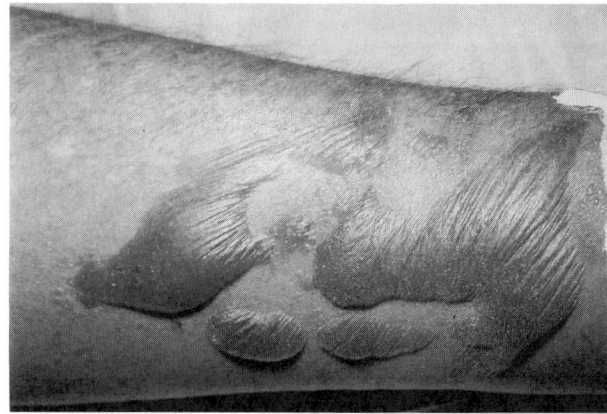

FIG. 1. Bullous skin lesions of a patient with *V. vulnificus* septicemia and hypotension. Photograph was taken approximately 48 hr after onset of symptoms.

symptoms of gastroenteritis, and *V. vulnificus* may cause gastroenteritis in the absence of bacteremia (143, 145–148).

Wound infections range from mild, self-limited lesions to rapidly progressive cellulitis and myositis that mimics clostridial myonecrosis in rapidity of spread and destructiveness (171,172). Up to 35% of patients with wound infections may become bacteremic. Mortality rates as high as 25% have been reported, with deaths (and bacteremia) concentrated in the same populations that are at risk for primary septicemia.

Patients who survive severe *V. vulnificus* infections often have some degree of residual disability. This does not appear to be related to the actual infection, which appears to clear readily with antibiotic therapy, but rather to the consequences of multiple organ system failure and the prolonged hospitalization associated with occurrence of a shock syndrome.

Diagnosis

Early diagnosis of *V. vulnificus* septicemia is essential, given its severity and the rapidity with which the disease progresses, and the possible benefit of early antimicrobial therapy (146). A presumptive clinical diagnosis can be made on the basis of (a) occurrence of shock or hypotension, or other signs suggesting sepsis (for wound infections, evidence of rapidly progressive cellulitis or myositis); (b) a history of cirrhosis, chronic alcoholism, immunosuppression, or hemochromatosis; (c) a history of recent consumption of raw oysters, or exposure of wounds to estuarine water; and (d) the presence of characteristic bullous skin lesions.

A definitive diagnosis requires isolation of *V. vulnificus* from blood; in some instances, skin bullae may also harbor the organism. Blood agar and other nonselective media, including media used in commercial blood culture systems, are adequate for isolation. As the organism is presumed to enter the body through the intestinal tract in cases of primary septicemia, stool cultures may be positive for *V. vulnificus* (173). TCBS is the preferred medium for isolation from feces; over 90% of strains produce blue–green (sucrose-negative) colonies. In the proper clinical setting, isolation of *V. vulnificus* from stool is highly suggestive of the diagnosis (although there is a possibility that such isolation reflects incidental, asymptomatic intestinal carriage of the organism).

Presumptive identification of *V. vulnificus* from cultures is based on standard biochemical tests. The identity of individual bacterial colonies can be further evaluated by immunological assays directed against various *V. vulnificus* surface antigens (174,175). As noted above, highly sensitive and specific DNA probes for the organism are also available on an experimental basis (149,150).

The immune response of patients infected with *V. vulnificus* tends to be variable (176,177). Because of this variability (and the associated lack of assay sensitivity and specificity), serological confirmation of infection is currently not possible.

Therapy

The early administration of antimicrobial agents is critical to successful treatment, with case fatality rates showing a significant increase with increasing time between onset of symptoms and initiation of therapy (146). *V. vulnificus* is susceptible to a wide range of agents *in vitro*, including ampicillin, tetracycline, chloramphenicol, trimethoprim-sulfamethoxazole, and ciprofloxacin; the minimum inhibitory concentration 90% to gentamicin is 8 μg/mL (25,84). Studies in mice indicate that tetracycline has the best efficacy against the organism (178), and there is a suggestion from a large series of cases from Florida that antimicrobial combinations that included tetracycline were more efficacious (146). Based on these data, and the experience with tetracycline with other *Vibrio* species, tetracycline is the drug of choice for *V. vulnificus* infections. In more severe infections, it may be desirable to add a second antimicrobial agent: based on *in vitro* susceptibilities, ciprofloxacin is recommended. As is true for any patient with gram-negative sepsis, persons in shock require careful monitoring and aggressive supportive care.

Prevention

As long as oysters and other shellfish are harvested from warm waters and eaten raw or with minimal cooking, there is risk of infection with *V. vulnificus*. Persons who are immunocompromised, have cirrhosis (or a history of heavy ingestion of ethanol), or have conditions predisposing them to increased saturation of their transferrin with iron should not eat raw oysters, particularly during the summer and early fall when water temperatures may exceed 20°C. Persons in these same risk groups also should try to minimize exposure of wounds to warmer estuarine or marine waters.

REFERENCES

1. Gardner AD, Venkatraman VK. The antigens of the cholera group of vibrios. *J Hyg* 1935;35:262–282.
2. Pollitzer R. *Cholera*. Geneva: WHO; 1959.
3. Aldova E, Laznickova K, Stepankova E, Lietava J. Isolation of nonagglutinating vibrios from an enteritis outbreak in Czechoslovakia. *J Infect Dis* 1968;118:25–31.
4. El-Shawi N, Thewaini AJ. Non-agglutinable vibrios isolated in the 1966 epidemic of cholera in Iraq. *Bull WHO* 1969;40:163–166.
5. Kamal AM. Outbreak of gastroenteritis by non-agglutinable (NAG) vibrios in the republic of the Sudan. *J Egyp Public Health Assoc* 1971;46:125–173.
6. McIntyre OR, Feeley JC, Greenough WB, Benenson AS, Hassan SI, Saad A. Diarrhea caused by non-cholera vibrios. *Am J Trop Med Hyg* 1965;14:412–418.
7. Yajnik BS, Prasad BG. A note on vibrios isolated in Kumbh Fair, Allahbad, 1954. *Ind Med Gazette* 1954;89:341–349.
8. Janda JM, Powers C, Bryant RG, Abbott SL. Current perspectives on the epidemiology and pathogenesis of clinically significant Vibrio species. *Clin Microbiol Rev* 1988;1:245–267.
9. Morris JG Jr, Black RE. Cholera and other vibrioses in the United States. *N Engl J Med* 1985;312:343–350.

10. Albert MJ, Siddique AK, Islam MS, et al. A large outbreak of clinical cholera due to *Vibrio cholerae* non-O1 in Bangladesh. *Lancet* 1993;341:704.
11. International Center for Diarrheal Disease Research, Bangladesh, Cholera Working Group. Large epidemic of cholera-like disease in Bangladesh caused by *Vibrio cholerae* O139 synonym Bengal. *Lancet* 1993;342:387–390.
12. Ramamurthy T, Garg S, Sharma R, et al. Emergence of novel strain of *Vibrio cholerae* with epidemic potential in southern and eastern India. *Lancet* 1993;341:703–704.
13. Chongsa-nguan M, Chaicumpa W, Moolasart P, et al. *Vibrio cholerae* O139 Bengal in Bangkok. *Lancet* 1993;342:430–431.
14. Shehabi AA, Abu Rajab AB, Shaker AA. Observations on the emergence of non-cholera Vibrios during an outbreak of cholera. *Jordan Med J* 1980;14:125–127.
15. Dutt AK, Alwi S, Velauthan T. A shellfish-borne cholera outbreak in Malaysia. *Trans R Soc Trop Med Hyg* 1971;65:815–818.
16. Morris JG Jr, Wilson R, Davis BR, et al. Non-O Group 1 *Vibrio cholerae* gastroenteritis in the United States. *Ann Intern Med* 1981;94:656–658.
17. Morris JG Jr, Takeda T, Tall BD, et al. Experimental non-O group 1 *Vibrio cholerae* gastroenteritis in humans. *J Clin Invest* 1990;85:697–705.
18. Morris JG JR, Miller HG, Wilson RA, et al. Illness caused by *Vibrio damsela* and *Vibrio hollisae*. *Lancet* 1982;1:1294–1297.
19. Bode RB, Brayton PR, Colwell RR, Russo FM, Bullock WE. A new *Vibrio* species, *Vibrio cincinnatiensis*, causing meningitis: successful treatment in an adult. *Ann Intern Med* 1986;104:55–56.
20. Pavia AT, Bryan JA, Maher KL, Hester TR, Farmer JJ III. *Vibrio carchariae* infection after a shark bite. *Ann Intern Med* 1989;111:85–86.
21. Jean-Jacques W, Rajashekaraiah KR, Farmer JJ III, Hickman FW, Morris JG Jr, Kallick CA. *Vibrio metschnikovii* bacteremia in a patient with cholecystitis. *J Clin Microbiol* 1981;14:711–712.
22. Farmer JJ III, Hickman-Brenner FW, Fanning GR, Gordon CM, Brenner DJ. Characterization of *Vibrio metschnikovii* and *Vibrio gazogenes* by DNA-DNA hybridization and phenotype. *J Clin Microbiol* 1988;26:1993–2000.
23. West PA, Brayton PR, Twilley RR, Bryant TN, Colwell RR. Numerical taxonomy of nitrogen-fixing "decarboxylase-negative" *Vibrio* species isolated from aquatic environments. *Int J Sys Bacteriol* 1985;35:198–205.
24. Morris JG Jr. Non-O group 1 *Vibrio cholerae:* a look at the epidemiology of an occasional pathogen. *Epidemiol Rev* 1990;12:179–191.
25. Farmer JJ III, Hickman-Brenner FW, Kelly MT. Vibrio. In: Lennette EH, Balows A, Hausler WJ, Shadomy HJ, eds. *Manual of clinical microbiology*. Washington, DC: American Society for Microbiology; 1985.
26. Stroeher UH, Karageorgios LE, Morona R, Manning PA. Serotype conversion in *Vibrio cholerae* O1. *Proc Natl Acad Sci USA* 1992;89:2566–2570.
27. Johnson JA, Salles CA, Panigrahi P, Albert MJ, Johnson RJ, Morris JG Jr. *Vibrio cholerae* O139 synonym Bengal is closely related to *Vibrio cholerae* O1 El Tor, but has important differences. *Infect Immun* 1994;62:2108–2110.
28. Smith HL Jr. Serotyping of non-cholera vibrios. *J Clin Microbiol* 1979;10:85–90.
29. Sakazaki R, Shimada T. Serovars of *Vibrio cholerae*. *Jpn J Med Sci Biol* 1977;30:279–282.
30. Momen H, Salles CA. Enzyme markers for *Vibrio cholerae:* identification of classical, El Tor, and environmental strains. *Trans R Soc Trop Med Hyg* 1985;79:773–776.
31. Salles CA, da Silva AR, Momen H. Enzyme typing and phenetic relationships in *Vibrio cholerae*. *Rev Brasil Genet* 1986;9:407–419.
32. Johnson JA, Panigrahi P, Morris JG Jr. Non-O1 *Vibrio cholerae* NRT36S produces a polysaccharide capsule that determines colony morphology, serum resistance, and virulence in mice. *Infect Immun* 1992;60:684–689.
33. Amaro C, Toranzo AE, Gonzalez EA, et al. Surface and viru-

34. Kaper JB, Lockman H, Colwell RR, Joseph SW. Ecology, serology, and enterotoxin production of *Vibrio cholerae* in Chesapeake Bay. *Appl Environ Microbiol* 1979;37:91–103.
35. Lee JV, Bashford DJ, Donovan TJ, Furniss AL, West PA. The incidence and distribution of *V. cholerae* in England. In: Colwell RR, ed. *Vibrios in the environment*. New York: John Wiley and Sons; 1984:427–450.
36. Roberts NC, Seibeling RJ, Kaper JB, Bradford HB. Vibrios in the Louisiana Gulf Coast environment. *Microb Ecol* 1982;8:299–312.
37. Colwell RR, West PA, Maneval D, Remmers EF, Elliot EL, Carlson NE. Ecology of pathogenic *Vibrios* in Chesapeake Bay. In: Colwell RR, ed. *Vibrios in the environment*. New York: John Wiley and Sons; 1984:367–387.
38. Rhodes JB, Smith HL Jr, Ogg JE. Isolation of non-O1 *Vibrio cholerae* serovars from surface waters in western Colorado. *Appl Environ Microbiol* 1986;51:1216–1219.
39. Mulder GD, Reis TM, Beaver TR. Non-toxigenic *Vibrio cholerae* wound infection after exposure to contaminated lake water. *J Infect Dis* 1989;159:809–811.
40. Pitrak DL, Gindorf JD. Bacteremia cellulitis caused by non-serogroup O1 *Vibrio cholerae* acquired in a freshwater inland lake. *J Clin Microbiol* 1989;27:2874–2876.
41. Twedt RM, Madden JM, Hunt JM, et al. Characterization of *Vibrio cholerae* isolated from oysters. *Appl Environ Microbiol* 1981;41:1475–1478.
42. Sack RB. A search for canine carriers of *Vibrio*. *J Infect Dis* 1973;127:709–712.
43. Sanyal SC, Singh SJ, Tiwari IC, et al. Role of household animals in maintenance of cholera infection in a community. *J Infect Dis* 1974;130:575–579.
44. Bisgaard M, Sakazaki R, Shimada T. Prevalence of non-cholera vibrios in cavum nasi and pharynx of ducks. *Acta Pathol Microbiol Scand, Sect B* 1978;86:261–266.
45. Rhodes JB, Schweitzer D, Ogg JE. Isolation of non-O1 *Vibrio cholerae* associated with enteric disease of herbivores in western Colorado. *J Clin Microbiol* 1985;22:572–575.
46. Lowry PW, McFarland LM, Peltier BH, et al. Vibrio gastroenteritis in Louisiana: a prospective study among attendees of a scientific congress in New Orleans. *J Infect Dis* 1989;160:978–984.
47. Zafari Y, Zarifi AZ, Rahmanzadeh S, Fakhar N. Diarrhea caused by non-agglutinable *Vibrio cholerae* (non-cholera Vibrio). *Lancet* 1973;2:429–430.
48. Klontz KC. Fatalities associated with *Vibrio parahaemolyticus* and *Vibrio cholerae* non-O1 infections in Florida (1981–1988). *South Med J* 1990;83:500–502.
49. Safrin S, Morris JG Jr, Adams M, Pons V, Jacobs R, Conte JE Jr. Non-O:1 *Vibrio cholerae* bacteremia: case report and review. *Rev Infect Dis* 1988;10:1012–1017.
50. Dakin WPH, Howell DJ, Sutton RGA, O'Keefe MF, Thomas P. Gastroenteritis due to non-agglutinable (non-cholera) vibrios. *Med J Aust* 1974;2:487–490.
51. Finch MJ, Valdespino JL, Wells JG, et al. Non-O1 *Vibrio cholerae* infections in Cancun, Mexico. *Am J Trop Med Hyg* 1987;36:393–397.
52. Taylor DN, Echeverria P, Pitarangsi C, et al. Application of DNA hybridization techniques in the assessment of diarrheal disease among refugees in Thailand. *Am J Epidemiol* 1988;127:179–187.
53. Varlea G, Olarte J, Perez-Miravete A, Filloy L. Failure to find cholera and non-cholera Vibrios in diarrheal disease in Mexico City, 1966–7. *Am J Trop Med Hyg* 1971;20:925–926.
54. Black RE, Merson MH, Brown KH. Epidemiological aspects of diarrhea associated with known enteropathogens in rural Bangladesh. In: Chen LC, Scrimshaw NS, eds. *Diarrhea and malnutrition*. New York: Plenum Press; 1983:73–86.
55. Hoge CW, Watsky D, Peeler RN, Libonati JP, Israel E, Morris JG Jr. Epidemiology and spectrum of vibrio infections in a Chesapeake Bay community. *J Infect Dis* 1989;160:985–993.
56. Levine WC, Griffin PM, Gulf Coast *Vibrio* Working Group.

Vibrio infections on the Gulf Coast: results of first year of regional surveillance. *J Infect Dis* 1993;167:479–483.

57. Datta-Roy K, Banerjee K, De SP, Ghose AC. Comparative study of expression of hemagglutinins, hemolysins, and enterotoxins by clinical and environmental isolates of non-O1 *Vibrio cholerae* in relation to their enteropathogenicity. *Appl Environ Microbiol* 1986;52:875–879.

58. Spira WM, Daniel RR, Ahmed QS, Huq A, Yusuf A, Sack DA. Clinical features and pathogenicity of O group 1 non-agglutinating *Vibrio cholerae* and other vibrios isolated from cases of diarrhea in Dacca, Bangladesh. In: Takeya J, Zinnaka Y, eds. *Symposium on cholera:* Karatsu 1978: Proceedings of the 14th Joint Conference U.S.–Japan Cooperative Medical Science Program Cholera Panel. Tokyo: Toho University: 137–153.

59. Yamamoto K, Takeda Y, Miwatani T, Craig JP. Evidence that a non-O1 *Vibrio cholerae* produces enterotoxin that is similar but not identical to cholera enterotoxin. *Infect Immun* 1983; 41:896–901.

60. Hanchalay S, Seriwatana J, Echeverria P, et al. Non-O1 *Vibrio cholerae* in Thailand: homology with cloned cholera toxin genes. *J Clin Microbiol* 1985;21:288–289.

61. Kaper JB, Nataro JP, Roberts NC, Siebeling R, Bradford HB. Molecular epidemiology of non-O1 *Vibrio cholerae* and *Vibrio mimicus* in the U.S. Gulf Coast region. *J Clin Microbiol* 1986; 23:652–654.

62. Arita M, Takeda T, Honda T, Miwatani T. Purification and characterization of *Vibrio cholerae* non-O1 heat-stable enterotoxin. *Infect Immun* 1986;52:45–49.

63. Honda T, Arita M, Takeda T, Yoh M, Miwatani T. Non-O1 *Vibrio cholerae* produces two newly identified toxins related to *Vibrio parahaemolyticus* hemolysin and *Escherichia coli* heat-stable enterotoxin. *Lancet* 1985;2:163–164.

64. Johnson JA, Salles CA, Morris JG Jr. Correlation of heat-stable enterotoxin and capsule type of non-O1 *Vibrio cholerae*. 32nd Interscience Conference on Antimicrobial Agents and Chemotherapy, Anaheim, California, October 11–14, 1992.

65. Hoge CW, Sethabutr O, Bodhidatta L, Echeverria P, Robertson DC, Morris JG Jr. Use of a synthetic oligonucleotide probe to detect strains of non-O1 *Vibrio cholerae* carrying the gene for heat stable enterotoxin (NAG-ST). *J Clin Microbiol* 1990; 28:1473–1476.

66. Gyobu Y, Kodama H, Sato S. Studies on the enteropathogenic mechanism of non-O1 *Vibrio cholerae*. III. Production of enteroreactive toxins. *Kansenshogaku Zasshi* 1991;65:781–787.

67. Ichinose Y, Yamamoto K, Nakasone N, et al. Enterotoxicity of El Tor-like hemolysin of non-O1 *Vibrio cholerae*. *Infect Immun* 1987;55:1090–1093.

68. McCardell BA, Madden JM, Shah DB. Isolation and characterization of a cytolysin produced by *Vibrio cholerae* serogroup non-O1. *Can J Microbiol* 1985;31:711–720.

69. Yamamoto K, Ichinose Y, Nakasone N, et al. Identify of hemolysins produced by *Vibrio cholerae* non-O1 and *V. cholerae* O1, biotype El Tor. *Infect Immun* 1986;51:927–931.

70. Levine MM, Kaper JB, Herrington D, et al. Volunteer studies of deletion mutants of *Vibrio cholerae* O1 prepared by recombinant techniques. *Infect Immun* 1988;56:161–167.

71. Alm RA, Mayrhofer G, Kotlarski I, Manning PA. Amino-terminal domain of the El Tor hemolysin of *Vibrio cholerae* O1 is expressed in classical strains and is cytotoxic. *Vaccine* 1991; 9:588–591.

72. Johnson JA, Panigrahi P, Russell RG, Morris JG Jr. Role of hemolysin in the pathogenesis of non-serogroup O1 *Vibrio cholerae*. 31st Interscience Conference on Antimicrobial Agents and Chemotherapy, Chicago, Illinois, September 29–October 2, 1991.

73. O'Brien AD, Chen ME, Holmes RK, Kaper JB, Levine MM. Environmental and human isolates of *Vibrio cholerae* and *Vibrio parahaemolyticus* produce a *Shigella dysenteriae* 1 (Shiga-like) cytotoxin. *Lancet* 1984;1:77–78.

74. Johnson JA, Morris JG Jr, Kaper JB. Gene encoding zonula occludens toxin (*zot*) does not occur independently from cholera enterotoxin genes (*ctx*) in *Vibrio cholerae*. *J Clin Microbiol* 1993;31:732–733.

75. Shehabi AA, Drexler H, Richardson SH. Virulence mecha-

76. Spira WM, Fedorka-Cray PJ, Pettebone P. Colonization of the rabbit small intestine by clinical and environmental isolates of non-O1 *Vibrio cholerae* and *Vibrio mimicus*. *Infect Immun* 1983;41:1175–1183.

77. Nakasone N, Iwanaga M. Pili of *Vibrio cholerae* non-O1. *Infect Immun* 1990;58:1640–1646.

78. Johnson JA, Joseph A, Panigrahi P, Morris JG Jr. Frequency of encapsulated versus unencapsulated strains of non-O1 *Vibrio cholerae* isolated from patients with septicemia or diarrhea, or from environmental strains. American Society for Microbiology Annual Meeting, New Orleans, Louisiana, May 26–30, 1992.

79. Bonner JR, Coker AS, Berryman CR, Pollock HM. Spectrum of *Vibrio* infections in a Gulf coast community. *Ann Intern Med* 1983;99:464–469.

80. Hughes JM, Hollis DG, Gangarosa EJ, Weaver RE. Non-cholera *Vibrio* infections in the United States: clinical, epidemiologic, and laboratory features. *Ann Intern Med* 1978;88: 602–606.

81. Black RE. The prophylaxis and therapy of secretory diarrhea. *Med Clin North Am* 1982;66:611–621.

82. Swerdlow DL, Ries AA. Cholera in the Americas: guidelines for the clinician. *JAMA* 1992;267:1495–1499.

83. Wallace CK, Anderson PN, Brown TC, et al. Optimal antibiotic therapy in cholera. *Bull WHO* 1968;39:239–245.

84. Morris JG Jr, Tenney JH, Drusano GL. In vitro susceptibility of pathogenic *Vibrio* species to norfloxacin and six other antimicrobial agents. *Antimicrob Agents Chemother* 1985;28: 442–445.

85. Northrup RS. Antibiotics in cholera therapy. *J Pakistan Med Assoc* 1969;19:363–365.

86. Davis BR, Fanning GR, Madden JM, et al. Characterization of biochemically atypical *Vibrio cholerae* strains and designation of a new pathogenic species, *Vibrio mimicus*. *J Clin Microbiol* 1981;14:631–639.

87. Chowdhury MA, Yamanaka H, Miyoshi S, Aziz KM, Shinoda S. Ecology of *Vibrio mimicus* in aquatic environments. *Appl Environ Microbiol* 1989;55:2073–2078.

88. Shandera WX, Johnston JM, Davis BR, Blake PA. Disease from infection with *Vibrio mimicus*, a newly recognized *Vibrio* species. *Ann Intern Med* 1983;99:169–171.

89. Spira WM, Fedorka-Cray PJ. Production of cholera toxin-like toxin by *Vibrio mimicus* and non-O1 *Vibrio cholerae*: batch culture conditions for optimal yields and isolation of hypertoxigenic lincomycin-resistant mutants. *Infect Immun* 1983;42: 501–509.

90. Gyobu Y, Isobe J, Kodama H, Sato S. Enteropathogenicity and enteropathogenic toxin production of *Vibrio mimicus*. *J Jpn Assoc Inf Dis* 1992;66:115–120.

91. Tamplon ML, Jalali R, Ahmed MK, Colwell RR. Variation in epitopes of the B subunit of *Vibrio cholerae* non-O1 and *Vibrio mimicus* cholera toxins. *Can J Microbiol* 1990;36:409–413.

92. Arita M, Honda T, Miwatani T, Takeda T, Takeo T, Shimonishi Y. Purification and characterization of a heat-stable enterotoxin of *Vibrio mimicus*. *FEMS Microbiol Lett* 1991;63: 105–110.

93. Yoshida H, Honda T, Miwatani T. Purification and characterization of a hemolysin of *Vibrio mimicus* that relates to the thermostable direct hemolysin of *Vibrio parahaemolyticus*. *FEMS Microbiol Lett* 1991;68:249–253.

94. Terai A, Shirai H, Yoshida O, Takeda Y, Nishibuchi M. Nucleotide sequence of the thermostable direct hemolysin gene 9tdh gene) of *Vibrio mimicus* and its evolutionary relationship with the tdh genes of *Vibrio parahaemolyticus*. *FEMS Microbiol Lett* 1990;59:319–323.

95. Joseph SW, Colwell RR, Kaper JB. *Vibrio parahaemolyticus* and related halophilic vibrios. *CRC Crit Rev Microbiol* 1983; 10:77–124.

96. Miwatani T, Takeda Y. Vibrio parahaemolyticus: a causative bacterium of food poisoning. Tokyo: Saikon; 1976.

97. Barker WH JR. *Vibrio parahaemolyticus* outbreaks in the United States. *Lancet* 1974;1:551–4.

nisms associated with clinical isolates of non-O1 *Vibrio cholerae*. *Zbl Bakt Hyg* 1986;A261:232–239.

98. Dadisman TA, Nelson R, Molenda JR, Gasber HJ. *Vibrio parahaemolyticus* gastroenteritis in Maryland. I. Clinical and epidemiologic aspects. *Am J Epidemiol* 1973;96:414–426.

99. Centers for Disease Control. *Vibrio parahaemolyticus* foodborne outbreak—Louisiana. *MMWR* 1978;27:345–346.

100. Sakazaki R, Tamura K, Kato T, Obara Y, Yamai S, Hobo K. Studies on the enteropathogenic, facultatively halophilic bacteria, *Vibrio parahaemolyticus*. III. Enteropathogenicity. *Jpn J Med Sci Biol* 1968;21:325–331.

101. Miyamoto Y, Kato T, Obara Y, Akiyama S, Kinjiro T, Yamai S. In vitro hemolytic characteristic of *Vibrio parahaemolyticus*: its close correlation with human pathogenicity. *J Bacteriol* 1969;100:1147–1149.

102. Sakazaki R, Balows A. The genus *Vibrio*, *Plesiomonas*, and *Aeromonas*. In: Starr MP, Stolp H, Truper HG, Balows A, Schlegel HG, eds. *The prokaryotes*. Berlin: Springer-Verlag; 1978:1272–1301.

103. Fujino T, Sakazaki R, Tamura K. Designation of the type strain of *Vibrio parahamolyticus* and description of 200 strains of the species. *Int J Syst Bacteriol* 1974;24:447–449.

104. Huq MI, Huber D, Kibryia G. Isolation of urease producing *Vibrio parahaemolyticus* strains from cases of gastroenteritis. *Ind J Med Res* 1979;70:549–553.

105. Kelly MT, Stroh EM. Urease-positive, Kanagawa-negative *Vibrio parahaemolyticus* from patients and the environment in the Pacific Northwest. *J Clin Microbiol* 1989;27:2820–2822.

106. Abbott SL, Powers C, Kaysner CA, et al. Emergence of a restricted bioserovar of *Vibrio parahaemolyticus* as the predominant cause of *Vibrio*-associated gastroenteritis on the west coast of the United States and Mexico. *J Clin Microbiol* 1989;27:2891–2893.

107. Magalhaes M, Magalhaes V, Antas MG, Tateno S. Isolation of urease-positive *Vibrio parahaemolyticus* from diarrheal patients in northeast Brazil. *Revista do Instituto de Medicina Tropical de Sao Paulo* 1991;33:263–265.

108. Kaysner CA, Abeyta C Jr, Stott RF, Lilja JL, Wekell MM. Incidence of urea-hydrolyzing *Vibrio parahaemolyticus* in Willapa Bay, Washington. *Appl Environ Microbiol* 1990;56:904–907.

109. Honda S, Matsumoto S, Miwatani T, Honda T. A survey of urease-positive *Vibrio parahaemolyticus* strains isolated from traveller's diarrhea, sea water and imported frozen sea foods. *Eur J Epidemiol* 1992;8:861–864.

110. DePaola A, Hopkins LH, Peeler JT, Wentz B, McPhearson RM. Incidence of *Vibrio parahaemolyticus* in U.S. coastal waters and oysters. *Appl Environ Microbiol* 1990;56:2299–2302.

111. Kumazawa NH, Fukuma N, Komoda Y. Attachment of *Vibrio parahaemolyticus* strains to estuarine algae. *J Vet Med Sci* 1991;53:201–205.

112. Thompson CA Jr, Vanderzant C, Ray SM. Serological and hemolytic characteristics of *Vibrio parahaemolyticus* from marine souces. *J Food Sci* 1976;41:204–205.

113. Sanyal SC, Sen PC. Human volunteer study on the pathogenicity of *Vibrio parahaemolyticus*. In: International Symposium on *Vibrio parahaemolyticus*. Tokyo, Japan, September 17–18, 1973. Tokyo: Saikon: 227–230.

114. Kaper JB, Campen RK, Seidler RJ, Baldini MM, Falkow S. Cloning of the thermostable direct or Kanagawa phenomenon-associated hemolysin of *Vibrio parahaemolyticus*. *Infect Immun* 1984;45:290–292.

115. Takeda Y, Taga S, Miwatani T. Evidence that thermostable direct hemolysin of *Vibrio parahaemolyticus* is composed of two subunits. *FEMS Microbiol Lett* 1978;4:271–274.

116. Twedt RM, Peeler JT, Spaulding PL. Effective ileal loop dose of Kanagawa-positive *Vibrio parahaemolyticus*. *Appl Environ Microbiol* 1980;28:567–576.

117. Nishibuchi M, Fasano A, Russell RG, Kaper JB. Enterotoxigenicity of *Vibrio parahaemolyticus* with and without genes encoding thermostable direct hemolysin. *Infect Immun* 1992; 60:3539–3545.

118. Honda T, Ni YX, Hata A, et al. Properties of a hemolysin related to the thermostable direct hemolysin produced by a Kanagawa phenpmeno negative, clinical isolate of *Vibrio parahaemolyticus*. *Can J Microbiol* 1990;36:395–399.

119. Yoh M, Miwatani T, Honda T. Comparison of *Vibrio parahaemolyticus* hemolysin (Vp-TRH) produced by clinical and environmental isolates. *FEMS Microbiol Lett* 1992;71:157–161.

120. Shirai H, Ito H, Hirayama T, et al. Molecular epidemiologic evidence for association of thermostable direct hemolysin (TDH) and TDH-related hemolysin of *Vibrio parahaemolyticus* with gastroenteritis. *Infect Immun* 1990;58:3568–3573.

121. Honda T, Honda S, Ni YX, Miwatani T. Development of application of enzyme-linked immunosorbent assay using monoclonal antibody against a hemolysin (Vp-TDH) of *Vibrio parahaemolyticus*-evidence that Vp-TDH producing Kanagawa phenomenon–negative *V. parahaemolyticus* is a human pathogen. *Kansenshogaku Zasshi* 1990;64:767–773.

122. Hughes JM, Boyce JM, Aleem ARMA, Wells JG, Rahman ASMM, Curlin GT. *Vibrio parahaemolyticus* enterocolitis in Bangladesh: report of an outbreak. *Am J Trop Med Hyg* 1978; 27:106–112.

123. Bolen JL, Zamiska SA, Greenough WB III. Clinical features in enteritis due to *Vibrio parahaemolyticus*. *Am J Med* 1974; 57:638–641.

124. Calia FM, Johnson DE. Bacteremia in suckling rabbits after oral challenge with *Vibrio parahaemolyticus*. *Infect Immun* 1975;11:1222–1225.

125. Nishibuchi M, Ishibashi M, Takeda Y, Kaper JB. Detection of the thermostable direct hemolysin gene and related DNA sequences in *Vibrio parahaemolyticus* and other *Vibrio* species by the DNA colony hybridization test. *Infect Immun* 1985;49:481–486.

126. Nishibuchi M, Hill WE, Zon G, Payne WL, Kaper JB. Synthetic oligodeoxyribonucleotide probes to detect Kanagawa phenomenon-positive *Vibrio parahaemolyticus*. *J Clin Microbiol* 1986;23:1091–1095.

127. Lee JV, Shread P, Furniss AL, Bryant TN. Taxonomy and description of *Vibrio fluvialis* sp. nov. (synonym group F Vibrios, group EF-6). *J Appl Bacteriol* 1981;50:73–94.

128. Seidler RJ, Allen DA, Colwell RR, Joseph SW, Daily OP. Biochemical characteristics and virulence of environmental group F bacteria isolated in the United States. *Appl Environ Microbiol* 1980;40:715–720.

129. Klontz KC, Desenclos JC. Clinical and epidemiological features of sporadic infections with *Vibrio fluvialis* in Florida, USA. *J Diarrh Dis Res* 1990;8:24–26.

130. Huq MI, Alam AKMJ, Brenner DJ, Morris GK. Isolation of Vibrio-like group, EF-6, from persons with diarrhea. *J Clin Microbiol* 1980;11:621–624.

131. Thekdi RJ, Lakhani AG, Rale VB, Panse MV. An outbreak of food poisoning suspected to be caused by *Vibrio fluvialis*. *J Diarrh Dis Res* 1990;8:163–165.

132. Lockwood DE, Kreger AS, Richardson SH. Detection of toxins produced by *Vibrio fluvialis*. *Infect Immun* 1982;35:702–708.

133. Tacket CO, Hickman F, Pierce GV, Mendoza LF. Diarrhea associated with *Vibrio fluvialis* in the United States. *J Clin Microbiol* 1982;16:991–992.

134. Brenner DJ, Hickman-Brenner FW, Lee JV, et al. *Vibrio furnissi* (formerly aerogenic biogroup of *Vibrio fluvialis*), a new species isolates from human feces and the environment. *J Clin Microbiol* 1983;18:816–824.

135. Yu C, Bassler BL, Roseman S. Chemotaxis of the marine bacterium *Vibrio furnissii* to sugars. A potential mechanism for initiating the chitin catabolic cascade. *J Biol Chem* 1993;268:9405–9409.

136. Centers for Disease Control. An outbreak of acute gastroenteritis during a tour of the orient—Alaska. *MMWR* 1969;18:150.

137. Centers for Disease Control. Follow-up outbreak of gastroenteritis during a tour of the orient—Alaska. *MMWR* 1969;18:168.

138. Hickman FW, Farmer JJ III, Hollis DG, et al. Identification of *Vibrio hollisae* sp. nov. from patients with diarrhea. *J Clin Microbiol* 1982;15:395–401.

139. Kothary MH, Richardson SH. Fluid accumulation in infant

mice caused by *Vibrio hollisae* and its extracellular enterotoxin. *Infect Immun* 1987;55:626–630.

140. Yamasaki S, Shirai H, Takeda Y, Nishibuchi M. Analysis of the gene of *Vibrio hollisae* encoding the hemolysin similar to the thermostable direct hemolysin of *Vibrio parahaemolyticus. FEMS Microbiol Lett* 1991;64:259–263.

141. Lowry PW, McFarland LM, Threefoot HK. *Vibrio hollisae* septicemia after consumption of catfish. *J Infect Dis* 1986;154: 730–731.

142. Rank EL, Smith IR, Langer M. Bacteremia caused by *Vibrio hollisae. J Clin Microbiol* 1988;26:375–376.

143. Blake PA, Merson MH, Weaver RE, Hollis DG, Heublein PC. Disease caused by a marine *Vibrio:* clinical characteristics and epidemiology. *N Engl J Med* 1979;300:1–5.

144. Farmer JJ III. *Vibrio (Beneckea) vulnificus,* the bacterium associated with sepsis, septicemia, and the sea. *Lancet* 1979;2: 903.

145. Tacket CO, Brenner F, Blake PA. Clinical features and an epidemiologic study of *Vibrio vulnificus* infections. *J Infect Dis* 1984;149:558–61.

146. Klontz KC, Lieb S, Schreiber M, Janowski HT, Baldy LM, Gunn RA. Syndromes of *Vibrio vulnificus* infections: Clinical and epidemiological features in Florida cases, 1981–1987. *Ann Intern Med* 1988;109:318–323.

147. Johnston JM, Becker SF, McFarland LM. *Vibrio vulnificus:* man and the sea. *JAMA* 1985;253:2850–2852.

148. Park SD, Shon HS, Joh NJ. *Vibrio vulnificus* septicemia in Korea: clinical and epidemiologic findings in seventy patients. *J Am Acad Dermatol* 1991;24:397–403.

149. Morris JG, Wright AC, Roberts DM, Wood PK, Simpson LM, Oliver JD. Identification of environmental *Vibrio vulnificus* isolates with a DNA probe for the cytotoxin-hemolysin gene. *Appl Environ Microbiol* 1987;53:193–195.

150. Wright AC, Miceli GA, Landry WL, Christy JB, Watkins WD, Morris JG Jr. Rapid identification of *Vibrio vulnificus* on non-selective media with an alkaline phosphatase-labeled oligonucleotide probe. *Appl Environ Microbiol* 1993;59:541–546.

151. Simpson LM, White VK, Zane SF, Oliver JD. Correlation between virulence and colony morphology in *Vibrio vulnificus. Infect Immun* 1987;55:269–272.

152. Yoshida SI, Ogawa M, Mizuguchi Y. Relation of capsular materials and colony opacity to virulence of *Vibrio vulnificus. Infect Immun* 1985;47:446–451.

153. Wright AC, Simpson LM, Oliver JD, Morris JG Jr. Phenotypic evaluation of acapsular transposon mutants of *Vibrio vulnificus. Infect Immun* 1990;58:1769–1773.

154. Reddy GP, Hayat U, Abeygunawardana C, et al. Purification and structure determination of *Vibrio vulnificus* capsular polysaccharide. *J Bacteriol* 1992;174:2620–2630.

155. Hayat U, Reddy GP, Bush CA, Johnson JA, Wright AC, Morris JG Jr. Capsular types of *Vibrio vulnificus:* an analysis of strains from clinical and environmental sources. *J Infect Dis* 1993;168: 758–762.

156. Oliver JD, Warner RA, Cleland DR. Distribution and ecology of *Vibrio vulnificus* and other lactose-fermenting marine Vibrios in coastal waters of the southeastern United States. *Appl Environ Microbiol* 1982;44:1404–1414.

157. Kaysner CA, Abeyta C Jr, Wekell MM, DePaola A Jr, Stott RF, Leitch JM. Virulent strains of *Vibrio vulnificus* isolated from estuaries of the United States west coast. *Appl Environ Microbiol* 1987;53:1349–1351.

158. Tamplin M, Rodrick GE, Blake NJ, Cuba T. Isolation and characterization of *Vibrio vulnificus* from two Florida estuaries. *Appl Environ Microbiol* 1982;44:1466–1470.

159. Kelly MT. Effect of temperature and salinity on *Vibrio (Be-

neckea) vulnificus* occurrence in a Gulf Coast environment. *Appl Environ Microbiol* 1982;44:820–824.

160. Centers for Disease Control. *Vibrio vulnificus* infections associated with raw oyster consumption—Florida, 1981–1992. *MMWR* 1993;42:405–407.

161. Brennt EC, Wright AC, Dutta SK, Morris JG Jr. Growth of *Vibrio vulnificus* in serum from alcoholics: association with high transferrin iron saturation (letter). *J Infect Dis* 1991;164: 1030–1032.

162. Morris JG Jr, Wright AC, Simpson LM, Wood PK, Johnson DE, Oliver JD. Virulence of *Vibrio vulnificus:* association with utilization of transferrin-bound iron, and lack of correlation with levels of cytotoxin or protease production. *FEMS Microbiol Lett* 1987;40:55–59.

163. Gray LD, Kreger AS. Purification and characterization of an extracellular cytolysin produced by *Vibrio vulnificus. Infect Immun* 1985;48:62–72.

164. Kothary MH, Kreger AS. Production and partial characterization of an elastolytic protease of *Vibrio vulnificus. Infect Immun* 1985;50:534–540.

165. Smith GC, Merkel JR. Collagenolytic activity of *Vibrio vulnificus:* potential contribution to its invasiveness. *Infect Immun* 1982;35:1155–1156.

166. Testa J, Daniel LW, Kreger AS. Extracellular phospholipase A$_2$ and lysophospholipase produced by *Vibrio vulnificus. Infect Immun* 1984;45:458–463.

167. Gray LD, Kreger AS. Mouseskin damage caused by cytolysin from *Vibrio vulnificus* and by *V. vulnificus* infection. *J Infect Dis* 1987;155:236–241.

168. Miyoshi N, Miyoshi S-I, Sugiyama K, Suzuki Y, Furuta H, Shinoda S. Activation of the plasma kallikrein-kinin system by *Vibrio vulnificus* protease. *Infect Immun* 1987;55:1936–1939.

169. Wright AC, Simpson LM, Oliver JD, Morris JG Jr. Phenotypic evaluation of acapsular transposon mutants of *Vibrio vulnificus. Infect Immun* 1990;58:1769–1773.

170. Wright AC, Simpson LM, Russell RG, Morris JG. *Vibrio vulnificus* protease: regulation and relationship to virulence. American Society for Microbiology Annual Meeting, Dallas, Texas, May 5–9, 1991.

171. Kelly MT, McCormick WF. Acute bacterial myositis caused by *Vibrio vulnificus. JAMA* 1981;246:72–73.

172. Castillo LE, Winslow DL, Pankey GA. Wound infection and septic shock due to *Vibrio vulnificus. Am J Trop Med Hyg* 1981;30:844–848.

173. Pollak SJ, Parrish EF III, Barrett TJ, Dretler R, Morris JG Jr. *Vibrio vulnificus* septicemia: isolation of organism from stool and demonstration of antibodies by indirect immunofluorescence. *Arch Intern Med* 1983;143:837–838.

174. Simonson J, Siebeling RJ. Rapid serological identification of *Vibrio vulnificus* by anti-H coaggluation. *Appl Environ Microbiol* 1986;52:1299–1304.

175. Tamplin ML, Martin AL, Ruple AD, Cook DW, Kaspar CW. Enzyme immunoassay for identification of *Vibrio vulnificus* in seawater, sediment, and oysters. *Appl Environ Microbiol* 1991; 57:1235–1240.

176. Lefkowitz A, Fout GS, Losonsky G, Wasserman SS, Israel E, Morris JG Jr. A serosurvey of pathogens associated with shellfish: prevalence of antibodies to *Vibrio* species and Norwalk agent in the Chesapeake Bay area. *Am J Epidemiol* 1992; 135:369–380.

177. Fiore A, Hayat U, Wright AC, Wasserman SS, Morris JG Jr. Infection with *Vibrio vulnificus* elicits an antibody response to capsular polysaccharide. *Clin Res* 1992;40:428A.

178. Bowdre JH, Hull JH, Cocchetto DM. Antibiotic efficacy against *Vibrio vulnificus* in the mouse: superiority of tetracycline. *J Pharmacol Exp Ther* 1983;225:595–598.

Infections of the Gastrointestinal Tract,
edited by M. J. Blaser, P. D. Smith, J. I. Ravdin,
H. B. Greenberg, and R. L. Guerrant
Raven Press, Ltd., New York © 1995.

CHAPTER 48

Types of *Escherichia coli* Enteropathogens

Richard L. Guerrant and Nathan M. Thielman

Within the versatile species of *E. coli* is practically the entire range of types of microbial enteropathogens and representative mechanisms by which microorganisms derange intestinal function to cause secretion and/or inflammation and thus diarrhea. As noted in Table 1, these include four different types of enterotoxins (LT/I, LT/II, STa, STb), SLT/I and/or SLT/II-producing enterohemorrhagic *E. coli* (EHEC), enteroinvasive *E. coli* (EIEC), classical (locally adherent) enteropathogenic *E. coli* (EPEC), enteroaggregative *E. coli* (EAggEC), diffusely adherent *E. coli* (DAEC), and enteric-colonizing *E. coli* for a total of ten different types of potential *E. coli* enteropathogens. Of these, the six underlined have their pathogenicity in humans established in either outbreaks or in volunteer studies [these include LT/I, STa, EHEC (SLTI/II), EIEC, EPEC, and EAggEC]. The roles of LT/II-, STb-, DAEC-, and enteric-colonizing *E. coli* remain to be definitively established as causes of diarrhea in humans (although STb-producing *E. coli* cause significant diarrhea in some animals). Because the genetic codes for many of these virulence traits reside on plasmids or phages (or on chromosomal elements regulated by plasmid-encoded products), the capacity to be a pathogen consequently may be transferred from one serotype of *E. coli* to another. Nevertheless, the serogroups listed in column 5 tend to predominate to a greater or lesser extent among the different types of *E. coli*. Indeed, for many years serotyping provided the only potential means to recognize classic "enteropathogenic serotypes" of *E. coli,* the specific virulence mechanisms of which are now being further distinguished by both biotype and DNA probe as local and aggregative adherence. Some suggest that we should move away from serotypical characterization of these organisms in favor of definition by virulence traits or by the presence of genetic elements that encode these traits.

Cholera-like LT/I-producing enterotoxigenic *E. coli* (ETEC), which activate adenylate cyclase and may act through additional pathways such as those that involve prostaglandin synthesis and PAF production (1–3), are well established in both field and volunteer studies as enteropathogens. In contrast, the other well-established ETEC produce the heat-stable enterotoxin STa, which is much smaller (16–18 amino acids), less antigenic, and promptly and reversibly activates guanylate cyclase rather than adenylate cyclase to cause chloride-dependent net secretion by elevating cyclic GMP instead of cyclic AMP (4–10). Furthermore, this guanylate cyclase–activating ST family of enterotoxins not only has been expanded to include STs produced by microoorganisms other than *E. coli* but has also uncovered the ST-like mammalian tissue products from intestine or kidney such as guanylin (11).

The methanol-insoluble heat-stable toxin recognized predominantly from animal isolates is much larger and causes cyclic nucleotide–independent bicarbonate secretion in piglet loops (12,13). Although Whipp et al. demonstrated that rabbit and mouse loops were not responsive to STb because of protease degradation which can be inhibited (14–16), an extensive search among *E. coli* isolates from Brazil and Bangladesh using a gene probe for STb as well as in vitro study of STb on human intestinal tissue in Ussing chambers failed to shown an effect of STb on human tissue or an association with diarrhea in humans (12,17).

EHEC that produce at least one or more of the Shiga-like toxins, or verocytotoxins (SLTI or SLTII), appear to be increasingly associated with rare hamburger ingestion in several outbreaks as well as fresh-pressed apple cider (18–21). This organism is recognized by its ability to produce the Shiga-like toxin (verocytotoxin). Indeed, the toxin may be found more often than the organism is cultured in some fecal specimens in outbreaks. Many of the recognized EHEC outbreaks have involved *E. coli* O157:H7, which is often (albeit not always) sorbitol-negative and can therefore be suspected by routinely culturing fecal specimens on sorbitol MacConkey agar plates as recommended by the Centers for Disease Control (22).

EIEC behave much like a fifth serogroup of *Shigella* to which *E. coli* are closely related, even to the point of

R. L. Guerrant and N. M. Thielman: Division of Geographic and International Medicine, University of Virginia School of Medicine, Charlottesville, Virginia.

TABLE 1. *Types of* E. coli *enteropathogens:*

	Genetic code	Mechanism	Model	Predominant O serogroups	Type of diarrhea
Enterotoxigenic (ETEC):					
LT	Plasmid	CFA/I-V-colonize	MRHA		
	Plasmid/chromosomal	Adenylate cyclase secretion	18th Rabbit ileal loop CHO/Y1 cells	1,6,7,8,9,11,15,20,25,27,60,63, 75,80,85,88,89,99,101,109, 114,128,139,153	Acute watery
STa	Plasmid	Guanylate cyclase secretion	4–8h Rabbit ileal loop suckling mice	11,12,15,20,25,27,60,63,75, 78,80,85,88,89,99,101,109,114, 115,139,148,149,153,159,166, 167	Acute watery
STb	Plasmid	Cyclic nucleotide-independent HCO₃ secretion	Piglet loop		
Enterohemorrhagic (EHEC)					
SLT	Phage/?plasmid (some also have eaeA; see below)	Glycosidase cleaves adenosine-4324 in 28SrRNA of 60S ribosomal subunits to halt protein synthesis	HeLa cell cytotoxicity	157,26,103,111,113 et al. 104,153,163	Bloody (±HUS)
Enteroinvasive (EIEC)	plasmid (140 MDa) + chromosomal	Cell invasion and spread 58- to 80-kDa EIET (chromosomal)	Sereny test	11,28,29,112,115,121,124, 138,143,144,147,152,164, 173	Acute dysenteric
Enteropathogenic (EPEC)	1. Plasmid (60 MDa; EAF, bfpA)	BFP-efficient localized adherence (LA)	LA to HEp-2 cells	18,26,44,55,86,111,114, 119,125,126,127,128,142, 157,158	Acute + persistent
	2. Chromosomal (cfm)	Tyrosine kinase and Intracellular Ca²⁺ dependent actin condensation	Fluorescence actin staining (FAS)		
	3. Chromosomal (eaeA)	94-kDa intimin →intimate-effacing adherence			
Enteroaggregative (EAggEC)	Plasmid (60 MDa;AA)	BFP-aggregative adherence (AA)	AA to HEp-2 cells	3(17-2), 15,44(042),51,77, 78,86,91,92(221)	Persistent (? Acute)
	Plasmid (60 MDa;AA)	2- to 5-KDa EAST-1, guanylate cyclase, EALT pore forming Ca²⁺ Ionophore	Ussing chambers	111,113,126,141,146, ?(346)	
Diffusely Adherent (DAEC)	Chromosomal (daaC probe)	Fimbrial adhesion (F1845)	Diffuse Adherence to HEp-2 cells	75(F1845), ?(189), 15(57-1),126(AIDA-I)	? Acute ?Persistent
	Plasmid	Afimbrial adhesin (hemologeous to Shigella IcsA			
Enteric Colonizing	Plasmid	CFA/I-V ↘ colonize ?Hydrophobic ↗	MRHA (NH₁)₂SO₄ hydrophobicity	—	?Persistent
GU/CNS/Normal flora	Chromosomal/plasmid	type I pill P—fimbriae S-fimbriae AFA—I	MSHA bind P blood gp. Ag.	1,2,4,6,7,25, 45,75,81	None

Underline signifies pathogenicity in humans established in outbreaks or volunteer studies. HUS, hemolytic-uremic syndrome. BFP, bundle-forming pili; LT, heat labile toxin; ST, heat stable toxin; SLT, shiga-like toxin.

sharing a similar 140-mDa plasmid and chromosomal elements responsible for cell invasion and spread as well as certain O-antigen cross-reactivity.

Beside ETEC, EHEC, and EIEC, a group of *E. coli* enteropathogens can be recognized by their ability to adhere in one of three or more characteristic patterns to HEp2 (and other) cells in tissue culture. These include the locally adherent classically recognized EPEC, EAggEC that adhere in a "stacked-brick" pattern to both HEp2 cells and glass slides, and the DAEC that adhere in a diffuse pattern to HEp2 cells only. The EPEC adherence factor (EAF), 60-mDa plasmid-encoded bundle forming pili [which cross-react with the bundle forming toxin co-regulated pili (TCP) on *Vibrio cholerae*], mediates the initial local adherence of EPEC seen in vitro as microcolonies on tissue culture cells. This is followed by an impressive pedestal formation by the host cell (HEp2 cells or intestinal epithelial cells) that now appear to involve tyrosine phosphorylation and intracellular calcium-dependent actin condensation encoded by a class four mutant (cfm) region on the chromosome as well as "intimin"-mediated intimate-effacing adherence encoded by an *eaeA* region on the chromosome (23–25). A functionally homologous *eae* gene in EHEC O157:H7 induces F-actin accumulation in HEp2 cells and facilitates intimate attachment to colonic epithelial cells in the newborn piglet model (24), although its role in the hemorrhagic colitis or other complications of this infection remain unclear (20). Thus the events leading to the localized adherence and attachment and effacement by EPEC (and perhaps other *E. coli* such as EHEC as well) appear to involve the orchestration of at least three separable plasmid and chromosomally encoded traits.

EAggEC that exhibit stacked-brick adherence have become increasingly recognized in recent years in association with persistent diarrhea in studies in India, Brazil, Chile, and Mexico (27–31). Strain 221 (O92:H33) isolated from a patient with traveler's diarrhea in Mexico, initially thought to be a DAEC, was subsequently shown to exhibit the aggregative pattern of adherence; probes positive with an aggregative adherence (AA) probe for AAF\1; and has variably caused diarrhea in volunteer studies in Houston but not in Maryland (32,33). In addition, strain 17-2 (O3:H2), isolated from a child with diarrhea in Chile, the strain from which the AA probe was developed, failed to cause diarrhea in 23 of 24 volunteers studied by Nataro et al. (34) at the University of Maryland, although both strains 221 and 172 as well as 042 (serotype O44:H18) have all shown colonization, epithelial disruption, and diarrhea in rabbit, rat, or gnotobiotic pig models (35,36). EAggEC strain 042 (serotype O44:H18) also caused diarrhea in three of five volunteers given this organism and a fourth patient in this group developed abdominal symptoms and loose stools. The roles of bundle-forming or other fimbriae, the heat-stable 2- to 5-kDa guanylate cyclase–activating enterotoxin (EAST), and the heat-labile pore-forming calcium ionophore in causing EAggEC diarrhea remain unclear. Scotland et al. further found that certain O44, O111, and O126 serogroups have exhibited aggregative rather than localized adherence to HEp2 cells and thus at least some of these organisms probably belong in the EAggEC group rather than EPEC (37). In addition, strain 34B has been shown to exhibit aggregative adherence. *EAggEC* strain O146:H39 studied by Enslava, Cravioto et al. (38) in an outbreak in Mexico appears to produce a 107-kDa protein product that is currently under study.

DAEC include well-characterized strains C1845 (O75:NM), 189 (O?:H33/35), and 57-1 (O15:HM), which have all been identified and characterized, and are probe-positive for either fimbriate or afimbriate adhesins but have failed to cause diarrhea in volunteer studies to date. In addition, DAEC strain O126:H7 exhibits the AIDA-I adhesin which was studied by Benz et al. (39). The role of DAEC in acute or persistent disease has been questioned in some studies in which these organisms are found in controls as often as in cases (29), but suggested by others with an increasing association in children over 18 months of age with acute or persistent diarrhea (40).

Enteric-colonizing *E. coli,* represented by strains such as 1392, which had previously been an ETEC but that now expresses only the colonization factor antigen (CFA/

II) without recognized enterotoxins, has caused diarrhea in human volunteers as well as in the reversible ileal tie adult rabbit diarrhea model (RITARD). In this model colonization by that organism was associated with an impairment of normal water and electrolyte absorption as well as impaired disaccharidase activity and diarrhea (41,42). The potential role for colonization, therefore, in causing persistent diarrhea in children in tropical developing areas (as well as possibly in diarrhea caused by genetically engineered colonizing live vaccine organisms) remains to be clarified, as does the mechanism by which these colonizing organisms may trigger diarrhea.

Finally, the "normal flora" *E. coli* tend to occur in yet a different range of serogroups and may sometimes include *E. coli* that produce type 1 pili or those that produce P or S fimbriae or AFA and may be associated with genitourinary or central nervous system infections (43–46).

In summary, it is clear that within the versatile species of *E. coli* are a range of lessons regarding virulence traits involved in the pathogenesis of bacterial diarrheas of many types, as reviewed in subsequent chapters.

REFERENCES

1. Peterson JW, Ochoa G. Role of prostaglandins and cAMP in the secretory effects of cholera toxin. *Science* 1989;245:857–859.
2. Peterson JW, Reitmeyer JC, Jackson CA, Ansare GAS. Protein synthesis is required for cholera toxin-induced stimulation or arachidonic acid metabolism. *Biochim Biophys Acta* 1991;1092:79–84.
3. Thielman N, Fang GD, Barrett LJ, Fonteles MC, Guerrant RL. Inhibition of choleratoxin effects on intestinal secretion and CHO cell elongation by platelet activating factor (PAF) antagonists. *Proc. 29th Joint Conference US–Japan Cholera Meeting, Monterey, CA.* 1993;172–176.
4. Hughes JM, Murad F, Chang B, Guerrant RL. Role of cyclic GMP in the action of heat-stable enterotoxins of *Escherichia coli. Nature* 1978;271:755–756.
5. Field M, Graf Jr LH, Mata LJ. Heat stable enterotoxin of *E. coli.* In vitro effects on guanylate cyclase activity, cyclic GMP concentration, and ion transport in small intestine. *Proc Natl Acad Sci USA* 1978;75:2800–2804.
6. Guerrant RL, Hughes JM, Chang B, Robertson DC, Murad F. Activation of intestinal guanylate cyclase by heat-stable enterotoxin of *E. coli:* studies of tissue specificity, potential receptors and intermediates. *J Infect Dis* 1980;142:220–228.
7. Chen LC, Rohde JE, Sharp GWG. Intestinal adenyl-cyclase activity in human cholera. *Lancet* 1971;1:939–941.
8. Kimberg DV, Field M, Johnson J, Henderson A, Gershon E. Stimulation of intestinal mucosal adenyl cyclase by cholera enterotoxin and prostaglandins. *J Clin Invest* 1971;50:1218–1230.
9. Guerrant RL, Chen LC, Sharp GWG. Intestinal adenyl-cyclase activity in canine cholera: Correlation with fluid accumulation. *J Infect Dis* 1972;125:377–381.
10. Guerrant RL, Ganguly U, Casper AGT, Moore EJ, Pierce NF, Carpenter CCF. Effect of *Escherichia coli* on fluid transport across canine small bowel: Mechanism and time-course with enterotoxin and whole bacterial cells. *J Clin Invest* 1973;52:1707–1714.
11. Currie MG, Fok KF, Kato J, et al. Guanylin: An endogenous activator of intestinal guanylate cyclase. *Proc Natl Acad Sci USA* 1992;89:947–951.
12. Weikel CS, Nellans HN, Guerrant RL. The in vivo and in vitro effects of a novel enterotoxin, STb, produced by *Escherichia coli. J Infect Dis* 1986;153:893–901.
13. Kennedy DJ, Greenberg RN, Dunn JA, Abernathy R, Ryerse JS, Guerrant RL. Effects of *Escherichia coli* heat-stable enterotoxin

STb on intestines of mice, rats, rabbits, and piglets. *Infect Immun* 1984;46:639–643.

14. Kupersztoch YM, Tachias K, Moomaw CR, et al. Secretion of methanol-insoluble heat-stable enterotoxin (ST_B): energy-and secA-dependent conversion of Pre-ST_B to an intermediate indistinguishable from the extracellular toxin. *J Bacteriol* 1990; 172(5):2427–2432.

15. Whipp SC. Protease degradation of *Escherichia coli* heat stable, mouse negative, pig positive enterotoxin. *Infect Immun* 1987; 55:2057–2060.

16. Whipp S. Assay for enterotoxigenic *Escherichia coli* heat-stable toxin b in rats and mice. *Infect Immun* 1990;58(4):930–934.

17. Weikel CS, Tiemans K, Moseley S, Guerrant RL. Species specificity and lack of production of sTb enterotoxin by *Escherichia coli* strains isolated from humans with diarrheal illness. *Infect Immun* 1986;52:323–325.

18. Anonymous. Preliminary report: foodborne outbreak of *Escherichia coli* O157:H7 infections from hamburgers—western United States, 1993. *MMWR* 1993;42:85–86.

19. Davis M, Osaki C, Gordon D, et al. Update: multistate outbreak of *E. coli* O157:H7 infections from hamburgers—W. U.S., 1992–1993. Centers for Disease Control. *MMWR* 1993;42: 258–263.

20. MacDonald KL, Osterholm MT. The emergence of *Escherichia coli* O157:H7 infection in the United States. The changing epidemiology of foodborne disease (editorial; comment). *JAMA* 1993; 269:2264–2266.

21. Besser RE, Lett SM, Weber JT. An outbreak of diarrhea and hemolytic uremic syndrome from *Escherichia coli* O157:H7 in fresh-pressed apple cider (see comments). *JAMA* 1993;269: 2217–2220.

22. Centers for Disease Control. Emerging infectious diseases. *MMWR* 1993;42:257–263.

23. Donnenberg MS, Tackett CO, James JP. Role of the eaeA gene in experimental enteropathogenic *Escherichia coli* infection. *J Clin Invest* 1993;92:1412–1417.

24. Donnenberg MS, Tzipori S, McKee ML, O'Brien AD, Alroy J, Kaper JB. The role of *eae* gene and of enterohemorrhagic *Escherichia coli* in intimate attachment in vitro and in a pocine model. *J Clin Invest* 1993;92:1418–1424.

25. Donnenberg MS, Kaper JB. Enteropathogenic *Escherichia coli*. *Infect Immun* 1992;60:3953–3961.

26. Schoolnik GK. Intimin and the intimate attachment of bacteria to human cells [editorial; comment]. *J Clin Invest* 1993;92: 1117–1118.

27. Bhan MK, Raj P, Levine MM. Enteroaggregative *Escherichia coli* associated with persistent diarrhea in a cohort of rural children in India. *J Infect Dis* 1989;159(6):1061–1064.

28. Bhan MK, Khoshoo V, Sommerfelt H, Pushker R, Sazawal S, Srivastava R. Enteroaggregative *Escherichia coli* and *Salmonella* associated with nondysenteric persistent diarrhea. *Pediatr Infect Dis J* 1989;8:499–502.

29. Wanke CA, Schorling JB, Barrett LJ, de Souza MA, Guerrant RL. Adherence traits of *Escherichia coli*, alone and in association with other stool pathogens: potential role in pathogenesis of persistent diarrhea in an urban Brazilian slum. *Pediatr J Infect Dis* 1991;10:746–751.

30. Fang GD, Lima AM, Wanke CA, Kaper JB, Levine MM, Guer-

rant RL. HEp-2 cell-adherent *E. coli*: potential causes of persistent diarrhea of multiple genotypes and different adherence phenotypes. *Clin Res* 1991;39(2):223A.

31. Cravioto A, Tello A, Navarro A, et al. Association of *Escherichia coli* HEp-2 adherence patterns with type and duration of diarrhoea. *Lancet* 1991;337:262–264.

32. Nataro JP, Yikang D, Giron JA, Savarino SJ, Kothary MH, Hall R. Aggregative adherence fimbria I expression in enteroaggregative *Escherichia coli* requires two unlinked plasmid regions. *Infect Immun* 1993;61(3):1126–1131.

33. Savarino SJ, Fasano A, Robertson DC, Levine MM. Enteroaggregative *Escherichia coli* elaborate a heat-stable enterotoxin demonstrable in an in vitro rabbit intestinal model. *J Clin Invest* 1991;87:1450–1455.

34. Nataro JP, Levine MM, Savarino S, Losonsky G, Guers L, Tacket CO. Volunteer studies of enteroaggregative *Escherichia coli*. General Meeting *Am Soc Microbiol* Abstract B315:82.

35. Vial P, Robins-Browne R, Lior H, et al. Characterization of enteroadherent-aggregative *Escherichia coli*, a putative agent of diarrheal disease. *J Infect Dis* 1988;158:70–79.

36. Tzipori S, Montanaro J, Robins-Browne RM, Vial P, Gibson R, Levine MM. Studies with enteroaggregative *Escherichia coli* in the gnotobiotic piglet gastroenteritis model. *Infect Immun* 1992; 60:5302–5306.

37. Scotland SM, Smith HR, Said B, Willshaw GA. Cheasty T, Rowe B. Identification of enteropathogenic *Escherichia coli* isolated in Britain as enteroaggregative or as members of a subclass of attaching-and-effacing *E. coli* not hybridising with the EPEC adherence-factor probe. *J Med Microbiol* 1991;35:278–283.

38. Enslava C, Villaseca J, Morales R, Navarro A, Cravioto A. Identification of a protein with toxigenic activity produced by aggregative *Escherichia coli*, General Meeting *Am Soc Microbiol* Abstract B105:44.

39. Benz I, Schmidt MA. Isolation and serologic characterization of AIDA-I, the adhesin mediating the diffuse adherence phenotype of the diarrhea-associated *Escherichia coli* strain 2787 (O126:H27). *Infect Immun* 1992;60(1):13–18.

40. Baqul AH, Sack RB, Black RE, et al. Enteropathogens associated with acute and persistent diarrhea in Bangladeshi children <5 years of age. *J Infect Dis* 1992;166:792–796.

41. Wanke C, Guerrant RL. Small bowel colonization alone is a cuase of diarrhea: a rabbit model. *Infect Immun* 1987;55: 1924–1926.

42. Schlager TA, Wanke CA, Guerrant RL. Net fluid secretion and impaired villous function induced by colonization of the small intestine by nontoxigenic colonizing *Escherichia coli*. *Infect Immun* 1990;58:1337–1343.

43. Svanborg C, Agace W, Hedges S, Svensson M. Bacterial adherence and mucosal inflammation in the bowel and the urinary tract. *Scand J Urol Nephrol* (Suppl) 1992;142:54.

44. Svanborg Eden C, Engberg I, Hedges S. Consequences of bacterial attachment in the urinary tract. *Biochem Soc Trans* 1989; 17:464–466.

45. Svanborg-Eden C, Hausson S, Jodal U, et al. Host–parasite interaction in the urinary tract. *J Infect Dis* 1988;157(3):421–426.

46. Hedges S, Svensson M, Svanborg C. Interleukin-6 response of epithelial cell lines to bacterial stimulation in vitro. *Infect Immun* 1992;60:1295–1301.

Infections of the Gastrointestinal Tract,
edited by M. J. Blaser, P. D. Smith, J. I. Ravdin,
H. B. Greenberg, and R. L. Guerrant
Raven Press, Ltd., New York © 1995.

CHAPTER **49**

Enterotoxigenic *Escherichia coli*

Mitchell B. Cohen and Ralph A. Giannella

Enterotoxigenic *Escherichia coli* (ETEC) are an important worldwide cause of diarrheal disease in humans and domestic animals. These organisms cause intestinal secretion by elaborating enterotoxin(s) without invading or damaging intestinal epithelial cells. Characteristically these organisms elaborate one or more enterotoxins that are either heat-stable (ST) or heat-labile (LT).

The ST group can be further subdivided into two categories. The first class of toxins are the STa (or STI) family. These are small methanol-soluble peptides that activate a transmembrane guanylate cyclase and lead to intestinal secretion. STa can also be abbreviated STp or STh to indicate strains of porcine or human origin. The second subset is designated STb (or STII). These toxins are methanol-insoluble and do not activate guanylate cyclase. However, they also cause intestinal secretion, most commonly in pigs.

The LT group can also be further subdivided. LT-I binds to a GM1 ganglioside receptor, activates adenylate cyclase, and is neutralized by antiserum to cholera toxin (CT). LT-I can also be designated LTp or LTh to indicate strains of porcine or human origin. LT-II, which was originally isolated from water buffalo, does not bind to a GM1 ganglioside and is not neutralized by anticholera toxin antisera. The LT-II toxins have been further categorized into LT-IIa and LT-IIb on the basis of chemical and antigenic properties.

ETEC also possess fimbrial attachments that enable these organisms to come in close contact with intestinal receptors for the elaborated enterotoxins. These proteinaceous structures on the surface of ETEC are also called colonization factor antigens (CFAs) (Fig. 1); they are almost always encoded by plasmids that also encode for ST and/or LT.

In this chapter we will review the history, epidemiology, pathogenesis, clinical features, treatment, and prevention of ETEC infections.

M. B. Cohen: Division of Pediatric Gastroenterology, Children's Hospital Medical Center, Cincinnati, Ohio 45229.

R. A. Giannella: Division of Digestive Diseases, University of Cincinnati, Ohio 25267.

HISTORY

The toxin-producing potential of *E. coli* was first discovered in the 1960s (2,3). Taylor and coworkers reported that certain *E. coli* isolated from children with diarrhea caused secretion in a ligated rabbit intestinal loop model (3). This was in contrast to strains that were isolated from the stools of healthy infants and urinary tract isolates of *E. coli* that did not cause secretion. Similar to cholera-producing organisms, the products of chloroform-inactivated ETEC were also found to provoke intestinal secretion thereby suggesting the presence of an enterotoxin (2).

The clinical importance of human infection with ETEC was outlined in the 1970s by investigators in Calcutta who identified these organisms as a major cause of endemic diarrhea (4,5). At approximately the same time, ETEC were also shown to be a major cause of diarrhea in swine (6,7).

EPIDEMIOLOGY

Although diarrheal disease caused by ETEC is usually less severe than that caused by cholera, ETEC-associated morbidity and mortality probably exceed that of cholera on a worldwide basis because of the high frequency of ETEC infection. The incidence of ETEC infection is greater than or comparable to that of rotavirus and these two organisms are the predominant cause of dehydrating diarrheal disease throughout the developing world (8–11). In developing countries, children under 2 or 3 years of age experience two to three episodes of diarrhea a year due to infections with ETEC; this represents >25% of all diarrheal illness (10,11). The incidence of ETEC infections then declines rapidly to reach a constant lower level of infection seen in adults (10,11).

In Naples, Italy, where sanitation conditions may be intermediate between developed and developing countries, ETEC infection accounts for approximately 5.4% of episodes of acute diarrhea (12). In contrast, in the United States, despite initial reports that ETEC were responsible

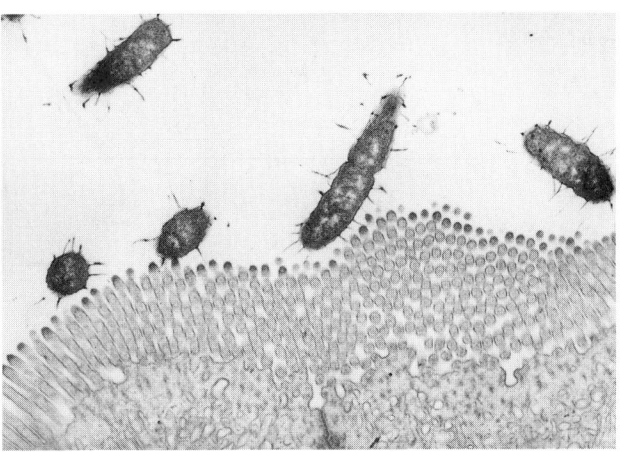

FIG. 1. Attachment of enterotoxigenic *Escherichia coli* (ETEC). Electron micrograph of porcine small intestine. ETEC must express both virulence factors of adherence and toxin elaboration to be fully pathogenic. Specific attachment factors (fimbriae or colony factory antigens) permit colonization of the intestine by ETEC. Unlike enteropathogenic *E. coli,* these organisms do not alter the architecture of the brush border membrane during attachment. (From ref. 1, with permission.)

for a significant portion of severe childhood diarrheal disease in Chicago (13), ETEC have not been isolated in prospective studies of urban childhood diarrhea in Boston and Baltimore (14,15). Several factors may explain the rarity of ETEC-mediated diarrhea in the United States: a large dose (10^8 organisms) is required for clinical illness (16,17), ETEC are not excreted during convalescence (18–20), and ETEC are not prevalent in the environment in developed countries (21,22). Host immunity probably does not play a significant factor in the rarity of ETEC infection in developed countries since ETEC are a common cause of diarrhea in adults from developed areas who visit endemic areas (18,23,24). In fact, in many studies, ETEC are the leading cause of traveler's diarrhea; in Kenya (25) and Mexico City (23) approximately three quarters of traveler's diarrhea in adults was due to ETEC infection. In addition, ETEC have been identified as an important cause of "traveler's diarrhea" in soldiers deployed to the Middle East (26,27).

ETEC are acquired by ingestion of contaminated water and food. In endemic areas, ETEC infection is more prominent in the wet season (28,29), possibly due to increased contamination of water sources due to runoff. ETEC have been isolated from water supplies in endemic areas including the White River Apache Reservation (30), and both river (29) and tank water (31) in Bangladesh. Children are at increased risk for ETEC infection at the time of weaning. More than 40% of food (milk, rice, water) fed to weaning children in Bangladesh has been shown to be contaminated with ETEC (28). In a prospective study involving physicians and their families attending a conference in Mexico, food and raw salad in particular were implicated in the transmission of disease (23). Although uncommon, foodborne and waterborne outbreaks have also been reported in the United States (19,32).

PATHOGENESIS

In order to be fully pathogenic, enterotoxigenic *E. coli* must express both the virulence factors of adherence and enterotoxin elaboration. The bacteria first colonize the small intestine with the aid of specific CFA attachment factors. Unlike enteropathogenic *E. coli,* ETEC do not alter the ultrastructure of the brush border membrane of the enterocyte during attachment (Fig. 1). Once these organisms colonize the small intestine, they elaborate ST and/or LT. Different combinations of these pathogenic factors probably account in part for the spectrum of illness associated with ETEC infection.

Adherence Factors and Serotypes

As is the case for the other categories of diarrheagenic *E. coli,* ETEC organisms generally belong to restricted serogroups (33). Although many other serotypes can be pathogenic, the major O serogroups associated with ETEC organisms are shown in Table 1. The serogrouping of these bacteria have allowed epidemiological investigation of ETEC infection. While serotyping alone does not identify a strain as toxigenic, serogrouping has helped to elucidate the pathogenesis of ETEC infection since the major O serogroups are also associated with certain fimbrial colonization factors (33). In the presence of mannose, most fimbrial antigens cause hemagglutination of various erythrocytes; this feature allows another classification schema based on the patterns of hemagglutination produced (34–37).

Initially two colonization factor antigens, CFA/I and CFA/II, were described for ETEC isolated from humans (34,35). The CFA/II antigens have been further divided into a family of three related coli surface factors (CS1–3) that are all expressed on the same plasmid genes (38). CS1 and CS2 are similar to CFA/I; they are well-ordered, rigid, 6- to 7-nm diameter, proteinaceous structures (39,40). CS3 is present in nearly all strains of certain serogroups, either alone or in combination with CS1 or CS2 (37). CS3, unlike CFA/I, CS1, and CS2, is a thin, flexible, 2- to 3-nm diameter, fibrillar structure (41,42). The plasmids that encode CFA/I and CFA/II often, but not always, encode ST and/or LT as well. More recently, several other colonization factor fimbriae have been identified, including CFA/III and a second family of antigens CFA/IV that includes CS4, CS5, and CS6 (33,43–45). CFA/III, CS4, and CS5 are rod-like fimbriae (45), whereas CS5 appears to be composed of two fine fibrils arranged in a double helix. These two antigens, similar to CFA/I

TABLE 1. *O serogroups associated with ETEC*

O6	O27	O850	O148
O8	O63	O115	O153
O15	O78	O128ac	O159
O20	O80	O139	O167
O25			

Modified from ref. 33.

and CFA/II, all promote adherence of ETEC to human small intestinal enterocytes and cultured human intestinal mucosa (46). In contrast, CS6 was difficult to characterize morphologically; furthermore, organisms that expressed only CS6, and no other CFA, were nonadherent (45). Most but not all traditional ETEC serogroups have been associated with at least one CFA (45,47–49). Consequently, a number of investigators have used the expression of CFA in immunization strategies to evoke a protective antibody response against ETEC. It is clear that an effective vaccine based on CFA will require multiple protective antigens.

Enterotoxins

By definition, ETEC elaborate ST and/or LT. Although many ETEC organisms elaborate both ST and LT, we will discuss these two groups separately for purposes of clarity.

STa

Structure and Physicochemical Characteristics

The heat-stable toxins are further divided into two major types: the STa (or STI) family and STb (or STII). The amino acid structure of the STa family of toxins is shown in Figure 2. An 18-amino-acid toxin of porcine origin is often described as STp. A 19-amino-acid toxin of human origin is often described as STh. These STa enterotoxins are small (MW approximately 2000) heat- and acid-stable toxins with no subunit structure containing three disulfide bonds that are important for biological activity. The carboxyl terminal amino acids of these two toxins are highly conserved with differences between them occurring largely in the amino terminus. Biological activity of these toxins is predominantly confined to the carboxyl terminus since peptides lacking the amino terminal four amino acids possess full, or nearly full, biological and immunological activity (60–62).

Although naturally occurring *E. coli* STa peptides purified from human, bovine, and porcine isolates are either 18 or 19 amino acids (50–52,63–65), the bacterial transposon that encodes for STa has an open reading frame that encodes for a pre-propeptide of 72 amino acids (66). This gene product is shortened by a combination of posttranslational removal of a hydrophobic leader sequence in the bacterial periplasm and further extracellular processing of the propeptide to yield a smaller mature toxin (66–68). In addition, the location of the STa gene on a transposon may explain the heterogeneity of ST plasmids. The family of STa peptides shares certain physicochemical properties presumably engendered by their primary and secondary structures (69,70): (a) they retain full biological activity when heated to 60°C for several hours or 100°C for 15 min; (b) they are stable in acid and not denatured by detergents; (c) they are soluble in water and, unlike STb, are soluble in methanol; (d) they are resistant to many proteases (pronase, trypsin, chymotrypsin) (71,72) but possibly sensitive to β-chymotrypsin (73); and (e) disruption of disulfide bonds destroys their biological activity (69). Several laboratories (74–76) have presented data that are consistent with a model of STa in which there is linkage of disulfide bonds between Cys-5/Cys-10, Cys-6/Cys-14, and Cys-9/Cys-17. In addition, substitution of individual amino acids can have a dramatic effect on the biochemical and pharmacological properties of STa further illustrating the importance of the primary and secondary structure of this peptide (62,77,78).

Biologic Actions

STa, like cholera toxin and LT, causes fluid and electrolyte secretion. However, as shown in Table 2, they differ in their mechanism of action. The biological effect of cholera toxin and LT has a lag phase, is irreversible, and is mediated by activation of adenylate cyclase. In contrast, STa has an immediate onset of action, is reversible, and activates guanylate cyclase (71,80–84).

An overall schema of the mechanism of action of STa is shown in Fig. 3. There is strong evidence that the action

	Amino terminus	Carboxyl terminus
E. coli STp		N–T–F–Y–**C–C–E–L–C–C–N–P–A–C**–A–**G–C**–Y
E. coli STh		N–S–S–N–Y–**C–C–E–L–C–C–N–P–A–C**–T–**G–C**–Y
Citrobacter freundi ST		N–T–T–Y–**C–C–E–L–C–C–N–P–A–C**–A–**G–C**
Y. enterocolitica ST		.....–D–**C–C**–D–Y–**C–C–N–P–A–C**–A–**G–C**
V. cholerae non-01 ST		–**D–C–C–E**–I–**C–C–N–P–A–C**–F–**G–C**–L–N
E. coli EAST–1		....A–S–S–Y–A–S–**C**–I–W–**C**–T– - - –T–**A–C**–A–S–**C**–H–G....
Guanylin		P–N–T–**C**–E–I–**C**–A–Y–A–**A–C**–T–**G–C**

FIG. 2. Comparison of the amino acid sequence of STp (50–52), STh (53), *Citrobacter freundi* ST (54) *Y. enterocolitica* ST (55), *V. cholerae* non-O1 ST (56,57), *E. coli* EAST-1 (58), and guanylin (59). Conserved amino acid sequences are highlighted in bold. STp (porcine) and STh (human) are both forms of *E. coli* STa.

TABLE 2. *Comparison of heat-labile and heat-stable toxins using cholera toxin and* Escherichia coli *STa as prototypes*

	Heat-labile toxin (Cholera toxin)	Heat-stable toxin (*Escherichia coli* STa)
Onset	Lag phase ≈ 1 hr	Rapid, maximal in 5 min
Duration	Prolonged	Short-lived, reversible
Molecular weight	86,000	≈2000
Antigenic	Yes	Haptenic
Tissue specificity	No	Relatively specific
Mechanism		
Toxin internalization required	Yes	No
Cytosolic factors required	Yes	No
Target enzyme	Adenylate cyclase	Guanylate cyclase
Covalent modification of target enzyme	Yes	No

From ref. 79, with permission.

of STa is mediated by increased concentration of cyclic GMP. In both rabbit ileum and T84 cells mounted in the Ussing chamber, the time course for STa-induced elevation of cyclic GMP concentration was identical to the onset of secretion measured by a rise in short circuit current (Isc) (80,85). In the suckling mouse bioassay, the time course of intestinal fluid accumulation was also immediately preceded by an increase in tissue levels of cyclic GMP (86,87). In addition, in this bioassay, the permeable cyclic GMP analog, 8-bromocyclic GMP, was able to stimulate fluid secretion (86,88). Initially, the intestinal receptor for STa was thought to be separate from but tightly coupled to particulate cyclase (89–91). Recently, the intestinal receptor for STa has been shown to be a particulate guanylate cyclase termed GC-C in the rat and STaR in the human (84,92–94). Incubation of STa with GC-C– or STaR–transfected COS cells resulted in a dose-dependent increase in the level of intracellular cGMP (84,92,94,95).

Despite the persuasive evidence that STa activates guanylate cyclase, there is also good evidence that alternate pathways, including protein kinase C, participate in

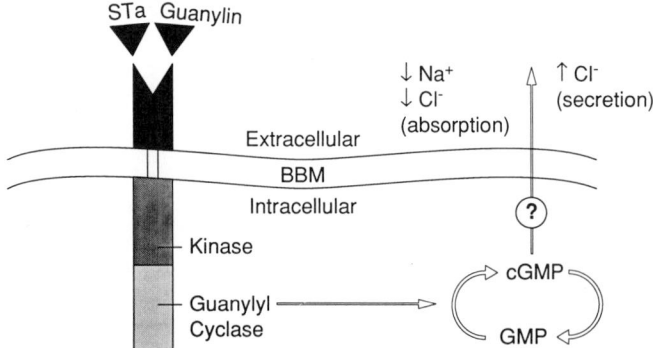

FIG. 3. Outline of the overall schema of action of STa. STa or guanylin, the endogenous mammalian homolog, binds to a receptor that includes extracellular, transmembrane, putative kinase, and guanyl cyclase domains. This results in increased intracellular levels of cyclic GMP, which leads to decreased absorption of sodium and increased chloride secretion.

the cyclic GMP response engendered by STa (96–98). Carbachol, a cholinergic agent, also acts synergistically with STa to produce an Isc response in T84 cells, suggesting that multiple intracellular mediators may influence the ability of STa to cause intestinal secretion (99). Other cofactors, including adenine nucleotides, may potentiate the action of STa on GC-C (95,100–102). ATP may interact directly with GC-C, stabilizing its active conformation (103).

STa has a dual effect on chloride transport, both reducing the mucosal to serosal flux and increasing the serosal to mucosal flux of chloride (80). STa also reduces the mucosal to serosal flux of sodium (104). The observation that both sodium and chloride flux from mucosa to serosa are inhibited suggests that, similar to theophylline, which increases cyclic AMP, STa inhibits neutral Na^+Cl^- absorption. The effects of STa and theophylline on neutral Na^+Cl^- absorption are equal and not additive suggesting a final common pathway.

Both the T84 and the Caco-2 human colonic carcinoma cell lines have proved useful in the study of the biological actions of STa. ETEC adhere to Caco-2 cells (105,106) and STa activates guanylate cyclase (GC-C) in both of these cell lines (72,94,107). T84 cells resemble small intestinal crypt epithelium and secrete Cl^- in response to various secretagogues (108–111). STa stimulates Cl^- secretion across T84 monolayers by elevating cyclic GMP and activating apical Cl^- and basolateral K^+ channels (85). It is thought that this cyclic GMP–mediated channel activation is similar to the cyclic AMP–mediated channel activation of Cl^- secretion (85). However, in contrast to the similar magnitude of effect by STa and theophylline on neutral chloride absorption, STa is less potent than cyclic AMP in stimulating electrogenic chloride secretion (85).

Furthermore, the *in vivo* STa–enterocyte interaction is likely to be at least as important on villus (absorptive) as on crypt (secretory) cells. Several additional lines of evidence are consistent with this interpretation: (a) Villus cells bind more STa and have more STa stimulatable guanylate cyclase activity (71,112–114). (b) Caco-2 cells, which spontaneously differentiate to resemble mature small intestinal enterocytes, express four- to fivefold greater STa binding and guanylate cyclase activity as they differentiate (94,107). (c) In the rat small intestine, the STa receptor GC-C is predominantly, if not exclusively, expressed in villus rather than crypt cells in jejunum and ileum (114). (d) Lastly, the rat IEC-6 crypt cell line does not express GC-C and STa does not activate guanylate cyclase in these cells (94). Although these observations suggest that STa-mediated transport effects are predominantly via its effect on neutral chloride absorption in villus cells, recent evidence suggests that villus as well as crypt cells are capable of electrogenic chloride secretion (115).

The intermediate steps by which cyclic GMP leads to these transport alterations are not known. Several studies have demonstrated STa stimulation of a "particulate" (116), or cyclic GMP–dependent (117–119), or cyclic AMP–dependent protein kinase (120). In addition, protein kinase inhibitors block the fluid accumulation induced by STa (121) and inhibit STa-mediated phosphorylation of rat brush border membrane proteins (122). These intracellular signaling mechanisms are discussed in the chapter by Crowe and Powell. Furthermore, although it is traditionally thought that enterotoxins do not alter the cytoskeletal architecture, recent data demonstrated that exposure of T84 cells to STa results in functional rearrangement of basolateral F-actin filaments (123,124), which, if inhibited, results in STa stimulated Na^+-K^+-$2Cl^-$ cotransport activity being reduced by approximately 60% (123). This suggests that the ability of STa to elicit a cytoskeletal rearrangement is an important intermediate in STa-induced electrogenic Cl^- secretion.

Interaction with Receptors

A cDNA encoding a protein with STa binding properties and guanylate cyclase activity was recently cloned by Schulz et al. (84) from rat, and by several groups from human (92–94) intestine. In the rat, the receptor has been designated GC-C, to indicate its similarity to the other particulate guanylate cyclases (GC-A, GC-B) that bind atrial natriuretic peptides (84,125). In the human, the homologous receptor has been designated STaR (92,94). Each cDNA encodes a 121-kDa transmembrane guanylate cyclase containing three domains: an extracellular domain linked through a single transmembrane region to an intracellular protein kinase–like region and a guanylyl cyclase catalytic domain (84) (Fig. 3). The intracellular portion of GC-C shows considerable homology to other particulate guanylate cyclases (GC-A, GC-B), but the extracellular domain has little amino acid similarity and does not bind the natriuretic peptide ligands (84). However, it is noteworthy that although the human and rat clones are considered homologs, there is only 70% amino acid homology in the extracellular putative binding domain between the human and rat clones.

Kinetic measurements of STa binding to recombinant cell lines (293-STaR) gives an association constant of 10^8 L/mol (84,92,94). However, in all transfected cell lines studied, there appears to be a discrepancy between the dose of STa required for inhibition of radiolabeled STa binding and STa-induced stimulation of guanylate cyclase activity. While the reasons for this discrepancy are not clear, it is probable that STa binding is necessary but not uniquely sufficient for guanylate cyclase activation and that some other event, e.g., receptor aggregation or receptor phosphorylation, is required for full expression of guanylate cyclase activity.

While the biological action of STa is rapidly and completely reversible (81,82), it has not been possible to demonstrate the reversibility of STa binding as clearly. A number of studies have demonstrated partial (>50%) reversibility of STa binding to rat intestinal cells and membranes (71,83,126) as well as T84 cells (72), whereas others have found minimal (2–5%) dissociation (113). The discrepancy between the complete reversibility of secretion and the incomplete reversibility of binding could be due to a dynamic interaction between STa and its receptor after binding occurs.

In the rat, the number of STa receptors and their affinity for STa are similar in jejunum and ileum (71). In the small intestine, STa receptors are primarily if not exclusively localized to the brush border membrane (BBM) rather than the basolateral membrane (BLM) (72). Furthermore, binding studies (113,114,127) as well as northern analysis and *in situ* hybridization studies (114) demonstrate that GC-C is localized to small intestinal villus rather than crypt epithelial cells. While it is thought that the principal site of action of bacterial enterotoxins is in the small intestine, recent studies in children have also demonstrated that both STa binding activity and STa-responsive guanyl cyclase are present in the human colon (128,129). In the rat, the number of receptors per colonocyte is even greater than the number of receptors per small bowel enterocyte (81). Furthermore, there may be site-specific effects of STa within the colon (130).

Immature humans and other animals are at increased risk for STa-mediated diarrheal disease. Immune mechanisms may play a major role in this increased susceptibility. In addition, there is increased age-specific colonization of the intestinal epithelium by piliated ETEC in pigs, calves, and mice (131,132). It is also likely that the number of intestinal STa receptors plays a role in the severity of STa-mediated diarrheal disease. For example, there is an absence of ST receptors in piglets that are refractory to the experimental induction of STa-mediated diarrhea (133). Some investigators have shown greater STa receptor density in the immature compared with the adult intestine of the rat, pig, and human (128,134–136). Other investigators have failed to show increased guanylate cyclase activation in the immature pig (137–139). However, the experimental design of these studies has not been identical. Furthermore, different investigators have shown age-dependent changes in patterns of affinity labeling of STa receptors (136,138).

The amino acid sequence of the STaR predicted by the cloned cDNA is 121 kDa with eight potential glycosylation sites (92). In both Caco-2 cells and human intestine crosslinking of radiolabeled STa results in a protein of 140–165 kDa (92,107). It is likely that differences between the predicted size of this protein and the size observed by crosslinking represent the addition of carbohydrate moieties as well as the additional 2 kDa of crosslinked STa. In addition, several smaller proteins are also consistently crosslinked to ^{125}I-STa (92,107). These proteins may represent degradation products of the larger STaR or other receptors for STa. Similarly, in the rat, a protein of approximately 120 kDa is seen with photoaffinity crosslinking (140). However, various studies have reported crosslinking of radiolabeled STa to several bands of 54–80 kDa (75,91,140,141). Recently, a 74-kDa STa-binding protein was affinity-purified from rat intestine (142,143). This protein, which could not be tested for guanylate cyclase activity, could represent either a novel STa receptor or a proteolytically cleaved portion of the extracellular domain of the larger (121-kDa) guanylate cyclase receptor. In addition, as suggested by deSauvage et al. (95), the occurrence of proteolytic receptor degradation could account for the earlier identification of separable STa-binding proteins and guanylate cyclase activity. In contrast to these observations, when immunopurified GC-C, stabilized with ATP and bovine serum albumin, was analyzed by sodium dodecyl sulfate–polyacrylamide gel electrophoresis (SDS-PAGE) under nonreducing conditions, in addition to the expected 120- to 130-kDa band, proteins with almost twice the molecular mass (220 and 245 kDa) of the monomer were demonstrated, suggesting that GC-C may also exist as a dimer (103).

Inactivation by Intestinal Receptor

Because sustained STa-induced secretion requires continuous receptor occupancy, diminishing the supply of biologically active toxin by toxin inactivation could be a mechanism by which the host limits the secretory response to STa (144). We have demonstrated that in the adult rat jejunum there is inactivation of STa and coordinate cessation of secretion (73). Although toxin modification occurred after exposure to luminal fluid, pancreatic fluid, and jejunal brush border membranes, a completely inactive toxin species was generated only after incubation with jejunal organ culture slices (73). Toxin inactivation was greater in the adult than in the immature rat suggesting that this mechanism plays a role in the increased response and sensitivity observed to STa in the immature jejunum.

Extraintestinal Receptors for STa

In contrast to cholera toxin, the effects of STa are relatively specific to the small and large intestine. Initial studies of the tissue specificity of the STa receptor in the rat demonstrated no STa receptor activity in the lung, liver, brain, heart, pancreas, and gastric antrum (88,145). Recent data demonstrate low levels of GC-C expression in rat adrenal gland, testis, liver, and placenta (146,147). Maximal expression of GC-C in the rat liver occurs in the perinatal period. The presence of GC-C in multiple tissues is analogous to the tissue distribution of other members of the guanylate cyclase family. Surprisingly, there is no evidence of GC-C expression in the kidney (146,147), an organ with structural and enzymatic homology to the intestine and from which an endogenous ligand for GC-C was recently isolated (59). Furthermore, STa binding also

occurs in the opossum kidney (148) and the OK cell line derived from opossum kidney (149). The function of the STa receptor in these tissues and cell lines is uncertain although it is possible that these extraintestinal receptors bind an endogenous peptide with some homology to STa.

We recently demonstrated expression of GC-C mRNA in the regenerating rat liver following either partial hepatectomy or CCl_4-induced hepatic necrosis (150). We have also shown that GC-C mRNA expression occurred in association with an acute phase reaction (150). Coordinate with the expression of GC-C mRNA, there was upregulation of radiolabeled STa binding to liver plasma membranes. Maximal binding occurred in preparations enriched for the canalicular domain (150). Although the function of GC-C in the liver is unknown, localization to the canalicular domain would be consistent with a role for GC-C in hepatic chloride secretion.

STa binding has also been demonstrated in rat basophilic leukemia cells (151); toxin binding to these cells results in histamine and intracellular calcium release (152). However, in contrast to the intestinal STa receptor, the STa-induced increase in cyclic GMP concentration is slow (20–30 min) and modest (less than twofold) (151).

Assays

Three whole-animal models have been used to detect STa. Initially, a rabbit ileal loop assay was performed (153), but this was replaced by a standardized suckling mouse bioassay (154,155). The suckling mouse assay tests for fluid accumulation in the intestine of newborn (1–4 days old) Swiss CD4 mice after percutaneous injection of culture supernatants from E. coli colonies isolated from fecal specimens (73,155). While this assay is reliable and reproducible, it is cumbersome, labor-intensive, and requires large numbers of suckling mice. A guinea pig ileal loop assay for ST was also described (156). This assay uses an intestinal dilation index to measure the secretory response, and compared to the suckling mouse assay a much larger minimum effective dose is required for STa. Furthermore, both STa and STb cause a positive assay.

Another bioassay was recently used by Currie and colleagues (59). This assay relies on the observation that STa activates particulate guanylate cyclase in intestinal cell tissue culture lines. A 30,000- to 100,000-fold increase in cGMP concentrations was seen in the T84 cell line after the addition of STa.

A number of radioimmunoassays have been developed to detect STa producing organisms (157,158). Several enzyme-linked immunosorbent assays (ELISA) using anti-STa antibody have shown complete correlation with the suckling mouse assay and radioimmunoassay (159–161). One of these assays is commercially available (161).

For mass screening approaches to detect STa-producing organisms, the best system has been the use of gene probe assays and the colony blot approach to detect one or more of the heat-stable enterotoxins (162–164). These assays are based on the cloned genes for STh and STp. There is a positive predictive value of greater than 95% when comparing alkaline phosphatase conjugated oligonucleotide probes, ^{32}P-labeled oligonucleotide probes, and/or cloned digoxigenin or ^{32}P-labeled polynucleotide probes with the suckling mouse bioassay (165). Commercial DNA hybridization assay kits are available (165,166). Trivalent probes that detect both heat-stable toxins and heat-labile toxins have also been described (167,168). Lastly, a combination of immunomagnetic separation of pili-expressing *E. coli* and a nested colorimetric polymerase chain reaction (PCR) was shown to identify genes encoding the heat-stable enterotoxin in porcine fecal specimens (169).

Related Bacterial Toxins

Other organisms that elaborate highly homologous heat-stable enterotoxins include *Y. enterocolitica* (55,170), *Citrobacter freundi* (54), and non-O1 vibrios (56,57). These enterotoxins, whose structure is shown in Fig. 2, seem to act in a manner similar to that of *E. coli* STa. There is direct evidence of interspecies transfer of the ST plasmid to other non–*E. coli* bacterial strains (171).

In addition, enteroaggregative *E. coli* were recently described to produce a low molecular weight, heat-stable enterotoxin that has been named EAST-1 (58,172). Enteroaggregative *E. coli* have been epidemiologically associated with infantile diarrhea in rural Chile (173) and with persistent diarrhea in children in India (174), Mexico (175) and Brazil (176). Other studies have shown no difference in the colonization by enteroaggregative *E. coli* from controls (177–180). The structural gene for EAST-1 shows significant homology with the enterotoxic domain of STa. However, unlike STa, which requires six cysteines and three disulfide linkages for full biological activity, EAST-1 contains four cysteine residues. Interestingly, this is similar to guanylin (*vide infra*), an endogenous ligand for the STa receptor that also contains four cysteines (59).

Endogenous Mammalian Ligands

An endogenous ligand that binds to and activates GC-C, termed guanylin, was recently isolated from rat intestine (59). It is composed of 15 amino acids (Fig. 2) and has approximately 50% homology to STa (59). The peptide is only biologically active when the first and third cysteines and the second and fourth cysteines are disulfide-bonded. Guanylin was found in human, rat, and mouse intestine (59,148,181) and a cDNA encoding a larger 115-amino-acid pre-prohormone was identified in each species (146,181–184). In the intestine, guanylin expression is greatest in the colon and ileum and less in the jejunum; there is no expression in the stomach. Expression of guanylin mRNA in the colon is limited to the superficial epithelial cells (185,186); in the ileum, guanylin is primarily expressed in villous enterocytes (186). It is therefore likely that guanylin is expressed in the same or near-neighbor enterocytes that express GC-C. Guanylin mRNA is also expressed in low levels in the adrenal, kidney, and uterus/oviduct of rat (146), and a larger form (10.3 kDa)

of circulating guanylin was identified in the blood of renal failure patients (187).

While guanylin interacts with GC-C and causes an increase in cyclic GMP concentration and Isc in the intestine (188), it is approximately 20-fold less potent than STa. This may reflect the existence of another receptor, more specific for guanylin. While it is thought that this ligand plays a role in modulating fluid and electrolyte flux in the intestine, this hypothesis has not yet been proven. Furthermore, there is a possibility that guanylin modulates other functions in the intestine as a result of increased intracellular levels of cyclic GMP (189).

STb

Moon and Whipp (190) identified a second type of heat-stable enterotoxin elaborated by diarrheagenic *E. coli*. This toxin, termed STb or STII, causes secretion in weaned pigs. STb is unlike STa in that STb is methanol-insoluble and is inactive in the suckling mouse assay (191). Although culture filtrates of STa cause no histological lesions, culture filtrates of STb result in loss of villus absorptive cells and partial atrophy (192,193). However, as shown in Table 3, both STa and STb are low molecular weight peptides that rapidly stimulate secretion (194,195). The actions of both are rapidly reversible (81,83,194).

STb was thought to cause fluid secretion only in piglets (191,194,196). Recently, Whipp demonstrated that the host response specificity of STb could be attributed to the susceptibility of STb to protease (197). Soybean trypsin inhibitor protected STb from proteolysis and resulted in positive responses of STb in intestinal segments of mice, rats, calves, and rabbits, demonstrating that the activity of STb is not species specific (197–199).

The gene for STb encodes a 71-amino-acid prohormone with a 32-amino-acid leader sequence (200,201). This is consistent with the observation that the toxin is found in the bacterial periplasm as an 8.1-kDa precursor, which is converted to a 5.2-kDa mature, active form that is secreted (202). Mature STb was recently purified and is composed of 48-amino-acid residues that contain two disulfide bonds (203,204). However, there is no amino acid homology with STa; antisera raised against each of these toxins do not recognize the other (158,205).

Exposure of pig intestine mounted in an Ussing chamber to STb results in an increase in Isc (195), but unlike STa there is no change in neutral sodium and chloride absorption or electrogenic chloride secretion (195). STb does effect the calculated net residual ion flux. This likely represents bicarbonate secretion and is consistent with the observation that STb raises luminal pH and the bicarbonate content of intestinal secretion *in vivo* (195). STb does not change cyclic AMP or cyclic GMP levels (194,206). Although initial reports suggested that the action of a crude STb is not affected by the presence of calcium ions in the bathing solution (207), more recent data demonstrate that pure STb induces a dose-dependent increase in intracellular calcium concentrations that is entirely dependent on a source of extracellular calcium (208). STb-mediated intracellular calcium elevation is not

TABLE 3. *Comparison of the properties of STa and STb*

	STa	STb
Similarities		
Rapid onset	Yes	Yes
Action reversible with rinsing	100%	≈80%
Histologic damage	No	Some
Low molecular weight	Yes	Yes
Differences		
Suckling mouse assay	Yes	No
Mechanism		
Toxin internalization required	No	?
Cytosolic factors required	No	?
Target enzyme	Guanylate cyclase	?
Intracellular messenger	Cyclic GMP	Not cyclic GMP or cyclic AMP; maybe Ca^{2+}
Covalent modification of target enzyme	No	?
Ion fluxes	Na^+, Cl^-	HCO_3

Modified from ref. 79.

inhibited by drugs that block voltage-gated calcium channels or agents that deplete and block internal calcium stores (208). These data suggest that STb opens a receptor-operated calcium channel in the plasma membrane. In addition, prostaglandins may play a role in the mechanism of STb action. The level of prostaglandin E_2 is increased in the secreted fluid accumulated as a result of STb and the prostaglandin synthesis inhibitors aspirin and indomethacin significantly reduce the response to STb (196).

Although STb is the most prevalent toxin associated with diarrheagenic *E. coli* of porcine origin (198), STb-producing *E. coli* are not thought to be a major cause of diarrheal illness in humans (209–211). However, recently STb-elaborating strains of *E. coli* have been isolated from humans with diarrhea in Canada and Japan (212,213).

Heat-Labile Toxins (LTI, LTII)

LTI is actually a family of high molecular weight proteins that are structurally and functionally similar to cholera toxin. The LTI family includes the subtypes LThI and LTpI, which designate antigenic variants of human and porcine origin (214). Checkerboard immunoblotting recently showed that there is also immunological heterogeneity within the LThI subtype (215). Similar to cholera toxin, LTI consists of a single enzymatically active (A) subunit surrounded by five binding (B) subunits (216). The mechanism of action of LTI and its relationship to cholera toxin is discussed in the chapter by Butterton and Calderwood. The deduced amino acid sequences of the A and B subunits are approximately 80% homologous between LTI and cholera toxin (217–222) and the action of LTI is neutralized by antisera against cholera toxin. Again, similar to cholera toxin, LTI induces intestinal secretion by activating adenylate cyclase in an NAD-dependent reaction (223,224). The A subunit of LTI contains an NAD binding site (225) and has structural homology to diphtheria toxin (226). However, in contrast to cholera toxin, LTI binds not only to a GM1 ganglioside receptor, but also to a 130- to 140-kDa glycoprotein receptor present on the

intestinal brush border membrane (227–232). This second binding site is 20–30 times more prevalent in intestinal brush border membranes than is the binding site for cholera toxin (230). Evidence for the full biological effectiveness of this second receptor comes from the fact that saturation of the GM1 ganglioside receptor by cholera toxin does not inhibit the secretory response to LTI in the rabbit and only partially blocks the effect of LTI in humans (229,231).

Heat-labile toxins that are not neutralized by antisera against cholera toxin are designated LTII (233). LTIIa can be distinguished from LTIIb based on antigenic determinants and chemical properties (234) and the ability to inhibit the binding of other enterotoxins to Y1 adrenal cells (235). The gene encoding the A subunit of LTIIa is 50% to 60% homologous with the corresponding genes encoding the A subunits of LThI and cholera toxin (236). However, there is no homology between the B subunits of LTIIa and LThI or cholera toxin (236). Consequently, LTIIa demonstrates binding characteristics to the glycoprotein receptor that are dissimilar to LThI or cholera toxin (237).

A number of other bacteria elaborate LT like toxins including *Klebsiella, Enterobacter, Aeromonas, hydrophila, Plesiomonas shigelloides, Campylobacter, Salmonella typhimurium,* and *Salmonella enteritidis* (238–247).

LT Assays

The two standard assays for LT are the Biken test and the Y1 adrenal cell test. In the Biken test, LT is detected by the appearance of a precipitin line between growth of the organism and antisera against LT (248,249). Although reagents for this test are commercially available, the test takes 5 days to complete (250). The standard LT tissue culture assay uses Y1 adrenal cells (251,252). The amount of LT present in a culture supernatant is titered by serial dilution to detect rounding of at least 50% of Y1 cells. Several different tests for LT using immunological methods including ELISA and passive hemagglutination have been described (253–255). However, the unavailability of reagents for these tests has limited their usefulness. More recently, an immunological assay that uses latex bead agglutination (256–258) as well as a commercially available reversed passive latex agglutination test (VET-RPLA) (259) and a staphylococcal coagglutination test (Phadebact ETEC-LT) (260) have been described. Both of the commercial tests are highly accurate (259–262). Both PCR-based assays (263) and gene probe assays for LT-producing organisms are also available (162–164, 264–266). At present all of these tests are difficult to perform in the field and are not generally available in clinical laboratories.

CLINICAL ILLNESS

Illness caused by enterotoxigenic *E. coli* is characterized by watery diarrhea. The spectrum of illness ranges from very mild to dehydrating cholera-like purging. In travelers, ETEC disease often occurs between 5 and 15 days after arrival in an endemic area, with an incubation period of 14–50 hr (267). Infection with ST-producing organisms cannot be differentiated from infection with LT-producing organisms although LT/ST disease is more severe than LT disease alone (268). Stools are watery, yellow, and devoid of mucus, pus, and fecal leukocytes. The illness is most often self-limited lasting less than 5 days with few cases persisting more than 3 weeks (25,269). Abdominal pain is modest or absent and fever is usually absent.

Infection with ETEC has also been specifically associated with short- and long-term adverse nutritional consequences in infants and children. Infection with ETEC not only caused acute diarrheal disease and the interruption of normal feeding patterns, but it also resulted in diminished long-term linear growth (10,11).

TREATMENT

Most diarrheal illness due to enterotoxigenic *E. coli* does not require antibiotic treatment since the illness is short-lived and oral rehydration therapy is safe, effective, and commercially available. The use of oral rehydration solutions containing between 35 and 90 meq sodium/L, with added glucose, potassium, and bicarbonate, has proven remarkably effective in underdeveloped countries and has prompted their use in developed countries as well (270). Three placebo-controlled studies have evaluated whether antibiotics are efficacious in the treatment of ETEC infection (268,271,272). Merson and coworkers showed that tetracycline slightly shortened the duration of diarrhea in adults with naturally acquired infection (268). Black and coworkers showed that early therapy (after the third loose stool) with trimethoprim-sulfamethoxazole significantly decreased the duration of diarrhea and the fecal excretion of enterotoxigenic *E. coli* in young adult volunteers who were experimentally infected with an LT/ST-producing strain (271). DuPont and coworkers demonstrated that trimethoprim-sulfamethoxazole and trimetho-

prim alone significantly reduced the duration of diarrhea, the number of loose stools, and the fecal excretion of enterotoxigenic *E. coli* in college students from the United States with natural infection acquired while in Mexico (272). However, since these studies were reported, there has been increasing resistance of *E. coli* to antimicrobials in developing countries (273,274).

Pepto-bismol and its active ingredient, bismuth subsalicylate, significantly inhibit fluid accumulation in experimental animals inoculated with *E. coli* producing ST, LT, or both (275); clinical studies with Pepto-bismol have also shown effectiveness in treating ETEC diarrhea (276). A number of studies have shown efficacy of bismuth subsalicylate, trimethoprim-sulfamethoxazole, and ciprofloxacin to prevent or treat traveler's diarrhea, which is commonly caused by ETEC (272,277,278).

Antidiarrheal drugs are generally not used in the treatment of infants with acute diarrhea. In adults, the use of antidiarrheal drugs such as loperamide or diphenoxylate dihydrochloride with atropine (Lomotil) decreases the stool volume and provide symptomatic relief. Therapy is more thoroughly discussed in the chapter by Snyder.

VACCINES

A number of approaches have been tried to develop effective vaccines against ETEC. These approaches have used nonliving oral antigens as well as live oral vaccines designed to stimulate anticolonization immunity and/or antitoxic immunity (279). The major problem associated with developing an efficacious vaccine against ETEC is the fact that ETEC are antigenically diverse, i.e., they are found in a number of O serogroups (Table 1), and they possess one of several possible CFAs. In addition, one of the important toxins they produce, ST, is not antigenic because of its small size.

One live oral vaccine approach involves the use of ETEC that express CFA but not ST or LT (279,280). A prototype vaccine was highly protective against experimental challenge with ETEC expressing the same CFA (281–283). This validates the concept but would provide immunity to only a fraction of ETEC. An ideal vaccine would contain all of the common CFA and would also contain the B subunit (immunogenic binding, nontoxic subunit) of LT and possibly an immunogenic nontoxic variant of ST and/or LT. Better understanding of the common ETEC serotypes and CFA involved in clinical infections will provide a guide to more effective candidate vaccines (27,47,48,284).

Another live oral vaccine strategy uses attenuated *S. typhi* strains that have been genetically engineered to produce the B subunit of LT and some CFA; these vaccines have been shown to be immunogenic (285,286). Nonliving oral toxoid vaccines consisting of synthetic ST linked to the B subunit of LT have also shown an immune response (287,288). Purified fimbriae have been used as vaccines but to date have not been protective against clinical infection in people possibly because of antigenic degradation in the stomach (33,280,289). New approaches using fimbrial adhesin antigens include the use of CFA encapsulated in biodegradable microspheres of poly(lactide-*co*-glycolide) (290). These microspheres protect CFA from degradation and deliver antigen to the enteric immune system (290,291). Clinical studies using these vaccines are underway. Fimbrial vaccines are routinely given parenterally to pregnant cattle, sheep, and swine to protect suckling newborn calves, lambs, and pigs against ETEC infections (292). However, the efficacy of these vaccines as well as the effect of these vaccines in selecting for novel or previously low-prevalence fimbrial antigen types has not been well studied (292). Alternative approaches using formalinized fimbriated *E. coli* and LT and ST toxoids given with killed fimbriated bacteria are also being pursued (293).

Finally the use of food substances (eggs and milk) to deliver passive protection against enteropathogens was recently explored. Oral ingestion of egg yolk immunoglobulin from hens immunized with an ETEC strain prevented diarrhea in rabbits challenged with the same strain (294,295). This leads to the speculation that hens or cows immunized with appropriate antigens may have usefulness as a source of passive immunity against ETEC.

Specific vaccine strategies are discussed more thoroughly in the chapter by Levine.

REFERENCES

1. Moon HW, Nagy B, Isaacson RE. Intestinal colonization and adhesion by enterotoxigenic *Escherichia coli*: ultrastructural observations on adherence to ileal epithelium of the pig. *J Infect Dis* 1977;136:S124–S129.
2. Taylor J, Bettelheim KA. The action of chloroform-killed suspension of enteropathogenic *Escherichia coli* on ligated rabbit-gut segments. *J Gen Microbiol* 1966;42:309–313.
3. Taylor J, Wilkins MP, Payne JM. Relation of rabbit gut reaction to enteropathogenic *Escherichia coli*. *Br J Exp Pathol* 1961;42:43–52.
4. Gorbach SL, Banwell JG, Chatterjee BD, Jacobs B, Sack RB. Acute undifferentiated human diarrhea in the tropics. I. alterations in intestinal microflora. *J Clin Invest* 1971;50:881–889.
5. Sack RB. Enterotoxigenic *Escherichia coli*: identification and characterization. *J Infect Dis* 1980;142:279–286.
6. Whipp SC, Moon HW, Lyon NC. Heat-stable *Escherichia coli* enterotoxin production in vivo. *Infect Immun* 1975;12:240–244.
7. Gyles CL. Heat labile and heat stable forms of the enterotoxin from *Escherichia coli* strains enteropathogenic for pigs. *Ann NY Acad Sci* 1971;176:314–322.
8. Sack RB. Human diarrheal disease caused by enterotoxigenic *Escherichia coli*. *Annu Rev Microbiol* 1975;29:333–353.
9. Lanata CF, Black RE, Gil A, et al. Etiologic agents in acute vs. persistent diarrhea in children under three years of age in peri-urban Lima, Peru. *Acta Paediatr* 1992;81(Suppl 381):32–38.
10. Black RE, Merson HM, Huq I, Aleim ARM, Yunus N. Incidence and severity of rotavirus and *Escherichia coli* in rural Bangladesh. *Lancet* 1981;1:141–143.
11. Black RE, Brown KH, Becker S, Abdul Alim ARM, Huq I. Longitudinal studies of infectious diseases and physical growth of children in rural Bangladesh. II. Incidence of diarrhea and association with known pathogens. *Am J Epidemiol* 1982;115:315–324.
12. Guarino A, Alessio M, Tarallo L, et al. Heat stable enterotoxin by *Escherichia coli* in acute diarrhoea. *Arch Dis Child* 1989;64:808–813.
13. Gorbach SL, Khurana CM. Toxigenic *Escherichia coli*: a cause of infantile diarrhea in Chicago. *N Engl J Med* 1972;287:791–796.
14. Echeverria P, Blacklow NR, Smith DH. Role of heat-labile toxigenic *Escherichia coli* and reovirus-like agent in diarrhea in Boston children. *Lancet* 1975;2:1113–1116.
15. Kotloff KL, Wasserman SS, Steciak JY, et al. Acute diarrhea in Baltimore children attending an outpatient clinic. *Pediatr Infect Dis J* 1988;7:753–759.
16. DuPont HL, Formal SB, Hornick RB, et al. Pathogenesis of *Escherichia coli* diarrhea. *N Engl J Med* 1971;285:1–9.
17. Levine MM, Caplan ES, Watermann D, Cash RA, Hornick RB, Snyder MJ. Diarrhea caused by *Escherichia coli* that produce only heat-stable enterotoxin. *Infect Immun* 1977;17:78–82.
18. Gorbach SL, Kean BH, Evans DG, Evan DJ Jr, Bessudo D. Traveller's diarrhea and toxigenic *Escherichia coli*. *N Engl J Med* 1975;292:933–936.
19. Rosenberg ML, Koplan JP, Wachsmuth IK, et al. Epidemic diarrhea at Crater Lake from enterotoxigenic *Escherichia coli*: a large waterborne outbreak. *Ann Intern Med* 1977;86:714–718.
20. Levine MM, Rennels MB, Cisneros L, Hughes TP, Nalin DR, Young CR. Lack of person-to-person transmission of enterotoxigenic *Escherichia coli* despite close contact. *Am J Epidemiol* 1980;111:347–355.
21. Brunton J, Hinde D, Langston C, Gross R, Rowe B, Gurwith M. Enterotoxigenic *Escherichia coli* in central Canada. *J Clin Microbiol* 1980;11:343–438.
22. Bäck E, Blomberg S, Wadstrom T. Enterotoxigenic *Escherichia coli* in Sweden. *Infection* 1977;5:2–5.
23. Merson MH, Morris GK, Sack DA, et al. Traveller's diarrhea in Mexico. A prospective study of physicians and family members attending a congress. *N Engl J Med* 1976;294:1299–1305.
24. Consensus Conference: Traveler's diarrhea. *JAMA* 1985;253:2700–2704.
25. Sack DA, Kaminsky DC, Sack RB et al. Enterotoxigenic *Escherichia coli* diarrhea of travelers: a prospective study of American Peace Corps volunteers. *Johns Hopkins Med J* 1977;141:63–70.
26. Hyams KC, Bourgeois AL, Merrell BR, et al. Diarrheal disease during Operation Desert Storm. *N Engl J Med* 1991;325:1423–1428.
27. Wolf MK, Taylor DN, Boedeker EC. Characterization of enterotoxigenic *Escherichia coli* isolated from US troops deployed to the Middle East. *J Clin Microbiol* 1993;31:851–856.
28. Black RE, Merson MH, Rahman ASMM, et al. A two year study of bacterial viral and parasitic agents associated with diarrhea in rural Bangladesh. *J Infect Dis* 1980;142:660–665.
29. Guerrant RL, Kirchhoff LV, Nations MK, et al. Prospective study of diarrhoeal illness in northeastern Brazil. *J Infect Dis* 1983;148:986–997.
30. Sack RB, Hirschorn N, Brownlee I, Cash RA, Woodward WE, Sack DA. Enterotoxigenic *Escherichia coli* associated diarrhoeal illness in Apache children. *N Engl J Med* 1975;292:1041–1045.
31. Ryder RW, Sack DA, Kapikian AZ, et al. Enterotoxigenic *Escherichia coli* and reovirus-like agent in rural Bangladesh. *Lancet* 1976;1:659–662.
32. Taylor WR, Schell WL, Wells JG, et al: A foodborne outbreak of enterotoxigenic *Escherichia coli* diarrhea. *N Engl J Med* 1982;306:1093–1095.
33. Levine MM. *Escherichia coli* that cause diarrhea: enterotoxigenic, enteropathogenic, enteroinvasive, enterohemorrhagic, enteroadherent. *J Infect Dis* 1987;155:377–389.
34. Evans DG, Evans Jr DJ. New surface-associated heat-labile colonization factor antigen (CFA/II) produced by enterotoxigenic *Escherichia coli* of serogroups 06 and 08. *Infect Immun* 1978;21:638–647.
35. Evans DG, Silver RP, Evans DJ Jr, Chase GG, Gorbach SL. Plasmid controlled colonization factor associated with virulence in *Escherichia coli* enterotoxigenic for humans. *Infect Immun* 1975;12:656–667.
36. Cravioto A, Scotland SM, Rowe B. Hemagglutination activity and colonization factor antigens I and II enterotoxigenic and nonenterotoxigenic strains of *Escherichia coli* isolated from humans. *Infect Immun* 1982;36:189–197.
37. Smyth CJ. Two mannose-resistant haemagglutinins on entero-

toxigenic *Escherichia coli* of serotype 06:K15:H16 or H-iso-lated from travellers' and infantile diarrhoea. *J Gen Microbiol* 1982;128:2081–2096.

38. Smith HR, Scotland SM, Rowe B. Plasmids that code for production of colonization factor antigen II and enterotoxin production of *Escherichia coli*. *Infect Immun* 1983;40:1236–1239.

39. Mullany P, Field AM, McConnell MM, Scotland SM, Smith HR, Rowe B. Expression of plasmids coding for colonization factor antigen II (CFA/II) and enterotoxin production in *Escherichia coli*. *J Gen Microbiol* 1983;129:3591–3601.

40. Smyth CJ. Serologically distinct fimbriae on enterotoxigenic *Escherichia coli* of serotype O6:K15:H16 or H-. *FEMS Lett* 1984;21:51–57.

41. Levine MM, Ristaino P, Marley G, et al. Coli surface antigens 1 and 3 of colonization factor antigen II-positive enterotoxigenic *Escherichia coli*: morphology, purification and immune responses in humans. *Infect Immun* 1984;44:409–420.

42. Knutton S, Lloyd Dr, Candy DCA, McNeish AS. Ultrastructural study of adhesion of enterotoxigenic *Escherichia coli* to erythrocytes and human intestinal epithelial cells. *Infect Immun* 1984;44:519–527.

43. Tacket CO, Maneval DR, Levine MM. Purification, morphology and genetics of a new fimbrial putative colonization factor of enterotoxigenic *Escherichia coli* O159:H4. *Infect Immun* 1987;55:1063–1069.

44. Thomas LV, Cravioto A, Scotland SM, Rowe B. New fimbrial antigenic type (E8775) that may represent a colonization factor in enterotoxigenic *Escherichia coli* in humans. *Infect Immun* 1982;35:1119–1124.

45. Knutton S, McConnell MM, Rowe B, McNeish AS. Adhesion and ultrastructural properties of human enterotoxigenic *Escherichia coli* producing colonization factor antigens III and IV. *Infect Immun* 1989;57:3364–3371.

46. Cheney CP, Boedeker EC. Adherence of enterotoxigenic *Escherichia coli* strain, serotype O78:H11, to purified human intestinal brush borders. *Infect Immun* 1983;39:1280–1284.

47. Binsztein N, Jouve MJ, Viboud GI, et al. Colonization factors of enterotoxigenic *Escherichia coli* isolated from children with diarrhea in Argentina. *J Clin Microbiol* 1991;29:1893–1898.

48. McConnell MM, Hibberd ML, Penny ME, Scotland SM, Cheasty T, Rowe B. Surveys of human enterotoxigenic *Escherichia coli* from three different geographic areas for possible colonization factors. *Epidemiol Infect* 1991;106:477–484.

49. Nagy B, Arp LH, Moon HW, Casey TA. Colonization of the small intestine of weaned pigs by enterotoxigenic *Escherichia coli* that lack known colonization factors. *Vet Pathol* 1992;29:239–246.

50. Takao T, Hitouji T, Aimoto S, et al. Amino acid sequence of a heat-stable enterotoxin isolated from enterotoxigenic *Escherichia coli* strain 18D. *FEBS Lett* 1983;152:1–5.

51. Chan S-K, Giannella RA. Amino acid sequence of heat-stable enterotoxin produce by *Escherichia coli* pathogenic for man. *J Biol Chem* 1981;256:7744–7746.

52. Thompson MR, Giannella RA. Revised amino acid sequence for a heat-stable enterotoxin produced by and *Escherichia coli* strain (18D) that is pathogenic for humans. *Infect Immun* 1985; 47:834–836.

53. Aimoto S, Takao T, Shimonishi Y, et al. Amino-acid sequence of a heat-stable enterotoxin produced by human enterotoxigenic *Escherichia coli*. *Eur J Biochem* 1982;129:257–263.

54. Guarino A, Giannella RA, Thompson MR. *Citrobacter freundii* produces an 18-amino acid heat-stable enterotoxin identical to the 18 amino acid *Escherichia coli* heat stable enterotoxin (ST Ia). *Infect Immun* 1989;57:649–652.

55. Takao T, Tominga N, Shimonshi Y. Primary structure of heat-stable enterotoxin produced by *Yersinia enterocolitica*. *Biochem Biophys Res Commun* 1984;125:845–851.

56. Takao T, Shimonishi Y, Kobayashi M, et al. Amino acid sequence of heat-stable enterotoxin produced by *Vibrio cholerae* non-01. *FEBS Lett* 1985;193:250–254.

57. Arita M, Takeda T, Honda T, Miwatani T. Purification and characterization of *Vibrio cholerae* non-O1 heat-stable enterotoxin. *Infect Immun* 1986;52:45–49.

58. Savarino SJ, Fasano A, Watson J, et al. Enteroaggregative

Escherichia coli heat-stable enterotoxin 1 represents another subfamily of *E. coli* heat-stable toxin. *Proc Natl Acad Sci USA* 1993;90:3093–3097.

59. Currie MG, Fok KF, Kato J, et al. Guanylin: an endogenous activator of intestinal guanylate cyclase. *Proc Natl Acad Sci USA* 1992;89:947–951.

60. Giannella RA, Luttrell M. Characteristics of the binding of pure human *Escherichia coli* heat-stable enterotoxin to rat intestine. In: Kuwahara S, Pierce NF, eds. *Advances in research on cholera and related diseases*. Tokyo: KTK; 1983:259–268.

61. Yoshimura S, Ikemura H, Watanabe H, et al. Essential structure for full enterotoxigenic activity of heat-stable enterotoxin produced by enterotoxigenic *Escherichia coli*. *FEBS Lett* 1985; 181:138–142.

62. Waldman SA, O'Hanley P. Influence of a glycine or proline substitution on the functional properties of a 14-amino-acid analog of *Escherichia coli* heat-stable enterotoxin. *Infect Immun* 1989;57:2420–2424.

63. Lazure C, Seidah N, Chrétien M, et al. Primary structure determination of *Escherichia coli* heat-stable enterotoxin of porcine origin. *Can J Biochem Cell Biol* 1983;61:287–292.

64. Ronnberg B, Wadstrom T, Jornvall H. Structure of a heat-stable enterotoxin produced by a human strain of *Escherichia coli*. *FEBS Lett* 1983;155:183–186.

65. Saeed A, Magnuson NS, Sriranganathan N, et al. Molecular homogeneity of heat-stable enterotoxins produced by bovine enterotoxigenic *Escherichia coli*. *Infect Immun* 1984;45:242–247.

66. So M, McCarthy BJ. Nucleotide sequence of the bacterial transposon TN1681 encoding a heat-stable enterotoxin (ST) and its identification in enterotoxigenic *Escherichia coli* strains. *Proc Natl Acad Sci USA* 1980;77:4011–4015.

67. Rasheed JK, Guzman-Verduzco LM, Kupersztoch YM. Two precursors of the heat-stable enterotoxin of *Escherichia coli*: evidence of extracellular processing. *Mol Microbiol* 1990;4:265–273.

68. Guzman-Verduzco LM, Kupersztoch YM. Export and processing of a fusion between the extracellular heat-stable enterotoxin and the periplasmic B subunit of the heat-labile enterotoxin in *Escherichia coli*. *Mol Microbiol* 1990;4:253–264.

69. Staples SJ, Asher SE, Giannella RA. Purification and characterization of heat-stable enterotoxin produced by a strain of *Escherichia coli* pathogenic for man. *J Biol Chem* 1980;255:4716–4721.

70. Rao MC. Toxins which activate guanylate cyclase: heat-stable *Escherichia coli* enterotoxin. In: Evered D, Whelan J, eds. *Microbial toxins and diarrhoeal disease*. Ciba Foundation Symposium 112. London: Pitman; 1985:74–93.

71. Giannella RA, Luttrell M, Thompson M. Binding of *Escherichia coli* heat-stable enterotoxin to receptors on rat intestinal cells *Am J Physiol* 1983;243:G36–G41.

72. Guarino A, Cohen MB, Overmann GJ, Thompson MR, Giannella RA. Binding of *E. coli* heat-stable enterotoxin to rat brush border and basolateral membranes. *Dig Dis Sci* 1987;32:1017–1026.

73. Cohen MB, Giannella RA. Jejunal inactivation regulates susceptibility of the immature rat to ST$_a$. *Gastroenterology* 1992; 102:1988–1996.

74. Houghton RA, Ostresh JM, Klipstein FA. Chemical synthesis of an octadecapeptide with the biological and immunological properties of human heat-stable *Escherichia coli* enterotoxin. *Eur J Biochem* 1984;145:157–162.

75. Gariépy J, Schoolnik GK. Design of a photoreactive analogue of the *Escherichia coli* heat-stable toxin STIb: use in identifying its receptor on rat brush border membranes. *Proc Natl Acad Sci USA* 1986;83:483–487.

76. Shimonshi Y, Hidaka Y, Koizumi M. Mode of disulfide bond formation by a heat-stable enterotoxin (STh) produced by a human strain of enterotoxigenic *Escherichia coli*. *FEBS Lett* 1987;215:165–170.

77. Kubota H, Hidaka Y, Ozaki H, et al. A long-acting heat-stable enterotoxin analogy of enterotoxigenic *Escherichia coli* with a single D-amino acid. *Biochem Biophys Res Commun* 1989;161:229–235.

78. Okamoto K, Jukitake J, Kawamoto Y, Miyama A. Substitutions of cysteine residues of *Escherichia coli* heat-stable enterotoxin by oligonucleotide-directed mutagenesis. *Infect Immun* 1987;55:2121–2125.

79. Schron CM, Giannella RA. Bacterial enterotoxins. In: Field M, ed. *Diarrheal diseases*. New York: Elsevier; 1991:115–138.

80. Field M, Graf LH, Laird WJ, Smith PL. Heat stable enterotoxin of *Escherichia coli:* in vitro effects on guanylate cyclase activity, cyclic GMP concentration, and ion transport in small intestine. *Proc Natl Acad Sci USA* 1978;75:2800–2804.

81. Mezoff AG, Giannella RA, Eade MN, Cohen MB. *Escherichia coli* enterotoxin (STa) binds to receptors, stimulates guanyl cyclase and impairs absorption in rat colon. *Gastroenterology* 1992;102:816–822.

82. Giannella RA, Walls D, Eade MN. Effect of pure *E. coli* heat-stable enterotoxin on small and large intestinal water and glucose absorption, mucosal histology and intestinal permeability. In: Kuwahara S, Pierce N, eds. *Advances in research on cholera and related diseases*. Tokyo: KTK; 1986;327–332.

83. Cohen MB, Thompson MR, Overmann GJ, Giannella RA. Association and dissociation of *Escherichia coli* heat-stable enterotoxin from rat brush border membrane receptors. *Infect Immun* 1987;55:329–334.

84. Schulz S, Green CK, Yuen PST, Garbers DL. Guanylyl cyclase is a heat-stable enterotoxin receptor. *Cell* 1990;63:941–948.

85. Huott PA, Liu W, McRoberts JA, Giannella RA, Dharmsathaphorn K. Mechanism of action of *Escherichia coli* heat stable enterotoxin in a human colonic cell line. *J Clin Invest* 1988;82:514–523.

86. Giannella RA, Drake KW. Effect of purified *Escherichia coli* heat-stable enterotoxin on intestinal cyclic nucleotide metabolism and fluid secretion. *Infect Immun* 1979;24:19–23.

87. Newsome PM, Burgess MN, Mullan NA. Effect of *Escherichia coli* heat-stable enterotoxin on cyclic GMP levels in mouse intestine. *Infect Immun* 1978;22:290–291.

88. Rao MC, Guandalini S, Smith PL, Field M. Mode of action of heat-stable *Escherichia coli* enterotoxin. Tissue and subcellular specificities and role of cyclic GMP. *Biochim Biophys Acta* 1980;632:35–46.

89. Waldman SA, Kuno T, Kamiskai Y, et al. Intestinal receptor for heat-stable enterotoxin is tightly coupled to a novel form of particulate guanylate cyclase. *Infect Immun* 1986;51:320–326.

90. ElDeib MMR, Parker CD, Veum TL, Zinn GM, White AA. Characterization of intestinal brush border guanylate cyclase activation by *Escherichia coli* heat-stable enterotoxin. *Arch Biochem Biophys* 1986;245:51–65.

91. Kuno T, Kamisaki Y, Waldman SA, Gariepy J, Schoolnik G, Murad F. Characterization of the receptor for heat-stable enterotoxin from *Escherichia coli* in rat intestine. *J Biol Chem* 1986;261:1470–1476.

92. deSauvage FJ, Camerato TR, Goeddel DV. Primary structure and functional expression of the human receptor for *Escherichia coli* heat-stable enterotoxin. *J Biol Chem* 1991;266:17912–17918.

93. Singh S, Singh G, Helm JM, Gerzer R. Isolation and expression of a guanylate cyclase-coupled heat stable enterotoxin receptor cDNA from a human colonic cell line. *Biochem Biophys Res Commun* 1991;179:1455–1463.

94. Mann EA, Cohen MB, Giannella RA. Comparison of receptors for *Escherichia coli* heat-stable enterotoxin: novel receptor present in IEC-6 cells. *Am J Physiol* 1993;264:G172–G178.

95. deSauvage FJ, Horuk R, Bennett G, Quan C, Burnier JP, Goeddel DV. Characterization of the recombinant human receptor for *Escherichia coli* heat-stable enterotoxin. *J Biol Chem* 1992;267:6479–6482.

96. Weikel CS, Spann CL, Chambers CP, Crane JK, Linden J, Hewlett EL. Phorbol esters enhance the cyclic GMP response of T84 cells to the heat-stable enterotoxin of *Escherichia coli* (STa). *Infect Immun* 1990;58:1402–1407.

97. Crane JK, Burrell LL, Weikel CS, Guerrant RL. Carbachol mimics phorbal esters in its ability to enhance cyclic GMP production by STa, the heat-stable enterotoxin of *Escherichia coli*. *FEBS Lett* 1990;274:199–202.

98. Crane JK, Wehner MS, Bolen EJ, et al. Regulation of intestinal guanylate cyclase by the heat stable enterotoxin of *Escherichia coli* (STa) and protein kinase C. *Infect Immun* 1992;60:5004–5012.

99. Levine SA, Donowitz M, Watson AJ, Sharp GW, Crane JK, Weikel CS. Characterization of the synergistic interaction of *Escherichia coli* heat-stable toxin and carbachol. *Am J Physiol* 1991;261:G592–G601.

100. Gazzano H, Wu HI, Waldman SA. Activation of particulate guanylate-cyclase by *Escherichia coli* heat-stable enterotoxin is regulated by adenine nucleotides. *Infect Immun* 1991;59:1552–1557.

101. Katwa LC, Parker CD, Dybing JK, White AA. Nucleotide regulation of heat-stable enterotoxin receptor binding and of guanylate cyclase activation. *Biochem J* 1992;283:727–735.

102. Hakki S, Crane M, Hugues M, O'Hanley P, Waldman SA. Solubilization and characterization of functionally coupled *Escherichia coli* heat-stable toxin receptors and particulate guanylate cyclase associated with the cytoskeleton compartment of intestinal membranes. *Int J Biochem* 1993;25:557–566.

103. Vaandrager AB, van der Wiel E, de Jonge HR. Heat-stable enterotoxin activation of immunopurified guanylyl cyclase C. Modulation by adenine nucleotides. *J Biol Chem* 1993;268:19598–19603.

104. Guandalini S, Rao MC, Smith PL, Field M. cGMP modulation of ileal ion transport: in vitro effects of *Escherichia coli* heat-stable enterotoxin. *Am J Physiol* 1982;243:G36–G41.

105. Darfeuille-Michaud A, Aubel D, Chauviere G, et al. Adhesion of enterotoxigenic *Escherichia coli* to the human colon carcinoma cell line Caco-2 in culture. *Infect Immun* 1990;58:893–902.

106. Kerneis S, Chauviere G, Darfeuille-Michaud A, et al. Expression of receptors for enterotoxigenic *Escherichia coli* during enterocytic differentiation of human polarized intestinal epithelial cells in culture. *Infect Immun* 1992;60:2572–2580.

107. Cohen MB, Jensen NJ, Hawkins JA, et al. Receptors for *Escherichia coli* heat stable enterotoxin in human intestine and in a human intestinal cell line (Caco-2). *J Cell Physiol* 1993;156:138–144.

108. Weymer A, Huott P, Liu W, McRoberts JA, Dharmsathaphorn K. Chloride secretory mechanism induced by prostaglandin E1 in a colonic epithelial cell line. *J Clin Invest* 1985;76:1828–1836.

109. Cartwright CA, McRoberts JA, Mandel KG, Dharmsathaphorn K. Synergistic action of cyclic adenosine monophosphate- and calcium mediated chloride secretion in a colonic cell line. *J Clin Invest* 1985;76:1837–1842.

110. Dharmsathaphorn K, Mandel KG, Masui H, McRoberts JA. Vasoactive intestinal polypeptide-induced chloride secretion by a colonic epithelial cell line. Direct participation of a basolaterally localized $Na+$, $K-$, $Cl-$ cotransport system. *J Clin Invest* 1985;75:462–471.

111. Dharmsathaphorn K, Pandol SJ. Mechanism of chloride secretion induced by carbachol in a colonic cell line. *J Clin Invest* 1986;77:348–354.

112. Dreyfus LA, Jaso-Freidman L, Robertson DC. Characterization of the mechanisms of action of *Escherichia coli* heat-stable enterotoxin. *Infect Immun* 1984;44:493–501.

113. Frantz JC Jaso-Friedman L, Robertson DC. Binding of *Escherichia coli* heat stable enterotoxin to rat intestinal cells and brush border membranes. *Infect Immun* 1984;43:622–630.

114. Cohen MB, Mann EA, Lau C, Henning SJ, Giannella RA. A gradient in expression of the *Escherichia coli* heat stable enterotoxin receptor exists along the villus-to-crypt axis of rat small intestine. *Biochem Biophys Res Commun* 1992;186:483–490.

115. Kockerling A, Fromm M. Origin of cAMP dependent Cl^- secretion from both crypts and surface epithelia of rat intestine. *Am J Physiol* 1993;254:C1294–C1301.

116. Knoop FC, Martig RJ, Boehm WJ. The effect of *Escherichia coli* heat-stable enterotoxin in protein kinase activity. *Toxicon* 1990;28:493–500.

117. deJonge HR. Cyclic nucleotide-dependent phosphorylation of intestinal epithelium proteins. *Nature* 1976;262:590–592.

118. deJonge HR. Cyclic GMP-dependent protein kinase in intes-

tinal brush borders. *Adv Cyclic Nucleotide Res* 1981;14: 315–333.

119. deJonge HR. The mechanism of action of *Escherichia coli* heat-stable enterotoxin. *Biochem Soc Trans* 1984;12:180–184.

120. Forte LR, Thorne PK, Eber SL, et al. Simulation of intestinal Cl⁻ transport by heat-stable enterotoxin: activation of cAMP-dependent protein kinase by cGMP. *Am J Physiol* 1992;263: C607–C615.

121. Hirayama T, Ito H, Takeda Y. Inhibition by the protein kinase inhibitors, isoquinolinesulfanamides, of fluid accumulation induced by *Escherichia coli* heat-stable enterotoxin, 8-bromo-cGMP and 8-bromo-cAMP in suckling mice. *Microbial Pathog* 1989;7:255–261.

122. Hirayama T, Noda M, Ito H, Takeda Y. Stimulation of phophorylation of rat brush-border membrane proteins by *Escherichia coli* heat-stable enterotoxin, cholera enterotoxin, and cyclic nucleotides, and its inhibition by protein kinase inhibitors, isoquinolinesulfonamides. *Microb Pathog* 1990;8:421–431.

123. Matthews JB, Awtrey CS, Thompson R, Hung T, Tally KJ, Madara JL. Na⁺-K⁺-2Cl⁻ cotransport and Cl⁻ secretion evoked by heat-stable enterotoxin is microfilament dependent in T84 cells. *Am J Physiol* 1993;265:G370–G378.

124. Matthews JB, Awtrey CS, Madara JL. Microfilament dependent activation of Na⁺/K⁺/Cl⁻ cotransport by cAMP in intestinal epithelial monolayers. *J Clin Invest* 1992;90:1608–1613.

125. Schulz S, Singh S, Bellet RA, et al. The primary structure of a plasma membrane guanylate cyclase demonstrates diversity within this new receptor family. *Cell* 1989;58:1155–1162.

126. Gariépy J, Lane A, Frayman F, et al. Structure of the toxic domain of the *Escherichia coli* heat-stable enterotoxin ST1. *Biochemistry* 1986;25:7854–7866.

127. Almenoff JS, Williams S, Scheving LA, Judd AK, Schoolnik GK. Ligand-based histochemical localization and capture of cells expressing heat-stable enterotoxin receptors. *Mol Microbiol* 1993;8:865–873.

128. Cohen MB, Guarino A, Shukla R, Giannella RA. Age-related differences in receptors for *Escherichia coli* heat-stable enterotoxin in the small and large intestine of children. *Gastroenterology* 1988;94:367–373.

129. Guarino A, Cohen MB, Giannella RA. Small and large intestinal guanylate cyclase activity in children: effect of age and stimulation by *Escherichia coli* heat-stable enterotoxin. *Pediatr Res* 1987;21:551–555.

130. Nobles M, Diener M, Rummel W. Segment-specific effects of the heat-stable enterotoxin of *E. coli* on electrolyte transport in the rat colon. *Eur J Pharmacol* 1991;202:201–211.

131. Dean EA, Whipp SC, Moon HW. Age-specific colonization of porcine intestinal epithelium by 987P-piliated enterotoxigenic *Escherichia coli*. *Infect Immun* 1989;57:82–87.

132. Runnels PL, Moon HW, Schneider RA. Development of resistance with host age to adhesion of K99+ *Escherichia coli* to isolated intestinal epithelial cells. *Infect Immun* 1980;28: 298–300.

133. Saeed AM, McMillan R, Huckelberry V, Greenberg RN. Specific receptor for *Escherichia coli* heat-stable enterotoxin (STa) may determine susceptibility of piglets to diarrheal disease. *FEMS Microbiol Lett* 1987;43:247–251.

134. Cohen MB, Moyer MS, Luttrell M, Giannella RA. The immature rat small intestine exhibits an increased response and sensitivity to *Escherichia coli* heat-stable enterotoxin. *Pediatr Res* 1986;20:555–560.

135. Guarino A, Cohen M, Thompson M, Dharmsathaphorn K, Giannella R. T84 cell receptor binding and guanylate cyclase activation by *E. coli* heat stable toxin. *Am J Physiol* 1987;253: G775–G780.

136. Mezoff AG, Jensen NJ, Cohen MB. Mechanisms of increased susceptibility of immature and weaned pigs to *Escherichia coli* heat-stable enterotoxin. *Pediatr Res* 1991;29:424–428.

137. Robertson DC. Pathogenesis and enterotoxins of diarrheagenic *Escherichia coli*. In: Roth JA, ed. *Virulence mechanisms of bacterial pathogens*. Washington, DC: American Society for Microbiology; 1988:241–263.

138. Katwa LC, Parker CD, White AA. Age-dependent changes in affinity-labeled receptors for *Escherichia coli* heat-stable

139. Jaso-Friedman L, Dreyfus LA, Whipp SC, Robertson DC. Effect of age on activation of porcine intestinal guanylate cyclase and binding of *Escherichia coli* heat-stable enterotoxin (STa) to porcine intestinal cells and brush border membranes. *Am J Vet Res* 1991;53:2251–2258.

140. Thompson MR, Giannella RA. Different crosslinking agents identify distinctly different putative *Escherichia coli* heat-stable enterotoxin rat intestinal cell receptor proteins. *J Receptor Res* 1990;10:97–117.

141. Hirayama T, Wada A, Iwata N, Takasaki S, Shimonishi Y, Takeda Y. Glycoprotein receptors for a heat-stable enterotoxin (STh) produced by enterotoxigenic *Escherichia coli*. *Infect Immun* 1992;60:4213–4220.

142. Hugues M, Crane M, Hakki S, O'Hanley P, Waldman SA. Identification and characterization of a new family of high-affinity receptors for *Escherichia coli* heat-stable enterotoxin in rat intestinal membranes. *Biochemistry* 1991;30:10738–10745.

143. Hugues M, Crane MR, Thomas BR, et al. Affinity purification of functional receptors for *Escherichia coli* heat-stable enterotoxin from rat intestine. *Biochemistry* 1992;31:16–20.

144. Giannella RA, Luttrell M, Thompson M. Receptor occupancy in intestinal secretion induced by *Escherichia coli* heat-stable enterotoxin. *Gastroenterology* 1985;88:1392.

145. Guerrant RL, Hughes JM, Chang B, Robertson DC, Murad F. Activation of intestinal guanylate cyclase by heat-stable enterotoxin of *Escherichia coli*: studies of tissue specificity, potential receptors, and intermediates. *J Infect Dis* 1980;142:220–228.

146. Schulz S, Chrisman TD, Garbers DL. Cloning and expression of guanylin. Its existence in various mammalian tissues. *J Biol Chem* 1992;267:16019–16021.

147. Laney Jr DW, Mann EA, Dellon SC, Perkins DR, Giannella RA, Cohen MB. Novel sites for expression of a *Escherichia coli* heat-stable enterotoxin receptor in the developing rat. *Am J Physiol* 1992;263:G816–G821.

148. Forte LR, Krause WJ, Freeman RH. *Escherichia coli* enterotoxin receptors: localization in opossum kidney, intestine and testis. *Am J Physiol* 1989;257:G874–G881.

149. Forte LR, Krause WJ, Freeman RH. Receptors and cGMP signalling mechanisms of *Escherichia coli* enterotoxin in opossum kidney. *Am J Physiol* 1988;255:F1040–F1046.

150. Laney Jr DW, Bezerra JA, Kosiba JL, Degen SJF, Cohen MB. Upregulation of the *Escherichia coli* heat stable enterotoxin receptor in the regenerating rat liver. *Am J Physiol* 1994;29: G899–G906.

151. Knoop FC, Thomas DD. Stimulation of calcium uptake and cyclic GMP synthesis in rat basophilic leukemia cells by *Escherichia coli* heat-stable enterotoxin. *Infect Immun* 1983;41: 971–977.

152. Thomas DD, Knoop FC. Effect of heat-stable enterotoxin of *Escherichia coli* on cultured mammalian cells. *J Infect Dis* 1983;147:450–459.

153. Evans DG, Evans DJ Jr, Pierce NF. Differences in the response of rabbit small intestine to heat-labile and heat-stable enterotoxins of *Escherichia coli*. *Infect Immun* 1973;7:873–880.

154. Dean AG, Ching Y, Williams RG et al. Test of *Escherichia coli* enterotoxin using infant mice: application in a study of diarrhea in children in Honolulu. *J Infect Dis* 1972;125:407–411.

155. Giannella RA. Suckling mouse model for detection of heat-stable *Escherichia coli* enterotoxin: characteristics of the model. *Infect Immun* 1976;14:95–99.

156. Choudry MA, Gupta S, Yadava JN. Guinea pig ileal loop assay: a better replacement of the suckling mouse assay for detection of heat-stable enterotoxins of *Escherichia coli*. *J Trop Med Hyg* 1991;94:234–240.

157. Giannella RA, Drake KW, Luttrell M. Development of a radioimmunoassay for *Escherichia coli* heat stable enterotoxin. *Infect Immun* 1981;33:186–192.

158. Frantz JC, Robertson DC. Immunological properties of *Escherichia coli* heat-stable enterotoxins: development of a radioimmunoassay specific for heat-stable enterotoxins with suckling mouse activity. *Infect Immun* 1981;33:193–198.

159. Thompson MR, Jordan RL, Luttrell MA, et al. Blinded, two-laboratory comparative analysis of *Escherichia coli* heat-stable

enterotoxin production by using monoclonal antibody enzyme-linked immunosorbent assay, radioimmunoassay, suckling mouse assay and gene probes. *J Clin Microbiol* 1986;24: 753–758.

160. Cryan B. Comparison of three assay systems for detection of enterotoxigenic *Escherichia coli* heat-stable enterotoxin. *J Clin Microbiol* 1990;28:792–794.

161. Scotland SM, Willshaw GA, Said B, Smith HR, Rowe B. Identification of *Escherichia coli* that produces heat-stable enterotoxin STa by a commercially available enzyme-linked immunoassay and comparison of the assay with infant mouse and DNA probe tests. *J Clin Microbiol* 1989;27:1697–1699.

162. Moseley SL, Echeverria P, Seriwatana J, et al. Identification of enterotoxigenic *Escherichia coli* by colony blot hybridization using three gene probes. *J Infect Dis* 1982;145:863–869.

163. Echeverria P, Taylor DN, Seriwatana J, et al. A comparative study of enterotoxin gene probes and tests for toxin production to detect enterotoxigenic *Escherichia coli*. *J Infect Dis* 1986; 153:255–260.

164. Gicquelais KG, Baldini MM, Martinez J, et al. Practical and economical method for using biotinylated DNA probes with bacterial colony blots to identify diarrhea-causing *Escherichia coli*. *J Clin Microbiol* 1990;28:2485–2490.

165. Bopp CA, Threatt VL, Moseley SL, Wells JG, Wachsmuth IK. A comparison of alkaline phosphatase and radiolabelled gene probes with bioassays for enterotoxigenic *Escherichia coli*. *Mol Cell Probes* 1990;4:193–203.

166. Cryan B. Comparison of the synthetic oligonucleotide gene probe and infant mouse bioassay for detection of enterotoxigenic *Escherichia coli*. *Eur J Clin Microbiol Infect Dis* 1990;9: 229–232.

167. Abe A, Komase K, Bangtrakulnonth A, Ratchtrachenchat OA, Kawahara K, Danbara H. Trivalent heat-labile and heat-stable enterotoxin probe conjugated with horseradish peroxidase for detection of enterotoxigenic *Escherichia coli* by hybridization. *J Clin Microbiol* 1990;28:2616–2620.

168. Saez-Llorens X, Guzman-Verduzco LM, Shelton S, Nelson JD, Kupersztoch YM. Simultaneous detection of *Escherichia coli* heat-stable and heat labile enterotoxin genes with a single RNA probe. *J Clin Microbiol* 1989;27:1684–1688.

169. Hornes E. Wasteson Y, Olsvik O. Detection of *Escherichia coli* heat-stable enterotoxin genes in pig stool specimens by immobilized, colorimetric, nested polymerase chain reaction. *J Clin Microbiol* 1991;29:2375–2379.

170. Rao MC, Guandalini S, Laird W, Field M. Effects of heat stable enterotoxin of *Yersinia enterocolitica* on ion transport and cyclic guanosine 3′,5′-monophosphate metabolism in rabbit ileum. *Infect Immun* 1979;26:875–879.

171. Alessio M, Albano F, Tarallo L, Guarino A. Interspecific plasmid transfer and modification of heat-stable enterotoxin expression by *Klebsiella pneumoniae* for infants with diarrhea. *Pediatr Res* 1993;33:205–208.

172. Savarino SJ, Fasano A, Robertson DC, Levine MM. Enteroaggregative *Escherichia coli* elaborate a heat-stable enterotoxin demonstrable in an in vitro rabbit intestinal model. *J Clin Invest* 1991;87:1450–1455.

173. Levine MM, Prado V, Robins-Browne R, et al. Use of DNA probes and HEp-2 cell adherence assay to detect diarrheagenic *Escherichia coli*. *J Infect Dis* 1988;158:224–228.

174. Bhan MK, Raj P, Levine MM, et al. Enteroaggregative *Escherichia coli* associated with persistent diarrhea in cohort of rural children in India. *J Infect Dis* 1989;159:1601–1604.

175. Cravioto A, Tello A, Navarro A, et al. Association of *Escherichia coli* HEp-2 adherence patterns with type and duration of diarrhea. *Lancet* 1991;337:262–264.

176. Wanke CA, Shorling JB, Barrett LJ, Desouza MA, Guerrant RL. Potential role of adherence traits of *Escherichia coli* in persistent diarrhea in an urban Brazilian slum. *Pediatr Infect Dis* 1991;10:746–751.

177. Echeverria P, Serichantalerg S, Changchawalit S, et al. Tissue culture-adherent *Escherichia coli* in infantile diarrhea. *J Infect Dis* 1992;165:141–143.

178. Giron JA, Jones T, Millan-Velasco F, et al. Diffuse adhering

179. Gomes TAT, Blake PA, Tabulsi LR. Prevalence of *Escherichia coli* strains with localized, diffuse and aggregative adherence to HeLa cells in infants with diarrhea and matched controls. *J Clin Microbiol* 1989;27:266–269.

180. Cohen MB, Hawkins JA, Weckbach LS, Staneck JL, Levine MM, Heck JE. Colonization by enteroaggregative *Escherichia coli* in travelers with and without diarrhea. *J Clin Microbiol* 1993;31:351–353.

181. deSauvage FJ, Keshav S, Kuang W-J, Gillett N, Henzel W, Goeddel DV. Precursor structure, expression and tissue distribution of human guanylin. *Proc Natl Acad Sci USA* 1992;89: 9089–9093.

182. Weigand RC, Kato J, Currie MG. Rat guanylin cDNA: characterization of the precursor of an endogenous activator of intestinal guanylate cyclase. *Biochem Biophys Res Commun* 1992; 185:812–817.

183. Weigand RC, Kato J, Huang MD, Fok KF, Kachur JF, Currie MG. Human guanylin: cDNA isolation structure, and activity. *FEBS Lett* 1992;311:150–154.

184. Kato J, Wiegand RC, Currie MG. Characterization of the structure of preproguanylin. In: Brown BL, Dobson PRM, eds. *Advances in second messenger and phosphoprotein research.* New York: Raven Press; 1993;28:139–142.

185. Li Z, Goy MF. Peptide-regulated guanylate cyclase pathways in rat colon: in situ localization of GCA, GCC, and guanylin mRNA. *Am J Physiol* 1993;265:G394–G402.

186. Lewis LG, Witte DP, Laney DW, Currie MG, Cohen MB. Guanylin mRNA is expressed in villous enterocytes of the rat small intestine and superficial epithelia of the rat colon. *Biochem Biophys Res Commun* 1993;196:553–560.

187. Kuhn M, Raida M, Adermann K, et al. The circulating bioactive form of human guanylin is a high molecular weight peptide (10.3 kDa). *FEBS Lett* 1993;318:205–209.

188. Forte LR, Eber SL, Turner JT, Freeman RH, Fok KF, Currie MG. Guanylin stimulation of Cl-secretion in human intestinal T84 cells via cyclic guanosine monophosphate. *J Clin Invest* 1993;91:2423–8.

189. Garbers DL. Guanylyl cyclase receptors and their endocrine, paracrine and autocrine ligands. *Cell* 1992;71:1–4.

190. Moon HW, Whipp SC. Development of resistance with age by swine intestine to effects of enteropathogenic *Escherichia coli*. *J Infect Dis* 1970;122:220–223.

191. Burgess MN, Bywater RJ, Cowley CM, et al. Biological evaluation of a methanol-soluble, heat-stable *Escherichia coli* enterotoxin in infant mice, pigs, rabbits and calves. *Infect Immun* 1978;21:526–531.

192. Whipp SC, Moseley SL, Moon HW. Microscopic alterations in jejunal epithelium of 3-week old pigs induced by pig-specific, mouse-negative, heat-stable *Escherichia coli* enterotoxin. *Am J Vet Res* 1986;47:615–618.

193. Rose R, Whipp SC, Moon HW. Effects of *Escherichia coli* heat-stable enterotoxin b on small intestinal villi in pigs, rabbits and lambs. *Vet Pathol* 1987;24:71–79.

194. Kennedy DJ, Greenberg RN, Dunn JA, et al. Effects of *Escherichia coli* heat-stable enterotoxin STb on intestines of mice, rats, rabbits and piglets. *Infect Immun* 1984;46:639–643.

195. Weikel CS, Nellans HN, Guerrant RL. In vivo and in vitro effects of a novel enterotoxin, STb, produced by *Escherichia coli*. *J Infect Dis* 1986;153:893–901.

196. Hitotsubashi S, Fujii Y, Yamanaka H, Okamoto K. Some properties of purified *Escherichia coli* heat-stable enterotoxin II. *Infect Immun* 1992;60:4468–4474.

197. Whipp SC. Protease degradation of *Escherichia coli* heat-stable, mouse-negative, pig-positive enterotoxin. *Infect Immun* 1987;55:2057–2060.

198. Whipp SC. Assay of enterotoxigenic *Escherichia coli* heat-stable toxin b in rats and mice. *Infect Immun* 1990;58:930–934.

199. Whipp SC. Intestinal responses to enterotoxigenic *Escherichia coli* heat-stable toxin b in non-porcine species. *Am J Vet Res* 1991;52:734–737.

200. Lee CH, Moseley SL, Moon HW, et al. Characterization of the gene encoding heat-stable toxin II and preliminary molecular

epidemiological studies of enterotoxigenic *Escherichia coli* heat-stable toxin II producers. *Infect Immun* 1983;42:264–268.

201. Picken RN, Mazaitis AJ, Maas WK, et al. Nucleotide sequence of the gene for heat-stable enterotoxin II of *Escherichia coli*. *Infect Immun* 1983;42:269–275.

202. Kupersztoch YM, Tachias K, Mooman CR, et al. Secretion of methanol-insoluble heat-stable enterotoxin (STb): energy and secA dependent conversion of pre-STb to an intermediate indistinguishable from the extracellular toxin. *J Bacteriol* 1990; 172:2427–2432.

203. Fujii Y, Hayashi M, Hitotsubashi S, Fuke Y, Tamanaka H, Okamato K. Purification and characterization of *Escherichia coli* heat-stable enterotoxin II. *J Bacteriol* 1991;173:5516–5522.

204. Dreyfus LA, Urban RG, Whipp SC, Slaughter C, Tachias K, Kupersztoch YM. Purification of the STb enterotoxin of *Escherichia coli* and the role of selected amino acids on its secretion, stability and toxicity. *Mol Microbiol* 1992;6:2397–2406.

205. Urban RG, Pipper EM, Dreyfus LA. Monoclonal antibodies specific for the *Escherichia coli* heat-stable enterotoxin STb. *J Clin Microbiol* 1991;29:1963–1968.

206. Greenberg RN, Chang B, Murad F, Guerrant RL. Lack of effect of porcine *Escherichia coli* enterotoxin (STb) on cyclic nucleotide metabolism. *Clin Res* 1980;28:830.

207. Weikel S, Guerrant RL. STb enterotoxin of *Escherichia coli*: cyclic nucleotide independent secretion. In: Evered D, Whelan J, eds. *Microbial toxins and diarrhoeal disease*. Ciba Foundation Symposium 112. London: Pitman; 1985:94–115.

208. Dreyfus LA, Harville B, Howard DE, Shaban R, Beatty DM, Morris SJ. Calcium influx mediated by the *Escherichia coli* heat-stable enterotoxin B (STB). *Proc Natl Acad Sci* USA 1993;90:3202–3206.

209. Weikel CS, Tiemens KM, Moseley SL, Huq IM, Guerrant RL. Species specificity and lack of production of STb enterotoxin by *Escherichia coli* strains isolated from humans with diarrheal illness. *Infect Immun* 1986;52:323–325.

210. Echeverria P, Seriwatana J, Patamaroj U, et al. Prevalence of heat-stable II enterotoxigenic *Escherichia coli* in pigs, water, and people at farms in Thailand as determined by DNA hybridization. *J Clin Microbiol* 1984;19:489–491.

211. Echeverria P, Seriwatana J, Taylor DN, et al. Identification by DNA hybridization of enterotoxigenic *Escherichia coli* in a longitudinal study of villages in Thailand. *J Infect Dis* 1985; 151:124–130.

212. Lortie LA, Dubreuil JD, Harel J. Characterization of *Escherichia coli* strains producing heat-stable enterotoxin b (STb) isolated from humans with diarrhea. *J Clin Microbiol* 1991;29: 656–659.

213. Okamoto K, Fujii Y, Akashi N, et al. Identification and characterization of heat-stable enterotoxin-II producing *Escherichia coli* from patients with diarrhea. *Microbiol Immunol* 1993;37: 411–414.

214. Honda T, Tsuji T, Takeda Y, Miwatani T. Immunological nonidentity of heat-labile enterotoxins from human and porcine enterotoxigenic *Escherichia coli*. *Infect Immun* 1981;33: 677–682.

215. Qu Z-H, Boesman-Finkelstein M, Kazemi M, Finkelstein RA. Heterogeneity of immunotypes of heat-labile enterotoxins of enterotoxigenic *Escherichia coli* of human origin. *J Infect Dis* 1991;164:796–799.

216. Gill DM, Clements JD, Robertson DC, Finkelstein RA. Subunit number and arrangement in *Escherichia coli* heat-labile enterotoxin. *Infect Immun* 1981;33:677–682.

217. Spicer EK, Kavanaugh WM, Dallas WS, et al. Sequence homologies between A subunits of *Escherichia coli* and *Vibrio cholerae* enterotoxins. *Proc Natl Acad Sci USA* 1981;78:50–54.

218. Spicer EK, Noble JA. *Escherichia coli* heat-labile enterotoxin. Nucleotide sequence of the A subunit gene. *J Biol Chem* 1982; 257:5716–5721.

219. Dallas WS, Falkow S. Amino acid sequence homology between cholera toxin and *Escherichia coli* heat-labile toxin. *Nature* 1980;288:499–501.

220. Lockman H, Kaper JB. Nucleotide sequence analysis of the A2 and B subunits of *Vibrio cholerae* enterotoxin. *J Biol Chem* 1983;258:13722–13726.

221. Mekalanos JJ, Swartz DJ, Pearson GD, et al. Cholera toxin genes; nucleotide sequence, deletion analysis and vaccine development. *Nature* 1983;306:551–557.

222. Yamamoto T, Nakazawa T, Miyata T, et al. Evolution and structure of two ADP-ribosylation enterotoxins: *Escherichia coli* heat-labile and cholera toxin. *FEBS Lett* 1984;169:241–246.

223. Evans DJ, Chen LC, Curlin GT, Evans DG. Stimulation of adenyl cyclase by *Escherichia coli* enterotoxin. *Nature* 1972; 236:137–138.

224. Gill DM, Evans DJ Jr, Evans DG. Mechanism of activation of adenylate cyclase in vitro by polymyxin-released, heat-labile enterotoxin of *Escherichia coli*. *J Infect Dis* 1976;133: S103–S107.

225. Sixma TK, Kalk KH, van Zanten BA, et al. Refined structure of *Escherichia coli* heat-labile enterotoxin, a close relative of cholera toxin. *J Mol Biol* 1993;230:890–918.

226. Sixma TK, Pronk S, Kalk KH, et al. Crystal structure of a cholera toxin-related heat-labile enterotoxin from *E. coli*. *Science* 1991;351:371–377.

227. Moss J. Garrison S, Fishman PH, Richardson SH. Gangliosides sensitize unresponsive fibroblasts to *Escherichia coli* heat-labile enterotoxin. *J Clin Invest* 1979;64:381–384.

228. Holmgren J. Comparison of the tissue receptors for *Vibrio cholerae* and *Escherichia coli* enterotoxins by means of gangliosides and natural cholera toxoid. *Infect Immun* 1973;8:851–859.

229. Holmgren J, Fredman P, Lindblad M, et al. Rabbit intestinal glycoprotein receptor for *Escherichia coli* heat-labile enterotoxin lacking affinity for cholera toxin. *Infect Immun* 1982;38: 424–433.

230. Griffiths SL, Critchley DR. Characterisation of the binding sites for *Escherichia coli* heat-labile toxin type I in intestinal brush borders. *Biochem Biophys Acta* 1991;1075:154–161.

231. Holmgren J, Lindblad M, Fredman P, Svennerholm L, Myrvold H. Comparison of receptors for cholera and *Escherichia coli* enterotoxins in human intestine. *Gastroenterology* 1985; 89:27–35.

232. Zemelman BV, Chu S-HW, Walker WA. Host response to *Escherichia coli* heat-labile enterotoxin via two microvillus membrane receptors in the rat intestine. *Infect Immun* 1989; 57:2947–2952.

233. Green BA, Neill RJ, Ruyechan WT, Holmes RK. Evidence that a new enterotoxin of *Escherichia coli* which activates adenylate cyclase in eucaryotic target cells is not plasmid mediated. *Infect Immun* 1983;41:383–389.

234. Chang PP, Moss J, Twiddy EM, Holmes RK. Type II heat-labile enterotoxin of *Escherichia coli* activates adenylate cyclase in human fibroblasts by ADP ribosylation. *Infect Immun* 1987;55:1854–1858.

235. Donta ST, Tomicic T, Holmes RK. Binding of class II *Escherichia coli* enterotoxins to mouse Y1 and intestinal cells. *Infect Immun* 1992;60:2870–2873.

236. Pickett CL, Weinstein DL, Holmes RK. Genetics of type IIa heat-labile enterotoxin of *Escherichia coli*: operon fusions, nucleotides sequence, and hybridization studies. *J Bacteriol* 1987; 169:5180–5187.

237. Fukuta S, Magnani JL, Twiddy EM, Holmes RK, Ginsburg V. Comparison of the carbohydrate-binding specificities of cholera toxin and *Escherichia coli* heat-labile enterotoxins LTh-1 and LT-IIb. *Infect Immun* 1988;56:1748–1753.

238. Guerrant RL, Moore RA, Kirschenfeld BA, Sande MA. Role of toxigenic and invasive bacteria in acute diarrhea of childhood. *N Engl J Med* 1975;293:567–573.

239. Back E, Molby R, Kaijser B, Stintzing G, Wadstrom T, Habte D. Enterotoxigenic *Escherichia coli* and other gram-negative bacteria of infantile diarrhea: surface antigens, hemagglutinins, colonization factor antigen, and loss of enterotoxigenicity. *J Infect Dis* 1980;142:318–326.

240. Schultz AJ, McCardell BA. DNA homology and immunological cross-reactivity between *Aeromonas hydrophila* cytotonic toxin and cholera toxin. *J Clin Microbiol* 1988;26:57–61.

241. Rose JM, Houston CW, Cappenhaver DH, Dixon JD, Kurosky A. Purification and chemical characterization of cholera toxin: cross-reactive cytolytic enterotoxin produced by a human iso-

late of *Aeromonas hydrophila. Infect Immun* 1989;57:
1165–1169.

242. Gardner SE, Fowiston SE, Geroge WL. In vitro production of cholera toxin-like activity by *Plesiomonas shigelloides. J Infect Dis* 1987;156:720–722.

243. Ruiz-Palacios GM, Torres J, Torres NI, et al. Cholera-like enterotoxin produced by *Campylobacter jejuni:* characteristics and clinical significance. *Lancet* 1983;2:250–253.

244. Walker RI, Caldwell MB, Lee EC, et al. Pathophysiology of *Campylobacter* enteritis. *Microbiol Rev* 1986;50:81–94.

245. Jiwa SFH. Probing for enterotoxigenicity among the salmonellae. *J Clin Microbiol* 1981;14:463–472.

246. Finkelstein RA, Marchlewicz BA, McDonald RJ, Boesman-Finkelstein M. Isolation and characterization of a cholera-related enterotoxin from *Salmonella typhimurium. FEMS Microbiol Lett* 1983;17:239–241.

247. Baloda SB, Faris A, Krovacek K, Wadstrom T. Cytotonic enterotoxins and cytotoxic factors produced by *Salmonella enteriditis* and *Salmonella typhimurium. Toxicon* 1983;21:785–796.

248. Honda T, Taga S, Takeda Y, Miwatani T. Modified Elek test for detection of heat-labile enterotoxin of enterotoxigenic *Escherichia coli. J Clin Microbiol* 1981;13:1–5.

249. Honda T, Arita M, Takeda Y, Miwatani T. Further evaluation of the Biken (modified Elek test) for detection of enterotoxigenic *Escherichia coli* producing heat-labile enterotoxin and application of the test to sampling of heat-stable enterotoxin. *J Clin Microbiol* 1982;16:60–62.

250. Sutton RGA, Merson M, Craig JP, et al. Evaluation of the Biken test for the detection of LT-producing *Escherichia coli.* In: Takeda Y, Miwatani T, eds. *Bacterial diarrheal diseases.* Tokyo: KTK; 1985:209–218.

251. Donta ST, Moon HW, Whipp SC. Detection of heat-labile *Escherichia coli* enterotoxin with the use of adrenal cells in tissue culture. *Science* 1974;183:334–336.

252. Scotland SM, Gross RJ, Rowe B. Laboratory tests for enterotoxin production, enteroinvasion and adhesion in diarrhoeagenic *Escherichia coli.* In: Sussman M, ed. *The virulence of Escherichia coli. Reviews and methods.* London: Academic Press; 1985:395–405.

253. Bongaerts GPA, Bruggeman-Ogle KM, Mouton RP. Improvements in the microtire GM1 ganglioside enzyme-linked immunosorbent assay for *Escherichia coli* heat-labile enterotoxin. *J Appl Bacteriol* 1985;59:443–449.

254. Evans Jr. DJ, Evans DG. Direct serological assay for the heat-labile enterotoxin of *Escherichia coli* using passive immune homolysis. *Infect Immun* 1977;16:604–609.

255. Yolken RH, Greenberg HB, Merson MH, Sack RB, Kapikian AZ. Enzyme-linked immunosorbent assay for detection of *Escherichia coli* heat-labile enterotoxin. *J Clin Microbiol* 1977;5:439–444.

256. Finkelstein RA, Yang Z. Rapid test for identification of heat labile enterotoxin of *Escherichia coli* colonies. *J Clin Microbiol* 1983;18:1417–1418.

257. Finkelstein RA, Yang Z, Moseley LS, Moon HW. Rapid latex particle agglutination test for *Escherichia coli* strains of porcine origin producing heat-labile enterotoxin. *J Clin Microbiol* 1983;18:1417–1418.

258. Ito T, Kuwahara S, Yokota T. Automatic and manual latex agglutination tests for measurement of cholera toxin and heat-labile enterotoxin of *Escherichia coli. J Clin Microbiol* 1983;17:7–12.

259. Scotland SM, Flowmen RH, Rowe B. Evaluation of a reversed passive latex agglutination test for detection of *Escherichia coli* heat-labile toxin in culture supernatants. *J Clin Microbiol* 1989;27:339–340.

260. Speirs J, Stavric S, Buchanan B. Assessment of two commercial agglutination kits for detecting *Escherichia coli* heat-labile enterotoxin. *Can J Microbiol* 1991;37:877–880.

261. Bettelheim KA, Hanna N, Smith DL, Dwyer BW. Evaluation of the Phadebact ETEC-LT test for the heat-labile enterotoxin of *Escherichia coli. Int J Med Microbiol* 1989;271:70–76.

262. Chapman PA, Daly CM. Comparison of Y1 mouse adrenal cell

and coagglutination assays for detection of *Escherichia coli* heat-labile enterotoxin. *J Clin Pathol* 1989;42:755–758.

263. Wernars K, Delfgou E, Soentoro PS, Notermans S. Successful approach for detection of low numbers of enterotoxigenic *Escherichia coli* in minced meat by using the polymerase chain reaction. *Appl Environ Microbiol* 1991;57:1914–1919.

264. Moseley SL, Huq I, Alim ARMA, So M, Samadpour-Motalebi M, Falkow S. Detection of enterotoxigenic *Escherichia coli* by DNA colony hybridization. *J Infect Dis* 1980;142892–142898.

265. Olive DM, Khalik DA, Sethi SK. Identification of enterotoxigenic *Escherichia coli* using alkaline phosphatase-labeled synthetic oligodeoxyribonucleotide probes. *Eur J Clin Microbiol Infect Dis* 1988;7:167–171.

266. Dallas WS, Gill DM, Falkow S. Cistrons encoding *Escherichia coli* heat-labile toxin. *J Bacteriol* 1979;139:850–858.

267. Nalin DR, McLaughlin JC, Rahaman M, Yunus M, Curlin G. Enteropathogenic *Escherichia coli* and idiopathic diarrhoea in Bangladesh. *Lancet* 1975;2:1116–1119.

268. Merson MH, Sack RB, Islam S, et al. Disease due to enterotoxigenic *Escherichia coli* in Bangladeshi adults: clinical aspects in a controlled trial of tetracycline. *J Infect Dis* 1980;141:702–708.

269. Echeverria P, Blacklow NR, Sanford LB, Cukor G. Travellers diarrhoea among peace corps volunteers in Thailand. *J Infect Dis* 1981;143:767–771.

270. Santosham M, Burns B, Nadkarni V, et al. Oral rehydration therapy for acute diarrhea in ambulatory children in the United States: a double-blind comparison of four different solutions. *Pediatrics* 1985;76:159–164.

271. Black RE, Levine MM, Clements ML, Cisnersos L, Daya V. Treatment of experimentally induced enterotoxigenic *Escherichia coli* with trimethoprim-sulfamethoxazole or a placebo. *Rev Infect Dis* 1982;4:540–545.

272. DuPont HL, Reves RR, Galindo E, Sullivan PS, Wood LV, Mediola JG. Treatment of travellers' diarrhea with trimethoprim/sulfamethoxazole and with trimethoprim alone. *N Engl J Med* 1982;307:841–844.

273. Lester SC, de Pilar-Pla M, Perez-Schael I, et al. The carriage of *Escherichia coli* resistant to antimicrobial agents in healthy children in Boston, in Caracas and in Qin Pu, China. *N Engl J Med* 1990;323:285–289.

274. Murray BE, Rensimer ER, DuPont HL. Emergence of high-level trimethoprim resistance in fecal *Escherichia coli* during oral administration of trimethoprim or trimethoprim-sulfamethoxazole. *N Engl J Med* 1982;306:130–135.

275. Ericsson CD, Tannenbaum C, Charles TT. Antisecretory and antiinflammatory properties of bismuth subsalicylate. *Rev Infect Dis* 1990;12:S16–S20.

276. DuPont HL, Sullivan P, Pickering LK, Haynes G, Ackerman PB. Symptomatic treatment of diarrhoea with bismuth subsalicylate among students attending a Mexican University. *Gastroenterology* 1977;73:715–718.

277. DuPont HL, Sullivan P, Evans DG, et al. Prevention of traveler's diarrhea: prophylactic administration of subsalicylate bismuth. *JAMA* 1980;243:237–241.

278. Ericsson CD, Johnson PL, DuPont HL, Morgan DR, Bitsura JM, Cabada FJ. Ciprofloxacin or trimethoprim-sulfamethoxazole as initial therapy for traveler's diarrhea. *Ann Intern Med* 1987;106:216–220.

279. Levine MM, Kaper JB, Black RE, Clements ML. New knowledge on pathogenesis of bacterial infections as applied to vaccine development. *Microbiol Rev* 1983;47:510–550.

280. Levine MM, Morris JG, Losonsky G, Boedeker E, Rowe B. Fimbriae (pili) adhesins as vaccines. In: Lark D, Normak S, Brent-Uhiln E, eds. *Protein–carbohydrate interactions in biological systems.* London: Academic Press; 1986:143–145.

281. Levine MM. Development of vaccines against bacteria. In: Farthing MJG, Keusch GT, eds. *Enteric infection: mechanisms, manifestations and management.* New York: Raven Press; 1989:495–508.

282. Levine MM, Kaper JB, Herrington D, et al. Volunteer studies of deletion mutants of *Vibrio cholerae* C1 prepared by recombinant techniques. *Infect Immun* 1987;56:161–167.

283. Sack RB, Kline RL, Spira WM. Oral immunization of rabbits with enterotoxigenic *Escherichia coli* protects against intraintestinal challenge. *Infect Immun* 1988;56:387–394.

284. Lopez-Vidal Y, Calva JJ, Trujillo A, et al. Enterotoxins and adhesins of enterotoxigenic *Escherichia coli:* are they risk factors for acute diarrhea in the community? *J Infect Dis* 1990; 162:442–447.

285. Clemens JD, El-Morshiday S. Construction of a potential live oral bivalent vaccine for typhoid fever and cholera—*Escherichia coli* related diarrheas. *Infect Immun* 1984;46:564–569.

286. Yamamoto T, Tamura Y, Yokota T. Enteroadhesion fimbriae and enterotoxin of *Escherichia coli:* genetic transfer to a streptomycin-resistant mutant of the *galE* oral-route live-vaccine *Salmonella typhi* Ty21a. *Infect Immun* 1985;50:925–928.

287. Klipstein FA, Engert RF, Houghton RA. Immunization of volunteers with a synthetic peptide vaccine for enterotoxigenic *Escherichia coli. Lancet* 1986;1:471–473.

288. Houghton RA, Engert RF, Osteresh JM, Hoffman SR, Klipstein FA. A completely synthetic toxoid vaccine containing *Escherichia coli* heat-stable toxin and antigenic determinants of the heat-labile toxin and antigenic determinants of the heat-labile toxin B subunit. *Infect Immun* 1985;48:735–740.

289. Evans DG, Graham DY, Evans DG. Administration of purified colonization factor antigens (CFA/I, CFA/II) of enterotoxigenic *Escherichia coli* to volunteers. *Gastroenterology* 1984; 87:934–940.

290. Edelman R, Russell RG, Losonsky G, et al. Immunization of rabbits with enterotoxigenic *Escherichia coli* colonization factor antigen (CFA/I) encapsulated in biodegradable microspheres of poly (lactide-co-glycolide). *Vaccine* 1993;11: 155–158.

291. Reid RH, Boedeker EC, McQueen CE, et al. Preclinical evaluation of microencapsulated CFA/II oral vaccine against enterotoxigenic *Escherichia coli. Vaccine* 1993;11:159–193.

292. Moon HW, Bunn TO. Vaccines for preventing enterotoxigenic *Escherichia coli* infections in farm animals. *Vaccine* 1993;11: 213–220.

293. Holmgren J, Svennerholm AM. Development of oral vaccines against cholera and enterotoxigenic *Escherichia coli* diarrhea. *Scand J Infect Dis* 1990;76:47–53.

294. O'Farrelly C, Branton D, Wanke CA. Oral ingestion of egg yolk immunoglobulin from hens immunized with an enterotoxigenic *Escherichia coli* strain prevents diarrhea in rabbits challenged with the same strain. *Infect Immun* 1992;60:2593–2597.

295. Yokoyama H, Peralta RC, Diaz R, Sendo S, Ikemori Y, Kodama Y. Passive protective effect of chicken egg yolk immunoglobulins against experimental enterotoxigenic *Escherichia coli* infection in neonatal piglets. *Infect Immun* 1992;60:998–1007.

Infections of the Gastrointestinal Tract,
edited by M. J. Blaser, P. D. Smith, J. I. Ravdin,
H. B. Greenberg, and R. L. Guerrant
Raven Press, Ltd., New York © 1995.

CHAPTER 50

Enteropathogenic *Escherichia coli*

Michael S. Donnenberg

Enteropathogenic *Escherichia coli* (EPEC) comprise a unique class of intestinal pathogen with remarkable characteristics. EPEC were the first group of *E. coli* shown to cause diarrhea and have been responsible for devastating outbreaks of nosocomial neonatal diarrhea with extraordinary mortality. They have been implicated by epidemiological studies as important etiological agents of infant diarrhea in virtually every corner of the globe. The mechanism by which EPEC strains cause disease, totally enigmatic until recently, is now yielding to experimental investigation and is currently appreciated as among the most fascinating examples of the host–parasite relationship under study.

Controversy as to the identity of this class of diarrheagenic *E. coli* has existed for decades and is rooted in our ignorance of the pathogenetic mechanisms by which EPEC cause diarrhea. However, recent advances described below allow a more precise categorization of the strains that make up this class of *E. coli*. The lack of information available on EPEC pathogenesis at the time led to the following definition of EPEC, issued as a result of a workshop held at the National Institutes of Health in September 1982: "[EPEC may be defined as] diarrheagenic *E. coli* belonging to serogroups epidemiologically incriminated as pathogens but whose pathogenic mechanisms have not been proven to be related to either heat-labile enterotoxins or heat-stable enterotoxins or *Shigella*-like invasiveness" (1). Although this definition is still in use, it is largely one of exclusion and obviously may embrace a heterogeneous group of pathogens. It can be argued that, because of new information discussed below, the time has come to describe EPEC on the basis of specific virulence characteristics. Thus EPEC may now be considered to be a class of diarrheagenic *E. coli,* pathogenic for humans, that attach intimately to and efface the microvilli of enterocytes but do not produce high levels of Shiga-like toxins. The attaching and effacing effect is characterized by intimate adherence of the bacteria to epi-

thelial cells with destruction of microvilli and disruption of the cytoskeleton beneath the adherent organisms (Fig. 1A). This definition is consistent with the most current data derived from molecular pathogenesis studies and is rooted in an understanding of the prototypic strains originally classified as EPEC. Moreover, this appellation excludes *E. coli* that cause diarrhea by other mechanisms, such as the enteroaggregative and diffuse adhering strains (see chapter by Nataro), and reduces the heterogeneity of the group.

An understanding of the role of EPEC in human diarrheal disease requires examination of these strains from a historical perspective. For greater detail than can be presented here, the reader is referred to excellent reviews of the subject (2,3). *E. coli* was first widely accepted as a cause of diarrhea on the basis of epidemiological investigations of outbreaks of community-acquired and nosocomial infantile gastroenteritis in the United Kingdom in the 1940s (4–7). These outbreaks were characterized by their explosive nature and extraordinary mortality rates, sometimes exceeding 50% (4,6,8). Investigations of these outbreaks depended on the recognition that strains of *E. coli* cultured from infants with diarrhea could be agglutinated by specific antiserum raised against isolates from index cases, whereas *E. coli* isolated from well children could not. Soon a number of serologically distinct strains had been isolated from outbreaks (7). With the advent of the serological typing system of Kauffmann, it was recognized that these early outbreak strains belonged to certain serogroups (especially O111 and O55) whereas these serogroups are rarely found among *E. coli* isolated from healthy individuals (9). Netter et al. coined the term *enteropathogenic* to refer specifically to the strains associated with infantile gastroenteritis long before it was appreciated that *E. coli* could cause diarrhea by more than one mechanism (10). Some investigators have voiced objections to the continued use of the term *enteropathogenic* to describe a single class of virulent strains because this designation is nonspecific and could apply to any member of the species capable of causing diarrhea. However, the tide of historical precedent is too strong to overturn at

M. S. Donnenberg: Department of Medicine, University of Maryland at Baltimore School of Medicine, and VA Medical Center, Baltimore, Maryland 21201.

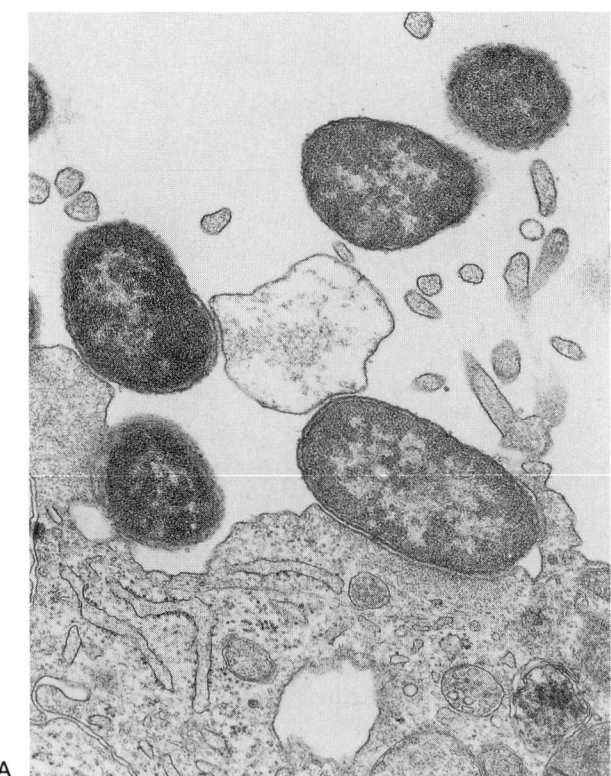 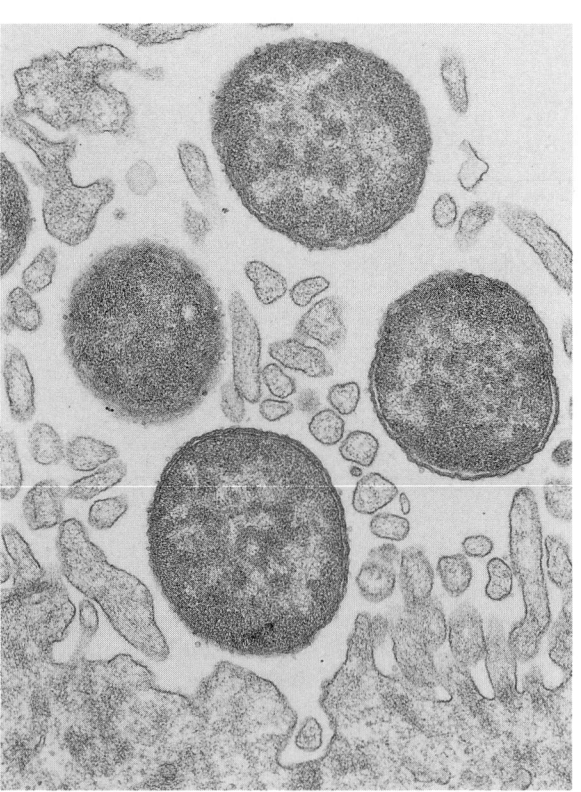

FIG. 1. Electron micrographs of Caco-2 intestinal tissue culture cells infected with a wild-type EPEC (**A**) or an isogenic mutant of that strain with an *eaeA* gene deletion (**B**). In (A) the attaching and effacing effect of EPEC upon intestinal tissue culture cells is shown. Bacteria are found intimately attached to the epithelial cell, which responds by forming cup-like pedestals composed of cytoskeletal proteins. In contrast, the mutant adheres at a distance from the cells, yet still damages microvilli (B). From ref. 76, with permission.

this point. Thus, the term *diarrheagenic* is often used generically, and *EPEC* is understood to refer specifically to strains that cause diarrhea by the mechanism common to the originally reported isolates. Recently, many of the isolates from the original investigations of infantile gastroenteritis have been resurrected and confirmed to possess the virulence genes currently under study that are characteristic of this group (see below), thus validating the relationship between classic EPEC strains and those used in recent genetic investigations (11).

During the 1950s additional serogroups were added to the list of those epidemiologically incriminated as causing diarrhea (2,3). Also during this period, human challenge studies confirmed the hypothesis that EPEC strains were pathogenic (12–14). However, with the discovery of the heat-labile and heat-stable enterotoxins of enterotoxigenic *E. coli* (ETEC) (see chapter by Cohen and Gianella) and of the invasive properties of enteroinvasive strains (EIEC) (see chapter by Acheson and Keusch), there ensued a period of confusion and doubt as to the pathogenic potential of EPEC strains. Investigators soon realized that strains belonging to EPEC serogroups lacked the virulence characteristics associated with ETEC and EIEC (15,16). Some suggested that most strains belonging to EPEC serogroups were not pathogenic (16), while others speculated that over the years the original EPEC strains

had lost plasmids necessary for virulence, accounting for their lack of definable virulence traits (17). These doubts were allayed when Levine et al. reported that strains belonging to traditional EPEC serogroups, confirmed to lack features characteristic of ETEC and EIEC, maintained their pathogenicity in volunteer studies (18). Thus new impetus was added to the search for pathogenic mechanisms of EPEC.

MICROBIOLOGY

EPEC Serotypes

Although EPEC were originally distinguished from other *E. coli* by serogroup [somatic lipopolysaccharide (O) antigen testing], identification is more accurately achieved by serotype [flagellar (H) antigen as well as O antigen testing] (2,3,19). Table 1 lists some of the most important serotypes considered to represent EPEC. Some serotypes, such as O111:H2, O55:H6, and O119:H6, are quite common and enjoy an association with diarrhea worldwide (20–23). Others originally thought to represent EPEC, such as O18:H7 and O18:H14, have rarely been associated with diarrhea and appear not to be pathogenic (19). Some serotypes consist of strains that lack the puta-

TABLE 1. *Serotypes commonly regarded to be enteropathogenic*

Serogroup	Flagellar antigens	Comments
O18	H7, H14	probably not EPEC (19,30)
O26	H−, H11	EHEC (24,25,155)
O44	H18, H34	O44:H18 often EAggEC (26)
O55	H−, **H6,** H7	O55:H7 often EAF-negative (26,33)
O86	**H34**	
O111	H−, **H2,** H7, H12, H21	Some O111:H− are EHEC (155)
O114	**H2**	
O119	**H6**	
O125	H21	
O126	H−, H2, H27	O126:H27 often EAggEC (26,33)
O127	H−, **H6,** H21	
O128	H2, H7, H12	
O142	**H6**	
O158	H23	

Data from refs. 2, 3, 9, and 19.
EPEC, enteropathogenic *E. coli;* EHEC, enterohemorrhagic *E. coli;* EAggEC, enteroaggregative *E. coli;* EAF, EPEC adherence factor. Shown in bold type are serotypes most closely associated with EPEC virulence factors.

tive virulence characteristics now known to be common to classic EPEC strains and therefore should no longer be considered to be members of this category. Included among these are serotypes now considered to consist of strains that belong to other pathogenic classes. For example O26:H11 is now considered to be an EHEC serotype (24,25), while O44:H18 and O126:H27 strains often belong to the enteroaggregative (EAggEC) category (26). It further complicates matters that strains from serotypes other than those commonly included with the EPEC have been isolated from children with diarrhea and shown to possess the putative virulence properties characteristic of EPEC (27,28).

Nataro et al. proposed in 1985 to consider two classes of EPEC (29). Class I would consist of strains from the most common serogroups, which share the ability to adhere to epithelial cells in a characteristic localized pattern and are positive with a DNA probe (see below). Class II strains belong to serogroups (O44, O86, O114) less frequently associated with diarrhea and may not share the adherence characteristics of class I strains. This separation no longer appears valid. O114:H2 and O86:H34 strains, the only EPEC serotypes within these serogroups, in fact display the adherence phenotypes characteristic of traditional EPEC (30–33). O44 strains do not appear to possess the putative EPEC virulence traits; many may actually be EAggEC (26,31) (Table 1).

CLONAL RELATEDNESS OF EPEC

From the point of view of the clinical microbiology laboratory, EPEC are similar in most respects to conventional *E. coli.* However, particular serotypes of EPEC tend to have certain biochemical idiosyncracies, principally in their ability to ferment sugars (34–36). This observation, and the observation that outer membrane protein profiles of EPEC correlate with serotyping, led to the suggestion that the EPEC population structure is clonal (34). The results of multilocus enzyme electrophoresis analysis, a technique for quantifying the genetic relatedness of microorganisms, has confirmed this hypothesis (37). The limited number of EPEC strains examined to date appear to compose two great lineages (37,38). One group includes serotypes O55:H6, O125:H6, O142:H6, and O86:H34. Also related was a single isolate of O127:H−, perhaps a nonmotile mutant of O127:H6. The other lineage includes serotypes O111:H2 and O128:H2. It appears from these experiments that the flagellar H antigen is more indicative of relatedness than the O antigen (37). Strains from the two lineages appear to be only distantly related to each other. The relationships among many other serotypes of EPEC remain to be elucidated.

A close examination of O114 strains indicates that a particular serogroup can be quite heterogeneous, composed of several lineages each containing closely related strains that are distantly related to each other (32). However, within the O114 serogroup, strains that fall into particular pathogenic categories, such as EPEC, ETEC, and P-fimbriated *E. coli,* share common H antigens and are quite closely related. Similar results have been obtained with other serogroups (38). These observations underscore the importance of determining the serotype of an isolate rather than merely its serogroup when performing diagnostic studies.

The EPEC share notable pathogenetic features with the enterohemorrhagic *E. coli* (EHEC); the latter are distinguished by the production of high levels of Shiga-like toxins. The most important EHEC serotype, O157:H7, seems to share a common ancestor with EPEC serotype O55:H7, which in turn is related to the H6 EPEC lineage (38). Interestingly, many strains of the O55:H7 serotype, like EHEC, commonly lack adherence features found in most other EPEC (26). In contrast, EHEC of serotypes O26:H11 and O111:H8 are more closely related to the H2 EPEC lineage. These observations suggest that horizontal transfer of Shiga-like toxin genes encoded by bacteriophages was an important step in the divergent evolution of EPEC and EHEC strains. It will be interesting to investigate the relationship between EPEC strains and animal *E. coli* pathogens such as rabbit pathogen RDEC-1, which cause diarrhea by mechanisms similar to EPEC.

EPIDEMIOLOGY

An understanding of the epidemiology of EPEC infection is hampered by the use in different studies of different criteria for the diagnosis of EPEC infections. Results may vary depending on whether EPEC were sought by serogroup, serotype, the results of DNA probe assays for putative virulence attributes, or the results of a fluorescent assay used as a surrogate for the attaching and effacing effect. Nevertheless, it is obvious that EPEC is an endemic diarrheal pathogen of considerable importance among infants in developing countries. Our knowledge of the incidence of EPEC in developed countries is less complete, however, due to the abandonment by clinical microbiology laboratories in the 1970s of efforts to diagnose EPEC infection.

The predominant mode of transmission of EPEC infection is not firmly established, but strong evidence suggests that person-to-person spread by the fecal–oral route is most important (3,39). Several outbreaks of nosocomial EPEC infection have been traced to an index case (8,40,41). EPEC may be isolated from asymptomatic children, especially those older than 6 months of age (42–44). Such carriers may represent the primary reservoir for infection. Occasionally asymptomatic infection in an adult is implicated as the source of an outbreak or sporadic case (40,45). Contamination of the hands of caretakers has been documented and suggested to be a major mode of nosocomial transmission (3,40). Handwashing effectively eliminates the organism (40). There is no evidence of an animal reservoir for EPEC infection, as attaching and effacing bacteria of animals generally belong to non-EPEC serotypes (46–48). Similarly, although environmental contamination occurs with EPEC (3,40), contaminated food and water is the cause of only rare EPEC outbreaks (49,50).

EPEC in the Developing World

The evidence that EPEC are an important cause of infant diarrhea in developing countries is very convincing. Prospective studies performed on six continents have demonstrated a higher rate of isolation of EPEC strains from infants with diarrhea than from matched controls. This association has been demonstrated in Mexico (21,23), Peru (29), Brazil (20,22,51,52), Chile (53), the former Yugoslavia (42), South Africa (54), Ethiopia (55), Thailand (43,56), China (57), India (58,59), New Caledonia (60), and Australia (44). Numerous uncontrolled studies support the case-control data. Studies showing an association between EPEC and diarrhea have included patients presenting to hospitals (22,43,51,52,54–58,60) and to outpatient clinics (20,42) as well as community-based longitudinal studies (21,23,29,44,59). The associa-

tion between EPEC and diarrhea is particularly strong among younger children (42,44), and strongest among infants less than 6 months of age (23,43,52). In the youngest children, EPEC may be the most common identifiable bacterial cause of diarrhea and in several studies has exceeded even rotavirus in incidence (23,51,52,54).

The possibility that bottle feeding is a risk factor for the development of EPEC infection has been suggested since the 1940s (6,8). More recent case-control studies have confirmed that breastfeeding is protective for the development of EPEC diarrhea (54,61). Both the immunoglobulin and the oligosaccharide fractions of breast milk have been shown to inhibit EPEC adherence to epithelial cells (62). A recent study has identified a heretofore unappreciated risk factor for EPEC diarrhea. Infants presenting to a hospital in São Paulo, Brazil with EPEC diarrhea were 12 times more likely than controls to have been hospitalized during the month prior to the onset of illness (61). This unexpected finding in outpatients reemphasizes the importance of EPEC as a nosocomial pathogen in developing as well as developed countries.

EPEC in Developed Countries

A reexamination of 93 *E. coli* strains submitted to the Centers for Disease Control and Prevention between 1934 and 1987 from 50 outbreaks in the United States of diarrhea in children under 2 years of age revealed that the majority of these strains were of EPEC serotypes and were positive when tested with an EPEC DNA probe (63). This study confirms the suspicion that most of these outbreaks were due to what are now regarded to be EPEC strains. While two outbreaks were from 1983, the majority of the EPEC outbreaks were from the 1950s and 1960s.

It is generally accepted that EPEC are no longer a common cause of diarrhea in the United States and other developed nations. However, the validity of this assumption is subject to debate. In Manitoba, Canada, EPEC were still an important cause of community-acquired diarrhea among infants in 1976 (45), and in a study conducted between 1983 and 1986 in the former West Germany, EPEC serotypes were found significantly more often in infants with diarrhea than controls (64). The abandonment in many hospitals of efforts to diagnose EPEC may have led to significant underappreciation of the prevalence of EPEC disease. The availability of improved methods for EPEC diagnosis based on putative virulence factors (see below) should prompt a reinvestigation of the role of EPEC in developed countries. Despite the fact that EPEC are not often sought, outbreaks and sporadic cases of EPEC infection in the United States, the United Kingdom, and Finland were recently reported (33,39,41,49,65–67). Two severe outbreaks were associated with child daycare centers, an increasingly popular environment with great potential for EPEC transmission (41,67). The AIDS epidemic may also provide a reservoir of susceptible hosts. A recent case report described attaching and effacing bacteria, possibly EPEC, in an AIDS patient with persistent diarrhea (68). Further studies on patients with diarrhea and HIV infection appear warranted.

PATHOGENESIS AND IMMUNITY

Pathology

The histopathology of severe natural EPEC infection has been studied in detail. Gross examination of the intestines rarely reveals abnormalities, even in fatal cases (8,69). However, on microscopic inspection of the jejunum, there is severe villus atrophy often accompanied by crypt hypertrophy (65,66,70,71). An inflammatory infiltrate is found in the lamina propria, which may be mononuclear (66,71) or composed of neutrophils as well as lymphocytes, plasma cells, and macrophages (39,65). Similar changes can be found in ileal and rectal biopsy of severe cases (66,72). On ultrastructural examination, bacteria are found intimately attached to epithelial cells, microvilli are effaced, and the cytoskeleton is damaged (see below). In addition, progressive loss of cytoplasmic organelles is observed (72), an observation consistent with cellular necrosis. The loss of microvilli is correlated with a loss of activity of enzymes associated with the brush border (71,73).

Molecular Pathogenesis

Application of the tools of recombinant DNA technology has greatly advanced our understanding of EPEC pathogenesis. The isolation of random mutants generated by transposon mutagenesis followed by screening for loss of a phenotype presumed to be involved in virulence has proved to be a very successful strategy for identifying EPEC genes (74,75). Once a mutant with loss of an interesting phenotype is identified, the gene into which the transposon has inserted can be recovered and character-

ized. In one application of this approach 339 transposon mutants of an O127:H6 EPEC strain were screened for the ability to invade tissue culture cells; 22 were found to be deficient (75). Analysis of these noninvasive mutants revealed that they could be classified on the basis of phenotypic and genotypic criteria into five categories. Study of mutants from each of these categories has led to the identification of putative virulence genes associated with pathogenesis, as will be discussed below. The composite picture that has emerged, based on analysis of mutants deficient in one or more features, indicates that the pathogenesis of EPEC infection may be viewed as encompassing at least three distinct stages (Fig. 2) (76). It is tempting to conceptualize these stages as occurring in a temporal sequence. However, there are no data to validate such a progression and in truth, the various stages may occur concurrently. Nevertheless, for ease of discussion, the pathogenesis of EPEC will be discussed in the context of a sequence of events. The major proposed virulence factors of EPEC are summarized in Table 2.

Localized Adherence

The first breakthrough in understanding the pathogenesis of EPEC infection was the observation by Cravioto et al. that, unlike most *E. coli*, EPEC adhere avidly to epithelial cells in tissue culture (77). Rather than covering the entire surface of the cells, EPEC bind as tight microcolonies (Fig. 3) in a pattern termed *localized adherence* (78). Other classes of diarrheagenic *E. coli* once considered to be EPEC, which bind in diffuse or aggregative patterns, are not capable of attaching and effacing and are therefore considered in the chapter by Nataro.

Pioneering work in the laboratory of James Kaper soon led to the realization that the localized adherence phenomenon was plasmid-encoded. EPEC strains representing a

TABLE 2. *Summary of proposed and confirmed virulence factors of EPEC*

Feature	Description	Associated proteins	Genetic loci
Localized adherence	Formation of adherent microcolonies on epithelial cells	I. Bundle-forming pilus II. Periplasmic disulfide bond oxidoreductase	I. Plasmid-encoded *bfpA* gene, other uncharacterized regions of plasmid II. Chromosomal *dsbA* gene
Intimate attachment	Attachment of bacteria within 10 nm of the epithelial cell	I. Intimin, a 94-kDa outer membrane protein II. The 39-kDa EaeB protein	The chromosomal *eae* gene cluster, including *eaeA* which encodes intimin, *eaeB*, and other uncharacterized loci
Signal transduction	Activation of epithelial cell signal pathways including protein tyrosine kinases, protein kinase C, and phospholipase C leading to cytoskeletal disruption	Unknown	Uncharacterized genetic loci tentatively termed *cfm* (for category four mutants)
Invasion	Entry of a subset of bacteria to an undefined intracellular compartment	Invasion-specific proteins not characterized	I. All loci noted above and additional uncharacterized loci not required for above processes II. Plasmid-encoded loci in some strains sufficient for invasion
Gene regulation	Activation of transcription of *eaeA* and *eaeB* genes	A 26-kDa regulator with sequence similarities to the AraC protein	Plasmid-encoded *perA* gene

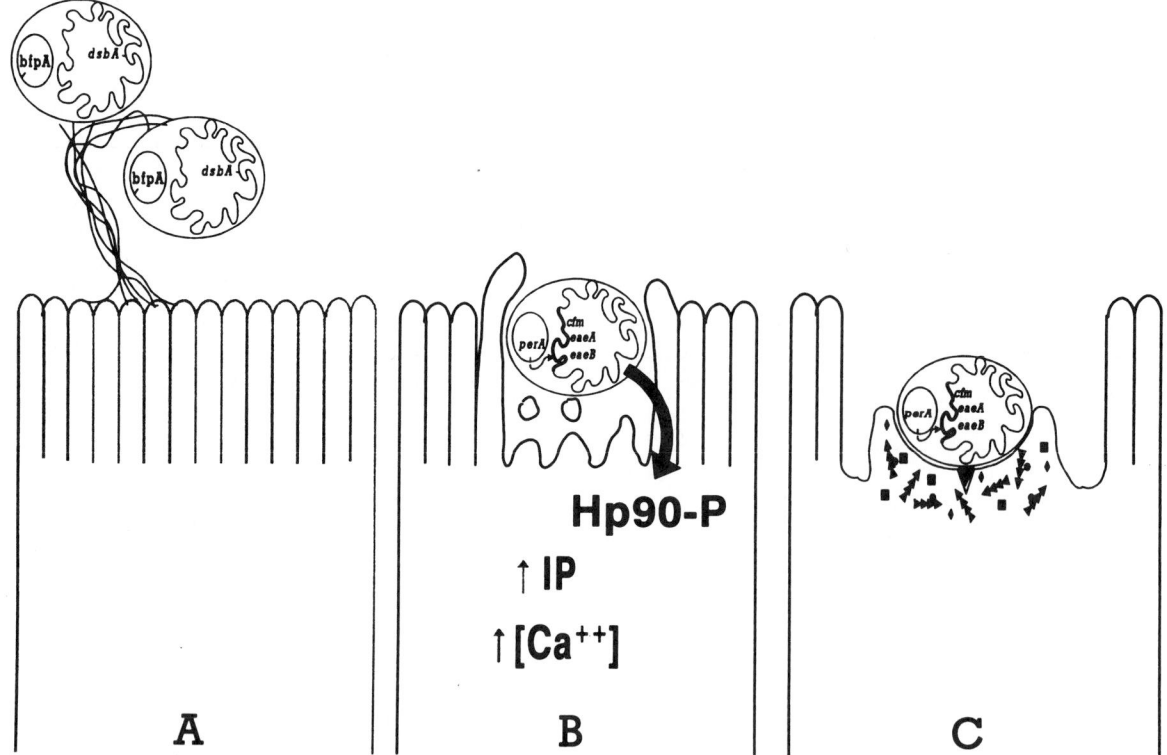

FIG. 2. A three-stage model of EPEC pathogenesis. The model does not imply a strict temporal relationship, but is based in the analysis of mutants deficient in specific stages of the infection. The first panel (**A**) depicts localized adherence, proposed to be mediated by the bundle-forming pilus, the major structural subunit of which is encoded by the *bfpA* gene. The chromosomal *dsbA* gene, encoding a periplasmic enzyme that catalyzes disulfide bond formation, is also required for this step. The second panel (**B**) depicts the signals transduced to the epithelial cell, which include activation of tyrosine kinases to phosphorylate a 90-kDa protein (HP-90-P), rises in inositol phosphates (IP), and elevations of intracellular calcium. The uncharacterized bacterial genes responsible are called *cfm*. Also depicted is transcriptional activation of the *eaeA* and *eaeB* loci by the plasmid-encoded *perA* regulator. The third panel (**C**) depicts intimate attachment of the bacterium to the epithelial cell mediated by intimin (*solid triangle*), the product of the *eaeA* gene. The epithelial cell embraces the bacterium in a cup-like pedestal, supported by cytoskeletal proteins such as actin, α-actinin, talin, and ezrin (*geometric shapes*). (Modified and reprinted from ref. 76, with permission.)

variety of serotypes were found to possess highly conserved high molecular weight plasmids associated with localized adherence (79–81). A link between this plasmid, localized adherence, and virulence was established when a volunteer study revealed that the attack rate for diarrhea was lower in individuals fed a plasmid-cured EPEC strain than in those fed the parental plasmid-containing wild-type strain (82). The term *EPEC adherence factor* (EAF) was used to describe the hypothetical ligand responsible for localized adherence. Efforts to identify the EAF resulted in the identification of two large regions of the plasmid necessary for localized adherence (80). A 1-kb DNA fragment from one of these regions, known as the EAF probe, is highly sensitive and specific in identifying EPEC strains (29) and has been widely used as an epidemiological tool to study the prevalence of EPEC infections (21,22,29,44,51,57,60,63,83,84).

The identification by Girón et al. of a plasmid-associated fimbria in EPEC was the next breakthrough in understanding localized adherence (85). Repetitive subculture on blood agar plates appears to be necessary for appreciation of these fimbriae. The fimbriae appear as flexible rope-like bundles that intertwine, linking individual bacteria. Transposon mutants from the first of the five noninvasive categories described above have insertions in the EAF plasmid and are deficient in localized adherence. Sequencing the DNA adjacent to the site of the transposon insertions in these mutants revealed the gene encoding the major structural subunit of this fimbriae (*bfpA*) (86). This gene was soon identified by another group using a different approach (87). The DNA sequence predicts a protein related to the type IV fimbriae family, which includes the pili of *Vibrio cholerae*, *Pseudomonas aeruginosa*, *Neisseria gonorrhoeae*, as well as other pathogens and confirms the amino acid sequence obtained from the purified fimbriae (85). The possibility that this fimbria is the EAF is supported by the lack of localized adherence by a mutant with an insertion in the *bfpA* locus (86) and

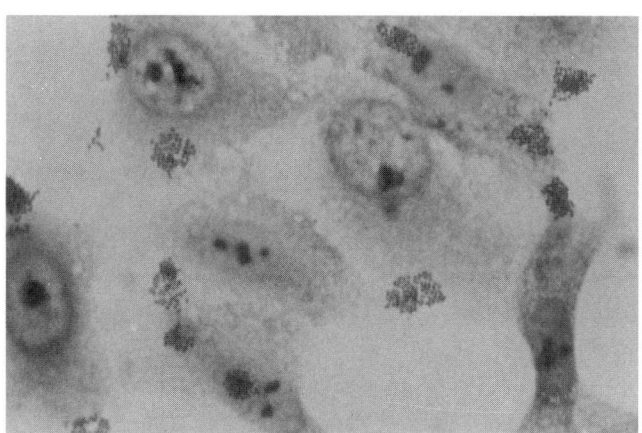

FIG. 3. HEp-2 tissue culture cells infected with an EPEC strain and stained with Geimsa. Bacteria adhere in discrete microcolonies characteristic of localized adherence.

by the inhibition of localized adherence with antiserum prepared against the purified pilus (85).

In addition to the *bfpA* locus, there is evidence that a number of other plasmid and chromosomal genes are required for localized adherence (75,80). Additional loci on the plasmid necessary for localized adherence may be involved in processing, export, assembly, and regulation of the fimbriae. Recently, a second category of the 22 noninvasive mutants deficient in localized adherence was shown to have insertions in the chromosomal *dsbA* gene (88). The ubiquitous *E. coli dsbA* locus encodes an oxidoreductase enzyme necessary for efficient disulfide bond formation in the periplasmic space (89,90) and required for proper function of a variety of exported virulence factors and other proteins that contain disulfide bonds (89,91–94). Presumably DsbA oxidizes cysteine residues required for function of the EPEC bundle-forming pilus (the major structural subunit itself possesses two cysteine residues), but this has yet to be demonstrated.

Several investigators have reported that certain strains, e.g., O55:H7 and some O111 and O128 serotypes, display less exuberant localized adherence to epithelial cells and are frequently negative upon testing with the EAF probe (26,33,95,96), yet are capable of attaching and effacing. Some but not all strains of these serotypes are negative when tested with a *bfpA* probe as well (97). It is not yet clear as to whether other adhesins might mediate this poor localized adherence (33) or whether indeed this pattern is due to attaching and effacing alone without additional adhesins.

Intimate Attachment to Epithelial Cells: The eae Gene Cluster

The hallmark of EPEC infection is the ability of the organism to attach intimately to epithelial cells and efface microvilli (Fig. 1). This effect was first described by Staley et al. in 1969 (98), although the term *attaching and*

effacing was coined by Moon et al. in 1983 (99). The lesion consists of bacteria in close proximity to the plasma membrane of enterocytes, separated by a distance of only 10 nm. Microvilli vesiculate early in the interaction between bacterium and epithelial cell, are absent directly beneath intimately attached bacteria, and are elongated adjacent to the organisms (100). The epithelial cell responds by forming cup-like pedestals, on which the bacteria rest. Directly beneath adherent organisms there is a reorganization of cytoskeletal elements including actin (30), a light chain of myosin (101), α-actinin, talin, and ezrin (102). These cytoskeletal elements are so sharply focused beneath the organisms that, when viewed by fluorescence microscopy using probes for these eukaryotic proteins, it appears as though the bacteria themselves are staining (Fig. 4).

Attaching and effacing activity has been observed with EPEC of classic serogroups (100) and with prototypic strains from the original outbreaks (11). The effect has been noted using animal models (98,99,103,104), tissue culture cells (74,105), and in pathological tissue from human infections (65,66,71,73,106). Unlike localized adherence, attaching and effacing activity does not require the presence of the EPEC plasmid, although the plasmid facilitates this effect (100,104,105). Attaching and effacing activity has also been observed in animal models of EHEC (107,108) and certain strains of *Hafnia alvei* (109) and *Citrobacter freundii* (110). *Helicobacter pylori* also exhibits some of the features of the attaching and effacing effect (111,112).

Jerse et al. were the first investigators to identify an EPEC gene involved in interactions with epithelial cells (74). The *eaeA* locus (for *E. coli a*ttaching and *e*ffacing gene *A*) was found by screening transposon mutants of a plasmid-cured EPEC strain for deficiency in inducing accumulations of filamentous actin in epithelial cells. The same gene was independently identified among yet another category of the 22 noninvasive transposon mutants (75). Mutants at the *eaeA* locus are incapable of attaching intimately to epithelial cells (Fig. 1B) (74,113), but retain the ability to transduce signals to the epithelial cell that result in cytoskeletal alterations and in accumulations of host cell tyrosine kinase substrates (see below) (114). Sequences of the *eaeA* gene have been detected in all EPEC, EHEC (115), *H. alvei* (116), and *C. fruendii* (117) strains capable of attaching and effacing. Gene sequences have also been detected in *E. coli* strains pathogenic for animals that display attaching and effacing effects (47,115,118). Sequences hybridizing with an *eaeA* gene probe have not been detected in *H. pylori* (112). A mutation of the EHEC *eaeA* locus has been engineered in a wild-type EHEC strain. This mutant fails to produce attaching and effacing lesions in newborn piglets. The ability to perform this function is restored upon introduction of the cloned *eaeA* genes of either EHEC or EPEC, demonstrating that these loci are functionally homologous (119). In all cases tested, the *eaeA* gene sequences have been found on the bacterial chromosome rather than on plasmids (115). The *eaeA* homologs of EHEC (120,121) and *C. freundii* (117) have been cloned and sequenced and are highly similar to the EPEC locus.

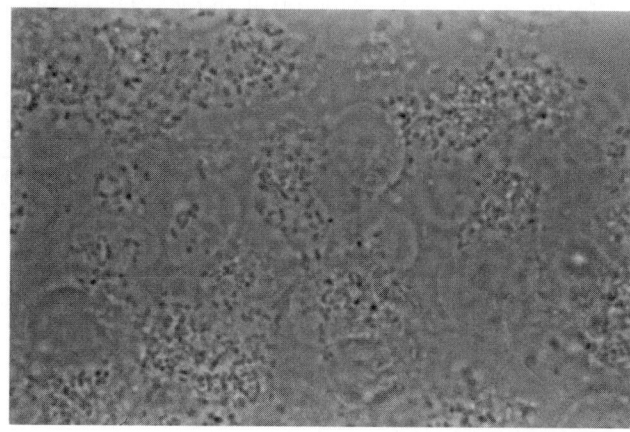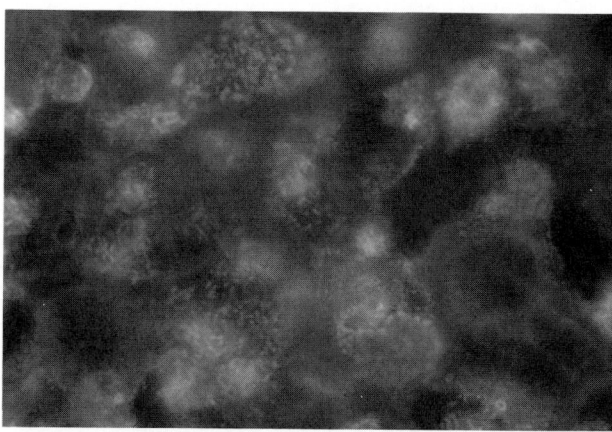

FIG. 4. Phase contrast (**A**) and fluorescent (**B**) views of the same field of HEp-2 cells infected with an EPEC strain and stained with fluorescein-labeled phalloidin, which binds to filamentous actin. Note the intense fluorescence at sites of bacterial adherence, indicating deposition of filamentous actin directly beneath bacterial attaching and effacing lesions.

The *eaeA* gene encodes a 94-kDa outer membrane protein known as intimin (122). Intimin was originally thought to be encoded by the EPEC plasmid, but it is now clear that plasmid loci regulate intimin expression (122,123). The amino acid sequence of intimin, deduced from the EPEC *eaeA* gene sequence, reveals a protein with a high degree of similarity to the invasin protein of *Yersinia pseudotuberculosis* and *Y. enterocolitica*. This latter protein confers on normally noninvasive *E. coli* strains the ability to enter epithelial cells with high efficiency (124). Invasin binds tenaciously to members of the β_1 class of integrins, receptors normally involved in interactions between eukaryotic cells and extracellular substrates and ligands (125). The sequence similarities between invasin and intimins of EPEC, EHEC, and *C. freundii* are concentrated near the amino terminus of the molecules (120), domains that are involved in the localization of invasin to the bacterial outer membrane (126). In contrast, the carboxyl termini of the proteins, the domain responsible for receptor binding and internalization of invasin (127), are much less similar. In addition, while all intimin sequences are nearly identical at their amino termini, at the carboxyl terminal 25% of the predicted proteins are only about 50% identical.

The precise function of intimin is not known. On the basis of sequence similarities with invasins, surface localization, and lack of intimate attachment by *eaeA* mutants, it is tempting to speculate that intimin is the intimate adhesin that binds to an epithelial cell receptor, as the name suggests. However, this has yet to be established.

A volunteer study has confirmed that the *eaeA* gene is indeed the first EPEC virulence gene to be identified (128). Volunteers were randomized under double-blind conditions to receive either a wild-type EPEC strain or an isogenic mutant differing only in that it had an internal deletion within the *eaeA* locus. Only 4 of 11 volunteers who received the mutant developed diarrhea in comparison with all 11 recipients of the wild-type strain. Fever was also more common in recipients of wild-type and titers of serum antibodies against the lipopolysaccharide

(LPS) of the infecting strain were higher in this group. Interestingly, the levels of secretory IgA in jejunal fluid did not differ between groups.

Intimin alone is not sufficient for intimate attachment or invasion when cloned into laboratory *E. coli* strains (74). Among the 22 noninvasive mutants are 5 with transposon mutations within *eaeA* and 2 with insertions that map downstream of *eaeA* and also interfere with intimate attachment of EPEC to epithelial cells (75). Recently a second locus necessary for intimate attachment was identified (129). The *eaeB* gene is located approximately 5 kb downstream of *eaeA*. A mutant engineered to have an internal in-frame deletion within this gene is unable to attach intimately to epithelial cells. The predicted product of the *eaeB* gene is a unique protein whose function is unknown at this time. In addition, indirect evidence suggests that additional loci between *eaeA* and *eaeB* are necessary for intimate attachment.

Intimin is not produced constitutively. Expression of intimin is influenced by growth conditions, and the presence of the EAF plasmid greatly enhances intimin production (122). Recently a plasmid locus (*perA* for *p*lasmid-*e*ncoded *r*egulator) has been identified that acts as a positive regulator of *eaeA* and *eaeB* expression at the transcriptional level (123). The predicted sequence of the protein identifies PerA as a member of the AraC family of transcriptional activators.

Signal Transduction

The dramatic effects of EPEC on the epithelial cell cytoskeleton are the result of the ability of the bacteria to interfere with normal pathways of signal transduction in epithelial cells. Several such pathways have been implicated. Using a phosphotyrosine-specific monoclonal as primary antibody for fluorescent microscopy, Rosenshine et al. demonstrated that tyrosine kinase substrates colocalize with the accumulated cytoskeletal products beneath adherent bacteria (114). Furthermore, a prominent 90-kDa host cell tyrosine kinase substrate is specifically detected in cells infected with EPEC. The identity of this protein is not yet known. Other investigators have demonstrated that a myosin light chain becomes phosphorylated upon infection of epithelial cells with EPEC, but the responsible kinases have not been identified (101). Protein kinase C has also been indirectly implicated in EPEC infection (130). Still other investigators have reported that vinculin and α-actinin become phosphorylated when cells infected with EPEC are broken open and then assayed for kinase activity (131).

In addition to or as a consequence of alterations of protein kinase/phosphatase pathways, EPEC infection *in vitro* causes calcium to be released from intracellular stores (132,133). The accumulation of actin beneath the EPEC organisms appears to be dependant on this calcium flux (134). Phospholipase C activity, detected by measuring rises in inositol phosphates (IPs); has also been detected in cells infected with EPEC (135). These observations suggest that EPEC induces host cell phospholipase C, the activation of which would result in elevations in IPs and diacylglycerol (136). The IP flux in turn may cause release of calcium from intracellular stores, while the diacylglycerol can activate protein kinase C. Diacylglycerol has also been shown to cause actin nucleation (137), which may be an additional factor in the cytoskeletal changes induced by EPEC. Interestingly, inhibition of tyrosine kinase activity blocks the rise in IPs, suggesting that tyrosine kinases are proximal in this signal transduction cascade.

Two EPEC mutants, belonging to a fourth category among the 22 noninvasive mutants, fail to induce the accumulation of filamentous actin in epithelial cells (75). In contrast, *eaeA* mutants retain the ability to influence cellular actin and to initiate signal transduction. Thus, the attaching and effacing lesion can be separated into two steps: intimate attachment and cytoskeletal damage. Interestingly, these are the only mutants among the five categories that do not induce the 90-kDa tyrosine-phosphorylated host cell protein (114). These mutants also fail to induce the accumulation of tyrosine kinase substrates beneath sites of attachment and fail to induce IP accumulation. Thus these appear to have mutations in loci required for transduction of the signal(s) to epithelial cells that result(s) in the cytoskeletal damage characteristic of EPEC infection. The genetic defects in these mutants have not yet been described, so the loci affected have been given the temporary moniker *cfm*, for *c*ategory *f*our *m*utants.

Cellular Invasion

There is no reason to believe that EPEC is primarily an invasive pathogen, at least in the way that *Shigella* and *Salmonella* are. EPEC does not cause dysentery or typhoidal syndromes. Sepsis or disseminated disease due to EPEC is rare, seemingly a near-terminal event in severe protracted cases (8,40,41). Although EPEC have been observed in the lamina propria and in distant sites in fatal cases (138), and crypt abscesses have been described in the small intestine (139), these reports may represent the extremes of pathology in the most severe cases. Yet more subtle aspects of EPEC infection, such as the capacity of EPEC to cause protracted infection, the fever seen in many patients, and the lactoferrin detected in stool samples (140), may be influenced by the ability of the organism to enter epithelial cells. Intracellular organisms have been observed, not only in tissue culture (141–143) and animal models (98,99,103,104) of EPEC infection, but in some (65,71) [though not all (66,106)] clinical specimens from patients with EPEC.

Considerable attention has recently been paid to EPEC's capacity for epithelial cell invasion *in vitro*. When tested in a quantitative gentamicin protection assay, EPEC invade at levels comparable to those seen with EIEC (141,144). However, when the number of intracellular organisms is divided by the total number of cell-associated bacteria, the ratio is much lower for EPEC than EIEC (144). Thus, only a minority of the adherent EPEC invade epithelial cells, but since EPEC adhere so avidly, the total number of intracellular organisms is large.

While the significance of EPEC cellular invasion is unclear, there can be no argument that invasion has proven to be a useful property for the study of EPEC pathogenesis. Initial adherence by the bacterium is necessary but not sufficient for efficient invasion by EPEC and EPEC-like organisms (141,145,146). The reduction of EPEC invasion by microtubule inhibitors may provide a clue to interactions between EPEC and the host cytoskeleton that has not yet been explored (145,147). Finally, the identification of noninvasive transposon mutants described above has led to the characterization of multiple genes involved in EPEC pathogenesis (75).

Fletcher et al. described a 4.5-kb restriction fragment cloned from an O111:H− strain that confers epithelial cell invasion on a noninvasive laboratory strain when present in high copy number (148). The fragment was cloned from a large plasmid of the EPEC strain on which neither the EAF nor the *eaeA* gene are found, but which reportedly confers attaching and effacing ability when introduced into a laboratory *E. coli* strain (149). The cloned locus does not encode attaching and effacing. Hybridization with the cloned fragment was detected in only 11 of 49 *E. coli* strains from EPEC serogroups tested. Only 4 of these 11 were also positive when tested with the EAF probe, suggesting that this locus is present in a minority of true EPEC. The genetic determinant from this clone has not yet been characterized.

Other Potential Virulence Factors

The restricted number of serogroups associated with EPEC strains has led to the hypothesis that LPS itself may be a virulence factor for EPEC. Of course the correlation between O antigens and EPEC virulence may not indicate a causal relationship. In one strain, the loss of O-antigen specificity does not result in a loss of attaching and effacing ability (150). Nevertheless, it has been pointed out that some O antigens, such as O111 and O114, are found in *E. coli* from multiple pathogenic classes, while many others are not found among pathogenic *E. coli*, suggesting that certain O-antigen types may contribute to pathogenesis (19,37).

The role of Shiga-like toxins in EPEC pathogenesis has been controversial. Low levels of toxin activity from sonic lysates of *E. coli* of EPEC serogroups as well as many other *E. coli* have been reported (151–153). In a minority of cases, this activity is neutralized by antiserum specific for Shiga toxin (151). In most of these studies, the strains were not characterized beyond serogrouping to determine whether they were truly EPEC. In studies in which this was done, Shiga-like toxin activity has been found in serotypes such as O26:H11 and O111:H− now considered to be EHEC (64). However, strains from some EPEC serotypes such as O119:H6 and O55:H6 can display Shiga-like toxin activity and localized adherence (64). Although the vast majority of EPEC strains that hybridize with the EAF probe do not hybridize with Shiga-like toxin gene probes, some do (154,155). It can be concluded that most EPEC do not produce high levels of Shiga-like toxins or possess the genes for Shiga-like toxins, and therefore Shiga-like toxins are not necessary for EPEC pathogenesis. While many EPEC are cytotoxic in tissue culture, the nature of this activity has eluded definition. A recent report suggests that cytotoxicity by whole organisms may be related to signal transduction and calcium elevation (134).

Mechanism of Diarrhea in EPEC Infection

The linkage between the dramatic effects that EPEC has on epithelial cells and the diarrhea seen in patients with EPEC infection remains to be elucidated. It has been proposed that the loss of microvilli that accompanies EPEC infection may result in malabsorption. Certainly in protracted cases of EPEC disease, both the small and large intestine may be heavily involved, perhaps resulting in loss of enough of the absorptive surface to cause diarrhea by this mechanism (72). Furthermore, in severe cases diarrhea may decrease following institution of total parenteral nutrition (TPN), again suggesting that malabsorption is contributory (66). Yet diarrhea can persist despite TPN (71). Furthermore, in volunteer studies, EPEC diarrhea usually begins within 12 hr, and in some cases the onset is less than 3 hr after ingestion (128). This suggests that secretory mechanisms operate as well. There is also some support for secretory mechanisms from studies of fecal electrolytes in children with EPEC infection (65). The elevations in intracellular calcium concentrations observed in epithelial cells infected with EPEC may be the cause of a secretory component of EPEC diarrhea through the activation of calcium-sensitive chloride channels. In a polarized tissue culture model, prolonged incubation of an intestinal epithelial cell line with EPEC results in an increase in transcellular tissue conductance (156). This increase in conductance is reversible and correlates with attaching and effacing activity, inasmuch as mutants deficient qualitatively or quantitatively in attaching and effacing fail to produce the effect. The increased conductance may be indicative of an increase in permeability that could contribute to diarrhea, or may be representative of the decreased surface area present in cells after effacement of microvilli. In cecal tissue removed from rabbits infected with the lapine attaching and effacing strain RDEC-1, tissue conductance also increases and sodium and chloride absorption is reduced, again consistent with loss of microvilli (157). In all probability both secretory and osmotic mechanisms are operative in severe EPEC infection.

Immune Response and Protection

EPEC disease is largely restricted to the very young. The highest incidence occurs in infants less than 6 months of age whereas infections in adults are rare. This observation may indicate that infants are exposed to EPEC early in life and develop protective immunity. Indeed, early studies have demonstrated that volunteers convalescent from EPEC infection develop increases in strain-specific antibodies directed against the O antigen (13). The incidence of such antibodies increases with increasing age; approximately 50% of children over the age of one year have hemagglutinating antibodies against O111, O55, and O26 LPS (10). Volunteers infected with EPEC develop responses to LPS, intimin, and type I fimbriae (12,82,128,158). The risk of diarrhea due to EPEC seems to decrease with previous infection. In a longitudinal study (159), 34 (64%) of 53 infants less than one year of age had diarrhea when first colonized by an EPEC strain. In comparison, only 2 of 8 infants had diarrhea during a second episode of EPEC colonization. The foregoing observations are consistent with the development of protective immunity against EPEC infection. On the other hand, infants may be inherently susceptible and older children and adults inherently resistant to EPEC infection, e.g., because of the loss with age of specific receptors. In a classic study, Mushin and Dubos reported that infant mice were readily colonized and often died following oral or intragastric administration of *E. coli* O26. In contrast, adult mice from the same colony were not colonized (160). Furthermore, colonized mice abruptly cleared their infection at 24–28 days of age, regardless of when they were infected. While O26 is no longer considered to be an EPEC serogroup, these studies clearly point to the possibility of age-specific differences in susceptibility. There is suggestive evidence that EPEC susceptibility also decreases with increasing age in humans. EPEC disease is not only more common but also more severe during the first 6 months of life (159). Volunteer studies (13,18) and common source outbreaks (49,50) have clearly demonstrated that it is possible for adults to be infected with EPEC; however, it appears that the inoculum required to cause illness in adults is large. On the other hand, the propensity for person-to-person spread of EPEC in hospital neonatal units (40) and daycare centers (41) strongly suggests that the inoculum required for natural infection in children may be lower than that needed for adults in experimental infection and common source outbreaks.

It has not been possible to demonstrate protective immunity to EPEC in experimental infection. In comparison to naive controls, volunteers previously given EPEC did not have a significant reduction in diarrheal attack rate when challenged with the homologous strain, but the power to detect a difference in this study was low (161). Also, the model of high inoculum adult experimental infection may not mimic natural infection in infants. Interestingly, an influence of prior infection on disease severity was suggested by a significant inverse correlation between prechallenge serum anti-LPS IgG titer and total stool output.

The association of EPEC infection with bottle feeding suggests a protective role for breast milk. Antibodies against EPEC LPS and specific EPEC antigens have been detected in breast milk (62,162) and breast milk has been shown to inhibit localized adherence of EPEC to epithelial cells *in vitro* (62,163). Thus passive immunity may have a role in protection against EPEC infection.

CLINICAL ILLNESS

It is ironic that with all of the progress that has recently been made in elucidating the molecular pathogenesis of EPEC infection, our knowledge of clinical aspects of the disease remains incomplete. There are no recent detailed descriptions of the clinical manifestations of EPEC infection. However, detailed reports from early outbreaks reveal that the disease as originally described was devastating. Infants with EPEC infection had profuse watery diarrhea. Vomiting and low-grade fever were common. Illness was often relentlessly progressive and staggering mortality rates of 25% to 70% were reported (6–8,69). More recent descriptions of disease in the outbreak setting have been comparable. Four of 13 infants infected with EPEC in a 1985 Kenyan preterm nursery outbreak died (83). In a 1987 outbreak in the United States involving infants in a daycare center with secondary cases in hospital and home contacts, there was an average of 8–12 stools passed per day (41). All infants had low-grade fever and symptoms lasted for a mean of 18 days. Four of 6 infants infected as outpatients required hospitalization and 1 of 4 secondary nosocomial infections was fatal. In another outbreak in a childcare center, 14 of 25 children developed watery diarrhea (67). EPEC serogroup O111 was isolated from 11 of 14 ill children and 2 of 11 well children. Five of 14 ill children had fever, 2 had vomiting, and 2 were hospitalized with dehydration. Rothbaum et al. described 15 infants hospitalized in Cincinnati, Ohio between 1979 and 1981 with severe EPEC infection and chronic diarrhea requiring TPN (66). Duration of hospitalization ranged from 25 to 120 days.

The foregoing studies are all retrospective; most are from developed countries and describe illness in the outbreak setting. These reports are therefore likely to overestimate the severity of EPEC infection. Unfortunately, there is little information regarding the clinical features of EPEC infection in developing countries. In a prospective study from São Paulo, Brazil where EPEC is the most common identifiable cause of diarrhea in young infants, fever was present in 59%, vomiting in 80%, and dehydration in 71% of infants with EPEC (52). In this study EPEC diarrhea was more severe than diarrhea due to rotavirus.

In Ethiopia, EPEC infection was characterized by watery diarrhea and fever. Dehydration was present in 3 of 10 infants. The clinical features of EPEC in Ethiopia were not distinctive in comparison to those of other pathogens (55). In a longitudinal community study in Mexico, which should be subject to less reporting and selection bias than hospital-based studies, EPEC diarrhea lasted a mean of 8 days, was associated with fever in 63% and vomiting in 48% of infants, and was more severe in infants less than 6 months of age than those between 6 months and 1 year of age (159).

EPEC can cause protracted diarrheal illness, an important factor in mortality due to diarrheal disease (164). In addition to numerous case reports of persistent diarrhea due to EPEC (39,41,65–67,70,71), case-control studies in some parts of the world (164,165), but not others (21,49), testify to the importance of EPEC in chronic diarrhea. Little is known regarding the proportion of EPEC infections that become chronic, but in one retrospective review of 26 children with EPEC admitted to Queen Elizabeth Hospital for Children in London between 1984 and 1987, 6 children developed persistent diarrhea (65).

In experimental infections of adult volunteers in which a large inoculum is given, watery diarrhea ensues approximately 7–16 hr after inoculation and lasts on average less than 2 days (12,18,128). The incubation period may be as short as 3 hr. Diarrhea on occasion is voluminous and may exceed 3.5 kg. Abdominal cramps, nausea, vomiting, malaise, and fever are common. Fecal leukocytes are sometimes seen (128).

DIAGNOSIS

Serogrouping and Serotyping

The most common procedure in use in clinical microbiology laboratories for the diagnosis of EPEC infection is slide agglutination of suspected colonies using commercial polyvalent antisera recognizing O antigens considered to represent EPEC. The advantage of this method is that it is extremely easy to perform. The disadvantages are legion. First, a positive result can be due to low-titer cross-reactivity between antigens. Second, some important EPEC serogroups are not included in the antisera. More importantly, some of the O antigens included in the sera, such as O18, O26, and O44, do not belong to EPEC (see Table 1). Even among serogroups that contain EPEC serotypes, many (e.g., O86) are also common among commensal *E. coli*. Thus, especially in situations where the prevalence of EPEC infection is low, such as sporadic cases of diarrhea in developed countries, the positive predictive value of commercial slide agglutination tests is almost nil. Thus serogrouping should be abandoned as an unreliable method for the diagnosis of EPEC. Unfortunately, despite such recommendations decades ago (166), serogrouping is still performed in some institutions and positive results are interpreted as evidence for EPEC.

The diagnostic accuracy of serological testing for EPEC can be improved considerably by performing complete serotyping for all 173 O antigens and all 56 H antigens, with tube dilutions of the test antigens to confirm the specificity of the reaction (19). Obviously, this is an extremely laborious exercise that is performed in a small and diminishing number of reference laboratories worldwide.

Identification of EPEC on the Basis of Putative Virulence Factors

Because of limitations in the predictive value of serogrouping, and because of impracticalities relating to the work required for serotyping, there is considerable interest in the use of markers for putative virulence factors for the diagnosis of EPEC infection. Such markers include tissue culture tests for adherence phenotypes, fluorescence microscopy with actin probes for cytoskeletal disruption, and radioactive and nonradioactive DNA probes. By definition the use of these tests provides more accurate diagnosis of EPEC infection than serogrouping or serotyping.

The localized adherence phenotype is easily tested and highly conserved among EPEC from the most common serotypes (35,167,168). This method requires only tissue culture facilities and a light microscope, and therefore can be used in virtually any microbiology laboratory. Transformed cell lines, such as HeLa or HEp-2 cells, are incubated with bacteria, fixed, stained, and examined for adherent microcolonies of bacteria. Virtually all *E. coli* strains that produce large microcolonies in this assay possess the *bfpA* and *eaeA* genes and do not produce high levels of Shiga-like toxins, and therefore can be considered EPEC. Problems associated with the use of this assay include the subjective nature of distinguishing localized adherence from other adherence patterns, the effect of incubation conditions on the pattern of adherence, and the fact that some serotypes, such as O55:H7, that are considered EPEC often produce small microcolonies (26). These problems can be overcome somewhat by performing the test under standard conditions and by establishing predefined objective criteria for localized adherence (169).

DNA probes provide a more objective method for EPEC diagnosis. The most experience by far has been gained with the EAF probe described by Nataro and colleagues (29). This probe is a 1-kb fragment of the EPEC adherence plasmid that is adjacent to a site into which insertions disrupt localized adherence. The probe correlates very well with localized adherence and has been used to study the epidemiology of EPEC infections worldwide (21,22,29,44,51,57,60,63,83,84). Refinements of the originally described probe include nonisotopic labeling to enhance its use in clinical laboratories (60,170) and the use of an oligonucleotide derived from within the EAF probe fragment to increase sensitivity and specificity and to reduce ambiguous results (171). Still, strains have been described that exhibit attaching and effacing activity, do not produce high levels of Shiga-like toxins, and produce at least modest localized adherence, yet are negative with the EAF probe (21,33,95,96,172). Some but not all of these strains are positive when tested with a *bfpA* DNA probe consisting of the gene for the major structural sub-

unit of the bundle-forming pilus (97). The latter probe has been proposed as an improvement over the EAF probe since it represents a known virulence factor, may have superior diagnostic accuracy, and is present on a higher copy number vector. However, the practical utility of these advantages has yet to be demonstrated. A fragment derived from within the *eaeA* coding sequences hybridizes with all EPEC and EHEC that exhibit attaching and effacing activity and may also prove useful for the diagnosis of EPEC infection in conjunction with tests to exclude EHEC (115).

A promising alternative to the use of DNA probes for the diagnosis of EPEC infection is the application of fluorescence microscopy to identify the concentrated filamentous actin in epithelial cells beneath the sites of EPEC attachment as a surrogate marker for the attaching and effacing effect (30). This fluorescence actin staining (FAS) test appears to correlate perfectly with electron microscopy for attaching and effacing. The FAS test has been applied to epidemiological studies with encouraging results (21,33,56,173). Some FAS-positive *E. coli*, of both EPEC– and non-EPEC–associated serotypes, are negative when tested with the EAF probe (21,33). The role of FAS-positive, EAF-negative strains needs to be further clarified as in some studies these strains have not been significantly associated with diarrhea (56). Disadvantages of the FAS test include the need for relatively expensive fluorescent microscopes and reagents and the need to combine the test with assays for Shiga-like toxin genes or activity to distinguish EPEC from EHEC, which are also FAS-positive.

Albert et al. recently described an enzyme-linked immunosorbent assay for the detection of EPEC using an antiserum raised against an EAF plasmid-containing strain and absorbed against a plasmid-cured strain (174). The test appears to be very accurate for identifying EAF-positive strains but has yet to be more widely applied.

What is the best test for the diagnosis of EPEC infection? The answer depends in part on the resources available. If a fluorescent microscope and tissue culture facilities are available, the FAS test combined with cytotoxicity assays for Shiga-like toxins (EPEC being positive for FAS and negative for Shiga-like toxins) appears to be accurate. An alternative would be DNA probe testing for *eaeA* and *bfpA*/EAF (EPEC being positive in both). The role in disease of strains positive for some but not all of the tests (for example strains that are FAS-positive, EAF-negative or EAF-positive, non-EPEC serotype) remains unresolved. A prospective case-control study of the various available tests, using the odds ratio for diarrhea as the gold standard, would be very helpful.

TREATMENT

As noted above, diarrhea due to EPEC is often severe and may be life threatening. The primary concern in caring for a patient with EPEC diarrhea is to correct and prevent fluid and electrolyte disturbances. This can be accomplished in most patients with oral rehydration therapy (see chapter by Snyder). However, a minority of patients with EPEC infection have severe vomiting or massive fluid losses that cannot be replaced by the oral route and require parenteral rehydration (65,66,175). In most cases of EPEC infection, early feeding should be instituted to prevent or reverse the rapid decline in nutritional status that can result from acute and chronic diarrhea. In young infants breast milk or lactose-free formula should be reinstituted as soon as the fluid deficit is corrected. In older infants and children, high-calorie foods should be used. In some cases of EPEC diarrhea, reducing substances are present in the stool and the volume of diarrhea increases with enteral feeding, suggesting that malabsorption due to extensive microvillus effacement is contributing an osmotic component to the diarrhea (39,66). In these cases, TPN should be initiated if available to prevent and reverse severe nutritional depletion.

In addition to nonspecific measures to correct and prevent fluid, electrolyte, and nutritional imbalance, consideration should be given to therapeutic measures to ameliorate the diarrhea. In a recent randomized placebo-controlled trial, bismuth subsalicylate, at a dosage of 100 mg/kg/day in divided doses every 4 hr, given in addition to oral rehydration and early feeding, reduced the duration of diarrhea, the duration of hospitalization, and the total stool output in infants and children less than 5 years old (176). The most common potential etiological agents identified in this study were rotaviruses and *E. coli* of EPEC serogroups. Furthermore, this regimen appeared to be free of toxicity or adverse effects.

The role of antibiotics in the therapy of EPEC infection is not well defined. The apparent beneficial effects of the initiation of antibiotic therapy in patients with prolonged diarrhea due to EPEC have been noted (39,65), but controlled clinical trials are uncommon. In one study conducted in Ethiopian children with diarrhea associated with EPEC serogroups, therapy for 5 days with trimethoprim-sulfamethoxasole or mecillinam resulted in a higher percentage of patients free of diarrhea at 3 days in comparison to children given no antibiotics (177). However, resistance to multiple antibiotics is the rule for EPEC, greatly limiting the available therapeutic options (40,52,63,70,178–181).

There is increasing interest in alternatives to antimicrobial therapy in the treatment of infectious diseases. Among the alternative approaches under investigation are therapeutic agents such as receptor and ligand analogs aimed at interfering with bacterial adhesion (see chapter by Banwell and Binion). As the ligands responsible for EPEC attachment are identified, this approach may become feasible. Another innovative strategy is passive immunotherapy. Preliminary data from a study of bovine milk immunoglobulin concentrate prepared from cows immunized with a mixture of formalin-killed organisms representing 14 EPEC serogroups suggest that this approach may have beneficial effects (182). Clearly more studies of this sort would be welcome.

PREVENTION

Strategies for the prevention of EPEC infection include efforts to improve social and economic conditions in de-

veloping countries, efforts to encourage breastfeeding, and efforts to prevent nosocomial transmission of infections. In addition to these laudable but elusive goals, the possibility of preventing EPEC infection through vaccination remains an attractive objective.

The impressive potential for protection against diarrheal disease by passive immunization was illustrated by the ability of a bovine milk immunoglobulin concentrate prepared by immunizing cows with a mixture of enterotoxigenic *E. coli* antigens to completely prevent diarrhea due to ETEC in a placebo-controlled volunteer trial (183). The inhibitory activity of human milk against EPEC adherence suggests that such an approach may be feasible for the protection of humans against this pathogen as well.

The evidence for the existence of protective immunity against EPEC infection has been summarized above. Attempts to develop an EPEC vaccine have met with some success. A killed oral vaccine consisting of a mixture of *E. coli* of O111, O55, and O86 serogroups has been administered in multiple doses to hospitalized infants. The vaccine had a protective efficacy of 31% to 74%, depending on the age of the infant, in preventing nosocomial diarrhea due to *E. coli* (184). The protective effect lasted only one month.

Rabbits infected with the RDEC-1 strain of attaching and effacing *E. coli* acquire protective immunity against recurrent disease. A subunit vaccine consisting of purified fimbriae from this strain incorporated into microspheres produced secretory IgA responses and provided protection against colonization, diarrhea, and weight loss (185). It would seem that a similar preparation composed of purified bundle-forming pili from human EPEC strains would be worthy of evaluation. An encouraging result in this regard is the fact that despite their distant evolutionary relationship (37), strains from O127:H6 and O111:H− serotypes have identical *bfpA* gene sequences (86,87).

The prospect of longer lasting immunity may be realized by using live attenuated vaccines. One candidate for such a formulation would be the previously constructed *eaeA* deletion mutant (113). Unfortunately, this strain was not fully attenuated and did not protect against challenge with the wild-type strain in the doses and conditions under which it was tested (161). Yet the inability to detect protective immunity even upon homologous rechallenge with wild-type strains suggests that the experimental model of adult EPEC infection may be flawed. However, the *eaeA* deletion mutant does not produce intimin, the 94-kDa antigen proposed to have a role in immunity (82), and elicited lower systemic immunoglobulin responses to LPS than the wild-type strain (128). The problems of insufficient attenuation and reduced antigenicity may be overcome by using strains with additional or alternative attenuating mutations. The *eaeB* locus or the genes involved in signal transduction would be attractive candidates because strains with these mutations still produce intimin. Any practical EPEC vaccine would likely consist of a mixture of strains from the predominant EPEC serotype from a given geographic region, each with similar attenuating mutations.

If the problems of developing an effective EPEC vaccine are overcome, the next issue would be identifying a population group to which the vaccine should be targeted. Since infants under 6 months of age suffer the brunt of the burden of EPEC infection, infants of this age group in countries with a high prevalence of EPEC infection would have the most to gain. An alternative strategy would be to immunize pregnant women to induce passive immunity in newborns conferred by both the transplacental and secretory (breast milk) routes. The goal of this approach would be to postpone EPEC infection beyond the period of greatest risk or to a time when active immunization by oral vaccination could be accomplished.

Progress in the elucidation of EPEC pathogenesis, agonizingly slow initially, has been accelerating exponentially. Further research will likely yield important insights into host–bacterium interactions in general and eventually will be translated into novel prophylactic and therapeutic interventions to reduce the affliction imposed by this common and serious pathogen.

ACKNOWLEDGMENTS

This work was supported by the Office of Research and Development, Medical Research Service, Department of Veterans Affairs and by Public Health Service award AI32074 from the National Institutes of Health.

REFERENCES

1. Edelman R, Levine MM. Summary of a workshop on enteropathogenic *Escherichia coli*. *J Infect Dis* 1983;147:1108–1118.
2. Robins-Browne RM. Traditional enteropathogenic *Escherichia coli* of infantile diarrhea. *Rev Infect Dis* 1987;9:28–53.
3. Levine MM, Edelman R. Enteropathogenic *Escherichia coli* of classic serotypes associated with infant diarrhea: epidemiology and pathogenesis. *Epidemiol Rev* 1984;6:31–51.
4. Bray J. Isolation of antigenically homogeneous strains of *Bact. coli neapolitanum* from summer diarrhoea of infants. *J Pathol Bacteriol* 1945;57:239–247.
5. Giles C, Sangster G. An outbreak of infantile gastroenteritis in Aberdeen. *J Hyg* 1948;46:1–9.
6. Taylor J, Powell BW, Wright J. Infantile diarrhea and vomiting: a clinical and bacteriological investigation. *Br Med J* 1949;2:117–141.
7. Smith J. The association of certain types (α and β) of *Bact. coli* with infantile gastro-enteritis. *J Hyg* 1949;47:221–226.
8. Giles C, Sangster G, Smith J. Epidemic gastroenteritis of infants in Aberdeen during 1947. *Arch Dis Child* 1949;24:45–53.
9. Kauffmann F, Dupont A. *Escherichia* strains from infantile epidemic gastroenteritis. *Acta Path* 1950;27:552–564.
10. Neter E, Westphal O, Lüderitz O, Gino RM, Gorzynski EA. Demonstration of antibodies against enteropathogenic *Escherichia coli* in sera of children of various ages. *Pediatrics* 1955;16:801–808.
11. Robins-Browne RM, Yam WC, O'Gorman LE, Bettelheim KA. Examination of archetypal strains of enteropathogenic *Escherichia coli* for properties associated with bacterial virulence. *J Med Microbiol* 1993;38:222–226.
12. Ferguson WW, June RC. Experiments of feeding adult volunteers with *Escherichia coli* 111, B₄, a coliform organism associated with infant diarrhea. *Am J Hyg* 1952;55:155–169.
13. June RC, Ferguson WW, Worfel MT. Experiments in feeding adult volunteers with *Escherichia coli* 55, B₅, a coliform organism associated with infant diarrhea. *Am J Hyg* 1953;57:222–236.
14. Koya G, Kosakai N, Kono M, Mori M, Fukasawa Y. Observations on the multiplication of *Escherichia coli* O-111 B4 in the intestinal tract of adult volunteers in feeding experiments: the intubation study with Miller–Abbott's double lumen tube. *Jap J Med Sci Biol* 1954;7:197–203.
15. Goldschmidt MC, DuPont HL. Enteropathogenic *Escherichia coli:* lack of correlation of serotype with pathogenicity. *J Infect Dis* 1976;133:153–156.
16. Echeverria P, Chang CP, Smith D, Anderson GL. Enterotoxigenicity and invasive capacity of "enteropathogenic" serotypes of *Escherichia coli*. *J Pediatr* 1976;89:8–10.
17. Sack RB. Human diarrheal disease caused by enterotoxigenic *Escherichia coli*. *Ann Rev Microbiol* 1975;29:333–353.
18. Levine MM, Bergquist EJ, Nalin DR, et al. *Escherichia coli* strains that cause diarrhoea but do not produce heat-labile or heat-stable enterotoxins and are non-invasive. *Lancet* 1978;1:1119–1122.
19. Ørskov F, Ørskov I. *Escherichia coli* serotyping and disease in man and animals. *Can J Microbiol* 1992;38:699–674.
20. Toledo MR, Alvariza M, Murahovschi J, Ramos SR, Trabulsi LR. Enteropathogenic *Escherichia coli* serotypes and endemic diarrhea in infants. *Infect Immun* 1983;39:586–589.
21. Cravioto A, Tello A, Navarro A, et al. Association of *Escherichia coli* HEp-2 adherence patterns with type and duration of diarrhoea. *Lancet* 1991;337:262–264.
22. Gomes TAT, Vieira MAM, Wachsmuth IK, Blake PA, Trabulsi LR. Serotype-specific prevalence of *Escherichia coli* strains with EPEC adherence factor genes in infants with and without diarrhea in São Paulo, Brazil. *J Infect Dis* 1989;160:131–135.
23. Cravioto A, Reyes R, Ortega R, Fernández G, Hernández R, López D. Prospective study of diarrhoeal disease in a cohort of rural Mexican children: incidence and isolated pathogens during the first two years of life. *Epidemiol Infect* 1988;101:123–134.
24. Levine MM, Xu J-G, Kaper JB, et al. A DNA probe to identify enterohemorrhagic *Escherichia coli* of O157:H7 and other serotypes that cause hemorrhagic colitis and hemolytic uremic syndrome. *J Infect Dis* 1987;156:175–182.
25. Scotland SM, Willshaw GA, Smith HR, Rowe B. Properties of strains of *Escherichia coli* O26:H11 in relation to their enteropathogenic or enterohemorrhagic classification. *J Infect Dis* 1990;162:1069–1074.
26. Scotland SM, Smith HR, Said B, Willshaw GA, Cheasty T, Rowe B. Identification of enteropathogenic *Escherichia coli* isolated in Britain as enteroaggregative or as members of a subclass of attaching-and-effacing *E. coli* not hybridising with the EPEC adherence-factor probe. *J Med Microbiol* 1991;35:278–283.
27. Albert MJ, Alam K, Ansaruzzaman M, et al. Localized adherence and attaching-effacing properties of nonenteropathogenic serotypes of *Escherichia coli*. *Infect Immun* 1991;59:1864–1868.
28. Pedroso MZ, Freymüller E, Trabulsi LR, Gomes TAT. Attaching-effacing lesions and intracellular penetration in HeLa cells and human duodenal mucosa by two *Escherichia coli* strains not belonging to the classical enteropathogenic *E. coli* serogroups. *Infect Immun* 1993;61:1152–1156.
29. Nataro JP, Baldini MM, Kaper JB, Black RE, Bravo N, Levine MM. Detection of an adherence factor of enteropathogenic *Escherichia coli* with a DNA probe. *J Infect Dis* 1985;152:560–565.
30. Knutton S, Baldwin T, Williams PH, McNeish AS. Actin accumulation at sites of bacterial adhesion to tissue culture cells: basis of a new diagnostic test for enteropathogenic and enterohemorrhagic *Escherichia coli*. *Infect Immun* 1989;57:1290–1298.
31. Chart H, Scotland SM, Willshaw GA, Rowe B. HEp-2 adhesion and the expression of a 94 kDa outer-membrane protein by strains of *Escherichia coli* belonging to enteropathogenic serogroups. *J Gen Microbiol* 1988;134:1315–1321.
32. Beutin L, Ørskov I, Ørskov F, et al. Clonal diversity and virulence factors in strains of *Escherichia coli* of the classic enteropathogenic serogroup O114. *J Infect Dis* 1990;162:1329–1334.
33. Knutton S, Phillips AD, Smith HR, et al. Screening for enteropathogenic *Escherichia coli* in infants with diarrhea by the fluorescent-actin staining test. *Infect Immun* 1991;59:365–371.

34. Stenderup J, Ørskov F. The clonal nature of enteropathogenic *Escherichia coli* strains. *J Infect Dis* 1983;148:1019–1024.

35. Scaletsky ICA, Silva MLM, Toledo MRF, Davis BR, Blake PA, Trabulsi LR. Correlation between adherence to HeLa cells and serogroups, serotypes, and bioserotypes of *Escherichia coli*. *Infect Immun* 1985;49:528–532.

36. Katouli M, Kühn I, Möllby R. Biochemical phenotypes of enteropathogenic *Escherichia coli* common to Iran and Sweden. *J Med Microbiol* 1991;35:270–277.

37. Ørskov F, Whittam TS, Cravioto A, Ørskov I. Clonal relationships among classic enteropathogenic *Escherichia coli* (EPEC) belonging to different O groups. *J Infect Dis* 1990;162:76–81.

38. Whittam TS, Wolfe ML, Wachsmuth IK, Ørskov F, Ørskov I, Wilson RA. Clonal relationships among *Escherichia coli* strains that cause hemorrhagic colitis and infantile diarrhea. *Infect Immun* 1993;61:1619–1629.

39. Clausen CR, Christie DL. Chronic diarrhea in infants caused by adherent enteropathogenic *Escherichia coli*. *J Pediatr* 1982; 100:358–361.

40. Wu S-X, Peng R-Q. Studies on an outbreak of neonatal diarrhea caused by EPEC 0127:H6 with plasmid analysis restriction analysis and outer membrane protein determination. *Acta Paediatr Scand* 1992;81:217–221.

41. Bower JR, Congeni BL, Cleary TG, et al. *Escherichia coli* O114:nonmotile as a pathogen in an outbreak of severe diarrhea associated with a day care center. *J Infect Dis* 1989;160: 243–247.

42. Cobeljić M, Mel D, Arsić B, et al. The association of enterotoxigenic and enteropathogenic *Escherichia coli* and other enteric pathogens with childhood diarrhoea in Yugoslavia. *Epidemiol Infect* 1989;103:53–62.

43. Chatkaeomorakot A, Echeverria P, Taylor DN, et al. HeLa cell-adherent *Escherichia coli* in children with diarrhea in Thailand. *J Infect Dis* 1987;156:669–672.

44. Gunzburg ST, Chang BJ, Burke V, Gracey M. Virulence factors of enteric *Escherichia coli* in young Aboriginal children in north-west Australia. *Epidemiol Infect* 1992;109:283–289.

45. Gurwith M, Hinde D, Gross R, Rowe B. A prospective study of enteropathogenic *Escherichia coli* in endemic diarrheal disease. *J Infect Dis* 1978;137:292–297.

46. Peeters JE, Geeroms R, Orskov F. Biotype, serotype, and pathogenicity of attaching and effacing enteropathogenic *Escherichia coli* strains isolated from diarrheic commercial rabbits. *Infect Immun* 1988;56:1442–1448.

47. Pohl PH, Peeters JE, Jacquemin ER, Lintermans PF, Mainil JG. Identification of *eae* sequences in enteropathogenic *Escherichia coli* strains from rabbits. *Infect Immun* 1993;61: 2203–2206.

48. Moxley RA, Francis DH. Natural and experimental infection with an attaching and effacing strain of *Escherichia coli* in calves. *Infect Immun* 1986;53:339–346.

49. Viljanen MK, Peltola T, Junnila SYT, et al. Outbreak of diarrhoea due to *Escherichia coli* O111:B4 in schoolchildren and adults: association of Vi antigen-like reactivity. *Lancet* 1990; 336:831–834.

50. Schtoeder SA, Caldwell JR, Vernon TM, White PS, Granger SI, Bennett JV. A waterborne outbreak of gastroenteritis in adults associated with enteropathogenic *Escherichia coli*. *Lancet* 1968;1:737–740.

51. Gomes TAT, Blake PA, Trabulsi LR. Prevalence of *Escherichia coli* strains with localized, diffuse, and aggregative adherence to HeLa cells in infants with diarrhea and matched controls. *J Clin Microbiol* 1989;27:266–269.

52. Gomes TAT, Rassi V, Macdonald KL, et al. Enteropathogens associated with acute diarrheal disease in urban infants in São Paulo, Brazil. *J Infect Dis* 1991;164:331–337.

53. Nataro JP, Kaper JB, Robins-Browne R, Prado V, Vial P, Levine MM. Patterns of adherence of diarrheagenic *Escherichia coli* to HEp-2 cells. *Pediatr Infect Dis J* 1987;6:829–831.

54. Robins-Browne R, Still CS, Miliotis MD, et al. Summer diarrhoea in African infants and children. *Arch Dis Child* 1980;55: 923–928.

55. Thorén A, Stintzing G, Tufvesson B, Walder M, Habte D. Aeti-ology and clinical features of severe infantile diarrhoea in Addis Ababa, Ethiopia. *J Trop Pediatr* 1982;28:127–131.

56. Echeverria P, Ørskov F, Ørskov I, et al. Attaching and effacing enteropathogenic *Escherichia coli* as a cause of infantile diarrhea in Bangkok. *J Infect Dis* 1991;164:550–554.

57. Kain KC, Barteluk RL, Kelly MT, et al. Etiology of childhood diarrhea in Beijing, China. *J Clin Microbiol* 1991;29:90–95.

58. Ghosh AR, Nair GB, Naik TN, Paul M, Pal SC, Sen D. Entero-adherent *Escherichia coli* is an important diarrhoeagenic agent in infants aged below 6 months in Calcutta, India. *J Med Microbiol* 1992;36:264–268.

59. Bhan MK, Raj P, Levine MM, et al. Enteroaggregative *Escherichia coli* associated with persistent diarrhea in a cohort of rural children in India. *J Infect Dis* 1989;159:1061–1064.

60. Begaud E, Jourand P, Morillon M, Mondet D, Germani Y. Detection of diarrheogenic *Escherichia coli* in children less than ten years old with and without diarrhea in New Caledonia using seven acetylaminofluorene-labeled DNA probes. *Am J Trop Med Hyg* 1993;48:26–34.

61. Blake PA, Ramos S, Macdonald KL, et al. Pathogen-specific risk factors and protective factors for acute diarrheal disease in urban Brazilian infants. *J Infect Dis* 1993;167:627–632.

62. Cravioto A, Tello A, Villafan H, Ruiz J, Del Vedovo S, Neeser J-R. Inhibition of localized adhesion of enteropathogenic *Escherichia coli* to HEp-2 cells by immunoglobulin and oligosaccharide fractions of human colostrum and breast milk. *J Infect Dis* 1991;163:1247–1255.

63. Moyenuddin M, Wachsmuth IK, Moseley SL, Bopp CA, Blake PA. Serotype, antimicrobial resistance, and adherence properties of *Escherichia coli* strains associated with outbreaks of diarrheal illness in children in the United States. *J Clin Microbiol* 1989;27:2234–2239.

64. Karch H, Heesemann J, Laufs R. Phage-associated cytotoxin production by and enteroadhesiveness of enteropathogenic *Escherichia coli* isolated from infants with diarrhea in West Germany. *J Infect Dis* 1987;155:707–715.

65. Hill SM, Phillips AD, Walker-Smith JA. Enteropathogenic *Escherichia coli* and life threatening chronic diarrhoea. *Gut* 1991;32:154–158.

66. Rothbaum R, McAdams AJ, Giannella R, Partin JC. A clinico-pathological study of enterocyte-adherent *Escherichia coli*: a cause of protracted diarrhea in infants. *Gastroenterology* 1982; 83:441–454.

67. Paulozzi LJ, Johnson KE, Kamahele LM, Clausen CR, Riley LW, Helgerson SD. Diarrhea associated with adherent enteropathogenic *Escherichia coli* in an infant and toddler center, Seattle, Washington. *Pediatrics* 1986;77:296–300.

68. Kotler DP, Orenstein JM. Chronic diarrhea and malabsorption associated with enteropathogenic bacterial infection in a patient with AIDS. *Ann Intern Med* 1993;119:127–128.

69. Bray J, Beavan TED. Slide agglutination of *Bacterium coli* var. *neapolitanum* in summer diarrhoea. *J Pathol Bacteriol* 1948; 60:395–401.

70. Khoshoo V, Bhan MK, Mathur M, Raj P. A fatal severe enter-opathy associated with enteropathogenic *E. coli*. *In Pediatr* 1988;25:308–309.

71. Ulshen MH, Rollo JL. Pathogenesis of *Escherichia coli* gastroenteritis in man—another mechanism. *N Engl J Med* 1980; 302:99–101.

72. Rothbaum RJ, Partin JC, Saalfield K, McAdams AJ. An ultrastructural study of enteropathogenic *Escherichia coli* infection in human infants. *Ultrastruct Pathol* 1983;4:291–304.

73. Taylor CJ, Hart A, Batt RM, McDougall C, McLean L. Ultrastructural and biochemical changes in human jejunal mucosa associated with enteropathogenic *Escherichia coli* (0111) infection. *J Pediatr Gastroenterol Nutr* 1986;5:70–73.

74. Jerse AE, Yu J, Tall BD, Kaper JB. A genetic locus of enteropathogenic *Escherichia coli* necessary for the production of attaching and effacing lesions on tissue culture cells. *Proc Natl Acad Sci USA* 1990;87:7839–7843.

75. Donnenberg MS, Calderwood SB, Donohue-Rolfe A, Keusch GT, Kaper JB. Construction and analysis of TnphoA mutants of enteropathogenic *Escherichia coli* unable to invade HEp-2 cells. *Infect Immun* 1990;58:1565–1571.

76. Donnenberg MS, Kaper JB. Minireview: enteropathogenic *Escherichia coli*. *Infect Immun* 1992;60:3953–3961.

77. Cravioto A, Gross RJ, Scotland SM, Rowe B. An adhesive factor found in strains of *Escherichia coli* belonging to the traditional infantile enteropathogenic serotypes. *Curr Microbiol* 1979;3:95–99.

78. Scaletsky ICA, Silva MLM, Trabulsi LR. Distinctive patterns of adherence of enteropathogenic *Escherichia coli* to HeLa cells. *Infect Immun* 1984;45:534–536.

79. Baldini MM, Kaper JB, Levine MM, Candy DC, Moon HW. Plasmid-mediated adhesion in enteropathogenic *Escherichia coli*. *J Pediatr Gastroenterol Nutr* 1983;2:534–538.

80. Nataro JP, Maher KO, Mackie P, Kaper JB. Characterization of plasmids encoding the adherence factor of enteropathogenic *Escherichia coli*. *Infect Immun* 1987;55:2370–2377.

81. McConnell MM, Chart H, Scotland SM, Smith HR, Willshaw GA, Rowe B. Properties of adherence factor plasmids of enteropathogenic *Escherichia coli* and the effect of host strain on expression of adherence to HEp-2 cells. *J Gen Microbiol* 1989; 135:1123–1134.

82. Levine MM, Nataro JP, Karch H, et al. The diarrheal response of humans to some classic serotypes of enteropathogenic *Escherichia coli* is dependent on a plasmid encoding an enteroadhesiveness factor. *J Infect Dis* 1985;152:550–559.

83. Senerwa D, Olsvik O, Mutanda LN, et al. Enteropathogenic *Escherichia coli* serotype O111:HNT isolated from preterm neonates in Nairobi, Kenya. *J Clin Microbiol* 1989;27:1307–1311.

84. Echeverria P, Taylor DN, Bettelheim KA, et al. HeLa cell-adherent enteropathogenic *Escherichia coli* in children under 1 year of age in Thailand. *J Clin Microbiol* 1987;25:1472–1475.

85. Girón JA, Ho ASY, Schoolnik GK. An inducible bundle-forming pilus of enteropathogenic *Escherichia coli*. *Science* 1991; 254:710–713.

86. Donnenberg MS, Girón JA, Nataro JP, Kaper JB. A plasmid-encoded type IV fimbrial gene of enteropathogenic *Escherichia coli* associated with localized adherence. *Mol Microbiol* 1992; 6:3427–3437.

87. Sohel I, Puente JL, Murray WJ, Vuopio-Varkila J, Schoolnik GK. Cloning and characterization of the bundle-forming pilin gene of enteropathogenic *Escherichia coli* and its distribution in *Salmonella* serotypes. *Mol Microbiol* 1993;7:563–575.

88. Zhang H-Z, Donnenberg MS. Localized adherence by enteropathogenic *Escherichia coli* (EPEC) requires the chromosomal *dsbA* locus, abstr. B-312, p. 81. In: *Abstracts of the 93rd General Meeting of the American Society for Microbiology*. Washington, DC: American Society for Microbiology; 1993.

89. Bardwell JC, McGovern K, Beckwith J. Identification of a protein required for disulfide bond formation in vivo. *Cell* 1991; 67:581–589.

90. Kamitani S, Akiyama Y, Ito K. Identification and characterization of an *Escherichia coli* gene required for the formation of correctly folded alkaline phosphatase, a periplasmic enzyme. *EMBO J* 1992;11:57–62.

91. Peek JA, Taylor RK. Characterization of a periplasmic thiol: disulfide interchange protein required for the functional maturation of secreted virulence factors of *Vibrio cholerae*. *Proc Natl Acad Sci USA* 1992;89:6210–6214.

92. Yu J, Webb H, Hirst TR. A homologue of the *Escherichia coli* DsbA protein involved in disulphide bond formation is required for enterotoxin biogenesis in *Vibrio cholerae*. *Mol Microbiol* 1992;6:1949–1958.

93. Tomb J-F. A periplasmic protein disulfide oxidoreductase is required for transformation of *Haemophilus influenzae* Rd. *Proc Natl Acad Sci USA* 1992;89:10252–10256.

94. Dailey FE, Berg HC. Mutants in disulfide bond formation that disrupt flagellar assembly in *Escherichia coli*. *Proc Natl Acad Sci USA* 1993;90:1043–1047.

95. Scotland SM, Smith HR, Rowe B. *Escherichia coli* 0128 strains from infants with diarrhea commonly show localized adhesion and positivity in the fluorescent-actin staining test but do not hybridize with an enteropathogenic *E. coli* adherence factor probe. *Infect Immun* 1991;59:1569–1571.

96. Scotland SM, Willshaw GA, Cheasty T, Rowe B. Strains of *Escherichia coli* 0157:H8 from human diarrhoea belong to at-

97. Girón JA, Donnenberg MS, Martin WC, Jarvis KG, Kaper JB. Distribution of the bundle-forming pilus structural gene (*bfpA*) among enteropathogenic *Escherichia coli*. *J Infect Dis* 1993; 168:1037–1041.

98. Staley TE, Jones EW, Corley LD. Attachment and penetration of *Escherichia coli* into intestinal epithelium of the ileum in newborn pigs. *Am J Pathol* 1969;56:371–392.

99. Moon HW, Whipp SC, Argenzio RA, Levine MM, Giannella RA. Attaching and effacing activities of rabbit and human enteropathogenic *Escherichia coli* in pig and rabbit intestines. *Infect Immun* 1983;41:1340–1351.

100. Knutton S, Lloyd DR, McNeish AS. Adhesion of enteropathogenic *Escherichia coli* to human intestinal enterocytes and cultured human intestinal mucosa. *Infect Immun* 1987;55:69–77.

101. Manjarrez-Hernandez HA, Amess B, Sellers L, et al. Purification of a 20 kDa phosphoprotein from epithelial cells and identification as a myosin light chain: phosphorylation induced by enteropathogenic *Escherichia coli* and phorbol ester. *FEBS Lett* 1991;292:121–127.

102. Finlay BB, Rosenshine I, Donnenberg MS, Kaper JB. Cytoskeletal composition of attaching and effacing lesions associated with enteropathogenic *Escherichia coli* adherence to HeLa cells. *Infect Immun* 1992;60:2541–2543.

103. Polotsky YE, Dragunskaya EM, Seliverstova VG, et al. Pathogenic effect of enterotoxigenic *Escherichia coli* and *Escherichia coli* causing infantile diarrhoea. *Acta Microbiol Acad Sci Hung* 1977;24:221–236.

104. Tzipori S, Gibson R, Montanaro J. Nature and distribution of mucosal lesions associated with enteropathogenic and enterohemorrhagic *Escherichia coli* in piglets and the role of plasmid-mediated factors. *Infect Immun* 1989;57:1142–1150.

105. Knutton S, Baldini MM, Kaper JB, McNeish AS. Role of plasmid-encoded adherence factors in adhesion of enteropathogenic *Escherichia coli* to HEp-2 cells. *Infect Immun* 1987;55: 78–85.

106. Sherman P, Drumm B, Karmali M, Cutz E. Adherence of bacteria to the intestine in sporadic cases of enteropathogenic *Escherichia coli*–associated diarrhea in infants and young children: a prospective study. *Gastroenterology* 1989;96:86–94.

107. Francis DH, Collins JE, Duimstra JR. Infection of gnotobiotic pigs with an *Escherichia coli* O157:H7 strain associated with an outbreak of hemorrhagic colitis. *Infect Immun* 1986;51: 953–956.

108. Tzipori S, Wachsmuth IK, Chapman C, et al. The pathogenesis of hemorrhagic colitis caused by *Escherichia coli* O157:H7 in gnotobiotic pigs. *J Infect Dis* 1986;154:712–716.

109. Albert MJ, Alam K, Islam M, et al. *Hafnia alvei,* a probable cause of diarrhea in humans. *Infect Immun* 1991;59:1507–1513.

110. Johnson E, Barthold SW. The ultrastructure of transmissible murine colonic hyperplasia. *Am J Pathol* 1979;97:291–314.

111. Smoot DT, Resau JH, Naab T, et al. Adherence of *Helicobacter pylori* to cultured human gastric epithelial cells. *Infect Immun* 1993;61:350–355.

112. Dytoc M, Gold B, Louie M, et al. Comparison of *Helicobacter pylori* and attaching-effacing *Escherichia coli* adhesion to eukaryotic cells. *Infect Immun* 1993;61:448–456.

113. Donnenberg MS, Kaper JB. Construction of an *eae* deletion mutant of enteropathogenic *Escherichia coli* by using a positive-selection suicide vector. *Infect Immun* 1991;59:4310–4317.

114. Rosenshine I, Donnenberg MS, Kaper JB, Finlay BB. Signal exchange between enteropathogenic *Escherichia coli* (EPEC) and epithelial cells: EPEC induce tyrosine phosphorylation of host cell protein to initiate cytoskeletal rearrangement and bacterial uptake. *EMBO J* 1992;11:3551–3560.

115. Jerse AE, Gicquelais KG, Kaper JB. Plasmid and chromosomal elements involved in the pathogenesis of attaching and effacing *Escherichia coli*. *Infect Immun* 1991;59:3869–3875.

116. Albert MJ, Faruque SM, Ansaruzzaman M, et al. Sharing of virulence-associated properties at the phenotypic and genetic levels between enteropathogenic *Escherichia coli* and *Hafnia alvei*. *J Med Microbiol* 1992;37:310–314.

117. Schauer DB, Falkow S. Attaching and effacing locus of a *Citro-*

bacter freundii biotype that causes transmissible murine colonic hyperplasia. *Infect Immun* 1993;61:2486–2492.

118. Barrett TJ, Kaper JB, Jerse AE, Wachsmuth IK. Virulence factors in Shiga-like toxin-producing *Escherichia coli* isolated from humans and cattle. *J Infect Dis* 1992;165:979–980.

119. Donnenberg MS, Tzipori S, McKee M, O'Brien AD, Alroy J, Kaper JB. The role of the *eae* locus of enterohemorrhagic *Escherichia coli* in intimate attachment in vitro and in a porcine model. *J Clin Invest* 1993;92:1418–1424.

120. Yu J, Kaper JB. Cloning and characterization of the *eae* gene of enterohemorrhagic *Escherichia coli* O157:H7. *Mol Microbiol* 1992;6:411–417.

121. Beebakhee G, Louie M, De Azavedo J, Brunton J. Cloning and nucleotide sequence of the *eae* gene homologue from enterohemorrhagic *Escherichia coli* serotype O157:H7. *FEMS Microbiol Lett* 1992;91:63–68.

122. Jerse AE, Kaper JB. The *eae* gene of enteropathogenic *Escherichia coli* encodes a 94-kilodalton membrane protein, the expression of which is influenced by the EAF plasmid. *Infect Immun* 1991;59:4302–4309.

123. Gómez O, Kaper JB. Plasmid encoded factors regulate the expression of *eae* gene of enteropathogenic *E. coli*, abstr. B-179, page 55. In: *Abstracts of the 92nd General Meeting of the American Society for Microbiology*. Washington, DC: American Society for Microbiology; 1992.

124. Isberg RR, Voorhis DL, Falkow S. Identification of Invasin: a protein that allows enteric bacteria to penetrate cultured mammalian cells. *Cell* 1987;50:769–778.

125. Tran Van Nhieu G, Isberg RR. The *Yersinia pseudotuberculosis* invasin protein and human fibronectin bind to mutually exclusive sites on the $\alpha_5\beta_1$ integrin receptor. *J Biol Chem* 1991;266:24367–24375.

126. Leong JM, Fournier RS, Isberg RR. Identification of the integrin binding domain of the *Yersinia pseudotuberculosis* invasin protein. *EMBO J* 1990;9:1979–1989.

127. Rankin S, Isberg RR, Leong JM. The integrin-binding domain of invasin is sufficient to allow bacterial entry into mammalian cells. *Infect Immun* 1992;60:3909–3912.

128. Donnenberg MS, Tacket CO, James SP, et al. The role of the *eaeA* gene in experimental enteropathogenic *Escherichia coli* infection. *J Clin Invest* 1993;92:1412–1417.

129. Donnenberg MS, Yu J, Kaper JB. A second chromosomal gene necessary for intimate attachment of enteropathogenic *Escherichia coli* to epithelial cells. *J Bacteriol* 1993;175:4670–4680.

130. Baldwin TJ, Brooks SF, Knutton S, Manjarrez Hernandez HA, Aitken A, Williams PH. Protein phosphorylation by protein kinase C in HEp-2 cells infected with enteropathogenic *Escherichia coli* [published erratum appears in *Infect Immun* 1990 Jun;58(6):2024]. *Infect Immun* 1990;58:761–765.

131. Riley L, Russell B, Agarwal S, Arruda S, Ho J. Phosphorylation of cytoskeletal proteins by enteropathogenic *Escherichia coli*, abstr. B-180, page 56. In: *Abstracts of the 92nd General Meeting of the American Society for Microbiology*. Washington, DC: American Society for Microbiology; 1992.

132. Baldwin TJ, Ward W, Aitken A, Knutton S, Williams PH. Elevation of intracellular free calcium levels in HEp-2 cells infected with enteropathogenic *Escherichia coli*. *Infect Immun* 1991;59:1599–1604.

133. Dytoc M, Fedorko L, Sherman P. Changes in cytosolic free calcium in HEp-2 cells infected with attaching and effacing *Escherichia coli*, abstr. B-108, page 43. In: *Abstracts of the 91st General Meeting of the American Society for Microbiology*. Washington, DC: American Society for Microbiology; 1991.

134. Baldwin TJ, Lee-Delaunay MB, Knutton S, Williams PH. Calcium-calmodulin dependence of actin accretion and lethality in cultured HEp-2 cells infected with enteropathogenic *Escherichia coli*. *Infect Immun* 1993;61:760–763.

135. Dytoc MT, Sherman PM, Fedorko L. Phospholipase C mediates attaching and effacing activities of gastrointestinal pathogens in vitro. *J Cell Biol* 1991;115:218a (Abst).

136. Berridge MJ. Inositol trisphosphate and calcium signalling. *Nature* 1993;361:315–325.

137. Shariff A, Luna EJ. Diacylglycerol-stimulated formation of

138. Drucker MM, Polliack A, Yeivin R, Sacks TG. Immunofluorescent demonstration of enteropathogenic *Escherichia coli* in tissues of infants dying with enteritis. *Pediatrics* 1970;46:855–864.

139. Boyd JF. Non-enterotoxin-producing, non-invasive enteropathogenic *Escherichia coli*. *Lancet* 1978;1:1309.

140. Miller JR, Barrett LJ, Kotloff K, Guerrant RL. Antilactoferrin antibody latex bead agglutination assay as a rapid diagnostic test for inflammatory enteritis: results from volunteer and hospital studies. *Arch Intern Med* (in press).

141. Donnenberg MS, Donohue-Rolfe A, Keusch GT. Epithelial cell invasion: an overlooked property of enteropathogenic *Escherichia coli* (EPEC) associated with the EPEC adherence factor. *J Infect Dis* 1989;160:452–459.

142. Miliotis MD, Koornhof HJ, Phillips JI. Invasive potential of noncytotoxic enteropathogenic *Escherichia coli* in an in vitro Henle 407 cell model. *Infect Immun* 1989;57:1928–1935.

143. Andrade JR, Da Veiga VF, De Santa Rosa MR, Suassuna I. An endocytic process in HEp-2 cells induced by enteropathogenic *Escherichia coli*. *J Med Microbiol* 1989;28:49–57.

144. Robins-Browne RM, Bennett-Wood V. Quantitative assessment of the ability of *Escherichia coli* to invade cultured animal cells. *Microb Pathog* 1992;12:159–164.

145. Francis CL, Jerse AE, Kaper JB, Falkow S. Characterization of interactions of enteropathogenic *Escherichia coli* O127:H6 with mammalian cells in vitro. *J Infect Dis* 1991;164:693–703.

146. Cantey JR, Moseley SL. HeLa cell adherence, actin aggregation, and invasion by nonenteropathogenic *Escherichia coli* possessing the *eae* gene. *Infect Immun* 1991;59:3924–3929.

147. Donnenberg MS, Donohue-Rolfe A, Keusch GT. A comparison of HEp-2 cell invasion by enteropathogenic and enteroinvasive *Escherichia coli*. *FEMS Microbiol Lett* 1990;57:83–86.

148. Fletcher JN, Embaye HE, Getty B, Batt RM, Hart CA, Saunders JR. Novel invasion determinant of enteropathogenic *Escherichia coli* plasmid pLV501 encodes the ability to invade intestinal epithelial cells and HEp-2 cells. *Infect Immun* 1992;60:2229–2236.

149. Fletcher JN, Saunders JR, Batt RM, Embaye H, Getty B, Hart CA. Attaching effacement of the rabbit enterocyte brush border is encoded on a single 96.5-kilobase-pair plasmid in an enteropathogenic *Escherichia coli* O111 strain. *Infect Immun* 1990;58:1316–1322.

150. Riley LW, Junio LN, Schoolnik GK. HeLa cell invasion by a strain of enteropathogenic *Escherichia coli* that lacks the O-antigenic polysaccharide. *Mol Microbiol* 1990;4:1661–1666.

151. Marques LRM, Moore MA, Wells JG, Wachsmuth K, O'Brien AD. Production of Shiga-like toxin by *Escherichia coli*. *J Infect Dis* 1993;154:338–341.

152. Cleary TG, Mathewson JJ, Faris E, Pickering LK. Shiga-like cytotoxin production by enteropathogenic *Escherichia coli* serogroups. *Infect Immun* 1985;47:335–337.

153. Echeverria P, Taylor DN, Donohue-Rolfe A, et al. HeLa cell adherence and cytotoxin production by enteropathogenic *Escherichia coli* isolated from infants with diarrhea in Thailand. *J Clin Microbiol* 1987;25:1519–1523.

154. Smith HR, Scotland SM, Stokes N, Rowe B. Examination of strains belonging to enteropathogenic *Escherichia coli* serogroups for genes encoding EPEC adherence factor and Vero cytotoxins. *J Med Microbiol* 1990;31:235–240.

155. Bitzan M, Karch H, Maas MG, et al. Clinical and genetic aspects of Shiga-like toxin production in traditional enteropathogenic *Escherichia coli*. *Zbl Bakt-Int J Med Microbiol* 1991;274:496–506.

156. Canil C, Rosenshine I, Ruschkowski S, Donnenberg MS, Kaper JB, Finlay BB. Enteropathogenic *Escherichia coli* decreases the transepithelial electrical resistance of polarized epithelial monolayers. *Infect Immun* 1993;61:2755–2762.

157. Tai YH, Gage TP, McQueen C, Formal SB, Boedeker EC. Electrolyte transport in rabbit cecum. I. Effect of RDEC-1 infection. *Am J Physiol* 1989;256:G721–G726.

158. Karch H, Heesemann J, Laufs R, Kroll HP, Kaper JB, Levine MM. Serological response to type 1-like somatic fimbriae in

actin nucleation sites at plasma membranes. *Science* 1992;256:245–247.

diarrheal infection due to classical enteropathogenic *Escherichia coli*. *Microb Pathog* 1987;2:425–434.

159. Cravioto A, Reyes RE, Trujillo F, et al. Risk of diarrhea during the first year of life associated with initial and subsequent colonization by specific enteropathogens. *Am J Epidemiol* 1990; 131:886–904.

160. Mushin R, Dubos R. Colonization of the mouse intestine with *Escherichia coli*. *J Exp Med* 1965;122:745–757.

161. Donnenberg MS, Tacket CO, Losonsky G, Nataro JP, Kaper JB, Levine MM. The role of the *eae* gene in experimental human enteropathogenic *Escherichia coli* (EPEC) infection. *Clin Res* 1992;40:214A (Abst).

162. Sussman S. The passive transfer of antibodies to *Escherichia coli* O111:B4 from mother to offspring. *Pediatrics* 1961;27: 308–313.

163. Silva MLM, Giampaglia CMS. Colostrum and human milk inhibit localized adherence of enteropathogenic *Escherichia coli* to HeLa cells. *Acta Paediatr Scand* 1992;81:266–267.

164. Lima AA, Fang G, Schorling JB, et al. Persistent diarrhea in northeast Brazil: etiologies and interactions with malnutrition. *Acta Paediatr Suppl* 1992;381:39–44.

165. Fagundes Neto U, Ferreira V, Patricio FRS, Mostaço VL, Trabulsi LR. Protracted diarrhea: the importance of the enteropathogenic *E. coli* (EPEC) strains and *Salmonella* in its genesis. *J Pediatr Gastroenterol Nutr* 1989;8:207–211.

166. Gangarosa E, Merson MH. Epidemiologic assessment of the relevance of the so-called enteropathogenic serogroups of *Escherichia coli* in diarrhea. *N Engl J Med* 1977;296:1210–1213.

167. Nataro JP, Scaletsky ICA, Kaper JB, Levine MM, Trabulsi LR. Plasmid-mediated factors conferring diffuse and localized adherence of enteropathogenic *Escherichia coli*. *Infect Immun* 1985;48:378–383.

168. Levine MM, Prado V, Robins-Browne R, et al. Use of DNA probes and HEp-2 cell adherence assay to detect diarrheagenic *Escherichia coli*. *J Infect Dis* 1988;158:224–228.

169. Vial PA, Mathewson JJ, DuPont HL, Guers L, Levine MM. Comparison of two assay methods for patterns of adherence to HEp-2 cells of *Escherichia-coli* from patients with diarrhea. *J Clin Microbiol* 1990;28:882–885.

170. Gicquelais KG, Baldini MM, Martinez J, et al. Practical and economical method for using biotinylated DNA probes with bacterial colony blots to identify diarrhea-causing *Escherichia coli*. *J Clin Microbiol* 1990;28:2485–2490.

171. Jerse AE, Martin WC, Galen JE, Kaper JB. Oligonucleotide probe for detection of the enteropathogenic *Escherichia coli* (EPEC) adherence factor of localized adherent EPEC. *J Clin Microbiol* 1990;28:2842–2844.

172. Senerwa D, Olsvik O, Mutanda LN, Gathuma JM, Wachsmuth K. Colonization of neonates in a nursery ward with enteropathogenic *Escherichia coli* and correlation to the clinical histories of the children. *J Clin Microbiol* 1989;27:2539–2543.

173. Shariff M, Bhan MK, Knutton S, Das BK, Saini S, Kumar R. Evaluation of the fluorescence actin staining test for detection of enteropathogenic *Escherichia coli*. *J Clin Microbiol* 1993; 31:386–389.

174. Albert MJ, Ansaruzzaman M, Faruque SM, Neogi PKB, Haider K, Tzipori S. An ELISA for the detection of localized adherent classic enteropathogenic *Escherichia coli* serogroups. *J Infect Dis* 1991;164:986–989.

175. Marin L, Aperia A, Zetterström R, et al. Unsuccessful oral rehydration therapy in an infant with enteropathogenic *E. coli* diarrhoea. Studies of fluid and electrolyte homeostasis. *Acta Paediatr Scand* 1985;74:477–479.

176. Figueroa-Quintanilla D, Salazar-Lindo E, Sack RB, et al. A controlled trial of bismuth subsalicylate in infants with acute watery diarrheal disease. *N Engl J Med* 1993;328:1653–1658.

177. Thorén A, Wolde-Mariam T, Stintzing G, Wadström T, Habte D. Antibiotics in the treatment of gastroenteritis caused by enteropathogenic *Escherichia coli*. *J Infect Dis* 1980;141:27–31.

178. Antai SP, Anozie SO. Incidence of infantile diarrhoea due to enteropathogenic *Escherichia coli* in Port Harcourt metropolis. *J Appl Bacteriol* 1987;62:227–229.

179. Thorén A. Antibiotic sensitivity of enteropathogenic *Escherichia coli* to mecillinam, trimethoprim-sulfamethoxazole and other antibiotics. *Acta Pathol Microbiol Scand [B]* 1980;88: 265–268.

180. Senerwa D, Mutanda LN, Gathuma JM, Olsvik O. Antimicrobial resistance of enteropathogenic *Escherichia coli* strains from a nosocomial outbreak in Kenya. *Acta Pathol Microbiol Scand [B]* 1991;99:728–734.

181. Lim YS, Ngan CCL, Tay L. Enteropathogenic *Escherichia coli* as a cause of diarrhoea among children in Singapore. *J Trop Med Hyg* 1992;95:339–342.

182. Mietens C, Keinhorst H, Hilpert H, Gerber H, Amster H, Pahud JJ. Treatment of infantile *E. coli* gastroenteritis with specific bovine anti-*E. coli* milk immunoglobulins. *Eur J Pediatr* 1979;132:239–252.

183. Tacket CO, Losonsky G, Link H, Hoang Y, Guesry P, Hilpert H, Levine MM. Protection by milk immunoglobulin concentrate against oral challenge with enterotoxigenic *Escherichia coli*. *N Engl J Med* 1988;318:1240–1243.

184. Kubinyi L, Kiss I, Lendvai KG. Epidemiological-statistical evaluation of oral vaccination against infantile *Escherichia coli* enteritis. *Acta Microbiol Acad Sci Hung* 1974;21:187–191.

185. McQueen CE, Boedeker EC, Reid R, et al. Pili in microspheres protect rabbits from diarrhoea induced by *E. coli* strain RDEC-1. *Vaccine* 1993;11:201–206.

Infections of the Gastrointestinal Tract,
edited by M. J. Blaser, P. D. Smith, J. I. Ravdin,
H. B. Greenberg, and R. L. Guerrant
Raven Press, Ltd., New York © 1995.

CHAPTER 51

Enteroaggregative and Diffusely Adherent *Escherichia coli*

James P. Nataro

Escherichia coli were first recognized as diarrheal pathogens in 1898, when Lesage demonstrated that serum from diarrhea patients agglutinated strains of *E. coli* isolated from other patients in the same outbreak but not those of control (1). In 1945, Bray discovered that *E. coli* strains of certain serogroups were the predominant cause of summer diarrhea in infants in the United Kingdom, coining the term *enteropathogenic E. coli* (EPEC) (1). EPEC were recognized as important causes of infant diarrhea in the 1950s and 1960s in the developed world, and subsequently have been shown to be common agents of gastroenteritis in the developing world (1).

In 1979, Cravioto et al. (2) observed that most EPEC isolates adhered to HEp-2 cells in cell culture. Baldini et al. (3) subsequently showed that this adherence trait was associated with the presence of a 60-MDa plasmid. Scaletsky et al. (4) and Nataro et al. (5) examined collections of *E. coli* from studies of diarrhea in the developing world and found, like Cravioto, that most EPEC adhered to HEp-2 cells. However, these investigators also showed that many *E. coli* that were not of EPEC serogroups adhered to HEp-2 cells, but that the adherence phenotype was clearly distinguishable from that of EPEC. The adherence pattern of EPEC was described as "localized" adherence, based on the presence of clusters or microcolonies on the surface of the HEp-2 cells (5). In contradistinction, non-EPEC did not adhere in the characteristic microcolonies, instead displaying a phenotype initially described as "diffuse adherence." A DNA probe specific for the 60-MDa adherence plasmid of EPEC (designated the EAF probe) was shown to correlate closely with localized, EPEC-type adherence, whereas HEp-2-adherent *E. coli* of non-EPEC serogroups were generally EAF probe–negative (6). Nataro et al. (5) reported that in one "diffuse-adherent" non-EPEC and

EAF probe–negative strain, *E. coli* 042 (O44:H18), HEp-2 adherence was associated with the presence of a 65-MDa plasmid. DNA hybridization studies of the plasmid from strain 042 with the EAF plasmid of EPEC revealed no significant homology (5). Thus, the diffuse adherence factor was hypothesized to be plasmid-mediated, yet to be genetically distinct from that conferring localized adherence. Of note, strain 042 was later shown to be an enteroaggregative *E. coli* (EAggEC) (7).

Mathewson et al. (8) concurrently observed that *E. coli* that were not of EPEC serotypes and that adhered to HEp-2 cells were associated with diarrheal disease in adult travelers to Mexico. Furthermore, these investigators demonstrated that one such strain was capable of causing diarrhea in adult volunteers (9). In these reports, diarrheagenic *E. coli* that adhered to HEp-2 cells but were not of EPEC serotypes were termed enteroadherent *E. coli* (EAEC).

Nataro et al. (10) examined the HEp-2 adherence properties of *E. coli* isolated in Santiago, Chile from the stools of 154 children with diarrhea and 66 healthy controls. In the course of this study, these investigators were able to divide the "diffuse" adherence phenotype into two further categories: aggregative and (true) diffuse (Fig. 1). Aggregative adherence (AA) was distinguished by the prominent autoagglutination of the bacterial cells to each other; often this occurred on the surface of the cells as well as on the glass coverslip free from the HEp-2 cells. The *sine qua non* of AA, however, was the characteristic layering of the bacteria, best described as a "stacked brick" configuration. In diffuse adherence (DA), bacteria were seen dispersed over the surface of the HEp-2 cell, with little aggregation and little adherence to the glass coverslip free from the cells. Of 253 EAF probe-negative *E. coli* from Chilean diarrhea patients, 84 (33%) exhibited the AA pattern of adherence. In contrast, only 20 (15%) of 134 probe-negative strains from asymptomatic controls were AA-positive ($p < 0.00001$). Recognizing a possible new category of diarrheagenic *E. coli,* these investigators coined

J. P. Nataro: Center for Vaccine Development, University of Maryland School of Medicine, Baltimore, Maryland 21201.

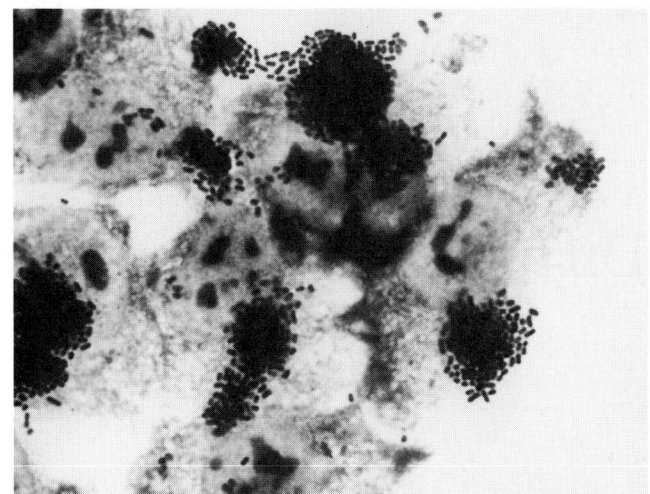
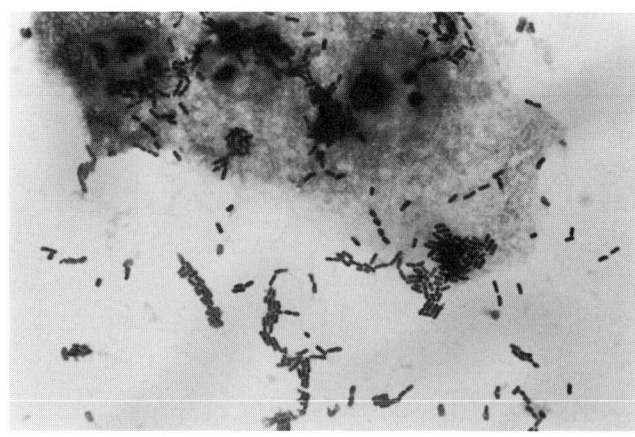
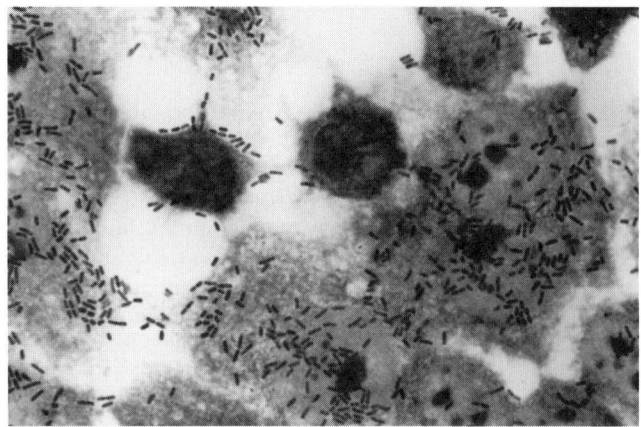

FIG. 1. Adherence patterns of *E. coli* to HEp-2 cells after 3 hr incubation according to the method of Cravioto et al (2). **A:** Localized adherence. Note clusters or microcolonies of bacteria on the surface of the HEp-2 cells. This pattern is typical of enteropathogenic *E. coli*. **B:** Aggregative adherence. Note aggregation of bacteria in typical "stacked brick" pattern on the surface of the cell as well as free from the cell. **C:** Diffuse adherence. Bacteria are scattered over the surface of the cell with little aggregation or adherence to the glass background.

the term "enteroadherent-aggregative *E. coli*" (later shortened to enteroaggregative *E. coli*, EAggEC) to describe organisms expressing AA. Diffusely adherent *E. coli* (DAEC) were not associated with diarrhea in this study.

Reports following the initial descriptions of enteroadherent, diffusely adherent, and enteroaggregative *E. coli* have suggested that these are diarrheal pathogens in many areas. However, a great deal of confusion surrounds the terminology of these strains. As discussed below, EAggEC and DAEC are distinct categories, with different epidemiological, clinical, and perhaps pathogenetic features. Thus, it is appropriate to designate these categories by their most descriptive names: enteroaggregative and diffusely adherent *E. coli*. The term *enteroadherent* is frequently used in ways other than as originally defined and should be discarded. If one wishes to select a term to group EPEC, EAggEC, and DAEC, "HEp-2–adherent" would be most accurate.

ENTEROAGGREGATIVE *E. COLI*

Enteroaggregative *E. coli* (EAggEC) are currently defined as *E. coli* that do not secrete enterotoxins LT or ST and that adhere to HEp-2 cells in an aggregative pattern. It is likely that this definition encompasses both pathogenic and nonpathogenic clones, which share a factor(s) conferring a common phenotype.

Microbiology

Each category of diarrheagenic *E. coli* is found to comprise its own characteristic serotypes (11). Serotypic markers most likely correlate with clones expressing a particular package of virulence determinants rather than the antigens themselves conferring virulence (the K1 antigen of systemic *E. coli* may be an exception). The serotypes characteristic of EAggEC are not thoroughly de-

TABLE 1. *Serotypes of EAggEC compiled from published reports[a]*

Serotype	Number reported	Site
O15:H18	21	Chile, Thailand
O44:H18	16	United Kingdom, Peru
O77:H18	15	India, Chile
O126:H27	14	United Kingdom
O3:H2	12	Chile
O111ab:H21	10	United Kingdom
O141:H49	7	Bangladesh
O51:H11	6	India
O?:H33	6	Chile, United Kingdom
O?:NM	6	Chile, India
O86:H2	6	Chile
O92:H33	4	India, United Kingdom
O113:NM	4	Bangladesh
Rough:H33	4	Chile
Rough:H2	3	Chile
O?:H21	3	Thailand, India

[a] Data from refs. 7, 21, 29, and 46.

scribed, although several serotypes are repeatedly found. Table 1 summarizes the serotypes of EAggEC from all studies in which serotyping was performed. The table illustrates the heterogeneity of EAggEC isolates; however, a few serotypes are isolated commonly and from multiple locations. As in EPEC, certain flagellar antigens are conserved across O serogroups and may signify a clonal relationship (12). The most frequently isolated serotypes may be the most virulent EAggEC. Evidence for the pathogenicity of O44:H18 is compelling (see below).

Table 1 also illustrates the finding of nontypable or rough *E. coli* expressing the AA phenotype. Vial et al. (7) characterized a collection of 40 EAggEC strains isolated from the stools of children in Santiago. Twenty-seven (68%) were found to exhibit rough-like properties, i.e., spontaneous agglutination in saline. Only 5 of the 27, however, were susceptible to rough-specific phages. Four such rough-resistant strains were selected for lipopolysaccharide (LPS) analysis; all four exhibited O antigen profiles characteristic of smooth *E. coli*. Thus, it is likely that some EAggEC share a surface factor that confers autoagglutination in saline, mimicking the behavior of rough strains. Lindberg et al. extensively characterized

the O antigen of one such rough-like EAggEC and found it to be most similar to that of *Salmonella thompson* (serogroup C1) (13).

EAggEC Volunteer Studies

Several EAggEC strains have been fed to adult volunteers in an effort to identify truly pathogenic strains. A summary of the studies reported to date is provided in Table 2.

Mathewson et al. fed two EAggEC strains to two groups of volunteers (9). EAggEC strain JM221, isolated from the stool of a diarrhea patient in Mexico, was fed to eight volunteers each at doses of 7×10^8 and 10^{10}. Of the volunteers fed the higher dose, three of eight experienced diarrhea, while two others reported "enteric" symptoms including borborygmi and cramps.

Nataro et al. (14) conducted volunteer studies using four different EAggEC strains isolated from different geographic locations and representing different serotypes. As seen in Table 2, of five volunteers fed 10^{10} EAggEC 042 (O44:H18), three met the study definition of diarrhea (>200 mL of loose stool). One other volunteer fed 042 developed enteric symptoms, including low-volume liquid stools and borborygmi. Of the 15 volunteers fed other EAggEC strains (including JM221), none met the study definition of diarrhea and only 1 of the 15 had stools looser than normal. These data support strongly the pathogenicity of EAggEC in humans and, moreover, suggest that the virulence of these strains varies according to as yet unknown properties.

Epidemiology of EAggEC

The first description of EAggEC implicated these organisms in diarrheal disease of children in Santiago, Chile (see above) (10). As shown in Table 3, subsequent studies have supported the association of EAggEC with diarrhea in other developing populations, most prominently in association with persistent diarrhea (> 14 days).

Bhan et al. conducted two separate studies in Indian children and first reported the association of EAggEC with persistent diarrhea. These investigators performed weekly household surveillance on a cohort of 452 children (<3 years of age) who lived in the rural village of Anapur-

TABLE 2. *Volunteer studies with EAggEC*

Strain	Dose	Number of volunteers	Number with diarrhea	Number with enteric symptoms[a]	Ref.
JM221	7×10^8	8	2	1	9
JM221	1×10^{10}	8	3	5	9
JM221	1×10^{10}	5	0	0	14
189	7×10^8	4	1	3	9
189	1×10^{10}	4	0	0	9
17-2	1×10^{10}	24	1	1	14
042	1×10^{10}	5	3	4	14
34b	1×10^{10}	5	0	0	14

[a] Includes abdominal pain, borborygmi, nausea, vomiting.

TABLE 3. *Studies implicating EAggEC as agents of diarrheal disease*

Study	Control (%)	Acute (%)	Persistent (%)	p Value
Nataro et al. (10)	20/134 (15)	81/253 (32)		<0.00001
Bhan et al. (15)	20/201 (9.9)	23/179 (12.8)	18/61 (29.5)	0.0006[a]
				0.03[b]
Bhan et al. (16)	6/92 (6.5)		18/92 (19.6)	0.016
Cravioto et al. (17)	5/100 (5)		29/57 (51)	0.001
Wanke et al. (18)	2/38 (5)	4/50 (8)	8/40 (20)	<0.05[a]
Henry et al. (20)		5/28 (18)	17/62 (27)	<0.05

[a] Persistent diarrhea vs. control.
[b] Persistent diarrhea vs. acute diarrhea.

Palla in northern India (15). Fecal specimens were obtained from 240 episodes of diarrhea and from age-matched asymptomatic controls in the same population. EAggEC (defined by AA in the HEp-2 assay) were found in the stools of 10% and 13% of controls and acute (<14 days) diarrhea patients, respectively. By contrast, 30% of those with persistent diarrhea yielded EAggEC isolates (p = 0.0052 vs. acute and p = 0.0006 vs. controls). Logistic regression was performed using acute/persistence as the dependent variable with independent variables of age, gender, breastfeeding, income, maternal education, season of occurrence, and antibiotic intake. The corrected odds ratio for association of EAggEC with persistence was 2.2 ($p < 0.05$). Patients with EAggEC diarrhea had a mean duration of illness of 17.0 days; fever was present in 12.2% and grossly bloody stools in 12.2%.

Bhan and coworkers (16) subsequently studied 92 children (<2 years of age) admitted to the All India Medical Institute with nondysenteric diarrhea for >14 days. Ninety-two children admitted for nondiarrheal diseases were selected as controls. Stools were collected from all subjects and tested for enteric pathogens, including analysis of five *E. coli* in the HEp-2 adherence assay. In patients, the most frequently isolated stool pathogen was EAggEC (18 of 92, or 19.6%); EAggEC were isolated from the stools of only 6/92 controls (6.5%; p = 0.016).

Cravioto et al. (17) followed a cohort of 75 infants and children under 2 years of age born in the Mexican village of Lugar Sobre la Tierra Blanca. Household visits were performed every 48 hr to assess children for the presence of diarrhea; when cases were detected, stool specimens were obtained from the patient and a matched control from the village. EAggEC were found in 29 (51%) of the 57 cases of diarrhea which persisted for >14 days. In contrast, EAggEC were found in only 49 (8%) of 579 acute cases and 5 (5%) of 100 nondiarrheal controls ($p < 0.001$). In this study, EAggEC were the most frequent pathogens associated with bloody diarrhea: 33% of those with EAggEC in the stool manifested gross blood.

Guerrant and coworkers have been conducting long-term surveillance of a cohort of infants and children (<5 years) in Fortaleza, Brazil. A number of studies published by these investigators have consistently found a high rate of isolation of EAggEC and have demonstrated a strong association between the presence of EAggEC and persistence of diarrhea past 14 days. Wanke et al. (18) reported the results of 27 months of surveillance in this population.

Household visits were conducted three times per week and specimens were collected from those with diarrhea as well as asymptomatic controls. EAggEC were found in 2 (5%) of 28 asymptomatic controls, 4 (8%) of 50 acute diarrhea cases, and 8 (20%) of 40 persistent cases ($p < 0.05$ persistent vs. acute and controls). EAggEC were found in 18% of persistent cases when cultured during the first 14 days of illness and 27% of such cases after 14 days. Working in the same population, Lima et al. found EAggEC in the stools of 10 (53%) of 19 with persistent diarrhea (19).

Henry et al. (20) followed a cohort of children <6 years of age in Mirzapoor, Bangladesh for a period of 2 years. Household visits were performed 5 days a week, assessing for diarrhea and obtaining stool specimens. Age- and sex-matched controls were selected for each diarrheal specimen. EAggEC (by HEp-2 assay) were isolated during the first 2 days of illness in 27% of the patients whose diarrhea eventually persisted for 14 days or more, compared with 18% of those whose diarrhea lasted 1–13 days ($p < 0.05$).

EAggEC are not strictly confined to the developing world. Scotland et al. (21) studied the adherence properties of several strains thought to be of EPEC serogroups but which proved negative with the EAF probe. Seven of 13 O44:H18 strains, all of 10 O111ab:H21, and 13 of 21 O126:H27 were found to display the AA pattern in the HEp-2 assay. Of note, three of the O44:H18 EAggEC strains were isolated in outbreaks, two in infants and one in hospitalized elderly patients.

In some studies, EAggEC have not been associated with diarrhea (22–24). EAggEC are commonly found in virtually all intensively studied populations; asymptomatic excretion rates can be as high as 28% (R. Dagan, *personal communication*). It is well documented that established enteropathogens are often found in asymptomatic individuals in developing populations and frequently cannot be statistically associated with diarrheal illness (15,18,25–27). Moreover, it is likely that the definition of EAggEC (AA in the HEp-2 assay) includes nonpathogenic *E. coli* that may be missing one or more necessary virulence determinants. This latter possibility is favored by the volunteer studies described above. Analysis of volunteer data and the serotyping data presented in Table 1 support pathogenicity for some serotypes, most notably O44:H18.

Pathogenesis of EAggEC Diarrhea

The study of EAggEC has been hampered by the fact that the virulence of different strains is apparently heterogeneous and that observations made in nonpathogenic isolates may not be relevant to the pathogenicity of virulent EAggEC.

Histopathology

Vial et al. studied the histopathology of infection with EAggEC strains 042 and 17-2 in rabbit and rat ileal loop models (7). Both organisms elicited a destructive lesion on light microscopy, characterized by shortening of the villi, hemorrhagic necrosis of the villous tips, and a mild inflammatory response with edema and mononuclear infiltration of the submucosa. Transmission electron microscopy showed normal microvillar architecture without invasion of enterocytes. Both light and electron microscopy revealed prominent adherence of bacteria to the mucosal surface.

Tzipori et al. fed JM221 and 17-2 to gnotobiotic piglets (28). Of six piglets fed strain 17-2, four developed severe enteric signs, two leading to death. Necropsy of all the piglets fed 17-2 revealed a histopathological lesion of the ileum similar to that described by Vial et al., but with more prominent edema and without necrosis of the villous tips. Bacteria adhered strongly to the mucosa in a stacked brick pattern. Two of six piglets fed JM221 became ill and three developed abnormalities of the ileal mucosa. Description of the EAggEC histopathological lesion and site of infection awaits data from affected humans.

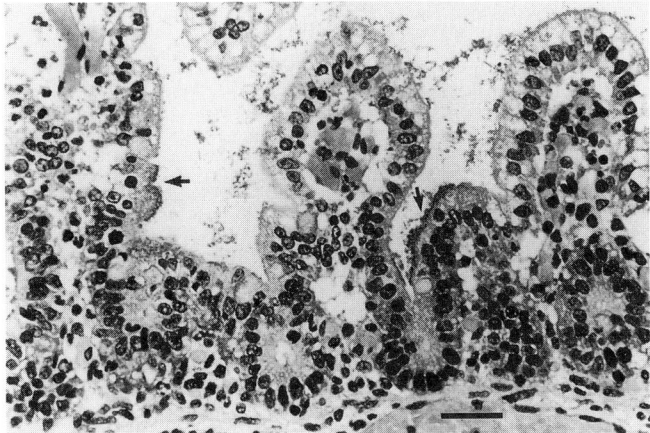

FIG. 2. Histopathology of EAggEC infection in the gnotobiotic piglet ileum. At 24 hr of age, piglets were fed a dose of 1 × 10^10 CFU of the inoculum strain 17-2 and observed for 3 days. The light photomicrograph is typical of the lesion seen in the ileum of piglets who experienced diarrhea. Enterocytes appear swollen; edema and vascular congestion are seen in the lamina propria, accompanied by coagulated erythrocytes. Arrows point to aggregates of bacteria on the mucosal surface (bar = 50 μm). From ref. 28, with permission.

Adherence

The earliest work on EAggEC pathogenesis fortuitously focused on the O44:H18 strain, 042. Both Nataro et al. (5) and Vial et al. (7) demonstrated that the AA property in this strain was associateed with the presence of the 65-MDa plasmid. Upon acquisition of the 65-MDa plasmid, *E. coli* HB101 was found to adhere to HEp-2 cells an AA pattern and to express surface fimbriae. In addition, HB101 that was transformed with the 65-MDa plasmid was found to have acquired a new LPS O-antigen profile.

Vial et al. (7) examined the surface of several wild-type EAggEC strains using electron microscopy. Eight of the strains were found to express surface fimbriae of a rod-like morphology, 6–7 nm in diameter, despite being negative for type 1 fimbrial expression. Antiserum raised against purified fimbriae from one strain reacted on immunoblot with the other seven, suggesting that some EAggEC share a common fimbria.

Knutton et al. (29) studied 44 strains producing characteristic AA to HEp-2 cells (organisms adhering to the glass coverslip but not the cells were excluded from analysis); all 44 were positive for the AA probe described below. These investigators found that all 44 strains possessed surface fimbriae, detectable by negative staining and transmission electron microscopy. The fimbrial structures were categorized according to four different morphologies: hollow rod, rod, fibrillar, and fibrillar bundles. All of the strains expressed the fibrillar bundle morphology and most expressed at least one of the other morphologies as well.

These investigators also studied the adherence of EAggEC to cells in tissue culture and to human and animal intestinal sections. EAggEC adherence to Caco-2 cell surfaces featured a distinct space between the bacterium and the cell, similar to that reported in animal models by Vial et al. (7), but in contrast to the intimate adherence seen with EPEC. In addition, it was shown that whereas EAggEC strains did not adhere to cultured duodenal mucosa, all 44 strains adhered markedly to cultured colonic mucosa.

Yamamoto et al. also studied the adherence of an EAggEC strain (O127a:H2) to explants of intestinal tissue (30). These investigators found marked adherence to colonic tissue from adults and children, significant adherence to the epithelium overlying ileal lymphoid follicles, and modest adherence to ileal and jejunal sections. These data agree with those of Knutton in suggesting a colonic localization of EAggEC colonization yet are in contrast to the ileal adherence observed in animal models.

The HEp-2 adherence of EAggEC strain 17-2 has been studied in great detail. Nataro et al. identified a flexible, bundle-forming fimbrial structure, with fibers of 2–3 nm diameter, designated aggregative adherence fimbriae I (AAF/I) (31,32), which mediates HEp-2 adherence and human erythrocyte hemagglutination (Fig. 3). The genes for AAF/I are organized as two separate gene clusters on the 17-2 plasmid, separated by 9 kb of intervening DNA (32). Region 1 encodes a cluster of genes require for fim-

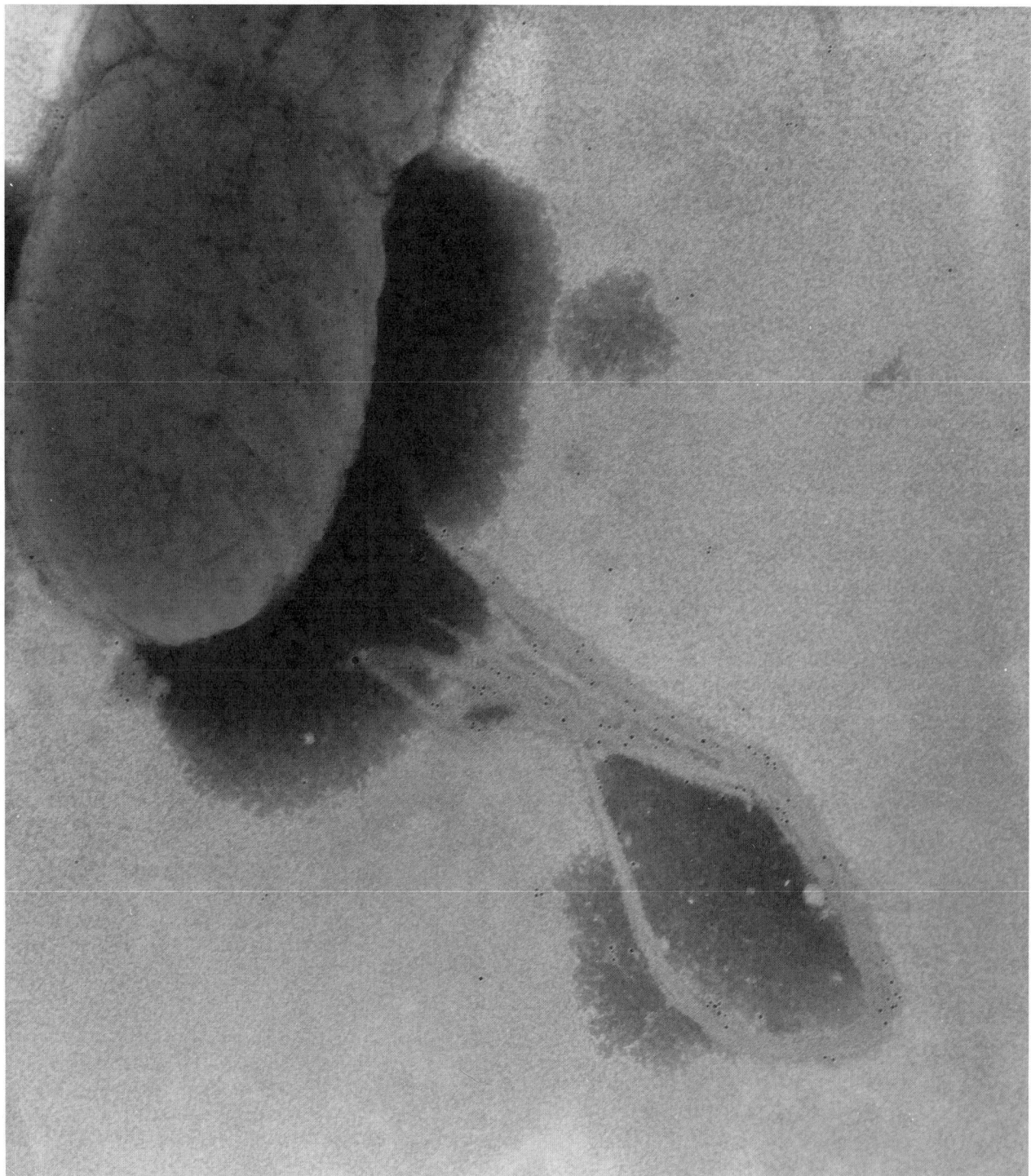

FIG. 3. Aggregative adherence fimbriae I (AAF/I) on strain 17-2. Bacteria were harvested from a static L-broth culture grown overnight at 37°C, then incubated with anti-AAF/I antiserum and secondary antibody labeled with 10-nm gold particles. Specimens were negative-stained and visualized under transmission electron microscopy at 25,000 ×. Note flexible bundle-forming morphology of the fimbriae; individual filaments are 2–3 nm in diameter. From ref. 32, with permission.

brial synthesis and assembly, including the structural subunit of the fimbria itself. Region 2 encodes a transcriptional activator of AAF/I expression that shows homology to members of the AraC family of DNA-binding proteins. The AAF/I fimbriae are morphologically similar to other bundle-forming fimbriae, including those belonging to the type 4 class. Members of the type 4 class of fimbriae have been shown to bear homology at the amino terminus of their fimbrial structural subunits (33,34); AAF/I lacks such conserved sequences.

Toxins

While studying the plasmid of strain 17-2, Savarino et al. identified an open reading frame encoding a 4100-kDa homolog of the heat-stable enterotoxin (ST), designated EAST1 (35,36). EAST1 is a 38-amino-acid protein that consists of four cysteine residues, unlike the six characteristic of E. coli ST. Of considerable interest is the observation that the eukaryotic membrane protein, guanylin, previously shown to have homology to ST, also contains four cysteine residues. The role of EAST1 in secretion has not yet been determined, although EAST1 clones yield net increases in short circuit current in the rabbit mucosal Ussing chamber model.

Baldwin et al. (37) reported that the supernatant of an O44:H18 EAggEC strain induces rises in the intracellular calcium level of HEp-2 cells. The increase in calcium was neutralizable with extracellular calcium chelators, such as EGTA. Moreover, these investigators were able to block the action of the supernatants using antibodies against the E. coli hemolysin. EAggEC supernatants also induced phosphorylation of several HEp-2 cytoplasmic proteins. A role for this putative toxin in EAggEC diarrhea has not yet been demonstrated.

Eslava et al. (38) studied an EAggEC strain (O146:H39) isolated from an outbreak in a Mexican village. Supernatants of this strain induced necrosis and edema in rat ileal loops. These investigators were able to purify a protein of MW 107 kDa that induced this pathology in the rat loop model. Furthermore, antibodies to the 107-kDa moiety were found in the sera of patients with diarrhea associated with this organism.

Pathogenetic Models

Available data do not permit a full description of EAggEC pathogenesis, yet several hypotheses can be entertained. Colonization of the bowel is a highly conserved feature of enteric pathogenesis and fimbrial adherence factors have been identified in most categories of diarrheagenic E. coli (11). AAF/I, and other fimbriae as described by Knutton and Vial, are candidates for factors that may facilitate initial colonization, most likely of the large bowel (or perhaps both large and small bowel sites). The putative enterotoxin EAST1 may contribute to watery diarrhea induced by EAggEC; however, the histopathological lesion seen in animal models and humans is much more destructive than that produced by ST-produc-

ing ETEC. In addition, volunteer studies with EAST1-producing EAggEC have not uniformly resulted in diarrhea despite intestinal colonization (14) (albeit in adults).

The histopathological lesion described for EAggEC suggests greater damage to villous tips than to crypts. This observation suggests the hypothesis that diarrhea may be due to damage of the tip absorptive cells, while leaving crypt secretory cells relatively unaffected. The mechanism of this cellular damage is as yet undetermined, yet the putative toxins described by Baldwin et al. and Eslava et al. are potential candidates.

The association of EAggEC with persistence deserves special attention. First, severe damage to mucosal cells implies that a longer time would be needed for regeneration of functional epithelium than is observed in secretory diarrheas; this regeneration would be further retarded in malnourished children. Second, it is tempting to speculate that EAggEC may directly affect the host immune response normally responsible for elimination of enteric pathogens, yet experimental support for this hypothesis is lacking. A third hypothesis to explain EAggEC persistence is that these organisms may act in concert with other pathogens, concurrently or perhaps sequentially.

Diagnosis of EAggEC

EAggEC infection is diagnosed by the isolation of E. coli from the stools of patients and the analysis of such isolates in the HEp-2 assay or by DNA probe. Analysis of small bowel aspirates has not increased yield (19). The number of E. coli isolates in each stool specimen that are tested in the HEp-2 assay has varied in published studies from two to five colonies per specimen. No formal data exist to suggest the minimum number of colonies needed for optimal diagnostic yield. However, analysis of data compounded in the author's laboratory suggests that in greater than 70% of cases in which three colonies are selected from each patient, the same E. coli category is found in at least two of the three isolates. Thus, including greater than three colonies per specimen is unlikely to provide substantially greater sensitivity.

HEp-2 Assay

The AA phenotype defines EAggEC, yet variations on this pattern can be readily discerned. Investigators (Ref. 29 and author's unpublished data) have noted that some EAggEC show a prominent adherence to the cell surface and little aggregation free from the cells; other strains preferentially adhere to each other and the glass coverslips, sparing the cells. Still other EAggEC adhere to both cells and glass equally well. These variations in phenotype are generally reproducible for a given isolate (29). No molecular mechanisms have yet been described to explain these variations; however, single-transposon insertions have been shown to change one such AA pattern to another pattern (31).

Several different methods for performing the HEp-2 assay have been described (39–41). The method used in the first description of the three HEp-2 adherence phenotypes is essentially the technique first described by Cravioto et al. (2), employing a single 3-hr incubation of bacteria and cells without a change in medium during the course of the assay. Mathewson et al. (42) reported a variation on this assay in which, after the first hour of incubation, the tissue culture medium was changed and replaced with fresh sterile medium, then incubated for an additional 2 hr. Vial et al. (39), in a collaborative study with Mathewson, compared the 3-hr incubation methods with and without a change of medium. These investigators determined that the method of Cravioto (also called the CVD method), without a change of medium, was best at differentiating all three patterns. Specifically, when the medium was changed, the method was unable to distinguish the AA pattern. It should also be stressed that AAF/I is maximally expressed in static L-broth cultures at 37°C (43), thus the author incubates all HEp-2 assay inocula under these conditions.

DNA Probe

Several lines of evidence suggest that the large plasmids present in most EAggEC strains share a high degree of DNA homology (7,44). Baudry et al. (44) selected a 1.0-kb Sau3a fragment from the plasmid of strain 17-2 that hybridized with a fragment of similar size from the 65-MDa plasmid of strain 042. This DNA probe was hybridized against a collection of EAggEC strains from various parts of the world (Table 4). In the initial report, of the 63 EAggEC strains (by HEp-2 assay), 56 (89%) were positive with the EAggEC probe. Of 376 strains representing normal flora and other diarrheagenic categories, only two hybridized with the probe. Subsequent experience with the EAggEC probe has revealed that the correlation of probe positivity with AA varies by location. In some studies the correlation approaches the 89% sensitivity reported by Baudry et al. (author's unpublished observations). In other studies, however, the sensitivity may be substantially lower. Fang et al. (45) reported that only 39% of the EAggEC strains isolated from a study in Fortaleza, Brazil were positive with the EAggEC probe. The epidemiological significance of probe-positive vs. probe-negative strains is as yet undetermined. Moreover, the precise gene recognized by the Baudry probe is as yet unidentified.

TABLE 4. *Testing of E. coli categories with EAggEC probe*

Category	Number	EAggEC probe positive (%)
EAggEC[a]	63	56 (89)
ETEC	84	0
EIEC	50	2 (4)
EHEC	143	0
EPEC[a]	57	0
DAEC[a]	43	0
Normal flora	62	0

Data from ref. 44.
[a] Defined by HEp-2 adherence pattern.

Other Tests for EAggEC

Methods other than the HEp-2 and DNA probe assays have been suggested to identify EAggEC. Albert et al. (46) have reported that EAggEC probe-positive organisms display an unusual pellicle formation in Mueller–Hinton broth. Similarly, growing EAggEC strains in polystyrene culture tubes or dishes at 37°C overnight without shaking produces a bacterial film on the polystyrene surface, easily visualized with Giemsa stain. Both phenotypes are likely due to high surface hydrophobicity of EAggEC. Either of these techniques is a convenient substitute for the DNA probe in assaying EAggEC. It should be emphasized, however, that until epidemiological studies show greater pathogenicity of probe-positive strains over probe-negative strains, the HEp-2 assay should remain the gold standard for EAggEC detection.

The critical question in the management of patients from whom EAggEC are isolated is whether or not the isolate is responsible for the patient's symptoms. It is wise to approach any such isolate with skepticism. The author currently accepts an EAggEC as a likely cause of the patient's diarrhea in only three situations: (a) when the patient presents in the course of a documented outbreak; (b) when the patient's isolate can be shown to belong to one of the common EAggEC serotypes associated with disease (eg. O44:H18); and/or (c) when the patient exhibits persistent diarrhea and stools repeatedly yield an EAggEC as the predominant flora in the absence of another enteric pathogen.

Treatment

No studies have been performed assessing the value of antibiotic treatment for EAggEC diarrhea. In studies in Thailand, Yamamoto et al. (43) have suggested that most EAggEC are resistant to antibiotics routinely used for the treatment of gastroenteritis, including amoxicillin and cotrimoxazole; most strains were sensitive to fluoroquinolones. Thus any study evaluating antibiotic therapy for EAggEC diarrhea would require the testing of antibiotic sensitivity patterns. The decision of whether or not to treat a patient from whom an EAggEC is isolated depends on the considerations of causality listed above, the antibiotic susceptibility of the isolate, and the severity of the patient's presentation. It should be emphasized that as yet no data support the efficacy of such treatment.

Prevention

The association of EAggEC with persistent disease makes this syndrome less amenable to management with oral rehydration therapy alone, and thus the development of preventive strategies, including vaccination, would be a high priority for areas in which this disease commonly occurs. Candidates under investigation as potential critical antigens include the AAF/I fimbriae.

DIFFUSELY ADHERING *E. COLI*

Description

The first descriptions of DA failed to distinguish this phenotype from AA. Thus several early papers describing DAEC actually include EAggEC strains (4,5). Little is known of the pathogenesis and clinical characteristics of what we now consider DAEC. No published reports allow characterization of characteristic serotypes, although the author's preliminary data suggest that nontypable and rough-like strains are characteristic of DAEC as they are for EAggEC.

Epidemiology

Early studies in which DAEC were found and clearly distinguished from EAggEC shared the common feature of failing to find an association between DAEC and diarrheal disease (10,15–18). However, more recent studies have succeeded in demonstrating such an association. Of interest is the fact that in such studies, the association is generally seen in children outside of infancy.

Giron et al. (23) performed a community-based, case-control study in a southern Mexican village covering 3 weeks during the peak diarrhea season. Among the 24 (of 58) cases from whom no recognized pathogen was identified, DAEC were significantly associated with diarrhea ($p < 0.02$). This study examined a population of children <6 years of age; stratification by age was not performed.

Gunzberg et al. (26) studied the adherence characteristics of 138 *E. coli* samples from the stools of aboriginal children from whom no recognized pathogen had been isolated. Twenty-five (36.8%) of 68 children with diarrhea and 32 (45.7%) of 70 without diarrhea had diffusely adherent isolates ($p > 0.25$). After age stratification, however, DAEC strains were found to be significantly associated with diarrhea in children >18 months of age ($p < 0.05$).

Levine et al. (47) performed a prospective cohort study of children in Santiago, Chile. Three hundred sixty children from the village of Santa Julia, all <4 years old, were recruited. Ninety children were chosen from each year of age. Each child was followed until the age of 60 months, at which time he or she was dropped from the study and replaced by a child <12 months old. Observation was continued for a total of 30 months. During this period, stool samples were obtained from 1081 cases of diarrhea and from case-matched controls from the same population. Table 5 illustrates that the frequency of isolation of DAEC in cases varied between 12.3% and 19.7% among the age strata. The association between DAEC and diarrheal disease increased with each year of age, maximizing at a relative risk of 2.1 at 48–60 months. In this study, the seasonal pattern of DAEC infection was similar to that of ETEC, occurring more commonly in the warm season.

Baqui et al. (22) followed a cohort of 705 children <5 years of age in rural Bangladesh, for a period of 13 months. Age-matched controls from the same cohort were chosen for each case of diarrhea; cases which persisted

TABLE 5. *Association of DAEC with diarrhea by age in a cohort of Chilean children*

Age (months)	Rate of DAEC in cases (%)	Rate of DAEC in controls (%)	Relative risk
0–11	20/162 (12.3)	18/159 (11.3)	1.1
12–23	51/281 (18.1)	41/275 (14.9)	1.2
24–35	44/251 (17.5)	31/249 (12.4)	1.4
36–47	33/230 (14.3)	21/223 (9.4)	1.5
≥48	31/157 (19.7)	15/157 (9.6)	2.1
Total	179/1081 (16.6)	126/1063 (11.9)	1.4

Data from ref. 47.

for >14 days were matched with both asymptomatic and acute diarrheal cases. In this study, DAEC were found in 16.4% of 177 cases of persistent diarrhea, 10.3% of matched acute diarrheal cases, and 8.2% of asymptomatic matched controls ($p < 0.05$ for persistent diarrhea vs. both acute and no diarrhea; no association was found comparing acute with asymptomatic patients). These data would suggest that not only is DAEC associated with the syndrome of persistent diarrhea, but that studies in which diarrheal cases are not stratified by duration may be less likely to demonstrate an association of DAEC with diarrhea.

Jallat et al. (48) characterized 262 strains of *E. coli* isolated from diarrhea patients of all ages hospitalized in Clermont-Ferrand, France. One-hundred strains (38.2%) exhibited the DA phenotype compared with 8.9% (8/90) of *E. coli* isolated from asymptomatic patients ($p < 0.0001$). This study demonstrates that whereas DAEC prevalence may be very much dependent on geography, these organisms may in fact be quite common in the developed world. Moreover, the high rate of isolation from hospitalized patients suggests a relatively severe clinical presentation.

Pathogenesis and Immunity

Little is known about the pathogenetic features of DAEC-induced diarrhea. Bilge et al. (49) have cited preliminary evidence that strain C1845 is capable of inducing inflammatory lesions in the ileum of gnotobiotic piglets. These investigators have described the cloning and characterization of a surface fimbria in this strain, which mediates the DA phenotype (49–51). The genes encoding these fimbriae (designated F1845) can be found either on the bacterial chromosome or on a plasmid. The fimbrial genes show homology to members of the Dr group of bacterial adhesins, so called because they mediate adherence to the Dr blood group antigen. Genetic characterization of the F1845 fimbrial genes has resulted in the description of novel means of RNA processing (51).

Benz et al. (52–54) have described a 100-kDa outer membrane protein that is associated with the DA phenotype in one strain of serotype O126:H27. The gene encoding this factor (designated AIDA-I) has been completely sequenced. Use of a DNA probe specific for AIDA-I suggests that this factor is expressed by a minority of DAEC isolates (author's unpublished observations).

DAEC Volunteer Studies

Tacket and coworkers (55) fed two different DAEC strains (57-1 and C1845) to two cohorts of volunteers at escalating doses as high as 10^{10} CFU. Despite fecal shedding of the challenge organisms, none of the volunteers experienced diarrhea. There are several possible explanations for the failure of the DAEC strains to cause diarrhea. The most obvious is that neither of the two strains fed are true pathogens. This does not preclude the possibility that other DAEC strains may be pathogenic, as was seen with the EAggEC volunteer study. Another possible explanation follows from the age specificity of DAEC attack rates in several studies cited above. It is possible that adults are as resistant to diarrhea from these strains as infants seem to be.

Diagnosis

Methods and considerations useful for diagnosing DAEC disease are similar to those used for EAggEC. Presence of the DA pattern in the HEp-2 assay defines DAEC. A DAEC DNA probe is available, which consists of a part of the daaC gene (49), necessary for expression of the F1845 fimbriae. Approximately 75% of DAEC strains from around the world are positive with the F1845 gene probe (author's unpublished observations). Due to the genetic relatedness of F1845 with other members of the Dr family of adhesins, false-positives with the DA probe occur, albeit with unknown frequency.

Treatment

No studies have yet been reported describing treatment of DAEC infections. Antibiotic susceptibility data for large numbers of isolates have similarly not been reported.

REFERENCES

1. Levine MM, Edelman R. Enteropathogenic *Escherichia coli* of classic serotypes associated with infant diarrhea: epidemiology and pathogenesis. *Epidemiol Rev* 1984;6:31–51.
2. Cravioto A, Gross RJ, Scotland SM, Rowe B. An adhesive factor found in strains of *Escherichia coli* belonging to the traditional infantile enteropathogenic serotypes. *Curr Microbiol* 1979;3:95–99.
3. Baldini MM, Kaper JB, Levine MM, Candy DC, Moon HW. Plasmid-mediated adhesion in enteropathogenic *Escherichia coli*. *J Pediatr Gastroenterol Nutr* 1983;2:534–538.
4. Scaletsky ICA, Silva MLM, Trabulsi LR. Distinctive patterns of adherence of enteropathogenic *Escherichia coli* to HeLa cells. *Infect Immun* 1984;45:534–536.
5. Nataro JP, Scaletsky ICA, Kaper JB, Levine MM, Trabulsi LR. Plasmid-mediated factors conferring diffuse and localized adherence of enteropathogenic *Escherichia coli*. *Infect Immun* 1985; 48:378–383.
6. Nataro JP, Baldini MM, Kaper JB, Black RE, Bravo N, Levine MM. Detection of an adherence factor of enteropathogenic *Escherichia coli* with a DNA probe. *J Infect Dis* 1985;152: 560–565.
7. Vial PA, Robins Browne R, Lior H, et al. Characterization of enteroadherent-aggregative *Escherichia coli*, a putative agent of diarrheal disease. *J Infect Dis* 1988;158:70–79.
8. Mathewson JJ, Oberhelman RA, DuPont HL, Javier de la Cabada F, Garibay EV. Enteroadherent *Escherichia coli* as a cause of diarrhea among children in Mexico. *J Clin Microbiol* 1987; 25:1917–1919.
9. Mathewson JJ, Johnson PC, DuPont HL. Pathogenicity of enteroadherent *Escherichia coli* in adult volunteers. *J Infect Dis* 1986; 154:524–527.
10. Nataro JP, Kaper JB, Robins Browne R, Prado V, Vial P, Levine MM. Patterns of adherence of diarrheagenic *Escherichia coli* to HEp-2 cells. *Pediatr Infect Dis* J 1987;6:829–831.
11. Levine MM. Escherichia coli that cause diarrhea: enterotoxigenic, enteropathogenic, enteroinvasive, enterohemorrhagic, and enteroadherent. *J Infect Dis* 1987;155:377–389.
12. Orskov F, Whittam TS, Cravioto A, Orskov I. Clonal relationships among classic enteropathogenic *Escherichia coli* (EPEC) belong to different O groups. *J Infect Dis* 1990;162:76–81.
13. Weintraub A, Leontein K, Widmalm G, Vial PA, Levine MM, Lindberg AA. Structural studies of the O-antigenic polysaccharide of an enteroaggregative *Escherichia coli* strain. *Eur J Biochem* 1993;213:859–864.
14. Nataro JP, Levine MM, Savarino S, Losonsky G, Guers L, Tacket CO. Volunteer studies of enteroaggregative *Escherichia coli*. *Abstr Gen Meeting Am Soc Microbiol* 1993;B315:82 (abstract).
15. Bhan MK, Raj P, Levine MM, et al. Enteroaggregative *Escherichia coli* associated with persistent diarrhea in a cohort of rural children in India. *J Infect Dis* 1989;159:1061–1064.
16. Bhan MK, Khoshoo V, Sommerfelt H, Raj P, Sazawal S, Srivastava R. Enteroaggregative *Escherichia coli* and *Salmonella* associated with nondysenteric persistent diarrhea. *Pediatr Infect Dis* J 1989;8:499–502.
17. Cravioto A, Tello A, Navarro A, et al. Association of *Escherichia coli* HEp-2 adherence patterns with type and duration of diarrhoea. *Lancet* 1991;337:262–264.
18. Wanke CA, Schorling JB, Barrett LJ, Desouza MA, Guerrant RL. Potential role of adherence traits of *Escherichia coli* in persistent diarrhea in an urban Brazilian slum. *Pediatr Infect Dis* J 1991;10:746–751.
19. Lima AAM, Fang G, Schorling JB, et al. Persistent diarrhea in Northeast Brazil: Etiologies and interactions with malnutrition. *Acta Paediatr Scand* 1992;81 Suppl. 381:39–44.
20. Henry FJ, Udoy AS, Wanke CA, Aziz KMA. Epidemiology of persistent diarrhea and etiologic agents in Mirzapur, Bangladesh. *Acta Paediatr Scand* 1992;81 Suppl. 381:27–31.
21. Scotland SM, Smith HR, Said B, Willshaw GA, Cheasty T, Rowe B. Identification of enteropathogenic *Escherichia coli* isolated in Britain as enteroaggregative or as members of a subclass of attaching-and-effacing *E. coli* not hybridising with the EPEC adherence-factor probe. *J Med Micro Biol* 1991;35:278–283.
22. Baqui AH, Sack RB, Black RE, et al. Enteropathogens associated with acute and persistent diarrhea in Bangladeshi children <5 years of age. *J Infect Dis* 1992;166:792–796.
23. Giron JA, Jones T, Millan Velasco F, et al. Diffuse-adhering *Escherichia coli* (DAEC) as a putative cause of diarrhea in Mayan children in Mexico. *J Infect Dis* 1991;163:507–513.
24. Lanata CF, Black RE, Maúrtua D, et al. Etiologic agents in acute vs persistent diarrhea in children under three years of age in peri-urban Lima, Perú. *Acta Paediatr Scand* 1992;81 Suppl. 381:32–38.
25. Gunzberg ST, Chang BJ, Elliott SJ, Burke V, Gracey M. Diffuse and enteroaggregative patterns of adherence of enteric *Escherichia coli* isolated from aboriginal children from the Kimberley region of western Australia. *J Infect Dis* 1993;167:755–758.
26. Kim K-H, Suh I-S, Kim JM, Kim CW, Cho Y-J. Etiology of childhood diarrhea in Korea. *J Clin Microbiol* 1989;27: 1192–1196.
27. Echeverria P, Taylor DN, Bettelheim KA, et al. HeLa cell-adherent enteropathogenic *Escherichia coli* in children under 1 year of age in Thailand. *J Clin Microbiol* 1987;25:1472–1475.
28. Tzipori S, Montanaro J, Robins-Browne RM, Vial P, Gibson R, Levine MM. Studies with enteroaggregative *Escherichia coli* in

the gnotobiotic piglet gastroenteritis model. *Infect Immun* 1992; 60:5302–5306.

29. Knutton S, Shaw RK, Bhan MK, et al. Ability of enteroaggregative *Escherichia coli* strains to adhere in vitro to human intestinal mucosa. *Infect Immun* 1992;60:2083–2091.

30. Yamamoto T, Endo S, Yokota T, Echeverria P. Characteristics of adherence of enteroaggregative *Escherichia coli* to human and animal mucosa. *Infect Immun* 1991;59:3722–3739.

31. Nataro JP, Deng Y, Maneval DR, German AL, Martin WC, Levine MM. Aggregative adherence fimbriae I of enteroaggregative *Escherichia coli* mediate adherence to HEp-2 cells and hemagglutination of human erythrocytes. *Infect Immun* 1992;60:2297–2304.

32. Nataro JP, Yikang D, Giron JA, Savarino SJ, Kothary MH, Hall R. Aggregative adherence fimbria I expression in enteroaggregative *Escherichia coli* requires two unlinked plasmid regions. *Infect Immun* 1993;61:1126–1131.

33. Donnenberg MS, Giron JA, Nataro JP, Kaper JB. A plasmid-encoded type IV fimbrial gene of enteropathogenic *Escherichia coli* associated with localized adherence. *Mol Microbiol* 1992; 6:3427–3437.

34. Shaw CE, Taylor RK. Vibrio cholerae 0395 tcpA pilin gene sequence and comparison of predicted protein structural features to those of type 4 pilins. *Infect Immun* 1990;58:3042–3049.

35. Savarino SJ, Fasano A, Robertson DC, Levine MM. Enteroaggregative *Escherichia coli* elaborate a heat-stable enterotoxin demonstrable in an in vitro rabbit intestinal model. *J Clin Invest* 1991;87:1450–1455.

36. Savarino SJ, Fasano A, Watson J, et al. Enteroaggregative *Escherichia coli* heat-stable enterotoxin 1 represents another subfamily of *E. coli* heat-stable toxin. *Proc Natl Acad Sci USA* 1993; 90:3093–3097.

37. Baldwin TJ, Knutton S, Sellers L, Hernandez HAM, Aitken A, Williams PH. Enteroaggregative *Escherichia coli* strains secrete a heat-labile toxin antigenically related to *E. coli* hemolysin. *Infect Immun* 1992;60:2092–2095.

38. Eslava C, Villaseca J, Morales R, Navarro A, Cravioto A. Identification of a protein with toxigenic activity produced by enteroaggregative *Escherichia coli*. *Abstr Gen Meet Am Soc Microbiol* 1993;B105:44 (abstract).

39. Vial PA, Mathewson JJ, DuPont HL, Guers L, Levine MM. Comparison of two assay methods for patterns of adherence to HEp-2 cells of *Escherichia coli* from patients with diarrhea. *J Clin Microbiol* 1990;28:882–885.

40. Scaletsky ICA, Milani SR, Trabulsi LR, Travassos LR. Isolation and characterization of the localized adherence factor of enteropathogenic *Escherichia coli*. *Infect Immun* 1988;56:2979–2983.

41. Haider K, Faruque SM, Albert MJ, Nahar S, Neogi PKB, Hossain A. Comparison of a modified adherence assay with existing assay methods for identification of enteroaggregative *Escherichia coli*. *J Clin Microbiol* 1992;30:1614–1616.

42. Mathewson JJ, Johnson PC, DuPont HL, et al. A newly recognized cause of traveler's diarrhea: enteroadherent *Escherichia coli*. *J Infect Dis* 1985;151:471–475.

43. Yamamoto T, Echeverria P, Yokota T. Drug resistance and adherence to human intestines of enteroaggregative *Escherichia coli*. *J Infect Dis* 1992;165:744–749.

44. Baudry B, Savarino SJ, Vial P, Kaper JB, Levine MM. A sensitive and specific DNA probe to identify enteroaggregative *Escherichia coli*, a recently discovered diarrheal pathogen. *J Infect Dis* 1990;161:1249–1251.

45. Fang GD, Lima AM, Martin CC, Barrett LJ, Nataro JP, Guerrant RL. Aggregative HEp-2 cell adherent *Escherichia coli* and Cryptosporidium: important pathogens in hospitalized children with persistent diarrhea in Northeast Brazil. *Abstr 32nd Intersci Conf Antimicrob Agents Chemother* 1992;Abstr. 686:(abstract).

46. Albert MJ, Qadri F, Haque A, Bhuiyan NA. Bacterial clump formation at the surface of liquid culture as a rapid test for identification of enteroaggregative *Escherichia coli*. *J Clin Microbiol* 1993;31:1397–1399.

47. Levine MM, Ferreccio C, Prado V, et al. Epidemiologic studies of *Escherichia coli* diarrheal infections in a low socioeconomic level peri-urban community in Santiago, Chile. *Am J Epidemiol* 1993;(in press)

48. Jallat C, Livrelli V, Darfeuille-Michaud A, Rich C, Joly B. *Escherichia coli* strains involved in diarrhea in France: high prevalence and heterogeneity of diffusely adhering strains. *J Clin Microbiol* 1993;31:2031–2037.

49. Bilge SS, Apostol JM, Jr., Fullner KJ, Moseley SL. Transcriptional organization of the F1845 fimbrial adhesin determinant of *Escherichia coli*. *Mol Microbiol* 1993;7:993–1006.

50. Bilge SS, Clausen CR, Lau W, Moseley SL. Molecular characterization of a fimbrial adhesin, F1845, mediating diffuse adherence of diarrhea-associated *Escherichia coli* to HEp-2 cells. *J Bacteriol* 1989;171:4281–4289.

51. Bilge SS, Apostol JM, Jr., Aldape MA, Moseley SL. mRNA processing independent of RNase III and RNase E in the expression of the F1845 fimbrial adhesin of *Escherichia coli*. *Proc Natl Acad Sci USA* 1993;90:1455–1459.

52. Benz I, Schmidt MA. Cloning and expression of an adhesin (AIDA-I) involved in diffuse adherence of enteropathogenic *Escherichia coli*. *Infect Immun* 1989;57:1506–1511.

53. Benz I, Schmidt MA. Isolation and serologic characterization of AIDA-I, the adhesin mediating the diffuse adherence phenotype of the diarrhea-associated *Escherichia coli* strain 2787 (O126:H27). *Infect Immun* 1992;60:13–18.

54. Benz I, Schmidt MA. AIDA-I, the adhesin involved in diffuse adherence of the diarrhoeagenic *Escherichia coli* strain 2787 (O126:H27), is synthesized via a precursor molecule. *Mol Microbiol* 1992;6:1539–1546.

55. Tacket CO, Moseley SL, Kay B, Losonsky G, Levine MM. Challenge studies in volunteers using *Escherichia coli* strains with diffuse adherence to HEp-2 cells. *J Infect Dis* 1990;162:550–552.

Infections of the Gastrointestinal Tract,
edited by M. J. Blaser, P. D. Smith, J. I. Ravdin,
H. B. Greenberg, and R. L. Guerrant
Published by Raven Press, Ltd., New York, 1995.

CHAPTER 52

Escherichia coli O157:H7 and Other Enterohemorrhagic *Escherichia coli*

Patricia M. Griffin, M.D.

In 1982, the Centers for Disease Control and Prevention (CDC) investigated two outbreaks of severe bloody diarrhea linked to the same fast food restaurant chain; *Escherichia coli* O157:H7, a serotype not then recognized to cause human illness, was isolated from ill persons but not controls (1). That same year, an outbreak of bloody diarrhea occurred in a nursing home in Canada, and *E. coli* O157:H7 was isolated from ill patients (2). These outbreak strains produced toxins active on Vero (green monkey kidney) and HeLa cells (3,4). At the same time, investigators in Canada who were examining stools from children with hemolytic-uremic syndrome (HUS) found that most contained *E. coli* strains that produced a toxin active on Vero cells (5). Two of the eight strains they isolated were serotype O157:H7. These investigators later clearly demonstrated the association between verotoxin-producing *E. coli* and HUS (6).

Further investigation of strains from the U.S. outbreaks demonstrated that those *E. coli* O157:H7 strains produced two toxins, one neutralized by antisera to Shiga toxin produced by *Shigella dysenteriae* type 1, the other not (4,7,8). This finding led to two parallel nomenclatures: verotoxin 1 or Shiga-like toxin (SLT) I for the toxin neutralized by antisera to Shiga toxin, and verotoxin 2 or SLT II for the other toxin. Thus, any *E. coli* that produces moderate or large amounts of either of these two toxins is called a Shiga-like toxin-producing *E. coli* (SLTEC), or a verotoxin-producing *E. coli*. Many other *E. coli,* as well as other bacteria, produce very low levels of a cell-associated toxin neutralized by antisera to Shiga toxin; these are not considered Shiga-like toxin-producing bacteria (9).

The initial studies demonstrating the association between SLTEC and both bloody diarrhea and HUS shed

light on the significance of earlier work that had demonstrated that *E. coli* in the stools of some persons with diarrhea produced a toxin active on Vero cells (10–13). Subsequent studies have led to the recognition of a new class of *E. coli,* the enterohemorrhagic *E. coli* (EHEC). EHEC were originally defined as those serotypes that cause a clinical illness similar to that caused by *E. coli* O157:H7, produce one or more phage-encoded SLTs, possess a 60-MDa virulence plasmid, and produce attaching–effacing lesions in an animal model (14,15).

In this chapter, the terms SLT and SLTEC are generally used even if the original report used the parallel nomenclature. Following convention, the term EHEC is used to refer to those SLTEC that can cause diarrhea or HUS. The term *E. coli* O157 is used only when the H type of some strains was not reported, or some strains were nonmotile; otherwise, the term *E. coli* O157:H7 is used. The abbreviation NM means nonmotile.

MICROBIOLOGY

E. coli O157:H7 is similar to most other *E. coli* in that it ferments lactose. However, unlike 80% to 95% of *E. coli* in human stool, it does not ferment sorbitol rapidly (16) and, unlike 92% to 96% of *E. coli,* does not produce β-glucuronidase (17). It also does not grow well at 44–45.5°C, the usual temperature for detecting *E. coli* in food and water (18,19). *E. coli* O157:H- strains that ferment sorbitol have been described only in Germany; however, they were isolated at different geographic locations in all years from 1988 to 1991 (20,21). Biochemical traits that would aid in screening have not been described for the other SLTEC.

Most *E. coli* O157:H7 strains are susceptible to ampicillin, trimethoprim-sulfamethoxazole, tetracycline, and quinolones, and resistant to erythromycin, metronidazole, and vancomycin (22–24). However, resistant strains have been reported, including one resistant to sulfisoxa-

P. M. Griffin: Foodborne Diseases Epidemiology Section, Foodborne and Diarrheal Diseases Branch, Division of Bacterial and Mycotic Diseases, Centers for Disease Control and Prevention, Atlanta, Georgia 30333.

zole, tetracycline, and streptomycin that caused a large waterborne outbreak (25).

E. coli O157 strains with H types other than H7 have never been shown to produce SLT; however, many non-motile isolates produce SLTs and may be *E. coli* O157:H7 strains that lost their flagellar antigens.

The SLT family consists of SLT I, SLT II, and variants of SLT II (26), some of which are still being described (27). SLT II has 56% nucleotide sequence homology to SLT I (28). The structural genes for SLTs are encoded on bacteriophages; in contrast, those for the Shiga toxin of *S. dysenteriae* type 1 are on the chromosome (8).

SLTs resemble Shiga toxin in structure and function (8). They are composed of a single A subunit and five B subunits (29); the B subunits bind the toxin to cells by interaction with a membrane glycolipid called globotrio-sylceramide (Gb3) (30). The toxin then appears to be en-docytosed from coated pits (31). The A subunit is an *N*-glycosidase enzyme that inactivates the 60S ribosomal subunits and thus blocks peptide elongation (32).

The vast majority of *E. coli* O157:H7 strains produce SLT II with or without SLT I. In a study of 88 sporadic *E. coli* O157:H7 isolates in the United States in 1987, 76% had both SLT I and II sequences, 20% had only SLT II, and 3% had only SLT I (33).

EPIDEMIOLOGY

The epidemiology of *E. coli* O157:H7 and non-O157 SLTEC infection is discussed in this section. For more detailed information on these topics and for specific information on the epidemiology of HUS, see Ref. 34.

Escherichia coli O157:H7

Modes of Transmission

Most information about modes of transmission and other aspects of *E. coli* O157:H7 infection has been derived from outbreak investigations. Table 1 lists outbreaks reported from the United States. Many more U.S. outbreaks have occurred but were incompletely investigated or not reported in the medical literature. Many outbreaks have also occurred in Canada, the United Kingdom, and Japan (29,34–36). Outbreak investigations have demonstrated that *E. coli* O157:H7 can be transmitted by food, water, and direct person-to-person spread.

In the United States, more outbreaks were caused by foods of bovine origin than any other foods. Among the 13 outbreaks reported in the United States between 1982 and 1993 with an identified food source, 7 were linked to ground beef, 2 to roast beef, and 1 to raw milk (Table 1). In addition, an outbreak in Canada was caused by raw milk consumed on a school trip to a dairy (37,38). An outbreak in England was caused by yogurt made from milk that was probably contaminated after pasteurization (39).

Nonbovine foods have also caused outbreaks, though

an original bovine source was suspected for many (Table 1). In the United States, implication of fresh-pressed apple cider in one outbreak (40) and of commercial mayonnaise in another (41) supports laboratory data showing that this organism is acid-tolerant (42). The first outbreak in Great Britain was among persons who prepared new potatoes that had been packed in peat that may have been contaminated with calf manure (43); similarly, the initial patient in an outbreak in the United States probably acquired illness from vegetables fertilized with manure from her cow and calf (44). Unrefrigerated sandwiches probably caused an outbreak in a nursing home in Canada (45); turkey roll, possibly cross-contaminated from raw beef, was suspected in an outbreak in Great Britain (46).

The spread of *E. coli* O157:H7 by water was clearly demonstrated by a large outbreak caused by unchlorinated municipal water; many pipes had burst during a freeze, and proper repair procedures had not been followed (25). Another outbreak was traced to swimming in a contaminated lake (Table 1).

Person-to-person transmission has been the mode of spread in every day care center outbreak (47,48); it caused a second wave of illness in an outbreak in a nursing home in Canada (45) and was the mode of transmission to staff in an outbreak in institutions for the retarded (49).

The modes of transmission for sporadic *E. coli* O157:H7 infections appear to be similar to those for outbreaks. In a study of 25 sporadic cases occurring over 1 year in Seattle, Washington, illness was associated with the eating of rare ground beef, and two patients had drunk raw milk shortly before their illness (50). In a study of 49 cases occurring in Canada during the warmer months, the eating of undercooked meat was associated with illness (51). Another study of 110 sporadic cases in Canada between the months of June and September found that illness was associated with the eating of pink ground beef and attending a picnic or special event (52). Sewage-contaminated water was the suspect source for two adults with *E. coli* O157:H7-associated HUS (53), and raw milk was the likely cause of *E. coli* O157:H7-associated HUS in two children (54). In a study of persons with HUS, most of whom had evidence of SLTEC infection, close contact with a person with diarrhea was the strongest risk factor for illness; the drinking of well water was also linked to illness (55).

Other factors affect the risk of infection. Several studies have reported that the youngest children in day care centers are at greatest risk of illness, as are the oldest nursing home patients (34). One report found increased risk associated with antimicrobial therapy before the onset of illness (45), and another found a trend in this direction (49); previous gastrectomy was a risk factor in one outbreak (45). A nurse caring for a child with HUS was infected by nosocomial person-to-person spread (56), and three cases of suspected laboratory-acquired infection have been reported (57–59). Persons with occupational or other exposure to cattle and ground beef may also be at increased risk (55,59,60).

Frequency of and Location of Isolation

Sporadic cases of *E. coli* O157:H7 infection appear to be more common in Canada than in the United States,

TABLE 1. *Reported outbreaks of* E. coli *O157:H7 infections in the United States, 1982–1993*

Month and year	State	Setting	No. affected	No. hospitalized	No. with HUS or TTP	No. dead	Likely vehicle or mode of spread	Ref.
February 1982	OR	Community	26	19	0	0	Ground beef	1
May 1982	MI	Community	21	14	0	0	Ground beef	1
September 1984	NE	Nursing home	34	14	1	4	Ground beef	86
September 1984	NC	Day care center	36	3	3	0	Person-to-person	47
October 1986	WA	Community	37	17	4	2	Ground beef/ranch dressing	90
June 1987	UT	Custodial institutions	51	8	8	4	Ground beef/person-to-person	49
May 1988	WI	School	61	2	0	0	Roast beef	a
August 1988	MN	Day care center	19	NR	3	0	Person-to-person	48
October 1988	MN	School	54	4	0	0	Precooked ground beef	92
December 1989	MO	Community	243	32	2	4	Municipal water	25
July 1990	ND	Community	65	16	2	0	Roast beef	91
November 1990	MT	School	10	2	1	0	School lunch	a
July 1991	OR	Community	28	7	3	0	Swimming water	281
November 1991	MA	Community	23	7	3	0	Apple cider	40
July 1992	NV	Day care center	57	1	0	0	Person-to person	a
September 1992	ME	Family	4	3	1	1	Vegetable/person-to-person	44
December 1992	OR	Community	8	2	0	0	Raw milk	282[b]
January 1993	WA, ID, NV, CA	Community	732	195	55	4	Ground beef	a
March 1993	OR	Community	48	12	0	0	Mayonnaise-containing dressing and sauces	41[b]
TOTAL			1557	358	86	19		

HUS, hemolytic uremic syndrome; TTP, thrombotic thrombocytopenic purpura; NR, not reported.
[a] Centers for Disease Control and Prevention, *unpublished data.*
[b] W. E. Keene, Oregon Health Division, *personal communication.*

and more common in western than in eastern Canada (34). In the United States, sporadic cases are more frequently reported from northern than southern states, and 9 of the 19 reported U.S. outbreaks occurred in states bordering Canada (Table 1) (34).

Few population-based studies have been performed to determine the incidence of *E. coli* O157:H7 infections. A study in a Seattle health maintenance organization in 1985–1986 in which all stools submitted were cultured for *E. coli* O157:H7 reported an incidence of 8 infections per 100,000 persons per year (50). In the United States, because few clinical laboratories routinely test stool specimens for *E. coli* O157:H7, most infections are not recognized (61,62). In Canada, where many clinical laboratories routinely culture stools for *E. coli* O157:H7, the rates of culture-confirmed infection per 100,000 population in 1989 were 29 for Calgary, 18.5 for Saskatoon, and 4 for Toronto (52).

Several large studies in the United States and Canada have compared the overall isolation rate for *E. coli* O157: H7 with that for other bacterial pathogens (Table 2). Studies from Washington and Minnesota have reported that *E. coli* O157:H7 was isolated more frequently than *Shigella* from routine stool specimens (50,63). In Canada, *E. coli* O157:H7 was the second most frequently isolated bacterial pathogen in two studies (64,65) and ranked third in another (66). Few such studies have been performed in other areas; in studies in England (67), Belgium (68), and Australia (69), the isolation rates for *E. coli* O157 were below those for *Shigella*.

Studies of bloody stool specimens have generally demonstrated high isolation rates for *E. coli* O157:H7. In Canada, isolation rates were 15% to 18% in three studies (16,23,70) and 39% in a study conducted in the warmer months in Alberta (51). In the latter study, the isolation rate for *E. coli* O157:H7 from persons with bloody diarrhea was more than threefold higher than for any other bacterial pathogen. Similarly, preliminary data from a U.S. multicenter study showed that *E. coli* O157:H7 was isolated more frequently from stool specimens with visible blood than was any other pathogen (71). Studies of bloody stools in the United Kingdom have reported widely varying isolation rates of 5% (72), 6% (73), 29% (74,75), and 75% (76).

E. coli O157:H7 has been isolated in many other countries, including Africa, Argentina, Chile, China, Czechoslovakia, France, Germany, India, Ireland, Italy, and Japan (34,77–81,88), but its frequency in comparison with other pathogens is not well studied. In addition, *E. coli* O157:NM caused a day care center outbreak in Israel (82) and an epidemic in South Africa and Swaziland (83).

Seasonality

Sporadic cases of *E. coli* O157:H7 peak during the warm months in the United States (59), Canada (64), the United Kingdom (35), and Japan (36). Of the 19 outbreaks reported in the United States between 1982 and 1993, two occurred from January to March, 3 from April to June,

TABLE 2. *Rank order of isolation of pathogens from stools submitted to microbiology laboratories in the United States and Canada, 1984–1991*[a]

Location	Year study began	Campylobacter	Salmonella	E. coli O157:H7	Shigella	Ref.
United States						
Washington	1985	1st	2nd	3rd	4th	50
Minnesota	1987	1st	2nd	3rd	4th	63
Ten medical centers	1990	1st	2nd	4th	3rd	71
Canada						
Alberta	1984	3rd	1st	2nd	4th	64
British Columbia	1984	1st	3rd	2nd	4th	65
Ontario	1986	1st	2nd	3rd	4th	66

[a] Only studies that analyzed at least 1000 specimens are included.

seven from July to September, and seven from October to December (Table 1).

Infectious Dose

Because studies of human ingestion of the organism have not been performed, the infectious dose for *E. coli* O157:H7 is not known. Person-to-person spread in outbreaks provided the initial evidence that *E. coli* O157:H7 has a low infectious dose (47,84). Transmission by water, which would tend to dilute organisms and not permit growth, substantiates these findings.

Carriage

Young children carry *E. coli* O157:H7 longer after resolution of symptoms than do older children and adults. In one study, 9 (53%) of 17 infected children ≤4 years old had positive stool cultures more than 3 weeks after onset of symptoms, compared with only 2 (8%) of 25 older children and adults ($p = 0.003$) (64). In a study of 24 children under 5 years old in day care center outbreaks, the median duration of shedding after onset of symptoms was 17 days, and 38% shed *E. coli* O157:H7 for over 20 days (48). The determinants of prolonged carriage other than age are unknown. No correlation was found with severity of illness in one study (48). In one cohort, the longest carriage (62 days) occurred in a child who received amoxicillin 26 days after onset of illness (48); in another, the longest carriage (71 days) occurred in a child who never had symptoms and had not received an antimicrobial agent (C. M. Whitman, *personal communication*). Intermittent shedding has also been reported (48). By comparison, the duration of shedding of *E. coli* O157:H7 is much shorter than that for *Salmonella* in both children and adults (85).

Although asymptomatic infection (2,37,48,64,86) and carriage occur, *E. coli* O157:H7 is clearly not part of normal human bowel flora. *E. coli* O157:H7 was not isolated from stool specimens from 530 healthy controls in 7 countries (6,15,20,73,81,87–90) (see Table 3).

Incubation Period

Outbreak investigations have determined that the usual incubation period for *E. coli* O157:H7 infections is 3 or 4 days (1,46,90,91). However, longer incubation periods of 5–8 days are not uncommon (37,45,49,86,92). Incubation periods for culture-positive cases as short as 1 or 2 days (37,46,90) have been reported.

Isolations from Food and Water

Investigations of human illnesses have led to isolation of *E. coli* O157:H7 from implicated ground beef (61,93,94), raw milk (54,95), and veal chops (96). Isolation rates of *E. coli* O157:H7 from ground beef samples from stores and restaurants in North America have varied from none (70,97) to 1.3% (98), 2.4% (99), 2.8% (100), and 3.7% (101). In one study, 10% of bulk raw milk samples contained *E. coli* O157:H7 (100). *E. coli* O157:H7 has also been isolated from foods that have not been linked to human illness, including lamb, chicken, turkey, pork, beef, venison, and veal kidneys (18,34,101). It has also been isolated from untreated surface water (102).

Animal Reservoir

Although the first reported isolation of *E. coli* O157:H7 from an animal was from a calf in Argentina with coli bacillosis in 1977 (103) and an isolate was obtained from a calf in Spain with diarrhea (104), *E. coli* O157:H7 has since been isolated from many healthy cattle and has not been shown to be a pathogen for cattle (105). It was isolated from calves on a farm where ill kindergarten children drank raw milk (37,38), from a heifer on a farm where a child with *E. coli* O157:H7-associated HUS drank raw milk (54,95), and from cattle manure used to fertilize vegetables eaten by the initial patient in an outbreak (44). CDC culture surveys on U.S. dairy farms (some linked to human illnesses), a stockyard, and a packing house in two northern states showed an overall fecal isolation rate for *E. coli* O157 of 0.15% from cows and 2.8% from heifers and calves (95). A U.S. Department of Agriculture study of fecal swabs from calves found no *E. coli* O157 (106). However, another study found similar proportions of *E. coli* O157:H7-positive dairy calves in all U.S. regions, and the investigators estimated that the proportion of dairy herds that have one or more carriers of *E. coli* O157:H7 is much higher than 1.8% (107). In Ontario, Canada, a survey of fecal samples from dairy cows and calves found no *E. coli* O157:H7 (108). However, in an Ontario slaughter plant, isolation rates of 0, 0.5%, and 1.5% were found among fecal samples from veal calves, dairy cows, and beef cattle, respectively (109). *E. coli* O157 has also been isolated from cattle in the United Kingdom (76,110) and from bulls in Germany (111). The paradox that *E. coli* O157:H7 is much more easily isolated from the feces of young animals than from the older animals that supply ground beef has not been explained.

It is not known whether dairy or beef cattle are more likely to carry *E. coli* O157:H7. Most fecal culture surveys have targeted dairy farms for various reasons: some dairy farms have supplied implicated raw milk; meat from dairy cattle can more easily be traced to its origin; and implicated ground beef often contains mostly lean meat, and meat from dairy cows is usually leaner than that from beef cattle.

Other Shiga-like Toxin-Producing *E. coli*

Frequency of Isolation

Over 100 non-O157 SLTEC serotypes have been isolated from humans, mostly from persons with HUS (H. Lior, *personal communication*). Some of those most frequently isolated from persons with diarrhea are O26:H11, O103:H2, O111:NM, and O113:H21 (34). Serotypes O26:H11 and O111:NM are also among the most common serotypes of classic enteropathogenic *E. coli* (EPEC) (14,112). However, only a small proportion of classic EPEC O111 and O26 strains produce SLT (113,114).

Because isolation of non-O157 SLTEC requires techniques not generally available in clinical laboratories, these organisms are rarely sought or detected in routine practice (115). In addition, few studies have sought virulence markers, which may help determine whether the non-O157 SLTEC isolated are pathogens (115). The paucity of reported outbreaks due to non-O157 SLTEC (116,117) suggests that, although the absence of a biochemical marker (such as slow sorbitol fermentation for *E. coli* O157:H7) likely leads to underrecognition, no single member of this group or the group as a whole is of nearly the public health importance as *E. coli* O157:H7 in North America at this time. The situation in other countries is less clear.

After the reports in the 1970s describing verotoxins (10,11), but before verotoxin-producing organisms were linked to human illness, investigators in the United Kingdom and India detected verotoxin-producing *E. coli* in the stools of children with diarrhea (12,13). The three isolates detected in the U.K. study were serotype O26 and were from children with bloody diarrhea (12).

In Alberta, Canada, in a 2-year study of stools from 5415 persons submitted to microbiology laboratories, 0.7% (36 stools) contained non-O157 SLTEC, compared with 2.5% with *E. coli* O157:H7 and 0.5% with *Shigella* (64). *E. coli* O26:H11 was the most frequently isolated non-O157 SLTEC, found in specimens from 11 persons. In British Columbia, Canada, 7 (0.07%) of 9449 stool specimens collected over a 16-month period contained non-O157 SLTEC, compared with 60 (0.6%) with *E. coli* O157. Five of the non-O157 isolates were O26 (118).

In Seattle, Washington, in a one-year prospective study of 445 children's stools submitted to a microbiology laboratory, non-O157 SLTEC were isolated from 5 (1.1%), compared with 2.9% for *E. coli* O157:H7 and 0.2% for *Shigella* (119). All non-O157 strains induced actin aggregation in HeLa cells. Two of the strains were serogroup O26. Only one of the five children with non-O157 SLTEC had bloody diarrhea, four had nonbloody diarrhea, and one of these also had mesenteric adenitis.

Studies in other areas have confirmed that non-O157 SLTEC are ubiquitous. In studies in Korea (89), Thailand (120), Chile (15), Argentina (87), and Switzerland (121), the isolation rate of non-O157 SLTEC from persons with diarrhea ranged from 0.6% to 2.3%. Other reports, including studies from Korea (122,123) and the United Kingdom (73), found none, whereas a high isolation rate of 7% was reported from Germany (20) (Table 3). Findings from a U.K group suggested that non-O157 SLTEC could play an important role in community-acquired diarrhea: 29 (18%) of 162 culture-negative stool samples from persons with diarrhea exhibited cytotoxicity neutralized by SLT II, and 9 (6%) showed cytotoxity neutralized by SLT I; none of 25 samples from healthy adults was cytotoxic (124).

Isolations from Food

Non-O157 SLTEC are more readily isolated from food than is *E. coli* O157:H7. In a Canadian study in which no *E. coli* O157:H7 was isolated, non-O157 SLTEC were isolated from 10% of ground beef, 4% of pork, and no chicken samples (97). In another Canadian study, slightly more non-O157 SLTEC strains than O157:H7 were isolated from ground beef (99). In a Thai study in which no *E. coli* O157:H7 was isolated, non-O157 SLTEC were isolated from 9% of beef samples, 1% of chicken samples, and 1% of pork samples (125). In a U.K. study in which no *E. coli* O157:H7 was isolated, non-O157 SLTEC were isolated from 11% of retail pork samples but not from retail chickens (126).

Animal Reservoir

Non-O157 SLTEC are much more readily isolated from animals than is *E. coli* O157:H7 (reviewed in Ref. 34). For example, in a U.S. study, fecal specimens from 19% of dairy heifers and calves and 8% of cows grew non-O157 SLTEC, compared with *E. coli* O157:H7 rates of 2.3% and 0.4%, respectively, from the same populations (34,95). In a Canadian study on 100 dairy farms, non-O157 SLTEC were isolated from 9% of calves and 3% of cows; most were serotypes that have not been isolated from humans, and *E. coli* O157:H7 was not isolated (108). The proportion of cattle on each farm that carried non-O157 SLTEC varied from none to over 50%. Other investigators have

TABLE 3. *Major prospective studies of the association between HUS and infection with Shiga-like toxin-producing E. coli (SLTEC) in the Americas and Europe, ordered by starting date*

Location	Years	Syndrome[a]	Patients No.	Patients ( )[b]	E. coli O157[c] No.	E. coli O157[c] %	Other SLTEC No.	Other SLTEC %	Total No.	Total %	Antibody to O157 LPS No.	Antibody to O157 LPS %	Total with evidence of SLTEC[d] No.	Total with evidence of SLTEC[d] %	Comments	Ref.
Canada	1980–83	HUS	40[e]		3	8	9	23	12	30	ND		30	75	17 had *Campylobacter* enteritis	6
		Controls	40		0	0	0	0	0	0			0	0		
U.K.	1983–85	HUS	66	(59)	15	23	4	6	19	29	ND		22	33		283
U.S.	1985–87	HUS	52[e]		33	63	ND[f]		33	63	ND		33	63	Four more patients were contacts of other children with HUS from whom *E. coli* O157:H7 was isolated	215
U.K.	1985–88	HUS	196	(185)	38	19	15	8	52	27	ND		58	30	One patient had *E. coli* O157:H7 and another SLTEC cultured	73
		Bloody diarrhea	50	(48)	3	6	0	0	3	6			4	8		
		Nonbloody diarrhea	62	(54)	1	2	0	0	1	2			3	5		
		Healthy	51	(46)	0	0	2	4	2	1			2	4		
Argentina	1986–88	HUS	51		1	2	0	0	1	2	ND		48	94		87
		Diarrhea	44		2	5	1	2	3	7			14	32		
		Controls	25		0	0	0	0	0	0			4	16		
Canada	1986–88	HUS	169		87	51	ND		87	51	ND		87	51		209
Germany	1986–89	HUS	22[e]		5	23	3	14	8	36	20	91	22	100	These patients were included in Ref. 216 The only test performed was measurement of antibody to O157 LPS. Some controls had diarrhea due to pathogens other than *E. coli*; others did not have diarrhea; one had pneumococcal-associated HUS	248
		Controls	32		ND		ND		ND		0	0	0	0		

Region	Years	Category	No.[b]											Comments	Ref.
Central Europe	1986–91	HUS	147	11	7	8	5	19	13	108	73	126	86	Includes 2 patients for whom SLTEC were isolated only from siblings. Includes patients in Ref. 248	216
Argentina	1988	HUS[b]	20	4	20	0	0	4	20	ND		9	45		284
Chile	1988–89	HUS	20[e]	3	10	3	10	6	30	ND		6	30		
		Controls	38	0	0	2	5	2	5			2	5		88
Italy	1988–91	HUS	49	1	2	1	2	2	4	25	51	37	76	Four had antibodies to O26 LPS, and 1 to O111 LPS. Nine of 14 patients without diarrhea had evidence of SLTEC infection.	81
Germany	1988–91	Controls	39	0	0	1	3	1	3	1	3	1	3		
		HUS	104[e]	26	25	7	7	33	32	ND		33	32	Fourteen (54%) O157 strains were nonmotile, sorbitol positive at 24 hr, and b-glucuronidase positive	20, 21
		Diarrhea	668	18	3	44	7	62	9			62	9	Patients were hospitalized. Three (17%) O157 strains were nonmotile, sorbitol positive at 24 hr, and b-glucuronidase positive	
Canada	1990	Controls	184	0	0	1	0.5	1	0.5	ND		1	0.5		
		HUS	34[e] (30)	26	76	2	6	28	82	ND		30	88	Includes one patient with E. coli O157:H7 isolated only from a sibling with HUS	217

[a] Those listed simply as controls had neither diarrhea nor HUS except if noted otherwise in comments.

[b] Number in parentheses indicates number of patients whose specimens had coliform growth.

[c] All strains were H7 except for the following: in ref. 283, one was nonmotile; in ref. 73, 3 were H−; in ref. 248, all were H−; in ref. 284, 3 were H7 and 1 was NM; in ref. 88, all were NM; in ref. 216, 6 were H− and for 2 others the H was not determined.

[d] By culture, fecal toxin, or serological testing.

[e] All had a prodrome of diarrhea, in some studies by definition, in others without preselection.

[f] ND, not done.

confirmed that non-O157 SLTEC are frequently shed in the feces of healthy calves (105,127).

Role in Disease

Several lines of evidence suggest that many of the non-O157 SLTEC are not human pathogens:

1. Some patients from whom non-O157 SLTEC are isolated also have evidence of *E. coli* O157:H7 infection, suggesting that in some patients isolation of a non-O157 SLTEC may be a marker for exposure to *E. coli* O157:H7 acquired from the same source (73,128). In one study, seven patients with non-O157 SLTEC also had *E. coli* O157:H7 in their stools (64). In other studies, HUS patients from whom non-O157 SLTEC were isolated had antibodies to O157 lipopolysaccharide (LPS) (81,129).
2. In a few studies the proportion of controls from whom non-O157 SLTEC were isolated was similar to that for HUS patients (20,81).
3. The proportion of healthy persons from whose stools non-O157 SLTEC can be isolated is similar to that reported above for persons with diarrhea. Summarizing data from healthy controls in seven countries (Table 3), non-O157 SLTEC were isolated from 1% of 530 stool specimens (6,15,20,73,81,87–89).
4. One group reported that non-O157 SLTEC isolated from humans were more likely to be *eae*-positive and CVD419-positive than those from animals, suggesting that many of the non-O157 SLTEC isolated from animals are not human pathogens (130). (See next section for information about *eae*.) In another study, only about two thirds of 38 non-O157, non-O126 SLTEC strains of human origin hybridized with the CVD419 probe, and only about one third hybridized with the *eae* probe (115).
5. Although non-O157 SLTEC are isolated more frequently from the feces of cattle (34,95) and from foods (97,99,125) than is *E. coli* O157:H7, making the opportunities for exposure greater than for O157, they cause fewer human illnesses.

Further studies are needed to determine which non-O157 SLTEC are human pathogens.

PATHOGENESIS AND IMMUNITY

EHEC have two well-recognized virulence attributes: production of one or more SLTs, and attaching and effacing adherence. In addition, all isolates of *E. coli* O157:H7 harbor a plasmid of about 60 MDa. Other factors may also confer virulence, and some SLTEC strains may possess virulence factors not present in others (131,132). That host factors must play a role is clear since *E. coli* O157:H7 is not pathogenic for cattle. In addition, any model of pathogenesis must take into account that many *E. coli* O157:H7 strains that cause human illness do not produce SLT I.

Attachment

Attachment to mucosal surfaces prevents loss of bacteria into the environment (133) and promotes the delivery of toxins to eukaryotic cell surfaces in a concentrated manner (32,134).

The 60-MDa plasmid of *E. coli* O157:H7 contains DNA sequences common to plasmids present in many other serotypes of SLTEC (15). This plasmid and a fimbrial adhesin are probably involved in adherence (135), but reports of their exact roles are conflicting (136–140). A DNA probe (CVD419) can detect this plasmid in *E. coli* O157:H7 and other SLTEC (15), but some SLTEC with a 60-MDa plasmid do not react with the probe, demonstrating that the plasmid is heterogeneous (130).

The type of adherence demonstrated by SLTEC to animal and tissue culture cells is referred to as "attaching and effacing." This is characterized by intimate adherence to the enterocyte and dissolution of the brush border at the site of attachment (141). Within the enterocyte, filamentous actin accumulates at the site of attachment and the enterocyte membrane may cup the bacteria, forming a pedestal-like structure that can be detected by fluorescent actin staining (142). Although adherence of EHEC to the human gastrointestinal mucosa has not been demonstrated, attaching and effacing lesions have been demonstrated in the gut of infants with diarrhea due to EPEC, which have a similar adherence mechanism (143).

The *eaeA* gene of *E. coli* O157:H7, which is homologous to the *eaeA* gene of EPEC, is necessary (144,145) but not sufficient (135,146) for the production of attaching and effacing lesions. The gene product is a 97-kDa protein, provisionally known as intimin$_{O157}$ (146); its role as an adhesin is supported by its predicted amino acid sequence having homology with the invasin protein of *Yersinia* (144), which is a known adhesin (147). In addition, antisera against a 94-kDa outer membrane protein (which is not a product of the *eaeA* gene) abolish attaching and effacing binding of *E. coli* O157:H7 to human embryonic lung (HEL) cells (135,146,148).

Shiga-like Toxins

The SLTs and Shiga toxin are cytotoxic for some cell lines; they are enterotoxic, mediating fluid accumulation in ligated ileal loops, and paralytic-lethal when injected intravenously in mice and rabbits (8).

Role of Shiga-like Toxin in Colonic Disease

The role of SLT in diarrheal illness is unknown; it may act both locally and systemically on the gut mucosa. Evidence suggesting that SLT has a role in the gut manifestations of EHEC infection includes the following:

1. Free SLT can be identified in the stools of persons with SLTEC infection (149).
2. Shiga toxin is cytotoxic to cultured epithelial cells from human colon and ileum (150).

3. Both Shiga toxin and toxin extracted from a strain that produces both SLT I and SLT II cause nonbloody fluid accumulation when applied directly to rabbit ileal loops, probably by destroying mature columnar absorptive epithelial cells (7,151).

4. Parenteral injection of SLT I or II in rabbits results in nonbloody diarrhea and lesions in the cecum resembling those of humans infected with *E. coli* O157:H7 (152,153). Parenteral injection of SLT II in mice results in bloody diarrhea and colonic lesions characterized by sloughing of surface and crypt epithelial cells (154).

5. Studies of *Shigella dysenteriae* type 1 infection suggest that Shiga toxin is not necessary for colonic disease but exacerbates it by damaging the microvasculature of the large intestine, resulting in edema, local ischemia, and an influx of inflammatory cells into the mucosa. In one study, monkeys fed a tox⁻ *S. dysenteriae* type 1 strain had diarrhea, bloody in some, that was indistinguishable from that seen with the parent strain; the tox⁻ strain also produced fever and dysentery in human volunteers, but the disease was milder than with the parent strain (155). In another study using genetically engineered tox⁻ mutants of *S. dysenteriae* 1 in monkeys, the presence of Shiga toxin was correlated with blood in the stools and destruction of capillary vessels in the colonic mucosa (156). Interpretation of these data for *E. coli* O157:H7 must take into account the fact that *S. dysenteriae* type 1, unlike *E. coli* O157:H7, is locally invasive, i.e., capable of epithelial penetration (155), and does not produce SLT II.

6. The histological pattern of human colonic injury in *E. coli* O157:H7 infection caused by strains producing SLT II with or without SLT I is similar to that of *Clostridium difficile* colitis, which is caused by a locally acting toxin (157). This similarity suggests that SLT II plays a role in colonic injury.

Tzipori and colleagues (138) found that monkeys fed a mutant strain of *E. coli* O157 that did not produce SLT developed diarrhea, and diarrhea was correlated with the strain's ability to produce attaching and effacing lesions. Overall the data suggest that SLT is not necessary for but can worsen the colonic disease due to SLTEC.

Role of Shiga-like Toxin in Hemolytic-Uremic Syndrome

Colonic vascular damage by SLT may provide access for SLT, LPS, and other inflammatory mediators to the circulation, thus initiating HUS. This possibility is supported by the finding that among persons with *E. coli* O157:H7 infection, those with bloody diarrhea are more likely than those with nonbloody stools to develop HUS (45). Bacterial factors such as LPS and Shiga toxin may elicit production of interleukin-1 (IL-1) and tumor necrosis factor (TNF) from macrophages (158,159). IL-1β, TNF-α, and LPS may then increase the sensitivity of endothelial cells to Shiga toxin by increasing expression of Gb3 on the cell surface (159–161). Shiga toxin then inhib-

its protein synthesis (8), and the endothelial cells may then detach, exposing platelets to the subendothelium, and initiating coagulation (159).

It is not known whether findings using Shiga toxin or SLT I would apply to SLT II. This is important because data on humans suggest that SLT II is a more important virulence factor than SLT I for progression of *E. coli* O157:H7 infection to HUS (33,35,162), and animal models support this (see below). Neither SLT I nor SLT II has been detected in human serum. These concerns stated, several lines of evidence suggest that SLT is the major virulence factor responsible for HUS caused by SLTEC:

1. The only other enteric pathogen well recognized to cause HUS is *Shigella dysenteriae* type 1, a pathogen encountered in areas with poor hygiene (163). This is also the only *Shigella* species that produces Shiga toxin. SLT I is antigenically identical to Shiga toxin and SLT II has 56% nucleotide sequence homology with it (28).

2. Many different SLT-producing *E. coli* have been isolated from patients with postdiarrheal HUS (29), suggesting that the common pathogenic mechanism is production of SLT.

3. Glomerular capillary endothelial cell injury is the most consistent renal finding in patients with HUS (164), and histopathological studies of patients with HUS have demonstrated microvascular angiopathy (165). Shiga toxin and SLT II are toxic for human endothelial cells *in vitro* (166,167).

4. Rabbits injected with SLT I develop thrombotic microvascular angiopathy similar to that seen in humans with HUS (although HUS is not produced in rabbits) (153).

5. Gb3, the receptor for SLT (30), is present in human renal tissue (168).

Immunity

It is not known whether circulating antibody to O157 LPS or to SLT may decrease the likelihood of infection or severe illness. The increased rate of infection and complications in children under 5 years old and the elderly (34) suggests some role for immunity. However, protective immunity has not been demonstrated in humans, and children without evident immunological abnormalities have been infected twice. Siegler and colleagues described a previously healthy child who developed postdiarrheal HUS twice within 18 months (169). During the first episode, serological studies demonstrated a greater than fourfold rise in antibody titer to O157 LPS, and polymerase chain reaction (PCR) assay demonstrated SLT I and II gene sequences in the stool; *E. coli* O157:H7 was isolated from the stool during the second episode. An older child had bloody diarrhea due to *E. coli* O157:H7 twice in 4 years; the first episode was complicated by HUS (170).

Animal Models

No animal model has reproduced the typical human colonic disease that progresses to HUS. However, animal models reproduce some features and provide a means to study putative virulence factors and to compare strains.

One type of model involves oral administration of the pathogen, which usually results in diarrhea. One group of investigators that inoculated infant rabbits orally with *E. coli* O157:H7 reported nonbloody diarrhea and intestinal lesions, most severe in the cecum and appendix; no lesions were observed in the kidneys (171). Another group that inoculated infant rabbits orally with *E. coli* O157:H7 demonstrated lesions mainly in the mid- and distal colon, which were duplicated by intragastric administration of SLT (172). *E. coli* O157:H7 inoculated orally into gnotobiotic piglets produced nonbloody diarrhea with abundant red blood cells in the lumen, and intestinal lesions, most severe in the distal ileum and cecum; renal lesions were minimal (173). Mice fed a plasmid-cured *E. coli* O157:H7 strain did not develop colonic lesions but died from renal cortical tubular necrosis (139).

Injection of SLT also produces some typical features of human infection along with features not seen in humans. Mice injected intraperitoneally with SLT II developed bloody diarrhea, with sloughing of surface and crypt colonic cells and vacuolization of renal tubular cells (154). SLT II injected into rabbits by continuous intraperitoneal infusion caused diarrhea with striking submucosal edema and hemorrhage in the cecum and proximal colon, similar to the findings in infected humans (152). Areas of hemorrhage and necrosis were observed in the central nervous system, but only minimal lesions developed in the kidneys, and glomeruli were normal (152). SLT I injected intravenously into rabbits produced nonbloody diarrhea with microvascular angiopathy, edema, and hemorrhage in the cecum, brain, and spinal cord; the kidneys were normal (153). In all of these models, lower extremity paresis was also observed.

The lack of glomerular damage, the hallmark of HUS (164), in animal models is likely due at least in part to the absence of the SLT receptor, Gb3. Its absence in rabbit kidneys has been documented (174).

Data on animals support human studies suggesting that SLT II is a more important virulence factor than SLT I. Streptomycin-treated mice fed *E. coli* K12 strains containing only SLT II genes died with acute renal tubular necrosis, but those fed a strain containing only SLT I genes did not die (175). Only strains that produced high levels of SLT II killed mice. Streptomycin-treated mice fed an *E. coli* strain that produced both SLT I and II were protected from renal tubular necrosis by passive transfer of antibodies to SLT II but not SLT I (175). The enhanced lethality of SLT II compared with SLT I in streptomycin-treated mice was also observed following injection of toxins (176). In another model, gnotobiotic piglets inoculated with *E. coli* O157:H7 strains that produced only SLT II or both SLT I and SLT II developed brain lesions, and loss of ability to produce SLT II resulted in loss of ability to cause brain lesions (177).

Edema disease of pigs, which is caused by SLTEC, predominantly serogroups O138, O139, and O141, serves as a natural model for human illness (178,179). Edema disease affect pigs shortly after weaning; clinical signs include edema of the eyelids, ataxia, and convulsions;

diarrhea may occur but is not characteristic (178). The histological lesion is microvascular angiopathy affecting many organs, most often the brain and intestine (178). A colonization factor and SLT IIv, which is neutralized by antiserum against SLT II, are the major virulence factors (178,180). The clinical signs and typical lesions can be reproduced by intravenous injection of SLT IIv (181).

Animal models suggest that LPS may play an important role in pathogenesis. In rabbits and mice, the effects of SLT II can be enhanced or inhibited by LPS, depending on the timing of its administration (182). The fact that most patients with severe illness develop an antibody response to the O157 LPS suggests that LPS is hematogenously disseminated from the gut (183).

Additional information on animal studies, including those on naturally occurring non-O157 SLTEC infection in calves (184,185) and on animal models using non-O157 SLTEC, can be found in other sources (172,186,187).

Human Gut Endoscopic and Histological Findings

By colonoscopy, the mucosa of patients with *E. coli* O157:H7 infection typically shows edema, erythema, and superficial ulceration, usually in a patchy distribution. Dusky-appearing mucosa or bleeding may also be observed. A gradient of severity of findings is typical, with the most severe disease in the cecum and right colon (157). Typical findings of pseudomembranous colitis are uncommon but have been reported (188).

Persons with bloody diarrhea due to *E. coli* O157:H7 may have colonic biopsy specimens that show only an ischemic pattern of injury, only an infectious pattern, both, or neither (157). In a series of patients with illness severe enough to warrant colonoscopy, most patients had hemorrhage and edema in the colonic lamina propria. Focal necrosis with hemorrhage and acute inflammation in the superficial mucosa but preservation of the deep crypts, similar to the findings in acute ischemic colitis (Fig. 1A), was common. Specimens from some patients had fibrin/platelet thrombi within mucosal capillaries (Fig. 1B), and some had deep apoptosis of colonic crypts. Neutrophilic infiltration of the lamina propria and crypts, similar to the findings in infectious colitis (Fig. 1C), was also common. Poorly formed pseudomembranes were observed (Fig. 1D). Nonspecific changes and occasional normal specimens have also been described; because the disease is often patchy, obtaining more than one biopsy specimen increases the likelihood of identifying an abnormality (157). In addition, because the gradient of injury is from right to left colon, rectal biopsy specimens are least likely to demonstrate abnormalities (157).

CLINICAL ILLNESS

E. coli O157:H7 causes nonbloody diarrhea, bloody diarrhea (hemorrhagic colitis), HUS, thrombotic thrombocytopenic purpura (TTP), and death (189). In reported U.S. outbreaks, 23% of affected persons were hospitalized, 6% developed HUS or TTP, and 1% died (Table

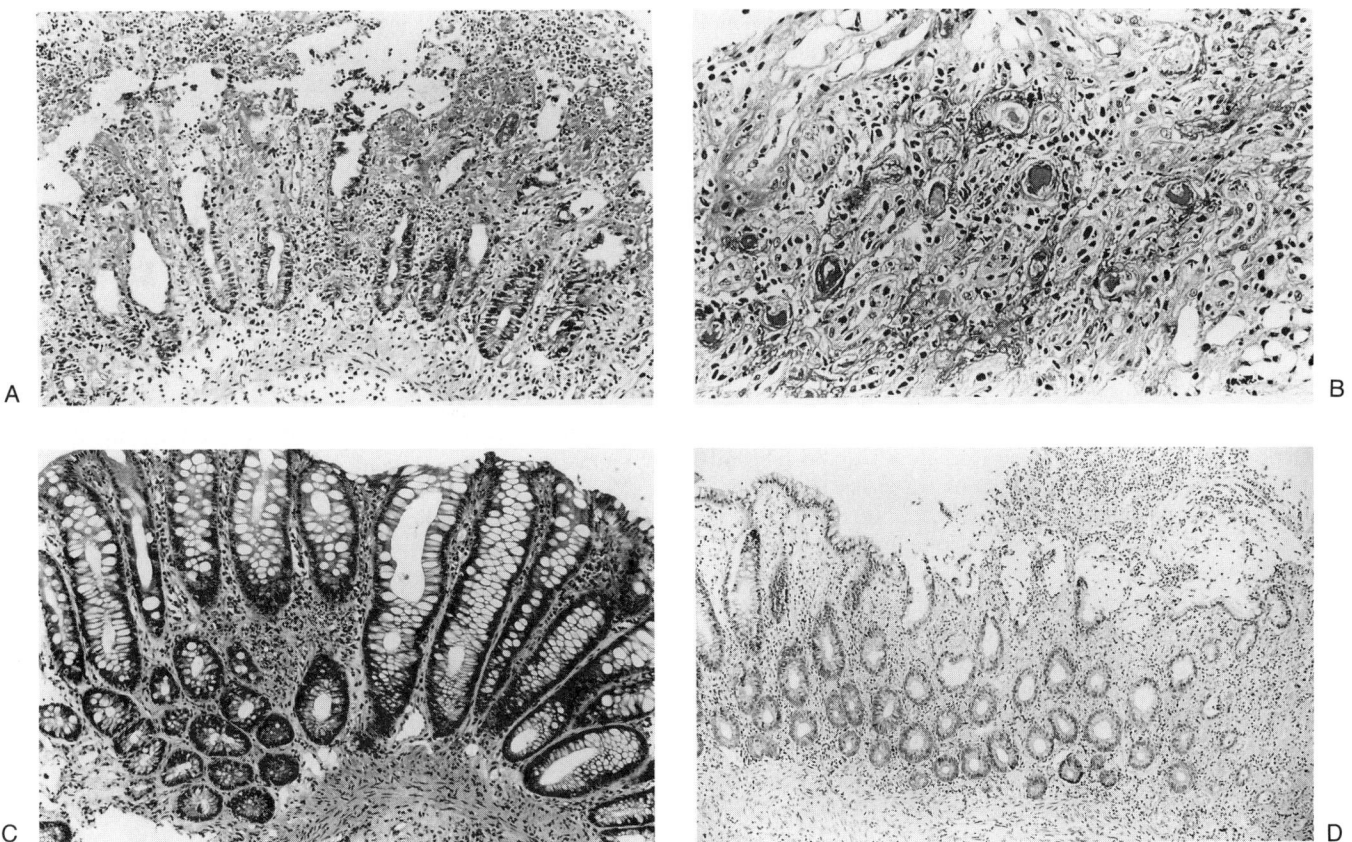

FIG. 1. Endoscopic mucosal biopsies from patients with *E. coli* O157:H7 infection. **A:** The ischemic pattern of injury with superficial necrosis, mucosal hemorrhage, an overlying pseudomembrane, and relative preservation of deep crypts. **B:** Small fibrin-platelet thrombi in mucosal capillaries. **C:** The infectious pattern of injury with an area of focal infiltration of the lamina propria by neutrophils. **D:** An inflammatory pseudomembrane. (From ref. 157, with permission.)

1). Some of the other SLTEC appear to have a similar spectrum of illness.

Diarrhea and Manifestations Other Than Hemolytic Uremic Syndrome

E. coli *O157:H7*

Illness with *E. coli* O157:H7 typically begins with nonbloody diarrhea. In one fourth to three quarters of patients, the diarrhea remains nonbloody and the illness is mild (34). However, in most cases that come to medical attention, the diarrhea becomes bloody on the second or third day of illness. About half of patients have vomiting; fever occurs in fewer than one third and is more common in those with severe illness. The illness typically resolves in about a week with no obvious sequelae, although long-term follow-up of infected persons has not been reported. *E. coli* O157:H7 has also been isolated from some persons with chronic diarrhea, but whether it caused the chronic diarrhea was not known (190,191).

Patients with *E. coli* O157:H7 infection have received mistaken diagnoses of appendicitis, intussusception, primary inflammatory bowel disease, and ischemic colitis, and unnecessary surgical procedures have been performed (34,188). Evidence of right-sided colonic inflammation by barium enema (49,86,192) or colonoscopy with histological changes suggesting ischemia and/or infectious injury (157) in a patient with a compatible clinical illness should strongly suggest *E. coli* O157:H7 infection. Without stool cultures, *E. coli* O157:H7 infection may be especially difficult to differentiate from ischemic colitis or pseudomembranous colitis in elderly patients (86). The finding of other persons with similar illness that suggests a common exposure, and the more common right- than left-sided involvement in *E. coli* O157:H7 infection, may provide clues.

As more cases of *E. coli* O157:H7 infection are recognized, many of the complications of HUS that have been long recognized may be observed in some patients whose infection has not progressed to HUS. These include bowel perforation, bowel necrosis, toxic megacolon, gastrointestinal tract stricture, myocardial dysfunction, pulmonary edema, pancreatitis, hepatitis, and neurological abnormalities (193,194). Intussusception (195), appendicitis (190), and rectal prolapse (P.I. Tarr, *personal communi-*

cation) have been reported in patients with *E. coli* O157:H7 infection without HUS. Inflammation of the small bowel, predominantly the terminal ileum, in addition to the colon has been described in a child with *E. coli* O157:H7 infection without HUS (196). Anal abnormalities have been described in children with *E. coli* O157:H7-associated HUS (197).

Extraintestinal isolations of *E. coli* O157:H7 have only been reported from persons who had diarrhea. These include one isolate from the glans penis (198), two urine isolates (198,199), and one blood isolate obtained 2 days before death (200).

Non-O157 Shiga-like Toxin-Producing E. coli

Non-O157 SLTEC have been isolated from both bloody and nonbloody diarrhea, although as a group they appear less likely to cause bloody diarrhea than *E. coli* O157:H7 (64,73,119). It is possible that some non-O157 SLTEC tend to produce bloody diarrhea, others produce nonbloody diarrhea, and others are not human pathogens. Complications possibly due to non-O157 SLTEC have been reported. *E. coli* O145, which may have produced SLT, was isolated from a child with bloody diarrhea and radiographic evidence of small bowel obstruction; at surgery, the distal ileum was severely inflamed, with a thickened wall causing near-total obstruction (201). SLT-producing *E. coli* O113:H21 and *E. coli* O111 involved other parts of the gut in addition to the colon in two children with HUS (165). *E. coli* O153:H2 containing genes for SLT I but not SLT II was isolated from the stool of a child operated on for possible appendicitis; the appendix was normal but a supurative mensenteric lymph node was removed (119).

Non-O157 SLTEC have been isolated from intestines of children with sudden infant death syndrome (202) and from patients with ulcerative colitis (203,204), but whether they have any role in these illnesses is unknown.

Hemolytic-Uremic Syndrome and Thrombotic Thrombocytopenic Purpura

Hemolytic-uremic syndrome is characterized by microangiopathic hemolytic anemia, thrombocytopenia, renal failure, and central nervous system symptoms (205). It was first well described in 1955 in Switzerland (206). About 90% of cases of HUS are preceded by diarrhea (87,207–209). *Shigella dysenteriae* type 1 was recognized as a major cause of HUS in developing countries long before *E. coli* O157:H7 was recognized as a pathogen (210). It is only in the past decade that the SLTEC, and *E. coli* O157:H7 in particular, have been recognized as the major cause of HUS in developed countries. HUS is a serious illness, with 3% to 5% of affected children dying acutely (207–209), and 12% having severe sequelae of renal impairment, neurological injury, or hypertension (211).

Thrombotic thrombocytopenic purpura includes all the clinical features of HUS; proposed distinctions between the two include less frequent renal failure but more frequent neurological involvement in TTP (212,213). However, in major case series of patients with TTP, diarrhea is not even mentioned as a preceding symptom (212,214). In clinical practice, TTP tends to be diagnosed in adults. The rare patient with a diagnosis of TTP whose illness was preceded by diarrhea is likely to be infected with *E. coli* O157:H7 or another SLTEC (34). In this chapter, the term HUS is used to include any hemolytic-uremic illness preceded by gastrointestinal illness in a person of any age. Studies of the incidence, etiology, clinical features, and outcome of postdiarrheal HUS have focused on children; studies of this complication of SLTEC infection in adults are needed.

E. coli O157:H7 has been consistently isolated from patients with HUS in prospective studies, all of which have been conducted in North and South America and Europe (Table 3). In none of these studies was it isolated from controls without diarrhea. The proportion of HUS patients from whom *E. coli* O157:H7 was isolated has varied widely among studies; the most important responsible factor is likely the length of time between the onset of diarrhea and culture of stool. Persons with HUS seek medical attention an average of 6.5 ± 2.8 days after the onset of diarrhea, when the numbers of pathogens in the stool are decreasing (215). The importance of timing in obtaining specimens was demonstrated by a study from Seattle in which, while *E. coli* O157:H7 was isolated from only 63% of all patients, 96% of those whose stools were cultured within 6 days of the onset of illness carried the organism (215). Other studies have also reported an important effect of timing (208,216). The highest isolation rate reported was from a recent Canadian study, in which *E. coli* O157:H7 was isolated from 76% of children with HUS; among those whose stool cultures yielded some growth and were performed within 6 days of the onset of gastrointestinal symptoms, 87% were infected with *E. coli* O157:H7 (217). Three of these studies, from Germany, Central Europe, and Italy, reported antibody responses to O157 LPS; the proportions of HUS patients with positive antibody titers were 91%, 73%, and 51%, much higher than the proportions whose stools yielded *E. coli* O157:H7. In addition, a study of 60 patients with HUS in the United Kingdom found antibodies to O157 LPS in 73%, including all nine whose stools grew *E. coli* O157:H7 (129). Together these data strongly suggest that *E. coli* O157:H7 is by far the most common cause of postdiarrheal HUS and is likely responsible for 85% to 95% of cases.

Non-O157 SLTEC are isolated from some HUS patients in most studies (Table 3). A few, particularly O26:H11, O111:NM, and O113:H21, appear to be isolated more frequently than others (34). The 1990 Canadian study may have the most accurate data on the proportion of HUS cases caused by non-O157 SLTEC because it reported the highest overall SLTEC isolation rate of any study (82%); non-O157 SLTEC were isolated from 7% of patients from whom any SLTEC was isolated (217).

The data suggest that HUS without a gastrointestinal prodrome (atypical HUS) is unlikely to be caused by SLTEC, although no prospective studies have focused on this type of HUS, and many studies include only patients with a diarrheal prodrome (Table 3). In a U.S. study, *E. coli* O157:H7 was not isolated from two patients without a diarrheal prodrome (218). In U.K. studies, none of 7 children without a diarrheal prodrome had SLTEC or free fecal toxin in their stools (208), and none of 3 without diarrhea had antibodies to O157 LPS (129). In a central European study, none of 11 patients with atypical HUS had elevated IgM antibodies to O157 LPS, but two had elevated IgA antibodies; the specificity of the enzyme-linked immunosorbent assays (ELISAs) in the study was not reported (216). In an Italian study, 9 of 14 HUS patients without diarrhea had laboratory evidence of SLTEC infection; however, SLTEC were not isolated from any of these patients (81). Moreover, the authors could not exclude the possibility that mild enteric symptoms were overlooked by parents. A few persons with SLTEC-associated HUS have had nondiarrheal gastrointestinal symptoms. A man with *E. coli* O157:H7-associated HUS had a prodrome of abdominal pain and hemorrhagic gastroduodenitis (219). *E. coli* O26-associated HUS preceded by abdominal pain and vomiting occurred in a person with AIDS (220).

Isolation of an enteric pathogen other than SLTEC from the stool of a patient with HUS does not prove it to be the cause of the illness. A child with *E. coli* O157:H7-associated HUS also had *Salmonella* and group A β-streptococcal bacteremia (221). *Campylobacter* was isolated from a patient with SLTEC-associated HUS (208). In a European study, *Salmonella* spp., rotavirus, corona virus, respiratory syncytial virus, and *Cryptosporidium* were isolated from HUS patients who also had evidence of SLTEC infection (216). No organisms other than *E. coli* isolated from patients with HUS have ever been shown to produce SLT (216; and J. G. Wells, *personal communication*).

The proportion of patients who develop HUS following *E. coli* O157:H7 infection has varied widely among studies and outbreaks (Table 1). Factors reported to increase the risk of HUS include being at the extremes of age, female gender, mental retardation, absent or weak P1 antigen expression by red cells, bloody diarrhea, fever, elevated leukocyte count, toxin type of the infecting strain, and treatment with an antimotility or antimicrobial agent (34). The rate of HUS appears to vary by which of these factors the infected population exhibits. For example, bloody diarrhea is an important predictor. In a community outbreak in which 97% of patients had bloody diarrhea, 11% developed HUS (90), whereas in a community outbreak in which only 35% of patients had bloody diarrhea, only 0.4% developed HUS (25). The overall rate of HUS in sporadic *E. coli* O157:H7 cases with bloody diarrhea is about 5% to 10% (34). The rate of HUS among persons with bloody diarrhea severe enough to present to an emergency room may be above 10%.

In retrospective analyses, persons infected with an *E. coli* O157:H7 strain that produces only SLT II were more likely to develop HUS than those infected with strains that produce both toxins or only SLT I (33,35,162). The reason for this has not been determined: in an animal model, the amount of SLT II produced was important in determining the severity of illness (175), but it is not known whether strains producing only SLT II produce more SLT II than strains that produce both toxins. Of interest, SLT I is almost completely cell-associated, and SLT II is found primarily in culture supernatants (9,175).

The P antigen, which is present on erythrocytes in most persons (222,223), has structural similarities to Gb3 (30). The role of P antigen in HUS, if any, has not been determined (224,225). Some have suggested that absent or weak P1 antigen expression by red blood cells may increase that risk of HUS (26,224,226).

The rate and risk factors for infection with non-O157 SLTEC in general, or for particular serotypes, progressing to HUS have not been determined.

LABORATORY DIAGNOSIS

Stool

Most patients with *E. coli* O157:H7 infection do not have fecal leukocytes, so that the presence of fecal leukocytes is not an appropriate criterion for culture. In one outbreak, two thirds of patients had fewer than one fecal leukocyte per high-power microscopic field (189).

Screening tests take advantage of the fact that although *E. coli* O157:H7 ferments lactose like most *E. coli,* it does not ferment sorbitol within 24 hr or produce β-glucuronidase (22). Sorbitol–MacConkey (SMAC) agar, in which lactose is replaced by sorbitol, is commercially available and is the medium of choice for screening (16). Traditional MacConkey agar is a poor screening medium because as many as 20 colonies may need to be tested biochemically for sorbitol fermentation to achieve a similar level of sensitivity as testing 3 colonies from SMAC agar (J. G. Wells, *personal communication*). Sorbitol-negative (clear) colonies should be selected from the SMAC plate and tested with commercially available *E. coli* O157 antiserum (227,228).

Most misidentifications of other organisms as *E. coli* O157 occur from failure to use a latex control reagent in conjunction with O157 antibody–coated latex reagent; most organisms that agglutinate in both are nonspecific agglutinators (229). Isolates that agglutinate in O157 antiserum must be confirmed biochemically as *Escherichia coli* because some other organisms cross-react with O157 antiserum, including *Brucella abortis, Salmonella* group N, *Vibrio cholerae, Yersinia enterocolitica* O9, *Francisella tularensis, Pseudomonas maltophilia* (230), *Citrobacter freundii* (231), and *Escherichia hermanii* (232). Whereas usual biochemical tests can differentiate most cross-reacting organisms from *E. coli,* special tests are required to distinguish *E. hermanii* from *E. coli* (233). Tests to exclude *E. hermanii* may not be cost-effective because it is rare in stool specimens (233) and because this false-positive would be detected during H7 testing.

Other properties of *E. coli* O157:H7 can also aid screening. Some laboratories screen for the enzyme β-glucuronidase, which *E. coli* O157:H7 lacks, using medium containing the substrate 4-methylumbelliferyl-β-D-glucuronide (MUG). When MUG is cleaved by this enzyme, a fluorescent product is produced that is detectable with long-wave ultraviolet light (17). Modifying SMAC medium by adding cefixime, rhamnose, and tellurite has also been reported to improve detection (234,235).

Presumptive identification of *E. coli* O157:H7 can be reported for any organism that is sorbitol-negative on SMAC agar, agglutinates in O157 antiserum, and is biochemically an *E. coli*. The H type of presumptive *E. coli* O157:H7 should be determined, usually in a reference laboratory, because *E. coli* O157 strains of other H types occur; however, they are uncommon and do not produce SLT (236–238). Some O157 strains are nonmotile; most of these produce SLT, suggesting that they previously carried the H7 antigen. Fewer than 2% of *E. coli* O157 strains isolated from sporadic diarrhea are nonmotile (51,64,118); a larger proportion have been reported from persons with HUS (Table 3). Toxin testing of sporadic *E. coli* O157:H7 isolates is generally not necessary because nontoxigenic strains are very rare (35). CDC has identified only 3 nontoxigenic strains of *E. coli* O157:H7 among over 1800 tested over 9 years (J. G. Wells, *personal communication*); one of these, isolated from a patient in an outbreak, had the same plasmid profile as SLT-producing strains isolated from other patients (90). This and evidence that *E. coli* can lose SLT genes upon subcultivation (239) suggest that nontoxigenic strains originally produced SLT. Toxin testing of nonmotile *E. coli* O157 should be performed because only toxin-producing strains have been linked to human illness. Subtyping of *E. coli* O157:H7 is useful in outbreaks; the methods include plasmid profiles, antibiograms, toxin typing, phage typing, and pulsed-field gel electrophoresis (236,240,241).

The development of commercially available, sensitive, specific, rapid tests for identification of *E. coli* O157 in stool specimens would be helpful in differential diagnosis, in conducting treatment trials, and in selecting patients for close monitoring (242).

Several techniques not generally available in clinical microbiology laboratories are useful for detecting both *E. coli* O157:H7 and non-O157 serotypes, and would also detect the rare sorbitol-fermenting *E. coli* O157. Free fecal toxin can be identified in stools of some infected persons (149,236). Adding this method to isolation on SMAC may increase the number of infections detected (118). Probes for the SLT I and II genes can be used to screen large numbers of colonies (236,243). PCR can be used to detect DNA sequences for SLT (244).

Serology

Antibodies to Lipopolysaccharide

Several investigators have devised methods to measure serum antibodies to O157 LPS. A British group has reported measuring immunoglobulin M and A, but not G, antibodies using ELISA and immunoblotting (245,246). German and Japanese groups have used indirect hemagglutination (77,247,248). A U.S. group examined sera from 26 persons with positive *E. coli* O157:H7 cultures and from 66 well controls using an IgG ELISA; 24 (92%) patients had a positive titer to IgG, compared with only

2 (3%) controls (183). The response peaked in the second and third week after onset of illness. However, only 19 (33%) of 57 culture-negative ill persons drawn from the same outbreaks had positive titers. Although some of these latter persons may not have been infected, it seems more likely that some infections do not elicit a marked IgG response. The height of the response may be related to the severity of illness: culture-positive patients with HUS developed higher titers than those without HUS (183). Age did not appear to affect the antibody response: all culture-confirmed patients <5 or >60 years old were seropositive (183). Measurement of several immunoglobulin class responses may improve sensitivity (246). A test for fecal IgA has also been reported (249).

Measurement of antibodies to O157 LPS is particularly useful in studies of groups of ill patients who may not have had stool cultures taken during their diarrheal illness. Serological findings in studies on patients with HUS are reported in the section on HUS and in Table 3. When these tests are applied to persons who are less likely to have been infected, the proportion of falsely positive tests increases. False-positive antibody titers to O157 LPS have also been reported among patients with yersiniosis and brucellosis (250,251). Conversely, patients with *E. coli* O157 infection developed antibodies that reacted with the O antigen of *B. abortus*, but not with *Y. enterocolitica* (250,251). In addition, five of nine volunteers given cholera vaccine developed borderline positive ELISA antibody titers to O157 LPS, which were confirmed by immunoblotting (252).

Several studies have measured the duration of the O157 LPS antibody response. In one study, five of seven patients who had blood samples drawn between 31 and 62 days after onset of diarrhea had positive IgG antibody titers (196). In a study of patients with HUS (most not culture-confirmed), mean IgM antibody titers to O157 LPS declined to near negative by 8 weeks after the onset of diarrhea, although some patients had positive titers at 7 months; IgA antibody titers declined to near negative by 4 weeks (216).

Some studies have attempted to measure antibodies against the LPS of other SLTEC. Among 48 Italian patients with HUS, 4 had serum antibodies to O26 LPS and 1 to O111 LPS; only 1 of 25 control sera was positive, a weak positive reaction against both O157 and O26 LPS (81). However, none of the infections were confirmed by stool culture. Another study failed to detect antibodies to the LPS of *E. coli* O111, O26, or O55 in three patients with HUS from whose stools these organisms were isolated (248).

Antibodies to Shiga-like Toxins

Barrett and colleagues demonstrated that a small proportion of patients infected with SLT I–producing *E. coli* O157:H7 produce antibody titers to SLT I but none produce antibodies to SLT II (183). They detected SLT I antibodies by ELISA in only 11 (23%) of 47 patients in an outbreak caused by an SLT I- and II-producing *E. coli* O157:H7 (183). Titers were also positive in 11% of well controls and in 14% of patients infected with a strain that produced only SLT II, but most titers were lower than those in patients. In the same study, none of 83 ill persons in two *E. coli* O157:H7 outbreaks (one caused by a strain that produced only SLT II, the other by a strain that produced both toxins) developed antibodies to SLT II by neutralization or ELISA (183). However, sera from all patients and controls exhibited nonspecific neutralization of SLT II. The reason for the lack of a measurable antibody response to SLT II is unclear but has been confirmed by others (216,253).

The proportion of patients with HUS who develop SLT I antibody titers has varied in different studies. These variations could be due to differences in methodologies as well as to differences in the proportion of infecting strains that produced SLT I; in many patients an SLTEC was not isolated. In the first major HUS study, 16 (59%) of 27 Canadian children with postdiarrheal HUS from whom acute and convalescent sera were obtained had a greater than fourfold rise in SLT-neutralizing antibody titer (6). In a later Canadian study, 12 (55%) of 22 children with HUS who were infected with *E. coli* O157:H7 strains that produced both SLT I and II had antibodies to SLT I (217). In Argentina, 45% of children with HUS had antibody titers to SLT I, compared with 14% for children with diarrhea alone and 5% for controls (87). Later studies reported a lower proportion with SLT I titers. In a central European study, 12 (9%) of 131 children with postdiarrheal HUS and 3% of controls had SLT I titers (216). In Italy, 9 (19%) of 48 children with HUS had SLT I neutralizing antibody titers (81).

TREATMENT

There is no proven specific therapy for infection with *E. coli* O157:H7 or other EHEC. However, only small retrospective analyses and one prospective study of treatment of *E. coli* O157:H7 diarrhea have been reported. Although the vast majority of *E. coli* O157:H7 strains are susceptible to antimicrobial agents (see microbiology section), these agents had no effect on the duration of diarrhea in three retrospective studies (59,189,254) and prolonged the duration of bloody stools in another (59). In the prospective study, trimethoprim-sulfamethoxazole did not decrease the duration of gastrointestinal symptoms, although treatment was begun relatively late in the illness (255).

Analyses of the effect of antimicrobial therapy on the risk of HUS following *E. coli* O157:H7 infection have been inconclusive—one prospective and two retrospective studies reported no benefit, whereas another retrospective study reported benefit. In one case series, treatment with trimethoprim-sulfamethoxazole or gentamicin was possibly associated with an increased risk of HUS or TTP (59). In an outbreak, all five patients who received trimethoprim-sulfamethoxazole but only two of seven who received no antimicrobial agent for bloody diarrhea developed HUS (49). However, in another case series, patients with HUS were less likely than those with only diarrhea to have received an "appropriate" antimicrobial

agent for >24 hr (256). Moreover, although the one prospective study showed no significant difference in outcome between the group that received trimethoprim-sulfamethoxazole and no antimicrobial, treatment was begun relatively late in illness and the proportion who developed HUS was higher in the group that did not receive the antimicrobial (255). It is perhaps relevant that a study of 117 children with HUS (most of whom had a prodrome of diarrhea but few of whom had culture-confirmed *E. coli* O157:H7 infection) found that those who had received an antimicrobial agent during the prodromal illness had a better outcome (48).

The retrospective analyses suggesting harm from antimicrobial agents are inconclusive for several reasons: they are small, patients were given a variety of agents at different times in their illness, and development of HUS could simply be a marker for a more severe illness that prompted the administration of an antimicrobial. However, antimicrobial agents can influence production of SLT *in vitro*. One group reported that subinhibitory concentrations of trimethoprim-sulfamethoxazole increased, and ciprofloxacin decreased, SLT production by *E. coli* O157:H7 (257,258). In contrast, others reported that ciprofloxacin induced a large increase in SLT I production by *E. coli* O157:H7 (259). Another study demonstrated that ciprofloxacin can cause rapid and sustained release of endotoxin from *Escherichia coli* (260). Whether these phenomena occur *in vivo* is unknown. Moreover, data from patients infected with *Shigella dysenteriae* type 1 support the possibility that antimicrobial agents can promote progression to HUS. Bangladeshi patients with *S. dysenteriae* type 1 infection who received an inappropriate antimicrobial agent in the hospital had an increased risk of developing HUS (163). Among U.S. travelers with *S. dysenteriae* type 1 infection, 3 of 9 who received an antimicrobial drug to which the organism was resistant, but none of 21 who received appropriate antimicrobial therapy, developed a hemolytic syndrome (261).

Although antimicrobial agents might worsen the course of *E. coli* O157:H7 diarrhea and the risk of complications, beneficial effects might depend on the agent given, the dose, the route of administration, the stage of infection at which it is administered, and other factors. Considering that both adherence to the gut mucosa and toxin production are major virulence factors, antimicrobial agents could help by killing the pathogen but harm by causing the resultant release and absorption of SLT and other bacterial products. It is possible that early initiation of treatment could be beneficial, as has been shown for *Campylobacter* diarrhea (262). Clearly, large prospective treatment trials with early institution of therapy are needed (24,255).

Antimotility agents are not indicated for persons with bloody diarrhea (263). In retrospective analyses, one group found that receiving an antimotility agent for >24 hr increased the risk of *E. coli* O157:H7 infection progressing to HUS and increased the risk of central nervous system manifestations in HUS (256,264). An increased risk of HUS was not demonstrated in another retrospective analysis (265).

Other promising therapies for infection with *E. coli*

O157:H7 include toxin-binding agents and SLT II antitoxin. Antibody to SLT may protect against infection or complications. When MacLeod and colleagues immunized pigs (some actively, some passively) against SLT IIv, then challenged them with intravenous SLT IIv, all immunized pigs survived, but those with the lowest titer of SLT IIv neutralizing antibody showed mild signs of edema disease; all control pigs died (266). *In vitro* studies have suggested that immunoglobulin G from normal adults may decrease platelet aggregation in HUS, but the mechanism and whether treatment improves outcome are unknown (267). Immune globulins are used to treat some bacterial infections (268), and specific immune globulin appears to shorten the clinical illness and improve the survival of patients with botulism (269). The timing of administration may be critical: human intravenous immune globulin protected infant rabbits against diarrhea when given 1 hr after intraperitoneal injection of SLT I, but not when given at 6 or 24 hr (270). Commercially available immune globulin preparations contain antibody to SLT I but not SLT II (253,271). Since SLT II appears to be a more important virulence factor than SLT I, treatment trials using specific anti-SLT II immune globulin should be considered.

Persons with diarrhea due to *E. coli* O157:H7 or with acute bloody diarrhea of unknown cause, especially children under 5 years old and the elderly, should be monitored for HUS (23,34,49,59,189,256). Clinical features suggesting an increased likelihood of developing HUS include bloody diarrhea, fever, and elevated leukocyte count (45,49,65). Monitoring of peripheral blood count, blood smear, serum creatinine, and urine sediment has permitted detection of mild or "subclinical" HUS in some patients (34).

Additional information on general supportive and investigational treatment of patients with HUS is provided in Ref. 267.

PREVENTION

Prevention of *E. coli* O157:H7 infection is a particular challenge because, like *Salmonella,* it lives in the intestines of healthy food animals and can survive and multiply in foods but, like *Shigella,* it is transmitted directly from person to person.

Control measures on farms and in slaughtering and processing plants are needed. Studies of host factors, farm practices, and environmental conditions that increase the risk of animals being colonized, and of farms having *E. coli* O157:H7-positive animals, are the first steps in developing control strategies. Similarly, studies of factors in slaughtering and processing that increase the risk of meat contamination are needed. In 1985, a report by the National Research Council found that "the number of . . . organisms that leave slaughtering establishments can be reduced considerably by improved dressing procedures to prevent fecal soilage of carcasses and carcass-to-carcass cross contamination" (272). However, the meat safety system in the United States remains antiquated and is still not based on risk assessment or microbiological data.

Unlike *Salmonella,* which colonizes many food animals, *E. coli* O157:H7 has not been clearly linked to meat from animals other than cattle, and natural infection of other animals with this pathogen has not been reported. However, *E. coli* O157:H7 can colonize chickens (18,273,274). A concerted effort now to understand the ecology and decrease the burden of *E. coli* O157:H7 in cattle could have future benefits in decreasing the likelihood of other food animal populations becoming carriers.

Proper processing and cooking of contaminated foods by industry is also needed. New regulations precipitated by outbreak investigations should be promulgated and enforced: these include requiring manufacturing plants to heat fully cooked meat patties sufficiently to kill pathogenic microorganisms (92,275) and recommendating that retail establishments cook ground beef to an internal temperature of at least 155°F (61). Lessons may be learned from the manner in which milk and ice cream, which were notorious sources of diarrhea until the 1930s, were made safe. Sir Graham Wilson introduced the concept of processing food for safety, using a series of steps including strict hygienic care of the raw material, thorough pasteurization, and prevention of adverse postprocess events (276). A similar approach, perhaps including surface disinfection (276) or irradiation (277) of some products, should now be considered for meat.

Because it is unlikely that the risk of infection with *E. coli* O157:H7 and other enteric pathogens will ever be completely eliminated, better education of consumers is needed about the risk of infection from consumption of foods of animal origin and about food preparation practices that increase risk. Consumers and food preparers should be taught that all raw foods of animal origin can harbor infectious agents. Ground beef that is not thoroughly cooked is a high-risk food because a single serving typically contains meat from many different animals that came from many different farms, and contaminants on the outside of meat can be mixed in when the meat is ground. Labels are one way of educating consumers. In 1973, the American Public Health Association sued the U.S. Department of Agriculture (USDA), charging that "Inspected for Wholesomeness" labels on meat and poultry were misleading, and that the USDA should affix a warning label with advice on how to avoid food poisoning (278). The court sided with the USDA's plan to substitute a consumer education program for labels. Twenty years later, in the wake of the large *E. coli* O157:H7 outbreak in the western United States (61), the USDA reconsidered this decision and initiated regulations to require warning labels (279).

However, improvements in meat production, processing, and cooking will not prevent transmission of *E. coli* O157:H7 by other foods and water. *E. coli* O157:H7 outbreaks have been linked to unpasteurized milk, unchlorinated municipal water, contaminated swimming water, fresh-pressed apple cider, uncooked vegetables fertilized with manure, and turkey probably cross-contaminated with beef. Thus, many infections could be prevented by simple precautions that also protect against other enteric infections. These include drinking only pasteurized milk and disinfected water, bacteriological monitoring of swimming water, careful washing or thorough cooking of fruits and vegetables, and avoidance of cross-contamination.

Prevention of person-to-person spread of *E. coli* O157:H7 is a challenge. An initial *E. coli* O157:H7 infection from contaminated food or water can cause a cascade of person-to-person spread, sometimes resulting in HUS and death (44,45). Spread in day care centers can be a particularly difficult problem. In Minnesota, health officials developed a policy requiring that both ill and well children from any day care center that has experienced transmission of *E. coli* O157:H7 be excluded from that and all other centers until two stool cultures are negative (48). Although this aggressive approach was considered justified because of the sometimes severe consequences of infection, it was costly. Many parents lost time from work staying home with their well children, and health department personnel spent much time ensuring that children were not taken to other centers. More research is needed to assess the optimal strategy for prevention and control of *E. coli* O157:H7 infections in child care centers.

CONCLUSION

Culturing stools for *E. coli* O157:H7 has important benefits for both the individual and the community. Diagnosis can be critical for individual patients, who may be spared unnecessary and even life-threatening diagnostic and surgical procedures and therapies performed for incorrect diagnoses. Infected patients and their families can be counseled to increase handwashing with soap to prevent the spread of infection within the home (44). Monitoring of patients with *E. coli* O157:H7 infection for HUS may result in earlier initiation of dialysis, which may improve survival (280). In addition, detecting individual cases is the first step in detecting outbreaks, investigation of which results in measures to prevent more cases, such as removing contaminated food from the market (61), closing contaminated lakes (281), or improving hygiene in child care facilities. Continued investigations of outbreaks are critical because their findings exert pressure on industry and on government regulators to increase the safety of the food supply.

ACKNOWLEDGMENTS

The author thanks Timothy J. Barrett and Joy G. Wells for critical review of the manuscript, Ethel Jordan for technical assistance, and Lynne McIntyre for editorial assistance.

REFERENCES

1. Riley LW, Remis RS, Helgerson SD, et al. Hemorrhagic colitis associated with a rare *Escherichia coli* serotype. *N Engl J Med* 1983;308:681–685.
2. Stewart PJ, Desormeaux W, Chene J, Lior H. Hemorrhagic colitis in a home for the aged—Ontario. *Can Dis Week Rep* 1983;9–8:29–32.
3. Johnson WM, Lior H, Bezanson GS. Cytotoxic *Escherichia coli* O157:H7 associated with haemorrhagic colitis in Canada (letter). *Lancet* 1983;1:76.
4. O'Brien AD, Lively TA, Chen ME, Rothman SW, Formal SB. *Escherichia coli* O157:H7 strains associated with haemorrhagic colitis in the United States produce a *Shigella dysenteriae* 1 (Shiga) like cytotoxin (letter). *Lancet* 1983;1:702.
5. Karmali MA, Steele BT, Petric M, Corazon L. Sporadic cases of haemolytic-uraemic syndrome associated with faecal cytotoxin and cytotoxin-producing *Escherichia coli* in stools. *Lancet* 1983;1:619–620.
6. Karmali MA, Petric M, Lim C, Fleming PC, Arbus GS, Lior H. The association between idiopathic hemolytic uremic syndrome and infection by verotoxin-producing *Escherichia coli*. *J Infect Dis* 1985;151:775–782.
7. Strockbine NA, Marques LRM, Newland JW, Smith HW, Holmes RK, O'Brien AD. Two toxin-converting phages from *Escherichia coli* O157:H7 strain 933 encode antigenically distinct toxins with similar biologic activities. *Infect Immun* 1986;53:135–140.
8. O'Brien AD, Holmes RK. Shiga-like toxins. *Microbiol Rev* 1987;51:206–220.
9. Marques LRM, Moore MA, Wells JG, Wachsmuth IK, O'Brien AD. Production of Shiga-like toxin by *Escherichia coli*. *J Infect Dis* 1986;154:338–341.
10. Konowalchuk J, Speris JI, Stavric S. Vero response to a cytotoxin of *Escherichia coli*. *Infect Immun* 1977;18:775–779.
11. Konowalchuk J, Dickie N, Stavric S, Speirs JI. Properties of an *Escherichia coli* cytotoxin. *Infect Immun* 1978;20:575–577.
12. Wade WG, Thom BT, Evans N. Cytotoxic enteropathogenic *Escherichia coli*. *Lancet* 1979;2:1235–1236.
13. Hardas UD, Jalgaonkar SV, Kulkarni VK. Cytotoxic effect of culture filtrate of enteropathogenic *Escherichia coli* from diarrhoea in children on Vero cell culture. *Indian J Med Res* 1982;76:86–88.
14. Levine MM, Edelman R. Enteropathogenic *Escherichia coli* of classic serotypes associated with infant diarrhea: epidemiology and pathogenesis. *Epidemiol Rev* 1984;6:31–51.
15. Levine MM, Xu J, Kaper JB, et al. A DNA probe to identify enterohemorrhagic *Escherichia coli* of O157:H7 and other serotypes that cause hemorrhagic colitis and hemolytic uremic syndrome. *J Infect Dis* 1987;156:175–182.
16. March SB, Ratnam S. Sorbitol-MacConkey medium for detection of *Escherichia coli* O157:H7 associated with hemorrhagic colitis. *J Clin Microbiol* 1986;23:869–872.
17. Thompson JS, Hodge DS, Borczyk AA. Rapid biochemical test to identify verocytotoxin-positive strains of *Escherichia coli* serotype O157. *J Clin Microbiol* 1990;28:2165–2168.
18. Doyle MP. *Escherichia coli* O157:H7 and its significance in foods. *Int J Food Microbiol* 1991;12:289–301.
19. Raghubeer EV, Matches JR. Temperature range for growth of *Escherichia coli* serotype O157:H7 and selected coliforms in *E. coli* medium. *J Clin Microbiol* 1990;28:803–805.
20. Gunzer F, Bohm H, Russmann H, Bitzan M, Aleksic S, Karch H. Molecular detection of sorbitol-fermenting *Escherichia coli* O157 in patients with hemolytic-uremic syndrome. *J Clin Microbiol* 1992;30:1807–1810.
21. Karch H, Bohm H, Schmidt H, Gunzer F, Aleksic S, Heesemann J. Clonal structure and pathogenicity of Shiga-like toxin-producing, sorbitol-fermenting *Escherichia coli* O157:H—. *J Clin Microbiol* 1993;31:1200–1205.
22. Ratnam S, March SB, Ahmed R, Bezanson GS, Kasatiya S. Characterization of *Escherichia coli* serotype O157:H7. *J Clin Microbiol* 1988;26:2006–2012.
23. Pai CH, Gordon R, Sims HV, Bryan LE. Sporadic cases of hemorrhagic colitis associated with *Escherichia coli* O157:H7: clinical, epidemiologic, and bacteriologic features. *Ann Intern Med* 1984;101:738–742.
24. Tarr PI, Neill MA, Christie DL, Anderson DE. *Escherichia coli* O157:H7 hemorrhagic colitis (letter). *N Engl J Med* 1988;318:1697.
25. Swerdlow DL, Woodruff BA, Brady RC, et al. A waterborne outbreak in Missouri of *Escherichia coli* O157:H7 associated

with bloody diarrhea and death. *Ann Intern Med* 1992;117: 812–819.

26. Lingwood CA. Verotoxins and their glycolipid receptors. *Adv Lipid Res* 1993;25:189–211.

27. Paton AW, Paton JC, Heuzenroeder MW, Goldwater PN, Manning PA. Cloning and nucleotide sequence of a variant Shiga-like toxin II gene from *Escherichia coli* OX3:H21 isolated from a case of sudden infant death syndrome. *Microb Pathog* 1992; 13:225–236.

28. Jackson MP, Neill RJ, O'Brien AD, Holmes RK, Newland JW. Nucleotide sequence analysis and comparison of the structural genes for Shiga-like toxin I and Shiga-like toxin II encoded by bacteriophages from *Escherichia coli* 933. *FEMS Microbiol Lett* 1987;44:109–114.

29. Karmali MA. Infection by verocytotoxin-producing *Escherichia coli*. *Clin Microbiol Rev* 1989;2:15–38.

30. Lingwood CA, Law H, Richardson S, et al. Glycolipid binding of purified and recombinant *Escherichia coli* produced verotoxin in vitro. *J Biol Chem* 1987;262:8834–8839.

31. Sandvig K, Olsnes S, Brown JE, Petersen OW, Van Deurs B. Endocytosis from coated pits of Shiga toxin: a glycolipid-binding protein from *Shigella dysenteriae*. *J Cell Biol* 1989;108: 1331–1343.

32. Tesh VL, O'Brien AD. The pathogenic mechanisms of Shiga-toxin and the Shiga-like toxins. *Mol Microbiol* 1991;5: 1817–1822.

33. Ostroff SM, Neill MA, Lewis JH, Hargrett-Bean N, Kobayashi JM. Toxin genotypes and plasmid profiles as determinants of systemic sequelae in *Escherichia coli* O157:H7 infections. *J Infect Dis* 1989;160:994–998.

34. Griffin PM, Tauxe RV. The epidemiology of infections caused by *Escherichia coli* O157:H7, other enterohemorrhagic *E. coli*, and the associated hemolytic uremic syndrome. *Epidemiol Rev* 1991;13:60–98.

35. Thomas A, Chart H, Cheasty T, Smith HR, Frost JA, Rowe B. Vero cytotoxin-producing *Escherichia coli*, particularly serogroup O157, associated with human infections in the United Kingdom: 1989–91. *Epidemiol Infect* 1993;110:591–600.

36. IASR. Verotoxin-producing enterohemorrhagic *Escherichia coli*, January 1992–July 1993. *Infec Ag Surv Rep* 1993;14:1–2.

37. Duncan L, Mai V, Carter A, Carlson JAK, Borczyk A, Karmali MA. Outbreak of gastrointestinal disease—Ontario. *Can Dis Week Rep* 1987;13-2:5–8.

38. Borczyk AA, Karmali MA, Lior H, Duncan LMC. Bovine reservoir for verotoxin-producing *Escherichia coli* O157:H7 (letter). *Lancet* 1987;1:98.

39. Morgan D, Newman CP, Hutchinson DN, Walker AM, Rowe B, Majid F. Verotoxin producing *Escherichia coli* O157 infections associated with the consumption of yoghurt. *Epidemiol Infect* 1993;111:181–187.

40. Besser RE, Lett SM, Weber JT, et al. An outbreak of diarrhea and hemolytic uremic syndrome from *Escherichia coli* O157: H7 in fresh-pressed apple cider. *JAMA* 1993;269:2217–2220.

41. Keene WE, McAnulty JM, Williams LP, Hoesly FC, Hedberg K, Fleming DW. A two-restaurant outbreak of *Escherichia coli* O157:H7 enteritis associated with consumption of mayonnaise. Program and Abstracts of the 33rd Interscience Conference on Antimicrobial Agents and Chemotherapy, New Orleans, LA; 1993:354.

42. Glass KA, Loeffelholz JM, Ford JP, Doyle MP. Fate of *Escherichia coli* O157:H7 as affected by pH or sodium chloride and in fermented, dry sausage. *Appl Environ Microbiol* 1992;58: 2513–2516.

43. Morgan GM, Newman C, Palmer SR, et al. First recognized community outbreak of haemorrhagic colitis due to verotoxin-producing *Escherichia coli* O157:H7 in the UK. *Epidemiol Infect* 1988;101:83–91.

44. Cieslak PR, Barrett TJ, Griffin PM, et al. *Escherichia coli* O157: H7 infection from a manured garden. *Lancet* 1993;342:367.

45. Carter AO, Borczyk AA, Carlson JAK, et al. A severe outbreak of *Escherichia coli* O157:H7-associated hemorrhagic colitis in a nursing home. *N Engl J Med* 1987;317:1496–1500.

46. Salmon RL, Farrell ID, Hutchinson JGP, et al. A christening party outbreak of haemorrhagic colitis and haemolytic uraemic

47. Spika JS, Parsons JE, Nordenberg D, Wells JG, Gunn RA, Blake PA. Hemolytic uremic syndrome and diarrhea associated with *Escherichia coli* O157:H7 in a day care center. *J Pediatr* 1986;109:287–291.

48. Belongia EA, Osterholm MT, Soler JT, Ammend DA, Braun JE, MacDonald KL. Transmission of *Escherichia coli* O157: H7 infection in Minnesota child day-care facilities. *JAMA* 1993; 269:883–888.

49. Pavia AT, Nichols CR, Green DP, et al. Hemolytic-uremic syndrome during an outbreak of *Escherichia coli* O157:H7 infections in institutions for mentally retarded persons: clinical and epidemiologic observations. *J Pediatr* 1990;116:544–551.

50. MacDonald KL, O'Leary MJ, Cohen ML, et al. *Escherichia coli* O157:H7, an emerging gastrointestinal pathogen. Results of a one-year study, prospective, population-based study. *JAMA* 1988;259:3567–3570.

51. Bryant HE, Athar MA, Pai CH. Risk factors for *Escherichia coli* O157:H7 infection in an urban community. *J Infect Dis* 1989;160:858–864.

52. Le Saux N, Spika JS, Friesen B, et al. Ground beef consumption in noncommercial settings is a risk factor for sporadic *Escherichia coli* O157:H7 infection in Canada. *J Infect Dis* 1993;167:500–502.

53. Neill MA, Agosti J, Rosen H. Hemorrhagic colitis with *Escherichia coli* O157:H7 preceding adult hemolytic uremic syndrome. *Arch Intern Med* 1985;45:2215–2217.

54. Martin ML, Shipman LD, Wells JG, et al. Isolation of *Escherichia coli* O157:H7 from dairy cattle associated with two cases of haemolytic uraemic syndrome (letter). *Lancet* 1986;2:1043.

55. Rowe PC, Orrbine E, Lior H, Wells GA, McLaine PN, CPKDRC Co-investigators. Diarrhoea in close contacts as a risk factor for childhood haemolytic uraemic syndrome. *Epidemiol Infect* 1993;110:9–16.

56. Karmali MA, Arbus GS, Petric M, Patrick ML, Roscoe M, Shaw J. Hospital-acquired *Escherichia coli* O157:H7 associated haemolytic uraemic syndrome in a nurse (letter). *Lancet* 1988;1:526.

57. Booth L, Rowe B. Possible occupational acquisition of *Escherichia coli* O157 infection. *Lancet* 1993;342:1298–1299.

58. Burnens AP, Zbinden R, Kaempf L, Heinzer I, Nicolet J. A case of laboratory acquired infection with *Escherichia coli* O157:H7. *Zentralbl Bakteriol* 1993;279:512–517.

59. Ostroff SM, Kobayashi JM, Lewis JH. Infections with *Escherichia coli* O157:H7 in Washington State: the first year of statewide disease surveillance. *JAMA* 1989;262:355–359.

60. Renwick SA, Wilson JB, Clarke RC, et al. Evidence of direct transmission of *Escherichia coli* O157:H7 infection between calves and a human. *J Infect Dis* 1993;168:792–793.

61. Centers for Disease Control. Update: Multistate outbreak of *Escherichia coli* O157:H7 infections from hamburgers—Western United States, 1992–1993. *MMWR* 1993;42:258–263.

62. Hedberg C, Belongia E, McFarland J, Soler J, Osterholm M, MacDonald K. Laboratory-based surveillance for *Escherichia coli* O157:H7 in Minnesota. Program and Abstracts of the 33rd Interscience Conference on Antimicrobial Agents and Chemotherapy, New Orleans, LA; 1993:353.

63. Marshall WF, McLimans CA, Van Scoy RE, Anhalt JP. Results of a 6-month survey of stool cultures for *Escherichia coli* O157:H7. *Mayo Clin Proc* 1990;65:787–792.

64. Pai CH, Ahmed N, Lior H, Johnson WM, Sims HV, Woods DE. Epidemiology of sporadic diarrhea due to verocytotoxin-producing *Escherichia coli*: a two-year prospective study. *J Infect Dis* 1988;157:1054–1057.

65. Gransden WR, Damm MAS, Anderson JD, Carter JE, Lior H. Further evidence associating hemolytic uremic syndrome with infection by verotoxin-producing *Escherichia coli* O157:H7. *J Infect Dis* 1986;154:522–524.

66. Cahoon FE, Thompson JS. Frequency of *Escherichia coli* O157:H7 isolation from stool specimens. *Can J Microbiol* 1987; 33:914–915.

67. Maher DP, Stanley PF. Verotoxin-producing *Escherichia coli*

infection in hospitalised patients with acute gastro-enteritis. *J Infect* 1991;24:220–221.

68. Pierard D, Van Etterijck R, Breynaert J, Moriau L, Lauwers S. Results of screening for verocytotoxin-producing *Escherichia coli* in faeces in Belgium. *Eur J Clin Microbiol Infect Dis* 1990;9:198–200.

69. Ong J, Zhe L, Robins-Browne R, Gapes M, O'Loughlin EV. Prevalence of verocytotoxigenic *Escherichia coli* serotype O157:H7 in children with diarrhoea attending a Sydney hospital. *J Paediatr Child Health* 1993;29:185–187.

70. Ratnam S, March SB. Sporadic occurrence of hemorrhagic colitis associated with *Escherichia coli* O157:H7 in Newfoundland. *Can Med Assoc J* 1986;134:43–46.

71. Ries A, Griffin P, Greene K, *Escherichia coli* O157:H7 study group. *Escherichia coli* O157:H7 diarrhea in the United States: a 10 center surveillance study. Program and Abstracts of the 33rd Interscience Conference on Antimicrobial Agents and Chemotherapy, New Orleans, LA; 1993:385.

72. Walker CW, Upson R, Warren RE. Haemorrhagic colitis: detection of verotoxin producing *Escherichia coli* O157 in a clinical microbiology laboratory. *J Clin Pathol* 1988;41:80–84.

73. Kleanthous H, Smith HR, Scotland SM, et al. Haemolytic uraemic syndromes in British Isles, 1985–8: association with verocytotoxin producing *Escherichia coli*. 2. Microbiological aspects. *Arch Dis Child* 1990;65:722–727.

74. Smith HR, Rowe B, Gross RJ, Fry NK, Scotland SM. Haemorrhagic colitis and verocytotoxin-producing *Escherichia coli* in England and Wales. *Lancet* 1987;1:1062–1064.

75. Kleanthous H, Fry NK, Smith HR, Gross RJ, Rowe B. The use of sorbitol–MacConkey agar in conjunction with a specific antiserum for the detection of Vero cytotoxin-producing strains of *Escherichia coli* O157. *Epidemiol Infect* 1988;101:327–335.

76. Chapman PA, Wright DJ, Norman P. Verotoxin-producing *Escherichia coli* infections in Sheffield: cattle as a possible source. *Epidemiol Infect* 1989;102:439–445.

77. Yamada S, Matsushita S, Kai A, et al. Detection of verocytotoxin from stool and serological testing of patients with diarrhea caused by *Escherichia coli* O157:H7. *Microbiol Immunol* 1993; 37:111–118.

78. Spriggs DR, Guerrant RL. Summary of the 27th United States–Japan joint conference on cholera and related diarrheal diseases. *J Infect Dis* 1992;167:1–6.

79. Verdier D, Mallet L, Terris G, Petite JP. Colite ischemique ''spontanee'': colite infectieuse ou medicamenteuse? *La Presse Medicale* 1992;23:891–894.

80. Gupta S, Soni NK, Kaur P, Sood DK. Verocytopathic activity of *Escherichia coli* O157 and other ''O'' serogroups isolated from patients of diarrhoea. *Indian J Med Res* 1992;95:71–76.

81. Capriolo A, Luzzi I, Rosmini F, et al. Hemolytic-uremic syndrome and Vero cytotoxin-producing *Escherichia coli* infection in Italy. *J Infect Dis* 1992;166:154–158.

82. Lerman Y, Cohen D, Gluck A, Ohad E, Sechter L. A cluster of cases of *Escherichia coli* O157 infection in a day-care center in a communal settlement (kibbutz) in Israel. *J Clin Microbiol* 1992;30:520–521.

83. Isaacson M, Canter PH, Effler P, Arntzen L, Bomans P, Heenan R. Haemorrhagic colitis epidemic in Africa. *Lancet* 1993; 341:961.

84. Ratnam S, March SB, Sprague WD, Severs D, Sullivan RM. Are humans a source of *Escherichia coli* O157:H7, the agent of hemorrhagic colitis? (letter). *N Engl J Med* 1986;315: 1612–1613.

85. Buchwald DS, Blaser MJ. A review of human salmonellosis. II. Duration of excretion following infection with nontyphi *Salmonella*. *Rev Infect Dis* 1984;6:345–356.

86. Ryan CA, Tauxe RV, Hosek GW, et al. *Escherichia coli* O157: H7 diarrhea in a nursing home: clinical, epidemiological, and pathological findings. *J Infect Dis* 1986;154:631–638.

87. Lopez EL, Diaz M, Grinstein S, et al. Hemolytic uremic syndrome and diarrhea in Argentine children: the role of Shiga-like toxins. *J Infect Dis* 1989;160:469–475.

88. Cordovez A, Prado V, Maggi L, et al. Enterohemorrhagic *Escherichia coli* associated with hemolytic-uremic syndrome in Chilean children. *J Clin Microbiol* 1992;30:2153–2157.

89. Kim K-H, Suh I-S, Kim JM, Kim CW, Cho Y-J. Etiology of childhood diarrhea in Korea. *J Clin Microbiol* 1989;27: 1192–1196.

90. Ostroff SM, Griffin PM, Tauxe RV, et al. A statewide outbreak of *Escherichia coli* O157:H7 infections in Washington State. *Am J Epidemiol* 1990;132:239–247.

91. Centers for Disease Control. Foodborne outbreak caused by *Escherichia coli* O157:H7—North Dakota. *MMWR* 1991;40: 265–267.

92. Belongia EA, MacDonald KL, Parham GL, et al. An outbreak of *Escherichia coli* O157:H7 colitis associated with consumption of precooked meat patties. *J Infect Dis* 1991;164:338–343.

93. Wells JG, Davis BR, Wachsmuth IK, et al. Laboratory investigation of hemorrhagic colitis outbreaks associated with a rare *Escherichia coli* serotype. *J Clin Microbiol* 1983;18:512–520.

94. Hockin J, Lior H, Mueller L, Davidson C, Ashton E, Wu F. An outbreak of *E. coli* O157:H7 diarrhea in a nursing home—Alberta. *Can Dis Week Rep* 1987;13–45:206.

95. Wells JG, Shipman LD, Greene KD, et al. Isolation of *Escherichia coli* serotype O157:H7 and other Shiga-like toxin-producing *E. coli* from dairy cattle. *J Clin Microbiol* 1991;29:985–989.

96. Lior H. Incidence of hemorrhagic colitis due to *Escherichia coli* in Canada. *Can Med Assoc J* 1988:1073–1074.

97. Read SC, Gyles CL, Clarke RC, Lior H, McEwen S. Prevalence of verocytotoxigenic *Escherichia coli* in ground beef, pork and chicken in southwestern Ontario. *Epidemiol Infect* 1990;105:11–20.

98. Kim MS, Doyle MP. Dipstick immunoassay to detect enterohemorrhagic *Escherichia coli* O157:H7 in retail ground beef. *Appl Envirn Microbiol* 1992;58:1764–1767.

99. Sekla L, Milley D, Stackiw W, Sisler J, Draw J, Sargent D. Verotoxin-producing *Escherichia coli* in ground beef in Manitoba. *Can Med Assoc J* 1990;143:519–521.

100. Padhye NV, Doyle MP. Rapid procedure for detecting enterohemorrhagic *Escherichia coli* O157:H7 in food. *Appl Envirn Microbiol* 1991;57:2693–2698.

101. Doyle MP, Schoeni JL. Isolation of *Escherichia coli* O157:H7 from retail fresh meats and poultry. *Appl Environ Microbiol* 1987;53:2394–2396.

102. McGowan KL, Wickersham E, Strockbine NA. *Escherichia coli* O157:H7 from water (letter). *Lancet* 1989;1:967–968.

103. Orskov F, Orskov I, Villar JA. Cattle as reservoir of verotoxin-producing *Escherichia coli* O157:H7 (letter). *Lancet* 1987;2: 276.

104. Gonzalez EA, Blanco J. Serotypes and antibiotic resistance of verotoxigenic (VTEC) and necrotizing (NTEC) *Escherichia coli* strains isolated from calves with diarrhoea. *FEMS Microbiol Lett* 1989;60:31–36.

105. Blanco M, Blanco J, Blanco JE, Ramos J. Enterotoxigenic, verotoxigenic, and necrotoxigenic *Escherichia coli* isolated from cattle in Spain. *Am J Vet Res* 1993;54:1446–1451.

106. Martin DR, Uhler PM, Okrend AJG, Chiu JY. Testing of bob calf fecal swabs for the presence of *Escherichia coli* O157:H7. *J Food Prot* 1994;57:70–72.

107. Hancock DD, Wells SJ, Thomas LA, et al. National prevalence study for *E. coli* O157:H7 in dairy calves. Abstracts of the Western States Food Animal Research Conference, Pullman Washington, March 1993(Suppl.).

108. Wilson JB, McEwen SA, Clarke RC, Leslie KE, Wilson RA, Waltner-Toews D. Distribution and characteristics of verocytotoxigenic *Escherichia coli* isolated from Ontario dairy cattle. *Epidemiol Infect* 1992;108:423–439.

109. Clarke R, McEwen S, Harnett N, Lior H, Gyles C. The prevalence of verotoxin—producing *Escherichia coli* (VETEC) in bovines at slaughter. Abstracts of the Annual Meeting of the American Society for Microbiology, Miami Beach, FL; 1988: 282.

110. Chapman PA, Siddons CA, Wright DJ, Norman P, Fox J, Crick E. Cattle as a possible source of verocytotoxin-producing *Escherichia coli* O157 infections in man. *Epidemiol Infect* 1993;111: 439–447.

111. Montenegro MA, Bulte M, Trumpf T, et al. Detection and characterization of fecal verotoxin-producing *Escherichia coli* from healthy cattle. *J Clin Microbiol* 1990;28:1417–1421.

112. Robins-Browne RM. Traditional enteropathogenic *Escherichia coli* of infantile diarrhea. *Rev Infect Dis* 1987;9:28–53.
113. Scotland SM, Willshaw GA, Smith HR, Rowe B. Properties of strains of *Escherichia coli* O26:H11 in relation to their enteropathogenic or enterohemorrhagic classification. *J Infect Dis* 1990;162:1069–1074.
114. Bitzan M, Karch H, Maas MG, et al. Clinical and genetic aspects of Shiga-like toxin production in traditional enteropathogenic *Escherichia coli*. *Zentralbl Bakteriol* 1991;274:496–506.
115. Willshaw GA, Scotland SM, Smith HR, Rowe B. Properties of Vero cytotoxin-producing *Escherichia coli* of human origin of O serogroups other than O157. *J Infect Dis* 1992;166:797–802.
116. Itoh T, Kai A, Saito K, et al. Gastroenteritis associated with verocytotoxin producing *Escherichia coli* O145:NM. In: Kuwahara S, Pierce NF, eds. *Advances in research on cholera and related diarrheas*. Tokyo: KTK; 1988:21–28.
117. Caprioli A, Luzzi I, Rosmini F, et al. Communitywide outbreak of hemolytic-uremic syndrome associated with non-O157 verocytotoxin-producing *Escherichia coli*. *J Infect Dis* 1994;169:208–211.
118. Ritchie M, Partington S, Jessop J, Kelly MT. Comparison of a direct fecal Shiga-like toxin assay and sorbitol–MacConkey agar culture for laboratory diagnosis of enterohemorrhagic *Escherichia coli* infection. *J Clin Microbiol* 1992;30:461–464.
119. Bokete TN, O'Callahan CM, Clausen CR, et al. Shiga-like toxin producing *Escherichia coli* in Seattle children: a prospective study. *Gastroenterology* 1993;105:1724–1731.
120. Bettelheim KA, Brown JE, Lolekha S, Echeverria P. Serotyes of *Escherichia coli* that hybridized with DNA probes for genes encoding Shiga-like toxin I, Shiga-like toxin II, and serogroup O157 enterohemorrhagic *E. coli* fimbriae isolated from adults with diarrhea in Thailand. *J Clin Microbiol* 1990;28:293–295.
121. Burnens AP, Boss P, Orskov F, et al. Occurrence and phenotypic properties of verotoxin producing *Escherichia coli* in sporadic cases of gastroenteritis. *Eur J Clin Microbiol Infect Dis* 1992;11:631–634.
122. Seriwatana J, Brown JE, Echeverria P, Taylor DN, Suthienkul O, Newland J. DNA probes to identify Shiga-like toxin I- and II-producing enteric bacterial pathogens isolated from patients with diarrhea in Thailand. *J Clin Microbiol* 1988;26:1614–1615.
123. Sunthadvanich R, Chiewsilp D, Seriwatana J, Sakazaki R, Echeverria P. Nationwide surveillance program to identify diarrhea-causing *Escherichia coli* in children in Thailand. *J Clin Microbiol* 1990;28:469–472.
124. Burke D, Al Jumaili BJ, Al Mardini H, Record CO. Culture negative cytotoxin positive stools in community acquired diarrhoea. *Gut* 1993;34:192–193.
125. Suthienkul O, Brown JE, Seriwatana J, Tienthongdee S, Sastravaha S, Echeverria P. Shiga-like toxin-producing *Escherichia coli* in retail meats and cattle in Thailand. *Appl Environ Microbiol* 1990;56:1135–1139.
126. Smith HR, Cheasty T, Roberts D, Thomas A, Rowe B. Examination of retail chickens and sausages in Britain for Vero cycotoxin-producing *Escherichia coli*. *Appl Environ Microbiol* 1991;57:2091–2093.
127. Tokhi AM, Peiris JSM, Scotland SM, Willshaw GA, Smith HR, Cheasty T. A longitudinal study of Vero cytotoxin producing *Escherichia coli* in cattle calves in Sri Lanka. *Epidemiol Infect* 1993;110:197–208.
128. Sramkova L, Bielaszewska M, Janda J, Blahova K, Hausner O. Vero cytotoxin-producing strains of *Escherichia coli* in children with haemolytic uraemic syndrome and diarrhoea in Czechoslovakia. *Infection* 1990;4:204–209.
129. Chart H, Smith HR, Scotland SM, Rowe B, Milford DV, Taylor CM. Serological identification of *Escherichia coli* O157:H7 infection in haemolytic uraemic syndrome. *Lancet* 1991;337:138–140.
130. Barrett TJ, Kaper JB, Jerse AE, Wachsmuth IK. Virulence factors in Shiga-like toxin-producing *Escherichia coli* isolated from humans and cattle. *J Infect Dis* 1992;165:979–980.
131. Beutin L, Montenegro MA, Orskov I, et al. Close association of verotoxin (Shiga-like toxin) production with enterohemolysin production in strains of *Escherichia coli*. *J Clin Microbiol* 1989;27:2559–2564.
132. Tzipori S, Gibson R, Montanaro J. Nature and distribution of mucosal lesions associated with enteropathogenic and enterohemorrhagic *Escherichia coli* in piglets and the role of plasmid-mediated factors. *Infect Immun* 1989;57:1142–1150.
133. Beachey EH. Bacterial adherence: adhesin-receptor interactions mediating the attachment of bacteria to mucosal surfaces. *J Infect Dis* 1981;143:325–345.
134. Zafriri D, Oron Y, Eisenstein BI, Ofek I. Growth advantage and enhanced toxicity of *Escherichia coli* adherent to tissue culture cells due to restricted diffusion of products secreted by the cells. *J Clin Invest* 1987;79:1210–1216.
135. Dytoc M, Soni R, Cockerill F, et al. Multiple determinants of verotoxin-producing *Escherichia coli* O157:H7 attachment-effacement. *Infect Immun* 1993;61:3382–3391.
136. Karch H, Heesemann J, Laufs R, O'Brien AD, Tacket CO, Levine MM. A plasmid of enterohemorrhagic *Escherichia coli* O157:H7 is required for expression of a new fimbrial antigen and for adhesion to epithelial cells. *Infect Immun* 1987;55:455–461.
137. Toth I, Barrett TJ, Cohen ML, Rumschlag HS, Green JH, Wachsmuth IK. Enzyme-linked immunosorbent assay for products of the 60-megadalton plasmid of *Escherichia coli* serotype O157:H7. *J Clin Microbiol* 1991;29:1016–1019.
138. Tzipori S, Karch H, Wachsmuth IK, et al. Role of a 60-megadalton plasmid and Shiga-like toxins in the pathogenesis of infection caused by enterohemorrhagic *Escherichia coli* O157:H7 in gnotobiotic piglets. *Infect Immun* 1987;55:3117–3125.
139. Wadolkowski EA, Burris JA, O'Brien AD. Mouse model for colonization and disease caused by enterohemorrhagic *Escherichia coli* O157:H7. *Infect Immun* 1990;58:2438–2445.
140. Ashkenazi S, Larocco M, Murray BE, Cleary TG. The adherence of verocytotoxin-producing *Escherichia coli* to rabbit intestinal cells. *J Med Microbiol* 1992;37:304–309.
141. Moon HW, Whipp SC, Argenzio RA, Levine MM, Giannella RA. Attaching and effacing activities of rabbit and human enteropathogenic *Escherichia coli* in pig and rabbit intestines. *Infect Immun* 1983;41:1340–1351.
142. Knutton S, Baldwin T, Williams PH, McNeish AS. Actin accumulation at sites of bacterial adhesion to tissue culture cells: basis of a new diagnostic test for enteropathogenic and enterohemorrhagic *Escherichia coli*. *Infect Immun* 1989;57:1290–1298.
143. Jerse AE, Yu J, Tall BD, Kaper JB. A genetic locus of enteropathogenic *Escherichia coli* necessary for the production of attaching and effacing lesions on tissue culture cells. *Proc Natl Acad Sci USA* 1990;87:7839–7843.
144. Yu J, Kaper JB. Cloning and characterization of the *eae* gene of enterohaemorrhagic *Escherichia coli* O157:H7. *Mol Microbiol* 1991;6:411–417.
145. Donnenberg MS, Tzoipori S, McKee ML, O'Brien AD, Alroy J, Kaper JB. The role of the *eae* gene of enterohemorrhagic *Escherichia coli* in intimate attachment in vitro and in a porcine model. *J Clin Invest* 1992;92:1418–1424.
146. Louie M, De Azavedo JCS, Handelsman MYC, et al. Expression and characterization of the *eaeA* gene product of *Escherichia coli* serotype O157:H7. *Infect Immun* 1993;61:4085–4092.
147. Isberg RR, Leong JM. Cultured mammalian cells attach to the invasin protein of *Yersinia pseudotuberculosis*. *Proc Natl Acad Sci* 1988;85:6682–6686.
148. Sherman P, Cockerill F, Soni R, Brunton J. Outer membranes are competitive inhibitors of *Escherichia coli* O157:H7 adherence to epithelial cells. *Infect Immun* 1991;59:890–899.
149. Karmali MA. Laboratory diagnosis of verotoxin-producing *Escherichia coli* infections. *Clin Microbiol Newslett* 1987;9:65–70.
150. Moyer MP, Dison PS, Rothman SW, Brown JE. Cytotoxicity of Shiga toxin for primary cultures of human colonic and ileal epithelial cells. *Infect Immun* 1987;55:1533–1535.
151. Keenan KP, Sharpnack DD, Collins H, Formal SB, O'Brien AD. Morphologic evaluation of the evaluation of Shiga toxin and *E. coli* Shiga-like toxin on the rabbit intestine. *Am J Pathol* 1986;125:69–80.
152. Barrett TJ, Potter ME, Wachsmuth IK. Continuous peritoneal

infusion of Shiga-like toxin II (SLT II) as a model for SLT II-induced diseases. *J Infect Dis* 1989;159:774–777.

153. Richardson SE, Rotman TA, Jay V, et al. Experimental verocytotoxemia in rabbits. *Infect Immun* 1992;60:4154–4167.

154. Padhye VV, Beery JT, Kittel FB, Doyle MP. Colonic hemorrhage produced in mice by a unique Vero cell cytotoxin from an *Escherichia coli* strain that causes hemorrhagic colitis. *J Infect Dis* 1987;155:1249–1253.

155. Levine MM, DuPont HL, Formal SB, et al. Pathogenesis of *Shigella dysenteriae* 1 (Shiga) dysentery. *J Infect Dis* 1973;127:261–270.

156. Fontaine A, Arondel J, Sansonetti PJ. Role of Shiga toxin in the pathogenesis of bacillary dysentery, studied by using a tox-negative mutant of *Shigella dysenteriae* 1. *Infect Immun* 1988;56:3099–3109.

157. Griffin PM, Olmstead LC, Petras RE. *Escherichia coli* O157:H7-associated colitis: a clinical and histological study of 11 cases. *Gastroenterology* 1990;99:142–149.

158. Barrett TJ, Potter ME, Strockbine NA. Evidence for macrophage participation in Shiga-like-toxin II-induced lethality in mice. *Microb Pathog* 1990;9:95–103.

159. Louise CB, Obrig TG. Shiga toxin-associated hemolytic-uremic syndrome: combined cytotoxic effects of Shiga toxin, interleukin-1 beta, and tumor necrosis factor alpha on human vascular endothelial cells in vitro. *Infect Immun* 1991;59:4173–4179.

160. van de Kar NCAJ, Monnens LAH, Karmali MA, van Hinsbergh VWM. Tumor necrosis factor and interleukin-1 induce expression of the verocytotoxin receptor globotriaosylceramide on human endothelial cells: implications for the pathogenesis of the hemolytic uremic syndrome. *Blood* 1992;80:2755–2764.

161. Kaye SA, Louise CB, Boyd B, Lingwood CA, Obrig TG. Shiga toxin-associated hemolytic uremic syndrome: interleukin-1B enhancement of Shiga toxin cytotoxicity toward human vascular endothelial cells in vitro. *Infect Immun* 1993;61:3886–3891.

162. Scotland SM, Willshaw GA, Smith HR, Rowe B. Properties of strains of *Escherichia coli* belonging to serogroup O157 with special reference to production of vero cytotoxins VT1 and VT2. *Epidemiol Infect* 1987;99:613–624.

163. Butler T, Islam MR, Azad MAK, Jones PK. Risk factors for development of hemolytic uremic syndrome during shigellosis. *Pediatrics* 1987;110:894–897.

164. Fong JSC, de Chadarevian J-P, Kaplan BS. Hemolytic-uremic syndrome. Current concepts and management. *Pediatr Clin North Am* 1982;29:835–856.

165. Richardson SE, Karmali MA, Becker LE, Smith CR. The histopathology of the hemolytic uremic syndrome associated with verocytotoxin-producing *Escherichia coli* infections. *Hum Pathol* 1988;19:1102–1108.

166. Obrig TG, Del Vecchio PJ, Brown JE, et al. Direct cytotoxic action of Shiga toxin on human vascular endothelial cells. *Infect Immun* 1988;56:2373–2378.

167. Tesh VL, Samuel JE, Perera LP, Sharefkin JB, O'Brien AD. Evaluation of the role of Shiga and Shiga-like toxins in mediating direct damage to human vascular endothelial cells. *J Infect Dis* 1991;164:344–352.

168. Boyd B, Lingwood C. Verotoxin receptor glycolipid in human renal tissue. *Nephron* 1989;51:207–210.

169. Siegler RL, Griffin PM, Barrett TJ, Strockbine NA. Recurrent hemolytic uremic syndrome secondary to *Escherichia coli* O157:H7 infection. *Pediatrics* 1993;91:666–668.

170. Robson WLM, Leung AK, Miller-Hughes DJ. Recurrent hemorrhagic colitis caused by *Escherichia coli* O157:H7. *Pediatr Infect Dis J* 1993;12:699–701.

171. Potter ME, Kaufmann AF, Thomason BM, Blake PA, Farmer JJ. Diarrhea due to *Escherichia coli* O157:H7 in the infant rabbit. *J Infect Dis* 1985;152:1341–1343.

172. Pai CH, Kelly JK, Meyers GL. Experimental infection of infant rabbits with verotoxin-producing *Escherichia coli*. *Infect Immun* 1986;51:16–23.

173. Tzipori S, Wachsmuth IK, Chapman C, et al. The pathogenesis of hemorrhagic colitis caused by *Escherichia coli* O157:H7 in gnotobiotic piglets. *J Infect Dis* 1986;154:712–716.

174. Zoja C, Corna D, Farina C, et al. Verotoxin glycolipid receptors determine the localization of micrangiopathic process in rabbits given verotoxin-1. *J Lab Clin Med* 1992;120:229–238.

175. Wadolkowski EA, Sung LM, Burris JA, Samuel JE, O'Brien AD. Acute renal tubular necrosis and death of mice orally infected with *Escherichia coli* strains that produce Shiga-like toxin type II. *Infect Immun* 1990;58:3959–3965.

176. Tesh VL, Burris JA, Owens JW, et al. Comparison of the relative toxicities of Shiga-like toxins type I and type II for mice. *Infect Immun* 1993;61:3392–3402.

177. Francis DH, Moxley RA, Andraos CY. Edema disease-like brain lesions in gnotobiotic piglets infected with *Escherichia coli* serotype O157:H7. *Infect Immun* 1989;57:1339–1342.

178. Imberechts H, De Greve H, Hernalsteens J-P, et al. The role of adhesive F107 fimbriae and of SLT-IIv toxin in the pathogenesis of edema disease in pigs. *Zentralbl Bakteriol* 1993;278:445–450.

179. Kausche FM, Dean EA, Arp LH, Samuel JE, Moon HW. An experimental model for subclinical edema disease (*Escherichia coli* enterotoxemia) manifest as vascular necrosis in pigs. *Am J Vet Res* 1992;53:281–287.

180. Marques LRM, Peiris JSM, Cryz SJ, O'Brien AD. *Escherichia coli* strains isolated from pigs with edema disease produce a variant of Shiga-like toxin II. *FEMS Microbiol Lett* 1987;44:33–48.

181. MacLeod DL, Gyles CL, Wilcock BP. Reproduction of edema disease of swine with purified Shiga-like toxin II variant. *Vet Pathol* 1991;28:66–73.

182. Barrett TJ, Potter ME, Wachsmuth IK. Bacterial endotoxin both enhances and inhibits the toxicity of Shiga-like toxin II in rabbits and mice. *Infect Immun* 1989;57:3434–3437.

183. Barrett TJ, Green JH, Griffin PM, Pavia AT, Ostroff SM, Wachsmuth IK. Enzyme-linked immunosorbent assay for detecting antibodies to Shiga-like toxin I, Shiga-like toxin II, and *Escherichia coli* O157:H7 lipopolysaccharide in human serum. *Curr Microbiol* 1991;23:189–195.

184. Sherwood D, Snodgrass DR, O'Brien AD. Shiga-like toxin production from *Escherichia coli* associated with calf diarrhoea. *Vet Rec* 1985;116:217–218.

185. Janke BH, Francis DH, Collins JE, et al. Attaching and effacing *Escherichia coli* infection as a cause of diarrhea in young calves. *JAMA* 1990;196:897–901.

186. Tzipori S, Wachsmuth IK, Smithers J, Jackson C. Studies in gnotobiotic piglets on non-O157:H7 *Escherichia coli* serotypes isolated from patients with hemorrhagic colitis. *Gastroenterology* 1988;94:590–597.

187. Lindgren SW, Melton AR, O'Brien AD. Virulence of enterohemorrhagic *Escherichia coli* O91:H21 clinical isolates in an orally infected mouse model. *Infect Immun* 1993;61:3832–3842.

188. Hunt CM, Harvey JA, Youngs ER, Irwin ST, Reid TM. Clinical and pathological variability of infection by enterohaemorrhagic (Vero cytotoxin producing) *Escherichia coli*. *J Clin Pathol* 1989;42:847–852.

189. Griffin PM, Ostroff SM, Tauxe RV, et al. Illnesses associated with *Escherichia coli* O157:H7 infections. *Ann Intern Med* 1988;109:705–712.

190. Cimolai N, Anderson JD, Bhanji NMF, Chen L, Blair GK. *Escherichia coli* O157:H7 infections associated with perforated appendicitis and chronic diarrhoea. *Eur J Pediatr* 1990;149:259–260.

191. MacDonald KL, O'Leary MJ, Cohen ML, et al. *Escherichia coli* O157:H7, an emerging gastrointestinal pathogen. Results of a one-year, prospective, population-based study. *JAMA* 1988;259(24):3567–3570.

192. Riley LW. The epidemiologic, clinical, and microbiologic features of hemorrhagic colitis. *Ann Rev Microbiol* 1987;41:383–407.

193. Levin M, Walters MDS, Barratt TM. Hemolytic uremic syndrome. In: Arnoff SC, Hughes WT, Kehl S, Speck WT, Wald ER eds. *Advances in pediatric infectious diseases*. Vol 4. Chicago: Year Book; 1989:51–81.

194. de la Hunt MN, Morris KP, Coulthard MG, Rangecroft L. Oesophageal and severe gut involvement in the haemolytic uraemic syndrome. *Br J Surg* 1991;78:1469–1472.

195. Lopez EL, Devoto S, Woloj M, Pickering LK, Cleary TG. Intussusception associated with *Escherichia coli* O157:H7. *Pediatr Infect Dis J* 1989;8:471–473.

196. Tarr PI, Weinberger E, Hatch EI, Christie DL. Bacterial ileocecitis caused by *Escherichia coli* O157:H7. *J Pediatr Gastroenterol Nutr* 1992;14:261–263.

197. Vickers D, Morris K, Coulthard MG, Eastham EJ. Anal signs in haemolytic uraemic syndrome (letter). *Lancet* 1988;1:998.

198. Gransden WR, Damm MAS, Anderson JD, Carter JE, Lior H. Haemorrhagic cystitis and balanitis associated with verotoxin-producing *Escherichia coli* O157:H7 (letter). *Lancet* 1985;2:150.

199. Harris AA, Kaplan RL, Goodman LJ, et al. Results of a screening method used in a 12-month stool survey for *Escherichia coli* O157:H7. *J Infect Dis* 1985;152:775–777.

200. Krishnan C, Fitzgerald VA, Dakin SJ, Behme RJ. Laboratory investigation of outbreak of hemorrhagic colitis caused by *Escherichia coli* O157:H7. *J Clin Microbiol* 1987;25:1043–1047.

201. Sonnino RE, Laberge J-M, Mucklow MG, Moir CR. Pathogenic *Escherichia coil*: a new etiology for acute ileitis in children. *J Pediatr Surg* 1989;24:812–814.

202. Bettelheim KA, Goldwater PN, Evangelidis H, Pearce JL, Smith DL. Distribution of toxigenic *Escherichia coli* serotypes in the intestines of infants. *Comp Immun Microbiol Infect Dis* 1992;15:65–70.

203. Ljungh A, Eriksson M, Eriksson O, Henter JI, Wadstrom T. Shiga-like toxin production and connective tissue protein binding of *Escherichia coli* isolated from a patient with ulcerative colitis. *Scand J Infect Dis* 1988;20:443–446.

204. Von Wulffen H, Russmann H, Karch H, et al. Verocytotoxin-producing *Escherichia coli* O2:H5 isolated from patients with ulcerative colitis (letter). *Lancet* 1989;1:1449–1450.

205. Parsonnet J, Griffin PM. Hemolytic uremic syndrome: clinical picture and bacterial connection. In: Remington JS, Swartz MN, eds. *Current clinical topics in infectious diseases.* Boston: Blackwell Scientific; 1993:172–187.

206. Gasser C, Gautier E, Steck A, Siebenmann RE, Oechslin R. Hamolytisch-uramische syndrome: bilaterale nierenrindennekrosen bei akuten erworbenen hamolytischen anamien. *Schweiz Med Wochenschr* 1955;85:205–209.

207. Martin DL, MacDonald KL, White KE, Soler JT, Osterholm MT. The epidemiology and clinical aspects of the hemolytic uremic syndrome in Minnesota. *N Engl J Med* 1990;323:1161–1167.

208. Milford DV, Taylor CM, Guttridge B, Hall SM, Rowe B, Kleanthous H. Haemolytic uraemic syndromes in the British Isles 1985–8: association with verocytotoxin producing *Escherichia coli.* 1. Clinical and epidemiological aspects. *Arch Dis Child* 1990;65:716–721.

209. Rowe PC, Orrbine E, Wells GA, McLaine PN, Members of the Canadian Pediatric Kidney Disease Reference Centre. Epidemiology of hemolytic uremic syndrome in Canadian children from 1986–1988. *J Pediatr* 1991;119:218–224.

210. Koster F, Levin J, Walker L, et al. Hemolytic-uremic syndrome after shigellosis. Relation to endotoxemia and circulating immune complexes. *N Engl J Med* 1978;298:927–33.

211. Siegler RL, Pavia AT, Christofferson RD, Milligan MK. A 20 year population-based study of post-diarrheal hemolytic uremic syndrome in Utah. *Pediatrics* 1994;94:35–40.

212. Amorosi EL, Ultmann JE. Thrombotic thrombocytopenic purpura: report of 16 cases and review of the literature. *Medicine* 1966;45:139–159.

213. Remuzzi G, Garella S. HUS and TTP: Variable expression of a single entity. *Kidney Int* 1987;32:292–308.

214. Ridolfi RL, Bell WR. Thrombotic thrombocytopenic purpura: report of 25 cases and review of the literature. *Medicine* 1981;60:413–428.

215. Tarr PI, Neill MA, Clausen CR, Watkins SL, Christie DL, Hickman RO. *Escherichia coli* O157:H7 and the hemolytic uremic syndrome: importance of early cultures in establishing the etiology. *J Infect Dis* 1990;162:553–556.

216. Bitzan M, Ludwig K, Klemt M, Konig H, Buren J, Muller-Wiefel DE. The role of *Escherichia coli* O157 infections in the classical (enteropathic) haemolytic uraemic syndrome: results of a Central European, multicentre study. *Epidemiol Infect* 1993;110:183–196.

217. Rowe PC, Orrbine E, Lior H, Wells GA, McLaine PN, CPKDRC co-investigators. A prospective study of exposure to verotoxin-producing *Escherichia coli* among Canadian children with haemolytic uraemic syndrome. *Epidemiol Infect* 1993;110:1–7.

218. Neill MA, Tarr PL, Clausen CR, Christie DL, Hickman RO. *Escherichia coli* O157:H7 as the predominant pathogen associated with the hemolytic uremic syndrome: a prospective study in the Pacific Northwest. *Pediatrics* 1987;80:37–40.

219. Windler F, Weh HJ, Hossfeld DK, et al. Verotoxin in thrombotic thrombocytopenic purpura. *Eur J Haematol* 1988;42:103.

220. Farina C, Gavazzeni G, Caprioli A, Remuzzi G. Hemolytic uremic syndrome associated with verocytotoxin-producing *Escherichia coli* infection in acquired immunodeficiency syndrome. *Blood* 1990;75:2465–2468.

221. Ornt DB, Griffin PM, Wells JG, Powell KR. Hemolytic uremic syndrome due to *Escherichia coli* O157:H7 in a child with multiple infections. *Pediatr Nephrol* 1992;6:270–272.

222. Henningsen K. Investigations on the bloodfactor P. *Acta Pathol Scand* 1949;26:639–654.

223. Sanger R. An association between the P and Jay systems of blood groups. *Nature* 1955;176:1163–1164.

224. Taylor CM, Milford DV, Rose PE, Roy TCF, Rowe B. The expression of blood group P1 in post-enteropathic haemolytic uraemic syndrome. *Pediatr Nephrol* 1990;4:59–61.

225. Boyd B, Tyrrell G, Maloney M, Gyles C, Brunton J, Lingwood C. Alteration of the glycolipid binding specificity of the pig edema toxin from globotetraosyl to globotriaosyl ceramide alters in vivo tissue targetting and results in a verotoxin 1-like disease in pigs. *J Exp Med* 1993;177:1745–1753.

226. Newburg DS, Chaturvedi P, Lopez EL, Devoto S, Fayad A, Cleary TG. Susceptibility to hemolytic-uremic syndrome relates to erythrocyte glycosphingolipid patterns. *J Infect Dis* 1993;168:476–479.

227. Chapman PA. Evaluation of commercial latex slide test for identifying *Escherichia coli* O157. *J Clin Pathol* 1989;42:1109–1110.

228. Tison DL. Culture confirmation of *Escherichia coli* serotype O157:H7 by direct immunofluorescence. *J Clin Microbiol* 1990;28:612–613.

229. Borczyk AA, Harnett N, Lombos M, Lior H. False-positive identification of *Escherichia coli* O157 by commercial latex agglutination tests. *Lancet* 1990;336:946–947.

230. Corbel MJ. Recent advances in the study of *Brucella* antigens and their serological cross-reactions. *Vet Bull* 1985;55:927–942.

231. Bettelheim KA, Evangelidis H, Pearce JL, Sowers E, Strockbine NA. Isolation of a *Citrobacter freundii* strain which carries the *Escherichia coli* O157 antigen. *J Clin Microbiol* 1993;31:760–761.

232. Lior H, Borczyk AA. False positive identifications of *Escherichia coli* O157 (letter). *Lancet* 1987;1:333.

233. Brenner DJ, Davis BR, Steigerwalt AG, et al. Atypical biogroups of *Escherichia coli* found in clinical specimens and description of *Escherichia hermannii* sp. nov. *J Clin Microbiol* 1982;15:703–713.

234. Chapman PA, Siddons CA, Zadik PM, Jewes L. An improved selective medium for the isolation of *Escherichia coli* O157. *J Med Microbiol* 1991;35:107–110.

235. Zadik PM, Chapman PA, Siddons CA. Use of tellurite for the selection of verocytotoxigenic *Escherichia coli.* *J Med Microbiol* 1993;39:155–158.

236. Smith HR, Scotland SM. Isolation and identification methods for *Escherichia coli* O157 and other Vero cytotoxin producing strains. *J Clin Pathol* 1993;46:10–17.

237. Scotland SM, Willshaw GA, Cheasty T, Rowe B. Strains of *Escherichia coli* O157:H8 from human diarrhoea belong to attaching and effacing class of *E. coli.* *J Clin Pathol* 1992;45:1075–1078.

238. Borczyk AA, Lior H, Thompson S. Sorbitol-negative *Escherichia coli* O157 other than H7. *J Infect* 1989;18:198–199.

239. Karch H, Meyer T, Russmann H, Heesemann J. Frequent loss

of Shiga-like toxin genes in clinical isolates of *Escherichia coli* upon subcultivation. *Infect Immun* 1992;60:3464–3467.

240. Khakharia R, Duck D, Lior H. Extended phage-typing scheme for *Escherichia coli* O157:H7. *Epidemiol Infect* 1990;105: 511–520.

241. Frost JA, Cheasty T, Thomas A, Rowe B. Phage typing of Vero cytotoxin-producing *Escherichia coli* O157 isolated in the United Kingdom: 1989–1991. *Epidemiol Infect* 1993;110: 469–475.

242. Park CH, Hixon DL, Morrison WL, Cook CB. Rapid diagnosis of enterohemorrhagic *Escherichia coli* O157:H7 directly from fecal specimens using immunofluorescence stain. *Am J Clin Pathol* 1994;101:91–94.

243. Newland JW, Neill RJ. DNA probes for Shiga-like toxins I and II and for toxin-converting bacteriophages. *J Clin Microbiol* 1988;26:1292–1297.

244. Read SC, Clarke RC, Martin A, et al. Polymerase chain reaction for detection of verocytotoxigenic *Escherichia coli* isolated from animal and food sources. *Mol Cell Probes* 1992;6:153–161.

245. Chart H, Scotland SM, Rowe B. Serum antibodies to *Escherichia coli* serotype O157:H7 in patients with hemolytic uremic syndrome. *J Clin Microbiol* 1989;27:285–290.

246. Chart H, Rowe B. Improved detection of infection by *Escherichia coli* O157 in patients with haemolytic uraemic syndrome by means of IgA antibodies to lipopolysaccharide. *J Infect* 1992;24:257–261.

247. Bitzan M, Karch H. Indirect hemagglutination assay for diagnosis of *Escherichia coli* O157 infection in patient with hemolytic-uremic syndrome. *J Clin Microbiol* 1992;30:1174–1178.

248. Bitzan M, Moebius E, Ludwig K, Muller-Wiefel DE, Heesemann J, Karch H. High incidence of serum antibodies to *Escherichia coli* O157 lipopolysaccharide in children with hemolytic-uremic syndrome. *J Pediatr* 1991;119:380–385.

249. Siddons CA, Chapman PA. Detection of faecal IgA in the diagnosis of infection by *Escherichia coli* O157 (letter). *J Infection* 1993;26:343–344.

250. Chart H, Cheasty T, Cope D, Gross RJ, Rowe B. The serological relationship between *Yersinia enterocolitica* O9 and *Escherichia coli* O157 using sera from patients with yersiniosis and haemolytic uraemic syndrome. *Epidemiol Infect* 1991;107: 349–356.

251. Notenboom RH, Borczyk A, Karmali MA, Duncan LMC. Clinical relevance of a serological cross-reaction between *Escherichia coli* O157 and *Brucella abortus*. *Lancet* 1987;2:745.

252. Chart H, Rowe B. Antibody cross-reactions with lipopolysaccharide from *E. coli* O157 after cholera vaccination. *Lancet* 1993;341:1282.

253. Bitzan M, Klemt M, Steffens R, Muller-Wiefel DE. Differences in verotoxin neutralizing activity of therapeutic immunoglobulins and sera from healthy controls. *Infection* 1993;21:140–145.

254. Cimolai N, Anderson JD, Morrison BJ. Antibiotics for *Escherichia coli* O157:H7 enteritis? *J Antimicrob Chemother* 1989; 23:807–808.

255. Prouix F, Turgeon JP, Delage G, Lafleur L, Chicoine L. Randomized, controlled trial of antibiotic therapy for *Escherichia coli* O157:H7 enteritis. *J Pediatr* 1992;121:299–303.

256. Cimolai N, Carter JE, Morrison BJ, Anderson JD. Risk factors for the progression of *Escherichia coli* O157:H7 enteritis to hemolytic-uremic syndrome. *J Pediatr* 1990;116:589–592.

257. Karch H, Goroncy-Bermes P, Opferkuch W, Kroll H-P, O'Brien A. Subinhibitory concentrations of antibiotics modulate amount of Shiga-like toxin produced by *Escherichia coli*. In: Adam D, Hahn H, Opferkuch W, eds. *The influence of antibiotics on the host–parasite relationship*. Vol 2. Berlin: Springer-Verlag; 1985.

258. Karch H, Strockbine NA, O'Brien AD. Growth of *Escherichia coli* in the presence of trimethoprim-sulfamethoxazole facilitates detection of Shiga-like toxin producing strains by colony blot assay. *FEMS Microbiol Lett* 1986;35:141–145.

259. Walterspiel JN, Ashkenazi S, Morrow AL, Cleary TG. Effect of subinhibitory concentrations of antibiotics on extracellular Shiga-like toxin I. *Infection* 1992;20:25–29.

260. Cohen J, McConnell JS. Release of endotoxin from bacteria exposed to ciprofloxacin and its prevention with polymyxin B. *Eur J Clin Microbiol Infect Dis* 1986;5:13–17.

261. Parsonnet J, Greene KD, Gerber RA, Tauxe RV, Aguilar OJV, Blake PA. *Shigella dysenteriae* type 1 infections in US travellers to Mexico. *Lancet* 1989;2:543–545.

262. Salazar-Lindo E, Sack RB, Chea-Woo E, et al. Early treatment with erythromycin of *Campylobacter jejuni* associated dysentery in children. *J Pediatr* 1986;109:355–360.

263. DuPont HL, Hornick RB. Adverse effect of Lomotil therapy in shigellosis. *JAMA* 1973;226:1525–1528.

264. Cimolai N, Morrison BJ, Carter JE. Risk factors for the central nervous system manifestations of gastroenteritis-associated hemolytic-uremic syndrome. *Pediatrics* 1992;90:616–621.

265. Ostroff SM, Kobayashi JM, Lewis JH. Epidemiology and complications of *Escherichia coli* O157:H7 infections (letter). *JAMA* 1989;262:3408.

266. MacLeod DL, Gyles CL. Immunization of pigs with a purified Shiga-like toxin II variant toxoid. *Vet Microbiol* 1991;29: 309–318.

267. Siegler RL. Management of hemolytic-uremic syndrome. *J Pediatr* 1988;112:1014–1020.

268. Stiehm ER, Ashida E, Kim KS, Winston DJ, Haas A, Gale RP. Intravenous immunoglobulins as therapeutic agents. *Ann Intern Med* 1987;107:367–382.

269. Tacket CO, Shandera WX, Mann JM, Hargrett NT, Blake PA. Equine antitoxin use and other factors that predict outcome in type A foodborne botulism. *Am J Med* 1984;76:794–798.

270. Havens PL, Dunne WM, Burd EM. Effects of human intravenous immune globulin on diarrhea caused by Shiga-like toxin I and Shiga-like toxin II in infant rabbits. *Microbiol Immunol* 1992;36:1077–1085.

271. Ashkenazi S, Cleary TG, Lopez E, Pickering LK. Anticytotoxin-neutralizing antibiodies in immune globulin preparations: potential use in hemolytic-uremic syndrome. *J Pediatr* 1988; 113:1008–1014.

272. Committee on the Scientific Basis of the Nation's Meat and Poultry Inspection Program. Meat and poultry inspection. The scientific basis of the nation's program. Washington, DC: National Academy Press; 1985:90.

273. Beery JT, Doyle MP, Schoeni JL. Colonization of chicken cecae by *Escherichia coli* associated with hemorrhagic colitis. *Appl Environ Microbiol* 1985;49:310–315.

274. Stavric S, Buchanan B, Gleeson TM. Intestinal colonization of young chicks with *Escherichia coli* O157:H7 and other verotoxin-producing serotypes. *J Appl Bacteriol* 1993;74:557–563.

275. USDA. 9 CFR parts 318 and 320. Heat processing, cooking, and cooling, handling and storage requirements for uncured meat patties; rule. *Fed Reg* 1993;58:41138–41152.

276. Mossel DAA, Struijk CB. Food-borne illness 1993: updating Wilson's triad. *Lancet* 1993;342:1254.

277. Thayer DW, Boyd G. Elimination of *Escherichia coli* O157:H7 in meats by gamma irradiation. *Appl Environ Microbiol* 1993; 59:1030–1034.

278. American Public Health Association v. Butz, 511 F.2d 331 (D.C. Cir. 1974).

279. USDA. 9 CFR parts 317 and 381. Mandatory safe handling, statements on labeling of raw meat and poultry products: final rule. *Fed Reg* 59:14528–14540.

280. Kaplan BS, Katz J, Krawitz S, Lurie A. An analysis of the results of therapy in 67 cases of the hemolytic-uremic syndrome. *J Pediatr* 1971;78:420–425.

281. Keene WE, McAnulty JM, Hoesly FC, et al. A swimming-associated outbreak of hemorrhagic colitis caused by *Escherichia Coli* O157:H7 and *Shigella sonnei*. *N Engl J Med* 1994; 331:579–584.

282. Oregon Health Division. *Escherichia coli* O157:H7 outbreak traced to raw milk. *CD Summary* 1993;42:1–2.

283. Scotland SM, Rowe B, Smith HR, Willshaw GA, Gross RJ. Vero cytotoxin-producing strains of *Escherichia coli* from children with haemolytic uraemic syndrome and their detection by specific DNA probes. *J Med Microbiol* 1988;25:237–243.

284. Rivas M, Voyer LE, Tous MI, et al. Deteccion de *Escherichia coli* O157 productor de verotoxina en pacientes con sindrome uremico hemolitico. *Medicina—Buenos Aires* 1990;50:571.

Infections of the Gastrointestinal Tract,
edited by M. J. Blaser, P. D. Smith, J. I. Ravdin,
H. B. Greenberg, and R. L. Guerrant
Raven Press, Ltd., New York © 1995.

CHAPTER 53

Shigella and Enteroinvasive *Escherichia coli*

David W. K. Acheson and Gerald T. Keusch

Shigella dysenteriae type I, originally known as Shiga's bacillus, was first isolated by Kiyoshi Shiga in 1898 (1) during an epidemic of severe dysentery in Japan in 1896, involving nearly 90,000 cases, with a mortality rate approaching 30%. The initial description of the distinctive gram-negative rod that now bears his name included the demonstration that infected patients developed agglutinating antibodies and thus superseded prior descriptions of what was probably the same organism. Other workers quickly confirmed the presence of *S. dysenteriae* type 1 in other parts of the world (2,3) and over the subsequent 40 years described related but antigenically and biochemically distinctive organisms, now known as *S. flexneri, S. boydii*, and *S. sonnei*.

In 1900 Flexner reported that injections of killed *Shigella* cultures were able to cause illness and death in animals and he concluded that the disease was caused by "a toxic agent rather than infection per se" (2). In retrospect Flexner was probably seeing the effects of lipopolysaccharide (LPS) endotoxin, and for many years thereafter contamination of protein "toxins" with LPS continued to confuse the interpretation of experiments using cell-free toxin preparations. In 1903 Conradi (4) demonstrated the presence of a "toxin" in autolysates of 18-hr cultures of *S. dysenteriae* type 1, which resulted in diarrhea, as well as paralysis and death, in rabbits within 48–72 hr following intravenous injection. Because of the latter manifestations, this activity became known as Shiga neurotoxin. Todd (5) found that *S. paradysenteriae* Flexner (*S. flexneri*) filtrates caused diarrhea but not paralysis, and suggested that the production of neurotoxin differed between members of the *Shigella* genus.

Over the subsequent 50 years the microbiology and epidemiology of *Shigella* species were clarified, culminating in the recommendations of the Congress of the International Association of Microbiologists Shigella Commission in 1950 that *Shigella* be adopted as the generic name (6). Since then, the mechanisms whereby *Shigella* cause

disease have been intensively investigated and the roles of cell invasion and toxins explored (7,8). Over the past decade in particular, there has been an explosion in our understanding of the genetic elements involved in *Shigella* virulence. In addition, the group of *Shigella*-like enteroinvasive *E. coli* (EIEC) has been identified and shown to possess a 140-MDa invasion plasmid encoding virulence genes that appear to be identical to *Shigella* virulence genes. This is not surprising since EIEC are taxonomically more closely related to *Shigella* than to other *E. coli*. For these reasons, EIEC are briefly considered in this chapter.

MICROBIOLOGY

Shigella belong to the family Enterobacteriaceae, tribe Escherichiae, and genus *Shigella*, and closely resemble *E. coli* at the genetic level. There are four species of *Shigella* (*S. dysenteriae, S. flexneri, S. boydii*, and *S. sonnei*), which are differentiated by group-specific polysaccharide antigens of LPS, designated A, B, C, and D respectively, biochemical properties (9) (Table 1), and phage or colicin susceptibility. *Shigella* do not possess flagella, are nonmotile, and express no H antigens useful for diagnosis or for the targeting of immunological interventions. *S. dysenteriae* consists of 10 antigenic types of which type 1, also known as *S. shigae* or Shiga's bacillus, produces a potent protein synthesis-inhibiting cytotoxin called Shiga toxin. *S. flexneri* is divided into 6 types and 14 subtypes, each possessing type- and subtype-specific antigens. *S. boydii* includes 18 serological types, and while there is only one *S. sonnei* serotype, there are at least 20 colicin types. *Shigella* are gram-negative, nonencapsulated bacilli and are typically non–lactose-fermenting, non–gas-producing (with rare exceptions), and lysine decarboxylase-, acetate-, and mucate-negative. The exceptions are *S. sonnei*, which ferments lactose slowly and can be mucate positive, and *S. flexneri* 6 and *S. boydii* 13, which produce gas from glucose. Because *Shigella* species are biochemically very similar, in practice differentiation among species depends on serological methods

D. W. K. Acheson and G. T. Keusch: Division of Geographic Medicine and Infectious Diseases, Tufts University School of Medicine–New England Medical Center, Boston, Massachusetts 02111.

TABLE 1. *Comparison of biochemical characteristics of* Shigella *and* Escherichia coli

Test or substrate	Result for *Shigella* (% positive)	Result for *E. coli* (% positive)
Acetate	−	+ (84)
Adonitol	−	−
Argine decarboxylase	− (8)	Variable (17)
Citrate	−	Variable (24)
DNase	−	−
Esculin	−	Variable (31)
Gas from glucose[a]	− (<1–2)	+ (91)
Hydrogen sulfide on TSI agar	−	−
Indole	Variable (38)	+ (99)
Inositol	−	−
KCN	−	−
Lactose fermentation[b]	− (<1–2)	+ (91)
Lysine decarboxylase	−	+ (90)
Malonate	−	−
Mannitol	+ (except *S. dysenteriae*)	+
Methyl red	+	+
Motility	−	+ (80)
Mucate	−	+ (92)
Ornithine decarboxylase[c]	Variable (20–23)	+ (63)
Phenylalanine deaminase	−	−
Salicin	−	+ (40)
Sucrose	− (<1–2)	+ (50)
Urease	−	−
Voges–Proskauer	−	−
Xylose	− (2–5)	+ (95)

Adapted from ref. 9.
[a] Some *S. flexneri* 6 produce gas from glucose.
[b] *S. sonnei* usually ferment lactose or sucrose after several days in culture.
[c] Some *S. sonnei* decarboxylate ornithine.

using group- and type-specific antisera. However, all commercially available antisera are not equally sensitive or specific, especially for detection of *S. flexneri* (10). Monoclonal antibodies offer a more reliable alternative but are not yet commercially available (11).

TABLE 2. *Biochemical characteristics of* Shigella *and EIEC*

Characteristic	*E. coli*[a] (% positive)	EIEC[b] (% positive)	*Shigella*[a] (% positive)
Lysine decarboxylase	89	0	0
Christensen citrate	95	8.3	0
Motility	69	7.2[c]	0
Lactose	90	30.9	0.3

[a] Data from ref. 13.
[b] Data from ref. 14.
[c] Primarily serotype O124.

Most EIEC serogroups share antigenic specificities with *Shigella* serovars (12), and are physiologically similar as well in that they are consistently lysine decarboxylase–negative, nonmotile (except for O124), and often lactose-negative (13–15) (Table 2).

EPIDEMIOLOGY

Shigellosis occurs throughout the world. The organisms are highly host-adapted and naturally infect only humans and some nonhuman primates. Although point source food- and water-associated outbreaks do occur, most transmission is via person-to-person contact (16). *S. flexneri* and *S. dysenteriae* type 1 are at present the predominant species causing disease in developing countries, whereas *S. sonnei* is the major isolate in developed countries, accounting for over three quarters of the isolates in the United States. The fourth species, *S. boydii*, is uncommonly encountered except in the Indian subcontinent, where it was first identified.

One of the most striking features of shigellosis, in contrast to other enteric pathogens, is the exceedingly small inoculum of organisms necessary to cause disease. As few as 10–100 organisms of the most virulent of the genus, *S. dysenteriae* type 1, are sufficient to cause clinical dysentery in an otherwise healthy adult (17). While the other species may require an inoculum 10–100 times greater, this is still readily transmitted directly, as by fecal contamination of the hands. As a consequence, approximately 20% of persons in a household acquire infection when an index case is identified in a family (18). For the same reason, person-to-person spread of shigellosis has been common in children institutionalized because of retardation or other handicaps that may impair maintaining adequate personal hygiene.

Although distributed worldwide, prevalence of shigellosis differs from place to place. It is prominently associated with poverty, overcrowding, poor personal hygiene, inadequate water supplies and malnutrition, conditions that characterize developing countries and disadvantaged populations of developed countries. In the former setting, the estimated incidence of shigellosis is 750–2000 per 1000 children per year compared with 0.22 cases per 1000 children per year in the United States (19), although estimates from the United States are based on cases voluntarily reported to the Centers for Disease Control (CDC) and significantly underestimate the real incidence. There are places in the United States where the incidence is known to be much higher, e.g., in the southwestern states and among native American populations. Endemic shigellosis is a pediatric disease, with the majority of patients being less than 10 years of age and most under 5 years old. The disease is uncommon in infants under 6 months of age, even in highly endemic settings. Severe shigellosis may occur in neonates, and is more frequent and more likely to be severe in the non–breast-fed infants (20). Endemic shigellosis also often exhibits seasonal peaks, but the specifics can vary from one country to another. For example, transmission peaks in the hot dry season in Bangladesh and Egypt but in the rainy season in Guatemala (19).

These may relate to the use of more contaminated water for consumption or decreased personal hygiene in times of water scarcity in the former, or water-washed transmission during heavy rains in the latter.

During this century major global sequential shifts in the predominant *Shigella* species have occurred, without adequate epidemiological explanation (21). Before World War I, *S. dysenteriae* type I was the most common *Shigella* isolate in the world, causing large epidemics as well as endemic illness. In the period between World Wars I and II, however, *S. flexneri* emerged as the predominant isolate, only to be replaced by *S. sonnei* after 1945 in industrialized nations such as the United States and England. Since 1969, however, epidemic *S. dysenteriae* type 1 infection has reemerged in Mexico and Central America (22); Central Africa including Zaire, Rwanda, and the Central African Republic; Asia including Burma, Vietnam, and Thailand; and the Indian subcontinent including India, Bangladesh, and Pakistan (23). As might be expected with the introduction of a serotype not in recent circulation in the community, acquired immunity was negligible and attack rates tended to be high across all age groups.

Two populations in developed countries are at particular risk of *Shigella* infection. First, the incidence rates among children in day care centers are reported to be as high as 669 per 1000 per year, attributable to the ease of person-to-person transmission of the organism and the lack of bowel control of young infants (24). In prospective studies, infection was introduced into the household in 26% of families with an affected child in day care. The second group of concern is homosexual males, in whom shigellosis can be sexually transmitted (25). Curiously, although *S. sonnei* is the predominant *Shigella* isolate in the U.S. population as a whole, *S. flexneri* is the most common isolate in male homosexuals (26). In fact, in the past decade the incidence of *S. flexneri* in the United States has, for the first time in the past 25 years, increased significantly. This increase occurred virtually exclusively among young adult males, while the rates in females and children continued to decrease. As a consequence, the average age of patients with *S. flexneri* has risen from around 5 to 25 years (27).

Shigellosis, especially among young infants, may be fatal. The recent epidemics of *S. dysenteriae* type 1 in Guatemala and Zaire were associated with minimum reported case fatality rates of 7.4% and 2.5%, respectively (28,29). While this already exceeds the death rate in the huge Latin America cholera epidemic of 1991, the estimate of the *Shigella* death rate is certainly too low as the result of incomplete case reporting. The *S. dysenteriae* type 1 epidemic in Bangladesh in 1984 was associated with a 42% increase in mortality in children aged 1–4 years (30). The mortality rate among inpatients with documented *S. dysenteriae* type 1 infection at the International Centre for Diarrhoeal Disease Research in Dhaka, Bangladesh is around 10%. Malnutrition is an important conditioning factor for lethal infection and may account for the similarly high mortality rates due to the other *Shigella* species in Bangladesh, including *S. sonnei,* which does not ordinarily terminate fatally in other populations. The

additional observation that dysentery mortality in Bangladesh is more than twice as high in female compared with male children probably reflects sociological factors and cultural practices, such as parental preference for male children over female children, as expressed in feeding patterns and the provision of medical care (30).

There are few published data on the epidemiology of EIEC. One of the first recognizable outbreaks probably occurred during World War II (31), before EIEC were distinguished as a separate group of diarrhea-causing *E. coli*. In this outbreak, Ewing and Gravatti identified *S. dysenteriae* type 3 as the cause of bloody diarrhea; however, the organism was subsequently found to be the invasive serogroup O124. In another study in 1947 (32), Hobbs and Thomas isolated an organism from a foodborne outbreak at an English school, which later turned out to be an EIEC. These retrospectively diagnosed outbreaks serve to illustrate that EIEC were around for decades prior to their full recognition in the early 1970s. *E. coli* O124 has remained the most prevalent serogroup isolated among the several EIEC serogroups now known. French camembert cheese imported to the United States was the source of an outbreak of bloody diarrhea due to *E. coli* O124 in 1973 (33) that brought attention to the distinctive illness caused by these organisms and identified their ability to invade mammalian cells, much like *Shigella*. EIEC account for only 1–2% of endemic disease episodes where they have been looked for, but they are now being reported from an increasing number of countries.

CLINICAL FEATURES

Shigellosis usually begins with generalized constitutional symptoms, including fever, fatigue, anorexia, and malaise. Soon thereafter watery diarrhea develops, which in some patients, in part depending on the infecting species, becomes bloody or progresses to dysentery within a few hours to a few days. In the latter patients, the watery phase may be brief or even absent altogether. While large volume fluid loss is not common during shigellosis, profound and prolonged hyponatremia can be a problem, apparently due to inappropriate secretion of antidiuretic hormone (34). The classic dysenteric stool consists of a small amount of blood and mucus, sometimes grossly purulent; however, more often patients with shigellosis pass partially formed stools mixed with blood, pus, and mucus. Clinical dysentery is defined as the frequent passage of dysenteric or bloody stools associated with abdominal cramps and tenesmus due to proctitis. The inflammatory response can also result in rectal prolapse secondary to the intense straining to pass stools, especially in the very young in whom the ligamentous support of the rectum is poorly developed.

Macroscopic and microscopic histological damage is most evident in the distal large bowel, becoming progressively milder in the transverse and descending colon (35). Death and sloughing of epithelial cells results in ulcerations, which may extend to the lamina propria, associated with an inflammatory infiltrate in the submucosa and exudate in the bowel lumen. Stool frequency is variably increased, typically at least 8–10 movements per day, but as often as 100 times per day in an occasional unfortunate patient. But because stool volume is small—usually no more than 30 mL/kg/day of fluid is lost (36)—severe dehydration is not a part of the typical picture of this infection. However, anorexia, prominent at the outset, may persist well into the convalescent period and contributes in a major way to the adverse effects of shigellosis on nutritional status.

In developed countries the incidence of *Shigella* infection is relatively low (37). But because the illness is usually mild, self-limiting, and does not precipitate a visit to a physician, the estimates are probably several orders of magnitude lower than the true frequency of infection. In developing countries, however, shigellosis is frequently a severe disease and may persist for weeks to months unless antibiotic therapy is given. Progression to clinical dysentery is uncommon in *S. sonnei* infection, occurs more often in *S. boydii* infection, is common in *S. flexneri*, and occurs in most patients when *S. dysenteriae* type I is the cause.

Shigellosis may cause both local intestinal and systemic complications that can be severe and life threatening. In the United States and other industrialized countries, intestinal obstruction and toxic megacolon during shigellosis are uncommon events but in developing countries they occur regularly and are associated with a high mortality rate, especially if perforation of the dilated intestine occurs (38,39). The pathogenesis of toxic megacolon remains obscure but its increased association with *S. dysenteriae* type 1 infection supports the concept that it is a direct consequence of the intensity of the inflammatory reaction in the mucosa, and presumably of the release of inflammatory mediators.

The inflammatory response in shigellosis results in a protein-losing enteropathy, which has been assessed in some studies by measuring stool excretion of the serum enzyme, α_1-antitrypsin, as a marker of the escape of serum proteins into the gut lumen. Mean stool excretion of α_1-antitrypsin is 50% greater in *S. dysenteriae* type 1 compared to all other *Shigella* infections and correlates with the number of erythrocytes in the stool (40). Because protein losses are cumulative during infection, protein-losing enteropathy contributes to the negative nitrogen balance during shigellosis and increases the risk of acute protein energy malnutrition. If uncorrected during convalescence, protein losses are manifested as growth retardation in children, which is associated with increased morbidity and mortality (19).

Documented *Shigella* bacteremia has been considered to be uncommon but when routinely looked for is not rare. For example, bacteremia due to the causative *Shigella* species was documented in 4% of a series of severely ill patients with shigellosis in Bangladesh, and an additional 4% were bacteremic with other Enterobacteriaceae (41). Bacteremic patients were more likely to die, and the mortality rate in *Shigella* sepsis was 21%, reaching 51% in patients with sepsis due to other gram-negative rods, compared to a mortality rate of 10% in the absence of bacteremia. Even without documented bacteremia, however, circulating endotoxin is commonly detected when looked for in hospitalized patients with *Shigella* infection in developing countries, with the highest levels recorded in *S. dysenteriae* type 1 infection.

Associated systemic complications are especially frequent in dysentery due to *S. dysenteriae* type 1, including toxic megacolon, leukemoid reactions, with leukocyte counts in excess of 50,000/dL, and hemolytic-uremic syndrome (HUS) (23). HUS is a microangiopathic hemolytic process, resulting from damage to the small vessels in the kidney and elsewhere, leading to hemolytic anemia, thrombocytopenia usually in the range of 30,000–100,000, and acute renal failure. Evidence that procoagulant activity is increased in HUS patients includes the reports of elevated circulating levels of von Willebrand factor multimers and plasminogen activator inhibitor-1 and reduced levels of prostacyclin (PGI_2), and elevated circulating and urinary levels of the vasoconstrictor factor endothelin. HUS usually becomes clinically manifest during the convalescent phase of illness, when the acute diarrheal or dysenteric episode is subsiding (42). This suggests that the initiating events in HUS occur early in the course of the illness, probably when both endotoxin (an important activator of endothelial cell synthesis of cytokines and other vasoactive mediators) and Shiga toxin or Shiga-like toxins (which are cytotoxic to endothelial cells) are circulating. The hemolysis may be dramatic, e.g., a drop in hematocrit of 10% or more within a 24-hr period, requiring immediate blood transfusion as a life-saving intervention. Uremia develops more slowly and often necessitates dialysis. In some patients dialysis may be avoided because the rise in creatinine is gradual. Ironically, the preexisting total body potassium deficiency associated with malnutrition and diarrhea among children in developing countries often precludes clinically significant hyperkalemia from developing and reduces the need for dialysis (23).

Neurological complications, especially seizures, are also well documented in shigellosis. Seizures are usually generalized, occur early in the course of disease due to any *Shigella* species, are often associated with a rapidly rising fever, usually do not recur, and are rarely associated with permanent sequelae. They resemble typical febrile seizures in children, except for the higher mean age in *Shigella* patients. Pathogenesis is unknown, and the suggestions that it may be due to Shiga toxin, or to a 100- to 125-kDa cytotoxin distinct from Shiga toxin, remain unproven (43). Encephalopathy independent of hypoglycemia may develop, especially during infection with *S. flexneri*, contributing to the overlap in clinical presentation between shigellosis and bacterial meningitis in some patients. Fatalities in HUS are often associated with central nervous system pathology and cerebral edema.

Other recognized complications include post-*Shigella* reactive arthritis or full-blown Reiter's syndrome, particularly, it seems, with *S. flexneri* infection. An immunological basis for this is suggested by the strong correlation between reactive arthritis and expression of the HLA-B27 histocompatibility antigen. Monoclonal antibodies against B27 epitopes cross-react with 36- and 23-kDa proteins of *S. flexneri* (44), and monoclonal antibodies raised against a 36-kDa *S. flexneri* outer membrane protein cross-react with lymphocytes expressing HLA-B27 (45). These findings suggest that molecular mimicry between organism and host may be the basis for the response. In addition, a 2-MDa plasmid containing genes with sequence homology with the α_1 domain of HLA-B27 has been identified in arthritogenic strains of *S. flexneri* (46). Nonetheless, the specific role of molecular mimicry in pathogenesis of Reiter's syndrome remains uncertain and unproven (47).

PATHOGENESIS

The molecular basis of shigellosis is complex and excellent reviews have been published (6,8,48). Virulence of *Shigella* is absolutely determined by the capacity of the organism to invade mammalian cells, often demonstrated in vivo by a positive Sereny test, the purulent keratoconjunctivitis that follows inoculation of the organism onto the cornea of a guinea pig or rabbit that results from microbial invasion of and replication within the corneal epithelium (49). However, this property does not explain the most unique characteristic of *Shigella* pathogenesis, i.e., the very small inoculum required to cause disease. Secretion of acid in the stomach is known to be a major barrier to infection due to a number of enteric pathogens, and gastric acid secretion is directly correlated with the infectious dose of acid-sensitive organisms such as *V. cholerae* and nontyphoidal salmonellae. Until recently, *Shigella* also was considered to be acid-sensitive in vitro although it behaved as if it were acid-resistant in vivo. That is, no increase in susceptibility was observed in hypochlorhydric patients nor did buffering affect the inoculum size in human infection models. By systematic study under controlled conditions of pH and time of exposure, however, Gorden and Small (50) recently demonstrated that *Shigella flexneri* is significantly more acid-resistant in vitro than are *Salmonella* or *E. coli*. Acid resistance was strikingly dependent on growth phase, becoming manifest first in late exponential growth and being fully expressed in stationary phase. It was also possible to genetically manipulate the organisms and select for acid-sensitive mutants. Genetic recombination experiments have demonstrated that a global regulatory system in which a putative stationary phase σ factor encoded by *rpo*s (formerly designated *katF*) plays an important role in acid resistance, along with other still unidentified genes (50,51).

Acid-exposed organisms, however, lose their ability to invade HEp-2 cells, and invasive properties are clearly required for shigellae to cause disease, so there may be a tradeoff for the ability to survive low pH. But when placed in an epidemiological context, these findings are not as paradoxical as they seem at first glance. Acid resistance is most useful when the organisms initially enter the host in order to help them pass the stomach barrier. That organisms in the environment will be acid-resistant is insured because the acid-resistant phenotype is associated with stationary phase of growth as occurs in environmental settings. Once past the gastric acid barrier, when they begin to multiply the organisms can express other critical virulence traits, such as the ability to invade host cells.

It is interesting that although *Shigella* and EIEC have identical virulence determinants, the infective dose for EIEC has been reported to be at least 1000-fold higher (52); the explanation for this is not readily apparent but may account in part for the relative infrequency of EIEC infections. Bloch et al. (53) suggested that the low infective dose for certain enteric pathogens could be due to initial colonization of the oropharynx. However, this does not seem consistent with the fact that most *Shigella* are nonpiliated, the organisms are not ordinarily isolated from the pharynx, a pharyngeal prodrome is absent in shigellosis, and invasion from the upper airway site would not explain localization to the colonic mucosa.

Shigella are a dramatic example of the polygenic nature of virulence, with necessary virulence genes present on both the chromosome and plasmids (6) (Fig. 1). Genetic studies using conjugal matings, transposon- and site-directed mutagenesis, and the construction of gene libraries has over a number of years resulted in the identification of multiple chromosomal loci associated with *Shigella* virulence (Table 3). Hale (6) classified these genes in three groups: (a) determinants such as siderophores, somatic antigens, and superoxide dismutase that affect survival of *Shigella* in the gastrointestinal lumen or in the mucosa; (b) cytotoxins; and (c) regulatory factors.

Siderophores

Biosynthetic and transport genes for aerobactin-type iron-binding proteins have been found in all *Shigella* species except *S. dysenteriae* type I and some strains of *S. sonnei* that usually express enterobactin siderophores. *S. flexneri* also possess enterobactin genes, but they are usually cryptic (6). As siderophores enable the organism to compete for iron in the in vivo setting in which virtually all iron is protein-bound, it is not surprising that tissue culture models fail to differentiate the virulence potential of siderophore phenotypes (54). However, subtle differences in the virulence of aerobactin mutants can be detected in vivo. In animal models, for example, an *iuc* aerobactin mutant produces a delayed-positive Sereny test (55). When the inoculum is increased this difference disappears, suggesting that a functional aerobactin gene facilitates the initial multiplication of *Shigella*, especially when the inoculum is small (6).

Group-Specific Somatic Antigen

One of the earliest indications of the importance of the O side chain of somatic antigens was the work of Gemski et al. (56), showing that conjugal transfer of the genes encoding *E. coli* somatic antigens 8 or 25 into *S. flexneri* 2a altered the virulence of the transconjugant. These O serotypes were chosen because O-25 resembles *flexneri* 2a in having a high mannose content, whereas O-8 is chemically distinctive. Whereas all O-8 hybrids were avirulent, some of the O-25 hybrids retained virulence by both Sereny test and oral challenge, suggesting that the chemical composition and structure of the O side chain affects *Shigella* virulence. Rough strains of *Shigella* lacking O side chains retain the ability to invade and multiply within

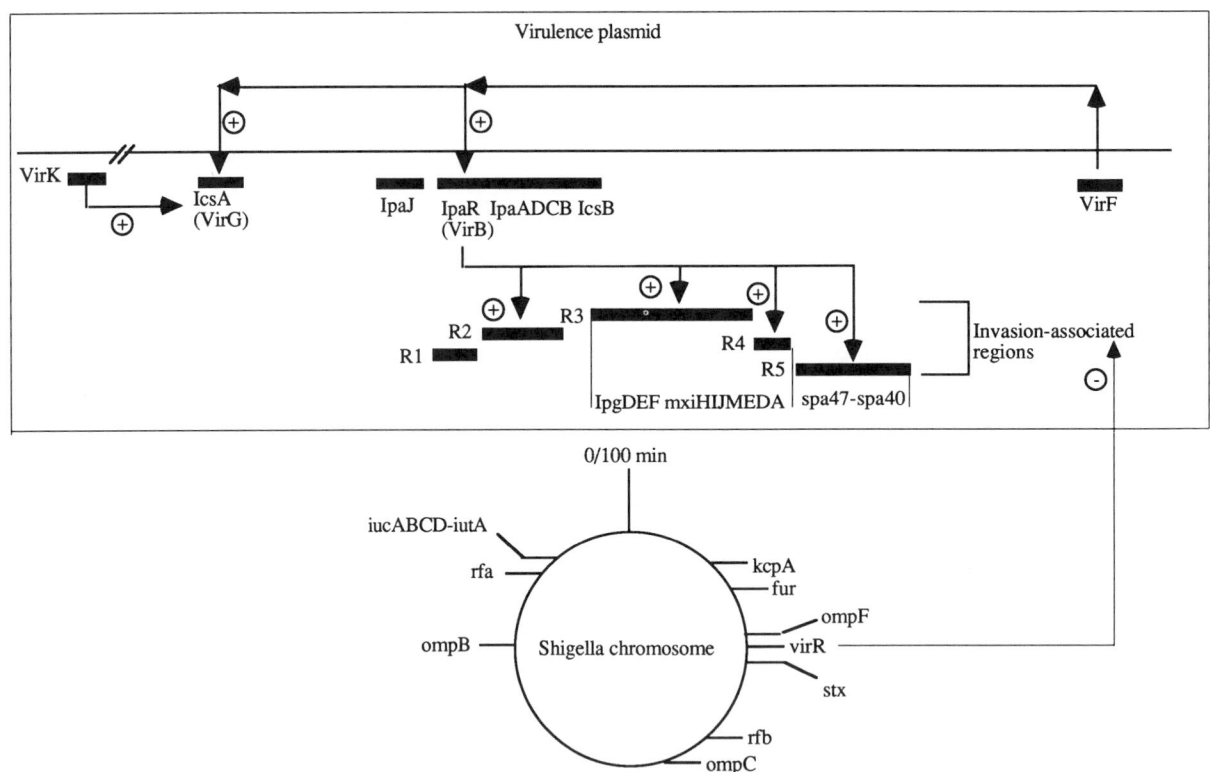

FIG. 1. Composite map of the *Shigella* chromosomal and invasion plasmid virulence genes, indicating the positive regulatory pathways (*heavy line arrow*) and negative regulatory pathways (*fine line arrow*). R1–R5 refer to regions in the invasion plasmid discussed in the text. (Courtesy of Dr. J. Buysse.)

TABLE 3. *Chromosomal loci associated with virulence in* S. flexneri

Locus	Virulence phenotype of mutants	Regulatory or effector function
T locus	Y variant expressing only group 3,4 somatic antigen may exhibit decreased virulence	Integration site for incorporation of lysogenic phage 4 encoding type specific somatic antigen
kcpA	Sereny-negative with limited intracellular and intercellular bacterial spread in tissue culture monolayers	Positive regulation of plasmid gene *virG (icsA)*
virR	Invasive in tissue culture when grown at 30°C	Repression of plasmid invasion loci, e.g., *ipaA,B,C,D,* in response to temperature
stx	Decrease in vascular damage in the colonic epithelium or orally challenged monkeys[a]	Synthesis of Shiga toxin
rfb	Sereny-negative, decreased intercellular spread in infected tissue culture monolayers	Synthesis of group-specific somatic antigen
ompR-envZ	Decreased invasion in tissue culture: Sereny-negative	Induction of plasmid invasion loci
rfa	Delayed or negative Sereny test, decreased intercellular spread in infected tissue culture monolayers	Synthesis of somatic antigen basal core
iucA,B,C,D-iutA	Delayed Sereny reaction, decreased mortality in orally challenged guinea pig; decreased histopathology and fluid response in ligated rabbit ileal loop; diminished virulence in orally challenged monkey model	Synthesis of aerobactin and 76-kDa aerobactin receptor protein
sodB	Sensitivity to oxygen-dependent killing by phagocytes; Sereny-negative; greatly decreased histopathology in ligated rabbit ileal loop	Superoxide dismutase inactivates superoxide radicals produced by phagocytes during respiratory burst

Modified from ref. 6, which should be consulted for a complete list of references.
[a] The *stx* gene is only present in the chromosome of *S. dysenteriae* type 1.

tissue culture cells but are not able to spread to adjacent cells, are avirulent in vivo in animal models (57,58), and do not cause infection in laboratory workers in contrast to smooth isolates which regularly result in laboratory acquired disease.

Together with the now extensive epidemiological evidence of type-specific resistance to *Shigella* infection, these data indicate the importance of LPS antigens in the pathogenesis of shigellosis. Evidence for this is slowly accumulating. For example, a Tn5 insertion into the *rfa* locus, necessary for the synthesis of the LPS basal core region, results in delayed plaque formation in cell culture and a delayed Sereny test reaction in vivo, both of which assess the ability of the organism to invade and spread from cell to cell (56). It is possible however, that alterations in LPS core composition do not directly affect virulence but rather exert an indirect effect on the expression, insertion, or conformation of outer membrane proteins involved in virulence (6). In contrast to *S. flexneri*, plasmid-encoded enzymes are required for somatic antigen biosynthesis in both *S. dysenteriae* type 1 and *S. sonnei*. For example, the galactose transferase gene (*rfp*) is located on a 9-kb plasmid in the former (59,60). While the precise role of LPS in virulence is not clear, it is possible to express O antigen biosynthesis genes from *Shigella* in various hosts, which may be useful both for studying its role in virulence and potentially for developing vaccines (61).

Superoxide Dismutase

Superoxide dismutase (*sodB*) may enhance the survival of *Shigella* in vivo by inhibiting the bactericidal effect of host-derived reactive oxygen radicals (6,62). Allelic exchange of the unmapped *S. flexneri* superoxide dismutase gene has been accomplished and the resulting *sodB* − *Shigella* mutant is extremely sensitive to oxygen stress and killing by either mouse peritoneal macrophages or human polymorphonuclear leukocytes. Such mutants cause little histopathological damage to the mucosa when inoculated into ligated rabbit ileal loops.

Shiga Toxin

Although the prototype *Shigella* species, *S. dysenteriae* type 1, was known to produce a potent toxin as early as 1903 (4), its precise role in *Shigella* pathogenesis remains uncertain to this day. After the 1972 report that Shiga toxin produced a fluid secretory response in the rabbit ileal loop model (63), there has been a remarkable increase in interest in this protein, with the discovery that closely related Shiga-like toxins (also known as verotoxins) are made by *E. coli* associated with a characteristic clinical disease, hemorrhagic colitis (64).

Shiga toxin consists of two noncovalently liked peptides, a 32-kDa enzymatically active A subunit and five 7- to 8-kDa B subunits responsible for binding toxin to a cell surface glycolipid receptor, globotriaosylceramide (Gb3). Like cholera toxin, the Shiga toxin A subunit is

activated by proteolytic processing and reduction of an internal disulfide linkage into an A1 fragment (27 kDa) and a carboxy terminal A2 fragment (4 kDa) (64). The A1 subunit possesses the identical N-glycosidase enzymatic activity as the toxic plant lectin, ricin, and by removing adenine from a single specific adenosine in the 28S component of the 60S ribosomal subunit it permanently inactivates that ribosome and ultimately stops protein synthesis completely in the affected cell, resulting in cell death (65).

Alteration of certain amino acids critically affects the enzymatic action of Shiga toxin. For example, Hovde et al. (66) reported that glutamic acid$_{167}$ is a critical active site residue of Shiga-like toxin I (SLT-I), which is almost identical to Shiga toxin. Even a conservative change of glutamic acid$_{167}$ to aspartic acid resulted in a 1000-fold reduction in enzymatic activity. The B subunit of Shiga toxin and SLT-I are identical, and the latter has been purified to homogeneity by several groups (67,68) and its X-ray crystallographic structure solved (69). Interestingly, the pentameric folding of SLT-I B is very similar to that of the B oligomer of heat-labile enterotoxin from *E. coli*. Stein et al. (69) speculated that a conserved carbohydrate binding site may be formed by the β-sheet interaction between adjacent B monomers, suggesting that there are five potential binding sites per pentamer, assuming a five-fold symmetry. Site-directed mutagenesis of Shiga toxin B subunit suggests that the aspartate residues at positions 16 and 17 may be part of the receptor binding site (70). Aspartate$_{17}$ is one of the amino acids lining the potential binding cleft described by Stein et al. (69), consistent with the notion that this is an important functional residue.

Shiga toxin has been purified to homogeneity using a variety of techniques (64). The toxin is cytotoxic to certain tissue culture cell lines (HeLa, Vero, certain intestinal epithelial cell lines, and low-passage primary vascular endothelial cell cultures) but not others (CHO, WI-38), it results in "neurotoxicity" (paralysis and delayed death) after parenteral inoculation in experimental animals, and it is an enterotoxin (i.e., it leads to intestinal fluid accumulation in rabbit ileal loops). The *stx* gene is unique to *S. dysenteriae* type I of all the *Shigella* species, and is located on the chromosome at 28 minutes near *pyrF*, a known hot spot for chlorate mutagenesis. The gene for Shiga toxin and the genes for the closely related *E. coli* SLT's encoded on transforming phage have been sequenced and show significant homology, ranging from 99% for SLT-I to 55% for SLT-II (64). The production of Shiga toxin is suppressed by anaerobiasis and by high levels of iron, due to regulation of the *stx* operon by the *fur* gene product, a DNA-binding protein that, when complexed with iron under high iron conditions, binds to the *stx* promoter and blocks transcription (71).

The glycolipid receptor for Shiga toxin was independently identified by two groups using two different approaches. Lindberg and colleagues demonstrated that toxin bound to purified erythrocyte Gb3 immobilized on a solid phase (72), whereas Jacewicz et al. (73) extracted a toxin-binding glycolipid from both HeLa cells and from microvillus membranes of rabbit small bowel and identified this as Gb3. The critical feature of toxin-binding glycolipids is a galactose-α1→4-galactose disaccharide, which for Shiga toxin and SLT-I and II is terminal and for SLT-II variant toxins is internal. The binding is highly specific; for example, alteration of the galactose-galactose linkage to $\alpha1\rightarrow3$ destroys toxin binding capacity. Several lines of evidence suggest that this binding site is a functional receptor. The most critical of these is the finding by Mobassaleh et al. (74,75) that the inability of infant rabbits younger than 16 days old to respond to the enterotoxic activity of Shiga toxin inoculated into the intestinal lumen was due to developmental regulation of Gb3 in this species. Increasing expression of Gb3 in the microvillus membrane of intestinal epithelial cells after day 16 of life (74) is accompanied by a progressive increase in the fluid response to toxin (75). Developmental regulation of Gb3 in rabbit small intestine has been shown to be related to an increase in activity of the biosynthetic enzyme, UDP-galactose:lactosylceramide galactosyltransferase, and a decrease in the activity of the degradative enzyme, α-galactosidase (76). It is not known as to whether or not the relative protection of human newborns and small infants against *Shigella* infection reflects developmental regulation of membrane glycolipids in intestinal epithelial cells or other biological characteristics of the host, or whether it is related to passive maternal protection via milk or limited exposure to the organisms in the environment.

The necessary role of Gb3 in cell cytotoxicity has been absolutely confirmed by studies in cell culture. Susceptibility to Shiga toxin is directly related to the cellular content and surface expression of Gb3 in cell culture lines (77), and cloning or selecting resistant cells actually selects for reduced activity of the synthetic Gb3-galactosyltransferase and Gb3 expression (78). In addition, direct manipulation of Gb3 levels with metabolic inhibitors, e.g., increasing Gb3 by blocking the degradative α-galactosidase activity or decreasing Gb3 by blocking the initial enzyme in neutral glycolipid synthesis, UDP-glucose:ceramide glucosyltransferase, results in an increase or decrease in the cytotoxic activity of the toxin, respectively (78). Even more convincing, however, is that resistant HeLa or Vero cells either selected for low Gb3 expression or blocked in Gb3 synthesis by incubation in the presence of a metabolic inhibitor can be made sensitive to toxin by the insertion of Gb3 delivered via liposomes, whereas other related glycolipids lacking the terminal galactose-$\alpha1\rightarrow4$-galactose disaccharide are ineffective (78).

However, Gb3 may not be all that is required for the action of Shiga toxin. Scatchard analysis of carefully conducted binding studies have revealed two classes of binding sites, one of which, a tunicamycin-sensitive low-capacity/high-affinity site, directly correlated with sensitivity to toxin (77). The nature of this site remains unknown, but its susceptibility to tunicamycin suggests that it might be an N-linked glycoprotein. Recent studies using Chinese hamster ovary (CHO) cells, which are naturally resistant to toxin because they lack the Gb3-specific galactosyltransferase activity and do not produce Gb3, suggest that Gb3 is required but not sufficient for susceptibility to Shiga toxin. When Gb3 was inserted into CHO cells using liposomes as the carrier, binding of toxin was restored but there was no cytotoxicity detected (78). This suggests that CHO cells not only fail to express the Gb3

receptor for toxin but also lack additional properties necessary for toxin uptake and/or trafficking within the cell.

In addition to developmental regulation of Shiga toxin receptors, luminal toxin reduces sodium absorption without altering chloride secretion by rabbit small bowel mucosa (79), suggesting that the physiological effect of toxin on intestinal electrolyte transport is primarily on the absorptive villus cells. Villus cells isolated from rabbit small bowel preferentially expressed Gb3 and were susceptible to the biochemical effect of toxin on protein synthesis, whereas crypt cells lacked Gb3 and were toxin-resistant. Recent studies using intestinal cell lines in vitro have confirmed that synthesis of Gb3 is correlated with state of differentiation. Thus, villus-like lines (CaCo-2 and HT-29) express Gb3 and respond to toxin whereas a crypt-like line (T-84) neither expresses Gb3 nor responds to toxin (80). Addition of butyrate, a differentiation stimulus in many cells, results in a significant upregulation of Gb3 galactosyltransferase, increased synthesis of Gb3 and markedly increased sensitivity to toxin in MDCK cells (81), and villus-like but not crypt-like intestinal cells in culture (80).

Following binding to its receptor, Shiga toxin is taken up by receptor-mediated endocytosis at clathrin-coated pits (82,83) and is transported within the cell to and beyond the Golgi apparatus where the A1 subunit probably reaches its target (81). The details of the transfer of the A chain across the vesicular membrane are not known; however, cell intoxication is blocked by brefeldin A, which disrupts the Golgi membrane, and by inhibitors of calcium transport, acting at an as yet undetermined site (64).

The lack of Shiga toxin production by non-*dysenteriae* type I strains of *Shigella* has questioned the primary role of toxin in pathogenesis, except as an accessory virulence factor in *S. dysenteriae* type 1. The dramatic local and systemic manifestations of enterohemorrhagic *E. coli* (EHEC), which resemble enteropathogenic *E. coli* and do not invade the mucosa, but rather produce large amounts of SLT in the bowel lumen, suggests the importance of toxin at the local and/or systemic sites of pathology. There is ample evidence that Shiga toxin acts as a cytotoxin on tumor-derived intestinal cells in vitro and on isolated human colonic cells in primary culture (84). To study the effect of Shiga toxin on pathogenesis in vivo, *stx*-negative mutants have been constructed. Because of the vulnerability of the region of the chromosome containing the *stx* operon to chemical mutagenesis with chlorate, selection for chlorate resistance selects toxin mutants. These strains (85,86) and a specific toxin deletion mutant in *S. dysenteriae* type I (87) retain the ability to produce intestinal disease in primates, although the clinical illness is less severe than disease caused by the wild-type organisms. In one study (87) the presence of a functional *stx* gene resulted in more extensive inflammatory lesions and capillary destruction in the colonic mucosa. Indeed, as discussed below, targeting of Shiga toxin to endothelial cells may be important in the pathogenesis of the local and systemic complications of shigellosis (88,89).

Shiga toxin and SLTs bind to endothelial cells and result in inhibition of protein synthesis and cell death (90).

This can be considerably enhanced by pretreatment of human umbilical vein endothelial cell monolayers with LPS, with the cytokines tumor necrosis factor-α (TNF-α) or interleukin-1β (IL-1β), or with LPS plus cytokine, with a resultant increase in the expression of Gb3 and cytotoxicity (91,92). Of interest, human renal endothelial cells appear to constitutively express high levels of Gb3 that are not further induced by LPS or these cytokines (93). In view of the strong association of endotoxemia with systemic complications in shigellosis and the well-known ability of LPS to upregulate cytokines, it is reasonable to propose that endotoxemia initially sensitizes some endothelial cell beds to the effects of Shiga toxin or SLTs absorbed from the gut lumen during infection (94). Species and regional endothelial cell differences in expression of Shiga toxin receptors or regulatory responses to LPS and TNF-α may be responsible for localized involvement of certain endothelial cell beds during infection with toxin-producing organisms, e.g., in the kidney in HUS or the central nervous system in thrombotic thrombocytopenic purpura. This is consistent with the finding of earlier studies that localized vascular damage in the spinal cord was responsible for the classical neurotoxicity due to parenteral injections of Shiga toxin in experimental animals (95,96). Parenteral administration of SLT-II or porcine SLT-II variant toxins to young piglets also reproduces both the central nervous system endothelial cell damage and clinical manifestations of edema disease in this species (97), indicating the role of toxin in pathogenesis of this syndrome and localizing its action to the endothelial cell resulting in thrombotic microangiopathy.

Although the structural genes for Shiga toxin are not present in species other than *S. dysenteriae* type 1, cytotoxic activity neutralized by antibodies to Shiga toxin has been reported in culture filtrates or sonicates of *S. flexneri* 2a and *S. sonnei* (98,99). Low-level cytotoxin production by species other than *Shigella* has been reported by many investigators, but the validity of these data and the significance of the observation remain uncertain. Fasano, Nataro, and colleagues have presented evidence that *Shigella* enterotoxins, distinct from the cytotoxic Shiga toxin, are produced by all species. The toxins, tentatively designated ShET-1 and ShET-2, alter electrolyte transport by rabbit small bowel tissue in vitro and cause fluid secretion in vivo in ligated rabbit ileal loops. ShET-1 appears to be encoded by a chromosomal gene (100), whereas ShET-2 is controlled by an iron-regulated plasmid gene and is highly homologous with a previously described EIEC enterotoxin (101). Their role, if any, in the pathogenesis of the watery diarrhea phase of shigellosis and diarrhea due to EIEC, is being investigated.

Cellular Invasion by *Shigella* and Enteroinvasive *E. coli*

The full invasive process of *Shigella* and EIEC may be divided into four stages: (a) initial entry into cells; (b) intracellular multiplication; (c) intra- and intercellular spread; and (d) host cell killing (102). Most studies of inva-

sion have been carried out with *S. flexneri* strains, and it is presumed that all other *Shigella* and EIEC enter cells by the same basic process.

Initial Entry

S. flexneri are internalized by epithelial cells via an endocytic process that involves formation of long host cell pseudopods (103) (Fig. 2) and internalization within a vesicle (104) (Fig. 3). This process resembles phagocytosis, is inhibited by cytochalasins B and D, and is active, requiring energy produced by both the bacterium and the host cell (105). Because the target cells involved are not normally phagocytic, the invasive process is to a large degree initiated and directed by bacterium-related factors. Using fluorescent-tagged probes for various cytoskeletal elements, accumulation of aggregated actin filaments and myosin has been demonstrated to occur beneath the plasma membrane in areas of the HeLa cell surface interacting with invading organisms (102,106). These changes

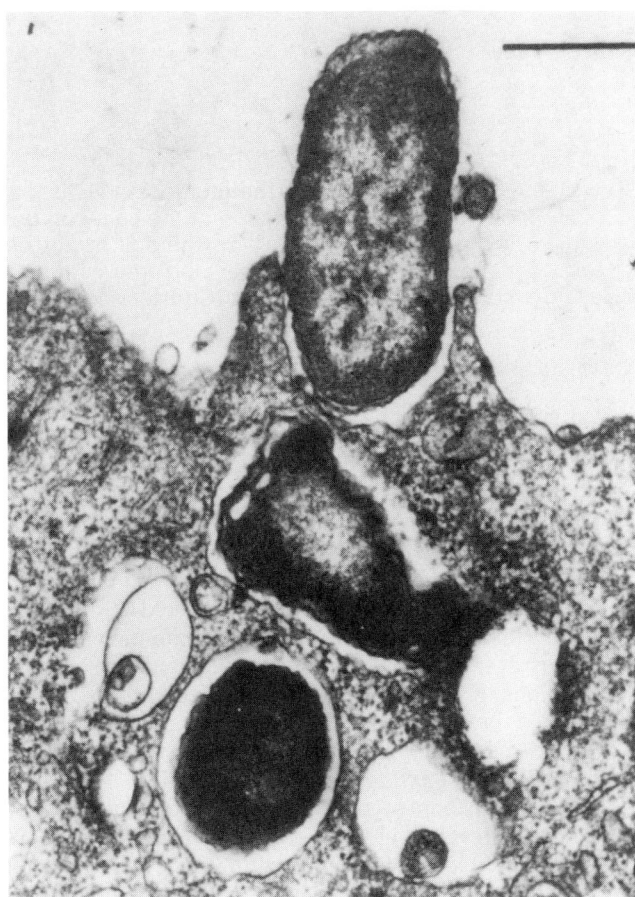

FIG. 2. *Shigella* invasion. Phagocytosis of virulent *Shigella flexneri* 2a by HeLa cells in culture. Note the host cell pseudopods beginning to engulf the organism at the top of the figure, which will ultimately fuse to form a phagocytic vesicle within the cytoplasm. In addition, several internalized bacteria are present within this cell. Bar = 1 μm. (From ref. 103, with permission.)

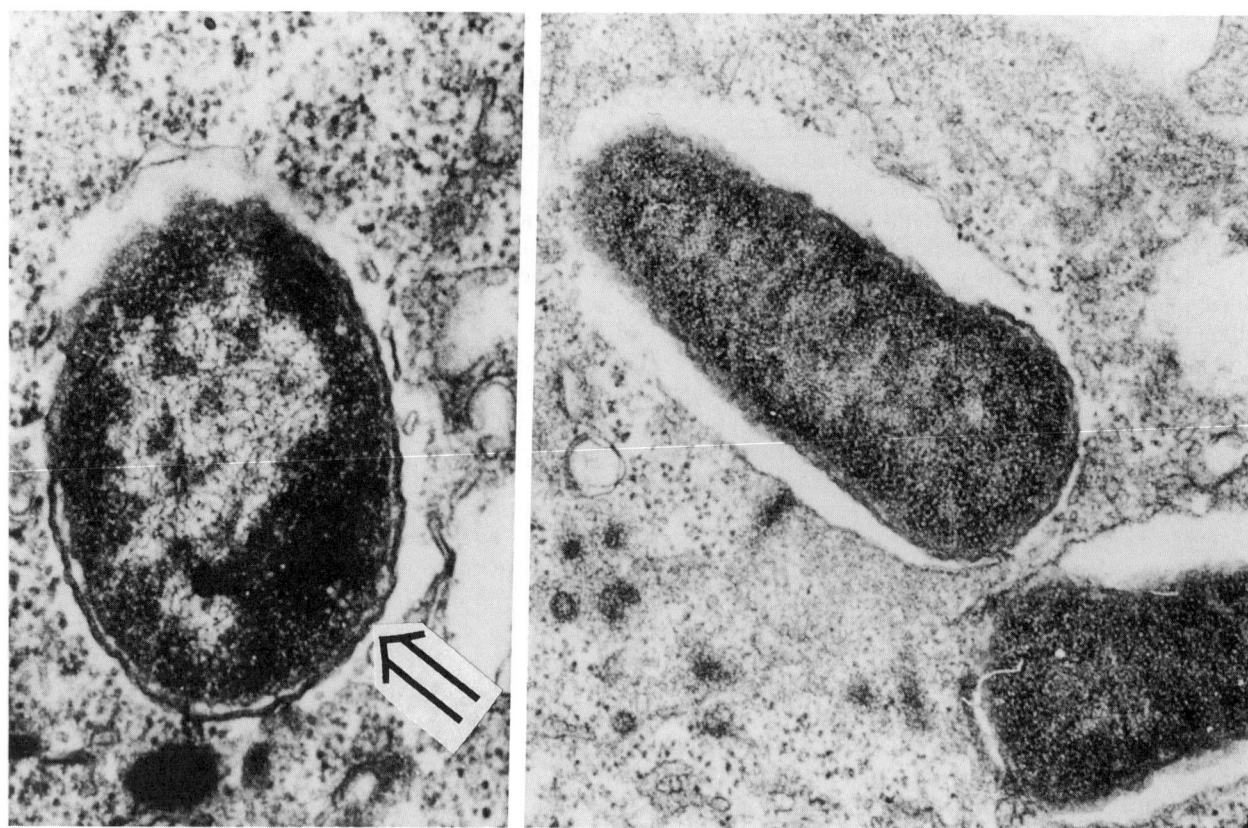

FIG. 3. Escape from the phagosome. Dissolution of the phagosomal vesical membrane, which occurs soon after invasion of the cell, can be seen over the upper portion of the organism in the left panel (arrow points to the still intact portion of the phagosomal membrane). In the right panel, two organisms are lying free within the cytoplasm after the phagosomal membrane has completely disintegrated. (Courtesy of Dr. P. J. Sansonetti.)

in cytoskeletal organization result in the formation of a host plasma membrane–derived "outside-in" vesicle within which the organism lies, wholly analogous to the phagosome within professional phagocytes.

The large 220-kb plasmid of *S. flexneri* is necessary for expression of the invasive phenotype and similar plasmids are present in virulent isolates of other *Shigella* species (107,108). A great deal is now known about these plasmids, and interested readers are referred to a recent review for more information and further references (109). By means of Tn5 mutagenesis, five independent contiguous regions (R1–R5) have been identified within a 30-kb segment of the large plasmid (Fig. 1). Region 1 contains a positive regulatory gene named *virB* in *S. flexneri* 2a (110), *ipaR* in *S. flexneri* 5a (111), and *invE* in *S. sonnei* (112). Under the control of *virF,* a second positive regulatory gene, *ipaR* (*virB*) induces several invasion genes contained in other loci, of which region 2, the most extensively studied, encodes the *ipa* genes for the synthesis of outer membrane *i*nvasion *p*lasmid *a*ntigens, or Ipa's. The *mxi* genes, encoding proteins required for *m*embrane *ex*port and *i*nsertion of the Ipa proteins, are located in regions 3 and 4 (113). The DNA sequence for *virF* encodes three proteins of 30, 27, and 21 kDa. The 30-kDa protein has partial amino acid homology with the AraC family of DNA-binding proteins (109).

Expression of the seven plasmid-encoded Ipa proteins, designated IpaA–G, in *S. flexneri* minicells (small anucleate cells resulting from aberrant cell division at the polar ends of the organism) enabled them to invade cultured HeLa cells (114). Western blot analysis using convalescent human sera demonstrated that four of these, IpaA–D, were antigenic in the host and that the sera reacted with the same proteins in all species of *Shigella,* as well as in EIEC (115). These proteins were clustered in a 6-kb segment of the invasion plasmid in the transcriptional order *ipaB/ipaC/ipaD/ipaA* (116) (Fig. 1), of which only Ipa B, C, and D are required for invasiveness. This 6-kb region consists of at least three operons coordinately regulated by the *ipaR* gene product through temperature-activated transcription (105). The Ipa proteins have not been purified but examination of their nucleotide sequences indicates that they are hydrophilic with few cysteine residues. Interestingly, the G + C content of the *ipa* gene region in *Shigella* is significantly lower than that of the chromosome, suggesting a different evolutionary origin and later acquisition of invasion antigens by *Shigella.*

The *mxi* genes, involved in export and secretion of the Ipa proteins, are necessary for invasion and are located downstream from the *ipa* locus. Secretion and surface presentation of IpaB and IpaC is abolished by transposon insertions in either *mxiA* or the nearby *spa* locus (*s*urface *p*resentation of invasion *p*lasmid *a*ntigens), which is downstream from *mxiA* in region 5 of the 30-kb segment of the virulence plasmid discussed above (117,118). The *mxiD* and *mxiJ* regions, located in the region between *ipa* and *mxiA,* also are required for secretion of Ipa proteins. Allaoui et al. (119) recently characterized three additional invasion *p*lasmid *g*enes, *ipgD, ipgE,* and *ipgF,* located in the 5′ end of the *mxi–spa* locus that appear to belong to the same operon. *ipgD* encodes a secreted protein of approximately 58–60 kDa, which is dependent on *mxi* gene products for secretion. Mutations in *ipgD* and *ipgF* do not affect invasion of cultured cells. Although the precise role of these three genes in virulence has yet to be determined, their association with *mxi* in the critical virulence region of the plasmid raises the possibility that they play a role in virulence that in vitro tests fail to reveal (118).

It is not known as to whether the actual mechanism for adherence of *Shigella* to eukaryotic cells prior to invasion is distinct from the invasion process itself; hence the molecular basis for selective invasion of the colon rather than the small bowel is not understood. There is some evidence that clathrin may be involved in bacterial uptake at the site of microbial entry, in addition to the formation of actin and myosin complexes (102). However, *S. flexneri* do not recognize receptors on the apical surface of polarized monolayers of CaCo-2 cells, but rather enter via the basolateral surface, suggesting that initial invasion does not occur at the epithelial cell surface. In situ studies in human tissues also suggest that colonocytes are not the primary site of invasion but rather that selective uptake of organisms occurs via M cells, with infection of adjacent enterocytes resulting from subsequent cell-to-cell spread (102). This sequence of events is supported by in vivo data from experimental shigellosis in rabbits (120).

Intracellular Multiplication

Following invasion, organisms multiply within the target cell. Using HeLa cells as a model, the phagocytic vacuole containing intracellular *S. flexneri* is lysed within 30 min of its formation and organisms come to lie freely in the cytoplasm (Fig. 3) where they multiply rapidly (102,104). Vacuolar lysis is associated with the expression of a contact hemolytic activity and it is necessary for virulence since hemolysin negative strains are avirulent (121). This also has been shown by growing virulent strains at 30°C, a temperature at which they neither express hemolysin nor multiply in host cells. The likelihood that hemolysin plays a role in the release of organisms from the phagocytic vacuole is further suggested by the observation that hemolysin activity increases 100- to 1000-fold as the pH drops from 7 to 5.5 (122), as is known to happen in phagocytic vesicles.

Mutations affecting intracellular growth also are attenuating. For example, blocking folic acid synthesis via the aromatic pathway impairs intracellular growth and such *aro* mutants are attenuated in vivo, which makes them

possible vaccine candidates. Mutations of the porins OmpC and OmpF and deletion mutants in the regulatory gene *ompB,* also result in slower intracellular growth rates and attenuation of virulence; *ompB* and *ompC* deletion mutants are defective in their ability to spread from cell to cell and kill epithelial cells (123). The *ompB* deletion mutant was restored to virulence by introducing a recombinant plasmid carrying the cloned *E. coli ompC* gene, indicating the requirement for a functional OmpC protein in virulence.

Intracellular Spread

The third phase in the invasion process is intracellular movement and cell-to-cell spread of organisms growing in the cytoplasm, a process that utilizes the host cell cytoskeleton (124). In an early study, *virG* (now generally termed *icsA*) was shown to be necessary for reinfection of adjacent cells in the Sereny test and production of keratoconjunctivitis (125). Movement of the nonmotile *Shigella* organisms within the cytoplasm of the host cell, and from cell to cell, depends on the interaction of the organism with the host cell cytoskeleton in a process inhibited by cytochalsin D (126). Within 2 hr of entry, *Shigella* become coated with polymerized actin, which is redistributed to one end of the bacterium (127) (Fig. 4). The continuous deposition of actin and myosin provides a propulsive force for the organisms to move toward the periphery of the cell, where they often cause a protrusion of the cytoplasm that reaches to the adjacent cell (127)

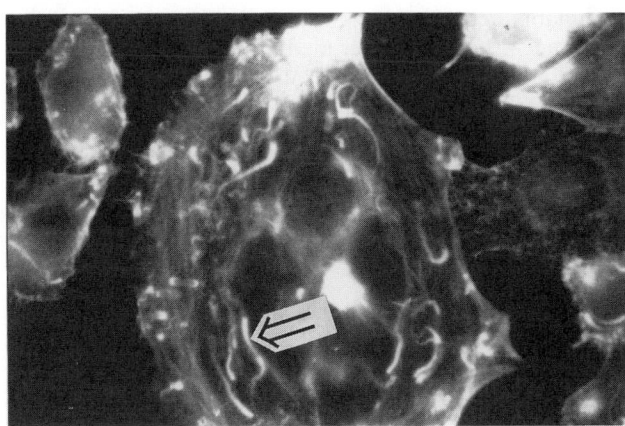

FIG. 4. Intracellular motility. In this photomicrograph, HeLa cells have been invaded by virulent *S. flexneri* 2a and then stained with fluorescein-conjugated phalloidin, a reagent that reacts specifically with polymerized actin. A brightly fluorescing, serpentine "comet's tail" can be appreciated, even in this black-and-white photograph, which represents polymerized actin accumulating at the posterior end of the organism. The organism lies just ahead of the brightest portion of the tail, where deposition of polymerized actin is occurring, and it is being propelled forward. The arrow points to an organism within the interior of a HeLa cell that is heading directly toward the top of the page. (From ref. 127, with permission.)

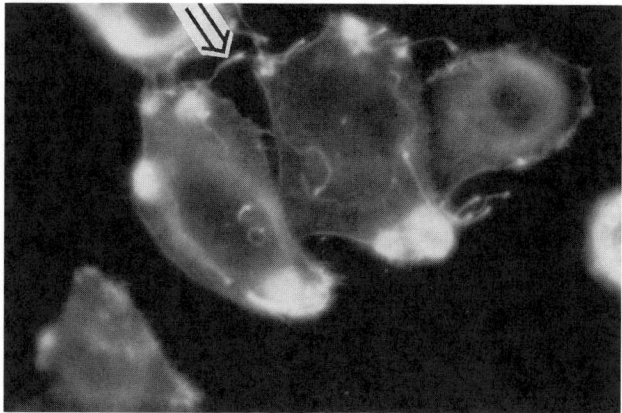

FIG. 5. Intercellular spread. HeLa cells exposed to invasive, virulent *Shigella flexneri* 2a, have been stained as in Fig. 4 with fluorescein-conjugated phalloidin, a reagent that reacts with polymerized actin. The arrow points to an organism that has been propelled to the periphery of the cell where it is projecting beyond the plane of the cell membrane, thus approaching the adjacent cell, which will be invaded by this organism when the membrane of the projection fuses with the membrane of the second cell. In this manner, the organism can infect from cell to cell without ever leaving the protected intracellular environment. (From ref. 127, with permission.)

(Fig. 5). This provides a convenient pathway for cell-to-cell invasion and the movement has been termed the Ics (intracellular spread) phenotype.

Shigella flexneri mutants containing a *TnphoA* insertion in a gene designated *icsA* are unable to move within the cell, or for that matter from cell to cell since the latter is presumably dependent on the former. These mutants fail to produce a 120-kDa outer membrane protein, IcsA, and do not induce actin polymerization (127,128). *icsA* deletion mutants have a very limited capacity to cause disease in vivo. In certain cells, such as chick embryo fibroblasts, *Shigella* also move within the cell by binding to actin stress fibers in a very organized manner in which they follow the cytoskeletal architecture (129). The intracellular movement and cell-to-cell spread of *Shigella* has been divided into two phenotypes: Ics (intracellular and intercellular spread) and Olm (organelle-like movement) (129). Movement of *S. flexneri* appears to result from the expression of both the Olm and Ics phenotypes. When intracellular motility of *S. flexneri* was examined in the intestinal cell line, CaCo-2, Olm movement was associated with colonization of organisms in the actin filament ring of the perijunctional area, and Ics movement was related to cell-to-cell spread of infection. Together the two provide a mechanism for a single organism to gain entry to a cell, to multiply, and to spread in a contiguous fashion in a monolayer without ever exiting from the intracellular milieu during the process (130).

d'Hauteville and Sansonetti (131) showed that IcsA is a major substrate for phosphorylation by cyclic nucleotide–dependent protein kinases from the host cell. Site-directed mutagenesis of a sequence encoding a phosphorylation consensus motif almost completely abolished the ability of IcsA to be phosphorylated by protein kinase A. This mutant expressed a "super Ics" phenotype, characterized by an increased capacity to spread from cell to cell. Thus host cell phosphorylation of microbial products may be an important defense mechanism (131).

Cell Death

The mechanism whereby *Shigella* induces cell death is also not fully elucidated. Macrophages are rapidly killed by phagocytosed *Shigella* organisms, independent of their capacity to produce the cytolethal protein, Shiga toxin. Invasion by *S. flexneri* induces apoptosis in the macrophage model (132), implicating apoptosis as the underlying mechanism by which the organisms induce eukaryotic cell death in other cells as well. However, recent data show that the binding of isolated Shiga toxin B subunit to Gb3, which is expressed in high amount on Burkitt lymphoma cells, also triggers apoptosis (133). The relevance of the findings in these two nontarget cells for events in intestinal epithelial cells or endothelial cells remains to be demonstrated.

Regulation of **Shigella** *virulence genes*

Regulation of virulence genes in vivo is critical to the success of pathogenic microorganisms surviving in their host and being transmitted to the next one. For example, a number of toxins, including Shiga toxin, are known to be iron-regulated via the *fur* gene system (71). Temperature and osmotic pressure also are known to have an effect on the expression of *Shigella* invasion genes (134). When grown at 30°C, virulent strains of *S. flexneri*, *S. sonnei*, and *S. dysenteriae* type 1 are neither able to invade epithelial cells in vitro nor able to induce a positive Sereny test. Reexpression of virulence, however, requires several generations of growth at 37°C and is dependent on the synthesis of new proteins. Temperature-regulated factors that may be important for virulence include the production of Shiga toxin, synthesis of *ipaA–D* gene products, synthesis of *mxi* gene products, contact hemolytic activity, and the expression of the positive regulators *virF* and *ipaR* (134). *virR*, a chromosomal gene located just in front of the *stx* gene, serves as a negative regulator of the temperature-regulated genes for Ipa proteins, and the *mxi/spa* gene products, as well as for Congo red binding (135) (Fig. 1).

One of the environmental changes that occurs when *Shigella* invade a mammalian host is a change in osmolarity in the lumen of the gastrointestinal tract. Two classes of genes in *Shigella* respond to changes in osmolarity (134). The first includes genes whose expression is required for the actual physiological adaption to osmotic stress, such as *proU*, *ompF*, *ompC*, and *kdp*. The second class includes genes not directly involved in physiological adaptation but whose expression is clearly optimized under conditions of high osmolarity; as such, these gene products may play a role in pathogenesis. Regulation of *ompC–ompF* expression in *Shigella* is controlled by *ompR–envZ,* which constitute the *ompB* locus. Regulation is similar to the system in *E. coli* in that high osmolarity favors the expression of OmpC in preference to OmpF (134). Deletion of *ompB* or an *envZ::*Tn10 mutation in *S. flexneri* 5a significantly inhibits the organisms' capability to invade HeLa cells and results in a delayed Sereny response in vivo.

A well-described phenotypic characteristic of invasive *Shigella* and EIEC is their ability to bind the dye Congo red (136). Failure to bind Congo red is generally due to the complete loss of, or deletions within, the 220-kb virulence plasmid. Binding to Congo red also is temperature-dependent. Although the precise relationship between Congo red binding and virulence is not known, recent data demonstrate that virulent *S. flexneri, S. dysenteriae* type 1, and EIEC grown in the presence of Congo red synthesize increased levels of membrane-associated proteins of 43, 58, and 63 kDa (137). Other environmental factors that may affect protein synthesis in *Shigella* include the intracellular environment itself as well as alterations in pH and levels of oxygen, all of which are dramatically changed as the organisms progress from the upper to the lower intestinal tract and, even further, as they invade mucosal cells.

DIAGNOSIS

There are at least three means to diagnose shigellosis or infection due to EIEC: clinical, microbiological, and serological.

Clinical Diagnosis

Patients presenting with a classical picture of dysentery, with frequent, small-volume, bloody stools, with abdominal cramps, and with tenesmus (spasms of pain associated with straining to pass stool), especially when febrile, and having large clumps of leukocytes in the stool, can be given a presumptive diagnosis of shigellosis or EIEC infection (19). Examination of stool for leukocytes has been used as a simple and rapid method to differentiate shigellosis and other invasive bacterial diarrheas from amebiasis and secretory bacterial diarrheas such as cholera (138). In Bangladesh, 85% of patients with documented shigellosis had greater than 50 leukocytes per high power field when stool was directly examined by light microscopy, compared to 28% of patients with diagnosed amebic dysentery, even though the latter is generally believed to be without much of an inflammatory exudate in stool because the parasite lyses neutrophils. This finding is not specific, of course; in a study in Thailand, fecal leukocytes were detected not only in shigellosis, but also as expected in patients with diarrhea due to EIEC, *Campylobacter,* and *Salmonella,* as well as in some patients with enteropathogenic or enterotoxigenic *E. coli,* and even rotavirus (139). However, the number of leukocytes was low in the non-*Shigella* cases; the presence of sheets of neutrophils in the stool remains a good clue for the diagnosis of *Shigella* infection. Patients with shigello-

sis can benefit from antimicrobial therapy (see below); however, drug resistance remains a major problem. Therefore, even when antibiotic treatment is begun empirically, laboratory confirmation of the specific etiology is important to guide continuing therapy; microbiological methods are the only way to rapidly confirm the diagnosis of shigellosis or EIEC infections.

Laboratory Diagnosis

Shigella are extremely fastidious and readily die off if the stool sample is not well handled. The best way to isolate them is to obtain stool and not rectal swabs, to rapidly inoculate specimens onto selective culture plates, preferably at the bedside, and to quickly incubate them at 37°C. If a delay in transporting specimens is expected, they should be inoculated directly into transport medium such as buffered glycerol saline (BGS), which appears to better preserve the organisms than Carey–Blair transport medium (140). BGS serves as a true transport medium, and it should be refrigerated after inoculation and used to plate on selective media as rapidly as possible when the specimen reaches the laboratory.

Although fecal samples are readily obtainable in the hospital or clinic setting, rectal swabs may be more practical in the field. *Shigella* isolation from anal swabs is not as good as from either rectal swabs or fecal samples and is not recommended (141). If *Shigella* is strongly suspected on clinical grounds, the fastidiousness of the organism makes it desirable to obtain several cultures to maximize chances of recovering the organism.

To optimize isolation of *Shigella,* more than one medium should be used (142). Ideally, these should include mildly selective media such as MacConkey agar (considered to be the standard), deoxycholate, and eosin–methylene blue (EMB), and highly selective media such as Hektoen-enteric (HE), salmonella–shigella (SS), and xylose–lysine–deoxycholate (XLD) agars. SS agar has the advantage of not requiring autoclaving in the field because it is so inhibitory to common contaminants; however, it is much better for isolation of *Salmonella* than *Shigella,* and is not very good at all for *S. dysenteriae* type 1. The choice of media is best determined by the experience of the microbiologist and the prevalent strains as well. For example, in the United States and United Kingdom, where *S. sonnei* accounts for most isolates, the optimal choice of media may be different from that in India, where *S. flexneri* and *S. dysenteriae* type 1 strains abound. Pitarangsi et al. (142) examined various media for the isolation of *Shigella* from 645 children with diarrhea in Bangkok. *Shigella* were isolated from 98 (15%) of the children, of which 50 isolates were *S. sonnei* and 48 isolates were *S. flexneri* and MacConkey was the best medium (Table 4). In the 1969 Guatemala epidemic, isolation of *S. dysenteriae* type 1 was facilitated by the use of tergitol-7-tetrazolium agar (143).

Enteroinvasive *E. coli* are more difficult to identify than *Shigella* because their biochemical reactions are more variable, distinctive flags such as the inability to ferment lactose are lacking, and they do not fall into classical

TABLE 4. *Comparison of media for the isolation of Shigella species from 645 fecal specimens in Bangkok*

Culture medium	Number of isolates (percent positive)	
	S. flexneri	S. sonnei
MacConkey	44 (6.8)	43 (6.7)
Teknaf enteric[a]	36 (5.6)	3 (0.4)
Hektoen	36 (5.6)	30 (4.6)
Salmonella–Shigella	34 (5.3)	40 (6.2)

Modified from ref. 139.

[a] Teknaf enteric is MacConkey supplemented with 1 mg of potassium tellurite/mL.

EPEC serotypes for which many laboratories have typing sera. While plasmid analysis for the large invasion plasmid or the Sereny test can be used to screen *E. coli* isolates, neither is practical for the routine laboratory (139). EIEC have usually been found to belong to a restricted number of O antigen serogroups, including O28, O29, O112, O124, O136, O143, O144, O147, O152, O164, and O167 (14,144). In addition, fully 10% of EIEC isolates in Thailand belonged to other serogroups, including a new serogroup of EIEC (O171) identified in the same study (145).

The development of molecular techniques using DNA probes or the polymerase chain reaction (PCR) has enabled investigators to determine the prevalence of both *Shigella* and EIEC in different populations (146–149). Although use of DNA probes is both more specific and sensitive than conventional microbiological techniques, this method is somewhat labor-intensive, time consuming, and costly, whether radioactive or the current nonradioactive detection systems are used. PCR allows the detection of very small numbers of organisms, is generally more sensitive than either conventional microbiological techniques or DNA probes (149), and is simple and quick, although direct PCR of stool may require processing to remove inhibitors of the PCR reaction. In addition, the results may be so sensitive as to raise the question of clinical relevance of finding one in a million organisms. The use of molecular diagnostic techniques also requires expertise, equipment, and separate clean laboratory areas to avoid contamination with exogenous DNA, which may not be readily available in developing countries. One outstanding advantage of PCR based diagnostics, however, is their potential use in diagnosing enteric pathogens, including *Shigella* and EIEC, in patients who have been taking antibiotics, since amplification of bacterial DNA can be achieved from nonreplicating organisms and even from dead bacteria present in the fecal sample. PCR techniques may also allow simultaneous detection of several virulence genes in a diarrheal stool sample (148).

Examination for fecal leukocytes can be used also to guide the laboratory in culturing stool. In the United States, the cost per positive stool culture can be markedly reduced if stools are first screened for leukocytes and cultured only if these cells are present (150), because this increases the likelihood of isolating *Shigella*, *Salmonella*, and *Campylobacter* species. The philosophy underlying this idea is to restrict the use of laboratory examinations to identify causes of diarrhea that require treatment other than rehydration. If this concept is adopted, then in addition to fecal leukocytes, the presence of erythrocytes in the stool should be another indicator for culture.

Serological Diagnosis

For epidemiological studies, detection of antibodies to *Shigella* LPS is an alternative method for diagnosis of past *Shigella* infection (151). This technology has been further developed recently as a consequence of the increasing knowledge of the LPS structure in *Shigella* (152,153), combined with the ability to isolate pure LPS (154) and the availability of simple and sensitive immunoassays (155). The LPS of *S. dysenteriae* type 1 has a unique repeating unit (156) that is thought to be shared only with *E. coli* O-antigenic groups 1 and 120, neither of which are common bacterial pathogens. The LPS of *S. flexneri* types 1a–5b, in contrast, is built by a repeating tetrasaccharide with extensive cross-reactions among the serotypes (157), whereas the LPS from *S. flexneri* type 6 is serologically distinctive (153). The O antigen of *S. sonnei* is a disaccharide of two unusual sugars, 2-acetamido-2-deoxy-L-altruronic acid linked 1→4 to 2-acetamido-4-amino-2,4,6-trideoxy-D-galactose, and is shared only with *Plesiomonas shigelloides* (153).

An LPS-EIA for *S. dysenteriae* type 1 has been developed and appears to provide sensitive and specific serodiagnosis when immunoglobulin class–specific determination of IgG or IgA anti-LPS is performed (151). Serotype-specific LPS-EIA for *S. flexneri* 1a–5 is a problem because of the presence of one or more common epitopes; however, a species-specific EIA works well for diagnosis of acute infection in countries where *S. flexneri* is uncommon and primary responses are expected in all patients regardless of age (151). In contrast, in *S. flexneri* endemic countries the EIA may be useful only for children under 3 years of age. EIA for *S. sonnei* LPS appears to be specific and reasonably sensitive, but would probably not be clinically useful in the United States since the illness would be over in the majority of patients by the time the EIA became positive.

Differentiating EIEC from culture-negative shigellosis in the clinical microbiology laboratory can be difficult, since serotyping for invasive *E. coli* strains is generally unavailable. However, in purely clinical terms it is of little consequence since the manifestations of the two diseases overlap, with EIEC usually the milder illness, and their clinical management will be the same and can be guided by clinical features.

TREATMENT

Dysentery or bloody diarrhea due to *Shigella* or EIEC infections are generally not severely dehydrating illnesses. Nonetheless the first therapy for these infections is to replace lost fluids and electrolytes because this is simple, helpful, and usually can be done by the oral route. In most patients in the United States, especially with infection due to *S. sonnei*, the disease is over in a few days to a week. In more severe *Shigella* infections, e.g., in children in Bangladesh, clinically significant hyponatremia occurs in many hospitalized patients infected with either *S. dysenteriae* type 1 or *S. flexneri*. In many of these patients, serum sodium levels drop to less than 120 mmol/L, resulting in central nervous system depression (158). As these findings are associated with increased mortality, some authorities recommend the infusion of hypertonic (3%) saline, 12 mL/kg over 2 hr, to raise the serum Na by around 10 mmol/L. This rapidly reverses the central nervous system manifestations. However, unless access to ad libitum water is restricted, hyponatremia will recur due to underlying inappropriate secretion of antidiuretic hormone (159).

Hypoglycemia, while not common in well-nourished patients with shigellosis or EIEC infection in the United States, can occur and is quite frequent in children in developing countries, usually associated with *S. dysenteriae* type 1 or *S. flexneri* infections (34). Current evidence indicates that this is due to an inadequate gluconeogenic response for the energy needs. Because the blood glucose levels may be less than 1 mmol/L, immediate correction is needed to prevent a fatal outcome. One way to do this is to rapidly infuse 1 g of glucose per kg body weight (5.6 mmol/kg) over 5–10 min, and then give a continuous infusion of fluid containing 50 g glucose/L (278 mmol/L), until the infection is controlled (34).

Shigellosis also represents a major nutritional insult, with catabolic stress during the infection due to fever and cytokine-mediated changes in host metabolism added onto a protein losing enteropathy due to the intestinal damage. As a rule of thumb, it takes around four times as long to repair such deficits as it takes to incur them, assuming unrestricted access to food of high protein quality and adequate energy density (160). It is especially important to ensure that nutritional rehabilitation is accomplished in children in developing countries, although this is usually difficult in the very patient population most affected because of continuing malnutrition, poverty, and inadequate health supervision.

Shigellosis is associated with seizures, which resemble typical febrile seizures except in somewhat older children. These are usually not recurrent and do not need anything other than the reduction of body temperature by the use of antipyretics. Only uncommonly is there an indication for anticonvulsive therapy with barbiturates or diazepam.

Specific therapy in shigellosis requires the administration of effective antimicrobial agents, and this is known to lower mortality and shorten the illness (161,162). Because *Shigella* has acquired multiple antibiotic resistance with apparent ease, the most difficult aspect has been to find drugs that are effective, affordable, and safe. The major problem is to select antimicrobials to which the organism remains sensitive (163,164). Virtually all *Shigellae* carry resistance for streptomycin, tetracycline, and chloramphenicol; many strains are now resistant to ampicillin; and, depending on geographic locale, a varying proportion also are resistant to trimethoprim-sulfamethoxazole (165). In the United States and other developed countries, it is possible to use an oral (166) or parenteral (167) third-generation cephalosporin or, in the case of adults, a new 4-fluoroquinolone (168) (Table 5). The latter drugs are presently not approved for use in those under 17 years of

TABLE 5. *Options for antimicrobial therapy of shigellosis*

Drug	Cost/5 days[a]	Dose		Comments
		Children	Adult	
First-line agents				
Ampicilin	0.48/kg; $3.00	100 mg/kg/d	500 mg qid	Resistance common in Sd, Sf, and Ss
TMP-SMZ	$0.15/kg; $1.40	10/50 mg/kg/d in two doses	1 ds tablet bid	Resistance common in Sd and Ss; variable for Sf
Ciprofloxacin	—; $29.23	Not recommended	500 mg bid	Resistance rare to date
Other new quinolones		Not recommended	Depends on the drug used	
Alternative agents				
Amdinocillin	Not available in U.S.	80 mg/kg/d	400 mg qid[b]	Resistance rare to date
Cefixime	$1.15/kg; $24.00	8 mg/kg/d	400 mg/day[b]	Effective in TMP-SMZ resistant strains
Ceftriaxone	$8.84/kg; $157–305	50 mg/kg IV qd	1–2 g/day[b]	2 days as effective as 5 days
Alternative for developing countries				
Naladixic acid	$1.10/kg; $20.50	55 mg/kg/d	1 g qid	Widely used to treat ampicillin- and TMP-SMZ–resistant Sd and Sf in developing countries but not FDA-approved for use in the US

Sd, *S. dysenteriae* type 1; Sf, *S. flexneri*; Ss, *S. sonnei*; TMP, trimethoprim-sulfamoxazole.

[a] Based on *Redbook* listing for average drug cost (generic when available) for pediatric patients per kg body weight using suspension formulations and total dose for adults for a 5-day course of treatment (does not include the cost of drug administration, if any, and does not include pharmacist markup). Cost for pediatric patients is also an underestimate because pharmacists will ordinarily dispense and charge for an entire commerical package of suspension, which may exceed the need for that child.

[b] Use not reported in adults.

age because of a concern that they will cause cartilage damage, as reported in young rodents exposed to chronic high levels of these drugs. It may be that single-dose treatment with a quinolone will prove to be adequate (169), and under these circumstances the likelihood of toxicity, already near the vanishing point, will diminish still further. Unless single-dose therapy is established, the cost of these drugs currently precludes their use in the developing countries, and instead the first-generation quinolone, naladixic acid, is commonly used, even though it is not licensed in the United States for this indication (170). Although likely to be true, it has not been demonstrated that early treatment with an effective agent will reduce the incidence of systemic complications, and a few retrospective studies have suggested that antibiotic treatment may be a risk factor for HUS (171). This seems to us to be improbable, as the most severely affected are the most likely to both receive antibiotics and to develop complications.

There are no clinical trials of antibiotic treatment of EIEC infection. These generally behave as mild "culture-negative" shigellosis. Antibiotics are often not needed, but should reduce the duration of illness as in shigellosis, except for the fact that resistance to commonly used agents may be a significant problem.

PREVENTION

Prevention of shigellosis falls under two headings: general preventative measures that apply to any disease transmitted by the fecal–oral route and the use of *Shigella*-specific vaccines. Common sense hygienic practices can reduce person-to-person transmission of *Shigella* infection. Simple measures such as separating food preparation and eating from the care of infected individuals and handling of objects potentially contaminated with feces can be very effective, both in the hospital setting and in day care centers. It has been shown under controlled conditions that handwashing with soap prevents transmission of shigellosis, even in a highly endemic area such as Bangladesh (172). The principle problem is how to motivate people to change age-old customs and wash hands adequately after defecation. When handwashing practices and perceptions of soap utilization were analyzed in Bangladesh (173), it was discovered that concepts of cleanliness generally were not based on any germ theory but were viewed in a socioreligious context. Handwashing served both physical and spiritual needs and was performed according to defined patterns that may not necessarily interrupt bacterial transmission routes.

Where flies are plentiful and have access to human feces, i.e., wherever flush toilets or water seal privies and sewage systems do not exist, infectious inocula of *Shigella* can be transmitted by flies from feces to food. Fly control can therefore reduce the incidence of infection (174). It should be noted that the habits of different flies are not identical, and only some species will go between feces in the environment and food in the house or market. Classic studies on fly control and shigellosis were done in the late 1940s (175) and have been repeated in modern

times using an ingenious simple baited fly trap, in which flies are drawn by sweetened bait beneath the trap, which has an entrance at the bottom and a screened hole at the top to allow sunlight to enter (176). Once in the region of the bait below the entrance, the flies are induced to enter the trap by their heliotropism (their tendency to fly toward light). Significant reduction in shigellosis rates, due primarily to *S. sonnei* in this setting, were achieved.

As far as specific vaccine protection is concerned, developing a satisfactory vaccine has proved to be both more difficult and time consuming than originally hoped. While it is likely that secretory IgA on mucosal surfaces and mucosal lymphocytes play important roles in the immunological defense against shigellosis, the actual protective immune responses are still uncertain, and the general strategy to use oral live vaccines may not be entirely on target. The only established principle is that in natural shigellosis protection is serotype-specific, and thus presumably related to the oligosaccharide structure of LPS. Thus, an individual convalescent after *S. flexneri* 2a infection is protected against reinfection only with the homologous serotype. This has been the basis for a resurgence in interest in LPS determinants for immunization, even by the parenteral route (177).

The major evidence that protective immunity to *Shigella* infection occurs is epidemiological. For example, the simple observation in endemic countries that shigellosis is a pediatric disease suggests that infection protection occurs early in life, although this could also be explained by age-related alterations in host susceptibility factors, such as developmentally regulated receptors, or behavioral changes that reduce exposure or improve personal hygiene practices. In addition, evidence from early vaccine trials using two mixtures of live streptomycin-dependent vaccine strains, each containing a different group of several serotypes, demonstrated protection against the serotypes in the vaccine administered, but not against the serotypes in the other vaccine (178). In addition, serotype-specific protection has been observed in humans or rhesus monkeys challenged with *S. flexneri* 2a and then rechallenged with either the same organism or *S. sonnei* (179,180).

The original *Shigella* vaccines were, like other bacterial vaccines, heat- or acetone-killed whole-cell preparations for parenteral administration, designed to induce circulating antibody. These failed to provide significant protection when administered either enterally or parenterally (181). With the advances in understanding mucosal immunity, attention focused on secretory immunoglobulin A and mucosal lymphocytes. A major role of secretory IgA bathing a mucosal surface is to prevent attachment of microorganisms to the mucosa, and secondarily to neutralize microbial products such as toxins. It is not certain that either mechanism is relevant to shigellosis, since secretory IgA collected from the gut of rabbits immunized with an invasive *E. coli–Shigella* hybrid vaccine strain failed to inhibit the invasion of cultured mammalian cells by *S. flexneri* 2a (181). In addition, no evaluation of antitoxin sIgA-based immunity has been carried out. Some evidence has been presented that antibody-dependent cellular cytotoxicity responses develops during shigellosis and may contribute to the control of the infection (182,183). The nature of the antibody, however, has been IgG and the antigens are unclassified. Classical cell-mediated immune responses have not been described in this infection.

Contemporary vaccine development for shigellosis has concentrated on use of living attenuated strains, broadly classified into three types, *Shigella* strains with attenuating chromosomal mutations, *Shigella* strains with attenuating plasmid mutations, and hybrid *Shigella* or *E. coli* strains expressing a limited set of *Shigella* virulence determinants (181). It is likely that an effective vaccine will induce immunity to several microbial antigens. A variety of chromosomal mutations have been studied including spontaneous mutations such as streptomycin dependence (SmD), a combination of spontaneous and chemical mutation (Pur$^-$/Rif), spontaneous and ultraviolet mutagenesis (TSF-21), or insertional mutagenesis (Sfl-114) (181). Problems have arisen with each. The SmD mutation proved to be unstable, with reversion to streptomycin independence occurring at a low but unacceptable rate. It offered marginal protection compared to side effects, and it required the administration of multiple doses of large numbers of organisms. The Pur$^-$/Rif mutants were found to elicit a high rate of reactions (tenesmus, meteorism, and diarrhea) and are not being investigated further. It is probable that the TSF-21 vaccine is functionally noninvasive and such noninvasive strains usually require multiple large doses that limit their practical usefulness. Its greatest fault is the lack of a precisely known mutation, which is no longer acceptable in vaccinology in the molecular biology era. The fourth example, Sfl-114, was constructed by transduction of an insertionally inactivated *aroD*::Tn10 gene of *E. coli* K-12 NK 5131 into *S. flexneri* serotype Y, strain Sfl-1 (184,185). The *aroD* insertion inhibits the biosynthesis of aromatic metabolites resulting in an inability of the organism to synthesis folic acid. Thus, although these strains are able to invade, their subsequent intracellular survival is very limited. Karnell et al. (186) studied the safety and immunogenicity of Sfl-114 in volunteers who were given either 10^9 or 10^{10} Sfl-114 by mouth. Mild transient intestinal discomfort was reported in 12% of the volunteers given 10^9 and in 54% given 10^{10}. Satisfactory immune responses were obtained; however, further work with *aroD* deletion mutants are required to reduce reactogenicity before protective efficacy will be evaluated.

Various vaccines based on attenuating plasmid mutations are being made (181). T$_{32}$Istrati was one of the earliest, being isolated in 1961 following 32 subcultures of *S. flexneri* 2a on nutrient agar. The nature of the attenuating alteration was characterized only later, when the genetics of virulence were better known, and it turns out that this strain contains a deletion eliminating both the invasion region and the *icsA* gene of the plasmid. This strain has been extensively tested (181) and vaccination is associated with greater than 80% reduction in the incidence of *S. flexneri* infection. However, it requires repeated inoculation of large doses and is therefore cumbersome and expensive. Other plasmid mutations of interest include a series of specifically designed mutants produced by Sansonetti et al. (187). These strains (SC560, SC570, SC5700) are invasive but fail to spread from cell to cell because

of *icsA* mutations. They elicit significant serum immune response in monkeys but are excessively reactogenic for testing in humans.

The early genetic approach used *E. coli–S. flexneri* hybrid vaccines in which genes have been moved back and forth to attenuate virulent *Shigella* or to introduce genes for protective *Shigella* antigens into *E. coli* (see Ref. 181 for review). One principle emerging from these experiments is that noninvasive hybrids are unlikely to generate a protective immune response, whereas invasive *aroD$^-$* *E. coli–S. flexneri* hybrids may eventually prove to be useful *Shigella* vaccines (181).

Other groups have continued to explore the use of killed vaccine preparations. For example, Russian investigators have been studying the use of ribosomal vaccines, with some experimental support for the approach (188). A radical alternative *Shigella* vaccine strategy has recently been suggested by Robbins et al. (177,189) in which O-specific side chains of *Shigella* LPS would be linked to a carrier protein, with the LPS–protein conjugate used as a parenteral vaccine. The idea is that enough IgG antibody would leak into the lumen to kill organisms at and within the mucosa, and that circulating antibody will be bactericidal for organisms gaining entrance to the circulation.

While progress is being made, it is unlikely that a safe, effective, and cost-efficient vaccine will become available in the near future. The role of such a vaccine would be to reduce morbidity and mortality in exposed populations, such as the children of the developing world, infants in day care, children in custodial care, the military, and other travelers to endemic countries. The importance of vaccine development is underscored by the unlikely probability that widespread implementation of protected water supplies and sanitary fecal disposal will happen soon in developing countries; this is simply unrealistic. For these reasons the most positive preventive strategies in the foreseeable future revolve around teaching and reinforcing behavioral modifications such as handwashing, protection of food and drinking water supplies, case containment, appropriate and restricted use of antibiotics, and the encouragement of breastfeeding (190).

REFERENCES

1. Shiga K. Ueber den Dysenteriebacillus (*Bacillus dysenteriae*). *Zentbl Bakt ParasitKde Abt I Orig* 1898;24:817–824.
2. Flexner S. On the etiology of tropical dysentery. *Bull Johns Hopkins Hosp* 1900;11:231–242.
3. Kruse W. Ueber die Ruhr als Volkskrankheit und ihrer Erreger. *Deutsch Med Wschr* 1900;26:637–639.
4. Conradi H. Uber losliche, durch aseptische Autolyse erhlatene Giftstoffe von Ruhrund Typhus bazillen. *Deutsch Med Wschr* 1903;20:26–28.
5. Todd C. On a dysentery toxin and antitoxin. *J Hyg* 1904;4: 480–494.
6. Hale TL. Genetic basis of virulence in *Shigella* species. *Microbiol Rev* 1991;55:206–224.
7. Keusch GT, Donohue-Rolfe A, Jacewicz M. *Shigella* toxin(s): description and role in diarrhea and dysentery. *Pharmacol Ther* 1982;15:403–438.
8. Sansonetti PJ. *Pathogenesis of shigellosis*. Berlin: Springer-Verlag; 1992. (*Current topics in microbiology and immunology*).

9. Keusch GT. Shigella. In: Gorbach SL, Bartlett JG, Blacklow NR, eds. *Infectious diseases*. Philadelphia: WB Saunders; 1992:1484–1489.
10. Evins GM, Ghessling LL, Tauxe RV. Quality of commercially produced *Shigella* serogrouping and serotyping antisera. *J Clin Microbiol* 1988;26:438–442.
11. Carlin NIA, Lindberg AA. Monoclonal antibodies specific for O-antigenic polysaccharides of *Shigella flexneri*: clones bind to II, II:3,4 and 7,8 epitopes. *J Clin Microbiol* 1983;18:1183–1189.
12. Cheasty T, Rowe B. Antigenic relationships between the enteroinvasive *Escherichia coli* O antigens O28ac, O112ac, O136, O143, O144, O152 and O164 and *Shigella* O antigens. *J Clin Microbiol* 1983;17:681–684.
13. Edwards PR, Ewing WH. In: *Identification of Enterobacteriaceae*. Minneapolis: Burgess; 1972.
14. Trabulsi LR, Fernandes MFR, Zuliani ME. Novas bacterias; pathogenicas para o intestino do homen. *Rev Inst Med Trop S Paolo* 1967;9:31–36.
15. Toledo MRF, Trabulsi LR. Correlation between biochemical and serological characteristics of *Escherichia coli* and results of the Sereny test. *J Clin Microbiol* 1983;17:419–421.
16. Mosley WH, Adams B, Lyman ED. Epidemiological and sociologic features of a large urban outbreak of shigellosis. *JAMA* 1962;182:1307–1311.
17. DuPont HL, Levine MM, Hornick RB, Formal SB. Inoculum size in shigellosis and implications for expected mode of transmission. *J Infect Dis* 1989;159:1126–1128.
18. Wilson R, Feldman RA, Davis J, LaVenture M. Family illness associated with *Shigella* infection: the interrelationship of age of the index patient and the age of household members in acquisition of illness. *J Infect Dis* 1981;143:130–132.
19. Keusch GT, Bennish ML. Shigellosis. In: Evans AS, Brachman P, eds. *Bacterial diseases of humans*. 2nd ed. New York: Plenum Press; 1989.
20. Clemens JD, Stanton B, Stoll B, Shahid NS, Banu H, Chowdhury A. Breast feeding as a determinant of severity in shigellosis. *Am J Epidemiol* 1986;123:710–718.
21. Kostrewski J, Stypulkowska-Misiurewicz H. Changes in the epidemiology of dysentery in Poland and the situation in Europe. *Arch Imuno Ther Exp Med* 1968;20:608–615.
22. Mata LJ, Gangarosa EJ, Caceres A, Perera DR, Mejicanos ML. Epidemic Shiga bacillus dysentery in Central America. I. Etiologic investigations in Guatemala, 1969. *J Infect Dis* 1969;122:170–180.
23. Keusch GT, Bennish ML. Shigellosis: recent progress, persisting problems and research issues. *Pediatr Infect Dis J* 1989;8:713–719.
24. Pickering LK, Bartlett AV, Woodward WE. Acute infectious diarrheas among children in day care: epidemiology and control. *Rev Infect Dis* 1986;8:539–547.
25. Dritz SK, Black AF. *Shigella* enteritis venereally transmitted. *N Engl J Med* 1974;291:1194.
26. Drusin LM, Genvert G, Topf-Olstein B, et al. Shigellosis: another sexually transmitted disease? *Br J Vener Dis* 1976;52:348–350.
27. Tauxe RV, McDonald RC, Hargrett-Bean N, Blake PA. The persistence of *Shigella flexneri* in the United States: the increased role of the adult male. *Am J Public Health* 1988;78:1432–1435.
28. Gangarosa EJ, Perera DR, Mata LJ, Mendizabal-Morris C, Cuzma G, Reller LB. Epidemic Shiga bacillus dysentery in Central America. II. Epidemiologic studies, 1969. *J Infect Dis* 1970;122:170–180.
29. Malengreau M, Molima-Kaba, Gillieaux M, deFeyter M, Kyele-Duibone, Mukolo-Ndjolo. Outbreak of *Shigella* dysentery in Eastern Zaire, 1980–1982. *Ann Soc Belge Med Trop* 1983;63:59–67.
30. Bennish ML. Wojtyniak BJ. Mortality due to shigellosis: community and hospital data. *Rev Infect Dis* 1991;13:S245–S251.
31. Ewing WH, Gravatti JL. *Shigella* types encountered in the mediterranean area. *J Bacteriol* 1947;53:191–195.
32. Hobbs BC, Thomas MEM. School outbreak of gastroenteritis associates with a pathogenic paracolon bacillus. *Lancet* 1949; 2:530–532.
33. Marier R, Wells JC, Swanson RC, Callahan W, Mehlman IJ. An outbreak of enteropathogenic *Escherichia coli* foodborne disease traced to imported French cheese. *Lancet* 1973;2:1376–1378.
34. Bennish ML, Azad AK, Rahman O, et al. Hypoglycemia during childhood diarrhea: prevalence, pathophysiology and outcome. *N Engl J Med* 1990;322:1357–1363.
35. Speelman P, Kabir I, Islam M. Distribution and spread of colonic lesions in shigellosis: a colonoscopic study. *J Infect Dis* 1984;150:899–903.
36. Butler T, Speelman P, Kabir I, Banwell J. Colonic dysfunction during shigellosis. *J Infect Dis* 1986;154:817–824.
37. Blaser MJ, Pollard RA, Feldman RA. *Shigella* infections in the United States 1974–1980. *J Infect Dis* 1983;147:771–775.
38. Azad MAK, Islam M, Butler T. Colonic perforation in *Shigella dysenteriae* type I infection. *Pediatr Infect Dis* 1986;5:103–104.
39. Bennish ML, Azad AK, Yousefzadeh D. Intestinal obstruction during shigellosis: incidence, clinical features, risk factors, and outcome. *Gastroenterology* 1991;101:626–634.
40. Bennish ML, Salam MA, Wahed MA. Enteric protein loss during shigellosis. *Am J Gastroenterol* 1993;88:53–57.
41. Struelens MJ, Pate D, Kabir I, Salam A, Nath SK, Butler T. *Shigella* septicemia: prevalence, presentation, risk factors, and outcome. *J Infect Dis* 1985;152:784–790.
42. Koster F, Levin J, Walker L, et al. Hemolytic-uremic syndrome after shigellosis: relation to endotoxemia and circulating immune complexes. *N Engl J Med* 1978;298:927–933.
43. Ashkenazi S, Cleary KR, Pickering LK, Murray BE, Cleary TG. The association of Shiga toxin and other cytotoxins with the neurologic manifestations of shigellosis. *J Infect Dis* 1990;161:961–965.
44. Raybourne RB, Williams KM. Monoclonal antibodies against an HLA-B27-derived peptide react with an epitope present on bacterial proteins. *J Immunol* 1990;145:2539–2544.
45. Williams KM, Raybourne RB. Demonstration of cross-reactivity between bacterial antigens and class I human leukocyte antigens by using monoclonal antibodies to *Shigella flexneri*. *Infect Immun* 1990;58:1774–1781.
46. Stieglitz H, Formal SB, Lipsky P. Identification of a 2-Md plasmid from *Shigella flexneri* associated with reactive arthritis. *Arthritis Rheum* 1989;32:937–946.
47. Kapasi K, Chui B, Inman RD. HLA-B27/microbial mimicry: an in vivo analysis. *Immunology* 1992;77:456–461.
48. Yoshikawa M, Sasakawa C. Molecular pathogenesis of shigellosis: a review. *Microbiol Immunol* 1991;35:809–824.
49. Sereny B. Experimental keratoconjunctivitis shigellosa. *Acta Microbiol Acad Sci Hung* 1957;4:367–376.
50. Gorden J, Small PLC. Acid resistance in enteric bacteria. *Infect Immun* 1993;61:364–367.
51. Small PLC, Falkow S. A genetic analysis of acid resistance in *Shigella flexneri*; the requirement for a *katF* homologue. *Abstr Gen Meet Am Soc Microbiol* 1992;B74:38.
52. DuPont HL, Formal SB, Hornick RB, et al. Pathogenesis of *Escherichia coli*. *N Engl J Med* 1971;285:1–9.
53. Bloch CA, Stocker BAD, Orndorff PE. A key role for type 1 pili in enterobacterial communicability. *Mol Microbiol* 1992;6:697–701.
54. Payne SM. Iron and virulence. *Mol Microbiol* 1989;3:1301–1306.
55. Nassif X, Mazert MC, Mouniew J, Sansonetti PJ. Evaluation with an *iuc*::Tn10 mutant of the role of aerobactin production in the virulence of *Shigella flexneri*. *Infect Immun* 1987;55:1963–1969.
56. Gemski P, Sheahan DG, Washington O, Formal SB. Virulence of *Shigella flexneri* hybrids expressing *Escherichia coli* somatic antigens. *Infect Immun* 1972;6:104–111.
57. Okada N, Sasakawa C, Tobe T et al. Virulence-associated chromosomal loci of *Shigella flexneri* identified by random Tn5 insertion mutagenesis. *Mol Microbiol* 1991;5:187–195.
58. Okamura N, Nagai T, Nakaya R, Kondo S, Murakami M, Hisatsune K. HeLa cell invasiveness and O antigen of *Shigella flexneri* as a separate and prerequisite attributes of virulence

to evoke keratoconjunctivitis in guinea pigs. *Infect Immun* 1983;39:505–513.

59. Watanabe H, Nakamura A, Timmis KN. Small virulence plasmid of *Shigella dysenteriae* 1 strain W30864 encodes a 41,000 dalton protein involved in formation of specific lipopolysaccharide side chains of serotype 1 isolates. *Infect Immun* 1984;46:55–63.

60. Watanabe H, Timmis KN. A small plasmid in *Shigella dysenteriae* I specifies one or more functions essential for O antigen production and bacterial virulence. *Infect Immun* 1984;43:391–396.

61. Brahmbhatt HN, Lindberg AA, Timmis KN. *Shigella* lipopolysaccharide: structure, genetics and vaccine development. In: Sansonetti PJ, ed. *Pathogenesis of shigellosis*. Berlin: Springer-Verlag; 1992:45–64. (*Current topics in microbiology and immunology*).

62. Franzon VL, Arondel J, Sansonetti PJ. Contribution of superoxide dismutase and catalase activities to *Shigella flexneri* pathogenesis. *Infect Immun* 1990;58:529–535.

63. Keusch GT, Grady GF, Mata LJ, McIver J. The pathogenesis of *Shigella* diarrhea I. Enterotoxin production by *Shigella dysenteriae* 1. *J Clin Invest* 1972;51:1212–1218.

64. O'Brien AD, Tesh VL, Donohue-Rolfe, et al. Shiga toxin: biochemistry, genetics, mode of action and role in pathogenesis. In: Sansonetti PJ, ed. *Pathogenesis of shigellosis*. Berlin: Springer-Verlag; 1992:65–94. (*Current topics in microbiology and immunology*).

65. Endo Y, Tsurugi K, Yutsudo K, Takeda T, Ogasawara T, Igararshi K. Site of action of Vero toxin (VT2) from *Escherichia coli* O157:H7 and of Shiga toxin on eukaryotic ribosomes. RNA N-glycosidase activity of the toxins. *Eur J Biochem* 1988;171:45–50.

66. Hovde CJ, Calderwood SB, Mekalanos JJ, Collier RJ. Evidence that glutamic acid 167 is an active-site residue of Shiga-like toxin I. *Proc Natl Acad Sci USA* 1988;85:2568–2572.

67. Ramotar K, Boyd B, Tyrrell G, Gariepy J, Lingwood C, Brunton J. Characterization of Shiga-like toxin I B subunit purified from overproducing clones of the SLT-I B cistron. *Biochem J* 1990;272:805–811.

68. Acheson DWK, Calderwood SB, Boyko SA, et al. Comparison of Shiga-like toxin I B-subunit expression and localization in *Escherichia coli* and *Vibrio cholerae* by using *trc* or iron-regulated promoter systems. *Infect Immun* 1993;61:1098–1104.

69. Stein PE, Boodhoo A, Tyrrell GJ, Brunton JL, Read RJ. Crystal structure of the cell-binding B oligomer of verotoxin-1 from *E. coli*. *Nature* 1992;355:748–750.

70. Jackson MP, Wadolkowski EA, Weinstein DL, Holmes RK, O'Brien AD. Functional analysis of the Shiga toxin and Shiga-like toxin type II variant binding subunits by using site-directed mutagenesis. *J Bacteriol* 1990;172:653–658.

71. Calderwood SB, Mekalanos JJ. Iron regulation of Shiga-like toxin expression in *Escherichia coli* is mediated by the *fur* locus. *J Bacteriol* 1987;169:4759–4764.

72. Lindberg AA, Brown JE, Stromberg N, Westling-Ryd M, Schultz JE, Karlsson KA. Identification of the carbohydrate receptor for Shiga toxin produced by *Shigella dysenteriae* type 1. *J Biol Chem* 1987;262:1779–1785.

73. Jacewicz M, Clausen H, Nudelman E, Donohue-Rolfe A, Keusch GT. Pathogenesis of *Shigella* diarrhea XI. Isolation of shigella toxin-binding glycolipid from rabbit jejunum and HeLa cells and its identification as globotriaosylceramide. *J Exp Med* 1986;163:1391–1404.

74. Mobassaleh M, Gross SK, McCluer RH, Donohue-Rolfe A, Keusch GT. Quantitation of the rabbit intestinal glycolipid receptor for Shiga toxin. Further evidence for the developmental regulation of globotriaosylceramide in microvillus membranes. *Gastroenterology* 1989;97:384–391.

75. Mobassaleh M, Donohue-Rolfe A, Jacewicz M, et al. Pathogenesis of *Shigella* diarrhea: evidence for a developmentally regulated glycolipid receptor for *Shigella* toxin involved in the fluid secretory response of rabbit small bowel. *J Infect Dis* 1988;157:1023–1031.

76. Mobassaleh M, Koul O, Mishra K, McClure RH, Keusch GT. Developmental regulation of intestinal Gb3 galactosyltransfer-

ase and α-galactosidase control shiga toxin receptors. *Am J Physiol*; in press.

77. Jacewicz M, Feldman HA, Donohue-Rolfe A, Balsubramanian KA, Keusch GT. Pathogenesis of *Shigella* diarrhea XIV. analysis of Shiga toxin receptors on cloned HeLa cells. *J Infect Dis* 1989;159:881–889.

78. Jacewicz MS, Mobassaleh M, Gross SK, et al. Pathogenesis of *Shigella* diarrhea. XVII. A mammalian cell membrane glycolipid, Gb3, is required but not sufficient to confer sensitivity to Shiga toxin. *J Infect Dis* 1994;169:538–546.

79. Kandel G, Donohue-Rolfe A, Donowitz M, Keusch GT. Pathogenesis of *Shigella* diarrhea. XVI. Selective targeting of Shiga toxin to villus cells or rabbit jejunum explains the effect of the toxin on intestinal electrolyte transport. *J Clin Invest* 1989;84:1509–1517.

80. Jacewicz MS, Mobassaleh M, Acheson D, et al. Butyrate induces receptors and increases sensitivity to Shiga toxin in intestinal cell lines. *Proceedings of the 33rd Interscience Conference on Antimicrobial Agents and Chemotherapy*. Abstract 1298A. 1993;357.

81. Sandvig K, Prydz K, Ryd M, van Deurs B. Endocytosis and intracellular transport of the glycolipid-binding ligand Shiga toxin in polarized MDCK cells. *J Cell Biol* 1991;113:553–562.

82. Jacewicz M, Keusch GT. Pathogenesis of *Shigella* diarrhea. VIII. Evidence for a translocation step in the cytotoxic action of Shiga toxin. *J Infect Dis* 1983;148:844–854.

83. Sandvig K, Olsnes S, Brown JE, Petersen OW, van Deurs B. Endocytosis from coated pits of Shiga toxin: a glycolipid-binding protein from *Shigella dysenteriae* I. *J Cell Biol* 1989;108:1331–1343.

84. Moyer MP, Dixon PS, Rothman SW, Brown JE. Cytotoxicity of Shiga toxin for primary cultures of human colonic and ileal epithelial cells. *Infect Immun* 1987;55:1533–1535.

85. Levine MM, DuPont HL, Formal SB, et al. Pathogenesis of *Shigella dysenteriae* I (Shiga) dysentery. *J Infect Dis* 1973;127:261–270.

86. Neill RJ, Gemski P, Formal SB, Newland JW. Deletion of the Shiga toxin gene in a chlorate-resistant derivative of *Shigella dysenteriae* type I that retains virulence. *J Infect Dis* 1988;158:737–741.

87. Fontaine A, Arondel J, Sansonetti PJ. Role of Shiga toxin in the pathogenesis of bacillary dysentery studied using a tox mutant of *Shigella dysenteriae* I. *Infect Immun* 1988;56:3099–3109.

88. Richardson SE, Karmali MA, Becker LE, Smith CR. The histopathology of the hemolytic uremic syndrome associated with verocytotoxin-producing *Escherichia coli* infections. *Hum Pathol* 1988;19:1102–1108.

89. Butler T, Rahman H, Al-Mahmud KA, Islam M, Bardhan P, Kabir I, Rahman MM. An animal model of haemolytic-uraemic syndrome in shigellosis: lipopolysaccharides of *Shigella dysenteriae* I and *S. flexneri* produces leucocyte-mediated renal cortical necrosis in rabbits. *Br J Exp Pathol* 1985;66:7–15.

90. Obrig TG, Del Vecchio PJ, Karmali MA, Petric M, Moran TP, Judge TK. Pathogenesis of haemolytic uraemic syndrome. *Lancet* 1987;2:687.

91. van de Kar NC, Monnens LA, Karmali MA, van Hinsbergh VW. Tumor necrosis factor and interleukin-1 induce expression of the verocytotoxin receptor globotriaosylceramide on human endothelial cells: implications for the pathogenesis of the hemolytic uremic syndrome. *Blood* 1992;80:2755–2764.

92. Kaye SA, Louise CB, Boyd B, Lingwood CA, Obrig TG. Shiga toxin-associated hemolytic uremic syndrome: interleukin-1b enhancement of Shiga toxin cytotoxicity toward human vascular endothelial cells in vitro. *Infect Immun* 1993;61:3886–3891.

93. Obrig TG, Louise CB, Lingwood CA, Boyd B, Barley-Maloney L, Daniel TO. Endothelial heterogeneity in Shiga toxin receptors and responses. *J Biol Chem* 1993;268:15484–15488.

94. Louise CB, Obrig TG. Shiga toxin-associated hemolytic uremic syndrome: combined cytotoxic effects of Shiga toxin and lipopolysaccharide (endotoxin) on human vascular endothelial cells in vitro. *Infect Immun* 1992;60:1536–1543.

95. Bridgewater FAJ, Morgan RS, Rowson KEK, Payling-Wright G. The neurotoxin of *Shigella shigae*. Morphological and func-

tional lesions produced in the central nervous system of rabbits. *Br J Exp Pathol* 1955;36:447–453.

96. Howard JG. Observations on the intoxication produced in mice and rabbits by the neurotoxin of *Shigella shigae. Br J Exp Pathol* 1955;36:439–446.

97. MacLeod DL, Gyles CL, Wilcock BP. Reproduction of edema disease of swine with purified Shiga-like toxin-II variant. *Vet Pathol* 1991;28:66–73.

98. Keusch GT, Jacewicz M. Pathogenesis of *Shigella* diarrhea. VI. Toxin and antitoxin in *S. flexneri* and *S. sonnei* infections in humans. *J Infect Dis* 1977;135:552–557.

99. O'Brien AD, Thompson MR, Gemski P, Doctor BP, Formal SB. Biological properties of *Shigella flexneri* 2a toxin and its serological relationship to *Shigella dysenteriae* 1 toxin. *Infect Immun* 1977;15:796–798.

100. Fasano A, Guandalini S, Russell RG, Rae B, Raimondi F, Levine MM. Enterotoxin production by *Shigella flexneri* 2a. *J Pediatr Gastroenterol Nutr* 1991;13:320.

101. Fasano A, Kay BA, Russell RG, Maneval Jr DR, Levine MM. Enterotoxin and cytotoxin production by enteroinvasive *Escherichia coli. Infect Immun* 1990;58:3717–3723.

102. Sansonetti PJ. Molecular and cellular biology of *Shigella flexneri* invasiveness: from cell assay systems to shigellosis. In: Sansonetti PJ, ed. *Pathogenesis of shigellosis.* Berlin: Springer-Verlag; 1992:1–19. (*Current topics in microbiology and immunology*).

103. Sansonetti PJ. Genetic and molecular basis of epithelial cell invasion by *Shigella* species. *Rev Infect Dis* 13 (Suppl 4);1991: S285–S292.

104. Sansonetti PJ, Ryter A, Clerc P, Maurelli AT, Mounier J. Multiplication of *Shigella flexneri* within HeLa cells: lysis of the phagocytic vacuole and plasmid mediated contact hemolysis. *Infect Immun* 1986;51:461–465.

105. Hale TL, Morris RE, Bonventre PF. *Shigella* infection of Henle intestinal epithelial cells: role of the host cell. *Infect Immun* 1979;24:887–894.

106. Clerc P, Sansonetti PJ. Entry of *Shigella flexneri* into HeLa cells: evidence for direct phagocytosis involving actin polymerization and myosin accumulation. *Infect Immun* 1987;55: 2681–2688.

107. Sansonetti PJ, Kopecko DJ, Formal SB. Involvement of a plasmid in the invasive ability of *Shigella flexneri. Infect Immun* 1982;35:852–860.

108. Sansonetti PJ, Hale TL, Dammin GI, Kapper C, Collins HH, Formal SB. Alterations in the pathogenesis of *Escherichia coli* K12 after transfer of plasmid and chromosomal genes from *Shigella flexneri. Infect Immun* 1983;39:1392–1402.

109. Sasakawa C, Buysse JM, Watanabe H. The large virulence plasmid of *Shigella*. In: Sansonetti PJ, ed. *Pathogenesis of shigellosis.* Berlin: Springer-Verlag; 1992:21–44. (*Current topics in microbiology and immunology*).

110. Adler B, Sasakawa C, Tobe T, Makino S, Komatsu K, Yoshikawa M. A dual transcriptional activation system for the 230kb plasmid genes coding for virulence associated antigens of *Shigella flexneri. Mol Microbiol* 1989;3:627–635.

111. Buysse JM, Venkatesan JA, Mills JA, Oaks EV. Molecular characterization of a trans-acting positive effector (*ipaR*) of invasion plasmid antigen synthesis in *Shigella flexneri* serotype 5. *Microb Pathog* 1990;8:197–211.

112. Watanabe H, Arakawa E, Ito K, Kato JI, Nakamura A. Genetic analysis of an invasion region by use of a Tn3-lac transposon and identification of a second positive regulator gene, *invE* for cell invasion of *Shigella sonnei*: significant homology of inv E with par B of plasmid Pl. *J Bacteriol* 1990;172:619–629.

113. Hromockyj AE, Maurelli AT. Identification of *Shigella* invasion genes by construction of temperature-regulated *inv::lacZ* operon fusions. *Infect Immun* 1989;57:2963–2970.

114. Gemski P, Griffin DE. Isolation and characterization of minicell-producing mutants of *Shigella* spp. *Infect Immun* 1980;30: 297–302.

115. Hale TL, Sansonetti PF, Schad PA, Austin S, Formal SB. Characterization of virulence plasmids and plasmid-associated outer membrane proteins in *Shigella flexneri, Shigella sonnei* and *Escherichia coli. Infect Immun* 1983;40:340–350.

116. Buysse JM, Stover CK, Oaks EV, Venkatesan M, Kopecko DJ. Molecular cloning of invasion plasmid antigen (ipa) genes from *Shigell flexneri:* analysis of *ipa* gene products and genetic mapping. *J Bacteriol* 1987;169:2561–2569.

117. Andrews GP, Hromockyj AE, Coker C, Maurelli AT. Two novel virulence loci, *mxiA* and *mxiB*, in *Shigella flexneri* 2a facilitate excretion of invasion plasmid antigens. *Infect Immun* 1991;59:1997–2005.

118. Venkatesan MM, Buysse JM, Oaks EV. Surface presentation of *Shigella flexneri* invasion plasmid antigens requires the products of the *spa* locus. *J Bacteriol* 1992;174:1900–2001.

119. Allaoui A, Menard R, Sansonetti, Parsot C. Characterization of the *Shigella flexneri ipgD* and *ipgF* genes, which are located in the proximal part of the *mxi* locus. *Infect Immun* 1993;61: 1707–1714.

120. Wassef JS, Keren DF, Mailloux JL. Role of M cells in initial bacterial uptake and in ulcer formation in the rabbit intestinal loop model in shigellosis. *Infect Immun* 1989;57:858–863.

121. Clerc P, Baudry B, Sansonetti PJ. Plasmid-mediated contact hemolytic activity in *Shigella* species: correlation with penetration into HeLa cells. *Ann Inst Pasteur Microbiol* 1986;137A: 267–278.

122. Clerc P, Ryter A, Mounier J, Sansonetti PJ. Plasmid mediated early killing of eucaryotic cells by *Shigella flexneri* as studied by infection of J774 macrophages. *Infect Immun* 1987;55: 521–527.

123. Bernardini ML, Sanna MG, Fontaine A, Sansonetti PJ. OmpC is involved in invasion of epithelial cells by *Shigella flexneri. Infect Immun* 1993;61:3625–3635.

124. Goldberg MB, Sansonetti PJ. *Shigella* subversion of the cellular cytoskeleton: a strategy for epitheial colonization. *Infect Immun* 1993;61:4941–4946.

125. Makino S, Sasakawa C, Kamata K, Kurata T, Yosikawa M. A genetic determinant required for continuous reinfection of adjacent cells on large plasmid in *Shigella flexneri* 2a. *Cell* 1986; 46:551–555.

126. Pal T, Newland JW, Tall D, Formal SB. Intracellular spread of *Shigella flexneri* associated with the kcpA locus and a 140-kilodalton protein. *Infect Immun* 1989;578:477–486.

127. Bernardini ML, Mounier J, d'Hauteville H, Coquis-Rondon M, Sansonetti PJ. Identification of *icsA*, a plasmid locus of *Shigella flexneri* that governs intra- and intercellular spread through interaction with F-actin. *Proc Natl Acad Sci USA* 1989;86: 3867–3871.

128. Lett MC, Sasakawa C, Okasa N, et al. *virG*, a plasmid coded virulence gene of *Shigella flexneri:* identification of the VirG protein and determination of the complete coding sequence. *J Bacteriol* 1989;171:353–359.

129. Vasselon T, Mounier J, Prevost MC, Hellio R, Sansonetti PJ. A stress fiber-based movement of *Shigella flexneri* within cells. *Infect Immun* 1991;59:1723–1732.

130. Vasselon T, Mounier J, Hellio R, Sansonetti PJ. Movement along actin filaments of the perijunctional area and de novo polymerization of cellular actin are required for *Shigella flexneri* colonization of epithelial Caco-2 cell monolayers. *Infect Immun* 1992;60:1031–1040.

131. d'Hauteville H, Sansonetti PJ. Phosphorylation of IcsA by cAMP-dependent protein kinase and its effect on intercellular spread of *Shigella flexneri. Mol Microbiol* 1992;6:833–841.

132. Zychlinsky A, Prevost MC, Sansonetti PJ. *Shigella flexneri* induces apoptosis in infected macrophages. *Nature* 1992;358: 167–169.

133. Mangeney M, Lingwood CA, Taga S, Caillou B, Tursz T, Wiels J. Apoptosis induced in Burkitt's lymphoma cells via Gb3/CD77, a glycolipid antigen. *Cancer Res* 1993;53:5314–5319.

134. Maurelli AT, Hromockyj AE, Bernardini ML. Environmental regulation of *Shigella* virulence. In: Sansonetti PJ, ed. *Pathogenesis of shigellosis.* Berlin: Springer-Verlag; 1992:85–116. (*Current topics in microbiology and immunology*).

135. Maurelli AT, Sansonetti PJ. Identity of a chromosomal gene controlling temperature regulated expression of *Shigella* virulence. *Proc Natl Acad Sci USA* 1988;85:2820–2824.

136. Payne SM, Finkelstein RA. Detection and differentiation of

iron-responsive avirulent mutants on Congo red agar. *Infect Immun* 1977;18:94–98.

137. Sankaran K, Ramachandran V, Subrahmanyam YVBK, Rajarathnam S, Elango S, Roy RK. Congo red-mediated regulation of levels of *Shigella flexneri* 2a membrane proteins. *Infect Immun* 1989;57:2364–2371.

138. Speelman P, McGlaughlin R, Kabir I, Butler T. Differences in clinical features and stool findings in shigellosis and amebic dysentery. *Trans R Soc Trop Med Hyg* 1987;81:549–551.

139. Echeverria P, Sethabutr O, Pitarangsi C. Microbiology and diagnosis of infections with *Shigella* and enteroinvasive *E. coli*. *Rev Infect Dis* 1991;13:S220–S225.

140. Wells JG, Morris GK. Evaluation of transport methods for isolating *Shigella* ssp. *J Clin Microbiol* 1981;13:789–790.

141. Adkins HJ, Santingo LT. Increased recovery of enteric pathogens by use of both stool and rectal swab specimens. *J Clin Microbiol* 1987;25:158–159.

142. Pitarangsi C, Taylor DN, Echeverria P, Johnson S. Media for the isolation of *Shigella*. *J Diarrh Dis Res* 1987;5:43.

143. Mata LJ, Gangarosa EJ, Caceres A, Perera DR, Mejicanos ML. Epidemic Shiga bacillus dysentery in Central America. I. Etiologic investigations in Guatemala. *J Infect Dis* 1969;123:25–38.

144. Taylor DN, Echeverria P, Sethabutr O, et al. Clinical and microbiologic features of *Shigella* and enteroinvasive *Escherichia coli* infections detected by DNA hybridization. *J Clin Microbiol* 1988;26:1362–1366.

145. Echeverria P, Taylor DN, Lexsomboon U, et al. Case-control study of endemic diarrheal disease in Thai children. *J Infect Dis* 1989;159:543–548.

146. Small PLC, Falkow S. Development of a DNA probe for the virulence plasmid of *Shigella* ssp. and enteroinvasive *Escherichia coli*. In: Leive L, Bonaventre PF, Morello JA, Silver SD, Wu WC, eds. *Microbiology—1986*. Washington, DC: American Society for Microbiology; 1986.

147. Sethabutr O, Hanchalay S, Echeverria P, Taylor DN, Leksomboon U. A nonradioactive DNA probe to identify *Shigella* and enteroinvasive *Escherichia coli* in stools of children with diarrhoea. *Lancet* 1985;2:1095–1097.

148. Frankel G, Giron JA, Valmassoi J, Schoolnik GK. Multi-gene amplification; simultaneous detection of three virulence genes in diarrhoeal stool. *Mol Microbiol* 1989;3:1729–1734.

149. Frankel G, Riley L, Giron A, et al. Detection of *Shigella* in feces using DNA amplification. *J Infect Dis* 1990;161: 1252–1256.

150. Guerrant RL, Shields DS, Thorson SM, Schorling JB, Groschel DH. Evaluation and diagnosis of acute infectious diarrhea. *Am J Med* 1985;78:91–98.

151. Lindberg AA, Cam PD, Chan N, et al. Shigellosis in Vietnam: seroepidemiologic studies with use of lipopolysaccharide antigens in enzyme immunoassays. *Rev Infect Dis* 1991;13: S231–S237.

152. Ewing WH, Lindberg AA. Serology of *Shigella*. In: Bergan T, ed. *Methods in microbiology*. London: Academic Press; 1984; 14:113–142.

153. Lindberg AA, Karnell A, Weintraub A. The lipopolysaccharide of *Shigella* bacteria as a virulence factor. *Rev Infect Dis* 1991; 13(Suppl 4):S279–S284.

154. Lindberg AA, Holme T. Evaluation of some extraction methods for the preparation of bacterial lipopolysaccharides for structural analysis. *Acta Pathol Microbiol Scand Sect B* 1972; 80:751–759.

155. Carlsson HE, Lindberg AA, Application of enzyme immunoassay for diagnosis of bacterial and mycotic infections. *Scand J Immunol* 1978;8(Suppl 7):97–110.

156. Dmitriev BA, Knirel YA, Kochetkov NK, Hofman IL. Somatic antigens of *Shigella*. Structural investigations of the O-specific polysaccharide chain of *Shigella dysenteriae* type I lipopolysaccharide. *Eur J Biochem* 1976;66:559–566.

157. Carlin NIA, Lindberg AA, Bock K, Bundle DR. The *Shigella flexneri* O-antigenic polysaccharide chain: nature of the biological repeating unit. *Eur J Biochem* 1984;139:189–194.

158. Samadi AR, Wahed MA, Islam MR, Ahmed SM. Consequences of hyponatremia and hypernatremia in children with acute diarrhoea in Bangladesh. *Br Med J* 1983;286:671–673.

159. Bennish ML, Harris JR, Wojtyniak BJ, Struelens M. Death in shigellosis: incidence and risk factors in hospitalized patients. *J Infect Dis* 1990;161:500–506.

160. Scrimshaw NS. Effect of infection on nutrient requirements. *Am J Clin Nutr* 1977;30:1536–1544.

161. Keusch GT. Antimicrobial therapy for enteric infections and typhoid fever: state of the art. *Rev Infect Dis* 1988;10: S199–205.

162. Salam MA, Bennish ML. Antimicrobial therapy of shigellosis. *Rev Infect Dis* 1991;13:S332–S341.

163. DuPont HL, Ericsson CD, Robinson A, Johnson RC. Current problems in antimicrobial therapy for bacterial enteric infections. *Am J Med* 1987;82:324–328.

164. Bennish ML, Salam MA, Hossain MA, et al. Antimicrobial resistance of *Shigella* isolates in Bangladesh, 1983–1990: increasing frequency of strains multiply resistant to ampicillin, trimethoprim-sulfamethoxazole, and naladixic acid. *Clin Infect Dis* 1992;14:1055–1060.

165. Bennish ML, Salam MA. Rethinking options for the treatment of shigellosis. *J Antimicrob Chemother* 1992;30:243–247.

166. Ashkenazi S, Amir J, Waisman Y, et al. A randomized double-blind study comparing cefixime and trimethoprim-sulfamethoxazole in the treatment of childhood shigellosis. *J Pediatr* 1993; 123:817–821.

167. Eidlitz T, Cohen YH, Nussimovitch M, Elian I, Varsana I. Comparative efficacy of two- and five-day courses of ceftriaxone for treatment of severe shigellosis in children. *J Pediatr* 1993;123:822–824.

168. Bennish ML, Salam MA, Haider R, Barza M. Therapy for shigellosis. II. Randomized, double-blind comparison of ciprofloxacin and ampicillin. *J Infect Dis* 1990;162:711–716.

169. Bennish ML, Salam MA, Khan WA, Khan AM. Treatment of shigellosis. III. Randomized, blinded comparison of one- or two-dose ciprofloxacin with standard five day therapy. *Ann Intern Med* 1992;117:727–734.

170. Salam MA, Bennish ML. Therapy for shigellosis. I. Randomized, double blind trial of nalidixic acid in childhood shigellosis. *J Pediatr* 1988;113:901–913.

171. Butler T, Islam MR, Azad MAK, Jones PK. Risk factors for development of hemolytic-uremic syndrome during shigellosis. *J Pediatr* 1987;100:894–897.

172. Khan MU. Interruption of shigellosis by hand washing. *Trans R Soc Trop Med Hyg* 1982;76:164–168.

173. Zeitlyn S, Islam F. The use of soap and water in two Bangladeshi communities: implications for the transmission of diarrhea. *Rev Infect Dis* 1991;13:S259–S264.

174. Levine OS, Levine MM. Houseflies (*Musca domestica*) as mechanical vectors of shigellosis. *Rev Infect Dis* 1991;13:688–696.

175. Watt J, Lindsay DR. Diarrheal disease control studies. I. Effect of fly control in a high morbidity area. *Public Health Rep* 1948; 63:1319–1334.

176. Cohen D, Green M, Block C, et al. Reduction of transmission of shigellosis by control of houseflies (*Musca domestica*). *Lancet* 1991;337:993–997.

177. Robbins JB, Chu C, Schneerson R. Hypothesis for vaccine development: protective immunity to enteric diseases caused by non-typhoidal *Salmonellae* and *Shigellae* may be conferred by serum IgG antibodies to the O-specific polysaccharide of their lipopolysaccharides. *Clin Infect Dis* 1992;15:346–361.

178. Mel DM, Arsic BL, Mikolic BD, Radovanovic ML. Studies on vaccination against bacillary dysentery. 4. Oral immunization with live monotypic and combined vaccines. *Bull WHO* 1968; 39:375–380.

179. DuPont HL, Hornick RB, Snyder MJ, Libonati JP, Formal SB, Gangarosa EJ. Immunity in shigellosis. II. Protection induced by oral live vaccine or primary infection. *J Infect Dis* 1972;125: 12–16.

180. Formal SB, Oaks EV, Olson RE, Wingfield-Eggleston M, Snoy PJ, Coggan JP. Effect of prior infection with virulent *Shigella flexneri* 2a on the resistance of monkeys to subsequent infection with *Shigella sonnei*. *J Infect Dis* 1991;164:533–537.

181. Hale TL, Kern DF. Pathogenesis and immunology in shigellosis: applications for vaccine development. In: Sansonetti PJ,

ed. *Pathogenesis of shigellosis*. Berlin: Springer-Verlag; 1992: 117–137. (*Current topics in microbiology and immunology*).

182. Lowell GH, McDermott RP, Sommers PL, Reeder AA, Bertovitch MJ, Formal SB. Antibody-dependent cell-mediated antibacterial activity: K lymphocytes, monocytes, and granulocytes are effective against *Shigella*. *J Immunol* 1980;125: 2778–2784.

183. Tagliabue A, Nencioni L, Villa L, Keren DF, Lowell GH, Boraschi D. Antibody-dependent cell-mediated antibacterial activity of intestinal lymphocytes with secretory IgA. *Nature* 1983; 306:184–186.

184. Lindberg AA, Karnell A, Stocker BAD, Katakura S, Sweiha H, Reinholt FP. Development of an auxotrophic oral live *Shigella flexneri* vaccine. *Vaccine* 1988;6:146–150.

185. Lindberg AA, Karnell A, Pal T, Sweiha H, Hultenby K, Stocker BAD. Construction of an auxotrophic *Shigella flexneri* strain for use as a live vaccine. *Microb Pathog* 1990;8:433–440.

186. Karnell A, Stocker BAD, Katakura S, et al. An auxotrophic live oral *Shigella flexneri* vaccine: development and testing. *Rev Infect Dis* 1991;13:S357–S361.

187. Sansonetti PJ, Arondel J. Construction and evaluation of a double mutant of *Shigella flexneri* as a candidate for oral vaccination against shigellosis. *Vaccine* 1989;7:443–450.

188. Levenson VI, Egorova TP, Belkin ZP, et al. Protective ribosomal preparation from *Shigella sonnei* as a parenteral candidate vaccine. *Infect Immun* 1990;59:3610–3618.

189. Robbins RB, Che C, Watson DC, et al. O-specific side-chain toxin-protein conjugates as parenteral vaccines for the prevention of shigellosis and related diseases. *Rev Infect Dis* 1991;13: S362–S365.

190. Kunstadter P. Social and behavioral factors in transmission and response to shigellosis. *Rev Infect Dis* 1991;13:S272–S278.

Infections of the Gastrointestinal Tract,
edited by M. J. Blaser, P. D. Smith, J. I. Ravdin,
H. B. Greenberg, and R. L. Guerrant
Raven Press, Ltd., New York © 1995.

CHAPTER 54

Salmonella Including *S. typhi*

David A. Pegues, Elizabeth L. Hohmann, and Samuel I. Miller

Salmonella is named for the pathologist Salmon who first isolated *S. cholerasuis* from porcine intestine (1). *Salmonella typhi* was isolated by Gaffkey in Germany in 1884 from the spleens of infected patients (2,3). Nontyphi salmonellae are widely dispersed in nature, including the gastrointestinal tracts of domesticated and wild mammals, reptiles, birds, and insects (4). They are effective commensals, as well as pathogens that cause a spectrum of diseases in man and animals. Some *Salmonella* serotypes, such as *S. typhi, S. paratyphi,* and *S. sendai,* are highly adapted to man and have no other known natural hosts (4). Other organisms, such as *S. typhimurium,* have a broad host range and can infect a wide variety of animal hosts and humans (5). Some *Salmonellae,* such as *S. dublin* (cattle) (6) and *S. arizonae* (reptiles) (7,8), are most adapted to an animal species but occasionally infect humans. *Salmonella* have fascinated physicians, microbiologists, epidemiologists, and geneticists for decades by virtue of their diversity and success in nature.

CLASSIFICATION AND TAXONOMY

Salmonella is a genus of the family of Enterobacteriaceae (9). Like other members of the family, they are gram-negative bacilli, 2–3 × 0.4–0.6 μm in size.

Before 1983 the existence of multiple *Salmonella* species was taxonomically accepted. Presently, as a result of experiments indicating a high degree of DNA similarity, all *Salmonella* isolates are classified in a single species, *Salmonella cholerasuis* (10–13). This single species includes organisms formerly designated *arizonae*. The species *Salmonella cholerasuis* can be subclassified into seven subgroups based on DNA similarity and host range. Subgroup I contains almost all of the serotypes pathogenic for man, except for rare human infections with group IIIa and IIIb formally designated *arizonae*. Previously, various serotypes and isolates that were formally known as

D. A. Pegues, E. L. Hohmann, and S. I. Miller: Infectious Disease Unit, Massachusetts General Hospital, Boston, Massachusetts 02114.

species were classified based on surface antigen structure, biochemical characteristics, and host range. Since these designations are in wide clinical use it is appropriate, though taxonomically incorrect, to refer to serotypes as species. Therefore the terminology *Salmonella cholerasuis* or *Salmonella typhi,* which seems to designate these organisms as separate species, is commonly used to distinguish these organisms though their correct taxonomical names would be *Salmonella cholerasuis* (group I), serotype *cholerasuis* and *Salmonella cholerasuis* (group I), serotype *typhi.*

Serotyping

Three kinds of surface antigens determine the organisms' reaction to specific antisera (13,14). After treatment with formaldehyde, antibodies to the flagellar or H antigen can be used to agglutinate the organism. After heat, acid, or acetone treatment abolishes the labile flagellar antigen, antibodies to the somatic or polysaccharide O antigen can be used to agglutinate the bacteria. In *S. typhi* and *S. paratyphi* C the polysaccharide Vi antigen can inhibit O antigen agglutination because it is so abundant. The Vi antigen is a homopolymer of *N*-acetylgalactosaminourionic acid and is identical to that of *Citrobacter freundii,* a highly related organism that causes opportunistic infection (15–18).

Kaufman and White utilized cross-absorption and antisera cross-reaction to different bacterial O and H antigens to classify a wide range of *Salmonella* (14). Specific serotypes were defined based on complex antigen variability resulting in the identification of over 2000 *Salmonella* serotypes, most named for the city in which they were defined (19). Most antigenic variability occurs in the O antigen that is composed of chains of oligosaccharide attached to a core oligosaccharide linked covalently to lipid A. This structure comprises the bacterial lipopolysaccharide (LPS). Hence, most serotypes have unique LPS structures (13).

Although serotyping of all surface antigens can be used for formal identification, most laboratories perform a few simple agglutination reactions that define specific O antigens into serogroups, designating group A, B, C$_1$, C$_2$, D, and E *Salmonella* (9). Although this grouping is useful in epidemiological studies and can be used to confirm genus identification, it cannot identify whether the organism is likely to cause enteric fever, as considerable cross-reactivity occurs among serogroups. For example, *S. enteritidis,* which typically causes gastroenteritis, and *S. typhi,* which causes enteric fever, are both group D. Similarly, another frequent cause of gastroenteritis, *S. typhimurium,* and some *S. paratyphi,* another cause of enteric fever, are both group B. Biochemical and serological determination are necessary to define the specific *Salmonella* serotype.

Phage Typing

In addition to serological and biochemical characterization, bacteriophage typing can be used to distinguish *Salmonella* within serotypes (20,21). This method has been most widely used for *S. typhi.* Despite the ability to distinguish *S. typhi* isolates by sensitivity to specific bacteriophages these organisms appear clonal by multilocus enzyme electrophoresis and DNA hybridization analysis (22). Thus the differences in phage typing likely reflect more recent evolutionary events, as prophage acquisition is all that is required to alter bacteriophage sensitivity.

CLINICAL MICROBIOLOGY

Salmonellae are gram-negative, non–spore-forming, facultatively anaerobic bacilli. Like other Enterobacteriaceae, they produce acid on glucose fermentation, reduce nitrates, and do not produce cytochrome oxidase (10,13). All organisms except *S. gallinarium-pullorum* are motile by peritrichous flagella and most do not ferment lactose. However, approximately 1% of organisms are able to ferment this sugar (10) and thus may not be detected by clinical laboratories that use MacConkey agar or other semiselective media to identify *Salmonella* based on colorometric assay for fermentation of lactose. The differential metabolism of sugars can be used to distinguish many *Salmonella* serotypes; *S. typhi* is the only organism that does not produce gas on sugar fermentation (10).

The isolation of *Salmonella* in stool cultures is ideally performed using freshly passed stools and not stool swabs. Stool is directly plated onto agar plates. Low-selectivity media such as MacConkey and deoxycholate agar and intermediate-selective agar such as salmonella-shigella (SS) or Hektoen are widely used by clinical laboratories to screen for *Salmonella* in primary stool cultures because they also screen for *Shigella* species. If laboratory resources permit, a highly *Salmonella*-selective medium, such as brilliant green, can be also used. Bismuth sulfite agar contains an indicator of hydrogen sulfite (H$_2$S) production and does not contain lactose. It is preferred for isolating *S. typhi* and can also be used for the detection of *Salmonella* strains that ferment lactose. *Salmonella* enrichment broths are highly selective and can be used to enhance the isolation of low numbers of organisms from stool specimens. The most widely used are tetrathionate broth, tetrathionate with brilliant green, and selenite F broth (23).

After primary isolation, possible *Salmonella* isolates can be tested in commercial identification systems or inoculated into screening media such as triple sugar iron (TSI) and lysine iron agar (10,23). Lysine iron agar detects decarboxylation or deamination of lysine and H$_2$S production. *Salmonella* strains most often are TSI alkaline/acid, gas-positive, and H$_2$S-positive. Rarely, strains that ferment lactose or sucrose will have an acid/acid slant and be H$_2$S-negative. The usual reaction on lysine iron agar is alkaline/alkaline and H$_2$S-positive. Isolates with typical biochemical profiles for *Salmonella* should be tested for slide agglutination with commercial polyvalent antisera specific for *Salmonella* O-group antigens and Vi antigen. *Salmonella* strains will not agglutinate with the commercial antisera when the antigens represented are not in the commercial profile. Such strains can only be detected by a more complete set of biochemical reactions. In the United States *Salmonella* isolates that have been confirmed by biochemical testing can be forwarded to most state health laboratories for more complete serotyping as part of the Nationwide Salmonella Surveillance System.

Salmonella can contain a wide variety of plasmids that encode virulence factors and antimicrobial resistance (24–26). Many strains of nontyphoidal *Salmonella,* especially *Salmonella typhimurium* and *S. dublin,* contain large 50- to 120-kDa plasmids that encode factors for animal virulence (27).

EPIDEMIOLOGY

S. typhi and *S. paratyphi*

S. typhi and *S. paratyphi* only colonize humans and therefore disease can only be acquired through close contact with a person who has had typhoid fever or is a chronic carrier. Most often, acquisition of organisms occurs by ingestion of food or water contaminated with human excreta. Although direct person-to-person transmission is rare, anal–oral transmission of *S. typhi* has been demonstrated (28). Laboratory accidents have also resulted in typhoid fever transmission to laboratory workers (29). Occasionally, health care workers can acquire the disease from infected patients as a result of poor handwashing technique (30). Sewage workers are not at higher risk of acquiring typhoid, although this is a theoretical concern (31).

Typhoid fever continues to be a global health problem. Based on surveys by the World Health Organization (WHO) Diarrhoeal Disease Control Programme and 1980 census data, it has been estimated that approximately 12.5 million cases occur per year (excluding China) with an annual incidence of 0.5% of the world population (3). Seven million cases are estimated to occur annually in South and East Asia alone. Africa and Latin America also have a high incidence of typhoid. Certain countries, including Indonesia, India, and Nigeria, report high typhoid fever mortality rates that range from 12% to 32% in different studies despite antibiotic therapy (3,32–34). These countries seem to share several characteristics including rapid population growth, increased urbanization, inadequate human waste treatment, limited water supply, and overburdened health care systems. In Indonesia the yearly incidence of typhoid fever is estimated to be 1%, and typhoid fever is among the five leading causes of death (3). A recent study comparing the mortality of native-born Israelis and Ethiopian immigrants with typhoid fever suggests that the high mortality rate in developing countries is more likely related to delayed hospitalization and treatment than host factors or differences in organism virulence (35).

In the United States, substantial progress has been made in the eradication of *S. typhi.* The incidence of typhoid fever in the United States decreased from 1 case per 100,000 population in 1955 to 0.2 case per 100,000 population in 1966 and since then has remained fairly stable (31). From 1968 to 1986, the number of *S. typhi* isolates reported to the U.S. Centers for Disease Control and Prevention (CDC) ranged from 458 in 1984 to 683 in 1973 (36) compared with 35,994 cases of typhoid fever in 1920. In 1991, 493 *S. typhi* isolates from human sources were reported (37). This progress is clearly related to improved food-handling practices and water treatment. However, contaminated food or water remains the source of most recent outbreaks. Usually, waterborne transmission involves the ingestion of fewer microorganisms and, as a result, has a longer incubation period and lower attack rate than foodborne transmission (31).

From 1974 to 1985, 62% of reported typhoid cases in the United States were associated with foreign travel (31). Persons with typhoid fever most frequently reported travel to Mexico (39%) or the Indian subcontinent (17%). Substantial numbers of cases were also acquired after travel to Peru, Central America, the Philippines, Chile, Egypt, Korea, and Haiti. However, the estimated attack rate for Mexican travel is small (20.2 cases/10^6 travelers) (39). The destinations with the highest estimated attack rates per 10^6 travelers were Peru (173.8), India (118.5), Pakistan (105.1), Chile (58.4), and Haiti (41.8).

In the United States most domestically acquired cases of typhoid can be traced to chronic carriers who contaminate foods. Although foodborne outbreaks of typhoid fever are rare today, the potential still exists for outbreaks related to food contamination by a chronic carrier such as "Typhoid Mary" Mallon. Three recent typhoid outbreaks have been reported in Maryland (38), Skagit County, Washington (39), and Sullivan County, New York (40), where a large outbreak occurred at a resort hotel in 1989. Forty-six confirmed and twenty-four probable cases of illness occurred among hotel guests and employees, including one case of secondary transmission. Twenty-one patients were hospitalized; two persons had bowel perforation requiring surgery. The food vehicle was most likely a large vat of orange juice prepared by an asymptomatic food handler from Central America. The financial costs of typhoid compared with nontyphoidal *Salmonella* outbreaks are considerable. Estimates vary from approximately $2500 to $4500 per person for typhoid illness compared with $645 per person for nontyphoidal illness (39).

In endemic areas the incidence of *S. typhi* infection is highest among children older than 1 year of age and likely reflects their lack of acquired immunity (40,41). When children less than 1 year of age acquire typhoid the disease is often more severe and is associated with a higher rate of complications (42). In addition, patients with immunosuppression, biliary and urinary tract abnormalities, and reticuloendothelial blockade, such as hemoglobinopathies, malaria, schistosomiasis, bartonellosis, and histoplasmosis, are at increased risk of severe disease (5,43–47).

Outbreaks of typhoid fever in developing countries can result in high morbidity and mortality, especially when caused by antimicrobial-resistant organisms (25,48–51). Antimicrobial resistance in developing countries may be promoted by the widespread use of over-the-counter antibiotics and transmigrant populations, as illustrated by a recent outbreak of multidrug-resistant *S. typhi* in the Indian subcontinent. Early in the outbreak typhoid fever mortality rates increased dramatically before the recognition that the outbreak strain phage type O biotype II *S. typhi* contained a 120-MDa plasmid encoding both chloramphenicol and trimethoprim-sulfamethoxizole resistance (47–51). The outbreak was subsequently controlled with the use of quinolone therapy.

Nontyphoidal *Salmonellae*

In contrast to *S. typhi,* the incidence of reported cases of nontyphoidal *Salmonella* has recently increased in the United States (Fig. 1) (36,37,52–53). Despite a substantial increase in isolation of *S. enteritidis, S. typhimurium* was still the most common serotype isolated from human sources reported in 1991 (Table 1) (37). However, in 1992, *S. enteritidis* probably exceeded *S. typhimurium* as the most frequent serotype isolated among humans (53). In the United States only an estimated 1–5% of cases of

TABLE 1. *The ten most frequently isolated* Salmonella *serotypes from human sources reported to the U.S. Centers for Disease Control and Prevention, 1991*

Rank	Serotype	Number of isolates	Percent
1	*S. typhimurium*[a]	8,878	22.2
2	*S. enteritidis*	7,712	19.3
3	*S. heidelberg*	2,927	7.3
4	*S. hadar*	1,945	4.9
5	*S. newport*	1,790	4.5
6	*S. agona*	988	2.5
7	*S. montevideo*	861	2.2
8	*S. poona*	787	2.0
9	*S. javiana*	780	1.9
10	*S. thompson*	705	1.8
	Subtotal	27,373	68.4
	Total	40,012	

[a] *S. typhimurium* includes variant Copenhagen.

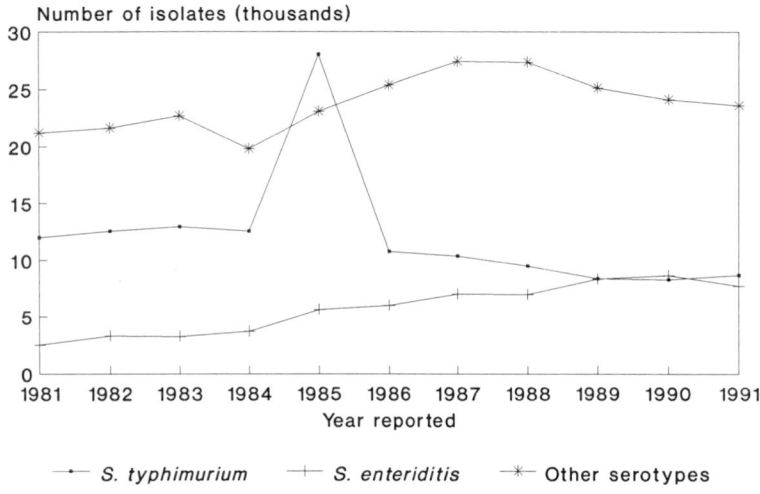

Number of isolates (thousands)

—•— *S. typhimurium*   —+— *S. enteriditis*   —*— Other serotypes

FIG. 1. Number of isolates of *Salmonella* and selected serotype reported to the U.S. Centers for Disease Control and Prevention, 1981–1991.

human salmonellosis are reported; the true incidence is estimated to be 0.8–3.7 million cases per year (52).

Unlike *S. typhi* and *S. paratyphi*, nontyphoidal *Salmonella* are widely disseminated in nature and are intimately associated with animal reservoirs. In specific geographic areas there is a close correlation between the serotypes present in animals and disease in man (24,36,37,54–56). In humans nontyphoidal *Salmonella* infections are most often associated with food products (54) and are the most frequent etiological agent of foodborne disease outbreaks in the United States (55) (Table 2). Recently described outbreaks have included *S. enteritidis* infection associated with eggs, especially in New England and the mid-Atlantic states (53,54,56), *S. hadar* infection associated with pet ducklings in Connecticut, Maryland, and Pennsylvania (57), *S. arizonae* infection associated with ingestion of contaminated rattlesnake meat sold as folk medicine (7,8), *S. muenchen* infection associated with contaminated marijuana (58), *S. dublin* infection associated with unpasteurized milk and injection of cow liver as an alternative treatment for malignancy (6), and *S. poona* (melons) (59), *S. chester* (cantaloupes) (60), and *S. javiania* (tomatoes) (61) infection related to fruits and vegetables.

The largest reported outbreak of *Salmonella* in the United States occurred in Illinois in 1984–1985. Approximately 200,000 persons acquired *S. typhimurium* from contaminated pasteurized milk (62). The outbreak was characterized by an organism with a plasmid carrying an unusual antimicrobial resistance pattern. Although the ac-

tual source of the contamination could not be pinpointed, it was hypothesized that contamination of milk postpasteurization with unpasteurized milk lead to the outbreak. In the developed world acquisition of salmonellosis is most often associated with consumption of poultry and eggs (52,56,63–65).

Salmonellosis has been associated with the practice of cooking poultry slowly at low temperature, especially when the bird cavity is stuffed with foodstuffs that may support growth of organisms. *Salmonella* can be passed transovarially from chickens to eggs; in the United States an estimated 0.01% of intact shell eggs contain *S. enteritidis* (66,67). Outbreaks of *S. enteritidis* infection in the United States and Great Britain have been associated with ingestion of raw or lightly cooked eggs (i.e., sunny side up) (67–69). Outbreaks have also been reported in restaurants associated with egg-containing food products, including caesar salad dressing and hollandaise sauce (63,67,70,71).

During 1985–1991, state and territorial health departments in the United States reported 375 *S. enteritidis* outbreaks, which accounted for 12,784 cases of illness, 1508 hospitalizations, and 49 deaths (53). In addition, a recent study of Minnesota adults with sporadic *S. enteritidis* and *S. typhimiurium* infection found that persons with infection were more likely to have consumed undercooked eggs or egg-containing food during the 3 days before onset of illness compared with controls (72). These findings support the hypothesis that most cases of nontyphoidal salmonellosis can be traced to contact with food contami-

TABLE 2. *Confirmed foodborne outbreaks, cases, and deaths, by etiological agent, United States, 1983–1987*

Etiological agent	Outbreaks		Cases		Deaths	
	No.	%	No.	%	No.	%
Salmonella	342	37.6	31,245	57.2	39	28.5
Other bacteria	258	28.4	19,060	35.0	93	67.9
Chemical	232	25.5	1,244	2.3	3	2.2
Parasitic	36	4.0	203	0.4	1	0.7
Viral	41	4.5	2,789	5.1	1	0.7
Total	909	100.0	54,541	100.0	137	100.0

nated with *Salmonella* from animal sources or during processing and suggest that human carriage plays a limited role in the transmission of nontyphoidal *Salmonella*.

Fecal–oral transmission has been reported in a health care facility (30), but in the absence of immunosuppression and/or reduced gastric acidity likely requires ingestion of a significant number of microorganisms. Despite the low risk of human-to-human transmission, health care workers and food handlers are frequently excluded from work because of convalescent carriage of *Salmonella*. However, the risk of person-to-person transmission in health care facilities appears to be low. No transmission to patients was documented during an outbreak of salmonellosis at a teaching hospital among nurses who ingested contaminated food served at Nurses Appreciation Day despite probable carriage among many of the nurses who worked after their illness (73).

In contrast to the low risk of transmission of nontyphoidal *Salmonella* by health care workers and food handlers, the risk of transmission to neonates and infants from chronically or recently infected family members is high (74). Neonates are at high risk for fecal–oral transmission of *Salmonella* because of their relative achlorhydria and the buffering capacity of ingested breast milk and formula (75). In addition, high-iron infant formula may increase the risk of infant salmonellosis compared with breastfeeding (76). Outbreaks in day care centers have also been reported (77). Controlling outbreaks of infant salmonellosis in institutional settings may be difficult because of the need for frequent diaper changes and the higher rate and longer duration of convalescent carriage seen in this age group (78).

PATHOGENESIS

Infectious Dose

Data on the number of *Salmonella* organisms required to cause disease come from volunteer studies and investigations of outbreaks in which numbers of bacteria in contaminated foodstuffs are known. Volunteer studies may not be generalizable because too few subjects are usually studied and laboratory-passaged bacterial strains may be less virulent than those found in nature. Also, higher doses of organisms are probably needed to infect healthy adult volunteers compared with populations at high risk of salmonellosis. The most important factor in decreasing the infectious dose appears to be a lack of gastric acidity (e.g., neonates, achlorhydria, gastric surgery, or antacid use) (75,79,80).

Between 1936 and 1970 nine studies were performed on volunteers administered a variety of *Salmonella* serotypes. In general, these studies found that the attack rate increased with increasing inoculum size (81–83). In addition, the number of organisms necessary to cause salmonellosis in volunteers varied with the host specificity of the organism. For example, ingestion of less than 10^5 organisms of *S. typhi* resulted in disease while 10^{10} *S. pullorum,* an organism that is highly adapted to fowl, was required to produce colonization and gastroenteritis.

Blaser and Newman reviewed data from outbreaks of salmonellosis for which counts of bacteria in the contaminated vehicle were determined (81). In both nontyphoidal *Salmonella* gastroenteritis and *S. typhi* infection, low inocula (less than 10^3 organisms) may produce human disease. Even lower inocula may cause disease in persons with deficiencies in host defenses.

Gastrointestinal Tract Host–Pathogen Interactions

Ingested *Salmonella* must transverse the acid barrier of the stomach—the first line of defense against enteric infections (81,82). Although *Salmonella* survive poorly at normal gastric pH (<1.5) (84), organisms survive well at pH ≥ 4.0 and have an adaptive acid tolerance response that may promote survival at low pH (85). After leaving the stomach, organisms move into the small intestine, where they interact with the intestinal wall. To result in infection *Salmonellae* must traverse the mucous layer overlying the intestinal epithelium and evade secretory products of the intestine, pancreas, and gallbladder, including pancreatic enzymes and bile salts. Antimicrobial peptides secreted by granule-containing Paneth cells located in the small intestinal crypts may represent an important second line of defense against *Salmonellae* and other enteric pathogens (86). These peptides are small cationic proteins of the defensin family that likely have a detergent-like action on bacterial membranes (87). Secretory IgA and intestinal mucus may also play a role in preventing *Salmonellae* penetration to the enterocytes that line the intestinal wall (88).

After crossing the small bowel mucous layer *Salmonellae* interact with both enterocytes and microfold cells (M cells). M cells are epithelial cells that overlie the Peyer's patches and are probably the initial target of *Salmonella* infection (89,90). On contact with M cells organisms are rapidly internalized and transported into the submucosal lymphoid tissue where they may enter the systemic circulation.

Salmonellae also have the ability to induce nonphagocytic cells, including intestinal cells, to internalize them (91,92). This process, termed bacterial-mediated endocytosis, is likely another important pathway for transcytosis across the intestinal mucosal barrier. In tissue culture of human and rodent epithelial cells internalization of *Salmonella* is associated with the formation of large membrane ruffles and cytoskeletal rearrangements similar to those induced by exposure of cells to growth factors (93,94). Exposure of a transformed epithelial cell line to *Salmonella* resulted in phosphorylation of the epidermal growth factor receptor and mitogen-associated kinase, and induction of phospholipase A2 (95,96). The induction of phospholipase A2 appears to result in an increase in leukotriene D4, which promotes *Salmonella* internalization, possibly through an increase in free intracellular calcium (95). *Salmonellae* are internalized by epithelial cells within membrane-bound vacuoles (92). In polarized tissue culture cells these organisms transcytose from the apical to basolateral surface (91). Although the efficiency of this process is low *in vitro,* this may be an important pathway for invasive *Salmonella* to reach deeper tissues.

After *Salmonellae* transcytose the intestinal epithelial barrier, the organisms rapidly interact with macrophages and lymphocytes in Peyer's patches and other lymphoid tissue located in the small intestinal submucosa (97). Peyer's patch enlargement may result from the recruitment of mononuclear cells and lymphocytes (5). After several weeks of infection, Peyer's patch enlargement and necrosis can be marked and are likely responsible both for the abdominal pain that is characteristic of typhoid fever and the rare reports of pseudoappendicitis associated with nontyphoidal *Salmonella* infection.

Survival Within Phagocytes

The ability of *Salmonella* to survive within macrophages is likely to be essential to typhoid fever pathogenesis and the spread of organisms beyond the bowel to the systemic circulation. In patients with typhoid fever and positive blood cultures almost all of the organisms are contained in the mononuclear cell fraction (98). Eventually, organisms are taken up by tissue macrophages in the bone marrow, liver, spleen, and Peyer's patches (5,83,99). During the asymptomatic incubation phase of typhoid fever, most organisms are localized intracellularly within macrophages and possibly epithelial cells (103). Symptoms of typhoid fever occur only when a critical number of organisms have replicated. These symptoms may result from the secretion of cytokines by macrophages in response to bacterial infection (3,83). The characteristic enlargement of the liver and spleen are likely related to *S. typhi* survival or replication within reticuloendothelial cells, the pathological recruitment of mononuclear cells, and the development of a cell-mediated immune response (5).

The morphology and cell biology of *S. typhimurium* infection of mouse macrophages has been studied. *Salmonella* induces membrane ruffling in macrophages similar to that observed in epithelial cells. Unlike other enteric bacteria, such as *Yersinia enterocolitica,* *Salmonellae* enter macrophages by induction of generalized macropinocytosis rather than by receptor-mediated endocytosis, even when they are opsonized with complement (100). *Salmonellae* are internalized in 2- to 5-μm membrane-bound vacuoles with a large amount of extracellular fluid termed macropinosomes that are formed by fusion of ends of membrane ruffles. After endocytosis, fusion with other macropinosomes can result in the formation of large vacuoles containing *Salmonella* termed spacious phagosomes (100). The ability of *Salmonella* to delay lysosomal fusion and to attenuate acidification of spacious phagosomes likely contributes to *Salmonella* survival within macrophages (100,101). In addition, the ability to induce phagocytosis by macrophages and epithelial cells may protect *Salmonella* from phagocytosis by neutrophils. *Salmonellae* are rapidly killed by neutrophils, with less than 10% of an initial inoculum surviving after phagocytosis (102). The finding that neutrophils from patients with chronic granulomatous disease are as effective at killing *S. typhi-*murium and almost as effective at killing *S. typhi* compared with normal neutrophils suggests that only oxygen-independent killing mechanisms are required to kill *Salmonella* within neutrophils (103). However, resistance to oxygen-dependent killing mechanisms may be more important within macrophages. This is supported by the finding that *S. typhimurium recA* and *recBC* mutants that are defective for recombination and DNA repair are attenuated in mouse virulence and survive only within macrophages that do not produce an oxidative burst (104).

The increase in generalized macropinocytosis demonstrated in the mouse model of typhoid fever may be important clinically in the development of neutropenia in typhoid fever. In a small study of children with typhoid fever and neutropenia, bone marrow examinations revealed the presence of histiocytes that had internalized neutrophils, red blood cells, and platelets (105). In addition, liver biopsies of patients with typhoid show Kupffer cell hyperplasia and erythrophagocytosis (106). These findings suggests that *Salmonella* stimulation of hemophagocytosis may be important mechanism in producing anemia, neutropenia, and thrombocytopenia.

Bacterial Factors

S. typhimurium infection of inbred, susceptible mice is a widely studied experimental model because the host specificity of *S. typhi* for man limits its study. There is good correlation between the ability of *S. typhimurium* to cause mouse typhoid fever and survival of organisms within cultured macrophages (107). In addition, sophisticated classical and molecular genetic techniques are available that facilitate the study of *S. typhimurium.* A number of genes have been identified as essential to the endocytosis of *Salmonella* by epithelial cells, although their protein products have not been defined (108–111).

Multiple bacterial factors are important to the pathogenesis of salmonellosis (Fig. 2). Many of the genes that are important to the virulence of *S. typhimurium* are regulatory proteins that control the synthesis of multiple proteins at the level of gene transcription. Examples include *phoP/phoQ,* which regulate acid phosphatase synthesis, proteins necessary to survival within macrophages and resistance to mammalian cationic antimicrobial proteins and acid pH, and factors necessary to invasion of epithelial cells (107,111–114); *crp/cya,* which regulate catabolite repression and surface proteins through adenylate cyclase (115); *ompR,* the regulators of porin gene transcription (116); and *katF,* an alternative bacterial σ factor which regulates catalase production (117). The *phoP/phoQ* system may function specifically to promote survival within macrophages as through this system *Salmonellae* are able to sense the macrophage intracellular environment and activate transcription of genes essential to survival (101). The *crp/cya* system appears important for human typhoid pathogenesis; when mutants deleted in *cya/crp* were fed to human volunteers virulence was attenuated (118).

The *Salmonella* virulence plasmid found in most nontyphoidal serotypes is important in the pathogenesis of typhoid fever in animals and bacteremia in man (26). The

BACTERIAL FACTOR

INGESTED DOSE

HOST SPECIFICITY

SURVIVAL WITHIN MACROPHAGES
- Induction of macropinocytosis
- Delayed lysosomal fusion
- Attenuated phagosome acidification

ACID RESISTANCE

INTRALUMINAL FACTORS
- Mucous layer penetration (e.g., motility)
- Cationic protein resistance (e.g., defensins)
- Bile salt resistance

MUCOSAL INVASION
- Microfold cell uptake
- Induction of endocytosis by epithelial cells
- Activation of eukaryotic cell signal transduction

ADDITIONAL FACTORS
- Regulatory proteins (e.g., PhoP/PhoQ)
- Virulence plasmids
- Surface molecules (e.g., LPS, Vi antigen)
- Cytotoxins (e.g., hemolysins)
- Stress response (e.g., DNA repair)
- Metabolic-enzymatic pathways (e.g., purine synthesis)

HOST FACTOR

AGE
- Neonates
- Elderly

CELL-MEDIATED IMMUNITY
- AIDS
- Organ transplantation
- Lymphoproliferative disease

PHAGOCYTIC FUNCTION
- Hemoglobinopathies
- Chronic granulomatous disease
- Bartonellosis
- Malaria
- Disseminated histoplasmosis
- Schistosomiasis

GASTRIC ACIDITY
- Antacids
- Achlorhydria
- Gastric resection

INTESTINAL FLORA
- Antimicrobials
- Bowel surgery

MUCOSAL INTEGRITY
- Inflammatory bowel disease
- Gastrointestinal malignancy

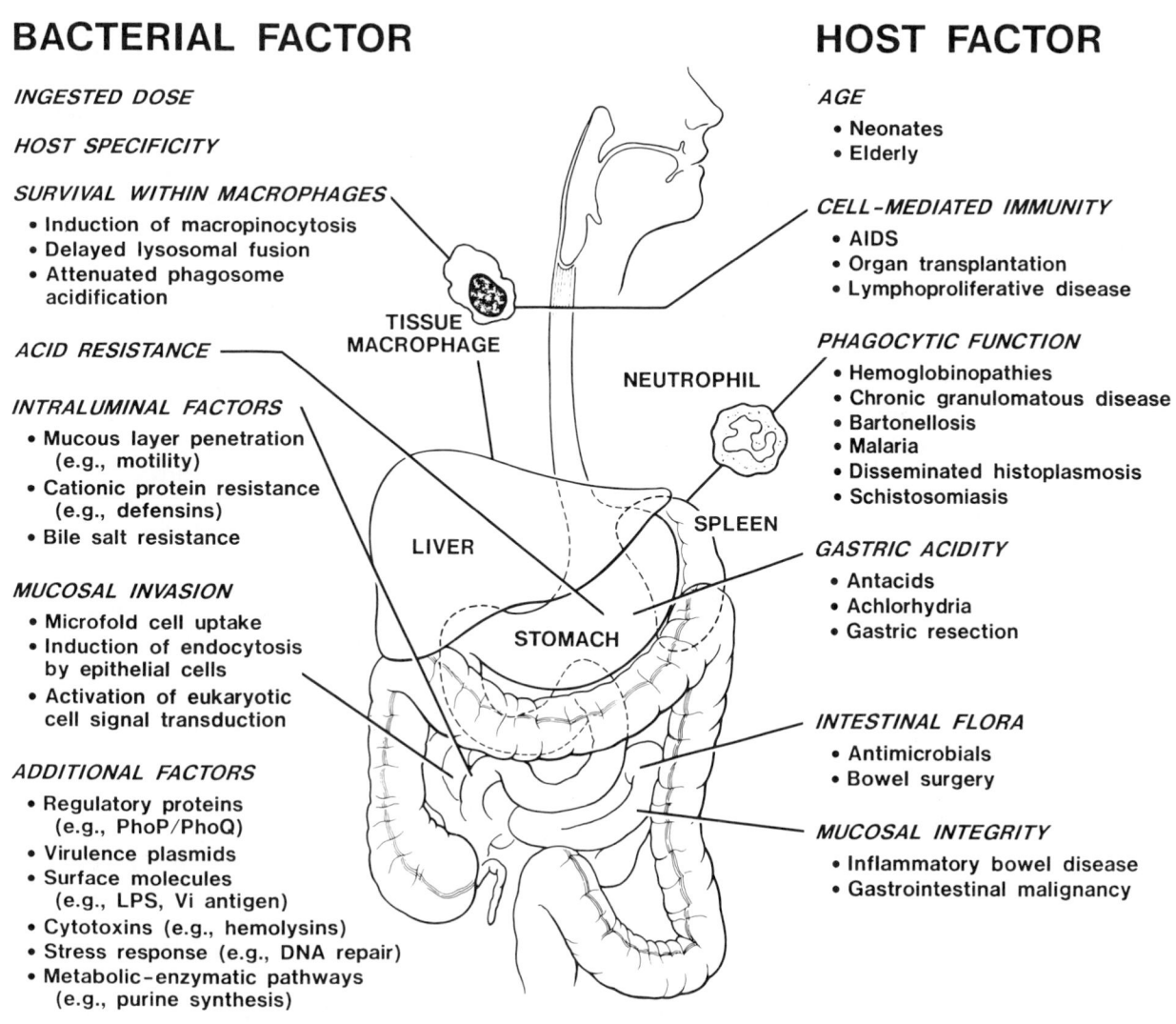

FIG. 2. Pathogenic bacterial properties and host factors conferring increased susceptibility to *Salmonella* infection.

plasmids of *S. typhimurium, S. dublin, S. cholerasuis,* and *S. enteritidis* all contain a 8-kb region that appears to be essential for most virulence functions. This plasmid also encodes factors that under some circumstances encode serum resistance.

The major surface carbohydrate-containing molecules of *Salmonella* appear to be important in pathogenesis. The lipid A component of LPS is a potent toxin for mammalian cells and LPS is an essential virulence determinant in *S. typhimurium* infections of mice (119). Both deep rough (missing the core polysaccharide) and rough mutants (missing the O-polysaccharide side chain) are avirulent (120). Mutants missing various O side chains also have increased susceptibility to complement-mediated serum killing (120). However, results obtained in the mouse model of typhoid fever are not always applicable to man. For example, *galE* (Vi antigen–negative) mutants of *S. typhi* that are missing the O side chain in the absence of exogenous galactose are fully virulent when fed to human volunteers (121). Different O side chains contrib-

ute to the virulence properties of nontyphoidal *Salmonella*. For example, strains with the O-6,7 side chain activate the alternate complement pathway and demonstrate increased phagocytosis and reduced virulence (120). On the other hand, strains with the O-4,12 side chain fail to activate the alternate complement pathway and demonstrate decreased internalization by phagocytes, a property that may be especially important in preventing neutrophil-mediated killing (102,120).

Other *Salmonella* cytotoxins have been described that are unrelated to LPS (122). None of these cytotoxins have been fully characterized. The recent identification and molecular characterization of a hemolysin that demonstrates hemolytic activity only immediately after human passage may be such a cytotoxin (123). A number of genes that encode the synthesis of essential nutrients are also important to *Salmonella* pathogenesis. Vaccine candidate strains with mutations in genes encoding for aromatic amino acid and purine synthesis have shown virulence attenuation in human volunteer studies (118,124).

The Vi antigen has protective properties for *S. typhi* (103). Vi antigen prevents antibody-mediated opsonization, increases peroxide resistance, and confers resistance to complement activation by the alternate pathway and to complement-mediated lysis. Vi antigen may therefore function to inhibit phagocytosis by neutrophils while not interfering with the ability of *Salmonella* to induce phagocytosis by more permissive macrophages and epithelial cells.

Pathophysiology of Gastroenteritis

The mechanisms by which nontyphoidal *Salmonella* causes gastroenteritis remain obscure despite extensive study. Although a number of enterotoxins antigenically similar to cholera toxin and *E. coli* heat-labile toxin have been described in *Salmonella* species, none have ever been purified or fully characterized biochemically (125–127). Because of the presence of multiple plasmids in *Salmonella* species, it is possible that the heat-labile toxin, which is carried on a plasmid, is occasionally transferred to *Salmonella* species. However, some of the enterotoxin-producing strains that cause fulminant watery diarrhea in humans produce this toxin activity after plasmid curing (125).

It seems more likely that *Salmonella* diarrhea is usually caused by bacterial entry into enterocytes and/or by the induction of an immune response in the intestine. The entrance of *Salmonella* into epithelial cells is associated with a number of biochemical alterations, including phosphorylation of the epidermal growth factor receptor and activation of leukotriene synthesis through phospholipase A2 (95,96). These or other epithelial cell signals mediated by *Salmonella* may result in diarrhea.

The pathology of nontyphoidal gastroenteritis in humans reveals massive neutrophil infiltration into both the large and small bowel mucosa (5). In contrast, infiltration of the small bowel mucosa with mononuclear cells is seen in typhoid fever. Degranulation and release of toxin substances by neutrophils could contribute to inflammation and result in tissue damage and subsequent fluid secretion or leakage across the bowel mucosa. Of note, *Salmonella* can induce epithelial cells to secrete interleukin-8, a potent neutrophil chemotactic factor (128). In an infectious model of *Salmonella* gastroenteritis using *S. typhimurium* and human intestinal T84 cells that form tight junctions, *Salmonella* localized to the apical surface can induce purified human neutrophils to transmigrate from the basolateral to apical surface through the tight junctions (128). This transmigration through the paracellular pathway may result in fluid leakage and diarrhea.

Host Factors

The virulence of any microorganism involves a complex interaction between the microorganism and the host's ability to limit infection (Fig. 2). In *Salmonella* infection, host specificity is extremely important to disease. For example, *S. typhi* causes potentially lethal typhoid fever in humans but is avirulent in mice (129). In contrast, *S. typhimurium*, the most common serotype to cause gastroenteritis in humans, causes lethal infection in mice. In inbred mice susceptibility to *S. typhimurium*, *Mycobacterium*, and *Leishmania* segregates in a dominant Mendelian pattern, and a locus (termed *Bcg*, *Lsh*, or *Ity*) identified on mouse chromosome 1 controls susceptibility to these infections through an alteration in macrophage function (130). A gene designated *nramp* has been identified within the *Ity* locus (131); this gene encodes an integral membrane protein with structural similarity to transport proteins and may function in macrophages to transport microbicidal substances into phagosomes.

Host susceptibility to salmonellosis is influenced by a variety of anatomical, pharmacological, and immunological factors (Fig. 2). A recent example is recurrent nontyphoidal *Salmonella* bacteremias occurring in patients with AIDS (132–134). This association and the increased severity of salmonellosis in patients with organ transplantation or lymphoproliferative disease emphasize the importance of cell-mediated immunity in controlling this intracellular pathogen (135–137). In addition, patients with chronic granulomatous disease or diseases causing phagocytic overload, such as bartonellosis, malaria, schistosomiasis, histoplasmosis, and sickle cell disease, have an increased incidence of salmonellosis (5,43,44, 46,47,138–140). Persons at the extremes of age are more likely to acquire severe illness; neonates who acquire the disease from mothers are at high risk for severe meningitis and septicemia (43,141).

Alterations in the gastrointestinal tract can increase susceptibility to salmonellosis. The risk of infection is increased and the infectious dose is decreased in the presence of gastric achlorhydria, antacids administration, or gastric resection (75,79,80). Alterations in the endogenous intestinal flora can also increase susceptibility to salmonellosis, although the mechanism is unknown; persons receiving antimicrobials (142) or those with intestinal surgery are also at increased risk (46,79). Normal bacterial flora may compete with *Salmonella* for nutrients or binding sites within the intestine. Chronic gastrointestinal diseases, such as inflammatory bowel disease and malignancies, also are associated with increased susceptibility to salmonellosis (137,139).

IMMUNITY

Immunity to *S. typhi* requires both cell-mediated and humoral immune responses and is achievable by vaccination (143). Although most individuals are immune after typhoid infection, reinfection can rarely occur and is often associated with early institution of antimicrobial therapy (144). Little is known about the immune response to nontyphoidal *Salmonella*, but its invasive nature and histology suggest that both cell-mediated and humoral immunity are important.

Although both serum and intestinal antibody responses have been documented after typhoid fever or vaccination (145), little is known about the protective antigens against which an immune response must be generated. Vaccine studies indicate that the Vi polysaccharide antigen should be an important immune target, since parenteral immunization with this antigen leads to increased protection in endemic areas (146). No data exist on whether immunization with this antigen can protect previously unexposed individuals. Chronic carriers of *S. typhi* are immune to active infection and have very high antibody titers to *Salmonella* surface proteins, including the Vi antigen (147). However, these high titers may reflect chronic exposure to the organism rather than affording protection against clinical disease. By extrapolation from animal studies, it seems likely that antibody to the O polysaccharide of LPS is also important (148). The importance of an intestinal immune response in suggested by an animal model of infection where a single monoclonal IgA antibody against O antigen secreted into the intestinal lumen provided measurable protection against *Salmonella* infection (88).

In addition to antibodies directed against the *Salmonella* surface proteins, lymphocyte proliferation assays have documented that a cell-mediated immune response occurs after *S. typhi* infection (149). Consistent with this observation are data from live vaccine studies indicating that a cell-mediated immune response against crude typhoid antigen correlated with the development of immunity after vaccination. In addition, cytotoxic CD4 T lymphocytes can be enhanced by vaccine-induced IgA antibodies (150).

CLINICAL MANIFESTATIONS

Specific *Salmonella* serotypes most often produce characteristic clinical manifestations that have been given the syndrome designations gastroenteritis, enteric fever, bacteremia and vascular infection, focal infections including osteomyelitis, and a chronic carrier state. Although dividing salmonellosis into these syndromes is clinically useful, many patients have signs and symptoms of more than one syndrome. For example, some patients with enteric fever have diarrhea and characteristics of gastroenteritis on presentation and others will present with localized infection with *S. typhi*, such as a splenic abscess. Some patients with gastroenteritis have positive blood cultures, abdominal pain, and high fever.

Gastroenteritis

Salmonella-induced gastroenteritis is indistinguishable from that due to many other gastrointestinal pathogens. Within 48 hr after ingestion of contaminated food or water, nausea, vomiting, and diarrhea occur (53,139). Diarrhea may vary in volume and frequency. In most cases the stools are loose and are of moderate volume without blood or mucus. Occasionally, stools can be of large volume and watery as is typical of severe cholera or toxigenic *E. coli*. Some patients present with dysentery with bloody stools and mucus. Fecal leukocytes are usually present. Fevers (38–39°C), abdominal cramping, nausea, vomiting, and chills are frequently reported. Headache, myalgias, and other systemic symptoms may also

occur in a substantial minority of cases. *Salmonella* can also cause a syndrome of pseudoappendicitis similar to that produced by *Y. enterocolitica* and other enteric bacteria; patients have severe abdominal pain and physical findings suggesting an acute abdomen (139).

Diarrhea is usually self-limited, lasting for 3–7 days (139); diarrhea persisting for more than 10 days should suggest another diagnosis. In a recent outbreak of *S. enteritidis* gastroenteritis the median duration of illness was 7 days (range 4–10 days) (53). If fever is present, it usually resolves within 48–72 hr. Occasionally, patients require intravenous hydration and hospitalization. Death occurs rarely; in the United States in 1991, only 49 (0.4%) of 12,748 outbreak-associated cases of *S. enteritidis* resulted in death (53).

Less than 5% of immunocompetent individuals with *Salmonella* gastroenteritis have positive blood cultures (46,139); the proportion is greater for persons who are at the extremes of age or who are immunosuppressed (43). In addition, persons with underlying illnesses, including inflammatory bowel disease, organ transplantation (135), malignancy (136,137), and malnutrition (46), may have more severe gastroenteritis and higher rates of bacteremia. Neonates have an increased risk of associated bacteremia and meningitis (43,151). Patients with human immunodeficiency virus (HIV) infection are at increased risk of *Salmonella* bacteremia, and recurrent *Salmonella* bacteremia is an AIDS-defining illness (132,134,152,153).

After resolution of gastroenteritis, the mean duration of carriage of nontyphoidal *Salmonella* in the stool is 4–5 weeks and varies by *Salmonella* serotype (78). Ninety percent of patients infected with *S. typhimurium* are culture negative at 9 weeks. In comparison, more than 20% of patients infected with other nontyphoidal *Salmonella* including *S. panama*, *S. muenchen*, and *S. newport*, are culture-positive at 20 weeks. Some studies have demonstrated that antimicrobial therapy may increase the duration of carriage (78,154). In addition, a higher proportion of neonates have prolonged carriage; in one study, 50% of neonates were still excreting *Salmonella* at 6 months (155). However, the delayed clearance of infection in neonates does not result in permanent carriage, as almost all chronic carriers are adults (78,155).

Enteric Fever

Human typhoid and paratyphoid fever are severe systemic illnesses characterized by fever and abdominal symptoms. In the preantibiotic era approximately 15% of patients with typhoid fever died (156,157). More recently, in some areas of Africa and Asia case fatality rates of 10–30% have been reported; in the United States less than 1% of persons with typhoid fever die (3,35,37). Higher case fatality rates are associated with delayed institution of treatment, especially when more than a week has elapsed from the onset of symptoms (35).

The syndrome of enteric fever is most often caused by *S. typhi*. A similar but less severe syndrome is caused by *S. paratyphi* A, *paratyphi* B (*S. schottmuelleri*), and *S. typhi* C (*S. hirschfeldii*) (83,157). When enteric fever is caused by *S. typhi* it is often referred to as typhoid fever and when caused by *S. paratyphi* it is referred to as paratyphoid fever. Although enteric fever is classically described as an acute illness with fever and abdominal tenderness, the symptoms are nonspecific and may be insidious in onset. The diagnosis of enteric fever should be considered strongly in the evaluation of travelers who return from tropical and subtropical areas with fever. The differential diagnosis of gradual onset of fever and abdominal pain with hepatosplenomegaly also includes malaria, amebic liver abscess, visceral leishmaniasis, and viral syndromes such as dengue fever.

The incubation period of *S. typhi* ranges from 5 to 21 days depending on the inoculum ingested and the health and immune status of the person. Following ingestion of the organism, persons may develop enterocolitis with diarrhea lasting several days; these symptoms usually resolve before the onset of fever. Diarrhea is more common in certain geographic areas, among patients with AIDS, and among children under 1 year old (42,133). In one study in Bangladesh the mean duration of diarrhea was approximately 6 days and all patients had fecal leukocytes present (42). Among patients with diarrhea, stool protein is often increased with a mean value of approximately 9 g/L. Constipation is present in 10–38% of patients (42). Although fever is a classic sign of typhoid fever, it does not always develop, and the pattern of fever is not clinically useful. In addition, only 20–40% of patients will have abdominal pain at presentation; the frequency of other abdominal symptoms varies widely in different clinical series.

Nonspecific symptoms such as chills, diaphoresis, headache, anorexia, cough, weakness, sore throat, dizziness, and muscle pains are frequently present before the onset of fever in typhoid (159). Neuropsychiatric manifestations, including psychosis and confusion, occur in 5–10% of patients with typhoid fever (34,157,160). This so-called typhoid state has been described as "muttering delirium" and "coma vigil" (160). Picking at the bedclothes and at imaginary objects and muscle twitching are characteristic. Seizures, lethargy, and coma can also occur; seizures are reported in less than 1% of persons and may represent febrile seizures of childhood. The cerebrospinal fluid (CSF) is usually normal in typhoid fever. Abnormal CSF studies or recurrent seizures suggest another diagnosis, such as bacterial meningitis due to typical central nervous system pathogens. The pathophysiology of the neuropsychiatric manifestations of typhoid fever is unknown but may be related to cytokine release from *S. typhi*–infected macrophages (3).

On physical examination, patients with typhoid fever usually appear acutely ill; however, persons with previous exposure to *S. typhi* or those who seek early medical attention can present with a milder illness. In some cases the pulse may be relatively slow for the degree of fever (157,158). However, relative bradycardia is neither a sensitive nor specific diagnostic sign of typhoid fever as it occurs in less than 50% of patients and is influenced by the physical conditioning and resting heart rate of the person. Approximately 30% of patients will have rose spots—a faint salmon-colored maculopapular rash on the trunk (158). Organisms can be cultured from punch biopsies of these lesions, and the pathology is characterized by a perivascular mononuclear cell infiltrate. The rash can be very subtle, especially in highly pigmented individuals, and frequently fades to small macules that appear to be resolving skin hemorrhages. Some patients develop cervical lymphadenopathy. Rales were frequently reported in patients in older series but are infrequently noted in more recent series (42,160). Chest radiographs are invariably normal. The examination of the abdomen usually reveals pain on deep palpation, and peristalsis is frequently increased. Approximately 50% of the patients have hepatosplenomegaly. Pain may localize to the right upper quadrant in approximately 3% of adults with typhoid fever who develop cholecystitis (157). Pancreatitis has also been described rarely (161).

Most symptoms resolve by the fourth week of infection without antimicrobial therapy in the approximately 90% of patients who survive. However, weakness, weight loss, and debilitation may persist for months, and 10% of patients will relapse (83,157,159). In the preantibiotic era, two thirds of pregnancies complicated by typhoid fever resulted in abortion (43).

Many of the complications of untreated enteric fever occur in the third or fourth week of infection (5). These include intestinal hemorrhage and perforation that are related to hyperplasia of the lymphoid tissue in the ileocecum followed by sloughing, ulceration, and necrosis, and focal infections, such as pericarditis, orchitis, and splenic or liver abscesses. In some series reported from the Indian subcontinent and other developing areas, up to 10% of patients required surgery for intestinal perforation (3,42). In other series these complications occurred in less than 3% of patients receiving antimicrobial therapy and even less frequently among children (35,40).

Some patients improve initially only to develop high fever and increasing abdominal pain from inflammation of Peyer's patches and intestinal microperforation followed by secondary bacteremia with normal enteric flora. In such a case, the patient's blood should be recultured and antimicrobial therapy broadened to cover aerobic and anaerobic enteric organisms.

Hematological abnormalities associated with typhoid include leukopenia and anemia. Leukocytosis can also be seen, most often in children and in the first 10 days of illness. Some patients develop thrombocytopenia and clotting abnormalities that usually resolve spontaneously. Elevated liver function tests and muscle enzymes are common; liver biopsies demonstrate focal Kupffer cell hyperplasia and mononuclear cell infiltration of the portal space (106). Rarely, patients develop proteinuria and immune complex glomerulonephritis. Creatinine clearance is usually normal and permanent loss of renal function has not been reported. Nonspecific ST- and T-wave electrocardiographic abnormalities are infrequently seen.

Enteric Fever Diagnosis

The definitive diagnosis of enteric fever requires the isolation of *S. typhi* or *S. paratyphi* from the patient. Cultures of blood, stool, urine, rose spots, blood mononuclear–cell–platelet fraction, bone marrow, and gastric or intestinal secretions may all be useful in establishing the diagnosis (162–164). The duodenal string test is especially useful as a noninvasive technique to sample duodenal secretions (163,165,166). The diagnosis is established in more than 90% of patients if blood, bone marrow, and intestinal secretions are all cultured (164,167). The sensitivity of blood culture alone is only 50–70% (168), probably because small quantities of *S. typhi* (i.e., <15 organisms/mL) are typically present in the blood of patients with typhoid fever (169,170). Oxgall media cultures may increase sensitivity from blood but not bone marrow cultures (3). Since almost all *S. typhi* in blood are associated with the mononuclear–cell–platelet fraction, centrifugation of blood and culture of this fraction can reduce the time to isolation of the organism but does not increase sensitivity (98).

The sensitivity of bone marrow culture is 90% and, unlike blood culture, is not reduced by prior antimicrobial therapy (164,167). In some patients with negative bone marrow cultures, duodenal string cultures have been positive (167). One study found that in children the combination of blood and duodenal string culture was as sensitive as bone marrow culture (165). Children also have a higher incidence of positive stool cultures than adults (60% vs. 27%) (3). Therefore, in both adults and children, blood, bone marrow, stool, and duodenal string cultures ideally should all be performed.

A number of serological tests including the classic Widal test have been developed to detect *S. typhi* antigen or antibody (3,171–175). None of these tests is sufficiently sensitive, specific, or rapid for clinical use. DNA probes for *S. typhi* and other *Salmonellae* have been developed, but these tests are not commercially available and may not be as sensitive as culture (169,176).

Bacteremia and Vascular Infection

Classically, *S. cholerasuis* and *S. dublin* produce a syndrome of sustained bacteremia with fever, but any *Salmonella* serotype can cause bacteremia (6,43,139). *Salmonellae* have a propensity for infection of vascular sites, and high-grade bacteremia (i.e., greater than 50% of blood cultures positive) suggests endovascular infection. *Salmonella* infection of the aorta is a well-recognized clinical syndrome and is occasionally complicated by aortoduodenal fistula formation (177). Most often endovascular infections result from bacteremic seeding of atherosclerotic plaques or aneurysms, and the risk increases with age and the prevalence of atherosclerosis. The estimated risk of endovascular infection complicating *Salmonella* bacteremia is 25% in patients >50 years of age (178,179).

Endocarditis

Endocarditis is an infrequent complication of *Salmonella* infection. Only 0.5% of cases from two autopsy series in the preantibiotic era had endocarditis as a pathological finding (180,181). In major reviews of nontyphoidal

Salmonella bacteremia, less than 5% of patients had endocarditis (43,139). Approximately 75% of these patients had underlying cardiac diseases, including rheumatic heart disease (33%), ventricular aneurysm (12%), or prosthetic valve (7%) (43). Endocarditis most frequently involved the mitral valve (40%), aortic valve (33%), and mural endocardium (24%). *Salmonella* infection of the endocardium is a highly destructive process. Serious complications include valve perforation (10%) and valve ring abscess (5%) (43), and mortality rates are high. In one series, 69% of patients died, and no patients with mural endocarditis survived (43). The mortality rate was greater for patients with nontyphoidal *Salmonella* than *S. typhi* endocarditis (43). A relapse rate of 20–25% among survivors was reported that may have been due in part to concurrent aortic infection. Early and aggressive surgery should be considered, especially in the management of mural endocarditis and infected mural thrombi, and patients may also require resection of aortic aneurysms to prevent relapse (43,178,182,183).

Arterial Infections

Although the abdominal aorta is the most frequent site of involvement, almost every arterial site in the body has been reported to be a focus of *Salmonella* infection (43,184). Patients with extraaortic arterial infection appear to have a better prognosis (43). The diagnosis of *Salmonella* aortic infection may be difficult. Rubin and Weinstein reported clinical findings that suggest the diagnosis: prolonged fever after gastroenteritis (especially with a known or palpable aneurysm); pain in the back, abdomen, or chest associated with *Salmonella* bacteremia; recurrent *Salmonella* bacteremia after appropriate therapy; vertebral osteomyelitis or a paravertebral mass associated with *Salmonella* bacteremia; and *Salmonella* bacteremia in patients with prosthetic grafts (5). Back pain and gastrointestinal bleeding due to aortoduodenal fistulas caused by rupture and erosion of the aortic aneurysm into the small bowel is a rare but well-described presentation (177).

The mortality of *Salmonella* aortic infection is high; in one review no patients survived with medical therapy alone (185). The prognosis is better with combined medical–surgical therapy with 18 (60%) of 30 patients surviving in another series (43). However, of survivors, seven (39%) had significant postoperative complications that likely were a result of recurrent infection. Six of those seven were corrected with extraanatomical bypass. The authors emphasized that successful surgical management depends on prompt surgical intervention with wide excision of the infected aneurysm and bed. Extraanatomical bypass through clean tissue planes (e.g., axillofemoral bypass) should be performed to decrease the high incidence of recurrent infection associated with reconstruction in the aneurysm bed. With these principles and improved surgical technique, the outcome of *Salmonella* arteritis may be better today than suggested by reported relapse and mortality rates. Patients should receive 6 weeks of antimicrobial therapy with a bactericidal agent, such as ampicillin or ceftriaxone; some patients who relapse may require prolonged suppressive oral antimicrobial therapy (43,179,184,186).

Localized Infections

Abdominal Infections

Salmonella abdominal infections can occur at any site but typically involve the hepatobiliary tract and the spleen. Many of the patients with biliary tract infections have underlying anatomical abnormalities, including biliary stones, cirrhosis, and chronic cholangitis (43). Patients present with symptoms referable to the involved organ and most have organomegaly or a palpable mass. Cholecystitis is the most frequent intraabdominal infection, occurring in up to 3% of patients with typhoid fever (157); most cases are associated with underlying cholelithiasis. The presentation of patients with *Salmonella* liver abscesses is similar to that of other patients with pyogenic liver infections; most patients have preexisting liver diseases, including amebic abscess (187), echinococcal cysts (188), and intrahepatic hematomas (189).

Other intraabdominal *Salmonella* infections have been reported, including splenic, subphrenic, pancreatic, adrenal, and perirectal abscesses (43). In addition, abdominal tumors can be the site of *Salmonella* seeding (136). Approximately 15% of pyogenic splenic abscesses are caused by *Salmonella* (190), and one third of such patients have sickle cell disease (43). Other conditions that predispose to splenic abscess formation include splenic hematomas and cysts, and *Salmonella* endocarditis. Some patients with *Salmonella* splenic abscesses develop left-sided pleural effusions that are culture-positive. The survival rate is high with splenectomy and antimicrobial therapy.

Soft Tissue Infections

Salmonella soft tissue infections are uncommon. In one series, most patients had underlying illnesses, such as malignancies, diabetes, transplants, burns, or sickle cell disease (43). Previous trauma at a site, including intramuscular injections or surgical incisions, were frequently identified, suggesting that disrupted tissue planes may serve as a nidus for bacteremic seeding. In one series, the most frequent manifestations of *Salmonella* soft tissue infection were pustular dermatitis and subcutaneous abscesses. *Salmonella dublin* cutaneous infections can also occur in veterinarians and farmers exposed to parturient cattle (191). Breast and thyroid abscesses and endophthalmitis have also been reported, and infants have acquired salmonellosis from mothers with *Salmonella* mastitis (43).

Urogenital Infections

Urinary tract infections with *Salmonella* are uncommon. In older series, approximately 1% of typhoid fever patients had pyelonephritis, but urine cultures often grew another, more typical urinary pathogen (192). In one series from the preantibiotic era, 81 (23%) of 346 patients with typhoid fever had positive urine cultures; however, none had chronic urinary carriage (157). Nontyphoidal *Salmonella* urinary tract infections are rare (139). In the antibiotic era, most reported cases are localized to the upper urinary tract, and most of these patients had a malignancy, renal transplant, nephrolithiasis, or structural urinary tract abnormality (43). More than half of the infections in renal transplant patients occurred after an episode of rejection. Symptoms, if present, are usually referable to the lower urinary tract. Blood cultures are frequently positive in immunosuppressed patients but are rarely positive in immunocompetent patients.

Most patients with chronic urinary carriage of *S. typhi* have an underlying abnormality such as nephrolithiasis, renal tuberculosis, or schistosomiasis. Although patients with urolithiasis and other urinary tract anatomical abnormalities may be cured by antimicrobial therapy, relapses occur frequently and approximately 50% of patients who relapse will require surgery for cure. In such cases a prolonged course of antimicrobial therapy and lithotomy or nephrectomy are necessary to eradicate carriage of *S. typhi* and to prevent recurrences. Structural abnormalities, such as bladder and ureteral fibrosis, and stone formation associated with concurrent *Schistosoma haematobium* infection also predispose to chronic *Salmonella* carriage. Prolonged administration of antibiotics as well as antischistosomal therapy is required (45).

Treatment of urinary tract infections in immunocompromised patients may be difficult, especially in renal transplant patients (135). These patients may have frequent relapses and chronic bacteriuria accompanied by recurrent focal infections. The initial treatment of such patients should include parenteral antimicrobial therapy for 1–2 weeks followed by at least 6 weeks of oral antimicrobial therapy. In men antimicrobials that penetrate the prostate, such as quinolones or trimethoprim-sulfamethoxizole, are recommended.

Salmonella genital infections are also rare. Orchitis occurs in less than 1% of patients with untreated typhoid fever in the convalescent stage (157). Ovarian abscesses, salpingitis, prostatitis, and epididymitis can also occur. Most genital infections require surgical drainage for cure, and often occur in immunocompromised patients or those with anatomical abnormalities (43).

Pneumonia and Empyema

Pneumonia is very rare in typhoid fever (157,193), and when pneumonia occurs it is most often due to a secondary infection with a different pathogen. Occasionally, patients with nontyphoidal *Salmonella* present with acute bacterial pneumonia associated with fever and abnormal chest radiograph (43,194). Many of these patients have positive stool and blood cultures suggesting a gastrointestinal source with hematogenous spread. *Salmonella* pneumonitis can be difficult to treat and requires at least 2 weeks of intravenous antimicrobial therapy. Complications of pneumonia frequently develop and can include lung abscess, empyema, and bronchopleural fistula. Lung abscesses require prolonged antimicrobial therapy. Empyema may also develop as a result of contiguous spread from a splenic abscess into the left pleural space and require surgical or percutaneous tube drainage.

Central Nervous System Infections

An estimated 0.14–0.9% patients with nontyphoidal salmonellosis develop meningitis (139,195), and meningitis is more common in neonates (43). In recent reviews *Salmonella* was the second most frequently isolated organism in children with gram-negative meningitis, occurring in 6% of the cases (195) and was the cause of 0–9% adult cases (196,197). Many cases of neonatal *Salmonella* meningitis result from vertical transmission from mothers with peripartum gastroenteritis or in association with nursery outbreaks (198,199). Neonatal *Salmonella* meningitis is associated with a high frequency of complications, including continued seizures, hydrocephalus, ventriculitis, abscess formation, and subdural empyema, and permanent disability, including mental retardation, hemiparesis, and seizures (151). The relapse rate is high, especially in children less than 2 months of age (43). In one review, the overall mortality rate was 43% among infants, 38% among children, and 57% among adults (43). Prolonged antimicrobial therapy (i.e., greater than 3 weeks) with a third-generation cephalosporin is recommended, in part because of reports of persistent positive spinal fluid cultures associated with chloramphenicol therapy (141). Intrathecal antimicrobials do not influence the outcome of therapy. Focal central nervous system infections including *Salmonella* brain abscess and subdural empyema have been reported (43,200). Recently, many of these patients have HIV infection (134). Most patients have done well with surgical drainage and antimicrobial therapy.

Osteomyelitis

Salmonella osteomyelitis most frequently occurs in children and is usually hematogenous in origin (43). In the antibiotic era osteomyelitis in adults is most often associated with sickle cell disease or other hemoglobinopathies, preexisting bone disease, or systemic lupus erythematosus. The femur, tibia, humerus, and lumbar vertebrae are most commonly involved (43). *Salmonella* infection of the lumbar vertebrae in an older adult should raise the concern of an infected aortic aneurysm (5). Most patients have fever, leukocytosis, elevated sedimentation rate, and diarrhea at presentation; most patients with diarrhea have positive stool cultures (43).

The association between *Salmonella* osteomyelitis and sickle cell disease is well described (140,201). In a review by Hook et al. in 1957, the three most common *Salmonella* serotypes causing osteomyelitis in persons with sickle cell disease were *S. typhimurium, S. paratyphi B,* and *S. cholerasuis* (201). The diagnosis of osteomyelitis can be difficult in patients with sickle cell disease because the signs

and symptoms are similar to those of sickle cell crisis. In one review, 71% of patients with *Salmonella* osteomyelitis had positive blood cultures, 45% had positive stool cultures, and 24% had positive urine cultures (52). Most patients are cured with medical or surgical therapy; acute *Salmonella* osteomyelitis is cured by antimicrobial therapy alone in 75% of cases (43). Relapses can occur, and approximately 20% of patients will develop chronic osteomyelitis. Prolonged therapy with a bactericidal antimicrobial agent for greater than 4 weeks is recommended. Historically, ampicillin has been used most effectively. Currently, third-generation cephalosporins may be especially useful.

Arthritis

Septic Arthritis

Most cases of septic arthritis occur in children, the immunosuppressed, or patients with sickle cell disease (43,202). Patients with sickle cell disease almost always have associated osteomyelitis. Only about half of patients with *Salmonella* septic arthritis give a history of a diarrheal illness. The knee, hip, and shoulder are most commonly affected. Infections of prosthetic joints and aseptic necrosis of the associated bone are also seen. Most patients have fever, joint pain and swelling, purulent synovial fluid, and radiographic evidence of adjacent bone disease (43). Most patients with infected joints without prosthetic material will have good outcome without surgical drainage if repeated needle aspirations are performed. Surgical drainage is required if needle aspiration fails to achieve adequate drainage.

Reactive Arthritis

Approximately 2% of episodes of *Salmonella* gastroenteritis are followed by symptoms of reactive arthritis (i.e. Reiter's syndrome) (203). *Salmonella* reactive arthritis is strongly associated with HLA-B27 antigen. In one study of patients with *Salmonella* gastroenteritis, 69% of patients with reactive arthritis were HLA-B27 positive compared with only 8% of patients without joint involvement (204). Symptoms can range from mild arthralgia to severe arthropathy and almost all patients report a preceding febrile diarrheal illness. Arthritis occurs an average of 10 days after the onset of diarrhea and lasts an average of 5½ months (43).

Eighty percent of patients have involvement of three or more joints, with the knee (66%), ankle (57%), and wrist (32%) most commonly involved (43). Radiographs show soft tissue swelling or periarticular decalcification in two thirds of patients; destructive changes are not seen (43). About 25% of patients will have the full triad of Reiter's syndrome—arthritis, conjunctivitis, and urethritis. Erythema nodosum and iritis have also been reported (205); iritis may develop months to years after the onset of arthritis. Unlike typical Reiter's syndrome, keratoderma, balanitis, or nail changes are not seen in *Salmonella*-associated cases. *Salmonella*-specific antibodies (206) and T-cell clones (207) have been identified in the serum and synovial fluid of persons with this syndrome, but their pathophysiological significance is unclear. Symptomatic therapy with nonsteroidal antiinflammatory agents is usually effective, and the prognosis is good.

Salmonella and HIV Infection

Salmonella infection occurs more frequently in persons with HIV infection than in the general population, and recurrent *Salmonella* bacteremia is an AIDS-defining illness (132,134,152,153). Based on a small study in an endemic area, the incidence of *S. typhi* infection in HIV-infected patients was estimated to be 60 times that of the general population (133). The incidence of recurrent bacteremia may have decreased since the introduction of zidovudine therapy (208); zidovudine has activity against *Salmonella in vitro* (209) and against *Salmonella*-infected macrophages (210). Patients with AIDS may have severe salmonellosis, with fulminant diarrhea, acute enterocolitis, rectal ulceration, recurrent bacteremia, and death despite antimicrobial therapy. In contrast, the severity of *Salmonella* infection in persons with AIDS-related complex or asymptomatic HIV infection is similar to infection in immunocompetent hosts.

Chronic Carrier State

The chronic carrier state is defined as the persistence of *Salmonella* in stool or urine for periods greater than a year. From 0.2% to 0.6% of patients with nontyphoidal salmonellosis (211) and from 1% to 4% of patients with *S. typhi* infection develop chronic carriage (43,157,159). The frequency of chronic carriage is higher in women and in persons with biliary abnormalities or concurrent bladder infection with *Schistosoma* (45). Serology for the Vi antigen can be useful in distinguishing chronic carriage from acute infection as chronic carriers will often have a high titer to this antigen (147).

IMMUNIZATION AGAINST *S. TYPHI*

Enteric fever can be prevented by immunization and several commercially available vaccines are available and approved for administration to travelers to typhoid endemic regions. These vaccines have been most extensively evaluated in endemic populations, require multiple doses to achieve approximately 70% efficacy, and confer protection that lasts only for several years (3).

Currently, the Immunizations Practice Advisory Committee recommends that typhoid vaccine should be administered to persons traveling to developing countries who may be exposed to contaminated food and drink, laboratory workers who work with *S. typhi,* and household contacts of known *S. typhi* carriers (212,213). Because vaccine protective efficacy can be overcome by high inocula that are common in foodborne exposure—the most frequent exposure among travelers (145,83,214,215)—it is controversial as to whether all travelers to areas with high rates of typhoid fever should be immunized with the currently available preparations (216). Immunization is not recommended for persons attending summer camps, persons residing in areas that have experienced floods or other natural disasters, sewer workers, or in the management of persons potentially exposed to a common source outbreak. Immunization is an adjunct and not a substitute for avoiding high-risk foods and beverages or utilizing good laboratory technique.

Since the nineteenth century the heat-killed whole-organism *S. typhi* vaccine has been the mainstay of immunization against typhoid fever. The heat-phenol–inactivated parenteral *S. typhi* vaccine is from 51–77% effective compared with tetanus placebo in studies in endemic populations (213,217–220). An acetone-inactivated vaccine provided greater protection (range 79–94%) in endemic populations (217,218,221); the higher efficacy was attributed to the preservation of Vi antigen in this preparation (216,220,222). However, the acetone-inactivated vaccine is associated with more frequent side effects, costs more than the heat-phenol–inactivated vaccine (215,223), and in the United States is only available to the military. Both preparations appear to result in equal protection in immunologically naive persons.

Local and systemic adverse reactions occur frequently with the heat-phenol–inactivated vaccine. Side effects include fever (17–29%), severe headache (10%), and significant local pain at the site of administration (35–60%) (217–219). More importantly, approximately 25% of individuals missed work or school as a result of vaccination. Reactions occur within hours after the vaccine and can persist for up to 72 hr. In general, reactions are milder with subsequent vaccine doses. Severe reactions to immunization can include anaphylaxis, chest pain, liver damage, neurological problems, and reactive arthropathy (224,225).

The Immunization Practices Advisory Committee recommends a primary immunization series of two doses administered subcutaneously at greater than 4-week intervals and booster doses administered every 3 years (212). The dose for primary and booster immunization is 0.25 mL administered subcutaneously for children age 6 months to 10 years and 0.5 mL for those more than 10 years old (212). Booster doses for persons age 6 months to adulthood can also be administered as 0.1 mL intradermally (212).

A live attenuated oral vaccine Ty21a (Vivotif Berna, Swiss Serum and Vaccine Institute, Bern, Switzerland) has been licensed in the United States since December 1989. The molecular basis of attenuation of Ty21a is unknown and is not related to the *galE* mutation present in the vaccine (121). Its main advantage is that it yields a markedly reduced incidence of side effects compared with parenteral vaccines (3,143,213). No serious adverse reactions have been observed in large-scale field trials or during postmarketing surveillance in Switzerland (226–229). Following administration of three doses of Ty21a vaccine containing 10^9 organisms on alternate days, the protective efficacy ranged from 43% to 96% in endemic populations (230,331).

The currently recommendation is that a total of four doses of Ty21a in an enteric-coated capsule should be taken 1 hr before meals every other day. The stored capsules must be refrigerated (212). Noncompliance with the multidose administration schedule and the requirement for home refrigeration has been reported (232). A booster series of four capsules is recommended every 5 years, although few data are available on the persistence of antibody titers against *S. typhi*. There is limited evidence for the efficacy of Ty21a in immunologically naive individuals; in some studies in travelers no efficacy was demonstrated (233,234). Nevertheless, based on studies in endemic populations it is likely that Ty21a is as effective as the heat-phenol–inactivated vaccine if compliance is adequate. Because of the possibility of illness associated with administration of a live attenuated vaccine, Ty21a is not recommended for children less than 6 years of age, the immunosuppressed, and those on antibiotic therapy (212). A Vi antigen vaccine has also been developed that shows promise in field studies.

In summary, none of the currently available typhoid vaccines has been demonstrated to have sufficient efficacy in travelers to recommend their widespread use. Because of its low frequency of side effects, it is reasonable to recommend the use of oral live vaccine Ty21a for travelers spending a prolonged period in a high-risk area, despite its limited efficacy and risk of noncompliance. The usefulness of the parenteral typhoid vaccine is limited by the high incidence of serious side effects and its failure to protect against high inocula. However, this vaccine is the only available option for persons less than 6 years old or with immunosuppression in whom prolonged exposure to *S. typhi* is anticipated (212). Existing and experimental typhoid vaccines are discussed further in the chapter by Skiest and Hill and Levine.

THERAPY FOR SALMONELLOSIS

Typhoid Fever

Chloramphenicol has been the treatment of choice for typhoid fever since its introduction in 1948 (235) and remains the standard against which newer antimicrobials must be compared. Chloramphenicol is inexpensive and is highly effective after oral administration. Treatment with chloramphenicol reduces typhoid fever mortality from approximately 20% to 1% and duration of fever from 14–28 days to 3–5 days (235,236). However, chloramphenicol therapy has been associated with emergence of resistance (49,50,237–239), a high relapse rate (10–25%) (83,236, 240,241), a high rate of continued and chronic carriage (83), bone marrow toxicity (242,243), and high mortality rates in some recent series from the developing world (34,50,240). If intravenous therapy is required a different antimicrobial agent should be administered because intravenous chloramphenicol succinate is cleared in the urine before conversion to chloramphenicol thus resulting in much lower serum concentrations than the equivalent oral dose (244,245). Although *in vitro* studies have not always correlated with *in vivo* efficacy, chloramphenicol is only bacteriostatic against clinical isolates (246,247) and against *S. typhi* within cultured human macrophages. In contrast, ceftriaxone, ampicillin, and quinolones are highly bactericidal for intracellular *S. typhi* (247).

Plasmid-mediated resistance to chloramphenicol emerged in the 1970s and has been associated with outbreaks in Latin America (237) and Asia (238,239,248,249). In South Vietnam during the 1970s more than 80% of strains were chloramphenicol-resistant (249). Although the frequency of isolation of chloramphenicol-resistant organisms subsequently decreased, these outbreaks prompted the use of amoxicillin (250,251) and trimethoprim-sulfamethoxizole (252,253) as alternatives to chloramphenicol for the treatment of typhoid fever. Despite several studies suggesting that ampicillin is inferior to chloramphenicol, these agents are probably equivalent to chloramphenicol when administered orally and may decrease the relapse rate (240).

Third-generation cephalosporins are effective in the treatment of typhoid fever (141,254–258). Ceftriaxone and cefoperazone administered either intravenously or intramuscularly for 10–14 days were shown to be equivalent to oral or intravenous chloramphenicol administered for the same duration in several studies (254–256). In one small study, ceftriaxone was effective when administered for only 5–7 days (255), but the relapse rate was not determined. After initial control of the symptoms typhoid fever with a parenteral third-generation cephalosporin, many practitioners switch to an oral agent to complete 10–14 days of therapy.

Several small studies have reported the successful treatment of typhoid fever with aztreonam (260,261). However, a prospective clinical trial in children in Malaysia was discontinued because of a high failure rate with aztreonam (262). First- and second-generation cephalosporins are also clinically ineffective and should not be used to treat typhoid fever or nontyphoidal salmonellosis, despite adequate *in vitro* killing activity (263–266). In addition, aminoglycosides are clinically ineffective, perhaps because they lack activity against intracellular *Salmonella* (267).

Quinolones are highly active against *Salmonella in vitro*, penetrate effectively into macrophages, and achieve high concentrations in the bowel and bile lumens, and thus have potential advantages over other antimicrobials in the treatment of typhoid fever (268,269). Oral ciprofloxicin (500 mg twice a day for 10–14 days) appears to be effective in treating patients with multidrug-resistant typhoid (49,270) and should be used initially in the treatment of patients from the Indian subcontinent or the Middle East where strains resistant to chloramphenicol, ampicillin, and trimethoprim-sulfamethoxizole have been reported (50,271,272). Recently, *S. typhi* isolates with nalidixic acid resistance and higher quinolone minimum inhibitory concentrations were identified from the Indian subcontinent (273). This finding suggests that persons who acquire typhoid in the Indian subcontinent should be treated with higher doses of ciprofloxacin (i.e., 10 mg/kg twice a day) while awaiting susceptibility results to prevent underdosing of relatively resistant strains (274,275). Other quinolones including ofloxacin, norfloxacin, and fleroxacin have been effective in small clinical trials (276–278).

Quinolones should be avoided in children less than 10 years old or pregnant women because of data demonstrating cartilage damage in young animals (279). The preferred treatment of known or suspected multidrug-resistant typhoid in children is a parenteral third-generation cephalosporin, especially ceftriaxone (50,255). However, quinolones have been used to treat multidrug-resistant typhoid in children and pregnant patients without adverse effects (287,288). For the initial or continued treatment of drug-sensitive organisms, oral therapies with chloramphenicol or trimethoprim-sulfamethoxazole appear to be equivalent.

The use of glucocococorticosteroids has been advocated in severe typhoid fever accompanied by altered mental status. A study in Jakarta showed a significant reduction in mortality among patients with severe typhoid fever (i.e., associated with delirium, obtundation, stupor, coma, or shock) treated with chloramphenicol and dexamethasone compared with chloramphenicol-treated control patients (case fatality rate: 10% vs. 56%; $p = 0.03$) (42). Although the case fatality rate in the control group was high and the study has never been repeated, based on this study dexamethasone 3 mg/kg intravenously followed by 8 doses of 1 mg/kg every 6 hr should be considered in the treatment of severe typhoid with altered mental status or shock. Steroid treatment beyond 48 hr may increase the relapse rate (282).

Nontyphoidal *Salmonella*

Antibiotic Resistance

In a recent study, investigators from the CDC found a significant increase in antimicrobial resistance among nontyphoidal *Salmonella* isolates from humans in 50 counties in the United States (283). Of 12 antimicrobials tested in 1989–1990, 32% of organisms were resistant to one or more antimicrobial compared with 16% of isolates in 1979–1980 and 24% of isolates in 1984–1985 (χ^2 test, $p < 0.001$) (283,284). In 1989–1990, 24% of isolates were resistant to tetracycline, 15% to sulfamethoxazole, 13% to ampicillin, 4% to chloramphenicol, and 4% to gentamicin (Fig. 3). Patients with resistant organisms were more likely to be infected with *S. typhimurium* or *S. hadar* than *S. enteritidis* and to have recently received antimicrobials. The available evidence suggests that resistance is increasing both inside and outside the United States with the widespread use of antimicrobial agents in animals (24,283–285).

Antibiotic-resistant *Salmonella* are associated with certain geographic areas worldwide and specific nontyphoidal serotypes (286–289). Therefore, pending susceptibility testing parenteral third-generation cephalosporins and oral quinolones (e.g., ciprofloxacin administered 10 mg/kg twice a day) are preferred for the empiric treatment if indicated for acutely ill patients with nontyphoidal *Salmo-*

nella infection. Recently, a strain of *Salmonella mbandaka* containing CTX-2, a novel cefotaximase, was isolated in an asymptomatic infant born in Algeria who was living in France (288). This enzyme confers resistance to extended spectrum third-generation cephalosporins. In addition, quinolone resistance has developed in patients receiving low-dose therapy or when the agent is administered to patients with undrained abscesses in which antimicrobial penetration may be poor (274,290). Therefore, in seriously ill individuals with nontyphoidal *Salmonella* infection, especially if the organism may have been acquired in a developing country, it is reasonable to administer more than one class of antimicrobial until susceptibilities are known.

Gastroenteritis

Salmonella gastroenteritis is usually a self-limited disease and therapy should primarily be directed to the replacement of fluid and electrolyte losses. Antimicrobial treatment of gastroenteritis does not appear to substantially improve symptoms or outcome (291,292). In one small study treatment of acute *Salmonella* gastroenteritis with ciprofloxacin significantly decreased the duration of diarrhea (292). The best study evaluating the efficacy of antimicrobials in the treatment of gastroenteritis was a double-blind prospective study in infants and children with uncomplicated gastroenteritis (291). Patients were randomized to receive ampicillin, amoxicillin, or placebo for 5 days. The mean duration of diarrhea was 8.8, 7.3, and 7.2 days in patients receiving ampicillin, amoxicillin, and placebo, respectively (291). In addition, antimicrobial therapy was associated with a higher clinical relapse rate compared with placebo (53% vs. 9%; $p = 0.03$). In two recent institutional outbreaks of nontyphoidal *Salmonella* gastroenteritis in England, ciprofloxacin (500 mg twice a day for 7 days) was administered in an attempt to reduce convalescent carriage (293). No person had stool carriage at 90 days, but there was no control group. A recent study at a military base in Sweden found that the rates of carriage following norfloxicin therapy (400 mg twice daily for one week) were similar to that of placebo (294). However, a study performed among health care workers with outbreak-associated *Salmonella* gastroenteritis found that bacteriological relapse occurred more frequently in those who were treated with 2 weeks of ciprofloxacin (750 mg twice daily) compared with placebo-treated controls (64% vs. 0%) (295). Therefore, antimicrobials should not be used routinely to treat gastroenteritis or to reduce convalescent stool excretion.

Although less than 5% of all patients with *Salmonella* gastroenteritis develop bacteremia, certain patients are at increased risk for bacteremia and metastatic infection and may benefit from "prophylactic" treatment during symptomatic *Salmonella* gastroenteritis. Prophylactic treatment should be considered for neonates and persons older than 50 and for patients with immunosuppression, cardiac valvular, or mural abnormalities, severe aortic atherosclerosis or aneurysm, or prostheses. Prophylaxis should consist of treatment with an oral or intravenous antimicrobial

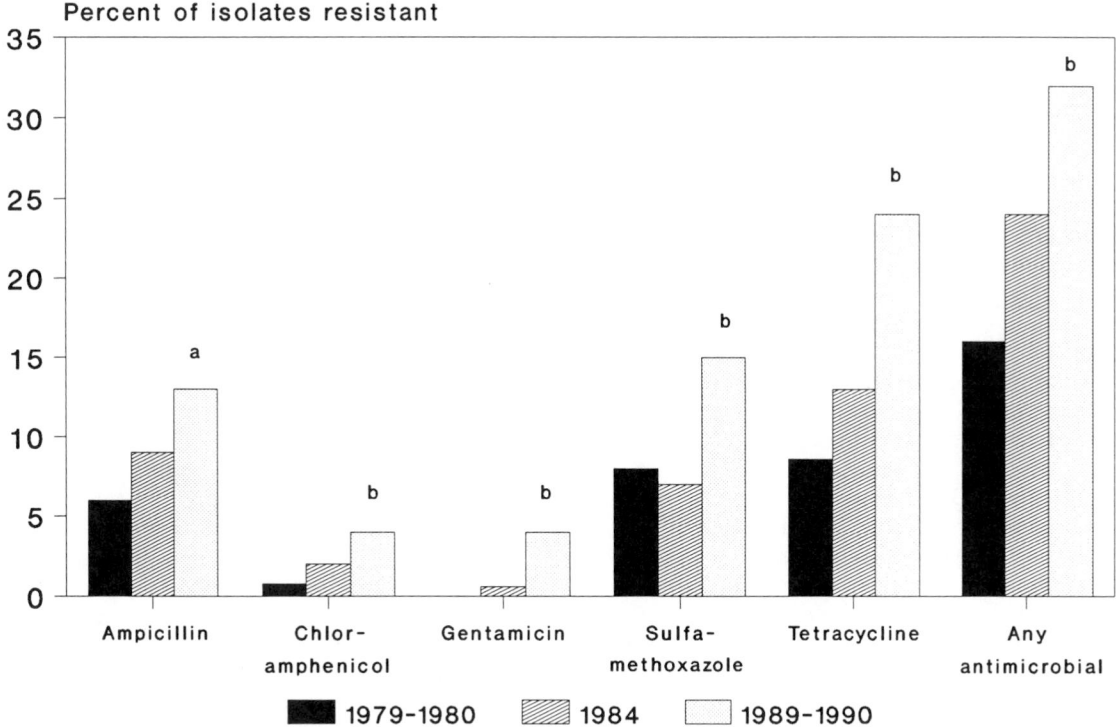

Percent of isolates resistant

FIG. 3. Rates of antimicrobial resistance for *Salmonella* isolated from humans in 50 U.S. counties in 1979–1980, 1984, and 1989–1990, by antimicrobial. (a) χ^2 for trend, $p < 0.01$; (b) χ^2 for trend, $p < 0.001$. Adapted from refs. 283 and 284.

for 48–72 hr or until the patient becomes afebrile. Longer treatment may result in a higher rate of chronic carriage and relapse. For susceptible organisms, prophylaxis with oral ciprofloxicin, trimethoprim-sulfamethoxizole, or amoxicillin is adequate. Occasionally, antimicrobial prophylaxis has been required to control institutional epidemics, especially in long-term care facilities or pediatric wards where compliance with infection control measures may be difficult. Furazolidone (2.5 mg/kg twice a day) has been used to control an outbreak in a pediatric unit (296).

Bacteremia

Because of the increased risk of endovascular infection complicating *Salmonella* bacteremia in older patients (178), it is important to document whether the bacteremia is high grade (i.e., greater than 50% of three or more blood cultures positive) and to search for endovascular abnormalities by echocardiogram or other techniques. Low-grade bacteremia not involving vascular structures should be treated with 7–14 days of intravenous antimicrobial therapy. Six weeks of intravenous therapy is required to treat documented or suspected intravascular infection. In addition, surgical resection of infected aneurysms or other infected endovascular sites is often required. Patients with infected prosthetic vascular grafts that could not be resected have been maintained on suppressive oral therapy for life (297). β-Lactam antibiotics are preferred for the treatment of endovascular infection (177,298); the

largest clinical experiences are with ampicillin and with ceftriaxone (43). Chloramphenicol should not be used to treat endovascular infection (179). Empiric therapy of nontyphoidal *Salmonella* bacteremia should include a third-generation cephalosporin and/or a quinolone because of the increasing possibility of antimicrobial resistance (274,288,290).

Recurrent *Salmonella* Bacteremia in Patients with AIDS

The treatment of *Salmonella* bacteremia in patients with AIDS can be difficult because of the high relapse rate. Jacobson et al. reported no breakthrough bacteremias in four patients with AIDS and recurrent *Salmonella* bacteremia who were treated with prolonged (i.e., 1–8 months) ciprofloxacin therapy (750 mg twice a day) (299). In persons with AIDS and a first episode of *Salmonella* bacteremia, 1–2 weeks of intravenous therapy followed by 4 weeks of oral quinolone therapy should be administered to attempt to eradicate the organism and to decrease the risk of recurrent bacteremia. Quinolones and zidovudine have a synergistic antibacterial effect against *Salmonella* (300); administration of both drugs may decrease the risk of recurrent infection. However, some patients relapse following 6 weeks of antimicrobial therapy and require long-term suppressive therapy. Trimethoprim-sulfamethoxazole may be preferred for long-term suppressive therapy if the organism is susceptible and because it is also an effective pneumocystis prophylaxis (301).

Chronic Carrier State (Typhoid and Nontyphoidal *Salmonella*

Antimicrobial agents are infrequently effective in eradicating the carrier state if anatomical abnormalities, such as biliary or kidney stones, are present (211,302). The largest clinical experience in treating chronic carriage is with amoxicillin (303) and trimethoprim-sulfamethoxizole (253,304). Both agents are effective in eradicating chronic carriage with cure rates of greater than 80% after 6 weeks of therapy. Good results have also been obtained with the use of ciprofloxacin and norfloxacin (268,304,305), including eradicating chronic carriage in a small number of patients with gallstones (304). The high concentration of amoxicillin and quinolones in bile and the superior intracellular penetration of quinolones are theoretical advantages compared with trimethoprim-sulfamethoxizole. Quinolones were effective in eliminating carriage when administered for only 4 weeks in several small studies (305,306), but cost substantially more than amoxicillin (268).

In patients with gallstones, eradication of long-term carriage with amoxicillin (6 g/day for 6 weeks with or without probenecid) or, alternatively, ciprofloxacin (500 mg twice a day) or norfloxacin (400 mg twice a day) each for 4 weeks should be attempted before proceeding to cholecystectomy. Patients who fail to respond may require cholecystectomy if eradication is necessary. Chronic suppressive antimicrobial therapy should be considered in those patients in whom no anatomical abnormality can be identified or who relapse after cholecystectomy. In patients with chronic urinary carriage, praziquantel should be administered if concurrent schistosomiasis is documented.

PREVENTION

Since 1962, the CDC in conjunction with the Association of State and Territorial Health Officers has maintained surveillance for *Salmonella* infections in the United States. Because this system relies on passive reporting of human cases or clinical isolates, the number of cases of salmonellosis in humans reported each year represents only 1–5% of the actual yearly incidence (54). Despite this limitation, ongoing surveillance is an important mechanism to characterize trends in *Salmonella* occurrence and to identify outbreaks.

The prevention and control of salmonellosis require an understanding of the complex cycles of transmission. As illustrated by the recent example of *S. enteritidis* infection in the United States, control of foodborne salmonellosis requires a coordinated effort on multiple levels, including the farm, food processors, and food handlers to identify specific control points. Recently, foodborne illness due to *S. enteritidis*–contaminated eggs has increased dramatically in the United States. During 1985–1989, 89 (82%) of 109 outbreaks in which a food vehicle was identified

were linked to shell eggs (71). Outbreaks were initially limited to New England and the mid-Atlantic states, but in 1991 45% of *S. enteritidis* outbreaks occurred outside these areas (53). In 1991, in response to these outbreaks the U.S. Food and Drug Administration and Department of Agriculture implemented a series of control measures, including investigation of egg-laying flocks whose eggs are implicated in *S. enteritidis* outbreaks and diverting eggs of infected flocks into pasteurization or, alternatively, destroying the flocks. The U.S. Congress also mandated refrigeration of eggs during interstate shipping. Commercial food service establishments can reduce the risk of foodborne *S. enteritidis* illness if they substitute pasteurized eggs for pooled eggs whenever possible and do not serve food containing raw or undercooked eggs.

Although most cases of *Salmonella* infection occur sporadically, large numbers of persons may potentially become infected when commercial kitchens serve *Salmonella*-contaminated foods that have not been sufficiently cooked or have been mishandled. The most cost-effective approach to the control of salmonellosis in food handlers is attention to good personal hygiene and maintenance of time–temperature standards for food handling. Potential human transmission appears to be overemphasized and routine screening of staff for carriage after gastroenteritis is common before allowing individuals to return to work. There seems to be little justification for this approach, as only 2% of 566 outbreaks in the United Kingdom were related to a specific food handler (65). Prolonged carriage in food handlers after gastroenteritis is rare and the amount of organisms present is small. Therefore, it seems reasonable to allow individuals to return to work after diarrhea is resolved, with instructions to follow careful hygienic practices. Three negative stool samples should be required only for high-risk individuals whose work involves touching unwrapped foods consumed raw or without further cooking.

Despite the risk of prolonged carriage, the risk of transmission of *Salmonella* from health care workers to patients appears to be very small. Once the health care worker is clinically recovered and passing formed stool there appears to be little risk of transmission and individuals should be allowed to return to work again with instructions to follow careful handwashing and hygienic practices. Patients excreting *Salmonella* should be managed with enteric isolation precautions. Control of *Salmonella* outbreaks in long-term care facilities or neonatal care areas may be difficult because of poor compliance with enteric isolation precautions and the increased susceptibility of these patients.

REFERENCES

1. Smith T. The hog-cholera group of bacteria. *US Bur Anim Ind Bull* 1894;6:6–40.
2. Schroeter J. Kryptogamenflora von Schlesien Bd. 3. Breslau. *J U Kern* 1885:1–814.
3. Edelman R, Levine MM. Summary of an international workshop on typhoid fever. *Rev Infect Dis* 1986;8:329–349.
4. Committee on *Salmonella*, Division of Biology and Agriculture of the National Research Council. *An evaluation of the* Salmo-

nella *problem*. Washington DC: National Academy of Science; 1969.

5. Rubin RH, Weinstein L. *Salmonellosis: microbiologic, pathologic, and clinical features.* New York: Stratton Intercontinental; 1977.

6. Fang FC, Fierer J. Human infection with *Salmonella dublin*. *Medicine* 1991;70:198–207.

7. Waterman SH, Juraez G, Carr SJ, Kilman L. *Salmonella arizona* infections in latinos associated with rattlesnake folk medicine. *Am J Public Health* 1990;80:286–289.

8. Bhatt BD, Zuckerman MJ, Foland JA, Polly SM, Marwah RK. Disseminated *Salmonella arizona* infection associated with rattlesnake meat ingestions. *Am J Gastroenterol* 1989;84:433–435.

9. Farmer JJ, Kelly MT. Enterobacteriaceae. In: *Manual of clinical microbiology*. 5th ed. Washington, DC: American Society for Microbiology; 1991:371–373.

10. Zinder ND, Lederberg J. Genetic exchange in *Salmonella*. *J Bacteriol* 1952;64:679–699.

11. Crosa JH, Brenner DJ, Ewing UH, Falkow S. Molecular relationships among *Salmonellae*. *J Bacteriol* 1973;115:307–315.

12. Stoleru L, Le Minor L, Lherithier AM. Polynucleotide sequence divergence among strains of *Salmonella subgenus IV* and closely related organisms. *Ann Microbiol* 1976;127:477–486.

13. Falkow S, Mekalanos JJ. Enteric bacilli. In: *Microbiology*. Philadelphia: JB Lippincott; 1990:561–587.

14. Kauffman F. *The diagnosis of* Salmonella *types*. Springfield, IL: Charles C Thomas; 1950.

15. Felix A, Pitt RM. A new antigen of *B. typhosus*. *Lancet* 1934; 2:186–191.

16. Baker EE, Whiteside RE, Derow MA. The Vi antigen of the *Enterobacteriaceae*. II. Immunologic and biologic properties. *J Immunol* 1959;83:680–686.

17. Daniels EM, Schneerson R, Egan WE, Szu SC, Robbins JB. Characterization of the *Salmonella paratyphi* C Vi polysaccharide. *Infect Immun* 1989;57:3159–3164.

18. Heyns K, Kiessling G. Strukturaufklarung des Vi-antigens aus *Citrobacter freundii* (*E. coli*) 5396/38. *Carbohydrate Res* 1967; 3:340–352.

19. World Health Organization, Centre for Reference and Research on *Salmonella*. Antigenic formulae of the *Salmonella*. WHO International *Salmonella* Center, Institute Pasteur, Paris, 1980.

20. Anderson ES, Wand LR, De Saxe MJ, De Sa JDH. Bacteriophage typing designations of *Salmonella typhimurium*. *J Hyg* 1977;78:297–300.

21. Gershman M. Single phage-typing set for differentiating *Salmonellae*. *J Clin Microbiol* 1977;5:302.

22. Reeves MW, Evins GM, Heiba AA, Plikaytis BD, Farmer JJ. Clonal nature of *Salmonella typhi* and its genetic relatedness to other *Salmonella* as shown by multilocus enzyme electrophoresis, and proposal of *Salmonella bongori* comb. nov. *J Clin Microbiol* 1989;27:313–320.

23. Le Minor L. Genus III. *Salmonella*. In: *Bergey's manual of systematic bacteriology*. Baltimore: Williams & Wilkins; 1984: 427–458.

24. O'Brien TF, Hopkins JD, Silleece ES, et al. Molecular epidemiology of antibiotic resistance in *Salmonella* from animals and human beings in the United States. *N Engl J Med* 1982;307: 1–6.

25. Goldstein FW, Chumpitaz JC, Guevara JM, Papadopoulou B, Acar JF, Vieu JF. Plasmid-mediated resistance to multiple antibiotics in *Salmonella typhi*. *J Infect Dis* 1986;153:261–266.

26. Gulig PA, Danbara H, Guiney DG, Lax A, Norel F, Rhen M. Molecular analysis of *spv* virulence genes of the *Salmonella* virulence plasmids. *Mol Microbiol* 1993;7:825–830.

27. Sanderson KE, Roth JR. Linkage map of *Salmonella typhimurium*, edition VII. *Microbiol Rev* 1988;52:485–532.

28. Dritz SK, Braff EH. Sexually transmitted typhoid fever. *N Engl J Med* 1977;296:1359.

29. Blaser MJ, Hickman FW, Farmer JJ, Benner DJ, Balows A, Feldman RA. *Salmonella typhi:* the laboratory as a reservoir of infection. *J Infect Dis* 1980;142:934–938.

30. Weikel CS, Guerrant RL. Nosocomial salmonellosis. *Infect Control* 1985;6:218–220.

31. Ryan CA, Hargrett-Bean NT, Blake PA. *Salmonella typhi* infections in the United States, 1975–1984: increasing role of foreign travel. *Rev Infect Dis* 1989;11:1–8.

32. Anderson ES, Joseph SW, Nasution R. Febrile illness resulting in hospital admission: a bacteriological and serological study in Jakarta, Indonesia. *Am J Trop Med Hyg* 1976;25:116–121.

33. Gulati PD, Saxena SN, Gupta PS, Chuttani HK. Changing pattern of typhoid fever. *Am J Med* 1968;45:544–548.

34. Hoffman SL, Punjabi NH, Kumala S, et al. Reduction of mortality in chloramphenicol-treated severe typhoid fever by high-dose dexamethasone. *N Engl J Med* 1984;310:82–88.

35. Carmeli Y, Raz R, Schapiro JM, Alkan M. Typhoid fever in Ethiopian immigrants to Israel and native-born Israelis: a comparative study. *Clin Infect Dis* 1993;16:213–215.

36. Martin SM, Hardgrett-Bean N, Tauxe RV. An atlas of *Salmonella* in the United States: serotype-specific surveillance 1968–1986. Atlanta, Georgia: U.S. Department of Health and Human Services, Public Health Service, Centers for Disease Control, 1987.

37. Centers for Disease Control and Prevention. *Salmonella* surveillance: annual summary, 1991. Atlanta: U.S. Department of Health and Human Services, Public Health Service, 1991.

38. Lin FYC, Becke JM, Groves C. Restaurant-associated outbreak of typhoid fever in Maryland: identification of carrier facilitated by measurement of serum Vi antibodies. *J Clin Microbiol* 1988;26:1194–1197.

39. Shandera WX, Taylor JP, Betz TG, Blake PA. An analysis of economic costs associated with an outbreak of typhoid fever. *Am J Public Health* 1985;75:71–73.

40. Birkhead GS, Morse DL, Levine WC, et al. Typhoid fever at a resort hotel in New York: a large outbreak with an unusual vehicle. *J Infect Dis* 1993;167:1228–1232.

41. Thikyakorn U, Mansuwan P, Taylor DN. Typhoid and paratyphoid fever in 192 children in Thailand. *Am J Dis Child* 1987; 141:862–865.

42. Butler T, Islam A, Kabir I, Jones PK. Patterns of morbidity and mortality in typhoid fever dependent on age and gender: review of 552 hospitalized patients with diarrhea. *Rev Infect Dis* 1991;13:85–90.

43. Cohen JI, Bartlett JA, Corey GR. Extra-intestinal manifestations of *Salmonella* infections. *Medicine* 1987;66:349–388.

44. Barrett-Connor E. Bacterial infection and sickle cell anemia: an analysis of 250 infections in 166 patients and a review of the literature. *Medicine* 1971;50:97–112.

45. Neves J, Raso P, Marinko PP. Prolonged septicemic salmonellosis intercurrent with *Schistosomiasis mansoni* infection. *J Trop Med Hyg* 1971;74:9.

46. Black PH, Kunz KL, Swartz MN. Salmonellosis—a review of some unusual aspects. *N Engl J Med* 1960;262:864–870, 921–927.

47. Wheat LJ, Rubin RH, Harris NL, et al. Systemic salmonellosis in patients with disseminated histoplasmosis. *Arch Intern Med* 1987;147:561–564.

48. Arand AC, Kataria VK, Singh W, Chatterjee SK. Epidemic multiresistant enteric fever in Eastern India. *Lancet* 1990;335: 352.

49. Sugandhi Rao P, Rajashekar V, Varghese GK, Shivananda PG. Emergence of multidrug-resistant Salmonella typhi in rural southern India. *Am J Trop Med Hyg* 1993;48:108–111.

50. Bhutta ZA, Naqvi SH, Razzaq RA, Farooqui BJ. Multidrug-resistant typhoid in children: presentation and clinical features. *Rev Infect Dis* 1991;14:832–836.

51. Vasquez V, Calderon E, Rodriquez R. Chloramphenicol-resistant strains of Salmonella typhosa. *N Engl J Med* 1972;286: 1220.

52. Chalker RB, Blaser MJ. A review of human salmonellosis: III. Magnitude of salmonella infection in the United States. *Rev Infect Dis* 1988;10:111–124.

53. Centers for Disease Control and Prevention. Outbreak of Salmonella enteritidis infection associated with consumption of raw shell eggs. *MMWR* 1992;267:3263–3264.

54. Parker-Baird AC. Foodborne salmonellosis. *Lancet* 1990;336: 1231–1235.

55. Bean NH, Griffin PM, Goulding JS, Ivey CB. Foodborne dis-

ease outbreaks, 5-year summary, 1983–1987. *MMWR* 1990;
39(SS-1):15–57.

56. Centers for Disease Control and Prevention. Increased rate of *Salmonella enteritidis* infections in the northeastern United States. *MMWR* 1987;36:10–11.

57. Centers for Disease Control and Prevention. *Salmonella hadar* associated with pet ducklings—Connecticut, Maryland, and Pennsylvania, 1991. *MMWR* 1992;41:185–187.

58. Taylor DN, Wachsmuth IK, Shangkuan YH, et al. Salmonellosis associated with marijuana. *N Engl J Med* 1982;306:1249–1253.

59. Centers for Disease Control and Prevention. Multistate outbreak of *Salmonella poona* infections—United States and Canada. *MMWR* 1991;40:549–552.

60. Ries AA, Zaza S, Langkop C, et al. A multistate outbreak of *Salmonella chester* linked to imported cantaloupe. Program and Abstracts of 30th Interscience Conference on Antimicrobial Agents and Chemotherapy, 1990;238.

61. Wood RC, Hedberg C, White K, et al. A multi-state outbreak of *Salmonella javiana* infections associated with raw tomatoes Epidemic Intelligence Service 40th Annual Conference, Atlanta, GA: U.S. Department of Health and Human Services, Public Health Service, Centers for Disease Control and Prevention, 1991:69.

62. Ryan CA, Nickels MK, Hargrett-Bean NT, et al. Massive outbreak of antimicrobial-resistant salmonellosis traced to pasteurized milk. *JAMA* 1987;258:3269–3274.

63. Mishu B, Griffin PM, Tauxe RV, Cameron DN, Hutcheson RH, Schaffner W. *Salmonella enteritidis* gastroenteritis transmitted by intact chicken eggs. *Ann Intern Med* 1991;115:190–194.

64. Wilder AN, MacCready RA. Isolation of *Salmonella* from poultry. *N Engl J Med* 1966;274:1453.

65. Mandal BK. Typhoid fever and other *Salmonellae*. *Curr Opin Infect Dis* 1988;1:84–87.

66. Omelettes without broken eggs? *Nature* 1988;336:699–700.

67. St Louis ME, Morse DL, Potter ME, et al. The emergence of Grade A eggs as a major source of *Salmonella enteritidis* infections. *JAMA* 1988;259:2103–2107.

68. Cowden JM. Salmonellosis and eggs: public health, food poisoning, and food hygiene. *Curr Opin Infect Dis* 1990;3:246–249.

69. Cowden JM, Lynch D, Jospeh CA, et al. Case-control study of infections with *Salmonella enteritidis* phage type 4 in England. *Br Med J* 1989;299:771–773.

70. Hedberg CW, White KE, Johnson JA, et al. An outbreak of *Salmonella enteritidis* infection at a fast-food restaurant: implications for foodhandler-associated transmission. *J Infect Dis* 1991;164:1135–1140.

71. Centers for Disease Control and Prevention. Update: *Salmonella enteritidis* infections—United States. *MMWR* 1990;50:909–912.

72. Hedberg CW, David MJ, White KE, MacDonald KL, Osterholm MT. Role of egg consumption in sporadic *Salmonella enteritidis* and *Salmonella typhimurium* infections in Minnesota. *J Infect Dis* 1993;167:107–111.

73. Tauxe RV, Hassan LF, Findeisen KO, Sharrar RG, Blake PA. Salmonellosis in nurses: lack of transmission to patients. *J Infect Dis* 1988;157:370–373.

74. Wilson R, Feldman RA, Davis J, LaVenture M. Salmonellosis in infants: the importance of intrafamilial transmission. *Pediatrics* 1982;69:436–438.

75. Agunod M, Yamaguchi N, Lopez R, Luhby AL, Glass GBJ. Correlative study of hydrochloric acid, pepsin, and intrinsic factor secretion in newborns and infants. *Am J Dig Dis* 1969;45:14–26.

76. Haddock RL, Cousens SN, Guzman CC. Infant diet and salmonellosis. *Am J Public Health* 1992;81:997–1000.

77. Chorba TL, Meriwether RA, Jenkins BR, Gunn RA, MacCormack JN. Control of a non-foodborne outbreak of salmonellosis: day care in isolation. *Am J Public Health* 1987;77:979–981.

78. Buchwald DS, Blaser MJ. A review of human salmonellosis. II. Duration of excretion following infection with nontyphi *Salmonella*. *Rev Infect Dis* 1984;6:345–356.

79. Waddell WR, Kunz LJ. Association of *Salmonella enteritis* with operation of stomach. *N Engl J Med* 1956;255:555–559.

80. Gianella RA, Broitman SA, Zamcheck N. Gastric acid barrier to ingested microorganisms in man: studies in vivo and in vitro. *Gut* 1972;13:251–256.

81. Blaser MJ, Neuman LS. A review of human salmonellosis. I. Infective dose. *Rev Infect Dis* 1982;4:1096–1106.

82. McCullough NB, Eisele CW. Experimental human salmonellosis. IV. Pathogenicity of strains of *Salmonella pullorum* obtained from spray-dried whole egg. *J Infect Dis* 1951;89:1540–1545.

83. Hornick RB, Greisman SE, Woodward TE, et al. Typhoid fever: pathogenesis and immunologic control. *N Engl J Med* 1970;283:686–691.

84. Gorden J, Small PLC. Acid resistance in enteric bacteria. *Infect Immun* 1993;61:364–367.

85. Foster JW, Hall HK. Adaptive acidification tolerance response of *Salmonella typhimurium*. *J Bacteriol* 1990;172:771–778.

86. Selsted ME, Miller SI, Henschen AH, Ouellette AJ. Enteric defensins: antibiotic peptide components of intestinal host defense. *J Cell Biol* 1992;118:929–936.

87. Lehrer RI, Ganz T, Selsted ME. Defensins, endogenous antibiotic peptides of animal cells. *Cell* 1991;64:229–230.

88. Michetti P, Mahan MJ, Slauch JM, Mekalanos JJ, Neutra MR. Monoclonal secretory immunoglobulin A protects mice against oral challenge with the invasive pathogen *Salmonella typhimurium*. *Infect Immun* 1992;60:1786–1792.

89. Brandtzaeg P. Overview of the mucosal system. *Curr Top Microbiol Immunol* 1989;146:13–25.

90. Kohbata S, Yokobata H, Yabuuchi E. Cytopathogenic effect of *Salmonella typhi* GIFU 10007 on M cells of murine ileal Peyer's patches in ligated ileal loops: an ultrastructural study. *Microbiol Immunol* 1986;30:1225–1237.

91. Finlay BB, Gumbiner B, Falkow S. Penetration of *Salmonella* through a polarized MDCK epithelial cell monolayer. *J Cell Biol* 1988;107:221–230.

92. Takeuchi A. Electron microscopic studies of experimental *Salmonella* infection 1. Penetration into the intestinal epithelium by *Salmonella typhimurium*. *Am J Pathol* 1967;50:109–136.

93. Francis CL, Starnbach MN, Falkow S. Morphological and cytoskeletal changes in epithelial cells occur immediately upon interaction with *Salmonella typhimurium* grown under low-oxygen conditions. *Mol Microbiol* 1992;6:3077–3087.

94. Finley BB, Falkow S. Comparison of the invasion strategies used by *Salmonella cholerae-suis*, *Shigella flexneri* and *Yersinia enterocolitica* to enter cultured animal cells: endosome acidification is not required for bacterial invasion or intracellular replication. *Biochimie* 1988;70:1089–1099.

95. Pace JH, Hayman MJ, Galan JE. Signal transduction and invasion of epithelial cells by *Salmonella typhimurium*. *Cell* 1993;72:505–514.

96. Galan JE, Pace JH, Hayman MJ. Involvement of the epidermal growth factor receptor in the invasion of cultured mammalian cells by *Salmonella typhimurium*. *Nature* 1992;357:588–589.

97. Hackett J, Kotlarski I, Mathan V, Rowley D. The colonization of Peyer's patches by a strain of *Salmonella typhimurium* cured of the cryptic plasmid. *J Infect Dis* 1986;153:1119–1125.

98. Rubin FA, McWhirter PD, Burr D, et al. Rapid diagnosis of typhoid fever through identification of *Salmonella typhi* within 18 hours of specimen acquisition by culture of the mononuclear cell-platelet fraction of blood. *J Clin Microbiol* 1990;28:825–827.

99. Greisman SE, Woodward TE, Hornick RB, Snyder MJ, Carozza FA Jr. Typhoid fever: a study of pathogenesis and physiologic abnormalities. *Trans Am Clin Climat Assoc* 1961;73:146–161.

100. Alpuche-Aranda CM, Racoosin EL, Swanson JA, Miller SI. *Salmonella* stimulate macrophage macropinocytosis and persist within spacious phagosomes. *J Exp Med* 1994;179:601–608.

101. Alpuche-Aranda CM, Swanson JA, Loomis WP, Miller SI. *Salmonella typhimurium* activates virulence gene transcription

within acidified macrophage phagosomes. *Proc Natl Acad Sci USA* 1992;89:10079–10083.

102. Weiss J, Stendhal O, Elsbach P. Killing of Gram negative bacteria by polymorphonuclear leukocytes: role of an O_2-independent system. *J Clin Invest* 1982;69:959–970.

103. Looney JR, Steigbigel RT. Role of the Vi antigen of *Salmonella typhi* in resistance to host defense in vitro. *J Lab Clin Med* 1986;108:506–516.

104. Buchmeier NA, Lipps CJ, So MYH, Heffron F. Recombination-deficient mutants of *Salmonella typhimurium* are avirulent and sensitive to the oxidative burst of macrophages. *Mol Microbiol* 1993;7:933–936.

105. Fame TM, Engelhard D, Riley HD Jr. Hemophagocytosis accompanying typhoid fever. *Pediatr Infect Dis* 1986;5:367–369.

106. Calva JJ, Ruiz-Palacios GM. *Salmonella hepatitis:* detection of *Salmonella* antigens in the liver of patients with typhoid fever. *J Infect Dis* 1986;154:373–374.

107. Miller SI. *PhoP/PhoQ:* macrophage-specific modulators of *Salmonella* virulence? Mol Microbiol 1991;5:2073–2078.

108. Galan JE, Curtiss R. Cloning and molecular characterization of genes whose products allow *Salmonella typhimurium* to penetrate culture cells. *Proc Natl Acad Sci USA* 1989;86:6383–6387.

109. Ginnochio C, Pace J, Galan JE. Identification and molecular characterization of a *Salmonella typhimurium* gene involved in triggering the internalization of *Salmonellae* into cultured epithelial cells. *Proc Natl Acad Sci USA* 1992;89:5976–5980.

110. Lee CA, Jones BD, Falkow S. Identification of a *Salmonella typhimurium* invasion locus by selection for hyperinvasive mutants. *Proc Natl Acad Sci USA* 1992;89:1847–1851.

111. Behlau I, Miller SI. A *PhoP* repressed gene promotes *Salmonella* invasion of epithelial cells. *J Bacteriol* 1993;175:4475–4484.

112. Fields PI, Swanson RV, Haidaris CG, Heffron F. Mutants of *Salmonella typhimurium* that cannot survive within the macrophage are avirulent. *Proc Natl Acad Sci USA* 1986;83:5189–5193.

113. Fields P, Groisman E, Heffron F. A *Salmonella* locus that controls resistance to microbicidal proteins from phagocytic cells. *Science* 1989;243:1059–1062.

114. Miller SI, Kukral AM, Mekalanos JJ. A two-component regulatory system (*phoP phoQ*) controls *Salmonella typhimurium* virulence. *Proc Natl Acad Sci USA* 1989;86:5054–5058.

115. Curtiss R III, Kelly SM. *Salmonella typhimurium* deletion mutants lacking adenylate cyclase and cyclic AMP receptor protein are avirulent and immunogenic. *Infect Immun* 1987;55:3035–3043.

116. Dorman CJ, Chatfield S, Higgins CF, Hayward C, Dougan G. Characterization of porin and *ompR* mutants of a virulent strain of *Salmonella typhimurium:* *ompR* mutants are attenuated in vivo. *Infect Immun* 1989;57:2136–2140.

117. Fang FC, Libby SJ, Buchmeier NA, et al. The alternative sigma factor KatF (RpoS) regulates *Salmonella* virulence. *Proc Natl Acad Sci USA* 1992;89:11978–11982.

118. Tacket GO, Hone DM, Curtiss RI, et al. Comparison of the safety and immunogenicity of *aroC, aroD,* and *cya crp Salmonella typhi* strains in adult volunteers. *Infect Immun* 1992;60:536–541.

119. Lindberg AA. Bacterial virulence factors—with particular reference to *Salmonella* bacteria. *Scand J Infect Dis* 1980;24 (Suppl):86–92.

120. Finlay BB, Falkow S. Virulence factors associated with *Salmonella* species. *Microbiol Sci* 1988;5:324–328.

121. Hone DM, Attridge SR, Forrest B, et al. A *galE via* (Vi antigen-negative) mutant of *Salmonella typhi* Ty2 retains virulence in humans. *Infect Immun* 1988;56:1326–1333.

122. Reitmeyer JC, Peterson JW, Wilson KJ. *Salmonella* cytotoxin: a component of the bacterial outer membrane. *Microbiol Pathog* 1986;1:503–510.

123. Libby S, Buchmeier N, Guiney D, Bowe F, Heffron F. A cytolytic toxin encoded by *Salmonella* is required for virulence and survival within macrophages. Program and Abstracts of the 93rd General Meeting of the American Society of Microbiology, 1993:39.

124. Levine MM, Herrington D, Murphy JR, et al. Safety, infectivity, immunogenicity, and in vivo stability of two attenuated auxotrophic mutant strains of *Salmonella typhi*, 541Ty and 543Ty, as live oral vaccines in humans. *J Clin Invest* 1987;79:888–902.

125. Aguero J, Faundez G, Nunez M, Wormser GP, Lieberman JP, Cabello FC. Choleriform syndrome and production of labile enterotoxin (CT/LT1)-like antigen by species of *Salmonella infantis* and *Salmonella haardt* isolated from the same patient. *Rev Infect Dis* 1991;13:420–423.

126. Peterson NJ. *Salmonella* toxins. In: *Pharmacology of bacterial toxins*. New York: Pergamon Press; 1986:227–234.

127. Chopra AK, Houston CW, Peterson JW, Prasad R, Mekalanos JJ. Cloning and expression of the *Salmonella* enterotoxin gene. *J Bacteriol* 1987;169:5095–5100.

128. McCormick BA, Colgan SP, Nelp-Archer C, Miller SI, Madara JL. *Salmonella typhimurium* attachment to human intestinal epithelial monolayers: transcellular signalling to subepithelial neutrophils. *J Cell Biol* 1993;123:895–907.

129. O'Brien A. Innate resistance of mice to *Salmonella typhi* infection. *Infect Immun* 1982;38:948–952.

130. Lissner CR, Swanson R, O'Brien A. Genetic control of the innate resistance of mice to *Salmonella typhimurium:* expression of the *Ity* gene in peritoneal and splenic macrophages isolated in vitro. *J Immunol* 1983;131:3006–3013.

131. Vidal SM, Malo D, Vogan K, Skamene E, Gros P. Natural resistance to infection with intracellular parasites: isolation of a candidate for *Bcg*. *Cell* 1993;73:469–485.

132. Levine WC, Buehler JW, Bean NH, Tauxe RV. Epidemiology of nontyphoidal *Salmonella* bacteremia during the human immunodeficiency virus epidemic. *J Infect Dis* 1991;164:81–87.

133. Gotuzzo E, Frisancho O, Sanchez J, et al. Association between the acquired immunodeficiency syndrome and infection with *Salmonella typhi* or *Salmonella paratyphi* in an area endemic for typhoid fever. Arch Intern Med 1991;151:381–382.

134. Sperber SJ, Schleupner CJ. Salmonellosis during infection with the human immunodeficiency virus. *Rev Infect Dis* 1987;9:925–934.

135. Mussche MM, Lameire NH, Ringoir SMG. *Salmonella typhimurium* infections in renal transplant patients. *Nephron* 1975;15:143–150.

136. Han T, Sokal JE, Neter E. Salmonellosis in disseminated malignant diseases: a seven year review 1959–1965. *N Engl J Med* 1967;276:1045–1052.

137. Wolfe MS, Armstrong D, Louria DB, et al. Salmonellosis in patients with neoplastic diseases: a review of 100 episodes at Memorial Cancer Center over a 13 year period. *Arch Intern Med* 1971;128:546.

138. Moellering RC, Weinberg AN. Persistant *Salmonella* infection in a female carrier for chronic granulomatous disease. *Ann Intern Med* 1970;73:595–601.

139. Saphra I, Winter JW. Clinical manifestations of salmonellosis in man: an evaluation of 7779 human infections identified at the New York Salmonella Center. *N Engl J Med* 1957;256:1128–1134.

140. Diggs LW. Bone and joint lesions in sickle cell disease. *Clin Orthop* 1967;52:119–143.

141. Kinsella TR, Yogev R, Shulman ST, Gilmore R, Chadwick EG. Treatment of salmonella meningitis and brain abscess with the new cephalosporins: two case reports and a review of literature. *Pediatr Infect Dis J* 1987;6:476–480.

142. Pavia AT, Shipman LD, Wells JG, et al. Epidemiologic evidence that prior antimicrobial exposure decreases resistance to infection by antimicrobial-sensitive *Salmonella*. *J Infect Dis* 1990;161:255–260.

143. Levine MM, Ferreccio C, Black RE, Tacket CO, Germanier R. Progress in vaccines against typhoid fever. *Rev Infect Dis* 1989;11:S552–S567.

144. Marmion DE, Naylor GRE, Stewart IO. Second attacks of typhoid fever. *J Hyg* 1953;51:260–267.

145. Forrest BD, LaBrooy JT, Breyer L, Dearlove CE, Shearman DJC. The human humoral immune response to *Salmonella typhi* Ty21a. *J Infect Dis* 1991;163:336–345.

146. Acharya IL, Lowe CU, Thapa R, et al. Prevention of typhoid

fever in Nepal with the Vi capsular polysaccharide of *Salmonella typhi*. *N Engl J Med* 1987;317:1101–1104.

147. Lanata CF, Levine MM, Ristori C, et al. Vi serology in detection of chronic *Salmonella typhi* carriers in an epidemic area. *Lancet* 1983;2:441–443.

148. Blanden RV, Mackaness MB, Collins FM. Mechanisms of acquired resistance in mouse typhoid. *J Exp Med* 1966;124:585–600.

149. Murphy J, Wasserman S, Baqar S, Schlesinger L, Lindberg A, Levine M. Immunity to *Salmonella typhi* considerations relevant to measurement of cellular immunity in typhoid-endemic regions. *Clin Exp Immunol* 1989;75:228–233.

150. Nencione L, Villa L, DeMagistris MT. Cellular immunity against *Salmonella typhi* after live oral vaccine. *Adv Exp Med Biol* 1987;216B:1669–1684.

151. Rabinowitz SG, MacLeod NR. *Salmonella* meningitis. A report of three cases and review of the literature. *Am J Dis Child* 1972;123:259–262.

152. Celum CL, Chairsson RE, Rutherford GW, et al. Incidence of salmonellosis in patients with AIDS. *J Infect Dis* 1987;156:998–1001.

153. Noskin GA, Clarke JT. *Salmonella arizonae* bacteremia as the presenting manifestation of human immunodeficiency virus infection following rattlesnake meat ingestion. *Rev Infect Dis* 1990;12:514–517.

154. Aserkoff B, Bennett JV. Effect of antibiotic therapy in acute salmonellosis on the fecal excretion of *Salmonellae*. *N Engl J Med* 1969;281:636–640.

155. Szanton VL. Epidemic salmonellosis. *Pediatrics* 1957;20:794–808.

156. Woodward TE, Smadel JE, Ley HL, Green R, Mankikar DS. Preliminary report on the beneficial effect of chloromycetin in the treatment of typhoid fever. *Ann Intern Med* 1948;131–134.

157. Stuart BM, Pullen RL. Typhoid: clinical analysis of three hundred and sixty cases. *Arch Intern Med* 1946;78:629–661.

158. Hoffman TA, Ruiz CJ, Counts GW. Water-borne typhoid fever in Dade County, FL: clinical and therapeutic evaluations of 105 bacteremic patients. *Am J Med* 1975;59:481–487.

159. Roland HAK. The complications of typhoid fever. *J Trop Med Hyg* 1961;64:143–150.

160. Verghese A. The "typhoid state" revisited. *Am J Med* 1985;79:370–372.

161. Hearne SE, Whigham TE, Brady CEI. Pancreatitis and typhoid fever. *Am J Med* 1989;86:471–473.

162. Khourieh M, Schlesinger M, Tabachnik E, Bibi H, Armoni M, Pollak S. Typhoid fever diagnosed by isolation of *S. typhi* from gastric aspirate. *Acta Pediatr Scand* 1989;78:653–655.

163. Avendano A, Herrera P, Horwitz I, et al. Duodenal string cultures: practicality and sensitivity for diagnosing enteric fever in children. *J Infect Dis* 1986;153:359–362.

164. Gilman RH, Terminel M, Hernandez-Mendoza P, Hornick RB. Relative efficacy of blood, urine, rectal swab, bone-marrow and rose-spot cultures for recovery of *Salmonella typhi* in typhoid fever. *Lancet* 1975;1:1211–1213.

165. Benavente L, Gotuzzo E, Guerra J, Grados O, Guerra H, Bravo N. Diagnosis of typhoid fever using a string capsule device. *Trans R Soc Trop Med Hyg* 1984;78:564–565.

166. Hoffman SL, Punjabi NH, Rockhill RC, Sutomo A, Pulungsih AR. Duodenal string-capsule culture compared with bone marrow, blood, and rectal swab cultures for diagnosing typhoid and paratyphoid fever. *J Infect Dis* 1984;149:157–161.

167. Guerra-Caceres JG, Gotuzzo-Herencia E, Crosby-Dagnino E, Miro-Quesada J, Carillo-Parodi C. Diagnostic value of bone marrow culture in typhoid fever. *Trans R Soc Trop Med Hyg* 1979;73:680–683.

168. Farooqui BJ, Khurshid M, Ashfaq MK, Khan MA. Comparative yield of *Salmonella typhi* from blood and bone marrow cultures in patients with fever of unknown origin. *J Clin Pathol* 1991;44:258–259.

169. Rubin FA, McWhirter PD, Punjabi NH, et al. Use of DNA probe to detect *Salmonella typhi* in the blood of patients with typhoid fever. *J Clin Microbiol* 1989;27:1112–1114.

170. Watson K. Isolation of *Salmonella typhi* from the blood stream. *J Lab Clin Med* 1959;47:329–332.

171. Isomaki O, Vuento R, Granfors K. Serological diagnosis of *Salmonella* infections by enzyme immunoassay. *Lancet* 1989;1:1411–1414.

172. Coovadia YM, Singh V, Bhana RH, Moodley N. Comparison of passive haemagglutination test with Widal agglutination test for serological diagnosis of typhoid fever in an endemic area. *J Clin Pathol* 1986;39:680–683.

173. Abraham G, Teklu B, Gedebu M, Selassie GH, Azene G. Diagnostic value of the Widal test. *Trop Geogr Med* 1981;33:329–333.

174. Wicks ACB, Cruickshank JG, Musewe N. Observations on the diagnosis of typhoid fever in an endemic area. *S Afr Med J* 1974;48:1368–1370.

175. Welch H, Mickle FL. A rapid slide test for the serological diagnosis of typhoid and paratyphoid fevers. *Am J Public Health* 1936;26:248–255.

176. Rubin FA. Nucleic acid probes for the identification of *Salmonella*. In: *Gene probes for bacteria*. New York: Academic Press; 1990:323–352.

177. Morrow C, Safi H, Beall AC Jr. Primary aortoduodenal fistula caused by *Salmonella* aortitis. *J Vasc Surg* 1987;6:415–418.

178. Cohen PS, O'Brien TF, Schoenbaum SC, Medieiros AA. The risk of endothelial infection in adults with *Salmonella* bacteremia. *Ann Intern Med* 1978;89:931–932.

179. Parsons R, Gregory J, Palmer DL. *Salmonella* infections of the abdominal aorta. *Rev Infect Dis* 1983;5:227–231.

180. Thayer WS. On the late effects of typhoid fever on the heart and vessels. *Am J Med Sci* 1904;127:391–422.

181. Tenbroeck C, Li CP, Yu H. Studies on paratyphoid C bacilli isolated in China. *J Exp Med* 1934;53:307–315.

182. Von Reyn CF, Levy BS, Arbeit RD, Friedland G, Crumpacker CS. Infective endocarditis: an analysis based on strict case definitions. *Ann Intern Med* 1981;94:505–518.

183. Alvarez-Elcoro S, Soto-Ramirez L, Mateos-Mora M. *Salmonella* bacteremia in patients with prosthetic heart valves. *Am J Med* 1984;77:61–63.

184. Zak FG, Strauss L, Saphra I. Rupture of diseased large arteries in the course of enterobacterial (*Salmonella*) infection. *N Engl J Med* 1958;258:824–828.

185. Jarrett F, Darling CR, Mundth E, Austen GW. Experience with infected aneurysms of the abdominal aorta. *Arch Surg* 1975;110:1281–1286.

186. Mantello MT, Panaccione JL, Moriarty PE, Espos WJ. Impending rupture of nonaneurysmal bacterial aortitis CT diagnosis. *J Comput Assist Tomogr* 1990;6:950–953.

187. Marr J, Haff R. Superinfection of an amoebic abscess by *Salmonella enteritidis*. *Arch Intern Med* 1971;128:291–294.

188. Matossian RM, Najjar F. Suppurative salmonellosis in human hepatic hydatid cysts. *Ann Trop Med Parasitol* 1968;62:143–146.

189. Hirschowitz B. Pyogenic liver abscess. A review with a case report of a solitary abscess caused by *Salmonella enteritidis*. *Gastroenterology* 1952;21:291–299.

190. Chulay J, Lankerani M. Splenic abscess. *Am J Med* 1976;61:513–522.

191. Carswell W, Magrath I. Skin ulceration caused by *Salmonella dublin*. *Br Med J* 1973;1:331–332.

192. Huckstep RL. Typhoid fever and other *Salmonella* infections. Edinburgh: E&S Livingstone; 1962.

193. Sharma AM, Sharma OP. Pulmonary manifestations of typhoid fever: two case reports and a review of the literature. *Chest* 1992;101:1144–1146.

194. Aguado JM, Obeso G, Cabanillas JJ, Fernandez-Guerrero M, Ales J. Pleuropulmonary infections due to nontyphoidal strains of *Salmonella*. *Arch Intern Med* 1990;150:54–56.

195. Wilson K, Feldman R. Reported isolates of *Salmonella* from cerebrospinal fluid in the United States, 1968–1979. *J Infect Dis* 1981;143:504–506.

196. Durand ML, Calderwood SB, Weber DJ, et al. Acute bacterial meningitis in adults: a review of 493 episodes. *N Engl J Med* 1993;328:21–28.

197. Cherubin C, Marr J, Sierra M, Becker S. *Listeria* and gram negative bacillary meningitis in New York City 1972–1979. *Am J Med* 1981;71:199–209.

198. Curbelo AJ, Martineq-Cruz JA. Historia de la *Salmonella habana. Arch Med Inf* 1941;10:170–175.

199. High R, Spaudling F. Human infections with *Salmonella panama. Am J Dis Child* 1946;72:181–188.

200. Dunn DW, McAllister J, Craft JC. Brain abscess and empyema caused by *Salmonella. Pediatr Infect Dis* 1984;4:394–398.

201. Hook BW, Campbell CG, Weens HS, Cooper GR. *Salmonella* osteomyelitis in patients with sickle cell anemia. *N Engl J Med* 1957;257:403–407.

202. David JR, Lack RL. *Salmonella* arthritis. *Medicine* 1960;39: 385–403.

203. Warren CPW. Arthritis associated with *Salmonella* infection. *Ann Rheum Dis* 1970;29:483–487.

204. Hakansson U, Eitrem R, Low B, Winblad S. HLA-antigen B27 in cases with joint affections in an outbreak of salmonellosis. *Scand J Infect Dis* 1976;8:245–248.

205. Steckelberg JM, Terrell CL, Edson RS. Laboratory-acquired *Salmonella typhimurium* enteritis: association with erythema nodosum and reactive arthritis. *Am J Med* 1988;85:705–707.

206. Maki-Ikola O, Leirisalo-Repo M, Kantele A, Toivanen P, Granfors K. *Salmonella*-specific antibodies in reactive arthritis. *J Infect Dis* 1991;164:1141–1148.

207. Hermann E, Mayet WJ, Poralla KH, Meyer zum Buschenfelde KH, Fleischer B. *Salmonella*-reactive synovial fluid T-cell clones in a patient with post-infectious *Salmonella* arthritis. *Scand J Rheumatol* 1990;19:350–355.

208. Salmon D, Detruchis P, Leport C, et al. Efficacy of zidovudine in preventing relapses of *Salmonella* bacteremia in AIDS. *J Infect Dis* 1991;163:415–416.

209. Keith BR, White G, Wilson HR. In vivo efficacy of zidovudine (3'-azido-3'-deoxythimidine) in experimental gram-negative bacterial infections. *Antimicrob Agents Chemother* 1989;33: 479–483.

210. Herrmann JL, Lagrange PH. Intracellular activity of zidovudine (3'-azido-3'deoxythymidine, AZT) against *Salmonella typhimurium* in the macrophage cell line J774-2. *Antimicrob Agents Chemother* 1992;36:1081–1085.

211. Musher DM, Rubenstein AD. Permanent carriers of nontyphosal *Salmonellae. Arch Intern Med* 1973;132:869–872.

212. Centers for Disease Control and Prevention. Typhoid immunization: recommendations of the Immunization Practices Advisory Committee (ACIP). *MMWR* 1990;39:1–5.

213. Woodruff BA, Pavia AT, Blake PA. A new look at typhoid vaccination. *JAMA* 1991;265:756–759.

214. Hornick RB, Woodward TE. Appraisal of typhoid vaccine in experimentally infected human subjects. *Trans Am Clin Climat* Assoc 1978;78:70–78.

215. Murphy JR, Grez L, Schlesinger L, et al. Immunogenicity of *Salmonella typhi* Ty21a for young children. *Infect Immun* 1991; 59:4291–4293.

216. Typhoid vaccination: weighing the options (editorial). *Lancet* 1992;340:341–342.

217. Yugoslav Typhoid Commission. A controlled field trial of the effectiveness of acetone-dried and inactivated and heat phenol-inactivated typhoid vaccines in Yugoslavia. *Bull WHO* 1964; 30:623–630.

218. Hejfec LB, Salmin LV, Lejtman MZ, et al. A controlled field trial and laboratory study of five typhoid vaccines in the USSR. *Bull WHO* 1966;34:321–339.

219. Ashcroft MT, Morrision RJ, Nicholson CC. Controlled field trial in British Guiana school children of heat-killed-phenolized and acetone-killed lyophilized typhoid vaccines. *Am J Hyg* 1964;79:196–206.

220. Ashcroft MT, Singh B, Nicholson CC, Ritchie JM, Sobryann E, Williams F. A seven-year field trial of two typhoid vaccines in Guyana. *Lancet* 1967;2:1056–1059.

221. Walter Reed Army Institute of Research. Preparation of dried acetone-inactivated and heat-phenol-inactivated typhoid vaccines. *Bull WHO* 1964;30:635–646.

222. Hejfec LB. Results of the study of typhoid vaccines in four controlled field trials in the USSR. *Bull WHO* 1965;32:1–14.

223. Edwards EA, Johnson DP, Pierce WE, Peckinpaugh RO. Reactions and serologic responses to monovalent acetone-inacti-

vated typhoid vaccine and heat-killed TAB when given by jet-injection. *Bull WHO* 1974;51:501–505.

224. Wilson GS. *The hazards of immunization*. London: Athlone Press; 1967.

225. Calin A, Goulding N, Brewerton D. Reactive arthropathy following *Salmonella* vaccination. *Arthritis Rheum* 1987;30:1197.

226. Gilman RH, Hornick RB, Woodward WE, DuPont HL, Levine MM, Libonati JP. Evaluation of a UDP-glucose-4-epimerase-less mutant of Salmonella typhi as a live oral typhoid vaccine. *J Infect Dis* 1977;136:716–723.

227. Wahdan MH, Serie C, Germanier R, et al. A controlled field trial of live oral vaccine Ty21a. *Bull WHO* 1980;58:469–474.

228. Black RE, Levine MM, Ferreccio C, et al. Efficacy of one or two doses Ty21a *Salmonella typhi* vaccine in enteric-coated capsules in a controlled field trial. *Vaccine* 1990;8:81–84.

229. Levine MM, Black RE, Ferreccio C, Germanier R. Large-scale field trial of Ty21a live oral typhoid vaccine in enteric-coated capsule formulation. *Lancet* 1987;1049–1052.

230. Wahdan MH, Serie C, Ceriser Y, Sallam S, Germanier R. A controlled field trial of live Salmonella typhi strain Ty21a oral vaccine against typhoid three year results. *J Infect Dis* 1982; 145:292–295.

231. Simanjuntak CH, Paleolog FP, Punjabi NH, et al. Oral immunization against typhoid fever in Indonesia with Ty21a vaccine. *Lancet* 1991;338:1055–1059.

232. Kaplan DT, Hill DR. Compliance with live, oral Ty21a a typhoid vaccine. *JAMA* 1992;267:1074.

233. Hirschel B, Wuethrich R, Somaini B, Steffen R. Inefficacy of the commercial live oral Ty21a vaccine in the prevention of typhoid fever. *Eur J Clin Microbiol Infect Dis* 1985;4:295–298.

234. Schwartz E, Shlim DR, Eaton M, Jenks N, Houston R. The effect of oral and parenteral typhoid vaccination on the rate of infection with *Salmonella typhi* and *Salmonella paratyphi* A among foreigners in Nepal. *Arch Intern Med* 1990;150:349–351.

235. Woodward TE, Smadel JE, Ley HL, Green R, Mankikar DS. Preliminary report on the beneficial effect of chloromycetin in the treatment of typhoid fever. *Ann Intern Med* 1948;29: 131–134.

236. El-Ramli A. Chloramphenicol in treatment of typhoid fever. *Lancet* 1950;1:618.

237. Olarte J, Galindo E. *S. typhi* resistant to chloramphenicol, ampicillin, and other antimicrobial agents: strains isolated and extensive typhoid fever epidemic in Mexico. *Antimicrob Agents Chemother* 1973;4:597–601.

238. Paniker CK, Vimala KN. Transferable chloramphenicol resistance in *Salmonella typhi. Nature* 1972;239:109–110.

239. Lampe PM, Mansuwan P, Duangmain C. Chloramphenicol-resistant typhoid. *Lancet* 1974;1:623–624.

240. Butler T, Rumans L, Arnold K. Response of typhoid-fever caused by chloramphenicol-susceptible and chloramphenicol-resistant strains of *Salmonella typhi* to treatment with trimethoprim-sulfamethoxazole. *Rev Infect Dis* 1982;4:551–561.

241. Bouquier Y, Hervonet D, Hilleritean H. Resultats du traitement par la chloromyceine de soixante fievres typhoides. *Bull Mem Soc Med Hop Paris* 1949;32:1396.

242. Erselv A. Hematopoietic depression induced by chloromycetin. *Blood* 1953;8:170–174.

243. Wallerstein RO, Condit PK, Kasper CK, Brown JW, Morrison FR. Statewide study of chloramphenicol therapy and fatal aplastic anemia. *JAMA* 1969;208:2045–2050.

244. Glazko AJ, Dill WA, Kinkel AW, Goulet JR, Halloway WJ, Buchanan RA. Absorption and excretion of parenteral doses of chloramphenicol sodium succinate (CMS) in comparison with peroral doses of chloramphenicol (CM). *Clin Pharmacol Ther* 1977;21:104.

245. Ti TT, Monteiro EH, Lam S, Lee HS. Chloramphenicol concentrations in sera of patients with typhoid fever being treated with oral or intravenous preparation. *Antimicrob Agents Chemother* 1990;34:1809–1811.

246. Rahal JJJ, Simberkoff MS. Bactericidal and bacteriostatic action of chloramphenicol against meningeal pathogens. *Antimicrob Agents Chemother* 1979;16:13–18.

247. Chang HR, Vladoianu IR, Pechere JC. Effects of ampicillin, ceftriaxone, chloramphenicol, pefloxacin and trimethoprim-

sulfamethoxazole on *Salmonella typhi* within human monocyte-derived macrophages. *J Antimicrob Chemother* 1990;26:
689–694.

248. Brown JD, Mo DH, Rhoades ER. Chloramphenicol-resistant *Salmonella typhi* in Saigon. *JAMA* 1975;231:162–166.
249. Linh NN, Arnold K. Treatment of typhoid fever and typhoid carriers in South East Asia—viewpoint from South Vietnam. *Drugs* 1975;9:241–246.
250. Pillay N, Adams EB, North-Coobes D. Comparative trial of amoxacyllin and chloramphenicol in treatment of typhoid fever in adults. *Lancet* 1975;2:332–334.
251. Scragg JN, Rubidge CJ. Amoxycillin in the treatment of typhoid fever in children. *Am J Trop Med Hyg* 1975;24:860–865.
252. Herzog C. Chemotherapy of typhoid fever. *Infection* 1976;4: 166–173.
253. Brodie J, MacQueen IA. Effect of trimethoprim-sulfamethoxazole on typhoid and *Salmonella* carriers. *Br Med J* 1970;3: 318–319.
254. Soe GB, Overturf GD. Treatment of typhoid fever and other systemic salmonelloses with cefotaxime, ceftriaxone, cefoperazone, and other newer cephalosporins. *Rev Infect Dis* 1987;9: 719–736.
255. Moosa A, Rubidge CJ. Once daily ceftriaxone vs. chloramphenicol for treatment of typhoid fever in children. *Pediatr Infect Dis J* 1989;8:696–699.
256. Pape JW, Gerdes H, Oriol L, Johnson WDJ. Typhoid fever: successful therapy with cefoperazone. *J Infect Dis* 1986;153: 272–276.
257. Lepage P, Bogaerts J, Goethem CV, Hitimana DG, Nsengumuremy F. Multiresistant *Salmonella typhimurium* systemic infection in Rwanda. Clinical features and treatment with cefotaxime. *J Antimicrob Chemother* 1990;26:53–57.
258. Islam A, Buter T, Nath SK, et al. Randomized treatment of patients with typhoid fever by using ceftriaxone or chloramphenicol. *J Infect Dis* 1988;158:742–747.
259. Bryan JP, Rocha H, Silva HR, et al. Comparisons of ceftriaxone and ampicillin plus chloramphenicol for the therapy of acute bacterial meningitis. *Antimicrob Agents Chemother* 1985; 28:361–368.
260. Tanaka Kido J, Ortega L, Santos JI. Comparative efficacies of aztreonam and chloramphenicol in children with typhoid fever. *J Pediatr Infect Dis* 1990;9:44–48.
261. Farid Z, Girgis NI, Kamal M, Bishay E, Kilpatrick ME. Successful aztreonam treatment of acute typhoid fever after chloramphenicol failure. *Scand J Infect Dis* 1990;22:505–506.
262. Choo KE, Ariffin WA, Ong KH, Sivakumaran S. Aztreonam failure in typhoid fever. *Lancet* 1991;337:498.
263. Cherubin CE, Eng RHK, Smith SM, Goldstein EJC. Cephalosporin therapy for salmonellosis. *Arch Intern Med* 1986;146: 2149–2152.
264. Preblud SR, Gill CJ, Campos JM. Bactericidal activities of chloramphenicol and eleven other antibiotics against *Salmonella spp. Antimicrob Agents Chemother* 1984;3:327–330.
265. Barros F, Korzeniowski OM, Sande MA, Martins K, Santos LC, Rocha H. In vitro antibiotic susceptibility of *Salmonellae. Antimicrob Agents Chemother* 1977;6:1071–1073.
266. De Carvalho EM, Martinelli R. Cefamandole treatment of *Salmonella* bacteremia. *Antimicrob Agents Chemother* 1982;21: 334–336.
267. Vaudaux P, Waldvogel FA. Gentamicin antibacterial activity in the presence of human polymorphonuclear leukocytes. *Antimicrob Agents Chemother* 1979;16:743–749.
268. Rodriquez-Norriega E, Andrade-Villanueva J, Amaya-Taipa G. Quinolones in the treatment of *Salmonella* carriers. *Rev Infect Dis* 1989;11:S1179–S1186.
269. Easmon CSF, Crane JP, Blowers A. Effect of ciprofloxacin on intracellular organisms: in-vitro and in-vivo studies. *J Antimicrob Chemother* 1986;18:43–48.
270. Stanley PJ, Flegg PJ, Mandal B, Geddes A. Open study of ciprofloxacin in enteric fever. *J Antimicrob Chemother* 1989; 23:789–791.
271. Mandal BK. Modern treatment of typhoid fever. *J Infect* 1991; 22:1–4.

272. Wallace M, Yousif AA. Spread of multiresistant *S. typhi*. *Lancet* 1990;336:1065–1066.
273. Lewin CS, Nandivada LS, Amyes SG. Multiresistant *Salmonella* and fluoroquinolones. *J Antimicrob Chemother* 1991;27: 47–49.
274. Piddock LJ, Whale K, Wise R. Quinolone resistance in *Salmonella:* clinical experience. *Lancet* 1990;335:1459.
275. Lewin CS. Treatment of multiresistant *Salmonella* infection. *Lancet* 1991;337:47.
276. Sabbour MS, Osman LM. Experience with ofloxacin in enteric fever. *J Chemother* 1990;2:113–115.
277. Sarma PS, Durairaj P. Randomized treatment of patients with typhoid and paratyphoid fevers using norfloxacin or chloramphenicol. *Trans R Soc Trop Med Hyg* 1991;85:670–671.
278. Arnold K, Hong CS, Nelwan R, et al. Randomized comparative study of fleroxacin and chloramphenicol in typhoid fever. *Am J Med* 1993;94:3A195S–3A200S.
279. Christ W, Lehner T, Ulbrich B. Specific toxicologic aspects of the quinolones. *Rev Infect Dis* 1988;10(Suppl 10):141–146.
280. Cheesbrough JS, Mwema JS, Green SDR. Quinolones in children with invasive salmonellosis. *Lancet* 1991;338:127.
281. Dawood ST, Uwaydah AK. Treatment of multiresistant *Salmonella typhi* with intravenous ciprofloxacin. *Pediatr Infect Dis* 1991;10:343.
282. Cooles P. Adjuvant steroids and relapse of typhoid fever. *J Trop Med Hyg* 1986;89:229–231.
283. Lee LA, Puhr ND, Bean NH, Tauxe RV. Antimicrobial resistance of *Salmonella* isolated from patients in the United States, 1989–1990. Program and Abstracts 31st Interscience Conference on Antimicrobial Agents and Chemotherapy, 1991:186.
284. MacDonald KL, Cohen ML, Hargrett BNT, et al. Changes in antimicrobial resistance of *Salmonella* isolated from humans in the United States. *JAMA* 1987;258:1496–1499.
285. Spika JS, Waterman SH, SooHoo GW, et al. Chloramphenicol-resistant *Salmonella newport* traced through hamburger to dairy farms. *N Engl J Med* 1987;316:565–570.
286. Farhoudi-Moghaddam AA, Katouli M, Jafari A, Bahavar MA, Parsi M, Malekzadeh F. Antimicrobial drug resistance and resistance factor transfer among clinical isolates of *Salmonella* in Iran. *Scand J Infect Dis* 1990;22:197–203.
287. Georges-Courbot MC, Wachsmuth IK, Bouquety JC, Siopathis MR, Cameron DN, Georges AJ. Cluster of antibiotic-resistant *Salmonella enteritidis* infection in the Central African Republic. *J Clin Microbiol* 1990;28:771–773.
288. Poupart CM, Chanal C, Sirot D, Labia R, Sirot J. Identification of CTX-2, a novel cefotxiimase from a *Salmonella mbandaka* isolate. *Antimicrob Agents Chemother* 1991;35:1498–1500.
289. Ward LR, Threlfall EJ, Rowe B. Multiple-drug resistance in Salmonellae in England and Wales: a comparison between 1981 and 1988. *J Clin Pathol* 1990;43:563–566.
290. Gibb AP, Lewin CS, Garden OJ. Development of quinolone resistance and multiple antibiotic resistance in *Salmonella bovismorbificans* in a pancreatic abscess. *J Antimicrob Chemother* 1991;28:318–321.
291. Nelson JD, Kusmiesz H, Jackson LH, Woodman E. Treatment of *Salmonella* gastroenteritis with ampicillin, amoxicillin or placebo. *Pediatrics* 1980;65:1125–1130.
292. Pichler HET, Dridl G, Stickler K, Wolf D. Clinical efficacy of ciprofloxacin compared with placebo in bacterial diarrhea. *Am J Med* 1987;82(Suppl 4A):329–332.
293. Lightfoot NF, Ahmad F, Cowden J. Management of institutional outbreaks of *Salmonella* gastroenteritis. *J Antimicrob Chemother* 1990;26:37–46.
294. Carlstedt G, Dahl P, Magnus Niklasson P, Gullberg K, Banck G, Kahlmeter G. Norfloxicin treatment of salmonellosis does not shorten the carrier stage. *Scand J Infect Dis* 1990;22: 553–556.
295. Neill MA, Opal SM, Heelan J, et al. Failure of ciprofloxicin to eradicate convalescent fecal excretion after acute salmonellosis: experience during an outbreak in health care workers. *Ann Intern Med* 1991;114:195–199.
296. Kassis I, Dagan R, Chipman M, Alkan M, Simo A, Gorodischer R. The use of prophylactic furazolidone to control a nosocomial

epidemic of multiply resistant *Salmonella typhimurium* in pediatric wards. *Pediatr Infect Dis J* 1990;9:551–555.

297. Donabedian H. Long-term suppression of *Salmonella* aortitis with an oral antibiotic. *Arch Intern Med* 1989;149:1452–1453.

298. Gabbi E, Rossi G, Ghidoni I. *Salmonella typhimurium* infection of thoracic aorta aneurysm in immunocompetent subject. Case report and literature review. *Infection* 1989;17:306–308.

299. Jacobson MA, Hahn SM, Gerberding JL, Lee B, Sande MA. Ciprofloxacin for salmonella bacteremia in the acquired immunodeficiency syndrome (AIDS). *Ann Intern Med* 1989;110: 1027–1029.

300. Lewin CS, Allen RA, Amyes SG. Antibacterial activity of fluoroquinolones in combination with zidovudine. *J Med Microbiol* 1990;33:127–131.

301. Centers for Disease Control. Recommendations for prophylaxis against *Pneumocystis carinii* pneumonia for adults and adolescents infected with human immunodeficiency virus. *MMWR* 1992;42(No. RR-4):1–11.

302. Freitag JL. Treatment of chronic typhoid carrier by cholecystectomy. *Public Health Rep* 1973;32:869.

303. Nolan CM, White PCJ. Treatment of typhoid carrier with amoxicillin. *JAMA* 1978;239:2352–2354.

304. Freerksen E, Rosenfield M, Freerksen R, et al. Treatment of chronic *Salmonella* carriers. Study of 40 cases of *S. typhi*, 19 cases of *S. paratyphi* b and 28 cases of *S. enteritidis* strains. *Chemotherapy* 1977;23:192–210.

305. Sammalkorpi K, Lahdevirta J, Makela R. Treatment of chronic *Salmonella* carriers with ciprofloxacin. *Lancet* 1987;2:164–165.

306. Ferrecio C, Morris GJ, Valivieso C, et al. Efficacy of ciprofloxacin in the treatment of chronic typhoid carriers. *J Infect Dis* 1988;157:1235–1239.

Infections of the Gastrointestinal Tract,
edited by M. J. Blaser, P. D. Smith, J. I. Ravdin,
H. B. Greenberg, and R. L. Guerrant
Published by Raven Press, Ltd., New York, 1995.

CHAPTER 55

Yersinia enterocolitica and *Yersinia pseudotuberculosis*

Timothy L. Cover

YERSINIA ENTEROCOLITICA

Description

Infection of humans with the enteric pathogen *Yersinia enterocolitica* most frequently results in diarrheal illness, but may be associated with a wide spectrum of other clinical manifestations, including abdominal pain, septicemia, arthritis, and erythema nodosum (1,2). The two other pathogenic species of the genus *Yersinia* are *Y. pestis*, the causative agent of plague, and *Y. pseudotuberculosis*. Several other *Yersinia* species, including *Y. bercovieri*, *Y. mollaretii*, *Y. intermedia*, *Y. kristensenii*, *Y. fredericksenii*, *Y. aldovae*, and *Y. rohdei*, are widespread in the environment but are rarely human pathogens. Like *Escherichia coli* and *Salmonellae*, *Y. enterocolitica* is a heterogeneous species, comprising more than 50 O-antigen serotypes and several biotypes and phage types (3). However, only a few pathogenic *Y. enterocolitica* serotypes commonly cause human disease (1,3).

Microbiology

Y. enterocolitica is a facultatively anaerobic gram-negative organism that is classified in the family *Enterobacteriaceae*. Isolates are characteristically urease-positive and citrate-negative, and most isolates reduce nitrates (4). *Y. enterocolitica* produces an acid slant and acid butt on triple sugar iron agar without hydrogen sulfide or gas. Metabolic and nutritional requirements and synthetic functions of the organism are regulated by temperature. At 25°C, the organism is motile and has minimal nutritional requirements, whereas at 37°C the organism is nonmotile, re-

quires additional nutrients for growth (3), and produces various plasmid-encoded proteins related to virulence.

Epidemiology

The frequency of *Y. enterocolitica* infection as a cause of diarrheal illness has been assessed in several studies in which stool cultures were collected from diarrheic persons. In Montreal, *Y. enterocolitica* was isolated from 2.8% of 6364 symptomatic children during a 15-month period (5). In similar studies in Finland, Belgium, the Netherlands, Italy, British Columbia, and Australia, the organism was cultured from 4.7%, 5.9%, 2.9%, 1.4%, 6.7%, and 0.7% of stool specimens, respectively (6–11). In three studies conducted in the United States, *Y. enterocolitica* was isolated from ≤0.4% of stool specimens (12–14), but recently (1988–1991), *Y. enterocolitica* was recovered from 1% of 7290 rectal swab specimens collected from patients in Atlanta, Georgia (15). Seasonal clustering of cases in fall and winter months occurs in Europe, and was recently described in the United States (9,15,16). There is general agreement that the incidence of *Y. enterocolitica* is higher in several northern countries, including Scandinavia, the Netherlands, Belgium, and Canada, than elsewhere (16). In areas of high incidence, *Y. enterocolitica* is isolated more commonly from stools than *Shigella*, and rivals both *Salmonella* and *Campylobacter* as a cause of acute bacterial enteritis (5,7,10).

The predominant serotypes of *Y. enterocolitica* isolated from symptomatic humans vary according to geographic location. In Europe and Japan, illness is most commonly caused by serotypes O:3 or O:9 (6–9,16,17), whereas serotypes O:8, O:4,32, O:13a,13b, O:18, O:20, and O:21 are isolated almost exclusively from American patients (18–21), and have been termed "American serotypes." Serotype O:3 was rarely isolated from ill persons in the United States prior to 1980, but has been steadily increasing in prevalence in several regions of the United States

---

T. L. Cover: Division of Infectious Diseases, Vanderbilt University School of Medicine and Veterans Affairs Medical Center, Nashville, Tennessee 37232-2605.

TABLE 1. *Selected outbreaks of* Yersinia enterocolitica *infection with identified sources*

Location (ref.)	Number of cases	Source or common vehicle	Predominant serotype
North Carolina (28)	16	Dog	O:8
Canada (31)	138	?Raw milk	O:5,27
New York (27)	38	Chocolate milk	O:8
Japan (32)	1051	Milk	O:3
New York (26)	159	Powdered milk, chow mein	O:8
Washington (29)	50	Tofu, spring water	O:8
Pennsylvania (33)	16	Bean sprouts, well water	O:8
Southern United States (30)	172	Pasteurized milk	O:13a,13b
Georgia (25)	15	Chitterlings	O:3

(15,22–25). Outbreaks of *Y. enterocolitica* infection have been reported commonly in the United States (1,25–33) (Table 1), whereas in European countries with a high incidence of *Y. enterocolitica* infection, outbreaks have rarely been reported and sporadic disease seems to predominate (1,16). These geographic differences may become less pronounced with time, in association with the introduction of American serotypes into Europe and Japan (8,34), and the dissemination of serotype O:3 in the United States (22–25).

Swine are a major reservoir for the pathogenic *Y. enterocolitica* serotypes O:3 and O:9 (35). *Y. enterocolitica* may be cultured from the tongue, throat, tonsils, cecal contents, and feces of swine, as well as from pork, ham, and butcher shop cutting boards (1,36). Serotype O:3 isolates from swine and symptomatic humans are indistinguishable by genetic analysis (37,38). In a Belgian case-control study, *Y. enterocolitica* infection with serotypes O:3 or O:9 was strongly associated with consumption of raw pork in the 2-week period prior to illness (16). Similarly, an outbreak of infection with serotype O:3 in Atlanta, Georgia in 1988 was associated with consumption or preparation of chitterlings (raw pork intestines) (25). Thus, swine and the consumption of undercooked pork products play a major role in the epidemiology of human *Y. enterocolitica* infections.

Several outbreaks of *Y. enterocolitica* infection have been attibuted to ingestion of contaminated milk products (26,27,30,31). *Y. enterocolitica* may commonly be cultured from cow feces (39), from raw milk, and occasionally from pasteurized milk or pasteurized milk products (40–42). The mechanisms whereby *Y. enterocolitica* survives pasteurization or contaminates milk after pasteurization are unclear. However, *Y. enterocolitica* can multiply in milk stored at 4°C (43,44) and thus small inocula potentially could proliferate during refrigerated storage.

In addition to swine and cows, *Y. enterocolitica* has been isolated from a wide array of other mammals, as well as birds, frogs, fish, flies, fleas, snails, crabs, and oysters (1,18,45). The organism also may be isolated from lakes, streams, well water, and soil (46,47), which presumably are seeded with fecally shed organisms. *Y. enterocolitica* occasionally has been transmitted from dogs to humans (28,48). In addition, the ingestion of unchlorinated water has resulted in sporadic cases and several outbreaks of *Y. enterocolitica* infection (49,50). However, *Y. enterocolitica* isolates from most animals and environ-

mental sources typically belong to nonpathogenic serotypes (18,45); hence most of these reservoirs have not been implicated commonly as sources of human infections.

Transmission of infection from person to person has been suggested by the sequential onset of illness in family members (5,17,28,51,52). In addition, there have been several reported incidents of nosocomial transmission of *Y. enterocolitica* infection (53–56). Although person-to-person transmission by a fecal–oral route probably occurs, it is likely that most human infections are acquired instead by consumption of contaminated food or beverages. In addition to fecal–oral transmission, person-to-person transmission occasionally occurs by transfusion of contaminated blood products (57–59).

Pathogenesis and Immunity

Prior to the development of molecular biological approaches for the study of bacterial pathogenesis, it was recognized that *Y. enterocolitica* constituted a heterogeneous collection of serotypes that differed significantly in virulence. Clinical and epidemiological studies identified pathogenic serotypes that were commonly isolated from symptomatic humans (5,6,19), and contrasted these with nonpathogenic serotypes, which were predominantly isolated from animals, environmental sources, or asymptomatic humans (7,42,60), but rarely caused human disease. Among the pathogenic serotypes, O:8 was identified as a highly virulent American strain that produced more severe disease in humans than O:3 or O:9 (28).

Experimental animal studies also indicated that *Y. enterocolitica* serotypes differ in virulence. Isolates from symptomatic humans typically caused disease in mice, rabbits, or guinea pigs, whereas environmental isolates were avirulent in these models (61,62). Among pathogenic strains, several highly virulent American strains, including O:8 and O:21, caused lethal infections in adult mice (63–66), whereas infections with serotypes O:3 and O:9 were nonlethal unless mice were pretreated with desferrioxamine or iron (3,67). In addition, serotype O:8 caused keratoconjunctivitis in guinea pigs (Sereny test), whereas serotypes O:3 and O:9 did not (64,68). Thus, clinical observations and experimental animal studies have utilized the natural heterogeneity that exists among *Y. enterocolitica* isolates to provide important clues to the pathogene-

TABLE 2. *Virulence factors of* Yersinia enterocolitica

Virulence factor	Size (kDa)	Established role in animal model	Function
Chromosomally encoded			
Invasin	92	Yes	Adherence and invasion
Ail	17	—	Adherence and invasion, resistance to serum killing
Myf fibrillae	21	—	? Adherence
Enterotoxin	30 amino acids	Yes	Activates guanylate cyclase
Siderophore	—	Yes	Iron acquisition
High molecular weight iron-regulated proteins	190, 240	Yes	? Iron acquisition
Lipopolysaccharides	—	Yes	? Serum resistance
Plasmid-encoded			
YadA	50	Yes	Inhibits complement activation; adherence and invasion
YpkA	82	Yes[b]	Protein kinase
YopB	42	—	Homology to RTX family of toxins
YopD	33	—	Facilitates entry of YopE into target cells
YopE	23	Yes[b]	Cytotoxin; resistance to phagocytosis
YopH	51	Yes[b]	Tyrosine phosphatase; resistance to phagocytosis
YopM	42	Yes[a]	Binds α-thrombin
V antigen	37–41	—	Resistance to host defenses; regulatory role in Yop expression

[a] Established in animal model for *Y. pestis* infection.
[b] Established in animal model for *Y. pseudotuberculosis* infection.

sis of this infection. The following discussion addresses the roles of various specific virulence factors in the pathogenesis of *Y. enterocolitica* infection (Table 2).

Adherence and Invasion

Gastrointestinal disease caused by *Y. enterocolitica* is initiated with binding of the bacteria to intestinal epithelial cells. Adhesion of *Y. enterocolitica* to host cells may be mediated by three different proteins: Inv (invasin), Ail (attachment invasion locus), and YadA. In addition, Myf fibrillae may play a role in adherence (69). Binding of the bacteria to eukaryotic cells via the former three adhesins is directly associated with subsequent internalization of the bacteria into cells. Thus, multiple independent pathways are available for entry of *Y. enterocolitica* into host cells.

The most efficient pathway for intracellular entry is promoted by invasin. The invasin of *Y. enterocolitica* is a 92-kDa outer membrane protein that is highly homologous to the 103-kDa invasin of *Y. pseudotuberculosis* (70–73). The role of invasin in the internalization process has been demonstrated by several means. First, a single *Y. pseudotuberculosis* or *Y. enterocolitica* chromosomal gene encoding invasin can confer to *E. coli* the ability to invade mammalian cells (72,73). Second, *Y. enterocolitica* strains harboring *inv* mutations are defective for entry into mammalian cells (74,75). Third, coating an inert particle with invasin is sufficient to mediate uptake of the particle into eukaryotic cells (76). Finally, monoclonal antibodies directed against bacterial surface–exposed epitopes of invasin inhibit attachment and penetration (77).

Ail is a 17-kDa *Y. enterocolitica* protein that shares no sequence homology with invasin (70,78). Sequences homologous to *ail* are present in *Y. pseudotuberculosis* and *Y. pestis,* but not in nonpathogenic *Yersinia* species (79). Like invasin, Ail mediates adhesion and invasion of *E. coli* into epithelial cells in vitro (70,80,81). In contrast to invasin, which promotes invasion of most tissue culture cell types, Ail promotes entry into only a few cell lines (70).

YadA is a plasmid-encoded protein, expressed maximally at 37°C, that forms multimeric fibrillae on the surface of pathogenic *Y. enterocolitica* strains (82) and mediates yersinial attachment and entry into host cells (82–85). YadA also mediates binding of *Y. enterocolitica* to collagen (86,87), fibronectin (88), and mucus (89), and mediates several other biological effects, including autoagglutination, hemagglutination (90), and inhibition of the antiinvasive effect of interferon (91).

Binding of *Y. enterocolitica* to eukaryotic cells is followed by internalization of the bacteria into endocytic vacuoles (74). Both invasin (92–94) and YadA (85) bind to β1-integrins on the cell surface, which mediate the internalization process. Agents such as cytochalasin D block internalization of *Y. enterocolitica,* which indicates that actin microfilament function is required for internalization (74). Tyrosine protein kinase inhibitors also block internalization (95), which suggests that bacterial uptake is dependent on the activity of this enzyme in host cells. Entry of *Y. enterocolitica* into cells is accompanied by cytoskeletal rearrangement (76), which is in contrast to the lack of cytoskeletal rearrangement associated with entry of *Salmonella typhimurium* into cells (96). Antiintegrin antibodies inhibit invasion of cells by *Y. enterocolitica,* but not invasion by *S. typhimurium;* similarly, protein kinase inhibitors prevent invasion by *Y. enterocolitica* but fail to inhibit *S. typhimurium* invasion (95). Thus, the mechanism whereby *Y. enterocolitica* invades eukaryotic cells is different from that utilized by *S. typhimurium.*

The differences in virulence among *Y. enterocolitica* serotypes may be explained in part by differences in expression of proteins that mediate epithelial cell adherence and invasion. *Y. enterocolitica* serotypes associated with human disease invade tissue culture cells in vitro, whereas nonpathogenic serotypes do not (97,98). These differences in invasiveness are attributable predominantly to differences in expression of invasin. Sequences homologous to *inv* can be detected in all species examined (79), but these sequences are functional only in pathogenic *Y. enterocolitica* serotypes (99). In addition, only invasive *Y. enterocolitica* contain DNA sequences homologous to probes derived from *ail* (79). Genetic differences between highly virulent American *Y. enterocolitica* serotypes and non-American serotypes have been detected at the *ail* locus (100). *E. coli* bearing the *ail* gene from American serotypes is five- to sixfold more invasive in vitro than *E. coli* bearing the *ail* gene from non-American strains (100). Finally, the *myfA* gene is present in pathogenic serotypes of *Y. enterocolitica* but is absent from nonpathogenic strains (69).

Resistance to Host Defense Mechanisms

Animal models indicate that after invading intestinal epithelial cells, *Y. enterocolitica,* like *Salmonella,* localize within lymphoid tissue such as Peyer's patches and mesenteric lymph nodes, and may thereafter multiply and disseminate throughout the host (62,101–104). Most multiplication of the organism is in extracellular sites (105–107), although the organism may also multiply within the phagocytic vacuoles of macrophages (62). The capacity of *Y. enterocolitica* to proliferate and disseminate is dependent on the ability of the organism to evade host defense mechanisms. The resistance of *Y. enterocolitica* to human host defenses is mediated predominantly by proteins encoded by a 70-kDa virulence plasmid (pYV) (3,108,109). The role of pYV has been demonstrated convincingly in animal models. When rabbits are infected with isogenic *Y. enterocolitica* strains differing only in the presence of pYV, only the plasmid-bearing strains proliferate and disseminate (110,111). Although pYV-negative strains can adhere to intestinal epithelium, invade, and colonize murine Peyer's patches, these organisms are rapidly cleared by host defenses (106).

All pathogenic strains of *Y. enterocolitica,* as well as *Y. pseudotuberculosis* and *Y. pestis,* harbor the 70-kb pYV, whereas most environmental, nonpathogenic *Y. enterocolitica* isolates do not (65,112). The pYV plasmids of *Y. pseudotuberculosis* and *Y. pestis* are almost identical and are functionally interchangeable, whereas the pYV plasmid of *Y. enterocolitica* is only about 50% homologous with those of the other two species (112–114). pYV plasmids encode proteins designated Yops (*Yersinia* outer membrane proteins), which are highly conserved among

Yersinia species (108,109). The structural genes encoding Yops are scattered on pYV, whereas genes that regulate Yop expression in response to environmental signals are localized within a 20-kb region of the plasmid. The expression of most Yops is regulated by a complex loop of multiple genes in response to environmental factors, including temperature and calcium concentration (108,109). The synthesis of Yops is strongly induced at 37°C in the absence of Ca^{2+} and downregulated at 37°C in the presence of 2.5 mM Ca^{2+}.

The resistance of pathogenic *Y. enterocolitica* to host defense mechanisms involves both resistance to the bactericidal action of serum (111) and resistance to phagocytosis (107,116). A major factor mediating resistance to killing by human serum is YadA, which inhibits complement activation (117,118). Ail, the 17-kDa *Y. enterocolitica* protein that mediates invasion of epithelial cells, and lipopolysaccharide side chains also contribute to serum resistance (81,82,119).

The specific functions of several Yops in mediating resistance to phagocytosis by macrophages and neutrophils are now known (Table 2) (120,121). YopE is cytotoxic when introduced intracellularly (121,122) and induces disruption of actin microfilament structures of eukaryotic cells (122). This cytotoxin may act locally on phagocytes and thereby inhibit phagocytosis. YopH is a tyrosine phosphatase that causes dephosphorylation of eukaryotic cell proteins (123,124). This protein may inhibit phagocytosis by subverting normal signal transduction within phagocytes. *Yersinia* strains with insertional mutations in YopE (125) and YopH (126) are significantly reduced in virulence.

Several other *Yersinia* proteins also contribute to evasion of host defenses. The 42-kDa YopM protein binds human α-thrombin and inhibits platelet aggregation (127), and may thereby provide an antiinflammatory effect. YopO (YpkA) is a serine-threonine protein kinase, which, like YopM, is an essential virulence determinant (127,128). The V antigen (LcrV) also contributes to the evasion of host defenses (129), although the specific actions of this protein are not known. In addition, the V antigen functions as a regulatory protein for synthesis of other Yops (130,131).

Other Virulence Determinants

Clinical isolates of *Y. enterocolitica,* but not *Y. pseudotuberculosis,* produce a 30-amino-acid heat-stable enterotoxin (Yst), which is similar in physical and immunological properties to the heat-stable enterotoxins of *E. coli,* non-01 *V. cholerae,* and *Citrobacter freundii* (132,133). Like the *E. coli* heat-stable enterotoxin, the *Y. enterocolitica* enterotoxin is an activator of guanylate cyclase (134). Nearly all freshly isolated pathogenic *Y. enterocolitica* isolates from humans produce the enterotoxin, compared to 14–39% of nonpathogenic strains (135,136). In one study, DNA sequences homologous with *yst* were identified in all 89 pathogenic *Y. enterocolitica* strains tested, but in none of 51 nonpathogenic strains (132). The *Y. enterocolitica* enterotoxin is not produced in vitro at temperatures exceeding 30°C (137), and therefore its clinical relevance has been questioned. However, a wild-type *yst⁺* *Y. enterocolitica* strain induced diarrhea in a rabbit, whereas an isogenic *yst*-negative mutant did not (138). Thus, the enterotoxin may contribute to diarrheal disease.

Iron is an essential growth factor for bacteria, but mammalian hosts typically withhold iron from invading microorganisms. One pathway whereby *Y. enterocolitica* acquires iron is by production of siderophores. Siderophore production has been detected for serotypes of *Y. enterocolitica* that are lethal for mice, but not in nonlethal serotypes such as O:3 and O:9 (139,140). A 65-kDa iron-repressible outer membrane protein (Irp65) that probably functions as a siderophore receptor has been identified in mouse-lethal strains (140). Irp65-negative or siderophore-negative mutants are nonlethal in mice (140), which indicates that iron acquisition via this siderophore-dependent pathway is an important virulence factor. In addition, serotype O:8 isolates synthesize high molecular weight outer membrane proteins under conditions of iron starvation, which may play a role in iron acquisition (141–143). Mutagenesis of the gene (*irp2*) encoding one of these proteins results in decreased virulence for mice (143).

Y. enterocolitica may also acquire iron via the use of exogenous siderophores. Several iron-repressible outer membrane proteins that function as receptors for exogenous siderophores have been identified (144,145). Desferrioxamine is a siderophore that is commonly used in clinical medicine for treatment of iron overload, and may be utilized by serotypes O:3 and O:9 for iron acquisition (67,146). Intraperitoneal inoculation with desferrioxamine reduces the median lethal dose of *Y. enterocolitica* O:3 for mice more than 100,000-fold (67). Similarly, desferrioxamine therapy is a predisposing factor for severe systemic *Y. enterocolitica* infection in humans. Finally, *Y. enterocolitica* possesses a hemin uptake system that enables the organism to utilize the host's heme-containing compounds as a source of iron (147).

Clinical Illness

Y. enterocolitica infection may be associated with a variety of syndromes, dependent in part on the age and physical state of the host (Table 3). Overall, illness occurs most commonly among children (16,17,29,30). Enterocolitis, the most common presentation, is characterized by diarrhea, low-grade fever, and abdominal pain (10,16, 17,24,149–151). In a prospective study of 181 Canadian children with symptomatic *Y. enterocolitica* infection (median age 24 months), diarrhea was present in 98%, fever in 88%, abdominal pain in 64%, and vomiting in 38% of cases (5). Grossly bloody stools are present in one fourth of patients (5,16,17,24) and apparently occur more commonly among young persons than adults (17). Leukocytes and erythrocytes are present in the stool in 10–50% of cases (10,28). Leukocytosis is typically present, frequently accompanied by marked left shifts with immature to total neutrophil ratios >0.5 (17,25). The mean duration of illness is typically 14–22 days (5,16,17), but symptoms occasionally persist for several months (17,149,152). The mean duration of excretion of organisms in stool is 6–7 weeks (5,17). Most infections are self-limited, but complications may include appendicitis, diffuse ulceration and inflammation of the small intestine and colon (28), intestinal perforation (153), peritonitis (30), ileocolic intussusception, toxic megacolon, cholangitis, and mesenteric vein thrombosis (1).

The pseudoappendicular syndrome occurs primarily in older children and adults (5,27,152,154,155). The cardinal features of this syndrome are fever, abdominal pain, tenderness of the right lower quadrant, and leukocytosis, with or without diarrhea. Due to the clinical similarities between this syndrome and appendicitis, laparotomy is frequently performed. Among patients in Scandinavia with suspected appendicitis, stool cultures or operative specimens from 50 (3.6%) of 1362 patients who underwent laparotomy yielded *Y. enterocolitica* (155). In other studies, *Y. enterocolitica* infection has been detected in 1.9%, 4.6%, or 5.4% of patients with suspected appendicitis (156–158). The operative findings in patients with this syndrome include marked mesenteric lymphadenopathy, terminal ileitis, and a normal or slightly inflamed appendix (27,149,154,155,159,160). Ultrasonography may be useful in distinguishing true appendicitis from *Y. enterocolitica* infection (160).

Pharyngitis, frequently associated with cervical adenpathy, may occur either in association with *Y. enterocolitica* enterocolitis or independent of gastrointestinal illness (16,17,28,30,152,161,162). Cutaneous infection may also occur, and is manifested as cellulitis, abscesses, or wound infection (1,28,29,163–165). Other focal suppurative infections that have occurred in the absence of detectable bacteremia include suppurative conjunctivitis (166), urinary tract infections (30), renal abscesses, pneumonia (167,168), and lung abscess (1).

Y. enterocolitica septicemia is typically a severe illness with case fatality rates of 7.5–50% (169–171). Pathological conditions associated with an iron-overloaded state are well-recognized predisposing factors for severe systemic *Y. enterocolitica* infection; these include hemochro-

TABLE 3. *Clinical manifestations of* Yersinia enterocolitics *infection*

Syndrome	Typical age of patient	Predisposing host factors
Enterocolitis	Child or adult	Young age
Pseudoappendicular syndrome	Older child or adult	None
Septicemia	Child or adult	Iron overload; deferoxamine therapy; immunocompromise
Reactive arthritis	Adult	HLA B27; residence in Scandinavia
Erythema nodosum	Adult	Residence in Scandinavia; female gender

matosis, acute iron poisoning, and transfusion-dependent blood dyscrasias (169–172). Other predisposing factors for *Y. enterocolitica* septicemia include desferrioxamine therapy, cirrhosis, immunosuppressive therapy, diabetes mellitus, alcoholism, and malnutrition (169,170).

The bacteremic spread of *Y. enterocolitica* to extraintestinal sites may result in abscess formation in the liver, spleen, or other sites (169,172–174). Other complications of *Y. enterocolitica* bacteremia include endocarditis (175), mycotic aneurysm (176), meningitis, osteomyelitis (177), septic arthritis, lung abscess, empyema (178), renal abscess, panophthalmitis, cutaneous pustules, and bullous skin lesions (1,30,175–178).

Y. enterocolitica septicemia occasionally results from the transfusion of contaminated blood products (57–59). This syndrome is characterized by the sudden onset of fever, hypotension, and generalized pain within 1 hr after the start of transfusion (57–59). Vomiting and explosive diarrhea may also occur. More than 50% of reported cases are fatal. The diagnosis may be made quickly by Gram stain of the untransfused blood. Donors of the implicated contaminated blood products have been healthy at the time of blood donation, but typically have reported a history of diarrheal illness during the 4 weeks prior to donation (57–59). The donors are presumed to have had asymptomatic bacteremia at the time of blood donation. The contaminated erythrocytes in these cases have typically been stored for longer than 25 days. After a lag phase of 10–20 days, low inocula of *Y. enterocolitica* can proliferate in blood stored at 4°C, resulting in bacterial counts of 10^7–10^8 CFU/mL (179). *Y. enterocolitica* is able to utilize hemin as an iron source (146,147) and therefore progressive hemolysis of stored blood may be required for bacterial proliferation to occur. The presence of *Y. enterocolitica* bacteremia in asymptomatic blood donors (57–59) supports the hypothesis that bacteremia occurs commonly among patients with *Y. enterocolitica* infection, but that transient bacteremia is typically self-limited among persons with normal host defenses.

Acute reactive arthritis accompanies *Y. enterocolitica* infection in 10–30% of cases in Scandinavia (149, 180–185). Arthritis occurs predominantly in adults (17) and is associated with the presence of the HLA B27 antigen (183–185). Arthritic symptoms may accompany acute illness (17) or occur weeks to months after gastrointestinal illness (17). Arthritic symptoms typically persist for one to several months, but chronic arthritis may develop (149). Synovial fluid cultures are sterile (149), but *Yersinia* antigens can be detected in synovial fluid cells from the majority of patients with *Yersinia*-triggered arthritis (186); synovial fluid cells from patients with other rheumatic diseases fail to react with the immunofluorescent antibodies used in these studies. Amplification of *Yersinia*-specific sequences from synovial fluid by polymerase chain reaction (PCR) methodology has not yet been successful (187). Arthritis can be induced experimentally in mice or rats by oral or parenteral adminstration of *Y. enterocolitica* (188–191). A purified 19-kDa *Y. enterocolitica* protein with strong homology to a urease subunit also induces arthritis in rats when injected intraarticularly (192,193).

Uveitis (194) and Reiter's syndrome (184) occur commonly in Scandinavia in association with *Y. enterocolitica* infection (149); the presence of the HLA B27 antigen is a risk factor for these conditions. In addition, erythema nodosum is reported in up to 30% of cases of *Y. enterocolitica* infection in Finland and occurs predominantly in adult women (149). In contrast to arthritis, there is no association between erythema nodosum and the presence of the HLA B27 antigen (183).

Numerous studies have reported that *Y. enterocolitica* infection is associated with a high incidence of subsequent inflammatory diseases (195,196), including ankylosing spondylitis (195), Reiter's syndrome, myocarditis (149,182,197), glomerulonephritis (198,199), and thyroid disease (200–202). The known capacity of *Y. enterocolitica* to induce inflammatory joint disease suggests that individual cases of many of these other inflammatory syndromes may indeed by precipitated by *Y. enterocolitica* infection. *Y. enterocolitica* produces antigens with T-cell superantigenic activity (203), which may play a role in the pathogenesis of these inflammatory syndromes. Although a temporal association between *Y. enterocolitica* infection and various nonsuppurative complications supports a causal relationship, in many reports, preceding *Y. enterocolitica* infections have been documented only by serological assays. False-positive serology results potentially could occur due to polyclonal immune activation in these inflammatory disorders and thus lead to erroneous conclusions. In addition, many studies that report a high prevalence of anti-*Yersinia* antibodies among patients with inflammatory diseases have not compared the prevalence of anti-*Yersinia* antibodies in properly matched healthy controls. The high prevalence in Scandinavia of both the HLA B27 antigen and *Y. enterocolitica* infection makes it imperative that these variables be assessed independently. The relationship between *Y. enterocolitica* and the many diseases with which it is potentially associated will be clarified in the future as prospective, well-controlled studies of patients with culture-proven *Y. enterocolitica* infection are performed.

Diagnosis

Y. enterocolitica may be isolated from stool on commonly used selective media, such as MacConkey agar, and appear as lactose-negative colonies after 48 hr of growth at 25–28°C. The use of cefsulodin-irgasin-novobiocin (CIN) agar (204) and cold enrichment techniques (7,205) may increase the rate of recovery from stool cultures. Nonpathogenic *Y. enterocolitica* may occasionally be isolated from stools, particularly if cold enrichment techniques are utilized (205), and therefore rapid clinical tests to distinguish between pathogenic and nonpathogenic *Y. enterocolitica* isolates are useful. Tests for calcium dependency and autoagglutination are useful indicators for the presence of the pYV plasmid (206). Other tests for pathogenicity include assays for Congo red absorption, crystal violet binding, pyrazinamidase activity, sialicin fermentation, and esculin hydrolysis (207–209). Detection of pathogenic *Y. enterocolitica* in stool by PCR methodology may be a useful diagnostic option in the future.

Serological testing is commonly utilized in countries where *Y. enterocolitica* infection is caused by a restricted number of serotypes (5,149,210). The use of serotype-specific serological assays in other areas is limited by the need to screen sera for reactivity with multiple separate antigens. Newer assays that utilize antigens that are not serotype-specific may eliminate this problem (211). Serological diagnosis is limited by false-positive reactions, related to the cross-reactivity of some *Y. enterocolitica* antigens with antigens of other gram-negative bacteria (6). Therefore, isolation of the organism from clinical specimens should be attempted whenever possible. In the future, as serological assays for *Y. enterocolitica* infection are improved and standardized by the use of well-defined unique antigens, serological testing may prove particularly valuable in the evaluation of postinfectious sequelae of *Y. enterocolitica* infection.

Treatment

Y. enterocolitica isolates are typically susceptible in vitro to tetracycline, chloramphenicol, aminoglycosides, trimethoprim-sulfamethoxazole, third-generation cephalosporins, ticarcillin-clavulanate, imipenem, aztreonam, and fluoroquinolones (212,213). Resistance to ampicillin and first-generation cephalosporins is mediated by β-lactamases (214). Despite the in vitro susceptibility of *Y. enterocolitica* to newer β-lactam agents, cefotaxime and imipenem were unsuccessful for treatment of *Y. enterocolitica* infection in mice, whereas doxycycline or gentamicin were active in inhibiting bacterial proliferation in this model (215). Fluoroquinolones are efficacious in the treatment of murine *Y. pseudotuberculosis* infection (216) and also have been utilized successfully for treatment of *Y. enterocolitica* infections in humans (171).

Uncomplicated cases of enterocolitis or pseudoappendicular syndrome due to *Y. enterocolitica* typically resolve spontaneously without antibiotics and therefore antimicrobial therapy is usually not required. In a placebo-controlled, double-blind evaluation of trimethoprim-sulfamethoxazole for *Y. enterocolitica* infection in children, treatment did not shorten the clinical or bacteriological course of the illness (217). However, in this study the mean duration of illness before the institution of therapy was 12 days. An apparent lack of treatment efficacy in other studies may also be attributable to delays in instituting therapy (17). Although antimicrobial therapy may reduce the period of postsymptomatic fecal shedding (17), this benefit is probably not clinically important. Localized suppurative infection, bacteremia in compromised hosts, and severe systemic infection in normal hosts should be treated with antibiotics, but controlled clinical trials to determine optimal therapies have not been performed. Until the results of antimicrobial susceptibility tests are available, institution of therapy with combinations of doxycycline, aminoglycosides, trimethoprim-sulfamethoxazole, or fluoroquinolone agents is appropriate. Cessation of desferrioxamine therapy is also recommended.

Prevention

The strongest known risk factor for *Y. enterocolitica* infection at present is the ingestion of uncooked pork products (16). Education of the public regarding the risks associated with raw pork or chitterling ingestion, and thorough cooking of the meat would be expected to reduce the incidence of infection with O:3 serotypes. Elimination of *Y. enterocolitica* colonization of swine is another potential approach, although effective measures for accomplishing this have not yet been clearly demonstrated. There are currently no vaccines available to prevent *Y. enterocolitica* infection in humans or swine.

YERSINIA PSEUDOTUBERCULOSIS

Y. pseudotuberculosis is an enteropathogen of a wide range of wild and domestic animals throughout the world, and occasionally causes human disease. Human infection with *Y. pseudotuberculosis* is less common than infection with *Y. enterocolitica* (6). *Y. pseudotuberculosis* and *Y. pestis* exhibit a high level of chromosomal DNA relatedness, whereas chromosomal DNA from *Y. enterocolitica* shows greater divergence (3). In contrast to *Y. pestis, Y. pseudotuberculosis* is motile at 25°C, hydrolyzes urea, and ferments adonitol, L-rhamnose, and melibiose (4). Unlike *Y. enterocolitica, Y. pseudotuberculosis* lacks ornithine decarboxylase activity and does not ferment D-sorbitol (4).

Epidemiology

Y. pseudotuberculosis has been isolated from many animal species, including cattle, horses, deer, sheep, goats, swine, hare, foxes, rodents, cats, dogs, and birds (218–223). In addition, *Y. pseudotuberculosis* has been isolated from environmental sources such as streams and lakes (219).

Human infection with *Y. pseudotuberculosis* occurs as both sporadic and epidemic disease (224–228) and occurs most frequently among children (229,230). In several countries there has been a clustering of human infections during winter months (231). Transmission of infection to humans has been possibly associated with ingestion of water or sand contaminated by an infected cat (232), ingestion of unpasteurized goat's milk (233), and ingestion of mountain stream water (219). However, the sources of most outbreaks of *Y. pseudotuberculosis* infection have not been successfully determined.

Pathogenesis

The pathogeneses of *Y. pseudotuberculosis* and *Y. enterocolitica* infections share many common features, and the reader is referred to the preceding discussion of *Y. enterocolitica* for a detailed discussion. However, there are several notable differences between these two organisms. First, *Y. pseudotuberculosis* is significantly more invasive in animal models than *Y. enterocolitica* O:3 or O:9 (3,61,67,108). Both invasin and YadA are expressed in *Y. pseudotuberculosis,* but mutants defective in production of YadA remain fully virulent (234–236). *Y. pseudotuberculosis* produces a pH 6 antigen, related to the Myf fibrillae of *Y. enterocolitica,* that may also play a role in adherence (108,237). Genetic sequences resembling Ail are present in *Y. pseudotuberculosis* (79), but expression of Ail by *Y. pseudotuberculosis* has not been demonstrated. Like *Y. enterocolitica, Y. pseudotuberculosis* harbors a 70-kb pYV, which contributes to the ability of the organism to resist host defenses. Production of siderophores by *Y. pseudotuberculosis* has been demonstrated (140) and may partially explain the increased invasiveness of this species compared to *Y. enterocolitica* O:3 and O:9.

Clinical Manifestations

The clinical manifestations of *Y. pseudotuberculosis* infection closely resemble those of *Y. enterocolitica* infection (238,239). Diarrheal illness, abdominal pain, and fever are the most common clinical features in normal hosts (149). At laparotomy, mesenteric lymphadenopathy is commonly noted (240). Complications of infection include sepsis (241), liver abscesses (242), erythema nodosum (227), and reactive arthritis (149,243,244). Several cases of hemolytic uremic syndrome and nephritis have been attributed to *Y. pseudotuberculosis* (149,245,246).

Y. pseudotuberculosis infection in Japan has been associated with clinical features different from those observed in the United States and Europe. Infected Japanese children frequently develop high fever, a desquamative rash, red or crusted lips, strawberry tongue, conjunctivitis, and lymphadenopathy (247,248). These symptoms are identical to those described in an epidemic Japanese illness known as Izumi fever (247). Thus, it is likely that *Y. pseudotuberculosis* infection is the cause of many cases formerly classified as Izumi fever. Production of antigens with superantigen activity (249,250) may be important in the pathogenesis of this syndrome, as well as other postinfectious nonsuppurative sequelae. Despite the clinical similarities between this syndrome and Kawasaki disease, no cases of Kawasaki disease associated with *Y. pseudotuberculosis* have been identified in the United States or Europe.

Diagnosis and Treatment

Y. pseudotuberculosis may be isolated from stools using methods appropriate for the isolation of *Y. enterocolitica.* Serological tests for *Y. pseudotuberculosis* also are available, but are associated with some of the same limitations described for *Y. enterocolitica* serological assays. Most uncomplicated cases of *Y. pseudotuberculosis* infection resolve without therapy. In one randomized trial, there was no clinical benefit associated with ampicillin treatment compared to placebo (251). Therapy with fluoroquinolones has shown efficacy in an animal model (216), and thus may be the treatment of choice for severe human infections.

ACKNOWLEDGMENT

The author thanks Dr. Susan Straley for critical review of the manuscript.

REFERENCES

1. Cover TL, Aber RC. *Yersinia enterocolitica. N Engl J Med* 1989;321:16–24.
2. Black RE, Slome S. *Yersinia enterocolitica. Infect Dis Clin North Am* 1988;2:625–641.
3. Brubaker RR. Factors promoting acute and chronic diseases caused by Yersiniae. *Clin Microbiol Rev* 1991;4:309–324.
4. Farmer JJ III, Kelly MT. Enterobacteriaceae. In: Hausler WJ Jr, Herrmann KL, Isenberg HD, Shadomy HJ, eds. *Manual of clinical microbiology.* 5th ed. Washington, DC: American Society for Microbiology; 1991.
5. Marks MI, Pai CH, Lafleur L, Lackman L, Hammerberg O. *Yersinia enterocolitica* gastroenteritis: a prospective study of clinical, bacteriologic, and epidemiologic features. *J Pediatr* 1980;96:26–31.
6. Ahvonen P. Human yersiniosis in Finland: bacteriology and serology. *Ann Clin Res* 1972;4:30–38.
7. Van Noyen R, Vandepitte J, Wauters G, Selderslaghs R. *Yersinia enterocolitica:* its isolation by cold enrichment from patients and healthy subjects. *J Clin Pathol* 1981;34:1052–1056.
8. Hoogkamp-Korstanje JAA, de Koning J, Samsom JP. Incidence of human infection with *Yersinia enterocolitica* serotypes O3, O8, and O9 and the use of indirect immunofluorescence in diagnosis. *J Infect Dis* 1986;153:138–141.
9. Mingrone MG, Fantasia M, Figura N, Guglielmetti P. Characteristics of *Yersinia enterocolitica* isolated from children with diarrhea in Italy. *J Clin Microbiol* 1987;25:1301–1304.
10. Mollee T, Tilse M. Yersinia enterocolitica: isolation from faeces of adults and children in Queensland. *Med J Aust* 1985; 143:488–489.
11. Barteluk RL, Noble MA. Routine culturing of stool specimens for *Yersinia enterocolitica. J Clin Microbiol* 1988;26: 1616–1617.
12. Dajani AS, Maurer MJ. Is *Yersinia enterocolitica* gastroenteritis a Canadian disease? *J Pediatr* 1980;97:165–166.
13. Marymont JH Jr., Durfee KK, Alexander H, Smith JP. *Yersinia enterocolitica* in Kansas: attempted recovery from 1,212 patients. *Am J Clin Pathol* 1982;77:753–755.
14. Kachoris M, Ruoff KL, Welch K, Kallas W, Ferraro MJ. Routine culture of stool specimens for *Yersinia enterocolitica* is not a cost-effective procedure. *J Clin Microbiol* 1988;26:582–583.
15. Metchock B, Lonsway DR, Carter GP, Lee LA, McGowan JE Jr. *Yersinia enterocolitica:* a frequent seasonal stool isolate from children at an urban hospital in the southeast United States. *J Clin Microbiol* 1991;29:2868–2869.
16. Tauxe RV, Vandepitte J, Wauters G, et al. *Yersinia enterocolitica* infections and pork: the missing link. *Lancet* 1987;1: 1129–1132.
17. Ostroff SM, Kapperud G, Lassen J, Aasen S, Tauxe RV. Clinical features of sporadic *Yersinia enterocolitica* infections in Norway. *J Infect Dis* 1992;166:812–817.
18. Shayegani M, DeForge I, McGlynn DM, Root T. Characteristics of *Yersinia enterocolitica* and related species isolated from human, animal, and environmental sources. *J Clin Microbiol* 1981;14:304–312.
19. Bissett ML. *Yersinia enterocolitica* isolates from humans in California, 1968–1975. *J Clin Microbiol* 1976;4:137–144.
20. Snyder JD, Christenson E, Feldman RA. Human *Yersinia enterocolitica* infections in Wisconsin: clinical, laboratory and epidemiologic features. *Am J Med* 1982;72:768–774.
21. Kay BA, Wachsmuth K, Gemski P, Feeley JC, Quan TJ, Bren-

ner DJ. Virulence and phenotypic characterization of *Yersinia enterocolitica* isolated from human in the United States. *J Clin Microbiol* 1983;17:128–138.

22. Bottone EJ. Current trends of *Yersinia enterocolitica* isolates in the New York City area. *J Clin Microbiol* 1983;17:63–67.

23. Bissett ML, Powers C, Abbott SL, Janda JM. Epidemiologic investigations of *Yersinia enterocolitica* and related species: sources, frequency, and serogroup distribution. *J Clin Microbiol* 1990;28:910–912.

24. Lee LA, Taylor J, Carter GP, et al. *Yersinia enterocolitica* O: 3: an emerging cause of pediatric gastroenteritis in the United States. *J Infect Dis* 1991;163:660–663.

25. Lee LA, Gerber AR, Lonsway DR, et al. *Yersinia enterocolitica* O:3 infections in infants and children, associated with the household preparation of chitterlings. *N Engl J Med* 1990;322: 984–987.

26. Shayegani M, Morse D, DeForge I, Root T, Parsons LM, Maupin PS. Microbiology of a major foodborne outbreak of gastroenteritis caused by *Yersinia enterocolitica* serogroup O:8. *J Clin Microbiol* 1983;17:35–40.

27. Black RE, Jackson RJ, Tsai T, et al. Epidemic *Yersinia enterocolitica* infection due to contaminated chocolate milk. *N Engl J Med* 1978;298:76–79.

28. Gutman LT, Ottesen EA, Quan TJ, Noce PS, Katz SL. An interfamilial outbreak of *Yersinia enterocolitica* enteritis. *N Engl J Med* 1973;288:1372–1377.

29. Tacket CO, Ballard J, Harris N, et al. An outbreak of *Yersinia enterocolitica* infections caused by contaminated tofu (soybean curd). *Am J Epidemiol* 1985;121:705–711.

30. Tacket CO, Narain JP, Sattin R, et al. A multistate outbreak of infections caused by *Yersinia enterocolitica* transmitted by pasteurized milk. *JAMA* 1984;251:483–486.

31. de Grace M, Laurin M-F, Belanger C, et al. *Yersinia enterocolitica* gastroenteritis outbreak—Montreal. *Can Dis Week Rep* 1976;2:41–44.

32. Maruyama T. *Yersinia enterocolitica* infection in humans and isolation of the microorganism from pigs in Japan. *Contr Microbiol Immunol* 1987;9:48–55.

33. Aber RC, McCarthy MA, Berman R, DeMelfi T, Witte E. An outbreak of *Yersinia enterocolitica* gastrointestinal illness among members of a Brownie troop in Centre County, Pennsylvania. Presented at the 22nd Interscience conference on antimicrobial agents and chemotherapy, Miami Beach, October 4–6, 1982.

34. Ichinohe H, Yoshioka M, Fukushima H, Kaneko S, Maruyama T. First isolation of *Yersinia enterocolitica* serotype O:8 in Japan. *J Clin Microbiol* 1991;29:846–847.

35. Toma S, Deidrick VR. Isolation of *Yersinia enterocolitica* from swine. *J Clin Microbiol* 1975;2:478–481.

36. Pedersen KB. Occurrence of *Yersinia enterocolitica* in the throat of swine. *Contr Microbiol Immunol* 1979;5:253–256.

37. Kapperud G, Nesbakken T, Aleksic S, Mollaret HH. Comparison of restriction endonuclease analysis and phenotypic typing methods for differentiation of *Yersinia enterocolitica* isolates. *J Clin Microbiol* 1990;28:1125–1131.

38. Blumberg HM, Kiehlbauch JA, Wachsmuth IK. Molecular epidemiology of *Yersinia enterocolitica* O:3 infections: use of chromosomal DNA restriction fragment length polymorphisms of rRNA genes. *J Clin Microbiol* 1991;29:2368–2374.

39. Davey GM, Bruce J, Drysdale EM. Isolation of *Yersinia enterocolitica* and related species from the faeces of cows. *J Appl Bacteriol* 1983;55:439–443.

40. Greenwood MH, Hooper WL. Excretion of *Yersinia* spp. associated with consumption of pasteurized milk. *Epidemiol Infect* 1990;104:345–350.

41. Greenwood MH, Hooper WL, Rodhouse JC. The source of *Yersinia* spp. in pasteurized milk: an investigation at a dairy. *Epidemiol Infect* 1990;104:351–360.

42. Hughes D. Repeated isolation of *Yersinia enterocolitica* from pasteurized milk in a holding vat at a dairy factory. *J Appl Bacteriol* 1980;48:383–385.

43. Schiemann DA. Association of *Yersinia enterocolitica* with the manufacture of cheese and occurrence in pasteurized milk. *Appl Environ Microbiol* 1978;36:274–277.

44. Olsvik O, Kapperud G. Enterotoxin production in milk at 22 and 4 degrees C by *Escherichia coli* and *Yersinia enterocolitica*. *Appl Environ Microbiol* 1982;43:997–1000.

45. Shayegani M, Stone WB, DeForge I, Root T, Parsons LM, Maupin P. *Yersinia enterocolitica* and related species isolated from wildlife in New York state. *Appl Environ Microbiol* 1986; 52:420–424.

46. Harvey S, Greenwood JR, Pickett MJ, Mah RA. Recovery of *Yersinia enterocolitica* from streams and lakes of California. *Appl Environ Microbiol* 1976;32:352–354.

47. Highsmith AK, Feeley JC, Skaliy P, Wells JG, Wood BT. Isolation of *Yersinia enterocolitica* from well water and growth in distilled water. *Appl Environ Microbiol* 1977;34:745–750.

48. Wilson HD, McCormick JB, Feeley JC. *Yersinia enterocolitica* infection in a 4-month-old infant associated with infection in household dogs. *J Pediatr* 1976;89:767–769.

49. Thompson JS, Gravel MJ. Family outbreak of gastroenteritis due to *Yersinia enterocolitica* serotype O:3 from well water. *Can J Microbiol* 1986;32:700–701.

50. Keet EE. *Yersinia enterocolitica* septicemia: source of infection and incubation period identified. *N Y State J Med* 1974; 74:2226–2230.

51. Martin T, Kasian GF, Stead S. Family outbreak of yersiniosis. *J Clin Microbiol* 1982;16:622–626.

52. Rose FB, Camp CJ, Antes EJ. Family outbreak of fatal *Yersinia enterocolitica* pharyngitis. *Am J Med* 1987;82:636–637.

53. McIntyre M, Nnochiri E. A case of hospital-acquired *Yersinia enterocolitica* gastroenteritis. *J Hosp Infect* 1986;7:299–301.

54. Cannon CG, Linnemann CC Jr. *Yersinia enterocolitica* infections in hospitalized patients: the problem of hospital-acquired infections. *Infect Control Hosp Epidemiol* 1992;13:139–143.

55. Ratnam S, Mercer E, Picco B, Parsons S, Butler R. A nosocomial outbreak of diarrheal disease due to *Yersinia enterocolitica* serotype O:5, biotype 1. *J Infect Dis* 1982;145:242–247.

56. Toivanen P, Toivanen A, Olkkonen L, Aantaa S. Hospital outbreak of *Yersinia enterocolitica* infection. *Lancet* 1973;1: 801–803.

57. Tipple MA, Bland LA, Murphy JJ, et al. Sepsis associated with transfusion of red cells contaminated with *Yersinia enterocolitica*. *Transfusion* 1990;30:207–213.

58. Bufill JA, Ritch PS. *Yersinia enterocolitica* serotype O:3 sepsis after blood transfusion. *N Engl J Med* 1989;320:810.

59. Woernle CH, Hoffman RE, Smith JD, et al. Update: *Yersinia enterocolitica* bacteremia and endotoxin shock associated with red blood cell transfusions—United States, 1991. *MMWR* 1991; 40:176–178.

60. Kapperud G. *Yersinia enterocolitica* and *Y. enterocolitica*-like bacteria isolated from healthy humans in Norway. *Acta Pathol Microbiol Scand Sect B* 1980;88:303–306.

61. Smith RE, Carey AM, Damare JM, et al. Evaluation of iron dextran and mucin for enhancement of the virulence of *Yersinia enterocolitica* serotype O:3 in mice. *Infect Immun* 1981;34: 550–560.

62. Une T. Studies on the pathogenicity of *Yersinia enterocolitica*. I. Experimental infection in rabbits. *Microbiol Immunol* 1977; 21:349–363.

63. Schiemann DA, Devenish JA, Toma S. Characteristics of virulence in human isolates of *Yersinia enterocolitica*. *Infect Immun* 1981;32:400–403.

64. Aulisio CCG, Hill WE, Stanfield JT, Sellers RL Jr. Evaluation of virulence factor testing and characteristics of pathogenicity in *Yersinia enterocolitica*. *Infect Immun* 1983;40:330–335.

65. Heesemann J, Keller C, Morawa R, Schmidt N, Siemens HJ, Laufs R. Plasmids of human strains of *Yersinia enterocolitica*: molecular relatedness and possible importance for pathogenesis. *J Infect Dis* 1983;147:107–115.

66. Kay BA, Wachsmuth K, Gemski P. New virulence-associated plasmid in *Yersinia enterocolitica*. *J Clin Microbiol* 1982;15: 1161–1163.

67. Robins-Browne RM, Prpic JK. Effects of iron and desferrioxamine on infections with *Yersinia enterocolitica*. *Infect Immun* 1985;47:774–779.

68. Mors V, Pai CH. Pathogenic properties of *Yersinia enterocolitica*. *Infect Immun* 1980;28:292–294.

69. Iriarte M, Vanooteghem J-C, Delor I, Diaz R, Knutton S, Cornelis GR. The Myf fibrillae of *Yersinia enterocolitica*. *Mol Microbiol* 1993;9:507–520.
70. Miller VL, Falkow S. Evidence for two genetic loci in *Yersinia enterocolitica* that can promote invasion of epithelial cells. *Infect Immun* 1988;56:1242–1248.
71. Pepe JC, Miller VL. The *Yersinia enterocolitica* inv gene product is an outer membrane protein that shares epitopes with *Yersinia pseudotuberculosis* invasin. *J Bacteriol* 1990;172:3780–3789.
72. Young VB, Miller VL, Falkow S, Schoolnik GK. Sequence, localization and function of the invasin protein of *Yersinia enterocolitica*. *Mol Microbiol* 1990;4:1119–1128.
73. Isberg RR, Falkow S. A single genetic locus encoded by *Yersinia pseudotuberculosis* permits invasion of cultured animal cells by *Escherichia coli* K-12. *Nature* 1985;317:262–264.
74. Isberg RR, Voorhis DL, Falkow S. Identification of invasin: a protein that allows enteric bacteria to penetrate cultured mammalian cells. *Cell* 1987;50:769–778.
75. Pepe JC, Miller VL. *Yersinia enterocolitica* invasin: a primary role in the initiation of infection. *Proc Natl Acad Sci USA* 1993;90:6473–6477.
76. Young VB, Falkow S, Schoolnik GK. The invasin protein of *Yersinia enterocolitica*: internalization of invasin-bearing bacteria by eukaryotic cells is associated with reorganization of the cytoskeleton. *J Cell Biol* 1992;116:197–207.
77. Leong JM, Fournier RS, Isberg RR. Mapping and topographic localization of epitopes of the *Yersinia pseudotuberculosis* invasin protein. *Infect Immun* 1991;59:3424–3433.
78. Miller VL, Bliska JB, Falkow S. Nucleotide sequence of the *Yersinia enterocolitica ail* gene and characterization of the Ail protein product. *J Bacteriol* 1990;172:1062–1069.
79. Miller VL, Farmer JJ III, Hill WE, Falkow S. The *ail* locus is found uniquely in *Yersinia enterocolitica* serotypes commonly associated with disease. *Infect Immun* 1989;57:121–131.
80. Bliska JB, Falkow S. Bacterial resistance to complement killing mediated by the Ail protein of *Yersinia enterocolitica*. *Proc Natl Acad Sci USA* 1992;89:3561–3565.
81. Pierson DE, Falkow S. The ail gene of *Yersinia enterocolitica* has a role in the ability of the organism to survive serum killing. *Infect Immun* 1993;61:1846–1852.
82. Kapperud G, Namork E, Skurnik M, Nesbakken T. Plasmid-mediated surface fibrillae of *Yersinia pseudotuberculosis* and *Yersinia enterocolitica*: relationship to the outer membrane protein Yop1 and possible importance for pathogenesis. *Infect Immun* 1987;55:2247–2254.
83. Heeseman J, Gruter L. Genetic evidence that the outer membrane protein Yop1 of *Yersinia enterocolitica* mediates adherence and phagocytosis resistance to human epithelial cells. *FEMS Microbiol Lett* 1987;40:37–41.
84. Yang Y, Isberg RR. Cellular internalization in the absence of invasin expression is promoted by the *Yersinia pseudotuberculosis* yadA product. *Infect Immun* 1993;61:3907–3913.
85. Bliska JB, Copass MC, Falkow S. The *Yersinia pseudotuberculosis* adhesin YadA mediates intimate bacterial attachment to and entry into HEp-2 cells. *Infect Immun* 1993;61:3914–3921.
86. Schulze-Koops H, Burkhardt H, Heesemann J, von der Mark K, Emmrich F. Plasmid-encoded outer membrane protein YadA mediates specific binding of enteropathogenic *Yersiniae* to various types of collagen. *Infect Immun* 1992;60:2153–2159.
87. Emody L, Heesemann J, Wolf-Watz H, et al. Binding to collagen by *Yersinia enterocolitica* and *Yersinia pseudotuberculosis*: evidence for yopA-mediated and chromosomally encoded mechanisms. *J Bacteriol* 1989;171:6674–6679.
88. Tertti R, Skurnik M, Vartio T, Kuusela P. Adhesion protein YadA of *Yersinia* species mediates binding of bacteria to fibronectin. *Infect Immun* 1992;60:3021–3024.
89. Paerregaard A, Espersen F, Jensen OM, Skurnik M. Interactions between *Yersinia enterocolitica* and rabbit ileal mucus: growth, adhesin, penetration, and subsequent changes in surface hydrophobicity and ability to adhere to ileal brush border membrane vesicles. *Infect Immun* 1991;59:253–260.
90. Skurnik M, Bolin I, Heikkinen H, Piha S, Wolf-Watz H. Virulence plasmid-associated autoagglutination in *Yersinia* spp. *J Bacteriol* 1984;158:1033–1036.
91. Bukholm G, Kapperud G, Skurnik M. Genetic evidence that the *yopA* gene-encoded *Yersinia* outer membrane protein Yop1 mediates inhibition of the anti-invasive effect of interferon. *Infect Immun* 1990;58:2245–2251.
92. Tran Van Nhieu G, Isberg RR. The *Yersinia pseudotuberculosis* invasin protein and human fibronectin bind to mutually exclusive sites on the $\alpha_5\beta_1$ integrin receptor. *J Biol Chem* 1991;266:24367–24375.
93. Leong JM, Fournier RS, Isberg RR. Identification of the integrin binding domain of the *Yersinia pseudotuberculosis* invasin protein. *EMBO J* 1990;9:1979–1989.
94. Isberg RR, Leong JM. Multiple beta₁ chain integrins are receptors for invasin, a protein that promotes bacterial penetration into mammalian cells. *Cell* 1990;60:861–871.
95. Rosenshine I, Duronio V, Finlay BB. Tyrosine protein kinase inhibitors block invasin-promoted bacterial uptake by epithelial cells. *Infect Immun* 1992;60:2211–2217.
96. Finlay BB, Ruschkowski S, Dedhar S. Cytoskeletal rearrangements accompanying *Salmonella* entry into epithelial cells. *J Cell Sci* 1991;99:283–296.
97. Kapperud G. Studies on the pathogenicity of *Yersinia enterocolitica* and *Y. enterocolitica*-like bacteria. *Acta Pathol Microbiol Scand Sect B* 1980;88:293–297.
98. Une T. Studies on the pathogenicity of *Yersinia enterocolitica*. II. Interaction with cultured cells in vitro. *Microbiol Immunol* 1977;21:365–377.
99. Pierson DE and Falkow S. Nonpathogenic isolates of *Yersinia enterocolitica* do not contain functional *inv*-homologous sequences. *Infect Immun* 1990;58:1059–1064.
100. Beer KB, Miller VL. Amino acid substitutions in naturally occurring variants of Ail result in altered invasion activity. *J Bacteriol* 1992;174:1360–1369.
101. Hanski C, Kutschka U, Schmoranzer HP, et al. Immunohistochemical and electron microscopic study of interaction of *Yersinia enterocolitica* serotype O8 with intestinal mucosa during experimental enteritis. *Infect Immun* 1989;57:673–678.
102. Skurnik M, Poikonen K. Experimental intestinal infection of rats by *Yersinia enterocolitica* O:3. *Scand J Infect Dis* 1986;18:355–364.
103. Carter PB, Collins FM. Experimental *Yersinia enterocolitica* infection in mice: kinetics of growth. *Infect Immun* 1974;9:851–857.
104. Pai CH, Mors V, Seemayer TA. Experimental *Yersinia enterocolitica* enteritis in rabbits. *Infect Immun* 1980;28:238–244.
105. Simonet M, Richard S, Berche P. Electron microscopic evidence for in vivo extracellular localization of *Yersinia pseudotuberculosis* harboring the pYV plasmid. *Infect Immun* 1990;58:841–845.
106. Hanski C, Naumann M, Hahn H, Riecken EO. Determinants of invasion and survival of *Yersinia enterocolitica* in intestinal tissue: an in vivo study. *Med Microbiol Immunol* 1989;178:289–296.
107. Lian C-J, Hwang WS, Pai CH. Plasmid-mediated resistance to phagocytosis in *Yersinia enterocolitica*. *Infect Immun* 1987;55:1176–1183.
108. Straley SC, Skrzypek E, Plano GV, Bliska JB. Yops of *Yersinia* spp. pathogenic for humans. *Infect Immun* 1993;61:3105–3110.
109. Straley SC, Plano GV, Skrzypek E, Haddix PL, Fields KA. Regulation by Ca^{2+} in the Yersinia low-Ca^{2+} response. *Mol Microbiol* 1993;8:1005–1010.
110. Lian C-J, Hwang WS, Kelly JK, Pai CH. Invasiveness of *Yersinia enterocolitica* lacking the virulence plasmid: an in-vivo study. *J Med Microbiol* 1987;24:219–226.
111. Pai CH, DeStephano L. Serum resistance associated with virulence in *Yersinia enterocolitica*. *Infect Immun* 1982;35:605–611.
112. Portnoy DA, Wolf-Watz H, Bolin I, Beeder AB, Falkow S. Characterization of common virulence plasmids in *Yersinia* species and their role in the expression of outer membrane proteins. *Infect Immun* 1984;43:108–114.
113. Wolf-Watz H, Portnoy DA, Bolin I, Falkow S. Transfer of the

virulence plasmid of *Yersinia pestis* to *Yersinia pseudotuberculosis*. *Infect Immun* 1985;48:241–243.

114. Portnoy DA, Falkow S. Virulence-associated plasmids from *Yersinia enterocolitica* and *Yersinia pestis*. *J Bacteriol* 1981; 148:877–883.

115. Portnoy DA, Moseley SL, Falkow S. Characterization of plasmids and plasmid-associated determinants of *Yersinia enterocolitica* pathogenesis. *Infect Immun* 1981;31:775–782.

116. Lian C-J, Pai CH. Inhibition of human neutrophil chemiluminescence by plasmid-mediated outer membrane proteins of *Yersinia enterocolitica*. *Infect Immun* 1985;49:145–151.

117. Pilz D, Vocke T, Heesemann J, Brade V. Mechanism of YadA-mediated serum resistance of *Yersinia enterocolitica* serotype O3. *Infect Immun* 1992;60:189–195.

118. Martinez RJ. Thermoregulation-dependent expression of *Yersinia enterocolitica* protein 1 imparts serum resistance to *Escherichia coli* K-12. *J Bacteriol* 1989;171:3732–3739.

119. Wachter E, Brade V. Influence of surface modulations by enzymes and monoclonal antibodies on alternative complement pathway activation by *Yersinia enterocolitica*. *Infect Immun* 1989;57:1984–1989.

120. Rosqvist R, Bolin I, Wolf-Watz H. Inhibition of phagocytosis in *Yersinia pseudotuberculosis:* a virulence plasmid-encoded ability involving the Yop2b protein. *Infect Immun* 1988;56: 2139–2143.

121. Rosqvist R, Forsberg A, Rimpilainen M, Bergman T, Wolf-Watz H. The cytotoxic protein YopE of Yersinia obstructs the primary host defence. *Mol Microbiol* 1990;4:657–667.

122. Rosqvist R, Forsberg A, Wolf-Watz H. Intracellular targeting of the *Yersinia* YopE cytotoxin in mammalian cells induces actin microfilament disruption. *Infect Immun* 1991;59: 4562–4569.

123. Bliska JB, Guan K, Dixon JE, Falkow S. Tyrosine phosphate hydrolysis of host proteins by an essential *Yersinia* virulence determinant. *Proc Natl Acad Sci USA* 1991;88:1187–1191.

124. Guan K, Dixon JE. Protein tyrosine phosphatase activity of an essential virulence determinant in *Yersinia*. *Science* 1990;249: 553–556.

125. Forsberg A, Wolf-Watz H. The virulence protein Yop5 of *Yersinia pseudotuberculosis* is regulated at transcriptional level by plasmid-p1B1-encoded trans-acting elements controlled by temperature and calcium. *Mol Microbiol* 1988;2:121–133.

126. Bolin I, Wolf-Watz H. The plasmid-encoded Yop2b protein of *Yersinia pseudotuberculosis* is a virulence determinant regulated by calcium and temperature at the level of transcription. *Mol Microbiol* 1988;2:237–245.

127. Leung KY, Reisner BS, Straley SC. YopM inhibits platelet aggregation and is necessary for virulence of *Yersinia pestis* in mice. *Infect Immun* 1990;58:3262–3271.

128. Galyov EE, Hakansson S, Forsberg A, Wolf-Watz H. A secreted protein kinase of *Yersinia pseudotuberculosis* is an indispensable virulence determinant. *Nature* 1993;361:730–732.

129. Brubaker RR. The V antigen of Yersiniae: an overview. *Contr Microbiol Immunol* 1991;12:127–133.

130. Price SB, Cowan C, Perry RD, Straley SC. The *Yersinia pestis* V antigen is a regulatory protein necessary for Ca^{2+}-dependent growth and maximal expression of low-Ca^{2+} response virulence genes. *J Bacteriol* 1991;173:2649–2657.

131. Bergman T, Hakansson S, Forsberg A, et al. Analysis of the V antigen lcrGVH-yopBD operon of *Yersinia pseudotuberculosis:* evidence for a regulatory role of LcrH and LcrV. *J Bacteriol* 1991;173:1607–1616.

132. Delor I, Kaeckenbeeck A, Wauters G, Cornelis GR. Nucleotide sequence of yst, the *Yersinia enterocolitica* gene encoding the heat-stable enterotoxin, and prevalence of the gene among pathogenic and nonpathogenic Yersiniae. *Infect Immun* 1990; 58:2983–2988.

133. Takao T, Tominaga N, Yoshimura S, et al. Isolation, primary structure and synthesis of heat-stable enterotoxin produced by *Yersinia enterocolitica*. *Eur J Biochem* 1985;152:199–206.

134. Robins-Browne RM, Still CS, Miliotis MD, Koornhof HJ. Mechanism of action of *Yersinia enterocolitica* enterotoxin. *Infect Immun* 1979;25:680–684.

135. Robins-Browne RM, Takeda T, Fasano A, et al. Assessment of enterotoxin production by *Yersinia enterocolitica* and identification of a novel heat-stable enterotoxin produced by a noninvasive *Yersinia enterocolitica* strain isolated from clinical material. *Infect Immun* 1993;61:764–767.

136. Pai CH, Mors V, Toma S. Prevalence of enterotoxigenicity in human and nonhuman isolates of *Yersinia enterocolitica*. *Infect Immun* 1978;22:334–338.

137. Pai CH, Mors V. Production of enterotoxin by *Yersinia enterocolitica*. *Infect Immun* 1978;19:908–911.

138. Delor I, Cornelis GR. Role of *Yersinia enterocolitica* Yst toxin in experimental infection of young rabbits. *Infect Immun* 1992; 60:4269–4277.

139. Heeseman J. Chromosomal-encoded siderophores are required for mouse virulence of enteropathogenic Yersinia species. *FEMS Microbiol Lett* 1987;48:229–233.

140. Heesemann J, Hantke K, Vocke T, Saken E, Rakin A, Stojiljkovic I, Berner R. Virulence of *Yersinia enterocolitica* is closely associated with siderophore production, expression of an iron-repressible outer membrane polypeptide of 65,000 Da and pesticin sensitivity. *Mol Microbiol* 1993;8:397–408.

141. Carniel E, Mazigh D, Mollaret HH. Expression of iron-regulated proteins in *Yersinia* species and their relation to virulence. *Infect Immun* 1987;55:277–280.

142. Carniel E, Mercereau-Puijalon O, Bonnefoy S. The gene coding for the 190,000-dalton iron-regulated protein of *Yersinia* species is present only in the highly pathogenic strains. *Infect Immun* 1989;57:1211–1217.

143. Carniel E, Guiyoule A, Guilvout I, Mercereau-Puijalon O. Molecular cloning, iron-regulation and mutagenesis of the irp2 gene encoding HMWP2, a protein specific for the highly pathogenic Yersinia. *Mol Microbiol* 1992;6:379–388.

144. Baumler AJ, Hantke K. Ferrioxamine uptake in *Yersinia enterocolitica:* characterization of the receptor protein FoxA. *Mol Microbiol* 1992;6:1309–1321.

145. Kobnik R, Baumler AJ, Heesemann J, Braun V, Hantke K. The TonB protein of *Yersinia enterocolitica* and its interactions with TonB-box proteins. *Mol Gen Genet* 1993;237:152–160.

146. Perry RD, Brubaker RR. Accumulation of iron by *Yersiniae*. *J Bacteriol* 1979;137:1290–1298.

147. Stojiljkovic I, Hantke K. Hemin uptake system of *Yersinia enterocolitica:* similarities with other TonB-dependent systems in Gram-negative bacteria. *EMBO J* 1992;11:4359–4367.

148. Al-Hendy A, Toivanen P, Skurnik M. Lipopolysaccharide O side chain of *Yersinia enterocolitica* O:3 is an essential virulence factor in an orally infected murine model. *Infect Immun* 1992;60:870–875.

149. Ahvonen P. Human yersinoisis in Finland. II. Clinical features. *Ann Clin Res* 1972;4:39–48.

150. Simmonds SD, Noble MA, Freeman HJ. Gastrointestinal features of culture-positive *Yersinia enterocolitica* infection. *Gastroenterology* 1987;92:112–117.

151. Vantrappen G, Agg HO, Ponette E, Geboes K, Bertrand PH. *Yersinia* enteritis and enterocolitis: gastroenterological aspects. *Gastroenterology* 1977;72:220–227.

152. Marriott DJE, Taylor S, Dorman DC. *Yersinia enterocolitica* infection in children. *Med J Aust* 1985;143:489–492.

153. Mazzoleni G, deSa D, Gately J, Riddell RH. *Yersinia enterocolitica* infection with ileal perforation associated with iron overload and deferoxamine therapy. *Dig Dis Sci* 1991;36: 1154–1160.

154. Olinde AJ, Lucas JF Jr, Miller RC. Acute yersiniosis and its surgical significance. *South Med J* 1984;77:1539–1544.

155. Van Noyen R, Selderslaghs R, Bekaert J, Wauters G, Vandepitte J. Causative role of *Yersinia* and other enteric pathogens in the appendicular syndrome. *Eur J Clin Microbiol Infect Dis* 1991;10:735–741.

156. Jepsen OB, Korner B, Lauritsen KB, et al. *Yersinia enterocolitica* infection in patients with acute surgical abdominal disease. A prospective study. *Scand J Infect Dis* 1976;8:189–194.

157. Nilehn B, Sjostrom B. Studies on *Yersinia enterocolitica:* occurrence in various groups of acute abdominal disease. *Acta Pathol Microbiol Scand* 1967;71:612–628.

158. Pai CH, Gillis F, Marks MI. Infection due to *Yersinia enterocol-*

itica in children with abdominal pain. *J Infect Dis* 1982;146: 705.

159. Bradford WD, Noce PS, Gutman LT. Pathologic features of enteric infection with *Yersinia enterocolitica. Arch Pathol* 1974;98:17–22.

160. Puylaert JBCM, Vermeijden RJ, van der Werf SDJ, Doornbos L, Koumans RKJ. Incidence and sonographic diagnosis of bacterial ileocaecitis masquerading as appendicitis. *Lancet* 1989; 2:84–86.

161. Tacket CO, Davis BR, Carter GP, Randoph JF, Cohen ML. *Yersinia enterocolitica* pharyngitis. *Ann Intern Med* 1983;99: 40–42.

162. Jaffe KM, Smith AL. *Yersinia enterocolitica* cervical lymphadenitis. *J Pediatr* 1980;97:937–939.

163. Lewis JF, Alexander J. Facial abscess due to *Yersinia enterocolitica. Am J Clin Pathol* 1976;66:1016–1018.

164. Karmali MA, Toma S, Schiemann DA, Ein SH. Infection caused by *Yersinia enterocolitica* serotype O:21. *J Clin Microbiol* 1982;15:596–598.

165. Krogstad P, Mendelman PM, Miller VL, et al. Clinical and microbiologic characteristics of cutaneous infection with *Yersinia enterocolitica. J Infect Dis* 1992;165:740–743.

166. Crichton EP. Suppurative conjunctivitis caused by *Yersinia enterocolitica. Can Med Assoc J* 1978;118:22–24.

167. Cropp AJ, Gaylord SF, Watanakunakorn C. Case report: cavitary pneumonia due to *Yersinia enterocolitica* in a healthy man. *Am J Med Sci* 1984;288:130–132.

168. Bigler RD, Atkins RR, Wing EJ. *Yersinia enterocolitica* lung infection. *Arch Intern Med* 1981;141:1529–1530.

169. Rabson AR, Hallett AF, Koornhof HJ. Generalized *Yersinia enterocolitica* infection. *J Infect Dis* 1975;131:447–451.

170. Bouza E, Dominguez A, Meseguer M, et al. *Yersinia enterocolitica* septicemia. *Am J Clin Pathol* 1980;74:404–409.

171. Gayraud M, Scavizzi MR, Mollaret HH, Guillevin L, Hornstein MJ. Antibiotic treatment of *Yersinia enterocolitica* septicemia: a retrospective review of 43 cases. *Clin Infect Dis* 1993;17: 405–410.

172. Mofenson HC, Caraccio TR, Sharieff N. Iron sepsis: *Yersinia enterocolitica* septicemia possibly caused by an overdose of iron. *N Engl J Med* 1987;316:1092–1093.

173. Viteri AL, Howard PH, May JL, Ramesh GS, Roberts JW. Hepatic abscess due to *Yersinia enterocolitica* without bacteremia. *Gastroenterology* 1981;81:592–593.

174. Leighton PM, MacSween HM. *Yersinia* hepatic abscesses subsequent to long-term iron therapy. *JAMA* 1987;257:964–965.

175. Appelbaum JS, Wilding G, Morse LJ. *Yersinia enterocolitica* endocarditis. *Arch Intern Med* 1983;143:2150–2151.

176. Plotkin GR, O'Rourke JN. Mycotic aneurysm due to *Yersinia enterocolitica. Am J Med Sci* 1981;281:35–42.

177. Thirumoorthi MC, Dajani AS. *Yersinia enterocolitica* osteomyelitis in a child. *Am J Dis Child* 1978;132:578–580.

178. Clarridge J, Roberts C, Peters J, Musher D. Sepsis and empyema caused by *Yersinia enterocolitica. J Clin Microbiol* 1983; 17:936–938.

179. Arduino MJ, Bland LA, Tipple MA, Aguero SM, Favero MS, Jarvis WR. Growth and endotoxin production of *Yersinia enterocolitica* and *Enterobacter agglomerans* in packed erythrocytes. *J Clin Microbiol* 1989;27:1483–1485.

180. Kingsley G, Panayi G. Antigenic responses in reactive arthritis. *Rheum Dis Clin North Am* 1992;18:49–66.

181. Granfors K. Do bacterial antigens cause reactive arthritis? *Rheum Dis Clin North Am* 1992;18:37–48.

182. Leino R, Kalliomaki JL. Yersiniosis as an internal disease. *Ann Intern Med* 1974;81:458–461.

183. Laitinen O, Leirisalo M, Skylv G. Relation between HLA-B27 and clinical features in patients with Yersinia arthritis. *Arthritis Rheum* 1977;20:1121–1124.

184. Aho K, Ahvonen P, Lassus A, Sievers K, Tiilikainen A. HL-A27 in reactive arthritis: a study of Yersinia arthritis and Reiter's disease. *Arthritis Rheum* 1974;17:521–526.

185. Dequeker J, Jamar R, Walravens M. HLA-B27, arthritis and *Yersinia enterocolitica* infection. *J Rheumatol* 1980;7:706–710.

186. Granfors K, Jalkanen S, von Essen R, et al. *Yersinia* antigens in synovial-fluid cells from patients with reactive arthritis. *N Engl J Med* 1989;320:216–221.

187. Nikkari S, Merilahti-Palo R, Saario R, et al. *Yersinia*-triggered reactive arthritis. *Arthritis Rheum* 1992;35:682–687.

188. de los Toyos JR, Vazquez J, Sampedro A, Hardisson C. *Yersinia enterocolitica* serotype O:3 is arthritogenic for mice. *Microb Pathog* 1990;8:363–370.

189. Merilahti-Palo R, Gripenberg-Lerche C, Soderstrom K-O, Toivanen P. Long term follow up of SHR rats with experimental yersinia associated arthritis. *Ann Rheum Dis* 1992;51:91–96.

190. Hill JL, Yu DTY. Development of an experimental animal model for reactive arthritis induced by *Yersinia enterocolitica* infection. *Infect Immun* 1987;55:721–726.

191. Gaede K, Mack D, Heesemann J. Experimental *Yersinia enterocolitica* infection in rats: analysis of the immune response to plasmid-encoded antigens of arthritis-susceptible Lewis rats and arthritis-resistant Fischer rats. *Med Microbiol Immunol* 1992;181:165–172.

192. Mertz AKH, Batsford SR, Curschellas E, Kist MJ, Gondolf KB. Cationic *Yersinia* antigen-induced chronic allergic arthritis in rats: a model for reactive arthritis in humans. *J Clin Invest* 1991;87:632–642.

193. Skurnik M, Batsford S, Mertz A, Schiltz E, Toivanen P. The putative arthritogenic cationic 19-kilodalton antigen of *Yersinia enterocolitica* is a urease beta-subunit. *Infect Immun* 1993;61: 2498–2504.

194. Wakefield D, Stahlberg TH, Toivanen A, Granfors K, Tennant C. Serologic evidence of *Yersinia* infection in patients with anterior uveitis. *Arch Ophthalmol* 1990;108:219–221.

195. Lindholm H, Visakorpi R. Late complications after a *Yersinia enterocolitica* epidemic: a follow up study. *Ann Rheum Dis* 1991;50:694–696.

196. Saebo A, Lassen J. A survey of acute and chronic disease associated with *Yersinia enterocolitica* infection. *Scand J Infect Dis* 1991;23:517–527.

197. Agner E, Larsen JH, Leth A. *Yersinia enterocolitica* carditis as a differential diagnosis and the prognosis of this disease. *Scand J Rheumatol* 1978;7:26–28.

198. Friedberg M, Denneberg T, Brun C, Larsen J Hannover, Larsen S. Glomerulonephritis in infections with *Yersinia enterocolitica* O-serotype 3. II. The incidence and immunological features of *Yersinia* infection in a consecutive glomerulonephritis population. *Acta Med Scand* 1981;209:103–110.

199. Denneberg T, Friedberg M, Samuelsson T, Winblad S. Glomerulonephritis in infections with *Yersinia enterocolitica* O-serotype 3. I. Evidence for glomerular involvement in acute cases of yersiniosis. *Acta Med Scand* 1981;209:97–101.

200. Shenkman L, Bottone EJ. Antibodies to *Yersinia enterocolitica* in thyroid disease. *Ann Intern Med* 1976;85:735–739.

201. Bech K, Nerup J, Larsen JH. *Yersinia enterocolitica* infection and thyroid diseases. *Acta Endocrinologica* 1977;84:87–92.

202. Tomer Y, Davies TF. Infection, thyroid disease, and autoimmunity. *Endocr Rev* 1993;14:107–120.

203. Stuart PM, Woodward JG. *Yersinia enterocolitica* produces superantigenic activity. *J Immunol* 1992;148:225–233.

204. Head CB, Whitty DA, Ratnam S. Comparative study of selective media for recovery of *Yersinia enterocolitica. J Clin Microbiol* 1982;16:615–621.

205. Pai CH, Sorger S, Lafleur L, Lackman L, Marks MI. Efficacy of cold enrichment techniques for recovery of *Yersinia enterocolitica* from human stools. *J Clin Microbiol* 1979;9:712–715.

206. Bhaduri S, Turner-Jones C, Lachica RV. Convenient agarose medium for simultaneous determination of the low-calcium response and congo red binding by virulent strains of *Yersinia enterocolitica. J Clin Microbiol* 1991;29:2341–2344.

207. Bhaduri S, Conway LK, Lachica RV. Assay of crystal violet binding for rapid identification of virulent plasmid-bearing clones of *Yersinia enterocolitica. J Clin Microbiol* 1987;25: 1039–1042.

208. Kandolo K, Wauters G. Pyrazinamidase activity in *Yersinia enterocolitica* and related organisms. *J Clin Microbiol* 1985;21: 980–982.

209. Riley G, Toma S. Detection of pathogenic *Yersinia enterocoli-*

tica by using congo red-magnesium oxalate agar medium. *J Clin Microbiol* 1989;27:213–214.

210. Paerregaard A, Shand GH, Gaarslev K, Espersen F. Comparison of crossed immunoelectrophoresis, enzyme-linked immunosorbent assays, and tube agglutination for serodiagnosis of *Yersinia enterocolitica* serotype O:3 infection. *J Clin Microbiol* 1991;29:302–309.

211. Maki-Ikola O, Heesemann J, Lahesmaa R, Toivanen A, Granfors K. Combined use of released proteins and lipopolysaccharide in enzyme-linked immunosorbent assay for serologic screening of *Yersinia enterocolitica* infections. *J Infect Dis* 1991;163:409–412.

212. Pham JN, Bell SM, Lanzarone JYM. Biotype and antibiotic sensitivity of 100 clinical isolates of *Yersinia enterocolitica*. *J Antimicrob Chemother* 1991;28:13–18.

213. Segreti J, Nelson JA, Goodman LJ, Kaplan RL, Trenhome GM. In vitro activities of lomefloxacin and temafloxacin against pathogens causing diarrhea. *Antimicrob Agents Chemother* 1989;33:1385–1387.

214. Pham JN, Bell SM, Lanzarone JYM. A study of the b-lactamases of 100 clinical isolates of *Yersinia enterocolitica*. *J Antimicrob Chemother* 1991;28:19–24.

215. Scavizzi MR, Alonso J-M, Philippon AM, Jupeau-Vessieres AM, Guiyoule A. Failure of newer beta-lactam antibiotics for murine *Yersinia enterocolitica* infection. *Antimicrob Agents Chemother* 1987;31:523–526.

216. Lemaitre BC, Mazigh DA, Scavizzi MR. Failure of b-lactam antibiotics and marked efficacy of fluoroquinolones in treatment of murine *Yersinia pseudotuberculosis* infection. *Antimicrobial Agents Chemother* 1991;35:1785–1790.

217. Pai CH, Gillis F, Tuomanen E, Marks MI. Placebo-controlled double-blind evaluation of trimethoprim-sulfamethoxazole treatment of *Yersinia enterocolitica* gastroenteritis. *J Pediatr* 1984;104:308–311.

218. Hubbert WT. Yersiniosis in mammals and birds in the United States. *Am J Trop Med Hyg* 1972;21:458–463.

219. Fukushima H, Gomyoda M, Shiozawa K, Kaneko S, Tsubokura M. *Yersinia pseudotuberculosis* infection contracted through water contaminated by a wild animal. *J Clin Microbiol* 1988;26:584–585.

220. Fukushima H, Gomyoda M, Kaneko S. Mice and moles inhabiting mountainous areas of Shimane peninsula as sources of infection with *Yersinia pseudotuberculosis*. *J Clin Microbiol* 1990;28:2448–2455.

221. Slee KJ, Skilbeck NW. Epidemiology of *Yersinia pseudotuberculosis* and *Yersinia enterocolitica* infections in sheep in Australia. *J Clin Microbiol* 1992;30:712–715.

222. Tsubokura M, Otsuki K, Sata K, et al. Special features of distribution of *Yersinia pseudotuberculosis* in Japan. *J Clin Microbiol* 1989;27:790–791.

223. Toma S. Human and nonhuman infections caused by *Yersinia pseudotuberculosis* in Canada from 1962 to 1985. *J Clin Microbiol* 1986;24:465–466.

224. Randall KJ. Family outbreak of *Pasteurella pseudotuberculosis* infection. *Lancet* 1962;1:1042–1043.

225. Nakano T, Kawaguchi H, Nakao K, Maruyama T, Kamiya H, Sakurai M. Two outbreaks of *Yersinia pseudotuberculosis* 5a infection in Japan. *Scand J Infect Dis* 1989;21:175–179.

226. Inoue M, Nakashima H, Ueba O, et al. Community outbreak of *Yersinia pseudotuberculosis*. *Microbiol Immunol* 1984;28:883–891.

227. Tertti R, Granfors K, Lehtonen O-P, et al. An outbreak of *Yersinia pseudotuberculosis* infection. *J Infect Dis* 1984;149:245–250.

228. Stahlberg TH, Tertti R, Wolf-Watz H, Granfors K, Toivanen A. Antibody response in *Yersinia pseudotuberculosis* III infection: analysis of an outbreak. *J Infect Dis* 1987;156:388–391.

229. Saari TN, Triplett DA. *Yersinia pseudotuberculosis* mesenteric adenitis. *J Pediatr* 1974;85:656–659.

230. Knapp W. Mesenteric adenitis due to *Pasteurella* pseudotuberculosis in young people. *N Engl J Med* 1956;259:776–778.

231. deGroote G, Vandepitte J, Wauters G. Surveillance of human *Yersinia enterocolitica* infections in Belgium: 1963–1978. *J Infect* 1982;4:189–197.

232. Fukushima H, Gomyoda M, Ishikura S, et al. Cat-contaminated environmental substances lead to *Yersinia pseudotuberculosis* infection in children. *J Clin Microbiol* 1989;27:2706–2709.

233. Prober CG, Tune B, Hoder L. *Yersinia pseudotuberculosis* septicemia. *Am J Dis Child* 1979;133:623–624.

234. Bolin I, Wolf-Watz H. Molecular cloning of the temperature-inducible outer membrane protein 1 of *Yersinia pseudotuberculosis*. *Infect Immun* 1984;43:72–78.

235. Rosqvist R, Skurnik M, Wolf-Watz H. Increased virulence of *Yersinia pseudotuberculosis* by two independent mutations. *Nature* 1988;334:522–524.

236. Kapperud G, Namork E, Skurnik M, Nesbakken T. Plasmid-mediated surface fibrillae of *Yersinia pseudotuberculosis* and *Yersinia enterocolitica*: relationship be the outer membrane protein Yop1 and possible importance for pathogenesis. *Infect Immun* 1987;55:2247–2254.

237. Lindler LE, Tall BD. *Yersinia pestis* pH 6 antigen forms fimbriae and is induced by intracellular association with macrophages. *Mol Microbiol* 1993;8:311–324.

238. Weber J, Finlayson NB, Mark JBD. Mesenteric lymphadenitis and terminal ileitis due to *Yersinia pseudotuberculosis*. *N Engl J Med* 1970;283:172–174.

239. Hubbert WT, Petenyi CW, Glasgow LA, Uyeda CT, Creighton SA. *Yersinia pseudotuberculosis* infection in the United States. Septicemia, appendicitis, and mesenteric lymphadenitis. *Am J Trop Med Hyg* 1971;20:679–684.

240. El-Maraghi NRH, Mair NS. The histopathology of enteric infection with *Yersinia pseudotuberculosis*. *Am J Clin Pathol* 1979;71:631–639.

241. Boelaert JR, van Landuyt HW, Valcke YJ, et al. The role of iron overload in *Yersinia enterocolitica* and *Yersinia pseudotuberculosis* bacteremia in hemodialysis patients. *J Infect Dis* 1987;156:384–387.

242. Farrer W, Kloser P, Ketyer S. Case report: *Yersinia pseudotuberculosis* sepsis presenting as multiple liver abscesses. *Am J Med Sci* 1988;295:129–132.

243. Chalmers A, Kaprove RE, Reynolds WJ, Urowitz MB. Postdiarrheal arthropathy of *Yersinia pseudotuberculosis*. *Can Med Assoc J* 1978;118:515–516.

244. Bignardi GE. *Yersinia pseudotuberculosis* and arthritis. *Ann Rheum Dis* 1989;48:518–519.

245. Davenport A, Finn R. Haemolytic uraemic syndrome induced by *Yersinia pseudotuberculosis*. *Lancet* 1988;1:358–359.

246. Okada K, Yano I, Kagami S, et al. Acute tubulointerstitial nephritis associated with *Yersinia pseudotuberculosis* infection. *Clin Nephrol* 1991;35:105–109.

247. Sato K, Ouchi K, Taki M. *Yersinia pseudotuberculosis* infection in children, resembling Izumi fever and Kawasaki syndrome. *Pediatr Infect Dis* 1983;2:123–126.

248. Chiba S, Kaneko K, Hashimoto N, Nakao T. *Yersinia pseudotuberculosis* and Kawasaki disease. *Pediatr Infect Dis* 1983;2:494.

249. Abe J, Takeda T, Watanbe Y, et al. Evidence for supernantigen production by *Yersinia pseudotuberculosis*. *J Immunol* 1993;151:4183–4188.

250. Uchiyama T, Miyoshi-Akiyama T, Kato H, Fujimake W, Imanishi K, Yan X-J. Superantigenic properties of a novel mitogenic substance produced by *Yersinia pseudotuberculosis* isolated from patients manifesting acute and systemic symptoms. *J Immunol* 1993;151:4407–4413.

251. Sato K, Ouchi K, Komazawa M. Ampicillin vs. placebo for *Yersinia pseudotuberculosis* infection in children. *Ped Infect Dis J* 1988;7:686–689.

Infections of the Gastrointestinal Tract,
edited by M. J. Blaser, P. D. Smith, J. I. Ravdin,
H. B. Greenberg, and R. L. Guerrant
Raven Press, Ltd., New York © 1995.

CHAPTER 56

Campylobacter jejuni

Martin B. Skirrow and Martin J. Blaser

It is surprising that *Campylobacter* enteritis, the commonest bacterial form of acute infective diarrhea in developed countries, was not recognized until the mid-1970s. How *Campylobacter jejuni* came to be overlooked by bacteriologists for so long is a matter for debate, but a too rigid adherence to traditional methods of culture and a failure to pick up ideas from the rich field of veterinary microbiology were certainly factors. Yet there were several points in history when the discovery might have been made.

As long ago as 1886, Theodor Escherich described and sketched spiral organisms that, with hindsight, must have been campylobacters in the colonic mucus of infants who had died of "cholera infantum," but they could not be cultured and he did not attach any great importance to them (1). Campylobacters were first isolated in culture by McFadyean and Stockman in 1909 in the United Kingdom from aborted sheep fetuses, but these were *C. fetus* (2). *C. jejuni,* which can also cause abortion in sheep, was first distinguished in 1931 as a cause of winter dysentery in calves by Jones Orcutt and Little (3), but it was not until 1957 that Elizabeth King described the group more fully (provisionally named "related vibrio") and observed an association with human diarrhea (4). The strains she studied were from blood, for at that time no one knew how to isolate them from feces. That crucial breakthrough was made some 15 years later by Butzler and his colleagues in Belgium (5) and it soon became apparent that campylobacters, far from being rare curiosities in man, were a common cause of diarrhea (6). A full historical account of the bacteriology of campylobacters is given by Karmali and Skirrow (7).

MICROBIOLOGY

Campylobacters are small, nonsporing, spiral, gram-negative bacteria that exhibit a rapid darting motility.

M. Skirrow: Public Health Laboratory Service, Gloucestershire Royal Hospital, Gloucester GL1 3NN, United Kingdom.

M. J. Blaser: Departments of Microbiology and Immunology, Vanderbilt University School of Medicine, Nashville, Tennessee 37232.

They were first placed in the genus *Vibrio,* but in 1963 were assigned to a new genus *Campylobacter* (Greek, curved rod) (8). Recent molecular techniques have shown that *Campylobacter* (11 species), *Helicobacter, Arcobacter,* and *Wolinella* belong to a distinct phylogenetic group far removed from other gram-negative bacteria (9). These bacteria have a spiral configuration and are motile by means of polar flagella—a single long unsheathed flagellum at each pole in the case of *C. jejuni.* This spiral shape and motility are adaptations to penetrating and colonizing mucus. Many of these organisms change into coccal forms when exposed to atmospheric oxygen.

C. jejuni, C. coli, and *C. lari* form a subgroup of the genus *Campylobacter* known as the "thermophilic" group on account of their relatively high optimum growth temperature of 42–43°C. Although "*Campylobacter jejuni*" is the title of this chapter, we also include *C. coli,* as the two species are closely related and both cause *Campylobacter* enteritis. Indeed the name *C. jejuni* is often used loosely to embrace both species, as differentiation between the two is seldom of clinical value and in most areas *C. coli* accounts for less than 10% of infections. In this chapter the anglicized "*Campylobacter*" refers to both species, and Latin names are used in their strict sense. *C. lari,* which can be confused with *C. jejuni* on primary isolation media, rarely causes *Campylobacter* enteritis—less than 0.1% of cases in a large British survey (10). There are two subspecies of *C. jejuni:* subsp. *jejuni* and subsp. *doylei.* The former is the typical one and the latter is a much less common, fastidious, and slow-growing organism considered, along with other *Campylobacter* species, in the next chapter. In this chapter we refer to *C. jejuni* subsp. *jejuni* simply as *C. jejuni.*

Metabolism and Growth Requirements

Campylobacters are strict microaerophiles: they need oxygen for growth, yet the oxygen concentration in air is toxic because they are unusually vulnerable to superoxides and free radicals. *C. jejuni* grow best in an atmosphere containing 5% to 10% oxygen and 1% to 10% carbon dioxide, which means that plate cultures have to be incubated in sealed containers charged with an appropriate gas mixture. *Campylobacter* culture media usually contain compounds that quench superoxides and free radicals, which increases their oxygen tolerance. Primary isolation media also contain antimicrobial agents that suppress coliforms and other fecal organisms, and plates are incubated at 42–43°C to give extra selectivity and more rapid *Campylobacter* growth.

Susceptibility to Physical and Chemical Agents

Campylobacters are more susceptible to physical and chemical agents than most pathogenic bacteria perhaps because they are well adapted for an *in vivo* existence. They are readily killed by pasteurization ($D \leq 1$ min at 60°C). They are damaged by freezing and thawing, which causes a 1–2 $\log_{10}$ fall in numbers, although once frozen they survive for many months at $-20°C$. They can survive in natural water for several weeks at 4°C but for only a few days at temperatures above 15°C (11) and it is possible that they can survive in a "nonculturable" form for much longer periods (12). While mice and chickens have been infected by ingestion of water from which campylobacters cannot be cultured in the laboratory (13,14), it is not certain as to whether this is due to a specific survival form or the simple fact that culture is a less sensitive method of detection.

Campylobacters are highly susceptible to drying and exposure to atmospheric oxygen and are at least as susceptible as coliforms, salmonellas, and other enterobacteria to ultraviolet light, γ radiation, and commonly used disinfectants such as hypochlorites, phenols, iodophors, and quaternary ammonium compounds. Campylobacters are progressively inactivated at pH values outside the range 5.0–9.0. However, they survive in 6.5% NaCl for 3 weeks at 4°C, so it is likely that they could survive in salted uncooked meats if initial contamination is heavy (15).

Strain Typing

There are several methods of typing campylobacters. Biotyping is not very discriminating, but it is useful in combination with other typing methods. The biotyping scheme of Lior (16) is well established. The scheme of Bolton and colleagues, which is an extension of the Lior scheme, combines identification and biotyping tests expressed as a four-figure numerical code for each type (17).

Serotyping is currently the most widely used form of typing. There are hundreds of serotypes of *C. jejuni* and *C. coli*. Several schemes have been described, but those of Penner and Hennessy (18) and Lior and colleagues (19) are the most widely used. They are complementary: the Penner scheme is based on heat-stable somatic lipopolysaccharide antigens forming >90 serogroups (the HS system); the Lior scheme is based on heat-labile surface protein antigens (flagellar and cellular) of which 112 have been defined, including 8 among *C. lari* strains (the HL system). The full serotype is given by identifying both

classes of antigen. As many of these antigens are rarely encountered, a common practice is to use a restricted panel of antisera from each scheme.

Phage typing, usually used in conjunction with serotyping, can detect differences between strains of one serotype and therefore gives greater discrimination. There are also several molecular typing methods that can give extremely fine discrimination within serotypes. They include protein profiling and analyses of various endonuclease digests of DNA and ribosomal RNA. Their main drawback is that the complex patterns produced usually require computer-assisted analysis and they are difficult to catalogue into universally recognized types. Polymer chain reaction (PCR)–based typing schemes also are emerging.

Typing is currently useful only for epidemiological purposes and is not recommended routinely (20). Review of the microbiology of campylobacters was provided by Skirrow (21).

EPIDEMIOLOGY

Campylobacter enteritis is an infection of worldwide distribution, but the pattern of disease differs greatly between developed and developing countries (22,23).

Campylobacter Enteritis in Developed Countries

Incidence and Costs

In developed countries campylobacters are the most frequently identified bacterial cause of acute infective diarrhea. In the USA the annual incidence of laboratory-diagnosed cases of *Campylobacter* enteritis is estimated to be 54–60/100,000 (24), but these figures represent only a fraction of all *Campylobacter* infections. Calculations based on medical consultation and stool sampling rates during a waterborne outbreak of *Campylobacter* enteritis placed the incidence at 1% (1000/100,000) per year, or 2.1–2.4 million cases per year (24). In the UK, national surveillance of laboratory reports shows a rising incidence (thought to be due mainly to increasing ascertainment), which reached 100/100,000 in 1993, but a survey of patients seeking treatment for acute diarrhea in a single medical practice (25) gave an estimated incidence of 1.1% (1100/100,000) per year (0.5 million cases per year), close to the U.S. incidence. Estimates of mortality are imprecise because they depend on extrapolations, but in the USA they have been placed in the range of 200–700 deaths per year (about 1–3/1 million) (24). In general the infection has a higher incidence in rural than urban communities; this was strikingly shown in a Yugoslavian study (26).

The cost of health care and lost productivity for *Campylobacter* enteritis was measured in the UK in 1986 and found to be £273 (about $400) per case; it was twice that sum if the costs of pain and suffering were included (27). The costs in the USA are likely to be higher. Thus, even if calculations are limited to laboratory-diagnosed cases, it is clear that *Campylobacter* enteritis costs society many millions of dollars annually.

Seasonal Variation

In temperate climates the incidence of *Campylobacter* enteritis is highest in summer. In the UK a remarkably constant pattern has been observed over 9 years: there is a sharp rise of incidence in early summer to about twice the mean and then it falls back gradually to a low winter level (28). A broadly similar pattern pertains in the USA, but there is a secondary peak in the late fall. Sporadic cases peak in the summer, whereas outbreak-associated cases peak in the spring and fall (24).

Distribution of Infection in the Population

Population-based studies show that *Campylobacter* enteritis affects people of all ages, but the infection has a unique bimodal age distribution with peaks of incidence in children below the age of 1 year and adults aged 15–24 years (10,24). The high incidence in young children may be partly due to high sampling rates at that age (10), although a survey of young children attending day nurseries in the UK gave an annual incidence of 169/1000; half of the infections were asymptomatic and most illnesses were mild (29). The reasons for the high incidence in young adults are unknown but may reflect primary exposures to important vehicles. In Britain there is a notable preponderance of reported cases in males (M/F ratio 1.7:1) in this age group (average for all ages 1.2:1), and this ratio rises during the summer peak (2.1:1) (10).

Most infections occur as single sporadic cases, or in family clusters of two or three cases. Family outbreaks are underreported; other infected persons (15% without symptoms) have been found in 40% of households of index cases (6). In most such instances the timing of illness suggests a common source, but secondary cases have been reported, particularly when the index case involves a young child. The prevalence of symptomless *Campylobacter* excretion in the general population of developed countries is substantially less than 1%.

Major outbreaks of *Campylobacter* enteritis are uncommon and are almost always waterborne or milkborne, but they can affect several thousand persons at a time (see below).

Campylobacter *Enteritis in Developing Countries*

Campylobacters are environmentally abundant in developing countries and infection is hyperendemic. Breastfed infants are largely protected against infection until weaned, and so infections begin to appear in the second 6 months of life. These early infections are often symptomatic, with diarrhea, but as children progress through their second and third years they develop immunity (30,31) and an increasing proportion of infections are asymptomatic (32). Apart from a high frequency of asymptomatic infection, children with *Campylobacter* enteritis in developing countries tend to have watery rather than inflammatory diarrhea and infection with multiple pathogens, including multiple *Campylobacter* strains.

Children over the age of 5 years (2 in some areas) and adults are immune and untroubled by *Campylobacter* infection. In general, *Campylobacter* enteritis does not cause as much serious dehydrating diarrhea as rotavirus and various pathogenic *Escherichia coli* in developing countries, but it remains a major contributor to childhood morbidity from diarrhea (33).

Sources of Human Infection

C. jejuni, C. coli, and *C. lari* live as commensals in the intestinal tracts of a wide variety of birds and mammals, including domestic pets and animals used for food production, notably poultry. *C. coli* is the predominant species in swine, and in some areas swine are believed to be the source of unusually high proportions of *C. coli* infection in humans (26). Both *C. jejuni* and *C. coli* can be pathogenic to lambs, calves, and puppies, and they are a common cause of epizootic abortion in ewes. Their optimum growth temperature of 42–43°C reflects an adaptation to birds. Thus, *Campylobacter* enteritis is a zoonosis and control depends largely on reducing transmission from animals to human via foods of animal origin and water, as described at the end of this chapter.

Transmission of Infection

Infection may be acquired from direct contact with infected animals or their products. Such contact is usually occupational, involving farmers, butchers, and workers in poultry-processing plants, but domestic infection from infected pets, usually a puppy or kitten with diarrhea, is well recognized. In one study it was estimated that 6.3% of *Campylobacter* enteritis cases were attributable to exposure to animals with diarrhea (34). Person-to-person spread is infrequent, but when it occurs it is usually from a young child to its mother or attendant. Conversely, babies who are born to mothers who are excreting campylobacters at the time of birth are at risk of infection. Homosexual men who engage in a variety of sexual practices are at increased risk of infection, not only from *C. jejuni* but from other *Campylobacter* species as well (35). A rare form of spread is via blood transfusion (36). Indirect transmission is more usual. The main vehicles of infection are water, milk, and raw meats, especially poultry.

Water and Milk

Virtually all surface waters contain campylobacters, even in remote regions where they are contaminated by wild birds. Waterborne outbreaks affecting as many as 3000 persons have arisen from the distribution of unchlorinated water (37,38). Sporadic infections from drinking untreated surface water in wilderness areas also occur, and *C. jejuni* may be a more common cause of "backpacker's" diarrhea than *Giardia* (39). Major outbreaks have arisen from the consumption of raw milk (40,41). In the USA infection has occurred in children and college students given raw milk to drink while on educational visits to farms (42). An unusual source of sporadic milkborne infection has been described in the UK where milk is delivered to the doorsteps of houses in aluminum foil–topped bottles. In certain areas, magpies (*Pica pica*) and jackdaws (*Corvus monedula*) have acquired the habit of pecking through the foil bottle tops and contaminating the contents with campylobacters (43). This activity is limited to early summer when the birds are feeding their young, and in affected areas it has accounted for up to 60% of infections at that time. Contaminated raw milk taken in tea or coffee can cause infection (44).

Raw Meats

Retailed fresh raw meats are contaminated with campylobacters to varying degrees: pork, beef, and lamb, 3% to 6% (means of 9 surveys); liver, kidney, and heart from the same animals, 22% (mean of 8 surveys); broiler chickens, 60% (mean of 17 surveys). Broiler chickens are by far the largest potential source. Not only are contamination rates high, but contamination is often heavy, with campylobacter counts of up to 1.5×10^6 per fresh bird and 2.4×10^7 in uneviscerated birds (45). Moreover, vast numbers of birds are consumed; in the USA, approximately 9 billion are sold annually (about 36 per capita). It is not easy to measure the proportion of infections that can be attributed to the consumption (and handling) of broiler chickens, but in a detailed case-control study in King County, Washington (Seattle), the proportion was calculated to be 48% of all cases (46).

Infection can be acquired from raw meats in three ways. First, bacteria may be transferred to the mouth when handling meat; inexperienced handlers are especially at risk. Second, the product may be consumed in the raw or undercooked state; barbecue- and fondue-cooked meats are liable to be undercooked (47). Third, other foods may become cross-contaminated from raw meats in the kitchen by means of hands or utensils. The latter is probably a frequent route, but it is the most difficult to substantiate, which may be why the source of many sporadic infections remains unknown (48). It is likely to be the main route by which nonimmune travelers to developing countries develop traveler's diarrhea due to *Campylobacter,* which is a common affliction. In contrast to *Salmonella* food poisoning, foodborne *Campylobacter* enteritis rarely takes the form of explosive outbreaks. This may be because campylobacters do not multiply in food as do salmonellas; they are more fastidious and slower growing, and do not grow below 30°C. Infections therefore tend to be due to the chance cross-contamination of odd food items resulting in sporadic cases or small family outbreaks.

PATHOGENESIS AND IMMUNITY

Pathogenesis

Initial Events

Experimental *C. jejuni* infection has been induced with as few as 500 organisms (49). In general, attack rates have been dose-dependent in volunteer studies (50). In these studies and in outbreaks the incubation period to onset of symptoms has ranged from about 1 day to 1 week. *C. jejuni* are susceptible to the low pH present in the gastric lumen (11), which is consistent with the dose effect. This phenomenon may help explain outbreaks involving vehicles such as milk or water, which may enhance survival through the gastric phase, by buffering or rapid wash-through, respectively. *C. jejuni* multiplies in the presence of bile, which may be a selective advantage in the bile-rich small intestine (11).

Intestinal Luminal Events

In animal models, motility of *C. jejuni* is critical for the establishment of colonization or infection (51). Spiral morphology undoubtedly contributes to the ability to move in the intestinal mucus gel. *C. jejuni* possess a single flagellum at one or both poles that is necessary for motility, and there is phase variation of expression of flagellation (21). The flagellar structural proteins are encoded by two highly related genes, *flaA* and *flaB* (with 98% homology) (52). In most strains, the products of both genes are expressed and the flagellar filament represents a complex of both proteins (53). However *flaA* mutants have only slight motility whereas *flaB* mutants retain motility, indicating the dominant role of the *flaA* product in flagellar biosynthesis and function (53); nevertheless, the presence of both gene products is necessary for maximal motility. The two structural genes are under the independent control of two different promotors, σ28 for *flaA* and σ54 for *flaB* (54). As with other genes under the control of σ54 promoters, *flaB* is subject to environmental regulation by pH, temperature, and concentrations of certain inorganic salts and divalent cations (54). Another gene, *flbA*, a homolog of *lcr* genes in *Yersinia*, may be involved in flagellar assembly and export because mutants deficient in its product are not motile (55).

Unlike the necessity for motility, the role of adherence to epithelial cells in *C. jejuni* pathogenesis is less clear-cut. Adherence has been assessed in a variety of tissue culture systems, and in general a pattern of diffuse adherence may be seen (56–58). The ability of *C. jejuni* strains to adhere to HeLa cells has been correlated with the severity of clinical infection in one study (58). Flagellation appears to enhance adherence, perhaps only by bringing the bacterial cells in contact with the mucosa, or the flagellae may be adhesins per se (56). However, Fla⁻ cells may adhere, especially if artificial motility is provided.

PATHOLOGY

From biopsies and occasional autopsies, it is evident that *C. jejuni* causes an acute inflammatory enteritis (59). Both the colon and the small intestine may be involved, but it is not clear as to which is the predominant site (60,61). Involved tissue shows infiltration of the lamina propria with neutrophils and mononuclear cells; edema is common and eosinophils also may be present. The inflammatory lesions may cause a cryptitis; and the presence of crypt abscesses has been mistaken for ulcerative colitis (60,61). Occasionally granulomata may be present and can mimic Crohn's disease (62). The mucosal epithelium also is disrupted with decreased mucus production, abnormal architecture of the epithelial glands, and occasionally ulceration. The findings are nonspecific; there are no pathognomonic features but trained pathologists should be able to distinguish infectious from idiopathic (inflammatory bowel disease) colitis (62). After appropriate antibiotic therapy, the lesions usually resolve within several weeks. Considering the pathology, the finding of leukocytes and erythrocytes commonly in fecal specimens from affected persons is not surprising (63,64).

Examination of tissues for organisms has not yielded an abundance of findings. The best data are from experimental infections of nonhuman primates, on which electron microscopy showed invasion of *C. jejuni* into epithelial cells (65). Other animal models generally support this notion, but owing to the paucity of organisms, the issue is not completely resolved. In a rabbit model, the organisms are taken up by M cells, but whether this represents nonspecific antigenic sampling or the usual route of invasion is not known (66).

TOXINS

A cholera-like enterotoxin produced by *C. jejuni* strains *in vitro* has been found by some investigators (67–69), but in other laboratories this activity could not be reproduced (70,71). Furthermore, analysis of fecal specimens from persons with *C. jejuni* enteritis did not reveal enterotoxic activity (72), and unlike for cholera or infections with enterotoxigenic (LT-producing) *E. coli*, affected persons do not produce serum antibodies to the putative toxin. Thus more than 10 years after its initial description, there is uncertainty as to whether the cholera-like enterotoxin of *C. jejuni* actually exists. Finally, since the predominant pathology is that of an inflammatory enteritis, the biological relevance of an enterotoxin, if present, would be limited. A cytolethal distending toxin (73) also has been described, but its role in pathogenesis is uncertain.

Conversely, cytotoxin activity would be more relevant to the pathology observed and several candidates have been described (74,75). Analysis of cultures for Shiga-like toxins have shown that a minority of strains produce a cytolethal toxin that is specifically neutralized by antiserum to *E. coli* shiga-like toxin 1 (SLT-1) (74). However, this activity is produced *in vitro* at very low titer (74), and fecal filtrates from infected persons and controls show no greater difference in cytotoxicity (72). Other cytotoxic activities may be present in *in vitro* culture supernatants but their biological relevance is uncertain.

TISSUE INVASION

Although apparently less common than *Salmonella* enteritis, *C. jejuni* infection can result in bacteremia (76,77). This phenomenon suggests that, at least for a subgroup

of strains, tissue invasion represents a part of the pathogenetic mechanism. Several investigations of *in vitro* invasion of tissue culture cell lines indicate that invasion occurs (78–80). However, the invasivity is low compared to other known enteroinvasive organisms. Since *C. jejuni* is a fastidious organism, lack of high-titer invasion *in vitro* is not surprising. It has been suggested that invasion of epithelial cells requires microtubule-dependent endocytosis mechanisms (81) rather than the microfilament-dependent mechanisms used by other enteric pathogens. After invasion of epithelial cells, or after passage of *C. jejuni* in ileal loops (82), proteins that are not expressed *in vitro* have been observed.

HOST RESPONSE

Antigens

Following *C. jejuni* infections there is a humoral response to a variety of *C. jejuni* proteins and to its lipopolysaccharide (LPS). The response to the LPS is both species-specific and type-specific (83). The anti-LPS response is important because type O19 shows antigenic cross-reactivity with host glycolipids; this may be a part of the basis of the pathogenesis of Guillain–Barré syndrome after O19 infections (84). Other important antigens include those of the flagellar proteins, the major outer membrane protein (a porin), and a group of antigens of approximately 28–32 kDa in size. One of these, PEB1, a conserved antigen among *C. jejuni* and *C. coli* strains to which most affected persons seroconvert (85), has been identified as a major adhesin to epithelial cells (86). This molecule may be a vaccine candidate.

Humoral Responses

Persons infected with *C. jejuni* develop both serum (50,87) and intestinal antibodies (88). The serum responses are in IgA, IgG, and IgM; they peak within 2–4 weeks and then rapidly decline (50,87). Hypogammaglobulinemic patients develop prolonged and severe infections, which they often cannot clear (see below); this phenomenon illustrates the central role of the humoral response in control of *C. jejuni* infections. In developing countries, where *C. jejuni* infections are hyperendemic and recurrent exposure occurs, healthy persons show a progressive increase in serum IgA (30,89). IgG responses rise in early childhood and then decline after high levels of IgA have been reached.

Cellular Responses

Little is known about the cellular immune response to *C. jejuni* infections. However, the increased frequency of this infection in persons infected with human immunodeficiency virus (HIV) (90) suggests that cell-mediated immunity also is important in determining whether or not an infection is clinically apparent. In HIV-infected patients, *C. jejuni* infections also may be recurrent, but this phenomenon may correlate with acquired hypogammaglobulinemia as well (91). In the presence of serum, *C. jejuni* induces a superoxide response by phagocytic cells (88), although intracellular survival has been reported (92).

Immunity

Most *C. jejuni* strains are susceptible to the nonspecific complement-mediated bactericidal activity present in normal human serum (93). This may help explain why bacteremia is uncommon except in immunodeficient hosts (94,95). Occasional strains are serum-resistant and have been isolated from cerebrospinal fluid of patients with meningitis (96).

There is an increasing body of evidence that specific immunity to intestinal *C. jejuni* infection may be acquired. Volunteer studies indicate that short-term immunity to homologous rechallenge occurs (50,88). In developing countries in which infection is common in early childhood, infection rates decline with age (33). Importantly, the case-to-infection ratio (32) as well as the duration and magnitude of convalescent carriage (31) also declines with age. These both are correlates of intestinal phase immunity. Studies of colony-raised nonhuman primates show similar phenomena (97). The basis of immunity is not known, but the serum IgA response may reflect this (30,89). Despite the marked heterogeneity of *C. jejuni* serotypes, the development of immunity under natural conditions implies that conserved antigens are present and that development of a vaccine is feasible. However, work on vaccine development currently is at an early stage.

CLINICAL ASPECTS

Incubation Period

In human volunteer studies, mean incubation periods were just under 3 days (68 hr) from ingestion of *C. jejuni*

to the onset of fever, and just under 4 days (88.5 hr) to the onset of diarrhea (50). With a more infective strain reported mean periods to the onset of diarrhea and fever were 53 and 67 hr, respectively. However, the range of incubation periods recorded in individual volunteers was 32 hr–7 days. Analysis of reports of 17 point source outbreaks of *Campylobacter* enteritis gave mean incubation periods ranging from 1.5 to 5.0 days (overall mean 3.2 days), with an extreme range of 18 hr–8 days among approximately 1700 individual victims.

Description of Illness

Campylobacter enteritis is essentially an acute diarrheal disease (Fig. 1) that in any one patient is clinically indistinguishable from that caused by *Salmonella*, *Shigella*, or another bacterial enteropathogen, although certain differences are evident when groups of patients are compared. The mean frequencies of the principal features of *Campylobacter* enteritis, summarized in Table 1, are derived from surveys of community outbreaks, which included patients who did not seek medical advice. Surveys of hospital patients show higher proportions with fever (63% vs. 53%), vomiting (28% vs. 15%), and blood in their stools (31% vs. 14%).

Prodrome

The illness usually starts abruptly with abdominal cramps and diarrhea, but about one third of patients suffer a prodromal period of fever, headache, dizziness, myalgia, and other nonspecific influenza-like symptoms lasting from a few hours to a few days. Prodromal symptoms appear to be associated with more severe illness, being reported in 50% of patients attending hospital (98), whereas 30% is a more typical figure for patients in the community (99). Rigors were found in 22% of patients in three surveys (63,100,101). Temperatures exceeding 40°C have been observed uncommonly [4% of patients (102)]

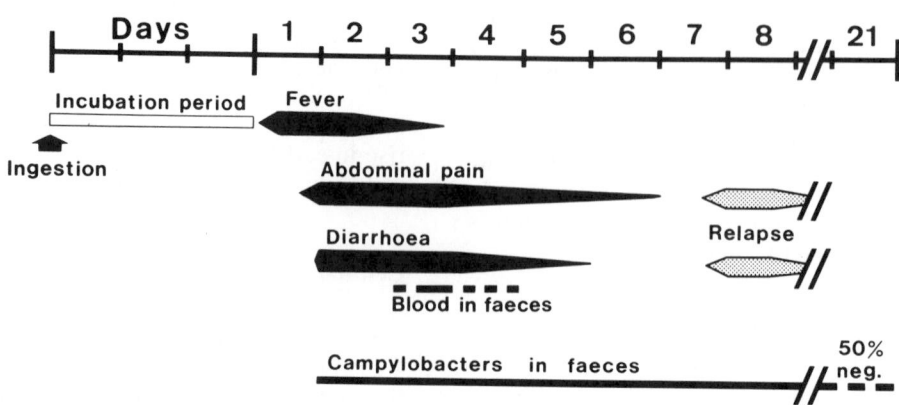

FIG. 1. Diagram illustrating the typical course of *Campylobacter* enteritis. (From ref. 9a, with permission.)

TABLE 1. *Frequency (percentage) of clinical features of* Campylobacter *enteritis derived from surveys of community outbreaks*[a]

	Diarrhea (44)	Abdominal pain (43)	Fever (42)	Headache (35)	Myalgia (8)	Vomiting (34)	Blood in feces (11)
Mean	86	78	53	39	40	15[b]	14
Range	27–100	39–100[c]	6–90	0–72	27–59	0–44	0.5–32

[a] Numbers in parentheses are numbers of outbreaks from which data are taken.
[b] Excluding waterborne outbreaks (see text).
[c] 39% recorded in nursery outbreak affecting children aged 1–5 years; lowest figure in patients old enough to complain of abdominal pain, 48%.

and may be associated with delirium in adults or convulsions in children. Some patients exhibit meningismus (103,104).

Gastrointestinal Symptoms

Abdominal pain is usually the first gastrointestinal symptom to appear, and tends to be more severe and last longer in *Campylobacter* enteritis than *Salmonella* enteritis (105). Although usually colicky and periumbilical, it may become continuous and radiate to the right iliac fossa, with the result that some patients end up under the surgeon's knife for suspected appendicitis (see below). In about 10% of patients the illness does not go beyond this stage and diarrhea is absent or slight. This pattern of illness has featured prominently in some school outbreaks: 30% of cases in a British boarding school involved pain without diarrhea (106) and in a Japanese school 83% of children were reported as having fever, 63% with abdominal pain, but only 27% with diarrhea (107). Nevertheless, diarrhea is usually the main complaint and it ranges from a few loose movements to profuse prostrating watery diarrhea. At least 50% of patients attending emergency rooms have ten or more bowel movements per day (60,63,100,108,109), but diarrhea may be less intense than that seen with *Salmonella* or *Shigella* diarrhea. However, the presence of blood in stools or bleeding per rectum is more frequent in *Campylobacter* than *Salmonella* or *Shigella* infection (64,110). If blood appears in stools, it is usually on or after the second day of diarrhea.

Although nausea is common, vomiting is not a major feature of *Campylobacter* infection. Analysis of 34 food- and milkborne outbreaks of *Campylobacter* enteritis show that on average only 15% of affected persons vomit (Table 1). Interestingly, the equivalent figure for seven waterborne outbreaks is significantly higher at 42%. A possible explanation is that undetected Norwalk-like viruses were also present in some of the waterborne outbreaks.

Resolution follows after a few days, but abdominal pain or discomfort often persists for longer, and short relapses of diarrhea have been reported in 15% to 25% of hospital patients (63,109,111). Any injudicious loading of the stomach during recovery is likely to precipitate a sharp return of symptoms. Weight loss of at least 5 kg is not unusual during the course of illness.

Skin rashes, notably urticaria appearing a few days after onset of illness, have occasionally been reported in association with *Campylobacter* enteritis (112–115). Some 10% of boys had urticaria toward the end of a large school outbreak of *Campylobacter* enteritis (113) and unspecified rash was listed as a feature in 2% of patients in a milkborne outbreak (116). Erythema nodosum is an uncommon late complication (see below).

Duration of Illness and Morbidity

The illness usually lasts 4–5 days. An analysis of nine outbreaks affecting about 1500 persons shows a mean of 4.6 days, but in two outbreaks 20% and 33% of victims were ill for more than 7 days (117,118). In a recent Norwegian study of 135 sporadic cases the mean duration of symptoms was 14.6 days (range 2–67 days) (102). There is an extraordinary case of a young man who apparently had *Campylobacter* diarrhea for 17 years; *C. jejuni* was isolated from his stools and he was completely cured by a course of erythromycin (119). Death is rare and usually due as much to underlying disease as to *Campylobacter* infection (76,120).

The proportion of patients admitted to hospital in nine community outbreaks ranged from 0.5% (121) to 22% (41) (mean 4.9%), and in four studies of sporadic cases they ranged from 9.4% to 32% (27,102,110,122). There is conflicting evidence as to the relative severity of symptoms due to *C. jejuni* and *C. coli* (123,124).

Convalescent Excretion of Campylobacters

The proportion of patients excreting campylobacters in their feces after the illness falls exponentially with time. Early studies showed that about 50% and 85% of patients are culture-negative after 3 and 5 weeks, respectively. Culture methods have since improved and in a more recent study the mean excretion period was 37.6 days (max. 69 days) (102). Long-term carriage has only been reported in patients with immune deficiency (see below). As discussed above, in developing countries, excretion is brief (33).

Campylobacter Enteritis in Children

In general, prepubertal children tolerate *Campylobacter* infection better than adults, but certain features are more pronounced. Fever is more common, except in infants, and this may be accompanied by convulsions (125–131). In a milkborne outbreak affecting an estimated 2500 children, 9 were admitted to hospital because of grand mal seizures; 7 had suffered a febrile seizure on a previous occasion (121,125). The average age of these children was higher than normally associated with febrile seizures, which raises the possibility that a neurotoxin may play a part, an idea supported by the fact that some children with *Campylobacter* enteritis experience hallucinations (126). A single case of acute encephalopathy associated with *Campylobacter* infection in a previously healthy 6-year-old boy has been reported (132).

The passage of blood via the rectum is more commonly seen in children than adults. In one series, 92% of children, mostly infants under the age of 1 year, admitted to a children's hospital with *Campylobacter* infection had frank blood in their stools (126). By contrast, abdominal pain and fever are less evident in young children, although about 50% vomit (126,133; PA Holt, unpublished). In developing countries, watery diarrhea is a more prominent feature of infection in children than in developed countries, but dehydration is less common than with enterotoxigenic *Escherichia coli* or rotavirus infection.

Neonatal Infection

Neonatal *Campylobacter* infections are usually sporadic and acquired at the time of birth from a mother who is excreting campylobacters in her feces—sometimes, but not always, with a history of recent diarrhea (133,134). Nosocomial outbreaks in neonatal units occur (135–139). In general, neonatal infection with *C. jejuni* or *C. coli* is surprisingly benign, although there are particular risks and exceptions. As the passage of blood per rectum, often in the absence of diarrhea and fever, is a common presenting feature, clinicians can be misled into thinking the infant has intussusception and laparotomy is performed (140). Severe illness with constitutional symptoms occasionally precedes or accompanies the passage of blood via rectum and mimics necrotizing enterocolitis (131). Systemic spread of infection rarely can cause meningitis (141). In a nosocomial outbreak in a maternity unit, 11 newborn infants developed meningitis due to the same serogroup (Penner O18) *C. jejuni* strain (136), which has been linked with systemic infection (76). Most cases of neonatal *Campylobacter* meningitis are caused by *C. fetus* (142). Hemolytic anemia requiring blood transfusion in a 3½-week-old boy with vomiting and diarrhea was believed to be due to *C. jejuni* (143).

Premature Labor and Septic Abortion

The predilection of campylobacters for the placentas of sheep, in which they commonly cause septic abortion, is not frequently paralleled in humans. Among 20 cases of *Campylobacter* abortion, half were due to *C. jejuni* or *C. coli* and half to *C. fetus* (144), but cases continue to be reported (145–147). A woman with acquired agammaglo-

bulinemia and *Campylobacter* diarrhea suffered recurrent early abortion (148). Placentitis probably arises from hematogenous spread from the gut. The few live-born infants often die soon after birth. Although septic abortion due to *Campylobacter* is apparently rare, it can easily be overlooked, unless specific cultures are done. Nevertheless, it is clear that most women who develop *Campylobacter* infection during pregnancy have no undue consequences (146,149,150).

ACUTE STAGE COMPLICATIONS

Colitis

The colon is affected in most patients with *Campylobacter* infection, but it is useful to consider *Campylobacter* colitis separately, as in some patients colitic symptoms dominate from the outset and mimic an acute attack of nonspecific inflammatory bowel disease (IBD) (60,61,98,151–158). Because the treatment in each condition is different it is important to make a correct diagnosis, especially as many patients with *Campylobacter* enteritis are young and at an age at which acute ulcerative colitis is unusually severe. Nonetheless, intercurrent *Campylobacter* infection can precipitate an acute exacerbation of IBD (151,152). The distinction of *Campylobacter* colitis from IBD is not easy, since findings overlap (62,159). Endoscopic appearances range from normal, through mild nonspecific colitis with intact epithelium, to mucosal granularity, friability, spontaneous bleeding, and patchy aphthous-type ulceration. Active colitis has been observed at least as far as the splenic flexure and one patient had ulcers up to 3 × 5 cm and "cobblestone" mucosa, albeit with "skip areas" of normal mucosa (157). The histological appearance on colonic biopsy is indistinguishable from *Salmonella* or *Shigella* colitis, but these may be distinguished from those of IBD (62). However, there are difficulties, especially in patients who have been ill for more than a week (98), and mistakes occur (62). *Campylobacter* antigens have been found in the mucosa of infected patients by immunohistochemical methods and IgG-containing plasma cells in the mucosa are increased in patients with IBD but not *Campylobacter* colitis (59). There is no evidence that *Campylobacter* colitis initiates IBD (161–163).

Toxic megacolon complicating *Campylobacter* colitis has been reported in three patients, all women aged 23–83 years (164–166). Such cases are best treated conservatively with an appropriate antibiotic unless there is perforation of the bowel. *Campylobacter* colitis including chronic colitis also has been described in children (167,168). Examples are pancolitis, diagnosed radiographically, in a 14-year-old boy (153), fatal infection superimposed on Crohn's disease in a 4-year-old girl (169), and bowel obstruction, colon distension and stasis, and aphthous ulceration in a 7-year-old boy (170).

Acute Appendicitis and "Pseudoappendicitis"

Campylobacters have been isolated from acutely inflamed appendices (171–174) and immunohistochemical and electron microscopic evidence of *Campylobacter* infection has been found in 3% of appendectomy specimens studied retrospectively (175). Although *Campylobacter*-associated appendicitis is seemingly rare and possibly a distinct disease, it is probably underreported, as surgically removed appendices are not usually cultured and when they are, specific culture for campylobacters may not be performed.

Patients with genuine *Campylobacter* appendicitis are far outnumbered by patients with pseudoappendicitis, in whom the symptoms of acute appendicitis are simulated by the severity of abdominal pain in *Campylobacter* enteritis, especially when it is present before the onset of diarrhea. Abdominal tenderness as well as pain in the right iliac fossa may be present, but true rebound tenderness and guarding are absent in uncomplicated disease. A survey of 251 children admitted to a surgical unit with suspected appendicitis showed that 6 (2.4%) had *Campylobacter* infection: 3 had acute appendicitis but 3 had mesenteric adenitis with normal appendices (171). In a similar survey of 533 older children and adults, campylobacters were isolated from 15 (2.8%), only 1 of whom had slight histological evidence of acute appendicitis; the others had ileocecitis and mesenteric adenitis diagnosed by ultrasonography (176). Pseudoappendicitis is most commonly diagnosed in children aged 6–15 years.

Estimates of the percentage of patients with *Campylobacter* enteritis who are referred with suspected appendicitis differ according to the population studied. They range from 0.1% of cases in a large milkborne outbreak in the UK (121), through 0.27% of routine laboratory reports in the UK (unpublished), to 2.7% and 5.3% of persons who are hospitalized because of their symptoms (109,177). An increased awareness of *Campylobacter* infection has possibly reduced the incidence of laparotomy in such patients.

Other Intestinal Problems

There is a single report of massive life-threatening hemorrhage from an ulcer in the terminal ileum of a previously healthy 24-year-old nurse with *Campylobacter* enteritis (178); emergency hemicolectomy was performed. Two patients with long-established ileostomies, both constructed after total colectomy for IBD, suffered extensive ulceration of their stomas apparently as a direct consequence of *Campylobacter* infection (179,180). Ulceration was thought to have been caused by partial strangulation resulting from gross edema and congestion. Ulceration lasted several weeks in both patients, but healing was complete. The mucosa of a continent ileostomy (Kock pouch) was observed to be friable and inflamed in another patient with *Campylobacter* enteritis (181). *C. jejuni* and *Citrobacter freundii* were isolated from a perirectal abscess in a 64-year-old woman 3 weeks after she had suffered diarrhea presumed to have been *Campylobacter* enteritis (182).

Cholecystitis

There are several reports of patients with acute, or acute on chronic, *Campylobacter* cholecystitis (183–186). Some patients gave a history of diarrhea shortly before they developed cholecystitis symptoms, but others did not. *Campylobacter* infection of the biliary tract is apparently uncommon; campylobacters were not found in over 280 cholecystectomy samples that were specifically cultured (184).

Hepatitis

Mildly raised serum transaminase concentrations have been found in 14% to 25% of *Campylobacter* enteritis patients admitted to hospital (98,109,111), but clinical hepatitis is rare. "Jaundice" and/or "hepatitis" are recorded in several of the routine reports of *Campylobacter* enteritis submitted in England and Wales during the last 10 years (unpublished). There are more detailed reports of five patients. A previously healthy 48-year-old man had *Campylobacter* bacteremia and hepatitis with necrosis and polymorphonuclear cell infiltration (187). A 48-year-old alcoholic man had diarrhea, bacteremia, and cholestatic hepatitis with lymphohistiocytic infiltration of portal tracts (188). A 52-year-old man was shown to have nonspecific reactive hepatitis with focal necrosis at the same time as a *Campylobacter* infection (189). Two young men had obvious clinical hepatitis with deranged liver function tests evident after a week of *Campylobacter* diarrhea; liver biopsy was not performed, but both men had enlarged livers, palpable below the costal margin, which shrank after antibiotic treatment (190). In rhesus monkeys experimentally infected with *C. jejuni*, the liver and gallbladder are the most consistently colonized extraintestinal sites (191). Some strains of *C. jejuni* may produce hepatotoxic factors; focal necrotic lesions of the liver with mononuclear cell infiltration were produced in mice by both experimental infection and the injection of extracts of whole-cell lysates (192).

Pancreatitis

Several cases of pancreatitis complicating *Campylobacter* enteritis have been described (193–196). In a Finnish study of hospital patients with *Campylobacter* enteritis, 11 (22%) of 50 were considered to have pancreatitis on the grounds of raised serum amylase or lipase values (109), but in another smaller series of patients, none had raised values (197). The pathogenic mechanism by which campylobacters cause pancreatitis is unknown.

Peritonitis

Campylobacter peritonitis, mostly due to *C. jejuni*, in patients on continuous ambulatory peritoneal dialysis (CAPD) has been well reported (198,199). Most patients are elderly, and diarrhea but not bacteremia usually precedes the onset of peritonitis. In most cases the infection was initially controlled by empirical intraperitoneal antimicrobial treatment, such as an aminoglycoside or vancomycin, but patients given sulfamethoxazole-trimethoprim or cefuroxime did not respond until treatment was changed to an appropriate agent. It is unknown as to whether the bacteria seed the peritoneum from the bloodstream, by transluminal migration from the gut, or by transfer to catheter fittings from the skin or other extraneous sources. *Campylobacter* peritonitis in patients on CAPD is probably underdiagnosed because typical protocols for the culture of CAPD fluid do not normally provide ideal conditions for isolating campylobacters. Diarrhea is the feature that should alert clinicians and microbiologists to the possibility of campylobacters in peritoneal fluid, particularly if no organisms are seen on Gram-stained smears—the usual finding in such cases. Spontaneous *Campylobacter* peritonitis is rare.

Urinary Tract Infections

Acute cystitis (200) and prostatitis (201) due to *Campylobacter* have been described. A history of diarrhea may not be present. As with other focal infections due to *Campylobacter* species, this is probably underdiagnosed.

Bacteremia and Focal Extraintestinal Infection

If rigors signify bacteremia, then bacteremia occurs in about 2% of all patients with bacteriologically confirmed *Campylobacter* infection, or about 20% of hospitalized *Campylobacter*-infected patients. Yet analysis of *Campylobacter* reports over 11 years in the UK showed a mean bacteremia rate of only 1.5 per 1000 infections (76). There are three explanations for these differences. First, blood cultures are seldom taken from patients with acute gastroenteritis, and virtually never at the time patients are having rigors early in the disease. Second, the sensitivity of methods for detecting campylobacters in blood is low. On the other hand, serial blood cultures on 30 ill volunteers were all negative, although only 11 had fever and there was no mention of rigors (50). Third, bacteremia due to species other than *C. fetus* is probably in actuality much less frequent than *Salmonella* bacteremia. In the UK survey, bacteremia rates rose steeply in patients over 55 years of age to a maximum rate of 5.9 per 1000 in patients aged 65 years or more (76); the lowest rate of 0.3 per 1000 was in children aged 1–4 years (Fig. 2). Of the bacteremic patients, 29% had immunodeficiency or another underlying disease. Bacteremia rates were nearly twice as high in males than females. *C. jejuni* strains belonging to serogroups O4 and O18 (Penner) were more frequent among blood than fecal isolates.

Bacteremia carries a risk of focal infection anywhere in the body, but in the case of campylobacters this is rare. With the exception of septic abortion, focal infection is virtually limited to patients with immune deficiency or a predisposing lesion (Table 2). Most adult cases of *Campylobacter* meningitis are due to *C. fetus*, although in the early reports it is not always possible to identify the responsible species (77). Focal infections are not always preceded by diarrhea.

Hemolytic-Uremic Syndrome

Nine patients have been reported, five of them children under the age of 5 years, who developed hemolytic-uremic

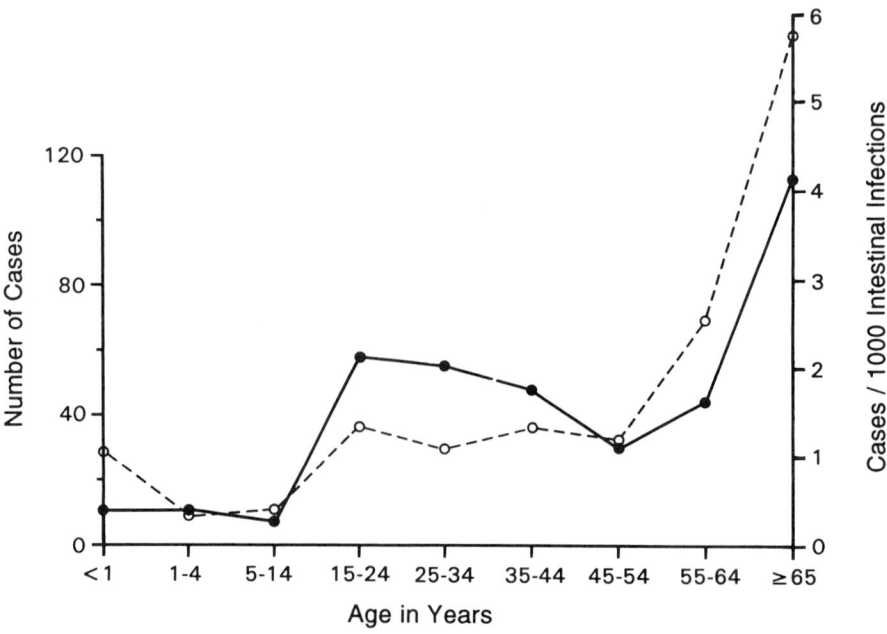

FIG. 2. Distribution of *Campylobacter* bacteremia cases by age in England and Wales 1981–1991. ○- - - -○, number of cases (*n* = 374); ●——● cases per 1000 intestinal infections. (From ref. 76, with permission.)

TABLE 2. *Focal infections due to* Campylobacter jejuni

Focus of infection	Age (y)/sex of patient	Predisposing condition	Organism	Ref.
Spontaneous peritonitis	56 M; 76 M	Alcoholic liver disease	*C. jejuni*	202–204
	46 M		*C. coli*	
	83 M	Liver cirrhosis from congestive cardiac failure	*C. jejuni/coli*	205
Chest wall abscess	72 F	Mastectomy scar, postirradiation	*C. jejuni*	206
Osteitis of foot	57 M	Site of previously removed histiocytoma	*C. jejuni*	207
Prosthetic hip sepsis	60 M	AIDS	*C. jejuni*	208
Septic arthritis of knee	51 F	Rheumatoid arthritis	*C. jejuni*	209
Septic arthritis of shoulder	90 M	NK	*Campylobacter* sp.	Unpublished[a]
Acute bursitis	81 M	Chronic bursitis	*C. jejuni*	210
Meningitis (nonneonatal)	34 M	Longstanding ventricular shunt	*C. jejuni*	211
Subdural sepsis	2½ F	Previous hemispherectomy	*C. jejuni*	212
Empyema	70 M	NK	*C. jejuni*	Unpublished[a]
	52 M	NK	*C. coli*	Unpublished[a]

NK, not known.
[a]Public Health Laboratory Service, United Kingdom.

syndrome (HUS) during the course of *Campylobacter* enterocolitis (213–220). The signs of HUS became apparent 3–10 days after the onset of bowel symptoms, except in one patient in whom the interval was 1 month. Frank blood was present at some time in the stools of most patients and the course of the disease was generally typical of HUS. Most patients recovered without apparent sequelae, but a 4-month-old infant in Bangladesh died (218). The possibility that some or all of these cases were due to coincident infection with verotoxin-producing *E. coli* or *Shigella* species cannot be excluded.

Nephritis

Mesangial IgA glomerulonephritis has been recorded in two patients, both males, aged 15 and 26 years (221; Skirrow, *unpublished data*). In both cases, hematuria was evident within 2 days of the onset of diarrhea. Acute glomerulonephritis may occur within a week of the onset of *Campylobacter* enteritis. In an 18-year-old man the disease was mild and renal biopsy was not performed (222). A 33-year-old man required hemodialysis but recovered completely; renal biopsy showed moderately severe diffuse proliferative endocapillary glomerulonephritis (223). A 5-year-old girl developed pulmonary hemorrhage and anemia with glomerulonephritis (Goodpasture's syndrome) 3–4 weeks after the onset of diarrhea (224). Renal biopsy showed immune complex–mediated crescentic glomerulonephritis, and *C. jejuni* antigen was identified in the glomeruli. She eventually suffered progressive renal failure. Self-limited tubulointerstitial nephritis was reported in a previously healthy 20-year-old man 8 days after an attack of *Campylobacter* enteritis (225).

Cardiorespiratory Disease

Two patients, both young men, are reported as having had infectious myocarditis arising 7 and 3 days after the

onset of *C. jejuni* enteritis (226,227). Transient atrial fibrillation in three *Campylobacter* enteritis patients, all over 50 years old, has also been reported (228). Endocarditis was diagnosed but not bacteriologically proven 2 weeks after the onset of *C. jejuni* enteritis (with reactive arthritis) in a young man (226). Mild bronchopneumonia has been reported in elderly patients during the acute stages of *Campylobacter* enteritis, but there was no direct evidence of pulmonary *Campylobacter* infection (229). Similarly, malnourished infants may develop pneumonia during *Campylobacter* infection.

LATE ONSET COMPLICATIONS

Reactive Arthritis and Reiter's Syndrome

Reactive (aseptic) arthritis is now a well-recognized sequelum to *Campylobacter* enterocolitis (230,231), and the syndrome appears no different from that following *Salmonella* or *Yersinia* enterocolitis. Pain and swelling of the joints typically appears 1–2 weeks (mean 11 days, range 3–42 days) after the onset of bowel symptoms (231). Ankles, knees, wrists, and the small joints of the hands and feet are most commonly affected, often in a migratory fashion. The arthritis, which may be incapacitating, usually lasts for 1–21 weeks (occasionally for as long as a year), but complete resolution is the rule. Conjunctivitis is common and full Reiter's syndrome has been observed in up to one fifth of patients with arthritis (231–233). Acute erosions of the hamate bone of the wrist and distal ends of the clavicles have been reported in one patient (234). Persons possessing the HLA B27 antigen have a strong predisposition to reactive arthritis, constituting about 60% of patients with this complication. The incidence of reactive arthritis depends on the prevalence of HLA B27 in a population, but 1% is an average figure. An incidence of 5% in hospital patients has been reported in Scandinavia where about 14% of the population are HLA B27–positive, but figures ranging from 0% to 1.7% have been found in community outbreaks of *Campylobacter* enteritis (37,118,121,235–237).

A long-term follow-up of a *C. jejuni* foodborne outbreak in Sweden suggested that nonspecific rheumatic disorders might be a relatively frequent sequel to infection. Four of the 66 infected persons, all of whom initially had asymptomatic infection, suffered chronic or relapsing rheumatic symptoms beginning 3–8 months after exposure and persisting for 5 years (238). However, in the absence of a control group, the significance of this finding is questionable. There also is a report of a tenuous association between *Campylobacter* infection and "irritable hip" in three boys aged 5–10 years (239).

Uveitis

Uveitis without arthritis has been reported in two patients with *Campylobacter* enteritis, both middle-aged women. One had hypogammaglobulinemia (240); the other had previously been healthy, and conjunctivitis preceded the uveitis by several weeks (241). Evidence of *Campylobacter* infection in Behçet's disease has been reported from Turkey, but the link may not be significant (242).

Guillain–Barré Syndrome

Reactive arthritis is the most frequent of the late onset "immunological" complications of *Campylobacter* enteritis, but Guillain–Barré syndrome (GBS), also known as postinfective polyneuronopathy or polyradiculopathy, is the most distressing and dangerous. The association had been reported in case reports since 1982 (243). Retrospective evidence of recent *Campylobacter* infection was found in 38% of a series of 56 Australian patients with GBS (244). Subsequent prospective studies in the UK and Japan confirmed this association with incidences of 14% (245), 35% (246), and 41% (247). Thus *Campylobacter* infection appears to be the most frequently identified antecedent event in GBS (248,249). A more recent retrospective case-control study of GBS patients in the USA gave an odds ratio for *Campylobacter* infection of 5.3 (95% CI 2.4–12.5) compared with controls and a conservatively estimated etiological fraction of 15% to 20% (250). Neurological symptoms appear 1–3 weeks after the onset of *Campylobacter* infection, which is usually manifested by diarrhea but is sometimes silent (247). Male patients outnumber female patients by 3:2, and persons with the HLA B35 antigen may be particularly associated with *Campylobacter*-induced GBS (249).

Five patients, all adults, had the Miller–Fisher variant of GBS, with external ophthalmoplegia, ataxia, and areflexia (251–254). A 12-year-old girl developed bilateral abducens paresis without any other neurological abnormality a few days after the onset of *Campylobacter* diarrhea (255).

The pathological processes operating in the disease are unknown, but there is evidence of immunological cross-reaction between certain *Campylobacter* antigens and peripheral nerve myelin proteins, which could trigger an autoimmune response (256). It is particularly significant that 10 of 12 *C. jejuni* strains isolated from a series of Japanese patients with GBS were of serogroup O19 (Penner), a serogroup found in less than 2% of sporadic cases of *Campylobacter* enteritis (247). Moreover, all of these O19 strains were of lectin type 8, whereas only 1 of 14 O19 strains from patients with sporadic enteritis were of this type. Strains of lectin type 8 are known to contain terminal β-N-acetylglucosamine residues in their cell surface. Recent work suggests that these particular LPS molecules may mimic host glycolipid structures (84).

Evidence of *Campylobacter* infection has also been found in patients with Chinese paralytic syndrome (257–259), a disorder similar to GBS (257), but the significance of this and its relation to GBS needs clarification (259).

Erythema Nodosum

Erythema nodosum associated with *Campylobacter* enteritis has been reported in five patients, all women (106,260–263). The lesions appeared within 1–2 weeks of onset of diarrhea and lasted 3–7 weeks. Terminal ileitis was present in one patient and her forearms and elbows were affected as well as her shins (260). Immune complex vasculitis with thrombophlebitis is described in a 51-year-old man (264).

Campylobacter Infection and Immune Deficiency

There are numerous reports of long-term carriage of campylobacters, sometimes with recurrent enteritis and bacteremia, in patients with immune deficiency (265). Hypogammaglobulinemia and AIDS are the two most commonly reported forms of immune deficiency. In a survey of 41 hypogammaglobulinemic patients, 5 were found to have experienced at least one episode of *C. jejuni* septicemia and 3 also had erysipelas-like cellulitis (266). Antimicrobial therapy is liable to fail, but success after initial failure has been achieved when combined with plasma infusions (266,267). Children with immunodeficiency are also prone to chronic *Campylobacter* infection (95).

Although no campylobacters were found in 36 patients with symptomatic HIV infection, including 27 with unexplained chronic diarrhea (268), the incidence of *Campylobacter* infection in such patients is much increased (90). When infection does arise the consequences can be severe and persistent (91,269).

LABORATORY DIAGNOSIS

Laboratory Diagnosis

A definitive diagnosis of *Campylobacter* enteritis can only be made by identifying campylobacters in a patient's stools. Therefore the laboratory plays an essential role both in the identification of individual patients and in the compilation of epidemiological statistics. Tests for *Campylobacter* should be included in all protocols for the examination of feces from patients being investigated for acute diarrhea; it is the most frequently identified pathogen.

Collection and Transport of Specimens

Feces in plain containers are satisfactory provided they are examined within a few hours of collection and preferably held in a refrigerator. Properly taken rectal swabs are also satisfactory, but they must be placed in a suitable semisolid transport medium. Transport medium should also be used for feces if a delay of more than a few hours is likely (270,271).

Microscopy and Direct Detection Methods

Simple methylene blue staining of wet or dried fecal smears is an easy way of detecting fecal leukocytes, which are present in 66% to 93% of *Campylobacter* enteritis cases (63,111,272–274). Some advocate using this method to select specimens for bacterial culture; they claim that very few patients with inflammatory bacterial diarrhea are missed if only feces containing leukocytes are cultured (273). It is also possible to identify campylobacters in fresh feces (voided within 2 hr) by dark field microscopy (275), or in dried smears stained with a strong stain such as carbol fuchsin. Compared with cultural methods, sensitivities range from 36% (dark field) to 44% to 94% for stained smears (272,276–278). Such methods can be useful in office laboratories where access to a full microbiological laboratory service is limited.

Detection of campylobacters by DNA probes and PCR (See chapter by Tompkins and Michelson) amplification show considerable promise, but are as yet insufficiently developed to be used for the direct detection of organisms in feces.

Culture

The isolation of campylobacters by cultural methods remains the mainstay of bacteriological diagnosis. Special dedicated media and cultural conditions are necessary. The details of these are beyond the scope of this chapter and are available elsewhere (279,280), but briefly, fecal suspensions are plated out on a medium containing one or more selective antimicrobial agents and then incubated in sealed containers under increased CO_2 and reduced oxygen tension at 42–43°C (the optimum temperature for *C. jejuni*, *C. coli*, and *C. lari*). Growth may be visible after overnight incubation, but in many laboratories plates are read after 2 days incubation. Enrichment culture, which increases sensitivity but costs more and delays results by a day, is found to be worthwhile by some but not by others (280). Much depends on variables such as the freshness

of samples, the quality of primary plating medium, and the gaseous conditions. However, enrichment culture is essential for environmental and food samples.

Recently, interest has been renewed in filtration as a means of selecting campylobacters from mixed bacterial flora, the method by which they were first isolated from human feces (5). Campylobacters are small enough to migrate through 0.45- to 0.65-μm pore sized filters, whereas other bacteria are retained. Its advantage is that filtrates can be cultured on plain media without antimicrobial agents. Occasional strains of *C. jejuni* and *C. coli* and several other *Campylobacter* species are inhibited by conventional selective media and can only be isolated by the filtration method (see chapter by Mishu, Blaser, and Lastovica). On the other hand, the sensitivity of the method for most *C. jejuni* and *C. coli* strains is less than that for selective media, so that it cannot be used as the sole method of culture; to use both methods in parallel would substantially increase costs.

Identification and Typing of Isolates

Identification of a culture as a *Campylobacter* takes only moments, but species identification by traditional methods takes 1 or 2 more days. Testing for hippurate and indoxyl acetate hydrolysis, and for susceptibility to nalidixic acid and cephalothin, is simple and presumptively identifies the relevant species. Latex agglutination tests capable of giving rapid identification are commercially available, but their cost does not justify their routine use; it is not necessary to identify every isolate, only those where special clinical or epidemiological circumstances demand it. In such cases it may be desirable to identify the strain as precisely as possible. Biotyping, serotyping, phage typing, molecular typing, or a combination of these methods are all used to this end, but they are only available at reference or specialist laboratories. The general subject of *Campylobacter* isolation and identification has been fully reviewed elsewhere (280).

Serodiagnosis

Serodiagnosis may occasionally be of value in patients with suspected late complications of infection, such as reactive arthritis or Guillain–Barré syndrome, in whom stool cultures are negative because of antimicrobial treatment or the lapse of time. There are two sorts of test: (a) those that provide a general screen for *Campylobacter* infection by detecting antibody to *Campylobacter* antigens common to all strains of *C. jejuni* and *C. coli;* (b) those that screen for infection only with a specific strain. Examples of the first sort of test are the complement fixation test (CFT) (281), which is reliable but somewhat insensitive, and enzyme-linked immunosorbent assays (ELISA), which are more complex but permit different classes of antibody (IgA, IgM, IgG) to be measured (87,282). A bactericidal test was the first strain-specific test to be used successfully (281), but ELISA can also be used. In general, serological tests for *Campylobacter* are available only in reference laboratories, but the bactericidal test can be done in any well-equipped diagnostic laboratory provided a culture of the suspected infecting strain is available. The sort of circumstance when it could be of great value is that of a culture-negative patient with GBS, which is particularly associated with *C. jejuni* strains of serogroup O19. Lastly, a minority of patients with *Campylobacter* enteritis show serological cross-reactions with *Legionella pneumophila* antigens (283). It is not yet clear as to what antigens are responsible for this (284,285).

SPECIAL INVESTIGATIONS

Hematology

The erythrocyte sedimentation rate is usually raised. Mean values of 25–30 mm/hr with occasional values in excess of 100 mm/hr have been reported in surveys of hospital inpatients. Leukocyte counts are usually normal or only mildly raised (109). In several series of patients, mean counts of 7.9×10^9/L (108), 8.9×10^9/L (100), and 10.0×10^9/L (286) have been reported, but the particular feature that distinguished *Campylobacter* enteritis from other forms of acute diarrhea (except shigellosis) was a relatively high band form count (mean 15.1%), especially in the presence of a modest total leukocyte count (286).

Biochemistry

In the absence of dehydration, biochemical values in *Campylobacter* enteritis are normal, although in one study metabolic acidosis was detected in 14 (32%) of 44 hospital patients (109). Mildly raised serum transaminases have been reported in 14% to 25% of hospital patients (98,109,111) and slightly raised alkaline phosphatase values were found in 10% (111). In one study, elevated C-reactive protein concentrations were reported in all patients in the acute diarrheal stage of illness (109).

Radiography

Plain radiographs of the abdomen in severely affected patients may show dilated loops of intestine with fluid levels. Such changes were observed in 5 of 20 hospital patients (112), but in none of 14 patients in another hospital series (100). Contrast radiography is usually normal, but gross changes have been observed in severe infections: pancolitis (61,153); multiple aphthous type ulceration, in one case highly suggestive of Crohn's disease (170); right-sided colonic ulceration and dilatation (164); nodular mucosal thickening of the terminal ileum (260). In two patients barium enema suggested colonic carcinoma: in a 46-year-old woman, a 3- to 4-cm intrinsic mass on the lateral wall of the ascending colon opposite the ileocecal valve looked so like a carcinoma that hemicolectomy was performed, although subsequent histology showed only edema, congestion, and lymphoid hyperpla-

sia (287); the other patient had a narrowed segment 8–10 cm long in his distal transverse colon with mucosal irregularity, but it resolved completely after treatment with erythromycin (288). Graded compression ultrasonography was used successfully to distinguish *Campylobacter* ileocolitis from acute appendicitis by Puylaert and colleagues in the Netherlands (176,289).

TREATMENT

General Measures

Most patients with *Campylobacter* enteritis require no more than simple oral rehydration and electrolyte replacement as described in the chapter by Snyder. In our view patients in hospital need not be isolated. The low infectivity of campylobacters is well illustrated by the case of a man who developed severe *Campylobacter* enteritis and infectious hepatitis after falling into a tank of concentrated sewage; despite having profuse diarrhea for 19 days, there was no spread of *Campylobacter* infection to his attendant nurses, yet seven of them contracted hepatitis A (290).

Antimicrobial Therapy

Controlled trials of antimicrobial therapy given at the time of bacteriological diagnosis show no clear benefit in terms of shortening illness, although the excretion of campylobacters in the stools is sharply curtailed (291–294). This is not to say that antimicrobial treatment is never of clinical value. In two of the trials cited above (291,293), the average duration of illness before antimicrobials were started, i.e., the time taken for patients to consult a doctor and fecal samples to be tested, was 6 days, and in another it was 4.5 days (294). As the average duration of illness is no longer than this, it is not surprising that no clinical effect was apparent; indeed many patients were recovering by the time treatment was started. However, trials in which antimicrobials (erythromycin, ciprofloxacin, norfloxacin) were given empirically when patients first presented demonstrated a shortening of illness (295–298). In developing countries, trials of this sort have not shown benefit, but results were confounded by patients infected with multiple pathogens (299) or antibiotic-resistant campylobacters (300). There are also clear instances of clinical benefit from antimicrobial treatment, usually with erythromycin, in patients with severe or chronic illness, often where other measures have failed (61,151,170,288).

Thus, appropriate antimicrobial therapy is worth giving if patients are still acutely ill at the time of bacteriological diagnosis or if they have complications, systemic infection, immunosuppression, or some other special circumstance. The ability of antimicrobials to eliminate campylobacters from the stools can be used to control the spread of infection where there is special risk. Erythromycin was used successfully in this way to control a persistent outbreak in a day nursery in Israel (301).

In Vitro Susceptibilities

First, campylobacters are inherently resistant to trimethoprim and most cephalosporins, except cefotaxime, ceftazidime, and cefpirone, to which they are moderately susceptible (302). Some activity is shown by penicillins, of which ampicillin and amoxicillin are the most active, although minimum inhibitory concentrations (MICs) are usually too high for them to be of much clinical use (MIC_{90} 15 mg/L, average of 16 surveys), even in combination with clavulanic acid, which neutralizes the β-lactamase produced by many strains (303). Some *C. coli* strains are sensitive to ampicillin (304).

The most consistently active agents are macrolides, quinolones, aminoglycosides, and nitrofurans, which are considered below (302,305–307). Tetracycline and chloramphenicol are also active and are occasionally useful when other agents are contraindicated because of strain resistance or idiosyncratic responses in patients. Almost all strains are sensitive to chloramphenicol, but up to 25% may be resistant to tetracyclines (plasmid-mediated). Nitroimidazole derivatives are active against some strains, but many are resistant (308).

Erythromycin

Erythromycin remains the antimicrobial of choice for the treatment of *Campylobacter* enteritis. It has low toxicity, a fairly narrow spectrum of activity, and relatively low cost. Most *Campylobacter* strains are inhibited by 2.7 mg/L (Table 3). Strains can develop high degrees of resistance, but rates are generally low (Table 4) and they have changed little over the past 15 years (307,309–313). The highest recorded resistance rate is 67%, which was found in an orphanage in Thailand (300). Erythromycin resistance is far more frequent in *C. coli* than *C. jejuni;* in fact, almost all erythromycin resistant strains in developed countries are *C. coli* (311,314–316). The use of the macrolide tylosin for growth promotion in swine, the principal host of *C. coli*, is thought to be the reason for this. The resistance mechanisms of erythromycin resistance in campylobacters are discussed by Taylor (317).

TABLE 3. *Susceptibility of* Campylobacter jejuni *and C. coli to commonly used antimicrobial agents*

Agent	No. of studies	Mic$_{90}$ in mg/L Mean value	Range
Erythromycin	23	2.7	0.5–8.0
Ciprofloxacin	9	0.5	0.2–1.0
Gentamicin	15	0.5	0.2–1.6
Chloramphenicol	16	5.8	1.8–12.5
Furazolidone	6	0.4	<0.1–0.8
Tetracycline	12[a]	0.8[a]	0.1–2.0[a]
Doxycycline	12[a]	0.4[a]	0.1–1.0[a]

Data taken from published studies.
[a] MIC$_{50}$.

TABLE 4. *Erythromycin resistance rates (%) among campylobacters (C. jejuni and C. coli combined) isolated from human sources around the world*

Canada	0.6–1.0
USA	2.4–4.0
UK	0.5–1.6
Denmark	2.0
Scandinavia	5.0–8.0
France	6.0
Germany	14.0
Italy	7.5–7.8
Spain	1.6
Israel	<1.0–12.6
Bangladesh	0
Thailand	19.0
Australia	0–2.0

There are theoretical grounds for choosing erythromycin stearate as the best preparation to give for *Campylobacter* enteritis, but there is no clinical evidence that it is superior to other forms of erythromycin. The stearate is acid-resistant, stable, and incompletely absorbed and therefore able to exert a contact effect throughout the bowel contents as well as a systemic effect. A suitable dose is 500 mg twice daily for 5 days; higher doses should not be given as they are liable to cause nausea and acute abdominal pain (318). Enteric-coated pills are not recommended for patients with diarrhea as they are likely to be passed intact without having released their contents. For children the recommended treatment is erythromycin ethyl succinate 40 mg/kg/day in divided doses for 5 days.

Other Macrolides

Clindamycin, rosaramicin, and josamycin have activities as good as or better than that of erythromycin (319,320). Oleandomycin, spiramycin, lincomycin, and pristinamycin are less active. Among the new macrolides azithromycin, clarithromycin, and rokitamycin have good activity, and the former two attain high intracellular concentrations (321,322). Unfortunately these new macrolides are ineffective against erythromycin-resistant strains as there is cross-resistance between erythromycin and other macrolides, except for pristinamycin, which has equal but poor activity against both erythromycin-sensitive and resistant strains (320,324). At present there is insufficient evidence of the superiority of these new macrolides over erythromycin to justify their cost for the treatment of *Campylobacter* enteritis.

Quinolones

The fluoroquinolones are highly active against most strains of *C. jejuni* and *C. coli* (307). At one time it looked as though ciprofloxacin was emerging as the agent of choice both for *Campylobacter* enteritis and acute bacterial diarrhea in general. Unfortunately, it soon became apparent that resistance can develop *in vivo,* not only in immunodeficient patients who need long courses of treatment (326,327) but in normal persons (298). Quinolone resistance rates among sporadic *Campylobacter* isolates have risen sharply since the late 1980s, mainly in places where there are few restrictions on the use of antibiotics (313). Thus in Britain and Finland most quinolone-resistant campylobacters were, until recently, isolated from patients who had returned from abroad (312,328), but there are now signs that they are becoming endemic in Britain (329). Another major source of quinolone-resistant strains is believed to be the extensive use of enrofloxacin in poultry. In the Netherlands the prevalence of quinolone resistance in campylobacters isolated from poultry products rose from 0% in 1982 to 14% in 1989, and in the same period the prevalence in humans rose from 0% to 11% (330). As the macrolide activity of quinolone-resistant campylobacters remains unchanged (323), erythromycin is to be preferred as a first-line drug. If a quinolone is given, we recommend ciprofloxacin 500 mg taken orally twice a day for 5–7 days.

Nitrofurans

Furazolidone is highly active against campylobacters (Table 3) and resistance is rare, but its activity is limited to the gut. Anxieties concerning toxicity have inhibited its use, but it has been used successfully to treat *Campylobacter* enteritis in Belgium.

Aminoglycosides and Imipenem

Aminoglycosides and imipenem are highly active against *Campylobacter,* and resistance rates consistently remain below 1%. Gentamicin, or imipenem for patients with renal damage, is therefore a drug of choice for patients with serious systemic infection. As gentamicin is ineffective against campylobacters in the gut, orthodox antimicrobial treatment must also be given (331).

PREVENTION

As campylobacters are so widely distributed in nature, there is no possibility of reducing the reservoir of infection. Prevention must be aimed at controlling infection in domestic animals and interrupting transmission from them.

Basic Hygiene

Handwashing and general hygiene affords protection against infection from handling animals, animal products, and patients with diarrhea. In general, there is only small risk of direct fecal–oral spread, but puppies and young children with *Campylobacter* enteritis pose a greater risk.

Flies can carry campylobacters and are a potential source of infection (332). Fly control and fly proofing of food premises are important in warm climates.

Treatment of Sewage and Water

The safe disposal of sewage and the protection and purification of water supplies are fundamental control measures. Conventional treatments remove nearly all campylobacters from sewage (333,334); less than 0.1% of the incoming campylobacters are likely to remain in the final effluent (333). Yet surface waters invariably contain campylobacters, mainly from the excreta of sheep, cattle, and wild and domestic birds. It is therefore essential that all surface water destined for drinking is chlorinated, a process that reliably inactivates campylobacters (335). In 14 of 20 recorded waterborne outbreaks of *Campylobacter* enteritis the implicated water was unchlorinated, in 2 it was only intermittently chlorinated, and in the remaining 4 there was a failure of chlorination or a fault in the distribution system.

Heat Treatment of Milk

A basic and unequivocally effective preventive measure is the pasteurization or other approved heat treatment of all milk sold for human consumption. Outbreaks of *Campylobacter* enteritis regularly occur where the sale of raw milk is still allowed (40,42). It has been shown that no amount of care during milking can prevent contamination with campylobacters (336), either from fecal contamination or from a cow with silent *Campylobacter* mastitis, so that heat treatment is the only answer. Milk that is doorstep-delivered in foil-topped bottles should be protected in areas where birds have developed the habit of pecking through the tops and contaminating the contents (43).

PRODUCTION AND HANDLING OF FOOD

Raw meats, especially poultry, are the main source of campylobacters in food. There are basically two points at which control can be applied: (a) in the source animal and its products; and (b) in the kitchen at the point of food preparation. If the former could be achieved there would be no need for the latter, but as campylobacters are such ubiquitous bacteria this is an unrealistic goal. Control must be exercised at both points.

Red Meat and Poultry

Red meats are not nearly as contaminated as poultry, even though carcasses often start out heavily contaminated through spillage of gut contents at slaughter. The reason is that conventional evaporative air chilling of large carcasses, which takes several hours, causes surface drying and destruction of campylobacters. Poultry, being of smaller size, cool quickly and remain moist, or are cooled by immersion in cold water, so that campylobacters survive well. Moreover, the high degree of mechanization required for processing birds at rates that satisfy public demand causes cross-contamination of gut contents that is difficult to control. There is a limit to what can be achieved and contaminated carcasses are inevitable as long as heavily infected flocks continue to be submitted for processing (337). Terminal irradiation is a promising solution that kills other pathogens as well as campylobacters, but there are problems of cost and public acceptability. The immediate aim should be to reduce infection in broilers. Some progress has been made, but control measures are still experimental and a long way from general application.

Campylobacters are not transmitted vertically via eggs, so they must be introduced into growing flocks from extraneous sources. Potential sources are the boots and clothing of attendants, small birds and animals, insects, and water supplies. Colonization rates have been reduced by the application of hygienic measures (338,339) and the cleansing and redesigning of water supplies to broiler houses (340). These are promising interventions, but they require cooperation among microbiologists, veterinarians, private industry, and government to research and implement. They will also increase costs, but this must be put into perspective. In a case-control study in Seattle (46), half of all *Campylobacter* enteritis cases were attributable to the consumption—and, by implication, handling—of poultry, so if this is representative of the rest of the USA, the costs of health care and lost productivity due to poultry-borne *Campylobacter* enteritis are likely to far outweigh the costs of reducing *Campylobacter* infection in poultry.

The various approaches to the control of *Campylobacter* infection and contamination of poultry are discussed by Stern (341).

Food Preparation

The consumption of raw or undercooked meats, including fish and shellfish, carries a risk of *Campylobacter* infection (46,342). Conventional cooking kills campylobacters (343), but barbecue and fondue cooking may not. Prevention depends on ensuring that meats are properly cooked. Probably the most frequent form of foodborne infection is the consumption of foods such as salads, bread, or cooked foods that have become cross-contaminated in the kitchen from raw meats. Campylobacters do not multiply in food like salmonellas, but few bacteria are needed to cause infection. The single most important rule in food preparation is to separate the storage and handling of all raw meats from all other foods, to use separate utensils for each, and to wash hands between the handling of each. This is mandatory for professional catering, but in the home it is sufficient to wash surfaces and utensils scrupulously with hot water and detergent between use for meats and other foods. Much could be done by way of public education. In the UK, a survey showed that less

than one third of respondents appreciated the need to handle raw meats separately from other foods.

Food handlers who have diarrhea (from whatever cause) should not be allowed to prepare food, but there is no evidence that symptomless campylobacter excreters pose a risk to consumers. No infections were found among children at a day center or members of a hospital who had eaten food prepared over a period of 10 days by two cooks who were excreting *C. jejuni* (344). We do not believe that normal responsible food handlers who happen to be excreting campylobacters should be excluded from their work.

Vaccination

Vaccination would be an appropriate form of control in developing countries and possibly for travelers to such countries. Common antigens that are good vaccine candidates have been identified, but a practical vaccine is still far away.

REFERENCES

1. Kist M. Wer entdeckte *Campylobacter jejuni/coli*? Eine Zusammenfassung bisher unberücksichtiger literaturguellen. [Who discovered *Campylobacter jejuni/coli*. A historical review.] *Zentralbl Bakt Hyg* 1986;A261:177–186.
2. McFadyean J, Stockman S. *Report of the Departmental Committee appointed by the Board of Agriculture and Fisheries to inquire into epizootic abortion. Part III. Abortion in sheep.* London: His Majesty's Stationary Office; 1913.
3. Jones FS, Orcutt M, Little RB. Vibrios (*Vibrio jejuni*, n. sp.) associated with intestinal disorders of cows and calves. *J Exp Med* 1931;53:853–863.
4. King EO. Human infections with *Vibrio fetus* and a closely related vibrio. *J Infect Dis* 1957;101:119–128.
5. Butzler JP, Dekeyser P, Detrain M, Dehaen F. Related vibrio in stools. *J Pediatr* 1973;82:493–495.
6. Skirrow MB. Campylobacter enteritis: a "new" disease. *Br Med J* 1977;2:9–11.
7. Karmali MA, Skirrow MB. Taxonomy of the genus *Campylobacter*. In: Butzler J-P, ed. *Campylobacter infection in man and animals*. Boca Raton: CRC Press; 1984:1–20.
8. Sebald M, Véron M. Teneur en bases de l'ADN et classification des vibrions. *Ann Inst Pasteur* 1963;105:897–910.
9. Vandamme P, Falsen E, Rossau R, et al. Revision of *Campylobacter, Helicobacter,* and *Wolinella* taxonomy: emendation of generic descriptions and proposal of *Arcobacter* gen. nov. *Int J Syst Bact* 1990;41:88–103.
9a. Skirrow MB. Campylobacter and helicobacter. In: Greenwood D, Slack R, Peutherer J, eds. *Medical microbiology. A guide to microbial infections: pathogenesis, immunity, laboratory diagnosis and control.* Edinburgh: Churchill Livingstone; 1992:351–359.
10. Skirrow MB. A demographic survey of *campylobacter, salmonella* and *shigella* infections in England. *Epidemiol Infect* 1987; 99:647–657.
11. Blaser MJ, Hardesty HL, Powers B, Wang W-LL. Survival of *Campylobacter fetus* subsp. *jejuni* in biological milieus. *J Clin Microbiol* 1980;11:309–313.
12. Rollins DM, Colwell RR. Viable but nonculturable stage of *Campylobacter jejuni* and its role in survival in the natural aquatic environment. *Appl Environ Microbiol* 1986;52:531–538.
13. Jones DM, Sutcliffe EM, Curry A. Recovery of viable but nonculturable *Campylobacter jejuni*. *J Gen Microbiol* 1991;137: 2477–2482.
14. Pearson AD, Greenwood M, Healing TD, et al. Colonization

of broiler chickens by waterborne *Campylobacter jejuni*. *Appl Environ Microbiol* 1993;59:987–996.

15. Abram DD, Potter NN. Survival of *Campylobacter jejuni* at different temperatures in broth, beef, chicken and cod supplemented with sodium chloride. *J Food Protect* 1984;47:795–800.

16. Lior H. New, extended biotyping scheme for *Campylobacter jejuni*, *Campylobacter coli*, and "*Campylobacter laridis*". *J Clin Microbiol* 1984;20:636–640.

17. Bolton FJ, Wareing DRA, Skirrow MB, Hutchinson DN. Identification and typing of campylobacters. In: Board RG, Jones D, Skinner FA, eds. *Identification methods in applied and environmental microbiology*. Oxford: Blackwell Scientific; 1992: 151–161.

18. Penner JL, Hennessy JN. Passive hemagglutination technique for serotyping *Campylobacter fetus* subsp. *jejuni* on the basis of soluble heat-stable antigens. *J Clin Microbiol* 1980;12:732–737.

19. Lior H, Woodward DL, Edgar JA, Laroche LJ, Gill P. Serotyping of *Campylobacter jejuni* by slide agglutination based on heat-labile antigenic factors. *J Clin Microbiol* 1982;15:761–768.

20. Patton CM, Wachsmuth IK. Typing schemes: are current methods useful? In: Nachamkin I, Blaser MJ, Tompkins LS. *Campylobacter jejuni: current status and future trends*. Washington DC: Am Soc Microbiol; 1992:110–118.

21. Skirrow MB. *Campylobacter, Helicobacter* and other motile curved gram-negative rods. In: Parker MT, Collier LH, eds. *Topley and Wilson's principles of bacteriology, virology and immunity*. vol 2. 8th ed. London: Edward Arnold; 1990: 531–549.

22. Blaser MJ, Taylor DN, Feldman RA. Epidemiology of *Campylobacter jejuni* infections. *Epidemiol Rev* 1983;5:157–176.

23. Skirrow MB. Epidemiology of *Campylobacter* enteritis. *Int J Food Microbiol* 1991;12:9–16.

24. Tauxe RV. Epidemiology of *Campylobacter jejuni* infections in the United States and other industrialized nations. In: Nachamkin I, Blaser MJ, Tompkins LS, eds. *Campylobacter jejuni: current status and future trends*. Washington DC: Am Soc Microbiol; 1992:9–19.

25. Kendall EJC, Tanner EI. Campylobacter enteritis in general practice. *J Hyg* (*Lond*) 1982;88:155–163.

26. Popovic-Uroic T. *Campylobacter jejuni* and *Campylobacter coli* diarrhoea in rural and urban populations in Yugoslavia. *Epidemiol Infect* 1989;102:59–67.

27. Sockett PN, Pearson AD. Cost implications of human campylobacter infections. In: Kaijser B, Falsen E, eds. *Campylobacter IV: Proceedings of the fourth international workshop on campylobacter infections*. Göteborg: University of Göteborg; 1988:261–264.

28. Skirrow MB. Foodborne illness: *Campylobacter*. *Lancet* 1990; 336:921–923.

29. Riordan T. Intestinal infection with *Campylobacter* in children. *Lancet* 1988;1:992.

30. Blaser MJ, Taylor DN, Echeverria P. Immune response to *Campylobacter jejuni* in a rural community in Thailand. *J Infect Dis* 1986;153:249–254.

31. Taylor DN, Perlman DM, Echeverria PD, Lexomboon U, Blaser MJ. *Campylobacter* immunity and quantitative excretion rates in Thai children. *J Infect Dis* 1993;168:754–758.

32. Calva JJ, Ruiz-Palacios GM, Lopez-Vidal AB, Ramos A, Bojalil R. Cohort study of intestinal infection with *Campylobacter* in Mexican children. *Lancet* 1988;1:503–506.

33. Taylor DN. *Campylobacter* infections in developing countries. In: Nachamkin I, Blaser MJ, Tompkins LS, eds. *Campylobacter jejuni: current status and future trends*. Washington DC: Am Soc Microbiol; 1992:20–30.

34. Saeed AM, Harris NV, DiGiacomo RF. The role of exposure to animals in the etiology of *Campylobacter jejuni/coli* enteritis. *Am J Epidemiol* 1993;137:108–114.

35. Totten PA, Fennell CL, Tenover FC, et al. *Campylobacter cinaedi* (sp. nov.) and *Campylobacter fennelliae* (sp. nov.): two new *Campylobacter* species associated with enteric disease in homosexual men. *J Infect Dis* 1985;151:131–139.

36. Pepersack F, Prigogyne T, Butzler JP, Yourassowsky E. *Campylobacter jejuni* post-transfusional septicaemia. *Lancet* 1979;2:911.

37. Mentzing L-O. Waterborne outbreaks of campylobacter enteritis in central Sweden. *Lancet* 1981;2:352–354.

38. Vogt RL, Sours HE, Barrett T, Feldman RA, Dickinson RL, Witherell L. Campylobacter enteritis associated with contaminated water. *Ann Intern Med* 1982;96:292–296.

39. Taylor DN, McDermott KT, Little JR, Wells JG, Blaser MJ. Campylobacter enteritis from untreated water in the Rocky Mountains. *Ann Intern Med* 1983;99:38–40.

40. Robinson DA, Jones DM. Milk-borne campylobacter infection. *Br Med J* 1981;282:1374–1376.

41. Potter ME, Blaser MJ, Sikes RK, Kaufmann AF, Wells JG. Human *Campylobacter* infection associated with certified raw milk. *Am J Epidemiol* 1983;117:475–483.

42. Wood RC, MacDonald KL, Osterholm MT. *Campylobacter* enteritis outbreaks associated with drinking raw milk during youth activities. *JAMA* 1992;268:3228–3230.

43. Hudson SJ, Lightfoot NF, Coulson JC, Russell K, Sisson PR, Sobo AO. Jackdaws and magpies as vectors of milkborne human campylobacter infection. *Epidemiol Infect* 1991;107: 363–372.

44. Hudson PJ, Vogt RL, Brondum J, Patton CM. Isolation of *Campylobacter jejuni* from milk during an outbreak of campylobacteriosis. *J Infect Dis* 1984;150:789.

45. Hood AM, Pearson AD, Shahamat M. The extent of surface contamination of retailed chickens with *Campylobacter jejuni* serogroups. *Epidemiol Infect* 1988;100:17–25.

46. Harris NV, Weiss NS, Nolan CM. The role of poultry and meats in the etiology of *Campylobacter jejuni/coli* enteritis. *Am J Public Health* 1986;76:407–411.

47. Istre G, Blaser MJ, Shillam P, Hopkins RS. Campylobacter enteritis associated with undercooked barbecued chicken. *Am J Public Health* 1984;74:1265–1267.

48. Brown P, Kidd D, Riordan T, Barrell RA. An outbreak of foodborne *Campylobacter jejuni* infection and the possible role of cross-contamination. *J Infect* 1988;17:171–176.

49. Robinson DA. Infective dose of *Campylobacter jejuni* in milk. *Br Med J* 1981;282:1584.

50. Black RE, Levine MM, Clements ML, Hughes TP, Blaser MJ. Experimental *Campylobacter jejuni* infection in humans. *J Infect Dis* 1988;157:472–479.

51. Caldwell MB, Guerry P, Lee EC, Burans JP, Walker RI. Reversible expression of flagella in *Campylobacter jejuni*. *Infect Immun* 1985;50:941–943.

52. Guerry P, Logan SM, Thornton S, Trust TJ. Genomic organization and expression of *Campylobacter* flagellin genes. *J Bacteriol* 1990;172:1853–1860.

53. Guerry P, Alm RA, Power ME, Logan SM, Trust TJ. Role of two flagellin genes in *Campylobacter* motility. *J Bacteriol* 1990; 173:4757–4764.

54. Alm RA, Guerry P, Trust TJ. Distribution and polymorphism of the flagellin genes from isolates of *Campylobacter coli* and *Campylobacter jejuni*. *J Bacteriol* 1993;175:3051–3057.

55. Miller S, Pesci EC, Pickett CL. A *Campylobacter jejuni* homolog of the LcrD/FlbF family of proteins is necessary for flagellar biogenesis. *Infect Immun* 1993;61:2930–2936.

56. McSweegan E, Walker RI. Identification and characterization of two *Campylobacter jejuni* adhesins for cellular and mucous substrates. *Infect Immun* 1986;53:141–148.

57. Lindblom GB, Cervantes LE, Sjögren E, Kaijser B, Ruiz-Palacios GM. Adherence, enterotoxigenicity, invasiveness, and sero-groups in *Campylobacter jejuni* and *Campylobacter coli* strains from adult humans with acute enterocolitis. *APMIS* 1990;98:179–184.

58. Fauchère JL, Kervella M, Rosenau A, Mohanna K, Veron M. Adhesion to HeLa cells of *Campylobacter jejuni* and *C. coli* outer membrane components. *Res Microbiol* 1989;140: 379–392.

59. Van Spreeuwel JP, Duursma GC, Meijer CJLM, Bax R, Rosekrans PCM, Lindeman J. Campylobacter colitis: histological immunohistochemical and ultrastructural findings. *Gut* 1985;26: 945–951.

60. Price AB, Jewkes J, Sanderson PJ. Acute diarrhoea: campylobacter colitis and the role of rectal biopsy. *J Clin Pathol* 1979; 32:990–997.

61. Blaser MJ, Parsons RB, Wang WLL. Acute colitis caused by *Campylobacter fetus ss. jejuni*. *Gastroenterology* 1980;78: 448–453.

62. Surawicz CM, Belic L. Rectal biopsy helps to distinguish acute self-limited colitis from idiopathic inflammatory bowel disease. *Gastroenterology* 1984;86:104–113.

63. Blaser MJ, Berkowitz ID, LaForce FM, Cravens J, Reller LB, Wang W-LL. Campylobacter enteritis: clinical and epidemiologic features. *Ann Intern Med* 1979;91:179–185.

64. Blaser MJ, Wells JG, Feldman RA, Pollard RA, Allen JR. *Campylobacter enteritis* in the United States. A multicenter study. *Ann Intern Med* 1983;98:360–365.

65. Russell RG, O'Donnoghue M, Blake DC Jr, Zulty J, DeTolla LJ. Early colonic damage and invasion of *Campylobacter jejuni* in experimentally challenged infant *Macaca mulatta*. *J Infect Dis* 1993;168:210–215.

66. Walker RI, Schmauder-Chock A, Parker JL, Burr D. Selective association and transport of *Campylobacter jejuni* through M cells of rabbit Peyer's patches. *Can J Microbiol* 1988;34:1143–1147.

67. Ruiz-Palacios GM, Torres J, Torres NI, Escamilla E, Ruiz-Palacios BR, Tamayo J. Cholera-like enterotoxin produced by *Campylobacter jejuni*. *Lancet* 1983;1:250–253.

68. Klipstein FA, Engert RF. Properties of crude *Campylobacter jejuni* heat-labile enterotoxin. *Infect Immun* 1984;45:314–319.

69. Klipstein FA, Engert RF. Purification of *Campylobacter jejuni* enterotoxin. *Lancet* 1985;1:1123–1124.

70. Olsvik O, Wachsmuth K, Morris G, Feeley JC. Genetic probing of *Campylobacter jejuni* for cholera toxin and *Escherichia coli* heat-labile enterotoxin. *Lancet* 1984;1:449.

71. Pérez-Pérez GI, Cohn DL, Guerrant RL, Patton C, Reller LB, Blaser MJ. Clinical and immunological significance of cholera-like toxin and cytotoxin production by Campylobacter species in patients with acute inflammatory diarrhea. *J Infect Dis* 1989;160:460–468.

72. Cover TL, Pérez-Pérez GI, Blaser MJ. Evaluation of cytotoxic activity in fecal filtrates from patients with *Campylobacter jejuni* or *Campylobacter coli* enteritis. *FEMS Microbiol Lett* 1990;70:301–304.

73. Johnson WM, Lior H. Cytotoxic and cytotonic factor produced by *Campylobacter jejuni, Campylobacter coli*, and *Campylobacter laridis*. *J Clin Microbiol* 1986;24:275–281.

74. Moore MA, Blaser MJ, Pérez-Pérez GI, O'Brien AD. Production of a shiga-like cytotoxin by *Campylobacter*. *Microb Pathog* 1988;4:455–462.

75. Guerrant RL, Wanke CA, Pennie RA, Barrett LA, Linva AAM, O'Brien AD. Production of a unique cytotoxin by *Campylobacter jejuni*. *Infect Immun* 1987;55:2526–2530.

76. Skirrow MB, Jones DM, Sutcliffe J, Benjamin J. Campylobacter bacteraemia in England and Wales, 1981–91. *Epidemiol Infect* 1993;110:567–573.

77. Guerrant RL, Lahita RG, Winn WC, Roberts RB. Campylobacteriosis in man: pathogenic mechanisms and review of 91 bloodstream infections. *Am J Med* 1978;65:584–592.

78. Konkel ME, Joens LA. Adhesion to and invasion of Hep-2 cells by *Campylobacter* spp. *Infect Immun* 1989;57:2984–2990.

79. De Melo MA, Gabbiani G, Pechère JC. Cellular events and intracellular survival of *Campylobacter jejuni* during infection of Hep-2 cells. *Infect Immun* 1989;57:2214–2222.

80. Fauchere JL, Rosenau M, Veron M, Moyen EN, Richard S, Pfister A. Association with HeLa cells of *Campylobacter jejuni* and *C. coli* isolated from human feces. *Infect Immun* 1986;54:283–287.

81. Oelshlager TA, Guerry P, Kopecko DJ. Unusual microtubule-dependent endocytosis mechanisms triggered by *Campylobacter jejuni* and *Citrobacter freundii*. *Proc Natl Acad Sci USA* 1993;90:6884–6888.

82. Konkel ME, Babakhani F, Joens LA. Invasion-related antigens of *Campylobacter jejuni*. *J Infect Dis* 1990;162:888–895.

83. Blaser MJ, Pérez-Pérez GI. Humoral immune response to lipopolysaccharide antigens of *Campylobacter jejuni*. In: Nachamkin I, Blaser MJ, Tompkins LS, eds. *Campylobacter jejuni. Current status and future trends*, Washington, DC: Am Soc Microbiol; 1992:230.

84. Yuki N, Taki T, Inagaki F, et al. A bacterium lipopolysaccharide that elicits Guillain–Barré syndrome has a GM1 ganglioside-like structure. *J Exp Med* 1993;178:1771–1775.

85. Pei Z, Ellison RT III, Blaser MJ. Identification, purification and characterization of major antigenic proteins of *Campylobacter jejuni*. *J Biol Chem* 1991;266:16363–16369.

86. Kervella M, Pagès J-M, Pei Z, Grollier G, Blaser MJ, Fauchere J-L. Isolation and characterization of two *Campylobacter* glycine-extracted proteins that bind to HeLa cell membranes. *Infect Immun* 1993;61:3440–3448.

87. Blaser MJ, Duncan D. Human serum antibody response to *Campylobacter jejuni* infection as measured in an enzyme-linked immunosorbent assay. *Infect Immun* 1984;44:292–298.

88. Black RE, Perlman D, Clements ML, Levine MM, Blaser MJ. Human volunteer studies with *Campylobacter jejuni*. In: Nachamkin I, Blaser MJ, Tompkins LS, eds. *Campylobacter jejuni: current status and future trends*. Washington, DC: Am Soc Microbiol; 1992:207.

89. Blaser MJ, Black RE, Duncan DJ, Amer J. *Campylobacter jejuni*-specific serum antibodies are elevated in healthy Bangladeshi children. *J Clin Microbiol* 1985;21:164–167.

90. Sorvillo FJ, Lieb LE, Waterman SH. Incidence of Campylobacteriosis among patients with AIDS in Los Angeles County. *J AIDS* 1991;4:598–602.

91. Perlman DM, Ampel NM, Schifman RB, et al. Persistent *Campylobacter jejuni* infections in patients infected with human immunodeficiency virus (HIV). *Ann Intern Med* 1988;108:540–546.

92. Kiehlbauch JA, Albach RA, Baum LL, Chang KP. Phagocytosis of *Campylobacter jejuni* and its intracellular survival in mononuclear phagocytes. *Infect Immun* 1985;48:446–451.

93. Blaser MJ, Smith PF, Kohler PA. Susceptibility of *Campylobacter* isolates to the bactericidal activity in human serum. *J Infect Dis* 1985;151:227–235.

94. Johnson RJ, Wang SP, Shelton WR, Nolan C, Blaser MJ. Persistent *Campylobacter jejuni* infection in an immunocompromised host. *Ann Intern Med* 1984;100:832–834.

95. Melamed A, Zakuth V, Schwartz D, Spirer Z. The immune system response to *Campylobacter* infection. *Microbiol Immunol* 1988;32:75–82.

96. Blaser MJ, Pérez-Pérez GI, Smith PF, et al. Extraintestinal *Campylobacter jejuni* and *Campylobacter coli* infections: host factors and strain characteristics. *J Infect Dis* 1986;153:552–559.

97. Russell RG, Blaser MJ, Sarmiento I, Fox J. Experimental *Campylobacter jejuni* infection in *Macaca nemestrina*. *Infect Immun* 1989;57:1438–1444.

98. McKendrick MW, Geddes AM, Gearty J. Campylobacter enteritis: a study of clinical features and rectal mucosal changes. *Scand J Infect Dis* 1982;14:35–38.

99. Wallace JM. Milk-associated campylobacter infection. *Health Bull (Edinb)* 1980;38:57–61.

100. Pentland B. Campylobacter enteritis: an in-patient study. *Scot Med J* 1979;24:299–301.

101. Pitkänen T, Pettersson T, Pönkä A, Kosunen TU. Clinical and serological studies in patients with *Campylobacter fetus* ssp. *jejuni* infection: I. Clinical findings. *Infection* 1981;9:274–278.

102. Kapperud G, Lassen J, Ostroff SM, Aasen S. Clinical features of sporadic campylobacter infections in Norway. *Scand J Infect Dis* 1992;24:741–749.

103. Wright EP. Meningism associated with *Campylobacter jejuni* enteritis. *Lancet* 1979;1:1092.

104. Williams GV, Deacon GJ. Campylobacter: common cause of enteritis in an infectious diseases hospital. *Med J Aust* 1980;2:268–271.

105. Jewkes J, Larson HE, Price AB, Sanderson PJ, Davies HA. Aetiology of acute diarrhoea in adults. *Gut* 1981;22:388–392.

106. Wilson PG, Davies JR, Hoskins TW, et al. Epidemiology of an outbreak of milk-borne enteritis in a residential school. In: Pearson AD, Skirrow MB, Rowe B, Davies JR, Jones DM, Eds. *Campylobacter II: proceedings of the Second International Workshop on Campylobacter Infections*. London: Public Health Laboratory Service; 1983:143.

107. Matsusaki S, Katayama A. Studies on outbreaks of food poisoning due to *Campylobacter jejuni* between 1980 and 1982 in Yamaguchi prefecture, Japan. *Yamaguchi J Vet Med* 1984;11:53–56.

108. Svedhem Å, Kaijser B. *Campylobacter fetus* subspecies *jejuni:* a common cause of diarrhea in Sweden. *J Infect Dis* 1980;142:353–359.

109. Pitkänen T, Pönkä A, Pettersson T, Kosunen TU. *Campylobacter* enteritis in 188 hospitalized patients. *Arch Intern Med* 1983;143:215–219.

110. Rao GG, Fuller M. A review of hospitalized patients with bacterial gastroenteritis. *J Hosp Infect* 1992;20:105–111.

111. Drake AA, Gilchrist MJR, Washington JA, Huizenga KA, Van Scoy RE. Diarrhea due to *Campylobacter fetus* subspecies *jejuni. Mayo Clin Proc* 1981;56:414–423.

112. Bradshaw MJ, Brown R, Swallow JH, Rycroft JA. *Campylobacter* enteritis in Chelmsford. *Postgrad Med J* 1980;56:80–84.

113. Hoskins TW. Campylobacter enteritis and erythema nodosum. *Br Med J* 1982;285:1661.

114. Bretag AH, Archer RS, Atkinson HM, Woods WH. Circadian urticaria: another *Campylobacter* association. *Lancet* 1984;1:954.

115. Lopez-Brea M, Fontelas PM, Baquero M, Aragon L. Urticaria associated with campylobacter enteritis. *Lancet* 1984;1:1354.

116. Porter IA, Reid TMS. A milk-borne outbreak of *Campylobacter* infection. *J Hyg (Lond)* 1980;84:415–419.

117. Blaser MJ, Checko P, Bopp C, Bruce A, Hughes JM. *Campylobacter* enteritis associated with foodborne transmission. *Am J Epidemiol* 1982;116:886–894.

118. Millson M, Bokhout M, Carlson J, et al. An outbreak of *Campylobacter jejuni* gastroenteritis linked to meltwater contamination of a municipal well. *Can J Public Health* 1991;82:27–31.

119. Paulet Ph, Coffernils M. Very long term diarrhoea due to *Campylobacter jejuni. Postgrad Med J* 1990;66:410–411.

120. Smith GS, Blaser MJ. Fatalities associated with *Campylobacter jejuni* infections. *JAMA* 1985;253:2873–2875.

121. Jones PH, Willis AT, Robinson DA, Skirrow MB, Josephs DS. Campylobacter enteritis associated with the consumption of free school milk. *J Hyg (Lond)* 1981;87:155–162.

122. Steingrimsson O, Thorsteinsson SB, Hjalmarsdottir M, Jonasdottir E, Kolbeinsson A. Campylobacter ssp. infections in Iceland during a 24-month period in 1980–1982. *Scand J Infect Dis* 1985;17:285–290.

123. Popovic-Uroic T. Gmajnicki B, Kalenic S, Vodopija I. Clinical comparison of *Campylobacter jejuni* and *C. coli* diarrhoea. *Lancet* 1988;1:176–177.

124. Figura N, Guglielmetti P. Clinical characteristics of *Campylobacter jejuni* and *C coli* enteritis. *Lancet* 1988;1:942–943.

125. Havalad S, Chapple MJ, Kahakachchi M, Hargreaves DB. Convulsions associated with campylobacter enteritis. *Br Med J* 1980;280:984–985.

126. Karmali MA, Fleming PC. *Campylobacter* enteritis in children. *J Pediatr* 1979;94:527–533.

127. Wright EP, Seager J. Convulsions associated with campylobacter enteritis. *Br Med J* 1980;281:454.

128. Malowany M, Lewin S, Geller M, Kittick J, Gertner M, Nicholas P. Seizures associated with *Campylobacter* enteritis. *Am J Dis Child* 1982;136:1028.

129. Buchta RM. *Campylobacter* enteritis associated with convulsions. *Am J Dis Child* 1983;137:919.

130. Lerner A, Ianco TC, Landoy Z, Schmilowitz M, Kretzer B. Seizures associated with *Campylobacter jejuni* enteritis. *Pediatr Infect Dis* 1984;3:281.

131. Colver AF, Pedler SJ, Hawkey PM. Severe campylobacter infection in children. *J Infect* 1985;11:217–220.

132. Levy I, Weissman Y, Sivan Y, Ben-Ari J, Scheinfeld T. Acute encephalopathy associated with campylobacter enteritis. *Br Med J* 1986;293:424.

133. Anders BJ, Lauer BA, Paisley JW. *Campylobacter* gastroenteritis in neonates. *Am J Dis Child* 1981;135:900–902.

134. Karmali MA, Norrish B, Lior H, Heyes B, Monteath A, Montgomery H. *Campylobacter* enterocolitis in a neonatal nursery. *J Infect Dis* 1984;149:874–877.

135. Terrier A, Altwegg M, Bader P, von Graevenitz A. Hospital epidemic of neonatal *Campylobacter jejuni* infection. *Lancet* 1985;2:1182.

136. Goossens H, Henocque G, Kremp L, et al. Nosocomial outbreak of *Campylobacter jejuni* meningitis in newborn infants. *Lancet* 1986;2:146–149.

137. Hershkowici S, Barak M, Cohen A, Montag J. An outbreak of *Campylobacter jejuni* infection in a neonatal intensive care unit. *J Hosp Infect* 1987;9:54–59.

138. Rusu V, Lucinescu S. The value of *Campylobacter jejuni/coli* serotyping for the evaluation of an enteritis outbreak in newborn infants. In: Kaijser B, Falsen E, eds. *Campylobacter IV: Proceedings of the Fourth International Workshop on Campylobacter Infections.* Göteborg: University of Göteborg; 1988:138–139.

139. Van Dijk WC, van der Straaten PJC. An outbreak of *Campylobacter jejuni* infection in a neonatal intensive care unit. *J Hosp Infect* 1988;11:91–99.

140. Begue P, Broussin B, Carros I, Thien HV. Pathologie intestinale à *Campylobacter. Méd Mal Infect* 1989;19:48–54.

141. Torphy DE, Bond WW. *Campylobacter fetus* infections in children. *Pediatrics* 1979;64:898–903.

142. Thomas K, Chan KN, Ribeiro CD. *Campylobacter jejuni/coli* meningitis in a neonate. *Br Med J* 1980;280:1301–1302.

143. Damani NN, Humphrey CA, Bell B. Haemolytic anaemia in campylobacter enteritis. *J Infect* 1993;26:109–110.

144. Simor AE, Karmali MA, Jadavji T, Roscoe M. Abortion and perinatal sepsis associated with campylobacter infection. *Rev Infect Dis* 1986;8:397–402.

145. Moscuna M, Gross Z, Korenblum R, Volfson M, Oettinger M. Septic abortion due to *Campylobacter jejuni. Eur J Clin Microbiol Infect Dis* 1989;8:800–801.

146. Simor AE, Ferro S. *Campylobacter jejuni* infection occurring during pregnancy. *Eur J Clin Microbiol Infect Dis* 1990;9:141–144.

147. Denton KJ, Clarke T. Role of *Campylobacter jejuni* as a placental pathogen. *J Clin Pathol* 1992;45:171–172.

148. Pines A, Goldhammer E, Bregman J, Kaplinsky N, Frankl O. Campylobacter enteritis associated with recurrent abortions in agammaglobulinemia. *Acta Obstet Gynecol Scand* 1983;62:279–280.

149. Youngs ER, Roberts C. *Campylobacter* carriage and pregnancy. *Brit J Obstet Gynaecol* 1985;92:541–542.

150. Wong S-K, Tam AY-C, Yuen K-Y. *Campylobacter* infection in the neonate: case report and review of the literature. *Pediatr Infect Dis* 1990;9:665–669.

151. Newman A, Lambert JR. Campylobacter jejuni causing flare-up in inflammatory bowel disease. *Lancet* 1980;2:919.

152. Goodman MJ, Pearson KW, McGhie D, Dutt S, Deodhar SG. Campylobacter and *Giardia lamblia* causing exacerbation of inflammatory bowel disease. *Lancet* 1980;2:1247.

153. Lambert ME, Schofield PF, Ironside AG, Mandal BK. Campylobacter colitis. *Br Med J* 1979;1:857–859.

154. Willoughby CP, Piris J, Truelove SC. Campylobacter colitis. *J Clin Pathol* 1979;32:986–989.

155. Lambert JR, Tischler ME, Karmali MA, Newman A. Campylobacter colitis: an inflammatory bowel disease. *Can Med Assoc J* 1979;121:1377–1379.

156. Colgan T, Lambert JR, Newman A, Luk SC. *Campylobacter jejuni* enterocolitis. *Arch Pathol Lab Med* 1980;104:571–574.

157. Loss RW, Mangla JC, Pereira M. *Campylobacter* colitis presenting as inflammatory bowel disease with segmental colonic ulcerations. *Gastroenterology* 1980;79:138–140.

158. Rutgeerts P, Geboes K, Ponette E, Coremans G, Vantrappen G. Acute infective colitis caused by endemic pathogens in western Europe. *Endoscopy* 1982;14:212–219.

159. Mee AS, Shield M, Burke M. Campylobacter colitis: differentiation from acute inflammatory bowel disease. *J R Soc Med* 1985;78:217–223.

160. Green ES, Parker NE, Gellert AR, Beck ER. Campylobacter infection mimicking Crohn's disease in an immunodeficient patient. *Br Med J* 1984;289:159–160.

161. Melby K, Kildebo S. Antibodies against *Campylobacter jejuni/coli* in patients suffering from campylobacteriosis or inflammatory bowel disease. *NIPH Ann* 1988;11:47–52.

162. Blaser MJ, Hoverson D, Ely IG, Duncan DJ, Wang WLL, Brown WR. Studies of *Campylobacter jejuni* in patients with inflammatory bowel disease. *Gastroenterol* 1984;86:33–38.

163. Blaser MJ, Miller RA, Lacher J, Singleton JW. Patients with active Crohn's disease have elevated serum antibodies to anti-

gens of seven enteric bacterial pathogens. *Gastroenterology* 1984;87:888–894.

164. McKinley MJ, Taylor M, Sangree MH. Toxic megacolon with campylobacter colitis. *Conn Med* 1980;44:496–497.

165. Stephenson TJ, Cotton DWK. Toxic megacolon complicating campylobacter colitis. *Br Med J* 1985;291:1242.

166. Gould SR. Toxic megacolon complicating campylobacter colitis. *Br Med J* 1985;291:1580.

167. Guandalini S, Cucchiara S, de Ritis G, et al. Campylobacter colitis in infants. *J Pediatr* 1983;102:72–74.

168. Heyman MB, Paterno VI, Ament ME. *Campylobacter* colitis: a cause of chronic diarrhea in children. *West J Med* 1982;137:243–245.

169. Coffin CM, L'Heureaux P, Dehner LP. Campylobacter-associated enterocolitis in childhood: report of a fatal case. *Am J Clin Pathol* 1982;78:117–123.

170. Bentley D, Lynn J, Laws JW. Campylobacter colitis with intestinal aphthous ulceration mimicking obstruction. *Br Med J* 1985;291:634.

171. Pearson AD, Drake DP, Brookfield D, et al. Campylobacter infections in patients presenting with diarrhoea, mesenteric adenitis and appendicitis. In: Newell DG, ed. *Campylobacter: epidemiology, pathogenesis and biochemistry.* Lancaster: MTP Press; 1982:147–151.

172. Megraud F, Tachoire C, Latrille J, Bondonny JM. Appendicitis due to *Campylobacter jejuni. Br Med J* 1982;285:1165–1166.

173. Chan FTH, Stringel G, Mackenzie AMR. Isolation of *Campylobacter jejuni* from an appendix. *J Clin Microbiol* 1983;18:422–424.

174. Morlet N, Glancy R. *Campylobacter jejuni* appendicitis. *Med J Aust* 1986;145:56–57.

175. Meijer CJLM, Lindeman J, Elbers JRJ, Sybrandy R, van Spreeuwel JP. Campylobacter associated appendicitis: prevalence, clinical and histological features. *Pathol Res* 1985;180:295 (Abstr).

176. Puylaert JBCM, Vermeijden RJ, van der Werf SDJ, Doornbos L, Koumans RKJ. Incidence and sonographic diagnosis of bacterial ileocaecitis masquerading as appendicitis. *Lancet* 1989;2:84–86.

177. Kist M. Campylobacter enteritis: epidemiological and clinical data from recent isolations in the region of Freiburg, West Germany. In: Newell DG, ed. *Campylobacter: epidemiology, pathogenesis and biochemistry.* Lancaster: MTP Press; 1982:138–142.

178. Michalak DM, Perrault J, Gilchrist MJ, Dozois RR, Carney JA, Sheedy PF. *Campylobacter fetus* ss. *jejuni:* a cause of massive lower gastrointestinal hemorrhage. *Gastroenterology* 1980;79:742–745.

179. Meuwissen SGM, Bakkar PJM, Rietra PJGM. Acute ulceration of ileal stoma due to *Campylobacter fetus* subspecies *jejuni. Br Med J* 1981;282:1362.

180. Skirrow MB. Acute ulceration of ileal stoma due to *Campylobacter fetus* subspecies *jejuni. Br Med J* 1981;282:1978.

181. Drake AA, Huizenga KA, Van Scoy RE. *Campylobacter fetus* subsp *jejuni:* a cause of diarrhea in a patient with a continent ileostomy. *Dig Dis Sci* 1982;27:1037–1038.

182. Krajden S, Burul CJ, Fuksa M. *Campylobacter jejuni* associated with a perirectal abscess. *Can J Surg* 1986;29:228.

183. Mertens A, De Smet M. Campylobacter cholecystitis. *Lancet* 1979;1:1092.

184. Darling WM, Peel RN, Skirrow MB, Mulira AEJL. Campylobacter cholecystitis. *Lancet* 1979;1:1302.

185. De Sa Pereira M. Lipton SD, Kim JK. Acute cholecystitis and *Campylobacter fetus. Ann Intern Med* 1981;94:821.

186. Drion S, Wahlen C, Taziaux P. Isolation of *Campylobacter jejuni* from the bile of a cholecystic patient. *J Clin Microbiol* 1988;26:2193–2194.

187. Ampelas M, Perez C, Jourdan J, et al. Hépatite à *Campylobacter coli. Nouv Presse Méd* 1982;11:593–595.

188. Nahum HD, Kaloustian E, Baumer Ph, Felten Papaiconomuo A, Lubetski J. Syndrome de rétention biliaire au cours d'une septicémie à *Campylobacter jejuni. Nouv Presse Méd* 1982;11:1805–1806.

189. Reddy KR, Thomas E. *Campylobacter jejuni* enterocolitis and hepatitis. *Gastroenterology* 1982;82:1156.

190. Humphrey KS. Campylobacter infection and hepatocellular injury. *Lancet* 1993;341:49.

191. Fitzgeorge RB, Baskerville A, Lander KP. Experimental infection of Rhesus monkeys with a human strain of *Campylobacter jejuni. J Hyg (Lond)* 1981;86:343–351.

192. Kita E, Nishikawa F, Kamikaidou N, Nakano A, Katsui N, Kashiba S. Mononuclear cell response in the liver of mice infected with hepatotoxigenic *Campylobacter jejuni. J Med Microbiol* 1992;37:326–331.

193. Gallagher P, Chadwick P, Jones DM, Turner L. Acute pancreatitis associated with campylobacter infection. *Br J Surg* 1981;68:383.

194. Pönkä A, Kosunen TU. Pancreas affection in association with enteritis due to *Campylobacter fetus* ssp. *jejuni. Acta Med Scand* 1981;209:239–240.

195. De Bois MHW, Schoemaker MC, van der Werf SDJ, Puylaert JBCM. Pancreatitis associated with *Campylobacter jejuni* infection: diagnosis by ultrasonography. *Br Med J* 1989;298:1004.

196. Ezpelata C, Rojo de Ursua P, Obregon F, Goñi, Cisterna R. Acute pancreatitis associated with *Campylobacter jejuni* bacteremia. *Clin Infect Dis* 1992;15:1050.

197. Murphy S, Beeching NJ, Rogerson SJ, Harries AD. Pancreatitis associated with *Salmonella* enteritis. *Lancet* 1991;338:571.

198. Pepersack F, D'Haene M, Toussaint C, Schoutens E. *Campylobacter jejuni* peritonitis complicating continuous ambulatory peritoneal dialysis. *J Clin Microbiol* 1982;16:739–741.

199. Wood CJ, Fleming V, Turnidge J, Thomson N, Atkins RC. *Campylobacter* peritonitis in continuous peritoneal dialysis: a report of eight cases and a review of the literature. *Am J Kidney Dis* 1992;19:257–263.

200. Feder HM, Rasoulpour M, Rodriquez AJ. *Campylobacter* urinary tract infection: value of the urine Gram's stain. *JAMA* 1986;256:2389.

201. Davies JS, Penfold JB. *Campylobacter* urinary infection. *Lancet* 1979;1:1091.

202. McNeil NI, Buttoo S, Ridgway GL. Spontaneous bacterial peritonitis due to *Campylobacter jejuni. Postgrad Med J* 1984;60:487–488.

203. Domingo P, Mirelis B, Gimeno A, Cabezas R. Peritonitis espontánea por *Campylobacter jejuni* en un paciento cirrótico. [Spontaneous peritonitis caused by *Campylobacter jejuni* in a cirrhotic patient]. *Med Clin (Barc)* 1985;84:416.

204. Ho H, Zuckerman MJ, Polly SM. Spontaneous bacterial peritonitis due to *Campylobacter coli. Gastroenterology* 1987;92:2024–2025.

205. Schmidt U, Chmel H, Kaminski Z, Sen P. The clinical spectrum of *Campylobacter fetus* infections: report of five cases and review of the literature. *Q J Med* (New Series) 1980;49:431–442.

206. Muytjens HL, Hoogenhout J. *Campylobacter jejuni* isolated from a chest wall abscess. *Clin Microbiol Newslett* 1982;4:166.

207. Pedler SJ, Bint AJ. Osteitis of the foot due to *Campylobacter jejuni. J Infect* 1984;8:84–85.

208. Peterson MC, Farr RW, Castiglia M. Prosthetic hip infection and bacteremia due to *Campylobacter jejuni* in a patient with AIDS. *Clin Infect Dis* 1993;16:439–440.

209. Pasticci MB, Baratta E, Del Favero A, Gillio A, Baldelli F, Pauluzzi S. *Campylobacter jejuni:* an unusual cause of infectious arthritis. *Postgrad Med J* 1992;68:150–152.

210. Schieven BC, Baird D, Leatherdale CL, Hussain Z. *Campylobacter jejuni* infected bursitis. *Diag Microbiol Infect Dis* 1991;14:507–508.

211. Norrby R, McCloskey RV, Zàckrisson G, Falsen E. Meningitis caused by *Campylobacter fetus* ssp *jejuni. Br Med J* 1980;280:1164.

212. Ritchie PMA, Forbes JC, Steinbok P. Subdural space *Campylobacter* infection in a child. *Can Med Assoc J* 1987;137:45–46.

213. Denneberg T, Freidberg M, Holmberg L, et al. Combined plasmapheresis and hemodialysis treatment for severe hemolytic-uremic syndrome following campylobacter colitis. *Acta Paediatr Scand* 1982;71:243–245.

214. Chamovitz BN, Hartstein AI, Alexander SR, Terry AB, Short P, Katon R. *Campylobacter jejuni*-associated hemolytic-ure-

mic syndrome in a mother and daughter. *Pediatrics* 1983;71: 253–256.

215. Shulman ST, Moel D. Campylobacter infection. *Pediatrics* 1983;72:437.

216. Dickgiesser A. Campylobakterinfektion und hämolytischurämisches Syndrom. *Immun Infect* 1983;11:71–74.

217. Delans RJ, Biuso JD, Saba SR, Ramirez G. Hemolytic uremic syndrome after *Campylobacter*-induced diarrhea in an adult. *Arch Intern Med* 1984;144:1074–1076.

218. Haq JA, Rahman KM, Akbar MS. Haemolytic-uraemic syndrome and campylobacter. *Med J Aust* 1985;142:662–663.

219. Morton AR, Yu R, Waldek S, Holmes AM, Craig A, Mundy K. *Campylobacter*-induced thrombocytopenic purpura. *Lancet* 1985;2:1133–1134.

220. May Th., Gerard A, Voiriot P, Schmit JL, Lion C, Canton Ph. Entérite à *Campylobacter jejuni* associée à un syndrome hémolytique et urémique. *Presse Méd* 1986;15:803–804.

221. Carter JE, Cimolai N. IgA nephropathy associated with *Campylobacter jejuni* enteritis. *Nephron* 1991;58:101–102.

222. Menck H. *Campylobacter jejuni* enteritis complicated by glomerulonephritis. *Ugeskr Laeger* 1981;143:1020–1021.

223. Maidment CGH, Evans DB, Coulden RA, Thiru S. *Campylobacter* enteritis complicated by glomerulonephritis. *J Infect* 1985;10:177–178.

224. Andrews PI, Kainer G, Yong LCJ, Tobias VH, Rosenberg AR. Glomerulonephritis, pulmonary hemorrhage and anemia associated with *Campylobacter jejuni* infection. *Aust NZ J Med* 1989;19:721–723.

225. Rautelin HI, Outinen AV, Kosunen TU. Tubulointerstitial nephritis as a complication *Campylobacter jejuni* enteritis. *Scand J Urol Nephrol* 1987;21:151–152.

226. Pönkä A, Pitkänen T, Pettersson T, Aittoniemi S, Kosunen TU. Carditis and arthritis with *Campylobacter jejuni* infection. *Acta Med Scand* 1980;208:495–496.

227. Florkowski CM, Ikram RB, Crozier IM, Ikram H, Berry ME. *Campylobacter jejuni* myocarditis. *Clin Cardiol* 1984;7: 558–560.

228. Kell RJA, Ellis ME. Transient atrial fibrillation in *Campylobacter jejuni* infection. *Br Med J* 1985;291:1542.

229. Pönkä A, Kosunen TU. Pneumonia associated with enteritis due to *Campylobacter fetus* ssp *jejuni*. *Ann Clin Res* 1982;14: 137–139.

230. Berden JHM, Muytjens HL, van der Putte LBA. Reactive arthritis associated with *Campylobacter jejuni* enteritis. *Br Med J* 1979;1:380–381.

231. Schaad UB. Reactive arthritis associated with campylobacter enteritis. *Pediatr Infect Dis* 1982;1:328–332.

232. Saari KM, Kauranen O. Ocular inflammation in Reiter's syndrome associated with *Campylobacter jejuni* enteritis. *Am J Ophthalmol* 1980;90:572–573.

233. Leung FY-K, Littlejohn GO, Bombardier C. Reiter's syndrome after *Campylobacter jejuni* enteritis. *Arthritis Rheum* 1980;23: 948–950.

234. Ebright JR, Ryan LM. Acute erosive reactive arthritis associated with *Campylobacter jejuni*-induced colitis. *Am J Med* 1984;76:321–323.

235. Eastmond CJ, Rennie JAN, Reid TMS. An outbreak of campylobacter enteritis: a rheumatological followup survey. *J Rheumatol* 1983;10:107–108.

236. Melby K, Dahl OP, Crisp L, Penner JL. Clinical and serological manifestations in patients during a waterborne epidemic due to *Campylobacter jejuni*. *J Infect* 1990;21:309–316.

237. Rautelin H, Koota K, von Essen R, Jahkola M, Siitonen A, Kosunen TU. Waterborne *Campylobacter jejuni* epidemic in a Finnish hospital for rheumatic diseases. *Scand J Infect Dis* 1990;22:321–326.

238. Bremell T, Bjelle A, Svedhem Å. Rheumatic symptoms following an outbreak of campylobacter enteritis: a five year follow up. *Ann Rheum Dis* 1991;50:934–938.

239. Jones DA. Irritable hip and campylobacter infection. *J Bone Joint Surg* 1989;71-B:227–228.

240. Lever AML, Dolby JM, Webster ADB, Price AB. Chronic campylobacter colitis and uveitis in patient with hypogammaglobulinaemia. *Br Med J* 1984;288:531.

241. Howard RS, Sarkies NJC, Sanders MD. Anterior uveitis associated with *Campylobacter jejuni* infection. *J Infect* 1987;14: 186–187.

242. Toivanen A, Lahesmaa-Rantala R, Meurman O, et al. Antibodies against *Yersinia, Campylobacter, Salmonella,* and *Chlamydia* in patients with Behçet's disease. *Arthritis Rheum* 1987; 30:1315–1316.

243. Rhodes KM, Tattersfield AE. Guillain–Barré syndrome associated with campylobacter infection. *Br Med J* 1982;285:173–174.

244. Kaldor J, Speed BR. Guillain–Barré syndrome and *Campylobacter jejuni*: a serological study. *Br Med J* 1984;288: 1867–1870.

245. Winer JB, Hughes RAC, Anderson MJ, Jones DM, Kangro H, Watkins RPF. A prospective study of acute idiopathic neuropathy. II. Antecedent events. *J Neurol Neurosurg Psychiatry* 1988;51:613–618.

246. Gregson NA, Koblar S, Hughes RAC. Antibodies to gangliosides in Guillain–Barré syndrome: specificity and relationship to clinical features. *Q J Med* 1993;86:111–117.

247. Kuroki S, Saida T, Nukina M, et al. *Campylobacter jejuni* strains from patients with Guillain–Barré syndrome belong mostly to Penner serogroup 19 and contain β-N-acetylglucosamine residues. *Ann Neurol* 1993;33:243–247.

248. Sovilla J-Y, Regli F, Francioli PB. Guillain–Barré syndrome following *Campylobacter jejuni* enteritis. *Arch Intern Med* 1988;148:739–741.

249. Mishu B, Blaser MJ. The role of *Campylobacter jejuni* in the initiation of Guillain–Barré syndrome. *Clin Infect Dis* 1993;17: 104–108.

250. Mishu B, Ilyas AA, Koski CL, et al. Serologic evidence of previous *Campylobacter jejuni* infection in patients with the Guillain–Barré syndrome. *Ann Intern Med* 1993;118:947–953.

251. Constant OC, Bentley CC, Denman AM, Lehane JR, Larson HE. The Guillain–Barré syndrome following *Campylobacter* enteritis with recovery after plasmapheresis. *J Infect* 1983;6: 89–91.

252. Wroe SJ, Blumhardt LD. Acute polyneuritis with cranial nerve involvement following *Campylobacter jejuni* infection. *J Neurol Neurosurg Psychiatry* 1985;48:593.

253. Roberts T, Shah A, Graham JG, McQueen IN. The Miller–Fisher syndrome following *Campylobacter* enteritis, report of two cases. *J Neurol Neurosurg Psychiatry* 1987;50: 1557–1558.

254. Kohler A, de Torrenté A, Inderwildi B. Fisher's syndrome associated with *Campylobacter jejuni* infection. *Eur Neurol* 1988; 28:150–151.

255. Van der Kruijk RA, Lampe AS, Endtz H Ph. Bilateral abducens paresis following *Campylobacter jejuni* enteritis. *J Infect* 1992; 24:215–216.

256. Fujimoto S, Amako K. Guillain–Barré syndrome and *Campylobacter jejuni* infection. *Lancet* 1990;335:1350.

257. McKhann GM, Cornblath DR, Ho T, et al. Clinical and electrophysiological aspects of acute paralytic disease of children and young adults in northern China. *Lancet* 1991;338:593–597.

258. Blaser MJ, Olivares A, Taylor DN, Cornblath DR, McKhann GM. Campylobacter serology in patients with Chinese paralytic syndrome. *Lancet* 1991;338:308.

259. McKhann GM, Cornblath DR, Griffin JW, et al. Acute motor axonal neuropathy: a frequent cause of acute flaccid paralysis in China. *Ann Neurol* 1993;33:333–342.

260. Lambert M, Marion E, Coche E, Butzler J-P. Campylobacter enteritis and erythema nodosum. *Lancet* 1982;1:1409.

261. Ellis ME, Pope J, Mokashi A, Dunbar E. Campylobacter colitis associated with erythema nodosum. *Br Med J* 1982;285:937.

262. Eastmond CJ, Reid TMS. Campylobacter enteritis and erythema nodosum. *Br Med J* 1982;285:1421–1422.

263. Ashworth J, English JSC. Recurrent erythema nodosum and prolonged *Campylobacter jejuni* excretion. *Br Med J* 1984;288: 830.

264. Nagaratnam N, Goh TK, Ghoughassian D. *Campylobacter jejuni*-induced vasculitits. *Br J Clin Pract* 1990;44:636–637.

265. Dworkin B, Wormser GP, Abdoo RA, Cabello F, Aguero ME, Sivak SL. Persistence of multiply antibiotic-resistant *Campylo-*

bacter jejuni in a patient with the acquired immune deficiency syndrome. *Am J Med* 1986;80:965–970.

266. Kerstens PJSM, Endtz HP, Meis JFGM, et al. Erysipelas-like skin lesions associated with *Campylobacter jejuni* septicemia in patients with hypogammaglobulinemia. *Eur J Clin Microbiol Infect Dis* 1992;11:842–847.

267. Hammarström V, Smith CIE, Hammarström L. Oral immunoglobulin treatment in *Campylobacter jejuni* enteritis. *Lancet* 1993;341:1036.

268. Wilcox CM, Byford BA, Forsmark CE, Hadley WK, Cello JP, Jacobson MA. *Campylobacter*-like organisms are uncommon pathogens in patients infected with the human immunodeficiency virus. *J Clin Microbiol* 1990;28:2370–2371.

269. Bernard E, Roger PM, Carles D, Bonaldi V, Fournier JP, Dellamonica P. Diarrhea and *Campylobacter* infections in patients with the human immunodeficiency virus. *J Infect Dis* 1989;159:143–144.

270. Sjögren E, Lindblom G-B, Kaijser B. Comparison of different procedures, transport media, and enrichment media for isolation of *Campylobacter* species from healthy laying hens and humans with diarrhea. *J Clin Microbiol* 1987;25:1966–1968.

271. Butt CJ, Whale MCJ. Implications of delay in culturing for campylobacter. *J Clin Pathol* 1990;43:962–963.

272. Sazie ESM, Titus AE. Rapid diagnosis of campylobacter enteritis. *Ann Intern Med* 1982;96:62–63.

273. Thorson SM, Lohr JA, Dudley S, Guerrant RL. Value of methylene blue examination, dark-field microscopy, and carbolfuchsin Gram stain in the detection of campylobacter enteritis. *J Pediatr* 1985;106:941–943.

274. Goodman LJ, Trenholme GM, Kaplan RL, et al. Empiric antimicrobial therapy of domestically acquired acute diarrhea in urban adults. *Arch Intern Med* 1990;150:541–546.

275. Paisley JW, Mirrett S, Lauer BA, Roe M, Reller LB. Darkfield microscopy of human feces for presumptive diagnosis of *Campylobacter fetus* subsp. *jejuni* enteritis. *J Clin Microbiol* 1982;15:61–63.

276. Ho DD, Ault MJ, Ault MA, Murata GH. *Campylobacter* enteritis. *Arch Intern Med* 1982;142:1858–1860.

277. Schwartz RH, Bryan C, Rodriguez WJ, Park C, McCoy P. Experience with the microbiologic diagnosis of *Campylobacter* enteritis in an office laboratory. *Pediatr Infect Dis* 1983;2:298–301.

278. Park C, Hixon DL, Polhemus AS, et al. A rapid diagnosis of *Campylobacter* enteritis by direct smear examination. *Am J Clin Pathol* 1983;80:388–390.

279. Morris GK, Patton CM. *Campylobacter*. In: Lennette EH, Balows A, Hausler WJ, Shodomy WJ, eds. *Manual of clinical microbiology*. 4th ed. Washington, DC: Am Soc Microbiol; 1985:302–308.

280. Goossens H, Butzler J-P. Isolation and identification of *Campylobacter* spp. In: Nachamkin I, Blaser MJ, Tompkins LS, eds. *Campylobacter jejuni: current status and future trends*. Washington, DC: Am Soc Microbiol; 1992:93–109.

281. Jones DM, Robinson DA, Eldridge J. Serological studies in two outbreaks of *Campylobacter jejuni* infection. *J Hyg (Lond)* 1981;87:163–170.

282. Herbrink P, van den Munckhof HAM, Bumkens M, Lindeman J, van Dijk WC. Human serum antibody response in *Campylobacter jejuni* enteritis as measured by enzyme-linked immunosorbent assay. *Eur J Clin Microbiol Infect Dis* 1988;7:388–393.

283. Boswell TCJ, Kudesia G. Serological cross-reaction between *Legionella pneumophila* and campylobacter in the indirect fluorescent antibody test. *Epidemiol Infect* 1992;109:291–295.

284. Boswell TCJ, Marshall LE, Kudesia G. Cross-reactions between *Legionella* and *Campylobacter* spp. *Lancet* 1992;340:551.

285. Fallon RJ, Abraham WH. Cross-reactions between *Legionella* and *Campylobacter* spp. *Lancet* 1992;340:551–552.

286. De Witt TG, Humphrey KF, Doern GV. White blood cell counts in patients with *Campylobacter*-induced diarrhea and controls. *J Infect Dis* 1985;152:427–428.

287. Doberneck RC. *Campylobacter* colitis mimicking colonic cancer during barium enema examination. *Surgery* 1983;93:508–509.

288. Noble CJ, Hibbert DJ, Patel GJ. Campylobacter colitis: a case with unusual radiological features. *J Infect* 1982;5:199–200.

289. Puylaert JBCM, Lalisang RI, van der Werf SDJ, Doornbos L. Campylobacter ileocolitis mimicking acute appendicitis: differentiation with graded-compression US. *Radiology* 1988;166:737–740.

290. Sumathipala RW, Morrison GW. Campylobacter enteritis after falling into sewage. *Br Med J* 1983;286:1356.

291. Anders BJ, Lauer BA, Paisley JW, Reller LB. Double-blind placebo controlled trial of erythromycin for treatment of campylobacter enteritis. *Lancet* 1982;1:131–132.

292. Pitkänen T, Pettersson T, Pönkä A. Effect of erythromycin on the fecal excretion of *Campylobacter fetus* subspecies *jejuni*. *J Infect Dis* 1982;145:128.

293. Pai CH, Gillis F, Tuomanen E, Marks MI. Erythromycin in treatment of *Campylobacter* enteritis in children. *Am J Dis Child* 1983;137:286–288.

294. Mandal BK, Ellis ME, Dunbar EM, Whale K. Double-blind placebo-controlled trial of erythromycin in the treatment of clinical campylobacter infection. *J Antimicrob Chemother* 1984;13:619–623.

295. Salazar-Lindo E, Sack RB, Chea-Woo E, et al. Early treatment with erythromycin of *Campylobacter jejuni*–associated dysentery in children. *J Pediatr* 1986;109:355–360.

296. Pichler HET, Diridl G, Stickler K, Wolf D. Clinical efficacy of ciprofloxacin compared with placebo in bacterial diarrhea. *Am J Med* 1987;82 (suppl 4A);329–332.

297. Goodman LJ, Trenholme GM, Kaplan RL, et al. Empiric antimicrobial therapy of domestically acquired acute diarrhea in urban adults. *Arch Intern Med* 1990;150:541–546.

298. Wiström J, Jertborn M, Ekwall E, et al. Empiric treatment of acute diarrheal disease with norfloxacin. *Ann Intern Med* 1992;117:202–208.

299. Robins-Browne RM, Coovadia HM. Bodasing MN, Mackenjee MKR. Treatment of acute nonspecific gastroenteritis of infants and young children with erythromycin. *Am J Trop Med Hyg* 1983;32:886–890.

300. Taylor DN, Blaser MJ, Echeverria P, Pitarangsi C, Bodhidatta L, Wang W-LL. Erythromycin-resistant *Campylobacter* infections in Thailand. *Antimicrob Agents Chemother* 1987;31:438–442.

301. Ashkenazi S, Danziger Y, Varsano Y, Peilan J, Mimouni M. Treatment of campylobacter gastroenteritis. *Arch Dis Child* 1987;62:84–85.

302. Van der Auwera, Scorneaux B. In vitro susceptibility of *Campylobacter jejuni* to 27 antimicrobial agents and various combinations of β-lactams with clavulanic acid or sulbactam. *Antimicrob Agents Chemother* 1985;28:37–40.

303. Lachance N, Gaudreau C, Lamothe F, Larivière LA. Role of the β-lactamase of *Campylobacter jejuni* in resistance to β-lactam agents. *Antimicrob Agents Chemother* 1991;35:813–818.

304. Lachance N, Gaudreau C, Lamonthe F, Turgeon F. Susceptibilities of β-lactamase-positive and -negative strains of *Campylobacter coli* to β-lactam agents. *Antimicrob Agents Chemother* 1993;37:1174–1176.

305. Vanhoof R, Goossens H, Coignau H, Stas G, Butzler JP. Susceptibility pattern of *Campylobacter jejuni* from human and animal origins to different antimicrobial agents. *Antimicrob Agents Chemother* 1982;21:990–992.

306. Lariviere LA, Gaudreau CL, Turgeon FF. Susceptibility of clinical isolates of *Campylobacter jejuni* to twenty-five antimicrobial agents. *J Antimicrob Chemother* 1986;18:681–685.

307. Sjögren E, Kaijser B, Werner M. Antimicrobial susceptibilities of *Campylobacter jejuni* and *Campylobacter coli* isolated in Sweden: a 10-year follow-up report. *Antimicrob Agents Chemother* 1992;36:2847–2849.

308. Bannatyne RM, Jackowski J, Karmali MA. Susceptibility of campylobacter species to metronidazole, its bioactive metabolites and tinidazole. *Infection* 1987;15:457–458.

309. Karmali MA, De Grandis S, Fleming PC. Antimicrobial susceptibility *Campylobacter jejuni* with special reference to resistance patterns of Canadian isolates. *Antimicrob Agents Chemother* 1981;19:593–597.

310. Andreasen JJ. In vitro susceptibility of *Campylobacter jejuni* and *Campylobacter coli* isolated in Denmark to fourteen antimicrobial agents. *Acta Pathol Microbiol Immunol Scand* 1987; 95 Sect B:189–192.

311. Varoli O, Gatti M, Montella MT, La Placa M. Observations on strains of *Campylobacter* spp. isolated in 1989 in northern Italy. *Microbiologica* 1991;14:31–35.

312. Rautelin H, Renkonen O-V, Kosunen TU. Emergence of fluoroquinolone resistance in *Campylobacter jejuni* and *Campylobacter coli* in subjects from Finland. *Antimicrob Agents Chemother* 1991;35:2065–2069.

313. Reina J, Borrell N, Serra A. Emergence of resistance to erythromycin and fluoroquinolones in thermotolerant *Campylobacter* strains isolated from feces 1987–1991. *Eur J Clin Microbiol Infect Dis* 1992;11:1163–1166.

314. Secker DA, Erythromycin resistance only found in *Campylobacter coli*. *J Antimicrob Chemother* 1983;12:414–415.

315. Wang W-L L, Reller LB, Blaser MJ. Comparison of antimicrobial susceptibility patterns of *Campylobacter jejuni* and *Campylobacter coli*. *Antimicrob Agents Chemother* 1984;26: 351–353.

316. Fliegelman RM, Petrak RM, Goodman LJ, Segreti J, Trenholme M, Kaplan RL. Comparative in vitro activities of twelve antimicrobial agents against *Campylobacter* species. *Antimicrob Agents Chemother* 1985;27:429–430.

317. Taylor DE. Antimicrobial resistance of *Campylobacter jejuni* and *Campylobacter coli* to tetracycline, chloramphenicol, and erythromycin. In: Nachamkin I, Blaser MJ, Tompkins LS, eds. *Campylobacter jejuni: current status and future trends.* Washington, DC: Am Soc Microbiol; 1992:74–86.

318. Butzler JP, Vanhoof R, Clumeck N, De Mol P, Vanderlinden MP, Yourassowsky E. Clinical and pharmacological evaluation of different preparations of oral erythromycin. *Chemotherapy* 1979;25:367–372.

319. Smith JA, Isaac-Renton JL, Jellett JF, Chow AW, Ngui-Yen J. Inhibitory and lethal activities of rosaramycin, erythromycin, and clindamycin against *Campylobacter fetus* subsp *jejuni* and *intestinalis*. *Am J Vet Res* 1983;44:1605–1606.

320. Elharrif Z, Mégraud F, Marchand A-M. Susceptibility of *Campylobacter jejuni* and *Campylobacter coli* to macrolides and related compounds. *Antimicrob Agents Chemother* 1985; 28:695–697.

321. Taylor DE, Chang N. In vitro susceptibilities of *Campylobacter jejuni* and *Campylobacter coli* to azithromycin and erythromycin. *Antimicrob Agents Chemother* 1991;35:1917–1918.

322. Miyake Y, Okada M, Sasaki M, Nagasaka N, Suginaka H. In vitro susceptibility of *Campylobacter jejuni* to rokitamycin. *Antimicrob Agents Chemother* 1990;34:1440–1441.

323. Endtz HP, Broeren M, Mouton RP. In vitro susceptibilty of quinolone-resistant *Campylobacter jejuni* to new macrolide antibiotics. *Eur J Clin Microbiol Infect Dis* 1993;12:48–50.

324. Burridge R, Warren C, Phillips I. Macrolide, lincosamide and streptogramin resistance in *Campylobacter jejuni/coli*. *J Antimicrob Chemother* 1986;17:315–321.

325. Segreti J, Nelson JA, Goodman LJ, Kaplan RL, Trenholme GM. In vitro activities of lomefloxacin and temafloxacin against

326. Adler-Mosca H, Altwegg M. Fluoroquinolone resistance in *Campylobacter jejuni* and *Campylobacter coli* isolated from human faeces in Switzerland. *J Infect* 1991;23:341–342.

327. Segreti J, Gootz TD, Goodman LJ, et al. High-level quinolone resistance in clinical isolates of *Campylobacter jejuni*. *J Infect Dis* 1992;165:667–670.

328. Bowler I, Day D. Emerging quinolone resistance in campylobacters. *Lancet* 1992;340:245.

329. McIntyre M, Lyons M. Resistance to ciprofloxacin in *Campylobacter* spp. *Lancet* 1993;341:188.

330. Endtz HP, Ruijs GJ, van Klingeren B, Jansen WH, van der Reyden T, Mouton RP. Quinolone resistance in *Campylobacter* isolated from man and poultry following the introduction of fluoroquinolones in veterinary medicine. *J Antimicrob Chemother* 1991;27:199–208.

331. Mawer SL, Smith BAM. Campylobacter infection of premature baby. *Lancet* 1979;1:1041.

332. Rosef O, Kapperud G. House flies (*Musca domestica*) as possible vectors of *Campylobacter fetus* subsp. *jejuni*. *Appl Environ Microbiol* 1983;45:381–383.

333. Arimi SM, Fricker CR, Park RWA. Occurrence of "thermophilic" campylobacters in sewage and their removal by treatment processes. *Epidemiol Infect* 1988;101:279–286.

334. Stampi S, Varoli O, De Luca G, Zanetti F. Occurrence, removal and seasonal variation of "thermophilic" campylobacters in in a sewage treatment plant in Italy. *Int J Med Microbiol* 1992;193:199–210.

335. Blaser MJ, Smith PF, Wang W-LL, Hoff JC. Inactivation of *Campylobacter jejuni* by chlorine and monochloramine. *Appl Environ Microbiol* 1986;51:307–311.

336. Humphrey TJ, Beckett P. *Campylobacter jejuni* in dairy cows and raw milk. *Epidemiol Infect* 1987;98:263–269.

337. Humphrey TJ. *Salmonella, Campylobacter* and poultry: possible control measures. *Abstr Hyg Commun Dis* 1989;64:R1–R8.

338. Van de Giessen A, Mazurier SI, Jacobs-Reitsma W, et al. Study on the epidemiology and control of *Campylobacter jejuni* in poultry broiler flocks. *Appl Environ Microbiol* 1992;58: 1913–1917.

339. Humphrey TJ, Henley A, Lanning DG. The colonization of broiler chickens with *Campylobacter jejuni*: some epidemiological investigations. *Epidemiol Infect* 1993;110:601–607.

340. Pearson AD, Greenwood M, Healing TD, et al. Colonization of broiler chickens by waterborne *Campylobacter jejuni*. *Appl Environ Microbiol* 1993;59:987–996.

341. Stern NJ. Reservoirs for *Campylobacter jejuni* and approaches for intervention in poultry. In: Nachamkin I, Blaser MJ, Tompkins LS, eds. *Campylobacter jejuni: current status and future trends.* Washington, DC: Am Soc Microbiol; 1992:49–60.

342. Deming MS, Tauxe RV, Blake PA, et al. *Campylobacter* enteritis at a university: transmission from eating chicken and from cats. *Am J Epidemiol* 1987;126:526–534.

343. Gill CO, Harris LM. Hamburgers and broiler chickens as potential sources of human *Campylobacter* enteritis. *J Food Protect* 1984;47:96–99.

344. Norkrans G, Svedhem Å. Epidemiological aspects of *Campylobacter jejuni* enteritis. *J Hyg (Lond)* 1982;89:163–170.

pathogens causing diarrhea. *Antimicrob Agents Chemother* 1989;33:1385–1387.

Infections of the Gastrointestinal Tract,
edited by M. J. Blaser, P. D. Smith, J. I. Ravdin,
H. B. Greenberg, and R. L. Guerrant
Raven Press, Ltd., New York © 1995.

CHAPTER 57

Atypical Campylobacters and Related Microorganisms

Ban Mishu Allos, Albert J. Lastovica, and Martin J. Blaser

Campylobacters are important causes of gastroenteritis in developing and developed countries and now are the most frequently identified bacterial causes of diarrhea in the United States. Worldwide more than 80% of *Campylobacter* isolates implicated in human disease are *C. jejuni*; however, culture media commonly used to identify Campylobacters may not support growth of other potentially pathogenic *Campylobacter* species. Although these "atypical" Campylobacters are not presently known to be common human gastrointestinal pathogens, as improved methods are developed to identify these organisms, it may be recognized that they play a larger role in causing human disease, perhaps in all populations but especially in immunocompromised persons (Table 1). This chapter will describe the microbiology, epidemiology, and clinical features associated with infections with campylobacters and related organisms other than *C. jejuni* or *C. coli*.

CAMPYLOBACTER FETUS

Campylobacters were recognized in 1909 as a cause of abortion in sheep. Because of the curved shape of these gram-negative rods, they were initially called *Vibrio fetus ovid* (1). The name was later shortened to *Vibrio fetus* when it was realized the organisms also caused septic abortion in cattle (2). Since 1947, *C. fetus* subsp. *fetus* has been recognized as a cause of a broad range of illnesses in humans; most manifestations of *C. fetus* subsp. *fetus*

B. Mishu Allos: Department of Medicine, Division of Infectious Diseases, Vanderbilt University School of Medicine, Nashville, Tennessee 37232.
A. J. Lastovica: Department of Medical Microbiology, Red Cross Children's Hospital, Cape Town, South Africa.
M. J. Blaser: Department of Medicine, Division of Infectious Diseases, Vanderbilt University School of Medicine, Nashville, Tennessee 37232.

infections are extraintestinal, but intestinal infection and symptoms also occur.

Another subspecies, *C. fetus* subsp. *venerealis,* is associated with infection of the reproductive tract in cattle (3). This organism was never considered a human pathogen, however, it now has been isolated from stools of two homosexual men in Australia and from two women with vaginosis (4,5). These isolates were confirmed as *C. fetus* subsp. *venerealis* by both conventional methods and by pulsed field gel electrophoresis (5). Future studies may better define the role *C. fetus* subsp. *venerealis* plays in causing disease in humans. In this chapter, *C. fetus* shall refer to *C. fetus* subsp. *fetus* unless otherwise indicated.

Microbiology

Like other Campylobacters, *C. fetus* grows best in a microaerobic atmosphere (5–10% oxygen) (6,7). The organisms are oxidase-, catalase-, and nitrate-positive; they do not ferment carbohydrates (Table 2). Unlike *C. jejuni,* most *C. fetus* strains do not grow at 42°C; they grow well at 25°C and 37°C (8). Other characteristics that distinguish *C. fetus* from *C. jejuni* include the resistance of *C. fetus* to nalidixic acid, susceptibility to cephalothin (9), and lack of pyrazinamidase activity (10).

C. fetus grows slowly and 3–25 days may be required for primary isolation from blood cultures (11,12). Detection in radiometric blood culture may be difficult; the aerobic bottles are superior to anaerobic bottles for *C. fetus* (12). Because other enteric flora grow more rapidly than Campylobacters, use of antibiotic-containing media is usually necessary for isolation of Campylobacters from stools. However, use of cephalothin-containing media will inhibit growth of *C. fetus* and many other non-*jejuni* Campylobacters. Because of the small size of Campylobacters (0.3–0.6 μm in diameter), filtration of stools using a 0.45- or 0.65-μm filter allows for isolation of Campylobacters on antibiotic-free media (13).

TABLE 1. *Clinical features associated with* Campylobacter *and related species implicated as causes of human illness*

Species	Commonly encountered clinical features	Less commonly encountered clinical features
C. jejuni	Fever, diarrhea, abdominal pain	Bacteremia
C. coli	Fever, diarrhea, abdominal pain	Bacteremia
C. fetus	Bacteremia, sepsis, meningitis, vascular infections	Diarrhea, relapsing fevers
C. upsaliensis	Watery diarrhea, low-grade fever, abdominal pain	Bacteremia, abscesses
C. lari	Gastroenteritis, abdominal pain, diarrhea	Colitis, appendicitis
C. hyointestinalis	Watery or bloody diarrhea, vomiting, abdominal pain	Bacteremia
H. fenneliae	Chronic, mild diarrhea, abdominal cramps, proctitis	Bacteremia in HIV-infected persons and children
H. cinaedi	Chronic, mild diarrhea, abdominal cramps, proctitis	Bacteremia in HIV-infected persons and children
C. jejuni subsp. doylei	Gastroenteritis	Chronic gastritis, bacteremia in children
A. cryaerophila	Gastroenteritis	Bacteremia
A. butzleri	Fever, diarrhea, abdominal pain, nausea	Bacteremia, appendicitis
C. sputorum	Lung, perianal, groin, axillary abscesses	
H$_2$-requiring Campylobacters[a]	Peridontal disease	Diarrhea, osteomyelitis, bacteremia in children

[a] Includes *C. rectus, C. curvus, C. consisus.*

TABLE 2. *Biochemical characteristics of* Campylobacter *and related species*

Organism	Cat[e]	Nit[f] red	Ind[g] ace	Aryl[h] sulf	Pyrazin[i]	Hipp[j]	Nal[k]	Ceph[l]	H$_2$S Rapid[m]	H$_2$S Lead[n] ace	TSI[o]	Growth at 25°C	Growth at 37°C	Growth at 42°C	H$_2$ required
C. jejuni bio 1	+	+	+	−	+	+	S	R	−	++	−	−	+	+	−
C. jejuni bio 2	+	+	+	+	+	+	S	R	+	++	−	−	+	+	−
C. coli	+	+	+	−	+	−	S	R	−	++	−	−	+	+	−
C. fetus	+	+	−	−	−	−	R	S	−	+	−	+	+	−	−
C. upsaliensis	(+)	+	+	−	+	−	S	S	−	(+)	−	−	+	(+)	d
C. lari	+	+	−	−	+	−	R	R	+	+	−	−	+	+	−
C. hyointestinalis	+	+	−	−	−	−	R	S	−	5+	3+	(+)	+	+	d
H. fenneliae[a,b]	+	−	+	+	−	−	S	(S)	−	+	−	−	+	−	−
H. cinaedi[a]	+	+	−	−	−	−	S	(S)	−	(+)	−	−	+	−	−
C. jejuni subsp. doylei	(+)	−	+	−	+	(+)	S	(S)	−	−	−	−	+	(+)	d
A. cryaerophilus[c]	+	+	+	−	−	−	S	(R)	−	−	−	+	+	−	−
A. butzleri[c]	(+)	+	+	−	−	−	S	(R)	−	−	−	−	+	(+)	−
C. sputorum bio. sputorum	−	+	−	+	+	−	R	S	+	5+	3+	−	+	+	−
C. sputorum bio. bubulis	−	+	−	+	−	−	R	S	+	5+	3+	−	+	(+)	−
C. sputorum bio. faecalis	+	+	−	+	+	−	R	S	+	5+	3+	−	+	+	−
C. concisus	−	+	−	+	+	−	(R)	S	−	3+	(+)	−	+	(−)	+
C. mucosalis	−	+	−	−	−	−	R	S	−	5+	+	(−)	+	(−)	+
C. curvus	−	+	+	+	+	−	R	S	−	5+	+	−	+	+	+
C. rectus	−	+	+	+	+	−	S	R	−	3+	+	−	+	+	+

+, positive; (+), most strains positive; −, negative; (−), most strains negative; R, resistant; (R), most strains resistant; S, susceptible; (S), most strains susceptible. [a] spreading, noncolonial growth; [b] hypochlorite odor; [c] aerobic growth occurs at 30°C; [d] some isolates grow much better in H$_2$-enhanced growth conditions; [e] catalase; [f] nitrate reduction; [g] indole acetate; [h] aryl sulfatase; [i] pyrazinamidase; [j] hippurate hydrolysis; [k] nalidixic acid resistance; [l] cephalothin resistance; [m] Rapid H$_2$S—method of Skirrow and Benjamin, *J Clin Pathol* 1980; 33: 1122; [n] lead acetate; [o] triple sugar iron. NB: *C. jejuni* subsp *jejuni* biotypes 1 and 2 refer to Skirrow's scheme. Susceptibilities are based on 30-μg disks.

Epidemiology

Between 1987 and 1989, 122 human *C. fetus* isolates were reported to the Centers for Disease Control and Prevention (CDC) *Campylobacter* surveillance system (14); of 66 isolates for which the source was known, 18 were from blood, 41 from stool, and 7 from other sites. The incidence of *C. fetus* infections peaks in late summer and early fall, although this is not as pronounced as with *C. jejuni* infections.

The source of *C. fetus* infections in humans is not known with certainty. However, it is likely that many infections are transmitted from animals. *C. fetus* has been isolated from sheep, cattle, poultry, reptiles, and swine (6). It is a major cause of septic abortion in cattle, sheep, and other domesticated animals (15). Feces from infected animals may contaminate soil or water. Meats from infected animals frequently become contaminated with intestinal contents during slaughter (16). Acquisition of infection in humans probably results from consumption of contaminated food and water. A nutritional supplement containing raw calve's liver caused an outbreak of *C. fetus* infection in California (17), and other cases also have been caused by ingestion of raw liver (18). Another outbreak of *C. fetus* infection occurred in Wisconsin among persons who drank unpasteurized (raw) milk (19). This outbreak was detected only because of the unusual ability of the *C. fetus* strains to grow at 42°C. Other cases of raw milk–related *C. fetus* infections have been reported (20).

Despite the evidence to suggest animal-to-human transmission of *C. fetus* infection, more than two thirds of patients with *C. fetus* bacteremia live in urban areas with no exposure to farm animals (21). Some of these patients may have been infected by consuming contaminated food or water. Venereal transmission of *C. fetus* subsp. *venerealis* occurs in cattle (3). Sexual transmission of *C. fetus* subsp. *fetus* has not been demonstrated in humans; however, reports of infection among homosexual men at least raise that possibility, although alternative modes of transmission also are likely (22,23).

Clinical Features

Uncomplicated diarrheal disease due to *C. fetus* infections occurs occasionally in healthy hosts (10,19,24). The diarrheal illness is similar to that produced by infection with *C. jejuni;* sequelae are uncommon. Most patients do well without antimicrobial treatment.

In contrast to *C. jejuni,* which usually causes illness in previously healthy persons, *C. fetus* infections usually occur in compromised patients. More than three fourths of affected patients have a serious medical condition such as diabetes mellitus, atherosclerosis, cirrhosis or other liver disease, chronic alcoholism, immune compromise, treatment with immunosuppressive agents, or malignancy (21,24). *C. fetus* infections also occur in patients with AIDS (11). Among adults with *C. fetus* infections, men outnumber women three to one (24).

C. fetus infections were previously thought to typically cause bacteremia in elderly men with chronic underlying illness, although now patients with AIDS may represent the most typical population with *C. fetus* infection. High fevers often occur but these are usually well tolerated; however, the overall mortality is about 20% (25,26). The bacteremia can be primary (presumably arising from the gastrointestinal tract) or may result from infection of another site. Patients with *C. fetus* bacteremia without a localizing site should be carefully evaluated for septic thrombophlebitis. *C. fetus* exhibits a tropism for vascular tissue; infections have been associated with thrombophlebitis, mycotic aneurysms, and endocarditis (27–30).

C. fetus also causes a prolonged relapsing illness characterized by fever, chills, and myalgia without an identified source of infection (21,24,31). Occasionally, secondary seeding to an organ will occur, leading to a more complicated and sometimes fatal outcome (31–33).

In the first decades of this century, *C. fetus* was recognized as a cause of septic abortions in animals and is now known to cause perinatal sepsis and fetal loss in humans as well. In pregnant animals, ingestion of *C. fetus* leads to intestinal infection followed by bacteremia and infection of the placenta and fetus (34). A similar mechanism—gastrointestinal colonization with or without enteritis, then hematogenous spread, then placental infection—likely occurs in women (35). *C. fetus* infection in pregnant women usually is recognized during the third trimester and although the illness is mild and self-limited in the mothers, outcome is usually poor in the infants. Neonates may be infected transplacentally or during delivery. The overall mortality of fetuses and neonates is 80% even when appropriate antimicrobial therapy is used (36,37). Whether or not *C. fetus* infection results in apparent miscarriage when women are infected earlier in their pregnancy has not been established.

C. fetus infections may affect the central nervous system (CNS) in both adults and neonates. The most common CNS manifestation in adults is meningoencephalitis (38). Brain abscesses, subarachnoid hemorrhages, and cerebral infarctions also occur. Although about two thirds of patients survive, neurological sequelae are common. In neonates, the prognosis is worse. As with adults, meningoencephalitis is the most common presentation of CNS *C. fetus* infection. The cerebrospinal fluid typically shows polymorphonuclear pleocytosis. Subdural effusions may complicate infection.

Other signs of *C. fetus* infection includes salpingitis, vertebral osteomyelitis, empyema, lung abscess, cellulitis, cholecystitis, and urinary tract infection (31,39–41). Peritoneal infection due to *C. fetus* in a peritoneal dialysis patient occurred as a result of direct contamination of a catheter (42). *C. fetus* peritonitis also has occurred in patients with alcoholic cirrhosis (43), probably as a result of impaired reticuloendothelial clearance of portal bacteremia. After bacteremic seeding, *C. fetus* can remain latent in a bony focus in immunocompromised hosts, only to reactivate years later (44); eradication of infection probably requires surgical excision of the infected focus. Postoperative prosthetic hip joint infection due to *C. fetus* has been reported (45).

Pathogenesis

Most reported *C. fetus* infections of humans involve bloodstream or systemic sites (46). The probable portal of entry is the gastrointestinal tract, with secondary bacteremia. Although *C. fetus* is rarely detected in stools, 40% of patients with *C. fetus* bacteremia have a preceding diarrheal illness (11,24). It is likely that whereas a normal host usually can confine *C. fetus* infection to the gut, the compromised host cannot.

The resistance of *C. fetus* to the bactericidal activity of normal human serum could account for the high proportion of *C. fetus* infections that results in bacteremias (47,48). Human *C. fetus* isolates are covered by a surface (S)–layer protein forming a paracrystalline surface array that functions as a capsule and strongly inhibits binding of C3b (49). Disruption of C3b binding explains both the serum and phagocytosis resistance that has been observed; S$^+$ strains are not recognized by the alternative pathway of complement. Oral inoculation of mice with *C. fetus* strains that carry the S-layer protein results in bacteremia, whereas inoculation with strains without the S-layer protein does not (50). *C. fetus* also is able to change the antigenic characteristics of the particular S-layer protein expressed (51). This antigenic variation, which apparently occurs at high frequency (52), favors long-term residence at mucosal sites in ungulates, its usual host. Whether or not antigenic variation plays a role in persistence of *C. fetus* in humans is not known (53). *C. fetus* organisms possess approximately eight homologs of the *sapA* gene which encode the major S-layer protein migrating at 97 kDa (54,55). Each homolog contains both conserved and divergent domains (55), which provides opportunities for homologous recombination as well as antigenic variation. Current evidence indicates that there is a single expression locus with recombination of homologs into that site.

Treatment and Outcome

C. fetus infections often are prolonged and relapsing. However, most patients will recover with appropriate antimicrobial treatment and drainage procedures. The prognosis depends largely on the severity of underlying medical illnesses and the rapidity with which appropriate antimicrobial therapy is started. *C. fetus* infections may be lethal in some debilitated patients and may hasten the demise of others. Healthy patients may have self-limited bacteremia with no sequelae. Immunocompetent patients with uncomplicated intestinal infections may not require antibiotics. In contrast, patients with systemic *C. fetus* infections usually require parenteral therapy.

Unlike most *C. jejuni* infections, erythromycin may not be sufficient to treat infections due to *C. fetus* (56). Patients with *C. fetus* endocarditis require at least 4 weeks of parenteral antibiotic therapy; gentamicin or another aminoglycoside may be included in the regimen. Ampicillin or third-generation cephalosporins also are usually effective against serious *C. fetus* infections (44). Patients with *C. fetus* infections of the CNS should be treated for 2–3 weeks with an aminoglycoside, ampicillin, or chloramphenicol. Similar agents may be used for serious *C. fetus* infections of other sites. Chronic (or possibly lifelong) antibiotic therapy may be required in patients with hypogammaglobulinemia and persistent *C. fetus* bacteremia. Intravenous immunoglobulins are not helpful in the treatment of immunodeficient persons with *C. fetus* infection, as the serum from normal persons usually does not contain opsonizing antibodies to *C. fetus* (44).

CAMPYLOBACTER UPSALIENSIS

C. upsaliensis is a recognized human pathogen, causing diarrhea and bacteremia in healthy and immunocompromised persons (57). The organism first was identified in 1983 in the stools of dogs whether or not they had diarrhea; DNA-DNA hybridization studies indicated this was a new species (58). The name "upsaliensis" was proposed after the Swedish town, Uppsala, where the organism first was isolated; the name was validated in 1991 (59).

Microbiology

C. upsaliensis is a thermotolerant *Campylobacter* that is catalase-negative or only weakly positive (60). The hippurate test is negative and these microorganisms usually grow well at 42°C but not at 25°C (Table 2). They are nitrate reductase– and indoxyl acetate–positive, and are sensitive to colistin. One of the distinguishing characteristics of this microorganism is its intense susceptibility to nalidixic acid and cephalothin, with zones of inhibition of up to 80 mm for cephalothin (61). Because cephalothin is a common component of media used to isolate *C. jejuni*, *C. upsaliensis* cannot be isolated with such media. One diagnostic laboratory only began to isolate *C. upsaliensis* from stool specimens when their isolation protocol was changed from using antibiotic-containing media to filtration onto antibiotic-free blood agar plates (62). *C. upsaliensis* can be coisolated with *C. jejuni* subsp. *jejuni*, *C. jejuni* subsp. *doylei*, *H. fennelliae*, and other Campylobacters (62,63).

Epidemiology

Identification of C. upsaliensis in Humans

C. upsaliensis was first identified in dogs and initially it was not certain that it was a human pathogen (58). However, in 1985 the organism was identified in the stools of 9 Australian patients with diarrhea; 8 patients were children aged less than 3 years and 1 was an adult (64). In France, 5 children, also with diarrhea, had *C. upsaliensis* cultured from their stools (65). Between 1980 and 1986, the CDC received 11 *Campylobacter* isolates identified as *C. upsaliensis* from patients aged 6 months to 87 years (66); 3 were from stool and 8 were from blood. A total of 17 blood isolates of *C. upsaliensis* were cultured from 16 patients, all with serious underlying illnesses, between 1985 and

1988 at a children's hospital in South Africa (61). At this same hospital, during a 30-month period, from October 1990 to March 1993, 337 *C. upsaliensis* strains (22% of all Campylobacters isolated) were recovered from the diarrheal stools of pediatric patients (62).

Source and Seasonality of C. upsaliensis Infections

Although the source of human *C. upsaliensis* infection is not known, transmission from animals is possible. *C. upsaliensis* has been isolated from the stools of dogs in Europe and the United States (58,67). Families of four of seven patients reported animal exposure (66). A 53-year-old man with bloody diarrhea and fever and his healthy 3-year-old dog had *C. upsaliensis* cultured from stools (68). Identical plasmid profile patterns have been detected in human and dog isolates, providing additional evidence of animal-to-human transmission (69). Cats with *C. jejuni* infection have been linked to illness in humans (70). *C. upsaliensis* has been isolated from stools of asymptomatic cats used in biomedical research (71) and from the nondiarrheal stools of Vervet monkeys (72). However, the overall importance of animal-to-human transmission of *C. upsaliensis* is unknown.

Onset of symptoms with *C. upsaliensis* infection occurs in all seasons. However, of 86 Campylobacter isolates at a pediatric hospital in Toronto, 6 (7%) were *C. upsaliensis* and all were isolated within 4 weeks during the fall (73). No evidence of person-to-person transmission has been found. Two of 8 bacteremic patients had had recent emergency abdominal surgery (66), and 8 of 16 children with *C. upsaliensis* bacteremia had gastrointestinal symptoms; suggesting that the bacteremias may have been secondary to intestinal infections (61).

Incidence of C. upsaliensis Infections and Differentiation of Isolates

The proportion of all Campylobacters that are *C. upsaliensis* is relatively high when all fecal samples are prospectively cultured for this organism. From 1990 to 1994, one South African medical center isolated 424 *C. upsaliensis* strains accounting for 22% of all Campylobacters isolated (Table 3). This high isolation rate of *C. upsaliensis* is attributed to filtration onto antibiotic-free blood agar plates (63,74). In a Belgian study, Campylobacters were the most frequent enteric pathogens identified; of 15,185 fecal samples cultured, 802 yielded *Campylobacter* species; 99 (12%) were identified as *C. upsaliensis* (75). In contrast, only 1 (1%) of 93 *Campylobacter* isolates from 631 Thai children with diarrhea was *C. upsaliensis* (76). Similarly, in the Netherlands, only 1 (0.6%) of 161 *Campylobacter* isolates from 1980 stool specimens was *C. upsaliensis*. Of 915 *Campylobacter* stool isolates obtained during a 3-year period in northern Alberta, only 7 (<1%) were identified as *C. upsaliensis* (77). Of these, 5 were from children less than 2 years of age (77). Among 394 *Campylobacter* strains isolated from the bloodstream of patients in England and Wales, 2 (0.8%) were *C. upsaliensis* (78).

TABLE 3. *Prevalence and distribution of the 1911 clinical* Campylobacter *isolates at the Red Cross Children's Hospital, Cape Town, October 1990–March 1994*[a]

Species	Numbers (%)
C. jejuni subsp. jejuni	781 (40.9)
C. coli	49 (2.6)
C. upsaliensis	424 (22.2)
C. hyointestinalis	30 (1.6)
C. lari	2 (0.1)
C. concisus	262 (13.7)
C. jejuni subsp. doylei	199 (10.4)
H. fennelliae	131 (6.8)
H. cinaedi	15 (0.8)
C. fetus	9 (0.5)
A. butzleri	6 (0.3)
C. curvus	3 (0.1)

[a] Ref. 171 (*n* = 1519) and unpublished data.

It is possible that methodological differences account for some of this wide variation in prevalence.

Unlike other *Campylobacter* species, *C. upsaliensis* strains frequently (approximately 90%) contain detectable plasmids (69,75,79,80); and 15 plasmid profile patterns have been identified (69,75). Using *Hae*III DNA digestion of chromosomal DNA, fewer than 20% of strains have identical patterns (80), but the epidemiological relatedness of these strains has not been studied. Serotyping (81) and sodium dodecyl sulfate–polyacrylamide gel electrophoresis (SDS-PAGE) profiles (82) also can be used to differentiate individual *C. upsaliensis* isolates.

Clinical Features

The principal symptoms associated with *C. upsaliensis* are gastrointestinal, including watery diarrhea, abdominal cramps, vomiting, and low-grade fevers (Table 1) (65,66,77). Although most patients recover quickly, others are ill for several weeks (65,66,73,77). In one study of 99 patients with *C. upsaliensis* in their stools, onset of symptoms was abrupt—92% had diarrhea, 14% had vomiting, and only 6% reported fever >38°C (74). Symptoms persisted for more than 1 week in 16% of patients. Unlike for *C. jejuni* infections, only 25% had blood in their stools; <10% had fecal leukocytes (74).

In a pediatric study (Table 4) the average age of *C. upsaliensis*–infected patients was 19.6 months (range 1 month–10 years). Stools were loose in 89%, watery in 10%, and formed in <1%. Symptoms of gastroenteritis were present in 91%, 8% reported vomiting, and 6% had fever of >38°C. Fewer than 4% had coinfection with *Salmonella* or *Shigella*; however, 10% of patients had *Ascaris, Tricuris, Giardia,* or *Cryptosporidium* detected in their stools. Underlying illnesses such as kwashiorkor, marasmus, protein-losing enteropathy, convulsions, hepatitis, tuberculosis, or anemia were noted in 13% of the children (62).

Patients with primary *C. upsaliensis* bacteremia frequently report gastrointestinal symptoms, especially diar-

TABLE 4. *Clinical features of infection with various* Campylobacter *species among children in Capetown, South Africa, 1990–1993*

Clinical feature	Percent of patients infected with pathogen							
	C. upsaliensis n = 337	*C. concisus* n = 186	*C. jejuni doylei* n = 159	*H. fennelliae* n = 100	*C. hyointestinalis* n = 23	*H. cinaedi* n = 11	*C. fetus fetus* n = 6	*A. butzleri* n = 5
Symptoms:								
Diarrhea	88	80	78	78	75	78	100	100
Vomiting	8	3	6	9	12	9	17	60
Fever >38°C	6	9	4	5	4	9	17	20
Coexisting enteric pathogens:								
Bacterial	<4	3	<5	5	7	9	17	20
Parasitic	10	6	<9	6	11	9	0	0
Preexisting conditions	13	15	12	21	39	27	100	40

rhea, suggesting an intestinal source of infection (61,66). Most patients with *C. upsaliensis* bacteremia have other serious underlying medical conditions (61,66,83). The organism also has been isolated from a breast abscess (84). The patient reported no contact with animals and had no gastrointestinal symptoms (84).

Diagnosis

Detection of *C. upsaliensis* in stool samples remains difficult. Because *C. upsaliensis* is susceptible to antibiotics that are standard components of *Campylobacter* media, ordinary efforts to detect Campylobacters will fail to detect *C. upsaliensis* (75). An antibiotic-free medium used in combination with a porous membrane to filter stool samples provides an essential adjunct to *Campylobacter*-selective media (85). The filtration method may require a high concentration (>10^5 colony-forming units per gram of feces) of the bacteria in stool.

In a study of 676 hospitalized gastroenteritis patients in Australia, 75 *Campylobacter* strains were isolated on blood-free medium with a selective supplement, but concurrent isolation onto blood agar overlaid with a membrane filter yielded 213 *Campylobacter* strains, and some *Campylobacter* species only were isolated by the membrane filter technique (63). Similar results were documented by South African workers (62). Technical considerations such as the viscosity of the fecal suspension, incubation time, and temperature may affect the efficiency of this method. While some studies recommend both membrane filtration and selective media for optimum *Campylobacter* isolation (63,86), others have found membrane filtration by itself to be extremely efficient (62). Membrane filtration has the added advantage of permitting isolation of antibiotic-susceptible *Campylobacter* species other than *C. upsaliensis*. Antibiotic-containing media have a very limited shelf life, and a selection of different media may be required for the isolation of the whole spectrum of *Campylobacter, Arcobacter,* and *Helicobacter* species.

Pathogenesis

The pathogenic mechanisms of *C. upsaliensis* have not been well characterized. *C. upsaliensis*, like other *Campylobacter* species, adheres to an endothelial cell monolayer (61). The occurrence of *C. upsaliensis* sepsis in a boy with hypogammaglobulinemia (83) suggests that antibody-mediated killing of *C. upsaliensis* is important. Bloodstream isolates of *C. upsaliensis* usually are serum-resistant, whereas fecal isolates usually are serum-susceptible (66,75).

Treatment

Fluoroquinolones are the most active antimicrobial agents available for treatment of *C. upsaliensis* (87). Erythromycin was once considered the treatment of choice in *Campylobacter* infections, but 4–18% of *C. upsaliensis* isolates are resistant to erythromycin (66,74,79). *C. upsaliensis* infections have been treated successfully with doxycycline, cefotaxime, and Augmentin (66,68,83). More studies may further define the antibiotic susceptibility of this organism and the clinical indications and efficacy of treatment with antimicrobial agents.

CAMPYLOBACTER HYOINTESTINALIS

C. hyointestinalis first was recognized as a cause of proliferative enteritis in swine, a disease in weaned pigs of all ages (88). The organism also may be a cause of diarrhea in humans and has been isolated from stools of homosexual men and compromised persons. The name *hyointestinalis* comes from the Latin word *hyo* meaning hog and *intestinalis* meaning pertaining to the intestines.

Microbiology and Diagnosis

C. hyointestinalis is most closely related to *C. fetus* and most distant from *C. jejuni*, based on phenotypic (89) and molecular (90) properties (Table 2). *C. hyointestinalis* grows under microaerobic conditions, but some strains have an additional H$_2$ requirement (91). These isolates can be differentiated from other Campylobacters with similar growth requirements for hydrogen by the catalase and nitrite reductase tests (91). *C. hyointestinalis* is an abundant producer of hydrogen sulfide in triple sugar iron media and often completely blackens lead acetate strips. Its hydrogenase activity, intolerance to 3% sodium chloride, and lack of activity in the aryl sulfatase test are useful diagnostic features (10,17,28). This microorganism is catalase- and nitrate reductase–positive and indoxyl acetate–negative. It is thermotolerant (not thermophilic) as it exhibits some growth at 42°C but grows most abundantly at 37°C (92). As cephalothin is a component of most *Campylobacter*-selective media, *C. hyointestinalis*, like other cephalothin-susceptible Campylobacters, is underdetected. Filtration onto antibiotic-free blood agar media and incubation under microaerobic or H$_2$-enhanced microaerobic atmospheres has been extremely efficient for the isolation of *C. hyointestinalis* (62). SDS-PAGE and gel electrophoresis pulsed field have proven useful in the differentiation of strains of *C. hyointestinalis* as well as for differentiating *C. hyointestinalis* from other *Campylobacter* species (93–95). Recently, 21 (72%) of 29 *C. hyointestinalis* strains isolated from swine with proliferative enteropathy were found to produce a cytotoxin, although its role in clinical illness is uncertain (96).

In swine with proliferative enteritis, DNA probes may be useful for detection of *C. hyointestinalis* (97). Similarly, in humans with acute enteric infections, enzyme-labeled oligonucleotide probes have been used to detect *C. hyointestinalis* (98).

Epidemiology

C. hyointestinalis is consistently isolated from the intestines of pigs with proliferative enteritis but not from asymptomatic pigs or pigs with other enteric diseases (99); its role in this disorder however, remains uncertain (88). In addition to pigs, *C. hyointestinalis* has been isolated from hamsters, cattle, and deer (88,100–103), as well as nonhuman primates (104).

The first description of *C. hyointestinalis* associated with human illness was reported in 1986 (105). *C. hyointestinalis* was cultured from the stools of a homosexual man with proctitis; no other pathogens were identified. The patient's symptoms resolved and the organism disappeared after treatment with antibiotics to which the strain was susceptible (105).

Clinical Characteristics

Published reports describe 13 persons from whom *C. hyointestinalis* was cultured, in each case from stools (91–93,106). Six patients had watery, nonbloody diarrhea, 1 had bloody diarrhea, 1 had proctitis, and 5 persons were asymptomatic. The patients with diarrhea also experienced vomiting or abdominal pain; 3 were febrile with mild leukocytosis but none had fecal leukocytes. Three of the patients were homosexual men, 2 were older than 70 years, 1 had leukemia, and 1 was an infant. The 5 asymptomatic persons belonged to 1 family and included children. All symptomatic persons responded to antimicrobial therapy, whether or not *C. hyointestinalis* caused the symptoms.

In a South African study, 23 strains of *C. hyointestinalis* were isolated from 6111 diarrheal stools from pediatric patients, and comprised 1.5% of all Campylobacters isolated during a 30-month period (Table 4) (62). The average age of the patients was 16 months (range 1 month–7 years). Stools were loose in 79%, watery in 19%, and formed in <5%. Blood was present in 13% of stools, and 18% had fecal leukocytes. Other associated clinical features are shown in Table 4. The only known extraintestinal isolation is from the blood culture of an adult after bone marrow transplantation.

Treatment

In vitro antimicrobial testing has demonstrated that *C. hyointestinalis* is susceptible to erythromycin, metronidazole, nitrofurantoin, ampicillin, and aminoglycosides (107). All clinical isolates tested have been susceptible to erythromycin (92).

CAMPYLOBACTER LARI

C. lari is a nalidixic acid–resistant, thermophilic *Campylobacter* first identified in 1980 (108). Initially, most strains were isolated from wild seagulls (genus *Larus*), hence the name proposed was *C. laridis;* the name was shortened to *C. lari* in 1990 (109). Up to 25% of healthy seagulls may be infected with *C. lari* (108); however, the organism is an infrequently identified human pathogen. Although the first human isolate was from an asymptomatic 6-year-old boy, it can produce an acute diarrheal illness in normal hosts and can cause bacteremia in immunocompromised persons (Table 1).

Microbiology

C. lari are microaerophilic (some isolates may require H$_2$-enhanced microaerobic growth conditions), thermophilic Campylobacters; they grow at 42°C but not 25°C (Table 2). They are resistant to nalidixic acid, cephalosporins, vancomycin, and trimethoprim. Most are oxidase- and catalase-positive and are able to reduce nitrate to nitrite. *C. lari* strains do not hydrolyze hippurate (110).

Epidemiology

C. lari may be isolated from a variety of environmental sources. Of 312 riverine samples collected in Lancastershire, England, 134 yielded Campylobacters; 7 (5%) of these were *C. lari* (111). In a survey of surface waters in

Norway, *C. lari* was isolated from 2 (2%) of 96 samples cultured (46). These isolations may be significant since water is an established vehicle for transmission of Campylobacters to humans (112,113). Of 1564 samples of fresh vegetables cultured in Canada, 3% yielded campylobacters; *C. lari* composed 8% of all *Campylobacter* isolates (114).

C. lari isolation rates are 25% from seagulls (109), 8% from herring gulls and 29% from kittiwakes (115), and 5–7% from crows (116,117). Unlike other Campylobacters, *C. lari* is only infrequently isolated from poultry. Of 90 *Campylobacter* isolates from broilers, layers, and free-range poultry, only 1 (2.2%) was *C. lari* (118). *C. lari* also is only infrequently isolated from dogs (116,119). In Sweden, *C. lari* was isolated from 8 (17%) of 47 pigs but in no humans or hens (120).

Clinical Features

C. lari is an enteric pathogen for both immunocompetent and immunocompromised hosts. The first human isolates of *C. lari* were in asymptomatic persons (108,121). However, bloodstream isolates (122,123) confirm its pathogenic potential. *C. lari* induced colitis in a 32-year-old HIV-positive woman (CD4 = 90/mm^3) who required more than 5 weeks of antimicrobial therapy before symptoms improved (124). Another HIV-infected patient, an intravenous drug user with *C. lari* bacteremia, had persistently positive blood cultures despite aminoglycoside treatment (125). *C. lari* was isolated from the stools of 5 immunocompetent persons (1 was pregnant) with diarrhea and abdominal pain that had lasted from 1 week to 4 months (110); none of the patients was febrile. Further support for the pathogenic role of *C. lari* was provided by a report of *C. lari* cultured from the stools of a 32-year-old man with diarrhea; he developed specific serum bactericidal antibody response to the *C. lari* strain which declined in the weeks following his acute illness (126). *C. lari* accounted for 2 (0.8%) of 394 *Campylobacter* strains isolated from the bloodstream of patients in England and Wales (78).

Urease-positive, nalidixic acid–susceptible variants of *C. lari* were isolated from the stools of two compromised (one was an alcoholic, the other had ovarian cancer) patients with diarrhea in France and from the inflamed appendix of an immunocompetent 10-year-old boy (127). A urinary tract infection caused by a urease-positive, nalidixic acid–susceptible *C. lari* variant was reported in an alcoholic man with cirrhosis (128).

In 1985, a waterborne outbreak of gastroenteritis occurred in Ontario (129). The treated drinking water supply became contaminated with surface water from Lake Ontario (an area frequented by large numbers of seagulls) (129). A total of 162 persons became ill; 87% reported diarrhea, 70% had abdominal pain, 51% had vomiting, 50% nausea, 26% malaise, 20% fever, 17% headache, and 8% dizziness (129). Only one patient reported bloody stools. The mean duration of illness was 4 days (range 1–10 days). Of 125 stool specimens cultured, 7 yielded *C. lari;* however, the specimens were transported in dry containers, which could have reduced the isolation rate. No other potential pathogens were identified.

Diagnosis

Because the spectrum of clinical disease described in association with *C. lari* is similar to that seen with other Campylobacters, diagnosis of *C. lari* depends on isolation and identification of the organisms from cultured specimens. Distinguishing *C. lari* from *C. jejuni* may be difficult because most clinical microbiology laboratories do not routinely test isolates for nalidixic acid resistance. Furthermore, several nalidixic acid–susceptible isolates of *C. lari* have been reported (111,127,128,130) as well as nalidixic acid–resistant *C. jejuni* strains (103,131). Hippurate hydrolysis (negative for *C. lari*, positive for *C. jejuni*) also may distinguish the strains (Table 2). *C. lari* can be distinguished from *C. jejuni* since all *C. jejuni* strains, even nalidixic acid–resistant ones, hydrolyze indoxylacetate whereas *C. lari* do not (132). Species-specific antibodies also distinguish *C. lari* from other thermophilic Campylobacters (133).

Treatment

C. lari infections that are limited to uncomplicated diarrheal disease do not require antimicrobial therapy. For patients with fever or more severe disease, antibiotics may be used. The organism also is susceptible to erythromycin, clindamycin, chloramphenicol, aminoglycosides, and imipenem (122,124,126). *C. lari* is resistant to first-, second-, and third-generation cephalosporins, penicillin, vancomycin, and trimethoprim-sulfamethoxazole (124, 126). Quinolone-resistant strains have been reported in HIV-infected persons (124).

HELICOBACTER CINAEDI AND *HELICOBACTER FENNELLIAE*

These organisms, formerly called *Campylobacter*-like organisms (CLOs), are a cause of enteritis and proctocolitis, especially in homosexual men, and sometimes also cause bacteremia (Table 1).

Microbiology

H. cinaedi and *H. fennelliae* grow well under microaerobic conditions at 37°C, but poorly or not at all at 25°C and 42°C (6,133) (Table 2). *H. fennelliae* may be differentiated from *H. cinaedi* by SDS-PAGE profile (134), serology (135), and aryl sulfatase activity (10). *H. fennelliae* colonies have an odor similar to that of hypochlorite (''Clorox''), which is absent in *H. cinaedi* and Campylobacters. While *Campylobacter* species form domed colonies on agar, both *H. fennelliae* and *H. cinaedi* produce flat, spreading growth without discrete colonies on freshly prepared agar plates (136); this growth may be missed on primary isolation plates, particularly if the domed colo-

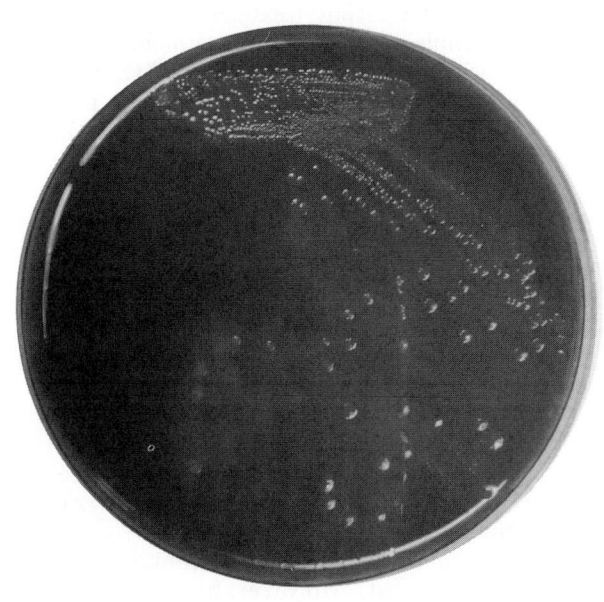

FIG. 1. Photomicrograph of culture plate showing the spreading noncolonial growth of *H. fennelliae* (**top**) and the domed colonies of *C. concisus* (**bottom**).

nies of *Campylobacter* sp. are present. *H. fennelliae* is often coisolated with *C. jejuni* subsp. *jejuni*, *C. jejuni* subsp. *doylei*, and *C. upsaliensis* (Fig. 1) (62,63).

Initially, CLOs were divided into three phenotypic groups: CLO1, CLO2, and CLO3. CLO1 was found to include two genetically distinct groups, CLO1A and CLO1B, that were phenotypically indistinguishable (137). CLO1A was initially called *Campylobacter cinaedi* for the Latin word *cinaedi* meaning "of a homosexual." CLO2 strains initially were called *C. fennelliae* for Cynthia Fennell, the microbiologist who first isolated the organisms from the rectal swabs of homosexual men. Only two CLO3 have been isolated from the stools of gay men with proctocolitis (137–139). In 1991, the names of the organisms were further amended to *Helicobacter cinaedi* and *Helicobacter fennelliae* (140).

Epidemiology and Clinical Features

CLOs were first recognized as human pathogens when they were isolated from the stools of 26 of 158 homosexual men with gastrointestinal symptoms seen at an STD clinic (141,142). The organisms were isolated from 6 of 75 asymptomatic homosexual men and from none of 150 heterosexual men and women (142).

Campylobacter or *Helicobacter* species were isolated from the diarrheal stools of 9 (27%) of 33 homosexual or bisexual men in Baltimore and Washington, DC; 2 had *H. cinaedi* infections; 1 was infected with an organism identified as CLO3 (138). CLOs may be isolated from up to 8% of stools from homosexual men with diarrhea or proctitis (143). In contrast, however, CLOs were not iden-

tified in the stools or colonic brushings of 27 homosexual men in California with chronic diarrhea (144).

In the initial descriptions of patients with gastrointestinal symptoms attributed to CLO infections, the clinical features were similar to those seen in patients infected with *C. jejuni* and included diarrhea, abdominal cramps, tenesmus, and hematochezia (142). CLO infections also were noted to produce fever and anal discharge and pain (142). Sigmoidoscopic examinations of infected patients showed ulcerations and mucosal bleeding. Fecal leukocytes were present in most patients and histopathologically, crypt abscesses and polymorphonuclear leukocytes were scattered throughout the lamina propria. Subsequent reports, however, have described HIV-infected patients with *H. cinaedi* in their stools who experienced more chronic but mild symptoms that lasted several weeks (145); blood and polymorphonuclear cells were absent from stools. The diarrhea consisted of three to four loosely formed bowel movements per day and was not associated with fever, chills, or other evidence of systemic illness.

In addition to gastrointestinal illness, *H. cinaedi* and *H. fennelliae* may cause bacteremia in HIV-infected patients. Of 14 Campylobacters isolated from the blood of 13 patients in Denver over a 6-year period, 6 were *H. cinaedi* (146); 5 patients were HIV-positive. Eleven other reports of *H. cinaedi* bacteremia have been published (147–150). Low-grade fevers, chills, lethargy, and malaise are generally present; many but not all patients with *H. cinaedi* bacteremia have preceding gastrointestinal symptoms. Other clinical features associated with *H. cinaedi* bacteremia include monoarticular arthritis and a skin rash resembling multifocal cellulitis (146). Hypotension or other signs of sepsis are not usually present.

A 32-year-old homosexual man with AIDS developed recurrent *H. cinaedi* bacteremia. He had had 2 months of intermittent diarrhea, tenesmus, and fecal incontinence. Paradoxically, his blood cultures subsequently yielded a second organism most closely resembling *H. fennelliae*; cultures remained positive despite treatment with ciprofloxacin and trimethoprim-sulfamethoxazole. The patient died 4 months later, although the role of *H. fennelliae* infection in causing his death was uncertain (150). Another case of bacteremia due to an *H. fennelliae*-like organism in an AIDS patient was reported (151). Of 394 bloodstream *Campylobacter* isolates from patients in England and Wales, 2 were *H. fennelliae* and 1 was *H. cinaedi* (78).

Recently, gastroenteritis due to *H. cinaedi* and *H. fennelliae* was reported in heterosexual men and in women and children (144,145,152–154). In a South African study, 100 strains of *H. fennelliae* and 11 strains of *H. cinaedi* were isolated from 6111 diarrheal stools of pediatric patients, and comprised 6.6% and 0.7% of all Campylobacters isolated during a 30-month period (62). The average age of the patients was 19 months (range 2 weeks–11 years). Seventy-two percent of the stools contained blood, and in 18% fecal leukocytes were present. Other clinical features are shown in Table 4. These reports suggest *H. cinaedi* and *H. fennelliae* infections may occur more frequently than previously thought in immunocompetent and heterosexual populations.

The source of human infection with these organisms is not known; however, transmission from animals has caused some human illness. *H. cinaedi* was isolated from the cerebrospinal fluid and blood of a 5-day-old girl whose mother had a mild diarrheal illness during her third trimester of pregnancy. The mother reported no contact with homosexual men but had cared for pet hamsters during the first two trimesters of pregnancy (155). *H. cinaedi* has been isolated from 54 (72%) of healthy hamsters obtained from two commercial sources (156). Introduction of gerbils into the rectum for sexual gratification reportedly has been done by some homosexual men; gerbils have not been studied for the presence of *H. cinaedi* or *H. fennelliae*. Organisms resembling *H. fennelliae* also have been isolated from fecal specimens from dogs with diarrhea (152).

Pathogenesis

The evidence that *H. cinaedi* and *H. fennelliae* are indeed pathogens of the gastrointestinal tract and causes of systemic infection comes from several sources. Their association with homosexual men who had proctitis and enteritis (but not with asymptomatic men) supports a causal relationship. The presence of bacteremia in immunocompromised patients as well as fecal leukocytes suggests the organisms may have a pathogenic role.

Animal studies also provide evidence for the pathogenicity of this organism. Flores and colleagues studied the effects of experimental *H. cinaedi* and *H. fennelliae* infections in infant macaques (157). Four monkeys were challenged with *H. cinaedi;* two of the animals developed diarrhea. The organism was subsequently isolated from stools and bloodstream from all four animals. Three monkeys challenged with *H. fennelliae* all became bacteremic, had the organism recovered from their stools, and two developed diarrhea. Prolonged rectal colonization was observed in all animals observed; fecal leukocytes were absent. Necropsy of one animal showed marked hyperplasia in Peyer's patches.

Treatment

No fatal outcomes resulting from *H. cinaedi* or *H. fennelliae* infections have been described, although some patients had slow clinical responses to antimicrobial therapy. Antimicrobial agents that demonstrated *in vitro* activity against 50 CLO strains include ampicillin, gentamicin, doxycycline, tetracycline, ceftriaxone, rifampin, streptomycin, nalidixic acid, and chloramphenicol (139). In contrast, 28% of strains were resistant to erythromycin and clindamycin, and 17% were resistant to sulfamethoxazole (139). Thirteen percent of *H. fennelliae* and *H. cinaedi* isolates from pediatric patients including bloodstream isolates were erythromycin-resistant (62). All CLOs are resistant to trimethoprim and most also are resistant to metronidazole. Two patients with persistent *H.*

cinaedi bacteremia despite treatment with erythromycin had a rapid clinical response to treatment with oral ciprofloxacin (500 mg every 12 hr) (148,149). Oral fluoroquinolones may be the best therapeutic option in patients with persistent or severe *H. cinaedi* or *H. fennelliae* infections.

ARCOBACTER CRYAEROPHILA AND *ARCOBACTER BUTZLERI*

Arcobacter cryaerophila and *Arcobacter butzleri* (previously *Campylobacter cryaerophila* and *Campylobacter butzleri*) differ from other *Campylobacter* species in that they can be cultured under aerobic conditions. In 1991, following DNA-DNA hybridization studies, these organisms were moved from the genus *Campylobacter* to *Arcobacter* (158).

A. cryaerophila first was isolated from pig fetuses and bovine feces (159–161). However, human isolates rarely have been reported, despite the high density of the organism in urban sewage, which may result from inflows from slaughterhouses (162). The first human isolate of a strain thought to be *A. cryaerophila* was from feces of an Australian traveler with gastroenteritis (163). However, later the organism was found to belong to group 2 aerotolerant *Campylobacter* species, i.e., *A. butzleri*. *A. cryaerophila* has been isolated from the blood of two patients who aspirated fecal contents and from the stools of a patient with gastroenteritis (164).

Like *A. cryaerophila*, *A. butzleri* grow poorly on blood agar plates and do not grow at 42°C (Table 2). *A. butzleri* are aerotolerant at 30°C and 36°C (*A. cryaerophila* is aerotolerant only at 30°C), grow on MacConkey agar, and are resistant to cephalothin (164). Restriction fragment length polymorphisms and ribotyping also may distinguish between *A. cryaerophila* and *A. butzleri* (165). *A. butzleri* was identified by Kiehlbach and colleagues during a study of aerotolerant *Campylobacter* presumed to be *C. cryaerophila* (164). Genetic studies showed the aerotolerant bacteria belonged to two groups; group 2 was called *C. butzleri* in recognition of Jean-Paul Butzler, a Belgian clinician and microbiologist.

Arcobacter butzleri may produce diarrhea and other gastrointestinal symptoms in humans (Table 1) and has been isolated from stool cultures from 43 patients with diarrhea, from 3 blood cultures, and from abdominal contents of 3 patients with appendicitis (164). More than 50% of these patients experienced abdominal pain and nausea. Many also had fever, chills, vomiting, and malaise. Of 631 Thai children with diarrhea, *A. butzleri* was the most frequent atypical "*Campylobacter*" isolated from stools (76). In contrast, during an outbreak of *A. butzleri* infection among ten children at an Italian elementary school, none had diarrhea but all had recurrent abdominal cramps (166). Attacks of abdominal cramps lasting 2 hr occurred two to three times per day for 5–10 days; the children felt well between attacks. Although the children's illnesses were self-limited, most children seroconverted. Furthermore, all the strains belonged to a single serogroup and had identical protein profiles, suggesting a common source (166).

A. butzleri may be enzootic in nonhuman primates. A. butzleri infection was found in 14 (6%) of 222 nonhuman primates with diarrhea. In addition, 3 (4%) colonic specimens obtained at necropsy from 76 macaques yielded A. butzleri; all 3 animals had chronic active colitis (167). Similarly, A. butzleri was isolated from the stools of 7 (39%) of 18 Macaca nemestrina monkeys cultured every week from birth to age 1 year (168).

CAMPYLOBACTER JEJUNI SUBSP. DOYLEI

C. jejuni has been separated into two subspecies: C. jejuni subsp. jejuni and C. jejuni subsp. doylei, as a result of DNA hybridization studies (64). C. jejuni subsp. doylei was named after L. P. Doyle, an American veterinarian who isolated vibrios in the intestines of pigs with swine dysentery (169). The pathogenic potential of this newly recognized microorganism in humans is just beginning to be appreciated.

Microbiology and Diagnosis

C. jejuni subsp. doylei does not reduce nitrate to nitrite (169), which distinguishes it from C. jejuni subsp. jejuni and all other Campylobacters (Table 2). While H. fennelliae also is nitrate reductase–negative, it has a spreading colony morphology on blood agar plates, a strong hypochlorite smell (136), and is resistant to polymyxin B (10). C. jejuni subsp. doylei grows poorly at 42°C and is usually catalase-negative and hippuricase-positive (Table 2). C. doylei is susceptible to nalidixic acid but, unlike C. jejuni subsp. jejuni, also is susceptible to cephalothin (170). Filtration of stools onto antibiotic-free blood agar plates is an efficient and simple method of obtaining these microorganisms (Fig. 2). Differences in colony morphology on primary isolation and subsequent confirmation by serological and biochemical characterization indicates that C. jejuni subsp. doylei can be isolated with C. jejuni subsp. jejuni, C. upsaliensis, H. fennelliae, and other campylobacters (62,63).

Epidemiology and Clinical Features

C. jejuni subsp. doylei may be present in the upper gastrointestinal tract (171–173). Urease-negative, Campylobacter-like organisms (initially called GCLO2 and later C. jejuni subsp. doylei) were identified in the gastric antral biopsy specimens of six patients (171,174). Four of these patients did not have H. pylori infection, yet all had gastric ulcer and active chronic gastritis. Identical microorganisms were identified in the feces of young Australian children hospitalized with gastroenteritis (64,175). Other studies (Table 3) also have shown that the microorganism may be associated with diarrhea in children (62,63, 74,76,176). Of 631 Thai children with diarrhea, 93 (15%) had Campylobacters isolated from their stools and 1

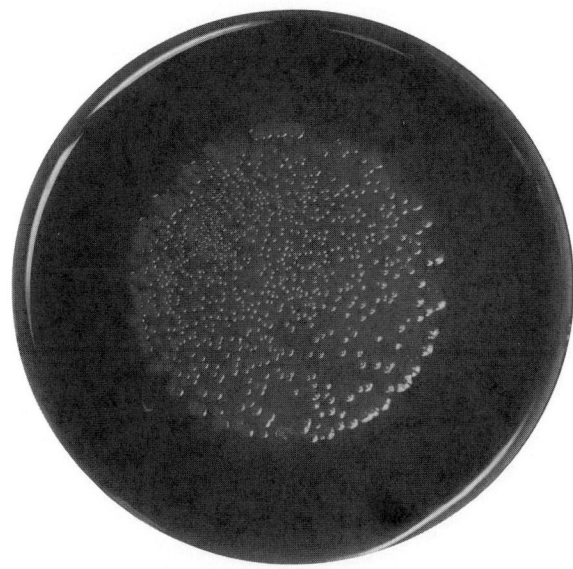

FIG. 2. Photomicrograph of a 5-day-old pure growth of C. jejuni subsp. doylei after filtration onto antibiotic-free blood-agar plate.

(1.1%) of these was C. jejuni subsp. doylei. C. jejuni subsp. doylei accounted for 4 (0.5%) of 802 Campylobacter isolates cultured from the stools of 15,185 patients in Belgium (74).

In a South African study (Table 4), C. jejuni subsp. doylei was isolated 159 times from 6111 diarrheal, pediatric stool specimens, and comprised 10.5% of all Campylobacters isolated during a 30-month period (62). These 159 isolates were obtained from 142 gastroenteritis patients whose average age was 21 months (range 1 month–11 years). Eighty-one percent had loose stools, 19% had watery stools, and <1% had formed stools. Fourteen percent of the patients had blood in their stools; 20% had fecal leukocytes. Other clinical features are shown in Table 4. Eleven blood culture isolates of C. jejuni subsp. doylei were obtained from 11 bacteremic children whose average age was 13 months (range 2–30 months). Seven of these 11 children had had diarrhea, suggesting that intestinal infection preceded systemic infection.

H₂-REQUIRING CAMPYLOBACTERS

Campylobacters that have a growth requirement for hydrogen are beginning to be appreciated as potential causative agents of gastrointestinal illness. C. concisus, [Latin: concisus meaning concise (177)]; C. rectus [Latin: rectus meaning straight (177)]; and C. curvus [Latin: curvus meaning curved (178)] are known to be implicated in human periodontal disease (177–180). C. mucosalis, formerly called C. sputorum subsp. mucosalis (181), is of considerable veterinary importance as it is associated with proliferative enteritis in pigs and lambs (182,183).

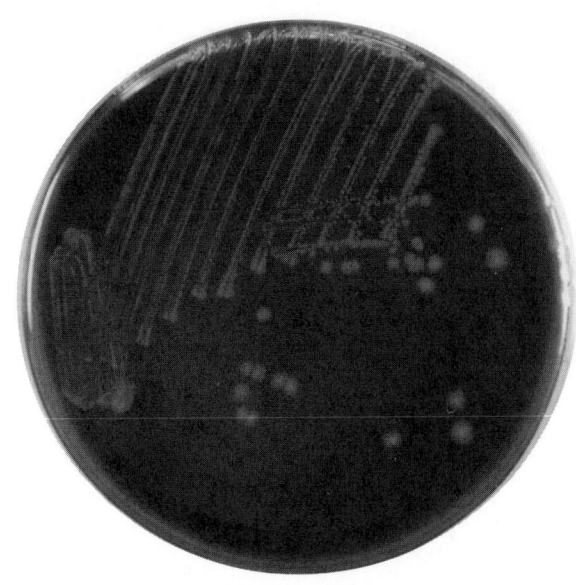

FIG. 3. Photomicrograph of a 5-day-old culture of *C. concisus.*

Microbiology and Diagnosis

Four species of *Campylobacter*—*concisus* (Fig. 3), *mucosalis, rectus* [formerly *Wolinella recta* (140)], and *curvus* [formerly *Wolinella curva* (140)]—are known to require H_2 for growth (Table 2). Many, but not all, isolates are susceptible to cephalothin and nalidixic acid (30-µg disks) with inhibitory zones up to 50 mm in diameter (62,91). *C. curvus* is difficult to differentiate from *C. concisus* as the indoxylacetate hydrolysis assay is not infallible (184) and serological (178) or electrophoretic (185) methods may be required. The occasional *C. hyointestinalis* isolate requires an H_2-enriched microaerobic atmosphere for growth but can be differentiated from the above four species by the catalase and nitrite reductase tests (91).

Epidemiology and Clinical Features

C. rectus has been isolated from 80% of 1654 adult and children with periodontitis in a 2-year longitudinal study (180). *C. rectus* also has been isolated from a lung infection (186) and from periodontitis patients with inflammatory bowel disease (187), HIV infection (188), or diabetes mellitus (189). *C. rectus* produces an extracellular cytotoxin (190). To date there is no report of *C. rectus* being implicated in gastrointestinal illness, which may be due to less than optimal isolation conditions since it is fastidious. *C. curvus* has been recovered from periodontal and septicemia patients (178). Recently, *C. curvus* has been isolated from the diarrheal stools of children in Belgium (184) and South Africa (62). The pathogenicity of *C. cur-*

vus in human gastrointestinal disease remains to be determined.

The association of *C. concisus* with periodontal disease in humans is well documented (177,179,191); however, a direct causal role has not been established. Osteomyelitis of the sacrum in a patient with diabetes and a sacral decubitus ulcer may have been due to *C. concisus* (192). Belgian investigators have isolated *C. concisus* from the feces, stomach, esophagus, duodenum, and blood of 22 patients with gastroenteritis (193). Another Belgian study of the stools of 3165 children and 1265 adults used filtration onto antibiotic-free blood agar plates and an H_2-enriched microaerobic (7% CO_2, 4.5% O_2, 7% H_2, and 81.5% N_2) atmosphere. Seventy-five (2.4%) and 19 (1.5%) of the *Campylobacter* isolates obtained from the stools of the children and adults, respectively, were *C. concisus* (184). Fifty-four percent of the children with *C. concisus* were <1 year old; only 9% were >5 years old. Seventy-two percent of the children had gastrointestinal symptoms; 62% had diarrhea and 22% vomiting. The mean age of the adults with *C. concisus* was 60 years (range 21–87 years), and all but two had diarrhea. Five patients had abdominal cramps and five had signs of colitis.

In a South African study of 1519 *Campylobacter* isolates, 187 (12.3%) required H_2 for growth (62,194). One hundred and eighty-four isolates were from pediatric diarrheal stools, one was from an adult diarrheal stool, one was from the blood culture of an 18-day-old infant, and one was from a duodenal biopsy from an adult. Ninety-two of the stool isolates were confirmed as *C. concisus* by DNA hybridization. The mean age of the gastroenteritis patients was 24 months (range 4 days–11 years). Twenty-one percent of the stools were watery, the rest were loose. Fourteen percent of the stools were bloody, and fecal leukocytes were detected in 27% of the stools (Table 4).

Thirty *C. concisus* isolates from pediatric stools were tested against eight antimicrobial agents (195). Ciprofloxacin was the most active agent examined. All strains were susceptible to tetracycline, ampicillin, and gentamicin, and all but one of the strains was resistant to erythromycin (minimum inhibitory concentration >1 mg/mL). Activity of the cephalosporins was variable.

In cases of porcine intestinal adenomatosis, *C. mucosalis* can be recovered at high concentrations (up to 10^8/g) from the diseased intestinal mucosa but experimental infection does not cause the disease (182). A *Campylobacter* isolate with the phenotypic characteristics of *C. mucosalis* has been isolated from the blood of a 71-year-old man with pneumonia (123). Stool cultures from this patient were negative and no gastrointestinal symptoms were reported. Two *C. mucosalis* isolates characterized by phenotypic criteria were isolated from the diarrheal stools of two children (196). However, these three *C. mucosalis* isolates were identified solely on phenotypic characteristics that are known to be variable.

MISCELLANEOUS *CAMPYLOBACTERS*

Several Campylobacters have been implicated as causes of human disease but their role as gastrointestinal pathogens has not been established. *C. sputorum* has three biovars (subspecies), which may be clinically relevant. *C. sputorum* subsp. *sputorum* is normally found in the human oral cavity and gastrointestinal tract and *C. sputorum* subsp. *bubulus* is normally found in the reproductive tract of cattle (197). Both have been isolated from human lung, perianal, groin, and axillary abscesses (197–199) but have not been reported as causes of diarrhea or other gastrointestinal illness. *C. sputorum* subsp. *faecalis* were first isolated from sheep feces (170), where they were described as "*V. faecalis*." Strains of this biovar are catalase-positive and abundant producers of H_2S. This organism has been isolated from bovine semen and the vagina (7), but to date there is no evidence to suggest that it is pathogenic for humans or animals.

CONCLUSIONS

New members of the genus *Campylobacter* and related genera are being identified with regularity. Furthermore, increasing numbers of these organisms have been isolated from humans with gastrointestinal illness, suggesting that "atypical" Campylobacters play a greater role in causing human disease than previously thought. Because methods to culture *C. jejuni* often will fail to support growth of other *Campylobacter* and related species, the number of human infections with these organisms likely is underdetected. However, even when atypical Campylobacters are isolated from symptomatic persons, the role they play in causing disease is not known with certainty. Future epidemiological and laboratory studies may better define the scope of human illness caused by infections with these organisms. Future investigations also will likely continue to uncover as yet unrecognized *Campylobacter* species that may produce disease in humans. Over time, as the genera expand, it is likely that the "atypical" Campylobacters and related organisms will be increasingly implicated in human gastrointestinal illnesses.

REFERENCES

1. McFadyean J, Stockman S. Report of the department of committee appointed by the Board of Agriculture and Fisheries to inquire into epizootic abortions. *Appendix to Part III: Abortion in sheep* 1913;1–29 (Abstr).
2. Smith T. The etiological relationship of spirilla (*Vibrio fetus*) to bovine abortion. *J Exp Med* 1919;30:313–322.
3. Garcia MM, Eaglesome MD, Rigby C. Campylobacters important in veterinary medicine. *Vet Bull* 1983;53:793–818.
4. Holst E, Schalen C, Mardh P-A. Isolation of *Campylobacter* spp. from the vagina, in *Campylobacter IV, 1988.* Gotenborg, Sweden, 1987:167–168.
5. Salama SM, Garcia MM, Taylor DE. Differentiation of the subspecies of *Campylobacter fetus* by genomic sizing. *Int J Syst Bacteriol* 1992;42:446–450.
6. Smibert RM. Genus *Campylobacter.* In: Krieg NR, Holt HG, eds. *Bergey's manual of systematic bacteriology. vol 1.* Baltimore: Williams and Wilkins; 1993:111–118.
7. Penner JL. *Campylobacter, Helicobacter,* and related spiral bacteria. In: Lennette EH, Balows A, Hausler WJ Jr, Truant JP, eds. *Manual of clinical microbiology.* Washington, DC: Am Soc Microbiol; 1991:402–409.
8. Edmonds P, Patton CM, Barrett TJ, Morris GK, Steigerwalt

AG, Brenner DJ. Biochemical and genetic characteristics of atypical *Campylobacter fetus* subsp. fetus strains isolated from humans in the United States. *J Clin Microbiol* 1985;21:936–940.
9. Kaplan RL. *Campylobacter.* In: Lennette EH, Balows A, Hausler WJ Jr, Truant JP, eds. *Manual of clinical microbiology.* Washington, DC: Am Soc Microbiol; 1980:235–241.
10. Burnens AP, Nicolet J. Three supplementary diagnostic tests for *Campylobacter* species and related organisms. *J Clin Microbiol* 1993;31:708–710.
11. Francioli P, Herztein J, Grob JP, Vallotton JJ, Mombelli G, Glauser MP. *Campylobacter fetus* subspecies fetus bacteremia. *Arch Intern Med* 1985;145:289–292.
12. Wang WL, Blaser MJ. Detection of pathogenic *Campylobacter* species in blood culture systems. *J Clin Microbiol* 1986;23:709–714.
13. Steele TW, McDermott JN. Technical note: the use of membrane filters applied directly to the surface of agar plates for the isolation of *Campylobacter jejuni* from feces. *Pathology* 1984;16:263–265.
14. U.S. Department of Health and Human Services Public Health Service: *Centers for Disease Control Campylobacter Annual Tabulation 1987–1989.* Washington, DC: U.S. Department of Health and Human Services; 1990:5–10.
15. Karmali MA, Allen AK, Fleming PC. Differentiation of catalase-positive Campylobacters with special reference to morphology. *Int J Syst Bacteriol* 1981;31:64–71.
16. Blaser MJ, Taylor DN, Feldman RA. Epidemiology of *Campylobacter jejuni* infections. *Epidemiol Rev* 1983;5:157.
17. Centers for Disease Control. *Campylobacter* sepsis associated with "nutritional therapy"—California. *MMWR* 1981;30:294–295.
18. Centers for Disease Control. Premature labor and neonatal sepsis caused by *Campylobacter fetus,* subsp. fetus-Ontario. *MMWR* 1984;33:483–489.
19. Klein BS, Vergeront JM, Blaser MJ, et al. *Campylobacter* infection associated with raw milk: an outbreak of gastroenteritis due to *Campylobacter jejuni* and thermotolerant *Campylobacter fetus* subsp. fetus. *JAMA* 1986;255:361–364.
20. Taylor PR, Weinstein WM, Bryner JH. *Campylobacter fetus* infection in human subjects: association with raw milk. *Am J Med* 1979;66:779.
21. Bokkenheuser V: *Vibrio fetus* infection in man. I. Ten new cases and some epidemiologic observations. *Am J Epidemiol* 1970;91:400.
22. Quinn TC, Stamm WE, Goodell SE, et al. The polymicrobial origin of intestinal infections in homosexual men. *N Engl J Med* 1983;309:576–582.
23. Devlin HR, McIntyre L. *Campylobacter fetus* subsp. fetus in homosexual males. *J Clin Microbiol* 1983;18:999–1000.
24. Guerrant RL, Lahita RG, Winn EC Jr, et al. *Campylobacter*iosis in man: pathogenic mechanisms and review of 91 bloodstream infections. *Am J Med* 1978;65:484.
25. Dickgiesser N, Kasper G, Kihm W. *Campylobacter fetus* ssp. fetus bacteremia: a patient with liver cirrhosis. *Infection* 1983;5:288.
26. Rao GG, Karim QN, Maddocks A, Hillman RJ, Harris JRW, Pinching AJ. *Campylobacter fetus* infections in two patients with AIDS. *J Infect* 1990;20:170–172.
27. Anolik JR, Mildvan D, Winter JW, Puttllitz D, Rubenstein S, Lozman H. Mycotic aortic aneurysm: a complication of *Campylobacter fetus* septicemia. *Arch Intern Med* 1983;143:609–610.
28. Carbone KM, Heinrich MC, Quinn TC. Thrombophlebitis and cellulitis due to *Campylobacter fetus* ssp. fetus. *Medicine* 1985;64:244–250.
29. Marty AT, Webb TA, Stubbs G, Penkava RR. Inflammatory abdominal aortic aneurysm infected by *Campylobacter fetus.* *JAMA* 1983;249:1190–1192.
30. Morrison VA, Lloyd BK, Chia JKS, Tuazon CU. Cardiovascular and bacteremic manifestations of *Campylobacter fetus* infection: case report and review. *Rev Infect Dis* 1990;12:387–392.
31. Franklin B, Ulmer DD. Human infection with *Vibrio fetus.* *West J Med* 1974;120:200.

32. Collins HS, Blevins A, Baxter E. Protracted bacteremia and meningitis due to *Vibrio fetus*. *Arch Intern Med* 1964;113:361.

33. Park CH, McDonald F, Twohig AM, et al. Septicemia and gastroenteritis due to *Vibrio fetus*. *South Med J* 1973;66:531.

34. Miller VA, Jenson R, Gilroy JJ. Bacteremia in pregnant sheep following oral administration of *Vibrio fetus*. *Am J Vet Res* 1959;20:677–679.

35. Lowrie DB, Pearce JH. The placental localisation of *Vibrio fetus*. *J Med Microbiol* 1970;3:607–614.

36. Eden AH. Perinatal mortality caused by *Vibrio fetus*. Review and analysis. *J Pediatr* 1966;68:297.

37. Simor AE, Karmali MA, Jadavji T, Roscoe M. Abortion and perinatal sepsis associated with *Campylobacter* infection. *Rev Infect Dis* 1986;8:397–402.

38. Gunderson CH, Sack GE. Neurology of *Vibrio fetus*. *Neurology (NY)* 1971;21:307.

39. Kilo C, Hagemann PO, Maryi J. Septic arthritis and bacteremia due to *Vibrio fetus*. *Am J Med* 1965;38:962.

40. Lawrence R, Nibbe AF, Levin S. Lung abscess secondary to *Vibrio fetus* malabsorption and syndrome and acquired agammaglobulinemia. *Chest* 1971;60:191.

41. Brown WJ, Sautter R. *Campylobacter fetus* septicemia with concurrent salpingitis. *J Clin Microbiol* 1977;6:72–75.

42. Wens R, Dratwa M, Potvliege C, Hansen W, Tielemans C, Collart F. *Campylobacter fetus* peritonitis followed by septicaemia in a patient on continuous ambulatory peritoneal dialysis. *J Infect* 1985;10:249–251.

43. Targan SR, Chow AW, Guze LB. Spontaneous peritonitis of cirrhosis due to *Campylobacter fetus*. *Gastroenterology* 1976;71:311–313.

44. Neuzil K, Wang E, Haas D, Blaser MJ. Persistence of *Campylobacter fetus* bacteremia associated with absence of opsonizing antibodies. *J Clin Microbiol* 1994;32:1718–1720.

45. Yao JDC, Ng HMC, Campbell I. Prosthetic hip joint infection due to *Campylobacter fetus*. *J Clin Microbiol* 1993;31:3323–3324.

46. Brennhoud O, Kapperud G, Langeland G. Survey of thermotolerant *Campylobacter* spp. and *Yersinia* spp. in three surface water sources in Norway. *Int J Food Microbiol* 1992;15:327–338.

47. Blaser MJ, Smith PF, Kohler PA. Susceptibility of *Campylobacter* isolates to the bactericidal activity in human serum. *J Infect Dis* 1985;151:227.

48. Blaser MJ, Smith PF, Hopkins JA, Bryner J, Heinzer I, Wang WLL. Pathogenesis of *Campylobacter fetus* infections. Serum-resistance associated with high molecular weight surface proteins. *J Infect Dis* 1987;155:696–706.

49. Blaser MJ, Smith PF, Repine JE, Joiner KA. Pathogenesis of *Campylobacter fetus* infections. Failure of C3b to bind explains serum and phagocytosis resistance. *J Clin Invest* 1988;81:1434–1444.

50. Pei Z, Blaser MJ. Pathogenesis of *Campylobacter fetus* infections. Role of surface array proteins in virulence in a mouse model. *J Clin Invest* 1990;85:1036–1043.

51. Wang E, Garcia MM, Blake MS, Pei Z, Blaser MJ. Shift in S-layer protein expression responsible for antigenic variation in *Campylobacter fetus*. *J Bacteriol* 1993;175:4979–4984.

52. Tummuru MKR, Blaser MJ. Rearrangement of *sapA* homologs with conserved and variable regions in *Campylobacter fetus*. *Proc Natl Acad Sci* 1993;90:7265–7269.

53. Blaser MJ. Role of the S-layer proteins of *Campylobacter fetus* in serum-resistance and antigenic variation: a model of bacterial pathogenesis. *Am J Med Sci* 1993;306:325–329.

54. Blaser MJ, Gotschlich EC. Surface array protein of *Campylobacter fetus*: cloning and gene structure. *J Biol Chem* 1990;265:14529–14535.

55. Tummuru MKR, Blaser MJ. Characterization of the *Campylobacter fetus* sapA promoter: evidence that the sapA promoter is deleted in spontaneous mutant strains. *J Bacteriol* 1992;174:5916–5922.

56. Francioli P, Herzstein J, Grob J-P, et al. *Campylobacter fetus* subspecies fetus bacteremia. *Arch Intern Med* 1985;145:289–292.

57. Mishu B, Patton C, Tauxe RV. Clinical and epidemiologic features of non-jejuni *Campylobacters*. In: Nachamkin I, Blaser MJ, Tompkins L, eds. *Campylobacter jejuni—current strategy and future trends*. Washington, DC: Am Soc Microbiol; 1992:31–41.

58. Sandstedt K, Ursing J, Walder M. Thermotolerant *Campylobacter* with no or weak catalase activity isolated from dogs. *Curr Microbiol* 1983;8:209–213.

59. International Union of Microbiological Societies. Validation of the publication of new names and new combinations previously effectively published outside the IJSB. *Int J Syst Bacteriol* 1991;41:331.

60. Sandstedt K, Ursing J. Description of *Campylobacter upsaliensis* sp. nov. previously known as the CNW group. *Syst Appl Microbiol* 1991;14:39–48.

61. Lastovica AJ, Le Roux E, Penner JL. "*Campylobacter upsaliensis*" isolated from blood cultures of pediatric patients. *J Clin Microbiol* 1989;27:657–659.

62. Lastovica AJ, Le Roux E. Prevalence and distribution of *Campylobacter* spp. in the diarrhoeic stools and blood cultures of pediatric patients. *Acta Gastroenterol Belg* 1993;56(Suppl):34.

63. Albert MJ, Tee W, Leach A, Asche V, Penner JL. Comparison of a blood-free medium and a filtration technique for the isolation of *Campylobacter* spp. from diarrhoeal stools of hospitalized patients in central Australia. *J Med Microbiol* 1992;37:176–179.

64. Steele TW, Sangster N, Lanser JA. DNA relatedness and biochemical features of *Campylobacter* spp. isolated in central and south Australia. *J Clin Microbiol* 1985;22:71–74.

65. Megraud F, Bonnet F. Unusual *Campylobacters* in human feces. *J Infect* 1986;12:275–276.

66. Patton CM, Shaffer N, Edmonds P, et al. Human disease associated with "*Campylobacter upsaliensis*" (catalase-negative or weakly positive *Campylobacter* species) in the United States. *J Clin Microbiol* 1989;27:66–73.

67. Davies AP, Beghart CJ, Meric SA. *Campylobacter* associated chronic diarrhea in a dog. *J Am Vet Med* 1984;184:469–471.

68. Goossens H, Vales L, Butzler JP, et al. *Campylobacter upsaliensis* enteritis associated with canine infections. *Lancet* 1991;337:1486–1487.

69. Owen RJ, Hernandez J. Occurrence of plasmids. In: "*Campylobacter upsaliensis*" (catalase negative or weak group) from geographically diverse patients with gastroenteritis or bacteremia. *Eur J Epidemiol* 1990;6:111–117.

70. Deming MS, Tauxe RV, Blake PA, et al. *Campylobacter enteritis* at a university: transmission from eating chicken and from cats. *Am J Epidemiol* 1987;126:526–533.

71. Fox JO, Maxwell KO, Taylor NS, Runsick CD, Edmonds P, Brenner DJ. "*Campylobacter upsaliensis*" isolated from cats as identified by DNA relatedness and biochemical features. *J Clin Microbiol* 1989;27:2376–2378.

72. Lastovica AJ, LeRoux E, Jooste M. "*Campylobacter upsaliensis*" isolated from vervet monkeys. *Microb Ecol Health Dis* 1991;4(S):S87.

73. Walmsley SL, Karmali MA. Direct isolation of thermophilic *Campylobacter* species from human feces on selective agar medium. *J Clin Microbiol* 1989;27:668–670.

74. Goossens H, Vlaes L, De Bobck M, et al. Is "*Campylobacter upsaliensis*" an unrecognized cause of human diarrhea? *Lancet* 1990;336:584–586.

75. Goossens H, Pot B, Vlaes L, et al. Characterization and description of *Campylobacter upsaliensis* isolated from human feces. *J Clin Microbiol* 1990;28:1039–1046.

76. Taylor DN, Diehlbauch JA, Tee W, Pitarangsi C, Echeverria P. Isolation of group 2 aerotolerant *Campylobacter* species from Thai children with diarrhea. *J Infect Dis* 1991;163:1062–1067.

77. Taylor DE, Hiratsuks K, Mueller L. Isolation and characterization of catalase-negative and catalase-weak strains of *Campylobacter* species, including "*Campylobacter upsaliensis*," from humans with gastroenteritis. *J Clin Microbiol* 1987;27:2042–2045.

78. Skirrow MB, Jones DM, Sutcliffe E, Benjamin J. *Campylobacter* bacteremia in England and Wales, 1981–91. *Epidemiol Infect* 1993;110:567–573.

79. da Silva-Tatley FM, Lastovica AJ, Steyn LM. Plasmid profiles of "*Campylobacter upsaliensis*" isolated from blood cultures and stools of pediatric patients. *J Med Microbiol* 1992;37:8–14.

80. Owen RJ, Hernandez J. Genotypic variation in "*Campylobacter upsaliensis*" from blood and feces of patients in different countries. *FEMS Microbiol Lett* 1990;72:5–10.

81. Lior H, Woodward D. A serotyping scheme for *Campylobacter upsaliensis*. *Microb Ecol Health Dis* 1991;4(S):S89.

82. Owen RJ, Morgan DD, Costas M, Lastovica A. Identification of "*Campylobacter upsaliensis*" and other catalase-negative *Campylobacters* from pediatric blood cultures by numerical analysis of electrophoretic protein patterns. *FEMS Microbiol Lett* 1989;58:145–150.

83. Chusid MJ, Wortmann DW, Dunne WM. "*Campylobacter upsaliensis*" sepsis in a boy with acquired hypogamaglobulinemia. *Diagn Microbiol Infect Dis* 1990;13:367–369.

84. Gaudreau C, Lamonthe F. *Campylobacter upsaliensis* isolated from a breast abscess. *J Clin Microbiol* 1992;30:1354–1356.

85. Aspinall ST, Wareing DRA, Hayward PG, Hutchinson DN. Selective medium for thermophilic campylobacters including *Campylobacter upsaliensis*. *J Clin Pathol* 1993;46:829–831.

86. Endtz HP, Ruijs GJHM, Zwinderman AH, van der Reijden T, Biever M, Mouton RP. Comparison of six media including a semisolid agar, for the isolation of various *Campylobacter* species from stool specimens. *J Clin Microbiol* 1991;29:1007–1010.

87. Preston MA, Simor AE, Walmsley SL, et al. In vitro susceptibility of "*Campylobacter upsaliensis*" to twenty-four antimicrobial agents. *Eur J Clin Microbiol Infect Dis* 1990;9:822–824.

88. Gebhart CJ, Ward GE, Chang K, Kurtz HJ. *Campylobacter hyointestinalis* (new species) isolated from swine with lesions of proliferative ileitis. *Am J Vet Res* 1983;44:361–367.

89. Waterman SR, Hackett J. Outer membrane components of *Campylobacter hyointestinalis*. *FEMS Microbiol Lett* 1992;92:279–284.

90. Vandamme P, Goossens H. Taxonomy of *Campylobacter, Arcobacter*, and *Helicobacter*: a review. *Zentralbl Bakteriologie* 1992;276:447–472.

91. Vandamme P, De Ley J. Proposal for a new family, *Campylobacteraceae*. *Int J Syst Bacteriol* 1991;41:451–455.

92. Edmonds P, Patton CM, Griffin PM, et al. *Campylobacter hyointestinalis* associated with human gastrointestinal disease in the United States. *J Clin Microbiol* 1987;25:685–691.

93. Salana SM, Tabor H, Richter M, Taylor DE. Pulsed-field gel electrophoresis for epidemiologic studies of *Campylobacter hyointestinalis* isolates. *J Clin Microbiol* 1992;30:1982–1984.

94. Costas M, Owen RJ, Jackman PJH. Classification of *Campylobacter sputorum* and allied *Campylobacters* based on numerical analysis of electrophoretic protein patterns. *Syst Appl Microbiol* 1987;9:125–131.

95. Vandamme P, Pot B, Falsen E, Kersters K, De Ley J. Intra- and interspecific relationships of veterinary *Campylobacters* revealed by numerical analysis of electrophoretic protein profiles and DNA:DNA hybridizations. *Syst Appl Microbiol* 1990;13:295–303.

96. Ohya T, Nakazawa M. Production and some properties of cytotoxins produced by *Campylobacter* species isolated from proliferative enteropathy in swine. *J Vet Med Sci* 1992;54:1031–1033.

97. Gebhart CJ, Murtaugh MP, Lin GF, Ward GE. Species-specific DNA probes for *Campylobacter* species isolated from pigs with proliferative enteritis. *Vet Microbiol* 1990;24:367–379.

98. Thorne GM, Macone A, Goldman DA. Enzymatically labelled nucleic acid probe assays for detection of *Campylobacter* spp. in human fecal specimens and in culture. *Mol Cell Probes* 1990;4:133–142.

99. Gebhart CJ, Edmonds P, Ward GE, Kurtz HJ, Brenner DJ. "*Campylobacter hyointestinalis*" sp. nov.: a new species of *Campylobacter* found in the intestines of pigs and other animals. *J Clin Microbiol* 1985;21:715–720.

100. Hill BD, Thomas RJ, Mackenzie AR. *Campylobacter hyointestinalis*–associated enteritis in moluccan rusa deer. *J Comp Pathol* 1987;97:687–694.

101. Lambert M, Jones JMW, Lister SA. Isolation of *Campylobacter hyointestinalis* from pigs in the United Kingdom. *Vet Rec* 1984;115:128–129.

102. Ursing J, Sandstedt K, Hansson E. Genetic and phenotypic characteristics of a new group of *Campylobacter* isolated from pigs and cattle. *Acta Pathol Microbiol Immunol Scand Sect* 1984;B92:71–72.

103. Walder M, Sandstedt K, Ursing J. Phenotypic characteristics of thermotolerant *Campylobacter* from human and animal sources. *Curr Microbiol* 1983;9:291–296.

104. Russell RG, Kiehlbauch JA, Gebhart CJ, De Tolla LJ. Uncommon *Campylobacter* species in infant Macaca nemestrina monkeys housed in a nursery. *J Clin Microbiol* 1992;30:3024–3027.

105. Fennell CL, Rompalo AM, Totten PA, Bruch KL, Flores BM, Stamm WE. Isolation of "*Campylobacter hyointestinalis*" from a human. *J Clin Microbiol* 1986;24:146–148.

106. Minet J, Grosbois B, Megraud F. *Campylobacter hyointestinalis*: an opportunistic enteropathogen? *J Clin Microbiol* 1988;26:2659–2660.

107. Gebhart CJ, Ward GE, Kurtz HJ. In vitro activities of 47 antimicrobial agents against three *Campylobacter* spp. from pigs. *Antimicrob Agents Chemother* 1985;27:55–59.

108. Skirrow MB, Benjamin J. "1001" *Campylobacters*: cultural characteristics of intestinal *Campylobacters* from man and animals. *J Hyg* 1980;85:427–442.

109. Von Graevenitz A. Revised nomenclature of *Campylobacter laridis, Enterobacter intermedium*, and "*Flavobacterium branchophilia*." *Int J Syst Bacteriol* 1990;40:211.

110. Tauxe RV, Patton CM, Edmonds P, Barrett TJ, Brenner DJ, Blake PA. Illness associated with *Campylobacter laridis*, a newly recognized *Campylobacter* species. *J Clin Microbiol* 1985;21:222–225.

111. Bolton FJ, Coates D, Hutchinson DN, Godfree AF. A study of thermophilic *Campylobacter* in a river system. *J Appl Bacteriol* 1987;62:167–176.

112. Taylor DN, McDermott KT, Little JR, Wells JG, Blaser MJ. *Campylobacter* enteritis from untreated water in the Rocky Mountains. *Ann Intern Med* 1983;99:38–40.

113. Vogt RL, Sours HE, Barrett T, Feldman RA, Dickinson RJ, Witherell L. *Campylobacter* enteritis associated with contaminated water. *Ann Intern Med* 1982;96:292–296.

114. Park CE, Sanders GW. Occurrence of thermotolerant *campylobacters* in fresh vegetables sold at farmers' outdoor markets and supermarkets. *Can J Microbiol* 1992;38:313–316.

115. Glunder G, Petermann S. The occurence and characterization of *Campylobacter* spp. in silver gulls (*Larus argentatus*), three-toed gulls (*Rissa tridactyla*), and house sparrows (*Passer domesticus*). *Zentralblatt Fur Veterinarmedizin Reihe B* 1989;36:123–130.

116. Kakkar M, Dogra SC: Prevalence of *Campylobacter* infections in animals and children in Haryana, India. *J Diarr Dis Res* 1990;8:34–36.

117. Maruyama S, Tanaka T, Katsube Y, Nakanishi H, Nukina M. Prevalence of thermophilic *Campylobacters* in crows (*Corvus lavaillantii, Corvus corne*) and serogroups of the isolates. *Jpn J Vet Sci* 1990;52:1237–1244.

118. Kazawala RR, Jiwa SF, Nkya AE. The role of management systems in the epidemiology of thermophilic *Campylobacters* among poultry in eastern zone of Tanzaria. *Epidemiol Infect* 1993;110:273–278.

119. Torre E, Tello M. Factors influencing fecal shedding of *Campylobacter jejuni* in dogs without diarrhea. *Am J Vet Res* 1993;54:260–262.

120. Lindblom GB, Johny M, Khalil K, Mazhar K, Ruiz-Palacios GM, Kaijser B. Enterotoxigenicity and frequency of *Campylobacter jejuni, C. coli* and *C. laridis* in human and animal isolates from different countries. *FEMS Microbiol Lett* 1990;54:163–167.

121. Benjamin J, Leaper S, Owen RJ, Skirrow MB. Description of *Campylobacter laridis*, a new species comprising the nalidixic acid resistant thermophilic *Campylobacter* (NARTC) group. *Curr Microbiol* 1983;8:231–238.

122. Nachamkin I, Stowell C, Skalina D, Jones AM, Hoop RM, Smibert RM. *Campylobacter laridis* causing bacteremia in an immunosuppressed patient. *Ann Intern Med* 1984;101:55–57.

123. Soderstrom C, Schalen C, Walder M. Septicaemia caused by

unusual *Campylobacter* species (*C. laridis* and *C. mucosalis*). *Scand J Infect Dis* 1991;23:369–371.

124. Evans TG, Riley D. *Campylobacter laridis* colitis in a human immunodeficiency virus–positive patient treated with a quinolone. *Clin Infect Dis* 1992;15:172–173.

125. Vargas J, Carzo JE, Perez MJ, Lazano F, Martin E. Enfermedades infecciosas. *Microbiologia Clinica* 1992;10:155–157.

126. Simor AE, Wilcox L. Enteritis associated with *Campylobacter laridis*. *J Clin Microbiol* 1987;25:10–12.

127. Megraud F, Chevrier D, Desplaces N, Sedallian A, Geusdon JL. Urease-positive thermophilic *Campylobacter* (*Campylobacter laridis* variant) isolated from an appendix and from human feces. *J Clin Microbiol* 1988;26:1050–1051.

128. Benzian MC, Ribou G, Barberis-Biletti C, Megraud F. Isolation of urease positive thermophilic variant of *Campylobacter lari* from a patient with urinary tract infection. *Eur J Clin Microbiol Infect Dis* 1990;9:895–897.

129. Borczyk A, Thompson S, Smith D, Lior H. Water-borne outbreak of *Campylobacter laridis*–associated gastroenteritis. *Lancet* 1987;1:164–165.

130. Owen RJ, Costas M, Sloss L, Bolton FJ. Numerical analysis of electrophoretic protein patterns of *Campylobacter laridis* and allied thermophilic *Campylobacters* from the natural environment. *J Appl Bacteriol* 1988;65:68–78.

131. Altwegg M, Burnens A, Zollinger-Iten J, Penner JL. Problems in identification of *Campylobacter jejuni* associated with acquisition of resistance to nalidixic acid. *J Clin Microbiol* 1987;25:1807–1808.

132. Popovic-Uroic T, Patton CM, Nicholson MA, Kiehlbauch JA. Evaluation of indoxylacetate hydrolysis test for rapid differentiation of *Campylobacter*, *Helicobacter*, and *Wolinella* species. *J Clin Microbiol* 1990;28:2335–2339.

133. Griffiths PL, Moreno GS, Park RW. Differentiation between thermophilic *Campylobacter* species by species-specific antibodies. *J Appl Bacteriol* 1992;72:467–474.

134. On SLW, Owen RJ, Lastovica A, Costas M, Lopez-Urquijo B. Taxonomic study of *Helicobacter* (*Campylobacter*) *fennelliae* from clinical material by numerical analysis of one-dimensional electrophoretic protein patterns. *Microb Ecol Health Dis* 1991;4(S):S103.

135. Flores BM, Fennell CL, Stamm WE. Characterization of *Campylobacter cinaedi* and *C. fennelliae* antigens and analysis of human immune response. *J Infect Dis* 1989;159:635–640.

136. Fennell CJ, Totten PA, Quinn TC, Patton CL, Holmes KK, Stamm WE. Characterization of *Campylobacter*-like organisms isolated from homosexual men. *J Infect Dis* 1984;149:58–66.

137. Totten PA, Fennell CL, Tenover FC, et al. *Campylobacter cinaedi* (sp. nov.) and *Campylobacter fennelliae* (sp. nov.): two new *Campylobacter* species associated with enteric disease in homosexual men. *J Infect Dis* 1985;151:131–139.

138. Laughon BE, Druckman DA, Vernon A, et al. Prevalence of enteric pathogens in homosexual men with and without acquired immunodeficiency syndrome. *Gastroenterology* 1988;94:984–993.

139. Flores BM, Fennell CL, Holmes KK, Stamm WE. In vitro susceptibility of *Campylobacter*-like organisms to twenty antimicrobial agents. *Antimicrob Agents Chemother* 1985;28:188–191.

140. Vandamme P, Falsen E, Rossau R, Hoste B, Tytgat R, De Ley J. Revision of *Campylobacter*, *Helicobacter*, and *Wolinella* taxonomy: emendation of generic descriptions and proposal of *Arcobacter* gen. nov. *Int J Syst Bacteriol* 1991;41:88–103.

141. Quinn TC, Stamm WE, Goodell SE, et al. The polymicrobial origin of intestinal infections in homosexual man. *N Engl J Med* 1983;309:76–82.

142. Quinn TC, Goodell SE, Fennell CL, et al. Infections with *Campylobacter jejuni* and *Campylobacter*-like organisms in homosexual men. *Ann Intern Med* 1984;101:187–192.

143. Laughon BE, Vernon AA, Druckman DA, et al. Recovery of *Campylobacter* species from homosexual men. *J Infect Dis* 1988;158:464–467.

144. Wilcox CM, Byford BA, Forsmark CE, Hadley WK, Cello JP, Jacobson MA. *Campylobacter*-like organisms are uncommon

145. Grayson ML, Tee W, Dwyer B. Gastroenteritis associated with *Campylobacter cinaedi*. *Med J Aust* 1989;150:214.

146. Burman WJ, Cohn DL, Reves RR, Wilson ML. Multifocal cellulitis and monoarticular arthritis as manifestations of *Helicobacter cinaedi* bacteremia. *Clin Infect Dis* 1995; (in press).

147. Pasternak J, Bolivar R, Hopper RL, et al. Bacteremia caused by *Campylobacter*-like organisms in two male homosexuals. *Ann Intern Med* 1984;101:339–341.

148. Sacks LV, Labriola AM, Gill VJ, Gordin FM. Use of ciprofloxacin for successful eradication of bacteremia due to *Campylobacter cinaedi* in a human immunodeficiency virus-infected patient. *Rev Infect Dis* 1993;13:1066–1068.

149. Decker CF, Martin GJ, Barham WB, Paparello SF. Bacteremia due to *Campylobacter cinaedi* in a patient infected with human immunodeficiency virus. *Clin Infect Dis* 1992;15:178–179.

150. Ng VL, Hadley WK, Fennell CL, Flores BM, Stamm WE. Successive bacteremias with *Campylobacter cinaedi* and *Campylobacter fennelliae* in a bisexual male. *J Clin Microbiol* 1987;25:2008–2009.

151. Kemper CA, Mickelson P, Morton A, Walton B, Deresinski SC. *Helicobacter* (*Campylobacter*) *fennelliae*-like organisms as an important but occult cause of bacteremia in a patient with AIDS. *J Infect* 1993;26:97–101.

152. Burnens AP, Angeloy-Wick B, Nicolet J. Comparison of *Campylobacter* carriage rates in diarrheic and healthy pet animals. *J Vet Med Ser B* 1992;39:175–180.

153. Tee W, Anderson BN, Ross BC, Dwyer B. Atypical *Campylobacters* associated with gastroenteritis. *J Clin Microbiol* 1987;25:1248–1252.

154. Burnens AP, Stanley J, Schaad VB, Nicolet J. Novel *Campylobacter*-like organism resembling *Helicobacter fennelliae* isolated from a boy with gastroenteritis and from dogs. *J Clin Microbiol* 1993;31:1916–1917.

155. Orlicek SL, Welch DF, Kuhls TL. Septicemia and meningitis caused by *Helicobacter cinaedi* in neonate. *J Clin Microbiol* 1993;31:569–571.

156. Gebhart CJ, Fennell CL, Murtaugh MP, Stamm WE. *Campylobacter cinaedi* is the normal intestinal flora in hamsters. *J Clin Microbiol* 1989;27:1692–1694.

157. Flores BM, Fennell CL, Kuller L, Brondson MA, Morton WR, Stamm WE. Experimental infection of pig-tailed macaques (*Macaca nemestrina*) with *Campylobacter cinaedi* and *Campylobacter fennelliae*. *Infect Immun* 1990;58:3947–3953.

158. Vandamme P, Falsen E, Rossau R, et al. Revision of *Campylobacter*, *Helicobacter*, and *Wolinella* taxonomy: emendations of generic descriptions and proposal of *Arcobacter* gen. nov. *Int J Syst Bacteriol* 1991;41:88–103.

159. Neill SD, Ellis WA, O'Brien JJ. The biochemical characteristics of *Campylobacter*-like organisms from cattle and pigs. *Res Vet Sci* 1978;25:368–372.

160. Ellis WA, Neill SD, O'Brien JJ, Ferguson HW, Hanna J. Isolation of spirillium/vibrio-like organisms from bovine fetuses. *Vet Rec* 1977;100:451–452.

161. Boudreau M, Higgins R, Mittal KR. Biochemical and serological characterization of *Campylobacter cryaerophila*. *J Clin Microbiol* 1991;29:54–58.

162. Stamp S, Varoli O, Zanetti F, DeLuca G. *Arcobacter cryaerophilus* and thermophilic *Campylobacters* in a sewage treatment plant in Italy: two secondary treatments compared. *Epidemiol Infect* 1993;110:633–639.

163. Tee W, Baird R, Dyall-Smith M, Dwyer B. *Campylobacter cryaerophila* isolated from a human. *J Clin Microbiol* 1988;26:2469–2473.

164. Keihlbauch JA, Brenner DJ, Nicholson MA, et al. *Campylobacter butzleri* sp. nov. isolated from humans and animals with diarrheal illness. *J Clin Microbiol* 1991;29:376–385.

165. Kiehlbauch JA, Plikaytis BD, Swaminathan B, Cameron CN, Wachsmuth IK. Restriction fragment length polymorphisms in the ribosomal genes for specific identification and subtyping of aerotolerant *Campylobacter* species. *J Clin Microbiol* 1991;29:1670–1676.

166. Vandamme P, Pugina P, Benzi G, et al. Outbreak of recurrent

abdominal cramps associated with *Arcobacter butzleri* in an Italian school. *J Clin Microbiol* 1992;30:2335–2337.

167. Anderson KF, Kiehlbauch JA, Anderson DC, McClure HM, Wachsmuth IK. *Arcobacter (Campylobacter) butzleri*–associated diarrheal illness in a non-human primate population. *Infect Immun* 1993;61:2220–2223.

168. Russell RG, Kiehlbauch JA, Gebhart CJ, DeTolla LJ. Uncommon *Campylobacter* species in infant *Macaca nemestrina* monkeys housed in a nursery. *J Clin Microbiol* 1992;30:3024–3027.

169. Steele TW, Owen RJ. *Campylobacter jejuni* subspecies *doylei* (subsp. nov.), a subspecies of nitrate-negative *Campylobacters* isolated from human clinical specimens. *Int J Syst Bacteriol* 1988;38:316–318.

170. Firehammer BD. The isolation of vibrios from ovine feces. *Cornell Vet* 1965;55:482–494.

171. Kasper G, Dickgiesser N. Isolation from gastric epithelium of *Campylobacter*-like bacteria that are distinct from *Campylobacter pyloridis*. *Lancet* 1985;1:111–112.

172. Goodwin S, Blincow E, Armstrong J, McCulloch R. *Campylobacter pyloridis* is unique: GCLO-2 is an ordinary *Campylobacter*. *Lancet* 1985;2:38–39.

173. Owen RJ, Beck A, Borman P. Restriction endonuclease digest patterns of chromosomal DNA from nitrate-negative *Campylobacter jejuni*-like organisms. *Eur J Epidemiol* 1985;1:281–287.

174. Owen RJ, Martin SR, Borman P. Rapid urea hydrolysis by gastric *Campylobacters*. *Lancet* 1985;2:111.

175. Steele TW, Lanser JA, Sangster N. Nitrate-negative *Campylobacter*-like organisms. *Lancet* 1985;1:394.

176. Lastovica AJ, Kirby R, Ambrosio RE. Clinical isolates of thermophilic *Campylobacter* spp. with no or weak catalase activity. In: Pearson AD, Skirrow MB, Lior H, Rowe B, eds. *Campylobacter*. vol 3. London: Public Health Laboratory Service; 1985: 201.

177. Tanner ACR, Badger S, Lai CH, Listgarten MA, Visconti RA, Socransky SS. *Wolinella* gen. nov., *Wolinella succinogenes* (*Vibrio succinogenes* Wolin et al.) comb. nov., and description of *Bacteroides gracilis* sp. nov., *Wolinella recta* sp. nov., *Campylobacter concisus* sp. nov., and *Eikenella corrodens* from humans with periodontal disease. *Int J Syst Bacteriol* 1981;31:432–435.

178. Tanner ACR, Listgarten MA, Ebersole JL. *Wolinella curva* sp. nov.: "*Vibrio succinogenes*" of human origin. *Int J Syst Bacteriol* 1984;34:275–282.

179. Tanner ACR, Dzink JL, Ebersole JL, Socransky SS. *Wolinella recta, Campylobacter concisus, Bacteroides gracilis,* and *Eikenella corrodens* from periodontal lesions. *J Periodont Res* 1987; 22:327–330.

180. Rams TE, Feik D, Slots J. *Campylobacter rectus* in human periodontitis. *Oral Microbiol Immunol* 1993;8:230–235.

181. Roop RMII, Smibert RM, Johnson JL, Krieg NR. *Campylobacter mucosalis* (Lawson, Leaver, Pettigrew, and Rowland). *Int J Syst Bacteriol* 1985;35:189–192.

182. Lawson GHK, Rowland AC. *Campylobacter sputorum* subsp. mucosalis. In: Butzler JP, ed. *Campylobacter infection in man and animals*. Boca Raton: CRC Press; 1984:207–225.

183. Megraud F, Elharrif Z. Isolation of *Campylobacter* species by filtration. *Eur J Clin Microbiol* 1985;4:437–438.

184. Lauwers S, Kevreker T, Van Etterijck R, et al. Isolation of *Campylobacter concisus* from human feces. *Microb Ecol Health Dis* 1991;4(S):S91.

185. Tanner ACR. Characterization of *Wolinella* spp., *Campylobacter concisus, Bacteroides gracilis,* and *Eikenella corrodens* by polyacrylamide gel electrophoresis. *J Clin Microbiol* 1986; 24:562–565.

186. Spiegel CA, Telford G. Isolation of *Wolinella recta* and *Actinomyces viscosus* from an actinomycotic chest wall mass. *J Clin Microbiol* 1984;20:1187–1189.

187. Van Dyke TE, Dowell VR, Offenbacher S, Snyder W, Hersh T. Potential role of micro-organisms isolated from periodontal lesions in the pathogenesis of inflammatory bowel disease. *Infect Immun* 1986;53:671–677.

188. Rams TE, Andriolo M, Feik D, Abel SN, McGivern TM, Slots J. Microbiological study of HIV-related periodontitis. *J Periodontol* 1991;62:74–81.

189. Zambon JJ, Reynolds H, Fisher HG, Schlossman M, Dunford R, Genco RJ. Microbiological and immunological studies of adult patients with non-insulin dependent diabetes mellitus. *J Periodontol* 1988;59:23–31.

190. Guillespie J, De Nardin E, Radel S, Kuracina J, Smutko J, Zambon J. Production of an extracellular toxin by the oral pathogen *Campylobacter rectus*. *Microb Pathogen* 1992;12: 69–77.

191. Badger SJ, Tanner ACR. Serological studies of *Bacteroides gracilis, Campylobacter concisus, Wolinella recta,* and *Eikenella corrodens,* all from humans with periodontal disease. *Int J Syst Bacteriol* 1981;31:446–451.

192. Johnson CC, Finegold SM. Uncommonly encountered motile, anaerobic gram-negative bacilli associated with infection. *Rev Infect Dis* 1987;9:1150–1162.

193. Vandamme P, Falsen E, Pot B, Hoste B, Kersters K, DeLey J. Identification of EF group 22 *Campylobacters* from gastroenteritis cases as *Campylobacter concisus*. *J Clin Microbiol* 1989; 27:1775–1781.

194. Lastovica AJ, Le Roux E, Warren R, Klump H. Clinical isolates of *Campylobacter mucosalis*. *J Clin Microbiol* 1993;31: 2835–2836.

195. Greig A, Hanslo D, Le Roux E, Lastovica A. In-vitro activity of eight antimicrobial agents against pediatric isolates of *C. concisus* and *C. mucosalis*. *Acta Gastroenterol Belg* 1993; 56(Suppl):12.

196. Figura N, Guglielmetti P, Zanchi A, et al. Two cases of *Campylobacter mucosalis* enteritis in children. *J Clin Microbiol* 1993; 31:727–728.

197. Raffi F, Derriennic M, Michault A, et al. Infections humaines a *Campylobacter sputorum*: a propos de deux observations. *Med Mal Infect* 1985;15:65–67.

198. Borczyk A, Lior H, McKeown A, Svendsen H. Isolations of *Campylobacter sputorum* associated with human infection, abstr. 211. In: Kaijser B, Falsen E, eds. *Campylobacter*. vol 4. Gothenburg: University of Gothenburg; 1987:166.

199. On SL, Ridgewell F, Cryan B, Azadian BS. Isolation of *Campylobacter* sputorum biovar sputorum from an axillary abscess. *J Infect* 1992;24:175–179.

Infections of the Gastrointestinal Tract,
edited by M. J. Blaser, P. D. Smith, J. I. Ravdin,
H. B. Greenberg, and R. L. Guerrant
Raven Press, Ltd., New York © 1995.

CHAPTER 58

Clostridium difficile

David M. Lyerly and Tracy D. Wilkins

The gastrointestinal tract contains an extremely complex ecosystem of microbes that acts as a natural barrier against colonization by enteropathogens. Once this barrier has been altered or broken down, a person becomes more susceptible to infection by enteric pathogens. Treatment with antibiotics is one way in which this barrier is altered. *Clostridium difficile,* which is a spore-forming anaerobe, is a major nosocomial pathogen for older patients in hospitals because of its ability to become established in the gastrointestinal tract once the natural microflora has been modified by antibiotic therapy. The organism causes intestinal disease ranging from mild diarrhea to fatal pseudomembranous colitis (PMC). *Clostridium difficile* is responsible for essentially (almost) all cases of pseudomembranous colitis. On the other hand, it is estimated to cause only 25% of antibiotic-associated diarrheas.

Even though we now recognize *C. difficile* as the single most common cause of bacterial diarrhea in hospitalized patients, the role of this organism as a pathogen had not been established as recently as the late 1970s. The first documented case of pseudomembranous colitis is attributed to a case history report by Dr. Albert Finney in 1893 (1), in which the presence of diphtheric lesions in the colon of a young woman was described. The organism was first described by Hall and O'Toole in 1935 (2), who named the organism *Bacillus difficilis* because of the difficulty in isolating the organism. The original isolates were from the feces of normal infants. The toxigenic nature of the organism was demonstrated in some of the original descriptions by Hall and O'Toole (2) and in subsequent studies, but the role of this organism as a major pathogen remained unknown until the late 1970s. In the 1950s and 1960s, *Staphylococcus aureus* was believed to cause pseudomembranous colitis, primarily because (a) this organism was beginning to be recognized as a major pathogen during this time and (b) large numbers of *Staphylococcus aureus* were reportedly observed in stools from patients with the disease. However, it is now believed

that *S. aureus* likely was not responsible for these cases because it could not be isolated routinely from patients with PMC and because it was present in high numbers in stool specimens from healthy persons. Much of the literature concerning the possible involvement of *S. aureus* has been reviewed by Dr. John Bartlett (3), one of the pioneers in the field, and it appears doubtful that *S. aureus* has caused many cases of PMC. The investigation that revived research on the cause of PMC was the landmark study by Tedesco et al. (4) published in 1974. In this report, an incidence of 10% was reported in patients who were treated with clindamycin. As a result of the high incidence, the disease was referred to as clindamycin-associated colitis. The article by Tedesco et al. served to further rule out any role of *S. aureus* by showing that the organism was not present in these patients with PMC.

In the mid to late 1970s, researchers detected, using tissue culture assay methods, cytotoxic activity in stool specimens from patients with antibiotic-associated pseudomembranous colitis (5–8). The effect, which consisted of rounding of the tissue culture cells, was neutralized by gas gangrene antitoxin and later by *C. sordellii* antitoxin, which was a component of the gas gangrene antitoxin. Scientists soon showed that *C. difficile* could be isolated from stool specimens of patients with pseudomembranous colitis and that filtrates prepared from broth cultures of these isolates produced the same rounding effect on tissue cultured cells which also was neutralized by *C. sordelli* antitoxin. These human isolates produced a similar disease in hamsters treated with antibiotics, providing more evidence implicating *C. difficile* as the cause of the disease. We now know that the neutralization of the rounding activity by *C. sordellii* antitoxin results from the fact that *C. sordellii* produces toxins similar to those of *C. difficile*.

At this time, it was believed that *C. difficile* produced only a single toxin that caused the rounding or cytotoxic effect. In 1980, however, Dr. John Bartlett and his research team at the Johns Hopkins University School of Medicine in Baltimore showed that *C. difficile* actually produces two toxins, A and B (9). Toxin A also is referred to as the enterotoxin and toxin B often is referred to as the cytotoxin. Both toxins are cytotoxic for mammalian cells. Toxin B, however, is 100 to 1000 times more cyto-

D. M. Lyerly and T. D. Wilkins: Department of Biochemistry and Anaerobic Microbiology and Center for Biotechnology, Virginia Polytechnic Institute and State University, Blacksburg, Virginia 24061.

toxic than toxin A against most cell lines. Toxin A is believed to cause most of the symptoms of the disease since it is highly active in the gastrointestinal tract whereas toxin B is not. This does not rule out a role for toxin B in disease. Both toxins are lethal at about the same dose when injected parenterally into experimental animals and there is some evidence indicating that the toxins may act synergistically in the intestine.

MICROBIOLOGY

Morphology

Clostridium difficile is a gram-positive anaerobe that forms subterminal spores. The ability to form spores makes this organism very difficult to remove from the hospital environment. Unlike some toxigenic clostridia, the production of spores is not associated with toxin production but toxin production is highest during the stationary growth phase. Some highly toxigenic strains are very poor spore formers whereas other strains that are only weakly toxigenic or nontoxigenic are much better spore producers. The germination of spores may be stimulated by the addition of sodium cholate and sodium taurocholate to media used to isolate the organism. Alternatively, the recovery of spores can be improved by treatment with sodium thioglycollate and lysozyme (10–16).

Some strains produce thin capsules (40–80 nm in thickness), the presence of which appears to be influenced by the level of glucose in the medium; however, there does not appear to be an association of capsule with virulence and there is no correlation with toxin production (17–19). Some strains produce structures that resemble fimbriae (20). The factors affecting the production of these structures have not been determined but they are not related to toxin production.

The cell wall of *C. difficile* consists of several proteins that have been partially characterized (21–25). Two of these proteins (M_r of 38 and 42 kDa) aggregate to form a regular array in the cell wall. Antisera against *C. difficile* cross-react with several other clostridia, including *C. sordellii* and *C. bifermentans*. A portion of this cross-reaction results from related cell wall antigens. One of these antigens consists of glucose, glucosamine, phosphate, and fatty acid, and constitutes about 40% by weight of the cell wall. Whether or not this antigen is distinct from the 38- and 42-kDa protein is not known. Two antigens that are extractable from the cell membrane and wall with the chelating agent ethylenediamine tetraacetate have been identified. One of these appears to be a membrane component that consists of glucose, mannose, galactosamine, and phosphate. The other is a 36-kDa protein that is located on the cell surface. This second antigen elicits antibodies in patients with *C. difficile* infections (26,27). Its function is not known, but it is not toxic or proteolytic and it does not bind to immunoglobulin as do some cell wall components from other clostridia (21).

In Vitro Growth Characteristics

The organism requires anaerobic conditions in order to grow; however, it is not as strict an anaerobe as some of the other clostridia such as *C. tetani*. Broth media that is reduced but not held under strict anaerobic conditions supports the growth of *C. difficile*. For the clinical isolation of the organism and for optimal growth conditions, however, it is important that anaerobic bacteriology be used. The organism exhibits several distinctive phenotypic properties such as fluorescence when grown on some types of agar media and the production of unusual metabolites. These properties are useful in the presumptive identification of *C. difficile* but they are not definitive because some other clostridia exhibit these properties. The organism gives a characteristic odor often referred to as "horse dung" odor, especially when grown on agar, but the odor is characteristic for many clostridia. The selective media most typically used is the cycloserine–cefoxitin–fructose agar (CCFA) originally described by George et al. (28). The original formulation, as reported by George et al., consists of egg yolk–fructose agar base (Difco Laboratories, Detroit, MI) supplemented with cycloserine (500 µg/mL, final concentration), cefoxitin (16 µg/mL, final concentration), and 5% egg yolk suspension. The medium serves as a selective and differential medium for *C. difficile* and detects as few as 2000 organisms in a total count of 6×10^{10} bacteria per gram (wet weight) of feces. The source of basal medium will affect the recovery and growth of the organism. In a study by Marler et al. (29), Carr-Scarborough CCFA with horse blood gave better recovery than CCFA medium from BBL and Remel *C. difficile* agar.

There have been several modifications of CCFA media since it was first described in 1979 and these modifications should be considered if increased recoveries are needed. The substitution of 0.1% sodium taurocholate in place of the egg yolk suspension improves the recovery of spores. This substitution is useful in improving the recovery of the organism from hospital environments. The recovery rates also are improved by using cycloserine mannitol blood agar (CMBA). Bartley and Dowell (30) compared the recovery rates of *C. difficile* on CMBA, cycloserine mannitol agar (CMA), and CCFA, and found in order of decreasing recovery: CMBA > CMA > CCFA. The formulation for CMBA is trypticase (30.0 g), yeast extract (5.0 g), sodium chloride (2.5 g), sodium sulfite (0.1 g), mannitol (6.0 g), agar (20.0 g), distilled water (1,000 mL), cycloserine (5%, 10.0 mL), and defibrinated sheep blood (50.0 mL). Levett (31) suggested that by decreasing the antibiotic concentration from 500 to 250 µg/mL of cycloserine and from 16 to 8 µg/mL of cefoxitin, the recovery rate increases about 30%. A recent modification consists of the use of a medium that uses the same basal agar as CCFA but utilizes cysteine hydrochloride as a growth supplement and norfloxacin (12 µg/mL, final concentration) and moxalactam (32 µg/mL, final concentration) as the selective agents (32). When compared with CCFA, this medium recovered 20% more *C. difficile* isolates and decreased contaminating isolates by 30%.

On selective medium, *C. difficile* gives flat colonies that are several millimeters in size and that exhibit yellow fluorescence under long-wavelength ultraviolet light. The fluorescence will vary, depending on the basal medium (33). Some of the basal CCFA media give only weak fluorescence that can be intensified by the addition of blood or brain-heart infusion. Nonspecific fluorescence may be reduced by adding blood to the CCFA media. Although this media is highly selective, other organisms, including some gram-negative anaerobes, lactobacilli, and some other clostridia, may grow. The organism does not form spores on CCFA. Colonies must be subcultured to nonselective media to induce spore formation.

In addition to the use of selective agar media, selective broths have been used with good recovery rates (34). CCF broth supplemented with 0.1% sodium taurocholate may be prepared according to the original formulation of George et al. by omitting the agar. Cooked meat-carbohydrate-selective broth containing cycloserine (500 μg/mL) and cefoxitin (16 μg/mL) was reported to work well for the isolation of *C. difficile*. We found that brain-heart infusion broth supplemented with cycloserine (500 μg/mL) and cefoxitin (16 μg/mL) is superior to CCFA for detecting *C. difficile* in stool specimens. Another advantage is that the broth cultures can be assayed for *C. difficile* toxin very easily if necessary. Clabots et al. (35), on the other hand, reported that CCFA is better than selective broth for the isolation of the organism. This discrepancy may reflect differences in how the selective media is used. In our studies in which we isolated the organism from stool specimens in patients with *C. difficile* disease, the organism was present in a vegetative state. In the study by Clabots et al., who were detecting the organism in environmental sites, the organism was present in the spore state.

Metabolic Products

Clostridium difficile grows fermentatively and produces high levels of acetic, isobutyric, butyric, and isocaproic acid. The production of isocaproic acid is unusual and its presence may serve as a presumptive marker for *C. difficile* when screening isolates. However, other clostridia, including *C. bifermentans*, *C. sordellii*, and *C. sporogenes*, produce isocaproic acid and the presence of this fatty acid cannot be used as a definitive identification for *C. difficile*. Growth of the organism in selective broth medium containing cefoxitin prior to performing analysis for volatile fatty acids by gas–liquid chromatography has been reported to improve the identification of the organism, and this approach has been suggested as an alternative method to the workup of specimens from patients with diarrhea (36). However, this procedure does not distinguish toxigenic isolates from nontoxigenic isolates that may be present in the patient and in the hospital environment.

Another unusual metabolic product of *C. difficile* is *p*-cresol, which is produced by the intracellular metabolism of tyrosine. The only other *Clostridium* known to produce *p*-cresol is *C. scatologenes* and it seldom is encountered in the clinical laboratory. The detection of *p*-cresol is useful in the presumptive identification of *C. difficile*, and it can be enhanced using media such as peptone yeast glucose broth supplemented with 0.1% *p*-hydroxyphenylacetic acid (37–40). However, as with isocaproic acid, the presence of *p*-cresol may be used only for the presumptive identification of *C. difficile* and it does not distinguish toxigenic from nontoxigenic strains.

Toxin Production

Toxigenic strains of *C. difficile* produce toxin A and toxin B. Highly toxigenic strains produce high levels of both toxins whereas weakly toxigenic strains produce low amounts of the toxins. Highly toxigenic strains may produce levels of toxin A and toxin B that are 100,000 higher than the levels produced by weakly toxigenic strains, indicating a wide variation in toxin production. Only one strain (CCUG strain 8864) has been reported to produce one toxin (41–43). Interestingly, this strain carries the toxin B gene but only the front portion of the toxin A gene. It produces high levels of toxin B but it is unclear if the fragment of toxin A is produced. The genes encoding the toxins are located in close proximity to each other (see "Toxin Genes," below) and their expression may be coregulated. The toxin levels in filtrates from highly toxigenic strains may comprise almost 5% of the total bacterial protein, indicating that the organism expends an enormous amount of energy producing the toxins.

The production of toxin is maximal when the organism grows slowly in a rich medium. This may be accomplished by growing toxigenic strains in dialysis flasks in which the organism grows within a sac of dialysis tubing initially containing water or saline (44). The sac is suspended in a medium such as brain-heart infusion. The small molecular weight components diffuse into the sac, resulting in slow growth of the organism and, consequently, high levels of toxins A and B. This method, which was originally described for large-scale production of botulinum toxin (45), also works well for other toxigenic clostridia. The amount of toxins A and B produced within the dialysis sac using these growth conditions is equivalent to the amount of toxin produced in 2 L of a typical broth culture. Therefore, the dialysis procedure actually results in a concentration of the toxin. In addition to this advantage, the high molecular weight components in the media outside of the sac do not diffuse into the sac and do not contaminate the toxins. Therefore, this method also simplifies the purification of toxins A and B. When grown in broth media, the amount of toxin produced is affected by the inoculum size. A small inoculum in broth inoculum results in slower growth and as a result higher levels of toxin are achieved. Some strains may produce higher levels of toxin in broth media supplemented with subinhibitory levels of clindamycin but the mechanism for this stimulation is not clear (46). It may result from more efficient release of the toxin from the cell.

Antibiotic Susceptibility and Inhibition by Other Bacteria

Most strains of *C. difficile* are susceptible in vitro to a variety of antibiotics, including penicillin, erythromycin, tetracycline, chloramphenicol, clindamycin, metronidazole, vancomycin, and cotrimoxazole (47–56). It is interesting that many isolates are susceptible to the antimicrobial agent that initiated the disease (48). Fortunately, all strains appear to be sensitive to vancomycin and metronidazole. There are certain strains that are resistant to chloramphenicol, rifampicin, erythromycin, clindamycin, and tetracycline, and serogroups having multiple resistances have been implicated in outbreaks. In one instance, a serogroup that caused a cluster of PMC cases was resistant to all five of the antibiotics listed above. Interestingly, there are both toxigenic and nontoxigenic strains within this particular group, and both types exhibit the same resistance profiles. The nontoxigenic strains were isolated primarily from asymptomatic infants whereas the toxigenic strains were from adults with the disease, suggesting some host specificity. Strains resistant to chloramphenicol also have been implicated in outbreaks (57–59). The resistance of *C. difficile* to erythromycin and clindamycin is believed to be chromosomal and the determinants responsible for the resistance show homology with the *S. aureus* transposon Tn551 (52). The resistance determinant for tetracycline may be part of a conjugative transposon and is more variable among different strains and serogroups (53).

The growth of *C. difficile* is inhibited in vitro by certain bacteria. Rolfe et al. (60) examined the inhibitory effect of 116 strains of aerobic bacteria (14 genera) and 285 strains of anaerobic bacteria (9 genera). They found that *S. aureus, Pseudomonas aeruginosa,* group D enterocci, and *Streptococcus mitis* inhibited *C. difficile*. *Bacteroides* species, *Bifidobacterium adolescentis, B. infantis,* and *B. longum,* and *Lactobacillus* species were anaerobes that inhibited the organism. Fecal streptococci also have been reported to inhibit the growth of *C. difficile* (61). The inhibition by these anaerobes possibly resulted from the large amount of lactic acid produced. Certain fatty acids such as acetate, propionate, and butyrate are produced in vivo by the colonic flora and these also are inhibitory in vitro for *C. difficile*. In hamster studies, it has been shown that the level of butyrate may become sufficiently high so that it inhibits the in vivo growth of *C. difficile,* possibly explaining part of the protective nature of the normal flora (62). *C. difficile* inhibits the growth of certain bacteria that occur in the normal colonic flora, including *Bacteroides, Peptococcus,* and *Peptostreptococcus,* but the nature of this inhibition and possible significance has not been determined.

EPIDEMIOLOGY

Typing Methods

Epidemiological studies on the transmission of *C. difficile* represent a major focus of study because of the prob-

lems associated with this nosocomial pathogen. There continue to be outbreaks of *C. difficile* disease at hospitals across the United States and around the world and the incidence continues to rise. An increased incidence has been noted in other parts of the world as well. In a study in southeastern Asia, the reported incidence of *C. difficile* disease was >12% and this incidence was considerably higher than that observed with other enteropathogens such as *Campylobacter, Shigella,* and *Salmonella* (D. M. Lyerly, *personal communication*). Whether the observed incidence rates represent true increases or whether the increased numbers result from an increased awareness of the disease is not clear. The fact remains, however, that *C. difficile* continues to be a major problem. An increase in incidence has been observed at large medical centers and Veterans Administration Hospitals because of the large numbers of highly susceptible patients at these facilities. However, the disease is not restricted to these larger centers. It occurs at all types of facilities and health care professionals need to be aware of the potential problems.

A number of methods have been developed for typing *C. difficile* isolates (63–77). These methods include restriction endonuclease mapping, serotyping by agglutination, electrophoretic profiles, bacteriophage typing, and plasmid and bacteriocin typing. Typing based on the presence of plasmids or sensitivity to bacteriophages and bacteriocins is restricted because not all isolates contain plasmids or are sensitive to bacteriophages or bacteriocins. Only about 60–70% of *C. difficile* isolates, for example, carry plasmids. In studies at Ann Arbor, Michigan (66,73), scientists typed more than 85% of isolates using bacteriophages but the remaining isolates could not be typed because of the lack of bacteriophages with appropriate specificities. Isolates also have been typed by their resistance to various antibiotics. One particular outbreak of *C. difficile* disease in a surgical ward was attributed to an isolate that was resistant to clindamycin, tetracycline, and rifampicin. All of these typing methods have been used to study the epidemiology of *C. difficile* and its disease, and a discussion of these findings is presented below.

Transmission of *Clostridium difficile*

One of the most important points that should be emphasized to the health care worker is the fact that *C. difficile* can spread from patient to patient. All of the typing methods described above have been used to document the spread of strains during nosocomial outbreaks of *C. difficile* disease. In addition to the study of outbreaks, the spread of the organism has been studied in endemic situations. McFarland et al. (78) studied the acquisition and spread of the organism in an endemic setting involving more than 400 patients over an 11-month period. In their study, they noted that patient-to-patient transmission was highly evident, based on the finding that certain strains appeared during clusters of outbreaks and that roommates of patients with *C. difficile* disease developed the disease more frequently and more quickly than other patients. At the anaerobe laboratory, we have analyzed isolates from several outbreaks and, like the results from other laboratories, our results demonstrate patient-to-patient transmission.

This organism has become a major problem because it persists in the environment by forming spores and because it has a very efficient mode of transmission—diarrhea. The organism is not only present in the infected patient and soiled linens, it can be isolated from bookshelves, curtains, and floors in rooms of infected patients (63,78,79). In one outbreak, the responsible strain was even found on medical equipment in a storage room. In a study published in 1981, a culture of an environmental isolate was spread onto the floor of an unused hospital room and persisted in the room for at least 5 months. These properties enhance the spread of the organism and exacerbate the problem facing many health care facilities. *Clostridium difficile* spores persist in the hospital environment for long periods and measures should be implemented to minimize the spread of the organism. The longer a patient is hospitalized, the higher the risk of developing *C. difficile* disease.

A major way (probably the primary way) by which the organism is spread is by the health care worker. Numerous studies have described the isolation of *C. difficile* from the hands, clothes, and shoes of health care workers. In the study by McFarland et al. (78), 59% of the health care workers attending patients with *C. difficile* disease had the organism on their hands and in almost all cases, the isolate from the worker was the same type as the patient's isolate. McFarland et al. noted also that the organism was picked up by the health care worker during procedures typically considered to be low risk such as the daily patient assessment, physical examinations, or charting. These findings raise the question of whether *C. difficile* from patients poses a risk to the health care worker. The risk is very low since the disease occurs primarily in debilitated elderly patients. There is an isolated report, however, of three nurses developing *C. difficile* disease after attending a symptomatic patient (80). All three nurses developed diarrhea and had *C. difficile* toxin in their feces. Each responded to vancomycin but it is puzzling why these health care workers, who were healthy and between the ages of 23 and 37, developed the infection. Following this incident, Dr. Michel Delmee in Belgium reported that of more than 1000 cases of *C. difficile* disease he had diagnosed over a 10-year period, only 1 case occurred in a health care worker. In that instance, the worker had been treated with clindamycin prior to the onset of disease (81).

Asymptomatic Carriers

The results of some recent epidemiological studies indicate that asymptomatic carriage may be higher than suggested from studies in the early 1980s. In the study by McFarland et al. (78), 7% of the patients were positive for *C. difficile* at admission and 21% of the patients who were negative upon admission became positive while in the hospital. Interestingly, of these patients, 63% remained asymptomatic even though the majority had received antibiotics. Similar results have been reported in other studies. It appears that asymptomatic patients tend to have low levels or undetectable levels of toxin even though there are high numbers of the organism present. The reasons for these low levels of toxin are not known but strains from asymptomatic patients can spread and cause disease in other patients. Unfortunately, preventive measures usually are not implemented until a patient has been identified as positive for toxigenic *C. difficile*. As a result, the spread of the organism from asymptomatic carriers goes unchecked. Elderly patients who are asymptomatic carriers represent an increasingly serious concern for health care professionals (82,83). Many elderly patients who have high numbers of *C. difficile* in their feces are admitted to long-term care facilities directly from hospitals. Long-term care facilities, of course, have a large susceptible population, many of whom are likely already colonized (84). Some nursing homes have refrained from admitting persons who have *C. difficile* in their fecal specimens, but this is a questionable practice.

Another factor associated with the spread of *C. difficile* in a hospital setting is the fact that many infants (possibly more than 50%) have toxigenic *C. difficile* in their feces and are asymptomatic. The resistance of infants has been known since the early 1980s and may relate to reduced toxin binding to infant mucosa (see "Toxin Receptors" below). Interestingly, the original *C. difficile* isolates described in the mid-1930s were from normal infants. Infants that are debilitated in some manner (e.g., premature birth, antibiotic treatment for sepsis, etc.) can develop *C. difficile* disease but, as in adults, there is almost always some type of predisposing condition. There have been isolated reports of *C. difficile* outbreaks in child care centers but these are rare. There is some indication that infants tend to be colonized with strains that are distinct from the strains responsible for outbreaks in adults and this possibility is described below. Even so, infants still can become colonized with highly toxigenic strains and remain asymptomatic, and precautionary measures are not used in hospital nurseries to limit the spread of the organism. Additional studies are needed to further examine the role of infants as a reservoir in the hospital.

Are Certain Epidemiological Groups of *C. difficile* Responsible for Disease?

The intestinal flora represents a complex ecosystem and when this ecosystem is altered, other organisms can gain a foothold and compete for nutrients. This is the way in which *C. difficile* disease is initiated. Many outbreaks of *C. difficile* disease have been traced to single strains and some hospitals have repeated outbreaks due to a single strain. However, patients can harbor multiple strains at the same time and there are some reports suggesting that multiple relapses in some *C. difficile* patients may be due to different strains. Relapses in *C. difficile* patients continue to be a major problem with relapse rates as high as 20% in some locations. Relapses probably occur in many instances because the therapy (usually vancomycin or metronidazole) also suppresses other normal flora and either does not completely eliminate the organism or the patient gets reinfected from the environment. As a result, during the weeks after therapy, the organism begins to grow and the disease process starts again.

Patients also can be infected simultaneously with a toxigenic and a nontoxigenic strain. The nontoxigenic strains have not been implicated in disease and they may actually be protective by competing with a toxigenic strain for an ecological niche in the intestine (85). Nontoxigenic strains, just like toxigenic strains, form spores and persist in the environment. As a result, they also are spread from patient to patient but they *do not* cause disease. For this reason, it is important to screen more than a single isolate from a patient for toxin production if isolation of the organism is performed as a diagnostic aid.

Based on some recent epidemiological data, it appears that *C. difficile* may exhibit host specificities. Toma et al. (76) showed that certain toxigenic serogroups were responsible for outbreaks of *C. difficile* disease in adults whereas other serogroups were prevalent in fecal specimens from infants. Analysis of the isolates from infants showed that the isolates were toxigenic but that they produced only low levels of toxin. Perhaps one reason for the resistance of infants to *C. difficile* disease is that infants are colonized primarily with weakly toxigenic strains. The host specificity reported by Toma et al. is supported by the results from other laboratories. In Italy, Pantosti et al. (72) showed that of 21 groups distinguished by their protein profile typing, group 2 isolates were primarily from hospital outbreaks whereas group 5 isolates were from healthy neonates and children. The group 2 isolates exhibited the same properties as the serogroup implicated in the outbreaks studied by Toma et al. in Belgium. As additional evidence, Tabaqchali et al. (74) noted that certain groups of *C. difficile* distinguished by their restriction endonuclease profiles were isolated predominantly from vaginal specimens of healthy mothers and fecal specimens of healthy infants. In addition, Depitre et al. (86) reported that serogroup F strains are very prevalent in infants. Interestingly, they reported that none of 44 serogroup F strains examined produced toxin A in vitro even when grown in brain-heart infusion dialysis flasks, although they did produce toxin B at levels of 10^2–10^4 and they do carry the toxin A gene. The resistance of infants to *C. difficile* disease is continuing to be studied because it may open new types of treatment once we understand the nature of the resistance. From an epidemiological perspective, infants represent a major reservoir for *C. difficile* in hospitals, but the implications at this time are not clear. There may be some selective advantage for toxigenic strains to produce only low or negligible levels of toxin, since in infants the toxins do not benefit the host and the production of toxin is a drain on energy.

There are several studies from the early 1980s suggesting that cystic fibrosis patients tend to be colonized with nontoxigenic strains (87). However, additional studies on this population have not been published. Typing of *C. difficile* isolates from AIDS patients has been reported and there appears to be some host specificity. Barbut et al. (88) compared *C. difficile* strains from 50 AIDS patients and 49 HIV-negative patients. Serogroup C was

found in 66% of the AIDS patients and only in 18.4% of the HIV-negative patients. The strains isolated from AIDS patients were significantly more resistant to tetracycline, chloramphenicol, erythromycin, rifampin, and clindamycin than strains from HIV-negative patients. The authors suggested that the selectivity of serogroup C in AIDS patients may result from the multiple antibiotic resistance since AIDS patients often receive multiple antibiotic therapy. An independent association of toxigenic *C. difficile* diarrhea with AIDS per se, however, has not been demonstrated.

PATHOGENESIS AND IMMUNITY

Virulence Factors

Biological Activities of Toxins A and B

Toxigenic strains produce two toxins designated toxin A and toxin B. Toxin A also is referred to as the enterotoxin and toxin B is commonly referred to as the cytotoxin. In addition to its enterotoxic activity, toxin A is cytotoxic and causes the same type of rounding observed with toxin B. There have been reports of other biologically active factors produced by *C. difficile*, but these have not been confirmed (89,90). In some of the reports on other biologically active factors, it appears that the activity resulted from contamination with small amounts of toxin A or B. These toxins tend to be "sticky" and precautions must be taken to ensure their complete removal. Both of the toxins, for example, bind some immunoglobulins (91) and this can lead to false-positive results in ELISA formats. A listing of the biological activities of toxins A and B is presented in Table 1. Both toxins cause the same type of rounding effect, although toxin B is considerably more active (1000-fold) than toxin A against most tissue cultured cells. The rounding effect is seen with a wide variety of cell lines, including cell lines that are transformed as well as untransformed cells. Cells from a variety of tissues, including lung, skin, ovary, brain, muscle, and intestine, exhibit the same "rounding" effect. In

TABLE 1. *Biological activities of toxins A and B*[a]

Biological activity	Minimum dose	
	Toxin A	Toxin B
Enterotoxic activity (in rabbit ileal loop assay)	1 μg	Negative
Cytotoxic activity (against CHO tissue culture cells)	10 ng (500 ng/mL)	1 pg (50 pg/mL)
Lethal activity (intraperitoneal injections in mice)	50 ng	50 ng

[a] Values in the table represent the minimum toxic dose.

addition, cell lines derived from different animal species exhibit this effect.

Both toxins are lethal when injected parenterally into animals and have similar lethal doses. Approximately 50 ng of either toxin is sufficient to kill a 25-g mouse if the toxin is injected intraperitoneally. Animals that die following the injection of either toxin do not exhibit any significant pathology. In rhesus monkeys, it has been shown that a general shutdown in physiological responses occurs (92).

The most striking activity of toxin A is its enterotoxic activity. The activity is distinct from the activity observed with other enterotoxins such as cholera toxin and *E. coli* heat-labile toxin. Toxin A causes a viscous hemorrhagic fluid response unlike the ricewater fluid elicited by these other toxins. The hemorrhage occurs following the tissue damage caused by toxin A. For this reason, toxin A is occasionally referred to as a histotoxin or tissue-damaging enterotoxin. This is the basis for protein-losing enteropathy that has been observed with *C. difficile* infections (93,94) and why toxin A is believed to the primary toxin in *C. difficile* disease. Approximately 1 μg of toxin A is sufficient to elicit this type of response when injected into ligated rabbit ileal loops. When compared on a molar basis, toxin A is at least as potent and effective as cholera toxin in eliciting a positive fluid response in this model (93). Toxin B is not active in the intestinal loop assay but this does not mean, however, that toxin B is not important in the disease. If toxin B is administered to hamsters intragastrically with small nontoxic doses of toxin A, the animal becomes lethargic and dies (95). Similarly, animals in which the cecum is bruised also die when administered toxin B intragastrically. Like animals injected parenterally with toxin, there is no obvious pathology in the intestinal tract in animals that die following the intragastric administration of toxin B mixed with low nontoxic doses of toxin A (95). These observations are intriguing because they suggest that toxin B can leave the intestine and act distally on other organs, and indicate some synergistic action between the toxins. These findings also have led to speculation on the possible role of *C. difficile* in sudden infant death syndrome (SIDS) in which there are no obvious symptoms. However, no correlations have been demonstrated in infants with SIDS and the presence of the organism and its toxin (96,97).

In addition to its toxic activities, toxin A is a lectin and agglutinates rabbit erythrocytes. The hemagglutinating activity is specific and occurs following the binding of the toxin to Galα1-3Galβ1-4GlcNAc residues (98). The agglutination is temperature-dependent and occurs at 4°C but not at room temperature or higher. This interesting phenomenon is easily illustrated by slide agglutination with rabbit erythrocytes. Clumping of the erythrocytes at 4°C is easily visible and the clumps are dispersed simply by warming the slide to room temperature or higher. Based on this phenomenon, Krivan and Wilkins (99) developed a simple purification procedure for toxin A. Bovine thyroglobulin, which contains Galα1-3Galβ1-4GlcNAc residues, is immobilized on agarose and is used to bind toxin from crude protein mixtures at 4°C. The

gel is washed and the bound toxin is eluted at 37°C. The procedure is mild and can be performed quickly.

Toxin A also binds to several carbohydrate antigens which occur on human cells and these may be biological receptors for the toxin in the colon (see "Toxin Receptors," below). Toxin B does not bind to such carbohydrates and this appears to be one of the reasons that toxin B cannot cause direct damage to the undisturbed intestinal epithelium.

Structure

Toxins A and B are the largest bacterial toxins known. Toxin A has an M_r of 308,000 and toxin B has an M_r of 269,000 (100–102). Both are produced as single polypeptides. There have been reports that intracellular toxin A is different from toxin released from the cell (103) but this has not been confirmed. However, neither toxin contains a signal sequence and neither is dependent on proteolytic nicking for activation. A comparison of the primary sequence of toxins A and B shows that the two toxins are highly related in their basic structure even though they show no significant immunological cross-reaction (104,105). The toxins exhibit an overall homology of >45% at the amino acid level. Both toxins contain a complex series of contiguous repeating units at the COOH terminus. The repeating units of toxins A and B exhibit an homology of about 41%. In each toxin, these repeating units comprise about one third of the molecule. There is a series of large repeating units and these large units, in turn, comprise smaller repeating units. A comparison of these units in toxins A and B is shown in Fig. 1. In toxin A, these repeating units function as the binding portion that recognizes the receptor (106). They possibly serve a similar function in toxin B, although specific receptors for toxin B have not been identified. These repeating units show extensive homology with the repeating units contained in the glucosyltransferases of *Streptococcus mutans* and *S. sobrinus* (designated *GtfB, GtfC,* and *GtfI*) (107,108). Like toxin A, the repeating units of the glucosyltransferases are responsible for binding to carbohydrate.

Based on immunological analyses (109), the repeating units comprise much of the exterior portion of the toxin A molecule. Toxin A is highly resistant to inactivation or degradation by trypsin, even at extremely high trypsin-to-toxin molar ratios. Therefore, in addition to recognizing the receptor, the repeating units may function by protecting the toxin against proteolysis. The repeating units represent the immunodominant portion of the molecule. They are highly immunogenic and elicit most of the antibody when the toxin is injected parenterally. Within the repeats there are at least two sites that are highly immunodominant. When these regions are blocked with monoclonal antibody, the binding of polyclonal antibody to the native toxin is competitively inhibited about 75%, indicating that most of the antibody elicited against the native toxin is directed against these sites. The repeating units are completely nontoxic but they retain the hemagglutinating activity of the molecule (106,110). The toxic activi-

Toxin A Gene

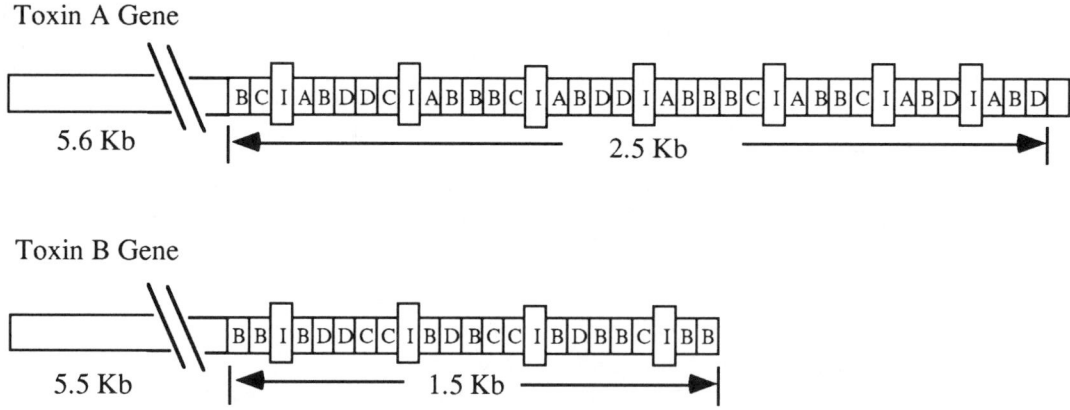

FIG. 1. Comparison of the repeating units of toxins A and B. Each block of repeating units comprises approximately one third of the molecule. The individual units are classified into class 1 and class 2 units. The class 1 units (I) are 30 amino acids in length. The class 2 units (A, B, C, D) are 20 amino acids in length and are categorized in order of decreasing homology. The A units, for example, are highly related to each other and their relationship to the other units in order of decreasing homology is B > C > D.

ties appear to be associated with active sites upstream of the repeating units. This observation and the fact that recombinant peptides comprising the repeating units elicit protective antibodies makes this portion of the molecule an attractive candidate for vaccine purposes. A monoclonal antibody, PCG-4, has been used to identify and characterize the regions involved in receptor binding. This antibody, which completely neutralizes the enterotoxic activity of toxin A, prevents the binding of the toxin to Galα-1-3Galβ1-4GlcNAc residues that bind the toxin (see "Toxin Receptors," below). The antibody has been used to identify two almost identical regions that are identical to or located near the immunodominant epitopes described above (111). A description of these regions is presented in Fig. 2.

There are additional features upstream of the repeating units that are conserved between the two toxins (Fig. 3). These features include four cysteine residues located in almost identical positions, a hydrophobic region located near the center of each toxin, and a putative ATP binding region. The conserved cysteines probably are integral in the structure of the toxins and the hydrophobic region, which is comprised of about 50 amino acids, may function

as a membrane spanning region during the intoxication process. Studies are now being performed to further examine the roles of these conserved regions and their involvement in the activity of these toxins. The regions of the toxins excluding the repeat section at the carboxyl end have a homology of almost 50%. Thus the two toxins appear to consist of gene repeats that have evolved different receptor binding properties.

Toxin Receptors

Toxin A binds to galactose-containing residues. In the hamster model, the binding is mediated through Galα1-3Galβ1-4GlcNAc residues located in the brush border membrane. The Galα1-3Galβ1-4GlcNAc residues also function as toxin A receptors in certain tissue cultured cell lines. F9 teratocarcinoma mouse cells, which have high numbers of this trisaccharide on the cell surface, are more than 100-fold more sensitive to toxin A than other cell lines that do not have the Galα1-3Galβ1-4GlcNAc moieties (112,113). As a result, F9 cells are almost as sen-

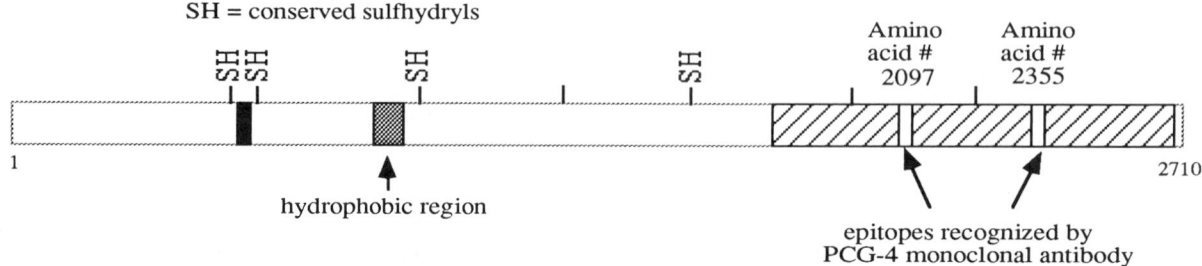

FIG. 2. Location of the epitopes on toxin A that are recognized by the monoclonal antibody PCG-4. There are two epitopes that have identical stretches of 42 amino acids. These epitopes are the immunodominant regions of the molecule and they are involved in the binding of the toxin to galactose-containing receptors.

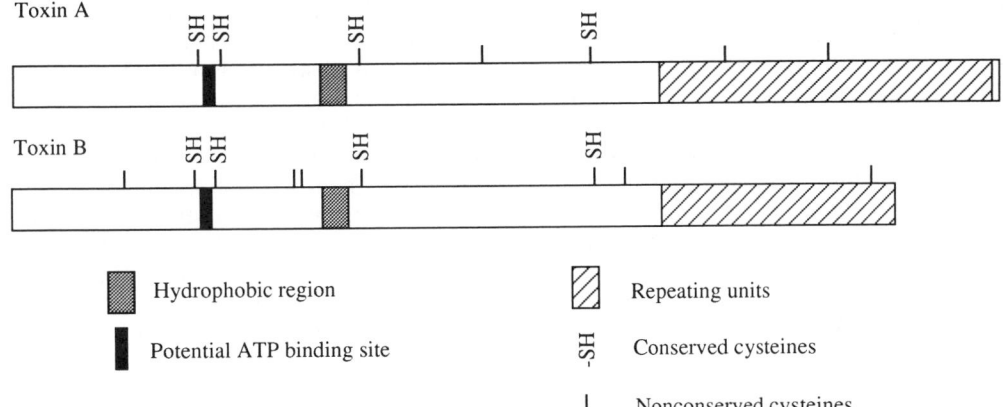

Toxin A

SH SH SH SH

Toxin B

SH SH SH SH

▨ Hydrophobic region   ▨ Repeating units

■ Potential ATP binding site   -SH Conserved cysteines

I Nonconserved cysteines

FIG. 3. Comparison of the conserved features of toxins A and B. The toxins exhibit >45% homology overall in their amino acid sequence, with the regions upstream of the repeating units exhibiting almost 50% homology. The potential ATP binding sites of the toxins contain an identical stretch of ten amino acids. The conserved cysteines are located in almost identical sites between the two toxins. They differ by a single amino acid position.

sitive to toxin A as they are to toxin B. As little as 5–10 pg of toxin A is sufficient to cause rounding of the cells.

Toxin A binds to human intestinal tissue. However, the binding is not due to the Galα1-3Galβ1-4GlcNAc as it is on hamster brush border membranes because this structure is not found on normal human cells. Additional studies have shown that the carbohydrate blood group antigens designated I, X, and Y, all of which exist on the intestinal epithelium of humans, bind toxin A (114). These antigens also are referred to as Lewis X (Le^x) and Lewis Y (Le^y) antigens, although they are not members of the Lewis blood group. The X antigen also is referred to as the My-1, VEP8-, and VEP9 antigen, and stage-specific embryonic antigen 1. All of these antigens are galactose-containing moieties and contain the type 2 core Galβ1-4GlcNAc that is present in the hamster brush border membrane receptor (Fig. 4). The binding to the I, X, and Y antigens is inhibited by the type 2 core but not by lactose, which is identical to the type 2 core except that it does not contain N-acetylamine. Therefore, the Galβ1-4GlcNAc structure appears to be the minimum structure needed for binding. The role of these antigens as receptors is intriguing because of their location on different proteins and lipids. The human glycoproteins carcinoembryonic antigen (CEA) and the secretory component of antibodies contain the X antigen and are present on intestinal epithelial cells. In addition, human granulocytes express high levels of the X antigen. Toxin A causes extensive inflammation and the possible targeting of the toxin to inflammatory cells via the X antigen may be a key step in the inflammatory response that occurs during the disease.

Human infants often have high levels of toxigenic *C. difficile* and toxins A and B in their feces and show no signs of disease. It was suggested previously by us that this resistance may result from the lack of receptors. Eglow et al. (115) also have suggested, using the rabbit model, that the absence of receptors may help to explain the resistance observed in infants. This is a plausible hypothesis in light of recent evidence indicating that the Shiga toxin receptor is nonfunctional in infant rabbits because it is developmentally regulated. However, human infant intestinal tissue contains the Y antigen and infant intestinal tissue binds toxin A as well as adult intestinal tissue (K. Tucker and T. Wilkins, personal communication). In addition, infant hamsters that are resistant to challenge with toxigenic *C. difficile* until they reach a cer-

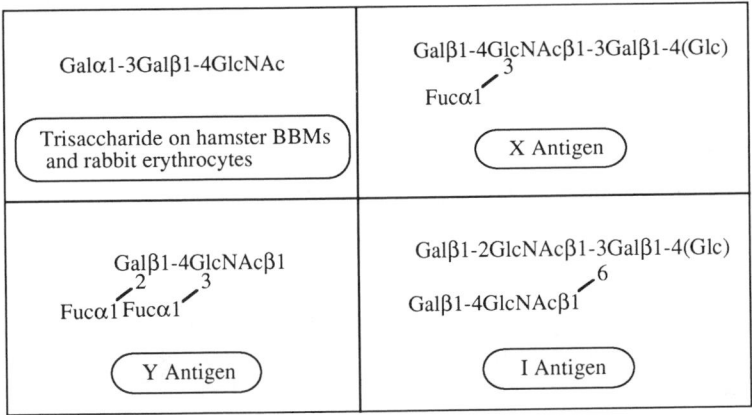

Galα1-3Galβ1-4GlcNAc (Trisaccharide on hamster BBMs and rabbit erythrocytes)	Galβ1-4GlcNAcβ1-3Galβ1-4(Glc) 3 Fucα1 (X Antigen)

Galβ1-4GlcNAcβ1
  2   3
Fucα1 Fucα1
 	
(Y Antigen)
	Galβ1-2GlcNAcβ1-3Galβ1-4(Glc)
	         6
	Galβ1-4GlcNAcβ1
	
	(I Antigen)

FIG. 4. Carbohydrates that bind toxin A. All of those shown in the figure contain the core Gal1β1-4GlcNAc. The X, Y, and I antigens are found on human cells, including those lining the intestinal tract.

tain age are still highly sensitive to the purified toxin (Tucker and Wilkins, *personal communication*). Therefore, the resistance of human infants and newborn animals appears to be more complicated than the simple absence of receptors.

Receptors for toxin B have not been identified. Our laboratory, in conjunction with Dr. Howard Krivan (MicroCarb, Gaithersburg, MD), examined the binding of toxin B to approximately 100 human carbohydrates found on eukaryotic cell surfaces and did not observe any binding to any of the carbohydrates. These results are puzzling in view of the fact that toxin B and toxin A are active against all cell lines that have been tested. Perhaps the toxin B molecule binds nonspecifically to lipid membranes.

Toxin Genes

The genes for toxins A and B and their general location relative to each other are illustrated in Fig. 5. The toxin B gene lies approximately 1 kb upstream of the toxin A gene. Both of the genes have been completely sequenced (100,101). A small open reading frame encoding a protein of about 17 kDa is located between the two genes. In addition, there is a small open reading frame located upstream of the toxin B gene and another downstream of the toxin A gene (Hammond and Johnson, *personal communication*). The role of these small open sequences is not known, but they do not appear to be involved in the activity of either toxin. This conclusion is based on studies showing that recombinant toxin, expressed by each toxin gene cloned independently of the small open reading frames, contains all the activities associated with native toxin. Recombinant toxin B is cytotoxic and lethal whereas recombinant toxin A is cytotoxic, lethal, and enterotoxic, and it agglutinates rabbit erythrocytes (116). Nontoxigenic strains do not carry either of the toxin genes or the small open reading frames (117).

The toxin genes, which are located on the chromosome, appear to be similarly controlled. The regulation of toxin production in *C. difficile* is poorly understood, although it appears to involve the region upstream of the toxin B gene. There appears to be some coregulation between the two toxins (118). Strains that produce high levels of one toxin produce high levels of the other toxin; strains that are weakly toxigenic produce low levels of both toxins. Highly toxigenic strains may have cytotoxic titers of 10^6 whereas weakly toxigenic strains may have titers of only

10^1 or 10^2. Thus, the amount of toxin produced varies tremendously between different clinical isolates. There is no clear-cut distinction in the association of these strains with increasing severity of disease. Only a single strain, CCUG 8864, has been described that produces only one of the toxins, in this instance toxin B (42–44). Attempts have been made to develop mutants that produce only one of the toxins but these attempts have not been successful. Interestingly, the CCUG strain carries the first portion of the toxin A gene but it is unclear if it is expressed. There is some heterogeneity among the toxin genes from various clinical isolates based on restriction endonuclease profiles. This heterogeneity reflects minor differences in the gene sequences. Toxin B from CCUG strain 8864 also exhibits some minor heterogeneity in its toxin B gene sequence compared to other well-characterized toxin B genes. Interestingly, the 8864 toxin B is more cytotoxic and exhibits low levels of enterotoxic activity, unlike toxin B from other highly toxigenic strains. In addition, it is about tenfold more lethal than toxin B from other strains. Several other isolates have been reported to produce only one of the toxins. However, these results must be interpreted carefully. In these instances, we have found these strains to be weakly toxigenic, and the detection of only a single toxin resulted from inadequate assays.

Mechanism of Action

The mechanism of action of these toxins at the molecular level is not known. However, some events leading to intoxication of tissue cultured cells by toxin A are known. The toxin binds to carbohydrates via its repeating units and enters cells via receptor-mediated endocytosis. The toxin is further processed in the endosome. The internalization of toxin A by receptor-mediated processes has been demonstrated by electron microscopy and is supported by the finding that agents such as monensin, chloroquin, and tetramethylamine, which interfere with receptor-mediated endocytosis and endosomal processing, inhibit both toxins (119,120). Both toxins, especially toxin B, bind very tightly to hydrophobic resins. Therefore, it is likely that both toxins bind in a nonspecific manner to mammalian cells via the hydrophobic cell membranes in this manner. Toxin A probably utilizes receptor binding as its primary means of entering cells but also enters cells by this other mechanism. This possibility is supported by electron microscopic analysis showing that toxin A enters

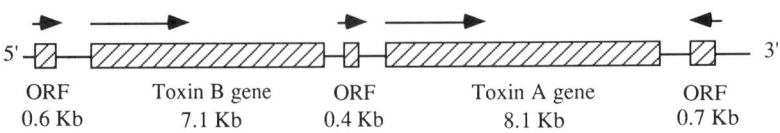

FIG. 5. Location of the toxin A and toxin B genes. The toxin B gene encodes a single polypeptide with an M_r of 279,000 and the toxin A gene encodes a single polypeptide with an M_r of 308,000. There are three small open reading frames associated with the toxin genes. The function of these small reading frames is not known, but they are not directly involved in the toxic activity of either toxin.

cells both by receptor-mediated endocytosis and by generalized pinocytosis.

At this point, the mechanism at the molecular level is unclear. The activity of both toxins results in cell rounding that eventually leads to cell death. This process likely is responsible for the in vivo toxicity of the toxins. The "cell rounding" phenomenon indicates that the cytoskeletal system is affected in some manner. The binary toxins produced by *C. botulinum* (C2 toxin, not the neurotoxin), *C. perfringens* (iota toxin), and *C. spiroforme* (iota toxin) cause cell rounding by transferring the ADP-ribose moiety of the cofactor NAD onto actin. In addition, cytochalasin B, which binds to actin filaments, causes a similar type of rounding. However, toxins A and B do not have ADP-ribosylating activity and they have not been shown to directly modify actin. The cytoskeletal system is very complex and actin exists in a dynamic state, fluctuating between globular (G) and filamentous (F) actin. There are numerous points that could be altered, thus affecting the dynamic actin pool and causing cell rounding, but any specific effect of the toxins has not been identified. The toxins have been examined for other types of activities associated with other bacterial toxins but these analyses have been negative. It appears that toxins A and B may have a new activity that has not been described for other bacterial toxins. There have been reports describing enolase activity in preparations of toxin B. However, the activity was due to contaminating enolase that copurified with the toxin (121).

The highly conserved structures and related cytotoxic activities of toxins A and B suggest that the toxin genes arose by gene duplication. This, in turn, suggests to us that the toxins likely have the same or a similar mechanism. The lack of enterotoxic activity in toxin B may simply reflect the absence of a suitable receptor for toxin B in the intestine, and other minor differences in levels of activity may reflect differences in binding affinity to receptors instead of suggesting different mechanisms. Additional studies are needed to confirm this hypothesis.

Events Leading to Clinical Illness

The initial step in the development of *C. difficile* disease involves disruption of the normal protective intestinal flora. In most instances, this modification occurs following therapy with some of the new wide-spectrum antibiotics. This organism causes disease in elderly compromised patients so the age and health are very important. Once the normal flora is disrupted, enteric pathogens such as *C. difficile* that are present in the hospital environment enter the intestine. When the amount of antibiotic in the colon drops below the level that inhibits *C. difficile,* the organism begins to grow. This occurs with toxigenic as well as nontoxigenic isolates, both of which form spores and exist in the environment. Once in the reduced environment of the colon with nutrients freely available due to lack of competition, the cells begin to grow to high number. Colony-forming counts of $>10^8$ are typical in patients with *C. difficile* disease. There has been speculation that *C. difficile* cells attach to specific receptors along

the colonic wall. These results, however, have not been confirmed and the evidence is not convincing. It appears more likely that the organism grows throughout the lumen of the colon and is not directly targeted to specific binding sites. Toxin A, on the other hand, is targeted to specific receptors once it is produced in the colon. The colonic mucus possibly interferes with the binding of the toxin to its receptor and it may have to be disrupted to get the disease. This may be one explanation why some but not all patients with *C. difficile* in their colon become ill.

Toxigenic strains begin to release toxin as they reach stationary phase. Like other large clostridial toxins such as the neurotoxins from *C. botulinum* and *C. tetani*, toxins A and B appear to be released during autolysis of the vegetative cells. Neither toxin has any N-terminal signal sequences that suggest secretion of processed toxin. In susceptible older patients, toxin A subsequently binds to galactose-containing receptors, possibly one of the galactose-containing moieties described above (see "Toxin Receptors," above), and is internalized and processed by receptor-mediated endocytosis and pinocytosis. This sequence of events ultimately leads to the action of the toxin on some target molecule inside the cell, leading to cell rounding and cell release. These events result in tissue damage, erosion of the microvilli, and extravasation of serous fluid into the lumen. These observations are based on results by Lima et al. (122), who showed that toxin A–induced damage to epithelial cells lining the mucosa preceded or coincided with the fluid response into the lumen. In addition to the direct tissue damage caused by toxin A, there is an inflammatory response that is very severe in PMC patients and that likely contributes to the severity of the disease. Studies by Triadafilopoulos et al. (123,124) showed that the injection of toxin A into ligated intestinal loops results in a severe inflammatory reaction in the lamina propria and necrosis of enterocytes. These changes are accompanied by increases in the levels of prostaglandin E_2 and leukotriene B_4, both of which are associated with the inflammation. There is some evidence that toxin A is chemotactic (125). This activity and the extensive tissue damage caused by toxin A to the microvilli exacerbate the disease process. The influx of serous fluid into the colon maintains the disruption of the intestinal flora and allows *C. difficile* to continue the disease process.

The role of toxin B in the disease process is poorly understood. Toxin B by itself is not active in the intestinal tract. However, if mixed with low nontoxic doses of toxin A, toxin B causes experimental animals to become lethargic and eventually die (95). These results indicate some synergy between the toxins and suggests that the initial tissue damage by toxin A allows toxin B to act. These results also indicate that toxin B and possibly toxin A disseminate from the intestinal tract once the initial tissue damage has occurred and then act distally on other target organs. This suggests to us that asymptomatic persons such as infants who have high levels of *C. difficile* toxin in their intestine might become ill and die from no apparent cause if the intestinal wall is damaged (e.g., colonization by other pathogens that tend to cause chronic intestinal illness, surgery, etc.). This possibility has been suggested as a cause for some cases of SIDS. However, any role of *C. difficile* and its toxins in SIDS has not been proven (96,97).

Antibodies in Patients with Disease

Antibodies against toxins A and B protect experimental animals against the disease and they likely are beneficial as part of our host defense against this pathogen. However, the immune response during *C. difficile* disease is only now beginning to be studied. There have been several studies describing the presence of IgG and IgM antibodies against toxins A and B in healthy children and adults (126–128). These results were obtained by ELISA using toxin immobilized on microtiter wells. Some of these results must be interpreted with caution because both toxins bind certain classes of immunoglobulins, especially IgM, in a nonimmune manner. As a result, elevated ELISA readings may be wrongly interpreted as positive reactions. In a more recent study, Johnson et al. (129) used ELISA to examine the mucosal and systemic antibody responses to toxin A in patients with *C. difficile* disease. Unlike the previous studies, however, these investigators determined if the antibodies in the specimens neutralized the toxin, providing another indication that the response they were observing resulted from specific toxin antibodies. They found that convalescent patients had considerably higher levels of mucosal and systemic antibodies against toxin A than acute patients, asymptomatic excretors, or control subjects. Four of 15 convalescent specimens neutralized toxin A but only 1 of 13 acute sera neutralized the toxin. Based on these results, they concluded that most convalescent patients develop systemic and mucosal antibodies against toxin A, but these antibodies do not appear to affect the clinical course of the disease.

CLINICAL ILLNESS

Criteria for Establishing Clinical Disease

The normal bacterial flora of the intestinal tract serves many functions. One of its key functions is its protective role against enteropathogens that enter the intestine. When antibiotics or other powerful drugs enter the intestine, they kill much of the protective flora. This is especially true with the new wide-spectrum antibiotics that are in use today. Some of the powerful anticancer drugs used today cause a similar effect. When this happens, enteropathogens that normally cannot grow in the intestine in healthy persons are able to effectively compete for nutrients and grow. *Clostridium difficile* represents a typical opportunistic pathogen that seldom is present in the intestinal tract of adults. The organism is commonly found in the intestine of infants and may be considered part of the normal flora, but this is not the case in adults. When persons, especially elderly patients who are hospitalized, begin antibiotic therapy, the protective flora is

drastically altered. If there are *C. difficile* spores in the environment, they infect the patient and begin to grow as the concentration of antibiotic decreases. The presence of toxin, however, does not mean that the patient has *C. difficile* disease. This is true in infants and there are many asymptomatic adults who have toxigenic *C. difficile* and toxin in their feces. Any antibiotic that disrupts the normal protective flora can predispose a patient to the disease. Antibiotics that are most commonly associated with the disease include clindamycin, cephalosporins, and ampicillin. Clindamycin, which binds to the 50S subunit of ribosomes of bacteria, is very active against anaerobic bacteria, especially *Bacteroides fragilis,* and is prescribed for many anaerobic infections. Ampicillin, like other penicillins, and cephalosporins inhibit cell wall synthesis in bacteria. Their high use and the fact that they have a broader spectrum than some of the other antibiotics probably explain the higher numbers of *C. difficile* cases associated with this antibiotic. *C. difficile* is usually susceptible to the inciting antibiotic, including those described above, but the organism may grow with the suppression of the competing flora as the concentration of antibiotic decreases toward the end of the therapy.

Clinical criteria as defined by Gerding and Brazier (130) include (a) diarrhea in which no other cause has been established, (b) loose or unformed stool that takes the shape of the container, (c) three or more bowel movements per day, (d) duration of at least 2 days, and (e) a prior history of antibiotic or antineoplastic agents in the preceding 4–6 weeks. Gerding noted that only 22% of their patients with *C. difficile* exhibited abdominal pain; 28% had fever; and very rarely did patients exhibit ileus and constipation. A positive response to treatment with metronidazole or vancomycin is considered confirmatory evidence although these antibiotics are not specific for *C. difficile* and will act on other etiological agents. There also has to be evidence for *C. difficile* toxin, either for toxin B by the tissue culture assay or toxin A by ELISA. A positive culture identification for *C. difficile* also may be performed, although there is some question about requiring culture. Peterson et al. (131,132) reported that isolation of the organism correlates more closely with *C. difficile*–associated disease, as defined by the clinical symptoms described above, than toxin detection. Bartlett (133), on the other hand, notes that stool cultures are not particularly useful for routine diagnosis of the disease. Instead, he notes that isolation is useful primarily in the management of epidemics. If isolation procedures are used, it is important that stringent methods be used for quality assurance of the isolation media since poor quality media will drastically lower the recovery rates.

Pathology

Pseudomembranous Colitis

The onset of *C. difficile* disease usually begins several days after starting antibiotic therapy up to 2 months following cessation of antibiotic therapy. Diarrhea and abdominal cramping usually are the first symptoms, followed by the development of fever and chills in severe cases. Occasionally there may be some bleeding. Pseudomembranes several millimeters in diameter appear as small, whitish yellow plaques along the colonic wall and these are diagnostic for pseudomembranous colitis. As the disease progresses, the pseudomembranes may coalesce to form larger plaques. Microscopically, the pseudomembranes appear as necrotic cells and debris, and usually numerous leukocytes are present. The leukocytes likely contribute significantly to the tissue damage that occurs during the disease because of the tissue-damaging substances they release. The infiltration of leukocytes results from the tissue damage caused by toxin A and by the chemotactic properties of the toxin (125). The presence of fecal leukocytes in stool specimens is not useful in the diagnosis of the disease. Guerrant et al. (134) noted that the presence of fecal leukocytes may be misleading. They suggested that leukocytes may be unstable in stool specimens, including those from C. difficile patients. This finding explains the absence of leukocytes in patients with high levels of C. difficile toxin. The insensitivity of fecal leukocytes in C. difficile diarrhea also was noted by Marx et al. (135), who showed the sensitivity and specificity of fecal leukocytes with C. difficile toxin results were 28% and 92%, respectively. The predictive positive and negative values, which were 27% and 93%, respectively, also were low.

Upon microscopic examination of biopsy tissue from C. difficile patients, the tips of the microvilli are eroded and cells are necrotic. Pseudomembranous colitis (PMC), as the name denotes, characteristically occurs in the colon. There have been some reports in which some involvement of the lower small intestine was noted. However, this is the exception. In a study by Pesce et al. (136), 27 cases of antibiotic-associated PMC were studied and in each instance the lesions were restricted to the colon. LaMont (137) also noted that in autopsies of PMC patients, the characteristic pseudomembrane lesions stopped at the ileocecal valve. This is expected because C. difficile is an obligate anaerobe that would grow best in the colon.

Antibiotic-Associated Diarrhea

Antibiotic-associated diarrhea is the most common form of the disease. Up to 25% of the diarrheal stools submitted for C. difficile testing have C. difficile toxin and are from hospitalized patients with this form of the disease. It is important that the physician be aware of the fact that the majority of antibiotic-associated diarrheas (i.e., the other 75%) are not caused by C. difficile. Essentially all cases of PMC, on the other hand, are caused by this organism. Newer and improved methods for the rapid diagnosis of the disease have enabled us to detect the disease earlier and initiate the proper therapy more quickly. As a result, cases of C. difficile disease do not progress as far, and fewer fatal cases of PMC are observed. It is unknown if milder forms of the disease are caused by weakly toxigenic strains whereas severe cases (i.e., PMC and cases that rapidly develop into life-threat-

ening conditions) are caused by highly toxigenic strains that produce much higher levels of toxins A and B. Generally, the diarrhea and abdominal cramping in cases of antibiotic-associated diarrhea due to C. difficile are less severe than that seen with colitis.

Relapse

C. difficile disease usually is effectively treated with oral vancomycin or metronidazole. A major problem, however, continues to be relapses following treatment with these agents. The relapse rates noted in the literature range from 10% to 20% in patients who initially respond to therapy. Relapses usually occur 1–5 weeks following treatment and multiple relapses can occur. The most likely explanation is that low numbers of spores remain in the patient or are picked up from the hospital environment and begin to grow when the vancomycin or metronidazole therapy is stopped. At this point, the normal microflora of the patient is still drastically altered and any spores that persist begin to grow, resulting in a relapse. Relapses may result from infection with a different strain although in most instances the initial infecting strain is responsible. Strains that are resistant to vancomycin and metronidazole have not been identified and relapses do not occur from the development of resistant strains.

Recurrent relapses represent a serious and debilitating predicament for the patient. The occurrence of several relapses is not uncommon and one patient reportedly had 18 relapses (138). It has been recommended that a patient undergoing a mild relapse not be treated with antibiotics since this inhibits the recolonization by the normal flora (138). Alternatively, Bartlett (139) used therapy with cholestyramine with some success in treating relapses. In this instance, the cholestyramine is not administered in conjunction with vancomycin since the cholestyramine also binds vancomycin. The cholestyramine therapy is begun following the vancomycin therapy and functions by binding the toxin as the normal flora becomes reestablished. Even with these alternatives, relapses continue to be a major problem and other methods need to be developed and evaluated. Hopefully, treatments such as immunoprophylaxis will soon be available as therapies.

Complications of C. difficile Disease Involving Other Intestinal Diseases

C. difficile is characteristically associated with intestinal disease in persons with predisposing conditions, primarily treatment with antibiotics and antineoplastic agents. However, there has been some speculation that C. difficile disease may complicate the diagnosis in patients with inflammatory bowel disease. In a study by Meyers et al. (140), C. difficile toxin was detected in 3 of 18 patients with ulcerative colitis and 1 of 26 patients with Crohn's disease. All of these persons had received antibiotics in the preceding 2 months, so that their normal flora was altered. In another study, LaMont and Trnka (141) demonstrated the presence of C. difficile toxin in six patients with chronic inflammatory bowel disease (IBD). All six patients improved with the disappearance of toxin in the stool, although they continued to have diarrhea or proctoscopic evidence of chronic colitis. As a result, it was suggested that patients with chronic colitis who do not respond to standard medical therapy should have stool specimens checked for toxin. In another study (142), 13% of the stools from patients (total of 109) with IBD were positive for *C. difficile* toxin. It was noted also that the frequency of a positive stool in patients with IBD was higher when the patients were in hospitals, indicating nosocomial acquisition. Other studies (143,144) also have noted higher incidences of *C. difficile* and toxin in stools from IBD patients. Therefore, it is recommended that stool specimens from patients with IBD be tested for *C. difficile* toxin, especially if the patient relapses and there is a history of recent antibiotic usage. Other complications include toxic megacolon and fulminant PMC (145–148). Fulminant PMC in the absence of toxic megacolon also has been reported (145).

DIAGNOSIS

Endoscopic Examination

Endoscopic examination revealing pseudomembranes is considered the diagnostic test for pseudomembranous colitis, signaling that the patient has severe *C. difficile* disease. This can be revealed by rigid proctoscopy or flexible sigmoidoscopy or by surgical exploration. Under these conditions, laboratory tests such as culturing, tissue culture assays, or immunoassays serve primarily to confirm the diagnosis. The results of laboratory tests become more critical when performed on patients with antibiotic-associated diarrhea since endoscopy is not performed routinely under these circumstances and because *C. difficile* is not the only organism that causes diarrhea under these conditions.

Some laboratories analyze only diarrheal specimens (i.e., specimens that retain the shape of the container) whereas other laboratories also analyze semisolid and formed stools. Occasionally, semisolid and formed stools from suspected patients can contain *C. difficile* toxin, and positive test results with the specimens can be indicative of *C. difficile* disease. Formed stool specimens are troublesome because they may give weak false-positive or false-negative results. This happens in both the tissue culture assay and ELISA. Because of these problems, some laboratories avoid the routine analysis of solid stool specimens. Fecal specimens containing blood also cause these types of problems so the clinical microbiologist should be aware of this potential problem. Under these circumstances, it is valuable to evaluate more than a single specimen. Many laboratories freeze specimens for several days and then process several days worth of specimens at one time for obvious economic and time saving reasons. Some stools, however, can lose their cytotoxic activity during a single freezing and thawing, or they may develop low levels of nonspecific cytotoxic activity and appear weakly positive, thus confusing the test results. Although this

happens only in a very low percentage of the specimens, best results are obtained using fresh specimens (usually diarrheal specimens) within 24 hr of collection, with the specimens held at 2–8°C until the assay is performed.

Diagnostic Tests

Clinical microbiologists face an array of methods and commercial tests when considering what procedures to perform for *C. difficile* and its toxins (Table 2). Fecal specimens are very complex and none of these tests is 100% accurate. For this reason, some clinical laboratories use two tests. It is important to remember that all of these tests serve as aids and that test results must be considered in conjunction with the patient history since toxins A and B can be present in specimens from healthy persons. If the incidence of toxin in fecal specimens is higher than 25%, the clinical microbiologist should check to ensure that weak false positives are not a problem.

Isolation of the Organism

Culturing for the organism, latex agglutination, tissue culture assay, and ELISA are used as aids in the diagnosis of *C. difficile*. A summary of the methods and tests available for the detection of *C. difficile* and its toxins is shown in Table 2. Culturing is the most difficult and may be the most inconsistent method due to variations in specimen storage, the type of enrichment procedures used, and the nature of the organism itself. Although *C. difficile* is not as strict an anaerobe as, for example, *C. tetani*, it can be difficult to recover from stool specimens and requires expertise in anaerobic bacteriology. In addition to these considerations, the source of media is critical and can affect recovery rates. Many laboratories prepare their own media because of the variable quality of some commercial media, and quality control must be done carefully. If culture is to be implemented, it is best to evaluate several types of procedures and sources of media before settling on a particular procedure and source. Inoculated media should be incubated at 37°C for a minimum of 3 days before tests are ruled negative.

The manner in which isolation is performed varies between laboratories. Some laboratories use a preliminary alcohol or heat-shock procedure for spore enrichment, whereas others plate fecal specimens directly onto selective media such as cycloserine-cefoxitin-fructose agar (CCFA) with good rates of success. Some laboratories use selective broth media for the isolation of *C. difficile* from stool specimens. Isolates of *C. difficile* vary in their ability to survive during culturing. Some are better spore formers than others and some will be more adaptable to plating on selective media (which represents a major shock for the organism going from the colonic environment to agar). As a result, recovery rates will vary among clinical laboratories. *Clostridium difficile* is presumptively identified on solid media by its colony morphology and fluorescence. However, other bacteria grow on CCFA and some of these, including some clostridia, flu-

TABLE 2. *Methods and tests for detecting* Clostridium difficile *and its toxins*

Method	Protein detected	Advantages	Limitations	Available tests
Culturing	Organism	Classical microbiology	Inconsistent; does not distinguish toxigenic and nontoxigenic isolates	Selective media from various sources
Latex agglutination/ELISA	Glutamate dehydrogenase	Rapid and simple	Not extremely sensitive; does not distinguish toxigenic and nontoxigenic isolates	Meritec/ImmunoCard (Meridian Diagnostics, Inc.) CDT (Becton Dickinson)
Tissue culture assay	Toxin B	Sensitive, specific, and adaptable	Requires 24 to 48 hr; noncommercial versions are not standardized; tedious; often done incorrrectly	Toxititer (Bartels Immunodiagnostics) Toxin/Antitoxin (TechLab, Inc.) Tox-B Test (TechLab, Inc.)
ELISA	Toxin A	Rapid, sensitive, and simple	Possibly higher number of indeterminate readings and unconfirmed positive results	Premier (Meridian Diagnostics, Inc.) Toxin A EIA (Bartels Immunodiagnostics) VIDAS-CDA (Vitek Systems) Tox-A Test (TechLab, Inc.) Toxin A Test (Becton Dickinson)
	Toxins A and B			Cytoclone A + B EIA (Cambridge Biotech)

oresce the same as *C. difficile*. The isolation of *C. difficile* from a stool specimen does not mean that it is toxigenic. Nontoxigenic isolates, which are not pathogenic, are often present in fecal specimens and are detected by culturing. Nontoxigenic isolates also form spores and are spread in a hospital environment like toxigenic isolates. In some hospitals, 25% of the isolates are nontoxigenic. It is advantageous to follow up the presumptive identification by growing the isolates in broth media and assaying filtrates for toxin using one of the toxin-detecting procedures described below. Several colonies should be screened because patients can be colonized with more than one type of isolate.

Latex Agglutination

There are two latex agglutination (LA) tests available as diagnostic aids for the direct testing of fecal specimens. The tests, which are essentially identical, detect the enzyme glutamate dehydrogenase, a nontoxic protein produced by all toxigenic and nontoxigenic isolates of *C. difficile* and by some other clostridia and anaerobes, including *C. sporogenes*, certain *C. botulinum*, and *Peptostreptococcus anaerobius* (149). The LA test was initially marketed as a test for toxin A (150), and there still are reports describing the "detection of toxin A" with the LA test. However, the glutamate dehydrogenase detected in the test has no relationship with either toxin A or toxin B and the LA tests do not distinguish between toxigenic and nontoxigenic isolates.

Reported values for the relative sensitivity and specificity for the commercial tests are at the 70–80% and 85–95%

levels, respectively, compared with culturing. The sensitivity and specificity values are low when the latex tests are compared to tissue culture assay because many of the isolates detected in some hospitals are nontoxigenic. Although these tests are rapid and simple, they are not extremely sensitive and they give false-positive reactions. The LA test is best used as a rapid screening test in hospitals and medical centers that have high rates (15–20%) of *C. difficile* disease. Fecal specimens that are positive by LA should be tested for toxin by tissue culture assay or ELISA. An alternative to the LA test is the ImmunoCard *C. difficile* marketed by Meridian Diagnostics. Like the LA format, the ImmunoCard test detects the glutamate dehydrogenase. The ImmunoCard is rapid and sensitive and does not require the preliminary centrifugation step needed to perform the LA test. The ImmunoCard reportedly offers improved sensitivity and specificity over the LA tests. Compared with culturing, the ImmunoCard has a sensitivity and specificity of 86.2% and 88.9%, respectively, compared with 79.3% and 86.7% for the LA test (151). As with the latex tests, additional testing must be done to detect the presence of toxin. The correlation of all of these tests with cytotoxicity or ELISA tests varies between hospitals depending on the number of patients with nontoxigenic strains. Thus, during a major disease outbreak, these assays appear to work better.

Tissue Culture Assay

The detection of toxin represents the best diagnostic test because it confirms the presence of toxigenic strains in the specimen. Two methods, tissue culture and ELISA, are used for this purpose. The tissue culture method was the first test to be developed and is considered the gold standard. Thus it is the method to which other tests are compared. The tissue culture assay detects toxin B, which masks the weaker cytotoxic activity of toxin A in fecal specimens. The primary advantage of the test, which can detect as little as 1 pg of toxin B, is its sensitivity. Even so, the test shows only a 70–80% correlation with culturing in patients with *C. difficile*–associated diarrhea in laboratories that are very successful at culturing the organism. This is one of the reasons why some laboratories who are very successful at isolating *C. difficile* from clinical specimens support the use of culture as a routine diagnostic aid. However, culture results should be interpreted with caution since many patients become asymptomatic carriers once they enter the hospital and may harbor so few organisms that significant toxin is not produced. The toxin produces the disease, not the bacterial cell.

The tissue culture test is somewhat tedious, requires 24–48 hr for results, and in-house methods are poorly standardized. An advantage, however, is that hospitals can produce and maintain their own cell lines for testing purposes, thereby keeping the cost of the test to a minimum. The cell lines that are used most commonly are WI-38, MRC-5, human foreskin, and Chinese hamster ovary (CHO) cells. All of these cell lines are comparable in sensitivity. Some cell lines have been advertised as more specific for toxin A, but toxin B is still the toxin detected by the cells. Tissue cell monolayers in tubes or microtiter plates can be used for the assay, with results being determined within 24–48 hr. Weakly positive specimens should be regarded suspiciously since the cytotoxic effect (i.e., cell rounding) occasionally may be caused by freezing and thawing of the specimen. Specimens from healthy individuals can have nonspecific titers of up to 10^2, so it is important that all test results, especially those that are weakly positive be considered in conjunction with patient history when making the diagnosis.

ELISA

There are now six commercial ELISAs available for *C. difficile* toxin (see Table 2). Five are specific for toxin A and the other ELISA detects both toxin A and toxin B. Five of the tests are performed manually and the other (VIDAS-CDA) is automated. All of these tests use a monoclonal antibody specific for toxin A. They are sensitive and can be completed in 2.5–3 hr. There are some differences in these ELISAs and these differences should be considered in the selection of a suitable test. Three of the tests, the Meridian Premier test, the TechLab Tox-A test, and the BD Toxin A test, require fewer steps and are simpler to perform than the other tests. The Meridian Premier and the TechLab Tox-A tests were initially marketed as 2-hr tests, but also can be done in 1-hr formats. The BD test requires about 75 min to perform. The VIDAS-CDA is automated but it requires expensive equipment. The advantage of detecting both toxins in the Cytoclone A + B EIA from Cambridge BioTech is still unclear because only a single strain has been described

that produces only toxin B. Toxin B also is more difficult to detect by ELISA.

These tests have sensitivity and specificity rates of 85–90% or higher and their overall performances are being studied in numerous laboratories. They appear highly suited as diagnostic aids. An advantage of the ELISA over the tissue culture test is that it detects inactive and active toxin whereas the tissue culture test requires biologically active toxin. As a result, some specimens that are positive by ELISA and negative by tissue culture (due to inactivation of toxin by proteases) are true positives. Washing the wells during the ELISA is very critical and must be done according to the manufacturer's instructions. Improper washing can result in weak false positives and indeterminate reactions. Laboratory technologists should note if weak reactions occur adjacent to strongly positive wells because splashover can occur. Specimens that test weakly positive or indeterminate should be retested, or a fresh specimen should be tested.

Other Methods

Methods such as gas–liquid chromatography have been used to detect *C. difficile* in stool specimens by detecting metabolic products such as volatile fatty acids and *p*-cresol (152–157). However, these methods are not specific and they do not distinguish toxigenic from nontoxigenic strains. As a result, they are not used routinely.

There are several commercial microsystems available that may be used as aids in the identification of *C. difficile* once the organism has been presumptively identified. These systems include the Minitek Anaerobe II from BBL Microbiology Systems, the API An-Indent System from Analytab Products, and the RapID ANA System from Innovative Diagnostic Systems. The results with the API ZYM and the RapID ANA System have been the most impressive (158–160). Both are completed within 4 hr. A drawback of these systems is that they rely on the detection of preformed enzymes in an aerobic environment. Therefore, even though the assays are performed within a short time, there is the possibility that some of the marker enzymes are inactive (161). Aspinall and Dealler (162) used five enzymes, prolyl aminopeptidase, galactosidase, leucine aminopeptidase, acid phosphatase, and indole, to identify *C. difficile* isolates. The majority of *C. difficile* are positive for prolyl aminopeptides and negative for the other four enzymes. In their test, substrates for these enzymes were impregnated into filter paper on plastic supports for the assay. The strips were inoculated and the results were read after 20 min. This method allowed 96.4% of the isolates to be confirmed within 30 min. The remaining isolates gave patterns similar to that observed with *C. sporogenes*. This shortened method looks promising but additional testing is needed for further development. Again, however, additional testing still must be performed to determine if the isolate is toxigenic.

Another method that looks promising but that is still in the developmental stage is the detection of toxigenic *C. difficile* using DNA probes specific for the toxin genes.

Wren et al. (163) used a 4.5-kb PstI fragment encoding a portion of the toxin A gene. This probe, which covered a portion of the repeating units of the gene, specifically hybridized with DNA from 58 toxigenic strains and did not hybridize with DNA from 17 nontoxigenic strains. The probe reacted with DNA from toxigenic strains of *C. sordellii* because of the similarity of toxin A with *C. sordellii* hemorrhage toxin (toxin HT).

In another study, Gumerlock et al. (164,165) used a set of primers to amplify a 399-bp fragment of the toxin B gene using polymerase chain reaction (PCR). They found that all 28 of the toxigenic strains were amplified with these primers and that DNA from *C. sordellii* and *C. bifermentans* were not amplified. They were able to detect the toxin B gene in as little as 1 pg of DNA from toxigenic strains. When applied to clinical specimens, 18 that were positive by tissue culture were positive by this method. In addition, 2 specimens that were negative by tissue culture but that were from patients who were suspected of having *C. difficile* disease were positive in the assay. This test was an improvement over their previous test based on a 16S rRNA PCR assay for *C. difficile* because it specifically detected toxigenic strains. Kato et al. (166,167) used primers to amplify a 252-bp DNA fragment of the toxin A gene. A probe based on the amplication product was specific for toxigenic *C. difficile* and did not react with DNA from nontoxigenic strains and with other enteropathogenic aerobes. However, when they applied the procedure in the analysis of stool specimens, they found that factors in the stools inhibited the PCR amplication step. This inhibitory activity was removed by ion exchange after phenol-chloroform extraction. Their results showed that 12 stools which were cytotoxic were positive by the PCR method, and 27 stools that were negative for cytotoxic activity were negative by PCR. Boondeekhun et al. (168) also used PCR primers to develop a 63-bp portion of the repeating units of the toxin A gene and found that their PCR method was more sensitive than culturing for the organism and showed a sensitivity comparable to that observed with the tissue culture test. These results using DNA probe methods are very encouraging but additional research and development is needed to further evaluate these methods for clinical testing. The need for DNA extraction or cleanup makes the current assays cumbersome and slow.

TREATMENT

Stopping the Inciting Agent

Most antibiotics and many anticancer agents have been implicated as initiators of *C. difficile* disease. In many instances, the disease may be self-limiting and the patient may respond simply by stopping the offending agent. This, of course, will depend on the condition of the patient. Supportive measures may be necessary to correct any fluid loss by the patient. If the patient has a mild form of the disease and is slowly improving, then additional therapy with vancomycin or metronidazole may not be necessary. In results noted by Dr. John Bartlett, 50 of 153

patients that had antibiotic-associated diarrhea or colitis and toxin in their stool specimens recovered without any additional therapy. Finegold and George (138) noted that if therapy is still needed for the initial infection, then switching to another antimicrobial agent that has less impact on the gut flora may be adequate. They also noted that on occasion it may be necessary to continue the initial offending agent and that it may be possible to begin vancomycin or metronidazole in addition to the offending agent. However, there has been little additional information in this area. Finegold and George (138) recommended that antiperistaltic drugs not be used, primarily because of increased exposure to toxin.

Antibiotic Therapy

The most common method of treating *C. difficile* disease is by oral administration of vancomycin or metronidazole. The most clinical experience has been reported with vancomycin (169–177). Other antibiotics have been used but not as commonly. Vancomycin kills the organism by inhibiting cell wall synthesis. The antibiotic exhibits a high affinity for precursors of the cell wall, possibly the D-alanylalanine portion. As a result, vancomycin is highly bactericidal for growing organisms. The drug does not kill spores and this is one reason why patients who respond favorably to vancomycin occasionally relapse.

Vancomycin is poorly absorbed in the intestinal tract. As a result, high concentrations are achieved in the intestine when it is administered orally, making the drug very effective at killing vegetative cells. The typical dose range is 125–500 mg every 6 hr. This range gives fecal levels in excess of 1 mg/mL and this is well above the normal minimal inhibitory concentration (MIC) value to *C. difficile*. Fekety et al. (178) compared two different dose regimens to determine if high doses (500 mg every 6 hr) are always warranted. In their study, they compared patients receiving 125 mg four times daily vs. those receiving 500 mg four times daily over a 10-day period. Their results showed the 125-mg dose to be adequate and concluded that unless the patient is critically ill, this dose should be used. This lower dosage also considerably lowers the cost of the treatment and this is an important consideration because of the high cost of the drug.

There have been several studies comparing two oral formulations for administering vancomycin (178–180). Vancomycin (vancomycin hydrochloride) typically is available in liquid form for oral administration. There also are capsules (Matrigel capsules) that were first introduced in 1985. The capsules combine the powdered drug with polyethylene glycol 6000, thus protecting it from environmental degradation. The capsule is slightly cheaper and does not have the bitter taste associated with liquid vancomycin. The capsules give similar fecal concentrations as the liquid. There is significant patient-to-patient variation in the concentrations achieved both with the liquid form and with the capsule. This variation also is noted with individual patients, presumably due to differences in the stool consistency and water content. Although the number of reported studies on the use of vancomycin capsules has been limited, the results show that the capsules have been as effective as the liquid form of vancomycin.

Metronidazole has selective toxicity for anaerobic and microaerophilic microorganisms and is highly active against *C. difficile* in vitro. This drug acts as an electron acceptor under certain conditions, leading to the development of biochemical lesions in the organism, resulting in cell death. There also is evidence that it interferes with or inhibits DNA synthesis in anaerobic bacteria. There have been some concerns about the use of metronidazole in the treatment of *C. difficile* disease because, unlike vancomycin, this drug is rapidly absorbed from the intestine and appropriate concentrations may not be achieved. However, in a study by Bolton and Culshaw (181), it was shown that fecal concentrations well exceeded the MICs of 0.25 μg to 1 μg/mL. Metronidazole is metabolized to hydroxymetronidazole in the body and this principle metabolite also is inhibitory, with MICs of 0.5–4 μg/mL. All nine patients in this study had effective antimicrobial concentrations of metronidazole, primarily during the acute phase of illness. These investigators noted also that the concentrations decreased during the recovery of the patient and this decrease was accompanied by a decrease in the mucosal inflammation and a return to normal stool consistency. Since this drug is destroyed inside the cells as it kills them, there appear to be lower amounts reaching the colon when the normal flora is present. There have been instances in which metronidazole has been administered intravenously with successful treatment of the patient, and it has been suggested that intravenous metronidazole may reduce complications that may develop in *C. difficile* disease (182,183). However, there are reports in which parenteral metronidazole as the initial treatment with this type of therapy was not successful (184), and parenteral administration of the drug is not considered the primary choice for treatment. The cost of metronidazole is considerably less than that of vancomycin and this is one reason for its extensive use. Many of the results on the use of metronidazole have been obtained with patients having mild or moderate disease and not severe pseudomembranous colitis, and it is very effective in patients who are not severely ill. However, in patients who have pseudomembranous colitis and/or those who are severely ill, oral vancomycin is still considered by some to be the drug of choice (176,185). A disadvantage that needs to be considered is the possible development of vancomycin-resistant enterococci. Both vancomycin and metronidazole are effective for the treatment of *C. difficile* disease in patients with AIDS (186).

There are some clinical data on the use of bacitracin for the treatment of *C. difficile* disease. In a study by Young et al. (187), bacitracin therapy was compared with vancomycin. For vancomycin treatment, patients were treated for 7 days with 125 mg administered orally every 6 hr. With bacitracin, 20,000 U was administered orally every 6 hr for 7 days. The symptoms were resolved in 16 patients (76%) treated with bacitracin compared with 18 patients (86%) receiving vancomycin. In another study (188), oral bacitracin vs. vancomycin was evaluated and it was concluded that oral bacitracin was as effective as vancomycin in resolving the clinical symptoms. In both studies, patients who received vancomycin had toxin-negative and culture-negative stools more frequently than did patients treated with bacitracin. Therefore, bacitracin is not as effective as vancomycin but it offers an alternative that is considerably less expensive. There are other disadvantages that should be considered. Isolates of *C. difficile* resistant to bacitracin have been reported, suggesting that the widespread use of this drug may lead to the development of resistant strains in hospitals. Bacitracin, like vancomycin and metronidazole, has a very disagreeable taste.

Teicoplanin, which is a relatively new glycopeptide antibiotic active in vitro against a wide spectrum of gram-positive aerobic and anaerobic organisms, has been evaluated in several studies. In one study (189), patients with PMC were given 200 mg teicoplanin orally on day 1 followed by 200 mg orally for the next 9 days. All of the patients were cured and only one still had the organism in their stool specimen after this treatment. In another study by de Lalla et al. (190), 47 patients with *C. difficile* disease were treated orally with either vancomycin or teicoplanin. In patients receiving vancomycin, 3 of 23 relapsed once the treatment stopped. In the group receiving teicoplanin, all of the patients remained asymptomatic after the treatment was completed and only one patient had *C. difficile* in their stool. These results are encouraging but additional randomized trials are needed to further examine the use of teicoplanin in the treatment of *C. difficile* disease. Fusidic acid, which is highly active against *C. difficile* in vitro, has been used as a treatment and has been given in doses of 0.5–1.5 g daily for 7–21 days (191). This drug is very cheap, but additional studies are needed to further examine its efficacy.

Anion Exchange Resins

The anion exchange resins cholestyramine and colestipol have been used with some success in treating *C. difficile* disease. Both are anion exchange resins that bind *C. difficile* toxin and other proteins (192). Both resins are available as a powder that must be mixed with water prior to ingestion. In a study by Bartlett (176), one packet containing 4 g of cholestyramine was administered orally on a daily basis and this dose was successful in treating some cases of *C. difficile* disease. However, Bartlett suggested that the resin may be most useful in treating patients that continue to relapse following therapy with vancomycin. Other studies (171,173) support the idea that these resins are not nearly effective as vancomycin or metronidazole but that they be used as alternative therapies when necessary, for example, in patients that continue to relapse. The basis for this approach is that the resin binds toxin and prevents any further tissue damage while the normal gut flora is being reestablished.

PROBIOTIC THERAPY

Treatment with *S. boulardii*

Saccharomyces boulardii is a nonpathogenic yeast that grows well at 37°C. It is used in Europe as a probiotic and is used to treat persons with gastrointestinal illness. The results of studies performed in several laboratories in the United States are encouraging for the use of the yeast as a treatment for *C. difficile* disease. The yeast is supplied as a lyophilized powder (Ultra-Levure) by Bio-Codex Laboratories (Montrouge, France) and is reconstituted with distilled water just before use. The yeast has been shown to prevent *C. difficile* in hamsters treated with clindamycin (193–195). Similar results were obtained in preventing the disease in gnotobiotic mice (196).

In a double-blind study performed at a hospital on the West Coast, a total of 180 patients were evaluated over a period of 23 months. In patients receiving a placebo, 31% developed diarrhea and were positive for *C. difficile*. In a second group receiving *S. boulardii* capsules (1 g of lyophilized organism per day), the incidence was 9.4%, suggesting that treatment with the yeast reduced the incidence of disease (197). In a follow-up case, a 67-year-old woman had recurrent diarrhea following various antibiotic regimens for *Campylobacter jejuni* enterocolitis (198). Of the eight episodes of recurrent diarrhea, five were associated with *C. difficile* toxin and a sixth was associated with the presence of the organism but no toxin. The patient received several regimens of vancomycin and metronidazole, and each time relapsed as the antibiotic therapy was completed. Prior to the last treatment with vancomycin, the patient began receiving *S. boulardii*. Two capsules (250 mg) were given to the patient daily and within a week, the diarrhea began to subside. The patient continued to receive *S. boulardii* over the following 2 months and had no recurrent bouts of diarrhea. These results are not clear-cut because of the involved treatment with vancomycin and because this was a single patient. However, taken together, the results suggest that probiotic therapy with this yeast may be useful in severe cases.

In another study, Buts et al. (199) administered 250-mg doses of *S. boulardii* two to four times daily to infants (median age 8 months) with persistent intestinal symptoms that appeared to be related to *C. difficile*. They noted that within 1 week the number of bowel movements decreased and the overall physical condition improved in 18 of 19 (95%) of the infants. In addition, within 15 days 85% of the infants no longer had detectable cytotoxic activity in their stool specimens and complete eradication of the organism was noted in 73% of the infants within 1 month. The yeast capsules currently are not available as approved for use in the United States and they were provided to scientists as investigational drugs for these studies.

Treatment with Lactobacillus

In a study reported by Gorbach et al. (200), five patients that continued to relapse following typical *C. difficile* therapy with antibiotics were given *Lactobacillus* GG, a human strain isolated by these scientists. The *Lactobacillus* was given in skim milk with a daily dose of 10^{10} over 7–10 days. Four of the patients gave an immediate response with negative or very low toxin titers in their stool specimens. The fifth patient responded initially but re-lapsed. However, a second regimen of metronidazole in this patient followed by *Lactobacillus* was successful.

Treatment with Fecal Enemas

Another alternative is the administration of nonpathogenic bacteria in patients who continue to relapse following vancomycin, metronidazole, or bacitracin. In a study by Wilson et al. (201), it was shown that the daily administration of cecal contents of healthy hamsters prevented the occurrence of *C. difficile* disease in hamsters. This is an important finding because these animals are very sensitive to *C. difficile*. It has been suggested that the administration of a single *C. difficile* cell to hamsters treated with clindamycin is sufficient to kill the animals. They develop acute fatal enterocolitis if treatment is not immediately initiated. Thus, methods or treatments that work in this animal model may be useful in treating humans with *C. difficile* disease.

Taking this approach, Bowden et al. (202) showed that human fecal enemas successfully treated 13 of 16 patients with PMC. In another study (203), two types of rectally instilled mixtures were evaluated in patients who did not respond to the normal treatment for *C. difficile*. In one part of the study, four patients received fecal enemas that consisted of 50 g of freshly passed stool from the patient's husband and child mixed in 500 mL saline. All four patients treated in this manner had normal bowel function within 24 hr coincident with the loss of *C. difficile* and toxin in the stool specimens. In the other part of the study, a bacterial mixture consisting of *S. faecalis*, *C. innocuum*, *C. ramosum*, *B. ovatus*, *B. vulgatus*, *B. thetaiotaomicron*, *E. coli*, *C. bifermentans*, and *P. productus* was rectally instilled into each of two patients. This approach was taken because previous studies showed that (a) *Bacteroides* species protected against invasive *E. coli*, (b) fatty acids from some anaerobes aided in reestablishing the colonic flora, and (c) *Bacteroides* species helped protect animals infected with *Salmonella* species (204). Both patients again had normal bowel movements within 24 hr and the level of *C. difficile* and toxin in the stool became negligible. Both patients remained healthy throughout the clinical follow-up over the following year. There are questions, however, on the selection of these 10 species out of the >400 species of bacteria in the human colon and it is unclear how this selective group provides protection. The instillation of fecal enemas as a method of treatment, which should be an excellent approach for reestablishing the normal flora, currently is not in use in the United States. There are considerable health risks such as the spread of other pathogens, and additional studies are needed for further evaluation.

In addition to these possibilities, there is some evidence from experimental animal studies that nontoxigenic strains may be protective. Clindamycin-treated hamsters that were administered nontoxigenic *C. difficile* prior to challenge with toxigenic *C. difficile* were protected (205). However, these studies have only been performed in animals and have not been attempted in humans.

Passive Immunotherapy

Antibodies against toxins A and B are protective against the disease because they neutralize the toxic activities. Experimental animals actively vaccinated against the toxins are completely protected against challenge with highly toxigenic strains of *C. difficile*. However, because the disease in humans is effectively treated with antibiotics, questions have been raised about the necessity of developing a parenteral vaccine for human use. An alternative possibility that is being examined is the passive immunization of humans by the oral administration of high-titered antibodies against the toxin and organism. In studies performed at the Anaerobe Laboratory at VPI & SU, we found that hamsters treated prophylactically with bovine colostral gamma globulin were protected against challenge with a toxigenic strain of the organism (206). Thus, the oral administration of antibodies, which has been used to protect against a variety of enteric pathogens, including bacteria and viruses, may be an effective treatment in *C. difficile* patients. Clinical trials are underway to further evaluate the efficacy of orally administered gamma globulin to patients with *C. difficile* disease. Patients who are at risk, including those undergoing prophylactic antibiotic therapy and/or those in endemic settings such as certain Veterans Administration hospitals, may benefit from the treatment. Other populations that may benefit would include patients who do not respond to other more commonly used treatments such as vancomycin or metronidazole and who continue to relapse from *C. difficile* disease.

PREVENTION

There are certain precautionary measures that should be implemented to minimize the spread of the disease. The use of vinyl disposable gloves, laboratory coats, and proper washing procedures is highly recommended (207–209). All items should be properly cleaned and disinfected. Rectal thermometers, for example, may represent a major fomite and the use of disposable thermometers has been reported to lower the incidence of the disease (210). Commodes and endoscopes, of course, must be cleaned properly. Isolation of the patient in single rooms with bathrooms is recommended, but this usually is not possible due to overcrowded conditions at most hospitals. Cleaning the rooms of *C. difficile* patients with disinfectants and sporicidal agents also may reduce the spread of the organism. In one study, aerosol application of phosphate-buffered hypochlorite (1600 ppm) reduced the number of *C. difficile* CFU by more than 98% in the room of a patient with antibiotic-associated colitis. The implementation of these measures, unfortunately, results in increased costs for patient care and this may limit the use of preventive measures at some facilities. It is very important that the health care worker be aware of how *C. difficile* is spread so that they can aid in minimizing transmission by using proper washing procedures. Gerding noted that soap and chlorhexidine worked equally well for this purpose. If possible, programs should be implemented to reduce the use of antibiotics, particularly clindamycin, ampicillin, and cephalosporins.

There is some question as to whether carriers should be treated prophylactically with antibiotics. The primary population would be the elderly who are at risk for the disease. Treatment of elderly asymptomatic carriers has been suggested but the results have been mixed. In one study, treatment with metronidazole along with limited antibiotic therapy and isolation of the patient did not lower the incidence of disease (82). In another study involving patients in a leukemia unit, treatment with vancomycin lowered the incidence (211). Currently, asymptomatic patients at medical facilities in this country usually are not sought or treated. An alternative to this approach may be to treat patients prophylactically with gamma globulin against *C. difficile*. The oral administration of antibodies against the organism may help eliminate the carrier status by lowering the number of organisms. However, clinical studies will be needed to investigate this possibility.

CONCLUSIONS

We now recognize *C. difficile* as a major nosocomial pathogen. It possibly is the primary cause of nosocomial diarrhea and it is important that precautionary measures are used to minimize the spread of the organism. These measures are especially important if a medical facility begins to see an increase in incidence of the disease. *C. difficile* will continue to be a major problem at medical facilities, and new ways of minimizing the spread of the organism and its disease in hospitals and long-term health care facilities will have to be developed. The new and improved typing methods will be very useful in studying the epidemiology of this disease and evaluating new methods of prevention. It is important that basic research at the molecular level continue on the toxins of *C. difficile* and new approaches for vaccines. These studies will lead to new and possibly better ways of treating patients, and give us a better understanding of this unusual pathogen and how it causes disease.

For additional information on *Clostridium difficile* and its toxins, the reader is referred to the chapter by Bartlett and to the following:

Levett PN. *Clostridium difficile* in habitats other than the human gastro-intestinal tract. *J Infect* 1986;12:253–263.
Rolfe RD, Finegold, SM, eds. Clostridium difficile: *its role in intestinal disease*. New York: Academic Press; 1988.

ACKNOWLEDGMENTS

The authors thank Dr. Lance Peterson and Dr. Lynn McFarland for supplying unpublished results. Some of the research on the molecular biology of toxins A and B of *Clostridium difficile* was supported by Public Health Service grant AI 15749 from the National Institute of Allergy and Infectious Diseases.

REFERENCES

1. Finney JMT. Gastro-enterostomy for cicatrizing ulcer of the pylorus. *Bull Johns Hopkins Hosp* 1893;4:53–55.
2. Hall JC, O'Toole E. Intestinal flora in new-born infants with a description of a new pathogenic anaerobe, *Bacillus difficilis*. *Am J Dis Child* 1935;49:390–402.
3. Bartlett JG. Introduction. In: Rolfe RE, Finegold SM, eds. *Clostridium difficile: its role in intestinal disease.* New York: Academic Press; 1988:1–13.
4. Tedesco FJ, Barton RW, Alpers DH. Clindamycin-associated colitis. *Ann Intern Med* 1974;81:429–433.
5. Larson HE, Parry JV, Price AB, Davies DR, Dolby J, Tyrrell DA. Undescribed toxin in pseudomembranous colitis. *Br Med J* 1977;1:1246–1248.
6. Rifkin GD, Fekety FR, Silva J, Sack RB. Antibiotic-induced colitis implication of a toxin neutralised by *Clostridium sordellii* antitoxin. *Lancet* 1977;2:1103–1106.
7. Bartlett JG, Gorbach SL. Pseudomembranous enterocolitis (antibiotic-related colitis). *Adv Intern Med* 1977;22:455–476.
8. Bartlett JG, Chang TW, Gurwith M, Gorbach SI, Onderdonk AB. Antibiotic-associated pseudomembranous colitis due to toxin-producing clostridia. *N Engl J Med* 1978;298(10):531–534.
9. Taylor NS, Thorne GM, Bartlett JG. Separation of an enterotoxin from the cytotoxin of *Clostridium difficile*. *Clin Res* 1980;28:285.
10. Clabots CR, Gerding SJ, Olson MM, Peterson LR, Gerding DN. Detection of asymptomatic *Clostridium difficile* carriage by an alcohol shock procedure. *J Clin Microbiol* 1989;27:2386–2387.
11. Kamiya S, Yamakawa K, Ogura H, Nakamura S. Recovery of spores of *Clostridium difficile* altered by heat or alkali. *J Med Microbiol* 1989;28:217–221.
12. Nakamura S, Yamakawa K, Izumi J, Nakashio S, Nishida S. Germinability and heat resistance of spores of *Clostridium difficile* strains. *Microbiol Immunol* 1985;29:113–118.
13. Riley TV, Brazier JS, Hassan H, Williams K, Phillips KD. Comparison of alcohol shock enrichment and selective enrichment for the isolation of *Clostridium difficile*. *Epidemiol Infect* 1987;99:355–359.
14. Wilson KH. Efficiency of various bile salt preparations for stimulation of *Clostridium difficile* spore germination. *J Clin Microbiol* 1983;18:1017–1019.
15. Wilson KH, Kennedy MJ, Fekety FR. Use of sodium taurocholate to enhance spore recovery on a medium selective for *Clostridium difficile*. *J Clin Microbiol* 1982;5:443–446.
16. Buggy BP, Wilson KH, Fekety R. Comparison of methods for recovery of *Clostridium difficile* from an environmental surface. *Clin Microbiol* 1983;18:348–352.
17. Davies HA, Borriello SP. Detection of capsule in strains of *Clostridium difficile* of varying virulence and toxigenicity. *Microb Pathog* 1990;9:141–146.
18. Strelau E, Wagner B, Wagner M, Karsch W. Demonstration of capsules on *Clostridium difficile*. *Zentral Bakteriol Hyg* 1989;270:456–461.
19. Baldassarri L, Donelli G, Cerquetti M, Mastrantonio P. Capsule-like structures in *Clostridium difficile* strains. *Microbiologica* 1991;14:295–300.
20. Borriello SP, Davies HA, Barclay FE. Detection of fimbriae amongst strains of *Clostridium difficile*. *FEMS Microbiol Lett* 1988;49:65–67.
21. Cerquetti M, Pantosti A, Stefanelli P, Mastrantonio P. Purification and characterization of an immunodominant 36 kDa antigen present on the cell surface of *Clostridium difficile*. *Microb Pathog* 1992;13:271–279.
22. Masuda K, Itoh M, Kawata T. Characterization and reassembly of a regular array in the cell wall of *Clostridium difficile* GAI 4131. *Microbiol Immunol* 1989;33:287–298.
23. Poxton IR, Byrne MD. Immunological analysis of the EDTA-soluble antigens of *Clostridium difficile* and related species. *J Gen Microbiol* 1981;122:41–46.
24. Poxton IR, Cartmill TDI. Immunochemistry of the cell-surface carbohydrate antigens of *Clostridium difficile*. *J Gen Microbiol* 1982;128:1365–1370.
25. Takumi K, Takeoka A, Kawata T. Purification and immunochemical properties of a wall protein antigen from *Clostridium difficile* ATCC 11011. *Microbiol Immunol* 1987;31:837–849.
26. Pantosti A, Cerquetti M, Viti F, Ortisi G, Mastrantonio P. Immunoblot analysis of serum immunoglobulin G response to surface proteins of *Clostridium difficile* in patients with antibiotic-associated diarrhoea. *J Clin Microbiol* 1989;27:2594–2597.
27. Pantosti A, Cerquetti M, Viti F, Ortisi G, Matrantonio P. Antibody response to *Clostridium difficile* determined by Western blot analysis. *Microecol Ther* 1989;18:303–309.
28. George WL, Sutter VL, Citron D, Finegold SM. Selective and differential medium for isolation of *Clostridium difficile*. *J Clin Microbiol* 1979;9:214–219.
29. Marler LM, Siders JA, Wolters LC, Pettigrew Y, Skitt GL, Allen SD. Comparison of five cultural procedures for isolation of *Clostridium difficile* from stools. *J Clin Microbiol* 1992;30:514–516.
30. Bartley SL, Dowell VR Jr. Comparison of media for the isolation of *Clostridium difficile* from fecal specimens. *Lab Med* 1991;22:335–338.
31. Levett PN. Effect of antibiotic concentration in a selective medium on the isolation of *Clostridium difficile* from faecal specimens. *J Clin Pathol* 1984;38:233–234.
32. Aspinall ST, Hutchinson DN. New selective medium for isolating *Clostridium difficile* from faeces. *J Clin Pathol* 1992;45:812–814.
33. Levett PN. Effect of basal medium upon fluorescence of *Clostridium difficile*. *Lett Appl Microbiol* 1985;1:75–76.
34. O'Farrell S, Wilks M, Nash JQ, Tabaqchali S. A selective enrichment broth for the isolation of *Clostridium difficile*. *J Clin Pathol* 1984;37:98–99.
35. Clabots CR, Bettin KM, Peterson LR, Gerding DN. Evaluation of cycloserine-cefoxitin-fructose agar and cycloserine-cefoxitin-fructose broth for recovery of *Clostridium difficile* from environmental sites. *J Clin Microbiol* 1991;29:2633–2635.
36. Johnson LL, McFarland LV, Dearing P, Raisys V, Schoenknecht FD. Identification of *Clostridium difficile* in stool specimens by culture-enhanced gas-liquid chromatography. *J Clin Microbiol* 1989;27:2218–2221.
37. D'Ari L, Barker HA. p-Cresol formation by cell-free extracts of *Clostridium difficile*. *Arch Microbiol* 1985;143:311–312.
38. Levett PN. Production of p-cresol by *Clostridium difficile* on different basal media. *Lett Appl Microbiol* 1987;5:71–73.
39. Sivsammye G, Sims HV. Presumptive identification of *Clostridium difficile* by detection of p-cresol in prepared peptone yeast glucose broth supplemented with p-hydroxyphenylacetic acid. *J Clin Microbiol* 1990;28:1851–1853.
40. Phillips KD, Rogers PA. Rapid detection and presumptive identification of *Clostridium difficile* by p-cresol production on a selective medium. *J Clin Pathol* 1981;34:642–644.
41. Borriello SP, Wren BW, Hyde S, et al. Molecular, immunological, and biological characterization of a toxin A-negative, toxin B-positive strain of *Clostridium difficile*. *Infect Immun* 1992;60:4192–4199.
42. Torres JF. Purification and characterization of toxin B from a strain of *Clostridium difficile* that does not produce toxin A. *J Med Microbiol* 1991;35:40–44.
43. Lyerly DM, Barroso LA, Wilkins TD, Depitre C, Corthier G. Characterization of a toxin A–negative, toxin B-positive strain of *Clostridium difficile*. *Infect Immun* 1992;60:4633–4639.
44. Sullivan NM, Pellett S, Wilkins TD. Purification and characterization of toxins A and B of *Clostridium difficile*. *Infect Immun* 1982;35:1032–1040.
45. Sterne M, Wentzel LM. A new method for the large-scale production of high-titre botulinum formol-toxoid types C and D. *J Immunol* 1950;65:175–183.
46. Nakamura S, Mikawa M, Tanabe N, Yamakawa K, Nishida S. Effect of clindamycin on cytotoxin production by *Clostridium difficile*. *Microbiol Immunol* 1982;26:985–992.
47. Clabots CR, Shanholtzer CJ, Peterson LR, Gerding DN. In vitro activity of efrotomycin, ciprofloxacin, and six other anti-

microbials against *Clostridium difficile. Diag Microbiol Infect Dis* 1987;6:49–52.

48. Dzink J, Bartlett JG. In vitro susceptibility of *Clostridium difficile* isolates from patients with antibiotic-associated diarrhoea or colitis. *Antimicrob Agents Chemother* 1980;17:695–698.

49. Levett PN. Antimicrobial susceptibility of *Clostridium difficile* determined by disc diffusion and breakpoint methods. *J Antimicrob Chemother* 1988;22:167–173.

50. Nakamura S, Nakashio S, Mikawa M, Yamakawa K, Okumura S, Nishida S. Antimicrobial susceptibility of *Clostridium difficile* from different sources. *Microbiol Immunol* 1982;26:25–30.

51. George WL, Kirby BD, Sutter VL, Finegold SM. Antimicrobial susceptibility of *Clostridium difficile. Am Soc Microbiol* 1979.

52. Hachler H, Berger-Bachi B, Kayser FH. Genetic characterization of a *Clostridium difficile* erythromycin-clindamycin resistance determinant that is transferable to *Staphylococcus aureus. Antimicrob Agents Chemother* 1987;31:1039–1045.

53. Hachler H, Kayser FH, Berger-Bachi B. Homology of a transferable tetracycline resistance determinant of *Clostridium difficile* with *Streptococcus (Enterococcus) faecalis* transposon Tn916. *Antimicrob Agents Chemother* 1987;31:1033–1038.

54. Ionesco H. Transfert de la resistance a la tetracycline chez *Clostridium difficile. Ann Microbiol* 1980;131:171–179.

55. Smith CJ, Markowitz SM, Macrina FL. Transferable tetracycline resistance in *Clostridium difficile. Antimicrob Agents Chemother* 1981;19:997–1003.

56. Wust J, Hardegger U. Transferable resistance to clindamycin, erythromycin, and tetracycline in *Clostridium difficile. Antimicrob Agents Chemother* 1983;23:784–786.

57. Wust J, Sullivan NM, Hardegger U, Wilkins TD. Investigation of an outbreak of antibiotic-associated colitis by various typing methods. *J Clin Microbiol* 1982;16:1096–1101.

58. Wren BW, Mullany P, Clayton C, Tabaqchali S. Molecular cloning and genetic analysis of a chloramphenicol acetyltransferase determinant from *Clostridium difficile. Antimicrob Agents Chemother* 1988;32:1213–1217.

59. Pierce PF, Wilson R, Silva J. Antibiotic-associated pseudomembranous colitis; an epidemic investigation of a cluster of cases. *J Infect Dis* 1982;145:269–274.

60. Rolfe RD, Helebian S, Finegold SM. Bacterial interference between *Clostridium difficile* and normal fecal flora. *J Infect Dis* 1981;143:470–475.

61. Malamou-Ladas H, Tabaqchali S. Inhibition of *Clostridium difficile* by faecal streptococci. *J Med Microbiol* 1980;15:569–574.

62. Rolfe RD. Role of volatile fatty acids in colonization resistance to *Clostridium difficile. Infect Immun* 1984;45:185–191.

63. Kaatz GW, Gitlin SD, Schaberg DR, et al. Acquisition of *Clostridium difficile* from the hospital environment. *Am J Epidemiol* 1988;127:1289–1294.

64. Delmee M, Avesani V. Correlation between serogroup and susceptibility to chloramphenicol, clindamycin, erythromycin, rifampicin and tetracycline among 308 isolates of *Clostridium difficile. J Antimicrob Chemother* 1988;22:325–331.

65. Delmee M, Verellen G, Avesani V, Francois G. *Clostridium difficile* in neonates: serogrouping and epidemiology. *Eur J Pediatr* 1988;147:36–40.

66. Bacon AE, Fekety R, Schaberg DR, Faix RG. Epidemiology of *Clostridium difficile* colonization in newborns: results using a bacteriophage and bacteriocin typing system. *J Infect Dis* 1988;158:349–354.

67. Devlin HR, Au W, Foux L, Bradburg WC. Restriction endonuclease analysis of nosocomial isolates of *Clostridium difficile. J Clin Microbiol* 1987;25:2168–2172.

68. Heard SR, Rasurn B, Matthews RC, Tabaqchali S. Immunoblotting to demonstrate antigenic and immunogenic differences among nine standard strains of *Clostridium difficile. J Clin Microbiol* 1986;24:384–387.

69. Kato H, Cavalloaro JJ, Kato N, et al. Typing of *Clostridium difficile* by western immunoblotting with 10 different antisera. *J Clin Microbiol* 1993;31:413–415.

70. Mahony DE, Clow J, Atkinson L, Vakharia N, Schlech WF. Development and application of a multiple typing system for *Clostridium difficile. Appl Environ Microbiol* 1991;57:1873–1879.

71. Mulligan ME, Peterson LR, Kwok RYY, Clabots CR, Gerding DN. Immunoblots and plasmid fingerprints compared with serotyping and polyacrylamide gel electrophoresis for typing *Clostridium difficile. J Clin Microbiol* 1988;26:41–46.

72. Pantosti A, Cerquetti M, Gianfrilli PM. Electrophoretic characterization of *Clostridium difficile* strains isolated from antibiotic-associated colitis and other conditions. *J Clin Microbiol* 1988;26:540–543.

73. Sell TL, Schaberg DR, Fekety FR. Bacteriophage and bacteriocin typing scheme for *Clostridium difficile. J Clin Microbiol* 1983;17:1148–1152.

74. Tabaqchali S, O'Farrell S, Holland D, Silman R. Method for the typing of *Clostridium difficile* based on polyacrylamide gel electrophoresis of [35S]methionine-labeled proteins. *J Clin Microbiol* 1986;23:197–198.

75. Guinet RM, Marlier H, de Barbeyrac G, Sabbagh I. *Clostridium difficile* electrophoretic typing. *FEMS Microbiol Lett* 1989;50:289–293.

76. Toma S, Lesiak G, Magus M, Lo H-L, Delmee M. Serotyping of *Clostridium difficile. J Clin Microbiol* 1988;26:426–428.

77. Wren BW, Tabaqchali S. Restriction endonuclease DNA analysis of *Clostridium difficile. J Clin Microbiol* 1987;25:2402–2404.

78. McFarland LV, Mulligan ME, Kwok RYY, Stamm WE. Nosocomial acquisition of *Clostridium difficile* infection. *N Engl J Med* 1989;320:204–210.

79. McFarland LV, Surawicz CM, Stamm WE. Risk factors for *Clostridium difficile* carriage and *C. difficile*—associated diarrhea in a cohort of hospitalized patients. *J Infect Dis* 1990;162:678–684.

80. Strimling MO, Sacho H, Berkowitz I. *Clostridium difficile* infection in health-care workers. *Lancet* 1989;1:866–867.

81. Delmee M. *Clostridium difficile* infection in health-care workers. *Lancet* 1989;2:1095.

82. Bender BS, Laughon BE, Gaydos C, et al. Is *Clostridium difficile* endemic in chronic-care facilities? *Lancet* 1986;1:11–13.

83. Monsieur I, Mets T., Lawers S, DeBock S, Delmee M. *Clostridium difficile* infection in a geriatric ward. *Arch Gerontol Geriatr* 1991;13:255–262.

84. Farber BR, Brennen C, Puntereri AJ, Brody JP. A prospective study of nosocomial infections in a chronic care facility. *J Am Geriatr Soc* 1984;32(7):499–502.

85. Borriello SP, Barclay FE. Protection of hamsters against *Clostridium difficile* ileocaecitis by prior colonisation with non-pathogenic strains. *J Med Microbiol* 1985;19:339–350.

86. Depitre C, Delmee M, Avesani V, L'Haridon R, Roels A, Popoff M, Corthier G. Serogroup F strains of *Clostridium difficile* produce toxin B but not toxin A. *J Med Microbiol* 1993;38:434–441.

87. Wu TC, McCarthy VP, Gill VJ. Isolation rate and toxigenic potential of *Clostridium difficile* isolates from patients with cystic fibrosis. *J Infect Dis* 1983;148:176.

88. Barbut F, Depitre C, Delmee M, Corthier G, Petit JC. Comparison of enterotoxin production, cytotoxin production, serogrouping, and antimicrobial susceptibilities of *Clostridium difficile* strains isolated from AIDS and human immunodeficiency virus-negative patients. *J Clin Microbiol* 1993;31:740–742.

89. Justus PG, Martin JL, Goldberg DA, Taylor NS, Bartlett JG, Alexander RW, Mathias JR. Myoelectric effects of *Clostridium difficile*: motility-altering factors distinct from its cytotoxin and enterotoxin in rabbits. *Gastroenterology* 1982;83:836–843.

90. Giuliano M, Piemonte F, Gianfrilli PM. Production of an enterotoxin different from toxin A by *Clostridium difficile. FEMS Microbiol Lett* 1988;50:191–194.

91. Lyerly DM, Carrig PE, Wilkins TD. Nonspecific binding of mouse monoclonal antibodies to *Clostridium difficile* toxins A and B. *Curr Microbiol* 1989;19:303–306.

92. Arnon SS, Mills DC, Day PA, Henrickson RV, Sullivan NM, Wilkins TD. Rapid death of infant rhesus monkeys injected with *Clostridium difficile* toxins A and B: physiologic and pathologic basis. *J Pediatr* 1984;101:34–40.

93. Lima AAM, Lyerly DM, Wilkins TD, Innes DJ, Guerrant RL. Effects of *Clostridium difficile* toxins A and B in rabbit small and large intestine in vivo and on cultured cells *in vitro. Infect Immun* 1988;56:582–588.

94. Rybolt AH, Laughon BE, Greenough WB III, Bennett RG, Thomas DR, Bartlett JG. Protein-losing enteropathy associated with *Clostridium difficile* infection. *Lancet* 1989;1:1353–1355.

95. Lyerly DM, Saum KE, MacDonald D, Wilkins TD. Effect of toxins A and B given intragastrically to animals. *Infect Immun* 1985;47:349–352.

96. Gurwith MJ, Langston C, Citron DM. Toxin-producing bacteria in infants. Lack of an association with sudden infant death syndrome. *Am J Dis Child* 1981;135:1104–1106.

97. Cooperstock MS, Steffen E, Yolken R, Onderdonk A. *Clostridium difficile* in normal infants and sudden infant death syndrome: an association with infant formula feeding. *Pediatrics* 1982;70:91–95.

98. Krivan HC, Clark GF, Smith DF, Wilkins TD. Cell surface binding site for *Clostridium difficile* enterotoxin: evidence for a glycoconjugate containing the sequence Galα1-3Galβ1-4GlcNAc. *Infect Immun* 1986;53:573–581.

99. Krivan HC, Wilkins TD. Purification of *Clostridium difficile* toxin A by affinity chromatography on immobilized thyroglobulin. *Infect Immun* 1987;55:1873–1877.

100. Barroso LA, Wang SZ, Phelps CJ, Johnson JL, Wilkins TD. Nucleotide sequence of *Clostridium difficile* toxin B gene. *Nucleic Acids Res* 1990;18:4004.

101. Dove CH, Wang SZ, Price SB, Phelps CJ, Lyerly DM, Wilkins TD, Johnson JL. Molecular characterization of the *Clostridium difficile* toxin A gene. *Infect Immun* 1990;58:480–488.

102. Eichel-Streiber C von, Laufenberg-Feldmann R, Sartingen S, Schulze J, Sauerborn M. Comparative sequence analysis of the *Clostridium difficile* toxins A and B. *Mol Gen Genet* 1992;233:260–268.

103. Meng XQ, Kamiya S, Yamakawa K, Ogura H, Nakamura S. Purification and characterisation of intracellular toxin A of *Clostridium difficile*. *J Med Microbiol* 1993;38:69–73.

104. Libby JM, Wilkins TD. Production of antitoxins to two toxins of *Clostridium difficile* and immunological comparison of the toxins by cross-neutralization studies. *Infect Immun* 1982;35:374–376.

105. Lyerly DM, Roberts MD, Phelps CJ, Wilkins TD. Properties of toxins A and B of *Clostridium difficile*. *FEMS Microbiol Lett* 1986;33:31–35.

106. Price SB, Phelps CJ, Wilkins TD, Johnson JL. Cloning of the carbohydrate-binding portion of the toxin A gene of *Clostridium difficile*. *Curr Microbiol* 1987;16:55–60.

107. Eichel-Streiber C von, Sauerborn M. *Clostridium difficile* toxin A carries a C-terminal repetitive structure homologous to the carbohydrate binding region of streptococcal glycosyltransferases. *Gene* 1990;96:107–113.

108. Eichel-Streiber C von, Sauerborn M, Kuramitsu HK. Evidence for a modular structure of the homologous repetitive C-terminal carbohydrate-binding sites of *Clostridium difficile* toxins and *Streptococcus mutans* glucosyltransferases. *J Bacteriol* 1992;174:6707–6710.

109. Lyerly DM, Johnson JL, Wilkins TD. Characterization of the binding portion of *Clostridium difficile* toxin A. *Microecol Ther* 1989;19:233–237.

110. Wren BW, Clayton CL, Mullany PP, Tabaqchali S. Molecular cloning and expressing of *Clostridium difficile* toxin A in *Escherichia coli* K12. *FEB* 1987;225:82–86.

111. Frey SM, Wilkins TD. Localization of two epitopes recognized by monoclonal antibody PCG-4 on *Clostridium difficile* toxin A. *Infect Immun* 1992;60:2488–2492.

112. Tucker KD, Carrig PE, Wilkins TD. Toxin A of *Clostridium difficile* is a potent cytotoxin. *J Clin Microbiol* 1990;28:869–871.

113. Wilkins TD, Tucker KD. *Clostridium difficile* toxin A (enterotoxin) uses Galα1-3Galβ1-4GlcNAc as a functional receptor. *Microecol Ther* 1989;19:225–227.

114. Tucker KD, Wilkins TD. Toxin A of *Clostridium difficile* binds to the human carbohydrate antigens I, X, and Y. *Infect Immun* 1991;59:73–78.

115. Eglow R, Pothoulakis C, Itzkowitz S, et al. Diminished *Clostridium difficile* toxin A sensitivity in newborn rabbit ileum is associated with decreased toxin A receptor. *J Clin Invest* 1992;90:822–829.

116. Phelps CJ, Lyerly DM, Johnson JL, Wilkins TD. Construction and expression of the complete *Clostridium difficile* toxin A gene in *Escherichia coli*. *Infect Immun* 1991;59:150–153.

117. Fluit AC, Wolfhagen MJHM, Verdonk GPHT, Jansze M, Torensma R, Verhoef J. Nontoxigenic strains of *Clostridium difficile* lack the genes for both toxin A and toxin B. *J Clin Microbiol* 1991;29:2666–2667.

118. Lyerly DM, Sullivan NM, Wilkins TD. Enzyme-linked immunosorbent assay for *Clostridium difficile* toxin A. *J Clin Microbiol* 1983;17:72–78.

119. Kushnaryov VM, Sedmak JJ, Lyerly DM, Wilkins TD. Reversibility of action of *Clostridium difficile* toxin A on CHO cells and intermediate filaments in nuclei. In: *Proc 46th Annu Meet Electron Microscopy Soc Am*. 1988:134–135.

120. Ball D, Van Tassell R, Roberts MD, Hahn P, Lyerly DM, Wilkins TD. Purification and characterization of the alpha-toxin of *Clostridium novyi*. *Infect Immun* 1993;61:2912–2918.

121. Fluit AC, Wolfhage MJHM, Jansze M, Torensma R, Verhoef J. Comment to Knoop et al. (1990) FEBS Letters 267, 9–12, toxin B of *Clostridium difficile* does not have enolase activity. *FEBS Lett* 1993;316:103–104.

122. Lima AAM, Innes DJ Jr, Chadee K, Lyerly DM, Wilkins TD, Guerrant RL. *Clostridium difficile* toxin A. Interactions with mucus and early sequential histopathologic effects in rabbit small intestine. *Lab Invest* 1989;61:419–425.

123. Triadafilopoulos G, Pothoulakis C, O'Brien MJ, LaMont JT. Differential effects of *Clostridium difficile* toxins A and B on rabbit ileum. *Gastroenterology* 1987;93:273–279.

124. Triadafilopoulos G, Pothoulakis C, Weiss R, Giampaolo C, LaMont JT. Comparative study of *Clostridium difficile* toxin A and cholera toxin in rabbit ileum. *Gastroenterology* 1989;97:1186–1192.

125. Pothoulakis H, Sullivan R, Melnick D, et al. *Clostridium difficile* toxin A stimulates intracellular calcium release and chemotactic response in human granulocytes. *J Clin Invest* 1988;81:1741–1745.

126. Aronsson B, Granstrom M, Mollby R, Nord CE. Serum antibody response to *Clostridium difficile* toxins in patients with *Clostridium difficile* diarrhoea. *Infection* 1985;13:97–101.

127. Bacon AE, Lyerly DM, Wilkins TD, Fekety R. Immunoglobulin G (IgG) against toxins A and B of *Clostridium difficile* in sera from the general population and patients with colitis. In: *Proc Annu Meet Am Soc Microbiol*. 1987.

128. Viscidi R, Laughon BE, Yolken R, et al. Serum antibody response to toxins A and B of *Clostridium difficile*. *J Infect Dis* 1983;148:93–100.

129. Johnson S, Gerding DN, Janoff EN. Systemic and mucosal antibody responses to toxin A in patients infected with *Clostridium difficile*. *J Infect Dis* 1992;166:1287–1294.

130. Gerding D, Brazier JS. Optimal methods for identifying *Clostridium difficile* infections. *Clin Infect Dis* 1993;16:S439–S442.

131. Peterson LR, Holter JJ, Shanholtzer CJ, Garrett CR, Gerding DN. Detection of *Clostridium difficile* toxins A (enterotoxin) and B (cytotoxin) in clinical specimens. *Am J Clin Pathol* 1986;86:208–211.

132. Peterson LR, Kelly PJ. The role of the clinical microbiology laboratory in the management of *Clostridium difficile*–associated diarrhea; submitted.

133. Bartlett JG. *Infect Dis Clin Pract* 1992;1:254–259.

134. Guerrant RL, Araujo V, Soares E, et al. Measurement of fecal lactoferrin as a marker of fecal leukocytes. *J Clin Microbiol* 1992;30:1238–1242.

135. Marx CE, Morris A, Wilson ML, Reller LB. Fecal leukocytes in stool specimens submitted for *Clostridium difficile* toxin assay. *Diagn Microbiol Infect Dis* 1993;16:313–315.

136. Pesce CM, Colacino R, Martelli M. Autopsy study of pseudomembranous colitis. Characteristics of the affected population and antibiotic involved. *Acta Gastroenterology* 1984;47:58–63.

137. LaMont JT. *Clostridium difficile* enterocolitis. In: Yamada T, Alpers DH, Owyang C, Powell DW, Silverstein FE, eds. *Textbook of gastroenterology*. New York: JB Lippincott, 1991:1756–1762.

138. Finegold SM, George WL. Therapy directed against *Clostridium difficile* and its toxins: complications of therapy. In: Rolfe

RD, Finegold SM, eds. *Clostridium difficile: its role in intestinal disease.* New York: Academic Press; 1988:342–357.

139. Bartlett JG. Treatment of *Clostridium difficile* colitis. *Gastroenterology* 1985;89:1192–1195.

140. Meyers S, Mayer L, Bottone E, Desmond E, Janowitz HD. Occurrence of *Clostridium difficile* toxin during the course of inflammatory bowel disease. *Gastroenterology* 1980;80:697–700.

141. LaMont JT, Trnka YM. Therapeutic implications of *Clostridium difficile* toxin during relapse of chronic inflammatory bowel disease. *Lancet* 1980;1:381–383.

142. Greenfield C, Aguilar Ramirez JR, Pounder RE, et al. *Clostridium difficile* and inflammatory bowel disease. *Gut* 1983;24:713–717.

143. Bolton RP, Sheriff RJ, Read AE. *Clostridium difficile* associated diarrhoea: a role in inflammatory bowel disease. *Lancet* 1980;1:383–384.

144. Keighley MRB, Youngs D, Johnson M, Allan RN, Burdon DW. *Clostridium difficile* toxin in acute diarrhoea complicating inflammatory bowel disease. *Gut* 1982;23:410–414.

145. Herman BE, Vargo J, Phillips WS, Sweeney WB, Volpe RJ. Antibiotic-associated fulminant pseudomembranous colitis without toxic megacolon. *Am J Gastroenterol* 1992;87:1816–1819.

146. Cone JB, Wetzel W. Toxic megacolon secondary to pseudomembranous colitis. *Dis Col Rectum* 1982;25:478–482.

147. Cummings JA, McCann BG, Ralphs DN. Fulminant pseudomembranous colitis with left hemicolon and rectal sparing. *Br J Surg* 1988;75:341.

148. Templeton JL. Toxic megacolon complicating pseudomembranous colitis. *Br J Surg* 1983;70:48.

149. Lyerly DM, Barroso LA, Wilkins TD. Identification of the latex-reactive protein of *Clostridium difficile* as glutamate dehydrogenase. *J Clin Microbiol* 1991;29:2639–2642.

150. Lyerly DM, Wilkins TD. Commercial latex test for *Clostridium difficile* toxin A does not detect toxin A. *J Clin Microbiol* 1986;23:622–623.

151. Kraft JA, Bechard RT, Rogers RK, Yi A, Willis DH. A rapid test for *C. difficile*. *Am Clin Lab* 1993;July:28–29.

152. Gianfrilli P, Pantosti A, Luzzi I. Evaluation of gas-liquid chromatography for the rapid diagnosis of *Clostridium difficile* associated disease. *J Clin Pathol* 1985;38:690–693.

153. Johnson LL, McFarland LV, Dearing P, Raisys V, Schoenknecht FD. Identification of *Clostridium difficile* in stool specimens by culture-enhanced gas-liquid chromatography. *J Clin Microbiol* 1989;27:2218–2221.

154. Levett PN. Detection of *Clostridium difficile* in faeces by direct gas liquid chromatography. *J Clin Pathol* 1984;37:117–119.

155. Levett PN, Phillips KD. Gas chromatographic identification of *Clostridium difficile* and detection of cytotoxin from a modified selective medium. *J Clin Pathol* 1985;38:82–85.

156. Makin T. Rapid identification of *Clostridium difficile* by direct detection of volatile organic acids from primary isolation media. *J Clin Pathol* 1984;37:711–712.

157. Pepersack F, Labbe M, Nonhoff C, Schoutens E. Use of gas-liquid chromatography as a screening test for toxigenic *Clostridium difficile* in diarrhoeal stools. *J Clin Pathol* 1983;36:1233–1236.

158. Bate G. Comparison of Minitek Anaerobe IIR, API An-IdentR, and RapID ANAR Systems for the identification of *Clostridium difficile*. *Am J Clin Pathol* 1986;85:716–718.

159. Head CB, Ratnam S. Comparison of API ZYM system with API AN-Ident, API 20A, Minitek Anaerobe II, and RapID-ANA systems for identification of *Clostridium difficile*. *J Clin Microbiol* 1988;26:144–146.

160. Levett PN. Identification of *Clostridium difficile* using the API ZYM system. *Eur J Clin Microbiol* 1985;4:505–507.

161. Peiffer S, Cox M. Enzymatic reactions of *Clostridium difficile* in aerobic and anaerobic environments with the RapID-ANA II identification system. *J Clin Microbiol* 1993;31:279–282.

162. Aspinall ST, Dealler SF. New rapid identification test for *Clostridium difficile*. *J Clin Pathol* 1992;45:956–958.

163. Wren BW, Clayton CL, Castledine NB, Tabaqchali S. Identification of toxigenic *Clostridium difficile* strains by using a toxin A gene-specific probe. *J Clin Microbiol* 1990;28:1808–1812.

164. Gumerlock PH, Tang YJ, Meyers FJ, Silva J Jr. Use of the polymerase chain reaction for the specific and direct detection of *Clostridium difficile* in human feces. *Rev Infect Dis* 1991;13:1053–1060.

165. Gumerlock PH, Tang YJ, Weiss JB, Silva J Jr. Specific detection of toxigenic strains of *Clostridium difficile* in stool specimens. *J Clin Microbiol* 1993;31:507–511.

166. Kato N, Ou CY, Kato H, et al. Identification of toxigenic *Clostridium difficile* by the polymerase chain reaction. *J Clin Microbiol* 1991;29:33–37.

167. Kato N, Ou CY, Kato H, et al. Detection of toxigenic *Clostridium difficile* in stool specimens by the polymerase chain reaction. *J Infect Dis* 1993;167:455–458.

168. Boondeekhun HS, Gurtler V, Odd ML, Wilson VA, Mayall BC. Detection of *Clostridium difficile* enterotoxin gene in clinical specimens by the polymerase chain reaction. *J Med Microbiol* 1993;38:384–387.

169. Batts DH, Martin D, Holmes R, Silva J Jr, Fekety FR. Treatment of antibiotic-associated *Clostridium difficile* diarrhea with oral vancomycin. *J Pediatr* 1980;97:151–153.

170. George WL, Rolfe RD, Finegold SM. Treatment and prevention of antimicrobial agent–induced colitis and diarrhea. *Gastroenterology* 1980;79:366–372.

171. Keighley MRB. Antibiotic-associated pseudomembranous colitis: pathogenesis and management. *Drugs* 1980;20:49–56.

172. Aronsson B, Mollby R, Nord CE. Antimicrobial agents and *Clostridium difficile* in acute enteric disease: epidemiological data from Sweden, 1980–1982. *J Infect Dis* 1985;151:476–481.

173. Tedesco FJ. Pseudomembranous colitis: pathogenesis and therapy. *Med Clin North Am* 1982;66:655–664.

174. Burdon DW. Treatment of pseudomembranous colitis and antibiotic-associated diarrheoa. *J Antimicrob Chemother* 1984;14:103–109.

175. Tedesco F, Markham R, Gurwith M, Christie D, Bartlett JG. Oral vancomycin for antibiotic-associated pseudomembranous colitis. *Lancet* 1987;2:226–228.

176. Bartlett JG. Treatment of antibiotic-associated pseudomembranous colitis. *Rev Infect Dis* 1984;6:S235–S241.

177. Teasley DG, Gerding DN, Olson MM, et al. Prospective randomised trial of metronidazole versus vancomycin for *Clostridium difficile*–associated diarrhoea and colitis. *Lancet* 1983;2:1043–1046.

178. Fekety R, Silva J, Kauffman C, Buggy B, Deery HG. Treatment of antibiotic-associated *Clostridium difficile* colitis with oral vancomycin: comparison of two dosage regimens. *Am J Med* 1989;86:15–19.

179. Baird DR. Comparison of two oral formulations of vancomycin for treatment of diarrhoea associated with *Clostridium difficile*. *J Antimicrob Chemother* 1989;23:167–169.

180. Lucas RA, Bowtle WJ, Ryden R. Disposition of vancomycin in healthy volunteers from oral solution and semi-solid matrix capsules. *J Clin Pharmacol Ther* 1987;12:27–31.

181. Bolton RP, Culshaw MA. Faecal metronidazole concentrations during oral and intravenous therapy for antibiotic colitis due to *Clostridium difficile*. *Gut* 1986;27:1169–1172.

182. Kleinfeld DI, Sharpe RJ, Donta ST. Parenteral therapy for antibiotic-associated pseudomembranous colitis. *J Infect Dis* 1988;157:389.

183. Johnson S, Peterson LR, Gerding DN. Intravenous metronidazole and *Clostridium difficile*–associated diarrhea or colitis. *J Infect Dis* 1989;160:1087.

184. Guzman R, Kirkpatrick J, Forward K, Lim F. Failure of parenteral metronidazole in the treatment of pseudomembranous colitis. *J Infect Dis* 1988;158:1146.

185. Caputo GM, Weitekamp MR. The treatment of *Clostridium difficile* colitis. *JAMA* 1993;269:1088.

186. Cozart JC, Kalangi SS, Clench MH, et al. *Clostridium difficile* diarrhea in patients with AIDS versus non-AIDS controls. *J Clin Gastroenterol* 1993;16(3):192–194.

187. Young GP, Ward PB, Bayley N, et al. Antibiotic-associated colitis due to *Clostridium difficile*: double-blind comparison of vancomycin with bacitracin. *Gastroenterology* 1985;89:1038–1045.

188. Dudley MN, McLaughlin JC, Carrington G, Frick J, Nightingale CH, Quintiliani R. Oral bacitracin vs vancomycin therapy for *Clostridium difficile*–induced diarrhea. *Arch Intern Med* 1986;146:1101–1104.

189. de Lalla F, Privitera G, Rinaldi E, Ortisi G, Santoro D, Rizzardini G. Treatment of *Clostridium difficile*–associated disease with teicoplanin. *Antimicrob Agents Chemother* 1989;33:1125–1127.

190. de Lalla F, Santoro D, Rinaldi E, et al. Teicoplanin in the treatment of infections by staphylococci, *Clostridium difficile* and other gram-positive bacteria. *J Antimicrob Chemother* 1989;23:131–142.

191. Cronberg S, Castor B, Thoren A. Fusidic acid for the treatment of antibiotic associated colitis induced by *Clostridium difficile*. *Infection* 1984;12:276–279.

192. Taylor NS, Bartlett JG. Binding of *Clostridium difficile* cytotoxin and vancomycin by anion-exchange resins. *J Infect Dis* 1980;141:92–97.

193. Massot J, Sanchez O, Couchy R, Astoin J, Parodi AL. Bacteriopharmacological activity of *Saccharomyces boulardii* in clindamycin induced colitis in the hamster. *Arzneimittelforschung* 1984;34:794–797.

194. Elmer GW, McFarland LV. *Saccharomyces boulardii* suppression of overgrowth of toxigenic *Clostridium difficile* following vancomycin treatment in the hamster. *Antimicrob Agents Chemother* 1987;31:129–131.

195. Toothaker RD, Elmer GW. Prevention of clindamycin-induced mortality in hamsters by *Saccharomyces boulardii*. *Antimicrob Agents Chemother* 1984;26:552–556.

196. Corthier G, Dubos F, Ducluzeau R. Prevention of *C. difficile* induced mortality in gnotobiotic mice by *Saccharomyces boulardii*. *Can J Microbiol* 1986;32:894–896.

197. Surawicz CM, Elmer GW, Speelman P, McFarland LV, Chinn J, van Belle G. Prevention of antibiotic-associated diarrhea by *Saccharomyces boulardii*: a prospective study. *Gastroenterology* 1989;96:981–988.

198. Kimmey MB, Elmer GW, Surawicz CM, McFarland LV. Prevention of further recurrences of *Clostridium difficile* colitis with *Saccharomyces boulardii*. *Dig Dis Sci* 1990;35:897–901.

199. Buts J-P, Corthier G, Delmee M. *Saccharomyces boulardii* for *Clostridium difficile*–associated enteropathies in infants. *J Pediatr Gastroenterol Nutr* 1993;16:419–425.

200. Gorbach SL, Chang T-W, Goldin B. Successful treatment of relapsing *Clostridium difficile* colitis with *Lactobacillus* GG. *Lancet* 1987;1:1519.

201. Wilson KH. Bacteriotherapy for *Clostridium difficile* colitis. *Lancet* 1989;1:1096.

202. Bowden TA Jr, Mansberger AR Jr, Lykins LE. Pseudomembranous enterocolitis: mechanism for restoring flora homeostasis. *Am Surg* 1981;47:178–183.

203. Tvede M, Rask-Madsen J. Bacteriotherapy for chronic relapsing *Clostridium difficile* diarrhoea in six patients. *Lancet* 1989;1:1156–1160.

204. Levison ME. Effect of colon flora and short-chain fatty acids on growth in vitro of *Pseudomonas aeruginosa* and Enterobactericeae. *Infect Immun* 1973;8:30–35.

205. Borriello SP, Barclay FE. Protection of hamsters against *Clostridium difficile* ileocaecitis by prior colonisation with nonpathogenic strains. *J Med Microbiol* 1986;19:339–350.

206. Lyerly DM, Bostwick E., Binion S, Wilkins TD. Passive immunization against *Clostridium difficile* disease in hamsters using bovine colostral antibodies. *Infect Immun* 1991;59:2215–2218.

207. Burdon DW. *Clostridium difficile:* the epidemiology and prevention of hospital-acquired infection. *Infection* 1982;10:203–204.

208. Delmee M., Michaux JL. Prevention of *Clostridium difficile* outbreaks in hospitals. *Lancet* 1986;1:350.

209. Johnson S, Gerdin DN, Olson MM, et al. Prospective, controlled study of vinyl glove use to interrupt *Clostridium difficile* nosocomial transmission. *Am J Med* 1990;88:137–140.

210. Brooks SE, Veal RO, Kramer M, Dore L, Schupf N, Adachi M. Reduction in incidence of *Clostridium difficile*–associated diarrhea in an acute care hospital and a skilled nursing facility following replacement of electronic thermometers with single-use disposables. *Infect Cont Hosp Epidemiol* 1992;13:98–103.

211. Delmee M, Michaux JL. Prevention of *Clostridium difficile* outbreaks in hospitals. *Lancet* 1986;1:350.

Infections of the Gastrointestinal Tract,
edited by M. J. Blaser, P. D. Smith, J. I. Ravdin,
H. B. Greenberg, and R. L. Guerrant
Raven Press, Ltd., New York © 1995.

CHAPTER 59

Antibiotic-Associated Diarrhea

John G. Bartlett

Diarrhea is one of the most common complications of antibiotic usage. Nearly all agents with an antibacterial spectrum of activity have been implicated. The purpose of this chapter is to review the current status of knowledge regarding the etiology, diagnosis, and management of antibiotic-associated diarrhea with particular emphasis on the major etiological agent, *Clostridium difficile*.

CLASSIFICATION

Most cases of antibiotic-associated diarrhea are due to *C. difficile* or are enigmatic. Occasional cases appear to involve alternative enteric pathogens such as *Salmonella* or enterotoxin-producing strains of *C. perfringens,* and possibly *Candida albicans* or *S. aureus*.

ANTIBIOTIC-ASSOCIATED DIARRHEA NOT CAUSED BY *C. DIFFICILE*

Salmonellosis

The frequency of salmonellosis as a cause of antibiotic-associated diarrhea has never been systematically studied, but the association is well established (1). A classic study by Bohnhoff et al. demonstrated that the inoculum size of *Salmonella* necessary to produce infection in mice was reduced 10,000-fold by pretreatment of the animals with oral streptomycin (2). More recent epidemics of salmonellosis have demonstrated that antibiotic exposure such as ampicillin treatment represents a distinct risk factor for symptomatic disease (1,3) as well as promoting the carrier state (4).

Clostridium perfringens

The role of enterotoxin-producing strains of *C. perfringens* was reported by a single investigator who noted

J. G. Bartlett: Department of Medicine; Johns Hopkins University School of Medicine, Baltimore, Maryland 21205.

C. perfringens enterotoxin in 15 (1.5%) of 940 specimens from persons with antibiotic-associated diarrhea (5). The diagnostic test used was Vero cell culture to demonstrate a cytotoxin that was neutralized by antitoxin to *C. perfringens* enterotoxin.

Candida albicans

A recent report suggested that *Candida albicans* may be responsible for some cases of diarrhea, particularly in elderly patients (6). The interpretation of this observation is confounded by the fact that *C. albicans* may be detected in the normal colonic flora in 20% to 30% of healthy persons and up to 80% of patients receiving antibiotics; concentrations often exceed 10^5/g in the absence of diarrhea (7,8). Supportive evidence for the presumed role in causing diarrhea in these cases was provided by the therapeutic response noted with orally administered nystatin, which was accompanied by a resolution of symptoms and decreased concentrations of *C. albicans;* recurrences occurred in some patients when nystatin was discontinued. However, others have noted that some patients with the same findings may have persistent diarrhea despite elimination of yeast forms in stool, so that the pathogenic role of *Candida* sp. remains speculative (9).

Staphylococcus aureus

This organism was the suspected agent of antibiotic-associated colitis or "pseudomembranous enterocolitis" (PMC) in the 1950s and 1960s (10). At that time, pseudomembranous lesions, primarily in the small bowel, became recognized as a relatively common complication of antibiotic use, especially after surgery in patients given prophylactic antibiotics. In some reports, rates were high as 14% or even 27% (11,12). *S. aureus* was the major nosocomial pathogen at the time and was implicated in this nosocomial complication on the basis of Gram stains and stool cultures (10-15). When vancomycin became available in 1959, orally administered vancomycin became standard treatment (15). During this period the terms "antibiotic-associated enterocolitis," "staphylococcal enterocolitis," and "pseudomembranous enterocolitis" were used interchangeably, and virtually all textbooks of medicine had chapters dealing with staphylococcal enterocolitis.

The etiological role of *S. aureus* was not seriously challenged until more recent studies in the 1970s when "clindamycin colitis" became a frequently recognized iatrogenic complication (16). *S. aureus* could not be recovered from stools of these patients despite the ease of culture using selective media, thus raising questions regarding its pathogenic role (16). It is not clear in retrospect if the case for *S. aureus* was ever clearly established. Some have argued that these were probably due to *C. difficile;* others conclude that staphylococcal enteritis was actually somewhat different from antibiotic-associated PMC as currently encountered because (a) the inducing agents were quite different (primarily tetracyclines, chloramphenicol, and bowel preparations with neomycin, all agents that are infrequently implicated at present), and (b) the distribution of anatomic lesions is quite different. The small bowel was frequently involved in cases from the 1950s; hence the term "pseudomembranous enteritis" as opposed to "pseudomembranous colitis." (Small bowel involvement is now considered extraordinary in patients with *C. difficile*–induced disease.) There continue to be occasional reports of staphylococcal enterocolitis, but they are rare (17). It appears that if *S. aureus* was once responsible for pseudomembranous lesions of the gut, it is rarely encountered at present (10,17). In our experience from 1977 to 1980, *C. difficile* toxin was detected in stool from 136 of 141 patients with PMC con-

firmed at endoscopy; specimens from the five exceptions failed to yield *S. aureus* despite attempts to culture it (18).

Enigmatic Cases

The great majority of patients with antibiotic-associated diarrhea or colitis with negative diagnostic studies for *C. difficile* have no established etiological agent or mechanism. Some believe that the explanation is "dysbiosis" of the colonic flora, which simply means disruption of the types and concentrations of bacteria that are presumably critical for homeostasis.

Clinical features of patients with *C. difficile* toxin–negative antibiotic-associated diarrhea show clinical features that never have been systematically studied but appear to be somewhat different (19,20) (Table 1). The antimicrobial agents involved are similar to those that cause *C. difficile*–associated disease. Especially common are the drugs that have a pronounced effect on the normal flora of the colon with local activity against the colonic flora due to reduced absorption when taken orally or by enterohepatic circulation. The spectrum of activity is obviously important, and drugs that have the greatest impact on the anaerobic component of the fecal flora at concentrations achieved in the colonic lumen seem to be associated with the highest rates. These include clindamycin, ampicillin, and cephalosporins. Rates of antibiotic-associated diarrhea will depend to a large extent on the diagnostic criteria for diarrhea, route of administration, and dosage. The best studied are clindamycin with diarrhea rates of 7% to 26%, oral ampicillin or amoxicillin with rates of 5% to 12%, tetracyclines with rates of 5% to 8%, cephalosporins with rates of 2% to 5%, and fluoroquinolones with rates of 1% to 2% (21–28).

TABLE 1. *Comparison of antibiotic-associated diarrhea/colitis due to* C. difficile *and enigmatic cases*

	Antibiotic-associated diarrhea/colitis	
Variable	Due to *C. difficile*	No clear cause
Implicated drugs: most common	Clindamycin, ampicillin, cephalosporins	Clindamycin, tetracycline, ampicillin, some cephalosporins
Relationship of illness to dose	Usually not dose-related	Dose-related
Response to drug withdrawal	Symptoms often persist	Symptoms usually resolve
Clinical features		
Intestinal	Watery diarrhea and cramps	Watery diarrhea
Constitutional	Fever and leukocytosis common	Occurrence of systemic symptoms unusual
History	Usually noncontributory	History of diarrhea with same or other antibiotics
Complications	Toxic megacolon, ileus, high fever, leukemoid reaction, dehydration, hypoalbuminemia with anasarca, arthritis (rare)	Rarely serious
Evidence of colitis	Cramps, white blood cells in feces; colitis or PMC evident with endoscopy or CT scan	Colitis uncommon
Epidemiology	Epidemic or endemic in hospitals and nursing homes	Sporadic
Treatment	Discontinue implicated drug; administer vancomycin or metronidazole	Discontinue implicated drug or reduce dose; some appear to respond to vancomycin

The frequency and severity of this enigmatic antibiotic-associated diarrhea appears to be dose-related. It is also more frequent with oral administration, but exceptions are parenterally administered drugs excreted in the bile to give high colonic levels such as clindamycin, ampicillin, cefoperazone, and nafcillin. Symptoms usually resolve within several days after the implicated drug has been discontinued or reduced in dose. By contrast, *C. difficile*–associated diarrhea or colitis does not appear to be a dose-related complication and symptoms may persist for months after discontinuation. Another factor that appears to distinguish these two forms of antibiotic-associated diarrhea or colitis is the fact that *C. difficile* is now generally recognized as a major nosocomial complication, whereas the enigmatic form seems to be sporadic with no apparent epidemiological pattern. Also of interest is the clinical impression that the patient's history may reveal similar symptoms with the same antibiotic on prior occasions, and often with other antibiotics as well. Patients with *C. difficile*–associated diarrhea usually get it once or have relapses; recurrent disease accounts for less than 2% of cases (18,20).

The major difference is the severity of the complication in terms of morbidity and potential mortality. Patients with enigmatic antibiotic-associated diarrhea rarely have systemic expression of disease with fever and leukocytosis. Stool exams and endoscopy are much less likely to indicate colitis and severe complications such as toxic megacolon, PMC, and chronic or debilitating diarrhea are all far less frequent.

Pseudomembranous Colitis

PMC was once considered synonymous with *S. aureus*–induced enteric disease, and *C. difficile* is now believed to be responsible for virtually all cases. Nevertheless, there are occasional exceptions including the observation that this complication was described long before the antibiotic era (29). The most common clinical setting for PMC not associated with antimicrobial agents is surgery, primarily colonic, gastric, or pelvic (10,30,31). Other risk factors include spinal fracture, intestinal obstruction, colonic carcinoma, leukemia, severe burns, shock, uremia, heavy metal poisoning, hemolytic-uremic syndrome, ischemic cardiovascular disease, Crohn's disease, shigellosis, severe infection, neonatal necrotizing enterocolitis, ischemic colitis, and Hirschsprung's disease (32–36). Occasional cases have been encountered in previously healthy individuals in whom there was no recent antibiotic exposure or other identifiable risk factor, and these cases are usually due to *C. difficile* (37–39).

ANTIBIOTIC-ASSOCIATED DIARRHEA AND COLITIS DUE TO *C. DIFFICILE*

Nearly all patients with enteric complications ascribed to *C. difficile* have diarrhea, although occasional patients present with toxic megacolon or ileus without diarrhea.

Nearly all patients have also had recent antibiotic exposure, although there are occasional exceptions (37–40).

With regard to antibiotics, virtually any antimicrobial agent with an antibacterial spectrum of activity has been implicated, and some antineoplastic compounds such as fluorouracil and methotrexate as well (19,20,41). There were multiple studies of antibiotic-associated PMC that came to be known as clindamycin colitis in the 1970s. The most quoted report was the study by Tedesco et al. at Barnes Hospital in 1974 (16). This was the first study in which endoscopy was routinely used in a prospective study of antibiotic-associated diarrhea. Results showed that 42 (21%) of 200 patients treated with clindamycin developed diarrhea and that 20 of these (10% of all clindamycin-recipients) had PMC at endoscopy. This report shocked the medical community because it implied an extraordinarily high rate of a life-threatening complication associated with a drug that had become the standard agent for the treatment of anaerobic infections. Subsequent studies on eight stool samples saved from that epidemic were tested in my laboratory in 1978 and all were found to contain both *C. difficile* and *C. difficile* toxin B (42); in retrospect, it appears that the high rate of *C. difficile* at Barnes Hospital in 1973 represented an epidemic of this complication. Subsequent studies by multiple other investigators in the 1970s also identified clindamycin as a common inducing agent for PMC, although frequency was variable due in part to the striking confounding variables not appreciated at the time, which included epidemic vs. sporadic disease and nosocomial infections vs. cases in outpatients (42–47). In the late 1970s and early 1980s it became widely recognized that many other antibiotics often caused this complication in both patients (18,19,48,49) and hamsters (50–55). In most studies at the present time, cephalosporins as a class are the most frequent offending agents followed by clindamycin or ampicillin (18,19,48,49).

The hamster model was the original means for detection of *C. difficile* as the putative agent of clindamycin-associated colitis and this has remained a useful model for study of the disease under controlled conditions. The following antibiotics are known to cause lethal hemorrhagic cecitis due to *C. difficile* in hamsters: ampicillin, carbenicillin, cefamandole, cefaclor, cefazolin, cefoxitin, cephalexin, cephalothin, cephridine, oral gentamicin, imipenem, metronidazole, nafcillin, penicillin, ticarcillin, and vancomycin (50–55). Antimicrobial agents that do not cause this complication or show inconsistent results in the hamster model include tetracyclines, chloramphenicol, and sulfonamides (55). These data are of interest because they support analogous observations in patients.

The clinical expression of *C. difficile* ranges from asymptomatic carriage to its most serious and characteristic form, PMC (18–20,42,56). The diarrhea is variable in severity ranging from a brief and self-limited bout of loose stools to cholera-like diarrhea with 20 or more watery stools per day. Severe diarrhea is often accompanied by crampy abdominal pain, fever, leukocytosis, dehydration, electrolyte imbalance, and protein loss with hypoalbuminemia. The average temperature in patients with colitis is 100–101°F, but may be above 105°F. The average pe-

TABLE 2. *Rates of* C. difficile *isolation and* C. difficile *cytotoxin in stools (%)*

Patient category	Culture positive rates	Toxin positive rates (tissue culture assay)
Antibiotic-associated diarrhea or colitis with positive toxin assay	95–100	—
Antibiotic-associated PMC	95–100	95–100
Antibiotic-associated diarrhea	15–25	10–25
Antibiotic-exposure without diarrhea	20	2–8
Hospitalized patients	10–25	?
Gastrointestinal disease unrelated to antibiotic exposure	2–3	0.5
Healthy adults	2–3	0
Healthy neonates	5–70	5–63

ripheral leukocyte count in patients with colitis is 12,000–20,000/mm^3, although it may reach 80,000/mm^3. Fecal leukocytes are found in about 30% to 50% of cases. Serious complications found in a minority include toxic megacolon, hyperpyrexia, leukemoid reaction, hypoalbuminemia with anasarca, and chronic diarrhea that may last for months despite discontinuation of the inducing agent. Reactive arthritis similar to that seen with other enteric infections was reported in ten patients (57).

The rate of *C. difficile* infection in patients with antibiotic-associated diarrhea depends to a large extent on associated findings. Positive toxin assays in stools submitted to laboratories when this diagnosis is suspected are usually reported in 10% to 25% of cases. Studies done systematically show that *C. difficile* is generally implicated in 15% to 25% of all cases of antibiotic-associated diarrhea without colitis; the frequency is 50% to 70% among patients with inflammation by endoscopic exam and approaches 100% in patients with PMC (Table 2) (58–63).

DIAGNOSTIC STUDIES

The two types of common diagnostic studies are those used to define anatomic changes and those used to identify the putative agent, primarily *C. difficile.*

ANATOMIC STUDIES

Major techniques for defining anatomic changes are endoscopy, x-ray, contrast studies, and CT scans.

Endoscopy

The preferred method to determine anatomic changes is endoscopy (16,45–50,64–67). Sigmoidoscopy is often adequate, but up to one third of cases of PMC may involve only the right side of the colon and consequently require colonoscopy (64,65). The most extensive studies of antibiotic-associated colitis detected with endoscopy were reported in the 1970s when clindamycin colitis was the subject of multiple reviews. Visualization of the colon and biopsies showed a spectrum of changes including a normal colonic mucosa, inflammation with a leukocytic infiltrate in the colonic mucosa, colonic erythema or ulceration, and the most characteristic form, PMC. Histological studies of the pseudomembrane typically show that it arises from a point of superficial ulceration and is accompanied by acute or chronic inflammatory infiltrates in the lamina propria (66,67). The pseudomembrane is composed of fibrin, mucin, sloughed mucosal epithelial cells, and acute inflammatory cells. The spectrum of changes have been classified in three categories by Price and Davis, and these appear to be rather uniform in individual patients (67). The earliest form consists of focal necrosis with polymorphonuclear infiltrates and eosinophilic exudate in the lamina propria. Spreading out from the necrotic focus is the characteristic "summit lesion" composed of fibrin and polymorphonuclear cells. The second category, which appears to represent a more advanced form of disease, shows glandular disruption and a focal infiltrate with acute inflammatory cells surmounted by typical pseudomembranes that may appear like a volcanic eruption. With both of these lesions there are intervening areas of normal mucosa. The third and most advanced form of disease shows complete structural necrosis with extensive involvement of the lamina propria that is overlayed by a thick, confluent pseudomembrane. Bacterial invasion of the bowel mucosa was not found in the earlier studies when PMC was commonly ascribed to *S. aureus,* nor is bacterial invasion found with *C. difficile.* This is a toxin-mediated disease in which studies in both experimental animals and patients show structural necrosis of the intestine following intraluminal challenge with cell-free supernatant or purified toxin A from *C. difficile* (19).

X-Rays

Radiological findings are often nonspecific, but may be helpful in specifically suggesting PMC in selected patients with advanced disease (68–71). Plain films of the abdomen often show a markedly edematous colon, distorted haustral markings, and distension of the colon. Occasionally there may be small irregularities representing pseudomembranous plaques in profile. Contrast studies often show rounded filling defects that outline the plaques, but findings are often nondiagnostic due to underpenetration of barium, confluence of the pseudomembrane, minimal involvement, or excessive mucous secretions (71). The diagnostic accuracy is improved with air contrast studies, which must be performed with caution due to the potential complication of colonic perforation.

CT Scans

These are the most useful of the nonendoscopic techniques and often show a thickened colon that may suggest idiopathic inflammatory bowel disease (72,73). A review of 26 cases by Fishman et al. (73) showed that 23 had increased thickness (average of 14.7 mm) of the colonic mucosa and contrast trapped in the thickened folds to give a characteristic "accordion sign." Additional features that specifically suggested *C. difficile*–associated enteric disease were the lack of small bowel involvement and the presence of ascites fluid.

Indications for these tests to define the anatomy of the lesion are arbitrary because the most important test is detection of *C. difficile* or its toxin since this provides the rationale for therapy. Disadvantages of endoscopy and CT scan with contrast are that both are expensive and unpleasant, and both fail to identify the putative agent of a treatable infectious disease. Nevertheless, the detection of PMC by endoscopy or the characteristic findings of CT scan are commonly considered sufficiently specific to proceed with a presumed diagnosis of *C. difficile*–associated disease. The best justification for these more invasive and high-priced procedures is clinical settings when immediate results are clinically important, alternative diagnostic possibilities are strongly considered, results of the *C. difficile* toxin assay are inconsistent with the clinical impression, or there is a failure to respond to therapeutic agents that are traditionally effective.

TESTS FOR *C. DIFFICILE*

C. difficile Cytotoxin Assay

The test that has traditionally been considered the gold standard is the tissue culture assay for detection of toxin B. This was originally described as a nonspecific cytotoxin in 1977 (74) and it became a highly specific test with the use of *C. sordelli*–antitoxin neutralization (75). The tissue culture assay is still considered the most accurate by many in the field in terms of sensitivity and specificity, but there are several concerns as follows:

1. The test has traditionally required tissue culture facilities that are not available in most diagnostic laboratories. (This problem has at least been partially obviated by the commercial availability of microtiter wells.)

2. Test results are often not available for 18–48 hr. Typical cytopathic changes are generally noted within 12–24 hr, but some laboratories do not report results for 48 hr and some test for neutralization by *C. sordellii* or *C. difficile* antitoxin only after cytopathic changes have been noted.

3. Some have reported unacceptably high rates of false-negative test results and consequently prefer the use of stool culture in combination with the toxin assay or alternative tests. In terms of sensitivity, it is noteworthy that the cytotoxin assay is universally positive as an early indicator of predictable death due to *C. difficile* in the hamster model of antibiotic-associated colitis (18–20,50,51). In terms of specificity, again the hamster model shows a perfect correlation. In addition, no other clostridial toxin is known to cause false-positive results (76). Our impression is that false-negative assay results usually reflect the use of inappropriately large dilutions of the specimen. The recommended process is to filter watery stools without dilution or use a 1:4 dilution of semisolid stools; some laboratories perform dilutions at 1:10 or even 1:40; this will introduce a 10% to 15% rate of false-negative results according to prior studies (76,77). Unfortunately, the reagents used for the tissue culture assay are not subject to FDA review and consequently there are no clearly defined standards.

4. False-positive test results are nil in the sense that positive results virtually always indicate the presence of *C. difficile* as indicated by near-uniform recovery rates of this organism in toxin-positive specimens and the failure to find any alternative microbial product that shows cross-reactivity (76). However, positive tests do not necessarily indicate that *C. difficile* is the cause of enteric symptoms. About 2% to 15% of antibiotic recipients will have toxin-positive specimens in the absence of diarrhea (18,60,61). In some studies of hospitalized patients with extensive sampling, the majority of patients with positive assays for *C. difficile* do not have diarrhea (78). This cannot be surprising since virtually all enteric pathogens show high rates of false-positive results in patients who harbor these organisms without clinical expression; this includes the standard tests for detection of *Salmonella, Shigella, Vibrio cholerae, Entamoeba histolytica*, and *Giardia*, among others. The observation simply calls attention to the need for appropriate clinical correlations with this as well as other tests for enteric pathogens. The one major exception is neonates since stool assays in this group give high yields of positive toxin assays in the absence of gut disease (18,61,79).

5. The tissue culture assay detects toxin B, although toxin A appears to be responsible for virtually all pathological changes and clinical expression (80,81). Although this is a theoretical concern, nearly all *C. difficile* strains that produced toxin A produce toxin B as well, and they seem to produce both toxins under identical conditions. The implication is that toxin B is an accurate indicator of toxin A with rare exceptions (82,83).

Alternative Tests for Toxin

Alternatives to the tissue culture assay are gaining increasing attention. These are summarized in Table 3 which shows their relative merits. Probably the preferred alternative test is the enzyme immunoassay (EIA) for detection of toxin A with or without toxin B as reported originally in 1984 (84). The reagents for this test have subsequently become commercially available from several suppliers. The initial experience shows sensitivity and

TABLE 3. *Diagnostic tests for* Clostridium difficile *toxins*

Variable	Tissue culture assay (18–20,40,56)	Latex particle agglutination (91–94)	Enzyme immunoassay (77, 84, 87–91)	Dot immunoblot (85)	PCR (95–98)	Culture (99–102)
Source	Microliter wells often preferred	Commercially available	Four suppliers	Commercially available	Experimental	CCFA media, etc.
Product detected	Toxin B	Glutamate dehydrogenase	Toxin A, or Toxin A plus Toxin B	Toxin A	Toxin B gene, Toxin A gene or both	Organism
Time required	28–48 hr	30 min	2–4 hr	30 min	2–4 hr	28–72 hr
Clinical correlations	Best sensitivity with proper dilutions; Good specificity	Least sensitive and specific	Good specificity; fair sensitivity	Initial studies promising	Good sensitivity; fair specificity	Good sensitivity; poor specificity

specificity rates that are somewhat variable but sufficiently promising for several labs to use it as a substitute for the tissue culture assay (84,86–90). This reflects the ease of performing EIA tests, rapid results that are generally available in 2–4 hr, and clinical studies showing acceptable rates of accuracy based on comparison with the tissue culture assay and/or clinical correlations. The latex agglutination assay was originally promoted as a rapid test for detection of toxin A (91–93), but subsequent work showed that it detects a nontoxic enzyme, glutamate dehydrogenase, that is produced by *C. difficile* and other organisms as well (94); not surprisingly, clinical trials have shown inconsistent results. The rapid test that is being pursued most aggressively in addition to EIA is polymerase chain reaction (PCR). This shows the expected high rate of sensitivity (95–98). The final rapid test for toxin A detection is the dot immunoblot, which is in the early stages of development (85).

Cultures for *C. difficile*

Some authorities have advocated cultures for C. *difficile* as the most sensitive method of detection. The preferred method is the use of antibiotic-incorporated agar media containing cycloserine and cefoxitin as originally described by George et al. (99) and subsequently modified to detect strains that are relatively sensitive to cefoxitin (100). Concerns about culture as a routine diagnostic test are the following: First, although the appropriate media are readily available and provide a high yield in research laboratories, the ability of clinical laboratories with less extensive experience to reproduce the published results is considered doubtful. Second, the rate of false-positive cultures is high; the carrier rate for C. *difficile* in healthy adults is approximately 3%, from hospitalized patients without diarrhea it is 10% to 20%, and for adults who recently received antibiotics without diarrhea it is 10% to 15% (18–20,61,101–104). It is the latter two groups who account for most tests done in clinical practice. Finally, cultures require 2–3 days, which is too long for therapeutic decision making. Perhaps the best justification for stool culture is its use in epidemics of C. *difficile*–associated

enteric complications where the information might be used to sequester carriers, as a guide for treatment to eradicate the carrier state, or to type isolates for purposes of epidemiological investigation.

Negative Assays

The need for repeat assays to confirm negative results for *C. difficile* toxin is arbitrary. As noted, *C. difficile* is generally the only enteric pathogen implicated in a great majority of cases of antibiotic-associated diarrhea and colitis; most patients with negative toxin assays have no etiological diagnosis. The diagnostic yield with duplicate testing using the same assay or different assays is presumably always greater than a single test, but how much better with the five different methods to detect *C. difficile* and its toxins is unknown. Nosocomial diarrhea is almost always due to *C. difficile* or is unrelated to cultivatable agents, so that the utility of attempting to detect other bacterial or parasitic agents is often questionable. In fact, the association is sufficiently strong for some laboratories to establish a procedural format in which additional diagnostic studies on stool for microbial agents are not done unless the *C. difficile* toxin assay first is shown to be negative (105). As noted above, *Salmonella* rarely causes antibiotic-associated diarrhea, most laboratories cannot test for *C. perfringens* enterotoxin, and the roles of *C. albicans* and *S. aureus* remain controversial.

Gram stain of stool to show large numbers of gram-positive cocci was a favored diagnostic technique when *S. aureus* was suspected (11–15). The problem is that the role of stool Gram stain for *S. aureus* in the light of present knowledge about *C. difficile* is unknown. Gram stains are not helpful in detecting *C. difficile* because the concentrations even with florid disease or high toxin titers ($\geq 10^{-5}$) usually account for less than 1% of the fecal flora (100). Fecal leukocyte exams are appropriate and positive results in specimens submitted for *C. difficile* toxin often correlate with a positive toxin assay; the problem is that the test is only about 30% sensitive among patients with *C. difficile*–associated disease (106).

TREATMENT

General Recommendations

Treatment of antibiotic-associated diarrhea or colitis begins with discontinuation of the implicated agent and any necessary supportive measures (Table 4). Supportive measures include fluid and electrolyte restoration orally or parenterally. There is no reason to limit oral intake, but electrolyte-rich fluids are suggested in patients with severe diarrhea. Before the discovery of C. difficile, some patients developed severe malnutrition with hypoalbuminemia (16,43–48). This is unusual at the present time due to earlier intervention with effective antibiotic treatment in cases involving C. difficile; cases of this severity that do not involve C. difficile are extraordinary. Antiperistaltic agents such as loperamide or diphenoxylate hydrochloride should be avoided since they appear to increase the incidence of antibiotic-associated diarrhea in patients receiving clindamycin and worsen symptoms among those patients with established disease (107,108). The systemic administration of corticosteroids is sometimes advocated for critically ill patients, but methylprednisolone in the animal model of antibiotic-induced colitis failed to delay death and the experience with patients is limited, anecdotal, and inconsistent (109–111).

In some patients, the indication for antibiotics that caused the complication is still present and may be compelling. The recommendation in this situation is to discontinue the inducing agent and substitute a drug that is unlikely to promote C. difficile. Antimicrobial agents in this category include quinolones, sulfonamides, parenteral aminoglycosides, trimethoprim-sulfamethoxazole, metronidazole, parenteral vancomycin, or tetracyclines (111).

Antibiotic Treatment

Antibiotics with established merit in antibiotic-associated diarrhea are usually limited to cases involving C. difficile. For rare cases that apparently involve S. aureus, the recommendation is for orally administered vancomycin in a dose of 250–500 mg four times daily (15). As noted, this is the dosage recommended in the 1960s when S. aureus was thought to be the putative agent of antibiotic-associated PMC, an association that is now disputed. The role of Candida sp. is also arbitrary, but some have suggested oral nystatin, 1 million units by mouth every 4 hr if concentrations of yeast exceed 10^5/g stool (6). The decision to treat patients with salmonellosis is often controversial since antibiotics, even those active against the implicated strain, appear to promote clinical expression and prolong the carrier state (1,3,4). Patients with severe disease and the compromised host should be treated with a fluoroquinolone, ampicillin, or trimethoprim-sulfamethoxazole.

Antibiotic treatment for cases involving C. difficile is readily available and probably abused. The drugs used most frequently are vancomycin and metronidazole; less frequent but also effective are fusidic acid, bacitracin, and teicoplanin. Comparative trials with all five drugs suggest they are therapeutically equivalent (18–20,56,111–120), although these trials often include large numbers of patients with relatively minor symptoms. Observation without antibiotic treatment after discontinuation of the implicated agent is often advised because many patients recover spontaneously and antimicrobial treatment incurs the risk of relapsing disease. Indications for antibiotic treatment include the following: (a) antibiotic treatment for the underlying condition must be continued; (b) the patient is seriously ill with evidence for colitis; (c) there is florid or devastating diarrhea; or (d) the patient has persistent diarrhea despite discontinuation of the inducing agent.

Oral vancomycin is generally considered the gold standard and is preferred for patients who are seriously ill (18,56,111). The usual dosage is 125 mg orally four times daily (56,121). Results with this treatment are impressive: fever usually resolves within 24 hr and diarrhea generally resolves over an average of 4–5 days (121). Response rates are usually reported at 95% to 100%. Vancomycin has ideal pharmacokinetic properties and in vitro activity. It is poorly absorbed with oral administration so that mean stool levels with 125-mg doses are 350–500 μg/g (111,122). In vitro susceptibility tests of over 200 strains of C. difficile indicate that all were susceptible at concentrations of 16 μg/mL or less (122–126). As noted, C. difficile does not invade the intestinal mucosa so that high fecal levels without tissue levels is an appropriate goal. Serum levels are negligible so that systemic toxicity is nil, although monitoring of blood levels is sometimes advised in patients with renal failure plus an inflamed bowel since small amounts of absorbed drug could conceivably accumulate in this setting. A review of our experience with 189 pa-

TABLE 4. *Treatment of* C. difficile–*associated diarrhea and colitis*

A. Nonspecific measures
   1. Discontinue implicated antimicrobial agent (alternatives is to change to another agent that is infrequently associated with this complication while giving oral vancomycin).
   2. Supportive measures.
   3. Avoid antiperistaltic agents.
   4. Enteric precautions for hospitalized patients (until diarrhea resolves).
B. Specific treatment: antimicrobial agents (advocated only if symptoms are severe or persist)
   1. Oral agent (preferred)
      a. Vancomycin: 125 mg po qid, 7–14 days (preferred for serious disease or patients who do not respond to metronidazole).
      b. Metronidazole: 250 mg po tid, 7–14 days (preferred for less serious disease, most outpatients and often preferred for inpatient treatment in hospitals where vancomycin-resistant E. faecium is problematic).
   2. Parenteral agents (to be used only until oral agents are tolerated): metronidazole: 500 mg IV q6h. Response rates are variable: oral treatment should be given concurrently or implemented as soon as possible; some advocate vancomycin by a long tube from above or by a catheter or enema from below).

tients showed that 183 (97%) responded (111). Major reasons for nonresponse are the presence of ileus, noncompliance, and concurrent presence of an alternative cause of intestinal disease.

The major alternative to oral vancomycin is metronidazole, which is advocated because it is less expensive and its preferential use in hospitals may limit the problem of vancomycin-resistant *E. faecium*. This drug has good *in vitro* activity vs. *C. difficile* (56,122–126) and comparative clinical trials in patients with mild to moderately severe disease show therapeutic responses comparable to those with vancomycin (117,118). A theoretical disadvantage is that metronidazole stool levels following oral administration are nil due to nearly complete absorption (127). The assumption is that in the presence of diarrhea a sufficient quantity reaches the colonic lumen for activity at the site of infection. Also disturbing is the observation that metronidazole has been implicated as a cause of *C. difficile*–associated colitis in at least ten reported patients (128,129). Nevertheless, it is cautioned that oral vancomycin might also be implicated if it was used by oral administration for other clinical indications. Both metronidazole and vancomycin cause lethal colitis in the hamster model when given by mouth (55) and it is possible that both drugs are inducing agents, which may be a factor in the pathogenesis of relapses following their use as treatment.

Other treatments for *C. difficile* include bacitracin by mouth, which appears to be as effective as vancomycin or metronidazole in two comparative trials (112,113). Disadvantages are the limited clinical experience, the fact that by *in vitro* testing some strains of *C. difficile* are highly resistant, and the relatively high cost of bacitracin compared to metronidazole. Cholestyramine was reportedly effective in antibiotic-associated PMC before the role of *C. difficile* was described (130). Subsequent studies have shown that this drug, like other anion exchange resins, binds toxin A and toxin B of *C. difficile* (131). The experience of different investigators has shown marked variation with these anion exchange resins with some reporting excellent response in virtually all patients (132) and others reporting high failure rates (133). Studies in the hamster model showed that cholestyramine was effective compared to placebo, but distinctly inferior to vancomycin (109,111,116). There is theoretical interest in combining cholestyramine with an antibiotic since the former would neutralize existing toxin and the antibiotic would presumably inhibit further toxin production. However, the resin binds vancomycin to produce a tenfold reduction in colonic levels (131). Interaction between cholestyramine and metronidazole or bacitracin has not been studied.

Relapses

The major complication of treatment is relapses, which are reported with a frequency of 5% to 50% (56,111–120,134). In the largest reported study of treatment, there were 46 relapses among 189 patients (24%) given oral vancomycin (111). These patients responded to a second course of vancomycin, but 22 (46%) suffered a second relapse (111). The typical sequence of events is for a patient to do well during therapy, but then suffer a recurrence with prior symptoms at 5–10 days following discontinuation of treatment. Some patients have suffered multiple relapses over a period of months or years with sequential courses of treatment. The incidence of relapses varies greatly and inexplicably in different reports, but comparative trials have shown no difference in frequency with comparative trials using vancomycin, metronidazole, or bacitracin (111–120). There is also no evidence that changing from one antimicrobial agent to another is likely to be more effective than simply readministering the previous drug, although cost and tolerance may be issues to consider. There also is no evidence that the dose or duration of treatment with these agents influences the frequency or severity of relapses. Stool assays at the time of relapse following vancomycin treatment are positive and cultures show organisms that are highly susceptible to vancomycin, thus eliminating acquisition of resistance as an issue (111,134).

The proposed mechanism of relapses is that the organism is not eradicated from the colonic lumen, and vegetative forms of *C. difficile* flourish when the antibiotic is discontinued. The alternative possibility is acquisition of a new strain of *C. difficile*, but this appears to apply to a relatively small number of patients. Studies supporting the first theory are from the monoassociated germ-free mice (135) that show that toxin production stops with vancomycin administration, but spores persist; when vancomycin is discontinued, vegetative forms return, replicate, and produce high concentrations of both toxin A and toxin B. Clinical studies also show that *C. difficile* can commonly be recovered from stool after vancomycin treatment despite stool levels that are several hundred fold higher than the minimum inhibitory concentration (134). These data support microbial persistence with sporulation as the mechanism of relapse; no antimicrobial agent kills spores and none has proven consistently successful in eliminating *C. difficile* from the colon. The two major agents used for treatment are also known to be inducing agents of this complication in the hamster model, to further confound the issue (111).

Suggested treatments of relapses include careful observation with no specific treatment, a second course of antimicrobial treatment, nonantibiotic treatments (cholestyramine, lactobacilli, fecal enema, etc.), or some combination of these (Table 5). Toxin assays are often positive at the completion of treatment even in patients who do not relapse (115,116). Thus, the decision to treat with an antibiotic should be based on clinical observations rather than results of the toxin assay. In many cases, it is appropriate to simply observe the patient and this may be mandatory in the most difficult cases.

The major therapeutic regimen used when tactics other than another course of vancomycin or metronidazole are considered necessary are based on the principal of sequential treatment using a standard course of antibiotics for 10–14 days to stabilize conditions in the gut and then follow with a 3- to 4-week course of alternative treatment designed to maintain homeostasis while the normal flora becomes reestablished. Vancomycin or metronidazole are generally used for the initial stage. Agents used for the second phase include cholestyramine, cholesty-

TABLE 5. *Methods to manage multiple relapses of* C. difficile–*associated diarrhea or colitis*

1. Metronidazole or vancomycin po × 10–14 days followed by cholestyramine (4 g tid) ± lactobacilli (as Lactinex, 1 g po qid) × 3 weeks (18–20,56,111,116).
2. Vancomycin, 125 mg po qid × 10–14 days followed by vancomycin 125 mg po every other day × 3 weeks (146).
3. Vancomycin, 125 mg po qid × 4–6 weeks, then taper over 4–8 weeks (134).
4. Vancomycin, 125 mg po qid plus rifampin, 600 mg po gd × 10–14 days (145)
5. Vancomycin, 125 po qid plus *Saccharomyces boulardii* × 10–14 days, then *Saccharomyces boulardii* for 4 weeks (141,142).
6. Intravenous gammaglobulin, 400 mg/kg q 3 weeks (reported in pediatric patients) (136)
7. Rectal instillation of feces: 50 g fresh stool from healthy donor in 500 mL saline delivered by enema (138,139).
8. Broth cultures of bacteria from healthy donors: stool culture using stool from healthy donor, 10 strains selected based on *in vitro* inhibition of *C. difficile* grown in broth culture 10⁹/mL, 2 mL of each mixed in anaerobic glovebox with 180 mL saline and given by enema (140).
9. Lactobacillus G-G (1 g po qid) × 3 weeks (143,144).

ramine combined with lactobacilli, very low-dose vancomycin, or oral administration of *Saccharomyces boulardii* (18–20,42,56,141–144).

Some have advocated the use of fecal enemas as the ultimate physiological mechanism to control the disease (138,139), but this approach lacks aesthetic appeal and there are concerns about transferable agents such as hepatitis viruses and retroviruses. An alterative is rectal instillation of components of the fecal flora using broth cultures (140) or attempted colonization with a nontoxigenic strain of *C. difficile* (137). Other strategies used with variable success are vancomycin combined with rifampin, tapering doses of vancomycin and immunoglobulin (Table 5) (56,145,146).

EPIDEMIOLOGY

Transmission of *C. difficile* in the hospital setting and in chronic care facilities is now a major concern (16,101,147–151). The organism and the disease it causes may be epidemic or endemic in many hospitals, long-term care facilities, and, to a lesser extent, day care centers. These are all settings in which there is clustering of people rendered vulnerable by high rates of exposure to antibiotics. Patients with *C. difficile*–associated diarrhea in hospitals and nursing homes should be placed on enteric precautions with assiduous attention to handwashing and glove use to prevent fecal–oral contamination (148). It is also appropriate to have patients assigned to private rooms with bathrooms in the early stages of disease, when there is severe diarrhea or when the patient is incontinent. Antibiotic control programs to limit unnecessary use of

clindamycin, ampicillin, and cephalosporins may be required.

Environmental cultures have shown increased rates of recovery of *C. difficile* in case-associated areas (152–155) and hospitalization per se is a notable risk for colonization (78,101,155). Evaluation of epidemics includes enhanced efforts in case detection with expanded use of toxin assays among patients with antibiotic-associated or nosocomial diarrhea, and a surveillance log by an infection control practitioner. This tactic is facilitated by authorizing nurses to order *C. difficile* toxin assays. Most epidemics are geographically limited to selected wards or services and some probably represent artifacts of enhanced recognition. A thorough investigation may require stool cultures to detect carriers, environmental cultures using selective media, and possibly strain typing of isolates using any of several methods that are currently available (155–161). However, most hospital laboratories do not offer *C. difficile* cultures or typing of strains and there are no clear guidelines of what to do with this information. Some have suggested treatment of carriers with vancomycin or metronidazole (150), but this does not have established merit, does not necessarily eliminate the carrier state (162), and may even promote disease. Thus, the following recommendations are generally accepted as a reasonable approach to nosocomial outbreaks: (a) Sequester patients. (b) Pay careful attention to enforcing enteric precautions. (c) Implement antibiotic control programs to reduce unnecessary use with particular attention to clindamycin, ampicillin, and cephalosporins. (d) Ensure cleansing of environmental sources with a sporicidal germicide.

REFERENCES

1. Sun M. In search of *salmonella*'s smoking gun. Science 1984; 226:30–32.
2. Bohnhoff M, Miller CP, Martin WR. Resistance of the mouse's intestinal tract to experimental salmonella infection. *J Exp Med* 1964;120:805–813.
3. Spika JS, Waterman SH, Soo Hoo GW, et al. Chloramphenicol-resistant *Salmonella newport* traced through hamburger to dairy farms. *N Engl J Med* 1987;316:565–570.
4. Neill MA, Opal SM, Heelan J, et al. Failure of ciprofloxacin to eradicate convalescent fecal excretion after acute salmonellosis: experience during an outbreak in health care workers. *Ann Intern Med* 1991;114:195–199.
5. Borriello SP, Larson HE, Welch AR. Enterotoxigenic *Clostridium perfringens:* a possible cause of antibiotic-associated diarrhoea. *Lancet* 1984;1:305.
6. Danna PL, Urban D, Bellin E, Rahall JJ. Role of candida in pathogenesis of antibiotic-associated diarrhoea in elderly patients. *Lancet* 1991;337:511–515.
7. Cohen R, Roth FJ, Delgado E, et al. Fungal flora of the normal human small and large intestine. *N Engl J Med* 1969;280:638.
8. Giuliano M, Barza M, Jacobus NV, Gorbach SL. Effect of broad spectrum antibiotics on composition of gastrointestinal microflora of humans. *Antimicrob Agents Chemother* 1987;31: 202.
9. Cooper TW. Secretary diarrhea and candidal overgrowth: cause and effect? *J Infect Dis* 1991;164:823.
10. Bartlett JB, Gorbach SL. Pseudomembranous enterocolitis (antibiotic-related colitis). In: Stollerman GH, ed. *Advances in internal medicine.* Chicago: Year Book; 1977;455–466.
11. Hummel RP, Altemeier WA, Hill EO. Iatrogenic staphylococcal enterocolitis. *Ann Surg* 1964;160:551.

12. Wakefield RD, Sommers SC. Fatal membranous staphylococcal enteritis in surgical patients. *Ann Surg* 1953;138:249.
13. Altemeier WA, Hummell RP, Hill EO. Staphylococcal enterocolitis following antibiotic-therapy. *Ann Surg* 1963;157:847.
14. Azar H, Drapanas T. Relationship of antibiotics to wound infection and enterocolitis in colon surgery. *Am J Surg* 1968;115:209.
15. Khan MY, Hall WH. Staphylococcal enterocolitis: treatment with oral vancomycin. *Ann Intern Med* 1966;65:1.
16. Tedesco FJ, Barton RW, Alpers DH. Clindamycin-associated colitis: a prospective study. *Ann Intern Med* 1974;81:429.
17. Wiesen S, Gregg PA, Kershenobich D, et al. Pseudomembranous enteritis: rediscovery of a previously well-described entity? *Am J Gatroenterol* 1992;87:1631–1633.
18. Bartlett JG, Taylor NW, Chang TW, Dzink JA. Clinical and laboratory observations in *Clostridium difficile* colitis. *Am J Clin Nutr* 1981;33:2521–2526.
19. Bartlett JG. *Clostridium difficile:* clinical considerations. *Rev Infect Dis* 1990;12:S244.
20. Bartlett JG. Antibiotic-associated diarrhea. *Clin Infect Dis* 1992;15:573.
21. Swartzberg JE, Maresca RM, Remington JW. Gastrointestinal side effects associated with clindamycin. *Arch Intern Med* 1976;136:876.
22. Neu HC, Prince A, Neu CO, Garvey GJ. Incidence of diarrhea and colitis associated with clindamycin therapy. *J Infect Dis* 1977;135:S120.
23. Gurwith M, Rabin HR, Love K. Diarrhea-associated with clindamycin and ampicillin therapy. *J Infect Dis* 1977;135:S104.
24. Lusk RH, Fekety R Jr, Silva J Jr, et al. Gastrointestinal side effects following clindamycin or ampicillin therapy. *J Infect Dis* 1977;135:S111–S119.
25. Brause BD, Romankiewicz JA, Gotz V, Franklin JE Jr. Comparative study of diarrhea associated with clindamycin and ampicillin therapy. *Am J Gastroenterol* 1980;73:244.
26. Leigh DA, Simmons K, Williams S. Gastrointestinal side effects following clindamycin and lincomycin treatment: a follow-up study. *J Antimicrob Chemother* 1980;6:639–645.
27. Tedesco FJ. Ampicillin-associated diarrhea: a prospective study. *Dig Dis Sci* 1975;20:295.
28. Fekety FR. Gastrointestinal complications of antibiotic therapy. *JAMA* 1968;203:144.
29. Finney JMT. Gastro-enterostomy for cicatrizing ulcer of the pylorus. *Bull Johns Hopkins Hosp* 1893;4:53.
30. Penner A, Bernheim A. Acute postoperative enterocolitis. *Arch Pathol* 1939;27:966.
31. Dixon CF, Weismann RE. Acute pseudomembranous enteritis or enterocolitis: a complication following intestinal surgery. *Surg Clin North Am* 1948;28:999.
32. Kelber M, Ament ME. *Shigella disenteriae.* I. A forgotten cause of pseudomembranous colitis. *J Pediatr* 1976;89:595.
33. Hardaway RM, McKay DG. Pseudomembranous enterocolitis. *Arch Surg* 1959;78:446.
34. Prolla JC, Kirsner JB. The gastrointestinal lesions and complications of the leukemias. *Ann Intern Med* 1964;67:1084.
35. Dosik GM, Luna M, Valdivieso M, McCredle KB. Necrotizing colitis in patients with cancer. *Am J Med* 1979;67:646.
36. Margaretten W, McKay DG. Thrombotic ulceration of the gastrointestinal tract. *Arch Intern Med* 1971;127:250.
37. Moskovitz M, Bartlett JG. Recurrent pseudomembranous colitis unassociated with prior antibiotic therapy. *Arch Intern Med* 1981;141:663.
38. Peikin SR, Galdibini J, Bartlett JG. Role of *Clostridium difficile* in a case of nonantibiotic-associated pseudomembranous colitis. *Gastroenterology* 1980;79:948.
39. Wald A, Mendelow H, Bartlett JG. Nonantibiotic-associated pseudomembranous colitis due to toxin-producing clostridia. *Ann Intern Med* 1980;923:798.
40. Aronsson B, Mollby R, Nord CE. Antimicrobial agents and *Clostridium difficile* in acute disease: epidemiological data from Sweden, 1980–1982. *J Infect Dis* 1985;151:476.
41. Anand A, Glatt AE. *Clostridium difficile* infection associated with antineoplastic chemotherapy: a review. *Clin Infect Dis* 1993;17:109.
42. Bartlett JG. *Clostridium difficile. Clin Infect Dis* 1994;18(Suppl. 4):S265.
43. Keusch GT, Present KH. Summary of workshop on clindamycin colitis. *J Infect Dis* 1976;133:578.
44. Totten MA, Gregg JA, Fremont-Smith P, Legg M. Clinical and pathologic spectrum of antibiotic-associated colitis. *Am J Gastroenterol* 1978;69:311.
45. LeFrock JL, Klainer AS, Chen S, et al. The spectrum of colitis associated with lincomycin and clindamycin therapy. *J Infect Dis* 1975;131:S108.
46. Slagle GW, Boggs HW. Drug induced pseudomembranous enterocolitis. *Dis Col Rect* 1976;19:253.
47. Ramirez-Ronda CH. Incidence of clindamycin-associated colitis. *Ann Intern Med* 1974;81:860.
48. Talbot RW, Walker RC, Beart WR. Changing epidemiology, diagnosis and treatment of *Clostridium difficile* toxin-associated colitis. *Br J Surg* 1986;73:452.
49. Silva J, Fekety R, Werk C, et al. Inciting and etiologic agents of colitis. *Rev Infect Dis* 1984;6:S214.
50. Bartlett JG, Onderdonk AB, Cisneros AB, Kapser DL. Clindamycin-associated colitis due to toxin producing species of clostridium in hamsters. *J Infect Dis* 1977;136:701–705.
51. Bartlett JB, Chang TW, Moon N, Onderdonk AB. Antibiotic-induced lethal enterocolitis in hamsters. *Am J Vet Res* 1978;39:1525.
52. Ebright JR, Fekety R, Silva J, Wilson KT. Evaluation of eight cephalosporins in hamster colitis model. *Antimicrob Agents Chemother* 1981;19:980.
53. Kemp G. Therapy of experimental leptospirosis. In: Sylvester JC, ed. *Antimicrobial agents and chemotherapy—1964.* Washington, DC: Am Soc Microbiol; 1965:746–750.
54. Fekety R, Silva J, Toshniwal R, et al. Antibiotic-associated colitis: effects of antibiotics on *Clostridium difficile* and the disease in hamsters. *Rev Infect Dis* 1979;1:386.
55. Small JD. Drugs used in hamsters with a review of antibiotic-associated colitis in the laboratory hamster. In: Van Hoosier GL Jr, McPherson CW, eds. *The laboratory hamster.* Orlando: Academic Press; 1987:179–199.
56. Fekety R, Shah AB. Diagnosis and treatment of *Clostridium difficile* colitis. *JAMA* 1993;269:71–75.
57. Mermel LA, Osborn TG. *Clostridium difficile* associated reactive arthritis in an HLA-B27 positive female: report and literature review. *J Rheumatol* 1989;16:133–135.
58. Mogg GM, Keighley M, Burdon D, et al. Antibiotic-associated colitis: a review of 66 cases. *Br J Surg* 1979;66:738–743.
59. Mulligan ME, Citron D, Gabay E, et al. Alterations in human fecal flora, including ingrowth of *Clostridium difficile,* related to cefoxitin therapy. *Antimicrob Agents Chemother* 1984;36:343.
60. George WL, Rolfe RD, Finegold SM. *Clostridium difficile* and its cytotoxin in feces of patients with antimicrobial agent-associated diarrhea and miscellaneous conditions. *J Clin Microbiol* 1982;15:1049.
61. Viscidi R, Willey S, Bartlett JG. Isolation rates and toxigenic potential for *Clostridium difficile* isolates from various patient populations. *Gastroenterology* 1981;81:5–9.
62. Gilligan PH, McCarthy LR, Genta VM. Relative frequency of *Clostridium difficile* in patients with diarrheal disease. *J Clin Microbiol* 1981;14:25.
63. Falsen E, Kaijser B, Nehls L, Nygren B. *Clostridium difficile* in relation to enteric bacterial pathogens. *J Clin Microbiol* 1980;12:297.
64. Tedesco FJ, Corless JK, Brownstein RE. Rectal sparing in antibiotic-associated pseudomembranous colitis: a prospective study. *Gastroenterology* 1982;83:1259.
65. Burbige EJ, Radigan JJ. Antibiotic-associated colitis with normal appearing rectum. *Dis Col Rect* 1981;23:198.
66. Summer HW, Tedesco FJ. Rectal biopsy in clindamycin-associated colitis. *Arch Pathol* 1975;99:237.
67. Price AB, Davies DR. Pseudomembranous colitis. *J Clin Pathol* 1977;30:1–12.
68. Stanley RJ, Melson GL, Tedesco FJ. The spectrum of radiographic findings in antibiotic-related pseudomembranous colitis. *Radiology* 1974;111:519.

69. Tully TE, Feinberg SBL. Those other types of enterocolitis. *Am J Roentgenol* 1974;121:291.

70. Stanley RJ, Melson GL, Tedesco FJ, Saylor JL. Plain-film findings in severe pseudomembranous colitis. *Radiology* 1976;118:7.

71. Rubesin SE, Levine MS, Glick SN, Herlinger H, Lauf I. Pseudomembranous colitis with rectosigmoid sparing on barium studies. *Radiology* 1989;170:811.

72. Merine DS, Fishman EK, Jones B. Pseudomembranous colitis: CT evaluation. *J Comput Assist Tomogr* 1987;2:1017.

73. Fishman E, Kavuru M, Kulzlman JE, et al. CT of pseudomembranous colitis: Radiologic, clinical and pathologic correlation. *Radiology* 1991;180:57–60.

74. Larson HE, Parry JV, Price AB, et al. Undescribed toxin pseudomembranous colitis. *Br Med J* 1977;1:1246–1248.

75. Rifkin GD, Fekety R, Silva J. Neutralization of *C. sordellii* antitoxin of toxins implicated in clindamycin-induced colitis in hamsters. *Gastroenterology* 1978;75:422.

76. Chang TW, Lauermann M, Bartlett JG. Cytotoxicity assay in antibiotic-associated colitis. *J Infect Dis* 1979;140:765–770.

77. Viscidi RP, Yolken RH, Laughon BE, Bartlett JG. Enzyme immunoassay for detection of antibody to toxin A and B of *Clostridium difficile*. *J Clin Microbiol* 1983;18:242–247.

78. Simor AE, Yake SL, Tsimidis K. Infection due to *Clostridium difficile* among elderly residents of long-term-care facility. *Clin Infect Dis* 1993;17:672–678.

79. Donta TS, Myers MG. *Clostridium difficile* toxin in asymptomatic neonates. *Pediatrics* 1982;100:431.

80. Taylor NS, Thorne GM, Bartlett JG. Comparison of two toxins produced by *Clostridium difficile*. *Infect Immun* 1981;34:1036–1043.

81. Lima AAM, Lyerly DM, Wilkins TD, et al. Effects of *Clostridium difficile* toxins A and B in rabbit small and large intestine in vivo and on cultured cells in vitro. *Infect Immun* 1988;56:582.

82. Lyerly DM, Barroso LA, Wilkins TD, et al. Characterization of a toxin A–negative, toxin B–positive strain of *Clostridium difficile*. *Infect Immun* 1992;60:4633–4639.

83. Borriello SP, Wren BW, Hyde S, et al. Molecular, immunological, and biological characterization of a toxin A–negative, toxin B–positive strain of *Clostridium difficile*. *Infect Immun* 1992;60:4192–4199.

84. Laughon BE, Viscidi RP, Gdovin SL, et al. Enzyme immunoassays for detection of *Clostridium difficile* toxins A and B in fecal specimens. *J Infect Dis* 1984;149:781–788.

85. Woods GL, Iwen PC. Comparison of a dot immunobinding assay, latex agglutination, and cytotoxin assay for laboratory diagnosis of *Clostridium difficile*–associated diarrhea. *J Clin Microbiol* 1990;28:855–857.

86. Gumerlock PH, Yajarayma JT, Weiss JB, Silva J Jr. Specific detection of toxigenic strains of *Clostridium difficile* in stool specimens. *J Clin Microbiol* 1993;31:507–511.

87. Barbut F, Kajzer C, Panas N, Petit JC. Comparison of three enzyme immunoassays, a cytotoxicity assay, and toxigenic culture for diagnosis of *Clostridium difficile*–associated diarrhea. *J Clin Microbiol* 1993;31:963–967.

88. Gilligan PH, Walden TP, Kelly WF, et al. The use of a commercially available enzyme immunoassay for the detection of *Clostridium difficile* toxin A. *Arch Pathol Lab Med* 1993;117(5):507–510.

89. Knapp CC, Sandin RL, Hall GS, et al. Comparison of vidas *Clostridium difficile* toxin-A assay and premier *C. difficile* toxin-A assay to cytotoxin-B tissue culture assay for the detection of toxins of *C. difficile*. *Diag Microbiol Infect Dis* 1993;17:7–12.

90. De Girolami PC, Hanff PA, Eichelberger K, et al. Multicenter evaluation of a new enzyme immunoassay for detection of *Clostridium difficile* enterotoxin A. *J Clin Microbiol* 1992;30:1085–1088.

91. Shanholtzer CJ, Willard KE, Holter JJ, et al. Comparison of the VIDAS *Clostridium difficile* toxin A immunoassay with *C. difficile* culture and cytotoxin and latex tests. *J Clin Microbiol* 1992;30:1837–1840.

92. Miles BL, Siders JA, Allen SD. Evaluation of a commercial

93. latex test for *Clostridium difficile* for reactivity with *C. difficile* and cross-reactions with other bacteria. *J Clin Microbiol* 1988;26:2452–2455.

93. Kelly MT, Champagne SG, Sherlock CH, et al. Commercial latex agglutination test for detection of *Clostridium difficile*–associated diarrhea. *J Clin Microbiol* 1987;25:1244–1247.

94. Lyerly DM, Barroso LA, Wilkins TD. Identification of the latex test-reactive protein of *Clostridium difficile* as glutamate dehydrogenase. *J Clin Microbiol* 1991;29:2639–2642.

95. Boondeekhun HS, Gurtler V, Odd ML, et al. Detection of *Clostridium difficile* enterotoxin gene in clinical specimens by the polymerase chain reaction. *J Med Microbiol* 1993;38(5):384–387.

96. Kato N, Cy O, Kato H, et al. Detection of toxigenic *Clostridium difficile* in stool specimens by the polymerase chain reaction. *J Clin Micro* 1991;29:343.

97. Gumerlock PH, Tan YJ, Weiss JB, Silva J Jr. Specific detection of toxigenic strains of *Clostridium difficile* in stool specimens. *J Clin Microbiol* 1993;31(3):507–511.

98. Wren BW, Heard SR, Al-Saleh AI, Tabaqchali S. Characterization of *Clostridium difficile* strains by polymerase chain reaction with toxin A- and B-specific primers. *J Med Microbiol* 1993;38(2):109–113.

99. George WL, Sutter VL, Citron D, Finegold SM. Selective and differential medium for isolation of *Clostridium difficile*. *J Clin Microbiol* 1979;9:214.

100. Willey SH, Bartlett JG. Cultures for *Clostridium difficile* in stools containing a cytotoxin neutralized by *Clostridium sordellii* antitoxin. *J Clin Microbiol* 1979;10:880.

101. McFarland LV, Stamm WE. Nosocomial *Clostridium difficile* infections. *N Engl J Med* 1989;321:190.

102. Bartlett JG. The pseudomembranous enterocolitis gastrointestinal disease. In: Sleisenger MH, Fordtran JS, eds. *Gastrointestinal disease*. 4th ed. Philadelphia: WB Saunders; 1989:1307.

103. Boriello SP. *Clostridium difficile* and its toxin in the gastrointestinal tract in health and disease. *Res Clin Forums* 1979;1:33–36.

104. Varki NM, Aquino T. Isolation of *C. difficile* from hospitalized patients without antibiotic-associated diarrhea or colitis. *J Clin Microbiol* 1982;16:659.

105. Asnis DS, Bresciani A, Ryan M, et al. Cost-effective approach to evaluation of diarrheal illness in hospitals. *J Clin Microbiol* 1993;31:1675.

106. Marx CE, Morris A, Wilson ML, Reller LB. Fecal leukocytes in stool specimens submitted for *Clostridium difficile* toxin assay. *Diag Microbiol Infect Dis* 1993;16(4):313–315.

107. Novak E, Lee JE, Seckman CE, et al. Unfavorable effect of atropine-diphenoxylate (Lomotil) therapy in lincomycin-caused diarrhea. *JAMA* 1976;235:1451.

108. Pittman EF. Lomotil and antibiotic colitis. *Ann Intern Med* 1975;83:124.

109. Bartlett JG, Chang TW, Onderdonk AB. Comparison of five regimens of treatment of experimental clindamycin-associated colitis. *J Infect Dis* 1978;138:81–86.

110. Viteri AL, Howard PH, Dyck WP. The spectrum of colitis associated with lincomycin and clindamycin therapy. *J Infect Dis* 1974;131:S1135.

111. Bartlett JG. Treatment of *Clostridium difficile* colitis. *Gastroenterology* 1985;89:1192.

112. Young GP, Ward PB, Bayley N. Antibiotic-associated colitis due to *Clostridium difficile:* double-blind comparison of vancomycin with bacitracin. *Gastroenterology* 1985;89:1038–1045.

113. Dudley MN, McLaughlin JC, Carrington G, et al. Oral bacitracin vs. vancomycin therapy for *Clostridium difficile*–induced diarrhea. *Arch Intern Med* 1986;146:1101.

114. Feketey R, Silva J, Armstrong J, et al. Treatment of antibiotic-associated enterocolitis with vancomycin. *Rev Infect Dis* 1981;3:S273.

115. Bartlett JG, Tedesco FJ, Shull S, et al. Symptomatic relapse after oral vancomycin therapy of antibiotic-associated pseudomembranous colitis. *Gastroenterology* 1980;78:431.

116. Bartlett JG. Treatment of antibiotic-associated pseudomembranous colitis. *Rev Infect Dis* 1984;6:S235.

117. Mogg GAG, Arabi Y, Youngs D, et al. Therapeutic trials of

antibiotic-associated colitis. *Scand J Infect Dis* 1980;23(Suppl): 41.

118. Teasley DG, Olson MM, Gebhard RL, et al. Prospective randomized trial of metronidazole versus vancomycin for *Clostridium difficile*–associated diarrhoea and colitis. *Lancet* 1983;2: 1444.

119. DeLalla F, Nicolin R, Rinaldi E, et al. Prospective study of oral teicoplanin vs oral vancomycin for therapy of pseudomembranous colitis and *Clostridium difficile*–associated diarrhea. *Antimicrob Agents Chemother* 1992;36:2192–2196.

120. Cronberg S, Castor B, Thoren A. Fusidic acid for the treatment of antibiotic-associated colitis induced by *Clostridium difficile*. *Infection* 1984;12:276.

121. Fekety R, Silva J, Kaufman C, et al. Treatment of antibiotic-associated *Clostridium difficile* colitis with oral vancomycin: comparison of two dosage regimens. *Am J Med* 1989;86:15–19.

122. Burdon DW, Brown JD, Youngs D, et al. Antibiotic susceptibility of *Clostridium difficile*. *J Antimicrob Chemother* 1979;5: 307.

123. George WL, Kirby BD, Sutter VL, Finegold SM. Antimicrobial susceptibility of *Clostridium difficile*. In: Schlessinger D, ed. *Microbiology 1979*. Washington DC: American Society for Microbiology; 1979:267–271.

124. George WL, Sutter VL, Finegold SM. Toxicity and antimicrobial susceptibility of *Clostridium difficile*, a cause of antimicrobial agent-associated colitis. *Curr Microbiol* 1978;1:55.

125. Dzink JA, Bartlett JG. In vitro susceptibility of *Clostridium difficile* isolates from patients with antibiotic-associated diarrhea or colitis. *Antimicrob Agents Chemother* 1980;17:695.

126. Shuttleworth R, Taylor M, Jones DM. Antimicrobial susceptibilities of *Clostridium difficile*. *J Clin Pathol* 1980;33:1002.

127. Bolton RP, Culshaw MA. Faecal metronidazole concentrations during oral and intravenous therapy for antibiotic associated colitis due to *Clostridium difficile*. *Gut* 1986;27:1169–1172.

128. Thompson G, Clark AH, Hare K, Spilg WGS. Pseudomembranous colitis after treatment with metronidazole. *Br Med J* 1981; 282:804.

129. Saginur R, Hawley CR, Bartlett JG. Colitis associated with metronidazole therapy. *J Infect Dis* 1980;141:772.

130. Burbige EJ, Milligan FD. Pseudomembranous colitis. *JAMA* 1975;213:1157.

131. Taylor NS, Bartlett JG. Binding of *Clostridium difficile* cytotoxin and vancomycin by anion exchange resins. *J Infect Dis* 1980;141:92.

132. Kreutzer EW, Milligan FD. Treatment of antibiotic-associated pseudomembranous colitis with cholestyramine resin. *Johns Hopkins Med J* 1978;143:67.

133. Tedesco FJ, Napier J, Gamble W, et al. Therapy of antibiotic associated pseudomembranous colitis. *J Clin Gastroenterol* 1979;1:51.

134. Walters BAJ, Roberts R, Stafford R, et al. Relapse of antibiotic associated colitis: endogenous persistence of *Clostridium difficile* during vancomycin therapy. *Gut* 1983;24:206.

135. Onderdonk AB, Cisnoeros RL, Bartlett JG. *Clostridium difficile* in gnotobiotic mice. *Infect Immun* 1980;28:277.

136. Leuong DYM, Kelly CP, Boguniewicz M, et al. Treatment with intravenously administered gamma globulin of chronic relapsing colitis induced by *Clostridium difficile* toxin. *J Pediatr* 1991; 118:633–637.

137. Seal D, Boriello SP, Barclay F, et al. Treatment of relapsing *Clostridium difficile* diarrhoea by administration of a non-toxigenic strain. *Eur J Clin Microbiol* 1987;6:51–53.

138. Bowden TA, Mansberger AR, Lykins LE. Pseudomembranous colitis: mechanism of restoring floral homeostasis. *Amer Surg* 1981;47:178.

139. Schwan A, Sjolin S, Trottestam U, et al. Relapsing *Clostridium difficile* enterocolitis cured by rectal infusion of normal feces. *Scand J Infect Dis* 1984;16:211.

140. Tvede M, Rask-Madsen J. Bacteriotherapy for chronic relapsing *Clostridium difficile* diarrhoea in six patients. *Lancet* 1989; 1:1156.

141. Surawicz CM, Elmer GW, Speelman P, et al. Prevention of antibiotic-associated diarrhea by *Saccharomyces boulardii*: a prospective study. *Gastroenterology* 1989;96:981–988.

142. Elmer GW, FcFarland LV. Suppression by *Saccharomyces boulardii* of toxigenic *Clostridium difficile* overgrowth after vancomycin treatment in hamsters. *Antimicrob Agents Chemother* 1987;31:129–131.

143. Gorbach S, Chang TW, Goldin B. Successful treatment of relapsing *C. difficile* colitis with *Lactobacillus GG*. *Lancet* 1987; 2:1519.

144. Siitonen S, Vapautalo H, Salminen S, et al. Effect of *Lactobacillus GG* yogurt in prevention of antibiotic-associated diarrhea. *Ann Med* 1990;22:57.

145. Buggy BP, Fekety R, Silva J. Therapy of relapsing *Clostridium difficile*–associated diarrhea and colitis with the combination of vancomycin and rifampin. *J Clin Gastroenterol* 1987;9(2): 155–159.

146. Tedesco FJ. Treatment of recurrent antibiotic-associated pseudomembranous colitis. *Am J Gastroenterol* 1982;77:220.

147. Silva J, Lezzi C. *Clostridium difficile* as a nosocomial pathogen. *J Hosp Infect II* 1988;(Suppl A):378.

148. Johnson S, Gerding DN, Olson MM, et al. Prospective, controlled study of vinyl glove use to interrupt *Clostridium difficile* nosocomial transmission. *Am J Med* 1990;88:137.

149. Bender BS, Laughon BE, Gaydos G, et al. Is *Clostridium difficile* endemic in chronic care facilities? *Lancet* 1986;2:11.

150. Delmee M, Vandercam B, Avesani V, Michaux JL. Epidemiology and prevention of *Clostridium difficile* infections in a leukemia unit. *Eur J Clin Microbiol* 1987;6:623.

151. Johnson S, Clabots CR, Linn FV, et al. Nosocomial *Clostridium difficile* colonisation and disease. *Lancet* 1990;336:97.

152. Fekety R, Kim KH, Brown D, et al. Epidemiology of antibiotic-associated colitis. *Am J Med* 1981;70:906–908.

153. Mulligan ME, Rolfe RD, Finegold SM, George WL. Contamination of a hospital environment by *Clostridium difficile*. *Curr Microbiol* 1979;3:173–175.

154. Clabots CR, Johnson S, Olson MM, et al. Acquisition of *Clostridium difficile* by hospitalized patients: evidence for colonized new admissions as a source of infection. *J Infect Dis* 1992;166: 561–567.

155. McFarland LV, Surawicz CM, Stamm WE. Risk factors for *Clostridium difficile*–associated diarrhea in a cohort of hospitalized patients. *J Infect Dis* 1990;162:678–684.

156. Wust J, Sullivan NM, Gardegger U, Wilkins TD. Investigation of an outbreak of antibiotic-associated colitis by various typing methods. *J Clin Microbiol* 1982;16:1096.

157. Pantosti A, Cerquetti M, Gianfrilli PM. Electrophoretic characterization of *Clostridium difficile* strains isolated from antibiotic-associated colitis and other conditions. *J Clin Microbiol* 1988;26:3:540.

158. Mulligan ME, Halebian S, Kwok RYY, et al. Bacterial agglutination and polyacrylamide get electrophoresis for typing *Clostridium difficile*. *J Infect Dis* 1986;153:267.

159. Tabaqchali S, O'Farrell S, Holland D, Silman R. Typing scheme for *Clostridium difficile*: its application in clinical and epidemiological studies. *Lancet* 1984;1:935.

160. Kuijper EJ, Oudbier JH, Stuifbergen WNHM, et al. Application of whole-cell DNA restriction endonuclease profiles to the epidemiology of *Clostridium difficile*–induced diarrhea. *J Clin Microbiol* 1987;25:751.

161. McFarland LV, Elmer GW, Stamm WE and Mulligan ME. Correlation of immunoblot type, enterotoxin production, and cytotoxin production with clinical manifestations of *Clostridium difficile* infection in a cohort of hospitalized patients. *Infect Immun* 1991;59:2456.

162. Johnson S, Homann SR, Bettin KM, et al. Treatment of asymptomatic *Clostridium difficile* carriers (fecal excretors) with vancomycin or metronidazole. *Ann Intern Med* 1992;117:297–302.

Infections of the Gastrointestinal Tract,
edited by M. J. Blaser, P. D. Smith, J. I. Ravdin,
H. B. Greenberg, and R. L. Guerrant
Raven Press, Ltd., New York © 1995.

CHAPTER 60

Aeromonas, Plesiomonas, and *Edwardsiella*

J. Michael Janda, Sharon L. Abbott, and J. Glenn Morris, Jr.

AEROMONAS

Description

Aeromonads are gram-negative, oxidase-positive bacteria that are presently included in the family Vibrionaceae along with two other genera pathogenic for humans (*Vibrio, Plesiomonas*). Although their existence has been known for over a century and their association with infectious processes in lower vertebrates recognized since the early 1900s, their role in causing illnesses in humans has only been recently appreciated (1). Some of the earliest studies of human illnesses attributed to members of the genus *Aeromonas* are the report of Rossner (2) describing a case of *Aeromonas*-associated gastroenteritis and the seminal review of von Graevenitz and Mensch (3) highlighting 30 cases of *Aeromonas* and *Plesiomonas* isolation from intestinal and extraintestinal sites in man. The role of *Aeromonas* as a cause of wound infections and septicemia in susceptible hosts is now well recognized (Table 1). Controversy still surrounds its role as a cause of gastroenteritis. Recent epidemiological studies suggest that the organism is indeed a pathogen, at least in certain settings; however, it likely that not all *Aeromonas* strains are able to cause illness, based on negative results obtained in volunteer studies.

Aeromonas species are routinely isolated from soil and freshwater samples. Though not as common as vibrios in the marine environment, aeromonads can be recovered from estuaries and on occasions from marine life such as shellfish. Ecological surveys in the late 1970s found *Aeromonas* species in virtually every freshwater source in the United States with the exception of hot springs

J. M. Janda and S. L. Abbott: Microbial Diseases Laboratory, Division of Communicable Disease Control, California Department of Health Services, Berkeley, California 94704-1011.

J. G. Morris, Jr.: Department of Veterans Affairs, Divisions of Geographic Medicine and Infectious Diseases, University of Maryland School of Medicine, Baltimore, Maryland 21201.

(4). Aeromonad densities peak during the summer months when warmer water temperatures lead to increased numbers of these microorganisms. This may lead to the introduction of aeromonads into fresh produce, meat products (beef, poultry, pork), and dairy (raw milk, ice cream) via contaminated water (5,6). The isolation of *Aeromonas* species from such a large number of foods and environmental sources, particularly during summer, has made it difficult to link *Aeromonas*-associated gastroenteritis to specific food vehicles or ecological niches.

The paramount association between *Aeromonas* and diseases of animals has concerned the fishing industry (7). Strains of *Aeromonas* that grow better at lower temperatures (25°C), termed psychrophilic strains, have been definitively linked to severe infections in fish such as furunculosis and motile *Aeromonas* septicemia. The fishing industry, particularly salmon and catfish farms, suffered enormous economic losses due to this genus. In addition, many sporadic cases or outbreaks of infection in a variety of animals have been reported over the past several decades; these include illnesses in frogs, pigs, cattle, birds, and marine animals such as seals and dolphins.

Probably the greatest difficulty in understanding the role of aeromonads in human disease concerns its taxonomy (1). Recent phylogenetic investigations indicate that members of the genus *Aeromonas* are not closely related to their phenotypically similar counterparts, the Vibrionaceae. This has lead to several proposals to remove *Aeromonas* from this family and to possibly establish these organisms in a family of their own, the Aeromonadaceae. For the present, they remain in the family Vibrionaceae. In regard to species designations, strains of *Aeromonas* were originally grouped together as *A. hydrophila*. Over the intervening years, it became apparent that psychrophilic strains that were associated with fish diseases were physiologically and biochemically distinct from mesophilic (grown at 37°C) strains and the former group became known as *A. salmonicida*. Then, in the mid- to late 1970s work by Popoff and others indicated that the genus was much more complex than previously believed (8,9). By virtue of these studies and those of Brenner and his

TABLE 1. Aeromonas, Plesiomonas, *and* Edwardsiella
species of potential medical significance

Genus and species	Disease associations
Aeromonas	
A. hydrophila	Gastroenteritis, wound infections, bacteremia, peritonitis, osteomyelitis
A. caviae	Gastroenteritis, bacteremia
A. veronii	Gastroenteritis, bacteremia, wound infections, peritonitis
A. schubertii	Wound infections, bacteremia
A. jandaei	Gastroenteritis, wound infections, bacteremia
A. trota	Gastroenteritis
Plesiomonas	
P. shigelloides	Gastroenteritis, bacteremia/meningitis
Edwardsiella	
E. tarda	Gastroenteritis, wound infections, abscesses, bacteremia

colleagues at the Centers for Disease Control (CDC) using DNA–DNA hybridization more than 13 species are now known to exist (10,11) (Table 1). Most of these species are named and can be identified by simple albeit extensive batteries of biochemical tests. Of particular importance to clinical disease is the fact that several molecular studies on the clinical distribution of *Aeromonas* have found that three species, represented by DNA hybridization groups (HGs) 1 (*A. hydrophila*), 4 (*A. caviae*), and 8 (*A. veronii* biotype *sobria*), account for >85% of all human infections (10–12). Whether this implies enhanced pathogenicity of these species for humans or relates to their predominance in nature is presently unknown since comparable studies of environmental strains have not yet been reported.

Microbiology

Morphological and Cultural Characteristics

Aeromonads are typical gram-negative, facultatively anaerobic bacilli measuring 1–3 μm in length by 0.3–1.0 μm in width; some studies indicate that *Aeromonas* strains may be encapsulated (10). Most aeromonads grow well on selective media such as MacConkey and Hektoen enteric (HE) agars and on nonselective media such as blood, nutrient, or heart infusion agars where they are buff in appearance; some strains elaborate a melanin-like pigment that produces a brownish discoloration to the agar surface. Such pigment-producing strains are most commonly associated with environmental species that infect fish, such as *A. salmonicida,* certain biogroups of *A. media,* and hybridization group 2 (HG2) isolates, a presently unnamed *Aeromonas* group that is most often recovered from animals and water sources.

Structural Features

Most aeromonads are motile via a single polar flagellum (Fig. 1). Pili, when present, can be of one of two morpho-

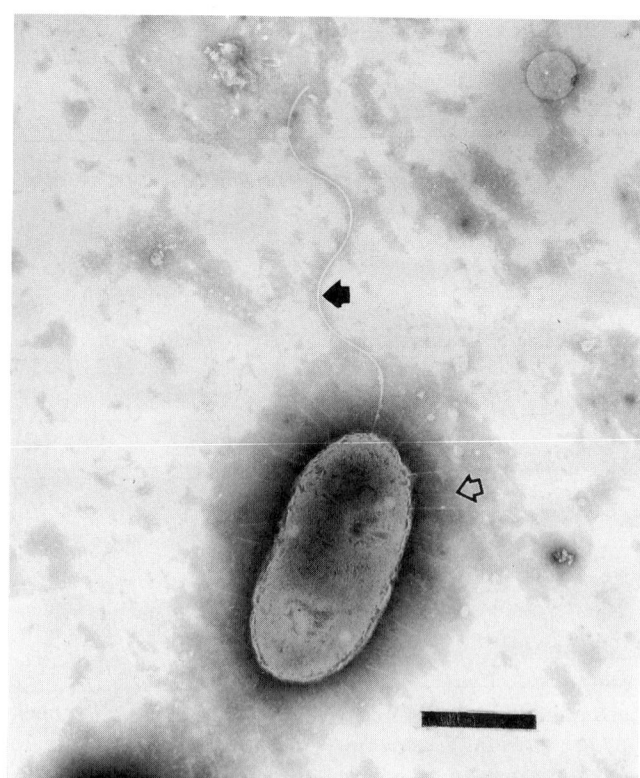

FIG. 1. Electron micrograph (negative stain) of *Aeromonas* with polar flagella (*solid arrow*) and numerous pili (*open arrow*); bar represents 1 μm.

logical varieties (rigid, flexible). Recently, several different *Aeromonas* species (*A. hydrophila, A. veronii*) in addition to *A. salmonicida* have been shown to possess a regular paracrystalline surface (or S) layer that is external to the outer membrane and is composed of protein subunits. These strains can be phenotypically recognized by their ability to autoagglutinate or aggregate in broth after boiling (12). Aeromonads also display 30–40 distinct whole-cell proteins by sodium dodecyl sulfate–polyacrylamide electrophoresis (SDS-PAGE); at least four to five major outer membrane proteins can be recognized in most isolates (13). The lipopolysaccharide (LPS) consists of a ladder-like construction of side chains as detected by PAGE and by silver staining, typical of gram-negative enteric organisms such as *Escherichia coli* and *Salmonella;* many different antigenic variations in LPS composition exist (14).

Biochemical Characteristics and Enzymatic Properties

One of the most interesting aspects of *Aeromonas* physiology is the vast array of substrates that the genus can utilize (15). Many isolates can ferment diverse groups of carbohydrates such as mono- and disaccharides, trisaccharides, and alcohol sugars. Their enzymatic machinery also is substantial since they elaborate >20 different extracellular enzymes including hemolysins, proteases,

TABLE 2. *Separation of pathogenic genera in the family* Vibrionaceae

| Characteristic | Vibrio | | Aeromonas | Plesiomonas |
	Nonhalophilic	Halophilic		
Growth on TCBS	+	+	−	−
Growth 0% NaCl	+	−	+	+
Growth 6% NaCl	+	+	−	−
O/129 (10 μg)	S[a]	V	R	S
O/129 (150 μg)	S[a]	V	R	S
String test	+	+	−	−
Ornithine decarboxylase	+	V	−[b]	+
Glucose (gas)	−	−[b]	+[b]	−

S, susceptible; V, variable (species-dependent); R, resistant.
[a] An increasing number of *V. cholerae* O1 and non-O1 strains are becoming resistant.
[b] For most species.

DNase, RNase, gelatinase, elastase, chitinase, amylase, chondroitinase, esterase, and fibrinolysin.

Possibly one of the most difficult identifications in the clinical laboratory involves the correct genus assignment of isolates phenotypically belonging to the family Vibrionaceae. This problem is particularly acute in regard to the separation of *Aeromonas* from nonhalophilic *Vibrio* species due to the emergence of *Vibrio cholerae* in Southeast Asia that are resistant to the vibriostatic agent O/129; this strain was recently introduced into the United States. In addition to this dilemma is the problem of phenotypically distinguishing *Aeromonas caviae* from *Vibrio fluvialis* (1). While aeromonads by far predominate over vibrios in clinical specimens in the United States, their actual laboratory identification is often incorrect (aeromonads

are misidentified as vibrios). Strains belonging to this family should be screened by a variety of biochemical techniques (salt tolerance, resistance to the vibriostatic agent O/129, string test, gas from glucose, growth on TCBS) to ensure their appropriate genus assignment (Table 2). For difficult strains or those possessing unusual properties, supplementary tests may be required.

Biochemical Identification and Species Designation

Because of the inherent taxonomic complexity of the genus *Aeromonas* and the large number of species found in association with human disease it is technically impractical to identify all such isolates to the genomospecies level

TABLE 3. *Major features of* Aeromonas *species associated with human disease*

	A. hydrophila[a]	A. caviae	A. veronii	A. jandaei	A. schubertii
DNA group	1	4	8,10	9	12
Phenospecies designation	hydrophila[b]	caviae	sobria	sobria	sobria
No. biotypes	1	1	2[c]	1	1
Biochemical:					
Lysine decarboxylase	+[d]	−	+	+	+
Ornithine decarboxylase	−	−	−	−	−
Arginine dihydrolase	+	+	+	+	+
Voges–Proskauer	+	−	+	+	+
Esculin	+	+	−	−	−
Arabinose	+	+	−	−	−
Salicin	+	+	−	−	−
Glucose (gas)	+	−	+	+	−
Sucrose	+	+	+	−	−
Mannitol	+	+	+	+	−
Disease Associations:					
Gastroenteritis	+ + +[e]	+ + +	+ + +	+	−
Wound infections	+ + +	+	+ +	+	+ +
Bacteremia	+ + +	+	+ + +	+	+ +

[a] Genomospecies (actual species identity) as determined by molecular assays or extensive biochemical methods.
[b] Phenospecies (a group of genetically distinct species that are phenotypically similar) as determined by a limited number of biochemical tests.
[c] Reactions are for the predominant clinical biotype (*sobria*); biotype *veronii* is ODC+.
[d] +, >85% positive; −, >85% negative.
[e] Relative association of individual species with disease process.

on a routine basis (Table 3). A further obstacle is the fact that many of the best tests for distinguishing among different *Aeromonas* species involve unusual phenotypic properties and are not included in most commercial identification systems. However, several approaches are possible. At a minimum, *Aeromonas* strains should be identified to phenospecies (a group of genetically distinct species that cannot be separated biochemically) level; this approach would result in the identification of >90% of all aeromonads as either *A. hydrophila*, *A. caviae*, and *A. sobria* (16). The number of tests required for such identification is small, usually five to six tests. Dichotomic approaches to such identifications were recently published (17). A rationale for such identifications stems from the higher likelihood of *A. hydrophila* and *A. sobria* as opposed to *A. caviae* to disseminate from the bowel of immunocompromised individuals and the association of enterotoxigenicity with phenotypic markers of these two species (hemolysin, lysine decarboxylase, Voges Proskauer). For the description of unusual cases for the medical literature, definitive genomospecies identification should be attempted, which normally requires more than 20 biochemical tests to be performed (18). At present, none of the currently available miniaturized or semi- to fully automated microbial identification systems from commercial suppliers have the inherent capacity to identify aeromonads to the correct species although individual biochemical tests in these panels may be useful in such identifications.

Isolation Methods

Aeromonads grow well on most selective and differential agars commonly used for fecal workups such as MacConkey, HE, xylose–lysine–deoxycholate, desoxycholate, and blood agars. Since some strains (or species) such as *A. hydrophila* and *A. veronii* have poor plating efficiencies on one or more selective media, a nonselective agar (such as blood) should be included in fecal workups to ensure recovery of aeromonads during the acute phase of an illness. Another problem relates to the fact that many strains of *Aeromonas* are sucrose-positive and some species (such as *A. caviae*) are lactose-positive (e.g., on MacConkey) making certain media, like HE, unsuitable for their recovery. Blood agar, with or without 20–30 µg/mL of ampicillin (to which most aeromonads are resistant), has gained favor as a common media to isolate these bacteria from diarrheal specimens (19). Blood agar has the additional advantage that individual colonies can be screened for oxidase and indole positivity directly. One recent finding is that one of the recently described species, *Aeromonas trota* (Table 1), is ampicillin-susceptible and therefore will not be isolated on ampicillin-containing media (20). It also has been suggested by in vitro susceptibility data that 5–10% of all aeromonads are susceptible to ampicillin and are likely to be missed. If blood agar is not used, lactose-negative colonies can be picked and screened to Kliger's iron agar (KIA) or triple sugar iron agar (TSI) and urea slants and subsequently worked up if appropriate reactions are recorded. Cefsulodin–irga-

san–novobiocin agar (CIN), commonly used to isolate *Yersinia enterocolitica* in the laboratory, also has been shown to be useful for the isolation of many *Aeromonas* strains (21). In our experience this medium gives results comparable to, or better than, ampicillin–sheep blood agar and its routine use in fecal exams may be warranted if the suspected incidence of *Yersinia enterocolitica* and *Aeromonas* species is sufficiently high to justify inclusion.

During the acute phase of the diarrheal illness isolation of aeromonads in a diagnostic setting should not be a difficult task since moderate to large numbers (10^4–10^{10}/g feces) of these bacteria should be present in the fecal specimens. However, after the peak of the gastrointestinal illness or in cases of subacute or chronic diarrhea, *Aeromonas* may be overlooked if enrichment procedures are not included. Both gram-negative and Selenite-F broths, primarily used for the recovery of *Salmonella* and *Shigella*, also can be used to enrich for aeromonads present in the sample; alkaline peptone water (APW, pH 8.5), used in the isolation of pathogenic *Vibrio* species, is also an excellent enrichment medium for the isolation of mesophilic aeromonads. Such enrichment broths may then be plated onto any of a number of media listed above to isolate *Aeromonas*. It should be noted, however, that concerns have been raised about the clinical significance of *Aeromonas* strains that are present in such low numbers that they can only be isolated with enrichment techniques.

Epidemiology

Although the association of *Aeromonas* with gastroenteritis is still somewhat controversial, experimental, clinical, and epidemiological evidence continues to lend credence to the assertion that at least certain strains (and maybe species) are etiologically involved in diarrheal illness (22). The highest attack rate appears to be in young children, particularly those under 3 years of age (23). These data may be somewhat misleading since children are probably more likely to require medical attention for gastrointestinal disease than adults. *Aeromonas* infections at any site are more likely to occur during the warmer months of the year (24) and the same seasonality of *Aeromonas*-associated gastroenteritis has been previously noted (25–27). The frequency of isolation of *Aeromonas* has ranged from a low of 0.7–0.9% in specimens submitted to reference public health laboratories or local hospitals in the Netherlands and France to a high of 50% in infants in Peruvian studies (28); the extremely high frequency with which *Aeromonas* was isolated from infants in this later study (28) is complicated by the fact that in at least 50% of these fecal specimens at least one additional coinfecting pathogen was present. Some of this variation may be due either to differences in sanitary conditions or to socioeconomic factors (such as diet) as reports from Japan (11%), Bali (15%), and the Ivory Coast (24%) tend toward higher isolation rates of this organism. Most U.S. studies have indicated an isolation rate of from 2.5–7.1%, depending on the study population, geographic location, and time of year in which *Aeromonas* was sought. Although vehicles of infection are poorly defined, one epidemiological survey by the CDC has linked the consumption of untreated well water to gastrointestinal infections with aeromonads (29) while in another retrospective survey both untreated water and prior antibiotic therapy were reported as risk factors for infection (24). Molecular analysis of fecal isolates of *Aeromonas* from symptomatic persons indicate that of more than ten named species, HG1 (*A. hydrophila*), HG4 (*A. caviae*), and HG8 (*A. veronii*), account for the vast majority of isolates (10–12,27).

Recent case-control investigations have shown a significant association between the isolation of *Aeromonas* on primary media and the presence of gastrointestinal symptoms (Table 4). In many of these studies, *Aeromonas* has ranked high on the list of reputed enteropathogens (28). Besides epidemiological reports, several studies have documented an immune response to gastrointestinal infection by *Aeromonas* in selected individuals or as part of cohort studies using a variety of techniques including enzyme-linked immunosorbent assay (ELISA) and immunoblotting (37–39). Kuijper et al. (37) evaluated the serum immune response in individuals with presumed acute or chronic gastroenteritis due to *Aeromonas* in individuals with diarrhea due to other recognized enteric pathogens and in healthy controls. Results significantly differed depending on the immunological assay used, which included ELISA (30% sensitivity, 74% specificity) and cytotoxin neutralization assays (46% sensitivity, 94% specificity). Positive ELISA results correlated with IgM and IgG responses to LPSs of homologous *Aeromonas* strains; tube agglutination tests were deemed unsatisfactory. Subsequent to this study, a fourfold rise in the fecal sIgA immune response (day 0 and day 5) to *Aeromonas* was detected in 11 of 12 U.S. students who developed diarrhea while in Mexico during summer studies (38); this immune response could be inhibited by preabsorption of the patient's fecal extract with the homologous strain. The major immune response appeared to be directed against the higher molecular weight bacterial LPS. Most recently, a specific IgG response to whole-cell proteins of an S layer–positive strain of *A. veronii* was observed in a 24-year-old-female suffering from ulcerative colitis (39); in addition to demonstration of the immune response, the infecting strain was isolated from feces and from the small intestine (in pure culture). An immune response to both the enterotoxin and cytolysin of an *A. veronii* strain associated with cholera-like diarrhea in a Thai woman has been previously reported (40). The effects of both microbial toxins on human embryonic fibroblasts and mouse Y1 adrenal tumor cells could be completely inhibited by the patient's acute (1:40) and convalescent (1:1280) phase sera. Gracey and colleagues (25,41) also found a significant higher rate of isolation of enterotoxigenic *Aeromonas* spp. (10.8%) from cases of diarrhea vs. controls (0.7%) in an epidemiological investigation of over 900 nonaboriginal Australian children. There also have been a number of cases of gastroenteritis (42) in which resolution of symptoms has been accompanied by the disappearance of aeromonads from feces following therapy with agents that were specifically directed against this group.

Despite these data, a number of troubling aspects regarding the association between *Aeromonas* and diarrhea remain unresolved. In contrast to other water- and food-borne pathogens, no clearly defined outbreaks of diarrheal illness due to *Aeromonas* have ever been reported (even though the organism is a frequent isolate from water, food, and other environmental sources). While many epidemiological studies have linked isolation of *Aeromonas* from stool with occurrence of disease, there are studies in which isolation rates of *Aeromonas* among

TABLE 4. *Recent investigations on the epidemiology of* Aeromonas-*associated gastroenteritis*

Country	Study design[a]	Population	*Aeromonas* isolated from:		Rank[b]	Major species	Ref.
			Symptomatic	Asymptomatic			
Nigeria	Active, clinic, unmatched	All ages	53/2350 (2.6%)[c]	2/5000 (4%)	2	ND	30
Djibouti	Active, community, matched	All ages	7/209 (3.3%)	0/100 (0%)	5[d]	ND	31
Israel	Active, hospital, unmatched	All ages	17/1005 (1.7%)	0/500 (0%)	ND	*A. veronii*	32
Peru	Active, hospital, unmatched	Infants <18 mo	205/391 (52.4%)	12/138 (8.7%)	1	*A. caviae*	28
Saudi Arabia	Passive, hospital, unmatched	All ages	58/15548 (0.4%)	0/1368 (0%)	4	ND	33
England	Active, hospital, unmatched	Children	2.5%[e]	ND	1	*A. caviae*	34
United States	Active, hospital, unmatched	Children	14/321 (3.2%)	2/380 (0.5%)	4	*A. caviae*	35
United States	Active, clinic, matched	Children <2 yr	15/246 (6%)	11/155 (7%)	1	*A. hydrophila*	43
Japan	Active, hospital, unmatched	Adults	29/262 (11.1%)	202/9104 (2.2%)	ND	*A. caviae*	6
India	Active, hospital, matched	All ages	45/2480 (1.8%)	0/512 (0%)	4	*A. hydrophila*	36

ND, not determined; AV, *Aeromonas veronii*; AC, *Aeromonas caviae*; AH, *Aeromonas hydrophila*.

[a] Type of surveillance, type of institution where study was conducted, and whether or not the controls were matched to the cases.

[b] Rank in frequency of *Aeromonas* among known bacterial enteropathogens in indicated survey.

[c] Number positive for *Aeromonas*/sample number (percent positive).

[d] Tie.

[e] Includes both symptomatic and asymptomatic individuals (not separated).

asymptomatic controls have been equal to or greater than rates of isolation among case patients (43), suggesting that *Aeromonas* could simply be a nonpathogenic "fellow traveler." Immune responses after infection do not prove pathogenicity: for example, in volunteer studies with non-O1 *V. cholerae*, immune responses were seen with strains that colonized the intestine but did not cause illness (44). Finally, volunteer studies have failed to establish *Aeromonas* spp. as bonafide enteropathogens despite the fact that high challenge doses were used (45). In summary, while the majority of evidence supports a role for aeromonads in diarrheal disease, there are still significant obstacles in unequivocally establishing which *Aeromonas* strains are genuine enteric pathogens.

Pathogenesis and Immunity

It is likely that aeromonads gain entry to the digestive tract via the ingestion of contaminated food or water. Although most affected persons appear to have normal immune and physiological mechanisms operative in the gut, George et al. (27) found that 30% of patients with *Aeromonas* infections had evidence of reduced or absent gastric acidity.

Attention has recently focused on potential colonization factors and enterotoxigenic molecules produced by *Aeromonas* (46) and their presumed relationship to intestinal disease. *Aeromonas* species have been shown to produce two morphologically distinct types of pili, termed straight (rigid) and flexible (wavy, curvilinear). Both molecules have a diameter of ~7–10 nm; the rigid pili are more numerous on the bacterial cell surface. However flexible pili bind to both human and rabbit intestine and agglutinate erythrocytes while rigid pili do not. The flexible minipilin (fxp) of Ho et al. (47) shows 91% amino acid sequence similarity to the core encoded pilin (cep) of *V. cholerae*, a molecule thought to play a role in intestinal colonization and associated with the core region of the CTX genetic element (48). Expression of this flexible pilin appears to be environmentally regulated by such factors as temperature and iron availability.

Enterotoxins also may play a role in the gastrointestinal pathophysiology of *Aeromonas*. Despite the fact that several different enterotoxins have been described, only one has been characterized to any significant extent. This enterotoxin, commonly referred to as the β-hemolysin or aerolysin, is a heat-labile protein that actively induces fluid accumulation in the gut of infant mice or in rabbit ileal loops (49). The aerolysin has been analyzed for amino acid sequence homology with other known bacterial toxins; it contains only two small regions of homology, one with the α toxin of *Staphylococcus aureus* and the other hemolysin (hly A) of *Escherichia coli* (50). Although there are immunologically and biochemically distinct versions of this molecule, most strains of *A. hydrophila* and *A. veronii* recovered from the feces of persons with diarrhea appear to produce this toxin (46); little is known about environmental strains. Some strains of *Aeromonas* produce a cytotonic enterotoxin (51). A cytolytic enterotoxin previously reported by Houston and colleagues (52) that cross-reacts with cholera toxin appears identical to the aerolysin molecule by N-terminal sequence analysis. Mesophilic aeromonads appear capable of invading tissue culture cells such as HEp-2 (53); however, these studies are difficult to evaluate since the potent β-hemolysin liberated by most isolates is cytotoxic to eukaryotic cell lines and masks any invasive characteristics of such strains.

Clinical Illness

Gastrointestinal illnesses caused by members of the genus *Aeromonas* span the spectrum of symptoms and syndromes associated with other classic bacterial enteric pathogens. *Aeromonas* spp. have been associated with several distinctive clinical syndromes, including (a) acute, watery diarrhea; (b) dysentery; and (c) subacute or chronic diarrhea (1). The acute, secretory diarrhea syndrome is most commonly described. The fecal specimen is typically loose in consistency and watery in appearance without the presence of red blood cells or leukocytes; mucus is occasionally observed (15–20%). The frequency of diarrhea in patients with this form ranges from 1 to 20 bowel movements a day (mean ~5–7). In most studies of pediatric patients with *Aeromonas*-associated gastroenteritis, watery diarrhea occurs at frequencies of 60–70% (24,54–56). Common symptoms associated with this type of gastroenteritis include abdominal pain (60–70%), fever (20–40%), nausea (40%), and vomiting (20–40%). Fever may exceed 39°C in some children (54). Approximately 10–15% of children with watery diarrhea from whom *Aeromonas* is isolated are coinfected with at least one other enteric pathogen. While this infection is usually self-limited (mean duration of <7 days), between 30% and 40% of children with secretory gastroenteritis may require hospitalization due to dehydration or persistent diarrhea (54,56). The most common *Aeromonas* species isolated in most of these studies is *A. caviae*. Some of these children experience additional complications subsequent to their diarrheal episodes including failure to thrive, gram-negative sepsis, and hemolytic-uremic syndrome (55). On rare occasions profuse, cholera-like diarrhea has been reported in association with *A. veronii* infections (1). Far fewer studies on adults with *Aeromonas*-induced secretory diarrhea have been reported. The acute, secretory form in adults appears similar to that seen in children with abdominal pain (60%), fever (20%), and nausea (20%) prominent symptoms (27); most of these infections are community-acquired with the mean duration of illness lasting 11 days. Half of these adults have fecal leukocytes in their stools and 15% harbor multiple enteric pathogens (27). In approximately 15–25% of all cases of *Aeromonas*-associated gastroenteritis a dysenteric-like illness resembling shigellosis occurs. Cardinal features of this infection include intense abdominal pain, bloody diarrhea, and mucus with fecal polymorphonuclear leukocytes; fever, nausea, and vomiting sometimes may be present. Particularly in children, the fulminant course of this illness can require hospitalization. Many persons who develop this type of diarrheal syndrome are initially suspected of having ulcerative, diffuse, or segmental colitis (57). In some instances, colonoscopy shows superficial ulceration, erythema, and friability of the mucosa (58) with biopsy revealing crypt abscesses and active colitis (57). One study has linked acute colitis caused by *Aeromonas* to chronic colonic inflammation that develops months to years later (59). A third manifestation of the infection is a subacute to chronic or intermittent condition in which the symptoms can persist for months to years (60). Although symptoms may vary, the chief complaint involves a simple nonresolving diarrhea that occurs at sporadic intervals.

Aside from the above-noted associations, there is not a clear correlation between any one species or HG and specific clinical manifestations. There also are conflicting data on the role of putative virulence factors, such as enterotoxins, in illness; some investigations have reported a strong link between occurrence of diarrheal disease and enterotoxin production (41), while others have found enterotoxin production among strains from both cases and asymptomatic controls (61).

Aeromonas species also cause a number of extraintestinal illnesses including wound infections and septicemia. Wound infections most commonly occur when freshwater sources that contain aeromonads come in contact with integument (62). Symptoms in such infected persons may range from a mild cellulitis to myonecrosis; those with more severe disease, especially when accompanied by positive blood cultures, have a much poorer prognosis. *Aeromonas* septicemia is most commonly observed in immunocompromised persons including those with hepatobiliary disease (e.g., cirrhosis), hematological malignancies, or solid tumors (1). On rare occasions *Aeromonas* sepsis has been noted in previously healthy or nonimmunocompromised persons. Fatality rates range from 30% to 50% in most surveys.

Diagnosis

Laboratory diagnosis of *Aeromonas* infections is primarily dependent on the isolation of aeromonads by culture. During the acute phase of a gastrointestinal illness, aeromonads should be present in moderate to large numbers (10^6–10^8 CFU/g feces). If aeromonads are suspected as the causative agent of subacute or chronic diarrhea, both enrichment cultures and selective media specifically designed for the isolation of *Aeromonas* may be required due to fluctuating bacterial concentrations. In the latter situations, the simple isolation of *Aeromonas* from feces is not sufficient to identify the cause of the infection. Rather, additional tests need to be performed such as tissue biopsy (for culture and the presence of bacilli in histological sections) and/or immunological investigations (immunoblots for fecal sIgA or serum IgM or IgG immune responses to the infecting strain). Several recent studies have detected specific immune responses to *Aeromonas* in the context of intestinal infections by finding sIgA responses directed against LPS components (38) or an immune response to whole-cell or outer membrane proteins of the homologous strain (37,39). Tube agglutination titers are less reliable since many healthy persons appear to possess antibody titers against *Aeromonas* (29).

In potential outbreaks in which multiple isolates of *Aeromonas* are isolated from different persons, relatedness of these isolates can be determined by a number of techniques. By far the simplest and least expensive method is to biochemically determine the genomospecies designation of each isolate (18); because aeromonads are so phenotypically diverse, such testing may also allow distinguishing between strains of the same species by biotype (15). If more advanced methods are required, serogrouping performed by one of several international reference centers would be practical (63,64). All aeromonads, regardless of species designation, fall into over 90 distinct serogroups based on the presence of unique somatic antigens; the likelihood that two given strains in the same outbreak would belong to the same species and have the same biotype and serogroup are extremely remote unless they are related. Present information indicates that no single serogroup accounts for more than 10–20% of all clinical strains so typed. Strains may also be distinguished by a variety of molecular methods including ribotyping, multilocus enzyme electrophoresis, and restriction endonuclease analysis (65–67); one recent case of *Aeromonas* gastroenteritis was traced to contaminated shrimp cocktail by the use of ribotyping (68). Plasmid analysis is not a useful technique since most strains (>70%) do not carry plasmids or lose them quickly upon subculture.

Treatment

Antimicrobial Susceptibility

Despite the fact that a major study on the susceptibility of *Aeromonas* spp. has not been undertaken since the advent of many newer species, aeromonads display a great consistency in their in vitro susceptibility profile (69–73). Most *Aeromonas* species are normally susceptible to tetracyclines, aminoglycosides, trimethoprim-sulfamethoxazole, third-generation cephalosporins and their analogs, and the quinolones (Table 5), but most (except *A. trota*) are resistant to ampicillin. For the first- and second-generation cephalosporins, results are variable and in some cases species-related (54). Nearly all aeromonads produce inducible β-lactamases, which may account for some therapeutic failures (74).

Treatment

The mainstay of therapy in *Aeromonas*-associated gastroenteritis, as in any diarrheal disease, is rehydration, via the oral or intravenous route. There are no controlled trials of antimicrobial therapy in *Aeromonas* gastroenteritis. Illness is usually self-limited, and previously healthy persons with acute illness who are not treated with antimicrobial agents appear to do well, with rapid resolution of symptoms and clearance of the organism from stool; there is no a priori reason to treat such cases. At the same time, there is no contraindication to antimicrobial therapy, and no indication that therapy prolongs intestinal carriage of the organism (29); there also are anecdotal reports that

TABLE 5. *In vitro susceptibility of* Aeromonas *phenospecies to selected antimicrobial agents*

Antibiotic	A. hydrophila		A. veronii		A. caviae	
	MIC$_{50}$[a]	MIC$_{90}$	MIC$_{50}$	MIC$_{90}$	MIC$_{50}$	MIC$_{90}$
Ampicillin	≥16–64	≥16–128	≥16–128	≥16–128	≥16–64	≥16–128
Carbenicillin	128	≥512	256	≥512	32	256
Piperacillin	2	4	0.5	32	2	8
Cephalothin	≥32	≥32	≤2	≥32	≥32	≥32
Cefotaxime	0.05–≤2	0.05–≤2	0.02–≤2	0.02–≤2	0.25–≤2	0.5–≤2
Cefaperazone	≤4	≤4	≤4	≤4	≤4	≤4
Aztreonam	≤0.02	≤0.02	≤0.02	≤0.02	≤0.02–≤0.06	≤0.02–0.25
Imipenem	0.25	1	0.5	1	0.1	0.1
Ciprofloxacin	≤0.01–≤0.06	≤0.01–≤0.06	≤0.01–≤0.06	≤0.01–≤0.06	≤0.01–≤0.06	.05–≤0.06
Gentamicin	≤0.5–1	1–2	≤0.5–1	1–2	≤0.5–2	0.5–4
Amikacin	≤2	≤2	≤2	≤2	≤2	≤2
Tetracycline	0.5–1	≤1–8	0.5–1	≤1–32	≤1–1	≤1–2
Chloramphenicol	0.5–1	0.5–4	0.5–1	0.5–4	≤1–2	≤1–4

[a] Minimum inhibitory concentration (MIC) of antibiotic to inhibit 50% (MIC$_{50}$) and 90% (MIC$_{90}$) of the strains tested in various investigations (53–56).

antimicrobial therapy results in "prompt" resolution of symptoms (22,23,29,75).

Data supporting antimicrobial therapy of chronic *Aeromonas*-associated diarrhea, while still anecdotal, are somewhat stronger. George and colleagues (27) documented clinical responses in three patients who had protracted diarrhea (21 days, 28 days, and 6 months, respectively). Similarly, Holmberg et al. (29) reported five patients who took antimicrobial agents to which their *Aeromonas* isolates were susceptible; within an average of 3.4 days all had marked alleviation or resolution of their gastrointestinal symptoms, which had lasted a mean of 47 days before treatment. Based on these observations, it would appear reasonable to administer antimicrobial agents to patients who have positive stool cultures for *Aeromonas* and who have had symptoms for at least 7–10 days. There also are very limited data suggesting that patients who are immunocompromised, who have malignancies or are receiving cancer chemotherapy, or who have underlying hepatobiliary disease have an increased susceptibility to septicemia (1,75). In these settings, it again would appear reasonable to treat affected patients with antimicrobial agents in an effort to minimize the risk of sepsis.

Based on very limited experience, trimethoprim-sulfamethoxazole may be considered as the drug of choice in cases of *Aeromonas* gastroenteritis (23,76). Tetracycline or doxycycline (23) might serve as alternatives in patients with allergies to sulfa drugs; aminoglycosides, such as gentamicin, are indicated in persons with septicemia. Based on antimicrobial susceptibility patterns, the quinolones also should have excellent activity against *Aeromonas* (69) as they do for enteric bacterial pathogens, including species of *Vibrio, Campylobacter, Salmonella, Shigella,* and diarrheagenic *E. coli.* While clinical efficacy data are lacking, ciprofloxacin would be a reasonable choice for emperic therapy before culture results are available.

PLESIOMONAS

Designated strain "C27" in 1947 by Ferguson and Henderson, *Plesiomonas shigelloides* was finally and de-

servedly placed in its own genus in 1962 (77). Although lacking many of the common characteristics associated with vibrios and aeromonads, it remains a member of the family Vibrionaceae; however, recent 5S rRNA sequencing data indicate that reassignment to the Enterobacteriaceae might be more appropriate (78).

Plesiomonas is primarily a freshwater organism with isolation rates increasing during warm months. Fish and shellfish, especially if associated with mud or sediment, frequently harbor plesiomonads; in a survey by Miller and Koburger (79), plesiomonads could be isolated from 58.7% of environmental samples including water, sediment, fish, crabs, and mollusks. *Plesiomonas* can be isolated from the feces of asymptomatic cold-blooded animals and warm-blooded animals including cats and dogs (80,81).

Plesiomonads are straight, facultatively anaerobic, gram-negative rods 0.8–1.0 μm wide to 3.0 μm long. They are motile by means of polar lophotrichous flagella. On noninhibitory media such as heart infusion or blood agar, colonies are nonhemolytic, 1–2 mm, opaque and convex with entire edges. The organism grows on and can be isolated from a variety of common differential or selective agars, generally appearing as a non–lactose-fermenting colony (77). However, approximately 30% of plesiomonads ferment lactose and would be overlooked on these media. Alternatively, colonies on nutrient or blood agar can be screened for oxidase and indole production and if positive tested further. When examining specifically for *Plesiomonas,* inositol–brilliant green–bile salts agar is useful since few enteric bacteria other than *Plesiomonas* can utilize inositol as a carbon source; white colonies with red coloration are likely to contain *Plesiomonas* (82). Enrichment broths are effective in the isolation of *Plesiomonas* from stools; a 1988 study by Rahim and Kay (83) found enrichment using bile peptone broth (BPB) or alkaline peptone broth to be superior to direct plating; 24-hr enrichment in BPB yielded 30 positive specimens vs. 5 by direct plating only (*n* = 423).

Once isolated, *P. shigelloides* is easily identified and separated from other Vibrionaceae and members of the Enterobacteriaceae. Key characteristics include positive oxidase, lysine and ornithine decarboxylase, and arginine dihydrolase activities; fermentation of inositol; lack of gas production from glucose; and susceptibility to O/129. As its name implies, *P. shigelloides* may antigenically cross-react with *Shigella,* most frequently with *S. sonnei* (84). Patients whose strains possess cross-reacting antigens do not necessarily have longer or more severe gastrointestinal illnesses (85).

Despite findings of little or no *P. shigelloides* enteropathogenicity in animal and human volunteer studies (86) and an inability to induce an sIgA immune response in colonized or infected students (38), there also is evidence to suggest a role as an enteropathogen (77). A pathogenic role is supported by a lessening in the severity and duration of symptoms by appropriate antibiotic therapy, an extremely low asymptomatic carriage rate (<0.1%) in humans, and outbreaks of diarrheal disease associated with contaminated water and oysters containing *Plesiomonas* (87,88). In two of these outbreaks reported from Japan (87), predominant serotypes (O17:H2, O22:H3) epidemiologically linked to each outbreak were recovered from 16 and 3 cases, respectively. Information from case studies indicates that all age groups may be affected; symptoms usually occur 24–48 hr postexposure. As for most enteric pathogens the incidence of *Plesiomonas*-associated gastroenteritis is highest in warm weather months. *Plesiomonas* infections have been linked to travel to the Far East and Mexico (85); consumption of raw or undercooked shellfish or contaminated water also is a risk factor for gastrointestinal infection (85).

Reports on virulence-associated characteristics in *Plesiomonas* are not conclusive. Sequences of heat-labile (89) and heat-stable (90) toxins demonstrated in *Plesiomonas* by animal and tissue culture cell systems show no homology with genes for these toxins in *E. coli* and *V. cholerae* O1 (91,92). Assays for invasiveness including production of conjunctivitis in the Sereny test, internalization in HEp-2 cells, or colony blot hybridization for detecting gene sequences have been negative, except for a study in which 31% (5 of 16) of freshly isolated strains of *P. shigelloides* from children with acute gastroenteritis were found to invade HeLa cells at frequencies similar to those of shigellae (93). Daskaleros et al. (94) recently reported on the production of an iron-regulated β-hemolysin that is produced by >90% of all *P. shigelloides* strains (95). This hemolysin may contain enterotoxigenic activity such as found with *Aeromonas* or alternatively may help release iron from erythrocytes. Colonization factors such as pili have not been described in *Plesiomonas* to date.

Although less frequently encountered in the United States, *P. shigelloides* is commonly isolated in other areas. One recent study from Bangladesh (96) listed *Plesiomonas* as the fourth leading cause of bacterial gastroenteritis (after *V. cholerae, Shigella,* and *Aeromonas*) when a single agent was involved (4% of these cases; 6.4% of cases including mixed infections); this study was limited by the lack of a control group. Features significantly associated with *Plesiomonas* enteric infection include travel to the tropics, abdominal pain, and gastrointestinal illness of ≥14 days duration (97). Intestinal infections associated with *P. shigelloides* can span the entire spectrum of symptoms and sequelae associated with enteric illnesses caused by other enteropathogens. Most gastrointestinal ailments associated with *Plesiomonas* last between 2 and 14 days and often include severe abdominal pain or cramping (56–100%). Other symptoms often associated with *P. shigelloides* gastroenteritis include nausea or vomiting (32–40%), fever (18–30%), and headaches (13%); approximately one third of the persons in one study were found to be dehydrated (85). In this study (85), 36% of infected individuals presented with frankly bloody stools, 36% described their abdominal pain as severe, and 18% had fever. Kain and Kelly (97) in a subsequent case-control investigation of 30 persons with acute gastrointestinal illnesses from which *Plesiomonas* was isolated found the chief features of infection to include abdominal pain (100%), nausea or vomiting (40%), and fever (30%). Besides presenting as a secretory or colitis/proctitis type of diarrhea, subacute to chronic infections with *P. shigelloides* also have been described (98). On occasion, intestinal infections with plesiomonads have preceded subsequent bacteremic episodes in apparently healthy hosts (99); fatal outcomes of severe gastrointestinal infections without apparent dissemination caused by *Plesiomonas* also have been described (100).

In vitro susceptibility data reveal that, like *Aeromonas,* most strains of *Plesiomonas* are resistant to ampicillin and susceptible to the cephalosporins, quinolones, trimethoprim-sulfamethoxazole, and chloramphenicol (69,101, 102). However, the susceptibility of plesiomonads to gentamicin (57–86%), tobramycin (36–97%), and amikacin (54–100%) has significantly varied among studies (101,102). Kain and Kelly (101) also found that unlike *Aeromonas* only 68% of the *Plesiomonas* stains tested were susceptible to tetracycline.

Observations from several studies suggest that the quinolones, trimethoprim, or trimethoprim-sulfamethoxazole may be the best oral agents for the treatment of uncomplicated cases of plesiomonad diarrhea. One recent retrospective study (97) suggested that treatment of *Plesiomonas* gastroenteritis with the appropriate antimicrobial agent shortens the course of diarrhea when compared to untreated infections or treatment with antibiotics to which the organism was not susceptible.

EDWARDSIELLA

The genus *Edwardsiella* was first described in the early 1960s when the species *E. tarda* was taxonomically defined from a group of biochemically distinct strains that had been previously referred to by a number of vernacular names including "the Asakusa group" and "the Bartholemew group." Since its initial description, *E. tarda* has been isolated from the feces of persons suffering from diarrheal ailments, the illness most often associated with this species (84). However, edwardsiellae also are found in the environment frequently being recovered from fish, freshwater ecosystems, and from those animals that inhabit these locales such as reptiles and amphibia. During the 1980s two other species (*E. ictaluri, E. hoshinae*) within this genus were described. To date, *E. tarda* is the only species in this genus consistently isolated from human specimens and associated with both intestinal and extraintestinal disease.

The genus *Edwardsiella* is composed of gram-negative, oxidase-negative rods that are facultatively anaerobic. *E. tarda,* which most closely resembles *Salmonella* biochemically, is motile by means of peritrichous flagella; fimbriae or other cell-associated structures have not been identified. In a study of 12 *E. tarda* strains, major outer membrane proteins of 36 and 46 kDa were consistently identified and protein profiles were quite similar (13). LPS analysis reveals a typical heterogeneous O polysaccharide side chain profile that is typical of other members of this family (103).

E. tarda fails to utilize a number of carbohydrate compounds typically oxidized as energy sources by other gram-negative bacteria. However, this species can be easily recognized in the clinical laboratory since its chief diagnostic feature, formation of H_2S, is usually a red flag for colonies isolated on media like xylose–lysine–deoxycholate (XLD), HE, and salmonella–shigella (SS). Reactions typically observed with this species include the ability to produce indole, acid, and gas from D-glucose, H_2S on triple sugar iron (TSI) slants, and lysine and ornithine decarboxylase activity. At present two biotypes of *E. tarda* are known to exist. The most common biotype, commonly known as "wild type," is associated with all human and most animal infections. Strains of the other biogroup (biogroup 1), isolated from freshwater and snakes, are biochemically more active producing acid from D-mannitol, L-arabinose, and sucrose. In addition, biogroup 1 strains fail to produce H_2S on TSI slants. Since *E. tarda* is only infrequently encountered in the clinical laboratory, detailed studies on the best enrichment and isolation methods have not been reported, although in our experience selenite produces excellent results.

Evidence supporting a definitive role for *E. tarda* as a causative agent of diarrheal illness continues to mount although such data are hampered by the relatively infrequent isolation of this species from human specimens. A retrospective analysis of most published literature on *E. tarda* indicates an approximately 3:1 ratio in the isolation rate of this organism from symptomatic vs. asymptomatic persons (104). Of asymptomatic persons from whom *E. tarda* has been recovered, most have occurred in those from tropical or subtropical regions of the world where *E. tarda* may be more common. In a recent cluster of *E. tarda* isolates from a day care center, most infected children were asymptomatic (105). Furthermore, the carrier rate for this organism in the general population appears to be <0.01% (104). In several well-described cases, serum agglutinating antibodies rose in *E. tarda*–infected individuals with fulminant or prolonged bouts of diarrheal disease (106,107). Risk factors associated with such infections include the handling of ornamental fish and turtles (107,108). Finally, recent laboratory studies have identified possible enteropathogenic mechanisms in *E. tarda* that may be operative in the gut.

There are a several candidate virulence factors associated with *E. tarda* gastrointestinal infections. Probably the best defined of these factors is the ability of most *E. tarda* strains to penetrate (invade) nonphagocytic cells such as HeLa or HEp-2 (109,110). This process is microfilament-dependent (inhibited by cytochalasin D) and invasion may correlate with the more severe gastrointestinal manifestations (colitis, dysenteric) often associated with enteric *Edwardsiella* infections (110). A second factor, production of a β-hemolysin, may be linked with invasive capabilities similar to that noted for *Shigella* and enteroinvasive *E. coli* (111). The β-hemolysin was originally detected on modified plate or broth assays and appeared cell-associated, but β-hemolysin may be released extracellularly in iron-deficient media (111). This molecule could facilitate intercellular spread by the release of replicated bacterial progeny or alternatively might have enterotoxigenic activity by itself.

E. tarda–associated gastroenteritis exists in two forms: either as a benign secretory diarrhea or in a more invasive process resembling dysentery or enterocolitis. In a study of ten persons with intestinal illnesses attributed to *E. tarda,* Kourany et al. (112) found the most common symptoms to include low-grade fever (38–38.5°C) and vomiting (70%) in addition to watery stools; only one of these ten subjects had a more severe gastrointestinal disorder, which included frankly bloody stools, fever, vomiting, and overt dehydration. Symptoms may be more severe (resembling pseudomembranous colitis and invasive enterocolitis) and include cramping abdominal pain, nausea, tenesmus, and up to 20 bowel movements per day. Proctoscopy/sigmoidoscopy examinations have revealed ulcerations of the mucosa and submucosal hemorrhages and, in the case of pseudomembranous colitis, hemorrhages with a green membranous mucous layer overlying the rectal mucosa. Occasionally, disseminated *E. tarda* infections (septicemia, hepatic abscesses) most frequently arise in persons with liver dysfunction and those with iron overload conditions (113,114).

Culture remains the diagnostic method of choice since edwardsiellae should be present in large numbers in fecal samples taken during the acute phase of an illness. In instances in which the numbers of *E. tarda* isolated are low, or the illness is in the subacute or chronic phase, acute and/or convalescent serum may be collected for tube agglutination assays (107). In outbreaks of gastrointestinal disease attributed to this bacterium, strains may be serotyped (somatic, flagellar) for epidemiological purposes (115).

Although only a limited number of studies on the in vitro susceptibility of *E. tarda* to antimicrobial agents have been performed, the results indicate that virtually all strains appear to be susceptible to a wide variety of antibiotics including β-lactams, aminoglycosides, and quinolones (116,117). In the absence of controlled clinical trials, it is not possible to make definite recommendations regarding antimicrobial therapy. In settings in which there is persistent diarrhea (>7 days) and *E. tarda* is regarded as the most likely pathogen, it would appear reasonable to undertake a course of therapy. Based on antimicrobial susceptibility patterns and the limited available patient data, ampicillin, trimethoprim-sulfamethoxazole, or ciprofloxacin all would be reasonable choices for antimicrobial therapy.

ACKNOWLEDGMENTS

We thank Dr. Lyndon S. Oshiro for help in the preparation of the *Aeromonas* electron micrograph.

REFERENCES

1. Janda JM, Duffey PS. Mesophilic aeromonads in human disease: current taxonomy, laboratory identification, and infectious disease spectrum. *Rev Infect Dis* 1988;10:980–997.
2. Rossner R. *Aeromonas hydrophila* as the etiologic agent in a case of severe gastroenteritis. *Am J Clin Pathol* 1964;42:402–404.
3. von Graevenitz A, Mensch AH. The genus *Aeromonas* in human bacteriology: report of 30 cases and review of the literature. *N Engl J Med* 1968;278:245–249.
4. Hazen TC, Fliermans CB, Hirsch RP, Esch GW. Prevalence and distribution of *Aeromonas hydrophila* in the United States. *Appl Environ Microbiol* 1978;36:731–738.
5. Buchanan RL, Palumbo SA. *Aeromonas hydrophila* and *Aeromonas sobria* as potential food poisoning species: a review. *J Food Safety* 1985;7:15–29.
6. Nishikawa Y, Kishi T. Isolation and characterization of motile *Aeromonas* from human, food and environmental specimens. *Epidemiol Infect* 1988;101:213–223.
7. Trust TJ. Pathogenesis of infectious diseases of fish. *Annu Rev Microbiol* 1986;40:479–502.
8. Popoff M, Veron M. A taxonomic study of the *Aeromonas hydrophila–Aeromonas punctata* group. *J Gen Microbiol* 1976;94:11–22.
9. Popoff MY, Coynault C, Kiredjian M, Lemelin M. Polynucleotide sequence relatedness among motile *Aeromonas* species. *Curr Microbiol* 1981;5:109–114.
10. Kuijper EJ, Steigerwalt AG, Schoenmakers BSCIM, Peeters MF, Zanen HC, Brenner DJ. Phenotypic characterization and DNA relatedness in human fecal isolates of *Aeromonas* spp. *J Clin Microbiol* 1989;27:132–138.
11. Altwegg M, Steigerwalt AG, Altwegg-Bissig R, Luthy-Hottenstein J, Brenner DJ. Biochemical identification of *Aeromonas* genospecies isolated from humans. *J Clin Microbiol* 1990;28:258–264.
12. Kokka RP, Janda JM, Oshiro LS, et al. Biochemical and genetic characterization of autoagglutinating phenotypes of *Aeromonas* species associated with invasive and noninvasive disease. *J Infect Dis* 1991;163:890–894.
13. Aoki T, Holland BI. The outer membrane proteins of the fish pathogens *Aeromonas hydrophila, Aeromonas salmonicida,* and *Edwardsiella tarda. FEMS Microbiol Lett* 1985;27:299–305.
14. Dooley JSG, Lallier R, Shaw DH, Trust TJ. Electrophoretic and immunochemical analyses of the lipopolysaccharides from various strains of *Aeromonas hydrophila. J Bacteriol* 1985;164:263–269.
15. Janda JM. Biochemical and exoenzymatic properties of *Aeromonas* species. *Diagn Microbiol Infect Dis* 1985;3:223–232.
16. Janda JM, Reitano M, Bottone EJ. Biotyping of *Aeromonas* as a correlate to delineating a species-associated disease spectrum. *J Clin Microbiol* 1984;19:44–47.
17. Carnahan AM, Behram S, Joseph SW. Aerokey II. a flexible key for identifying clinical *Aeromonas* species. *J Clin Microbiol* 1991;29:2843–2849.
18. Abbott SL, Cheung WKW, Kroske-Bystrom S, Malekzadeh T, Janda JM. Identification of *Aeromonas* strains to the genospecies level in the clinical laboratory. *J Clin Microbiol* 1992;30:1262–1266.
19. Kelly MT, Stroh EMD, Jessop J. Comparison of blood agar, ampicillin blood agar, MacConkey-ampicillin-Tween agar, and modified cefsulodin-irgasan-novobiocin agar for isolation of *Aeromonas* spp. from stool specimens. *J Clin Microbiol* 1988;26:1738–1740.
20. Carnahan AM, Chakraborty T, Fanning GR, et al. *Aeromonas trota* sp. nov., an ampicillin-susceptible species isolated from clinical specimens. *J Clin Microbiol* 1991;29:1206–1210.
21. Altorfer R, Altwegg M, Zollinger-iten J, von Graevenitz A. Growth of *Aeromonas* spp. on cefsulodin-irgasan-novobiocin agar selective for *Yersinia enterocolitica. J Clin Microbiol* 1985;22:478–480.
22. Holmberg SD, Farmer III JJ. *Aeromonas hydrophila* and *Plesiomonas shigelloides* as causes of intestinal infections. *Rev Infect Dis* 1984;6:633–639.
23. Cohen MB. Etiology and mechanisms of acute infectious diarrhea in infants in the United States. *J Pediatr* 1991;118:S34–S39.
24. Moyer NP. Clinical significance of *Aeromonas* species isolated from patients with diarrhea. *J Clin Microbiol* 1987;25:2044–2048.
25. Gracey M, Burke V, Robinson R. *Aeromonas*-associated gastroenteritis. *Lancet* 1982;2:1304–1306.
26. Janda JM, Bottone EJ, Reitano MR. *Aeromonas* species in clinical microbiology: significance, epidemiology, and speciation. *Diagn Microbiol Infect Dis* 1983;1:221–228.
27. George WL, Nakata MM, Thompson J, White ML. *Aeromonas*-related diarrhea in adults. *Arch Intern Med* 1985;145:2207–2211.
28. Pazzaglia G, Sack RB, Salazar E, et al. High frequency of coinfecting enteropathogens in *Aeromonas*-associated diarrhea of hospitalized Peruvian infants. *J Clin Microbiol* 1991;29:1151–1156.
29. Holmberg SD, Schell WK, Fanning GR, et al. *Aeromonas* intestinal infections in the United States. *Ann Intern Med* 1986;105:683–689.
30. Alabi SA, Odugbemi T. Occurrence of *Aeromonas* species and *Plesiomonas shigelloides* in patients with and without diarrhoea in Lagos, Nigeria. *J Med Microbiol* 1990;32:45–48.
31. Mikhail IA, Fox E, Haberberger RL, Ahmed MH, Abbatte EA. Epidemiology of bacterial pathogens associated with infectious diarrhea in Djibouti. *J Clin Microbiol* 1990;28:956–961.
32. Golik A, Modai D, Gluskin I, Schechter I, Cohen N, Eschar J. *Aeromonas* in adult diarrhea: an enteropathogen or an innocent bystander? *J Clin Gastroenterol* 1990;12:148–152.
33. Qadri SMH, Zafar M, Lee GC. Can isolation of *Aeromonas hydrophila* from human feces have any clinical significance? *J Clin Gastroenterol* 1991;13:537–540.
34. Wilcox MH, Cook AM, Eley A, Spencer RC. *Aeromonas* spp. as a potential cause of diarrhoea in children. *J Clin Pathol* 1992;45:959–963.
35. San Joaquin VH, Pickett DA. *Aeromonas*-associated gastroenteritis in children. *Pediatr Infect Dis J* 1988;7:53–57.
36. Deodhar LP, Saraswathi K, Varudkar A. *Aeromonas* spp. and their association with human diarrheal disease. *J Clin Microbiol* 1991;29:853–856.
37. Kuijper EJ, van Alphen L, Peeters MF, Brenner DJ. Human serum antibody response to the presence of *Aeromonas* spp. in the intestinal tract. *J Clin Microbiol* 1990;28:584–590.
38. Jiang ZD, Nelson AC, Mathewson JJ, Ericsson CD, DuPont HL. Intestinal secretory immune response to infection with *Aeromonas* species and *Plesiomonas shigelloides* among students from the United States in Mexico. *J Infect Dis* 1991;164:979–982.
39. Kokka RP, Velji AM, Clark RB, Bottone EJ, Janda JM. Immune response to S layer–positive O:11 *Aeromonas* associated with intestinal and extraintestinal disease. *Immunol Infect Dis* 1992;2:111–114.
40. Champsaur H, Andremont A, Mathieu D, Rottman E, Auzepy P. Cholera-like illness due to *Aeromonas sobria. J Infect Dis* 1982;145:248–254.
41. Burke V, Gracey M, Robinson J, Peck D, Beaman J, Bundell C. The microbiology of childhood gastroenteritis: *Aeromonas* species and other infective agents. *J Infect Dis* 1983;148:68–74.
42. del Val A, Moles J-R, Garrigues V. Very prolonged diarrhea associated with *Aeromonas hydrophila. Am J Gastroenterol* 1990;85:1535.
43. Kotloff KL, Wasserman SS, Steciak JY, et al. Acute diarrhea in Baltimore children attending an outpatient clinic. *Pediatr Infect Dis J* 1988;7:753–759.

44. Morris JG Jr, Takeda T, Tall BD, et al. Experimental non-O group 1 *Vibrio cholerae* gastroenteritis in humans. *J Clin Invest* 1990;85:697–705.

45. Morgan DR, Johnson PC, DuPont HL, Satterwhite TK, Wood LV. Lack of correlation between virulence properties of *Aeromonas hydrophila* and enteropathogenicity for humans. *Infect Immun* 1985;50:62–65.

46. Janda JM. Recent advances in the study of the taxonomy, pathogenicity, and infectious syndromes associated with the genus *Aeromonas*. *Clin Microbiol Rev* 1991;4:397–410.

47. Ho ASY, Mietzner TA, Smith AJ, Schoolnik GK. The pili of *Aeromonas hydrophila*: identification of an environmentally regulated "mini pilin." *J Exp Med* 1990;172:795–806.

48. Pearson GDN, Woods A, Chiang SL, Mekalanos JJ. CTX genetic element encodes a site-specific recombination system and an intestinal colonization factor. *Proc Nat Acad Sci* 1993;90:3750–3754.

49. Asao T, Kinoshita Y, Kozaki S, Uemura T, Sakaguchi G. Purification and some properties of *Aeromonas hydrophila* hemolysin. *Infect Immun* 1984;46:122–127.

50. Husslein V, Huhle B, Jarchau T, Lurz R, Goebel W, Chakraborty T. Nucleotide sequence and transcriptional analysis of the aerCaerA region of *Aeromonas sobria* encoding aerolysin and the regulatory region. *Mol Microbiol* 1988;2:507–517.

51. Chakraborty T, Montenegro MA, Sanyal SC, Helmuth R, Bulling E, Timmis KN. Cloning of enterotoxin gene from *Aeromonas hydrophila* provides conclusive evidence of production of a cytotonic enterotoxin. *Infect Immun* 1984;46:435–441.

52. Rose JM, Houston CW, Coppenhaver DH, Dixon JD, Kurosky A. Purification and chemical characterization of a cholera toxin-cross reactive cytolytic enterotoxin produced by a human isolate of *Aeromonas hydrophila*. *Infect Immun* 1989;57:1165–1169.

53. Krovacek K, Faris A, Mansson I. In vitro invasion of *Aeromonas* spp. to HEp-2 tissue culture cells. *Acta Vet Scand* 1991;32:139–143.

54. Agger WA, McCormick JD, Gurwith MJ. Clinical and microbiological features of *Aeromonas hydrophila*-associated diarrhea. *J Clin Microbiol* 1985;21:909–913.

55. San Joaquin VH, Pickett DA. *Aeromonas*-associated gastroenteritis in children. *Pediatr Infect Dis J* 1988;7:53–57.

56. Challapalli M, Tess BR, Cunningham DG, Chopra AK, Houston CW. *Aeromonas*-associated diarrhea in children. *Pediatr Infect Dis J* 1988;7:693–698.

57. Farraye FA, Peppercorn MA, Ciano PS, Kavesh WN. Segmental colitis associated with *Aeromonas hydrophila*. *Am J Gastroenterol* 1989;84:436–438.

58. Doman DB, Golding MI, Goldberg HJ, Doyle RB. *Aeromonas hydrophila* colitis presenting as medically refractory inflammatory bowel disease. *Am J Gastroenterol* 1989;84:83–85.

59. Willoughby JMT, Rahman AFMS, Gregory MM. Chronic colitis after *Aeromonas* infection. *Gut* 1989;30:686–690.

60. del Val A, Moles J-R, Garrigues V. Very prolonged diarrhea associated with *Aeromonas hydrophila*. *Am J Gastroenterol* 1990;85:1535.

61. Kindschuh M, Pickering LK, Cleary TG, Ruiz-Palacios G. Clinical and biochemical significance of toxin production by *Aeromonas hydrophila*. *J Clin Microbiol* 1987;25:916–921.

62. Voss LM, Rhodes KH, Johnson KA. Musculoskeletal and soft tissue *Aeromonas* infection: an environmental disease. *Mayo Clin Proc* 1992;67:422–427.

63. Sakazaki R, Shimada T. O-serogrouping scheme for mesophilic *Aeromonas* strains. *Jpn J Med Sci Biol* 1984;37:247–255.

64. Shimada T, Kosako Y. Comparison of the two O-serogrouping systems for mesophilic *Aeromonas* spp. *J Clin Microbiol* 1991;29:197–199.

65. Moyer NP, Martinetti G, Luthy-Hottenstein J, Altwegg M. Value of rRNA gene restriction patterns of *Aeromonas* spp. for epidemiologic investigations. *Curr Microbiol* 1992;24:15–21.

66. Kuijper EJ, van Alphen L, Leenders E, Zanen HC. Typing of *Aeromonas* strains by DNA restriction endonuclease analysis and polyacrylamide gel electrophoresis of cell envelopes. *J Clin Microbiol* 1989;27:1280–1285.

67. Altwegg M, Reeves MW, Altwegg-Bissig R, Brenner DJ. Multilocus enzyme analysis of the genus *Aeromonas* and its use for species identification. *Zbl Bakt* 1991;275:28–45.

68. Altwegg M, Martinetti Lucchini G, Luthy-Hottenstein J, Rohrbach M. *Aeromonas*-associated gastroenteritis after consumption of contaminated shrimp. *Eur J Clin Microbiol Infect Dis* 1991;10:44–45.

69. Reinhardt JF, George WL. Comparative in vitro activities of selected antimicrobial agents against *Aeromonas* species and *Plesiomonas shigelloides*. *Antimicrob Agents Chemother* 1985;28:151–153.

70. Motyl MR, McKinley G, Janda JM. In vitro susceptibilities of *Aeromonas hydrophila*, *Aeromonas sobria*, and *Aeromonas caviae* to 22 antimicrobial agents. *Antimicrob Agents Chemother* 1985;28:151–153.

71. Kuijper EJ, Peeters MF, Schoenmakers BSC, Zanen HC. Antimicrobial susceptibility of sixty fecal isolates of *Aeromonas* species. *Eur J Clin Microbiol Infect Dis* 1989;8:248–250.

72. Burgos A, Quindos G, Martinez R, Rojo P, Cisterna R. In vitro susceptibility of *Aeromonas caviae*, *Aeromonas hydrophila* and *Aeromonas sobria* to fifteen antibacterial agents. *Eur J Clin Microbiol Infect Dis* 1990;9:413–417.

73. Koehler JM, Ashdown LR. In vitro susceptibilities of tropical strains of *Aeromonas* species from Queensland, Australia, to 22 antimicrobial agents. *Antimicrob Agents Chemother* 1993;37:905–907.

74. Bakken JS, Sanders CC, Clark RB, Hori M. β-Lactam resistance in *Aeromonas* spp. caused by inducible β-lactamases active against penicillins, cephalosporins, and carbapenems. *Antimicrob Agents Chemother* 1988;32:1314–1319.

75. Trust TJ, Chipman DC. Clinical involvement of *Aeromonas hydrophila*. *Can Med Assoc J* 1979;120:942–946.

76. Namdari H, Bottone EJ. Microbiologic and clinical evidence supporting the role of *Aeromonas caviae* as a pediatric enteric pathogen. *J Clin Microbiol* 1990;28:837–840.

77. Brenden RA, Miller MA, Janda JM. Clinical disease spectrum and pathogenic factors associated with *Plesiomonas shigelloides*. *Rev Infect Dis* 1988;10:303–316.

78. East AK, Allaway D, Collins MD. Analysis of DNA encoding 23S rRNA and 16-23S rRNA intergenic spacer regions from *Plesiomonas shigelloides*. *FEMS Microbiol Lett* 1992;95:57–62.

79. Miller ML, Koburger JA. Evaluation of inositol brilliant green bile salts and *Plesiomonas* agars for recovery of *Plesiomonas shigelloides* from aquatic samples in a seasonal survey of the Suwannee river estuary. *J Food Protect* 1986;49:274–277.

80. Miller ML, Koburger JA. *Plesiomonas shigelloides*: an opportunistic food and waterborne pathogen. *J Food Protect* 1985;48:449–457.

81. Arai T, Ikejima N, Itoh T, Sakai S, Shimada R. A survey of *Plesiomonas shigelloides* from aquatic environments, domestic animals, pets and humans. *J Hyg Camb* 1980;84:203–211.

82. von Graevenitz A, Bucher C. Evaluation of differential and selective media for isolation of *Aeromonas* and *Plesiomonas* spp. from human feces. *J Clin Microbiol* 1983;17:16–21.

83. Rahim Z, Kay BA. Enrichment for *Plesiomonas shigelloides* from stools. *J Clin Microbiol* 1988;26:789–790.

84. Shimada T, Sakazaki R. On the serology of *Plesiomonas shigelloides*. *Jpn J Med Sci Biol* 1978;31:135–142.

85. Holmberg SD, Wachsmuth K, Hickman-Brenner FW, Blake PA, Farmer III JJ. *Plesiomonas* enteric infections in the United States. *Ann Intern Med* 1986;105:690–694.

86. Herrington DA, Tzipori S, Robins-Browne RM, Tall BD, Levine MM. In vitro and in vivo pathogenicity of *Plesiomonas shigelloides*. *Infect Immun* 1987;55:979–985.

87. Tsukamoto T, Kinoshita Y, Shimada T, Sakazaki R. Two epidemics of diarrhoeal disease possibly caused by *Plesiomonas shigelloides*. *J Hyg Camb* 1978;80:275–280.

88. Rutala WA, Sarubbi Jr FA, Finch CS, MacCormack JN, Steinkraus GE. Oyster-associated outbreak of diarrhoeal disease possibly caused by *Plesiomonas shigelloides*. *Lancet* 1982;1:739.

89. Gardner SE, Fowlston SE, George WL. In vitro production of

cholera toxin-like activity by *Plesiomonas shigelloides*. *J Infect Dis* 1987;156:720–722.

90. Matthews BG, Douglas H, Guiney DG. Production of a heat stable enterotoxin by *Plesiomonas shigelloides*. *Microb Pathog* 1988;5:207–213.

91. Olsvik O, Wachsmuth K, Kay B, Birkness KA, Yi A, Sack B. Laboratory observations on *Plesiomonas shigelloides* strains isolated from children with diarrhea in Peru. *J Clin Microbiol* 1990;28:886–889.

92. Abbott SL, Kokka RP, Janda JM. Laboratory investigations on the low pathogenic potential of *Plesiomonas shigelloides*. *J Clin Microbiol* 1991;29:148–153.

93. Binns MM, Vaughan S, Sanyal SC, Timmis KN. Invasive ability of *Plesiomonas shigelloides*. *Zbl Bakt Hyg* 1984;257: 343–347.

94. Daskaleros PA, Stoebner JA, Payne SM. Iron uptake in *Plesiomonas shigelloides:* cloning of the genes for the heme–iron uptake system. *Infect Immun* 1991;59:2706–2711.

95. Janda JM, Abbott SL. Expression of hemolytic activity by *Plesiomonas shigelloides*. *J Clin Microbiol* 1993;31:1206–1208.

96. Zeaur R, Akbar A, Bradford AK. Prevalence of *Plesiomonas shigelloides* among diarrhoeal patients in Bangladesh. *Eur J Epidemiol* 1992;8:753–756.

97. Kain KC, Kelly MT. Clinical features, epidemiology, and treatment of *Plesiomonas shigelloides* diarrhea. *J Clin Microbiol* 1989;27:998–1001.

98. DuPont HL. Subacute diarrhea: to treat or to wait? *Hosp Pract* 1989;24:111–118.

99. Ingram CW, Morrison Jr AJ, Levitz RE. Gastroenteritis, sepsis, and osteomyelitis caused by *Plesiomonas shigelloides* in an immunocompetent host: case report and review of the literature. *J Clin Microbiol* 1987;25:1791–1793.

100. Sinnott IV JT, Turnquest DG, Milam MW. *Plesiomonas shigelloides* gastroenteritis. *Clin Microbiol Newslett* 1989;11: 103–104.

101. Kain KC, Kelly MT. Antimicrobial susceptibility of *Plesiomonas shigelloides* from patients with diarrhea. *Antimicrob Agents Chemother* 1989;33:1609–1610.

102. Clark RB, Lister PD, Arneson-Rotert L, Janda JM. In vitro susceptibilities of *Plesiomonas shigelloides* to 24 antibiotics and antibiotic-β-lactamase-inhibitor combinations. *Antimicrob Agents Chemother* 1990;34:159–160.

103. Hitchcock PJ, Leive L, Makela PH, Rietschel ET, Strittmatter W, Morrison DC. Lipolysaccharide nomenclature—past, present, and future. *J Bacteriol* 1986;166:699–705.

104. Janda JM, Abbott SL. Infections associated with the genus *Edwardsiella:* the role of *E. tarda* in human disease. *Clin Infect Dis* 1993;17:742–748.

105. Desenclos J-CA, Conti L, Junejo S, Klontz KC. A cluster of *Edwardsiella tarda* infection in a day-care center in Florida. *J Infect Dis* 1990;162:782–783.

106. Gilman RH, Madasamy M, Mariappan M, Davis CE, Kyser KA. *Edwardsiella tarda* in jungle diarrhoea and a possible association with *Entamoeba histolytica*. *Southeast Asian J Trop Med Public Health* 1971;2:186–189.

107. Vandepitte J, Lemmens P, De Swert L. Human edwardsiellosis traced to ornamental fish. *J Clin Microbiol* 1983;17:165–167.

108. Nagel P, Serritella A, Layden TJ. *Edwardsiella tarda* gastroenteritis associated with a pet turtle. *Gastroenterology* 1982;82: 1436–1437.

109. Marques LRM, Toledo MRF, Silva NP, Magalhaes M, Trabulsi LR. Invasion of HeLa cells by *Edwardsiella tarda*. *Curr Microbiol* 1984;10:129–132.

110. Janda JM, Abbott SL, Oshiro LS. Penetration and replication of *Edwardsiella* spp. in HEp-2 cells. *Infect Immun* 1991;59: 154–161.

111. Janda JM, Abbott SL. Expression of an iron-regulated hemolysin from *Edwardsiella tarda*. *FEMS Microbiol Lett* 1993;111: 275–280.

112. Kourany M, Vasquez MA, Saenz R. Edwardsiellosis in man and animals in Panama: clinical and epidemiologic characteristics. *Am J Trop Med Hyg* 1977;26:1183–1190.

113. Wilson JP, Waterer RR, Wofford JD, Chapman SW. Serious infections with *Edwardsiella tarda:* a case report and review of the literature. *Arch Intern Med* 1989;149:208–210.

114. Zighelboim J, Williams Jr TW, Bradshaw MW, Harris RL. Successful management of a patient with multiple hepatic abscesses due to *Edwardsiella tarda*. *Clin Infect Dis* 1992;14: 117–120.

115. Tamura K, Sakazaki R, McWhorter AC, Kosako Y. *Edwardsiella tarda* serotyping scheme for international use. *J Clin Microbiol* 1988;26:2343–2346.

116. Reinhardt JF, Fowlston S, Jones J, George WL. Comparative in vitro activities of selected antimicrobial agents against *Edwardsiella tarda*. *Antimicrob Agents Chemother* 1985;27: 966–967.

117. Clark RB, Lister PD, Janda JM. In vitro susceptibilities of *Edwardsiella tarda* to 22 antibiotics and antibiotic-β-lactamase-inhibitor agents. *Diag Microbiol Infect Dis* 1991;14:173–175.

Infections of the Gastrointestinal Tract,
edited by M. J. Blaser, P. D. Smith, J. I. Ravdin,
H. B. Greenberg, and R. L. Guerrant
Published by Raven Press, Ltd., New York, 1995.

CHAPTER 61

Whipple's Disease

David A. Relman

Whipple's disease is a systemic infectious disorder first described in 1907 (1) that affects primarily the intestinal tract and its lymphatic drainage. Despite its apparent rarity, this disease continues to capture the attention of clinicians throughout the developed countries of the world. One of the fascinating aspects of this disorder is the presumed causative agent, an enigmatic bacterium that has defied laboratory cultivation and was only recently identified by molecular methods as a previously uncharacterized actinomycete (2,3). The principal clinical features of Whipple's disease are migratory polyarthralgias, weight loss, diarrhea with evidence of malabsorption, and abdominal pain. Lymphadenopathy and skin hyperpigmentation are also prominent findings. Accompanying these features is an unusual and in some situations diagnostic pattern of tissue pathology involving most often the proximal small intestines, the mesenteric lymphatics, and, less often, the heart and central nervous system. This clinical syndrome was described with remarkable accuracy by George Whipple in his initial case report.

On April 12, 1907 a 36-year-old medical missionary was admitted to Johns Hopkins Hospital with a 5-year history of migratory arthralgias and arthritis, cough, fever, diarrhea, evidence of fat malabsorption, weight loss, and abdominal pain. The clinical diagnosis was tuberculosis. A palpable abdominal mass prompted an exploratory laparotomy with the subsequent finding of massively enlarged mesenteric lymph nodes and a revised diagnosis of sarcoma or Hodgkins' disease. At autopsy 3 days later George Whipple found swollen small intestinal mucosa "flecked . . . with pin-point yellowish grains," with refractile "fat" deposits within mucosa and submucosa, and numerous "foamy" mononuclear cells containing vacuoles, especially within the lamina propria. Elsewhere there was pleuritis, pericarditis, aortic endocarditis, and diffuse chronic lymphadenitis. Whipple suspected altered fat metabolism as an etiological factor and named this

disorder "intestinal lipodystrophy"; however, he also raised the possibility of a microbial agent (see "Microbiology" below).

In 1949, Black-Schaffer applied Schiff's periodic acid stain (PAS) to sections of small intestinal and lymph node tissues from patients with intestinal lipodystrophy, with the goal of characterizing the unusual refractile tissue and cellular deposits (4). The intense "deep scarlet" staining of intracellular vacuoles indicated that this material was glycoprotein. Having raised doubts about the etiological importance of lipid metabolism in this disorder, Black-Schaffer argued for the use of the eponym "Whipple's disease." Alternative designations such as lipophagic intestinal granulomatosis (5) fell out of favor and the PAS stain became an important diagnostic tool. Retrospective use of this stain confirmed that macrophage vacuoles from Whipple's case in 1907 were PAS-positive (6) but that, in addition, a case published in 1895 may have represented unrecognized Whipple's disease (7).

Two fundamental observations concerning the causation of Whipple's disease occurred in the 1950s and early 1960s. Both suggested a bacterial etiology. The first was the observation that antibiotics significantly improved the outcome of what was otherwise an often fatal disease (8). The second was the detection of unusual-appearing monomorphic bacillary structures within many different tissues affected by this disease, using electron microscopy (9–11). George Whipple's early speculation of an infectious etiology was thus confirmed. Studies by Silva et al. and others (12,13) showed that a portion of the bacterial cell wall reacted with the PAS stain, and the PAS-positive macrophage vacuoles contained partially degraded remnants of this wall. Further evidence of bacterial causation followed: clinical response to antibacterial therapy was accompanied by disappearance of the bacilli, and reappearance of the bacilli heralded clinical relapse (14). Nonetheless, the organism could not be cultivated or purified in the laboratory. Hence, it remained unidentified until the application of an approach based on amplification of bacterial ribosomal RNA (rRNA) gene sequences directly from infected human tissue and the analysis of these

D. A. Relman: Department of Medicine, and Microbiology & Immunology, Stanford University School of Medicine, Stanford, California, and Palo Alto Department of Veterans Affairs Medical Center, Palo Alto, California 94304.

sequences for phylogenetic studies (15). The proposed name of the Whipple's disease bacillus is "*Tropheryma whippelii*" (2).

Between 1907 and 1986, approximately 700 patients with Whipple's disease were described in the medical literature (16). However, the true number of individuals with clinical manifestations of infection by this organism is probably at least several fold greater (17). Clinical symptoms and syndromes that are less well defined than "classical" Whipple's disease may often go unrecognized as manifestations of *T. whippelii* infection, e.g., chronic arthralgia, chronic uveitis, fever of unknown origin, and dementia with cerebellar ataxia. The recently acquired ability to detect this organism with great sensitivity and specificity should help define its natural ecology and the spectrum of human disease with which this bacterium is associated.

MICROBIOLOGY

Whipple's disease is clearly associated with a bacterium, and this organism is most probably the causal agent. However, the Koche–Henle postulates (18) have not been and will not be satisfied for this disorder unless or until this bacterium is purified or propagated in a biological system aside from the human host. The evidence favoring a bacterial etiology for Whipple's disease is circumstantial but compelling, and includes the consistent observation of a uniform, sometimes dividing, bacillary organism in many different affected tissues; the correlation of visible organisms with clinical disease activity; their disappearance with antibacterial therapy and subsequent clinical improvement; and the return of these organisms with clinical relapse (14). There is no known reservoir or animal host for this bacterium, although there are some animal diseases such as *Rhodococcus equi* enteritis in foals (19) that resemble Whipple's disease. In short, the natural biology of the Whipple's disease bacillus remains largely uncharacterized.

In the original description of the disease Whipple noted "great numbers of a rod-shaped organism (?)" that "closely resemble the tubercle bacillus" in a silver-stained lymph node (1). They were found within the foamy mononuclear cells and adjacent to them in a distribution that suggested to Whipple that they might play an etiological role. Electron microscopy has greatly facilitated the morphological characterization of this bacillus (9–13). Many independent investigators have described an organism of unusual but similar appearance in numerous patients with syndromes and pathology suggestive of Whipple's disease (Fig. 1). It has been thought that there is one bacterial species present in all of these tissues (16), but the means to prove this have not been available. The Whipple bacillus is 0.15–0.25 μm in diameter and 1–2 μm in length. There is no evidence of flagella. A 20-nm-thick cell wall lies external to the trilaminar cytoplasmic membrane (12,13). This cell wall thickness is typical of many gram-positive bacteria, and in fact the Whipple bacillus appears weakly gram-positive with the Brown and Brenn tissue stain. However, an additional, thin trilaminar membrane

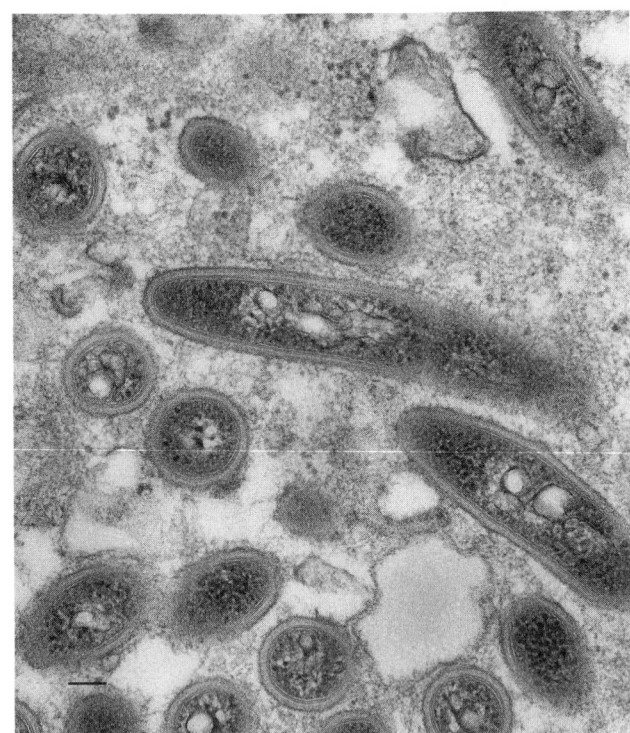

FIG. 1. Electron micrograph of the Whipple's disease bacillus ("*Tropheryma whippelii*"). These extracellular bacilli are abundant within the lamina propria of patients with untreated disease. The thick cell wall has a distinctive structure, more easily appreciated at higher magnifications. bar = 0.1 μm. Courtesy of Dr. William O. Dobbins III.

bilayer encompasses the cell wall. This outer membrane has symmetrical phospholipid leaflets that are devoid of lipopolysaccharide, unlike the surface membranes of gram-negative bacteria. Silva et al. postulated that the outer bacterial membrane may be of host origin (13). A bacillus with a cell wall of similar appearance was observed by Archer et al. in a febrile, asplenic patient with lymphadenopathy (20). An inner, electron-dense, polysaccharide-containing cell wall layer is thought to account for the PAS-positive staining properties of the Whipple bacillus; accumulations of this cell wall layer within macrophage vacuoles represent remnants of partially digested intracellular bacteria and explain the PAS-positive staining properties of the vacuoles. PAS reactivity by the Whipple bacillus is resistant to treatment with diastase. The Whipple bacillus is revealed by the Giemsa stain and by some silver stain procedures (e.g., Gomori), but it is not acid-fast.

Whipple bacilli are most prominent in the proximal small intestinal lamina propria, just below the epithelial basement membrane (see "Pathology"). Most intact organisms are free in the intercellular spaces, sometimes forming clusters; some are seen to undergo binary fission. On the other hand, most intracellular bacteria are found in various stages of degradation. From these observations, it is thought that the Whipple bacillus replicates preferentially in an extracellular environment but that it may survive for prolonged periods of time within host cells.

Numerous efforts to cultivate the Whipple bacillus in the laboratory, beginning with those of George Whipple, have failed to yield any particular organism in a reproducible and consistent manner. Methods have included the use of various intact animals (some were germ-free) as well as animal and human tissue culture cell lines (16). Two of the more prominent bacterial isolates were a cell wall–deficient *Streptococcus dysgalactiae* (21) and *Corynebacterium bovis* (22), each from one patient; however, these results were not reproducible. Cultivation of infected tissue with murine macrophage cell lines (23) and human fresh peripheral monocyte-derived macrophages, including supplementation with various macrophage inhibitory cytokines (Relman DA, Kornbluth RS, unpublished data), have not been helpful. In all likelihood, many more unsuccessful attempts to cultivate this organism have taken place than are represented in the medical literature.

Antigenic characterization of the Whipple bacillus has been approached with an *in situ* tissue immunofluorescence procedure. Among a diverse group of antibacterial polyclonal antisera, Keren and colleagues found that only those elicited by group A, B, and G streptococci and by group B *Shigella flexneri* generated significant fluorescence from jejunal macrophage vacuoles in Whipple's disease tissues (24). The pattern of tissue fluorescence was distinct, reproducible, and consistent from case to case. Although these staining patterns were cross-reactions with heterologous bacteria, the results suggested that different patients are infected with antigenically related if not identical organisms (25). This procedure has had limited use as a diagnostic test (26); however, it offered few if any specific clues concerning the nature of the Whipple bacillus. More precise antigenic or compositional analyses have been hindered by the lack of purified bacterial cell material.

The advent of molecular phylogeny and the use of rRNA sequences to infer evolutionary relationships has paved the way for the identification of uncultured microbial pathogens (27). Broad-range polymerase chain reaction (PCR) primers are designed from known conserved bacterial 16S rRNA sequence regions and then used to amplify corresponding gene fragments directly from infected host tissue (28). In an initial investigation, Wilson et al. studied one duodenal mucosal biopsy tissue from a patient with Whipple's disease (3). From this sample they amplified and sequenced a fragment of a previously uncharacterized bacterial 16S rRNA gene. Relman et al. analyzed duodenal and extraintestinal tissues from 5 unrelated patients with the "classical" form of Whipple's disease, as well as 14 tissues from 10 unrelated control patients without the disease (2). A 1321-base bacterial 16S rDNA sequence (approximately 90% of the gene) (GenBank sequence accession number M87484) was compiled from PCR-amplified fragments using digested tissue samples from one of the Whipple's disease patients; using PCR primers specific for this Whipple's disease-associated 16S rRNA sequence, the sequence was detected in all five patients and in none of the control tissues. In sub-

sequent work, the Whipple bacillus sequence has been detected in duodenal tissues from approximately six additional patients with Whipple's disease (Relman DA, unpublished data; 29) as well as within peripheral blood mononuclear cells and pleural effusion cells (30). With limited data available, 16S rDNA sequence heterogeneity between PCR-amplified products from unrelated Whipple's disease tissues occurs at approximately 0.14% (2). This degree of heterogeneity is similar to the intrinsic error rate of *Taq* DNA polymerase (31).

Phylogenetic analysis using amplified 16S rDNA sequences indicates that the Whipple bacillus is a previously uncharacterized member of the actinomycete subdivision of the "gram-positive" division of bacteria (Fig. 2). This subdivision is also known by the relatively "high G + C" (guanine plus cytosine) chromosomal composition of the member organisms. Most of the known bacteria that are PAS-positive after diastase digestion are also members of the gram-positive division (32). However, the Whipple bacillus sequence is no more than 92.5% similar to any known 16S rRNA sequence (2). Thus, this bacillus is not closely related to any previously characterized organism by the usual molecular phylogenetic standards. Although criteria for taxon boundaries are difficult to formulate in the absence of culture-based phenotypes, it seems apparent that the Whipple bacillus defines a new genus and species. Each of the several most closely related bacteria belong to a separate genus, and none of these bacteria is significantly more closely related to the Whipple bacillus than any other. The name "*Tropheryma whippelii*" has been proposed, from the Greek *trophe*, for nourishment, and *eryma*, for barrier, because malabsorption is a key feature of the syndrome with which it is associated, and from the name of George Whipple (2). There is no molecular evidence for multiple species in the Whipple's disease tissues studied to date.

What microbiological information can be inferred from the evolutionary relationships of *T. whippelii*? Many of the more closely related bacteria are common soil or water saprophytes (*Arthrobacter, Terrabacter, Streptomyces*). Some of them are skin or mucosa commensal organisms in animals (*Dermatophilus, Micrococcus*) and in humans (*Micrococcus, Actinomyces, Rothia, Mycobacterium*). All of these skin and mucosal commensals can cause invasive disease in humans when normal anatomic barriers are breached and/or host immune defenses are compromised. In fact, *Mycobacterium avium* complex and *Rhodococcus equi* both cause syndromes similar to Whipple's disease in HIV-seropositive individuals (33–38), *M. paratuberculosis* causes Johne's disease of cattle with histology that resembles Whipple's disease (39–41), and *R. equi* causes a granulomatous enteritis in foals with a PAS-positive macrophage infiltrate (19). Although this notion is speculative, *T. whippelii* may be a common soil or water commensal that gains access to humans via the gastrointestinal tract. Those that develop classical Whipple's disease may be particularly susceptible by virtue of a subtle immune defect. In support of this theory, Dobbins previously showed that farmers are disproportionately represented among patients with Whipple's disease (16) (see "Epidemiology").

GRAM POSITIVE BACTERIA

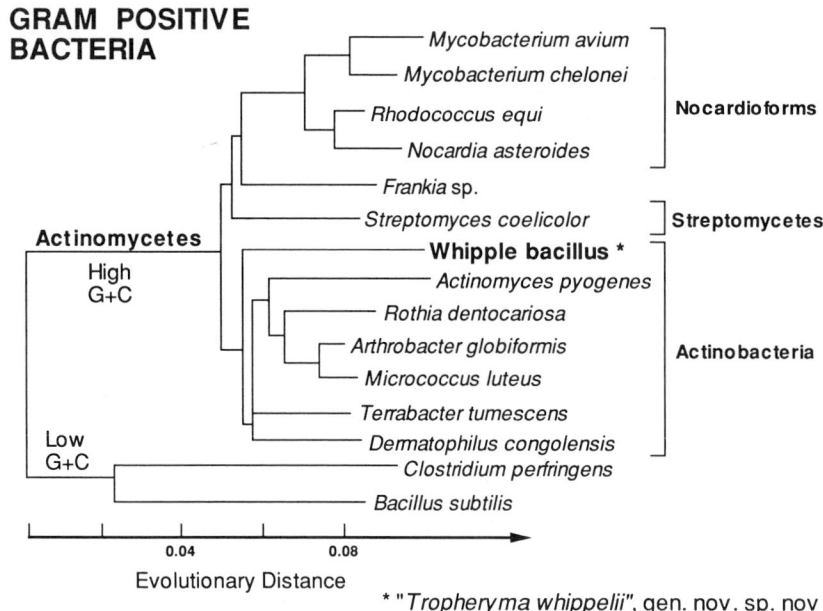

FIG. 2. Evolutionary tree indicating the phylogenetic relationships of the Whipple's disease bacillus ("*Tropheryma whippelii*"). This bacterium is a novel actinomycete that is not closely related to any other characterized organism. This tree is based on comparative analysis of 16S rRNA sequences; evolutionary distance (*abscissa*) is proportional to the sum of the horizontal line segments connecting any two organisms (point mutations per sequence position).

* "*Tropheryma whippelii*", gen. nov. sp. nov

Many soil microorganisms have the capacity to degrade natural organic compounds for nutrient acquisition. One potentially useful approach for further characterization of *T. whippelii* would be to attempt amplification of putative genes encoding these degradative enzymes based on consensus sequences found in known homologs. Other gene sequences that encode essential bacterial structures (*rpoB*, RNA polymerase subunit) or enzyme activities (ATPases) may also be useful targets for study, since these sequences contain reliable phylogenetic information. However, until more information can be gathered concerning biochemical or growth requirements, or natural habitat, one can only conclude that the morphology and staining properties of *T. whippelii* are consistent with its phylogenetic placement within the actinomycete subdivision.

EPIDEMIOLOGY

A number of curious and unusual features help to define the epidemiology of Whipple's disease. Although the data are limited because of the relatively low numbers of cases, it is clear that there is a striking gender bias, as well as probable predispositions based on age, race, and geography. In a review of 664 patients from the world's medical literature Dobbins found that 86.4% were male (16). The average age at the time of diagnosis was similar for males and females, 49.1 and 51.0 years, respectively. Only 4.1% of all cases occurred in persons 30 years of age or younger. In the same case review, caucasians accounted for 97.8% of Whipple's disease patients (16). Geography may partially explain this finding. Whipple's disease is recognized primarily in developed countries of Western Europe and North America, and seems to be less common in major urban population centers. No doubt limited disease awareness and availability of diagnostic techniques influence case ascertainment disproportionately in some

countries. But two thirds of all cases worldwide have been reported from the United States, Germany, and France. Few if any cases have been recognized in the Far East. In the United States, individuals from 39 states have been diagnosed with Whipple's disease. There is a suggestion of greater disease prevalence in portions of the northern central and mid-Atlantic states; however, the numbers are too few from which to conclude obvious regional clustering. In addition, academic tertiary care facilities with a longstanding interest in Whipple's disease may draw patients from other regions and distort this geographic distribution. There are no reliable data from which to calculate accurate disease prevalence and incidence rates.

Patient occupation, as an epidemiological parameter, yields interesting insights into Whipple's disease. In Dobbins's compilation of reported cases, farmers were the most commonly represented occupational group (22.5% of all patients), and all members of the farming trades accounted for 34% of the total group (16). During the same period of time the average proportion of farmers in the general workforce (e.g., United States, Britain, France, and Germany) was approximately 10%. Workers in the farming trades are more frequently and intensively exposed to soil and water than are workers in other trades. This feature of the Whipple's disease patient population is consistent with the natural ecology of most actinomycetes and, in particular, the actinobacteria grouping within which *T. whippelii* seems to be most closely aligned (see "Microbiology").

The mode of transmission is still largely an area of speculation in Whipple's disease. The propensity of this disease for causing intestinal pathology and the nature of the occupations at greatest risk would suggest an oral route of entry by the causative agent. The infrequent reporting of skin and lung parenchymal lesions argues against a significant role for percutaneous inoculation and aerosol transmission. Several disease clusters have been reported during the past 40 years. Some of these clusters involved as many as seven unrelated individuals living in a confined geographic area, e.g., within a 20-mile radius, or in a single village (42,43). In a few instances, more than one case has occurred in the same family (16,44).

PATHOLOGY, IMMUNITY, AND PATHOGENESIS

Pathology

The gastrointestinal tract and its mesenteric lymphatic drainage is the most common site of pathology in Whipple's disease (5,16,43,46), and is often involved in the absence of specific clinical manifestations related to that organ. While the disease can lead to tissue pathology in any portion of the intestinal tract, it is most often found in the small intestine, and especially within the lamina propria. Whipple commented on the "pink or red velvety swollen mucosa [of the jejunum] . . . flecked over thickly with little pin-point yellowish grains" (1). Enzinger and Helwig described the small intestines as distended, with thickened and "doughy" walls, "stippled by countless yellowish-white, frondlike villi" (45). The ileum and jejunum may be more frequently abnormal by gross inspection than the duodenum. Endoscopic evaluation of the small intestinal lining often reveals patchy areas of pale, shaggy mucosa as well as areas of erythematous, erosive, or friable mucosa (46); however, these grossly visible changes may not be evident in patients with subclinical gastrointestinal involvement. Whipple's disease very rarely involves the stomach or colon (16).

In "classical" Whipple's disease the "most severe and consistent [histologic] changes are seen in the proximal small intestine" (43). By microscopic examination, the small intestines often demonstrate thickened or clubbed villi, distorted by the mononuclear cell infiltrate within the lamina propria (45). Epithelial cells usually appear normal, although they may be somewhat flattened or vacuolated. Some investigators have noted atrophy of the microvilli (9). But the most dramatic aspects of Whipple's disease pathology are found beneath an intact basement membrane, in the lamina propria. Numerous large or plump macrophages fill this layer of the mucosa (Fig. 3; Plate 7). These "foamy" cells contain PAS-positive vacuoles that may sometimes appear as globules or as collections of fine rod- or sickle-shaped particles (Fig. 4; Plate 8). Sieracki and Fine suggested that this particle morphology was specific for Whipple's disease and coined the term *sickleform particle-containing (SPC) cells* (47). The particles correspond to intact or partially degraded bacteria. These particles are more prominent in early untreated disease (48). Other inflammatory cells within the lamina propria include moderate numbers of lymphocytes, eosinophils, and fewer neutrophils and plasma cells. Large neutral lipid droplets populate the lamina propria and sometimes elicit a local neutrophil response. In this circumstance, one may observe neutrophils within the epithelial layer. In addition, lymphatic channels within the lamina propria are usually dilated. These lacteals are thought to contain chylomicrons but not the neutral lipid that accumulates in nearby sites. PAS-positive macro-

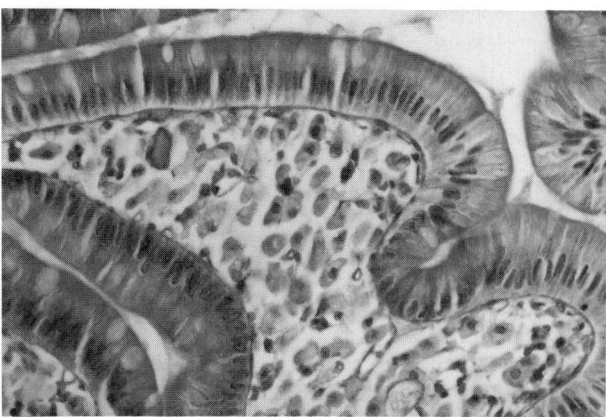

FIG. 3. Typical histology of the duodenal mucosa in a patient with Whipple's disease. Numerous vacuolated macrophages crowd the lamina propria. (H&E, ×300.) (Courtesy of Dr. Donald Regula.) (From ref. 2, with permission.) (See Plate 9.)

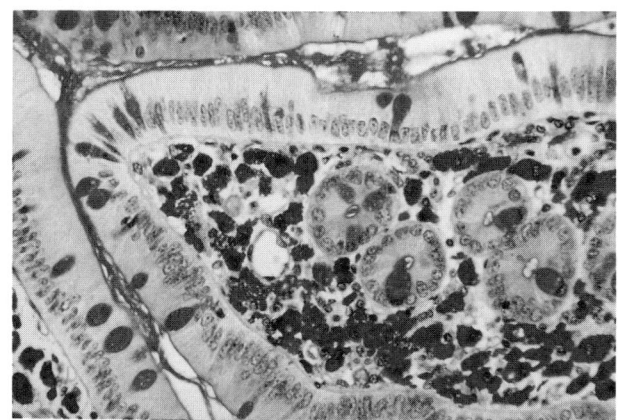

A

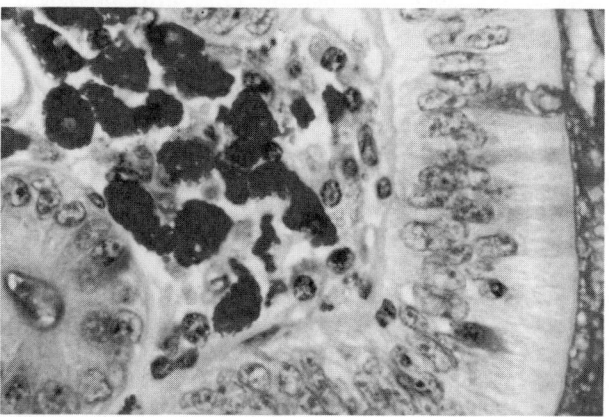

B

FIG. 4. A: Duodenal mucosa of same patient as mentioned in Fig. 2, stained with periodic acid–Schiff (PAS) reagent. Vacuoles of the macrophages within the lamina propria react intensely and appear purple, indicating the presence of glycoprotein (in this case, bacterial cell wall). Epithelial goblet cells are also PAS-positive. (×300). (From ref. 2, with permission.) **B:** Same tissue, higher magnification. (×750). (Courtesy of Dr. Donald Regula.) (See Plate 10.)

phages can also be detected in deeper portions of the mucosa and less often within the submucosa. In at least one patient with Whipple's disease, intestinal pathology was confined to the submucosa, although there had been a prior history of antimicrobial therapy (49). It is also important to recognize that intestinal pathology may be patchy and/or mild (50). As a result, endoscopically guided biopsies may miss areas of pathology.

Several more recent studies have confirmed and expanded on the initial electron microscopic observations of bacillary structures within the intestinal wall of Whipple's disease patients (9–11,14,51). In untreated patients most bacilli are extracellular within the stroma of the lamina propria. In most cases the density of bacilli is highest just below the epithelial basement membrane and progressively decreases from the villus tip toward the submucosa. Few bacteria are observed in the submucosa. Although most intracellular bacilli are found within macrophages, in one study they were seen within intestinal epithelial cells in 11 of 13 patients (12). The route and mechanism of bacterial entry into these nonprofessional phagocytes are unclear; Dobbins proposed that the bacilli may enter epithelial cells from the basolateral surface (51). In keeping with this hypothesis, bacilli can be observed within the epithelial intercellular space (12). Bacteria of typical appearance have also been identified within lymphatic and capillary endothelial cells, neutrophils, plasma cells, intraepithelial lymphocytes, and intestinal smooth muscle cells. They rarely if ever localize to capillary, lacteal, or intestinal lumen.

The pathology of Whipple's disease outside of the small intestines shares many of the features described above. PAS-positive, diastase-resistant macrophages are common in all anatomic sites of involvement and should raise the possibility of Whipple's disease; however, this finding alone is nonspecific. Cells of this type may accompany histoplasmosis, macroglobulinemia, and disseminated atypical mycobacterial disease (16). Morphological or molecular evidence of the characteristic intra- and extracellular Whipple's bacilli should be sought in cases with extraintestinal pathology. In addition, granulomatous responses may predominate in a number of anatomic sites, especially in lymph nodes and in the liver, and are found in approximately 9% (62/696) of Whipple's disease patients (16). Mesenteric lymph nodes are very frequently enlarged and matted together with an average individual diameter of 2–3 cm (45). These nodes are often homogeneously cystic and spongy, and contain an oily material of unknown composition. "Lipogranulomas" are often reported, as well as interstitial fibrosis (Fig. 5; Plate 9). One case of granulomatous gastritis has been attributed to Whipple's disease, but documentation of Whipple bacilli was not provided (52). PAS-positive macrophages in the stomach or rectum are likely to represent lipophages or muciphages, and alone do not constitute proof of Whipple's disease (53). Conversely, PAS-negative macrophages in the context of extraintestinal granulomatous inflammation do not rule out Whipple's disease. Sarcoid-like, epithelioid, noncaseating granulomata with negative PAS staining occur in Whipple's disease, primarily in

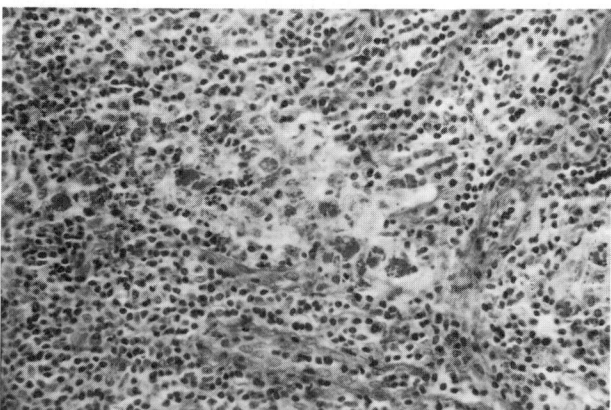

FIG. 5. Lymph node from a patient with Whipple's disease. Dark, PAS-positive clumps correspond to macrophage vacuoles. There is also a pronounced fibrotic reaction that stains less intensely, in a streak-like pattern. ×250. Periodic acid–Schiff reaction. (Courtesy of Dr. Donald Regula and Dr. Mark Feldman.) (See Plate 11).

lymph nodes, liver, spleen, and lungs, as well as in the intestines (54–56) (see "Clinical Illness").

Immunity

Host immune responses in Whipple's disease appear to be relatively intact, with a few exceptions (16,26,57). The available data are derived from immunohistological studies and the evaluation of humoral and cellular immune function in small numbers of patients. Circulating and mucosal antibody levels are usually within normal limits, and plasma cells of the lamina propria, although usually decreased in number in untreated patients, return to normal levels after treatment. On the other hand, in all Whipple's disease patients studied so far, there are no circulating antibodies directed against the PAS-positive material in the intestinal wall (24,58,59,60). Silva et al. speculated that the T. whippelii outer membrane is of host origin and that it may block the organism from eliciting a host humoral immune response (13).

Limited evidence suggests that there may be subtle underlying defects in the function of cellular immune elements in patients with Whipple's disease. Clearly, malnutrition contributes to cellular immune depression during clinically active phases of this disease. Poor lymphocyte mitogenic responses and cutaneous anergy (61–63) probably reflect nutritional status to a large extent. However, with antimicrobial therapy and clinical remission, mitogenic and delayed hypersensitivity responses improve only partially. Peripheral lymphocytopenia is common and persists in these patients, but the ratio of helper (CD4+) to suppressor (CD8+) T lymphocytes is normal. Of interest is an investigation of monocyte function in one patient with Whipple's disease, who was studied at five time points during the 4 years following diagnosis (64,65). Monocyte and macrophage phagocytic and intracellular microbicidal activities did not differ significantly from those cells from control, antibiotic-treated patients; however, they did exhibit impaired ability to degrade ingested bacteria and zymosan. This impairment persisted through a 4-year period comprising initial treatment with clinical remission, subsequent relapse, and then retreatment with a second remission. Granulocytes from this patient behaved normally, and patient serum did not impair functions of monocytes from control individuals. Although these types of studies have not been reported in other Whipple's disease patients, the results suggest that there is a subtle defect in monocytes and macrophages from these patients (64). These results are consistent with the widespread histological observations of partially degraded Whipple bacilli within macrophages (see above). It is not clear as to what extent this may be a preexisting host defect as opposed to an acquired defect, induced by *T. whippelii* and perhaps by other related bacteria (33,37,38) (see below).

Tissue-based characterization of cellular immune responses to *T. whippelii* have not yielded substantial insight into pathogenic mechanisms or clinical manifestations. In the small intestinal epithelium of patients with Whipple's disease intraepithelial lymphocytes (IELs) appear to be activated and have a CD8$^+$, major histocompatibility complex (MHC) class I$^+$ phenotype. The number of IELs per 100 epithelial cells is probably not increased in these patients compared with normal individuals (66), but at least one study demonstrated otherwise in 15 patients at the time of diagnosis (48). In the lamina propria of Whipple's disease patients there are relatively few lymphocytes and the CD4/CD8 ratio of these cells is reduced. Surface IgM$^+$ cells are more numerous in the lamina propria relative to IgA$^+$ cells, and the numerous plump macrophages express normal levels of MHC class II protein on their surface (48).

In the search for a genetic predisposition to Whipple's disease, most investigators have focused on human leukocyte antigen (HLA) antigen profiles. Retrospective analysis of selected cases reveals a greater representation of HLA-B27 than might be expected, even in the absence of sacroiliitis (16,67,68). However, the rarity of this disease hinders statistically meaningful population-based studies; in addition, HLA profiles may have been used for diagnostic purposes. A more recent, small study of a homogeneous population showed no association between Whipple's disease and any class I or class II HLA antigen (69). If Whipple's disease patients do indeed bear an intrinsic immune defect, then it would seem to be subtle. These patients are not at clear increased risk for other infections or for neoplastic disorders (16). Several case reports describe an association between Whipple's disease, giardiasis, and other intestinal parasitic infections (70–72). The numbers of cases are too few from which to draw conclusions about causality and, in particular, conclusions regarding the possibility of impaired intestinal mucosal immunity.

Pathogenesis

Microbial pathogenesis can be conceptualized as a staged process by which a microorganism establishes itself within a host and then ensures its eventual transmission to other hosts (73). The common steps to this process include entry into a susceptible host, acquisition of a suitable niche, multiplication, avoidance or evasion of host immune defenses, and transmission to a new susceptible host. Establishment usually entails microbial multiplication, which often results in tissue damage and pathophysiology. In the case of Whipple's disease the details of many of these steps are poorly understood.

The phylogenetic relationships of *T. whippelii* suggest that this organism may be found in aquatic or terrestrial environments (see "Microbiology"). Since gastrointestinal colonization is such a frequent feature of Whipple's disease, even in the absence of gastrointestinal symptoms or pathology (16,74), one might speculate that bacterial entry into the human host occurs by the oral route. Nonetheless, a scenario consisting of percutaneous inoculation, systemic dissemination, and tropism for the intestinal lamina propria cannot be ruled out. Electron microscopic studies of infected intestinal mucosa raise the possibility that *T. whippelii* penetrates epithelial tight junctions, gains access to epithelial intercellular spaces, and then either enters epithelial cells through the basolateral surface or directly penetrates the basement membrane. The lamina propria seems to offer preferred growth conditions to this organism. At this site, a strong macrophage response is elicited. It is unknown as to whether this cellular response to microbial colonization is the rule or the exception, since a PAS-positive macrophage infiltrate is the most frequently used diagnostic criterion for the disease, and hence the infection.

A number of mechanisms have been proposed to account for intestinal malabsorption in Whipple's disease. Earliest theories focused on the role of abnormal fat metabolism, leading to fat or fatty acid depositions within the intestinal mucosa (1,5); these theories soon gave way to an emphasis on lymphatic obstruction (45). Obstruction was presumed to follow from compression of lacteals by the macrophages and neutral fat deposits, and from fibrosis in the mesenteric lymphatics and lymph nodes. More recent observations of epithelial cell invasion and morphological alterations implicate epithelial cell dysfunction in the pathogenesis of malabsorption (12,43). In addition to all of these potential mechanisms, one must consider the possible toxic effects of substances secreted by *T. whippelii* or of bacterial breakdown products.

Binary division of Whipple's disease bacilli appears to take place almost exclusively in extracellular tissue spaces. On this basis, the organism has been defined as an extracellular pathogen (12,13). However, intracellular survival may also be an important feature of the host–pathogen relationship and may allow prolonged survival of the bacillus in some hosts. There are two basic explanations as to why this is a rare disease. First, exposure to sufficient numbers of the causative agent may be uncommon. For example, the bacillus may occupy an unusual environmental niche or survive only in low numbers in the external environment. Second, a putative defect in macrophage intracellular microbial killing may select rare human hosts for more severe local or systemic disease. While classical forms of the disease may be rare, it is important to remember that atypical disease or asymptomatic infection may be much more frequent.

Dissemination of the bacillus from the intestinal mucosa may occur initially by lymphatic or bloodborne routes. Detection of *T. whippelii* DNA in peripheral blood monocytes argues that bloodborne dissemination of this organism may indeed take place (30). The frequency of disease and visible organisms in various extraintestinal sites suggests bacterial tropism, especially for the central nervous system, the heart, and the reticuloendothelial system. Extraintestinal organ dysfunction probably stems largely from the mononuclear inflammatory cell response elicited by the Whipple bacillus. Later in the course of the disease remnants of *T. whippelii* cell wall may be sufficient for continuing the inflammatory response. Circulating immune complexes have been detected in a few patients but are of unclear significance (75,76). The similarity of Whipple's disease pathology to sarcoidosis in some cases argues that certain microorganisms, including *T. whippelii* and mycobacteria, may share cell wall components capable of stimulating a common host tissue response (77–79). Delineation of *T. whippelii* natural habitats and disease associations is now possible with the use of a specific PCR assay (2,28,80).

CLINICAL ILLNESS

Whipple's disease is a chronic, progressive systemic disorder with features most often referable to the gastrointestinal tract and its lymphatic drainage. The illness described by George Whipple illustrates many of the salient clinical features borne out by subsequent case reviews and analysis. "The . . . illness began insidiously five and a half years ago. . . . The first symptoms were (transient) attacks of arthritis coming on in various joints. . . . These attacks were associated with a gradual loss of weight and strength. In the course of a year he developed a cough which has continued ever since. . . . A slight evening fever developed (and) there were occasional night sweats." The physical examination at that point was unremarkable. Four months prior to admission, "a diarrhoea set in . . . the stools, from three to four a day, of fluid or semi-solid character. . . . (Several weeks later) the patient observed a swelling of the abdomen. . . . Soon after this, a mass became palpable below and to the right of the umbilicus. . . . There has been some tenderness on pressure in this region" (1).

In 1963, Enzinger reviewed the literature on Whipple's disease and described three clinical stages in the untreated patient (45). The first is "an early and indeterminate stage, with insidious onset marked by arthralgia, weight loss, fatigue, and anemia." This is followed by a second stage with "abdominal pain and distention followed by diarrhea and steatorrhea." Finally, there comes "a short terminal stage dominated by various manifestations of malnutrition, disturbed electrolyte balance, cachexia, and often cardiac failure."

The "classical" or typical clinical presentation of Whipple's disease is characterized by weight loss in 95% of patients, diarrhea in 78%, arthralgias in 65%, and abdominal pain in 60% (43). The first two symptoms are less common in patients less than 40 years of age. Arthralgias often predate other manifestations, usually by 3–24 years (81); they are migratory, usually involve large joints, and are only infrequently accompanied by evidence of joint inflammation. Among the physical signs reported in these patients, weight loss is most common (70% of patients), followed by lymphadenopathy (52%), abdominal tenderness (48%), skin hyperpigmentation (47%), and fever (38%) (43). With progressive malnutrition and subsequent hypoalbuminemia, signs of extracellular fluid accumulation, electrolyte imbalances, and anemia become more pronounced. These latter findings have become less common with early diagnosis and treatment. Laboratory investigations are relatively nonspecific; they most often reveal a normochromic-normocytic anemia (90% of patients), a normal or slightly elevated peripheral leukocyte count, thrombocytosis, and hypoalbuminemia.

Intestinal Disease

The known proclivity of Whipple's disease to cause pathology in the small intestines leads one to expect related clinical manifestations in nearly all patients. In fact, diarrhea is reported in approximately three quarters of all patients, although the true denominator is probably unknown, i.e., there may be many other individuals with no history of diarrhea and undiagnosed *T. whippelii* infection. The diarrhea may be watery or steatorrheic. In one review of Whipple's disease (43), 93% of the patients exhibited abnormally high stool fat content. D-Xylose absorption was deficient in 78%, although only 13% of patients had impaired vitamin B_{12} absorption. In a more recent study, 19 of 20 patients had a decreased serum carotene level (82). While it is not commonly appreciated, occult gastrointestinal bleeding is common in Whipple's disease. As many as 86% of patients in some series provide evidence of bleeding (45); in some cases, melena or hematochezia are reported (83). Bleeding sources can arise in both small and large intestines. Endoscopic examination may reveal erosions with friable mucosa or frank ulcerations. The anemia that is so common in Whipple's disease patients may be partially due to blood loss; however, the mean erythrocyte corpuscular volume in patients varies between 83 and 92 fL (43). The etiology of the mucosal erosive changes is unclear. Vascular insufficiency due to distal capillary compression (see "Pathology") or vasculitis (84) as well as nutritional factors may play a role. With respect to the latter possibility, scurvy has been a complication of Whipple's disease (85). Interestingly, weight loss may occur without any history of diarrhea or signs of malabsorption. Patients commonly experience a decrease of 20–30 pounds (82), usually in the later stages of the disease; but a 100-pound weight loss has been described in one patient (86). The abdominal pain in patients with Whipple's disease tends to be epigastric and intermittent.

Radiographic investigations of the gastrointestinal tract frequently reveal many of the nonspecific abnormalities that are associated with malabsorption syndromes. The most common finding with barium studies is prominent and edematous duodenal and jejunal mucosal folds (seen in 51% to 100% of patients) (43,82). Sometimes dilatation of the duodenum and jejunum accompany this picture. In addition, extensive paraaortic and retroperitoneal lymphadenopathies are sometimes first discovered with the use of computerized tomography or abdominal ultrasonography (82) (see "Lymph Nodes" below).

Extraintestinal Disease

The clinical manifestations of Whipple's disease tend to be protean and, because this is a rare disorder, extraintestinal disease may not be recognized as such. Most of the data on involvement of various anatomic sites in Whipple's disease derive from small autopsy series and retrospective case reviews (5,43,45,82,87,88). Thus, these data do not give an accurate picture of relative frequencies of different organ involvement. Nonetheless, some general impressions may be reliable (16). Excluding the gastrointestinal tract and its lymphatic drainage, the most commonly involved anatomic sites are the central nervous system—particularly later in the course of the disease—and the heart. Inflammation of various serosal surfaces is also common, including the pleura, pericardium, and peritoneum, and is often accompanied by a fluid exudate. Lymphadenopathy is relatively common and may be a sign of either localized or diffuse disease. In addition, numerous case reports have provided evidence of Whipple's disease in nearly all other types of tissue, organs, and anatomic compartments. Noteworthy among these relatively less frequently affected sites are the eye and lungs.

Central Nervous System

Whipple's disease involves the central nervous system in approximately 10% of patients based on clinical manifestations, but histological changes (PAS-positive macrophages) were found in 10 of 11 patients in an autopsy series (45). Neurological manifestations of Whipple's disease are particularly protean, reflecting lesions at diverse locations (89). In the pre- and early antibiotic periods, neurological disease became evident late in the course of the clinical illness, or not until autopsy (90). In the past 10–20 years a greater proportion of cases of Whipple's disease present initially with neurological manifestations and often show no clinical signs of intestinal disease (91–93). It is hypothesized that the increasing societal use of antibiotics for unrelated diseases has partially treated or masked intestinal and other well-recognized forms of Whipple's disease, leaving neurological disease to emerge at a later time (94). It is clear that drugs with poor penetration of the blood–brain barrier put patients with Whipple's disease at high risk for disease relapse in the central nervous system (95–97) (see "Treatment and Prophylaxis").

The three most common neurological manifestations of Whipple's disease are dementia, ophthalmoplegia (usually external), and myoclonus (16). The dementia includes memory loss, confusion, inappropriate behavior, and apathy (97); it tends to progress inexorably if not treated. Personality changes, hemiparesis, and seizures also indicate cortical disease. Hypothalamic symptoms feature prominently in many cases of neurological Whipple's disease, especially disruption of sleep patterns, hyperphagia, and polydipsia (95). Cerebellar ataxia and meningeal signs are less common. A rare but particularly important neurological manifestation of Whipple's disease is known as oculomasticatory myorhythmia (OMM) (98). OMM consists of pendular, periodic convergent oscillations of the eyes with concurrent contractions of the masticatory muscles. These oscillations occur at a frequency of approximately one per second. Patients usually also suffer from vertical gaze paralysis. The anatomic lesion is postulated to be a collection of inflammatory nodules in the rostral midbrain and brainstem. This syndrome is believed to be unique to patients with Whipple's disease and is the only pathognomonic clinical finding in this disease. As with other neurological forms of Whipple's disease, OMM may occur in the absence of gastrointestinal disease (98).

Histological changes in the central nervous system include widespread inflammatory nodules up to 2 mm in diameter, consisting of PAS-positive, sickleform particle–containing macrophages (90). They are located in cerebral and cerebellar, cortical and subcortical grey matter, hypothalamus, brainstem, and occasionally in subependymal tissue (16,45). Perivascular lymphocytic infiltrates may accompany these findings. One patient who presented with signs of increased intracranial pressure was found to have multiple, ring-enhancing intracerebral mass lesions (89). Brain tissue from one lesion revealed PAS-positive, diastase-resistant vacuolated macrophages and typical Whipple bacilli. Jejunal biopsies were normal. In general, it is not uncommon for extraintestinal Whipple's disease to occur in the absence of either clinical or histological intestinal manifestations. This is especially true of neurological Whipple's disease (91,99,100). In a variation on this theme, the diagnosis of Whipple's disease was made in one patient with OMM at laparotomy (101). Despite numerous negative small intestinal biopsies, characteristic pathology was found in mesenteric lymph nodes.

Cardiovascular System

The history of Whipple's disease is replete with descriptions of cardiac pathology and the resulting clinical manifestations. The autopsy on Whipple's original patient disclosed fibrinous pericarditis and aortic valve endocarditis (1). These two processes have been surprisingly common in autopsy-based studies. Plummer and colleagues reviewed 34 cases of Whipple's disease and found histological evidence of pericarditis in 71% and "verrucous" endocarditis in 50% (5). Upton was the first to document typical Whipple's disease pathology in the heart (102). He also noted eosinophils and mast cells in the pericardial exudate and a myocardial lymphocytic arteritis. Interstitial lymphocytic myocarditis was reported again in a patient with Whipple's disease more recently (103) and the notion of large-vessel arteritis discussed by James and

Bulkley (104). In a wider application of the PAS reaction, Enzinger and Helwig identified PAS-positive macrophages in the pericardium of 8 of 13 autopsy cases, the myocardium of 6 of 15 cases, and intense staining of the endocardium of 6 of 8 cases (45). In all of these cardiac sites, fibrosis becomes a dominant feature in later stages of disease. The pathogenesis of cardiac lesions in Whipple's disease was later clarified by two studies in which typical Whipple bacilli (some in the process of dividing) were revealed by electron microscopy in all three types of cardiac tissue (105,106).

Clinical evidence of cardiac disease in Whipple's disease appears to be less common than the tissue-based findings described above. However, isolated cardiac findings in the setting of nonspecific systemic signs and symptoms would probably rarely, if ever, raise the possibility of Whipple's disease in a differential diagnosis. In a series of 19 patients 79% had gross pathological abnormalities attributable to Whipple's disease at autopsy, but only 56% had had clinical manifestations (106). The latter included 22% with systolic murmurs, 11% with a percardial friction rub, 6% with congestive heart failure, and 33% with electrocardiographic abnormalities. Cardiac disease may be the initial manifestation of Whipple's disease. One patient presented with aortic insufficiency; typical pathology and microorganisms were found in her native valve at surgery, but it was only at autopsy soon thereafter that evidence of intestinal involvement was discovered (107). In a separate case, mitral valve endocarditis developed in a patient with previously diagnosed intestinal Whipple's disease (108). Two years after mitral valve replacement with a Carpentier–Edwards glutaraldehyde-fixed porcine prosthesis, this patient suffered recurrent congestive heart failure and required a second mitral valve replacement. The removed porcine prosthesis leaflets were covered with and infiltrated by PAS-positive macrophages; extra- and intracellular Whipple bacilli were detected by electron microscopy. The authors of this report suggested that these findings constituted a ''reverse'' application of Koch's postulates to the Whipple bacillus. Molecular phylogenetic analysis of bacilli from this case has not been reported.

Musculoskeletal System

Musculoskeletal involvement in Whipple's disease is much more often clinically apparent than is cardiac involvement, but documentation of tissue pathology is much less available. Arthralgias are one of the most consistent complaints in these patients (see above); they usually occur in acute attacks lasting less than several days and predate the onset of intra-abdominal symptomatology in more than 50% of patients (16). The mean duration of this symptom is approximately 7 years (45). Arthralgias tend to be migratory and involve most commonly the ankles, knees, shoulders, and wrists (43). Fluid accumulation, signs of inflammation, and radiographic or histological evidence of joint destruction are rare. In these cases, however, PAS-positive macrophages and typical bacilli can be detected in the synovial membrane (109). Whip-

ple's disease was diagnosed in one of these cases only following arthroplasty (110). In addition to the syndrome of seronegative inflammatory arthropathy, Whipple's disease may also present as sacroiliitis or spondylitis. The latter may be more common than clinically appreciated (111); one study detected spondylitis retrospectively in nearly 20% of those Whipple's disease patients in whom radiographs were performed, but ankylosing disease in only 10% of those with positive findings (112). The majority of these patients test negative for HLA-B27 antigen.

In the setting of Whipple's disease, skeletal muscle abnormalities are relatively uncommon. Sieracki and Fine first identified PAS-positive macrophages in skeletal muscle at autopsy (47). One patient developed a proximal myopathy in association with arthralgias, diarrhea, fever, and weight loss (113). There was type 2 fiber atrophy, variability in fiber size and shape, and PAS-positive macrophages in the endomysial connective tissue, but no convincing intact bacillary structures. Muscle weakness and atrophic changes are nonspecific and may also reflect malnutrition.

Eye

Ocular manifestations of Whipple's disease are diverse and reflect the potential for this disease to involve all portions of the eye and orbit. Although approximately 40 cases of ocular Whipple's disease have been reported in the literature, the clinical manifestations tend to be nonspecific; therefore, it is likely that many more cases occur and escape diagnosis. The majority of patients with ocular signs and symptoms have concurrent, clinically apparent central nervous system disease. In one review of ocular Whipple's disease, 30 of 36 cases were assigned to this category (114). In fact, many of the ocular findings in these patients, e.g., ophthalmoplegias, nystagmus, and gaze palsies, are due to central neuropathology. Although there have been cases reported of Whipple's disease with neurological manifestations in the absence of gastrointestinal pathology, nearly all patients with ocular manifestations have had either clinical or histological evidence of intestinal involvement (16). Intestinal disease may become clinically manifest well after development of ocular disease, at which time it may be mild or inapparent (83,115). Often intestinal involvement is discovered only at autopsy, as is the case in some patients who are thought to have disease of only the central nervous system. One exception is a case of chronic uveitis due to Whipple's disease, in which multiple small intestinal biopsy tissues were normal by microscopic examination; however, *T. whippelii* rDNA was detected in one of these tissues with the PCR (74).

The intraocular clinical manifestations of Whipple's disease most commonly include visual loss, with evidence of uveitis, vitritis, retinitis (often accompanied by retinal hemorrhage), and optic neuritis (16,114). Some patients have only anterior ocular disease, such as keratitis and corneal ulcers. The pathology of the eye and that of other extraintestinal tissues with Whipple's disease share common characteristics, suggesting similar pathogenic mechanisms. The vitreous and inner retina commonly contain cellular infiltrates consisting primarily of "foamy" macrophages with vacuoles that stain intensely PAS-positive and are diastase-resistant (116,117). Electron microscopy reveals intact and degenerating rod-shaped bacteria within the macrophage vacuoles (117) similar to those reported in numerous studies in other affected tissues. *T. whippelii* rRNA gene sequence has been detected in the vitreous of a patient with chronic uveitis due to Whipple's disease; this sequence was essentially identical to that which was amplified from duodenal tissue of the same patient (74). These findings suggest that the ocular manifestations of Whipple's disease result from the local presence of *T. whippelii*. One might speculate that the route by which this organism gains entry into the eye may involve passage through the intestinal mucosa.

Whipple's disease should always be suspected in patients with chronic bilateral retinitis and uveitis, especially when accompanied by a history of arthralgias, intestinal symptoms, or neurological disease. The differential diagnosis in these settings may include rheumatoid arthritis, ulcerative colitis, sarcoidosis, Lyme disease, and reticulum cell sarcoma. Since most of the ocular manifestations of Whipple's disease are nonspecific, a definitive diagnosis usually involves vitrectomy with light and electron microscopy of the vitreous. PCR may offer an alternative diagnostic method for examination of vitreous and may be more sensitive than traditional approaches.

Respiratory Tract

Chronic cough was a clinical feature of the illness described by Whipple in 1907 (1) and continues to be reported in approximately one half of patients (45). Respiratory manifestations do not usually occur without other concurrent clinical findings and tend not to be severe. Pleuritic chest pain and mild exertional dyspnea are not uncommon (118). In one study, adventitial lung parenchymal sounds and pleural friction rub were appreciated on physical examination in 13% and 15% of patients, respectively (119). In the same study, chest radiographs revealed pulmonary infiltrates in 17%, pleural changes in 19%, and hilar lymphadenopathy in 4% of patients. Pleuritis is found in approximately 72% of patients who complain of cough (45). In a series of 15 autopsies of patients with Whipple's disease, 14 had pleuritis and 6 had a pleural effusion (45). Winberg et al. visualized Whipple bacilli in the lung parenchyma of one patient (120) and *T. whippelii* 16S rDNA has been detected with the PCR in pleural effusion cells (30). However, the pathology of pleuropulmonary disease is variable; it includes pulmonary nodular disease on radiographs, and noncaseating granulomatous pneumonitis or pleuritis by microscopic examination (118,119) (see below). The relative importance of replicating or intact microorganisms vs. immune responses to bacterial cell wall continues to be disputed in the context of pleuropulmonary Whipple's disease.

Skin

Increased skin pigmentation was noted in many of the early descriptions of Whipple's disease. A review of the literature and of their own group of patients by Maizel et al. found hyperpigmentation in 47% and 36% of these populations (43). In their review, Fleming et al. calculated the prevalence of this sign to be 54% (82). This and other features of Whipple's disease has prompted some consideration of adrenal insufficiency in the pathogenesis of the disorder (5). Nonetheless, despite documentation of PAS-positive macrophages in the adrenal capsule, cortex, and medulla (45,47), adrenal functional deficiency does not occur. Other data concerning this issue are scant; thus, the mechanism of hyperpigmentation remains unknown. It tends to occur in exposed areas of skin and in scars.

Lymph Nodes

Peripheral lymphadenopathy occurs in 41% to 71% of Whipple's disease patients (5,43,45,82). Based on physical examination, axillary and cervical lymphatic systems are involved most often (82). Lymph nodes may measure as large as 3–4 cm in diameter. Nodal tenderness is unusual. Diffuse lymphadenopathy may dominate the clinical presentation of Whipple's disease (121), but the latter is of course a rare etiology among all causes of abdominal lymphadenopathy (122). Computerized tomography and ultrasonography may be helpful in detecting subclinical central lymphadenopathy. A few reports suggest that the high fat content of Whipple's disease lymph nodes may be responsible for a distinctive diffuse echogenic appearance (123). As with other forms of extraintestinal disease, lymph node involvement may occur in the absence of intestinal pathology (124).

Reactive hyperplasia, fibrosis, as well as PAS-positive macrophages are common in the enlarged peripheral lymph nodes of Whipple's disease. This picture is nonspecific, however (43). In some cases of Whipple's disease a granulomatous inflammatory response predominates in the peripheral lymph nodes, similar to that sometimes found in lungs and pleura (see "Respiratory Tract"), and liver (see below). Typical Whipple bacilli have been detected with electron microscopy in noncaseating, PAS-negative lymph node granulomata (56). As discussed elsewhere, this pathology can be indistinguishable from that of sarcoidosis (125).

Less Common Extraintestinal Sites

Whipple's disease is truly a systemic disorder. Like syphilis, Lyme disease, and tuberculosis, Whipple's disease can occasionally involve any anatomic site. Among those sites less commonly affected and so far not discussed, the liver, spleen, and kidney bear mention. Hepatomegaly and splenomegaly are detected on physical examination in fewer than 20% of patients but at autopsy are described in approximately 50% and 40% of patients, respectively (43,45). Elevated serum aspartate amino-transferase levels were found in 38% of patients in one study (82); in this situation one must rule out passive hepatic congestion secondary to congestive heart failure. One of the more common forms of hepatosplenic pathology is capsular fibrosis (45). In addition, as discussed earlier, granulomatous disease is relatively more frequent in the liver and spleen than it is in most other organs in patients with Whipple's disease. In this setting, granulomata are composed of epithelioid cells, are noncaseating, and may contain PAS-positive or PAS-negative macrophages (126). Renal complications of Whipple's disease are rarely reported, although approximately 60% of patients demonstrate an abnormal urinalysis (82). Proteinuria and microscopic hematuria are most common. The spectrum of renal disorders associated with Whipple's disease encompasses chronic interstitial nephritis sometimes with granulomata, glomerulonephritis, and IgA nephropathy (16,22,127). The Whipple bacillus has been visualized within the kidney parenchyma (127).

Other Systemic Syndromes Associated with Whipple's Disease

When a patient presents with arthralgias, followed by weight loss, diarrhea, abdominal pain, lymphadenopathy, and fever, Whipple's disease is usually included in the differential diagnosis. This presentation might be considered "classical" or typical Whipple's disease. But probably less than half of all individuals who are ultimately given this diagnosis present with this classical picture. And it is likely that there is a large unrecognized subpopulation of individuals with either asymptomatic or mild ill-defined syndromes due to *T. whippelii* infection.

Dobbins summarized a group of diverse clinical syndromes that deserve to be considered within a more broad definition of Whipple's disease (16). Intestinal signs and symptoms are not features of these nonclassical Whipple's disease syndromes. These syndromes include (a) fever of unknown origin, sometimes accompanied by peripheral lymphadenopathy or arthralgias; (b) dementia, otherwise unexplained, sometimes accompanied by ophthalmoplegias, myoclonus, or hypothalamic symptoms; (c) chronic migratory arthropathy, (d) generalized lymphadenopathy; (e) chronic bilateral uveitis or retinitis, especially when accompanied by the neurological manifestations listed above; (f) chronic pleuritis or pericarditis, accompanied by effusion and sometimes cough or chest pain; and (g) granulomatous hepatitis.

Sarcoidosis has been mentioned several times in previous discussions and deserves to be considered again here. Multiple patients with noncaseating PAS-negative granulomata in lungs, lymph nodes, liver, and spleen have been given a diagnosis of sarcoidosis; and then only later do more traditional and specific findings of Whipple's disease appear, e.g., PAS-positive macrophage infiltrates and electron microscopic documentation of Whipple bacilli (52,54–56,118,124–126,128–131). Are individuals with certain genetic backgrounds more likely to develop sarcoid-like pathology? Are certain *T. whippelii* strains or

closely related species specifically associated with this particular host inflammatory reaction? Is sarcoidosis simply a generic host inflammatory response to a variety of different microorganisms that all share specific cell wall components (78)? Two studies have suggested a role for mycobacteria in a subset of sarcoidosis tissues (77,79), although these results raise some issues concerning the diagnostic criteria used for sarcoidosis. These questions can now be approached with the same experimental techniques that have already revealed the nature of the visible bacillus associated with classical Whipple's disease (2,28).

Beginning in the early 1980s, patients with AIDS were discovered who suffered from syndromes resembling Whipple's disease (33–37). These individuals had chronic diarrhea, fever, weight loss, and abdominal pain; the small bowel mucosa was covered with yellowish grains and infiltrated by PAS-positive "foamy" macrophages. But these cells were also acid-fast and *Mycobacterium avium* complex (MAC) was cultivated from these tissues. MAC and *Rhodococcus equi* (38) may duplicate many of the features of Whipple's disease in immunocompromised hosts; both organisms are members of the actinomycete subdivision of gram-positive bacteria. Chronic diarrhea is a common problem in patients with AIDS and in only approximately 50% is the etiology defined (132,133). In the remaining patients, one might speculate that microorganisms that are currently uncultured, poorly characterized, or difficult to detect could play a role. The similarity between classical Whipple's disease and this syndrome in AIDS patients has prompted current studies that are designed to determine whether *T. whippelii* is involved in other chronic diarrhea syndromes such as this.

DIAGNOSIS

Whipple's disease is recognized and diagnosed infrequently (134). There are three potential explanations. First, the disease and its variant clinical presentations may in fact occur rarely. Second, there may be gross underrecognition of the disease with its protean features and its perhaps more common yet ill-defined nonclassical manifestations. Third, diagnosis of Whipple's disease has required tissue-invasive procedure. This last situation may be changing. In order to diagnose Whipple's disease accurately one must appreciate the diseases and syndromes that mimic it, and vice versa.

Classical Whipple's disease resembles in its clinical presentation a number of chronic systemic infectious, inflammatory, and neoplastic disorders. The original differential diagnosis for George Whipple's patient included Hodgkin's disease and gastrointestinal tuberculosis (1). Although these two diseases are less difficult diagnostic entities today than they were in 1907, two other very similar disorders still create substantial confusion in the interpretation of Whipple's-like clinical presentations, i.e., non-Hodgkin's lymphoma and disseminated MAC infection in HIV-infected hosts (see above). Intestinal lymphoma often generates abdominal symptoms, signs, and radiographic findings similar to those of Whipple's disease

(135). Other disorders that duplicate many of the clinical aspects of Whipple's disease are nontropical sprue, sarcoidosis (see above), and some collagen vascular diseases.

Extraintestinal presentations of Whipple's disease may raise questions concerning a variety of other disease entities. Central nervous system involvement is often nonspecific but may resemble, in particular, multiple sclerosis and Wernicke's encephalopathy. Features that distinguish these from Whipple's disease are the usual absence of supranuclear ophthalmoplegia, myoclonus, and seizures in the former (16), and a history of alcohol abuse and response to thiamine in the latter (97). OMM can be confused with palatal myoclonus, acquired pendular nystagmus, and segmental spinal myoclonus (98), and hypothalamic manifestations may suggest Kleine–Levin syndrome (95). Cerebrospinal fluid in neurological Whipple's disease may be normal or may contain small numbers of leukocytes. Some of these cells are PAS-positive. In most cases, however, the diagnosis of central nervous system involvement requires tissue. The differential diagnosis of chronic uveitis and retinitis includes rheumatoid arthritis, ulcerative colitis, sarcoidosis, Lyme disease, syphilis, tuberculosis, and reticulum cell sarcoma (see above).

The diagnosis of Whipple's disease most often requires peroral endoscopic biopsy of the duodenal mucosa. Hematological, chemical, and radiological tests and procedures are nonspecific and hence not helpful. Dobbins and others have emphasized the usefulness of small intestinal mucosal biopsy in Whipple's disease (16,45,136). Strongly PAS-reactive, diastase-resistant, acid-fast-negative macrophages in the small intestinal lamina propria are considered sufficient for the diagnosis of this disease, in the context of the other typical histological features in this tissue. (Periodic acid oxidizes glycol groups or their amino or alkylamino derivatives to dialdehydes, which then combine with Schiff's reagent to form a magenta compound that is insoluble.) Electron microscopy is usually not necessary in this circumstance. Because Whipple's disease pathology can be patchy in the small intestinal mucosa, multiple biopsies may be required (50). Another cause of false-negative endoscopically obtained histology is the infrequent occurrence of Whipple's disease pathology only in the submucosa (49) or only in extraintestinal tissues (see "Clinical Illness"). Amarenco et al. pointed out the potential diagnostic utility of laparotomy and intra-abdominal lymph nodes in patients with extraintestinal disease (101). Granulomata in any tissue that stains PAS-negative should not exclude the diagnosis of Whipple's disease. In terms of false-positive small intestinal histology, there are several other diseases in which one finds PAS-positive macrophages (16). MAC and R. equi infections can be ruled out with the acid-fast stain. In macroglobulinemia, the macrophages only stain weakly with PAS; and histoplasmosis can be distinguished by the observation of typical encapsulated intracellular yeast. It has already been mentioned that PAS-positive macrophages in the stomach, colon, or rectum may correspond to lipophages or muciphages, and thus are nonspecific and cannot be used as a basis for Whipple's disease diagnosis.

In the case of putative extraintestinal Whipple's disease, PAS-positive diastase-resistant macrophages are again nonspecific. In lymph nodes, for example, mast cells, Russell bodies (cytoplasmic immunoglobulin globules in plasma cells), and other structures may generate a similar staining pattern. Therefore, electron microscopic detection of typical Whipple bacilli morphology is usually required to confirm a diagnosis of Whipple's disease in extraintestinal tissues. Dobbins recommends sample fixation in modified Karnovsky's glutaraldehyde (2.5%) and paraformaldehyde (3%), and then treatment with osmium (16). Accurate discrimination between T. whippelii and other actinomycetes, e.g., MAC, by electron microscopy may require extensive experience.

Partial molecular characterization of the Whipple bacillus, T. whippelii, offers several new alternative diagnostic approaches to this disease. PCR-based detection of T. whippelii has been demonstrated in digested tissue using primers W3FE and W2RB, designed from specific regions of the 16S rRNA gene (2,80). The technique has been applied to fresh-frozen and paraffin-embedded duodenal mucosal biopsy tissues, lymph nodes, pleural fluid cells, peripheral blood mononuclear cells, and ocular vitreous (2,29,30,74). These primers fail to amplify a visible product from other actinomycetes, such as M. avium complex and R. equi. Visible DNA bands of the appropriate size (280 base pairs) in an ethidium-stained agarose gel should be characterized by probe hybridization, DNA sequence analysis, or DNA heteroduplex mobility assay (137). Studies so far have demonstrated that products of the expected size, generated with W3FE and W2RB, are either identical or nearly identical with the original published T. whippelii 16S rDNA sequence (M87484) (D. A. Relman, unpublished data; 2). Without cultivated organisms available, it is difficult to establish the sensitivity of this PCR assay; however, in experiments using paraffin-embedded negative tissue sections and serial dilutions of cloned T. whippelii 16S rDNA, one can detect approximately 100 gene copies (74).

PCR-based tissue assays are probably more sensitive than histological or electron microscopic tissue inspection, given that this assay has revealed T. whippelii in histologically normal duodenal tissue from a patient with extraintestinal Whipple's disease (74). Fresh-frozen tissue provides more sensitive detection with PCR than fixed tissue. It is currently unclear as to whether peripheral blood or cerebrospinal fluid will prove to be more useful targets for T. whippelii detection. However, PCR technology is fraught with the dangers of DNA cross-contamination (138) and can be technically demanding for many clinical microbiology laboratories. While not yet available, in situ tissue hybridization (139,140) with a specific T. whippelii DNA probe may also offer improved specificity and sensitivity over traditional approaches, and at the same time be a more appropriate procedure for widespread clinical application.

TREATMENT AND PREVENTION

Whipple's disease was uniformly fatal prior to the development of antibiotics. While some partial responses have been reported following the use of corticosteroids and adrenocorticotropic hormone (ACTH) (141), these responses have been only temporary and nearly all patients so treated have ultimately succumbed to this disease (43,136). Paulley in 1952 was the first to report the efficacy of antimicrobial therapy in Whipple's disease (8). Treatment of his patient with chloramphenicol resulted in elimination of fever and diarrhea within a week and disease remission lasting at least a year. Antibiotic therapy of Whipple's disease did not become common practice until the early 1960s when it became clear that these drugs could dramatically alter the natural history of the illness (136,142). A variety of antibiotics besides chloramphenicol are thought to have some efficacy in the treatment of Whipple's disease (96), including penicillin, ampicillin, tetracycline, streptomycin (in combination with penicillin), trimethoprim-sulfamethoxazole, erythromycin, and, more recently, ceftriaxone (143) and pefloxacin (101). Prolonged oral tetracycline was a common therapy in the 1960s. Early regimens then began to include an initial parenteral course of penicillin sometimes accompanied by streptomycin, followed by tetracycline for approximately a year (43).

In the late 1970s and early 1980s it became increasingly apparent that clinical relapse was a frequent problem in Whipple's disease patients (95,97,144). Most of these relapses were manifest by neurological disease. Keinath and coworkers reviewed the response to treatment in 88 patients with at least 1-year follow-up (96). Thirty-one (35%) patients suffered a relapse, at a mean of 4 years following initial diagnosis; 11 of these relapses were of a neurological form and occurred relatively late. The most common clinical findings in patients with neurological relapse were dementia and ataxia. Among risk factors for relapse, tetracycline therapy was most significant; 42% of patients treated with tetracycline alone suffered relapse, and they accounted for nearly all relapses involving the central nervous system. Patients with disease relapse outside of the central nervous system did well on any of a variety of antibiotic regimens, while those with central nervous system relapse had a poor response to retreatment. With encouraging reports on the use of trimethoprim-sulfamethoxazole to treat neurologic Whipple's disease, it became apparent that penetration of the blood–brain barrier is an important feature of drugs used for the initial treatment of this disorder (16,96,145,146). More recently, case reports have described the successful treatment of neurological disease with ceftriaxone followed by doxycycline (143), and with pefloxacin (101).

Recommendations for the treatment of Whipple's disease are based on empiric observations and retrospective reviews of the literature. No controlled trials have been published on this subject. Since the causative agent cannot be cultivated *in vitro*, no susceptibility tests can be performed in the laboratory. Can the phylogenetic relationships of the Whipple bacillus, *T. whippelii*, be used to guide the selection of antibiotics in a meaningful manner? Most of the other pathogenic members of the actinobacteria group are susceptible to penicillin, aminoglycosides, trimethoprim-sulfamethoxazole, dapsone, and the tetracyclines, many of which have been used successfully to treat Whipple's disease. Unfortunately, no known organism is closely related to *T. whippelii;* therefore, few inferences can be made regarding drug susceptibility. The current recommendation for the treatment of patients with Whipple's disease is the combination of procaine penicillin G, 1.2 million units IM/day and streptomycin, 1 g IM/day for 14 days, followed by trimethoprim-sulfamethoxazole 160 mg/800 mg PO two to three times a day for at least a year (16,82,96). Folinic acid dietary supplementation should be provided. Some investigators would treat patients with neurological disease for at least 2 years, and perhaps indefinitely.

Clinical response to antibiotic therapy is more dramatic than is the histological response. Approximately 90% of treated patients experience symptomatic relief (82). Diarrhea commonly resolves within 7 days, arthralgias within 1–3 weeks, and significant weight gain within 1 month (43,142). As early as 1 week following institution of therapy, the small intestinal epithelium begins to revert to normal, i.e., return of epithelial cell height, loss of intraepithelial cell bacilli, and the beginning restoration of villus architecture (14). Extracellular bacilli in the lamina propria become degraded and are usually eliminated between 2 and 9 weeks into therapy, and the PAS staining pattern of the macrophage vacuoles becomes more homogeneous (14,16,147). While PAS-positive macrophages become more sparse and patchy in their distribution, these cells usually persist for at least 1 and sometimes for as many as 8 years despite clinical remission (14,82,147). Other mucosal histological changes usually improve or resolve after approximately a year with successful treatment, although lipid deposits and some neutrophils often remain in the lamina propria (16,82). Endoscopic examination reveals the disappearance of gross mucosal changes after 6 months of treatment (46). Correction of the small bowel radiographic appearance occurs after a mean of 10 months (82). Neurological disease is the most recalcitrant to treatment. Gaze palsies and confusion respond most effectively, with eventual improvement or resolution (99). Dementia and long-tract signs may stabilize but usually do not improve. Hypothalamic signs may be the least responsive to treatment. In all forms of Whipple's disease relapse is associated with a return of previous tissue pathology and the reappearance of extracellular bacilli (14).

PCR-based detection of *T. whippelii* may facilitate studies of treatment response, as well as studies on the natural habitat and other disease associations of this organism. These investigations might then have implications for disease prevention. Quantitative PCR assays allow estimations of original target number (148). If these techniques were applied to detection of *T. whippelii,* direct estimations of bacterial burden in various infected anatomical compartments might be feasible. One would then be able to measure *in vivo* antibiotic effects more precisely over time. Likewise, sensitive PCR-based assays for *T. whippelii* in natural aquatic and soil environments might lead to an appreciation of the reservoir for this organism and, subsequently, to strategies for reducing human exposure to it. PCR-based detection of *T. whippelii* in patients with Whipple-like clinical syndromes would suggest the potential usefulness of antibiotic therapy for these patients. In a general sense, further molecular characterization of this microorganism may enhance our understanding of Whipple's disease pathogenesis and the means by which this process may be interrupted.

ACKNOWLEDGMENTS

I acknowledge the helpful discussions of Dr. William O. Dobbins III. D.A.R. is supported by the Lucille P. Markey Charitable Trust (D.A.R. is a Lucille P. Markey Scholar) and Stanford University PMGM Director's Research Fund, sponsored by SmithKline Beecham.

REFERENCES

1. Whipple GH. A hitherto undescribed disease characterized anatomically by deposits of fat and fatty acids in the intestinal and mesenteric lymphatic tissues. *Johns Hopkins Hosp Bull* 1907;18:382–391.
2. Relman DA, Schmidt TM, MacDermott RP, Falkow S. Identification of the uncultured bacillus of Whipple's disease (see comments). *N Engl J Med* 1992;327:293–301.
3. Wilson KH, Blitchington R, Frothingham R, Wilson JA. Phylogeny of the Whipple's-disease-associated bacterium. *Lancet* 1991;338:474–475.
4. Black-Schaffer B. The tinctoral demonstration of a glycoprotein in Whipple's disease. *Proc Soc Exp Biol Med* 1949;72:225–227.
5. Plummer K, Russi S, Harris WHJ, Caravati CM. Lipophagic intestinal granulomatosis (Whipple's disease). Clinical and pathologic study of thirty-four cases, with special reference to clinical diagnosis and pathogenesis. *Arch Intern Med* 1950;86:280–310.
6. Yardley JH, Flemming WH. Whipple's disease: a note regarding PAs-positive granules in the original case. *Johns Hopkins Hosp Bull* 1961;109:76–79.
7. Morgan AD. The first recorded case of Whipple's disease? *Gut* 1961;2:370–372.
8. Paulley JW. A case of Whipple's disease (intestinal lipodystrophy). *Gastroenterology* 1952;22:128–133.
9. Chears WCJ, Ashworth CT. Electron microscopic study of the intestinal mucosa in Whipple's disease: demonstration of encapsulated bacilliform bodies in the lesion. *Gastroenterology* 1961;41:129–138.
10. Cohen AS, Schimmel EM, Holt PR, Isselbacher KJ. Ultrastructural abnormalities in Whipple's disease. *Proc Soc Exp Bio Med* 1960;105:411–414.
11. Yardley JH, Hendrix TR. Combined electron and light microscopy in Whipple's disease: demonstration of "bacillary bodies" in the intestine. *Bull Johns Hopkins Hosp* 1961;109:80–98.
12. Dobbins WO, Kawanishi H. Bacillary characteristics in Whipple's disease: an electron microscopic study. *Gastroenterology* 1981;80:1468–1475.
13. Silva MT, Macedo PM, Nunes JFM. Ultrastructure of bacilli and the bacillary origin of the macrophagic inclusions in Whipple's disease. *J Gen Microbiol* 1985;131:1001–1013.
14. Trier JS, Phelps PC, Eidelman S, Rubin CE. Whipple's disease: light and electron microscope correlation of jejunal mucosal histology with antibiotic treatment and clinical status. *Gastroenterology* 1965;48:684–707.
15. Relman DA, Loutit JS, Schmidt TM, Falkow S, Tompkins LS. The agent of bacillary angiomatosis. An approach to the identification of uncultured pathogens (see comments). *N Engl J Med* 1990;323:1573–1580.
16. Dobbins WO. *Whipple's disease*. Springfield, IL: Charles C Thomas. 1987.
17. Dobbins WO III. Whipple's disease: an historical perspective. *Q J Med* 1985;56:523–531.
18. Evans AS. Causation and disease: the Henle-Koch postulates revisited. *Yale J Biol Med* 1976;49:175–195.
19. Cimprich RE, Rooney JR. *Corynebacterium equi* enteritis in foals. *Vet Pathol* 1977;14:95–102.
20. Archer GL, Coleman PH, Cole RM, Duma RJ, Johnston CJ. Human infection from an unidentified erythrocyte-associated bacterium. *N Engl J Med* 1979;301:897–900.
21. Clancy RL, Tomkins WA, Muckle TJ, Richardson H, Rawls WE. Isolation and characterization of an aetiological agent in Whipple's disease. *Br Med J* 1975;3:568–570.
22. Gupta S, Pinching AJ, Onwubalili J, Vince A, Evans DJ, Hodgson HJ. Whipple's disease with unusual clinical, bacteriologic, and immunologic findings. *Gastroenterology* 1986;90:1286–1289.
23. Sherris JC, Roberts CE, Porus RL. Microbiological studies of intestinal biopsies taken during active Whipple's disease. *Gastroenterology* 1965;48:708–710.
24. Keren DF, Weisburger WR, Yardley JH, Salyer WR, Arthur RR, Charache P. Whipple's disease: demonstration by immunofluorescence of similar bacterial antigens in macrophages from three cases. *Johns Hopkins Med J* 1976;139:51–59.
25. Bhagavan BS, Hofkin GA, Cochran BA. Whipple's disease: morphologic and immunofluorescence characterization of bacterial antigens. *Hum Pathol* 1981;12:930–936.
26. Keren DF. Whipple's disease: a review emphasizing immunology and microbiology. *Crit Rev Clin Lab Sci* 1981;14:75–108.
27. Woese CR. Bacterial evolution. *Microbiol Rev* 1987;51:221–271.
28. Relman DA. The identification of uncultured microbial pathogens. *J Infect Dis* 1993;168:1–8.
29. vonHerbay A, Otto HF. Whipple's disease: a report of 22 patients. *Klin Wochenschr* 1988;66:533–539.
30. Muller C, Stain C, Burghuber O. Tropheryma whippelii in peripheral blood mononuclear cells and cells of pleural effusion (letter). *Lancet* 1993;341:
31. Ennis PD, Zemmour J, Salter RD, Parham P. Rapid cloning of HLA-A,B cDNA by using the polymerase chain reaction: frequency and nature of errors produced in amplification. *Proc Natl Acad Sci USA* 1990;87:2833–2837.
32. Khavari PA, Bolognia JL, Eisen R, Edberg SC, Grimshaw SC, Shapiro PE. Periodic acid-Schiff-positive organisms in primary cutaneous *Bacillus cereus* infection. Case report and an investigation of the periodic acid–Schiff staining properties of bacteria. *Arch Dermatol* 1991;127:543–546.
33. Gillin JS, Urmacher C, West R, Shike M. Disseminated *Mycobacterium avium-intracellulare* infection in acquired immunodeficiency syndrome mimicking Whipple's disease. *Gastroenterology* 1983;85:1187–1191.
34. Maliha GM, Hepps KS, Maia DM, Gentry KR, Fraire AE, Goodgame RW. Whipple's disease can mimic chronic AIDS enteropathy. *Am J Gastroenterol* 1991;86:79–81.
35. Roth RI, Owen RL, Keren DF. AIDS with *Mycobacterium avium–intracellulare* lesions resembling those of Whipple's disease (letter). *N Engl J Med* 1983;309:1324–1325.
36. Roth RI, Owen RL, Keren DF, Volberding PA. Intestinal infection with Mycobacterium avium in acquired immune deficiency syndrome (AIDS). Histological and clinical comparison with Whipple's disease. *Dig Dis Sci* 1985;30:497–504.
37. Strom RL, Gruninger RP. AIDS with *Mycobacterium avium-intracellulare* lesions resembling those of Whipple's disease (letter). *N Engl J Med* 1983;309:1323–1324.
38. Wang HH, Tollerud D, Danar D, Hanff P, Gottesdiener K, Rosen S. Another Whipple-like disease in AIDS? (letter). *N Engl J Med* 1986;314:1577–1578.
39. Chiodini RJ, Van KH, Merkal RS. Ruminant paratuberculosis (Johne's disease): the current status and future prospects. *Cornell Vet* 1984;74:218–262.
40. Cornelius CE. Animal models—a neglected medical resource. *N Engl J Med* 1969;281:934–944.
41. Thoen CO, Baum KH. Current knowledge on paratuberculosis. *J Am Vet Med Assoc* 1988;192:1609–1611.
42. Capron JP, Thevenin A, Delamarre J, et al. Whipple's disease: study of three cases and epidemiological and radiological remarks. *Lille Med* 1975;20:842–845.
43. Maizel H, Ruffin JM, Dobbins W III. Whipple's disease: a re-

view of 19 patients from one hospital and a review of the literature since 1950. *Medicine (Baltimore)* 1970;49:175–205.

44. Puite RH, Tesluk H. Whipple's disease. *Am J Med* 1955;19:383–400.

45. Enzinger FM, Helwig EB. Whipple's disease: a review of the literature and report of 15 patients. *Virchows Arch Pathol Anat* 1963;336:238–269.

46. Geboes K, Ectors N, Heidbuchel H, Rutgeerts P, Desmet V, Vantrappen G. Whipple's disease: endoscopic aspects before and after therapy. *Gastrointest Endosc* 1990;36:247–252.

47. Sieracki JC, Fine G. Whipple's disease-observations on systemic involvement. II. gross and histologic observation. *Arch Pathol* 1959;67:81–93.

48. Ectors N, Geboes K, De VR, et al. Whipple's disease: a histological, immunocytochemical and electronmicroscopic study of the immune response in the small intestinal mucosa. *Histopathology* 1992;21:1–12.

49. Kuhajda FP, Belitsos NJ, Keren DF, Hutchins GM. A submucosal variant of Whipple's disease. *Gastroenterology* 1982;82:46–50.

50. Moorthy S, Nolley G, Hermos JA. Whipple's disease with minimal intestinal involvement. *Gut* 1977;18:152–155.

51. Dobbins WI, Ruffin JM. A light- and electron-microscopic study of bacterial invasion in Whipple's disease. *Am J Pathol* 1967;51:225–242.

52. Ectors N, Geboes K, Wynants P, Desmet V. Granulomatous gastritis and Whipple's disease. *Am J Gastroenterol* 1992;87:509–513.

53. Gear EVJ, Dobbins WOI. Rectal biopsy: a review of its diagnostic usefulness. *Gastroenterology* 1968;55:522–544.

54. Cho C, Linscheer WG, Hirschkorn MA, Ashutosh K. Sarcoid-like granulomas as an early manifestation of Whipple's disease. *Gastroenterology* 1984;87:941–947.

55. Spapen HDM, Segers O, DeWit N, et al. Electron microscopic detection of Whipple's bacillus in sarcoidlike periodic acid-Schiff-negative granulomas. *Dig Dis Sci* 1989;34:640–643.

56. Wilcox GM, Tronic BS, Schecter DJ, Arron MJ, Righi DF, Weiner NJ. Periodic acid-Schiff-negative granulomatous lymphadenopathy in patients with Whipple's disease. Localization of the Whipple bacillus to noncaseating granulomas by electron microscopy. *Am J Med* 1987;83:165–70.

57. Dobbins WOI. Is there an immune deficit in Whipple's disease? *Dig Dis Sci* 1981;26:247–252.

58. Groll A, Valberg LS, Simon JB, Eidinger D, Wilson B, Forsdyke DR. Immunological defect in Whipple's disease. *Gastroenterology* 1972;63:943–950.

59. Kent TH, Layton JM, Clifton JA, Schedl HP. Whipple's disease: light and electron microscopic studies combined with clinical studies suggesting an infective nature. *Lab Invest* 1963;12:1163–1178.

60. Kirkpatrick PJ, Kent SP, Mihas A, Pritchett P. Whipple's disease: case report with immunological studies. *Gastroenterology* 1978;75:297–301.

61. Feurle GE, Dorken B, Schopf E, Lenhard V. HLA B27 and defects in the T-cell system in Whipple's disease. *Eur J Clin Invest* 1979;9:385–389.

62. Martin FF, Vilseck J, Dobbins W3, Buckley C3, Tyor MP. Immunological alterations in patients with treated Whipple's disease. *Gastroenterology* 1972;63:6–18.

63. Veloso FT, Vaz SJ, Baptista F, Ribeiro E. Whipple's disease. Report of a case with clinical immunological studies. *Am J Gastroenterol* 1981;75:419–425.

64. Bjerknes R, Laerum OD, Odegaard S. Impaired bacterial degradation by monocytes and macrophages from a patient with treated Whipple's disease. *Gastroenterology* 1985;89:1139–1146.

65. Bjerknes R, Odegaard S, Bjerkvig R, Borkje B, Laerum OD, Whipple's disease. Demonstration of a persisting monocyte and macrophage dysfunction. *Scand J Gastroenterol* 1988;23:611–619.

66. Austin LL, Dobbins WO III. Intraepithelial leukocytes of the intestinal mucosa in normal man and in Whipple's disease: a light- and electron-microscopic study. *Dig Dis Sci* 1982;27:311–320.

67. Dobbins WO III. HLA antigens in Whipple's disease. *Arthritis Rheum* 1987;30:102–105.

68. Feurle GE. Association of Whipple's disease with HLA-B27 (letter). *Lancet* 1985;1:1336

69. Bai JC, Mota AH, Maurino E, et al. Class I and class II HLA antigens in a homogeneous Argentinian population with Whipple's disease: lack of association with HLA-B27. *Am J Gastroenterol* 1991;86:992–994.

70. Bassotti G, Pelli MA, Ribacchi R, et al. Giardia lamblia infestation reveals underlying Whipple's disease in a patient with long-standing constipation. *Am J Gastroenterol* 1991;86:371–374.

71. Meier WH, Maiwald M, von Herbay A. [Whipple's disease associated with opportunistic infections]. *Dtsch Med Wochenschr* 1993;118:854–860.

72. Oliver-Pascual E, Galan J, Oliver-Pascual A, Castillo E. Un caso de lipodistrofia intestinal con lesions ganglionares mesentericas de granulomatosis lipofagica (Enfermedad de Whipple). *Rev Esp Enferm Apar Dig Nutr* 1947;6:213–226.

73. Relman DA, Falkow S. A molecular perspective of microbial pathogenicity. In: Mandell GL, Douglas RG, Bennett JE, eds. *Principles and practice of infectious diseases.* Fourth Edition. New York: Churchill Livingstone; 1994:19–29.

74. Rickman LS, Freeman WR, Green WR, et al. Uveitis caused by *Tropheryma whippelii*. 1994:submitted.

75. Farr M, Morris C, Hollywell CA, Scott DL, Walton KW, Bacon PA. Amyloidosis in Whipple's arthritis. *J R Soc Med* 1983;76:963–965.

76. Kwitko AO, Shearman DJ, McKenzie PE, La BJ, Rowland R, Woodroffe AJ. Whipple's disease: a case with circulating immune complexes. *Gastroenterology* 1980;79:1318–1323.

77. Mitchell IC, Turk JL, Mitchell DN. Detection of mycobacterial rRNA in sarcoidosis with liquid-phase hybridisation. *Lancet* 1992;339:1015–1017.

78. Rook GA, Stanford JL. Slow bacterial infections or autoimmunity? *Immunol Today* 1992;13:160–164.

79. Saboor SA, Johnson NM, McFadden J. Detection of mycobacterial DNA in sarcoidosis and tuberculosis with polymerase chain reaction. *Lancet* 1992;339:1012–1015.

80. Relman DA. PCR-based detection of the uncultured bacillus of Whipple's disease. In: Persing DH, Smith TF, Tenover FC, White TJ, eds. *Diagnostic molecular microbiology: principles and applications.* Washington, DC: American Society for Microbiology; 1993:496–500.

81. Miksche LW, Blumcke S, Fritsche D, Kuchemann K, Schuler HW, Grozinger K-H. Whipple's disease: etiopathogenesis, treatment, diagnosis, and clinical course. *Acta Hepato-Gastroenterol* 1974;21:307–326.

82. Fleming JL, Wiesner RH, Shorter RG. Whipple's disease: clinical, biochemical, and histopathologic features and assessment of treatment in 29 patients. *Mayo Clin Proc* 1988;63:539–551.

83. Feldman M, Price G. Intestinal bleeding in patients with Whipple's disease. *Gastroenterology* 1989;96:1207–1209.

84. James TN, Bulkley BH, Kent SP. Vascular lesions of the gastrointestinal system in Whipple's disease. *Am J Med Sci* 1984;288:125–129.

85. Berger ML, Siegel DM, Lee EL. Scurvy as an initial manifestation of Whipple's disease. *Ann Intern Med* 1984;101:58–59.

86. Chears WCJ, Hargrove MD, Verner JV, Smith AG, Ruffin JM. Whipple's disease-a review of twelve patients from one service. *Am J Med* 1961;30:226–234.

87. Comer GM, Brandt LJ, Abissi CJ. Whipple's disease: a review. *Am J Gastroenterol* 1983;78:107–114.

88. Feldman M. Whipple's disease. *Am J Med Sci* 1986;291:56–67.

89. Wroe SJ, Pires M, Harding B, Youl BD, Shorvon S. Whipple's disease confined to the CNS presenting with multiple intracerebral mass lesions. *J Neurol Neurosurg Psychiatry* 1991;54:989–992.

90. Sieracki JC, Fine G, Horn RCJ, Bebin J. Central nervous system involvement in Whipple's disease. *J Neuropathol Exp Neurol* 1960;19:70–75.

91. Finelli PF, McEntee WJ, Lessell S, Morgan TF, Copetto J. Whipple's disease with predominantly neuroophthalmic manifestations. *Ann Neurol* 1977;1:247–252.

92. Kitamura T. Brain involvement in Whipple's disease: a case report. *Acta Neuropathol* 1975;33:275–278.
93. Knox DI, Bayless TM, Yardley JH, Charache P. Whipple's disease presenting with ocular inflammation and minimal intestinal symptoms. *Johns Hopkins Med J* 1968;123:175–182.
94. Riggs JE. The evolving natural history of neurologic involvement in Whipple disease: a hypothesis (letter). *Arch Neurol* 1988;45:830.
95. Feurle GE, Volk B, Waldherr R. Cerebral Whipple's disease with negative jejunal histology. *N Engl J Med* 1979;300:907–908.
96. Keinath RD, Merrell DE, Vlietstra R, Dobbins WOI. Antibiotic treatment and relapse in Whipple's disease. Long-term follow-up of 88 patients. *Gastroenterology* 1985;88:1867–1873.
97. Knox DL, Bayless TM, Pittman FE. Neurologic disease in patients with treated Whipple's disease. *Medicine (Baltimore)* 1976;55:467–476.
98. Schwartz MA, Selhorst JB, Ochs AL, et al. Oculomasticatory myorhythmia: a unique movement disorder occurring in Whipple's disease. *Ann Neurol* 1986;20:677–683.
99. Pollock S, Lewis PD, Kendall B. Whipple's disease confined to the nervous system. *J Neurol Neurosurg Psychiatry* 1981;44:1104–1109.
100. Romanul FC, Radvany J, Rosales RK. Whipple's disease confined to the brain: a case studied clinically and pathologically. *J Neurol Neurosurg Psychiatry* 1977;40:901–909.
101. Amarenco P, Roullet E, Hannoun L, Marteau R. Progressive supranuclear palsy as the sole manifestation of systemic Whipple's disease treated with pefloxacine (letter). *J Neurol Neurosurg Psychiatry* 1991;54:1121–1122.
102. Upton AC. Histochemical investigation of the mesenchymal lesions in Whipple's disease. *Am J Clin Pathol* 1952;22:755–764.
103. Pelech T, Fric P, Huslarova A, Jirasek A. Interstitial lymphocytic myocarditis in Whipple's disease (letter). *Lancet* 1991;337:553–554.
104. James TN, Bulkley BH. Abnormalities of the coronary arteries in Whipple's disease. *Am Heart J* 1983;105:481–491.
105. Lie JT, Davis JS. Pancarditis in Whipple's disease: electronmicroscopic demonstration of intracardiac bacillary bodies. *Am J Clin Pathol* 1976;66:22–30.
106. McAllister HJ, Fenoglio JJ. Cardiac involvement in Whipple's disease. *Circulation* 1975;52:152–156.
107. Bostwick DG, Bensch KG, Burke JS, et al. Whipple's disease presenting as aortic insufficiency. *N Engl J Med* 1981;305:995–998.
108. Ratliff NB, McMahon JT, Naab TJ, Cosgrove DM. Whipple's disease in the porcine leaflets of a Carpentier–Edwards prosthetic mitral valve. *N Engl J Med* 1984;311:902–903.
109. Rubinow A, Canoso JJ, Goldenberg DL, Cohen AS, Shirahama T. Arthritis in Whipple's disease. *Isr J Med Sci* 1981;17:445–450.
110. Farr M, Hollywell CA, Morris CJ, Struthers GR, Bacon PA, Walton KW. Whipple's disease diagnosed at hip arthroplasty. *Ann Rheum Dis* 1984;43:526–529.
111. Scheib JS, Quinet RJ. Whipple's disease with axial and peripheral joint destruction. *South Med J* 1990;83:684–687.
112. Canoso JJ, Saini M, Hermos JA. Whipple's disease and ankylosing spondylitis simultaneous occurrence in HLA-B27 positive male. *J Rheumatol* 1978;5:79–84.
113. Swash M, Schwartz MS, Vandenburg MJ, Pollock DJ. Myopathy in Whipple's disease. *Gut* 1977;18:800–804.
114. Avila MP, Jalkh AE, Feldman E, Trempe CL, Schepens CL. Manifestations of Whipple's disease in the posterior segment of the eye. *Arch Ophthalmol* 1984;102:384–390.
115. Finelli PF, McEntee WJ, Lessell S, Morgan TF, Copetto J. Whipple's disease with predominantly neuroophthalmic manifestations. *Ann Neurol* 1977;1:247–252.
116. Durant WJ, Flood T, Goldberg MF, Tso MO, Pasquali LA, Peyman GA. Vitrectomy and Whipple's disease. *Arch Ophthalmol* 1984;102:848–851.
117. Font RL, Rao NA, Issarescu S, McEntee WJ. Ocular involvement in Whipple's disease: light and electron microscopic observations. *Arch Ophthalmol* 1978;96:1431–1436.
118. Symmons DP, Shepherd AN, Boardman PL, Bacon PA. Pulmonary manifestations of Whipple's disease. *Q J Med* 1985;56:497–504.
119. Pequignot H, Morin Y, Grandjouan MS, et al. [Sarcoidosis and Whipple's disease. Association? Relation?]. *Ann Med Interne (Paris)* 1976;127:797–806.
120. Winberg CD, Rose ME, Rappaport H. Whipple's disease of the lung. *Am J Med* 1978;65:873–880.
121. Aubert L, Quilichi R, Gharbi G, Daumas B. Adenopathies in Whipple's disease (letter). *Nouv Presse Med* 1979;8:2986.
122. Deutsch SJ, Sandler MA, Alpern MB. Abdominal lymphadenopathy in benign diseases: CT detection. *Radiology* 1987;163:335–338.
123. Davis SJ, Patel A. Case report: distinctive echogenic lymphadenopathy in Whipple's disease. *Clin Radiol* 1990;42:60–62.
124. Mansbach C II, Shelburne JD, Stevens RD, Dobbins W III. Lymph-node bacilliform bodies resembling those of Whipple's disease in a patient without intestinal involvement. *Ann Intern Med* 1978;89:64–66.
125. Rodarte JR, Garrison CO, Holley KE, Fontana RS. Whipple's disease simulating sarcoidosis: a case with unique clinical and histologic features. *Arch Intern Med* 1972;129:479–482.
126. Giradin M-F S-M, Zafrani ES, Chaumette M-T, Delchier J-C, Metreau J-M, Dhumeaux D. Hepatic granulomas in Whipple's disease. *Gastroenterology* 1984;86:753–756.
127. Stoll T, Keusch G, Jost R, Burger H, Oelz O. IgA nephropathy and hypercalcemia in Whipple's disease. *Nephron* 1993;63:222–225.
128. Diaz LS, Gonzalez RJ, Granado S, et al. [Sarcoidosis and Whipple's disease: an association or a relationship?]. *Rev Clin Esp* 1992;190:184–186.
129. Frenk E, Merot Y, Perez I, Chamot AM, Gerster JC. Maladie de Whipple a presentation cutanee sarcoidosique. *Ann Dermatol Venereol* 1991;118:115–118.
130. Saint, Marc GM, Zafrani ES, et al. Hepatic granulomas in Whipple's disease. *Gastroenterology* 1984;86:753–756.
131. Southern JF, Moscicki RA, Magro C, Dickersin GR, Fallon JT, Bloch KJ. Lymphedema, lymphocytic myocarditis, and sarcoidlike granulomatosis. Manifestations of Whipple's disease. *JAMA* 1989;261:1467–1470.
132. Greenson JK, Belitsos PC, Yardley JH, Bartlett JG. AIDS enteropathy: occult enteric infections and duodenal mucosal alterations in chronic diarrhea (see comments). *Ann Intern Med* 1991;114:366–372.
133. Smith PD, Quinn TC, Strober W, Janoff EN, Masur H. NIH conference. Gastrointestinal infections in AIDS. *Ann Intern Med* 1992;116:63–77.
134. Donaldson RJ. Whipple's disease—rare malady with uncommon potential (editorial comment). *N Engl J Med* 1992;327:346–348.
135. Chetelat CA, Bruhlmann W, Ammann RW. Malignoma-like lymphography findings retroperitoneally in Whipple's disease: a possible source of misdiagnosis. *Schweiz Med Wochenschr* 1985;115:364–368.
136. Ruffin JM, Roufail WM. The diagnosis and treatment of Whipple's disease. *Am J Dig Dis* 1965;10:887–891.
137. Delwart EL, Shpaer EG, Louwagie J, et al. Genetic relationships determined by a DNA heteroduplex mobility assay: analysis of HIV-1 env genes. *Science* 1993;262:1257–1261.
138. Kwok S, Higuchi R. Avoiding false positives with PCR [published erratum appears in *Nature* 1989 Jun 8;339(6224):490]. *Nature* 1989;339:237–238.
139. Brigati DJ, Myerson D, Leary JJ, et al. Detection of viral genomes in cultured cells and paraffin-embedded tissue sections using biotin-labeled hybridization probes. *Virology* 1983;126:32–50.
140. Burns J, Graham AK, Frank C, Fleming KA, Evans MF, McGee JO. Detection of low copy human papilloma virus DNA and mRNA in routine paraffin sections of cervix by non-isotopic in situ hybridisation. *J Clin Pathol* 1987;40:858–864.
141. Radding J, Fiese MJ. Whipple's disease (intestinal lipodystrophy): review of the literature and report of a case successfully treated with adrenocorticotropin (ACTH) and cortisone. *Ann Intern Med* 1954;41:1066–1075.
142. Ruffin JM, Kurtz SM, Roufail WM. Intestinal lipodystrophy

(Whipple's disease): the immediate and prolonged effect of antibiotic therapy. *JAMA* 1966;195:476–478.

143. Adler CH, Galetta SL. Oculo-facial-skeletal myorhythmia in Whipple disease: treatment with ceftriaxone. *Ann Intern Med* 1990;112:467–469.

144. Feldman M, Hendler RS, Morrison EB. Acute meningoencephalitis after withdrawal of antibiotics in Whipple's disease. *Ann Intern Med* 1980;93:709–711.

145. Ryser RJ, Locksley RM, Eng SC, Dobbins WO III, Schoenknecht FD, Rubin CE. Reversal of dementia associated with Whipple's disease by trimethoprim-sulfamethoxazole, drugs that penetrate the blood-brain barrier. *Gastroenterology* 1984; 86:745–752.

146. Viteri AL, Greene JJ, Chandler JJ. Whipple's disease, successful response to sulfamethoxazole-trimethoprim. *Am J Gastroenterol* 1981;75:309–310.

147. Denholm RB, Mills PR, More IA. Electron microscopy in the long-term follow-up of Whipple's disease. Effect of antibiotics. *Am J Surg Pathol* 1981;5:507–516.

148. Wang AM, Doyle MV, Mark DF. Quantitation of mRNA by the polymerase chain reaction [published erratum appears in *Proc Natl Acad Sci USA* 1990 Apr;87(7):2865]. *Proc Natl Acad Sci USA* 1989;86:9717–9721.

Infections of the Gastrointestinal Tract,
edited by M. J. Blaser, P. D. Smith, J. I. Ravdin,
H. B. Greenberg, and R. L. Guerrant
Published by Raven Press, Ltd., New York, 1995.

CHAPTER 62

Mycobacterial Disease of the Gastrointestinal Tract

C. Robert Horsburgh, Jr. and Ann Marie Nelson

Mycobacteria are among the most ancient of bacteria, and mycobacterial diseases are among the most ancient of human diseases. Tuberculosis was prevalent in Egypt of the pharaohs, India of the Rig Veda, Persia of the Zoroastrians, and pre-Columbian Mesoamerica (1). The classical Greeks recognized the clinical entity of cough, fevers, and wasting, which they called "phthisis." Hippocrates noted the grave prognosis of gastrointestinal (GI) involvement with tuberculosis; he observed that "diarrhea attacking a person with phthisis is a mortal symptom" (2). The Greeks also recognized chronic cervical lymphadenitis, or scrofula (3), which in the middle ages became known as the "king's evil," since the king's touch was reputedly curative (4). The relationship between pulmonary tuberculosis and scrofula was not appreciated until the nineteenth century (3).

As rates of tuberculosis in the developed countries decreased in the mid-twentieth century, other mycobacterial diseases of the gastrointestinal tract were recognized. The foremost of these is infection with organisms of the *Mycobacterium avium* complex (MAC). This agent has replaced *Mycobacterium tuberculosis* as the commonest cause of scrofula in children. More recently, the severe immune suppression seen in patients with acquired immune deficiency syndrome (AIDS) has led to an upsurge in cases of MAC infection of the alimentary canal.

GASTROINTESTINAL DISEASE DUE TO *M. TUBERCULOSIS* COMPLEX

Epidemiology

Human tuberculosis (TB) is acquired either by ingestion or inhalation of organisms of the *M. tuberculosis* complex.

C. R. Horsburgh, Jr.: Division of Infectious Diseases, Department of Medicine, Emory University School of Medicine, Altanta, Georgia 30303.
A. M. Nelson: Division of AIDS Pathology, Armed Forces Institute of Pathology, Washington, D.C. 20306.

The major reservoirs for this infection are humans and cattle. Human-to-human transmission occurs when a person with active TB exhales or expectorates droplet nuclei containing organisms, which are then inhaled and cause a localized pulmonary process in the susceptible host. Transmission of TB from cattle to humans occurs when mycobacteria from infected cattle are excreted into milk, which when ingested (as milk or milk products) may then cause localized infection of the GI tract, mostly in the terminal ileum, cecum, colon, and rectum (5,6). "Secondary" infection of the GI tract also may occur; this term refers to GI involvement as a result of swallowing organisms from sputum in persons with active pulmonary TB or to GI involvement secondary to hematogenous dissemination of TB from any other site (5).

In the preantibiotic era, secondary GI TB in persons with advanced pulmonary TB was by far the most common form of GI TB. The overwhelming numbers of cases involved the lung, and 65–90% of pulmonary TB patients eventually developed secondary TB of the GI tract (5). In an autopsy series of patients with pulmonary tuberculosis reported in 1928, 184 (80%) of 230 had secondary TB of the GI tract (7); isolated GI TB was rare. More severe cases of pulmonary TB were more likely to develop into GI TB; 5–8% of "early pulmonary TB" had radiographic evidence of GI TB, compared to 14–18% of "moderately advanced" and 70–80% of "far advanced" cases (8). In the United States, GI TB was decreasing in frequency as TB cases overall decreased throughout the twentieth century. After the introduction of antibiotic therapy for TB in 1946, the incidence of GI TB dropped markedly. The prevalence of GI TB detected radiographically declined from 10% to 1% between 1924 and 1949 (9). By 1969–1973, the rate of nonperitoneal abdominal tuberculosis in a sample of the U.S. population was 0.08% of all TB cases, or 0.01 cases per 100,000 persons (10). Recent reports from India, Finland, and South Africa report less than 5% of TB cases with GI tract involvement (6,11,12).

This decrease has several probable causes. First,

prompt treatment of pulmonary TB may prevent GI TB. As noted, GI involvement is uncommon in persons with acute TB (either primary or reactivated) but increases in frequency with duration and severity of the pulmonary disease (5,8,13). Second, since GI TB responds to antibiotic therapy for pulmonary TB, many cases of GI TB go undiagnosed and resolve with treatment of the pulmonary focus. Third, to the extent that GI TB was related to the presence of *M. tuberculosis* or *M. bovis* in unpasteurized milk, such disease decreased with control of TB in cattle in the United States prior to 1946. Recent series of GI TB from developed countries have shown a predominance of isolated GI TB over GI TB secondary to pulmonary TB (14–18); series from developing countries continue to show that the majority of cases are secondary (6,19).

Much speculation has occurred regarding the relationship between the two most common pathogens in the *M. tuberculosis* complex—*M. tuberculosis* and *M. bovis*—and isolated vs. secondary TB of the GI tract. Early authors suggested that isolated infection, most likely due to exposure to contaminated milk or milk products, would be caused most commonly by *M. bovis,* while secondary GI TB, resulting from the more common *M. tuberculosis* disease of the lung, would usually be due to *M. tuberculosis* (5). Control of tuberculous cattle should have resulted in a rarity of isolated GI TB. However, in countries where disease of cattle is not well controlled, *M. bovis* is rare as a cause of either isolated or secondary GI TB (6). Therefore, it appears that both species are capable of producing either isolated or the secondary GI TB, depending on the route of exposure. Since *M. tuberculosis* is much more common than *M. bovis* worldwide, it now causes the overwhelming majority of cases of either presentation (6,20–22).

In the preantibiotic era, isolated GI TB was felt to be more common in children than adults, whereas secondary GI TB was more common in adults (5). More recent studies have shown both forms to be more common in older individuals; in the United States and Europe, the mean age of cases of both types appears to be 50–75 years, while in the developing countries the mean age is most often 20–40 years (6,23). This is most likely a reflection of the overall age distribution of active TB in those areas. Despite some reports showing higher rates in women, most data show the sexes to be equally affected (6,24,25). Racial and ethnic distribution of GI TB in the United States also mirrors that of TB overall, with fewer cases in whites than in nonwhites (10,26).

Although we generally include only disease in the alimentary canal itself under the rubric of GI TB, tuberculous scrofula is undoubtedly the sequelum of an oral exposure to mycobacteria. Infection in these cases was probably contained by the host in the paragastrointestinal lymphoid tissue. Scrofula should therefore be thought of as part of the spectrum of mycobacterial infection of the GI tract. This entity was formerly quite common, representing up to 25% of cases of tuberculosis in some areas, but became rare in the United States with pasteurization of milk and testing and elimination of tuberculous cows in the 1920s (3). Scrofula is still common in some developing countries, although *M. tuberculosis* is more commonly

the causative agent than *M. bovis* (27). Tuberculous scrofula occurs in all age groups but is more frequent in children; for unknown reasons, this entity is seen more commonly in females than in males (28).

Persons with human immunodeficiency virus (HIV) infection are uniquely susceptible to disease due to *M. tuberculosis,* both primary acquisition and reactivation disease. This susceptibility is in part responsible for recent increases in the incidence of tuberculosis in countries where HIV infection has become established. As might be expected, GI TB occurs in patients with AIDS, including TB of the stomach, jejunum, ileum, and rectum (29–31); both isolated and secondary GI TB cases have been reported. In patients with dual infection of HIV and *M. tuberculosis* who have disseminated tuberculosis, the rate of GI tract involvement ranged from 20% in Ivory Coast to 26% in Zaire (32). Tuberculous scrofula also occurs in HIV-infected persons (33).

Microbiology

Mycobacteria are considered transitional forms between eubacteria and actinomycetes, and so are classed in the order Actinomycetales, family Mycobacteriaceae. Mycobacteria are slender, sometimes curved, rod-shaped organisms. They are aerobic, non–spore-forming, nonmotile, and measure 0.2–0.6 by 1.0–4.0 μm. The cell walls of mycobacteria contain mycosides that are mycolic acid–containing long-chain glycolipids and/or phospholipoglycans that protect these facultative intracellular parasites from lysosomal attack. Between 25% and 60% of dry weight is lipid, compared to 0.5% for gram-positive and 3% for gram-negative organisms.

Mycosides retain red basic fuchsin dye after acid rinsing; this quality of acid fastness can be strong or weak. Organisms often appear beaded. Although highly specific, these stains are not very sensitive and are positive in sputa in only 25–50% of early or miliary cases of tuberculosis. Concentrations of at least 10,000 bacilli/mL are required for detection by this method. The auramine-rhodamine fluorescence stain is more sensitive but less specific than the carbol-fuchsin stains. The bacilli fluoresce bright orange–yellow with blue light (34–39).

The tuberculosis complex consists of four organisms: *M. tuberculosis hominis, M. bovis, M. africanum,* and *M. microti. M. tuberculosis hominis* and *M. bovis* are the strains most commonly associated with human disease in the United States.

Mycobacterium tuberculosis hominis

Humans are the primary reservoir of this organism. It is the most common species of mycobacteria found in tuberculosis of the GI tract (20,22). Growth is favored in 5–10% CO_2 but inhibited by pH < 6.5 and long-chain fatty acids. In vitro, bacilli grow at 35–37°C. Three weeks or more is required for culture because of the long doubling time (12–20 hr compared to <1 hr for most bacteria). In liquid media, organisms form cords, a factor associated with virulence. *M. tuberculosis* is niacin-positive, reduces nitrate, is usually sensitive to isoniazid, and will produce disease in guinea pigs.

Mycobacterium bovis

M. bovis causes tuberculosis in cattle and is highly virulent in man. Prior to use of pasteurization, milk from infected cows was an important source of human GI and oropharyngeal tuberculosis (5). *M. bovis* cannot be distinguished by disease manifestations or purified tuberculin (PPD) reaction, but demonstrates different culture characteristics. It is slightly smaller than *M. tuberculosis* and is slower growing. It is niacin-negative, does not reduce nitrates, and does not produce disease in guinea pigs (38,39). An attenuated strain of *M. bovis* was used to produce the BCG (bacille Calmette Guérin) vaccines.

Pathogenesis and Immunity

Virulence Factors

There are genetic and phenotypic differences in the ability of mycobacteria to produce disease (40); some strains from Africa and India produce attenuated disease in guinea pigs (39). Repeated passage through subcultures, exposure to ultraviolet light, and air drying decrease the virulence of most mycobacteria.

No exotoxins, endotoxins, or tissue-necrotizing enzymes of *M. tuberculosis* have been discovered in intact tubercle bacilli. Some toxic components (e.g., cord factor) may be released when the mycobacteria disintegrate. Glycolipids and peptides such as wax D and muramyl dipeptide enhance delayed-type hypersensitivity—one of the major causes of cell death (see below). Another mechanism that allows mycobacteria to multiply within macrophages (histiocytes) of the nonimmune host is their ability to block phagolysosomal fusion. Sulfatides modify lysosome membranes to prevent fusion with phagosomes (34,35,37).

Though morphology is not consistently related to virulence, virulent strains tend to produce rough colonies. The formation of serpentine cords in either liquid or solid media is associated with increased virulence in guinea pigs. Cord factor (trehalose 6,6'-dimycolate) inhibits polymorphonuclear leukocyte (PMN) migration in vitro, is lethal to mice, and has been related to profound disturbances of microsomal enzymes, mitochondria, and lipid metabolism in livers of mice by attacking the mitochondrial membranes (39,41).

The exact infective dose for humans is not known but is estimated at 5–200 organisms in the respiratory tract (40). The size of the inoculum is important for two reasons (a) larger numbers of organisms may overwhelm the host's immune system and (b) there is a higher probability of exposure to more virulent or drug-resistant organisms.

Pathophysiology

Many swallowed or ingested bacilli are destroyed in the acid environment of the stomach, but some pass through

TABLE 1. *Location of lesions of tuberculosis of the gastrointestinal tract in 184 cases*

Location	Number (%)
Tongue	1 (0.6)
Stomach	1 (0.6)
Duodenum	7 (3.8)
Jejunum	39 (21.2)
Ileum	153 (83.2)
Cecum	160 (87.0)
Appendix	72 (39.1)
Colon	132 (71.7)
Sigmoid/rectum	30 (16.3)

Data from ref. 7.

the mucosa where they are phagocytized and carried to Peyer's patches, lymphoid follicles in the mucosa, or the mesenteric lymph nodes. The most common sites of infection are located in areas with the greatest concentration of lymphoid tissue and the slowest transit time. Most infections occur in the ileocecal region, where 50–90% of lesions are observed (20). Lesions involve both sides of the valve and may extend into the appendix. Multiple lesions are common, but occur with decreasing frequency in the proximal portions of the small intestine (Table 1). Esophageal, pyloric, and anal lesions are rare and usually occur as secondary lesions.

Textbooks from the preantibiotic era provide the best gross descriptions of tuberculous enteritis (5), when this was "one of the most common conditions found in the intestines" (42). Three anatomic forms were described: acute ulcerative, miliary, and hyperplastic. This classification has been modified slightly: a combined ulcerohypertrophic form has replaced miliary. The ulcerative form is the most common (60%) and has the highest associated mortality, followed by the ulcerohypertrophic (30%). Only 10% of cases are hypertrophic (43). Miliary tuberculosis still occurs in the GI tract but is considered part of a disseminated disease. In any form, healing may result in fibrosis, strictures, or stenosis (43).

In the author's (A.M.N.) experience in Zaire, miliary disease was the most common form of GI tuberculosis seen at autopsy in patients with AIDS. Thirty of 70 (43%) patients with AIDS had tuberculosis. Of these, eight (26%) had involvement of the GI tract. No cases of primary GI tuberculosis were seen. Ulcers were present in about half the cases, but none were hypertrophic. In all but one case there was also involvement of the liver. The stomach was involved in two cases, and the esophagus in one (44).

The esophagus may be involved by direct extension from subcarinal lymph nodes or from swallowing bacilli. Lesions usually occur in the middle third of the esophagus. The ulcerative form is the most common and is a rare cause of hematemesis (45). Healing and scar formation are associated with traction diverticulae, and hyperplastic lesions may cause stricture (46,47).

In gastric and duodenal tuberculosis, lesions usually occur as a complication of disseminated disease or due to spread from celiac nodes. Antral and pyloric ulceration, stenosis (48), gastric outlet obstruction, upper GI bleeding, and pyeloduodenal fistulas have all been reported (49). Preexisting mucosal lesions are thought to be important in the pathogenesis of both esophageal and gastric tuberculosis (50).

Tuberculosis of the appendix is often ulcerative and occurs as a local extension of ileocecal or pelvic tuberculosis. Less frequently, it may represent an isolated extrapulmonary site of infection. Tuberculous colitis is usually segmental and associated with ileocecal disease. It can be ulcerative or hypertrophic; pipestem fibrosis and aphthous ulcers of the colon have been described (51,52). In their review of intestinal tuberculosis, Paustian and Monto (20) cite several cases of concurrent colonic tuberculosis and either carcinoma or ulcerative colitis. *M. tuberculosis* was thought to be a secondary invader.

Anorectal abscesses and fistulas were more common before antituberculosis therapy (20). There have been recent reports in the literature of tuberculous lesions with and without fistula formation (53).

Acute Pathology (Ulcerative)

Although acute ulcerative enteritis may occur as either isolated or secondary tuberculosis, the majority of cases occur as a complication of pulmonary tuberculosis (5). Ingested bacilli penetrate the mucosa and establish the initial lesion in lymphoid follicles of a Peyer's patch. Retrograde spread of bacilli from regional nodes and hematogenous spread in miliary tuberculosis are other sources of secondary GI infection. Subsequent follicular hyperplasia presents as a small submucosal nodule that is often associated with edema of the overlying mucosa (43,43,54).

Caseous necrosis develops as a result of delayed-type hypersensitivity to mycobacterial antigens. The center of the lesions becomes soft and yellow and the necrotic center sloughs, forming a small ulcer with raised borders. As the infection spreads via the lymphatics, small satellite nodules appear which in turn ulcerate. The lesions eventually coalesce to form a large ulcer. Multiple ulcers may form at several sites that appear as skip lesions radiographically (42,43,54).

The ulcers have a characteristic appearance with irregular, infiltrated borders and a necrotic base. They are initially round to oval with transverse or circumferential spread. The cut surface may be white and friable (Fig. 1). Multiple tuberculous nodules are often within and around the ulcer and in the adjacent serosa. Pseudopolyps may form. There is often involvement of the adjacent lymph nodes. Focal peritonitis is also common (5,42,43).

Histologically the early lesions show nonspecific inflammation with edema and mixed acute and chronic inflammatory cells. As the lesions progress, there is local accumulation of epithelioid macrophages and foci of central caseous necrosis develop. Sections of the ulcers reveal typical necrosis and granulation tissue with chronic inflammation, with macrophages and loosely formed granulomas in the surrounding tissue. PMNs may be present in and adjacent to areas of ulceration. Bowel involve-

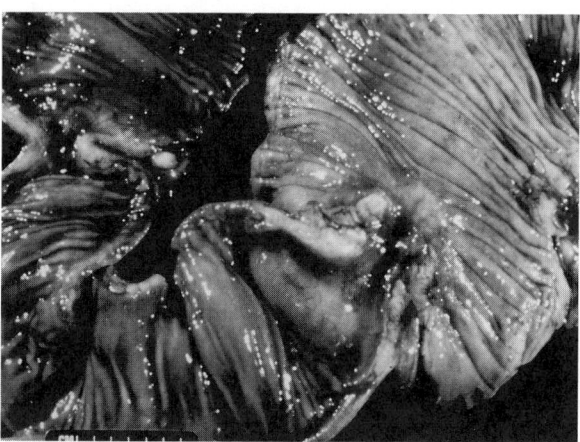

FIG. 1. Tuberculous enteritis, ulcerative, ileocolostomy specimen. Multiple ulcerations are present with focal thickening, especially at the ileocecal junction. (Courtesy of Mount Sinai Hospital, Miami.) (See Plate 12.)

ment is often transmural. Acid-fast bacilli may be found in areas of granuloma or in the ulcer bed (Fig. 2).

Delayed-type hypersensitivity-associated cellular killing and tissue destruction is increased in this form due to the greater number of acid-fast bacilli present (55) (see "Host Response" below). In the immunocompromised host, the ulceration may extend over a larger area of the bowel and deeper into the tissue in response to the large number of bacilli. The disease process seems to be accelerated and there is usually less fibrosis, more necrosis, and a variable inflammatory response (A.M.N., personal observations). Cases of intestinal perforation due to transmural multibacillary lesions have been reported in HIV-associated GI TB (30).

Chronic Pathology (Hypertrophic)

Chronic infection leads to extensive granuloma formation, fibrosis, and often a palpable mass (tuberculoma) in

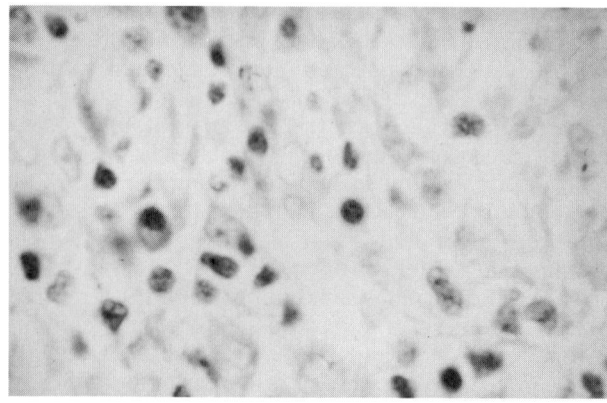

FIG. 2. Tuberculous enteritis, acute (×600). Ziehl–Neelsen–stained section of intestinal wall (see Fig. 1) reveals a loosely formed granuloma with numerous acid-fast bacilli. (Courtesy of Mount Sinai Hospital, Miami.) (See Plate 13.)

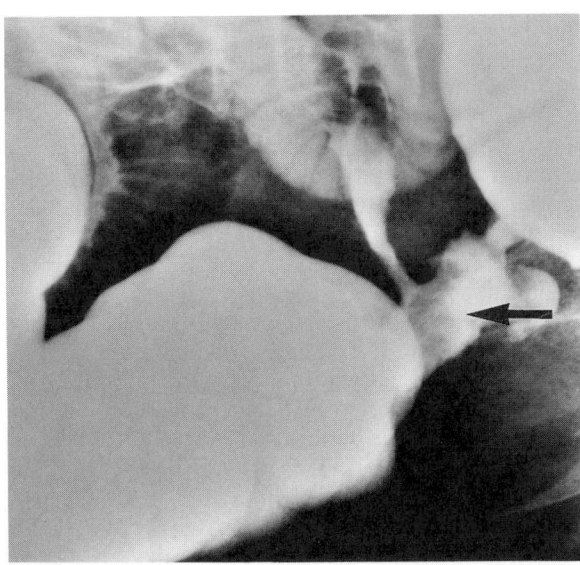

FIG. 3. Radiograph of hypertrophic tuberculous enteritis with marked thickening of the wall. Note stricture and proximal dilatation of the bowel.

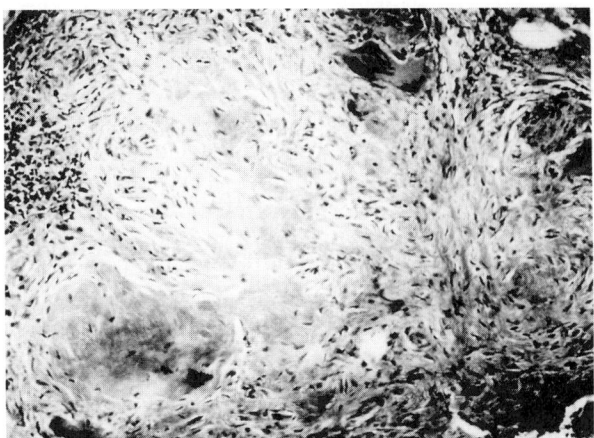

FIG. 5. Histological section of hypertrophic tuberculous enteritis (×200) (Fig. 4) showing granulomatous inflammation with abundant Langhans giant cells and fibrosis (H&E stain).

the ileocecal or other area of the gut. This so-called chronic productive or hyperplastic form of intestinal tuberculosis is usually circumferential (napkin ring) and is often mistaken for a neoplasm. The bowel wall may measure 1 cm or more in thickness. These strictures can be multiple and vary considerably in length. The overlying surface is often ulcerated (ulcerohypertrophic) or sclerotic (20,42,54). In cases of severe stenosis dilatation of the proximal bowel can be significant (Figs. 3 and 4) and in rare cases can result in perforation (30).

Peritonitis may occur with or without perforation (5,20,43). Occasionally, fibrous adhesions of one or more bowel loops develop. Fistulization usually occurs in the ulcerohypertrophic form. It is sometimes due to secondary bacterial invasion and can involve the adjacent bowel, the female adnexa, or the abdominal wall (20). Involvement of regional mesenteric lymph nodes is common.

On section there are caseating granulomas with varying

degrees of fibrosis; lesions are transmural. Peyer's patches and regional lymph nodes are almost invariably involved. These features are important in the differential diagnosis with Crohn's disease, but the presence of acid-fast bacilli in the tissue is the most important single feature in confirming the diagnosis of tuberculosis (20). Acid-fast bacilli are in areas of granuloma in active cases, both in the bowel wall and in the affected regional lymph nodes. Caseous material can be cultured for mycobacteria. Old, healed lesions are fibrotic, sometimes calcified, with few active granulomata; acid-fast bacilli are extremely rare and often impossible to find (Figs. 4 and 5).

Host Immune Response

Four stages of infection and disease are described (55). The first or primary infection occurs in the immunologically naive host. Inhaled or ingested viable mycobacteria are phagocytized by the resident macrophages (usually in the pulmonary alveoli). Whether the infection progresses or not depends on the microbicidal abilities of resident macrophages and on the virulence of the infecting agent.

If the mycobacteria are able to survive and multiply, they destroy the macrophage and the infection passes to the second or symbiotic stage. The mycobacterial antigens along with complement component C5a and cytokines (e.g., monocyte chemotactic protein–1) induce chemotaxis and macrophages (monocytes) are recruited from the peripheral blood. Bacilli are phagocytosed and then multiply logarithmically within these immature macrophages (55).

The infection advances to the third stage with the onset of acquired cellular resistance (cellular immunity); this occurs 4–8 weeks after the initial infection. Stage 3 is characterized by local accumulation of large numbers of macrophages and lymphocytes and a local activation of these cells. An indurated reaction to the intradermal injection of PPD indicates the presence of cell-mediated immu-

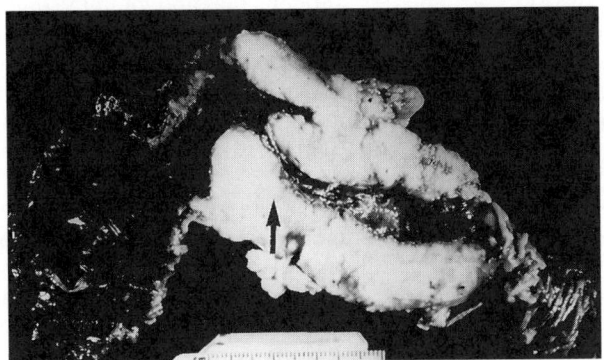

FIG. 4. Photograph of hypertrophic tuberculous enteritis with marked thickening of the wall. Note stricture and proximal dilatation of the bowel *(arrow).*

nity (CMI) to tuberculosis. CMI occurs with specific clonal proliferation of T cells and results in the activation of macrophages and enhanced intracellular killing of mycobacteria. Delayed-type hypersensitivity (DTH) causes cell killing with formation of caseous necrosis (55).

The fourth stage refers primarily to pulmonary tuberculosis and the formation of cavities. This stage of lung disease is important in enteric tuberculosis because it corresponds to the greatest release of mycobacteria into the sputum and subsequently into the alimentary tract. The reduction in cavitary tuberculosis by early treatment is probably the most important reason for the great decline in intestinal disease.

The stages of tuberculosis in the immunocompetent host seem to be reversed as HIV infection progresses to AIDS. Patients with early HIV disease and CD4+ counts above 400×10^6/L have good CMI and lesions remain well circumscribed and paucibacillary. Qualitative and quantitative defects in CD4+ cells allow increased proliferation of bacilli with a switch to DTH-mediated necrosis and subsequent expansion of the lesions. With increased immune suppression, DTH weakens and the host is unable to control the infection. This would presumably coincide with loss of DTH response to PPD.

In patients with advanced immunosuppression, macrophages continue to be recruited into the area. The lesion resembles the early tubercle. There is intracellular proliferation of bacilli within nonactivated (nonepithelioid) macrophages. Finally, PMNs are recruited into the area in a final attempt to control the infection. Suppurative necrosis and increased extracellular proliferation of mycobacteria are seen (56).

CMI–DTH interactions vary with changes in host immunity and mycobacterial concentration. CMI predominates when antigen levels are low, and DTH when large concentrations of bacilli are present or macrophage activation is impaired (55). In the immunocompromised host, bacilli that escape from the caseous centers are phagocytized by poorly activated macrophages, which in turn are destroyed by cytotoxic lymphocytes and other DTH mechanisms. There is centrifugal extension of the caseous necrosis when bacillary growth is no longer controlled by CMI as seen in HIV-infected patients. The ratio of CMI-to DTH-mediated responses is probably an important determinant of the morphology of lesions found in the GI tract.

High titers of antibodies to various antigens of *M. tuberculosis* develop following infection (57), but their significance in human tuberculosis is not known. Humoral response was shown to be greater to certain protein fractions of a culture filtrate than T-cell blastogenesis in patients with clinical disease; the reverse was true for healthy tuberculin reactors (58).

The histological patterns of tuberculosis reflect the integrity of the cellular immune response of the patient. Very little has been described in the literature regarding the specific pathology of enteric tuberculosis in the HIV-infected host. However, the host response to pulmonary tuberculosis probably serves as an adequate model.

Patients with relatively intact cellular immunity will have a typical granulomatous response (32,56,59). Immu-

nostaining shows clustering of CD4+ lymphocytes around epithelioid macrophages and Langhans giant cells. The majority of macrophages have abundant cytoplasm that stains intensely with KP-1 (CD68) macrophage markers (probably indicating activation) (56). As the CD4+ lymphocyte count drops, cellular immunity decreases. There is a loss of Langhans giant cells followed by a decrease in epithelioid macrophages. This decrease in activated macrophages results in poor intracellular killing of mycobacteria and a concomitant increase in levels of mycobacterial antigen. The immune response shifts toward DTH-mediated necrosis. Necrosis is mixed suppurative and caseous. Acid-fast bacilli are numerous, both in the areas of necrosis and within macrophages. In the gut this probably is associated with ulcerative lesions and increased incidence of perforations.

In the final stages of AIDS, there is a diffuse inflammatory response composed of immature macrophages and PMNs. Suppuration and coagulative necrosis have replaced the typical caseating granulomatous response. Acid-fast bacilli are myriad. The large number of acid-fast bacilli within macrophages is reminiscent of proliferation in the naive host (32,56).

Susceptibility Factors

Most persons infected by *M. tuberculosis* do not develop active tuberculosis but rather control the pathogen without eliminating it, a condition known as *tuberculosis infection (without disease)*. For practical purposes, this is the condition of having a positive PPD skin test without evidence of active disease anywhere in the body. In the United States 10–50% of exposed persons may acquire infection, depending on the intensity and duration of exposure. Of these, 5–10% develop disease within the first 2 years after exposure and another 5–10% will develop disease later in life (60). Most of these persons will have pulmonary tuberculosis, while a small fraction will be unable to localize the process and will have disseminated or miliary tuberculosis. Immunosuppressed persons, such as those with AIDS, are at increased risk for failure to control primary tuberculosis infection.

Caucasians and Mongolians are more resistant to infection than Africans, indigenous Americans, and Polynesians (61). Certain HLA antigens (62) and vitamin D deficiency have been associated with increased rates of disease (35). Partial immunity is afforded by BCG vaccine or exposure to nontuberculosis mycobacteria in the environment (41). The nonimmune host is most susceptible to infection, but reinfection with new strains of *M. tuberculosis* occurs (63,64).

Reactivation tuberculosis is the term used to describe development of active tuberculosis in a person who has had quiescent tuberculous infection; the active disease results from "reactivation" of a previously contained focus rather than from reacquisition of TB from an external source. Reactivation usually occurs as the result of a decline in host immune status, such as with intercurrent illness, malnutrition, alcoholism, or corticosteroid therapy. Persons coinfected with HIV and *M. tuberculosis* have the highest rates of developing reactivation tuberculosis, from 5–10% per year (65,66).

Clinical Manifestations

TB in the GI tract may occur in a single or in multiple sites. Table 1 shows the relative distribution of lesions in a United States autopsy series of 1928 (7). Bhansali in India in 1977 (6) and Novis et al. in South Africa in 1973 (24) report remarkably similar findings. Disease of the esophagus and stomach are rare, and the vast majority of involvement is in the small intestine, cecum, or both. Thus it is not surprising that the symptoms and signs manifested by patients with this entity are nonspecific. In a series of 58 cases reported by Hoon et al. in 1950, abdominal pain was reported in 88% of patients, weight loss in 77%, nausea in 52%, vomiting in 48%, anorexia in 41%, fever in 38%, diarrhea in 36%, and constipation in 24% (67). Disease of the esophagus may present with dysphagia or pain in the throat (45–47,68). Anorectal disease may be accompanied by perianal ulcers and/or fistulas (53,69,70).

In the preantibiotic era, pulmonary TB was usually present concurrently, aiding in establishing the diagnosis of GI TB. However, with the increasing proportion of GI TB that is isolated (i.e., not resulting from chronic autoingestion of infected sputum) this finding can no longer be expected. Tuberculous peritonitis is also uncommonly associated with GI TB, presumably because tuberculous peritonitis is usually the result of hematogenous spread rather than of direct extension from an enteric focus of TB (26). When GI TB disease is advanced, symptoms and signs of obstruction predominate, with nausea, vomiting, and pain; an abdominal mass may frequently be palpated (6,23), especially if the cecum is involved.

Pancreatic abscess due to M. tuberculosis is a rare complication and has a high mortality rate (71–73). It occurs as an isolated lesion or can be a complication of miliary disease. Reported presentations include multicystic lesions, abscesses, tumors, or miliary foci. Late complications of GI TB include biliary obstruction, malabsorption, perforation with secondary bacterial peritonitis, and, less commonly, GI hemorrhage or fistula formation (6,20, 26,72–74). Severe diarrhea is a rare but serious complication of GI TB; although it was referred to as "dysenteric tuberculosis," it is secretory rather than hemorrhagic (75).

Perforation of GI TB is rare in the HIV-uninfected host but has been reported with increasing frequency in HIV-seropositive patients with impaired cellular immunity (30,76). This is probably due to the large numbers of organisms and the full-thickness involvement of the bowel by active, necrotizing disease. Patients with longstanding chronic untreated GI TB may manifest abnormalities associated with all forms of chronic tuberculosis, such as inanition, anemia, amyloidosis, and Addison's disease.

Scrofula due to TB may present as asymptomatic swelling or with associated fevers, night sweats, and weight loss. The most commonly involved nodes are the anterior and posterior cervical, followed by the submental (77). A

thorough search should be made for signs of active tuberculosis in other sites, particularly in the HIV-infected patient (33). Complications include abscess formation and local sinus tracts (28).

Diagnosis

Diagnosis of GI TB is notoriously difficult. Confirmation of the diagnosis requires isolation of M. tuberculosis from affected tissue, or evidence of TB elsewhere with caseating granulomata in GI tissue samples. Hoon in 1950 proposed the following criteria: (a) growth of the organism from affected tissue, or (b) histologic demonstration of mycobacteria in tissue, or (c) histological demonstration of granulomata with caseation necrosis, or (d) typical gross pathological findings in the bowel with histological findings of granulomata with caseation necrosis in associated lymph nodes (67). These criteria must be somewhat modified today with the advent of MAC involvement of the gut in patients with AIDS. Current histological techniques do not permit differentiation of mycobacterial species by histological or microscopic techniques. Additionally, the increasing frequency of TB in AIDS patients, who often do not form granulomata with caseation necrosis in response to TB, makes criterion 3 less useful.

Traditionally, tissue for diagnosis was obtained on surgical exploration. While this may be required when obstruction occurs, many cases of GI TB may now be diagnosed by endoscopic biopsy (78,79). Endoscopic appearance may reveal deep ulcerative lesions, masses, or strictures, but these are not diagnostic. Biopsy specimens should have routine histology to look for granulomas and special strains to identify acid-fast organisms in addition to mycobacterial culture. Endoscopic biopsies should be taken from the nodular lesions or from the borders of ulcers to include as much submucosal material as possible. Superficial biopsies of epithelium may show only nonspecific inflammation and not the diagnostic granulomatous lesions or acid-fast bacilli.

Because acid-fast bacilli are commonly isolated from the stool in patients with pulmonary tuberculosis and probably represent swallowed organisms from sputum rather than infection of the GI tract, feces are usually not cultured (80). When it is necessary to speciate mycobacteria, as in patients with AIDS or in isolated GI infections, feces or other collections of GI contents should first be examined by microscopy to detect the presence of acid-fast bacilli. In the past, cultures were recommended only if smears were positive. However, a recent article reported that smears had only a 34% sensitivity. The authors recommend that feces be cultured for mycobacteria if GI involvement is suspected (81). AIDS patients with TB often have mycobacteremia, and blood cultures may be used as a means of detecting disseminated infection.

Routine culture techniques include a decontamination procedure and must be done using a biological safety cabinet (37). Several methods of decontamination of stool have been reported; most require longer decontamination than sputum (82,83). Feces should be frozen if processing cannot be done soon after collection. A nonselective egg medium, such as Lowenstein–Jensen, is used for primary isolation; Middlebrook agar (7H10 or 7H11, with or without antibiotics) can be used for primary recovery. Species are identified by pigmentation, growth characteristics, biochemical tests, and ability to produce disease in laboratory animals.

Radiometric and other rapid detection methods have been developed to reduce the long incubation period of standard techniques. The Bactec (Becton–Dickinson Diagnostic Instruments, Sparks, MD) and Isolator (Du Pont, Wilmington, DL) systems can detect *M. tuberculosis* within 8–10 days and some nontuberculous mycobacteria in as few as 5 days. NAP (ρ-nitro-α-acetylamino-β-hydroxypropriophenone) inhibition can be used to differentiate *M. tuberculosis* and *M. bovis* from other mycobacteria. GenProbe (San Diego, CA) uses specific DNA probes to the ribosomal RNA of mycobacteria to speciate clinically significant organisms (41). Gas–liquid chromatography and high-pressure liquid chromatography can be used to identify organisms in clinical isolates (84–86) but these techniques are not widely available.

PCR techniques are able to detect small numbers of mycobacteria in clinical specimens or in tissue sections (87). PCR techniques lack adequate sensitivity (88) and have not been approved for diagnostic use. DNA fingerprinting using restriction fragment length polymorphism (RLFP) is a useful epidemiological tool and may provide a rapid method for identifying multidrug-resistant strains (89). Cost and technical difficulty make current PCR methods impractical for routine use.

Radiological investigation can be very useful when GI TB is suspected; patients with a normal barium study of the upper GI tract (with small intestinal follow-through) and lower GI tract (with ileal reflux procedure) are unlikely to have GI TB. Special attention should be paid to signs of impaired motility (such as accelerated transit time and hypersegmentation), as these may be the earliest defects that can be appreciated radiographically. Stierlin's sign (localized failure to retain barium), the "string sign" (persistence of a thin line of barium), discrete filling defects, or distorted GI architecture suggesting tumor all may be seen but none are diagnostic (18–20,90,91). Newer radiographic techniques, such as CAT scan and magnetic resonance imaging, have not been shown to be of additional value in localizing affected areas or establishing a diagnosis of tuberculosis in the GI tract.

Tuberculin skin testing can be quite helpful in patients who have not received BCG and in areas, such as the United States, where tuberculous infection is uncommon. Early series showed a high proportion of anergy to skin testing in patients later shown to have GI TB (5). However, this was likely due to advanced tuberculosis and malnutrition, both of which may lead to failure to respond to a skin test in the face of active disease. In the postchemotherapy era, this clinical situation is less common, and recent reports show positive TB skin tests in 50–97% of patients with GI TB (6,15,22,92). When the TB skin test is negative, control skin tests should be placed to exclude anergy, which is often seen in TB patients with advanced HIV infection (80,93).

Routine laboratory tests may show anemia and stool examination will occasionally show pus, mucus, fat glob-

ules, or blood, but these are not common (6). Chest X ray should be performed to search for signs of TB elsewhere, and abdominal films may be indicated to identify air-fluid levels in cases of suspected obstruction or free air under the diaphragm in cases of suspected perforation. Plain abdominal films may also reveal calcifications in abdominal lymph nodes in cases of reactivation TB.

Differential diagnosis of GI TB includes ulcerative colitis, Crohn's disease, irritable bowel syndrome, malignancy, and other infectious processes, including bacterial abscess, diverticulitis, fungal enteritis, amebiasis, and schistosomiasis. The most common problems are differentiation of GI TB from intestinal lymphoma or Crohn's disease. Such decisions can only be made with adequate histological examination.

Tuberculous scrofula is diagnosed by histological examination and culture of the resected lymph node or fine-needle aspirate of its contents (27,28,77). The differential diagnosis is large and includes lymphadenitis due to nontuberculous mycobacteria, streptococci, staphylococci, cat-scratch disease, mumps, Epstein–Barr virus infection, lymphoma and other neoplasms, sarcoidosis, collagen vascular disease, thyroglossal duct cyst, and branchial cleft cyst.

Treatment

GI TB responds well to antimycobacterial chemotherapy. Regimens for GI TB are the same as those currently recommended for pulmonary TB (Table 2). Patients should be started on three or preferably four agents to speedily decrease the load of organisms and to minimize the chances of therapeutic failure due to drug-resistant organisms. These should include isoniazid, rifampin, pyrazinamide, and either ethambutol or streptomycin (94,95).

Drug resistance is occurring with increasing frequency among mycobacteria and can result in failure of therapy. Drug resistance occurs for two reasons: first, genetic resistance to each of the antimycobacterial agents is present at a frequency of 1 in 10^6 to 1 in 10^9 organisms. If the bacterial load in the patient exceeds this number, as is often the case, resistant organisms will be present and will soon replace the susceptible ones. Thus therapy with at least two agents concurrently is essential in any patient with tuberculosis. Second, in many areas of the world, including the United States, patients are exposed to organisms that are all highly resistant to one or more antimycobacterial agents. Since it is usually not possible to know the susceptibility pattern of the patient's isolate at the time of diagnosis, four agents are recommended as the best way to ensure therapy with at least two drugs to which the patient's isolate is susceptible.

The results of in vitro susceptibility testing should be available by the eighth week of therapy (96), and those results should be used to guide the selection of drugs for the individual patient at that time. If therapy is not interrupted, a 6-month course will be adequate to affect a cure. HIV-infected patients can also be cured of TB, but treatment should be prolonged if the clinical response is not prompt (94,95). All efforts should be made to ensure that

TABLE 2. *Agents for treatment of* M. tuberculosis *disease*

Agent	Adult dose	Pediatric dose
First-Line Drugs		
Isoniazid	300 mg PO qd	10–20 mg/kg/d PO
Rifampin	600 mg PO qd	10–20 mg/kg/d PO
Ethambutol	15–25 mg/kg/d PO	15–25 mg/kg/d PO[a]
Pyrazinamide	2 g PO qd	15–30 mg/kg/d PO
Streptomycin	1 g IM qd	20–40 mg/kg/d IM
Amikacin	1 g IV qd	20–40 mg/kg/d IV
Alternative Drugs		
Para-aminosalicylic acid	3 g PO qid	150 mg/kg/d PO
Cycloserine	250–500 mg PO bid	15–20 mg/kg/d PO
Ethionaimide	250–500 mg PO bid	15–20 mg/kg/d PO
Kanamycin	1 g IM qd	15–30 mg/kg/d IM
Capreomycin	1 g IM qd	15–30 mg/kg/d IM

[a] Not recommended for children <6 years of age.

therapy is not interrupted, and that if interruption is necessary, the patient not be kept on single-agent therapy during any period of time, as this is liable to foster additional drug resistance (97). It is critical that patients adhere to the regimen. Care providers must monitor adherence; this may require observation of medication ingestion by the patient ("directly observed therapy" DOT). Twice- and thrice-weekly dosing schedules have been formulated to aid in adherence to DOT (95).

If the patient's TB isolate shows resistance in vitro to two or more of the first-line antimycobacterial agents (usually isoniazid and rifampin), it is said to be "multiply drug resistant" (MDR). Patients with MDR TB can be successfully treated with alternate regimens, but success is achieved in less than two thirds of cases (98). Not only are agents other than isoniazid and rifampin less potent, but they are less well tolerated (see chapter by Morrow and Neuzil). Because treatment of MDR TB is less effective than treatment of drug-susceptible TB and most MDR TB is the result of failure of previous therapy, it is essential to achieve a cure with the first course of therapy.

The host immune response to TB is a balance between being too feeble, such that the pathogen is not controlled, and being too exuberant, such that vital host tissue is destroyed. Many investigators have attempted to use immunosuppressive or immunostimulatory therapies to maximize elimination of the organism while minimizing immune-mediated damage to the host. Prednisone has been successfully used to minimize pulmonary inflammation in panlobar TB, but there is no indication for such therapy in the treatment of GI TB in the absence of overwhelming pulmonary disease. Transfer factor and γ-interferon have been proposed for treatment of the patient with overwhelming TB who is anergic; indomethacin also may reverse anergy caused by mycobacterial infection (99). However, the benefit of such therapies remains to be established.

The most important therapeutic measure to restore immune function in the anergic TB patient is assurance of adequate nutrition. Many patients with chronic TB are visibly malnourished, but in others the signs are less obvious. Particularly in patients with GI TB when malabsorption is present, oral nutritional supplementation may

be inadequate, and parenteral nutrition is necessary. Because clinical malnutrition may not be apparent, parenteral hyperalimentation should be considered whenever weight loss does not respond to appropriate antimycobacterial therapy.

Surgical therapy is essential when GI TB is complicated by perforation, obstruction, or uncontrollable hemorrhage. Such cases are often far advanced and have a poor prognosis (6,23). In addition, by analogy with pulmonary TB, surgical therapy may have an adjunctive role in the treatment of TB of the GI tract that has not responded adequately to antimycobacterial therapy. This is most common when the burden of organisms is large or when large areas of poorly perfused tissue are involved. In such cases, resection of necrotic material may improve the clinical response to antimycobacterial agents.

Tuberculous scrofula is treated with the same antimycobacterial regimen as other forms of tuberculosis. In some cases, surgical resection, if not performed for diagnosis, may be necessary (28,77).

Prevention

GI TB can be prevented by avoiding exposure to *M. tuberculosis,* by vaccination, or by prevention of reactivation TB. Minimizing exposure has been accomplished in the United States by pasteurization of milk and by tuberculin testing of cattle with elimination of infected animals (4). This latter strategy was employed on a large scale in the United States in the 1920s and subsequently in Europe. As a result of these two measures, bovine TB is a rare source of TB for humans in these countries. Other animal species not normally thought to be hosts for TB can acquire the infection and transmit it to humans, including primates, seals, elk, and rhinoceroses (100–103). Avoidance of such infected animals is, in general, not difficult.

Prevention of GI TB secondary to pulmonary TB can be accomplished by prevention of pulmonary TB through active public health programs of prompt case identification and appropriate therapy, combined with contact tracing and identification of secondary cases. Prompt therapy of cases of pulmonary TB will also reduce the incidence of GI TB since, as noted, secondary GI TB increases with the duration of untreated pulmonary TB (8,13).

An additional effective strategy for prevention of TB, particularly in countries with a low incidence of active TB, such as the United States, is tuberculin skin testing with prophylactic therapy of persons with a positive skin test (indicating tuberculous infection). This therapy, consisting of isoniazid alone for 12 months and known as isoniazid preventive therapy (IPT), is 90% effective in preventing reactivation TB in persons with tuberculous infection without disease (104).

Vaccination is an alternative prevention strategy. *M. bovis*, strain BCG, has been used as a vaccine to prevent infection or disease due to *M. tuberculosis* since the early twentieth century. Its efficacy in prevention of disseminated TB in children is widely accepted, but some doubt exists about its efficacy in preventing pulmonary TB in adults (105,106). No data are available to address its use in prevention of GI TB, but prevention of pulmonary TB would logically prevent cases of secondary GI TB. In the United States, BCG is recommended for use only in infants and children who have prolonged, unavoidable exposure to persons with active tuberculosis (105).

GASTROINTESTINAL DISEASE DUE TO *M. AVIUM* COMPLEX

Epidemiology

The clinical entity of GI *M. avium* (MAC) disease was rare until the pandemic of AIDS, beginning in the 1980s (107–109). A localized MAC GI process progresses to disseminated disease within a few months (110,111), and disseminated disease due to MAC is largely the result of spread from a GI focus, although the GI focus may be unrecognized until dissemination has occurred. Not only have cases of disseminated MAC infection increased with the number of AIDS cases, but the frequency of disseminated MAC infection as a percentage of AIDS cases also has increased each year (107). Currently, from 15% to 24% of persons with AIDS can be expected to acquire MAC infection. In the United States in 1992 there were 47,000 new AIDS cases; if 20% of these have MAC infection, then 9400 MAC cases occurred (an annual incidence of 3.5 per 100,000 persons).

The major risk factor for MAC disease is the level of immune dysfunction, assessed by the CD4+ T-lymphocyte count. Most patients do not become at risk for MAC infection until the CD4+ cell count drops below 100 cells/mm³. Since CD4+ cell count declines continuously in HIV-infected persons, the risk of acquiring MAC also increases with duration of HIV infection; the overall incidence of MAC in AIDS patients is about 20% per year, and persons surviving for 30 months after a clinical AIDS diagnosis have a 50% chance of acquiring MAC infection (112).

After controlling for CD4+ cell counts, there are no differences in the frequency of disseminated MAC infection between males and females, and the rates of disease are similar in persons acquiring HIV through homosexual/bisexual activity, intravenous drug use, receipt of blood or blood products, heterosexual contact, or in persons acquiring HIV through vertical transmission (109). Risks are similar for children and adults (113). There is little variation in the frequency of the disease in various geographic locations in the United States, and rates are similar in Europe and Australia; however, MAC infection is rarely seen in Africa, even in patients with advanced AIDS (114,115). Reasons for this absence may include the high prevalence of TB in Africa and differences in environmental exposures to MAC. In an autopsy series of AIDS cases in Cote d'Ivoire, Lucas reported only one case of GI mycobacteriosis that was histologically consistent with MAC (53).

Specific information about the epidemiology of GI MAC is limited. Clinical and autopsy studies have shown that GI involvement is present in 58–78% of AIDS patients with MAC (116,117). Lesions in the GI tract are most common in the duodenum and rectum; however, esophagus, stomach, jejunum, ileum, and colon also may be affected (110,115–120). MAC in the GI tract is thought to be acquired from the environment by ingestion. The organisms occur in a wide variety of environmental sites, including animals, food, water, and soil (121–128), but specific risk behaviors and reservoirs for human disease have not been identified. Preliminary studies have suggested that disease may be acquired through ingestion of contaminated water or foods (129,130), but these results remain to be confirmed.

In persons without HIV infection, MAC as a cause of disease in the GI tract is almost unknown (131). The only clinical entity associated with MAC in such persons is cervical lymphadenitis (nontuberculous scrofula). This disease is presumed to be acquired through the GI tract by ingestion of MAC, but, as with tuberculous scrofula, no pathological evidence of disease is found in the GI tract, and the process is confined solely to the affected lymph nodes. MAC scrofula also may be seen in HIV-infected persons, but this is rare in the absence of disseminated disease (132).

Scrofula due to MAC is largely a disease of children without HIV infection, being most common in those under the age of 5 years (133–135); cases in persons over the age of 11 years are rare. No racial, ethnic, or geographic predilection is known. Cases are seen at similar rates in boys and girls (133,134). It is estimated that there are no more than 1000 cases annually in the United States (136). An intriguing observation is the increased number of cases occurring in the winter and spring when compared to the summer and fall (134,137). Several reports have indicated that its incidence appears to be increasing, both in the United States and other developed countries, such as Australia, Sweden, England, and Canada (138–141).

Microbiology

The term *Mycobacterium avium* complex, or MAC, refers to the species *M. avium* and *M. intracellulare;* some authors also include *M. scrofulaceum* in the complex, a grouping known as "MAIS." *M. avium* causes disease similar to tuberculosis in chickens, birds, and swine. Disease in humans usually occurs in patients with a preexisting parenchymal disease or in immunosuppressed hosts. *M. intracellulare* was previously known as the Battey bacillus; it is usually not pathogenic for man or animals, but patients with AIDS may acquire disease due to this organism. These organisms are found in soil, water, and tissues of domestic animals. They are acid-fast and periodic acid–Schiff (PAS)–positive. In culture, they are thermophilic (grow at 41°C) and some strains develop a pale yellow pigment with age (Runyon group III, nonchromogens). They are niacin-negative, do not reduce nitrates, and do not produce disease in guinea pigs. *M. scrofulaceum* is a common cause of lymphadenitis in children. It is classified as a scotochromagen (Runyon group II) because of the yellow–orange pigment produced, even in the dark. The organisms are not thermophilic but have other characteristics similar to those of MAC, such as the inability to reduce nitrate and a negative niacin test (1,38,39).

The staining characteristics of MAC are the same as those of *M. tuberculosis* and the two cannot be differentiated by microscopy. Specimen collection, preparation, and culture conditions for MAC are the same as for *M. tuberculosis* (see section on microbiology of *M. tuberculosis,* above).

Pathogenesis and Immunity

Virulence Factors

MAC organisms are ubiquitous in the environment and relatively avirulent in the normal host. There are usually no clinical manifestations of disease in immunocompetent individuals. Certain MAC serovars (4 and 8) are uncommon in the environment yet cause most cases of disseminated disease in AIDS patients (107,108). These serovars probably are associated with unidentified virulence factors or are able to overcome host defenses more easily

than other serovars (108). Differing abilities to adhere to intestinal epithelial cells may be important virulence factors (142,143); differences in the ability to produce catalase have also been described and linked to invasiveness (144).

Clinical isolates from patients with disseminated disease are always of the smooth, transparent colony type rather than the domed or opaque type (145). Colonies that are smooth and transparent are more likely to replicate in vivo than those that have a domed shape (146). They are also more likely to induce the cytokines tumor necrosis factor–α (TNF-α) and interleukin-1 (IL-1) (147). Smooth, transparent colonies usually have decreased susceptibility to antimycobacterial agents in vitro. The relationship between these two phenotypes is complicated by the ability of isolates to transform from one to the other and back, depending on culture conditions.

Pathophysiology

The GI tract is often the portal of entry of nontuberculous mycobacteria in the immunocompromised host. Similar to GI TB, GI MAC disease may be acquired through ingestion of MAC from the environment, the swallowing of organisms shed in sputum from pulmonary disease, or hematogenous dissemination. Direct GI acquisition from the environment is thought to cause most cases (107). There may be colonization of the GI tract prior to dissemination of the infection (111,148). Reactivation of a previously contained MAC infection has not been described.

Like *M. tuberculosis,* MAC invades Peyer's patches and mesenteric lymph nodes. Most infections occur in the small bowel and associated mesenteric lymph nodes. Histologically, one sees foamy macrophages within the lamina propria of the intestinal mucosa and in lymphoid tissue, often in sheets or clusters (Fig. 6). With severe infection, sheets of large, foamy macrophages expand the villi to such an extent that there is flattening of the microvilli, similar to that seen in Whipple's disease (149,150). True granulomas with Langhans giant cells, epithelioid

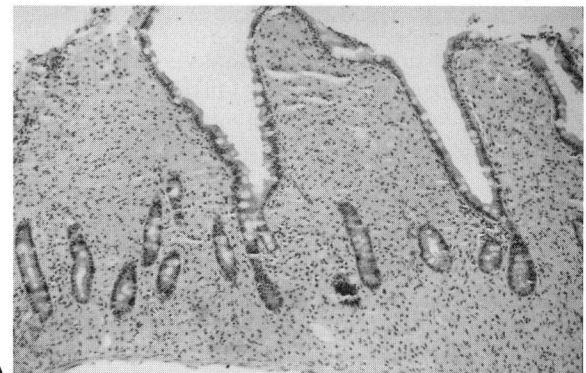
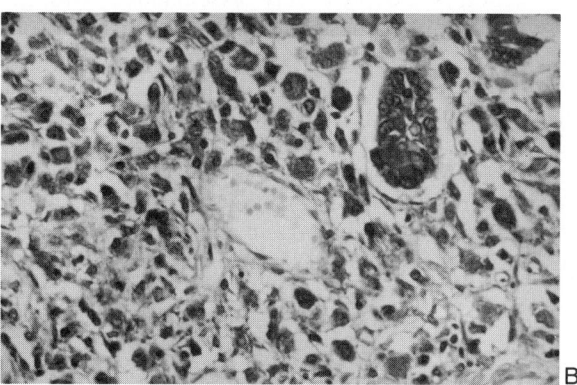

FIG. 6. *Mycobacterium avium* complex (MAC) disease. **A:** Histological section of intestine with marked expansion of villi and submucosa by a diffuse infiltrate of foamy histiocytes (H&E stain) (×100). (Courtesy of Dr. Charles M. Wilcox.) **B:** Ziehl–Neelsen stained section shows histiocytes stuffed with acid-fast bacilli (×300). (See Plate 14.)

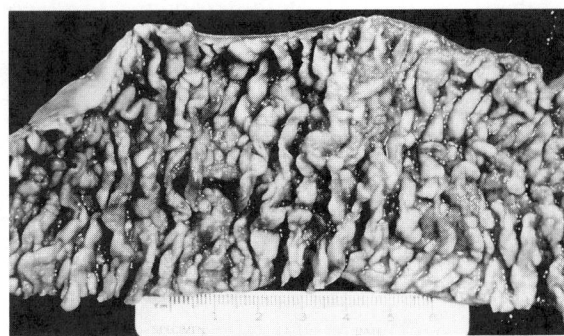

FIG. 7. *Mycobacterium avium* complex (MAC) disease. Gross specimen of intestine with diffuse thickening of mucosal folds. (Courtesy of Dr. Charles M. Wilcox.)

macrophages, and caseous necrosis are not typically seen in MAC infections of the gut (116). Enterocytes are usually intact; the luminal surface may show mild inflammatory changes, but ulceration is rare. On hematoxylin and eosin–stained tissue or in Giemsa-stained imprints and smears, the mycobacteria are negatively stained. Klatt describes these as "straited blue histiocytes" on Giemsa stain (116). Acid-fast and PAS stains and silver impregnation techniques reveal masses of bacilli.

MAC infection of the colon occurs as part of disseminated infection of the gastrointestinal tract or as a primary focus. There is edema and erythema of the mucosa (Figs. 6 and 7). In acute cases the mucosa is often friable with multiple erosions and ulceration—findings that explain the occurrence of bloody diarrhea (43). In tissue section, the organisms are located within foamy macrophages in the lamina propria. Typically, there are no Langhans giant cells or granulomas. There is sparing of the glands, but surface epithelium may show congestion and focal acute inflammation with erosions or ulcerations (43,151).

Patients with MAC disease of the GI tract manifest marked wasting. While diarrhea, malabsorption, and elevated circulating TNF all have been reported in these patients, none of these processes alone can explain the marked weight loss (152). It appears that the weight loss is multifactorial.

The infection is usually widely disseminated, with involvement of lymph nodes, liver, and spleen being the most common sites (116,117). Abdominal lymph node involvement varies from tiny foci of infection to marked lymphadenopathy with replacement of the normal architecture by sheets of foamy macrophages containing masses of mycobacteria. Because MAC infection occurs in patients with severe immunodeficiency, the normal architecture of the node is altered and often shows follicular atrophy. Mycobacterial spindle cell lesions similar to histioid leprosy have been reported with MAC infection (153), but pseudotumors in the GI tract have not been reported.

Host Immune Response

MAC infections of the GI tract are reported primarily in patients with advanced HIV disease and severe immu-

nosuppression. In most patients the mycobacteria are phagocytized by macrophages and other reticuloendothelial cells. However, these cells are unable to kill the organisms, and eventually the cells rupture, releasing the mycobacteria. In the final stages, the tissues are laden with huge numbers of mycobacteria, but tissue destruction is minimal due to the impaired cellular immune response, and cellular architecture may be preserved. Surprisingly, some patients are able to mount a granulomatous response (116). Such granulomas vary from well-formed granulomas with giant cells to loose collections of lymphocytes. Caseation is rare.

The specific defect that leads to the inability of these cells to kill MAC has not been defined. Recent evidence indicates that some cytokines inhibit growth of MAC that are contained within phagocytic cells (e.g., TNF-α, and migration inhibition factor, MIF), while other cytokines [e.g., Il-1α, IL-6) (154) and possibly the gp120 envelope protein of HIV] may also enhance replication of *M. avium* (155). Imbalances of these cytokines may contribute to the inability of the host to control MAC infection. Natural killer (NK) cell function also is impaired (156).

Humoral factors may contribute to the inability of the host to control MAC infection as well. Antibodies against MAC are produced in response to MAC infection in persons without AIDS, but not by AIDS patients (157,158). While these antibodies are not known to have a role in protection against MAC disease, they have been related to increased MAC killing in vitro (159). Deficiency of the HIV-infected host in lactoferrin has also been observed to enhance growth of MAC by increasing the availability of iron, an essential nutrient for MAC (160), and serum factors that support macrophage resistance to MAC may be absent in patients with AIDS (161).

Host Susceptibility Factors

The major risk for GI MAC infection is advanced HIV infection, usually when the CD4+ T-lymphocyte counts have fallen well below 100 cells/mL (112). This suggests that the intracellular killing of these organisms is very sensitive to CD4+-mediated immunity. However, at this late stage of HIV infection, CD8+ cell function, NK cell function, and humoral antibody production also are severely impaired. Other conditions that cause severe immunosuppression also may predispose to disseminated MAC infection, notably hairy cell leukemia (131,158).

Clinical Manifestations

GI MAC disease may present with fever, night sweats, abdominal pain, diarrhea, and/or weight loss. Physical examination of the abdomen may reveal hepatomegaly, splenomegaly, or both; abdominal lymphadenopathy is rarely palpable, while enlarged peripheral lymph nodes are uncommon. Laboratory findings may include severe anemia and a markedly elevated serum alkaline phosphatase, usually without a corresponding elevation in other hepatic enzymes. The frequency of these symptoms and signs in

GI MAC disease is not known, but of all persons with disseminated MAC disease, 97% have fevers, 96% have severe anemia, 62% have night sweats, 59% have weight loss of 10% or greater, 56% have abdominal pain, 54% have diarrhea, 47% have an elevated serum alkaline phosphatase, 39% have hepatomegaly, and 29% have splenomegaly (162). Severe anemia is a hallmark of this disease and should prompt a search for MAC (162–164).

MAC disease of the abdomen is often diffuse and widespread. In one series, 88% of patients had duodenal involvement and 64% had rectal involvement, while the esophagus was affected in only 6% (110). In some cases, a discrete clinical picture may be seen, such as a syndrome resembling Whipple's disease (118,119) or a terminal ileitis suggesting Crohn's disease (120). Although no studies of the clinical presentation of MAC in the GI tract in HIV-infected children have been reported, the clinical features of disseminated MAC in children are similar to those of the disease in adults (113,165,166).

Routine radiographs of the abdomen are rarely remarkable, but abdominal CT scan may often show multiple enlarged retroperitoneal lymph nodes or thickening of the bowel wall (Fig. 8). A large retrospective study showed that an abdominal CT scan may help differentiate MAC disease of the abdomen from TB of the abdomen in AIDS patients (167). MAC of the abdomen was characterized by hepatomegaly, splenomegaly, jejunal wall thickening, and abdominal lymph nodes with homogeneous soft tissue density. TB of the abdomen, on the other hand, was characterized by focal visceral lesions and abdominal lymph nodes with diffuse low attenuation.

Endoscopy frequently reveals abnormalities, either focal or diffuse. The most characteristic lesions are 2- to 4-mm white nodules; however, these are seen in only one third of patients (110,168). Endoscopy also may show thickened folds of bowel wall and/or a yellow mucosal discoloration (Fig. 9) (110). This yellow, granular appearance is similar to that seen in Whipple's disease (43,118,119). Ulceration or masses are rarely seen; in many cases the bowel appears normal despite massive infiltration with mycobacteria (110). Massive adenopathy

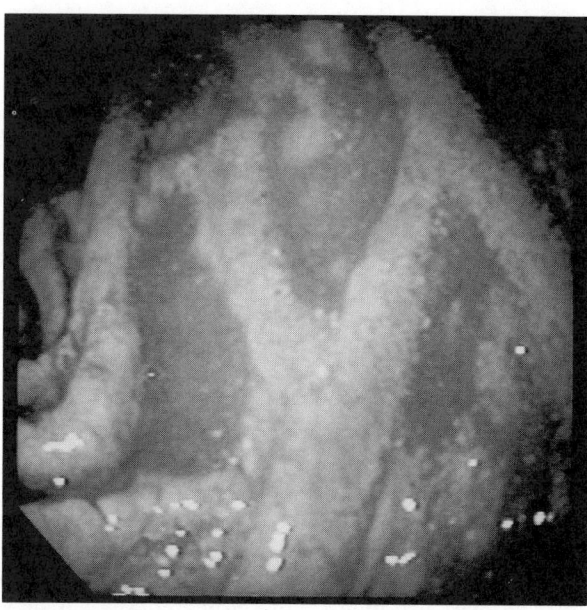

FIG. 9. Endoscopic appearance of the duodenal mucosa of a patient with disseminated *Mycobacterium avium* complex (MAC) disease. There are markedly thickened intestinal folds and multiple/plaques yellow. (Courtesy of Dr. Charles M. Wilcox.) (See Plate 15.)

and the thickening of the bowel wall can lead to intussusception with consequent GI hemorrhage, or can cause obstruction (120,169,170). As infection progresses, the bowel wall, liver, spleen, and abdominal lymph nodes become more and more densely laden with mycobacteria. Eventually, host tissue is replaced and decreased organ function results. This may include absorptive defects of the bowel; abnormal D-xylose tests have been reported in 50% of these patients (110). Abdominal pain becomes increasingly severe over the course of the illness, and often opiate analgesia is needed to control symptoms. Weight loss is inexorable, and patients progress to resemble victims of severe malnutrition. In contrast to GI TB, obstruction, perforation, and GI bleeding are rare.

If antimycobacterial therapy is not instituted, survival of such patients is markedly shortened, with death in a median of 4 months (171). With therapy, survival is longer, but progression to the advanced stages of the disease occurs eventually if death from other causes does not supervene. At autopsy, death is seldom attributed directly to MAC; in most cases death in patients with MAC is due to superinfection or inanition (116,117).

Scrofula due to MAC presents as asymptomatic or minimally tender enlargement of the submental, cervical, periauricular, or submandibular lymph nodes, usually of several months duration (135,172,173). The submental nodes are the most commonly involved. Erythema is rare, and nodes may be matted or discrete. Spontaneous drainage with sinus tract formation may occur, although this is more often the result of misguided attempts to manage the disease without total excision. If untreated, the disease may last for months to years.

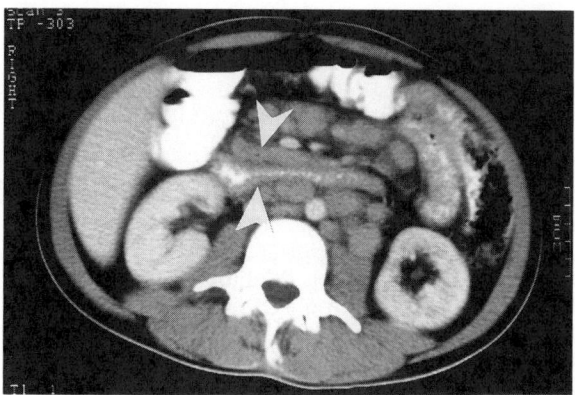

FIG. 8. Abdominal CAT scan of a patient with disseminated *Mycobacterium avium* complex (MAC) disease. Note multiple enlarged abdominal lymph nodes and thickening of the duodenal wall (*arrows*).

Diagnosis

Diagnosis of GI MAC disease is made by histological examination of GI tissue and culture of the organism from tissue samples. Since abdominal surgery is rarely indicated, endoscopic visualization and biopsy are required to establish the diagnosis in most cases. Stool smear and culture are alternatives, but smear is nonspecific and culture is insensitive; they are usually positive only when disease is far advanced (81,111,148). The time delay in culturing MAC (up to 6 weeks) results in a prolonged period of clinical uncertainty for many patients and physicians. For this reason, efforts are being made to develop more rapid diagnostic techniques. The most promising among these is PCR detection of mycobacterial DNA. However, at this time, no such assays for detection of MAC are commercially available.

Diagnosis of disseminated MAC disease is usually made by a positive blood culture. Positive cultures of other normally sterile sites, such as bone marrow, lymph node, or liver biopsy, also indicate disseminated MAC disease. Because mycobacteremia is continuous, a single positive blood culture is adequate to confirm the diagnosis, and two properly performed negative cultures can exclude the diagnosis (174,175). Blood culture should include lysis of the cellular fraction to release mycobacteria, and culture on solid or liquid mycobacterial media.

Since localized GI MAC disease may precede dissemination by several months (110,111), endoscopy is indicated when GI involvement is suspected on clinical grounds but blood cultures are negative. Multiple biopsies of all areas of the bowel should be taken, since endoscopic appearance may be normal despite extensive mycobacterial disease. Acid-fast smears of such biopsies may provide an immediate presumptive diagnosis of mycobacterial infection and accelerate the institution of appropriate therapy. Abdominal CT scan may be suggestive but is not adequate to establish the diagnosis.

Patients with advanced HIV infection rarely respond to skin tests; these are therefore not helpful in establishing a diagnosis of GI MAC disease. Serological testing for antimycobacterial antibodies is similarly unrewarding. CT scan or other radiological techniques are nonspecific and therefore can only be used to raise suspicion and recommend definitive diagnostic procedures.

A diagnosis of scrofula due to MAC is usually made by culture and histological examination of the affected node. In older children and in patients who have had lymphadenitis for a longer time, cultures may not be positive (173). Previously, a presumptive diagnosis could be made when chronic nonsuppurative lymphadenitis was seen in a child in conjunction with a positive skin test with PPD-B, a skin test reagent made from *M. intracellulare* (176,177). However, this skin test preparation is no longer available (178). The differential diagnosis is large and includes lymphadenitis due to *M. tuberculosis,* streptococci, staphylococci, cat-scratch disease, mumps, Epstein–Barr virus infection, lymphoma and other neoplasms, sarcoidosis, collagen vascular disease, thyroglossal duct cyst, and branchial cleft cyst.

Treatment

Early reports of antimycobacterial therapy of MAC disease showed no effect of therapy; however, more recent reports of three- and four-drug regimens have shown clinical responses and, in some cases, prolonged survival (162,171,179,180). The emergence of clarithromycin and azithromycin, two new and related antimycobacterial agents with excellent in vitro activity against MAC, has improved the efficacy and tolerance of anti-MAC regimens (181–184).

Treatment should be initiated with at least two, and preferably three, antimycobacterial agents, including one of the macrolide/azalide group (185) (Table 3). As with TB, single-agent therapy is contraindicated, due to the emergence of resistant organisms and subsequent clinical failure of the regimen (181). At least one additional agent should be administered with the macrolide to attempt to prevent emergence of resistance, although this may still occur despite combination therapy. Ethambutol is the preferred second agent, with the third to be selected from among the other oral agents (rifampin, rifabutin, clofazimine, ciprofloxacin, or ofloxacin). Amikacin is also effective, but is not demonstrably better than the oral agents while possessing greater potential for toxicity and requiring intravenous access. For patients who do not tolerate a macrolide or whose MAC isolate is not susceptible to macrolides, a four-drug regimen of rifampin, ethambutol, ciprofloxacin, and clofazimine should be used (179). Therapy is continued for the life of the patient.

There is currently no role for routine in vitro susceptibility testing of MAC isolates. No standardized method for such testing has been widely accepted and, with the exception of clarithromycin testing, none have been shown to correlate with clinical outcome. De novo infection with clarithromycin-resistant MAC has not been reported, although such resistance has been reported after clarithromycin monotherapy (181), and in vitro clarithromycin susceptibility testing of isolates from patients with clinical relapse while on clarithromycin is warranted (185).

GI MAC disease is a chronic process with a prolonged course. It is therefore not necessary to begin therapy before culture results are obtained, although some clinicians

TABLE 3. *Agents for treatment of* M. avium *complex (MAC) disease*

Agent	Adult dose	Pediatric dose
First-Line Drugs		
Azithromycin	600 mg PO qd	15 mg/kg/d PO
Clarithromycin	500 mg PO bid	15 mg/kg/d PO
Ethambutol	400 mg PO bid	10 mg/kg/d PO
Clofazimine	100 mg PO qd	1.5 mg/kg/d PO
Rifabutin	300 mg PO bid	10 mg/kg/d PO
Rifampin	300 mg PO bid	10 mg/kg/d PO
Alternative Drugs		
Amikacin	1 g IV qd	15 mg/kg/d IV
Ciprofloxacin	500 mg PO bid	Not recommended
Ofloxacin	400 mg PO bid	Not recommended

prefer to treat presumptively, pending the results of culture. Presumptive treatment without culture is to be avoided, since many other conditions may mimic the symptoms of MAC and could be missed. Patients with MAC rarely require hospitalization for treatment of their illness and may be followed as outpatients.

Patients should be followed with monthly blood cultures; cultures should become negative in 1–3 months. Blood cultures that become positive after having been negative are associated with clinical relapse and suggest a need for a different antimycobacterial regimen. For patients who do not respond to initial therapy or who relapse, there may be a role for intravenous therapy, at least for a limited time.

Anemia should be treated symptomatically; many patients will require transfusions when the hematocrit is less than 24% (164). Some authors have suggested a role for erythropoietin in treatment of anemia in these patients, although endogenous erythropoietin levels are often markedly elevated (163). Nonetheless, in some patients erythropoietin may decrease transfusion requirements.

The marked weight loss seen in these patients suggests a role for nutritional supplementation. However, in contrast to patients with GI TB, patients with AIDS and GI MAC have other metabolic and immunological defects that are not reversed by nutritional supplementation (152). Thus, intravenous hyperalimentation does not benefit these patients. Abdominal surgery, when necessary to treat obstruction, perforation, or bleeding, should be performed expeditiously (186).

MAC scrofula is effectively managed by surgical excision, and this is the therapy of choice (135,172). In general, antibiotics are not warranted; however, in cases where total excision might lead to damage of facial nerves, a trial of antimicrobial agents (including a macrolide or azalide), combined with partial excision, may be preferred.

Prevention

Since MAC disease is acquired from the environment, prevention by avoidance is a potential preventive strategy. However, the widespread presence of MAC in the environment makes such avoidance impractical. If specific reservoirs could be defined that accounted for a substantial portion of MAC infections, avoidance could be recommended, but while several have been suggested, none have yet been identified (129,130). Screening cultures to detect early disease are not useful (148).

On theoretical grounds, BCG vaccination might provide protection against MAC disease, but no data exist to support such a strategy, particularly in HIV-infected patients, whose responses to vaccines are often suboptimal. Moreover, BCG (since it is a live vaccine) may itself cause disease in AIDS patients (187,188). BCG should therefore not be used for protection against MAC in HIV-infected persons.

The only strategy with demonstrated effectiveness in preventing MAC disease is antimycobacterial prophylaxis. Such prophylactic therapy, with rifabutin 300 mg daily, was associated with a 50% reduction in MAC bacteremia in two recent trials (189). Antimycobacterial prophylaxis with other agents is currently being evaluated. Such therapy should be considered for persons with HIV infection and fewer than 100 CD4+ cells, although the risk for MAC disease is still relatively small for persons with 50–100 CD4+ cells (112). The benefits of administration of such therapy should be weighed against the potential for decreased adherence to other medications and increased numbers of drug interactions in patients receiving a large number of pharmacological agents.

REFERENCES

1. Calmette A. *Tubercle bacillus infection and tuberculosis in man and animals*. Translated by Soper WB, Smith GH. Baltimore: Williams and Wilkins; 1923.
2. Walsh J. Diagnosis of intestinal tuberculosis. *Trans Natl Assoc Prev Tuberc London* 1909;5:217.
3. Phillips B. *Scrofula: its nature, its causes, its prevalence, and the principles of treatment*. London: Bailliere; 1846.
4. Miller RH. *Tuberculosis of the lymphatic system*. New York: Macmillan; 1934.
5. Goldberg B. Tuberculous enterocolitis. In: Goldberg B, ed. *Clinical tuberculosis*. Vol 2. 5th ed. Philadelphia: FA Davis; 1947:H3–H33.
6. Bhansali SK. Abdominal tuberculosis. *Am J Gastroenterol* 1977;67:324–337.
7. Goldberg B, Sweany HC, Brown RW. Pathological studies on tuberculous enteritis. *Am Rev Tuberc* 1928;18:744–766.
8. Blumberg A. Pathology of intestinal tuberculosis. *J Clin Lab Med* 1928;13:405.
9. Mitchell RS. The prognosis of bilateral symmetrical diffuse nodular pulmonary tuberculosis and its possible relation to intestinal tuberculosis. *Dis Chest* 1956;29:669–674.
10. Farer LS, Lowell AM, Meador MP. Extrapulmonary tuberculosis in the United States. *Am J Epidemiol* 1979;109:205–217.
11. Fraki O, Peltokallio P. Intestinal and peritoneal tuberculosis: report of two cases. *Dis Colon Rectum* 1975;18:685–693.
12. Segal I. Intestinal tuberculosis, Crohn's disease and ulcerative colitis in an urban Black population. *South Afr Med J* 1984; 655:37–44.
13. Mitchell RS, Bristol LJ. Intestinal tuberculosis: an analysis of 346 cases diagnosed by routine intestinal radiography on 5,529 admissions for pulmonary tuberculosis. 1924–1949. *Am J Med Sci* 1954;227:241–251.
14. Schulze K, Warner HA, Murray D. Intestinal tuberculosis experience at a Canadian teaching institution. *Am J Med* 1977; 63:735–745.
15. Palmer KR, Patil DH, Basran GS, Riordan JF, Silk DBA. Abdominal tuberculosis in urban Britain—a common disease. *Gut* 1985;26:1296–1305.
16. Carrera GF, Young S, Lewicki. Intestinal tuberculosis. *Gastrointest Radiol* 1976;1:147–155.
17. Moshal MG, Spitaels JM. Gastrointestinal and peritoneal tuberculosis. *South Afr Med J* 1973;47:675–679.
18. Werbeloff L, Novis BH, Marks IN. The radiology of tuberculosis of the gastro-intestinal tract. *Br J Radiol* 1973;46:329–336.
19. Lewis EA, Kolawole TM. Tuberculous ileo-colitis in Ibadan: a clinicoradiological review. *Gut* 1972;13:646–653.
20. Paustian FF, Monto GL. Tuberculosis of the intestines. In: Bokus HL, ed. *Gastroenterology*. Vol 1. 3rd ed. Philadelphia: WB Saunders; 1976:750–776.
21. Tandon HD, Prakash A. Pathology of intestinal tuberculosis and its distinction from Crohn's disease. *Gut* 1972;13:260–269.
22. Homan WP, Grafe WR, Dineen P. A 44-year experience with tuberculous enterocolitis. *World J Surg* 1977;1:245–250.
23. Hill GS, Tabrisky J, Peter ME. Tuberculous enteritis. *West J Med* 1976;124:440–445.
24. Novis BH, Bank S, Marks IN. Gastrointestinal and peritoneal

tuberculosis. A study of cases at Groote Schuur Hospital 1962–1971. *South Afr Med J* 1973;47:365–372.

25. Freant LJ, Sawyers JL. Surgical management of tuberculous enteritis. *South J Med* 1970;63:711–714.

26. Abrams JS, Holden WD. Tuberculosis of the gastrointestinal tract. *Arch Surg* 1964;89:283–293.

27. Summers GD, McNicol MW. Tuberculosis of superficial lymph nodes. *Br J Dis Chest* 1980;74:369–373.

28. Huhti E, Brander E, Paloheimo S, Sutinen S. Tuberculosis of the cervical lymph nodes: a clinical pathological and bacteriological study. *Tubercle* 1975;56:27–36.

29. Lax JD, Haroutiounian G, Attia A, et al. Tuberculosis of the rectum in a patient with acquired immune deficiency syndrome. *Dis Colon Rectum* 1988;31:394–397.

30. Friedenberg KA, Draguesku JO, Kiyabu M, Valenzuela JE. Intestinal perforation due to *Mycobacterium tuberculosis* in HIV-infected individuals: report of two cases. *Am J Gastroenterol* 1992;88:604–607.

31. Brody JM, Miller DK, Zeman RK et al. Gastric tuberculosis: a manifestation of acquired imunodeficiency syndrome. *Radiology* 1986;159:347–348.

32. Lucas S, Nelson AM. Pathogenesis of tuberculosis in human immunodeficiency virus-infected people. In: Bloom BR, ed. Tuberculosis: pathogenesis, protection and control. Washington, DC: American Society of Microbiology; in press.

33. Shriner KA, Mathisen GE, Goetz MB. Comparison of mycobacterial lymphadenitis among persons infected with human immunodeficiency virus and seronegative controls. *Clin Infect Dis* 1992;15:601–605.

34. Warren J. Mycobacterial infections. In: Shulman ST, Phair JP, Sommers HM, eds. *The biological and clinical basis of infectious diseases*. 4th ed. Philadelphia: WB Saunders; 1992: 190–207.

35. Fox E. Mycobacterial infections. In: Strickland GT, ed. *Hunter's tropical medicine*. 7th ed. Philadelphia: WB Saunders; 1991:458–481.

36. von Lichtenberg F. Mycobacterial diseases. In: *Pathology of infectious diseases*. New York: Raven Press; 1991:173–187.

37. Musial CE, Roberts GD. Tuberculosis and other mycobacteriosis. In: Wentworth BB, et al., eds. *Diagnostic procedures for bacterial infections*. 7th ed. Washington, DC: American Public Health Association; 1987:539–580.

38. Wayne LG, Willet HP. Mycobacteria. In: Sneath PHA, et al., eds. *Bergey's manual of systemic bacteriology*. Vol 2. Baltimore: Williams and Wilkins; 1986:1435–1457.

39. Willet HP. Mycobacteria. In: Joklik WK, Willett HP, Amos DB, Wilfert CM, eds. *Zinsser Microbiology*. 20th ed. Norwalk, CT: Appleton and Lange; 1992:497–525.

40. Dannenberg AM. Pathogenesis of tuberculosis: native and acquired resistance in animals and humans. In: Leive L, Schlessinger D, eds. *Microbiology*. Washington DC: American Society of Microbiology; 1984:344–354.

41. Edwards D, Kirkpatrick CH. The immunology of mycobacterial diseases. *Am Rev Resp Dis* 1986;134:1062–1071.

42. Adami JG, Nicholls AG. *Principles of pathology*. Vol 2. Philadelphia: Lea and Febiger; 1909:439–442.

43. Fenoglio-Preiser CM, Lantz PE, Listrom MB, Davis M, Rilke FO. *Gastrointestinal pathology: an atlas and text*. New York: Raven Press; 1989:58,144,299–300,663–667,803.

44. Nelson AM, Kalengayi MMR. The pathology of AIDS in Africa. In: Essex ME et al, eds. *AIDS in Africa*. New York: Raven Press; 1994:283–323.

45. Newman RM, Fleshner PR, Lajam F, Kim U. Esophageal tuberculosis: a rare presentation with hematemesis. *Am J Gastroenterol* 1991;86:751–755.

46. Gordon AH, Marshall JB. Esophageal tuberculosis: definitive diagnosis by endoscopy (case report). *Am J Gastroenterol* 1990;85:174–177.

47. Damtew B, Frengley D, Wolinski, et al. Esophageal tuberculosis: mimicry of gastrointestinal malignancy. *Rev Infect Dis* 1987;9:140–146.

48. Tromba JL, Inglese R, Rieders B, Todaro R. Primary gastric tuberculosis presenting as pyloric outlet obstruction. *Am J Gastroenterol* 1991;86:1820–1822.

49. Nair KV, Pai CG, Rajagopal KP, Bhat VN, Thomas M. Unusual presentations of duodenal tuberculosis. *Am J Gastroenterol* 1991;86:756–760.

50. Palmer E. Tuberculosis of the stomach and the stomach in tuberculosis. *Am Rev Tuberc* 1950;61:116–118.

51. Kolawole TM, Lewis EA. A radiologic study of tuberculosis of the abdomen (gastrointestinal tract). *Am J Roentgenol* 1975; 123:348–358.

52. Downey DB, Nakielny RA. Aphthoid ulcers in colonic tuberculosis. *Br J Radiol* 1985;58:561–562.

53. Harland RW, Varkey B. Anal tuberculosis: report of two cases and literature review. *Am J Gastroenterol* 1992;87:1488–1491.

54. Morson BC, Dawson IMP. *Gastrointestinal pathology*. Oxford: Blackwell Scientific; 1972:246–250,449–450,613.

55. Dannenberg AM. Delayed-type hypersensitivity and cell-mediated immunity in the pathogenesis of tuberculosis. *Immunol Today* 1991;12:228–232.

56. Lewin-Smith MR, Nelson AM, Meyers WM. A semi-quantitative assessment of cellular immune response to tuberculosis in HIV-infected patients. *Int J Leprosy* 1993;61:123A.

57. Ivanyi J, Bothamley GH, Jackett PS. Immunodiagnostic assays for tuberculosis and leprosy. *Br Med Bull* 1988;4:634–649.

58. Havlir DV, Wallis RS, Boom WH, Daniel TM, Chervenak K, Ellner JJ. Human immune response to *Mycobacterium tuberculosis* antigens. *Infect Immun* 1991;59:665–670.

59. Nambuya A, Sewankambo N, Mugerwa J, Goodgame R, Lucas S. Tuberculous lymphadenitis associated with human immunodeficiency virus (HIV) in Uganda. *J Clin Pathol* 1988;41:93–96.

60. CDC. Management of persons exposed to multidrug-resistant tuberculosis. *MMWR* 1992;41(No.RR-11):61–71.

61. Stead WW, Senner JW, Reddick WT, Lofgren JP. Racial differences in susceptibility to infection by *Mycobacterium tuberculosis*. *N Engl J Med* 1990;322:422–427.

62. Hwang C-H, Khan S, Ende N, Mangura BT, Reichman LB, Chou J. The HLA-1, -B, and -DR phenotypes and tuberculosis. *Am Rev Resp Dis* 1985;132:382–385.

63. Small PM, Shafer RW, Hopewell PC, et al. Exogenous reinfection with multidrug-resistant *Mycobacterium tuberculosis* in patients with advanced HIV infection. *N Engl J Med* 1993;328: 1137–1144.

64. Nardell E, McInnis B, Thomas B, Weidhaas S. Exogenous reinfection with tuberculosis in a shelter for the homeless. *N Engl J Med* 1986;315:1570–1575.

65. Braun MM, Badi M, Ryder R, et al. A retrospective cohort study of the risk of tuberculosis amongst women of childbearing age with HIV infection in Zaire. *Am Rev Resp Dis* 1991;143: 601–604.

66. Selwyn P, Hartel D, Lewis V, et al. A prospective study of the risk of tuberculosis among intravenous drug users with human immunodeficiency virus infection. *N Engl J Med* 1989;320: 545–550.

67. Hoon JR, Dockerty MB, Pemberton JdeJ, et al. Ileocecal tuberculosis including comparison of this disease with nonspecific regional enterocolitis and noncaseous tuberculated enterocolitis. *Int Abstr Surg* 1950;91:417–440.

68. Rubinstein BM, Pastrana T, Jacobson HG. Tuberculosis of the esophagus. *Radiology* 1958;70:401–403.

69. Logan VD. Anorectal tuberculosis. *Proc R Soc Med* 1969;62: 1227–1230.

70. Martin CL. Anorectal tuberculosis. In: Goldberg B, ed. *Clinical tuberculosis*. 5th ed. Philadelphia: FA Davis; 1947.

71. Cappell MS, Javeed M. Pancreatic abscess due to mycobacterial infection associated with the acquired immunodeficiency syndrome. *J Clin Gastroenterol* 1990;12:423–429.

72. Koduri VG, Janardhanan R, Hagan P, Brodmerkel GJ Jr. Pancreatic TB: diagnosis by needle aspiration. *Am J Gastroenterol* 1992;87:1206–1208.

73. Desai DC, Santhi S, Mohandas KM, Borges A, et al. Tuberculosis of the pancreas: report of three cases. *Am J Gastroenterol* 1991;86:761–763.

74. Prout WG. Multiple tuberculous perforations of ileum. *Gut* 1968;9:381–382.

75. Davis G, Corbett DB, Krejs GJ. Ileal chloride secretion as a cause of secretory diarrhea in a patient with primary intestinal tuberculosis. *Gastroenterology* 1976;76:829–835.

76. Senise JF, Hamrick PA, Guidugli RB, et al. Ileal loop perforation caused by tuberculosis in patients with the acquired immunodeficiency syndrome. *Rev Paul Med* 1991;109:61–64.

77. Powell DA. Tuberculous lymphadenitis. In: Schlossberg D, ed. *Tuberculosis*. 2nd ed. New York: Springer-Verlag; 1988: 99–107.

78. Moshal MG, Baker LW, Lautre G, Bader G. Colonoscopy: 100 examinations. *South Afr J Surg* 1973;11:73–78.

79. Bhargava DK, Tandon HD. Ileocaecal tuberculosis diagnosed by colonoscopy and biopsy. *Aust N Z J Surg* 1980;50:583–585.

80. Barnes PF, Block AB, Davidson PT, Snider DE. Tuberculosis in patients with human immunodeficiency virus infection. *N Engl J Med* 1991;23:1644–1650.

81. Morris A, Reller LB, Salfinger M, Jackson K, Sievers A, Dwyer B. Mycobacteria in stool specimens: the nonvalue of smears for predicting culture results. *J Clin Microbiol* 1993;31: 1385–1387.

82. Damsker B, Bottone EJ. *Myobacterium-avium–Mycobacterium intracellulare* from the intestinal tracts of patients with the acquired immunodeficiency syndrome: concepts regarding acquisition and pathogenesis. *J Infect Dis* 1985;151:179–181.

83. Yajko DM, Nassos PS, Sanders CA, et al. Comparison of four decontamination methods for recovery of *Mycobacterium avium* complex from stools. *J Clin Microbiol* 1993;31:302–306.

84. Tisdall PA, Roberts GD, Anhalt JP. Identification of clinical isolates of mycobacteria with gas-liquid chromatography alone. *J Clin Microbiol* 1979;10:506–514.

85. Tisdall PA, DeYoung DR, Roberts GD, Anhalt JP. Identification of clinical isolates of mycobacteria with gas-liquid chromatography: a 10-month follow-up study. *J Clin Microbiology* 1982;16:400–402.

86. Butler WR, Kilburn JO. Identification of major slowly growing pathogenic mycobacteria and *Mycobacteria gordonae* by high-performance liquid chromatography of their mycolic acids. *J Clin Microbiol* 1988;26:50–53.

87. Eisenbach KD, Cave MD, Bates JH, Crawford JT. Polymerase chain reaction amplification of repetitive DNA sequence specific for *Mycobacterium tuberculosis*. *J Infect Dis* 1990;161: 977–981.

88. Noordhoek GT, Kolk AHJ, Bjune G, Catty D, et al. Sensitivity and specificity of PCR for detection of *Mycobacterium tuberculosis:* a blind comparison study among seven laboratories. *J Clin Microbiol* 1994;32:277–284.

89. Haas WH, Butler WR, Woodley CL, Crawford JT. Mixed-linker polymerase chain reaction: a new method for rapid fingerprinting of isolates of the *Mycobacterium tuberculosis* complex. *J Clin Microbiol* 1993;31:1293–1298.

90. Thoeni RF, Margulis AR. Gastrointestinal tuberculosis. *Sem Roentgenol* 1979;14:283–294.

91. Tabrisky J, Lindstrom RR, Peters R, Lachman RS. Tuberculous enteritis. Review of a protean disease. *Am J Gastroenterol* 1975;63:49–57.

92. Gilinsky NH, Marks IN, Kottler RE, Price SK. Abdominal tuberculosis, a ten year review. *South Afr Med J* 1983;64: 849–857.

93. Horsburgh CR, Pozniak A. Epidemiology of tuberculosis in the era of HIV. *AIDS* 1993;7:S109–114.

94. CDC. Initial therapy for tuberculosis in the era of multidrug resistance. *MMWR* 1993;42(No. RR-7):1–8.

95. Control of Tuberculosis in the United States. *Am Rev Resp Dis* 1992;146:1623–1633.

96. Tenover FC, Crawford JT, Huebner RE, et al. The resurgence of tuberculosis: is your laboratory ready? *J Clin Microbiol* 1993;31:767–770.

97. Mahmoudi A, Iseman MD. Pitfalls in the care of patients with tuberculosis. *JAMA* 1993;270:65–68.

98. Goble M, Iseman MD, Madsen LA, et al. Treatment of 171 patients with pulmonary tuberculosis resistant to isoniazid and rifampin. *N Engl J Med* 1993;328:527–532.

99. Horsburgh CR. Mycobacterial infections in the immunocompromised host. *Sem Resp Med* 1989;10:61–67.

100. CDC. Tuberculosis in imported nonhuman primates—United States, June 1990–May 1993. *MMWR* 1993;42:572–576.

101. Thompson PJ, Cousins DV, Gow BL, et al. Seals, seal trainers, and mycobacterial infection. *Am Rev Resp Dis* 1993;147: 164–167.

102. Dalovisio JR, Stetter M, Mikota-Wells S. Rhinoceros' rhinorrhea: cause of an outbreak of infection due to airborne *Mycobacterium bovis* in zookeepers. *Clin Infect Dis* 1992;15: 598–600.

103. Fanning A, Edwards S. *Mycobacterium bovis* infection in human beings in contact with elk *(Cervus elaphus)* in Alberta, Canada. *Lancet* 1991;338:1253–1255.

104. CDC. The use of preventive therapy for tuberculous infection in the United States. *MMWR* 1990;39(No. RR-8):9–12.

105. CDC. Use of BCG vaccines in the control of tuberculosis: a joint statement by the ACIP and the Advisory Committee for Elimination of Tuberculosis. *MMWR* 1988;37:663–675.

106. Clemens JD, Chuong JH, Feinstein AR. The BCG controversy. *JAMA* 1983;249:2362–2369.

107. Horsburgh CR. *Mycobacterium avium* complex infection in the acquired immunodeficiency syndrome. *N Engl J Med* 1991;324: 1332–1338.

108. Ellner JJ, Goldberger MJ, Parenti DM. AIDS comentary. *M. avium* infection and AIDS: a therapeutic dilemma in rapid evolution. *J Infect Dis* 1992;165:1082–1085.

109. Horsburgh CR, Selik RM. The epidemiology of disseminated nontuberculous mycobacterial infection in the acquired immunodeficiency syndrome (AIDS). *Am Rev Resp Dis* 1989;139: 4–7.

110. Gray JR, Rabeneck L. Atypical mycobacterial infection of the gastrointestinal tract in AIDS patients. *Am J Gastroenterol* 1989;12:1521–1524.

111. Chin DP, Hopewell PC, Yajko DM, et al. *Mycobacterium avium* complex (MAC) in the respiratory or gastrointestinal tract precedes MAC bacteremia (abstract). *Am Rev Resp Dis* 1993;147:A393.

112. Nightingale SD, Byrd LT, Southern PM, et al. Incidence of *Mycobacterium avium-intracellulare* complex bacteremia in human immunodeficiency virus–positive patients. *J Infect Dis* 1992;165:1082–1085.

113. Horsburgh CR, Caldwell MB, Simonds RJ. Epidemiology of disseminated nontuberculous mycobacterial disease in children with acquired immunodeficiency syndrome. *Pediatr Infect Dis* 1993;12:219–222.

114. Okello DO, Sewankambo N, Goodgame R, et al. Absence of bacteremia with *Mycobacterium avium-intracellulare* in Ugandan patients with AIDS. *J Infect Dis* 1990;162:208–210.

115. Lucas SB, Hounnou A, Peacock C, Beaumel A, et al. The mortality and pathology of HIV infection in a West African City. *AIDS* 1993;7:1569–1579.

116. Klatt EC, Jensen DF and Meyer PR. Pathology of *Mycobacterium avium-intracellulare* infection in acquired immunodeficiency syndrome. *Hum Pathol* 1987:709–714.

117. Wallace JM, Hannah JB. *Mycobacterium avium* complex infection in patients with the acquired immunodeficiency syndrome. *Chest* 1988;93:926–932.

118. Roth RI, Owen RL, Keren DF, Volberding PA. Intestinal infection with *Mycobacterium avium* in acquired immune deficiency syndrome (AIDS). Histological and clinical comparison with Whipple's disease. *Dig Dis Sci* 1985;30:497–504.

119. Gillin JS, Urmacher C, West R, Shike M. Disseminated *Mycobacterium avium-intracellulare* infection in acquired immunodeficiency syndrome mimicking Whipple's disease. *Gastroenterology* 1983;85:1187–1191.

120. Schneebaum CW, Novick DM, Chabon AB, Strutynsky N, Yancovitz SR, Freund S. Terminal ileitis associated with *Mycobacterium avium-intracellulare* infection in a homosexual man with acquired immune deficiency syndrome. *Gastroenterology* 1987;92:1127–1132.

121. Goslee S, Wolinsky E. Water as a source of potentially pathogenic mycobacteria. *Am Rev Resp Dis* 1976;113:287–292.

122. Meissner G, Anz W. Sources of *Mycobacterium avium* complex infection resulting in human diseases. *Am Rev Resp Dis* 1977;116:1057–1064.

123. du Moulin GC, Stottmeier KD, Pelletier PA, Tsang AY, Hedley-Whyte J. Concentration of *Mycobacterium avium* by hospital hot water systems. *JAMA* 1988;260(11):1599–1601.

124. Falkinham III JO, Parker BC, Gruft H. Epidemiology of infection by nontuberculous mycobacteria. *Am Rev Resp Dis* 1980; 121:931–937.

125. Hosty TS, McDurmont CI. Isolation of acid-fast organisms from milk and oysters. *Health Lab Sci* 1975;12(1):16–19.

126. Chapman JS, Bernard JS, Speight M. Isolation of mycobacteria from raw milk. *Am Rev Resp Dis* 1965;91:351–355.

127. Prichard WD, Thoen CO, Himes EM, Muscoplat CC, Johnson DW. Epidemiology of mycobacterial lymphadenitis in an Idaho swine herd. *Am J Epidemiol* 1977;106(3):222–227.

128. Wolinsky E, Rynearson TK. Mycobacteria in soil and their relation to disease-associated strains. *Am Rev Resp Dis* 1968; 97:1032–1037.

129. von Reyn CF, Arbeit RD, Gilks CF, et al. Risk factors for mycobacteremia among patients with AIDS in developed and developing countries (abstract). Abstracts of the Ninth International Conference on AIDS. Berlin: 1993;PO-B07-1186.

130. Horsburgh CR, Chin DP, Yajko DM, et al. Environmental risk factors for acquisition of *Mycobacterium avium* complex in persons with HIV infection (abstract). Abstracts of the first national conference on human retroviruses and related infections. Washington, DC: American Society for Microbiology; 1993: 190.

131. Horsburgh CR, Mason UG, Farhi DC, Iseman MD. Disseminated infection with *Mycobacterium avium-intracellulare*. *Medicine* 1985;64:36–48.

132. Barbaro DJ, Orcutt VL, Coldiron BM. *Mycobacterium avium–Mycobacterium intracellulare* infection limited to the skin and lymph nodes in patients with AIDS. *Rev Infect Dis* 1989;11:625–628.

133. Pransky SM, Reisman BK, Kearns DB, Seid AB, Collins DL, Krous HF. Cervicofacial mycobacterial adenitis in children: endemic to San Diego? *Laryngoscope* 1990;100:920–925.

134. Altman RP, Margileth AM. Cervical lymphadenopathy from atypical mycobacteria: diagnosis and surgical treatment. *J Pediatr Surg* 1975;10:419–422.

135. Margileth AM, Chandra R, Altman RP. Chronic lymphadenopathy due to mycobacterial infection. Clinical features, diagnosis, histopathology, and management. *Am J Dis Child* 1984; 138:917–922.

136. O'Brien RJ, Geiter LJ, Snider DE. The epidemiology of nontuberculous mycobacterial diseases in the United States. Results from a national survey. *Am Rev Resp Dis* 1987;135:1007–1014.

137. Saitz EW. Cervical lymphadenitis caused by atypical mycobacteria. *Ped Clin North Am* 1981;28:823–839.

138. Romanus V. Experience in Sweden 15 years after stopping general BCG vaccination at birth. *Bull Int Union Against Tuberc Lung Dis* 1990;65:2–3.

139. Martin T, Hoeppner VH, Ring ED. Clinical and community studies. Superficial mycobacterial lymphadenitis in Saskatchewan. *Can Med Assoc J* 1988;138:451–434.

140. Grange J, Collins C, Yates M. Bacteriological survey of tuberculous lymphadenitis in south-east England: 1973–80. *J Epidemiol Commun Health* 1982;36:157–161.

141. Llewelyn DM, Dorman D. Mycobacterial lymphadenitis. *Aust Pediatr J* 1971;7:97–102.

142. Mapother ME, Songer JG. In vitro interaction of *Mycobacterium avium* with intestinal epithelial cells. *Infect Immun* 1984; 45:67–73.

143. Brown ST. Epithelial cell invasion by *Mycobacterium avium* complex (abstract). Frontiers in mycobacteriology: *M. avium*, the modern epidemic. Denver, CO: National Jewish Center for Immunology and Respiratory Medicine; 1992:22.

144. Pethel ML, Falkinham JO III. Plasmid-influenced changes in *Mycobacterium avium* catalase activity. *Infect Immun* 1989; 57:1714–1718.

145. Prinzis S, Rivoire B, Brennan PJ. Comparative study of the protein profiles of smooth-domed, smooth-transparent, and rough variants of *M. avium* (abstract). Frontiers in mycobacteriology: *M. avium*, the modern epidemic. Denver, CO: National Jewish Center for Immunology and Respiratory Medicine; 1992:37.

146. Schafer WB, Davis CL, Cohn ML. Pathogenicity of transparent, opaque, and rough variants of *M. avium* in chicken and mice. *Am Rev Resp Dis* 1970;102:499–501.

147. Shiratsuchi H, Toosi Z, Mettler MA, Ellner JJ. Colonial morphotype as a determinate of cytokine expression by human monocytes infected with *M. avium*. *J Immunol* 1993;150: 2945–2954.

148. Havlik JA, Metchock B, Thompson SE, Barrett K, Rimland D, Horsburgh CR. A prospective evaluation of *Mycobacterium avium* complex colonization of the respiratory and gastrointestinal tracts of persons with HIV infection. *J Infect Dis* 1993; 168:1045–1048.

149. Strom RL, Gruninger RP. AIDS with *Mycobacterium avium-intracellulare* lesions resembling those of Whipple's disease. *N Engl J Med* 1983;309:1323–1324.

150. Sohn CC, Schroff RW, Kliewer KE, Lebel DM, Fligiel S. Disseminated *Mycobacterium avium-intracellulare* infection in homosexual men with acquired cell-mediated immunodeficiency: A histologic and immunologic study of two cases. *Am J Clin Pathol* 1983;79:247–252.

151. Waisman J, Rotterdam H, Niedt GN, Lewin K, Racz P. AIDS: an overview of the pathology. *Pathol Res Pract* 1987;182: 729–754.

152. Grunfeld C, Kotler DP. The wasting syndrome and nutritional support in AIDS. *Sem Gastrointest Dis* 1991:2:25–36.

153. Wood C, Nickeloff BJ, Todes-Taylor NR. Pseudo-tumor resulting from atypical mycobacterial infection: a "histoid" variety of *Mycobacterium avium-intracellulare* complex infection. *Am J Clin Pathol* 1985;83:524–527.

154. Shiratsuchi H, Johnson JL, Ellner JJ. Bidirectional effects of cytokines on growth of *M. avium* in human monocytes. *J Immunol* 1991;146:3165–3170.

155. Shiratsuchi H, Johnson JJ, Ellner JJ. Modulation of the effector function of human monocytes for *Mycobacterium avium* by human immunodeficiency virus-1 envelope protein gp120. *J Clin Invest* 1994;93:885–891.

156. Bermudez LE, Young LS. Natural killer cell-dependent mycobacteriostatic and mycobactericidal activity in human macrophages. *J Immunol* 1986;146:265–270.

157. Wayne WG, Young LS, Bertram M. Absence of mycobacterial antibody in patients with acquired immune deficiency syndrome. *Eur J Clin Microbiol* 1991;5:363–365.

158. Winter SM, Bernard EM, Gold JWM, Armstrong D. Humoral response to disseminated infection with *Mycobacterium avium–Mycobacterium intracellulare* in acquired immunodeficiency syndrome and hairy cell leukemia. *J Infect Dis* 1985; 151:523–527.

159. Schnittman S, Lane HC, Witebsky FG, et al. Host defense against *Mycobacterium avium* complex. *J Clin Immunol* 1988; 8:234–243.

160. Douvas GS, May MH, Crowle AJ. Transferrin, iron, and serum lipids enhance or inhibit *Mycobacterium avium* replication in human macrophages. *J Infect Dis* 1993;167:857–864.

161. Crowle AJ, Cohn D, Poche P. Defects in sera from acquired immunodeficiency syndrome (AIDS) patients and from non-AIDS patients with *Mycobacterium avium* infection which decrease macrophage resistance of *M. avium*. *Infect Immun* 1989; 57:1445–1451.

162. Horsburgh CR, Metchock B, Gordon SM, et al. Clinical syndromes and predictors of survival of patients with AIDS and disseminated *Mycobacterium avium* complex disease (abstract). Abstracts of the Annual Meeting of the Infectious Diseases Society of America. Washington, DC: Infectious Disease Society of America, 1993:18-A.

163. Sathe SS, Gascone P, Lo W, Pinto R, Reichman LB. Severe anemia is an important negative predictor for survival with disseminated *Mycobacterium avium-intracellulare* in acquired immunodeficiency syndrome. *Am Rev Resp Dis* 1990;142: 1306–1312.

164. Jacobson MA, Peiperi L, Volberding PA, et al. Red cell transfusion therapy for anemia in patients with AIDS and ARC: incidence, associated factors, and outcome. *Transfusion* 1990;30: 133–137.

165. Hoyt L, Connor E, Oleske J. Non-tuberculosis mycobacteria in children with acquired immunodeficiency syndrome. *Pediatr Infect Dis J* 1992;11:354–360.

166. Lewis LL, Butler KM, Husson RN, et al. Defining the popula-

tion of human immunodeficiency virus-infected children at risk for *Mycobacterium avium-intracellulare* infection. *J Pediatr* 1992;121:677–683.

167. Radin DR. Intraabdominal *Mycobacterium* tuberculosis vs *Mycobacterium avium-intracellulare* infections in patients with AIDS: distinction based on CT findings. *Am J Roentgenol* 1991; 156:487–491.

168. Monsour Jr HP, Quigley EMM, Markin RS, Dalke DD, Goldsmith JC, Harty RF. Endoscopy in the diagnosis of gastrointestinal *Mycobacterium avium-intracellulare* infection. *J Clin Gastroenterol* 1991;13:20–24.

169. Cappell MS, Hassan R, Rosenthal S, Mascarenhas M. Gastrointestinal obstruction due to *Mycobacterium avium-intracellulare* associated with the acquired immunodeficiency syndrome. *Am J Gastroenterol* 1992;12:1823–1827.

170. Cappell MS, Gupta A. Gastrointestinal hemorrhage due to gastrointestinal *Mycobacterium avium-intracellulare* or esophageal candidiasis in patients with the acquired immunodeficiency syndrome. *Am J Gastroenterol* 1991;87:224–229.

171. Horsburgh CR, Havlik JA, Ellis DA, et al. Survival of AIDS patients with disseminated *Mycobacterium avium* complex infection with and without antimycobacterial chemotherapy. *Am Rev Resp Dis* 1991;144:557–559.

172. Taha AM, Davidson PT, Bailey WC. Surgical treatment of atypical mycobacterial lymphadenitis in children. *Pediatr Infect Dis* 1985;4:664–667.

173. Spark RP, Fried ML, Bean CK, Figueroa JM, Crowe Jr CP, Campbell DP. Nontuberculous mycobacterial adenitis of childhood. The ten-year experience at a community hospital. *Am J Dis Child* 1988;142:106–108.

174. Yagupsky P, Menegus MA. Cumulative positivity rates of multiple blood cultures for *Mycobacterium avium-intracellulare* and *Cryptococcus neoformans* in patients with the acquired immunodeficiency syndrome. *Arch Pathol Lab Med* 1990;114: 923–925.

175. Barnes PF, Arevalo C. Blood culture positivity patterns in bacteremia due to *Mycobacterium avium-intracellulare*. *South Med J* 1988;81:1059–1060.

176. Alessi DP, Dudley JP. Atypical mycobacteria-induced cervical adenitis. *Arch Otolaryngol Head Neck Surg* 1988;114:664–666.

177. Levin-Epstein AA, Lucente FE. Scrofula—the dangerous masquerader. *Laryngoscope* 1982;92:938–943.

178. Huebner RE, Schein MF, Cauthen GM, Geiter LJ, O'Brien

RJ. Usefulness of skin testing with mycobacterial antigens in children with cervical adenopathy. *Pediatr Infect Dis J* 1992; 11:450–456.

179. Kemper CA, Meng TC, Nussbaum J et al. Treatment of *Mycobacterium avium* complex bacteremia with a four-drug oral regimen: rifampin, ethambutol, clofazimine and ciprofloxacin. *Ann Intern Med* 1992;116:466–472.

180. Kerlikowske KM, Katz MH, Chan AK, Stable EJ. Antimycobacterial therapy for disseminated *Mycobacterium avium* complex infection in patients with acquired immunodeficiency syndrome. *Arch Intern Med* 1992;152:813–817.

181. Chaisson RE, Benson C, Dube M, et al. Clarithromycin therapy for disseminated *Mycobacterium avium* complex in AIDS (abstract). Abstracts of the 32nd Interscience Conference on Antimicrobial Agents and Chemotherapy. Washington, DC: American Society for Microbiology; 1992:259.

182. Neu HC. New macrolide antibiotics: azithromycin and clarithromycin. *Ann Intern Med* 1992;116:517–519.

183. Young LS, Wiviott L, Wu M, et al. Azithromycin for treatment of *Mycobacterium avium-intracellulare* complex infection in patients with AIDS. *Lancet* 1991;338:1107–1109.

184. Dautzenberg B, Truffot C, Legris S, et al. Activity of clarithromycin against *Mycobacterium avium* infection in patients with the acquired immune deficiency syndrome. *Am Rev Resp Dis* 1991;144:564–569.

185. Masur H, and the U.S. Public Health Service task force. Recommendations on prophylaxis and therapy for disseminated *Mycobacterium avium* complex for adults and adolescents infected with human immunodeficiency virus. *N Engl J Med* 1993;329:898–904.

186. Deziel DJ, Hyser MJ, Doolas A, Bines SD, Blaauw BB, Kessler HA. Major abdominal operations in acquired immunodeficiency syndrome. *Am Surgeon* 1990;56:445–450.

187. Lumb R, Shaw D. Mycobacterium bovis (BCG) vaccination. Progressive disease in a patient asymptomatically infected with the human immunodeficiency virus. *Med J Aust* 1992;156: 286–287.

188. Smith E, Thybo S, Bennedsen J. Infection with *Mycobacterium bovis* in a patient with AIDS: a late complication of BCG vaccination. *Scand J Infect Dis* 1992;24:109–110.

189. Nightingale SD, Cameron DW, Gordin FM, et al. Two placebo controlled trials of rifabutin prophylaxis against *Mycobacterium avium* complex infection in AIDS patients. *N Engl J Med* 1993;329:828–833.

Infections of the Gastrointestinal Tract,
edited by M. J. Blaser, P. D. Smith, J. I. Ravdin,
H. B. Greenberg, and R. L. Guerrant
Published by Raven Press, Ltd., New York, 1995.

CHAPTER 63

Deep Mycoses

Ronald G. Washburn and John E. Bennett

Mycoses of the gastrointestinal (GI) tract may be divided into two broad categories: (a) those caused by transmucosal inoculation (e.g., *Candida* species) and (b) those that disseminate to the GI tract following primary pulmonary infection (e.g., *Histoplasma capsulatum*). An important concept is that fungal cultures must be interpreted in light of their anatomic sources. For example, a superficial swab or brushing from virtually any portion of the gut might be expected to grow *Candida* even in the absence of true pathology because it is a normal commensal. In contrast, isolation of that organism on culture would be clinically significant if yeast-like forms were seen in the submucosa of an intestinal or gastric biopsy.

Morphologically, the fungi can be divided into molds (fuzzy mycelial growth), yeasts (pasty colonies), and dimorphic fungi (mycelia at 30°C, yeast at 37°C). All fungi can be stained with Gomori methenamine silver (dark gray) or periodic acid–Schiff stain (pink).

Molds that cause GI disease include *Aspergillus* species and agents of mucormycosis (e.g., *Mucor, Rhizopus*). Tissue forms of those filamentous fungi are elongated hyphae that invade blood vessels. The hyphae of *Aspergillus* species are narrow and septated, with a tendency to dichotomous branching; for agents of mucormycosis, the hyphae are wide, irregular, aseptate, and tend to branch at right angles. *Candida* species grow in tissue as budding yeast and, except for *Candida glabrata*, they also may appear as hyphae or pseudohyphae. Pseudohyphae are defined as elongated structures possessing constrictions at areas of septae. The other yeast that causes GI disease is *Cryptococcus neoformans*. Dimorphic fungi discussed in this chapter are *Histoplasma capsulatum, Blastomyces dermatitidis,* and *Paracoccidioides brasiliensis*. These organisms all grow as budding yeast at 37°C in human tissues. Mean diameters of tissue phase yeast may overlap; for

that reason, Mayer's mucicarmine staining can be useful because, among the above-named species, only *C. neoformans* stains rose pink with that agent.

There is no human-to-human transmission of GI mycoses. Rather, *Candida* are resident flora, and the remaining fungi are acquired chiefly through inhalation.

Therapy for GI mycoses ranges from topical agents (e.g., nystatin or clotrimazole) for uncomplicated oral candidiasis to more potent systemic agents. The topical agents have very limited clinical utility in mycoses of the GI tract. A variety of azole compounds are available for systemic use, including ketoconazole, itraconazole, and fluconazole. Those agents act by inhibiting synthesis of the fungal membrane sterol ergosterol. Their major toxicities include drug-induced hepatitis, nausea, vomiting, and a variety of drug interactions. Patients infected with azole-unresponsive fungi (e.g., agents of mucormycosis) and those who are critically ill require therapy with intravenous amphotericin B. That amphophilic drug acts by intercalating itself between ergosterol molecules in fungal cell membranes, rendering the organisms leaky. Major toxicities of amphotericin B include reversible nephrotoxicity and anemia as well as fever, chills, nausea, and vomiting. A more complete discussion of the antifungal agents is provided in the chapter by Morrow and Neuzil.

CANDIDIASIS

Mycology

Candida species colonize the human GI tract, but they also are capable of invading the mucosa and beyond, under appropriate clinical circumstances. In the syndrome of superficial candidiasis, invasion is limited to mucosa and submucosa. In contrast, deep candidiasis does not respect anatomic barriers and is capable of producing severe tissue destruction, e.g., with perforation of the bowel wall or distant seeding of target organs such as eye, liver, and spleen.

R. G. Washburn: Division of Infectious Diseases, Bowman Gray School of Medicine, Wake Forest University, Winston-Salem, North Carolina.

J. E. Bennett: Clinical Mycology Section, National Institute of Allergy and Infectious Diseases, National Institutes of Health, Bethesda, Maryland.

Epidemiology and Predisposing Factors

Intact T-lymphocyte function contributes to defense of the squamous mucosa in superficial candidiasis, evidenced by the high incidence of oropharyngeal and esophageal candidiasis in patients with AIDS. Additionally, patients with chronic mucocutaneous candidiasis, an inborn defect in T-lymphocyte function, develop disfiguring mucosal and skin lesions.

Normal host defenses against deep candidiasis include intact mucosal surfaces and phagocytic host defenses. Therefore, key predisposing factors are (a) disruption of mucosal integrity (e.g., due to bowel surgery or cancer chemotherapy) and (b) diminished neutrophil numbers or function (e.g., cancer chemotherapy and chronic high-dose glucocorticoid therapy). Gastric and duodenal ulcers may serve as foci for superficial invasion.

Pathogenesis and Pathology

Hematogenously disseminated candidiasis can affect virtually any organ system, particularly the eyes, with characteristic focal white retinal lesions and abscesses in the liver and spleen. Invasive candidiasis usually elicits a neutrophilic inflammatory response, and there may be extensive tissue destruction. There is experimental evidence to suggest that the tissue destruction might be mediated, at least in part, by *Candida* proteases.

Clinical Manifestations

Oropharyngeal and esophageal candidiasis are discussed in detail in chapters concerning HIV infection and malignancy (see the chapters by Smith and Sepkowitz and Armstrong). Therefore, the present discussion focuses instead on disease distal to the esophagus. The "chronic *Candida* syndrome" has received publicity as an entity in which individuals have symptoms attributed to *Candida* colonization. The symptoms are protean, including fatigue, headache, and nausea, but no causal relationship has been established between *Candida* and the symptoms, leading authorities to doubt whether *Candida* has any role in the symptom complex.

The stomach is the second most commonly infected site after the esophagus, in patients with involvement of only a single site (1). It is important to differentiate between invasive disease and superficial colonization because *Candida* are clearly capable of colonizing benign gastric ulcers without invading deeply into the submucosa (2). Those colonized ulcers can be healed with conventional antiulcer therapy, without use of antifungal agents. Rarely, locally invasive gastric candidiasis may complicate peptic ulcer disease, producing mucosal microabscesses (3).

Autopsy data indicate that the small bowel is affected in about 20% of patients with multiple sites of GI candidia-

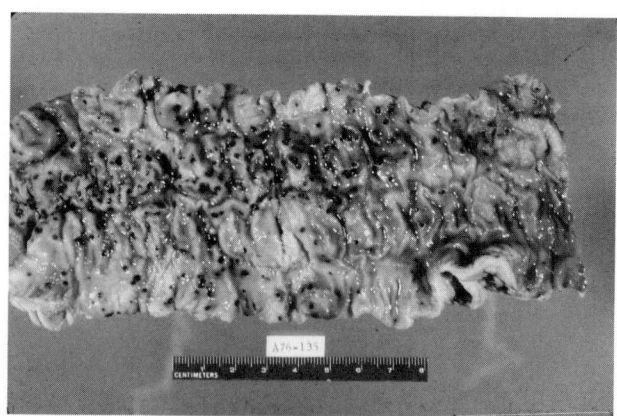

FIG. 1. Numerous shallow mucosal lesions due to *Candida* in the small intestine of a patient with acute leukemia and fatal disseminated candidiasis.

sis, usually in neutropenic hosts (Fig. 1) (1). Watery diarrhea and perforation have been attributed to intestinal candidiasis (4), but the contribution of the fungus remains unclear. Endoscopically, multiple mucosal ulcerations may be seen in the stomach or intestines. Intestinal ulcerations are a likely source of disseminated candidiasis in the neutropenic patient, and ulcerated tumor masses also have been described (1).

Diagnosis

The diagnosis of GI candidiasis should be made by finding fungi in brushings, biopsies, or surgical specimens from mucosal ulcerations (5). The organism can sometimes be recovered in pure culture on antibiotic-containing medium, but histological evidence of invasion is essential in assigning a causative role to *Candida*.

Therapy

Treatment for invasive GI candidiasis in the febrile neutropenic patient should usually include a prolonged course of intravenous amphotericin B. Fluconazole is useful in esophageal candidiasis and may prove to be effective for superficial mucosal disease lower in the GI tract. Topical therapy such as clotrimazole troches is best reserved for oropharyngeal candidiasis.

CRYPTOCOCCOSIS

Mycology

Cryptococcus neoformans is an opportunistic fungus that grows as a yeast form at both 30°C and 37°C. The organism usually is heavily encapsulated in human tissue, and budding is narrow-based, with the daughter cell typically smaller than the mother cell at the time of separation.

Mayer's mucicarmine stain usually stains the capsule reddish pink in histological section.

Epidemiology and Predisposing Factors

Cryptococcus neoformans var. *neoformans* (serotype A and D) can be recovered from a variety of different bird excreta, especially pigeon guano. In tropical and subtropical climates, *Cryptococcus neoformans* var. *gattii* (serotype B and C) is found in association with the *Eucalyptus* tree, *E. camaldulensis*. Desiccated yeasts are believed to be the infectious particles. Gastrointestinal lesions seem to represent manifestations of disseminated disease.

Normal host defenses against cryptococcosis are principally cell-mediated. Mononuclear phagocytes, natural killer (NK) cells, and cytotoxic T cells all are fungicidal or fungistatic against the organism. Thus, patients with defective cellular immunity are at risk for invasive cryptococcosis, including patients with AIDS, solid organ transplantation, Hodgkin's disease, other lymphomas, and sarcoidosis, as well as patients taking daily high-dose glucocorticoids.

Pathogenesis and Pathology

The usual mode of infection is through inhalation. In immunologically intact individuals, the majority of primary pulmonary infections are probably asymptomatic, but a subset of individuals develops progressive pulmonary disease and/or extrapulmonary dissemination. The most commonly affected target is the central nervous system, but the infection also can disseminate to skin, bone, prostate, and kidney; GI lesions are very rare.

Inflammatory response in tissues of normal hosts is granulomatous. Organisms may be intracellular, within large mononuclear phagocytes. Granulomas are only rarely found in AIDS patients, and there is usually a paucity of inflammation in central nervous system lesions even in normal hosts.

Clinical Manifestations

Gastrointestinal involvement has been described in all major areas of the GI tract, from the oral cavity to the anus (6). The GI lesions almost always are manifestations of disseminated disease, and pulmonary cryptococcosis may still be present when the GI disease becomes clinically apparent.

There are several reports about oral manifestations (7–10). Before the AIDS epidemic, the most recent previous report of oral cryptococcosis was in a patient with chronic lymphocytic leukemia (11). Recently, the majority of reports concern patients with AIDS. Oral lesions manifest as persistent ulcerations of the tongue or palate (10). A mucosal lesion contiguous with erosion of the hard palate has been reported as the first manifestation of disseminated cryptococcosis in AIDS (9). AIDS patients also may present with ulceration at dental extraction sites.

There also are a few case reports of esophageal cryptococcosis. A patient with Job's syndrome (hyper-IgE) pre-

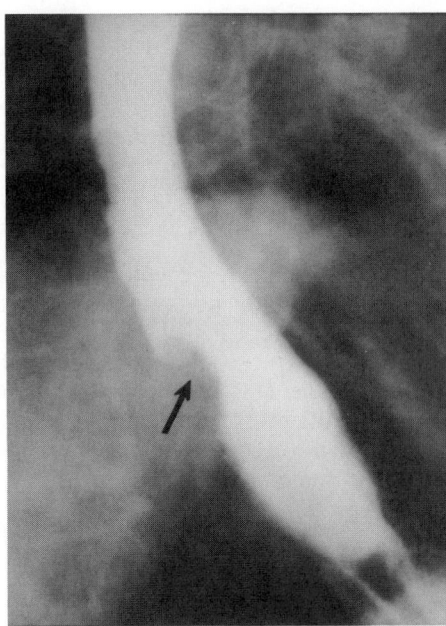

FIG. 2. Cryptococcal lesion of the esophagus in a patient with Job's syndrome. From Ref. 12, with permission.

sented with massive hematemesis due to esophageal cryptococcosis (Fig. 2) (12). Cultures of blood, urine, sputum, and spinal fluid were negative, as were cryptococcal antigen tests of the serum and spinal fluid, findings that suggested the disease was localized to the esophagus. A patient with chronic lymphocytic leukemia had cryptococcal esophagitis and fungal destruction of the colonic muscularis (13).

Gastrointestinal cryptococcosis distal to the esophagus has been reported as a manifestation of disseminated cryptococcosis in AIDS, with involvement of stomach, duodenum, pancreas, colon, and liver (14), as well as multiple sites outside the GI tract. Kovacs's original series of AIDS patients with cryptococcosis included a patient with a cryptococcal omental mass (15).

A patient with Job's syndrome presented with a constricting lesion of the ascending colon and a chronic perirectal abscess (16); similar to the patient with Job's syndrome who had esophageal involvement (12), this patient appeared to have localized disease. Several other patients with colonic tumor-like cryptococcal masses have been described (17–19). The lesions may be nodular, friable, or ulcerated. Finally, anal ulceration has been described in an AIDS patient with obvious disseminated disease (20).

Liver involvement is common in AIDS patients, with mass lesions containing little or no inflammation (14).

Diagnosis

The diagnosis of GI cryptococcosis can be made by deep biopsy specimens that show invading yeast with typical morphological appearance and a positive culture. When cultures are not available, mucicarmine staining is helpful because, among fungi of the appropriate diameter, *C. neoformans* is the sole organism that stains rose pink.

The organism may be difficult to recover in pure culture because of associated GI flora. However, the presence of suspicious lesions in the GI tract, combined with positive blood, spinal fluid, or urine cultures, or an elevated serum cryptococcal antigen supports the diagnosis.

Treatment

Treatment for disseminated cryptococcosis should include a full course of intravenous amphotericin B in most cases. Extirpative surgery for obstructive cryptococcal mass lesions of the GI tract could be considered if dissemination can be excluded (18), but a course of amphotericin B would still be prudent. Patients with AIDS and cryptococcosis are known to require lifelong suppressive therapy, usually with fluconazole.

ASPERGILLOSIS

Mycology

Aspergillus species grow as fluffy molds and reproduce by generating infectious conidia that are 2–3 μm in diameter. In tissue, the organisms grow as septate hyphae 2–3 μm wide, even in diameter, with a tendency to dichotomous branching.

Epidemiology and Predisposing Factors

Aspergillus conidia are ubiquitous in nature; for example, the organism grows in decaying organic material, and due to its thermophilicity, it can be found in high concentrations in compost heaps.

The human host has efficient defenses against invasive aspergillosis, mediated against conidia and hyphae by neutrophils and monocytes. Therefore, the most susceptible hosts are those with decreases in phagocyte numbers or function. For that reason, GI aspergillosis is primarily a disease of patients with prolonged neutropenia, e.g., those receiving bone marrow–suppressive chemotherapy.

Pathogenesis and Pathology

Due to the fact that the conidia are inhaled, primary infection is found either in the upper airways (e.g., paranasal sinuses) or in the lungs. Hyphae invade tissue, especially blood vessels, producing distal infarction and necrosis. In disseminated disease, the destructive process may affect a variety of different organ systems, including the GI tract, producing necrotic perforating ulcers, pseudomembranes, or pyogenic abscesses.

Clinical Manifestations

In Young's summary of invasive aspergillosis (21), GI involvement was found in the following order of fre-

quency in 32 patients with disseminated aspergillosis: 16 intestine, 12 liver, 10 esophagus, 5 stomach, 4 tongue, and 2 with palate lesions. Among patients with intestinal disease, the large intestine was most commonly involved.

In a summary of 93 cases with aspergillosis complicating neoplastic disease, nine patients had GI tract involvement (22). Eight of the 9 patients showed significant gastrointestinal blood loss during the last 2 weeks of their illness. In general, bowel infarction is a late manifestation of disseminated aspergillosis, but bowel infarction rarely may be the earliest manifestation of disseminated invasive aspergillosis (23).

Liver lesions may be either solitary or multiple abscesses, and they give rise to elevations in alkaline phosphatase and/or bilirubin.

Treatment

A full course of amphotericin B should be given (at least 35–50 mg/kg total dose). Mortality is unacceptably high, in many cases due to failure of predisposing factors (e.g. neutropenia) to resolve.

MUCORMYCOSIS

Mycology

The agents of mucormycosis include the following genera: *Mucor, Rhizopus, Rhizomucor, Cunninghamella, Saksenaea, Apophysomyces, Cokeromyces, Syncephalastrum,* and *Absidia.* The organisms are ubiquitous in nature and are opportunistic molds that usually infect immunocompromised patients. The infectious particles are inhaled spores produced by sporangiophores. In culture, the organisms grow as fluffy molds.

Epidemiology and Predisposing Factors

The usual route of infection is through inhalation of spores; thus, the most common clinical presentations are in the airways, with rhinocerebral or pulmonary disease.

Neutrophils and monocytes ingest and kill spores from species of the order *Mucorales,* and they also damage hyphae. Thus, neutropenic patients are at risk for invasive mucormycosis. Other conditions that predispose to mucormycosis are poorly controlled diabetes mellitus, chronic renal insufficiency, burns, deferoxamine therapy, and aplastic anemia. Rhinocerebral mucormycosis has been documented in African children with malnutrition (7,24), and there also is a strong association between gastric mucormycosis and protein-calorie malnutrition. Rarely, GI mucormycosis may be associated with amebic colitis (25) or penetrating abdominal trauma (26).

Pathogenesis and Pathology

After the spores are inhaled, they germinate into wide, irregular, aseptate hyphae with a tendency to right-angle branching. These elongated structures invade blood vessels, producing distal necrosis and infarction, and in diabetics there may be a neutrophilic inflammatory response. In neutropenic hosts, however, there is very little associated cellular response.

Clinical Manifestations

All major portions of the GI tract can be involved with GI mucormycosis, including the mouth, esophagus, stomach, and intestines. However, the most frequently involved organs are the stomach and colon (27). Gastrointestinal involvement usually represents a manifestation of disseminated disease (25). Although the portal is usually the lung, a radiologically visible pulmonary infiltrate is not always visible. In some of these patients with GI lesions, the portal of entry might be the gut.

Patients with esophageal disease present with dysphagia and odynophagia (28), and may have extensive areas of involvement (29). All patients with esophageal mucormycosis also have involvement elsewhere in the GI tract.

The most common site of GI mucormycosis is the stomach. Rarely patients may have peptic ulcer disease that is only colonized with the organisms (30). However, in patients at risk, the fungi invade stomach wall, leading to tissue necrosis and perforation that is highly lethal (29–31).

There are numerous reports of intestinal involvement, e.g., with shallow ulcerations or inflammatory masses that can extend into the retroperitoneal space (25,32). In pediatric patients, gastric involvement is most common, followed by large bowel, small bowel, and esophagus; disease may extend into adjacent organs (e.g., liver, kidney) due to intestinal perforation (28).

Diagnosis

Unfortunately, GI mucormycosis is usually diagnosed postmortem (25). Antemortem diagnosis rests on biopsy of suspicious lesions in the appropriate clinical setting. characteristic invasion of blood vessels by broad, nonseptate branching hyphae supports the diagnosis. The causative organism may sometimes be cultured from biopsy tissue, but the yield is low. There is no acceptable noninvasive means for establishing a diagnosis of mucormycosis.

Treatment

Several authorities advocate that infected portions of the alimentary tract should be surgically resected, and a full course of amphotericin B (at least 35–50 mg/kg total dose) is required for a successful outcome. Mortality remains unacceptably high.

HISTOPLASMOSIS

Mycology

Histoplasma capsulatum is a dimorphic fungus that grows in its mycelial form at 30°C and as budding yeast in the human host and *in vitro* at 37°C. The mycelial form produces both microconidia and characteristic tuberculate macroconidia (10–15 μm diameter) that possess prominent papillary excrescences. The yeast are tiny (2–3 μm diameter), oval-shaped, and reproduce by narrow-based budding.

Epidemiology and Predisposing Factors

In the United States, histoplasmosis is endemic in the Mississippi and Ohio River basins. The disease may also be found as far east as northern Maryland and as far west as California. The mycelial form of *H. capsulatum* is found in soil enriched by bird droppings, and the human host becomes infected by inhaling conidia.

Normal human defenses against *H. capsulatum* are primarily cellular as opposed to humoral, with mononuclear phagocytes playing a central role. Fungistatic activity of macrophages is enhanced by cytokines such as interferon-γ that are secreted by T lymphocytes. Therefore, patients with impaired numbers or function of macrophages or T lymphocytes (e.g., AIDS patients or individuals taking daily high-dose glucocorticoids) are at increased risk for severe histoplasmosis.

Pathogenesis and Pathology

Most inhalation exposures to *H. capsulatum* are thought to result in asymptomatic primary pulmonary infection, or mild flu-like illness, with nonproductive cough, fever, chills, sweats, myalgias, and arthralgias. Most mildly symptomatic cases of primary pulmonary histoplasmosis probably never reach a physician's attention because they resolve spontaneously without specific antifungal therapy. A small subset of patients develops more symptomatic pulmonary infection, leading to evaluation by a physician. However, even the majority of those more highly symptomatic cases resolve without specific antifungal therapy. In a very small proportion of patients, the organism escapes the normal defenses of human lung tissue and gives rise to disseminated disease, including GI manifestations, discussed below.

In human disease, *H. capsulatum* typically grows intracellularly within mononuclear phagocytes. In the previously normal adult, the organism elicits a granulomatous inflammatory response, with characteristic Langhans giant cells, palisading histiocytes, and round cell infiltrates with lymphocytes and plasmacytes. Granulomatous inflammation may be exuberant in chronic disseminated histoplasmosis. In the immunosuppressed patient, large numbers of organisms are found inside macrophages with minimal lymphocytic response.

Clinical Manifestations

Gastrointestinal histoplasmosis is probably always a manifestation of disseminated histoplasmosis rather than a primary site of infection. The most easily recognizable lesions of GI histoplasmosis are found in the mouth or larynx. One large series reported that 66% of patients with chronic disseminated histoplasmosis presented with such lesions, as did 31% of patients with subacute disseminated histoplasmosis and 18% of those with acute disseminated histoplasmosis (33). Patients with small and large bowel involvement often have other clinical manifestations that prove, in retrospect, to be due to disseminated histoplasmosis, including hepatosplenomegaly, adrenal insufficiency, and pancytopenia.

There is a wealth of dental literature about oral manifestations of disseminated histoplasmosis (34–36). The most common lesions are painful periodontal or gingival ulcerations (Fig. 3) that develop over a period of weeks or months (37). Periodontal ulcerations can lead to loosening of dentition, prompting dentists to perform extractions.

In addition to gingivae, the oral lesions also may be located on the lips (7,38), tongue (36,39), hard palate, larynx (40), or buccal mucosa. Lesions outside the gingiva are indurated, well circumscribed, and often elevated. Oropharyngeal and laryngeal lesions are commonly mistaken for squamous carcinoma. Histological evidence of pseudoepitheliomatous hyperplasia due to histoplasmosis can resemble squamous cell carcinoma in a superficial biopsy.

Oral lesions of disseminated histoplasmosis are being reported with increasing frequency as the first manifestation of AIDS (34), and the lesions may be very destructive. For example, one AIDS patient had a perforation of the hard palate (41), and another had a perioral herpetiform rash (42).

There are numerous reports of esophageal involvement. Patients present with dysphagia or odynophagia, and the esophageal mucosa may be ulcerated (40), or there may be esophageal compression by mediastinal granulomata (43,44) (Fig. 4) or fibrosing mediastinitis. Finally, esophageal abscesses may arise as a consequence of erosion of infected mediastinal nodes into the esophagus (45).

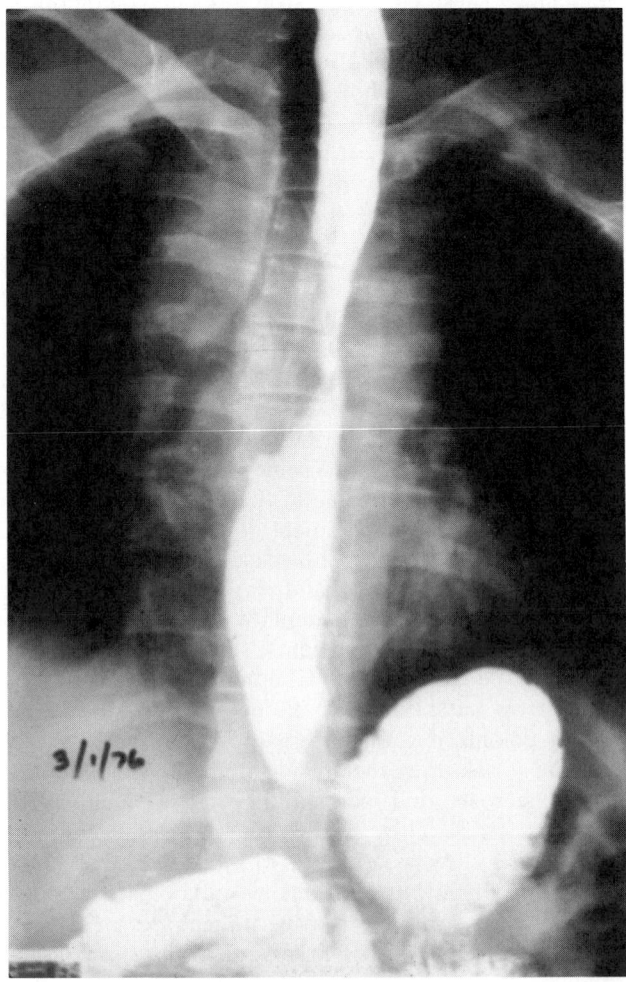

FIG. 4. Esophagogram in a patient with histoplasmosis and dysphagia from esophageal compression by massive mediastinal lymphadenopathy.

Severe esophagitis with friable mucosa and numerous umbilicated submucosal nodules has been observed in a patient with AIDS (46).

Gastric ulceration with hemorrhage (47) and bowel involvement by histoplasmosis have been known since the earliest descriptions of the disease; in his autopsy reports, Darling described superficial ulcerations in the small bowel, ileum, and cecum (48). A large autopsy series from Vanderbilt showed that 75% of patients with disseminated disease had histopathological evidence of small or large bowel involvement, though clinically obvious GI symptoms were less common: only 24% of patients with disseminated disease in that series had clinically apparent GI disease (33). In previously normal hosts, the typical clinical presentation of small and large bowel involvement is subacute onset of diarrhea (49,50) and cramping abdominal pain over a period of months or years, which, if left untreated, may progress to life-threatening bloody diarrhea. Fluid loss can be as high as 7 L/day (51), leading to marked weight loss; true malabsorption with steatorrhea also has been reported (52).

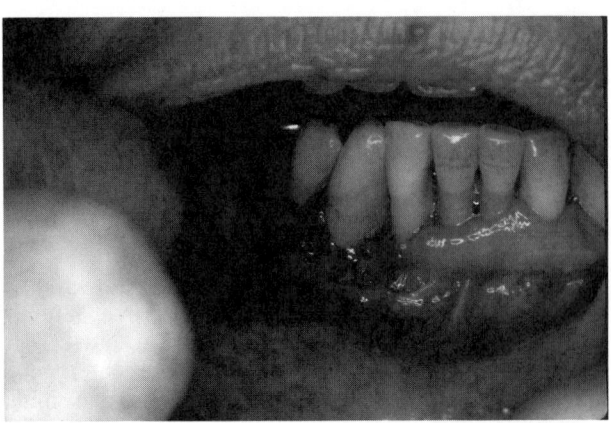

FIG. 3. Gingival lesion due to disseminated histoplasmosis.

The abdominal examination may reveal diffuse tenderness; rebound tenderness can be observed when secondary peritonitis follows intestinal perforation. Occasionally, a mass can be palpated in the right lower quadrant due to granulomatous disease in the ileocecal area (53,54). Indeed, obstruction can arise from such masses or from enlarged retroperitoneal nodes. Barium contrast studies of small and large bowel disclose a variety of different findings, including elongated constricting lesions (55) or polypoid lesions (51,53). Colonoscopy may reveal either superficial ulcerations or nodular granulomatous areas that partially obstruct the lumen, particularly in the region of the ileocecal valve.

Often patients with small or large bowel involvement are sufficiently ill to warrant exploratory laparotomy (56). Surgical specimens and autopsy tissues show mucosal ulcerations or cecal masses, sometimes with perforation and peritonitis (50,57,58). In previously normal hosts, microscopic examination shows mucosal granulomatous inflammation with tiny intracellular budding yeast within mononuclear phagocytes. One patient presented with protein-losing enteropathy, and jejunal biopsy showed "giant" villi engorged with yeast (59); another had intestinal lymphangiectasia due to *H. capsulatum* (40).

More than 100 cases of disseminated histoplasmosis have been reported in HIV-infected patients (60), and the mycosis is included in the Centers for Disease Control case definition for AIDS. In certain areas of the country (e.g., Kansas City) (61), disseminated histoplasmosis affects up to one third of patients with AIDS, being the second most common case-defining infection after *Pneumocystis carinii* pneumonia. Gastrointestinal histoplasmosis in patients with AIDS deserves special mention because the clinical manifestations can be unusually severe (61–63). For example, Graybill (64) described four patients with colonic involvement, including life-threatening bloody diarrhea and severe weight loss. One patient presented with involvement of the greater omentum (65). Ileal and duodenal perforation occur (66,67), and a recent report emphasized that colonic histoplasmosis should be suspected in any AIDS patient with bloody diarrhea who has ever resided in an endemic area (61).

A large autopsy series from the pre-AIDS era documented common hepatic involvement in patients with chronic disseminated histoplasmosis, with elevations of alkaline phosphatase and glutamic-oxaloacetic transaminase in 55% and 61% of patients, respectively (33). Indeed, hepatic infection may be the only sign of dissemination in some patients with disseminated histoplasmosis. Hepatic histoplasmosis is being reported with increasing frequency in patients with AIDS, with hepatomegaly being found in approximately 26% of patients with disseminated disease (68).

Diagnosis

Scrapings or biopsy tissues from GI lesions that contain tiny, oval, intracellular yeast support the diagnosis of GI histoplasmosis. Cultures on antibiotic-containing media may yield a pure growth of *H. capsulatum*. However, one must often resort to indirect methods for establishing the diagnosis of GI histoplasmosis, including blood cultures by the isolator technique and bone marrow cultures. The *H. capsulatum* serum complement fixation test is highly sensitive and specific for anti-*Histoplasma* antibodies, and a single titer of ≥1:32 or a four-fold rise in titer strongly suggests the diagnosis in the appropriate clinical setting. Unfortunately, AIDS patients are generally unable to mount specific antibody responses; in that population, diagnostic confirmation can be obtained with a commercially available antigen test (69). Testing for urinary antigen is most sensitive.

Treatment

In the normal host with non–life-threatening disseminated histoplasmosis, itraconazole is the treatment of choice (70). Doses should be at mealtime to enhance absorption. The drug requires normal gastric acidity for reliable absorption and therefore is not optimal for patients with achlorhydria or for those taking antacids or H_2 blockers. For such patients, an acceptable alternative would be intravenous amphotericin B, to a total dose of 1.5–2.0 g in adults (71). In patients with AIDS who are seriously ill, initial therapy should be with amphotericin B, followed by itraconazole maintenance therapy. The ideal maintenace therapy for meningitis has not been established; successes have been reported with itraconazole, and there is reason to believe fluconazole would be useful because it efficiently penetrates into cerebrospinal fluid. In those who are less ill, primary therapy with itraconazole is effective when given according to the following schedule: 600 mg/day for 3 days, followed by 400 mg/day for 12 weeks, and finally lifetime maintenance with 400 mg/day if the serum itraconazole concentration on that dose is <4 μg/mL. For patients in whom serum itraconazole concentration is ≥4 μg/mL, the dose may be decreased to 200 mg/day for lifetime maintenance therapy. Fluconazole appears to be less active than itraconazole, even at a dose of 800 mg/day, but would be an acceptable alternative for patients with poor gastrointestinal absorption of intraconazole.

BLASTOMYCOSIS

Mycology

Blastomyces dermatitidis is a dimorphic fungus that grows in its mycelial phase at 30°C and in the yeast phase in the host and *in vitro* at 37°C. The mycelial phase bears the microconidia that are the infectious particles. In human tissue the organism grows as large budding yeast (6–15 μm diameter) that may be either intracellular or extracellular. Budding is broad-based, and the single daughter cell is almost as large as the mother cell at the time of separation.

Epidemiology and Predisposing Factors

Recent epidemiological studies that examined outbreaks of blastomycosis following group exposures along

964 / CHAPTER 63

river banks (72) led to the discovery that the organism grows in moist soil, and microconidia are thought to be sporadically aerosolized when soil is disturbed, e.g., by rainstorms.

Normal host defenses against *Blastomyces dermatitidis* include growth inhibition by mononuclear phagocytes. The organism is a pathogen that infects normal hosts and no clear-cut predisposing factors have been identified, though disease severity appears to be increased in patients with AIDS.

Pathogenesis and Pathology

The infectious microconidia germinate in lung tissue and then reproduce by budding in the human host. The primary pneumonitis may be self-limited; however, a subset of patients with untreated pulmonary blastomycosis subsequently develops disseminated disease, with prominent skin and bone involvement, and in males, infection of the prostate and epididymis. Gastrointestinal manifestations are rare, as outlined below.

Skin lesions are typically raised, indurated, well-circumscribed and verrucous or ulcerative, with heaped-up advancing borders. Fresh pustules along the borders contain large budding yeast whose presence supports the diagnosis. The organism elicits pyogranulomatous inflammation and pseudoepitheliomatous hyperplasia, and the yeast may be found either intracellularly within Langhans giant cells, or extracellularly, surrounded by neutrophils.

Clinical Manifestations

Oral, nasal, and laryngeal lesions of *B. dermatitidis* are well described (73,74). Lesions can be found from the level of the oral cavity through the distal esophagus. There are no reports of intestinal or colonic blastomycosis.

Oral lesions are usually asymptomatic masses that resemble squamous cell carcinoma; alternatively, they may be ulcerative, sessile, plaque-like, or verrucous. The tongue, palate, larynx, parotid gland, or nasal cavity may be involved. Oral lesions may originate in the mucosa itself, or they may arise instead by extension from bony lesions in the mandible or maxilla (73). Mandibular or maxillary involvement may be mistaken for cervicofacial actinomycosis until appropriate smears and cultures reveal *B. dermatitidis*. Esophageal involvement rarely may be a prominent manifestation of disseminated blastomycosis (75,76).

Diagnosis

Diagnosis of GI blastomycosis is supported by biopsies that show typical broad-based budding yeast. Definitive identification is made by growing the organism in culture.

Treatment

The treatment of choice for non–life-threatening blastomycosis is oral itraconazole, 200 mg twice daily (70). Oral ketoconazole 400 mg once daily is somewhat more toxic but is less expensive and has roughly equal efficacy to itraconazole. Both drugs require gastric acidity for optimal absorption. Patients who receive ≥2 months of daily therapy have a 95% success rate with either oral agent. Toxicities of itraconazole, mild nausea, and transaminasemia, are less pronounced than those caused by ketoconazole. Critically ill hospitalized patients and all patients with AIDS should receive initial therapy with amphotericin B; patients with AIDS should then receive oral follow-up therapy with either itraconazole or ketoconazole.

PARACOCCIDIOIDOMYCOSIS

Mycology

Paracoccidioides brasiliensis is a dimorphic fungus that is endemic in many areas of Latin America. The mold grows in its mycelial form at 30°C and as budding yeast in the host and *in vitro* at 37°C. The budding yeast sometimes give the appearance of a "pilot's wheel" because multiple small daughter cells surround a large central mother cell. The pore between mother and daughter cell is very small, a helpful feature in identification.

Epidemiology and Predisposing Factors

The infection is acquired through inhalation of infectious conidia. Paracoccidioidomycosis of adults affects predominantly males, with a nearly 50-fold excess over females. Some authorities believe that the male predilection is due to increased exposure because the organism is found on plantations, where most workers are males. However, there also is *in vitro* evidence that *P. brasiliensis* is inhibited by estrogens, suggesting that adult females may possess increased natural resistance. Normal host defenses are both neutrophilic and monocytic, and there is also a suggestion that normal T-cell function plays a role in host defense against paracoccidioidomycosis, because the infection is being reported with increasing frequency in patients with AIDS (77).

Pathogenesis and Pathology

Following inhalation of infectious conidia, a primary pneumonitis ensues. If left untreated, the infection often disseminates, producing destructive exophytic lesions of the mucosa and skin, particularly around the nose. Disseminated infection also may involve the GI tract, distant skin sites, and bones.

The organism reproduces by budding in tissue, sometimes with the classic pilot's wheel appearance. Inflammation is pyogranulomatous, with pseudoepitheliomatous hyperplasia.

Clinical Manifestations

Oral manifestations of paracoccidioidomycosis are protean (78–80). The lesions may represent the first sign of disseminated disease, and pulmonary involvement may not necessarily be obvious at the time of presentation (81). Lesions are painful and may be either ulcerative or proliferative; the latter may be mulberry-like, with pinpoint hemorrhages. The frequency with which lesions are found in various areas of the mouth include 78% over the alveolar process or gingiva, 47% over the palate, 36% lip, 25% buccal mucosa, 11% oropharynx, and 11% tongue or floor of the mouth (80). Lesions of paracoccidioidomycosis also commonly involve the nasal mucosa, facial skin, and maxilla (82). If left untreated, oral lesions may spread to cervical lymph nodes, rarely producing palsies of vagus or hypoglossal nerves (83). More distal lesions beyond the mouth include involvement of the uvula, glottis, epiglottis, and larynx (79); ulcerated or nodular lesions of the small and large bowel also occur. Rarely, hepatic granulomata are seen.

Diagnosis

Paracoccidioidomycosis may be diagnosed by recovery of multiple-budding yeast forms in pus from scrapings or biopsies. Cultures are confirmatory. Serum antibody assays, including complement fixation and agar gel immunodiffusion tests, support the diagnosis (79).

Treatment

Imidazoles are the mainstay of therapy for non–life-threatening paracoccidioidomycosis. Ketoconazole, 200 mg daily for at least 6 months, is curative in many cases. Itraconazole also is effective, and studies are underway to identify the ideal dosage. In life-threatening cases or in patients with disease that progresses despite imidazole therapy, amphotericin B is usually effective at a total dose of 1–2 g in adults. Sulfadiazine has been used as chronic suppressive therapy because of its low cost, but recrudescence of symptoms during or after sulfonamide therapy is common.

REFERENCES

1. Joshi SN, Garvin PJ, Sunwoo YC. Candidiasis of the duodenum and jejunum. *Gastroenterology* 1981;80:829–833.
2. Minoli G, Terruzzi V, Ferrara A, et al. A prospective study of relationships between benign gastric ulcer, candida, and medical treatment. *Am J Gastroenterol* 1984;79:95–97.
3. Minoli G, Terruzzi V, Rossini A. Gastroduodenal candidiasis occurring without underlying disease (primary gastroduodenal candidiasis). *Endoscopy* 1979;1:18–22.
4. Eras P, Goldstein MJ, Sherlock P. Candida infection of the gastrointestinal tract. *Medicine* 1972;51:367–379.
5. Young JA, Elias E. Gastro-oesophageal candidiasis: diagnosis by brush cytology. *J Clin Pathol* 1985;38:293–296.
6. Washington K, Gottfried MR, Wilson ML. Gastrointestinal cryptococcosis. *Mod Pathol* 1991;4:707–711.
7. de Almeida OP, Scully C. Oral lesions in the systemic mycoses. *Curr Opin in Dent* 1991;1:423–428.
8. Dodson TB, Perrott DH, Leonard MS. Nonhealing ulceration of oral mucosa. *J Oral Maxillofac Surg* 1989;47:849–852.
9. Glick M, Cohen SG, Cheney RT, Crooks GW, Greenberg MS. Oral manifestations of disseminated *Cryptococcus neoformans* in a patient with acquired immunodeficiency syndrome. *Oral Surg Oral Med Oral Pathol* 1987;64:454–459.
10. Lynch DP, Naftolin LZ. Oral *Cryptococcus neoformans* infection in AIDS. *Oral Surg Oral Med Oral Pathol* 1987;64:449–453.
11. Newman CW, Rosenbaum D. Oral cryptococcosis. *J Periodontol* 1962;33:266–269.
12. Jacobs DH, Macher AM, Handler R, Bennett JE, Collen MJ, Gallin JI. Esophageal cryptococcosis in a patient with the hyperimmunoglobulin E-recurrent infection (Job's) syndrome. *Gastroenterology* 1984;87:201–203.
13. Hurd DD, Staub DB, Roelofs RI, Dehner LP. Profound muscle weakness as the presenting feature of disseminated cryptococcal infection. *Rev Infect Dis* 1989;11:970–974.
14. Bonacini M, Nussbaum J, Ahluwalia C. Gastrointestinal, hepatic, and pancreatic involvement with *Cryptococcus neoformans* in AIDS. *J Clin Gastroenterol* 1990;12:295–297.
15. Kovacs JA, Kovacs AA, Polis M, et al. Cryptococcosis in the acquired immunodeficiency syndrome. *Ann Intern Med* 1985;103:533–538.
16. Hutto JO, Bryan CS, Greene FL, White CJ, Gallin JI. Cryptococcosis of the colon resembling Chrohn's disease in a patient with the hyperimmunoglobulinemia E-recurrent infection (Job's) syndrome. *Gastroenterology* 1988;94:808–812.
17. Daly JS, Porter KA, Chong FK, Robillard RJ. Disseminated, nonmeningeal gastrointestinal cryptococcal infection in an HIV-negative patient. *Am J Gastroenterol* 1990;85:1421–1424.
18. Unat EK, Pars B, Kosyak JP. A case of cryptococcosis of the colon. *Br Med J* Nov. 19, 1960;1:1501–1502.
19. Zelman S, O'Neil RH, Plaut A. Disseminated visceral torulosis without nervous system involvement. *Am J Med* Nov. 1951;658–664.
20. Van Calck M, Motte S, Rickaert F, Serruys RE, Adler M, Wybran J. Cryptococcal anal ulceration in a patient with AIDS. *Am J Gastroenterol* 1988;83:1306–1308.
21. Young RC, Bennett JE, Vogel CL, Carbone PP, DeVita VT. Aspergillosis: the spectrum of the disease in 98 patients. *Medicine* 1970;49:147–173.
22. Meyer RD, Young LS, Armstrong D, Yu B. Aspergillosis complicating neoplastic disease. *Am J Med* 1973;54:6–15.
23. Cohen R, Heffner JE. Bowel infarction as the initial manifestation of disseminated aspergillosis. *Chest* 1992;101:877–879.
24. Hauman CHJ, Raubenheimer EJ. Orofacial mucormycosis. *Oral Surg Oral Med Oral Pathol* 1989;68:624–627.
25. Lyon DT, Schubert TT, Mantia AG, Kaplan MH. Phycomycosis of the gastrointestinal tract. *Am J Gastoenterol* 1979;72:379–394.
26. Taams M, Bade PG, Thomson SR. Post-traumatic abdominal mucormycosis. *Injury* 1992;23:413–415.
27. Smith JMB. Mycoses of the alimentary tract. *Gut* 1969;10:1035–1040.
28. Mooney JE, Wanger A. Mucormycosis of the gastrointestinal tract in children: report of a case and review of the literature. *Pediatric Infect Dis J* 1993;12:872–876.
29. Kahn LB. Gastric mucormycosis: report of a case with a review of the literature. *S Afr Med J* Dec. 14, 1963;1265–1269.
30. Thomson SR, Bade PG, Taams M, Chrystal V. Gastrointestinal mucromycosis. *Br J Surg* 1991;78:952–954.
31. Satir AA, Alla MD, Mahgoub S, Musa AR. Systemic phycomycosis. *Br Med J* 1971;1:440.
32. Nolan RL, Carter III RR, Griffith JE, Chapman SW. Case report: subacute disseminated mucormycosis in a diabetic male. *Am J Med Sci* 1989;298:252–255.
33. Goodwin RA, Shapiro JL, Thurman GH, Thurman SS, DesPrez

RM. Disseminated histoplasmosis clinical and pathologic correlations. *Medicine* 1980;59:1–33.

34. Oda D, McDougal L, Fritsche T, Worthington P. Oral histoplasmosis as a presenting disease in acquired immunodeficiency syndrome. *Oral Surg Oral Med Oral Pathol* 1990;70:631–636.

35. Cobb CM, Shultz RE, Brewer JH, Dunlap CL. Chronic pulmonary histoplasmosis with an oral lesion. *Oral Surg Med Oral Pathol* 1989;67:73–76.

36. Huber MA, Hall EH, Rathbun, WA. The role of the dentist in diagnosing infection in the AIDS patient. *Milt Med* 1989;154:315–318.

37. Hammarsten JE, Hammarsten JF. Histoplasmosis recognition and treatment. *Hosp Pract* June 15, 1990;95–126.

38. Smith JW, Utz JP. Progressive disseminated histoplasmosis. *Ann Intern Med* 1972;76:557–565.

39. Hiltbrand JB, McGuirt WF. Oropharyngeal histoplasmosis. *South Med J* 1990;83:227–230.

40. Wheat LJ, Slama TG, Eitzen HE, Kohler RB, French MLV, Biesecker JL. A large urban outbreak of histoplasmosis: clinical features. *Ann Intern Med* 1981;94:331–337.

41. Fowler CB, Nelson JF, Henley DW, Smith BR. Acquired immune deficiency syndrome presenting as a palatal perforation. *Oral Surg Oral Med Oral Pathol* 1989;67:313–318.

42. Bundy AT, Simjee S, Ray M, Ristow H-J. Psoriatic patient presenting with perioral herpetiform lesions. *Arch Dermatol* 1989;125:1440–1441.

43. Fifer, et al. Mediastinal histoplasmosis. *Diseases of the Chest* 1965;47:518.

44. Peabody JW Jr, Brown RB, Davis EW, Katz S, Cannon A. Surgical implications of mediastinal granulomas. *Amer Surg* 1959;25:357–368.

45. Jenkins DW, Fish DE, Byrd RB. Mediastinal histoplasmosis with esophageal abscess: two case reports. *Gastroenterology* 1976;70:109–111.

46. Forsmark CE, Wilcox DM, Darragh TM, Cello JP. Disseminated histoplasmosis in AIDS: an unusual case of esophageal involvement and gastrointestinal bleeding. *Gastrointest Endosc* 1990;36:604–605.

47. Fitzpatrick TJ, Neiman BH. *Histoplasma capsulatum* infection associated with gastric ulcer and fatal hemorrhage. *Arch Intern med* 1953;91:49.

48. Darling ST. A protozoan general infection producing pseudo tubercles in the lungs and focal necrosis in the liver, spleen and lymph nodes. *JAMA* 1906;46:1283.

49. Cappell MS, Mandell W, Grimes MM, Neu HC. Gastrointestinal histoplasmosis. *Dig Dis Sci* 1988;33:353–360.

50. Henderson RG, Pinkerton H, Moore LT. *Histoplasma capsulatum* as a cause of chronic ulcerative enteritis. *JAMA* 1942;118:885–889.

51. Kirk ME, Lough J, Warner HA. Histoplasma colitis: an electron microscopic study. *Gastroenterology* 1971;61:46–54.

52. Orchard JL. Malabsorption due to gastrointestinal histoplasmosis. *Am J Med* 1992;93:237–238.

53. Sturim HS, Kouchoukos NT, Ahlvin RC. Gastrointestinal manifestations of disseminated histoplasmosis. *Am J Surg* 1965;110:435–440.

54. Haggerty CM, Britton MC, Dorman JM, Marzoni FA, Gastrointestinal histoplasmosis in suspected acquired immunodeficiency syndrome. *West J Med* 1985;143:244–246.

55. Miller DP, Everett ED. Gastrointestinal histoplasmosis. *J Clin Gastroenterol* 1979;1:233–236.

56. Brett MT, Kwan JTC, Bending MR. Caecal perforation in a renal transplant patient with disseminated histoplasmosis. *J Clin Pathol* 1988;41:992–995.

57. Lee SH, Barnes WG, Hodges GR, Dixon A. Perforated granulomlatous colitis caused by *Histoplasma capsulatum*. *Dis Colon Rectum* 1985;28:171–176.

58. Shull HJ. Human histoplasmosis: a disease with protean manifestations often with digestive system involvement. *Gastroenterol* 1953;25:582–594.

59. Bank S, Trey C, Gans I, Marks IN, Groll A. Histoplasmosis of the small bowel with "giant" intestinal villi and secondary protein-losing enteropathy. *Am J Med* 1965;39:492–501.

60. Ankobiah WA, Vaidya K, Powell S, Carrasco M, Allam A, Chechani V, Kamholz SL. Disseminated histoplasmosis in AIDS. Clinicopathologic features in seven patients from a nonendemic area. *NY State J Med* 1990;90:234–238.

61. Graham BD, McKinsey DS, Driks MR, Smith DL. Colonic histoplasmosis in acquired immunodeficiency syndrome. *Dis Colon Rectum* 1991;34:185–190.

62. Gerstein HC, Fanning MM, Read SE, Shepherd FA, Glynn MFX. AIDS in a patient with hemophilia receiving mainly cryoprecipitate. *Can Med Assoc J* 1984;131:45–47.

63. Basgoz N, Mattia AR. A 38-year-old man with AIDS and the recent onset of diarrhea, hematochezia, fever, and pulmonary infiltrates. *N Engl J Med* 1994;330:273–280.

64. Graybill JR. Histoplasmosis and AIDS. *J Infect Dis* 1988;158:623–626.

65. Alterman DD, Cho KC. Histoplasmosis involving the omentum in an AIDS patient: CT demonstration. *J Comp Assist Tomogr* 1988;12:664–665.

66. Henghan SJ, Li J, Petrossian E, Bizer LS. Intestinal perforation from gastrointestinal histoplasmosis in acquired immunodeficiency syndrome. *Arch Surg* 1993;128:464–466.

67. Johnson PC, Khardori N, Najjar AF, Butt F, Mansell PWA, Sarosi GA. *Am J Med* 1988;85:152–158.

68. Wheat LJ, Connolly-Stringfield PA, Baker RL, et al. Disseminated histoplasmosis in the acquired immune deficiency syndrome: clinical findings, diagnosis, and treatment, and review of the literature. *Medicine* 1990;69:361–374.

69. Wheat LJ, Kohler RB, Tewari RP. Diagnosis of disseminated histoplasmosis by detection of *Histoplasma capsulatum* antigen in serum and urine specimens. *N Engl J Med* 1986;314:83–88.

70. Dismukes WE, Bradsher RW, Jr., Cloud GC, et al. Itraconazole therapy for blastomycosis and histoplasmosis. *Am J Med* 1992;93:489–497.

71. McKinsey DS, Gupta MR, Riddler SA, Driks MR, Smith DL, Kurtin PJ. Long-term amphotericin B therapy for disseminated histoplasmosis in patients with the acquired immunodeficiency syndrome (AIDS). *Ann Intern Med* 1989;111:655–659.

72. Klein BS, Vergeront JM, Weeks RJ. Isolation of *Blastomyces dermatitidis* in soil associated with a large outbreak of blastomycosis in Wisconsin. *N Engl J Med* 1986;314:529–534.

73. Mikaelian AJ, Varkey B, Grossman TW, Blatnik DS. Blastomycosis of the head and neck. *Otolaryngol Head Neck Surg* 1989;101:489–495.

74. Witorsch P, Utz JP. North American blastomycosis: a study of 40 patients. *Medicine* 1968;47:169–200.

75. Cherniss EI, Waisbren BA. North American blastomycosis: A clinical study of 40 cases. *Ann Intern Med* 1956;44:105–123.

76. Khandekar A, Moser D, Fidler WJ. Blastomycosis of the esophagus. *Ann Thorac Surg* 1980;30:76–79.

77. Goldani LZ, Coelho ECB, Machado AA, Martinez R. Paracoccidioidomycosis and AIDS. *Scand J Infect Dis* 1991;23:393.

78. Diaz M, Negroni R, Montero-Gei F, et al. A Pan-American 5-year study of fluconazole therapy for deep mycoses in the immunocompetent host. *Clin Infect dis* 1992;14(suppl 1):S68–76.

79. Restrepo A, Robledo M, Gutiérrez F, Sanclemente M, Castañeda E, Calle G. Paracoccidioidomycosis (South American blastomycosis): a study of 39 cases observed in Medellín, Columbia. *Am J Trop Med Hyg* 1970;19:68–76.

80. Sposto MR, Scully D, de Almeida OP, Jorge J, Graner E, Bozzo L. Oral paracoccidioidomycosis: a study of 36 South American patients. *Oral Surg Oral Med Oral Pathol* 1993;75:461–465.

81. de Almeida OP, Jorge J, Scully C, Bozzo L. Oral manifestations of paracoccidioidomycosis (Sourth American blastomycosis). *Oral Surg Oral Med Oral Pathol* 1991;72:430–435.

82. Lazow SK, Seldin RD, Solomon MP. South American blastomycosis of the maxilla: report of a case. *J Oral Maxillofac Surg* 1990;71:68–71.

83. de Freitas MRG, Nascimento OJM, Chimelli L. Tapia's syndrome caused by *Paracoccidioides brasiliensis*. *J Neurol Sci* 1991;103:179–181.

Infections of the Gastrointestinal Tract,
edited by M. J. Blaser, P. D. Smith, J. I. Ravdin,
H. B. Greenberg, and R. L. Guerrant
Raven Press, Ltd., New York © 1995.

CHAPTER 64

Group A Rotaviruses

Dorsey M. Bass and Harry B. Greenberg

DESCRIPTION

Introduction and Historical Perspective

Since its discovery as a human pathogen approximately 20 years ago, rotavirus has been recognized as an important agent of gastroenteritis in infants. In many studies throughout the world, rotavirus is the single most important cause of dehydrating diarrhea in young children. In the United States alone, rotavirus is estimated to account for $352 million in hospitalization cost (1) and as many as 500 pediatric deaths per year (2). In the developing world, rotavirus may account for 1 million childhood deaths each year as well as enormous morbidity (3).

Although it had long been known that a filterable agent was responsible for most childhood diarrhea, attempts to isolate such a virus via tissue culture in the 1950s and 1960s were unsuccessful. Rotaviruses had previously been identified by electron microscopy only in mice with diarrhea (4). In 1971 Mebus and co-workers (5) succeeded in isolating and propagating in tissue culture a bovine rotavirus from calves with scours (diarrhea). Bishop and co-workers (6) first described a similar agent in thin sections of duodenal mucosa from a child with acute gastroenteritis in 1973. Although several other animal rotaviruses were tissue culture adapted, it was not until 1980 that the first human strain was successfully passaged in tissue culture (7). Eventually, it was recognized that appropriate quantities of trypsin and the use of serum-free media allowed the tissue culture adaptation of large numbers of rotaviruses.

During the 1980s and 1990s monoclonal antibody and recombinant deoxyribonucleic acid (DNA) technologies were applied to the study of rotavirus with a rapid increase of our understanding about the virus, its replication cycle,

epidemiology, pathogenesis, and the nature of host resistance to rotavirus disease. This rapid increase in knowledge about rotaviruses is illustrated by a recent review, which listed more than 780 references (8).

Virus Structure and Physicochemical Properties

Rotaviruses are members of the Reoviridae family and consist of a three-layered protein capsid encasing a segmented double-stranded ribonucleic acid (dsRNA) genome. The complete virion observed with standard negative staining by electron microscopy has a distinct appearance, resembling a short-spoked wheel. The name rotavirus (*rota*, Latin for wheel) is derived from this appearance (9). The particle size is measured as approximately 70 nM by negative stained electron microscopy and 100 nM by cryoelectron microscopy. The outer capsid has icosahedral symmetry with T = 13 (10). The outer shell of the capsid consists of two viral proteins, VP7 and VP4, which form 132 capsomeres. The inner shell consists of trimerized VP6. A core shell of rotavirus consists largely of viral proteins VP2, VP1, and VP3.

Our understanding of the three-dimensional structure of the rotavirus particle has been greatly enhanced by the technique of cryoelectron microscopy with computer-assisted image enhancement (11,12). These studies have shown that the surface of rotavirus particles has 60 spike-like projections 10 nm in length, consisting of the VP4 protein, while the smooth outer capsid surface is made up of VP7. This smooth surface is perforated by 132 aqueous channels, which penetrate the virion to reach the viral core (Fig. 1).

The three forms of rotavirus particle (double-shelled, single-shelled, and cores) can be observed readily in stool samples and tissue culture supernatents. Of the three, only double-shelled particles are infectious under normal conditions (13). The outer capsid of double-shelled particles may be released from the particle by calcium chelation with ethylenediamine-tetraacetic acid (EDTA) or ethyleneglycol-tetraacetic acid (EGTA) (14,15). The resultant single-shelled particles, which are transcription-

D. M. Bass: Department of Pediatrics, Stanford University, Stanford, California 94305-5119.

H. B. Greenberg: Departments of Medicine and Microbiology and Immunology, Stanford University, Stanford, California 94305.

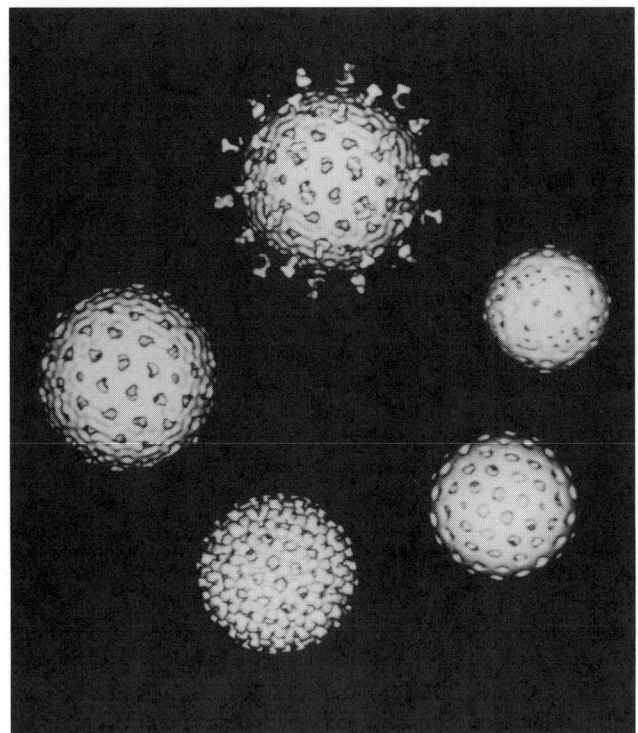

FIG. 1. Three-dimensional structure of rhesus monkey rotavirus by cryoelectron microscopy. The structures are as follows, anti-clockwise from the top: (a) complete double-shelled, infectious particle with 60 surface spikes consisting of VP4; (b) the smooth outer surface, attributed to VP7, is shown with the perforating aqueous channels; (c) the inner capsid consisting of VP6 trimers; (d) the VP6 trimers merge with a smooth inner capsid shell that is perforated by channels in register with those in the outer capsid; (e) a third protein shell, the core, made up of VP1, VP2, and VP3, which contains the double-stranded, segmented, RNA genome. (Courtesy of Dr. M. Yeager.)

ally active, may be converted to core particles by treatment with chaotropic agents. Single-shelled particles can be reconstituted to double-shelled particles in the presence of VP7, VP4, and appropriate free calcium ion (16).

Infectious rotavirus particles (double-shelled) have a density of 1.36 g/cm³ in cesium chloride gradients and sediment at 520 to 530 S in sucrose. Single-shelled (noninfectious) particles have a density of 1.38 g/cm³ and sediment at approximately 390 S. Core particles have a density of 1.44 g/cm³ and sediment at 280 S.

Infectious double-shelled rotavirus particles are relatively stable under a variety of environmental conditions. They are resistant to fluorocarbons, ether, chloroform, and nonionic detergents, reflecting the lack of a lipid membrane on the virion (15). Infectivity is maintained in the pH range of 4 to 9. At high pH, VP4 is selectively lost from the virion (17), while very low pH results in disassociation of the entire particle (18,19). Rotaviruses remain infectious for months at room temperature but repeated freezing and thawing will decrease titers. Sodium dodecyl sulfate destroys infectivity, presumably by dis-

rupting the capsid structure. Other disinfectants that are effective against rotavirus include 95% ethanol, phenols, chlorine, and formalin (20–24).

MICROBIOLOGY

Rotavirus Classification

Rotaviruses are classified by group, subgroup, and serotype. Viruses are identified as rotaviruses by their characteristic size and morphology and by the presence of 11 double strands of RNA in their genome. The distinct groups of rotaviruses designated A, B, and C bear little or no immunologic relationship with each other and on a genomic basis share only limited homology. The group antigen is VP6, the major inner capsid protein. Most of the commercial rotavirus stool immunoassays are based on this antigen and therefore detect only group A rotaviruses. This chapter discusses only group A rotaviruses, which are the most common cause of severe watery diarrhea in infancy and early childhood. Group B and C rotaviruses are discussed in the chapter by Mackow.

Subgrouping of group A rotaviruses is also based on antigenic characteristics of the inner capsid protein VP6 (25). Monoclonal antibodies can be used in an enzyme-linked immunoadsorbent assay (ELISA) to distinguish samples as either subgroup I or II (26). A small percentage of samples are not typeable or contain both subgroup I and II reactivities. With few exceptions, all human subgroup I rotaviruses belong to G serotype 2 while subgroup II strains may belong to G serotypes 1, 3, or 4.

Rotavirus serotypes were first identified based on classical cross-neutralization studies employing sera from animals hyperimmunized with purified rotaviruses. Over ten rotavirus serotypes have been identified to date. Of these, only serotypes 1 through 4 are felt to be epidemiologically important human pathogens in all areas of the world. Genetic studies have identified the viral gene encoding VP7 as the primary determinant of serotype (25). The development of anti-VP7 monoclonal antibodies (MABs) with serotype specificity has allowed workers to determine the serotypes of large numbers of rotaviruses in prospective and retrospective studies (27–32).

Recently, a new approach to serotyping rotaviruses has been proposed. The previously described VP7-based serotypes are now referred to as G types (for glycoprotein as in VP7). Because it is known that the other major outer capsid protein, VP4, also contains neutralizing epitopes, it has been proposed that rotaviruses also be categorized according to VP4 amino acid similarity into P types (33–36). The P represents the "protease" sensitivity of VP4. To date, four major P types for human viruses have been described but only two are frequently encountered. As noted, most of the P typing has been based on deduced amino acid sequence or hyperimmune sera to expressed proteins rather than virions. It is unclear whether immune responses to these different P or G types are significant predictors of protection from disease.

Genome Structure, Protein Coding Assignments, and Rotavirus Protein Function

Genome Structure

The rotavirus genome consists of 11 segments of dsRNA, which range in molecular weight (MW) from 2 × 105 to 2.2 × 10⁶ daltons (37). With one exception (gene 11) (38), the segments encode one polypeptide each. The segmented genome is significant in two regards. First, the genomic RNA segments can be resolved on polyacrylamide gels relatively easily. The pattern of the segments (known as the electropherotype) is quite variable among rotaviruses and has been used as a marker for rotavirus strain variation in epidemiologic studies. The second important feature of the segmented genome is that it facilitates the development of reassortant viruses when cells are coinfected with different rotavirus strains. Because the source of individual RNA segments in progeny viruses from such "matings" can be identified either by migration on polyacrylamide gel electrophoresis (PAGE) or by hybridization, reassortant viruses have proved to be a powerful genetic tool for assigning phenotypic characteristics such as virulence, growth in tissue culture, or hemagglutination to specific rotavirus genes. Reassortant rotaviruses have also played an important role in rotavirus vaccine strategy (see chapter by Offit and Clark). Reassortment occurs in nature as well and plays a role in rotavirus strain variations.

The nucleotide sequences of all 11 of the rotavirus RNA segments have been determined. Each RNA segment begins at the 5' end with a guanidine followed by conserved noncoding sequences (39,40). The noncoding sequences are followed by the sequences encoding the protein, which terminate with a stop codon. The 3' end consists of another set of noncoding sequences without polyadenylation. The dsRNA segments are completely base paired and the 5″ end of the positive strand contains a cap structure similar to that found in other members of the Reoviridae family.

Rotavirus Protein Coding Assignments and Protein Function

The coding assignments and properties of rotavirus proteins have been determined by *in vitro* translation of viral RNA, immunological analyses with MABs, expression of rotaviral proteins via recombinant DNA, and the study of reassortant viruses (41–46). Table 1 lists the genome segments and protein products for simian SA11 virus. Both the gene segments and structural proteins are numbered from the slowest migrating on PAGE to the fastest. It should be noted that RNA segments 7, 8, and 9 are usually closely grouped on PAGE and the proteins encoded by these three segments may vary by rotavirus strain. Cognate RNA segments may be identified by hybridization or direct sequence analysis. It should also be noted that in papers published prior to 1988, when the

core protein VP3 was identified, the viral hemagglutinin (now known as VP4) was referred to as VP3.

The rotavirus inner core proteins (VP1, VP2, VP3) are the products of gene segments 1, 2, and 3, respectively. Collectively, the three proteins probably function as the transcriptional machinery of the virus. VP2 expressed in a baculovirus system spontaneously forms core-like particles (47). VP2 has also been shown to be a RNA binding protein (48). VP1 has recently been shown to have RNA polymerase activity (49) and VP3 to have guanylyltransferase activity necessary for RNA replicase activity (50). VP6 forms the inner capsid of the virus and accounts for approximately 50% of the total virion protein. The VP6 protein is hydrophobic and spontaneously forms trimers and higher order multimers (51,52). When VP6 is coexpressed with VP2 in a baculovirus system, particles quite similar to native rotavirus single-shelled particles spontaneously assemble (47). VP6 is the group and subgroup antigen as noted above and the protein is highly immunogenic. Antibodies directed against VP6 are not protective, however.

VP4 is one of the two outer capsid proteins of rotavirus and constitutes the spike-like projections noted in cryoelectron microscopic photographs. Genetic and biochemical studies have shown that it functions as the viral hemagglutinin (53,54), mediates permissivity for tissue culture growth, protease-enhanced plaque formation (25), and is a determinant of virulence of rotaviruses in mice (55). Both its structural role in the rotavirus particle (12) and studies employing MABs (56) have suggested that VP4 may function as the rotavirus viral attachment protein, mediating binding to target cells. Cleavage of VP4 by trypsin results in enhanced infectivity of rotaviruses, probably by facilitating membrane penetration (57). The cleavage products known as VP5* (approximately 60 kDa) and VP8* (approximately 28 kDa) remain virion associated (58). The trypsin cleavage sites for SA11 rotavirus have been shown to be at amino acids 241 and 247 with 247 being the preferred site (59). These sites are conserved in all rotavirus strains although some human strains have a third upstream cleavage site (60,61). Unlike the ortho- and paramyxoviruses, the trypsin cleavage does not expose a new hydrophobic amino terminus. The cleavage may allow a conformational change to occur, exposing amino acids 384 to 401 of VP5*, which share homology with alpha virus fusion proteins (62). VP4 is immunogenic and contains strain-specific neutralization antigens in the VP8* portion and cross-reactive neutralization regions in the VP5* portion (62).

VP7 is an outer capsid glycoprotein, which constitutes the smooth portion of the outer capsid, beneath the VP4 spikes. Approximately 30% of the virion protein is VP7. VP7 is the primary determinant of rotavirus serotype as measured by cross-neutralization studies (46). The importance of VP7 as a neutralization antigen and its unique cell biology as a model glycoprotein have led to intense study of this protein and its intracellular processing. The nucleotide sequence of VP7 predicts an open reading frame of 326 amino acids with two in-frame start codons separated by 30 codons (63). The initiation codons are followed by two stretches of hydrophobic amino acids,

970 / Chapter 64

TABLE 1. *Rotavirus proteins*

Genome segment	Protein	Molecular weight	Modification	Location in virion	Function	Percent capsid protein
1	VP1	125,000	—	Core	RNA polymerase	2
2	VP2	94,000	—	Core	RNA binding	15
3	VP3	88,000	—	Core	Guanyl transferase	0.5
4	VP4	88,000	Extracellular trypsin cleavage to VP5* and VP8*	Outer capsid	Hemagglutinin, membrane penetration, cell attachment protein, neutralization	1.5
5	NS53 (NSVP1)	58,700	—	Nonstructural	Zinc finger, RNA binding	
6	VP6	44,800	—	Inner capsid	Hydrophobic trimer, group and subgroup antigen	51
7	NS34 (NSVP2)	34,600	—	Nonstructural	RNA binding	
8	NS35 (NSVP3)	36,700	—	Nonstructural	RNA binding	
9	VP7	33,900	High mannose glycosylation, ER retention		Major outer capsid structure, neutralization	30
10	NS28 (NSVP4)	28,000	High mannose glycosylation, ER retention	Nonstructural	"Receptor" for single-shelled particles on surface of ER membrane	
11	NS26 (NSVP5)	26,000	Phosphorylated and O-glycosylation, two open reading frames	Nonstructural	??	

either of which may serve as signal sequences to direct the nascent peptide into the endoplasmic reticulum (ER) (64–66). These sequences are cleaved at amino acid 51. VP7 is retained in the ER until assembled onto complete virions and is not transported to the Golgi or the cell surface. Two sets of amino-terminal amino acids have been shown to be responsible for this retention (67). The protein is apparently an integral protein in the ER membrane with a luminal orientation (68). Glycosylation is of the high mannose type and VP7 from various rotavirus strains has one to three potential glycosylation sites although no more than two are apparently used (69,70).

During rotavirus infection at least five nonstructural proteins are produced. Although not components of purified, fully infectious, double-shelled rotavirus particles, these proteins undoubtedly play essential roles in virion replication and morphogenesis. Perhaps the best studied is NS28 (segment 10), which is a 28-kDa transmembrane ER glycoprotein that has been proposed as a receptor for single-shelled particles as they bud through the ER membrane (71–74). NS53 (RNA segment 5), NS34 (RNA segment 7), and NS35 (RNA segment 8) bind RNA and have been associated with intermediate replicase particles (75,76). NS34 has been shown to bind specifically to the 3″ untranslated sequences in rotavirus messenger ribonucleic acids (mRNAs) (77). In recent genetic studies, NS53 has been linked to virulence in the murine model of rotavirus disease (78). NS26, the product of the 11th gene is both phosphorylated and O-glycosylated (38). Its role in replication is unknown.

Viral Replication Cycle

Rotavirus replication has been studied rather extensively in tissue culture systems. Important features of the replicative cycle are that (a) replication is strictly cytoplasmic; (b) the viral particle contains enzymatic machinery to transcribe the dsRNA genome; (c) initial + RNA transcripts serve as both mRNA for peptide synthesis and as templates for negative strand synthesis; (d) newly synthesized dsRNA strands associate with viral peptides to form subviral particles, which gain their outer capsid by budding through the ER with a transient enveloped stage; and (e) progeny virions are released by cell lysis.

Cell Attachment

The process of target cell binding by viruses is a critical step in viral pathogenesis and can be an important determinant of cellular and host susceptibility to infection. Viral attachment may be a primary determinant of cell and tissue tropism and host range. There are two obvious components to the virus–cell interaction: a viral structure that serves as a ligand (viral attachment protein or VAP) and a cellular receptor. Most studies to date have used tissue culture conditions to examine this interaction but they may be relevant to *in vivo* conditions. Studies have shown that only double-shelled particles attach to cells and that neither proteolytic activation by cleavage of the VP4 outer capsid protein (79,80) nor glycosylation of VP7

(81) is required for attachment. The demonstration by immunocryoelectron microscopy that the outer capsid protein VP4 forms spike-like projections on the rotavirus particle has led to speculation that VP4 is the viral attachment protein (12). Recent studies of the mechanism by which MABs neutralize rotavirus demonstrated that antibodies against the smaller trypsin fragment of rhesus rotavirus VP4 (VP8*), but not the other major surface protein, VP7, neutralize virus by inhibition of binding to target cells (56). Previous studies had shown that a 35-kDa rotavirus protein bound to target cells (79,82). Although initially thought to be VP7, this cell-binding viral protein was later shown to be NS35, which is not thought to be present in mature virus particles (83). Thus studies to date have not unequivocally determined the nature of the rotavirus cell attachment protein. It is possible that no single protein functions as the cell attachment protein but that a structure composed of components of several outer capsid proteins serves this purpose as has been shown for poliovirus and the rhinoviruses (84).

Studies on cellular receptors for rotavirus have shown that simian SA11 rotavirus binding to MA104 cells is saturable (approximately 13,000 binding sites/cell), sodium dependent, relatively pH independent, and sensitive to neuraminidase (80). Sialic acid-containing compounds such as fetuin and mucin inhibit binding of SA11 rotavirus to tissue culture cells (80,85). However, similar studies on human viruses have shown that virus attachment to cells and subsequent infection bear no relation to sialic acid (86,87). Large molecular weight, highly glycosylated surface proteins isolated from suckling murine enterocytes have been shown to specifically bind rhesus rotavirus in a sialic acid-dependent fashion (88) Other studies have suggested that sialic acid-containing gangliosides (89) or asialogangliosides (90) may function as rotavirus receptors. Studies in which highly polarized cells were grown on filter devices have shown that, unlike some viruses, rotavirus infects cells from either the basolateral or apical pole with equal efficiency (91). Further studies in this area are needed to determine the role of receptors in rotavirus pathogenesis and tissue tropism.

Penetration

After binding to an appropriate target cell, the viral genome must then be introduced into the cytoplasm in order for viral replication to proceed. Rotavirus entry is blocked at 4° due to either a block in endocytosis or decreased fluidity of the cellular plasma membrane. The mechanism of penetration is somewhat controversial.

Early ultrastructural studies suggested that rotavirus enters cells via endocytosis and that the viral particles were transported to lysosome-like structures (92). Some studies have shown clear evidence of viral entry via coated pits and vesicles, indicating that receptor-mediated endocytosis is the major route of rotavirus entry (93). Other ultrastructural studies of a human rotavirus strain suggested that treatment of rotavirus with trypsin allowed the virus to directly penetrate the plasma membrane in a fashion analogous to bacteriophage injection

of nucleic acid into bacteria (94,95). Virus that had not been treated with trypsin entered cells by endocytosis. Kinetic studies of the rate of entry of trypsin treated (infectious) versus untreated (noninfectious) rotavirus have supported the direct entry hypothesis (57). Recently, studies from our laboratories have shown that penetration of target cell plasma membrane is the restrictive step in some tissue culture cells that are resistant to rotavirus infection (96). Virus binds these nonpermissive cells to a comparable level to permissive cells and is efficiently internalized, but the internalized virus fails to uncoat and enter the eclipse phase. If intact rotavirus particles are transfected into nonpermissive cells via cationic liposomes, full viral replication ensues. Whatever the route of membrane penetration may be, it is clear from a number of studies that, unlike many viruses, rotavirus does not require acidification of endosomes for productive infection (57,93,97).

Uncoating

After penetration of the host cell plasma membrane, the infecting rotavirus must activate its RNA polymerase to begin replicating. In vitro this may be accomplished by the use of chelating agents such as EDTA, which remove the outer capsid of the virus and activate polymerase activity (14). It is thought that the low calcium concentration in the intracellular cytoplasmic microenvironment induces similar events (93).

Transcription and Translation

As noted earlier, the initiation of transcription is thought to be simultaneous with uncoating. The mechanism and precise cytoplasmic location of transcriptional activation is not known. It may be that the outer capsid serves as a barrier to the free movement of RNA templates past an active catalytic site. All initial transcripts are positive sense, full length single-stranded ribonucleic acid (ssRNA) molecules derived from the parental strands and require adenosine triphosphate (ATP) for their synthesis (98). The positive sense RNA transcripts may then serve as templates for translation, using cellular free ribosomes for most of the rotavirus proteins and/or function as templates for negative sense RNA synthesis. Newly synthesized negative RNA strands are immediately associated with complementary positive strands within nascent subviral particles, which have been termed replicase particles (75). The formation of these single-shelled particles occurs in cytoplasmic electron dense bodies referred to as viroplasm (99).

While little is known about the mechanism of rotavirus capsid assembly in mammalian cells, it is known that baculovirus-expressed VP2 spontaneously forms core-like particles (47). Baculovirus-expressed VP6 self-assembles into oligomeric structures similar to single-shelled particles (51). Coexpression of VP6 and VP7 with or without VP4 leads to the spontaneous assembly of particles similar to double-shelled particles (100,101). During rotavirus infection of mammalian cells, the two viral glycoproteins, VP7 and NS28, are synthesized in ribosomes associated with the ER and are cotranslationally inserted into the ER membrane due to hydrophobic amino acid signal sequences (68). Here they undergo N-linked glycosylation. The single-shelled particles then bind to the ER membrane via NS28 and bud through the ER, presumably gaining the outer capsid protein VP7 in the process. By an unknown mechanism the particles lose their transiently acquired envelope within the ER cisternae.

The infectious cycle ends with cell lysis and release of the progeny virions. A significant portion of released virus remains associated with cell debris, suggesting a possible role for the cellular cytoskeleton in virus assembly and/or transport (102). *In vivo* the virus is released into the intestinal lumen, where it may infect other villous enterocytes.

Effects on Host Cells

As noted earlier, rotavirus is a lytic virus and infection results in death of the host cell. Observed cytopathic effects include cytoplasmic vacuolization and small cytoplasmic inclusions. Biochemical studies have shown that host protein synthesis is shut down by 4 hr (103). Other studies have shown host DNA and RNA synthesis is greatly reduced (104). It is unknown whether specific rotavirus gene products are responsible for these alterations in cellular metabolism. As early as 4 hr postinfection, infected cell membranes become increasingly permeable to calcium, sodium, and potassium (105). In certain tissue culture conditions, nonlytic persistent infections have been established (106). These infections could be relevant to the occasional persistent infection in immunocompromised children (107–109).

EPIDEMIOLOGY

Rotaviruses are ubiquitous and infect almost all mammalian species throughout the world. Although rotavirus may infect humans or other mammals at any age, rotavirus disease occurs mainly in the very young. The burden of rotavirus diarrhea in both the developed and developing worlds is staggering. In a recent analysis it was estimated that each year over 125 million children in developing countries contract rotavirus gastroenteritis, with 18 million severe cases resulting in an estimated 873,000 deaths (110). In the United States alone, 1 million cases per year are estimated to occur with an estimated hospital expenditure in excess of $300 million (1). Of course, the costs of outpatient therapy and lost parental productivity would greatly increase the cost estimate. Diarrhea accounts for approximately 500 childhood deaths per year in the United States (2) and perhaps half of these are rotavirus associated. Although rotaviruses are not always found to be the most common cause of diarrhea among children, they are usually the most common cause of severe, dehydrating disease requiring inpatient therapy. In 8 years 34.5% of infants admitted to a Washington, DC, hospital

for diarrhea had rotavirus infections (111). Similarly, in Bangladesh rotavirus was detected in less than 4% of all pediatric diarrheal episodes but was associated with 39% of all diarrhea cases with significant dehydration (112).

Age

Greater than 90% of children have antibody directed against rotavirus by 3 years of age. In most studies the peak incidence of rotavirus diarrhea is between 6 and 24 months of age, although recent studies from the developing world suggest that rotavirus can be an important pathogen in infants less than 6 months of age (113), a finding that has significant implications for vaccine strategy. Most rotavirus infections in older children and adults produce minimal to no symptoms, possibly because of the acquisition of immunity. Paradoxically, neonates less than 1 month of age often exhibit minimal symptoms with rotavirus infection. This finding may be partially explained by preexisting maternal-derived immunity and/or the presence in some hospital nurseries of apparently attenuated rotavirus strains (114). It has been suggested that certain sequence variations in the vp4 protein of these strains may account for their attenuation (61).

Region and Season

Like any other fecal–orally transmitted pathogen, rotavirus spreads most easily under conditions of overcrowding and poor hygiene. Thus children in developing countries and those in crowded day care centers may be exposed to the virus many times in infancy, with many of the infections being asymptomatic. In the developed world, waves of rotavirus infection occur in regular seasonal patterns with peaks of symptomatic infection occurring in the cooler winter months (111,115). In the United States, it appears that the peak incidence of rotavirus disease begins in the fall in the Southwest and spreads eastward so that by late winter and spring infection peaks in the Northeast (2). This wave of infection, however, does not represent the spread of a single strain or group of rotavirus strains as observed during influenza epidemics. The seasonality of rotavirus infection is less appreciable in tropical countries.

Serotype

In many communities a variety of human rotavirus strains are in circulation at any one time. The strains vary by both electropherotype and serotype. Often a particular strain will be predominant for 1 or 2 years before a new dominant strain emerges, perhaps due to immune selection. It may be that the strain diversity is most pronounced in the developing world. In a recent study of rotavirus isolates from rural Bangladesh during one year, a remarkable diversity of eletropherotypically distinct strains distributed throughout the four major serotypes was observed (116). There have been few reports of animal rotaviruses being transmitted directly to humans. In a study of cattle ranchers in Panama, no evidence of cross-infection between humans and cattle could be detected (117). On the other hand, widespread asymptomatic neonatal infection with a bovine-like strain has been observed in India (118,119). The basis of the host species specificity of rotavirus strain is not known. Likewise, the epidemiologic significance of reassortment events between human and animal rotaviruses, which may occur occasionally *in vivo,* is not known.

The precise relationship of rotavirus serotype (both P and G types) to protective immunity is a topic of some controversy. Although the total number of distinct P and G types in humans is large, the great majority of isolates fall into four G types and two P types. Most children appear to undergo only one or two symptomatic rotavirus infections during childhood, so it is likely that some form of heterotypic immunity develops after infection.

Transmission

Most evidence suggests that rotaviruses are transmitted by the fecal–oral route. Although respiratory transmission has been suggested, no convincing evidence supports this mechanism. It is clear that under appropriate circumstances as little as one infectious particle can initiate disease in animal models (78,120). During rotavirus infection, large numbers of viral particles are shed in the stool. The high environmental stability of rotavirus, the low infectious dose, and the large number of virions passed during infection seem to guarantee the observed infection of virtually all children as well as occurrence of large nosocomial and day care outbreaks.

PATHOGENESIS

Rotavirus is a lytic virus and causes diarrhea primarily by destruction of intestinal villous epithelial cells. A number of studies of experimentally infected animals have demonstrated both morphologic and biochemical changes in the rotavirus-infected small intestine.

The pathology of the small intestine in acute viral gastroenteritis has been described in a variety of species infected naturally or experimentally with a variety of viral agents (5,121–126). Human studies have been more limited but demonstrate similar features (6,126–129). Generally, the pathology of acute viral enteritis is characterized by variable shortening of the villi, a moderate round cell infiltrate in the lamina propria, and elongation of crypts (see Fig. 2). Early in the infection vacuolization and shedding of enterocytes from the apical portion of villi may be observed. Lesions are often patchy in nature and symptoms may occur in the absence of a lesion demonstrable by light microscopy. In a recent study of 40 infants with acute rotavirus gastroenteritis, only two had definitely abnormal duodenal biopsies (129).

A critical concept in the pathogenesis of rotavirus disease is that of cell and tissue tropism. Although occasional reports have described rotavirus antigen in the upper re-

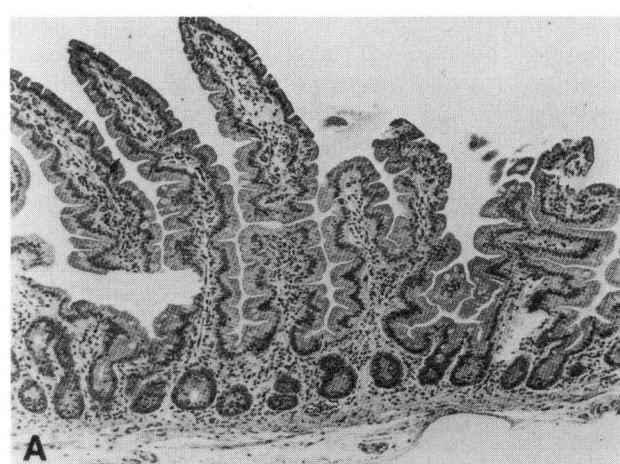

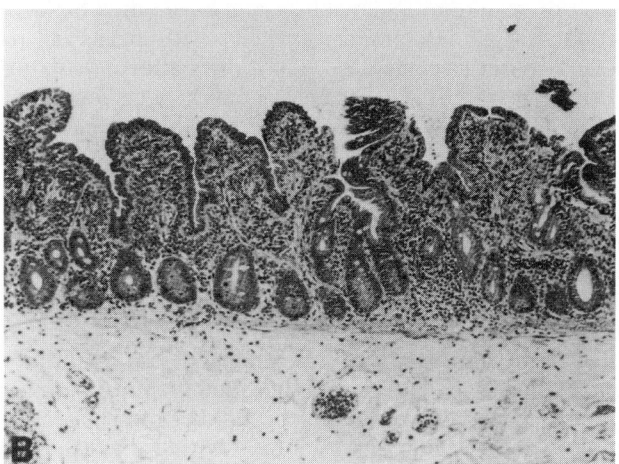

FIG. 2. A: Normal jejunal biopsy from a volunteer prior to experimental infection with Norwalk virus (×100). **B:** Jejunal biopsy from the same volunteer after experimental infection with Norwalk virus, showing shortened villi and increased lymphoid cell infiltrate (×100). (From ref. 127, with permission.)

spiratory tract (130,131), under normal circumstances rotavirus infects only the epithelium of the small intestine. Hepatic infection has been described in immunocompromised hosts and under certain experimental conditions in mice but does not appear to be clinically important in human disease (132–134). A single report described renal and hepatic rotavirus infection in several severely immunocompromised children (135). Low levels of colonic infection may occur but are not important in the pathophysiology of rotavirus disease. Within the small intestine, rotavirus selectively infects enterocytes on the upper villi, sparing the crypt cells. Chronologically, it seems that the proximal small intestine is initially infected with subsequent spread to the distal bowel. The strongest immunofluorescence of the infected apical villous enterocytes in the proximal small bowel precedes the onset of diarrhea.

In the generally accepted view of rotavirus diarrhea pathophysiology, the lytic infection of large numbers of highly differentiated absorptive villous enterocytes and sparing of undifferentiated crypt cells results in both (a) loss of absorptive capacity for water and sodium without impairment of crypt cell secretion and (b) loss of brush border hydrolase activity (e.g., lactase). Morphologic and biochemical studies of experimentally infected animals provide evidence to support this view.

Time course studies of histopathologic changes in experimentally infected animals have shown that in the early hours after rotavirus or coronavirus infection villous cells in the proximal small intestine are infected and produce viral antigen, followed by infection of the distal intestine (122,123). The infected cells become vacuolated, often containing abnormal collections of lipid-like material in their cytoplasm (136). Ultimately, the infected cells are sloughed into the intestinal lumen. It is only at this point that serious diarrhea appears. Thus relatively little intestinal epithelial viral antigen may be demonstrable after the onset of symptoms. Some observers have noted biphasic production of infectious rotavirus, with peaks of recovered virus occuring at 2 and 4 days after inoculation of suckling mice (137). The uninfected crypt cells are stimulated by the injury to proliferate rapidly to replace the shed villous cells. These replacement cells may appear cuboidal, with poorly developed microvilli. The increased migration rate of these crypt epithelial cells is reflected in strikingly shortened cell replacement times for villi. In one study of piglets with viral enteritis, this replacement time was reduced from 11 to 2 days (138). Age-related differences in susceptibility to viral diarrhea may be related to the normally longer replacement and maturation times for villous enterocytes in young mammals than in older animals. For example, the normal life span of an enterocyte as it migrates from the crypt to a villus tip in a newborn pig is 7 to 10 days, while by 3 weeks of age the same journey requires only 3 days (139,140).

Biochemical correlates of this pattern of destruction of differentiated villus epithelium and its subsequent replacement by relatively undifferentiated crypt-like epithelium have been demonstrated (126,141–144). Levels of brush border enzymes characteristic of differentiated cells such as sucrase, alkaline phosphatase, and lactase are decreased in most studies. Sodium-coupled glucose transport and sodium–potassium ATPase are likewise reduced while markers for proliferative crypt cells, such as thymidine kinase, are increased in the intestinal epithelia of animals with viral gastroenteritis. Thus normal absorptive processes are lost and the inherent secretory capacity of the crypt-like epithelium results in excessive losses of water and salts into the gut lumen. The loss of brush border hydrolases complicates the situation as the osmotic load of undigested nutrients draws yet more fluid into the lumen (126,143). The marked reduction in glucose-coupled sodium transport might theoretically diminish the efficacy of oral rehydration solutions originally designed for treatment of cholera, but in actual clinical practice this does not seem to be a problem (145).

Other models for the mechanism of diarrhea associated with viral gastroenteritis have been proposed. One group of investigators has proposed that initial viral infection of a small number of enterocytes leads to release of an unidentified vasoactive agent that induces local intestinal ischemia resulting in damage to villous enterocytes (122).

In subsequent studies, these investigators have observed alternating ischemic and hyperemic phases of villous circulation during rotavirus gastroenteritis, which they hypothesize are important in the imbalance between water absorption and secretion during rotaviral diarrhea in the mouse (146–148). They have also hypothesized that rapidly proliferating crypt cells may have pleomorphic junctional complexes, with resultant abnormal paracellular fluxes of salt and water (142). When mice are infected with very high doses of certain rotavirus strains from other species, diarrhea may occur with minimal evidence for productive viral replication (149,150). To date, there has been no evidence for any toxin-like activity in viral gastroenteritis. Levels of adenylate and guanylate cyclases have been normal in experimental viral gastroenteritis (142–144), as have endogenous cytokines such as tumor necrosis factor (TNF) and interleukin-6 (IL-6) (151). Systemic interferon-α (IFN-α) levels in children hospitalized with rotavirus gastroenteritis have been noted to be elevated during the first few days of illness (152).

A number of studies have demonstrated increased small intestinal permeability to macromolecules during rotavirus gastroenteritis (153–157). It has been proposed that this decrease in mucosal barrier function may lead to abnormal host immune responses to luminal antigens such as the development of food allergy (158,159).

IMMUNITY AND HOST RESISTANCE

Many studies have investigated the immune response to rotavirus in experimental animals and in humans. Several studies have used viral reassortants and monoclonal antibodies to show that antibodies directed against VP4 and VP7 can neutralize rotaviruses in vitro assays and protect animals from disease (reviewed in ref. 160). Neutralizing antibodies against VP7 are generally serotype specific while those directed against the VP5* portion of VP4 are able to neutralize a broad range of rotaviruses. Several studies have suggested that mucosal antibody protection is much more efficacious than serum antibody in preventing symptomatic disease (161–163). Measurements of both serum and intestinal antibody levels have been only fair predictors of susceptibility to rotavirus disease (164,165). Rotavirus does elicit a cytotoxic T cell response (166–171) and passive transfer of these cells can prevent or clear rotavirus infection in both normal mice and severe combined immunodeficient (SCID) mice (172–174). It is also known that nude mice clear rotavirus infection normally (175). Passive immunity from both transplacentally acquired immunoglobulin and breast milk immunoglobulin may provide some degree of protection. In the developed world, infants under 3 months of age are infrequently symptomatically infected. Although some targets of cellular and humoral immunity have been identified in model systems, it is not known which type of immune response is the best predictor of protection from disease in the field. Likewise, it is not clear which viral antigens best stimulate protective immunity in the context of vaccine development. The chapter by Offit and Clark discusses the immune response to rotavirus in relation to vaccination, so the remainder of this section focuses primarily on nonimmune mechanisms of host resistance.

Host factors that may protect against rotavirus disease include diet and nutritional status, gastric secretions, mucus, intestinal flora, and age. Although colostrum feeding is a significant immunologic resistance factor in many animals (176–178), in humans the protective effect of breast-feeding on rotavirus disease is not consistently strong (179–184). Nonimmunologic protective factors in breast milk such as protease inhibitors have been proposed, but one study failed to confirm their role in ameliorating rotavirus disease (180). Recently, mucin-like glycoproteins in human breast milk have been described, which inhibit rotavirus infection (185). Malnutrition, including specific micronutrient deficiencies, predisposes animals and probably humans to severe illness (186–194). Pepsin and acid secreted by the stomach are effective in neutralizing rotaviruses (18,19) and studies have shown that the "take" rate of orally administered live rotavirus vaccine candidates is greatly improved if the stomach contents are buffered (195,196). Intestinal mucins are inhibitors of rotavirus infection *in vitro* although the strongest activity is directed against nonhuman sialic acid-dependent rotaviruses such as those used in most current candidate vaccine strains (86). As noted earlier, intestinal proteases such as trypsin greatly enhance rotavirus replication efficiency both *in vitro* and *in vivo* by cleaving VP4.

Human breast-fed infants with a predominance of bifidobacteria were resistant to severe rotavirus disease, suggesting a role of intestinal flora in susceptibility to rotavirus diarrhea (197). Experimental rotavirus infection caused greater growth failure in previously germ-free mice than in conventional mice (198). In animal models, dual infections with enterotoxigenic *Escherichia coli* and rotavirus appear to act synergistically to produce severe diarrhea (199,200).

CLINICAL ILLNESS

Many if not most rotavirus infections are asymptomatic (201–208). Such infections occur in neonates, older children, and adults and provide a reservoir that helps facilitate the transmission of rotavirus to susceptible hosts, infants, and toddlers. Symptomatic rotavirus infection follows an incubation period of 1 to 3 days followed by the onset of fever, vomiting, and watery diarrhea. Fever and vomiting usually remit within the first 2 to 3 days of illness while diarrhea frequently persists for 5 to 8 days. Laboratory tests typically show mild to moderate elevation of the blood urea nitrogen (BUN) level and mild metabolic acidosis (209). Minimal elevations of liver function tests during rotavirus enteritis have been noted although their significance is uncertain (210). In a study comparing rotavirus diarrhea with other diarrheal illness, vomiting and dehydration were significantly more common in rotavirus diarrhea (209). Stools in rotavirus gastroenteritis are watery and do not contain blood or white blood cells. Although the majority of cases of rotavirus disease result in only mild to moderate dehydration, fulminant cases

occur. Over a 5-year period in Toronto, the deaths of 21 children were attributed to rotavirus disease (211). Over 80% of these children were seen by a physician during the early phase of the illness, yet all the deaths occurred within the first 3 days of symptoms.

Although a variety of clinical conditions have been associated with rotavirus infection, the frequency of rotavirus infection makes it likely that many of these are coincidental associations. There is some evidence that rotavirus may cause some outbreaks of necrotizing enterocolitis in intensive care nurseries (212–214). Rotavirus infections in immunocompromised infections can be atypically long (months) and severe. Rotaviruses recovered from such patients often have bizarre electropherotypes due to gene segment rearrangements (107). There have been reports of rotavirus replication in the liver and kidney of severely immunocompromised hosts (135).

DIAGNOSIS

As noted earlier, the clinical syndrome associated with rotavirus is relatively nonspecific. Although the average clinician facing a child with acute gastroenteritis has little need for diagnostic testing, confirmation of rotavirus infection is vital for epidemiologic and vaccine studies and for the control of outbreaks of enteric illness. Therefore a variety of diagnostic methods have been developed including electron microscopy, solid phase immunoassays, RNA electrophoresis, nucleic acid hybridization (with and without polymerase chain reaction amplification), and direct cultivation of rotavirus from clinical samples in primary simian renal cell lines (see the chapter by Yolken). Historically, the first diagnostic test used was electron microscopy (6). The abundance of rotavirus particles shed in the stool and their distinctive morphology result in high sensitivity and specificity with this technique. Another advantage of electron microscopy in the diagnosis of diarrheal disease is the fact that other enteric viruses or atypical rotaviruses (non-group A rotaviruses) may be identified. The obvious disadvantages are the need for both equipment and expertise. A variety of immunoassays have been developed with several commercial kits available for detecting group A rotavirus antigen in stools (215–218). Most immunoassays have sensitivities and specificities in the 90% range. It is also possible to determine subgroup and G serotype with immunoassays employing MABs (26,29). Comparable sensitivity to electron microscopy and immunoassays can be obtained by simple protocols for isolating genomic RNA directly from stool, resolving it on polyacrylamide gels, and staining with silver to visualize the characteristic 11 segments of dsRNA (219–221). Nucleic acid hybridization tests have also been developed to not only detect rotaviruses but to serotype them as well (222–224). Recently, investigators have reported successful cultivation of human rotaviruses from greater than 90% of antigen-positive stools using primary African green monkey kidney cells (116).

TREATMENT

Treatment of rotavirus diarrhea is supportive. The primary objective of therapy is to treat and prevent dehydration, which is the major cause of morbidity and mortality in infants with rotavirus disease. A worthy secondary objective is treatment and prevention of malnutrition, which is both a contributing factor in disease severity and a frequent result of moderate to severe disease.

Two major technological advances of the 20th century have greatly decreased rotavirus mortality in the developed world. In the 1930s, the use of intravenous fluid for rehydration of infants dramatically reduced the mortality of infantile diarrhea. In the developing world, where facilities, equipment, and expertise in this form of therapy are lacking, great efforts have gone into developing low-cost electrolyte solutions for oral rehydration (225–228). Knowledge of sodium/glucose cotransporters in the intestine led eventually to solutions that had equal molar ratios of these solutes as well as potassium and bicarbonate salts for repletion of stool losses. Oral rehydration solution (ORS) has been used successfully throughout the world in infants and children of all ages with a variety of dehydrating diarrheal illnesses and electrolyte abnormalities. Treatment failures occur only in the face of severe vomiting and frank shock. Protocols for oral rehydration differ from those for intravenous rehydration in that deficits are corrected rapidly with the oral solutions (4 to 6 hr) compared to intravenous rehydration (24 to 48 hr). The standard World Health Organization (WHO) ORS solution contains 3.5 g sodium chloride, 2.5 g sodium bicarbonate, 1.5 g potassium chloride, and 20 g glucose in 1 L of water. Similar solutions with somewhat lower sodium levels (40 to 60 mEq/L versus 90 mEq/L) are available commercially in the United States. Currently, efforts are under way to improve these solutions by the addition of amino acids (to utilize amino acid/sodium cotransporters) or rice starch as a low osmolality carbohydrate source (229–234). To date none of these newer formulations have proved more efficacious than the standard WHO formula for treatment of viral diarrhea (229,231,234). A more complete discussion of ORS can be found in the chapters by Pickering and Snyder.

Traditional dietary management of diarrheal illness has consisted mainly of withholding food. While this may reduce the number of stools passed, the ensuing acute malnutrition prolongs recovery from gastroenteritis (235,236). Current recommendations are to begin refeeding with a complete diet as soon as oral rehydration is complete. Breast-feeding should continue through the rehydration process. Although secondary biochemical lactase deficiency is common in rotavirus infection, many children can be fed unrestricted diets without apparent ill effect (235–238). Likewise, the use of starchy diets low in fat and protein (BRAT or ABC diets) is without any known benefit.

Passive immunotherapy has been used in several situations. Attempts have been made to use milk antibody concentrates from rotavirus-immunized cows to treat infants with acute rotavirus infection (239,240). Although the duration of viral shedding was reduced, little effect was noted on the clinical illness. Oral immunoglobulins and colostrum have been given to immunocompromised children with chronic symptomatic rotavirus disease with resolution of their symptoms (241).

Drug therapy in rotavirus gastroenteritis is generally ill advised. Antibiotics are ineffective and may lead to untoward side effects. Opiates and loperamide may reduce visible stool output but carry the risk of causing ileus and/or vomiting, which may preclude the use of ORS. Severe complications of such medications given to young children have been reported both in the developing and developed world (242–244) and have been observed in our own practices. Clinical trials of loperamide at the recommended doses have shown little or no benefit in children with gastroenteritis (245,246). The WHO recommendation for treatment of diarrhea in children is that "antidiarrheal drugs should never be used. None has any proven practical value and some are dangerous" (247).

Specific antiviral therapy for rotavirus disease has also been studied. A variety of nucleoside analogs have been reported to inhibit rotavirus infection *in vitro* (248–251). Others have proposed the use of protease inhibitors to prevent intestinal trypsin from cleaving VP4 (252,253). Glycoproteins such as mucins, which can function as pseudoreceptors if given orally, have also been suggested as candidate therapies for rotavirus disease (85,90,185). Given the fact that much of the intestinal damage in rotavirus infection occurs prior to symptoms, antivirals will probably not have a large impact on rotavirus disease.

PREVENTION

The substantial morbidity and mortality associated with group A rotavirus disease clearly suggests the need for a vaccine. The status of current vaccine development is described in the chapter by Offit and Clark.

REFERENCES

1. Matson DO, Estes MK. Impact of rotavirus infection at a large pediatric hospital. *J Infect Dis* 1990;162(3):598–604.
2. Ho MS, Glass RI, Pinsky PF, Anderson LJ. Rotavirus as a cause of diarrheal morbidity and mortality in the United States. *J Infect Dis* 1988;158(5):1112–1116.
3. Institute of Medicine. Prospects for immunizing against rotavirus. In: *New vaccine development. Establishing priorities,* vol II. Washington, DC: National Academy Press, 1986;308–318.
4. Adams WR, Kraft LM. Electron microscopic study of the intestinal epithelium of mice infected with the agent of epizootic diarrhea of infant mice (EDIM virus). *Am J Pathol* 1967;(51):39–47.
5. Mebus CA, Stair EL, Underdahl NR, Twiehaus MJ. Pathology of neonatal calf diarrhea induced by a reo-like virus. *Vet Pathol* 1971;(8):490–496.
6. Bishop RF, Davidson GP, Holmes IH, Ruck BJ. Virus particles in epithelial cells of duodenal mucosa from children with viral gastroenteritis. *Lancet* 1973;2:1281–1283.
7. Wyatt RG, James WD, Bohl EH. Human rotavirus type 2: cultivation in vitro. *Science* 1980;207:189–191.
8. Kapikian AZ, Chanock RM. Rotaviruses. In: Fields BN, ed. *Virology,* vol 2, 2nd ed. New York: Raven Press, 1990; 1353–1404.

9. Flewett TH, Bryden AS, Davies H, Woode GN, Bridger JC, Derrick JM. Relation between viruses from acute gastroenteritis of children and newborn calves. *Lancet* 1974;2:61–63.
10. Ludert JE, Gil F, Liprandi F, Esparza J. The structure of the rotavirus inner capsid studied by electron microscopy of chemically disrupted particles. *J Gen Virol* 1986;67:1721–1725.
11. Yeager M, Dryden KA, Olson NH, Greenberg HB, Baker TS. Three-dimensional structure of rhesus rotavirus by cryoelectron microscopy and image reconstruction. *J Cell Biol* 1990; 110(6):2133–2144.
12. Prasad BV, Burns JW, Marietta E, Estes MK, Chiu W. Localization of VP4 neutralization sites in rotavirus by three-dimensional cryo-electron microscopy. *Nature* 1990;343(6257): 476–479.
13. Bridger JC, Woode GN. Characterization of two particle types of calf rotavirus. *J Gen Virol* 1976;31:245–250.
14. Cohen J, Laporte J, Charpilienne A, Scherrer R. Activation of rotavirus RNA polymerase by calcium chelation. *Arch Virol* 1979;60:177–186.
15. Estes MK, Graham DY, Smith EM, Gerba CP. Rotavirus stability and inactivation. *J Gen Virol* 1979;43:403–408.
16. Chen D, Ramig RF. Rescue of infectivity by in vitro transcapsidation of rotavirus single-shelled particles. *Virology* 1993; 192(2):422–429.
17. Anthony ID, Bullivant S, Dayal S, Bellamy AR, Berriman JA. Rotavirus spike structure and polypeptide composition. *J Virol* 1991;65(8):4334–4340.
18. Bass DM, Baylor M, Broome R, Greenberg HB. Molecular basis of age-dependent gastric inactivation of rhesus rotavirus in the mouse. *J Clin Invest* 1992;89(6):1741–1745.
19. Weiss C, Clark HF. Rapid inactivation of rotaviruses by exposure to acid buffer or acidic gastric juice. *J Gen Virol* 1985;66: 2725–2731.
20. Chen YS, Vaughn JM. Inactivation of human and simian rotaviruses by chlorine dioxide. *Appl Environ Microbiol* 1990;56(5): 1363–1366.
21. Rodgers FG, Hufton P, Kurzawska E, Molloy C, Morgan S. Morphological response of human rotavirus to ultra-violet radiation, heat and disinfectants. *J Med Microbiol* 1985;20(1): 123–130.
22. Narang HK, Codd AA. Action of commonly used disinfectants against enteroviruses. *J Hosp Infect* 1983;4(2):209–212.
23. Tan JA, Schnagl RD. Rotavirus inactivated by a hypochlorite-based disinfectant: a reappraisal. *Med J Aust* 1983;1(12):550.
24. Sattar SA, Springthorpe VS, Karim Y, Loro P. Chemical disinfection of non-porous inanimate surfaces experimentally contaminated with four human pathogenic viruses. *Epidemiol Infect* 1989;102(3):493–505.
25. Greenberg HB, Flores J, Kalica AR, Wyatt RG, Jones R. Gene coding assignments for growth restriction, neutralization and subgroup specificities of the W and DS-1 strains of human rotavirus. *J Gen Virol* 1983;64:313–320.
26. Greenberg H, McAuliffe V, Valdesuso J, et al. Serological analysis of the subgroup protein of rotavirus, using monoclonal antibodies. *Infect Immun* 1983;39(1):91–99.
27. Ahmed MU, Taniguchi K, Kobayashi N, et al. Characterization by enzyme-linked immunosorbent assay using subgroup- and serotype-specific monoclonal antibodies of human rotavirus obtained from diarrheic patients in Bangladesh. *J Clin Microbiol* 1989;27(7):1678–1681.
28. Birch CJ, Heath RL, Gust ID. Use of serotype-specific monoclonal antibodies to study the epidemiology of rotavirus infection. *J Med Virol* 1988;24(1):45–53.
29. Taniguchi K, Urasawa T, Morita Y, Greenberg HB, Urasawa S. Direct serotyping of human rotavirus in stools by an enzyme-linked immunosorbent assay using serotype 1-, 2-, 3-, and 4-specific monoclonal antibodies to VP7. *J Infect Dis* 1987; 155(6):1159–1166.
30. Beards GM. Serotyping of rotavirus by NADP-enhanced enzyme-immunoassay. *J Virol Methods* 1987;18(2–3):77–85.
31. Coulson BS, Unicomb LE, Pitson GA, Bishop RF. Simple and specific enzyme immunoassay using monoclonal antibodies for serotyping human rotaviruses. *J Clin Microbiol* 1987;25(3): 509–515.
32. Flores J, Taniguchi K, Green K, et al. Relative frequencies of rotavirus serotypes 1, 2, 3, and 4 in Venezuelan infants with gastroenteritis. *J Clin Microbiol* 1988;26(10):2092–2095.
33. Larralde G, Gorziglia M. Distribution of conserved and specific epitopes on the VP8 subunit of rotavirus VP4. *J Virol* 1992; 66(12):7438–7443.
34. Li B, Larralde G, Gorziglia M. Human rotavirus K8 strain represents a new VP4 serotype. *J Virol* 1993;67(1):617–620.
35. Larralde G, Li BG, Kapikian AZ, Gorziglia M. Serotype-specific epitope(s) present on the VP8 subunit of rotavirus VP4 protein. *J Virol* 1991;65(6):3213–3218.
36. Gorziglia M, Larralde G, Kapikian AZ, Chanock RM. Antigenic relationships among human rotaviruses as determined by outer capsid protein VP4. *Proc Natl Acad Sci USA* 1990;87(18): 7155–7159.
37. Estes MK, Cohen J. Rotavirus gene structure and function. *Microbiol Rev* 1989;53(4):410–449.
38. Welch SK, Crawford SE, Estes MK. Rotavirus SA11 genome segment 11 protein is a nonstructural phosphoprotein. *J Virol* 1989;63(9):3974–3982.
39. Imai M, Akatani K, Ikegami N, Furuichi Y. Capped and conserved terminal structures in human rotavirus genome double-stranded RNA segments. *J Virol* 1983;47(1):125–136.
40. McCrae MA, McCorquodale JG. Molecular biology of rotaviruses. V. Terminal structure of viral RNA species. *Virology* 1983;126(1):204–212.
41. McCrae MA, McCorquodale JG. Genetic heterogeneity within individual bovine rotavirus isolates. *J Virol* 1983;44(3): 813–822.
42. Mason BB, Graham DY, Estes MK. Biochemical mapping of the simian rotavirus SA11 genome. *J Virol* 1983;46(2):413–423.
43. Both GW, Siegman LJ, Bellamy AR, Atkinson PH. Coding assignment and nucleotide sequence of simian rotavirus SA11 gene segment 10: location of glycosylation sites suggests that the signal peptide is not cleaved. *J Virol* 1983;48(2):335–339.
44. Kantharidis P, Dyall SM, Holmes IH. Completion of the gene coding assignments of SA11 rotavirus: gene products of segments 7, 8, and 9. *J Virol* 1983;48(1):330–334.
45. Both GW, Mattick JS, Bellamy AR. Serotype-specific glycoprotein of simian 11 rotavirus: coding assignment and gene sequence. *Proc Natl Acad Sci USA* 1983;80(10):3091–3095.
46. Greenberg HB, Flores J, Kalica AR, Wyatt RG, Jones R. Gene coding assignments for growth restriction, neutralization and subgroup specificities of the W and DS-1 strains of human rotavirus. *J Gen Virol* 1983;64:313–320.
47. Labbe M, Charpilienne A, Crawford SE, Estes MK, Cohen J. Expression of rotavirus VP2 produces empty corelike particles. *J Virol* 1991;65(6):2946–2952.
48. Boyle JF, Holmes KV. RNA-binding proteins of bovine rotavirus. *J Virol* 1986;58(2):561–568.
49. Valenzuela S, Pizarro J, Sandino AM, et al. Photoaffinity labeling of rotavirus VP1 with 8-azido-ATP: identification of the viral RNA polymerase. *J Virol* 1991;65(7):3964–3967.
50. Vasquez M, Sandino AM, Pizarro JM, Fernandez J, Valanzuel S, Spencer E. Function of rotavirus VP3 polypeptide in viral morphogenesis. *J Gen Virol* 1993;74:937–941.
51. Estes MK, Crawford SE, Penaranda ME, et al. Synthesis and immunogenicity of the rotavirus major capsid antigen using a baculovirus expression system. *J Virol* 1987;61(5):1488–1494.
52. Gorziglia M, Larrea C, Liprandi F, Esparza J. Biochemical evidence for the oligomeric (possibly trimeric) structure of the major inner capsid polypeptide (45K) of rotaviruses. *J Gen Virol* 1985;66:1889–1890.
53. Kalica AR, Flores J, Greenberg HB. Identification of the rotaviral gene that codes for hemagglutination and protease-enhanced plaque formation. *Virology* 1983;125(1):194–205.
54. Mackow ER, Barnett JW, Chan H, Greenberg HB. The rhesus rotavirus outer capsid protein VP4 functions as a hemagglutinin and is antigenically conserved when expressed by a baculovirus recombinant. *J Virol* 1989;63(4):1661–1668.
55. Offit PA, Blavat G, Greenberg HB, Clark HF. Molecular basis of rotavirus virulence: role of gene segment 4. *J Virol* 1986; 57(1):46–49.
56. Ruggeri FM, Greenberg HA. Antibodies to the tyrpsin cleavage

peptide vp8* neutralize rotavirus by inhibiting binding of virions to target cells in culture. *J Virol* 1991;65:2211–2219.

57. Kaljot KT, Shaw RD, Rubin DH, Greenberg HB. Infectious rotavirus enters cells by direct cell membrane penetration, not by endocytosis. *J Virol* 1988;62(4):1136–1144.

58. Estes MK, Graham DY, Mason BB. Proteolytic enhancement of rotavirus infectivity: molecular mechanisms. *J Virol* 1981; 39(3):879–888.

59. Lopez S, Arias CF, Bell JR, Strauss JH, Espejo RT. Primary structure of the cleavage site associated with trypsin enhancement of rotavirus SA11 infectivity. *Virology* 1985;144(1):11–19.

60. Lopez S, Arias CF, Mendez E, Espejo RT. Conservation in rotaviruses of the protein region containing the two sites associated with trypsin enhancement of infectivity. *Virology* 1986; 154(1):224–227.

61. Gorziglia M, Hoshino Y, Buckler WA, et al. Conservation of amino acid sequence of VP8 and cleavage region of 84-kDa outer capsid protein among rotaviruses recovered from asymptomatic neonatal infection. *Proc Natl Acad Sci USA* 1986; 83(18):7039–7043.

62. Mackow ER, Shaw RD, Matsui SM, Vo PT, Dang MN, Greenberg HB. The rhesus rotavirus gene encoding protein VP3: location of amino acids involved in homologous and heterologous rotavirus neutralization and identification of a putative fusion region. *Proc Natl Acad Sci USA* 1988;85(3):645–649.

63. Chan WK, Penaranda ME, Crawford SE, Estes MK. Two glycoproteins are produced from the rotavirus neutralization gene. *Virology* 1986;151(2):243–252.

64. Stirzaker SC, Whitfeld PL, Christie DL, Bellamy AR, Both GW. Processing of rotavirus glycoprotein VP7: implications for the retention of the protein in the endoplasmic reticulum. *J Cell Biol* 1987;105:2897–2903.

65. Stirzaker SC, Both GW. The signal peptide of the rotavirus glycoprotein VP7 is essential for its retention in the ER as an integral membrane protein. *Cell* 1989;56(5):741–747.

66. Stirzaker SC, Poncet D, Both GW. Sequences in rotavirus glycoprotein VP7 that mediate delayed translocation and retention of the protein in the endoplasmic reticulum. *J Cell Biol* 1990; 111(4):1343–1350.

67. Poruchynsky MS, Atkinson PH. Primary sequence domains required for the retention of rotavirus VP7 in the endoplasmic reticulum. *J Cell Biol* 1988;107(5):1697–1706.

68. Kabcenell AK, Atkinson PH. Processing of the rough endoplasmic reticulum membrane glycoproteins of rotavirus SA11. *J Cell Biol* 1985;101(4):1270–1280.

69. Kouvelos K, Petric M, Middleton PJ. Comparison of bovine, simian and human rotavirus structural glycoproteins. *J Gen Virol* 1984;65:1211–1214.

70. Kouvelos K, Petric M, Middleton PJ. Oligosaccharide composition of calf rotavirus. *J Gen Virol* 1984;65:1159–1164.

71. Au KS, Chan WK, Burns JW, Estes MK. Receptor activity of rotavirus nonstructural glycoprotein NS28. *J Virol* 1989;63(11):4553–4562.

72. Maass DR, Atkinson PH. Rotavirus proteins VP7, NS28, and VP4 form oligomeric structures. *J Virol* 1990;64(6):2632–2641.

73. Taylor JA, Meyer JC, Legge MA, et al. Transient expression and mutational analysis of the rotavirus intracellular receptor: the C-terminal methionine residue is essential for ligand binding. *J Virol* 1992;66(6):3566–3572.

74. Chan WK, Au KS, Estes MK. Topography of the simian rotavirus nonstructural glycoprotein (NS28) in the endoplasmic reticulum membrane. *Virology* 1988;164(2):435–442.

75. Patton JT, Gallegos CO. Structure and protein composition of the rotavirus replicase particle. *Virology* 1988;166(2):358–365.

76. Gallegos CO, Patton JT. Characterization of rotavirus replication intermediates: a model for the assembly of single-shelled particles. *Virology* 1989;172(2):616–627.

77. Poncet D, Aponte C, Cohen J. Rotavirus protein NSP3 (NS34) is bound to the 3' end consensus sequence of viral mRNAs in infected cells. *J Virol* 1993;67(6):3159–3165.

78. Broome RL, Vo PT, Ward RL, Clark HF, Greenberg HB. Murine rotavirus genes encoding outer capsid proteins VP4 and VP7 are not major determinants of host range restriction and virulence. *J Virol* 1993;67(5):2448–2455.

79. Fukuhara N, Yoshie O, Kitaoka S, Konno T. Role of VP3 in human rotavirus internalization after target cell attachment via VP7. *J Virol* 1988;62(7):2209–2218.

80. Keljo DJ, Smith AK. Characterization of binding of simian rotavirus SA-11 to cultured epithelial cells. *J Pediatr Gastroenterol Nutr* 1988;7(2):249–256.

81. Petrie BL, Estes MK, Graham DY. Effects of tunicamycin on rotavirus morphogenesis and infectivity. *J Virol* 1983;46(1):270–274.

82. Sabara M, Babiuk LA. Identification of a bovine rotavirus gene and gene product influencing cellular attachment. *J Virol* 1984; 51(2):489–496.

83. Bass DM, Mackow ER, Greenberg HB. NS35 and not vp7 is the soluble rotavirus protein which binds to target cells. *J Virol* 1990;64(1):322–330.

84. Colonno RJ, Condra JH, Mizutani S, Callahan PL, Davies ME, Murcko MA. Evidence for the direct involvement of the rhinovirus canyon in receptor binding. *Proc Natl Acad Sci USA* 1988;85(15):5449–5453.

85. Yolken RH, Willoughby R, Wee SB, Miskuff R, Vonderfecht S. Sialic acid glycoproteins inhibit in vitro and in vivo replication of rotaviruses. *J Clin Invest* 1987;79(1):148–154.

86. Chen CC, Baylor M, Bass DM. Murine intestinal mucins inhibit rotavirus infection. *Gastroenterology* 1993;105(1):84–92.

87. Fukudome K, Yoshie O, Konno T. Comparison of human, simian, and bovine rotaviruses for requirement of sialic acid in hemagglutination and cell absorption. *Virology* 1989;172:196–205.

88. Bass DM, Mackow ER, Greenberg HB. Identification and partial characterization of a rhesus rotavirus binding glycoprotein on murine enterocytes. *Virology* 1991;183(2):602–610.

89. Superti F, Donelli G. Gangliosides as binding sites in SA-11 rotavirus infection of LLC-MK2 cells. *J Gen Virol* 1991;72:2467–2474.

90. Willoughby RE, Yolken RH, Schnaar RL. Rotaviruses specifically bind to the neutral glycosphingolipid asialo-GM1. *J Virol* 1990;64:4830–4835.

91. Svensson L, Finlay BB, Bass D, von BC, Greenberg HB. Symmetric infection of rotavirus on polarized human intestinal epithelial (Caco-2) cells. *J Virol* 1991;65(8):4190–4197.

92. Quan CM, Doane FW. Ultrastructural evidence for the cellular uptake of rotavirus by endocytosis. *Intervirology* 1983;20(4):223–231.

93. Ludert JE, Michelangeli F, Gil F, Liprandi F, Esparza J. Penetration and uncoating of rotaviruses in cultured cells. *Intervirology* 1987;27(2):95–101.

94. Suzuki H, Kitaoka S, Konno T, Sato T, Ishida N. Two modes of human rotavirus entry into MA 104 cells. *Arch Virol* 1985; 85(1–2):25–34.

95. Suzuki H, Kitaoka S, Sato T, et al. Further investigation on the mode of entry of human rotavirus into cells. *Arch Virol* 1986;91(1–2):135–144.

96. Bass DM, Baylor MR, Chen C, Mackow EM, Bremont M, Greenberg HB. Liposome-mediated transfection of intact viral particles reveals that plasma membrane penetration determines permissivity of tissue culture cells to rotavirus. *J Clin Invest* 1992;90(6):2313–2320.

97. Keljo DJ, Kuhn M, Smith A. Acidification of endosomes is not important for the entry of rotavirus into the cell. *J Pediatr Gastroenterol Nutr* 1988;7(2):257–263.

98. Spencer E, Arias ML. In vitro transcription catalyzed by heat treated human rotavirus. *J Virol* 1981;(40):1–10.

99. Petrie BL, Greenberg HB, Graham DY, Estes MK. Ultrastructural localization of rotavirus antigens using colloidal gold. *Virus Res* 1984;1(2):133–152.

100. Sabara M, Parker M, Aha P, et al. Assembly of double-shelled rotaviruslike particles by simultaneous expression of recombinant VP6 and VP7 proteins. *J Virol* 1991;65(12):6994–6997.

101. Redmond MJ, Ijaz MK, Parker MD, et al. Assembly of recombinant rotavirus proteins into virus-like particles and assessment of vaccine potential. *Vaccine* 1993;11(2):273–281.

102. Musalem C, Espejo RT. Release of progeny virus from cells infected with simian rotavirus SA11. *J Gen Virol* 1985;66:2715–2724.

103. McCrae MA, Faulkner-Valle GP. Molecular biology of rotaviruses: I. Characterization of basic growth parameters and pattern of macromolecular synthesis. *J Virol* 1981;39:490–496.

104. Carpio MM, Babiuk LA, Misra V, Blumethal RM. Bovine rotavirus-cell interactions: effect of rotavirus infection on cellular integrity and macromolecular synthesis. *Virology* 1981;114: 86–93.

105. Michelangeli F, Ruiz MC, Del CJ, Ludert JE, Liprandi F. Effect of rotavirus infection on intracellular calcium homeostasis in cultured cells. *Virology* 1991;181(2):520–527.

106. Chiarini A, Arista S, Giammanco A, Sinatra A. Rotavirus persistence in cell cultures: selection of resistant cells in the presence of foetal calf serum. *J Gen Virol* 1983;64:1101–1110.

107. Eiden J, Losonsky GA, Johnson J, Yolken RH. Rotavirus RNA variation during chronic infection of immunocompromised children. *Pediatr Infect Dis* 1985;4(6):632–637.

108. Pedley S, Hundley F, Chrystie I, McCrae MA, Desselberger U. The genomes of rotaviruses isolated from chronically infected immunodeficient children. *J Gen Virol* 1984;65:1141–1150.

109. Wood DJ, David TJ, Chrystie IL, Totterdell B. Chronic enteric virus infection in two T-cell immunodeficient children. *J Med Virol* 1988;24(4):435–444.

110. Institute of Medicine. The prospects for immunizing against rotavirus disease. In: *New vaccine development. Establishing priorities. Diseases of importance in developing countries,* vol II. Washington, DC: National Academy Press, 1986;308–318.

111. Brandt CD, Kim HW, Rodriguez WJ, et al. Pediatric viral gastroenteritis during eight years of study. *J Clin Microbiol* 1983; 18(1):71–78.

112. Black RE, Greenberg HB, Kapikian AZ, Brown KH, Becker S. Acquisition of serum antibody to Norwalk virus and rotavirus in relation to diarrhea in a longitudinal study of young children in rural Bangladesh. *J Infect Dis* 1982;145:483–489.

113. Huilan S, Zhen LG, Mathan MM, et al. Etiology of acute diarrhoea among children in developing countries: a multicentre study in five countries. *Bull World Health Organ* 1991;69(5): 549–555.

114. Haffejee IE. Neonatal rotavirus infections. *Rev Infect Dis* 1991; 13(5):957–962.

115. Konno T, Suzuki H, Katsushima N, et al. Influence of temperature and relative humidity on human rotavirus infection in Japan. *J Infect Dis* 1983;147(1):125–128.

116. Ward RL, Clemens JD, Sack DA, et al. Culture adaptation and characterization of group A rotaviruses causing diarrheal illnesses in Bangladesh from 1985 to 1986. *J Clin Microbiol* 1991;29(9):1915–1923.

117. Ryder RW, Yolken RH, Reeves WC, Sack RB. Enzootic bovine rotavirus is not a source of infection in Panamanian cattle ranchers and their families. *J Infect Dis* 1986;153(6):1139–1144.

118. Das M, Dunn SJ, Woode GN, Greenberg HB, Rao CD. Both surface proteins (VP4 and VP7) of an asymptomatic neonatal rotavirus strain (I321) have high levels of sequence identity with the homologous proteins of a serotype 10 bovine rotavirus. *Virology* 1993;194(1):374–379.

119. Dunn SJ, Greenberg HB, Ward RL, et al. Serotypic and genotypic characterization of human serotype 10 rotaviruses from asymptomatic neonates. *J Clin Microbiol* 1993;31(1):165–169.

120. Graham DY, Dufour GR, Estes MK. Minimal infective dose of rotavirus. *Arch Virol* 1987;92(3–4):261–271.

121. Snodgrass DR, Angus KW, Gray EW. Rotavirus in lambs: pathogenesis and pathology. *Arch Virol* 1977;55:263–271.

122. Osborne MP, Haddon SJ, Spencer AJ, et al. An electron microscopic investigation of time-related changes in the intestine of neonatal mice infected with murine rotavirus. *J Pediatr Gastroenterol Nutr* 1988;7(2):236–248.

123. Mebus CA, Stair EL, Underdahl NR, Twiehaus MJ. Pathology of neonatal calf diarrhea induced by a reo-like virus. *Vet Pathol* 1971;8:490–496.

124. Mebus CA, Wyatt RG, Kapikian AZ. Pathology of diarrhea in gnotobiotic calves induced by the human reovirus-like agent infantile gastroenteritis. *Vet Pathol* 1977;14:273–282.

125. Hall GA. Comparative pathology of infection by novel diarrhoea viruses. *Ciba Found Symp* 1987.

126. Davidson GP, Barnes GL. Structural and functional abnormalities of the small intestine in infants and children with rotavirus enteritis. *Acta Paediatr Scand* 1979;68:181–188.

127. Agus SG, Dolin R, Wyatt RG, Tousimas AJ, Northrup RJ. Acute infectious nonbacterial gastroenteritis: intestinal pathology and enzyme alterations during illness produced by the Norwalk agent in man. *Ann Intern Med* 1973;79:18–25.

128. Schreiber DS, Blacklow NR, Trier JS. The small intestinal lesion induced by the Hawaii agent in infectious nonbacterial gastroenteritis. *J Infect Dis* 1974;124:705–708.

129. Kohler T, Erben U, Wiedersberg H, Bannert N. Histologische Befunde der Dunndarmschleimhaut bei Rotavirusinfektionen im Sauglings- und Kleinkindalter. *Kinderarztl Prax* 1990;58(6): 323–327.

130. Fragoso M, Kumar A, Murray DL. Rotavirus in nasopharyngeal secretions of children with upper respiratory tract infections. *Diagn Microbiol Infect Dis* 1986;4(1):87–88.

131. Novikova NA, Al'tova EE, Noskova NV, Epifanova NV, Tamoikina NA. The detection of rotavirus RNA in nasopharyngeal smears by molecular hybridization. *Zh Mikrobiol Epidemiol Immunobiol* 1991;24:142–145.

132. Grunow JE, Dunton SF, Waner JL. Human rotavirus-like particles in a hepatic abscess. *J Pediatr* 1985;106(1):73–76.

133. Geme GS, Hyman D. Hepatic injury during rotavirus infections. *J Pediatr* 1988;113(5):952–953.

134. Uhnoo I, Riepenhoff TM, Dharakul T, et al. Extramucosal spread and development of hepatitis in immunodeficient and normal mice infected with rhesus rotavirus. *J Virol* 1990;64(1): 361–368.

135. Gilger MA, Matson DO, Conner ME, Rosenblatt HM, Finegold MJ, Estes MK. Extraintestinal rotavirus infections in children with immunodeficiency. *J Pediatr* 1992;120(6):912–917.

136. Wolf JL, Cukor G, Blacklow NR, Dambrauskas R, Trier JS. Susceptibility of mice to rotavirus infection: effects of age and corticosteroid administration. *Infect Immun* 1981;33:565–574.

137. Riepenhoff TM, Dharakul T, Kowalski E, Sterman D, Ogra PL. Rotavirus infection in mice: pathogenesis and immunity. *Adv Exp Med Biol* 1987;216B:1015–1026.

138. Thake DC, Moon HW, Lambert G. Epithelial cell dynamics in transmissible gastroenteritis of neonatal pigs. *Vet Pathol* 1973; 10:330–341.

139. Moon HW. Epithelial cell migration in the alimentary mucosa of the suckling pig. *Proc Soc Exp Biol Med* 1971;137:151–159.

140. Moon HW, Joel DD. Epithelial cell migration in the small intestine of sheep and calves. *Am J Vet Res* 1975;36:187–194.

141. Davidson GP, Gall DG, Petric M, Butler DG, Hamilton JR. Human rotavirus enteritis induced in conventional piglets: intestinal structure and transport. *J Clin Invest* 1977;60: 1402–1409.

142. Collins J, Starkey WG, Wallis TS, et al. Intestinal enzyme profiles in normal and rotavirus-infected mice. *J Pediatr Gastroenterol Nutr* 1988;7(2):264–272.

143. Graham DY, Sackman JW, Estes MK. Pathogenesis of rotavirus-induced diarrhea. Preliminary studies in miniature swine piglet. *Dig Dis Sci* 1984;29(11):1028–1035.

144. Hamilton JR, Gall DG, Butler DG, Middleton PJ. Viral gastroenteritis: recent progress, remaining problems. In: Elliot K, Knight J, eds. *Acute diarrhea in childhood.* Ciba Foundation Symposium; vol 42. Amsterdam: Elsevier/Excerpta Medica/North-Holland, 1976;209–219.

145. Sack DA, Chodhury AMAK, Eusof A, et al. Oral rehydration in rotavirus diarrhea: a double blind comparison of sucrose with glucose electrolyte solution. *Lancet* 1978;2:280–283.

146. Osborne MP, Haddon SJ, Worton KJ, et al. Rotavirus-induced changes in the microcirculation of intestinal villi of neonatal mice in relation to the induction and persistence of diarrhea. *J Pediatr Gastroenterol Nutr* 1991;12(1):111–120.

147. Starkey WG, Collins J, Candy DC, Spencer AJ, Osborne MP, Stephen J. Transport of water and electrolytes by rotavirus-infected mouse intestine: a time course study. *J Pediatr Gastroenterol Nutr* 1990;11(2):254–260.

148. Starkey WG, Candy DC, Thornber D, et al. An in vitro model to study aspects of the pathophysiology of murine rotavirus-induced diarrhoea. *J Pediatr Gastroenterol Nutr* 1990;10(3): 361–370.

149. Offit PA, Clark HF, Kornstein MJ, Plotkin SA. A murine model for oral infection with a primate rotavirus (simian SA11). *J Virol* 1984;51(1):233–236.

150. Ramig RF. The effects of host age, virus dose, and virus strain on heterologous rotavirus infection of suckling mice. *Microb Pathog* 1988;4(3):189–202.

151. de Silva DG, Mendis LN, Sheron N, et al. Concentrations of interleukin 6 and tumour necrosis factor in serum and stools of children with *Shigella dysenteriae* 1 infection. *Gut* 1993;34(2): 194–198.

152. De Boissieu D, Lebon P, Badoual J, Bompard Y, Dupont C. Rotavirus induces alpha-interferon release in children with gastroenteritis. *J Pediatr Gastroenterol Nutr* 1993;16(1):29–32.

153. Heyman M, Corthier G, Petit A, Meslin JC, Moreau C, Desjeux JF. Intestinal absorption of macromolecules during viral enteritis: an experimental study on rotavirus-infected conventional and germ-free mice. *Pediatr Res* 1987;22(1):72–78.

154. Uhnoo IS, Freihorst J, Riepenhoff TM, Fisher JE, Ogra PL. Effect of rotavirus infection and malnutrition on uptake of a dietary antigen in the intestine. *Pediatr Res* 1990;27(2): 153–160.

155. Jalonen T, Isolauri E, Heyman M, Crain DA, Sillanaukee P, Koivula T. Increased beta-lactoglobulin absorption during rotavirus enteritis in infants: relationship to sugar permeability. *Pediatr Res* 1991;30(3):290–293.

156. Isolauri E, Juntunen M, Wiren S, Vuorinen P, Koivula T. Intestinal permeability changes in acute gastroenteritis: effects of clinical factors and nutritional management. *J Pediatr Gastroenterol Nutr* 1989;8(4):466–473.

157. Johansen K, Stintzing G, Magnusson KE, et al. Intestinal permeability assessed with polyethylene glycols in children with diarrhea due to rotavirus and common bacterial pathogens in a developing community. *J Pediatr Gastroenterol Nutr* 1989; 9(3):307–313.

158. Firer MA, Hosking CS, Hill DJ. Possible role for rotavirus in the development of cows' milk enteropathy in infants. *Clin Allergy* 1988;18(1):53–61.

159. Ogra PL, Welliver RC, Riepenhoff TM, Faden HS. Interaction of mucosal immune system and infections in infancy: implications in allergy. *Ann Allergy* 1984.

160. Matsui SM, Mackow ER, Greenberg HB. Molecular determinants of rotavirus neutralization and protection. *Adv Virus Res* 1989;36:181–214.

161. Ward RL, Bernstein DI, Shukla R, et al. Effects of antibody to rotavirus on protection of adults challenged with a human rotavirus. *J Infect Dis* 1989;159(1):79–88.

162. Offit PA, Clark HF. Protection against rotavirus-induced gastroenteritis in a murine model by passively acquired gastrointestinal but not circulating antibodies. *J Virol* 1985;54(1):58–64.

163. Offit PA, Shaw RD, Greenberg HB. Passive protection against rotavirus-induced diarrhea by monoclonal antibodies to surface proteins vp3 and vp7. *J Virol* 1986;58(2):700–703.

164. Ward RL, Bernstein DI, Shukla R, et al. Protection of adults rechallenged with a human rotavirus. *J Infect Dis* 1990;161(3): 440–445.

165. Ward RL, McNeal MM, Sheridan JF. Evidence that active protection following oral immunization of mice with live rotavirus is not dependent on neutralizing antibody. *Virology* 1992; 188(1):57–66.

166. Offit PA, Dudzik KI. Rotavirus-specific cytotoxic T lymphocytes cross-react with target cells infected with different rotavirus serotypes. *J Virol* 1988;62(1):127–131.

167. Offit PA, Dudzik KI. Noninfectious rotavirus (strain RRV) induces an immune response in mice which protects against rotavirus challenge. *J Clin Microbiol* 1989;27(5):885–888.

168. Offit PA, Svoboda YM. Rotavirus-specific cytotoxic T lymphocyte response of mice after oral inoculation with candidate rotavirus vaccine strains RRV or WC3. *J Infect Dis* 1989;160(5): 783–788.

169. Offit PA, Dudzik KI. Rotavirus-specific cytotoxic T lymphocytes appear at the intestinal mucosal surface after rotavirus infection. *J Virol* 1989;63(8):3507–3512.

170. Offit PA, Hoffenberg EJ, Pia ES, Panackal PA, Hill NL. Rotavirus-specific helper T cell responses in newborns, infants, children, and adults. *J Infect Dis* 1992;165(6):1107–1111.

171. Offit PA, Cunningham SL, Dudzik KI. Memory and distribution of virus-specific cytotoxic T lymphocytes (CTLs) and CTL precursors after rotavirus infection. *J Virol* 1991;65(3): 1318–1324.

172. Dharakul T, Rott L, Greenberg HB. Recovery from chronic rotavirus infection in mice with severe combined immunodeficiency: virus clearance mediated by adoptive transfer of immune CD8+ T lymphocytes. *J Virol* 1990;64(9):4375–4382.

173. Dharakul T, Labbe M, Cohen J, et al. Immunization with baculovirus-expressed recombinant rotavirus proteins VP1, VP4, VP6, and VP7 induces CD8+ T lymphocytes that mediate clearance of chronic rotavirus infection in SCID mice. *J Virol* 1991;65(11):5928–5932.

174. Offit PA, Dudzik KI. Rotavirus-specific cytotoxic T lymphocytes passively protect against gastroenteritis in suckling mice. *J Virol* 1990;64(12):6325–6328.

175. Eiden J, Lederman HM, Vonderfecht S, Yolken R. T-cell-deficient mice display normal recovery from experimental rotavirus infection. *J Virol* 1986;57(2):706–708.

176. Leece JG, King MW, Dorsey WE. Rearing regimen producing piglet diarrhea (rotavirus) and its relevance to acute infantile diarrhea. *Science* 1978;199:776–778.

177. Snodgrass DR, Fahey KJ, Well PW, Campbell I, Whitelaw A. Passive immunity in calf rotavirus infections: maternal vaccination increases and prolongs immunoglobulin G antibody secretion. *Infect Immun* 1980;28:344–349.

178. Snodgrass DR, Nagy LK, Sherwood D, Campbell I. Passive immunity in calf diarrhea: vaccination with K99 antigen of enterotoxigenic *Escherichia coli* and rotavirus. *Infect Immun* 1982;37(2):586–591.

179. Totterdell BM, Chrystie IL, Banatvala JE. Cord blood and breast milk antibodies in neonatal rotavirus infection. *Br Med J* 1980;280:828–830.

180. Totterdell BM, Nicholson KG, MacLeod J, Chrystie IL, Banatvala JE. Neonatal rotavirus infection: role of lacteal neutralising alpha1-anti-trypsin and nonimmunoglobulin antiviral activity in protection. *J Med Virol* 1982;10(1):37–44.

181. Totterdell BM, Banatvala JE, Chrystie IL. Studies on human lacteal rotavirus antibodies by immune electron microscopy. *J Med Virol* 1983;11(2):167–175.

182. Gurwith M, Wenman W, Gurwith D, Brunton J, Feltham S, Greenberg H. Diarrhea among infants and young children in Canada: a longitudinal study in three northern communities. *J Infect Dis* 1983;147(4):685–692.

183. Glass RI, Stoll BJ, Wyatt RG, Hoshino Y, Banu H, Kapikian AZ. Observations questioning a protective role for breast-feeding in severe rotavirus diarrhea. *Acta Paediatr Scand* 1986; 75(5):713–718.

184. Glass RI, Stoll BJ. The protective effect of human milk against diarrhea. A review of studies from Bangladesh. *Acta Paediatr Scand Suppl* 1989;351:131–136.

185. Yolken RH, Peterson JA, Vonderfecht SL, Fouts ET, Midthun K, Newburg DS. Human milk mucin inhibits rotavirus replication and prevents experimental gastroenteritis. *J Clin Invest* 1992;90(5):1984–1991.

186. Morrey JD, Sidwell RW, Noble RL, Barnett BB, Mahoney AW. Effects of folic acid malnutrition on rotaviral infection in mice. *Proc Soc Exp Biol Med* 1984;176(1):77–83.

187. Noble RL, Sidwell RW, Mahoney AW, Barnett BB, Spendlove RS. Influence of malnutrition and alterations in dietary protein on murine rotaviral disease. *Proc Soc Exp Biol Med* 1983; 173(3):417–426.

188. Black RE, Merson MH, Eusof A, Huq I, Pollard R. Nutritional status, body size and severity of diarrhoea associated with rotavirus or enterotoxigenic *Escherichia coli*. *J Trop Med Hyg* 1984;87(2):83–89.

189. Offor E, Riepenhoff TM, Ogra PL. Effect of malnutrition on rotavirus infection in suckling mice: kinetics of early infection. *Proc Soc Exp Biol Med* 1985;178(1):85–90.

190. Riepenhoff TM, Offor E, Klossner K, Kowalski E, Carmody PJ, Ogra PL. Effect of age and malnutrition on rotavirus infection in mice. *Pediatr Res* 1985;19(12):1250–1253.

191. Riepenhoff TM, Uhnoo I, Chegas P, Ogra PL. Effect of nutritional deprivation on mucosal viral infections. *Immunol Invest* 1989;18(1–4):127–139.
192. Ahmed F, Jones DB, Jackson AA. The interaction of vitamin A deficiency and rotavirus infection in the mouse. *Br J Nutr* 1990;63(2):363–373.
193. Ahmed F, Jones DB, Jackson AA. Effect of vitamin A deficiency on the immune response to epizootic diarrhoea of infant mice (EDIM) rotavirus infection in mice. *Br J Nutr* 1991;65(3):475–485.
194. Uhnoo IS, Freihorst J, Riepenhoff TM, Fisher JE, Ogra PL. Effect of rotavirus infection and malnutrition on uptake of a dietary antigen in the intestine. *Pediatr Res* 1990;27(2):153–160.
195. Pichichero ME, Losonsky GA, Rennels MB, et al. Effect of dose and a comparison of measures of vaccine take for oral rhesus rotavirus vaccine. The Maryland Clinical Studies Group. *Pediatr Infect Dis J* 1990;9(5):339–344.
196. Ing DJ, Glass RI, Woods PA, et al. Immunogenicity of tetravalent rhesus rotavirus vaccine administered with buffer and oral polio vaccine. *Am J Dis Child* 1991;145(8):892–897.
197. Duffy LC, Riepenhoff TM, Byers TE, et al. Modulation of rotavirus enteritis during breast-feeding. Implications on alterations in the intestinal bacterial flora. *Am J Dis Child* 1986;140(11):1164–1168.
198. Heyman M, Corthier G, Petit A, Meslin JC, Moreau C, Desjeux JF. Intestinal absorption of macromolecules during viral enteritis: an experimental study on rotavirus-infected conventional and germ-free mice. *Pediatr Res* 1987;22(1):72–78.
199. Stiglmair HM, Pospischil A, Hess RG, Bachmann PA, Baljer G. Enzyme histochemistry of the small intestinal mucosa in experimental infections of calves with rotavirus and enterotoxigenic *Escherichia coli*. *Vet Pathol* 1986;23(2):125–131.
200. Tzipori S, Chandler D, Smith M. The clinical manifestation and pathogenesis of enteritis associated with rotavirus and enterotoxigenic *Escherichia coli* infections in domestic animals. *Prog Food Nutr Sci* 1983;7(3–4):193–205.
201. Pickering LK, O'Ryan M. Serotypes of rotavirus that infect infants symptomatically and asymptomatically. *Adv Exp Med Biol* 1991;310:241–247.
202. Abiodun PO, Ihongbe JC, Ogbimi A. Asymptomatic rotavirus infection in Nigerian day-care centres. *Ann Trop Paediatr* 1985;5(3):163–165.
203. Araya M, Figueroa G, Espinoza J, Zarur X, Brunser O. Acute diarrhoea and asymptomatic infection in Chilean preschoolers of low and high socio-economic strata. *Acta Paediatr Scand* 1986;75(4):645–651.
204. Barron RB, Barreda GJ, Doval UR, Zermeno ELJ, Huerta PM. Asymptomatic rotavirus infections in day care centers. *J Clin Microbiol* 1985;22(1):116–118.
205. Champsaur H, Henry AM, Goldszmidt D, et al. Rotavirus carriage, asymptomatic infection, and disease in the first two years of life. II. Serological response. *J Infect Dis* 1984;149(5):675–682.
206. Eiden JJ, Verleur DG, Vonderfecht SL, Yolken RH. Duration and pattern of asymptomatic rotavirus shedding by hospitalized children. *Pediatr Infect Dis J* 1988;7(8):564–569.
207. Losonsky GA, Reymann M. The immune response in primary asymptomatic and symptomatic rotavirus infection in newborn infants. *J Infect Dis* 1990;161(2):330–332.
208. Walther FJ, Bruggeman C, Daniels BM, et al. Symptomatic and asymptomatic rotavirus infections in hospitalized children. *Acta Paediatr Scand* 1983;72(5):659–663.
209. Rodriguez WJ, Kim HW, Brandt CD, et al. Fecal adenoviruses from a longitudinal study of families in metropolitan Washington, D.C.: laboratory, clinical, and epidemiologic observations. *J Pediatr* 1985;107(4):514–520.
210. Geme JS, Hyman D. Hepatic injury during rotavirus infections. *J Pediatr* 1988;113(5):952–953.
211. Carlson JAK, Middleton PJ, Shaw RD, Petric M. Fatal rotavirus gastroenteritis. An analysis of 22 cases. *Am J Dis Child* 1978;132:477–479.
212. Rotbart HA, Levin MJ, Yolken RH, Manchester DK, Jantzen J. An outbreak of rotavirus-associated neonatal necrotizing enterocolitis. *J Pediatr* 1983;103(3):454–459.
213. Rotbart HA, Nelson WL, Glode MP, et al. Neonatal rotavirus-associated necrotizing enterocolitis: case control study and prospective surveillance during an outbreak. *J Pediatr* 1988;112(1):87–93.
214. Keller KM, Schmidt H, Wirth S, Queisser LA, Schumacher R. Differences in the clinical and radiologic patterns of rotavirus and non-rotavirus necrotizing enterocolitis. *Pediatr Infect Dis J* 1991;10(10):734–738.
215. Christy C, Vosefski D, Madore HP. Comparison of three enzyme immunoassays to tissue culture for the diagnosis of rotavirus gastroenteritis in infants and young children. *J Clin Microbiol* 1990;28(6):1428–1430.
216. Yolken RH, Leggiadro RJ. Immunoassays for the diagnosis of viral enteric pathogens. *Diagn Microbiol Infect Dis* 1986;4(suppl. 3):S61–S69.
217. Honma H, Ushijimma H, Takagi M, Kitamiura T. Evaluation of a new enzyme immunoassay (TESTPACK ROTAVIRUS) for diagnosis of viral gastroenteritis. *Kansenshogaku Zasshi* 1990;64(2):174–178.
218. Chernesky M, Castriciano S, Mahony J, DeLong D. Examination of the Rotazyme II enzyme immunoassay for the diagnosis of rotavirus gastroenteritis. *J Clin Microbiol* 1985;22(3):462–464.
219. Herring AJ, Inglis NF, Ojeh CK, Snodgrass DR, Menzies JD. Rapid diagnosis of rotavirus infection by direct detection of viral nucleic acid in silver-stained polyacrylamide gels. *J Clin Microbiol* 1982;16(3):473–477.
220. Avendano LF, Dubinovsky S, James HJ. Comparison of viral RNA electrophoresis and indirect ELISA methods in the diagnosis of human rotavirus infection. *Bull Pan Am Health Organ* 1984;18(3):245–249.
221. Chudzio T, Kasatiya S, Irvine N, Sankar MP. Rapid screening test for the diagnosis of rotavirus infection. *J Clin Microbiol* 1989;27(10):2394–2396.
222. Flores J, Green KY, Garcia D, et al. Dot hybridization assay for distinction of rotavirus serotypes. *J Clin Microbiol* 1989;27(1):29–34.
223. Flores J, Sears J, Schael IP, et al. Identification of human rotavirus serotype by hybridization to polymerase chain reaction-generated probes derived from a hyperdivergent region of the gene encoding outer capsid protein VP7. *J Virol* 1990;64(8):4021–4024.
224. Fernandez J, Sandino A, Yudelevich A, et al. Rotavirus detection by dot blot hybridization assay using a non-radioactive synthetic oligodeoxynucleotide probe. *Epidemiol Infect* 1992;108(1):175–184.
225. Sack DA, Chodhury AMAK, Eusof A, et al. Oral rehydration in rotavirus diarrhea: a double blind comparison of sucrose with glucose electrolyte solution. *Lancet* 1978;2:280–283.
226. Marin L, Gunoz H, Sokucu S, et al. Oral rehydration therapy in malnourished infants with infectious diarrhoea. *Acta Paediatr Scand* 1986;75(3):477–482.
227. Sokucu S, Marin L, Gunoz H, Aperia A, Neyzi O, Zetterstrom R. Oral rehydration therapy in infectious diarrhoea. Comparison of rehydration solutions with 60 and 90 mmol sodium per litre. *Acta Paediatr Scand* 1985;74(4):489–494.
228. Farthing MJ. History and rationale of oral rehydration and recent developments in formulating an optimal solution. *Drugs* 1988;8:16–21.
229. Sazawal S, Bhatnagar S, Bhan MK, et al. Alanine-based oral rehydration solution: assessment of efficacy in acute noncholera diarrhea among children. *J Pediatr Gastroenterol Nutr* 1991;12(4):461–468.
230. Rhoads JM, Keku EO, Quinn J, Woosely J, Lecce JG. L-Glutamine stimulates jejunal sodium and chloride absorption in pig rotavirus enteritis. *Gastroenterology* 1991;100(3):683–691.
231. Khin MU, Myo K, Nyunt NW, Mu MK, Mya T, Thein TM. Comparison of glucose/electrolyte and maltodextrin/glycine/glycyl-glycine/electrolyte oral rehydration solutions in acute diarrhea in children. *J Pediatr Gastroenterol Nutr* 1991;13(4):397–401.

232. Farthing MJ. Studies of oral rehydration solutions in animal models. *Clin Ther* 1990;23:72–81.

233. Bhan MK, Sazawal S, Bhatnagar S, Bhandari N, Guha DK, Aggarwal SK. Glycine, glycyl-glycine and maltodextrin based oral rehydration solution. Assessment of efficacy and safety in comparison to standard ORS. *Acta Paediatr Scand* 1990;79(5):518–526.

234. Santosham M, Burns BA, Reid R, et al. Glycine-based oral rehydration solution: reassessment of safety and efficacy. *J Pediatr* 1986;109(5):795–801.

235. Hjelt K, Paerregaard A, Petersen W, Christiansen L, Krasilnikoff PA. Rapid versus gradual refeeding in acute gastroenteritis in childhood: energy intake and weight gain. *J Pediatr Gastroenterol Nutr* 1989;8(1):75–80.

236. Armitstead J, Kelly D, Walker-Smith J. Evaluation of infant feeding in acute gastroenteritis. *J Pediatr Gastroenterol Nutr* 1989;8(2):240–244.

237. Quak SH, Low PS, Quah TC, Teo J. Oral refeeding following acute gastro-enteritis: a clinical trial using four refeeding regimes. *Ann Trop Paediatr* 1989;9(3):152–155.

238. Haffejee IE. Cow's milk-based formula, human milk, and soya feeds in acute infantile diarrhea: a therapeutic trial. *J Pediatr Gastroenterol Nutr* 1990;10(2):193–198.

239. Brussow H, Hilpert H, Walther I, Sidoti J, Mietens C, Bachmann P. Bovine milk immunoglobulins for passive immunity to infantile rotavirus gastroenteritis. *J Clin Microbiol* 1987;25(6):982–986.

240. Hilpert H, Brussow H, Mietens C, Sidoti J, Lerner L, Werchau H. Use of bovine milk concentrate containing antibody to rotavirus to treat rotavirus gastroenteritis in infants. *J Infect Dis* 1987;156(1):158–166.

241. Guarino A, Guandalini S, Albano F, Mascia A, De Ritig G, Rubino A. Enteral immunoglobulins for treatment of protracted rotaviral diarrhea. *Pediatr Infect Dis J* 1991;10(8):612–614.

242. Schwartz RH, Rodriquez WJ. Toxic delirium possibly caused by loperamide. *J Pediatr* 1991;118(4 Pt 1):656–657.

243. Minton NA, Henry JA. Loperamide poisoning in children. *Lancet* 1990;335(8692):788.

244. Bhutta TI, Tahir KI. Loperamide poisoning in children. *Lancet* 1990;335(8685):363.

245. Kassaem AS, Madkour AB, Massoub BS, Mehanna ZB. Loperamide in acute childhood diarrhea. *J Diarrhoeal Dis Res* 1983;1:10–16.

246. Owens JR, Broadhead R, Hendrickse RG, Jaswal OP, Gangal RN. Loperamide in the treatment of acute gastroenteritis in children: report on a two centre double-blind controlled clinical trial. *Ann Trop Paediatr* 1981;1:135–141.

247. World Health Organization (WHO). *The rational use of drugs in the management of acute diarrhea in children.* Geneva: WHO, 1990.

248. De Clercq E, Bergstrom DE, Holy A, Montgomery JA. Broad-spectrum antiviral activity of adenosine analogues. *Antiviral Res* 1984;4(3):119–133.

249. De Clercq E, Cools M, Balzarini J, et al. Broad-spectrum antiviral activities of neplanocin A, 3-deazaneplanocin A, and their 5'-nor derivatives. *Antimicrob Agents Chemother* 1989;33(8):1291–1297.

250. Kitaoka S, Konno T, De Clerq E. Comparative efficacy of broad-spectrum antiviral agents as inhibitors of rotavirus replication in vitro. *Antiviral Res* 1986;6(1):57–65.

251. Linhares RE, Wigg MD, Lagrota MH, Nozawa CM. The in vitro antiviral activity of isoprinosine on simian rotavirus (SA-11). *Braz J Med Biol Res* 1989;22(9):1095–1103.

252. Ebina T, Tsukada K. Protease inhibitors prevent the development of human rotavirus-induced diarrhea in suckling mice. *Microbiol Immunol* 1991;35(7):583–588.

253. Vonderfecht SL, Miskuff RL, Wee SB, et al. Protease inhibitors suppress the in vitro and in vivo replication of rotavirus. *J Clin Invest* 1988;82(6):2011–2016.

Infections of the Gastrointestinal Tract,
edited by M. J. Blaser, P. D. Smith, J. I. Ravdin,
H. B. Greenberg, and R. L. Guerrant
Published by Raven Press, Ltd., New York, 1995.

CHAPTER 65

Group B and C Rotaviruses

Erich R. Mackow

Group A rotaviruses are the most common cause of diarrheal disease in infants and young children. However, the identification of genetically and antigenically distinct human group B and C rotaviruses has stimulated interest in their contribution to diarrheal disease in various populations. Group C rotaviruses, like group A strains, cause diarrhea in young children age 4 months to 4 years. Recent reports implicate group C rotaviruses as the cause of clinical disease primarily in older children (older than 4 years) and in some adults (1). Recently, group C rotaviruses have been identified as the causative agents of foodborne institutional diarrheal outbreaks in Japanese and British elementary schools (2–4).

In contrast to other human rotaviruses, group B rotaviruses are responsible for predominantly adult diarrheal disease (5,6). Group B rotaviruses were first identified as the cause of human disease in 1983 (5). At that time a group B rotavirus named adult diarrheal rotavirus (ADRV) was identified as the causative agent of severe "cholera-like" diarrheal outbreaks in large portions (5% to 45%) of the rural Chinese population (5–10). Contamination of water supplies during the outbreaks suggest that ADRV was introduced via drinking water. Outbreaks of ADRV-induced diarrhea have continued to appear in China but have not been widely encountered elsewhere. There is only one report of a group B rotavirus outbreak in the United States (11). However, recent epidemiologic studies suggest that approximately 5% of the U.S. population is seropositive for ADRV and all those identified are adults (12). The presence of human group B rotavirus antibodies has also been documented in other parts of the world including Japan, Thailand, Mexico, Australia, and the United Kingdom, suggesting that ADRV may be a more widespread cause of adult diarrhea than previously estimated (8,9,13–17).

One caveat to the infrequent detection of both group B and C rotaviruses is that standardized diagnostic assays for these viruses are not yet widely available. The rota-zyme assay is the only available clinical diagnostic assay for rotavirus and this assay detects exclusively group A strains. Another consideration for the infrequent detection of these viruses is that adults rarely report diarrheal incidents. Recent progress on the study of group B and C rotavirus strains promises the development of clinical diagnostic tests for these viruses in the near future.

Rotaviruses from groups A, B, and C cause disease in both human and animal populations (5,7,11,18–47). In animals, rotavirus infections are endemic and provide a reservoir of virus for potential human infections. Further suggesting the potential for zoonotic infections in humans is the fact that U.S. pigs are 70% to 99% seropositive for groups A, B, and C rotaviruses (14). Additionally, rotaviruses contain a segmented ribonucleic acid (RNA) genome and individual gene segments can be reassorted upon mixed infection (48). Segmented viruses like influenza and rotavirus permit for rapid genetic shifts and, as a result, the potential for rapid development of new viral strains with altered host range restrictions and virulence characteristics. One possibility for the recent outbreaks of human group B rotavirus disease in China is the reassortment of normally benign human viruses to new, more virulent, strains. Alternatively, the reassortment or genetic drift of zoonotic group B rotaviruses may have altered viral host ranges to include humans.

Studies of group B and C rotaviruses in human populations are only beginning to shed light on their contributions to diarrheal disease. The role of group B and C rotavirus strains in worldwide human disease should soon unfold with the implementation of newly developing diagnostic tests, the recent cultivation of group C strains, and the increasing use of recombinant DNA techniques to study the viruses.

HISTORY

Atypical Rotaviruses

Historically, rotaviruses were identified by their electron microscopic morphology and by their genetic content

E. R. Mackow: Departments of Medicine and Microbiology, SUNY at Stony Brook, Stony Brook, New York and Northport VA Medical Center, Northport, New York 11768.

of 11 double-stranded RNA (dsRNA) segments (49,50). Rotaviruses that were antigenically distinct or contained a unique electrophoretic pattern of dsRNA segments were referred to as atypical rotavirus strains, pararotaviruses, novel rotaviruses, or rotavirus-like viruses, since they differed from the predominantly encountered group A rotavirus strains (5,20,31,44,47,51–62). In 1983, Pedley et al. (56) proposed the classification of rotaviruses into serologically related groups A, B, and C. In 1984 avian serogroup D was defined and in 1986 serogroup E rotaviruses were identified (57). With more specific serogroup definitions, still more rotavirus groups were identified by their antigenic similarity to other rotavirus strains. Antigenically distinct rotavirus groups A to G have now been defined (63,64). Each group is also genetically distinct and gene reassortment, which occurs between rotavirus strains of the same group, has not been observed to occur between strains of different groups (65).

Among rotavirus groups, only group A, B, and C strains have been identified as clinical pathogens in humans (5,16,49,50,52,62,66). However, there are recent reports of new human rotavirus isolates that are not from serogroups A, B, C, or D and have unique electrophoretic patterns. These viruses may define new serogroups that cause human disease.

ADRV

A group B rotavirus was first identified as a human pathogen in 1983 following epidemic outbreaks of severe dehydrating diarrhea in the Chinese population (5–7). Interestingly, these outbreaks primarily occurred in individuals age 15 and older with the highest infection rate occurring in individuals over age 30 (1.6% to 2.3%) (8–10). Of those infected, 85% were over 15 years of age and only 2.8% were 0 to 4 years of age (8). As a result, the rotavirus agent was dubbed the adult diarrheal rotavirus or ADRV. Initially, ADRV was referred to as "rotavirus-like" or "novel" because its morphology resembled other rotavirus strains, it lacked serologic cross-reactivity with group A and C rotavirus strains, and it contained a unique dsRNA electrophoretic pattern (5). It was later confirmed to be antigenically related to group B rotavirus strains (7). Another epidemic outbreak of ADRV occurred in 1987 in China and reports of continued sporadic ADRV outbreaks in China have persisted since then (8,9,67).

IDIR

In 1984 a group B rotavirus was detected as the cause of infectious diarrhea of infant rats (IDIR) (47). This virus caused the formation of syncytia in the villous epithelium of the infected animals, which contained 80-nm rotavirus-like particles (47). The viral dsRNAs were distinct from group A strains and were later demonstrated to be antigenically related to group B rotaviruses (47,68). The RNA electrophoretic pattern of IDIR is not identical to ADRV but they are similar. The two viruses have since been found to be related both antigenically and genetically (68).

IDIR and ADRV are also able to fuse cells forming multinucleate syncytia in the infected cell monolayer (47,69). Syncytia are hallmarks of group B rotavirus strains and absent from all other rotaviruses (21,31,47,51,61,69,70).

There is one report of a rat group B rotavirus infecting humans (11). In 1985 IDIR infections were reported during an analysis of non-group A rotavirus infections of children and adults in Baltimore, Maryland. Six fecal specimens from three children and three adults were able to confer IDIR infections to rats (11). Since the three adults were physicians at the same hospital and one physician worked with IDIR-infected rats, there is some question as to whether the virus was inadvertently introduced into others by contact or whether the children were the source of the virus (71). Of the three children infected, one was a child of one of the doctors, one was admitted with diarrhea, and one developed diarrhea after admission (11). Regardless of the source of the inoculum, this study indicates the ability of IDIR to infect humans and that it is a potential source of human disease.

Group C Rotavirus

Group C rotaviruses were originally referred to as pararotaviruses for their similarity to typical group A rotavirus strains (55,72). The first report of human pararotaviruses appeared in 1982 in the infection of an infant in Australia (38). Two additional reports of human group C rotaviruses in Brazil and France also appeared in 1983 (55,58). In each case a single infant was infected with a group C rotavirus. Since then many clinical diarrheal cases of infants and adults have been attributed to group C rotavirus infections (1,3,4,22,52,54,66,73–82). In contrast to other rotaviruses, group C rotavirus infections have only been reported in humans and pigs. A high percentage of pigs are seropositive in both North America and the United Kingdom (13,39).

Human group C rotavirus infections have now been reported in Argentina, Australia, Brazil, Bulgaria, Chile, China, Ecuador, England, Finland, France, Germany, India, Italy, Japan, Mexico, Nepal, South Africa, and Thailand (1,3,4,22,38,52,54,55,58,66,73–85). Recent epidemic outbreaks of group C rotavirus infections were reported in both England and Japan in 1989 (2,81). In each case large numbers of school children became ill, with vomiting being the primary symptom of the infection. In the Japanese outbreak both children and adults were infected (ages 7 to 54) and the outbreak included 22% (675 children) of the elementary school students (81). In the British outbreak, 28 of 130 school children, 4 to 10 years of age, became ill (2). In both outbreaks a school lunch was a common factor. The Japanese outbreak involved seven separate schools, which were served by a common regional food preparation service, although the cause of the outbreak was not linked to a common food source. Others have also indicated that group C rotavirus infections occur in adults and children and that group C infections are the most common cause of gastroenteritis in children between 4 and 7 years of age (1).

CLASSIFICATION AND VIRAL STRUCTURE

Rotaviruses are members of the family Reoviridae by virtue of their icosahedral double-protein capsid structure and the presence of a segmented dsRNA genome. Complete rotavirus particles are approximately 70 nm in diameter and indistinguishable from group A rotaviruses by electron microscopy (EM) (63,86–88). Rotaviruses are not enveloped, and, as a result, they are resistant to lipid solvents (89). The IDIR group B rotavirus is reported to be labile at pH 3 but stable to ether or pH 5 (47). ADRV viral particles are reported to be 70 nm in diameter (5,7,8,90); however, more often than not, ADRV virions are found as degraded 45- to 52-nm viral core-like particles (8,91). ADRV is also reported to be more stable at 4°C than at $-20°C$ (8).

Treatment of viral particles with calcium chelators, ethyleneglycol tetraacetic acid (EGTA) or ethylenediamine tetraacetic acid (EDTA), results in the production of single-shelled particles approximately 55 nm in diameter and activates the viral transcriptase (92). Core-like particles of 48 to 52 nm are predominant in ADRV preparations, although at least part of this finding may be attributable to preparative treatments of the virus for EM. Group C rotaviruses are reported to be insensitive to 1.5 M $CaCl_2$ treatments, which disrupt double-shelled group A rotavirus particles (93).

All Reoviridae are transcriptionally active and contain a dsRNA-dependent RNA polymerase within their viral cores (63). The RNA polymerase complex synthesizes capped but not polyadenylated mRNAs, which exit pores in the single-shelled virus particle into the cell's cytoplasm. Virus replication is fully cytoplasmic and genomic dsRNAs are synthesized within replicase particles, which include the viral proteins VP1, VP2, and VP3 and 11 single-stranded template RNAs (63).

SEROGROUPS

Rotaviruses are distinguished serologically into groups A to G (64). Viruses from a single rotavirus group are antigenically unique and are not recognized by infection serum from other rotavirus groups. Cross-reactive epitopes present on the major inner capsid protein, VP6, are primarily involved in differentiating rotavirus groups and subgroups since this highly antigenic protein comprises approximately 50% of the viruses mass (63,94–97). The VP6 protein is also the target of most diagnostic virus and serum antibody detection assays. Although tests for the group specificity of rotaviruses have been used for many years in research laboratories, the wide availability of standardized tests for group B and C rotaviruses is just beginning. Newly developed group B and C diagnostic assays have been reported using recombinant VP6 proteins and monoclonal antibodies (MABs) to the VP6 antigen (12,98–106). These tests should offer the same rapid diagnostic testing currently available for group A rotaviruses.

GROUP B AND C ROTAVIRUS SEROTYPES

Two proteins of the rotavirus outer capsid have been shown to be involved in neutralization specificity. The VP4 and VP7 proteins of the outer capsid are recognized by antibodies that neutralize rotaviruses (63,107–110). Within each rotavirus group are a variety of different interactive VP4 and VP7 neutralization antigens, which form the basis of rotavirus serotypes (64,111,112). Infection sera from viruses of the same serotype are able to prevent or neutralize the infectivity of each other. Within group A rotaviruses, serotyping nomenclature has been developed based on these two proteins. The VP4 protein, which is proteolytically cleaved, defines the P serotype of the virus and the VP7 glycoprotein defines the G serotype (107,108,113–115).

Serotypes have not been defined for group B rotavirus strains largely due to the inability to cultivate these viruses and as a result develop neutralization tests. The ability of antibodies to the ADRV VP4 protein to neutralize ADRV has recently been demonstrated using a focus reduction neutralization (FRN) test in a transient infection assay (69). This initial neutralization assay demonstrates that the VP4 protein plays a role in viral neutralization and that at least one P type exists for group B strains. However, multiple group B rotavirus P types are likely to exist because of the low level of identical amino acids between the VP4 proteins of ADRV and IDIR (58%) (116,117) and due to the the low level of antibody cross-reactivity between the VP4 proteins of ADRV, IDIR, and a porcine strain, SRV-1 (116,118; E. R. Mackow, *unpublished data*).

The serotypic diversity of the VP7 protein of group B strains has not been investigated but is likely to turn up multiple serotypes similar to that of group A rotaviruses. The low level of homology between the IDIR and ADRV VP7 proteins (52% identical amino acids) (119,120) is much less than the 85% homology of group A VP7 proteins, which define different serotypes (121). The genes encoding the VP4 and VP7 proteins of ADRV and IDIR strains have recently been cloned and expressed (116,117,119,120). These reagents will provide investigators the means to study the serotypic diversity of group B rotaviruses.

It now appears that more than one ADRV isolate has been derived from the outbreaks in China (5,8,69). At least one ADRV-like virus with a distinct morphological plaquing phenotype has been observed in transient infection assays of tissue culture cells. This small plaque-forming virus, designated ADRV-2, forms syncytia in 48 hr rather than 12 to 18 hr. Interestingly, this isolate came from the outbreak in the northeast Heilongjiang province of China as opposed to ADRV-1, which was derived from the northwest Gansu province. The reduced rate of syncytia formation could be caused by reduced rates of transcription, translation, or viral assembly by these viruses. Alternatively, differences in potential fusion proteins of ADRV-1 and ADRV-2 isolates could account for differences in the rate of cell–cell fusion during syncytia formation. The serotypic relationships of these two human strains have yet to be investigated.

GROUP C SEROTYPES

The serotypic evaluation of group C rotaviruses has also been hampered by the inability to cultivate group C strains. However, this obstacle has recently been overcome and there are now several reports of group C rotaviruses that have been adapted to growth in tissue culture (122–125). In addition, the cloning of human group C rotavirus genes encoding the VP6, VP7, and NS26 proteins have been reported and the VP4 protein has been cloned from animal strains (126–135). With these developments the tools for evaluating the serotypic diversity of human and animal group C rotavirus strains are nearly ready. Initial studies with hyperimmune sera to human (Ehime 86-542) (81), porcine (Cowden) (122), and bovine (Shintoku) (124) strains of group C rotavirus have indicated that at least two different serotypes exist (136). Hyperimmune or convalescent sera to the Ehime strain and two porcine strains are able to neutralize the Cowden group C rotavirus, while they have no effect on the bovine, Shintoku, or porcine, HF, rotavirus strains (136). The human Bristol strain was not tested in this study (3).

Although these studies were not able to consider the two different neutralization antigens on the virus, it is unlikely that there will be only one G or P serotype for group C strains since there are so many different group C isolates and infected species (human, porcine, and bovine) (136). Defining the serotypes that exist in humans and animals will help us to resolve the source of human infections and to devise preventative measures for group C rotaviruses.

ELECTROPHEROTYPES

Group B and C rotaviruses each have unique electrophoretic RNA profiles from group A rotavirus strains (Fig. 1). Each virus contains 11 dsRNA segments in its genome; however, the length of the gene segments and their migration by neutral polyacrylamide gel electrophoresis (PAGE) vary between groups (13,75,137). The gel electrophoretic migration of the genes is a characteristic of the virus and is also similar within rotavirus groups. Because of this the electrophoretic profile of dsRNAs or

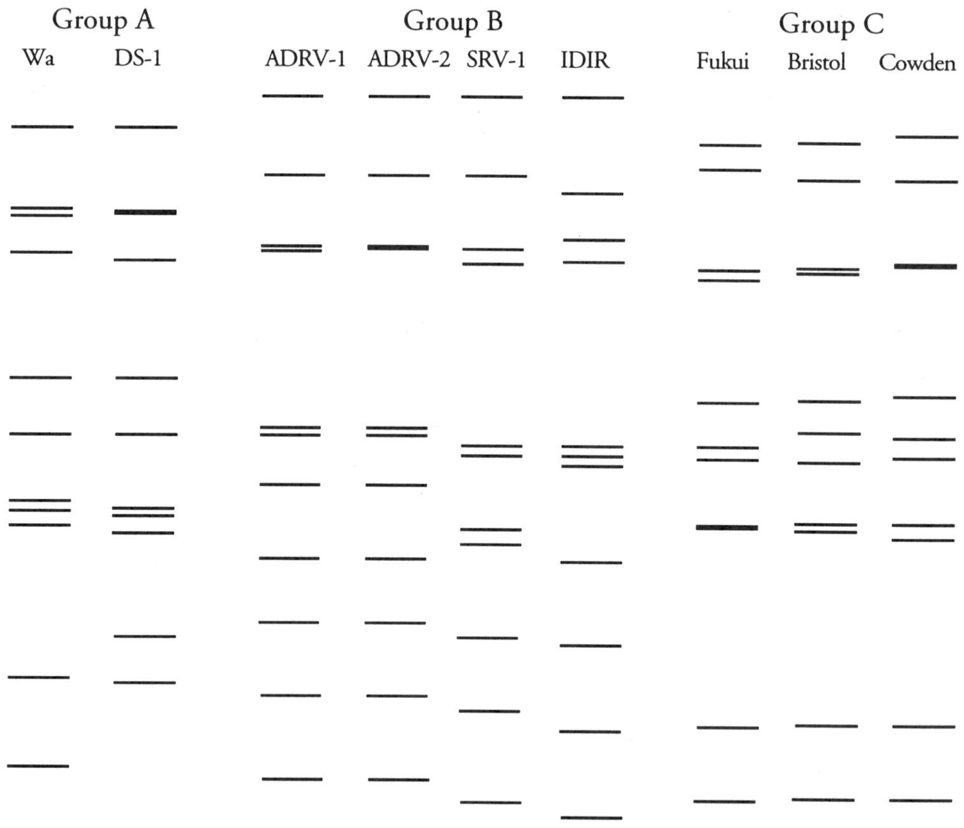

FIG. 1. Electropherotypes of group A, B, and C rotaviruses. Genomic dsRNA is extracted from rotavirus isolates and separated by 7.5% to 12% polyacrylamide gel electrophoresis (PAGE) under neutral conditions. Gels are fixed and silver stained in order to visualize dsRNA segments. This figure diagrammatically represents the position of dsRNA segments separated from human group A, B, and C rotaviruses by PAGE. All strains listed are human rotaviruses except for the IDIR, rat group B rotavirus strain, and the Cowden, porcine group C rotavirus. dsRNA patterns are referred to as "electropherotypes" since patterns are fingerprints of individual viruses and often can be used to designate their group specificity.

their "electropherotype" has been used to characterize strains and to preliminarily specify their rotavirus group (138–141). However, as described below, substantial nucleic acid sequence differences between viruses of the same group may not result in changes in gene migration patterns and therefore electropherotyping patterns of viruses are not definitive determinants of viral groups.

Group A genes fall into four size classes from top to bottom of the gel in a pattern 4-2-3-2. Group B and C rotaviruses also contain several patterns of gene segments with common elements. ADRV is a 4-2-1-1-1-1-1 pattern, IDIR is 4-3-1-1-1-1, while bovine and porcine group B rotaviruses have a pattern of 4-2-2-3. Common elements are the four large RNA segments and the equal distribution of the smallest three gene segments with variation occurring in gene segments 5 to 8. Group C rotaviruses have a 4-3-2-2 pattern (13,39).

The gross electropherotyping patterns of rotaviruses also contain subtle differences between rotavirus groups. Within the four largest gene segments of groups A, B, and C rotaviruses, there are unique electrophoretic patterns. In group A strains, gene segments 2 and 3 are usually close together in contrast to group B strains, where gene segments 3 and 4 comigrate, and group C rotaviruses, which tend to have the four large gene segments more equally distributed. Group B strains also have the largest gene segment 2. Gene segments 5 and 6 of group B strains migrate close together or comigrate in contrast to A or C strains, where these genes are discrete. In addition, the size of dsRNA gene segment pairs and triplets are specific to each rotavirus group. Most rotaviruses can tentatively be classified by their electropherotype, although final serogrouping is dependent on serologic testing.

Variations in the electropherotype of rotaviruses often reflect minor changes in the RNA, which affect their migration on the gel. These changes may not reflect antigenic differences between viruses and/or differences in the size of the RNA segments. Most notable in this respect is the variable migration of group A gene segments 7 to 9. Nearly all these gene segments are the same length and the apparant differences in their electrophoretic mobility are only the result of sequence-induced differences, which change the migration of their RNA segments on PAGE. Another example of this migrational anomaly is the apparent sizes of gene segments 5 and 6 of ADRV. Sequencing full-length clones of these segments has revealed that gene 6 is actually 7 bases longer than gene 5, even though gene 6 migrates below that of gene 5 on electropherotyping gels and therefore appears smaller (142). Numbering of electrophoretically separated RNAs rather than their sequence length has conventionally been used in the naming of Reoviridae RNA segments.

During ADRV outbreaks in different parts of China, a variety of group B isolates were compared electrophoretically (8,9). These isolates were mostly identical by electropherotype but slight variations in genome profiles were detected (Fig. 1). In the two most distant outbreaks in Lanzhou and Jinzhou, China, 1100 miles apart, electrophoretic RNA profiles were very similar but oligonucleotide mapping of the RNA segments suggested substantial differences in these viruses (8,9). As described earlier, viruses from Jinzhou are now referred to as ADRV-2 since they also differ from ADRV-1 by having a small plaque size phenotype.

HYBRIDIZATION

Hybridization of nucleic acids between rotavirus strains has also been used to define group specificity (68,97,131,132,143–147). In general, RNA from rotaviruses of one group hybridize only to viruses within the group and do not cross-hybridize with those from other rotavirus groups (97,131,132,145,147). This distinction can be used as a way of grouping rotaviruses and has also been used to detect group B strains in a dot blot hybridization format (68,131,145). Group B ADRV cross-hybridizes with both porcine and rat group B strains and does not hybridize with the group A or C strains tested (13,132,145,148). It has been reported that gene segment 1 of groups A and B or A and C rotaviruses hybridize but that probes to group B or C do not cross-hybridize with each other (39).

More recently, recombinant approaches to the study of group A, B, and C rotaviruses have led to the development of gene-specific probes for these viruses. Clones for each RNA segment of the group B ADRV were reported in 1990 as indicated in Fig. 2 (92). Since then, probes for the IDIR and porcine strains have been developed. Virtually all group C rotavirus genes have also been cloned and probes have been made for their detection. Porcine and human group C rotavirus RNA segments are highly conserved by hybridization analysis. The least homologous gene segment reported in group C rotaviruses is the gene segment 7. These new additions to rotavirus detection have also led to rapid progress in viral detection via the polymerase chain reaction (PCR) (149,150). The sensitivity of PCR nucleic acid detection is a dramatic improvement in our ability to identify and type rotaviruses from minute quantities of sample. However, PCR diagnostics are dependent on the identification of absolutely conserved nucleic acid sequences within the highly variable rotavirus RNA genome. Sensitive PCR diagnostics using group-specific conserved nucleic acid sequences should enhance progress in identifying group B and C rotavirus-induced disease.

VIRAL STABILITY

Group C rotaviruses are purified by techniques used for group A rotaviruses (39). However, ADRV is purified by ammonium sulfate (18%) fractionating the virus from specimens (92,151). After resuspending the viral concentrate, ADRV is pelleted through a 20% to 40% sucrose gradient for 2 hr onto a 1.5 g/mL CsCl cushion. Virus at the interface is applied directly to 1.37 g/mL CsCl gradients and banded by isopycnic centrifugation (92). A visible virus band is present at 1.385 g/mL CsCl and harvested by pelleting (47,92).

We have analyzed some parameters affecting the viability of infectious ADRV using the ability of the virus to

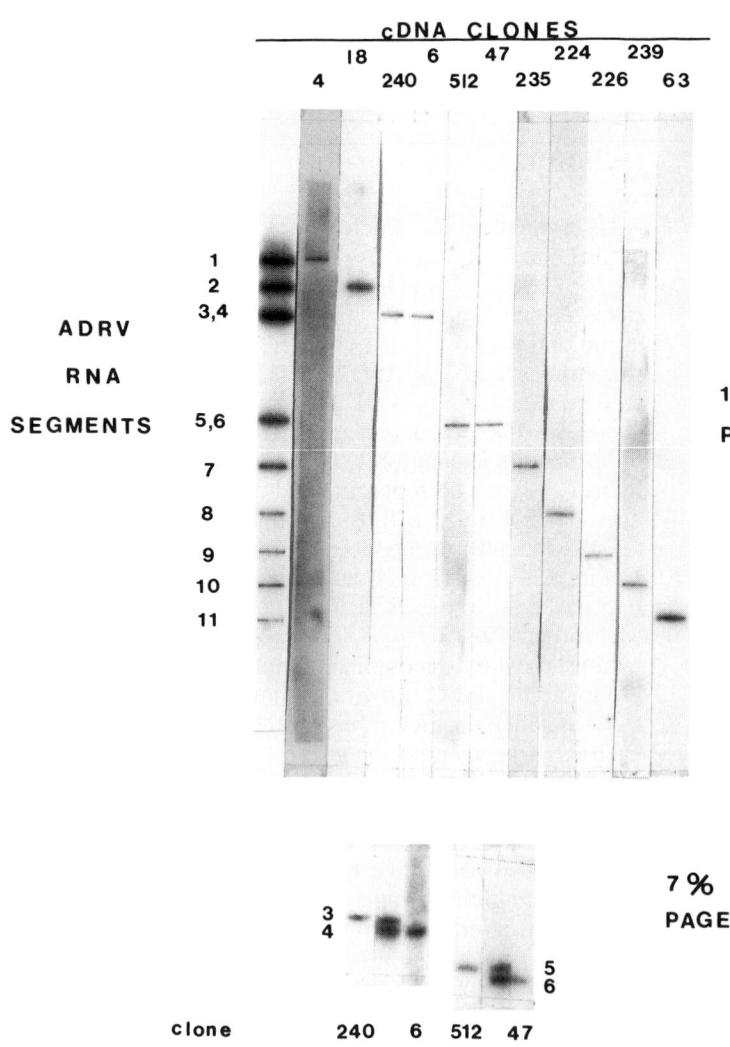

FIG. 2. Hybridization of group B rotavirus clones to ADRV viral dsRNAs. ADRV virion dsRNAs were separated by PAGE and blotted onto nitrocellulose. cDNA clones of ADRV gene segments were used to probe strips of the nitrocellulose blot in order to determine their genetic specificity. RNA segments 3,4 and 5,6, which comigrate on 10% gels, were resolved by 7% PAGE and are shown below. Each clone hybridizes to a single dsRNA segment and is compared to a control hybridization (lane 1) to all 11 segments. Representative clones from each ADRV RNA segment have been identified.

transiently infect Ma104 cells in tissue culture. Interestingly, group A and C rotaviruses are completely resistant to many agents that inactivate ADRV (39,87,89,90). ADRV infectivity is inactivated by many of the manipulations used for purification such as hydrocarbon extraction (trichloro-trifluoroethane, genetron; chloroform; ether) and detergents (deoxycholate, sodium dodecyl sulfate, Triton X-100, Tween 20), and titers appear to be reduced by even brief sonication (E. R. Mackow, *unpublished data*). Trypsin, chymotrypsin, and pancreatin at a variety of concentrations also appear to completely inactivate ADRV for infecting Ma104 cells (E. R. Mackow, *unpublished data*). Calcium chelators EDTA and EGTA, reducing agents, pH < 6, heat (42°C or 50°C), and freezing and thawing all inactivate ADRV as assayed by transient infection of tissue culture cells (69).

GENE STRUCTURE

All rotaviruses contain a genome of 11 dsRNA segments within the core of the virus (49,63). Genomic RNA serves as a template for messenger ribonucleic acid (mRNA) synthesis by the endogenous dsRNA-dependent RNA polymerase present within the core particle (63,152,153). In addition, replication of genomic dsRNA from cytoplasmic mRNAs occurs within replicase particles, which self-assemble in the cytoplasm during infection (154–157).

Rotavirus dsRNAs have short conserved sequences at their 5' and 3' termini (63). Group A, B, and C rotaviruses differ in the sequence of their genomic end-terminal RNAs and these differences may be the prime factor that prevents different rotavirus groups from reassorting gene segments between them (65). The sequence at the ends of nine out of eleven ADRV gene segments have been determined and provide consensus sequences for human group B rotavirus strains (see Fig. 3). There is a substantial sequence difference in many ADRV RNA segments in comparison with reported IDIR end-terminal RNA sequences (158,159), which demonstrates the divergence of these two group B rotavirus strains.

The 5' consensus sequence is extremely short GG(C/U)A and precedes six A or U residues at the beginning

Gene 5'   3'

```
2  GGCAAUUGUCGUGAUGG                                                        GACAUGAUAUUUUAAAAAACCC

4  GGCAAUAUAUUUGCUAUGU                                                      UGCAAAUACAUAUAAAAAACCC
5  GGUUUAAAUAGCCCAACCGGUGAUUCAAGCAUGG                                       AAAAAAUAAGCAAUAAAAACCC
6  GGUAUAAUUAGAUUGUCAGUAUCCAGGUUUGGGAAACCUAUGG                              UACAUAUCUAAAUAAAAAACCC
7  GGUAUAAUUACGUUUGAUUCAGAUAGUACUUCGGGUUACUGAGAAACAAACGUAAUGG                CAACCAAAGUAAUAAAAACCC
8  GGUAGAAAUUAAUCUAUUCAGUGUGUCGUGAGAGGGCUCCAUCACCCUGGUCACCAUGA               UAACGGCUAUUUUUAAAAACCC
9  GGCAAUAAAAUGG                                                           UAGCCGAAGCUGUAAAAACCC
10 GGCAAUUAAAAAGUCCAGUUAUGG                                                 UGAUCAAACUGAUAAGGACCC
11 GGUAUAUAAAAAGUCAGUAGACGGCUGGAAACGUUGCACGUACUACUCACUACCCAGAGAUGG           UGAGUUAUAUUUUAAAAAACCC
```

Consensus

```
        U AAAAAA                                    AAA
5'     GGCAUUUUUU                                  UUUAAAACCC   3'
```

FIG. 3. End-terminal RNA sequences of ADRV. cDNA clones and viral mRNAs were sequenced and the end-terminal sequences of known gene segments are presented. Each 5'- and 3'-terminal RNA sequence maintains a small consensus sequence, which is common to each RNA segment. 5'-Terminal sequences differ widely in the position of their methionine initiation codons, AUG. Gene segment 9 initiates at base 10 from the 5' end and contains the shortest noncoding 5'-terminal sequence.

of each gene segment. A longer region of nine nucleotides are conserved at the 3' end of ADRV gene segments. Only gene segment 10 contains any mismatches with the consensus sequences for the first seven nucleotide residues from the 3' end. The eighth and ninth residues from the 3' end are AU, respectively, in seven out of nine of the ADRV genes. The 3' terminal conservation identified in these genes could represent a mechanism by which viral mRNAs are recognized and assembled into replicase particles prior to negative-strand RNA synthesis or they could be required for polymerase initiation during viral replication. Hairpin structures at the 3' end of RNA segments may also be required to stabilize and prevent the degradation of positive-strand RNAs and/or as gene-specific viral replication signals, which allow the virus to select 11 different RNA segments for replication within viral particles. The 5' end of each gene segment also contains large hairpin structures that extend well into the coding sequences of the viral genes and thus could be used as gene-specific recognition sequences for viral RNA packaging. In addition, the 5' and 3' end-terminal structures can base pair to each other and thus provide gene-specific bilobed cruciform or panhandle structures that could be used for RNA packaging and for initiation of transcription within replicase particles (92).

Group C rotaviruses contain even less conservation at their RNA termini than group B rotaviruses. The 5' sequence 5'-G(GCU)(AC)AU occurs in each gene segment thus sequenced. As in group B rotaviruses the 3' end is more highly conserved than the 5' end having a unique UGUGGCU-3' sequence. The only discrepancy in this sequence is from some sequences that reportedly lack the terminal CU or U residues, although these may represent incomplete end-terminal sequence determinations. Consensus sequences may change as larger numbers of terminal sequences are determined for group C rotavirus genes. To date, group C strains are the only rotaviruses reported to lack CC at their 3' termini.

Transcription

Rotaviruses contain an endogenous transcriptase that permits them to transcribe capped mRNAs either *in vivo* or *in vitro* (152,153,160–162). Virus purification has been used as a means of generating large amounts of viral mRNA. Purified double-shelled viral particles are transcriptionally activated by chelating calcium or by brief heat treatment of the virus or both (142,153,162,163). These treatments result in the dissolution of the outer caspid and produce single-shelled particles that are capable of transcription (63). Single-shelled particles are permeable to buffer and nucleotide triphosphates needed for transcription and at the correct pH the particles synthesize mRNAs, which are extruded from the particle into the cell or test tube (153,162).

Group B and C rotaviruses are activated in roughly the same way as group A strains although each may have slightly different pH or nucleotide concentration optima (142,160,163,164; E. R. Mackow, *unpublished data*). Both group B and C rotaviruses have been used to generate mRNAs in order to amplify virus-specific nucleic acids. Optimized transcription from the ADRV RNA polymerase includes viral activation by a combination of heating at 55°C for 1 min and the presence of 5 mM EGTA (142; E. R. Mackow, *unpublished data*). RNA transcription is maximally active at pH 8.5 and the temperature optimum is 42°C (116,142; E. R. Mackow, *unpublished data*). Transcription is inhibited by magnesium ion concentrations that deviate from 2mM and is optimized in 8 mM rXTPs (E. R. Mackow, *unpublished data*). *In vitro* synthesized mRNAs can be used to *in vitro* express ADRV proteins for the purpose of determining gene coding assignments and for obtaining full-length clones of gene segments (116,142,164,165; E. R. Mackow, *unpublished data*).

Two methods for determining gene coding assignments have been used for ADRV RNA segments

TABLE 1. *ADRV gene coding assignments[a]*

ADRV gene		ADRV protein		Group A rotavirus			
Segment	Length (bases)	Number of amino acids (kDa)	Capsid location if determined	Protein equivalent (kDa)	Group A gene	ADRV equivalency determined by	ADRV protein attributes
1	Incomplete	(?) Incomplete		VP1 (125?)	1	AA alignment	
2	2844	933 (105)	Inner	VP2 (103)	2	AA alignment Viral comp./IgG	GTP binding domain
3	Incomplete	(?) Incomplete		VP3 (88?)	3	AA alignment	
4	2303	749 (84)	Outer	VP4 (86.5)	4	AA alignment Viral comp./IgG	Neutralization, spike Trypsin cleavage sites
5	1269	391 (44)	Inner	VP6 (45)	6	AA alignment Viral comp./IgG	Trimer, hexamer formation
6	1276	107 AAs. (11.7) ORF 40-360	?	None			Fusion, myristoylated AD6F1 frame 1
		321 (37) ORF 257-1219		NS53 (58.5)	5	NBRF FastA	Zinc finger AD6F2 frame 2
7	1179	324 (37.5)		NS34 (36)	7	AA alignment	Acidic
8	1006	279 (32)		NS35 (36.5)	8	AA alignment	Basic
9	814	249 (28.5)	Outer	VP7 (34)	9	AA alignment Viral comp./IgG	Glycosylated to 36 kDa ? Neutralization
10	751	219 (25.4)		NS28 (28)	10	Hydrophilicity and AA comp.	Glycosylated
11	631	170 (20)		NS26 (22)	11	AA alignment	

[a] ADRV gene segments have been cloned and sequenced and are available from Genbank at the following accession numbers: M91433, M91434, M55982, M91435, M91436, M91437, X56143, M33872, and M33873.
AA, amino acid.

(92,116,119,142,165–167). The first method used to determine gene coding assignments is to isolate individual dsRNA from agarose or acrylamide gels, to denature the double strands, which renders them single-stranded, and to translate the single strands in *in vitro* translation reactions (166–168). This method extracts the RNA from large amounts of a rotavirus in order to translate their encoded proteins. It is difficult to use this method for group B strains, which can neither be cultivated in tissue culture nor regenerated from animal infection models. A second caveat is that if gene segments comigrate they cannot be separated well by preparative PAGE. A second way of determining gene coding assignments is to clone individual gene segments, to analyze the nucleic acid and deduced polypeptide sequences, to determine the RNA segment from which the clone is derived, and to express encoded proteins from the complementary deoxyribonucleic acid (cDNA) clones *in vitro* or via baculovirus re-

TABLE 2. *Group C gene coding assignments[a]*

Group C gene		Protein		Group A rotavirus					
Segment	Length (bases)	Number of amino acids (kDa)	Capsid location if determined	Protein equivalent (kDa)	Percentage amino acid identity	Equivalency group A gene	Determined by	Source	Protein attributes
1	3313	1082 (125)		VP1 (125)	48.2	1	Hybridization/AA	Porcine	Polymerase
2	2655	873 (101)	Core	VP2 (103)	43.6	2	Hybridization/AA	Porcine	GTP binding domain
3	2646	736 (83)	Outer	VP4	33.2	4	Hybridization/AA	Porcine	Neutralization, spike
4	2145	692 (81)		VP3	34.5	3	Hybridization/AA	Porcine	
5	1352	395 (44.5)	Inner	VP6	41.3	6	Alignment	Hum/Por/Bov	Major viral antigen
6	1348	402 (39)		NS34	23	7	Alignment	Por/Bov	
7	1235	393 (46.4)		NS53	15	5	Alignment	Porcine	Zinc finger
8	1063	332 (37.3)	Outer	VP7	<30	9	Alignment	Hu/Por	Glycosylation
9	995	312 (35.8)		NS35	37	8	Alignment	Porcine	Basic
10	693	210–212 (923.4)		NS26	16	11	Alignment	Hu/Por/Bov	
11	ND	ND		ND	ND	ND			

[a] Gene segments have been cloned and sequenced and the sequences are available from Genbank at the following accession numbers: L12390, L12391, M29287, M81488, M74216, M74217, M74218, M74219, M88768, M61100, M61101, X60546, X65938, and X65939.
AA, amino acid; ND, not determined.

combinants (116,142,165,166,169–172). The latter technique has the additional advantage of generating a renewable source of viral nucleic acid for further genetic manipulation.

Tables 1 and 2 compile features of ADRV and group C rotavirus genes along with their gene coding assignments and the similarity of their encoded proteins to those of group A rotavirus.

Cloning and Expression of ADRV Genes and Proteins

Molecular Analysis of Group B Strains

Group B rotaviruses have been isolated from humans and from a variety of animals (5–7,19–21,31,44,47,51,53, 70,122,170,173,174). The genes from human (ADRV) and rat (IDIR) group B rotavirus strains have been cloned, sequenced, and expressed (92,98,116,118,119,120,142, 165,171,175–177). ADRV gene segments 2, 4, 5, and 9 encoding structural proteins VP2, VP4, VP6, and VP7 have been expressed via baculovirus recombinants (99,116,118,165,177; E. R. Mackow, *unpublished data*). Baculovirus coexpression of these four structural proteins may produce ADRV-like particles similar to what has been accomplished with expressed structural proteins from bluetongue virus and group A rotaviruses (178–182). The recombinant assembly of group B rotavirus particles may be more useful than for other Reoviridae since they will provide virus-like antigens and immunogens, which cannot be obtained from other sources.

The nucleic acid sequences and encoded polypeptides of group B rotaviruses, IDIR and ADRV, are dramatically different from group A and C rotavirus strains (92,98,116, 118,119,120,142,165,171,175–177). Each ADRV protein contains low-level amino acid identity (18% to 28%) with corresponding group A rotavirus proteins (E. R. Mackow, *unpublished data*). Although group A equivalent proteins are likely to be involved in analogous ADRV functions, very little has been presented to verify the function of group B rotavirus proteins.

Structural Proteins

ADRV gene segments 2, 4, 5, and 9 encode the major structural proteins of the viral capsid (92,116,119, 142,165). Gene segment 5 of ADRV encodes the major inner capsid protein, VP6 (142). The *in vitro* expressed gene 5 polypeptide comigrates with the 44-kD protein present on EDTA-treated, iodinated ADRV virions. The baculovirus-expressed VP6 protein is oligomeric and multimerizes to apparent trimer, hexamer, and greater molecular mass products as assayed by SDS-PAGE (99). Antibodies made to the expressed protein recognize ADRV virions (12,99) and should prove useful as diagnostic reagents.

The ADRV VP6 equivalent protein contains 25% and 20% identical amino acids to the group C and group A

rotavirus VP6 proteins (142). The similarity of these proteins suggests an evolutionary relationship between the three, which distantly relates ADRV to both group A and C rotaviruses and suggests that group B rotaviruses are more closely related to group C rotaviruses (142).

The ADRV (gene 5) and IDIR (gene 6) VP6 encoding genes and proteins are highly related (142,175). IDIR and ADRV genes contain 73% identical nucleic acid sequences. Cloned IDIR and porcine group B genes encoding the VP6 protein have permitted amino acid comparisons of three group B rotavirus VP6 proteins (142,175; E. R. Mackow, *unpublished data*). Sequence comparisons indicate that these proteins share about 80% to 84% identical and 92% to 95% similar VP6 amino acids. This is the most homology among IDIR and ADRV proteins compared thus far. The similarity between group B VP6 proteins can be used as a reference point for the dramatic divergence of outer capsid proteins VP4 and VP7 discussed later.

The baculovirus-expressed VP6 protein can be used as a reagent for ADRV detection and for seroprevalence studies of human populations (12,118). The ADRV VP6 equivalent protein is recognized by hyperimmune serum to ADRV or the porcine group B rotavirus, human ADRV convalescent serum from Chinese or U.S. adults, by group B-specific monoclonal antibodies, and by some but not all IDIR-specific antibodies (8,12,99,142,177,183; E. R. Mackow, *unpublished data*). The group B VP6 protein is not recognized by group A hyperimmune sera. This is a predictable finding since VP6 is the predominant antigen confering serogroup specificity to rotaviruses. The baculovirus-expressed VP6 protein promises to provide better reagents for ADRV detection and for seroprevalence studies of human populations (12).

Gene segment 2 of ADRV encodes a single 105-kDa protein that is similar to the group A rotavirus VP2 protein and present in the viral core (165). The gene 2 protein has been expressed both *in vitro* and in baculovirus and the expressed protein has the same molecular mass as a 105-kDa protein present on single-shelled ADRV virions. The protein is recognized by anti-ADRV hyperimmune and convalescent serum and does not cross-react with group A rotavirus sera (165).

Although expression of the VP2 protein of group A strains results in the formation of core-like particles, similar structures have not yet been identified for the baculovirus expressed ADRV VP2 protein (165). ADRV VP2 assembled core-like particles have not been identified by sucrose density centrifugation, by electron microscopy, or by mobility shifts of the protein analyzed by PAGE under varying conditions (165; E. R. Mackow, *unpublished data*). However, it is still possible that the conditions for self-assembly of expressed VP2 into ADRV cores have not been determined. Alternatively, the ADRV VP2 protein may require other viral structural proteins for assembly.

Viral Glycoprotein

The *gene 9*-encoded protein shares similar amino acids throughout its length (48% similarity, 28% identity) with the group A rotavirus outer capsid protein VP7 (119,184–186). The gene 9-encoded protein contains three potential N-linked glycosylation sites and an amino-terminal signal sequence that could be used to translocate the protein into the lumen of the endoplasmic reticulum (ER) or associate it with plasma membranes (119). Interestingly, early observations of intracellular group B rotaviruses suggest that they are associated with smooth ER membranes in contrast to the rough ER association of group A rotavirus particles (70). It is unknown if VP7 protein translocation, viral budding through the ER, or both are specific to smooth ER membranes in group B rotaviruses; however, this could represent a fundamental difference in group B rotavirus assembly.

The gene 9-encoded protein also contains a conserved A/Q cleavage site, which is used in group A rotavirus strains to cleave the amino-terminal signal sequence from the VP7 protein (63,107,119,187). The *in vitro* translated gene 9 protein has demonstrated that the expressed protein is glycosylated and increases in size from 29 to 37 kDa in the presence of canine microsomes. In fact, the glycosylated gene 9 protein comigrates with a protein present on iodinated ADRV virions (142; E. R. Mackow, *unpublished data*). As a result, gene segment 9 encodes the major virion outer capsid glycoprotein and is likely to be the VP7 equivalent protein in ADRV. In group A strains, antibodies to the VP7 protein neutralize the virus and protect animals from disease. It will be interesting to determine whether the VP7 protein of group B strains is involved in similar protein processing and neutralization.

The VP7 protein from the IDIR group B strain is substantially different from ADRV, only 52% identical (119,120). In group A strains different serotypes are defined by VP7 proteins with approximately 85% identical amino acids (121). The low level of identity between these proteins is greater than that of any two group A VP7 proteins and suggests at the very least that they represent different group B rotavirus glycoprotein serotypes. These differences are about the same as observed between the VP4 amino acid sequences (see later discussion) and suggest that these viruses may have entirely different outer capsid neutralization components.

VP4 Protein Conservation

Group A, B, and C strains appear to share additional amino acid identity among their VP4 polypeptides (approximately 20% identical and 42% similar amino acids) (116–118,127,188). Expression and sequencing studies determined that gene segment 4 encodes an 84-kDa protein and that the encoded protein comigrates with a protein present on the ADRV outer capsid (116). In group A strains the VP4 protein is the viral spike protein (86.5 kDa), which is proteolytically cleaved to activate virus for infection (107,113,189,190). The group A VP4 protein is also the viral hemagglutinin, a determinant of viral neutralization, and confers to the virus one of its serotypes, the P type (107,108,191–195).

There is no evidence that group B rotaviruses agglutinate erythrocytes or that the baculovirus-expressed VP4 protein is capable of hemagglutination. However, there are several potential proteolytic cleavage sites on the VP4 protein at approximately the same point in the sequence as the group A VP4 protein (116,196). The importance of proteolytic processing of group B rotavirus VP4 proteins has not been demonstrated. Similar to group A rotavirus VP4 proteins, antibodies to the baculovirus-expressed ADRV VP4 protein neutralize ADRV and the porcine rotavirus in focus reduction neutralization assays described later (69,116; E. R. Mackow, *unpublished data*). The baculovirus-expressed VP4 protein should be useful for developing N-MAbs, diagnostic tests and neutralization tests for human group B rotaviruses (172,193,197).

The ADRV and IDIR VP4 proteins are only 58% identical at the amino acid level (116,118). In group A rotaviruses, amino acid differences of only 8% define different serotypes (198). By analogy, the substantial differences between the rat and human VP4 proteins suggests that they are distantly related and likely to define unique group B rotavirus P types. In contrast, the VP4 proteins from ADRV and the porcine group B rotavirus strains are immunologically cross-reactive and may be more closely related to each other than to the rat strain (E. R. Mackow, *unpublished data*).

In group A rotaviruses the VP8 portion of VP4 functions as the viral hemagglutinin (191,193). There is one report of a group B rotavirus isolated from a Chinese infant that hemagglutinates rhesus monkey erythrocytes (199). However, no further reports of group B rotavirus hemagglutination have appeared. This includes studies on ADRV, IDIR, or other group B rotaviruses as well as recombinant baculovirus-expressed ADRV VP4 preparations.

Potential Fusion Protein

Gene 6 of ADRV encodes two proteins in two different overlapping reading frames (ORFs) (171). The encoded proteins have been termed AD6F1 and AD6F2 for their origin in ADRV gene segment 6 and the open reading frame from which they are derived. The first ORF, called AD6F1, is a 107 amino acid protein. AD6F1 does not share amino acid similarity with any group A rotavirus protein (171). However, AD6F1 shares significant amino acid similarity with the respiratory syncytial virus (RSV) and Newcastle disease virus (NDV) fusion (F) proteins (171; E. R. Mackow, *unpublished data*). This finding is interesting since both RSV and NDV fuse cells and form syncytia via the F protein (200,201). An NBRF database search for proteins with similarities to AD6F1 revealed that the NDV F protein contains 24% identical and 43% similar amino acids while the RSV F protein is 22% identical and 53% similar to AD6F1 (over 91 amino acids) (171,202–206). The region of similarity comprises nearly the entire length of the 107 amino acid long AD6F1 protein (Fig. 4).

During RSV and NDV infections antibodies against the F protein are neutralizing and prevent syncytia formation (207–211). The AD6F1 protein has recently been expressed via a baculovirus recombinant and immunopre-

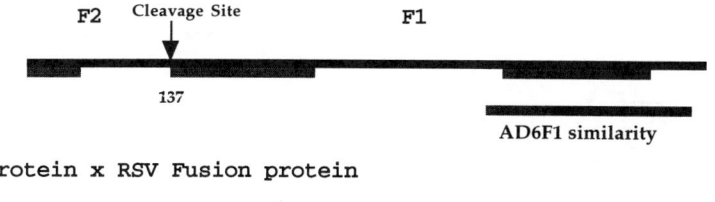

```
Ad61 protein x RSV Fusion protein

AD6F1    6  SSAQLNSHLTHINS..QNSNLFISDSKTAVFH......TQHILLAAGVGI  47
            .|.::::. :.::|.  ..|  .||. |.. : :    | :|::.  .|
RSV    484  PSDEFDASISQVNEKINQSLAFIRRSDELLHNVNTGKSTTNIMIT...TI  530


AD6F1   48  IATLLVLLLCSCVLNCYLCRRLKRTNGVSSLLERNLRQNGSSAK  91
            |  .::|:||:  ..:. .|: :  |.|  ..  |  : .  .|  ..|
RSV    531  IIVIIVVLLSLIAIGLLLYCKAKNTPVTLSKDQLSGINNIAFSK  574
```

FIG. 4. Similarity of the respiratory syncytial virus fusion protein and the AD6F1 protein of group B rotaviruses. AD6F1 was aligned to the NBRF protein database and found to contain significant amino acid similarity to fusion (F) proteins of paramyxoviruses, respiratory syncytial virus, and Newcastle disease virus. As illustrated, similarity of the proteins is confined to the carboxy-terminal end of the F protein but encompasses nearly all of the group B rotavirus protein AD6F1. Additional hydrophobic domains present in the F protein, which are implicated in cell fusion, are highlighted. The AD6F1 protein contains no similarity to any known rotavirus protein and only group B rotaviruses fuse cells and form syncytia during infection. The similarity of the AD6F1 protein with F proteins, which have been demonstrated to induce cell fusion, suggests a possible role for the protein in ADRV-induced cell fusion.

cipitated with hyperimmune anti-ADRV serum, peptide sera, and human convalescent serum, suggesting that AD6F1 is a structural protein of the virus (E. R. Mackow, *unpublished data*). AD6F1 is precipitated as a monomer of 11 kDa and multimers of 44, 66, and approximately 180 kDa. It will be interesting to determine if antibodies to the AD6F1 protein neutralize ADRV or inhibit syncytium formation.

The AD6F1 protein contains a potential N-terminal myristoylation site and several potential proteolytic cleavage sites (Fig. 5) (171,212). AD6F1 also contains one long, potentially membrane spanning, hydrophobic domain. Within this domain are alpha helical heptad repeats, which form a hydrophobic face on the protein and a leucine zipper (213,214). Each of these transmembrane elements could be involved in protein oligomerization or membrane integration (213–216). Interestingly, the NDV fusion protein is acylated, containing a fatty acid moiety at its carboxy terminus (217,218). Although the role of acylation has not been defined for NDV cell fusion, it could serve to associate the protein with cell membranes similar to a myristoyl group on the group B rotavirus AD6F1 protein (212). This interesting finding may suggest a role for myristoylation in icosahedral virus-induced cell fusion.

The AD6F1 protein is also similar in size and hydrophobic arrangement to the influenza virus M2 and NB proteins, which are 97 and 100 amino acids in length and have a single internal hydrophobic domain (219–221). In addition, some M2 proteins are palmitoylated, further suggesting their similarity with the AD6F1 protein (222). The M2 protein is an oligomeric integral membrane protein that forms an ion channel involved in the pH-dependent entry of influenza virus from lysosomes into cells (223,224). One hypothetical role for AD6F1 is that it could

similarly mediate group B rotavirus-induced cell fusion by its insertion into membranes via the concomitant creation of an ion channel between cellular plasma membranes.

AD6F1 contains two N/G cleavage sites that are associated with the proteolytic cleavage of myristoylated poliovirus and human immunodeficiency virus (HIV) polyproteins and the reovirus μ1 protein to produce mature myristoylated structural proteins (225–233). Proteolytic processing of AD6F1 at the N/G cleavage site or several adjacent trypsin or chymotrypsin sites would yield a mature amino-terminal polypeptide of 7 kDa (Fig. 5). These potential cleavages of AD6F1 would contain both the N-terminal myristoyl group and a carboxy-terminal transmembrane domain, which could associate the protein with one or more cell membranes in order to induce cell fusion.

The potential myristoylation of AD6F1, its recognition by virus-specific serum, and its similarities to other fusion and ion channel proteins together suggest that AD6F1 could be a viral outer capsid protein involved in viral neutralization and cell fusion. Another possibility is that proteolytic cleavage of AD6F1 may be required for enhanced cell fusion, viral maturation, or subsequent viral entry. The function of AD6F1 protein in these processes is under investigation. The second ORF in gene 6, AD6F2, tentatively encodes a protein similar to the NS53 protein of group A rotavirus strains (E. R. Mackow, *unpublished data*).

Other Group B Rotavirus Genes

Gene 11 of ADRV is 631 bases long and encodes a 20-kDa protein (92). The gene 11 protein from group A rotavirus (NS26) shares 40% similar amino acids (25% identical)

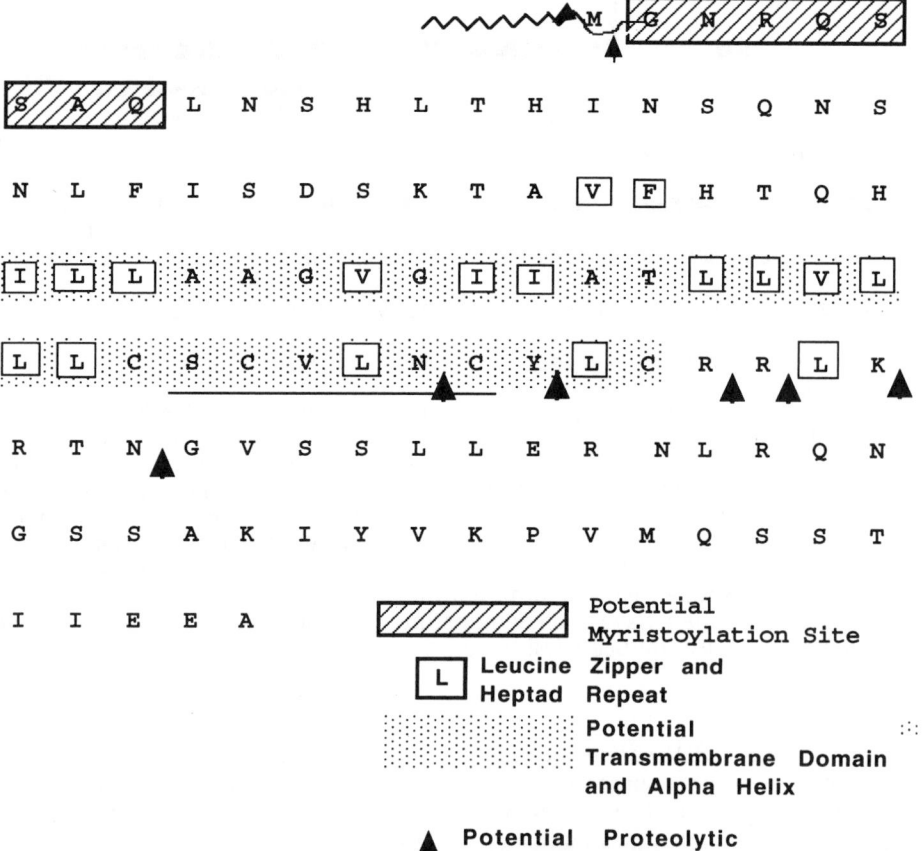

FIG. 5. AD6F1 protein attributes. The AD6F1 protein contains a consensus sequence for N-terminal myristoylation and one long hydrophobic, potentially membrane spanning, domain downstream. Each of these attributes can associate proteins with membranes. Within the hydrophobic domain is an alpha-helical heptad repeat with a leucine zipper-like sequence which is often associated with protein oligomerization and with integral membrane proteins. Several potential proteolytic cleavage sites are present just downstream of the hydrophobic domain, including trypsin and chymotrypsin sites as well as two sites similar to those used to cleave myristoylated poliovirus, reovirus, and HIV polyproteins.

with the ADRV gene 11 product. A comparison of IDIR and ADRV gene 11 sequences indicates that they are 72% and 66.5% identical at the nucleic acid and amino acid levels, respectively (92,120).

Gene segments 7, 8, and 10 are likely to encode nonstructural proteins NS34, NS35, and NS28 based on amino acid similarities with group A strains (E. R. Mackow, *unpublished data*). Gene segment 7 of ADRV and gene 5 of IDIR encode homologous NS34 protein equivalents to group A rotaviruses (175; E. R. Mackow, *unpublished data*). It has been reported that the IDIR gene segment 8-encoded protein is immunoprecipitated by three human (IDIR-specific) sera but not by ADRV-specific sera, suggesting variation in this gene product between group B rotavirus strains (164). It has not been demonstrated that any nonstructural ADRV protein provides to group B strains the same functions demonstrated in group A rotaviruses.

The gene encoding the VP1 protein equivalent in IDIR has been cloned and sequenced and appears to contain a polypeptide equivalent to the group A rotavirus protein present in transcriptionally active viral cores (176). The gene segment 1-encoded protein is 27.6% identical and 50% similar to the group A rotavirus VP1 protein and contains RNA polymerase-specific domains including a GDD amino acid sequence (177).

Group C Gene Coding Assignments

Two genes (encoding VP6 and NS26) from human group C rotaviruses have been presented (128,134,234). However, 10/11 group C rotavirus gene segments from porcine or bovine strains have been cloned and sequenced (126,127,130–135,235,236). A summary of group C rotavirus gene coding assignments is presented in Table 2 and detailed descriptions of animal group C rotaviruses have been reviewed by Saif and Bridger (13,14,39,52).

Group C rotaviruses, are highly related to group A rotavirus strains. An indication of this is the ability of gene segment 1 of group C rotaviruses to hybridize to group A gene segment 1 (39,68). Antigenic cross-reactivity between group C and A rotavirus VP6 proteins has also been noted (105). Along with hybridization, amino acid alignments have been used to define protein homologies between group C and A rotaviruses as described earlier for group B rotavirus proteins.

Structural Proteins

There are two reports that describe the structural proteins of group C rotaviruses (238,239). Each study reports the identification of six structural proteins of the group C rotavirus virion. In one study, 52,000- and 39,000-kDa virion proteins of the outer shell are lost by EDTA treatment of the virus (237). The 39,000-kDa protein is reported to be glycosylated since it is sensitive to endoglycosidase F and likely represents the viral VP7 protein. It has been further suggested that 44- and 93-kDa proteins are likely to be the group C rotavirus VP6 and VP2 proteins of the inner capsid (237). Another report describes four inner shell structural proteins of 125, 93, 74, and 41 kDa, two nonstructural proteins of 39 and 35 kDa, and 37- and 33-kDa outer shell proteins (238). The 37-kDa protein is glycosylated and there is some question about the association of a 25-kDa protein with the virion and whether this protein is also glycosylated (238).

Within group C rotaviruses nucleic acid and amino acid comparisons have been performed between individual genes and proteins. The VP6 proteins from the bovine (Shintoku), porcine (Cowden), and three recently studied human strains (Bristol, Belem, and Preston) of group C rotavirus have been compared (127,129,130,235). The bovine, porcine, and Bristol VP6 proteins share 88% to 92% identical amino acids. In group A rotaviruses, antigenic subgroups of viruses are defined by differences within their VP6 proteins. The differences between group C rotavirus strains are greater than any two subgroups of group A rotaviruses. This suggests that these viruses are likely to define their own subgroups and that they are antigenically quite discrete.

Within human group C rotavirus strains the VP6 genes are 97.9% to 99.6% identical with 100% identical amino acid sequence (128,234). Even Brazilian and U.K. isolates share 100% identical amino acid sequences, suggesting similar and recent origins for these human group C rotavirus strains (234). Table 3, a list of human group C rotavirus

nucleic acid and amino acid homologies with the porcine Cowden strain, illustrates the relatedness of group C rotavirus strains.

Porcine and human group C rotavirus VP7 proteins have also been compared and found to contain 83% nucleic acid identity and 88% amino acid identity (134). Differences of this magnitude between group A VP7 proteins often define viruses of different serotypes (121). This suggests that human and porcine group C strains may also comprise their own group C rotavirus glycoprotein-specific serotype. In contrast, the Cowden and a second human group C rotavirus strain, Ehime 86-542, are probably within the same group C serotype since antibodies to the Cowden strain neutralize the human strain (136). Similar to group B homologies, the group C rotavirus VP7 protein shares less than 30% amino acid identity with group A rotavirus VP7 protein.

Nonstructural Proteins

Nonstructural proteins of group C strains have also been analyzed by amino acid comparison. Porcine and bovine NS34 proteins share 81% identical amino acids, while NS26 proteins from bovine and human group C strains share only 68% identical amino acids but both have a relatively constant (78%) nucleic acid homology (130,135). As in group A strains, viral nonstructural proteins are more divergent than their structural protein counterparts.

Homology between group C and group A rotavirus strains are listed in Table 2. Identical amino acids shared between these two rotavirus groups are approximately 15% to 20% greater for most proteins (except for VP7) than comparable group B to group A protein homologies. This indicates that group C and A strains are more closely related and that group B strains are distant relatives to other rotavirus groups. However, the NS26, NS53, and NS34 proteins share a mere 15% to 23% amino acid identity and are almost completely different for group A, B, and C rotaviruses.

Protein Functions

As with group B strains very little has been done to define functional properties of group C rotavirus proteins. The proteins involved in group C rotavirus neutralization

TABLE 3. *Group C rotavirus VP6 gene and protein homology*

Virus	Cowden NA	Cowden AA	Bristol NA	Bristol AA	Belem NA	Belem AA	Preston NA	Preston AA
Cowden (porcine)	—	—	84%	92%	83%	92%	84%	92%
Bristol (human)			—	—	98%	100%	99.6%	100%
Belem (human)					—	—	98%	100%
Preston (human)							—	—

NA and AA are the percentages of identical nucleic acids and amino acids between group C rotavirus VP6 proteins.

and serotype specificity have not been defined but are presumed to be the VP7 and VP4 equivalent proteins of group C strains.

Hemagglutination

Group C rotaviruses have been determined to agglutinate human and sheep erythrocytes (239). In group A rotaviruses this function has been attributed to the VP8 proteolytic cleavage fragment of the outer capsid spike protein VP4 (191,240). It is likely that the VP4 protein of group C strains is also the viral hemagglutinin in group C rotaviruses.

Coexpression Studies

The function of the group C rotavirus VP6 protein has been defined by baculovirus coexpression of the protein with the group A rotavirus VP2 protein (241). In group A strains coexpression of VP2 and VP6 proteins results in the assembly of single-shelled like particles (179). When the VP6 protein of group C rotavirus was coexpressed with the group A rotavirus VP2 protein, similar single-shelled like particles were obtained (241). This result demonstrates the similarity of these two viruses since it defines structural protein homologies with nearly identical viral functions. The ability of both VP6 proteins to bind the group A rotavirus VP2 protein suggests conservation of VP2-binding domains by both proteins. Differences between the group A and C rotavirus VP6 proteins were demonstrated during coexpression studies by their inability to form mixed trimers or hexamers. This finding suggests that there are substantial differences in the way in which VP6 monomers oligomerize to form single-shelled particles.

Investigations into other functional correlates between group C and group A proteins are being pursued. Baculovirus expression of many of the group C rotavirus structural proteins are under way and these reagents will dramatically change our ability to study human group C rotavirus capsid assembly and to detect group C rotavirus infections.

HOST RANGE: ANIMAL AND HUMAN INFECTION

There are a variety of hosts for both group B and C rotavirus infections (1,3–7,11,13,15,18–41,43–47,52,54, 60,61,70,73,74,77–82,174,242,243). Thus far, group B rotavirus infections have been identified in humans, rats, swine, calves, and sheep. Interestingly, the only rotavirus group to infect rats is the group B rotavirus IDIR (47). Pigs in particular are reported to be seropositive for group A, B, and C rotaviruses at 99%, 86%, and 77% levels in the United States, suggesting the possibility of zoonotic infections of humans from endemic porcine strains (14–16,93,174). Serological evidence of animal and human group B rotavirus infections in the United States, United

Kingdom, and China suggests that these viruses are not geographically limited. Group C rotaviruses have been identified predominantly in humans (Bristol), swine (Cowden), and calves (Shintoku) and evidence of group C rotavirus infections have been documented throughout the world in animal and human populations (1,3,4,52,73, 74,77–82,242,243).

ANIMAL MODELS

Attempts have been made to infect rats and pigs with the human group B rotavirus strain ADRV but none of these trials has resulted in infection or viral shedding. With the large differences reported in the outer capsid proteins of group B rotaviruses, it is not surprising that viral isolates are host restricted and fail to infect other mammalian species.

Studies on the human group B rotavirus ADRV have been severely limited by the inability to study the virus in tissue culture or animal models. In contrast, the rat (IDIR) strain, the porcine (Ohio and SRV-1) strains, and bovine (Ohio) strain have been studied in animal models (39,44,47,61,174,244). Rat and porcine systems are viable animal models for the study of group B rotavirus infections (21,44,47).

Rats and pigs infected with group B rotavirus shed small amounts of virus by group A rotavirus standards (44,47). In the rat model the infected animal must also be sacrificed in order to harvest high titer virus from washes of the small intestine (47). Very little virus is shed into the animal's stool and virus that is obtained from stool is less infectious than virus from gut washes. Porcine rotavirus infection also produces only a small amount of virus even though it induces acute transient diarrhea in the animal (44,174). A small amount of high titer virus has been obtained from porcine, rat, and human group B rotavirus infections. These preparations have permitted much of the molecular biology of group B rotavirus strains.

Group C rotaviruses can be passed serially to new animals for the purposes of generating more virus and for studying viral pathogenesis. Representative strains exist for each species infected by group C rotaviruses but the Cowden porcine strain has been studied the most and has also been grown in tissue culture (122–125). A complete discussion of animal group C rotavirus strains has been presented in a review by Saif (39).

TISSUE CULTURE PROPAGATION OF GROUP B AND C ROTAVIRUSES

In an attempt to infect tissue culture cell lines, porcine group B rotavirus strains were originally added to cells in tissue culture monolayers (174). The presence of infected cells was detected by immunofluorescence and by the formation of syncytia in the monolayer (174). The formation of syncytia is characteristic of group B rotavirus strains and syncytia were used to screen for new group B rotavirus isolates. Rat, bovine, and ovine rotaviruses were all identified as group B rotavirus strains by their ability to form syncytia in infected cell monolayers and by their reactivity with antisera by immunofluorescence or immunostaining (21,31,47,53,61,70,174). Attempts to cultivate group B rotaviruses did not lead to the productive infection of tissue culture cells. Virus particles were detected by electron microscopy; however, the particles were abnormal, lacking a viral core and containing only a single shell (70). In contrast to group A rotavirus particles, the group B particles were associated with smooth rather than rough ER membranes (70). The use of proteases, which activate group A and C rotaviruses for infection, have been found to inactivate human and animal group B rotavirus for tissue culture infection (69,113,119,174,245).

A diethylaminoethyl dextran (DEAE-D) technique has been reported for the propagation of group B rotavirus strains (244). In this method rotaviruses are treated with EDTA and then bound to DEAE-D before being incubated with tissue culture cells. This transfection-like method for introducing group B porcine strain SRV-1 into cells has been used to passage group B rotaviruses. Titers of progeny virus are reported to be 10^3 to 10^5 focus forming units/mL and the progeny remains infectious to pigs (244). The ability to cultivate SRV-1 should simplify studies of group B rotavirus assembly and permit the use of gene reassortment to study the neutralization determinants of currently noncultivable human group B rotavirus strains.

Several reports have now appeared describing the cultivation of group C rotavirus strains. Porcine and human group C rotaviruses have been adapted to growth in tissue culture on primary AGMK cell lines, Ma104 cells, or ST cells (122–125). Essential to the growth process was the use of roller tubes and high concentrations of proteolytic enzymes trypsin or pancreatin in the maintenance medium (122–125). Infection of monolayers was monitored by immunofluorescence of infected cells and virus was passed 16 times until 10^7 focus forming units were obtained. The origin of the virus was confirmed by immune electron microscopy and electropherotyping, demonstrating that the input viral dsRNA was the same as that of the isolated progeny virus.

PATHOGENESIS

Rotaviruses of all groups infect the epithelium of the small intestine. Differences in the location of infection have been reported, indicating that group B rotavirus infections occur primarily in the distal small intestine while group A and C rotaviruses infect primarily the proximal small intestinal epithelium (70). The mechanism by which these viruses induce watery diarrhea is still unclear and may be the result of tissue injury or responses to epithelial damage, toxin-like effects, increased luminal solute concentrations that cause the efflux of water into the intestinal lumen, or failure to absorb water from the lumen. Group B rotaviruses have an additional pathogenic effect on the epithelial cells they infect. Group B rotaviruses cause the formation of giant cells or syncytia, which result from the fusion of adjacent infected cells (19,21,31,44,47, 51,61,69,70,174,246). Syncytium formation enhances the

pathogenesis of the virus for several reasons. Syncytium formation allows the virus to spread rapidly to adjacent cells without the need for viral assembly, exit, and infection of the neighboring cell. As a result, direct cell to cell spread of virus evades normal immunological surveillance mechanisms. Additionally, cell fusion is rapid and it can damage large contiguous portions of the intestinal epithelium, which may enhance diarrheal mechanisms.

SYNCYTIUM FORMATION

There are few icosahedral viruses that have been demonstrated to fuse infected cells. However, group B rotaviruses, avian reoviruses, and Nelson Bay virus are all icosahedral viruses of the Reoviridae family, which fuse cells and form syncytia during infection (20,21,31,44,70, 247–251). Syncytia formation during animal group B rotavirus infections has been demonstrated for some time (19,21,31,44,47,61,69,70,174) and recently the human group B rotavirus, ADRV, was shown to form syncytia in infected Ma104 cells (Fig. 6) (69). Syncytium formation is a hallmark of group B rotavirus infections and has not been demonstrated in other rotavirus groups. It is not clear how icosahedral viruses form syncytia, what proteins cause fusion, or whether presumed fusion proteins are structural or nonstructural viral components.

Transient Infection of Ma104 Cells by ADRV

ADRV is currently noncultivable and no animal model has been developed for the growth of ADRV. Many attempts to grow ADRV in tissue culture have only resulted in the transient infection of Ma104 cells, a continuous rhesus monkey kidney cell line (69; E. R. Mackow, *unpublished data*). The infected cells are present as focal plaques of fused cells or syncytia, each containing approximately 20 to 50 cells at 18 hr postinfection (PI) (Fig. 6) (69; E. R. Mackow, *unpublished data*). Similar syncytia were previously reported by several investigators using animal group B rotaviruses and intestinal epithelium or tissue culture cells (19,21,31,44,70,174).

A study of the time course of ADRV infection demonstrated that single cells were found to contain ADRV-specific antigens 3 to 6 hr PI and larger foci are found at subsequent times (69). This finding and the fact that 0.22-μm filtered ADRV is infectious indicate that syncytia are formed from single infection events and not as a result of the binding of ADRV aggregates. Although adjacent cells are fused, syncytia do not continue to spread and fuse the whole monolayer. In fact, fusion stops and the syncytium detaches from the monolayer, leaving a hole with no signs of the ADRV infection (69). The monolayer eventually grows over the syncytial hole and produces an intact monolayer without further ADRV infection or passage of the virus. The inability to passage ADRV indicates that an abortive transient infection of tissue culture cells occurs and that blocks to ADRV propagation exist under these conditions.

In addition to Ma104 cells, AGMK, HNK, Vero,

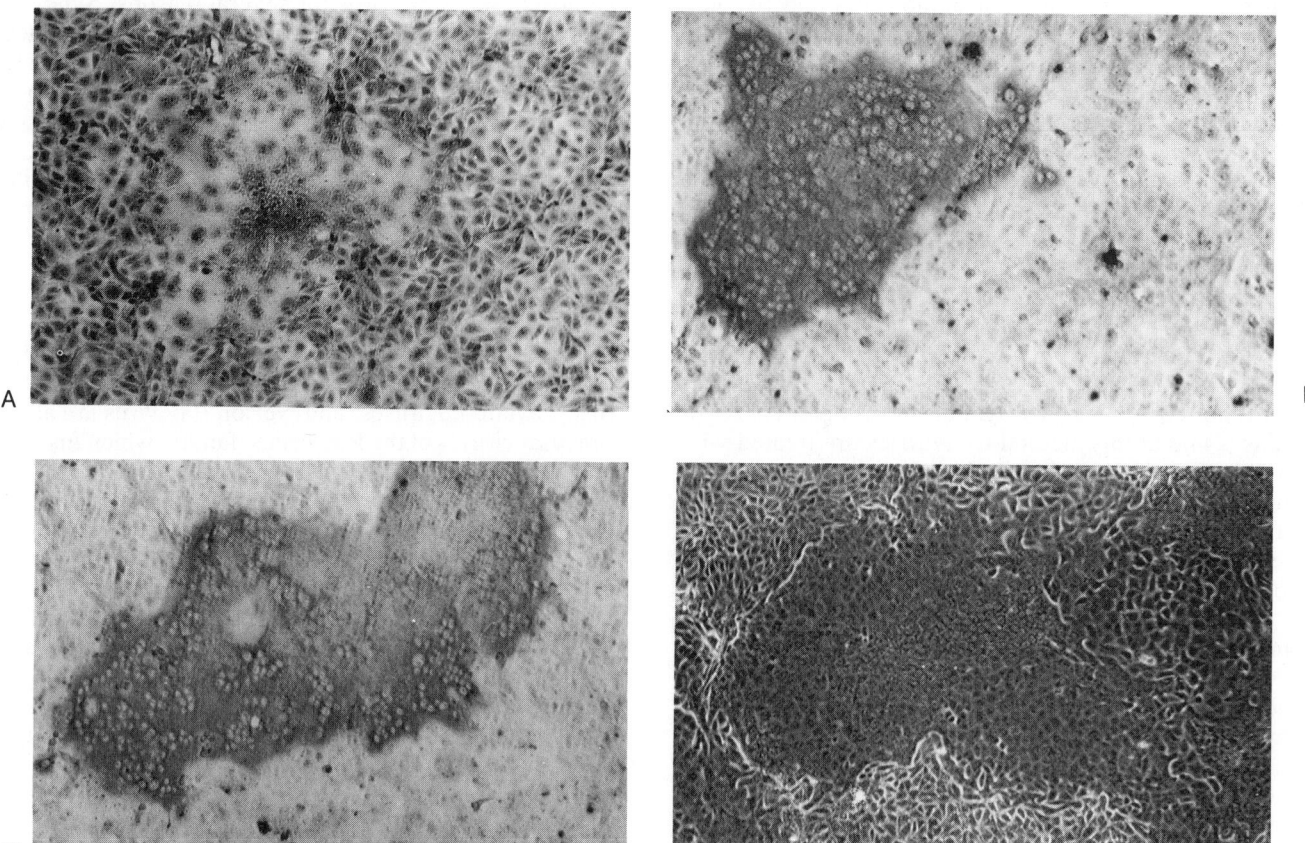

FIG. 6. ADRV-induced syncytia. Cells transiently infected with ADRV cause the formation of syncytia by fusing adjacent cells. Shown are syncytia formed from the infection of (**A**) Ma104 cells (H&E stain) and (**B,C,D**) AGMK cells (B,C, immunoperoxidase stain; D, visualized by phase contrast microscopy).

LLCMK-2, CaCo, Henle, HT-29, WI-38 and HEp-2 cell lines have also been transiently infected with ADRV (69; E. R. Mackow, *unpublished data*). Two interesting findings have emerged from the infection of different cell lines. First, the size of ADRV syncytia in AGMK cells is larger than any other cell line including 100 to 200 cells (69; E. R. Mackow, *unpublished data*). Syncytia within the AGMK cells appear to continue to spread to adjacent cells even though these syncytia also are self-limited and detach from the monolayer 18 to 48 hr PI. Second, there is no sign of cell fusion and syncytium formation during the infection of Henle cells (E. R. Mackow, *unpublished data*). These interesting observations provide research directions for further understanding ADRV tissue culture restrictions and a means of defining the mechanism of ADRV-induced cell fusion in the future.

A phenotypic variant of ADRV virus has also been identified, which forms small syncytial plaques 18 to 24 hr PI and full-size plaques at 48 hr PI (69). This isolate, which was collected from the northern part of China has been designated ADRV-2 for its unique syncytial phenotype. This virus cross-hybridizes with ADRV-1 and is antigenically highly related to ADRV-1. However, ADRV-2 may have distinct neutralization and fusion phenotypes from ADRV-1 (E. R. Mackow, *unpublished data*).

ADRV Tissue Culture Restriction

Further studies to determine the nature of the block to ADRV replication in tissue culture cells have looked for the ability of virus to synthesize protein and nucleic acids intracellularly. Immunostaining of infected cells as well as radiolabeling and immunoprecipitation of ADRV proteins have determined that viral proteins (VP2, VP4, and VP6) are being synthesized within the infected cell (69). However, it has not been determined if a full complement of proteins are being synthesized intracellularly. The replication of dsRNA within infected cells has also been detected (69). This latter finding suggests that additional ADRV proteins required for dsRNA replication are being made within infected cells. Since group A rotavirus strains synthesize dsRNA within assembled replicase particles (154,156,157), these data also suggest that ADRV replicase particles are being assembled within the infected cells. Further blocks to the maturation of ADRV in infected cells are unknown and the subject of current studies.

Neutralization of ADRV

The transient infection of Ma104 cells has recently been used as the basis of FRN assays (69; E. R. Mackow, *unpublished data*). ADRV-1 and ADRV-2 have been treated with hyperimmune serum to ADRV virus (1/1600) or anti-VP4 hyperimmune serum (1/400) prior to infecting tissue culture monolayers. In each case virus is neutralized by anti-ADRV-specific sera while VP6-specific and group A-specific hyperimmune sera have no effect (69; E. R. Mackow, *unpublished data*). Since high concentrations of anti-VP4 sera are required for neutralization, it is possible that other neutralization antigens besides VP4 are present on the virion or that most of the VP4 in the sample is dissociated from virion. The fusion protein and VP7 protein of ADRV are other likely neutralization targets.

EPIDEMIOLOGY

ADRV

The human group B rotavirus, ADRV, was initially isolated in 1982 and 1983 from epidemic gastroenteritis outbreaks in Chinese adults (5–8). The outbreaks were unique in their host range since infection was limited primarily to adults. ADRV predominantly infects individuals over the age of 15 and results in a low level of mortality (0.1%) in elderly or infirm individuals (5,9). Interestingly, the incidence of ADRV disease in individuals aged 20 to 29 years was ten times those of infants and young children (0 to 4 years of age) (5,9). In, fact 85% of those infected were over 15 years of age. Even among families where the virus spread through familial contacts, infants and young children were often spared from the disease (5,9). However, infection of infants and young children has been documented from studies of hospitalized individuals during the Chinese ADRV outbreaks (199).

In 1982 and 1983 the People's Republic of China experienced nationwide outbreaks of severe adult diarrheal disease caused by ADRV. Outbreaks originated in the northeast of China in the Heilongjiang province in the spring of 1982 (8,9). In the initial outbreak a quarter of all counties were affected with a very low mortality rate associated with elderly and infirm individuals. The incidence of ADRV-induced disease continued into 1983 and included approximately one-half of the counties and in excess of 1 million people (8).

In the fall of 1982 and spring of 1983, a separate epidemic outbreak of adult diarrheal disease was reported in the distant northwest of China in Gansu province (8,9). This outbreak began in a coal mining area near Lanzhou City and spread rapidly to the city. The prevalence of ADRV in Lanzhou included as many as 3.45% of the city population (8).

A third epidemic appearance of ADRV occurred in the south of China in Guangxi province as two discrete outbreaks (91). One report discusses the 19,000 patients affected by the outbreaks (91). The first outbreak occurred from April to September in 1983 and the second occurred in June 1984 in a different county 700 kilometers from the first. The first epidemic involved 12 cities and resulted in 37.5% seroconversion of convalescent sera by complement fixation. The second outbreak occurred in a village in which 122 of 136 families using the same well water were affected with an incidence of 45%. Incubation periods were 1 to 3 days and resulted in an average of 5 to 10 bowel movements per day with some patients experiencing dehydration due to diarrheal episodes up to 30 times per day (91). Immunoelectron microscopy (IEM) examination showed virus particles in 15 of 34 fecal samples from the two outbreaks and nine samples were positive for rotavirus RNA by PAGE (91). Electropherotypes are identical to those of ADRV reported by Hung in the northern China epidemics (5,6,8,91).

In each of these initial outbreaks it was demonstrated that the water was either fecally contaminated (230 *E. coli*/mL *E. coli*), common to those afflicted, or the water system was not chlorinated for several days prior to the outbreak and that the causative agent, ADRV, was probably transmitted as a waterborne pathogen (8,91,252). Subsequent to primary infections from drinking water, ADRV spread via close personal contacts. Epidemics quickly subsided following chlorination of the water supply.

The incidence of disease during the Chinese ADRV outbreaks was of epidemic proportions and ranged from 5% to 44% of the local population (8). ADRV-induced diarrhea is severe and has been described as "cholera-like" in its ability to induce voluminous diarrhea (5,6,8). The average incubation period for ADRV infection is 56 hr followed by the sudden onset of severe and frequent cramping diarrhea (100%). Vomiting is associated with 80% of cases reported and nearly half the cases demonstrated signs of dehydration (5,6,8). Fever is not normally associated with ADRV infections since only 1% of affected persons had low-grade fevers. Symptoms lasted 1 to 14 days and averaged 6 days in duration. There is a very low mortality rate associated with the infection and this may be the result of secondary complications in elderly or infirm individuals (8).

High titer virus is shed in human stools approximately 24 hr following ADRV infection at a time when diarrhea is minimal (5,6,8). By the time large quantities of watery diarrhea are observed (approximately 48 hr) shedding is diminished. Stools from outbreaks of ADRV-induced diarrhea in China are in fact the only source of high titer ADRV virus in the world.

In contrast to other rotavirus groups, ADRV disease does not appear to have a seasonal distribution. Chinese outbreaks occurred in the winter in the northwest and northeast of China and in the early summer in southern provinces (8–10). Outbreaks are not likely to represent the first human infections by group B rotaviruses since gamma globulin pools that precede the outbreak contain antibodies to ADRV (253). Epidemic outbreaks have continued to be reported periodically in China (8,67). In one report an epidemic of diarrhea was associated with ADRV in Qinhuangdao City, China, in 1987 (67). This outbreak affected in excess of 200 persons and was reportedly associated with two deaths. It is suggested that the outbreak was initiated by the return of a person from an ADRV epidemic area (67). Initially, ADRV spread to family members and this family remains the point source of the infection to the rest of the community. ADRV was identified as the cause of the outbreak by enzyme-linked immunoadsorbent assay (ELISA) and EM. A blocking ELISA was used to detect serum antibodies to ADRV and this assay detected the seroconversion of six out of seven individuals (67).

Antibodies to group B rotaviruses are common in China (254) and have been detected in 5% to 15% of human serum samples from India, Australia, Baltimore (Maryland) (8,9), and England (16). A study of ADRV seroprevalence in the general Chinese population detected antibodies to ADRV in 10% of healthy adults ($N = 1380$) (255). In a separate study, antibody to group B rotavirus was detected much less frequently in serum from individuals from the United States (1/155), Kenya (1/10), Thailand (1/20), and Canada (1/15) (102) Recent studies using recombinant ADRV antigens are just beginning to define the prevalence of group B rotavirus disease in human populations; however, these studies demonstrate that about 4% to 8% of the worldwide human population has been exposed to some form of group B rotavirus and that the exposure rates are highest in adults (12).

IDIR

In contrast to human strains, animal group B strains are primarily pathogens of the young (19,20,44,47,53,70). The rat group B rotavirus strain IDIR is named for its ability to infect infant rats (47). There is one report that the IDIR strain infected humans, children, and adults, which was described earlier (11). However, the infection was linked to physicians and their families who were directly involved in IDIR research and other cases of IDIR infections of humans have not been documented. In contrast to humans, watery diarrhea is not seen during IDIR infection of rats (47,61,255). This is presumably the result of particularly efficient water scavenging by the rat's cecum.

GROUP C EPIDEMIOLOGY

Human and animal group C rotavirus infections have now been documented in Africa, Australia, Europe, North and South America, Japan, and Thailand (2–4,52,55,59,66,73,74,80–82,84,85,138,256). It is therefore likely that group C rotaviruses are endemic in human populations throughout the world as they are for porcine and bovine populations. However pre-1984 pooled immunoglobulins from the United Kingdom, Belgium, the United States, Canada, and Japan indicate no signs of group C rotavirus in human population (52). Sera since 1984 have demonstrated an 8% prevalence rate for group

C rotavirus in the United Kingdom and a worldwide prevalence of 6% to 29% (14).

Human group C rotavirus outbreaks of gastroenteritis have now been documented in several institutional settings. Group C rotavirus infections are the most frequent among children aged 4 to 7 years of age but the virus has also been documented in infants and adults (2,4,257). The frequency of group C rotavirus disease, however, is much lower than that for group A strains. The most dramatic outbreak of group C rotavirus infection is a Japanese outbreak in which 675 out of 3102 (21.8%) school children were infected with the virus (4). A foodborne origin is suspected in this outbreak since all affected children had lunch from one particular food preparation center and since the outbreak encompassed seven different elementary schools. A common food source for the infection was not identified. Virus was determined to be group C specific by IEM and did not react with group A- or group C-specific reference sera (4).

Of the children infected, 46% presented with abdominal pain, 44.6% with acute vomiting, 41.3% with nausea, 41.1% with fever greater than 37°C, and only 27.6% with diarrhea (4). Thus vomiting and fevers are the main clinical symptoms for group C rotavirus infections and diarrhea was less associated with group C rotavirus infections than with group A or B rotaviruses.

There is one report of group C rotavirus infection among adults. In this report 23 college students on a college trip came down with severe diarrhea. Samples from the students were EM positive for rotavirus and subsequently found to contain group C rotavirus electropherotypes. Further analysis identified the viruses immunologically as group C by IEM (258).

IMMUNITY, DIAGNOSIS, AND PREVENTION

The determinants of group B and C rotavirus immunity and protection are currently based on presumptions from group A rotavirus studies. From group A rotavirus studies the outer capsid VP4 and VP7 proteins of group B and C rotavirus strains are likely to be involved in viral neutralization and host immunity to rotavirus disease. In the case of group B rotaviruses, antibodies to the recombinant VP4 protein reportedly neutralize the virus, suggesting that these presumptions are likely to hold true. In group C rotavirus, recent progress has also defined at least two serotypes based on one-way neutralization assays of cultivable strains (137). Serotypically similar porcine and human strains may already provide the basis for host-attenuated vaccines for the prevention of group C rotavirus disease.

Diagnostic Assays

The cause of approximately 50% of all clinical diarrheal cases remain unresolved (259). Group B and C rotavirus infections are among the causes of undiagnosed human diarrheal disease (259,260). Except for the general detection of rotavirus particles by EM, clinical diagnostic assays for group B and C rotaviruses have not been established, although there is one report of a MAb-based assay for detecting dsRNA of group A and non-group A rotaviruses (261). Outside research laboratories there is no way of diagnosing infections caused by these agents or determining the seroprevalence of group B and C rotavirus infections. Detection of group B and C rotaviruses has traditionally been approached by electropherotyping assays in which atypical patterns of nucleic acids are detected on polyacrylamide gels (39,49,50,64). Another assay that is used to differentiate group A, B, and C rotavirus infections is IEM. This technique uses hyperimmune sera to aggregate viruses from specific viral groups and aggregates are detected visually by EM.

Initial ELISA assays to detect group-specific antibodies in serum have also been performed (17,81,254). Some of these assays have suffered from the poor sensitivity and high background problems associated with the use of virus in stool as the antigen coat on ELISA plates (67,102). Assays using MAbs to detect group B-specific viral antigens in stools have also been developed and presented (8,102,106,262). ELISA and MAb diagnostic assays for ADRV have also been reported and in one study three MAbs to ADRV were prepared to outer capsid proteins (8–10,101,106,150,262). One of these MAbs has since been reported to immunoprecipitate the ADRV VP4 protein expressed from baculovirus recombinants (116,262). There are also two reports of MAbs made to the group B rotavirus VP6 protein, which have been used in ELISA and immunofluorescence assays (8,106).

Antibodies to the recombinant ADRV VP6 protein have also been used in an ADRV antigen detection assay using a rabbit anti-ADRV capture serum and detected with an ADRV VP6-specific MAb (12,99; E. R. Mackow, unpublished data). The development of MAb reagents to group B strains is very important for clinically detecting group B rotaviruses. With the advent of recombinant viral antigens for group B and C rotaviruses, the development of sensitive ELISA diagnostic assays are in progress.

There is one report of a counter-immunoelectrophoresis (CIE) assay for group B rotavirus detection. In this study 47% of rats, 36% of pigs, less than 1% of chickens, and 0% of horses were seropositive for group B rotaviruses in China (8). CIE was also used to assess the prevalence of group B rotavirus disease in some human populations (8). In China, 12% to 41% of persons surveyed were seropositive for group B rotavirus. However, only 15% of Australians, 9.5% of Americans, and 12.5% of Canadians surveyed were group B rotavirus positive by this assay. There is also one report of a latex agglutination assay for the rapid detection of ADRV using MAbs bound to latex beads although no further reports of this assay have been presented (8).

The recombinant baculovirus-expressed ADRV VP6 protein has been used to develop a standardized ELISA assay for serum antibodies to group B rotavirus (12). From this test and the screening of over 1100 serum samples the seroprevalence rates for U.S. adults and veterans have been determined to be about 5%. In 88 other human serum samples from adults varying from 18 to 69 years of age, a 4.5% (4/88) prevalence of group B rotavirus anti-

bodies was detected. Group B-positive sera were only obtained from individuals over age 40 (14% in this subset) in the U.S. who were sera tested (12). These data suggest either a preference of the virus for this age group or the prior exposure of a cohort of individuals age 40 and over to the agent at an early time in life when the rate of group B rotavirus infections was high. Sera from Thailand and Mexico were also determined to have group B-specific seroprevalence rates of 6% and 8%, respectively. Two hundred group A-positive sera from Mexican and U.S. children (under 2 years of age) screened by this assay were all seronegative for group B rotaviruses (12; E. R. Mackow, unpublished data).

In two studies, the seroprevalence of group B rotavirus infections was investigated using IDIR as the target antigen in human serum ELISAs (11,263). The study analyzed human serum antibodies to IDIR and determined that 43.4% of U.S. children less than 1 year old were seropositive for IDIR. Children under 2 years of age had an IDIR seroprevalence rate of 51.4%, and 87.9% of individuals over age 20 were determined to have serum antibodies to IDIR (11). These percentages represent the highest seroprevalence rates reported for group B rotavirus disease in any human cohort and may represent false-positive results.

Group C Rotavirus Diagnostics

Several reports of group C rotavirus MAbs and ELISAs have recently appeared. In one report three MAbs to the porcine group C rotavirus were generated, which immunoprecipitate the VP6 protein of group C strains and do not cross-react with group A or B strains (103). In another report five MAbs were generated that cross-react with both group A and C rotaviruses in cell culture immunofluorescence tests (105). These MAbs recognized the VP6 protein of each strain in Western blot assays. This report suggested that three overlapping epitopes within a single antigenic domain are shared by the MAbs (105). There are no further reports of cross-reactive epitopes between the VP6 proteins of group A and C rotavirus strains.

Several other group C rotavirus studies have made use of MAbs in diagnostic assays for group C rotaviruses (76,93,103–105,264,265). A majority of these diagnostics have relied on sandwich ELISAs in which MAbs are used to capture group C rotavirus antigens and the antigen is subsequently detected with a polyclonal serum. These tests are 63% to 100% accurate for the detection of group C rotaviruses (76,93,103–105,264,265). However, tests with reported 100% positivity have not tested their assays on a diverse set of group C rotavirus isolates used in other assays.

There is one report of a rapid diagnostic assay for group C rotaviruses using a reverse passive hemagglutination assay (RHPA) and a latex agglutination test (264). In these tests sheep erythrocytes or latex beads are coated with group C-specific MAbs and used to assay samples containing group C rotaviruses. In the presence of group C-specific antigen the erythrocytes or latex beads agglutinate and precipitate from the diagnostic solution (264).

These tests are reported to be 96% and 100% accurate at detecting group C rotavirus antigens and the latex agglutination test is complete in 2 min (264). With a number of MAbs and other reagents for group C strains already developed, clinical diagnostic assays for these viruses should soon be widely available.

Nucleic acid-based assays have also been used to detect viral groups by hybridization and by electropherotyping (39,132,139,257). Group C rotavirus hybridization studies have been used to categorize similar group C rotavirus strains. The similarities identified by hybridization have subsequently been shown to be significant by cross-neutralization studies performed on hybridization-related viruses. One report used viral electropherotypes to diagnose and determine the prevalence of group A, B, and C rotaviruses in diarrheic pigs. In this study 68% to 76% of pigs contained group A rotavirus while 7.4% to 10% contained group B or group C RNA electropherotypes (139). In weaned pigs 41% were group A infections while 18% to 22% were group B or C infections (139).

The polymerase chain reaction has also been used to detect group B and C viruses and promises the best sensitivity of any assay to date (150). However, since RNA viruses are inherently inaccurate during RNA replication and since nucleic acid sequences can be even more variable than protein sequences, the oligonucleotide primers chosen to detect virus by PCR are extremely important and must be complementary to highly conserved nucleic acid sequences in order for this strategy to be used successfully. Thus this technique is limited for the detection of new viral isolates since it may only detect very similar viral strains. Although group-specific PCR assays have been proposed, the ability of these assays to detect all viruses of a group have not been tested adequately. In addition, fairly large amounts (2 ng to 0.008 pg) of rotavirus RNA are required for positive PCR results in these reports (149,150). With the sequencing of more and more group B and C rotavirus genes, comparative sequence analysis may at some point define extremely conserved sequences, which can be used reliably as group-specific virus screens.

ELISAs for serum antibodies to group B or C viruses or for viral antigens still represent the best diagnostic choice for the specific and sensitive detection of rotaviruses. With the development of cultivable viruses that can be purified and recombinant expressed proteins, assays for group B and C rotaviruses should soon appear and be added to the existing group A-specific rotazyme assay for the routine detection of human rotaviruses.

CONCLUSIONS

Group B and C rotaviruses are emerging as important human pathogens worldwide. The development of MAbs, cultivated viral strains, and recombinant diagnostic reagents will soon allow the detection of these viruses in many clinical laboratories. Diagnostic assays for group B and C rotaviruses should permit more accurate assessments of their contribution to human disease and help to define the cause of some of the 50% of diarrheal cases that remain undiagnosed each year (259,260). We are only beginning to discover the functions of group B and C rotavirus proteins. Defining the means in which similar viral functions can be performed from dissimilar proteins among group A, B, and C rotaviruses will assist our general understanding of how all rotaviruses function. Unique group B and C rotavirus proteins will also allow us to define new mechanisms of rotavirus pathogenesis. The mechanism of icosahedral virus cell fusion has not been studied and could be substantially different from that of enveloped viruses. Group B rotavirus-induced cell fusion and the enhanced pathogenesis accompanying epithial syncytia are particularly interesting biologic problems that will be addressed in the coming years. Analysis of the antigenic diversity among human group B and C rotaviruses is also in its infancy. The ability to antigenically discriminate viral isolates will soon allow us to establish subgroups and serotypes for group B and C rotaviruses. Establishing antigenic differences of circulating group B and C rotaviruses will permit us to rationally approach questions concerning the necessity and feasibility of preventative measures for human group B and C rotavirus disease.

REFERENCES

1. Ishimaru Y, Nakano H, Oseto M, Yamashita Y, Kobayashi N, Urasawa S. Group C rotavirus infection and infiltration. *Acta Paediatr Jpn (Overseas Ed)* 1990;32:523–529.
2. Brown DW, Campbell L, Tomkins DS, Hambling MH. School outbreak of gastroenteritis due to atypical rotavirus [letter]. *Lancet* 1989;2:737–738.
3. Caul EO, Ashley CR, Darville JM, Bridger JC. Group C rotavirus associated with fatal enteritis in a family outbreak. *J Med Virol* 1990;30:201–205.
4. Matsumoto K, Hatano M, Kobayashi K, et al. An outbreak of gastroenteritis associated with acute rotaviral infection in schoolchildren. *J Infect Dis* 1989;160:611–615.
5. Hung T, Chen GM, Wang CG, et al. Rotavirus-like agent in adult non-bacterial diarrhoea in China [Letter]. *Lancet* 1983; 2:1078–1079.
6. Hung T, Chen GM, Wang CG, et al. Waterborne outbreak of rotavirus diarrhoea in adults in China caused by a novel rotavirus. *Lancet* 1984;1:1139–1142.
7. Chen CM, Hung T, Bridger JC, McCrae MA. Chinese adult rotavirus is a group B rotavirus [letter]. *Lancet* 1985;2: 1123–1124.
8. Hung T. *Rotavirus and adult diarrhea,* Advances in virus research, vol 35. Orlando, FL: Academic Press, 1988;193–218.
9. Hung T, Chen GM, Wang CG, et al. Seroepidemiology and molecular epidemiology of the Chinese rotavirus. *Ciba Found Symp* 1987;128:49–62.
10. Hung T, Fan RL, Wang CA, et al. Seroepidemiology of adult rotavirus [letter]. *Lancet* 1985;2:325–326.
11. Eiden J, Vonderfecht S, Yolken RH. Evidence that a novel rotavirus-like agent of rats can cause gastroenteritis in man. *Lancet* 1985;2:8–11.
12. Mackow ER, Wang Z, Gallo F, Fay ME, Hung T, Chen GM. Development of an ELISA assay for detecting group B rotavirus antibodies using a recombinant VP6 protein. [*Submitted*].
13. Bridger JC. *Novel rotaviruses in animals and man. Novel diarrhoea viruses.* Ciba Foundation Symposium, vol 128. Chichester: Wiley, 1987;5–23.
14. Bridger JC, Farthing MJ. New and emerging gut viruses: structure, pathophysiology and clinical manifestations. *Non-Group-A Rotaviruses* 1988;79–82.

15. Bridger JC, Brown JF. Prevalence of antibody to typical and atypical rotaviruses in pigs. *Vet Rec* 1985;116:50.

16. Brown DW, Beards GM, Chen GM, Flewett TH. Prevalence of antibody to group B (atypical) rotavirus in humans and animals. *J Clin Microbiol* 1987;25:316–319.

17. Ushijima H, Shinozaki T, Fang ZY, Glass RI. Group B rotavirus antibody in Japanese children [letter]. *J Diarrhoeal Dis Res* 1992;10:41.

18. Bellinzoni R, Mattion N, Vallejos L, La TJ, Scodeller EA. Atypical rotavirus in chickens in Argentina. *Res Vet Sci* 1987; 43:130–131.

19. Chasey D, Banks J. The commonest rotaviruses from neonatal lamb diarrhoea in England and Wales have atypical electropherotypes. *Vet Rec* 1984;115:326–327.

20. Chasey D, Davies P. Atypical rotaviruses in pigs and cattle. *Vet Rec* 1984;114:16–17.

21. Chasey D, Higgins RJ, Jeffrey M, Banks J. Atypical rotavirus and villous epithelial cell syncytia in piglets. *J Comp Pathol* 1989;100:217–222.

22. Dimitrov DH, Estes MK, Rangelova SM, Shindarov LM, Melnick JL, Graham DY. Detection of antigenically distinct rotaviruses from infants. *Infect Immun* 1983;41:523–526.

23. Echeverria P, Burke DS, Blacklow NR, Cukor G, Charoenkul C, Yanggratoke S. Age-specific prevalence of antibody to rotavirus, *Escherichia coli* heat-labile enterotoxin, Norwalk virus, and hepatitis A virus in a rural community in Thailand. *J Clin Microbiol* 1983;17:923–925.

24. Gatti MS, Hara NH, Ferraz MM, Pestana de Castro A. Presence of group A and non-A rotaviruses in neonatal piglets in Campinas, SP, Brazil. *Med Microbiol Immunol* 1989;178: 347–349.

25. Gough RE, Wood GW, Spackman D. Studies with an atypical avian rotavirus from pheasants. *Vet Rec* 1986;118:611–612.

26. Kang SY, Nagaraja KV, Newman JA. Electropherotypic analysis of rotaviruses isolated from turkeys. *Avian Dis* 1986;30: 794–801.

27. Liprandi F, Garcia D, Botero L, Gorziglia M, Cavazza ME, Perez SI, Esparza J. Characterization of rotaviruses isolated from pigs with diarrhoea in Venezuela. *Vet Microbiol* 1987;13: 35–45.

28. Magar R, Robinson Y, Morin M. Identification of atypical rotaviruses in outbreaks of preweaning and postweaning diarrhea in Quebec swine herds. *Can J Vet Res* 1991;55:260–263.

29. Mattion NM, Bellinzoni RC, Blackhall JO, La TJ, Scodeller EA. Antigenic characterization of swine rotaviruses in Argentina. *J Clin Microbiol* 1989;27:795–798.

30. McNulty MS, Allan GM, McFerran JB. Prevalence of antibody to conventional and atypical rotaviruses in chickens. *Vet Rec* 1984;114:219.

31. Mebus CA, Rhodes MB, Underdahl NR. Neonatal calf diarrhea caused by a virus that induces villous epithelial cell syncytia. *Am J Vet Res* 1978;39:1223–1228.

32. Morilla A, Arriaga C, Ruiz A, Martinez AG, Cigarroa R, Valazquez A. Association between diarrhoea and shedding of group A and atypical groups B to E rotaviruses in suckling pigs. *Ann Rech Vet* 1991;22:193–200.

33. Morin M, Magar R, Robinson Y. Porcine group C rotavirus as a cause of neonatal diarrhea in a Quebec swine herd. *Can J Vet Res* 1990;54:385–389.

34. Nagesha HS, Hum CP, Bridger JC, Holmes IH. Atypical rotaviruses in Australian pigs. *Arch Virol* 1988;102:91–98.

35. Pipittajan P, Kasempimolporn S, Ikegami N, Akatani K, Wasi C, Sinarachatanant P. Molecular epidemiology of rotaviruses associated with pediatric diarrhea in Bangkok, Thailand. *J Clin Microbiol* 1991;29:617–624.

36. Puerto MF, Avendano L, Esparza J, Caul EO. Antigenic variation in Latin American human pararotaviruses (a typical rotaviruses) [Letter]. *J Clin Pathol* 1984;37:1416–1417.

37. Reynolds DL, Saif YM, Theil KW. A survey of enteric viruses of turkey poults. *Avian Dis* 1987;31:89–98.

38. Rodger SM, Bishop RF, Holmes IH. Detection of a rotavirus-like agent associated with diarrhea in an infant. *J Clin Microbiol* 1982;16:724–726.

39. Saif LJ. NonGroup A rotaviruses. In: Saif LJ, Theil KW, eds.

Viral diarrheas of man and animals. Boca Raton, FL: CRC Press, 1989;73–95.

40. Sigolo de San Juan C, Bellinzoni RC, Mattion N, La TJ, Scodeller EA. Incidence of group A and atypical rotaviruses in Brazilian pig herds. *Res Vet Sci* 1986;41:270–272.

41. Szucs G, Kende M, Uj M. Atypical rotaviruses in Hungary. *Ann Inst Pasteur/Virol* 1987;138:391–395.

42. Szucs G, Kende M, Uj M, Deak J, Koller M, Szarka E, Csik M. Different electrophoretypes of human rotaviruses in Hungary. *Acta Virol* 1987;31:369–373.

43. Takase K, Uchimura T, Katsuki N, Yamamoto M. A survey of chicken sera for antibody to atypical avian rotavirus of duck origin, in Japan. *Nippon Juigaku Zasshi* 1990;52:1319–1321.

44. Theil KW, Saif LJ, Moorhead PD, Whitmoyer RE. Porcine rotavirus-like virus (group B rotavirus): characterization and pathogenicity for gnotobiotic pigs. *J Clin Microbiol* 1985;21: 340–345.

45. Theil KW, Saif YM. Age-related infections with rotavirus, rotaviruslike virus, and atypical rotavirus in turkey flocks. *J Clin Microbiol* 1987;25:333–337.

46. Torres MA. Isolation of an atypical rotavirus causing diarrhea in neonatal ferrets. *Lab Anim Sci* 1987;37:167–171.

47. Vonderfecht SL, Huber AC, Eiden J, Mader LC, Yolken RH. Infectious diarrhea of infant rats produced by a rotavirus-like agent. *J Virol* 1984;52:94–98.

48. Greenberg HB, Kalica AR, Wyatt RG, Jones RW, Kapikian AZ, Chanock RM. Rescue of noncultivatable human rotavirus by gene reassortment during mixed infection with ts mutants of a cultivatable bovine rotavirus. *Proc Natl Acad Sci USA* 1981;78:420–424.

49. Estes MK, Palmer EL, Obijeski JF. Rotaviruses: a review. *Curr Top Microbiol Immunol* 1983;105:123–184.

50. Holmes I. Rotaviruses. In: Joklik WK, ed. *The Reoviridae*. New York: Plenum Press, 1983;359–423.

51. Askaa J, Bloch B. Infection in piglets with a porcine rotavirus-like virus. Experimental inoculation and ultrastructural examination. *Arch Virol* 1984;80:291–303.

52. Bridger JC, Pedley S, McCrae MA. Group C rotaviruses in humans. *J Clin Microbiol* 1986;23:760–763.

53. Chasey D, Bridger JC, McCrae MA. A new type of atypical rotavirus in pigs. *Arch Virol* 1986;89:235–243.

54. Espejo RT, Puerto F, Soler C, Gonzalez N. Characterization of a human pararotavirus. *Infect Immun* 1984;44:112–116.

55. Nicolas JC, Cohen J, Fortier B, Lourenco MH, Bricout F. Isolation of a human pararotavirus. *Virology* 1983;124:181–184.

56. Pedley S, Bridger JC, Brown JF, McCrae MA. Molecular characterization of rotaviruses with distinct group antigens. *J Gen Virol* 1983;64:2093.

57. Pedley S, Bridger JC, Chasey D, McCrae MA. Definition of two new groups of atypical rotaviruses. *J Gen Virol* 1986;67: 131.

58. Pereira HG, Leite JP, Azeredo RS, de Farias V, Sutmoller F. An atypical rotavirus detected in a child with gastroenteritis in Rio de Janeiro, Brazil. *Mem Inst Oswaldo Cruz* 1983;78: 245–250.

59. Snodgrass DR, Herring AJ, Campbell I, Inglis JM, Hargreaves FD. Comparison of atypical rotaviruses from calves, piglets, lambs and man. *J Gen Virol* 1984;65:909.

60. Thouless ME, DiGiacomo RF, Neuman DS. A new type of atypical rotavirus in pigs. *Arch Virol* 1986;89:235–243.

61. Vonderfecht SL, Eiden JJ, Torres A, Miskuff RL, Mebus CA, Yolken RH. Identification of a bovine enteric syncytial virus as a nongroup A rotavirus. *Am J Vet Res* 1986;47:1913–1918.

62. Willoughby RE, Wee SB, Yolken RH. Non-group A rotavirus infection associated with severe gastroenteritis in a bone marrow transplant patient. *Pediatr Infect Dis J* 1988;7:133–135.

63. Estes MK. Rotaviruses and their replication. In: Fields BN, Knipe DM, eds. *Fields Virology*. New York: Raven Press, 1990;1329–1352.

64. Kapikian AZ, Chanock RM. Rotaviruses. In: Fields BN, Knipe DM, Chanock RM, Hirsch MS, Joseph LM, Monath TP, Roizman B, eds. *Virology*, vol 2, 2nd ed. New York: Raven Press, 1990;1353–1404.

65. Yolken R, Arango JS, Eiden J, Vonderfecht S. Lack of genomic

reassortment following infection of infant rats with group A and group B rotaviruses. *J Infect Dis* 1988;158:1120–1123.

66. Beards GM, Desselberger U, Flewett TH. Temporal and geographical distributions of human rotavirus serotypes, 1983 to 1988. *J Clin Microbiol* 1989;27:2827–2833.

67. Fang ZY, Ye Q, Ho MS, et al. Investigation of an outbreak of adult diarrhea rotavirus in China. *J Infect Dis* 1989;160:948–953.

68. Eiden J, Vonderfecht S, Theil K, Torres MA, Yolken RH. Genetic and antigenic relatedness of human and animal strains of antigenically distinct rotaviruses. *J Infect Dis* 1986;154:972–982.

69. Mackow ER, Wang Z, Chou RH, Fay ME, Chen GM. Syncytia formation during transient infection of Ma104 cells with the human group B rotavirus ADRV. [*Submitted*].

70. Chasey D, Banks J. Replication of atypical ovine rotavirus in small intestine and cell culture. *J Gen Virol* 1986;67:567–576.

71. Graham DY, Estes MK. Rotavirus-like agent, rats, and man [Letter]. *Lancet* 1985;2:886.

72. Bohl EH, Saif LJ, Theil KW, Agnes AG, Cross RF. Porcine pararotavirus: detection, differentiation from rotavirus, and pathogenesis in gnotobiotic pigs. *J Clin Microbiol* 1982;15:312–319.

73. Bothig B, Schulze P, Schreier E, Diedrich S, Michel S. Atypical human rotaviruses in the G.D.R. *Acta Virol* 1989;33:320–326.

74. Brown DW, Mathan MM, Mathew M, Martin R, Beards GM, Mathan VI. Rotavirus epidemiology in Vellore, south India: group, subgroup, serotype, and electropherotype. *J Clin Microbiol* 1988;26:2410–2414.

75. Dimitrov DH, Graham DY, Lopez J, Muchinik G, Velasco G, Stenback WA, Estes MK. RNA electropherotypes of human rotaviruses from North and South America. *Bull World Health Organ* 1984;62:321–329.

76. Fujii R, Kuzuya M, Hamano M, Yamada M, Yamazaki S. Detection of human group C rotaviruses by an enzyme-linked immunosorbent assay using monoclonal antibodies. *J Clin Microbiol* 1992;30:1307–1311.

77. Gabbay YB, Mascarenhas JD, Linhares AC, Freitas RB. Atypical rotavirus among diarrhoeic children living in Belem, Brazil. *Mem Inst Oswaldo Cruz* 1990;84:5–8.

78. Ishimaru Y, Nakano S, Nakano H, Oseto M, Yamashita Y. Epidemiology of group C rotavirus gastroenteritis in Matsuyama, Japan. *Acta Paediatr Jpn* (*Overseas Ed*) 1991;33:50–56.

79. Maunula L, Svensson L, von BC. A family outbreak of gastroenteritis caused by group C rotavirus. *Arch Virol* 1992;124:269–278.

80. Penaranda ME, Cubitt WD, Sinarachatanant P, Taylor DN, Likanonsakul S, Saif L, Glass RI. Group C rotavirus infections in patients with diarrhea in Thailand, Nepal, and England. *J Infect Dis* 1989;160:392–397.

81. Ushijima H, Honma H, Mukoyama A, et al. Detection of group C rotaviruses in Tokyo. *J Med Virol* 1989;27:299–303.

82. Von Bonsdorf C-H, Svensson L. Human serogroup C rotavirus in Finland. *Scand J Infect Dis* 1988;20:475–478.

83. Dimitrov DH, Shindarov LM, Rangelova S. Occurrence of antigenically distinct rotaviruses in infants in Bulgaria. *Eur J Clin Microbiol* 1986;5:471–473.

84. Sorrentino A, Scodeller EA, Bellinzoni R, Muchinik GR, La TJ. Detection of an atypical rotavirus associated with diarrhoea in Chaco, Argentina. *Trans R Soc Trop Med Hyg* 1986;80:120–122.

85. Suzuki H, Sato T, Kitaoka S, et al. Epidemiology of rotavirus in Guayaquil, Ecuador. *Am J Trop Med Hyg* 1986;35:372–375.

86. Prasad BV, Wang GJ, Clerx JP, Chiu W. Three-dimensional structure of rotavirus. *J Mol Biol* 1988;199:269–275.

87. Suzuki H, Chen GM, Hung T, Beards GM, Brown DW, Flewett TH. Effects of two negative staining methods on the Chinese atypical rotavirus. *Arch Virol* 1987;94:305–308.

88. Yeager M, Dryden KA, Olson NH, Greenberg HB, Baker TS. Three-dimensional structure of rhesus rotavirus by cryoelectron microscopy and image reconstruction. *J Cell Biol* 1990;110:2133–2144.

89. Estes M, Graham DY, Smith EM, Gerba CP. Rotavirus stability and inactivation. *J Gen Virol* 1979;43:403–409.

90. Nakata S, Petrie BL, Calomeni EP, Estes MK. Electron microscopy procedure influences detection of rotaviruses. *J Clin Microbiol* 1987;25:1902–1906.

91. Wang SS, Cai RF, Chen J, Li RJ, Jiang RS. Etiologic studies of the 1983 and 1984 outbreaks of epidemic diarrhea in Guangxi. *Intervirology* 1985;24:140–146.

92. Chen GM, Hung T, Mackow ER. cDNA cloning of each genomic segment of the group B rotavirus ADRV: molecular characterization of the 11th RNA segment. *Virology* 1990;175:605–609.

93. Terrett LA, Saif LJ, Theil KW, Kohler EM. Physicochemical characterization of porcine pararotavirus and detection of virus and viral antibodies using cell culture immunofluorescence. *J Clin Microbiol* 1987;25:268–272.

94. Both GW, Siegman LJ, Bellamy AR, Atkinson PH. Coding assignment and nucleotide sequence of simian rotavirus SA11 gene segment 10: location of glycosylation sites suggests that the signal peptide is not cleaved. *J Virol* 1983;48:335–339.

95. Estes MK, Crawford SE, Penaranda ME, et al. Synthesis and immunogenicity of the rotavirus major capsid antigen using a baculovirus expression system. *J Virol* 1987;61:1488–1494.

96. Greenberg H, McAuliffe V, Valdesuso J, et al. Serological analysis of the subgroup protein of rotavirus, using monoclonal antibodies. *Infect Immun* 1983;39:91–99.

97. Lin M, Imai M, Ikegami N, et al. cDNA probes of individual genes of human rotavirus distinguish viral subgroups and serotypes. *J Virol Methods* 1987;15:285–289.

98. Eiden JJ, Nataro J, Vonderfecht S, Petric M. Molecular cloning, sequence analysis, in vitro expression, and immunoprecipitation of the major inner capsid protein of the IDIR strain of group B rotavirus (GBR). *Virology* 1992;188:580–589.

99. Mackow ER, Fay ME, Werner-Eckert R, Hung T, Wang ZJ, Chen G. Baculovirus expression of the ADRV gene 5 encoded protein produces an oligomerized, antigenic, and immunogenic VP6 protein. *Virology* 1993;193:537–542.

100. Mnisi YN, Williams MM, Steele AD. Subgroup and serotype epidemiology of human rotaviruses recovered at Ga-Rankuwa, southern Africa. *Central Afr J Med* 1992;38:221–225.

101. Nakata S, Estes MK, Graham DY, et al. Antigenic characterization and ELISA detection of adult diarrhea rotaviruses [published erratum appears in *J Infect Dis* 1987;155(1):162]. *J Infect Dis* 1986;154:448–455.

102. Nakata S, Estes MK, Graham DY, Wang SS, Gary GW, Melnick JL. Detection of antibody to group B adult diarrhea rotaviruses in humans. *J Clin Microbiol* 1987;25:812–818.

103. Ojeh CK, Jiang BM, Tsunemitsu H, Kang SY, Weilnau PA, Saif LJ. Reactivity of monoclonal antibodies to the 41-kilodalton protein of porcine group C rotavirus with homologous and heterologous rotavirus serogroups in immunofluorescence tests. *J Clin Microbiol* 1991;29:2051–2055.

104. Ojeh CK, Tsunemitsu H, Simkins RA, Saif LJ. Development of a biotin-streptavidin-enhanced enzyme-linked immunosorbent assay which uses monoclonal antibodies for detection of group C rotaviruses. *J Clin Microbiol* 1992;30:1667–1673.

105. Tsunemitsu H, Ojeh CK, Jiang B, Simkins RA, Weilnau PA, Saif LJ. Production and characterization of monoclonal antibodies to porcine group C rotaviruses cross-reactive with group A rotaviruses. *Virology* 1992;191:272–281.

106. Yolken R, Wee SB, Eiden J, Kinney J, Vonderfecht S. Identification of a group-reactive epitope of group B rotaviruses recognized by monoclonal antibody and application to the development of a sensitive immunoassay for viral characterization. *J Clin Microbiol* 1988;26:1853–1858.

107. Estes MK, Cohen J. Rotavirus gene structure and function. *Microbiol Rev* 1989;53:410–449.

108. Estes MK, Conner ME, Gilger MA, Graham DY. Molecular biology and immunology of rotavirus infections. *Immunol Invest* 1989;18:571–581.

109. Matsui SM, Mackow ER, Greenberg HB. Molecular determinant of rotavirus neutralization and protection. *Adv Virus Res* 1989;36:181–214.

110. Shaw RD, Vo PT, Offit PA, Coulson BS, Greenberg HB. Antigenic mapping of the surface proteins of rhesus rotavirus. *Virology* 1986;155:434–451.

111. Chen DY, Estes MK, Ramig RF. Specific interactions between rotavirus outer capsid proteins VP4 and VP7 determine expression of a cross-reactive, neutralizing VP4-specific epitope. *J Virol* 1992;66:432–439.

112. Greenberg HB, Flores J, Kalica AR, Wyatt RG, Jones R. Gene coding assignments for growth restriction, neutralization and subgroup specificities of the W and DS-1 strains of human rotavirus. *J Gen Virol* 1983;64:313–320.

113. Estes MK, Graham DY, Mason BB. Proteolytic enhancement of rotavirus infectivity: molecular mechanisms. *J Virol* 1981; 39:879–888.

114. Snodgrass DR, Hoshino Y, Fitzgerald TA, Smith M, Browning GF, Gorziglia M. Identification of four VP4 serological types (P serotypes) of bovine rotavirus using viral reassortants. *J Gen Virol* 1992;73:2319–2325.

115. Wyatt RG, James HJ, Pittman AL, et al. Direct isolation in cell culture of human rotaviruses and their characterization into four serotypes. *J Clin Microbiol* 1983;18:310–317.

116. Mackow ER, Werner-Eckert R, Fay ME, Tao H, Chen G. Identification and baculovirus expression of the VP4 protein of the human group B rotavirus ADRV. *J Virol* 1993;67:2730–2738.

117. Sato S, Yolken RH, Eiden JJ. The complete nucleic acid sequence of gene segment 3 of the IDIR strain of group B rotavirus. *Nucleic Acids Res* 1989;17:10113.

118. Lindsay DA, Vonderfecht SS, Willoughby R, Betenbaugh MJ, Eiden JJ. Identification and expression of the outer capsid protein (VP4) of the IDIR strain of group B rotavirus. *Virology* 1993;194:724–733.

119. Chen GM, Hung T, Mackow ER. Identification of the gene encoding the group B rotavirus VP7 equivalent: primary characterization of the ADRV segment 9 RNA. *Virology* 1990;178: 311–315.

120. Petric M, Mayur K, Vonderfecht S, Eiden JJ. Comparison of group B rotavirus genes 9 and 11. *J Gen Virol* 1991;72: 2801–2804.

121. Green KY, Sears JF, Taniguchi K, et al. Prediction of human rotavirus serotype by nucleotide sequence analysis of the VP7 protein gene. *J Virol* 1988;62:1819–1823.

122. Saif LJ, Terrett LA, Miller KL, Cross RF. Serial propagation of porcine group C rotavirus (pararotavirus) in a continuous cell line and characterization of the passaged virus. *J Clin Microbiol* 1988;26:1277–1282.

123. Terrett LA, Saif LJ. Serial propagation of porcine group C rotavirus (pararotavirus) in primary porcine kidney cell cultures. *J Clin Microbiol* 1987;25:1316–1319.

124. Tsunemitsu H, Saif LJ, Jiang BM, et al. Isolation, characterization, and serial propagation of a bovine group C rotavirus in a monkey kidney cell line (MA104). *J Clin Microbiol* 1991;29: 2609–2613.

125. Welter MW, Welter CJ, Chambers DM, Svensson L. Adaptation and serial passage of porcine group C rotavirus in ST-cells, an established diploid swine testicular cell line. *Arch Virol* 1991; 120:297–304.

126. Bremont M, Chabanne VD, Vannier P, McCrae MA, Cohen J. Sequence analysis of the gene (6) encoding the major capsid protein (VP6) of group C rotavirus: higher than expected homology to the corresponding protein from group A virus. *Virology* 1990;178:579–583.

127. Bremont M, Juste LP, Chabanne VD, Charpilienne A, Cohen J. Sequences of the four larger proteins of a porcine group C rotavirus and comparison with the equivalent group A rotavirus proteins. *Virology* 1992;186:684–692.

128. Cooke SJ, Lambden PR, Caul EO, Clarke IN. Molecular cloning, sequence analysis and coding assignment of the major inner capsid protein gene of human group C rotavirus. *Virology* 1991; 184:781–785.

129. Jiang B, Tsunemitsu H, Gentsch JR, Glass RI, Green KY, Qian Y, Saif LJ. Nucleotide sequence of gene 5 encoding the inner capsid protein (VP6) of bovine group C rotavirus: comparison with corresponding genes of group C, A and B rotaviruses. *Virology* 1992;190:542–547.

130. Jiang B, Tsunemitsu H, Gentsch JR, Saif LJ, Glass RI. Nucleotide sequences of genes 6 and 10 of a bovine group C rotavirus. *Nucleic Acids Res* 1993;21:2250.

131. Jiang BM, Qian Y, Tsunemitsu H, Green KY, Saif LJ. Analysis of the gene encoding the outer capsid glycoprotein (VP7) of group C rotaviruses by Northern and dot blot hybridization. *Virology* 1991;184:433–436.

132. Jiang BM, Tsunemitsu H, Qian Y, Green KY, Oseto M, Yamashita Y, Saif LJ. Analysis of the genetic diversity of genes 5 and 6 among group C rotaviruses using cDNA probes. *Arch Virol* 1992;126:45–56.

133. Lambden PR, Cooke SJ, Caul EO, Clarke IN. Cloning of noncultivatable human rotavirus by single primer amplification. *J Virol* 1992;66:1817–1822.

134. Qian YA, Jiang BM, Saif LJ, et al. Sequence conservation of gene 8 between human and porcine group C rotaviruses and its relationship to the VP7 gene of group A rotaviruses. *Virology* 1991;182:562–569.

135. Qian YA, Jiang BM, Saif LJ, Kang SY, Ojeh CK, Green KY. Molecular analysis of the gene 6 from a porcine group C rotavirus that encodes the NS34 equivalent of group A rotaviruses. *Virology* 1991;184:752–757.

136. Tsunemitsu H, Jiang B, Yamashita Y, Oseto M, Ushijima H, Saif L. Evidence of serologic diversity within group C rotaviruses. *J Clin Microbiol* 1992;30:3009–3012.

137. Laemmli UK. Cleavage of structural proteins during the assembly of the head of bacteriophage T4. *Nature* 1970;227:680–685.

138. Arista S, Giovannelli L, Pistoia D, Cascio A, Parea M, Gerna G. Electropherotypes, subgroups and serotypes of human rotavirus strains causing gastroenteritis in infants and young children in Palermo, Italy, from 1985 to 1989. *Res Virol* 1990;141: 435–448.

139. Janke BH, Nelson JK, Benfield DA, Nelson EA. Relative prevalence of typical and atypical strains among rotaviruses from diarrheic pigs in conventional swine herds. *J Vet Diagn Invest* 1990;2:308–311.

140. Lipson SM, Kaplan MH. Atypical rotavirus genomic patterns identified by polyacrylamide gel electrophoresis. *J Diarrhoeal Dis Res* 1992;10:97–100.

141. Pocock DH. Characterisation of rotavirus isolates from subclinically infected calves by genome profile analysis. *Vet Microbiol* 1987;13:27–34.

142. Chen GM, Werner ER, Tao H, Mackow ER. Expression of the major inner capsid protein of the group B rotavirus ADRV: primary characterization of genome segment 5. *Virology* 1991; 182:820–829.

143. Dimitrov DH, Graham DY, Estes MK. Detection of rotaviruses by nucleic acid hybridization with cloned DNA of simian rotavirus SA11 genes. *J Infect Dis* 1985;152:293–300.

144. Eiden J, Sato S, Yolken R. Specificity of dot hybridization assay in the presence of rRNA for detection of rotaviruses in clinical specimens. *J Clin Microbiol* 1987;25:1809–1811.

145. Eiden JJ, Firoozmand F, Sato S, Vonderfecht SL, Yin FZ, Yolken RH. Detection of group B rotavirus in fecal specimens by dot hybridization with a cloned cDNA probe. *J Clin Microbiol* 1989;27:422–426.

146. Mason BB, Graham DY, Estes MK. Biochemical mapping of the simian rotavirus SA11 genome. *J Virol* 1983;46:413–423.

147. Rosen BI, Saif LJ, Jackwood DJ, Gorziglia M. Serotypic differentiation of group A rotaviruses with porcine rotavirus gene 9 probes. *J Clin Microbiol* 1990;28:2526–2533.

148. McCrae MA. Nucleic acid-based analyses of non-group A rotaviruses. *Ciba Found Symp* 1987;128:24–48.

149. Eiden JJ, Wilde J, Firoozmand F, Yolken R. Detection of animal and human group B rotaviruses in fecal specimens by polymerase chain reaction. *J Clin Microbiol* 1991;29:539–543.

150. Gouvea V, Allen JR, Glass RI, et al. Detection of group B and C rotaviruses by polymerase chain reaction. *J Clin Microbiol* 1991;29:519–523.

151. Fang ZY, Glass RI, Penaranda M, et al. Purification and characterization of adult diarrhea rotavirus: identification of viral structural proteins. *J Virol* 1989;63:2191–2197.

152. Flores J, Myslinski J, Kalica AR, Greenberg HB, Wyatt RG, Kapikian AZ, Chanock RM. In vitro transcription of two human rotaviruses. *J Virol* 1982;43:1032–1037.

153. Spencer E, Arias ML. In vitro transcription catalyzed by heat-treated human rotavirus. *J Virol* 1981;40:1–10.

154. Gallegos CO, Patton JT. Characterization of rotavirus replication intermediates: a model for the assembly of single-shelled particles. *Virology* 1989;172:616–627.

155. Mansell EA, Patton JT. Rotavirus RNA replication: VP2, but not VP6, is necessary for viral replicase activity. *J Virol* 1990;64:4988–4996.

156. Patton JT, Gallegos CO. Structure and protein composition of the rotavirus replicase particle. *Virology* 1988;166:358–365.

157. Patton JT, Gallegos CO. Rotavirus RNA replication: single-stranded RNA extends from the replicase particle. *J Gen Virol* 1990;71:1087–1094.

158. Eiden JJ, Vonderfecht S, Petric M. Terminal sequence conservation among the genomic segments of a group B rotavirus (IDIR strain). *Virology* 1992;191:495–497.

159. Eiden JJ, Yolken RH, Vonderfecht SL, Tao H, McCrae MA. Terminal fingerprint analysis of group B rotaviruses [Letter]. *J Infect Dis* 1988;158:657–658.

160. Jashes M, Sandino AM, Faundez G, Avendano LF, Spencer E. In vitro transcription of human pararotavirus. *J Virol* 1986;57:183–190.

161. Sandino AM, Jashes M, Faundez G, Spencer E. Role of the inner protein capsid on in vitro human rotavirus transcription. *J Virol* 1986;60:797–802.

162. Spencer E, Garcia BI. Effect of S-adenosylmethionine on human rotavirus RNA synthesis. *J Virol* 1984;52:188–197.

163. Jiang BM, Saif LJ. In vitro transcription and translation of genomic RNA from a porcine group C rotavirus. *Arch Virol* 1992;124:181–185.

164. Eiden JJ, Wee SB, Vonderfecht SL. In vitro transcription and translation of group B rotavirus strain IDIR gene 8 and immunoprecipitation by human sera. *J Clin Microbiol* 1992;30:440–443.

165. Mackow ER, Fay ME, Hung T, Shaw R, Chen GM. Cloning, sequencing and expression of the gene encoding the VP2 protein of the human group B rotavirus, ADRV. *Virology* [in press].

166. Fang ZY, Monroe SS, Dong H, et al. Coding assignments of the genome of adult diarrhea rotavirus. *Arch Virol* 1992;125:53–69.

167. Smith ML, Lazdins I, Holmes IH. Coding assignments of double-stranded RNA segments of SA 11 rotavirus established by in vitro translation. *J Virol* 1980;33:976–981.

168. Ericson BL, Graham DY, Mason BB, Estes MK. Identification, synthesis, and modifications of simian rotavirus SA11 polypeptides in infected cells. *J Virol* 1982;42:825–839.

169. Devereaux J, Haeberli P, Smithies O. A comprehensive set of sequence analysis programs for the VAX. *Nucleic Acids Res* 1984;12:387–395.

170. Eiden JJ, Allen JR. Identification of cognate genes among heterologous strains of group B rotavirus. *J Virol* 1992;66:1232–1235.

171. Mackow ER, Chou RH, Dowling W, Fay ME, Dowling W, Chen GM. Gene segment 6 of ADRV encodes a putative fusion protein of group B rotaviruses. [*Submitted*].

172. Mackow ER, Yamanaka MY, Dang MN, Greenberg HB. DNA amplification-restricted transcription-translation: rapid analysis of rhesus rotavirus neutralization sites [published erratum appears in *Proc Natl Acad Sci USA* 1990;87(11):4411]. *Proc Natl Acad Sci USA* 1990;87:518–522.

173. Theil KW, McCloskey CM. Rabbit syncytium virus is a Kemerovo serogroup orbivirus. *J Clin Microbiol* 1991;29:2059–2062.

174. Theil KW, Saif LJ. In vitro detection of porcine rotavirus-like virus (group B rotavirus) and its antibody. *J Clin Microbiol* 1985;21:844–846.

175. Eiden JJ. Gene 5 of the IDIR agent (group B rotavirus) encodes a protein equivalent to NS34 of group A rotavirus. *Virology* 1993;196:298–302.

176. Eiden JJ, Hirshon C. Sequence analysis of group B rotavirus gene 1 and definition of a rotavirus-specific sequence motif within the RNA polymerase. *Virology* 1993;192:154–160.

177. Lindsay DA, Vonderfecht SL, Betenbaugh MJ, Eiden JJ. Baculovirus expression of gene 6 of the IDIR strain of group B rotavirus (GBR): coding assignment of the major inner capsid protein. *Virology* 1993;193:367–375.

178. French TJ, Marshall JA, Roy P. Assembly of double-shelled, viruslike particles of bluetongue virus by the simultaneous expression of four structural proteins. *J Virol* 1990;64:5695–5700.

179. Labbe M, Charpilienne A, Crawford SE, Estes MK, Cohen J. Expression of rotavirus VP2 produces empty corelike particles. *J Virol* 1991;65:2946–2952.

180. Liu HM, Booth TF, Roy P. Interactions between bluetongue virus core and capsid proteins translated in vitro. *J Gen Virol* 1992;73:2577–2584.

181. Loudon PT, Roy P. Assembly of five bluetongue virus proteins expressed by recombinant baculoviruses: inclusion of the largest protein VP1 in the core and virus-like particles. *Virology* 1991;180:798–802.

182. Sabara M, Parker M, Aha P, Cosco C, Gibbons E, Parsons S, Babiuk LA. Assembly of double-shelled rotaviruslike particles by simultaneous expression of recombinant VP6 and VP7 proteins. *J Virol* 1991;65:6994–6997.

183. Vonderfecht SL, Schemmer JK. Purification of the IDIR strain of group B rotavirus and identification of viral structural proteins. *Virology* 1993;194:277–283.

184. Both GW, Mattick JS, Bellamy AR. Serotype-specific glycoprotein of simian 11 rotavirus: coding assignment and gene sequence. *Proc Natl Acad Sci USA* 1983;80:3091–3095.

185. Estes MK, Mason BB, Crawford S, Cohen J. Cloning and nucleotide sequence of the simian rotavirus gene 6 that codes for the major inner capsid protein. *Nucleic Acids Res* 1984;12:1875–1887.

186. Mackow ER, Shaw RD, Matsui SM, Vo PT, Benfield DA, Greenberg HB. Characterization of homotypic and heterotypic VP7 neutralization sites of rhesus rotavirus. *Virology* 1988;165:511–517.

187. Stirzaker SC, Both GW. The signal peptide of the rotavirus glycoprotein VP7 is essential for its retention in the ER as an integral membrane protein. *Cell* 1989;56:741–747.

188. Mackow ER, Shaw RD, Matsui SM, Vo PT, Dang MN, Greenberg HB. The rhesus rotavirus gene encoding protein VP3: location of amino acids involved in homologous and heterologous rotavirus neutralization and identification of a putative fusion region. *Proc Natl Acad Sci USA* 1988;85:645–649.

189. Anthony ID, Bullivant S, Dayal S, Bellamy AR, Berriman JA. Rotavirus spike structure and polypeptide composition. *J Virol* 1991;65:4334–4340.

190. Prasad BV, Burns JW, Marietta E, Estes MK, Chiu W. Localization of VP4 neutralization sites in rotavirus by three-dimensional cryo-electron microscopy. *Nature* 1990;343:476–479.

191. Fiore L, Greenberg HB, Mackow ER. The VP8 fragment of VP4 is the rhesus rotavirus hemagglutinin. *Virology* 1991;181:553–563.

192. Kalica AR, Flores J, Greenberg HB. Identification of the rotaviral gene that codes for hemagglutination and protease-enhanced plaque formation. *Virology* 1983;125:194–205.

193. Mackow ER, Barnett JW, Chan H, Greenberg HB. The rhesus rotavirus outer capsid protein VP4 functions as a hemagglutinin and is antigenically conserved when expressed by a baculovirus recombinant. *J Virol* 1989;63:1661–1668.

194. Offit PA, Blavat G. Identification of the two rotavirus genes determining neutralization specificities. *J Virol* 1986;57:376–378.

195. Offit PA, Blavat G, Greenberg HB, Clark HF. Molecular basis of rotavirus virulence: role of gene segment 4. *J Virol* 1986;57:46–49.

196. Lopez S, Arias CF, Bell JR, Str AJ, Espejo RT. Primary structure of the cleavage site associated with trypsin enhancement of rotavirus SA11 infectivity. *Virology* 1985;144:11–19.

197. Mackow ER, Vo PT, Broome R, Bass D, Greenberg HB. Immunization with baculovirus-expressed VP4 protein passively protects against simian and murine rotavirus challenge. *J Virol* 1990;64:1698–1703.

198. Gorziglia M, Larralde G, Kapikian AZ, Chanock RM. Antigenic relationships among human rotaviruses as determined by outer capsid protein VP4. *Proc Natl Acad Sci USA* 1990;87:7155–7159.

199. Dai GZ, Sun MS, Liu SQ, et al. First report of an epidemic of diarrhoea in human neonates involving the new rotavirus and

biological characteristics of the epidemic virus strain (KMB/R85). *J Med Virol* 1987;22:365–373.

200. Spear PG. Virus-induced cell fusion. In: Sowers AE, ed. *Cell fusion*. New York: Plenum Press, 1987;3–31.

201. White J. Membrane fusion. *Science* 1992;258:917–924.

202. Collins PL, Huang YT, Wertz GW. Nucleotide sequence of the gene encoding the fusion (F) glycoprotein of human respiratory syncytial virus. *Proc Natl Acad Sci USA* 1984;81:7683–7687.

203. Hsu M, Choppin P. Analysis of Sendai virus mRNAs with cDNA clones of viral genes and sequences of biologically important regions of the fusion protein. *Proc Natl Acad Sci USA* 1984;81:7732–7736.

204. McGinnes LW, Morrison TG. Nucleotide sequence of the gene encoding the Newcastle disease virus fusion protein and comparison with other paramyxovirus fusion protein sequences. *Virus Res* 1986;5:343–356.

205. Portner A, Scroggs R, Naeve C. The fusion glycoprotein of Sendai virus: sequence analysis of an epitope involved in fusion and virus neutralization. *Virology* 1987;157:556–559.

206. Richardson C, Hull D, Greer P, et al. The nucleotide sequence of the mRNA encoding the fusion protein of measles virus: a comparison of fusion proteins from several different paramyxoviruses. *Virology* 1986;155:508–523.

207. Horvath C, Paterson R, Shaughnessy M, Wood R, Lamb R. Biological activity of paramyxovirus fusion proteins: factors influencing formation of syncytia. *J Virol* 1992;66:4564–4569.

208. Horvath CM, Lamb RA. Studies on the fusion peptide of a paramyxovirus fusion glycoprotein: roles of conserved residues in cell fusion. *J Virol* 1992;66:2443–2455.

209. Iorio R, Glickman R, Sheehan J. Inhibition of fusion by neutralizing monoclonal antibodies to the haemagglutinin–neuraminidase glycoprotein of Newcastle disease virus. *J Gen Virol* 1992;73:1167–1176.

210. Richardson CD, Choppin PW. Oligopeptides that specifically inhibit membrane fusion by paramyxoviruses: studies on the site of action. *Virology* 1983;131:518–532.

211. Taylor G, Stott E, Furze J, Ford J, Sopp P. Protective epitopes on the fusion protein of respiratory syncytial virus recognized by murine and bovine monoclonal antibodies. *J Gen Virol* 1992;73:2217–2223.

212. Gordon JI, Duronio RJ, Rudnick DA, Adams SP, Gokel GW. Protein N-myristoylation. *J Biol Chem* 1991;266:8647–8650.

213. Buckland R, Malvaoisin E, Beauverger P, Wild F. A leucine zipper structure in the measles virus fusion protein is not required for tetramerization but is essential for fusion. *J Gen Virol* 1992;73:1703–1707.

214. Chen S, Lee C, Lee W, McIntosh K, Lee T. Mutational analysis of the leucine zipper-like motif of the HIV type 1 envelope transmembrane glycoprotein. *J Virol* 1993;67:3615–3619.

215. Eisenberg D. Three-dimensional structure of membrane and surface proteins. *Ann Rev Biochem* 1984;53:595–623.

216. Helseth E, Olshevsky U, Gabuzda D, Ardman B, Haseltine W, Sodroski J. Changes in the transmembrane region of the human immunodeficiency virus type 1 gp41 envelope glycoprotein affect membrane fusion. *J Virol* 1990;64:6314–6318.

217. Schmidt MFG. Acylation of viral spike glycoproteins: a feature of enveloped RNA viruses. *Virology* 1982;116:327–338.

218. Towler DA, Gordon JI, Adams SP, Glaser L. The biology and enzymology of eukaryotic protein acylation. *Annu Rev Biochem* 1988;57:69–99.

219. Lamb RA, Choppin PW. Identification of a second protein (M2) encoded by RNA segment 7 of influenza virus. *Virology* 1981;112:729–737.

220. Lamb RA, Zebedee SL, Richardson CD. Influenza virus M2 protein is an integral membrane protein expressed on the infected-cell surface. *Cell* 1985;40:627–633.

221. Shaw MW, Lamb RA, Choppin PW. A previously unrecognized influenza B virus glycoprotein from a bicistronic mRNA that also encodes the viral neuraminidase. *Proc Natl Acad Sci USA* 1984;80:4879–4883.

222. Sugrue RJ, Belshe RB, Hay AJ. Palmitoylation of the influenza A virus M2 protein. *Virology* 1990;179:51–56.

223. Pinto LH, Holsinger LJ, Lamb RA. Influenza virus M2 protein has ion channel activity. *Cell* 1992;69:517–528.

224. Sugrue RJ, Hay AJ. Structural characteristics of the M2 protein of influenza A viruses: evidence that it forms a tetrameric channel. *Virology* 1991;180:617–624.

225. Bryant M, Heuckeroth R, Kimata J, Ratner L, Gordon J. Replication of HIV 1 and Maloney murine leukemia virus is inhibited by different deteroatom containing analogs of myristic acid. *Proc Natl Acad Sci USA* 1989;86:8655–8659.

226. Bryant M, Ratner L, Duronio R, Kishore N, Devadas B, Adams S, Gordon J. Incorporation of 12-methoxydodecanoate into the HIV 1 gag polyprotein precursor inhibits its proteolytic processing and virus production in a chronically infected human lymphoid cell line. *Proc Natl Acad Sci USA* 1991;88:2055–2059.

227. Hsu M, Scheid A, Choppin PW. Activation of the Sendai virus fusion protein (F) involves a conformational change with exposure of a new hydrophobic region. *J Biol Chem* 1981;256:3557–3563.

228. Krausslich HG, Holscher C, Reuer Q, Harber J, Wimmer E. Myristoylation of the poliovirus polyprotein is required for proteolytic processing of the capsid and for viral infectivity. *J Virol* 1990;64:2433–2436.

229. Moscufo N, Chow M. Myristate–protein interactions in poliovirus: interactions of VP4 threonine 28 contribute to the structural conformation of assembly intermediates and the stability of assembled virions. *J Virol* 1992;66:6849–6857.

230. Nibert M, Fields BN. A carboxy-terminal fragment of protein μ is present in infectious subvirion particles of mammalian reoviruses and is proposed to have a role in penetration. *J Virol* 1992;66:6408–6418.

231. Nibert ML, Schiff LA, Fields BN. Mammalian reoviruses contain a myristoylated structural protein. *J Virol* 1991;65:1960–1967.

232. Tillotson L, Shatkin AJ. Reovirus polypeptide sigma 3 and N-terminal myristoylation of polypeptide μ1 are required for site-specific cleavage to μ1c in transfected cells. *J Virol* 1992;66:2180–2186.

233. Wang C, Barklis E. Assembly, processing, and infectivity of HIV type 1 Gag mutants. *J Virol* 1993;67:4264–4273.

234. Cooke SJ, Clarke IN, Freitas RB, Gabbay YB, Lambden PR. The correct sequence of the porcine group C/Cowden rotavirus major inner capsid protein shows close homology with human isolates from Brazil and the U.K. *Virology* 1992;190:531–537.

235. Bremont M, Chabanne-Vautherot D, Cohen J. Sequence analysis of three non structural proteins of a porcine group C (Cowden strain) rotavirus. *Arch Virol* 1993;130:85–92.

236. Bremont M, Juste LP, Chabanne VD, Charpilienne A, Cohen J. Erratum: Sequences of the four larger proteins of a porcine group C rotavirus and comparison with the equivalent group A rotavirus proteins. *Virology* 1992;189:402.

237. Bremont M, Cohen J, McCrae MA. Analysis of the structural polypeptides of a porcine group C rotavirus. *J Virol* 1988;62:2183–2185.

238. Jiang BM, Saif LJ, Kang SY, Kim JH. Biochemical characterization of the structural and nonstructural polypeptides of a porcine group C rotavirus. *J Virol* 1990;64:3171–3178.

239. Svensson L. Group C rotavirus requires sialic acid for erythrocyte and cell receptor binding. *J Virol* 1992;66:5582–5585.

240. Bastardo JW, Holmes IH. Attachment of SA-11 rotavirus to erythrocyte receptors. *Infect Immun* 1980;29:1134–1140.

241. Tosser G, Labbe M, Bremont M, Cohen J. Expression of the major capsid protein of group C rotavirus and synthesis of chimeric single-shelled particles by using recombinant baculoviruses. *J Virol* 1992;66:5825–5831.

242. Alpers D, Sanders RC, Hampson DJ. Rotavirus excretion by village pigs in Papua New Guinea. *Aust Vet J* 1991;68:65–67.

243. Noel JS, Beards GM, Cubitt WD. Epidemiological survey of human rotavirus serotypes and electropherotypes in young children admitted to two children's hospitals in northeast London from 1984 to 1990. *J Clin Microbiol* 1991;29:2213–2219.

244. Welter M, Chambers DM, Horstman MP, Welter CJ, Mackow ER. Development of a neutralization assay for the evaluation of human and porcine serogroup B antibodies. Double-Stranded RNA Virus Meeting Scottsdale, Arizona, 1992, p 35.

245. Estes MK, Graham DY, Gerba CP, Smith EM. Simian rotavirus SA11 replication in cell cultures. *J Virol* 1979;31:810–815.
246. Huber AC, Yolken RH, Mader LC, Strandberg JD, Vonderfecht SL. Pathology of infectious diarrhea of infant rats (IDIR) induced by an antigenically distinct rotavirus. *Vet Pathol* 1989; 26:376–385.
247. Gard G, Compans RW. Structure and cytopathic effects of Nelson Bay virus. *J Virol* 1970;6:100–106.
248. Kawamura H, Shimizu F, Maeda M, Tsubahara H. Avian reovirus: its properties and serological classification. *Natl Inst Anim Health Q (Tokyo)* 1965;5:115–124.
249. Ni Y, Ramig RF. Characterization of avian reovirus-induced cell fusion: the role of structural proteins. *Virology* 1993;194: 705–714.
250. Wilcox GE, Compans RW. Cell fusion induced by Nelson Bay virus. *Virology* 1982;123:312–322.
251. Wilcox GE, Compans RW. Characterization of Nelson Bay virus and virus-induced cell fusion. Bishop RWC, Bishop DHL, eds. *Double-stranded RNA viruses.* New York: Elsevier Science Publishing, 1983;391–403.
252. Ramia S. Transmission of viral infections by the water route: implications for developing countries. *Rev Infect Dis* 1985;7: 180–188.
253. Penaranda ME, Ho MS, Fang ZY, et al. Seroepidemiology of adult diarrhea rotavirus in China, 1977 to 1987. *J Clin Microbiol* 1989;27:2180–2183.
254. Qiu FX, Tian Y, Liu JC, Zhang XS, Hao YP. Antibody against adult diarrhoea rotavirus among healthy adult population in China. *J Virol Methods* 1986;14:127–132.
255. Vonderfecht SL, Eiden JJ, Miskuff RL, Yolken RH. Kinetics of intestinal replication of group B rotavirus and relevance to diagnostic methods. *J Clin Microbiol* 1988;26:216–221.
256. Besselaar TG, Rosenblatt A, Kidd AH. Atypical rotavirus from South African neonates. Brief report. *Arch Virol* 1986;87: 327–330.
257. Qian Y, Saif LJ, Kapikian AZ, et al. Comparison of human and porcine group C rotaviruses by Northern blot hybridization analysis. *Arch Virol* 1991;118:269–277.
258. Oishi I, Yamazaki K, Minekawa Y. An occurrence of diarrheal cases associated with group C rotavirus in adults. *Microbiol Immunol* 1993;37:505.
259. Lebaron CW, Furutan NP, Lew JF, Allen JR, Gouvea V, Moe C, Monroe SS. Viral agents of gastroenteritis. *MMWR Morb Mortal Wkly Rep* 1990;39:1–24.
260. Flewett TH, Beards GM, Brown DW, Sanders RC. The diagnostic gap in diarrhoeal aetiology. *Ciba Found Symp* 1987;128: 238–249.
261. Kinney JS, Viscidi RP, Vonderfecht SL, Eiden JJ, Yolken RH. Monoclonal antibody assay for detection of double-stranded RNA and application for detection of group A and non-group A rotaviruses. *J Clin Microbiol* 1989;27:6–12.
262. Burns JW, Welch SK, Nakata S, Estes MK. Characterization of monoclonal antibodies to human group B rotavirus and their use in an antigen detection enzyme-linked immunosorbent assay. *J Clin Microbiol* 1989;27:245–250.
263. Vonderfecht SL, Miskuff RL, Eiden JJ, Yolken RH. Enzyme immunoassay inhibition assay for the detection of rat rotavirus-like agent in intestinal and fecal specimens obtained from diarrheic rats and humans. *J Clin Micro* 1985;22:726–730.
264. Kuzuya M, Fujii R, Hamano M, et al. Rapid detection of human group C rotaviruses by reverse passive hemagglutination and latex agglutination tests using monoclonal antibodies. *J Clin Microbiol* 1993;31:1308–1311.
265. Tsunemitsu H, Jiang B, Saif LJ. Detection of group C rotavirus antigens and antibodies in animals and humans by enzyme-linked immunosorbent assays. *J Clin Microbiol* 1992;30: 2129–2134.

Infections of the Gastrointestinal Tract,
edited by M. J. Blaser, P. D. Smith, J. I. Ravdin,
H. B. Greenberg, and R. L. Guerrant
Raven Press, Ltd., New York © 1995.

CHAPTER 66

Norwalk Virus and Other Enteric Caliciviruses

Mary K. Estes and Michele E. Hardy

Acute infectious nonbacterial gastroenteritis is a common illness that frequently occurs in young children and in epidemics involving older children and adults (1). Epidemic viral gastroenteritis usually occurs in family or community-wide outbreaks, affecting adults, school-age children, family contacts, and some young children as well. Epidemic viral gastroenteritis is usually mild and self-limited, generally distinguishing it from infantile gastroenteritis caused by rotaviruses, which is associated with severe (often life-threatening) diarrheal illness in infants and young children.

The first virus identified as a cause of gastroenteritis was the agent known as Norwalk virus (NV). This virus originated from an outbreak of epidemic gastroenteritis in an elementary school in Norwalk, Ohio, in 1968. During this outbreak, 50% of the students and teachers became ill and secondary spread to 32% of family contacts was documented (2). Ultimately, NV was visualized using immunoelectron microscopy (IEM) and described as a filterable agent 27-nm × 32-nm (3). This report provided definitive proof that viruses can cause diarrhea, a hypothesis based on many studies performed during the 1940s and 1950s in which filterable infectious agents were able to be passaged serially in volunteers, yet no virus was successfully cultivated using the tissue culture techniques developed during the 1950s. Administration of a bacteria-free fecal filtrate of NV to volunteers resulted in the first clear description of the basic virologic, clinical, and immunologic responses to nonbacterial infections (4) (see later discussion). The history of these early investigations leading to visualization of the agent by IEM provides an excellent example of the fact that major scientific advances often require and parallel new technologic opportunities. The subsequent application of IEM to other diarrheal stool samples ultimately led to the discovery of many other viral agents of gastroenteritis (see later discussion

and chapters by Greenberg, Bass and Greenberg, Mackow, Matsui, Herrmann and Blacklow, and Glass).

MORPHOLOGY AND CLASSIFICATION

After the initial description of NV in 1972 and until 1990, it was difficult to study NV and related agents for several reasons. First, these viruses remained refractory to cultivation and there are no animal models to produce virus particles. These complications resulted in limiting study of these agents to a few research laboratories or to public health or hospital laboratories, which were able to identify viruses by relatively sophisticated methods such as IEM. This method of virus detection was necessitated by the extremely low concentrations of virus present in stool samples. In addition, the initial tests for virus detection, which utilized reagents from human volunteer studies, had limited availability and sensitivity.

While the ability to characterize many of these viruses remained limited, once NV was recognized in stools by IEM, an explosion of studies rapidly reported many similar agents, including the Hawaii agent (5), Snow Mountain agent (6), Montgomery County agent (7), Taunton agent (8), and Otofuke, Sapporo, and Osaka agents (9–11). Thus visualization of NV opened a new era in characterization of viral agents associated with diarrheal disease, and in a seemingly short time, the relatively large-sized rotaviruses, enteric adenoviruses, coronaviruses, toroviruses and the smaller-sized viruses (caliciviruses and astroviruses) possessing a reproducible classic surface morphology were identified. The rotaviruses were quickly recognized to be the major viral agents responsible for life-threatening diarrheal illness in young children and animals (see chapters by Bass and Greenberg and Mackow).

Viruses of smaller size with an amorphous surface structure and a ragged ill-defined edge were increasingly identified but were difficult to classify. Historically, NV and related viruses were classified based on morphology.

M. K. Estes and M. E. Hardy: Division of Molecular Virology, Baylor College of Medicine, Houston, Texas 77030.

TABLE 1. *Interim classification of small round fecal viruses according to morphology by electron microscopy*

Morphology	Type of virus	Morphologic/biophysical properties/genome	Examples	Comment
Featureless (no surface structure; smooth outer edge)	Picornavirus	BD 1.34 g/cm³ Size ~23–30 nm RNA genome	Poliovirus, coxsackievirus, hepatitis A virus	
	Parvovirus	BD 1.38–1.46 g/cm³ Size ~18–26 nm ssDNA	Mink enteritis virus, feline/canine/bovine parvoviruses	
	Small round viruses	BD 1.38–1.40 g/cm³ Size ~22–26 nm DNA?	Wollan, Parramatta, Ditchling, cockle agents	May be parvoviruses or bacteriophage heads carried in feces and unrelated to gastroenteritis. Ditchling virus originally classified here later shown to be an astrovirus.
Structured (surface structure and/or ragged edge)	Astrovirus	5–6 pointed surface star BD 1.36–1.38 g/cm³ Size ~28–30 nm RNA	Lamb, human astroviruses (five serotypes)	
	Calicivirus	Surface hollows, ragged outline, "Star of David" configuration BD 1.36–1.39 g/cm³ Size ~30–38 nm RNA	Human (UK1–4 and Sapporo), Newbury (bovine), porcine	
	Small round structured virus (SRSV)	Amorphous surface, ragged outline; BD 1.36–1.41 g/cm³ Size ~30–35 nm RNA	Norwalk, Hawaii, Snow Mountain, Montgomery County, Taunton, Otofuke, Sapporo, Osaka, minireoviruses	Norwalk, Hawaii, Snow Mountain, and most SRSVs now shown to be human caliciviruses based on sequence analysis; others still not tested (see text)

Adapted from ref. 13.
BD, buoyant density.

Geographical names were used to denote the location of the outbreak of gastroenteritis as a way to describe these morphologically ill-defined particles. In the absence of being able to cultivate these agents, they were divided into two morphological groups (Table 1) as one means of classifying them. In this interim classification system, viruses were first characterized according to whether they had visible structural features, and NV was classified as a small round structured virus (SRSV) (12,13). This system helped researchers and electron microscopists compare agents, but it suffered from being simply a morphologic system with its success dependent on the timing and quality of samples collected and given to the microscopists and on the skill and interpretation of individual electron microscopists. These inherent difficulties were compounded for stool samples, which are not clear or easy samples to study, and which may contain fecal immunoglobulins or other factors (proteolytic enzymes, mucins, etc.) that may obscure or degrade the surface structure of viruses. In spite of these limitations, this interim classification system served a need with the recognized caveat

that conclusions based on EM classification alone must be regarded as tentative. Recent studies in which new methods have been applied to samples previously characterized by EM alone have highlighted this point and demonstrated that some agents previously classified solely by morphology have been incorrectly identified (14). Similarly, recent studies using molecular methods have shown that many particles previously characterized as other agents (e.g., minireoviruses) are actually Norwalk-like viruses, and viruses with or without typical calicivirus morphology also may be Norwalk-like agents (see later discussion).

Definitive virus classification is based on virus morphology, biophysical and biochemical properties, and on properties of the organization of a viral genome and its strategy of expression (15). Early biochemical studies on the proteins of NV isolated from stools of infected volunteers predicted this agent to be a calicivirus based on the presence of a single virion-associated protein of approximately 59K (16). This characteristic was consistent with the prototypical caliciviruses having a single structural protein with molecular weights ranging from 60K to 71K (17–19). Molecular cloning and characterization of the NV genome allowed this virus to be unequivocally classified as a member of the family Caliciviridae (20). The name caliciviruses comes from the Latin *calyx,* meaning "cup" or "goblet" from cup-shaped depressions observed by EM. Caliciviruses are nonenveloped icosahedral particles with a capsid made up of a single polypeptide. The calicivirus genome contains a single-stranded ribonucleic acid (RNA) genome of positive polarity, approximately 7.7 kilobases in size.

The NV genome characteristics and organization showed that it is a calicivirus, and new structural studies confirm that this virus contains cup-shaped depressions. However, these depressions are not very apparent in negative-stain electron micrographs. Thus NV, the previous prototype SRSV, is a human calicivirus and it has now been proposed to be the prototype human calicivirus by the International Committee on Taxonomy of Viruses (ICTV). Many other SRSVs (over 50) that have been characterized recently also have been shown to be human caliciviruses.

Currently, it remains unknown whether all previously characterized SRSVs will ultimately be shown to be human caliciviruses, or whether another type of virus will be identified from the group of SRSVs. To facilitate communication among researchers, it has been proposed that these viruses be denoted by a cryptogram that includes the following information: type of virus/name of virus/ strain designation/year of isolation/country of isolation. Once this information is provided, for simplicity, one can subsequently refer to the virus by the virus name or the strain designation. In this system, the prototype human calicivirus NV would be denoted HuCV/NV/8FIIa/68/US and, subsequently, NV. Agents initially identified by EM as SRSVs would be denoted SRSV in the cryptogram and

this designation would be changed to HuCV providing the viruses are found to be caliciviruses (Table 2). As serotypes are understood and defined, the serotype designation could be added after the HuCV. Thus it can be anticipated that NV will be HuCV-1 to designate serotype 1.

Knowing NV is a human calicivirus, it is of interest to compare the properties of this prototype virus with other known caliciviruses (Table 3). Three key features come from this comparison: (a) the only cultivatable caliciviruses have been strains from animals; (b) animal caliciviruses cause a spectrum of diseases, in addition to diarrheal disease; and (c) some caliciviruses have a broad host range and infect more than one species. It should be noted that human caliciviruses remain relatively poorly studied compared to some of the animal caliciviruses. It seems likely that additional human illnesses and possibly crosstransmission of viruses between species will be discovered as the human caliciviruses become better characterized. This idea is fortified by the rapid changes being observed in the epidemiology of NV-induced disease now that new methods of virus detection are available (see later discussion.)

VIRUS STRUCTURE

Norwalk virus was classically described as a 27-nm particle based on analysis of particles obtained from stools that were aggregated with antibody (3). One limitation to the EM structural analysis of particles from stool has been the necessity to perform IEM due to the low numbers of particles present in most stool preparations. However, based on these micrographs, it was rare to see particles with typical calicivirus structure, having distinct cup-like indentations in the surface of particles (see Fig. 1A,B).

TABLE 2. *Cryptogram and genogroups of NV and NV-related viruses*

Virus	Previous morphologic designation	Cryptogram	Genogroup[a]	References
Norwalk virus	SRSV/NV	HuCV/NV/8FIIa/68/US	I	3,20
Southampton agent	SRSV/SHV	HuCV/SHV/9/UK	I	28
Desert Shield virus	SRSV/DSV	HuCV/DSV/395/90/KU	I	30
Hawaii agent	SRSV/HV	HuCV/HV/71/US	II	5,31
Snow Mountain agent	SRSV/SMA	HuCV/SMA/76/US	II	35
Minireovirus	Minireovirus	HuCV/TV/24/77/Can	II	29
Human calicivirus Sapporo	HuCV/Sapporo or HuCV/Japan	HuCV/SV/strain/82/J	III	10,37
SRSVs	Many different strains	HuCV/strain/yr/country	I, II, III	28,32–35
SRSVs UK1–4	SRSV/UK1–4	HuCV/strain/yr/UK	I or II	32,33
Japanese SRSV1–9	SRSV/J1–9	HuCV/strain/yr/J	I or II	32
Human caliciviruses UK1, UK2, UK3, UK4	HuCV/UK1–4	HuCV/strain/yr/UK	II*. Many not yet typed	154
Otofuke agent	SRSV/Otofuke	Currently unknown	ND	9

ND, not determined.

[a] Grouping is based on nucleotide/amino acid sequence homologies in the polymerase region and the capsid region of the calicivirus genome. For the capsid region, viruses within a genogroup show >80% amino acid similarity. For the polymerase region, viruses within a genogroup show >92% amino acid similarity. The cutoff value for genetic grouping is at present arbitrary. (See Figs. 4 and 5.)

TABLE 3. *Comparison of human calicivirus (Norwalk) with animal caliciviruses*

Virus strain	Host range origin (secondary hosts)	Designation	Disease	Typical calicivirus structure	Cultivated	Other comments
Norwalk virus	Humans	HuCV/NV/8FIIa/68/US	Diarrhea	No	No	Prototype human calicivirus; several genogroups (see Table 2)
Porcine enteric calicivirus	Pigs	PEC	Diarrhea	Yes	Yes	Cultivation required adding large intestinal content fluids
Bovine enteric calicivirus	Calves	Newbury agent 1 and 2	Diarrhea	Yes	No	
Feline calicivirus	Cats, dogs (humans?)	FCV	Respiratory illness, arthritis	Yes	Yes	One serotype with many variants, persistent infections
Rabbit hemorrhagic disease virus	Rabbits	RHDV	Hemorrhagic diarrheal disease—often lethal; liver infected	Yes	No	Not yet isolated in United States; found in Europe, China, Mexico
San Miguel sea lion virus	Sea lions (humans)	SMSV	Abortions, vesicular lesions	Yes	Yes	Possibly the same virus as VESV
Vesicular exanthema of swine virus	Pigs (fish; sea lions?)	VESV	Skin lesions, glossitis, diarrhea	Yes	Yes	Possibly the same virus as SMSV
Primate calicivirus	Pigmy chimpanzees	PrCV-Pan 1/82	None	Yes	Yes	Persistent infections
Chicken enteric calicivirus	Chickens	ChCV	Diarrhea	Yes	No	

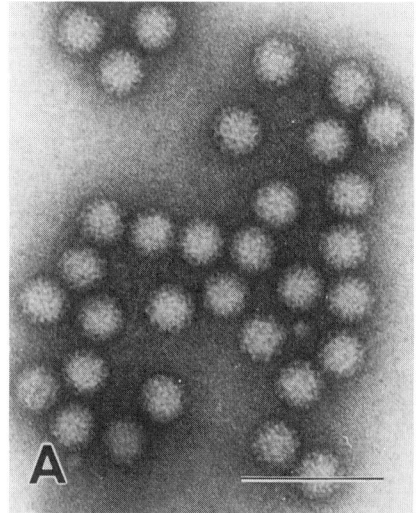 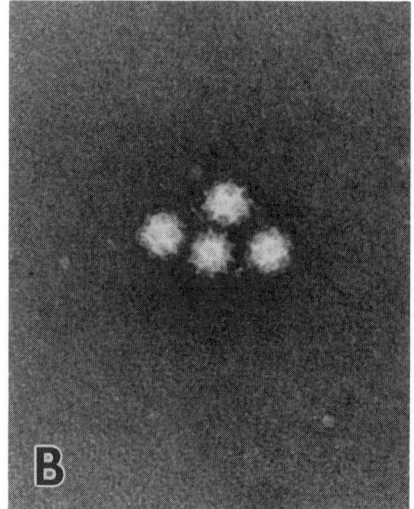 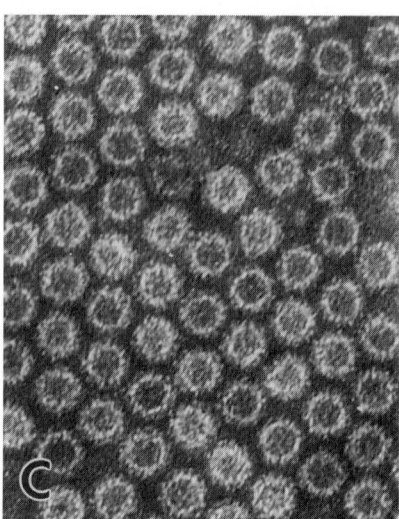

FIG. 1. Electron micrographs of caliciviruses. Negative-stain electron micrographs of (**A**) Norwalk virus from the stool of a volunteer given HuCV/NV/8FIIa; (**B**) a human calicivirus with typical structure including distinct cup-like indentations in the surface of particles, taken from the stool of a child containing HuCV/Sapporo; and (**C**) rNV particles produced and purified from insect cells infected with a baculovirus recombinant that expresses the NV ORF2. Bar, 50 nm.

Instead, the NV appeared to have a feathery outer edge that lacked a definitive surface substructure (Fig. 1A); in certain orientations, NV appeared to have minor surface indentations.

A more precise description of the structure of NV is now available based on the analysis of recombinant Norwalk virus (rNV) particles produced in insect cells by a baculovirus recombinant expressing the cDNA that encodes the capsid protein (21). The NV capsid is unusual among animal viruses in that it is composed of a single polypeptide. While this property is common among plant viruses, it is unusual among animal viruses and the only other known animal viruses to share this feature, apart from caliciviruses, are the nodaviruses (22,23). By negative-stain EM, rNV particles have a similar morphology to the native NV (Fig. 1A,C). Analysis of these rNV particles by electron cryomicroscopy and computer image processing has shown the rNV particles have a distinct architecture and exhibit T = 3 icosahedral symmetry (Fig. 2A) (24). The capsid is made of 90 dimers of the capsid protein that form a shell domain from which arch-like capsomers protrude (Fig. 2B–D). These arches are arranged in such a way that there are large hollows at the icosahedral 5- and 3-fold positions (Fig. 2B). These hollows are what appear as the cup-like structures in typical caliciviruses. The three-dimensional structure of a typical calicivirus (the primate PrCV Pan-1) also has been determined (25); this typical calicivirus structure differs from that of NV primarily in the length and shape of the protruding arch-like domains. That is, the protruding domain in the typical calicivirus is longer than that for NV and the shape of the top of the arch also differs in such a way that the NV would show a feathery appearance by negative-stain EM.

These three-dimensional structures are valuable as they provide independent evidence of the similarities of these two distinct types of caliciviruses. It is tantalizing to speculate about where antigenic epitopes and where the cellular attachment site in the virus capsid might be located. It is possible that the virus binds to a cellular receptor either by recognition sites on the top of the protruding arches or by the receptor fitting into the hollow of the cup-like depressions on the virus surface. Clearly, interest is high to determine which domain in the linear structure of the capsid protein makes up each domain in the three-dimensional virus structure.

GENOME ORGANIZATION

The NV genome was not characterized until it was cloned from virus partially purified from stools obtained from volunteer studies (26,27). Because the virus used for cloning came from feces, it was critical and not straightforward to detect and prove the specificity of the first cloned DNAs (cDNAs) for NV. Early critics argued that any cDNA made from unpurified stool-derived material, and tested on stool material, would never be able to detect a specific pathogen. In spite of these recognized difficulties, specificity of cDNA was accomplished by preparing individual probes from putative cDNA inserts excised from plasmid DNA. Each probe was tested with nucleic

acid from stool samples (taken before and after infection) of volunteers different from the individual from whom the virus was purified for cloning. While such testing was labor intensive, the 953rd probe tested was found to react with post- but not preinfection stools from volunteers. Specificity of the first cDNA was shown by demonstrating that the probe (a) reacted with post- but not preinfection stools from volunteers, (b) reacted with the fractions of a CsCl gradient where virus in stool was found to peak, (c) reacted with highly purified NV particles electrophoresed on an agarose gel, (d) did not react with other enteric viruses such as rotavirus and hepatitis A virus, and (e) was able to identify additional overlapping cDNAs from the initial and subsequent libraries that also were shown to be specific for the NV genome. In addition, the sequence from the cDNA did not show any significant homology with other sequences in the GenBank. The sequence of the entire genome also was found to contain the sequence of a cDNA identified independently as encoding an immunoreactive protein (20,27), and cloning of the genome of multiple strains of SRSVs has subsequently been successful based on using primers designed from the original NV sequence (28–39). Currently, the genome organization predicted from the sequences of full-length cDNAs is known for NV and another SRSV initially obtained from a 2-year-old child during a family outbreak that occurred in Southampton, United Kingdom, in 1991 (HuCV/SHV/91/UK) (20,28).

Characterization of the genome of NV, using single-stranded RNA probes of opposite polarity made from the initial cDNA, and partial sequence information first showed that the NV genome is a positive-sense polyadenylated single-stranded RNA of 7642 nucleotides (nt), excluding the 3' polyadenylated tail (20,26). The NV genome is predicted to encode three open reading frames (ORFs) (Fig. 3A).

The first and longest ORF (ORF1) is predicted to encode a polyprotein precursor to nonstructural proteins based on identification of sequences similar to the picornavirus 2C helicase, 3C protease, and 3D RNA-dependent RNA polymerase. While the first AUG initiation codon is found at nt 146, seven in-frame AUG codons are located in the first 1100 nt of the genome, and only the first, fifth (nt 953–955), and seventh AUGs are favored codons based on Kozak's rules (40). It is possible that an internal AUG is used for initiation of ORF1 (as in picornaviruses and other positive-stranded RNA viruses) as the observed size of the protein made from synthetic RNAs (transcribed from a full-length cDNA) in cell-free systems is approximately 160K, i.e., smaller than the 193K polypeptide predicted if the first AUG was used for initiation. In addition, expression in insect cells of a cDNA in a baculovirus recombinant that contained nt 1 to nt 2535 resulted in the production of a single protein band of 57K after immunoprecipitation of the proteins with the serum of a volunteer obtained after infection with NV. These results are consistent with internal initiation of translation being used for NV, and with the fifth AUG being used to initiate translation. If internal initiation of translation of ORF1 is confirmed, the mechanism for this may be of interest, as a typical oligopyrimidine tract reported for the

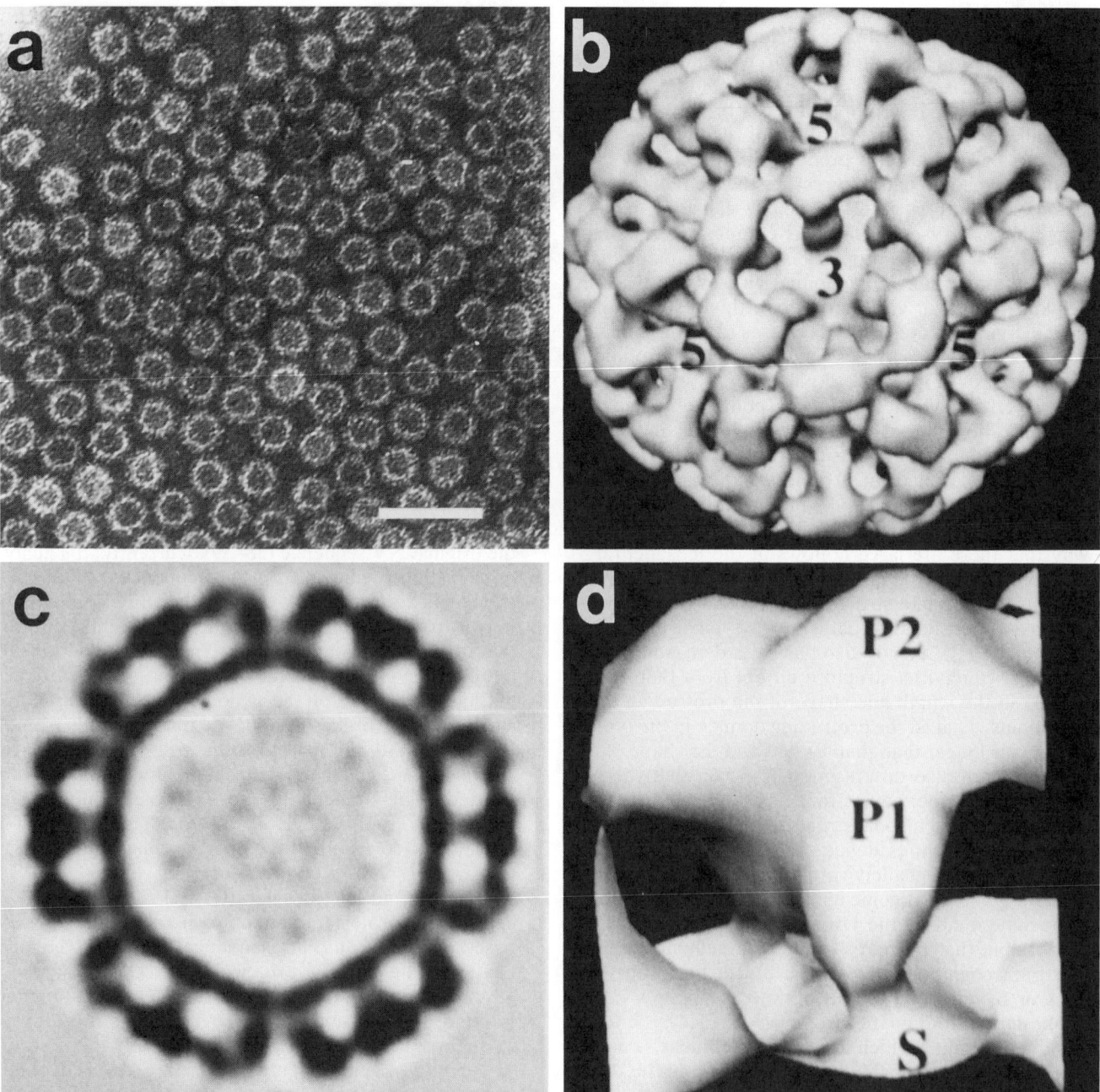

FIG. 2. The structure of NV particles. (**A**) Negative-stain electron micrographs of rNV particles and (**B**) the three-dimensional structure of rNV particles viewed along the icosahedral 3-fold axis. This structure was determined by image processing of the rNV particles shown in panel A. The rNV particles have a distinct architecture and they exhibit T = 3 icosahedral symmetry; the 3-fold and 5-fold axes of symmetry are shown and the cup-like depressions are evident at the 3-fold and 5-fold axes. The capsid structure is made up of 90 dimers of a single protein that form a shell domain from which arch-like capsomers protrude (see Fig. 1B and D). **C:** A central section of the particle perpendicular to the icosahedral 3-fold axis. In this panel, the *dark regions* correspond to the regions of higher scattering density (i.e., proteins) and the *lighter regions* represent the regions of lower scattering density (i.e., solvent). **D:** A side of an arch is shown. The three domains of the arch, protruding domain 1 (P1), protruding domain 2 (P2), and the shell domain (S) are indicated. Adapted from (24). (Panels B–D courtesy of B.V.V. Prasad.)

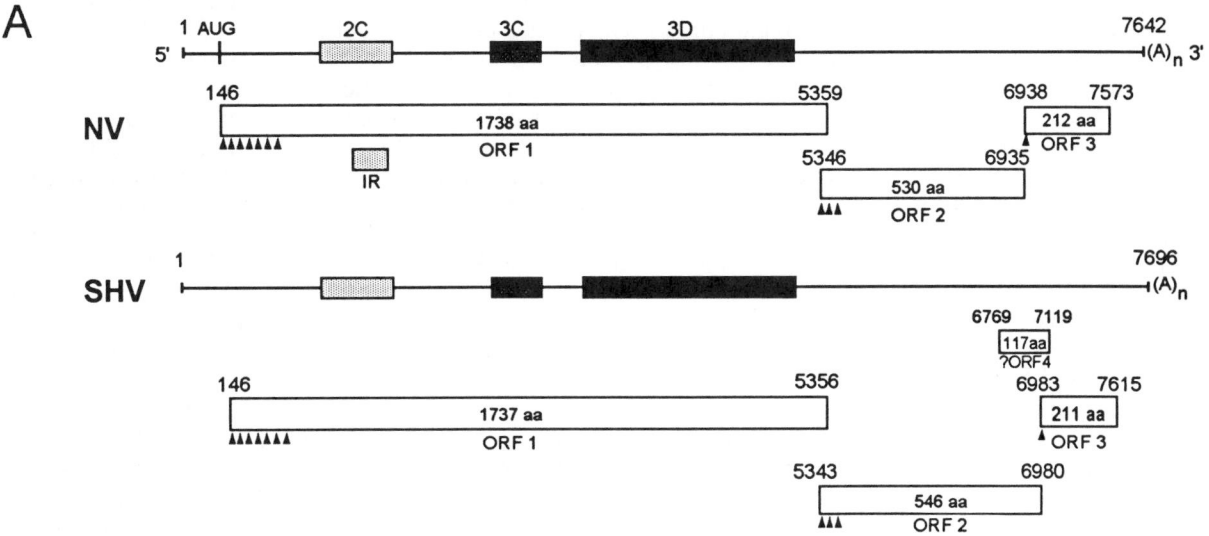

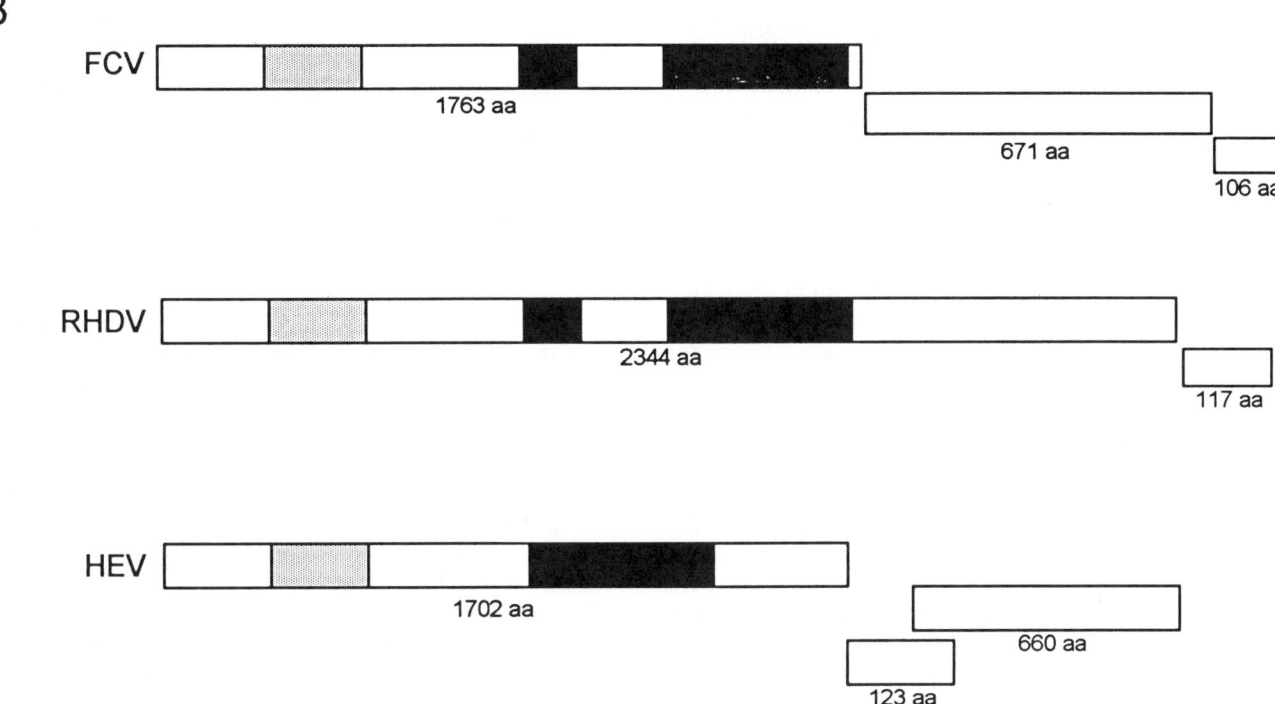

FIG. 3. A: Genomic organization of NV and other NV-like caliciviruses. Schematic of the genomic organization of NV and Southampton virus (SHV) based on analyses of the nucleotide sequence. Three predicted ORFs include: ORF1, a polyprotein that contains regions of amino acid similarity with the picornavirus 2C helicase, 3C protease, and the 3D RNA-dependent RNA polymerase of most RNA viruses; ORF2, the capsid protein; and ORF3 that codes for a protein of unknown function. A fourth ORF is predicted for SHV that is not present in NV. *Arrowheads* (▲) show locations of AUG initiation codons, and IR denotes an immunoreactive region in ORF1 of NV reported by Matsui et al. (27). (Adapted from ref. 20 with information compiled from ref. 28.) **B:** Genomic organization of two animal caliciviruses and hepatitis E virus. The feline calicivirus (FCV), rabbit hemorrhagic disease virus (RHDV), and hepatitis E virus (HEV) are shown for comparison to the NV genome organization. This information was compiled from GenBank sequences M86370 (FCV), M67473 (RHDV), and D10330 (HEV).

internal ribosome entry site of enteroviruses and rhinoviruses (41) is not present in the 5′ nontranslated region of the NV genome.

The ability to immunoprecipitate a protein from expressed ORF1 confirms the immunoreactivity of a cDNA produced using sequence-independent single primer amplification (SISPA) followed by immunodetection of a fusion protein expressed in a λgt11 library (27). These results are important as they indicate that infected individuals make antibodies to proteins other than the capsid protein. This must be remembered when one reanalyzes early data on the antigenic relatedness of these viruses determined by radioimmunoassay (RIA) or enzyme-linked immunoadsorbent assay (ELISA) using viruses in stool and sera from adult volunteers.

The second ORF is predicted to encode a protein of 530 aa with a molecular weight of 56,571, similar in size to the viral capsid protein (Fig. 3A). The NV ORF2 protein contains a conserved amino acid motif of PPG that also is found in the picornavirus capsid protein VP3 (42). Expression of ORF2 and ORF3 in insect cells infected with a baculovirus recombinant containing this gene, and the expression of ORF2 alone in cell-free translation systems producing a product similar in size to that observed for the capsid protein of native NV particles, confirmed that ORF2 encodes the capsid protein that self-assembles into virus-like particles (Fig. 1C).

ORF3 at the 3′ end of the genome is predicted to encode a small protein of 212 aa with a molecular weight of 22.5K and a very basic charge (isoelectric point of 10.99). ORF3 does not have any sequence similarity with other proteins in the GenBank and its function remains unknown. Expression of ORF3 was not detected in insect cells infected with a baculovirus recombinant (that contained a cDNA of both ORF2 and ORF3). This could indicate that (a) ORF3 was not expressed at sufficiently high levels to be detected; (b) ORF3 was not expressed at all due to dominance of translation by the upstream ORF2, which prevented internal translation from the initiation codon for ORF3; (c) a subgenomic RNA may be necessary for the expression of ORF3; or (d) other viral proteins or cellular proteins may be required for translation of ORF3. The conservation of this ORF in other human and animal caliciviruses indicates that it most likely has a function. It has been suggested to be involved in nucleic acid binding because it is basic and is located at the 3′ terminus of the genome in a manner similar to small cysteine-rich nucleic acid binding proteins of plant RNA viruses. However, the NV ORF3 protein is not cysteine-rich and therefore may not bind RNA in the same manner.

The overall genome organization of NV is conserved in another Norwalk-like virus, the Southampton virus (SHV) (Fig. 3A), and is similar to that reported for other caliciviruses (Fig. 3B). The first and third ORFs in NV and SHV are in the same reading frames. This occurs because of a 17 nt overlap from the stop codon of ORF1 to the first AUG codon of ORF2, creating a −2 frameshift. A 1 nt overlap between the ORF2 stop and the ORF3 start codons results in a −1 frameshift.

There also are several notable differences among the NV and SHV genome organization and between these viruses and those of the other caliciviruses. First, the SHV has a predicted additional fourth ORF; this has not been seen in other Norwalk-like viruses sequenced recently and so its significance remains unclear. Second, the sizes of the predicted capsid protein in ORF2 are different, with the ORF2 of feline calicivirus (FCV) (43), rabbit hemorrhagic disease virus (RHDV) (44), hepatitis E virus (HEV) (45), and San Miguel sea lion virus serotypes 1 and 4 (SMSV, not shown) (46) being longer than that of the NV ORF2. This large size of the predicted ORF2 protein is due to the presence of additional amino acids at the N terminus of ORF2 of these other viruses; in some cases, these sequences have been shown to be removed by cleavage of a capsid protein precursor, so that the mature capsid protein is smaller. However, the mature capsid proteins of these viruses also are larger than the capsid protein of NV. Third, the RHDV genome only contains two predicted ORFs because the RHDV capsid protein sequence is fused to ORF1. This RHDV genome organization has been confirmed in more than one strain of virus so it is not simply the result of a sequencing error. Fourth, the relative sizes of the capsid proteins and the small 3′-terminal (ORF3) proteins are distinctly different among these different caliciviruses. Thus the N terminus of ORF2 is larger and ORF3 is smaller for the animal caliciviruses when compared to ORF3 of NV. Finally, the feline calicivirus genome has a −1 frameshift at both ORF1/2 and ORF2/3 junctions with the result that all three ORFs are in different reading frames. Possible mechanisms for expression of ORF3 by frameshifting are discussed later under replication strategies.

GENETIC AND ANTIGENIC VARIABILITY OF NORWALK AND NORWALK-LIKE AGENTS

The availability of the first NV sequence opened a new era in the characterization of Norwalk and Norwalk-related viruses, including many agents previously characterized as SRSVs. This was made possible by two technological advances. First, the initial sequencing of the NV genome allowed primers to be selected to amplify similar and more heterologous agents. Second, new methods were developed to reduce the presence of inhibitors in stool and allow small amounts of nucleic acid from similar agents to be detected and characterized. Several methods have been described but one employed extensively uses the cationic detergent cetyltriammonium bromide (CTAB) to remove inhibitors (47). These advances have resulted in the sequence analysis of at least 50 different SRSVs in the past two years (28–39,48,49). Most of these studies have only characterized a portion of the viral genome in the RNA polymerase region because this region of the genome was the first published and was expected to be conserved; consistent with this idea, many viruses could be amplified with primers designed based on the NV polymerase sequence. These studies have been useful to answer a number of important questions related to the classification, genetic relatedness, detection ability, mo-

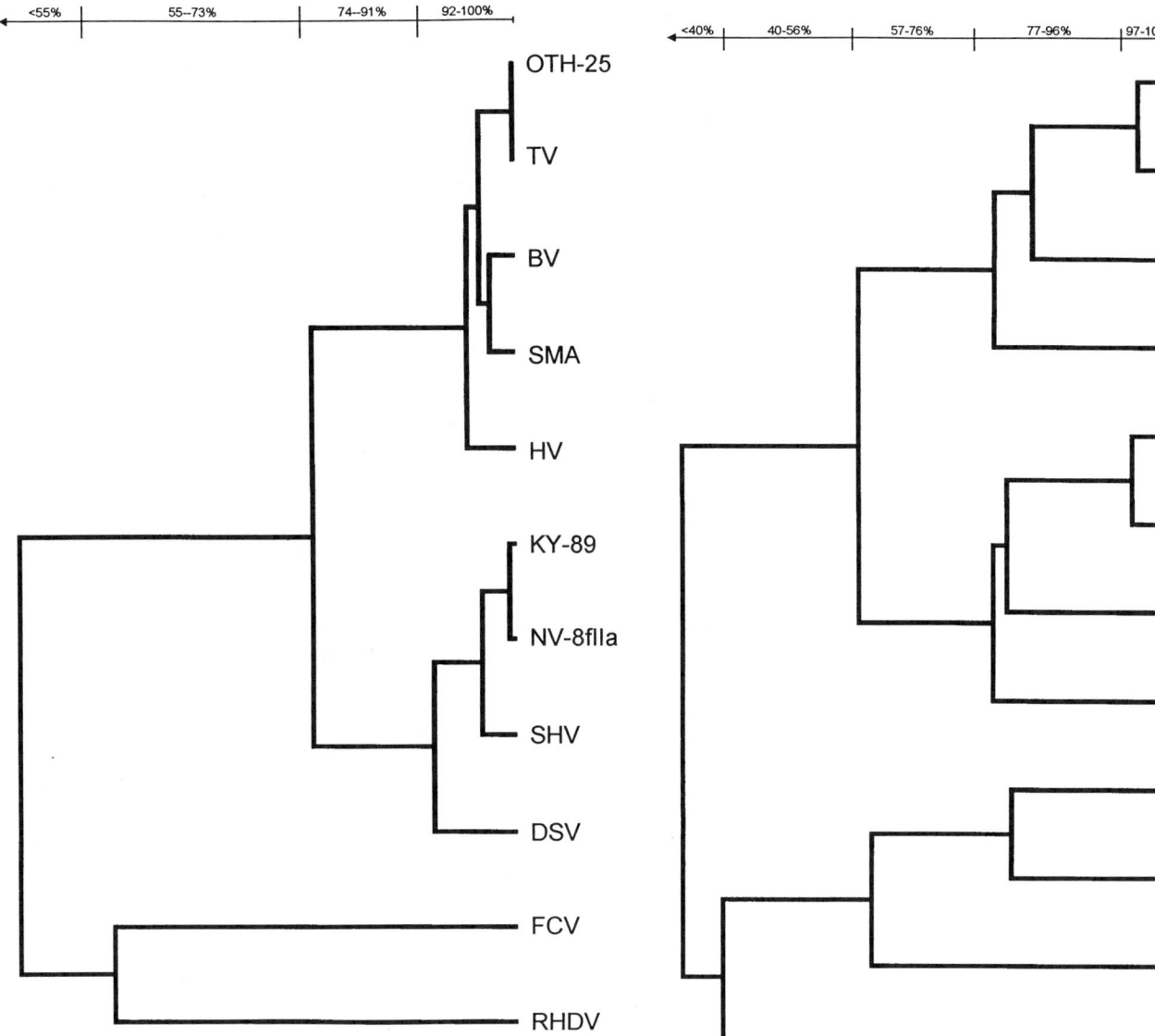

FIG. 4. Dendrogram of predicted genetic relationships among the different human and animal caliciviruses by comparison of a part of the polymerase region within ORF1. Sequences from amino acids 1473 to 1572 of the polymerase region of ORF1 of the NV genome were used to determine the order of the pairwise alignments. The vertical branch lengths are proportional to the similarities of the sequences. The scale at the top represents an analysis of the genetic distances among sequences generated by the DISTANCES program of GCG using a threshold of 0.6. The data were compiled from sequences whose GenBank accession numbers are as follows: L23830 (OTH-25), U02030 (TV), X76716 (BV), L23830 (SMA), XXXXX (HV), L23828 (KY-89), M87661 (NV-8flla), L07418 (SHV), U04538 (DSV), M86379 (FCV), and M67473 (RHDV). The distribution of these viral sequences into three genogroups (I for NV, II for SMA and HV, and III for FCV and RHDV) is evident.

FIG. 5. Dendrogram of predicted genetic relationships among the different human and animal caliciviruses by comparison of the capsid regions. The 530 amino acids of the predicted capsid protein of the NV genome were used to determine the order of the pairwise alignments. The vertical branch lengths are proportional to the similarities of the sequences. The scale at the top represents an analysis of the genetic distances among sequences generated by the DISTANCES program of GCG using a threshold of 0.6. The heterologous viruses used for comparison are the same as in Fig. 4 with the addition of sequences from two San Miguel sea lion viruses SMSV1 and SMSV4 (GenBank accession numbers M87481 and M87482, respectively). Additional accession numbers for capsid regions are L23827 (KY-89), L23829 (OTH-25), and U04469 (DSV).

lecular epidemiology, and evolution of NV and Norwalk-related viruses.

Different approaches were taken to address the genetic relationship between NV and other Norwalk-like agents. First, previously well-characterized NV-like strains

[Snow Mountain agent (SMA) (6,50) and Hawaii agent (HV) (7)] were amplified and sequenced and their relatedness to NV was determined (31,35). These studies are important in that they provide a foundation for genetic comparison based on previous antigenic relationships de-

TABLE 4. *Sequence similarities of the RNA polymerase region among SRSVs*

	NV-8fIIa	KY-89	SHV	DSV	SMA	OTH-25	TV	HV	BV
NV-8fIIa		88	77	72	63	62	62	62	60
KY-89	99		77	72	80	78	78	60	87
SHV	98	97		73	62	64	60	62	61
DSV	92	92	92		60	59	60	61	62
SMA	76	76	76	77		80	80	84	85
OTH-25	78	78	78	78	99		97	78	85
TV	78	78	78	78	99	100		78	78
HV	76	76	76	79	95	96	96		87
BV	77	77	77	80	97	97	97	97	

Sequences from nucleotides 4562 to 4921 (aa 1473 to 1572) of ORF1 of the NV-8fIIa genome were aligned with similar sequences of indicated SRSVs. Numbers in the upper right triangle are percent nucleotide similarities, and numbers in the lower left triangle are percent amino acid similarities. NV-8fIIa and KY-89 both were reactive in the rNV antigen ELISA. SMA, OTH-25, DSV, TV, and HV were negative in the rNV antigen ELISA. BV and SHV were not tested.

fined either by human volunteer cross-challenge studies or IEM, using well-characterized sera from human volunteer studies. Thus the Hawaii agent (HV) had previously been shown to be distinct from NV based on finding that human volunteers initially challenged with NV were not protected from subsequent challenge with Hawaii agent, and these distinct biologic differences were confirmed by IEM studies (7). In addition, the Snow Mountain agent was characterized as being antigenically distinct from NV and HV based on IEM experiments (50). Comparisons of the sequences of these viruses showed initially that the NV and SMA represented two genogroups (I and II) based on analysis of nucleotide or predicted amino acid sequences from part of the polymerase region, the entire capsid region (see Figs. 4 and 5 and Tables 2 and 4), and ORF3 (data not shown). Subsequent analysis of the HV found that this virus also falls in genogroup II, regardless of whether the predicted sequences from the polymerase or the capsid regions were compared; this result was unexpected because it had been assumed that SMA and HV were distinct viruses based on previous IEM data. Within a genogroup, the aa similarity between two different strains ranges from 80% to 96% for the polymerase region and from 77% to 98% for the capsid region. The HV shows only 85% to 86% similarity with the predicted capsid proteins of two other viruses [Toronto virus (TV) and OTH-25], which are identical to SMA; this difference is sufficiently large that the HV and these other two SMA-like viruses may still fall within different serotypes. Currently, it remains unknown what cutoff of sequence similarity will reflect serotype differences.

Analysis of the predicted amino acid sequences of the capsid protein of these different viruses shows that regions of sequence conservation and variability are easily identified. These regions of sequence variability are of interest as they often represent regions where neutralization epitopes are present on viral capsid proteins. The NV capsid protein can be divided into three domains based on sequence comparisons (29) (Figs. 6 and 7). Region 1 is relatively conserved and it contains the region predicted to form the shell domain of the capsid (24). This region corresponds essentially to the relatively conserved B domain described for animal caliciviruses (46). A second

region (aa 281–404 for NV) shows relatively high sequence variability and this corresponds to variable domains C to E described for animal caliciviruses by Neill (46). The third region (aa 405 to the C terminus for NV) is more conserved but still shows some variability. Regions 2 and 3 are those predicted to form the protruding arch-like capsomeres (24). Future studies can be expected to confirm which of these domains represents the sides and the surfaces of these arches.

A second approach taken to understand the genetic relationship between NV and other Norwalk-like agents or SRSVs involved sequencing SRSVs from multiple outbreaks and from different geographic locations (35). These studies also sequenced virus strains (called UK types 1 to 4) previously characterized as SRSVs using a solid phase immunosorbent method (32,34,51). The results from many studies show that all the SRSVs examined to date and able to be sequenced can be divided first into the two genogroups described above. In addition, viruses previously classified as UK2 that were thought to be related to NV have been shown to fall into genogroup I. In contrast, viruses classified as UK1, 3, and 4 generally fell into genogroup II, and viruses simply classified as SRSVs fell into either I or II. A striking result from the analyses of multiple viruses is that, even within the RNA polymerase region, there is a high degree of genomic variation (Table 4). Taken together and based on the extensive sequence database of a relatively short region of the polymerase, it is unlikely that one set of universal conserved primers will be found to amplify all SRSVs. Instead, either multiple sets of primers or degenerate primers will be needed to assure that any SRSV will be detected.

Sequence analysis of NV and other morphologically typical human and animal caliciviruses is beginning to unravel the genetic relationships between these viruses. Sequence analysis of the polymerase region initially was done on a limited number (three) of morphologically typical human caliciviruses all previously characterized by EM and obtained from infants and young children; the sequences of these viruses were found to be closely related to SMA and they would cluster in genogroup II (36). Thus at least some morphologically typical human caliciviruses are genetically related to SMA. It was a great sur-

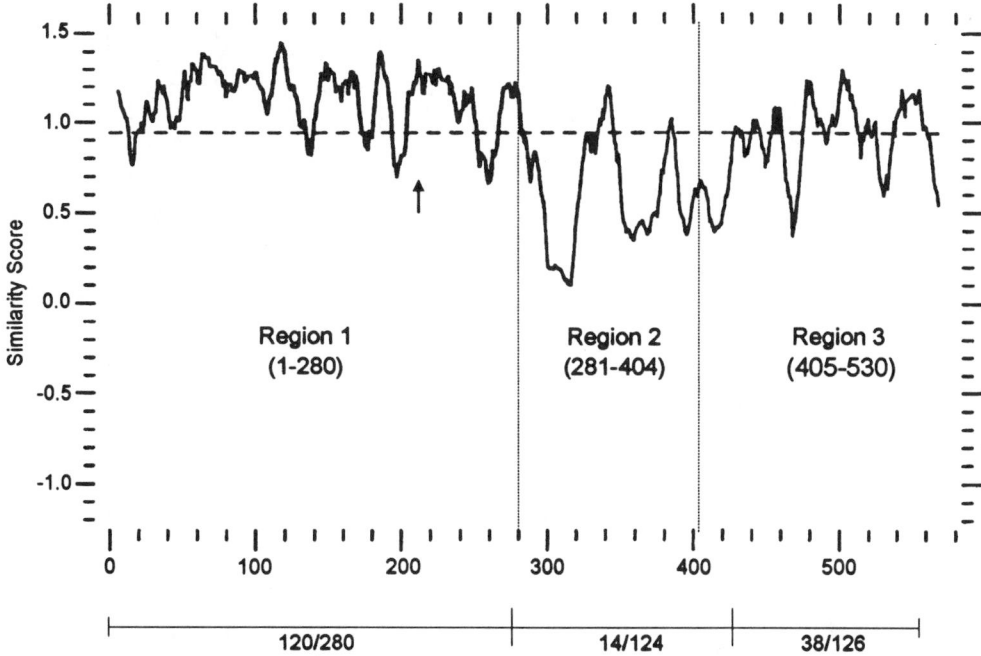

FIG. 6. Similarity plot of eight sequences of the capsid protein of NV and related viruses. The average similarity among the capsid proteins was calculated using a 10 amino acid window and the Dayhoff table of amino acid similarities. The *horizontal dotted line* corresponds to the average similarity, that is, the sum of the separate window similarities divided by the number of windows. Three regions have been defined, with region 2 being the most variable. The position of the cleavage observed in rNV capsids expressed in insect cells is marked by an *arrow*. The amino acid residue numbers given for each region are for NV. The line at the bottom shows the number of consensus amino acids in each region among these human caliciviruses. These data were analyzed using the PILEUP and PLOTSIMILARITY programs of GCG for multiple sequence alignments using a gap weight of 3. The sequences compared (and their accession numbers) were M87661 (NV), LO7418 (SHV), L23930 (OTH-25), L23830 (SMA), L23828 (KY-89), X76716 (BV), U02030 (TV), U04469 and U04538 (DSV), and U07611.

prise when a previously uncharacterized agent, called minireovirus, found in stool samples from children hospitalized in Toronto was studied and also shown to be a human calicivirus with a polymerase sequence similar to SMA (29). If these HuCVs also prove to be antigenically similar to SMA, then physical or chemical factors must be the reason for the morphological differences between viruses previously called HuCVs and SRSVs. This would not be surprising since it is known that other caliciviruses—that is, vesicular exanthema of swine virus (52), hepatitis E virus (53), and amyelosis chronic stunt virus (54)—are degraded by adverse physical conditions and/or proteolytic enzymes.

Different results have recently been obtained from the study of other morphologically typical human caliciviruses. Analysis of the predicted sequence of the polymerase region of the HuCV Sapporo virus and of other antigenically uncharacterized viruses with typical calicivirus morphology has indicated that these viruses are more closely related to feline caliciviruses (37,38). Thus there is at least a third genogroup of human caliciviruses. The significance of this finding remains unknown, and it may simply indicate that some human caliciviruses have evolved from animal caliciviruses. The sequence similarity observed in the short regions of genome studied is

not extremely high (less than 40%) when compared to the limited number of FCV sequences currently available. Therefore it is not possible with our current knowledge to know if direct transmission of virus from cats to humans occurred sometime in the past, followed by virus mutation as it became adapted to growth in humans. It is of interest that transmission of animal caliciviruses to humans has been suggested previously (55, 55a), and transmission of caliciviruses likely occurs among animals (56,57). Transmission of viruses among animals is supported by recent sequence analyses that have shown that several SMSV serotypes, VESV, and a newly isolated skunk calicivirus appear to be closely related (56). These results raise interesting epidemiologic and evolutionary questions that will need to be answered in future studies.

Some of the new sequence studies included a preliminary analysis of whether these RNA viruses undergo rapid mutation, resulting in continual appearance of new serotypes. This question was addressed by determining whether currently circulating viruses are very similar to the prototype NV, SMA, and HV. Comparisons of the sequences of viruses found to have similar antigenic reactivity, but isolated at different times and geographic locations, indicate that the amino acid sequences are not rapidly changing.

Multiple sequence alignment (rows: NV-8fIIa, KY-89, SHV, DSV, OTH-25, TV, HV, BV, Consensus)

```
                    1                                                                                                          120
NV-8fIIa   MMMASKDATS SVDGASGAGQ LVPEVNASDP LAMDPVAGSS TAVATAGQVN PIDPWIINNF VQAPGEFTI  SPNNTPGDVL FDLSLGPHLN PFLLHLSQMY NGWGNMRVR  IMLAGNAFTA
KY-89      MMMASKDATS SVDGASASVQ LVPEVNASDP LAMDPVAGSS TAVATAGQVN PIDPWIINNF VQAPGEFTI  SPNNTPGDVL FDLSLGPHLN PFLLHLSQMY NGWGNMRVR  IMLAGNAFTA
SHV        MMMASKDAPQ SADGASGAGQ LVPEVNTADP LEMEPVAGPT TAVATAGQVN MIDPWIMSNY VQSPQGEFTI SPNNTPGDIL FDLQLGPHLN PFLSHLSQMY NGWGNMRVR  ILLAGNAFSA
DSV        MMMASKDAPT NMDGTSGAGQ LVPEANTAEP ISMEPVAGAA TAAATAGQVN MIDPWIMSNY VQAPQGEFTI SPNNTPGDIL FDLQLGPHLN PFLSHLAQMY NGWGNMRVK  VLLAGNAFTA
OTH-25     MKMASNDAAP SNDGAAG... LVPEIN.NEA MALDPVAGAA IAAPLTGQQN IIDPWIMNNF VQAPGGEFTV SPRNSPGEVL LNLELGPEIN PYLAHLARMY NGYAGGFEVQ VLLAGNAFTA
TV         MKMASNDAAP SNDGAAC... LVPEIN.NEA MALEPVAGSA IAAPLTGQQN IIDPWIMNNF VQAPGGEFTV SPRNSPGEVL LNLELGPEIN PYLAHLARMY NGYAGGFEVQ VVLAGNAFTA
HV         MKMASNDAAP SNDGAAG... LVPEVN.NET MALEPVAGAS IAAPLTGQNN VIDPWIRMNF VQAPNGEFTV SPRNSPGEIL LNLELGPELN PFLAHLSRMY NGYAGGFEVQ VLLAGNAFTA
BV         MKMASNDANP SDGSAAN... LVPEVN.NEV MALEPVVGAA IAAPVAGAQN VIDPWIRNNF VQAPGGEFTV SPRNAPGEIL WSAPLGPDLN PYLSHLSRMY NGYAGGFEVQ VILAGNAFTA
Consensus  M-MAS-DA-- ---------- LVPE-N---- ----PV-G-- -A---GQ-N  -IDPWI--N- VQ-P-GEFT  SP-N-PG--L ---LGP--N  P-L-HL--MY NG--G---Y- --LAGNAF-A
```

Region 1

```
                    121                                                                                          238
NV-8fIIa   GKIIVSCIPP GFGSHNLTIA QATLFPHVIA DVRTLDPIEV PLEDVRNVLF HNNDRNQQTM RLVCMLYTPL RTGGGTG..D SFVVAGRVMT CPSPDFNLF  LVPPTVEQKT RPFTLPNLPL
KY-89      GKIIVSCIPP GFGSQQLTIA QATLFPHVIA DVRTLDPIEV PLEDVRNVLF HNNDRNQQTM RLVCMLYTPL STGGGTG..D SFVVAGRVMT CPSPDFNLF  LVPPTVEQKT RPFTLPNLPL
SHV        GKIIVCCVPP GFTSSSLTIA QATMFPHVIA DVRTLEPIEM PLEDVRNVLY HTND.NQPTM RLVCMLYTPL RTGGGSGNSD SFVVAGRVLT APSDFSFLF  LVPPTIEQKT RAFTVPNIPL
DSV        GKIIISCIPP GFAAQNISIA QATMFPHVIA DVRVLEPIEV PLEDVRNVLY HNNDS.PTM  RLVCMLYTPL RASGSSSGTD PFVIAGRVLT CPSPDFSFLF LVPPNVEQKT KPFSVPNLPL
OTH-25     AKVIFAAIPP NFPIDNLSAA QITMCPHVIV DVRQLEPINL PMPDVRNNFF HYNQGSDSRL RLIAMLYTPL RANNSGD..D VFTVSCRVLT RPSPDFSFNF LVPSTMESKT KPFTLPILTI
TV         GKIFAAIPP  NFPIDNLSAA QITMCPHVIV DVRQLEPINL PMPDVRNNFF HYNQGSDSRL RLIAMLYTPL RANNSGD..D VFTVSCRVLT RPSPDFSFNF LVPPTVESKT KPFTLPLTI
HV         GKLVFAAIPP HFPLENLSPG QITMFPHVII DVRTLEPVLL PLPDVRNNFF HYNQQEPRM  RLVAMLYTPL RSNGSGD..D VFTVSCRVLT RPSPDFDFNY LVPPTVESKT KPFTLPILTI
BV         GRVIFAAVPP NFPTEGLSPS QVTMFPHIIV DVRQLEPVLI PLPDVRNNFY HYNQANDSTL KLIAMLYTPL RANNAGD..D VFTVSCRVLT RPSPDFDFIF LVPPTVESRT KPFTVPVLTV
Consensus  -K-------PP -F-------- Q-T--PH-I- DVR-L-P--- P--DVRN--- H-N------ -L--MLYTPL ---------- -F----RV-T -PS-DF-F-- LVP----E-T --F-F----
                                                                                      ↓
```

Region 2

```
                    239                                                                                  337
NV-8fIIa   SSLSNSRAPL PISSIGISPD NVQSVQFQNG RCTLDGRLVG TTPVSLSHVA KIRGT..... .....SNGTV INLTELDGTP FHPFEG.PAP IGFPDLGGCD WHINMTQFGH
KY-89      SSLSNSRAPL PISWGISPD  NVQSVQFQNG RCTLDGRLVG TTPVSLSHVA KIRGT..... SN..GTV    INLTELDGTP FHPFEG.PAP IGFPDLGGCD WHINMTQFGH
SHV        QTLSNSRFPS LIQKMILSPD ASQVVQFQNG RCLIDGQLLG TTPATSGQLF RVRGK..... ..INQGART  LNLTEVDGKP FMAFDS.PAP VGFPDFGKCD WHMRISKTPN
DSV        NTLSNSRVPS LINAMMISRD HGQMVQFQNG RVTLDGQLQG TTPTSLSQLC KIRGKVFHAS GGNG...... LNLTELDGSA YHAFES.PAP IGFPDIGDCD WHMSATATNN
OTH-25     SEMSNSRFPV PIDSLHTSPT ESIVVQCQNG RVTLDGELMG TTQLLPNQIC AFRGTLRST  NRASDQADTA IQLDNLNGTP YDPAEDIPAP LGTPDFRGKV FGVA...GQR
TV         SEMSNSRFPV PIDSLHTSPT ESIVVQCQNG RVTLDGELMG TTQLLPSQIC AFRGTLRST  SRASDQADTP IQLDNLNGTP YDPAEDIPAP LGTPDFRGKV FGVA...SQR
HV         GELSNSRPV  PIDELYTSPN EGVIVQQNG  RSTLDGELLG TTQLVSNVIC ALRG...RIN AQVPDD.... LQDTNLNGTP FDPTEDVPAP LGTPDFLANI YGVT...SQR
BV         EEMSNSRFPI PLEKLYTGPS SAFVVQFQNG RCTTDGVLLG TTQLSAVNIC NFRGDVTHIA G......... MNLASQNWSN YDPTEEIPAP LGTPDFVGKI QGLLTQTTR.
Consensus  --SNSR-P-  ---------- --VQ-QNG   R---DG-L-G TT-------- -RG------- ---------- ---------- --------PAP -G-PD----- ----------
                                                                     [          T
```

Region 3

```
                    338                                                                                              *  440
NV-8fIIa   SSQTQ..... YDVDTTPDTF VPHLGSIQA. ....NGI... GSGNVGVLS  WISPPSHPSG SQVDLWKIPN YGSSITEATH LAPSVYPPGF GEVLVFFMSK MPGP....GA YNLPCLLPQE
KY-89      SSQTQ..... YDVDTTPDTS VPHLGSIQA. ....NGI... GSGNYIGVLS WSPPSHPSG  SQVDLWKIPN YGSSITEATH LAPSVYSPGF GEVLVFFMSK IPGP....GG DSLPCLLPQG
SHV        NTGSGDPMRS VSVQTNVQGF VPHLGSIQF. ....DEVFNH PTGDYIGTIE WISQPSTPPG TDINLWEIPD YGSSLSQAAN LAPPVFPPGF GEALVYFVSA FPGPNNRSAP NDVPCLLPQE
DSV        FTGSSNEYQI LIKQES..AF APHLGHVQA. ....DNLSAG ANTDLIVSLS WISPVSDQHR HDVDPWVIPR YGSSLTEAAQ LAPIYPPGF  GEAIVFFMSD .RIPCTLPQE .RIPCTLPQE
OTH-25     NPDSTTRAHE AKVDTTSGRF TPKLGSLEIT T.ESDDFDPN QSTKFTPVG. ...I..GVDNE ADFQQWSLPD YSGQFTHNMN LAPAVAPNFP GEQLLFFRSQ LPSSGGRSNG I.LDCLVPQE
TV         NPDSTTRAHE AKVDTTSGRF TPKLGSLEIT T.ESDDFDPN QPTKFTPVG. ..V..GVDNE AEFQQFTHNMN YSGQFTHNMN LAPAVAPNFP GEQLLFFRSQ V.LDCLVPQE V.LDCLVPQE
HV         NPNNTCRAHD GVLATWSPKF TPKLGSVILG TWEESDLDLN .LF..NTDH. ..FDQWALPS YSGRLTLNMN YSGRLTLNMN LAPSVSPLFP LEQLLFFRSH IPLKGGTSDG A.IDCLLPQE
BV         .ADGSTRAHK ATVSTGSVHF TPKLGSVQFT TDTNNDFQAG .VIQDGDHHQ NEPQQWLLPN YSGRTGHNVH YSGRTGHNVH LAPAVAPTFP GEQLLFFRST MPGCSGYPN. MNLDCLLPQE
Consensus  ---------- ---------- -P-LG----- ---------- ---------  --W--P---- Y----      Y--------- LAP------- -E--F----- ---------- ---C--LPQE
```

Region 3

```
                    441                                                          530
NV-8fIIa   YISHLASEQA PTVGEAALLH YDVPDTGRNL GEFKAYPDGF LTCVPNGASS GPQQLPINGV FVFVSWVSRF YQLKPVGTAS SARGRLGLRR
KY-89      YISHLASEQA PTVGEGPLLH YDVPDTDRNL GEFKAYPDGF LTCVPNGASS GPQQLPINGV FVFVSWVSRF YQLKPVGTAS TARGRLGLRR   530
SHV        YITHFVSEQA PTMGDAALLH YVDPDTNRNL GEFKLYPGGY LTCVPNGGSS GPQQLPLNGV FLFVSWVSRF YQLKPVGTAS TARGRLGVRRI 546
DSV        YVAHFVNEQA PTRGEAALLH YVNPDTGRVL GEFKMYPGGF MTCVPNSSGS GPQTLPHRNL FTFVSWVSRF YQLKPVGTAG PAR.RLGIRRS 545
OTH-25     WQHFYQESA  PAQTQVALVR YVNPDTGRVL FEAKLHKLGF MTIAKNGDS. .PITVPPNGY FRFESWVNPF YTLAPMGTGN .GRRRIQ...  548
TV         WQHFYQESA  PAQTQVALVR YVNPDTGRVL FEAKLHKLGF MTIAKNGDS. .PITVPPNGY FRFESWVNPF YTLAPMGTGN .GRRRIQ :   549
HV         WIQHFYQESA PAATDVALIR YTNPDTGRVL FEAKLHRQGF ITVANSGSR. .PIVVPPNGY FRDSWVNQF  YSLAPMGTGN .GRRRVQ :   536
BV         WVIHFYQEAA PAQSDVALLR FVNPDTGRVL FECKLHKSGY ITVAHTGP.. YDLVLPPNGY FRDSWVNQF  YTLAPMGNGT GRRRAL...   540
Consensus  --H--E-A   P-------L- ---PDT-R-L --E-K---G- --T------- -------P-- F-F-SWV--F Y-L-P-G--- --R--------
```

Viruses with very similar sequences to prototype NV have been found. Thus a virus (HuCV/KY-89/89/J) was found to be antigenically similar to prototype NV based on its reactivity in an ELISA that uses polyclonal antibody to the baculovirus-expressed rNV, but this virus was isolated 21 years later in Japan (58). Sequence analysis of KY-89 and comparison with NV showed 87.2% nt similarity over 2516 continuous nucleotides amounting to 96% to 98% amino acid similarity in two ORFs (35). Distinct strains related to SMA but isolated 13 to 16 years later in Japan or the United Kingdom also have shown 80% nucleotide and 88% to 92% amino acid similarity to the prototype strain. Thus viruses antigenically similar to the prototype viruses are still circulating, and these have been found to show relatively good conservation of amino acid sequences over long periods of time. Although variable regions in the capsid protein have been identified, it is noteworthy that these did not change more dramatically within a specific antigenic virus type than did other regions of the genome. A larger sequence database over larger regions of the genome is needed to permit extensive analysis of the evolutionary relationships of these viruses. This can be expected to be obtained in the near future.

A number of the viruses whose sequences have been characterized were initially identified as NV based on the NV ELISA with convalescent serum from volunteers. A subset of these SRSVs also have been tested by the new NV ELISA that uses hyperimmune antiserum made to the baculovirus-expressed rNV particles. Unexpectedly, only some of the viruses positive using the human reagent ELISA also were positive using the rNV antigen ELISA. Sequence analysis of the strains showing different reactivities in each test was of interest to determine the basis for this different reactivity. The results showed that viruses that were positive in both the human and the rNV antigen ELISA were genetically very similar to the prototype NV within the polymerase region, with similarities ranging from between 80% to 87% nt and 89% to 99% amino acid, respectively. In contrast, viruses that were positive in the human ELISA but negative in the rNV antigen test showed polymerase similarities with prototype NV of 71% to 75% nucleotide and 82% to 87% amino

acid, respectively (Table 4) (summarized in ref. 59). Because the rNV ELISA only detects the capsid protein, these results indicate either (a) there are other proteins in stool samples that are cross-reactive with human convalescent serum, or (b) human convalescent serum contains antibodies that detect a different form of the capsid protein that contains more cross-reactive epitopes, while the hyperimmune antiserum made to rNV particles is highly specific for conformationally specific epitopes on virus particles. Production of monoclonal antibodies to the distinct regions of the capsid protein may help distinguish between these possibilities.

NORWALK VIRUS REPLICATION STRATEGIES

Because a cell culture system is not available for NV, a description of the replication strategy of this and other NV-like viruses remains speculative. However, a few predictions can be made based on genome homology with viruses for which mechanisms of replication have been described. The similarities in genome organization between NV and the animal caliciviruses that have been propagated in cell culture suggest that NV may use a replication strategy similar to these animal viruses. For example, it is clear that other caliciviruses make at least one major species of subgenomic RNA during virus replication (60,61). Multiple species of subgenomic RNA were observed in FCV-infected cells by Carter (62), and preliminary evidence indicates that NV also may produce a subgenomic RNA. This is based on hybridization of viral RNA with a NV cDNA probe. Besides the genomic RNA, a major species of subgenomic RNA (over 2 kb) was observed in stools of a volunteer infected with NV (X. Jiang and M. K. Estes, *unpublished data*). In addition, cell-free translation of viral RNA synthesized by *in vitro* transcription of a plasmid that contained a full-length NV cDNA resulted in the production of only a single large protein from ORF1; no protein products from the downstream ORF2 and ORF3 were observed. These results indicate a separate message might be required for the expression of the two downstream ORFs.

FIG. 7. Alignment comparing the deduced amino acid sequences of the capsid protein of NV and other human caliciviruses. This alignment compares the capsid sequence of NV, OTH-25, a virus similar to SMA (35), Toronto virus [TV, previously called minireovirus (29)], Hawaii virus (HV, 31), Bristol virus (BV, 48), Southampton virus (SHV, 28), and Desert Shield virus (DSV, 30). Alignment of these sequences was obtained using the GAP and PILEUP programs of GCG. The two bottom lines show consensus sequences. *Dots* correspond to a deletion or insertion. *Dashes* indicate the absence of consensus. The first line of the consensus sequence represents consensus amino acids among human caliciviruses. The second line of the consensus shows consensus amino acids among these human caliciviruses and animal caliciviruses including FCV, RHDV, and SMSV1 and SMSV4. The numbers shown correspond to the amino acid sequence number of the NV capsid protein, which is shown first because it is the prototype virus; however, note that the NV capsid protein sequence is not the longest. The sequence accession numbers used from the GenBank are as indicated in Figs. 3 and 6. The highly conserved region (called region B by Neill, ref. 46) of animal caliciviruses would span aa 1 to 280 (region 1). Regions C to E, which were characterized as variable, would correspond to aa 281 to 404 (region 2), and the conserved C-terminal domains would correspond to aa 405 to 530 (region 3). The conserved PP similar to that in VP3 of picornaviruses is highlighted by a *bar*, the cleavage site detected for NV in insect cells is shown by an *arrow*, and one conserved cysteine is highlighted by an *asterisk*.

ORF1 of the NV genome and of other caliciviruses shows regions of amino acid similarity with picornavirus P2 and P3 precursor proteins, suggesting that some of the replication strategies of picornaviruses may be followed by NV as well. Comparison of amino acid sequences in this region shows a significant homology to the 2C helicase and 3C protease of picornaviruses, and RNA-dependent RNA polymerase found in other RNA viruses. These data suggest that the first ORF encodes a long polyprotein that is post-translationally processed into the nonstructural proteins required for complete genome expression and replication. By analogy to the picornaviruses, it is possible that all the necessary information to produce functional nonstructural proteins is virus encoded, and that the initial proteolytic cleavage events probably occur in *cis* in the nascent polyprotein.

Post-translational cleavage also is apparent for the structural proteins of some caliciviruses such as FCV and SMSV, because the mature capsid protein is smaller than the predicted capsid precursor encoded by the genome. Post-translational cleavage of the viral capsid protein encoded in ORF2 does not seem to be required for NV. Baculovirus-expressed NV capsid protein self-assembles into virus-like particles, and the predicted size of the capsid protein matches the apparent size of the purified expressed protein. Amino acid sequencing of the viral capsid protein purified from rNV particles showed that the N terminus of the protein is blocked, suggesting this protein might not be processed from a polyprotein as reported for other caliciviruses (21).

A subcapsid protein of 34K was observed in baculovirus recombinant-infected insect cells, and this protein was confirmed to be a cleavage product of the capsid protein (21). This is consistent with the previous observation that a soluble viral antigen of approximately 30K is excreted in the stools of volunteers infected with NV (16). Recently, trypsin treatment of rNV particles has been shown to result in the specific cleavage of the capsid protein with an approximately 32K product being produced that has the same N terminus as the soluble protein detected in the stools of volunteers given NV (63). Because specific proteolytic cleavages have been associated with viral pathogenesis in several viruses that infect the mucosal surfaces, it will be of interest to determine whether this specific cleavage results in activation of infectivity or altered immunogenicity for these viruses.

The function of the third ORF is unknown, but this ORF is conserved in the available sequences of each calicivirus. Sequence comparisons showed that NV ORF3, like that of the other four caliciviruses, is basic, suggesting potential involvement of this protein in nucleic acid binding (61). Analysis of ORF3 from the three complete sequences currently available suggests that this protein may have three conserved domains. A mechanism of ribosomal frameshifting for expression of this ORF has been proposed for FCV (64), but no specific RNA structure similar to the stem–loop structures associated with frameshifting in other systems is present in the NV genome sequence. Strong AUG initiation codons for ORF3 suggest that it may be expressed independently.

Three double-stem RNA loops are predicted in the 5′ end (nt 20 to 98) and upstream of ORF2 (nt 5268 to 5344) and ORF3 (nt 6836 to 6929) in the NV genome. These structures may be important not only for synthesis of viral genomic but also for subgenomic RNA replication. A consensus sequence also is located at the 5′ end of the viral genome and upstream of ORF2 (nt 5288 to 5357), suggesting this may be a packaging signal for genomic and subgenomic RNA.

Until an *in vitro* replication system for NV is established, confirmation of these potential replication strategies may be possible by expression of NV cDNAs in eukaryotic cells.

DIAGNOSTIC ASSAYS

It is not possible to make a specific diagnosis of infection with the NV group on the sole basis of clinical findings. However, a provisional diagnosis of infection during outbreaks of gastroenteritis is possible if the following criteria are met: (a) absence of bacterial or parasitic pathogens, (b) vomiting in more than 50% of cases, (c) duration of illness (mean or median ranges) from 12 to 60 hr, and (d) an incubation period of 24 to 48 hr. These criteria were met in 81% to 100% of ill individuals in 38 NV outbreaks (65) and have been used successfully in several epidemiologic studies. A definitive diagnosis desirable for both clinical and epidemiologic studies requires the availability of detection methods for antigen or antibody responses. Because previous and current epidemiologic studies rely on detection of infection based on available diagnostic assays, it is pertinent to begin by briefly discussing the various assays for detection of NV and human calicivirus infections (Table 5).

Because none of these agents has been grown in cell culture, and particle-positive stools were not readily available, initial assays for viral diagnosis were developed using reagents (pre- and postinfection serum and stool) from volunteer studies. The first immunologic test developed for NV diagnosis was IEM (3). This method (in addition to direct EM) has remained the most widely used and applicable test for the examination of fecal samples for the presence of NV and other human caliciviruses in diagnostic laboratories worldwide. While EM methods only detect particulate antigen, they have been an extremely effective method for virus detection in stool because EM is not biased to detect a specific type of virus; thus its open-ended nature has resulted in the detection of all types of enteric calicivirus (and other enteric viruses) shed in stool (66). Interestingly, direct EM often has been successful in detecting human caliciviruses or SRSVs in fecal samples from children, while IEM has generally been required for detection of NVs in adults. With the current recognition that most, if not all, of the detected SRSVs and Norwalk-like agents are human caliciviruses, and that adults shed large amounts of soluble antigen that is derived from the viral capsid, it is likely that different intestinal factors (such as antibody, proteases, pH, etc.) affect the form of antigen shed by different individuals rather than the fact that infected adults simply excrete less virus. It is not yet proved that children shed such large amounts

TABLE 5. *Methods to detect NV and other human calicivirus infections*

Methods to detect infection using					
Human reagents (stool and pre- and postinfection serum)	Purified virus, recombinant virus, or genomic sequences	Method to detect antibody	Method to detect antigen in stools	Method to detect viral genome	References
IEM		Yes	Yes, particulate antigen only, specific [a]	No	3
RIA		Yes	Yes, particulate and soluble antigen	No	69
ELISA		Yes	Yes, particulate and soluble antigen	No	70–72
IAHA		Yes	No	No	91
Blocking ELISA or RIA		Yes	No	No	3,75,155
SPIEM		Yes	Yes, particulate antigen	No	51
Western blot		Yes, broadly reactive	No	No	79
	RT-PCR	Yes	Yes	Yes, specific or more broadly reactive[b]	33,35,39, 47,81
	Hybridization	Yes	Yes	Yes	27,59,84
	ELISA	Yes, broadly reactive	Yes, highly specific	No	47,59,83, 84,101
	IEM	Yes	Yes, particulate antigen	No	83
	RIA	Yes	Yes	No	47,59,84

[a] Specificity obtained using selected paired reference sera.
[b] Specificity depends on choice of primers.

of soluble antigen, although some samples from children have been reported to contain a 33K protein (58).

IEM has been used to detect both antigen and seroresponses following infection and it is an extremely effective method if performed with the proper controls and standardized reference sera (67). One disadvantage of this method is that it can obscure the characteristic surface morphology of HuCVs, making them indistinguishable from antibody-coated astroviruses. If antibody is present in excess, the virus may be totally masked, resulting in a failure of detection. The use of solid-phase immunosorbent immunoelectron microscopy (SPIEM), which essentially is a capture ELISA performed on an EM grid (51,68), or immunogold labeling has facilitated visualization of particles, although these methods still require the availability of expensive equipment and highly skilled personnel.

The first immunologic assay developed that was more amenable to large-scale use was RIA (69). This solid-phase assay was developed in formats to detect antigen and to measure serologic responses using a blocking RIA. Subsequently, ELISAs of different formats were developed using human volunteer reagents to detect both antibody and virus for Norwalk, Snow Mountain agent, and Hawaii agent (70–75). All these solid-phase assays are based on the differential binding of NV antigen (present in stool) to microtiter wells coated with convalescent-phase or preinfection serum. These assays are more sensitive and more efficient than EM-based assays for virus detection, partly because they were found to detect both

particulate and soluble antigen. In fact, the presence of a large amount of soluble antigen in stools of volunteers infected with NV was first predicted based on results from a RIA, where stool samples from volunteers were positive for NV antigen by RIA, but negative by EM (69). A RIA and an ELISA to detect the Sapporo strain of human calicivirus also were developed but they differed from the assays for Norwalk and related agents in that the HuCV Sapporo ELISA used hyperimmune antiserum made against purified virus (obtained from the stools of young children) as the capture and detector antibodies (76,77). The ELISA to detect HuCV Sapporo antigen was found to be quite specific and it did not detect virus in all stools containing particles with typical human calicivirus morphology by EM (76,78). Similarly, the ELISAs to detect NV, SMA, or HV were specific for detection of these agents, although in certain cases they could detect anamnestic antibody responses or some cross-reactivity. In contrast, the HuCV Sapporo assay only detected antibody to the homologous virus (78). A Western blot assay also has been developed to detect SRSVs and antibody responses but this has not been used extensively (79).

The cloning, sequencing, and expression of the NV capsid protein have permitted a number of new assays to be developed that are quickly replacing the assays that used reagents from volunteers. The new assays for virus detection include reverse transcriptase–polymerase chain reaction (RT-PCR) to detect the viral genome and new ELISAs to detect both antibody responses and viral antigen.

The usefulness of each of these assays to detect infections with specific viruses is summarized briefly here.

The first new molecular assays developed to detect NV were based on detection of the viral genome. Nucleic acid hybridization assays and RT-PCR assays to amplify the small amount of nucleic acid found in many stools were shown to be about as sensitive as RIA to detect virus in stools of volunteers and in oysters seeded with NV (33,47,59,80–82). Two key points must be considered for the success of using RT-PCR as a routine diagnostic method. First, the availability of universal primers to detect all human caliciviruses would facilitate their use in diagnostic settings. Second, the exquisite sensitivity of these assays is both an asset and a problem in that extreme caution must be taken to assure that any results obtained are not false positives caused by contamination within a laboratory. The use of primers initially developed to detect the polymerase region of the NV genome proved useful for obtaining amplification and subsequent sequence information of a broad range of human caliciviruses (59). These results and the sequence data obtained from a relatively large number of studies indicate that it may not be possible to select a single set of primer pairs that will detect a broad range of viruses. Instead, it is likely that either (a) several sets of primer pairs that detect the polymerase region of viruses in the distinct genogroups, (b) possibly degenerate primers, or (c) primers from another region of the genome will be needed to detect all enteric caliciviruses. Currently, it does not appear that primers from the 5' untranslated region of the human caliciviruses will be useful for universal virus detection, as has been successful for the relatively sequence variable hepatitis C viruses (82a).

ELISAs to detect virus antigen and antibody responses also have been developed to detect NV. These assays were developed following the successful expression and self-assembly of the NV capsid protein into stable virus-like particles (21). The rNV particles were first used to develop an ELISA to detect antibody responses and, in this assay, rNV particles are used to coat the wells of microtiter plates (21). Initially, this assay was developed and validated using samples from human volunteers and well-characterized samples tested with previous assays (83–85). These studies showed that the rNV ELISA to detect antibody was as specific, sensitive, and efficient as previously described methods for detecting NV infection, and often more sensitive. The increased test sensitivity can be attributed to the very low assay background, which enables sera lacking antibody or containing very low levels of antibody to be detected, and these test results can easily be documented by use of the readily available rNV antigen for antibody absorption (84). In addition, higher antibody titers are obtained using the rNV antibody ELISA (83). The rNV antibody assay also has been shown to be broadly reactive in that it is able to detect seroresponses in volunteers given NV, HV, or SMA, although the highest increases in antibody titer are in NV-infected individuals (85). This assay has already been used in several small and large scale epidemiologic studies (83,86–88).

The rNV particles also were used to produce the first hyperimmune antiserum to NV and antiserum produced in guinea pigs, mice, and rabbits contains high titered antibodies to the immunogen and to native NV in stool (21,83,84). These results show that the previous lack of success of producing high titered antiserum was not due to any inherent poor antigenicity of NV, but rather to the paucity of pure antigen. The hyperimmune antisera were subsequently used to develop an antigen ELISA, which has been shown to be a highly sensitive and specific assay for NV antigen (59,84). The test sensitivity of the standard antigen ELISA was determined to be 1.4×10^6 virions without using any enhanced methods of signal amplification (84), and antigen was detected in the stools of volunteers diluted as much as 1:10,000. Comparison of the sensitivity of the ELISA, RT-PCR, dot blot hybridization, and RIA (using human volunteer reagents) to detect NV in stool showed that the sensitivity of the ELISA was similar to RT-PCR, and the ELISA was more sensitive than dot blot hybridization and RIA. The rNV antigen ELISA can detect both virus particles and soluble protein, and the presence and detection of such large amounts of soluble protein in stools likely explain the comparable sensitivities of the ELISA and RT-PCR.

Because of the relative simplicity of performing an ELISA, this theoretically is the assay of choice for virus detection. This asset currently is offset by the finding that the NV antigen ELISA is specific for NV, and many of the human caliciviruses (SRSVs, Norwalk-related viruses) do not react in this simple, sensitive, and specific assay. A compilation of testing of stool samples from 451 patients involved in volunteer studies, 26 outbreaks, and approximately 175 sporadic cases of acute gastroenteritis using the ELISA and RT-PCR showed that the NV antigen ELISA detected relatively few samples and only a subset of outbreak samples previously identified as NV origin based on testing with the human reagent ELISAs (59). RT-PCR detection of these same samples using primers specific for NV also identified a low number of positives. However, RT-PCR testing of these samples with more broadly reactive primers and subsequent sequence analysis indicated that viruses with a wide range of variable genomic sequences (44% to 87% nucleotide and 31% to 99% amino acid similarity to the 8fIIa NV genome polymerase sequence) were responsible for the outbreaks not detected with the NV antigen ELISA. All viruses positive in the rNV antigen ELISA had the highest sequence similarity to NV [over 81% nucleotide and over 90% amino acid within the polymerase region (59)]. Several recent outbreaks from the United States, Japan, and the United Kingdom were related to the SMA by sequence analysis. Thus detection of these non-NV viruses (i.e., probably viruses in other serotypes) currently requires either RT-PCR or the development of new specific or more commonly reactive antigen ELISAs. Based on these results, it can be expected that new methods will continue to be developed to detect common and specific epitopes of human caliciviruses. By combining these techniques, it is promising that sensitive and specific tests will be available in the near future for the diagnosis, basic research, epidemiology, and environmental monitoring of all human caliciviruses.

ANTIBODY PREVALENCE AND INCIDENCE

At the time of writing this chapter, our knowledge of the epidemiology of NV and human calicivirus infections is changing rapidly. This is because the cloning and expression of the NV genome have permitted large scale epidemiologic studies to begin to be performed and the results from such studies are indicating that infection with NV or Norwalk-like viruses is much more widespread than previously recognized. Here, we briefly review the previous understanding of NV epidemiology, which has been reviewed extensively elsewhere (1,89,90), and summarize how some of this previous dogma is changing with results from new studies based on widespread use of more sensitive molecular assays.

Norwalk virus antibody prevalence initially was studied using a RIA or immune adherence hemagglutination assay (IAHA) in relatively large studies (91–93). One classic study examined acquisition of antibody in the United States to NV or rotavirus, the virus known to cause severe life-threatening disease in young children (91). In this study, NV antibody was acquired gradually, beginning slowly in childhood and accelerating in adult years, so that 50% of adults possessed Norwalk antibody by age 50. Similar observations have been made in the United Kingdom and Japan using recombinant NV capsid antibody (87,93a,94). This pattern of antibody acquisition was similar to that observed for hepatitis A in similar populations and it contrasted with antibody acquisition to rotavirus, which occurs more rapidly with 90% of children possessing rotavirus antibody by age 3 (91). Other studies showed the rate of antibody acquisition varied between locations, with antibody acquisition occurring earlier in less developed countries (93). Thus it was found that in countries such as Bangladesh and Ecuador most people had antibody to NV by the age of 5 years, whereas in the United States and the former Yugoslavia, antibody acquisition occurs gradually over the first two decades of life (92,93,95–97). A recent study on the seroprevalence of NV antibody in isolated communities in the Amazon region using the new rNV antibody assay showed a range of antibody prevalence from 38% to 100% for different communities (98). In addition, children aged 6 to 10 years had NV antibody levels similar to that of adults. Taken together, these data suggested that transmission occurs largely by the fecal–oral route and exposure risks decrease as sanitary conditions improve. However, this may not be the only route of NV transmission as some evidence suggests that certain hospital outbreaks may be due to airborne or fomite transmission (99,100).

The lack of detection of antibodies to NV in infants and young children in the United States and other developed countries (using the original antibody assays with reagents from human volunteers) suggested that this virus was not an important cause of severe infantile diarrhea (reviewed in ref. 90). However, this role of NV and other related agents in diarrheal illness in infants or young children deserves further attention because, in certain studies, SRSVs have been detected in stool specimens in this age group, and these SRSVs probably all represent different types of human caliciviruses. In addition, in a recent longitudinal study, infection with the NV detected by ELISA using the rNV antigen was observed in 49% of 154 infants and young children in Finland over a period of almost 2 years (83,86). There are several explanations for the lack of detection of antibody in the earlier studies. First, the new rNV assay is more sensitive than the previous human reagent assays (83–85,101). In addition, the sensitivity of detecting low avidity antibody following primary infections in young children remains unknown and it is not yet clear how well the rNV antibody assay will detect seroresponses in young children infected with viruses in other serotypes. Thus similar assays based on the expression of antigens from viruses in the other genogroups need to be developed and compared for their respective abilities to detect responses in children infected with different serotypes of virus. It is known that the rNV assay is broadly reactive and it does detect antibody responses in adults who were infected with SMA or HV, but the magnitude of responses in individuals with heterologous infections generally was not as great as the responses seen in volunteers given NV (85). Responses to rNV antigen in children with heterologous infections may be even weaker.

The discovery that the minireovirus (TV) is a human calicivirus most closely related to the SMA is one example that highlights the possible importance of human caliciviruses in causing more than mild diarrhea in young children (29). Minireoviruses originally were detected by EM and described as second to rotavirus in causing young children to be hospitalized for diarrheal illness in Toronto (102,103). TV originally was only able to be detected using EM and more recently by other molecular techniques such as RT-PCR. TV does not react in the new antigen ELISA that uses hyperimmune antiserum made to the rNV that detects NV and closely related viruses (29,59,84). This result illustrates that the hyperimmune antiserum made to the rNV is very specific, and detection of other virus types will require the development of similar antigen ELISAs using particles expressed from the other virus types, or the development of other assays that can detect more broadly reactive antigenic epitopes. The type specificity of the rNV antigen assay and the broader reactivity of the rNV antibody assay is reminiscent of the results obtained in the early studies using the first human calicivirus ELISA developed to detect the HuCV Sapporo strain (76,78).

Given the current new information concerning the relatedness between different human caliciviruses, it is clear that our understanding of the epidemiology of these infections is just beginning. Antibody prevalence data available to date based on previous and possibly even new assays appear to measure primarily group-reactive antibodies; therefore we really have little idea of the relative importance of any given strain or serotype in different geographic locations. Because of the apparent broader reactivity of the rNV antibody assay, data with these new assays also may not provide serotype-specific information. However, further clarification of these issues is likely to come as the domains containing common and serotype-specific antigenic epitopes are characterized, and as new tests are developed and used based on this more precise information.

IMPORTANCE OF THE ENTERIC CALICIVIRUSES IN CAUSING DISEASE

Norwalk and related viruses have been well documented as the major causes of epidemic gastroenteritis in both developed and developing countries. These viruses have been documented on all continents where they have been sought, and it is expected that they will be found worldwide, as have rotaviruses, once diagnostic assays are readily available. Because of the limited availability of diagnostic assays to date, our current understanding of the importance of NV disease comes primarily from studies from a few laboratories that have had access to these diagnostic reagents.

Current information shows that these viruses cause outbreaks of waterborne and foodborne gastroenteritis and previous studies have estimated that at least 42% of outbreaks of nonbacterial gastroenteritis in the United States are caused by such infections (104). In fact, these are certainly minimal estimates because we know that the diagnostic methods used to study these outbreaks had limited sensitivity and did not detect all known virus strains. In the United Kingdom, where EM has been used extensively as an effective diagnostic tool, SRSVs have been considered to cause the majority of foodborne outbreaks of gastroenteritis, accounting for over 90% of outbreaks in which a virus is recognized (105). Similarly, in Japan, SRSVs are recognized as being the major cause of foodborne outbreaks of gastroenteritis and, in many outbreaks, oysters were the vehicle of transmission (106). In fact, the largest outbreak of foodborne illness affecting more than 2000 persons resulted from consumption of shellfish in Australia (107). Outbreaks have occurred in recreational camps, cruise ships, communities, hospitals, schools (elementary or college), nursing homes, and families, and they have been associated with contaminated drinking water, swimming water, consumption of uncooked or poorly cooked shellfish, ice, and bakery products (frosting), various types of salads (potato, fruit, tossed), and cold foods (celery, melon, vermicelli consommé, sandwiches, and cold cooked ham). Outbreaks have occurred year round and have affected primarily young children (4 years and older) and adults.

The spectrum of infections is widened when one includes the outbreaks associated with morphologically typical human caliciviruses. Infections with these viruses have been documented almost exclusively by EM and with a worldwide distribution in Europe, North America, Africa, Asia, and Australia (reviewed in ref. 108). Infections with these morphologically typical human caliciviruses were first detected among infants with gastroenteritis (109), and such infections among infants and young children have been confirmed and extended to adults and the elderly; they have been associated with outbreaks in orphanages, day care centers, schools, and hospital wards (108). Because it is now recognized that human caliciviruses now can be distinguished into distinct genogroups

(I, II, and III), it will be of interest to determine whether viruses in these specific groups have a different relative importance in causing infections among different age groups. Again, this will require the development of specific diagnostic assays for these distinguishable genogroups, and ultimately for specific virus serotypes. The information on the importance of the morphologically typical caliciviruses is particularly rudimentary because much of it relied on direct EM studies. These studies have indicated that caliciviruses are found in a low rate (0.2% to 6%) of stools associated with diarrhea from a variety of centers around the world. However, it is difficult to have confidence in these data because it is known that EM is relatively insensitive and samples known to contain HuCV detected by ELISA have not been detected by EM (68).

Nosocomial infection with HuCV has been documented (102) and may be quite common, and asymptomatic infections can occur (110). The high rate of nosocomial infection in children in Toronto often was associated with immunocompromised children (102,103). While NV has been found in the stools of HIV-positive patients, its role in the etiology of gastroenteritis or infection in this group has not been reported to be greater than in non-HIV infected controls (111,112). Because of the discovery that the minireovirus in many immunocompromised children is a NV-like agent (29), it may be worthwhile to reevaluate the role of these infections in other immunocompromised populations using the new assays.

The types of clinical manifestations caused by enteric animal caliciviruses are important to consider because, historically, comparative virology has shown that human viral infections ultimately are found to mimic previously described animal virus infections. The best studied animal calicivirus is FCV, which causes respiratory infections, conjunctivitis, pneumonia, vesicles, diarrhea, and possibly an arthritic-like limping disease in infected kittens (reviewed in ref. 113). Infected cats may become persistently infected with virus remaining in the tonsils (114). These viruses are interesting in that they appear to fall into one serotype with many variants that give one-way reactions in cross-neutralization assays (113,115). In spite of this, a vaccine composed of one serotype appears to provide broad protection. The marine caliciviruses (SMSVs) are of interest because they may have a broader host range, and feeding of uncooked fish containing caliciviruses to piglets resulted in epidemic outbreaks of vesicular exanthema of swine virus infections (VESV) in pigs (reviewed in refs. 116 and 117). The clinical manifestations were indistinguishable from foot and mouth disease, including vesicles in the mouth, tongue, lips, and snout and between the toes (118–120). In addition, VESV may cause encephalitis, myocarditis, fever, diarrhea, failure of infected animals to survive, and pregnant sows and sea lions to abort (121).

Porcine enteric caliciviruses have been found to cause diarrhea in pigs and this is one of the few enteric viruses successfully cultivated (122,123). Cultivation required the addition of large intestinal fluid contents from pigs to the tissue culture system (124). A devastating but relatively recently recognized disease in rabbits, RHDV, is noteworthy because it causes a hemorrhagic diarrheal disease, with hemorrhagic septicemia, infectious necrosis of the liver in rabbits, and high mortality in adult animals (125–127). While this virus cannot be cultivated in tissue culture, it has been cloned and rRHDV capsids expressed using baculovirus recombinants in a manner similar to NV have been shown to be an effective vaccine (127a). A chicken calicivirus also causes diarrhea in infected animals (128,129), while other caliciviruses, such as the primate calicivirus, have been reported to cause no detectable illness although they do cause persistent infections (130). A final possible member of the family is hepatitis E virus, which produces hepatitis in humans with a high mortality (approximately 20%) in pregnant women (131).

CLINICAL FEATURES OF INFECTION, PATHOGENESIS, AND TREATMENT

The clinical manifestations of NV infections have been reported both from natural outbreaks and from volunteer studies. The illness is generally mild and self-limited, with symptoms lasting 12 to 24 hr, with a mean incubation time of 48 hr. The main clinical features include the sudden onset of vomiting and/or diarrhea, and a wide spectrum of disease may be seen in individual volunteers. For example, in one study, within a 24-hr period, one volunteer vomited 20 times and required parenteral fluid therapy, while other volunteers had no vomiting but had diarrhea with up to 8 stools (4). The diarrheal stools are often liquid, without mucus, blood, or leukocytes (132). It has been estimated that about 50% of people exposed to NV become ill and secondary cases often occur. Hospitalization or rehydration is rarely required for adults and the major impact of this disease has been morbidity and loss of time from work and school. However, as noted earlier, because of the previous difficulty in diagnosing many infections, the real impact of these infections is certainly underestimated and still poorly understood.

A recent analysis of the clinical, virologic, and immunologic responses in a volunteer study using the newly developed diagnostic assays has confirmed and extended conclusions about NV infection of adults (84) (Table 6). Specifically, this study shows a higher infection rate, more subclinical infections, and longer virus excretion following NV inoculation than previously recognized. Of 50 volunteers administered NV, 41 (82%) became infected; of these infections, 68% were symptomatic and 32% were asymptomatic. The peak of virus shedding was between 25 and 72 hr and virus first appeared in stool 15 hr after virus administration. Surprisingly, stool specimens collected 7 days after inoculation remained ELISA positive for both individuals with symptomatic and asymptomatic infection . These new data add to our understanding of the clinical manifestations of NV-induced acute gastroenteritis and have implications for the diagnosis of NV infections and the natural history and epidemiology of NV. For example, the findings of prolonged virus shedding and a higher rate of subclinical infections are important for understanding virus transmissions and for planning intervention measures to control disease spread. Previously, it had been thought that virus shedding began with the onset of clinical illness and usually did not last more than 72 hr (4,133). These new results indicate that while virus excretion peaks at 3 days, virus antigen is still being shed in the latest samples available for testing (7 days postinoculation). The high rate of asymptomatic infection, with one individual still shedding virus at day 6, also may facilitate virus transmission, and this could help explain those foodborne epidemics where food handlers report no previous illness (134). It will be important to determine the maximal time of virus shedding, and whether the viral antigen excreted at late times is infectious (and not simply soluble antigen); if infectious virus is routinely shed for long times, this information will need to be considered in planning outbreak control efforts in hospitals, in nursing homes, and in the food industry.

Illnesses induced in volunteers with the Hawaii, Mont-

TABLE 6. *Clinical status in relation to magnitude of seroresponse to Norwalk virus*

Antibody response (-fold)	No. of cases	No. antigen positive	Diarrhea (38 [15–55])	Vomiting[a] (24 [23–31])	Nausea[b] (25 [15–51])	Cramps (28 [7–55])	Headache/ body ache[c] (29 [3–55])	Chills (27 [19–55])	Fever >37.8°C)[d] (33 [15–55])
0	10[e]	1[e] (10)	1[e] (10)	0	1 (10)	0	4 (40)	0	0
4	3	0	0	0	0	1 (33)	0	0	0
16	15	13 (87)	9 (60)	4 (27)	10 (67)	10 (67)	11 (73)	4 (27)	3 (20)
64	17	17 (100)	11 (65)	9 (53)	13 (76)	12 (71)	12 (71)	5 (29)	3 (18)
256	5	5 (100)	3 (60)	3 (60)	4 (80)	4 (80)	4 (80)	1 (20)	3 (60)
Total	50[f]	36 (88)	24 (59)	16 (39)	27 (66)	27 (66)	27 (66)	10 (24)	9 (22)

Symptom headings show (median h of incubation [range]).
[a] $P = .02$, χ^2 for trend = 5.4.
[b] $P \leq .02$, χ^2 for trend = 5.9.
[c] $P = .04$, χ^2 for trend = 4.2.
[d] $P = .08$, χ^2 for trend = 3.2.
[e] Includes 1 infected subject with no antibody response but who had watery diarrhea and excreted virus and had antibody titers of 1:2560. Norwalk infection was confirmed in 41 subjects by either antigen excretion or seroconversion; %s were calculated on 41 as total.
(From ref. 84, with permission.)

gomery County, Snow Mountain agents, and one strain of morphologically typical HuCV, as well as naturally occurring illnesses with the morphologically typical HuCV in infants, older children, and adults, appear clinically indistinguishable from those observed with the NV (reviewed in refs. 90 and 108). Abdominal pain has been noted as a symptom that accompanies the vomiting and diarrhea in older children and adults and, in some outbreaks, symptoms have been described as "flu-like," with aching limbs, headache, malaise, and fever being noted. With the new tests available for diagnosis, it will be of interest to monitor flu-like illnesses not attributable to influenza and determine whether a significant percentage of these illnesses are actually due to HuCV infections.

The pathogenesis of NV and HV illness has been examined in volunteer studies where proximal intestinal biopsies were taken (135–138). Histologic changes were seen in jejunal biopsies from ill volunteers. Symptomatic illness was correlated with a broadening and blunting of the intestinal villi, crypt cell hyperplasia, cytoplasmic vacuolization, and infiltration of polymorphonuclear and mononuclear cells into the lamina propria, but the mucosa itself remained intact. Histologic changes were not seen in the gastric fundus, antrum, or colonic mucosa (138) or in convalescent phase biopsies. The extent of small intestinal involvement remains unknown because studies have only examined the proximal small intestine and the site of virus replication has not been identified. Clinical studies also showed that small intestinal brush border enzymatic activities (alkaline phosphatase, sucrase, and trehalase) were decreased, resulting in mild steatorrhea and transient carbohydrate malabsorption (135). Jejunal adenylate cyclase activity was not elevated (139), gastric secretion of HCl, pepsin, and intrinsic factor was associated with these histologic changes, and gastric emptying was delayed (140). It has been suggested that reduced gastric motility may be responsible for the nausea and vomiting associated with this gastroenteritis. Attempts to detect interferon in sera, jejunal aspirates, or jejunal biopsy specimens from volunteers inoculated with NV or HV were not successful; however, it is unclear whether these viruses do not induce interferon production in the gut, or if there are alternative physiological explanations for lack of detection (141).

It is of interest to consider data on the pathogenesis of porcine enteric calicivirus infections in piglets, and infection of calves with Newbury agent (a bovine enteric calicivirus), as the consequences of calicivirus infection in the gut by these viruses appears similar to what is known about HuCV (122,142–145). Oral inoculation in piglets and/or calves resulted in diarrhea and anorexia 2 to 4 days postinoculation and loss of digestive and absorptive function. Mature enterocytes were infected, villi were stunted, and lesions were restricted to the anterior portion of the small intestine. In calves, histologic changes in the stomach, large intestine, liver, or lungs were not observed. It may be that calicivirus infection in these animals is similar enough to HuCV infections that supportive evidence for the mechanisms of calicivirus pathogenesis in humans can be provided by these models.

As discussed earlier, the illnesses caused by these en-

teric caliciviruses are generally mild and self-limited, and resolution occurs without sequelae (108,146). Treatment involves symptomatic therapy with oral rehydration generally being sufficient. In rare cases, parenteral administration of intravenous fluids is required. Deaths in the elderly infected with NV and in immunocompromised children infected with HuCV have been reported, but these have generally been attributable to other primary causes (104; D. O. Matson and M. K. Estes, *unpublished data*).

IMMUNITY, PREVENTION, AND CONTROL

Studies of viral immunity have been relatively limited and have monitored the clinical resistance to infection or illness as correlated with preinfection antibody status of volunteers administered NV, SMA, or HV, and of individuals involved in outbreaks (7,147,148). The development of immunity also has been monitored in similar settings by characterizing the seroresponses of individuals exposed to virus and with various clinical or infection outcomes. The assays used for most analyses of immunity have been the first generation tests such as IEM, RIAs, and ELISAs that used human reagents. The inability to cultivate NV and other enteric human caliciviruses has hampered studies of viral immunity because *in vitro* neutralization assays are not available. Thus the analyses of immunity in volunteers are complicated by several factors, including the following: (a) the preinfection exposure status to any of the HuCV agents of any adult volunteer is not known so interpretation of results is never completely clear; and (b) neutralization assays with well-characterized cultivated viruses are not available; therefore the results of available assays may reflect responses to common or shared nonneutralizing epitopes.

Few studies have examined immunity to typical calicivirus infections in young children. However, one study that measured immunity to the HuCV Sapporo strain using a RIA with hyperimmune antiserum and apparently measured type-specific antibodies found that the presence of serum antibody was clearly correlated with resistance to illness, but not infection (149). These results are of interest with the knowledge that this virus strain appears to fall into a separate genogroup, and that children become infected with other virus serotypes (149a).

Studies of clinical immunity in volunteers to NV and the other SRSVs have resulted in a more complex picture. Initial studies indicated that at least 50% of adult volunteers are susceptible to illness following administration of NV, HV, or SMA, or a strain of HuCV. Early volunteer studies also showed that short-term homologous immunity develops, as volunteers who became ill following an initial NV challenge failed to become ill on rechallenge 6 to 14 weeks later with the same agent (148). It would be interesting to determine if any of these individuals actually had asymptomatic infections using the new more sensitive assays. Several volunteer studies were unable to correlate elevated preexisting levels of serum or intestinal antibody to NV with long-term resistance to illness but, instead, observed an unexpected reciprocal relationship between prechallenge NV antibody levels and susceptibility to illness (148,150). In other volunteer studies, short-term resistance to infection was induced by prior homologous infection and was correlated with high antibody levels (7,150). Other potentially conflicting data were obtained from epidemiology studies where, in some cases, the level of antibody has not been correlated with protection (151,152).

The recent analysis of volunteers given NV using the new molecular assays has confirmed that 50% of volunteers are susceptible to illness, but a larger number (80%) of volunteers may be infected, with many of these infections being asymptomatic (84). Analysis of the preinfection serum antibody levels confirmed and extended the conclusions summarized earlier about clinical immunity. In this study, the volunteers were divided into five groups based on infection status and clinical outcome and severity of the infection (Fig. 8). Uninfected individuals were more likely to have lower preexisting antibody titers compared to any of the infected groups ($P < 0.001$). In addition, individuals who got watery diarrhea but no vomiting had significantly higher preexisting antibody titers when compared to uninfected individuals. For all the infected groups, there were significant increases in the geometric mean titers after infection, and among the groups of infected volunteers, the rises in antibody titers in the convalescent sera were significantly higher in volunteers who vomited (groups 3 and 5 versus groups 2 and 4) and in volunteers who vomitted and had diarrhea (group 5 versus groups 2, 3, and 5). This result suggests that volunteers who vomit have high titer antibody responses and these could be prolonged responses. If true, this could explain the association of diarrheal disease with vomiting with seroresponses to NV in epidemiology studies.

An analysis of the infection outcome of volunteers relative to their preexisting antibody status also showed that individuals lacking antibody were not resistant to infection or illness (Table 7). Instead, there was a 60% seroconversion in volunteers lacking preexisting serum antibody (titers < 10), so the lack of detectable serum antibody did not fully correlate with protection from infection. While some volunteers with preexisting serum antibody titers of less than 1:50 (determined by the human reagent RIA) previously had been reported to become ill (92), it was not clear if these individuals really lacked antibody or simply possessed low titers. The lack of antibody in our volunteers was able to be confirmed by adsorption of the prechallenge sera with rNV particles. However, individuals who excreted virus had significantly higher preexisting antibody titers and there was a trend for higher preexisting antibody titers in those who seroconverted.

Taken together, these results suggest that our knowledge about immunity to human calicivirus infections remains incomplete and the conflicting data may be clarified once assays that measure neutralizing epitopes become available. Currently, it appears that short-term resistance to illness can be induced by infection and this immunity appears to correlate with the level of serum antibody. On the other hand, long-term resistance to illness appears to be more complicated and may be influenced by other

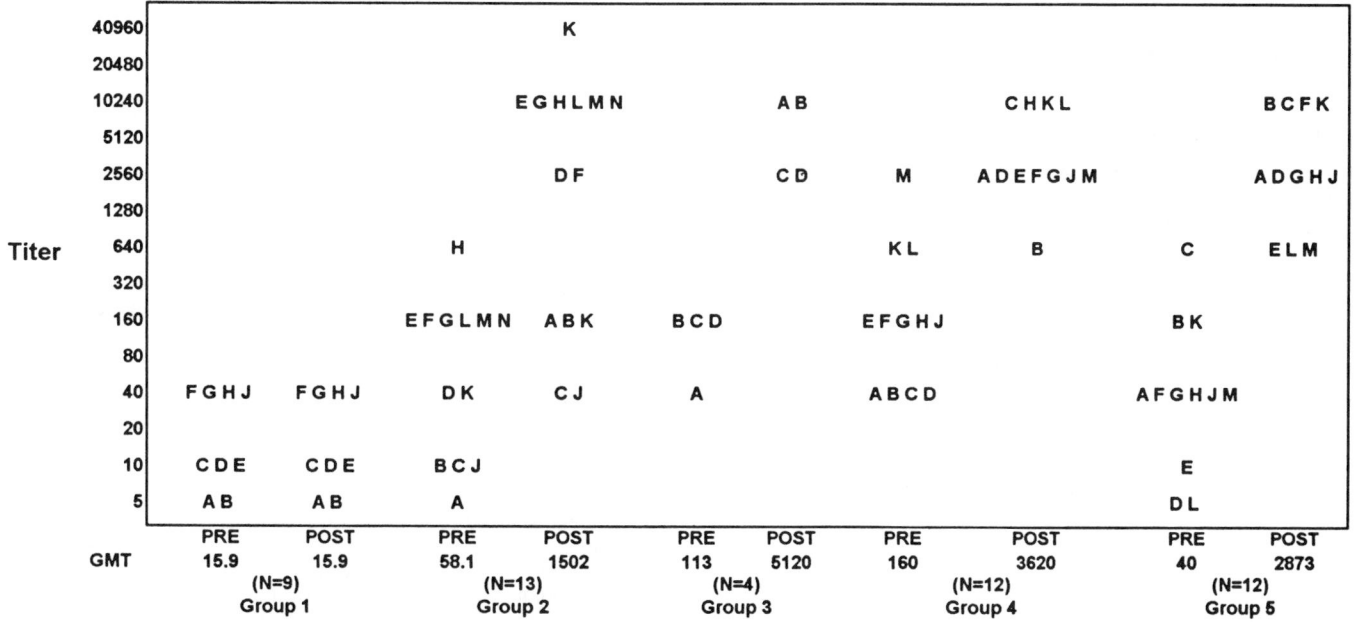

FIG. 8. Serologic status of volunteers inoculated with NV relative to clinical illness. Group 1, uninfected (no seroconversion and no antigen shedding); group 2, asymptomatic or mild symptomatic infection (no vomiting and no diarrhea); group 3, symptomatic infection (vomiting, no diarrhea); group 4, symptomatic infection (no vomiting but watery diarrhea); group 5, symptomatic infection (vomiting and watery diarrhea). Preinoculation and postinoculation titers for each subject are shown (individual letters); geometric means (GMT) are at bottom. Cutoff was A_{414nm} of 0.1. (From ref. 84, with permission.)

TABLE 7. *Infection outcome relative to preexisting Norwalk virus antibody status*

Serum titers	Number of cases	Number of volunteers (%) who had								
		Sero-conversion[a]	Virus shedding[b]	Diarrhea	Vomiting	Nausea[a]	Cramps	Headache	Chills	Fever
<10[c]	5	3 (60)	2 (40)	2 (40)	2 (40)	2 (40)	2 (40)	4 (80)	1 (20)	1 (20)
10	7	4 (57)	2 (29)	1 (14)	1 (14)	1 (14)	1 (14)	3 (42)	0 (0)	0 (0)
40	17	13 (76)	12 (70)	10 (59)	7 (41)	11 (65)	12 (70)	12 (70)	5 (29)	4 (23)
160	16	16 (100)	16 (100)	7 (44)	5 (31)	10 (62)	10 (62)	9 (56)	3 (19)	3 (19)
640	4	4 (100)	3 (75)	3 (75)	1 (25)	4 (100)	2 (50)	3 (75)	1 (25)	1 (25)
2560	1	0 (0)	1 (100)	1 (100)	0 (0)	0 (0)	0 (0)	0 (0)	0 (0)	0 (0)

[a] $P = 0.065$, χ^2 for trend $= 3.4$.
[b] $P = 0.0012$, χ^2 for trend $= 10.5$.
[c] Subjects did not have preexisting antibody; blocking also was consistent with lacking antibody.
From ref. 84, with permission.

factors; for example, there may be a genetic susceptibility to infection determined by the presence or absence of a specific virus receptor. It has been suggested that there is a subset of individuals who are relatively resistant to NV infection, and these individuals tend to have lower levels of antibody to NV, probably because they are less frequently infected (148). Whether these individuals would be resistant to infections with all human caliciviruses or only to a subset of such agents remains to be determined. Again, cultivation of these agents will facilitate answering these questions and likely will lead to resolution of whether individual serotypes of these viruses use distinct receptors to infect the gastrointestinal tract.

Because of our incomplete understanding of protective immunity to NV and other human caliciviruses, currently it is unclear whether vaccination strategies will be able to prevent such illnesses. Vaccines might prove effective, if the evidence for widespread and broad immunity to the morphologically typical caliciviruses is correct, and if the results in less-developed countries reflect the ability to induce protection, possibly with repeated exposure. Some of these data are reminiscent of early reports for poliovirus exposure and resistance. It clearly is important to determine the number of serotypes of human caliciviruses and the relationship of serotypes to specific syndromes. It is possible that repeated immunization will be required to induce long-lasting immunity, but the availability of large amounts of stable recombinant particles makes it feasible if these induce a prolonged immunity. The rNV particles are safe and immunogenic when given to volunteers (153), and it is likely that evaluation of the immune response to these particles will help us understand immunity to these enteric infections.

SUMMARY

In the last 3 years, significant advances in our knowledge about NV and related viruses have come from the cloning, sequencing and expression of cDNAs of the genomes of these viruses. The availability of new diagnostic assays based on unlimited recombinant antigen and molecular assays based on knowledge of the sequence of the genome are allowing large scale epidemiologic studies and

characterization of the similarity and diversity of virus strains to proceed. The new information already obtained indicates that the epidemiology of infections with these viruses is not yet well understood and can be expected to continue to change. There is little doubt that further studies of the molecular biology and epidemiology of these viruses will reveal unexpected and exciting new information about the interactions of these viruses with a diversity of cells of the gastrointestinal tract and possibly extraintestinally, as have similar studies with the rotaviruses over the past 20 years. We predict that as the human caliciviruses are studied, they will be found to play significant role(s) in both acute and chronic human illness whose etiologies currently are unknown.

ACKNOWLEDGMENTS

We gratefully acknowledge support for our research on Norwalk virus and human caliciviruses provided by the FDA, Thrasher Research Fund, NOAA, and the NIH.

REFERENCES

1. Kapikian AZ, Chanock RM. Norwalk group of viruses. In: Fields BN, ed. *Virology,* 2nd ed. New York: Raven Press, 1990; 671–693.
2. Adler I, Zickl R. Winter vomiting disease. *J Infect Dis* 1969; 119:668–673.
3. Kapikian AZ, Wyatt RG, Dolin R, Thornhill TS, Kalica AR, Chanock RM. Visualization by immune electron microscopy of a 27 nm particle associated with acute infectious nonbacterial gastroenteritis. *J Virol* 1972;10:1075–1081.
4. Dolin R, Blacklow NR, DuPont H, et al. Transmission of acute infectious nonbacterial gastroenteritis to volunteers by oral aministration of stool filtrates. *J Infect Dis* 1971;123:307–312.
5. Thornhill TS, Wyatt RG, Kalica AR, Dolin R, Chanock RM, Kapikian AZ. Detection by immune electron microscopy of 26–27 nm virus-like particles associated with two family outbreaks of gastroenteritis. *J Infect Dis* 1977;135:20–27.
6. Morens DM, Zweighaft RM, Vernon TM, et al. A waterborne outbreak of gastroenteritis with secondary person-to-person spread: association with a viral agent. *Lancet* 1979;1:964–966.
7. Wyatt RG, Dolin R, Blacklow NR, et al. Comparison of three agents of acute infectious nonbacterial gastroenteritis by crosschallenge in volunteers. *J Infect Dis* 1974;127:709–714.
8. Caul EO, Ashley C, Pether JV. "Norwalk"-like particles in

the epidemic gastroenteritis in the U.K. [Letter]. *Lancet* 1979; 2:1292.

9. Taniguchi K, Urasawa S, Urasawa T. Virus-like particle, 35 to 40 nm, associated with an institutional outbreak of acute gastroenteritis in adults. *J Clin Microbiol* 1979;10:730–736.

10. Kogasaka R, Nakamura S, Chiba S, Sakuma Y, Terashima H, Yokoyama T, Nakao T. The 33- to 39-nm virus-like particles, tentatively designed as Sapporo agent, associated with an outbreak of acute gastroenteritis. *J Med Virol* 1981;8:187–193.

11. Oishi I, Yamazaki K, Minekawa Y, Nishimura H, Kitaura T. Three-year survey of the epidemiology of rotavirus, enteric adenovirus, and some small spherical viruses including "Osaka-agent" associated with infantile diarrhea. *Biken J* 1985;28:9–19.

12. Caul EO, Appleton H. The electron microscopical and physical characteristics of small round human fecal viruses: an interim scheme for classification. *J Med Virol* 1982;9:257–265.

13. Appleton H. Small round viruses: classification and role in food-borne infections. In: *Novel diarrhoea viruses*. Ciba Foundation Symposium 128. Chichester: Wiley, 1987;108–125.

14. Herrmann JE, Hudson RW, Blacklow NR. Marin County agent, an astrovirus [letter]. *Lancet* 1987;2:743.

15. Murphy FA, Kingsbury DW. Virus taxonomy. In: Fields BN, Knipe DM, eds. *Virology*, 2nd ed. New York: Raven Press, 1990;9–35.

16. Greenberg HB, Valdesuso JR, Kalica AR, Wyatt RG, McAuliffe VJ, Kapikian AZ, Chanock RM. Proteins of Norwalk virus. *J Virol* 1981;37:994–999.

17. Burroughs JN, Brown F. Physico-chemical evidence for the reclassification of the caliciviruses. *J Gen Virol* 1974;22:281–286.

18. Schaffer FL, Soergel ME. Single major polypeptide of a calicivirus: characterization by polyacrylamide gel electrophoresis and stabilization of virions by cross-linking with dimethyl suberimidate. *J Virol* 1976;19:925–931.

19. Bachrach HL, Hess WR. Animal picornaviruses with a single major species of capsid protein. *Biochem Biophy Res Commun* 1973;55:141–149.

20. Jiang X, Wang M, Wang K, Estes MK. Sequence and genomic organization of Norwalk virus. *Virology* 1993;195:51–61.

21. Jiang X, Wang M, Graham DY, Estes MK. Expression, self-assembly, and antigenicity of the Norwalk virus capsid protein. *J Virol* 1992;66:6527–6532.

22. Hendry DA. Nodaviridae in invertebrates. In: Kurstak E, ed. *Viruses of invertebrates*. New York: Marcel Dekker;1991; 227–276.

23. Hosur MV, Schmidt T, Rucker RC, Johnson JE, Gallagher RM, Selling BH, Rueckert RR. Structure of an insect virus at 3.0 Å resolution. *Proteins* 1987;2:167–176.

24. Prasad BVV, Rothnagel R, Jiang X, Estes MK. Three-dimensional structure of baculovirus-expressed Norwalk virus capsids. *J Virol* 1994;68:5117–5125.

25. Prasad BVV, Matson DO, Smith AJ. Three-dimensional structure of calicivirus. *J Mol Biol* 1994;240:256–264.

26. Jiang X, Graham DY, Wang K, Estes MK. Norwalk virus genome cloning and characterization. *Science* 1990;250: 1580–1583.

27. Matsui SM, Kim JP, Greenberg HB, et al. The isolation and characterization of a Norwalk virus-specific cDNA. *J Clin Invest* 1991;87:1456–1461.

28. Lambden PR, Caul EO, Ashley CR, Clarke IN. Sequence and genome organization of a human small round-structured (Norwalk-like) virus. *Science* 1993;259:516–519.

29. Lew JF, Petric M, Kapikian AZ, Jiang X, Estes MK, Green KY. Identification of "minireovirus" as a Norwalk-like virus in pediatric patients with gastroenteritis. *J Virol* 1994;68: 3391–3396.

30. Lew JF, Kapikian AZ, Jiang X, Estes MK, Green KY. Molecular characterization and expression of the capsid protein of a Norwalk-like virus recovered from a Desert Shield troop with gastroenteritis. *Virology* 1994;200:319–325.

31. Lew JF, Kapikian AZ, Valdesuso J, Green KY. Molecular characterization of Hawaii virus and other Norwalk-like viruses: evidence for genetic polymorphism among human caliciviruses. *J. Infect Dis* 1994;170:535–542.

32. Ando T, Mulders MN, Lewis DC, Estes MK, Monroe SS, Glass RI. Comparison of the polymerase region of small round structured virus strains previously characterized in three serotypes by solid-phase immune electron microscopy. *Arch Virol* 1994;135:217–226.

33. Green J, Norcott JP, Lewis D, Arnold C, Brown WG. Norwalk-like viruses: demonstration of genomic diversity by polymerase chain reaction. *J Clin Microbiol* 1991;31:3007–3012.

34. Norcott JP, Green J, Lewis D, Estes MK, Brown DWG. Genomic diversity of small round structured viruses in the UK. *J Med Virol (in press)*.

35. Wang J, Jiang X, Madore HP, et al. Sequence diversity of small round structured viruses. *J Virol* 1994;68:5982–5990.

36. Cubitt WD, Jiang XJ, Wang J, Estes MK. Sequence similarity of human caliciviruses and small round structured viruses. *J Med Virol* 1994;43:252–258.

37. Matson DO, Zhong W, Nakata S, et al. Molecular characterization of a human calicivirus with closer sequence relatedness to animal caliciviruses than other known human caliciviruses. *J Med Virol (in press)*.

38. Lambden PR, Caul EO, Ashley R, Clarke IN. Human enteric caliciviruses are genetically distinct from small round structured viruses. *Lancet* 1994;343:666–667.

39. Moe CL, Gentsch J, Grohmann G, et al. Application of PCR to detect Norwalk virus in fecal specimens from outbreaks of gastroenteritis. *J Clin Microbiol* 1994;32:642–648.

40. Kozak M. Possible role of flanking nucleotides in recognition of the AUG initiator codon by eukaryotic ribosomes. *Nucleic Acids Res* 1981;9:5233–5252.

41. Pestova TV, Hellen CUT, Wimmer E. Translation of poliovirus RNA: role of an essential cis-acting oligopyrimidine element within the 5' nontranslated region and involvement of a cellular 57-kilodalton protein. *J Virol* 1991;65:6194–6204.

42. Palmenberg AC. Sequence alignments of picornaviral capsid proteins. In: Semler BL, Ehrenfeld E, eds. *Molecular aspects of picornavirus infection and detection*. Washington, DC: American Society for Microbiology, 1989;211–241.

43. Carter MJ, Milton ID, Meanger J, Bennett M, Gaskell RM, Turner PC. The complete nucleotide sequence of a feline calicivirus. *Virology* 1992;190:443–448.

44. Meyers G, Wirblich C, Thiel HJ. Rabbit hemorrhagic disease virus—molecular cloning and nucleotide sequencing of a calicivirus genome. *Virology* 1991;184:664–676.

45. Tam AW, Smith MM, Guerra ME, Huang CC, Bradley DW, Fry KE, Reyes GR. Hepatitis E virus (HEV): molecular cloning and sequencing of the full-length viral genome. *Virology* 1991;185:120–131.

46. Neill JD. Nucleotide sequence of the capsid protein gene of two serotypes of San Miguel sea lion virus: identification of conserved and non-conserved amino acid sequences among calicivirus capsid proteins. *Virus Res* 1992;24:211–222.

47. Jiang X, Wang J, Graham DY, Estes MK. Detection of Norwalk virus in stool by polymerase chain reaction. *J Clin Microbiol* 1992;30:2529–2534.

48. Green SM, Dingle KE, Lambden PR, Caul EO, Ashley CR, Clarke IN. Human enteric caliciviridae; a new prevalent SRSV group defined by RNA-dependent RNA polymerase and capsid diversity. *J Gen Virol* 1994;75:1883–1888.

49. Moussa A, Chasey D, Lavazza A, et al. Haemorrhagic disease of lagomorphs: evidence for a calicivirus. *Vet Microbiol* 1992; 33:375–381.

50. Dolin R, Reichman RC, Roessner KD, Tralka TS, Schooley RT, Gary W, Morens D. Detection by immune electron microscopy of the Snow Mountain agent of acute viral gastroenteritis. *J Infect Dis* 1982;146:184–189.

51. Lewis DC. Three serotypes of Norwalk-like virus demonstrated by solid-phase immune electron microscopy. *J Med Virol* 1990;30:77–81.

52. Oglesby AS, Schaffer FL, Madin SH. Biochemical and biophysical properties of vesicular exanthema of swine virus. *Virology* 1971;44:329–331.

53. Bradley DW, Purdy MA, Reyes GR. Hepatitis E virus genome. Molecular features, expression of immunoreactive proteins and sequence divergence. *J Hepatol* 1991;13(Suppl 4):S152–S154.

54. Hillman B, Morris TJ, Kellen WR, Hoffman D, Schlegl DE.

An invertebrate calici-like virus. Evidence for partial virion disintegration in host excreta. *J Gen Virol* 1982;60:115–123.

55. Smith AW, Prato C, Skilling DE. Caliciviruses infecting monkeys and possibly man. *Am J Vet Res* 1978;39:287–289.

55a. Humphrey TJ, Cruickshank JG, Cubitt WD. An outbreak of calcivirus associated gastroenteritis in an elderly person's home. A possible zoonosis? *J Hyg* 1984;93:293–299.

56. Neill JD, Meyer R, Seal BS. Genetic relatedness of the caliciviruses: PCR amplification and sequence analysis of specific regions to the genomic RNAs of San Miguel sea lion and vesicular exanthema of swine viruses. Abstract: American Society for Virology 13th Annual Meeting, Madison, Wisconsin, July 10–14, 1994.

57. Barlough JE, Berry ES, Skilling DE, Smith AW, Fay FH. Antibodies to marine caliciviruses in the Pacific walrus (*Odobenus rosmarus divergens Illiger*). *J Wildl Dis* 1986;22:165–168.

58. Oishi I, Yamazaki K, Kimoto T, Minekawa Y. Demonstration of low molecular weight polypeptides associated with small, round-structured viruses by Western immunoblot analysis. *Microbiol Immunol* 1992;36:1105–1112.

59. Jiang X, Wang J, Estes MK. Characterization of SRSVs using RT-PCR and a new antigen ELISA: a short communication. *Arch Virol (in press)*.

60. Neill JD, Mengeling WL. Further characterization of the virus-specific RNAs in feline calicivirus infected cells. *Virus Res* 1988;11:59–72.

61. Meyers G, Wirblich C, Thiel HJ. Genomic and subgenomic RNAs of rabbit hemorrhagic disease virus are both protein-linked and packaged into particles. *Virology* 1991;184:677–686.

62. Carter MJ. Transcription of feline calicivirus RNA. *Arch Virol* 1990;114:143–152.

63. Hardy ME, White LJ, Ball JM, Estes MK. Specific proteolytic cleavage of the Norwalk virus capsid protein. (*submitted*).

64. Neill JD, Reardon IM, Heinrikson RL. Nucleotide sequence and expression of the capsid protein gene of feline calicivirus. *J Virol* 1991;65:5440–5447.

65. Kaplan JE, Feldman R, Campbell DS, Lookabaugh C, Gary GW. The frequency of a Norwalk-like pattern of illness in outbreaks of acute gastroenteritis. *Am J Public Health* 1982;72:1329–1332.

66. Kapikian AZ, Feinstone SM, Purcell RH, Wyatt RG, Thornhill TS, Kalica AR, Chanock RM. Detection and identification by immune electron microscopy of fastidious agents associated with respiratory illness, acute nonbacterial gastroenteritis, and hepatitis A. *Perspect Virol* 1975;9:9–47.

67. Kapikian AZ, Yolken RH, Greenberg HB, Wyatt RG, Kalica AR, Chanock RM, Kim HW. Gastroenteritis viruses. In: Lennette EH, Schmidt NJ, eds. *Diagnostic procedures for viral, rickettsial, and chlamydial infections*, 5th ed. Washington, DC: American Public Health Association, 1979;927–995.

68. Matson DO, Estes MK, Glass RI, et al. Human calicivirus-associated diarrhea in children attending day care centers. *J Infect Dis* 1989;159:71–78.

69. Greenberg HB, Wyatt RG, Valdesuso J, Kalica AR, London WT, Chanock RM, Kapikian AZ. Solid-phase microtiter radioimmunoassay for detection of the Norwalk strain of acute nonbacterial, epidemic gastroenteritis virus and its antibodies. *J Med Virol* 1978;2:97–108.

70. Herrmann JE, Nowak NA, Blacklow NR. Detection of Norwalk virus in stools by enzyme immunoassay. *J Med Virol* 1985;17:127–133.

71. Herrmann JE, Kent GP, Nowak NA, Brondum J, Blacklow NR. Antigen detection in the diagnosis of Norwalk virus gastroenteritis [Letter]. *J Infect Dis* 1986;154:547–548.

72. Gary GW Jr, Kaplan JE, Stine SE, Anderson LJ. Detection of Norwalk virus antibodies and antigen with a biotin-avidin immunoassay. *J Clin Microbiol* 1985;22:274–278.

73. Cukor G, Nowak NA, Blacklow NR. Immunoglobulin M responses to the Norwalk virus of gastroenteritis. *Infect Immun* 1982;37:463–468.

74. Erdman DD, Gary GW, Anderson LJ. Development and evaluation of an IgM capture enzyme immunoassay for diagnosis of recent Norwalk virus infection. *J Virol Methods* 1989;24:57–66.

75. Madore HP, Treanor JJ, Pray KA, Dolin R. Enzyme-linked immunosorbent assays for Snow Mountain and Norwalk agents of viral gastroenteritis. *J Clin Microbiol* 1986;24:456–459.

76. Nakata S, Estes MK, Chiba S. Detection of human calicivirus antigen and antibody by enzyme-linked immunosorbent assays. *J Clin Microbiol* 1988;26:2001–2005.

77. Nakata S, Chiba S, Terashima H, Sakuma Y, Kogasaka R, Nakao T. Microtiter solid-phase radioimmunoassay for detection of human calicivirus in stools. *J Clin Microbiol* 1983;17:198–201.

78. Cubitt WD, Blacklow NR, Herrmann JE, Nowak NA, Nakata S, Chiba S. Antigenic relationships between human caliciviruses and Norwalk virus. *J Infect Dis* 1987;156:806–814.

79. Hayashi Y, Ando T, Utagawa E, et al. Western blot (immunoblot) assay of small, round-structured virus associated with an acute gastroenteritis outbreak in Tokyo. *J Clin Microbiol* 1989;27:1728–1733.

80. Atmar RL, Metcalf TG, Neill FH, Estes MK. Detection of enteric viruses in oysters by using the polymerase chain reaction. *Appl Environ Microbiol* 1993;59:631–635.

81. De Leon R, Matsui SM, Baric RS, Herrmann JE, Blacklow NR, Greenberg HB, Sobsey MD. Detection of Norwalk virus in stool specimens by reverse transcriptase–polymerase chain reaction and nonradioactive oligoprobes. *J Clin Microbiol* 1992;30:3151–3157.

82. Wilcocks JJ, Silcock JG, Carter MJ. Detection of Norwalk virus in the UK by the polymerase chain reaction. *FEMS Microbiol Lett* 1993;112:7–12.

82a. Okamoto H, Okada S, Sugiyama Y, et al. Nucleotide sequence of the genomic RNA of hepatitis C virus isolated from a human carrier: comparison with reported isolates for conserved and divergent regions. 1991.

83. Green KY, Lew JF, Jiang X, Kapikian AZ, Estes MK. Comparison of the reactivities of baculovirus-expressed recombinant Norwalk virus capsid antigen with those of the native Norwalk virus antigen in serologic assays and some epidemiologic observations. *J Clin Microbiol* 1993;31:2185–2191.

84. Graham DY, Jiang X, Tanaka T, Opekun AR, Madore HP, Estes MK. Norwalk virus infection of volunteers: new insights based on improved assays. *J Infect Dis* 1994;170:34–43.

85. Treanor JJ, Jiang X, Madore HP, Estes MK. Subclass-specific serum antibody responses to recombinant Norwalk virus capsid antigen (rNV) in adults infected with Norwalk, Snow Mountain, or Hawaii virus. *J Clin Microbiol* 1993;31:1630–1634.

86. Lew JF, Valdesuso J, Vesikari T, Kapikian AZ, Jiang X, Estes MK, Green KY. Detection of Norwalk virus infection in Finnish infants and young children. *J Infect Dis* 1994;169:1364–1367.

87. Gray JJ, Jiang X, Morgan Capner P, Desselberger U, Estes MK. Prevalence of antibodies to Norwalk virus in England: detection by enzyme-linked immunosorbent assay using baculovirus-expressed Norwalk virus capsid antigen. *J Clin Microbiol* 1993;31:1022–1025.

88. Khan AS, Moe CL, Glass RI, et al. Norwalk virus-associated gastroenteritis traced to ice consumption aboard a cruise ship in Hawaii: application of molecular-based assays. *J Clin Microbiol* 1994;32:318–322.

88a. Parker SP, Cubitt WD, Jiang X, Estes MK. The efficacy of a recombinant Norwalk virus protein enzyme immunoassay for the diagnosis of infections with Norwalk virus and other human "candidate" caliciviruses. *J Med Virol* 1993;41:179–184.

89. Blacklow NR, Greenberg HB. Viral gastroenteritis. *N Engl J Med* 1991;325(4):252–264.

90. Kapikian AZ, Estes MK. The Norwalk and related viruses of acute gastroenteritis. In: Webster RG, Granoff A, eds. *Encyclopedia of virology*. New York: Academic Press, 1994.

91. Kapikian AZ, Greenberg HB, Cline WL, et al. Prevalence of antibody to the Norwalk agent by a newly developed immune adherence hemagglutination assay. *J Med Virol* 1978;2:281–294.

92. Blacklow NR, Cukor G, Bedigian MK, Echeverria P, Greenberg HB, Schreiber DS, Trier JS. Immune response and prevalence of antibody to Norwalk enteritis virus as determined by radioimmunoassay. *J Clin Microbiol* 1979;10:903–909.

93. Greenberg HB, Valdesuso J, Kapikian AZ, et al. Prevalence

of antibody to the Norwalk virus in various countries. *Infect Immun* 1979;26:270–273.

93a. Parker SP, Cubitt WD, Jiang X, Estes MK. Seroprevalence studies using a recombinant Norwalk virus protein immunoassay. *J Med Virol* 1994;42:146–150.

94. Numata K, Nakata S, Jiang X, Estes MK, Chiba S. Epidemiological study on Norwalk virus infection in Japan and Southeast Asia using enzyme-linked immunosorbent assays with baculovirus-expressed Norwalk virus capsid protein. *J Clin Microbiol* 1994;32:121–126.

95. Cukor G, Blacklow NR, Echeverria P, Bedigian MK, Puruggan H, Basaca Sevilla V. Comparative study of the acquisition of antibody to Norwalk virus in pediatric populations. *Infect Immun* 1980;29:822–823.

96. Echeverria P, Burke DS, Blacklow NR, Cukor G, Charoenkul C, Yanggratoke S. Age-specific prevalence of antibody to rotavirus, *Escherichia coli* heat-labile enterotoxin, Norwalk virus, and hepatitis A virus in a rural community in Thailand. *J Clin Microbiol* 1983;17:923–925.

97. Black RE, Greenberg HB, Kapikian AZ, Brown KH, Becker S. Acquisition of serum antibody to Norwalk virus and rotavirus and relation to diarrhea in a longitudinal study of young children in rural Bangladesh. *J Infect Dis* 1982;145:483–489.

98. Gabbay YB, Glass RI, Monroe SS, et al. Prevalence of antibodies to Norwalk virus among Amerindians in isolated Amazonian communities. *Am J Epidemiol* 1994;139(7):728–733.

99. Sawyer LA, Murphy JJ, Kaplan JE, et al. 25- to 30-nm virus particle associated with a hospital outbreak of acute gastroenteritis with evidence for airborne transmission. *Am J Epidemiol* 1988;127:1261–1271.

100. Ho MS, Glass RI, Monroe SS, et al. Viral gastroenteritis aboard a cruise ship. *Lancet* 1989;2:961–965.

101. Monroe SS, Stine SE, Jiang X, Estes MK, Glass RI. Detection of antibody to recombinant Norwalk virus antigen (rNV) in specimens from outbreaks of gastroenteritis. *J Clin Microbiol* 1993;31:2866–2872.

102. Spratt HC, Marks MI, Gomersall M, Gill P, Pai CH. Nosocomial infantile gastroenteritis associated with minirotavirus and calicivirus. *J Pediatr* 1978;93:922–926.

103. Middleton PJ, Szymanski MT, Petric M. Viruses associated with acute gastroenteritis in young children. *Am J Dis Child* 1977;131:733–737.

104. Kaplan JE, Gary GW, Baron RC, Singh N, Schonberger LB, Feldman R, Greenberg HB. Epidemiology of Norwalk gastroenteritis and the role of Norwalk virus in outbreaks of acute nonbacterial gastroenteritis. *Ann Intern Med* 1982;96:756–761.

105. PHLS Working Party on Viral Gastroenteritis. Foodborne viral gastroenteritis: an overview (with a brief comment on hepatitis A). *PHLS Microbiol Dig.* 1988;5:69–75.

106. Okada S, Sekine S, Ando T, et al. Antigenic characterization of small, round-structured viruses by immune electron microscopy. *J Clin Microbiol* 1990;28:1244–1248.

107. Murphy AM, Grohmann GS, Christopher PJ, Lopez WA, Davey GR, Millsom RH. An Australia-wide outbreak of gastroenteritis from oysters caused by Norwalk virus. *Med J Aust* 1979;2:329–333.

108. Cubitt WD. Diagnosis, occurrence and clinical significance of the human "candidate" caliciviruses. *Prog Med Virol* 1989;36:103–119.

109. Madeley CR, Cosgrove BP. Caliciviruses in man [Letter]. *Lancet* 1976;1:199–200.

110. Matson DO, Estes MK, Tanaka T, Bartlett AV, Pickering LK. Asymptomatic human calicivirus infection in a day care center. *Pediatr Infect Dis J* 1990;9:190–196.

111. Kaljot KT, Ling JP, Gold JW, et al. Prevalence of acute enteric viral pathogens in acquired immunodeficiency syndrome patients with diarrhea. *Gastroenterology* 1989;97:1031–1032.

112. Cunningham AL, Grohman GS, Harkness J, Law C, Marriott D, Tindall B, Cooper DA. Gastrointestinal viral infections in homosexual men who were symptomatic and seropositive for human immunodeficiency virus. *J Infect Dis* 1988;158:386–391.

113. Studdert MJ. Caliciviruses. Brief review. *Arch Virol* 1978;58:157–191.

114. Dick CP, Johnson RP, Yamashiro S. Sites of persistence of feline calicivirus. *Res Vet Sci* 1989;47:367–373.

115. Kalunda M, Lee KM, Holmes DF, Gillespie JH. Serologic classification of feline caliciviruses by plaque-reduction neutralization and immunodiffusion. *Am J Vet Res* 1975;36:353–356.

116. Barlough JE, Berry ES, Skilling DE, Smith AW. The marine calicivirus story—part I. *Comp Contin Ed Pract Vet* 1986;8(9):F5–F14.

117. Barlough JE, Berry ES, Skilling DE, Smith AW. The marine calicivirus story—part II. *Comp Contin Ed Pract Vet* 1986;8(10):F75–F82.

118. Mohler JR, Snyder R. The 1932 outbreak of foot and mouth disease in South California. *US Dept Agric Misc Publ* 1933;163:1–10.

119. Smith AW, Akers TG. Vesicular exanthema of swine. *J Am Vet Med Assoc* 1976;169:700–703.

120. Smith AW, Akers TG, Madin SH, et al. San Miguel sea lion virus isolation, preliminary characterization and relationship to vesicular exanthema of swine virus. *Nature* 1973;244:108–110.

121. Sawyer JC. Vesicular exanthema of swine and San Miguel sea lion virus. *J Am Vet Med Assoc* 1976;169:707–709.

122. Saif LJ, Bohl EH, Theil KW, Cross RF, House JA. Rotavirus-like, calicivirus-like, and 23-nm virus-like particles associated with diarrhea in young pigs. *J Clin Microbiol* 1980;12:105–111.

123. Parwani AV, Flynn WT, Gadfield KL, Saif LJ. Serial propagation of porcine enteric calicivirus in a continuous cell line. Effect of medium supplementation with intestinal contents or enzymes. *Arch Virol* 1991;120:115–122.

124. Flynn WT, Saif LJ. Serial propagation of porcine enteric calicivirus-like virus in primary porcine kidney cell cultures. *J Clin Microbiol* 1988;26:206–212.

125. Liu SJ, Xue HP, Pu BQ, Qian NH. A new viral disease in rabbits. *Anim Husb Vet Med* 1984;16:253–255.

126. Parra F, Prieto M. Purification and characterization of a calicivirus as the causative agent of a lethal hemorrhagic disease in rabbits. *J Virol* 1990;64:4013–4015.

127. Ohlinger VF, Haas B, Thiel HJ. Rabbit hemorrhagic disease (RHD): characterization of the causative calicivirus. *Vet Res* 1993;24:103–116.

127a. Laurent S, Vautherot J-F, Madelaine M-F, Le Gall G, Rasschaert D. Recombinant rabbit hemorrhagic disease virus capsid protein expressed in baculovirus self-assembles into viruslike particles and induces protection. *J Virol* 1994;68:6794–6798.

128. Cubitt WD, Barrett AD. Propagation and preliminary characterization of a chicken candidate calicivirus. *J Gen Virol* 1985;66:1431–1438.

129. Wyeth JP, Chettle NJ, Labram J. Avian calicivirus [Letter]. *Vet Rec* 1981;109:477.

130. Smith AW, Skilling DE, Ensley PK, Benirschke K, Lester TL. Calicivirus isolation and persistence in a pygmy chimpanzee (*Pan paniscus*). *Science* 1983;221:79–81.

131. Hollinger FB. Non-A, non-B hepatitis viruses. In: Fields BN, Knipe DM, eds. *Virology*, 2nd ed. New York: Raven Press, 1990;2239–2273.

132. Dolin R, Reichman RC, Fauci AS. Lymphocyte populations in acute viral gastroenteritis. *Infect Immun* 1976;14:422–428.

133. Thornhill TS, Kalica AR, Wyatt RG, Kapikian AZ, Chanock RM. Pattern of shedding of the Norwalk particle in stools during experimentally induced gastroenteritis in volunteers as determined by immune electron microscopy. *J Infect Dis* 1975;132:28–34.

134. Hedberg CW, Osterholm MT. Outbreaks of food-borne and waterborne viral gastroenteritis. *Clin Microbiol Rev* 1993;6:199–210.

135. Agus SG, Dolin R, Wyatt RG, Tousimis AJ, Northrup RS. Acute infectious nonbacterial gastroenteritis: intestinal histopathology. Histologic and enzymatic alterations during illness produced by the Norwalk agent in man. *Ann Intern Med* 1973;79:18–25.

136. Schreiber DS, Blacklow NR, Trier JS. The small intestinal lesion induced by Hawaii agent acute infectious nonbacterial gastroenteritis. *J Infect Dis* 1974;129:705–708.

137. Schreiber DS, Blacklow NR, Trier JS. The small intestinal le-

sion induced by Hawaii agent acute infectious nonbacterial gastroenteritis. *J Infect Dis* 1974;129(6):705–708.

138. Widerlite L, Trier JS, Blacklow NR, Schreiber DS. Structure of the gastric mucosa in acute infectious bacterial gastroenteritis. *Gastroenterology* 1975;68:425–430.

139. Levy AG, Widerlite L, Schwartz CJ, et al. Jejunal adenylate cyclase activity in human subjects during viral gastroenteritis. *Gastroenterology* 1976;70:321–325.

140. Meeroff JC, Schreiber DS, Trier JS, Blacklow NR. Abnormal gastric motor function in viral gastroenteritis. *Ann Intern Med* 1980;92:370–373.

141. Dolin R, Baron S. Absence of detectable interferon in jejunal biopsies, jejunal aspirates, and sera in experimentally induced viral gastroenteritis in man. *Proc Soc Exp Biol Med* 1975;150: 337–339.

142. Bridger JC. Detection by electron microscopy of caliciviruses, astroviruses and rotavirus-like particles in the faeces of piglets with diarrhoea. *Vet Rec* 1980;107:532–533.

143. Flynn WT, Saif LJ, Moorhead PD. Pathogenesis of porcine enteric calicivirus-like virus in four-day-old gnotobiotic pigs. *Am J Vet Res* 1988;49:819–825.

144. Woode GN, Bridger JC. Isolation of small viruses resembling astroviruses and caliciviruses from acute enteritis of calves. *J Med Microbiol* 1978;11:441–452.

145. Hall GA, Bridger JC, Brooker BE, Parsons KR, Ormerod E. Lesions of gnotobiotic calves experimentally infected with a calicivirus-like (Newbury) agent. *Vet Pathol* 1984;21:208–215.

146. Blacklow NR, Cukor G. Viral gastroenteritis. *N Engl J Med* 1981;304:397–406.

147. Dolin R, Blacklow NR, DuPont H, et al. Biological properties

148. Parrino TA, Schreiber DS, Trier JS, Kapikian AZ, Blacklow NR. Clinical immunity in acute gastroenteritis caused by Norwalk agent. *N Engl J Med* 1977;297:86–89.

149. Nakata S, Chiba S, Terashima H, Yokoyama T, Nakao T. Humoral immunity in infants with gastroenteritis caused by human calicivirus. *J Infect Dis* 1985;152:274–279.

149a. Cubitt WD, McSwiggan DA. Seroepidemiological survey of the prevalence of antibodies to a strain of human calicivirus. *J Med Virol* 1987;21:361–368.

150. Johnson PC, Mathewson JJ, DuPont HL, Greenberg HB. Multiple-challenge study of host susceptibility to Norwalk gastroenteritis in US adults. *J Infect Dis* 1990;161:18–21.

151. Baron RC, Greenberg HB, Cukor G, Blacklow NR. Serological responses among teenagers after natural exposure to Norwalk virus. *J Infect Dis* 1984;150:531–534.

152. Ryder RW, Singh N, Reeves WC, Kapikian AZ, Greenberg HB, Sack RB. Evidence of immunity induced by naturally acquired rotavirus and Norwalk virus infection on two remote Panamanian islands. *J Infect Dis* 1985;151:99–105.

153. Ball JM, Hardy ME, Barone C, Conner ME, Estes MK. Oral immunization of recombinant Norwalk particles. Abstract: American Society for Virology, 13th Annual Meeting, Madison, WI, July 10–14, 1994.

154. Cubitt WD. Caliciviruses. In: Kapikian AZ, ed. *Viral infections of the gastrointestinal tract,* 2nd ed. New York: Marcel Dekker, 1994;549–568.

155. Treanor JJ, Madore HP, Dolin R. Development of an enzyme immunoassay for the Hawaii agent of viral gastroenteritis. *J Virol Methods* 1988;22:207–214.

of Norwalk agent of acute infectious nonbacterial gastroenteritis. *Proc Soc Exp Biol Med* 1972;140:578–583.

Infections of the Gastrointestinal Tract,
edited by M. J. Blaser, P. D. Smith, J. I. Ravdin,
H. B. Greenberg, and R. L. Guerrant
Published by Raven Press, Ltd., New York, 1995.

CHAPTER 67

Astroviruses

Suzanne M. Matsui

Astrovirus was first described in association with gastroenteritis in 1975 (1,2). Appleton and Higgins (1) examined fecal samples from 14 newborn infants with diarrhea and vomiting and visualized by electron microscopy (EM) 29- to 30-nm diameter viral particles in the specimens from eight babies. These particles differed morphologically from rotavirus and Norwalk virus and were subsequently confirmed to be astrovirus (3). In the same year, Madeley and Cosgrove (2) reported finding a 28-nm diameter, small round structured virus (SRSV) with distinctive surface features in the stools of infants with diarrhea. This virus was named astrovirus for the characteristic five- or six-pointed star configuration that was evident on the surface of approximately 10% of the viral particles examined (4). A major breakthrough in the study of these viruses occurred in 1981 when Lee and Kurtz (5) demonstrated serial passage of astrovirus in cell culture with the use of trypsin. This has enabled more detailed characterization of the virus, in terms of its epidemiology, pathogenesis, and, more recently, its molecular biology. Astrovirus has emerged as a medically important pathogen with notable features (described later) and, as such, has now been assigned its own viral family, the Astroviridae.

In addition to the five serotypes of human astrovirus (6,7), morphologically indistinguishable, but serologically distinct, astroviruses have been found by EM in the feces of cats (8), calves (9), deer (10), dogs (11,12), mice (13), pigs (14,15), lambs (16), turkeys (17,18), and ducks (19). Infection with astroviruses appears to be species specific (20), and, as a consequence, no animal model for human infection currently exists. In general, astrovirus infection results in diarrhea, but a fatal hepatitis has been observed in 3- to 6-week-old ducklings (19).

ASTROVIRUS PHYSICAL FEATURES

In an effort to facilitate classification of small round viruses found in feces, Caul and Appleton (3) proposed a

scheme based on the physical and electron microscopic features of these viruses (Table 1). In this scheme, astroviruses comprise a unique subgroup of SRSVs, separate from other SRSVs such as the classic human caliciviruses and Norwalk virus (Fig. 1). Astroviruses visualized by EM display a smooth circular border, triangular surface hollows, and a characteristic five- or six-pointed surface star with a stain-displacing center that appears white on negatively stained micrographs (4,21). While the stellate surface configuration is its most distinct feature, it is not present on all particles (3,4) and may be obscured by antibody coating of viral aggregates in stool (20,22) or in preparations for immune EM (IEM) (23). "Bridging structures" between astrovirus particles have been observed occasionally and may represent surface extensions of the virus (4,16).

The viral particles are stable at pH 3 and chloroform resistant. Human astrovirus remains active after 5 min at 60°C but is inactivated after 10 min at that temperature (20). Characteristic astrovirus morphology has been shown to be retained in infected fecal specimens that were stored at ultralow temperatures of $-70°C$ to $-85°C$ for 6 to 10 years (24). Repeated freezing and thawing, however, may disrupt astrovirus particles.

The diameter of astrovirus particles may vary depending on the species of origin and method of fixation. Average diameters in the range of 27 to 34 nm have been reported. Madeley (21) systematically measured over 1000 negatively stained (3% potassium phosphotungstate) astroviruses from stool specimens of infected infants and found a mean viral diameter of 28 ± 1.6 nm. At the other end of the spectrum, bovine astrovirus 2, shed by experimentally infected gnotobiotic calves and prepared for EM with glutaraldehyde/1% osmium tetroxide, ranged in diameter from 30 to 37 nm and averaged 34 nm (25).

Human astroviruses have typically been reported to band at a buoyant density of 1.35 to 1.37 g/mL in cesium chloride (CsCl) (3,20,26). In outbreaks of astrovirus gastroenteritis at a school in Japan (27) and a convalescent home in the United States (28), the buoyant density of the astrovirus particles was slightly higher, 1.39 to 1.40 g/mL. In animal infections, buoyant densities of astrovirus

S. M. Matsui: Department of Medicine, Division of Gastroenterology, Stanford University School of Medicine, Stanford, California; and Center for Molecular Biology and Medicine, VA Medical Center, Palo Alto, California 94304.

TABLE 1. *Physical features*

27–34 nm diameter, spherical, nonenveloped particles
Characteristic star-like surface appearance by EM
Particles may be sensitive to CsCl, repeated freezing/thawing
Buoyant density: 1.35–1.38 g/mL (CsCl), 1.32 g/mL (potassium tartrate)
Single-stranded, plus-sense, poly(A)+, 6.8 kb RNA genome
2.4 kb, poly(A)+, subgenomic RNA produced during infection
M_r 87K structural protein produced in infected cells
    Encoded by subgenomic RNA
    Likely a precursor to 3–5 smaller capsid proteins
Seven serotypes by IEM

have ranged from 1.34 g/mL in beagle pups (11) to 1.38 to 1.40 g/mL in lambs (29). It has been observed that astrovirus morphology may be disrupted after viral particles are pelleted from a cesium chloride density gradient (30). Substantially better recovery of intact astrovirus particles has been reported when astrovirus in fecal extracts is separated on a potassium tartrate–glycerol density gradient, then concentrated by pelleting. The buoyant density for human astrovirus in this medium is 1.32 g/mL (30).

In a recent description of human astrovirus adapted to growth in CaCo-2 cells (see later discussion), Willcocks et al. (31) found astrovirus particles at two densities in a CsCl gradient. They speculated that the fraction with density 1.35 g/mL likely represented complete viral particles, while the fraction with density 1.32 g/mL possibly represented empty particles. The particles had identical polypeptide profiles, but no attempt was made to determine the nature of the nucleic acid contained within these particles. A similar observation was made by Matsui et al. (26) for astrovirus serotype 1 grown in LLCMK2 cells. Enzymeimmunoassay (EIA) (32,33) performed on CsCl gradient fractions identified two peaks of astrovirus antigen activity, one at density 1.37 g/mL (major peak) and the other at 1.33 g/mL (minor peak). Ribonucleic acid (RNA) extracted from the major peak fraction hybridized with

probes from two different regions of the viral genome, while that extracted from the minor peak did not hybridize to either probe. This suggests that the lower density particles do not contain viral nucleic acid. From these limited experiments, there does not appear to be a subpopulation of viral particles that contain subgenomic RNA only, as is the case for rabbit hemorrhagic disease virus (RHDV), a calicivirus (34).

MICROBIOLOGY

Growth in Cell Culture

The progress made in adapting human astroviruses to growth in cell culture has paralleled, to a large degree, the strides made in cultivating rotaviruses during the late 1970s (35,36). Both viruses are now cultivatable in continuous lines of monkey kidney epithelial cells, in the presence of trypsin. In rotaviruses, trypsin facilitates viral uncoating by cleaving the outer capsid protein VP4. Although trypsin is definitely required for astrovirus infection to occur in cell culture, the mechanism by which trypsin influences viral infectivity is not known at this time.

Two years after the identification of astroviruses in human fecal specimens, Lee and Kurtz (37) described the detection of astrovirus antigen in primary cells by immunofluorescence. For these studies, primary human embryonic kidney (HEK) cells were incubated for 24 hr with 10% fecal extracts, then washed and fixed. The fixed cells were subsequently incubated with convalescent serum from an astrovirus-infected individual followed by a sheep antihuman immunoglobulin conjugate. Specific fluorescence was detectable with the convalescent serum, but not with acute serum from the same person or convalescent serum that had been adsorbed with astrovirus-containing fecal extracts. Furthermore, convalescent sera from other individuals who had been ill with astrovirus gastroenteritis reacted specifically with infected HEK cells, as demonstrated by IEM and immunofluorescence.

In 1981, these investigators reported the successful serial passage of astrovirus in tissue culture with trypsin in the growth medium (5). Trypsin at a concentration of 10 μg/mL was reported to be the optimal concentration required for productive infection. Increasing the trypsin concentration to 50 μg/mL did not enhance viral growth. Lower trypsin concentrations, such as the 0.5-μg/mL concentration used for rotavirus propagation, were not sufficient for astrovirus. The greatest number of viral particles were detected in the cell-free supernatant of primary HEK cell monolayers after 48 hr of growth in trypsin-containing medium. Viral titers of 10^5 to 10^7/mL were observed. Primary baboon kidney (PBK) cells and a continuous line of LLCMK2 cells were infectable with astrovirus (originally from feces) after six passages in HEK cells, but direct inoculation of either PBK and LLCMK2 cells with fecal extracts was not successful. Viral yield was significantly reduced by diminishing the concentration of trypsin in the medium of LLCMK2 cells in which serial passage had been established. All five serotypes of astrovirus de-

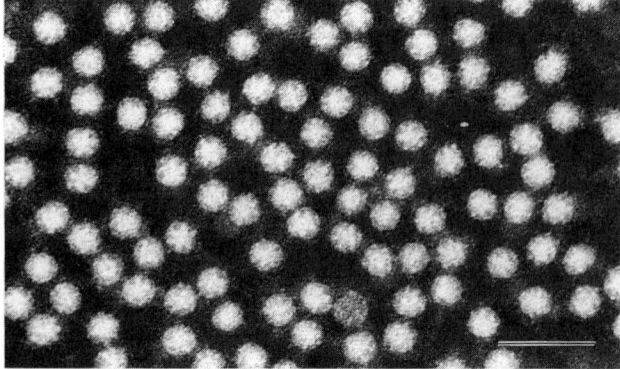

FIG. 1. Astroviruses. Electron micrograph of astrovirus particles in a human fecal specimen. Bar marker represents 100 nm. (Courtesy of Dr. Charles D. Humphrey.)

scribed by Kurtz and Lee (6,7) have been adapted to growth in LLCMK2 cells. Astrovirus serotype 3, however, has been difficult to maintain at high titer in cell culture (J. E. Herrmann, *personal communication*). Although cytopathic effect is not demonstrated easily in LLCMK2 cells, assays to quantify astrovirus infectivity and study viral neutralization have been developed for at least three serotypes (types 1, 2, and 5) (38).

More recently, a continuous line of human colon carcinoma cells, CaCo-2, have been directly infected with an astrovirus-containing fecal extract, isolate A88/2 (Newcastle), from a 1988 outbreak of gastroenteritis in the United Kingdom (31). Trypsin, at a concentration of 5 μg/mL, was required for growth of the virus. Cytopathic effect was apparent at 2 days postinfection and progressed substantially over the next 2 days. After five passages in CaCo-2 cells, astrovirus particles were indistinguishable from astroviruses derived from feces. This may prove to be an expedient way to adapt wild-type astroviruses to cell culture without first having to pass the virus in primary HEK cells.

Astrovirus Serotypes

To date, seven serotypes of human astrovirus have been identified by immunofluorescence and IEM (6,7,39,39a). Each of the prototype (Oxford) strains was isolated from natural infections and adapted to growth in cell culture by Kurtz and Lee (5). In the Oxford region of the United Kingdom, where community-acquired strains of astrovirus were monitored between 1975 and 1987, serotype 1 emerged as the most common serotype found and accounted for 72%. Each of the other serotypes were responsible for 6% to 8% of the community-acquired astrovirus strains in this region. Similar results were obtained by other investigators in the United Kingdom who found that 55% of the 40 astrovirus-positive stools tested in their population were serotype 1 by IEM (20,40).

Hyperimmune sera to each of the reference strains of human astrovirus have been produced and appear to be largely serotype specific when used in immunofluorescence tests and IEM (20,32). Herrmann et al. have produced a monoclonal antibody that recognizes all seven serotypes of human astrovirus (33,39). This monoclonal antibody has proved useful in developing an EIA to detect astrovirus antigen (see later discussion and ref. 33). While this monoclonal antibody appears to be directed to a viral structural protein (41), the specific epitope that is recognized by this antibody has not been elucidated.

Molecular Biology and Genome Organization

The astrovirus genome consists of single-stranded, positive-sense RNA that is approximately 6800 nucleotides long, excluding the poly(A) tail at the 3′ end. Of the seven astrovirus serotypes described to date (6,7,39a), the complete nucleotide sequences of two serotypes are now available. Two serotype 1 strains, the prototype Oxford strain adapted to growth in LLCMK2 cells and the Newcastle strain recently isolated and adapted to growth in CaCo-2 cells, have been cloned and sequenced (41–43). Limited 3′-end sequence (118 nt) from another serotype 1 strain is also available (44) and corroborates serotype 1 sequence determined earlier (45). In addition, the complete sequence of the reference Oxford serotype 2 astrovirus has been reported recently (46). Astrovirus serotype 3 has been difficult to maintain in cell culture, and, as a consequence, virtually no molecular information is available about this astrovirus serotype. Partial sequences of serotypes 4 and 5 (described later) are available at present (41).

During infection of susceptible cells, two populations of positive-sense astrovirus RNA that are coterminal at the 3′ end are produced: (a) full-length, 6.8-kb genomic RNA and (b) a 2.4-kb subgenomic RNA (Fig. 2) (26,47). The astrovirus genome consists of three long open reading frames (ORFs). The 5′-most ORF, designated ORF1a by the International Committee on the Taxonomy of Viruses (ICTV) (48) [also called *orf-1* (41)], is preceded by a 5′-untranslated region of 82 (serotype 2) to 85 (serotype 1)

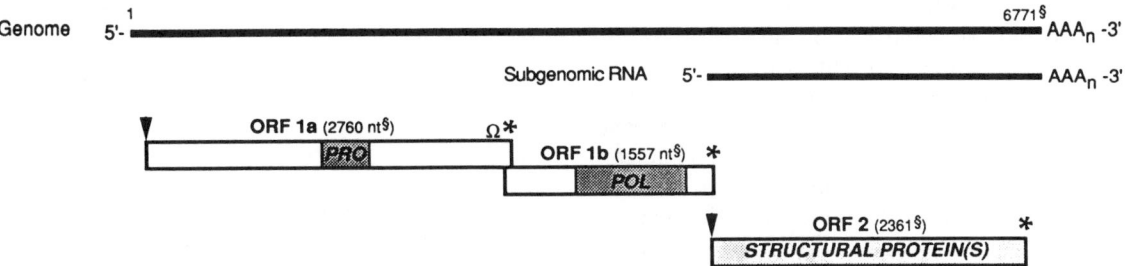

FIG. 2. Genome organization for astrovirus serotype 1 (Oxford reference strain) is shown. Genome and ORF lengths vary slightly, depending on the strain of astrovirus examined (§). For example, in another strain of serotype 1 astrovirus (CaCo-2-adapted) (31), the genome is 6813 nt, ORF1a is 2805 nt, ORF1b is the same as shown and ORF2 is 2358 nt. For serotype 2 (Oxford reference strain), the genome is 6797 nt, ORF1a and ORF1b are the same as shown and ORF2 is 2388 nt (42). The *arrowhead* indicates an initiation codon and the *asterisk* a termination codon. The ribosomal frameshift region is found toward the 3′ end of ORF1a (Ω). The locations of the protease (*PRO*) and RNA-dependent RNA polymerase (*POL*) motifs are *shaded* (▨).

nucleotides (nt). ORF1a ranges in length from 2760 to 2805 nt and overlaps the second ORF, designated ORF1b [also called *orf-2* (41)] by 70 nt. ORF1b is 1557 nt in length for all three astrovirus strains studied thus far (41,43,46). ORF1b overlaps the third, 3'-most ORF, designated ORF2 [also called *orf-3* (41)] by 5 nt. ORF2 is encoded in both genomic and subgenomic RNAs. Its length differs for each of the three strains sequenced thus far, ranging from 2358 (43) to 2388 (46) nt in length. The 3'-untranslated region consists of 83 nt that precede the poly (A) tail.

Nucleotide sequence analysis indicates that all regions of the genome are 95% to 100% conserved between the two serotype 1 strains sequenced to date. ORF1a, ORF1b, and the 3'-untranslated region are also highly conserved (92% to 95%) among the two serotype 1 and one serotype 2 strains examined. General features of the 3'-untranslated region, such as distance to the poly (A) tail and predicted secondary structure, suggest similarities between astrovirus and picornaviruses (45). However, sequence identity in this region is minimal. The 5'-untranslated region is 95% conserved between the two serotype 1 strains, but only 78% to 80% conserved between the serotype 1 and serotype 2 strains.

The greatest variation in sequence between serotype 1 and serotype 2 strains is observed in ORF2. Comparison of nucleotide sequence of the serotype 1 and serotype 2 strains shows that there is 97% identity between the two serotype 1 strains, but only 68% identity between the serotype 1 and serotype 2 strains. At the amino acid (aa) level, there is 80% similarity and 69% to 70% identity between the serotype 1 strains and serotype 2. The slight differences found between the two serotype 1 strains may be influenced by passage number and viral adaptation to different host cells.

Sequence analysis of the polypeptides encoded by the ORFs indicates that viral nonstructural proteins are encoded by the 5'-end ORFs 1a and 1b. ORF1a encodes a polypeptide of 920 (41,46) to 935 (43) aa that contains a viral serine protease motif, while ORF1b encodes a polypeptide of 786 (43) to 796 (46) aa that contains an RNA-dependent RNA polymerase motif. The polymerase motif is highly conserved (85% to 94% nt and 91% to 97% aa) among four of five astrovirus serotypes (Oxford reference serotypes 1, 2, 4, and 5) examined. Comparisons of a 600-nt fragment containing the pertinent sequences of the motif indicate that astrovirus serotypes 1 and 2 are the most closely related, while serotypes 4 and 5 are the least related in this region (41). Sequences suggesting a nuclear localization signal and potential transmembrane helices have been found in ORF1a (46,49–51), but the significance of these observations remains speculative at present. A clear VPg domain has not been identified. The region between the putative transmembrane domain and the protease motif contains one serine at position 420 that may link the hypothetical astrovirus VPg to its genomic RNA (46).

The mechanism by which ORF1b is translated is not immediately evident from routine sequence analysis, since the first AUG codon occurs at nt 454 to 456 of ORF1b and is in a suboptimal context for initiation according to Kozak's rules (52). With more detailed analysis, however, it has been possible to identify highly conserved sequences (in three available astrovirus serotypes that were examined) that strongly suggest a (−1) ribosomal frameshifting mechanism for translation of ORF1b (41,43,46). These sequences include a heptameric shift sequence (A AAA AAC) and downstream stem–loop structure that resemble the required elements for the translation of retrovirus protease and polymerase (53–56) and coronavirus polymerase (57). Recent data indicate that this translational mechanism is operative in astrovirus (57a,57b). The subsequent processing and cleavage of the ORF1a–ORF1b polyprotein product has not been investigated to date.

Since ORF2 is encoded by both the genomic and subgenomic RNA, it was hypothesized that ORF2 encodes a structural protein (58). Other viruses, such as the enveloped alphaviruses, use their subgenomic RNA to produce large quantities of the structural proteins that are required for assembly of intact progeny viruses (59). Recently, the role of the astrovirus subgenomic RNA was proved by immunoprecipitation of the M_r 87K ORF2 product (Oxford serotype 1) with antibodies produced to purified astrovirus particles (41). This protein is likely the precursor of the three to five, M_r 20K to 40K structural proteins that were identified in earlier analyses of human and animal astroviruses (see later discussion and refs. 41 and 47). The subgenomic RNA of astrovirus serotype 1 (Newcastle) (42) has a 5' noncoding region that is 3 to 19 nt longer than that described for astrovirus serotype 2 (Oxford) (58).

The astrovirus genome is thus organized with nonstructural proteins encoded by the 5'-end ORFs 1a and 1b and a structural protein by ORF2 at the 3' end. While this general genome organization is similar to that found in caliciviruses (60), some of the key features that distinguish astroviruses from caliciviruses include the size and number of structural proteins and the strategies used to translate the viral RNA-dependent RNA polymerase as well as the M_r 87K structural protein. Based on these distinctive characteristics, the ICTV recently recommended the classification of astroviruses in a new, separate viral family, the Astroviridae (48,58).

Structural Proteins

The size and number of astrovirus structural proteins described have varied from study to study. To date, the polypeptide profiles of ovine, porcine, and several serotypes of human astrovirus have been examined. Ovine astrovirus was studied first. Herring et al. (29) purified astrovirus particles shed by experimentally infected lambs and found two polypeptides that migrated at M_r ~33K. Five proteins have been described for porcine astrovirus. They range in mass from 13K to 39K (15). The studies of human astrovirus have been done on tissue culture-adapted strains of the virus. Kurtz and Lee (20) described four proteins with M_r 36.5K, 34K, 33K, and 32K for astrovirus serotype 4 that was grown in cell culture in the presence of trypsin. They postulated that the faint M_r 36.5K band might be a precursor protein that is processed to one of the smaller proteins, in a manner analogous to the enterovirus VP0 protein (61). In a more recent report, Kurtz (62) identified two additional proteins (M_r 24K and 5.2K) in astrovirus serotype 1-infected cells. Willcocks et al. (31) studied the astrovirus-specific polypeptides in purified astrovirus serotype 1-infected CaCo-2 cells. Three proteins with M_r 33.5K, 31.5K, and 24K were consistently detected in purified astrovirus particles by astrovirus serotype 1-specific antiserum. The M_r 24K polypeptide was sensitive to treatment with sodium dodecyl sulfate (SDS) and was hypothesized to be a protein that is not securely attached to the viral particle. An additional M_r 27K polypeptide was seen in some preparations, and it was suggested that this may be a proteolytic digestion product of one of the larger proteins. In studies of astrovirus serotype 5 [Marin County strain (28)] proteins, a single structural protein with M_r 30K was immunoprecipitated.

Monroe et al. (47) used a different approach to examine the protein composition of astrovirus particles. Protein synthesis in astrovirus-infected LLCMK2 cells was examined in the absence of trypsin. With this strategy, a single, M_r ~90K protein was immunoprecipitated from infected cell lysates. If the infected cell lysates were pretreated with trypsin, a predominant M_r 29K protein and two other proteins (M_r 31K and 20K) were immunoprecipitated. This suggested that the M_r ~90K protein might be a precursor protein that is proteolytically cleaved to yield the smaller proteins described in previous studies. This hypothesis has not been rigorously proved, nor has it been determined whether astrovirus particles are initially assembled with a single, large structural protein and modified upon release.

EPIDEMIOLOGY

Role in Disease

Astrovirus infections occur worldwide, as evidenced by reports from far-reaching parts of the globe (1,2,27,30,31,63–97). These infections may be community-acquired (73,74,82,87,98) or nosocomial (1,2,30,68,69,74,75,83,87,99) (Table 2). While astrovirus, like rotavirus, primarily causes disease in young children, it is also a cause of outbreaks of gastroenteritis among elderly patients (70,79,90; S. M. Matsui, *unpublished data*) and immunocompromised adults (65,72). Peak incidence is in the winter months in temperate regions (64,71,77,86,87,100) and in the rainy season in tropical areas (66), similar to human rotavirus infections. Viral transmission occurs through the fecal–oral route with spread via person-to-person contacts, contaminated food or water, and possibly fomites (22,101).

The true incidence of astrovirus gastroenteritis and its role in disease have been difficult to assess for a variety

TABLE 2. *Epidemiologic features*

Worldwide distribution
Primarily a pediatric pathogen
    Outbreaks in elderly and immunocompromised patients also
Antibody acquisition in childhood
Antibody prevalence 75% by age 10
    Antibody to serotypes 1–5 in U.S. gamma globulin pools
    Serotype 1 predominance in Oxford region of United Kingdom
Fecal–oral transmission (person-to-person, contaminated food/water, ?fomites)
Peak incidence in winter in Northern temperate regions

of reasons. Astrovirus gastroenteritis is generally a mild, self-limiting illness that does not routinely lead to hospitalization, extensive outpatient evaluation, or clinic visits. The virus may be difficult to detect by EM since only about 10% of the viral particles exhibit the characteristic star-like ultrastructure. Newer detection methods have been devised (32,33,85,102), but not implemented, until recently.

Herrmann et al. (32,33) developed an EIA for detecting astrovirus antigen in fecal specimens. The EIA uses a monoclonal antibody that recognizes all seven serotypes of astrovirus as a capture antibody and rabbit polyclonal antiserum as the detector antibody (33). With this EIA, they performed controlled studies in Thailand (73) to determine the incidence of astrovirus gastroenteritis in the pediatric outpatient setting and its importance as a pathogen, relative to rotavirus and enteric adenovirus. Rotavirus, as expected, was the most frequently detected viral pathogen and was found in 19% of patients with gastroenteritis. Of particular note, astrovirus was the second most frequently detected virus, found in 8.6% of patients with diarrhea. Enteric adenovirus was found in only 2.6% of these patients with diarrhea. In a similar study of rural Guatemalan children, astrovirus was found in 7.3% of those with diarrhea (66). These findings are in contrast to hospital-based EM studies that indicate enteric adenovirus is the second most common cause of viral diarrhea in young children (64,77,82,103) and typically quote the incidence of astrovirus diarrhea to be in the 1% to 4% range (64,67,77,82,94,103).

Adult volunteer studies have helped to evaluate astrovirus pathogenicity. The first study (104), conducted in the United Kingdom, administered fecal extracts containing astrovirus from a child to eight adults who had little or no astrovirus-specific antibody at entry. Only one volunteer developed overt illness. Fecal filtrates containing large numbers of astrovirus from this individual were administered to nine other volunteers. Five of the nine developed mild symptoms, but no vomiting or diarrhea. Of the 17 volunteers in the two phases of the study, viral shedding was documented in four, with the largest number of viral particles shed by the most symptomatic volunteer. In 16 of the volunteers, seroconversion was demonstrated in 13 (by immunofluorescence) and 10 (by IEM).

A second study (28) by investigators in the United

States administered serotype 5 astrovirus (from an outbreak at a northern California elderly care facility) to 19 adult volunteers. One of the volunteers became ill on day 5–6 and had a serologic response, while seven others were asymptomatic but developed a serologic response. These studies demonstrate that astrovirus, unlike Norwalk virus, is of relatively low pathogenicity in adults.

Antibody Prevalence

Antibody to human astrovirus has been found in U.S. (100) and Japanese (27) gamma globulin pools, indicating that astrovirus infection is common. Detecting these astrovirus infections, however, is a more difficult task (see earlier discussion). Antibodies to astrovirus serotypes 1 to 5 are detectable in U.S. gamma globulin preparations (100).

Antibody acquisition occurs in early childhood in the majority of cases. In a survey of 87 children less than 10 years old in Oxford, United Kingdom, Kurtz and Lee (105) found that antibody prevalence rises from 7% in 6- to 12-month-old infants to 70% by the time children enter school. Seventy-five percent of children 10 years of age had such antibodies, a level comparable to that found in nursing students (77%) who were concurrently tested.

The characteristics of immunity to astrovirus are not well understood at present. Symptomatic astrovirus infection involves primarily two age groups, young children and elderly patients, suggesting that antibody acquired in childhood may afford protection from illness during early adulthood. In one volunteer study (104), those with detectable anti-astrovirus antibody in serum did not develop diarrhea after ingesting the inoculum. Studies by Wilson and Cubitt (40) demonstrated both immunoglobulin M (IgM) and immunoglobulin G (IgG) responses to serotype 1 astrovirus in a volunteer infected with the Marin County agent, a serotype 5 astrovirus. They speculated that the anamnestic response observed in this individual was due to prior infection with astrovirus serotype 1 and the antigenic relatedness of these two serotypes. The specifics of immunity to astrovirus infection and the determinants of astrovirus infectivity require further investigation.

VIRAL PATHOGENESIS

Astrovirus pathogenesis in humans is not well studied. In the only study reported to date, astrovirus shedding in diarrheal feces was correlated with the visualization of astrovirus particles in intestinal epithelial cells by EM (93). This suggests that the intestine is the site of viral replication in humans. Small intestinal biopsy from one of the patients demonstrated astrovirus in epithelial cells located in the lower part of the villus. In the other patient, astrovirus was found in "exposed" surface epithelial cells. Both children described in this report had a history of gastrointestinal problems including chronic diarrhea, sucrase-isomaltase deficiency or cow's milk sensitive enteropathy, and prior shedding of *Escherichia coli* 086 or rotavirus in the stool. Neither of the human volunteer

studies (described earlier) (28,104) were designed to examine histologic effects of the infection.

Viral pathogenesis has been studied more extensively in lambs and calves. Gnotobiotic lambs infected with an outbreak strain of ovine astrovirus developed illness on day 4 and shed astrovirus in feces from day 3 to day 9 postinoculation (16,106,107). Histologic examination of the intestines indicated that only mature enterocytes and subepithelial macrophages in the small intestine were infected and resulted in transient villus atrophy and crypt hypertrophy. Some enterocytes contained aggregates of virus particles along the microvilli and in lysosomes and autophagic vacuoles. Other enterocytes demonstrated only indirect evidence of infection such as intracytoplasmic inclusions and vacuoles and degenerate nuclei.

Bovine astroviruses are antigenically distinct from ovine astroviruses (108). Although bovine astroviruses are among several small round viruses isolated from feces of calves with diarrhea, they are generally considered nonpathogenic since inoculation with bovine astrovirus alone does not result in diarrhea in gnotobiotic calves (9,109). Bovine astroviruses, in contrast to ovine astroviruses, preferentially infect M cells and absorptive enterocytes overlying the dome villi of small intestinal Peyer's patches (9,110). When bovine astrovirus infection accompanies infection with bovine rotavirus or Breda virus 2, more severe diarrhea (than with either virus alone), more extensive infection of the dome epithelial cells, and an active inflammatory reaction are noted (9).

Viral Infection *in Vitro*

Given the above observations, it seems reasonable to expect that astroviruses enter cells through the apical surface. However, in polarized CaCo-2 cells, wild-type human astroviruses appear to enter through the basolateral surface (31). Willcocks et al. (51) have suggested that this may be an artifact of the *in vitro* cell culture system and that differentiated intestinal epithelial cells may well have receptors for astrovirus infection on the apical surface.

Entry of astrovirus has also been studied in Graham 293 cells, a transformed line of primary human embryonal kidney cells (111). Graham 293 cell monolayers were infected with astrovirus serotype 1 and treated with lysosomotropic agents (ammonium chloride, methylamine, dansylcadaverine) or the ionophore monensin. These agents inhibited the early stages of infection, distal to viral attachment to the cell membrane, and did not appear to have a direct virucidal effect. In these experiments, all the chemicals at nontoxic levels inhibited viral infection, suggesting that the endocytic pathway may be critical to delivery of the astrovirus genome into the cytoplasm. Ultrastructural analysis corroborated these biochemical results. Viral particles attached at various sites on the cell membrane, and after about 10 min, they were internalized by membrane invagination at coated pits. After about 30 min, larger smooth vacuoles containing multiple viral particles were observed. In other studies, flavanoids that inhibit early steps in picornavirus replication have been shown to inhibit astrovirus antigen synthesis in LLCMK2 cells in a dose-dependent fashion (112). The precise mechanism by which these chemicals act is not known.

A cell culture model of bovine astrovirus infection has been achieved also. In this system, bovine astrovirus serotype 2 (US2) was adapted to growth in primary neonatal bovine kidney (NBK) cells in the presence of 50 μg/mL of trypsin (25). By using immunofluorescent probes to track the expression of viral antigens, the following was observed. The first indication of viral infection and production of viral antigens was at 7 hr postinfection when viral antigen was first observed in the cytoplasm. Soon thereafter, two or three brilliant immunofluorescent granules were seen in the nucleus, in a pattern that suggested nucleolar involvement. Subsequently, dense immunofluorescent granules were seen in the perinuclear region of the cytoplasm, followed by diffuse cytoplasmic staining. Typically ≤2%, and occasionally 10% to 20%, of the cells were infected when administered an inoculum with a multiplicity of infection (MOI) level of more than 1. The role of the nucleus and nucleoli in astrovirus replication is not known. Since astrovirus infection was not inhibited by the addition of the deoxyribonucleic acid (DNA) transcription inhibitor, these investigators concluded that either the nucleoli are not affected by actinomycin D or that they are not essential for viral replication.

CLINICAL ILLNESS

Astrovirus gastroenteritis is primarily a disease that affects pediatric populations throughout the world (Table 3). Its medical importance was established recently when it was shown to be the second most common viral agent in young children with diarrhea who were evaluated in an outpatient setting (73). While serotype 1 appears to be the most common human astrovirus (20,40), severe infections with astrovirus serotype 4 have been noted in young adults (39).

The incubation period determined by adult human volunteer studies is 3 to 4 days (28,104). A shorter incubation period of 24 to 36 hr was extrapolated from the secondary spread characteristics during an outbreak of gastroenteritis in a kindergarten (27). In general, the illness caused by human astrovirus consists of a mild, watery diarrhea, 2 to 3 days in duration, with vomiting, fever, anorexia, abdominal pain, and various constitutional symptoms that last ≤4 days (20,22,100,113,114). Diarrhea lasting 7 to 14 days and prolonged viral shedding occur in some individu-

TABLE 3. Clinical features

Incubation period: 3–4 days
Duration of illness: 1–4 days
Self-limiting disease in otherwise normal individuals
    May be prolonged in immunocompromised patients
Signs and symptoms: watery diarrhea, anorexia, fever, vomiting
Symptomatic infection in young children, elderly patients, and immunocompromised individuals

als (20). In children, the diarrhea due to astrovirus may be indistinguishable from that due to rotavirus (20,66), but it is frequently milder (75,87). Astrovirus diarrhea, however, does not cause significant dehydration typically and may contribute to fewer hospitalizations (73). Certain patients may develop prolonged lactose intolerance (68,75,87). Deaths associated with astrovirus infection are rare but have been reported (94).

Astrovirus appears to be an important cause of diarrhea in immunocompromised patients. In a recent case–control study of human immunodeficiency virus (HIV)-infected individuals with diarrhea (72), astrovirus was found in 13 of 109 (12%) fecal specimens from 65 patients with diarrhea and 2 of 113 (2%) fecal specimens from 65 controls without diarrhea. To place these figures in perspective, it should be noted that seven different types of viruses were identified in 35% of patients with diarrhea, single agents were detected in most cases, and bacteria and parasite detections were far less common. In a similar study of bone marrow transplant recipients with diarrhea (65), an enteric pathogen was found in 13% of cases. Among the enteric pathogens, astrovirus was most frequently identified and accounted for 7 of 150 (4.7%) episodes of diarrhea. In these patients, diarrhea developed in the hospital between days 21 and 65 and lasted 2 to 31 days. In a separate case (20), a child with combined immunodeficiency developed chronic astrovirus diarrhea with viral shedding for more than 4 months following bone marrow transplantation. This illness persisted until the child's death.

DIAGNOSIS

Traditionally, direct EM has been the cornerstone of astrovirus detection in fecal specimens. Patients with acute astrovirus diarrhea have been noted to shed as many as 10^{10} virus particles/mL (or 10^8 viable particles) (20). IEM has also been described for the detection of astrovirus and evaluation of immune responses (27,115,116). This technique may be useful in evaluating specimens that contain fewer viral particles or may help to establish etiology if paired acute and convalescent sera are available.

Although the virus has distinctive surface features (described earlier), only about 10% of the particles display these features and identification may require an experienced microscopist (117). A retrospective study of fecal viruses, previously identified as small round featureless viruses (SRVs) by EM alone, revealed that many of the viruses had been misclassified (89). By using complementary techniques, these investigators found that astroviruses, in particular, were prone to misclassification. Fourteen of 53 (26%) "SRV" samples were shown to be astrovirus by careful reexamination of the morphological features and IEM with convalescent human serum as well as astrovirus serotype 1-specific rabbit antiserum. Two caliciviruses and one Norwalk-like virus were also found to be misclassified. Another example of misclassification is the Marin County virus, which was isolated from a nursing home outbreak in 1981 and initially identified as a "Norwalk-like" virus (90). It was later proved to be an astrovirus (118,119) and is now considered to be the astrovirus serotype 5 prototype strain.

An EIA that uses a group reactive monoclonal antibody to capture viral antigen and polyclonal antiserum as the detector antibody has been developed by Herrmann et al. (32,33). A biotinylated detector antibody has been incorporated into the modified EIA described by Moe et al. (85). Both EIAs have comparable sensitivity (91%) and specificity (98%) when compared to IEM. Neither is available commercially, but several recent studies have relied on these tests for rapid identification of astrovirus infection (66,73,78,85).

Detection strategies using molecular probes and reverse transcriptase–polymerase chain reaction (RT-PCR) have also been described (85,102,120,121). Complete sequence information of three astrovirus strains, representing two serotypes, is available at present (see earlier discussion). Primers derived from the 3' end of the genome reportedly have been successful in amplifying astrovirus-specific products from all five reference serotypes (58). Other primers derived from the RNA-dependent RNA polymerase motif are also suitable candidates for RT-PCR amplification of different human astrovirus serotypes (41). In recent studies, good correlation has been observed when RT-PCR was used to confirm EIA diagnosis of astrovirus (65,72,84).

Regions encoding immunoreactive viral epitopes may be important in the future development of recombinant antigens and more specifically targeted antibodies that can be produced in large quantities. While tests to detect astrovirus antibody may be useful in epidemiologic investigations, tests that rapidly and accurately identify astrovirus antigen are likely to be preferable in the clinical setting.

TREATMENT AND PREVENTION

Astrovirus gastroenteritis is generally a mild, self-limiting illness that may disrupt one's normal activities for a few days but does not require specific therapy. Dehydration, requiring fluid resuscitation, may develop in those patients with underlying gastrointestinal disease, poor nutritional status, severe mixed infection, or prolonged illness (20,66).

In order to prevent astrovirus infection, its transmission must be interrupted. This is particularly important in hospitals and other institutions, day care centers, as well as families, where person-to-person transmission is likely to occur. Strict implementation of universal hygienic procedures is essential. The virus is relatively resistant to alcohols, including isopropanol, ethanol, and methanol (122). Of these alcohols, methanol was shown to be the most effective in reducing astrovirus infectivity. Seventy percent methanol reduced astrovirus infectivity by 3 $\log_{10}$, while 90% methanol reduced viral titers to less than 10 infective units/mL.

For foodhandlers, it is important to keep in mind that viral shedding in feces may begin a day before symptoms and continue for several days after diarrhea resolves. A rapid diagnostic test that detects astrovirus in stool may be useful in this setting. Careful selection and preparation of foods, such as shellfish, that have been implicated in outbreaks of astrovirus gastroenteritis are advisable.

The feasibility of developing a vaccine to prevent astrovirus illness has not been fully evaluated. Recent epidemiologic studies have demonstrated the medical importance of astrovirus. More work is required to understand the fundamentals of immunity to astrovirus.

SUMMARY

Astrovirus gastroenteritis is largely a disease of childhood but is also found among immunocompromised individuals and elderly institutionalized patients. Human astrovirus, a member of the new viral family Astroviridae, has many unique characteristics that range from its ultrastructural appearance to its strategies for viral protein expression. As our ability to detect this virus has improved, it has been possible to establish its medical importance, identify outbreaks due to this agent, and study its cell localization. Important information regarding viral replication and morphogenesis, as well as mechanisms of immunity, remain to be elucidated.

REFERENCES

1. Appleton H, Higgins PG. Viruses and gastroenteritis in infants. *Lancet* 1975;1:1297.
2. Madeley CR, Cosgrove BP. Viruses in infantile gastroenteritis. *Lancet* 1975;2:124.
3. Caul EO, Appleton H. The electron microscopical and physical characteristics of small round human fecal viruses: an interim scheme for classification. *J Med Virol* 1982;9:257–265.
4. Madeley CR, Cosgrove BP. 28 nm particles in faeces in infantile gastroenteritis. *Lancet* 1975;2:451–452.
5. Lee TW, Kurtz JB. Serial propagation of astrovirus in tissue culture with the aid of trypsin. *J Gen Virol* 1981;57:421–424.
6. Kurtz JB, Lee TW. Human astrovirus serotypes. *Lancet* 1984; 2:1405.
7. Lee TW, Kurtz JB. Human astrovirus serotypes. *J Hyg (Camb)* 1982;89:539–540.
8. Hoshino Y, Zimmer JF, Moise NS, Scott FW. Detection of astroviruses in faeces of a cat with diarrhoea. *Arch Virol* 1981; 70:373–376.
9. Woode GN, Bridger JC. Isolation of small viruses resembling astroviruses and caliciviruses from acute enteritis of calves. *J Med Microbiol* 1978;11:441–452.
10. Tzipori S, Menzies JD, Gray EW. Detection of astroviruses in the faeces of red deer. *Vet Rec* 1981;108:286.
11. Williams FP Jr. Astrovirus-like, coronavirus-like, and parvovirus-like particles detected in the diarrheal stools of beagle pups. *Arch Virol* 1980;66:216–226.
12. Marshall JA, Healey DS, Studder MJ, et al. Viruses and virus-like particles in the faeces of dogs with and without diarrhoea. *Aust Vet J* 1984;61:33–38.
13. Kjeldsberg E, Hem A. Detection of astroviruses in gut contents of nude and normal mice. *Arch Virol* 1985;84:135–140.
14. Bridger JC. Detection by electron microscope of caliciviruses, astroviruses and rotavirus-like particles in the faeces of piglets with diarrhoea. *Vet Rec* 1980;107:532–533.
15. Shimizu M, Shirai J, Narita M, Yamane T. Cytopathic astrovirus isolated from porcine acute gastroenteritis in an established cell line derived from porcine embryonic kidney. *J Clin Microbiol* 1990;28:201–206.
16. Snodgrass DR, Gray EW. Detection and transmission of 30 nm

virus particles (astroviruses) in faeces of lambs with diarrhoea. *Arch Virol* 1977;55:287–291.

17. McNulty MS, Curran WL, McFerran JB. Detection of astroviruses in turkey faeces by direct electron microscopy. *Vet Rec* 1980;106:561.

18. Reynolds DL, Saif YM. Astrovirus: a cause of an enteric disease in turkey poults. *Avian Dis* 1986;30:728–735.

19. Gough RE, Collins MS, Borland E, Keymer IF. Astrovirus-like particles associated with hepatitis in ducklings. *Vet Rec* 1984;114:279.

20. Kurtz JB, Lee TW. Astroviruses: human and animal. In: Bock G, Whelan J, eds. *Novel diarrhoea viruses*. Ciba Foundation Symposium 128. Chichester: Wiley, 1987;92–107.

21. Madeley CR. Comparison of the features of astroviruses and caliciviruses seen in samples of feces by electron microscopy. *J Infect Dis* 1979;139:519–523.

22. Kurtz J, Cubitt WD. Astroviruses and caliciviruses. In: Farthing MJG, Keusch GT, eds. *Enteric infection: mechanisms, manifestations, and management*. New York: Raven Press, 1989;205–215.

23. Ashley CR, Caul EO, Paver WK. Astrovirus-associated gastroenteritis in children. *J Clin Pathol* 1978;31:939–943.

24. Williams FP Jr. Electron microscopy of stool-shed viruses: retention of characteristic morphologies after long-term storage at ultralow temperatures. *J Med Virol* 1989;29:192–195.

25. Aroonprasert D, Fagerland JA, Kelso NE, Zheng S, Woode GN. Cultivation and partial characterization of bovine astrovirus. *Vet Microbiol* 1989;19:113–125.

26. Matsui SM, Kim JP, Greenberg HB, et al. Cloning and characterization of human astrovirus immunoreactive epitopes. *J Virol* 1993;67:1712–1715.

27. Konno T, Suzuki H, Ishida N, Chiba R, Mochizuki K, Tsunoda A. Astrovirus-associated epidemic gastroenteritis in Japan. *J Med Virol* 1982;9:11–17.

28. Midthun K, Greenberg HB, Kurtz JB, Gary GW, Lin FC, Kapikian AZ. Characterization and seroepidemiology of a type 5 astrovirus associated with an outbreak of gastroenteritis in Marin County, California. *J Clin Microbiol* 1993;31:955–962.

29. Herring AJ, Gray EW, Snodgrass DR. Purification and characterization of ovine astrovirus. *J Gen Virol* 1981;53:47–55.

30. Ashley CR, Caul EO. Potassium tartrate–glycerol as a density gradient substrate for separation of small, round viruses from human feces. *J Clin Microbiol* 1982;16:377–381.

31. Willcocks MM, Carter MJ, Laidler FR, Madeley CR. Growth and characterisation of human faecal astrovirus in a continuous cell line. *Arch Virol* 1990;113:73–81.

32. Herrmann JE, Hudson RW, Perron-Henry DM, Kurtz JB, Blacklow NR. Antigenic characterization of cell-cultivated astrovirus serotypes and development of astrovirus-specific monoclonal antibodies. *J Infect Dis* 1988;158:182–185.

33. Herrmann JE, Nowak NA, Perron-Henry DM, Hudson RW, Cubitt WD, Blacklow NR. Diagnosis of astrovirus gastroenteritis by antigen detection with monoclonal antibodies. *J Infect Dis* 1990;161:226–229.

34. Meyers G, Wirblich C, Thiel H-J. Genomic and subgenomic RNAs of rabbit hemorrhagic disease virus are both protein-linked and packaged into particles. *Virology* 1991;184:677–686.

35. Banatvala JE, Totterdell BM, Chrystie IL, Woode GN. In vitro detection of human rotaviruses. *Lancet* 1975;2:821.

36. Graham DY, Estes MK. Proteolytic enhancement of rotavirus infectivity: biologic mechanisms. *Virology* 1980;101:432–439.

37. Lee TW, Kurtz JB. Astroviruses detected by immunofluorescence. *Lancet* 1977;2:406.

38. Hudson RW, Herrmann JE, Blacklow NR. Plaque quantitation and virus neutralization assays for human astroviruses. *Arch Virol* 1989;108:33–38.

39. Cubitt WD. Human, small round structured viruses, caliciviruses and astroviruses. *Bailliere's Clin Gastroenterol* 1990;4: 643–656.

39a. Lee TW, Kurtz JB. Prevalence of human astrovirus serotypes in the Oxford region 1976–92, with evidence for two new serotypes. *Epidemiol Infect* 1994;112:187–193.

40. Wilson SA, Cubitt WD. The development and evaluation of radioimmune assays for the detection of immune globulins M and G against astrovirus. *J Virol Methods* 1988;19:151–160.

41. Lewis TL, Greenberg HB, Herrmann JE, Smith LS, Matsui SM. Analysis of astrovirus serotype 1 RNA, identification of the viral RNA-dependent RNA polymerase motif, and expression of a viral structural protein. *J Virol* 1994;68:77–83.

42. Willcocks MM, Carter MJ. Identification and sequence determination of the capsid protein gene of human astrovirus serotype 1. *FEMS Microbiol Lett* 1993;114:1–8.

43. Willcocks MM, Brown TDK, Madely CR, Carter MJ. The complete sequence of a human astrovirus. *J Gen Virol* 1994;75: 1785–1788.

44. Major ME, Eglin RP, Easton AJ. 3′ Terminal nucleotide sequence of human astrovirus type 1 and routine detection of astrovirus nucleic acid and antigens. *J Virol Methods* 1992;39: 217–225.

45. Willcocks MM, Carter MJ. The 3′ terminal sequence of a human astrovirus. *Arch Virol* 1992;124:279–289.

46. Jiang B, Monroe SS, Koonin EV, Stine SE, Glass RI. RNA sequence of astrovirus: distinctive genomic organization and a putative retrovirus-like ribosomal frameshifting signal that directs the viral replicase synthesis. *Proc Natl Acad Sci USA* 1993;90:10539–10543.

47. Monroe SS, Stine SE, Gorelkin L, Herrmann JE, Blacklow NR, Glass RI. Temporal synthesis of proteins and RNAs during human astrovirus infection of cultured cells. *J Virol* 1991;65: 641–648.

48. Monroe SS, Carter MJ, Herrmann JE, Kurtz JB, Matsui SM. Astroviridae. In: *Sixth Report of the International Committee on the Taxonomy of Viruses. (In press)*.

49. Willcocks MM, Carter MJ. Sequence analysis of a human astrovirus (Abstract P7-10). In: *Abstracts of the IXth International Congress of Virology*. Glasgow, Scotland, UK. 8–13 Aug 1993;138.

50. Willcocks MM, Carter MJ, Sequence analysis of a human astrovirus (Abstract P2-47). In: *Abstracts of the Third International Symposium on Positive Strand RNA Viruses*. Clearwater, FL. 19–24 Sept 1992;49.

51. Willcocks MM, Carter MJ, Madeley CR. Astroviruses. *Rev Med Virol* 1992;2:97–106.

52. Kozak M. An analysis of 5′-noncoding sequences from 699 vertebrate messenger RNAs. *Nucleic Acid Res* 1987;15: 8125–8148.

53. Chamorro M, Parkin N, Varmus HE. An RNA pseudoknot and an optimal heptameric shift site are required for highly efficient ribosomal frameshifting on a retroviral messenger RNA. *Proc Natl Acad Sci USA* 1992;89:713–717.

54. Jacks T, Madhani HD, Masiarz FR, Varmus HE. Signals for ribosomal frameshifting in the rous sarcoma virus. *Cell* 1988; 55:447–458.

55. Jacks T, Power MD, Masiarz FR, Luciw PA, Barr PJ, Varmus HE. Characterization of ribosomal frameshifting in HIV-1 gag-pol expression. *Nature* 1988;331:280–283.

56. Wilson W, Braddock M, Adams SE, Rathjen PD, Kingsman SM, Kingsman AJ. HIV expression strategies: ribosomal frameshifting is directed by a short sequence in both mammalian and yeast systems. *Cell* 1988;55:1159–1169.

57. Brierley I, Digard P, Inglis SC. Characterization of an efficient coronavirus ribosomal frameshifting signal: requirement for an RNA pseudoknot. *Cell* 1989;57:537–547.

57a. Lewis TL, Greenberg HB, Dormitzer PR, Matsui SM. In vitro characterization of a ribosomal frameshifting signal that may be involved in regulation of the astrovirus polymerase gene. In: *Scientific Program and Abstracts, American Society for Virology, 13th annual meeting*. University of Wisconsin, Madison, WI. July 9–13, 1994.

57b. Marczinke B, Bloys AJ, Brown TDK, Willcocks MM, Carter MJ, Brierley I. The human astrovirus RNA-dependent RNA polymerase coding region is expressed by ribosomal frameshifting. *J Virol* 1994;68:5588–5595.

58. Monroe SS, Jiang B, Stine SE, Koopmans M, Glass RI. Subgenomic RNA sequence of human astrovirus supports classification of Astroviridae as a new family of RNA viruses. *J Virol* 1993;67:3611–3614.

59. Strauss JH, Strauss EG. Replication of the RNAs of alphaviruses and flaviviruses. In: Domingo E, Holland JJ, Ahlquist P, eds. *RNA genetics. Volume 1: RNA-directed virus replication.* Boca Raton, FL: CRC Press, 1988;71–90.

60. Studdert MJ. Caliciviruses. *Arch Virol* 1978;58:157–191.

61. Semler BL, Kuhn RJ, Wimmer E. Replication of the poliovirus genome. In: Domingo E, Holland JJ, Ahlquist P, eds. *RNA genetics. Volume 1: RNA-directed virus replication.* Boca Raton, FL: CRC Press, 1988;23–48.

62. Kurtz JB. Astroviruses. In: Farthing MJG, ed. *Viruses and the Gut, Proceedings of the Ninth British Society of Gastroenterology.* Smith Kline and French International Workshop, Windsor, Berks, UK. 2–4 Oct 1988;84–87.

63. Avery RM, Shelton AP, Beards GM, Omotade OO, Oyejide OC, Olaleye DO. Viral agents associated with infantile gastroenteritis in Nigeria: relative prevalence of adenovirus serotypes 40 and 41, astrovirus, and rotavirus serotypes 1 to 4. *J Diarrhoeal Dis Res* 1992;10:105–108.

64. Bates PR, Bailey AS, Wood DJ, Morris DJ, Couriel JM. Comparative epidemiology of rotavirus, subgenus F (types 40 and 41) adenovirus, and astrovirus gastroenteritis in children. *J Med Virol* 1993;39:224–228.

65. Cox GJ, Matsui SM, Lo RS, et al. Etiology and outcome of diarrhea after marrow transplantation: a prospective study. *Gastroenterology* (in press).

66. Cruz JR, Bartlett AV, Herrmann JE, Caceres P, Blacklow NR, Cano F. Astrovirus-associated diarrhea among Guatemalan ambulatory rural children. *J Clin Microbiol* 1992;30:1140–1144.

67. Donelli G, Ruggeri FM, Tinari A, et al. A three-year diagnostic and epidemiological study on viral infantile diarrhoea in Rome. *Epidemiol Infect* 1988;100:311–320.

68. Esahli H, Breback K, Bennet R, Ehrnst A, Eriksson M, Hedlund K-O. Astroviruses as a cause of nosocomial outbreaks of infant diarrhea. *Pediatr Infect Dis J* 1991;10:511–515.

69. Ford-Jones EL, Mindorff CM, Gold R, Petric M. The incidence of viral-associated diarrhea after admission to a pediatric hospital. *Am J Epidemiol* 1990;131:711–718.

70. Gray JJ, Wreghitt TG, Cubitt WD, Elliot PR. An outbreak of gastroenteritis in a home for the elderly associated with astrovirus type 1 and human calicivirus. *J Med Virol* 1987;23:377–381.

71. Grohmann G. Viral diarrhoea in children in Australia. In: Tzipori S, ed. *Infectious diarrhoea in the young.* Amsterdam:Elsevier, 1985;25–32.

72. Grohmann GS, Glass RI, Pereira HG, et al. Enteric viruses and diarrhea in HIV-infected patients. *N Engl J Med* 1993;329:14–20.

73. Herrmann JE, Taylor DN, Echeverria P, Blacklow NR. Astroviruses as a cause of gastroenteritis in children. *N Engl J Med* 1991;324:1757–1760.

74. Kotloff KL, Herrmann JE, Blacklow NR, et al. The frequency of astrovirus as a cause of diarrhea in Baltimore children. *Pediatr Infect Dis J* 1992;11:587–589.

75. Kurtz JB, Lee TW, Pickering D. Astrovirus associated gastroenteritis in a children's ward. *J Clin Pathol* 1977;30:948–952.

76. Leite JPG, Barth OM, Schatzmayr HG. Astrovirus in faeces of children with acute gastroenteritis in Rio de Janeiro, Brazil. *Mem Inst Oswaldo Cruz* 1991;86:489–490.

77. Lew JF, Glass RI, Petric M, et al. Six-year retrospective surveillance of gastroenteritis viruses identified at ten electron microscopy centers in the United States and Canada. *Pediatr Infect Dis J* 1990;9:709–714.

78. Lew JF, Moe CL, Monroe SS, et al. Astrovirus and adenovirus associated with diarrhea in children in day care settings. *J Infect Dis* 1991;164:673–678.

79. Lewis DC, Lightfoot NF, Cubitt WD, Wilson SA. Outbreaks of astrovirus type 1 and rotavirus gastroenteritis in a geriatric in-patient population. *J Hosp Infect* 1989;14:9–14.

80. Maass G, Baumeister HG, Hergemoller R, Jansen P, Schumacher H. Visualization by electronmicroscopy of 28 nm virus-particles (astroviruses) in faeces of newborns with acute nonbacterial gastroenteritis (author's transl). *Zentralbl Bakt Parasit Infekt Hyg* 1978;242:423–430.

81. Marshall JA, Birch CJ, Williamson HG, et al. Coronavirus-like particles and other agents in the faeces of children in Efate, Vanatu. *J Trop Med Hyg* 1982;85:213–215.

82. McLean DM, Wong KSK, Bergman SKA. Virions associated with acute gastroenteritis in Vancouver, 1976. *Can Med Assoc J* 1977;117:1035–1036.

83. Middleton PJ, Szymanski MT, Petric M. Viruses associated with acute gastroenteritis in young children. *Am J Dis Child* 1977;131:733–737.

84. Mitchell DK, Van R, Morrow AL, Monroe SS, Glass RI, Pickering LK. Outbreaks of astrovirus gastroenteritis in day care centers. *J Pediatr* 1993;123:725–732.

85. Moe CL, Allen JR, Monroe SS, et al. Detection of astrovirus in pediatric stool samples by immunoassay and RNA probe. *J Clin Microbiol* 1991;29:2390–2395.

86. Monroe SS, Glass RI, Noah N, et al. Electron microscopic reporting of gastrointestinal viruses in the United Kingdom, 1985–1987. *J Med Virol* 1991;33:193–198.

87. Nazer H, Rice S, Walker-Smith JA. Clinical associations of stool astrovirus in childhood. *J Pediatr Gastroenterol Nutr* 1982;1:555–558.

88. Nozawa CM, Vaz MGS, Guimaraes MAAM. Detection of astrovirus-like in diarrhoeic stool and its coexistence with rotavirus. *Rev Inst Med Trop Sao Paulo* 1985;27:238–241.

89. Oliver AR, Phillips AD. An electron microscopical investigation of faecal small round viruses. *J Med Virol* 1988;24:211–218.

90. Oshiro LS, Haley CE, Roberto RR, et al. A 27-nm virus isolated during an outbreak of acute infectious nonbacterial gastroenteritis in a convalescent hospital: a possible new serotype. *J Infect Dis* 1981;143:791–795.

91. Pavone R, Schinaia N, Hart CA, Getty B, Molyneux M, Borgstein A. Viral gastroenteritis in children in Malawi. *Ann Trop Paediatr* 1990;10:15–20.

92. Peigue H, Beytout-Monghal M, Laveran H, Bourges M. Coronavirus and ''astrovirus'' observed in stools of children with gastroenteritis (author's transl). *Ann Microbiol* 1978;129B:101–106.

93. Phillips AD, Rice SJ, Walker-Smith JA. Astrovirus within human small intestinal mucosa. *Gut* 1982;23:A923–A924.

94. Singh PB, Sreenivasan MA, Pavri KM. Viruses in acute gastroenteritis in children in Pune, India. *Epidemiol Infect* 1989;102:345–353.

95. Spence IM. Astrovirus in South Africa: a case report. *S Afr Med J* 1983;64:181–182.

96. Stewien KE, Durigon EL, Tanaka H, Gilio AE, Baldacci ER. Occurrence of human astrovirus in Sao Paulo City, Brazil. *Rev Saude Publica* 1991;25:157–158.

97. Xu AY, Wan XB, Qiu FX, Pang QF. Astrovirus in autumn infantile gastroenteritis. *Chin Med J (Engl Ed)* 1981;94:659–662.

98. Madeley CR, Cosgrove BP, Bell EJ, Fallon RJ. Stool viruses in babies in Glasgow; 1. Hospital admissions with diarrhoea. *J Hyg (Camb)* 1977;787:261–273.

99. Riepenhoff-Talty M, Saif LJ, Barret HJ, Suzuki H, Ogra PL. Potential spectrum of etiological agents of viral enteritis in hospitalized infants. *J Clin Microbiol* 1982;17:352–356.

100. LeBaron CW, Furutan NP, Lew JF, et al. Viral agents of gastroenteritis. *MMWR Morb Mortal Wkly Rep* 1990;39 (RR-5):1–24.

101. Appleton H. Small round viruses: classification and role in food-borne infections. In: Bock G, Whelan J, eds. *Novel diarrhoea viruses.* Ciba Foundation Symposium 128. Chichester: Wiley, 1987;108–125.

102. Jonassen TO, Kjeldsberg E, Grinde B. Detection of human astrovirus serotype 1 by the polymerase chain reaction. *J Virol Methods* 1993;44:83–88.

103. Kapikian AZ. Viral gastroenteritis. *JAMA* 1993;269:627–630.

104. Kurtz JB, Lee TW, Craig JW, Reed SE. Astrovirus infection in volunteers. *J Med Virol* 1979;3:221–230.

105. Kurtz J, Lee T. Astrovirus gastroenteritis age distribution of antibody. *Med Microbiol Immunol* 1978;166:227–230.

106. Gray EW, Angus KW, Snodgrass DR. Ultrastructure of the small intestine in astrovirus-infected lambs. *J Gen Virol* 1980;49:71–82.

107. Snodgrass DR, Angus KW, Gray EW, Menzies JD, Paul G. Pathogenesis of diarrhoea caused by astrovirus infections in lambs. *Arch Virol* 1979;60:217–226.

108. Woode GN, Pohlenz JF, Kelso Gourley NE, Fagerland JA. Astrovirus and Breda virus infections of dome cell epithelium of bovine ileum. *J Clin Microbiol* 1984;19:623–630.

109. Bridger JC, Hall GA, Brown JF. Characterization of a calici-like virus (Newbury agent) found in association with astrovirus in bovine diarrhea. *Infect Immun* 1984;43:133–138.

110. Hall GA. Comparative pathology of infection by novel diarrhoea viruses. In: Bock G, Whelan J, eds. *Novel diarrhoea viruses*. Ciba Foundation Symposium 128. Chichester: Wiley, 1987;192–217.

111. Donelli G, Superti F, Tinari A, Marziano ML. Mechanism of astrovirus entry into Graham 293 cells. *J Med Virol* 1992;38: 271–277.

112. Superti F, Seganti L, Orsi N, et al. In vitro effect of synthetic flavanoids on astrovirus infection. *Antiviral Res* 1990;13: 201–208.

113. Greenberg HB, Matsui SM. Astroviruses and caliciviruses: emerging enteric pathogens. *Infect Agents Dis* 1992;1:71–91.

114. Blacklow NR, Greenberg HB. Viral gastroenteritis. *N Engl J Med* 1991;325:252–264.

115. Kjeldsberg E. Small spherical viruses in faeces from gastroenteritis patients. *Acta Pathol Microbiol Immunol Scand B* 1977; 85B:351–354.

116. Berthiaume L, Alain R, McLaughlin B, Payment P, Trepanier P. Rapid detection of human viruses in faeces by a simple and routine immune electron microscopy technique. *J Gen Virol* 1981;55:223–227.

117. Madeley D. Viruses and diarrhoea—where are we now? *APMIS* 1993;101:497–504.

118. Herrmann JE, Cubitt WD, Hudson RW, Perron-Henry DM, Oshiro LS, Blacklow NR. Immunological characterization of the Marin County strain of astrovirus. *Arch Virol* 1990;110: 213–220.

119. Herrmann JE, Hudson RW, Blacklow NR. Marin County agent, an astrovirus. *Lancet* 1987;2:743.

120. Willcocks MM, Carter MJ, Silcock JG, Madeley CR. A dot-blot hybridization procedure for the detection of astrovirus in stool samples. *Epidemiol Infect* 1991;107:405–410.

121. Willcocks MM, Silcock JG, Carter MJ. Detection of Norwalk virus in the UK by the polymerase chain reaction. *FEMS Microbiol Lett* 1993;112:7–12.

122. Kurtz JB, Lee TW, Parsons AJ. The action of alcohols on rotavirus, astrovirus and enterovirus. *J Hosp Infect* 1980;1: 321–325.

Infections of the Gastrointestinal Tract,
edited by M. J. Blaser, P. D. Smith, J. I. Ravdin,
H. B. Greenberg, and R. L. Guerrant
Raven Press, Ltd., New York © 1995.

CHAPTER 68

Enteric Adenoviruses

John E. Herrmann and Neil R. Blacklow

Two distinct serotypes of adenovirus, types 40 and 41, now categorized as subgroup F adenoviruses, have been commonly identified in the stools of infants and young children with gastroenteritis in temperate countries (1–12). These viruses have been isolated from cases of diarrhea in Asia, Africa, and South America as well (13–18). The percentage of cases of pediatric gastroenteritis found to be due to enteric adenoviruses has ranged from 1.5% to 12.0%.

Other types of adenoviruses have also been isolated from stools, and some have been associated with gastroenteritis (19,20), but only types 40 and 41 have been consistently associated with gastroenteritis. These enteric types also appear in higher concentrations in stools than other adenovirus types as determined by electron microscopy (EM) studies (21). The number of particles shed, like rotavirus, may exceed 10^{11} particles/g feces in children with diarrhea (22).

Enteric adenoviruses were originally described as being noncultivatable or fastidious viruses, because they could be seen in large numbers by EM in stools (6,7,23) but could not be cultivated in cell lines generally used to isolate other adenovirus types. In 1981, Takiff et al. (24) showed that these viruses could be cultivated in Graham 293 cells, a line of human embryonic kidney (HEK) cells transformed with sheared adenovirus type 5 deoxyribonucleic acid (DNA). Subsequently, it has been found that some subgroup F adenoviruses can be isolated in HEp-2 cells, Chang conjunctiva cells (25–27), or PLC/PRF/5 cells (28) as well as Graham 293 cells, and can be propagated in HeLa, HI407 cells (29) KB, or A549 cells.

DESCRIPTION OF THE VIRUSES

Morphology and Physical Properties

Like other adenoviruses, enteric adenoviruses are non-enveloped, icosahedral, double-stranded DNA viruses of

J. E. Herrmann and N. R. Blacklow: Division of Infectious Diseases and Immunology, University of Massachusetts Medical School, Worcester, Massachusetts 01655.

80-nm diameter. They have 252 capsomeres, which consist of 20 equilateral triangular sides and 12 vertices, and no morphological differences are seen by EM between the enteric and nonenteric types (Fig. 1). Complete enteric adenovirus particles form a band at a density of 1.34 g/mL and incomplete particles form a band at a density of 1.30 g/mL in cesium chloride. The enteric serotypes (40 and 41) share the adenovirus group antigen and are distinguished from each other and from the nonenteric serotypes serologically, and by their genome profiles after cleavage with restriction endonucleases followed by gel electrophoresis. The two serotypes collectively have been designated as subgroup F adenoviruses, but each of the two enteric serotypes gives an electrophoretic pattern distinct from any of the other adenovirus serotypes (22).

Stability studies of adenoviruses, specifically relating to the two enteric types, have not been reported. It can be assumed, based on their biophysical and biochemical properties, that they are no different from the other adenovirus types.

Propagation in Cell Cultures

The subgroup F adenoviruses, unlike other adenoviruses, cannot be serially cultivated on primary HEK cells. Takiff et al. (24) found that these viruses could be cultivated in a HEK cell line transformed by adenovirus type 5, Graham 293 cells. Because of this, they postulated that the adenovirus 41 strain, which they examined in detail, was similar in action to an adenovirus host-range mutant deficient in early gene functions (30). It was further suggested by Van Loon et al. (31) that the inability of adenovirus types 40 and 41 to be cultivated on cell lines normally supportive for other adenovirus types was due to the relative inability of the adenovirus 41 E1A gene to transactivate other adenovirus 41 early genes. Thus these reports indicated that the enteric adenoviruses required early gene products from other adenovirus types for efficient growth.

Studies by Pieniazek et al. (29) questioned the conclusions of Van Loon et al. (31). In their study, the prototype

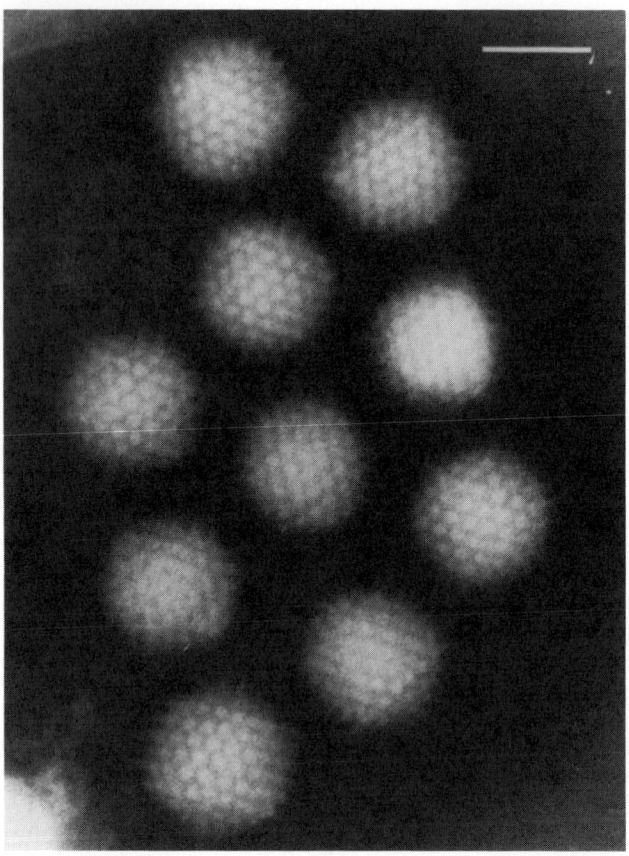

FIG. 1. Electron micrograph of enteric adenovirus type 40, isolated from a stool specimen in Graham 393 cells. Negatively stained with phosphotungstic acid. Bar, 50 nm. (Courtesy of W. D. Cubitt.)

strain of adenovirus, strain TAK, lost over 90% of its infectivity on the first passage in Graham 293 cells and lost 100% by the second passage. In contrast to these results, adenovirus 41 strain TAK was able to be serially cultivated to high titer in HeLa, HI407, or HEp-2 cells. The basis for the loss of infectivity of this virus strain in Graham 293 cells was found to be due to a defect in assembly of the virion. In Graham 293 cells, only traces of adenovirus protein V could be found by Western blot analysis, whereas in adenovirus 41 strain TAK virions obtained from HEp-2-infected cells, a strong band in the position of protein V was found.

Grabow et al. (28) have also reported a cell line that showed greater efficiency for propagating laboratory strains of adenovirus types 40 and 41 than Graham 293 cells or Chang conjunctiva cells. The cell line used was PLC/PRF/5, a cell line derived from a human hepatocellular carcinoma. The reason for the high susceptibility of the cell line was not determined.

Immunotypes

There are currently 47 serotypes (32) of human adenoviruses, subdivided into six subgenera (or subgroups) A through F. All serotypes share a cross-reacting common antigen. There are several antigens associated with the major structural proteins, proteins that have been resolved by polyacrylamide gel electrophoresis. The most abundant, the hexon (polypeptide II), contains both the common genus, species-specific, and subgenus-specific antigens. The penton base (polypeptide III) and the fiber antigens (polypeptide IV) have genus and species reactivities, respectively, as well as subgenus specificity. There are also core proteins (polypeptides V and VII) and other virion polypeptides IIIa and IX (33). The molecular weights of the internal polypeptides of adenovirus 40 and 41 were sufficiently different from subgroups A through E to establish them as group F and G (22), now collectively classified as subgenus F adenoviruses.

A comparison of the predicted amino acid sequence of the adenovirus 40 hexon with that of adenovirus 41 revealed an overall identity of 88% (34). The regions in the hexon protein that varied between adenovirus 40 and adenovirus 41 were the same regions that varied between adenovirus 2 and adenovirus 5 (subgroup C), suggesting that these are the areas of the protein that represent type-specific determinants.

Cross reactions between adenoviruses 40 and 41 are seen with antiserum raised to either type, and a one-way cross reaction has been noted between antisera to type 4 and type 40 (35). Monoclonal antibodies have been prepared that are specific for each type (36–41), antibodies that may or may not neutralize virus infectivity. Various DNA variants of adenovirus 41 have been described, which may not be neutralized by some monoclonal antibodies that neutralize prototype strains (36). Variants of adenovirus 40 have also been detected but have not been found to differ in their ability to be neutralized by adenovirus 40 monoclonal antibodies (36).

Genome Profiles

Adenoviruses contain double-stranded DNA of approximately 2.3×10^7 daltons. DNA restriction patterns for adenoviruses in subgenera A to F have been published for restriction endonucleases BamHI, BgIII, BstE11, HindIII, and SamI (42). Both adenoviruses 40 and 41 give genome profiles distinct from the other known adenovirus serotypes. Genome variants have also been described for adenoviruses 40 and 41 (43–46). An extensive study of variants among 48 strains of adenovirus 40 and 128 strains of adenovirus 41, using nine and ten different restriction endonucleases, respectively, has been reported by van der Avoort et al. (47). Variants among both adenoviruses 40 and 41 were found, but variants that resulted in detectable antigenic changes, which could be detected by neutralization studies with monoclonal antibodies or later by monoclonal antibody enzyme-linked immunoadsorbent assay (ELISA) (36,47), seemed to be among adenovirus 41 strains only. In some studies, strains of adenovirus 40 or adenovirus 41 did not show variation after treatment with SmaI (44), but in other studies variants have been detected with this enzyme as well (47).

EPIDEMIOLOGY

Studies on the incidence of infection with the enteric types of adenoviruses, as determined by detection of viruses in stool samples and by seroepidemiologic studies, indicate that these viruses cause infections worldwide. Unlike rotavirus infection, most studies do not indicate seasonal variation, although increased numbers of cases during the summer in Sweden (48) and in a rural area of South Africa (18) have been noted. A slight peak of incidence was also observed in the cool, dry months in a study in Bangladesh (17). Most infections (approximately 95%) occur in infants less than 2 years of age.

Where extensive studies have been done, it appears that enteric adenoviruses may be proportionately more important as causes of diarrhea in developed countries than in developing countries. The incidence of infection reported for children with acute gastroenteritis in developed countries has usually been between 4% and 10%, and these viruses are often considered to be second in importance only to rotaviruses. The incidence from year to year in the same geographic area, however, may be highly variable. For example, Brandt et al. (49), in an EM study of stools from children in the Washington, DC area with gastroenteritis, detected adenovirus (all serotypes) from a low of 1.4% to a high of 10.7% during eight successive years of study.

In developing countries, the incidence of enteric adenovirus gastroenteritis has generally been low, 2% to 3%. In a study of Thai children, 2% (22/1114) with gastroenteritis were found to have enteric adenoviruses. In a study in rural Bangladesh, the incidence was 2.8% (125/4409) of children less than 5 years old with diarrhea (16). In India, there was no significant difference in the infection rate with enteric adenoviruses for children with and without gastroenteritis in a 1-year survey (50). In Australian aboriginal children, a 1-year survey on stools from children with gastroenteritis showed that only 1.3% (18/1343) harbored enteric adenoviruses, compared with 6.8% (91/1343) who were positive for group A rotaviruses and 5.5% (74/1343) who were positive for astroviruses (51).

There have been reports of higher rates in some developing countries. In a 1-year survey of children in rural Guatemala (13), children had a greater incidence of enteric adenoviruses associated with diarrheal episodes (14.0%; 54/385) than rotaviruses (4.7%; 18/385). A 1-year survey in a rural African area (18) found that 13.2% (41/432) were positive for enteric adenoviruses by a dot-blot hybridization test, although only 3 of these 41 were positive by EM or isolation in cell culture, and 9/432 (2.1%) were positive by ELISA.

Seroepidemiologic studies also indicate that infection with enteric adenoviruses is widespread and occurs in both developed and developing countries. In a serological survey (52), more than one-third of the sera from the United Kingdom, New Zealand, Hong Kong, and Gambia were positive for neutralizing antibodies against a strain of enteric adenovirus that could be neutralized by antisera to both serotypes 40 and 41. None of 16 sera from Guatemala were positive and 15% of Kuwaiti sera were positive.

It was noted that the proportion of positive sera increased with age, generally being more than double in children 2 to 4 years old, than in children aged 2 years or less.

PATHOGENESIS

Adenovirus particles have been seen within the nucleus of small intestinal mucosal cells in a fatal case of adenovirus gastroenteritis and enteric adenoviruses have been recovered from fluids in the small intestine (53). The high number of enteric particles shed (up to 10^{11} particles/g) in stools also indicates these viruses actively multiply in the intestinal tract. Detailed studies regarding mechanisms of enteric adenovirus gastroenteritis have not been reported.

Adenoviruses have also been frequently isolated from acquired immunodeficiency syndrome (AIDS) patients and immunocompromised patients (32,54–57). However, there does not seem to be a major involvement of the enteric types or of any other particular serotype. In a study of 67 adenovirus isolates from 48 patients with AIDS, there were isolates from subgenera A, B, C, and D, including five new serotypes (types 43 to 47) of subgenus D (32). Because of the variety of serotypes obtained from liver, lung, blood, urine, and stool samples, the authors could not assign any epidemiologic significance to a particular serotype. Chronic diarrhea is also common in AIDS patients. Adenoviruses have been associated with this chronic diarrhea in some studies (55,57), but diarrhea has not been specifically associated with the enteric types, 40 and 41 (55,57). Whether further studies on adenovirus-induced diarrhea in AIDS patients will implicate specific serotypes remains to be determined.

Transmission of these viruses appears to be by person-to-person spread, as with rotaviruses, and no waterborne or foodborne outbreaks have been reported to date. It has also been suggested that nosocomial infections occur (58). Spread to adults is uncommon. Asymptomatic infections may occur in approximately 2% of those studied in one report (48), and up to 8% (59) and 17% (60) in studies done in day care centers.

CLINICAL ILLNESS

The clinical course of gastroenteritis caused by enteric adenoviruses is similar to that caused by rotavirus, with diarrhea being the most frequent symptom. Vomiting is also a common finding. Fever and respiratory symptoms may also be present. The age groups mainly affected are infants and young children. The illness is usually mild and asymptomatic infections are known to occur, but the disease can also be severe and fatal cases have been reported (53). The incubation period is approximately 7 days and virus excretion in stools lasts 10 to 14 days (61).

Detailed studies of enteric adenovirus gastroenteritis have been reported by Uhnoo et al. (61). The characteristics of patients with gastroenteritis caused by enteric ad-

TABLE 1. *Comparison of clinical features of children infected with enteric adenoviruses or rotaviruses*

Clinical feature	Number infected (% infected)	
	Enteric adenovirus (*N* = 32)	Rotavirus (*N* = 168)
Diarrhea	31 (97)	164 (98)
Diarrhea >10 times daily	7 (22)	36 (21)
Vomiting	25 (78)	146 (87)
Fever	14 (44)	141 (84)
Fever >39°C	1 (3)	71 (42)
Abdominal pain	8 (25)	31 (18)
Blood in stools	1 (3)	2 (1)
Mucus in stools	6 (19)	28 (17)
Respiratory symptoms	6 (19)	56 (33)
Admission to hospital	9 (28)	65 (39)
Duration (mean days)		
Hospital stay	3.6	2.4
Diarrhea	10.8	5.9
Vomiting	3.2	2.5

Table adapted from data presented in ref. 61.

enoviruses and rotaviruses are shown in Table 1. These data were obtained in a prospective 1-year study, comprising children with acute gastroenteritis admitted to hospital or treated as outpatients. Significant differences between group A rotavirus and enteric adenovirus gastroenteritis were found for fever over 39°C, where 42% of the rotavirus patients showed fever over 39°C compared to 3% of the enteric adenovirus patients, and for duration of diarrhea. Those infected with enteric adenoviruses had diarrhea for a mean duration of 10.8 days compared to 5.9 days for the rotavirus patients.

In an earlier study by Uhnoo et al. (48), a follow-up study of three children who recovered from enteric adenovirus gastroenteritis showed that they had lactose intolerance for up to 5 to 7 months after recovery. Evidence of malabsorption using the D-xylose absorption test during acute enteric adenovirus disease was shown by Mavromichalis et al. (62). A possible role for adenoviruses in celiac disease, characterized by small intestinal mucosal injury and malabsorption, has also been suggested (63).

The clinical picture for infants in developing countries is similar to that seen in developed countries. In a study of infants less than 5 years of age in Bangladesh, who had enteric adenovirus gastroenteritis, the symptoms experienced by 80 children examined were similar to symptoms in infants infected with group A rotaviruses (17). The most common clinical features were watery diarrhea (88%; 69% had bowel movements more than eight times per day), vomiting (80%), abdominal pain (76%), and low-grade fever (95%). Mild to moderate dehydration was also commonly found. There was no significant difference in the degree of dehydration seen in patients with enteric adenovirus gastroenteritis and those with gastroenteritis caused by group A rotaviruses.

DIAGNOSIS

Electron Microscopy

The enteric adenoviruses were first associated with diarrheal disease based on EM studies, and the viral particles are generally seen in high numbers, up to 10^{11} per gram of feces. Because they occur in higher numbers than other nonenteric types, Brandt et al. (21) has reported that the likelihood of detecting the enteric types by EM alone was increased when one or more particles were detected per minute of viewing. For definitive identification, however, immune EM, using type-specific antisera, is required (64,65).

Enzyme-Linked Immunoadsorbent Assay

In earlier studies, ELISAs specific for each of the enteric types (40 and 41) were developed with polyclonal sera that had been absorbed with adenovirus antigens from other subgenera (66,67). Since then, ELISA tests have been described, utilizing monoclonal antibodies specific for types 40 and 41 (36–41). For direct detection in stool samples, we developed an indirect ELISA that utilizes a polyclonal capture antibody directed against adenovirus group antigen, and murine monoclonal antibody to each enteric type as detector antibodies (39). Monoclonal antibody-based ELISA tests for group F adenoviruses are now commercially available as well and have been evaluated in epidemiologic and other studies (13,60,68). Because of the ease of performance, commercial availability, and the high sensitivity and specificity obtained, monoclonal antibody ELISA is at present the method of choice for routine diagnosis of enteric adenovirus infections.

Detection of Viral DNA

Detection of viral DNA has been applied to both adenovirus type 40 and type 41. In earlier studies, cloned DNA fragments used by Takiff et al. (69) in a dot-blot hybridization system were found to detect less than 20 pg of enteric adenovirus DNA. A hybridization test was also described that had a similar sensitivity to a radioimmunoassay (RIA) for enteric adenoviruses (70). Later studies have concentrated on polymerase chain reaction (PCR) techniques (71). By use of primers from genes encoding early regions E1A and E1B of subgroup F adenoviruses, PCR was found effective for detecting enteric adenoviruses at a level of 10^3 virus particles (380 fg). Although this PCR was not tested extensively on stool samples known to contain enteric adenoviruses, preliminary studies (71) and a later study concerning specificity of PCR (72) suggested PCR was potentially an effective means for diagnosing enteric adenovirus infection. No commercial PCR assays are available at this writing.

Detection of enteric adenoviruses with synthetic oligonucleotide probes has also been described (73). When tested on clinical stool samples, hybridization with the probes was found to have a sensitivity approximately equal to that obtained with a commercial monoclonal antibody ELISA but was less specific than the ELISA.

Isolation in Cell Culture

For isolation of enteric adenoviruses, stool samples are prepared by dilution in phosphate-buffered saline (PBS) and clarification by centrifugation. The clarified stool suspensions are inoculated onto monolayers of Graham 293 cells, maintenance medium is added (Eagle's MEM plus 2% fetal calf serum and antibiotics), and the cells are held for 7 to 10 days at 37°C. Cultures should be passaged at least once if no cytopathic effect is evident on the first passage. Adenoviruses can be identified as enteric types by ELISA with monoclonal antibodies, as discussed earlier, or by examination of the DNA patterns obtained on agarose gels after the DNA is treated with restriction endonucleases (22,74). Several different enzymes have been used to classify adenoviruses, but Sma1 has been favored for identification of the enteric types. The procedure for preparation and treatment of the virus samples has been described (74).

Electrophoresis can be done in polyacrylamide gels (74) or in agarose minigels (75). The bands are visualized with an ultraviolet illuminator or a silver stain can be used (74). The bands are compared with those obtained with known prototype strains of type 40 and 41 viruses. Additional, unclassified types may also be found in adenovirus-associated gastroenteritis (19) but their significance remains to be established.

Other Methods

Other methods for the direct detection of enteric adenoviruses in stools have been described, most of which have now been replaced by monoclonal antibody ELISAs. Extraction of DNA directly from stools followed by treatment with restriction endonucleases and electrophoresis in agarose (75) or polyacrylamide gels (76) has been reported. A latex agglutination test has also been applied to detection of enteric adenoviruses in stools. However, this test detects adenoviral group antigen and is not specific for the enteric types (77).

TREATMENT AND PREVENTION

There is presently no specific antiviral therapy for treatment of enteric adenovirus infection. As with diarrheal diseases caused by rotaviruses and other viral agents, treatment is directed at prevention of severe dehydration and electrolyte imbalance. Use of oral rehydration salt solutions containing glucose or sucrose has been shown in recent years to be as effective as intravenous fluid therapy for mild to moderately severe dehydrating rotavirus gastroenteritis, and presumably this would apply to dehydrating enteric adenovirus gastroenteritis as well. The

standard World Health Organization formula consists of the following per liter of water: glucose 20 g, sodium chloride 3.5 g, sodium bicarbonate 2.5 g, and potassium chloride 1.5 g. Oral rehydration solutions are also commercially available. Intravenous therapy must be administered if oral rehydration is unsuccessful in replacing fluids and electrolytes, or if the patient is in shock or is severely dehydrated.

Little is known about immune responses, immunity, or duration of immunity should it occur. Clinical or epidemiologic studies regarding immunity to reinfection with either of the enteric adenoviruses have not been reported. Persistence of neutralizing antibodies, as seen in seroepidemiologic studies, and the successful development of vaccines against adenoviral acute respiratory disease suggest the possibility for development of vaccines against enteric adenovirus infection. However, because enteric adenoviruses do not as yet appear to be of high importance in developing countries, where diarrheal diseases are major causes of morbidity and mortality, development of a vaccine would not appear to be of high priority. Whether further epidemiologic studies will demonstrate a greater need for vaccine development remains to be determined.

REFERENCES

1. Brandt CD, Kim HW, Rodriguez WJ, et al. Adenoviruses and pediatric gastroenteritis. *J Infect Dis* 1985;151:437–443.
2. Albert MJ. Enteric adenoviruses. *Arch Virol* 1986;88:1–17.
3. Yolken RH, Lawrence F, Leister F, Takiff HE, Strauss SE. Gastroenteritis associated with enteric type adenovirus in hospitalized infants. *J Pediatr* 1982;101:21–26.
4. Wood DJ. Adenovirus gastroenteritis. *Br Med J* 1988;296:229–230.
5. Wood DJ, Longhurst D, Killough RI, David TJ. One-year prospective cross-sectional study to assess the importance of group F adenovirus infections in children under 2 years admitted to hospital. *J Med Virol* 1988;26:429–435.
6. Brandt CD, Kim HW, Yolken RH, et al. Comparative epidemiology of two rotavirus serotypes and other viral agents associated with pediatric gastroenteritis. *Am J Epidemiol* 1979;110:243–254.
7. Gary GW Jr, Hierholzer JC, Black RE. Characteristic of noncultivable adenoviruses associated with diarrhea in infants: a new subgroup of human adenoviruses. *J Clin Microbiol* 1979;10:96–103.
8. Uhnoo I, Wadell G, Svensson L, Johansson M. Two new serotypes of enteric adenovirus causing infantile diarrhoea. *Dev Biol Stand* 1983;53:311–318.
9. Madeley CR. The emerging role of adenoviruses as inducers of gastroenteritis. *Pediatr Infect Dis* 1986;5:S63–S74.
10. Schoenemann W. The importance of infections with adenoviruses in infancy. *Monatsschr Kinderheilkd* 1988;136:680–685.
11. Cevenini R, Mazzaracchio R, Rumpianesi F, Donati M, Moroni A, Sambri V, LaPlace M. Prevalence of enteric adenovirus from acute gastroenteritis: a five year study. *Eur J Epidemiol* 1987;3:147–150.
12. Richmond SJ, Dunn SM, Caul EO, Ashley CR, Clarke SKR. An outbreak of gastroenteritis in young children caused by adenoviruses. *Lancet* 1979;1:1178.
13. Cruz JR, Caceres P, Cano F, Flores J, Bartlett A, Torun B. Adenovirus types 40 and 41 and rotaviruses associated with diarrhea in children from Guatemala. *J Clin Microbiol* 1990;28:1780–1784.
14. Oishi I, Yamazaki K, Minekawa Y, Nishimura H, Kitaura T. Three-year survey of the epidemiology of rotavirus, enteric ade-

novirus, and some small spherical viruses including "Osaka-agent" associated with infantile diarrhea. *Biken J* 1985;28:9–19.

15. Shinozaki, Arakf K, Fujita Y, Kobayashi M, Tajima T, Abe T. Epidemiology of enteric adenoviruses 40 and 41 in acute gastroenteritis in infants and young children in the Tokyo area. *Scand J Infect Dis* 1991;23:543–547.

16. Herrmann JE, Blacklow NR, Perron-Henry DM, Clements E, Taylor DN, Echeverria P. Incidence of enteric adenoviruses among children in Thailand and the significance of these viruses in gastroenteritis. *J Clin Microbiol* 1988;26:1783–1786.

17. Jarecki-Khan K, Tzipori SR, Unicomb LE. Enteric adenovirus infection among infants with diarrhea in rural Bangladesh. *J Clin Microbiol* 1993;31:484–489.

18. Tiemessen CT, Wegerhoff MJ, Erasmus MJ, Kidd AH. Infection by enteric adenoviruses, rotaviruses, and other agents in a rural African environment. *J Med Virol* 1989;28:176–182.

19. Bishai FR, Yolken RH, Chernesky MA, Johnston S, Rossier E. Studies on fastidious adenoviruses in Ontario: a distinct strain associated with gastroenteritis. *J Clin Microbiol* 1986;23:398–400.

20. Brown M. Laboratory identification of adenoviruses associated with gastroenteritis in Canada from 1983 to 1986. *J Clin Microbiol* 1986;28:1525–1529.

21. Brandt CD, Rodriguez WJ, Kim HW, Arrobis JO, Jeffries BC, Parrott RH. Rapid presumptive recognition of diarrhea-associated adenoviruses. *J Clin Microbiol* 1984;20:1008–1009.

22. Wadell G. Molecular epidemiology of human adenoviruses. *Curr Top Microbiol Immunol* 1984;110:191–220.

23. Madeley CR, Cosgrove BP, Bell EJ, Fallon RJ. Stool viruses in babies in Glasgow. 1. Hospital admissions with diarrhea. *J Hyg (Camb)* 1977;261–273.

24. Takiff HE, Straus SE, Garon CF. Propagation and in vitro studies of previously non-cultivable enteral adenoviruses in 293 cells. *Lancet* 1981;2:832.

25. Kidd AH, Madeley CA. In vitro growth of some fastidious adenoviruses from stool specimens. *J Clin Pathol* 1981;34:213–316.

26. de Jong JC, Wigand R, Kidd AH, et al. Candidate adenoviruses 40 and 41: fastidious adenoviruses from human infant stool. *J Med Virol* 1983;11:215–231.

27. Perron-Henry DM, Herrmann JE, Blacklow NR. Isolation and propagation of enteric adenoviruses in HEp-2 cells. *J Clin Microbiol* 1988;26:1445–1447.

28. Grabow WOK, Puttergill DL, Bosch A. Propagation of adenovirus types 40 and 41 in the PLC/PRF/5 primary liver carcinoma cell line. *J Virol Methods* 1992;37:201–208.

29. Pieniazek D, Pieniazek N, Macejak D, Coward J, Rayfield M, Lufting RB. Differential growth of human enteric adenovirus 41 (TAK) in continuous cell lines. *Virology* 1990;174:239–249.

30. Takiff HE, Straus SE. Early replicative block prevents the efficient growth of fastidious diarrhea-associated adenovirus in cell culture. *J Med Virol* 1982;9:93–100.

31. van Loon AE, Maas R, Vaessen RTMJ, Reemst AMCB, Sussenbach JS, Rozijn ThH. Cell transformation by the left terminal regions of the adenovirus 40 and 41 genomes. *Virology* 1985;147:227–230.

32. Hierholzer JC, Wigand R, Anderson LJ, Adrian T, Gold JWM. Adenoviruses from patients with AIDS: a plethora of serotypes and a description of five new serotypes of subgenus D (types 43–47). *J Infect Dis* 1988;158:804–813.

33. Philipson L. Structure and assembly of adenoviruses. *Curr Top Microbiol Immunol* 1983;109:1–52.

34. Toogood CIA, Murali R, Burnett RM, Hay RT. The adenovirus type 40 hexon: sequence, predicted structure and relationship to other adenovirus hexons. *J Gen Virol* 1989;70:3203–3214.

35. Svensson L, Wadell G, Uhnoo I, Johansson M, Von Bonsdorff C-H. Cross-reactivity between enteric adenoviruses and adenovirus type 4: analysis of epitopes by solid-phase immune electron microscopy. *J Gen Virol* 1983;64:2517–2520.

36. de Jong JC, Bijlsma K, Wermenbol AG, et al. Detection, typing and subtyping of enteric adenoviruses 40 and 41 from fecal samples and observation of changing incidence of infections with these types and subtypes. *J Clin Microbiol* 1993;31:1562–1569.

37. Wood DJ, deJong JC, Bijlsma K, van der Avoort HGAM. Development and evaluation of monoclonal antibody-based immune electron microscopy for diagnosis of adenovirus types 40 and 41. *J Virol Methods* 1989;25:241–250.

38. Herrmann JE, Perron-Henry DM, Stobbs-Walro D, Blacklow NR. Preparation and characterization of monoclonal antibodies to enteric adenovirus types 40 and 41. *Arch Virol* 1987;94:259–265.

39. Herrmann JE, Perron-Henry DM, Blacklow NR. Antigen detection with monoclonal antibodies for the diagnosis of adenovirus gastroenteritis. *J Infect Dis* 1987;155:1167–1171.

40. Singh-Naz N, Naz RK. Development and application of monoclonal antibodies for specific detection of human enteric adenoviruses. *J Clin Microbiol* 1986;23:840–842.

41. Singh-Naz N, Rodriguez WJ, Kidd AH, Brandt CD. Monoclonal antibody enzyme-linked immunosorbent assay for specific identification and typing of subgroup F adenoviruses. *J Clin Microbiol* 1988;26:297–300.

42. Adrian T, Wadell G, Hierholzer JC, Wigand R. DNA restriction analysis of adenovirus prototypes 1 to 41. *Arch Virol* 1986;91:277–290.

43. Willcocks MM, Carter MJ, Laidler FR, Madeley CR. Restriction enzyme analysis of faecal adenoviruses in Newcastle upon Tyne. *Epidemiol Infect* 1988;101:445–458.

44. Kidd AH. Genome variants of adenovirus 41 (subgroup G) from children with diarrhoea in South Africa. *J Med Virol* 1984;14:49–59.

45. Shinozaki T, Araki K, Kobayashi M, Fujita Y, Abe T, Ushijima H. Genome variants of human adenovirus types 40 and 41 (subgroup F) in Japan. *J Clin Microbiol* 1988;26:2567–2571.

46. Kidd AH, Berkowitz FE, Blaskovic PJ, Schoub BD. Genome variants of human adenovirus 40 (subgroup F). *J Med Virol* 1984;14:235–246.

47. van der Avoort HGAM, Wermenbol AG, Zomerdijk TPL, et al. Characterization of fastidious adenovirus types 40 and 41 by DNA restriction enzyme analysis and by neutralizing monoclonal antibodies. *Virus Res* 1989;12:139–158.

48. Uhnoo I, Wadell G, Svensson L, Johansson ME. Importance of enteric adenoviruses 40 and 41 in acute gastroenteritis in infants and young children. *J Clin Microbiol* 1984;20:365–372.

49. Brandt CD, Kim HW, Rodgriguez WJ, et al. Pediatric viral gastroenteritis during eight years of study. *J Clin Microbiol* 1983;18:71–78.

50. Bhan MK, Raj P, Bhandari N, et al. Role of enteric adenoviruses and rotaviruses in mild and severe acute enteritis. *Pediatr Infect Dis J* 1988;7:320–323.

51. Herrmann JE, Henry DM, Albert MJ, Erlich J, Blacklow NR. Incidence of astroviruses in Australian aboriginal children and comparison with other gastroenteritis viruses. *Abstr IXth Int Congress Virol* 1993;P7-6:138.

52. Kidd AH, Banatvala JE, de Jong JC. Antibodies to fastidious faecal adenoviruses (species 40 and 41) in sera from children. *J Med Virol* 1983;11:333–341.

53. Whitelaw A, Davies H, Parry J. Electron microscopy of fatal adenovirus gastroenteritis. *Lancet* 1977;1:361.

54. Grohmann GS, Glass RI, Pereira HG, et al. Enteric viruses and diarrhea in HIV-infected patients. *N Engl J Med* 1993;329:14–20.

55. Smith PD, Quinn TC, Strober W, Janoff EN, Masur H. Gastrointestinal infection in AIDS. *Ann Intern Med* 1992;116:63–67.

56. Smith PD, Saini SS, Orenstein JM. Infections of the large intestine in the immunocompromised host. In: Philips SF, Pemberton JH, Shorter RG, eds. *The large intestine: physiology, pathophysiology, and disease.* New York: Raven Press, 1991;437–444.

57. Janoff EN, Orenstein JM, Manischewitz JF, Smith PD. Adenovirus colitis in the acquired immunodeficiency syndrome. *Gastroenterology* 1991;100:976–979.

58. Kotloff KL, Losonsky GA, Morris JG Jr, Wasserman SS, Singh-Naz N, Levine MM. Enteric adenovirus infection and childhood diarrhea: an epidemiologic study in three clinical settings. *Pediatrics* 1989;84:219–225.

59. Lew JF, Moe CL, Monroe SS, et al. Astrovirus and adenovirus associated with diarrhea in children in day care settings. *J Infect Dis* 1991;164:673–678.

60. Van R, Wun C-C, O'Ryan ML, Matson DO, Jackson L, Picker-

ing LK. Outbreaks of human enteric adenovirus types 40 and 41 in Houston day care centers. *J Pediatr* 1992;120:516–521.

61. Uhnoo I, Olding-Stenkvist E, Kreuger A. Clinical features of acute gastroenteritis associated with rotavirus, enteric adenoviruses, and bacteria. *Arch Dis Child* 1986;61:732–738.

62. Mavromichalis J, Evans N, McNeish AS, Bryden AS, Davis HA, Flewett TH. Intestinal damage in rotavirus and adenovirus gastroenteritis assessed by D-xylose malabsorption. *Arch Dis Child* 1977;52:589–591.

63. Kagnoff MF, Austin RK, Hubert JJ, Bernardin JE, Kasarda DD. Possible role for a human adenovirus in the pathogenesis of celiac disease. *J Exp Med* 1984;160:1544–1557.

64. Leite JPG, Pereira HG, Azeredo RS, Schatzmayr HG. Adenoviruses in faeces of children with acute gastroenteritis in Rio De Janeiro, Brazil. *J Med Virol* 1985;15:203–209.

65. Wood DJ, Bailey AS. Detection of adenovirus types 40 and 41 in stool specimens by immune electron microscopy. *J Med Virol* 1987;21:191–199.

66. Johansson ME, Uhnoo I, Svensson L, Pettersson C-A, Wadell G. Enzyme-linked immunosorbent assay for detection of enteric adenovirus 41. *J Med Virol* 1985;17:19–27.

67. Johansson ME, Uhnoo I, Kidd AH, Madeley CR, Wadell G. Direct identification of enteric adenovirus, a candidate new serotype, associated with infantile gastroenteritis. *J Clin Microbiol* 1980;12:95–100.

68. Wood DJ, Bijlsma K, de Jong JC, Tonkin C. Evaluation of a commercial monoclonal antibody-based enzyme immunoassay for detection of adenovirus types 40 and 41 in stool specimens. *J Clin Microbiol* 1989;27:1155–1158.

69. Takiff HE, Seidlin M, Krause P, et al. Detection of enteric adenoviruses by dot-blot hybridization using a molecularly cloned viral DNA probe. *J Med Virol* 1985;16:107–118.

70. Stalhandske P, Hyypia T, Allard A, Halonen P, Pettersson U. Detection of adenoviruses in stool specimens by nucleic acid spot hybridization. *J Med Virol* 1985;16:213–218.

71. Allard A, Girones R, Juto P, Wadell G. Polymerase chain reaction for detection of adenoviruses in stool samples. *J Clin Microbiol* 1990;28:2659–2667.

72. Allard A, Albinsson B, Wadell G. Detection of adenoviruses in stools from healthy persons and patients with diarrhea by two-step polymerase chain reaction. *J Med Virol* 1992;37:149–157.

73. Scott-Taylor TH, Ahluwalia G, Dawood M, Hammond GW. Detection of enteric adenoviruses with synthetic oligonucleotide probes. *J Med Virol* 1993;41:328–337.

74. Brown M, Petric M, Middleton PJ. Silver staining of DNA restriction fragments for the rapid identification of adenovirus isolates: application during nosocomial outbreaks. *J Virol Methods* 1985;10:39–44.

75. Buitenwerf J, Louwerens JJ, de Jong JC. A simple and rapid method for typing adenoviruses 40 and 41 without cultivation. *J Virol Methods* 1985;10:39–44.

76. Moosai RB, Carter MJ, Madeley CR. Rapid detection of enteric adenovirus and rotavirus: a simple method using polyacrylamide gel electrophoresis. *J Clin Pathol* 1984;37:1404–1408.

77. Grandien M, Pettersson CA, Svensson L, Uhnoo I. Latex agglutination test for adenovirus diagnosis in diarrheal disease. *J Med Virol* 1987;23:311–316.

Infections of the Gastrointestinal Tract,
edited by M. J. Blaser, P. D. Smith, J. I. Ravdin,
H. B. Greenberg, and R. L. Guerrant
Published by Raven Press, Ltd., New York, 1995.

CHAPTER 69

Other Viral Agents of Gastroenteritis

Roger I. Glass

More than 15 different groups of viruses encompassing more than 100 serotypes can be found in the gut. The continual turnover of this massive epithelial cell pool provides a constant supply of new tissue to support the propagation or passage of a wide variety of viruses. However, while many viruses are present in the gut, relatively few are causative agents of diarrhea. Some are either not pathogenic to the gut epithelium or cause other unrelated illnesses; these include hepatitis A virus, reoviruses, nonenteric adenoviruses, poliovirus, coxsackieviruses A and B, echovirus, and most if not all of the other human enteroviruses (1). Others, such as cytomegalovirus, varicella zoster, measles, mumps, parainfluenza, papillomavirus, herpes simplex virus, and perhaps human immunodeficiency virus (HIV), commonly infect other parts of the body but can occasionally cause opportunistic infections in the gut. When these viruses opportunistically infect epithelial cells at different sites in the gastrointestinal tract from the mouth to the rectum, they cause illnesses such as malabsorption, esophagitis, proctitis, and colitis, which may have gastrointestinal signs and symptoms but for which diarrhea is usually only a secondary problem (see chapter by Greenberg).

In fact, a relatively small group of viruses have been incriminated as causes of acute gastroenteritis in humans and fewer have proved to be true etiologic agents. Before the 1970s, viruses were suspected to be the cause of a majority of diarrheal episodes because the recognized bacterial and parasitic agents could be found in only a small fraction of diarrheal specimens (2,3). Volunteer studies in the 1940s and 1950s supported this hypothesis since bacteria-free stool filtrates from patients with gastroenteritis were found to cause diarrhea in volunteers and could be passaged serially in volunteers, suggesting that viruses and not toxins were the causative agents (4,5).

The identification of specific viruses and their associa-

tion with gastroenteritis were boosted with each major advance in diagnostic virology (Table 1). In the 1950s and 1960s, the development of tissue culture techniques led to the cultivation and identification of echoviruses, adenoviruses, coxsackieviruses A and B, and reovirus from stool and led to their identification as putative diarrheal pathogens. The development of electron microscopic (EM) methods in the 1970s and their application to screening fecal specimens led to breakthroughs in the identification of new enteric viruses that were difficult to culture, including the Norwalk agent (6), rotavirus (7), caliciviruses, coronavirus (8,9), parvovirus (10,11), torovirus (12), and other small round structured viruses (SRSVs) that looked like the Norwalk agent but were antigenically distinct by immunoelectron microscopy (IEM). While many viruses could be identified in fecal specimens from patients with diarrhea, not all these agents were necessarily etiologic agents of gastroenteritis.

This chapter begins with a review of the types of evidence required to establish that a virus is a causative agent of gastroenteritis, and then describes a collection of viruses not discussed elsewhere in this book that have been implicated as etiologic agents, but for which a causal relationship is still unproved (Table 1). Much research is ongoing to establish whether these agents actually cause gastroenteritis.

WHEN IS A NOVEL VIRUS AN ENTERIC PATHOGEN?

Evidence to Establish a Causal Relationship

The observation of a virus in a fecal specimen from a patient with diarrhea raises two questions: (a) What is the true identity of the virus seen by EM or grown in culture? and (b) Can the virus be implicated as the causative agent of the patient's diarrhea? The first question relates to virus detection and characterization (Table 2). Some viruses, such as the coronaviruses or toroviruses, have a pleomorphic structure as seen by EM that can often be

R. I. Glass: Viral Gastroenteritis Section, Respiratory and Enteric Viruses Branch, Division of Viral and Rickettsial Diseases, National Center for Infectious Diseases, Centers for Disease Control and Prevention (CDC), Atlanta, Georgia 30333.

TABLE 1. *History of the identification of viral agents associated with diarrhea*

Time	Recognized agents	Putative pathogens
Cultivation period		
1940–1950s		Transmissible agents
1958		Echovirus 14, 18, 19 and others
1960		Adenovirus (1, 2, 3, 4, 5, 7) and others
1970		Coxsackievirus A and B
EM period		
1972	Norwalk	Parvovirus
1973	Rotavirus—group A	
1975	Enteric adenoviruses 40 and 41	Coronavirus
	Astrovirus	
	Calicivirus	
1980s	Rotavirus—groups B and C	
1974 to present	SRSVs, Norwalk, SMA, Hawaii, Taunton, Paramatta	
1984		Toroviruses (Berne/Breda)
1988		Picobirnavirus

confused with other membranous material from the patient's gut that is seen in fecal specimens. Similarly, viruses that produce cytopathic effect (CPE) in cell culture, such as enteroviruses and adenoviruses, may be enteric agents that are easy to cultivate but not necessarily the cause of disease. With the exception of the enteroviruses and reoviruses, the enteric viral pathogens described in this chapter either are noncultivatable or grow poorly in cell culture and have only a single principal method for identification, usually EM.

When possible, one way to avoid problems in virus identification is to establish more than one detection method. The development or availability of alternative assay systems to EM and IEM, such as immunoassays, molecular-based detection techniques, or cultivation methods, can help confirm the identity of a viral agent seen initially by EM. For example, work to establish the pathogenic role of coronaviruses as agents of gastroenteritis has been inhibited by the lack of alternative, confirmatory assays that are needed to distinguish particles that appear to be coronaviruses from cellular debris with comparable morphologic features. Consequently, the observation of a fringed agent with crown-like appearance and size in a stool specimen is often termed a "coronavirus-like particle" since no method is available to confirm this observation.

TABLE 2. *Requirements for a novel virus to be considered an etiologic agent*

1. Strength/consistency of the association: more common in cases with diseases than in controls.
2. Documented immune response to the agent.
3. Consistency/temporality:
   onset of disease corresponds to onset of infection; termination of disease corresponds to termination of infection.
4. Biologically *plausible/analogy* (e.g., evidence from animal models).
5. Specificity.
6. Biological gradient—dose response (A. B. Hill, 1965).
7. Volunteer studies (Koch's postulates).

Once an agent has been found in a fecal specimen from a patient with diarrhea, the establishment of its role as the etiologic agent can be difficult. For an individual patient, one first would have to rule out the presence of more than two dozen other etiologic agents and toxins that are known to cause gastroenteritis, a very difficult task. The issue is less problematic in an epidemic since one assumes that all patients were infected with the same agent, and therefore the finding of an etiologic agent in most of these patients and the failure to identify the same agent among controls without illness provide strong epidemiologic evidence of causality. To establish that the agent is not only present in the intestine but actually replicating and causing disease, one would like to document an immune response, which can be measured by a difference in antibody titers between acute- and convalescent-phase sera. For example, the pathogenicity of parvoviruses was questioned early on by difficulty in documenting an immune response to this agent, whereas the immune response to the Norwalk agent could be clearly demonstrated.

Most of the novel viral agents found in diarrheal specimens from humans are known to be agents of gastroenteritis in different animal species. Toroviruses and coronaviruses were established pathogens in animals, and picobirnaviruses were originally associated with diarrhea in pigs and passaged in the same species. The fact that a virus can cause diarrhea in another animal model provides a measure of biological plausibility and affirms that the virus can home to gut cells in the animal, replicate in a mammalian host, and is not a pathogen of another microorganism in the gut (e.g., parasite, helminth, or bacteria). Consequently, while phages can be seen in many fecal specimens, they have never been associated with diarrhea in animals or humans, cause no immune response in the host, and are recognized pathogens of bacteria rather than the human host.

In establishing causality, several other lines of evidence are helpful although often difficult to establish (13,14). In general, one would expect the onset of disease to correspond with the onset of infection and the termination of disease to correspond with the termination of infection. At the period of most intense diarrhea, the virus is often shed in its highest concentration. For all viral pathogens that have been intensively studied, asymptomatic infections can occur although virus is often present in substantially lower titers than in patients with acute diarrhea. Of note, new diagnostic tests like polymerase chain reaction (PCR) and cultivation may detect very low titers of virus that may be normally present in the gut but not be pathogenic. As more sensitive assays are employed, we will learn more about the normal viral flora of the gut and what level of virus might be associated with illness. Finally, many different microorganisms, as well as toxins, drugs, allergies, and other conditions, have been associated with gastroenteritis. In establishing the pathogenicity of a new viral agent, one would like to make certain that these other etiologic agents or conditions are not present simultaneously. These requirements for a novel agent to be considered an etiologic agent are similar to those postulates outlined by Robert Koch for infectious agents and A. B. Hill for use with epidemiologic data (14).

Review of Agents

Table 3 provides a listing of viruses that may cause gastroenteritis in humans, which includes details on their sizes and morphology. Illustrations are shown in Figure 1.

Picobirnavirus

Picobirnaviruses are small (pico), bisegmented (bi), double-stranded (ds) ribonucleic acid (RNA) viruses that were first identified by Pereira et al. in 1988 (15). The virus was first found by polyacrylamide gel electrophoresis (PAGE) analysis of RNA extracted from the intestinal contents of a rat. The bands were determined to be dsRNA with lengths of approximately 2.6 and 1.5 kb, respectively. The virus has a density of 1.38 to 1.40 g/mL and appears as a 35-nm discrete small round virus without distinctive surface structure. Since the original description of the virus, picobirnaviruses have been detected in fecal specimens of a variety of animal species, including guinea pigs (16), pigs (17,18), calves (19), rabbits (20), birds (21), and humans (22), and have varied with some strains having two segmented dsRNA bands and others with three distinct dsRNA bands (trirnaviruses) (23). Gatti et al. (17) observed that the virus was more common in pigs with diarrhea than in control animals, thereby linking the presence of the picobirnaviruses with diarrhea. Picobirnaviruses have been propagated in mammalian cell cultures as well (24).

In humans, picobirnaviruses have been identified in fecal specimens collected in various settings. After the original identification from fecal specimens in Brazil, these viruses were identified in fecal specimens from children or adults with gastroenteritis in Venezuela (23), England (20), and the United States (25), and in people without diarrhea in England (20). Only in an American study of a cohort of HIV-infected patients was picobirnavirus significantly linked with diarrhea (25). Six of 65 HIV-infected patients with diarrhea excreted picobirnavirus compared with 1 of 65 HIV-infected patients without diarrhea ($P = 0.11$). Nonetheless, these patients had ten distinct episodes of diarrhea from which picobirnavirus was detected compared with only two episodes in a control group without diarrhea ($P = 0.02$). Infected patients tended to excrete the virus for prolonged periods of time and one patient excreted the virus for 8 months. No immune response could be detected in the sera of these pa-

TABLE 3. *Viruses that may cause gastroenteritis in humans*

		Virus description			Enteric disease in	
Virus	Family	Size (nm)	Nucleic acid	Morphology—EM	Animals	Humans
Coronavirus	Coronaviridae	60–2200	+ ssRNA	Enveloped, pleomorphic, fringed	Diarrhea in cows and other animals	? diarrhea, ? NEC, ? tropical sprue
Torovirus	Coronaviridae genus *Torovirus*	100–150	+ ssRNA	Enveloped, pleomorphic, fringed	Diarrhea in cows (Breda)	?Diarrhea in children
Picobirnavirus	Not classified	35	dsRNA, two segments	SRV	Diarrhea in pigs; infections in pigs, hamsters, rabbits, and birds	?Diarrhea in HIV-infected humans
Reovirus	Reoviridae	70–75	dsRNA, ten segments	Spoked wheel-shape, double capsid		?Diarrhea, no confirmed disease, ?biliary atresia
Enterovirus	Picornaviridae	26–28	ssRNA	SRV		?Outbreaks of diarrhea due to select types
Parvovirus	Parvoviridae	20–30	ssDNA	SRV	Diarrhea in cows, cats, mink, and dogs	?Diarrhea

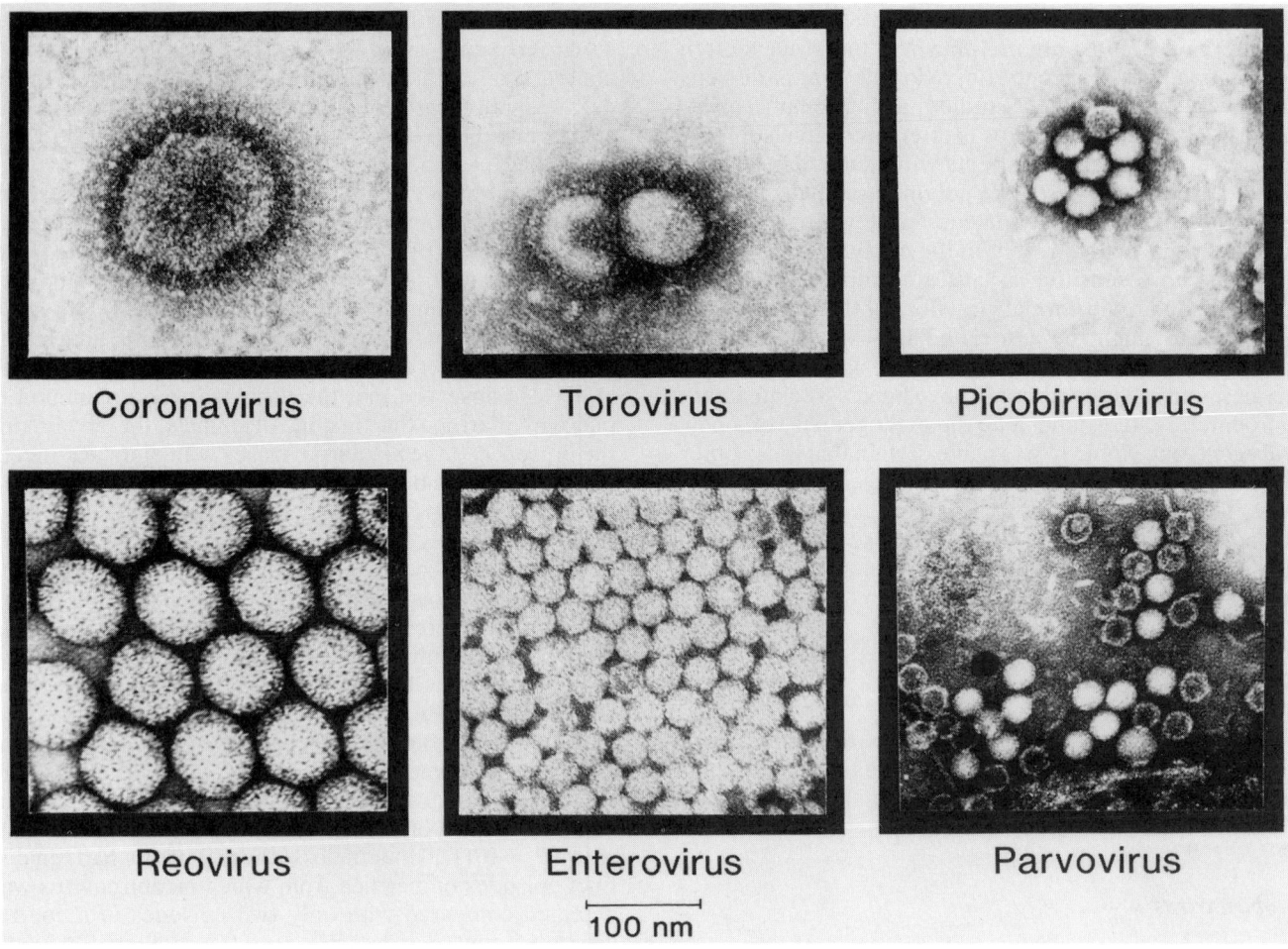

FIG. 1. Viruses that may cause gastroenteritis in humans.

tients by IEM, an observation that was difficult to assess given the severe stage of disease of these immunocompromised patients. Similar rates of detection have been found among HIV-infected persons in Australia and Venezuela (G. S. Grohmann and F. Liprandi, *personal communications*).

While no immune response could be documented in these HIV-infected patients, an immune response could be documented by solid-phase IEM in rabbits experimentally infected with picobirnavirus. The demonstration of an immune response that was associated in time with the period of virus excretion and the ability to culture an animal strain in a mammalian cell line both suggest that picobirnavirus is a virus of vertebrates.

Diagnosis of picobirnavirus rests with the identification of two segments by PAGE examination of RNA extracted from fecal specimens. Recent evidence suggests that the sensitivity of detection can be increased at least fourfold if the RNA is first concentrated (25). The role of the virus as a pathogen in humans remains in question, and improvements in diagnostic assays are needed to examine the epidemiology and association of this novel agent with diarrhea (20).

Toroviruses

Toroviruses are enveloped, positive-strand RNA viruses that cause enteric infections and diarrhea in animals and, perhaps, humans (26–28). The virus was first identified in Berne, Switzerland, from the rectal swab of a horse with pseudomembranous enteritis attributed to *Salmonella* as well as the prototype strain-Berne virus (BEV) (29). The enteropathogenic role of toroviruses was supported by studies of Woode et al. (30) in Breda, Iowa, who found a bovine torovirus (the Breda agent, BRV) to be present in stool specimens obtained from calves with severe diarrhea during an outbreak in a dairy herd. The discovery and description of toroviruses as enteric pathogens in cows and their finding in a broad group of higher vertebrates (e.g., pigs, cats, and mice) led to an intense search to ascertain whether torovirus was also a cause of diarrhea in humans.

Studies of animals led to a broader understanding of the pathogenicity, clinical features, and epidemiology of toroviruses that has helped guide the search for human disease. While the importance of BEV as an etiologic agent of diarrhea in horses is unclear, BRV strains cause watery diarrhea in gnotobiotic calves, 24 to 48 hr after experimental infection (31). This diarrhea is accompanied by dehydration, weakness, and malabsorption measured as a reduction in xylose resorption. Infection occurs primarily in the crypt cells of the intestinal villi, particularly in the large intestine. Koopmans and co-workers (26,32) have described a high attack rate of torovirus-associated diarrhea under field conditions in The Netherlands when colostrum-fed calves were monitored prospectively. Diarrhea occurred in nine of ten calves, lasted 2 to 13 days, and caused dehydration in four animals. Symptoms were similar to those of calf rotavirus and coronavirus. Toroviruses appeared to cause respiratory or generalized infections as well and have been identified in respiratory secretions and the respiratory tract on postmortem examination. The intestines of experimentally infected cows examined on postmortem show involvement from the midjejunum to the lower small intestine, with thinning of the wall, villus fusion, atrophy, and epithelial disorientation.

Virologic studies of animal toroviruses have provided diagnostic tools that have helped in the search for toroviruses in humans. The virus, which belongs to the genus *Torovirus* and the family Coronaviridae, has an unusual, pleomorphic structure by EM (28). The viruses often appear like a misshaped donut (torus) that can be deformed to biconcave disks, or membranous particles with a wide variety of intermediate forms that make them difficult to identify except to the alert and motivated electron microscopist (33). They are 100 to 150 nm in length and have 20-nm peplomers that project from the surface like clubs or fringe. BEV is the only strain successfully adapted to grow in tissue culture.

Torovirus contains a single positive strand of RNA 25 to 30 kb long that is polyadenylated and has six open reading frames, which encode for a variety of proteins that have not been fully characterized. Several of these proteins are antigenic and lead to an immune response in experimentally infected calves (34). An immunoglobulin M (IgM) response can be measured early after infection and seroconversion by IgG occurs subsequently. Serosurveys of herds of cows indicate that most adult cows from various countries surveyed have IgG antibodies; maternal antibody is present in most newborn calves, disappears after 3 to 4 months, and is replaced by 2 years of age with antibody acquired through natural infection (35). In serosurveys, most adult horses also have antibodies to toroviruses (BEV) (36). The observation that antibodies to BEV and BRV are partially cross-reactive is based on experiments in which assays for these viruses detected antibodies in other species (i.e., goats, sheep, pigs, rabbits, and mice), suggesting that these assays might be used for serosurveys in humans (37). However, serosurveys of veterinarians and farm workers in Great Britain (37) and Switzerland, and in Indians with tropical sprue (38), were negative for antibodies to BRV, indicating either that humans have little exposure to the virus or that the human strain does not cross-react with the animal strains (37,38).

Work with animal torovirus has also led to the development of assays to detect torovirus antigen in fecal specimens. Besides EM and IEM, an enzyme-linked immu-

noadsorbent assay (ELISA) has been developed using bovine reagents (37), as well as cDNA probes for hybridization made from the BEV strain (39). Finally, reverse transcription–polymerase chain reaction (RT-PCR) has been used to detect RNA from the conserved 3' ends of the virus, and this method can detect both equine (BEV) and bovine (BRV) strains (40). These assays have not been used extensively to search for toroviruses in human fecal specimens.

The role of toroviruses as a cause of diarrhea in humans remains unanswered. Torovirus-like particles (TVLPs) have been seen by EM in fecal specimens from children and adults with diarrhea in Great Britain, France (12), and The Netherlands. However, no other assays were applied to confirm the identity of the particle or assess its etiologic role as the cause of diarrhea. Koopmans et al. (39) identified toroviral RNA by using a hybridization assay with a cDNA probe prepared from BEV, but the results were not unequivocal due to high background levels and rapid degradation of RNA in stool specimens. In Toronto, a recent survey of patients with diarrhea whose fecal specimens were screened by EM identified torovirus-like particles in 224 (8%) of 2800 specimens screened, suggesting that TVLPs may be more common in human fecal specimens than was previously determined (40). Koopmans and co-workers tested a subset of these specimens with a variety of additional diagnostic tests to determine the true identity of these particles. While molecular assays used previously gave inconclusive results, an ELISA using bovine torovirus reference reagents distinguished between those stools found to be positive for TVLPs by EM and those that were negative. This finding suggested that a two-way antigenic cross-reactivity existed between human TVLPs and bovine TVLPs and led to the use of human reagents from which human TVLP-specific antiserum was raised, and this antiserum was found to be more specific than antiserum to the bovine strain. These assays and reagents need to be applied further to other surveys to detect TVLPs.

In summary, toroviruses have been found in human stools by EM and their presence has been confirmed by immunoassay based on reagents to bovine toroviruses. Their role as etiologic agents of diarrhea in the human population remains to be determined and will rest, in part, upon finding an immune response, which is a *sine qua non* of infection (37). Improved diagnostics, particularly molecular assays based on sequence information of human TVLPs, will assist in confirming those specimens that appear to be positive by EM. The availability of new assays for TVLPs should lead rapidly to more information about their etiologic role in humans.

Coronavirus

Coronaviruses are large, enveloped, positive-strand RNA viruses belonging to the family Coronaviridae that cause gastroenteritis in many animal species but are most commonly associated with respiratory infections in humans (41). They were first reported to cause explosive diarrhea in adults (8) and were later found to be associated with tropical sprue in Indian children and adults (9). The regular finding of coronaviruses in the feces of patients with nonbacterial gastroenteritis and the recognition that coronaviruses are a common cause of diarrhea in other animal species has led many investigators to seek an etiologic role for the human enteric coronaviruses (HECVs) as an agent of gastroenteritis in humans (42,43). Despite two decades of research to test this association, the findings have been inconclusive, leaving this question unanswered.

The virus can be detected in human feces by direct EM with negative stain and appears as a pleomorphic particle 60 to 2200 nm in diameter, covered with a distinct, crownlike (corona) fringe made up of regularly spaced, clubshaped projections approximately 20 nm long (44). This fringe is often disrupted, leaving a particle that could easily be confused with cellular debris in the stool (45). In the absence of any confirmatory assay, all particles found in fecal specimens are referred to as "coronavirus-like particles" (CVLPs). These are distinct from the coronaviruses present in the human respiratory tract that are a recognized cause of acute infections and for which confirmatory diagnostic assays are available. Human respiratory coronaviruses cross-react with enteric coronaviruses by IEM (46,47), but not by ELISA or immunoblots (48,49).

Since EM is the only method routinely used to search for coronaviruses in fecal specimens and since the particles are pleomorphic, variations in the prevalence of infection observed in epidemiologic studies may reflect more the ability of and the criteria used by the electron microscopist than the true prevalence of infection. The prevalence of CVLPs observed in a recent 3-year survey of more than 50,000 stool examinations conducted by electron microscopists in England indicated that about 0.7 CVLPs were detected for every 100 rotaviruses, and this rate varied from 0% to 2.3% (50). A similar 6-year survey of electron microscopists at ten centers in the United States indicated that from more than 50,000 EM examinations, CVLPs were detected in about 6% of specimens and detection rates ranged from 0% at three centers to 13% at one center, where rates have always been reported high (51–53). CVLPs had no distinct seasonality and were found in both children and adults. Given the variable range and prevalence within a single country, the results obtained from surveys in many other countries are hard to interpret. What is clear is that CVLPs appear to have a global distribution (54–58), are more commonly found in the stools of infants and children than in adults, and do not appear to have a distinct seasonality in their distribution or known mode of transmission. Fewer studies have compared the rates of CVLPs among patients with diarrhea and among controls or have monitored the duration of viral shedding. Some investigators have found more CVLPs in patients with diarrhea than in controls (46,59). Others have found CVLPs to be as common in patients with diarrhea as in controls without diarrhea (44,56,60), raising doubts about their etiologic role. Since asymptomatic shedding is common, and since CVLPs can be excreted for long periods in healthy people, it may

be difficult to prove pathogenicity merely by comparing prevalence in patients with and without diarrhea.

Several investigators have identified CVLPs in stools of infants with necrotizing enterocolitis and tried to implicate this virus as the causative agent (61,62). In 1985, Resta et al. (48) reported the first successful propagation of one such CVLP and the development of confirmatory assays for this infection. In the subsequent decade, efforts to reproduce these results have been unsuccessful, raising doubts about their initial validity. Others have found CVLPs in intestinal lesions of patients with necrotizing enterocolitis (NEC), but in the absence of confirmatory assays the virus could not be distinguished from other cellular material with similar morphologic features (63). In 1975, Mathan et al. (9) found CVLPs to be more common in fecal specimens from patients with tropical sprue. They later described virus-like particles in the cisternae of the smooth endoplasmic reticulum of damaged crypt cells (64). Despite these observations, the etiology of tropical sprue remains unknown and the association with coronavirus has not been confirmed.

In summary, CVLPs are found in fecal specimens from humans and are most frequently detected in specimens from infants and young children by EM. It is often difficult to distinguish CVLPs from other cellular debris present in stool, and no independent culture method or antigenic or molecular-based assays are currently available to confirm the identity of the virus. Hence any attempt to prove the association of CVLPs with human disease must await the development of diagnostic reagents prepared from fecal specimens or cultures of virus of human origin.

Enteroviruses

The enteroviruses were among the first viral agents suggested to be causative agents of nonbacterial gastroenteritis in humans (65). These viruses were among the first to be successfully cultivated from stools, and their considerable antigenic diversity with multiple serotypes perhaps ensured that at least some might be implicated as an agent of gastroenteritis in humans. Some of these viruses appeared to cause respiratory infections or viral syndrome in which gastroenteritis might be an associated symptom rather than the prime presentation of infection. In many early studies, individual serotypes of enteroviruses (echoviruses 4, 11, 14, 18, 19) were tentatively associated with gastroenteritis even though full evidence for causality was lacking (1,66). Over time, these associations have been put aside and, today, enteroviruses are not generally considered to be causative agents of gastroenteritis in humans, even though several serotypes may well be diarrheal pathogens.

The enteroviruses are positive-strand RNA viruses that combine the polioviruses, coxsackieviruses, and echoviruses, all of which are found in the human intestine. Enteroviruses are small (20 to 30 nm), nonenveloped viruses that appear as small round viruses (SRVs) or small round featureless viruses by EM since they have none of the distinct morphologic features of the SRSVs, which include both the caliciviruses and astroviruses (67). More than 70 serotypes of enteroviruses have been identified, and in humans these are associated with a wide variety of clinical illnesses, ranging from acute respiratory infections, hemorrhagic conjunctivitis, aseptic meningitis, and encephalitis, to carditis. Because of the great antigenic diversity of this group, neutralization tests are required to characterize the agent and to detect a type-specific immune response in infected patients. Detection is by cultivation of stool specimens, EM detection of SRVs, or hybridization using oligonucleotide probes common to all enteroviruses, and subsequent typing by neutralization (68).

Epidemiologic studies to examine whether enteroviruses cause diarrhea have rested either on the investigation of specimens collected from longitudinal studies or case–control studies of diarrhea in children or on the examination of fecal specimens collected in outbreaks of nonbacterial gastroenteritis. In outbreaks, one assumes that a single serotype would be involved and that this serotype would be detected more frequently among cases with diarrhea than controls who were well. Eichenwald and colleagues (69) identified echovirus 18 among premature infants with diarrhea in a nursery and in sick infants less than 5 months of age on a hospital ward. Investigations of other outbreaks have implicated serotypes 1, 2, 6, 7, 11, 14, 19, 20, and 22 to be associated with diarrhea (66,70–77). Here, the finding of the same organism in more than one child with symptoms supported an etiologic role but did not confirm it. Moreover, the virus was often identified in other children who did not have diarrhea. At the time of these studies, many other diarrheal pathogens that are currently recognized had not yet been discovered and could therefore not be ruled out.

Case–control and longitudinal studies have compared detection rates and serotypes of enteroviruses in children with diarrhea and in those without diarrhea. Ramos-Alvarez and Sabin (77) implicated enterovirus types 2, 6, 7, 8, 10, 11, 12, 14, 18, and 19 as the agents of summer diarrhea in 42% of young children with diarrhea compared with 13% of those without diarrhea. Sommerville (78) isolated echovirus strains 6, 7, 9, 11, and 13 from 8.5% of 338 children with diarrhea but only 2.5% of 115 children the same age with respiratory infections. Other investigators have failed to support these findings. Yow et al. (79), for example, isolated enteroviruses in 5.6% of 390 infants with diarrhea compared with 4.4% of 380 controls, giving numbers too small to establish an etiologic role for all enteroviruses or for any individual serotype. Since many of these serotypes are common respiratory pathogens in children, it is difficult to determine whether these were primary enteric infections or whether the diarrheal illness was secondary to a respiratory infection, possibly mediated by use of medications or altered diet.

Despite the wealth of early studies implicating enteroviruses as potential causes of diarrhea, the large number of types and the low frequency of any single type have made it difficult to unequivocally implicate individual strains as a cause of diarrhea (70). In outbreaks, a number of enteroviruses have been identified from patients with gastroenteritis, suggesting that they may have an etiologic role in some settings. Nonetheless, given the large number

of serotypes and a relatively small contribution of any individual serotype, very large longitudinal studies or more outbreak investigations would be required to arrive at a conclusion concerning causality. Even then, it may be difficult to separate infections for which diarrhea is the prime illness from those where gastrointestinal symptoms were secondary to other infections.

Reoviruses

The first reoviruses were identified in the early 1950s from fecal specimens of persons who clinically did not have a gastrointestinal illness (80). While these viruses were initially thought to be in the enterovirus group, they were later distinguished by their larger size (75 nm), cytoplasmic inclusions produced in monkey kidney tissue cells, patterns of hemagglutination of human type O erythrocytes, and pathogenicity for newborn mice. Sabin proposed the name reovirus to emphasize that they were respiratory and enteric isolates that were not associated with disease (orphan). Later, the virus was found to contain ten segments of dsRNA that was specific for this virus group, and these viruses were reclassified in a new family, Reoviridae.

Members of the Reoviridae family are found in a wide host of animals from insects and crustaceans to vertebrates, including mammals. In mammals other than humans, they produce a range of upper respiratory and enteric symptoms, with diarrhea occurring as one of the many presentations in mice, infant and adult cows, sheep, pigs, and dogs. While reoviruses have been periodically implicated as etiologic agents of diarrhea in humans (75,77,81,82), studies so far have been inconclusive, and they are currently not considered causative agents of diarrhea. Reoviruses have also been implicated in biliary atresia (83–86), but this association has never been confirmed. Despite the availability of good diagnostic assays for detecting these agents in humans, the reoviruses are only occasionally identified in a human fecal specimen and are probably unrelated to diarrhea.

Parvovirus

Parvoviruses are small (20 to 30 nm), round, featureless single-stranded DNA viruses that can be distinguished from the enteroviruses by their different buoyant density in cesium chloride, from the Norwalk viruses by their featureless surface and slightly smaller size, and from both of these RNA viruses by their nucleic acids (87). Several animal parvoviruses, including strains from cows, cats, mink, and dogs, have been well characterized and appear to cause gastroenteritis in these species (88). In humans, the search for a comparable pathogenic strain has been elusive.

Several outbreaks of gastroenteritis have been identified in which a SRV was seen by EM that could not be cultivated but resembled parvovirus in morphology, size, or buoyant density (10,11,89). These SRVs were often found with other established pathogens (e.g., astroviruses, caliciviruses, or SRSVs). In the absence of alternative immune or nucleic acid based assays to characterize the strain, no final identification was made. No distinct seroconversion could be observed in paired sera collected from patients involved in these outbreaks, raising questions about their true infectious potential. B19, the only recognized parvovirus in humans, causes aplastic anemia, erythema infectiosum (fifth disease), and possible birth defects but is not associated with gastroenteritis. B19 is distinct from the enteric candidate parvoviruses based on the lack of antigenic cross-reactivity and failure to cross-hybridize, using nucleic acid probes. Both the identity of the fecal parvoviruses and their role in gastroenteritis remain in question.

SUMMARY

While many viruses inhabit the gut, relatively few directly cause diarrhea. Some agents, such as the reoviruses and enteroviruses, survive well in the human intestine, can easily be identified and characterized by culture, and probably cause little, if any, diarrhea. Others that grow poorly, like toroviruses, picobirnaviruses, and coronaviruses, cause diarrhea in animals and may well cause diarrhea in humans, although this may not be common. Finally, a third group of viruses are generally found elsewhere in the body but can be opportunists in the gut and are infrequently, if ever, even secondarily associated with gastroenteritis. When a virus is identified in a stool of a patient with gastroenteritis, its identity must be confirmed, other common agents of gastroenteritis must be ruled out, and an immune response must be documented before any thought can be given to its role as the causative agent.

REFERENCES

1. Madeley CR. Epidemiology of gut viruses, p. 5–15. In: Farthing, MJG, ed. *Viruses and the gut*. London: Smith Kline and French Laboratories Ltd, 1989.
2. Kapikian AZ, Chanock RM. Norwalk group of viruses, p. 671–693. In: Fields BN, Knipe DM, Chanock RM, Hirsch MS, Melnick JL, Monath TP, Roizman B, eds. *Virology*, vol 1, 2nd ed. New York: Raven Press, 1990.
3. Yow MD, Melnick JL, Blattner RJ, Stephenson WB, Robinson NM, Burkhardt MA. The association of viruses and bacteria with infantile diarrhea. *Am J Epidemiol* 1970;92:33–39.
4. Reiman HA, Price AH, Hodges JH. The cause of epidemic diarrhea, nausea and vomiting (viral dysentery?). *Proc Soc Exp Biol Med* 1945;59:8–9.
5. Gordon I, Ingraham HS, Korns RF. Transmission of epidemic gastroenteritis to human volunteers by oral administration of fecal filtrates. *J Exp Med* 1947;86:409–422.
6. Kapikian AZ, Wyatt RG, Dolin R, Thornhill TS, Kalica AR, Chanock RM. Visualization by immune electron microscopy of a 27 nm particle associated with acute infectious nonbacterial gastroenteritis. *J Virol* 1972;10:1075–1081.
7. Bishop RF, Davidson GP, Holmes IH, Ruck BJ. Virus particles in epithelial cells of duodenal mucosa from children with viral gastroenteritis. *Lancet* 1973;1:1281–1283.
8. Caul EO, Paver WK, Clarke SK. Coronavirus particles in faeces from patients with gastroenteritis [Letter]. *Lancet* 1975;1:1192.
9. Mathan M, Mathan VI, Swaminathan SP, Yesudoss S, Baker SJ. Pleomorphic virus-like particles in human faeces. *Lancet* 1975;1:1068–1069.
10. Appleton H, Higgins PG. Viruses and gastroenteritis in infants [Letter]. *Lancet* 1975;1:1297.
11. Clarke SKR, Cook GT, Egglestone SI, et al. A virus from epidemic vomiting disease. *Br Med J* 1972;3:86–89.
12. Beards GM, Green J, Hall C, Flewett TH, Lamouliatte F, Du-Pasquier P. An enveloped virus in stools of children and adults with gastroenteritis that resembles the Breda virus of calves. *Lancet* 1984;1:1050–1052.
13. Huebner RJ. Criteria for etiologic association of prevalent viruses with prevalent diseases. *Ann NY Acad Sci* 1957;67:430–438.
14. Hill AB. The environment and disease: association or causation. *Proc R Soc Med* 1965;58:295–300.
15. Pereira HG, Flewett TH, Candeias JAN, Barth OM. A virus with a bisegmented double-stranded RNA genome in rat (*Oryzomys nigripes*) intestines. *J Gen Virol* 1988;69:2749–2754.
16. Pereira HG, de Araujo HP, Fialho AM, de Castro L, Monteiro SP. A virus with bi-segmented double-stranded RNA genome in guinea pig intestines. *Mem Inst Oswaldo Cruz* 1989;84:137–140.
17. Gatti MSV, Pestana de Castro AF, Ferraz MMG, Fialho AM, Pereira HG. Viruses with bisegmented double-stranded RNA in pig faeces. *Res Vet Sci* 1989;47:397–398.
18. Chasey D. Porcine picobirnavirus in UK? *Vet Rec* 1990;126:465.
19. Vanopdenbosch E, Wellemans G. Bovine birna type virus: a new etiological agent of neonatal calf diarrhoea? *Vlaams Diergeneeskd Tijdschr* 1990;59:1–4.
20. Gallimore C, Lewis D, Brown D. Detection and characterization of a novel bisegmented double-stranded RNA virus (picobirnavirus) from rabbit faeces. *Arch Virol* 1993;133:63–73.
21. Leite JPG, Monteiro SP, Fialho AM, Pereira HG. A novel avian virus with trisegmented double-stranded RNA and further observations on previously described similar viruses with bisegmented genome. *Virus Res* 1990;16:119–126.
22. Pereira HG, Fialho AM, Flewett TH, Teixeira JMS, Andrade ZP. Novel viruses in human feces. *Lancet* 1988;2:103–104.
23. Ludert JE, Liprandi F. Identification of viruses with bi- and trisegmented double-stranded RNA genome in faeces of children with gastroenteritis. *Inst Pasteur/Elsevier* 1993;144:219–224.
24. Pereira HG. Double-stranded RNA viruses. *Semin Virol* 1991;2:39–53.
25. Grohmann GS, Glass RI, Pereira HG, Monroe SS, Hightower AW, Weber R, Bryan RT. Enteric viruses and diarrhea in HIV-infected patients. *N Engl J Med* 1993;329:14–20.
26. Koopmans M, Horzinek M. *Toroviruses of animals and humans*. 1993:1–68.
27. Horzinek MC, Flewett T, Saif L, Spaan WJM, Weiss M, Woode GN. A new family of vertebrate viruses: toroviridae. *Intervirology* 1987;27:17–24.
28. Weiss M, Horzinek M. The proposed family Toroviridae: agents of enteric infections. *Arch Virol* 1987;92:1–15.
29. Weiss M, Steck F, Horzinek MC. Purification and partial characterization of a new enveloped RNA virus (Berne virus). *J Gen Virol* 1983;64:1849.
30. Woode GN, Reed DE, Runnels PL, Herig MA, Hill HT. Studies with an unclassified virus isolated from diarrheic calves. *Vet Microbiol* 1982;7:221–240.
31. Pohlenz JFL, Cheville NF, Woode GN, Mokresh AH. Cellular lesions in intestinal mucosa of gnotobiotic calves experimentally infected with a new unclassified bovine virus (Breda virus). *Vet Pathol* 1984;21:407.
32. Koopmans M, van Wuijckhuise-Sjouke L, Schukken YH, Cremers H, Horzinek MC. Association of diarrhea in cattle with torovirus infections on farms. *Am J Vet Res* 1991;52:1769–1773.
33. Fagerland JA, Pohlenz JFL, Woode GN. A morphologic study of the replication of Breda virus (proposed family Toroviridae) in bovine intestinal cells. *J Gen Virol* 1986;67:1293–1304.
34. Koopmans M, van den Boom U, Woode G, Horzinek MC. Seroepidemiology of Breda virus in cattle using ELISA. *Vet Microbiol* 1989;19:223–243.
35. Koopmans M, Cremers H, Woode G, Horzinek MC. Breda virus (Toroviridae) infection and systemic antibody response in sentinel calves. *Am J Vet Res* 1990;51:1443–1448.

36. Weiss M, Steck F, Kaderli R, Horzinek MC. Antibodies to Berne virus in horses and other animals. *Vet Microbiol* 1984;9: 523–531.

37. Brown DWG, Beards GM, Flewett TH. Detection of Breda virus antigen and antibody in humans and animals by enzyme immunoassay. *J Clin Microbiol* 1987;24:637–640.

38. Brown DWG, Selvakumar R, Daniel DJ, Mathan VI. Prevalence of neutralizing antibodies to Berne virus in animals and humans in Vellore, South India. *Arch Virol* 1988;98:267–269.

39. Koopmans M, Snijder EJ, Horzinek MC. cDNA probes for the detection of bovine torovirus (Breda virus) infections. *J Clin Microbiol* 1991;29:493–497.

40. Koopmans M, Petric M, Glass RI, Monroe SS. Enzyme-linked immunosorbent assay reactivity of torovirus-like particles in fecal specimens from humans with diarrhea. *J Clin Microbiol* 1993;31:2738–2744.

41. McIntosh K. Coronaviruses. In: Fields BN, Knipe DM, Chanock RM, Hirsch MS, Melnick JL, Monath TP, Roizman B, eds. *Virology,* vol 1, 2nd ed. New York: Raven Press, 1990; 857–864.

42. Macnaughton MR, Davies HA. Human enteric coronaviruses. *Arch Virol* 1981;70(4):301–313.

43. Clarke SK, Caul EO, Egglestone SI. The human enteric coronaviruses. *Postgrad Med J* 1979;55:135–142.

44. Saif LJ, Heckert RA. Enteric coronaviruses. In: Saif LJ, Theil KW, eds. *Viral diarrheas of man and animals.* Boca Raton, FL: CRC Press, 1990;185–252.

45. Dourmashkin RR, Davies HA, Smith H, Bird RG. Are coronavirus-like particles seen in diarrhoea stools really viruses? *Lancet* 1980;2:971.

46. Gerna G, Passarani N, Battaglia M, Revello MG, Torre D, Cereda PM. Coronaviruses and gastroenteritis: evidence of antigenic relatedness between human enteric coronavirus strains and human coronavirus OC43. *Microbiologica* 1984;7:315.

47. Gerna G, Passerani N, Cereda PM, Battaglia M. Antigenic relatedness of human enteric coronavirus strains to human coronavirus OC43: a preliminary report. *J Infect Dis* 1984;150:618.

48. Resta S, Luby JP, Rosenfeld CR, Siegel JD. Isolation and propagation of a human enteric coronavirus. *Science* 1985;229: 978–981.

49. Battaglia M, Passarani N, Di Matteo A, Gerna G. Human enteric coronaviruses: further characterizations and immunoblotting of viral proteins. *J Infect Dis* 1987;155:140–143.

50. Monroe SS, Glass RI, Noah N, et al. Electronmicroscopic reporting of gastrointestinal viruses in the United Kingdom, 1985–87. *J Med Virol* 1991;33:193–198.

51. Lew JF, Glass RI, Petric M, et al. Six year retrospective surveillance of gastroenteritis viruses identified at ten electron microscopy centers in the United States and Canada. *Pediatr Infect Dis J* 1990;9:709–714.

52. Payne CM, Ray CG, Bourdin V, Minnich LL, Lebowitz MD. An eight-year study of the viral agents of acute gastroenteritis in humans: ultrastructural observations and seasonal distribution with a major emphasis on coronavirus-like particles. *Diagn Microbiol Infect Dis* 1986;5:39–54.

53. Mortensen ML, Ray CG, Payne CM, Friedman AD, Minnich LL, Rousseau C. Coronavirus-like particles in human gastrointestinal disease. *Am J Dis Child* 1985;139:928.

54. Schnagl RD, Morey R, Homes IH. Rotavirus and coronavirus-like particles in aboriginal and non-aboriginal neonates in Kalgoorlie and Alice Springs. *Med J Aust* 1979;2:178.

55. Yongnian H, Wang NL, Lo HN, Nie AG, Li A. A finding of coronavirus particles in feces of patients with diarrhea. *Chin J Epidemiol* 1987;8:25.

56. Bennett PH, Gust ID. Coronavirus-like particles and other agents in the faeces of children in Efate, Vanuatu. *J Trop Med Hyg* 1982;85:213.

57. Simhon A, Mata L. Fecal rotaviruses, adenoviruses, coronavirus-like particles, and small round viruses in a cohort of rural Costa Rican children. *Am J Trop Med Hyg* 1985;34:931.

58. Sitbon M. Human-enteric-coronavirus-like particles (CVLP) with different epidemiological characteristics. *J Med Virol* 1985; 16:67.

59. Vaucher YE, Ray CG, Minnich LL, Payne CM, Beck D, Lowe

60. Maass G, Baumeister HG. Coronavirus-like particles as aetiolgical agents of acute non-bacterial gastroenteritis in humans. In: Karger S, Basel M, eds. *Developments in Biological Standardization: International Symposium on Enteric Infection in Man and Animals: Standardization of Immunology Proceedings,* vol 5. Dublin: 1982;319.

61. Siegel JD, Luby JP, Laptook AR, Butler S. Identification of coronavirus (CRNV) in a premature nursery during an outbreak of necrotizing enterocolitis (NEC) and diarrhea (D). *Pediatr Res* 1983;17:181A.

62. Chany C, Moscovici O, Lebon P, Rousset S. Association of coronavirus-like infection with neonatal necrotizing enterocolitis. *Pediatrics* 1982;69:209.

63. Moscovici O, Chany C, Lebon P, Rousset S, Laporte J. Association d'infection a coronavirus avec l'enterocolite hemorragique du nouveau-ne. *C R Acad Sci Paris* 1980;290:869–872.

64. Baker SJ, Mathan M, Mathan VI, Jesudoss S, Swaminathan SP. Chronic enterocyte infection with coronavirus: one possible cause of the syndrome of tropical sprue? *Dig Dis Sci* 1982;27: 1039–1043.

65. Melnick JL. Enteroviruses: polioviruses, coxsackieviruses, echoviruses, and newer enteroviruses. In: Fields BN, Knipe DM, Chanock RN, Hirsch MS, Melnick JL, Monath TP, Roizman B, eds. *Virology,* vol 1, 2nd ed. New York: Raven Press, 1990;549–605.

66. Kibrick S. Current status of coxsackie and ECHO viruses in human disease. *Prog Med Virol* 1964;6:27–70.

67. Caul EO, Appleton H. The electron microscopical and physical characteristics of small round human fecal viruses: an interim scheme for classification. *J Med Virol* 1982;9:257–265.

68. Morens DM, Pallansch MA, Moore M. Polioviruses and other enteroviruses. In: Belshe RB, ed. *Textbook of human virology,* 2nd ed. St Louis: Mosby Year Book, 1991;484–494.

69. Eichenwald HF, Ababio A, Arky AM, Hartmen AP. Epidemic diarrhea in premature and older infants caused by ECHO virus type 18. *JAMA* 1958;166:1563–1566.

70. Melnick JL. Enteroviruses. In: Evans AS, ed. *Viral infections of humans, epidemiology and control.* New York: Plenum Press, 1978.

71. Wenner HA. The ECHO viruses. *Ann NY Acad Sci* 1991;101: 398–412.

72. McAllister RM. Echovirus infections. *Pediatr Clin North Am* 1960;7:927–945.

73. Parrott RH. The clinical importance of group A coxsackie viruses. *Ann NY Acad Sci* 1957;67:230–240.

74. Sanford JP, Sulkin SE. The clinical spectrum of echovirus infection. *N Engl J Med* 1959;261:1113–1122.

75. Ramos-Alvarez M. Cytopathogenic enteric viruses associated with undifferentiated diarrheal syndromes in early childhood. *Ann NY Acad Sci* 1957;67:326–331.

76. Klein JO, Lerner AM, Finland M. Acute gastroenteritis associated with ECHO virus, type 11. *Am J Med Sci* 1960;240:749–753.

77. Ramos-Alvarez M, Sabin AB. Enteropathogenic viruses and bacteria. Role in summer diarrheal diseases of infancy and early childhood. *JAMA* 1958;167:147–156.

78. Sommerville RG. Enteroviruses and diarrhoea in young persons. *Lancet* 1958;2:1347–1349.

79. Yow MD, Melnick JL, Blattner RJ, Rasmussen LE. Enteroviruses in infantile diarrhea. *Am J Hyg* 1963;77:283–292.

80. Tyler KL, Fields BN. Reoviruses. In: Fields BN, Knipe DM, Chanock RM, Hirsch MS, Melnick JL, Monath TP, Roizman B, eds. *Virology,* vol 2, 2nd ed. New York: Raven Press, 1990; 1307–1328.

81. Ramos-Alvarez M, Sabin AB. Characteristics of poliomyelitis and other enteric viruses recovered in tissue culture from healthy American children. *Proc Soc Exp Biol Med* 1954;87: 655–661.

82. Rosen L, Hovis JF, Mastrota FM, Bell JA, Huebner RJ. An outbreak of infection with a type 1 reovirus among children in an institution. *Am J Hyg* 1960;71:266–274.

83. Bangaru B, Morecki R, Glaser JH, Gartner LM, Horwitz MS. Comparative studies of biliary atresia in human newborn and

reovirus-induced cholangitis in weanling mice. *Lab Invest* 1980; 43:456–462.

84. Glaser JH, Balistreri WF, Morecki R. Role of reovirus type 3 in persistent infantile cholestasis. *Pediatrics* 1984;105:912–915.

85. Glaser JH, Morecki R. Reovirus type 3 and neonatal cholestasis. *Semin Liver Dis* 1987;7:100–107.

86. Morecki R, Glaser JH, Cho S, Balistreri WF, Horwitz MS. Biliary atresia and reovirus type 3 infection. *N Engl J Med* 1982; 307:481–484.

87. Pattison JR. Parvoviruses: medical and biological aspects. In: Fields BN, Knipe DM, Chanock RN, Hirsch MS, Melnick JL, Monath TP, Roizman B, eds. *Virology,* vol 2, 2nd ed. New York: Raven Press, 1990;1766–1784.

88. Bridger JC. Small viruses associated with gastroenteritis in animals. In: Saif LJ, Thiel KW, eds. *Viral diarrheas of man and animals.* Boca Raton, FL: CRC Press, 1989;161–182.

89. Appleton H. Small round viruses: classification and role in foodborne infections. In: *Novel diarrhoea viruses.* Ciba Foundation Symposium 128. New York: Wiley, 1987;108–125.

Infections of the Gastrointestinal Tract,
edited by M. J. Blaser, P. D. Smith, J. I. Ravdin,
H. B. Greenberg, and R. L. Guerrant
Raven Press, Ltd., New York © 1995.

CHAPTER 70

Amebiasis

Sharon L. Reed and Jonathan I. Ravdin

Amebiasis, colitis, and invasive extraintestinal disease due to *Entamoeba histolytica* are some of the great parasitic diseases of humans. This enteric protozoan is the third leading parasitic cause of death worldwide (1); currently there is no vaccine or form of chemoprophylaxis available. The organism spreads by direct fecal–oral contact or contamination of food and water due to poor sanitary facilities and practices; therefore the disease burden is concentrated in the poorest, least-developed regions. Recent investigations of the parasite's pathogenic mechanisms and the host's immune response provide promise for vaccine development.

BIOLOGY

The life cycle of *E. histolytica* is relatively straightforward, in comparison to the nematodes and cestodes that parasitize the gut (Fig. 1). The cyst is the infective form due to its chitinous cell wall (a polymer of *N*-acetyl-D-glucosamine) (2). Cysts can survive for weeks at an appropriate temperature and humidity. Following ingestion of the cyst, stimulation by stomach acid apparently induces excystation in the small bowel. Trophozoites go on to colonize the large bowel, feed on bacteria, and multiply or encyst depending on local conditions. The infective dose can be as little as a single cyst; the incubation period appears to diminish with the size of the infective dose (from weeks to a few days) (3). Trophozoites are not transmissible due to their rapid disintegration outside the body and susceptibility to the low pH environment of the stomach.

Entamoeba histolytica belongs to the pseudopod-forming protozoan superclass Rhizopoda within the subphylum Sarcodina (4). There is now definitive evidence that distinct pathogenic and nonpathogenic strains of *Entamoeba* exist. Studies of zymodeme analysis, the pattern of electrophoretic mobility of certain parasite isoenzymes, revealed an association of distinct zymodemes with symptomatic invasive amebic disease (5). Studies with ribonucleic acid (RNA) and deoxyribonucleic acid (DNA) probes demonstrated genetic differences between pathogenic and nonpathogenic *E. histolytica* (6–8). Ribosomal RNA probes have indicated strain specificity, further distinguishing the pathogenic from nonpathogenic isolates (6). Reports of phenotypic transformation *in vitro* due to the influence of bacterial associates were apparently flawed by inadvertent contamination of the cultures. Recently, it has been proposed that the nonpathogenic *Entamoeba* zymodemes be reclassified as *Entamoeba dispar* (9).

Entamoeba histolytica has been demonstrated to have numerous antigenic differences from *E. dispar*. Distinct epitopes of the 170-kDa heavy subunit of the galactose-inhibitable adherence protein exist in pathogenic *E. histolytica* isolates (10). Murine monoclonal antibodies have been produced that distinguish between *E. histolytica* and *E. dispar* isolates by immunofluorescence (11,12) and immunoblotting (13). For example, antibodies to a recombinant form of the 29-kDa amebic surface antigen differentiated *E. histolytica* from *E. dispar* (14), despite the fact that the gene encoding the protein was present in all isolates. The first demonstration of genomic DNA differences was made by screening a complementary DNA (cDNA) library with pooled human immune sera to identify a cDNA clone unique to *E. histolytica* (15). Southern blotting of the cDNA probe and hybridization with an actin cDNA probe revealed significant genomic DNA differences between strains (15). The restriction fragment patterns of specific polymerase chain reaction (PCR) amplified genomic DNA fragments were also able to differentiate *E. histolytica* and *E. dispar* isolates; additional strain-specific cDNA clones have been produced (16,17). Studies of amebic ribosomal RNA were successful in differentiating strains (6,18), and genetic distance analysis also supports the existence of two distinct groups within the species previously referred to as *E. histolytica* (19).

S. L. Reed: Department of Medicine, Division of Infectious Diseases, University of California at San Diego Medical Center, San Diego, California 92103-9981.

J. I. Ravdin: Department of Medicine, Case Western Reserve University School of Medicine, and the Cleveland Veterans Affairs Medical Center, Cleveland, Ohio 44106.

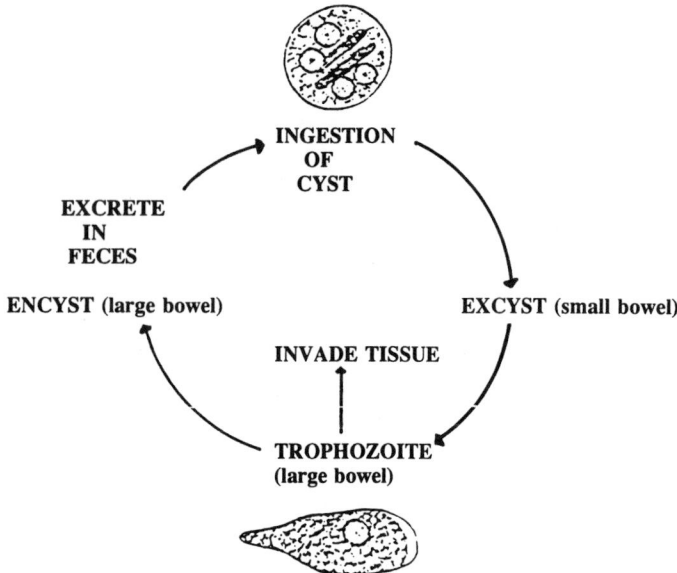

FIG. 1. Life cycle of *Entamoeba histolytica.*

The *E. dispar* and *E. histolytica* trophozoites range in size from 10 to 60 μm with a single 3- to 5-μm nucleus containing fine peripheral chromatin and a central nucleolus. The *E. histolytica* trophozoites may contain ingested erythrocytes. The amebic cytoplasm consists of a clear ectoplasm with a granular endoplasm and numerous vacuoles. Cysts of *E. dispar* and *E. histolytica* average 12 μm in diameter (range, 5 to 20 μm) and contain one to four nuclei dependent on maturity; nuclei are morphologically identical to that in trophozoites. Young cysts contain chromatoid bodies with smooth, rounded edges; these are composed of ribosome particles in crystalline arrays (20). Immature cysts often contain clumps of glycogen that stain with iodine.

To recognize patients with amebiasis, clinicians should have an in-depth knowledge of the epidemiology of the organism (Table 1). Epidemiologic surveys are difficult to interpret due to the insensitivity of a single stool examination (21,22), frequent laboratory errors made in identification of *E. dispar* (23), and the variability in detection of serum anti-amebic antibodies (*E. dispar* does not elicit a

humoral immune response). It is estimated that 10% of the world's population is infected by *E. dispar* or *E. histolytica* (1). Excluding the People's Republic of China, each year, worldwide, approximately 50 million cases of invasive disease occur, resulting in up to 100,000 deaths (1). The prevalence of infection may be as high as 50% in certain underdeveloped areas (24,25). Serologic studies in Mexico City indicate that up to 9% of the population were infected with pathogenic *E. histolytica* in the last 5 to 10 years (8,26). The prevalence of amebic infection depends on cultural habits, age (increased in school-age children), level of sanitation, crowding, and socioeconomic status (24,26). Asymptomatic intestinal infection occurs in 90% to 99% of infected individuals (21,22,27–29); usually, the parasite is eliminated from the gut within 12 months, possibly due to competition with the host's intestinal flora or as yet undefined mucosal immune mechanisms (30).

In Durban, South Africa, a 10% combined prevalence of *E. dispar* and *E. histolytica* infection resulted in 0.1% of the population suffering invasive amebiasis annually (31,32). In another study, there was a 10% risk per year of developing symptomatic invasive amebiasis following acquisition of *E. histolytica* (32). The percentage of asymptomatic intestinal infections that are pathogenic (*E. histolytica*) range from 10% in Durban, South Africa, to a surprising 96% in southeastern Mexico (33). In the latter study, PCR methodology revealed a high prevalence of mixed infection with *E. dispar* and *E. histolytica* (56%). The occurrence of asymptomatic infection in endemic areas with pathogenic *E. histolytica* accounts for the high prevalence of serum anti-amebic antibodies observed. As mentioned, and of clinical relevance, *E. dispar* infection does not elicit a serum anti-amebic antibody response (34,35).

In the United States the combined prevalence of *E. dispar* and *E. histolytica* infection is approximately 4%; however, certain high-risk groups have a high incidence of

TABLE 1. *Epidemiologic risk factors that apparently predispose to* E. histolytica *infection and increased severity of disease*

Prevalence	Increased severity
Lower socioeconomic status in an endemic area, including crowding and lack of indoor plumbing	Children, especially neonates
	Pregnancy and postpartum states
Immigrants from endemic area	
Institutionalized population, especially mentally retarded	Corticosteroid use
	Malignancy
Communal living	Malnutrition
Promiscuous male homosexuals	

From ref. 179, with permission.

infection and disease. Institutionalized populations, especially the mentally retarded, have a very high rate of infection concomitant with invasive amebiasis and significant mortality (36–38). Mass therapy or isolation of stool carriers has been unsuccessful in the long-term prevention of amebiasis within institutions (36,39). Improved housing conditions and staffing of health care personnel appear to make a substantial impact (40). In the late 1970s, there was a markedly increased prevalence of amebic infection among sexually promiscuous male homosexuals. The prevalence of *Entamoeba* infection in the gay male population of New York City and San Francisco approached 40% to 50%; however, this only resulted in occasional cases of amebic colitis, as most of the men were infected with *E. dispar* (41–45). The prevalence of *E. histolytica* infection in this population has now declined due to the changes in sexual practices that resulted from the fear of acquisition of the human immunodeficiency virus (HIV) (46). Nevertheless, a continued high index of clinical suspicion is indicated (47–49). Amebiasis is one of the causes of diarrhea in individuals with the acquired immunodeficiency syndrome (AIDS) (49a). Potential consequences of coinfection of *E. histolytica* with HIV may be enhanced HIV replication as suggested by Petri and Ravdin (49b). *Entamoeba histolytica* contains a potent T cell mitogen (49c); stimulation of HIV-infected T helper cells *in vitro* with the plant mitogen phytohemagglutinin accelerates HIV expression and T cell death (50). Croxsan and coworkers (51) demonstrated that amebic antigen increased HIV replication in a subset of subjects *in vitro;* however, there is as yet no evidence that asymptomatic infection with *E. dispar* results in systemic antigenic exposure to the host. Axenic *E. histolytica* trophozoites take up the HIV *in vitro* but do not transfer it to uninfected human cells (52). Some risk factors for amebic infection are unanticipated, such as colonic irrigation without proper sterilization of equipment at a chiropractic clinic in Colorado (53). Recent immigrants or migrant workers from endemic areas such as Mexico are an important foci of disease in the United States. The majority of cases of invasive amebiasis reported from academic institutions in the southwestern United States actually occurred in Mexican-Americans (54–59). Foreign travel to any endemic area in the world is associated with increased risk of amebiasis, especially without taking precautions to avoid enteric infection (60). The acquisition of *E. dispar* and *E. histolytica* is associated with long-term (greater than 1 month) residence in endemic areas and is usually detected only when symptomatic disease results (61,62).

PATHOGENESIS AND HOST IMMUNITY

Entamoeba histolytica is named for its lytic effect on tissue. Trophozoites appear to invade the colonic epithelium directly with diffuse mucosal damage before amebic invasion (63–65). An amorphous, granular, eosinophilic material surrounds trophozoites in tissue, whether in colon, liver, or lung (63,65,66). Inflammatory cells are found only at the periphery of established amebic lesions (63,65) due to the contact-dependent amebic lysis of neu-

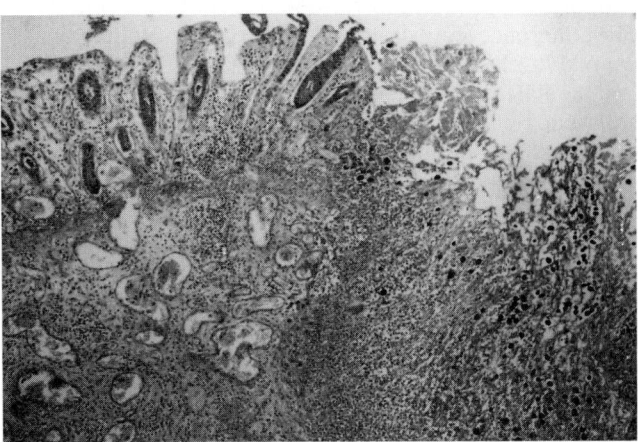

FIG. 2. Pathology of amebic colitis. Undermined colonic ulcer with trophozoites on periphery of lesion (*arrow*). H&E stain, ×100. (From ref. 178, with permission.)

trophils (67,68). This results in the release of toxic nonoxidative neutrophil products that contribute to the destruction of host tissues (69,70).

Colonic amebic lesions may manifest as nonspecific thickening of the mucosa or the classic flask-shaped ulcer (3,65) (Fig. 2). The *E. histolytica* trophozoites in tissue can be recognized by a surrounding clear halo due to fixation artifact, the presence of characteristic nuclear morphology and ingested erythrocytes, and intense staining with periodic acid–Schiff stain or detection of ingested erythrocytes by Gridley stain (71). The amebic liver "abscess" contains acellular, proteinaceous debris rather than white cells with trophozoites invading tissue in the surrounding rim (63,66). Amebae establish hepatic infection by ascending the portal venous system; triangular areas of hepatic necrosis may occur, apparently due to ischemia from amebic obstruction of portal vessels (63,72,73). Liver enzyme abnormalities, frequently present with intestinal amebiasis, are associated with periportal inflammation without demonstrable trophozoites (66,74). Periportal fibrosis has been reported and may reflect past trophozoite invasion or host reaction to amebic antigens and toxins.

The development of an axenic culture medium for *E. histolytica* stimulated a rapid expansion of research into the pathogenic mechanisms of the parasite. The pathogenesis of invasive amebiasis commences with the adherence of trophozoites to the mucins lining the luminal surface of the large bowel, followed by proteolytic degradation of the basement membrane of the mucosa, direct amebic cytolytic and proteolytic effects on tissue, and, lastly, the resistance of the parasite to host luminal and cellular defense mechanisms (75). Adherence of *E. histolytica* trophozoites to Chinese hamster ovary (CHO) cells and human colonic mucins *in vitro* is mediated by the parasite's galactose inhibitable adherence lectin (76–79). The lectin participates in adherence of *E. histolytica* trophozoites to human leukocytes (68,80), rat and human colonic mucosa and submucosa (79), human erythrocytes (76,81), opsonized bacteria or bacteria with galactose-containing lipopolysaccharide, and rat colonic epithelial cells (78). The adherence lectin is a 260-kDa surface protein, consisting of 170-kDa and 35-kDa subunits (77). The heavy subunit mediates attachment as indicated by recognition with adherence-inhibitory monoclonal antibodies (82,83) and direct galactose-binding activity of recombinant heavy subunit produced by expression-PCR methodology (84). A multigene family encodes the lectin's heavy and light subunits (85,86). The heavy subunit has a short cytoplasmic domain, a transmembrane domain, and a large extracellular portion with a highly antigenic distinct cysteine-rich area. The light subunit, in contrast, attaches to the membrane via a glycosyl-phosphatidylinositol anchor (86). There are at least seven discrete epitopes in the heavy subunit as found by monoclonal immunoglobulin G (IgG) antibody mapping (83); all are located in the cysteine-rich domain. Binding by monoclonal antibodies to the 170-kDa subunit can abrogate amebic resistance to the lytic effect of the human complement, apparently by blocking the lectin's interference with the C5b-9 membrane attack complex at the steps of C8 and C9 assembly. The lectin has sequence and antigenic similarities to the human CD59 inhibitor of C8 and C9 (87).

Axenic *E. histolytica* trophozoites kill target cells only upon direct contact in a calcium-dependent manner (78,88,89). Adherence mediated by the galactose-inhibitable lectin is absolutely required for the *in vitro* lysis of target cells. Target cell death occurs up to 20 min after attachment by trophozoites; a lethal hit can be delivered within seconds (88,89). Amebic cytolytic activity is dependent on parasite microfilament function (76,88), calcium (89,90), Ca^{2+}-dependent parasite phospholipase A (PLA) enzyme activity (90,91), and maintenance of an acid pH in amebic endocytic vesicles (92). Adherence of *E. histolytica* trophozoites is followed by a sustained elevation of target cell-free intracellular calcium concentration ($[Ca^{2+}]_i$), which contributes to, but may not be totally sufficient for, target cell death (89). The purified *E. histolytica* lectin induces a rapid but nonlethal, reversible increase in target cell $[Ca^{2+}]_i$ (93). Phorbol esters and protein kinase C activators specifically augment parasite cytolytic activity (94). *Entamoeba histolytica* contains an ionophore-like protein of 77 amino acids, with sequence homology to the saposins and to surfactant-associated protein B, that induces lipid bilayers or vesicles to leak Na^+, K^+, and, to a lesser degree, Ca^{2+} (95–97). This ionophore is packaged in dense intracellular aggregates; purified preparations can depolarize erythrocytes (98). Unfortunately, there is as yet no direct evidence that the pore-forming protein mediates parasite cytolysis of target cells following lectin binding. Recently, a number of *E. histolytica* hemolysins were found to be encoded by plasmid ribosomal DNA (99). Hemolysins were cytotoxic to an intestinal mucosal cell line, CaCo-2, and the hemolysin gene was found associated only with a more pathogenic strain (99). *Entamoeba histolytica* contains numerous proteolytic enzymes, including a cathepsin B proteinase, an acidic proteinase (100), a collagenase (101), and a well characterized major neural proteinase (102). Proteinases appear to be involved in dissolution of the extracellular matrix anchoring cells and tissue structure by invading trophozoites.

Kelsall and Ravdin (103) recently demonstrated that parasite cysteine proteinases degrade human secretory IgA molecules, a possible means of immune evasion. The 56-kDa cysteine proteinase activates complement by cleavage of C3 (104); pathogenic organisms were found to release greater amounts of the enzyme (105). Reed and co-workers (106) recently succeeded in cloning the amebic cysteine proteinase genes, demonstrating that a unique cysteine proteinase gene is present in pathogenic isolates. Amebic glycosidases, such as β-glucosaminidase (107) and a surface membrane-associated neuraminidase (108), may be involved in the degradation of colonic mucins or alteration of target cell surface membrane glycoproteins. *Entamoeba histolytica* sonicate or whole trophozoites demonstrate enterotoxigenic activity (109–111); whether this factor contributes to the diarrheal symptoms observed in intestinal amebiasis is unknown.

Host polymorphonuclear leukocytes constitute the initial host response to *E. histolytica* (69,70). Neutrophils chemotax to trophozoites (112); however, their lysis by the ameba enhances the destruction of host tissues. A further understanding of the biochemical and molecular basis for the pathogenicity of *E. histolytica* is necessary for development of an amebiasis vaccine or other intervention strategies.

Cure of amebic colitis or liver abscess apparently results in a level of immunity to recurrence of invasive amebiasis. In a 5-year follow-up of 1021 subjects in Mexico City with amebic liver abscess, only five recurrences developed. In a study of 982 subjects in a highly endemic area of India, the presence of serum anti-amebic antibodies was associated with a lower rate of intestinal infection (25). As discussed, asymptomatic infection with nonpathogenic *E. histolytica* spontaneously clears within 8 to 12 months (30). Specific human immune responses to *E. histolytica* have been well characterized, mainly following treatment of amebic liver abscess.

Patients with amebic liver abscess develop high titers of serum anti-amebic antibodies (56) by the seventh day of illness, which persist for up to 10 years. However, amebic liver abscess is a progressive, unremitting disease despite the presence of serum antibodies that are capable of inhibiting amebic adherence *in vitro* (113). By immunoblotting human sera to total parasitic protein, a set of highly conserved *E. histolytica* antigens of approximately 37, 43, 59, 90, 110, and 170 kDa has been defined (114,115). The 170-kDa antigen, the heavy subunit of the galactose-inhibitable lectin, has been recognized by antibodies in over 95% of sera from hundreds of subjects with invasive amebiasis (35). Serum antibodies from subjects residing in India, Mexico, Zaire, Egypt, South Africa, and the United States all recognize the lectin heavy subunit as purified from a single clone of an axenic strain originally isolated in Mexico City (strain HMI:IMSS), indicating a high degree of conserved antigenicity (35,116). Additional amebic antigens that have been cloned and well characterized include the 29-kDa surface antigen (117), a 125-kDa surface antigen (118), and the major cysteine proteinase (105). Sera from both healthy controls and infected patients (with high antibody titers to *E. histolytica*) are amebicidal to trophozoites through activation of the alternate and classic complement pathways (119,120). However, strains isolated from a liver abscess or colonic lesions are resistant to complement-mediated lysis (120); complement-resistant amebae can be selected *in vitro* by culture in normal human serum (121). Complement activation occurs at least in part via cleavage of C3 by the parasite's 56-kDa neutral cysteine proteinase (104). As mentioned, the lectin 170-kDa subunit inhibits assembly of C8 and C9 into the membrane attack complex, contributing to the parasite's resistance to complement-mediated lysis (87).

Recently, investigations of the mucosal immune responses to *E. histolytica* revealed that anti-amebic sIgA is produced during natural infection (122,123). Colostral anti-amebic sIgA antibodies are found during asymptomatic intestinal infection without serum anti-amebic IgA or IgG antibodies being present, suggesting mucosal immune responses to *E. dispar*. Study of salivary IgA responses to *E. histolytica* infection yielded conflicting results (124–126). Initially, an infrequent association was found between salivary anti-amebic IgA and intestinal infection (124), with none to only 36% being positive. In contrast, a strikingly positive correlation was reported between anti-*E. histolytica* IgA in whole clarified saliva and amebic infection in asymptomatic school children in Mexico (125). This study has been criticized for the possible misidentification of the smaller, identical-appearing *E. hartmanni* as *E. histolytica*, but it again suggests that a sIgA response to *E. dispar* infection does occur.

It is highly unlikely that all these asymptomatic children had pathogenic infections, although zymodeme analysis and serum antibody studies were not performed. In contrast, a follow-up study of subjects with seropositive invasive amebiasis, asymptomatic intestinal infection, and uninfected controls demonstrated that salivary anti-amebic IgA was found exclusively during invasive amebiasis (126).

Cell-mediated immune defense mechanisms clearly have an important role in limiting invasive disease and resisting a recurrence after appropriate therapy. The cell-mediated response consists of antigen-specific lymphocyte blastogenesis with production of lymphokines (including interferon-γ) capable of activating monocyte-derived macrophages to kill *E. histolytica* trophozoites *in vitro* (80,127). In addition, incubation of immune T cells with *E. histolytica* antigen *in vitro* elicits cytotoxic T lymphocyte activity against trophozoites (128). Purified 260-kDa galactose-inhibitable lectin is a highly conserved T as well as B cell antigen, eliciting lymphocyte responses in seropositive subjects (129). However, in acute disease the T lymphocyte responses to *E. histolytica* appear to be specifically depressed by a parasite-induced serum factor (130). The lack of an increased incidence of severe invasive amebiasis in AIDS patients (46) suggests that host resistance to the initial amebic invasion of the colonic mucosa does not involve cell-mediated mechanisms. Clinical correlations of the severity of established invasive disease with cell-mediated immune function include the depression of T cell numbers and delayed hypersensitivity in patients with an amebic liver abscess (112,131), the

severe exacerbation of intestinal amebiasis with the occurrence of toxic megacolon during corticosteroid therapy (132,133), and the fulminant amebic disease found in young infants and pregnant women (134–136).

Nonimmune host defenses are crucial for resistance to symptomatic invasive amebiasis. In animal models, mucous trapping of *E. histolytica* trophozoites occurs (137), and depletion of the colonic mucous blanket is always seen before parasite invasion (138). Chadee et al. (78,139) demonstrated that purified rat and human colonic mucins, rich in terminal galactose residues, act as high-affinity receptors for the *E. histolytica* lectin. Colonic mucins inhibit amebic adherence to and lysis of colonic epithelial cells *in vitro* (78). Apparently, relevant to depletion of the protective mucous blanket, *E. histolytica* trophozoites release a potent mucous secretagogue (140). Therefore colonic mucin glycoproteins act as an important host defense by binding to the parasite's adherence lectin; however, this interaction probably facilitates intestinal colonization, thus promoting parasitism by *E. histolytica*.

Interruption of transmission of *E. histolytica* requires addressing complex socioeconomic problems or inducing changes in human behavior. Clearly, the application of our knowledge of disease pathogenesis and host immunity to vaccine development would be the most efficient and cost effective means of disease prevention. The native galactose-inhibitable lectin has been demonstrated by Petri and Ravdin (141) to be highly effective as a subunit vaccine in an experimental model of amebic liver abscess in the gerbil. Numerous research groups are now working on development of recombinant vaccines to induce amebicidal cell-mediated immunity, adherence-inhibitory secretory IgA responses, or humoral immunity that contributes to protection against invasive amebiasis.

Clinical Syndromes of Amebiasis

Intestinal Amebiasis

Intestinal infection with *E. histolytica* causes a wide spectrum of disease. The major clinical syndromes fall into four groups: asymptomatic cyst passers, acute colitis, fulminant colitis, and ameboma (reviewed in refs. 142 and 143).

Asymptomatic Cyst Passers. Since an estimated 90% of patients infected with *E. histolytica* are asymptomatic (1), cyst passers are the most common presentation physicians will encounter worldwide, particularly in developed countries. Interpretation of most of the early clinical studies is difficult because they predated isoenzyme techniques and thus probably involved mixed populations of carriers of pathogenic and nonpathogenic strains. Banerjee et al. (144) followed 167 patients for 1 to 5 years following treatment with metronidazole or diloxanide furoate (a luminal agent). A number of patients (5.8%) treated only with diloxanide furoate went on to develop amebic liver abscesses and thus were probably colonized or subsequently exposed to pathogenic strains. Nanda et al. (30) performed amebic cultures, rectal biopsies, and amebic serologies on patients presenting to gastrointestinal clinics with a variety of intestinal disorders in India. Nineteen percent were culture positive for *E. histolytica* and had no evidence of invasive disease on biopsy. Fifteen patients were followed for a mean of 9 months without therapy and found to spontaneously stop shedding within 5 months, although many had only one follow-up culture.

In developed countries, a physician is most likely to encounter *E. histolytica* cysts in homosexual men, with colonization rates on routine stool exams as high as 30% (145). Several large studies from London have characterized the prevalence and clinical impact of infection in homosexual patients (42,43,49). All 100 patients who were culture positive were carriers of nonpathogenic zymodemes, had negative amebic serology, and no histologic evidence of invasive amebiasis (42,49). Since T cell-mediated immunity is an important defense against amebiasis (128–130), one might anticipate that colonization, even with nonpathogenic strains, might cause significant disease in these patients. Instead, a benign clinical course was found in follow-up of 19 AIDS patients (146). All were colonized with nonpathogenic strains, none had positive amebic serology, and all untreated patients became culture-negative in an average of 11 weeks. A majority of the symptomatic patients (64%) had other potential pathogens isolated at the same time, suggesting that a search for other causes is always appropriate in a symptomatic AIDS patient with diarrhea and *E. histolytica* cysts.

A variable percentage of asymptomatic patients will be carriers of pathogenic zymodemes of *E. histolytica,* however. In South Africa, Gathiram and Jackson (32) identified 20 asymptomatic carriers with pathogenic strains (10% of all infections, incidence of 1%). Within 1 year, 10% had developed amebic colitis, and the rest remained asymptomatic with spontaneous cure. Studies in Mexico and other regions have found that a higher percentage of asymptomatic infections may be due to pathogenic organisms (33). These patients would be particularly important to identify and treat as they are a potential source of disease transmission.

Acute Colitis. Patients with acute amebic colitis usually present with the gradual onset of abdominal pain and frequent, loose, watery stools containing blood and mucus. Associated symptoms may include back pain, tenesmus, or flatulence (see Table 2). Most patients have symptoms for 1 to 2 weeks before presentation, but the occasional patient may have profuse diarrhea leading to rapid dehydration. A minority of patients are febrile, in contrast to patients with bacterial dysentery. Most patients have abdominal tenderness on examination, often localized to the lower abdomen. The characteristic appearance of the punctate, hemorrhagic ulcers with relatively normal intervening mucosa on rectal or sigmoidoscopic examination may be helpful in the diagnosis (Fig. 3).

Fulminant Colitis. Fulminant colitis is an unusual complication of amebic dysentery, which carries a grave prognosis with survival rates rarely greater than 40% (147). Clinically, patients present with more severe bloody diarrhea and fever, followed by rapid progression to diffuse abdominal tenderness. The progression may be so rapid,

TABLE 2. *Presenting symptoms and signs of patients with amebic colitis*

Presentation	Percentage
Symptoms	
Diarrhea	100
Dysentery	99
Abdominal pain	85
Low back pain	66
Signs	
Fever	38
Abdominal tenderness	83
Localized	42
Generalized	41
Dehydration	5
Length of symptoms	
0–1 week	48
2–4 weeks	37
>4 weeks	15

Adapted from ref. 149.

however, that only 25% of adults who ultimately had perforations detected at surgery presented with a rigid abdomen (147) (Table 3). Young children appear to be at increased risk for fulminant colitis (148). The clinical development of fulminant colitis is associated with the pathologic progression from superficial ulceration of the bowel to transmural necrosis (Table 3).

Ameboma. Ameboma is an unusual presentation of amebic intestinal infection, occurring in less than 1% of patients with invasive intestinal disease (149). The majority of patients present with an abdominal mass, which may be tender, but are otherwise asymptomatic. The appearance on radiographic studies mimics a carcinoma pre-

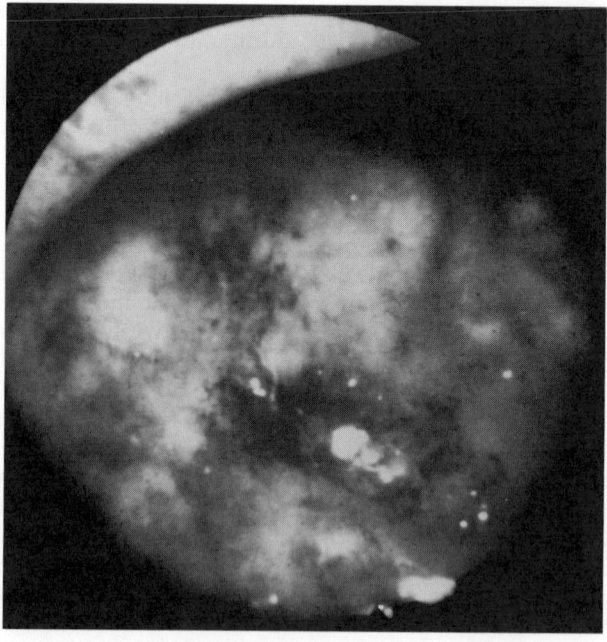

FIG. 3. Patient with amebic colitis at colonoscopy. Note punctate hemorrhagic ulcers with normal appearing mucosa. (See Plate 16.) (Courtesy of H. Jinich, UCSD Medical Center.)

TABLE 3. *Findings at laparotomy in patients with fulminant amebic colitis*

Finding	Percentage
Multiple perforations	60
Colonic gangrene	16
Single perforation	10
Perforated ameboma	2
Microscopic perforation	12

Adapted from ref. 147.

senting as an "apple core-like" lesion (150) (Fig. 4). A positive amebic serology or biopsy by colonoscopy can prevent an unnecessary surgical procedure, although an ameboma and carcinoma may coexist (151).

Other Syndromes. The clinical significance of persistent diarrhea following adequate therapy of intestinal amebic infection, called chronic nondysenteric colitis (149) or ulcerative postdysenteric colitis (151), is unclear. Recurrent amebic infection cannot be identified, and these patients do not respond to additional antiparasitic therapy.

Complications

The most common complication of acute amebic colitis is peritonitis. Patients usually develop slow leakage with a delay in clinical signs of peritonitis, but fulminant colitis

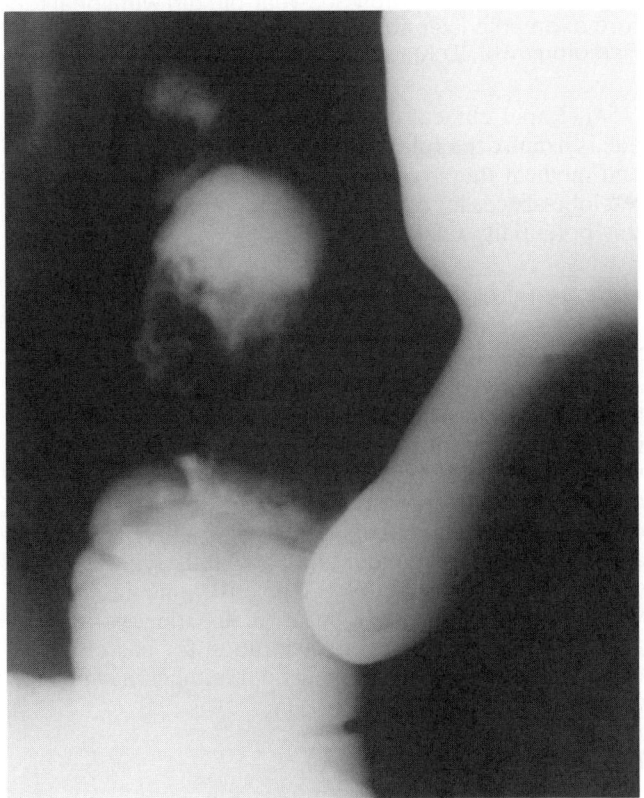

FIG. 4. Barium enema examination on 26-year-old Filipino man with asymptomatic left lower quadrant mass. (Courtesy of Department of Radiology, UCSD Medical Center.)

and acute perforation may also occur (149). Less frequent complications include sudden hemorrhage requiring transfusion and amebic strictures of the anus, rectum, or sigmoid colon (149). Cutaneous amebiasis results from direct spread of intestinal infection. These lesions are usually painful ulcers, which are easily confused with squamous cell carcinoma (152). Amebic trophozoites are usually apparent on biopsy, and patients respond well to medical therapy alone. Cutaneous amebiasis and carcinomas may coexist so a follow-up biopsy of any nonresolving lesion is important (152).

Differential Diagnosis

Acute amebic colitis must be distinguished from bacterial causes of dysentery, including *Shigella*, *Campylobacter*, *Salmonella*, *Vibrio*, *Salmonella*, and enteroinvasive *Escherichia coli*. One clinical clue to amebiasis is the relative lack of fever or possible absence of fecal leukocytes; however, examination of stool for parasites, cultures, and amebic serology are usually required to make the definitive diagnosis. It is particularly important to exclude amebic colitis before treating any patient with presumptive inflammatory bowel disease with steroids (153), as potentially fatal toxic megacolon may develop.

Amebic Liver Abscess

Amebic liver abscess is the most common complication of invasive amebiasis (reviewed in refs. 142 and 143). Diagnosis is hindered by the nonspecific nature of the symptoms and the potential for presentation months after leaving an endemic area. The majority of patients present acutely with less than 10 days of fever and abdominal pain (Table 4) (56,154). Dull, right upper quadrant pain, which may radiate to the shoulder, is the most common symptom, but diffuse epigastric or pleuritic pain may also occur. An enlarged, painful liver is the most useful sign but is not diagnostic. Most patients are febrile (>80%), and a minority of patients (10%) may actually present with a fever of unknown origin (154). Although all patients have had intestinal infection preceding development of a

TABLE 4. *Signs and symptoms of amebic liver abscess*

Presentation	Adams and MacLeod (154) (N = 2074)	Katzenstein et al. (56) (N = 67) Acute	Katzenstein et al. (56) (N = 67) Chronic
Symptom			
Fever	75	85	32
Diarrhea	14	30	30
Weight loss	NR	20	60
Cough	11	5	7
Sign			
Tender liver	80	90	90
Hepatomegaly	80	25	60
Rales/rhonchi	47	27	60

NR, not reported.

liver abscess, less than 30% have active diarrhea at any time before presentation. A subset of patients have a more chronic course with subacute symptoms for more than 2 weeks (154). These patients are more likely to present as a wasting disease with hepatomegaly, weight loss, and anemia. Atypical presentations may include shortness of breath and cough secondary to pleural effusions or rupture into the pleural space.

Complications of Amebic Liver Abscess

Death from uncomplicated amebic liver abscess is less than 1%, but mortality increases at least tenfold with rupture (154,155) (Table 5).

Pleuropulmonary Complications. Pleuropulmonary complications of amebic abscess, including localized rupture, empyema, and hepatobronchial fistulas, are most common, occurring in approximately 10% of patients. Up to half of patients may have a small to moderate, serous pleural effusion, which may be the first radiographic clue to underlying liver disease. Localized rupture by contiguous spread into the pleural cavity is usually quite benign and responds to medical therapy alone (Fig. 5). Formation of an empyema is much more serious and is usually heralded by sudden pleuritic pain and shortness of breath, necessitating aggressive drainage and medical therapy. The development of an hepatobronchial fistula is potentially the most dramatic complication of an amebic abscess with the patient coughing up large amounts of necrotic debris which may contain trophozoites. This complication usually responds well to medical therapy unless aspiration of the abscess contents into the lungs occurs.

Peritoneal Rupture. Rupture of amebic liver abscesses into the peritoneum occurs in 2% to 5% of patients (154). Because the contents are sterile, the prognosis is much better than with rupture of infected bowel. Mortality from this complication has fallen dramatically following the advent of percutaneous catheter drainage (156).

Pericardial Rupture. Rupture of an amebic liver abscess into the pericardium is the most serious complication, with a mortality of more than 70% if not recognized early (157). Rupture into the pericardium may occur even when the patient is on adequate medical therapy and is usually preceded by the development of a serous effusion

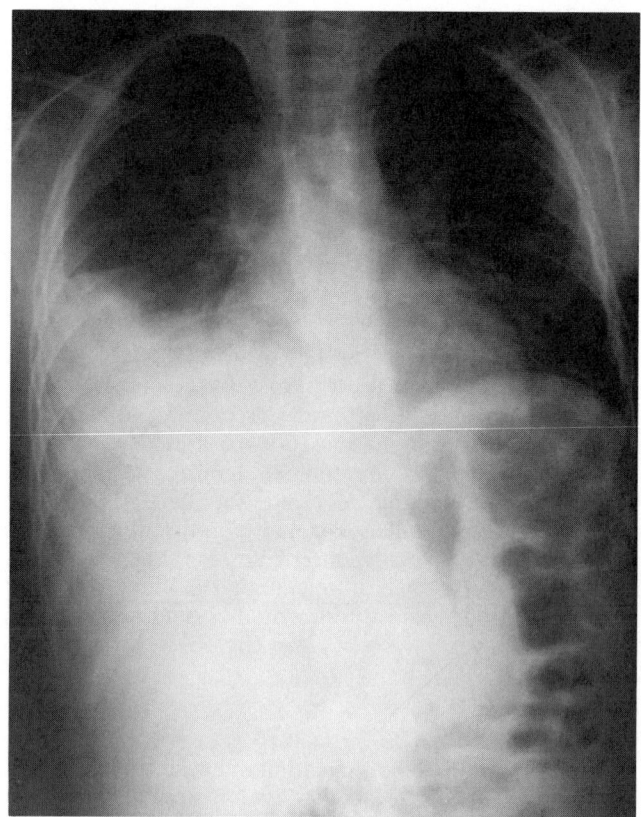

FIG. 5. Chest radiograph of 8-year-old girl with local rupture of amebic liver abscess. (Courtesy of Department of Radiology, UCSD Medical Center.)

(154). Rapid clinical deterioration from cardiac tamponade is usually the rule (154), although aggressive drainage and medical therapy may be curative. Early drainage of left lobe abscesses of the liver is recommended to prevent this potentially fatal complication (158).

Differential Diagnosis of Amebic Liver Abscess

The diagnosis of an amebic liver abscess should be considered in any patient from an endemic area with fever and right upper quadrant abdominal tenderness. Although infection of the biliary tract may be suspected initially, with the advent of modern imaging techniques the differential diagnosis is usually limited to a pyogenic abscess or necrotic tumor. Patients with pyogenic liver abscesses are more likely to be older and have underlying gallbladder or bowel disease (159). A positive amebic serology will confirm the diagnosis, but in an ill patient with multiple abscesses, percutaneous aspiration for bacterial cultures, pathologic examination, and treatment may be indicated.

Diagnosis of Amebic Infection

Microscopic Diagnosis

Early diagnosis is critical for successful treatment of invasive amebiasis. Intestinal infection is diagnosed by

TABLE 5. *Complications of amebic liver abscesses*

Complications	Cases	Percentage	Mortality (%)
Pulmonary	146	7.8	6.2
Pleural effusion and empyema		29	
Hepatobronchial fistula		47	
Lung abscess		14	
Consolidation		10	
Abdominal rupture	38	2.0	18.4
Pericardial rupture	27	1.4	29.6

Adapted from ref. 154.

the presence of the distinct cysts or hematophagous trophozoites of *E. histolytica* on wet mount or trichrome stain of stool concentrates (see Fig. 4 in the chapter by Oberhelman and Krogstad). Shedding of cysts may be intermittent so examination of at least three stools is recommended. Although patients with frank colitis usually have a large number of motile trophozoites in their stool, specimens must be examined immediately as the trophozoites are rapidly killed by drying, water, urine, barium, or a number of antibiotics. Biopsy or scrapings from the edge of bowel ulcers may increase the diagnostic yield but should be avoided in patients with fulminant colitis. Cysts of pathogenic *E. histolytica* and nonpathogenic *E. dispar* cannot be distinguished microscopically. Amebic cultures are more sensitive than standard stool examinations (160) but are not available in most microbiology laboratories.

Less than 30% of patients with amebic liver abscess have symptomatic intestinal infection, but recent studies in which daily stool cultures were performed on patients with amebic liver abscesses suggest that more than 70% may have asymptomatic colonization (160). Trophozoites are rarely seen in aspirates of the necrotic debris, which forms the bulk of amebic liver abscesses.

Laboratory Tests

Routine hematology or chemistry tests are rarely helpful in the diagnosis of invasive amebiasis. Sixty percent of patients with an amebic liver abscess will have a white blood cell count greater than 15,000. It is important to remember that invasion with *E. histolytica* does not cause eosinophilia. An elevated alkaline phosphatase was the most consistent biochemical indicator of an amebic liver abscess, increased in 84% (56). Transaminases were only elevated in 50% of patients, and abnormal values were more frequent in patients with acute infection and complications such as rupture (56).

Serologic Tests

Amebic serology is very useful in the diagnosis of invasive amebiasis. The most commonly used tests, counterimmunoelectrophoresis (CIE), agar gel diffusion (AGD), indirect hemagglutination (IHA), and enzyme-linked immunoadsorbent assay (ELISA), are positive in 85% to 95% of patients with amebic colitis or liver abscesses (161). The titer correlates with the duration of illness rather than severity of disease. Serologic tests were initially negative in 10% of patients who presented acutely with an amebic liver abscess, but all were positive within 2 weeks (56). Caution must be taken with the interpretation of IHA titers as they may remain elevated for several years following successful treatment (161). In contrast, CIE and AGD usually revert to negative within months. Asymptomatic carriers of pathogenic *E. histolytica* develop a serum antibody response that serves as a useful marker of both active and potential disease (34).

Radiographic Studies

Barium studies are relatively contraindicated in the workup of a patient with acute dysentery because of the risk of perforation. Patients with amebomas rarely have acute diarrhea, however, and the lesions are usually identified on barium studies to define an abdominal mass.

Noninvasive radiographic studies, including ultrasound, computed tomography (CT) scan, and magnetic resonance imaging (MRI), have dramatically improved the early diagnosis of amebic liver abscesses. The classic ultrasound appearance is a round or cystic mass with well-defined borders (Fig. 6). The majority of patients (75%) have single abscesses of the right lobe of the liver (162), but up to 50% of patients who present acutely may have multiple lesions, which may be difficult to distinguish from a pyogenic abscess (56) (Fig. 7). The time for complete resolution of abscesses is very variable, ranging from 1½ to 23 months (163). Abscesses may actually increase in size early in the course of successful therapy so it is important not to obtain follow-up studies too early (31). CT scans have also enhanced the detection of early rupture (Figure 8).

Pathology

Amebic trophozoites invade the colonic epithelium forming an ulcer that progresses through the lamina propria to the muscularis mucosa and extends laterally under normal appearing mucosa, forming a "flask-shaped ulcer" (63). Significant tissue necrosis is detected with a relative paucity of inflammation. Amebic trophozoites are

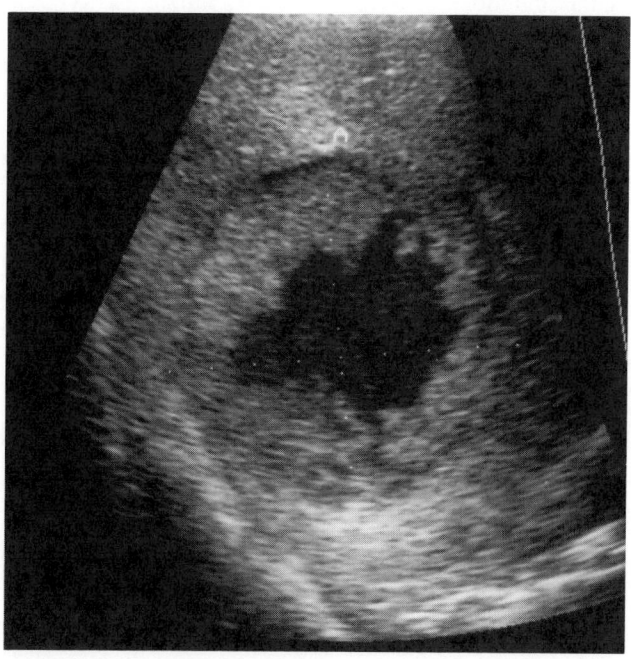

FIG. 6. Liver ultrasound of same 8-year-old girl as in Fig. 5 showing a large cystic mass. (Courtesy of Department of Radiology, UCSD Medical Center.)

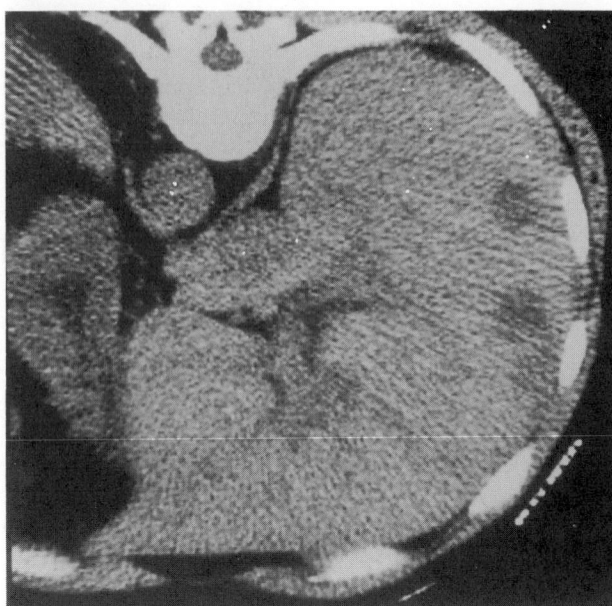

FIG. 7. CT scan of patient with multiple liver abscesses. Liver aspirate grew *E. histolytica* on culture. (Courtesy of Department of Radiology, UCSD Medical Center.)

usually seen in clusters in the periphery of necrotic areas (63) (Fig. 9). Although trophozoites are detectable by standard hematoxylin–eosin (H&E) staining of tissues, the distinct pink color seen with periodic acid–Schiff (PAS) stain helps differentiate trophozoites from phagocytic cells (reviewed in ref. 164).

In an amebic liver abscess, the liver parenchyma is completely replaced with necrotic debris with a paucity of inflammatory cells or amebic trophozoites (63). The color of the fluid may range from yellow to brown and has been described as "anchovy paste" from its consis-

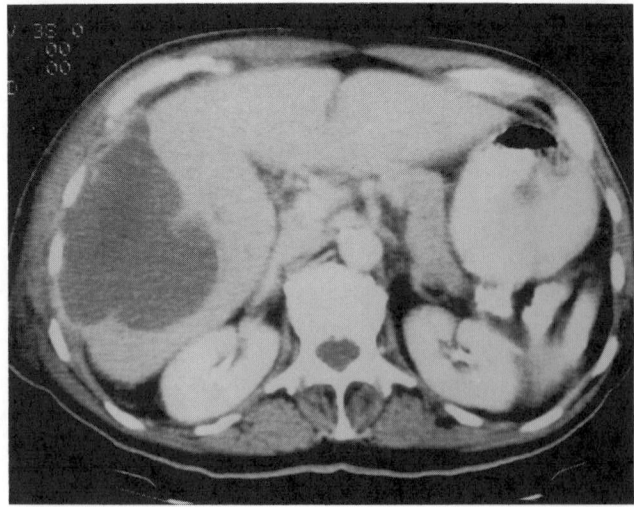

FIG. 8. Patient with localized rupture of amebic liver abscess detected by CT scan. (Courtesy of Department of Radiology, UCSD Medical Center.)

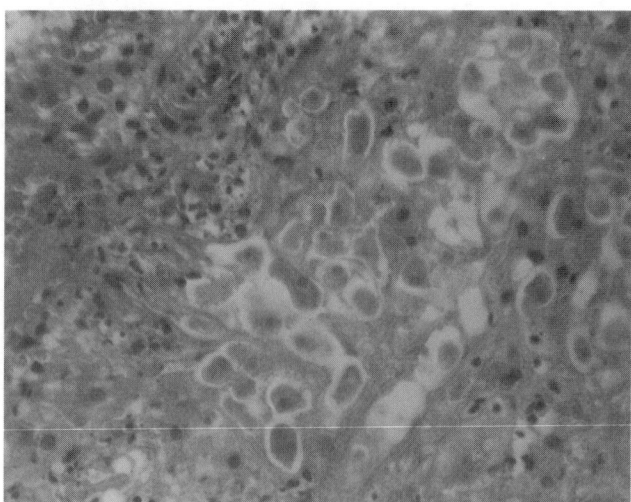

FIG. 9. Pathology of amebic liver abscess. Trophozoites seen on edge of necrotic liver abscess. H&E stain, ×100.

tency and color when it is mixed with blood. Trophozoites are usually only found near the capsule of the abscess (Fig. 9).

Future Diagnostic Tests

A number of new tests may be available in the near future to aid with the early diagnosis of invasive amebiasis. Detection of specific IgA in saliva correlated well with standard serum ELISAs (125). Several different approaches have been used to differentiate potentially invasive *E. histolytica* from noninvasive *E. dispar* directly in stool samples. A number of monoclonal antibodies have been made to epitopes unique to pathogenic isolates (10,11,165,166). Pathogen-specific epitopes of the galactose adhesin have formed the basis of a very sensitive (100%) and specific (97%) stool ELISA (167,168). A unique approach has focused on the release of a cysteine proteinase by potentially invasive strains of *E. histolytica*. The proteinase is immunoadsorbed from stool samples and enzymatic activity is detected by a color reaction (169). Other groups have exploited conserved unique nucleotide sequences that differentiate pathogenic and nonpathogenic entamoeba, particularly in rRNA, to develop nucleotide probes (7) or PCR amplification (33) to differentiate *E. histolytica* from *E. dispar* in stool samples.

Treatment of Amebic Infection

Treatment of Cyst Passers

Two main classes of drugs are used to treat amebiasis: luminal agents that are poorly absorbed in tissues and agents with good tissue penetration. Three major luminal agents are available: iodoquinol, diloxanide furoate, and paromomycin (Table 6). All have efficacy rates of 85% to 95% for the eradication of cyst passage (170). Iodoquinol,

TABLE 6. *Treatment of amebiasis*

Syndrome	Adult dose
Asymptomatic cyst passer, luminal agent	
Iodoquinol (650 mg tablets)	650 mg tid × 20 days
Paromomycin (250 mg tablets)	500 mg tid × 7 days
Diloxanide furoate (500 mg tablets)[a]	500 mg tid × 10 days
Acute colitis	
Metronidazole (250 or 500 mg tablets)	750 mg tid × 5–10 days
+	
Luminal agent (above)	
Amebic liver abscess	
Metronidazole	750 mg tid iv or po × 5–10 days
Tinidazole[b]	2 g po
Ornidazole[b]	2 g po
+	
Luminal agent (above)	

[a] Available only from Centers for Disease Control (Telephone: 404-639-3356).
[b] Not available in the United States.

a halogenated hydroxyquinoline, is effective but must be given for a 20-day course. Diloxanide furoate, a substituted acetanilide, has been widely used outside the United States but is only available from the Centers for Disease Control (171). Paromomycin is a nonabsorbable aminoglycoside that is active against both trophozoites and cysts (172). The most important indication for use of a luminal agent is adjunctive therapy in all patients with invasive amebiasis; metronidazole is not effective therapy for cysts. Although all three luminal active drugs are very effective, the treatment of asymptomatic cyst passers is perhaps the biggest dilemma in the management of amebiasis. If the patient is asymptomatic, has a negative serology, and the infecting strain can be characterized as *E. dispar*, follow-up without treatment is advised (43,49). If serologic tests or amebic cultures are not available to identify carriers of pathogenic strains, it is most prudent to treat all patients. The treatment of pregnant patients is particularly a difficult issue because of anectdotal evidence that invasive amebiasis is more severe and the theoretical teratogenic risk of metronidazole. Some authors would argue that an asymptomatic woman with a negative amebic serology should be carefully followed without therapy and treatment with metronidazole reserved for those with invasive disease (142). Others would advise that all pregnant women with "mild-to-moderate" intestinal disease be treated with paromomycin (170).

Intestinal Amebiasis

The therapy of invasive amebiasis has dramatically improved since the introduction of imidazoles, particularly metronidazole. Metronidazole is the most effective amebicide for treatment of both colonic and extracolonic disease. Standard oral doses of 750 mg (10 mg/kg) three times a day for 5 to 10 days are indicated, followed by a luminal agent to prevent recurrence. The main side effects of metronidazole are nausea, vomiting, and a disulfiram-like effect with alcohol. Potential teratogenic effects of metronidazole have been noted *in vitro,* but long-term follow-up

of several thousand women inadvertently given therapy for trichomoniasis during pregnancy failed to reveal any problems (173).

Amebic Liver Abscess

Mortality from uncomplicated amebic liver abscesses has decreased to less than 1% with early therapy with imidazoles. Single-dose therapies with metronidazole, tinidazole, and ornidazole have efficacies greater than 80%, but only metronidazole is available in the United States. Follow-up therapy with a luminal agent is very important even in patients without active diarrhea because asymptomatic colonization rates of up to 72% were detected in patients with amebic liver abscesses (160). Although all 50 patients in the South African study with amebic liver abscesses responded rapidly to metronidazole, cysts were not eradicated in 55% by metronidazole alone, creating potential sources for recurrence of invasive amebiasis or transmission (160).

The majority of patients respond dramatically within 72 hr of instituting metronidazole therapy (174). In patients who do not, evaluation for possible rupture should be instituted. Some authors advocate the addition of emetine 65 mg im qd and chloroquine 600 mg po followed by 300 mg qd (174), but we have found this unnecessary as all patients responded to percutaneous drainage (158). The primary indications for drainage include the following (158): (a) for initial diagnosis to exclude a pyogenic liver abscess, (b) for imminent rupture (usually >12 cm); (c) failure to respond to medical therapy after 72 hr, (d) to drain a left lobe abscess and prevent pericardial rupture, and (e) to drain a ruptured abscess (156). Open surgery is relatively contraindicated except for bowel perforation.

Prevention of Amebiasis

Transmission of amebiasis, like all fecally spread infections, could be completely prevented with adequate sanitation. The four critical areas to limit infection are adequate sanitation, health education, early treatment of potentially infectious cases, and surveillance and control programs (reviewed in ref. 175). Effective prevention through sanitation requires both adequate disposal of human stools and sterilization of water. Asymptomatic carriers may excrete up to 15 million cysts a day, which can survive in water for several weeks and are resistant to levels of chlorination used in water purification. Although filtration and precipitation will usually eliminate cysts, recontamination must be prevented. Infected food handlers are major sources of transmission, and health education emphasizing basic sanitation is required. Early treatment of patients with invasive disease and those shedding pathogenic cysts is critical. In the future, such targeted therapy will be helped significantly by more sensitive diagnostic tests. Mass chemotherapy trials for high-risk populations, such as in chronically institutionalized, mentally challenged populations, have been disappointing (176). Targeted surveillance in endemic areas, particularly utilizing serologic testing and identification of pathogenic strains, will be important, particularly when integrated into programs for control of diarrheal diseases. For the individual traveler, no effective chemoprophylaxis for amebiasis exists. Risk of infection is best minimized by avoiding unpeeled fruits and vegetables and using bottled water. Boiling water or disinfection by iodination (tetraglycine hydroperiodide) is most effective (177).

REFERENCES

1. Walsh JA. Prevalence of *Entamoeba histolytica* infection. In: Ravdin JI, ed. *Amebiasis: human infection by* Entamoeba histolytica. New York: Churchill Livingstone, 1988;93–105.
2. Chayen A, Avron B, Nuchamowitz Y, et al. Appearance of sialoglycoproteins in encysting cells of *Entamoeba histolytica*. *Infect Immun* 1988;56:673–681.
3. Walker EL, Sellards AW. Experimental entamoebic dysentery. *Philippine J Sci B Trop Med* 1913;8:253–330.
4. Levine ND, Corliss JO, Cox FEG. A newly revised classification of the protozoa. *J Protozool* 1980;27:37–58.
5. Sargeaunt PG, Williams JE, Grene JD. The differentiation of invasive and non-invasive *Entamoeba histolytica* by isoenzyme electrophoresis. *Trans R Soc Trop Med Hyg* 1978;72:519–521.
6. Clark CG, Diamond LS. Ribosomal RNA genes of "pathogenic" *Entamoeba histolytica* are distinct. *Mol Biochem Parisitol* 1991;49:297–302.
7. Garfinkel LI, Gilandi M, Huber M, et al. DNA probes specific for *Entamoeba histolytica* possessing pathogenic and nonpathogenic zymodemes. *Infect Immun* 1989;57:926–931.
8. Tannich E, Burchard GD. Differentiation of pathogenic from nonpathogenic *Entamoeba histolytica* by restriction fragment analysis of a single gene amplified *in vitro*. *J Clin Microbiol* 1991;29:250–255.
9. Diamond LS, Clark CG. A redescription of *Entamoeba histolytica* Schaudinn. 1903 (Emended Walker, 1911) separating it from *Entamoeba dispar* (Brumpt, 1925). *J Eukaryotic Microbiol* 1993;40:340–344.
10. Petri WA Jr, Jackson TFHG, Gathiram V, et al. Pathogenic and nonpathogenic strains of *Entamoeba histolytica* can be differentiated by monoclonal antibodies to the galactose-specific adherence lectin. *Infect Immun* 1990;58:1802–1806.
11. Strachan WD, Spice WM, Chiodini PL, et al. Immunological differentiation of pathogenic and nonpathogenic isolates of *Entamoeba histolytica*. *Lancet* 1988;1:561–562.
12. Tachibana H, Kobayashi S, Nagakura K. Reactivity of monoclonal antibodies to species-specific antigens of *Entamoeba histolytica*. *J Protozool* 1991;38:329–334.
13. Bhattacharya, Bhattacharya S, Sharma MP, et al. Metabolic labeling of *Entamoeba histolytica* antigens: characterization of a 28-kDa major intracellular antigen. *Exp Parasitol* 1990;70:255–263.
14. Reed SL, Flores BM, Batzer MA, et al. Molecular and cellular characterization of the 29-kilodalton peripheral membrane protein of *Entamoeba histolytica*: differentiation between pathogenic and nonpathogenic isolates. *Infect Immun* 1992;60:542–549.
15. Tannich E, Horstmann RD, Knobloch J, et al. Genomic DNA differences between pathogenic and nonpathogenic *Entamoeba histolytica*. *Proc Natl Acad Sci USA* 1989;86:5118–5122.
16. Tachibana H, Kobayashi S, Paz KC, et al. Analysis of pathogenicity by restriction-endonuclease digestion of amplified genomic DNA of *Entamoeba histolytica* isolated in Pernambuco, Brazil. *Parasitol Res* 1992;78:433–436.
17. Burch DJ, Li E, Reed S, et al. Isolation of a strain-specific *Entamoeba histolytica* cDNA clone. *J Clin Microbiol* 1991;29:696–701.
18. Que X, Reed SL. Nucleotide sequence of a small subunit ribosomal RNA (16S-like rRNA) gene from *Entamoeba histolytica*: differentiation of pathogenic from nonpathogenic isolates. *Nucleic Acids Res* 1991;19:5438.
19. Blanc DS. Determination of taxonomic status of pathogenic and nonpathogenic *Entamoeba histolytica* zymodemes using isoenzyme analysis. *J Protozool* 1992;39:471–479.
20. Barker DC. Differentiation of *Entamoeba*. Patterns of nucleic acids and ribosomes durng encystation and excystation. In: Van den Bossche H, ed. *Biochemistry of parasites and host–parasite relationships*. Amsterdam: Elsevier Biomedical, 1976;253.
21. Healy GR. Diagnostic techniques for stool samples. In: Ravdin JI, ed. *Amebiasis: human infection of* Entamoeba histolytica. New York: Churchill Livingstone, 1988;635–649.
22. Mathur TN, Kaur J. The frequency of excretion of cysts of *Entamoeba histolytica* in known cases of nondysenteric amoebic colitis based on 21 stool examinations. *Indian J Med Res* 1973;61:330–334.
23. Krogstad DJ, Spencer HC, Healy GR, et al. Amebiasis: epidemiologic studies in the United States, 1971–1974. *Ann Intern Med* 1978;88:89–97.
24. Bray RS, Harris WG. The epidemiology of infection with *Entamoeba histolytica* in The Gambia, West Africa. *Trans R Soc Trop Med Hyg* 1977;71:401–407.
25. Choudhuri G, Prakash V, Kumar A, et al. Protective immunity to *Entamoeba histolytica* infection in subjects with antiamoebic antibodies residing in a hyperendemic zone. *Scand J Infect Dis* 1991;23:771–776.
26. Caballero-Salcedo A, Viveros-Rogel M, Salvatiena B, et al. Seroepidemiology of amebiasis in Mexico. *Am J Trop Med Hyg* 1994;50:412–419.
27. Walsh JA. Transmission of *Entamoeba histolytica* infection. In: Ravdin JI, ed. *Amebiasis: human infection by* Entamoeba histolytica. New York: Churchill Livingstone, 1988;106–119.
28. Gutierez G, Ludlow A, Espinos G, et al. National serologic survey II. Search for antibodies against *Entamoeba histolytica* in Mexico. In: Proceedings of the International Conference on Amebiasis. Sepulveda B, Diamond LS, eds. *Amebiasis*. Mexico City: Instito Mexicano del Seguro Social, 1976;609–618.
29. Abdel-Hafez MM, el-Kady N, Bolbol AS, et al. Prevalence of intestinal parasitic infections in Riyadh district, Saudi Arabia. *Ann Trop Med Parasitol* 1986;80:631–634.
30. Nanda R, Baveja U, Anand BS. *Entamoeba histolytica* cyst passers: clinical features and outcome in untreated subjects. *Lancet* 1984;2:301–303.
31. Gathiram V, Jackson TFHG. Frequency distribution of *Entamoeba histolytica* zymodemes in a rural South African population. *Lancet* 1985;1:719–721.
32. Gathiram V, Jackson TFHG. A longitudinal study of asymp-

tomatic carriers of pathogenic zymodemes of *Entamoeba histolytica. S Afr Med J* 1987;72:669–672.

33. Acuna-Soto R, Samuelson J, De Girolami P, et al. Application of the polymerase chain reaction to the epidemiology of pathogenic and nonpathogenic *Entamoeba histolytica. Am J Trop Med Hyg* 1993;48:58–70.
34. Jackson TFHG, Gathiram V, Simjee AE. Seroepidemiological study of antibody responses to the zymodemes of *Entamoeba histolytica. Lancet* 1985;1:716–719.
35. Ravdin JI, Jackson TF, Petri WA Jr, et al. Association of serum antibodies to adherence lectin with invasive amebiasis and asymptomatic infection with *Entamoeba histolytica. J Infect Dis* 1990;162:768–772.
36. Thacker SB, Simpson S, Gordon TJ, et al. Parasitic disease control in a residential facility for the mentally retarded. *Am J Public Health* 1979;69:1279–1281.
37. Sexton DJ, Krogstad DJ, Spencer HC, et al. Amebiasis in a mental institution: serologic and epidemiologic studies. *Am J Epidemiol* 1974;100:414–423.
38. Petri WA, Ravdin JI. Amebiasis in institutionalized populations. In: Ravdin JI, ed. *Amebiasis: human infection by* Entamoeba histolytica. New York: Churchill Livingstone, 1988.
39. Thacker SB, Kimball AM, Wolfe M, et al. Parasitic disease control in a residential facility for the mentally retarded: failure of selected isolation procedures. *Am J Public Health* 1981;71:303.
40. Brooke MM. Epidemiology and control of amebiasis in institutions for the mentally retarded. *Am J Ment Defic* 1963;68:187.
41. Kean BH, William DC, Luminais SK. Epidemic of amoebiasis and giardiasis in a biased population. *Br J Vener Dis* 1979;55:375–378.
42. Goldmeier D, Sargeaunt PG, Billington O, et al. Is *Entamoeba histolytica* in homosexual men a pathogen? *Lancet* 1986;1:641–644.
43. Allason-Jones E, Mindel A, Sargeaunt P, et al. *Entamoeba histolytica* is a commensal intestinal parasite in homosexual men. *N Engl J Med* 1986;515:353–356.
44. Markell EK, Havens RF, Kuritsubo RA, et al. Intestinal protozoa in homosexual men of the San Francisco Bay area: prevalence and correlates of infection. *Am J Trop Med Hyg* 1984;33:239–245.
45. Ortega HB, Borchardt KA, Hamilton R, et al. Enternic pathogenic protozoa in homosexual men from San Francisco. *Sex Transm Dis* 1983;11:59.
46. Druckman DA, Quinn TC. *Entamoeba histolytica* infection in homosexual men. In: Ravdin JI, ed. *Amebiasis: human infection by* Entamoeba histolytica. New York: Churchill Livingstone, 1988;563–575.
47. Peters CS, Sable R, Janda WM, et al. Prevalence of enteric parasites in homosexual patients attending an outpatient clinic. *J Clin Microbiol* 1986;24:684–685.
48. Sorvillo FJ, Strassburg MA, Seidel J, et al. Amebic infections in asymptomatic homosexual men, lack of evidence of invasive disease. *Am J Public Health* 1986;76:1137–1139.
49. Allason-Jones E, Mindel A, Sargeaunt PG, Katz D. Outcome of untreated infection with *Entamoeba histolytica* in homosexual men with and without HIV antibody. *Br Med J* 1988;297:654–657.
50. Zagury D, Bernard J, Leonard R, et al. Long-term cultures of HTLV-III-infected T cells: a model of cytopathogenicity of T cell depletion in AIDS. *Science* 1986;231:850–853.
51. Croxson S, Mildvan D, Matthews H, et al. *Entamoeba histolytica* antigen-specific induction of human immunodeficiency virus replication. *J Clin Microbiol* 1988;26:1304–1308.
52. Brown M, Reed S, Levy JA, et al. Detection of HIV-1 in *Entamoeba histolytica* without evidence of transmission to human cells. *AIDS* 1991;5:93–96.
53. Istre GR, Kriess K, Hopkins RS, et al. An outbreak of amebiasis spread by colonic irrigation at a chiropractic clinic. *N Engl J Med* 1982;309:339–342.
54. Sabot JM, Patterson M. Amebic liver abscess: 1966–1976. *Dig Dis* 1978;23:110.

55. Abuabara SF, Barrett JA, Hau T, et al. Amebic liver abscess. *Arch Surg* 1982;117:239–244.
56. Katzenstein D, Rickerson V, Braude A. New concepts of amebic liver abscess derived from hepatic imaging, serodiagnosis, and hepatic enzymes in 67 consecutive cases in San Diego. *Medicine (Baltimore)* 1982;61:237–246.
57. Thompson JE Jr, Forlenza S, Verma R. Amebic liver abscess: a therapeutic approach. *Rev Infect Dis* 1985;7:171–179.
58. Barnes PF, DeCock KM, Reynolds TN, et al. A comparison of amebic and pyogenic abscess of the liver. *Medicine (Baltimore)* 1987;66:472–483.
59. Thompson JE Jr, Glasser AJ. Amebic abscess of the liver. Diagnostic features. *J Clin Gastroenterol* 1986;8:550–554.
60. Pearson RD, Hewlett EL. Amebiasis in travelers. In: Ravdin JI, ed. *Amebiasis: human infection by* Entamoeba histolytica. New York: Churchill Livingstone, 1988;556–562.
61. Pehrson PO. Amoebiasis in a non-endemic country. *Scand J Infect Dis* 1983;15:207–214.
62. Merson MH, Morris GK, Sack DA, et al. Traveler's diarrhea in Mexico: a prospective study. *N Engl J Med* 1976;294:1299.
63. Brandt H, Perez Tamayo R. Pathology of human amebiasis. *Hum Pathol* 1970;1:351–385.
64. Griffin JL, Juniper K Jr. Ultrastructure of *Entamoeba histolytica* from human amebic dysentery. *Arch Pathol* 1971;91:271–280.
65. Prahap K, Gilman R. The histopathology of acute intestinal amebiasis. *Am J Pathol* 1970;60:229–239.
66. Chatgidakis CB. The pathology of hepatic amoebiasis as seen on the Witwatersrand. *S Afr J Clin Sci* 1953;4:230.
67. Guerrant RL, Brush J, Ravdin JI, et al. Interaction between *Entamoeba histolytica* and human polymorphonuclear neutrophils. *J Infect Dis* 1981;143:83–93.
68. Ravdin JI, Murphy CF, Salata RA, et al. The N-acetyl-D-galactosamine-inhibitable adherence lectin of *Entamoeba histolytica*. I. Partial purification and relation to amoebic virulence *in vitro. J Infect Dis* 1985;151:804–815.
69. Tsutsumi V, Mena-Lopez R, Anaya-Velazquez F, et al. Cellular basis of experimental amebic liver abscess formation. *Am J Pathol* 1984;117:81–91.
70. Salata RA, Ravdin JI. The interaction of human neutropils and *Entamoeba histolytica* increases cytopathogenicity for liver cell monolayers. *J Infect Dis* 1986;154:19–26.
71. Joyce MP, Ravdin JI. Pathology of human amebiasis. In: Ravdin JI, ed. *Amebiasis: human infection by* Entamoeba histolytica. New York: Churchill Livingstone, 1988;129–146.
72. Aikat BK, Bhusnurmath SR, Pal AK, et al. The pathology and pathogenesis of fatal hepatic amoebiasis: a study based on 79 autopsy cases. *Trans R Soc Trop Med Hyg* 1979;73:188–192.
73. Gulati PD, Gupta DN, Chuttani HK. Amoebic liver abscess and disturbances of portal circulation. *Am J Med* 1967;45:852–854.
74. Tandon BN, Tandon HD, Puri BK. An electron microscopic study of liver in hepatomegaly presumably caused by amebiasis. *Exp Mol Pathol* 1975;22:118.
75. Ravdin JI. *Entamoeba histolytica*: pathogenic mechanisms, human immune response, and vaccine development. *Clin Res* 1990;38:215–225.
76. Ravdin JI, Guerrant RL. Role of adherence in cytopathogenic mechanisms of *Entamoeba histolytica. J Clin Invest* 1981;68:1305–1313.
77. Petri WA, Smith RD, Schlesinger PH, et al. Isolation of the galactose-binding lectin which mediates the *in vitro* adherence of *Entamoeba histolytica. J Clin Invest* 1987;80:1238–1244.
78. Chadee K, Petri WA, Innes DJ, et al. Rat and human colonic mucins bind to and inhibit the adherence of lectin of *Entamoeba histolytica. J Clin Invest* 1987;80:1245–1254.
79. Ravdin JI, John JE, Johnston LI, et al. Adherence of *Entamoeba histolytica* trophozoites to rat and human colonic mucosa. *Infect Immuun* 1985;48:292–297.
80. Salata RA, Pearson RD, Ravdin JI. Interaction of human leukocytes with *Entamoeba histolytica*: killing of virulent amebae by the activated macrophage. *J Clin Invest* 1985;76:491–499.
81. Orozco ME, Rodriguez M, Murphy CF, et al. *Entamoeba histo-*

lytica: cytopathogenicity and lectin activity of avirulent mutants. *Exp Parasitol* 1987;63:157–165.

82. Petri WA Jr, Chapman MD, Snodgrass T, et al. Subunit structure of the galactose and *N*-acetyl-D-galactosamine-inhibitable adherence lectin of *Entamoeba histolytica. J Biol Chem* 1989; 264:3007–3012.

83. Mann BJ, Chung CY, Dodson JM, et al. Neutralizing monoclonal antibody epitopes of the *Entamoeba histolytica* galactose adhesin map to the cysteine-rich extracellular domain of the 170-kilodalton heavy subunit. *Infect Immun* 1993;61: 1772–1778.

84. Kain KC, Ravdin JI. Galactose-specific adherence mechanisms of *Entamoeba histolytica,* a model for the study of enteric pathogens. *Methods in Enzymology (in press)*

85. Tannich E, Ebert F, Horstmann RD. Primary structure of the 170-kDa surface lectin of pathogenic *Entamoeba histolytica. Proc Natl Acad Sci USA* 1991;88:1849–1853.

86. McCoy JJ, Mann BJ, Vedvick T, Pak Y, Heimark DB, Petri WA Jr. Structural analysis of the light subunit of the *Entamoeba histolytica* adherence lectin. *J Biol Chem* 1993;24: 223–231.

87. Braga LL, Ninomiya H, McCoy JJ, et al. Inhibition of the complement membrane attack complex by the galactose-specific adhesion of *Entamoeba histolytica. J Clin Invest* 1992;90: 1131–1137.

88. Ravdin JI, Croft BY, Guerrant RL. Cytopathogenic mechanisms of *Entamoeba histolytica. J Exp Med* 1980;152:377–390.

89. Ravdin JI, Moreau F, Sullivan JA, et al. The relationship of free intracellular calcium ions to the cytolytic activity of *Entamoeba histolytica. Infect Immun* 1988;56:1505–1502.

90. Ravdin JI, Murphy CF, Guerrant RL, et al. Effect of calcium and phospholipase A antagonists on the cytopathogenicity of *Entamoeba histolytica. J Infect Dis* 1985;152:542–549.

91. Long-Krug SA, Hysmith RM, Fischer KJ, et al. The phospholipase A enzymes of *Entamoeba histolytica:* description and subcellular localization. *J Infect Dis* 1985;152:536–541.

92. Ravdin JI, Schlesinger PH, Murphy CF, et al. Acid intracellular vesicles and the cytolysis of mammalian target cells by *Entamoeba histolytica* trophozoites. *J Protozool* 1986;33:478–486.

93. Aucott JN, Scarpa A, Ravdin JI. Mechanisms of *Entamoeba histolytica* cytotoxicity, identification of amebic programming for Ca²⁺ dependent target cell death. *Clin Res* 1991;39:243A.

94. Weikel CS, Murphy CF, Orozco ME, et al. Phorbol esters specifically enhance the cytolytic activity of *Entamoeba histolytica. Infect Immun* 1988;56:1485–1491.

95. Young JE, Young TM, Lu LP, et al. Characterization of a membrane pore-forming protein from *Entamoeba histolytica. J Exp Med* 1982;156:1677–1690.

96. Lynch EC, Rosenberg IM, Gitler C. An ion-channel forming protein produced by *Entamoeba histolytica. EMBO J* 1982;1: 801–804.

97. Leippe M, Tannich E, et al. Primary and secondary structure of the pore-forming peptide of pathogenic *Entamoeba histolytica. EMBO J* 1992;11:3501–3506.

98. Young JD-E, Cohn ZA. Molecular mechanisms of cytotoxicity mediated by *Entamoeba histolytica:* characterization of a pore-forming protein (PFP). *J Cell Biochem* 1985;29:299–308.

99. Jansson A, Gillin F, Kagardt U, Hagblom P. Coding of hemolysins within the ribosomal RNA repeat on a plasmid in *Entamoeba histolytica. Science* 1994;263:1440–1443.

100. Scholze H, Werries E. A weakly acidic protease has a powerful proteolytic activity in *Entamoeba histolytica. Mol Biochem Parasitol* 1984;11:293–300.

101. Munoz MDL, Calderon J, Rojkind M. The collagenase of *Entamoeba histolytica. J Exp Med* 1982;155:42–51.

102. Keene WE, Petitt MG, Allen S, et al. The major neutral proteinase of *Entamoeba histolytica. J Exp Med* 1986;163:536–549.

103. Kelsall BL, Ravdin JI. Proteolytic degradation of human IgA by *Entamoeba histolytica. J Infect Dis* 1993;168:1319–1322.

104. Reed SL, Gigli I. Lysis of complement-sensitive *Entamoeba histolytica* by activated terminal complement components. *J Clin Invest* 1990;86:1815–1822.

105. Reed SL, Keene WE, McKerrow JH. Thiol proteinase expression and pathogenicity of *Entamoeba histolytica. J Clin Microbiol* 1989;27:2772–2777.

106. Reed S, Bouvier J, Pollack AS, et al. Cloning of a virulence factor of *Entamoeba histolytica. J Clin Invest* 1993;91: 1532–1540.

107. Werries E, Nebinger P, Franz A. Degradation of biogene oligosaccharides by beta-*N*-acetylglucosaminidase secreted by *Entamoeba histolytica. Mol Biochem Parasitol* 1983;7:127–140.

108. Udezulu IA, Leitch GJ. A membrane-associated neuraminidase in *Entamoeba histolytica* trophozoites. *Infect Immun* 1981;36:795–801.

109. Udezulu IA, Leitch GJ, Bailey GB. Use of indomethacin to demonstrate enterotoxic activity in extracts of *Entamoeba histolytica* trophozoites. *Infect Immun* 1981;36:795–801.

110. McGowan K, Kane A, Asarkof N, et al. *Entamoeba histolytica* causes intestinal secretion: role of serotonin. *Science* 1983;221: 762–764.

111. Feingold C, Bracha R, Wexler A, et al. Isolation, purification, and partial characterization of an enterotoxin from extracts of *Entamoeba histolytica* trophozoites. *Infect Immun* 1985;48: 211–218.

112. Salata RA, Ahmed P, Ravdin JI. *Entamoeba histolytica* chemoattractant activity of human polymorphonuclear neutrophils. *J Parasitol* 1989;75:644–646.

113. DeLeon A. Prognostico tardio en el absceso hepatico amibiano. *Arch Invest Med (Mex)* 1970;1(Suppl 1):205–6.

114. Petri WA, Joyce MP, Broman J, et al. Recognition of the galactose- or *N*-acetylgalactosamine-binding lectin of *Entamoeba histolytica* by human immune sera. *Infect Immun* 1987;55: 2327–2331.

115. Joyce MP, Ravdin JI. Antigens of *Entamoeba histolytica* recognized by immune sera from liver abscess patients. *Am J Trop Med Hyg* 1988;38:74–80.

116. Abd-Alla M, El-Hawey AM, Ravdin JI. Use of an enzyme-linked immunosorbent assay to detect anti-adherence protein antibodies in sera of patients with invasive amebiasis in Cairo, Egypt. *Am J Trop Med Hyg* 1992;47:800–804.

117. Torian BE, Flores BM, Stroeher VL, et al. cDNA sequence analysis of a 29kDa cysteine-rich surface antigen of pathogenic *Entamoeba histolytica. Proc Natl Acad Sci USA* 1990;87: 6358–6362.

118. Edman U, Meraz MA, Agabian N, et al. Characterization of an immuno-dominant variable surface antigen from pathogenic and nonpathogenic *E. histolytica. J Exp Med* 1990;172: 879–888.

119. Ortiz-Ortiz L, Capin R, Capin NR, et al. Activation of the alternative pathway of complement by *Entamoeba histolytica. Clin Exp Immunol* 1978;34:10–18.

120. Reed SL, Sargeaunt PG, Braude AI. Resistance to lysis by human serum of pathogenic *Entamoeba histolytica. Trans R Soc Trop Med Hyg* 1983;77:248–253.

121. Calderon J, Tovar R. Loss of susceptibility to complement lysis in *Entamoeba histolytica* HM1 by treatment with human serum. *Immunology* 1986;58:467–471.

122. Grundy MS, Cartwright TL, Lundin L, et al. Antibodies against *Entamoeba histolytica* in human milk and serum in Kenya. *J Clin Microbiol* 1983;17:753–758.

123. Islam A, Stoll BJ, Ljungstrom I, et al. The prevalence of *Entamoeba histolytica* in lactating women and in their infants in Bangladesh. *Trans R Soc Trop Med Hyg* 1988;82:99–103.

124. Speelman P, Ljungstrom I. Protozoal enteric infections among expatriates in Bangladesh. *Am J Trop Med Hyg* 1986;35: 1140–1145.

125. del Muro R, Acosta E, Merino E, Glender W, Ortiz-Ortiz L. Diagnosis of intestinal amebiasis using salivary IgA antibody detection. *J Infect Dis* 1990;162:1360–1364.

126. Aceti A, Pennica A, Celestino D, et al. Salivary IgA antibody detection in invasive amebiasis and in asymptomatic infection. *J Infect Dis* 1991;164:613–615.

127. Salta RA, Murray HW, Rubin BY, et al. The role of gamma interferon in the generation of human macrophages and T lym-

phocytes cytotoxic for *Entamoeba histolytica*. *Am J Trop Med Hyg* 1987;37:72–78.

128. Salata RA, Martinez-Palomo A, Murphy CF, et al. Patients treated for amebic liver abscess develop a cell-mediated immune response effective *in vitro* against *Entamoeba histolytica*. *J Immunol* 1986;136:2633–2639.

129. Schain DS, Salata RA, Ravdin JI. Human T-lymphocyte proliferation, lymphokine production, and amebicidal activity elicited by the galactose-inhibitable adherence protein of *Entamoeba histolytica*. *Infect Immun* 1992;60:2143–2146.

130. Salata RA, Martinez-Palomo A, Conales L, Ravdin JI. Immune sera suppresses the antigen specific proliferative response in T lymphocytes from patients cured of amebic liver abscess. *Infect Immun* 190;58:3941–3946.

131. Sepulveda B, Martinez-Palomo A. Immunology of amoebiasis by *Entamoeba histolytica*. In: Cohen S, Warren VS, eds. *Immunology of parasitic infections,* vol 1, 2nd ed. Oxford: Blackwell Scientific Publications, 1982;70–91.

132. Kanani SR, Knight R. Relapsing amoebic colitis of 12 years' standing exacerbated by corticosteroids. *Br Med J* 1969;2:613–614.

133. Balikian JP, Bitar JG, Rishani KI, et al. Fulminating necrotizing amebic colitis in children. *Am J Proctol* 1977;28:69.

134. Tucker PC, Webster PD, Kilpatrick ZM. Amebic colitis mistaken for inflammatory bowel disease. *Arch Intern Med* 1975;135:681.

135. Lewis EA, Anitia AU. Amoebic colitis: review of 295 cases. *Trans R Soc Trop Med Hyg* 1969;63:633–638.

136. Fuchs G, Ruiz-Palacios G, Pickering LK. Amebiasis in the pediatric population. In: Ravdin JI, ed. *Amebiasis: human infection by* Entamoeba histolytica. New York: Churchill Livingstone, 1988;594–613.

137. Leitch GJ, Dickey AD, Udezulu IA, et al. *Entamoeba histolytica* trophozoites in the lumen and mucus blanket of rat colons studied *in vivo*. *Infect Immun* 1985;47:68–73.

138. Chadee K, Meerovitch E. *Entamoeba histolytica:* early progressive pathology in the cecum of the gerbil (*Meriones unguiculatus*). *Am J Trop Med Hyg* 1985;34:283–291.

139. Chadee K, Petri WA, Johnson M, et al. Binding and internalization of purified rat colonic mucins by the Gal/GalNAc adherence lectin of *Entamoeba histolytica*. *J Infect Dis* 1988;158:398–406.

140. Chadee K, Innes DJ, Ravdin JI. Mucin and nonmucin secretagogue activity of *Entamoeba histolytica* and cholera toxin in rat colon. *Gastroenterology* 1991;100:986–997.

141. Petri WA Jr, Ravdin JI. Protection of gerbils from amebic liver abscess by immunization with the galactose-specific adherence lectin of *Entamoeba histolytica*. *Infect Immun* 1991;59:97–101.

142. Reed SL. Amebiasis: an update. *Clin Infect Dis* 1992;14:385–393.

143. Bruckner DA. Amebiasis. *Clin Microbiol Rev* 1992;5:356–369.

144. Banerjee RN, Sahani AL, Nag AK. A longitudinal study of intestinal amoebiasis. *J Assoc Physicians India* 1976;24:83.

145. Quinn TC, Stamm WE, Goodell SE, et al. The polymicrobial origin of intestinal infections in homosexual men. *N Engl J Med* 1983;309:576–582.

146. Reed SL, Wessel DW, Davis CE. *Entamoeba histolytica* infection and AIDS. *Am J Med* 1991;90:269–270.

147. Aristizabal H, Acevedo J, Botero M. Fulminant amebic colitis. *World J Surg* 1991;15:216–221.

148. Fuchs G, Ruiz-Palacios G, Pickering LK. Amebiasis in the pediatric population. In: Ravdin JI, ed. *Amebiasis: human infection by* Entamoeba histolytica. New York: Churchill Livingstone, 1988;594–613.

149. Adams EB, MacLeod IN. Invasive amebiasis. I. Amebic dysentery and its complications. *Medicine (Baltimore)* 1977;56:315–323.

150. Radke RA. Ameboma of the intestine: an analysis of the disease as presented in 78 collected and 41 previously unreported cases. *Ann Intern Med* 1955;43:1048–1066.

151. Powell SJ, Wilmot AJ. Ulcerative post-dysenteric colitis. *Gut* 1966;7:438–443.

152. Mhlanga BR, Lanoie LO, Norris HJ, Lack EE, Connor DH. Amebiasis complicating carcinomas: a diagnostic dilemma. *Am J Trop Med Hyg* 1992;759:764.

153. Patel AS, DeRidder PH. Amebic colitis masquerading as acute inflammatory bowel disease: the role of serology in its diagnosis. *J Clin Gastroenterol* 1989;11:407–410.

154. Adams EB, MacLeod IN. Invasive amebiasis. II. Amebic liver abscess and its complications. *Medicine (Baltimore)* 1977;56:325–334.

155. Ibarra-Perez C. Thoracic complications of amebic abscess of the liver. Report of 501 cases. *Chest* 1981;79:672–677.

156. Ken JG, vanSonnenberg E, Casola G, Christensen R, Polansky AM. Perforated amebic liver abscesses: successful percutaneous treatment. *Radiology* 1989;170:195–197.

157. Ibarra-Perez C, Green L, Calvillo-Juarez M, Vargas de la Cruz J. Diagnosis and treatment of rupture of amebic abscess of the liver into the pericardium. *J Thorac Cardiovasc Surg* 1972;64:11–17.

158. vanSonnenberg E, Mueller PR, Schiffman HR, et al. Intrahepatic amebic abscesses: indications for and results of percutaneous catheter drainage. *Radiology* 1985;156:631–635.

159. Barnes PF, DeCock KM, Reynolds TR, Ralls PW. A comparison of amebic and pyogenic abscess of the liver. *Medicine (Baltimore)* 1987;66:472–483.

160. Irusen EM, Jackson TFHG, Simjee AE. Asymptomatic intestinal colonization by pathogenic *Entamoeba histolytica* in amebic liver abscess: prevalence, response to therapy, and pathogenic potential. *Clin Infect Dis* 1992;14:889–893.

161. Healy GR. Immunologic tools in the diagnosis of amebiasis: epidemiology in the United States. *Rev Infect Dis* 1986;8:239–245.

162. Ahmed L, El Rooby A, Kassem MI, Salama ZA, Strickland GT. Ultrasonography in the diagnosis and management of 52 patients with amebic liver abscess in Cairo. *Rev Infect Dis* 1990;12:330–337.

163. Ralls PW, Quinn MF, Boswell WD, Colletti PM, Radin TR, Halls J. Patterns of resolution in successfully treated hepatic amebic abscess: sonographic evaluation. *Radiology* 1983;149:541–543.

164. Joyce MP, Ravdin JI. Pathology of human amebiasis. In: Ravdin JI, ed. *Amebiasis: human infection by* Entamoeba histolytica. New York: Churchill Livingstone, 1988;129–146.

165. Reed SL, Flores BM, Batzer MA, et al. Molecular and cellular characterization of the 29-kDa peripheral membrane protein of *Entamoeba histolytica:* differentiation between pathogenic and nonpathogenic isolates. *Infect Immun* 1992;60:542–549.

166. Tachibana H, Kobayashi S, Kato Y, Nagakura K, Kaneda Y, Takeuchi T. Identification of a pathogenic isolate-specific 30,000-Mr antigen of *Entamoeba histolytica* by using a monoclonal antibody. *Infect Immun* 1990;58:955–960.

167. Haque R, Kress K, Wood S, et al. Diagnosis of pathogenic *Entamoeba histolytica* infection using a stool ELISA based on monoclonal antibodies to the galactose-specific adhesin. *J Infect Dis* 1993;167:247–249.

168. Abd-Alla M, Jackson TFHG, Gathirim V, El-Hawey AM, Ravdin JI. Differentiation of pathogenic from nonpathogenic *Entamoeba histolytica* infection by detection of galactose-inhibitable adherence protein antigen in sera and feces. *J Clin Microbiol* 1993;31:2845–2850.

169. Luaces AL, Pico T, Barrett AJ. The ENZYMEBA test: detection of intestinal *Entamoeba histolytica* infection by immunoenzymatic detection of histolysin. *Parasitology* 1992;105:203–205.

170. McAuley JB, Juranek DD. Luminal agents in the treatment of amebiasis. *Clin Infect Dis* 1992;14:1161–1162.

171. McAuley JB, Herwaldt BL, Stokes SL, et al. Diloxanide furoate for treating asymptomatic *Entamoeba histolytica* cyst passers: 14 years' experience in the United States. *Clin Infect Dis* 1992;15:464–468.

172. Sullam PM, Slutkin G, Gottlieb AB, Mills J. Paromomycin therapy of endemic amebiasis in homosexual men. *Sex Transm Dis* 1986;13:151–155.

173. Beard CM, Noller KL, O'Fallon WM, Kurland LT, Dockerty

MB. Lack of evidence for cancer due to use of metronidazole. *N Engl J Med* 1979;301:519–522.

174. Thompson JE, Forlenza S, Verma R. Amebic liver abscess: a therapeutic approach. *Rev Infect Dis* 1985;7:171–179.

175. Martinez-Palomo A, Martinez-Baez M. Selective primary health care: strategies for control of disease in the developing world. X. Amebiasis. *Rev Infect Dis* 1983;5:1093–1102.

176. Sexton DJ, Krogstad DJ, Spencer HC, et al. Amebiasis in a mental institution: serologic and epidemiologic studies. *Am J Epidemiol* 1974;100:414–423.

177. Backer H. Field water disinfection. In: Auerbach PS, Geehr EC, eds. *Management of wilderness and environmental emergencies*. St Louis: CV Mosby, 1989;805–829.

178. Ravdin JI, Guerrant RL. A review of the parasite cellular mechanisms involved in the pathogenesis of amebiasis. *Rev Infect Dis* 1982;4:1185–1207.

179. Ravdin JI. Intestinal disease caused by *Entamoeba histolytica*. In: Ravdin JI, ed. *Amebiasis: human infection by* Entamoeba histolytica. New York: Churchill Livingstone, 1988;495–509.

Infections of the Gastrointestinal Tract,
edited by M. J. Blaser, P. D. Smith, J. I. Ravdin,
H. B. Greenberg, and R. L. Guerrant
Raven Press, Ltd., New York © 1995.

CHAPTER 71

Giardia lamblia

Michael J. G. Farthing

Giardia lamblia is the most common intestinal protozoan enteropathogen worldwide. For more than half a century there was debate as to whether this organism was a pathogen or merely a harmless commensal. There is now compelling evidence to indicate that *Giardia* is an important cause of acute and chronic diarrhea, which may be associated with intestinal malabsorption and growth retardation in infants and young children (1–3). Recent analysis of ribosomal ribonucleic acid (rRNA) indicates that *Giardia* has a unique place in evolution, being the missing link between prokaroytes and eukaroytes (4). Despite rapid progress in our understanding of the biology of *Giardia*, several questions remain unanswered. There is still no adequate explanation for the diverse clinical spectrum associated with giardiasis, which ranges from asymptomatic carriage to acute self-limiting diarrhea or sometimes persistent diarrhea that may fail to respond to appropriate therapy, even in immunocompetent individuals. In addition, the mechanisms by which *Giardia* produces diarrhea and malabsorption are poorly understood, although several theories have been put forward. Finally, despite extensive study in animal models and in humans, the key immunological determinants of clearance of acute infection and the development of protective immunity remain ill-defined.

DESCRIPTION

Anton van Leeuwenhoek wrote a letter to Robert Hooke, Secretary of the Royal Society, London, dated November 4, 1681 in which he gives what most scientists believe to be the first account of the identification of *Giardia*, using one of his own hand lenses and a specimen of his own diarrheal stools (5). Vilem Lambl in 1859 rediscovered the parasite in the diarrheic stools of children and named the organism *Cercomonas intestinalis*, again making the link between the presence of this organism

and diarrhea. The name *Lamblia* was first applied to the genus by Blanchard in 1888. Kunstler in 1882 discovered a similar organism in tadpoles and named it *Giardia agilis*, after his teacher and mentor Professor Alfred Giard. As far as can be ascertained, Giard had no direct involvement in the discovery of this organism or in the description of its biology. Although discovery of the cyst form of the parasite is often attributed to Grassi in 1879, cysts are present in the sketches of Vilem Lambl, which he published in 1860 (Fig. 1).

Taxonomy

Phylum to Family

Giardia has traditionally been placed in the subphylum Sarcomastigophora, in the superclass Mastigophora, and in the order Diplomonadida. In addition, *Giardia* belongs to the family Hexamitidae, which contains six genera, three of which, including *Giardia,* are exclusively parasitic (6).

Genus, Species, and Race

Organisms in the genus *Giardia* possess an adhesive disc on the ventral surface, which distinguishes it from other members of the family Hexamitidae. All members of this genus are vertebrate parasites, although only one of the three morphological types of *Giardia* are known to infect humans. This is sometimes referred to as the genus *Lamblia.*

Different *Giardia* species were initially assigned on the basis of the host from which they were derived, which produced more than 40 *Giardia* "species." Filice (7) in 1952 considered host specificity unreliable and emphasized the shape of the median body as an approach to distinguish between the three major morphological types: *Giardia agilis* from amphibians, *Giardia muris* from mice, and *Giardia intestinalis* (*duodenalis*) from humans and

M. J. G. Farthing: Department of Gastroenterology, St. Bartholomew's Hospital, London ECIA 7BE, United Kingdom.

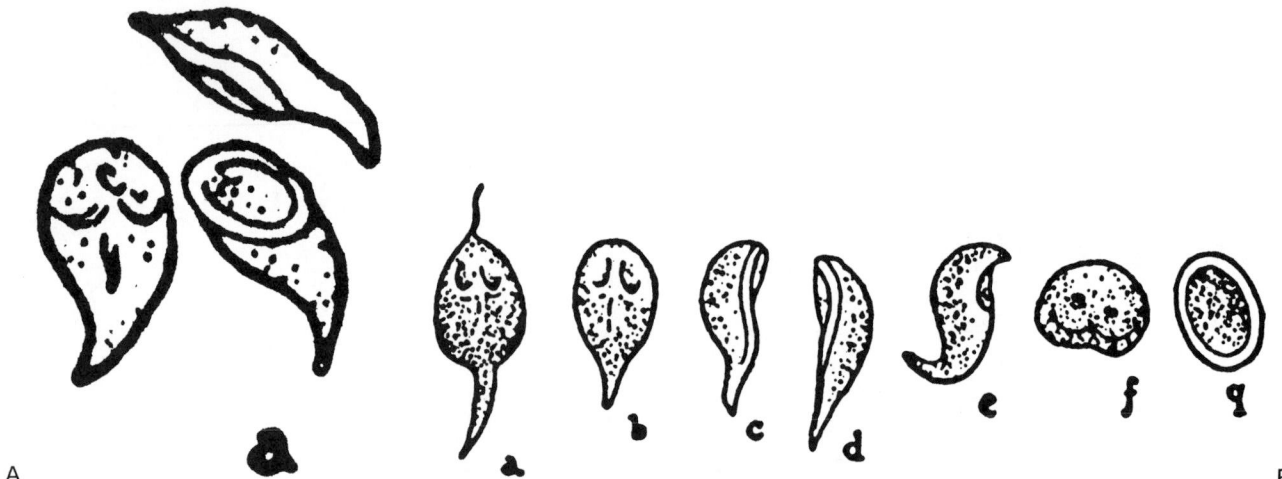

FIG. 1. Vilem Lambl's drawings of *Giardia* trophozoites and cysts from 1859 (**A**) and 1860 (**B**).

some other vertebrates (Fig. 2). Trophozoites of the *G. agilis* group have a long club-shaped median body situated parallel to the longitudinal axis of the cell, trophozoites of the *G. muris* group have small round median bodies, and those of the *G. duodenalis* group are claw hammer-shaped and lie transversely across the trophozoite body. In addition to these three major morphological subtypes, two other *Giardia* isolates have been described and have been assigned to separate species: *G. psittaci,* an isolate from a budgerigar that has median bodies of the *G. intestinalis* type but lacks the ventrolateral flange and thus the marginal groove bordering the adhesive disc; and *G. ardeae,* an isolate from the Great blue heron, that has a median body similar to those of *G. muris* and *G. intestinalis* but a ventral disc and single caudal flagellum more similar to *G. muris* (7).

Chemotaxonomy

A variety of techniques, including antigen analysis, iso-enzyme determinations, and deoxyribonucleic acid (DNA) analysis have been used to confirm the morphological species described previously and to determine whether subspecies or races exist within these morphological types.

Antigen Analysis

Recent studies have shown that there are antigenic differences between *Giardia* isolates in axenic culture, but these data are almost exclusively limited to the *G. intestinalis* group (8,9). No typing system has emerged that

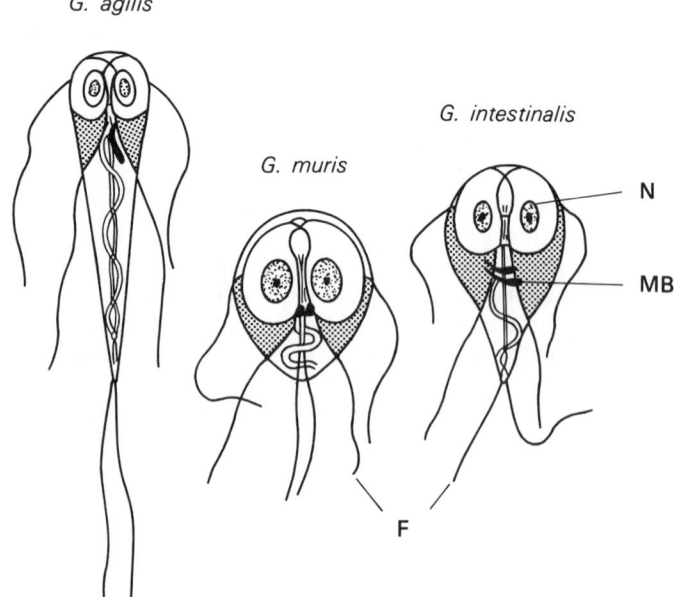

FIG. 2. Morphological types of *Giardia*. Diagrammatic representations of light microscopic appearances of *G. agilis, G. muris,* and *G. intestinalis*. N, nucleus; MB, median body; F, flagella.

can routinely be used for classifying *Giardia* isolates, and this probably relates to the finding that *Giardia* isolates in axenic culture are "mixed" and may not have a single antigenic profile. In addition, cloned *Giardia* isolates can vary their surface antigens *in vitro* and *in vivo*, possibly as a result of immune or other host pressures (10). It has also been suggested that bacterial endosymbionts and *Giardia* RNA viruses may also modulate surface antigens and thus interfere with chemotaxonomic determination (11). This observation suggests that antigenic analysis is unlikely to emerge as a widely applicable typing system for *Giardia*.

Isoenzymes

This approach has been highly successful in distinguishing pathogenic from nonpathogenic *Entamoeba histolytica* isolates. Up to ten different enzymes have been studied and thirteen different zymodemes identified in *Giardia* species (12). It has been possible to show clear differences between isolates of *Giardia intestinalis* and attempts have been made to group isolates according to their zymodeme patterns. However, as yet there are insufficient data to use this approach to assign specific zymodeme patterns to *G. intestinalis* subspecies and there is no clear association between the isoenzyme profile and biotype. In some instances, isolates from human and animal origins have been shown to have the same isoenzyme profiles, suggesting that giardiasis may be a zoonosis (12).

DNA Analysis

Pulsed-field separations of intact chromosomes have shown that *Giardia* possesses at least five distinct sets of chromosomes varying in size between 1×10^6 and 4×10^6 bp (13,14). Using this technique, differences between human isolates have been detected and similarities and differences between human and animal isolates are also apparent (15). Heterogeneity between isolates can also be demonstrated by restriction fragment length polymorphism analysis and DNA fingerprinting using the bacteriophage M13 genome as a probe (16,17). However, as yet no universally accepted typing system has emerged that will reliably distinguish any particular human or animal subspecies of the *G. intestinalis* type, and thus at present the consensus of opinion indicates that further attempts to phenotype or genotype *Giardia* isolates should not be made until they can be related to differences in subspecies biology.

A Unique Place in Evolution

The rRNAs of *G. duodenalis* are unique in that they are smaller than those of eukaryotes and the eubacteria (18). Sequence analysis of the gene encoding the small subunit rRNA of *Giardia* has shown that *Giardia* is more closely related to the archebacteria than to other eukaryotes. These findings suggest that *Giardia* species is the first organism to evolve from the prokaryote state and is thus the missing link between prokaryotes and eukaryotes.

Structure and Ultrastructure of *Giardia* Species

Giardia species exists in two forms: the motile trophozoite, which exists exclusively within the intestinal tract and which produces diarrheal disease, and the cyst, which can survive outside the host in appropriate conditions and which transmits the infection.

Trophozoite

The trophozoite measures approximately 12 to 15 μm in length and 5 to 9 μm in width. It has two nuclei and four symmetrically placed flagella originating from basal bodies at the anterior pole of the nuclei. The prominent dark staining median body is found in the posterior portion of the organism and has a different form depending on the morphological type of *Giardia* (Fig. 2). Scanning electron microscopy clearly shows the convex dorsal surface of the trophozoite and the concave ventral surface containing the attachment organelle, the ventral disc (Fig. 3). The disc is a rigid structure consisting of a platform of microtubules, 50- to 60-nm cross-bridges attached to the microtubules, and microribbons that run perpendicularly to both the cross-bridges and microtubules and appear unique to *Giardia*. These *Giardia*-specific proteins have been called giardins, which range in size from 29 to 38 kDa (19–23). Two giardins, α and β giardin, have been cloned and sequenced and the secondary structure predicted (Table 1). The rim of the disc contains contractile

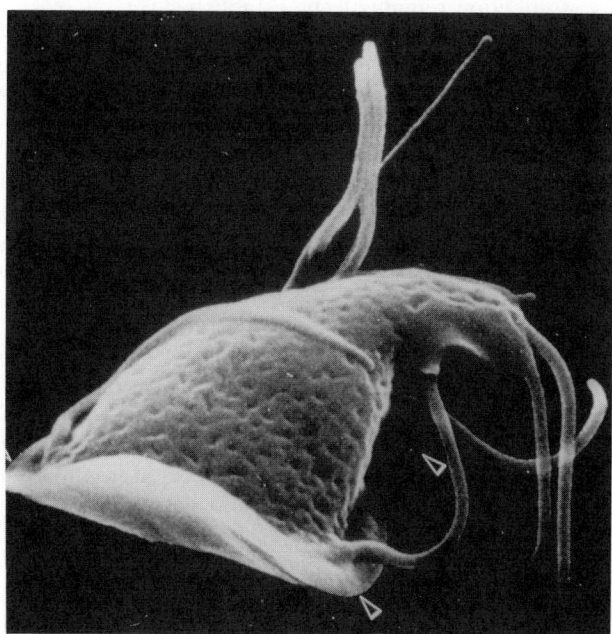

FIG. 3. Scanning electron micrograph of *G. intestinalis* trophozoites. (×1680). (Courtesy Stanley Erlandsen.)

TABLE 1. *Giardins: structure and sequence*

Giardin	Molecular weight (kDa)	Secondary structure	Sequence at probable site of translocation initiation	Length of 5' untranslated sequence	3' untranslated sequence[a]	G + C content of protein coding portion (%)
α_1-Giardin	33.8	α Helical	TTAAAA<u>ATG</u>CCG	3	TAGGGG<u>TTTAGTGAA</u>CGTC<u>TTTAG</u>	60
α_2-Giardin			TAGAAA<u>ATG</u>CCG	3	<u>TAG</u>GCGCCTTTACTGCGGGG<u>TTTCC TTTCGCT</u>AGTGAATGCCTAGCGGGT	57
β-Giardin	29.4	α Helical	CCGTCT<u>ATG</u>TTC	—	<u>TAA</u>CGCCTCGAG<u>TAAA</u>	59
γ-Giardin			AAGAAA<u>ATG</u>AAG	—	<u>TAA</u>GGGGCTGGGCTGGTG<u>AGTAAAT TTCCCTATAGC</u>	53

Adapted from ref. 2.
[a] Stop codon and possible polyadenylation signal (AGTPuAAP$_y$) are underlined.

proteins, actin, α-actinin, myosin, and tropomyosin, which give the outer portion of the disc its flexibility and are presumed to be involved in attachment to the intestinal epithelium (24). The flagella have the usual eukaryotic pattern of nine pairs and two central single microtubules. Flagella contain axonemal proteins and an additional set of polypeptides of approximately 30 kDa. These are not giardins and await further characterization.

The median body appears to contain giardins, actin, and α-actinin, suggesting that the median body may be involved in disc synthesis during cell division or possibly acting as a reservoir or nucleating template for new disc fibers (24).

Giardia contains few defined cytoplasmic organelles and has no mitochondria. However, there are multiple ovoid vacuoles 0.1 to 0.4 μm in diameter, usually situated immediately beneath the plasma membrane. These vacuoles appear to be lysosomal in function in that they contain a variety of hydrolyses, including acid phosphatase, thiol-dependent and thiol-independent proteinases, DNAses, and RNAses (25–28). The function of these structures in the parasite's life cycle and in the pathogenesis of infection remains to be established.

Although no classic Golgi apparatus has been described in *Giardia*, a structure containing encystation-specific antigens has been detected in encysting trophozoites (29). Evidence has been presented that these structures are involved in protein sorting and it seems likely that they will also be present in nonencysting trophozoites.

Bacterial endosymbionts were first observed by Boeck in 1917 (30). These observations have been confirmed by a number of ultrastructural studies of both *G. muris* and *G. intestinalis*. Mycoplasma-like structures have also been identified in *Giardia* cysts and trophozoites from a variety of vertebrate sources (11). A 33-nm double-stranded (ds) RNA virus, which appears to impair *Giardia* adherence and reduce its rate of growth, has been found in a number of human isolates (31). It has been possible to transfer this virus to previously uninfected trophozoites by electroporation. The relationship between this virus and parasite virulence *in vivo* has not been established.

Cysts

Giardia intestinalis cysts are ovoid or elliptical in shape and measure approximately 7 to 10 μm in length. The cyst

wall is composed of a layer of fibrils arranged as a felt-like web (Fig. 4). The chemical structure of the cyst wall remains controversial. Lectin-binding studies have suggested that *N*-acetyl glucosamine was the major cyst wall sugar (31) and the finding that encysting trophozoites contained chitin synthetase activity suggested that chitin was a major component of the cyst wall (32,33). Subsequent studies, however, have suggested that galactosamine is the major cyst wall sugar accompanied by glucose, probably in the form of glycogen (34). *N*-acetyl-D-galactosamine (GalNAc) is not detected in trophozoites, but a biosynthetic pathway operates during encystation. Uridine-diphospho-*N*-acetylglucosamine (UDP-GlcNAc) 4'-epi-

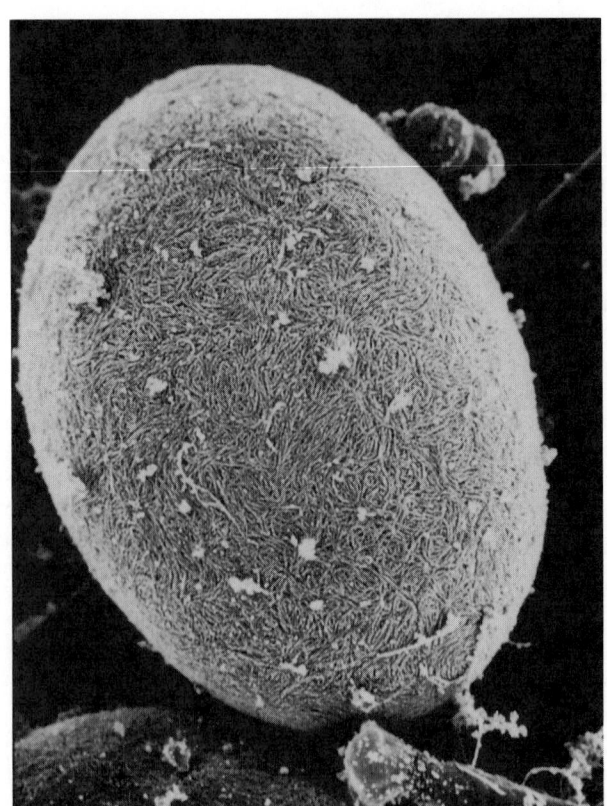

FIG. 4. High-resolution, low-voltage scanning electron micrograph of *G. intestinalis* cyst (×7700). (Courtesy of Stanley Erlandsen.)

merase is detectable during the encystation process and is involved in the synthesis of GalNAc from glucose. Cyst wall proteins (29 to 102 kDa) have been detected by immunostaining (35), but their final structure remains to be determined.

Within the cyst two or four nuclei can be detected together with the median body and cytoskeletal components.

MICROBIOLOGY

Life Cycle

Infection is initiated by ingestion of *Giardia* cysts generally through contaminated water or food, although direct person-to-person transfer does occur. Infection can be initiated with as few as 10 to 100 cysts (36). Excystation occurs in the proximal small intestine where the newly formed trophozoites emerge and multiply. As trophozoites pass distally along the small intestine, encystation occurs, and in humans 150 to 20,000 cysts per gram feces are excreted daily (37). The pattern of cyst excretion is highly variable such that on some days cyst counts may be below the detection limit of light microscopy. Cysts can survive in a cool, moist environment for several weeks and possibly months (38). The cycle is completed when cysts are ingested by another human or animal host.

Colonization Mechanisms

Colonization of the small intestine is an essential component of *Giardia*'s life cycle and is essential for production of diarrheal disease. Colonization occurs as a three-step process: (a) excystation, (b) attachment to intestinal epithelium, and (c) multiplication.

Excystation

Excystation of *G. intestinalis* and *G. muris* has been achieved *in vitro* by exposure of cysts to low pH, 1.3 to 2.7 (38) or 4.0 (39) followed by transfer to neutral pH. This mimics the situation *in vivo* when the cysts move from the acid environment of the stomach into the near neutral pH of duodenal and jejunal fluids. However, excystation of *G. intestinalis* and *G. muris* can occur at neutral pH (39,40), and *G. muris* has been shown to exist following exposure to sodium bicarbonate at pH 7.5 (40), consistent with a role for duodenal and pancreatic bicarbonate secretion in the excystation process. Excystation begins within 5 to 10 min of exposure to a suitable excystation environment, flagella movement being the first sign of activity. The intracellular vacuoles are thought to discharge their contents during excystation (41), suggesting a role for hydrolase activity in the process.

Attachment

Giardia attaches intimately to the intestinal epithelium and also to a variety of other inert substrates such as glass and plastic. The ventral disc is thought to be the primary organelle of attachment. It has been suggested that hydrodynamic forces generated beneath the disc by the continuous activity of the ventral flagella mediate the attachment process (42). It also has been proposed that flagella activity causes a low-pressure area under the ventral disc due to fluid fluxes around the ventral and marginal grooves. However, attachment occurs in *G. psittaci* in which the ventrolateral flange is incomplete (6), thus making it unlikely that hydrodynamic forces can be the sole explanation for disc-mediated attachment. The presence of contractile proteins in the peripheral regions of the ventral disc suggests that they participate in attachment (24). Inhibitors of microfilament function such as cytochalasin-B and low calcium concentration inhibit attachment (43,44).

Many enteropathogens possess lectin or lectin-like substances on surface structures. These sugar-binding proteins, which recognize oligosaccharide receptors on the intestinal epithelium, are now considered to have a central role in mediating attachment. A mannose-binding surface lectin has been described on *G. lamblia* using the classic approach of mixed-cell agglutination with mammalian erythrocytes (45). This lectin is distributed throughout the parasite surface and is not specifically localized to the ventral disc (46). It is present within the trophozoite as a prolectin, which can be activated by trypsin (47). *Giardia* lectin has been purified and thought to have a molecular weight of 28 to 30 kDa (48). *Giardia* has been shown to adhere to isolated mammalian intestinal epithelial cells *in vitro* by mechanisms that are consistent with lectin-mediated attachment (49). *Giardia* also attach to CaCo-2 cells, the small intestinal epithelial cell line, by mechanisms that incorporate both contractile proteins and surface lectin-mediated processes (50). The relative importance of mechanical and lectin-mediated attachment mechanisms has not been established. The surface lectin may operate in the initial attachment between *Giardia* and the epithelium, since, unlike ventral disc-related attachment, the parasite does not need to be in a specific orientation to the mucosa. Subsequently, the parasite may reorientate in a ventral surface-down position when mechanical forces may be more effective.

Multiplication

Giardia trophozoites divide by binary fission. There is no evidence that a sexual stage is involved in parasite replication. *Giardia* is essentially a luminal parasite and is thus predominantly dependent on factors within the intestinal lumen for growth and multiplication. Bile promotes growth of *Giardia* both *in vivo* and *in vitro* (51–54) and seems relatively specific for *Giardia* since other related protozoa and intestinal bacteria do not exhibit a similar dependence (55). The mechanism by which bile promotes growth appears to be related to the organism's requirement for preformed phospholipid, which is plentiful in bile, its uptake being facilitated by the presence of conjugated bile salts (56). *Giardia* is unable to synthesize its own membrane phospholipid from precursors and thus the availability of phospholipid and sterols in the proximal small intestine may be the main reason why the parasite has a predilection to colonize this region of the intestine. Other luminal nutrients, notably carbohydrates, are important for parasite growth, as is the relatively low oxgyen tension that is present in the intestinal lumen (57).

Encystation

Encystation is vital for completing the life cycle of *Giardia* and probably occurs in the distal half of the small intestine. Encystation has been achieved *in vitro* by exposing trophozoites to high concentrations of conjugated bile salts and myristic acid at approximately neutral pH (33,58,59). Specific encystation antigens appear during the first 6 to 18 hr (21 to 39 kDa) followed at 24 hr by other antigens of higher molecular weight (66 to 103 kDa), which bind the GlcNAc binding lectin, wheat germ agglutinin. These antigens are transported to the cyst wall and are probably involved in wall structure.

In vitro Culture

The biology of *Giardia* began to unfold when methods become available for *in vitro* cultivation. Karapetyan (60) first described methods for *in vitro* cultivation of *Giardia* using complex media with the addition of *Candida* species and chick fibroblasts. The chick fibroblasts gradually died, the culture system becoming monoaxenic. In 1970, Meyer (61) described a method for axenically culturing *Giardia* trophozoites from rabbit, chinchilla, and cat using Hank's solution, serum, yeast extract, and cysteine. Since then, a variety of modifications have been made, the most commonly used medium currently being TYI-S-33, which includes a casein digest (trypticase), yeast extract, iron (ferric ammonium citrate), dextrose, bovine serum, ascorbic acid, bile salts, and cysteine (54). Cultures are usually maintained in screw-capped glass tubes or flasks containing a very limited air space to maintain a low oxgyen concentration.

Metabolism

Information on the biochemistry and metabolism of *Giardia* was extremely limited until 1980 when axenic cultivation of *G. intestinalis* trophozoites became widely available (57).

Carbohydrate Metabolism

Giardia is an aerotolerant anaerobe and thus differs from most eukaryotes, which have a predominantly aerobic metabolism; other notable exceptions are the protozoan pathogens *Entamoeba histolytica* and *Trichomonas* species. *Giardia* lacks mitochondria and mitochondrial enzymes and respires in the presence of oxygen by a flavin, iron–sulfur protein-mediated electron transport system. Glucose is the major energy source, which is converted to pyruvate by Embden-Meyerhof and hexose monophosphate shunt pathways (62,63). Glucose and possibly other carbohydrate substrates (64) are metabolized incompletely to carbon dioxide, ethanol, and acetate. The predominant oxidative metabolic pathway appears to vary depending on the oxygen concentration. In a strictly anaerobic environment, alanine is produced from pyruvate and ketoglutarate, whereas in the presence of low oxygen concentrations ethanol production increases and alanine production is reduced (65,66).

Lipid Metabolism

Giardia predominantly acquires membrane and other lipids from the culture medium, since the parasite appears to have little or no capacity for *in vivo* synthesis (64). There is evidence, however, that trophozoites can use exogenous arachidonic acid for phosphatidylinositol synthesis (67). Biliary lipids may be an extremely important source of membrane phospholipid for *Giardia*, the uptake of phospholipid and cholesterol being facilitated by conjugated bile salts (55,56).

Nucleic Acid Metabolism

Similar to some protozoan parasites, *Giardia* is unable to synthesize purines and pyrimidines, which distinguishes it from most other eukaryotes (57,68,69). *Giardia* is therefore dependent on salvage pathways for both of the nucleic acids, which must be synthesized exogenously. Pyrimidines appear to be taken up by active transport mechanisms, one site being used for uridine and cytosine and another for thymidine (70).

Calcium Metabolism

The calcium binding protein, calmodulin, has been detected in *Giardia* trophozoites and probably has a similar function in maintaining intracellular calcium homeostasis as it does in eukaryotes (71,72).

Genetics

Genetic analysis of *Giardia* has been hindered by lack of a defined growth medium with nutritional auxotrophs or drug-resistant mutants. A stable transformation with foreign DNA is also not easy to achieve in protozoa. Information on the genetics of *Giardia* derives predominantly from analysis of the few genes that have been cloned.

Chromosomes

Light microscopy has suggested the presence of four chromosomes while pulse-field gel electrophoresis indicates at least five sets of chromosomes, often with additional minor bands (73). Chromosome size varies between 1×10^6 and 4×10^6 bp, giving the total of 1.2×10^7 bp for the five chromosomes. Densitometric scanning of restriction endonuclease digests of *Giardia* DNA produces a similar genome size (73). Current evidence suggests that *Giardia* nuclei are haploid and that genetic diversity from *Giardia* isolates is explained on the basis of clonal divergence.

DNA Content

The G + C content of the *G. intestinalis* genome has been estimated to be 42% to 48%, of the protein-coding gene sequences to be 49% to over 60%, and of the rDNA gene to be 75% (74–76). The noncoding regions are relatively A + T rich.

rRNA

Giardia rRNAs are smaller than other eukaryotes and eubacteria (75,77). The rRNA gene is only 5566 bp in *G. intestinalis* and slightly larger at 7.5 kb in *G. muris* and *G. ardeae* because of larger intergenic spacer regions. Sequence analysis of the 16S-like RNA has demonstrated *Giardia*'s intermediate position between prokaryotes and eukaryotes (18).

Translation

Sequences reported from cDNA clones and confirmed by RNA sequencing of the 5' and/or S1 mapping indicate that the messenger ribonucleic acid (mRNA) leader sequences are only 1 to 6 bases, which is very much shorter than those usually found in higher vertebrates (2). Nevertheless, translation of *Giardia* mRNA has been achieved in the rabbit reticulocyte lysate system.

Transcription

Detailed information on *Giardia* species is limited, although available evidence suggests that it conforms more closely with transcription in other eukaryotes. Of the genomic clones that have been sequenced, a possible TAA box has been identified, 9 to 134 bases upstream from the initiation codon, although it is uncertain whether these represent recognition sites for RNA polymerase (78–80). A 6 to 19 nucleotide interval separates AGTPuAAPy from the stop codon, which is separated by 7 to 10 bases from the start of the poly(A) tail. AGTPuAA is thought to be the polyadenylation signal for *Giardia*. Introns have not been reported in *Giardia* species to date. Codon usage by *Giardia* is similar to that of the archebacteria, confirming *Giardia*'s intermediate position between prokaryote and eukaryote states (81).

EPIDEMIOLOGY

Giardiasis is the most common protozoal infection of the human intestine worldwide. It occurs throughout temperate and tropical locations, prevalence varying between 2% and 5% in the industrialized world and up to 20% to 30% in the developing world (82–90). One of the earliest systematic surveys of prevalence was carried out by Clifford Dobell and reported in 1921 in a report for the Medical Research Council of Great Britain (91). Giardiasis was found to be endemic at this time with prevalence rates from 3.8% to 9.3%. Dobell also made the highly relevant observation that infection was two to three times more common in children. Nevertheless, he remained unconvinced of the importance of *Giardia* as a cause of diarrheal disease at this time. It is now well recognized that giardiasis is common in children in the developing world. In rural Guatemala, 45 children were followed from birth through the first 3 years of life, and all were found to have had giardiasis during this period, many having had recurrent infections (85). Prevalence in Peruvian children reached 40% by the age of 6 months, whereas stool examination confirmed prevalence rates of about 20% in children in Zimbabwe and Bangladesh (86). Age-specific prevalence of giardiasis continues to rise through infancy and childhood and only begins to decline after adolescence (83).

High-Risk Groups

Infants and young children have increased susceptibility to giardiasis, although infection is rare during the first 6 months of life when breast-feeding is common (85). Nutritional insufficiency in children may be an additional risk factor, possibly contributing to chronicity of disease and a downward spiral in the infection–undernutrition cycle. A recent study of 31 Gambian children with chronic diarrhea and malnutrition showed that 14 (45%) had giardiasis compared with only 4 of 33 (12%) of healthy age- and sex-matched control children (90). The study indicates that *Giardia* is highly prevalent in children with chronic diarrhea and malnutrition and supports the view that chronic infection is strongly associated with persistent diarrhea and undernutrition.

Giardiasis has long been recognized to be a disease of travelers (92). British soldiers returning from northern France and the eastern Mediterranean during World War I were among the first well-documented cases (93). Subsequently, attention focused on European and North American tourists to the Soviet Union, particularly, St. Petersburg (94–96), and then locations within the developing world (92). Overall, the risk of acquiring giardiasis in the traveler is relatively low, usually accounting for less than 5% of cases of traveler's diarrhea. However, 30% of travelers to the Soviet Union acquired *Giardia* and more than 40% of Scandinavian visitors to St. Petersburg acquired the infection. It is not essential to move from the industrialized to the developing world to acquire the infection, since visitors to ski resorts and national parks in the United States can acquire the infection (97).

Immunodeficiency predisposes to infection and appears to be a major contributor to the persistence of symptoms (98,99). The classic descriptions occur in individuals with common variable immunodeficiency, predominantly with varying degrees of hypo- or agammaglobulinemia. Chronic giardiasis, both as the carrier state and symptomatic chronic diarrhea, is found in higher prevalence in male homosexuals with and without HIV infection than would be expected in the general population (100–102). However, this prevalence probably relates to increased transmission rather than immunodeficiency, since the prevalence is similar in male homosexuals with and without HIV/AIDS (102). *Giardia* coexists with other enteropathogens such as *Cryptosporidium parvum* and thus its role in the etiology of diarrhea is often unclear.

Although animal studies suggest that genetic factors are important in determining the host response to *Giardia,* whether such factors contribute to human infection is uncertain. However, the frequency of HLA antigens A1, A2, B8, and B12 is higher than expected in patients with giardiasis (1). No other genetic markers of host susceptibility have as yet been identified.

Transmission

The cyst is the infective form of the parasite and is able to survive for long periods in a suitable environment outside the host. Survival in freshwater has enabled *Giardia* to achieve the reputation as the most common cause of epidemic waterborne diarrheal disease. Epidemics have been well characterized in North America and Europe (103,104) and have usually been associated with inadequate water treatment, since reliance on chlorination alone will not guarantee cyst inactivation. Waterborne transmission in swimming pools has also been reported (105). Despite the public health importance of waterborne giardisis, numerically it may represent a small proportion of the total infections worldwide.

Direct person-to-person spread by fecal–oral transmission is another major mechanism by which the disease is transmitted. Outbreaks of giardiasis are well recognized in day care centers, residential institutions, and schools, where prevalence may be as high as 35% (106,107). Many infections are asymptomatic but spread can occur to other members of the family. Transmission of the parasite also occurs during sexual activity, particularly as a result of intimate oro-anal contact (108).

Survival of cysts in food and the contribution of foodborne transmission of giardiasis have not been well characterized. However, there have been a number of reports where food has clearly been identified as the source in several outbreaks of giardiasis (109,110). In most cases an infected food handler has been implicated, presumably transmitting cysts to freshly prepared food.

Reservoirs

The most important defined reservoir of *Giardia* is infected humans. However, surface water supplies are known to be contaminated with *Giardia* cysts and it has been suggested that this reservoir is replenished by cysts from infected humans. However, there is compelling evidence that many wild and domestic animals carry *Giardia* species, which are morphologically, phenotypically, and genotypically indistinguishable from isolates from humans. There is circumstantial evidence to suggest that wild animals might serve to maintain contamination levels of surface water supplies and that farm and domestic animals might act as reservoirs for direct transmission of *Giardia* species to humans (111,112). Direct evidence that giardiasis is a zoonosis is still awaited, but it seems highly likely that this will eventually be shown to be the case (112).

PATHOGENESIS AND IMMUNITY

Expression of intestinal disease following infection with an enteropathogen depends on a series of host–parasite interactions. In giardiasis, the variation in disease expression is extensive, ranging from symptom-free carriage of the organism to chronic diarrhea with malabsorption and weight loss and, in infants and young children, growth retardation. This variation may be due to (a) host factors, which may be genetically or environmentally determined, and (b) variable virulence of *Giardia* isolates.

Pathogenesis of Diarrhea

The mechanisms by which *Giardia* causes diarrhea and intestinal malabsorption remain controversial and probably multifactorial. Early ideas on pathogenesis suggested that *Giardia* trophozoites act as a mechanical barrier to absorption or competed for host nutrients. The enormous functional reserve of the small intestine and the relatively small metabolic mass of the parasite make these hypotheses untenable. There is evidence, however, that *Giardia* can produce varying degrees of mucosal injury and at the same time influence conditions in the intestinal lumen, which could impair nutrient digestion and absorption (113).

Mucosal Factors

Morphology

A variety of structural and functional abnormalities of the small intestinal mucosa occur during human infection and in animal models of giardiasis. In humans, *Giardia* can produce the complete repertoire of abnormalities of villous architecture, ranging from normal through partial to subtotal villous atrophy (114–123). However, the majority of individuals have either normal or relatively mild villous shortening, usually associated with an increase in

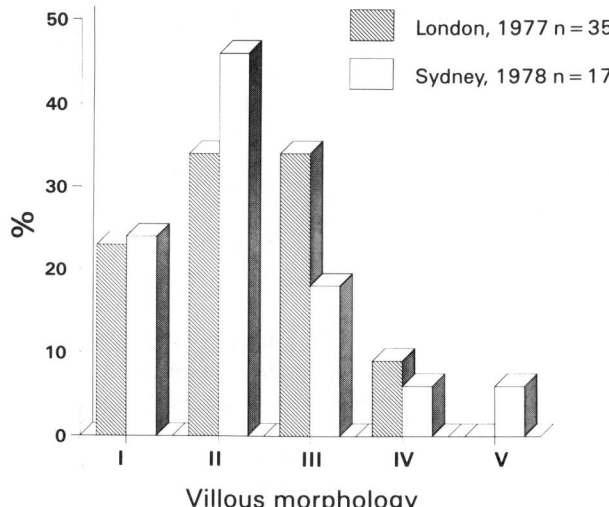

FIG. 5. Percentage of subjects with villous architectural abnormalities (normal, I; mild partial villous atrophy, II; moderate partial villous atrophy, III; severe partial villous atrophy, IV; and subtotal villous atrophy, V). Data are from studies in London (118) and Sydney (119).

crypt depth (Fig. 5). Experimental infections in gerbils, mice, and rats can produce similar abnormalities of mucosal architecture, and, like human infection, the abnormalities are generally mild (124). The gerbil provides a particularly good model to study small intestinal structure and function, as weanling gerbils develop diarrhea and have significant morphological abnormalities on the sixth day of infection, with villous shortening in the duodenum and increase in crypt depth throughout the small intestine (125,126). In the ileum there is a small but significant increase in villous height. These changes in crypt morphology occur in the absence of any inflammatory infiltrate in the lamina propria and without an increase in the number of intraepithelial lymphocytes.

Ultrastructural changes such as shortening and disruption of microvilli have been reported in human giardiasis even when villous architecture appears normal by light microscopy (115,127,128). Reduction in microvillous membrane surface area in both jejunum and ileum also has been reported in the gerbil model (126), although these abnormalities were extremely transient and their importance in the pathogenesis of diarrhea has been questioned (129). The decrease in microvilli is not found uniformly in the small intestine and is not specifically related to sites of trophozoite attachment. In human infection evidence suggests that the extent of mucosal abnormality relates to the severity of diarrhea (118,119).

Disaccharidase Activity

These morphological abnormalities in human giardiasis and in experimental infections in animals have been associated with reduction in lactase, sucrase, and maltase activities in the microvillous membrane (119,125,130–134).

In animal models, reductions in disaccharidase activities are maximal when diarrhea and villous morphological abnormalities are most severe.

Disruption of Intestinal Function

There is increasing evidence to suggest that there are functional consequences of the disturbances of structure and reduction in disaccharidase activity in the small intestine. In gerbils, basal transport of sodium and chloride ions was similar to noninfected controls, but glucose-stimulated sodium absorption was significantly reduced in stripped jejunal mucosal segments mounted in Ussing chambers (126). *In vivo* perfusion studies in animals have also shown impaired water, sodium, and chloride absorption in response to glucose, although basal transport was similar to controls (126). In the neonatal rat model of infection, basal transport of water, sodium ions, and chloride ions was impaired with some animals showing net secretion of sodium and chloride ions (134). Perfusion of a lactose-containing solution (lactose is the major carbohydrate source for 10-day-old neonatal rats) further exaggerated these transport abnormalities. Studies with brush-border membrane vesicles from infected mice provide further support for an impairment of glucose and amino acid transport (135,136).

Mechanisms of Mucosal Damage

From the foregoing discussion it is likely that structural and functional abnormalities in the small intestine are responsible, at least in part, for the diarrhea and malabsorption associated with giardiasis. The mechanisms by which these abnormalities occur, however, are poorly defined. Although there have been a few reports of epithelial invasion (137,138), *Giardia* is predominantly a luminal parasite, and thus invasive episodes must be regarded as exceptional and cannot be evoked as a major mechanism for disrupting mucosal structure and function. *Giardia* trophozoites, however, do attach to the epithelium and have been shown by electron microscopy to disrupt and distort microvilli at the site where the ventral adhesive disc interfaces with the microvillous membrane (139). In the mouse model of giardiasis, ventral disc imprints are particularly marked; similar but less impressive attachment imprints have been reported in infected human small intestine. It seems unlikely, however, that the localized attachment sites can account for the widespread changes in microvillous membrane surface area observed in the small intestine (126).

There is some experimental evidence to suggest that *Giardia* might produce and possibly release cytopathic substances into the intestinal lumen (136), although as yet none have been identified to account for the abnormalities in the small intestine. *Giardia* does contain both thiol-dependent and thiol-independent proteinases (27,28,140), which might attack surface glycoproteins and disrupt microvillous membrane integrity. In addition, *Giardia* has been shown to express a surface mannose-binding lectin, which may contribute to the attachment process (45–50). Dietary plant lectins can directly damage intestinal epithelial cells and produce microvillous membrane abnormalities similar to those seen in giardiasis (141,142). It remains to be determined whether any of these parasite products are directly injurious to host enterocytes. An alternative explanation might be that the increase in crypt depth observed in human infection and in experimental infections in animals is associated with increased crypt cell production rate and more rapid migration of enterocytes along the villus. In other conditions where this occurs, such as celiac disease, this results in the villus becoming populated by relatively immature enterocytes with reduced absorptive capacity. Increased proliferation has been confirmed in the gerbil model, but using thymidine kinase activity as a marker of maturity, there was no evidence in the jejunum or ileum that the cells repopulating the villus were less mature than those in noninfected controls (126). It seems likely therefore that the structure and functional abnormalities observed in the microvillous membrane relate to direct injury rather than another secondary mechanism that is causing crypt cell proliferation.

In human giardiasis, there is a variable immune response within the mucosa, although infection is often associated with an increase in lymphocytes in the lamina propria and in the epithelium (119,122,143,144). These changes have been more difficult to reproduce in experimental models. However, there is compelling evidence that T cell activation alone can produce villous atrophy. The enteropathy occurring in intestinal graft-versus-host disease and rejection of transplanted intestinal allografts is characterized by villous atrophy, crypt cell hyperplasia, and a lymphocytic infiltrate. Using human fetal small intestinal explants, it has been possible to partly characterize the mechanisms involved, by activating T cells either with pokeweed mitogen or with an anti-CD3 antibody; both approaches produce villous atrophy, crypt cell hyperplasia, and increased interleukin-2 (IL-2) production, confirming T cell activation (145). Further support for this hypothesis has been obtained from studies of experimental G. muris infection in athymic nu/nu mice. Despite prolonged infection, the alteration of villous/crypt cell ratio is less severe in the T cell deficient mice compared to immunocompetent controls (146). When lymphocytes from the spleen of immunologically intact mice were injected in athymic infected mice, histological abnormalities in the small intestine became more apparent. However, reduction in the villous/crypt cell ratio did occur in the immunocompromised mice before reconstitution, and thus it seems likely that T cell-independent mechanisms are also involved. In addition, immunosuppression in mice results in more profound effects on disaccharidase activities in conventional animals, indicating that epithelial damage is not solely dependent on immune function (132). Furthermore, although intraepithelial lymphocytes are frequently increased in giardiasis, a study in the mouse model indicated that intraepithelial lymphocyte numbers increased *after* villous shortening and the reduction in brush-border disaccharidases (131). Whether *Giardia* lectin can act as a mitogen and directly activate mucosal T cells remains to be established.

However, challenge of mice (previously infected with *G. muris*) with *G. muris* trophozoite extract resulted in a rapid decrease of disaccharidase activity, which might be immune mediated. The effect was most marked in the genetically susceptible C3H/HeN mouse (147).

Luminal Factors

Bacterial Overgrowth

Symptomatic giardiasis has been associated with increased numbers of aeroboic and/or anaerobic bacteria in the proximal small intestine. In one study from India, 8 of 17 (47%) patients with steatorrhea had more than 10^4 aerobic bacteria cultured from duodenal fluid, whereas none from a giardiasis control group without steatorrhea had bacterial overgrowth. Three of the patients with steatorrhea also had anaerobes present (148). Tomkins et al. (149) in 1978 found increased numbers of aerobic bacteria in 9 of 14 (64%) symptomatic overland travelers with giardiasis returning to the United Kingdom, two of whom also had anaerobes present. Bacterial overgrowth can produce architectural abnormalities in the small intestine similar to those seen in giardiasis, and thus it may have a role in producing mucosal injury.

Bile Salt Deconjugation

The removal of the glycine or taurine conjugate from bile salts reduces bile salt solubility in aqueous solution and thus reduces their efficacy for micelle formation within the intestinal lumen. In addition, free bile salts are membranotoxic and can cause intestinal secretion, thus potentially contributing to the pathogenesis of diarrhea. Tandon et al. (148) in 1977 found evidence of bile salt deconjugation in all of their Indian patients with bacterial overgrowth and in 40% of giardiasis controls without malabsorption, but another study of patients in the United Kingdom failed to confirm this observation (55). *Giardia* does not itself have the ability to deconjugate bile salts (55,150).

Bile Salt Uptake by Giardia

Bile and bile salts have important roles in the parasite's life cycle. At low concentrations bile salts stimulate parasite growth and thus may be an important colonization factor (54–56). High concentrations of bile salts trigger parasite encystation (58,59). More recently, it has been shown that parasites grown in bile are larger than those grown in a bile-free medium and that the presence of bile alters antigen expression by the parasite (151).

During the course of bile stimulation experiments, it became apparent that the parasite was consuming conjugated bile salts (56). Further studies showed that this was relatively specific for *Giardia* (55) and that uptake appeared to occur by a carrier-mediated, active transport process. A metabolic advantage of bile uptake for the parasite has not been defined, although bile salts do appear to be fully internalized into the cytoplasm and not sequestered in the surface membrane. Theoretically, consumption of host bile salts in chronic diarrhea could deplete the bile salt pool and thus contribute to fat malabsorption by impairing micellar solubilization of ingested fats and decreasing the effectiveness of pancreatic lipase, whose action is bile salt-dependent.

Inhibition of Hydrolytic Enzymes

Duodenal concentrations of trypsin, chymotrypsin, and lipase have been shown to be reduced in symptomatic patients with giardiasis (152–154). There is no evidence that this is due to a failure of pancreatic exocrine secretion but could be related to the more recent observation that live *Giardia* trophozoites and trophozoite sonicates inhibit trypsin activity and lipolysis *in vitro* (150,155,156). The mechanism by which the parasite inhibits these enzyme activities has not been established but could be related to the direct interaction between a parasite product, such as its own proteinases, and the host enzyme. However, the pancreas has a large functional reserve and the magnitude of the reduction observed in clinical studies is itself unlikely to account for malabsorption but could contribute to the cascade of abnormalities that together impair the absorptive mechanisms of the gut and contribute to diarrhea and malabsorption.

Thus there is no unifying hypothesis to explain the production of diarrhea and intestinal malabsorption in giardiasis. From the evidence presented, it seems likely that a number of factors are operating, which include varying degrees of mucosal injury in combination with disruption of the luminal phases of digestion and absorption.

Immunity

Increasing evidence suggests a central role for the immune system in determining the natural history of infection with *Giardia*, both with respect to eradicating acute infection and in the development of protective immunity (9). Epidemiologic evidence indicates that age-specific prevalence of giardiasis rises during childhood and only begins to decline during early adolescence, presumably as protective immunity is required (83,85). Further evidence for the development of protective immunity comes from studies of the prevalence of symptomatic giardiasis following waterborne epidemics. Prevalence is lower in the indigenous population compared to individuals who had recently arrived in an endemic area. Individuals who have recurrent or chronic exposure to the parasite appear more likely to have asymptomatic infections than those who are exposed to the parasite for the first time or at infrequent intervals (157). This probably accounts for the relative infrequency of symptomatic infections in homosexual men, those living in developing countries, and residents of high prevalence areas in the industrialized world such as Colorado mountain towns. All these studies sug-

gest that exposure to the parasite does produce immune protection, albeit not always complete (158,159).

Clinical evidence for the importance of immune host defense mechanisms in giardiasis is suggested by the apparent increased prevalence of giardiasis in some immunodeficiency states, notably common variable immunodeficiency and hypogammaglobulinemia.

Antibodies

Serum Antibody

Presence of complement-fixing antibody was first demonstrated in patients with giardiasis in 1946 (160) and the presence of specific anti-*Giardia* antibody was demonstrated by indirect immunofluorescence in 1976 using trophozoites obtained from a human intestinal aspirate (161). Subsequently, anti-*Giardia* antibodies were demonstrated by immunofluorescence and immunodiffusion using *Giardia* cysts prepared from human fecal specimens (162–164). The availability of axenic *Giardia* trophozoites provided a source of antigen that allowed the development of enzyme-linked immunoadsorbent assay (ELISA) for detecting antibody responses in serum (165).

Anti-*Giardia* immunoglobulin G (IgG) can be detected in more than 80% of patients with symptomatic infection and antibody titers may remain elevated for months or even years after primary infection (166). IgG titers are often raised in noninfected individuals in endemic areas, indicating previous exposure to the parasite (84,167). The relationship between the presence of anti-*Giardia* IgG and protective immunity has not been established. Anti-*Giardia* IgM titers increase early in infection and then decline within about 3 weeks (167,168). Specific IgM antibodies have been detected in naturally infected individuals in India, The Gambia, and United Kingdom (167,169) and also during experimental human infection (168).

Several studies have reported the presence of anti-*Giardia* IgA in serum from patients with giardiasis, although recent studies from India and The Gambia suggest that only about 30% of patients with active infection have detectable anti-*Giardia* IgA (170,171). Occasionally, giardiasis has been associated with an increase in total serum IgE. In one case the increase in IgE was not specific anti-*Giardia* IgE, and the authors suggested that infection had increased intestinal permeability, allowing entry of food antigens, which then became the target of the IgE response (172).

Specific anti-*Giardia* antibodies have been detected in sera of mice during experimental infection with *G. muris*. IgG and IgA were detected 2 to 3 weeks after initiation of infection, but no measurable IgM response was detected (173,174).

Secretory Antibody

There is relatively little information on the role of secretory immunoglobulin in human giardiasis, although there is evidence to suggest that individuals with secretory IgA (sIgA) deficiency are more susceptibile to infection (175). S-IgA has been demonstrated on the surface of *G. lamblia* trophozoites in human jejunal biopsies (176), and specific anti-*Giardia* S-IgA has been shown to be present in human duodenal fluid by ELISA. Total S-IgA concentration in duodenal fluid from infected patients has been found in two studies to be within the normal range (177,178). Specific anti-*Giardia* S-IgA has been identified in human milk and saliva and epidemiologic studies suggest that these antibodies may protect breast-fed infants from giardiasis (85,179,180).

Studies in murine giardiasis support a role for secretory immunoglobulin in eradication and prevention of infection (173,174). S-IgA and IgG antibodies have been demonstrated on the surface of *G. muris* trophozoites (173) and termination of infection was closely related to increased concentrations of specific S-IgA in intestinal fluid (181). Not all studies have been able to detect anti-*Giardia* S-IgA during experimental infection in mice. Profound reduction of S-IgA by chronic administration of anti-IgM to mice resulted in chronic giardiasis (174). The protective effect of immune milk has also been demonstrated in suckling mice (182).

However, specific anti-*Giardia* S-IgA concentrations in intestinal fluid are normal in C3H/He mice, although they develop chronic infection (8). Similarly, specific S-IgA concentrations were normal or even increased in mice with X chromosome-linked immunodeficiency, which again was associated with prolonged infection. This raises the issue of antibody quality, namely, antibody affinity and the ability of the mucosal immune system to produce antibody against "clearance" antigens.

Giardia Antigens and Antigenic Variation

The *Giardia* antigens studied so far are largely determinants of the IgG response, although some progress has been made in characterizing the antigenic profiles of specific IgM and IgA responses. Surface antigen profiles differ between *Giardia* isolates and, although certain major immunogens appear to be common to all isolates, considerable variation exists between human isolates. Thus, when examining the antigenic repertoire of serum or secretory antibodies during human or experimental infection, the same isolate should be used as antigen source for antigen analysis by immunoblotting or immunoprecipitation. Few human studies, however, have been able to achieve this goal.

A variety of antigens, measuring 24 to 225 kDa, have been detected by immunoprecipitation and immunoblotting techniques using polyclonal antisera, monospecific antisera, and monoclonal antibodies (1,2,8,9). A number of *Giardia* antigens have been studied in more detail. The WB isolate has been used to study a 170-kDa surface antigen, which has been partly cloned and sequenced (183). The gene encodes a cysteine-rich (12%) protein (CRP 170), which appears on sodium dodecyl sulfate–polyacrylamide gel electrophoresis (SDS-PAGE) as a 170-kDa doublet following metabolic labeling of trophozoites with cysteine. Other cysteine-rich proteins, including TSA 417, BSP 1267, and CRP 72 (2,184), have also been cloned.

Also, 82- and 88-kDa surface antigens have been detected by surface iodination followed by Western blotting or immunoprecipitation, respectively (185,186). Serum antibodies to the 88-kDa antigen have been detected during natural human infection (186).

A 65-kDa antigen has been identified in trophozoites and in cysts from infected humans (187). This protein appears to be a glycoprotein containing galactose residues (188). A 57-kDa antigen has been identified by mouse monoclonal antibody and shown to be immunogenic during human infection (171). This antigen is predominantly cytoplasmic but also is expressed in surface membrane. In children with *acute* giardiasis, IgG and IgA antibodies to the 57-kDa antigen were detected in seram, but in Gambian children with *chronic* giardiasis and undernutrition, an IgG and IgM response was detected but not an IgA response (189–191). These findings indicate that this antigen may be involved in parasite clearance; the failure to develop an IgA response suggesting that there may be a failure to switch from IgM to IgA production in the intestinal mucosa.

Lower molecular weight antigens include a 49-kDa glycoprotein (GP49), which is present in a variety of isolates from different geographic locations, and a 31-kDa antigen, which probably represents the giardins that seem to be immunogenic during human infection (192).

Relatively little is known about the function of these antigens during natural infection. However, antibodies to the 170-kDa antigen of *G. intestinalis* and to the 36.2- and 30.3-kDa antigens of *G. muris* are known to be cytotoxic to the parasite (193,194). Some *Giardia* surface antigens are excreted/secreted during *in vitro* growth (195).

Variation of the surface antigen profile is an established mechanism by which parasites may evade the host immune response, most characteristically demonstrated by the African trypanosomes. Antigenic variation has been shown *in vitro* in experimentally infected humans, in gerbils, and in neonatal mice (196–199). A 72-kDa antigen of a cloned *Giardia* isolate was lost during experimental infection in mice and humans at approximately 3 weeks, at which time specific antibody to this antigen was detected (199).

Failure to express certain surface proteins, particularly the cysteine-rich proteins, may offer a survival advantage to the parasite. WB trophozoites expressing CRP 70 were susceptible to the host enzymes trypsin and chymotrypsin but were relatively resistant when this surface protein was no longer expressed (200).

Cellular Immune Response

An inflammatory cell infiltrate in the small intestinal mucosa often accompanies human infection with *Giardia* (119,122,131,143). There is an increase in the lymphocyte numbers in both the lamina propria and the epithelium, which, when associated with partial or subtotal villous atrophy, can be so severe as to resemble untreated celiac disease. Intraepithelial lymphocyte numbers decrease when infection resolves. However, there have been no detailed studies of lymphocyte phenotypes in human giardiasis.

T Lymphocytes

The role of T lymphocytes, however, has been studied in detail in the murine model of giardiasis. Hypothymic nude (nu/nu) T cell-deficient mice experience markedly prolonged infection with *G. muris* compared to immunocompetent strains (145,201). Infection may be eradicated by reconstitution with lymphocytes from syngeneic mice with normal immune function and this may be accelerated if the donor mice have already acquired protective immunity against *Giardia* (145,201,202). In hypothymic mice the number of L3,T4+ (CD4) cells are profoundly reduced, whereas CD8 cells and macrophages are relatively preserved (203). It has therefore been suggested that CD4 cells are critically important for the ability of mice to clear *G. muris* infection and may be involved in switching B cell IgM to IgA production during infection. Natural killer cells seem relatively unimportant since depleted mice are still able to clear infection.

Genetic factors are also important in determining the ability of mice to clear experimental infection (9). Normal inbred strains of mice such as BALB/c and C3H/He have different susceptibilities to *G. muris,* the former being relatively resistant while the latter experience prolonged infection (204). C3H/He mice are not obviously immunodeficient, but it has been proposed that *G. muris* can suppress host-protective responses in chronically infected mice of this strain.

As in some human infections, *G. muris* induces increased numbers of lymphocytes in the small intestinal epithelium by 2 weeks, which closely parallels reduction in parasite numbers in the intestinal lumen (8,131). Intraepithelial lymphocytes are predominantly T cells, whereas in the lamina propria there is an increase in both B and T cells. Lymphocyte numbers in Peyer's patches more than double in number during the course of experimental infection with *G. muris* but return to normal following parasite eradication. Although there is an increase in the absolute numbers of Peyer's patch lymphocytes, the CD4/CD8 ratio remains unchanged (203). There is preliminary evidence to suggest that mucosal T lymphocytes from infected mice are sensitized to *Giardia* antigens (205).

B Lymphocytes

Intestinal mucosal B cells are important in secretory antibody production in the intestine. Plasma cell numbers increase in the intestinal mucosa of humans infected with *G. intestinalis,* IgM-bearing cells being the predominant subtype (162). IgM cells are prominent early in infection and in nodular lymphoid hyperplasia of the small intestine, which occurs in some patients with giardiasis (206,207). One study, however, failed to confirm the presence of IgM-bearing cells and found only IgA and IgG

cells (122), although this may reflect differences in sampling time since it would be expected that during the later stages of infection IgM-producing cells would switch to IgA production.

Mast Cells

Mast cell-deficient mice (W_fW_f) have prolonged experimental infections lasting 8 weeks or more compared with BALB/c mice, which clear infection in 4 to 5 weeks (208). Further support for a role for mast cells in controlling infection is the observation that administration of cyproheptadine, a drug that is a histamine and serotonin antagonist, also prolongs experimental infection. Degranulating mast cells might release mediators that are directly toxic to the parasite or that improve access of other effector cells into the mucosa.

Macrophages

Tissue macrophages and the group of related cells including dendritic and veiled cells have a critical role in the mucosal immune response as antigen-presenting cells. There is also evidence that macrophages act as effector cells for clearance of the parasite during experimental *G. muris* infection (209,210). Tissue macrophages engulf *Giardia* trophozoites and rabbit peritoneal macrophages will take up opsonized trophozoites *in vitro.* Mouse peritoneal macrophages will kill *G. muris* trophozoites *in vitro;* this effect is enhanced by immune serum or milk containing anti-*Giardia* IgG and IgA. Spontaneous cytotoxicity by macrophages may explain the relative susceptibility of C3H/HeJ mice to *G. muris* infection (211), although another study failed to confirm this (212). Peripheral blood monocytes also exhibit spontaneous cytotoxicity against *G. intestinalis,* although these findings were not confirmed by others, apparently due to a defect in the experimental design of the earlier studies (213).

Polymorphonuclear Leukocytes

Neutrophils from patients with giardiasis exhibit antibody-dependent cell-mediated cytotoxicity (ADCC) against *G. intestinalis in vitro.* Anti-*Giardia* IgG was the predominant antibody responsible for sensitization (214). ADCC was not observed with peripheral blood monocytes or lymphocytes.

Immune Function in Giardiasis

Parasite Clearance

The evidence presented suggests that both antibody- and cell-mediated mechanisms are involved in parasite eradication. The appearance of increasing concentrations of S-IgA in intestinal fluid and its association with clearance of *Giardia* in the mouse model strongly support the role for S-IgA in eradication. Anti-*Giardia* S-IgA agglutinates trophozoites *in vitro* and thus may interfere with motility and cell division. A mouse monoclonal antibody directed against a trophozoite surface 88-kDa antigen inhibited attachment to isolated mammalian intestinal epithelial cells *in vitro* (49), and a monoclonal antibody directed toward a 170-kDa surface protein was directly cytotoxic (193). ADCC and the direct effect of neutrophils and macrophages may also be important within the intestinal lumen.

Control of Mucosal Invasion

Although invasion is a rare event, potential pathways for preventing this include cytotoxic intraepithelial lymphocytes and ADCC by lamina propria lymphocytes (215). Activation of the classic complement pathway and a unique pathway involving calcium and complement components C1 and factor B will also effect trophozoite lysis within the mucosa (216,217).

Protective Immunity

Immune milk appears to passively prevent giardiasis both in experimental models and humans (179,182,204). Active immunity does appear to be acquired, although this may not be complete or long lasting. Continued exposure to the parasite may be required to maintain effective protective immunity. It is unclear as to exactly which pathways are involved in immune protection although secretion of *Giardia*-specific S-IgA would seem to be the first line of defense. The antigens involved in the production of protective immunity have not been defined although preliminary evidence suggests that a 57-kDa antigen, so-called *Giardia* heat shock antigen (GHSA), may be involved (189,190).

Nonimmune Defense Mechanisms

Although secretory antibody in immune human milk appears important for protection against giardiasis in neonates, nonimmune human milk is also cytolethal to trophozoites due to the release of free fatty acids from milk triglycerides following exposure to host intestinal lipase activity (218–221). Other protective factors may include intestinal mucus and intestinal motility.

CLINICAL ILLNESS

The clinical spectrum of giardiasis is extensive, ranging from asymptomatic infection to severe chronic diarrhea with intestinal malabsorption. As discussed previously, this probably relates to a combination of factors, including host susceptibility and response to infection and possibly parasite virulence (1).

Asymptomatic Infection

This most common form of infection occurs in both adults and children and predominates in those parts of the world where *Giardia* is highly endemic. Whether chronic carriers had a transient diarrheal illness that passed unnoticed or whether infection was acquired without producing any symptoms is unclear.

Acute Giardiasis

The clinical syndrome of acute giardiasis has been well characterized in travelers moving from an area of low to high endemicity (95,97) (Table 2). Symptoms usually begin within 3 to 20 days (mean of 7 days) of arrival in the high-risk area and, for the vast majority, the illness is over within a 2- to 4-week period. However, in up to 25% of infected travelers symptoms may persist for 7 weeks or more. The major symptom of acute giardiasis is diarrhea, which is usually initially watery but can progress to an illness characterized by steatorrhea, nausea, abdominal discomfort, bloating, and often weight loss.

Chronic Giardiasis

Although infection is self-limiting in the majority of healthy individuals, a proportion possibly as high as 30% to 50% will go on to have persistent diarrhea, often with the features of steatorrhea. Weight loss can be profound under these circumstances with losses of 10% to 20% of the usual or ideal body weight. Since the early absorption studies are Veghelyi (222) a number of reports confirm that intestinal malabsorption occurs in patients with giardiasis, with about 50% of symptomatic patients having biochemical evidence of fat malabsorption (115–118,121,223–229) (Table 3). Malabsorption of other nutrients such as vitamin A and B_{12} are also reported. Severe macrocytic anemia due to folate deficiency may occur infrequently. Indirect evidence of carbohydrate and malabsorption is suggested by reduced D-xylose absorption, although it is now considered that this test is only a reliable marker of glucose absorption at low concentration

TABLE 2. *Symptoms of acute giardiasis in travelers*

Clinical features	Aspen, Colorado (ref. 97) (n = 324) (%)	Soviet Union (ref. 95) (n = 56) (%)
Diarrhea	96	93
Weakness	72	80
Weight loss	62	73
Abdominal pain	61	77
Nausea	60	59
Steatorrhea	57	55
Flatulence	35	—
Vomiting	29	—
Fever	17	—

TABLE 3. *Intestinal malabsorption in giardiasis*

Study	Reference	Location	Number of subjects	Percentage of subjects with abnormal results				
				D-Xylose	Lactose	Fat	Vitamin B_{12}	Vitamin A
Veghelyi, 1939	222	Hungary	14	—	—	71	—	—
Katsampes et al., 1944	223	U.S.A.	15	—	—	—	—	100
Cantor et al., 1967	224	Argentina	20	—	—	25	—	—
Hoskins et al., 1967	115	U.S.A.	6	50	100	40	100	—
Alp and Hislop, 1969	116	Australia	5	20	20	100	—	—
Barbieri et al., 1970	225	Brazil	11[a]	27	—	82	—	—
Ament and Rubin, 1972	117	U.S.A.	77	—	—	66	100	—
Cowen and Campbell, 1973	226	U.S.A.	3	100	—	66	100	—
Tewari and Tandon, 1974	227	India	30	23	—	50	6	—
Rabassa et al., 1975	228	Cuba	50	62	27	34	—	—
Wright et al., 1977	118	U.K.	40	45	—	35	—	—
Tandon et al., 1977	148	India	63	4	—	27	0	—
Hartong et al., 1979	121	U.S.A.	12	55	—	64	60	—
Mahalanabis et al., 1979	229	India	4	79	—	50	—	100
Mean (%)				47	49	55	61	100

[a] Asymptomatic children.

and probably reflects a combination of active and passive transport. D-Xylose is metabolized by intestinal bacteria and thus results are difficult to interpret in the presence of bacterial overgrowth. Secondary lactase deficiency with lactose malabsorption is, however, well recognized to occur in giardiasis and may take several weeks to recover, even after clearance of the parasite (230,231).

Clinical Sequelae of Giardiasis

Growth Impairment

Nutritional insufficiency is a major complication of giardiasis, which in adults can result in a variety of problems associated with macro- and micronutrient deficiency. However, in children it is well established that recurrent gastrointestinal infection can retard growth and development, and several lines of evidence suggest that *Giardia* may be a candidate enteropathogen, since (a) it occurs commonly in infants and children, with peak prevalence

in the preschoool years; (b) it is known to damage the small intestine and cause intestinal malabsorption; (c) it is not always self-limiting and may persist for many weeks or months; and (d) it causes impaired growth in some young animals (232). Since the early 1920s, a number of hospital-based studies have shown the deleterious effects of giardiasis on growth in infants and young children (233–241) (Table 4). However, these studies are highly biased toward more severely affected children and do not give clear indications as to the impact of giardiasis in the community. A few reports have emerged that attempt to tackle this key question; these suggest that *Giardia* may have an independent growth inhibitory effect in poor communities in the developing world (Table 5), although it is difficult to separate out *Giardia* from other growth-retarding influences, such as other enteric infections, respiratory infections, and viral exanthemata (85,242–244). Studies of well-nourished children in day care centers have not found evidence of growth failure in this population. Pickering et al. (245) studied children with *Giardia* in a day care center but found no association between the oc-

TABLE 4. *Giardiasis: impact on child growth*

Hospital-based study	Year	Reference	Location	Number studied	Patients (%) growth retarded		
					Weight	Height	Not specified
Perkins	1921	233	U.K.	7	—	—	14
Miller	1926	234	U.K.	23	39	+	—
Veghelyi	1938	235	Hungary	93	86	13	—
Boe and Rinvik	1943	236	Norway	22	—	—	9
Cortner	1959	237	U.S.A.	4	100	75	—
Court and Anderson	1959	238	Australia	13	92	—	—
Burke	1975	239	U.S.A.	7	100	—	—
Kay et al.	1977	240	Australia	154	—	—	31
Pugh and Newton	1980	241	U.K.	17	—	—	41

TABLE 5. *Giardiasis: impact on child growth*

Community-based study	Year	Reference	Location	Number studied	Summary of findings
Rowland et al.	1977	242	The Gambia	152	No effect
Cole and Parkin	1977	243	The Gambia	152	↓ Weight gain ($p < 0.05$)
Gupta and Urrutia	1982	244	Guatemala	159	↑ Growth with metronidazole
Farthing et al.	1986	85	Guatemala	45	↓ Weight gain 2nd year of life

currence of the parasite and diarrhea and found no evidence of growth failure in those with the parasite. Ish-Horowicz et al. (246) found *Giardia* in 33 of 89 (37%) children aged 3 months to 3 years during a 12-month period in a day care center. Infection was usually asymptomatic and there was no evidence of impaired weight gain or linear growth. These two studies may reflect differences between relatively healthy urban children and the poor, underprivileged in rural parts of the developing world.

Allergic and Inflammatory Phenomena

Although immediate-type hypersensitivity is a relatively common association with helminthic infections, it is rare with the protozoa. However, urticaria, arthralgia, and other allergic phenomena have been described in patients with giardiasis. Acute urticaria in one case was associated with increased serum IgE concentrations, although there was no increase in anti-*Giardia* IgE (172). Lymphoid nodular hyperplasia has been associated with both chronic giardiasis and immune deficiency (206,247,248). Several studies have examined the prevalence of giardiasis in patients with hypogammaglobulinemia and found it to occur in 29% to 71% of cases. However, in one study from India, 25 patients were described, all of whom had giardiasis and lymphoid hyperplasia, but none had immunoglobulin deficiency (207). Thus the relationships between lymphoid nodular hyperplasia, hypogammaglobulinemia, and giardiasis remain unclear, although it would appear that any two can occur in combination without any direct implications for pathogenesis. There are no clear indications as to the pathogenesis of lymphoid nodular hyperplasia although several studies have shown a predominance of IgM-producing B cells within the mucosa and lymphoid nodules, suggesting there might be immune "overactivity" to a luminal antigen, possibly with failure to switch from IgM to IgA production within the intestine.

Protein-Losing Enteropathy

There have been several case reports of protein-losing enteropathy in children with giardiasis associated with severe undernutrition and edema (249,250). In a recent survey of children in The Gambia, it would appear that this is uncommon and rarely of a degree that has a major clinical impact (251). The precise mechanisms of protein-losing enteropathy in giardiasis have not been defined.

DIAGNOSIS

Clinical

Clinical diagnosis of giardiasis is often suggested by a typical history, particularly if there has been recent foreign travel. For the traveler, diarrhea usually begins toward the end of the holiday and persists on return, unlike most other forms of traveler's diarrhea that occur early and resolve rapidly. Many clinicians will treat empirically at this stage even without knowing the results of fecal examinations.

Microscopy

Light microscopic detection of *Giardia* forms (cysts and less frequently trophozoites) continues to be the mainstay of diagnosis. Stool specimens are examined either fresh or fixed with polyvinyl alcohol formalin and then stained with trichrome or iron hematoxylin. Cyst detection can be improved by using formalin–ethyl acetate or zinc sulfate methods. Cyst detection can be assisted by use of an immunofluorescent antibody to cyst protein. Examination of a single stool specimen may detect up to 70% of cases of giardiasis rising to 85% following examination of three separate specimens (252). Cyst excretion varies from day to day, and thus it is important that different specimens on different days should be examined (37). Trophozoites are usually only found in watery diarrhea and stools should be examined as a saline wet mount immediately after they have been passed.

Trophozoites may also be detected in duodenal fluid, and although some studies have suggested that this is a more reliable approach to diagnosis than fecal examination, only 44% of 74 South Indian patients with giardiasis had a positive duodenal aspirate (252). Stool positivity in these subjects was only 85%, indicating that the two diagnostic approaches are complementary. Trophozoites may also be identified by endoscopic brush cytology (253), in mucosal impression smears of duodenal or jejunal biopsies, and in histopathological sections.

Immunodiagnosis

Fecal Antigen ELISA

Giardia antigens in feces have been detected by a variety of methods, the most widely used being ELISA. A variety of assays have been developed using polyclonal antisera or monclonal antibodies (254–259). Sensitivity and specificity of these assays range from 87% to 100% and several of these assays have been commercialized. Further studies on their evaluation are awaited to determine whether their use can be recommended widely in routine diagnostic laboratories. Interpretation of "false-positive" results are, however, difficult. Enthusiasts will regard this as "microscopy negative" giardiasis, while the pessimist will merely regard this as a true false positive, possibly due to the presence of cross-reacting fecal antigens. It seems likely, however, that microscopy negative cases of giardiasis do exist and that more sensitive methods of detection such as ELISA or DNA-based diagnostic techniques will eventually show this to be the case.

Serology

Specific antibody detection in body fluids has not proved to be a highly rewarding approach to diagnosis. Anti-*Giardia* IgG is found in infected and noninfected individuals in endemic areas, presumably because of continued exposure to the parasite, and is thus unhelpful in distinguishing past from current infection (166,167). However, specific anti-*Giardia* IgM titers are usually only elevated in individuals with current infection, antibody concentrations falling rapidly once the infection has been cleared. Anti-*Giardia* IgM has been shown to be useful in identifying individuals with acute giardiasis even in endemic areas such as India and The Gambia (167,169). However, sensitivity and specificity decrease in children with persistent diarrhea, although even a proportion of children with symptoms that have persisted for several months continue to have elevated specific anti-*Giardia* IgM in serum (169). Approximately one-third of patients develop a specific serum anti-*Giardia* IgA response, which like IgM is relatively short-lived and thus may be of value in the diagnosis of ongoing infection in those patients with raised IgA titers (169,170). A negative result clearly does not exclude infection.

DNA-Based Approaches

With the development of specific DNA probes for *Giardia* it should be possible to develop DNA-based fecal detection assays (260). Preliminary studies suggest that this approach is feasible (261), although there are difficulties in liberating DNA from *Giardia*, which may be overcome by increasing sensitivity of the assay by using amplification techniques such as the polymerase chain reaction.

TREATMENT

There are three major classes of drug that are widely used in the treatment of giardiasis but none are ideal because of associated adverse effects and none can be regarded as safe in pregnancy. Treatment failures occur with all the standard drugs and the development of sensitivity testing for *Giardia* has allowed investigation of some of the mechanisms of treatment failure including drug resistance.

Standard Therapeutic Regimens

The three major classes of drugs used to treat giardiasis are the nitroimidazole derivatives, the acridine dyes such as mepacrine (quinacrine), and the nitrofurans such as furazolidone (2,262). The recommended doses for adults and children and an estimate of efficacy are outlined in Table 6. Metronidazole and tinidazole are probably the drugs of choice, since the treatment period is brief and compliance is generally good (262). However, the latter agent is not approved for the treatment of giardiasis in the United States. Mepacrine is of similar efficacy to the nitroimidazole derivatives, but some studies suggest that it is less well tolerated. Of particular concern is the reversible toxic psychosis seen in adults and skin problems, particularly in patients with underlying skin disorders such as psoriasis. Furazolidone appears to be a less effective drug in giardiasis but is widely used in children in the United States, partly because it is available as a suspension (263,264). None of these drugs can be regarded as safe during pregnancy. Paromomycin has some activity against *Giardia* and, since it is poorly absorbed, has been suggested as a possible drug for use in pregnancy. Adverse effects of these agents are summarized in Table 7.

The mechanisms of action of these drugs in giardiasis have not been examined in detail although exposure of metronidazole to bacterial or protozoal nitroreductase produces cytotoxic compounds that disrupt the helical structure of DNA (265). Quinacrine interferes with flavin enzymes, causing depression in oxygen consumption, and is an intercalating drug and thus may be incorporated into DNA (266). Furazolidone and other nitrofurans form su-

TABLE 6. *Drug treatment of giardiasis*

| Drug | Treatment regimen | | Efficacy |
	Adults	Children	
Metronidazole	2 g (single dose) daily, for 3 days or 400 mg three times daily for 5 days	15 mg/kg/day (max 750 mg) for 10 days	>90%
Tinidazole	2 g single dose	50–75 mg/kg in a single dose	>90%
Mepacrine (quinacrine)	100 mg three times daily for 5–7 days	2 mg/kg three times daily for 5–7 days	>90%
Furazolidone	100 mg four times daily for 7–10 days	2 mg/kg three times daily for 7–10 days	>80%

TABLE 7. *Adverse effects of antigiardial drugs*

Drugs	Adverse effects
Metronidazole and tinidazole[a]	Nausea, vomiting, metallic taste, gastrointestinal disturbances, rashes, urticaria, and angioedema *Rarely* drowsiness, headache, dizziness, and ataxia *Prolonged* use, peripheral neuropathy Disulfiram-like reaction with alcohol *Avoid* in pregnancy and breast-feeding
Mepacrine (Quinacrine)	Gastrointestinal disturbances, dizziness, headache, nausea, and vomiting Occasionally toxic psychosis *Prolonged* use, yellow discoloration of skin, sclerae, and urine; chronic dermatoses; hepatitis; and aplastic anemia *Avoid* in pregnancy, hepatic impairment, psoriasis, the elderly, and history of psychosis
Furazolidone	Nausea, vomiting Hemolysis in glucose-6-phosphate dehydrogenase

[a] These two drugs are not approved by the Food and Drug Administration for giardiasis.

peroxides and other toxic radicals, which may be relevant to its antigiardial effects (267).

New Antigiardial Agents

Recent studies suggest that benzoimidazoles, drugs with broad spectrum antihelminthic activity, may also be useful in the treatment of giardiasis (268–270). Their anti-*Giardia* activity probably relates to their interaction with β-tubulin and their ability, at least *in vitro,* to inhibit attachment. Mebendazole has *in vitro* activity against *Giardia* and was effective in one clinical study (268), although these findings were not confirmed in a further study using a much shorter treatment regimen (269). Albendazole also has *in vitro* activity against *Giardia* (270) and clinical trials have confirmed its efficacy in human giardiasis. Albendazole may be particularly useful in children in the developing world when treatment for intestinal helminths and *Giardia* can be administered at the same time.

Other drugs have been shown to have anti-*Giardia* activity including some antidepressants (271), sodium fusidate (272), D- and DL-propranolol (273,274), mefloquine, doxycycline, and rifampicin (275). Drug combinations may be more effective than single-agent therapy, although this has not been widely investigated in the clinical setting (275).

Drug Sensitivity Testing

A variety of approaches have been developed to measure *in vitro* drug sensitivity profiles of *Giardia* isolates in axenic culture (276–280). These may be categorized into assays that (a) quantitate parasite growth and (b) evaluate inhibition of adherence. Growth has been measured morphometrically in liquid culture or as a clonal growth assay in semisolid medium (276). Growth radiometric assays have been developed to measure incorporation of [^{3}H]thymidine both in standard liquid cultures and miniaturized 96-well tissue culture plates (277,280). These assays have clearly shown that *Giardia* isolates vary in their sensitivity to standard antigiardial drugs and that drug resistance can develop *in vitro* following long-term exposure to a nitroimidazole derivative (281,282). The development of resistance has also been described *in vivo* in a chronically infected individual who was treated repeatedly but unsuccessfully with a nitroimidazole derivative (17). Sensitivity to metronidazole decreased 40-fold during the 3-month treatment period. Furazolidone-resistant *Giardia* isolates have also been obtained from patients refractory to furazolidone.

Mechanisms of Drug Resistance

There is a negative correlation between pyuvate:ferredoxin oxidoreductase reactivity (PFOR) and metronidazole sensitivity in *G. intestinalis* (283). PFOR is presumed to be related to the decreased production of toxic radicals from metronidazole. There is also evidence that chromosomal rearrangement occurs in drug-resistant *Giardia* isolates. Deletion of one particular gene that encodes for a membrane-associated protein correlates with aberrant growth of the organism.

PREVENTION

Giardia species is widely distributed throughout the animal kingdom and may survive for extended periods outside a suitable host. The increasing evidence that giardiasis is a zoonosis makes it unlikely that the organism will ever be eliminated either from the environment or from human or animal reservoirs. Strenuous public health measures are clearly required to ensure that water supplies are *Giardia*-free and that methods are available to monitor the presence of the parasite in drinking water. Similarly, attention to personal hygiene should minimize person-to-person transmission, particularly in high-risk situations such as day care centers, residential institutions, and during sexual contact.

The question remains as to whether giardiasis can be prevented by the administration of an appropriate vaccine. Experimental infection in human volunteers (36) and epidemiologic studies (9) suggest that protective immunity is acquired following exposure to *Giardia*. It seems likely that protective immunity does not necessarily develop following a single infection, since in rural Guatemala many infants and children experienced multiple infections during the first 3 years of life (85), and age-specific prevalence is known to rise throughout childhood and only begins to fall to adult levels during adolescence (83). The question as to why the development of protective immunity during natural infection appears to be a lengthy process is intriguing. One possible explanation may relate to the presence of many different immunological subtypes of the parasite. *Giardia* is antigenically complex with antigenic profiles varying between isolates (284,285). Even within a single isolate antigen expression can vary (286). A large number of parasite antigens of 43 to 200 kDa have been identified as determinants of the antibody response (8,9). It seems likely that specific anti-*Giardia* S-IgA within the gut lumen will be an important component for the development of protective immunity. As yet, the biological relevance of these antigens to parasite clearance and protective immunity has not been determined. However, Gambian children with persistent diarrhea failed to mount an IgA response to a 56-kDa antigen, although there was an IgM response to this antigen (190). One might speculate that there existed a subtle immunoregulatory disorder in the intestinal mucosa with failure to switch from IgM to S-IgA production. The role of other *Giardia* antigens in determining antibody-directed clearance of the parasite and the development of protective immunity needs to be established.

FUTURE CHALLENGES IN GIARDIASIS

The relationship between animal and human infection needs to be further characterized, probably by careful community studies in regions where the parasite is present but not hyperendemic. Such studies will have important implications for local control programs, the administration of antigiardial chemotherapy for asymptomatic carriers, and possibly vaccine development.

Many questions remain as to how *Giardia* produces intestinal disease and diarrhea. Current views suggest that the process is multifactorial, although the most profound effects of the parasite appear to be on the enterocyte microvillus membrane, disrupting the digestive–absorptive complex. Progress in understanding pathogenesis, however, is restricted by a complete lack of knowledge of specific virulence factors. Characterization of these could influence the development of new antigiardial drugs and possibly guide vaccine strategies.

Despite clear evidence that *Giardia* promotes both a systemic and local immune response during natural infection, it is unclear as to why protective immunity does not appear to develop following a single infection, at least as far as children are concerned in the developing world. A more detailed evaluation of immune responses during human infection is required, with the identification of immunodominant antigens that direct both T cell-mediated and S-IgA responses. Identification, cloning, and "packaging" of suitable antigens could be valuable in the development of a *Giardia* vaccine.

REFERENCES

1. Farthing MJG. Host–parasite interactions in human giardiasis. *J Med* 1989;70:191–204.
2. Adam RD. The biology of *Giardia* spp. *Microbiol Rev* 1991; 55:706–732.
3. Farthing MJG. Giardiasis as a disease. In: Reynoldson JA, Thompson RCA, Lymbery AJ, eds. *Giardia: from molecules to disease and beyond*. Oxford: CAB International, 1993;15–37.
4. Kabnick KS, Peattie DA. *Giardia*: a missing link between prokaryotes and eukaryotes. *Am Scientist* 1991;79:34–43.
5. Dobell CA. The discovery of intestinal protozoa in man. *Proc R Soc Med* 1920;13:1–15.
6. Meyer EA. Taxonomy and nomenclature. In: Meyer EA, ed. *Giardiasis*. Amsterdam: Elsevier Science Publications, 1990; 51–60.
7. Filice PP. Studies on the cytology and life history of *Giardia* from the laboratory rat. *Univ Calif Publ Zool* 1952;57:53–143.
8. Den Hollander N, Riley D, Befus D. Immunology of giardiasis. *Parasitol Today* 1988;4:124–131.
9. Farthing MJG. Immunopathology of giardiasis. *Springer Semin Immunopathol* 1990;12:269–282.
10. Nash T. Surface antigen variability and variation in *Giardia lamblia*. *Parasitol Today* 1992;8:229–234.
11. Feely DE, Chase DG, Hardin EL, Erlandsen SL. Ultrastructural evidence for the presence of bacteria, viral-like particles, and mycoplasma-like organisms associated with *Giardia* spp. *J Parasitol* 1988;35:151–158.
12. Meloni BP, Lymbery AJ, Thompson RCA. Isoenzyme electrophoresis of 30 isolates of *Giardia* from humans and felines. *Am J Trop Med Hyg* 1988;38:65–73.
13. Upcroft JA, Boreham PFL, Upcroft P. Geographic variation in *Giardia* karyotypes. *Int J Parasitol* 1989;19:519–527.
14. Korman SH, LeBlancq SM, Deckelbaum RJ, Van Der Ploeg LHT. Investigation of human giardiasis by karyotype analysis. *J Clin Invest* 1992;89:1725–1733.
15. Nash TE, McCutchan T, Keister D, Dame JB, Conrad JD, Gillin FD. Restriction-endonuclease analysis of DNA from 15 *Giardia* isolates from humans and animals. *J Infect Dis* 1985; 152:64–73.
16. Upcroft P, Mitchell R, Boreham FP. DNA fingerprinting of the intestinal parasite *Giardia duodenalis* with the M13 phage genome. *Int J Parasitol* 1990;20:319–323.
17. Butcher PD, Cevallos AM, Carnaby S, Alstead ET, Farthing MJG. Phenotypic and genotypic variation in *Giardia lamblia* isolates during chronic infection. *Gut* 1993;34:35: 51–54.
18. Sogin ML, Gunderson JH, Elwood HJ, Alonso RA, Peattie DA. Phylogenetic meaning of the kingdom concept: an unusual ribosomal RNA from *Giardia lamblia*. *Science* 1989;243:75–77.
19. Holberton DV. Arrangements of subunits in microribbons from *Giardia*. *J Cell Sci* 1981;47:167–185.
20. Crossley R, Holberton DV. Characterization of proteins from the cytoskeleton of *Giardia lamblia*. *J Cell Sci* 1983;59:81–103.
21. Crossley R, Holberton D. Assembly of 2.5nm filaments from giardin, a protein associated with cytoskeletal microtubules in *Giardia*. *J Cell Sci* 1985;78:205–231.
22. Holberton D, Baker DA, Marshall J. Segmented alpha-helical coiled-coil structure of the protein giardin from the *Giardia* cytoskeleton. *J Mol Biol* 1988;204:789–795.
23. Peattie DA, Alonso RA, Hein A, Caulfield JP. Ultrastructural localization of giardins to the edges of disk microribbons of *Giardia lamblia* and the nucleotide and deduced protein sequence of alpha-giardin. *J Cell Biol* 1989;109:2323–2335.
24. Feely DE, Schollmeyer JV, Erlandsen SL. *Giardia* spp.: Distribution of contractile proteins in the attachment organelle. *Exp Parasitol* 1982;53:145–154.
25. Feely DE, Dyer JK. Localization of acid phosphatase activity in *Giardia lamblia* and *Giardia muris* trophozoites. *J Protozool* 1987;34:80–83.
26. Lindmark DG. *Giardia lamblia*: localization of hydrolyase activities in lysosome-like organelles of trophozoites. *Exp Parasitol* 1988;65:141–147.
27. Hare DF, Jarroll EL, Lindmark DG. *Giardia lamblia*: charac-

terization of proteinase activity in trophozoites. *Exp Parasitol* 1989;68:168–175.

28. Parenti DM. Characterization of a thiol proteinase in *Giardia lamblia*. *J Infect Dis* 1989;160:1076–1080.

29. Reiner DS, McCaffery M, Gillin FD. Sorting of cyst wall proteins to a regulated secretory pathway during differentiation of the primitive eukaryote, *Giardia lamblia*. *Eur J Cell Biol* 1990; 53:142–153.

30. Boeck WC. Mitosis in *Giardia lamblia*. *Univ Calif Publ Zool* 1917;18:1–26.

31. Wang AL, Wang CC. Discovery of a specific double-stranded RNA virus in *Giardia lamblia*. *Mol Biochem Parasitol* 1986; 21:269–276.

32. Ward HD, Alroy J, Lev BI, Keusch GT, Pereira MEA. Identification of chitin as a structural component of *Giardia* cysts. *Infect Immun* 1985;49:629–634.

33. Gillin FD, Reiner DS, Gault MJ, Douglas H, Das S, Wunderlich A, Sauch JF. Encystation and expression of cyst antigens by *Giardia lamblia in vitro*. *Science* 1987;235:1040–1043.

34. Jarroll EL, Manning P, Lindmark DG, Coggins JR, Erlandsen SL. *Giardia* cyst wall-specific carbohydrate: evidence for the presence of galactosamine. *Mol Biochem Parasitol* 1989;32: 121–132.

35. Erlandsen SL, Bemrick WJ, Schupp DE, Shields JM, Jarroll EL, Sauch JF, Pawley JB. High resolution immunogold localization of *Giardia* cyst wall antigens using field emission SEM with secondary and backscatter electron imaging. *J Histochem Cytochem* 1990;38:625–632.

36. Rendtorff RC. The experimental transmission of human intestinal protozoan parasites: II *Giardia lamblia* cysts given in capsules. *Am J Hyg* 1954;59:209–220.

37. Porter A. An enumerative study of the cysts of *Giardia* (*lamblia*) *intestinalis* in human dysenteric faeces. *Lancet* 1916;1: 1166–1169.

38. Bingham AK, Meyer EA. *Giardia* excystation can be induced *in vitro* in acidic solutions. *Nature* 1979;277:301–302.

39. Boucher SEM, Gillin FD. Excystation of *in vitro*-derived *Giardia lamblia* cysts. *Infect Immun* 1990;58:3516–3522.

40. Feely DE, Gardner MD, Hardin EL. Excystation of *Giardia muris* induced by a phosphate-bicarbonate medium: localization of acid phosphatase. *J Parasitol* 1991;77:441–448.

41. Coggins JR, Schaefer FW III. *Giardia muris*: ultrastructural analysis of *in vitro* excystation. *Exp Parasitol* 1986;61:219–228.

42. Holberton DV. Attachment of *Giardia*—a hydrodynamic model based on flagellar activity. *J Exp Biol* 1974;60:207–221.

43. Feely DE, Erlandsen SL. Effect of cytochalasin-B, low Ca++ concentration, iodoacetic acid and quinacrine-HCl on the attachment of *Giardia* trophozoites *in vitro*. *J Parasitol* 1982;68: 869–873.

44. Erlandsen SL, Feely DE. Trophozoite motility and the mechanism of attachment. In: Meyer EA, Erlandsen SL, eds. *Giardia and giardiasis*. New York: Plenum Press, 1984;33–60.

45. Farthing MJG, Pereira MEA, Keusch GT. *Giardia lamblia*—red cell interreactions: a model system for parasite adherence. In: Keusch GT, Wadstrom T, eds. *Experimental bacterial and parasitic infections*. Amsterdam: North-Holland/ Elsevier, 1983;333–341.

46. Farthing MJG, Pereira MEA, Keusch GT. Description and characterization of a surface lectin from *Giardia lamblia*. *Infect Immun* 1986;51:661–667.

47. Lev B, Ward H, Keusch GT, Pereira MEA. Lectin activation of *Giardia lamblia* by host protease: a novel host–parasite interaction. *Science* 1986;232:71–73.

48. Ward HD, Lev BI, Kane AU, Keuch GT, Pereira MEA. Identification and characterization of Taglin, a mannose-6-phosphate binding, trypsin-activated lectin from *Giardia lamblia*. *Biochemistry* 1987;26:8669–8675.

49. Inge PMG, Edson CM, Farthing MJG. Attachment of *Giardia lamblia* to mammalian intestinal cells. *Gut* 1988;29:795–801.

50. Katelaris PH, Naeem A, Farthing MJG. An *in vitro* model of attachment of *Giardia lamblia* to an intestinal cell line and potential use as an assay of drug sensitivity. *Gut* 1992;33(Suppl): S45.

51. Hegner RW, Eskridge L. The influence of bile salts on *Giardia* infection in rats. *Am J Hyg* 1939;26:186–192.

52. Bemrick WJ. The effect of bile flow on *Giardia duodenalis* race *Simoni* in the intestine of a laboratory strain of *Rattus norvegicus*. *J Parasitol* 1963;49:956–959.

53. Farthing MJG, Varon SR, Keusch GT. Mammalian bile promotes growth of *Giardia lamblia* in axenic culture. *Trans R Soc Trop Med Hyg* 1983;77:467–469.

54. Keister DB. Axenic culture of *Giardia lamblia* in TYI-S-33 medium supplemented with bile. *Trans R Soc Trop Med Hyg* 1983; 77:487–488.

55. Halliday CEW, Inge PMG, Farthing MJG. *Giardia* bile salt interactions *in vitro* and *in vivo*. *Trans R Soc Trop Med Hyg* 1988;82:428–432.

56. Farthing MJG, Keusch GT, Carey MC. Effects of bile and bile salts on growth and membrane lipid uptake by *Giardia lamblia*: possible implications for pathogenesis of intestinal disease. *J Clin Invest* 1985;76:1727–1732.

57. Jarroll EL, Manning P, Berrada A, Hare D, Lindmark DG. Biochemistry and metabolism of *Giardia*. *J Protozool* 1989;36: 190–197.

58. Gillin FD, Reiner DS, Boucher SE. Small intestinal factors promote encystation of *Giardia lamblia in vitro*. *Infect Immun* 1988;56:705–707.

59. Gillin FD, Boucher SE, Reiner DS. *Giardia lamblia*: the roles of bile, lactic acid, and pH in completion of the life cycle *in vitro*. *Exp Parasitol* 1989;69:164–174.

60. Karapetyan A. *In vitro* cultivation of *Giardia duodenalis*. *J Parasitol* 1962;46:337–340.

61. Meyer EA. *Giardia lamblia*: isolation and axenic cultivation. *Exp Parasitol* 1976;39:101–105.

62. Lindmark DG. Energy metabolism of the anaerobic protozoon *Giardia lamblia*. *Mol Biochem Parasitol* 1980;1:1–12.

63. Jarroll EL, Muller PJ, Meyer EA, Morse SA. Lipid and carbohydrate metabolism of *Giardia lamblia*. *Mol Biochem Parasitol* 1981;2:187–196.

64. Schofield PJ, Edwards MR, Kranz P. Glucose metabolism in *Giardia lamblia*. *Mol Biochem Parasitol* 1991;45:39–48.

65. Paget TA, Raynor MH, Shipp DWE, Lloyd D. *Giardia lamblia* produces alanine anaerobically but not in the presence of oxygen. *Mol Biochem Parasitol* 1990;42:63–68.

66. Paget TA, Kelly ML, Jarroll EL, Lindmark DG, Lloyd D. The effects of oxygen on fermentation in the intestinal protozoal parasite *Giardia lamblia*. *Mol Biochem Parasitol* 1993;57: 65–72.

67. Blair RJ, Weller PF. Uptake and esterification of arachidonic acid by trophozoites of *Giardia lamblia*. *Mol Biochem Parasitol* 1987;25:11–18.

68. Lindmark DG, Jarroll EL. Pyrimidine metabolism in *Giardia lamblia* trophozoites. *Mol Biochem Parasitol* 1982;5:291–296.

69. Wang CC, Aldritt S. Purine salvage networks in *Giardia lamblia*. *J Exp Med* 1983;158:1703–1712.

70. Jarroll EL, Hammond MM, Lindmark DG. *Giardia lamblia*: uptake of pyrimidine nucleosides. *Exp Parasitol* 1987;63: 152–156.

71. De Lourdes Munoz M, Weinbach EC, Wieder SC, Claggett CE, Levenbook L. *Giardia lamblia*: detection and characterization of calmodulin. *Exp Parasitol* 1987;63:42–48.

72. De Lourdes Munoz M, Claggett CE, Weinbach EC. Calcium transport and catabolism of adenosine triphosphate in the protozoan parasite *Giardia lamblia*. *Comp Biochem Physiol* 1988; 91B:137–142.

73. Adam RD, Nash TE, Wellems TE. The *Giardia lamblia* trophozoite contains sets of closely related chromosomes. *Nucleic Acids Res* 1988;16:4555–4567.

74. Nash TE, McCutchan T, Keister DB, Dame JB, Conrad JD, Gillin FD. Restriction-endonuclease analysis of DNA from 15 *Giardia* isolates obtained from humans and animals. *J Infect Dis* 1985;152:64–73.

75. Boothroyd JC, Wang A, Campbell DA, Wang CC. An unusually compact ribosomal DNA repeat in the protozoan *Giardia lamblia*. *Nucleic Acids Res* 1987;26:4065–4084.

76. Healey A, Mitchell R, Upcroft JA, Boreham PFL, Upcroft P. Complete nucleotide sequence of the ribosomal RNA tandem

repeat unit from *Giardia intestinalis. Nucleic Acids Res* 1990; 18:4006.

77. Edlind TD, Chakraborty PR. Unusual ribosomal RNA of the intestinal parasite *Giardia lamblia. Nucleic Acids Res* 1987;15: 7889–7901.

78. Kirk-Mason KE, Turner MJ, Chakraborty PR. Evidence for unusually short tubulin in RNA leaders and characterization of tubulin genes in *Giardia lamblia. Mol Biochem Parasitol* 1989; 36:87–100.

79. Gillin FD, Hagblom P, Harwood J, et al. Isolation and expression of the gene for a major surface protein of *Giardia lamblia. Proc Natl Acad Sci USA* 1990;87:4463–4467.

80. Aggarwal A, De La Cruz VF, Nash TE. A heat shock protein gene in *Giardia lamblia* unrelated to HSP70. *Nucleic Acids Res* 1990;18:3409.

81. Char S, Farthing MJG. Codon usage in the protozoan *Giardia lamblia. J Protozool* 1992;39:642.

82. Petersen H. Giardiasis (lambliasis). *Scand J Gastroenterol* 1972;7(Suppl 14):7–44.

83. Oyerinde JPO, Ogunbi O, Alonge AA. Age and sex distribution of infections with *Entamoeba histolytica* and *Giardia intestinalis* in the Lagos population. *Int J Epidemiol* 1977;6:231–234.

84. Gilman RH, Brown KH, Visvesvara GS, et al. Epidemiology and serology of *Giardia lamblia* in a developing country: Bangladesh. *Trans R Soc Trop Med Hyg* 1985;79:469–473.

85. Farthing MJG, Mata L, Urrutia JJ, Kronmal RA. Natural history of *Giardia* infection of infants and children in rural Guatemala and its impact on physical growth. *Am J Clin Nutr* 1986; 43:393–403.

86. Mason PR, Patterson BA. Epidemiology of *Giardia lamblia* infection in children: cross-sectional and longitudinal studies in urban and rural communities in Zimbabwe. *Am J Trop Med Hyg* 1987;37:277–282.

87. Sullivan PS, Du Pont HL, Arafat RR, Thornton SA, Selwyn BJ, El Alamay MA, Zaki AM. Illness and reservoirs associated with *Giardia lamblia* infection in rural Egypt: the case against treatment in developing world environments of high endemicity. *Am J Epidemiol* 1988;127:1272–1280.

88. Grimmond TR, Radford AJ, Brownridge T, Farshid A, Harris C, Turton P, Wordsworth K. *Giardia* carriage in aboriginal and non-aboriginal children attending urban daycare centres in South Australia. *Aust Paediatr J* 1988;24:304–305.

89. Shetty N, Narasimha M, Raghuveer TS, Elliott EJ, Farthing MJG, Macaden R. Intestinal amoebiasis and giardiasis in Southern Indian infants and children. *Trans R Soc Trop Med Hyg* 1990;84:382–384.

90. Sullivan PB, Marsh MN, Phillips MB, et al. Prevalence and treatment of giardiasis in chronic diarrhoea and malnutrition. *Arch Dis Child* 1991;66:304–306.

91. Dobell C. *A report on the occurrence of intestinal protozoa in the inhabitants of Britain.* Medical Research Council Special Report Series No. 59, 1921.

92. Farthing MJG. Giardiasis: a cause of travellers' diarrhoea. *Trav Traff Med Int* 1984;2:3–10.

93. Fantham HB. Remarks on the nature and distribution of the parasites observed in the stools of 1,305 dysenteric patients. *Lancet* 1916;190:1165–1166.

94. Jokipii L, Jokipii AM. Giardiasis in travelers: a prospective study. *J Infect Dis* 1974;30:295–299.

95. Brodsky RE, Spencer HC, Schultz MG. Giardiasis in American travelers to the Soviet Union. *J Infect Dis* 1974;130:319–323.

96. Brandborg LL. Giardiasis and traveler's diarrhea. *Gastroenterology* 1980;78:1602–1614.

97. Moore GT, Cross WM, McGuire D, Mollohan CS, Gleason NN, Healy GR, Newton LH. Epidemic giardiasis at a ski resort. *N Engl J Med* 1969;281:402–407.

98. Zinneman HH, Kaplan AP. The association of giardiasis with reduced intestinal secretory immunoglobulins. *Am J Dig Dis* 1972;17:793–797.

99. Webster ADB. Giardiasis and immunodeficiency diseases. *Trans R Soc Trop Med Hyg* 1980;74:440–448.

100. Phillips SC, Mildvan D, William DC, Gelb AM, White MC. Sexual transmission of enteric protozoa and helminths in a venereal disease clinic population. *N Engl J Med* 1981;305: 603–606.

101. Smith PD, Lane C, Gill VJ, Manischewitz JF, Quinnan GV, Fauci AS, Masur H. Intestinal infections in patients with acquired immunodeficiency syndrome (AIDS). Etiology and response to therapy. *Ann Intern Med* 1988;108:328–333.

102. Laughon BE, Druckman DA, Vernon A, et al. Prevalence of enteric pathogens in homosexual men with and without acquired immunodeficiency syndrome. *Gastroenterology* 1988; 94:984–993.

103. Craun GF. Waterborne outbreaks of giardiasis. Current status. In: Erlandsen SL, Meyer EA, eds. Giardia and *giardiasis.* New York: Plenum Press, 1984;243–261.

104. Jephcott AE, Begg NT, Baker IA. Outbreak of giardiasis associated with mains water in the United Kingdom. *Lancet* 1986; 1:730–732.

105. Porter JD, Ragazzoni HP, Buchanon JD, Waskin HA, Juranek DD, Parkin WE. *Giardia* transmission in a swimming pool. *Am J Public Health* 1988;78:659–662.

106. Sealy DP, Schuman SH. Endemic giardiasis and daycare. *Pediatrics* 1983;72:154–158.

107. Thacker SB. Parasitic disease control in a residential facility for the mentally retarded: failure of selected isolation procedures. *Am J Public Health* 1981;71:303–305.

108. Owen RL. Direct fecal–oral transmission of giardiasis. In: Erlandsen SL, Meyer EA, eds. Giardia and *giardiasis.* New York: Plenum Press, 1984;329–339.

109. Osterholm MT, Forgang JC, Ristinen TL, et al. An outbreak of foodborne giardiasis. *N Engl J Med* 1981;304:24–28.

110. Petersen LR, Cartter ML, Hadler JL. A foodborne outbreak of *Giardia lamblia. J Infect Dis* 1988;157:846–848.

111. Winsland JKD, Nimmo S, Butcher PD, Farthing MJG. Prevalence of *Giardia* in dogs and cats in the United Kingdom: survey of an Essex veterinary clinic. *Trans R Soc Trop Med Hyg* 1989;83:791–792.

112. Buret A, den Hollander N, Wallis PM, Befus D, Olsen ME. Zoonotic potential of giardiasis in domestic ruminants. *J Infect Dis* 1990;162:231–237.

113. Katelaris PH, Farthing MJG. Diarrhoea and malabsorption in giardiasis: a multifactorial process. *Gut* 1992;33:295–297.

114. Yardley JH, Takano J, Hendrix TR. Epithelial and other mucosal lesions of the jejunum in giardiasis. Jejunal biopsy studies. *Bull Johns Hopkins Hosp* 1964;115:389–406.

115. Hoskins LC, Winawer SY, Broitman SA, Gottlieb LS, Zamcheck N. Clinical giardiasis and intestinal malabsorption. *Gastroenterology* 1967;53:265–279.

116. Alp MH, Hislop IG. The effect of *Giardia lamblia* infestation on the gastrointestinal tract. *Aust Ann Med* 1969;18:232–237.

117. Ament ME, Rubin CE. Relation of giardiasis to abnormal intestinal structure and function in gastrointestinal immunodeficiency syndromes. *Gastroenterology* 1972;62:216–226.

118. Wright SG, Tomkins AM, Ridley DS. Giardiasis: clinical and therapeutic aspects. *Gut* 1977;18:343–350.

119. Duncombe VM, Bolin TD, Davis AE, Cummins AG, Crouch RL. Histopathology in giardiasis: a correlation with diarrhoea. *Aust N Z J Med* 1978;8:392–396.

120. Levinson JD, Nastro LJ. Giardiasis with total villous atrophy. *Gastroenterology* 1978;74:271–275.

121. Hartong WA, Gourley WK, Arvanitakis C. Giardiasis: clinical spectrum and functional–structural abnormalities of the small intestinal mucosa. *Gastroenterology* 1979;77:61–69.

122. Rosekrans PCM, Lindeman J, Meijer CJLM. Quantitative histological and immunohistochemical findings in jejunal biopsy specimens in giardiasis. *Virchows Arch A Pathol Anat Histopathol* 1981;393:145–151.

123. Oberhuber G, Stolte M. Giardiasis: analysis of histological changes in biopsy specimens of 80 patients. *J Clin Pathol* 1990; 43:641–643.

124. Faubert GM, Belosevic M. Animal models for *Giardia duodenalis* type organisms. In: Meyer EA, ed. *Giardiasis.* Amsterdam: Elsevier Science Publishers, 1990;77–90.

125. Buret A, Gall DG, Olson ME. Growth, activities of enzymes in the small intestine and ultrastructure of the microvillus bor-

der in gerbils infected with *Giardia duodenalis*. *Parasitol Res* 1991;77:109–114.

126. Buret A, Hardin JA, Olson ME, Gall DG. Pathophysiology of small intestinal malabsorption in gerbils infected with *Giardia lamblia*. *Gastroenterology* 1992;103:506–513.

127. Takano J, Yardley JH. Jejunal lesions in patients with giardiasis and malabsorption. An electron microscopic study. *Bull Johns Hopkins Hosp* 1965;116:413–429.

128. Morecki R, Parker JG. Ultrastructural studies of the human *Giardia lamblia* and subjacent jejunal mucosa in a subject with steatorrhea. *Gastroenterology* 1967;52:151–164.

129. Cevallos AM, Katelaris PK, Farthing MJG. *Gastroenterology* 1993;105:306–307.

130. Hartong WA, Gourley WK, Arvanitakis C. Giardiasis: clinical spectrum and functional–structural abnormalities of the small intestinal mucosa. *Gastroenterology* 1979;77:61–69.

131. Gillon J, Al Thamery D, Ferguson A. Features of small intestinal pathology (epithelial cell kinetics, intraepithelial lymphocytes, disaccharidases) in a primary *Giardia muris* infection. *Gut* 1982;23:498–506.

132. Khanna R, Vinayak VK, Mehta S, KumKum, Nain CK. *Giardia lamblia* infection in immunosuppressed animals causes severe alterations to brush border membrane enzymes. *Dig Dis Sci* 1988;33:1147–1152.

133. Belosevic M, Faubert GM, MacLean JD. Disaccharidase activity in the small intestine of gerbils (*Meriones unguiculatus*) during primary and challenge infections with *Giardia lamblia*. *Gut* 1989;30:1213–1219.

134. Cevallos AM, Farthing MJG. Differences in functional mucosal damage between *Giardia lamblia* isolates. *Gut* 1992;33:S44.

135. Samra HK, Garg UC, Ganguly NK, Mahajan RC. Effect of different *Giardia lamblia* inocula on glucose and amino acids transport in the small brush border membrane vesicles of infected mice. *Ann Trop Med Parasitol* 1987;81:367–372.

136. Samra HK, Ganguly NK, Garg UC, Goyal J, Mahajan RC. Effect of excretory–secretory products of *Giardia lamblia* on glucose and phenylalanine transport in the small intestine of Swiss albino mice. *Biochem Int* 1988;17:801–812.

137. Brandborg LL, Tankersley CB, Gottlieb S, Barancik M, Sartor VE. Histological demonstration of mucosal invasion of *Giardia lamblia* in man. *Gastroenterology* 1967;52:143–150.

138. Saha TK, Ghosh TK. Invasion of small intestinal mucosa by *Giardia lamblia*. *Gastroenterology* 1977;72:402–405.

139. Erlandsen SL, Chase DG. Morphological alterations in the microvillus border of villous epithelial cells produced by intestinal micro-organisms. *Am J Clin Nutr* 1974;27:1277–1286.

140. North MJ, Mottram JC, Coombs GH. Cysteine proteinases of parasitic protozoa. *Parasitol Today* 1990;6:270–275.

141. Lorenzsonn V, Olsen WA. *In vivo* responses of rat intestinal epithelium to intraluminal dietary lectins. *Gastroenterology* 1982;82:838–848.

142. Dobbins JW, Laurenson JP, Gorelick FS, Banwell JG. Phytohemagglutinin from red kidney bean (*Phaseolus vulgaris*) inhibits sodium and chloride absorption in the rabbit ileum. *Gastroenterology* 1986;90:1907–1913.

143. Wright SG, Tomkins AM. Quantification of the lymphocytic infiltrate in jejunal epithelium in giardiasis. *Clin Exp Immunol* 1977;29:408–412.

144. Gillon J. Clinical studies in adults presenting with giardiasis to a gastrointestinal unit. *Scott Med J* 1985;30:89–95.

145. Roberts-Thomson IC, Mitchell FG. Giardiasis in mice. I Prolonged infections in certain mouse strains and hypothymic (nude) mice. *Gastroenterology* 1978;75:42–46.

146. MacDonald TT, Spencer J. Evidence that activated mucosal T cells play a role in the pathogenesis of enteropathy in human small intestine. *J Exp Med* 1988;167:1341–1349.

147. Daniels CW, Belosevic M. Disaccharidase activity in the small intestine of susceptible and resistant mice after primary and challenge infections with *Giardia muris*. *Am J Trop Med Hyg* 1992;46:382–390.

148. Tandon BN, Tandon RK, Satpathy BK, Shriniwas. Mechanism of malabsorption in giardiasis: a study of bacterial flora and bile salt deconjugation in upper jejunum. *Gut* 1977;18:176–181.

149. Tomkins AM, Drasar BS, Bradley AK, Williamson WA. Bacterial colonization of jejunal mucosa in giardiasis. *Trans R Soc Trop Med Hyg* 1978;72:33–36.

150. Smith PD, Horsburgh CR, Brown WR. *In vitro* studies on bile acid deconjugation and lipolysis inhibition by *Giardia lamblia*. *Dig Dis Sci* 1981;26:700–704.

151. Katelaris PH, McHugh TD, Carnaby S, Cevallos AM, Char S, Farthing MJG. Bile modulates genotypic and phenotypic characteristics of *Giardia lamblia*. *Gut* 1991;32:A1260.

152. Gupta RK, Mehta S. Giardiasis in children: a study of pancreatic functions. *Indian J Med Res* 1973;61:743–748.

153. Chawla LS, Sehgal AK, Broor SL, Verma RS, Chhuttani PN. Tryptic activity in the duodenal aspirate following a standard test meal in giardiasis. *Scand J Gastroenterol* 1975;10:445–447.

154. Okada M, Fuchigami T, Ri S, Kohrogi N, Omae T. The BTPABA pancreatic function test in giardiasis. *Postgrad Med J* 1983;59:79–82.

155. Katelaris PH, Seow F, Ngu MC. The effect of *Giardia lamblia* trophozoites on lipolysis *in vitro*. *Parasitology* 1991;103:35–39.

156. Seow F, Katelaris PH, Ngu M. The effect of *Giardia lamblia* trophozoites on trypsin, chymotrypsin and amylase *in vitro*. *Parasitology* 1993;106:233–238.

157. Istre GR, Dunlop TS, Gaspard B, Hopkins RS. Waterborne giardiasis at a mountain resort: evidence for acquired immunity. *Am J Public Health* 1984;74:602–604.

158. Ament ME, Ochs HD, Davis SD. Structure and function of the gastrointestinal tract in primary immunodeficiency syndromes, a study of 39 patients. *Medicine (Baltimore)* 1973;52:227–248.

159. Webster ADB. Giardiasis and immunodeficiency diseases. *Trans R Soc Trop Med Hyg* 1980;74:440–443.

160. Halita M, Isaicu L. Reactia de fixare a complementului, in lambliaza intestinula. *Ardealul Med* 1946;6:154.

161. Radulescu S, Iancu L, Simionescu O, Meyer EA. Serum antibodies in giardiasis [Letter]. *J Clin Pathol* 1976;29:863.

162. Ridley MJ, Ridley DS. Serum antibodies and jejunal histology in giardiasis associated with malabsorption. *J Clin Pathol* 1976; 29:30–34.

163. Vinayak UK, Jain P, Naik SR. Demonstration of antibodies in giardiasis using the immunodiffusion technique with *Giardia* cysts as antigen. *Ann Trop Med Parasitol* 1978;72:581–582.

164. Visvesvara GS, Smith PD, Healy GR, Brown WR. Serum antibodies to *Giardia lamblia* demonstrated by immunofluorescence. *Ann Intern Med* 1980;93:802–805.

165. Smith PD, Gillin FD, Brown WR, Nash TE. IgG antibody to *Giardia lamblia* detected by enzyme-linked immunosorbent assay. *Gastroenterology* 1981;80:1476–1480.

166. Farthing MJG, Goka AKJ, Butcher PD, Arvind AS. Serodiagnosis of giardiasis. *Serodiag Immunother* 1987;1:233–238.

167. Goka AKJ, Rolston DDK, Mathan VI, Farthing MJG. Diagnosis of giardiasis by specific IgM antibody enzyme-linked immunosorbent assay. *Lancet* 1986;2:184–186.

168. Nash TE, Herrington DA, Losonsky GA, Levine MM. Experimental human infections with *Giardia lamblia*. *J Infect Dis* 1987;156:974–984.

169. Sullivan PB, Neale G, Cevallos AM, Farthing MJG. Evaluation of specific serum anti-*Giardia* IgM antibody response in diagnosis of giardiasis. *Trans R Soc Trop Med Hyg* 1991;85: 748–749.

170. Goka AKJ, Rolston DDK, Mathan VI, Farthing MJG. Serum IgA response in human *Giardia lamblia* infection. *Serodiag Immunother* 1989;3:273–277.

171. Char S, Shetty N, Elliott EJ, Narashimha M, Macaden R, Farthing MJG. Serum antibody response in children with *Giardia lamblia* infection and identification of an immunodominant 57-kilodalton antigen. *Parasite Immunol* 1991;13:329–337.

172. Farthing MJG, Chong S, Walker-Smith JA. Acute allergic phenomena in giardiasis. *Lancet* 1984;2:1428.

173. Snider DP, Gordon J, McDermott MR, Underdown BJ. Chronic *Giardia muris* infection in anti-IgM-treated mice. I. Analysis of immunoglobulin and parasite specific antibody in normal and immunoglobulin deficient animals. *J Immunol* 1985; 135:4153–4162.

174. Snider DP, Underdown BJ. Quantitative and temporal analyses of murine antibody response in serum and gut secretions to infection with *Giardia muris*. *Infect Immun* 1986;52:271–278.

175. Popovic O, Pendic B, Paljm A, Andrejevic M, Trpkovic D. Giardiasis: local immune defence and responses. *Eur Soc Clin Invest* 1974;4:380.

176. Briaud M, Morichau-Beauchant M, Matuchansky C, Touchard G, Babin P. Intestinal immune response in giardiasis. *Lancet* 1981;2:358.

177. Jones EG, Brown WR. Serum and intestinal fluid immunoglobulin in patients with giardiasis. *Am J Dig Dis* 1974;19:291–296.

178. Naik SR, Kumar L, Sehgal S, Rau NF, Vinayak VK. Immunological studies in giardiasis. *Ann Trop Med Parasitol* 1979;73: 291.

179. Miotti PG, Gilmore RH, Pickering LK, Ruiz-Palacios G, Park HS, Yolken RH. Prevalence of serum and milk antibodies to *Giardia lamblia* in different populations of lactating women. *J Infect Dis* 1985;152:1025–1031.

180. Speelman P, Ljungstrom I. Protozoal enteric infections among ex-patriates in Bangladesh. *Am J Trop Med* 1986;35:1140–1145.

181. Heyworth MF. Intestinal IgA responses to *Giardia muris* in mice depleted of helper T lymphocytes and in immunocompetent mice. *J Parasitol* 1989;75:246–251.

182. Andrews JS, Hewlett EL. Protection against infection with *Giardia muris* by milk containing antibody to *Giardia*. *J Infect Dis* 1981;143:242–246.

183. Adam RD, Aggarwal A, Lal AA, de la Cruz VF, McCutchan T, Nash TE. Antigenic variation of a cysteine-rich protein in *Giardia lamblia*. *J Exp Med* 1988;167:109–118.

184. Gillin FD, Hagblom P, Harwood J, et al. Isolation and expression of a gene for a major surface protein of *Giardia lamblia*. *Proc Natl Acad Sci USA* 1990;87:4463–4467.

185. Einfeld DA, Stibbs HH. Identification and characterization of a major surface antigen of *Giardia lamblia*. *Infect Immun* 1984; 46:377–383.

186. Edson CM, Farthing MJG, Thorley-Lawson DA, Keusch GT. An 88,000-Mr *Giardia lamblia* surface protein which is immunogenic in humans. *Infect Immun* 1986;54:621–625.

187. Rosoff JD, Stibbs HH. Isolation and identification of a *Giardia lamblia*-specific stool antigen (GSA 65) useful in coprodiagnosis of giardiasis. *J Clin Microbiol* 1986;23:905–910.

188. Rosoff JD, Stibbs HH. Physical and chemical characterization of a *Giardia lamblia*-specific antigen useful in coprodiagnosis of giardiasis. *J Clin Microbiol* 1986;24:1079–1083.

189. Char S, Cevallos AM, Farthing MJG. An immunodominant antigen of *Giardia lamblia* is a heat shock protein. *Biotechnol Ther* 1992;3:151–157.

190. Char S, Cevallos AM, Yamson P, Sullivan PB, Neale G, Farthing MJG. Impaired IgA response to *Giardia* heat shock antigen in children with persistent diarrhoea and giardiasis. *Gut* 1992;34:38–40.

191. Char S, Farthing MJG. *Giardia lamblia*: amino acid composition of *Giardia* heat shock antigen. *Exp Parasitol* 1993;77: 254–256.

192. Taylor GD, Wenman WM. Human immune response to *Giardia lamblia* infection. *J Infect Dis* 1987;155:137–140.

193. Nash TE, Aggarwal A. Cytotoxicity of monoclonal antibodies to a subset of *Giardia* isolates. *J Immunol* 1986;136:2628–2632.

194. Butscher WG, Faubert GM. The therapeutic action of monoclonal antibodies against a surface glycoprotein of *Giardia muris*. *Immunology* 1988;64:175–180.

195. Nash TE, Keister DB. Differences in excretory–secretory products and surface antigens among 19 isolates of *Giardia*. *J Infect Dis* 1985;152:1166–1171.

196. Aggarwal A, Nash TE. Antigenic variation of *Giardia lamblia* in vivo. *Infect Immun* 1988;56:1420–1423.

197. Aggarwal A, Merritt JW, Nash TE. Cysteine-rich variant of surface proteins of *Giardia lamblia*. *Mol Biochem Parasitol* 1989;32:39–48.

198. Nash TE. Antigenic variation in *Giardia lamblia*. *Exp Parasitol* 1989;68:238–241.

199. Nash TE, Herrington DA, Levine MM, Conrad JT, Merritt JW. Antigenic variation of *Giardia lamblia* in experimental human infections. *J Immunol* 1990;144:4362–4369.

200. Nash TE, Merritt JW, Conrad JT. Isolate and epitope variability in susceptibility of *Giardia lamblia* to intestinal proteases. *Infect Immun* 1991;59:1334–1340.

201. Stevens DP, Frank DM, Mahmoud AAF. Thymus dependency of host resistance to *Giardia muris* infection: studies in nude mice. *J Immunol* 1978;120:680–682.

202. Vinayak VK, Aggarwal A, Bhatia A, Naik SR, Chakravarti RN. Adoptive transfer of immunity of *Giardia lamblia* infection in mice. *Ann Trop Med Parasitol* 1981;75:265–267.

203. Carlson JR, Heyworth MF, Owen RL. T-lymphocyte subsets in nude mice with *Giardia muris* infection. *Thymus* 1987;9: 189–196.

204. Underdown BJ, Roberts-Thomson IC, Anders RF, Mitchell GF. Giardiasis in mice: studies on the characteristics of chronic infection of C3H/He mice. *J Immunol* 1981;126:669–672.

205. Kanwar SS, Ganguly NK, Walia BNS, Mahajan RC. Enumeration of small intestinal lymphocyte population in *Giardia lamblia* infected mice. *J Diarrhoeal Dis Res* 1984;2:243–248.

206. Webster ADB, Kenwright S, Ballard J, et al. Nodular lymphoid hyperplasia of the bowel in primary hypogammaglobulinaemia. *Gut* 1977;18:364–372.

207. Ward H, Jalan KN, Maitra TK, Aggarwal SK, Mahalanabis D. Small intestinal nodular lymphoid hyperplasia in patients with giardiasis and normal serum immunoglobulins. *Gut* 1983;24: 120–126.

208. Mitchell GF, Anders RF, Brown GV, et al. Analysis of infection characteristics and anti-parasite immune responses in resistant compared with susceptible hosts. *Immunol Rev* 1982; 61:137–188.

209. Owen RL, Allen CL, Stevens DP. Phagocytosis of *Giardia muris* by macrophages in Peyer's patch epithelium in mice. *Infect Immun* 1981;33:591–601.

210. Radulescu S, Meyer EA. Opsonization in vitro of *Giardia lamblia* trophozoites. *Infect Immun* 1981;32:852–856.

211. Smith PD, Keister DB, Wahl SM, Meltzer MS. Defective spontaneous but normal antibody dependent cytotoxicity for an extracellular protozoan parasite *Giardia lamblia* C3H/Hej mouse macrophages. *Cell Immunol* 1984;895:244–251.

212. Belosevic M, Faubert GM. Killing of *Giardia muris* trophozoites in vitro by spleen, mesenteric lymph node and peritoneal cells from susceptible and resistant mice. *Immunology* 1986; 59:267–275.

213. Smith PD, Elson CE, Keister DB, Nash TE. Human host response to *Giardia lamblia*. I. Spontaneous killing by mononuclear leukocytes in vitro. *J Immunol* 1982;128:1372–1376.

214. Smith PD, Keister DB, Elson CO. Human host response to *Giardia lamblia*. II. Antibody-dependent killing in vitro. *Cell Immunol* 1983;82:308–315.

215. Kanwar SS, Ganguly NK, Walia BNS, Mahajan RC. Direct and antibody dependent cell mediated cytotoxicity against *Giardia lamblia* by splenic and intestinal lymphoid cells in mice. *Gut* 1986;27:73–77.

216. Hill DR, Burge JJ, Pearson RD. Susceptibility of *Giardia lamblia* trophozoites to the lethal effect of human serum. *J Immunol* 1984;132:2046–2051.

217. Deguchi M, Gillin FD, Gigli I. Mechanism of killing of *Giardia lamblia* trophozoites by complement. *J Clin Invest* 1987;79: 1296–1302.

218. Gillin FD, Reiner DS, Wang C-S. Human milk kills parasitic infectional protozoa. *Science* 1983;221:1290–1292.

219. Reiner DS, Wang C-S, Gillin FD. Human milk kills *Giardia lamblia* by generating toxic lipolytic products. *J Infect Dis* 1986;154:825–832.

220. Gillin FD. *Giardia lamblia*: the role of conjugated and unconjugated bile salts in killing by human milk. *Exp Parasitol* 1987; 63:74–83.

221. Hernell O, Ward H, Blackberg L, Pereira MEA. Killing of *Giardia lamblia* by human milk lipases: an effect mediated by lipolysis of milk lipids. *J Infect Dis* 1986;153:715–720.

222. Veghelyi P. Absorption studies in children with *Giardia lamblia* infection. *Arch Dis Child* 1939;14:155–158.

223. Katsampes CP, McCoord AB, Phillips WA. Vitamin A absorption test in cases of giardiasis. *Am J Dis Child* 1944;67:189–193.

224. Cantor D, Biempica L, Toccalino H, O'Donnell JC. Small intestine studies in giardiasis. *Am J Gastroenterol* 1967;47: 134–141.

225. Barbieri D, DeBrito T, Hoshino S, Nascimento OB, Martins

Campos JV, Quarentii G, Marcondes E. Giardiasis in childhood. Absorption tests and biochemistry, histochemistry, light and electron microscopy of jejunal mucosa. *Arch Dis Child* 1970;45:466–472.

226. Cowen AE, Campbell CB. Giardiasis—a cause of vitamin B^{12} malabsorption. *Am J Dig Dis* 1973;18:384–390.

227. Tewari SG, Tandon BN. Functional and histological changes of small bowel in patients with *Giardia lamblia* infestation. *Indian J Med Res* 1974;62:689–695.

228. Rabassa EB, Arbelo TF, Guillot CL, Gonzales ES. Malabsorion por *Giardia lamblia*. *Rev Cubana Pediatr* 1975;47:247–263.

229. Mahalanabis D, Simpson TW, Chakrorty ML, Ganguli C, Battacharjee AK, Mukherjee KL. Malabsorption of water miscible vitamin A in children with giardiasis and ascariasis. *Am J Clin Nutr* 1979;32:313–318.

230. Tolboom JJM. Milk intolerance due to lactose and giardiasis. *Am J Clin Nutr* 1988;48:178–179.

231. Mantovani MP, Guandalini S, Ecuba P, Corvino C, Di Martino L. Lactose malabsorption in children with symptomatic *Giardia lamblia* infection: feasibility of yogurt supplementation. *J Pediatr Gastroenterol Nutr* 1989;9:295–300.

232. Farthing MJG, Mata LJ, Urrutia JJ, Kronmal RA. Giardiasis: impact on child growth. In: Walker-Smith JA, McNeish AS, eds. *Diarrhea and malnutrition in childhood*. London: Butterworths, 1986;68–78.

233. Perkins H. Giardiasis in children. *Br Med J* 1921;i:364.

234. Miller R. Lambliasis as a cause of chronic enteritis in children. *Arch Dis Child* 1926;1:93–98.

235. Veghelyi P. Giardiasis in children. *Am J Dis Child* 1938;56:1231–1241.

236. Boe J, Rinvik R. Infection with *Lamblia intestinalis* in children: its clinical significance and treatment. *Acta Paediatr* 1943;31:125–146.

237. Cortner JA. Giardiasis: a cause of celiac syndrome. *Am J Dis Child* 1959;98:311–316.

238. Court JM, Anderson CM. The pathogenesis of *Giardia lamblia* in children. *Med J Aust* 1959;46:436–438.

239. Burke JA. Giardiasis in childhood. *Am J Dis Child* 1975;129:1304–1310.

240. Kay R, Barnes GL, Townley RRW. *Giardia lamblia* infestation in 154 children. *Aust Paediatr J* 1977;13:98–104.

241. Pugh RJ, Newton RW. Giardiasis in infancy and childhood. *Practitioner* 1980;224:393–397.

242. Rowland MGM, Cole TJ, Whitehead RG. A quantitative study into the role of infection in determining nutritional status in Gambian village children. *Br J Nutr* 1977;37:441–450.

243. Cole TJ, Parkin JM. Infection and its effect on the growth of young children: a comparison of The Gambia and Uganda. *Trans R Soc Trop Med Hyg* 1977;71:196–198.

244. Gupta MC, Urrutia JJ. Effect of periodic anti-*Ascaris* and anti-*Giardia* treatment on nutritional status of pre-school children. *Am J Clin Nutr* 1982;36:79–86.

245. Pickering LK, Woodward WE, Du Pont HL, Sullivan P. Occurrence of *Giardia lamblia* in children in day care centers. *J Pediatr* 1984;104:522–536.

246. Ish-Horowicz M, Korman SH, Shapiro M, Har-Even U, Tamir I, Strauss N, Deckelbaum RJ. Asymptomatic giardiasis in children. *Pediatr Infect Dis J* 1989;8:773–779.

247. Ajdukiewicz AB, Youngs GR, Bouchier IAD. Nodular lymphoid hyperplasia and hypogammaglobulinaemia. *Gut* 1972;13:589–595.

248. Nagura H, Kohler PF, Brown WR. Immunocytochemical characterisation of lymphocytes in nodular lymphoid hyperplasia of the bowel. *Lab Invest* 1979;40:66.

249. Sherman P, Liebman WM. Apparent protein-losing enteropathy associated with giardiasis. *Am J Dis Child* 1980;134:893–894.

250. Korman SH, Bar-Oz B, Mandelberg A, Matoth I. Giardiasis with protein-losing enteropathy: diagnosis by fecal α$_1$-antitrypsin determination. *J Pediatr Gastroenterol Nutr* 1990;10:249–252.

251. Sullivan PB, Lunn PG, Northrop-Clewes CA, Farthing MJG. Parasitic infection of the gut and protein-losing enteropathy. *J Pediatr Gastroenterol Nutr* 1992;15:404–407.

252. Goka AKJ, Rolston DDK, Mathan VI, Farthing MJG. The relative merits of faecal and duodenal juice microscopy in the diagnosis of giardiasis. *Trans R Soc Trop Med Hyg* 1990;84:66–67.

253. Bendig DW. Diagnosis of giardiasis in infants and children by endoscopic brush cytology. *J Pediatr Gastroenterol Nutr* 1989;8:204–206.

254. Ungar BLP, Yolken RH, Nash TE, Quinn TC. Enzyme-linked immunosorbent assay for detection of *Giardia lamblia* in fecal specimens. *J Infect Dis* 1984;149:90–97.

255. Green EL, Miles MA, Warhurst DC. Immunodiagnostic detection of *Giardia* antigen in faeces by a rapid visual enzyme-linked immunosorbent assay. *Lancet* 1985;2:691–693.

256. Janoff EN, Craft JC, Pickering LK, Novotny T, Blaser MJ, Knisley CV, Reller LB. Diagnosis of *Giardia lamblia* infections by detection of parasite-specific antigens. *J Clin Microbiol* 1989;27:431–435.

257. Wiencka J, Olding-Stenkvist E, Schroder H, Huldt G. Detection of *Giardia* antigen in stool samples by a semi-quantitative enzyme immunoassay (EIA) test. *Scand J Infect Dis* 1989;21:443–448.

258. Rosoff JD, Sanders CA, Sonnad SS, et al. Stool diagnosis of giardiasis using a commercially available enzyme immunoassay to detect *Giardia*-specific antigen 65 (GSA 65). *J Clin Microbiol* 1989;27:1997–2002.

259. Addiss DG, Mathews HM, Stewart JM, et al. Evaluation of a commercially available enzyme-linked immunosorbent assay for *Giardia lamblia* antigen in stool. *J Clin Microbiol* 1991;29:1137–1142.

260. Char S, Farthing MJG. DNA probes for diagnosis of enteric infection. *Gut* 1991;32:1–3.

261. Butcher PD, Farthing MJG. DNA probes for the faecal diagnosis of *Giardia lamblia* infections in man. *Biochem Soc Trans* 1988;17:363–364.

262. Davidson RA. Issues in clinical parasitology: the treatment of giardiasis. *Am J Gastroenterol* 1984;79:256–261.

263. Mendelson R. The treatment of giardiasis. *Trans R Soc Trop Med* 1980;74:438–439.

264. Quiros-Buelna E. Furazolidone and metronidazole for treatment of giardiasis in children. *Scand J Gastroenterol* 1989;24(Suppl 169):65–69.

265. Feingold SM. Metronidazole. *Ann Intern Med* 1980;93:585–587.

266. Paget TA, Jarroll EL, Manning P, Lindmark DG, Lloyd D. Respiration in the cysts and trophozoites of *Giardia muris*. *J Gen Microbiol* 1989;135:145–154.

267. Crouch AA, Seow WK, Thong YH. Effect of twenty-three chemotherapeutic agents on the adherence and growth of *Giardia lamblia* in vitro. *Trans R Soc Trop Med Hyg* 1986;80:893–896.

268. Al-Waili NS, Al-Waili BH, Saloom KY. Therapeutic use of mebendazole in giardial infections. *Trans R Soc Trop Med Hyg* 1988;82:438.

269. Gascon J, Abos R, Valls ME, Corachan M. Mebendazole and metronidazole in giardial infections. *Trans R Soc Trop Med Hyg* 1990;84:694.

270. Meloni BP, Thompson RCA, Reynoldson JA, Seville P. Albendazole: a more effective anti-giardial agent in vitro than metronidazole or tinidazole. *Trans R Soc Trop Med Hyg* 1990;84:375–379.

271. Weinbach EC, Costa JL, Wieder SC. Antidepressant drugs suppress growth of the human pathogenic protozoan *Giardia lamblia*. *Res Commun Chem Pathol Pharmacol* 1985;47:145–148.

272. Farthing MJG, Inge PMG. Anti-giardial activity of the bile salt-like antibiotic sodium fusidate. *J Antimicrob Chemother* 1986;17:165–171.

273. Farthing MJG, Inge PMG, Pearson RM. Effect of D-propranolol on growth and motility of flagellate protozoa. *J Antimicrob Chemother* 1987;20:519–522.

274. Popovic OS, Milovic V. Propranolol and metronidazole for the treatment of metronidazole-resistant giardiasis. *J Clin Gastroenterol* 1990;12:604–605.

275. Crouch AA, Seow WK, Whitman LM, Thong YH. Sensitivity in vitro of *Giardia intestinalis* to dyadic combinations of

azithromycin, deoxycline, mefloquine, tinidazole and furazolidone. *Trans R Soc Trop Med Hyg* 1990;84:246–248.

276. Gillin FD, Diamond LS. Inhibition of clonal growth of *Giardia lamblia* and *Entamoeba histolytica* by metronidazole, quinacrine and other antimicrobial agents. *J Antimicrob Chemother* 1981;8:305–316.

277. Boreham PF, Phillips RE, Shepherd RW. The sensitivity of *Giardia intestinalis* to drugs *in vitro*. *J Antimicrob Chemother* 1984;14:449–461.

278. Gordts B, Hemelhof W, Asselman C, Butzler J. *In vitro* susceptibility of 25 *Giardia lamblia* isolates of human origin to six commonly used anti-protozoal agents. *Antimicrob Agents Chemother* 1985;28:378–380.

279. Hoyne GF, Boreham PFL, Parsons PG, Ward C, Biggs B. The effect of drugs on the cell cycle of *Giardia intestinalis*. *Parasitology* 1989;99:333–339.

280. Inge PMG, Farthing MJG. A radiometric assay for anti-giardial drugs. *Trans R Soc Trop Med Hyg* 1987;81:345–347.

281. Boreham PF, Phillips RE, Shepherd RW. Heterogeneity in the responses of clones of *Giardia intestinalis* to anti-giardial drugs. *Trans R Soc Trop Med Hyg* 1987;81:406–407.

282. Boreham PF, Phillips RE, Shepherd RW. Altered uptake of metronidazole *in vitro* by stocks of *Giardia intestinalis* with different drug sensitivities. *Trans R Soc Trop Med Hyg* 1988;82:104–106.

283. Upcroft JA, Upcroft P. Drug resistance and *Giardia*. *Parasitol Today* 1993;9:187–190.

284. Smith PD, Gillin FD, Kaushal NA, Nash TE. Antigenic analysis of *Giardia lamblia* from Afghanistan, Puerto Rico, Ecuador and Oregon. *Infect Immun* 1982;36:714–719.

285. Udezulu IA, Visvesvara GS, Moss DM, Leitch GJ. Isolation of two *Giardia lamblia* (WB strain) clones with distinct surface protein and antigenic profiles and differing infectivity and virulence. *Infect Immun* 1992;60:2274–2280.

286. Nash T. Surface antigen variability and variation in *Giardia lamblia*. *Parasitol Today* 1992;8:229–243.

Infections of the Gastrointestinal Tract,
edited by M. J. Blaser, P. D. Smith, J. I. Ravdin,
H. B. Greenberg, and R. L. Guerrant
Raven Press, Ltd., New York © 1995.

CHAPTER 72

Cryptosporidium and Related Species

Karim A. Adal, Charles R. Sterling, and Richard L. Guerrant

Cryptosporidium parvum is a small protozoan parasite that has recently become the focus of increased attention. Although it has long been recognized as a veterinary pathogen, widespread interest in this organism as a human pathogen was fueled by patients with the acquired immunodeficiency syndrome (AIDS) and other immunosuppressed patients, in whom it causes a debilitating chronic diarrhea. We now know, however, that it is also an important cause of diarrheal illness in immunocompetent people, and it is increasingly recognized as a cause of diarrhea in children in developing areas worldwide, and as a difficult waterborne pathogen.

HISTORICAL ASPECTS

In 1907 Tyzzer (1) described clearly for the first time a new protozoan genus that he identified in the gastric epithelium of laboratory mice and named *Cryptosporidium*. The name *Cryptosporidium,* meaning "hidden spore" in Greek, reflects the unusual absence of sporocysts surrounding the sporozoites. In 1912 he identified and named *Cryptosporidium parvum* (2). Until recently, *Cryptosporidium* species were mainly of interest to the veterinary profession as etiologic agents of avian and bovine diarrheal disease. However, in 1976, infections in humans were first reported in an immunocompetent child with enterocolitis in whom it was diagnosed by rectal biopsy (3), and in an adult with bullous pemphigoid treated with cyclophosphamide and prednisolone (4). With an additional six case reports over the ensuing 5 years, including five patients with immune compromise [one with congenital hypogammaglobulinemia and one with immunoglobulin A (IgA) deficiency], only eight human cases (six immunocompromised) were reported before 1982 (5–10). Nevertheless, it was not until the advent of

K. A. Adal and R. L. Guerrant: Department of Medicine, Division of Infectious Diseases, University of Virginia School of Medicine, Charlottesville, Virginia 22908.

C. R. Sterling: Department of Veterinary Science, University of Arizona, Tucson, Arizona 85721.

AIDS that the medical profession really took notice of this organism (11), and it is considered an AIDS-defining illness (12). Most of our knowledge of the clinical significance and presentation, pathogenesis, epidemiology, and treatment of cryptosporidial infection has been accumulated in the last decade.

MICROBIOLOGY

Taxonomy

The classification of the genus *Cryptosporidium,* along with recognized species, is presented in Table 1. Characteristics that account for this classification include: an anterior polar complex with apical rings, micronemes, and subpellicular microtubules [phylum Apicomplexa]; locomotion by flexion, gliding, or undulation [class Sporozoasida]; a life cycle with merogony (asexual multiplication), gametogony (sexual multiplication), and sporogony (sporozoite formation) [subclass Coccidiasina]; merogony occurring within vertebrate hosts [order Eucoccidiorida]; independent development of male and female gametes [suborder Eimeriorina]; and a one host life cycle (homoxenous development) where the parasite develops just under the surface membrane of host cells, possesses microgametes without flagella, and oocysts with four naked sporozoites [family Cryptosporidiidae] (13).

The early belief that *Cryptosporidium* was host specific led to the naming of numerous species according to the host from which they were described. At least 21 species have been reported (14). Studies involving cross-transmission and more careful morphometric analysis, however, have either invalidated species distinctions or placed the validity of many in doubt. The currently recognized valid species of *Cryptosporidium* include *C. muris* from mice and cattle, *C. parvum* from a wide variety of mammalian species including humans, *C. wrairi* from guinea pigs, *C. baileyi* from chickens, *C. meleagridis* from turkeys, *C. serpentis* from snakes, and *C. nasorum* from a fish (14). The validity of the latter requires confirmation.

TABLE 1. *Taxonomic classification of* Cryptosporidium

Classification	Name	Author
Phylum	Apicomplexa	Levine, 1970
Class	Sporozoasida	Leuckart, 1879
Subclass	Coccidiasina	Leuckart, 1879
Order	Eucoccidiorida	Leger and Duboscq, 1910
Suborder	Eimeriorina	Leger, 1911
Family	Cryptosporidiidae	Leger, 1911
Genus	*Cryptosporidium*	Tyzzer, 1907
Species	*C. muris*	Tyzzer, 1907
	C. parvum	Tyzzer, 1912
	C. wrairi	Chrisp et al., 1992
	C. baileyi	Current et al., 1986
	C. meleagridis	Slavin, 1955
	C. serpentis	Levine, 1981
	C. nasorum	Hoover et al, 1981

Additional species may yet be identified due to the intense interest in organisms of this genus.

Cryptosporidium parvum is responsible for producing infection and disease in humans. There is one report of *C. baileyi* infecting an immunodeficient individual (15). Subspecies and strains of *C. parvum* are not yet recognized even though biological and molecular differences have been noted among isolates. There is much interest in this area because of the spectrum of disease seen in animals and humans infected with *C. parvum*.

Life Cycle and Morphology

The oocyst is the final development stage in the life cycle of *Cryptosporidium,* can be found in the feces of an infected host, and must be ingested or inhaled to initiate infection of a new susceptible host (Fig. 1). Oocysts of *C. parvum* measure 4 to 6 μm in diameter and are fully sporulated (contain four free fully developed and infectious sporozoites) when they leave their host. *Isospora* and *Toxoplasma*, coccidian relatives of *Cryptosporidium* that also infect humans, must sporulate in the environment before becoming infective and have eight sporozoites, which develop within sporocysts inside the oocyst.

Approximately 80% of the oocysts formed within an infected host are thick-walled. This oocyst population constitutes the environmentally resistant infectious forms that must find their way into a new host to initiate infection. The remaining 20% are referred to as thin-walled oocysts and are only rarely encountered within the feces of an infected host. These forms, which are enveloped by a single limiting membrane and can excyst spontaneously within the intestine or at extraintestinal sites, presumably account for the persistent infections frequently encountered in immunocompromised hosts (16). Spherical bodies resembling oocysts and referred to as atypical oocysts have been reported from patients with diarrhea (17). They do not stain with modified acid-fast, auramine-phenol, or safranin-methylene blue stains. They also do not react to commercially available monoclonal antibody-based im-

munofluorescence tests. It has been suggested that such forms may not be oocysts at all, but may represent a life cycle stage of an unidentified protozoon or fungus (18).

Upon ingestion, oocysts must undergo a process of excystation (release of infective sporozoites) for the life cycle to continue. This necessary step normally occurs in the environment of the small intestine of a susceptible host (13). Exposure to reducing conditions, enzymes, and bile salts are all important factors of this process within the host. Artificial exposure of oocysts to these conditions outside the host also can bring about a high level of excystation (19–21). The process of excystation results from the dissolution of a suture at one end of the oocyst wall. Sporozoites then escape through the opening created by the breakdown of this suture (22).

Newly excysted sporozoites must attach to and invade appropriate susceptible host cells to initiate the ensuing asexual merogonic cycle. Enterocytes of the terminal ileum appear to be preferentially invaded by *C. parvum* sporozoites in many mammalian hosts. In addition, parasite development has been reported at such extraintestinal sites as the conjunctiva of the eye and within cells of the respiratory and biliary tree of immune compromised human hosts. *Cryptosporidium* sporozoites are unique among the coccidia in that they invade cells only to the level of the extracytoplasmic compartment beneath the infected cell's outer limiting membrane.

Sporozoite attachment and subsequent internalization have been described in detail (23). The process is very much like that described for cell invasion by malaria and other apicomplexan parasites. Sporozoite probing and the release of contents from apical end organelles (micronemes) cause an indentation and folding of the host cell limiting membrane, which ultimately encompasses the parasite within a parasitophorous vacuole of host cell origin. Membrane junctions form at the vacuole base nearest the sporozoite apical end and this region ultimately differentiates into a complex "feeder organelle." The membranous folds of this organelle tremendously increase the available surface area between host cell and parasite, possibly to facilitate the exchange of materials.

Each sporozoite that has successfully invaded a cell dedifferentiates and rounds up within the parasitophorous vacuole to become a uninucleate trophozoite. Trophozoites undergo a complex cycle of growth and differentiation (merogony) to become type I meronts with six to eight merozoites. Studies in mice indicate that this process, which includes three successive synchronous nuclear divisions resulting in the production of eight nuclei that migrate to the parasite's periphery to form merozoite buds, occurs between 8 and 16 hr after the infection (24). Type I meronts persist throughout an infection and likely contribute to the severity of disease manifested in patients with AIDS.

Type I meronts rupture releasing six to eight merozoites to invade adjacent susceptible host cells. Parasites developing from these merozoites can become type I meronts again or type II meronts. The latter have been described from animals 24 hr after the infection. The persistence of type II meronts seen in infections is presumably the result

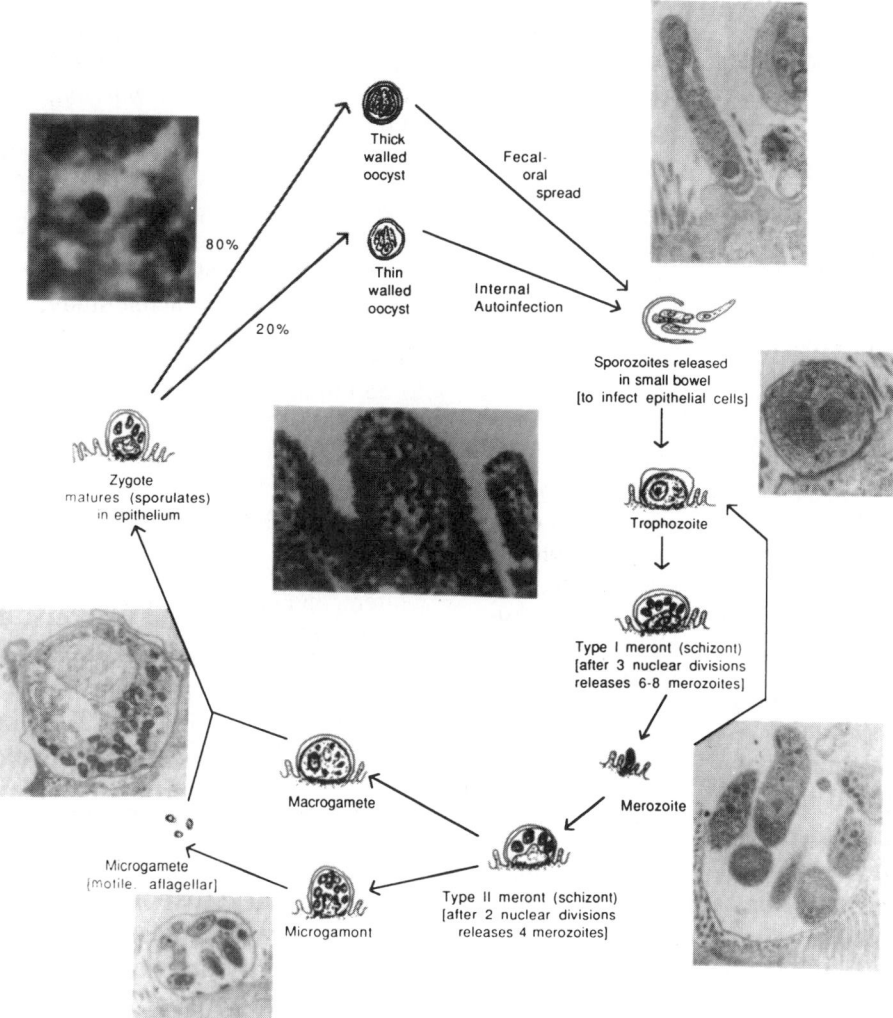

FIG. 1. Life Cycle of *Cryptosporidium*.

of a cycle involving the continued production of autoinfective thin-walled oocysts. Four merozoites are produced in type II meronts and presumably are destined only to become gamonts. Merozoites of type I and type II meronts are morphologically similar and measure approximately 5.0 × 1.0 μm. They are comma shaped, invested in a complex pellicle consisting of a plasmalemma plus a double inner membrane complex, have an apical complex consisting of rings and micronemes, and possess subpellicular microtubules, ribosomes, and a nucleus.

Merozoites from type II meronts invade host cells to become micro-(male) or macro-(female) gamonts. The majority differentiate into the latter. Gamonts have been seen at 36 (microgamont) and 48 (macrogamont) hr after the infection of animals.

Microgamonts show a more extensive nuclear division than observed in meronts and as many as 16 nuclei have been observed. These migrate to the periphery of the microgamont cytoplasm and bud to form the bullet-shaped microgametes, which measure about 1.4 × 0.4 μm. Mi-

crogametes have a centrally located nucleus that is surrounded by microtubules derived from a conical structure at one end. They lack flagella and mitochondria seen in the microgametes of other coccidia. Macrogamonts possess numerous amylopectin-like granules and two types of peripherally located wall-forming bodies.

Fertilization with ensuing zygote formation occurs when microgametes attach to and fuse with mature macrogametes. The fusion of male and female pronuclei has not been observed.

Zygotes develop into either thick-walled or thin-walled oocysts having four naked sporozoites. The process of sporogony is similar to that of merogony except that the first nuclear division is meiotic, restoring the haploid genomic complement of sporozoites. Sporulated oocysts can be observed in infected animals at 72 hr and subsequently during the course of an infection (24). Factors that influence the development of the two discrete oocyst forms are unknown. Those having thin walls, however, lack wall-forming bodies.

Sporozoites are structurally similar to merozoites except they possess a more tapered anterior end, centrally located amylopectin granules, and a posteriorly situated nucleus.

Cultivation

The complete growth and development of *C. parvum* apart from animals of its normal host range have been accomplished using *in ovo* and *in vitro* cultivation systems. In the former, inoculation of purified sporozoites from calf and human isolates of *C. parvum* into the chorioallantoic membrane (CAM) of chicken embryos results in parasite multiplication in endoderm cells with the eventual release of oocysts into the chorioallantoic fluid (25).

Parasite development in eggs appears similar to what has been reported in the ileum of experimentally infected neonatal mice. Drawbacks to the use of eggs are that not all eggs from different types or even the same type of chicken are equally susceptible to infection and that oocysts are not easily released from the CAM into the chorioallantoic fluid, making large-scale recovery difficult.

The *in vitro* development of *C. parvum* has been accomplished within a variety of cell lines. These include differentiated human enterocyte CaCo-2 and T84 carcinoma and HT29 cells and human fetal lung, human endometrial carcinoma, human rectal tumor, human foreskin, rat LGA carcinoma, Madin–Darby bovine and canine kidney, primary chicken kidney, porcine kidney, and mouse L929 cells (23,26–37). The extent of parasite multiplication within the various cell lines tested varies widely and is typically far less than what is encountered in experimentally infected animals. Individual laboratories often use different techniques to initiate infection of cell cultures. Some have utilized purified sporozoites while others have simply added oocysts to cell cultures and relied on spontaneous excystation to initiate infection. Such differences of technique could obviously affect further parasite development since success at infecting permissive cell lines appears to be dependent on appropriate presentation of sporozoites to the cells. Claims of complete development from sporozoite to infectious oocyst have been made but have been difficult to reproduce. It has been hypothesized that a major reason for this lies in the inability of the parasite to produce thin-walled autoinfective oocysts *in vitro* (27). What is clear is that much greater attention needs to be given to defining appropriate conditions under which this parasite can be propagated in reasonable numbers and in a reproducible way. This shortcoming, which is being addressed by a number of laboratories, has impeded studies on the meront and sexual life cycle stages of *C. parvum*.

EPIDEMIOLOGY

Environmental Transmission

Cryptosporidium species are ubiquitous and infect a wide variety of hosts, from fish, reptiles, and birds, to rodents, primates, and other mammals (13,38). Except for one reported case of infection with *C. baileyi* in a renal transplant patient with AIDS (15), human infections are due to *Cryptosporidium parvum,* a species that is infectious for most mammals and that is especially prevalent in ruminants. Calves are a source of human infection (39–45), with up to 44% of dairy farmers in one study having serologic evidence of past infection (46), and contact with farm animals is frequently reported in sporadic cases (47–50). Drinking unpasteurized milk has been implicated (50–52), and in one study, 14.6% of people working in the food industry were asymptomatic carriers of *Cryptosporidium* (53). Other animal species also believed to be important as potential reservoirs include rodents, sheep (49,54,55), and housepets such as cats and dogs, especially kittens and puppies (56–62). Many infections are therefore the result of zoonotic transmission; however, there is growing evidence that person-to-person transmission from fecal–oral spread is an important means of transmission in urban settings (63), day care centers, and nosocomial outbreaks, and there is evidence for transmission during male homosexual intercourse (64,65). In a recent study from Brazil, the majority of susceptible (seronegative) family members in the households of children with cryptosporidial diarrhea became secondarily infected (66). The organism has also been found in the stool of a 3-day-old infant whose mother had diarrhea several days prior to vaginal delivery (67), and in asymptomatic babies whose mothers had cryptosporidial diarrhea at the time of delivery (52,68). *Cryptosporidium* infection is also becoming more prominent in the differential diagnosis of traveler's diarrhea.

The 1993 waterborne outbreak of diarrheic illness in Wisconsin with an estimated 403,000 cases of diarrhea over the span of 2 months (69,69a), of which more than 600 were confirmed cases of cryptosporidiosis, provides another unfortunate reminder that routine chlorination of drinking water is relatively ineffective at killing the *Cryptosporidium* oocysts. They are several-fold more resistant to disinfectants than *Giardia lamblia* cysts and, because of their small size, are not well filtered by routine filtering devices (70) or totally removed by activated-sludge treatment of sewage (71,72). A number of waterborne outbreaks have been documented in recent years, including a large outbreak in Georgia in 1987 (73–83). Most outbreaks are due to contamination of the drinking water supply by raw sewage and runoff from dairies and grazing lands (84), or a breakdown in the filtering system of water purification plants. The detection of *Cryptosporidium* oocysts in water samples is obviously an important issue. It is more difficult than detection in stool, but as more sensitive techniques are developed, the prevalence of *Cryptosporidium* oocysts in nature and drinking water is becoming increasingly recognized (70,71,84–90). Outbreaks of swimming pool-associated cryptosporidiosis are further evidence of the highly infective nature of the organism and its resistance to disinfection and filtering (91–93).

The interplay between the numerous environmental

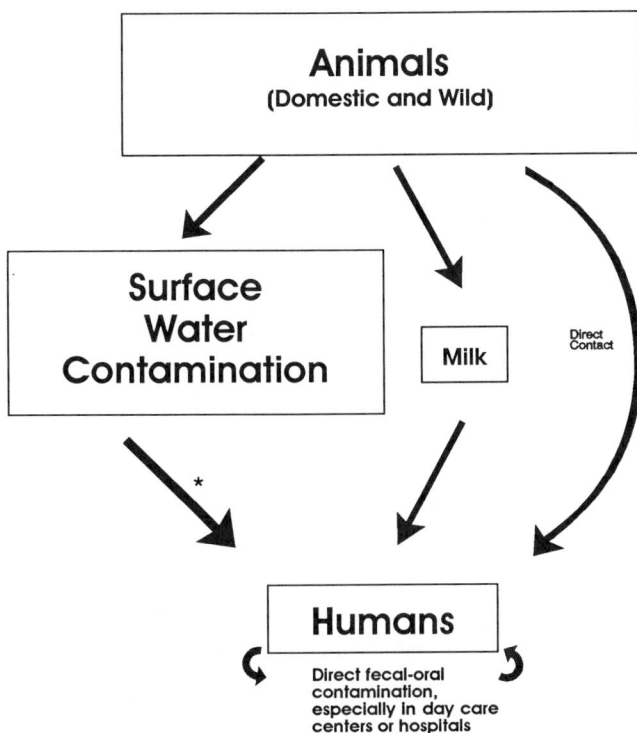

Animals
(Domestic and Wild)

**Surface
Water
Contamination**

Milk

Direct
Contact

*

Humans

Direct fecal-oral
contamination,
especially in day care
centers or hospitals

*Drinking untreated or inadequately treated water
(including swimming pools) or possibly via foods.

FIG. 2. Reservoirs (□) and routes of spread of *Cryptosporidium.*

TABLE 2. *Frequencies of* Cryptosporidium *infection in presumably immunocompetent patients with sporadic diarrheal illness and controls from 43 studies in developing countries (Asia, Africa, and Latin America) and 35 studies in developed countries (Europe, North America, and Australia)*

Area	Cryptosporidium cases/total diarrhea patients screened (% positive)	Positive controls/total control patients screened (% positive)
Developing countries	1486/24,269 (6.1%)	61/4146 (1.5%)
Developed countries	2232/107,329 (2.1%)	3/1941 (0.15%)

upper endoscopy (169). In another similarly designed study (170), no *Cryptosporidium* oocysts were found in any of the duodenal aspirates of 131 patients. Whether these differences are due to different patient populations, home environments, or ethnic groups is yet to be determined.

Developing Countries

In poorly developed regions where standards of sanitation and water treatment technology are low, and crowded living conditions predominate, the prevalence of cryptosporidiosis is much higher. While less than 20% of persons acquire serologic evidence of cryptosporidiosis by young adulthood in developed areas, less developed areas have seroprevalence rates that exceed 60% by 10 years of life in China and 95% by 2 years of life in northeastern Brazil (171). There is often a seasonal pattern of increased infections during warmer and rainy seasons (60,95,99,102,103, 106,116,118,123,131,132), although other studies have found an increased prevalence during the dry and warm season (38,98,109,172). Other risk factors include weaning and younger age (less than 2 years old), and breastfeeding seems to have a protective effect with significantly lower rates of cryptosporidiosis in breast-fed infants (94,99,103,105,106,112,115,118,121,126,128,130). Despite earlier speculations, the transfer of passive immunity via milk to the infant is apparently not the mechanism responsible for the lower incidence (173). Decreased exposure to the parasite in breast-fed infants may be a potential explanation. There is a significant association of cryptosporidiosis with malnutrition and a higher mortality rate.

Patients in developing countries who have AIDS have a higher incidence of chronic diarrhea than patients with AIDS in developed countries, and seem to have a higher rate (up to 48%) of *Cryptosporidium* infection as the etiology of their diarrhea (Table 3 compiled from refs. 174–182 and 149, 151, and 183–193).

reservoirs and hosts of *Cryptosporidium* is complex and the interactions and transmission patterns are not yet fully understood (Fig. 2).

Demographics

Cryptosporidium is associated with diarrheal illness in most areas of the world. Numerous studies have documented its presence in more than 40 countries spanning all six continents. Prevalence rates in patients with diarrhea have varied from as low as 1% in Europe and North America to up to 30% on other continents. If one pools data from multiple studies, an average of 6.1% of diarrheal illnesses in developing countries is due to *Cryptosporidium,* compared to 2.1% in developed countries (Table 2 compiled from refs. 94–136 and 50–52, 67, and 137–167). The prevalence in control patients averages 1.5% and 0.2%, respectively, suggesting that asymptomatic infections occur. Serologic studies confirm these results, with a higher seroprevalence in developing countries than in developed countries (168). An asymptomatic carrier state has now been clearly demonstrated in numerous patients. One study from the United States reports a prevalence of 12.7% in immunocompetent patients undergoing routine

TABLE 3. *Frequencies of* Cryptosporidium *infection in HIV-positive patients with diarrhea and HIV-positive controls without diarrhea from 9 studies in developing countries (Africa and Latin America) and 13 studies in developed countries (Europe, North America, and Australia)*

Area	Cryptosporidium cases/total diarrhea patients screened (% positive)	Positive controls/ total control patients screened (% positive)
Developing countries	120/503 (24%)	5/101 (5%)
Developed countries	148/1074 (13.8%)	0/35

Developed Countries

In the immunocompetent host in developed countries, disease outbreaks have been reported in a variety of groups, including day care center staffs and children (155,194–206), veterinary students and animal caretakers (39,40,207–210), and health care workers. Rates of infection during outbreaks in day care centers may reach as high as 43%, with significant secondary spread in family contacts (196,203). Asymptomatic cryptosporidiosis in day care centers has also been reported (211–213). A report of a nosocomial outbreak described serologic evidence for the transmission of *Cryptosporidium* to 31% of hospital personnel who came in contact with an infected patient with diarrhea (214). Other nosocomial outbreaks have been documented, some in immunocompromised patients and patients with AIDS (214–220). *Cryptosporidium* is becoming an increasingly recognized cause of traveler's diarrhea in people traveling to areas with an increased prevalence of cryptosporidiosis (137,151, 221–232). It is also the etiologic organism in sporadic cases in patients with gastroenteritis (197), and children are again most vulnerable (140,150), with transmission to other family members (142,151,155,203).

In the immunocompromised host, most cases of cryptosporidiosis are being reported in patients with AIDS, in whom it is being recognized as a leading etiology of chronic diarrhea (183–189,233). Recent data suggest that up to 15% of patients with AIDS in the United States are infected with *Cryptosporidium* (184–186), and homosexual males seem to have higher rates of infection than heterosexual patients (64). However, other patient populations are also at increased risk, such as patients with various forms of hypogammaglobulinemia including selective IgA deficiency (8,9,234–239), patients taking corticosteroids and other immunosuppressive agents (4,240), as well as patients with malignancies or undergoing chemotherapy (57,241–249), organ transplant recipients (10,250–252), and bone marrow transplant recipients (218,219,244,246,253–256). Diarrhea due to *Cryptosporidium* has also been reported in a patient with insulin-dependent diabetes mellitus, in whom it lasted for 4 months

(257), and in a patient with thalassemia (258). The disease proved fatal in a patient with Sheehan's syndrome (259).

PATHOLOGY AND PATHOGENESIS

Pathologic manifestations of cryptosporidiosis appear to be similar in all infected animal species and are largely a function of where infection occurs. In immunocompetent hosts, parasite replication is principally confined to the apical border of enterocytes in the lower jejunum and ileum. The entire gastrointestinal tract as well as ancillary extraintestinal sites including biliary and pancreatic ducts and portions of the respiratory tract may become infected in immunocompromised hosts. Mild to severe intestinal villous atrophy is observed. Villous stunting, broadening, and fusion may occur (7,10). Inflammation, accompanied by plasma cell, neutrophil, macrophage, and lymphocyte infiltration into the subepithelial lamina propria, has been noted (4,7). Crypts may appear enlarged and hyperplastic and Peyer's patches appear reactive (260,261). At the ultrastructural level, infected cells lack microvilli at the site of parasite attachment and the cytoplasm may appear excessively vacuolated. Mitochondria may also appear swollen and vacuolated (4,262). Similar changes are seen in epithelial cells of the respiratory tree and may be accompanied by hypertrophy, loss of cilia, and excess mucus production.

Pathogenic mechanisms operative during cryptosporidiosis still remain poorly defined. Much of what has been learned has come from animal models. Malabsorption in both the small and large intestine and impaired digestion in the small intestine underlie diarrhea in germ-free calves infected with *C. parvum* (263). Similar malabsorption, involving impairment to glucose-stimulated sodium and water absorption, has been reported in a neonatal pig model (264). D-Xylose and vitamin B_{12} malabsorption has been described in infected patients with AIDS (265). The end result may include bacterial overgrowth, osmotic pressure changes across the gut wall, and an excessive release of fluid into the intestinal lumen (18). The often described cholera-like diarrhea also suggests enterotoxin-like activity. Such activity, which has been reported in cell-free extracts from *C. parvum*-infected tissue (266), has not been confirmed by others (267). Additional studies demonstrate enterotoxic activity on human jejunum by stool filtrates from infected calves (268), but the source and mechanism of this effect may be of host or parasite origin (269).

Alterations in cellular enzyme activities also have been noted in association with *C. parvum* infections. Marked reductions in the brush border enzymes lactase and alkaline phosphatase have been reported from infected athymic rats (270). Decreases in these enzymes along with sucrase have been observed in neonatal pig models of infection (267). Lactase deficiency along with xylose malabsorption has been reported from infected calves (271). Epithelial barrier dysfunction, which is the site of parasite replication, is documented but may involve transcellular as well as paracellular pathways (26,269).

IMMUNITY

Overview of Animal Models

On the basis of clinical data from humans and experimental data from animals, a role for both humoral and cellular responses in resolving *C. parvum* infections has been accepted (171). Several reports note that either hypogammaglobulinemic or anergic patients have presented with severe protracted diarrhea with *Cryptosporidium* infection (4,8,234,235). Animal models, particularly those utilizing mice of different strains and genetic backgrounds, have focused largely on the role of cell-mediated responses. The use of athymic (272), CD4 (helper T cell) and interferon-γ (IFN-γ) depleted (273,274), severe combined immunodeficient (SCID) (275–277) and murine retrovirus infected (278) mouse models and the athymic rat model (270) demonstrate that a loss of T cell function leads to a variable, but persistent, cryptosporidiosis similar to what might be seen in patients with AIDS. Resolution of an established infection in reconstituted SCID mice was shown to be dependent on CD4 cells and IFN-γ. It has been argued, however, that since patients with AIDS show increasing levels of IFN-γ as their disease progresses, the models rendering mice deficient in CD4 and IFN-γ may not resemble what is seen in patients with AIDS and cryptosporidiosis (279). Cytotoxic CD8 cells appear to have little or no role in recovery from infection (274,277). A role for natural killer (NK) cells in resolving cryptosporidiosis has been suggested but also appears to be minimal (280,281).

While it is clear that different animal species can mount antibody responses of all subclasses to a variety of cryptosporidial antigens, their role in conferring protection is unclear. Neonatal BALB/c mice exhibit antibody responses that do not correlate with either the severity or duration of infection (282). Furthermore, if these mice were depleted of B cells, they did not differ from controls in the onset, peak, or duration of infection. Also, adult B cell-depleted mice were impossible to infect regardless of the infectious dose given, further suggesting that the development of anti-parasite antibody plays a less important role than CD4 cells in resolving this murine infection. Specific anti-parasite antibody, however, might prove of value in therapeutic regimens for controlling cryptosporidiosis (see Anticryptosporidial Therapy section).

While animal models have been useful in studying immune parameters involved in cryptosporidiosis, it must be kept in mind that they do not show all the clinical and immunological abnormalities associated with cryptosporidiosis in the AIDS population. Because of this, we constantly have to evaluate and question the meaning of results coming from such models. In this context it is perhaps relevant to exploit models such as monkeys infected with human immunodeficiency virus (HIV) or the simian immunodeficiency virus (SIV).

Humoral Immunity

Much of our current knowledge concerning immune responses to cryptosporidial infection in humans derives from serologic surveys and clinical case reports of immunocompetent and immunocompromised populations. The notion that humoral responses play a role in *C. parvum* infections comes from observations of persistent infections in congenitally immunodeficient patients with hypo- or agammaglobulinemias (8,39,283).

Initial insight into human anticryptosporidial humoral responses was provided using an immunofluorescence assay against cryostat sections of infected versus uninfected tissue of lamb origin. Immunofluorescence assays have also been used to demonstrate seroconversion in immunocompetent patients, a lack of responsiveness in hypogammaglobulinemic patients, low-level responses in patients with AIDS (283), and isotype-specific seroconversion responses in immunocompetent patients (284).

Enzyme-linked immunoadsorbent assays (ELISAs) also have been used to detect humoral responses to cryptosporidial infections. Elevated and persistent (up to 10 months) IgG responses have been detected in immunocompetent and immunocompromised patients. IgM responses in the same patients usually were detectable for only 4 months following infection (285). Subsequent studies centered on populations living in areas endemic for cryptosporidiosis have demonstrated persistently elevated titers for IgG and, in some cases, IgM and IgA (108,168,225,286). It could be argued that antibody persistence in these instances may be indicative of constant or recurrent parasite exposure.

The sera of infected patients also have been used in immunoblotting techniques to study antigen-specific immunoglobulin responses to *C. parvum*. A large number of antigens ranging from 3 to over 200 kDa react with human sera (287,288). Prominent among them is reactivity to an antigen of 20 to 23 kDa, which is localized on the surface of sporozoites. Immunoblot studies employing animal sera also have identified a number of other immunodominant antigens (289–294). The extent to which any demonstrable antibodies play a role in protective immunity remains unclear.

Cellular Immunity

Even fewer studies have been performed in humans to assess the role of cellular immunity in relation to *Cryptosporidium* infection. The association of *C. parvum* infection and disease in the HIV-infected population, however, underscores the role of cellular responses in controlling this infection. Patients with underlying lymphocyte malignancies have also proved highly susceptible to persistent cryptosporidiosis (242,244,246–248).

The results of two studies in patients with HIV infection clearly demonstrate that the severity of disease associated with cryptosporidiosis is a function of CD4 lymphocyte counts (295,296). Transient disease conditions were noted in patients with a wide range of lymphocyte counts and infections usually resolved when CD4 counts were greater than 180 cells/mm^3. Fulminating disease, resulting in death, was usually seen in patients with CD4 counts of less than 50 cells/mm^3. Treatment of some patients with AIDS with zidovudine (AZT) has resulted in clinical improvement and even complete recovery from cryptosporidiosis (297,298). The drug's activity, in these instances, was postulated to stimulate the patients' immune systems sufficiently to bring about termination of the infection. In another study, patients on zidovudine treatment and with CD4 counts of greater than 140 cells/mm³ were able to clear infection (295). This treatment, however, did not prevent *C. parvum* infection in patients with CD4 counts of less than 140 cells/mm³.

Further studies to define the role of cellular immunity in humans, such as *in vitro* antigen-induced lymphocyte proliferative assays, are just now receiving attention. Along with appropriately designed animal studies, a clearer understanding of the role of accessory cells and products (cytokines) in controlling cryptosporidial infection may emerge. Ultimately, and in consort with well-defined humoral studies, more efficient treatment strategies for control of this infection may be developed.

CLINICAL ILLNESS

The clinical manifestations of *Cryptosporidium* infection are influenced by the immune status of the host. After an incubation period of approximately 1 week (229,299), the disease becomes manifest by a watery, noninflammatory, foul-smelling diarrhea. However, the severity and duration of the disease will vary greatly depending on the status of the host's immune system. Patients at either end of the age spectrum or patients with nutritional deficiencies may behave similar to immunocompromised patients (123,300). Cryptosporidiosis has been reported in association with measles, probably due to the transient immune suppression associated with the acute phase of this disease (124). There is an important interplay between cryptosporidial infection and malnutrition, as it is becoming apparent that malnutrition predisposes to a more prolonged and severe diarrheal illness, while failure to thrive can be a significant manifestation of the disease in younger patients (97,108,123,128,136,172,301).

Immunocompetent Host

In immunocompetent patients, *C. parvum* causes a self-limited diarrheal illness that typically lasts 10 to 14 days, but may last anywhere from 3 days to longer than 1 month. The diarrhea is characteristically profuse and watery, sometimes containing mucus. Patients often complain of crampy abdominal pain, flatulence, nausea, and vomiting and may have constitutional symptoms (anorexia, malaise, weakness, myalgias, and headaches). The diarrhea and abdominal pain are often exacerbated by eating. Fever is rarely significant. The disease can rarely be protracted, severe, and associated with significant weight loss (59,142,232,302). Mortality is rare, usually only occurring in severely malnourished children (128). Spontaneous complete recovery is the rule. Protective immunity seems to develop as there have been no reported cases of recurrent infections. Now that therapeutic options are becoming available, it will be of interest to study in the future whether treated immunocompetent patients will

fail to develop protective immunity as we alter the natural history of the disease.

Interestingly, respiratory symptoms are significantly more frequent in children with cryptosporidial diarrhea than in patients with diarrhea of a different etiology (51,52,98,102,105,302), raising the issue that *Cryptosporidium* may indeed be a pulmonary pathogen as well. *Cryptosporidium* infection was documented by the demonstration of organisms in a tracheal aspirate of an immunocompetent child with laryngotracheitis and cryptosporidial diarrhea (303) and, as discussed later, is now recognized as a cause of pneumonia in the immunocompromised host. *Cryptosporidium* was the etiology of acute pancreatitis in a 14-year-old farmer's daughter who drank unpasteurized milk (304) and caused symptoms mimicking acute appendicitis in one case (305). It was associated with recurrent urticaria and angioedema in one patient (306) and reactive arthritis in several others (307–309).

Immunocompromised Host

In contrast to the presentation and course in the immunocompetent patient, *Cryptosporidium* infection in the immunocompromised patient usually presents as a more severe, prolonged, cholera-like illness that can be life-threatening, with as many as 71 stools/day and up to 17 L/day reported (11,310). Two to 3 L of diarrheic stool is common, and malabsorption can become a serious problem in these patients, with significant resulting dehydration and malnutrition and profound weight loss [up to 20 kg reported in one patient (311)]. Patients may complain of cramping upper abdominal pain. Uncontrolled disease may contribute or lead to the death of patients (216,235,241,244,265,312–314). Spontaneous clinical recovery occurs, with or without clearing of the stool (216,247,312,315–317), and seems to correlate with higher CD4 counts in patients with AIDS (216,295,318). Some patients have mild disease or are asymptomatic (246,252,319–322). Most often the disease is chronic in nature, with symptoms waxing and waning depending on a multiplicity of factors, including therapy, nutritional status, and variations in the immunologic status of the patient. In a recent study of 128 HIV-positive patients (296), four clinical patterns of disease were identified: transient in 28.7%, chronic in 59.7%, fulminant (more than 2 L of stool per day) in 7.8%, and asymptomatic in 3.9%. Fulminant disease only occurred in patients with a CD4 count less than 50 cells/mm³, who survived only 5 weeks on average, compared with 20 weeks for those with chronic diarrhea and 36 weeks for those with transient infection.

All segments of the gastrointestinal tract have been reported to be involved, including the pharynx, esophagus, stomach, duodenum, jejunum, ileum, appendix, colon, and rectum (9,323–327). Pancreatic duct involvement has been reported, with or without resultant pancreatitis (328,329), and cryptosporidial enteritis was associated with an enterovesical fistula in one patient (330). *Cryptosporidium* infection of the gallbladder and biliary tract is not uncommon [10% to 26% of patients with cryptosporidiosis in various studies (318,331)], resulting in acalculous cholecystitis, extrahepatic bile duct stenosis, and sclerosing cholangitis (238,296,318,332–343). Biliary duct involvement appears to predict a worse prognosis (312). The gallbladder may play a role as a reservoir of organisms, leading to persistent diarrhea, and in one patient cholecystectomy resulted in resolution of the diarrhea (344).

Although the literature debates whether respiratory tree involvement reflects true infection versus colonization or contamination, respiratory tract infection is now becoming increasingly recognized and well documented (sometimes at autopsy), often presenting as pneumonia (234,245,246,248,253,296,345–357). In one patient, *Cryptosporidium* was the only pathogen found during the workup of sinusitis (355). Infection at these extraintestinal sites is felt to occur via mucosal luminal spread rather than systemic dissemination or direct tissue invasion.

DIAGNOSIS

Laboratory Studies

Routine blood tests are usually unrevealing unless the diarrhea is very severe with resulting volume depletion and hypokalemia. With gallbladder involvement there can be abnormalities in liver function tests (mainly alkaline phosphatase and aspartate transaminase), and when malabsorption is significant, it may lead to abnormal values of nutritional parameters (e.g., albumin) and to abnormalities in specific malabsorption tests when these are performed (134,188,193,265,310,314,358,359).

Serologic testing (46,108,168,214,225,283–286,360) is mainly used for epidemiologic purposes and has little diagnostic application. Antibodies to *Cryptosporidium* can be detected by indirect immunofluorescence assay, ELISA, and other methods. Elevated serum IgM and/or IgG titers can be detected within 2 weeks of onset of symptoms in most patients. IgG and even IgM titers persist for long periods in a majority of patients, the latter suggesting possible reexposure in highly endemic areas.

Radiographic findings are nonspecific (361). Pneumatosis intestinalis was associated with cryptosporidiosis in one case (362). Computer tomographic scanning in one patient revealed marked thickening of the gastric antrum with possible ulceration (363). In a series of 16 patients (324), 13 had subtle to marked inflammatory changes in the mucosa of the proximal or entire small bowel on barium study. Two also had narrowing and irregularity of the gastric antrum. Similar changes of the gastric antrum were seen in other studies (364,365). Sonographic or computed tomographic examination may be helpful for the diagnosis of cryptosporidial cholangitis (192,366,367), and endoscopic retrograde cholangiography is often necessary for diagnosis and therapeutic intervention (328,338,368). Infection at extraintestinal sites usually requires biopsy for diagnosis, although it may be achievable by staining of bile, sputum, or bronchial washings.

Fecal blood and leukocytes are rarely found in cryptosporidial diarrhea, but some studies report their presence in a significant number of patients (103,177,369). When present, copathogens may be more likely to be found. The mainstay of diagnosis is the identification of the oocysts in stool specimens. Three or more specimens are sometimes needed for the diagnosis as oocyst excretion varies throughout the day and from day to day (370). Aspiration of duodenal fluid (180) or small intestinal brushing (371) can be used for diagnosis when upper gastrointestinal endoscopy is performed, especially if biopsies are contraindicated. There is little need anymore for routinely performing intestinal biopsies or electron microscopy for the diagnosis of cryptosporidiosis as noninvasive laboratory methods have become more sensitive (372). Concentration of stool specimens is mainly necessary in epidemiologic studies and evaluation of contacts of infected patients, where the number of parasites may be small, but it is usually unnecessary for the evaluation of the patient with diarrhea. A variety of methods (most commonly the formalin–ethyl acetate method) are used, including the use of a disposable parasite concentrator (373), and various fecal concentration devices (374). Newer concentration techniques are more sensitive, lowering the threshold of detection of oocysts in formed stool specimens to 5000 oocysts per gram of stool (375).

The most effective, convenient, and widely used method for identifying oocysts in stool samples is the acid-fast stain, which imparts a diagnostic red color to the oocysts (Fig. 3) (376–379). Other staining techniques include Giemsa stain, methenamine silver stain, periodic acid–Schiff stain, trichrome stain, and multiple other methods that stain the oocysts or act as negative stains (reviewed in refs. 13, 380, and 381). New staining methods are often proposed (382), but the acid-fast stain currently

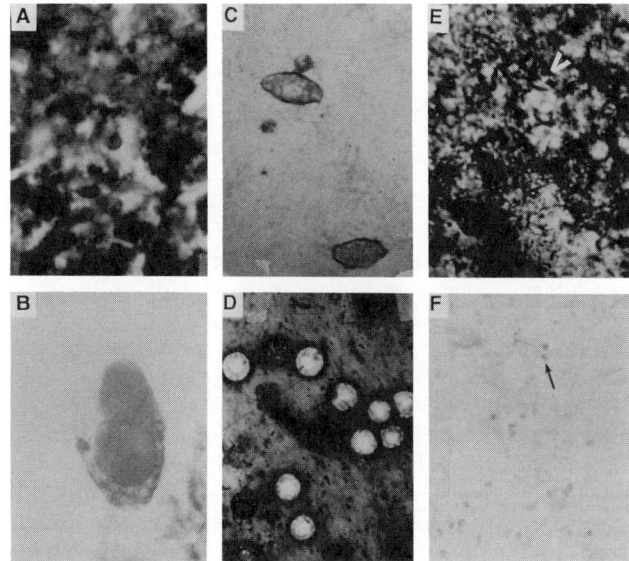

FIG. 3. Causes of diarrhea in AIDS patients. **A:** *Cryptosporidium* oocysts in fecal specimen. **B:** *Isospora belli* oocyst with bilobed nuclei. **C:** *I. belli* and *Cryptosporidium* together in the stool of a patient with AIDS. **D:** *Cyclospora* (formerly called "cyanobacterium-like organism") in the stool of a patient with AIDS and diarrhea. **E:** *M. avium* complex organisms (*arrow*) in the stool of a patient with AIDS and protracted fever and diarrhea. F: *Microsporidia*. A-E, acid-fast stain; F, chromotrope stain. (See Plate 17.) (Courtesy of Rosemary Soave, Cynthia Sears, Earl Long, Madeline Boucy, and Ralph Bryan.)

remains the technique of choice for the clinical microbiology laboratory (383). Fluorescent stains have also been used successfully (377,379,384–387).

Other approaches include immunofluorescence staining with fluorescein-labeled polyclonal or monoclonal antibody. The monoclonal antibody method is available commercially (Meridian Diagnostics, Inc., Cincinnati, Ohio) and is remarkably sensitive and specific (388–392), allowing for the detection of asymptomatic carriers and the identification of contaminated environmental sources.

ELISA kits are now commercially available for the detection of *Cryptosporidium* oocysts in stool. The IDEIA *Cryptosporidium* kit (Dako Diagnostics, Ltd.) has been found to be 100% sensitive and specific compared with immunofluorescence (393). The LMD Laboratories kit (Carlsbad, California) has recently been found to be 87.9% sensitive and 100% specific for the detection of *Cryptosporidium* in stool samples of individuals with diarrhea (394). However, it is not sensitive enough for use in epidemiologic studies.

Newer methods using molecular techniques are becoming available. A newly developed assay using the polymerase chain reaction is capable of detecting as little as one parasite and is highly specific (395,396). Tools such as this one may be helpful in improving our understanding of *Cryptosporidium* and its environmental and clinical epidemiology. They may revolutionize our laboratory diagnosis techniques, especially in light of recent evidence that our routine laboratory methods used for detection of *Cryptosporidium* in stool samples are not very sensitive, requiring at least 50,000 and 500,000 oocysts per gram of stool for their detection by immunofluorescence and acid-fast staining, respectively (397).

Differential Diagnosis

Other causes of noninflammatory diarrhea must obviously be considered during the workup. It is also important to realize that *Cryptosporidium* will sometimes be one of two or more organisms found during a workup for diarrhea, likely secondary to similar environmental transmission profiles. Careful epidemiologic questioning may help guide the clinician as to the most likely pathogen. In the normal host, enterotoxigenic *Escherichia coli,* viral infections (rotavirus and Norwalk virus), as well as other parasitic infections such as giardiasis should be considered. In immunocompromised patients, one also has to consider *Campylobacter, Salmonella, Clostridium difficile,* adenovirus, cytomegalovirus, and *Mycobacterium avium-intracellulare* as potential etiologies, as well as *Isospora belli* and other protozoa such as *Giardia, Entamoeba,* and microsporidia.

TREATMENT

Over the last few years, numerous compounds have been screened *in vitro* and *in vivo* for anticryptosporidial activity or tried empirically, mostly with negative results (5,7,11,29,216,234,265,311,313,314,346,359,398–409). More than 100 agents have been found to be ineffective,

including sulfonamides, clindamycin, metronidazole, and other antiprotozoal agents. Nevertheless, some promising results have recently been obtained as more drugs are being screened for anticryptosporidial activity. Guidelines for study designs have been recommended (410). In the immunocompromised host, specific antiparasitic therapy is extremely important since the patients are otherwise unlikely to clear the infection, but great care must be paid in these patients to supportive therapy, fluid balance, and nutritional status.

Some patients will present with significant volume loss and will need hospitalization for intravenous fluid repletion. Oral rehydration also needs to be encouraged. Careful attention to electrolytes is necessary. In immunocompromised patients, malabsorption may be significant and may contribute to severe malnutrition and weight loss. Nutritional supplementation intravenously may be needed, and total parenteral nutrition is occasionally used (226,238).

Drugs that affect gut motility (e.g., loperamide, diphenoxylate, opiates) should be used in an attempt to slow the increased peristalsis of the intestinal tract and the resulting volume loss and decreased transit time of nutrients. Somatostatin and octreotide, a long-acting synthetic somatostatin analog, have been used successfully in a few case reports (407,411–414), but a recent multicenter prospective trial showed octreotide to be minimally effective for the treatment of AIDS-associated diarrhea with an identifiable pathogen (415). It is very expensive and requires parenteral administration. Vapreotide, another somatostatin analog, was also found to be mostly ineffective in cryptosporidial diarrhea (191). Oral agents such as acetorphan, an enkephalinase inhibitor, are currently being investigated and appear to hold some promise (416).

Treatment with zidovudine is sometimes associated with resolution of the diarrhea and clearing of the oocysts from the stool, probably due to improvement in the immunologic status of the patients (187,297,298,417,418). In patients with exogenous immune suppression, immunosuppressive therapy should ideally be discontinued or tapered (4,57,244). In gallbladder disease, papillotomy may be helpful when there is evidence of obstruction due to papillary stenosis (335,368).

Anticryptosporidial Therapy

In some *in vitro* experiments as well as in animal models of the disease (419–422), hyperimmune bovine colostrum shows promise as a therapeutic agent for severe cryptosporidiosis. Oral administration has been attempted in a few immunosuppressed patients with relief of their symptoms and partial clearing of the infection in most cases, and occasional apparently complete eradication of the organisms (341,342,423). Differences in the immunologic composition of the colostrum preparations could account for the various responses. In fact, in one study, the administration of colostrum had no effect, although that preparation was obtained from cows from infected herds and not from immunized cows (424). In addition, the presence of *Cryptosporidium* oocysts in the gallbladder may prevent total eradication of the infection by the colostrum and provide a reservoir for continued reinfection. In some studies, the use of oral bovine transfer factor was variably effective in patients with AIDS and cryptosporidial diarrhea, with temporary or more sustained amelioration of symptoms (425,426), while in one case report of a single patient it had no effect (239). The clinical use of these immunologic therapies remains to be determined.

The search for a chemotherapeutic anticryptosporidial agent finally appears to have led to a somewhat promising drug. Paromomycin, an old antiamebic medication, is a nonabsorbable aminoglycoside that is at least partially effective against Cryptosporidium (370,427–433). In some patients it appears to eradicate the disease; however, in others, the symptoms recur while on therapy. Most of the time, after the completion of a course of therapy, a maintenance dose of the drug is necessary to prevent relapse in immunocompromised patients (434). The usual dose is 500 mg four times daily with a maintenance dose of 500 mg twice a day, and it appears to be well tolerated except for minor side effects such as nausea and abdominal discomfort. One should be aware that malabsorption can apparently be a side effect of paromomycin (435). Oral administration of paromomycin does not achieve systemic levels of the drug, and it is therefore ineffective in extraintestinal disease.

Many case reports or small series suggest that spiramycin, a macrolide antibiotic not available in the United States, is effective; however, in some patients and, more importantly, in controlled studies, it was not found to be of any benefit, although questions regarding dosing and suboptimal drug absorption have been raised (219, 232, 237, 246, 253, 255, 297, 300, 306, 355, 418, 436–443). Preliminary data in humans indicate that newer macrolides (e.g., azithromycin) in high dosages may be effective (444–446), corroborating previous results in animal models (447–449). Other potential therapies are also being evaluated, such as the use of letrazuril, but significant side effects have been reported (450–453).

PREVENTION

Environmental Eradication

Cryptosporidium oocysts are very resistant to a wide variety of environmental conditions and disinfection methods. They can survive for months when kept cold and moist. They are killed by exposure to temperatures greater than 60°C or less than −20°C for longer than 30 min (38). One study subjected the oocysts to conditions similar to milk pasteurization specifications and found effective neutralization of their infectivity (454). Most common disinfectants used routinely in hospitals and clinical laboratories do not kill Cryptosporidium oocysts when used at the usual recommended dilutions. Exposure to 5% ammonia or 10% formol saline for 18 hr is needed to kill the cysts (48). Routine chlorination and various water treatment processes used for water purification are not very effective at killing Cryptosporidium oocysts (455), especially when there is a sudden discharge of oocysts into the water, such as after a heavy rainfall. Recent studies indicate that ozone, chlorine dioxide, and sand filtra-

tion are partially effective in eradicating the oocysts from drinking water (71,456–458), giving some hope that a practical solution may be within reach. Ultraviolet light has been shown to adequately disinfect water contaminated with Cryptosporidium but is not a practical option (459). Both technical and financial problems for the commercial application of effective systems in the developing world remain a formidable challenge.

An important issue is the decontamination of the instruments used for gastrointestinal and pulmonary endoscopies. As mentioned earlier, one study found a high prevalence of Cryptosporidium oocysts in patients undergoing upper endoscopy for presumably unrelated diagnoses (169), raising a valid concern about the potential for patient-to-patient transmission by means of contaminated endoscopes. The need for and difficulty of disinfection have been addressed in some publications and the reader is referred to them for further information (460,461).

Enteric Precautions

Careful hand washing is of utmost importance in preventing spread in hospitals and day care centers, and the use of gowns and gloves and appropriate disposal of contaminated feces are necessary for caretakers of hospitalized patients. These patients should ideally be in private rooms. Contaminated equipment should be autoclaved, and contaminated surfaces should be washed with commercial bleach that, ideally, is left on to soak for at least 15 min. Shedding of oocysts usually stops 1 to 2 weeks after the onset of symptoms in immunocompetent patients (462), but a small number of oocysts may remain present in feces for 2 weeks or longer after the resolution of diarrhea (58,94,95,130,194,199,202,206,211,250,299,463,464). These persons and asymptomatic carriers are likely to be important reservoirs of infection.

Travelers should follow routine recommendations of avoiding unboiled or uncooked drinks and foods when traveling to endemic areas. Immunocompromised patients who go camping or undergo trips to endemic areas should be especially careful in avoiding any potentially contaminated water or foods.

Education

Health care professionals need to educate the medical community about the importance of including cryptosporidiosis in the differential diagnosis of diarrheal diseases, even in immunocompetent hosts and in developed countries and urban settings. The public needs to be educated about diarrheal diseases in general and routine precautions that need to be followed when a family member has a diarrheal illness. Immunocompromised patients should be advised to avoid, when possible, contact with animals with diarrhea.

RELATED SPECIES

A new protozoan parasite has recently been described and is now being increasingly recognized as a pathogen

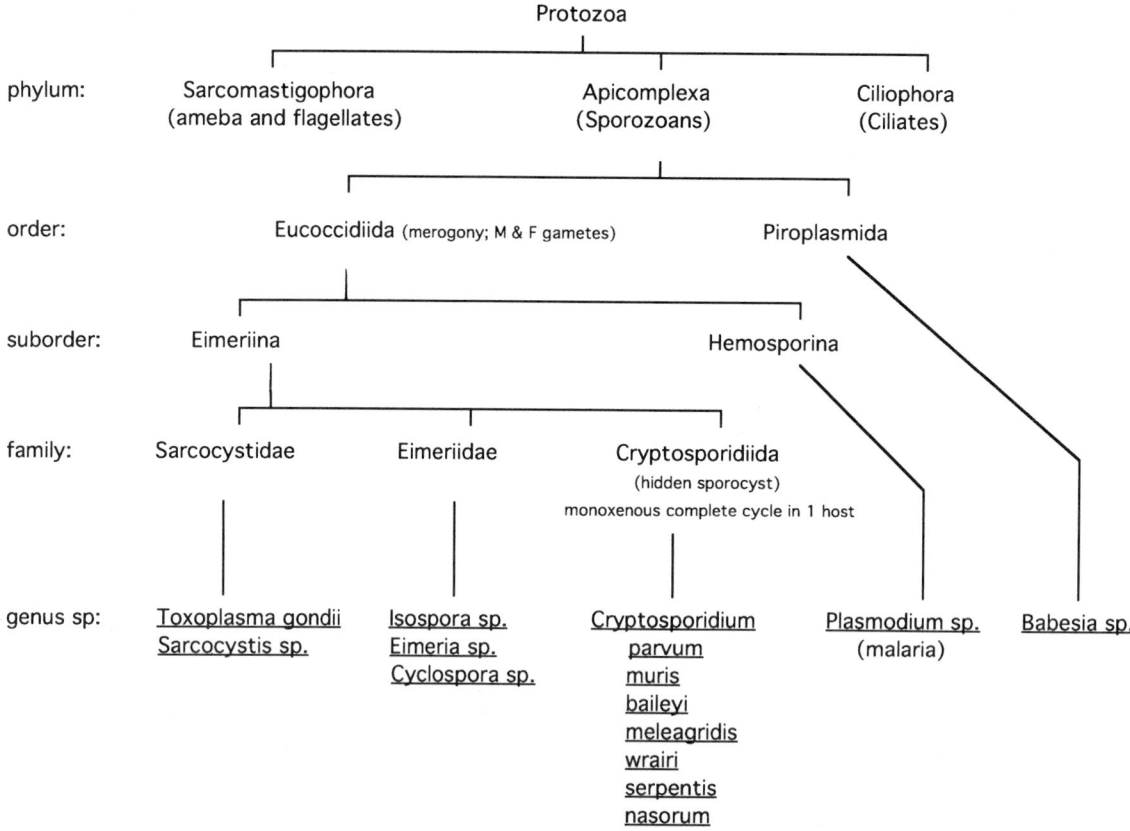

FIG. 4. Taxonomy of *Cryptosporidium* and related protozoa.

in humans with diarrhea. The first cases of infection with this organism were reported in 1986 (465). Since then it has been variably classified as a coccidian body or *Cryptosporidium*-like oocyst, flagellate, and blue-green alga (cyanobacterium-like body). Most recently, it was classified as a coccidian (phylum Apicomplexa), belonging to the genus *Cyclospora* as shown in Fig. 4 (466). *Cyclospora cayetanensis* is spherical, measuring 8 to 10 μm in diameter, stains variably with acid-fast staining or phenosafranin, and autofluoresces under ultraviolet light, appearing as neon-blue circles (466,467).

It causes a self-limiting diarrhea in immunocompetent patients, mostly children from developing countries (466) and travelers to, or foreign residents of, these countries (465,468–471). Most outbreaks have occurred in Southeast Asia, Eastern Europe, Central and South America, and the Caribbean islands, but it has been reported to occur in the United States as well (470,472). It has been associated with chronic diarrhea in a few patients with AIDS (468,470,473). Exposure to a contaminated water source has been described in an outbreak among hospital employees (472). Contact with water from a saltwater aquarium in one case and swimming in a lake in another case were thought to be temporally related exposures (470). Studies from Peru show a seasonal prevalence similar to that of *Cryptosporidium,* with most cases occurring between April and June (466).

The diarrhea is usually explosive, watery, and accompanied by fatigue, nausea, vomiting, abdominal cramping, anorexia, myalgias, and weight loss. It may remit in a few days but can last for 6 weeks or longer and can have a relapsing pattern (469,472). The pathologic basis of the diarrhea appears to be small bowel injury, with acute and chronic inflammation, surface epithelial disarray, villous atrophy, and crypt hyperplasia (471,474). The parasites are intracytoplasmic and contained within a vacuole located toward the luminal end of the cell (471). Some patients produce antibodies against the organism. So far no antimicrobial therapy has been found to be consistently effective, although a recent report describes successful response to co-trimoxazole therapy in five patients (475).

REFERENCES

1. Tyzzer EE. A sporozoan found in the peptic glands of the common mouse. *Proc Soc Exp Biol Med* 1907;5:12–13.
2. Tyzzer EE. *Cryptosporidium parvum* (sp. nov.), a coccidium found in the small intestine of the common mouse. *Arch Protistenkd* 1912;26:394–412.
3. Nime FA, Burek JD, Page DL, Holscher MA, Yardley JH. Acute enterocolitis in a human being infected with the protozoan *Cryptosporidium*. *Gastroenterology* 1976;70:592–598.
4. Meisel JL, Perera DR, Meligro C, Rubin CE. Overwhelming watery diarrhea associated with a *Cryptosporidium* in an immunosuppressed patient. *Gastroenterology* 1976;70:1156–1160.
5. Weinstein L, Edelstein SM, Madara JL, Falchuk KR, McManus BM, Trier JS. Intestinal cryptosporidiosis complicated by disseminated cytomegalovirus infection. *Gastroenterology* 1981;81:584–591.
6. Tzipori S, Angus KW, Campbell I, Sherwood D. Vomiting and

diarrhea associated with cryptosporidial infection. *N Engl J Med* 1980;303:818.

7. Stemmermann GN, Hayashi T, Glober GA, Oishi N, Frankel RI. Cryptosporidiosis: report of a fatal case complicated by disseminated toxoplasmosis. *Am J Med* 1980;69:637–642.

8. Lasser KH, Lewin KJ, Ryning FW. Cryptosporidial enteritis in a patient with congenital hypogammaglobulinemia. *Hum Pathol* 1979;10:234–240.

9. Booth CC, Slavin G, Dourmashkin RR, et al. Immunodeficiency and cryptosporidiosis. Demonstration at the Royal College of Physicians of London. *Br Med J* 1980;281:1123–1127.

10. Weisburger WR, Hutcheon DF, Yardley JH, Roche JC, Hillis WD, Charache P. Cryptosporidiosis in an immunosuppressed renal-transplant recipient with IgA deficiency. *Am J Clin Pathol* 1979;72:473–478.

11. Centers for Disease Control. Cryptosporidiosis: an assessment of chemotherapy of males with acquired immune deficiency syndrome (AIDS). *MMWR Morb Mortal Wkly Rep* 1982;31:589–592.

12. Centers for Disease Control. 1993 Revised classification for HIV infection and expanded surveillance case definition for AIDS among adolescents and adults. *MMWR Morb Mortal Wkly Rep* 1993;41:1–19.

13. Fayer R, Ungar BLP. *Cryptosporidium* spp. and cryptosporidiosis. *Microbiol Rev* 1986;50:458–483.

14. Fayer R, Speer CA, Dubey JP. General biology of *Cryptosporidium*. In: Dubey JP, Speer CA, Fayer R, eds. *Cryptosporidiosis of man and animals*. Boca Raton, FL: CRC Press, 1990;1–29.

15. Ditrich O, Palkovic L, Sterba J, Prokopic J, Loudová J, Giboda M. The first finding of *Cryptosporidium baileyi* in man. *Parasitol Res* 1991;77:44–47.

16. Crawford FG, Vermund SH. Human cryptosporidiosis. *CRC Crit Rev Microbiol* 1988;16:113–159.

17. Baxby D, Blundell N. Recognition and laboratory characteristics of an atypical oocyst of *Cryptosporidium*. *J Infect Dis* 1988;158:1038–1045.

18. Current WL, Garcia LS. Cryptosporidiosis. *Clin Microbiol Rev* 1991;4:325–358.

19. Current WL. Techniques and laboratory maintenance of *Cryptosporidium*. In: Dubey JP, Speer CA, Fayer R, eds. *Cryptosporidiosis of man and animals*. Boca Raton, FL: CRC Press, 1990;31–49.

20. Reduker DW, Speer CA. Factors influencing excystation in *Cryptosporidium* oocysts from cattle. *J Parasitol* 1985;71:112–115.

21. Woodmansee DB. Studies of in vitro excystation of *Cryptosporidium parvum* from calves. *J Protozool* 1987;34:398–402.

22. Reduker DW, Speer CA, Blixt JA. Ultrastructure of *Cryptosporidium parvum* oocysts and excysting sporozoites as revealed by high resolution scanning electron microscopy. *J Protozool* 1985;32:708–711.

23. Lumb R, Smith K, O'Donoghue PJ, Lanser JA. Ultrastructure of the attachment of *Cryptosporidium* sporozoites to tissue culture cells. *Parasitol Res* 1988;74:531–536.

24. Current WL, Reese NC. A comparison of endogenous development of three isolates of *Cryptosporidium* in suckling mice. *J Protozool* 1986;33:98–108.

25. Current WL, Long PL. Development of human and calf *Cryptosporidium* in chicken embryos. *J Infect Dis* 1983;148:1108–1113.

26. Adams RB, Guerrant RL, Zu S, Fang G, Roche JK. *Cryptosporidium parvum* infection of intestinal epithelium: morphologic and functional studies in an in vitro model. *J Infect Dis* 1994;169:170–177.

27. Current WL, Haynes TB. Complete development of *Cryptosporidium* in cell culture. *Science* 1984;224:603–605.

28. Buraud M, Forget E, Favennec L, Bizet J, Gobert J-G, Deluol A-M. Sexual stage development of cryptosporidia in the Caco-2 cell line. *Infect Immun* 1991;59:4610–4613.

29. McDonald V, Stables R, Warhurst DC, et al. In vitro cultivation of *Cryptosporidium parvum* and screening for anticryptosporidial drugs. *Antimicrob Agents Chemother* 1990;34:1498–1500.

30. Gut J, Petersen C, Nelson R, Leech J. *Cryptosporidium par-*

vum: in vitro cultivation in Madin–Darby canine kidney cells. *J Protozool* 1991;38:72S–73S.

31. Rasmussen KR, Larsen NC, Healey MC. Complete development of *Cryptosporidium parvum* in a human endometrial carcinoma cell line. *Infect Immun* 1993;61:1482–1485.

32. Upton SJ, Tilley M, Mitschler RR, Oppert BS. Incorporation of exogenous uracil by *Cryptosporidium parvum* in vitro. *J Clin Microbiol* 1991;29:1062–1065.

33. Flanigan TP, Aji T, Marshall R, Soave R, Aikawa M, Kaetzel C. Asexual development of *Cryptosporidium parvum* within a differentiated human enterocyte cell line. *Infect Immun* 1991;59:234–239.

34. Woodmansee DB, Pohlenz JFL. Development of *Cryptosporidium* sp. in a human rectal tumor cell line. In: *Proceedings of the IVth International Symposium on Neonatal Diarrhea*. Saskatoon, Saskatchewan, Canada, 1984;306–319.

35. Naciri M, Yvore P, de Boissieu C, Esnault E. Multiplication de *Cryptosporidium muris* (Tyzzer 1907) *in vitro* entretien d'une souche sur oeufs embryonnés. *Rec Med Vet* 1986;162:51–56.

36. Wagner ED, Prabhu Das M. *Cryptosporidium* in cell culture. *Jpn J Parasitol* 1986;35:253–255.

37. Bonnin A, Salimbeni I, Dubremetz JF, Harly G, Chavanet P, Camerlynck P. Mise au point d'un modèle expérimental de culture *in vitro* des stades asexués de *Cryptosporidium sp. Ann Parasitol Hum Comp* 1990;65:41–43.

38. Tzipori S. Cryptosporidiosis in animals and humans. *Microbiol Rev* 1983;47:84–96.

39. Current WL, Reese NC, Ernst JV, Bailey WS, Heyman MB, Weinstein WM. Human cryptosporidiosis in immunocompetent and immunodeficient persons: studies of an outbreak and experimental transmission. *N Engl J Med* 1983;308:1252–1257.

40. Anderson BC, Donndelinger T, Wilkins RM, Smith J. Cryptosporidiosis in a veterinary student. *J Am Vet Med Assoc* 1982;180:408–409.

41. Holten-Andersen W, Gerstoft J, Henriksen SA. Human cryptosporidiosis. *N Engl J Med* 1983;309:1325–1326.

42. Nouri M, Toroghi R. Asymptomatic cryptosporidiosis in cattle and humans in Iran. *Vet Rec* 1991;128:358–359.

43. Pohjola S, Jokipii AMM, Jokipii L. Sporadic cryptosporidiosis in a rural population is asymptomatic and associated with contact to cattle. *Acta Vet Scand* 1986;27:91–102.

44. Miron D, Kenes J, Dagan R. Calves as a source of an outbreak of cryptosporidiosis among young children in an agricultural closed community. *Pediatr Infect Dis J* 1991;10:438–441.

45. Rahman ASMH, Sanyal SC, Al-Mahmud KA, Sobhan A, Hossain KS, Anderson BC. Cryptosporidiosis in calves and their handlers in Bangladesh. *Lancet* 1984;2:221.

46. Lengerich EJ, Addiss DG, Marx JJ, Ungar BLP, Juranek DD. Increased exposure to cryptosporidia among dairy farmers in Wisconsin. *J Infect Dis* 1993;167:1252–1255.

47. Shield J, Baumer JH, Dawson JA, Wilkinson PJ. Cryptosporidiosis—an educational experience. *J Infect* 1990;21:297–301.

48. Campbell I, Tzipori S, Hutchison G, Angus KW. Effect of disinfectants on survival of *Cryptosporidium* oocysts. *Vet Rec* 1982;111:414–415.

49. Casemore DP. Sheep as a source of human cryptosporidiosis. *J Infect* 1989;19:101–104.

50. Public Health Laboratory Service Study Group. Cryptosporidiosis in England and Wales: prevalence and clinical and epidemiological features. *BMJ* 1990;300:774–777.

51. Egger M, Mäusezahl D, Odermatt P, Marti H-P, Tanner M. Symptoms and transmission of intestinal cryptosporidiosis. *Arch Dis Child* 1990;65:445–447.

52. Thomson MA, Benson JWT, Wright PA. Two year study of *Cryptosporidium* infection. *Arch Dis Child* 1987;62:559–563.

53. García P, Cataño MA. Importancia de los manipuladores de alimentos en la transmisión de la criptosporidiosis. *Enferm Infecc Microbiol Clin* 1991;9:583–584.

54. Nouri M, Karami M. Asymptomatic cryptosporidiosis in nomadic shepherds and their sheep. *J Infect* 1991;23:331–333.

55. Nouri M, Mahdavi Rad S. Effect of nomadic shepherds and their sheep on the incidence of cryptosporidiosis in an adjacent town. *J Infect* 1993;26:105–106.

56. Egger M, Mai Nguyen X, Schaad UB, Krech T. Intestinal cryptosporidiosis acquired from a cat. *Infection* 1990;18:177–178.
57. Lewis IJ, Hart CA, Baxby D. Diarrhoea due to *Cryptosporidium* in acute lymphoblastic leukaemia. *Arch Dis Child* 1985; 60:60–62.
58. Hart CA, Baxby D, Blundell N. Gastro-enteritis due to *Cryptosporidium:* a prospective survey in a children's hospital. *J Infect* 1984;9:264–270.
59. Edelman MJ, Oldfield EC. Severe cryptosporidiosis in an immunocompetent host. *Arch Intern Med* 1988;148:1873–1874.
60. Newman RD, Wuhib T, Lima AAM, Guerrant RL, Sears CL. Environmental sources of *Cryptosporidium* in an urban slum in northeastern Brazil. *Am J Trop Med Hyg* 1993;49:270–275.
61. Mtambo MMA, Nash AS, Blewett DA, Smith HV, Wright S. *Cryptosporidium* infection in cats: prevalence of infection in domestic and feral cats in the Glasgow area. *Vet Rec* 1991;129: 502–504.
62. Koch KL, Shankey TV, Weinstein GS, et al. Cryptosporidiosis in a patient with hemophilia, common variable hypogammaglobulinemia and the acquired immunodeficiency syndrome. *Ann Intern Med* 1983;99:337–340.
63. Brown EAE, Casemore DP, Gerken A, Greatorex IF. Cryptosporidiosis in Great Yarmouth—the investigation of an outbreak. *Public Health* 1989;103:3–9.
64. Navin TR, Hardy AM. Cryptosporidiosis in patients with AIDS. *J Infect Dis* 1987;155:150.
65. Weber J, Philip S. Human cryptosporidiosis. *N Engl J Med* 1983;309:1326.
66. Newman RD, Zu S-X, Wuhib T, Lima AAM, Guerrant RL, Sears CL. Household epidemiology of *Cryptosporidium* infection. *Ann Intern Med* 1994;120:500–505.
67. Bossen An, Britt EM. Cryptosporidiosis in immunocompetent patients. *N Engl J Med* 1985;313:1019.
68. Lähdevirta J, Jokipii AMM, Sammalkorpi K, Jokipii L. Perinatal infection with *Cryptosporidium* and failure to thrive. *Lancet* 1987;1:48–49.
69. Edwards DD. Troubled waters in Milwaukee. *ASM News* 1993; 59:342–345.
69a.MacKenzie WR. A massive outbreak in Milwaukee of *Cryptosporidium* infection transmitted through the public water supply. *N Engl J Med* 1994;331:161–167.
70. LeChevallier MW, Norton WD, Lee RG. *Giardia* and *Cryptosporidium* spp. in filtered drinking water supplies. *Appl Environ Microbiol* 1991;57:2617–2621.
71. Madore MS, Rose JB, Gerba CP, Arrowood MJ, Sterling CR. Occurrence of *Cryptosporidium* oocysts in sewage effluents and selected surface waters. *J Parasitol* 1987;73:702–705.
72. Villacorta-Martinez de Maturana I, Ares-Mazás ME, Duran-Oreiro D, Lorenzo-Lorenzo MJ. Efficacy of activated sludge in removing *Cryptosporidium parvum* oocysts from sewage. *Appl Environ Microbiol* 1992;58:3514–3516.
73. Richardson AJ, Frankenberg RA, Buck AC, et al. An outbreak of waterborne cryptosporidiosis in Swindon and Oxfordshire. *Epidemiol Infect* 1991;107:485–495.
74. Rush BA, Chapman PA, Ineson RW. *Cryptosporidium* and drinking water. *Lancet* 1987;2:632–633.
75. Rush BA, Chapman PA, Ineson RW. A probable waterborne outbreak of cryptosporidiosis in the Sheffield area. *J Med Microbiol* 1990;32:239–242.
76. Smith HV, Girwood RWA, Patterson WJ, et al. Waterborne outbreak of cryptosporidiosis. *Lancet* 1988;2:1484.
77. Smith HV, Patterson WJ, Hardie R, et al. An outbreak of waterborne cryptosporidiosis caused by post-treatment contamination. *Epidemiol Infect* 1989;103:703–715.
78. D'Antonio RG, Winn RE, Taylor JP, et al. A waterborne outbreak of cryptosporidiosis in normal hosts. *Ann Intern Med* 1986;103:886–888.
79. Joseph C, Hamilton G, O'Connor M, et al. Cryptosporidiosis in the Isle of Thanet; an outbreak associated with local drinking water. *Epidemiol Infect* 1991;107:509–519.
80. Gallaher MM, Herndon JL, Nims LJ, Sterling CR, Grabowski DJ, Hull HF. Cryptosporidiosis and surface water. *Am J Public Health* 1989;79:39–42.
81. Hayes EB, Matte TD, O'Brien TR, et al. Large community

82. outbreak of cryptosporidiosis due to contamination of a filtered public water supply. *N Engl J Med* 1989;320:1372–1376.
82. Weinstein P, Macaitis M, Walker C, Cameron S. Cryptosporidial diarrhoea in South Australia: an exploratory case–control study of risk factors for transmission. *Med J Aust* 1993;158: 117–119.
83. McNaulty JM, Keene WE, Fleming DW. A water system in one town causing an outbreak of cryptosporidiosis in another town [Abstract 1463]. In: *Program and Abstracts of the 33rd Interscience Conference on Antimicrobial Agents and Chemotherapy.* New Orleans, LA: American Society for Microbiology, 1993;387.
84. Hansen JS, Ongerth JE. Effects of time and watershed characteristics on the concentration of *Cryptosporidium* oocysts in river water. *Appl Environ Microbiol* 1991;57:2790–2795.
85. Musial CE, Arrowood MJ, Sterling CR, Gerba CP. Detection of *Cryptosporidium* in water by using polypropylene cartridge filters. *Appl Environ Microbiol* 1987;53:687–692.
86. Ongerth JE, Stibbs HH. Identification of *Cryptosporidium* oocysts in river water. *Appl Environ Microbiol* 1987;53:672–676.
87. Rose JB. Occurrence and significance of *Cryptosporidium* in water. *J Am Water Works Assoc* 1988;80:53–58.
88. LeChevallier MW, Norton WD, Lee RG. Occurrence of *Giardia* and *Cryptosporidium* spp. in surface water supplies. *Appl Environ Microbiol* 1991;57:2610–2616.
89. Isaac-Renton JL, Fogel D, Stibbs HH, Ongerth JE. *Giardia* and *Cryptosporidium* in drinking water. *Lancet* 1987;1: 973–974.
90. Stetzenbach LD, Arrowood MJ, Marshall MM, Sterling CR. Monoclonal antibody based immunofluorescent assay for *Giardia* and *Cryptosporidium* detection in water samples. *Water Sci Technol* 1988;20:193–198.
91. Sorvillo FJ, Fujioka K, Nahlen B, Tormey MP, Kebabjian R, Mascola L. Swimming-associated cryptosporidiosis. *Am J Public Health* 1992;82:742–744.
92. Joce RE, Bruce J, Kiely D, et al. An outbreak of cryptosporidiosis associated with a swimming pool. *Epidemiol Infect* 1991; 107:497–508.
93. Centers for Disease Control. Swimming-associated cryptosporidiosis—Los Angeles County. *MMWR Morb Mortal Wkly Rep* 1990;39:343–345.
94. Addy PA-K, Aikins-Bekoe P. Cryptosporidiosis in diarrhoeal children in Kumasi, Ghana. *Lancet* 1986;1:735.
95. Højlyng N, Mølbak K, Jepsen S, Hansson AP. Cryptosporidiosis in Liberian children. *Lancet* 1984;1:734.
96. Soave R, Ruiz J, Garcia-Saucedo V, Garrocho C, Kean BH. Cryptosporidiosis in a rural community in Central Mexico. *J Infect Dis* 1989;159:1160–1162.
97. Sallon S, Deckelbaum RJ, Schmid II, Harlap S, Baras M, Spira DT. *Cryptosporidium,* malnutrition, and chronic diarrhea in children. *Am J Dis Child* 1988;142:312–315.
98. Sallon S, El Showwa R, El-Masri M, Khalil M, Blundell N, Hart CA. Cryptosporidiosis in children in Gaza. *Ann Trop Paediatr* 1990;11:277–281.
99. Pal S, Bhattacharya SK, Das P, et al. Occurrence and significance of *Cryptosporidium* infection in Calcutta. *Trans R Soc Trop Med Hyg* 1989;83:520–521.
100. Zu S-X, Zhu S-Y, Li J-F. Human cryptosporidiosis in China. *Trans R Soc Trop Med Hyg* 1992;86:639–640.
101. Fang G-D, Lima AAM, Martins CV, Nataaro JP, Guerrant RL. Etiology and epidemiology of persistent diarrhea in northeastern Brazil: a hospital-based, prospective, case–control study. *J Ped Gastro Nutr* (in press).
102. Shahid NS, Rahman ASMH, Anderson BC, Mata LJ, Sanyal SC. Cryptosporidiosis in Bangladesh. *Br Med J* 1985;290: 114–115.
103. Shahid NS, Rahman ASMH, Sanyal SC. *Cryptosporidium* as a pathogen for diarrhoea in Bangladesh. *Trop Geogr Med* 1987; 39:265–270.
104. Taylor DN, Echeverria P. When does *Cryptosporidium* cause diarrhoea? *Lancet* 1986;1:320.
105. Weikel CS, Johnston LI, De Sousa MA, Guerrant RL. Cryptosporidiosis in northeastern Brazil: association with sporadic diarrhea. *J Infect Dis* 1985;151:963–965.

106. Mata L, Bolaños H, Pizarro D, Vives M. Cryptosporidiosis in children from some highland Costa Rican rural and urban areas. *Am J Trop Med Hyg* 1984;33:24–29.
107. Perez-Schael I, Boher Y, Mata L, Perez M, Tapia FJ. Cryptosporidiosis in Venezuelan children with acute diarrhea. *Am J Trop Med Hyg* 1985;34:721–722.
108. Janoff EN, Mead PS, Mead JR, et al. Endemic *Cryptosporidium* and *Giardia lamblia* infections in a Thai orphanage. *Am J Trop Med Hyg* 1990;43:248–256.
109. Dagan R, Bar-David Y, Kassis I, et al. *Cryptosporidium* in Bedouin and Jewish infants and children in southern Israel. *Isr J Med Sci* 1991;27:380–385.
110. Dan M, Gutman R. Prevalence of cryptosporidiosis in Israeli children with diarrhoea. *J Infect* 1990;21:139–141.
111. Guderian RH, Sandoval CA, Mackenzie CD. Cryptosporidiosis in Ecuadorian children with acute diarrhoea. *J Trop Pediatr* 1986;32:290–292.
112. Guessous-Idrissi N, Essadki O, Bennis M, el Kadioui F. Prévalence des cryptosporidies dans les diarrhées infantiles à Casablanca. *Presse Med* 1990;19:379.
113. Daoud AS, Zaki M, Pugh RNH, Al-Mutairi G, Al-Ali F, El-Saleh Q. *Cryptosporidium* gastroenteritis in immunocompetent children from Kuwait. *Trop Geogr Med* 1990;42:113–118.
114. Das P, Pal S, Dutta D, Bhattacharya MK, Pal SC. Cryptosporidiosis in Bengali children with acute diarrhoea. *Trans R Soc Trop Med Hyg* 1987;81:241.
115. Das P, Sengupta K, Dutta P, Bhattacharya MK, Pal SC, Bhattacharya SK. Significance of *Cryptosporidium* as an aetiologic agent of acute diarrhoea in Calcutta: a hospital based study. *J Trop Med Hyg* 1993;96:124–127.
116. Moodley D, Jackson TFHG, Gathiram V, Van den Ende J. *Cryptosporidium* infections in children in Durban: seasonal variation, age distribution and disease status. *S Afr Med J* 1991;79:295–297.
117. Moodley D, Jackson TFHG, Gathiram V, Van den Ende J. A comparative assessment of commonly employed staining procedures for the diagnosis of cryptosporidiosis. *S Afr Med J* 1991;79:314–317.
118. Mølbak K, Højlyng N, Ingholt L, Da Silva APJ, Jepsen S, Aaby P. An epidemic outbreak of cryptosporidiosis: a prospective community study from Guinea Bissau. *Pediatr Infect Dis J* 1990;9:566–570.
119. Black RE, Lopez de Romaña G, Brown KH, Bravo N, Grados Bazalar O, Creed Kanashiro H. Incidence and etiology of infantile diarrhea and major routes of transmission in Huascar, Peru. *Am J Epidemiol* 1989;129:785–799.
120. Berkowitz FE, Vallabh W, Buqwana A, Heney C. Cryptosporidiosis in black South African children. *S Afr Med J* 1988;74:272–273.
121. Carstensen H, Hansen HL, Kristiansen HO, Gomme G. The epidemiology of cryptosporidiosis and other intestinal parasitoses in children in southern Guinea-Bissau. *Trans R Soc Trop Med Hyg* 1987;81:860–864.
122. Højlyng N, Mølbak K, Jepsen S. *Cryptosporidium* spp., a frequent cause of diarrhea in Liberian children. *J Clin Microbiol* 1986;23:1109–1113.
123. Bogaerts J, Lepage P, Rouvroy D, Vandepitte J. *Cryptosporidium* spp., a frequent cause of diarrhea in Central Africa. *J Clin Microbiol* 1984;20:874–876.
124. DeMol P, Mukashema S, Bogaerts J, Hemelhof W, Butzler J-P. *Cryptosporidium* related to measles diarrhea in Rwanda. *Lancet* 1984;2:42–43.
125. Weitz JC, Tassara R, Mercado R. Cryptosporidiosis in Chilean children. *Trans R Soc Trop Med Hyg* 1987;82:335.
126. Smith G, Van den Ende J. Cryptosporidiosis among black children in hospital in South Africa. *J Infect* 1986;13:25–30.
127. Lanata CF, Black RE, Maúrtua D, et al. Etiologic agents in acute vs persistent diarrhea in children under three years of age in peri-urban Lima, Peru. *Acta Paediatr* 1992;81(Suppl 381):32–38.
128. MacFarlane DE, Horner-Bryce J. Cryptosporidiosis in well-nourished and malnourished children. *Acta Paediatr* 1987;76:474–477.
129. Mikhail IA, Hyams KC, Podgore JK, et al. Microbiologic and clinical study of acute diarrhea in children in Aswan, Egypt. *Scand J Infect Dis* 1989;21:59–65.
130. Pape JW, Levine E, Beaulieu ME, Marshall F, Verdier R, Johnson WD Jr. Cryptosporidiosis in Haitian children. *Am J Trop Med Hyg* 1987;36:333–337.
131. Rahman M, Shahid NS, Rahman H, Sack DA, Rahman N, Hossain S. Cryptosporidiosis: a cause of diarrhea in Bangladesh. *Am J Trop Med Hyg* 1990;42:127–130.
132. Steele AD, Gove E, Meewes PJ. Cryptosporidiosis in white patients in South Africa. *J Infect* 1989;19:281–285.
133. Simwa JM, Chunge RN, Kinoti SN, Karumba PN, Wamola I, Kabiru P. Cryptosporidiosis and childhood diarrhoea in a rural community in Kenya. *East Afr Med J* 1989;66:520–525.
134. Handousa AE, El-Shazly AM, El-Nashaar NM, Hamouda MM. Malabsorption syndrome in patients with cryptosporidiosis. *J Egypt Soc Parasitol* 1991;21:791–796.
135. Reinthaler FF, Link G, Klem G, Mascher F, Sixl W. Cryptosporidiosis in children with diarrhoea from slum areas in San Salvador. *Ann Trop Med Parasitol* 1988;82:209–210.
136. Sarabia-Arce S, Salazar-Lindo E, Gilman RH, Naranjo J, Miranda E. Case–control study of *Cryptosporidium parvum* infection in Peruvian children hospitalized for diarrhea: possible association with malnutrition and nosocomial infection. *Pediatr Infect Dis J* 1990;9:627–631.
137. Atterholm I, Castor B, Norlin K. Cryptosporidiosis in southern Sweden. *Scand J Infect Dis* 1987;19:231–234.
138. Casemore DP, Jackson B. Sporadic cryptosporidiosis in children. *Lancet* 1983;2:679.
139. Casemore DP, Armstrong M, Jackson B. Screening for *Cryptosporidium* in stools. *Lancet* 1984;1:734–735.
140. Hunt DA, Shannon R, Palmer SR, Jephcott AE. Cryptosporidiosis in an urban community. *Br Med J* 1984;289:814–816.
141. Montessori GA, Bischoff L. Cryptosporidiosis: a cause of summer diarrhea in children. *Can Med Assoc J* 1985;132:1285.
142. Issacs D, Hunt GH, Phillips AD, Price EH, Raafat F, Walker-Smith JA. Cryptosporidiosis in immunocompetent children. *J Clin Pathol* 1985;38:76–81.
143. Hart CA, Baxby D. Cryptosporidiosis in immunocompetent patients. *N Engl J Med* 1985;313:1018–1019.
144. Arnaud-Battandier F, Naciri M, Maurage C. Cryptosporidiosis in immunocompetent patients. *N Engl J Med* 1985;313:1019.
145. Holten-Andersen W, Gerstoft J, Henriksen SA, Pedersen NS. Prevalence of *Cryptosporidium* among patients with acute enteric infection. *J Infect* 1984;9:277–282.
146. Te Wiata I, Lennon D. *Cryptosporidium* infestation in hospitalised urban children. *N Z Med J* 1985;98:349.
147. Tzipori S, Smith M, Birch C, Barnes G, Bishop R. Cryptosporidiosis in hospital patients with gastroenteritis. *Am J Trop Med Hyg* 1983;32:931–934.
148. Lumb R, Erlich S, Davidson GP. Cryptosporidia detection. *Med J Aust* 1985;142:329–330.
149. Baron EJ, Schenone C, Tanenbaum B. Comparison of three methods for detection of *Cryptosporidium* oocysts in a low-prevalence population. *J Clin Microbiol* 1989;27:223–224.
150. Baxby D, Hart CA. The incidence of cryptosporidiosis: a two-year prospective study in a children's hospital. *J Hyg* 1986;96:107–111.
151. Biggs B-A, Megna R, Wickremesinghe S, Dwyer B. Human infection with *Cryptosporidium* spp.: results of a 24 month survey. *Med J Aust* 1987;147:175–177.
152. Caprioli A, Gentile G, Baldassarri L, Bisicchia R, Romoli E, Donelli G. *Cryptosporidium* as a common cause of childhood diarrhoea in Italy. *Epidemiol Infect* 1989;102:537–540.
153. Carson JWK. Changing patterns in childhood gastroenteritis. *Ir Med J* 1989;82:66–67.
154. Carter MJ. *Cryptosporidium:* an important cause of gastrointestinal disease in immunocompetent patients. *N Z Med J* 1986;99:101–103.
155. Cruickshank R, Ashdown L, Croese J. Human cryptosporidiosis in north Queenland. *Aust N Z J Med* 1988;18:582–586.
156. Corbett-Feeney G. *Cryptosporidium* among children with acute diarrhoea in the west of Ireland. *J Infect* 1987;14:79–84.
157. El-Ahraf A, Tacal JV Jr, Sobih M, Amin M, Lawrence W, Wilcke BW. Prevalence of cryptosporidiosis in dogs and human

beings in San Bernardino County, California. *J Am Vet Med Assoc* 1991;198:631–634.

158. Heidl M, Hering L, Scholz H. Cryptosporidiosis in children. *Infection* 1986;14:173–176.

159. Desgrandchamps D, Munzinger J. Infektiose gastroenteritis beim immunokompetent en kind. Bedeutung von *Cryptosporidium* spp. and *Aeromonas* spp. *Schweiz Med Wochenschr* 1989; 119:276–281.

160. Vuorio A, Jokipii AMM, Jokipii L. *Cryptosporidium* in asymptomatic children. *Rev Infect Dis* 1991;13:261–264.

161. Lopez-Brea M, Garcia-Picazo L, Del Rey M, Jimenez ML. *Cryptosporidium* in stool specimens in Madrid. *Trans R Soc Trop Med Hyg* 1985;79:422–423.

162. White WL, Picklo J. Human cryptosporidiosis. *N Engl J Med* 1983;309:1325.

163. Kern W, Mayer S, Kreuzer P, Vanek E. Low prevalence of intestinal cryptosporidiosis among immunocompetent and immunocompromised patients with and without diarrhoea in southern Germany. *Infection* 1987;15:440–443.

164. Mai Nguyen X. Cryptosporidial diarrhoea in children. *Infection* 1987;15:444–446.

165. Marshall AR, Al-Jumaili IJ, Fenwick GA, Bint AJ, Record CO. Cryptosporidiosis in patients at a large teaching hospital. *J Clin Microbiol* 1987;25:172–173.

166. Mann ED, Sekla LH, Nayar GPS, Koschik C. Infection with *Cryptosporidium* spp. in humans and cattle in Manitoba. *Can J Vet Res* 1986;50:174–178.

167. Steeb S, Hagedorn H-J, Krone J-R. Cryptosporidiosis in immune-competent patients: epidemiology and clinical aspects. *Dtsch Med Wochenschr* 1987;112:990–994.

168. Ungar BLP, Gilman RH, Lanata CF, Perez-Schael I. Seroepidemiology of *Cryptosporidium* infection in two Latin American populations. *J Infect Dis* 1988;157:551–556.

169. Roberts WG, Green PHR, Ma J, Carr M, Ginsberg AM. Prevalence of cryptosporidiosis in patients undergoing endoscopy: evidence for an asymptomatic carrier state. *Am J Med* 1989; 87:537–539.

170. Ramirez FC, Clarridge JE, Heiser MC, et al. A study of the frequency of recovery of unexpected *Giardia lamblia* and *Cryptosporidium* from duodenal aspirates taken during routine upper endoscopy. *Am J Gastroenterol* 1993;88:552–554.

171. Zu S-X, Li J-F, Barrett LJ, et al. Seroepidemiologic study of *Cryptosporidium* infection in children from rural communities of Anhui, China and Fortaleza, Brazil. *Am J Trop Med Hyg:* 1994;51:1–10.

172. Cruz JR, Cano F, Càceres P, Chew F, Pareja G. Infection and diarrhea caused by *Cryptosporidium* sp. among Guatemalan infants. *J Clin Microbiol* 1988;26:88–91.

173. Sterling CR, Gilman RH, Sinclair NA, Cama V, Castillo R, Diaz F. The role of breast milk in protecting urban Peruvian children against cryptosporidiosis. *J Protozool* 1991;38: 23S–25S.

174. Colebunders R, Francis H, Mann JM, et al. Persistent diarrhea, strongly associated with HIV infection in Kinshasa, Zaire. *Am J Gastroenterol* 1987;82:859–864.

175. Colebunders RK, Lusakumuni K, Nelson AM, et al. Persistent diarrhoea in Zairian AIDS patients: an endoscopic and histological study. *Gut* 1988;29:1687–1691.

176. Wuhib T, Silva TMJ, Newman RD, et al. Cryptosporidial and microsporidial infections in HIV-infected patients in northeastern Brazil. *J Infect Dis (in press)*.

177. Chacin-Bonilla L, Guanipa N, Cano G, Raleigh X, Quijada L. Cryptosporidiosis among patients with acquired immunodeficiency syndrome in Zulia state, Venezuela. *Am J Trop Med Hyg* 1992;47:582–586.

178. Conlon CP, Pinching AJ, Perera CU, Moody A, Luo NP, Lucas SB. HIV-related enteropathy in Zambia: a clinical, microbiological, and histological study. *Am J Trop Med Hyg* 1990;42: 83–88.

179. Malebranche R, Arnoux E, Guérin JM, et al. Acquired immunodeficiency syndrome with severe gastrointestinal manifestations in Haiti. *Lancet* 1983;2:873–878.

180. Floch JJ, Laroche R, Kadende P, Nkurunziza T, Mpfizi B. Les parasites, agents étiologiques des diarrhées du SIDA: intérêt de l'examen du liquide d'aspiration duodénale. *Bull Soc Pathol Exot Filiales* 1989;82:316–320.

181. Henry MC, De Clerq D, Lokombe B, et al. Parasitological observations of chronic diarrhoea in suspected AIDS adult patients in Kinshasa (Zaire). *Trans R Soc Trop Med Hyg* 1986; 80:309–310.

182. Sewankambo N, Mugerwa RD, Goodgame R, et al. Enteropathic AIDS in Uganda. An endoscopic, histological, and microbiological study. *AIDS* 1987;1:9–13.

183. Dryden MS, Shanson DC. The microbial causes of diarrhoea in patients infected with the human immunodeficiency virus. *J Infect* 1988;17:107–114.

184. Antony MA, Brandt LJ, Klein RS, Bernstein LH. Infectious diarrhea in patients with AIDS. *Dig Dis Sci* 1988;33:1141–1146.

185. Laughon BE, Druckman DA, Vernon A, et al. Prevalence of enteric pathogens in homosexual men with and without acquired immunodeficiency syndrome. *Gastroenterology* 1988; 94:984–993.

186. Smith PD, Lane HC, Gill VJ, et al. Intestinal infections in patients with the acquired immunodeficiency syndrome (AIDS): etiology and response to therapy. *Ann Intern Med* 1988;108: 328–333.

187. Connolly GM, Dryden MS, Shanson DC, Gazzard BG. Cryptosporidial diarrhoea in AIDS and its treatment. *Gut* 1988;29: 593–597.

188. Connolly GM, Forbes A, Gazzard BG. Investigation of seemingly pathogen-negative diarrhoea in patients infected with HIV1. *Gut* 1990;31:886–889.

189. René E, Marche C, Regnier B, et al. Intestinal infections in patients with acquired immunodeficiency syndrome: a prospective study in 132 patients. *Dig Dis Sci* 1989;34:773–780.

190. Dworkin B, Wormser GP, Rosenthal WS, et al. Gastrointestinal manifestations of the acquired immunodeficiency syndrome: a review of 22 cases. *Am J Gastroenterol* 1985;80:774–778.

191. Girard PM, Goldschmidt E, Vittecoq D, et al. Vapreotide, a somatostatin analogue, in cryptosporidiosis and other AIDS-related diarrhoeal diseases. *AIDS* 1992;6:715–718.

192. McCarty M, Choudhri AH, Helbert M, Crofton ME. Radiological features of AIDS related cholangitis. *Clin Radiol* 1989;40: 582–585.

193. Whiteside ME, Barkin JS, May RG, Weiss SD, Fischl MA, MacLeod CL. Enteric coccidiosis among patients with the acquired immunodeficiency syndrome. *Am J Trop Med Hyg* 1984; 33:1065–1072.

194. Stehr-Green JK, McCaig L, Remsen HM, Rains CS, Fox M, Juranek DD. Shedding of oocysts in immunocompetent individuals infected with *Cryptosporidium*. *Am J Trop Med Hyg* 1987; 36:338–342.

195. Ferson MJ, Young LC. *Cryptosporidium* and coxsackievirus B5 causing epidemic diarrhoea in a child-care centre. *Med J Aust* 1992;156:813.

196. Alpert G, Bell LM, Kirkpatrick CE, et al. Outbreak of cryptosporidiosis in a day-care center. *Pediatrics* 1986;77:152–157.

197. Wolfson JS, Richter JM, Waldron MA, Weber DJ, McCarthy DM, Hopkins CC. Cryptosporidiosis in immunocompetent patients. *N Engl J Med* 1985;312:1278–1282.

198. McNabb SJN, Hensel DM, Welch DF, Heijbel H, McKee GL, Istre GR. Comparison of sedimentation and flotation techniques for identification of *Cryptosporidium* sp. oocysts in a large outbreak of human diarrhea. *J Clin Microbiol* 1985;22: 587–589.

199. Melo Christino JAG, Carvalho MIP, Salgado MJ. An outbreak of cryptosporidiosis in a hospital day-care centre. *Epidemiol Infect* 1988;101:355–359.

200. Skeels MR, Sokolow R, Hubbard CV, Andrus JK, Baisch J. *Cryptosporidium* infection in Oregon public health clinic patients 1985–88: the value of statewide laboratory surveillance. *Am J Public Health* 1990;80:305–308.

201. Centers for Disease Control. Cryptosporidiosis among children attending day care centers—Georgia, Pennsylvania, Michigan, California, New Mexico. *MMWR Morb Mortal Wkly Rep* 1984; 33:599–601.

202. Combee CL, Collinge ML, Britt EM. Cryptosporidiosis in a

hospital-associated day care center. *Pediatr Infect Dis* 1986;5: 528–532.

203. Heijbel H, Slaine K, Seigel B, et al. Outbreak of diarrhea in a day care center with spread to household members: the role of *Cryptosporidium. Pediatr Infect Dis J* 1987;6:532–535.

204. Nwanyanwu OC, Baird JN, Reeve GR. Cryptosporidiosis in a day-care center. *Tex Med* 1989;85:40–43.

205. Taylor JP, Perdue JN, Dingley D, Gustafson TL, Patterson M, Reed LA. Cryptosporidiosis outbreak in a day-care center. *Am J Dis Child* 1985;139:1023–1025.

206. Walters IN, Miller NM, Van den Ende J, et al. Outbreak of cryptosporidiosis among young children attending a day-care centre in Durban. *S Afr Med J* 1988;74:496–499.

207. Reif JS, Wimmer L, Smith JA, Dargatz DA, Cheney JM. Human cryptosporidiosis associated with an epizootic in calves. *Am J Public Health* 1989;79:1528–1530.

208. Pohjola S, Oksanen H, Jokipii L, Jokipii AMM. Outbreak of cryptosporidiosis among veterinary students. *Scand J Infect Dis* 1986;18:173–178.

209. Levine JF, Levy MG, Walker RL, Crittenden S. Cryptosporidiosis in veterinary students. *J Am Vet Med Assoc* 1988;193: 1413–1414.

210. Højlyng N, Holten-Andersen W, Jepsen S. Cryptosporidiosis: a case of airborne transmission. *Lancet* 1987;2:271–272.

211. Tangermann RH, Gordon S, Wiesner P, Kreckman L. An outbreak of cryptosporidiosis in a day-care center in Georgia. *Am J Epidemiol* 1991;133:471–476.

212. Crawford FG, Vermund SH, Ma JY, Deckelbaum RJ. Asymptomatic cryptosporidiosis in a New York City day care center. *Pediatr Infect Dis J* 1988;7:806–807.

213. Diers J, McCallister GL. Occurrence of *Cryptosporidium* in home daycare centers in West-Central Colorado. *J Parasitol* 1989;75:637–638.

214. Koch KL, Phillips DJ, Aber RC, Current WL. Cryptosporidiosis in hospital personnel: evidence for person-to-person transmission. *Ann Intern Med* 1985;102:593–596.

215. Heald AE, Bartlett JA. *Cryptosporidium* spread in a group residential home. *Ann Intern Med* 1994;121:647–648

216. Ravn P, Lundgren JD, Kjaeldgaard P, et al. Nosocomial outbreak of cryptosporidiosis in AIDS patients. *BMJ* 1991;302: 277–280.

217. Navarrete S, Stetler HC, Avila C, Garcia Aranda JA, Santos-Preciado JI. An outbreak of *Cryptosporidium* diarrhea in a pediatric hospital. *Pediatr Infect Dis J* 1991;10:248–250.

218. Martino P, Gentile G, Captrioli A, et al. Hospital-acquired cryptosporidiosis in a bone marrow transplantation unit. *J Infect Dis* 1988;158:647–648.

219. Collier AC, Miller RA, Meyers JD. Cryptosporidiosis after marrow transplantation: person-to-person transmission and treatment with spiramycin. *Ann Intern Med* 1984;101:205–206.

220. Baxby D, Hart CA, Taylor C. Human cryptosporidiosis: a possible case of hospital cross infection. *Br Med J* 1983;287: 1760–1761.

221. Ma P, Kaufman DL, Helmick CG, D'Souza AJ, Navin TR. Cryptosporidiosis in tourists returning from the Caribbean. *N Engl J Med* 1985;312:647–648.

222. Soave R, Ma P. Cryptosporidiosis: traveler's diarrhea in two families. *Arch Intern Med* 1985;145:70–72.

223. Sterling CR, Seegar K, Sinclair NA. *Cryptosporidium* as a causative agent of traveler's diarrhea. *J Infect Dis* 1986;153: 380–381.

224. Taylor DN, Houston R, Shlim DR, Bhaibulaya M, Ungar BLP, Echeverria P. Etiology of diarrhea among travelers and foreign residents in Nepal. *JAMA* 1988;260:1245–1248.

225. Ungar BLP, Mulligan M, Nutman TR. Serologic evidence of *Cryptosporidium* infection in US volunteers before and during Peace Corps service in Africa. *Arch Intern Med* 1989;149: 894–897.

226. Flegg PJ. *Cryptosporidium* in travellers from Pakistan. *Trans R Soc Trop Med Hyg* 1987;81:171.

227. Jokipii L, Pohjola S, Jokipii AMM. *Cryptosporidium:* a frequent finding in patients with gastrointestinal symptoms. *Lancet* 1983;2:358–361.

228. Jokipii L, Pohjola S, Jokipii AMM. Cryptosporidiosis associated with traveling and giardiasis. *Gastroenterology* 1985;89: 838–842.

229. Jokipii AMM, Hemilä M, Jokipii L. Prospective study of acquisition of *Cryptosporidium, Giardia lamblia,* and gastrointestinal illness. *Lancet* 1985;2:487–489.

230. Gatti S, Cevini C, Bruno A, Bernuzzi AM, Scaglia M. Cryptosporidiosis in tourists returning from Egypt and the island of Mauritius. *Clin Infect Dis* 1993;16:344–345.

231. Elsser KA, Moricz M, Proctor EM. *Cryptosporidium* infections: a laboratory survey. *Can Med Assoc J* 1986;135:211–213.

232. Fafard J, Lalonde R. Long-standing symptomatic cryptosporidiosis in a normal man: clinical response to spiramycin. *J Clin Gastroenterol* 1990;12:190–191.

233. Kotler DP, Francisco A, Clayton F, Scholes JV, Orenstein JM. Small intestinal injury and parasitic diseases in AIDS. *Ann Intern Med* 1990;113:444–449.

234. Kocoshis SA, Cibull ML, Davis TE, Hinton JT, Seip M, Banwell JG. Intestinal and pulmonary cryptosporidiosis in an infant with severe combined immune deficiency. *J Pediatr Gastroenterol Nutr* 1984;3:149–157.

235. Sloper KS, Dourmashkin RR, Bird RB, Slavin G, Webster ADB. Chronic malabsorption due to cryptosporidiosis in a child with immunoglobulin deficiency. *Gut* 1982;23:80–82.

236. Jacyna MR, Parkin J, Goldin R, Baron JH. Protracted enteric cryptosporidial infection in selective immunoglobulin A and saccharomyces opsonin deficiencies. *Gut* 1990;31:714–716.

237. Heaton P. Cryptosporidiosis and acute leukaemia. *Arch Dis Child* 1990;65:813–814.

238. Davis JJ, Heyman MB, Ferrell L, Kerner R, Kerlan R Jr, Thaler MM. Sclerosing cholangitis associated with chronic cryptosporidiosis in a child with a congenital immunodeficiency disorder. *Am J Gastroenterol* 1987;82:1196–1202.

239. Chng HH, Shaw D, Klesius P, Saxon A. Inability of oral bovine transfer factor to eradicate cryptosporidial infection in a patient with congenital dysgammaglobulinemia. *Clin Immunol Immunopathol* 1989;50:402–406.

240. Holley HP, Thiers BH. Cryptosporidiosis in a patient receiving immunosuppressive therapy: possible activation of latent infection. *Dig Dis Sci* 1986;31:1004–1007.

241. Mead GM, Sweetenham JW, Ewins DL, Furlong M, Lowes JA. Intestinal cryptosporidiosis: a complication of cancer treatment. *Cancer Treat Rep* 1986;70:769–770.

242. Miller RA, Holmberg RE Jr, Clausen CR. Life-threatening diarrhea caused by *Cryptosporidium* in a child undergoing therapy for acute lymphocytic leukemia. *J Pediatr* 1983;103:256–259.

243. Oh SH, Jaffe N, Fainstein V, Pickering LK. Cryptosporidiosis and anticancer chemotherapy. *J Pediatr* 1984;104:963–964.

244. Foot ABM, Oakhill A, Mott MG. Cryptosporidiosis and acute leukaemia. *Arch Dis Child* 1990;65:236–237.

245. Gentile G, Baldassarri L, Caprioli A, et al. Colonic vascular invasion as a possible route of extraintestinal cryptosporidiosis. *Am J Med* 1987;82:574–575.

246. Gentile G, Venditti M, Micozzi A, et al. Cryptosporidiosis in patients with hematologic malignancies. *Rev Infect Dis* 1991; 13:842–846.

247. Stine KC, Harris J-AS, Lindsey NJ, Cho CT. Spontaneous remission of cryptosporidiosis in a child with acute lymphocytic leukemia. *Clin Pediatr* 1985;24:722–724.

248. Travis WD, Schmidt K, MacLowry JD, Masur H, Condron KS, Fojo AT. Respiratory cryptosporidiosis in a patient with malignant lymphoma. *Arch Pathol Lab Med* 1990;114:519–522.

249. Borowitz SM, Saulsbury FT. Treatment of chronic cryptosporidial infection with orally administered human serum immune globulin. *J Pediatr* 1991;119:593–595.

250. Roncoroni AJ, Gomez MA, Mera J, Cagnoni P, Davalos Michel M. *Cryptosporidium* infection in renal transplant patients. *J Infect Dis* 1989;160:559.

251. Ona ET. Early pitfalls in renal transplantation. *Transplant Proc* 1992;24:1280–1282.

252. Vajro P, di Martino L, Scotti S, Barbati C, Fontanella A, Pettoello Mantovani M. Intestinal *Cryptosporidium* carriage in two liver-transplanted children. *J Pediatr Gastroenterol Nutr* 1991; 12:139.

253. Kibbler CC, Smith A, Hamilton-Dutoit SJ, Milburn H, Pat-

tinson JK, Prentice HG. Pulmonary cryptosporidiosis occurring in a bone marrow transplant patient. *Scand J Infect Dis* 1987;19:581–584.

254. Manivel C, Filipovich A, Snover DC. Cryptosporidiosis as a cause of diarrhea following bone marrow transplantation. *Dis Colon Rectum* 1985;28:741–742.

255. Portnoy D, Whiteside ME, Buckley E III, MacLeod CL. Treatment of intestinal cryptosporidiosis with spiramycin. *Ann Intern Med* 1984;101:202–204.

256. Blakey JL, Barnes GL, Bishop RJ, Ekert H. Infectious diarrhea in children undergoing bone-marrow transplantation. *Aust N Z J Med* 1989;19:31–36.

257. Chan AW, MacFarlane IA, Rhodes JM. Cryptosporidiosis as a cause of chronic diarrhoea in a patient with insulin-dependent diabetes mellitus. *J Infect* 1989;19:293.

258. Gledhill JA, Porter J. Diarrhoea due to *Cryptosporidium* infection in thalassaemia major. *BMJ* 1990;301:212–213.

259. Tompkins DS, Batman PA. Fatal cryptosporidiosis in association with Sheehan's syndrome. *Br J Gen Pract* 1991;41:519.

260. Fletcher A, Sims TA, Talbot IC. Cryptosporidial enteritis without general or selective immune deficiency. *Br Med J* 1982;285:22–23.

261. Petras RE, Carey WD, Alanis A. Cryptosporidial enteritis in a homosexual male with acquired immunodeficiency syndrome. *Cleve Clin Q* 1983;50:41–45.

262. Bird RG, Smith MD. Cryptosporidiosis in man: parasite life cycle and fine structural pathology. *J Pathol* 1980;132:217–233.

263. Heine J, Pohlenz JFL, Moon HW, Woode GN. Enteric lesions and diarrhea in calves monoinfected with *Cryptosporidium* species. *J Infect Dis* 1984;150:768–775.

264. Argenzio RA, Liacos JA, Levy ML, Meuten DJ, Lecce JG, Powell DW. Villous atrophy, crypt hyperplasia, cellular infiltration, and impaired glucose–Na absorption in enteric cryptosporidiosis of pigs. *Gastroenterology* 1990;98:1129–1140.

265. Modigliani R, Bories C, Le Charpentier Y, et al. Diarrhoea and malabsorption in acquired immune deficiency syndrome: a study of four cases with special emphasis on opportunistic protozoan infestations. *Gut* 1985;26:179–187.

266. Garza DH, Fedorak RN, Soave R. Enterotoxin-like activity in cultured cryptosporidia: role in diarrhea. *Gastroenterology* 1986;90:1424.

267. Guerrant RL, Petri WA, Weikel CS. Parasitic causes of diarrhea. In: Lebenthal E, Duffey M, eds. *Textbook of secretory diarrhea*. New York: Raven Press, 1990;273–280.

268. Guarino A, Canani RB, Pozio E, Terracciano L, Albano F, Mazzeo M. Enterotoxic effect of stool supernatant of *Cryptosporidium*-infected calves on human jejunum. *Gastroenterology* 1994;106:28–34.

269. Sears CL, Guerrant RL. Cryptosporidiosis: the complexity of intestinal pathophysiology. *Gastroenterology* 1994;106:252–254.

270. Gardner AL, Roche JK, Weikel CS, Guerrant RL. Intestinal cryptosporidiosis: pathophysiologic alterations and specific cellular and humoral immune responses in rnu/+ and rnu/rnu (athymic) rats. *Am J Trop Med Hyg* 1991;44:49–62.

271. Moon HW, Pohlenz JFL, Woodmansee DB, et al. Intestinal cryptosporidiosis: pathogenesis and immunity. *Microecol Ther* 1985;15:103–120.

272. Heine J, Moon HW, Woodmansee DB. Persistent *Cryptosporidium* infection in congenitally athymic (nude) mice. *Infect Immun* 1984;43:856–859.

273. Ungar BLP, Burris JA, Quinn CA, Finkelman FD. New mouse models for chronic *Cryptosporidium* infection in immunodeficient hosts. *Infect Immun* 1990;58:961–969.

274. Ungar BLP, Kao T-C, Burris JA, Finkelman FD. *Cryptosporidium* infection in an adult mouse model. Independent roles for IFN-gamma and CD4+ T lymphocytes in protective immunity. *J Immunol* 1991;147:1014–1022.

275. Mead JR, Arrowood MJ, Healey MC, Sidwell RW. Cryptosporidial infections in SCID mice reconstituted with human or murine lymphocytes. *J Protozool* 1991;38:59S–61S.

276. Mead JR, Arrowood MJ, Sidwell RW, Healey MC. Chronic *Cryptosporidium parvum* infections in congenitally immunodeficient SCID and nude mice. *J Infect Dis* 1991;163:1297–1304.

277. Chen W, Harp JA, Harmsen AG. Requirements for CD4+ cells and gamma interferon in resolution of established *Cryptosporidium parvum* infection in mice. *Infect Immun* 1993;61:3928–3932.

278. Darban H, Enriquez J, Sterling CR, et al. Cryptosporidiosis facilitated by murine retroviral infection with LP-BM5. *J Infect Dis* 1991;164:741–745.

279. Petersen C. Cryptosporidiosis in patients infected with the human immunodeficiency virus. *Clin Infect Dis* 1992;15:903–909.

280. Enriquez FJ, Sterling CR. *Cryptosporidium* infections in inbred strains of mice. *J Protozool* 1991;38:100S–102S.

281. Harp JA, Moon HW. Susceptibility of mast cell-deficient W/Wᵛ mice to *Cryptosporidium parvum*. *Infect Immun* 1991;59:718–720.

282. Taghi-Kilani R, Sekla L, Hayglass KT. The role of humoral immunity in *Cryptosporidium* spp. infection. Studies with B cell-depleted mice. *J Immunol* 1990;145:1571–1576.

283. Campbell PN, Current WL. Demonstration of serum antibodies to *Cryptosporidium* sp. in normal and immunodeficient humans with confirmed infections. *J Clin Microbiol* 1983;18:165–169.

284. Casemore DP. The antibody response to *Cryptosporidium*: development of a serological test and its use in a study of immunologically normal persons. *J Infect* 1987;14:125–134.

285. Ungar BLP, Soave R, Fayer R, Nash TE. Enzyme immunoassay detection of immunoglobulin M and G antibodies to *Cryptosporidium* in immunocompetent and immunocompromised persons. *J Infect Dis* 1986;153:570–578.

286. Laxer MA, Alcantara AK, Javato-Laxer M, Menorca DM, Fernando MT, Ranoa CP. Immune response to cryptosporidiosis in Philippine children. *Am J Trop Med Hyg* 1990;42:131–139.

287. Ungar BLP, Nash TE. Quantification of specific antibody response to *Cryptosporidium* antigens by laser densitometry. *Infect Immun* 1986;53:124–128.

288. Mead JR, Arrowood MJ, Sterling CR. Antigens of *Cryptosporidium* sporozoites recognized by immune sera of infected animals and humans. *J Parasitol* 1988;74:135–143.

289. Tilley M, Upton SJ, Fayer R, et al. Identification of a 15-kilodalton surface glycoprotein on sporozoites of *Cryptosporidium parvum*. *Infect Immun* 1991;59:1002–1007.

290. Reperant J-M, Naciri M, Chardes T, Bout DT. Immunological characterization of a 17-kDa antigen from *Cryptosporidium parvum* recognized early by mucosal IgA antibodies. *FEMS Microbiol Lett* 1992;99:7–14.

291. Whitmire WM, Harp JA. Characterization of bovine cellular and serum antibody responses during infection by *Cryptosporidium parvum*. *Infect Immun* 1991;59:990–995.

292. Lumb R, Lanser JA, O'Donoghue PJ. Electrophoretic and immunoblot analysis of *Cryptosporidium* oocysts. *Immunol Cell Biol* 1988;66:369–376.

293. Hill BD, Blewett DA, Dawson AM, Wright S. Analysis of the kinetics, isotype and specificity of serum and coproantibody in lambs infected with *Cryptosporidium parvum*. *Res Vet Sci* 1990;48:76–81.

294. Tilley M, Upton SJ. Electrophoretic characterization of *Cryptosporidium parvum* (KSU-1 isolate) (Apicomplexa: Cryptosporidiidae). *Can J Zool* 1990;68:1513–1519.

295. Flanigan T, Whalen C, Turner J, et al. *Cryptosporidium* infection and CD4 counts. *Ann Intern Med* 1992;116:840–842.

296. Blanshard C, Jackson AM, Shanson DC, Francis N, Gazzard BG. Cryptosporidiosis in HIV-seropositive patients. *Q J Med* 1992;85:813–823.

297. Greenberg RE, Mir R, Bank S, Siegal FP. Resolution of intestinal cryptosporidiosis after treatment of AIDS with AZT. *Gastroenterology* 1989;97:1327–1330.

298. Sogni P. Treatment of intestinal cryptosporidiosis in AIDS. *Gastroenterology* 1990;99:602–603.

299. Jokipii L, Jokipii AMM. Timing of symptoms and oocyst excretion in human cryptosporidiosis. *N Engl J Med* 1986;315:1643–1647.

300. Bannister P, Mountford RA. *Cryptosporidium* in the elderly: a cause of life-threatening diarrhea. *Am J Med* 1989;86:507–508.

301. Lima AAM, Fang G, Schorling JB, et al. Persistent diarrhea in

northeast Brazil: etiologies and interactions with malnutrition. *Acta Paediatr* 1992;81(Suppl 381):39–44.

302. Keren G, Barzilai A, Barzilay Z, Goldschmied-Reouven A, Bogokowsky B, Rubinstein E. Life-threatening cryptosporidiosis in immunocompetent infants. *Eur J Pediatr* 1987;146:187–189.

303. Harari MD, West B, Dwyer B. *Cryptosporidium* as a cause of laryngotracheitis in an infant. *Lancet* 1986;1:1207.

304. Hawkins SP, Thomas RP, Teasdale C. Acute pancreatitis: a new finding in *Cryptosporidium* enteritis. *Br Med J* 1987;294:483–484.

305. Ramsden K, Freeth M. Cryptosporidial infection presenting as an acute appendicitis. *Histopathology* 1989;14:209–211.

306. Merino FJ, López-Serrano MC, Velasco AC. Diarrea por *Cryptosporidium* asociada a urticaria y angioedema. *Enferm Infecc Microbiol Clin* 1989;7:78.

307. Hay EM, Winfield J, McKendrick MW. Reactive arthritis associated with *Cryptosporidium* enteritis. *Br Med J* 1987;295:248.

308. Shepherd RC, Sinha GP, Reed CL, Russell FE. Cryptosporidiosis in the West of Scotland. *Scott Med J* 1988;33:365–368.

309. Shepherd RC, Smail PJ, Sinha GP. Reactive arthritis complicating cryptosporidial infection. *Arch Dis Child* 1989;64:743–744.

310. Andreani T, Modigliani R, le Charpentier Y, et al. Acquired immunodeficiency with intestinal cryptosporidiosis: possible transmission by Haitian whole blood. *Lancet* 1983;1:1187–1191.

311. Cooper DA, Wodak A, Marriot DJE, et al. Cryptosporidiosis in the acquired immune deficiency syndrome. *Pathology* 1984;16:455–457.

312. Gérard L, Daleine G, Longuet P, Le Bras J, Leport C, Vildé JL. Intestinal cryptosporidiosis in 37 HIV infected patients: prognostic significance of biliary tract involvement [Abstract WS-B13-4]. In: *IXth International Conference on AIDS*, Berlin, 1993;56.

313. Pitlik SD, Fainstein V, Garza D, et al. Human cryptosporidiosis: spectrum of disease. *Arch Intern Med* 1983;143:2269–2275.

314. Soave R, Danner RL, Honig CL, et al. Cryptosporidiosis in homosexual men. *Ann Intern Med* 1984;100:504–511.

315. Saltzberg DM, Kotloff KL, Newman JL, Fastiggi R. *Cryptosporidium* infection in acquired immunodeficiency syndrome: not always a poor prognosis. *J Clin Gastroenterol* 1991;13:94–97.

316. Berkowitz CD, Seidel JS. Spontaneous resolution of cryptosporidiosis in a child with acquired immunodeficiency syndrome. *Am J Dis Child* 1985;139:967.

317. Lerner CW, Tapper ML. Opportunistic infection complicating acquired immune deficiency syndrome: clinical features of 25 cases. *Medicine (Baltimore)* 1984;63:155–164.

318. Mc Gowan I, Hawkins AS, Weller IVD. The natural history of cryptosporidial diarrhoea in HIV-infected patients. *AIDS* 1993;7:349–354.

319. Scaglia M, Senaldi G, Di Perri G, Minoli L. Unusual low-grade cryptosporidial enteritis in AIDS: a case report. *Infection* 1986;14:87–88.

320. Janoff EN, Limas C, Gebhard RL, Penley KA. Cryptosporidial carriage without symptoms in the acquired immunodeficiency syndrome (AIDS). *Ann Intern Med* 1990;112:75–76.

321. Gentile G, Caprioli A, Donelli G, Venditti M, Mandelli F, Martino P. Asymptomatic carriage of *Cryptosporidium* in two patients with leukemia. *Am J Infect Control* 1990;18:127–128.

322. Zar F, Geiseler PJ, Brown VA. Asymptomatic carriage of *Cryptosporidium* in the stool of a patient with acquired immunodeficiency syndrome. *J Infect Dis* 1985;151:195.

323. Godwin TA. Cryptosporidiosis in the acquired immunodeficiency syndrome: a study of 15 autopsy cases. *Hum Pathol* 1991;22:1215–1223.

324. Berk RN, Wall SD, McArdle CB, et al. Cryptosporidiosis of the stomach and small intestine in patients with AIDS. *AJR Am J Roentgenol* 1984;143:549–554.

325. Kazlow PG, Shah K, Benkov KJ, Dische R, LeLeiko NS. Esophageal cryptosporidiosis in a child with acquired immune deficiency syndrome. *Gastroenterology* 1986;91:1301–1303.

326. Oberhuber G, Lauer E, Stolte M, Borchard F. Cryptospori-

diosis of the appendix vermiformis: a case report. *Z Gastroenterol* 1991;29:606–608.

327. Zambrano Nuñez MR, Sakai P, Ishioka S, Laudanna AA. Erosive gastroduodenitis with cryptosporidiosis in a patient with acquired immunodeficiency syndrome. *Rev Hosp Clin Fac Med Sao Paulo* 1990;45:188–189.

328. Gross TL, Wheat J, Bartlett M, O'Connor KW. AIDS and multiple system involvement with *Cryptosporidium*. *Am J Gastroenterol* 1986;81:456–458.

329. Orenstein J, Steinberg W, Simon G. Cryptosporidiosis of the pancreas [Abstract 1224]. In: *Program and Abstracts of the 33rd Interscience Conference on Antimicrobial Agents and Chemotherapy*. New Orleans, LA: American Society for Microbiology, 1993;344.

330. Meyers SA, Kuhlman JE, Fishman EK. Enterovesical fistula in a patient with cryptosporidiosis and AIDS: CT demonstration. *Clin Imaging* 1990;14:143–145.

331. Soave R, Johnson WD Jr. *Cryptosporidium* and *Isospora belli* infections. *J Infect Dis* 1988;157:225–229.

332. Lee JG, Grech P, Edwards P, Wilson JAP. AIDS cholangiopathy as the first sign of HIV infection. *N C Med J* 1993;54:16–17.

333. Kahn DG, Garfinkle JM, Klonoff DC, Pembrook LJ, Morrow DJ. Cryptosporidial and cytomegaloviral hepatitis and cholecystitis. *Arch Pathol Lab Med* 1987;111:879–881.

334. Pitlik SD, Fainstein V, Rios A, Guarda L, Mansell PWA, Hersh EM. Cryptosporidial cholecystitis. *N Engl J Med* 1983;308:967.

335. Dowsett JF, Miller R, Davidson R, et al. Sclerosing cholangitis in acquired immunodeficiency syndrome: case reports and review of the literature. *Scand J Gastroenterol* 1988;23:1267–1274.

336. Hasan FA, Jeffers LJ, Dickinson G, et al. Hepatobiliary cryptosporidiosis and cytomegalovirus infection mimicking metastatic cancer to the liver. *Gastroenterology* 1991;100:1743–1748.

337. Hinnant K, Schwartz A, Rotterdam H, Rudski C. Cytomegaloviral and cryptosporidial cholecystitis in two patients with AIDS. *Am J Surg Pathol* 1989;13:57–60.

338. Forbes A, Blanshard C, Gazzard B. Natural history of AIDS related sclerosing cholangitis: a study of 20 cases. *Gut* 1993;34:116–121.

339. Blumberg RS, Kelsey P, Perrone T, Dickersin R, Laquaglia M, Ferruci J. Cytomegalovirus- and *Cryptosporidium*-associated acalculous gangrenous cholecystitis. *Am J Med* 1984;76:1118–1123.

340. Cello JP. Acquired immunodeficiency syndrome cholangiopathy: spectrum of disease. *Am J Med* 1989;86:539–546.

341. Tzipori S, Roberton D, Chapman C. Remission of diarrhoea due to cryptosporidiosis in an immunodeficient child treated with hyperimmune bovine colostrum. *Br Med J* 1986;293:1276–1277.

342. Tzipori S, Roberton D, Cooper DA, White L. Chronic cryptosporidial diarrhoea and hyperimmune cow colostrum. *Lancet* 1987;2:344–345.

343. Margulis SJ, Honig CL, Soave R, Govoni AF, Mouradian JA, Jacobson IM. Biliary tract obstruction in the acquired immunodeficiency syndrome. *Ann Intern Med* 1986;105:207–210.

344. Amiel C, May T, Mansuy L, Laurent J, Guibert C, Canton P. *Cryptosporidium* cholangitis treated by celioscopic cholecystectomy and sphincterotomy [Abstract PO-B10-1460]. In: *IXth International Conference on AIDS*, Berlin, 1993;378.

345. Ma P, Villanueva TG, Kaufman D, Gillooley JF. Respiratory cryptosporidiosis in the acquired immune deficiency syndrome: use of modified Kinyoun and Hemacolor stains for rapid diagnoses. *JAMA* 1984;252:1298–1301.

346. Miller RA, Wasserheit JN, Kirihara J, Coyle MB. Detection of *Cryptosporidium* oocysts in sputum during screening for mycobacteria. *J Clin Microbiol* 1984;20:1192–1193.

347. Moore JA, Frenkel JK. Respiratory and enteric cryptosporidiosis in humans. *Arch Pathol Lab Med* 1991;115:1160–1162.

348. Forgacs P, Tarshis A, Ma P, et al. Intestinal and bronchial cryptosporidiosis in an immunodeficient homosexual man. *Ann Intern Med* 1983;99:793–794.

349. Fripp PJ, Bothma MT, Crewe-Brown HH. Four years of cryptosporidiosis at GaRankuwa Hospital. *J Infect* 1991;23:93–100.

350. Højlyng N, Jensen BN. Respiratory cryptosporidiosis in HIV-positive patients. *Lancet* 1988;1:590–591.

351. Goodstein RS, Colombo CS, Illfelder MA, Skaggs RE. Bronchial and gastrointestinal cryptosporidiosis in AIDS. *J Am Osteopath Assoc* 1989;89:195–197.

352. Jensen BN, Gerstoft J, Højlyng N, et al. Pulmonary pathogens in HIV-infected patients. *Scand J Infect Dis* 1990;22:413–420.

353. Jensen BN, Gerstoft J, Skinhøj P. The prognosis in HIV-infected patients with pneumonia. Relation to microbiological diagnoses. *Dan Med Bull* 1991;38:468–470.

354. Brady EM, Margolis ML, Korzeniowski OM. Pulmonary cryptosporidiosis in acquired immune deficiency syndrome. *JAMA* 1984;252:89–90.

355. Davis JJ, Heyman MB. Cryptosporidiosis and sinusitis in an immunodeficient adolescent. *J Infect Dis* 1988;158:649.

356. Martín Sánchez AM, Rodríguez Hernández J, Fuertes Martín A, Canut Blasco A. Criptosporidiasis respiratoria: a propósito de un nuevo caso. *Rev Clin Esp* 1991;189:300–301.

357. Rodríguez Pérez R, Fernández Pérez B, Domínguez Alvarez LM, Naval Calviño G. Criptosporidiasis respiratoria en pacientes VIH. Descripción de dos casos. *Rev Clin Esp* 1992;190: 210–211.

358. Bjarnason I, Keating J, Smith T, Macpherson A, Posniac A, Gazzard BG. Ileal function in HIV infection patients: a comparison with Crohn's disease [Abstract PO-B19-1831]. In: *IXth International Conference on AIDS,* Berlin, 1993;440.

359. Cohen JD, Ruhlig L, Jayich SA, Tong MJ, Lechago J, Snape WJ Jr. *Cryptosporidium* in acquired immunodeficiency syndrome. *Dig Dis Sci* 1984;29:773–777.

360. Gomez Morales MA, Pozio E, Croppo GP. Serodiagnosis of cryptosporidiosis in Italian HIV-positive patients by means of an oocyst soluble antigen in an ELISA. *J Infect* 1992;25: 229–236.

361. Blacklow NR. Case records of the Massachusetts General Hospital: case 39-1985. *N Engl J Med* 1985;313:805–815.

362. Collins CD, Blanshard C, Cramp M, Gazzard B, Gleeson JA. Case report: pneumatosis intestinalis occurring in association with cryptosporidiosis and HIV infection. *Clin Radiol* 1992;46: 410–411.

363. Soulen MC, Fishman EK, Scatarige JC, Hutchins D, Zerhouni EA. Cryptosporidiosis of the gastric antrum: detection using CT. *Radiology* 1986;159:705–706.

364. Cersosimo E, Wilkowske CJ, Rosenblatt JE, Ludwig J. Isolated antral narrowing associated with gastrointestinal cryptosporidiosis in acquired immunodeficiency syndrome. *Mayo Clin Proc* 1992;67:553–556.

365. Falcone S, Murphy BJ, Weinfeld A. Gastric manifestations of AIDS: radiographic findings on upper gastrointestinal examination. *Gastrointest Radiol* 1991;16:95–98.

366. Bonato C, Vigano MG, Nicoletti R, Balconi G, Finazzi R, Del Maschio A. Sonographic diagnosis of cholangitis in AIDS patients [Abstract PO-B10-1437]. In: *IXth International Conference on AIDS,* Berlin, 1993;375.

367. Teixidor HS, Godwin TA, Ramirez EA. Cryptosporidiosis of the biliary tract in AIDS. *Radiology* 1991;180:51–56.

368. Schneiderman DJ, Cello JP, Laing FC. Papillary stenosis and sclerosing cholangitis in the acquired immunodeficiency syndrome. *Ann Intern Med* 1987;106:546–549.

369. Huicho L, Sanchez D, Contreras M, et al. Occult blood and fecal leukoytes as screening tests in childhood infectious diarrhea: an old problem revisited. *Pediatr Infect Dis J* 1993;12: 474–477.

370. Goodgame RW, Genta RM, Clinton White A, Chappell CL. Intensity of infection in AIDS-associated cryptosporidiosis. *J Infect Dis* 1993;167:704–709.

371. Silverman JF, Levine J, Finley JL, Larkin EW, Norris HT. Small-intestinal brushing cytology in the diagnosis of cryptosporidiosis in AIDS. *Diagn Cytopathol* 1990;6:193–196.

372. Connolly GMM, Ellis DS, Williams JE, Tovey G, Gazzard BG. Use of electron microscopy in examination of faeces and rectal and jejunal biopsy specimens. *J Clin Pathol* 1991;44:313–316.

373. Zierdt WS. Concentration and identification of *Cryptosporidium* sp. by use of a parasite concentrator. *J Clin Microbiol* 1984;20:860–861.

374. Perry JL, Matthews JS, Miller GR. Parasite detection efficiencies of five stool concentration systems. *J Clin Microbiol* 1990; 28:1094–1097.

375. Weber R, Bryan RT, Juranek DD. Improved stool concentration procedure for detection of *Cryptosporidium* oocysts in fecal specimens. *J Clin Microbiol* 1992;30:2869–2873.

376. Smith HV, McDiarmid A, Smith AL, Hinson AR, Gilmour RA. An analysis of staining methods for the detection of *Cryptosporidium* spp. oocysts in water-related samples. *Parasitology* 1989;99:323–327.

377. Garcia LS, Bruckner DA, Brewer TC, Shimizu RY. Techniques for the recovery and identification of *Cryptosporidium* oocysts from stool specimens. *J Clin Microbiol* 1983;18: 185–190.

378. Garza D, Hópfer RL, Eichelberger C, Eisenbach S, Fainstein V. Fecal staining methods for screening *Cryptosporidium* oocysts. *J Med Technol* 1984;1:560–563.

379. Ma P, Soave R. Three-step stool examination for cryptosporidiosis in 10 homosexual men with protracted watery diarrhea. *J Infect Dis* 1983;147:824–828.

380. Garcia LS, Current WL. Cryptosporidiosis: clinical features and diagnosis. *Crit Rev Clin Lab Sci* 1989;27:439–460.

381. Casemore DP. ACP Broadsheet 128: June 1991, Laboratory methods for diagnosing cryptosporidiosis. *J Clin Pathol* 1991; 44:445–451.

382. Chichino G, Bruno A, Cevini C, Atzori C, Gatti S, Scaglia M. New rapid staining methods of *Cryptosporidium* oocysts in stool. *J Protozool* 1991;38:212S–214S.

383. MacPherson DW, McQueen R. Cryptosporidiosis: multiattribute evaluation of six diagnostic methods. *J Clin Microbiol* 1993; 31:198–202.

384. Casemore DP, Sands RL, Curry A. *Cryptosporidium* species a "new" human pathogen. *J Clin Pathol* 1985;38:1321–1336.

385. Casemore DP, Armstrong M, Sands RL. Laboratory diagnosis of cryptosporidiosis. *J Clin Pathol* 1985;38:1337–1341.

386. Payne P, Lancaster LA, Heinzman M, McCutchan JA. Identification of *Cryptosporidium* in patients with the acquired immunodeficiency syndrome. *N Engl J Med* 1983;309:613–614.

387. Ungureanu EM, Dontu GE. A new staining technique for the identification of *Cryptosporidium* oocysts in faecal smears. *Trans R Soc Trop Med Hyg* 1992;86:638.

388. Garcia LS, Brewer TC, Bruckner DA. Fluorescence detection of *Cryptosporidium* oocysts in human fecal specimens by using monoclonal antibodies. *J Clin Microbiol* 1987;25:119–121.

389. Garcia LS, Brewer TC, Bruckner DA. Incidence of *Cryptosporidium* in all patients submitting stool specimens for ova and parasite examination: monoclonal antibody IFA method. *Diagn Microbiol Infect Dis* 1989;11:25–27.

390. Garcia LS, Shum AC, Bruckner DA. Evaluation of a new monoclonal antibody combination reagent for direct fluorescence detection of *Giardia* cysts and *Cryptosporidium* oocysts in human fecal specimens. *J Clin Microbiol* 1992;30:3255–3257.

391. Arrowood MJ, Sterling CR. Comparison of conventional staining methods and monoclonal antibody-based methods for *Cryptosporidium* oocyst detection. *J Clin Microbiol* 1989;27: 1490–1495.

392. Rusnak J, Hadfield TL, Rhodes MM, Gaines JK. Detection of *Cryptosporidium* oocysts in human fecal specimens by an indirect immunofluorescence assay with monoclonal antibodies. *J Clin Microbiol* 1989;27:1135–1136.

393. Siddons CA, Chapman PA, Rush BA. Evaluation of an enzyme immunoassay kit for detecting *Cryptosporidium* in faeces and environmental samples. *J Clin Pathol* 1992;45:479–482.

394. Newman RD, Jaeger KL, Wuhib T, Lima AAM, Guerrant RL, Sears CL. Evaluation of an antigen capture enzyme-linked immunosorbent assay for detection of *Cryptosporidium* oocysts. *J Clin Microbiol* 1993;31:2080–2084.

395. Laxer MA, Timblin BK, Patel RJ. DNA sequences for the specific detection of *Cryptosporidium parvum* by the polymerase chain reaction. *Am J Trop Med Hyg* 1991;45:688–694.

396. Laxer MA, D'Nicuola ME, Patel RJ. Detection of *Cryptosporidium parvum* DNA in fixed, paraffin-embedded tissue by the polymerase chain reaction. *Am J Trop Med Hyg* 1992;47: 450–455.

397. Weber R, Bryan RT, Bishop HS, Wahlquist SP, Sullivan JJ, Juranek DD. Threshold of detection of *Cryptosporidium* oocysts in human stool specimens: evidence for low sensitivity of current diagnostic methods. *J Clin Microbiol* 1991;29: 1323–1327.

398. Angus KW, Hutchison G, Campbell I, Snodgrass DR. Prophylactic effects of anticoccidial drugs in experimental murine cryptosporidiosis. *Vet Rec* 1984;114:166–168.

399. Brasseur P, Lemeteil D, Ballet J-J. Anti-cryptosporidial drug activity screened with an immunosuppressed rat model. *J Protozool* 1991;38:230S–231S.

400. Lemeteil D, Roussel F, Favennec L, Ballet JJ, Brasseur P. Assessment of candidate anticryptosporidial agents in an immunosuppressed rat model. *J Infect Dis* 1993;167:766–768.

401. Rehg JE, Hancock ML, Woodmansee DB. Anticryptosporidial activity of sulfadimethoxine. *Antimicrob Agents Chemother* 1988;32:1907–1908.

402. Rehg JE. Anticryptosporidial activity is associated with specific sulfonamides in immunosuppressed rats. *J Parasitol* 1991; 77:238–240.

403. Kim CW. Chemotherapeutic effect of arprinocid in experimental cryptosporidiosis. *J Parasitol* 1987;73:663–666.

404. Menichetti F, Moretti MV, Marroni M, Papili R, Di Candilo F. Diclazuril for cryptosporidiosis in AIDS. *Am J Med* 1991; 90:271–272.

405. Rolston KVI, Fainstein V, Bodey GP. Intestinal cryptosporidiosis treated with eflornithine: a prospective study among patients with AIDS. *J Acquir Immune Defic Syndr* 1989;2: 426–430.

406. Brites C, Moreira ED Jr, Bina JC, Johnson WD Jr, Badaró R. Multiple drug regimen for severe diarrhea associated with *Cryptosporidium* in AIDS patients. *Rev Soc Bras Med Trop* 1991;24:117.

407. Cook DJ, Kelton JG, Stanisz AM, Collins SM. Somatostatin treatment for cryptosporidial diarrhea in a patient with the acquired immunodeficiency syndrome (AIDS). *Ann Intern Med* 1988;108:708–709.

408. Moon HW, Woode GN, Ahrens FA. Attempted chemoprophylaxis of cryptosporidiosis in calves. *Vet Rec* 1982;110:181.

409. Tzipori SR, Campbell I, Angus KW. The therapeutic effect of 16 antimicrobial agents on *Cryptosporidium* infection in mice. *Aust J Exp Biol Med Sci* 1982;60:187–190.

410. Cooperstock M, DuPont HL, Corrado ML, Fekety R, Murray DM. Evaluation of new anti-infective drugs for the treatment of diarrhea caused by *Cryptosporidium*. *Clin Infect Dis* 1992; 15(Suppl 1):S249–S253.

411. Katz MD, Erstad BL, Rose C. Treatment of severe *Cryptosporidium*-related diarrhea with octreotide in a patient with AIDS. *Drug Intell Clin Pharm* 1988;22:134–136.

412. Kreinik G, Burstein O, Landor M, Bernstein L, Weiss LM, Wittner M. Successful management of intractable cryptosporidial diarrhea with intravenous octreotide, a somatostatin analogue. *AIDS* 1991;5:765–767.

413. Romeu J, Miró JM, Sirera G, et al. Efficacy of octreotide in the management of chronic diarrhoea in AIDS. *AIDS* 1991;5: 1495–1499.

414. Simon D, Weiss L, Tanowitz HB, Wittner M. Resolution of *Cryptosporidium* infection in an AIDS patient after improvement of nutritional and immune status with octreotide. *Am J Gastroenterol* 1991;86:615–618.

415. Cello JP, Grendell JH, Basuk P, et al. Effect of octreotide on refractory AIDS-associated diarrhea: a prospective, multicenter clinical trial. *Ann Intern Med* 1991;115:705–710.

416. Beaugerie L, Baumer P, Bérard H, Rozenbaum W, Pialoux G, Lecomte JM. Treatment of refractory diarrhea in AIDS with acetorphan and octreotide: a randomized crossover study [Abstract WS-B21-6]. In: *IXth International Conference on AIDS,* Berlin, 1993;64.

417. Sogni P, Coutarel P, Chaussade S, et al. Effet de l'azidothymidine sur la diarrhée par cryptosporidies chez un sujet atteint du syndrome d'immunodéficience acquise. *Gastroenterol Clin Biol* 1989;13:1087–1088.

418. Chandrasekar PH. "Cure" of chronic cryptosporidiosis during treatment with azidothymidine in a patient with the acquired immune deficiency syndrome. *Am J Med* 1987;83:187.

419. Fayer R, Andrews C, Ungar BLP, Blagburn B. Efficacy of hyperimmune bovine colostrum for prophylaxis of cryptosporidiosis in neonatal calves. *J Parasitol* 1989;75:393–397.

420. Fayer R, Perryman LE, Riggs MW. Hyperimmune bovine colostrum neutralizes *Cryptosporidium* sporozoites and protects mice against oocyst challenge. *J Parasitol* 1989;75:151–153.

421. Fayer R, Guidry A, Blagburn BL. Immunotherapeutic efficacy of bovine colostral immunoglobulins from a hyperimmunized cow against cryptosporidiosis in neonatal mice. *Infect Immun* 1990;58:2962–2965.

422. Flanigan T, Marshall R, Redman D, Kaetzel D, Ungar B. In vitro screening of therapeutic agents against *Cryptosporidium:* hyperimmune cow colostrum is highly inhibitory. *J Protozool* 1991;38:225S–227S.

423. Ungar BLP, Ward DJ, Fayer R, Quinn CA. Cessation of *Cryptosporidium*-associated diarrhea in an acquired immunodeficiency syndrome patient after treatment with hyperimmune bovine colostrum. *Gastroenterology* 1990;98:486–489.

424. Saxon A, Weinstein W. Oral administration of bovine colostrum anti-cryptosporidia antibody fails to alter the course of human cryptosporidiosis. *J Parasitol* 1987;73:413–415.

425. Louie E, Borkowsky W, Klesius PH, et al. Treatment of cryptosporidiosis with oral bovine transfer factor. *Clin Immunol Immunopathol* 1987;44:329–334.

426. McMeeking A, Borkowsky W, Klesius PH, Bonk RS, Holzman S, Lawrence HS. A controlled trial of bovine dialyzable leukocyte extract for cryptosporidiosis in patients with AIDS. *J Infect Dis* 1990;161:108–112.

427. Marshall RJ, Flanigan TP. Paromomycin inhibits *Cryptosporidium* infection of a human enterocyte cell line. *J Infect Dis* 1992;165:772–774.

428. Armitage K, Flanigan T, Carey J, et al. Treatment of cryptosporidiosis with paromomycin: a report of five cases. *Arch Intern Med* 1992;152:2497–2499.

429. Bryan CK, Bryan RT, Stewart JM, Shulman JA, Thompson SE III. Decreased diarrhea frequency and *Cryptosporidium* oocyst excretion in AIDS patients treated with paromomycin [Abstract PO-B10-1446]. In: *IXth International Conference on AIDS,* Berlin, 1993;376.

430. Walmsley S, Phillips J, Loeb M, et al. Effectiveness of paromomycin in cryptosporidiosis in AIDS [Abstract PO-B10-1473]. In: *IXth International Conference on AIDS,* Berlin, 1993;381.

431. Kanyok TP, Novak RM, Danziger LH. Preliminary results of a randomized, blinded, control study of paromomycin (PRM) vs. placebo (PLC) for the treatment of *Cryptosporidium* diarrhea (CD) in AIDS patients (P) [Abstract PO-B10-1508]. In: *IXth International Conference on AIDS,* Berlin, 1993;386.

432. Fichtenbaum CJ, Ritchie DJ, Powderly WG. Use of paromomycin for treatment of cryptosporidiosis in patients with AIDS. *Clin Infect Dis* 1993;16:298–300.

433. Clezy K, Gold J, Blaze J, Jones P. Paromomycin for the treatment of cryptosporidial diarrhoea in AIDS patients. *AIDS* 1991; 5:1146–1147.

434. Bissuel F, Cotte L, Rabodonirina M, Rougier P, Piens MA, Trepo C. Paromomycin therapy for cryptosporidial diarrhoea in 24 AIDS patients [Abstract WS-B13-6]. In: *IXth International Conference on AIDS,* Berlin, 1993;56.

435. Keusch GT, Troncale FJ, Buchanan RD. Malabsorption due to paromomycin. *Arch Intern Med* 1970;125:273–276.

436. White AC Jr, Chappell CL, Hayat CS, Kimball KT, Flanigan TP, Goodgame RW. Paromomycin for cryptosporidiosis in AIDS: a prospective double-blind trial [Abstract 100]. In: *Program and Abstracts of the 33rd Interscience Conference on Antimicrobial Agents and Chemotherapy.* New Orleans, LA: American Society for Microbiology, 1993;138.

437. Sáez-Llorens X. Spiramycin for treatment of *Cryptosporidium* enteritis. *J Infect Dis* 1989;160:342.

438. Sáez-Llorens X, Odio CM, Umaña MA, Morales MV. Spiramycin vs. placebo for treatment of acute diarrhea caused by *Cryptosporidium*. *Pediatr Infect Dis J* 1989;8:136–140.

439. Wittenberg DF, Miller NM, Van den Ende J. Spiramycin is not effective in treating *Cryptosporidium* diarrhea in infants: results

of a double-blind randomized trial. *J Infect Dis* 1989;159:131–132.

440. Sánchez-Mejorada G, Ponce-de-León S, Santiago Y, Carranza D. Efficacy of combined spiramycin and metronidazole in diarrheas due to *Cryptosporidium* or with unidentified cause in patients with AIDS [Abstract PO-B19-1847]. In: *IXth International Conference on AIDS,* Berlin, 1993;443.

441. Centers for Disease Control. Update: treatment of cryptosporidiosis in patients with acquired immunodeficiency syndrome (AIDS). *MMWR Morb Mortal Wkly Rep* 1984;33:117–119.

442. Buhl MR, White JM. Spiramycin-induced thrombocytopenia in a HIV-infected patient. *Scand J Infect Dis* 1992;24:115.

443. Moskovitz BL, Stanton TL, Kusmierek JJE. Spiramycin therapy for cryptosporidial diarrhoea in immunocompromised patients. *J Antimicrob Chemother* 1988;22(Suppl B):189–191.

444. Dunne MW. Open label azithromycin in the treatment of cryptosporidiosis [Abstract PO-B10-1500]. In: *IXth International Conference on AIDS,* Berlin, 1993;385.

445. Sperber SJ, Gornish N. New macrolide antibiotics. *Ann Intern Med* 1992;117:533–534.

446. Soave R, Havlir D, Lancaster D, et al. Azithromycin (AZ) therapy of AIDS-related cryptosporidial diarrhea (CD): a multicenter, placebo-controlled, double-blind study [Abstract 405]. In: *Program and Abstracts of the 33rd Interscience Conference on Antimicrobial Agents and Chemotherapy.* New Orleans, LA: American Society for Microbiology, 1993;193.

447. Kimata I, Uni S, Iseki M. Chemotherapeutic effect of azithromycin and lasalocid on *Cryptosporidium* infection in mice. *J Protozool* 1991;38:232S–233S.

448. Rehg JE. Activity of azithromycin against cryptosporidia in immunosuppressed rats. *J Infect Dis* 1991;163:1293–1296.

449. Rehg JE. Anti-cryptosporidial activity of macrolides in immunosuppressed rats. *J Protozool* 1991;38:228S–230S.

450. Harris M, Deutsch G, MacLean JD, Tye L, Tsoukas CM. A phase I study of letrazuril in AIDS related cryptosporidiosis [Abstract WS-B13-5]. In: *IXth International Conference on AIDS,* Berlin, 1993;56.

451. Rubbert A, Schwab J, Kalden JR, Nüblein H. Myositis, fever, rash and thrombopenia after letrazuril treatment of intestinal cryptosporidiosis: a case report [Abstract PO-B10-1430]. In: *IXth International Conference on AIDS,* Berlin, 1993;373.

452. Walach C, Loeb M, Phillips J, et al. Use of letrazuril in refractory cryptosporidiosis in AIDS [Abstract PO-B10-1472]. In: *IXth International Conference on AIDS,* Berlin, 1993;380.

453. Victor GH, Conway B, Hawley-Foss NC, Manion D, Sahai J. Letrazuril therapy for cryptosporidiosis: clinical response and pharmacokinetics. *AIDS* 1993;7:438–440.

454. Anderson BC. Moist heat inactivation of *Cryptosporidium* sp. *Am J Public Health* 1985;75:1433–1434.

455. Robertson LJ, Campbell AT, Smith HV. Survival of *Cryptosporidium parvum* oocysts under various environmental pressures. *Appl Environ Microbiol* 1992;58:3494–3500.

456. Peeters JE, Mazás EA, Masschelein WJ, Martinez de Maturana IV, Debacker E. Effect of disinfection of drinking water with ozone or chlorine dioxide on survival of *Cryptosporidium parvum* oocysts. *Appl Environ Microbiol* 1989;55:1519–1522.

457. Chapman PA, Rush BA. Efficiency of sand filtration for removing *Cryptosporidium* oocysts from water. *J Med Microbiol* 1990;32:243–245.

458. Korich DG, Mead JR, Madore MS, Sinclair NA, Sterling CR. Effects of ozone, chlorine dioxide, chlorine, and monochloramine on *Cryptosporidium parvum* oocyst viability. *Appl Environ Microbiol* 1990;56:1423–1428.

459. Lorenzo-Lorenzo MJ, Ares-Mazas ME, Villacorta-Martinez de Maturana I, Duran-Oreiro D. Effect of ultraviolet disinfection of drinking water on the viability of *Cryptosporidium parvum* oocysts. *J Parasitol* 1993;79:67–70.

460. Weller IVD, Williams CB, Jeffries DJ, et al. Cleaning and disinfection of equipment for gastrointestinal flexible endoscopy: interim recommendations of a Working Party of the British Society of Gastroenterology. *Gut* 1988;29:1134–1151.

461. Casemore DP, Blewett DA, Wright SE. Cleaning and disinfection of equipment for gastrointestinal flexible endoscopy: interim recommendations of a Working Party of the British Society of Gastroenterology. *Gut* 1989;30:1156–1157.

462. Shepherd RC, Reed CL, Sinha GP. Shedding of oocysts of *Cryptosporidium* in immunocompetent patients. *J Clin Pathol* 1988;41:1104–1106.

463. Ratnam S, Paddock J, McDonald E, Whitty D, Jong M, Cooper R. Occurrence of *Cryptosporidium* oocysts in fecal samples submitted for routine microbiological examination. *J Clin Microbiol* 1985;22:402–404.

464. Baxby D, Hart CA. Cryptosporidiosis. *Br Med J* 1984;289:1148.

465. Soave R, Dubey JP, Ramos LJ, Tummings M. A new intestinal pathogen? *Clin Res* 1986;34:533A.

466. Ortega YR, Sterling CR, Gilman RH, Cama VA, Díaz F. *Cyclospora* species—a new protozoan pathogen of humans. *N Engl J Med* 1993;328:1308–1312.

467. Long EG, White EH, Carmichael WW, et al. Morphologic and staining characteristics of a cyanobacterium-like organism associated with diarrhea. *J Infect Dis* 1991;164:199–202.

468. Long EG, Ebrahimzadeh A, White EH, Swisher B, Callaway CS. Alga associated with diarrhea in patients with acquired immunodeficiency syndrome and in travelers. *J Clin Microbiol* 1990;28:1101–1104.

469. Shlim DR, Cohen MT, Eaton M, Rajah R, Long EG, Ungar BLP. An alga-like organism associated with an outbreak of prolonged diarrhea among foreigners in Nepal. *Am J Trop Med Hyg* 1991;45:383–389.

470. Wurtz RM, Kocka FE, Peters CS, Weldon-Linne CM, Kuritza A, Yungbluth P. Clinical characteristics of seven cases of diarrhea associated with a novel acid-fast organism in the stool. *Clin Infect Dis* 1993;16:136–138.

471. Bendall RP, Lucas S, Moody A, Tovey G, Chiodini PL. Diarrhoea associated with cyanobacterium-like bodies: a new coccidian enteritis of man. *Lancet* 1993;341:590–592.

472. Centers for Disease Control. Outbreaks of diarrheal illness associated with cyanobacteria (blue-green algae)-like bodies—Chicago and Nepal, 1989 and 1990. *MMWR Morb Mortal Wkly Rep* 1991;40:325–327.

473. Hart AS, Ridinger MT, Soundarajan R, Peters CS, Swiatlo AL, Kocka FE. Novel organism associated with chronic diarrhoea in AIDS. *Lancet* 1990;335:169–170.

474. Connor BA, Shlim DR, Scholes JV, Rayburn JL, Reidy J, Rajah R. Pathologic changes in the small bowel in nine patients with diarrhea associated with a coccidia-like body. *Ann Intern Med* 1993;119:377–382.

475. Madico G, Gilman RH, Miranda E, Cabrera L, Sterling CR. Treatment of cyclospora infections with co-trimoxazole. *Lancet* 1993;342:122–123.

Infections of the Gastrointestinal Tract,
edited by M. J. Blaser, P. D. Smith, J. I. Ravdin,
H. B. Greenberg, and R. L. Guerrant
Raven Press, Ltd., New York © 1995.

CHAPTER 73

Microsporidia

Donald P. Kotler and Jan M. Orenstein

DESCRIPTION

Microsporidia are protozoa that exist as obligate intracellular parasites. They are ubiquitous in nature, infecting species in all five classes of vetebrates as well as invertebrates, including arthropods and fish. The phylum Microspora is large, containing approximately 100 genera and 1000 species. They are primitive eukaryotes, containing nuclear membranes, but lack mitochondria, peroxisomes, and Golgi apparatus. Molecular taxonomic methods, based on sequence analysis of ribosomal ribonucleic acid (rRNA), show that microsporidia are similar to prokaryotes and have little homology to other eukaryotes (1). It is speculated that microsporidia branched off early from prototype eukaryotes.

Microsporidia have a unique mode of transmission (2). Microsporidial spores contain an extrusion apparatus consisting of a coiled polar filament and an anchoring disc. Cellular infection occurs through extrusion of the polar filament, followed by ejection of the sporoplasm through the hollow tube. The process of filament extrusion appears to involve an influx of calcium and water into the spore, with a rise in internal pressure. If the plasma membrane of a target cell is breached during this process, the sporoplasm is passed into the cell cytoplasm to continue its life cycle.

Microsporidia were first described in tissue sections about 70 years ago (3) and were recognized as a cause of tissue injury and disease about 30 years ago (4). Microsporidia have been identified as a cause of disease in several species of mammals. Most infections occur in young animals or in association with immune deficiencies. Six genera have been identified as pathogens in humans, three related to species causing disease in animals. *Encephalito-*

D. P. Kotler: Gastrointestinal Division, Department of Medicine, St. Luke's–Roosevelt Hospital Center, New York, and College of Physicians and Surgeons, Columbia University, New York, New York 10032.

J. M. Orenstein: Department of Pathology, George Washington University School of Medicine, Washington, DC 20037.

zoon cuniculi was the first microsporidian shown to cause infection in humans, and its occurrence was originally thought to be rare (5).

Several clinical syndromes are associated with microsporidiosis in patients with AIDS, including diarrhea, keratoconjunctivitis, nephritis, hepatitis, and myositis. Diarrhea and malabsorption are the most common clinical problems associated with microsporidial infection in this immunocompromised population. The aim of this chapter is to describe the clinical features, diagnostic modalities, and treatment of intestinal disease produced by the two species of microsporidia known to infect patients with AIDS.

ENTEROCYTOZOON BIENEUSI

Intestinal microsporidiosis in patients with AIDS was recognized almost simultaneously in different areas of the world. *Enterocytozoon bieneusi* were first observed in 1982 in small intestinal biopsies from AIDS patients in Texas and Washington, DC (6). The first cases were published about the same time (1985) from the United States and France, the latter in a Haitian patient (7,8). Several case reports from the United States and Europe followed these initial reports (9–13), until a series of 20 cases was published (14). By late 1991, almost 100 cases were known, with over 500 cases recognized by the middle of 1993. Cases of *E. bieneusi* have been reported from all continents with prevalence rates comparable to other AIDS-associated opportunistic enteric infections, such as *Cryptosporidium* (15). A recent report identified *E. bieneusi* in an immunocompetent individual with a self-limited diarrheal illness (16), suggesting that infection may be more widespread than previously suspected.

Microbiology

Taxonomy

The initial study of enteric microsporidiosis in an AIDS patient (7) demonstrated characteristics different from all other microsporidia known at the time, allowing its identification as a new genus and species. The characteristic features of *E. bieneusi* are its development as a multinucleate plasmodium in intimate contact with the cell cytoplasm, cleft-like structures called electron-lucent inclusions, and electron-dense discs that fuse to form the polar tubule. Other distinctive features include precocious development of the injection apparatus within the intact plasmodium, six turns of the polar tubule arranged in two layers, and mononuclear spores (1×1.5 μm) that are the smallest of all known microsporidia.

A recent report described a second species of *Enterocytozoon* that infects lymphocyte nuclei in a salmon species (*E. salmonis*) (17).

Life Cycle

The different stages in the life cycle of *E. bieneusi* have been characterized by transmission electron microscopy in several laboratories (6,18). Since no experimental system for *in vitro* culture of *E. bieneusi* is available, the various developmental stages have been characterized in clinical specimens and their sequence inferred from studies of other microsporidia. A single infected enterocyte may contain microsporidial forms in different stages of development. Whether this occurs as a result of multiple infections in the same cell, binary or multiple fission of plasmodial forms, or variable rates of maturation of infectious sporoplasm is unclear.

The earliest stage identified in clinical material is the proliferating plasmodium, or meront (Fig. 1A). These are small (1 μm in diameter), oval, membrane-bound inclusions, usually seen in the apical cytoplasm and usually associated with cellular mitochondria. The meront is more electron lucent than the surrounding cytoplasm and contains free ribosomes but no other recognizable structures. A nucleus is the next structure to be identified, with subsequent development indicated by nuclear division, emergence of rough endoplasmic reticulum, and development of electron-lucent inclusions (Fig. 1B). The electron-lucent inclusions are lined by electron-dense material (best demonstrated by ferric osmium staining) that is destined to form the polar tubule. Later in this stage, electron-dense disc-like structures begin to develop from the clefts (Fig. 1C) as the parasite enters sporogony. Future spores are defined by progressive development and association of the polar tube with its anchoring plate, polaroplast membrane, nucleus, and posterior vacuole. Through a complicated process of membrane invaginations, the sporogonial plasmodium divides into multiple sporonts. With development of the endospore and ectospore, first the sporoblast and then the mature electron-dense egg-shaped spore are formed.

The electron-dense discs, whose appearance indicates the beginning of sporogony, increase in number and size and form flat stacks within the plasmodia (Fig. 1C). In some sections, the discs appear ring-like. Interconnections develop, both end-to-end as well as in a syncytial-like pattern, leading to the coiled tubule. The coiled tube contains six turns in *E. bieneusi* and appears organized into two tiers of three turns each. Furthermore, the two tiers are consistently out of register by about 45 degrees.

Mature spores have been identified during eruption through the lysing enterocyte membrane. Other sections have shown sloughing of dying cells containing mature spores and plasmodia (Fig. 1D). However, some cells retain viability for a period of time after sloughing. For this reason, it is possible that spore maturation could proceed after the enterocyte has been extruded into the intestinal lumen.

Epidemiology

Although *E. bieneusi* was initially regarded as an uncommon pathogen, it is recognized now as a common enteric infection in patients with AIDS. Prevalence rates among AIDS patients have varied between 2% and 50% (19–25) depending on the study group and methods of diagnosis. Our own series of 250 consecutive HIV-infected individuals revealed an incidence of 33% in AIDS patients with diarrhea (25). A recent prospective study of HIV-infected patients with and without diarrhea showed *E. bieneusi* prevalence rates of over 20% for each group, irrespective of CD4 lymphocyte count, coinfections, or other clinical parameters (24). If confirmed, these results suggest that *E. bieneusi* infection is not necessarily associated with diarrhea but may be present in a clinically latent form for long periods of time.

The mode of transmission of *E. bieneusi* has not been defined. Most investigators suspect the parasite is acquired by ingestion of contaminated food and water and not by sexual activity. Although the majority of cases have been diagnosed in homosexual males, we have diagnosed *E. bieneusi* in two heterosexual women and in one 12-year-old girl, consistent with transmission by a nonsexual route.

Several studies have examined the development of symptomatic microsporidiosis as a function of the level of immune deficiency (25–28). The results demonstrated that microsporidiosis typically was diagnosed in patients with severe depletion of CD4 lymphocytes (18 to 30 cells/mm^3). The one study finding similar prevalence rates in patients with and without diarrhea showed mean CD4 lymphocyte counts of 113 and 192 cells/mm^3 in patients with and without diarrhea, respectively (24).

Pathogenesis and Immunity

Current understanding of disease pathogenesis related to *E. bieneusi* infection is based on clinicopathologic correlations and the pattern of intestinal injury. After passage of ingested spores into the intestinal lumen, the polar filament is extruded, possibly in response to the higher pH in the small intestinal lumen and other local factors (2). The polar filament likely facilitates infection of epithelial cells, which are eventually destroyed. The sloughed cells release mature spores into the lumen, and the infection continues via autoinfection. The life cycle of other microsporidia has been measured *in vitro* and is complete within

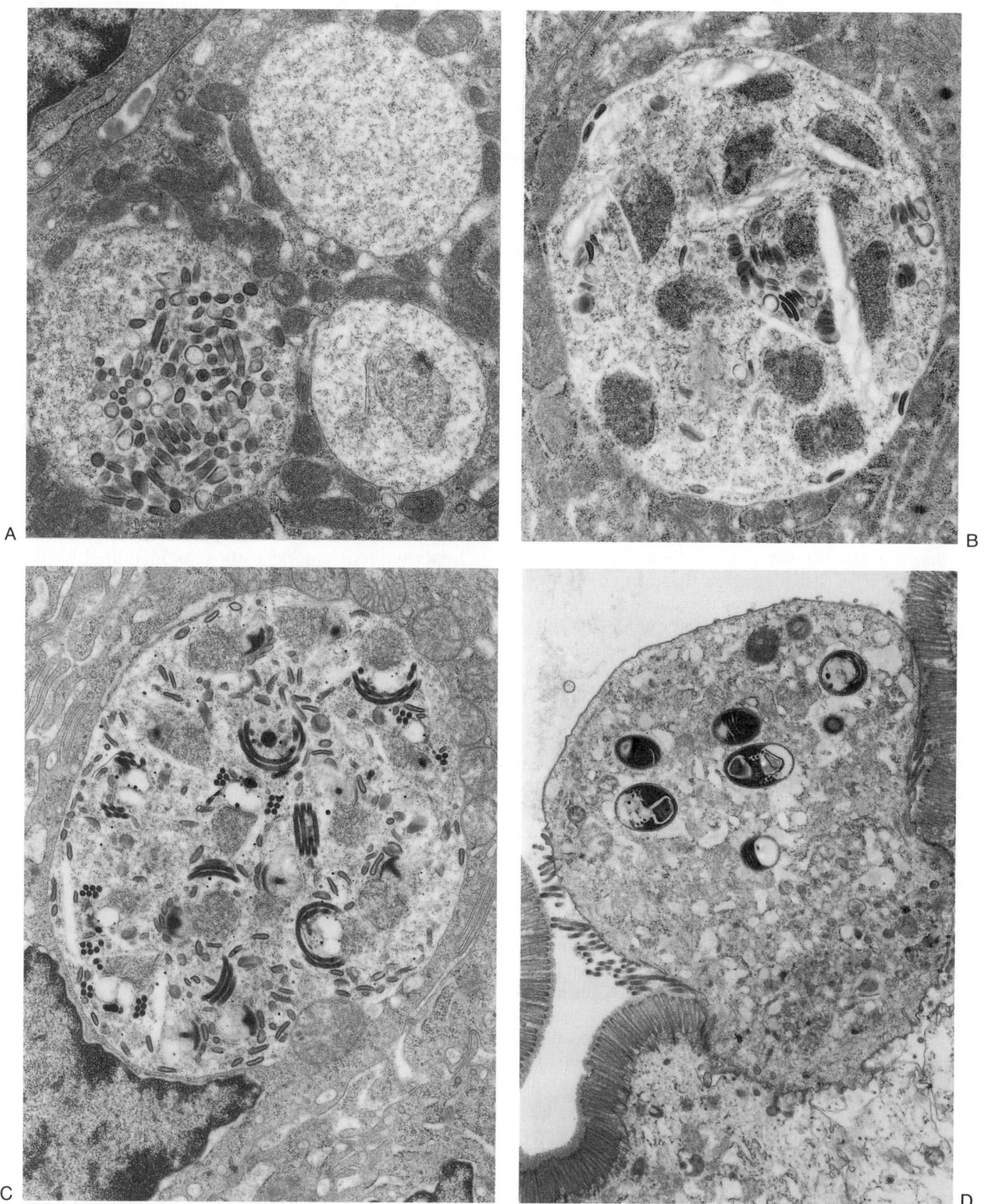

FIG. 1. Transmission electron microscopy of *E. bieneusi*. **A:** Two proliferative plasmodia, a very early one without a nucleus (**upper right**) and one with a single nucleus (**lower right**), and a sporogonial plasmodium (**lower left**) containing electron-dense disc and rod-shaped precursors of polar tubes. Note the intimate association of the cell's electron-dense mitochondria with the plasmodia. (×14850). **B:** An early sporogonial plasmodium with several electron-dense nuclei and discs and prominent electron-lucent clefts. (×13950). **C:** A single late sporogonial plasmodium molding the apical nuclear pole. Future spores are identified by the polar tubes coiling around nuclei and polar vacuoles. When cut on-end, the double layer of three turns is visible. (×13140). **D:** A shedding cell, with few microvilli, contains several spores with polar vacuoles. (×7200).

TABLE 1. *Effect of microsproidiosis on intestinal structure and function*

	Villous height[a]	Crypt depth[b]	Sucrase[a]	Lactase[c]	Maltase	D-Xylose[c]
Micro	50 ± 3	92 ± 11	140 ± 10	40 ± 10	1300 ± 430	16.1 ± 1.3
AIDS controls	86 ± 15	71 ± 8	500 ± 100	210 ± 30	2050 ± 310	31.2 ± 3.8
Controls	85 ± 8	52 ± 5	530 ± 130	190 ± 10	2040 ± 310	20–50

Adapted from ref. 34.
[a] $P < 0.01$.
[b] $P < 0.005$.
[c] $P < 0.001$.
Micro, patients with microsporidiosis; AIDS controls, AIDS patients with no pathogens detected by transmission electron microscopy of jejunal biopsies. Data as mean ± SE; villous heights and crypt depth in microns; sucrase, lactase, and maltase in units/mg protein; D-xylose as 1-hr serum value after 25-g oral dose.

a few hours (29). Spores may travel from cell to cell beneath the mucous layer, infecting contiguous cells, or may enter the luminal fluid and potentially infect a noncontiguous cell. It is unclear which mechanism is more important or if alternative mechanisms of cell-to-cell transmission occur.

The development of clinical disease is based on the continuous excess loss of epithelial cells. Although the specific pathogenic mechanisms differ, intestinal dysfunction in *E. bieneusi* infection resembles that of patients with tropical sprue and celiac disease, two diseases characterized by excess losses of villous enterocytes (30). Functional homeostasis in the intestine is regulated, in part, by coordinated modulation of cell proliferation and loss (31). The average turnover time for an epithelial cell is approximately 72 hr, during which time cell maturation and senescence occur. Different amounts of time are required for maturation of various enterocyte enzymes. For example, the specific activities of the brush border disaccharidases, maltase and sucrase, are roughly equivalent along the length of the villus while the specific activities of lactase and the enzymes of fatty acid esterification are absent in the lower villus and peak in the upper villus (32–33).

The rates of cell proliferation and loss are affected by many physiologic and pathologic stimuli. In addition, cell proliferation is affected by the rate of cell loss and *vice versa*. Under conditions of increased cell loss, such as during infections, compensatory crypt hyperplasia occurs and returns villous architecture toward normal, resulting in partial villous atrophy and crypt hyperplasia. The migration rate of newly formed enterocytes may be increased, leaving insufficient time for full functional maturation. For this reason, there are greater deficits in lactose and fat absorption than in starch and sucrose absorption in diseases producing villous atrophy and crypt hyperplasia.

The relationships between *E. bieneusi* infection and intestinal structure and function have been examined in patients with AIDS (34). Partial villous atrophy and crypt hyperplasia were present in AIDS patients with microsporidiosis and cryptosporidiosis but not in those without enteric pathogens (Table 1). Similarly, decreased levels of sucrase, lactase, and maltase were found in biopsies from AIDS patients with cryptosporidiosis and microsporidiosis, whereas normal levels were present in those without enteric pathogens. The ratios of sucrase to lactase (S/L) and maltase to lactase (M/L) are higher in the patients with parasitoses, implying a disproportionate loss of lactase. D-Xylose malabsorption also was prevalent in patients with parasitoses, but not in those without infections. Finally, small intestinal structure and function were fully preserved at the ultrastructural level in many patients without enteric pathogens identified by transmission electron microscopy (34).

Little is known about immunity to *E. bieneusi* infection. Two groups have detected antibodies to microsporidia using antigens derived from other microsporidia (35,36). There is no published information on the role of cell-mediated immunity in microsporidiosis, although clinical specimens often show increased numbers of intraepithelial mononuclear cells in areas containing *E. bieneusi*.

Clinical Illness

The clinical features of *E. bieneusi* enteritis are characteristic but vary in intensity (37). Typically, three to ten nonbloody bowel movements of variable volume and consistency occur at irregular intervals. The bowel movements tend to be clustered during one portion of the day, usually late evening or early morning. Nocturnal diarrhea is uncommon. Some of the bowel movements are watery and of large volume, while formed stools may occasionally be passed. Although diarrhea may not be present in every patient with *E. bieneusi* infection, evidence of enteropathy has been found in all in whom it has been sought. Excessive flatus and an alteration in the odor of feces and flatus are often present. The infection is not accompanied by fever. Patients with mild disease may describe intolerance to lactose and fat, whereas those with more severe disease are affected by almost all food intake. When severe, the diarrhea is associated with dehydration and electrolyte abnormalities, predominantly hypokalemia and hypomagnesemia. Serum bicarbonate concentrations may be subnormal, reflecting fecal losses.

No studies of resting energy expenditure in patients with microsporidiosis have been reported, although we observed subnormal resting energy expenditure in malnourished AIDS patients with malabsorption irrespective of cause (38). Patients note that appetite is preserved, but calorie counts often reveal inadequate food intake. Clinically, a prolonged satiety phase is observed, similar to that of other clinical and experimental malabsorption syndromes (39). Typically, the patient eats a normal breakfast and small lunch but is unable to eat any dinner. This eating pattern may be related to the presence of unabsorbed nutrients in the lower intestine, changes in gastric and pancreatic secretion, and disturbances in gastric emptying and small intestinal transit (40–42). Weight loss occurs slowly, and its rate may diminish over time. Rapid changes in weight usually are related to alterations in fluid balance associated with a change in the intensity of diarrhea. Studies of hydration status have shown that patients with microsporidiosis are chronically dehydrated compared to normal subjects and AIDS patients without malabsorption (43).

Microsporidiosis is associated with biliary tract disease (44–46) and is a potential cause of the cholangiopathy that may accompany AIDS (47). Involvement of the biliary tract often resembles primary sclerosing cholangitis (48), similar to the cholangiopathy associated with cryptosporidiosis and cytomegalovirus infection. Sclerosing cholangitis may be the final result of bile duct epithelial injury due to many causes. The syndrome is characterized biochemically by progressive elevations in serum activities of alkaline phosphatase and gamma glutamyl transpeptidase; bilirubin concentration usually is normal and transaminases are only mildly affected. Some patients complain of epigastric or right upper quadrant discomfort or pruritis; others are asymptomatic. Abdominal pain appears to be related to papillitis and papillary stenosis. AIDS cholangiopathy has been associated with progressive liver disease and liver failure in a few patients (D. P. Kotler, *unpublished data*), although it has not been reported in patients with *E. bieneusi* cholangiopathy. The authors have seen a case of subacute pancreatitis associated with chronic pain in a pediatric patient with *E. bieneusi* infection, although histologic examination of the pancreas or pancreatic ducts was not performed.

Diagnosis

The ability to diagnose *E. bieneusi* has undergone remarkable changes over the past several years. Initially, the diagnosis was based exclusively on transmission electron microscopy. The recognition that the parasite can be identified in tissue sections by light microscopy (49–51), coupled with confirmatory special stains (52,53), coincided with a marked increase in the number of cases that were diagnosed. More recently, techniques for the diagnosis of microsporidiosis have been applied to fecal specimens, broadening the pool of patients in whom a search for microsporidiosis is possible. Studies to correlate the sensitivities, specificities, and predictive values for the various diagnostic modalities will allow standardization of these techniques. Development of molecular techniques for the identification of *E. bieneusi* carries the promise of increased diagnostic sensitivity.

Electron Microscopy

The diagnosis of *E. bieneusi* infection by transmission electron microscopy is based on detection of the developing forms within enterocytes (see earlier discussion). Ultrastructural studies can be performed without regard to tissue orientation. All forms are readily detected except the early meronts, which may resemble tangential sections of intraepithelial mononuclear cells. The key difference is that the meronts are intracellular while intraepithelial mononuclear cells are intercellular in location. Enterocyte injury can be seen, but it is nonspecific.

Light Microscopy

Routine light microscopic diagnosis of *E. bieneusi* infection is difficult since the developing forms do not stain well with standard hematoxylin and eosin preparations. Detection of *E. bieneusi* is aided by its association with a characteristic pattern of tissue injury and cytopathology. As previous studies have indicated that the distal duodenum and proximal jejunum may have a higher parasite burden than the proximal duodenum (54), the endoscopist is advised to take biopsies from the most distal site possible. In addition, since biopsies may contain villi denuded of enterocytes, possibly due to cellular injury, several biopsies (usually six to eight) should be taken to ensure that sufficient numbers of intact villi are available for review. While a well-oriented specimen is not a requirement for proper identification, it greatly assists the observer in diagnosis. Biopsies containing long, slender villi and short crypts are very unlikely to harbor *E. bieneusi*.

Enterocytozoon bieneusi infection is associated with variable degrees of villous atrophy and crypt hyperplasia (Fig. 2A). In some cases, villous height is nearly normal and marked crypt hyperplasia is present. In other cases, significant villous atrophy is associated with less marked crypt hyperplasia. The reason for this variation is unknown but may reflect differences in parasite burden or endogenous factors, such as nutritional status. The degree of injury usually is similar in different biopsies obtained from the same area. Microsporidial infection of colonic epithelium has been reported (55), although the parasite burden is much lower than in the small intestine.

Enterocytozoon bieneusi causes cellular injury predominantly in the upper third of the villus. Typically, the numbers of intraepithelial mononuclear cells are increased. Infiltration with neutrophils or eosinophils does not occur. Infected epithelium shows disarray, atrophy, increased basophilia, and pleomorphism (Fig. 2B). The villous tips show piling up of cells, many of which are infected and in the process of being sloughed from the surface. Individual sloughing cells appear as teardrop-shaped cells, invariably containing refractile spores (Fig. 2C). This finding is characteristic of microsporidiosis and is its most readily recognized diagnostic feature.

The villous enterocytes demonstrate cytopathic changes, including pleomorphism, hyperchromatic nuclei, and loss of the basal orientation of nuclei. Entero-

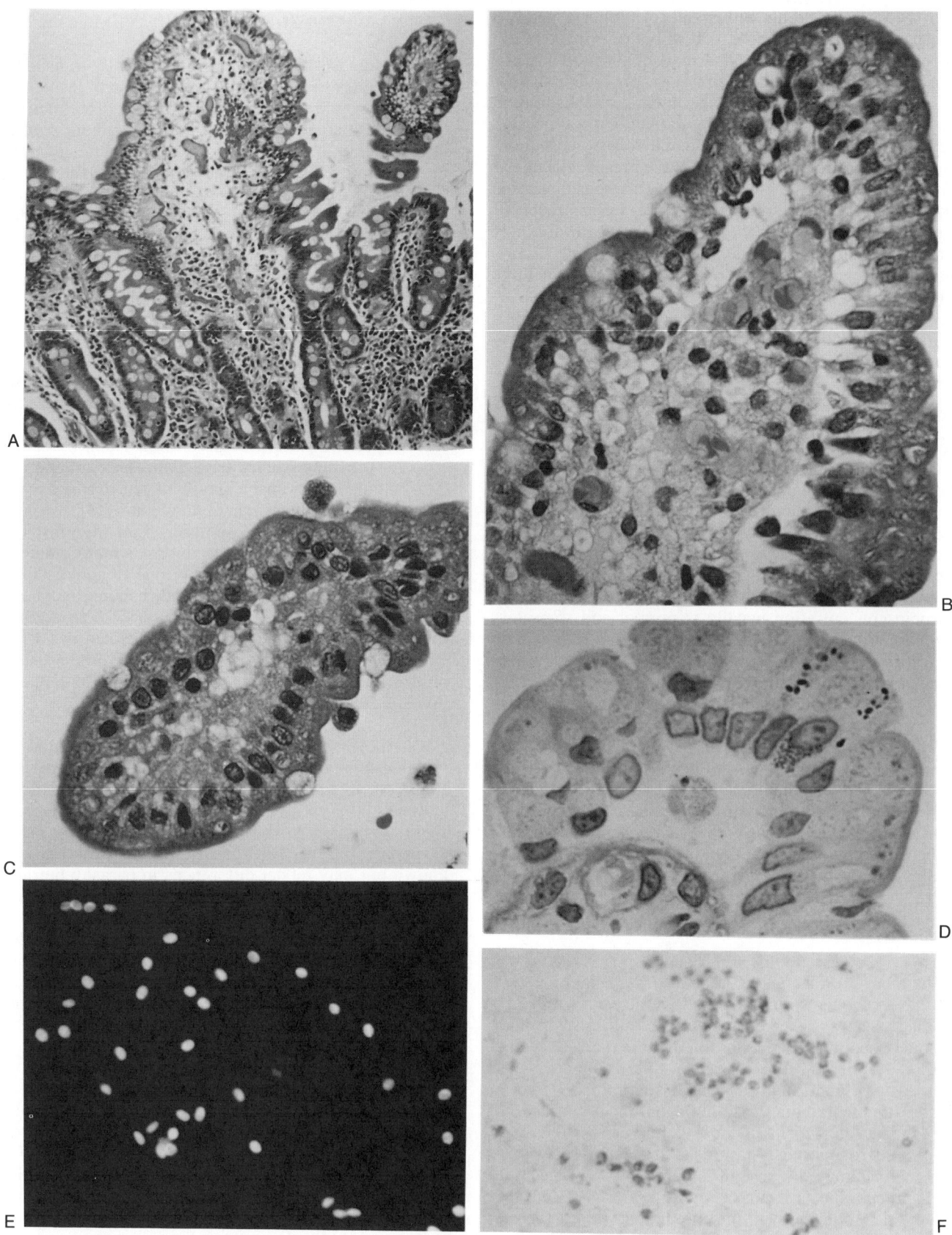

FIG. 2. Light microscopy of *E. bieneusi*. **A:** A distorted villus and elongated crypts typical of microsporidia infection. Several shed enterocytes are visible. (×152, H&E). **B:** Clear clefts are visible in some of the many bluish supranuclear plasmodia at the tip of a villus. Note the characteristic vacuolization and separation of enterocytes at the basement membrane. (×608, H&E). **C:**

TABLE 2. *Diagnosis of microsporidiosis by light microscopy*

Measurement	H&E	Gram	Giemsa	Chromotrope	Touch
Sensitivity (%)	83	77	57	83	83
Specificity (%)	95	100	100	100	100
(±) Predictive value (%)	94	100	100	100	100
(−) Predictive value (%)	88	88	75	88	88

Adapted from ref. 58.
H&E, hematoxylin and eosin; Gram, Brown–Hopp's tissue Gram stain; Chromotrope, chromatrope 2R modified trichrome stain; Touch, Giemsa stain of mucosal touch preparations.

cytes may show increased numbers of lysosomes, vesiculation, vacuolization, and occasional lipid accumulation. The epithelial layer contains an excess of cellular debris. The lamina propria may contain increased numbers of plasma cells and macrophages, but not neutrophils.

The various stages of *E. bieneusi* do not stain well or predictably with hematoxylin and eosin (H&E). Light microscopy of 1-μm, plastic-embedded sections stained with either toluidine blue or trichrome (methylene blue, basic fuchsin, azure II) stain are ideal for identifying *E. bieneusi*, increasing the sensitivity for detecting the organism to that of transmission electron microscopy. As the organisms develop in the supranuclear and apical cytoplasm, they may affect nuclear shape, producing a flattening or cupping of the apical pole (Fig. 2D). Electron-lucent clefts also may be visible, especially when flanked by material that picks up the hematoxylin stain. The result is a cat's-eye appearing structure in the apical portion of the cell. Although it is an artifact, plasmodia can appear to be within a vacuole. Rarely, spores may be detected as clusters of negatively staining or refractile granular material in the cytoplasm of individual, but especially sloughing, cells (Fig. 2C). Examination under polarized light is another effective means of detecting *E. bieneusi*, as the spores are birefringent, particularly in Gram-stained sections.

Special Preparations and Procedures

Special stains and preparations may enhance the ease of diagnosis or allow confirmation in a suspicious case, especially when transmission electron microscopy is not readily available. The stains include Gram, Giemsa, acid-fast, Warthin–Starry, and a modified tissue trichrome chromotrope 2R stain, as described for examination of fecal specimens (56). In addition, Giemsa-stained touch preparations of fresh mucosal biopsies may be helpful (56,57). We prospectively evaluated the sensitivities, specificities, and predictive values for these stains compared to transmission electron microscopy (Table 2)(58). The sensitivities and negative predictive values of the different techniques ranged from 57% to 88% while the specificities and positive predictive values ranged from 94% to 100%. As part of this study, methods for quantitating parasite burden were devised. The parasite burden was lower in cases with false-negative results than in those diagnosed correctly by any of the methods, suggesting that a false-negative diagnosis is related to a low parasite burden. Gram and Giemsa stains showed spores and some visualization of other intracellular forms, whereas the chromotrope stains and touch preparations demonstrated only spores. A surprising finding was the excellent sensitivity of diagnosing *E. bieneusi* in H&E-stained sections, albeit by observers with extensive clinical experience. The ability to correctly diagnose microsporidiosis by H&E-stained sections has been noted by several investigators (49,50,51,55,57).

Luminal fluid obtained by aspiration or lavage, or mucosal cytobrush preparations, also may be helpful in detecting microsporidia (59). Spores are readily identified in duodenal brush specimens with Giemsa, Gram, Diff-Quik, and modified trichrome stains. The chromotrope 2R stain allows differentiation between microsporidial spores and bacteria, since bacteria (light green counterstain) do not take up the chromotrope stain.

Stool Examination

The use of special stains and light microscopy has increased the ability to diagnose *E. bieneusi* infection, but they are of limited value since endoscopy with biopsy, or passage of a small intestinal tube for fluid aspiration or capsule biopsy, is required. The use of fecal specimens for diagnosis would greatly simplify diagnosis. Several techniques have been applied successfully. Giemsa staining of a fecal preparation that was homogenized, sieved, centrifuged, and extensively washed revealed *E. bieneusi* spores (60). The chromotrope 2R modified trichrome stain

The spores in one (**upper**) of the two shedding enterocytes are slightly refractile. Many bluish supranuclear plasmodia are visible. (×608, H&E). **D:** The spores stain dark blue while the plasmodia stain lighter than the cytoplasm in semithin plastic sections. The darker "dots" within the plasmodia are nuclei. There is a spore in a shed cell within the space created by the sloughing enterocytes. ×950; methylene-blue, basic fuchsin, azure II). **E:** The spores fluoresce white to pink using the Calcifluor whitening agent. (Courtesy of Dr. Elizabeth Didier.) (Duodenal fluid, ×1520). **F:** The spores stain pink and the background light blue in the modified trichrome, chromotrope 2R stain (61). The polar vacuole and a central band can be seen in several of the spores. (×1425). (See Plate 18.)

also has been used to detect spores in stool, staining *E. bieneusi* spores pink and most other material green (61)(Fig. 2F). Occasional yeast forms or bacteria take up the chromotrope stain, but they differ from *E. bieneusi* in size and shape. The advantage of this stain is that specimens without special preparation or formalin-fixed stool may be used. However, attention to the staining conditions, especially decolorization, is required. A further modification of this method, staining at 56°C, decreases the time required for the parasite to take up the stain (62). An alternative method for studying fecal specimens is based on binding of the fluorochrome, Uvitex 2B of Calcifluor, to chitin, which is a component of the microsporidial cell wall (63). This technique is quite sensitive and works well with fresh or concentrated preparations (Fig. 2E). Although prior formalin fixation reduces the staining, it is still within acceptable diagnostic levels.

Treatment

Drug Therapy

Few studies of drug therapy of *E. bieneusi* infection have been published. Symptomatic response to antiparasitic agents, such as metronidazole, has been reported, although histologic evidence of infection persists (64). A group from London reported their preliminary experience in the treatment of intestinal microsporidiosis using albendazole, an antitubulin drug (65). All six patients studied had a complete symptomatic response, although follow-up biopsies were still positive (B. Gazzard, *personal communication*). A prospective, published study of 29 patients and observations in a total of 66 patients with *E. bieneusi* confirmed that albendazole therapy leads to symptomatic improvement and weight stabilization (66). However, follow-up biopsies continued to show evidence of infection and follow-up D-xylose absorption tests failed to show evidence of improvement. Confirmation of the beneficial effect of albendazole awaits the completion of a double-blind, placebo-controlled trial.

Other antimicrobials such as humatin and trimethoprim–sulfamethoxazole have been used anecdotally (67). Despite symptomatic improvement, the use of these agent is associated with continued infection, intestinal injury, and malabsorption.

Fluid, Electrolyte, and Nutritional Therapies

Patients with *E. bieneusi* infection are chronically dehydrated (44) and may be depleted of both macronutrients and micronutrients. Electrolyte and mineral deficits, particularly K^{2+}, Ca^{2+}, and Mg^{2+}, may be severe (68). Diet modification may be helpful in patients with mild-to-moderate disease. A lactose-free, low-fat diet with calorie-rich fluid supplements containing extra protein may be well tolerated. Elemental diets also may be well tolerated but their efficacy in maintaining or repleting body mass has not been established. Parenteral nutritional therapy resulted in nutritional repletion in some patients (69). Hydrophilic bulking agents are variably effective, depending on the level of malabsorption. Opiates such as diphenoxy-late, paregoric, or tincture of opium may be effective, although the dose required sometimes causes excessive sedation. Formulas containing substantial quantities of long-chain fats and high concentrations of sugar are not recommended, as they often cause bloating and increased diarrhea, leading to decreased intake for fear of precipitating symptoms.

Prevention

Recommendations for prevention of microsporidiosis are not available, since the reservoirs and routes of transmission of *E. bieneusi* have not been elucidated.

SEPTATA INTESTINALIS

The first 40 cases of microsporidiosis reported in patients with AIDS were due to infection with *E. bieneusi*. In 1988, we identified a microsporidium by transmission electron microscopy that differed ultrastructurally from *E. bieneusi* (70). Two years later, three additional cases were identified. Since then, identification of the second microsporidium, named *Septata intestinalis* (71), with a prevalence one-tenth that of *E. bieneusi*, has been made in the United States, Europe, and Australia.

Microbiology

Taxonomic analysis permitted the classification of the organism within a new genus and species. Distinctive morphologic features include a unique development of individual cells within separate chambers of a parasitophorous vacuole (Fig. 3A). The developing organisms are separated by septa of parasite origin. Other distinguishing features include completion of merogony prior to development of the polar tubule, the lack of electron-lucent inclusions or electron-dense discs, the polar tubule with a single tier of five to six turns, and spores of 2.2×1.2 μm (Fig. 3B).

Epidemiology, Pathogenesis, and Immunity

The epidemiology, pathogenesis, and immunity of *S. intestinalis* have not been studied but are presumed to be the same as for *E. bieneusi*. Transmission likely is via the fecal–oral route. In contrast to infection with *E. bieneusi*, *S. intestinalis* infection is not limited to small intestinal enterocytes but also infects lamina propria macrophages. Renal involvement has been confirmed by the identification of spores, both free and within cells, in urinary sediment (Fig. 3B). Ultrastructural analysis of cell preparations revealed infection of both tubule cells (microvilli) and transitional cells (elongated cells with prominent cytokeratin). Autopsy material from a patient showed a granulomatous interstitial nephritis, with *S. intestinalis* in the proximal and distal convoluted tubule. Parasites also were found in the liver, both free and within cells of the portal vein, and endothelial and Kupffer cells, as well as in the gallbladders and biliary epithelium of three other

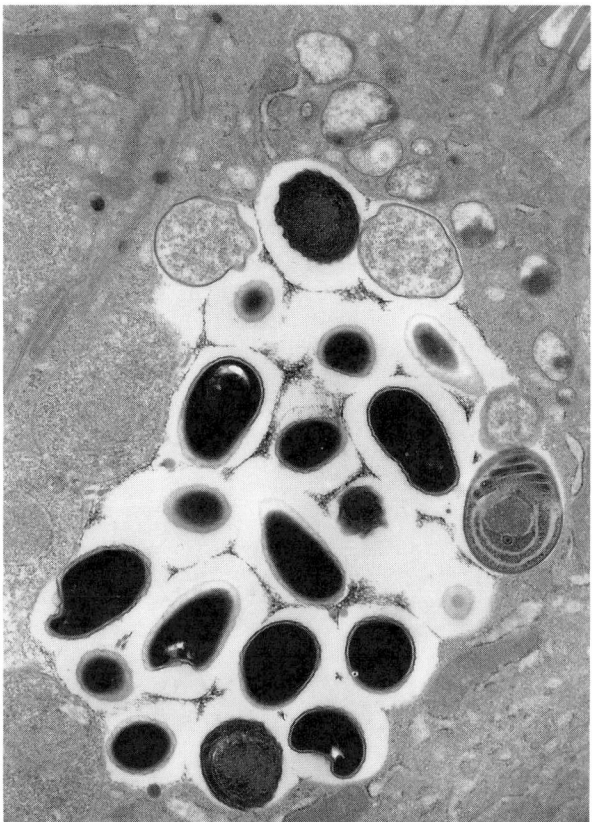

A

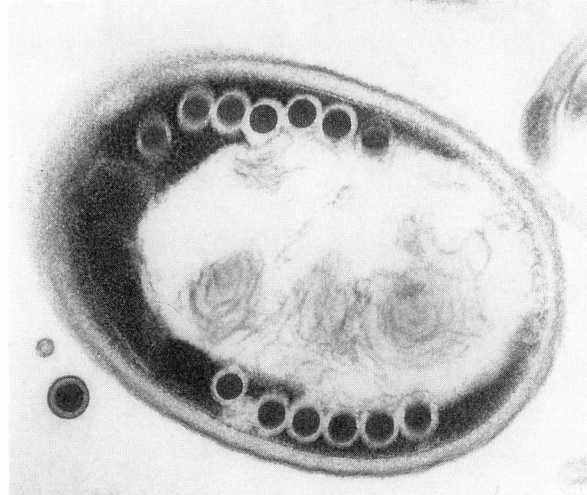

B

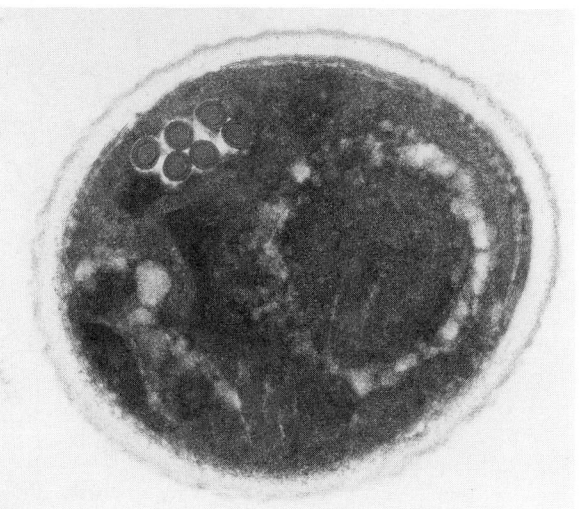

C

FIG. 3. Transmission electron microscopy of *Septata intestinalis.* **A:** Electron-dense fibrillar material divides the parasitophorous vacuole into chambers containing irregular light-staining meronts (on the vacuole edge) and oval sporoblasts/sporonts (coils visible in one), and more central electron-dense spores. (×9900). **B:** Spores of *S. intestinalis* have a single row of five to seven coils. Note the prominent polar vacuole. (Urine, ×54000). **C:** Spores of *E. bieneusi* have a double row of three turns each. Note the single nucleus and the ectospore and endospore layers. (Stool, ×69,300.)

patients (72). Recently, *S. intestinalis* was identified in the upper respiratory tract (73). Thus, in contrast to *E. bieneusi*, *S. intestinalis* disseminates widely to extraintestinal sites.

Clinical Illness

Clinically, intestinal infection with *S. intestinalis* is similar to *E. bieneusi* infection and is consistent with malabsorption. AIDS cholangiopathy also has been associated with *S. intestinalis* infection (72). Although patients with spores in urine sediment may be asymptomatic, some have flank pain and symptoms of urethritis. Parasites have been associated with a rectal ulcer as well as chronic sinusitis. It will be important to determine if this organism

infects the central nervous system and causes neurological syndromes in AIDS patients, like *E. cuniculi* in animals. Interestingly, the first patient reportedly (70) died from sudden multiorgan system failure, including encephalopathy.

Diagnosis

Septata intestinalis is diagnosed by the same techniques as *E. bieneusi*. The organism is usually easier to detect, due to its larger size, greater refractility, birefringence, staining qualities, and greater parasite burden. The electron microscopic features were noted earlier. As with *E. bieneusi*, the parasite and its associated pathology localize to the distal villus. Individual cell shedding is less

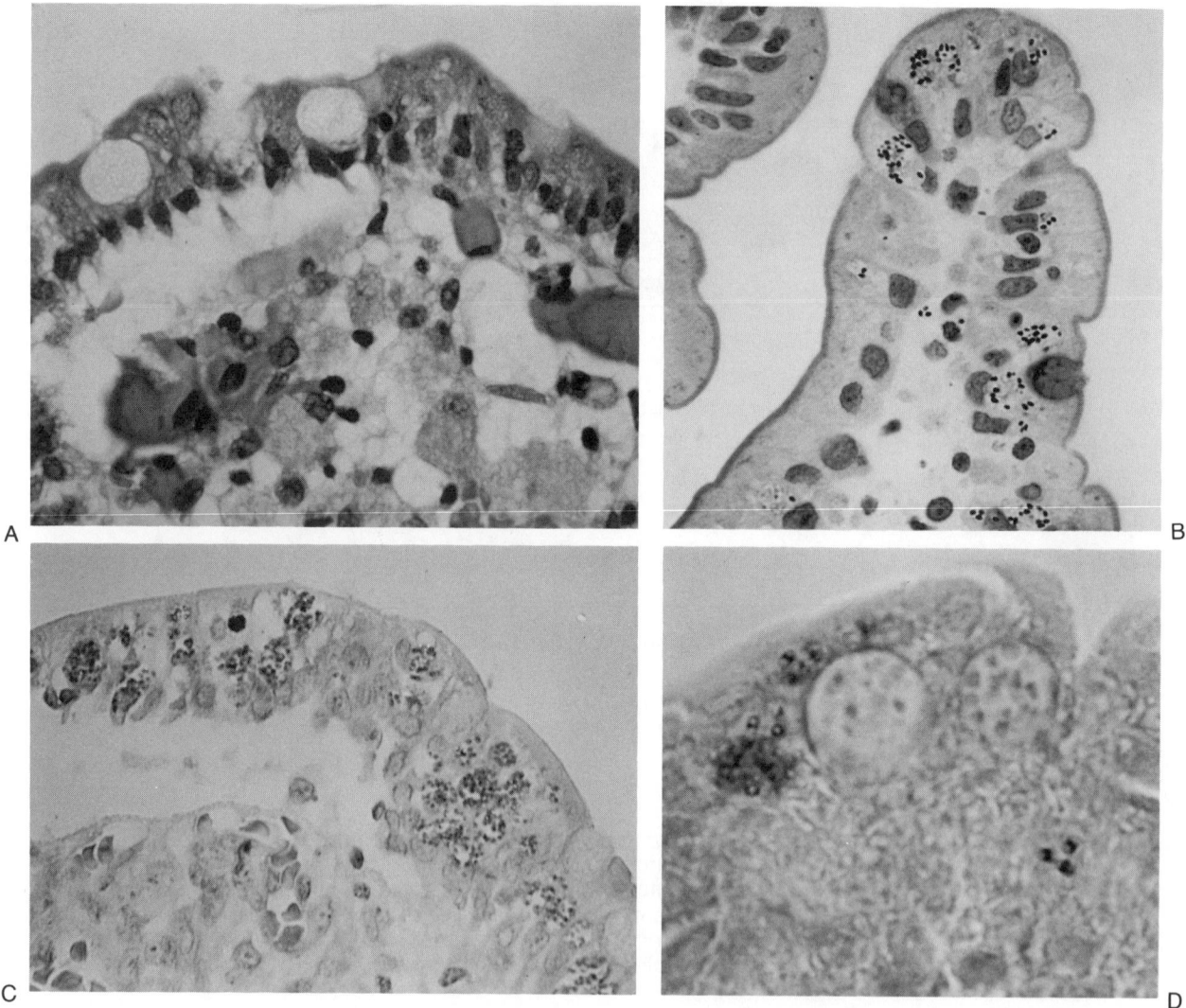

FIG. 4. Light microscopy of *S. intestinalis*. **A:** In H&E-stained sections the spores appear as supranuclear collections of refractile bluish bodies. Strips of enterocytes are frequently seen shedding. Some of the prominent lamina propria macrophages contain spores. (×576). **B:** In plastic sections the spores stain dark blue. (×576). **C:** A partially polarized Brown–Brenn, Gram stain showing the pink birefringence of some of the dark red-staining spores. (×576). **D:** A characteristic dark-staining central band is visible in some of the spores. Brown–Brenn-stained paraffin section. (×1080) (See Plate 19.).

frequent than sloughing of whole groups of attached enterocytes. Epithelial disarray is also present. The spores are brightly birefringent and stain to a much greater degree than *E. bieneusi* spores (Fig. 4). As is typical for microsporidia, the spores are gram-positive (something not easily demonstrated with *E. bieneusi*). Macrophages (even endothelial cells and fibroblasts) containing spores can be seen in the lamina propria. As noted earlier, free spores and cells containing spores can be found in urinary sediment, and spores can be detected in stool.

Treatment

Septata intestinalis differs from *E. bieneusi* in its uniformly good response to albendazole therapy (73,74). Although relatively few cases have been studied, all have responded clinically with a decrease or disappearance of diarrhea and a clearing of spores from the urine and stool. Follow-up biopsies have shown disappearance of spores and only ghosts of spores within macrophage lysosomes. Improvement in D-xylose absorption has been noted (73). Whether or not viable sporoplasm and spores are being sequestered in some location is unknown.

Management of fluid and electrolyte status and nutritional therapy are similar to those for *E. bieneusi* infection.

CONCLUSION

Despite recognition that microsporidiosis is a potentially important cause of intestinal disease in HIV-infected individuals, major gaps in our understanding of the transmission, life cycle, and immunobiology of microsporidia remain. Molecular techniques (75) and the ability to propagate the organism *in vitro* should be helpful in addressing these issues and, ultimately, developing effective therapies for *E. bieneusi* and *S. intestinalis*.

REFERENCES

1. Vossbrinck CR, Maddox JV, Friedman S, Debrunner-Vossbrinck BA, Woese CR. Ribosomal RNA sequence suggests microsporidia are extremely ancient eukaryotes. *Nature* 1987;326: 411–414.
2. Canning EU, Hollister WS. Microsporidia of mammals—widespread pathogens or opportunistic curiosities? *Parasitol Today* 1987;3:267–273.
3. Levaditi C, Nicolau S, Schoen R. L'etiologie de l'encephalite. *C R Acad Sci* 1923;177:985–988.
4. Matsubayashi H, Koike T, Mikata I, Takei H, Hagiwara S. A case of *Encephalitozoon*-like infection in man. *Arch Pathol* 1959; 67:181–187.
5. Bergquist NR, Waller T, Mravak S, Meyer U. Report of two recent cases of human microsporidiosis [Abstract]. Annual Meeting, American Society of Tropical Medicine and Hygeine, San Antonio, Texas, 1983.
6. Orenstein JM. Microsporidiosis in the acquired immunodeficiency syndrome. *J Parasitol* 1991;77:843–864.
7. Desportes I, Le Charpentier Y, Galian A, et al. Occurrence of a new microsporidian: *Enterocytozoon bieneusi* n.g., n.sp., in the enterocytes of a human patient with AIDS. *J Protozool* 1985; 32:250–254.
8. Dobbins W, Weinstein WM. Electron microscopy of the intes-

tine and rectum in acquired immunodeficiency syndrome. *Gastroenterology* 1985;88:738–749.
9. Curry A, McWilliam LJ, Haboubi NY, Mandal BK. Microsporidiosis in a British patient with AIDS. *Br Med J* 1988;41:477–478.
10. Bernard E, Michiels JF, Durant J, et al. Intestinal microsporidiosis due to *Enterocytozoon bieneusi:* a new case report in an AIDS patient. *AIDS* 1991;5:606–607.
11. Michiels JF, Hofman P, Saint Paul MC, Giorsetti V, Bernard E, Vinti H, Loubiere R. Microsporidiose intestinale: 3 cas chez des sujets seropositifs pour le VIH. *Ann Pathol* 1991;11: 169–175.
12. Ullrich R, Zeitz M, Bergs C, Janitschke K, Riecken EO. Intestinal microsporidiosis in a German patient with AIDS. *Klin Wochenschr* 1991;69:443–445.
13. Modigliani R, Bories C, Le Charpentier Y, et al. Diarrhoea and malabsorption in acquired immune deficiency syndrome: a study of four cases with special emphasis on opportunistic protozoan infestations. *Gut* 1985;26:179–187.
14. Orenstein JM, Chiang J, Steinberg W, Smith PD, Rotterdam H, Kotler DP. Intestinal microsporidiosis as a cause of diarrhea in human immunodeficiency virus-infected patients: a report of 20 cases. *Hum Pathol* 1990;21:475–481.
15. Kotler DP, Francisco A, Clayton F, Scholes J, Orenstein JM. Small intestinal injury and parasitic disease in AIDS. *Ann Intern Med* 1990;113:444–449.
16. Sandfort J, Hannamen A, Stark D, Gelderblom H. *Enterocytozoon bieneusi* in a patient not infected with HIV. Presented at *Microsporidiosis and cryptosporidiosis in immunodeficient patients*, Ceska Budejovice, Czech Republic, 9/29–10/1/93.
17. Chilmonczyk S, Cox WT, Hedrick RP. *Enterocytozoon salmonis* n. sp.: an intranuclear microsporidium from salmonid fish. *J Protozool* 1991;38:264–269.
18. Cali A, Owen RI. Intracellular development of *Enterocytozoon*, a unique microsporidian found in the intestine of AIDS patients. *J Protozool* 1990;37:145–155.
19. Canning EU, Hollister WS. *Enterocytozoon bieneusi* (Microspora): prevalence and pathogenicity in AIDS patients. *Trans R Soc Trop Med* 1990;84:181–186.
20. Greenson J, Belitsos P, Yardley J, Bartlett J. AIDS enteropathy: occult enteric infections and duodenal mucosal alterations in chronic diarrhea. *Ann Intern Med* 1991;114:366–372.
21. Swenson J, MacLean JD, Kokoskin-Nelson E, Szabo J, Lough J, Gill MJ. Microsporidiosis in AIDS patients. *Can Commun Dis Rep* 1993;19:13–15.
22. Cotte L, Rabodonirina M, Piens A, Perreard M, Mofon M, Trepo C. Prevalence of intestinal protozoons in French patients infected with HIV. *J Acquir Immune Defic Syndr* 1993;6: 1024–1029.
23. Simon D, Weiss L, Wittner M, Cello J, Basuk P, Rood R, Cali A. Prevalence of microsporidia in AIDS patients with refractory diarrhea. *Am J Gastroenterol* 1991;86:1348 (abst).
24. Rabeneck L, Gyorkey F, Genta R, Gyorkey P, Foote L, Risser JMH. The role of microsporidia in the pathogenesis of HIV-related chronic diarrhea. *Ann Intern Med* 1993;119:895–899.
25. Kotler DP, Orenstein JM. Prevalence of enteric pathogens in HIV-infected individuals referred for gastrointestinal evaluation. *Gastroenterology* 1994;106:714 (abst).
26. Molina JM, Sarfati C, Beauvais B, et al. Intestinal microsporidiosis in human immunodeficiency virus-infected patients with chronic unexplained diarrhea: prevalence and clinical and biologic features. *J Infect Dis* 1993;167:217–221.
27. Eeftinck Schattenkerk JKM, van Gool T, van Ketel RJ, Bartelsman JFWM, Kuiken C, Terpstra WJ, Reiss P. Clinical significance of small-intestinal microsporidiosis in HIV-1-infected individuals. *Lancet* 1991;337:895–898.
28. Field AS, Hing M, Milliken ST, Marriott DJ. Microsporidia in the small intestine of HIV-infected patients. *Med J Aust* 1990; 158:390–394.
29. Canning EU, Lom J. *The microsporidia of vertebrates.* Orlando, FL: Academic Press, 1986.
30. Brunner O, Edelman S, Klipstein FA. Intestinal morphology of rural Haitians: a comparison between overt tropical sprue and asymptomatic subjects. *Gastroenterology* 1970;58:655–672.
31. Johnson LR. Regulation of gastrointestinal mucosal growth. *Physiol Rev* 1988;68:456–469.

32. Boyle JT, Celano P, Koldovsky O. Demonstration of a difference in expression of maximal lactase and sucrase activity along the villus in the adult rat jejunum. *Gastroenterology* 1980;79:503–507.

33. Shiau YF, Kotler DP, Levine GM. Can normal small bowel morphology be equated with normal function? *Gastroenterology* 1979;76:1246A.

34. Kotler DP, Reka S, Chow K, Orenstein JM. Effects of enteric parasitoses and HIV infection upon small intestinal structure and function in patients with AIDS. *J Clin Gastroenterol* 1993;16:10–15.

35. Didier ES, Kotler DP, Dieterich DT, et al. Serologic studies in human microsporidiosis. *AIDS* 1993;7(Suppl 3):S8–S11.

36. Weiss LM, Cali A, Levee E, Laplace D, Tanowitz H, Simon D, Wittner M. Diagnosis of *Encephalitozoon cuniculi* infection by Western blot and the use of cross-reactive antigens for the possible detection of microsporidiosis in humans. *Am J Trop Med Hyg* 1992;47:456–462.

37. Kotler DP. Gastrointestinal complications of the acquired immunodeficiency syndrome. In: Yamada T, ed. *Textbook of gastroenterology*, vol 20. Philadelphia: Lippincott, 1991;86–103.

38. Kotler DP, Tierney AR, Brenner SK, Couture S, Wang J, Pierson RN Jr. Preservation of short-term energy balance in clinically stable patients with AIDS. *Am J Clin Nutr* 1990;57:7–13.

39. Sclafani A, Koopmans HS, Vasselli J, Reichman M. Effects of intestinal bypass surgery on appetite, food intake, and body weight in obese and lean rate. *Am J Physiol* 1978;234:E389–E398.

40. Spiller RC, Trotman IF, Higgins BE, et al. The ileal brake—inhibition of jejunal motility after ileal fat perfusion in man. *Gut* 1984;25:365–374.

41. Owyang C, Green L, Rader D. Colonic inhibition of pancreatic and biliary secretion. *Gastroenterology* 1983;84:470–475.

42. Burn-Murdoch RA, Fischer M, Hunt JN. The slowing of gastric emptying by proteins in test meals. *J Physiol* 1978;274:477–485.

43. Babameto G, Kotler DP, Burastero S, Wang J, Pierson RN. Alterations in hydration in HIV-infected individuals. *Clin Res* 1994;42:279A (abst).

44. McWhinney PHM, Nathwani D, Green ST, Boyd JF, Forrest JAH. Microsporidiosis detected in association with AIDS-related sclerosing cholangitis. *AIDS* 1991;5:1394–1395.

45. Beaugerie L, Teilhac M-F, Deluol A-M, et al. Cholangiopathy associated with *Microsporidia* infection of the common bile duct mucosa in a patient with HIV infection. *Ann Intern Med* 1992;117:401–402.

46. Pol S, Romana CA, Richard S, et al. Microsporidia infection in patients with the human immunodeficiency virus and unexplained cholangitis. *N Engl J Med* 1993;328:95–99.

47. Cello J. Acquired immunodeficiency syndrome cholangiopathy: spectrum of disease. *Am J Med* 1989;86:539–546.

48. Chen LY, Goldberg H. Sclerosing cholangitis. Broad spectrum of radiographic features. *Gastrointest Radiol* 1984;9:39–46.

49. Peacock CS, Blanshard C, Tovey DG, Ellis DS, Gazzard BG. Histological diagnosis of intestinal microsporidiosis in patients with AIDS. *J Clin Pathol* 1991;44:558–563.

50. Lucas SB, Papadaki L, Conlon C, Sewankambo N, Goodgame R, Serwadda D. Diagnosis of intestinal microsporidiosis in patients with AIDS. *J Clin Pathol* 1989;42:885–887.

51. Simon D, Weiss L, Tanowitz H, Cali A, Jones J, Wittner M. Light microscope diagnosis of human microsporidiosis and variable response to octreotide. *Gastroenterology* 1991;100:271–273.

52. Giang T, Kotler DP, Garro ML, Orenstein JM. Tissue diagnosis of intestinal microsporidiosis using the chromotrope-2R trichrome stain. *J Clin Pathol* 1993;117:1249–1253.

53. Bryan RT, Weber R. Microsporidia. Emerging pathogens in immunodeficient persons [Editorial]. *Arch Pathol Lab Med* 1993;117:1243–1245.

54. Orenstein JM, Tenner M, Kotler DP. Localization of infection by the microsporidian *Enterocytozoon bieneusi* in the gastrointestinal tract of AIDS patients with diarrhea. *AIDS* 1992;6:195–197.

55. Weber R, Muller A, Spycher MA, Opravil M, Ammann R, Briner J. Intestinal *Enterocytozoon bieneusi* microsporidiosis in an HIV-infected patient: diagnosis by ileo-colonoscopic biopsies and long-term follow-up. *Clin Invest* 1992;70:1019–1023.

56. Verre J, Marriott D, Hing M, Field A, Harkness J. Evaluation of light microscopic detection of microsporidial spores in faeces from HIV infected patients [Abstract]. In: *Program and Abstracts from the Workshop on Intestinal Microsporidia in HIV Infection*. Dec 15–16, 1992, Paris, France.

57. Rijpstra AC, Canning EU, Van Ketel RJ, Eeftinck Shattenkerk JKM, Laarman JJ. Use of light microscopy to diagnose small-intestinal microsporidiosis in patients with AIDS. *J Infect Dis* 1988;157:827–831.

58. Kotler DP, Giang TT, Garro ML, Orenstein JM. Light microscopic diagnosis of microsporidiosis in patients with AIDS. *Am J Gastroenterol* 1994;89:540–544.

59. Orenstein JM, Zierdt W, Zierdt C, Kotler DP. Identification of spores of the Microspora, *Enterocytozoon bieneusi*, in stool and duodenal fluid from AIDS patients with diarrhea. *Lancet* 1991;336:1127–1128.

60. van Gool T, Hollister WS, Schattenkerk JE, et al. Diagnosis of *Enterocytozoon bieneusi* microsporidiosis in AIDS patients by recovery of spores from faeces. *Lancet* 1990;2:697–698.

61. Weber R, Bryan RT, Owen RL, Wilcox CM, Gorelkin L, Visvesvara GS. Improved light-microscopical detection of microsporidia spores in stool and duodenal aspirates. *N Engl J Med* 1992;326:161–166.

62. Bryan RT, Weber R, Stewart JM, Angritt P, Visvesvara GS. New manifestations and simplified diagnosis of human microsporidiosis. *Am J Trop Med Hyg* 1991;45:133–134.

63. van Gool T, Snijders F, Reiss P, et al. Diagnosis of intestinal and disseminated microsporidial infections in patients with HIV by a new rapid fluorescence technique. *J Clin Pathol* 1993;46:694–699.

64. Field HM, Harkness A, Marriott D. Enteric microsporidiosis: incidence and response to albendazole or metronidazole [Abstract PoB 3344]. In: *VII International Conference on AIDS*, Amsterdam, 1992.

65. Blanshard C, Ellis DS, Tovey DG, Dowell S, Gazzard BG. Treatment of intestinal microsporidiosis with albendazole in patients with AIDS. *AIDS* 1992;6:311–313.

66. Dieterich DT, Lew E, Kotler DP, Poles M, Orenstein JM. Treatment with albendazole for intestinal disease due to *Enterocytozoon bieneusi* in patients with AIDS. *J Infect Dis* 1994;169:173–183.

67. Dieterich DT, Lew E, Kotler DP, Poles M, Orenstein JM. Divergence between clinical and histologic responses during treatment of *Enterocytozoon bieneusi* infection with albendazole: prospective study and review of the literature. *AIDS* 1993;7(Suppl 3):S43–S44.

68. Kotler DP, Tierney AR, Dilmanian A, Wang J, Pierson RN Jr, Weber D. Comparison of the losses of total body potassium and total body nitrogen in patients with AIDS. *Am J Clin Nutr* (in press).

69. Kotler DP, Tierney AR, Wang J, Pierson RN Jr. Effect of home total parenteral nutrition upon body composition in AIDS. *J Parenter Enteral Nutr* 1990;14:454–458.

70. Orenstein JM, Tenner M, Cali A, Kotler DP. A microsporidian previously undescribed in humans, infecting enterocytes and macrophages and associated with diarrhea in an AIDS patient. *Hum Pathol* 1992;23:722–728.

71. Cali A, Kotler DP, Orenstein JM. *Septata intestinalis*, n.g.,n.sp., an intestinal microsporidian associated with chronic diarrhea and dissemination in AIDS patients. *J Euk Microbiol* 1993;40:101–112.

72. Orenstein JM, Dieterich DT, Kotler DP. Systemic dissemination by a newly recognized microsporidia species in AIDS. *AIDS* 1992;6:1143–1150.

73. Orenstein JM, Dieterich DT, Lew EA, Kotler DP. Albendazole as a treatment for disseminated microsporidiosis due to *Septata intestinalis* in AIDS patients. *AIDS* 1993;7(Suppl 3):S40–S42.

74. Case Records of the Massachusetts General Hospital. *N Engl J Med* 1993;329:1946–1954.

75. Zhu X, Wittner M, Tanowitz H, Kotler DP, Cali A, Weiss LM. Small subunit rRNA sequence of *Enterocytozoon bieneusi* and its potential diagnostic role with use of the polymerase chain reaction. *J Infect Dis* 1993;168:1570–1575.

Infections of the Gastrointestinal Tract,
edited by M. J. Blaser, P. D. Smith, J. I. Ravdin,
H. B. Greenberg, and R. L. Guerrant
Raven Press, Ltd., New York © 1995.

CHAPTER 74

Intestinal Infection With Other Protozoa

Including *Isospora belli, Blastocystis hominis,* and *Dientamoeba fragilis*

Kevin C. Kain and Jay S. Keystone

This chapter focuses on other intestinal protozoa, that are either proven or probable human pathogens, and the nonpathogenic protozoa from which they must be differentiated (Table 1, Figs. 1 and 2). Most of these protozoa have two forms: a motile trophozoite that replicates in the bowel lumen and a nonreplicating infective cyst that resists the external environment.

The optimal laboratory diagnosis of intestinal protozoa generally requires the examination of at least three stool specimens collected over several days. However, recent studies suggest that one or two stool samples will detect up to 90% of the protozoa present (2). Any examination for parasites in fecal samples must include the use of a permanent stained smear and a micrometer. The identification of intestinal protozoa is based on unique characteristics of the trophozoite and cyst stages, including size and shape, nuclei number and structure, nuclear characteristics, motility (trophozoites), inclusions, and chromatoidal bodies. These features are most readily demonstrated using permanently stained fecal smears (trichrome or iron hematoxylin for amebae; modified acid-fast stain for coccidia), together with wet mounts and iodine-stained smears of direct and concentrated stool samples.

ISOSPORIASIS

Isosporiasis is caused by the intestinal sporozoan *Isospora belli,* related to cryptosporidia and sarcocystis. *Isospora belli* was first described by Virchow in 1860 but named in 1923 (3). Isosporiasis is an important cause of

protracted diarrhea in immunocompromised hosts, particularly in patients with acquired immunodeficiency syndrome (AIDS), and occasionally a cause of traveler's diarrhea (4,5).

Microbiology

Isospora belli is an obligate intracellular, coccidian protozoon of the phylum Apicomplexa (sporozoa). The life cycle of *I. belli* is similar to cryptosporidia and other coccidia with alternating asexual (schizogony) and sexual (sporogony) cycles in the enterocytes of the proximal small bowel (6,7). Human infection follows ingestion of mature sporulated oocysts containing two sporocysts, each of which has four sporozoites (Figs. 3 and 4). The sporulated oocyst is the infective stage that excysts in the small bowel and releases sporozoites. Liberated sporozoites invade the small bowel enterocytes and initiate asexual reproduction. The sexual cycle follows soon after and produces oocysts that are not infectious since they pass unsporulated in the feces approximately 9 to 15 days after ingestion. For sporulation to occur, a period of 24 to 48 hr is required outside the host depending on environmental conditions. For this reason exogenous autoinfection with *I. belli* is less likely than with cryptosporidia.

Epidemiology

Isosporiasis has a worldwide distribution but is most prevalent in the tropics and subtropics (8,9). Humans are the only recognized source of infection (10,11). The true prevalence in humans is unknown. As an opportunistic pathogen in HIV-1 infected individuals in the United

K. C. Kain and J. S. Keystone: Tropical Disease Unit, Department of Medicine, The Toronto Hospital and the University of Toronto, Toronto, Ontario M5G 2C4, Canada.

TABLE 1. *Commonly identified intestinal protozoa of humans*

Organism	Potentially pathogenic
Coccidia	
Cryptosporidium species	+
Isospora belli	+
Cyclospora[a] species	+
Sarcocystis species	+
Amebae	
Entamoeba histolytica	+
E. polecki	?
E. hartmanni	−
E. coli	−
Iodamoeba bütschlii	−
Endolimax nana	−
Flagellates	
Giardia duodenalis[b]	+
Dientamoeba fragilis[c]	+
Chilomastix mesnili	−
Pentatrichomonas hominis	−
Retortamonas intestinalis	−
Enteromonas hominis	−
Cilates	
Balantidium coli	+
Other	
Blastocystis hominis	?

[a] A coccidian-like protozoon; proposed name: *Cyclospora cayetanensis.*
[b] Formerly *Giardia lamblia.*
[c] An ameba-like flagellate.

States, *I. belli* remains an unusual cause of chronic diarrhea; it is identified in approximately 0.2% of patients. However, prevalence rates are much higher in the tropics. In some studies over 15% of AIDS patients in Africa and Haiti were infected with *I. belli* (9,11,12).

The mode of transmission is by ingestion of food or water contaminated with mature sporulated oocysts. Direct person-to-person transmission is also possible but likely less common (13). The incubation period is approximately 7 days. Like other coccidia, *I. belli* oocysts are highly resistant to common disinfectants and to changes in environmental conditions; oocysts may remain viable for months if kept moist and cool (11). Sporadic outbreaks have occurred in institutions and day care centers in the United States (14,15).

Pathogenesis and Immunity

Little is known about the pathogenesis of isosporiasis. Infection is associated with villous atrophy and increased inflammatory cells in the lamina propria of the proximal small bowel (6). Developmental stages of *I. belli* may be found within the epithelial cells and occasionally in the lamina propria. Lymph node involvement has been reported in AIDS patients.

The mechanisms of host immunity to *I. belli* are unknown. However, individuals with depressed cellular immunity are at greatest risk of developing persistent diarrhea. Isosporiasis associated with persistent diarrhea (lasting more than 1 month) is an AIDS-indicator condition in HIV-1 infected individuals. There is some evidence that *I. belli* oocysts may occasionally sporulate within the intestine, excyst, and reinitiate the endogenous cycle (autoinfection). Autoinfection and recycling of schizonts may, at least in part, be responsible for the prolonged diarrhea observed in immune deficient hosts.

Clinical Presentation

The clinical presentation of isosporiasis often resembles cryptosporidiosis or giardiasis. In immunocompetent hosts, isosporiasis is characterized by the acute onset of watery diarrhea, colicky abdominal pain, and low-grade fever. In almost all immunologically intact hosts it is a self-limited infection, lasting less than 1 month in duration. In immunodeficient hosts, particularly in patients with AIDS, infection is associated with protracted watery diarrhea, abdominal pain, nausea, weight loss, and malabsorption. If left untreated infection may persist for years.

Diagnosis

The diagnosis of isosporiasis can be made by demonstrating oocysts in stool samples or by finding developmental stages of the parasite in small bowel biopsy specimens. Oocysts are most commonly identified in fecal samples using wet preps, auramine-rhodamine, or modified acid-fast stains (11,16). Oocysts are elliptical (20 to 30 μm by 10 to 20 μm) and like the oocysts of cryptosporidia stain bright red with modified acid-fast stains (Figs. 3 and 4). Oocysts may not be detected in the feces at presentation but may be shed for up to 120 days following recovery. Unlike cryptosporidia, small numbers of *I. belli* oocysts may be shed intermittently and may easily be overlooked in standard ova and parasite examinations. Identification of isosporiasis may be facilitated by the examination of several stool samples (at least four) collected over several days (12), the use of a concentration technique such as Sheather's sugar flotation (11), and the use of a wet prep. Occasionally, small bowel biopsies will yield a positive result when stool samples are negative.

Treatment

Unlike cryptosporidia, *I. belli* responds promptly to appropriate antimicrobial therapy. The treatment of choice is trimethoprim (160 mg) and sulfamethoxazole (800 mg) (TMS) four times per day for 10 days, followed by TMS twice daily for 21 days (12,17). Approximately 50% of immunosuppressed patients will have a recurrence of symptomatic isosporiasis unless they receive maintenance therapy. Pyrimethamine (25 mg daily) and folinic

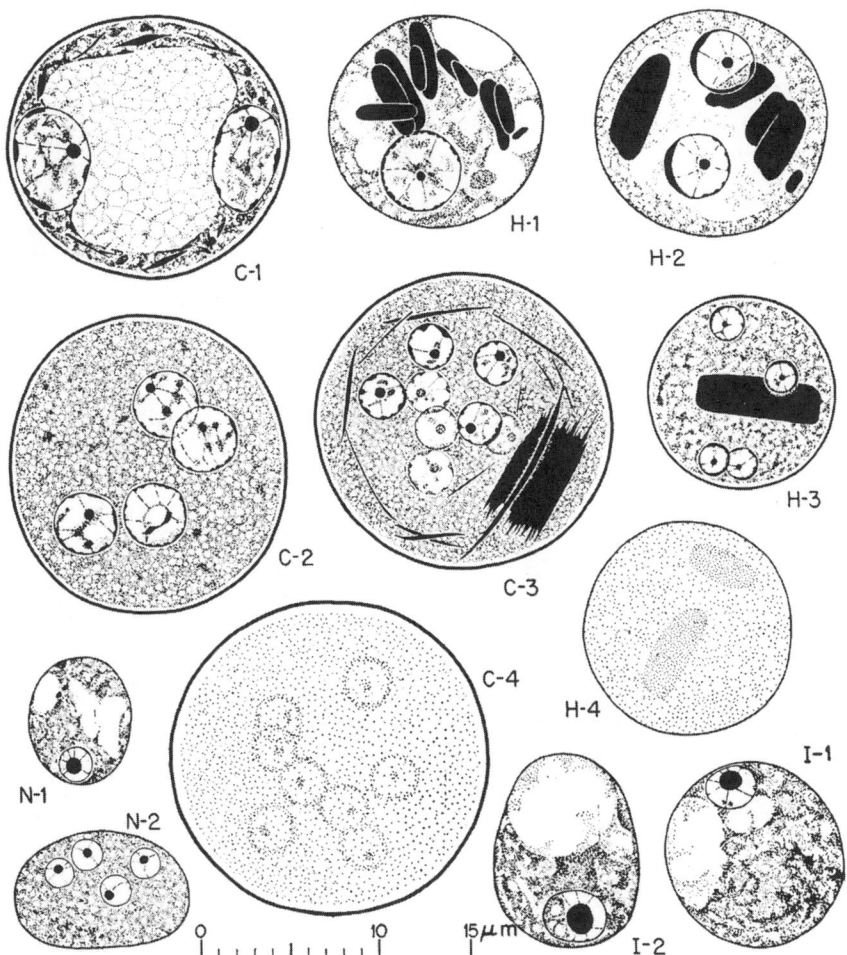

FIG. 1. Cysts of intestinal amebae. **C1–C3:** Cysts of *Entamoeba coli* (iron hematoxylin stain). **C-4:** Mature cyst of *E. coli* (unstained). **H-2, H-3:** Cysts of *E. histolytica* (iron hematoxylin stain). **H-4:** Unstained cyst of *E. histolytica* showing chromatoidal bars. **N-1, N-2:** Cysts of *Endolimax nana* (iron hematoxylin stain). **I-1, I-2:** cysts of *Iodamoeba bütschlii* (iron hematoxylin stain). (From ref. 1, with permission.)

acid (5 to 10 mg daily), TMS three times per week, or sulfadoxine/pyrimethamine (500/25 mg weekly) have all been used successfully to prevent relapses. In sulfa-intolerant individuals, pyrimethamine (75 mg daily) and folinic acid (10 mg daily) for 14 days followed by maintenance doses of pyrimethamine have been effective in treating isosporiasis (18). There have been anecdotal reports of responses to roxithromycin (19), metronidazole, quinacrine, diclazuril (20), and furazolidone.

SARCOCYSTOSIS

Sarcocystosis is a rare zoonotic infection of humans that was first described by Kartoulis in 1893 (21). *Sarcocystis* species are unique among coccidian infections in that humans can act both as the intermediate and the definitive host. This section focuses on the sexual stage of

infection (human as definitive host) as this stage is associated with gastrointestinal infection and may result in intestinal symptoms. For a review of extra intestinal disease caused by sarcocytosis the reader is referred to Beaver et al. (22).

Microbiology

Sarcocystis species are intracellular coccidian protozoa of the phylum Apicomplexa. The life cycle requires two hosts—a predator and a prey—generally a carnivore and a herbivore, respectively. The sexual stages develop in the intestinal tract of the definitive host (the predator) and the asexual stages in the tissues of the intermediate host (the prey). Humans become definitive hosts of sarcocystosis by ingesting inadequately cooked meat that contains tissue cysts (sarcocysts) of two species, *S. bovihominis* (beef) or *S. suihominis* (pork). Zoites (also called

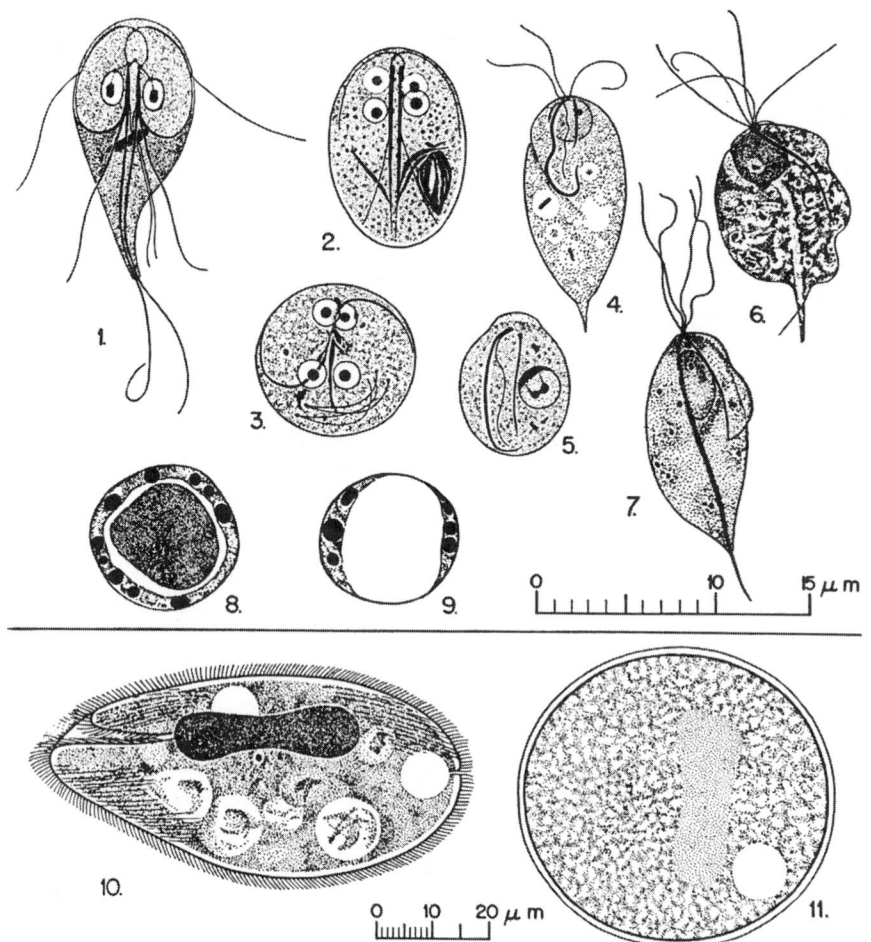

FIG. 2. Intestinal flagellates and ciliates. **1:** Trophozoite of *Giardia duodenalis* (iron hematoxylin stain). **2, 3:** Cysts of *G. duodenalis* (iron hematoxylin stain). **4:** Trophozoite of *Chilomastix mesnili* (iron hematoxylin stain). **5:** Cysts of *C. mesnili* (iron hematoxylin stain). **6:** Trophozoite of *Pentatrichomonas hominis* (iron hematoxylin stain). **7:** Trophozoite of *Trichomonas vaginalis* (iron hematoxylin stain). **8:** *Blastocystis hominis* (iron hematoxylin stain). **9:** *Blastocystis hominis* (unstained). **10:** Trophozoite of *Balantidium coli*. **11:** Cyst of *B. coli* (unstained). (From ref. 1, with permission.)

bradyzoites or cystozoites) contained in the sarcocysts are released by digestive enzymes and penetrate the enterocytes of the small bowel. Zoites invade to the lamina propria and differentiate into microgametocytes (male) and macrogametocytes (female). Fertilization of macrogametocytes by microgametocytes occurs in approximately 24 hr and the resulting zygotes undergo oocyst wall formation and sporulation. Sporulated oocysts consist of a thin wall containing two sporocysts, each of which contains four sporozoites (Fig. 5). Oocyst walls are thin and easily ruptured so that free sporocysts are the form most commonly seen in the feces, approximately 2 to 3 weeks after ingestion of infected meat.

Tissue cysts develop in intermediate hosts, including humans, who become infected by ingesting oocysts or free sporocysts. Sporozoites excyst from the sporocysts and enter vascular endothelium where they develop into schizonts that produce merozoites. These in turn enter striated muscle cells and produce sarcocysts. Tissue sar-

cocystosis is more common than previously recognized, particularly in Southeast Asia, where up to 21% of individuals were infected in some recent series (24,25). Sarcocysts, however, rarely produce symptoms (22,26,27).

Epidemiology (Human as Definitive Host)

Sarcocystosis is found worldwide but its prevalence and incidence are unknown. It is speculated that many infections go unrecognized (28). In two recent surveys, 10% of Laotians (29) and 22% of Tibetans (30) were found to be excreting oocysts; most were asymptomatic. A higher prevalence of infection may be found in agricultural societies or where inadequately cooked beef, pork, and occasionally caribou are consumed (31). Nonhuman primates may also serve as definitive hosts, but their importance as reservoirs for human infection is unknown (32).

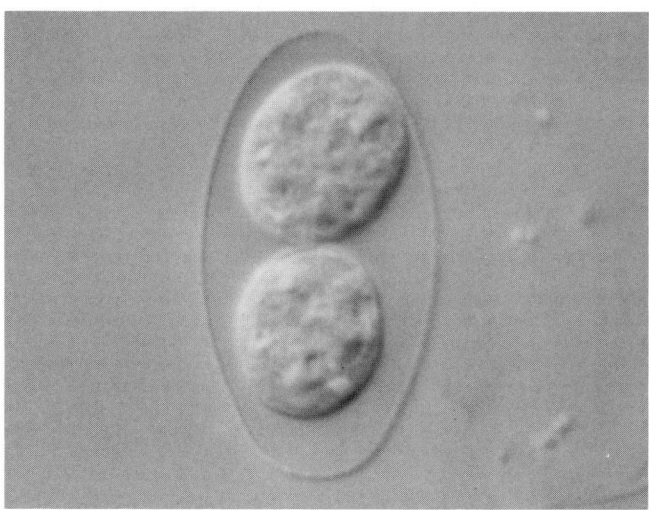

FIG. 3. Oocyst of *Isospora belli*. A mature sporulated oocyst containing two sporocysts, using Nomarski optics (×1250). (Courtesy of Dr. Murray Wittner.) (See Plate 20.)

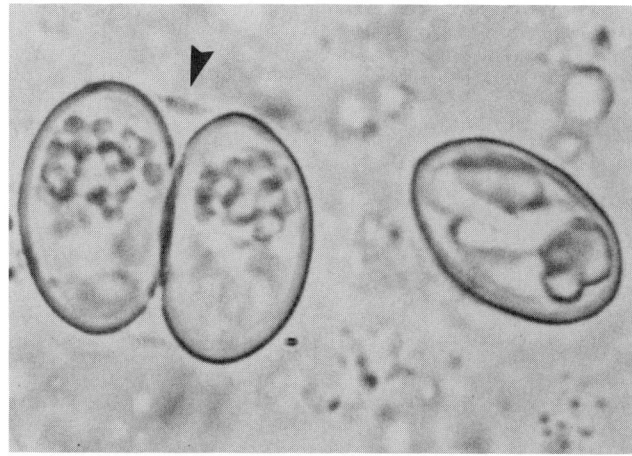

FIG. 5. Oocyst and free sporocyst of *Sarcocystis* species. The thin-walled (*arrow*) oocyst usually ruptures so that individual sporocysts are more commonly seen. In the oocyst, residual bodies are seen in each sporocyst overlying the individual sporozoites (formalin-fixed wet preparation, ×800). (From ref. 23, with permission.) (See Plate 22.)

Pathology

The histology of intestinal sarcocystosis ranges from segmental eosinophilic enteritis to necrotizing enteritis (28). In contrast to cryptosporidia and *I. belli* infections, there is no villous blunting observed with intestinal infection. Developmental stages of *Sarcocystis* species are occasionally identified in the lamina propria and submucosa on small bowel biopsy.

Clinical (Intestinal) Presentation

Sarcocystis species are generally not pathogenic to carnivores; however, humans may develop severe intestinal symptoms. The spectrum of disease ranges from asymp-

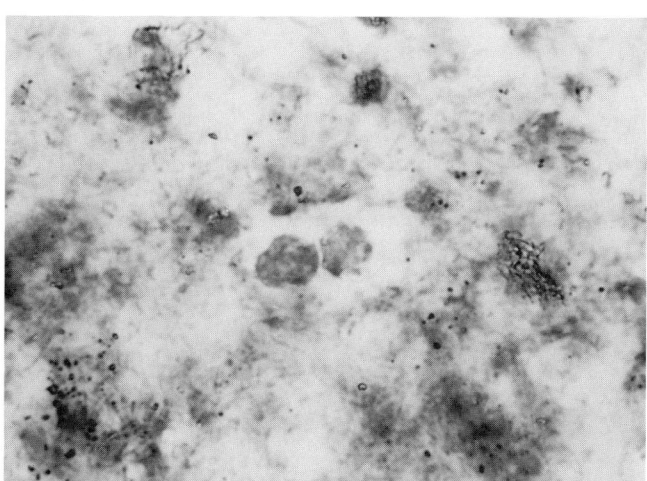

FIG. 4. Direct smear of stool sample from a patient with isosporiasis (modified acid-fast stain, ×600). (Courtesy of Dr. Jim Yang.) (See Plate 21.)

tomatic to necrotizing enteritis with intestinal obstruction. Volunteers who ingested *Sarcocystis*-infected beef and pork developed, 3 to 6 hr after consumption, abdominal pain, nausea, and diarrhea, which lasted approximately 48 hr and appeared to coincide with zoite invasion of enterocytes of the small bowel (33). Milder pain and diarrhea were associated with sporocyst appearance in the stool approximately 2 to 3 weeks after consumption of infected meat. Severe disease is occasionally reported; six patients in Thailand who consumed *Sarcocystis*-infected raw beef developed severe abdominal pain, fever, and intestinal obstruction (28). All six were improved by small bowel resection, which demonstrated multiple organisms. This report also noted that local market beef was infected with sarcocysts and speculated that there may be many unrecognized milder cases.

Diagnosis

The diagnosis of intestinal sarcocystosis is confirmed by the demonstration of oocysts or, more likely, free sporocysts (approximately 16 × 10 μm) in fresh stool samples or by finding developmental sexual stages of the parasite in biopsy specimens or resected tissue (Fig. 5). Oocysts and sporocysts are shed sporadically and optimal diagnosis requires the use of a concentration technique, such as Sheather's sugar flotation method, and the examination of several stool samples collected over several days (11). Diagnostic stages in the stool may take 2 to 3 weeks to appear after the patient first develops gastrointestinal symptoms. Oocysts and sporocysts may be identified in wet preps or by modified acid-fast or auramine staining. Oocysts stain bright red with modified acid-fast stains similar to the oocysts of cryptosporidia and *I. belli*.

Treatment

The optimal therapy for intestinal sarcocystosis is unknown. Many mild infections appear to be self-limited. However, severe infections may require bowel resection.

ENTAMOEBA POLECKI

Entamoeba polecki is a frequent intestinal protozoon of monkeys and pigs that in rare instances causes human infections. The pathogenic potential of *E. polecki* in humans is at present unresolved.

Microbiology

Both the trophozoite and cyst stages of *E. polecki* have been identified in human stool samples but the cyst is the form most frequently recognized. *Entamoeba polecki*, particularly the trophozoite stage, morphologically resembles both *E. histolytica* and *E. coli* and may frequently be misdiagnosed unless careful examination of permanently stained fecal smears is performed. The cyst stage is most helpful in differentiating *E. polecki* from other amebae and is characterized by the presence of a single nucleus with a prominent karyosome and large numbers of chromatoid bodies of varied morphology (Fig. 6). The isoenzyme patterns of *E. polecki* are almost identical to those of nonpathogenic *E. histolytica*, placing some doubt on the validity of this species (34) and on its pathogenicity for humans.

Epidemiology

Entamoeba polecki has a worldwide distribution but most human infections have been reported from Papua

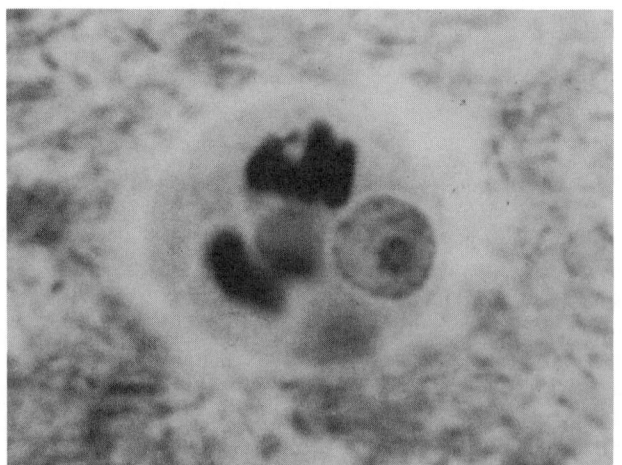

FIG. 6. Cyst of *Entamoeba polecki.* This photograph illustrates some of the morphologic features that distinguish *E. polecki* from other intestinal ameba. Uninucleate cysts that have large numbers of chromatoid bodies of varied morphology strongly suggest *E. polecki* infection (iron hematoxylin stain). (From ref. 23, with permission.) (See Plate 23.)

New Guinea, where up to 19% of children were infected (35). The most common mode of transmission appears to be the ingestion of cysts in food or water contaminated by infected monkey or pig feces. Human to human transmission has also been reported.

Clinical Presentation

The vast majority of infected individuals are asymptomatic, which is not surprising in view of the nonpathogenic isoenzyme patterns of this parasite. However, gastrointestinal symptoms including diarrhea, cramps, anorexia, and malaise have been reported in patients with heavy *E. polecki* infections.

Diagnosis

Many *E. polecki* infections may go unrecognized because of the difficulty in identifying this protozoon. Differentiating *E. polecki* cysts and trophozoites from *E. histolytica* and *E. coli* requires careful examination of permanently stained fecal smears (Fig. 6). The presence of uninucleate cysts with many chromatoid bodies should strongly suggest *E. polecki* infection.

Treatment

To date, there is no convincing evidence that *E. polecki* is pathogenic for humans; hence routine treatment is not warranted. In a limited number of anecdotal reports in which *E. polecki* was implicated in human disease, patients responded to treatment with metronidazole 750 mg tid for 5 to 10 days. Furamide (diloxanide furoate) 500 mg tid for 10 days combined with metronidazole has also been used successfully to eradicate *E. polecki* infection.

DIENTAMOEBA FRAGILIS

Dientamoeba fragilis is a protozoan parasite of the large intestine, which was first discovered by Wenyon in 1909; however, it was not until 1918 that Jepps and Dobell (36) described the parasite as a new species.

Microbiology

Dientamoeba fragilis was initially classified with the Sarcodina, but more recent electron microscopy and immunofluorescent studies suggest that it is a flagellate (without a flagellum) of the genera *Histomonas* and *Trichomonas* (37,38). The trophozoite may contain from one to four nuclei but is normally seen in the typical binucleate

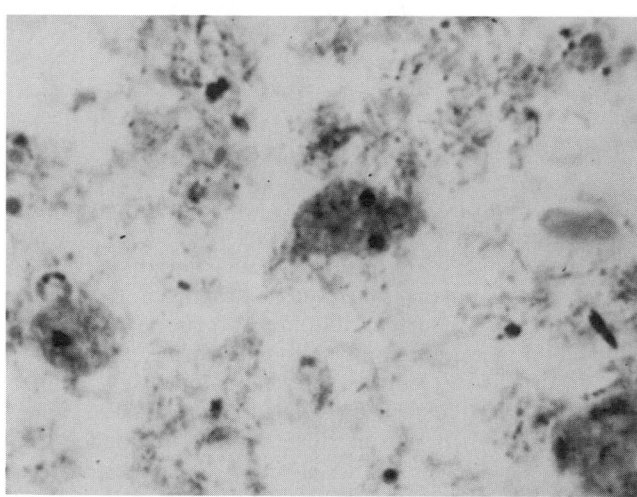

FIG. 7. Trophozoites of *Dientamoeba fragilis*. Uninucleate and more typical binucleate trophozoites of *D. fragilis*. A typical nucleus with a karyosome in the form of a tetrad is observed in the binucleate organism (iron hematoxylin stain, ×600). (See Plate 24.)

form (Fig. 7). It usually measures 5 to 12 μm in diameter but shows considerable variation in size. The nuclei contain four to six large granules clumped in the center and the cytoplasm may contain numerous food vacuoles. No cyst form has been described. The organism is usually found in the cecum and proximal large intestine. Its life span is unknown, but infection appears to persist for years.

Epidemiology

Dientamoebiasis is found worldwide with prevalence rates of 1.4% to 19% from population-based surveys (39–43). However, the actual prevalence may be higher since in many of these early studies stools were not preserved or examined with permanently stained smears (44,45). The highest prevalence of infection (8% to 69%) has been found in children, the institutionalized, native Americans, day care centers, and those with poor personal hygiene (46–51). It is interesting to note that the parasite is not seen with greater frequency in sexually active male homosexuals (52–54). Although the mode of transmission has not been determined, several observations suggest that transmission is likely by direct fecal–oral transmission by means of pinworm eggs, which contain the organism. Several studies have shown an 8- to 20-fold higher association of pinworm and *D. fragilis* than expected (55–57). The protozoon is not associated with other helminth infections. Two investigators have accidentally or deliberately infected themselves with one parasite and subsequently noted a coinfection with the other (55,58) However, attempts to infect a human volunteer with *D. fragilis* alone have failed (59,60). The parasite does not survive in water or in simulated gastric juice (57,59). Finally, Burrows and Swendlow (55) did find structures resembling *D. fragilis* in the eggs of pinworms,

but this study has not been confirmed by means of electron microscopy.

Pathogenesis and Immunity

Little is known about the pathogenesis of dientamoebiasis. To date, no studies have ever documented tissue invasion by this parasite although the authors of a single case report propose, without proof, that their patient's colitis was caused by *D. fragilis* (61). Clinical experience with dientamoebiasis suggests that immunity to infection is incomplete since individuals may be reinfected and may become symptomatic with subsequent infections.

Clinical Presentation

For many years *D. fragilis* was felt to be a harmless commensal although the literature contained many reports of illness associated with infection (62–64). In 1966 Kean and Malloch (65) published for the first time a large case series of 100 patients with symptomatic infections. Spencer and co-workers (66,67) brought the infection to the attention of physicians once again with two retrospective case series in 1978 and 1982 in which they reviewed the clinical picture and response to therapy of children and adults infected with *D. fragilis* alone.

Most symptomatic patients have abdominal pain (45% to 78%), diarrhea (46% to 68%), nausea (42%), or anorexia (20% to 31%). Less frequently, vomiting (17% to 22%), bloating/flatulence (16%), weight loss (22% to 26%), fatigue (6% to 13%), headache (24%), fever (12% to 26%), and irritability (12% to 20%) have also been described. Diarrhea occurs most often during the first week or two of illness and abdominal pain appears to predominate after 1 or 2 months. The incidence of symptomatic infection is unclear since most retrospective studies suffer from referral bias in that they are more likely to review symptomatic individuals. In a prospective study of children in 22 Canadian day care nurseries, only 10% of 72 infected children were symptomatic (49). This compares with 42% to 58% reported in retrospective studies (44). The most convincing evidence that *D. fragilis* is a human pathogen was shown by the results of a randomized, placebo-controlled treatment trial of individuals infected with *D. fragilis* alone (68). Eradication of the parasite resulted in significantly greater amelioration of gastrointestinal symptoms in infected children than did placebo therapy. Although the same benefit of therapy was not seen in adults, the number of patients in this group was too small for statistical significance to be reached.

Diagnosis

A high index of suspicion for dientamoebiasis should be present when someone with symptomatic enterobiasis presents with abdominal pain or diarrhea, two symptoms that do not usually accompany the latter infection. The corollary, pruritus ani in someone with dientamoebiasis, should suggest the likelihood of coinfection with pinworm.

Dientamoebiasis has been associated with peripheral eosinophilia in up to 50% of infected individuals (62,66,67). However, these reports require confirmation since absolute counts were not assessed and enterobiasis was not excluded. Absolute eosinophilia was detected in only 2 out of 29 patients with dientamoebiasis in whom enterobiasis had been ruled out (68).

The diagnosis depends largely on proper collection and processing techniques. Several stool samples taken at intervals of one day or more should be examined because excretion in stool is variable (57). Samples must be examined soon after defecation or be preserved in a suitable fixative immediately after passage (44). Appropriate fixatives include polyvinyl alcohol (PVA) (69), modified Schaudinn's (70), or sodium acetate–acetic acid–formalin (SAF) (71). A permanent stain of fecal films from fresh or preserved material is essential because concentration procedures alone are not reliable diagnostic techniques for this infection (44). Permanent stains may be done with hematoxylin (44), trichrome (72), or celestine blue B (73).

Treatment

In view of the high prevalence of dientamoebiasis in the community and the apparent low incidence of symptomatic infections, treatment is recommended only for symptomatic individuals. The most effective therapy for dientamoebiasis was a pentavalent arsenical, diphetarsone, which until recently was available in Europe and Canada. The drug showed a 95% efficacy in eradicating the infection (74). Iodoquinol, metronidazole, tetracycline, and paromomycin clear infection in a majority of cases, but efficacy data are lacking. When patients with dientamoebiasis complain of pruritus ani, a search for or presumptive treatment of enterobiasis is indicated.

Screening and treating all infected individuals in institutions or day care centers are likely to only temporarily reduce the prevalence of infection (75).

BALANTIDIASIS

Balantidiasis is caused by the protozoon *Balantidium coli*. It is the only ciliate known to parasitize humans. In rare instances *B. coli* invades the large bowel mucosa and produces intestinal symptoms.

Microbiology

Balantidium coli is the largest protozoon that infects humans. Both the cyst and trophozoite stages are found. The trophozoite is a large (50 to 200 μm), oval protozoon that moves with a rapid rotary motion by means of the synchronized beating of its cilia. It has a pointed anterior end with a cytostome. The cyst stage is spherical to oval shaped and measures 50 to 70 μm. Both trophozoite and cyst stages have a characteristic well-visualized macronu-

cleus and a smaller micronucleus that is difficult to discern even in stained organisms.

Epidemiology

Balantidium coli has a worldwide distribution and frequently inhabits the intestinal tract of insects, fish, and mammals, particularly primates and swine; however, balantidiasis in humans is infrequently reported. Pigs appear to be the major reservoir of human infection in both tropical and temperate regions. Most cases of *B. coli* infection are described in Central America, Papua New Guinea, and Asia, particularly in areas of poor hygiene where swine and humans are in close contact. Incidence rates in swine farmers or slaughterhouse employees may approach 30%. Contact with pigs was reported in approximately 50% of cases in Papua New Guinea. Human infection is rarer in temperate areas, but epidemics have been described in institutions in which overcrowding and poor personal hygiene were found (76). Transmission occurs by ingestion of the infective cyst stage, which may remain viable for weeks in moist feces or soil. Upon ingestion, cysts excyst and release trophozoites that reside in the lumen of the large bowel or invade the colonic mucosa.

Pathogenesis

Balantidium coli trophozoites may invade the colonic mucosa, in part facilitated by parasite-derived hyaluronidase. They multiply in the submucosa, producing necrosis and ulceration similar to that observed with *E. histolytica*. Typically, the resulting ulcers are flask-shaped, with undermined edges, and may involve the entire thickness of the colon. Secondary bacterial infection may follow mucosal invasion by the parasite, thereby increasing the inflammatory response. Rarely, balantidiasis is complicated by colonic perforation and metastatic spread to liver, bladder, or vagina.

Clinical Presentation

Balantidiasis represents a spectrum of disease from the silent carrier state to fulminant dysentery, but most infections are asymptomatic. Symptomatic infection may resemble amebiasis with symptoms ranging from chronic intermittent diarrhea, abdominal pain, and weight loss to a fulminant dysenteric form with blood and mucus per rectum, colonic tenderness, and fever. The dysenteric presentation is occasionally complicated by colonic hemorrhage and perforation. Rarely, extraintestinal spread to liver, lungs, and lymph nodes and appendix has been reported (77,78). Eosinophilia is not a feature of infection.

Diagnosis

Unlike other intestinal protozoan infections, the diagnosis of balantidiasis is dependent on the identification of

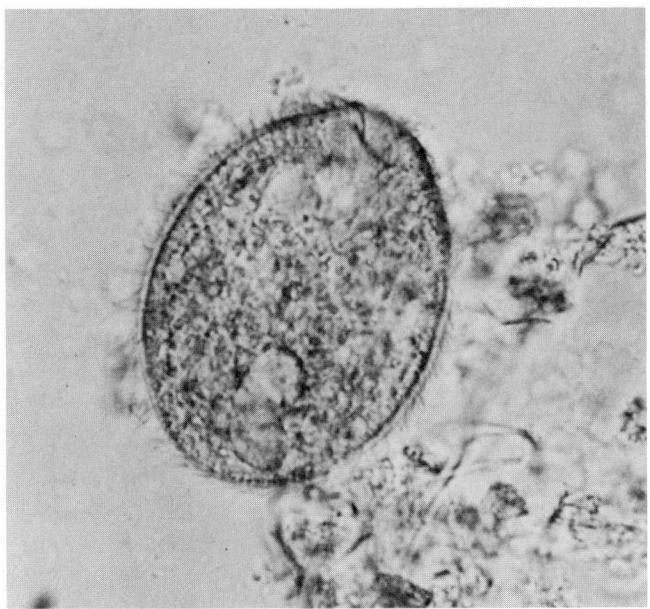

FIG. 8. *Balantidium coli* trophozoite in stool. These organisms can be recognized by their large size, ciliated surface, prominent cytosome, and large kidney bean-shaped macronucleus (formalin-preserved wet mount). (From ref. 23, with permission.) (See Plate 25.)

trophozoites (50 to 200 μm by 40 to 70 μm) in stool samples, in biopsies, or resected material. Cysts, measuring 50 to 70 μm, are rarely identified in feces. In direct wet preps, viable trophozoites show rapid rotary motion. The large size of this parasite makes identification possible by low-power microscopy. Both unstained and stained fecal preparations frequently demonstrate the characteristic kidney bean-shaped macronucleus and prominent cytostome of the trophozoite (Figs. 8 and 9).

Treatment

Tetracycline, 500 mg qid for 10 days, is the treatment of choice for balantidiasis. Alternatives include iodoquinol 650 mg tid for 20 days, metronidazole 750 mg tid for 5 days, or paromomycin.

BLASTOCYSTIS HOMINIS

Blastocystis hominis, initially described by Alexieff in 1911, is a common inhabitant of the human gastrointestinal tract. It was named by Brumpt (79) in 1912, who considered it to be a yeast. At present, *B. hominis* is an organism of uncertain taxonomic classification. Zierdt (80) recently classified *B. hominis* as a protozoon and placed it in the suborder Blastocystina, order Amoebida, pending confirmation at a molecular level (80,81). The role of *B. hominis* as a human pathogen is controversial and at present unresolved.

Microbiology

Blastocystis hominis is a strict anaerobic protozoon of variable size (5 to 40 μm), which resides primarily in the cecum and large bowel. It lacks a cell wall, divides by binary fission, and has three morphologic forms: vacuolated, ameba-like, and granular (81). The vacuolated form, characterized by a large membrane-bound central body, is most commonly identified in human fecal samples (Fig. 10). A cyst-like stage has recently been reported (82,83); however, it is unknown if this stage can survive adverse environmental conditions to represent the infective stage of the parasite. At least two demes or genetic groups of *B. hominis* exist, but it is not clear whether these are epidemiologically or clinically significant (84).

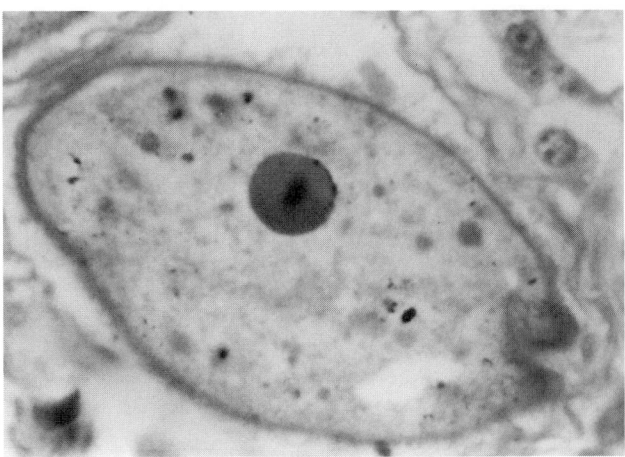

FIG. 9. Colonic biopsy showing trophozoite of *Balantidium coli*. Trichrome stain shows the prominent cytosome and the usual kidney bean-shaped macronucleus that has been bisected in this tissue section. (Courtesy of Dr. Jim Yang.) (See Plate 26.)

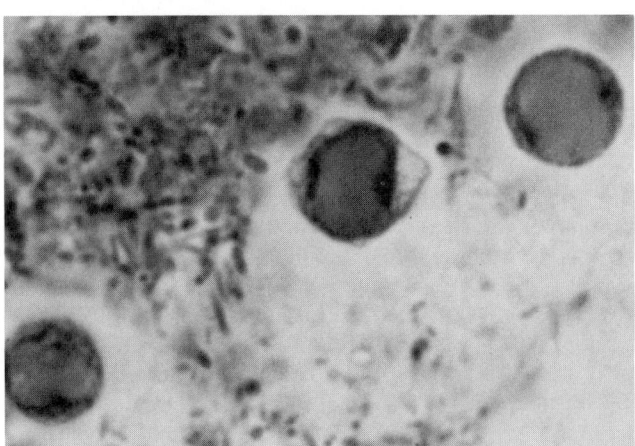

FIG. 10. *Blastocystis hominis.* Direct smear of stool sample from patient infected with *B. hominis* showing the typical vacuolated form of this parasite (iron hematoxylin stain, ×750).

Epidemiology

Blastocystis hominis has a worldwide distribution but some evidence suggests that it may be more common in the tropics and subtropics (85–89). Prevalence rates range from 3% to 20% in samples submitted to microbiology laboratories to 52% in homosexual males. Recent studies have not demonstrated a significant difference in the prevalence of infection between symptomatic and asymptomatic individuals (90,91). The mode of transmission of *B. hominis* has not been determined but is presumed to be fecal–oral because of the association of infection with consumption of untreated water and tropical travel (87,89,92). Rare outbreaks of blastocystosis have been reported (93,94). Also, infection appears to be widely distributed in the animal kingdom and has been reported in pigs, monkeys, reptiles, poultry, and rodents (81). However, it is not known whether animals are significant reservoirs of human infection.

Pathogenesis

Pathogenic mechanisms for *B. hominis* have not been identified. Attempts to infect gnotobiotic guinea pigs did not provide convincing evidence of pathogenicity unless large numbers of organisms were inoculated together with enteric flora. Twenty-two percent of these germ-free guinea pigs developed symptomatic infection and superficial invasion of cecal mucosa (95). Properly controlled prospective studies for pathogenicity of *B. hominis* in humans have not been performed.

Clinical Presentation

Infections with *B. hominis* have been increasingly reported in the 1980s and 1990s in both immunocompromised and immunologically intact hosts. In the absence of other identified microorganisms, several authors consider *B. hominis* to be a possible pathogen (80,81). Symptoms attributed to infection include diarrhea, abdominal pain, flatus, nausea, vomiting, anorexia, and malaise. However, virtually all the studies that have evaluated the clinical significance of blastocystosis have been retrospective case series from which a definitive answer has not been forthcoming. Earlier reports of a correlation between the presence of gastrointestinal symptoms and the number of *B. hominis* organisms identified in stool samples have not been confirmed by more recent studies (89–91). Peripheral eosinophilia has been reported in some cases; however, alternative causes of eosinophilia were often not excluded. Fecal leukocytes are rarely observed with *B. hominis* infection. Endoscopic, histopathologic, and radiologic studies of infected patients are usually normal (89,94).

Diagnosis

The diagnosis of blastocystosis is made by demonstrating the organism in unstained or permanently stained stool smears (Fig. 10). The vacuolated form is most often identified and stains well with iron hematoxylin or trichrome. Concentration techniques may result in lysis of the organism. Heavy infections may obscure the identification of other intestinal protozoa in stool specimens (96).

Treatment

Controlled prospective treatment trials for *B. hominis* have not been performed. No antimicrobial agents have been demonstrated to reliably eradicate *B. hominis* infection but metronidazole is frequently prescribed. However, it has not been convincingly shown to alter the natural history of infection. Limited *in vitro* susceptibility testing has shown activity against *B. hominis* by emetine, metronidazole, furazolidone, co-trimoxazole, quinacrine, and pentamidine (in order of efficacy) (97). Ketoconazole and iodoquinol are less active *in vitro* than metronidazole (98). Some reports indicate that iodoquinol and co-trimoxazole may have activity *in vivo* (87,99,100).

In summary, *B. hominis* is a frequently recognized colonic protozoon of uncertain pathogenic potential. Clarification of its role in human disease will require properly controlled prospective studies for pathogenicity and specific therapy. There is at present little evidence to support the routine use of antimicrobial therapy for blastocystosis.

NONPATHOGENIC INTESTINAL PROTOZOA

Nonpathogenic amebae and flagellates are frequently found on stool examination (Figs. 1 and 2) and need to be differentiated from potentially pathogenic protozoa. They are usually distinguished from known pathogens such as *E. histolytica* on the basis of (a) the number of nuclei present and the nuclear detail (best seen with permanent stains like iron hematoxylin), (b) the size and shape of cysts and trophozoites, (c) characteristic chromatoidal or inclusion bodies, and (d) the lack of rapid directional motility and erythrocyte ingestion by trophozoites.

The presence of these organisms may imply host consumption of fecally contaminated water or food. However, there is no evidence that any of these protozoa have pathogenic potential, even in immunocompromised hosts; hence therapy directed at eradicating carriage is not indicated. In symptomatic individuals that have nonpathogenic amebae identified, further investigation should be undertaken to search for recognized pathogens.

Amoeba

Entamoeba Hartmanni

Entamoeba hartmanni is found worldwide and was once considered to be a small race of *E. histolytica*. However, *E. hartmanni* has a unique isoenzyme pattern and is now considered to be a separate species (101). *Entamoeba hartmanni* is morphologically similar to *E. histolytica* but the cysts (<10 μm on wet prep; <9 μm on permanent stained smear) and trophozoites (<12 μm on wet prep; <11 μm on permanent stained smear) of *E. hartmanni* are smaller.

Entamoeba Coli

Entamoeba coli is a common gut protozoon that is also widely distributed. *Entamoeba coli* trophozoites and cysts are usually distinguished from *E. histolytica* on the basis of nuclear morphology. The *E. coli* nucleus generally has a larger and often eccentric karyosome. In addition, most mature cysts have more than five nuclei and are ≥15 μm in diameter compared to *E. histolytica* cysts, which have four or less nuclei and are 10 to 15 μm in diameter.

Endolimax Nana

Endolimax nana is a small nonpathogenic ameba that is at least as prevalent as *E. coli*. The cysts and trophozoites of *E. nana* are smaller than *E. histolytica* and have characteristic nuclear structure including the lack of peripheral chromatin on the nuclear membrane and a large central or eccentric karyosome.

Iodamoeba Bütschlii

This nonpathogenic ameba is less commonly encountered than *E. coli* or *E. nana*. The cysts of *I. bütschlii* have a characteristic large glycogen vacuole, which stains with iodine on a wet prep. The trophozoites have vacuolated cytoplasm.

Flagellates

Chilomastix mesnili is the most common nonpathogenic flagellate observed in fecal specimens. It is differentiated from *Giardia duodenalis* by its lemon-shaped cysts and the presence of a single nucleus. Other nonpathogenic flagellates such as *Enteromonas hominis*, *Retortamonas intestinalis*, and *Pentatrichomonas hominis* are rarely encountered.

REFERENCES

1. Strickland GT, ed. *Hunter's tropical medicine*, 7th ed. Philadelphia: Saunders, 1991.
2. Senay H, MacPherson D. Parasitology: diagnostic yield of stool examination. *Can Med Assoc J* 1989;140:1329–1331.
3. Wenyon CM. Coccidiosis of cats and dogs and the status of the *Isospora* of man. *Ann Trop Med Parasitol* 1923;17:231–239.
4. Godiwala T, Yaeger R. *Isospora* and traveler's diarrhea. *Ann Intern Med* 1987;106:909–910.
5. Shaffer N, Moore L. Chronic traveler's diarrhea in a normal host due to *Isospora belli*. *J Infect Dis* 1989;159:596–597.
6. Brandborg LL, Goldberg SB, Breidenbach WC. Human cocci-diosis—a possible cause of malabsorption. *N Engl J Med* 1970;283:1306–1313.
7. Trier JS, Moxey PC, Schimmel EM, Robles E. Chronic intestinal coccidiosis in men: intestinal morphology and response to treatment. *Gastroenterology* 1974;66:923–935.
8. Faust EC, Giraldo LE, Caicedo G, Bonfante R. Human isosporiosis in the Western Hemisphere. *Am J Trop Med Hyg* 1961;10:343–349.
9. Soave R, Johnson WD Jr. *Cryptosporidium* and *Isospora belli* infections. *J Infect Dis* 1988;157:225–229.
10. Kirkpatrick CE. Animal reservoirs of *Cryptosporidium* spp. and *Isospora belli*. *J Infect Dis* 1988;158:909.
11. Current WL. Human enteric coccidia. II. *Isospora belli* and *Sarcocystis* spp. *Clin Microbiol Newslett* 1985;7:175–182.
12. DeHovitz JA, Pape JW, Boncy M, Johnson WD. Clinical manifestations and therapy of *Isospora belli* infection in patients with the acquired immunodeficiency syndrome. *N Engl J Med* 1986;315:87–90.
13. Forthal DN, Guest SS. *Isospora belli* enteritis in three homosexual men. *Am J Trop Med Hyg* 1984;33:1060–1064.
14. Jeffery GM. Epidemiologic considerations of isosporiasis in a school for mental defectives. *Am J Hyg* 1958;67:251–255.
15. Current WL, Reese NC, Ernst JV, Bailey WS, Heyman MB, Weinstein WM. Human cryptosporidiosis in immunocompetent and immunodeficient persons: studies of an outbreak and experimental transmission. *N Engl J Med* 1983;308:1252–1257.
16. Ng E, Markell EK, Fleming RI, Fried M. Demonstration of *Isospora belli* by acid-fast stain in a patient with acquired immune deficiency syndrome. *J Clin Microbiol* 1984;20:384–386.
17. Pape JW, Verdier RI, Johnson WD Jr. Treatment and prophylaxis of *Isospora belli* infection in patients with the acquired immunodeficiency syndrome. *N Engl J Med* 1989;320:1044–1047.
18. Weiss LM, Perlman DC, Sherman J, Tanowitz H, Wittner M. *Isospora belli* infection: treatment with pyrimethamine. *Ann Intern Med* 1988;109:474–475.
19. Musey KL, Chidiac C, Beaucaire G, Houriez S, Fourrier A. Effectiveness of roxithromycin for treating *Isospora belli* infection. *J Infect Dis* 1988;158:646.
20. Kayembe K, Desmet P, Henry MC, Stoffels P. Diclazuril for *Isospora belli* infection in AIDS. *Lancet* 1989;1:1397–1398.
21. Kartulis S. Ueber pathogene protozoen bei dem Menschen. I. Gregarinose der Leber und der Bauchmuskeln. II. Amoben bei Knochennekrose (Osteomyelitis) der Unterkiefers. *Z Hyg Infectionskr* 1893;13:1–14.
22. Beaver PC, Gadgill K, Morera P. *Sarcocystis* in man: a review and report of five cases. *Am J Trop Med Hyg* 1979;28:819–844.
23. Ash LR, Orihel TC. *Atlas of human parasitology*, 3rd ed. Chicago: American Society of Clinical Pathologists, 1990.
24. Wong KT, Pathmanathan R. High prevalence of human skeletal muscle sarcocystosis in Southeast Asia. *Trans R Soc Trop Med Hyg* 1992;86:631–632.
25. Kan SP, Pathmanathan R. Review of sarcocystosis in Malaysia. *Southeast Asian J Trop Med Public Health* 1991;22(Suppl):129–134.
26. Kimmig P, Piekarski G, Heydorn AO. Sarcosporidiosis (*Sarcocystis suihominis*) in man. *Immunol Infect* 1979;7:170–177.
27. Piekarski G, Heydorn AO, Aryeetey ME, Hartiapp JH, Kimmig P. Clinical, parasitological and serological investigations in sarcosporidiosis (*Sarcocystis suihominis*) of man. *Immunol Infect* 1978;6:153–159.
28. Bunyaratvej S, Bunyawongwiroj P, Nitiyanant P. Human intestinal sarcosporidiosis: report of six cases. *Am J Trop Med Hyg* 1982;31:36–41.
29. Giboda M, Ditrich O, Scholz T, Viengsay T, Bouaphanh S. Current status of food-borne parasitic zoonoses in Laos. *Southeast Asian J Trop Med Public Health* 1991;22(Suppl):56–61.
30. Yu S. Field survey of *Sarcocystis* infection in the Tibet autonomous region. *Chung Kuo I Hsueh Ko Hsueh Yuan Hsueh Pao* 1991;13:29–32.
31. Khan RA, Fong D. *Sarcocystis* in caribou (*Rangifer tarandus terraenorae*) in Newfoundland. *Southeast Asian J Trop Med Public Health* 1991;22(Suppl):142–143.
32. Fayer R, Heydorn AO, Johnson AJ, Transmission of *Sarco-*

cystis suihominis from humans to swine to nonhuman primates. *Z Parasitenkd* 1979;59:15–20.

33. Dubey JP, Fayer R. Sarcocystosis. *Br Vet J* 1983;139:371–377.
34. Sargeaunt PG, Williams JE, Neal RA. A comparative study of *Entamoeba histolytica*, "*E. histolytica*-like" and other morphologically identical amoebae using isoenzyme electrophoresis. *Trans R Soc Trop Med Hyg* 1980;74:469–474.
35. Desowitz RS, Barnish G. *Entamoeba polecki* and other intestinal protozoa in Papua New Guinea highland children. *Ann Trop Med Parasitol* 1986;80:399–402.
36. Jepps MW, Dobell C. *Dientamoeba fragilis,* n.g., n.sp., a new intestinal amoeba from man. *Parasitology* 1918;10:352–367.
37. Dwyer DM. Analysis of the antigenic relationships among *Trichomonas, Histomonas, Dientamoeba* and *Entamoeba.* III. Immunoelectrophoresis techniques. *J Protozool* 1974;21:139–145.
38. Camp RR, Mattera CFT, Honigberg BM. Study of *Dientamoeba fragilis.* Jepps and Dobell. I. Electronmicroscopic observations of the binucleate stages II. Taxonomic position and revision of the genus. *J Protozool* 1974;21:69–82.
39. Svensson RM. A survey of human intestinal protozoa in Sweden and Finland. *Parasitology* 1928;20:237–249.
40. Wenrich DH, Stabler RM, Arnelt JH. *Entamoeba histolytica* and other intestinal protozoa in 1060 college freshmen. *Am J Trop Med* 1935;15:331–345.
41. Miller MJ. The intestinal protozoa of man in midwestern Canada. *J Parasitol* 1939;25:355–357.
42. Boe J. The occurrence of human intestinal protozoa in Norway. *Acta Med Scand* 1943;113:321–328.
43. Mackie TT, Larsh JE Jr, Mackie JW. A survey of intestinal parasitic infections in the Dominican Republic. *Am J Trop Med* 1951;31:825–832.
44. Scholten TH, Yang J. Evaluation of unpreserved and preserved stools for the detection and identification of intestinal parasites. *Am J Clin Pathol* 1974;62:563–567.
45. Garcia LS, Brewer TC, Bruckner DA. A comparison of the formalin–ether concentration and trichrome-stained smear methods for the recovery and identification of intestinal protozoa. *Am J Med Technol* 1979;45:932–935.
46. Weiner D, Brooke MM, Witkow A. Investigation of parasitic infections in the central area of Philadelphia. *Am J Trop Med Hyg* 1959;8:625–629.
47. Melvin DM, Brooke MM. Parasitologic surveys on Indian reservations in Montana, South Dakota, New Mexico, Arizona and Wisconsin. *Am J Trop Med Hyg* 1962;11:765–772.
48. Millet VE, Spencer MJ, Chapin MR, Garcia LS, Yatabe JH, Stewart ME. Intestinal protozoan infection in a semicommunal group. *Am J Trop Med Hyg* 1983;32:54–60.
49. Keystone JS, Yang J, Grisdale D, Harrington M, Pillon L, Andreychuk R. Intestinal parasites in metropolitan Toronto day-care centres. *Can Med Assoc J* 1984;131:733–735.
50. Spencer MJ, Millet VE, Garcia LS, Rhee L, Masterson L. Parasitic infections in a pediatric population. *Pediatr Infect Dis* 1983;2:110–113.
51. Naiman HK, Sckla L, Albritton WL. Giardiasis and other intestinal parasitic infections in a Manitoba residential school for the mentally retarded. *Can Med Assoc J* 1980;122:185–188.
52. Keystone JS, Keystone DL, Proctor EM. Intestinal parasitic infections in homosexual men: prevalence, symptoms and factors in transmission. *Can Med Assoc J* 1980;123:512–514.
53. Peters CS, Sable R, Janda WM, Chittom AL, Kocka TE. Prevalence of enteric parasites in homosexual patients attending an out-patient clinic. *J Clin Microbiol* 1986;24:684–685.
54. Ortega HB, Borchardt KA, Hamilton R, Ortega P, Mahood J. Enteric pathogenic protozoa in homosexual men from San Francisco. *Sex Transm Dis* 1984;11:59–63.
55. Burrows RB, Swerdlow MA. *Enterobias verminularis* as a probable vector of *Dientamoeba fragilis. Am J Trop Med Hyg* 1956;5:258–265.
56. Chang SL. Parasitization of the parasite. *JAMA* 1973;223:1510.
57. Yang J, Scholten TH. *Dientamoeba fragilis:* a review with notes on the epidemiology, pathogenicity, mode of transmission and diagnosis. *Am J Trop Med Hyg* 1977;26:16–22.
58. Ockert G. Zur Epidemiologic von *Dientamoeba fragilis* II Mit-

teilung: Versuch der Ubertragungdee der Art mit Enterobius. *Eur J Hyg Epidemiol Microbiol Immunol* 1972;16:222–225.
59. Wenrich DH. Studies on *Dientamoeba fragilis* (protozoa). IV. Further observations, with an outline of present day knowledge of this species. *J Parasitol* 1944;30:322–338.
60. Knoll EW, Howel KM. Studies on *Dientamoeba fragilis:* its incidence and possible pathogenicity. *Am J Clin Pathol* 1945;15:178–183.
61. Skein R, Gelb A. Colitis due to *Dientamoeba fragilis. Am J Gastroenterol* 1983;78:634–636.
62. Hood M. Diarrhea caused by *Dientamoeba fragilis. J Lab Clin Med* 1940;25:914–918.
63. Hakansoon EG. *Dientamoeba fragilis,* a cause of illness. *Am J Trop Med Hyg* 1936;16:175–183.
64. Yoeli M. A report of intestinal disorders accompanied by large numbers of *Dientamoeba fragilis. J Trop Med Hyg* 1955;58:38–41.
65. Kean BH, Malloch CL. The neglected amoeba: *Dientamoeba fragilis:* a report of 100 "pure" infections. *Am J Dig Dis NS* 1966;11:735–746.
66. Spencer MJ, Garcia LS, Chapin MR. *Dientamoeba fragilis:* an intestinal pathogen in children. *Am J Dis Child* 1979;133:390–393.
67. Spencer MJ, Chapin MR, Garcia LS. *Dientamoeba fragilis:* a gastrointestinal protozoan infection in adults 1982. *Am J Gastroenterol* 1982;77:565–569.
68. Keystone JS, MacPherson D, Navas L. The clinical significance of dientamoebiasis [Abstract]. Presented at the *41st Annual Meeting of the American Society of Tropical Medicine,* Seattle, WA, Nov 15–19, 1992.
69. Goldman M, Brooke MM. Protozoans in stools unpreserved and preserved in PVA fixative. *Public Health Rep* 1953;68:703–706.
70. Scholten T. An improved technique for the recovery of intestinal protozoa. *J Parasitol* 1972;58:633–634.
71. Yang J, Scholten T. An alternative to Schaudinn's fixative for the recovery and identification of intestinal parasites. *Can J Public Health* 1976;67:138.
72. Alger N. A simple, rapid, precise stain for intestinal protozoa. *Am J Clin Pathol* 1966;45:361–362.
73. Yang J, Scholten T. Celestin blue B stain for intestinal protozoa. *Am J Clin Pathol* 1976;65:715–718.
74. Keystone JS, Proctor EM, Glenn C, McIntyre L. Safety and efficacy of diphetarsone in the treatment of amoebiasis, nonpathogenic amoebiasis and trichiuriasis. *Trans R Soc Trop Med Hyg* 1983;77:84–86.
75. Thacker SB, Kimball AM, Wolfe M, Keewhan C, Gilmore L. Parasitic control in a residential facility for the mentally retarded: failure of selected isolation procedure. *Am J Public Health* 1981;71:303–305.
76. Walzer PD, Judson FN, Murphy KB, et al. Balantidiasis outbreak in Truk. *Am J Trop Med Hyg* 1973;22:33.
77. Dodd LG. *Balantidium coli* infestation as a cause of acute appendicitis. *J Infect Dis* 1991;163:1392.
78. Dorfman S, Rangel O, Bravo LG. Balantidiasis: report of a fatal case with appendicular and pulmonary involvement. *Trans R Soc Trop Med Hyg* 1984;78:833–834.
79. Brumpt E. *Blastocystis hominis* n. sp. et formes voisines. *Bull Soc Pathol Exot Filiales* 1912;5:725–730.
80. Zierdt CH. *Blastocystis hominis,* a long misunderstood intestinal pathogen. *Parasitol Today* 1988;4:15–17.
81. Zierdt CH. *Blastocystis hominis*—past and future. *Clin Microbiol Rev* 1991;4:61–79.
82. Stenzel DJ, Boreham PF. A cyst-like stage of *Blastocystis hominis. Int J Parasitol* 1991;21:613–615.
83. Stenzel DJ, Boreham PF, McDougall R. Ultrastructure of *Blastocystis hominis* in human stool samples. *Int J Parasitol* 1991;21:807–812.
84. Boreham PF, Upcroft JA, Dunn LA. Protein and DNA evidence for two demes of *Blastocystis hominis* from humans. *Int J Parasitol* 1992;22:49–53.
85. Yakimoff WL. Sur la question des *Blastocystis. Bull Soc Pathol Exot Filiales* 1923;161:326.

86. Sangiorgi G. Pathogenicity of *Blastocystis hominis*. *Pathologica* 1930;22:173.
87. Taylor DN, Echeverria P, Blaser MJ, Pitaranssi C, Blacklow N, Cross J, Weniser BO. Polymicrobial aetiology of traveller's diarrhoea. *Lancet* 1985;1:381.
88. Sheehan DJ, Raucher BC, McKitrick JC. Association of *Blastocystis hominis* with signs and symptoms of human disease. *J Clin Microbiol* 1986;24:548.
89. Kain KC, Noble MA, Freeman HJ, Barteluk RL. Epidemiology and clinical features associated with *Blastocystis hominis* infection. *Diagn Microbial Infect Dis* 1987;8:235–244.
90. Senay H, MacPherson D. *Blastocystis hominis:* epidemiology and natural history. *J Infect Dis* 1990;162:987–990.
91. Udkow MP, Markell EK. *Blastocystis hominis:* prevalence in asymptomatic versus symptomatic hosts. *J Infect Dis* 1993;168:242–244.
92. O'Gorman MA, Orenstein SR, Proujansky R, Wadowsky RM, Putnam PE, Kocoshis SA. Prevalence and characteristics of *Blastocystis hominis* infection in children. *Clin Pediatr (Phila)* 1993;32:91–96.
93. Gugliemetti P, Cellesi C, Figura N, Rossolini A. Family outbreak of *Blastocystis hominis* associated with gastroenteritis. *Lancet* 1989;3:1394.
94. Editorial: *Blastocystis hominis:* a commensal or pathogen? *Lancet* 1991;337:521–522.
95. Phillips BP, Zierdt CH. *Blastocystis hominis:* pathogenic potential in human patients and gnotobiotes. *Exp Parasitol* 1976;39:358–364.
96. Markell EK, Udkow MP. *Blastocystis hominis:* pathogen or fellow traveller? *Am J Trop Med Hyg* 1986;35:1023–1026.
97. Zierdt CH. In vitro response of *Blastocystis hominis* to antiprotozoal drugs. *J Protozool* 1983;30:332–334.
98. Dunn LA, Boreham PF. The in-vitro activity of drugs against *Blastocystis hominis*. *J Antimicrob Chemother* 1991;27:507–516.
99. Grossman I, Weiss LM, Simon D, Tanowitz HB, Wittner M. *Blastocystis hominis* in hospital employees. *Am J Gastroenterol* 1992;87:729–732.
100. Schwartz E, Houston R. Effect of co-trimoxazole on stool recovery of *Blastocystis hominis*. *Lancet* 1992;339:428.
101. Sargeaunt PG, Williams JE. Electrophoretic isoenzyme patterns of pathogenic and nonpathogenic intestinal amoebae of man. *Trans R Soc Trop Med Hyg* 1979;73:225–227.

Infections of the Gastrointestinal Tract,
edited by M. J. Blaser, P. D. Smith, J. I. Ravdin,
H. B. Greenberg, and R. L. Guerrant
Raven Press, Ltd., New York © 1995.

CHAPTER 75

Cestodes

Michele Barry and Michael Cappello

Cestodes (class Cestoidea in the phylum Platyhelminthes) include the parasitic flat tapeworms that have been described since the times of Aristotle (1). Tapeworms of the gastrointestinal tract of mammals have flat, segmented bodies consisting of a head or scolex and a series of segments (proglottids), which do not possess a true body cavity. The growth of the worm occurs in the anterior end by a process called *strobilation* or formation of new proglottids with the most posterior proglottids becoming mature and then gravid (2–4). These tapeworms can range in size from 25 to 35 mm in length (*Hymenolepis nana*) to 25 to 30 m (*Taenia saginata*) and are parasitic in the gastrointestinal tract of vertebrates. Cestodes lack a true digestive tract and absorb all nutrient molecules from the host through a surface membrane, a syncytial surface layer with minute projections, which usually abuts the host's intestinal villi (5). Tapeworms are hermaphroditic with proglottids containing both ovary and testes and the life cycles of all but one cestode (*H. nana*) require development in one or more intermediate hosts before development can occur in the final definitive host.

Of the four main groups of cestodes, only two groups are important parasites of humans: the order Pseudophyllidea, characterized by parasites with a scolex containing two sucking grooves (e.g., *Diphyllobothrium latum*), and the order Cyclophyllidea, characterized by the parasites with a scolex having four suckers (e.g., *T. saginata, T. solium, Echinococcus* species, *H. nana, H. diminuta, Mesocestoides,* and *Dipylidium caninum*) (2). Clinical manifestations of tapeworm infection may be due to infection with the adult or larval stage and some cestodes only infect humans in the larval stage. Humans are the only obligatory final host of two species (*T. saginata* and *T. solium*) but are accidentally involved in the life cycles of the others. This chapter reviews adult cestode infections

that involve the gastrointestinal tract of humans, excluding *Echinococcus* species.

TAENIA SAGINATA

Epidemiology

Taenia saginata, the beef tapeworm, is a parasite with highly endemic foci in Latin America and Africa, moderate prevalence in Europe, South Asia, and Japan, and low prevalence but still present in Australia, Canada, and the United States. Its prevalence exceeds 5% in such places as Ethiopia, where eating undercooked or raw beef is common and has been described in over 90% of certain tribes of Kenya where local habits enforce the life cycle (5). The geographic distribution of *T. saginata* reflects cattle husbandry where human excreta are not disposed of in a hygienic fashion.

Life Cycle

Humans are the definitive hosts for the adult tapeworm, which may live as long as 20 years. It is one of the largest of human parasites and attaches by its scolex to the intestinal mucosa of the small intestine. Infection is acquired by eating undercooked beef ("measly beef") containing living larval (cysticerci) forms of *T. saginata.* The larva evaginates in the small intestine, attaches to the surface with the aid of four suckers on the scolex, and then grows by segment differentiation (proglottid formation) to lengths up to 10 to 25 m (Fig. 1). The worm reaches adulthood and then begins to shed distal (six to ten) proglottids daily with up to 80,000 eggs per proglottid. These segments can actively migrate through the large intestine, rectum, and out the anus. Rarely, some of the eggs may burst from the segments but in general *T. saginata* proglottids are passed in intact form in the feces or migrate via independent muscular activity. After segments are ingested by the intermediate host (cattle), the hexacanth

M. Barry: Department of Medicine, and International Health Program, Yale University School of Medicine, New Haven, Connecticut 06504.

M. Cappello: Medical Helminthology Laboratory, Department of Pediatrics, Yale University School of Medicine, New Haven, Connecticut 06504.

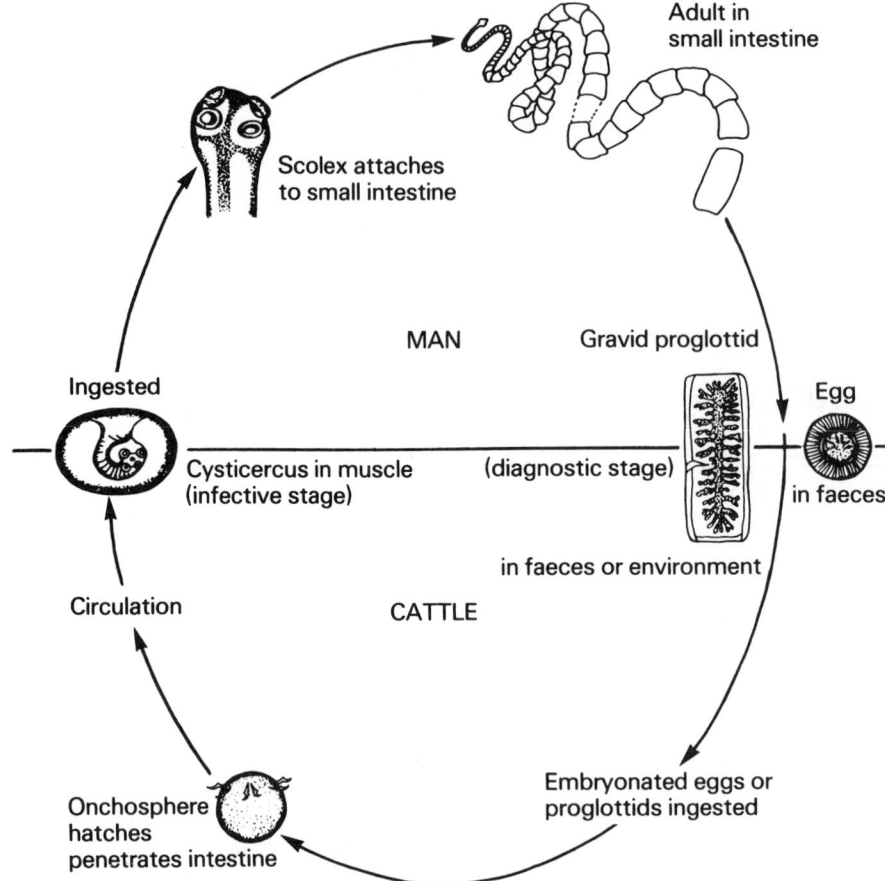

FIG. 1. Life cycle of *Taenia saginata*. (From ref. 6, with permission.)

embryos emerge from the eggs and pass by blood or lymph to muscle, subcutaneous tissue, or viscera of cattle, where the cycle will restart when humans eat undercooked larval contaminated beef. Only by eating contaminated cysticerci-infected undercooked beef can a human be infected by the adult tapeworm. Eggs of *T. saginata* when ingested by humans do not result in larval infection.

Clinical Manifestations

The incubation period from the time of infection to the passage of segments is 5 to 12 weeks (4). The majority of patients infected with *T. saginata* are usually infected with a single tapeworm (Fig. 2). At times mild gastrointestinal symptoms such as nausea, postprandial fullness, or vague epigastric pain are described. Rarely, vomiting, diarrhea, or intestinal obstruction have been described (2–4). The majority of patients are asymptomatic until they become aware of passage of tapeworm segments in feces. Occasionally, proglottids emerge from the anus and migrate actively down the thigh causing pruritus along the proglottid's pathway. Asymptomatic passage of proglottids or characteristic eggs in feces are more common. In a survey in Kenya, Hall et al. (7) noted that unless proglottids are actively crawling out of the anal sphincter, most

tapeworm proglottids are excreted with feces asymptomatically. Kaminsky (8), in a study of rural populations in Honduras, noted more than half of all patients infected were unaware of being infected. Rarely, proglottid segments can be vomited or enter the appendix or common bile duct and mimic appendicitis or gallstone disease (4) (Fig. 3). There is usually no malabsorption or weight loss described. Moderate eosinophilia can occur with initial infection but is rarely a feature of established tapeworm infections (4).

Diagnostic Tests

Definitive diagnosis depends on the identification of proglottids, which should be collected in water or saline (Fig. 4). Proglottids can be pressed between two microscope slides and then injected with India ink through the lateral pore to count lateral uterine branches in order to distinguish *T. saginata* proglottids from proglottids of *T. solium*. Gravid proglottids can also be fixed in 10% formalin for permanent carmine staining. *Taenia saginata* has 12 or more uterine branches on one side from the central core, while *T. solium* has usually fewer than 10 uterine branches per side. Eggs from both species are identical and are only irregularly present in feces (Fig. 5). Coproan-

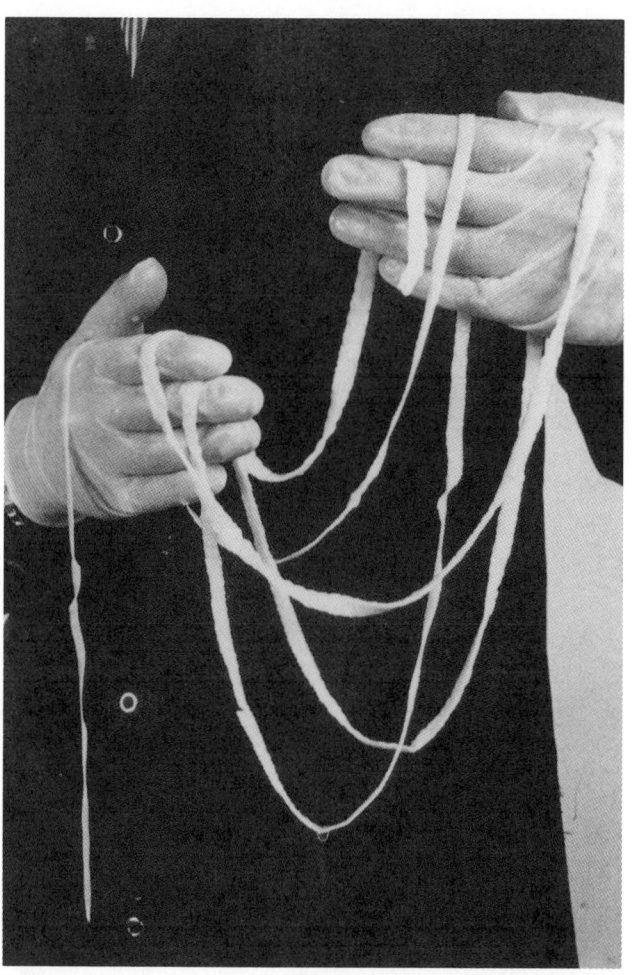

FIG. 2. Adult *T. saginata* tapeworm. (From ref. 4, with permission.)

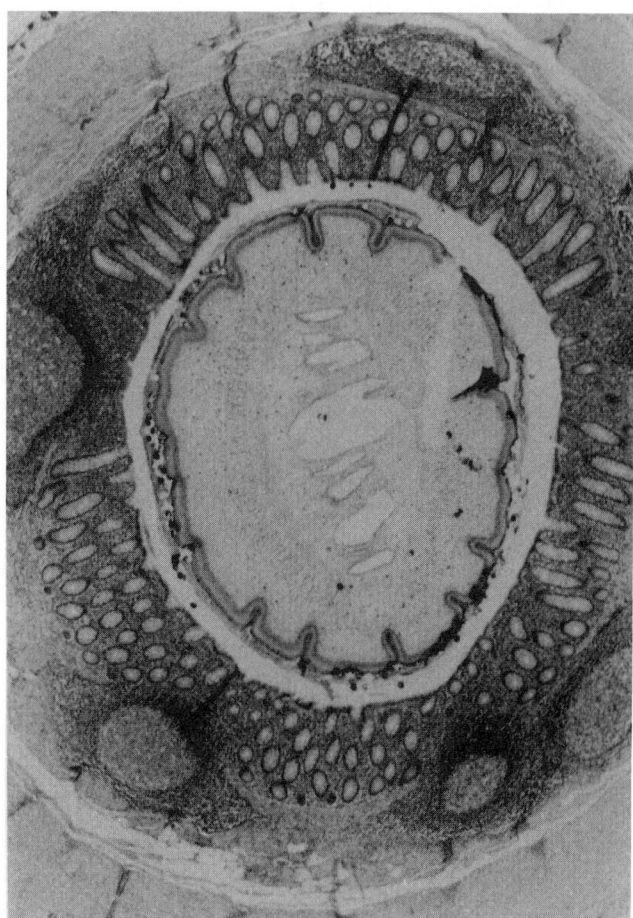

FIG. 3. Low-power view of appendix with a cross section of *T. saginata* proglottid filling lumen. (From ref. 3, with permission.)

tigen detection of *Taenia*-specific antigen in feces may prove to be a sensitive diagnostic tool (11). Scotch tape perianal swabs (STPS) have been used to collect eggs deposited in the perianal area or stools can be collected for egg examination by formalin–ether concentration.

Treatment

Antihelminthic drug therapy has been almost 100% effective with either praziquantel 10 to 20 mg/kg single dose or albendazole 400 mg daily for 3 days (8,12). An alternative drug therapy is niclosamide given as a single 2-g well-chewed dose for adults (pediatric dose: 11 to 34 kg, single dose 1.0 g); (34 to 57 kg, single dose of 1.5 g). Niclosamide tablets should be chewed well and taken after a day of light meals and only liquids the evening prior to treatment because failures have been described (13). Paromomycin 75 mg/kg (4 g maximum) after a meal produces good cure rates (93%) but mild side effects such as diarrhea occur commonly and make it a less attractive drug (13,14). Paromomycin does have the advantage of being a nonabsorbable drug and therefore considered safer in pregnancy although no studies have been conducted in pregnant women.

Passage of intact or disintegrating segments containing eggs may continue for days after treatment. Although a purge is not usually necessary after antihelminthic therapy, one may recover a scolex if a purge is administered within 2 hr of niclosamide treatment. Treatment with other antihelminthics, which disintegrate segments, may make scolex retrieval unlikely. Stools should be collected for 3 days after purge if recovery of the scolex is desired. Scolex recovery is the only total assurance that worm regeneration will not occur. Alternatively, a second stool examination for proglottids or eggs should be done 3 months after antihelminthic therapy (regeneration period for the scolex) to ensure that cure has been accomplished.

Prevention and Control

Since sociocultural factors such as requiring the consumption of raw meat for local ceremonial practices or the eating of raw meat as a traditional treatment for anemia can play a role in *T. saginata* infection, culturally

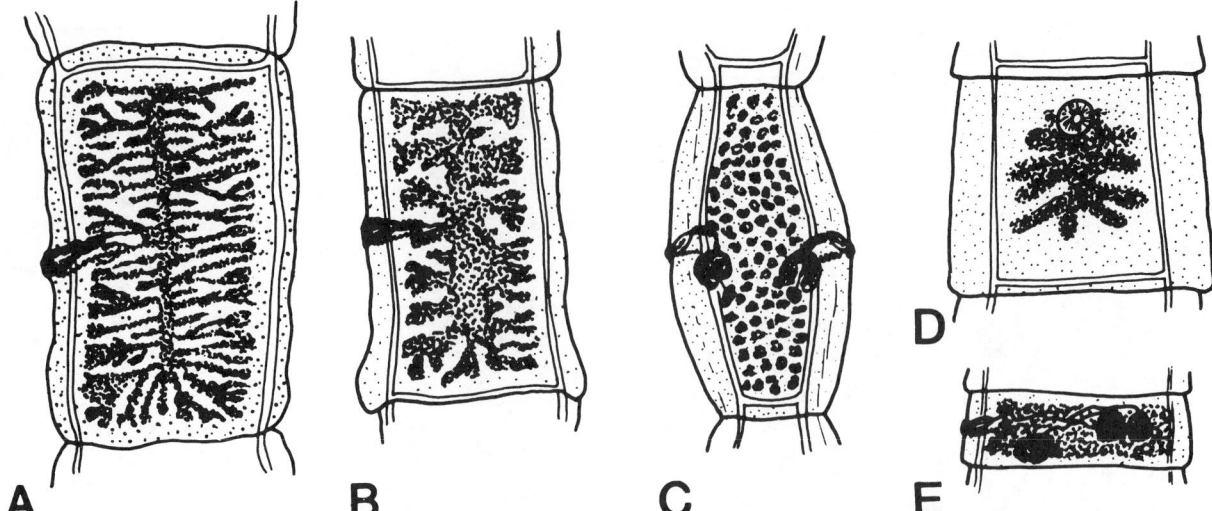

FIG. 4. Schematic representation (not to scale) of gravid proglottids of some common intestinal tapeworms of humans. **A:** *Taenia saginata* (12 or more uterine branches). **B:** *Taenia solium* (10 or less uterine branches). **C:** *Dipylidium caninum.* **D:** *Diphyllobothrium.* **E:** *Hymenolepis.* (From ref. 9, with permission.)

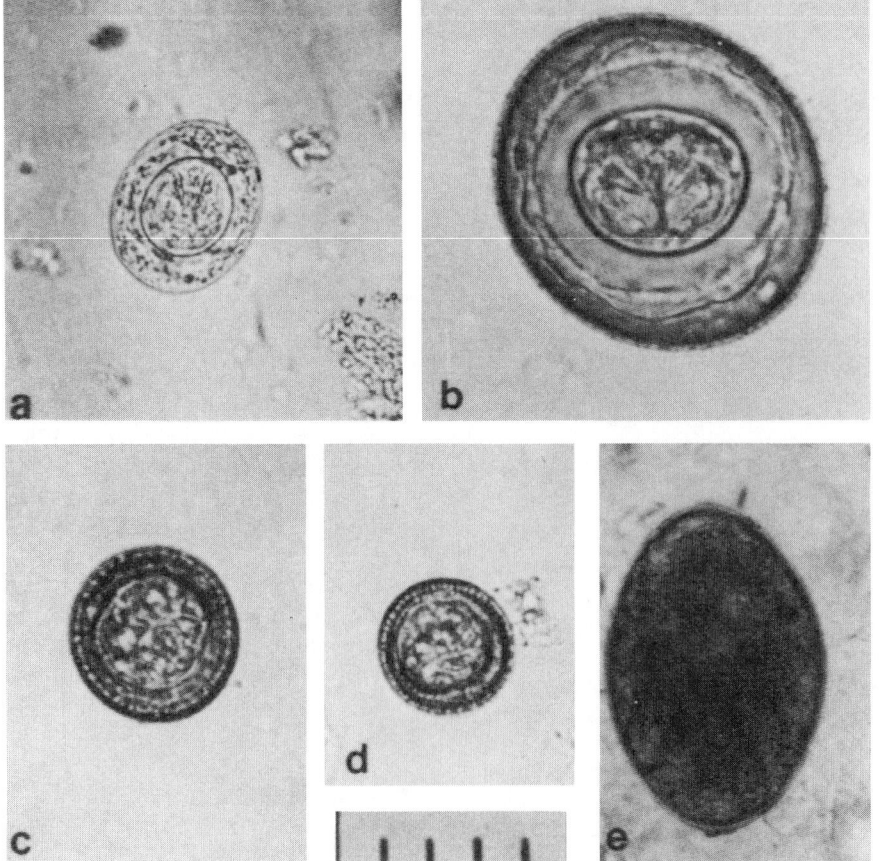

FIG. 5. Cestode eggs: (**a**) *Hymenolepis nana,* (**b**) *H. diminuta,* (**c, d**) *Taenia* species, and (**e**) *Diphyllobothrium latum.* All eggs photographed at same magnification; scale equals 50 μm. (From ref. 10, with permission.)

sensitive educational control programs are important. Thorough cooking of meat is a key individual preventive measure. Public health measures such as sanitary disposal of human feces and restriction of cattle from land contaminated by human feces will prevent transmission. Although freezing of beef at −20°C for 10 days will kill cysticerci, this is often not practical in endemic areas (5). Regional mass chemotherapy of human infections has had some success in interrupting the human to animal cycle.

TAENIA SOLIUM

Taenia solium, the pork tapeworm, is a flat tapeworm that also causes intestinal taeniasis in humans. Unlike *T. saginata*, the larval stage (cysticercal stage) can also invade humans and cause infection of the central nervous system (neurocysticercosis), subcutaneous tissue, muscle, myocardium, or, rarely, other viscera. Intestinal taeniasis is caused by the adult stage of *T. solium* and tapeworm carriers can contribute significantly to the transmission of the larval stage of the cysticercal stage in humans.

Epidemiology

Taenia solium is distributed throughout the world and coincides with pig-raising, especially when human ma-

nure is used. Highly endemic areas are Southeast Asia, Central and South America, Mexico, the Philippines, Micronesia, Africa, India, and Eastern Europe. Transmission has been described in the United States (18). There is no predilection for infection by sex or race (15).

Life Cycle

Adult *T. solium* closely resembles adult *T. saginata;* however, its scolex possesses two rows of rostellar hooks, which it uses along with its four suckers to attach to the small intestine of a human (Fig. 6). Ingestion of undercooked or raw cysticerci-infected pork results in the release of cysticerci in the human duodenum. The scolex develops into an adult worm in 2 months and daily sheds egg-filled proglottids. Unlike *T. saginata*, these proglottids, which contain 50,000 to 100,000 eggs, rarely crawl and remain mostly in feces. Pigs, the intermediate hosts, are coprophagic. After segments are ingested, hexacanth embryos emerge and penetrate the pig's intestinal wall, where they migrate to muscle, subcutaneous tissue, or viscera. Humans complete the cycle by eating larval-contaminated pork.

Larval invasion of humans (cysticercosis) can occur primarily by accidental ingestion of eggs in human feces by either anal–oral autoinfection or by the ingestion of *T. solium* eggs in fecally contaminated water or food. A recent outbreak of neurocysticercosis in an Orthodox Jew-

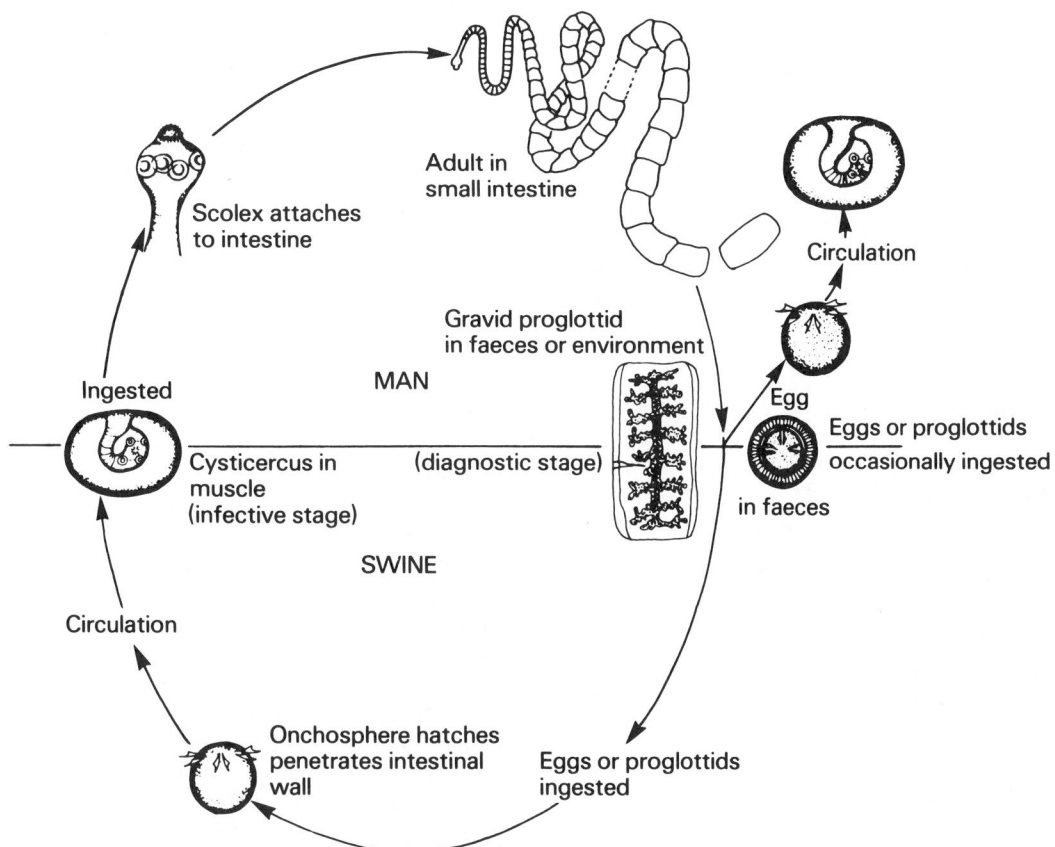

FIG. 6. Life cycle of *Taenia solium.* (From ref. 6, with permission.)

ish community that does not eat pork underscores that pork ingestion is not necessary for the larval infection of *T. solium* (16).

Clinical Manifestations: Intestinal Taeniasis

As *T. solium* is somewhat smaller than *T. saginata*, patients tend to be mostly asymptomatic and not aware of tapeworm infection until proglottids are passed in their stools. Infection with multiple tapeworms has been noted. Proglottid segments do not independently crawl out of the anus like *T. saginata* segments, and often patients just note proglottids in feces. Anal pruritus and urticaria have been described with heavy infections and eosinophilia may be present in early infection.

Diagnostic Tests

Diagnosis is made by either proglottid passage or egg identification. Discrimination between *T. saginata* and *T. solium* is critical for evaluation of possible concomitant cysticercosis. Proglottid examination is the best way to discriminate species and is performed as described for *T. saginata* (Fig. 4). A gravid proglottid of *T. solium* should have fewer than ten uterine branches on each side. Egg excretion is sporadic as proglottids are usually passed intact; eggs can be collected in fecal smears, stool concentrates, or by perianal swabs. Although egg identification cannot be species specific, recent coproantigen testing with a capture-type enzyme-linked immunoadsorbent assay (ELISA) for *Taenia* genus-specific fecal antigen has been attempted with some success, even in patients with low fecal egg counts (11). Work is now being conducted to try to develop a species-specific monoclonal probe for *T. solium* and *T. saginata* coproantigen (J. C. Allan, *personal communication*). Serodiagnostic testing for intestinal taeniasis has not been helpful, although immunologic testing with indirect hemagglutination antibody (IHA), ELISA, and specific serologic markers in immunoblot assays have been utilized for disseminated human cysticercosis (17).

Treatment

Intestinal taeniasis with *T. solium* is similar to *T. saginata*. Use of purgatives is controversial as there is a theoretical risk of regurgitation of eggs of *T. solium* into the stomach with purgatives and thus a risk of autoinfection and larval cysticercosis. Others have suggested purge to avoid the theoretical but not proved possibility of eggs hatching following proglottid disintegration (5,18). We do not use purgatives but do recheck the feces of patients several months after treatment. Treatment of larval invasion by *T. solium* has been recently reviewed (17).

Prevention and Control

Taenia solium intestinal infection is totally preventable by protection of pig feed from contamination of human feces. Individual maneuvers to protect oneself from infection are by thorough cooking of pork or by freezing pork at −20°C for 10 days. Abattoir inspection of pig carcasses may miss lightly infected pork and thus mass chemotherapy of villages where intestinal *T. solium* infection is prevalent may interrupt the cycle (17). Control of human fecal contamination of household environment, drinking water, and food when there is a *T. solium* tapeworm carrier in the house is imperative in order to prevent household cases of human cysticercosis.

DIPHYLLOBOTHRIUM LATUM

Epidemiology

Diphyllobothriasis is caused by infection with adult fish tapeworms of the genus *Diphyllobothrium*. While the majority of cases are caused by *D. latum*, other species are capable of infecting humans, including *D. dendriticum*, *D. pacificum*, *D. alascence*, and *D. ursi* (19). The disease is most common in northern Europe and Scandinavia, although isolated cases have been reported from throughout most areas of the world. In North America, diphyllobothriasis has frequently been described in the Great Lakes region, probably having been introduced to that area by Scandinavian settlers. Native American populations in northern Canada and Alaska also carry these tapeworms (20).

The practice of eating raw fish is perhaps the greatest risk factor for acquiring this infection. As such, cultures that rely heavily on this tradition tend to have an increased prevalence of diphyllobothriasis. Frequent cases have been reported in women who prepare gefilte fish, a popular Jewish delicacy that is often sampled prior to cooking to test for proper flavoring (5). Also, the rising popularity of sushi has increased the risk of *D. latum* infection in the United States over the past two decades (21). Overall, however, the incidence of diphyllobothriasis worldwide, even in areas of traditionally high endemicity, has fallen dramatically in recent years (19).

Life Cycle

Diphyllobothrium latum requires at least two intermediate hosts prior to completing its life cycle in humans (Fig. 7). When eggs passed in feces are deposited in freshwater streams or ponds, they must hatch and be eaten by suitable species of copepods. These freshwater crustaceans allow the eggs to develop from ciliated coracidia into procercoid larvae. When a small fish feeds on an infected copepod, the procercoids invade the stomach wall and penetrate the secondary host's musculature. Here the procercoid matures into a plerocercoid, growing from 500 μm to 5 mm in length over a 4-week period. Humans become infected by eating a fish that harbors a viable plerocercoid larva, which then matures into an adult tapeworm and attaches by its scolex to the wall of the small intestine. Species of fish known to carry *D. latum* include

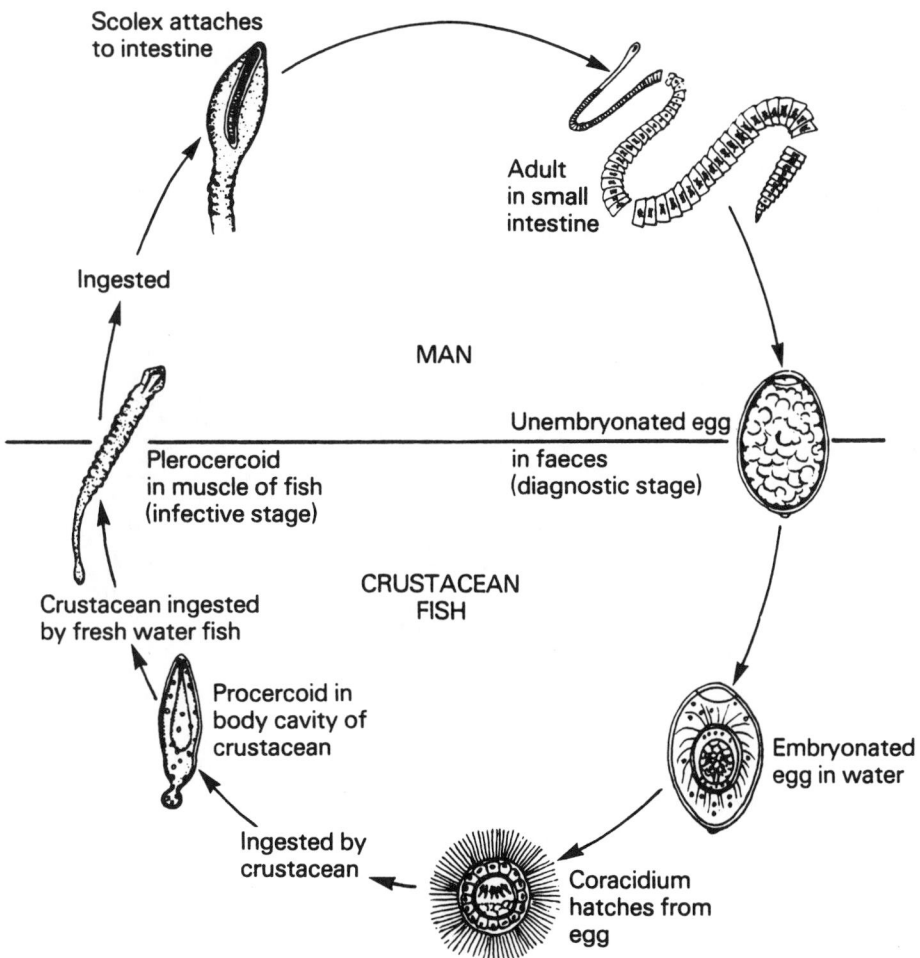

FIG. 7. Life cycle of *Diphyllobothrium latum*. (From ref. 6, with permission.)

pike, turbot, perch, and occasionally salmon. Eggs appear in the stool approximately 3 weeks after infection. The adult *D. latum* can grow at a rate of 5 cm/day and reach lengths of greater than 20 m. The scolex is rounded, with dorsal and ventral sucking grooves (Fig. 8). Each tapeworm can release up to one million eggs per day, which must be deposited in suitable fresh water (high oxygen content and a temperature below 22°C) to remain viable. A single parasite can survive many years within its human host. Other mammals, including bears, wolves, foxes, and cats, are capable of serving as definitive hosts to many species of *Diphyllobothrium,* including *D. latum.*

Clinical Manifestations

Despite the large size of this tapeworm, the majority of *D. latum* infections are asymptomatic. In a controlled trial, however, certain symptoms were found to be more common in otherwise healthy tapeworm carriers than noninfected controls, including diarrhea, fatigue, dizziness, distal paresthesias, and a sensation of hunger (22). Abdominal pain, while not a common feature of diphyllobothriasis, can occur in those with large tapeworm burdens or multiple infections.

A rare but striking clinical sequela of *D. latum* infection is tapeworm-associated pernicious anemia. This entity is virtually indistinguishable from the idiopathic form, with decreased serum levels of vitamin B_{12}, megaloblastosis, glossitis, and peripheral neuropathy. Although only 2% of infected individuals develop this anemia, subclinical vitamin B_{12} deficiency can be detected in a much higher percentage of nonanemic persons with diphyllobothriasis than uninfected controls (23). It has been demonstrated that the tapeworm actively absorbs free vitamin B_{12} from the small intestine and appears capable of dissociating the host intrinsic factor–vitamin B_{12} complex as well (19).

Diagnostic Tests

The diagnosis of diphyllobothriasis relies on identification of ova in the stool of an infected individual. These eggs measure approximately 60×40 μm and have a characteristic operculum at one pole (Fig. 5). The proglottids, which may be passed in the stool or occasionally vomited, can also be used for identification. These segments are wider than they are long and contain both male and female reproductive organs (Fig. 4). An egg-filled uterus leads to a midventral genital pore, through which the ova are

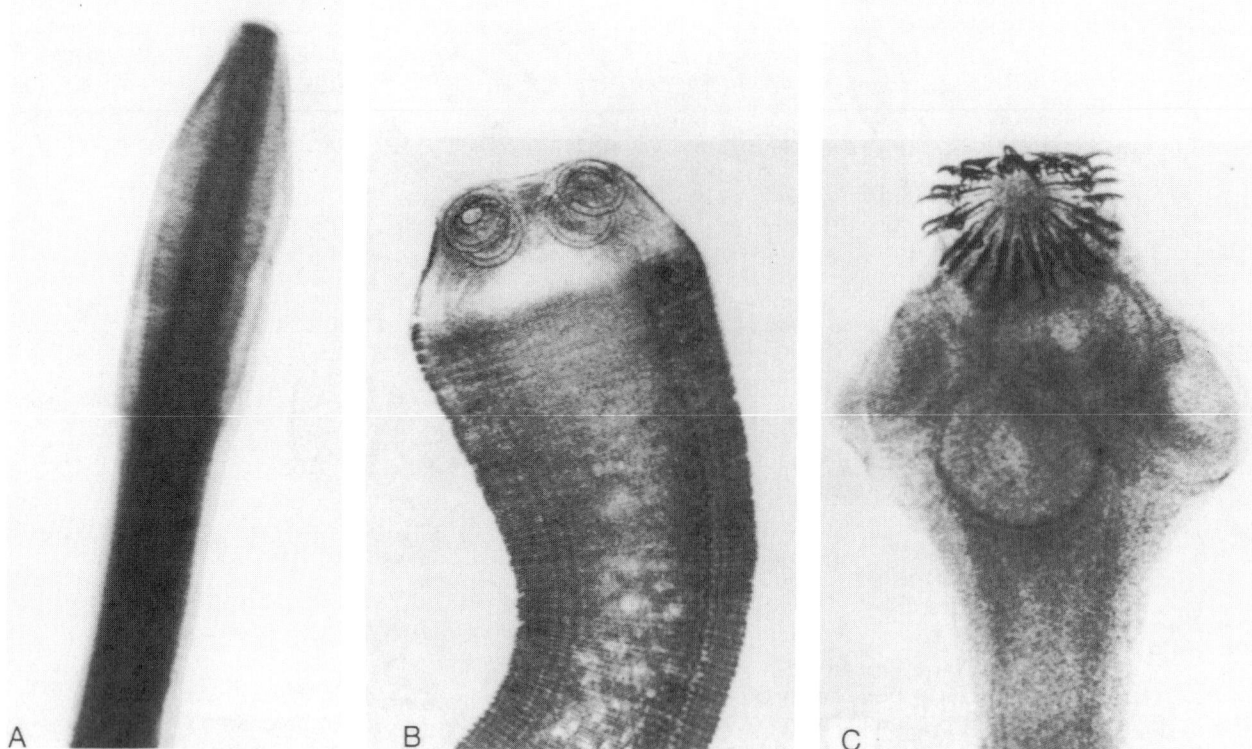

FIG. 8. Scolices of various tapeworms. **A:** *Diphyllobothrium latum.* **B:** *Taenia saginata.* **C:** *Taenia solium.* (From ref. 10, with permission.)

expelled into the small intestine (Fig. 4). It may be necessary to collect multiple stool samples to detect sporadic egg output. Serum B_{12} levels may be diminished even in the absence of megaloblastic anemia. To date, there is no serologic test to detect infection with *D. latum.*

Individuals with pernicious anemia or vitamin B_{12} deficiency who have a history of eating raw fish should be examined for fecal excretion of *Diphyllobothrium* eggs. In addition, those who have lived in highly endemic areas, particularly Scandinavia or the Great Lakes region of North America, may also be at increased risk of developing this infrequent but treatable complication of diphyllobothriasis.

Treatment

Praziquantel (10 mg/kg) and niclosamide (2 g for adults) are both effective in a single dose at treating diphyllobothriasis. Children under 34 kg should receive 1 g of niclosamide, while those weighing more than 34 kg should receive 1.5 g (12). The majority of the strobila is usually evacuated quickly, although the scolex itself may not be recovered. A post-treatment purge is not required. Follow-up stool examinations are recommended 6 to 8 weeks following therapy.

Tapeworm-associated pernicious anemia generally resolves with eradication of the parasite. However, supplemental vitamin B_{12} therapy is warranted in those cases

of symptomatic B_{12} deficiency associated with tapeworm infection.

Prevention

The most reliable means of preventing diphyllobothriasis is to adequately prepare all types of seafood prior to eating. Fish and hard roe should be thoroughly cooked to ensure that all viable procercoids are killed. Raw fish can be eaten safely only if it has been frozen at −18°C for at least 24 hr, or −10°C for 72 hr (21).

As stated, numerous mammalian species appear to be suitable hosts for the development of *D. latum.* Therefore it is unlikely that preventive measures will succeed in eradicating diphyllobothriasis. However, proper disposal and treatment of sewage should help to significantly reduce the transmission of this tapeworm in endemic areas.

HYMENOLEPIS NANA

Epidemiology

Hymenolepis nana, the dwarf tapeworm, is the most common cestode to infect humans, with up to 50 million cases estimated worldwide (24). The geographic distribution of *H. nana* is extensive and includes Europe, Africa, Asia, and the Americas. Transmission occurs most commonly via the fecal–oral route, so that high rates of disease spread are generally found in places where poor sanitary conditions exist. In the United States, outbreaks of hymenolepiasis have been reported most frequently in chronic care facilities, where poor hygiene and crowded living conditions likely facilitate transmission of the parasite (25).

Life Cycle

Hymenolepis nana is the only human tapeworm whose life cycle does not require an intermediate host (Fig. 9) When infective eggs are ingested, they hatch in the duodenum, releasing a double membraned oncosphere. After penetrating the intestinal mucosa, the oncosphere develops into a cysticercoid larva within the lymphatics of the intestinal villi. In 4 to 7 days, the cysticercoid migrates back into the lumen of the small bowel, attaches by its scolex to the intestinal wall, and eventually matures into an egg-laying adult. Importantly, this life cycle can be repeated within the same host, a phenomenon referred to as internal autoinfection. It takes approximately 3 to 4 weeks from the time of infection for eggs to appear in the

stool. The adult worm measures approximately 20 to 40 mm in length and up to 1 mm in width. There are four suckers on its scolex, with a retractable rostellum containing approximately 25 hooks. The proglottids are wider than they are long, with three testes and one ovary (Fig. 4). When gravid, each proglottid may contain up to 200 eggs.

Clinical Manifestations

While the majority of infections are asymptomatic, heavy infestation with *H. nana* can cause significant intestinal inflammation. Diarrhea, abdominal cramping, and anorexia are the most frequent gastrointestinal symptoms noted. Systemic illness, characterized by dizziness, irritability, and even generalized seizures, has been associated with hymenolepiasis, although the etiology of these central nervous system sequelae remains unknown. In addition, there is an interesting association between intestinal *H. nana* infection and phlyctenular keratoconjunctivitis, an allergic inflammatory condition of the eye, perhaps mediated by a parasite-released toxin (26). Also, immune suppression due to an underlying illness or systemic

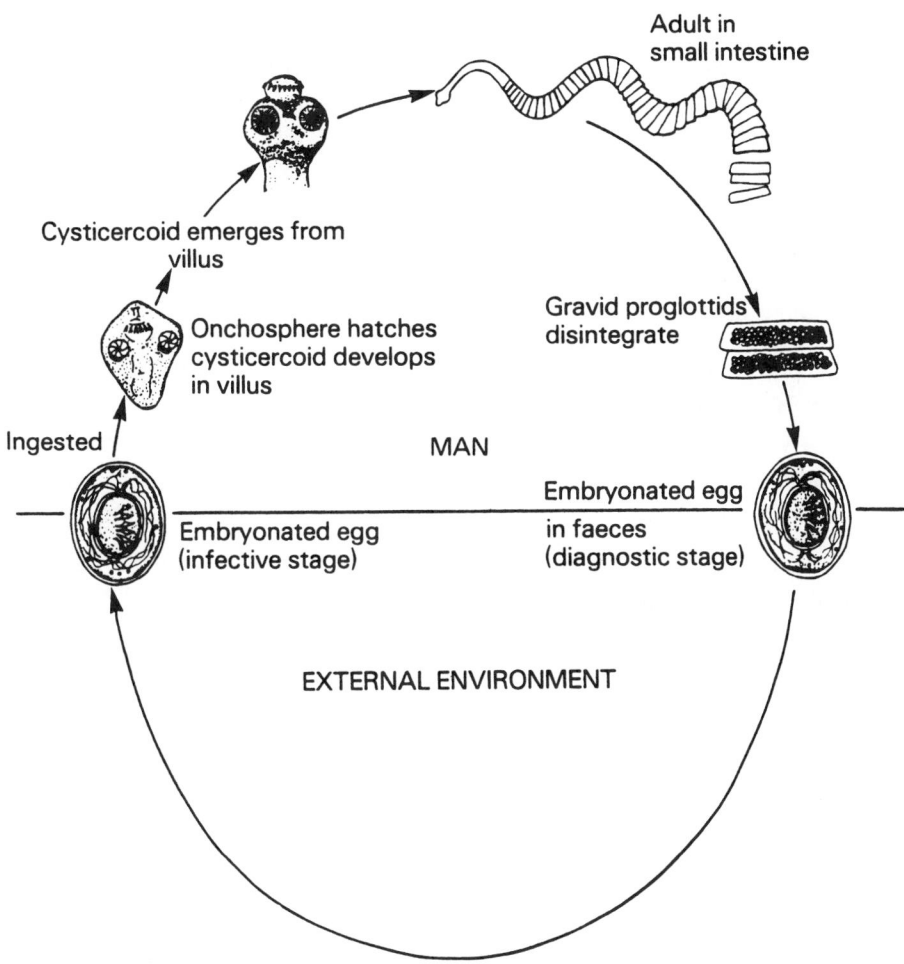

FIG. 9. Life cycle of *Hymenolepis nana*. (From ref. 6, with permission.)

chemotherapy may lead to overwhelming intestinal worm burdens caused by increased levels of *H. nana* autoinfection in certain compromised hosts. Lastly, disseminated hymenolepiasis, characterized by systemic tissue invasion of larvae, is an infrequent complication of *H. nana* infection (27).

Diagnostic Tests

The diagnosis of hymenolepiasis is made by identifying the characteristic double-membraned eggs in the stool of an infected individual.(Fig. 5). These ova are small, measuring approximately 40 μm in diameter, and samples should be handled carefully during processing to preserve their morphology. Multiple stool examinations using concentrating techniques may be necessary to detect light infections, as egg output can be irregular. ELISA has been used to detect antibodies to *H. nana* in the serum of infected individuals (28,29). However, this test has poor specificity due to frequent false-positive results in individuals with cysticercosis or hydatid disease. Therefore it is not recommended for routine clinical use in the diagnosis of hymenolepiasis.

Treatment

The drug of choice for hymenolepiasis is praziquantel, given in a single oral dose of 25 mg/kg. Cure rates of greater than 90% have been reported (30,31). Although niclosamide is also effective against the adult worm, it will not affect encysted larvae in the intestinal villi. Therefore a 7-day course of therapy (2 g/day for adults; 1 g/day for children weighing less than 34 kg, 1.5 g/day for those weighing between 34 and 57 kg, and 2 g/day for those weighing more than 57 kg) must be completed when niclosamide is chosen for the treatment of *H. nana* infection. A post-treatment purge is not necessary, although repeat stool examinations should be performed 8 to 12 weeks after therapy to confirm successful elimination of the parasite.

Prevention

Efforts aimed at interrupting the spread of *H. nana* should be directed at preventing fecal–oral contamination in populations at risk for infection, particularly young children. In addition, proper hygienic conditions must be rigidly maintained in those chronic care facilities found to harbor this tapeworm.

HYMENOLEPIS DIMINUTA

Epidemiology

Hymenolepis diminuta, the rodent tapeworm, can also cause disease in humans (32,33). The majority of infections occur in children, often in urban settings associated with impoverished living conditions and rodent infestation.

Life Cycle

The life cycle of *H. diminuta* begins with the ingestion of eggs by any one of a number of arthropod species, including fleas, cockroaches, and beetles. The eggs develop into cysticercoid larvae within the intestine of the intermediate host (Fig. 10). Most infections in humans occur when an insect harboring *H. diminuta* is inadvertently eaten, usually after having contaminated a source of cereal or grain. The larvae then attach to the mucosa of the small intestine, where they mature into adults. The adult scolex bears four suckers, yet lacks an armed rostellum. The mature proglottids are similar in appearance to those of *H. nana*. Adult worms can grow to 90 cm in length and up to 4 mm in width. Eggs are deposited in the stool when gravid proglottids are released into the bowel lumen and can generally be detected 2 to 3 weeks after infection.

Clinical Manifestations

The symptoms of *H. diminuta* infection are similar to those associated with *H. nana*, including diarrhea, abdominal pain, and anorexia. Most infections, however, appear to be asymptomatic.

Diagnostic Tests

Identification of *H. diminuta* eggs in stool confirms the diagnosis of infection. These characteristic ova measure approximately 60 μm in diameter (nearly twice the size of *H. nana*), with a thick outer membrane (Fig. 5).

Treatment

Single-dose therapy with either niclosamide (2 g for adults, 1 g for children weighing less than 34 kg, 1.5 g for those between 34 and 57 kg) or praziquantel (10 mg/kg) is recommended for individuals with *H. diminuta* infection (5). Of note, segments of somewhat larger tapeworms may continue to be passed in the stool for several days following successful treatment. Purgative therapy is not necessary.

Prevention

Prevention of *H. diminuta* infection requires careful storage of dried food products, particularly grains and cereals, to avoid contamination by rodents and insects.

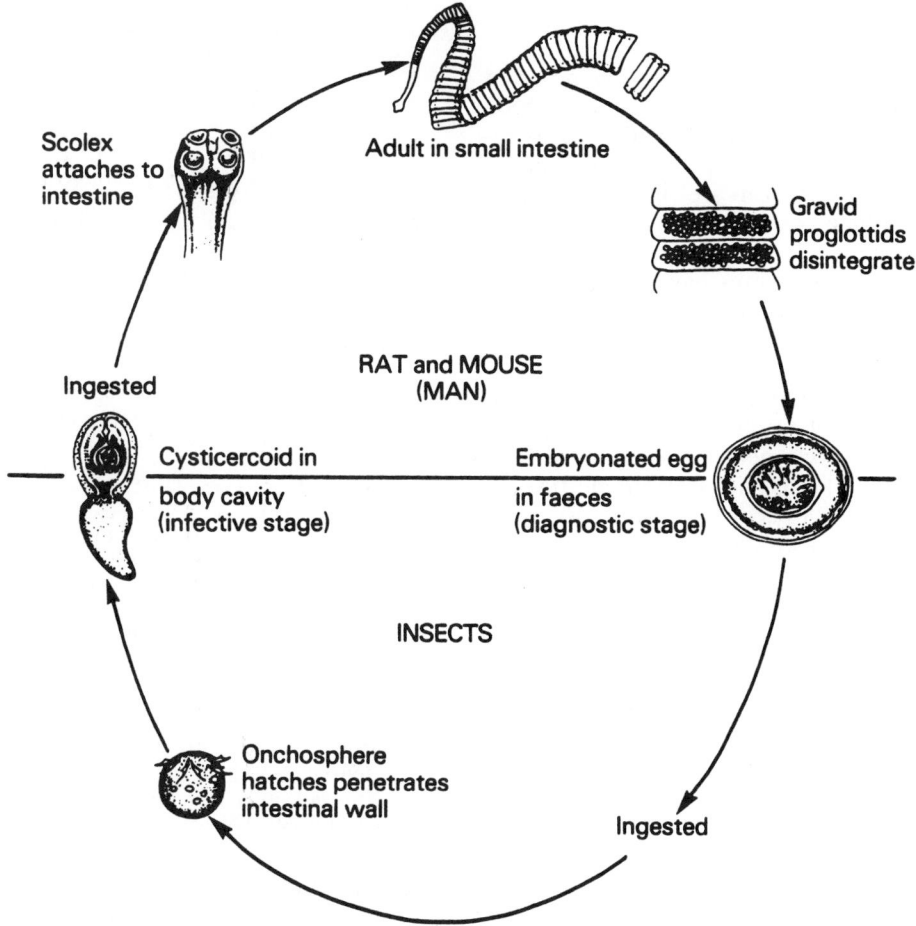

FIG. 10. Life cycle of *Hymenolepis diminuta*. (From ref. 6, with permission.)

LESS COMMON CESTODES CAUSING GASTROINTESTINAL DISEASE

Dipylidium caninum

Dipylidium caninum is the commonest tapeworm of domestic dogs and cats distributed worldwide (34). Infection in the United States usually occurs in children under 8 and in the southern states (35). Infection of a human requires ingestion of the intermediate host, the dog or cat flea (*Ctenocephalides canis* and *Ctenocephalides felis*) containing the larvae (cysticercoids) of *D. caninum*. Only rarely does the flea (*Pulex irritans*) of humans or the dog louse (*Trichodectis canis*) serve as an intermediate host (16). The life cycle is completed when a child ingests the cysticercoid-infected flea (34,35). An adult tapeworm develops measuring 6 to 30 in. in length and attaches to the wall of the intestine. Although most infections are probably asymptomatic, actively mobile gravid proglottids, the size and shape of cucumber seeds, can migrate out the anus or be passed in feces (34) (Fig. 4). In clinically recognized infections a transient diarrhea can occur as well as abdominal pain, anal pruritus, and irritability (36). Urticaria and eosinophilia have been described (37). Par-

ents have observed proglottids in children's diapers or feces. Praziquantel, 10 to 20 mg/kg in a single dose for adults or children, has been described as the drug of choice. Infection can also be effectively treated with single-dose niclosamide, children weighing less than 34 kg receive 1.0 g, those weighing 34 to 57 kg are given 1.5 g and for those weighing more than 57 kg a 2.0-g dose is required (37). Prevention can be accomplished by deworming pet dogs and cats and combating flea infestation on pets.

Bertiella studeri

Bertiella studeri is a tapeworm of nonhuman primates. Close association with primates is essential for access to the infecting agents (orbatid mites), which need to be ingested carrying the cysticercoid stage of the parasite (38). Monkeys have been implicated in the rare dozen or so human infections reported. Diarrhea, abdominal pain, and anorexia have been associated with the passage of proglottids and eggs. Treatment has been described with use of praziquantel (39).

Mesocestoides

Mesocestoides infections have rarely been reported from Asia, Africa, and North America. There have been 22 cases of human infection worldwide with 6 cases reported in children in the United States (40). The normal definitive hosts of these tapeworms are birds or mammals with the first intermediate host a coprophagic arthropod and larval tetrathyridial stage carried by dogs, cats, birds, reptiles, and amphibia. Tapeworms have been acquired by drinking the blood of snakes or turtles or eating the viscera from birds. A recent case describing infection in a 22-month-old child in a day care setting could not identify the route of infection, although a wide variety of reptiles and amphibians were housed as pets in the center, thus suggesting the life cycle needs further study (40). Again definite identification has been from proglottid passage. Niclosamide has been used successfully as treatment when proglottids are identified.

REFERENCES

1. Katz M, Despommier DD, Gwadz R. The cestodes. In: *Parasitic diseases,* 2nd ed. New York: Springer-Verlag, 1989.
2. Tanowitz H, Wittner M. Cestode infections. In: Strickland T, ed. *Hunter's tropical medicine.* Philadelphia: Saunders, 1991; 831–843.
3. Gutierrez Y. Introduction to cestodes. In: *Diagnostic pathology of parasitic infections with clinical correlations.* Philadelphia: Lea & Febiger, 1990;23–431.
4. Manson-Bahr PEC, Bell DR. Tapeworms (Cestoids). In: *Manson's tropical diseases.* London: Baillière Tindall, 1987; 521–557.
5. Schantz P. Cestode diseases. In: Goldsmith R, Heyneman D, eds. *Tropical medicine and parasitology.* East Norwalk, CT: Appleton & Lange, 1989;485–518.
6. Zaman V. *Atlas of medical parasitology,* 2nd ed. Balguwah, Australia: ADIS Health Science Press, 1984.
7. Hall A, Latham MC, Cromptom DWT, Stephensen L. *Taenia saginata* (Cestoda) in western Kenya: reliability of faecal examination in diagnosis. *Parasitology* 1981;83:91–101.
8. Kaminsky RG. Albendazole treatment in human *taeniasis. Trans R Soc Trop Med Hyg* 1991;85:648–650.
9. Smith JW, Gutierrez Y. Medical parasitology. In: Henry JB, Todd, Sanford, Davidsohn, eds. *Clinical diagnosis and management by laboratory methods,* 17th ed. Philadelphia, Saunders, 1984.
10. Markett EK, Voge M, John DT. *Medical parasitology,* 5th ed. Philadelphia: Saunders, 1981.
11. Allan JC, Noval JC, Flisser A, Craig, PS. Immunodiagnosis of taeniasis by coproantigen detection. *Parasitology* 1990;101: 473–477.
12. Drugs for parasitic infections. *Med Lett* 1992;34(865):17–26.
13. Vermund SH, MacLeod S, Goldstein RE. *Taeniasis* unresponsive to a single dose of niclosamide: case report of persistent infection with *Taenia saginata* and a review of therapy. *Rev Infect Dis* 1986;8:423–426.
14. Botero D. Paromomycin as effective treatment of taenia infections. *Am J Trop Med Hyg* 1970;19:234–237.
15. Botero D. Taeniasis. In: Goldsmith R, Heyneman D, eds. *Tropical medicine and parasitology.* East Norwalk, CT: Appleton & Lange, 1989;490–496.
16. Schantz PM, Moore AC, Muñoz JL, et al. Neurocysticercosis in an orthodox Jewish community in New York City. *N Engl J Med* 1992;327(10):692–695.
17. Barry M, Kaldjian L. Neurocysticercosis. *Semin Neurol* 1993; 13(2):131–143.
18. Richards F, Schantz P. Dogma disputed. Treatment of *Taenia solium* infection. *Lancet* 1985;1:1264–1265.
19. Von Bonsdorf B. *Diphyllobothriasis in man.* London: Academic Press, 1977.
20. Rausch RL, Scott EM, Rausch VR. Helminths in Eskimos in western Alaska, with particular reference to *Diphyllobothrium* infection and anaemia. *Trans R Soc Trop Med Hyg* 1967;61: 351–357.
21. Centers for Disease Control. Diphyllobothriasis associated with salmon—United States. *MMWR Morb Mortal Wkly Rep* 1981; 30:331–332,337–338.
22. Saarni M, Nyberg W, Grasbeck R, von Bonsdorff B. Symptoms in carriers of *Diphyllobothrium latum* and in non-infected controls. *Acta Med Scand* 1963;173:147–154.
23. Nyberg W, Grasbeck R, Saarni M, von Bonsdorff B. Serum vitamin B_{12} levels and incidence of tapeworm associated anemia in a population heavily infected with *Diphyllobothrium latum. Am J Clin Nutr* 1961;9:606–612.
24. Pawlowski ZS. Cestodiases: taeniasis, cysticercosis, diphyllobothriasis, hymenolepiasis, and others. In: Warren KS, Mahmoud A, eds. *Tropical and geographic medicine.* New York: McGraw-Hill, 1990;490–504.
25. Yoeli M, Most H, Hammond J, Scheinesson GP. Parasitic infections in a closed community: results of a 10-year survey in Willowbrook state school. *Trans R Soc Trop Med Hyg* 1972;66: 764–776.
26. Al-Hussaini MK, Khalifa R, Al-Ansary ATA, Hussain GH, Moustafa AKM. Phlyctenular eye disease in association with *Hymenolepis nana* in Egypt. *Br J Ophthalmol* 1979;63:627–631.
27. Gamal-Eddin FM, Aboul-Atta AM, Hassounah OA. Extraintestinal nana cysticercoidiasis in asthmatic and filarised Egyptian patients. *J Egypt Soc Parasitol* 1986;16:517–520.
28. Gomez-Priego A, Godinez-Hana AL, Gutierrez-Quiroz M. Detection of serum antibodies in human *Hymenolepis* infection by enzyme immunoassay. *Trans R Soc Trop Med Hyg* 1991;85: 645–647.
29. Castillo RM, Grados P, Carcamo CC, et al. Effect of treatment on serum antibody to *Hymenolepis nana* detected by enzyme-linked immunosorbent assay. *J Clin Microbiol* 1991;29:413–414.
30. Schenone H. Praziquantel in the treatment of *Hymenolepis nana* infections in children. *Am J Trop Med Hyg* 1980;29:320–321.
31. Groll E. Praziquantel for cestode infections in man. *Acta Trop (Basel)* 1980;37:293–296.
32. Hamrick HJ, Bowdre JH, Church SM. Rat tapeworm (*Hymenolepis diminuta*) infection in a child. *Pediatr Infect Dis J* 1990;9: 216–219.
33. Edelman MH, Spingarn CL, Nauenberg WG, Gregory C. *Hymenolepis diminuta* (rat tapeworm) infection in man. *Am J Med* 1965;38:951–953.
34. Marx M. Parasites, pets and people. *Primary Care* 1991;18(1): 153–165.
35. Turner JA. Human *Dipylidium* in the United States. *J Pediatr* 1962;61:763–768.
36. Raitiere C. Dog tapeworm (*Dipylidium caninum*) infestation in a 6-month-old infant. *J Fam Pract* 1992;34:101–102.
37. Neafie R, Marty A. Unusual infections in humans. *Clin Microbiol Rev* 1993;6:37–39.
38. Banyopadhyah AK, Manna B. The pathogenic and zoonotic potential of *Bertiella studeri. Ann Trop Med Parasitol* 1987;81(4): 465–466.
39. Conder GA, Roehm PA, Duprey DA, Johnson SS, Pagano PJ. Treatment of bertiellosis in *Macaca-fascicularis* with praziquantel. *J Helminthol Soc Wash* 1991;58(1):128.
40. Schultz L, Hummet B, Lubell I. Mesocestoides (cestoda) infection in a California child. *Pediatr Infect Dis J* 1992;11:332–333.

Infections of the Gastrointestinal Tract,
edited by M. J. Blaser, P. D. Smith, J. I. Ravdin,
H. B. Greenberg, and R. L. Guerrant
Raven Press, Ltd., New York © 1995.

CHAPTER 76

Ascariasis, Trichuriasis, and Enterobiasis

Ramya Gopinath and Jay S. Keystone

Human helminth infections are a major cause of morbidity and mortality, particularly in developing countries. It is estimated that greater than one billion people worldwide are infected with the four major geohelminths—*Ascaris, Trichuris,* hookworm, and *Strongyloides.* Ascariasis is the most common helminthic infection globally, but enterobiasis is the most common in the United States and Europe. All three are ancient human parasites, and eggs have been identified in animal and human coprolites from thousands of years ago (1). The prevalence and intensity of these infections depend more on socioeconomic standards and development than on regional ecological conditions.

ASCARIASIS

Ascaris is the largest intestinal helminth, with an estimated prevalence of one billion million cases globally and an annual mortality of 10,000 to 30,000 cases, due mainly to intestinal complications (2). In Bangladesh, where the overall prevalence of *Ascaris* infection is about 80%, it is the sixth leading cause of hospitalization. In Burma and Kenya, 3% and 2.6%, respectively, of all hospitalizations were due to ascariasis (3). *Ascaris lumbricoides* is specific for humans and has been found accidentally in other animals, such as the primates, and domestic animals. It was recognized as a distinct parasite by ancient cultures; in China, it was known to cause intestinal obstruction and was even used as a "catheter" to cure impotence. Since *Ascaris* is not a natural parasite of apes or humans, it is postulated that humans acquired infection from wild or domestic pigs. *Ascaris suum,* the helminth of pigs, is almost identical to *A. lumbricoides* except for a few minor differences in morphology and biochemistry which may have enabled its adaptation to humans. *Ascaris suum* has been found in humans but usually does not reach maturity (4). *Toxocara canis* and *T. cati,* roundworms of dogs and cats, are the cause of cutaneous and visceral larva migrans and may rarely live as adults in the human intestine.

Epidemiology

Ascariasis is most prevalent in Asia; it is estimated that 73% of the global pool is found there, followed by 12% in Africa, and 8% in Latin America (5). *Ascaris lumbricoides* and *T. trichiura* have closely related distributions and a high incidence of coinfection. In tropical climates, there is continuous transmission of infective eggs, while in temperate climates, a seasonal predilection is found. The distribution of the infection appears to be proportional to human population density, standards of education, levels of sanitation, and agricultural development, as well as regional climatic conditions. The majority of adult worms are harbored in a small proportion of the population, particularly in children. It is unclear whether this age-dependent intensity is due to reduced exposure or increased immunity in adults. In common with other helminths, there appears to be individual variation in predisposition to acquisition and intensity of infection; this is likely related to a variety of host factors (3,6).

Adult ascarids live in the small intestine with 88% found in the jejunum and 12% in the ileum. Sexual dimorphism is well expressed with the females being larger than males. On average, females are 20 to 49 cm long, males are 15 to 30 cm long, and both measure 3 to 6 mm in diameter. The body is cylindrical, unsegmented, and flesh-colored with lateral excretory canals. Anteriorly, three prominent lips are common to both sexes; the female has a vulvar opening ventrally one-third of the distance down the body, and the male has two copulatory spicules and numerous papillae on the curved posterior end. *Ascaris* feeds on the intestinal contents of humans and ingests barium. It is a facultative anaerobic organism, with a high glycogen consumption of 1.3 g per 100 g of body weight per day. The female has a prodigious reproductive potential, producing approximately 200,000 eggs per day. This accounts for a very high infection rate for soil in endemic areas.

R. Gopinath and J. S. Keystone: Tropical Diseases Unit, Division of Infectious Diseases, The Toronto Hospital, and University of Toronto, Toronto, Ontario M5G 2C4, Canada.

Life Cycle

Ascaris is a geohelminth; soil is necessary for development of eggs and acts as a reservoir. Humans, the definitive hosts for *Ascaris*, excrete fertilized eggs in feces (Fig. 1). These develop into first-stage larvae in 10 to 14 days in shaded soil. The optimal temperature is 28°C to 32°C, with a moisture level of greater than 80%. High temperature and desiccation readily kill eggs, but they may survive in soil for as long as 6 years in temperate zones. When embryonated eggs are ingested and reach the intestine, second-stage larvae develop and penetrate the mucosa of the small intestine. The extraintestinal stage then begins, with larval migration via lymphatics and blood vessels through the liver to the lungs. By day 14, larvae pass through the alveolar walls of the lung, migrate through the upper respiratory tract, are swallowed, and return to

the small bowel. During migration, larvae grow to about 2.2 mm in length and molt twice. Egg production begins about 60 to 75 days after ingestion of embryonated eggs. The mean life span of *Ascaris* is about 12 to 18 months.

Pathogenesis

The clinical picture and host response vary according to the stage of the infection. The tissue phase, in which larval migration occurs, is marked by various immunologic and inflammatory reactions, most notably an exuberant eosinophilic response with granuloma formation. Masses of acidophilic material are concentrated around the larvae (the Splendore–Hoeppli phenomenon), suggesting a hypersensitivity reaction. The eosinophilic response that occurs in the lung is responsible for the pulmo-

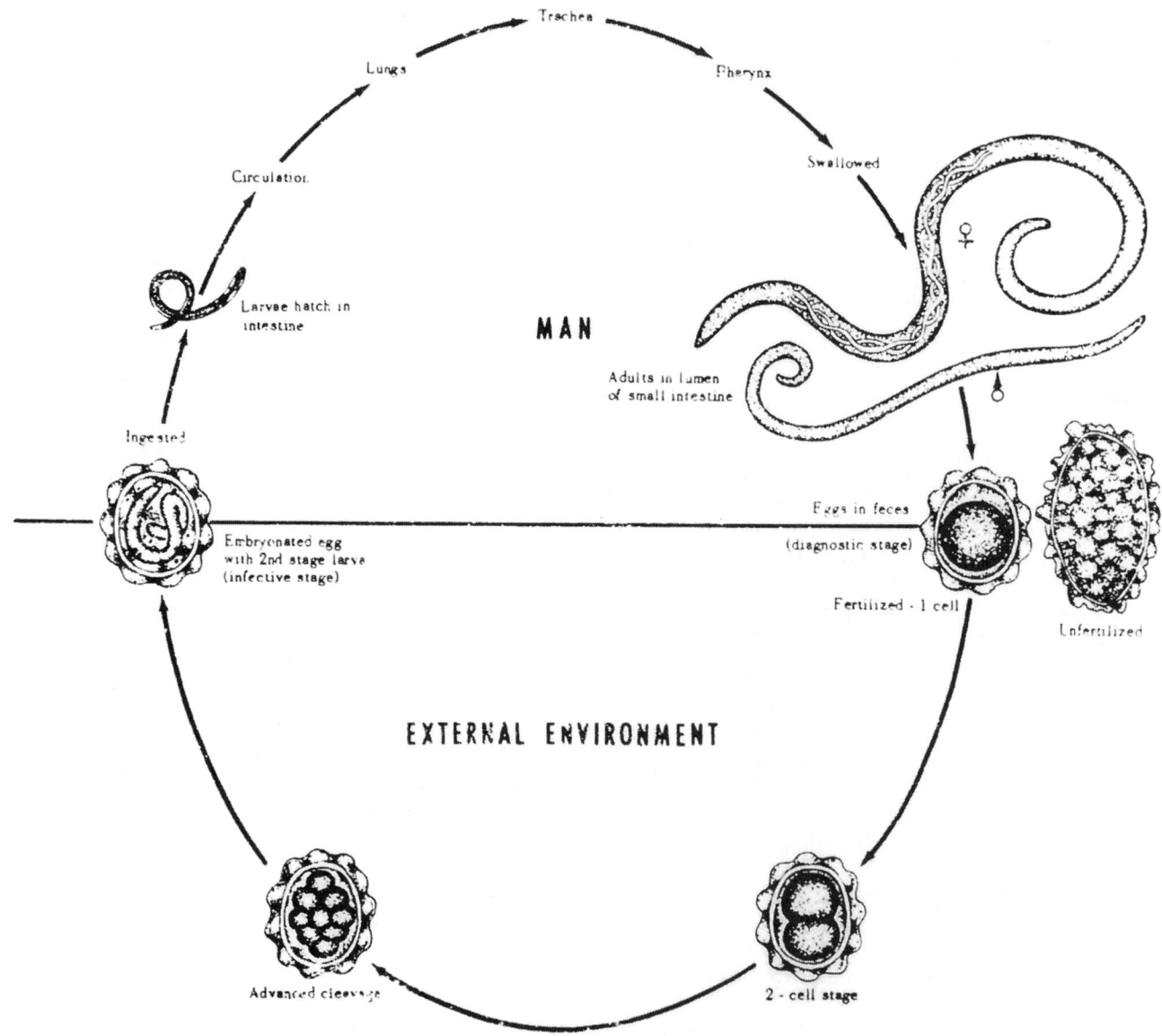

FIG. 1. Life cycle of *Ascaris lumbricoides*

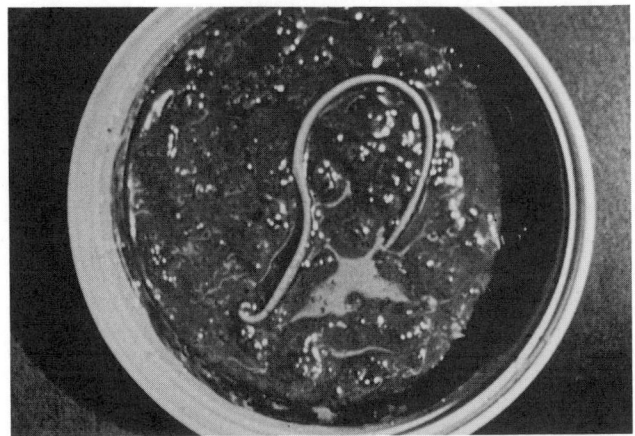

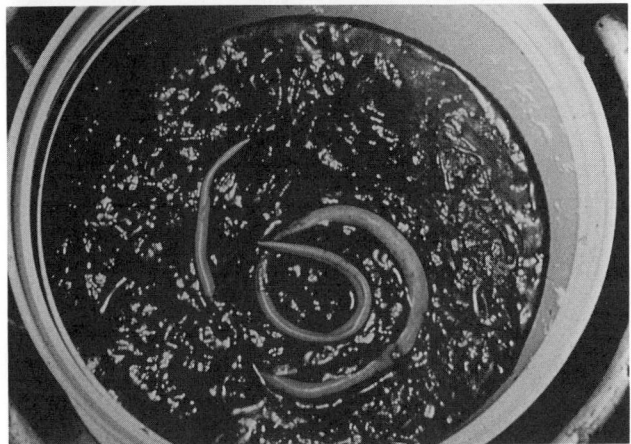

FIG. 2. Adult ascaris.

nary manifestations of Löffler's syndrome. The intensity of the host response to migrating larvae varies greatly, often is proportional to the number of larvae destroyed during migration, and seems to be greatest in populations sensitized by repeated exposure (7). Clinically, this may present as seasonal asthma in children.

The intestinal phase, by contrast, is often asymptomatic. Adult worms (Fig. 2) brace themselves against the intestinal wall and can migrate in the lumen, showing a tendency to enter small openings such as the appendix or ampulla of Vater. The association of ascariasis with protein-energy malnutrition has been noted for some time. Recent and controlled studies suggest that the effect of this infection on nutrition is probably important only in those on a marginal diet, with a heavy worm burden, and poor access to health care (8). Children appear to be the most seriously affected.

Immunity

Ascariasis stimulates the production of a variety of antibodies, including parasite-specific and nonspecific immunoglobulin E (IgE). A number of ascaris antigens act as potent allergens, particularly the internal antigen, a 14-kDa protein that is released by larval molting and disinte-

gration (9). Other antigens, including excretory–secretory products, also appear to elicit antibody responses. Interestingly, people infected with *Ascaris* vary considerably in the intensity and specificity of their antibody responses, even to the major internal antigen. This heterogeneity in response appears to be intrinsic to the host. In H-2-congenic mice infected with *A. suum,* it was demonstrated that the specificity of antibody response is major histocompatibility complex (MHC) restricted, while background genes may control its level or intensity (10). If MHC control of the response to ascariasis is proved to be of similar importance in humans, it would have implications in approaches to management and serodiagnosis. In addition, this would partially explain the long-observed predisposition of some individuals to heavy or light infections and perhaps provide the rationale for the targeting of chemotherapy. A study of class I histocompatibility locus antigens (HLAs) in Nigerian school children with varying levels of infection showed that uninfected children did not possess the A30/31 antigen in contrast to infected children who did (11).

The role of IgE in helminthic infections is still intensely debated. The control of IgE synthesis is complex and is influenced by the opposing effects of interleukin-4 (IL-4) and interferon-γ (IFN-γ), IgE-binding factors, and soluble CD23, which is the low-affinity receptor for IgE. Helminths stimulate the production of both parasite-specific and nonspecific IgE. The participation of IgE in immediate hypersensitivity reactions, although occasionally severe or fatal, appears, at a population level, to have evolved as a specific immune defense against helminths. In a Gambian study, high levels of specific IgE were clearly associated with resistance to reinfection with *Schistosoma haematobium* (12); whether this relationship can be extrapolated to other helminth infections remains to be proved.

The role of nonspecific IgE remains unclear. Pritchard (13) argues that large amounts of nonspecific IgE may actually benefit the parasite by effectively blocking IgE receptors on macrophages, mast cells, eosinophils, and B lymphocytes. This would limit the ability of parasite-specific IgE to provoke a hypersensitivity response and compromise antibody-dependent cellular cytotoxicity or expansion of antigen-specific T cell clones. The counterargument suggests that nonspecific IgE may reduce the risk of anaphylaxis, thereby protecting the host from a potentially lethal hypersensitivity response to parasite antigens (14). Much work remains to be done to clarify these issues.

Clinical Features

Ascariasis is often completely asymptomatic; however, when clinical manifestations do occur, the lungs are involved early and the gastrointestinal tract later. The pulmonary form, which begins within 1 to 2 weeks of infection, may present with a mild, self-limited cough, or acute illness characterized by low-grade fever, nonproductive cough, wheeze, dyspnea, eosinophilia, and bilateral transient fluffy infiltrates on chest radiograph. This illness

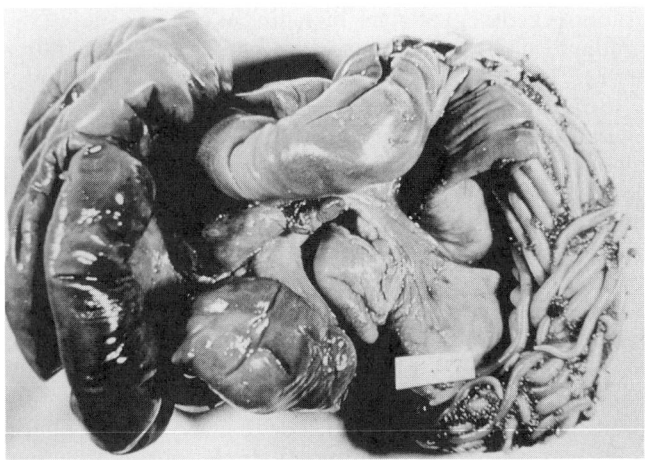

FIG. 3. Resected bowel obstructed by *Ascaris lumbricoides.*

usually lasts less than 1 week. Seasonal pneumonia due to *Ascaris* is well described in areas of the world where this infection is highly endemic (7). *Ascaris suum* infection has been known to cause respiratory failure in infected humans (4). The intestinal stage is often asymptomatic but may be marked by vague abdominal pain, nausea, and anorexia. The complications of ascariasis may be attributed to the large size of the worm and its propensity to migrate. The latter may be stimulated by fever, medications, anesthesia, or a change in diet. *Ascaris* is one of the worms that may be coughed or vomited up or extruded from the nose. Rarely, migrating worms may cause asphyxia due to upper airway obstruction. In endemic areas, 1% to 35% of all intestinal obstructions are due to adult ascarids. These may be partial or complete depending on worm burden and location of the obstruction (usually the terminal ileum) (Fig. 3). Intussusception, volvulus, infarction, or perforation may occur. A retrospective analysis of 1090 *Ascaris*-induced acute abdominal emergencies in South Africa found that 623 (57%) were caused by intestinal complications, 424 (39%) by biliary ascariasis, and 43 (4%) by pancreatic ascariasis (15).

Biliary and hepatic ascariasis are also common, usually presenting as biliary colic, cholangitis, or pancreatitis. In a large study of 507 patients from Srinagar, India, five major presentations were recognized for hepatobiliary ascariasis—acute cholecystitis (12.6%), acute cholangitis (23.9%), biliary colic (55.2%), acute pancreatitis (7.5%), and hepatic abscess (0.7%) (16). Contact with *Ascaris* allergens may cause hypersensitivity reactions in the skin, lungs, conjunctiva, and intestinal mucosa.

Diagnosis

The diagnosis of ascariasis is made by finding the adult worms, larvae, or eggs. The adults may be directly visualized when they are spontaneously expelled through the nose or anus, at surgery, or by endoscopy. In radiological contrast studies, worms may be outlined by barium,

which is also seen in the intestinal tract of the parasite (Fig. 4). Larvae may be found in sputum or gastric washings between 8 and 16 days following exposure, or occasionally in liver or lung biopsies. Eggs are detected by microscopic examination of concentrated or unconcentrated stool. Fertile eggs are ovoid and brown, measure 45 to 70 μm by 35 to 50 μm, and have a thick, multilayered outer shell. Infertile eggs, irregular, longer and narrower in shape, have a thinner shell and contain an amorphous material. The Kato–Miura technique (17) is commonly used for diagnosis of *Ascaris* eggs. Indirect methods of diagnosis include the demonstration of IgM antibodies to *Ascaris* by agar-gel diffusion or immunoelectrophoresis. Solid-phase radioimmunoassay (RIA), indirect immunofluorescence, or hemagglutination using both larval and adult ascaris antigen are also available but of limited practical use because of false-positive results with blood group antibodies, or cross-reaction with coexisting *Toxocara* infections. In general, the role of serodiagnosis is limited to the detection of early *Ascaris* infections (before egg production) or to epidemiologic studies. Eosinophilia may be marked (greater than 3000/mm³) during the larval migration phase but is not associated with adult infection.

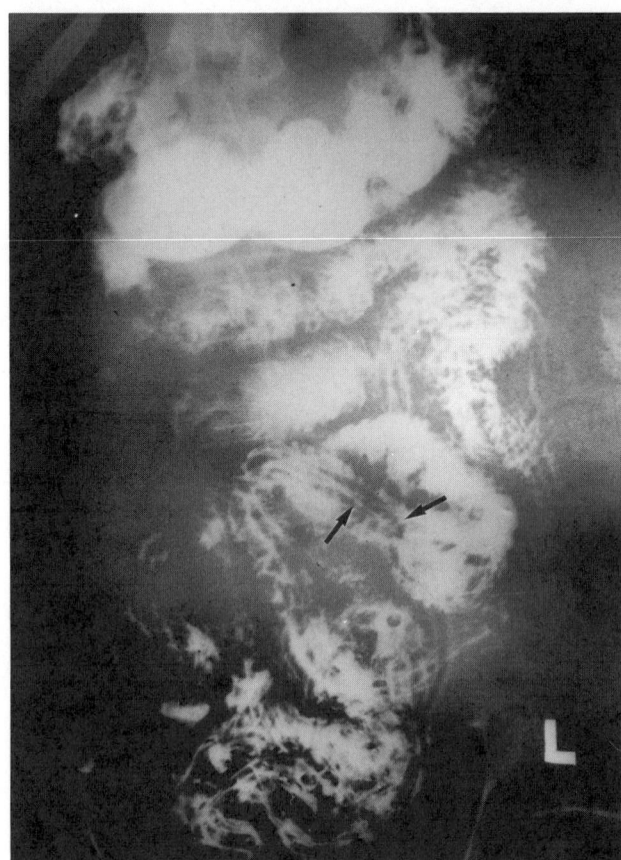

FIG. 4. Small bowel follow-through outlining an adult ascaris: barium within gut of the worm (*arrow on left*); and barium outlining the worm (*arrow on right*).

Treatment

Regardless of the worm burden, the intestinal form of ascariasis should always be treated in order to avert possible complications. The drugs of choice are pyrantel pamoate or the benzimidazole compounds such as mebendazole or albendazole. Pyrantel paralyzes the adult worm by acting on neuromuscular transmission. A single dose of 11 mg/kg is over 90% effective for lone infections with *Ascaris;* for mixed infections with hookworm and *Ascaris,* treatment is continued for 3 days. Pyrantel is well tolerated; when they occur, gastrointestinal side effects are mild and transient. However, in a recent case report, this drug was described to have possibly worsened preexisting myasthenia gravis (18). Mebendazole inhibits mitochondrial phosphorylation leading to death of the worm. A single dose of 200 mg, regardless of age, has an efficacy of 84% to 100% (19). Mixed infections require 400 to 600 mg as a single dose, or 200 mg daily for 3 days. Albendazole has over 90% efficacy in a dose of 200 mg in single infections; 400 mg is recommended for all age groups with mixed infections. The benzimidazoles are contraindicated in pregnancy. Other medications such as piperazine derivatives, levamisole, and ivermectin are also effective. In one study, ivermectin in a single dose for onchocerciasis appeared to be more effective than a single dose of benzimidazole in decreasing *Trichuris* egg burdens, equally effective against *Ascaris* and *Strongyloides* (100%), and less effective against hookworm (20). The pulmonary phase requires only supportive treatment; steroids may be indicated in severe cases. If intestinal obstruction is partial, piperazine or pyrantel may be given by nasogastric tube in an attempt to clear the obstruction. The treatment for complete obstruction or other intestinal complications is surgery with removal of the worm bolus or devitalized bowel. Biliary ascariasis may be treated conservatively with pyrantel or piperazine and/or by attempting to remove the worm by ERCP.

Prevention

Prevention must be practiced by individuals and on a community-wide basis. Individual prevention consists of thorough hand-washing, boiling water, attention to hygienic food preparation, and, particularly, supervision of children. In many communities in the developing world, children play and defecate in the same location, thus contributing to a continuing cycle of reinfection. Aspects of prevention at the community level include education, improved sanitation, provision of water for washing, and changes in agricultural practices (i.e., discouraging the use of night soil for fertilizer). Since these changes often occur slowly and are dependent on general socioeconomic development, mass chemotherapy has been investigated and appears to have a place in reducing transmission of infection, particularly in areas with a high prevalence (21,22). Initial mass treatment followed by targeted treatment of preschool and school children at 3-month intervals has been found to significantly reduce worm burden and soil contamination. A comparison of mass (all), targeted (children), and selective (heavily infected people) chemotherapy with levamisole for ascariasis was done in Nigeria (23). Significant differences in egg count were demonstrated after treatment in both treated and untreated individuals in the targeted population, and in all persons in the mass treatment populations, while no differences were found in the selective population. This and other studies (24) support the hypothesis that mass chemotherapy, at least initially, is more likely than selective chemotherapy to reduce worm burden and egg output and thereby to reduce morbidity.

TRICHURIASIS

Trichuris trichiura is a nematode responsible for intestinal syndromes of varying severity. Its common name, whipworm, is derived from the morphology of the adult worm. It differs from other geohelminths in that its life cycle lacks a pulmonary phase, and the adults are located in the large bowel.

Morphology

Humans are the primary host for *T. trichiura,* but many other species of the genus infect domestic animals. The pig whipworm, *T. suis,* is morphologically identical but rarely infects humans. *Trichuris vulpis,* a species whose primary host is the dog, has also occasionally been found in humans. The whip-like anterior end of this round worm makes up about three-fifths of the worm's length, with a thicker posterior end containing the intestine and reproductive organs. The female measures 30 to 50 mm in length, has an uncoiled posterior extremity, and lays between 3000 and 20,000 eggs per day. The male is slightly smaller, measuring 30 to 45 mm, and has a coiled caudal extremity with a copulatory spicule (Fig. 5). The eggs are barrel-shaped, measure 52 × 22 μm, and have plug-like prominences at either end.

Life Cycle

Eggs that are passed in stool mature best in warm, moist soil and require about 3 weeks to become infective. Under ideal conditions they can survive up to 1 year. When the embryonated egg is ingested, first-stage larvae hatch in the distal small bowel (Fig. 6). After a period of maturation, larvae migrate to the cecum, where the slender anterior end penetrates the intestinal mucosa while the posterior end protrudes into the lumen. The cycle, from egg ingestion through development to egg excretion, takes approximately 60 to 70 days; the life span of the adult may range from 1 to 8 years.

Epidemiology

It is estimated that about 800 million people are infected worldwide, primarily in the tropics. However, trichuriasis

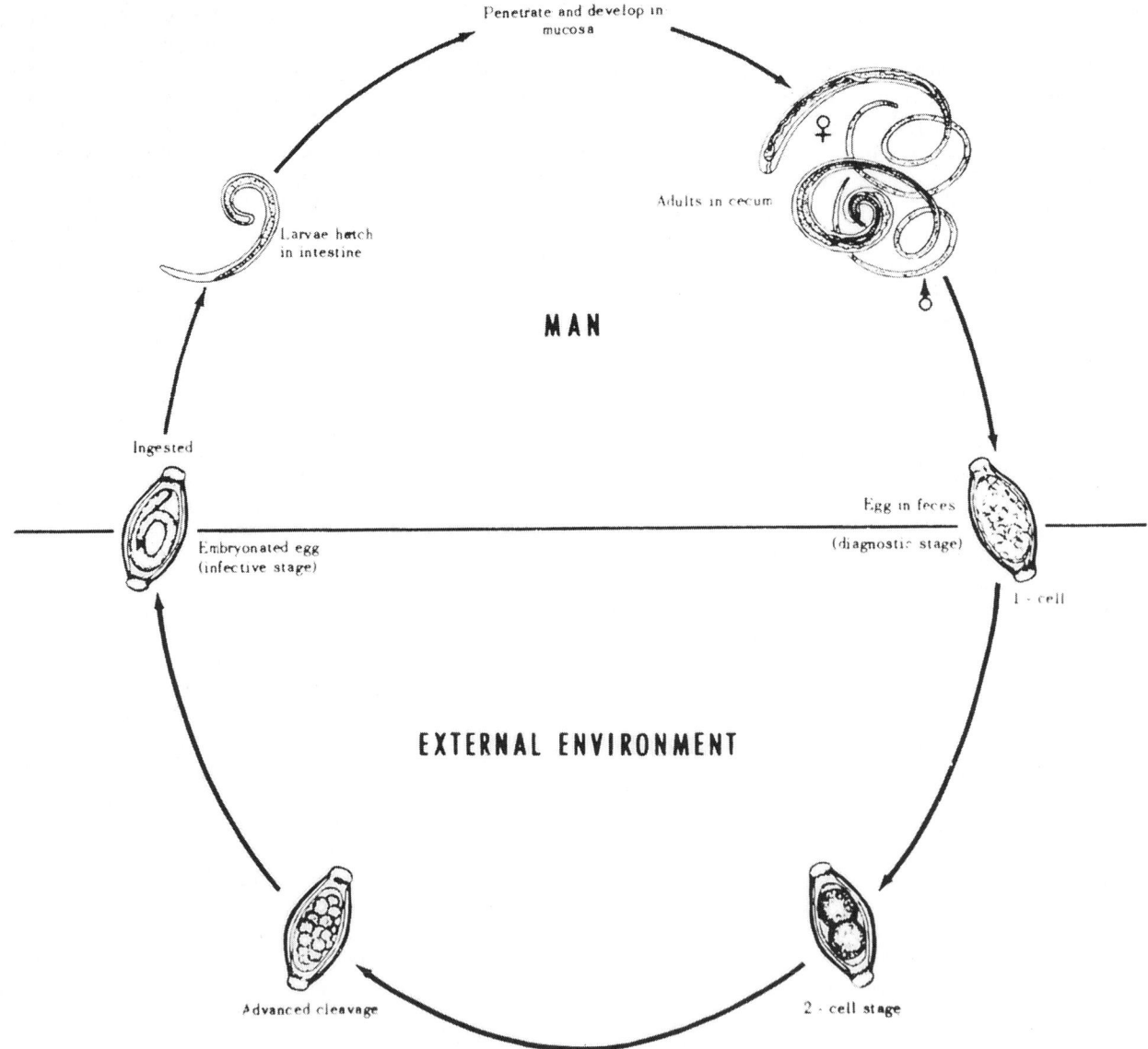

Penetrate and develop in mucosa

Adults in cecum

MAN

Larvae hatch in intestine

Ingested

Egg in feces

(diagnostic stage)

Embryonated egg
(infective stage)

1 - cell

EXTERNAL ENVIRONMENT

Advanced cleavage

2 - cell stage

FIG. 5. Life cycle of *Trichuris trichiura.*

is also endemic in temperate climates, with about 2.2 million people infected in the United States alone (25). The prevalence of *Trichuris* infection closely follows that of *Ascaris,* and both demonstrate an age-dependent density. Intensities of infection with both parasites are also strongly correlated, suggesting that individuals may be predisposed to infection with both species (26). As with the other geohelminths, its distribution appears to be predicated more on poor sanitation, overcrowding, and the practice of using night soil as fertilizer, than on climate. In endemic areas, children are often infected by age 2, with maximum infection rates occurring between the ages of 5 and 10 (25). There is usually a major reduction in worm burden in adults; this may be related to a decrease in exposure, or possibly to intrinsic individual susceptibility to reinfection. Worm burdens vary significantly and are highly aggregated with familial clustering; about 65%

of the worm population is found in less than 15% of the population (27). Person-to-person transmission does not occur because eggs require an incubation period in the soil before becoming infective.

Pathogenesis

The thin anterior end of the adult remains buried in the intestinal mucosa of the cecum and proximal large bowel throughout its life. In heavy infections, worms may be found from the terminal ileum to the rectum (Fig. 7). Mucosal abnormalities are usually seen only at the site of attachment of the worm and consist of small petechial or subepithelial hemorrhages, mucosal cell destruction, and a superficial infiltration with eosinophils, lymphocytes, and plasma cells. In heavy infections, the mucosa may be γ-producing) predominated (28). Rapid expulsion is not seen in human infections, and reinfection is the rule. *Trichuris* elicits a local immediate hypersensitivity reaction in the colonic mucosa, which may be involved in the pathogenesis of the *Trichuris* dysentery syndrome (TDS) (29). Compared with controls, children with TDS had significantly greater numbers of mast cells and cells with surface IgE in the subepithelial mucosa. Studies in humans have demonstrated a strong humoral immune response, primarily IgG (subclasses IgG1 and IgG4), IgA, and IgE (30). However, in spite of a high concentration of specific antibodies, a significant degree of immunity does not develop. There is an inverse age-dependent relationship between infection with *Trichuris* and parasite-specific antibody levels. A rapid increase in antibody levels is observed during the first infection in childhood, followed by a marked decline in these levels in adulthood, correlating with a decrease in the intensity of infection (31). This age-dependent immunorecognition also occurs in infections with *Ascaris*. By contrast, in schistosomiasis, an increase in parasite-specific IgE is seen with age in endemic areas and correlates with resistance to reinfection even when the level of exposure is constant (12). Interestingly, intense infection with *T. trichiura* appears to be associated with HLA class 1 B14/BW65 antigen, a marker for a haplotype associated with IgA deficiency (32).

Clinical Features

Depending on the worm burden, trichuriasis may be asymptomatic or associated with chronic diarrhea, dysentery, or growth retardation. Light infections are invariably asymptomatic. Moderate worm burdens may produce a picture of chronic colitis with lower abdominal pain, diarrhea, distention, anorexia, and weight loss. Children may also demonstrate pica and short stature for age, although they are not wasted (33,34). *Trichuris*-induced dysentery classically occurs in children with a heavy worm burden. They may have profuse bloody diarrhea, abdominal cramps, tenesmus, urgency, and rectal prolapse, which is a classic feature of this syndrome. They are often stunted in growth and underweight, anemic, and malnourished. Clubbing has been described in association with dysentery, and coinfection with *Shigella* and *Entamoeba histolytica* has also been reported (33). Treatment of trichuriasis in heavily infected children results in improvement in cognitive function, specifically in both short- and long-term memory (35).

Diagnosis

The diagnosis is made by finding adult worms or the characteristic barrel-shaped eggs in stool, which may also contain Charcot–Leyden crystals. Proctoscopy or colonoscopy may demonstrate hyperemic, friable mucosa, usually at the sites of attachment of the adult worms. The worms themselves may be noted hanging into the lumen of the intestine. Air-contrast barium enemas may demonstrate the worms as linear or coiled translucencies. Blood

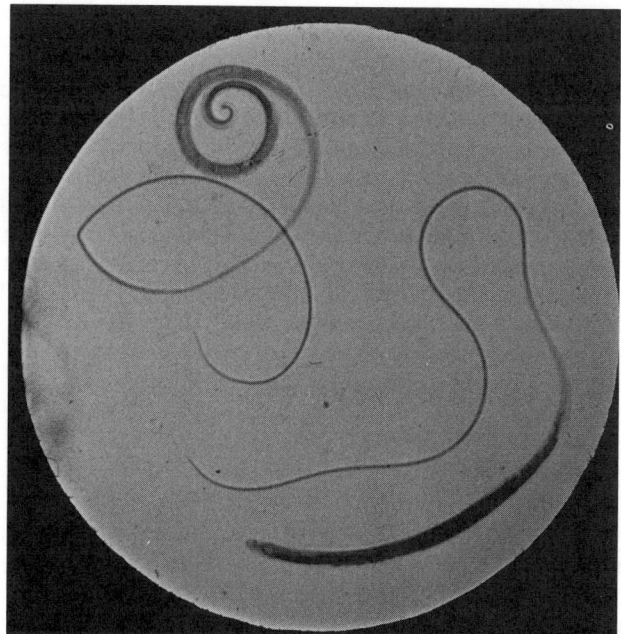
FIG. 6. Adult trichuris worms.

edematous and friable and tends to bleed easily. Anemia, when it occurs, is thought to be due to chronic occult blood loss in people with a marginal intake of iron. Opinion varies as to whether active blood ingestion by the parasite occurs.

Immunity

The immune response to trichuriasis in humans is the subject of ongoing study. In murine trichuriasis, an initial antibody-mediated phase and a subsequent lymphoid cell-mediated phase are involved in worm expulsion. In addition, mice resistant to infection with *T. muris* exhibited a T helper cell type 2 (Th2) dominated (IL-5, IL-9) response in contrast to susceptible mice, in whom Th1 cells (IFN-

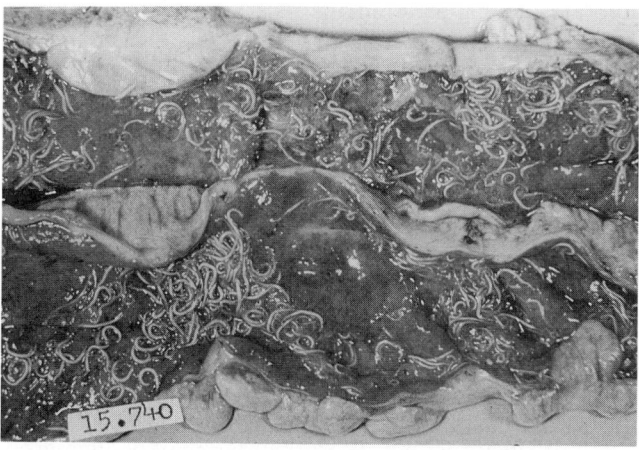
FIG. 7. *Trichuris trichiura* in resected colon.

tests are usually normal except for iron deficiency anemia in heavy infections and eosinophilia (usually 5% to 15%), which does not correlate with worm burden or symptoms.

Treatment

Treatment of trichuriasis is more difficult than it is for other geohelminths, partly because immature worms are less susceptible to antihelminthics. Asymptomatic infections require no treatment as they are self-limited and do not result in direct person-to-person transmission. For heavier infections, mebendazole at a dose of 100 mg twice a day for 3 days has resulted in cure rates of 60% to 80%; treatment may need to be repeated. Adverse reactions to therapy are rare and consist of nausea, vomiting, and diarrhea. Both mebendazole and albendazole in single doses have been used in mass chemotherapy trials; the former has shown about a 70% efficacy rate in clearing the infection. Stephenson et al. (36) reported the effect of a single 400-mg dose of albendazole on egg counts and anthropometric measurements in a group of children infected with multiple species. She found that treatment resulted in a highly significant increase in weight, height, and arm circumference. The effect of albendazole on egg counts was most pronounced for *Ascaris* followed by hookworm, and then *Trichuris*.

Oxantel pamoate as a single oral dose of 15 mg/kg, or as the same dose on two consecutive days, has a cure rate of 88%. Diphetarsone, 500 mg/day three times daily for 10 days, has also shown excellent cure rates, but in 5% of those treated, may be associated with mild GI side effects and transient elevations of liver enzymes. This compound has recently been withdrawn from production and is no longer available.

Prevention

Proper sanitation is the prime method of control for trichuriasis. However, even in areas with lavatories, infection may be maintained if night soil is used for fertilizer. On an individual basis, washing or peeling of fruit and vegetables and scrupulous personal hygiene will help to prevent transmission. Mass chemotherapy has been shown to reduce worm burden, and hence morbidity and transmission.

ENTEROBIASIS

Enterobius vermicularis, formerly called *Oxyuris,* is a nematode of the large bowel which has a worldwide distribution and a high prevalence of infection. Its common names are pinworm or threadworm based on the morphology of the adult worm. Alexander of Tralles in the 6th century ascribed them "the privilege over other helminths of being tormentors of any people of any age."

Morphology

Humans are the only host for *E. vermicularis*. Although dogs, cats and other domestic animals have been implicated in transmission, their role is limited to the carriage of eggs on their fur. There is marked sexual dimorphism between adult worms. The female, 8–13 mm long and about 0.5 mm wide, has a pointed tail and a ventral vulvar opening one-third of the body length from the anterior end. The male is much smaller, measuring 2.5 mm × 0.2 mm, and has a curved posterior end with a single copulatory spicule. The life span of the female is about 3–6 weeks; the male lives only 1–2 weeks.

Life Cycle

Eggs of *Enterobius* are embryonated when laid and require only 4–6 hours of oxygenation outside the intestine to mature and become infective. Its life cycle requires neither an intermediate host nor a period of incubation in the soil (Fig. 8). In the presence of high humidity and low temperature the eggs may remain viable for 2–3 weeks outside the host. Once the eggs are ingested, first-stage larvae hatch in the duodenum. They molt twice while passing down to the cecum where they develop into adults and mate. The time from egg ingestion to egg excretion is usually 2–4 weeks. The gravid female crawls out of the anus at night to deposit sticky eggs on the perianal skin. Egg deposition usually occurs by uterine contractions or actual rupture of the worm. Up to 11,000 eggs may be produced by a single female worm. The eggs are oval and have a double layered shell. Characteristically, they are flattened on one side and measure 50–60 × 20–30 um.

Epidemiology

E. vermicularis enjoys a worldwide distribution and is somewhat more common in temperate than tropical climates. There are an estimated 42 million infected persons in the United States alone (25). Enterobiasis occurs among all socioeconomic and age groups, although infection rates among children age 5–10 are highest and range from 10–50% (37). Recent studies, however, seem to indicate a decline in incidence and prevalence of this infection in areas in the United States (37,38). Transmission is favored by close proximity and overcrowding. Prevalence rates in institutionalized individuals may be close to 100%. Infection is also common in members of the same household and may occur as a sexually-transmitted disease among male homosexuals. Rapid infectivity of eggs, their adherence to the perianal region, and pruritus ani are factors in its transmission by the fecal-oral route. Transfer of eggs via fomites such as contaminated blankets, sheets, clothing, and even the fur of household pets may be an important factor in transmission. In some infected houses, more than 90% of dust samples had Enterobius eggs of which half were viable. Worm burden may be increased by autoinfection, when infected persons ingest eggs from

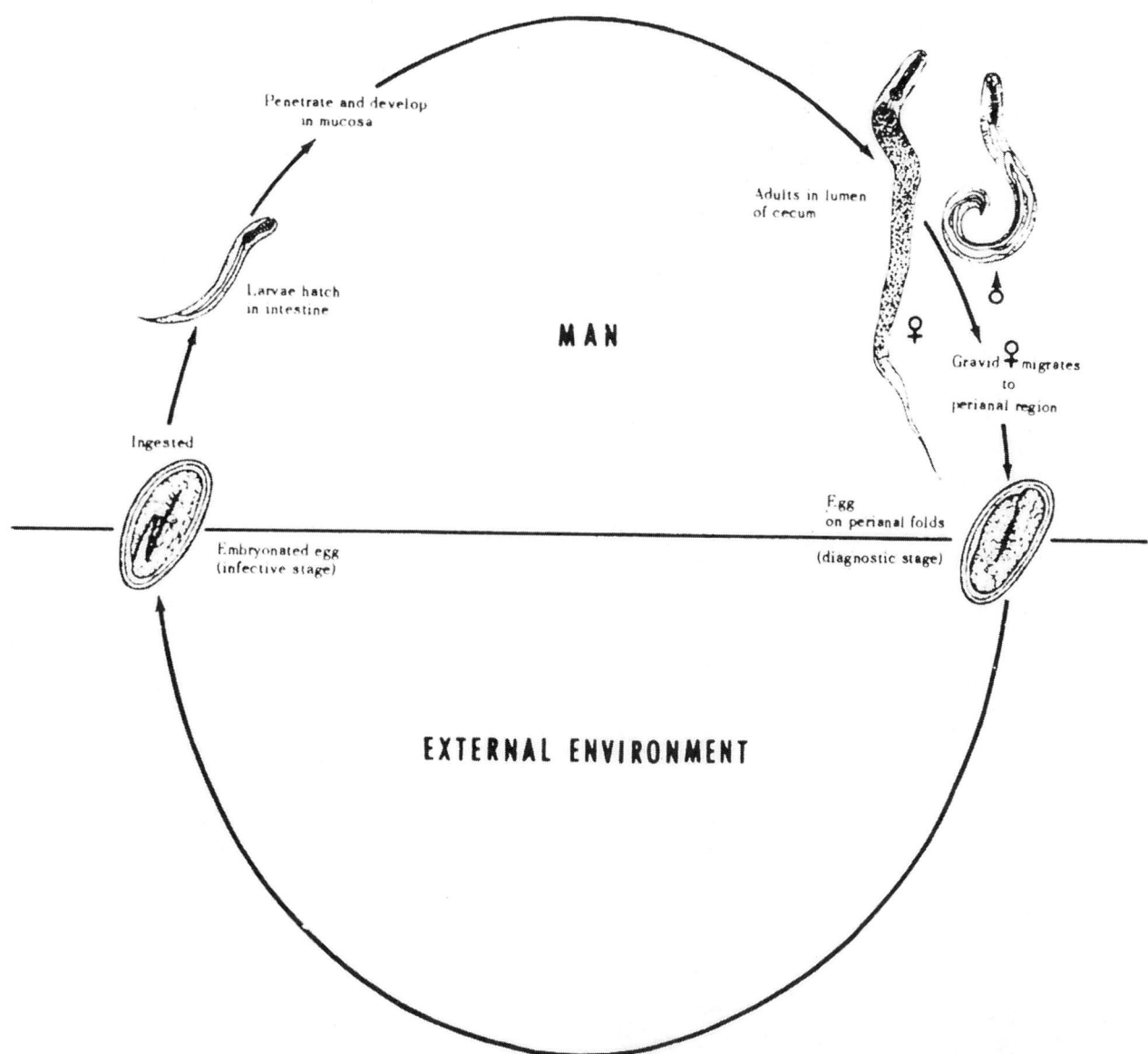

FIG. 8. Life cycle of *Enterobius vermicularis*.

their own fecally-contaminated fingers—this is enhanced by the perianal pruritus that commonly accompanies infection.

Pathogenesis and Immunity

E. vermicularis is found in the lumen of the cecum, appendix and adjacent portions of small and large bowel. The worm causes little mechanical injury and there is no well-developed allergic response or potent IgE-stimulating effect. *E. vermicularis* may cause acute, subacute, or chronic appendicitis; the prevalence of infection in surgically removed appendices varies from 1–38%. The adult worm has been associated with extraintestinal disease in the form of vulvovaginitis, endometriosis, prostatitis, and fallopian tube lesions. It is widely believed that *Dienta-*

meba fragilis, a large bowel protozoan, is transmitted within pinworm eggs; coinfection rates range as high as 50% (39).

Clinical Features

The majority of infections are aymptomatic. The most common symptom, which occurs in about one-third of infected patients, is perianal pruritus caused by the female worm or its eggs. Insomnia, irritability, and restlessness may be attributed to disturbed sleep due to nocturnal itching. Complications of pruritus ani include eczematous perianal skin lesions, which may become secondarily infected and rarely lead to local abscess formation. Although it appears to be uncommon, the incidence of abdominal pain is unclear since most studies have not controlled for duration or intensity of infection or coexisting conditions such as dientamebiasis. Children occasionally demonstrate anorexia and weight loss. In females, worms may migrate through the vagina and uterus, leading to vulvovaginitis, endometritis, salpingitis, or, rarely, a peritoneal granulomatous reaction. Enuresis and recurrent urinary tract infection have also been reported with enterobiasis, particularly in young girls (40).

Diagnosis

As with many other intestinal parasites, the diagnosis is made by visualization of adult worms or eggs. The adult may be seen on inspection of the perianal region, especially at night, or on proctoscopy. The most reliable test is the cellulose acetate (scotch tape) test for the demonstration of eggs on the perianal skin either during the night or on awakening in the morning (Fig. 9). This test is done by pressing a wooden tongue depressor, draped with a length of tape with the sticky side out, firmly against the skin of the perianal region. The tape is removed in the lab, placed sticky-side down on a slide, and examined microscopically for eggs. A flexible, sticky, plastic applicator has been found to be very practical (37). Multiple tests on consecutive days have a high likelihood of identifying the infection—with three tests detecting 90%, five tests detecting 99%, and seven tests 100% of infections (41).

Examination of the stool for pinworm eggs is a low-yield procedure since in only about 5% of infections will stool exams be positive. Identification of *Dientamoeba fragilis* in stool should prompt a search for enterobiasis given the high coinfection rate. Similarly, when patients with enterobiasis complain of abdominal pain or diarrhea,

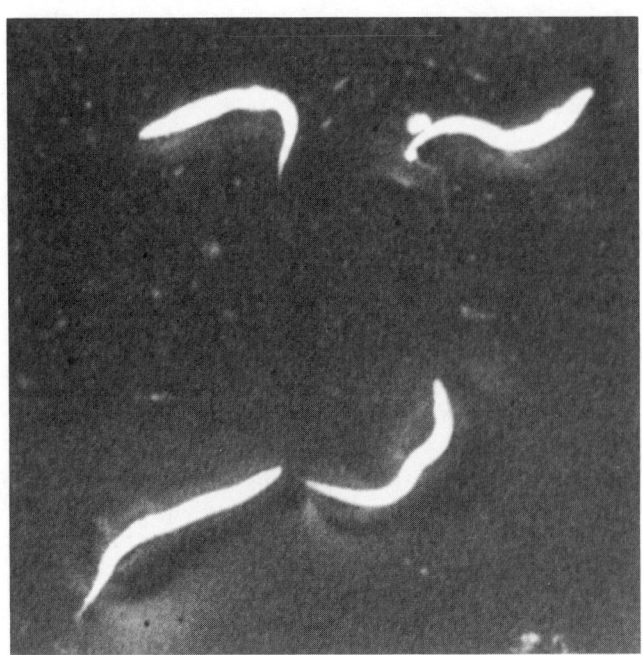

FIG. 9. *Enterobius vermicularis* on cellulose acetate.

a search for *D. fragilis* should be undertaken. Eosinophilia is rare.

Treatment

Unless reinfection or autoinfection occurs, primary infections usually clear spontaneously in 30 to 45 days. However, treatment is recommended for both symptomatic as well as asymptomatic individuals due to the risk of transmission to others. Particularly in households with small children, it is recommended that all members be treated at the same time as the index case. Treatment is not recommended in pregnancy unless absolutely necessary. A number of well-tolerated and effective medications are available for the treatment of enterobiasis, of which mebendazole and pyrantel pamoate are the most frequently used. Albendazole or mebendazole may be given in a one-time dose of 100 mg to those over 2 years of age; the dose of pyrantel is 11 mg/kg, also as a single dose (maximum 1 g). Since these drugs appear to be more effective against mature worms and less so against developing larvae and newly ingested eggs, it is recommended that both drugs be repeated in 2 weeks. With these regimens, cure rates are generally 90% to 100%. Although pyrvinium pamoate in a dose of 5 mg/kg is also effective, it tends to stain stools and underwear a deep red. Piperazine has also been used, but a 7-day course of therapy repeated in 2 weeks is required. Recurring infections should be treated at least four times at 2-week intervals, with concurrent treatment of all members of the household. Additional hygienic measures may be needed to break the transmission cycle; these include changing bed linen weekly, changing underwear daily, wearing underwear and pyjamas during sleep, attention to handwashing, and bathing in the morning.

Prevention

The measures adopted for prevention and control vary somewhat depending on whether the infection is confined to the individual or is circulating in the family or an institution. In preschools and schools a few children with enterobiasis may be the source of infection for many others. It may be possible to identify these children by questioning and/or examination, but periodic mass chemotherapy is more effective and certainly more practical. Although personal hygiene must be emphasized, family members should be reassured that this infection is common and occurs in all strata of society. This may be particularly relevant in developed countries where there is often a social stigma attached to pinworm infections. In the developing world, mass chemotherapy for ascariasis and other parasites is also likely to be effective for enterobiasis.

REFERENCES

1. Ferreira LF, Araujo A, Confalonieri U, Chame M, Gomes DC. *Trichuris* eggs in animal coprolites dated from 30,000 years ago. *J Parasitol* 1991;77(3):491–493.

2. Walsh JA, Warren KS. Selective primary health care; an interim strategy for disease control in developing countries. *N Engl J Med* 1979;301:967–974.
3. World Health Organization. *Prevention and control of intestinal parasitic infections.* WHO Technical Report Series no 749. Geneva, WHO, 1987.
4. Phills JA, Harrold AJ, Whiteman GV, Perelmutter L. Pulmonary infiltrates, asthma, and eosinophilia due to *Ascaris suum* infestation in man. *N Engl J Med* 1972;286:965–970.
5. Peters W. Medical aspects—comments and discussion II. *Symp Br Soc Parasitol* 1978;16:25–40.
6. Croll NA, Ghadirian E. Wormy persons: contribution to the nature and patterns of over dispersion with *Ascaris lumbricoides, Ancylostoma duodenale, Necator americanus,* and *Trichuris trichiura. Trop Geog Med* 1981;33:241–248.
7. Gelpi AP, Mustafa A. Seasonal pneumonia with eosinophilia. A study of larval ascariasis in Saudi Arabia. *Am J Trop Med Hyg* 1967;16:646–657.
8. Thein-Hlaing, Thane-Toe, Than-Saw, Myat-Lay-Kyin, Myint-Lwin. A controlled chemotherapeutic intervention trial on the relationship between *Ascaris lumbricoides* infection and malnutrition in children. *Trans R Soc Trop Med Hyg* 1991;85(4):523–528.
9. McGibbon AM, Christie JF, Kennedy MW, Lee TD. Identification of the major ascaris allergen and its purification to homogeneity by HPLC. *Mol Biochem Parasitol* 1990;39:163–171.
10. Kennedy MW, Tomlinson LA, Fraser EM, Christie JF. The specificity of the antibody response to internal antigens of *Ascaris:* heterogeneity in infected humans, and MHC (H-2) control of the repertoire in mice. *Clin Exp Immunol* 1990;80:219–224.
11. Holland CV, Crompton DW, Asaolu SO, Crichton WB, Torimiro SE, Walters DE. A possible genetic factor influencing protection from infection with *Ascaris lumbricoides* in Nigerian children. *J Parasitol* 1992;78(5):915–916.
12. Hagan P, Blumenthal OJ, Dunn D, Simpson AJG, Wilkins HA. Human IgE, IgG4 and resistance to reinfection with *Schistosoma hematobium. Nature* 1991;349:243–245.
13. Pritchard DI. Immunity to helminths: is too much IgE parasite-rather than host-protective? *Parasite Immunol* 1993;15:5–9.
14. Hagan P. IgE and protective immunity to helminth infections. *Parasite Immunol* 1993;15:1–4.
15. Davies MRQ, Rode H. Biliary ascariasis in children. *Prog Pediatr Surg* 1982;15:55–74.
16. Khuroo MS, Zarger SA, Mahajan R. Hepatobiliary and pancreatic ascariasis in India. *Lancet* 1990;335:1503–1506.
17. Kato K, Miura M. Comparative examinations. *Jpn J Parasitol* 1954;3:29.
18. Bescansa E, Nicolas M, Aguado C, Toledano M, Vinals M. Myasthenia gravis aggravated by pyrantel pamoate. *J Neurol Neurosurg Psychiatry* 1991;54(6):563.
19. Abadi K. Single dose mebendazole therapy for soil-transmitted nematodes. *Am J Trop Med Hyg* 1985;34:129–133.
20. Freedman DO, Zierdt WS, Lujan A, Nutman TB. The efficacy of ivermectin in the chemotherapy of gastrointestinal helminthiasis in humans. *J Infect Dis* 1989;159(6):1151–1153.
21. Anderson RM, Medley GF. Community control of helminth infections of man by mass and selective chemotherapy. *Parasitology* 1985;90:629–660.
22. Haswell-Elkins M, Elkins D, Anderson RM. The influence of individual, social group, and household factors on the distribution of *Ascaris lumbricoides* within a community and implications for control strategies. *Parasitology* 1989;98:125–134.
23. Asaolu SO, Holland CV, Crompton DWT. Community control of *Ascaris lumbricoides* in rural Oyo State, Nigeria: mass, targeted, and selected treatment with levamisole. *Parasitology* 1991;103(Pt 2):291–298.
24. Hall A, Anwar KS, Tomkins AM. Intensity of reinfection with *Ascaris lumbricoides* and its implications for parasite control. *Lancet* 1992;339(8804):1253–1257.
25. Warren KS. Helminthic diseases endemic in the United States. *Am J Trop Med Hyg* 1974;23:723–730.
26. Chan L, Kan SP, Bundy DA. The effect of repeated chemotherapy on age-related predisposition to *Ascaris lumbricoides* and *Trichuris trichiura. Parasitology* 1992;104(Pt 2):371–377.
27. Bundy DAP, Cooper ES, Thompson DE, Anderson RM, Didier JM. Age-related prevalence and intensity of *Trichuris trichiura* infection in a St. Lucian community. *Trans R Soc Trop Med Hyg* 1987;81:85–94.
28. Else KJ, Hultner L, Grencis RK. Modulation of cytokine production and response phenotypes in murine trichuriasis. *Parasite Immunol* 1992;14(14):441–449.
29. Cooper ES, Spencer J, Whyte-Alleng CAM, et al. Immediate hypersensitivity in colon of children with chronic *Trichuris trichiura* dysentery. *Lancet* 1991;338:1104–1107.
30. Lillywhite JE, Bundy DAP, Didier JM, Cooper ES, Bianco AE. Humoral immune responses in human infection with the whipworm *Trichuris trichiura. Parasite Immunol* 1991;13:491–507.
31. Bundy DAP, Lillywhite JE, Didier JM, Simmons I, Bianco AE. Age-dependency of infection status and serum antibody levels in human whipworm (*Trichuris trichiura*) infection. *Parasite Immunol* 1991;13:629–638.
32. Bundy DAP. Population ecology of intensity of helminth infections in human communities. *Philos Trans R Soc Lond B* 1986;321:405.
33. Gilman RH, Chong YH, Davis C, et al. The adverse consequences of heavy *Trichuris trichiura* infection. *Trans R Soc Trop Med Hyg* 1983;77(4):432–438.
34. Cooper ES, Bundy DAP. Trichuriasis in St. Lucia. In: McNeish AS, Walker-Smith JA, eds. *Diarrhea and malnutrition in childhood.* London: Butterworths; 1986;91–96.
35. Nokes C, Grantham-McGregor SM, Sawyer AW, Cooper ES, Robinson BA, Bundy DAP. Moderate to heavy infections of *Trichuris trichiura* affect cognitive function in Jamaican school children. *Parasitology* 1992;104(Pt 3):539–547.
36. Stephenson LS, Latham MC, Kurz KM, Kinoti SN, Brigham H. Treatment with a single dose of albendazole improves growth of Kenyan school children with hookworm, *Trichuris trichiura,* and *Ascaris lumbricoides* infections. *Am J Trop Med Hyg* 1989;41(1):78–87.
37. Wagner ED, Eby WC. Pinworm prevalence in California elementary school children and diagnostic methods. *Am J Trop Med Hyg* 1983;32:998–1001.
38. Vermund SH, Macleod S. Is pinworm a vanishing infection? *Am J Dis Child* 1988;142:566–568.
39. Yang J, Scholten T. *Dientameba fragilis:* a review with notes on its epidemiology, pathogenicity, mode of transmission, and diagnosis. *Am J Trop Med Hyg* 1977;26:16–22.
40. Sachdev YV, Howards SS. *Enterobius vermicularis* infestations and secondary enuresis. *J Urol* 1975;113:143–144.
41. Keystone JS. Enterobiasis. In: Goldsmith R, Heyneman D, eds. *Tropical medicine and parasitology.* Norwalk, CT: Appleton and Lange, 1989.

Infections of the Gastrointestinal Tract,
edited by M. J. Blaser, P. D. Smith, J. I. Ravdin,
H. B. Greenberg, and R. L. Guerrant
Raven Press, Ltd., New York © 1995.

CHAPTER 77

Trichinella spiralis

Dickson D. Despommier

Trichinella spiralis was first observed by Richard Owen, the director of the British Museum, and James Paget, a first-year medical student from St. Bartholmew's Hospital. With the aid of a borrowed microscope, they saw the larval stage in a piece of skeletal muscle (Fig. 1) taken from a 51-year-old Italian bricklayer who had died earlier that same day of tuberculosis (1). Within several years following its discovery, the essentials of the life cycle were derived from a series of experiments by Virchow in Germany (2), who determined that it could infect many different animal species, including human, and that its primary mode of transmission was by eating raw or under-cooked meat. He also deduced from surveys of various species of wild and domestic animals that, in nature, the cycle was maintained by scavenging. Virchow's microscopic method for detecting the larvae, in which a piece of diaphragmatic tissue is squashed between two glass slides and then microscopically observed, is still used today to inspect pork products in many parts of Europe (3). Human disease was first described by Zenker (4), also in Germany, who recognized muscle pain and fever as the dominant symptoms.

Today, all salient features of its life cycle (Fig. 2) are known (5), while many fundamental studies on its molecular and biochemical aspects still remain to be carried out. Up to several years ago, only one species of trichinella was generally recognized by the scientific community. However, there is a growing body of evidence from deoxyribonucleic acid (DNA) fingerprinting (7) and other biologically derived data strongly suggesting that there are several species in the genus *Trichinella* (8) and several subspecies as well (9,10). This chapter deals only with the most commonly occurring form of human infection, namely, that caused by *Trichinella spiralis*.

BIOLOGY AND LIFE CYCLE

Trichinella spiralis is an ubiquitously distributed para-sitic nematode (11) belonging to the family Trichurata,

which includes *Trichuris trichiura* and *Capillaria* species. It parasitizes a surprisingly wide variety of host species (12). The adult female (measuring 3 mm × 36 μm) and male (measuring 1.5 mm × 36 μm) (Fig. 3) live as intracel-lular parasites in a row of enterocytes in the small intestine (Fig. 4) (13), while the infective L1 larva (1 mm × 36 μm) occupies a unique intracellular spatial (i.e., physical) niche in a modified muscle cell termed the Nurse cell (Fig. 5) (14,15). The fact that trichinella lives most of its larval and adult life intracellularly, and that the first stage larva is the infective stage, makes this parasitic nematode unique among helminth infections of humans.

Infection begins with the ingestion of the first-stage larva and its Nurse cell within striated skeletal muscle tissue (16). Once freed from their host tissue in the stom-

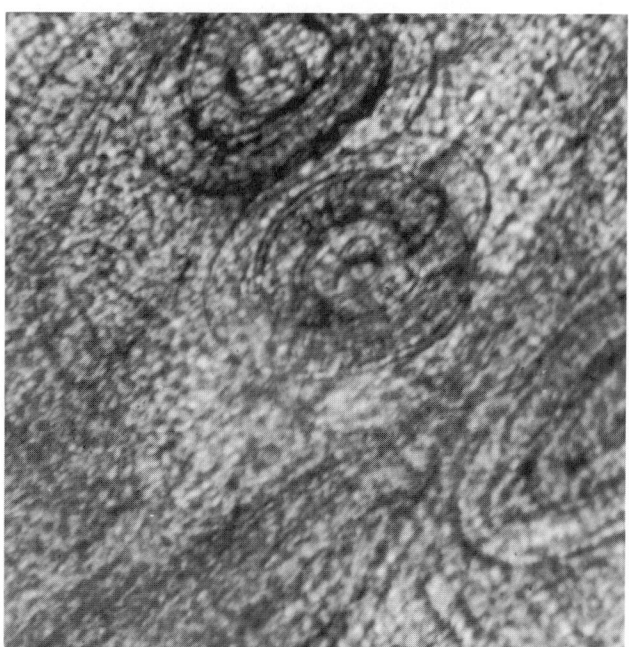

FIG. 1. Unstained muscle biopsy with three larvae of *Trichinella spiralis* (×235)

D. Despommier: Division of Environmental Sciences and Department of Microbiology, Columbia University, New York, New York 10032.

ENTERAL

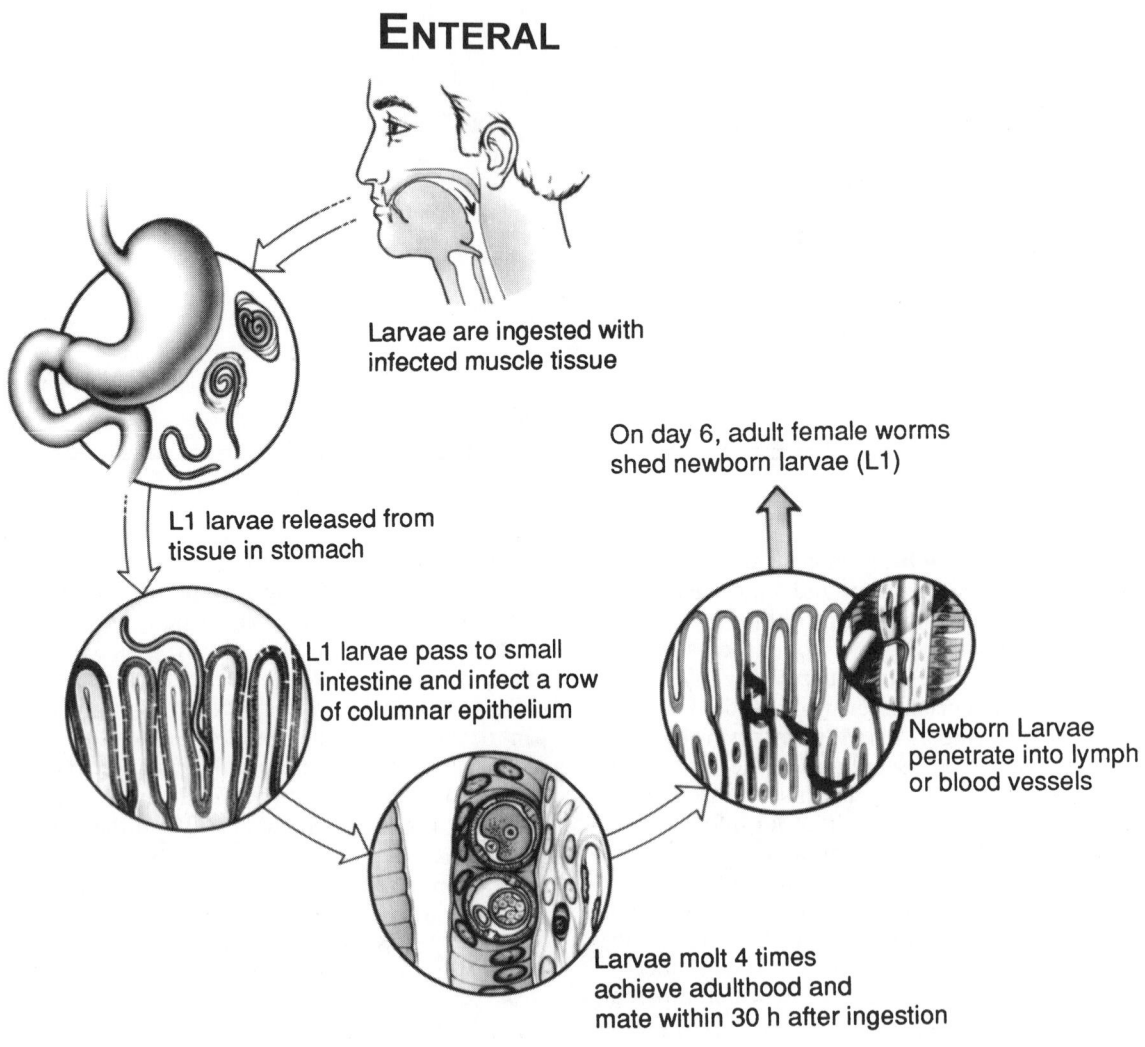

Larvae are ingested with infected muscle tissue

L1 larvae released from tissue in stomach

L1 larvae pass to small intestine and infect a row of columnar epithelium

Larvae molt 4 times achieve adulthood and mate within 30 h after ingestion

On day 6, adult female worms shed newborn larvae (L1)

Newborn Larvae penetrate into lymph or blood vessels

FIG. 2. Life cycle of *Trichinella spiralis*. (Adapted from ref. 6.)

ach, larvae (Fig. 6) pass into the small intestine and almost at once are "activated" by a combination of bile, proteases (e.g., trypsin and chymotrypsin), and the environment provided by a basic pH (17). This set of cues (18) triggers behavioral changes in the parasite that lead to the establishment of infection in the small intestine. The larva invades a row of columnar epithelium in the jejunum or ileum (Fig. 4). The mechanism of cellular invasion is not known, but any stage of the worm (i.e., first through fourth stage larvae and adult parasites) can enter and reenter columnar cells. For example, in experimental infections, *T. spiralis* can infect the epithelium of the large intestine and of the uteri of rats in estrus (19). Following entry into its multicellular spatial niche, the parasite develops to adulthood by molting four times in rapid succession (20). This developmental aspect of its life takes a mere 30 hr, thus making *T. spiralis* one of the world's fastest molting organisms.

During the first 48 hr *T. spiralis* induces many changes in its enteral niche (21,22), which presumably favors short-term survival, facilitating maturation and reproduction of the parasite. The mechanisms through which the

parasite accomplishes these goals have not yet been determined. The enteral stages are aerobic in their metabolism, while the infective L1 larva in the muscle tissue is a strict anaerobe (16). During the first 20 hr of life in its enteral niche, the worm secretes a battery of some 20 proteins, most of which are heavily glycosylated (23), which diffuse out and around the worm (24). Some of the secreted proteins contain a rare sugar, tyvelose, which confers group-specific antigenicity to that family of macromolecules (25). These secretions aid the worm in achieving its developmental cycle. Clinical symptoms are presumably elicited by epithelial cell destruction as the result of exposure to the secretions of the parasite. The latter emanate from a collection of secretory cells in the anterior part of the worm's esophagus known as stichocytes (Greek for "part of a row"). The organ is called the stichosome and is typical for all members of the order Trichuroidea (26).

Five days after the worms mate, the females begin to produce offspring termed newborn larvae (80 μm × 7 μm) (Fig. 7). Each female worm produces hundreds to thousands of newborns depending on the strength and nature of the immune responses mounted against it; that is,

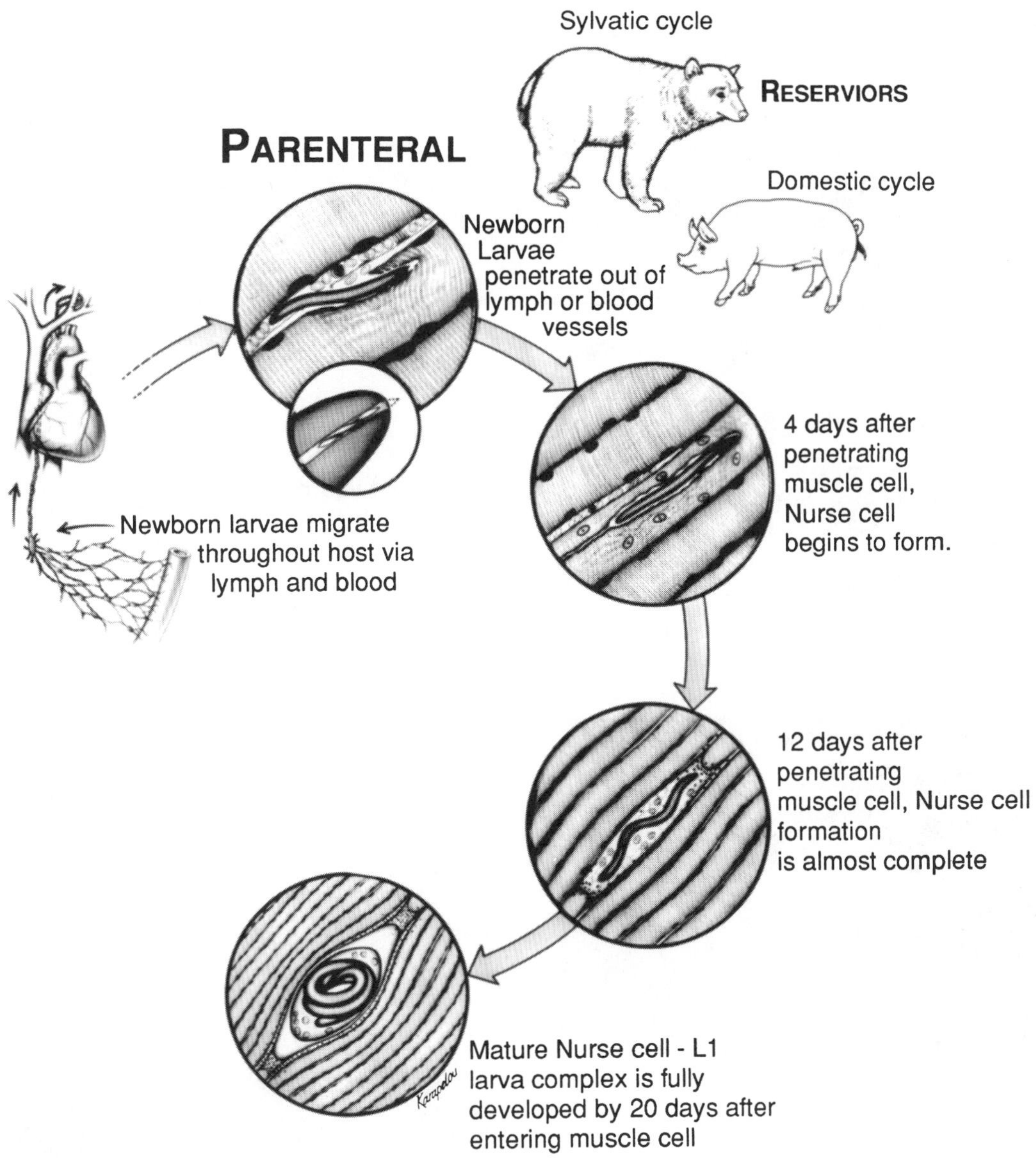

Sylvatic cycle

RESERVIORS

PARENTERAL

Domestic cycle

Newborn
Larvae
penetrate out of
lymph or blood
vessels

4 days after
penetrating
muscle cell,
Nurse cell
begins to form.

Newborn larvae migrate
throughout host via
lymph and blood

12 days after
penetrating
muscle cell, Nurse cell
formation
is almost complete

Mature Nurse cell - L1
larva complex is fully
developed by 20 days after
entering muscle cell

FIG. 2. *Continued.*

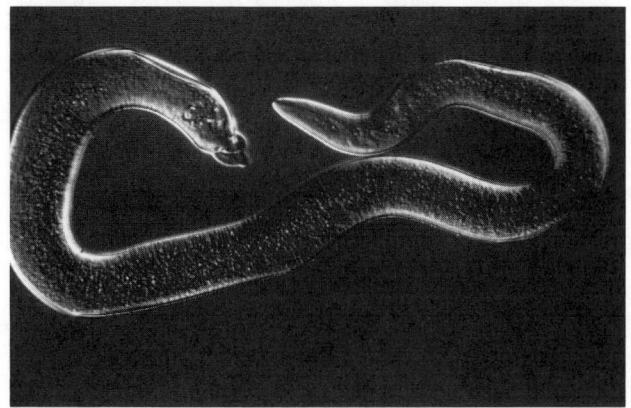

FIG. 3. Adult male *Trichinella spiralis*, 1.5 mm × 36 μm: Nomarski-phase interference photomicrograph (×300). (Courtesy of Eric Grave.)

the weaker the responses, the more larvae produced (27). The immature larva migrates systemically via blood and lymphatic vessels (28,29) and leaves them whenever it encounters a capillary. *Trichinella spiralis* indiscriminately penetrates various host cells, killing them in the process. The worm will only remain in striated skeletal muscle cells (Fig. 8) and exits from nonpermissive cells to renew its search. A parasite entering a striated skeletal muscle cell remains in that spatial niche. Experimental infections have shown that larvae find their correct host cells in less than two cycles of blood passage through the heart (29).

Once in the muscle cell, the worm initiates changes in contiguous host tissue, resulting in the transformation over 20 days of that portion of the cell into the Nurse cell (Fig. 5). The worm and its modified host cell can remain as such for up to 30 years in the human host (30). The development of the Nurse cell is paralleled by development of the larva, culminating in the worm achieving in-

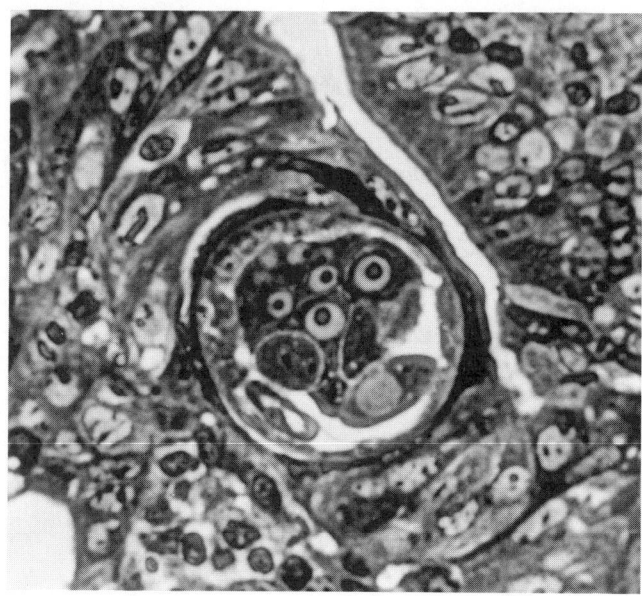

FIG. 4. Adult *Trichinella spiralis in situ* (×715).

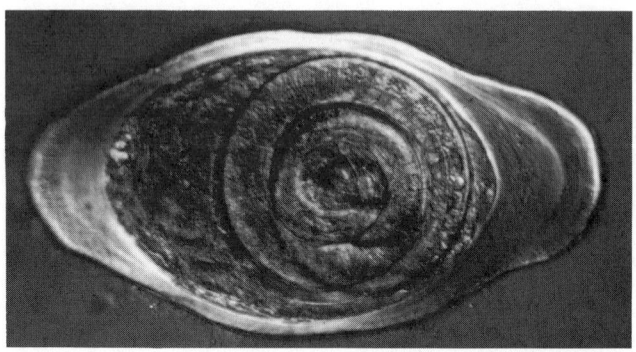

FIG. 5. Nurse cell–parasite complex: Nomarski-phase photomicrograph (×200). (Courtesy of Eric Grave.)

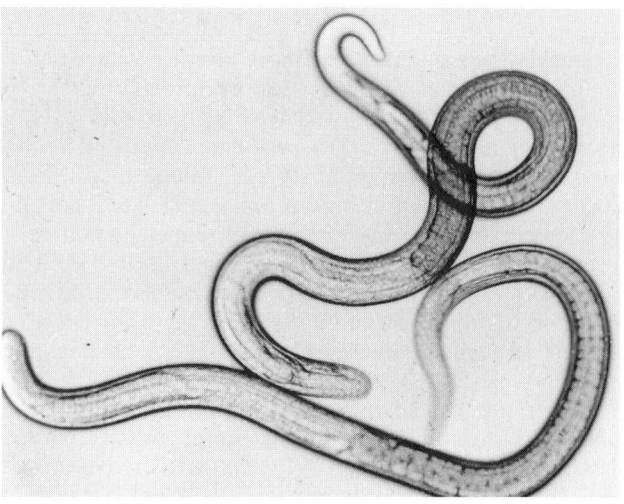

FIG. 6. Infective L1 larvae of *Trichinella spiralis* isolated from an infected animal by digesting muscle tissue for 1 hr at 37°C in pepsin–HCl (×180).

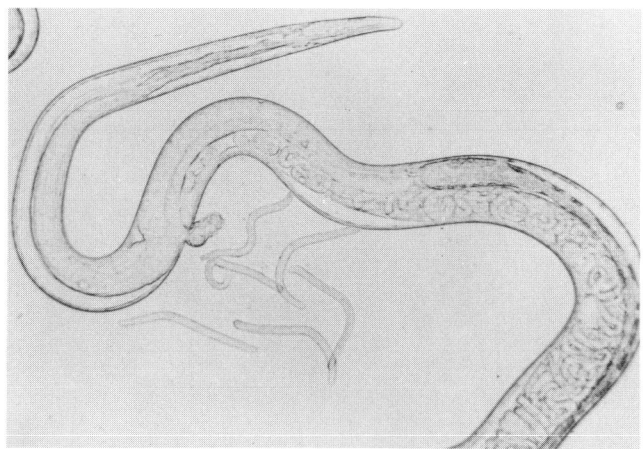

FIG. 7. Newborn larvae (80 μm × 7 μm) *in utero* and expressed from a female adult *Trichinella spiralis* (×250).

fectivity on the 14th day after entering its intracellular niche. The Nurse cell represents an altered state of cellular development and differentiation. In the mouse the genes for collagen (31), probably a mixture of type IV and VI (C. Kabbash, *personal communication*), are overexpressed, forming the capsule that surrounds the Nurse cell cytoplasm and the larva. Additionally, the Nurse cell acquires a circulatory rete (32–34), which abuts the outer surface of the capsule. No contractile elements typical for striated skeletal muscle cell can be detected in the Nurse cell after the fifth day of intracellular infection (35). Rather, its cytoplasm consists of whorls of smooth membranes and clusters of dysfunctional mitochondria (Fig. 9) (15). At the molecular level, Nurse cell formation involves

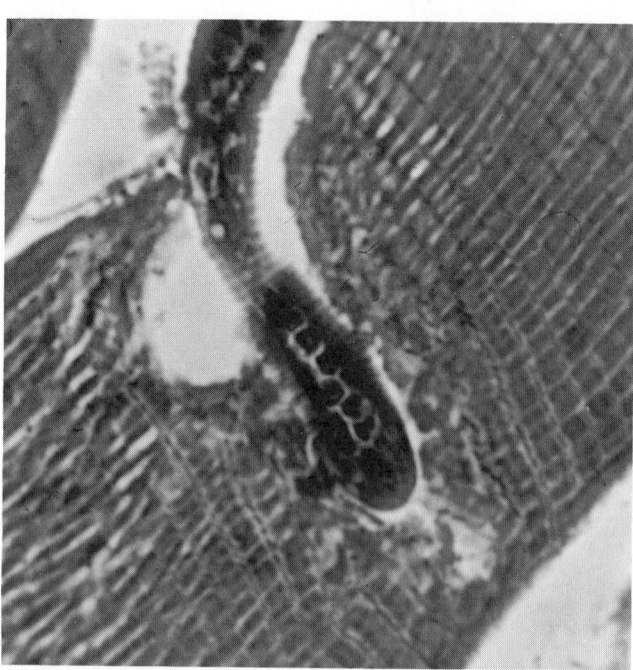

FIG. 8. Newborn larva of *Trichinella spiralis* penetrating a muscle fiber (×1760).

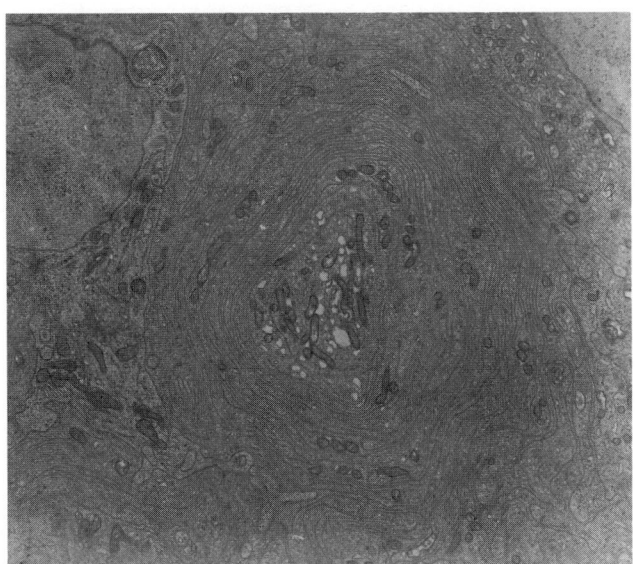

FIG. 9. The cytoplasm of the mature Nurse cell–parasite complex consists of whorls of smooth membranes and collections of dysfunctional mitochondria. Electron micrograph (×4800).

downregulation of the myogenic program. There are decreased levels of expression of Myo D-1, myogenin, and other known muscle transcription factors (35) and upregulation of an as yet undefined Nurse cell program (36). The control of these cellular modifications is parasite-based and most likely involves secreted proteins.

EPIDEMIOLOGY

Trichinella spiralis occurs worldwide, infecting many species of mammalian hosts, from polar bears to tropical bush pigs, and is endemic in unsuspected places, such as Egypt (37) and New Zealand. In Egypt, for example, Copts (there are some six million in Cairo alone) consume large quantities of pork. The pigs are fed on garbage and are allowed to roam freely among the refuse dumps of the city. Unofficial estimates indicate that over 30% of the pigs in that city are infected with *T. spiralis*.

The dominant mode of transmission to humans is through the ingestion of commercially available raw or undercooked meat, particularly pork products (85). Animals killed by hunting (e.g., bear) have also been responsible for significant outbreaks (38). In nature, scavenging is the most common way in which animals acquire infection, although predation, as well, is a popular mode (12). Human infections are mostly point source epidemics in which a single carcass contributes the infective larvae. More than one person is usually infected and the contaminated meat has often been traced back to its source. Several examples will serve to illustrate this point.

One outbreak was traced to a farm in New York State (D. Murrell, *personal communication*). This was determined only after much questioning of the butcher, whose shop was in New York City and to whom the infected

meat was traced. He had sold the meat to two families in the city and some members of each had become infected with *T. spiralis* and experienced clinical disease. The butcher then revealed the source of his pork, a farm in Duchess County in upstate New York. Upon questioning the farmer there, the epidemiologists learned that no uncooked garbage, scraps of meat, or debris from the local slaughterhouse was fed to his pigs. After further questioning, the farmer admitted feeding them carcasses of game animals he had trapped for fur. He did not realize that infection could and did exist in wild animals native to his farmland (e.g., fox, raccoon, opossum). Hence he felt justified in using every part of the trapped animal—skin and meat.

While carnivores are the usual source of infection, herbivores are also susceptible (39,40), and they acquire it by accidentally ingesting infected carcasses of small animals (e.g., mice and rats) while feeding on hay and grains. An outbreak of trichinellosis in Paris, France, in 1985 involved more than 1500 people, all of whom acquired the infection by ingesting portions of infected meat from the same horse (41,42). The horse was traced back to the state of Texas. It was assumed that the horse had eaten infected rodents by accident, which may have occurred if the hay meal that contained the carcasses was bailed on farmland adjacent to a slaughterhouse specializing in pigs. This epidemic led to the microscopical inspection of all horse meat shipped to France from Texas. To date, not one of the tens of thousands of animals examined thereafter was positive (G. Stewart, *personal communication*). *Trichinella spiralis* infection continues to occur in sporadic epidemic outbreaks among humans and is endemic among woodland scavengers; thus it must be considered in the differential diagnosis when a patient presents with signs and symptoms consistent with this pathogen, regardless of where that individual is from.

PATHOGENESIS AND IMMUNITY

The major pathological consequences of infection relate to the migratory behaviors of the newborn larvae. Cell destruction results from parasite penetration (Fig. 8); in heavy infection death of the host can occur because of heart and/or central nervous system failure (43,44). An intense mixed cell granulomatous reaction and edema accompany cell destruction (Fig. 10), affecting the surrounding normal tissue as well. The use of steroid-based drugs during this time often alleviates symptoms and favors survival of the host (45). The late stage inflammatory process (i.e., weeks 6 to 12) is characterized by an eosinophilic infiltrate that surrounds the fully developed Nurse cell but is most intense at its poles (46).

Hypersecretion (47), increased gut motility (48), loss of wheat germ agglutinin sites (49), disruption of the myoelectric potential (50), reduced glucose transport (51), altered sodium pump channels (52), and altered patterns of release of gut-specific hormones (53,54) are a few of the physiological correlates of gut infection. Malabsorption syndrome, while not a major clinical correlate, nonethe-

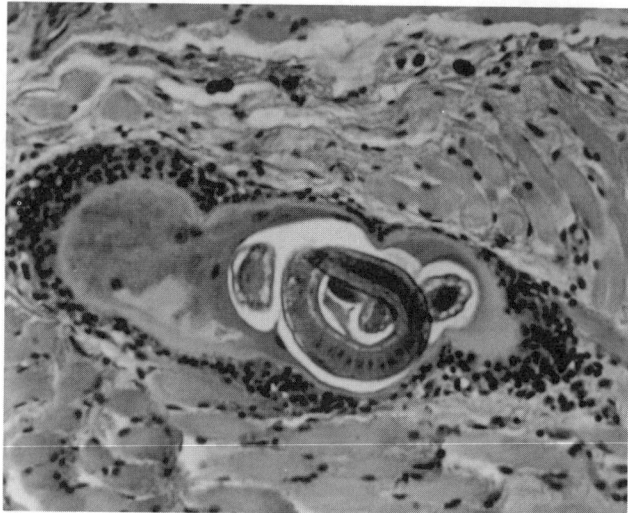

FIG. 10. The Nurse cell–parasite complex elicits an intense mixed cellular inflammatory response during the first 40 to 50 days after the parasite enters the host cell (×200).

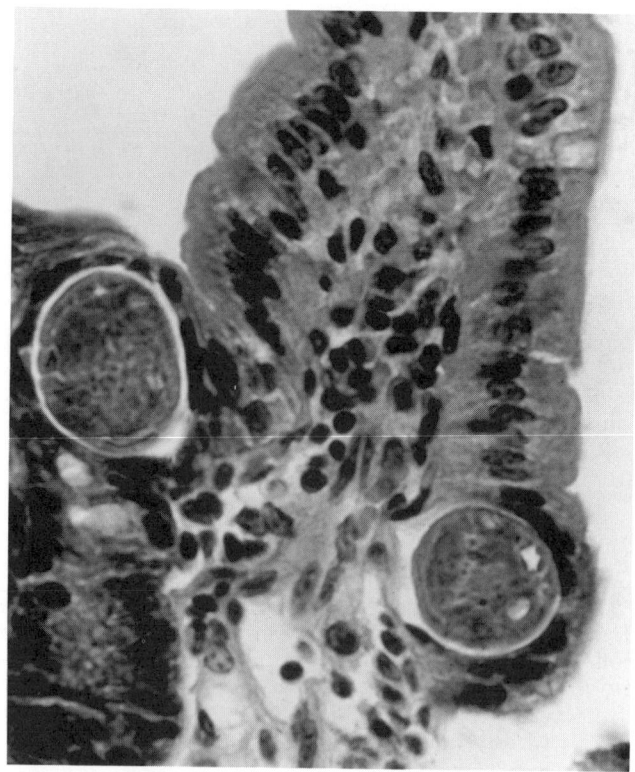

FIG. 11. The enteral phase of the infection elicits an intense mixed cellular inflammatory response that is thought to be the dominant immune mechanism that expels the worms from the host. This reaction is thought to be elicited by the adult worms during a primary infection (×565).

less adequately describes the state of intestinal distress during the height (i.e., weeks 2 to 6) of the infection.

In experimental infection, animals repeatedly infected via the oral route acquire immunity against larvae within their Nurse cells (i.e., those produced in the initial infection), resulting in parasite death (55). Hence it is likely that during a primary infection, larvae in their Nurse cells exert an immunosuppressive effect on the host. The only host species to successfully mount a lethal immune attack against the larvae in their Nurse cells during a primary infection is the golden hamster (56); this immunity can be suppressed by radiation or steroids.

Morphologically, infected villi are flattened (57) and the lamina propria is hyperinfiltrated with white cells (Fig. 11) that reflect an intense set of specific and nonspecific immune responses (58,59). It is hypothesized that inflammation together with specific humoral immune responses results in the egression of the adult parasites from the small intestine (60–62). With low-dose infection (i.e., 200 or less larvae) in mice homozygous at the H-2 locus, adult worm expulsion is correlated with the major histocompatibility complex (MHC) (62). For example, mice of the H-2^k haplotype are more resistant to a primary infection compared to mice of an H-2^q haplotype (63). However, these results were not consistently obtained when similar groups of mice were challenged with a higher dose of infective L1 larvae (64).

The protective effector mechanism(s) also varies between host species and strains within a given species. In mice, elevated levels of immunoglobulin E (IgE), eosinophils, and mast cells (65) have been shown to be important effector mechanisms, while rat pups suckling on immune mothers' milk expel incoming larvae during challenge infection (66). Withholding vitamin A from the diet causes a shift in the T cell responses, going from predominantly T helper cell type 2 (Th2) to T helper cell type 1 (Th1), but mice that are vitamin A deficient are still able to reject

their adult worm burdens as efficiently as their nondeficient counterparts (67). Hence even within the same strain of host, alternate protective responses are effective. Until the molecular targets of the parasite that result in protection are known, such data cannot be properly interpreted. The protective immune mechanism(s) in humans is not known.

CLINICAL DISEASE

The typical pattern of clinical signs and symptoms (i.e., diarrhea, vomiting, muscle pain, fever, edema, especially noticeable around the orbits, and splinter hemorrhages under the nail beds) is associated with moderate to heavy infection with *T. spiralis* (45), whereas most light infections go undetected due to the lack of symptoms. These "classic" signs and symptoms mimic a wide variety of other disease states (68), including food poisoning, influenza and other common viral infections, arthritis, allergic diseases associated with increased levels of eosinophils, and many other more rarely encountered pathologic conditions (45). *Trichinella spiralis* infections that result in patient death often present in a clinical atypical pattern, due to the severity of systemic involvement. It is important to stress that clinical signs and symptoms vary greatly from individual to individual and are dependent on the dose of larvae ingested, the immunological status of the individual, and the infectivity of the parasite. Thus for each documented epidemic, there is a spectrum of signs and symptoms from which an overall general pattern of disease can be derived.

After the ingestion of larvae the appearance of signs and symptoms occurs in three phases, which correlate with the parasite's life cycle. In the first 2 to 3 weeks of infection, patients experience intestinal symptoms including diarrhea, nausea, and, in severe infection, vomiting. As mentioned, destruction of enterocytes by developing parasites is thought to be the basis of these symptoms. As newborn larvae are produced over the next several weeks (i.e., weeks 3 to 8), the entire body becomes involved due to the indiscriminant penetration of cells by this stage. Petechiae in the fingernail beds (i.e., "splinter" hemorrhages), conjunctival inflammation, and bilateral periorbital edema are typically recorded signs during this phase (45). Fever accompanies this phase of illness and is present in more than 90% of clinical cases (69). As infection wanes due to the acquisition of immunity, symptoms abate and most patients recover uneventfully. Immunity is thought to be lifelong and is most likely due to the periodic death of a small population of larvae in the tissues with consequent release of protection-inducing antigens.

In severe infection that does not result in death, patients may experience unusual symptoms including photophobia (70), delirium, and confusion (44). Residual side effects of intense infection include dull muscle pain (71), most probably due to the ongoing calcification of Nurse cell–parasite complexes in muscle tissue (72). In a retrospective study of 128 persons infected 10 years previously, no residual effects of infection were found although many suffered from severe disease at the time of their active infection (73).

DIAGNOSIS

Microscopic identification of Nurse cells containing larvae within infected muscle tissue is still the only definitive method of diagnosis (Figs. 1 and 10), although experimental methods for the detection of circulating antigen (74,75) and *Trichinella*-specific DNA sequences (76) have been reported. Muscle biopsy, usually a 3- to 5-mm³ piece of tissue, is dissected from deltoid or gastrocnemius muscle and, in moderate to heavy infection, is often positive for larvae late in the infection (i.e., at 20 days or more after ingestion of infected meat; Fig. 12B). A portion of the same tissue may be minced into small pieces (i.e., 1 to 2 mm³), placed between two microscope slides, squashed, and examined microscopically, `a la Owen and Paget (Fig. 12A). Digestion of the whole biopsy specimen for 1 hr in a solution of 1% pepsin–1% HCl improves the chances of microscopically identifying the larvae by releasing them from the tissues (Fig. 6) (45). Biopsies taken at earlier times throughout infection may also be positive, but young larvae are difficult to recognize due to the fact that they have yet to assume their classic spiral configuration. Hence most larvae appear as small straight tubes and are often passed over as "muscle debris." Furthermore, young larvae are susceptible to digestion in pepsin–HCl and are lost to examination if the tissue is subjected to this procedure.

Since rapid diagnosis of severe infection is critical, indirect diagnostic approaches are also often useful. The most widely employed of these is serology, in particular, the enzyme-linked immunoadsorbent assay (ELISA)-based tests (77). Antigens from the infective L1 larval stichocyte secretions (23,78,79) are responded to by most infected individuals within the first several weeks after ingestion of parasites (77,80). These antigens are easily collected *in vitro* and have been applied successfully to ELISAs to reveal early infection (weeks 2 to 4 after ingestion of infected meat). Other serological modalities have been used with good results, including the bentonite flocculation (81) and passive hemagglutination tests (82).

During experimental infection, IgM antibodies are first to appear, followed soon thereafter by IgG class antibodies (83). IgE antibodies are also produced (84). However, most commercial ELISAs are designed to detect IgG class

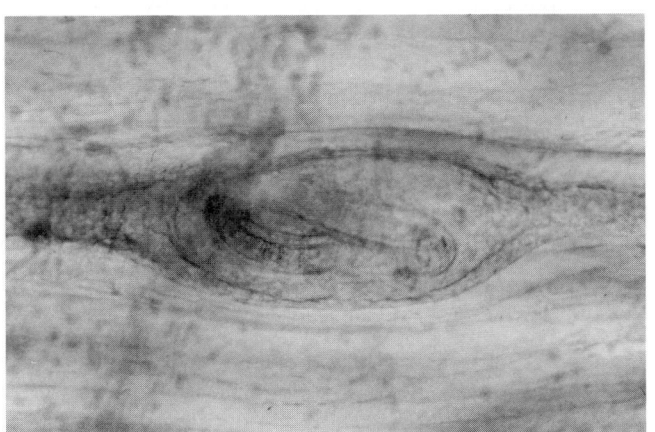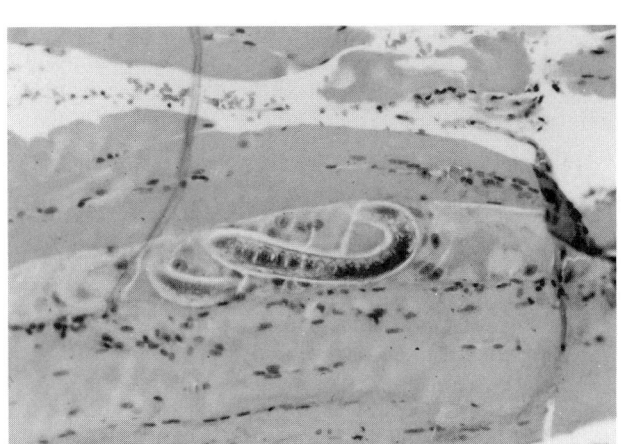

FIG. 12. Muscle biopsy from two infected individuals who suffered from clinical trichinellosis. **A:** The larva is mature, indicating that the biopsy was taken 25 days or more after the patient ate infected larvae. (×170). **B:** The larva has yet to achieve its full length, suggesting that the patient was recently infected (i.e., 15 to 20 days previous to the biopsy) (×175).

antibodies. As infection progresses, titers of IgG class antibodies rise then stabilize (85). However, IgM antibody titers may also remain high for some time after initial infection. Individuals remain serologically positive for most of the remainder of their lives, again probably due to the death of some larvae in the tissues throughout infection.

Evidence of recent infection can also be deduced from a combination of (a) a differential white cell determination, in which circulating eosinophil levels rise (weeks 2 to 6), plateau (weeks 7 to 12), and fall (weeks 13 to 20) throughout the acute and convalescent phases of disease (45); (b) physical findings such as muscle pain, fever, splinter hemorrhages, and conjunctivitis-like signs; and (c) a history of having recently eaten raw or undercooked meat, especially pork products. In most instances, other individuals besides the patient are also infected and the attending physician should therefore enquire if others also consumed portions of contaminated meat.

TREATMENT

If infection is detected early on (i.e., weeks 2 to 5), then benzimidazoles, particularly thiabendazole, are useful (86). Thiabendazole depolymerizes microtubules of the worm (87), thus directly or indirectly preventing further production of newborn larvae by interference with the mitotic spindle apparatus. Adult worms are also directly affected by the drug and egress from the small intestine shortly after its administration. The problem with the use of thiabendazole is not its efficacy against *T. spiralis,* but rather its untimely application, since most patients are diagnosed too late in their infection (i.e. during the "plateau" of clinical disease—weeks 5 to 9) for the drug to be used against the adults. In most cases, the adults are forced out of their intestinal niche by weeks 6 to 8 due to the development of immunity (62).

Since a large component of clinical disease is the result of inflammation due to cell damage and repair, use of steroids such as prednisolone (88) has a decidedly positive effect in relieving symptoms and increasing the chances for survival in heavy infection situations. Paradoxically, steroids prolong the life of the adult worms in the gut by interfering with the development of acquired immunity (89) and thus may even result in the production of more newborn larvae.

PREVENTION

The simplest way of preventing infection with *T. spiralis* is to avoid eating raw or undercooked meat. However, since most individuals occasionally dine at places other than their own homes, food preparation is often not under their control. Hence point source infections due to food served at restaurants sometimes occur. At home, an individual can prevent infection with *T. spiralis* by solidly freezing all fresh pork products (90,91). Larvae in commercial meats such as pork and beef are killed by ice crystal formation upon being frozen. Unfortunately, larvae in the muscle tissue of wild animals such as bear, fox,

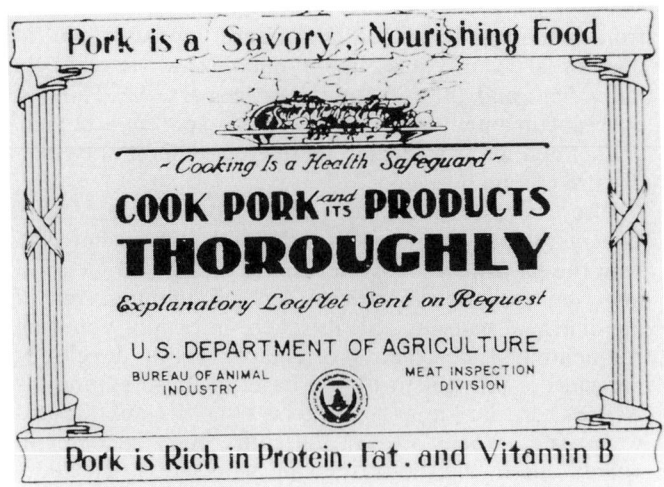

FIG. 13. A statement issued by the U.S. Department of Agriculture indicating that undercooked pork products may be unhealthy. The "explanatory leaflet" probably contained information on how to avoid infection with *Trichinella spiralis* and perhaps adult tapeworm due to *Taenia solium.*

raccoon, and opossum are not killed by this process (92), and it is believed that the tissues of these animals are protected from freezing by special proteins that prevent formation of ice crystals should temperatures fall below freezing.

While freezing cannot always ensure that transmission of infection will not occur, thoroughly cooking meat does (Fig. 13) (93). Raising the temperature above 137°F for 10 min has been shown to kill all worms *in situ.* It is important to note that the entire piece of meat must be kept at this temperature in order to kill all worms. The use of microwave ovens for cooking pork is not recommended due to the fact that the microwave beam is uneven and does not affect all parts of the meat the same (44).

At the community level, inspection for *T. spiralis* occurs in many parts of Europe. Several methods are in use today, including the one originated by Virchow in the 1870s; namely, trichinoscopy, in which large pieces of diaphragmatic muscle are pressed between two thick slides and viewed through a microscope (94). The use of the pooled sample digest method, in which pieces of diaphragmatic tissue from many pigs are minced together, then digested for a given time in 1% pepsin–1% HCl, has facilitated the inspection of hundreds of pigs a day at slaughterhouses throughout many of the Common Market countries of Europe (95). This method would not allow the inspection of the thousands of pigs slaughtered daily at regional abattoirs throughout the United States. Automated ELISA as a survey tool (96), again in use in Europe, has identified herds of infected pigs on large farms. There are no on-line serological procedures in use anywhere in the world today, but the technology for doing so has existed for at least 10 years. This approach would allow for inspecting large numbers of animals in a very short time. The reasons often given for not doing so have largely been based on political and economic principles, not public health concerns.

REFERENCES

1. Campbell WC. Historical introduction. In: Campbell WC, ed. *Trichinella and trichinosis*. New York: Plenum Press, 1983; 1–28.
2. Virchow R. Recherches sur le development du *Trichina spiralis*. *C R Acad Sci* 1859;49:660–662.
3. Zimmerman WJ. Surveillance in swine and other animals by muscle examination. In: Campbell WC, ed. *Trichinella and trichinosis*. New York: Plenum Press, 1983;515–528.
4. Zenker FA. Uber die Trichinen-krankheit des Menchen. *Virchows Arch A Pathol Anat* 1860;18:561–572.
5. Despommier DD. Biology. In: Campbell WC, ed. *Trichinella and trichinosis*. New York: Plenum Press, 1983;75–142.
6. Despommier DD, Karapelou JW. *Parasite life cycles*. New York: Springer-Verlag, 1987.
7. Soule C, Guillou J-P, Dupony-Camet J, et al. Differentiation of *Trichinella* isolates by polymerase chain reaction. *Parasitol Res* 1993;79:461–465.
8. Dick TA, Curran J, Klassen G. Genetics and molecular biology of *Trichinella*. In: Kim CW, ed. *Trichinellosis*. Albany: State University of New York Press, 1985;118–128.
9. Pozio E, La Rosa G, Murrell KD, Lichtenfeld JR. Taxonomic revisions of the genus *Trichinella*. *J Parasitol* 1992;78:654–659.
10. DiBari C, Schiraldi O. Epidemiological and clinical aspects in two outbreaks of trichinellosis caused by *Trichinella nelsoni* in southern Italy. In: Kim CW, ed. *Trichinellosis*. Albany: State University of New York Press, 1988;337–342.
11. Kim CW. Epidemiology II. Geographic distribution and prevalence. In: Campbell WC, ed. *Trichinella and trichinosis*. New York: Plenum Press, 1983;445–500.
12. Campbell WC. Epidemiology I. Modes of transmission. In: Campbell WC, ed. *Trichinella and trichinosis*. New York: Plenum Press, 1983;425–444.
13. Wright K. *Trichinella spiralis:* an intracellular parasite in the intestinal phase. *J Parasitol* 1979;65:441–445.
14. Despommier DD. *Trichinella spiralis* and the concept of niche. *J Parasitol* 1993;79:472–482.
15. Purkerson M, Despommier DD. Fine structure of the muscle phase of *Trichinella spiralis* in the mouse. In: Kim CW, ed. *Trichinellosis*. New York: Intext Educational Publishing, 1974; 7–23.
16. Ferguson JD, Castro GA. Metabolism of intestinal stages of *Trichinella spiralis*. *Am J Physiol* 1973;255:85–89.
17. Stewart GL, Despommier DD, Burnham J, et al. *Trichinella spiralis:* behavior, structure and biochemistry of larvae following exposure to components of the host enteric environment. *Exp Parasitol* 1987;63:195–204.
18. Despommier DD. Behavioral cues in migration and location of parasitic nematodes, with special emphasis on *Trichinella spiralis*. In: Bailey WS, ed. *Cues that influence the behavior of internal parasites*. Washington, DC: Agricultural Research Service (Southern Region), USDA, 1981;86–126.
19. McCoy OR. The development of trichinae in abnormal environments. *J Parasitol* 1936;22:54–59.
20. Kozek WJ. The molting pattern in *Trichinella spiralis*. I. A light microscope study. *J Parasitol* 1971;57:1015–1028.
21. Russell DA, Castro GA. Physiology of the gastrointestinal tract in the parasitized host. In: Johnson LR, Christianson J, Jackson MJ, Walsh JH, eds. *Physiology of the gastrointestinal tract*. New York: Raven Press, 1987;1749–1780.
22. Castro GA, Olson LJ, Baker RD. Glucose malabsorption and intestinal histopathology in *Trichinella spiralis*-infected guinea pigs. *J Parasitol* 1967;53:595–612.
23. Silberstein DS. Antigens. In: Campbell WC, ed. *Trichinella and trichinosis*. New York: Plenum Press, 1983;309–334.
24. Capo V, Silberstein DS, Despommier DD. Immunocytolocalization of two protective antigens of *Trichinella spiralis* during its

25. Wisnewski N, Mcneil M, Grieve RB, et al. Characterization of novel fucosyl-containing and tyvelosyl-containing glycoconjugates from *Trichinella spiralis* muscle stage larvae. *Mol Biochem Parasitol* 1993;61:25–36.
26. Chitwood BG. The structure of the esophagus in the Trichuroidea. *J Parasitol* 1930;17:35–42.
27. Despommier DD, Campbell WC, Blair LS. The in vivo and in vitro analysis of immunity to *Trichinella spiralis* in mice and rats. *Parasitology* 1977;74:109–119.
28. Harley JP, Gallicchico V. *Trichinella spiralis:* migration of larvae in the rat. *Exp Parasitol* 1971;30:11–12.
29. Wang CH, Bell RG. *Trichinella spiralis:* vascular recirculation and organ retention of newborn larvae in rats. *Exp Parasitol* 1986;62:430–441.
30. Frocher W, Gullotta F, Saatof M, et al. Chronic trichinosis. Clinical bioptic, serologic, and electromyographic observations. *Eur Neurol* 1989;28:221–226.
31. Ritterson AL. Nature of the cyst of *Trichinella spiralis*. *J Parasitol* 1966;52:157–161.
32. Pagenstecher HA. Die Trichinen. Leipzig: Engelsmanns, 1865; 116pp.
33. Humes AG, Ackers RP. Vascular changes in the cheek pouch of the golden hamster during infection with *Trichinella spiralis* larvae. *Anat Rec* 1952;114:103–113.
34. Baruch AM, Despommier DD. Blood vessels in *Trichinella spiralis* infection: a study using vascular casts. *J Parasitol* 1991; 77:99–103.
35. Jasmer DP. *Trichinella spiralis:* altered expression of muscle proteins in trichinosis. *Exp Parasitol* 1990;70:452–465.
36. Despommier DD. The worm that would be virus. *Parasitol Today* 1990;6:193–195.
37. El-Nawawi FA. Swine trichinellosis in Egypt. *Arch Lebensmittehyg* 1981;32:156–158.
38. Clark PS, Brownsberger KM, Saslow AR, et al. Bear meat trichinosis: epidemiologic, serologic and clinical observations from two Alaskan outbreaks. *Ann Intern Med* 1972;76:951–956.
39. Beck JW. Trichinosis in domesticated and experimental animals. In: Gould SE, ed. *Trichinosis in man and animals*. Springfield, IL: Charles C Thomas, 1970;61–80.
40. Bellani L, Mantovani A, Filippini I. Observations on an outbreak of human trichinellosis in northern Italy. In: Kim CW, Pawlowski ZS, eds. *Trichinellosis*. Hanover, NH: University Press of New England, 1978;535–539.
41. Van Knapen F, Franchimont JH. *Trichinella spiralis* infection in horses. In: Tanner CE, Martinez-Fernandez AR, Bolas-Fernandez F, eds. Madrid, Spain: Consejo Superior de Investigaciones Cientificas Press, 1988;376–381.
42. Bouree P, Leymarie JL, Anbe C. Epidemiological study of two outbreaks of trichinosis in France, due to horse meat. In: Tanner CE, Martinez-Fernandez AR, Bolas-Frenandez F, eds. *Trichinellosis*. Madrid, Spain, Consejo Superior de Investigaciones Cientificas Press, 1988;382–391.
43. Andy JJ, O'Connell JP, Daddario RC, et al. Trichinosis causing extensive ventricular mural endocarditis with superimposed thrombosis. *Am J Med* 1977;63:824–829.
44. Kramer MD, Aita JF. Trichinosis. In: Vinken PJ, Bruyn GW, eds. *Infections of the nervous system, Part III*. Amsterdam: North-Holland, 1978;267–290.
45. Pawlowski ZS. Clinical aspects in man. In: Campbell WC, ed. *Trichinella and trichinosis*. New York: Plenum Press, 1983; 367–401.
46. Weatherby NF. Anatomical pathology. In: Campbell WC, ed. *Trichinella and trichinosis*. New York: Plenum Press, 1983; 173–208.
47. Castro GA, Hessell JJ, Whalen G. Altered intestinal fluid movement in response to *Trichinella spiralis* in immunized rats. *Parasite Immunol* 1979;1:259–266.
48. Castro GA, Badial-Aceves F, Smith JW, et al. Altered small bowel propulsion associated with parasitism. *Gasteroenterology* 1976;71:620–625.
49. Harari Y, Castro GA. Sialic acid deficiency in lectin-resistant intestinal brush border membranes from rats following the intes-

tinal phase of trichinellosis. *Mol Biochem Parasitol* 1983;9:73–81.

50. Schanbacher LM, Nations JK, Weisbrodt NW, et al. Intestinal myoelectric activity in paralyzed dogs. *Am J Physiol* 1978;234:R188–R195.
51. Bullick GR, Frizzell RA, Castro GA. *Trichinella spiralis:* rapid, immunologically influenced reduction of intestinal sodium-coupled sugar transport in the rat. *Exp Parasitol* 1984;57:104–109.
52. Kahn I, Collins SM. Altered expression of sodium pump isoforms in the inflamed intestine of *Trichinella spiralis*-infected rats. *Am J Physiol* 1993;264:G1160–G1168.
53. Demlinski AB, Johnson LR, Castro GA. Influence of enteric parasitism on secretin-inhibited gastric secretion. *Am J Physiol* 1979;28:854–859.
54. Demlinski AB, Johnson LR, Castro GA. Influence of enteric parasitism on hormone-regulated pancreatic secretion in dogs. *Am J Physiol* 1979;237:R232–R238.
55. Madden KB, Murrell KD, Lunney JK. *Trichinella spiralis:* major histocompatibility complex-associated elimination of encysted muscle larvae in swine. *Exp Parasitol* 1990;70:443–451.
56. Ritterson AL. Innate resistance of a species of hamster to *Trichinella spiralis* and its reversal by cortisone. *J Infect Dis* 1959;105:253–266.
57. Lin T-M, Olson LJ. Pathophysiology of reinfection with *Trichinella spiralis* in guinea pigs during the intestinal phase. *J Parasitol* 1970;56:529–539.
58. Larsh JE Jr, Race GJ. A histopathologic study of the anterior small intestine of immunized and nonimmunized mice infected with *Trichinella spiralis. J Infect Dis* 1954;94:262–272.
59. Ruitenberg EJ, Perrudet-Badoux A, Boussac-Aron Y, et al. *Trichinella spiralis* infection in animals genetically selected for high and low antibody production: studies on intestinal pathology. *Int Arch Allergy Appl Immunol* 1980;62:104–110.
60. McCoy OR. Immunity of rats to reinfection with *Trichinella spiralis. Am J Hyg* 1931;14:484–494.
61. Love RJ, Ogilvie BM, McLaren DJ. The immune mechanism which expels the intestinal stage of *Trichinella spiralis* from rats. *Immunology* 1976;30:7–15.
62. Wakelin D, Denham DA. The immune response. In: Campbell WC, ed. *Trichinella and trichinosis.* New York: Plenum Press, 1983;265–308.
63. Wassom DL, David CS, Gleich GJ. MHC-linked genetic control of the immune response to parasites: *Trichinella spiralis* in the mouse. In: Sakemene E, Kongshaven PAL, Landy M, eds. *Genetic control of natural resistance to infection and malignancy.* New York: Academic Press, 1980;75–82.
64. Bell RG, Adams LS, Wilson RW. A single gene determines rapid expulsion of *Trichinella spiralis* in mice. *Infect Immun* 1984;45:273–275.
65. Grencis RK, Else KJ, Nishikawa SI. The in vivo role of stem cell factor (*c-kit* ligand) on mastocytosis and host protective immunity to the intestinal nematode, *Trichinella spiralis,* in mice. *Parasite Immunol* 1993;15:55–59.
66. Appleton JA, McGregor DD. Rapid expulsion of *Trichinella spiralis* in suckling rats. *Science* 1984;226:70–72.
67. Curman JA, Pond L, Nashold F, et al. Immunity to *Trichinella spiralis* infection in vitamin A-deficient mice. *J Exp Med* 1992;175:111–120.
68. Altus P, Blanco R, Chazal R. Trichinosis masquerading as a penicillin allergy. *JAMA* 1980;243:767–768.
69. Oppenheim JM, Whims CB, Frisch AW. Trichinosis. Clinical and laboratory observations in a group of 256 cases. *Mil Surg* 1947;101:294–301.
70. Stoll HF. Trichinosis. Report of two cases presenting diplopia and one polyserositis. *JAMA* 1929;92:791–793.
71. Gould SE. Clinical manifestations. A. Symptomatology. In: Gould SE, ed. *Trichinosis in man and animals.* Springfield, IL: Charles C Thomas, 1970;269–306.
72. Bullock WL. Phosphates in experimental *Trichinella spiralis* infections in the rat. *Exp Parasitol* 1953;2:150–162.
73. Harms G, Binz P, Feldmeier H, et al. Trichinosis: a prospective controlled study of patients ten years after acute infection. *Clin Infect Dis* 1993;17:637–643.
74. Gomez-Garcia V, Rodriguez-Perez J, Rodriguez-Orosins M, et al. Use of monoclonal antibodies for the detection of *Trichinella* circulating antigens. In: Tanner CE, Martinez-Fernandez AR, Bolas-Frenandez F, eds. *Trichinellosis.* Madrid, Spain: Consejo Superior Investigaciones Cientificas Press, 1988;188–193.
75. Candalfi E, Frache PH, Laince M, et al. Detection of circulating antigen in trichinellosis by immunoenzymology. Comparative results in mice, rats and humans. In: Tanner CE, Matrinez-Frenandez AR, Bolas-Feranadez F, eds. *Trichinellosis,* Madrid, Spain: Consejo Superior Investigaciones Cientificas Press, 1988;194–201.
76. Soule C, Guillou J-P, Dupouy-Camet J, et al. Differentiation of *Trichinella* isolates by the polymerase chain reaction. *J Parasitol* 1993;79:461–465.
77. Ljungstrom I. Immunodiagnosis in man. In: Campbell WC, ed. *Trichinella and trichinosis.* New York: Plenum Press, 1983;403–425.
78. Oliver-Gonzalez J. The in vitro action of immune serum on the larvae and adults of *Trichinella spiralis. J Infect Dis* 1940;67:292–300.
79. Despommier DD, Muller M. The stichosome and its secretion granules in the mature muscle larva of *Trichinella spiralis. J Parasitol* 1976;62:775–785.
80. Despommier DD, Muller M, Jenks B, et al. Immunodiagnosis of human trichinosis using counterimmunoelectrophoresis and agar gel diffusion techniques. *Am J Trop Med Hyg* 1974;23:41–44.
81. Bozichevich J, Tobie JE, Thomas EH, et al. A rapid flocculation test for the diagnosis of trichinosis. *Public Health Rep* 1951;66:806–814.
82. Price SG, Weiner LM. Use of hemagglutination in the diagnosis of trichinosis. *Am J Clin Pathol* 1956;26:1261–1269.
83. Crandall RB, Crandall CA. *Trichinella spiralis:* immunologic response to infection in mice. *Exp Parasitol* 1972;31:378–398.
84. Stumpf J, Undeutsch K, Landcraf H. Results of the clinical and serological diagnosis of an epidemic of *Trichinella spiralis.* In: Kim CW, Ruitenberg EJ, Teppema JS, eds. *Trichinellosis.* Chertsey, England: Reedbooks, 1981;279–282.
85. Olaison L, Ljungstrom I. An outbreak of trichinosis in Lebanon. *Trans R Soc Trop Med Hyg* 1992;86:658–660.
86. Gerwel C, Pawlowski Z, Kociecka W, et al. Probable sterilization of *Trichinella spiralis* by thiabendazole: further clinical observation of human infection. In: Kim CW, ed. *Trichinellosis.* New York: Intext Educational Publishing, 1974;471–475.
87. Lacey E. Mode of action of benzimidazoles. *Parasitol Today* 1990;4:112–115.
88. Anti-microbial therapies. *Med Lett Drugs Ther* Feb 1992.
89. Markell EK. The effect of cortisone upon the longevity and productivity of *Trichinella spiralis* in the rat. *J Infect Dis* 1958;102:158–161.
90. Leighty JC. Control I. Public health aspects (with special reference to the United States). In: Campbell WC, ed. *Trichinella and trichinosis.* New York: Plenum Press, 1983;501–513.
91. Ransom BH. Effects of refrigeration upon the larvae of *Trichinella spiralis. J Agric Res* 1916;5:819–853.
92. Dick TA. Infectivity of isolates of *Trichinella* and the ability of an arctic strain to survive freezing temperatures in the racoon, *Procyon lotor,* under experimental conditions. *J Wildl Dis* 1983;19:333–336.
93. Ransom BH, Schwartz B. Effects of heat on trichinae. *J Agric Res* 1919;17:201–221.
94. Lehmensick R. Inspection of pork and control of trichinosis in Germany. In: Gould SE, ed. *Trichinosis in man and animals.* Springfield, IL: Charles C Thomas, 1970;437–448.
95. Thomasen DU. "Stomacher" trikinkontrol-metoden. *Dansk Vet Tidsskr* 1976;59:481–490.
96. Ruitenberg EJ, Ljungstrom I, Steerenberg PA, et al. Application of immunofluorescence and immunoenzyme methods in the serodiagnosis of *Trichinella spiralis* infection. *Ann NY Acad Sci* 1975;254:296–303.

Infections of the Gastrointestinal Tract,
edited by M. J. Blaser, P. D. Smith, J. I. Ravdin,
H. B. Greenberg, and R. L. Guerrant
Raven Press, Ltd., New York © 1995.

CHAPTER 78

Hookworm Infections

Peter J. Hotez

Approximately one billion individuals are thought to harbor one or more species of hookworms, which cause intestinal blood loss leading to iron deficiency and anemia. Children and women of childbearing age are particularly susceptible to the effects of chronic hookworm anemia. In the former, hookworm anemia leads to deficits in physical, intellectual, psychomotor, and cognitive development (1). Because it occurs insidiously, hookworm infection is frequently overlooked as a major cause of global morbidity.

Hookworms were not recognized as etiologic agents of disease until the middle of the 19th century and did not receive widespread attention until they were implicated as the cause of "miners' anemia" among Italian laborers constructing the Saint Gothard railway tunnel in the Swiss Alps (2). The life cycle of *Ancylostoma duodenale* was elucidated by Looss (3), a German scientist working in Egypt, while the life cycle of *Necator americanus* was elucidated by Stiles (4), a U.S. government scientist. At one time hookworm infection was common throughout the southeastern United States. In the early part of this century, the South was targeted by a vigorous hookworm control campaign carried out by the Rockefeller Sanitary Commission (5).

MICROBIOLOGY AND LIFE CYCLE

Hookworms are bursate nematodes (order Strongylida) of the family Ancylostomidae, which are distinguished by their highly cuticularized buccal capsules provided with teeth or cutting plates (6). *Ancylostoma* and *Necator* are the only medically important genera (Fig. 1).

Necator

Necator americanus is the only human pathogen of this genus. It is known as the "New World" hookworm be-

cause of its widespread distribution in the Caribbean and the Americas. Small foci still remain in North America, particularly in Mexico and the southeastern United States. Despite its "New World" designation, *N. americanus* is also a major pathogen in Sub-Saharan Africa, Southeast Asia, and the Pacific Islands. It is presumed to have been introduced to the Americas by slaves and colonists from Africa (6). *Necator americanus* has only a single route of infection—by percutaneous entry of third-stage infective larvae (Fig. 2). Upon host entry, the larvae are swept from lymphatics and venules in the skin and are carried passively to the right side of the heart and then to pulmonary capillaries. The larvae enter the lung parenchyma, ascending the alveoli, bronchioles, bronchi, and trachea before being coughed and swallowed. The larvae molt twice and sexually differentiate into male (7 to 9 mm in length) and female (9 to 11 mm in length) adults, which live for 5 to 6 years (8). *Necator americanus* has a relatively small buccal capsule, which is armed with cutting plates that facilitate attachment to the intestinal mucosa (Fig. 3). A single female *N. americanus* produces 6000 to 11,000 eggs/day (after a prepatent period of 45 to 60 days), which, when deposited in feces onto moist soil, develop at an optimum temperature of 25°C to 28°C (6). The resulting first-stage larva undergoes two successive molts to become an infective filariform larva (Fig. 4). The third larval stage is nonfeeding and capable of considerable vertical movement, migrating to the soil surface or low vegetation in order to facilitate human contact and renew the life cycle (9).

Ancylostoma

Three members of the genus *Ancylostoma* have been described as parasites of humans (Fig. 5). Of these, *A. duodenale* is by far the most important human pathogen, while *A. ceylonicum* and the dog hookworm *A. caninum* have been described from human patients in restricted geographic areas.

Ancylostoma duodenale is known as the "Old World" hookworm, referring to its predominant distribution in the

P. Hotez: Departments of Pediatrics (Infectious Diseases Division) and Epidemiology and Public Health, Yale University School of Medicine, New Haven, Connecticut 06510.

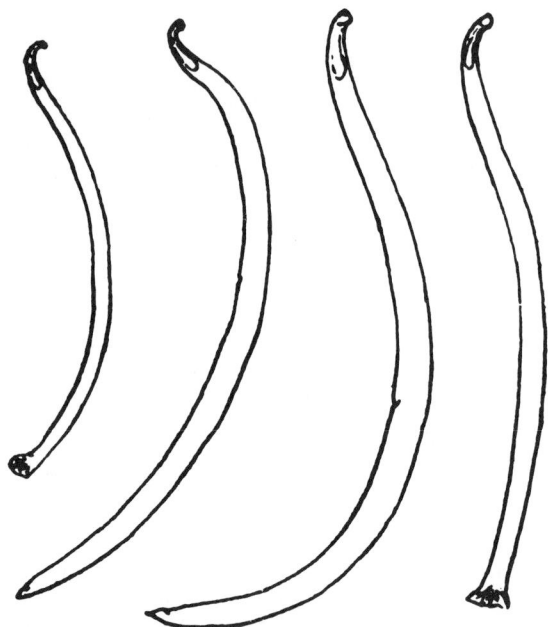

FIG. 1. Outline drawings showing relative length and shape of *Necator americanus* and *Ancylostoma duodenale*. **Left to right:** *N. americanus* male, *N. americanus* female, *A. duodenale* female, *A. duodenale* male (×10). (From ref. 7, with permission.)

Mediterranean regions of Africa and Europe and in India and China. Focal pockets of distribution also occur in Latin America (10). *Ancylostoma duodenale* has a number of features to distinguish it from *N. americanus,* including its larger size (8 to 11 mm for adult male, 10 to 13 mm for adult female), greater fecundity (10,000 to 30,000 eggs/day), greater virulence (the adults cause greater blood loss), and shortened life span. These features led Hoagland and Schad (11) to postulate that *A. duodenale* is the more "opportunistic species." Like *N. americanus, A. duodenale* larvae can infect humans percutaneously. However, *A. duodenale* larvae are also infective via the oral route. In some geographic areas oral ingestion may be the predominant route of transmission. Another unusual feature of *A. duodenale* larvae is their ability to undergo arrested development in the tissues after host entry (12). It has been suggested that the phenomenon of arrested development explains why humans with *A. duodenale* infection exhibit seasonal variation in their egg output (12). It has been further hypothesized that the arrested larvae can mobilize from the tissues to the colostrum and breast milk, thereby resulting in vertical transmission of ancylostomiasis to infants (1,13,14). The mechanism by which hookworm larvae remain in arrest is not known, although there is a phenotypic similarity between arrested hookworm larvae and the "dauer" larval stage of the free-living nematode *Caenorhabditis elegans* (15). Conceivably, similar environmental cues and signal transducing molecules have a role in this phenomenon.

Ancylostoma ceylonicum is a minor parasite of humans (as well as dogs and cats) in India and Southeast Asia,

which causes insignificant blood loss (16), while the canine hookworm *A. caninum* has been shown to cause eosinophilic enteritis (see later discussion) in a focal region of northern Queensland, Australia (17). The dog and cat hookworm, *A. braziliense,* cannot complete its life cycle in humans, but instead migrates aberrantly in the skin to cause cutaneous larva migrans (18).

EPIDEMIOLOGY

Because appropriate soil conditions are needed to facilitate egg development and to permit survival of the larval stages, the epidemiology of hookworm infection is intimately connected to the soil and to human agricultural pursuits. In general, favorable transmission requires moist soil (either through rainfall or irrigation), humidity, warm temperatures, and shade. These conditions can also be frequently met in mines and tunnels. In contrast, unshaded open areas, salinity, compacted, and water-logged soils are unfavorable for transmission (9).

With the appropriate climactic and soil conditions, a community will suffer from high-intensity hookworm infection wherever its members have a high likelihood of coming into contact with human feces. This generally occurs in one of three settings (9): (a) in areas lacking appropriate sanitation or where indiscriminate defecation occurs, (b) in areas where inadequately composted human excreta are used as fertilizer, or (c) in highly focal areas of human defecation such as in mines and tunnels and on plantations. Certain agricultural pursuits such as growing coffee beans, tea, mulberry leaves, and sugar cane are notorious for facilitating high rates of hookworm transmission.

In any given endemic area, the distribution of infection in a community will often vary widely (9). Most individuals will usually harbor light infections, whereas only a few will harbor heavy infections. Curiously, the subset of individuals who harbor large numbers of worms will, if treated, reacquire heavy worm burdens if left to live in the same endemic area (19). This predisposition to infection has been noted with other human helminth infections: its basis is unknown.

PATHOGENESIS AND IMMUNITY

Migratory Phase

Infective hookworm larvae elicit two types of histopathology depending on their mode of host entry.

Third-stage larvae that infect percutaneously cause mechanical, chemical, and inflammatory damage to all layers of the skin. In the epidermis, the larvae separate epidermal keratinocytes, a process facilitated by the release of a parasite hyaluronidase that breaks the hyaluronan bridges connecting these cells (20). Epidermal entry is usually followed by penetration through the basement membrane into the dermis. A zinc metalloprotease released by invading larvae (21,22) may also help to chemically dissolve

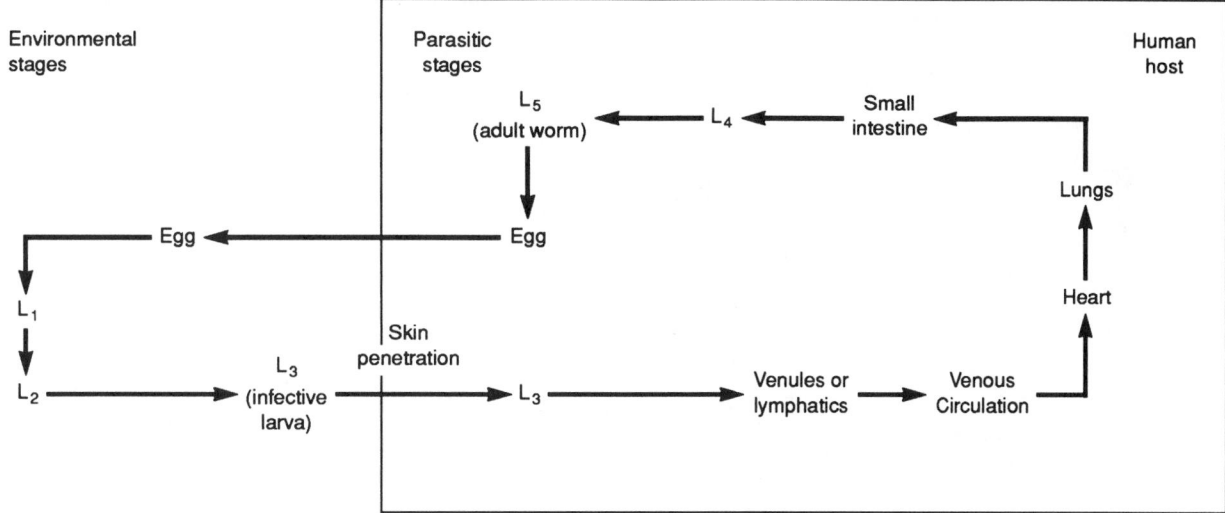

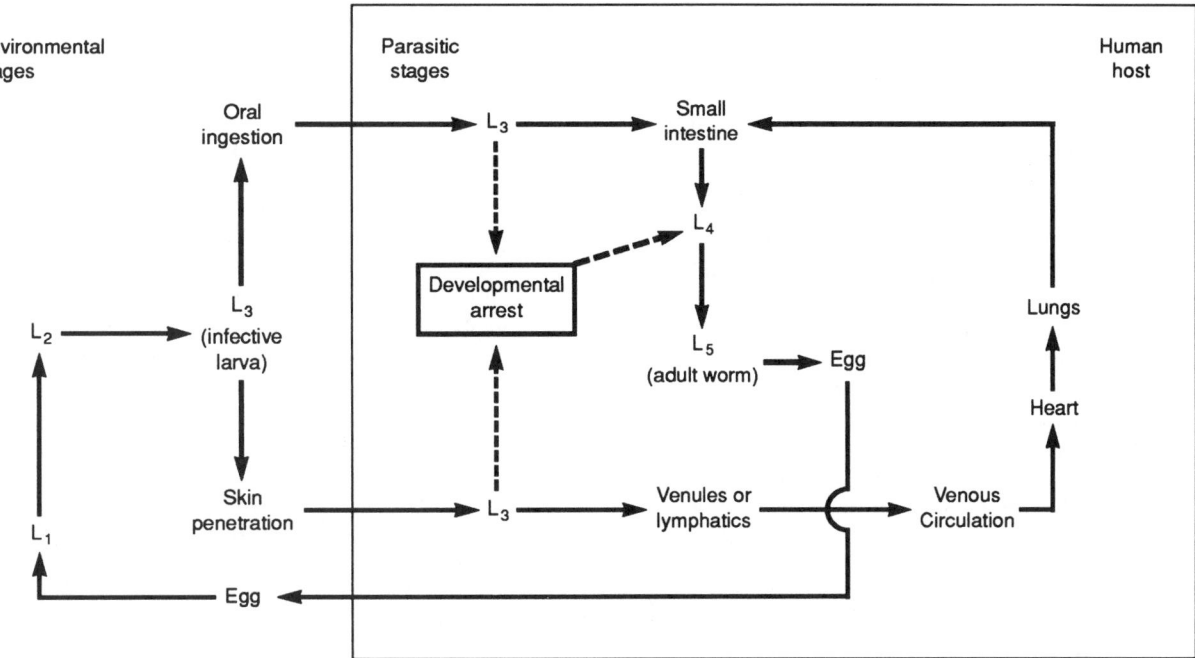

FIG. 2. Life cycles of *Necator americanus* and *Ancylostoma duodenale,* showing environmental and parasitic stages.

the major connective tissue macromolecular barriers. The host responds to hookworm larval skin invasion by mounting an intense inflammatory response, known as "ground itch." Ground itch has features that resemble a delayed-type hypersensitivity and probably results from the elaboration of cytokines by keratinocytes and infiltrating immunocompetent cells in the skin. Eicosanoids released by hookworm larvae may also contribute to cutaneous inflammation (23).

As noted earlier, hookworm larvae of the species *A. duodenale* may also directly enter the gastrointestinal

tract by host ingestion. When large numbers of larvae enter at once, a second type of hookworm-associated hypersensitivity syndrome, known as "Wakana disease" may occur (24).

Gastrointestinal Phase

Adult hookworms attach to the intestinal mucosa where they elicit mechanical and chemical damage. Mechanical damage occurs when the buccal capsule of the parasite

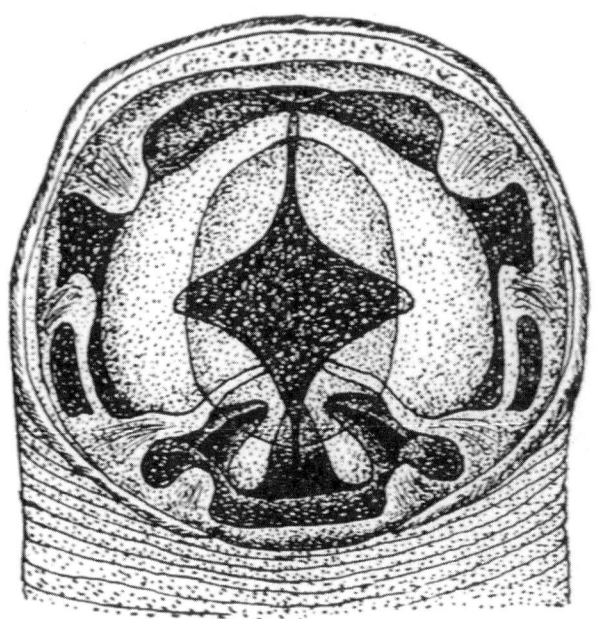

FIG. 3. Mouth capsule of *Necator americanus.* (From ref. 7, with permission.)

surrounds a bolus of intestinal mucosa and holds onto it by a combination of specialized teeth *(A. duodenale)* or cutting plates *(N. americanus).* As the parasite's esophageal muscles contract, a small vacuum is created that fixes the mucosa in the buccal capsule as a bolus (25,26) (Fig. 6). Chemical damage to the intestinal mucosal bolus subsequently occurs via the action of several parasite-derived hydrolytic enzymes, which presumably are released into the buccal capsule. Some of these hydrolases released include a protease (28–30), a hyaluronidase (31), and an acetylcholinesterase (29). Ultimately, the ingested bolus is degraded (25,26).

One consequence of mucosal degradation caused by hookworm attachment is the ultimate rupture and destruction of capillaries contained within the lamina propria, resulting in blood extravasation (25,26). Some blood leaks at the site of attachment, although much of it is ingested by the worm. A continuous flow of blood is guaranteed by the release of parasite-derived anticoagulants (32–35), including a small polypeptide that inhibits factor Xa (36,37) and a platelet antiaggregating factor. The amount of hookworm-associated blood loss is species dependent with the greatest amount caused by *A. duodenale,* approximately tenfold less caused by *N. americanus,* and almost none caused by *A. ceylonicum* (16,38). The differences in blood loss between species can usually account for the magnitude of hookworm anemia, although the onset of anemia is also dependent on dietary iron intake and host iron reserves (39). Even iron deficiency that does not result in clinical anemia, however, can severely impair the host. For instance, iron is essential for the development and function of dopaminergic neurons and as a prosthetic group in biosynthetic enzymes for neurotransmitters (40); its deficiency may account for the observed deficits in intellectual and cognitive development associated with

hookworm infection. Plasma protein losses also occur in association with hookworm-derived blood loss and mucosal edema, leading to hypoalbuminemia (41). Changes in gastric acidity (41) and peristalsis (42) may also contribute to the gastrointestinal pathology of hookworm infection.

Immunity

There is no strong evidence that humans mount an effective immune response to naturally acquired hookworm infections. This is in contrast to other geohelminths, in which age-acquired resistance can be demonstrated (43). Hookworm-infected individuals have demonstrable circulating antibodies to hookworm antigens, but they do not appear to correlate with resistance (44). The absence of clear-cut immunity has led a number of investigators to postulate the existence of different means of immune evasion and escape (29).

CLINICAL DISEASE

Migratory Phase

Ground itch is an intensely pruritic papular dermatitis, usually on the hands and feet. A distinct cutaneous manifestation, known as cutaneous larva migrans or "creeping eruption" occurs when canine or feline hookworm larvae (especially *A. braziliense*) enter the epidermis and migrate laterally to elicit long, serpiginous tracks that become raised and crusted (18). Both of these cutaneous manifestations are frequently accompanied by secondary bacterial invasion.

Lung involvement secondary to the pulmonary migration of hookworm larvae is not usually severe but may result in a pneumonitis associated with dyspnea, cough, and wheezing. Wakana disease is a gastrointestinal syndrome associated with the ingestion of large numbers of *A. duodenale* infective larvae, which is characterized by the presence of nausea, vomiting, cough, dyspnea, and eosinophilia (24).

Gastrointestinal Phase

The hallmark of the gastrointestinal phase of hookworm infection is iron deficiency and iron deficiency anemia resulting from intestinal blood loss. This phase usually begins 10 to 20 weeks after the initial exposure to infective hookworm larvae. However, for strains of *A. duodenale* larvae that are prone to undergo arrest, the gastrointestinal phase may not occur for several months (45).

A variety of gastrointestinal symptoms have been described in naturally infected patients and in human volunteers, including postprandial epigastric pain, nausea, and mild diarrhea (46,47). Patients with gastrointestinal symptoms from hookworm infection often report some relief after eating clay or other bulky substances.

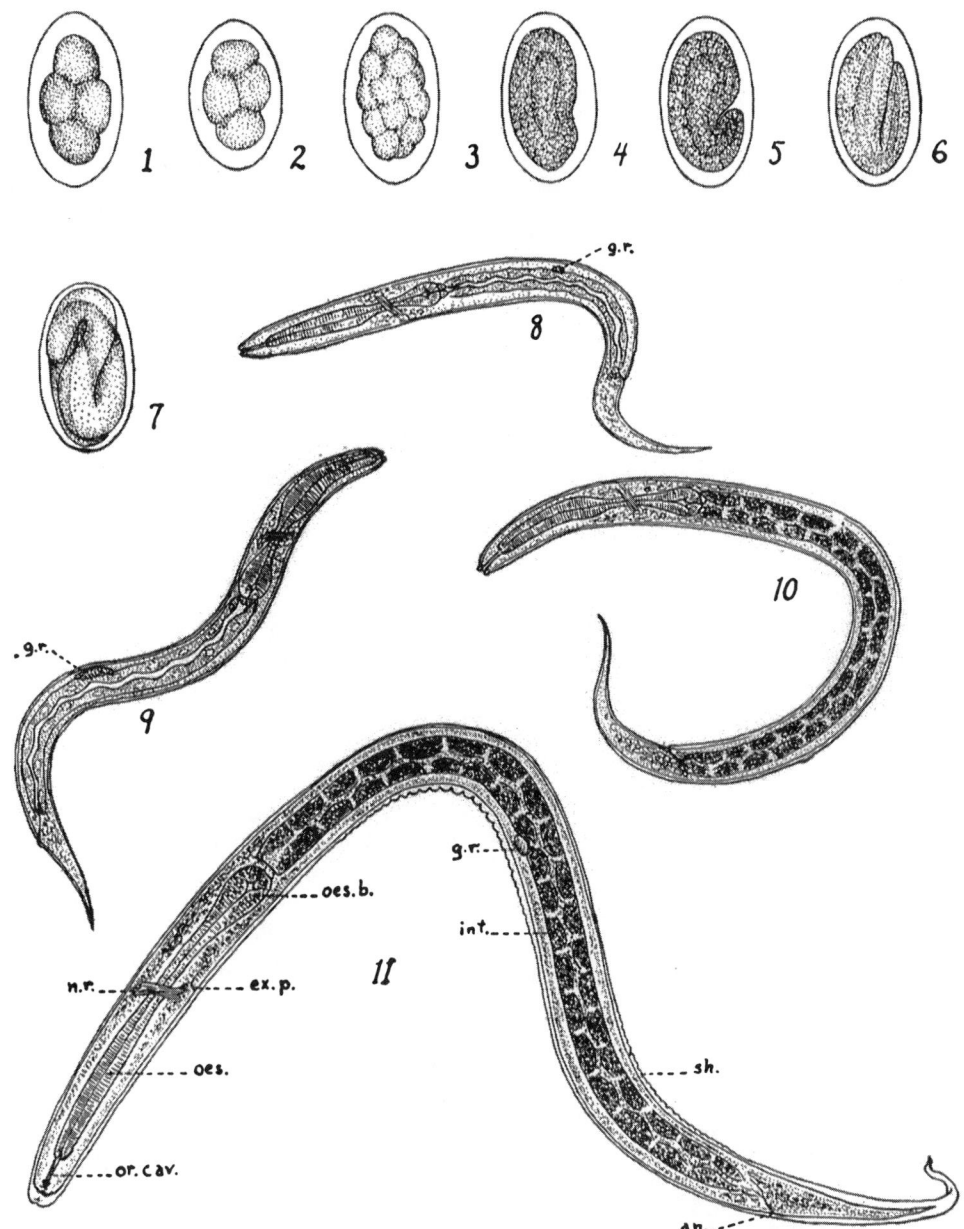

FIG. 4. Developmental stages of hookworms outside the body. 1, Four-celled egg of *Necator americanus*; 2, same of *Ancylostoma duodenale*; 3, morula stage of about 16 cells; 4, late morula stage; 5, early tadpole stage; 6, late tadpole stage; 7 developed embryo in egg; 8, newly hatched embryo; 9, newly hatched *Strongyloides* embryo for comparison; 10, larva after first moult; 11, infective larva (×500). (From ref. 7, with permission.)

Hookworm anemia can be severe enough to cause exertional dyspnea, lassitude, palpitations, and even high output heart failure. The physical signs of hookworm anemia include pale sclera, koilonychia, and cardiac flow murmurs. An extreme form of hookworm anemia with high mortality has been described in infants suffering from ancylostomiasis who develop melena, extreme paleness, diarrhea, and anorexia (14,15).

More commonly, however, heavily infected individuals suffer from chronic hookworm anemia, which is often exacerbated by underlying malnutrition (Fig. 7). Children especially can manifest signs and symptoms of moderate kwashiorkor (1). Curiously, the skin of these individuals often acquires a yellow-green pallor known as "chlorosis" (48) or, in dark-skinned patients, areas of depigmentation. Probably, the most devastating components of chronic hookworm anemia in childhood are the long-term effects on intellectual and physical growth. Although growth retardation is most apparent at the time of puberty (49), it is probably a continuous process throughout childhood. Moreover, it is partly reversible with interventions that use either specific anthelmintic chemotherapy (50,51)

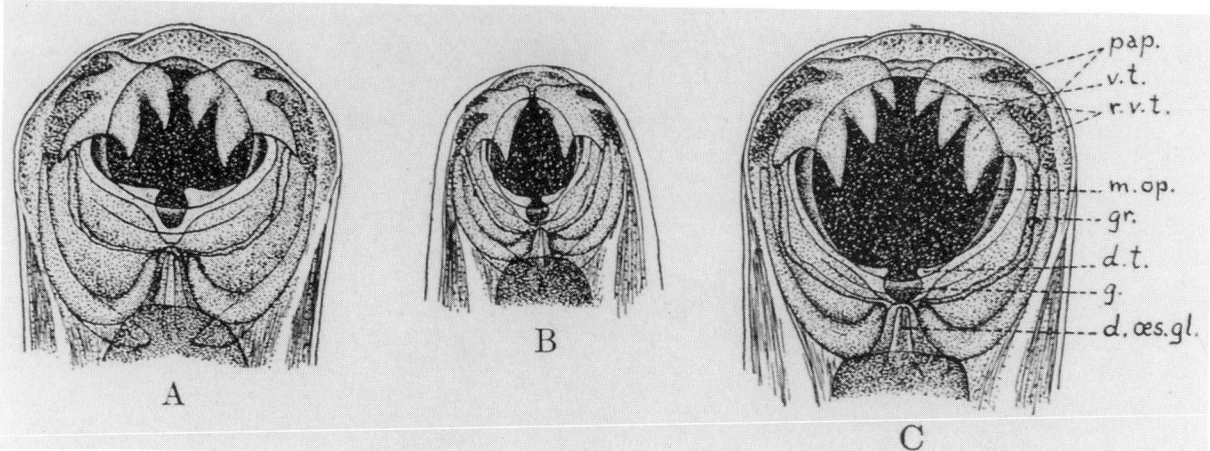

FIG. 5. Buccal capsules of three species of *Ancylostoma:* **(A)** *A. duodenale,* **(B)** *A. braziliense,* and **(C)** *A. caninum.* (From ref. 7, with permission.)

or oral iron supplementation (52). Delays in intellectual, cognitive, and psychomotor development also occur in association with chronic hookworm anemia (53), probably directly as a consequence of long-standing iron deficiency (1,52). Unlike "catch-up" growth, these mental delays may be permanent when they occur in infancy and early childhood.

Eosinophilic Enteritis

This syndrome has been described recently in a series of patients from northern Queensland, Australia, who harbor the adult dog hookworm, *A. caninum* (17). These patients presented with severe abdominal pain, weight loss,

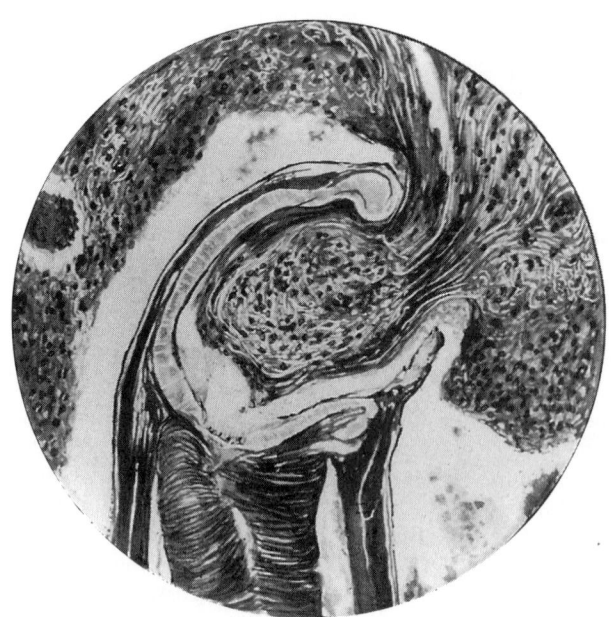

FIG. 6. Photomicrograph of *Necator americanus* attached to intestinal mucosa. (From ref. 27, with permission.)

and melena, in association with elevated serum immunoglobulin E (IgE) and eosinophilia. Eosinophilic enteritis from *A. caninum* has not been reported elsewhere.

DIAGNOSIS

Hookworm infection is diagnosed by identifying the characteristic eggs in the stools. Because only heavy hookworm infections are associated with anemia, it has been argued that there is no point to carrying out concentration techniques in order to identify individuals with very light infections. A number of quantitative egg counting techniques are available, which allow for indirect estimates of worm burden, including the Kato–Katz technique, Beaver's direct egg-count technique, Stoll's dilution egg-count technique, and the McMaster technique (9). All these techniques assume that the fecundity of the female hookworm population is constant, whereas in reality fecundity is strongly affected by worm crowding and host resistance (54,55). In addition, because of arrested development, there can be marked seasonal fluctuations in the egg counts for *A. duodenale* (12).

Because the eggs of *N. americanus* and *A. duodenale* have highly similar morphologies, it usually is necessary to differentiate the two species on the basis of differences between third-stage larvae (9). Currently, there is no reliable means of immunodiagnosis to differentiate these two species.

A specific diagnosis of eosinophilic enteritis has been made by recovering *A. caninum* at colonoscopy from the terminal ileum of a patient (17).

TREATMENT

A large number of anthelmintic agents are available, which can remove adult hookworms from the small intestine (56). The benzimidazole anthelmintics, mebendazole (100 mg bid for 3 consecutive days) or albendazole (400 mg as a single dose or sometimes administered for 3 con-

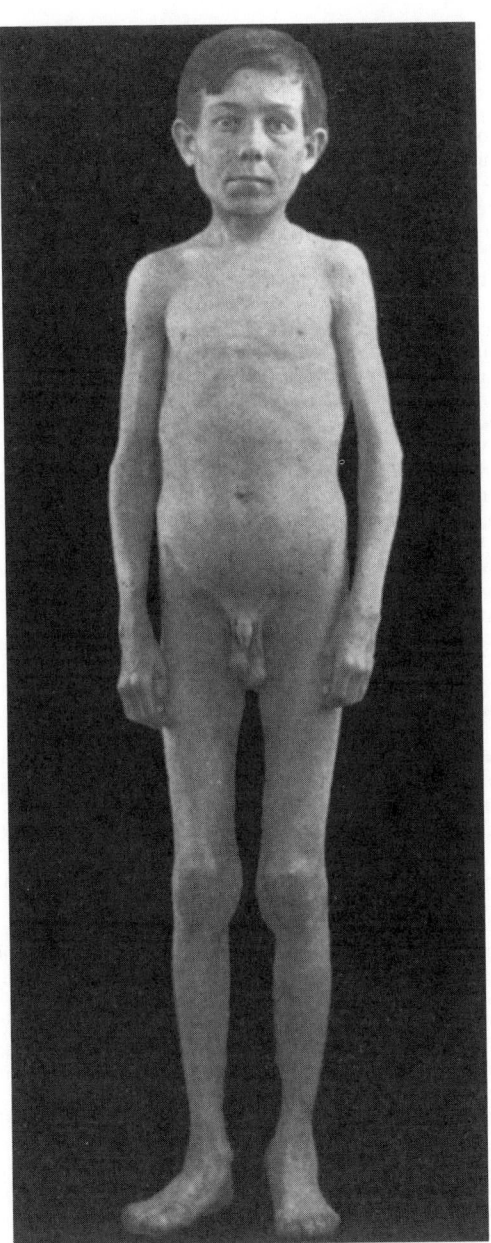

FIG. 7. Hookworm subject, 22 years old. Three hundred hookworms were expelled from this patient 2 years ago, but he is now reinfected. (From ref. 27, with permission.)

secutive days to ensure complete removal, are the major drugs of choice. The benzimidazoles have both theoretical and actual toxicities, including embryotoxicity and teratogenicity in laboratory animals, and are contraindicated in patients with blood dyscrasias, leukopenia, and liver disease. Because of the former, and the fact that the safety of benzimidazoles has not been established in infants, pyrantel pamoate in suspension (11 mg/kg/day, not to exceed 1 g) has been suggested as an alternative for young children. However, many thousands of children from Papua New Guinea were recently reported to have received mebendazole and albendazole with no side effects (57). Many anthelmintics are poorly absorbed and there is no

evidence that they eradicate populations of arrested *A. duodenale* larvae in the tissue.

In addition to specific anthelmintic therapy, dietary supplementation with iron in the form of ferrous sulfate can ameliorate many of the short-term and long-term effects of hookworm anemia (9,52).

PREVENTION

General improvements in quality of life and living standards and its associated improvements in sanitation and water supplies have been one of the most effective means of control human hookworm infection (9). This probably more than anything else accounted for the widespread eradication of hookworm infection in the United States, although pockets of infection still remain in socioeconomically depressed areas of the rural South. General improvements in living standards are not always possible, however, and in these cases combination programs consisting of sanitation with appropriate disposal of feces, health education, oral iron supplementation, and mass or targeted chemotherapy have been effective in the control of human hookworm infection. These efforts, however, can be expensive and require large investments of human energy. In many parts of the developing world this has proved to be extremely difficult. Better understanding of the biochemistry and molecular biology of human hookworm infection may ultimately provide the basis for rational vaccine development (58).

REFERENCES

1. Hotez PJ. Hookworm disease in children. *Pediatr Infect Dis J* 1989;8:516–520.
2. Peduzzi R, Piffaretti JC. *Ancylostoma duodenale* and the Saint Gothard anemia. *Lancet* 1983;287:1942–1945.
3. Looss A. On the penetration of *Ancylostoma* larvae into the human skin. *Centralblatt Bakteriol Parasitenkd* 1901;29: 733–739.
4. Stiles CW. A new species of hookworm (*Uncinaria americana*) parasitic in man. *Am Med* 1902;3:777–778.
5. Ettling J. *The germ of laziness, Rockefeller philanthropy and public health in the New South.* Cambridge, MA: Harvard University Press, 1981.
6. Anderson RC. *Nematode parasites of vertebrates, their development and transmission.* Wallingford, UK: CAB International, 1992.
7. Chandler AC. *Hookworm disease, its distribution, biology, epidemiology, pathology, diagnosis, treatment and control.* New York: Macmillan, 1929.
8. Kendrick JF. The length of life and rate of loss of hookworms, *Ancylostoma duodenale* and *Necator americanus. Am J Trop Med Hyg* 1934;14:363–379.
9. Pawlowski ZS, Schad GA, Stott GJ. *Hookworm infection and anemia, approaches to prevention and control.* Geneva: World Health Organization, 1991.
10. Soper FL. The report of a nearly pure *Ancylostoma duodenale* infestation in native South American Indians and a discussion of its ethnological significance. *Am J Hyg* 1927;7:174–184.
11. Hoagland KE, Schad GA. *Necator americanus* and *Ancylostoma duodenale:* life history parameters and epidemiological implications of two sympatric hookworms on humans. *Exp Parasitol* 1978;44:36–49.
12. Schad GA, Chowdhury AF, Dean CG, Kochar VK, Nawalinski TA, Thomas J, Tonascia JA. Arrested development in human

hookworm infections: an adaptation to a seasonally unfavorable external environment. *Science* 1973;180:502–504.

13. Schad GA. Hypobiosis and related phenomena in hookworm infection. In: Schad GA, Warren KS, eds. *Hookworm disease, current status and new directions.* London: Taylor and Francis, 1990.

14. Sen-hai Y, Wei-xia S. Hookworm infection and disease in China. In: Schad GA, Warren KS, eds. *Hookworm disease, current status and new directions.* London: Taylor and Francis, 1990.

15. Hotez PJ, Hawdon J, Schad GA. Hookworm larval infectivity, arrest and amphiparatenesis: the *Caenorhabditis elegans* Daf-c paradigm. *Parasitol Today* 1993;9:23–26.

16. Rep BH, Van Joost KS, Vetter JCM. Pathogenicity of *Ancylostoma ceylonicum. Trop Geogr Med* 1971;23:183–192.

17. Prociv P, Croese J. Human eosinophilic enteritis caused by dog hookworm *Ancylostoma caninum. Lancet* 1990;335:1299–1302.

18. Sulica VI, Berberian B, Kao GF. Histopathologic findings of cutaneous larva migrans. *J Cutan Pathol* 1988;15:346.

19. Schad GA, Anderson RM. Predisposition to hookworm infection. *Science* 1985;228:1537–1540.

20. Hotez PJ, Narasimhan S, Haggerty J, Bhopale V, Milstone L, Schad GA, Richards FF. Hyaluronidase from infective *Ancylostoma* hookworm larvae and its possible function as a virulence factor in tissue invasion and in cutaneous larva migrans. *Infect Immun* 1992;60:1018–1023.

21. Hotez PJ, Haggerty J, Hawdon J, Milstone L, Schad GA, Richards FF. Infective *Ancylostoma* hookworm larval metalloproteases and their functions in tissue invasion and ecdysis. *Infect Immun* 1990;58:3883–3892.

22. Kumar S, Pritchard DI. Secretion of metalloproteases by living infective larvae of *Necator americanus. J Parasitol* 1992;78: 917–919.

23. Salafsky B, Fusco AC, Siddiqui A. *Necator americanus:* factors influencing skin penetration by larvae. In: Schad GA, Warren KS, eds. *Hookworm disease, current status and new directions.* London: Taylor and Francis, 1990.

24. Yoshida Y, Nakanishi Y, Mitani W. Experimental studies on the infection modes of *Ancylostoma duodenale* and *Necator americanus* to the definitive host. *Jpn J Parasitol* 1958;7: 102–112.

25. Kalkofen UP. Attachment and feeding behavior of *Ancylostoma caninum. Z Parasitenkd* 1970;33:339–354.

26. Kalkofen UP. Intestinal trauma resulting from feeding activities of *Ancylostoma caninum. Am J Trop Med Hyg* 1974;23: 1046–1053.

27. Dock G, Bass CC. *Hookworm disease, etiology, pathology, diagnosis, prognosis, prophylaxis, and treatment.* St. Louis, MO: Mosby, 1910.

28. Hotez PJ, Trang NL, McKerrow JH, Cerami A. Isolation and characterization of a protease from the hookworm *Ancylostoma caninum. J Biol Chem* 1985;260:7343–7348.

29. Pritchard DI. *Necator americanus:* antigens and immunological targets. In: Schad GA, Warren KS, eds. *Hookworm disease, current status and new directions.* London: Taylor and Francis, 1990.

30. Pandey VC, Misra A, Agarwal A, Ghaatak S, Katiyar JC. Hydrolases of preparasitic and parasitic stages of *Ancylostoma ceylonicum* and *Nippostrongylus brasiliensis*—a comparative study. *Helminthologia* 1991;28:37–39.

31. Hotez PJ, Beckers C, Perregaux MA, Sakanari J. The hyaluronidase from the "sushi parasite" *Anisakis simplex* and the hookworm *Ancylostoma caninum:* biochemical properties reflect their enzymatic function in gastrointestinal invasion [IDSA abst.]. *Clin Infect Dis* 1993;17:544.

32. Carroll SM, Howse DJ, Grove DI. The anticoagulant effects of the hookworm, *Ancylostoma ceylonicum:* observations on human and dog blood in vitro and infected dogs in vivo. *Thromb Haemost* 1984;51:222–227.

33. Spellman GG, Nossel HL. Anticoagulant activity of dog hookworm. *Am J Physiol* 1971;220:922–927.

34. Hotez PJ, Cerami A. Secretion of a proteolytic anticoagulant by *Ancylostoma* hookworms. *J Exp Med* 1983;157:1594–1603.

35. Loeb L, Smith AJ. The presence of a substance inhibiting coagulation of blood in *Ancylostoma. Proc Pathol Soc Philos* 1904;7: 173–178.

36. Cappello M, Clyne L, MacPhedran P, Hotez PJ. *Ancylostoma* factor Xa inhibitor: partial isolation and identification as the predominant hookworm anticoagulant. *J Infect Dis* 1993;167: 1474–1477.

37. Cappello M, Vlasuk GP, Hawdon JM, Hotez PJ. The hookworm anticoagulant: a novel tissue factor pathway inhibitor [ASTMH/ ASP abst.] *Am J Trop Med Hyg* 1993;49:462.

38. Roche M, Layrisse M. Nature and causes of hookworm anemia. *Am J Trop Med Hyg* 1966;15:1029–1102.

39. Gilles HM. Selective primary health care: strategies for control of disease in the developing world. XVII. Hookworm infection and anemia. *Rev Infect Dis* 1985;7:111–118.

40. Scrimshaw NS. Iron deficiency. *Sci Am* 1991;265:46–52.

41. Miller TA. Hookworm infection in man. *Adv Parasitol* 1979;17: 315–384.

42. Castro GA, Behnke JM, Weisbrodt NW. Hookworm infection and malabsorption: a critical review. In: Schad GA, Warren KS, eds. *Hookworm disease, current status and new directions.* London: Taylor and Francis, 1990.

43. Schad GA, Soulsby EJL, Chowdhury AB, Gilles H. In: *Nuclear techniques in helminthological research.* Vienna: International Atomic Energy Agency, 1975;41–54.

44. Pritchard DI, Quinnell RJ, Slater AFG, McKean PG, Dale DDS, Raiko AE, Keymer AE. Epidemiology and immunology of *Necator americanus* infection in a community in Papua New Guinea: humoral responses to excretory–secretory and cuticular collagen antigens. *Parasitology* 1990;100:317–326.

45. Nawalinski TA, Schad GA. Arrested development in *Ancylostoma duodenale:* course of self-induced infection in man. *Am J Trop Med Hyg* 1974;23:895–898.

46. Maxwell C, Hussain R, Nutman TB, Little MD. Schad GA, Ottesen EA. Clinical and immunologic responses of normal volunteers to low dose hookworm *(Necator americanus)* infection. *Am J Trop Med Hyg* 1987;37:126–134.

47. Carroll SM, Grove DI. Experimental infections of humans with *Ancylostoma ceylonicum:* clinical, parasitological, haematological and immunological findings. *Trop Georg Med* 1986;38:38–45.

48. Crosby W H. What became of chlorosis? *JAMA* 1987;257: 2799–2800.

49. Smillie WG, Augustine DL. Hookworm infestation: the effect of varying intensities on the physical condition of school children. *Am J Dis Child* 1926;31:151–168.

50. Stephenson LS, Latham MC, Kurz KM, Kinoti SN, Brigham H. Treatment with a single dose of albendazole improves growth of Kenyan schoolchildren with hookworm, *Trichuris trichiura,* and *Ascaris lumbricoides* infections. *Am J Trop Med Hyg* 1989; 41:78–87.

51. Stephenson LS, Latham MC, Kinoti SN, Kurz KM, Brigham H. Improvements in physical fitness of Kenyan schoolboys infected with hookworm, *Trichuris trichiura,* and *Ascaris lumbricoides* following a single dose of albendazole. *Trans R Soc Trop Med Hyg* 1990;84:277–282.

52. Crompton DWT, Stephenson LS. Hookworm infection, nutritional status and productivity. In: Schad GA, Warren KS, eds. *Hookworm disease, current status and new directions.* London: Taylor and Francis, 1990.

53. Smillie WG, Spencer CR. Mental retardation in school children with hookworm. *J Educ Psychol* 1926;17:314–321.

54. Krupp IM. Effects of crowding and of superinfection on habitat selection and egg production in *Ancylostoma caninum. J Parasitol* 1961;47:957–961.

55. Miller TA. Vaccination against the canine hookworm disease. *Adv Parasitol* 1971;9:153–183.

56. Rossignol JF. Chemotherapy: present status. In: Schad GA, Warren KS, eds. *Hookworm disease, current status and new directions.* London: Taylor and Francis, 1990.

57. Biddulph J. Mebendazole and albendazole for infants. *Pediatr Infect Dis J* 1990;9:373.

58. Hotez PJ, Trang NL, Cerami A. Hookworm antigens: the potential for vaccination. *Parasitol Today* 1987;3:247–249.

Infections of the Gastrointestinal Tract,
edited by M. J. Blaser, P. D. Smith, J. I. Ravdin,
H. B. Greenberg, and R. L. Guerrant
Raven Press, Ltd., New York © 1995.

CHAPTER 79

Strongyloides stercoralis

Robert M. Genta

DESCRIPTION

Strongyloidiasis is an intestinal infection caused by the nematode *Strongyloides stercoralis*. In some parts of the world, notably Africa and New Guinea, human infections caused by *S. fuelleborni* have been reported (1–3). The growing importance of strongyloidiasis is related to the unique ability of this nematode to replicate within its host and behave as a potentially fatal opportunistic pathogen in immunocompromised patients, particularly in those receiving corticosteroids.

MICROBIOLOGY

Taxonomy

The family Strongyloidea (class Secernentasida, order Rhabditoidea) is formed by only one genus, *Strongyloides* Grassi, 1879. The members of this genus, also called threadworms, are heterogenetic, with free-living and parasitic generations, and comprise 38 named species. Most of these are parasites of mammals, but some can be found in birds, reptiles, and amphibians. The only species described in this chapter is *Strongyloides stercoralis* Bavay, 1876 (synonyms: *Anguillula stercoralis, S. intestinalis, S. canis, S. felis*). *Strongyloides fuelleborni* von Listow, 1905, is a parasite of primates that may also infect humans (1,2). Several other species are also important because they can cause disease in livestock (*S. ransomi, S. westeri, S. papillosus*) (4) or can be used as models of human strongyloidiasis (*S. ratti*) (5–9).

Morphology

The parasitic female, rarely identified in the stools of infected patients but present in tissue sections of the small

R. M. Genta: Departments of Pathology, Medicine, and Microbiology and Immunology, Baylor College of Medicine, and Center for Infectious Diseases, University of Texas School of Public Health, Houston, Texas 77030.

intestine, measures 1.5 to 10 mm in length and 27 to 95 μm in width. Its cuticle is finely striated and often wrinkled. In cross sections, muscular esophagus, intestine, ovaries, and eggs can be identified. Rhabditiform larvae are identified most commonly in the stools. They measure approximately 400 μm in length and 20 to 25 μm in diameter and are characterized by a bulbar esophagus and a thinner, longer intestine. In tissue sections, they are often present in the intestinal submucosa and small intestinal crypts and, rarely, in the lungs; they cannot specifically be identified based on their morphologic characteristics. Filariform (third stage) larvae are the stage most frequently identified in extraintestinal tissues and fluids (most often the sputum) in patients with disseminated infections. They are long and slender (400 to 700 μm in length and 12 to 20 μm in width) with a cylindrical esophagus that occupies one-half the body length. In transverse sections, the cuticle shows four characteristic lateral alae, which can be used for species identification (10).

Life Cycle and Pathophysiology

The life cycle of *S. stercoralis* begins when filariform larvae penetrate the intact skin of a susceptible host (Fig. 1). After entering a venous or lymphatic channel, the larvae are passively transported to the lungs (10–12). Here they break out of the capillaries into the alveoli, migrate up the trachea as they mature, and are eventually swallowed. Males have been identified in the stools of infected patients and dogs (10), but these findings have largely been ignored. In the duodenum and first part of the jejunum, parasitic adult females enter the lamina propria, where they deposit a small number of eggs per day. After the eggs hatch, rhabditiform larvae emerge and migrate into the intestinal lumen, eventually passing with the feces into the external environment. Here, depending on poorly understood conditions of temperature and humidity, the rhabditiform larvae either molt directly into infective filariform larvae, which are capable of repenetrating the skin of a suitable host (direct cycle), or pass through four ecdyses (molts) to become adult male and female worms,

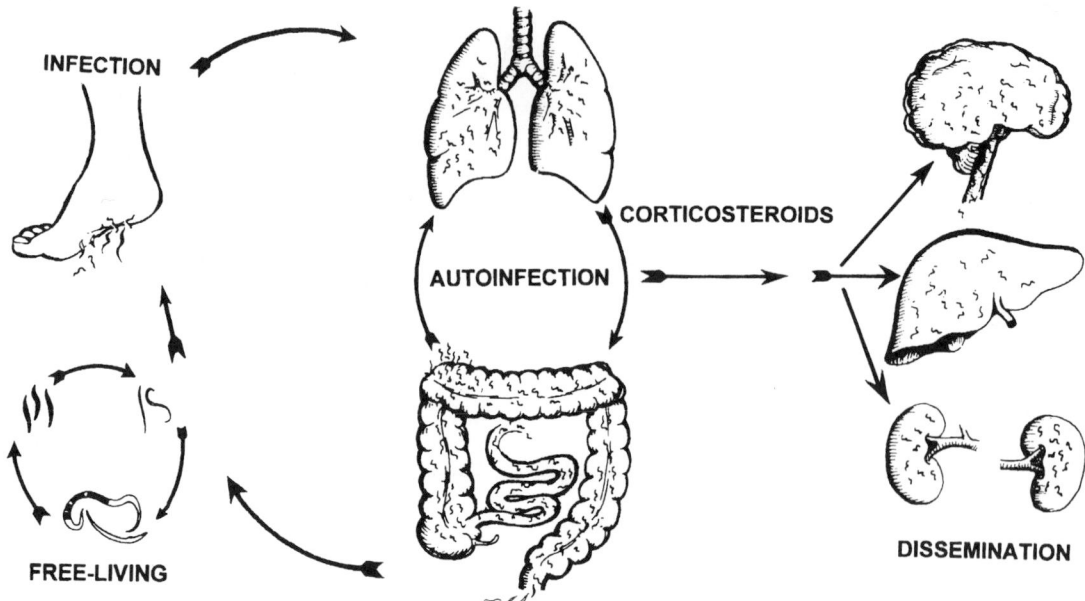

FIG. 1. The life cycle of *Strongyloides stercoralis.* The administration of corticosteroids disrupts the usually well-regulated autoinfection, resulting in the dissemination of larvae throughout the body. Steroids may act by depressing certain host immune responses or by directly stimulating parasite ecdysis.

which mate and produce offspring that develop into filariform larvae and reenter parasitic life (indirect or heterogonical cycle).

A small portion of the rhabditiform larvae that hatch from the eggs deposited in the intestine are believed to molt within the intestine into the filariform stage. These larvae penetrate the colonic wall or the perianal skin, complete the internal cycle, and establish themselves as mature adult females in the small intestine. This process, known as autoinfection, is believed to represent the mechanism by which *S. stercoralis* can persist virtually indefinitely in infected hosts (12,13).

EPIDEMIOLOGY

Although information regarding the worldwide prevalence of strongyloidiasis is fragmentary, 3 to 100 million are estimated to be infected worldwide (1,14). The unreliability of these estimates is reflected in the wide range of prevalence rates, varying between less than 1% and 85%, of populations living in adjacent regions of the same country (15–17). With these limitations in mind, one can assume that *S. stercoralis* is present in virtually all tropical and subtropical regions of the world. Pockets of low endemicity (less than 1% to 3%) exist in several industrialized countries of western Europe (e.g., Italy, France, and Switzerland) (15–24), eastern Europe (e.g., Poland and many parts of the former Soviet Union) (25–27), the United States (the Appalachian region and the Southern states) (28,29), Japan (Okinawa) (30), and Australia (aboriginal populations) (31,32). Significant prevalence rates of strongyloidiasis have been found in institutionalized

patients, even in Pennsylvania and British Columbia, where the parasite is not known to be endemic in the general population (33–35). Considering the long persistence of this parasite in its host and its relatively high prevalence among some populations, physicians practicing in industrialized countries should consider strongyloidiasis in immigrant or refugee patients born in tropical or subtropical regions as well as in persons from local areas of endemicity.

Strongyloidiasis and the Acquired Immunodeficiency Syndrome

Since cell-mediated immunity is thought to regulate *S. stercoralis* autoinfection, patients with the acquired immunodeficiency syndrome (AIDS) initially were expected to have more frequent and severe *S. stercoralis* infections. However, in areas of the world where both *S. stercoralis* and AIDS are endemic, there does not appear to be a higher incidence of chronic strongyloidiasis in patients with AIDS (36). This has led several authors to speculate that strongyloidiasis is regulated by other factors and that it may remain one of the "missing" infections in AIDS (1,37–39). During the past few years, a very limited number of patients, almost exclusively from Western countries, with AIDS and extraintestinal strongyloidiasis have been reported (40–44). Although most of these patients had conditions that required corticosteroid treatment, in several the development of *S. stercoralis* hyperinfection was apparently spontaneous. Thus, although it is unlikely that strongyloidiasis will become an important opportunistic infection associated with AIDS, *S. stercoralis* should be searched for in human immunodeficiency virus (HIV)-infected patients with an appropriate geographic history and suspected of having the infection.

PATHOGENESIS AND IMMUNITY

According to the life cycle outlined earlier, chronic infections are sustained by a relatively low and stable number of adult worms, which reside in harmony within their host's intestine and survive by means of well-regulated autoinfection (11). The rate of autoinfection is believed to be regulated by the host's cell-mediated immunity (12,45,46). When this regulatory function becomes impaired during immunosuppression, increasing numbers of autoinfective larvae complete the cycle, and the population of parasitic adult worms increases (hyperinfection). Eventually, the extraordinary numbers of migrating larvae deviate from the presumed route (intestine → venous bed → lungs → trachea → intestine) and disseminate to other organs, including meningeal spaces and brain, liver, kidneys, lymph nodes, and cutaneous and subcutaneous tissues. In these organs the larvae cause hemorrhage by breaking capillaries, elicit inflammatory responses, and implant gram-negative bacteria carried from fecal material. The resulting syndrome, known as disseminated strongyloidiasis, is nearly always fatal (45,46).

The validity of the above model has been questioned by Schad et al. (47,48), who used an experimental canine model of disseminated strongyloidiasis to show that only a few larvae could be recovered from the lungs of dogs with massive hyperinfection. Later, in a series of experiments based on the compartmental analysis of radio labeled larvae and mathematical modeling, they presented convincing evidence that the tracheobronchial route in the dog was not used by the majority of the migrating larvae (49). According to their model, larvae that began their migration in the skin (primary infection) or in the distal ileum (autoinfection) were not more likely to pass through the lungs than through any other organ, suggesting that the migratory pathway involved random dissemination throughout the body. However, this conclusion has not been fully accepted, because large numbers of larvae are frequently identified in bronchoalveolar lavage fluid from hyperinfected patients (50,51).

Determining the migratory pathway involved in autoinfection is important for understanding the biology of S. stercoralis and the host mechanisms that regulate internal infection. Recently, the accepted paradigm that host mechanisms regulate hyperinfection and dissemination has been challenged (11). The theory that host immunity controls infection fails to consider the role that parasites may play in this regulation. In this regard, the adverse impact of increased parasite density on egg production and growth ("crowding effect") has been demonstrated for several intestinal nematodes. Although distinguishing between host resistance and direct parasite-to-parasite effects may be difficult, it seems clear that in a normal host–parasite relationship, the parasite may reach a particular population size or a critical biomass, after which

yet unknown regulatory mechanisms intervene to limit the population (52).

We have proposed that during the parallel evolution of humans and their parasites, S. stercoralis developed the ability to reach an optimal population size in the duodenum of a human. If the initial infective dose of larvae is low, a higher rate of intraluminal molting occurs until the "optimal" size of the adult population is reached. In this model, it is assumed that S. stercoralis, similar to other nematodes, transmit their molting signal by molting hormones (ecdysteroids) (53,54). As the size of the parasite population reaches a certain level, adult females decrease their production of ecdysteroids, resulting in a lowered molting rate sufficient to replace the dying adults. During the initial phase of infection, the host mounts humoral and cellular immune responses directed at all tissue stages of the parasite. These well-characterized responses (16,20,55–65) do not eradicate all the parasites, but limit the size of the parasite population. Impaired immune responses may allow the growth of larger numbers of parasites, as reported in agammaglobulinemic patients (66,67), but total dysregulation of the parasite population does not occur since worms, in part, regulate their own growth. Conversely, the presence of intact immune responses is not sufficient to prevent dissemination should the parasites' own regulatory mechanisms fail (68).

The level of ecdysteroid-like substances are generally negligible in healthy subjects (53,54). The administration of corticosteroids may result in increased amounts of ecdysteroid-like substances in the host's tissues, including in the intestinal wall, where adult females reside. These substances may act as molting signals for the eggs or rhabditiform larvae, which transform intraluminally into excessive numbers of filariform larvae. Available data are not sufficient to prove a dose-dependent effect, but it is remarkable that patients who develop fulminating hyperinfection after only a few days of steroid administration are usually those who have received intravenous methylprednisone (69–73). Once the worm population has become large (100,000 adult worms), it may continue to expand rapidly, even at low molting rates, and the discontinuation of steroids may not be sufficient to arrest the relentless growth process that leads to the host's death.

Pathology

The pathologic lesions associated with chronic, uncomplicated S. stercoralis have received little attention, because only rarely have patients with such lesions come to autopsy. However, pathologic descriptions of the lesions in a few patients in whom strongyloidiasis was an incidental finding indicate that the worms can exist in the intestinal mucosa without causing significant inflammatory responses or tissue damage. The classic description of the pathology of strongyloidiasis was made by De Paola et al. (74) in 1962 and later updated by Genta and Caymmi-Gomes (75). These authors proposed the subdivision of the intestinal lesions into three distinct forms.

In "catarrhal enteritis" (presumably associated with

light infections), the small intestine is congested, the mucosa is covered with abundant mucoid secretions, and scattered petechial hemorrhages are present. The most remarkable histologic feature is an increased mononuclear infiltrate in the submucosa, although parasites are rare. In the more advanced form, "edematous enteritis," the intestinal wall is grossly thickened, the mucosal folds are flattened, and the affected intestinal segments assume a rubbery consistency. Submucosal edema, flattening of the villi, and parasites scattered throughout the lamina propria are observed microscopically. The most severe form, "ulcerative enteritis," occurs almost exclusively with hyperinfection. The intestinal walls may be rigid due to the edema and fibrosis resulting from long-standing inflammation and the mucosa may show atrophy, erosions, and ulcerations. An abundant inflammatory infiltrate, most often consisting of neutrophils, and all stages of *S. stercoralis* are present throughout the intestinal mucosa. Jejunal perforation has been reported in patients with the ulcerative enteritis form of strongyloidiasis (76). Uncommonly, the mucosal damage occurs predominantly in the large intestine, simulating ulcerative colitis and pseudopolyposis (77,78). *Strongyloides stercoralis* larvae have

been found in the appendix, and eosinophilic appendicitis apparently caused by this parasite has been reported (79–81). In patients with disseminated strongyloidiasis, the intestinal lesions reflect the large number of worms dwelling within the small intestinal mucosa and penetrating the intestinal walls (Fig. 2). In addition, the stomach (82) and the peritoneal cavity (13,83) may be invaded by migrating parasites. However, because most of these patients are receiving immunosuppressive doses of corticosteroids, inflammatory responses are often minimal in spite of extensive tissue damage. The gastrointestinal pathology is often overshadowed by the presence of lesions in other organs, particularly in patients who receive anthelmintic therapy before developing disseminated strongyloidiasis.

Migrating parasites may cause mechanical damage as well as inflammation. In human patients, the extraintestinal organ most commonly affected by this migratory damage is the lung. In severe disseminated infection, when hundreds of thousands of adult parasites dwell in the intestine and millions of larvae migrate throughout the body, alveolar microhemorrhages may result in massive pulmonary bleeding. As larvae penetrate the large intes-

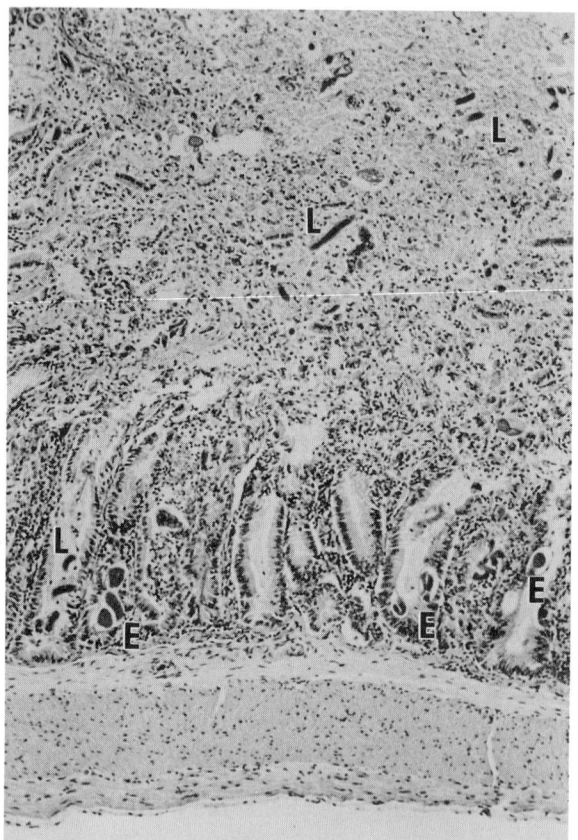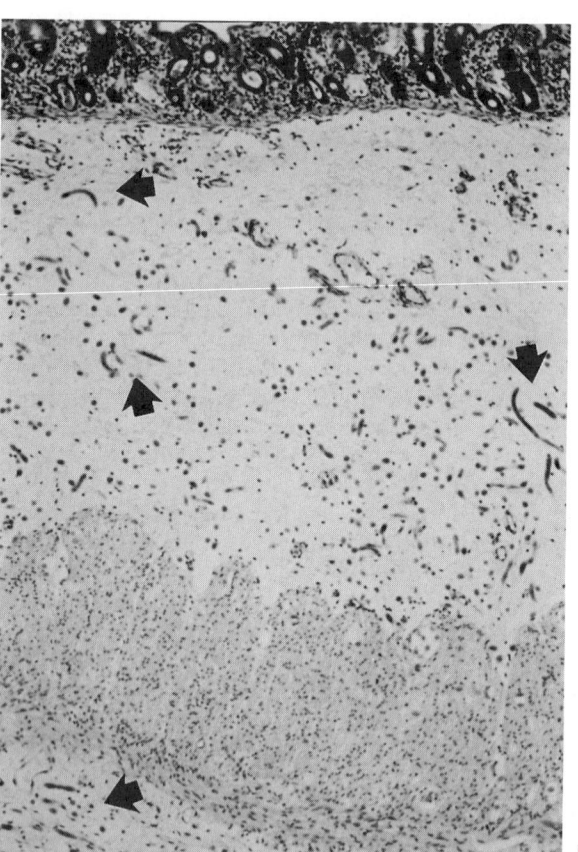

FIG. 2. Sections from the intestine of a host who died of disseminated strongyloidiasis following high-dose corticosteroid therapy. The architecture of the jejunal mucosa (**left**) is completely effaced and large numbers of larvae (L) and eggs (E) of *Strongyloides stercoralis* are visible on the surface and within the mucosa. The colonic wall (**right**) shows preservation of the mucosa and a high degree of submucosal edema. Innumerable migrating filariform larvae (*arrows*) are present within the edematous spaces.

tine, they create small breaks in the mucosa that facilitate the invasion of the bloodstream by enteric bacteria. The larvae themselves carry bacteria on their cuticle to distant sites. Regardless of the mechanism, the widespread dissemination of larvae is frequently associated with polymicrobial sepsis, diffuse or patchy bronchopneumonia, pulmonary and cerebral abscesses, and meningitis. Filariform larvae, and occasionally rhabditiform larvae and adult worms, also may disseminate to mesenteric lymph nodes, the biliary tract, as well as the liver, pancreas, spleen, heart, endocrine glands, and ovaries (75). In these locations the parasite frequently induces a granulomatous response (84).

CLINICAL ILLNESS

No other nematode has been associated with as broad a spectrum of manifestations or implicated as the cause of so many different clinical syndromes as *S. stercoralis*. Although some of these manifestations are dramatic, the majority of persons with chronic infection are either asymptomatic or have mild, nonspecific symptoms.

Gastrointestinal Manifestations

The gastrointestinal manifestations of chronic strongyloidiasis are usually nonspecific (16,85). Epigastric abdominal pain, postprandial fullness or bloating, and heartburn are among the symptoms most commonly reported (86,87). Brief episodes of diarrhea alternating with constipation may also occur. The diarrhea usually consists of semiformed, nonbloody stools (17). Occult bloody stools occasionally occur in persons with chronic infections (77), and even massive colonic hemorrhage has been reported (88). A severe, cholera-like diarrhea with electrolyte imbalance and cardiac arrest has been reported, but this is exceedingly uncommon (89,90).

Physical examination of chronically infected patients is normal or reveals only mild abdominal tenderness on palpation. Less commonly, chronic strongyloidiasis resembles inflammatory bowel disease, particularly ulcerative colitis, and the endoscopic appearance may be that of pseudopolyposis (77). Rarely, patients have undergone surgery for "chronic colitis," the correct diagnosis being established by pathological examination of the resected colon (78). Malabsorption frequently occurs in patients with strongyloidiasis (91–93). The majority of these patients, however, are from areas of the world where tropical sprue and sprue-like conditions are widespread, making a clear relationship of cause and effect between *S. stercoralis* infection and malabsorption difficult to determine. Garcia et al. (94) have convincingly argued that malnutrition was the cause rather than the effect of severe strongyloidiasis in a group of Colombian patients. Experimental work in rodents seems to support this conclusion (95).

In contrast to the asymptomatic nature of chronic strongyloidiasis, the gastrointestinal manifestations of disseminated strongyloidiasis are dramatic and often cata-

strophic. Hyperinfection is often heralded by profuse diarrhea, which may be watery, mucoid, and bloody. The diarrhea is a consequence of the erosions, ulcerations, and edema caused by millions of adult worms and filariform larvae in the mucosa of the small and large intestine (45,46,53). These mucosal changes predispose the patient to bacterial enterocolitis (96) and, after variable periods of diarrhea, paralytic ileus (73,97). Polymicrobial (predominantly gram-negative) sepsis may occur, probably due to the large number of larvae migrating from the large intestine into the circulation, leading to local infection and abscess in virtually any organ (45,46). Larvae have been identified in other gastrointestinal organs, including the liver, stomach, and pancreas of patients with overwhelming infections (53), but the presence of parasites in these locations does not cause characteristic symptoms.

Pulmonary Manifestations

Although patients with chronic obstructive pulmonary disease may have an increased risk of strongyloidiasis (98), no respiratory signs or symptoms are associated with acute or chronic strongyloidiasis. In these infections the number of larvae passing through the lungs is probably negligible. Chronic obstructive pulmonary disease has been associated with strongyloidiasis in some series of American patients (85,98,99). Although peculiar microcalcifications have been observed in the lungs of chronically infected dogs (100), a direct effect of parasites on the pulmonary parenchyma has not been documented in humans and appears unlikely. Occasionally, patients who presented with asthma have later developed disseminated strongyloidiasis (101–108), but these patients are often on low-dose steroid therapy, which predisposes to strongyloidiasis (85).

Among patients with disseminated strongyloidiasis, pulmonary manifestations are common, particularly diffuse bronchopneumonia (45,109–111). Pulmonary abscesses have also been reported (112). Intra-alveolar hemorrhage, often sufficiently severe to cause death, is a frequent event during the course of disseminated strongyloidiasis. In some cases, fatal pulmonary hemorrhages occur a few days after the apparently successful treatment of the parasite, suggesting an immunologically mediated mechanism of vascular damage (113,114).

Neurologic Manifestations

Gram-negative polymicrobial meningitis is the most frequent central nervous system manifestation of disseminated strongyloidiasis (115–121). In some cases, larvae have been identified in the cerebrospinal fluid. Rarely, larvae have been found in the central nervous system in the absence of bacteria in patients with signs of meningeal involvement, suggesting a parasitic (aseptic) meningitis (122–124). A less common form of central nervous system involvement is the formation of cerebral and cerebellar abscesses containing *S. stercoralis* larvae (125).

Other Systemic Manifestations

Arthritis is a rare manifestation of strongyloidiasis and is associated with the local deposition of immune complexes containing S. stercoralis antigens (126–129). Even more rare are cardiac arrhythmias and arrest, which have been attributed to direct myocardial damage from migrating larvae (130) or electrolyte imbalance due to severe intestinal strongyloidiasis (89,90). Depression and neurosis have been associated with chronic strongyloidiasis (131), but they likely represent reaction to the long duration of symptoms. The passage of larvae in the sperm and the presence of genital lesions in association with strongyloidiasis have also been described (132).

Cutaneous Manifestations

Three types of cutaneous manifestations have been described in patients with chronic strongyloidiasis. Urticarial rashes, possibly caused by a sensitization to parasite antigens, occur sporadically in patients from all parts of the world (29,56,133–135). In contrast, a characteristic dermatitis caused by the subcutaneous migration of filariform larvae (larva currens) has been reported almost exclusively in Caucasian patients who acquired the infection in Southeast Asia (89,135–141). In many of these patients, larva currens was the only sign of strongyloidiasis, and therapy with thiabendazole cured the dermatitis (141–144). Finally, generalized cutaneous purpura has been described in several patients with leukopenia, thrombocytopenia, and disseminated infection (135,145–147); the purpuric lesions appear to be due to the migration of filariform larvae in the dermis (135,147).

DIAGNOSIS

Radiographic features of S. stercoralis infection of the gastrointestinal tract are nonspecific. However, certain radiologic patterns may suggest strongyloidiasis in patients at risk for the infection (148–152). When malabsorption is present, the radiographic findings are similar to those of tropical sprue and include increased diameter of the small intestinal lumen, generalized hypotonia, and edema. Edema and fibrosis may be associated with severe, long-standing infections. In hyperinfection and dissemination, complete disruption of the mucosal patterns, ulcerations, and paralytic ileus have been observed. In the presence of dissemination, pulmonary involvement may be heralded by bilateral edema and patchy, often rapidly changing, infiltrates (146,153–155).

The stage of S. stercoralis most commonly identified in feces is the rhabditiform larva, but filariform larvae, adult females, and even eggs also may be present. The sensitivity of a single stool examination for the detection of S. stercoralis ranges between 30% and 60% (87,156,157). The method of Baermann allows a larger volume of feces (up to several grams) to be examined and is more sensitive than direct microscopy (158). Culturing

feces mixed with charcoal or peat moss also increases the sensitivity of fecal examination. However, these procedures are not suited for routine diagnosis. A detection method recently proposed by Koga involves the use of agar plates and appears to be very sensitive and easy to perform (159). Although the examination of a duodenal aspirate is reportedly very sensitive, this usually requires an invasive technique and is recommended only in the pediatric patient requiring a rapid diagnosis, such as an immunocompromised child with suspected overwhelming infection. The "string test," a gelatine capsule containing a string swallowed by the patient and retrieved after a few hours, enjoyed a brief moment of popularity a few years ago, but currently it is used infrequently (160). In disseminated infections larvae of all stages and adult parasites have been found in specimens of sputum and bronchoalveolar lavage, ascitic fluid, pancreatic aspirates, and cerebrospinal fluid (118,161–164). In summary, stool examination is currently the primary technique for the detection of S. stercoralis. If special techniques are not available, several specimens collected on different days should be examined when the diagnosis is strongly suspected.

The only hematologic abnormality associated with chronic, uncomplicated strongyloidiasis is eosinophilia. Although eosinophils may rarely exceed 30% of the total white blood cells, most patients have 6% to 15% eosinophils (between 500 and 1500 cells/mm^3) (16,165–168). Since considerable day-to-day variation in the degree of eosinophilia occurs, infected subjects may have normal eosinophil counts when studied at a single point in time. Patients with disseminated strongyloidiasis usually have normal eosinophil counts, most frequently due to concurrent immunosuppressive therapy.

Total serum immunoglobulin E (IgE) levels are elevated (over 200 IU/mL) in 50% to 70% of the patients with strongyloidiasis (16,20,62,68,169,170). The other classes of immunoglobulins are not affected by the presence of S. stercoralis, except in infected children with malnutrition and protein-losing enteropathy in whom levels may be reduced (171).

Several immunoassays for the detection of serum antibodies against filariform larvae or larval antigens are now available. The most commonly used tests include an indirect immunofluorescence test (65,172), which detects serum IgG antibodies to surface antigens on fresh or formalin-fixed filariform larvae, and an enzyme-linked immunoadsorbent assay (ELISA) (173–175) which also detects parasite-specific IgG antibodies. The former has a sensitivity of less than 85% and a specificity approaching 100%, while the latter has a sensitivity of approximately 90% and a similar specificity. Serum from patients with Filaria species and Ascaris lumbricoides infections rarely may be falsely positive for S. stercoralis. Assays for the detection of parasite-specific antibodies of the IgG4 subclass (58) and assays utilizing purified antigens are being developed (176–179). Although immunoserology appears to be a promising tool for the diagnosis of strongyloidiasis, its widespread use has been limited by the insufficient availability of suitable antigens.

TREATMENT

The drug of choice for strongyloidiasis is thiabendazole. The recommended dose is 25 mg/kg/day for 2 days (180,181), which appears to be effective in 80% to 90% of patients with chronic, uncomplicated infections. Multiple courses of therapy may be necessary to eradicate the parasite in certain cases. Immunocompromised patients may require higher doses of thiabendazole (up to 50 mg/kg/day) for longer periods (46,69). For patients unable to take oral medications, thiabendazole has been administered per rectum (182). Thiabendazole side effects include nausea, vomiting, foul-smelling urine, and dizziness in a high percentage of patients (180). In countries where thiabendazole is not available and in patients in whom thiabendazole therapy was unsuccessful, eradication of the parasites has been achieved with albendazole and mebendazole (183–186). However, because the efficacy of these two agents is not always satisfactory and the regimens are not well standardized, the use of albendazole and mebendazole should only be considered in selected cases. Ivermectin, recently introduced for the treatment of onchocerciasis, has been used to successfully treat strongyloidiasis in several trials conducted in Latin America, Asia, and Africa (187–190). In the United States, ivermectin is not approved for the treatment of uncomplicated S. stercoralis. Compassionate use has occasionally been approved in patients with life-threatening disseminated infection, but the data are presently insufficient to determine whether it is more effective than thiabendazole.

PREVENTION

The transmission of S. stercoralis can be prevented by implementing public health measures aimed at ensuring proper waste disposal and preventing skin contact with contaminated soil. In patients from endemic areas who may harbor asymptomatic chronic strongyloidiasis, life-threatening disseminated hyperinfection may be prevented by seeking and eradicating the parasite before corticosteroid, immunosuppressive, or antineoplastic therapy is started.

ACKNOWLEDGMENT

This work was supported by the Office of Medical Research of the Department of Veterans Affairs, Washington, DC.

REFERENCES

1. Genta RM. Global prevalence of strongyloidiasis: critical review with epidemiologic insights into the prevention of disseminated disease. *Rev Infect Dis* 1989;11:755–767.
2. Barnish G, Ashford RW. *Strongyloides fuelleborni* in Papua New Guinea: epidemiology in an isolated community, and results of an intervention study. *Ann Trop Med Parasitol* 1989;83:499–506.
3. Hira PR, Patel BG. Human strongyloidiasis due to the primate species *Strongyloides fuelleborni*. *Trop Geogr Med* 1980;32:23–29.
4. Little MD. Comparative morphology of six species of *Strongyloides* (Nematoda) and redefinition of the genus. *J Parasitol* 1966;48:41–47.
5. Abe T, Nawa Y, Yoshimura K. Protease resistant interleukin-3 stimulating components in excretory and secretory products from adult worms of *Strongyloides ratti*. *J Helminthol* 1992;66:155–158.
6. Grove DI, Northern C. Dissociation of the protective immune response in the mouse to *Strongyloides ratti*. *J Helminthol* 1989;63:307–314.
7. Genta RM, Ottesen EA, Gam AA, Neva FA. Immunologic responses to experimental strongyloidiasis in rats. *Z Parasitenkd* 1983;69:667–675.
8. Grove DI, Dawkins HJ. Effects of prednisolone on murine strongyloidiasis. *Parasitology* 1981;83:401–409.
9. Genta RM, Ward PA. The histopathology of experimental strongyloidiasis. *Am J Pathol* 1980;99:207–220.
10. Schad GA. Morphology and life history of *Strongyloides stercoralis*. In: Grove DI, ed. *Strongyloidiasis: a major roundworm infection of man*. London: Taylor and Francis, 1989;85–104.
11. Genta RM. Dysregulation of strongyloidiasis: a new hypothesis. *Clin Microbiol Rev* 1992;5:345–355.
12. Neva FA. Biology and immunology of human strongyloidiasis. *J Infect Dis* 1986;153:397–406.
13. Lintermans JP. Fatal peritonitis, an unusual complication of *Strongyloides stercoralis* infestation. *Clin Pediatr (Phila)* 1975;14:974–975.
14. Pawlowski ZS. Epidemiology, prevention and control. In: Grove DI, ed. *Strongyloidiasis: a major roundworm infection of man*. London: Taylor and Francis 1989;233–249.
15. Subbannayya K, Babu MH, Kumar A, Rao TS, Shivananda PG. *Entamoeba histolytica* and other parasitic infections in south Kanara district, Karnataka. *J Commun Dis* 1989;21:207–213.
16. de Messias IT, Telles FQ, Boaretti AC, Sliva S, Guimarres LM, Genta RM. Clinical, immunological and epidemiological aspects of strongyloidiasis in an endemic area of Brazil. *Allergol Immunopathol (Madr)* 1987;15:37–41.
17. Carvalho Filho E. Strongyloidiasis. *Clin Gastroenterol* 1978;7:179–200.
18. Poirriez J, Becquet R, Dutoit E, Crepin M, Cousin J. Autochthonous strongyloidiasis in the north of France. *Bull Soc Pathol Exot Filiales* 1992;85:292–295.
19. Doury P. Autochthonous anguilluliasis in France. *Bull Soc Pathol Exot Filiales* 1993;86:116.
20. Genta RM, Gatti S, Linke MJ, Cevini C, Scaglia M. Endemic strongyloidiasis in northern Italy: clinical and immunological aspects. *Q J Med* 1988;68:679–690.
21. Cadi Soussi M, Kerkeb O, Mellouki W. Autochthonous anguilluliasis. Apropos of 3 cases. *Maroc Med* 1986;8:476–480.
22. Eyckmans L, Van Landuyt H, Vermylen J, Vandepitte J, Bollens W. Autochthonous strongyloidiasis in Belgium. *Ann Soc Belg Med Trop* 1967;47:265–270.
23. Castelli D, Vercellino E. On strongyloidiasis endemy in Piedmont. *G Mal Infett Parassit* 1967;19:453–455.
24. Berthoud F, Berthoud S. 18 Cases of anguilluliasis diagnosed at Geneva. *Schweiz Med Wochenschr* 1975;105:1110–1115.
25. Shimanskaia GA. Strongyloidiasis in the population of Vladimir-Volynsk district of the Volynsk region. *Med Parazitol (Mosk)* 1973;42:612.
26. Borisenko VS. Strongyloidiasis in psychoneurological boarding houses of Dniepropetrovsk region. *Vrach Delo* 1974;140–143.
27. Prokhorov AF, Isupov Iul, Golovan' TV, Strikhanova EV, Fuki AD. Epidemiology of strongyloidiasis in the northern Caucasus. *Med Parazitol (Mosk)* 1983;52:34–38.
28. Genta RM, Weesner R, Douce RW, Huitger-O'Connor T, Walzer PD. Strongyloidiasis in US veterans of the Vietnam and other wars. *JAMA* 1987;258:49–52.
29. Walzer PD, Milder JE, Banwell JG, Kilgore G, Klein M, Parker R. Epidemiologic features of *Strongyloides stercoralis* infection in an endemic area of the United States. *Am J Trop Med Hyg* 1982;31:313–319.

30. Arakaki T, Kohakura M, Asato R, Ikeshiro T, Nakamura S, Iwanaga M. Epidemiological aspects of *Strongyloides stercoralis* infection in Okinawa, Japan. *J Trop Med Hyg* 1992;95: 210–213.

31. Fisher D, McCarry F, Currie B. Strongyloidiasis in the Northern Territory. Under-recognised and under-treated? *Med J Aust* 1993;159:88–90.

32. Prociv P, Luke R. Observations on strongyloidiasis in Queensland aboriginal communities. *Med J Aust* 1993;158: 160–163.

33. Braun TI, Fekete T, Lynch A. Strongyloidiasis in an institution for mentally retarded adults. *Arch Intern Med* 1988;148: 634–636.

34. Proctor EM, Muth HA, Proudfoot DL, Allen AB, Fisk R, Isaac-Renton J, Black WA. Endemic institutional strongyloidiasis in British Columbia. *Can Med Assoc J* 1987;136: 1173–1176.

35. Sargent RG. Parasitic infection among residents of an institution for mentally retarded persons. *Am J Ment Defic* 1983;87: 566–569.

36. Dias RM, Mangini AC, Torres DM, et al. Ocorrencia de *Strongyloides stercoralis* em pacientes portadores da sindrome de imunodeficiencia adquirida (AIDS). *Rev Inst Med Trop Sao Paulo* 1992;34:15–17.

37. Hunter G, Bagshawe AF, Baboo KS, Luke R, Prociv P. Intestinal parasites in Zambian patients with AIDS. *Trans R Soc Trop Med Hyg* 1992;86:543–545.

38. Lucas SB. Missing infections in AIDS. *Trans R Soc Trop Med Hyg* 1990;84(Suppl1):34–38.

39. Petithory JC, Derouin F. AIDS and strongyloidiasis in Africa [Letter]. *Lancet* 1987;1:921.

40. Kramer MR, Gregg PA, Goldstein M, Llamas R, Krieger BP. Disseminated strongyloidiasis in AIDS and non-AIDS immunocompromised hosts: diagnosis by sputum and bronchoalveolar lavage. *South Med J* 1990;83:1226–1229.

41. Maayan S, Wormser GP, Widerhorn J, Sy ER, Kim YH, Ernst JA. *Strongyloides stercoralis* hyperinfection in a patient with the acquired immune deficiency syndrome. *Am J Med* 1987; 83:945–948.

42. Makris AN, Sher S, Bertoli C, Latour MG. Pulmonary strongyloidiasis: an unusual opportunistic pneumonia in a patient with AIDS. *AJR Am J Roentgenol* 1993;161:545–547.

43. Schainberg L, Scheinberg MA. Recovery of *Strongyloides stercoralis* by bronchoalveolar lavage in a patient with acquired immunodeficiency syndrome. *Am J Med* 1989;87:486.

44. Vieyra Herrera G, Becerril Carmona G, Padua Gabriel A, Jessurun J, Alonso de Ruiz P. *Strongyloides stercoralis* hyperinfection in a patient with the acquired immune deficiency syndrome. *Acta Cytol* 1988;32:277–278.

45. Igra-Siegman Y, Kapila R, Sen P, Kaminski ZC, Louria DB. Syndrome of hyperinfection with *Strongyloides stercoralis*. *Rev Infect Dis* 1981;3:397–407.

46. Scowden EB, Schaffner W, Stone WJ. Overwhelming strongyloidiasis: an unappreciated opportunistic infection. *Medicine (Baltimore)* 1978;57:527–544.

47. Schad GA, Hellman ME, Muncey DW. *Strongyloides stercoralis:* hyperinfection in immunosuppressed dogs. *Exp Parasitol* 1984;57:287–296.

48. Genta RM, Schad GA, Hellman ME. *Strongyloides stercoralis:* parasitological, immunological and pathological observations in immunosuppressed dogs. *Trans R Soc Trop Med Hyg* 1986; 80:34–41.

49. Schad GA, Aikens LM, Smith G. *Strongyloides stercoralis:* is there a canonical migratory route through the host? *J Parasitol* 1989;75:740–749.

50. Berk SL, Verghese A. Parasitic pneumonia. *Semin Respir Infect* 1988;3:172–178.

51. Genta RM, Miles P, Fields K. Opportunistic *Strongyloides stercoralis* infection in lymphoma patients. Report of a case and review of the literature. *Cancer* 1989;63:1407–1411.

52. Schad GA, Smith G, Megyeri Z, Bhopale VM, Niamatali S, Maze R. *Strongyloides stercoralis:* an initial autoinfective burst amplifies primary infection. *Am J Trop Med Hyg* 1993;48: 716–725.

53. Koolman J, Moeller H. Diagnosis of major helminthic infections by RIA detection of ecdysteroids in urine and serum. *Insect Biochem* 1986;16:287–291.

54. Koolman J, Walter J, Zahner H. Ecdysteroids in helminths. In: Hoffmann J, Porchet M, eds. *Metabolism and mode of action of invertebrate hormones.* Berlin: Springer-Verlag, 1984;323–330.

55. Sato Y, Shiroma Y. Peripheral lymphocyte subsets and their responsiveness in human strongyloidiasis. *Clin Immunol Immunopathol* 1989;53:430–438.

56. Sato Y, Inoue F, Matsuyama R, Shiroma Y. Immunoblot analysis of antibodies in human strongyloidiasis. *Trans R Soc Trop Med Hyg* 1990;84:403–406.

57. Northern C, Grove DI. *Strongyloides stercoralis:* antigenic analysis of infective larvae and adult worms. *Int J Parasitol* 1990;20:381–387.

58. Genta RM, Lillibridge JP. Prominence of IgG4 antibodies in the human responses to *Strongyloides stercoralis* infection. *J Infect Dis* 1989;160:692–699.

59. Badaro R, Carvalho EM, Santos RB, Gam AA, Genta RM. Parasite-specific humoral responses in different clinical forms of strongyloidiasis. *Trans R Soc Trop Med Hyg* 1987;81: 149–150.

60. Northern C, Grove DI. Western blot analysis of reactivity to larval and adult *Strongyloides ratti* antigens in mice. *Parasite Immunol* 1988;10:681–691.

61. Genta RM, Frei DF, Linke MJ. Demonstration and partial characterization of parasite-specific immunoglobulin A responses in human strongyloidiasis. *J Clin Microbiol* 1987;25:1505–1510.

62. McRury J, de Messias IT, Walzer PD, Huitger T, Genta RM. Specific IgE responses in human strongyloidiasis. *Clin Exp Immunol* 1986;65:631–638.

63. Genta RM, Ottesen EA, Neva FA, Walzer PD, Tanowitz HB, Wittner M. Cellular responses in human strongyloidiasis. *Am J Trop Med Hyg* 1983;32:990–994.

64. Genta RM, Ottesen EA, Poindexter R, Gam AA, Neva FA, Tanowitz HB, Wittner M. Specific allergic sensitization to *Strongyloides* antigens in human strongyloidiasis. *Lab Invest* 1983;48:633–638.

65. Genta RM, Weil GJ. Antibodies to *Strongyloides stercoralis* larval surface antigens in chronic strongyloidiasis. *Lab Invest* 1982;47:87–90.

66. Shelhamer JH, Neva FA, Finn DR. Persistent strongyloidiasis in an immunodeficient patient. *Am J Trop Med Hyg* 1982;31: 746–751.

67. Brandt de Oliveira R, Voltarelli JC, Meneghelli UG. Severe strongyloidiasis associated with hypogammaglobulinaemia. *Parasite Immunol* 1981;3:165–169.

68. Genta RM, Douce RW, Walzer PD. Diagnostic implications of parasite-specific immune responses in immunocompromised patients with strongyloidiasis. *J Clin Microbiol* 1986;23: 1099–1103.

69. Morgan JS, Schaffner W, Stone WJ. Opportunistic strongyloidiasis in renal transplant recipients. *Transplantation* 1986;42: 518–524.

70. DeVault GA Jr, Brown ST, Montoya SF Jr, King JW, Rohr MS, McDonald JC. Disseminated strongyloidiasis complicating acute renal allograft rejection. Prolonged thiabendazole administration and successful retransplantation. *Transplantation* 1982;34:220–221.

71. Weller IV, Copland P, Gabriel R. Strongyloides stercoralis infection in renal transplant recipients. *Br Med J (Clin Res Ed)* 1981;282:524.

72. Scoggin CH, Call NB. Acute respiratory failure due to disseminated strongyloidiasis in a renal transplant recipient. *Ann Intern Med* 1977;87:456–458.

73. Hakim SZ, Genta RM. Fatal disseminated strongyloidiasis in a Vietnam War veteran. *Arch Pathol Lab Med* 1986;110:809–812.

74. De Paola D, Braga-Dias L, da Silva JR. Enteritis due to *Strongyloides stercoralis.* *Am J Dig Dis* 1962;7:1086–1098.

75. Genta RM, Caymmi-Gomes M. Pathology. In: Grove DI, ed. *Strongyloidiasis: a major roundworm infection of man.* London: Taylor and Francis, 1989;105–132.

76. Kennedy S, Campbell RM, Lawrence JE, Nichol GM, Rao DM. A case of severe *Strongyloides stercoralis* infection with

jejunal perforation in an Australian ex-prisoner-of-war. *Med J Aust* 1989;150:92–93.

77. Carp NZ, Nejman JH, Kelly JJ. Strongyloidiasis. An unusual cause of colonic pseudopolyposis and gastrointestinal bleeding. *Surg Endosc* 1987;1:175–177.

78. Berry AJ, Long EG, Smith JH, Gourley WK, Fine DP. Chronic relapsing colitis due to *Strongyloides stercoralis*. *Am J Trop Med Hyg* 1983;32:1289–1293.

79. Nadler S, Cappell MS, Bhatt B, Matano S, Kure K. Apprendiceal infection by *Entamoeba histolytica* and *Strongyloides stercoralis* presenting like acute appendicitis. *Dig Dis Sci* 1990; 35:603–608.

80. Shakir AA, Youngberg G, Alvarez S. *Strongyloides* infestation as a cause of acute appendicitis. *J Tenn Med Assoc* 1986;79: 543–544.

81. Noodleman JS. Eosinophilic appendicitis. Demonstration of *Strongyloides stercoralis* as a causative agent. *Arch Pathol Lab Med* 1981;105:148–149.

82. Williford ME, Foster WL Jr, Halvorsen RA, Thompson WM. Emphysematous gastritis secondary to disseminated strongyloidiasis. *Gastrointest Radiol* 1982;7:123–126.

83. Olurin EO. Strongyloidiasis causing fatal peritonitis. *West Afr Med J Niger Pract* 1970;19:102–104.

84. Poltera AA, Katsimbura N. Granulomatous hepatitis due to *Strongyloides stercoralis*. *J Pathol* 1974;113:241–246.

85. Davidson RA, Fletcher RH, Chapman LE. Risk factors for strongyloidiasis. A case–control study. *Arch Intern Med* 1984; 144:321–324.

86. Davidson RA. Strongyloidiasis: a presentation of 63 cases. *N C Med J* 1982;43:23–25.

87. Milder JE, Walzer PD, Kilgore G, Rutherford I, Klein M. Clinical features of *Strongyloides stercoralis* infection in an endemic area of the United States. *Gastroenterology* 1981;80: 1481–1488.

88. Dellacona S, Spier N, Wessely Z, Margolis IB. Massive colonic hemorrhage secondary to infection with *Strongyloides stercoralis*. *N Y State J Med* 1984;84:397–399.

89. Cunliffe WJ, Garcia S. Linear urticaria due to larva currens—strongyloidiasis. *Br J Dermatol* 1968;80:108–110.

90. Kane MG, Luby JP, Krejs GJ. Intestinal secretion as a cause of hypokalemia and cardiac arrest in a patient with strongyloidiasis. *Dig Dis Sci* 1984;29:768–772.

91. Milner PF, Irvine RA, Barton CJ, Bras G, Richards R. Intestinal malabsorption in *Strongyloides stercoralis* infestation. *Gut* 1965;6:574–581.

92. Laudanna AA, Polack M, Betarello A, Kieffer J. Evidence of protein-losing enteropathy in strongyloidiasis. *Rev Inst Med Trop Sao Paulo* 1973;15:222–226.

93. Alam SZ, Purohit D. A case report. Malabsorption secondary to *S. stercoralis* infestation. *Med J Zambia* 1982;16:85.

94. Garcia FT, Sessions JT, Strum WB, et al. Intestinal function and morphology in strongyloidiasis. *Am J Trop Med Hyg* 1977; 26:859–865.

95. Weesner RE, Kolinjivadi J, Giannella RA, Huitger OT, Genta RM. Effect of *Strongyloides ratti* on small bowel function in normal and immunosuppressed host rats. *Dig Dis Sci* 1988;33: 1316–1321.

96. Genta RM. Diarrhea in helminthic infections. *Clin Infect Dis* 1993;16(Suppl 2):S122–S129.

97. Cookson JB, Montgomery RD, Morgan HV, Tudor RW. Fatal paralytic ileus due to strongyloidiasis. *Br Med J* 1972;4: 771–772.

98. Davidson RA. Infection due to *Strongyloides stercoralis* in patients with pulmonary disease. *South Med J* 1992;85:28–31.

99. Berk SL, Verghese A, Alvarez S, Hall K, Smith B. Clinical and epidemiologic features of strongyloidiasis. A prospective study in rural Tennessee. *Arch Intern Med* 1987;147: 1257–1261.

100. Caceres MH, Genta RM. Pulmonary microcalcifications associated with *Strongyloides stercoralis* infection. *Chest* 1988;94: 862–865.

101. Kaslow JE, Novey HS, Zuch RH, Spear GS. Disseminated strongyloidiasis: an unheralded risk of corticosteroid therapy [Letter]. *J Allergy Clin Immunol* 1990;86:138.

102. Prociv P. Verminous asthma [Letter; Comment]. *Med J Aust* 1993;158:69.

103. Sadowska H, Konieczny B. Przypadek hiperinwazji *Strongyloides stercoralis* w przebiegu dychawicy oskrzelowej. *Pol Tyg Lek* 1990;45:628–629.

104. Sim TC, Alam R, Grant JA. Refractory wheezing and septicemia in a 57-year-old man with asthma [clinical conference]. *Ann Allergy* 1990;65:180–184.

105. Nwokolo C, Imohiosen EA. Strongyloidiasis of respiratory tract presenting as "asthma." *Br Med J* 1973;2:153–154.

106. Ujda J. Case of bronchial asthma in the course of infestation with *Strongyloides stercoralis*. *Wiad Lek* 1972;25:1089–1091.

107. Klein A, Kaufman H, Most H. Intestinal parasites and asthma. *N Engl J Med* 1971;285:179.

108. Quiox E, Hardy A, Kouao-Bile I, Rempp M, Gerszo I, Petitjean R. Bronchial asthma associated with anguilluliasis. *Rev Pneumol Clin* 1984;40:385–387.

109. Marsan C, Marais MH, Sollet JP, Le Turdu F, Guerin PH, Garcia R, Bleichner G. Disseminated strongyloidiasis: a case report. *Cytopathology* 1993;4:123–126.

110. Cook GA, Rodriguez H, Silva H, Rodriguez-Iturbe B, Bohorquez de Rodriguez H. Adult respiratory distress secondary to strongyloidiasis. *Chest* 1987;92:1115–1116.

111. Dwork KG, Jaffe JR, Lieberman HD. Strongyloidiasis with massive hyperinfection. *N Y State J Med* 1975;75:1230–1234.

112. Ford J, Reiss-Levy E, Clark E, Dyson AJ, Schonell M. Pulmonary strongyloidiasis and lung abscess. *Chest* 1981;79:239–240.

113. Genta RM, Harper JS, Gam AA, London WI, Neva FA. Experimental disseminated strongyloidiasis in *Erythrocebus patas*. II. Immunology. *Am J Trop Med Hyg* 1984;33:444–450.

114. Thompson JR, Berger R. Fatal adult respiratory distress syndrome following successful treatment of pulmonary strongyloidiasis. *Chest* 1991;99:772–774.

115. Thompson AJ, Brown MM, Ridley A. *Escherichia coli* meningitis and disseminated strongyloidiasis [Letter]. *J Neurol Neurosurg Psychiatry* 1988;51:1596–1597.

116. Tabacof J, Feher O, Katz A, Simon SD, Gansl RC. *Strongyloides* hyperinfection in two patients with lymphoma, purulent meningitis, and sepsis. *Cancer* 1991;68:1821–1823.

117. Schindzielorz A, Edberg SC, Bia FJ. *Strongyloides stercoralis* hyperinfection and central nervous system involvement in a patient with relapsing polychondritis. *South Med J* 1991;84: 1055–1057.

118. Chirgwin K. Meningitis and an unusual pathogen. *Hosp Pract* 1990;25:47–48, 51.

119. Furuya N, Shimozi K, Nakamura H, et al. A case report of meningitis and sepsis due to *Enterococcus faecium* complicated with strongyloidiasis. *Kansenshogaku Zasshi* 1989;63: 1344–1349.

120. Saito A, Aragaki T, Kinjou F. *Strongyloides* infection and bacterial meningitis in immunocompromised host, especially anti-HTLV-1 antibody positive patients. *Kansenshogaku Zasshi* 1988;62(Supp):71–72.

121. Vishwanath S, Baker RA, Mansheim BJ. *Strongyloides* infection and meningitis in an immunocompromised host. *Am J Trop Med Hyg* 1982;31:857–858.

122. Neefe LI, Pinilla O, Garagusi VF, Bauer H. Disseminated strongyloidiasis with cerebral involvement. A complication of corticosteroid therapy. *Am J Med* 1973;55:832–838.

123. Meltzer RS, Singer C, Armstrong D, Mayer K, Knapper WH. Case report: antemortem diagnosis of central nervous system strongyloidiasis. *Am J Med Sci* 1979;277:91–98.

124. Owor R, Wamukota WM. A fatal case of strongyloidiasis with *Strongyloides* larvae in the meninges. *Trans R Soc Trop Med Hyg* 1977;70:497–499.

125. Masdeu JC, Tantulavanich S, Gorelick PP, et al. Brain abscess caused by *Strongyloides stercoralis*. *Arch Neurol* 1982;39: 62–63.

126. Forzy G, Dhondt JL, Leloire O, Shayeb J, Vincent G. Reactive arthritis and *Strongyloides* [Letter]. *JAMA* 1988;259: 2546–2547.

127. Akoglu T, Tuncer I, Erken E, Gurcay A, Ozer FL, Ozcan K. Parasitic arthritis induced by *Strongyloides stercoralis*. *Ann Rheum Dis* 1984;43:523–525.

128. Doury P. Parasitic rheumatism [Letter]. *Arthritis Rheum* 1981; 24:638–639.

129. Bocanegra TS, Espinoza LR, Bridgeford PH, Vasey FB, Germain BF. Reactive arthritis induced by parasitic infestation. *Ann Intern Med* 1981;94:207–209.

130. Becquet R, Dutoit E, Poirriez J, Dutoit A, Vernes A. Cardiac form of anguillulosis [Letter]. *Presse Med* 1983;12:1366–1367.

131. Haggerty JJ Jr, Sandler R. Strongyloidiasis presenting as depression: a case report. *J Clin Psychiatry* 1982;43:340–341.

132. Agbo K, Deniau M. Anguillospermia resistant to treatment. Apropos of a case diagnosed in Togo. *Bull Soc Pathol Exot Filiales* 1987;80:271–273.

133. Corsini AC. Strongyloidiasis and chronic urticaria. *Postgrad Med J* 1982;58:247–248.

134. Leighton PM, MacSween HM. *Strongyloides stercoralis*. The cause of an urticarial-like eruption of 65 years' duration. *Arch Intern Med* 1990;150:1747–1748.

135. von Kuster LC, Genta RM. Cutaneous manifestations of strongyloidiasis. *Arch Dermatol* 1988;124:1826–1830.

136. Flensted-Jensen J. Cutaneous strongyloidiasis. *Ugeskr Laeger* 1982;144:721–722.

137. Lapierre J. Often unrecognized cutaneous manifestations of strongyloidosis: linear dermatitis or larva currens. *Sem Hop* 1980;56:409–413.

138. Orecchia G, Pazzaglia A, Scaglia M, Rabbiosi G. Larva currens following systemic steroid therapy in a case of strongyloidiasis. *Dermatologica* 1985;171:366–367.

139. Pelletier LL Jr, Baker CB, Gam AA, Nutman TB, Neva FA. Diagnosis and evaluation of treatment of chronic strongyloidiasis in ex-prisoners of war. *J Infect Dis* 1988;157:573–576.

140. Stone OJ, Newell GB, Mullins JF. Cutaneous strongyloidiasis: larva currens. *Arch Dermatol* 1972;106:734–736.

141. Verburg GP, de Geus A. Strongyloidiasis bij voormalige krijgsgevangenen en geinterneerden die tijdens de Tweede Wereldoorlog in Zuidoost-Azie verbleven. *Ned Tijdschr Geneeskd* 1990;134:2529–2533.

142. Pelletier LL Jr. Chronic strongyloidiasis in World War II Far East ex-prisoners of war. *Am J Trop Med Hyg* 1984;33:55–61.

143. Grove DI. Strongyloidiasis in Allied ex-prisoners of war in south-east Asia. *Br Med J* 1980;280:598–601.

144. Gill GV, Bell DR. *Strongyloides stercoralis* infection in former Far East prisoners of war. *Br Med J* 1979;2:572–574.

145. Bank DE, Grossman ME, Kohn SR, Rabinowitz AD. The thumbprint sign: rapid diagnosis of disseminated strongyloidiasis. *J Am Acad Dermatol* 1990;23:324–326.

146. Berenson CS, Dobuler KJ, Bia FJ. Fever, petechiae, and pulmonary infiltrates in an immunocompromised Peruvian man. *Yale J Biol Med* 1987;60:437–445.

147. Kalb RE, Grossman ME. Periumbilical purpura in disseminated strongyloidiasis. *JAMA* 1986;256:1170–1171.

148. Medina LS, Heiken JP, Gold RP. Pipestem appearance of small bowel in strongyloidiasis is not pathognomonic of fibrosis and irreversibility. *AJR Am J Roentgenol* 1992;159:543–544.

149. Adetiloye VA. A case of fatal gastrointestinal strongyloidiasis in an otherwise healthy Nigerian, masquerading as gastric outlet obstruction. *Trop Geogr Med* 1992;44:60–62.

150. Berkmen YM, Rabinowitz J. Gastrointestinal manifestations of strongyloidiasis. *Am J Roentgenol Radium Ther Nucl Med* 1972;115:306–311.

151. Dallemand S, Waxman M, Farman J. Radiological manifestations of *Strongyloides stercoralis*. *Gastrointest Radiol* 1983;8: 45–51.

152. Drasin GF, Moss JP, Cheng SH. *Strongyloides stercoralis* colitis: findings in four cases. *Radiology* 1978;126:619–621.

153. Rassiga AL, Lowry JL, Forman WB. Diffuse pulmonary infection due to *Strongyloides stercoralis*. *JAMA* 1974;230:426–427.

154. Pettersson T, Stenström R, Kyrönseppa H. Disseminated lung opacities and cavitation associated with *Strongyloides stercoralis* and *Schistosoma mansoni* infection. *Am J Trop Med Hyg* 1974;23:158–162.

155. Bruno P, McAllister K, Matthews JI. Pulmonary strongyloidiasis. *South Med J* 1982;75:363–365.

156. Nielsen PB, Mojon M. Improved diagnosis of *Strongyloides stercoralis* by seven consecutive stool specimens. *Zentralbl Bakteriol Mikrobiol Hyg [A]* 1987;263:616–618.

157. Genta RM. Immunobiology of strongyloidiasis. *Trop Geogr Med* 1984;36:223–229.

158. Pereira-Lima J, Delgado PG. Diagnosis of strongyloidiasis: importance of Baermann's method. *Am J Dig Dis* 1961;6:899–904.

159. Koga K, Kasuya S, Khamboonruang C, et al. A modified agar plate method for detection of *Strongyloides stercoralis*. *Am J Trop Med Hyg* 1991;45:518–521.

160. Beal CB, Viens P, Grant RG, Hughes JM. A new technique for sampling duodenal contents: demonstration of upper small-bowel pathogens. *Am J Trop Med Hyg* 1970;19:349–352.

161. Chaudhuri B, Nanos S, Soco JN, McGrew EA. Disseminated *Strongyloides stercoralis* infestation detected by sputum cytology. *Acta Cytol* 1980;24:360–362.

162. Kenney M, Webber CA. Diagnosis of strongyloidiasis in Papanicolaou-stained sputum smears. *Acta Cytol* 1974;18:270–273.

163. Wang T, Reyes CV, Kathuria S, Strinden C. Diagnosis of *Strongyloides stercoralis* in sputum cytology. *Acta Cytol* 1980; 24:40–43.

164. Williams J, Nunley D, Dralle W, Berk SL, Verghese A. Diagnosis of pulmonary strongyloidiasis by bronchoalveolar lavage. *Chest* 1988;94:643–644.

165. Gill GV, Bailey JW. Eosinophilia as a marker for chronic strongyloidiasis—use of a serum ELISA test to detect asymptomatic cases. *Ann Trop Med Parasitol* 1989;83:249–252.

166. Bhattacharyya DN. Eosinophilia due to multiple parasitic infection. *J Infect* 1985;10:172–173.

167. Reddy KR, Laurain AR, Thomas E. Strongyloidiasis. When to suspect the wily nematode. *Postgrad Med* 1983;74:273–275, 279–282.

168. Pierce JR Jr, Dyer EL. Extreme eosinophilia and strongyloidiasis: an uncommon manifestation of a common disease. *South Med J* 1981;74:995–996.

169. Carneiro Leao R, de Toledo Barras MM, Mendes E. Immunological study of human strongyloidiasis. I. Analysis of IgE levels. *Allergol Immunopathol (Madr)* 1980;8:31–34.

170. Bezjak B. Immunoglobulin studies in strongyloidiasis with special reference to raised serum IgE levels. Preliminary communication. *Am J Trop Med Hyg* 1975;24:945–948.

171. Purtilo DT, Riggs RS, Evans R, Neafie RC. Humoral immunity of parasitized, malnourished children. *Am J Trop Med Hyg* 1976;25:229–232.

172. Carroll SM, Karthigasu KT, Grove DI. Serodiagnosis of human strongyloidiasis by an enzyme-linked immunosorbent assay. *Trans R Soc Trop Med Hyg* 1981;75:706–709.

173. Gam AA, Neva FA, Krotoski WA. Comparative sensitivity and specificity of ELISA and IHA for serodiagnosis of strongyloidiasis with larval antigens. *Am J Trop Med Hyg* 1987;37: 157–161.

174. Genta RM. Predictive value of an enzyme-linked immunosorbent assay (ELISA) for the serodiagnosis of strongyloidiasis. *Am J Clin Pathol* 1988;89:391–394.

175. Sato Y, Takara M, Otsuru M. Detection of antibodies in strongyloidiasis by enzyme-linked immunosorbent assay (ELISA). *Trans R Soc Trop Med Hyg* 1985;79:51–55.

176. Conway DJ, Bailey JW, Lindo JF, Robinson RD, Bundy DA, Bianco AE. Serum IgG reactivity with 41-, 31-, and 28-kDa larval proteins of *Strongyloides stercoralis* in individuals with strongyloidiasis. *J Infect Dis* 1993;168:784–787.

177. Conway DJ, Atkins NS, Lillywhite JE, et al. Immunodiagnosis of *Strongyloides stercoralis* infection: a method for increasing the specificity of the indirect ELISA. *Trans R Soc Trop Med Hyg* 1993;87:173–176.

178. Lal RB, Ottesen EA. Phosphocholine epitopes on helminth and protozoal parasites and their presence in the circulation of infected human patients. *Trans R Soc Trop Med Hyg* 1989;83: 652–655.

179. Brindley PJ, Gam AA, Pearce EJ, Poindexter RW, Neva FA. Antigens from the surface and excretions/secretions of the filariform larva of *Strongyloides stercoralis*. *Mol Biochem Parasitol* 1988;28:171–180.

180. Grove DI. Treatment of strongyloidiasis with thiabendazole:

an analysis of toxicity and effectiveness. *Trans R Soc Trop Med Hyg* 1982;76:114–118.

181. Leapman SB, Rosenberg JB, Filo RS, Smith EJ. *Strongyloides stercoralis* in chronic renal failure: safe therapy with thiabendazole. *South Med J* 1980;73:1400–1402.

182. Boken DJ, Leoni PA, Preheim LC. Treatment of *Strongyloides stercoralis* hyperinfection syndrome with thiabendazole administered per rectum. *Clin Infect Dis* 1993;16:123–126.

183. Diaz Jidy M, Fernandez Abascal H, Millan Marcelo JC, Ruiz Perez A. Levamisol, mebendazol, tiabendazol. Su efectividad como helminticidas en pacientes africanos recien arribados a Cuba. Periodo 1987–1988. *Rev Cubana Med Trop* 1990;42:240–246.

184. Grove DI, Northern C. The effects of thiabendazole, mebendazole and cambendazole in normal and immunosuppressed dogs infected with a human strain of *Strongyloides stercoralis*. *Trans R Soc Trop Med Hyg* 1988;82:146–149.

185. Archibald LK, Beeching NJ, Gill GV, Bailey JW, Bell DR. Albendazole is effective treatment for chronic strongyloidiasis. *Q J Med* 1993;86:191–195.

186. Coulter C, Walker DG, Gunsberg M, Brown IG, Bligh JF, Prociv P. Successful treatment of disseminated strongyloidiasis. *Med J Aust* 1992;157:331–332.

187. Mansfield LS, Schad GA. Ivermectin treatment of naturally acquired and experimentally induced *Strongyloides stercoralis* infections in dogs. *J Am Vet Med Assoc* 1992;201:726–730.

188. Shikiya K, Kinjo N, Uehara T, et al. Efficacy of ivermectin against *S. stercoralis*. *Intern Med* 1992;31:310–312.

189. Naquira C, Jimenez G, Guerra JG, Bernal R, Nalin DR, Neu D, Aziz M. Ivermectin for human strongyloidiasis and other intestinal helminths. *Am J Trop Med Hyg* 1989;40:304–309.

190. Whitworth JA, Morgan D, Maude GH, McNicholas AM, Taylor DW. A field study of the effect of ivermectin on intestinal helminths in man. *Trans R Soc Trop Med Hyg* 1991;85:232–234.

Infections of the Gastrointestinal Tract,
edited by M. J. Blaser, P. D. Smith, J. I. Ravdin,
H. B. Greenberg, and R. L. Guerrant
Raven Press, Ltd., New York © 1995.

CHAPTER 80

Schistosomiasis

Christopher King and Adel A. F. Mahmoud

Human infection with several species of schistosomes may result in significant morbidity in the gastrointestinal tract and liver. Furthermore, mortality due to the subsequent hemodynamic changes in the portal circulation and liver failure is considerable. Infection is usually acquired in endemic areas early in life as children experience contact with freshwater bodies that contain the infective cercariae. Peak prevalence and intensity are generally seen in young adults 15 to 20 years of age, while disease sequelae may be seen in association with peak intensity of infection or later in life (1). Gastrointestinal and liver diseases are caused by infection with either *Schistosoma mansoni* or *S. japonicum*. In the Far East the less prevalent *S. mekongi* resembles *S. japonicum* infection and disease. There is controversy whether liver disease may occur in *S. haematobium* infection. For residents of nonendemic areas such as the United States, exposure to infection usually occurs during foreign travel. Infection acquired overseas should be preventable if proper travel advice is given. There is, however, a segment of our population who may be unable to avoid infection such as those involved in military operations.

Infection with *S. mansoni* is endemic in the northern area of South America and in the Caribbean, including Puerto Rico. *Schistosoma mansoni* is also prevalent in most African countries and all through the Middle East. In contrast, *S. japonicum* is limited in its geographic distribution to China, the Philippines, and Indonesia. *Schistosoma mekongi* is found in sporadic foci in Southeast Asia.

BIOLOGY

The schistosomes are flat worms (Platyhelminth). They differ from all other flukes that infect humans in differentiating into separate sex adult worms in the definitive host

(Fig. 1). The complicated life cycle of schistosomes alternates between parasitic and free-living forms, and between an intermediate and a definitive host (Fig. 2). Humans (definitive hosts) acquire infection while in contact with fresh water contaminated with cercariae. The free-living schistosome forms are capable of penetrating intact human skin and transforming into the first stage of parasitic life in the definitive host. Following skin penetration, the cercariae transform into schistosomula, which adapt to the hostile environment of the host through a series of membrane, biochemical, and antigenic changes (2). Schistosomula remain in the subcutaneous tissues for 2 to 3 days and then travel via the venous system to the lungs, where they reside for approximately 1 week. The worms migrate to the liver where they attain sexual maturity in 4 to 6 weeks and descend into the portal venous system. Adult worms mate and the females travel downstream to deposit eggs (Figs. 1 and 2). *Schistosoma mansoni* ova are usually deposited as single eggs while *S. japonicum* eggs are deposited as nests of multiple ova. The schistosome ova attempt to migrate from the small ven-

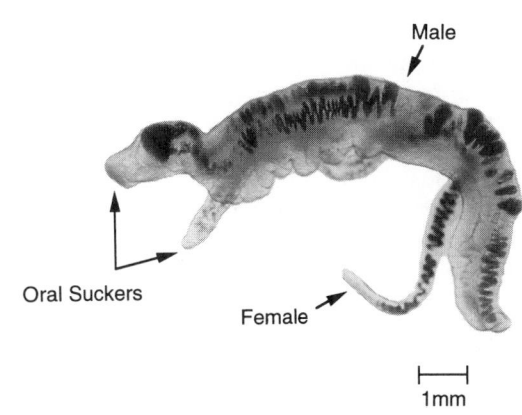

FIG. 1. Male and female schistosomes. Female worm (thinner worm) rests in the gynecophoral canal of the male. ×35.

C. King and A. A. F. Mahmoud: Division of Geographic Medicine, Department of Medicine, Case Western Reserve University and University Hospitals, Cleveland, Ohio 44106.

1209

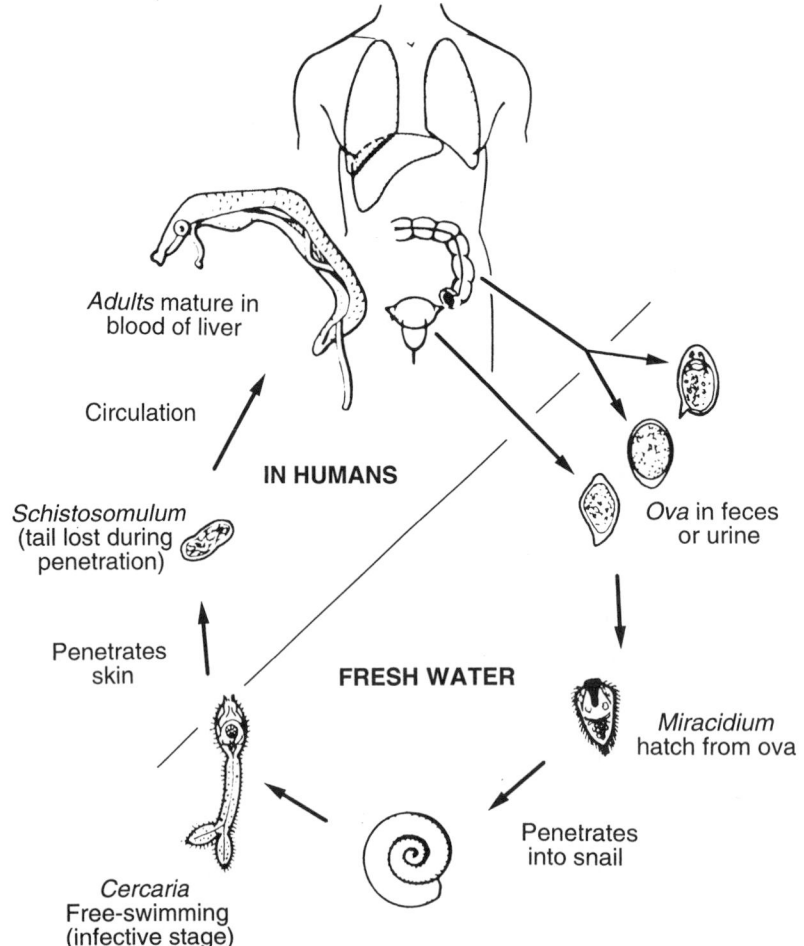

FIG. 2. Life cycle of schistosomiasis.

ules, where they were deposited, to the lumen of the gut. In the process, some ova are retained in the tissues, others are carried up to the liver in the portal system, while the remainder succeed in reaching the gut lumen and the outside environment via feces. Due to promiscuous defecation in the canals and water bodies of endemic areas, eggs reach fresh water, hatch, and release free-living miracidia. The miracidia search for their specific intermediate host, a snail, where they penetrate the snail's internal structures and undergo tremendous multiplication and, finally, transform into cercariae. These forms are shed into the fresh water, completing the life cycle of the helminth.

Human infection results in exposure of the host to a multitude of schistosome stages and antigens during the life cycle of the parasite. Disease may occur at each of the major steps of the parasite life cycle: cercarial invasion, schistosomula migration and maturation, and finally egg retention in tissues. Furthermore, the host immunopathological responses and attempts toward healing result in the major chronic sequelae of disease.

EPIDEMIOLOGY

The epidemiology of schistosomiasis in nonendemic areas such as North America or Europe differ from its features in endemic communities. Individuals (usually adults) from nonendemic areas are exposed to infection because of a lack of understanding of its mode of transmission. Contact with freshwater bodies in endemic areas whether stationary, slow, or fast flowing is the source of transmission. This mode of transmission results in infection of individual travelers or, rarely, a group traveling together, most of them with no previous exposure. Under such circumstances, the disease sequelae have a characteristic pattern. Invariably these manifestations will occur upon return to the nonendemic area, thus providing a diagnostic and management challenge to an unfamiliar medical profession. Occasionally, several individuals are exposed simultaneously, resulting in a "mini" epidemic presenting with the acute manifestations of disease.

In endemic areas, exposure to infection usually occurs at a younger age. The prevalence and intensity of infection increase with age up to 15 to 20 years (3). Beyond 30 years of age, the prevalence may decline; however, the intensity of infection decreases significantly. This age-specific pattern of intensity raises important issues related to the ecology of schistosomiasis, patterns of water contact, and the role of acquired immunity in regulating parasite burdens in infected individuals.

Similar to other worm infections, the distribution of parasite load in an endemic community does not follow a bell-shaped curve (4). Rather, there is overdispersion of the parasite in the human population with a majority of infected individuals harboring low worm burdens while only a small minority demonstrate high worm and egg counts. This pattern of distribution of infection in individuals in endemic areas poses several important clinical, biological, and epidemiologic issues. Because disease in schistosomiasis is related to the intensity of infection, the group with a heavy worm load is at exceptionally high risk for developing disease. Furthermore, this group is responsible for the major contamination of the environment with parasite eggs and perpetuation of the endemicity of the parasite. Finally, the reasons for such an aggregation of infection is unclear; whether it is due to the pattern of exposure, variable host susceptibility to infection and disease, or a combination of both factors remains an unanswered question (1).

PATHOGENESIS: DYNAMICS OF GRANULOMA FORMATION AND MODULATION

The parasite eggs, produced by the adult worms that live in the mesenteric plexus, are the principal cause of pathology in humans. Daily, each female worm deposits hundreds of eggs into the bloodstream. Although the parasite does not self-replicate within the host, it produces eggs continuously throughout the course of infection. Deposited eggs lodge in the intestinal wall or are carried by venous blood to liver, lung, and so on. The live embryo within each egg secretes antigenic material through ultramicroscopic pores in the shell. These antigens, continually released for 2 to 4 weeks, induce host sensitization and recruitment of macrophages, lymphocytes, epithelioid and occasional giant cells, fibroblasts, and numerous eosinophils to comprise the host granulomatous response (Figs. 3 and 4). The antigenic secretion stops when the embryo within the egg dies; granulomas then undergo a healing process with deposition of fibrous tissue. Fibrosis of the liver or other tissues can cause portal hypertension, varices, cor pulmonale, and other complications.

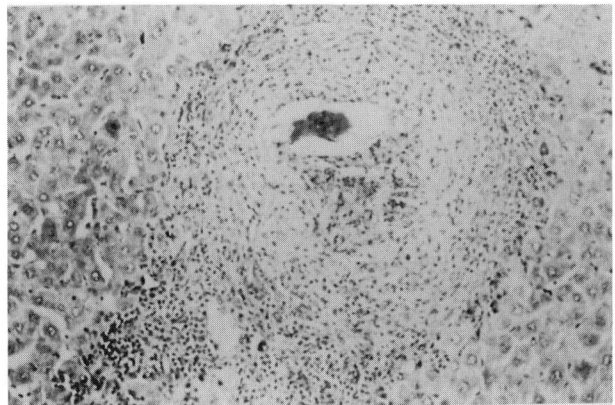

FIG. 3. Schistosome granuloma in liver *(Schistosoma mansoni)*. The structureless mass in the center is an ovum.

The function of the granuloma has been postulated to encase the egg and prevent secretion of potentially deleterious antigenic substances by the ova (5). Alternatively, it has been proposed that induction of an inflammatory response by the intravascularly laid schistosome eggs may facilitate their crossing tissue barriers (6,7). Thus the host's own inflammatory response either increases vascular permeability or destroys adjacent tissues sufficiently to allow egg passage into the gut or bladder lumen.

MURINE MODELS OF SCHISTOSOME GRANULOMA

Granuloma formation in naturally infected mice occurs after maturation and onset of egg deposition at approximately 8 weeks in *S. mansoni* infection. Granulomas reach maximal size and cellularity by 12 weeks and then shrink in size by 20 to 24 weeks (8). A similar pattern of granuloma formation and modulation is observed with murine infections with *S. japonicum;* however, the kinetics are accelerated by several weeks because of the earlier maturation of *S. japonicum* worms (Fig. 5) (9). Importantly, portal pressure elevates with the increase in granuloma size and diminishes as the granulomas are downmodulated. Initially, studies of the mechanism of granuloma formation were hindered by the long duration before granulomas appeared after infection and their asynchronous development. To avoid these difficulties, a model was developed where viable eggs were isolated from the livers of infected animals and then injected intravenously into normal mice (10). This procedure evoked well-delineated primary granulomas in the lung by 16 days, which could easily be stained and measured. Granuloma formation was found to be T cell mediated and could be accelerated and enhanced by sensitizing mice to egg antigens prior to intravenous challenge with viable ova (11). In this model, granulomas developed within the lung by 48 hr and reach peak size by 8 days. The accelerated granulomatous response was adoptively transferred by lymphocytes and not by serum. The pulmonary model has been widely used to study the immune regulation of schistosome granuloma formation. However, care must be made in extrapolating these findings to granulomas formed in the liver or intestine, since immune cells resident in any particular tissue may have important influences on the mechanisms and dynamics of granuloma formation. For example, both the size and composition of granulomas vary based on the anatomic site of deposition (12,13). Granulomas in the ileum are much smaller and are made primarily of macrophages compared to the much larger T- and B-cell-rich granulomas of liver and colon.

The hypersensitivity granuloma elicited by schistosome eggs is a complex orchestration of different cell types directed by T cells. As eggs become trapped in tissues, inflammatory cells are detectable within 48 hr (14). At this point the granuloma contains multiple populations of rapidly proliferating cells. The initial cell types in the granuloma are phagocytic cells followed by T cells, eosinophils, and finally B cells (Fig. 6). The predominant cell type within the maturing granuloma are CD4+ cells although

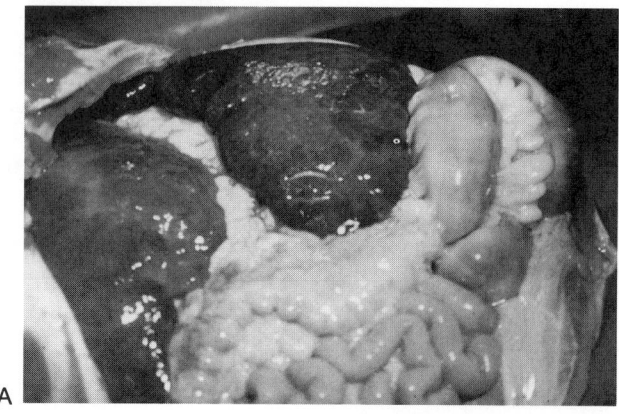
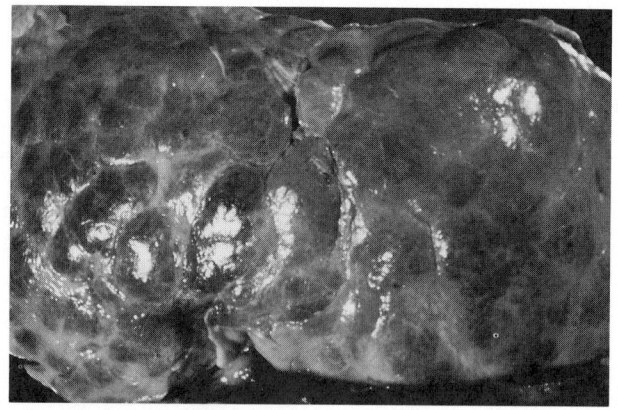
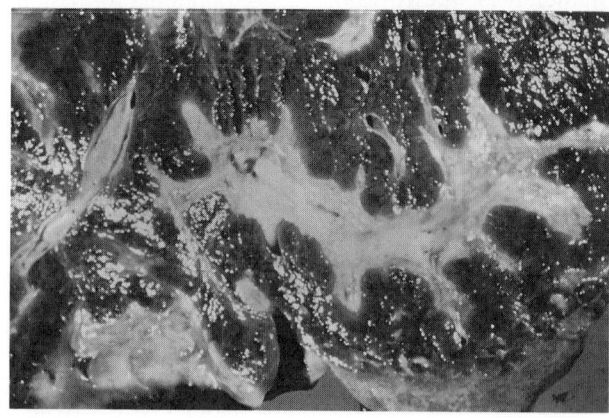

FIG. 4. Hepatosplenomegaly (liver, *red;* spleen, *purple*) at autopsy in patient with *Schistosoma mansoni* **(A).** Nodular changes on the surface of the liver **(B)** and the presinusoidal (Symmers' pipe-stem) fibrosis of the liver in cross section **(C)** (Courtesy of M. Mittermeyer.) (See Plate 27.)

some CD8+ cells are present (15). Neutrophils are also observed in the schistosome granuloma, but never exceed 10% of the cellular population. The sequential influx of cells into the granuloma likely reflect both the antigens secreted by the parasite embryo and the cytokines and chemokines produced by immune cells in the granuloma.

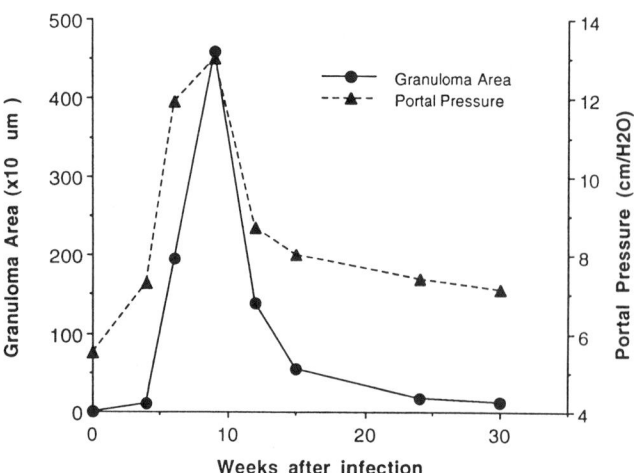

FIG. 5. Relationship of granuloma size with portal pressure in mice infected with *Schistosoma japonicum.*

Several hypotheses have emerged to account for the induction and modulation of schistosome granulomas. Initially, granuloma formation was thought to be regulated by macrophage inhibitory factors (MIFs) (14,16) and eosinophil chemotactic/stimulatory lymphokines (ESP/ECP) (17). Spleen and granuloma cells produced increased MIF synthesis with granuloma induction (16), which subsequently diminished by 20 weeks, suggesting MIFs played a major role in the granulomatous response. Eosinophil chemotactic lymphokines include the hematopoietic growth factors interleukin-5 (IL-5) and granulocyte–macrophage colony-stimulating factor (GM-CSF), which are produced by CD4+ cells within the granuloma (17,18).

Recently, it has been postulated that sequential induction of T helper (Th) subsets regulate granuloma formation (19,20). This concept has emerged from a key finding that CD4+ T lymphocytes can be divided into two distinct subsets—Th1 and Th2—which have different patterns of cytokine production (21). Th1 clones generate predominantly IL-2 and interferon-γ (IFN-γ) (in addition to IL-3 and GM-CSF), which promote cellular immunity, whereas Th2 clones secrete IL-4, IL-5, and IL-10, which provide help for B cell differentiation and humoral immune responses. A dynamic balance of cross-regulatory cytokines associated with activation of Th1 and Th2 subsets of CD4+ cells can regulate the outcome of immune

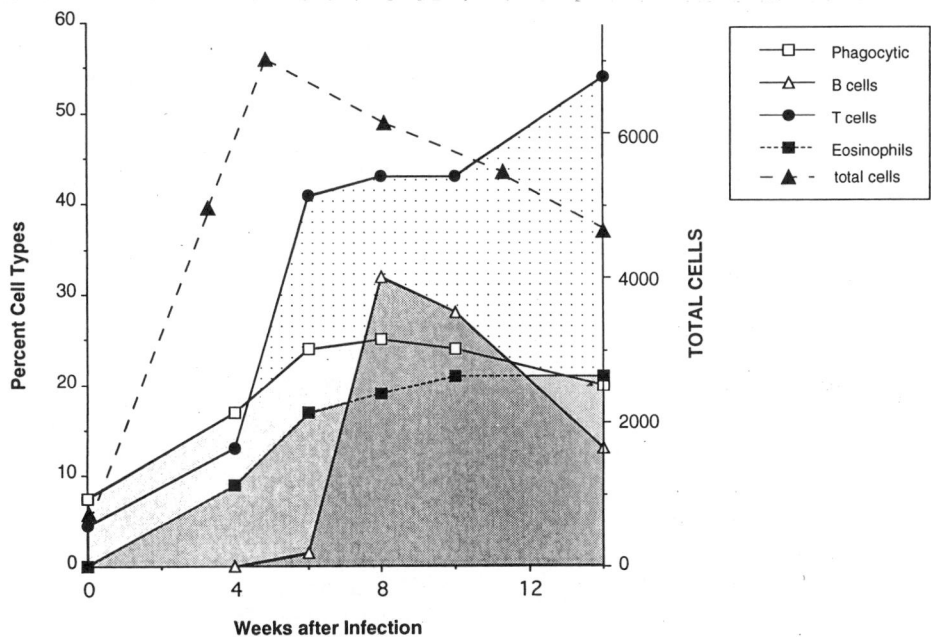

FIG. 6. Kinetics, cell composition, and cell number of the liver granuloma during the course of murine *Schistosoma japonicum* infection.

responses (22,23). Th1 responses predominate during schistosomula maturation; however, with peak granuloma formation Th-2-associated cytokines are expressed (19,20). Because Th subsets have been observed to cross-regulate one another by mutually inhibitory cytokines, the enhanced Th2 response has been postulated to suppress egg antigen-induced Th1 functions through enhanced production of IL-10 (24). IL-4 is essential for granuloma formation and modulation; neutralizing monoclonal antibodies against IL-4 blocks granuloma development (25). Treatment of chronically infected mice with recombinant IL-4 enhanced the size of the downmodulated granuloma but had little effect on granuloma size in acutely infected mice (26). IL-2 has also been shown to be critical in the generation of granulomas (25,27). In contrast, the Th1-associated cytokine IFN-γ suppresses granuloma formation (28–30). Recently, a phagocytic- and B-cell-derived cytokine, IL-12, has been shown to influence granuloma formation in mice (30). IL-12 is very potent and active in picomolar concentrations and promotes Th1 subset differentiation while suppressing Th2 responses (31,32). Administration of recombinant IL-12 to sensitized mice markedly suppressed granuloma formation and IL-4 messenger ribonucleic acid (mRNA) transcript levels while increasing IFN-γ production (30). Blocking endogenous IL-12 by administering neutralizing antibodies markedly enhanced granuloma size (28,30). IL-12 regulates granuloma development by suppressing Th2 responses and promoting IFN-γ production. An exciting implication of these experiments is that IL-12 could be used as a vaccine adjuvant to prevent schistosome egg-induced pathology. Interestingly, monoclonal egg antigen-specific Th1 clones can also mediate granuloma formation (33). This was demonstrated when these clones were transferred to naive mice. Upon intravenous challenge, vigorous granulomas

were observed around schistosome eggs embolized to the lung. This suggests that granuloma formation may not always be an exclusively Th2-mediated phenomenon. Moreover IL-2, IL-4, IFN-γ, and IL-12 affect many inflammatory cells and may regulate granulomatous inflammation by pathways other than Th subset differentiation.

Most studies describing cytokine production by schistosome granuloma lymphocytes examined the *in vitro* recall responses of isolated lymphocytes to egg antigens; little detectable spontaneous cytokine production is detected (34–37). However, antigenic stimulation of lymphocytes may bias findings. For example, generation of cross-regulatory molecules *in vitro* may lead to either enhanced or suppressed cytokine responses that may not reflect the ongoing cytokine production in the granuloma cells themselves. To circumvent these problems, cytokine mRNA levels have been measured *in vivo*. Northern blots of RNA extracted from granulomatous liver, spleen, and lymph nodes during the course of primary infection and modulation demonstrate that peak IL-4 and IFN-γ mRNA levels are coincident with acute granuloma formation and that the levels of both messengers decline as the infection becomes chronic (38,39). Interestingly, no IL-2 mRNA was found throughout the infection, indicating that increased Th1 cell activity during chronic infection was unlikely to account for the modulation (39). Measurement of cytokine transcript levels by an even more sensitive technique of reverse-transcriptase polymerase chain reaction (RT-PCR) demonstrated increased mRNA levels for IL-1, IL-6, IFN-γ, IL-2, IL-4, IL-10, IL-5, and tumor necrosis factor-α (TNF-α) that reached maximal levels by day 6 in the pulmonary granuloma model (29). Message levels for most cytokines (except IL-2 and IFN-γ) displayed a marked decrease by days 14 to 16. Increased numbers of IL-4-secreting CD4 + cells were found in liver granulomas to coincide with peak granuloma formation by using a technique of intracytoplasmic immunofluorescence (A. Stavitsky, *personal communication*). The number of IL-4-secreting CD4+ cells was diminished in chronically infected animals. Unlike the RT-PCR studies, however, consistently elevated counts of IL-2- and IL-10-secreting T cells were found throughout the course of granuloma formation and modulation. Overall modulation of the granuloma appears to be affected by a suppression of lymphokine secretion, although the mechanisms that lead to this suppression remain unclear.

The immune regulation of granuloma formation in murine models of *S. japonicum* is similar in many respects to that observed with *S. mansoni*, yet additional mechanisms have been observed. Transfer of the immunoglobulin (Ig) fraction of serum from chronically infected animals can suppress granuloma size in acutely infected mice (40). The critical component appears to be the murine IgG1 isotype (40).

There is evidence supporting other hypotheses to account for the modulation of granuloma formation with chronic infection. Immune complexes, formation of anti-idiotypic antibodies (41,42) prostaglandin production (43), CD8+ T cells (44), and the mammalian tachykinins, vasoactive intestinal peptide (VIP) and substance P (45), have all been convincingly demonstrated to modulate granuloma formation. Recent studies have established a critical role of monokines in granuloma formation. IL-1 (46,47), TNF-α (46,48,49), macrophage inhibitory protein-1α (MIP-1α) (50), and the endogenous IL-1 receptor antagonist protein (IRAP) (51) are secreted by macrophages in the schistosome egg granuloma. In particular, TNF-α appears to play an essential role in granuloma formation. TNF-α injected into schistosome-infected severe combined immunodeficient (SCID) mice restored granuloma formation (48). These observations have been supported in immunologically intact animals where injection of anti-

TNF-α antiserum to acutely infected mice suppressed the size of developing liver granulomas (49). Table 1 summarizes our understanding of the role of various substances in modulation of granuloma formation.

IMMUNE REGULATION OF GRANULOMAS IN HUMANS

Patients with acute schistosome infections develop fever, abdominal and pulmonary symptoms associated with brisk lymphocyte proliferative responses (52), and the onset of IL-2, IFN-γ, IL-4, and IL-5 production in response to egg antigens by peripheral blood mononuclear cells (PBMCs) (53). As the infection becomes chronic, egg antigen-induced lymphocyte blastogenesis and IL-2 and IFN-γ production are suppressed (36,52). Most chronically infected individuals remain asymptomatic. Approximately 10% to 15% of infected patients, mainly with heavy worm burdens, develop hepatosplenic disease with accompanying fibrosis and ultimately liver failure (1). Such patients frequently have higher lymphocyte proliferative responses to egg antigen compared to asymptomatic individuals, suggesting that failure to modulate egg-antigen-induced inflammatory responses results in enhanced granulomatous responses and fibrosis (54). Limited studies of rectal and liver biopsies indicate that granuloma modulation occurs in humans and that the magnitude of the granulomatous response positively correlated with egg-antigen-induced lymphocyte proliferative responses (55).

Development of an *in vitro* granuloma model using human PBMCs supports the indirect studies that demonstrate immunomodulation in humans (55). PBMCs obtained from recently infected individuals produce a strong *in vitro* granulomatous response to egg antigens compared with PBMCs obtained from chronically infected subjects (55). In vitro, granulomas contain lymphocyte subpopulations representative of those observed in murine schistosomiasis models and are Th cell dependent in their formation (55). In this model, idiotypic antibodies or immunocomplexes contribute to *in vitro* granuloma modulation (56,57).

Although granuloma formation and modulation have similarly been observed in the murine model and in human disease, significant differences do exist. Egg-antigen-induced proinflammatory responses characterized by augmented lymphocyte proliferation and IL-2 production are associated with more severe pathology in chronically infected humans (54). This contrasts with the murine model in which egg-antigen Th2 responses promote granuloma formation. Indeed, we have observed that egg antigens promoted mixed Th1 and Th2 responses and, in some individuals, primarily Th1 responses *(personal observations)*. In contrast, adult worm antigens favor a Th2 cytokine pattern by PBMCs from chronically infected individuals.

DYNAMICS AND REGULATION OF FIBROSIS

Liver fibrosis and intestinal fibrosis are the major sequelae of granulomatous reactions in *S. mansoni* or *S.*

TABLE 1. *Effect of cytokines, chemokines, and other bioactive molecules on granuloma formation*

Molecule	Effect on granuloma size and/or formation
Th1 cytokines	
IFN-γ	↓
IL-2	↑
IL-12	↓
Th2 cytokines	
IL-4	↑
IL-5	Induces eosinophil influx, but no effect on granuloma size
IL-6, IL-10	Unknown
Monokines	
TNF-α	↑
IRAP	↓
IL-1	↑
MIF	↑
Other molecules	
MIP-1α	↑
MCP	↑
Tachykinins	↑
Prostaglandins	↑

japonica infection. In addition to the T-cell-mediated inflammatory focus that occurs around schistosome eggs, the fibrous healing contributes to the portal and periportal fibrosis (58). Initially, fibrosis was viewed as a static consequence of the dying embryo within the schistosome egg. It is now recognized that fibrogenesis is a dynamic process involving mesenchymal cells that respond to a series of molecular signals generated by a variety of cell types (59,60). The fundamental process of scar formation that occurs in parallel to that of lymphocyte infiltration into the granuloma includes (a) hyperplasia of the fibroblast population (61); (b) increased synthesis and deposition of extracellular matrix constituents, particularly collagen (62); and (c) remodeling of the extracellular matrix by degradative enzymes. Changes in the relative production of collagen isotypes also occur as the infection progresses (63,64). As infection progresses, collagen deposition becomes more pronounced with increased amounts of type I relative to type III, and by 20 weeks high levels of both types I and III collagen as well as some type IV collagen are present. Type I collagen is more heavily cross-linked and degradation resistant and may correlate with enhanced morbidity. Conversely, in animals that modulate granuloma formation, a shift from a predominantly type I to type III collagen is observed (64). These changes in the quantity and makeup of extracellular collagen may ameliorate or exacerbate disease and enhance or diminish the potential of reversing fibrosis (65–67).

It is currently believed that granuloma-derived inflammatory cells generate fibrogenic cytokines that regulate hepatic fibrogenesis in schistosomiasis. Congenitally athymic (nude) mice, deficient in mature T cells, generate small granulomas and develop minimal hepatic fibrosis compared to a vigorous granulomatous response in their littermates with intact thymus glands (68). Specific cytokines within the granuloma that stimulate fibrogenesis are now being recognized. The production of transforming growth factor-β (TGF-β), which promotes collagen production *in vitro* in the granuloma, correlates with fibrosis (69). In contrast, IFN-γ suppresses fibrosis around the granuloma both *in vitro* and *in vivo* (70). These studies are, however, correlative. Recently, a CD4+ cell-derived protein termed fibroblast-stimulating factor-1 (FsF-1) has been isolated from granulomas and is a potent stimulant of fibroblast production (71). This molecule has been isolated to homogeneity and is postulated to be a novel lymphokine (72). Additional fibroblast-stimulating factors observed in the granuloma are likely to be of monocyte origin. Although there is a similarity in the dynamics of fibrogenesis and inflammation, these responses may be independently regulated (64). For example, peak synthesis rates for matrix deposition do not coincide with peak granuloma size (71). In addition, different strains of mice infected with *S. mansoni* develop different degrees of hepatic fibrosis that do not correlate with the relative magnitude of the granulomatous response, as determined by granuloma size (73).

Other mechanisms may contribute to fibrosis. Schistosome egg secretions themselves may act directly on fibroblasts to induce collagen synthesis (74). Live schistosome eggs or soluble egg antigen (SEA) cultured with normal human fibroblasts directly stimulated collagen production and decreased collagenase activity.

Like granuloma formation, factors that regulate hepatic fibrogenesis may have important clinical implications. Since only a small subpopulation of individuals infected with *S. mansoni* progress to severe liver fibrosis, spontaneous downregulation may occur in the majority. Those at greatest risk for developing extensive liver fibrosis may have an impaired ability to generate immunoregulatory mechanisms that restrict fibrosis (54). This may be related to genetic background of the individual as suggested by studies of inbred mice (73,75) and the recent finding that increased fibrosis is associated with certain HLA haplotypes in a population endemic for schistosomiasis in Brazil and Egypt (76).

IMMUNITY

During the course of natural infection in fully permissive animal models (mice, baboons) and the semipermissive rat model, acquired immunity develops to reinfection (reviewed in ref. 77). Acquired immunity also develops in chronically infected humans; however, the magnitude and duration of this immunity remain controversial (see below). Although these studies provided an impetus for production of a vaccine, an acceptable candidate vaccine has yet to be developed. This failure in developing a human vaccine results from an inadequate understanding of the mechanisms inducing acquired immunity in humans. Moreover, it has been difficult to extrapolate the multiplicity of immune mechanisms identified in the different animal models to humans.

Immunity in schistosomiasis appears to be CD4+ cell dependent and involves both humoral and cell-mediated responses (78,79). Since eosinophilia and IgG production are major immunologic hallmarks of schistosome infections in humans and in many animal models, it has been postulated that these responses are important effector mechanisms in immunity against parasite worms. However, other effector cells such as neutrophils, platelets, mast cells, and macrophages may participate in parasite killing.

The most completely studied models for schistosome infections are mice. Two forms of acquired immunity have been studied: (a) acquired resistance in the presence of a primary infection and (b) a vaccine model where animals are inoculated with radiation attenuated larvae that die prior to sexual maturation. Infected animals with concomitant immunity resist further infection, but the immune response does not affect established parasites.

In the concomitant immunity model, chronically infected mice develop partial resistance at the onset of egg deposition (80). Immunity requires the presence of adult worms and/or viable eggs. This immunity can be induced by transfer of adult worms to naive mice. However, single-sex infections do not induce immunity in mice (81), further demonstrating the need for the presence of eggs. An immune basis for concomitant immunity is reflected in several observations. Thymectomized mice fail to develop immunity to reinfection (82,83); however, this immunity can be restored by transfer of antibodies from infected mice (84,85). In addition, removal of neutrophils or eosinophils (86) with specific neutralizing monoclonal or polyclonal antibodies, respectively, inhibits concomitant immunity.

Mice vaccinated with irradiated cercariae develop much higher levels of resistance to reinfection (50% to 90%) than occurs with natural infections (79). Resistance to infection is CD4+ cell dependent (87). However, if mice are hyperimmunized with multiple vaccinations, the IgG or IgM fractions of immune serum can transfer resistance to naive mice (87,88). The IgE component in mice has failed to show a role in protective immunity (89). Recent studies in the mouse suggest that Th1-induced responses (IFN-γ) may be important in the development of acquired immunity (20,90). Administration of neutralizing anti-IFN-γ antibodies at 3 to 5 days after challenge resulted in complete abrogation of acquired immunity (91). Later treatment with anti-IFN-γ (at 1 week after challenge) resulted in a small, but significant, reduction in vaccine-induced immunity (92). Based on these studies it was hypothesized that the major site of elimination of parasites after challenge is the lung as schistosomula migrate through the lung 3 to 5 days after skin penetration (93,94).

The role of eosinophils in murine models have been controversial. *In vivo* depletion using a polyvalent antisera demonstrated a role for eosinophils in the development of acquired immunity in mice (86,95). Moreover, antibody-independent cell-mediated immunity appears to play an important role in murine immunity (96). Recent developments in cytokine research have demonstrated that IL-4 and IL-5 are the primary molecules for induction of IgE production and eosinophilia, respectively. Administration of specific neutralizing anti-monoclonal antibodies to each of these cytokines during the course of schistosome infection blocked induction of IgE production or eosinophilia but failed to affect immunity against *S. mansoni* infection in the mouse (92,97). However, IL-4 and IL-5 have effects on immune responses independent of induction of immediate hypersensitivity.

Studies of immunity in humans have been more difficult and initially relied on detailed epidemiologic studies. A striking feature of the epidemiology of schistosomiasis is the linear rise (with increasing age) in both prevalence and intensity of infection, up to the time of early adolescence, after which the average infection intensity and prevalence decline (98,99) (Fig. 7). In an attempt to demonstrate the presence of acquired immunity in humans, passive transfer of immune serum was obtained from infected adults and administered to young children that were either lightly infected or uninfected in hyperendemic

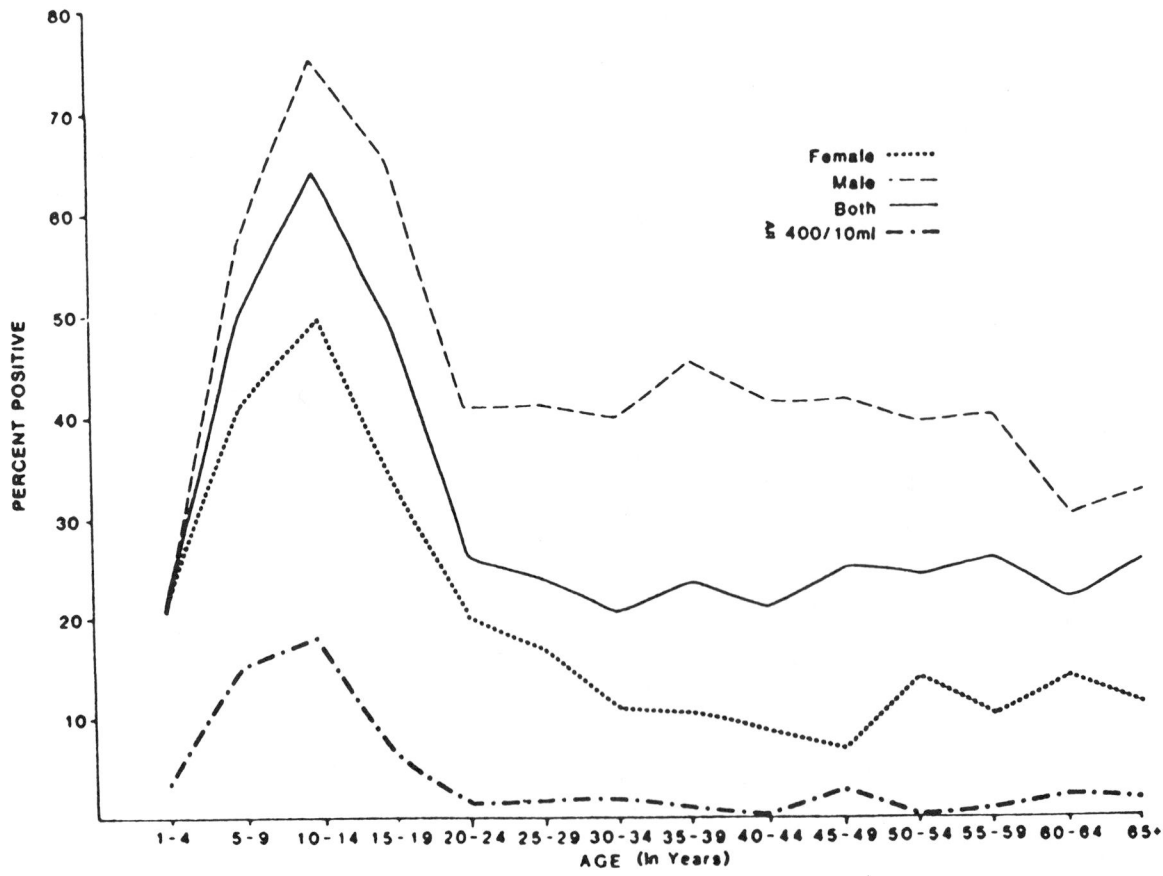

FIG. 7. The prevalence and intensity of infection in 6000 individuals from Upper Egypt endemic for *Schistosoma haematobium*. Heavy infections are considered to have more than 400 eggs per 10 mL of urine.

areas (100,101). The anti-schistosome immunoglobulin neither reduced output of eggs nor prevented the development of new infection in uninfected children. Extensive studies of changes in water contact patterns with age indicate that age and total duration of water exposure are independent predictors of *S. mansoni* infection. These observations have supported the notion that acquired immunity develops with repeated exposure to the parasite. Prospective cohort studies in humans based on evaluating rates of reinfection after parasitologic cure (102–106) provide evidence that acquired immunity develops in humans. Following treatment, the extent to which reinfection subsequently occurs is strongly age dependent. In areas of continued transmission, young children (12 years or less) rapidly become heavily reinfected; in some cases the children develop infections that reach 50% of pretreatment within 1 year. Moreover, children that are heavily infected prior to treatment generally reacquire heavy infections and those with light infections become lightly infected again. In contrast, older children and adults become reinfected, if at all, only at very low intensity.

The components of the human immune response that seem to play a role in host protection remain poorly defined. Studies indicate a variety of effector molecules capable of killing schistosomula *in vitro* primarily by antibody-dependent cell-mediated killing. Macrophages, platelets, neutrophils, and eosinophils all kill schistosomula in the presence of parasite-specific IgG and in some circumstances IgE antibodies (77,107–110). However, these *in vitro* studies may bear little relationship to human immunity *in vivo*. Recent epidemiologic studies demonstrate that serum levels of parasite-specific IgE are higher in immune subjects compared to susceptible individuals (103–105). Conversely, serum parasite-specific IgG4 levels are higher among susceptible individuals (103–105). Since IgG4 recognizes many of the same antigenic epitopes that IgE does, it may act as a blocking antibody to prevent engagement of effector cells coated with IgE (111). Schistosomula-specific IgG2 and IgM antibodies are also higher in sera from susceptible compared to resistant individuals, suggesting that these isotypes may also act as blocking antibodies (112,113). Based on the understanding of immune mechanisms in animal models and humans, efforts are underway to induce resistance against schistosomiasis using defined antigens that could be suitable for human use. Recombinant antigens have been identified that provide levels of protection in experimental animals similar to that produced by irradiation-attenuated cercariae. Five putative vaccine candidate molecules have tentatively been selected by the TDR/World Health Organization Steering Committee on Schistosomiasis Vaccines for human trials (Table 2).

CLINICAL FEATURES

Infection with *S. mansoni* or *S. japonicum* may result in gastrointestinal and/or hepatic disease (1). These manifestations are seen in association with the established chronic stages of infection. Most infections are asymptomatic. Disease is usually appreciated in a small group of infected individuals, usually the young with heavy infection or genetic susceptibility (120). In contrast, individuals from nonendemic areas often present early with signs and symptoms related to acute schistosomiasis (121). Physicians in North America, Europe, and other nonendemic areas also may encounter disease due to established infection in immigrants and rarely in individuals who had casual exposure.

Pathology of the gastrointestinal tract is found in most infected individuals. Eggs of *S. mansoni* are mainly deposited in the veins of the inferior mesenteric system while those of *S. japonicum* are usually seen in the distribution of the superior mesenteric vein. Granuloma formation, subsequent scarring, and occasionally colonic polyposis are the main pathologic features. Clinically, infection may be associated with nonspecific symptoms such as crampy abdominal pain, diarrhea, and passage of blood with stools. In endemic areas, it has been difficult to prove the specificity and causality of these symptoms (3). Colonic polyposis is a specific syndrome described in Egypt (122) but not in other *S. mansoni* endemic areas. Similar lesions have been described in China in association with *S. japonicum* infection. Colonic polyposis may cause bleeding but the association with colorectal carcinoma is not known. In individuals with chronic infection and portal hypertension due to liver fibrosis, porto-systemic varices may develop at the lower end of the esophagus and rectum and around the umbilicus (caput medusa). Esophageal varices may result in considerable bleeding, which may be the first serious manifestation of hepatic schistosomiasis and its hemodynamic sequelae. Usually, patients with schistosomal portal hypertension tolerate several bleeding episodes from esophageal varices without going into hepatic encephalopathy. This is because of the retention of a reasonable oxygenation level of hepatocytes due to arterialization of the blood supply of the liver.

In cases of moderate or heavy exposure, an acute febrile reaction can occur lasting for several days to weeks, which has been referred to as *Katayama fever*. This is most often seen with *S. japonicum* infection and less often with *S. mansoni*. Although rarely reported, similar acute episodes may occur with *S. haematobium* infection. The fever occurs at the time of egg deposition and results from immune complex formation between egg and adult worm

TABLE 2. *Experimental vaccine molecules demonstrated to protect animals from infection*

Molecule	Antigen size	Species studied	Percent protection	Reference
Sm28/GST	28 kDa	Mice, rats, baboons	40%–90%	114
Paramyosin	97 kDa	Mice, baboons	0%–39%	115
Triose phosphate isomerase (TPI)		Mice	32%–48%	116
IrV5	62 kDa	Mice, baboons	25%–75%	117,118
Sm23	23 kDa	Mice	30%–42%	119

antigens that complex with the rapidly rising antibody levels.

Liver disease in schistosomiasis mansoni or japonica represents the major pathological impact (123,124). Schistosome eggs are carried by portal blood flow and become trapped at the presinusoidal level. They are then encircled with granulomas and finally result in fibrosis and its hemodynamic sequelae. The first manifestation of liver disease is hepatomegaly, which may be seen in most individuals with heavy infection as well as in others (3). The association between hepatomegaly and intensity of infection has been repeatedly demonstrated in several endemic areas. It is, however, not an exact association since hepatomegaly in adults is not usually associated with high intensity of infection. With hepatomegaly there is very little change in liver function tests. As fibrosis develops it may take the form of diffuse or clay pipe stem patterns. The nature and dynamics of fibrosis follow a slow course that preserves liver parenchymal architecture and total hepatic blood flow. This occurs because of the shift of total hepatic blood flow from portal to arterial, thus maintaining hepatocyte oxygenation and function. Decompensation occurs late in the course of disease or it may result from additional insults due to viral infections or nutritional deficiencies that lead to hepatic encephalopathy. Portal hypertension is related to presinusoidal obstruction. It results in congestive splenomegaly, ascites (in late stages), and development of porto-systemic varices. Evaluations of these patients may demonstrate normal hepatic wedge pressure. In the late stages of liver disease, enlargement of the organ may not be detected because of extensive fibrosis. In most of these patients, extensive splenomegaly, esophageal varices, and ascites may be appreciated.

Although gastrointestinal manifestations are the predominant features of schistosome infections, other organs are affected. Although *S. haematobium* worms remain in the gastrointestinal tract, the majority of the symptoms occur in the venous plexus surrounding the bladder and ureters where most adult worms live. The ova cause mucosal and submucosal granulomatous lesions of the bladder and ureters. Small papules form on the bladder mucosa and often progress to polyp formation and ulceration, ultimately causing fibrosis, scarring, and calcifications. When granulomas are situated near ureters or the opening of the ureter into the bladder lumen, the inflammation and polyps can cause an obstructive uropathy. This can ultimately lead to hydronephrosis and renal failure. Cancer of the bladder has also been associated with chronic *S. haematobium* infections. Other complications that can occur with any of the schistosome species is pneumonitis, lesions in the cerebrum or spinal cord, and glomerulonephritis. The pneumonitis is associated with a hypersensitivity reaction to larvae as they migrate through the lung. Lesions in the central nervous system can be devastating and result from ova (usually *S. japonicum,* but also *S. mansoni*) deposited in small arterioles that can infarct and cause granulomatous lesions. Transverse myelitis may occur if ova deposit in critical areas of the spinal cord. Renal lesions are common with *S. mansoni* infection. Immune complexes deposit in glomeruli to cause membranoproliferative lesions with focal mesangial thickening and

crescent formation. These lesions do not resolve with treatment.

Other less common schistosome species also infect humans. *Schistosoma intercalatum,* found in Central Africa, causes a milder disease than *S. mansoni* but also involves the large intestine and liver. *Schistosoma mekongi,* found primarily in the Mekong River basin, is related to *S. japonicum* and causes a similar disease but milder. *Schistosoma mattheei* and *S. bovis* are primarily found in animals; however, humans infrequently become infected. *Schistosoma mattheei* generates a similar clinical picture to *S. mansoni,* whereas most patients infected with *S. bovis* (very common in cattle) are asymptomatic, but hematuria has been observed.

DIAGNOSIS AND MANAGEMENT

Individuals suspected of having schistosomal gastrointestinal or hepatic disease should be evaluated for geographic history and duration and intensity of infection. A thorough physical examination and laboratory evaluation are mandatory. Definitive diagnosis depends on demonstrating parasite eggs in stool specimens (Fig. 8). In rare occasions, rectal or liver biopsies may demonstrate the eggs and surrounding granulomatous response. Serologic testing may be helpful, especially in individuals suspected to have schistosomiasis who are living in nonendemic areas. Interpretation of serologic testing in endemic areas is difficult because of the frequent exposure to the parasite. Furthermore, once schistosome eggs are demonstrated in feces, quantification of infection and determination of the viability of eggs are recommended (125).

Chemotherapy of schistosomiasis has undergone tremendous development with the discovery of several effective oral compounds. Currently, praziquantel is the drug of choice (126). For *S. mansoni* infection, 40 mg/kg body weight as a single oral dose is recommended. For *S. japonicum* infection, the dose is increased to 60 mg/kg body weight, given in divided doses. The side effects of praziquantel are minimal and do not usually interfere with the delivery of the drug to individual patients. Praziquantel administration will result in parasitological cure in approximately 80% of cases and an approximately 95% to 99% decrease in fecal egg counts. When given to adolescents and young adults, praziquantel will reverse pathology and diminish hepatomegaly. In patients with chronic sequelae, specific chemotherapy does not reverse pathological lesions. Patients with portal hypertension, esophageal varices, or liver failure are treated with the standard surgical and medical regimens. Care should be taken in prescribing immediate surgical intervention for the first bleeding episode from esophageal varices. These patients usually tolerate several bleeding episodes and do not go into hepatic encephalopathy from one or two hematemesis attacks. Since surgery is associated with major complications and will not reverse the pathological sequences, it should be reserved for selected cases of recurrent bleeding. Recently, introduction of the trans-intrahepatic percutaneous shunt (TIPS) may offer a less invasive ap-

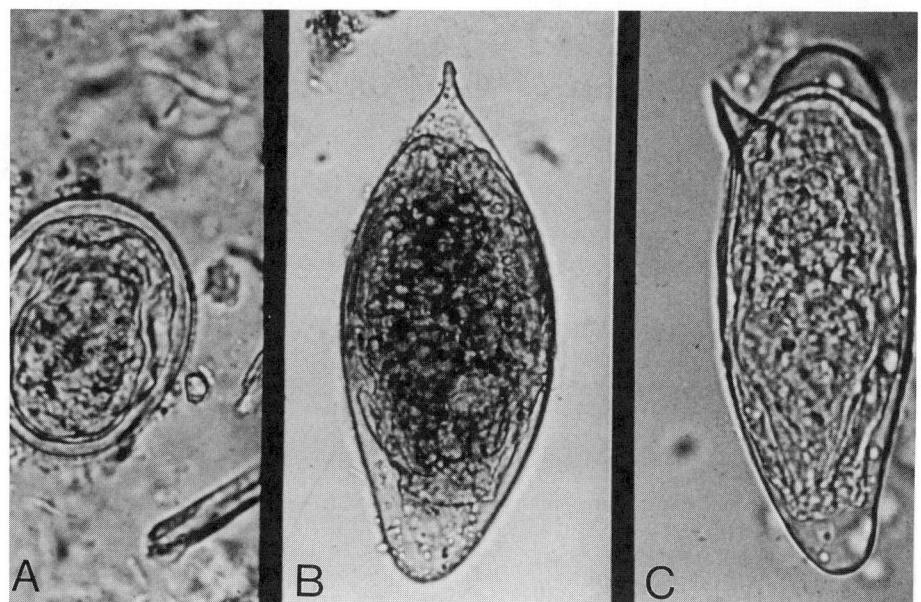

FIG. 8. *Schistosoma japonicum* **(A)**, *S. haematobium* **(B)**, and *S. mansoni* **(C)** ova in the stool or urine. (See Plate 28.)

proach to deal with the consequences of portal hypertension (127).

Prevention and control of schistosomiasis are complex medical, social, and economic problems. For the individual who is traveling to an endemic area, avoidance of contact with freshwater bodies is sufficient. No other practical protective measure exists as yet. When control programs attempted to eradicate infection, very little success was achieved. A more realistic goal may be reduction in transmission and morbidity. This may be accomplished by using targeted chemotherapy (128) and focal molluscidity when appropriate (129). Such approaches have shown good results that can be maintained. The ultimate control strategy should be educational and economic development. An efficacious vaccine would certainly make an impact, but one will not be available in the immediate future.

REFERENCES

1. Mahmoud AAF, Wahab MFA. Schistosomiasis. In: Warren KS, Mahmoud AAF, eds. *Tropical and geographical medicine*, 2nd ed. New York: McGraw-Hill, 1990;458.
2. Wiest PM, Tartakoff AM, Aikawa M, Mahmoud A. Inhibition of surface membrane maturation in schistosomula of *Schistosoma mansoni*. *Proc Natl Acad Sci USA* 1988;85:3825.
3. Arap Siongok TK, Mahmoud AA, Ouma JH, et al. Morbidity in schistosomiasis mansoni in relation to intensity of infection: study of a community in Machakos, Kenya. *Am J Trop Med Hyg* 1976;25:273.
4. Anderson RM, May RM. *Infectious disease of humans: dynamics and control*. Oxford: Oxford University Press, 1991.
5. Von Lichtenberg F. Studies on granuloma formation. III. Antigen sequestration and destruction in the schistosome pseudotubercle. *Am J Pathol* 1964;45:75.
6. Doenhoff M, Hassounah O, Murare H, Bain J, Lucas S. The schistosome egg granuloma: immunopathology is the cause of

host protection or parasite survival? *Trans R Soc Trop Med Hyg* 1986;80:503.
7. Damian R. The exploitation of host immune responses by parasites. *J Parasitol* 1987;73:1.
8. Boros DL, Pelley RP, Warren KS. Spontaneous modulation of granulomatous hypersensitivity in schistosomiasis mansoni. *J Immunol* 1976;114:1437.
9. Olds GR, Olveda R, Tracy JW, Mahoud AAF. Adoptive transfer of modulation of granuloma formation and hepatosplenic disease in murine schistosomiasis japonica by serum from chronically infected animals. *J Immunol* 1982;128:1391.
10. Von Lichtenberg F. Host response to eggs of *S. mansoni*. I. Granuloma formation in the unsensitized laboratory mouse. *Am J Pathol* 1962;41:711.
11. Warren KS, Domingo EO, Cohen RBT. Granuloma formation around schistosome eggs as a manifestation of delayed hypersensitivity. *Am J Pathol* 1967;51:735.
12. Weinstock JV, Boros DL. Heterogeneity of the granulomatous response in the liver, colon, ileum, and ileal Peyer's patches to schistosome eggs in murine schistosomiasis mansoni. *J Immunol* 1981;127:1906.
13. Weinstock JV, Boros DL. Organ-dependent differences in composition and function observed in hepatic and intestinal granulomas isolated from mice with schistosomiasis mansoni. *J Immunol* 1983;130:418.
14. Boros DL, Warren KS. Delayed hypersensitivity-type granuloma formation and dermal reaction induced and elicited by a soluble factor isolated from *Schistosoma mansoni* eggs. *J Exp Med* 1970;132:488.
15. Remick DG, Chensue SW, Hiserodt JC, Higashi GH, Kunkel SL. Flow-cytometric evaluation of lymphocyte subpopulations in synchronously developing *Schistosoma mansoni* egg and Sephadex bead pulmonary granulomas. *Am J Pathol* 1988;131:298.
16. Boros DL, Pelley RP, Warren KS. Spontaneous modulation of granulomatous hypersensitivity in schistosomiasis mansoni. *J Immunol* 1975;114:1437.
17. Colley D. Eosinophils and immune mechanisms. I. Eosinophil stimulation promoter (ESP): a lymphokine induced by specific antigen of phytohemagglutinin. *J Immunol* 1973;110:1419.
18. Owhashi M, Ishii A. Fractionation and characterization of allergens extracted from eggs of *Schistosoma japonicum*. *Int Arch Allergy Appl Immunol* 1981;64:146.

19. Grzych JM, Pearce EJ, Cheeve A, et al. Egg deposition is the major stimulus for the production of Th2 cytokines in murine schistosomiasis mansoni. *J Immunol* 1991;146:1322.

20. Pearce EJ, Caspar P, Grzych J-M, Lewis FA, Sher A. Down-regulation of Th1 cytokine production accompanies induction of Th2 responses by a parasitic helminth, *Schistosoma mansoni*. *J Exp Med* 1991;173:159.

21. Mosmann TR, Cherwinski H, Bond MA, Giedlin I, Coffman RL. Two types of murine helper T cell clones. I. Definition according to the profiles of lymphokine activities and secreted proteins. *J Immunol* 1986;136:2348.

22. Salgame P, Abrams JS, Clayberger C, et al. Differing lymphokine profiles of functional subsets of human CD4 and CD8 T cell clones. *Science* 1991;254:279.

23. Heinzel FP, Sadick MD, Holaday BJ, Coffman RL, Locksley RM. Reciprocal expression of interferon gamma or interleukin 4 during the resolution or progression of murine leishmaniasis. Evidence for expansion of distinct helper T cell subsets. *J Exp Med* 1989;169:59.

24. Sher A, Fiorentino D, Casper P, Pearce E, Mosmann T. Production of IL-10 by CD4+ lymphocytes correlates with down-regulation of Th1 cytokine synthesis in helminth infection. *J Immunol* 1991;147:2713.

25. Chensue SW, Terebuh PD, Warmington KS, et al. Role of IL-4 and IFN-γ in *Schistosoma mansoni* egg-induced hypersensitivity granuloma formation. Orchestration, relative contribution, and relationship to macrophage function. *J Immunol* 1992; 148:900.

26. Yamashita T, Boros DL. IL-4 influences IL-2 production and granulomatous inflammation in murine schistosomiasis mansoni. *J Immunol* 1992;149:3659.

27. Mathew RC, Ragheb S, Boros DL. Recombinant IL-2 therapy reverses diminished granulomatous responsiveness in anti-L3T4, *Schistosoma mansoni*-infected mice. *J Immunol* 1990; 144:4356.

28. Lukas NW, Boros DL. Lymphokine regulation of granuloma formation in murine schistosomiasis mansoni. *Clin Immunol Immunopathol* 1993;68:57.

29. Wynn TA, Eltoum I, Cheever AW, Lewis FA, Gause WC, Sher A. Analysis of cytokine mRNA expression during primary granuloma formation induced by eggs of *Schistosoma mansoni*. *J Immunol* 1993;151:1430.

30. Wynn T, Eltoum I, Oswald I, Cheever A, Sher A. Endogenous interleukin (IL)12 regulates granuloma formation induced by eggs of *Schistosoma mansoni* and exogenous IL-12 both inhibits and prophylactically immunizes against egg pathology. *J Exp Med* 1994;179:1551–1561.

31. Hsieh CS, Macatonia S, Tripp C, Wolf S, O'Garra A, Murphy K. Development of Th1 CD4+ T cells through IL-12 produced by *Listeria*-induced macrophages. *Science* 1993;260:547.

32. Sypek JP, Chung C, Mayor S, et al. Resolution of cutaneous leishmaniasis: interleukin 12 initiates a protective T helper type immune response. *J Exp Med* 1993;177:1797.

33. Chikunguwo S, Kanazawa T, Dayal Y, Stadecker MJ. The cell-mediated response to schistosomal antigens at the clonal level. In vivo functions of cloned murine egg antigen-specific CD4+ T helper type 1 lymphocytes. *J Immunol* 1991;147:3921.

34. Stavitsky AB. Immune regulation in schistosoma japonica. *Immunol Today* 1987;8:228.

35. Boros DL. Granulomatous inflammations. *Prog Allergy* 1978; 24:183.

36. Colley D. Dynamics of the human immune response to schistosomes. In: Mahmoud A, ed. *Clinical tropical medicine and communicable diseases*. London: Bailliere Tindel, 1987;315.

37. Phillips S, Lammie P. Immunopathology of granuloma formation and fibrosis in schistosomiasis. *Parasitol Today* 1986;2: 296.

38. Henderson GS, Conary JT, Summar M, McCurley TL, Colley DG. In vivo molecular analysis of lymphokines involved in the murine immune response during *Schistosoma mansoni* infection. I. IL-4 mRNA, not IL-2 mRNA, is abundant in the granulomatous livers, mesenteric lymph nodes, and spleens of infected mice. *J Immunol* 1991;147:992.

39. Henderson GS, Lu X, McCurley TL, Colley DG. In vivo molecular analysis of lymphokines involved in the murine immune response during *Schistosoma mansoni* infection. II. Quantification of IL-4 mRNA, IFN-gamma mRNA, and IL-2 mRNA levels in the granulomatous livers, mesenteric lymph nodes, and spleens during the course of modulation. *J Immunol* 1992;148: 2261.

40. Olds GR, Stavitsky AB. Mechanism of in vivo modulation of granulomatous inflammation in murine schistosomiasis japonica. *Infect Immun* 1986;52:512.

41. Montesano MA, Freeman J, Gazzinelli G, Colley DG. Expression of cross-reactive, shared idiotypes on anti-SEA antibodies from human and mice with schistosomiasis. *J Immunol* 1990; 145:1002.

42. Olds GR, Kresina TF. Network interactions in *Schistosoma japonicum* infection. Identification and characterization of a serologically distict immunoregulatory auto-antiidiotype antibody population. *J Clin Invest* 1985;76:2338.

43. Chenusue SW, Remick DG, Higashi GI, Boros DL, Kunkel SL. Modulation of murine schistosomiasis by exogenously administered prostaglandins. *Am J Pathol* 1986;125:28.

44. Chensue SW, Warmington KS, Hershey SD, Terebuh PD, Othman M, Kunkel SL. Evolving T cell responses in murine schistosomiasis. Th2 cells mediate secondary granulomatous hypersensitivity and are regulated by CD8+ T cell in vivo. *J Immunol* 1993;151:1391.

45. Weinstock JV. The pathogenesis of granulomatous inflammation and organ injury in schistosomiasis: interactions between the schistosome ova and the host. *Immunol Invest* 1992;21:455.

46. Chensue SW, Otterness IG, Higashi GI, Forsch GS, Kunkel SL. Monokine production by hypersensitivity (*Schistosoma mansoni* egg) and foreign body (Sephadex bead)-type granuloma macrophages: evidence for sequential production of IL-1 and tumor necrosis factor. *J Immunol* 1989;142:1281.

47. Elliot DE, Righthand VF, Boros DL. Characterization of regulatory (interferon α-β) and accessory (LAF-IL-1) monokine activities from liver granuloma macrophages of *Schistosoma mansoni*-infected mice. *J Immunol* 1987;138:2653.

48. Amiri P, Locksley RM, Parslow TG, et al. Tumor necrosis factor-alpha restores granulomas and induces parasite egg-laying in schistosome-infected SCID mice. *Nature* 1992;356:604.

49. Joseph AL, Boros DL. Tumor necrosis factor plays a role in *Schistosoma mansoni* egg-induced granulomatous inflammation. *J Immunol* 1993;151:5461.

50. Lukas NW, Kunkel SL, Strieter RM, Warmington K, Chensue SW. The role of macrophage inflammatory protein 1-alpha in *Schistosoma mansoni* egg-induced granulomatous inflammation. *J Exp Med* 1993;177:1551.

51. Chensue SW, Bienkowski M, Eessalu T, et al. Endogenous IL-1 receptor antagonist protein (IRAP) regulates schistosome egg granuloma formation and the regional lymphoid response. *J Immunol* 1993;151:3654.

52. Ottesen EA, Hiatt RA, Cheever AW, Sotomayor ZR, Neva FA. The acquisition and loss of antigen-specific cellular immune responsiveness in acute and chronic schistosomiasis in man. *Clin Exp Immunol* 1978;33:38.

53. King CL, Nutman TB. Biological role of helper T-cell subsets in helminth infections. *Chem Immunol* 1992;54:136.

54. Colley DG, Garcia AA, Lambertucci JR, et al. Immune responses during human schistosomiasis. XII. Differential responsiveness in patients with hepatosplenic disease. *Am J Trop Med Hyg* 1986;35:793.

55. Doughty BL, Phillips SM. Delayed hypersensitivity granuloma formation around *Schistosoma mansoni* eggs *in vitro*. *J Immunol* 1982;128:30.

56. Goes AM, Gazzinelli G, Rocha R, Katz N, Doughty B. Granulomatous hypersensitivity to *Schistosoma mansoni* egg antigens in human schistosomiasis. III. In vitro granuloma modulation induced by immune complexes. *Am J Trop Med Hyg* 1991; 44:434.

57. Parra JC, Gazzinelli G, Goes A, Rocha R, Colley D, Doughty B. Granulomatous hypersensitivity to *Schistosoma mansoni* egg antigens in human schistosomiasis. II. In vitro granuloma modulation induced by polyclonal idiotypic antibodies. *J Immunol* 1991;147:3949.

58. Warren KS. Pathophysiology and pathogenesis of hepatoplenic schistosomiasis mansoni. *Bull NY Acad Med* 1968;44: 280.

59. Evered DJW. *Fibrosis.* London: Pitman, 1985.

60. Wyler DJ. Schistosomes, fibroblasts, and growth factors: how a worm causes liver scarring. *N Biol* 1991;3:734.

61. Albini A, Adelmann-Grll BC, Muller PK. Fibroblast chemotaxis. *Cool Relat Res* 1985;5:283–286.

62. Procop DJ, Kivirikko KI, Tuderman L, Guzman NA. The biosynthesis of collagen and its disorders. *N Engl J Med* 1979; 301:77.

63. Grimaud JA, Boros DL, Takiya C, Mathew RC, Emonard H. Collagen isotypes, laminin, and fibronectin in granulomas of the liver and intestines of *Schistosoma mansoni*-infected mice. *Am J Trop Med Hyg* 1987;37:335.

64. Olds GR, El Meneza S, Mahmoud AAF, Kresina TF. Differential immunoregulation of granulomatous inflammation, portal hypertension, and hepatic fibrosis in murine schistosomiasis mansoni. *J Immunol* 1989;142:3605.

65. Marcos S, Khayyal M, Mansour M, et al. Reversal of hepatic fibrosis after praziquantel therapy of murine schistosomiasis. *Am J Trop Med Hyg* 1985;34:314.

66. Olds G, Griffith A, Kresina T. Dynamics of collagen accumulation and polymorphism in murine *Schistosoma japonicum*. *Gastroenterology* 1985;89:617.

67. Al Adnani M. Concomitant immunohistochemical localization of fibronectin and collagen in schistosome granuloma. *J Pathol* 1985;147:663.

68. Cheever AW, Byram JE, von Lichtenberg F. Immunopathology of *Schistosoma japonicum* infection in athymic mice. *Parasite Immunol* 1985;7:387.

69. Czaja MJ, Weiner FR, Flander KC, et al. In vitro and in vivo association of transforming growth factor-β1 with hepatic fibrosis. *J Cell Biol* 1989;108:2477.

70. Czaja MJ, Weiner FR, Takahashi S, et al. γ-Interferon treatment inhibits collagen deposition in murine schistosomiasis. *Hepatology* 1989;10:795.

71. Prakash S, Wyler DJ. Fibroblast stimulation in schistosomiasis. XII. Identification of CD4 + lymphocytes within schistosomal egg granulomas as a source of an apparently novel fibroblast growth factor (FsF-1). *J Immunol* 1992;11:3583.

72. Prakash S, Wyler DJ. Fibroblast stimulation in schistosomiasis. XI. Purification to apparent homogeneity of fibroblast-stimulating factor-1, an acidic heparin-binding growth factor produced by schistosomal egg granulomas. *J Immunol* 1991;146:1679.

73. Cheever AW, Duvall RH, Hallack TA Jr. Differences in hepatic fibrosis and granuloma size in several strains of mice infected with *Schistosoma japonicum*. *Am J Trop Med Hyg* 1984;33: 602.

74. Boros DL, Lande MA. Induction of collagen synthesis in cultured human fibroblasts by live *Schistosoma mansoni* eggs and soluble egg antigens (SEA). *Am J Trop Med Hyg* 1983;32:78.

75. Cheever A, Duvall R, Hallack TJ, Minker R, Malley J, Malley K. Variation of hepatic fibrosis and granuloma size among mouse strains infected with *Schistosoma mansoni*. *Am J Trop Med Hyg* 1987;37:85.

76. Dessein AJ, Couissinier P, Demeure C, et al. Environmental, genetic and immunological factors in human resistance to *Schistosoma mansoni*. *Immunol Invest* 1992;21:423.

77. Capron A, Dessaint JP, Capron M, Ouma JH, Butterworth AE. Immunity to schistosomes: progress toward vaccine. *Science* 1987;238:1065.

78. McLaren DJ, Smithers SR. The immune response to schistosomes in experimental hosts. In: Rollinson D, Simpson AJG, eds. *The biology of schistosomes: from genes to latrines.* London: Academic Press, 1987;233.

79. McLaren D. Will the real target of immunity to schistosomiasis please stand up. *Parasitol Today* 1989;5:279.

80. Smithers SR, Simpson AJ, Yi X, Omer-Ali P, Kelly C, McLaren DJ. The mouse model of schistosome immunity. *Acta Trop Suppl* 1987;12:21.

81. Bickle Q, Bain J, McGregor A, Doenhoff M. Factors affecting the acquisition of resistance against *Schistosoma mansoni* in the mouse: III. The failure of primary infections with cercariae of one sex to induce resistance to reinfection. *Trans R Soc Trop Med Hyg* 1979;73:37.

82. Doenhoff M, Long E. Factors affecting the acquisition of resistance against *Schistosoma mansoni* in the mouse. IV. The inability of T-cell-deprived mice to resist reinfection, and other in vivo studies on the mechanisms of resistance. *Parasitology* 1979;78:171.

83. Doenhoff MJ, Leuchars E, Kerbel RS, Wallis V, Davies AJ. Adult and pre-adult thymectomy of mice: contrasting effects on immune responsiveness, and on numbers of mitogen-responsive and Thy-1 + lymphocytes. *Immunology* 1979;37:397.

84. Sher A, Smithers SR, Mackenzie P. Passive transfer of acquired resistance to *Schistosoma mansoni* in laboratory mice. *Parasitology* 1975;3:347.

85. Sher A, Smithers SR, MacKenzie P, Broomfield K. *Schistosoma mansoni*: immunoglobulins involved in passive immunization of laboratory mice. *Exp Parasitol* 1977;41:160.

86. Mahmoud AA, Warren KS, Peters PA. A role for the eosinophil in acquired resistance to *Schistosoma mansoni* infection as determined by antieosinophil serum. *J Exp Med* 1975;142:805.

87. Kelly EA, Colley DG. In vivo effects of monoclonal anti-L3T4 antibody on immune responsiveness of mice infected with *Schistosoma mansoni*. Reduction of irradiated cercariae-induced resistance. *J Immunol* 1988;140:2737.

88. Mangold BL, Dean DA. Passive transfer with serum and IgG antibodies of irradiated cercariae-induced resistance against *Schistosoma mansoni* in mice. *J Immunol* 1986;136:2644.

89. Sher A, Correa-Oliveira R, Hieny S, Hussain R. Mechanisms of protective immunity against *Schistosoma mansoni* infection in mice vaccinated with irradiated cercariae. IV. Analysis of the role of IgE antibodies and mast cells. *J Immunol* 1983;131: 1460.

90. Sher A, Coffman RL. Regulation of immunity to parasites by T cells and T cell-derived cytokines. *Annu Rev Immunol* 1992; 10:385.

91. Smythies LE, Coulson PS, Wilson RA. Monoclonal antibody to IFN-gamma modifies pulmonary inflammatory responses and abrogates immunity to *Schistosoma mansoni* in mice vaccinated with attenuated cercariae. *J Immunol* 1992;149:3654.

92. Sher A, Coffman RL, Hieny S, Cheever AW. Ablation of eosinophil and IgE responses with anti-IL-5 or anti-IL-4 antibody fails to affect immunity against *Schistosoma mansoni* in the mouse. *J Immunol* 1990;145:3911.

93. Coulson PS, Smythies LE, Wilson RA. Functional and phenotypic properties of the CD4 + T cell population in a murine pulmonary delayed-type hypersensitivity response. *Chest* 1993;103 (Suppl. 2):S138.

94. Mountford AP, Coulson PS, Pemberton RM, Smythies LE, Wilson RA. The generation of interferon-gamma-producing T lymphocytes in skin-draining lymph nodes, and their recruitment to the lungs, is associated with protective immunity to *Schistosoma mansoni*. *Immunology* 1992;75:250.

95. Mahmoud AA, Warren KS, Graham R Jr. Antieosinophil serum and the kinetics of eosinophilia in schistosomiasis mansoni. *J Exp Med* 1975;142:560.

96. James SL, Sher A. Cell-mediated immune response to schistosomiasis. *Curr Top Microbiol Immunol* 1990;155:21.

97. Sher A, Coffman RL, Hieny S, Scott P, Cheever AW. Interleukin 5 is required for the blood and tissue eosinophilia but not granuloma formation induced by infection with *Schistosoma mansoni*. *Proc Natl Acad Sci USA* 1990;87:61.

98. Clarke VDV. Evidence of the development in man of acquired resistance to infection of *Schistosoma* spp. *Cent Afr J Med* 1966;12:1.

99. King CL, Miller FD, Hussein M, Barkat R, Monto AS. Prevalence and intensity of *Schistosoma haematobium* infection in six villages of upper Egypt. *Am J Trop Med Hyg* 1982;31:320.

100. Warren KS, Cook JA, Jordan P. Passive transfer of immunity in human schistosomiasis mansoni: effect of hyperimmune antischistosome gamma globulin on early established infections. *Trans R Soc Trop Med Hyg* 1972;66:65.

101. Cook JA, Warren KS, Jordan P. Passive transfer of immunity in human schistosomiasis mansoni: attempt to prevent infection

by repeated injections of hyperimmune antischistosome gamma globulin. *Trans R Soc Trop Med Hyg* 1972;66:777.

102. Hagan P, Blumenthal UJ, Chaudri M. Resistance to reinfection with *Schistosoma haematobium* in Gambian children: analysis of their immune responses. *Trans R Soc Trop Med Hyg* 1987; 81:938.

103. Hagan P, Blumenthal UJ, Dunn D, Simpson AJG, Wilkins HA. Human IgE, IgG4 and resistance to reinfection with *Schistosoma haematobium*. *Nature* 1991;349:243.

104. Rihet P, Demeure CE, Dessein AJ, Bourgois A. Strong serum inhibition of specific IgE correlated to competing IgG4, revealed by a new methodology in subjects from a *S. mansoni* endemic area. *Eur J Immunol* 1992;22:2063.

105. Dunne DW, Butterworth AE, Fulford AJC, et al. Immunity after treatment of human schistosomiasis: association between IgE antibodies to adult worm antigens and resistance to reinfection. *Eur J Immunol* 1992;22:1483.

106. Wilkins HA, Blumenthal UJ, Hagan P, Hayes RJ. Tulloch S. Resistance to reinfection after treatment of urinary schistosomiasis. *Trans R Soc Trop Med Hyg* 1987;81:29.

107. Capron A, Dessaint J, Capron M, Bazin H. Specific IgE antibodies in immune adherence of normal macrophages to *Schistosoma mansoni* schistosomules. *Nature* 1975;253:474.

108. Capron A, Dessaint JP, Capron M, Joseph M, Torpier G. Effector mechanisms of immunity to schistosomes and their regulation. *Immunol Rev* 1982;61:41.

109. Capron M, Spiegelberg HL, Prin L, et al. Role of IgE receptors in effector function of human eosinophils. *J Immunol* 1984;132: 462.

110. Capron M, Capron A. Effector functions of eosinophils in schistosomiasis. *Mem Inst Oswaldo Cruz* 1992;4:167.

111. Hussain R, Ottesen EA. IgE responses in human filariasis. IV. Parallel antigen recognition by IgE and IgG4 subclass antibodies. *J Immunol* 1986;136:1859.

112. Butterworth AE, Dunne DW, Fulford AJC, et al. Immunity in human schistosomiasis: cross-reactive IgM and IgG2 antibodies block the expression of immunity. *Biochimie* 1988;70: 1053–1063.

113. Butterworth AE, Bensted-Smith R, Capron A, et al. Immunity in human schistosomiasis: prevention by blocking antibodies of the expression of immunity in young children. *Parasitology* 1987;94:281–300.

114. Capron A, Dessaint JP, Capron M, Pierce RJ. Vaccine strategies against schistosomiasis. *Immunobiology* 1992;184:282.

115. Pearce EJ, James SL, Hieny S, Lanar DE, Sher A. Induction of protective immunity against *Schistosoma mansoni* by vaccination with schistosome paramyosin (Sm97), a nonsurface parasite antigen. *Proc Natl Acad Sci USA* 1988;85:5678.

116. Shoemaker C, Gross A, Geremichael A, Harn D. cDNA cloning and functional expression of the *Schistosoma* mansoni protective antigen triose phosphate isomerase. *Proc Natl Acad Sci USA* 1992;89:1842.

117. Soisson L, Masterson C, Tom T, McNally M, Lowell G, Strand M. Induction of protective immunity in mice using a 62-kDa recombinant fragment of a *Schistosoma mansoni* surface antigen. *J Immunol* 1992;149:3612.

118. Soisson L, Reid G, Farah I, Nyindo M, Strand M. Protective immunity in baboons vaccinated with a recombinant antigen or radiation-attenuated cercarae of *Schistosoma mansoni* is antibody-dependent. *J Immunol* 1993;151:4782.

119. Richter D, Reynolds S, Harn D. Candidate vaccine antigens that stimulate the cellular immune response of mice vaccinated with irradiated cercariae of *Schistosoma mansoni*. *J Immunol* 1993;151:256.

120. Abdel-Salam E, Khalik A, Abdel-Meguid A, Barakat W, Mahmoud A. Association of HLA class I antigens (A1, B5, B8 and CW2) with disease manifestations and infection in human schistomiasis in Egypt. *Tissue Antigens* 1986;27:142.

121. Lambertucci JR. Acute schistosomiasis: clinical, diagnostic and therapeutic features. *Ref Inst Med Trop Sao Paulo* 1983; 35:399–404.

122. Abdel-Wahab MF, Mahmoud AAF. Schistosomiasis mansoni in Egypt. In: Mahmoud AAF, ed. *Baillière's clinical tropical medicine and communicable diseases* vol 2. London: Baillière Tindall, 1987;371.

123. Prata A. Schistosomiasis mansoni in Barzil. In: Mahmoud AAF, ed. *Baillière's clinical tropical medicine and communicable diseases,* vol 2. London: Baillière Tindall, 1987;349.

124. Olveda RM, Domingo EO. Schistosomiasis japonica. In: Mahmoud AAF, ed. *Baillière's clinical tropical medicine and communicable diseases,* vol 2. London: Baillière Tindall, 1987;397.

125. Peters PA, Kazura JW. Update on diagnostic methods for schistosomiasis. In: Mahmoud AAF, ed. *Baillière's clinical medicine and communicable diseases,* vol 2. London: Baillière Tindall, 1987;419.

126. King CH, Mahmoud AAF. Drugs five years later: praziquantel. *Ann Intern Med* 1989;110:290.

127. Adams L, Soulen MC. TIPS: a new alternative for the variceal bleeder. *Am J Crit Care* 1993;2:196.

128. Mahmoud AAF, Siongok TK, Arp Ouma J, et al. Effect of targeted mass treatment on intensity of infection and morbidity in schistosomiasis mansoni: 3-year follow-up of a community in Machakos, Kenya. *Lancet* 1983;16:849–851.

129. *Control of schistosomiasis. A report of a WHO expert committee.* Technical Report Series #728. Geneva: WHO, 1985.

Infections of the Gastrointestinal Tract,
edited by M. J. Blaser, P. D. Smith, J. I. Ravdin,
H. B. Greenberg, and R. L. Guerrant
Raven Press, Ltd., New York © 1995.

CHAPTER 81

Use of the Bacteriology and Mycology Laboratories to Diagnose Gastrointestinal Infections

Patricia A. Mickelsen and Lucy S. Tompkins

This chapter has been organized to be useful to the clinician, particularly at the time of the initial assessment of the patient suspected of having a gastrointestinal (GI) tract infection, and to the microbiologist. An overview of laboratory methods employed to identify bacteria and fungi is provided in the context of the clinical presentation and other clinical or epidemiological features that suggest a particular microbiological differential diagnosis. Additional references (1–10) and chapters in this book should be consulted for more comprehensive discussion. This organization has limitations in that most infectious agents may also cause infections that defy the norm. The importance of communicating clinical information to the laboratory by the clinician and the equally important role of the laboratory in making certain that the list of microorganisms that the laboratory routinely identifies, as compared with those that require a special request, is underscored. Emphasis is also placed on specimen collection and transport to the laboratory. Some fastidious bacterial pathogens may not survive when the collection or transport system is suboptimal, and since the majority of infectious disease agents affecting the GI tract are identified by culture methods, the appropriate diagnosis may depend on compliance with the laboratory's requirement. In most instances specimens are not collected by physicians per se; therefore, the clinician must consider inadequate handling of the specimen as a possibility to account for a negative culture result.

The etiology of only a portion of cases of sporadic acute gastroenteritis can be identified even when extensive testing for a wide variety of known infectious agents is performed. The incidence of disease, as well as the spectrum of viral, parasitic, or bacterial agents implicated in infections, varies in different populations depending on age, geographic area, sanitary conditions, and other risk factors. Bacterial pathogens generally account for one third to one half of infections of known etiology (11–13).

Culture of fecal material is often the means by which diagnosis is made. Culture methodology is slow (frequently 48–72 hr) in generating clinically relevant information, and it is also labor and reagent-intensive, and thus expensive. Currently only about one half of the bacteria that are etiological agents of GI illness routinely are sought by even the more sophisticated clinical laboratories (Table 1). Molecular methods based on detection of specific DNA or RNA sequences have provided very sensitive and specific means to identify many of the enteric organisms not routinely cultivated in the laboratory. However, at the present time these methods are primarily used as epidemiological tools and are rarely offered by clinical laboratories because of the additional expense in material and labor costs incurred. Molecular technology is evolving and methods will increasingly be incorporated into diagnostic laboratories as procedures become more sensitive, more practical, and less expensive. We have included a section that briefly summarizes principles of some molecular methods used in diagnosis and epidemiology. In both developed and developing countries there is increasing emphasis on the practice of cost-effective laboratory medicine. We have therefore included some simple, inexpensive procedures that may be useful for the identification of pathogens.

P. A. Mickelsen: Clinical Microbiology Laboratory, Stanford University Hospital, and Division of Infectious Diseases and Geographic Medicine, Department of Medicine, Stanford University, Stanford, California 94305.

L. S. Tompkins: Clinical Microbiology Laboratory, Stanford University Hospital, and Division of Infectious Diseases and Geographic Medicine, and Departments of Medicine and Microbiology and Immunology, Stanford University, Stanford, California 94305.

TABLE 1. *Availability of laboratory studies for bacterial pathogens associated with diarrheal syndromes*

Syndrome	Risk factors	Bacterial or fungal agents	Specimens for lab evaluation[a–c]	Availability of testing, comments
Food Poisoning				
Nausea, vomiting, diarrhea (toxin-mediated)	Colonized food handler—poor refrigeration (ham, meat, poultry, cream-filled pastry)	*S. aureus*	Diagnosis usually clinical. Stool Vomitus Food (Special studies by public health labs)	Public health labs: quantitative culture, strain typing, and/or toxin testing in outbreaks
	Reheated rice, cereals	*B. cereus* (emetic form)		
	Soups, custards, meatloaf	*B. cereus* (diarrheal form)		
	Cooked meats held at improper temperature (cooked meat, poultry, gravy, stew)	*C. perfringens*		
Paralysis	Anaerobic conditions in food processing; home-made preserved food	*C. botulinum*	Stool Vomitus Serum (gastric aspirates) (Special studies by public health labs)	Public health labs will perform culture or toxin testing with appropriate history and symptoms
Diarrhea				
Dysentery (infammatory)	Poor santiation, travel; day care institutions	*Shigella*	Stool culture Fecal leukocytes	Organism detected in routine stool culture
	Poultry, water, raw milk	*Campylobacter jejuni*		
	Poultry, beef, eggs, and other foods	*Salmonella*		
	Developing countries	Enteroinvasive *E. coli* (EIEC)	Stool (special studies)	Assays currently not available in diagnostic labs. DNA probe or PCR on fecal sample or *E. coli* isolates
Pseudoappendicitis (mesenteric adenitis	Ingestion undercooked pork sausage, chitterlings, contaminated water	*Yersinia entercolytica* (*Y. pseudotuberculosis*)	Stool (rule out *Yersinia*) Lymph node	Inquire; some labs routinely culture for *Yersinia*, others upon request only
Enteric fever (systemic)	In typhoid endemic area Immunocompromised/ HIV	*S. typhi* *S. paratyphi* *S. choleraguis* *Salmonella enteritidis* *Salmonella species*	Stool Blood × 3 Urine Bone marrow	Routinely cultured
		Campylobacter fetus	Blood × 3 (special culture studies)	May require blind stains and subculture to detect in blood cultures. Notify lab
Hemorrhagic grossly bloody stools (hemolytic-uremic syndrome)	Undercooked ground beef	Enterohemorrhagic *E. coli* (EHEC)	Stool (special studies)	Inquire; only some laboratories routinely culture for 0157:H7 serotype. DNA probe, PCR or toxin assay for other verotoxin producing *E. coli* not routinely available
			Fecal verotoxin	Verotoxin assay is more sensitive and specific than culture, but not usually available in diagnostic labs
	Poultry, etc.	*C. jejuni*	Stool Culture	Gross blood seen occasionally. Routinely cultured
Mixed inflammatory or secretory diarrhea (often has WBC/RBC)	Marine exposure, shellfish ingestion	*V. paraherolytics* *Vibrio* species	Stool Culture (rule out *Vibrio*)	Notify lab to culture for vibrios

TABLE 1. *Continued*

Syndrome	Risk factors	Bacterial or fungal agents	Specimens for lab evaluation[a–c]	Availability of testing, comments
Mixed inflammatory or secretory diarrhea (continued)	Tropical countries Shellfish, marine exposure	*Plesiomonas* *Aeromonas*	Stool culture (special studies?)	Inquire; some labs routinely culture for these organisms if predominant flora; otherwise request
	Nosocomial Recent antibiotics Nursing home	*C. difficile*	Stool for *C. difficile* toxin	ELISA assay usually used. May need to specifically request cytotoxin, assay in limited circumstances
			Stool culture: usually reserved for epidemiologic investigation	Not performed by most labs because of poor specificity. (*C. difficile* may be present in absence of disease)
Watery-secretory diarrhea	Cholera epidemic area; ingestion of seafood, shellfish from endemic area	*V. cholera* 01	Stool Culture (rule out *Vibrio*)	Outside cholera epidemic areas request special culture for *Vibrio* sp. Agglutination or ELISA on feces may be available.
	Ingestion of shellfish, marine exposure	*V. cholera* non-01	Stool (rule out *Vibrio*)	Request culture for *Vibrio* sp.
		Aeromonas (*Plesiomonas*)		Inquire; routinely detected by only some labs. Optimum detection requires special media
	Children in developing countries Travelers to developing countries	Enterotoxigenic *E. coli* (ETEC)	Stool (special studies)	Assays currently not available in diagnostic labs. DNA probe, PCR or ELISA on stool or *E. coli* isolates
		(*Salmonella*) (*Shigella*) (*C. jejuni*)		Routinely cultured
Persistent diarrhea	Developing countries: infants	Enteroaggregative *E. coli* (AggEC)	Stool (special studies)	Tissue culture attachment bioassay. Not currently for diagnostic use (DNA probe or amplification?)
		Enteropathogenic *E. coli* (EPEC)	Stool (special studies)	Inquire; assays not routinely available in many laboratories. Often problems with specificity of serogrouping. DNA probe, amplification, tissue culture bioassay in reference labs. Contact public health for possible outbreak
	Elderly men—Whipples' disease	*Tropheryma whippelii*	Small bowel biopsy: histopathology	DNA probe or PCR not routinely available. Bacteria cannot be cultured
	HIV/AIDS	*Chlamydia trachomatis*	Rectal swab/biopsy (*Chlamydia*)	Culture or FA for *Chlamydia*
		Mycobacterium avium-intracellular	AFB blood culture Biopsy lesion: histopathology and AFB smear and culture on tissue Stool—AFB smear	Studies routinely available[c]
		(*C. difficile*) (*C. jejuni*) (*Salmonella*) (*Shigella*)	See above	

continues

TABLE 1. *Continued*

Syndrome	Risk factors	Bacterial or fungal agents	Specimens for lab evaluation[a–c]	Availability of testing, comments
Persistent diarrhea (continued)				
	Underlying GI problems	Bacterial overgrowth	Aspirate of upper small bowel for quantitative aerobic and anaerobic culture	Available only in some labs
Evidence of systemic disease: pain, abdominal and other lesions	Immunocompromised HIV	*P. brasilienis* (S. America) *H. capsulatum*	Biopsy lesion: Fungal culture and histopathology on tissue	Studies routinely available. Notify lab if histoplasmosis suspected
		M. avium-intracellulare	See above	
	Gumma	*T. pallidum*	Biopsy for histopathology Syphillis serology	Routinely available
Proctitis	Rectal Intercourse	*N. gonorrhea*	Rectal swab or biopsy for *N. gonorrhea* culture	Routinely available
		C. trachomatis	Rectal swab or biopsy for *Chlamydia* culture or FA	Routinely available
		T. pallidum	Syphilis serology. Biopsy for histopathology. Darkfield or FA	Routinely available. Darkfield may be difficult to interpret and, if negative, serology should be done.
Esophagitis	Immunocompromised HIV/AIDS	*Candida albicans*	Biopsy KOH and histopathology	Routinely available
Gastritis or Peptic Ulcer Disease		*Heliobacter pylori*	Biopsy: histopathology Urease assay	Some labs perform cultures. However, other tests are adequate unless susceptibility testing is indicated

[a] Stool samples are preferable to rectal swabs. Specimens should be cultured within 2 hr. If longer delay is anticipated, select portions of stool with pus, mucus, or blood; emulcify in fecal transport medium, and refrigerate. Rectal swabs should be immediately placed in fecal transport medium. Even for samples in transport medium, delays in culturing compromise recovery of most bacterial enteropathogens and should be avoided.

[b] Smears for fecal leukocytes are rapid, inexpensive, and may suggest possible etiologies.

[c] Acid-fast stain of stool will detect mycobacteria. *Cryptosporidium, Isospora,* and *Cyclospora* also may be detected; however, concentration and staining methods for optimum detection of these organisms by parasitology labs are different from those used for mycobacteria.

COMMUNICATION BETWEEN THE LABORATORY AND THE CLINICIAN

Exchange of relevant information is essential to good patient care, is required for cost-effective practice of medicine, and is a responsibility of both the clinician and the laboratory. As obvious as this might seem, communication failures may account for a significant proportion of instances in which patients are not optimally managed and unnecessary costs are incurred. Clinicians need to be aware of the spectrum of organisms routinely detected by the laboratory(ies) to which they send specimens for routine stool culture. The culture report should indicate not only enteric pathogens that were present in the specimen but also specify those microorganisms that are routinely screened but were found to be absent. Physicians need to notify the laboratory when the patient history or clinical presentation suggests an etiology that would re-

quire special procedures. For example, many laboratories do not routinely use selective media for isolation of *Vibrio* sp. but should be prepared to do so when informed that the patient has a history of travel to an endemic area or has ingested potentially contaminated shellfish or seafood. Laboratory request slips or computer order forms should solicit such information. Laboratories should expedite testing and reporting of significant results to the clinician and public health authorities to ensure that this information can be of maximum benefit to patient management and community infection control efforts.

The current cost of a positive stool culture in developed countries where prevalence of enteric pathogens is low is approximately $1000 when expense for all samples tested are considered (12,14–16). Laboratory workup of a single specimen from an intraabdominal source that contains several aerobes and anaerobes and that involves procedures for isolation, identification, and susceptibility testing costs several hundred dollars. Thus, efforts to promote cost effective utilization of laboratory resources have increasingly resulted in rejection of test requests that are usually not appropriate. Examples include policies not to perform stool culture for conventional pathogens if the patient has been hospitalized for more than 3 days, to reject samples that are not diarrheal (e.g., formed stool), or to reject multiple samples collected on the same day (14,17,18). Specimens for anaerobic culture that may be contaminated with flora of mucosal surfaces or have not been transported properly will be rejected for culture (1,6). In most instances, these policies have successfully decreased unnecessary or inappropriate testing; however, important and legitimate exceptions must be respected.

Accurate diagnosis of infections by communicable enteric pathogens is important not only to the clinician and patient but also to the community. Communication and cooperativity between physicians, public health laboratories, and diagnostic laboratories is essential to ensure that communicable diseases can be promptly diagnosed and, when necessary, public health interventions initiated. The mission and resource of diagnostic laboratories and public health laboratories are different. Diagnostic laboratories usually are not equipped or staffed to investigate community-based outbreaks of GI disease or to perform studies to evaluate cases of toxin-mediated food poisoning. Most diagnostic laboratories refer cultures of enteric pathogens to public health laboratories for purposes of confirmation and notification, and notification of certain species is required in most states. Diagnostic laboratories also may depend on public health laboratories to test for unusual agents for diagnostic purposes.

OVERVIEW OF METHODS FOR LABORATORY DIAGNOSIS

Culture

Culture methods extract and amplify bacteria present in clinical material by inoculation of the material onto a growth medium and incubation. Most *Enterobacteriaceae* have short generation times (10–15 min) and within a period of 18–24 hr one bacterial cell will have divided to produce $>10^8$ progeny, which are visible as colonies on solid medium or turbidity in broth. Selective media that often contain inhibitory substances such as antibiotics are used to suppress growth of some species likely to be present in a sample while enabling amplification of other potential pathogens. Differential media contain various substrates and color indicators, and metabolic activity of organisms has traditionally been an important means of identification. Technologists can often presumptively identify organisms based on Gram stain, growth, and colony morphology on selective or differential media within 18 hr after a specimen has been obtained. Unfortunately, this information is not often conveyed in preliminary culture reports.

Identification of organisms is usually based on phenotypic characteristics such as presence of enzymes and metabolic profiles or, occasionally, on the basis of charac-

teristic antigens detected with immunological reagents and can usually be completed within 4–18 hr, depending on the need to incubate tests. Commercial identification systems that are used by many laboratories are essentially miniaturized versions of a battery of conventional biochemical tests composed of small wells or cupules containing dehydrated substrates into which a liquid suspension of colonial growth is inoculated. After incubation, the pattern of positive reactions for various substrates in the battery is read, either manually or by instrumentation; this information is then translated into a code number consisting of several digits. An identification database that correlates each species with a particular biocode is then accessed to produce a species identification based on probability calculations. Supplemental tests may be indicated if the probability of identification is low. In some cases, commercial database systems may provide incorrect identification, although, overall, widespread use of commercial systems has standardized and greatly improved the accuracy of identification. Various systems may employ automated or semiautomatic reading and interface with laboratory computer systems. Continuous automated reading and use of modified substrates, such as those linked to fluorogenic compounds, may reduce time for identification to several hours. Pure cultures are required for identification and susceptibility testing. Therefore delays may be expected in cultures that contain numerous organisms, which is often the case with intraabdominal or wound infections, because of the need to isolate each organism prior to further testing. Some organisms, particularly anaerobes, fastidious organisms, fungi, and mycobacteria, simply do not grow quickly, and therefore both detection and additional testing may take much longer than the 24–48 hr required for identification and susceptibility determination of most common bacterial pathogens.

Because traditional culture methods are slow, Gram stain of clinical material that has a sensitivity of detecting $\approx 10^4$–10^5 bacteria/mL remains a useful rapid test. Often material from infections contains very high numbers of organisms, and reading of smears by skilled technologists can often provide presumptive identification to genus level based on appearance of organisms in the Gram stain. When possible presumptive identification of organisms seen in smears should be conveyed in laboratory reports.

Susceptibility Testing

Resistance to antibiotics of choice for treatment of many GI tract infections is increasingly a problem (19). Clinicians rely on these test results but often have questions about test limitations. Reference methods for determination of antibiotic susceptibility are agar and broth dilution procedures. These are standardized procedures in which a suspension of organisms is inoculated onto agar plates or into broth media in either tubes or microtiter plate wells that contain twofold dilutions of antibiotic. After incubation, usually overnight, the lowest concentration (μg/mL) of antibiotic that inhibits growth is reported as the minimum inhibitory concentration (MIC). Organisms are reported as susceptible, moderately susceptible, intermediate, or resistant to antibiotic based on interpretative breakpoints. In the United States interpretative guidelines for susceptibility recommended by the National Committee for Laboratory Standards (20,21) are usually used. In general, organisms categorized as susceptible can be successfully treated using doses of antibiotic recommended for systemic infections due to the species. Often the MIC of organisms classified as susceptible is one half to one fourth of achievable peak serum level of antibiotic using parenteral dosage. Obviously different levels of active antibiotic are achieved at various body sites including gut, urine, or intraabdominal abcess and depend on the dose, route of administration, and a number of other pharmacokinetic parameters. Whether these criteria used for systemic infections are also appropriate for many enteropathogens has not been established. When tested repeatedly the MICs for any given isolate may vary plus or minus one twofold dilution because of inherent imprecision of the test. Organisms that have MICs close to the interpretive breakpoints may on sequential testing be classified differently although the difference is usually only between susceptible and intermediate (or moderately susceptible) or resistant and intermediate (or moderately susceptible).

Disk diffusion (22) testing is commonly used in many laboratories for susceptibility testing because it is relatively inexpensive, simple, flexible, and usually provides adequate information for clinical management decisions. The test is standardized and involves inoculating the surface of Mueller–Hinton agar with a suspension of organism, dropping on paper disks containing appropriate concentration of antibiotic, incubating the plates overnight, and measuring diameter of zones of growth inhibition around each antibiotic disk. For rapidly growing nonfastidious organisms such as the Enterobacteriaceae, there is good correlation between MIC and zone size, which enables zone diameters to be translated into susceptible or resistant categories. This procedure has not been validated for fastidious organisms such as *Campylobacter* species, or for organisms such as *Yersinia* and *Vibrio*. The E test is similar to disk diffusion but employs a strip impregnated with an antibiotic gradient rather than a single potency disk. This system allows MIC determination and has been found to be an acceptable means of testing some fastidious organisms (23). Many rapid automated tests monitor growth curves of organisms in the presence and absence of antibiotic using turbidity or indicators of bacterial metabolism. The reliability of these systems for testing many of the enteric pathogens has not been validated, particularly for β-lactam antibiotics.

The need for antimicrobial susceptibility information is dependent on the nature of the infection and the pathogen (24). When possible, laboratories should use selective reporting of results and interpretative comments to assist physicians in making appropriate therapeutic choices. Providing susceptibility results for organisms that should not be treated is a waste of resources and, perhaps more importantly, may actually prompt some physicians to treat patients unnecessarily. When therapy is indicated, timely reporting of susceptibility results enables the physician to choose antibiotics likely to be effective for the pathogen. However, some antibiotics that may appear to be highly effective against the organism *in vitro* may not be effective clinically, and reporting such results may encourage the clinician to make an inappropriate choice of drug. Therefore, laboratories should attempt to confine susceptibility reporting to antibiotics indicated for treatment of the pathogen or add a comment to reports such as ''*in vitro* susceptibility may not predict clinical efficacy.'' Often treatment of some pathogens, e.g., *Salmonella* or *Yersinia,* depends on the nature of infection or the patient's underlying illness. In such cases the laboratory may suggest consultation with infectious disease or other specialists for assistance in management decisions. Periodically laboratories should meet with infectious diseases specialists and gastroenterologists to review national and local resistance trends as well as protocols for testing and reporting of susceptibility results.

Detection of Bacterial Pathogens by Nonculture Methods

Molecular Techniques

Some enteric pathogens, particularly pathogenic *E. coli* strains, can only be identified on the basis of genotypic characteristics. With the exception of *E. coli* O157:H7, which exhibits a distinct fermentation pattern, conventional biochemical tests cannot discriminate among enterotoxigenic (ETEC), enteropathogenic (EPEC), enteroinvasive (EIEC), enterohemorrhagic (EHEC), and enteroaggregative (EAgg) *E. coli*. Each of these pathogenic types contains unique genes that are usually important pathogenic determinants. Therefore, nucleic acid probes designed to be complementary to these genes can be employed to distinguish commensal *E. coli* and pathogenic strains with high specificity and sensitivity by the technique of nucleic acid hybridization (25) (Fig. 1). Labeled probes complementary to a nucleic acid sequence within the target microorganism are able to hybridize with nucleic acid in the specimen, whereas if there are no complementary sequences in the specimen the probe remains unbound. A variety of labels have been used to tag the probe, including radioactivity, biotin, alkaline phosphatase, and others. Following a wash step to eliminate unbound probe molecules, hybrids that formed are detected by methods that specifically identify the label on the probe.

DNA hybridization techniques were first used in epidemiological studies of ETEC in developing countries where the limits of sensitivity of hybridization were found to be approximately 10^3–10^5 bacteria per gram (mL) of stool (26–28). Because the concentration of ETEC in stool samples is very high, and therefore the number of gene targets is also high, it was possible to detect them by direct hybridization methods. However, it has not been possible to identify other enteric pathogens excreted in smaller amounts by direct hybridization because of the relatively low sensitivity of the method. Instead, the sensitivity is enhanced by testing colonies arising after amplification

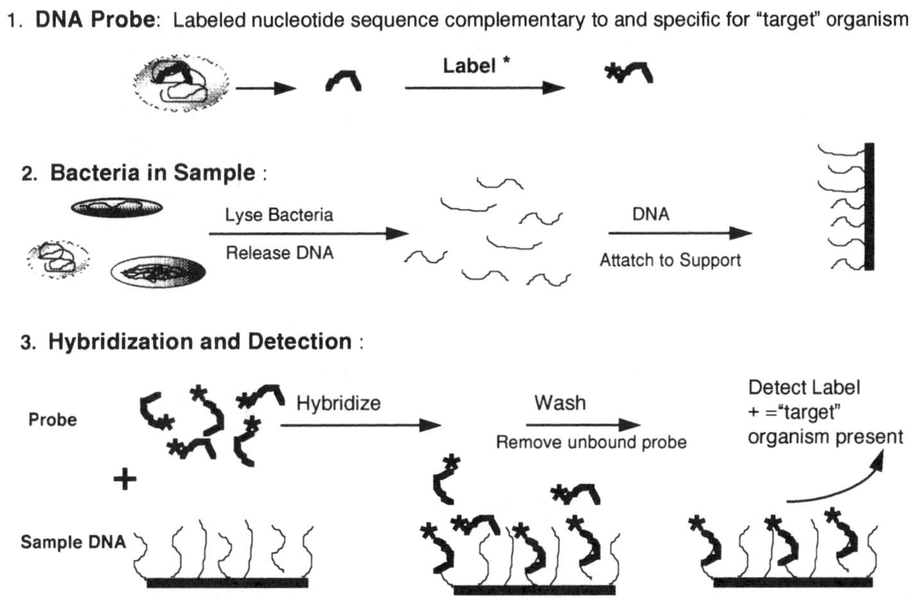

1. **DNA Probe**: Labeled nucleotide sequence complementary to and specific for "target" organism

2. **Bacteria in Sample** :

Lyse Bacteria
Release DNA

DNA
Attach to Support

3. **Hybridization and Detection** :

Probe

Hybridize

Wash
Remove unbound probe

Detect Label
+ ="target"
organism present

Sample DNA

FIG. 1. DNA hybridization.

on culture plates. Problems with sensitivity, specificity, turnaround time, the need for separate hybridizations to detect each pathogen, and expense have made DNA hybridization methods to detect enteric pathogens impractical for use by diagnostic laboratories. However, DNA hybridization methods have become widely employed to study the epidemiology of enteric infectious agents.

Various techniques have been devised to amplify the target genes prior to hybridization, usually by inoculating the specimen into an enrichment broth. For example, detection of enteric pathogens in food often requires an amplification step by growth prior to hybridization. The advent of procedures to amplify gene targets, as compared with growth enhancement of viable microorganisms, has provided a biochemical method of increasing the number of targets in clinical specimens, thereby enhancing the sensitivity by several orders of magnitude (25). One of these methods, polymerase chain reaction (PCR) amplification has been widely used. As compared with nucleic acid probes, PCR amplification utilizes single-stranded nucleic acid chains called *primers*. These molecules are designed to be complementary to DNA sequences flanking the target gene on each strand (Fig. 2). The primers bind to complementary nucleotides on each end of the target gene, thereby "priming" the polymerization of double-stranded DNA bounded by the primers, in the presence of a polymerase enzyme and nucleotides. If the target sequence is contained within the specimen, PCR amplification can increase the number of these sequences by a million fold. Subsequently, the amplified target sequences can be identified by electrophoresis or hybridization with a specific probe.

There are numerous modifications of the PCR procedure and a variety of alternative strategies for either amplification of nucleic acid in sample or to amplify hybridization signals. Examples of the latter two approaches include transcription-based amplification system (TAS),

self-sustaining sequence replication (SSR), strand displacement amplification (SDA), Q-β replicase, ligase chain reaction (LCR), or use of compound and branched probes (25). Although DNA amplification techniques offer sufficient sensitivity to detect enteric microorganisms often present in very low numbers, these methods cannot be used at present to determine the antibiotic susceptibility pattern and thus have not replaced conventional culture methods. Other inherent problems including the problem of nucleic acid contamination, inhibitors of polymerization enzymes present within GI tract material, clinical utility of results, and expense must be overcome before clinical laboratories routinely utilize these methods.

"Noncultivatable" Pathogens

A molecular approach (30) has been used to identify pathogens that have been seen in tissue but have not previously (or only rarely) been isolated in culture. For example, the microorganism "*Gastrospirillum hominis*" is not cultivatable, and therefore its presence would not be detected using conventional protocols. However, it is possible to assign a novel bacterial species to a position on the phylogenetic "family tree" based on the relationship of its ribosomal genes to other bacterial species (31). PCR amplification of noncultivatable bacteria is based on the carriage of ribosomal genes by all bacteria. Using highly conserved eubacterial ("universal") primers, it has now been possible to PCR-amplify 16S ribosomal genes of noncultivatable bacteria from tissue. Ribosomal genes contain nucleotide sequences that are highly conserved among all species, but each species has unique nucleotide sequences interspersed among these. Many bacteria have been classified in this way, and the RNA sequences have been deposited in large genetic libraries accessible by

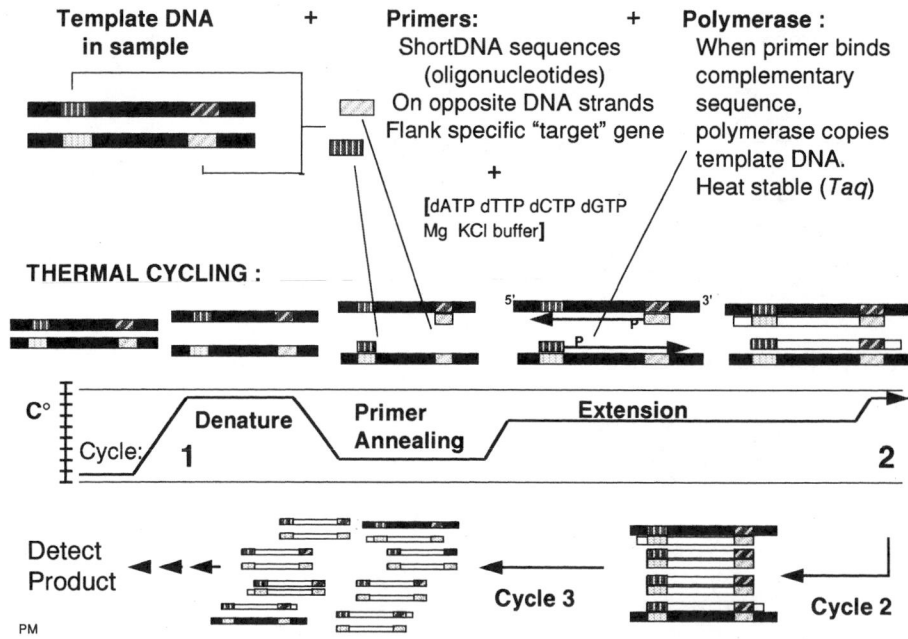

FIG. 2. DNA amplification: polymerase chain reaction (PCR).

computer. The PCR-amplified ribosomal genes of noncultivatable organisms can be sequenced and compared to rRNA gene sequences of other bacteria. Species-specific primers or DNA probes for detection of the new organism can then be developed. Such methodology is currently available only in research and reference laboratories. Diseases due to these "noncultivatable" pathogens that have been investigated include bacillary angiomatosis/peliosis hepatis/cat scratch syndromes that can be caused by the same organism (32–35), Whipples's disease (36), and gastritis associated with a *Helicobacter*-like microorganism (31). Possible infectious etiology for Crohn's disease also has been explored using a molecular approach (37–40).

Strain Typing for Epidemiological Investigation

One of the most important aspects of the epidemiological analysis of an outbreak of GI tract infection is to collect isolates recovered from clinical samples and to "fingerprint" them (41). Typing isolates makes it possible to determine whether all the cases were infected by the same strain, for example, or whether the strain isolated from patients was identical to the isolate recovered from the incriminated vehicle, i.e., food, etc. Bacterial phenotyping methods examine biochemical patterns, antibiotic resistance patterns, or antigenic typing by serological methods. *Salmonella* sp. are serotyped based on the expression of somatic ("O") and flagellar ("H") antigens. Certain serotypes are associated with the city of isolation, e.g., *S. heidelberg, S. derby, S. dublin,* etc. Serotyping requires access to a large number of antibody reagents and is usually done in reference or public health laboratories.

Even though different strains of a particular bacterial species might share common phenotypic characteristics, they might still be genetically different and therefore represent unique strains, or clones. As an example, two *Shigella flexneri* isolates expressing species-specific biochemical patterns might still be genetically different. While this might not have any importance for management of an individual patient, it would be extremely important to distinguish isolates if they had been recovered during an outbreak of infection. Generally, during an outbreak of GI tract infections, a single strain is responsible, and this information most often reflects a common source, such as a lot of contaminated beef in the case of some EHEC outbreaks, for example. On the other hand, if multiple strains are isolated, this tends to suggest that there is no single common source and that several factors are responsible for the increased infection rate.

Phenotyping methods are based on the expression of certain proteins, including antigens, surface-exposed proteins, enzymes, etc., all of which are encoded by specific genes. Protein patterns, therefore, most often reflect the genes encoding them; however, expression of the genetic potential may be affected by environmental or other factors. Even though it is not feasible to examine the entire genome of a bacterial strain, it is possible to genotype bacteria using molecular methods initially developed to clone and sequence genes. The first method of molecular typing, or fingerprinting, was based on the carriage of specific plasmids by strains of enteric bacteria; thus the designation "plasmid profiles." Plasmids are extrachromosomal DNA molecules carried by many bacteria. It was discovered that among isolates of the same enteric species, each strain tended to have a unique complement of plasmid molecules. Each strain could be distinguished from others by isolating the plasmid DNA as covalently closed, double-stranded circular molecules, followed by separation during gel electrophoresis. The relative molecular size of each plasmid can be calculated on its relative rate of migration through the gel. Smaller plasmids mi-

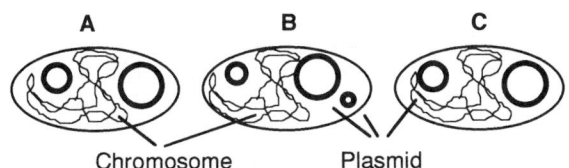

Lyse bacteria. Differentially precipitate chromosomal DNA, then plasmid DNA.

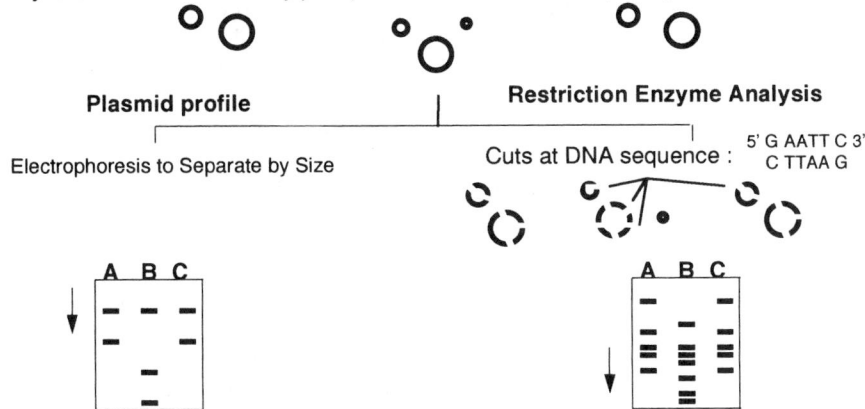

FIG. 3. Strain typing: plasmid analysis.

grate more quickly through the gel than large ones. The fingerprint consists of an enumeration of the number of plasmids and their relative molecular mass (Fig. 3).

Occasionally, two genetically different bacterial isolates may contain a plasmid of similar size. These may be distinguished by examining the manner in which restriction endonucleases cut each one. This depends on the distribution of endonuclease restriction sites, consisting of four to six nucleotide sequences that are recognized specifically by each type of restriction endonuclease. For

example, the enzyme *Eco*R1 cuts each strand of DNA at the site (reading 5' to 3') GAATTC. The effect of restriction endonuclease cleavage of plasmid DNA or chromosomal DNA is to form linear fragments, the length of each being determined by the relative position of the restriction sites. Therefore, *Eco*R1 digestion of two unique plasmids would produce two different sets of linear fragments that can be resolved by gel electrophoresis, producing two distinct restriction endonuclease digestion fingerprints (Fig. 3).

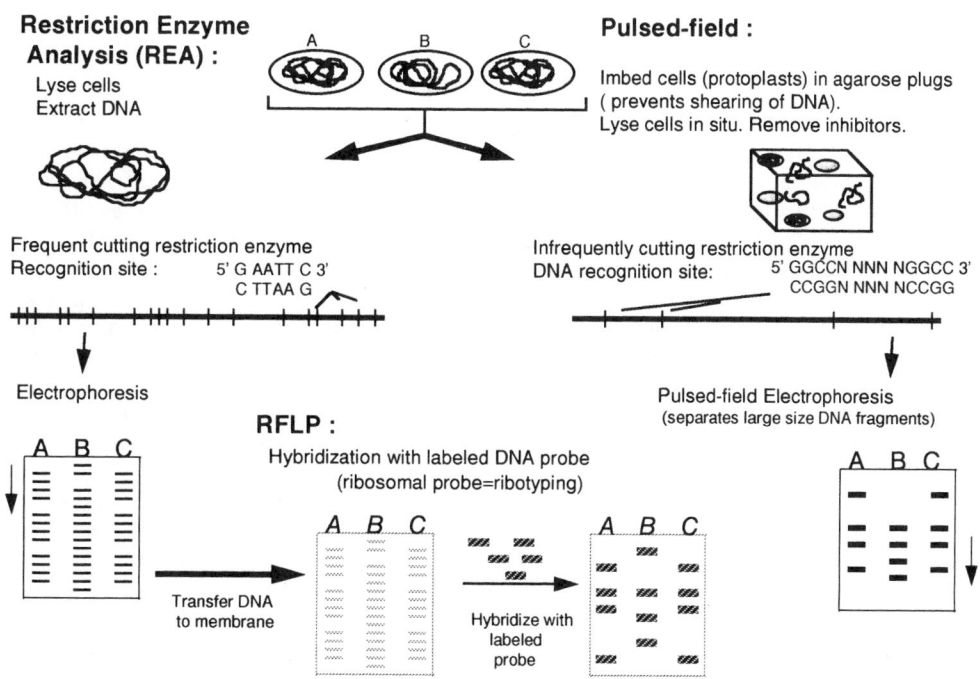

FIG. 4. Strain typing: chromosomal restriction length polymorphisms (RFLPs).

Restriction endonuclease digestion fingerprinting has been employed to examine bacterial isolates that lack plasmids, although the method works equally well to distinguish strains containing plasmids. The principle is the same as for restriction digestion fingerprinting of plasmid molecules, the difference being that the total genomic DNA content of the bacterial cell is exposed to the restriction enzyme.

Even though restriction endonuclease fingerprinting is a very specific method, the number of restriction fragments created by cleavage is very large and the fingerprint is therefore complex (Fig. 4). Restriction endonuclease analysis (REA) is generally done by comparing patterns of isolates by visual inspection. Thus, comparison of a large number of isolates by this method is cumbersome. Methods that highlight differences by limiting the number of bands to be compared facilitate visual inspection and provide a coding system. One way to accomplish this is to react the linear fragments with a nucleic acid probe that will hybridize only to a limited number of specific fragments. Thus, ribotyping is a molecular epidemiological method in which labeled ribosomal RNA is used as a probe to highlight the DNA fragments on the gel that encode rDNA. Another method of producing a discreet number of fragments is to use "rare" cutting restriction endonucleases that cleave bacterial chromosomes into a limited number of very large fragments. These fragments are best resolved by pulse gel electrophoresis. PCR has also been used for strain typing in a variety of ways including use of specific as well as "arbitrary primers" that enable generation of amplification products that elucidate genetic differences among strains. Procedures for strain typing may be found in Refs. 1, 9, and 25.

LABORATORY DIAGNOSIS OF GASTROINTESTINAL TRACT INFECTIONS

Diarrheal Syndromes

The clinical laboratory evaluation of GI tract specimens, particularly stool and rectal samples, is more complex, costly, and time consuming than any other specimen category. Therefore, each laboratory must adopt protocols to detect and identify the enteric pathogens that experience has established to be most prevalent in the population served. In addition to the usual battery of methods needed to detect common pathogens, laboratories should develop protocols to identify less frequently encountered microorganisms. These protocols may be activated when information provided by the physician suggests that additional procedures are warranted. The clinician's assessment of the patient with diarrhea, for example, is most often based on the patient's history, including travel, exposure to particular foodborne pathogens, occupation, antibiotic usage, and other epidemiological risk factors, and upon clinical findings including the characteristics of the diarrhea (11,12,42–45). The laboratory evaluation is particularly relevant to the diagnosis of diarrheal disease, since several bacterial pathogens may produce the same syndrome. For example, dysenteric diarrhea may be pro-

duced by *Campylobacter, Salmonella, Shigella,* or other enteric pathogens. Selective and differential media and a battery of biochemical assays are required to identify these bacterial species. These are routinely used in virtually all diagnostic laboratories in the United States and should not require a specific request from the clinician. However, if less common microorganisms are included within the differential diagnosis, it is important for this information to be communicated to the laboratory. Optimum detection of various enteric pathogens requires use of a variety of media and techniques (Fig. 5). It has also become clear in recent years that many of the bacterial enteric pathogens that are prevalent in developing countries now appear more commonly in the United States as a result of travel, immigration, and the importation of food, particularly fresh fruit and vegetables. It seems certain that the "routine" laboratory repertoire will continue to expand as more unusual microorganisms are recognized to cause epidemic and endemic infections. Technological advances may enable more widespread and reliable detection of organisms such as diarrheagenic *E. coli* strains, which are important pathogens but not identified by most clinical laboratories. Public health laboratories traditionally have been responsible for evaluating epidemics in the community, in processing specimens from patients with specified enteric illnesses, and in characterizing isolates of suspected enteropathogenic bacteria. These laboratories also should be consulted periodically to determine prevalence of enteric pathogens in the community to determine whether "routine" laboratory protocols need revision to enable to detect additional pathogens. However, resources for many public health functions have diminished and surveillance by clinical laboratories is essential for the early recognition of emergent unusual enteric pathogens in the community.

Appropriate Specimens

Number of Samples

The sensitivity of one vs. two or more stool cultures for laboratory diagnosis of GI tract infection has not been systematically evaluated. In one study (46) that compared recovery of pathogens from rectal swabs and stool specimens cultured in parallel and processed within 30 min, almost half of the bacterial pathogens were recovered with a single sample, although 25% of positive cultures would have been missed had only one specimen been cultured. In early stages of untreated acute illness the number of organisms, such as *Campylobacter, Salmonella, Vibrio cholerae,* and *Shigella,* may be quite high (10^5–10^9/g or mL of feces), and a single culture is usually adequate. Circumstances in which the number of organisms in a fecal sample would be low and associated with low sensitivity include prior or partial treatment with antibiotics or other antibacterial agents such as bismuth subsalicylate (*Helicobacter pylori*); during convalescence or later stages of illness (usually 3–7 days into the illness); chronic or asymptomatic carriage; enteric fever; inadequate sample; or suboptimum transport conditions. Two or three

SMEARS :   Methylene blue -Fecal leukocytes (large numbers of yeast post antibiotics)
                Gram stain - Occasional *C. jejuni* or *S. aureus* PMC (Not usually helpful.)
                AFB stain - Mycobacteria (Parasitology procedures best for *Cryptosporidium*, *Isospora*
                                Cyclospora in chronic diarrhea]

DIRECT ASSAYS : Toxin-   *C. difficile* (ELISA or cytotoxicity)
                        EHEC   (cytotoxicity for verotoxin) (a)
                        V. cholerae
            Antigen -   *V. cholerae* ⌐ ELISA or Agglutination   (a)

DNA Amplification (PCR) - Requires extraction and primers specific for each pathogen (a)

CULTURE :   Special media or testing often required for each pathogen. Examples:

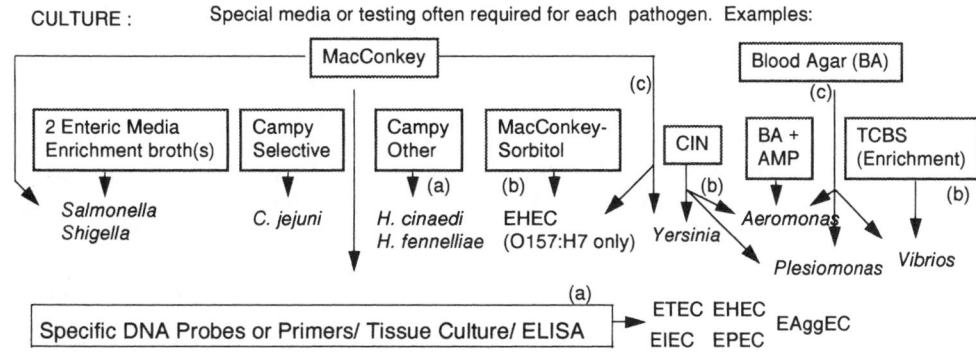

a) Not routinely available (b) Inquire; if not routine, usually available by request.   (c) Not optimum for detection.

FIG. 5. Laboratory detection of bacterial enteric pathogens.

separate sequential cultures may be indicated if the patient is severely ill or suspected to have a chronic bacterial infection. Communication with the laboratory is indicated when several cultures are contemplated to ensure that procedures are optimized for recovery of agents strongly suspected on the basis of symptoms and history.

Collection of Samples

Appropriate collection and transport of specimens is at least as important for the recovery of enteric pathogens as the procedures used by the laboratory to isolate and identify the organisms. It is important to collect good samples early in the acute phase of illness prior to antibiotic therapy, to ensure that specimens are properly and expeditiously transported to the laboratory, and to notify the laboratory if organisms not routinely cultured are suspected. Among the infectious agents affecting the intestine, the number of organisms in fecal material is greatest early in the acute phase of illness and may rapidly decrease even prior to clinical convalescence. *Salmonella typhi* and other enteric fever *Salmonella* are a notable exception. Antibiotics, even those that may not be clinically effective, may nonetheless diminish the viability or numbers of organisms present in feces. Some organisms, notably shigellae that are well adapted to the human host, are delicate and lose viability quickly upon drying swabs or in the acid environment of stool held at room temperature. Since bedside inoculation of culture media is rarely feasible, stool samples or rectal swabs should be sent to the laboratory and processed within 1–2 hr whenever possible.

Stool samples are generally preferred over rectal swabs

because they provide more material for culture studies and hence greater potential sensitivity. In addition, gross examination of stool can be performed, providing the clinician with valuable information relevant to the diarrheal syndrome. Stool samples are also better than rectal swabs for evaluating presence of fecal leukocytes, and the technologist can select portions of the sample likely to contain pathogens by picking areas for culture that contain mucus, blood, or pus. Samples may be collected from a bed pan or plastic wrap draped over the toilet and should be transferred to a leakproof waxed cardboard container or a clean jar for transport. Those collecting the specimen should be advised of the importance of not contaminating the sample with residual disinfectant or soaps from bed pans, with urine, or with toilet paper, which frequently has additives that can inhibit the growth of organisms. Patients should be cautioned about not contaminating the outside of the collection container that subsequently will be handled by numerous other individuals. Material the size of a walnut is usually sufficient for most laboratory studies. If delay of over 2 hr in culturing is unavoidable, portions of specimens containing mucus, pus, or blood should be selected and inoculated into transport medium for bacterial culture. Stool to be tested for *C. difficile* toxin may be refrigerated for up to 48 hr or frozen; however freezing may reduce toxin titer resulting in some false-negative tests.

Although stool is usually considered to be the best sample for culture of enteric pathogens, in some circumstances it is only feasible to obtain rectal swabs. Overall yields of bacterial pathogens from the two types of specimens were found to be comparable when specimens collected in parallel were cultured within 30 min (46). Rectal swabs rather than anal swabs should be obtained. The swab should be passed through the anal sphincter several centimeters into the rectum and gently rotated. Taking more than one sample will provide more material for culture studies. The swab(s) must be placed immediately in transport medium to avoid drying of the specimen.

Transport Media

Cary–Blair transport medium is widely used for stool cultures because it preserves viablilty of most enteric pathogens. One to two grams (mL) of stool can be emulsified in the medium and the sample refrigerated. When samples placed in Cary–Blair were cultured within 3 days of collection, only 12% of those stored at room temperature were positive for *Shigella* whereas 63% of refrigerated samples were positive (47). *C. jejuni* also survives in Cary–Blair better at 4°C than at room temperature; however, viability may decrease in samples held over 2 hr (48–51). Inclusion of a pH indicator into the medium will enable timely identification of specimens that are acidic (7,10) and unlikely to yield *Shigella*. Particularly if samples are refrigerated, buffered glycerol saline (BGS) is a better transport medium for *Shigella* than is Cary–Blair, although recovery of shigellae from either transport medium is diminished at room temperature (47). *Vibrio* and *Campylobacter* do not survive well in buffered glycerol saline; thus other kinds of transport medium may be appropriate if optimum recovery of a specific organism(s) is indicated.

Initial Evaluation

Visual Examination of Specimens

Visual examination of stool samples not only confirms the patient's history but may also provide clues as to etiology. For example, the presence of blood, mucus, or pus suggests infection by an "invasive" enteric pathogen, such as *Shigella* sp., whereas a thin, watery fecal specimen lacking these elements is characteristic of "secretory" diarrhea produced by an enterotoxigenic species.

Detection of Fecal Leukocytes and Blood

Fecal leukocytes signify intestinal inflammation and provide an essential diagnostic clue to the type of diarrheal syndrome and thereby provide a rational microbiological differential diagnosis. The presence, amount, and type of leukocyte can easily be determined by microscopy and should be ordered on all patients with diarrhea. Infection with *Shigella*, enteroinvasive *E. coli*, *Salmonella*, *Campylobacter*, and *V. parahemolyticus* is usually associated with the presence of granulocytes; while helpful if present (12), the absence of inflammatory cells does not always exclude one of these pathogens. It has been reported that 70% to 90% of patients with shigellosis may have >15 WBC per high-power field (HPF), and 60% to 95% of patients with *Salmonella*, *C. jejuni*, or *E. histolyt-*

ica infection may have >1 WBC/HPF (42,52–55). However, fecal samples fiom approximately 20% to 30% of patients with infection due to typically noninflammatory etiologies, including rotavirus, enterotoxigenic *E. coli*, and *V. cholerae*, also may contain >1 WBC/HPF. The negative predictive value of the test is better than the positive predictive value, which may be quite low in some populations. Polymorphonuclear leukocytes (PMNs) may also be seen in pseudomembranous colitis associated with *C. difficile*. A mononuclear response may be seen with typhoid fever, *Yersinia* or *E. histolytica* infection.

Methylene blue staining of fecal smears is the most widely accepted method of determining presence of leukocytes. The presence and number of WBC per high power field (HPF = $400\times$ magnification) should be reported and the presence of large numbers of yeast (or obvious parasites). Threshold values between >1 to >15 WBC/HPF have been used to indicate inflammation. A higher cutoff value may be useful in some settings such as tropical countries (54,56). Interpretation is by no means standardized and performance of the test is highly dependent on specimen quality and on skill of the microscopist. Reports of the sensitivity and specificity values obtained have varied considerably. If a differential is to be done, the sample should be thinly smeared, stained with trichrome or Wright's stain and approximately 300 cells counted. Fecal material should be examined as soon as possible. Specimens that cannot be examined within 1–2 hr should be refrigerated or smears prepared and fixed for later staining. PMNs deteriorate even under refrigeration and specimens older than 24 hr should not be tested. Fresh stool samples are more than twice as sensitive as swab or diaper specimens for detection of fecal leukocytes (57,58). Other methods have also been used to enumerate fecal leukocytes, including a latex test that detects lactoferrin liberated from the specific granules of PMNs (58). Such a test has the potential to circumvent some of the problems with methylene blue staining including lack of standardization and instability of cells.

The presence of fecal blood is determined by visual inspection, microscopy, or occult blood assays. Tests for occult blood that specifically detect human blood are available. One third of patients with *Shigella* infection may not have visible blood in feces (42) and blood may be found less frequently in infections caused by *S. sonnei* than by other shigellae (56). Grossly bloody stools can be caused by enterohemmorhagic *E. coli* (EHEC) and *Campylobacter*, although many patients may have only microscopic amounts or blood-tinged stools.

Stains and Smears to Detect Bacterial and Fungal Enteric Pathogens

Gram stain is generally not a particularly useful test in the diagnosis of gastroenteritis. WBCs stain pink when treated with the Gram stain and should be reported even though the methylene blue stain is more sensitive. *Campylobacter* sp. appear as faintly pink-staining, thin, gull-wing–shaped, gram-negative rods by the conventional Gram stain; these bacteria are better visualized when a basic fuchsin counterstain is used. *Campylobacter* sp. have polar flagella and spiral shape that provide a characteristic motility pattern that can be readily distinguished from other motile enteric bacilli by microscopy exam of a wet mount of fecal material. This technique has been used to screen fecal samples from patients living in areas where *Vibrio* infection is rare (*V. cholerae* exhibits similar motility). The sensitivity of wet mount and stain for *Campylobacter* sp. has ranged from 30% to 75% with higher values obtained when testing is limited to samples with fecal/WBC (59,60). Even though *Campylobacter* sp. have a distinctive morphology and motility, positive predictive value is highly dependent on skill of persons reading the smear, and most diagnostic laboratories do not perform this test. In epidemic situations or endemic areas where *V. cholerae* 01 infections are frequently seen, direct examination of "ricewater" stool demonstrating curved gram-negative rods may provide rapid presumptive diagnosis. However, due to the variable morphology and possible confusion with other curved or pleomorphic rods, this procedure is not recommended in most settings (61,62). In unusual cases of pseudomembranous colitis due to *Staphylococcus aureus,* sheets of staphylococci may be seen. However, this is more reliable when smears are made from material from lesions rather than from stool.

KOH or fluorescent stains of a variety of clinical materials may be used to presumptively diagnose some fungal infections; however, KOH of stool specimens is not indicated. The role of *Candida* overgrowth in diarrheal disease of patients treated with antibiotics is controversial. However, yeast can be visualized on methylene blue smears used for fecal leukocytes. The number of yeast per HPF should be reported.

Acid-fast smears may be useful for AIDS or severely immunocompromised patients with chronic diarrhea, and may need to be specifically requested. The presence of high numbers of mycobacteria detected by acid-fast stain of feces has correlated with disseminated *M. avium-intracellulare* infection and GI involvement in patients with AIDS or other severe immunocompromising conditions (see below). *Cyclospora* are protozoa that have been referred to as blue–green algae or *Cyanobacterium*-like bodies and have been implicated as a cause of diarrhea in travelers to tropical countries as well as in outbreaks associated with water consumption in the United States (63–66). *Cyclospora* demonstrate autofluorescence and, along with *Cryptosporidium* and *Isospora belli,* also can be detected by acid-fast staining. However, a modified acid-fast stain and concentration techniques used for ova and parasite exam are more sensitive for detection of these organisms than methods for detection of mycobacteria in feces. Additional studies are required to detect parasitic or viral causes of gastroenteritis.

Dysenteric Diarrhea

As shown in Table 1, the dysentery syndrome consisting of fever, abdominal cramps, rectal tenesmus, and diarrheal stools containing blood, pus, and/or mucus is most commonly caused by *Shigella,* enteric *Salmonella* sp., and *Campylobacter,* although other bacterial enteric pathogens, including *Y. enterocolitica,* some noncholera vibrios, *Aeromonas, Plesiomonas,* enterohemorrhagic *E. coli,* and *C. difficile* may provoke a similar inflammatory response. Infection due to agents that typically cause secretory diarrhea may sometimes manifest with characteristics of an inflammatory diarrheal syndrome, and vice versa. Therefore, syndromic categorization of agents is useful but not necessarily reliable for all cases.

Salmonella *and* Shigella

Salmonella, Campylobacter, and *Shigella* are among the most frequently isolated etiological agents of gastroenteritis in the United States. In many industrialized nations such as the United States, the frequency of isolation of *Salmonella* and *Campylobacter* is relatively similar, while *Shigella* is isolated much less frequently. In developing countries where sanitary conditions are poor or where *Shigella* infections may be more common, transmission of *Shigella* most often occurs by direct fecal-oral inoculation. Risk factors include exposure to young children in day care centers and to adults residing in institutions where hygiene may be poor (e.g., nursing homes, institutions for the mentally retarded, or psychiatric institutions) or exposures in developing countries where sanitation is poor. Contaminated food is the vehicle most implicated in salmonellosis, apart from *S. typhi* and *S. paratyphi* which are host-restricted to higher primates and humans, gastroenteritis caused by other *Salmonella* species is usually caused by ingestion of contaminated food of animal origin, including poultry, eggs, beef, unpasteurized milk, or cheese. Salmonellosis associated with tomatoes and watermelon has been reported. Salmonellosis is most common in developed countries that mass-produce and process animals for food although drinking or washing uncooked foods in water contaminated by sewage or animal waste can be mechanisms of transmission.

Culture. *Salmonella* and *Shigella* are easily grown on routine laboratory media. However, selective and differential media are usually employed to aid in the initial detection of these enteric pathogens in feces. Use of a combination of media with various selective properties is recommended (7,9,67,68) and includes a differential medium of low selectivity such as MacConkey agar, deoxycholate, or eosin-methylene blue (EMB), as well as two media of intermediate or high selectivity. Moderately selective media include salmonella-shigella (SS), deoxycholate citrate, xylose lysine (XLD), and Hektoen agar. The latter two media are better for recovery of *Shigella* (67,68). In a recent comparison (69) of MacConkey, Taknaf enteric agar (MacConkey supplemented with potassium telluride), Hektoen, and SS agar, MacConkey was found to be significantly better than SS agar for recovery of *S. flexneri* and for *S. sonnii.* Overall, MacConkey and SS agar performances were similar but significantly better than Hektoen and all media were superior to Taknaf enteric agar. Isolation of *Salmonella* sp. can be improved by inclusion of highly selective plating media, including brilliant green agar and bismuth sulfite agar, which is the medium of choice to isolate *S. typhi*. It should be noted that performance of these media may be affected by preparation and storage procedures (68). Rambach agar and SM-ID may not be as sensitive for isolation of nontyphae salmonellae as Hektoen (70).

Inoculation of feces into enrichment broth with subsequent subculture to selective media can significantly improve recovery of *Shigella* and particularly *Salmonella* (71–74). Gram negative broth is used primarily for *Shigella* enrichment; selenite F is used for *Salmonella* and *S. sonnei;* and medium containing tetrathionate is highly selective for *Salmonella*. Because *Salmonella* species causing enteric fever may be differentially inhibited by various enrichment broths, the choice of media for *Salmonella* isolation may depend on organisms likely to be found in the local population and on the clinical presentation (68). In acute disease, the number of *Salmonella* or *Shigella* are usually sufficiently high to be detected by direct plating methods. However, the number of organisms may be lower in samples collected later in the course of illness, in convalescent or carrier states, after partial treatment with antibiotics, or if rectal swabs are submitted, as is common with pediatric patients or in epidemiological studies. In such cases, broth enrichment procedures are likely to significantly improve detection. The cost effectiveness of routine broth enrichment procedures in some settings has been questioned (75). Antibody-coated latex reagents that may permit detection of *Salmonella* and *Shigella* in enrichment broths without subculture have been found to be sensitive in many but not all settings (71–73,76). This procedure is not adequately sensitive to replace direct plating; furthermore, the low positive predictive value precludes reporting presumptive results.

Identification. Colonies that develop on enteric selective and differential media that are suspect are picked for biochemical or serological tests to confirm the identification of enteric pathogens. Most laboratories perform a short battery of initial biochemical tests, including growth pattern on TSI or Kligler slants, on lysine iron agar and urea agar. *Shigella* species are lactose-, sucrose-, and lysine-negative, anaerogenic, acetate- and mucate-negative, and are nonmotile because they do not produce flagella. *S. sonnei* differs from other members of the serogroup species A–C by producing ornithine decarboxylase and β-galactosidase (ONPG-positive). Some shigellae including *S. flexneri* serotype 6, *S. boydii* 13, and some *S. sonnei* may have atypical reactions for gas production as well as mucate and lactose fermentation that can result in missing these strains with screening procedures (77). *Salmonella* sp. usually are lactose- and sucrose-negative, lysine-positive, and produce H_2S. However, many strains of *S. cholarasuis* are H_2S-negative, and *S. paratyphi A* is usually H_2S- and lysine-negative, which may result in overlooking these organisms with some screening procedures. Alternative approaches for screening suspicious colonies include using commercially available enteric pathogen screening batteries (78,79), agglutination of isolates subcultured to nonselective media using polyvalent anti-*Salmonella* or anti-*Shigella* antibody-coated particles

(78), and *in situ* testing of H_2S-positive colonies using a fluorogenic methylumbelliferone-conjugated C8 esterase substrate (80,81).

Isolates that are positive in biochemical screening tests and that agglutinate with *Shigella* polyvalent antiserum or with *Salmonella* Vi or polyvalent antiserum are presumptively reported to expedite appropriate patient management. The *S. typhi* capsular or virulence antigen (Vi: *N*-acetylgalactosaminuronic acid) may block agglutination with lipopolysaccharide somatic O antigens or flagellar H antigens. Therefore, biochemically suspect isolates of *Salmonella* or *Shigella* that do not agglutinate with polyvalent antiserum or *Salmonella* isolates that react with Vi antiserum should be heated in a 100°C waterbath for 15–30 min and retested. Isolates suspected of being *Salmonella* or *Shigella* should be subjected to a more extensive battery of biochemical tests (67,82,83).

Rare isolates of *Salmonella* or *Shigella* have O antigens not recognized by commercially available antisera, and other Enterobacteriaceae may have antigens that cross-react with antisera. For example, some strains of *Citrobacter* may react with *Salmonella* polyvalent antiserum but may be quickly differentiated from *Salmonella* by positive reaction with L-pyrrolidonyl-β-naphthylamide (PYR) spot test (used for identification of enterococci and group A streptococci) using inoculum from blood agar or alkaline TSI slant (84). *Salmonella typhi*, *S. paratyphi A*, and *S. cholerasuis*, which are associated with enteric fever and bacteremia, may be presumptively separated from other *Salmonella* species using readily available biochemical tests (67). By criteria of DNA-DNA hybridization *Shigella* and *E. coli* are essentially the same species. Some *E. coli* isolates including EIEC may react with *Shigella* antiserum and it may be very difficult to determine whether an isolate is an "inactive" *E. coli* or a *Shigella*. EIEC also share many characteristics with *Shigella* and some strains may be negative for lactose fermentation and often differ from most *E. coli* found in the intestine by being negative for lysine decarboxylase and motility (67,69). Isolates that are presumptively identified as *Salmonella* or *Shigella* should be promptly forwarded to a public health laboratory for more extensive biochemical characterization, serotype identification, and possibly strain typing analysis. Isolates resembling EIEC should be discussed with the clinician and sent to a reference laboratory.

Shigella species can be serogrouped into groups A, B, C, and D using commercially available antisera and thus identified as *S. dysenteriae*, *S. flexneri*, *S. boydii*, and *S. sonnei*, respectively. Serotyping of *Shigella* is restricted to public health reference laboratories and research settings.

Salmonella classification and nomenclature has changed over the years. Strains in the *Salmonella-Arizona* group are sufficiently related genetically to be regarded as a single species. There are seven DNA subgroups, although the great majority of isolates of clinical importance in humans belong to subgroup 1 (proposed *S. cholerasuis* subspecies). Some clinical laboratories may use commercially available antiserum for preliminary classification of *Salmonella* as groups A, B, C1, C2, D, and E, and more than 95% of strains causing human disease belong to these serotypes. Public health reference laboratories perform extensive serotype determinations of major and minor O antigens and phase 1 and 2 H antigens. Isolates with a particular antigenic formula are given a name and, in common parlance, *Salmonella* serotype *typhimurium* or *Salmonella* serotype *enteritidis* would be referred to as *S. typhimurium* or *S. enteritidis,* respectively.

Other Methods. Other approaches for detecting *Salmonella* or *Shigella* have included DNA probes (69,85–88), PCR (89–93), antigen detection in serum, urine, or stool (94,95). Currently these methods do not appear to be sufficiently sensitive, specific, or practical for application to routine diagnosis of *Salmonella* or *Shigella* GI infections.

Serology. At present there are no serological assays that reliably identify *Shigella* infection (93,96). Serological assays for *Salmonella* infection apply primarily to enteric fever rather than uncomplicated gastrointestinal infection (see below).

Campylobacter *and* Helicobacter

Campylobacter jejuni infection occurs worldwide and is one of the commonest causes of bacterial gastroenteritis (97–99). Depending on geographic area sampled, the incidence of *Salmonella* and *Campylobacter* infection may be similar, and *Campylobacter* is isolated far more often than *Shigella* in the United States and in other developed countries. *Campylobacter* species have a variety of mammalian hosts, including cows, pigs, commercially raised poultry, and wild birds. In developed countries that raise poultry in large enclosed facilities and that process massive quantities, *C. jejuni* may be isolated from a high proportion (50% to 100%) of carcasses tested. Other meats can also serve as vehicles of transmission in developed countries. Infection in the United States and Great Britain has also been acquired through ingestion of unpasteurized milk and contaminated water. Infected household pets can transmit infection occasionally, and person-to-person transmission can occur through fecal-oral contact.

Illness due to *C. jejuni* infection may present as brief self-limiting diarrhea, entercolitis, relapsing colitis resembling Crohn's disease or ulcerative colitis, or with other complications including mesenteric adenitis or appendicitis-like syndrome. Typically, infection with *C. jejuni* is associated with signs and symptoms of colonic inflammation, including fever, abdominal pain, frequent loose stools containing fecal leukocytes and microscopic blood, features also common to salmonellosis and shigellosis. Therefore, the diagnosis of *Campylobacter* enteritis depends on laboratory tests. Aspects of the history may suggest *Campylobacter* infection, especially ingestion of undercooked poultry. However, other risk factors for infection are also commonly associated with infection by *Salmonella*. Occasionally, infection may be associated with hemorrhagic colitis or gross hemorrhage. In industrialized nations, asymptomatic infection is rare, and in developing countries, infants with positive stool cultures are usually symptomatic. Therefore, culture is the major

means of establishing the diagnosis of infection and has a high degree of accuracy. Conversely, symptoms due to infection in older children and adults in some developing countries may be mild, and asymptomatic excretion is common (up to 40%). In such a setting, the positive predictive value of a positive culture for disease due to *C. jejuni* is low.

Campylobacter coli causes symptoms similar to those of *C. jejuni,* is generally less prevalent than *C. jejuni* and is most often associated with pork products (100). *Campylobacter lari* (*C. laridis*) may also cause diarrhea; other less frequently encountered species, including *C. upsaliensis, C. butzerli,* and possibly *C. jejuni* subsp. *doylei* are also suspected enteropathogens (99–104). Infection with nonthermotolerant campylobacters, including *C. fetus* subsp. *fetus* may be associated with GI symptoms (102–105), although *C. fetus* more commonly causes an enteric fever syndrome in immunocompromised hosts and blood cultures are usually positive. *Helicobacter cinaedi* and *H. fennelliae* and (formerly classified as *Campylobacter* species) have been associated with proctocolitis in homosexual men, but isolated on rare occasions from symptomatic women and children, and, on rare occasions, have been isolated from blood cultures (106–108). *H. pylori* is a cause of gastritis and is discussed below.

Culture. Culture is currently the best means of diagnosing *Campylobacter* infections, and methods for recovery of *C. jejuni* should be an integral part of a routine stool culture. *Campylobacter* species are nutritionally fastidious, require a microaerophilic atmosphere, and are relatively slow growing in comparison with other fecal flora (48,99,100). To recover these organisms in culture requires special procedures, including special atmosphere and selective media for isolation. *C. jejuni* strains grow better at 42°C than at 37°C, and incubation of cultures at the higher temperature provides a means of preventing overgrowth by commensal flora.

A variety of methods have been used to achieve an atmosphere of approximately 5% oxygen, 10% carbon dioxide, and 85% nitrogen required for growth of *Campylobacter*. The presence of low amounts of H_2 may be stimulatory for some strains or species. These atmospheric conditions can be provided by evacuation of anaerobe jars or polyethylene bags followed by replacement with an appropriate gas mixture; use of commercially available disposable gas generator systems; preparation of a "home-made" gas-generating system using steel wool, copper sulfate, sodium bicarbonate, and water; or use of the Fortner principal, in which plates for isolation of *Campylobacter* are incubated in a candle jar together with a plate(s) inoculated with rapidly growing facultative anaerobes that consume oxygen and produce CO_2 (48,100). The latter methods are inexpensive and use materials that may be accessible even in remote areas; however, these methods to generate a microaerobic environment may be less consistent than the former alternatives, and culture plates may require longer incubation. Some laboratories use anaerobic gas-generating packs in jars without catalyst (109) and this atmosphere provides H_2 stimulatory growth of *H. cinaedi* and *H. fennelliae* (106). However, this is not recommended by the manufacturer of these products because of concerns about explosiveness of accumulated H_2.

In comparison with other GI tract flora, *Campylobacter* sp. are more nutritionally fastidious and slower growing. For isolation of *C. jejuni,* many laboratories use enriched blood agar containing antibiotics to inhibit growth of other fecal flora. Formulations containing charcoal rather than blood may be more practical in some settings and have been shown to be equivalent or superior recovery for organisms (48,109–111). Media supplemented with cefoperazone has generally shown improved recovery of *Campylobacter* species and exhibited fewer problems with contamination by enteric flora than media containing cephalothin, polymyxin, or colistin. *Campylobacter* can be isolated on semisolid agar containing antibiotics by virtue of the ability of these highly motile organisms to swarm through the agar (112). Performance of this agar may be variable and specific lots suitable for this application should be requested (109,113,114).

A technique that does not require specialized medium containing antibiotics has been developed for *Campylobacter* isolation based on the ability of motile bacteria to pass through a 0.65-μm cellulose acetate filter placed on the surface of the agar plates incubated for 30–60 min at 37°C or 42°C (115,116). Incubation of plates at 42°C inhibits growth of most fecal flora thereby enhancing recovery of thermotolerant campylobacters (*C. jejuni, C. coli, C. lari, C. upsaliensis*), which includes most of the recognized enteropathogenic species. This technique may improve recovery of some *Campylobacter* sp. other than *C. jejuni* that are inhibited by antibiotics in the medium; however, the filtration method may be less sensitive for recovery of *C. jejuni* compared to use of some selective media because only a small proportion of cells present in feces pass through the membrane (104,109,116). Charcoal media and 37°C temperature can be employed to isolate thermosensitive campylobacters (*C. fetus* subsp. *fetus,* many strains of *C. jejuni* subsp. *doylei*) or when a 42°C incubator isn't available. Incubation for 72 hr rather than 48 hr has been reported to increase the isolation rate in some studies (48,109). Since no single medium or method is optimum for recovery of all campylobacters, significant improvement in the isolation rate may be provided when more than a single medium or system is used (109).

Campylobacter fetus isolates are susceptible to some cephalosporins and therefore *C. fetus* in fecal samples will not grow on selective agar containing cephalothin. Bacteremia may be caused by *C. fetus, C. jejuni, H. fenellelliae,* and *H. cinaedi.* Nonselective media should be used for subculture from blood culture media containing curved, gram-negative rods resembling campylobacters. *Helicobacter cinaedi* and *H. fennelliae* also do not grow under conditions ususally employed to detect *C. jejuni/coli,* grow at 37°C but not at 42°C, and are inhibited by some cephalosporin antibiotics. They may be detected in fecal specimens by use of the nonselective media and filtration technique or most efficiently using special selective media containing *Brucella* agar, 10% blood, and antibiotics, with incubation in anaerobic gas-pack jar without catylist (or appropriate gas mixture) for 7 days (106).

Identification. *Campylobacter* sp. that grow at 42°C can be presumptively identified as *C. jejuni/coli* on the basis of oxidase and catalase positivity, typical Gram stain morphology (e.g., thin-curved, spiral, or gull-wing–shaped gram-negative rods with coccoid shapes present in older cultures), darting motility on wet mounts prepared using saline or broth (not water), susceptibility to nalidixic acid, and resistance to cephalothin (48,100,102). This level of identification has been sufficient for most clinical purposes. Development of quinolone resistance is associated with resistance to nalidixic acid; under these conditions, *C. jejuni* may be mistakenly identified as *C. lari* (117,118). *Campylobacter jejuni* may be distinguished from *C. coli* by testing hippurate hydrolysis; however, atypical strains of *C. jejuni* may be hippurate-negative (119). Since both species cause similar clinical syndromes, most diagnostic laboratories do not distinguish between these. A battery of other tests including thermotolerance, nitrate reduction, H_2S and urease production, which are available in most laboratories, can be used to further characterize isolates of *Helicobacter* and *Campylobacter* when warranted (48,100). Polymyxin susceptibility is a simple test that may distinguish *H. cinaedi* and *H. fennelliae* from most nonthermotolerant *Campylobacter* sp. (120). A simple commercially available disk test for indoxyl acetate hydrolysis may be useful for distinguishing nalidixic acid resistant strains of *C. jejuni* from *C. lari* and for separation of *H. fennelliae* from *H. cinaedi* (121).

Other Methods of Detection and Identification. Species identification of *C. jejuni/coli* can be made using latex agglutination kits (122,123). Species-specific DNA probes have been developed that are useful for species identification in the reference laboratory setting (48). A commercially available, nonradioactive, DNA hybridization method specific for *C. jejuni-coli-lari* has been reported to be quite reliable for identification of *Campylobacter* in culture (124). Serological testing has not been employed to diagnose *Campylobacter* infection but is useful as a epidemiological tool.

Direct detection of *C. jejuni* in fecal samples by DNA hybridization has not been achieved. Even though the quantity of microorganisms that are excreted is relatively high (10^6–10^9 CFU/g of stool), direct hybridization on nitrocellulose is relatively insensitive, in part due to substances within feces that are inhibitory. Growth amplification prior to hybridization does enhance sensitivity but is not practical in routine diagnostic laboratories. PCR methods may detect 500–1000 organisms per gram of stool but the DNA must first be extracted from the fecal sample (125). Currently, there are no nucleic acid–based detection systems that are commercially available to detect *Campylobacter* sp. in stool.

Susceptibility Testing. Until recently, susceptibility testing was not routinely performed on *C. jejuni* isolates since resistance to antibiotics was rare and a standardized method had not been developed. However, resistance to macrolides and quinolone antibiotics is no longer rare (126), and relapse with resistant strains has been shown to occur, particularly in immunocompromised patients treated for prolonged periods. Therefore, susceptibility testing should be done in selected instances, including relapse of infection. A commercially available method that employs the use of strips impregnated with an antibiotic gradient, the E test (A. B. Biodisk), has been shown to compare favorably with agar dilution MIC for detection of erythromycin, ciprofloxacin, and tetracycline resistance, as defined by NCCLS breakpoints (23). Using this method, minor categorical errors (primarily difference in classification of susceptible vs. intermediate) were observed with erythromycin. Results obtained with the E test for other antibiotics did not correlate well with conventional methods. Most susceptibility breakpoints are based on achievable serum (not GI tract) levels of antibiotics, and the clinical predictive value of "low-level resistance" for some GI pathogens has not been established. Nonetheless, stepwise mutations may result in highly resistant isolates (127).

Enteroinvasive E. Coli (EIEC)

Enteroinvasive *E. coli* (EIEC) strains contain the large 140-MDa virulence plasmid, also carried by all virulent shigellae, which encodes the relevant virulence property of invasiveness thereby promoting dysentery (128). EIEC appear to be relatively uncommon causes of dysentery in both developed and developing countries, although it is possible that the true incidence of infection has been underestimated (85,87,129,130). Since there are no commercially available systems to detect them, EIEC strains are not identified in clinical laboratories. EIEC are confined to a limited number of serotypes. Unlike other *E. coli,* some EIEC strains are lysine-negative and nonmotile, characteristics typical of *Shigella.* However, many strains cannot be recognized on the basis of biochemical tests (67,69,131). In fact, at the DNA level, EIEC and *Shigella* sp. are virtually identical. EIEC and *Shigella* O antigens cross-react, sometimes making it difficult to distinguish them by this method (67). Like *Shigella,* EIEC are also Sereney test–positive and enter (invade) cultured epithelial cells. This assay has been used as a screening method to identify EIEC. An ELISA assay that specifically identifies outer membrane proteins has also been described (94). DNA probes that hybridize with plasmid-mediated invasion genes, *ipaBCD,* or with *ipaH,* a chromosomal determinant, have high specificity and have been useful in epidemiological studies (132). Spontaneous loss or deletion of the plasmid may cause false-negative results. Such probes also hybridize with shigellae, and since the clinical syndromes are identical, there is little impetus to distinguish EIEC from *Shigella* for clinical purposes.

Yersinia

Yersinia enterocolitica infection may present as acute or chronic diarrhea associated with fecal leukocytes and blood (133–140). Mesenteric adenitis, terminal ileitis, and pseudoappendicitis are less common and seen primarily in older children and adults. Localized infections including pharyngitis may develop at extraintestinal sites and bacteremia with a high mortality rate has been observed in some patients, particularly those with iron overload or other predisposing risk factors. Asymptomatic blood donors with *Y. enterocolitica* infection have been implicated as the source in transfusion-related bacteremia (133,141); asymptomatic carriage may occur with low frequency (142,143). Nosocomial aquisition unrelated to transfusion has been reported (144).

Y. enterocolitica infections occur worldwide but are rare in tropical countries and more common in cooler areas of temperate zones such as Scandinavia, Canada, northern Europe, Japan, South Africa, New Zealand, and some parts of South America (142–145). In the United States, the frequency of *Y. enterocolitica* infections appears to be increasing, particularly in black children and others who have consumed undercooked or uncooked pork (135,146,147). Pork products, particularly those prepared from organs containing lymphoid tissue, including intestines, neck, jaws, or head of the pig, may be an important source of *Y. enterocolitica;* however, contaminated water and other foods also have been implicated (133,142,147). The incidence of sporadic cases is seasonal, occurring primarily in colder months, although outbreaks may occur in any period. Certain serotypes are associated with disease as compared to environmental isolates. Serotype O:3, which was formerly dominant in northern Europe and infrequently seen in the United States, is now common in the United States, indicating a change in the epidemiology of infections.

Human infection with *Y. pseudotuberculosis* are much less common than those due to *Y. enterocolitica;* however, the clinical manifestations of infection by both may be similar and their geographic distribution is similar (142). Nonpathogenic *Y. enterocolitica* strains or other *Yersinia* species formerly classified as *Y. enterocolitica* or *Y. enterocolitica*-like (*Y. frederiksenii, Y. kristensenii, Y. ruckeri,* and *Y. aldovae*) can be recovered from a variety of environmental sources, animals, and foods, and, with the possible exception of *Y. intermedia,* are not considered to be GI pathogens (148).

Demonstration of virulent *Y. enterocolitica* (or *Y. pseudotuberculosis*) in clinical material is the most reliable means to diagnose infection (133). In temperate climates, particularly in cooler months, laboratories serving a population at risk for *Y. enterocolitica* infection should use media selective for recovery of *Y. enterocolitica* (135). In other circumstances, periodic surveillance should be conducted in conjunction with other clinical laboratories or public health facilities to monitor occurrence of *Y. enterocolitica* infections. At a minimum, laboratories should have protocols for recognition of *Y. enterocolitica* from routine cultures of stool or material submitted from biopsy of intestinal or cervical lymphatic tissue. In chronic infection, stool cultures may not be sensitive (133,149,150). Serology may be useful in some settings but has limitations.

Culture. Stool and fecal samples should be plated onto selective media for recovery of *Y. enterocolitica.* Cefsulodin-irgasan-novobiocin agar (CIN), a selective medium for *Y. enterocolitica* that also permits growth of *Aeromo-*

nas and *Plesiomonas,* is more sensitive than other enteric plating media (67,142). Inoculated CIN agar plates should be incubated at 32°C for 24 hr or at 22–25°C for 48 hr. Suspicious colonies should be tested with appropriate screening or identification systems.

Yersinia enterocolitica is readily isolated on nonselective media commonly used for culture of most specimen types (blood and chocolate agar), and colonies can grow on relatively noninhibitory enteric media, such as MacConkey agar, that is used to culture other enteric pathogens. Growth may be inhibited on more selective enteric plating agars such as SS, Hektoen or XLD. In order to recover *Y. enterocolitica* without use of specific selective media, some laboratories pick small colonies isolated on MacConkey incubated at 35–37°C for 24 hr and those that become larger after additional 24 hr incubation at 25°C for further analysis. Although extensive comparative studies have not been done, compared to use of CIN agar, this approach may detect 60% of patients with *Y. enterocolitica* in a low-prevalence population (0.2% of stool cultures positive) (151).

Identification. Conventional screening tests routinely employed for *Yersinia* identification include motility at 25°C but not at 37°C, citrate utilization, hydrolysis of urea, and reactions on TSI slants. It should be noted that reactions of different strains of *Y. enterocolitica* may vary, and only 75% of strains are urease positive (67). *Yersinia enterocolitica* colonies are often described as having a "plastic" odor on MacConkey agar. Commercially available biochemical test panels for screening potential enteric pathogens have not been evaluated with a large number of strains (79). *Yersinia enterocolitica* is less metabolically active at 37°C than at 22–28°C; therefore, results of conventional or commercial identification systems are more rapid and reliable when tests are incubated at lower temperature (67,82,152,153).

Since avirulent serotypes of *Y. enterocolitica* may be recovered from human feces, it has been suggested that the pathogenic potential of isolates recovered from stool be determined using phenotyping methods before a report is given (67). Virulent vs. avirulent environmental strains can be genotypically differentiated on the basis of carriage of plasmid genes encoding outer membrane proteins associated with attachment, resistance to phagocytosis, calcium-dependent growth at 37°C, iron storage, and uptake of the dye congo red (67,154). Two chromosomal loci, *inv* and *ail,* encode determinants that mediate invasion, attatchment, and serum resistance, which are also involved in virulence (155–157). Negative tests for pyrazinamidase, esculin hydrolysis, salicin fermentation, and plasmid-mediated uptake of the dye congo red at 37°C in the presence of a chelator (CR-MOX agar) are phenotypic assays that have been used to distinguish avirulent *Y. enterocolitica* serotypes or isolates lacking the virulence plasmid from isolates likely to be pathogenic (67,158). However, some investigators have found that such assays do not reliably correlate with clinical significance of isolates (146,159). The virulence plasmid may be unstable at 37°C; therefore, isolates that are to be further characterized should be passaged a minimum number of times at cooler temperatures.

Cold enrichment techniques, in which stool sample is placed in phosphate-buffered saline held at 4°C for up to 3 weeks before subculture, increases recovery of *Y. enterocolitica* and is especially useful to document asymptomatic carriage or persistent shedding in convalescent patients (67,133,142). At this temperature, *Y. enterocolitica* continue to grow while numbers of other bacteria in the stool remain stable or decline. Most diagnostic laboratories do not perform this method on a routine basis because of the limited impact of results on patient care and questionable virulence potential or clinical significance of isolates recovered.

Susceptibility Testing. In cases of uncomplicated enterocolitis or the pseudoappendicitis syndrome, antibiotic treatment may not be warranted and susceptibility testing is not indicated (133). GI isolates from patients at high risk for systemic infection or isolates from other normally sterile sources should be tested for susceptibility, preferably using a broth or agar dilution method. Susceptibility reports should include a cautionary statement indicating that some antibiotics to which the organism may appear susceptible *in vitro* may not be clinically effective.

DNA Probes. DNA probes have been used to differentiate among virulent and avirulent strains and to detect *Y. enterocolitica* in environmental samples (160–162). Although many of the determinants of virulence are plasmid-encoded, the instability of the plasmid and presence of homologous sequences in *Y. pseudotuberculosis* and *Y. pestis* pose potential problems with sensitivity and specificity. PCR procedure using primers for the chromosomally encoded *yst* gene (*Y. enterocolitica* heat-stable enterotoxin) has been employed to detect *Y. enterocolitica* in extracted fecal samples (163).

Serology. Serological assays are useful only in limited clinical situations, and results must be interpreted with a number of caveats in mind. An agglutination test using whole bacterial cells as antigen that detects primarily IgM has been used as a standard assay, although interpretation of results is not necessarily standardized. A fourfold increase or decrease in titer of paired specimens or a titer of $\geq 1:128$ in a single specimen has been considered presumptive evidence of recent infection by some investigators but not others (138,145,164). Serotype specificity of the lipopolysaccharide (LPS) antigens included In the preparation determines the sensitivity of the test. In Scandinavia or northern Europe where serotypes O:3 and O:9 are common, tests using these antigens alone may be acceptable, whereas in the United States or regions where other serotypes are common, such assays would enable detection of only a portion of the infected population. The test is negative in approximately 80% of cases of chronic infection, and false-positive tests due to cross-reactivity of shared antigens (145,149,150,165) are not uncommon in patients with other bacterial infections. In some populations, a high proportion of asymptomatic persons may have positive titers. ELISA assays using LPS antigen share many of these same problems but may be simpler to perform and enable determination of titers to IgG, IgM, and IgA. Detection of IgA antibodies may be useful in detecting chronic infection (150). ELISA using *Yersinia* outer membrane proteins (Yops) offer the potential of improved specificity; however, the sensitivity may be lower than the anti-LPS assay and have not been extensively evaluated (164–166). Immunoblotting may offer both sensitivity and specificity; however, this is expensive, not readily available, and interpretation is not standardized. Therefore, the diagnosis of *Y. enterocolitica* infection usually should be made by isolation of the organism from clinical specimens rather than reliance on serology alone (133).

Clostridium difficile

Clostridium difficile has been implicated in approximately 95% of cases of pseudomembranous colitis, and 15% to 25% of cases of antibiotic-associated colitis or diarrhea (167,168). It has been included with the group of enteric bacteria causing inflammation, since fever, abdominal pain, and microscopic blood are typically present in pseudomembranous colitis, even though the gross and microscopic appearance of the colonic mucosa differs from shigellosis, campylobacteriosis, and salmonellosis. Over one half of patients with pseudomembranous colitis have fecal WBC, although fecal leukocytes and fever are usually absent with antibiotic-associated diarrhea due to *C. difficile*.

In developed countries, nosocomial diarrhea (onset greater than 3 days after hospital admission) is usually caused by *C. difficile* in adults or by rotavirus or enteric adenoviruses in children less than 2 years of age (12,14,17,18). The major risk factor for acquisition of disease is prior antibiotic therapy (within 6–8 weeks), which may include short courses given as surgical prophylaxis. Other factors such as treatment with cytotoxic drugs and advanced age may enhance susceptibility to acquisition of disease (168,169). Disease in the absence of prior antibiotics or outside hospitals and nursing homes occurs but is unusual. Disease is caused by *C. difficile* colonizing the intestine that may be present upon admission to an institution or, more likely, acquired from the environment or via hands of hospital personnel (170). Approximately 75% to 95% of strains of *C. difficile* recovered from feces are toxigenic and only those that produce toxin have been associated with disease (171). With rare exceptions, toxigenic isolates produce toxin A and toxin B, both of which may have a role in pathogenesis of disease. Toxin A is an enterotoxin that causes fluid accumulation in rabbit ileal loops and is produced in much higher amounts (>1000×) than toxin B. Toxin B is a potent cytotoxin detected in the fecal cytotoxin assay.

Infection with *C. difficile* is often associated with significant complications. Conversely, there also can be adverse consequences when disease due to other underlying problems is ascribed incorrectly to *C. difficile*. Therefore, accurate diagnosis is important. However, no laboratory test is completely sensitive or specific for *C. difficile*–associated disease. Diagnosis and empiric therapy should be based on clinical findings with laboratory tests serving as an adjunct to diagnosis. The predictive value of each *C. difficile* test should be known, and this value should be weighed in making a diagnosis. Cytotoxicity of fecal filtrates for tissue culture remains the most sensitive and specific correlate of *C. difficile*–associated disease. Commercial ELISA assays for toxin that are currently available are less sensitive and specific than cytotoxicity. Culture is generally recommended only for epidemiological studies due to poor specificity, expense, and slow turnaround. If ELISA methods are used for screening, availability of cytotoxicity (or culture) has been recommended (167,168). Because of high rates of both *C. difficile* carriage and positive toxin asays in healthy infants, results of tests for *C. difficile* are of questionable significance and not recommended in patients less than one year of age (167,168).

Cytotoxicity Assay. The best correlate of disease and the most sensitive and specific method to detect toxin B is based on observation of specific cytotoxicity for tissue-cultured cells using fecal filtrates as a source of toxin. The cytotoxicity assay detects as little as 0.2–1.0 pg of toxin B and sensitivity for detection of *C. difficile*–mediated disease is 85% to 95% depending on criteria used for defining cases. Lower values were reported in some studies, particularly when tests other than positive culture or cytotoxicity were included in the case definition (167,168,172–177). Specificity is usually greater than 99%. Commercial ELISA assays for toxin that are currently available are less sensitive and specific than the cytotoxicity assay. Although toxin titer does not correlate with severity of disease, a higher proportion of patients with severe manifestations of disease (pseudomembranous colitis) are likely to be positive than those with milder disease. Athough widely used, the test is not completely standardized, and choice of tissue culture cells, age of cells, dilution of feces, incubation times, and technologist skill may affect test performance. Commonly used cell lines include WI-38, HeLa, Hep-2, NRC-5, human foreskin, and Chinese hamster ovary (CHO) cells. Although some investigators have found most of these cell lines to give comparable sensitivity results (178), differences among cell types have been reported (179–183). Neutralization by specific antisera of cytopathic effect is required to demonstrate that cytotoxicity is due to *C. difficile* toxin. Commercially available antiserum to *C. sordelli* that cross-reacts with *C. difficile* toxin B is used for neutralization studies (184,185). Commercially available systems for cytotoxicity testing compare favorably with conventional assays (180,184), and may offer advantage of standardization. When neutralization is performed concurrently with cytotoxicity testing, a large proportion of positive results may be detected within a day; however, other tests may not be positive in the first 48 hr of incubation and some may require 72 hr for positivity (180). Some tests require repeat testing or may not be interpretable due to sample toxicity or contamination. Cytotoxicity testing should be available to confirm positive results obtained with alternative screening assays that have low specificity or positive predicive value and to test samples from patients highly suspected of *C. difficile* disease in whom screening tests having only moderate sensitivity are negative. Cytotoxicity assay may be positive in a small proportion (2% to 8%) of patients without diarrhea who have been exposed to antibiotics (167,168,174,179). The test may remain positive in treated or recovering patients, and therefore it is not useful for following clinical response (167,168). Generally, one fecal sample is considered to be adequate for testing; however, there is limited information on sensitivity of one or more sequential tests for diagnosis.

Other Methods to Detect Toxin. A latex test that was shown to react with glutamate dehydrogenase of *C. difficile* and that reacted with toxigenic and nontoxigenic strains of *C. difficile,* as well as *C. sporogenes, C. botulinum,* and other anaerobic bacteria (186), has largely been replaced by more sensitive and specific ELISA assays. ELISA assays for detection of toxin A or toxins A and B are being used in many laboratories as screening tests because testing can be done within several hours as compared with cytotoxicity assays requiring up to 48–72 hr incubation. Performance of commercially available ELISA assays varied (sensitivity ranging from approximately 65% to 85%) compared to that of tissue culture cytotoxicity in these same studies (93% to 99%) (172,176,177). Specificity ranged from approximately 85% to 99%, depending on the method and the prevalence of disease in the population. Indeterminant or uninterpretable results may occur in approximately 2% to 5% of samples. These tests should be supplemented by cytotoxicity testing, or possibly culture (168,172) in selected cases, and reporting of ELISA results should include interpretative comments including sensitivity, specificity, and predictive values of the tests.

Organism Detection. Culture is generally recommended only for epidemiological studies due to poor specificity and is primarily reserved in epidemiological investigations for identification of *C. difficile* carriers. Although this is test is very sensitive, 30% to 70% of healthy neonates, 2% to 5% of healthy adults, and 10% to 20% of hospitalized adults and persons exposed to antibiotics but without disease may be culture-positive, thereby resulting in poor specificity and positive predictive values (167,168,170,179). Furthermore, delays in culturing specimens compromise recovery of *C. difficile,* and specimens should be cultured within 2 hr or frozen at −20°C or −70°C. Cycloserine-cefoxitin-fructose agar (CCFA) is the medium of choice for culture; however, differences in performance have been observed in formulations obtained from different manufacturers (187,188). Decreasing amounts of cycloserine and cefoxitin in CCFA have been found to increase isolation rates of *C. difficile* (179). Culture plates should be inoculated and incubated anaerobically 48 hr prior to examination. Colonies may be presumptively identified by Gram stain, typical colony morphology, *p*-creosol (horse manure) odor, and chartreuse fluorescence under long-wave ultraviolet light (5,179,184). *C. innocuum,* which also demonstrates the same yellow–green fluorescence and grows on this medium, has different colonial morphology and, in most cases, presumptive identification is adequate. For definitive identification, isolates should be tested for the presence of a characteristic pattern of short-chain fatty acid metabolic products using gas–liquid chromatography, and when necessary be characterized by conventional or some commercially available biochemical tests. Because a sig-

nificant proportion of isolates are nontoxigenic and have no clinical significance, *C. difficile* recovered in culture should be tested for presence of toxin using ELISA or cytotoxicity. Isolation rates of *C. difficile* may be increased by using enrichment broth and some investigators have used presumptive identification based on gas–liquid chromatography of enrichment broth (179). PCR amplification of *C. difficile* targets present in feces has been described (189); however, clinical performance and utility of the assay require evaluation.

Watery (Secretory) Diarrhea

Bacteria that usually are associated with a watery, secretory diarrhea include *V. cholerae,* enterotoxigenic *E. coli* (ETEC), *Aeromonas,* and sometimes enteropathogenic *E. coli* (EPEC) and enteroaggregative *E. coli* (EAggEC). *V. parahemolyticus* and *Plesiomonas* frequently cause inflammatory diarrheal syndromes. Although bacterial agents have been classified by diarrheal syndrome with which they are usually associated, this association is by no means absolute. *V. parahemolyticus* and *V. cholerae* as well as *Aeromonas* and *Plesiomonas* have been placed together in this section to expedite discussion of laboratory methods.

Vibrios

The current cholera pandemic has spread to Africa, Asia, Europe, Oceania, and to most of South and Central America (190). In the United States exposure to *V. cholerae* 01 strains has occurred in travelers to developing countries affected by the global pandemic. However, some cases have been reported in the United States among patients who ingested contaminated food imported from Asia and South America (191). Although not associated with epidemics, occasional strains of non-01 *V. cholerae* may produce cholera toxin and cause disease clinically indistinguishable from cholera (192–194). In the United States endemic infection by *V. cholerae* non-01 and occasionally by endemic *V. cholerae* 01 strains via ingestion of shellfish taken from Gulf Coast waters has been well documented (192–194). *V. parahemolyticus* has caused outbreaks and sporadic cases of acute gastroenteritis worldwide, including the United States and Japan (195–198). Less frequently *V. mimicus, V. fluvialis, V. furnissi,* and *V. hollisae* have been implicated as causes of diarrhea (195–203). *Vibrio* species including *V. cholerae* 01 naturally occur in marine and estuarine environments throughout the world and are isolated in larger numbers in warmer climates or in summer months when water temperatures are higher. Pathogenic *Vibrio* sp. are commonly found in seafood, particularly shellfish, and were recovered from a large proportion of cooked and uncooked samples of oysters, shrimp, and crab sampled in New Orleans restaurants (198). *Vibrio* species, particularly *V. vulnificus,* also can cause wound infections and septicemia, usually following exposure to marine or tidal waters. Although prior studies in coastal endemic areas of the United States have suggested that routine use of media specifically designed to optimize isolation of *Vibrio* species is not cost-effective (194,197), in view of current trends such methods would be appropriate in epidemic areas or in nonendemic areas for patients with compatible clinical presentation and a recent history indicating probability of *Vibrio* infection, e.g., travel to epidemic areas, consumption of seafood, particularly oysters, or exposure to marine waters. Communication of pertinent history to the laboratory is therefore quite important.

Culture. Pathogenic *Vibrio* sp. grow on blood agar, on chocolate agar, and in standard blood culture media, which usually contain 0.5% NaCl (202,203). Therefore, routine culture procedures for specimen types other than feces will recover these organisms. Screening for *Vibrio* sp. in fecal samples can be performed by oxidase testing. Routine inoculation of stool cultures on a blood agar plate without antibiotics (204) with subsequent screening colonies for oxidase positivity is a simple procedure for detection of vibrios as well as other oxidase-positive enteric pathogens such as *Aeromonas* and *Plesiomonas*. This will detect these organisms present in large numbers or as predominating flora and is not as sensitive as using *Vibrio*-selective media. Additionally, most pathogenic *Vibrio* sp. grow on MacConkey or MacConkey-sorbitol agar, which are standard plating media for enteric pathogens. *Vibrio* sp. other than *V. vulnificus* usually do not ferment lactose, and some vibrios, including *V. parahemolyticus,* do not ferment sucrose; therefore, these may be detected by routinely performing oxidase testing of nonlactose (nonsucrose) fermenting colonies subcultured to TSI, KIA slants, or blood agar plates.

Thio-citrate-bile salt-sucrose (TCBS) is recommended as a selective medium for recovery of *V. cholerae* and most other vibrios implicated in human GI infections. Batch-dependent plating efficiency has been reported for *V. parahemolyticus* as well as poor growth of some *Vibrio* species that can cause disease (202,203). On TCBS, *Vibrio* species such as *V. cholerae, V. fluvialis,* and *V. furnissi* produce yellow colonies, while non–sucrose fermenters such as *V. parahemolyticus, V. mimicus,* and *V. hollisae* appear as green or blue–green colonies. In most areas of North America or other locations where *Vibrio* infections occur primarily in the summer months or are seasonal, inclusion of TCBS as a part of routine stool culture workup during these months should be considered. Alkaline peptone water (pH 8.5) may increase recovery of vibrios. After incubation of 5–8 hr, surface growth should be subcultured to selective media such as TCBS as well as to less selective media such as blood agar or MacConkey for optimal recovery of organisms. This medium also serves as an excellent transport medium for *Vibrio* and *Aeromonas.*

Identification. Vibrio must be differentiated from *Aeromonas* and *Plesiomonas,* which are also oxidase-positive fermentative gram-negative rods that grow on MacConkey and other enteric media. Useful tests include growth in nutrient broth with 0% and 6% NaCl, growth on TCBS, ornithine decarboxylase activity, and susceptibility to the vibriostatic compound O/129 (202,203). In contrast to previous reports (202) that O/129 resistance is rare among *Vibrio* sp., 62% of *V. cholerae* 01 in Bangla-

desh were found to be O129-resistant indicating that the test may have limited reliability for identification, particularly among *V. cholerae* isolates resistant to ampicillin or trimethoprim-sulfamethoxazole (204). To accurately identify *Vibrio,* particularly halophilic species, both standard tube media and commercially available systems should be supplemented with adequate Na^+ by adding NaCl to media or suspending inoculum in NaCl or marine salts solution (202,205). Databases for commercial identification reagents may incorrectly identify organisms. Therefore it is recommended that standard identification tables such as in Ref. 202 be used. *V. vulnificus,* which causes wound infections and septicemia, may be misidentified as *V. parahemolyticus* because of false-negative ONPG results (205) and *V. fluvialis* may be confused with *Aeromonas* (202). *V. parahemolyticus* does not grow in 0% NaCl, is arginine dehydrolase–negative, lysine- and ornithine decarboxylase–positive. *V. cholerae* and *V. mimicus* can be separated biochemically from other vibrios by their ability to grow in medium without salt supplementation, negative arginine dehydrolase and sucrose fermentation, positive lysine and ornithine decarboxylase. Suspected *V. cholerae* isolates should be immediately reported to public health reference laboratories.

In epidemic and endemic areas, many larger diagnostic laboratories (202) may use polyvalent antiserum or *V. cholerae* coagglutination reagents (206) for rapid presumptive identification of *V. cholerae* 01. This may be done by subculturing heavy inoculum of suspicious colonies growing on TCBS or other selective media to nonselective medium for 5–8 hr. Oxidase-positive organisms growing on the blood agar or other nonselective medium may be tested directly for agglutination with polyvalent *V. cholerae* 01 antiserum or other suitable assay. Public health laboratories will subtype *V. cholerae* 01 on the basis of O antigens as Ogawa, Inaba, or Hikojima. Biogrouping *V. cholerae* is also done using a battery of tests that are not routinely available. Some simple tests may presumptively identify biotype; most isolates of the classical biotype that is now recovered in a limited number of areas show a zone of growth inihibition around a disk containing 50 μg polymyxin B and are Voges-Proskauer-negative while the predominant El Tor biotype is polymyxin B–resistant and Voges-Proskauer-positive and may be β-hemolytic (202).

Toxin Testing. Isolates of *V. cholerae* should be tested for toxin production and detection of toxin in fecal material may enable rapid diagnosis of cholera. Occasional toxigenic non-01 strains may cause disease clinically indistinguishable from cholera. Strains of *V. cholerae* 01 that do not produce toxin and are not pathogenic have been recovered from humans, sewage, oysters, and surface water (192,194,202,203,207). A relatively simple commercially available latex assay for cholera toxin (or *E. coli* LT) (Oxoid) has a sensitivity and a specificity of 97% and 100%, respectively, when compared to results obtained by ELISA, genetic probe, or bioassay (207), and may be employed in smaller labs.

Initial studies suggest that detection of *V. cholerae* antigen or cholera toxin in feces using commercially available agglutination (206,208) or bead ELISA (209), respectively, may be used in endemic areas or outbreak situations to facilitate diagnosis, and further evaluation of these assays is warranted. Approximately half of stools positive for cholera toxin may have <1 ng/mL of free toxin (209) and currently available ELISA assays may be more sensitive than latex tests or bioassay but not as sensitive as culture. Heat-labile toxin of ETEC is antigenically similar to cholera toxin, and whether positive tests due to ETEC infection may be a problem in some settings remains to be determined.

Susceptibility Testing. Susceptibility testing of *V. cholerae* by clinical or reference laboratories identifies resistance to antibiotics useful for treatment, which may include doxycycline, tetracycline, trimethoprim-sulfamethoxazole, erythromycin, and furzolidone (24,210). Performance of disk diffusion and automated systems has not been extensively evaluated for other vibrios, and reference methods such as broth or agar dilution should be used when possible. The literature should be consulted for antibiotics found to be clinically effective for specific infections due to other *Vibrio* species. Reports should indicate that *in vitro* susceptibility for some antibiotics may not predict clinical efficacy.

Enterotoxigenic E. coli (ETEC)

ETEC strains expressing heat-labile toxin (LT), which resembles cholera toxin, heat-stable toxin (ST), or both, are leading causes of secretory diarrhea in infants and children residing in developing countries and in travelers to these areas (12,13,128). Although outbreaks of ETEC have occurred in the United States or other industrialized nations, the incidence of sporadic ETEC infections is thought to be quite low. As with other pathogenic *E. coli* strains, practical assays have not been available for clinical laboratories to differentiate ETEC strains from commensal *E. coli*. ETEC strains belong to a limited number of *E. coli* serotypes (67). However, other assays that detect virulence determinants are preferred for identification of ETEC. Bioassays such as rabbit ileal loop and cytotoxicity for Y1 adrenal cells have been used to detect LT-producing strains, and the infant suckling mouse assay may be employed to identify ST-producing strains (128). Latex and EIA reagents are commercially available for LT toxin (and cholera toxin) determination (67,207,209,211), and ELISA assays for ST toxin have also been developed (212–214). These reagents may be useful in some settings. The most widely used method to identify ETEC for epidemiological purposes employs DNA probes derived from the toxin-encoding genes. DNA probes have been developed for use in direct hybridization assays, with or without dilution and/or amplification, and for screening colonies isolated on conventional media (26,85,86,89,215,216). Depending on the method, sensitivity and specificity of hybridization and bioassays for LT and ST are more or less comparable, and hybridization assays are far less cumbersome than bioassays. Simultaneous PCR amplification of an LT gene and a *Shigella* virulence gene has been successfully applied to extracted stool samples obtained from patients in Mexico (89).

Aeromonas *and* Plesiomonas

Aeromonas species (217–224) and *Plesiomonas shigelloides* (225–228) have been implicated as causes of both secretory diarrhea and invasive diarrhea. *Aeromonas* more often is associated with the former presentation and *P. shigelloides* with the latter symptoms. *P. shigelloides* has been associated with persistent diarrhea. Both *Aeromonas* sp. and *P. shigelloides* occur in aquatic habitats. Human infections are associated with water exposure and are most often associated with warm seasons in temperate climates or with tropical and subtropical geographic regions. Gastroenteritis due to *P. shigelloides* in the United States has most often been associated with travel to tropical countries, although up to 30% of cases appear to have been endemic and been associated with ingestion of shellfish, particularly raw oysters, or contaminated water (224,226,227). GI carriage rates in humans appear to be low (<0.1%) for *Plesiomonas* (although exceptions have been reported), and recovery of the organism is usually associated with GI illness. Carriage rates for *Aeromonas* have varied considerably (0.2% to 27%), with highest rates generally found in tropical developing countries. *Aeromonas* sp. found most frequently in the environment or in clinical material have shown geographic variation. *Aeromonas hydrophila, A. veronii* bv. *sobria* (formerly *A. sobria*), and *A. caviae* are most commonly associated with human infection although the role of the latter as a cause of gastroenteritis is somewhat more controversial. *Aeromonas* sp. have also been associated with extraintestinal infections, including wound infections and cellulitis in normal hosts, often resulting from traumatic exposure to soil and water. Septicemia usually has been associated with underlying illnesses, including hepatic, biliary, or pancreatic disease, or malignancy, particularly aplastic anemia and acute leukemia. Extraintestinal *P. shigelloides* infections are rare.

Although the etiological role of *Aeromonas* sp. and, to a lesser extent, *P. shigelloides* in GI disease has been controversial, sufficient evidence has accumulated suggesting that at a minimum the laboratory should consider using readily available reagents to detect them when stool cultures are performed (217,229). Currently many laboratories use methods for isolation that permit recovery of these species only when present in stool in relatively large numbers, and therefore these procedures are not specifically designed to optimize detection of small numbers of organisms as might occur with states of convalescence, chronic disease, carriage, or following antibiotic treatment. The rationale for this approach has included considerations such as questionable clinical significance of low numbers of *Aeromonas* in feces, relative infrequency of *Plesiomonas* infections, and low cost effectiveness of additional procedures for recovery of pathogens that do not exhibit person-to-person transmission and usually cause relatively mild self-limited disease.

Culture. *Aeromonas* and *Plesiomonas* are facultatively anaerobic gram-negative rods that grow readily on most commonly used nonselective bacteriological media such as blood agar. The simplest approach to isolation is to screen colonies isolated on blood agar with the oxidase test (217,229–231). *Aeromonas, Plesiomonas,* and *Vibrio* sp. are oxidase-positive, whereas Enterobacteriaceae are oxidase-negative. Unlike most enteric organisms, *A. hydrophila* and *A. veronii* bv. *sobria* (and some vibrios) are usually β-hemolytic and have colony morphology different from that of *P. aeroginosa,* which may aid in selection of suspect colonies for testing. The disadvantage of this approach is that these species will be detected only if they are present in relatively large numbers and may be overgrown by swarming *Proteus.* Use of blood agar containing 10 µg/mL of ampicillin may increase sensitivity of isolation of *Aeromonas* (217); however, not all strains of *Aeromonas* or *Plesiomonas* are ampicillin-resistant, and some *Vibrio* species are ampicillin-susceptible. Blood agar is less inhibitory to these species than conventional enteric media. Most strains of *Aeromonas, Plesiomonas,* and *Vibrio* appear as non–lactose fermenters, as are *Salmonella* and *Shigella. Aeromonas* can also be recovered with reasonable efficiency on cefsulodin-irgasan-novobiocin (CIN) agar, a selective medium commonly used to recover *Yersinia* sp. if CIN contains 4 µg/mL of cefsulodin (and not 15 µg/mL); plates are incubated at 25–30°C (217,218,231–233). The oxidase test may be falsely negative if growth from selective agars is tested. Inositol–bile salts brilliant green agar is selective for both *Aeromonas* and *Plesiomonas.* Pril-xylose-ampicillin and xylose-sodium desoxycholate-citrate agars are alternative selective agars for *Aeromonas.*

Identification. Aeromonas, Plesiomonas, and *Vibrio* are readily distinguished from nonfermentative oxidase-positive organisms, such as *Pseudomonas* sp., by the fermentative pattern. *Aeromonas* and *Plesiomonas* do not grow on media selective for *Vibrio* sp. (TCBS). Diagnostic laboratories should have the capability of providing rapid presumptive identification to the genus level of oxidase-positive fermentative organisms that grow on MacConkey (or similar media). Tests that are useful for separation of halophilic and nonhalophilic *Vibrio, Aeromonas,* and *Plesiomonas* include testing ability to grow in the presence of 0% and 6% NaCl, growth on *Vibrio*-selective media such as TCBS, ability to decarboxylate ornithine, and susceptibility to the vibriostatic compound O129 (2,4 diamino-6,7-diisopropylpteridine (Oxoid)(61) (231,232). Identification to the species level can be undertaken by most laboratories using seven commonly available tests and antibiotic susceptibility patterns (234), and results show good correlation with DNA hybridization groups (235). *Aeromonas* most frequently encountered in clinical material are found in DNA hybridization groups 1, 4, and 8 which correlate, respectively, with phenospecies *A. hydrophila, A. caviae,* and *A. veronii* bv. *sobria* (clinical isolates formerly identified as *A. sobria*). Currently, the databases provided by most commercial systems are not reliable for identification of *Aeromonas* and *Vibrio.*

Susceptibility Testing. Susceptibility testing using a broth or agar dilution method should be attempted when isolates are considered clinically significant and treatment is being considered (217,218,224–226). Susceptibility testing using rapid systems is not recommended because of problems with detection of inducible β-lactamases (236).

Hemorrhagic Diarrhea

Although enterohemorrhagic *E. coli* strains are the most commonly reported cause of frankly bloody or hemorrhagic stools, *C. jejuni* infection may also cause gross hemorrhage. The pathogenic mechanism involved is not known, but apparently does not involve secretion of a verotoxin.

Enterohemorrhagic E. coli (EHEC)

The spectrum of illness associated with EHEC infection includes watery diarrhea, grossly bloody diarrhea, and hemorrhagic colitis (128,237–239). In addition, EHEC infection is also closely linked to the subsequent development of the hemolytic-uremic syndrome or thrombocytopenia purpura (240–244). Severe disease and sequellae occur most frequently in children and the elderly. Asymptomatic infection may also occur but is unusual (242,245). Sources of EHEC infection have been ascribed to ingestion of undercooked ground beef, but also to poultry, lamb, and pork products. Person-to-person transmission may also occur and has been reported in day care centers and nursing homes (243,244). Distribution is worldwide although infections are quite common in some geographic areas including parts of Canada, the United States, Argentina, and Chile, and infrequently seen in some geographic regions. EHEC are confined to a limited number of *E. coli* serotypes (67). Serotype O157:H7 is the predominant serotype in North America although other serotypes may be more prevalent in some populations. EHEC strains produce bacteriophage-mediated toxins resembling Shiga toxin that are cytotoxic for vero cells in tissue culture and thought to be important in the pathogenesis of hemorrhagic diarrhea associated with EHEC infection (246). In addition to the toxins referred to as Shiga-like (SLT) or vero toxins (VT), EHEC strains also contain a 60-MDa plasmid containing a gene encoding a eukaryotic cell adhesion.

Laboratory methods to detect and differentiate EHEC with sufficient sensitivity and specificity are based on the following features of infection. First, although early on in the course of the illness EHEC may be present in large numbers in feces, the sensitivity of culture decreases over time such that positivity rates of >90% seen at the onset of illness decline to one third or less after 4–6 days (241,247). Second, between 17% and 30% of infected individuals studied in outbreaks and 5% of sporadic cases may not have bloody diarrhea or hemorrhagic colitis (248,249). Also, bloody diarrhea usually does not develop until the second or third day although this is usually (90%) present by day 5. Therefore, laboratories that use methods to detect EHEC from bloody stools only will miss some EHEC infections. Third, although *E. coli* O157:H7, the cause of several well-documented outbreaks associated with ingestion of undercooked hamburger, ferments sorbitol slowly and is often β-glucuronidase–negative, lysine decarboxylase– and ornithine decarboxylase–positive, and can be distinguished from commensal *E. coli* on differential agar and by biochemical methods, other vero toxin–producing

EHEC strains do not express unique biochemical patterns or this serotype (67,239,242,245–247,250–254). Finally, hemolytic-uremic syndrome often occurs about a week after onset of diarrhea, which may be resolving, and thus a stool sample obtained when hemolytic-uremic syndrome is manifested is frequently to be culture-negative (239–241,246). In some cases cultures of household contacts of the hemolytic-uremic syndrome patient may be positive when the patient has become culture-negative (241).

Culture. Some clinical laboratories in the United States employ MacConkey sorbitol agar to screen diarrheal stools for the presence of suspected *E. coli* O157:H7 (67,229,254). EHEC may represent only a small proportion of *E. coli* in the fecal sample (245,254), and this agar has been shown to be more sensitive and efficient than sorbitol testing 5–10 *E. coli* colonies isolated on regular MacConkey or other enteric agar. Sorbitol-negative *E. coli* should be tested with commercially available antisera for serogroup O157 and H7, and reagents that permit direct testing from MacConkey media are available (67). In some settings only a small proportion (10%) of sorbitol-negative colonies may be serotype O157:H7 and screening isolates for decarboxylation of lysine and ornithine or β-glucuronidase may decrease unnecessary serotyping (251,252); however, not all EHEC or O157 strains have "typical" phenotypic characteristics and may be overlooked. In one study from Germany (250) a large proportion of SLT-positive *E. coli* from patients with hemolytic-uremic syndrome or diarrhea in serogroup O157 had atypical characteristics and fermented sorbitol rapidly, were positive for β-glucuronidase, were nonmotile, and lacked the H antigen. Conversely, not all serogroup O157 or serotype O157:H7 strains produce SLTs necessary for virulence. Screening for EHEC using phenotypic characteristics may enable detection of a majority of EHEC strains. However, limitations of sensitivity and specificity should be appreciated by those relying on this methodology for diagnosis of EHEC infection. Cultures of suspected EHEC should be sent to a reference laboratory for serotype confirmation, testing of virulence determinants, and possible strain typing. Frequent loss of SLT genes in subcultured isolates has been demonstrated (255); therefore, isolates suspected of being EHEC should be passaged a minimum number of times before testing for cytotoxicity or assaying for virulence determinants using other methods. Susceptibility testing is usually not indicated because the benefit of antimicrobial therapy is controversial (239). Toxin testing of stool is more sensitive and specific than detection of isolates using biochemical or serological screening assays (239,240).

Toxin Testing. Reference and research laboratories utilize vero toxin assays to identify EHEC producing SLTs (246,256,257). Toxin is produced in the GI tract and can be extracted from fecal samples and assayed by a cytotoxicity assay on cultured vero or HeLa cells but not CHO or Y-1 adrenal cells. Specific cytotoxicity must be confirmed by neutralization studies. The sensitivity of culture alone when compared to the combination of cytotoxin assay and culture was 74%, compared to 93% for fecal cytotoxicity alone (245). Free fecal cytotoxin may be harder to detect early in the disease but may be more useful later in the disease when the number of EHEC in the stool declines. Because of the complexity, lack of commercially available reagents, and the many nuances of interpretation, few clinical laboratories offer cytotoxicity assay, although this may be used increasingly where prevalence of disease, particularly that due to strains other than O157:H7, is high. To facilitate testing, laboratories that do testing may use microtiter tissue culture wells and, when screening cultures, colony sweeps (246,256,257).

Other Assays. In addition to producing SLTs, EHEC strains also contain a plasmid encoding eukaryotic cell adhesins (128,246). Therefore, DNA probes derived from toxin genes and from the plasmid have been employed in hybridization assays to detect EHEC. Such methods are at least as sensitive as free fecal cytotoxin assays and are more sensitive than sorbitol MacConkey agar cultures (246,250,258). The significance of isolates that are adhesin gene probe–positive and toxin gene probe–negative is unclear (85). Preliminary studies have been done using DNA amplification to detect SLT gene sequences in stool (259). ELISAs have been used (239,246,260–262); however, their accuracy has not been adequately assessed and none are commercially available. Serological assays for the presence of antibodies directed against toxin or LPS antigens have been developed (239,257,263,264) but are not considered to be reliable for routine clinical diagnosis at present.

Persistent Bacterial Diarrhea

In addition to infections with enteropathogenic *E. coli* (EPEC) and enteroaggregative *E. coli* (EAggEC), which may cause persistent infections particularly in the very young, diarrhea lasting more than 2 weeks may occur with infection due to *Y. entercolytica* and *Plesiomonas*. Particularly in compromised hosts or AIDS patients, *Salmonella*, *Shigella*, *Campylobacter*, and *C. difficile* may cause prolonged illness or relapse. Chronic diarrhea has also been ascribed to bacterial overgrowth due to a variety of underlying problems. Symptoms also may be a manifestation of GI infection with pathogens usually associated with systemic disease such as mycobacteria or fungi. Protozoa such as *Giardia*, *Cryptosporidium*, or *Cyclospora* may also cause diarrhea lasting longer than 2 weeks.

Enteropathogenic E. coli (EPEC)

EPEC strains have traditionally been defined as specific serotypes (based on somatic LPS O and flagellar H antigens) epidemiologically associated with disease (3,67, 128,265,266). These strains were initially recognized to be a major cause of infantile diarrhea in newborn nurseries that occurred in industrialized countries in the 1940s and 1950s. EPEC strains appear to a major cause of diarrhea in infants and young children in developing countries (128,267–273).

Although EPEC apparently rarely cause sporadic cases of diarrhea in the United States, outbreaks have been reported. Acute infection may present as watery diarrhea with prominant amounts of mucus but not gross blood and usually is accompanied by fever, malaise, and vomiting. Diarrhea may be severe in infants and may persist for more than 14 days. Biopsies taken from the small bowel reveal characteristic attaching and effacing lesions of the mucosal epithelium. Serogrouping, serotyping, and, more recently, tissue culture, ELISA, and DNA-based assays have been used to distinguish EPEC from other *E. coli* present in feces. The definition of EPEC appears to be evolving and will probably be based on virulence determinants associated with disease. Currently reliable and standardized procedures for identification are not available in U.S. clinical laboratories; however, public health laboratories should be contacted for assistance in evaluating isolates obtained from patients with suspected EPEC infection.

At present, there are a dozen recognized EPEC serogroups (O antigens) and almost twice as many classical serotypes (O and H antigens) (3,67,128,268). Some serogroups are more frequently associated with outbreaks and are more common. However, the prevalence of serotypes may vary in different settings. EPEC strains associated with disease in epidemiological and volunteer studies, belong to classical EPEC serotypes and exhibit microcolony formation (localized adherence, LA) on HEp-2 and HeLa cells (267,268). Strains with somewhat different phenotypic properties have also been included as EPEC, although the importance of these as diarrheal pathogens is not as well established. There is still disagreement as to which serotypes compose the EPEC group (128,274). Furthermore, it has been shown that in some settings, a large proportion of isolates identified by serogrouping by clinical laboratories may not be EPEC serotypes (67,275–277). Serogrouping overestimates isolates that are pathogenic, particularly in low-prevalence settings (275,278,279), and it is generally not recommended for use in the United States and United Kingdom, except perhaps in outbreaks. Some isolates with putative virulence factors are not classical EPEC serotypes and some classical serotypes lack these determinants (266–272). Isolates suspected of being EPEC should be referred to reference laboratories for confirmation and further characterization.

EPEC strains can be identified by their phenotypic adherence properties. The assay requires multiple colonies to be picked from primary culture plates. Bacterial cells are grown in broth and inoculated onto epithelial cells, followed by staining and examination by light microscopy to define the type of adherence pattern. A good correlation between presence of the LA pattern and EPEC serogroup has been demonstrated (128,267–272,280). However, a proportion of isolates are LA-positive but do not express the classical EPEC serogroup antigens, and are of questionable significance. Another problem is that variations in the methods or interpretation of patterns used in different laboratories may result in strains being classified differently (277,281,282). Although fluorescent actin staining (FAS) may make it easier to visualize the characteristic cytoskeletal rearrangments associated with LA, this stain is hazardous and not suitable for routine use in clinical laboratories. Furthermore, EHEC as well

as some strains which are EPEC adherence factor (EAF), LA-negative, and strains not belonging to classical EPEC serotypes may be FAS-positive. Therefore, additional testing may be needed in order to characterize isolates. DNA probes derived from the plasmid-encoded EAF gene required for expression of localized adherence (128,265,270–272,283–287) have been used to identify EPEC, and an *eae* gene probe used to identify isolates capable of causing attaching and effacing lesions (287,288).

Another group of adherent *E. coli* that attach to HEp-2 or HeLa cells with a uniform distribution have been referred to as diffuse adhering *E. coli* (DAEC) (128,271,272,283,289,290). Some DAEC belong to classical EPEC serotypes differ from traditionally defined EPEC by tissue culture adherence pattern and failure to hybridize with with EAF probe and, based on hybridization with either fimbrial or membrane adhesin probes used in epidemiological studies, may be heterogeneous (267,269,291). DAEC have been implicated in diarrheal disease in some studies but not others.

Enteroaggregative E. coli *(EAggEC)*

EAggEC belong to a newly defined group of EPEC implicated as a cause of persistent diarrhea in children (267,269,292). However, not all studies have shown a significant association with disease (271,292). The characteristic aggregative adherence (AA) pattern consists of bacteria adhering to HEp-2 cells in "stacked-brick" aggregates (267). Classification of isolates as EAggEC may be dependent on tissue culture methodology and interpretation (277,281). A ~60-MDa plasmid has been associated with virulence and encodes bundle-forming fimbriae (AAF/I) the presence of which correlates with an aggregative adherence pattern (293). The plasmid in some strains of EAggEC also encodes a low molecular weight heat-stable toxin (EAST-1) (294). DNA probes derived from the plasmid that correlates with the AA phenotype have been used with varying success (271,295), and it is possible that isolates classified as EAggEC are heterogeneous (272,294). Preliminary studies using reference strains showed a good correlation between the AA phenotype and formation of bacterial clumps that were visible as scum at the surface of Mueller–Hinton broth cultures (296). This relatively simple assay warrants further evaluation.

Immunocompromised Patients

Bacteria. An established pathogen can be identified in AIDS patients with chronic diarrhea in approximately 70% to 85% of cases in developing countries and 40% to 50% of cases in tropical countries (11,44,297). Diagnostic approaches for the most appropriate workup of diarrhea in patients with AIDS are evolving (44,298–301). In patients with AIDS, infections with common enteric pathogens such as *Salmonella* sp., *Shigella* sp., *C. jejuni*, *Yersinia*, and *C. difficile* may be more severe, protracted, or relapsing than in the normal host. Up to three routine stool cultures and an assay for *C. difficile* toxin have been recommended in the diagnostic evaluation of patients with AIDS who have diarrhea (44). Special procedures are required for detection of the "*Campylobacter*-like organisms," *Helicobacter fenelliae,* and *Helicobacter cinaedi* associated with proctocolitis (11,302,303). The importance of spirochetes as causes of diarrhea (303) and appropriate methodology for identification has not been established.

Campylobacter fetus, C. jejuni, H. fenelliae, and *H. cinaedi* are among organisms that are associated with diarrhea and that are not readily detected with routine blood culture systems. To detect these or other slow-growing or fastidious organisms in blood cultures, special procedures are required.

In addition to fecal cultures, blood cultures should be obtained from febrile, immunocompromised patients with persistent diarrhea. Blood cultures may also be warranted in the immunocompetent individual who has fever and diarrhea.

Mycobacteria. Disseminated *M. avium-intracellulare* infection in patients with AIDS and occasionally other immunocompromising conditions often involves the intestine and has been associated with chronic diarrhea, abdominal pain, malabsorption, and marked wasting (44,298). Mycobacteria may be detected in feces by acid-fast smear and, although not highly sensitive (<35%) (304,305) compared to a culture, a positive smear has been correlated with disseminated infection, intestinal lesions, and chronic diarrhea (11,44,298,304,306). The most sensitive specific methods of diagnosing disseminated disease are acid-fast bacillus (AFB) culture of blood or demonstration of organisms in involved organs (lymph nodes, liver, spleen, bone marrow) by histopathology and culture. Smear and culture of respiratory secretions is neither as sensitive (33%) nor as specific. However, 65% of patients with a positive respiratory culture may later develop disseminated infection (307). The value of culturing stool in the absence of a positive AFB smear is not well established. *M. avium-intracellulare* is found in water, soil, and foods, and in some cases the significance of very low numbers of *Mycobacterium* recovered in stool may be difficult to assess.

Two or three AFB blood cultures can be used to rule out disseminated *M. avium-intracellulare* infection, and broth or lysis centrifugation methods appear to be comparable. For other types of specimens, use of both radiometric and conventional culture media may improve sensitivity and average time to detection for mycobacteria (approximately ≤2 weeks). DNA probes for identification of *M. tuberculosis* and *M. avium* or *M. intracellulare* are rapid and accurate means of identifying mycobacteria. Commercially available DNA amplification procedures for detection of mycobacteria in clinical samples are being evaluated. For culture of mycobacteria from stools, decontamination of specimens using oxalic acid or *N*-acetylcysteine–sodium hydroxide may be preferable to other methods (308).

Fungi. Esophagitis due to *C. albicans* occurs in immunocompromised patients including AIDS patients and is best diagnosed by biopsy and visualization of organisms in tissue (44). Due to frequent contamination of samples with *Candida* sp. in saliva from oropharyngeal colonization, fungal culture is usually not warranted unless other fungal pathogens are in the differential. KOH examination may enable rapid presumptive confirmation of esophagitis but is not as sensitive or specific as histopathology. In other circumstances biopsied lesions of the GI tract should be examined histologically as well as cultured for fungi unless appearance is completely incompatible with fungal etiology. Hepatosplenic abcesses secondary to disseminated candidiasis or intraabdominal infections may sometimes be culture-negative although organisms appear on smear. Biopsies for fungal culture should be obtained from the leading edge of the lesion and are more likely to contain viable organisms than samples obtained from the necrotic center of the lesion. Disseminated disease due to fungi including histoplasmosis and *Paracoccidioides brasiliensis* may involve the intestine and, in some patients, may cause intestinal symptoms.

A variety of selective media are used to culture fungi and usually include plates or tubes of media containing antibiotics to inhibit bacterial growth and compounds such as cyclohexamide, which permits growth of systemic dimorphic pathogens but inhibits growth of other opportunistic fungal species. Cultures are usually incubated at 30°C for 4–6 weeks. Many fungal pathogens will grow quickly within a few days and may be recovered on routine bacterial cultures. *H. capsulatum* may grow quite slowly and the laboratory should be notified to hold cultures at least 8 weeks if histoplasmosis is suspected.

Bacterial Overgrowth

A variety of predisposing conditions may lead to abnormal colonization of the upper small bowel, which has been associated with chronic malabsorption or noninflammatory diarrheal syndromes. Aspirates from the duodenum normally have relatively few (<10^5/mL) organisms composed primarily of gram-positive oral flora whereas aspirates from patients with overgrowth syndrome may be colonized by >10^5/mL of species such as Enterobacteriaceae and anaerobes that are usually found lower in the intestinal tract (309–311). Non–culture-based evaluations may be helpful in indicating bacterial overgrowth. However, if there are cases where culture is needed for diagnosis, single-dilution quantitative cultures with presumptive identification of isolates usually provides sufficient information for diagnosis. Because cultures are quantitative and delay in processing may effect colony counts, the duodenal aspirate should be placed immediately in an anaerobic transport vial, transported quickly to the laboratory, and processed promptly. The sample may be diluted 1:1000 in thioglycollate or similar broth, mixed by brief vortexing, and 0.1 mL of the dilution plated and spread on plates containing blood agar, MacConkey or similar medium, an anaerobic blood plate, and, if available, a selective-differential medium for anaerobic gram-negaive rods. More than 10 colonies or more than 100 colonies represent colony counts of >10^5 and >10^6 per mL, respectively. Approximate colony count and identification of predominant organisms based on colonial appearance may be reported. The report should convey the predominant organism, approximate total colony count, and a comment as to whether flora is primarily that normally observed in the oropharynx (gram-positive organisms such as viridans streptococci, lactobacilli, coagulase-negative staphylococci, and fastidious anaerobes) or the lower intestine (Enterobacteriaceae and gut anaerobes). The reliability of simple alternatives to culture such as Gram stain, which has a sensitivity of $10^4–10^5$ organisms/mL, or urine dip-stick tests, which detect the presence of enzymes produced by Enterobacteriaceae, has not been evaluated in terms of their use as an alternative method of ascertaining overgrowth using duodenal aspirates. Age, nutritional status, environmental factors including season and fecal contamination of foods, or presumably other risk factors such as hospitalization may affect both quantity and nature of flora colonizing the upper intestine (312–315). Disease does not always correlate with quantitation or predominance of lower GI tract flora.

The importance of altered intestinal flora as occurs with antibiotic treatment as a cause of diarrhea is unknown (316). Routine stool cultures only detect selected organisms and these normally represent only a small fraction of the normal intestinal flora. Culture reports that indicate absence of usual enteric organisms on stool culture or predominance of organisms such as *Candida, Pseudomonas,* or *S. aureus* verify changes in the gut flora and heavy colonization with these organisms (229,317,318).

Diagnostic Problems and Additional Procedures

Bacterial Agents. It may be necessary to order up to two or three stool cultures obtained from the patient with persistent diarrhea in order to detect presence of some bacterial pathogens, especially when previous cultures have been negative. *Salmonella* sp., *Shigella* sp., and *C. jejuni* may occasionally cause persistant diarrhea, although a single "routine" fecal culture is usually sufficient. One should be aware that not all laboratories employ enrichment procedures to enhance recovery of *Salmonella* or *Shigella,* and some do not routinely set up specimens to detect *Campylobacter* species, in particular those that are not thermotolerant or resistant to the antibiotics contained in *Campylobacter*-selective media. In instances in which the initial set of cultures for "routine" enteric bacteria are negative, clinicians are advised to request the laboratory to use additional procedures to isolate *Yersinia, Plesiomonas, Vibrio, Aeromonas,* and diarrheagenic *E. coli.* Suspicion of these agents should prompt consultation with the clinical laboratory about current availability of assays for diagnostic purposes.

Clostridium difficile may cause chronic or relapsing diarrhea. This occurs infrequently in the absence of prior antibiotic exposure. The cytotoxicity assay is most sensitive in comparison to immunological assays, although many laboratories do not utilize it. In unusual cases in which *C. difficile* toxin-mediated disease is suspected even though the immunoassay is negative, a specific request for cytotoxicity testing may be required.

Mycobacteria. Mycobacterial and fungal infections may involve the GI tract either as primary infections or secondary to disseminated disease. Special procedures are needed for isolation from GI tract specimens. Infections caused by *M. tuberculosis* or *M. bovis* although rare may be manifested as primarily a GI syndrome. Diagnosis is made by histological examination and AFB culture of biopsied lesions. Definitive diagnosis is based on culture and species identification. If epidemiology suggests that *M. bovis* infection is a possibility, the laboratory should be notified since commercially available DNA probes that are commonly employed in identification do not distinguish between these species. AFB culture or smear of feces is not a sensitive method to detect *M. tuberculosis* and *M. bovis* infection and is not indicated for this purpose.

Fungi. Although a variety of fungi may occasionally involve the GI tract in disseminated disease, persistent diarrhea is rarely a presenting complaint. Culture is required for definitive diagnosis. Infections caused by *P. brasiliensis* (South American blastomycosis) are limited to areas of South America and Central America. These may present as lesions involving respiratory tract, skin, oral mucosa, or intestinal tract. Disseminated histoplasmosis occasionally may present as a primarily GI syndrome. Diagnosis may be made by culture of the organism from biopsy of lesions and histopathology.

Candida sp. may cause systemic disease involving the GI tract. Dissemination may lead to hepatosplenic microabscesses. Documentation of infection of mucosal sites is made by observing hyphae, pseudohyphae, and occasional budding yeast forms in tissue and by culture of biopsy material to confirm identification. *Candida* sp. can be recovered from feces of normal individuals but heavy growth may signify abnormal GI tract colonization in patients treated with antibiotics (316). The etiological role of *Candida* colonization in diarrhea in such circumstances is controversial (317–319). Fungal cultures of stool usually are not indicated because of low specificity. Nonetheless, large numbers of yeast can be detected by methylene blue exam for fecal leukocytes. Normally $<10^3$/mL yeasts of stool are present and yeast or mycelial forms are infrequent in microscopic exam (316–318).

Food Poisoning: Intoxication Due to Bacterial Contamination of Foods

In contrast to enteric disease caused by infection and replication of pathogenic microorganisms, *S. aureus, B. cereus, C. botulinum,* and *C. perfringens* cause illness by producing toxins in improperly prepared foods that are subsequently ingested. Therefore the clinical hallmarks of staphylococcal enterotoxin-mediated food poisoning are predominant nausea and vomiting, with or without diarrhea, and a short incubation period (1–7 hr). Similarly, *B. cereus* emetic toxin produced in cooked rice also produces vomiting shortly after eating. The diarrheal syndromes associated with *B. cereus* and *C. perfringens* are characterized by a somewhat longer incubation period (8–12 hr), watery diarrhea with severe abdominal cramps, and little or no vomiting. Diagnosis is usually based on clinical features of the illness (320,321).

When outbreaks of foodborne intoxication are suspected, or in especially severe cases, appropriate samples, including stool, vomitus, and serum, should be collected and stored for transmission to public health laboratories (322). Clinical samples and suspected foods should be refrigerated immediately or stored in a freezer if already frozen. Physicians and the clinical laboratory should contact public health departments for diagnostic support and investigative follow-up. Special media and testing procedures are not available in clinical laboratories, whereas public health laboratories are able to do specific culture studies, toxin assays, and strain typing (322–326).

Since *B. cereus, S. aureus,* and *C. perfringens* may be found in fecal samples of healthy individuals and may be present in small amounts in food, isolation of these organisms is not diagnostic per se (320–323). Usually, high numbers of microorganisms ($>10^5$/g), which may sometimes be seen on Gram stain, presumptively implicates a food source. If the same strain is found in the suspected food vehicle and in clinical samples, this provides additional evidence suggesting illness due to a specific strain. Demonstration of the toxin in food and clinical material and toxin production by the putative strain *in vitro* may be attempted depending on the circumstances.

When botulism is suspected, samples of stool, serum, and, if available, gastric aspirates should be referred to public health laboratories for culture and toxin testing. Specimens should be collected as early in the course of disease as possible. Toxin assays are more likely to be positive earlier (<3 days), while cultures of stool may be helpful later on (327).

Gastritis/Peptic Ulcer Disease

Helicobacter pylori

Helicobacter pylori, the human-adapted member of the genus composed of spiral-shaped gram-negative bacilli, is the major cause of type B (type II) gastritis diagnosed by histopathological examination of gastric mucosa (328,329). There is also a substantial, if not overwhelming, amount of epidemiological, clinical, and histopathological evidence supporting the causal role of *H. pylori* in peptic ulcer disease. Several methods are available to detect *Helicobacter* infection, including culture by biopsy via endoscopy, urease reaction of biopsy material, Warthin–Starry or Giemsa stain on histopathological examation, nucleic acid hybridization/PCR of gastric aspirates, serology, and urea-breath test (330). The former three methods require an invasive procedure and biopsy. The histological diagnosis of chronic active gastritis and detection of urease activity of a biopsy are sufficiently sensitive and specific that culture may not be cost-effective. However, development of antimicrobial resistance during therapy has been reported (331–334), providing a rationale for culture in this setting.

Another *Helicobacter*-like spiral-shaped bacterium, initially called "*Gastrospirillum hominis,*" now known to be a member of the *Helicobacter* genus (31), has also been associated with gastritis (see below). *Helicobacter felis,* which has been associated with gastritis in cats, dogs, and other mammals, may rarely infect humans. These species can be differentiated from *H. pylori* on the basis of their morphological appearance as revealed by microscopy. Since "*G. hominis*" has not been successfully cultured and infection by *H. felis* is probably rare, species identification of these must be based on the microscopic appearance and the sophistication of the pathologist.

Culture. Helicobacter pylori is a fastidious microorganism, and success of culture methods depends on the number of samples, method of sample collection, proper transport, and laboratory methods. Because *H. pylori* are not evenly distributed throughout the gastric mucosa, at least two biopsy samples from the antrum and one from the gastric corpus should be obtained (330). Material submitted for culture should be placed into transport medium (20% glucose), bacteriological media, or Stuart's medium (335) on ice and taken immediately to the laboratory. Delays in transport, particularly when specimens are held at room temperature, may substantially decrease the viability of organisms. To ensure optimum recovery, the laboratory should process the specimen immediately, usually by grinding, and incubate agar plates promptly.

Helicobacter sp. are microaerophilic and grow well in the same atmospheric conditions employed for *Campylobacter* isolation e.g., 5% O_2, 10% CO_2, and 85% N (335). Humidity is important for good growth. A variety of blood-containing media can be utilized, including chocolate agar, blood agar, and *Brucella* agar. Use of selective media incorporating vancomycin, amphotericin, trimethoprim, and colistin or cefsulodin may significantly improve recovery by preventing overgrowth of gastric flora. A differential medium can be used to distinguish *H. pylori* from other organisms (336), and media that do not contain blood or serum may also be employed. Inoculated agar plates should be incubated at 37°C, even though some strains of *H. pylori* are able to grow at 42°C. Colonies usually develop within 3–4 days; plates should be held for 7 days before being discarded as culture-negative. *Helicobacter* colonies may lose viability within 45 min to 2 hr if held on the laboratory bench due to oxygen sensitivity.

Identification. Helicobacter pylori may be identified on the basis of the source of the culture (the stomach normally contains only transient bacteria), typical morphology on stained smear, and positive oxidase, catalase, and urease reactions. In most cases presumptive identification is adequate. Other reactions that help to distinguish *Helicobacter* and *Campylobacter* include negative nitrate and hippurate reactions, cephalothin susceptibility and nalidixic acid resistance, failure to grow at 25°C, negative indoxyl acetate hydrolysis, polymixin susceptibility, and others (99,100,120,121).

Susceptibility Testing. Metronidazole resistance appears to play a role in failure to eradicate *H. pylori* infections even with triple therapy (331–334,337). Agar dilution, bactericidal tests, disk diffusion, and E test have been used for susceptibility testing (331,332,338–340); however, a standardized method and appropriate interpretive breakpoints for resistance have not been established (331). Results of E tests compare favorably with those of agar dilution.

Serology. Persistent infection by *H. pylori* is associated with an IgG humoral response; IgM antibodies are produced following acute infection, and IgA antibody titers remain elevated through the duration of infection (330). A number of serology assay kits have recently been commercially produced. The sensitivity and specificity of these compared with other methods to detect *H. pylori* infection are variable; some, but not all, appear to have high predictive values (341–346). Several factors should be considered when considering an assay: The gold standard used as the reference method against which the serological assay was compared (culture sensitivity among laboratories may vary); the choice of study population and control groups evaluated; the quality and number of independent studies done to validate the product; and the setting in which the product is to be used. High IgG titers to *H. pylori* may be observed for some patients and antibody titers may fall relatively slowly following successful therapy. The reliability of serology for monitoring outcome of therapy may depend on observation of falling titer in paired pre- and posttreatment sera rather than testing of posttreatment sera using a predetermined cutoff (346). Specificity of serology (appropriately identifying treatment success) may be dependent on time interval from initiation of treatment and follow-up serological testing.

Molecular Methods. PCR amplification has been used to detect *H. pylori* in biopsy material (347) and in gastric aspirates (348), which frequently are culture-negative because the majority of bacteria are caught in the mucous gel. Although not routinely available, this method offers many advantages and would be useful to elucidate the reservoirs of infection, to further define the epidemiology of infection, and to identify noncultivatable bacteria.

"Gastrospirillum hominis" (Helicobacter *sp.*)

An uncultivated bacterium morphologically resembling *Helicobacter felis* called "*Gastrospirillum hominis*," has been identified in human gastric mucosa in association with gastritis. "*Gastrospirillum hominis*" is longer and the bacilli are relatively straight with more spiral turns than *H. pylori*. "*Gastrospirillum*" has not been cultivated *in vitro* and therefore the only means of identifying it and differentiating it from *H. pylori* is by Warthin–Starry stain of fixed tissue. The nature of this microorganism has been demonstrated using eubacterial primers and PCR amplification techniques to isolate and sequence the 16S rDNA "*Gastrospirillum*" gene from infected gastric tissue (36). By DNA sequence analysis, "*G. hominis*" was shown to be a member of the *Helicobacter* genus, most closely related to *H. felis*. The prevalence of "*G. hominis*" infection in humans is relatively low; however, the distinction between *H. pylori* and "*G. hominis*" can currently be made only by morphological criteria on Warthin–Starry–stained gastric biopsies. Therefore, the true incidence of infection may be greater than this. Like *H. py-*

lori, "*G. hominis*" also secretes urease, which may be detected by the CLO disk test.

Gastric Fluids and Biopsies for Other Studies

Gastric aspirates cultured from septic newborns are generally not cultured anaerobically and can be placed in a sterile screw-cap tube or container such as that used for collection of urine or sputum samples. Acidity of gastric aspirates cultured for AFB may decrease the viability of mycobacteria; therefore samples should be quickly transported to the laboratory for neutralization.

Whipple's Disease

Noncultivatable intracellular bacteria have been observed in small intestinal biopsy samples from patients with Whipple's disease. In recent reports, the identification of this bacillus has been made based on the sequence of the 16S rDNA gene that was obtained by PCR amplification using eubacterial primers (36,349). The proposed name for the Whipple's disease bacillus is *Tropheryma whippelii*. This organism is an actinomycete most closely related to soil or water saprophytes and oral or skin commensals of warm-blooded animals. Currently, traditional methods of histological diagnosis are indicated and identification of the organism using molecular methods is confined to research and reference laboratories.

Crohn's Disease

The possibility of an infectious etiology for Crohn's disease is controversial (36,350). Cell wall–deficient spheroplasts and DNA sequences of *M. paratuberculosis* or other mycobacteria have been detected in material of some patients with Crohn's disease; however, similar forms have been isolated from samples obtained from patients without disease (37–40). Attempts to implicate mycobacteria by serological methods have been unsuccessful (350,351). Traditional histological and clinical criteria should be used for diagnosis.

Proctitis

Neisseria gonorrhoeae, *Chlamydia trachomatis*, and *Treponema pallidum* are the most common bacterial causes of proctitis. Infections with *C. trachomatis* lymphogranuloma venerium (LGV) serotypes, *Helicobacter fennellii*, and *Helicobacter cinadei* (formerly in the genus *Campylobacter* or referred to as *Campylobacter*-like organisms; see above), and *S. flexneri* may also cause proctocolitis.

Neisseria gonorrhoeae

Both culture and Gram stain of exudate obtained at anoscopy are useful in diagnosis. Compared to culture, the sensitivity of Gram stain for samples obtained at proctoscopy is approximately 80% (352). However, interpretation may be a problem, particularly if bipolar-staining enteric gram-negative rods are present in the sample. Gram stains of material obtained from asymptomatic individuals are not worthwhile.

Cultures may also be obtained by insertion of the swab 2–3 cm into the anus and swabbing the mucosal surface, taking care to minimize fecal contamination of the swab as much as possible. The sensitivity of a single rectal swab for detection of gonococcal infection has not been ascertained, but has been estimated to be comparable to that of a single endocervical culture in women (80%) (352). Cotton swabs and some wooden or metal swab handles may be toxic for gonococci and other organisms; therefore, dacron or nylon swabs with plastic handles are recommended.

The most sensitive means of culturing for *N. gonorrhoeae* is to inoculate agar medium designed for culture the gonococcus directly (353), especially if a delay in transport to the laboratory is anticipated. The swab should be rolled over the surface of approximately one third of the agar medium and then a sterile loop or stick used to dilute the sample by streaking over the uninoculated surface of the agar. The culture should be immediately incubated at 35–37°C in a candle jar, or a system that results in an atmosphere of approximately 5%. After incubation for 18–24 hr, cultures may be transported to an off-site laboratory for further evaluation. There are several commercial culture kits suitable for this purpose. It is important that media used for culture be warmed to room temperature prior to inoculation and that plates be fresh and properly stored to prevent drying. Gonococci are fragile and highly susceptible to oxidation, desiccation, or significant temperature changes, including refrigeration. Swabs that are to be sent directly to a laboratory should be placed in either Amies or modified Stuart's transport medium. Holding samples in transport medium decreases sensitivity of culture (5% to 10% loss after 24 hr and 50% decrease after 48 hr); therefore, effort must be made to process samples within a minimum amount of time.

Gonococci are cultured on enriched selective media supplemented with antibiotics designed to suppress growth of other microorganisms. Appropriate culture media include New York City medium, Modified Thayer–Martin Agar, Martin–Lester medium, or GC-Lect (BBL). Selective media containing vancomycin (3–4 μg/mL) may inhibit some strains of the gonococcus. Therefore, the false-negative rate depends on selectivity of medium employed and prevalence of such strains in the population.

Gonococcal colonies from some specimen types may be identified presumptively by (a) growth on selective medium; (b) typical Gram stain and colony morphology; and (c) a positive oxidase test. Samples from nongenital sites require further biochemical and phenotypic tests for speciation. The usual methods of identification include carbohydrate assimilation, immunological techniques, and by commercially available DNA hybridization kits, the latter being highly sensitive and specific (354). Particularly in

low-risk populations, identification using more than one method may be advisable. Isolates from minors or patients who may be involved in legal or criminal proceedings should be frozen and also sent to a reference laboratory for confirmation.

Currently in the United States susceptibility testing of *N. gonorrhoeae* is not done in some laboratories because of recommendations for treatment with ceftriaxone to which resistance is rare (355,356). Nonetheless, gonococci may be easily tested for β-lactamase production using a chromagenic cephalosporin. So-called intrinsic or chromosomal resistance is mediated by changes in penicillin-binding proteins (PBPs) and may be measured by disk diffusion assay using special media and interpretative breakpoints (22). Resistance to ceftriaxone, tetracycline, and spectinomycin is also measured using this modified disk diffusion assay.

Gonococci also may be detected in clinical specimens by non–culture-based methods. These include ELISA, although it is less sensitive and specific than culture, particularly in some asymptomatic or low-risk populations (353), and commercially available nucleic acid probes or DNA ampification kits, the latter of which are currently being evaluated. Noncultural methods of detection are not indicated for rectal specimens.

Chlamydia trachomatis

Chlamydia trachomatis in genital samples can be detected by culture, fluorescent antibody staining, ELISA, commercially available nucleic acid probe or DNA probe, and PCR (357). Currently only fluorescent antibody staining or culture can be used for diagnosis of rectal *Chlamydia* infection. *C. trachomatis* is an obligate intracellular pathogen; therefore, sensitivity of detection correlates with the number of infected epithelial cells collected in the specimen. Anoscopy provides the most suitable opportunity to select infected areas for sampling (352,357). Cytobrush samples are excellent for cervical samples. However, dacron- or rayon-tipped swabs with a plastic handle may be more acceptable for collection of rectal samples. Samples for fluorescent antibody staining should be promptly spread on slides provided in a collection kit, and samples obtained for culture should be placed immediately in *Chlamydia* transport medium that contains antibiotics. A second sample should be obtained simultaneously for culture of *N. gonorrhoeae*. Samples for *Chlamydia* culture (but not for gonococcal culture) should be refrigerated and transported to the laboratory promptly. Viability significantly decreases after 24 hr refrigeration and samples that cannot be inoculated immediately onto tissue culture cells should be frozen at −70°C.

Culture is most sensitive when dram vials containing coverslips are used rather than microtiter plates, although the latter is more convenient and less costly (357,358). Cyclohexamide-treated McCoy cells or BGMK cells are most commonly employed to cultivate *Chlamydia*. Increased sensitivity and faster time to initial detection are provided by centrifugation of the sample onto the cells and use of fluorescent antibody, rather than iodine, to detect inclusions. Culture is warranted in instances that may involve legal action. Culture has been the reference method to which newer assays have been compared; however, studies have indicated a less than 100% sensitivity for culture using a single sample. Higher positivity rates may result when samples from more than one site are obtained. Pooling of cervical and urethral swab material obtained from women is recommended.

FAS has shown relatively good sensitivity and specificity when compared to culture, and like other nonculture assays is particularly suited to situations where specimen transport is a problem (357,358). ELISA, and particularly those that detect protein rather than LPS antigen, have shown high specificity in populations in which the prevalence of infection exceeds 10%. This method has low sensitivity to detect *Chlamydia* in male urethral samples, and ELISA is also not adequate to detect *Chlamydia* in genital samples from patients where the prevalence of infection is low. Kits designed for the detection of *C. trachomatis* in physicians offices have become available; however, sensitivity and positive predictive values of many of these has not been extensively evaluated in asymptomatic and low-prevalence populations. DNA probes have appeared to perform at least as well as ELISA and FAS in some populations and preliminary evaluations suggest that PCR is more sensitive than culture. Serological diagnosis is limited to detection of only some infections by LGV serotypes (Stamm) and is usually not indicated.

Treponema pallidum *(Syphilis)*

Anorectal syphilis is best detected in biopsies by routine histology and silver stain or fluorescent antibody staining to reveal treponemes (352,359). In some cases, it may be difficult to distinguish spirochetes from artifacts using a silver stain; FAS with specific antiserum is more specific, but availability of reagents varies. If a dark field examination is contemplated, the laboratory should be contacted for instructions and to obtain a specimen collection kit. Analysis of some rectal lesions using this method may not be worthwhile. The lesion should be cleaned with nonbacteriostatic saline and, if necesary, gently abraded to provoke oozing. The best sample consists of serous fluid free of red blood cells collected from the depths of the lesion. The material should be collected on one or more slides or coverslips directly; a small-bore pipet or loop also may be used. The coverslipped slide should immediately be placed in a petri dish containing moist gauze to prevent drying and examined using dark field microscopy.

Identification of spirochetes depends on viability since the criteria used depend on type of motility, shape of cells, length, width, number and amplitude of spirals (359,360). Commensal treponemes that may be found in the mouth may be difficult to distinguish from *T. pallidum,* and treponemes also are found in feces. Therefore, rectal samples contaminated by intestinal flora may be difficult to interpret. Fluorescent antibody stain provides an alternative to dark field exam. PCR procedures for *T. pallidum* have been described (25) and offer advantages of sensitiv-

ity and specificity compared to dark field exam. The sensitivity of these methods is such that the absence of treponemes does not rule out syphilis, and therefore so-called nontreponemal serology (VDRL or RPR) should also be obtained. If the test is negative, it should be followed by repeat testing at 1 week, 1 month, and 3 months (352,359). Serology is negative in 30% to 50% of cases of primary syphilis, and although the FTA-ABS treponemal test is more sensitive at this stage of the disease, approximately 1% of the population in the United States may have a false-positive test. Therefore, treponemal tests are not recommended for screening in the absence of a positive nontreponemal test (359,361).

EXTRAGASTROINTESTINAL INFECTIONS

Intraabdominal Infections

Proper collection of infectious material from extraintestinal tract sources is important, and each specimen should be accompanied by a laboratory slip containing appropriate clinical information. Only certain specimens require anaerobic cultures, and because of the sensitivity to oxygen, these must be properly collected and transported in an anaerobic system in order for the subsequent culture to yield meaningful results. For example, specimens contaminated by mucosal secretions or intestinal contents that normally harbor high concentrations of anaerobes should therefore not be cultured anaerobically (1,5,6, 362,363). On the other hand, intraabdominal or other infections that arise as a result of mucosal breakdown are frequently polymicrobial and involve both facultatively aerobic enteric gram-negative rods, particularly *E. coli* and *Proteus* in intestinal tract infections, *Klebsiella* and enterococci in biliary tract disease, and anaerobes, including *B. fragilis, B. fragilis* group (*B. distasonis, B. ovatus, B. thetaiotaomicron, B. vulgatus, B. uniformis*), *C. perfringens* and other clostridial species, and peptostreptococci. Particularly in nosocomial infections, these bacteria often are more antibiotic resistant microbes such as *Enterobacter, Citrobacter, Serratia, Pseudomonas,* and *Candida.* Gram stain of clinical material with a sensitivity of $\approx 10^4$ to -10^5/mL is a rapid test that may give valuable clues as to identification of organisms present. With the exception of anaerobes, "routine" methods of culture usually recover most pathogens within 18–24 hr of culture. Skilled technologists may be able to presumptively identify not only whether lactose-fermenting gram-negative rods such as *E. coli, Citrobacter, Klebsiella* (and most *Enterobacter* species) are present but, on the basis of colonial morphology and other rapid tests, may give a reasonably accurate guess of the genus. Such information provided in preliminary reports may be useful. Although *Candida* sp. will grow on routine bacteriological media, fungal media may be required in order to detect low numbers of fungi in mixed cultures.

Laboratories often have procedures to detect pathogens associated with specific disease syndromes and culture material from different sources accordingly. Diagnostic specimens obtained by invasive procedure are uncomfortable for the patient, costly to obtain, and cannot be readily recollected. Many of such specimens should be cultured for a wide range of potential pathogens whether or not requests to do so accompany the sample. Recovery of mycobacteria, fungi, or fastidious organisms requires specific culture procedures. For example, cholecystitis may be a complication of *Salmonella* infection and carriage of *Salmonella* may be due to infection of the bile duct. Since samples of infected gallbladder frequently contain several enteric gram-negative rods, laboratories should strongly consider routine inoculation of a selective medium for recovery of *Salmonella*. Lymph nodes should be routinely cultured for mycobacteria and fungi because these organisms are most frequently isolated from this sample. Mesenteric nodes and biopsy should be cultured so as to recover enteric pathogens such as *Yersinia;* liver or bone marrow should be cultured to recover AFB, fungi, as well as fastidious organisms including *Brucella* and *Rochalimea*. Most biopsies, particularly those from tissues contiguous to mucous membranes, should be cultured for anaerobes because of the frequency of anaerobic infections at such sites. Additionally, most specimens should be routinely Gram-stained because this is a rapid way to access specimen quality and inflammatory response, and presumptively to identify organisms when present.

Appropriate Specimens

Collection

Use of a swab is the least satisfactory means of collecting material for stains and culture. Biopsy material provides the best sample from which to culture relevant microorganisms, while aspirates are acceptable substitutes. Swab cultures are particularly insensitive because they provide a limited amount of material for laboratory evaluation. Therefore, a negative culture report may merely reflect an inadequate amount of infected clinical material. When used, more than one swab should be obtained; these should be combined by the laboratory to avoid possible problems with sample heterogeneity. Other inherent problems with swab culture are that they may result in both false-negative results (inadequate sample) and as false-positive results due to collection of organisms of little clinical significance that may be colonizing wound surfaces.

Aspirates and fluids may be collected by needle and syringe or by catheter. If the volume of the aspirate is small, it should be placed in an anaerobic transport tube or vial. Specimens with a volume of >5–10 mL should be placed in a sterile tube or urine container. Larger volume specimens may be split, using approximately one third to inoculate blood culture bottles (follow blood culture instructions for maximum amounts that should be added) and the remainder placed in a sterile cup or tube for concentration, preparation of stains, and plating onto appropriate media. It has been suggested that anaerobic pathogens of major importance (*B. fragilis* and *C. perfringens*) may survive for several hours in aerobic transport systems. This is more likely to be the case with larger biopsies

or larger volumes of aspirate or fluid; however, delay does compromise recovery of these less fastidious organisms and significantly affects the viability of more fastidious bacteria such as peptostreptococci, *Actinomyces* sp., fusobacteria, and other anaerobes including former *Bacteroides* species. (Many *Bacteroides* have been reclassified, e.g., *Porpheromonas melaninogenica,* formerly *Bacteroides melaninogenicus; Prevotella bivia,* formerly *Bacteroides bivius*). Biopsies or aspirates not transported in an anaerobic environment must be rapidly processed, and inoculated media must be placed in an anaerobic environment immediately to avoid further loss of viability.

Because anaerobes are extremely abundant in the small and large bowel and other mucosal surfaces, clinical specimens that are contaminated with intestinal flora or other mucosal secretions should not be evaluated for the presence of anaerobes. The significance of aerobes that might be isolated in such circumstances may be doubtful. Several references provide more detailed descriptions of specimen collection and transport procedures (1,5,6,9, 10,362).

Anaerobic Cultures

Anaerobic bacteria are typically involved in intraabdominal infections, most often as part of a polymicrobial infection (6,364). An average of 2.5–5.0 organisms are involved in intraabdominal infections, and anaerobes are usually recovered as frequently as aerobes or facultative anaerobes. Diagnostic samples should be collected so as to minimize contamination by flora normally colonizing musosal surfaces and secretions, placed in an anaerobic transport device, and transported to the laboratory promptly (within 10–30 min) (1,5,6,362). A Gram stain of the clinical material is often quite helpful and will presumptively identify anaerobes on the basis of their distinctive morphology and their association with other bacteria. The laboratory may report this with comments such as "*Clostridium/Bacillus* morphotype present" or "morphotype compatible with anaerobic gram-negative rods/ *Haemophilus*."

Anaerobes are relatively slow growing and usually are oxygen-intolerant, precluding an early (<48 hr) evaluation of inoculated plates or broth. (In selected clinical situations when Gram stain of clinical material suggests predominance of an anaerobes such as *Clostridium* sp. or *Bacteroides*, additional plates may be inoculated and read at 24 hr for identification of rapidly growing anaerobic pathogens.) Specimens likely to contain several organisms are usually plated onto selective and differential media (*Bacteroides*-bile-esculin agar; laked blood agar containing kanamycin and vancomycin) to prevent overgrowth by facultative bacteria and allow more rapid identification of *B. fragilis* group organisms (1,5). Characteristic colonies that develop are subsequently picked for definitive identification tests. Part of the explanation for the slow pace of the identification process in the laboratory is the requirement to first passage anaerobic isolates to obtain sufficient amounts of pure culture for subsequent verification that the isolate is an anaerobe and for biochemical tests. Gram stain, colony morphology, selective and differential media, and simple spot or disk tests should be used to enable relatively rapid, inexpensive presumptive identification of most anaerobes (5,365,366). When appropriate, laboratories additionally may utilize commercially available identification systems that also permit relatively rapid identification of anaerobes. However, these systems may not accurately characterize all species. Some isolates must be speciated by gas–liquid chromatographic analysis of fatty acids. DNA hybridization or amplification procedures for detection and identification of anaerobes currently are not commercially available, and FAS is infrequently used. The level of information provided about the identification of anaerobic isolates depends on the sophistication of the laboratory, the source of the specimen, the number of species present, and the clinical situation.

A minimalist approach to identification and susceptibility testing of anaerobes is used by many laboratories. Rationale has been that the expense and labor involved in completing species identification or susceptibility testing may not be clinically useful. This may change if new methods and technology are developed that allow a more rapid and less costly testing. Anaerobes are significant pathogens in most intraabdominal infections and antibiotic resistance is an increasing problem. However, the contribution of various species to a mixed infection is unclear, and often species identification and susceptibility testing results may not be required for effective therapy. Definitive identification to species level and susceptibility testing procedures are currently reserved for cultures obtained from normally sterile sources when specific antimicrobial therapy is pivotal to outcome, such as situations where antibiotic resistance might be associated with therapeutic failure, and in other situations where a cogent argument can be made (1,5,367–369). For example, central nervous system infections, recurrent or refractory bacteremia, osteomyelitis, infections of prosthetic devices or vascular grafts, and treatment failure possibly due to antibiotic resistance are instances in which species identification and susceptibility testing are warranted. In other clinical situations, presumptive identification of organisms to group or genus level is appropriate (365). Occasionally, the only information that may be needed is verification that anaerobes are present. Organisms that may warrant identification because they express important virulence determinants include *C. septicum, C. perfringens,* and those that commonly express antibiotic resistance, including the *B. fragilis* group, *C. ramosum, C. inocuum, C. clostridioforme,* anaerobic cocci, and fusobacteria.

Susceptibility testing of anaerobes has been fraught with difficulties, including limited correlation of *in vitro* susceptibility results with clinical response, problems with reproducability, inability to grow some pathogens, cumbersome methodology, slow turnaround, cost and controversy about clinically relevant breakpoints between susceptibility and resistance, and which organisms in mixed infections should be tested (367–370). Antibiotic resistance among anaerobes is increasing in some settings; however, resistance profiles in one institution may not be the same as those in another (370–372) indicating

the need for local monitoring. Broth microdilution and agar dilution are acceptable methods, whereas the less complex method of broth disk elution is no longer recommended (367). The E test has been found to be reliable for some organisms or drugs but not for others, but may circumvent some problems with current procedures (373,374).

Blood Cultures. Depending on the nature of the infection, 20% to 70% of patients with intraabdominal infections may have a positive blood culture (375). Bacteremia also may occur in salmonellosis, especially in immunocompromised patients, and in typhoid fever, and less frequently during enteric infections caused by *Yersinia, Campylobacter,* and *Shigella.* When bacteremia or sepsis is suspected, two or three blood cultures should be obtained (376–378). The sensitivity of a single blood culture (15 mL) is approximately 90%, and sensitivity of two or more cultures is >99%. Obtaining three blood cultures improves specificity and is particularly recommended in septic patients, for patients with indwelling lines or prosthetic devices, and for patients with suspected endocarditis. Obtaining a single blood culture may result in a false-negative result, and it is generally not productive to obtain more than three blood cultures during a single febrile episode. In cases of overwhelming sepsis, infections with intravascular foci such as endocarditis, or in patients with infected sites in close contiguity to vasculature, bacteremia is usually continuous, whereas in most other situations it is intermittent. Antimicrobial therapy significantly compromises the ability to isolate microorganisms, even when antibiotic removal devices are used; therefore, cultures should be obtained prior to starting antibiotics whenever this is clinically feasible. In medically urgent cases, simultaneous blood cultures should be obtained by separate venipunctures prior to starting therapy. In less urgent circumstances, collection of blood cultures can be spaced over a period of time, up to 24 hr prior to starting antibiotics.

For 30% to 50% of patients with a positive blood culture, the isolate is a coagulase-negative *Staphylococcus* and usually a single positive specimen. These are most often falsely positive and result from contamination by skin flora during venipuncture or during handling. False-positive cultures due to contamination may result in unnecessary treatment and additional testing. Therefore, it is important to use good technique for culture collection.

Streptococcus bovis I (379) and *Clostridium septicum* bacteremia (380) have been strongly associated with GI malignancy. Similarly, isolation of *S. bovis* II (variant) from a blood culture suggests hepatic or pancreatic disease (379), and isolation of *S. anginosis* (*S. milleri*) is often associated with abscesses in liver, brain, or lung (381,382). Bacteremia with *E. coli* or anaerobes is often associated with intraabdominal or GI disease. Although rates vary depending on patient population, approximately 10% to 15% of patients with positive cultures have polymicrobial bacteremia. The nature of the species comprising the polymicrobial infection can be a helpful clue as to the source; for example, polymicrobial cultures containing enteric facultative bacilli and *B. fragilis,* in the absence of decubitus ulcers, strongly suggests a possible focus of infection in the GI tract.

Anaerobic Bacteremia. The frequency of anaerobic bacteremias is often low and may only account for 3% to 7% of patients having a positive blood culture in some settings (383,384). Anaerobic blood culture media may be reserved only for patients at highest risk for anaerobic bacteremia in some institutions. In addition, the sensitivity of aerobic blood cultures may improve if all of the blood sample is used for aerobic culture. This is especially true for the isolation of *Pseudomonas, Acinetobacter, Candida,* and staphylococci. Broth-type blood culture systems have been found to be superior to lysis centrifugation systems (Isolator) for the isolation of anaerobes and streptococci. Physicians who care for patients at high risk for anaerobic bacteremia (GI and gynecologic patients) need to be aware if special procedures for detection of anaerobic bacteremia are required within their own institutions.

Fungal Blood Cultures. Fungal blood cultures may be indicated in some situations, particularly for patients who have received prolonged administration of broad-spectrum antibiotics. Using optimum methods, sensitivity of blood culture is approximately 80% for detection of disseminated candidiasis. Although some commercial broth blood culture systems may recover yeast, especially *C. albicans* (385), with moderately high sensitivity, the Isolator system, which employs lysis centrifugation to concentrate microorganisms and direct plating to solid media, appears to have greater sensitivity (386). A new broth-based blood culture system designed to isolate fungi has compared favorably with lysis centrifugation for recovery of fungi other than *Histoplasma capsulatum* (387). With current technology, usually bacterial pathogens can be recovered by fungal blood cultures and many fungi may be recovered from routine blood cultures. Therefore, it is not usually necessary to obtain more than two fungal blood cultures and two routine cultures.

Mycobacterial Blood Cultures. Special methods are required to isolate mycobacteria from blood (388). Mycobacterial blood cultures are most commonly used to isolate *M. avium-intracellulare* from patients with HIV infection. One or two blood cultures are adequate for diagnosis. Occasionally, *M. tuberculosis* may be found alone or with *M. avium.*

Blood Cultures for Fastidious Microorganisms. Slow-growing or nutritionally fastidious organisms, including *Rochalimaea* sp. and *Brucella,* may infect extraintestinal tract organs (primarily liver and spleen). In suspected cases of disseminated bacillary angiomatosis, disseminated cat-scratch disease, trench fever syndrome, bacillary peliosis hepatis (*Rochalimaea henselae, R. quintana*), and brucellosis, special blood cultures procedures are required; therefore, the laboratory should be contacted if such pathogens are suspected on the basis of clinical presentation or history.

Peritonitis

The species of bacteria causing peritonitis depend on underlying conditions and source of infection. Routine

and anaerobic cultures of peritoneal fluid are adequate for recovery of usual pathogens although sensitivity may be improved by bedside inoculation of a portion of the material directly into blood culture media (389) and anaerobic transport vials. Patients on chronic ambulatory peritoneal dialysis (CAPD) who develop peritonitis most commonly are infected by coagulase-negative staphylococci, which normally colonize the skin and are common culture contaminants. In CAPD-associated peritonitis, the number of organisms in dialysate also may be low. Techniques used to collect and transport specimens to the laboratory have an important effect on specificity and sensitivity of culture. If patients are to collect samples, they should be properly instructed in the appropriate method to collect dialysate cultures and rapid transport of sample to the laboratory should be encouraged. Direct inoculation of a blood culture system with dialysate is more sensitive than centrifugation and subsequent culture of 50 mL of dialysate (390–392). A portion of the sample should be placed in a blood culture system, either a lysis centrifugation (Isolator) tube or broth blood culture media. The remainder of the sample should be sent to the laboratory for cytocentrifuge prepared Gram stain, concentration, and plating onto appropriate media for rapid detection of organisms. Peritonitis due to anaerobes, fungi, and mycobacteria are uncommon (393–395). Usually *Candida* can be detected within 3 days with bacteriological culture. Fungal or AFB culture, respectively, may be needed to detect infections due to more slowly growing fungi and mycobacteria. In patients at risk for peritonitis involving anaerobes, the specimen additionally should be inoculated into an anaerobic blood culture medium and an anaerobic transport medium.

Hepatosplenic Bacillary Peliosis (Bartonella Rochalimaea)

Infection due to the recently recognized bacterium *Bartonella henselae* (formerly *Rochalimaea henselae*) may manifest as a variety of syndromes including bacillary angiomatosis, parenchymal bacillary peliosis, most cases of cat-scratch disease, and a bacteremic syndrome (trench fever) (32–35,396). Exposure to cats, particularly traumatic exposures involving scratches or bites or exposure to cat fleas, is associated with cat-scratch disease, bacillary angiomatosis, and bacillary peliosis hepatis (397,398). *Bartonella quintana,* the agent of trench fever, can also cause bacillary angiomatosis and bacteremia syndrome (394,399–401). Although infection by *Bartonella* sp. usually occurs in immunocompromised patients, particularly those with HIV infection, bacillary angiomatosis and trench fever caused by *B. henselae* have been described in immunocompetent individuals. Bacillary peliosis hepatis caused by *B. henselae* is most frequently documented in patients with HIV infection, and may present as a prolonged febrile illness with hepatic enlargement and tenderness associated with elevated hepatic enzymes. The diagnosis may be made by histopathological exam of liver or spleen biopsy material or by blood culture using special protocols. Bacilli may be visualized using Warthin–Starry silver stain of biopsies, although it is relatively insensitive.

Because special protocols are required to cultivate these organisms, the laboratory should be contacted when *Rochalimaea* infection is suspected.

Culture

Bartonella sp. may be isolated from blood using the lysis centifugation system (Isolator) by inoculating fresh chocolate or blood agar plates and incubation in 5% to 10% CO_2 and a humid environment for a minimum of 2 weeks (400,402,403). In addition to blood cultures, lymph node, liver, or splenic tissue cultures can be attempted. However, cultivation of *Bartonella* from tissue is more difficult (404) and may require cocultivation with endothelial cells (395). Colonies from positive blood cultures usually appear within 10–14 days, although some isolates may require longer for positivity. *B. henselae* colonies are cauliflower-like and embedded in agar; however, colonial variants that are smooth and mucoid and that resemble *B. quintana* colonies develop upon passage.

Identification

On Gram stain, *B. henselae* appear as curved, gram-negative bacilli resembling *Campylobacter*. Acid-fast stains should be performed to distinguish them from *Mycobacterium* sp., which also may be isolated under these conditions. Fresh clinical isolates of *B. henselae* also exhibit autoagglutination, pellicle formation in broth, and twitching motility, characteristics that have been associated with type 4 pili. *Bartonella* sp. are relatively inert in biochemical tests (400–402); they are oxidase-, catalase-, urease-, and esculin-negative, and unreactive with carbohydrate substrates. They demonstrate X factor (heme) dependence. Peptidase reactions with commercially available kits that are used for identification of other organisms may be useful for presumptive identification of *Bartonella* even though these organisms are not a part of the identification database for most systems, and this will not differentiate *B. henselae* from *B. quintana*. It was recently reported that the MicroScan Rapid Anaerobe Panel (Baxter Diagnostics, Deerfield, Il) can be used to speciate *Bartonella*; *B. henselae* is positive for bis-*para*-nitrophenylphosphatase and L-lysinearylamidase activity, whereas *B. quintana* is negative (400). Definitive identification of *Bartonella* species by a reference laboratory may involve cell wall fatty acid analysis, quantitative citrate synthetase, PCR–restriction length polymorphism analysis, DNA hybridization (400–402,405), and antibody-based identification (400,406).

Other Tests

DNA probes or PCR procedures for detection of *Rochalimaea* in tissue currently are not available outside reference and research laboratories, and antibody reagents for antigen detection are not commercially available. An indirect fluorescent antibody test directed

against *B. henselae* antigens has shown good sensitivity and specificity for diagnosis of cat-scratch disease (397,407).

Enteric Fever

Patients with suspected enteric fever should have stool, urine, blood, and possibly bone marrow cultured (408). Blood cultures obtained in the absence of antibiotic treatment will be positive in the majority (80%) of cases of typhoid fever in the first week of illness. Lower rates of positivity (20% to 30%) are seen by the third week. Rubin et al. (409) found that the use of lysis centrifugation blood culture or plating of the mononuclear cell platelet layer in density gradient–separated blood samples was as sensitive and provided more rapid detection of *S. typhi* than conventional broth blood culture media. Stool cultures have an overall sensitivity of approximately 50% and may become positive during the latter half of illness. Urine should be cultured when typhoid fever is suspected, even though it is frequently culture-negative; urine cultures become positive within the second or third week of illness. Treatment with antibiotics will considerably diminish the likelihood of obtaining positive cultures. Unfortunately, use of antibiotic-inactivating blood culture media is likely to provide only marginally improved recovery in treated patients. Bone marrow culture is a highly sensitive means to diagnose typhoid fever; bone marrow and rose spots remain infected longer following treatment than other material.

Initial studies suggest that PCR using blood samples may be a sensitive and specific means of diagnosing some cases of typhoid fever but requires further evaluation (410). Other approaches for organism detection have included DNA probes and antigen detection in serum, urine, or stool (411).

Serology

The current role of serological testing in diagnosis of typhoid or enteric fever is problematic. Problems with *Salmonella* serology (sensitivity, specificity, and practicality) are based on cross-reactivity of test antigens used with antigens of other infecting salmonellae or Enterobacteriaceae, suppression of antibody titer rise with early treatment, positive antibody titers in persons with prior infection, rapidly increasing titers in persons with prior infection such that fourfold increase in titer occurs early in the illness, expense and difficulty in obtaining paired acute and convalescent sera to document titer changes, as well as limited practical utility of the latter approach for patient management (412–419).

The Widal agglutination test lacks sensitivity and specificity and is of diagnostic utility only in unusual settings. Alternative serological tests including ELISA, radioimmunoassay, indirect hemagglutination, FAS and western blot assays have been described for Vi, LPS, and protein antigens. Anti-LPS ELISAs have been most extensively evaluated (411–413); sensitivity was found to be 77% to

94% in patients with culture-proven *S. typhi,* and 60% in paratyphoid fever. Specificity of 92% to 95% was reported; however, in one study (413) approximately 20% of patients with GI or urinary tract infections or malaria had positive anti-LPS antibodies, indicating the lack of specificity in populations experiencing other infectious diseases. Currently, there is no standardized procedure with well-established interpretive criteria that can be applied equally well to patients from endemic and nonendemic areas.

Necrotizing Enterocolitis

Neutropenic enterocolitis is a complication of chemotherapy for malignant disease and also occurs in other immunosuppressed patients (420). This is a diagnosis of exclusion. Microorganisms usually implicated in infection are normal inhabitants of the intestine. Laboratory tests that may be useful include toxin assay to rule out *C. difficile*–mediated disease and two or three blood cultures ordered to rule out bacteremia.

Necrotizing enterocolitis in newborns may result from injury to the immature GI mucosa. However, there is considerable controversy regarding the relative importance of factors that may contribute to or initiate disease (421–425). An infectious etiology for some cases of necrotizing entercolitis has been suggested by (a) the occurrence of outbreaks within nurseries and clusters of cases in a community, (b) the positive impact of initiating stringent infection control practices on occurrence of cases; and (c) the effect of antibiotic choices on incidence of disease (420,421,425). No single organism or virulence factor has been consistently identified as a causative agent. Therefore, the value of routine stool cultures for sporadic cases of necrotizing enterocolitis is questionable. During an outbreak of necrotizing enterocolitis, individuals with expertise in pertinent disciplines including pediatric infectious diseases should develop a rational strategy for investigation. Cultures should be done to rule out the occurrence of enteric pathogens likely to cause transmissible GI disease in infants such as *Salmonella, Shigella, C. jejuni,* and possibly *Aeromonas* and *Plesiomonas.* Ten *E. coli* colonies should be picked for further characterization by a reference laboratory to determine whether these may be EPEC or other strains of *E. coli* with known pathogenic potential. For investigational purposes only, laboratories can presumptively identify predominate isolates from outbreak and control patients to determine if a certain organism is associated with disease.

ACKNOWLEDGMENTS

We thank Sue Leamons, Pam Verducci, and Janet Payne for their valuable assistance.

REFERENCES

1. Balows A, Hausler Jr WJ, Herrmann KL, Isenberg HD, Shadomy HJ. *Manual of clinical microbiology.* 5th ed. Washington, DC: American Society for Microbiology; 1991.
2. Wentworth BB, ed. *Diagnostic procedures for bacterial infections.* 7th ed. Washington, DC: American Public Health Association; 1987.
3. World Health Organization. *Manual for laboratory investigations of acute enteric infections. programme for control of diarrheal diseases.* CDD/83.3 Rev 1. Geneva: World Health Organization; 1987.
4. Balows A, Hausler WJ Jr, Ohashi M, Turano A, eds. *Laboratory diagnosis of infectious diseases: principles and practice. Bacterial, mycotic, and parasitic diseases.* I. New York: Springer-Verlag; 1988.
5. Summanen P, Baron EJ, Citron DM, Strong C, Wexler HM, Finegold SM. *Wadsworth anaerobic bacteriology manual.* 5th ed. Belmont, CA: Star; 1993.
6. Finegold SM, George WL. *Anaerobic infections in humans.* San Diego: Academic Press; 1989.
7. Sack RB, Tilton RC, Weissfeld AS, Rubin SJ. *CUMITECH 12: laboratory diagnosis of bacterial diarrhea.* Washington, DC: American Society for Microbiology; 1980.
8. Rose NR, de Macario EC, Fahey JL, Friedman H, Penn GM. *Manual of clinical laboratory immunology.* 4th ed. Washington, DC: American Society for Microbiology; 1992.
9. Isenberg HD, ed. *Clinical microbiology procedures handbook.* II. Washington, DC: American Society for Microbiology; 1992.
10. Isenberg HD, Schoenknecht FD, von Graevenitz A, Rubin SJ. *CUMITECH 9: collection and processing of bacteriological specimens.* Washington, DC: American Society for Microbiology; 1979.
11. Smith PD, Lane HC, Gill VJ, et al. Intestinal infections in patients with the acquired immunodeficiency syndrome (AIDS): etiology and response to therapy. *Ann Intern Med* 1988;108: 328–333.
12. Guerrant RL, Bobak DA. Bacterial and protozoal gastroenteritis. *N Engl J Med* 1991;325:327–340.
13. Guerrant RL, Hughes JM, Lima NL, Crane J. Diarrhea in developed and developing countries: magnitude, special settings, and etiologies. *Rev Infect Dis* 1990;12:S41–S50.
14. Siegel DL, Edelstein PH, Nachamkin I. Inappropriate testing for diarrheal diseases in the hospital. *JAMA* 1990;263:979–982.
15. Koplan JP, Fineberg HV, Ferraro MJB, Rosenberg ML. Value of stool cultures. *Lancet* 1980;2:413–416.
16. Guerrant RL, Shields DS, Thorson SM, Schorling JB, Groschel DHM. Evaluation and diagnosis of acute infectious diarrhea. *Am J Med* 1985:78:91–98.
17. Brady MT, Pacini DL, Budde CT, Connell MJ. Diagnostic studies of nosocomial diarrhea in children: assessing their use and value. *Am J Infect Control* 1989:17:77–82.
18. Bowman RA, Bowman JM, Arrow SA, Riley TV. Selective criteria for the microbiological examination of faecal specimens. *J Clin Pathol* 1992;45:838–839.
19. Murray BE. Resistance of *Shigella, Salmonella,* and other selected enteric pathogens to antimicrobial agents. *Rev Infect Dis* 1986;8:S172–S181.
20. National Committee for Clinical Laboratory Standards. *Performance standards for antimicrobial susceptibility testing.* 4th Information Supplement. NCCLS vol 12, no 20, Doc M100-S4. Villanova, PA: NCCLS; 1992.
21. National Committee for Clinical Laboratory Standards. *Methods for dilution antimicrobial susceptibility tests for bacteria that grow aerobically.* 2nd ed. Approved standard. NCCLS vol 10, no 8, Doc M7-A2. Villanova, PA: NCCLS; 1990.
22. National Committee for Clinical Laboratory Standards. *Performance standards for antimicrobial disk susceptibility tests.* 4th ed. Approved standard. NCCLS vol 10, no 7, Doc M2-A4. Villanova, PA: NCCLS; 1990.
23. Huang MB, Baker CN, Banerjee S, Tenover FC. Accuracy of the E test for determining antimicrobial susceptibilities of staphylococci, enterococci, *Campylobacter jejuni,* and gram-negative bacteria resistant to antimicrobial agents. *J Clin Microbiol* 1992;30:3243–3248.
24. Levine MM. Antimicrobial therapy for infectious diarrhea. *Rev Infect Dis* 1986;8:S207–S216.
25. Persing DH, Smith TF, Tenover FC, White TH, eds. *Diagnos-*

tic molecular microbiology: principles and applications. Washington, DC: American Society for Microbiology; 1993.

26. Tompkins LS, Mickelsen PA, Troup N. DNA technology applied to the detection and epidemiology of enteric pathogens. In: Habermehl KO, ed. *Rapid methods and automation in microbiology and immunology.* New York: Springer-Verlag; 1985:68–72.

27. Tompkins LS. Nucleic acid probes in infectious disease. In: Remington JS, Shwartz M, eds. *Current topics in infectious diseases.* Vol 10. Boston: Blackwell Scientific; 1989:174–193.

28. Tompkins LS, Falkow SF. Molecular biology of virulence and epidemiology. In: Gorbach SL, Bartlett JG, Blacklow NR. *Infectious diseases.* Philadelphia: WB Saunders; 1992:30–37.

29. Tenover FC. Molecular methods for the clinical microbiology laboratory. In: Balows A, Hausler Jr WJ, Herrmann KL, Isenberg HD, Shadomy HJ, eds. *Manual of clinical microbiology.* 5th ed. Washington, DC: American Society for Microbiology; 1991:199–127.

30. Relman DA. The identification of uncultured microbial pathogens. *J Infect Dis* 1993:168:1–8.

31. Solnick JV, O'Rourke J, Lee A, Paster BJ, Dewhirst FE, Tompkins LS. An uncultured gastric spiral organism is a newly identified *Helicobacter* in humans. *J Infect Dis* 1993;168: 379–385.

32. Relman DA, Loutit JS, Schmidt TM, Falkow S, Tompkins LS. The agent of bacillary angiomatosis: an approach to the identification of uncultured pathogens. *N Engl J Med* 1990;323: 1573–1580.

33. Relman DA, Falkow S, LeBoit PE, et al. The organism causing bacillary angiomatosis, peliosis hepatis, and fever and bacteremia in immunocompromised patients [letter]. *N Engl J Med* 1991;324:1514.

34. Perkocha LA, Geaghan SM, Yen TSB, et al. Clinical and pathological features of bacillary peliosis hepatis in association with human immunodeficiency virus infection. *N Engl J Med* 1990; 323:1581–1586.

35. Slater MD, Welch DF, Hensel D, Coody DW. A newly recognized fastidious gram-negative pathogen as a cause of fever and bacteremia. *N Engl J Med* 1990;23:1587–1600.

36. Relman DA, Schmidt TM, MacDermott RP, Falkow S. Identification of the uncultured bacillus of Whipple's disease. *N Engl J Med* 1992;327:293–301.

37. McFadden JJ, Collins J, Beaman B, Arthur M, Gitnick G. Mycobacteria in Crohn's disease: DNA probes identify the wood pigeon strain of *Mycobacterium avium* and *Mycobacterium paratuberculosis* from human tissue. *J Clin Microbiol* 1992;30: 3070–3073.

38. Moss MT, Sanderson JD, Tizard MLV, Hermon-Taylor J, El-Zaatari FAK, Markesich DC, and Graham DY. Polymerase chain reaction detection of *Mycobacterium paratuberculosis* and *Mycobacterium avium* subsp. *silvaticum* in long term cultures from Crohn's disease and control tissues. *Gut* 1992;34: 1209–1213.

39. Sanderson JD, Moss MT, Tizard MLV, Hermon-Taylor J. *Mycobacterium paratuberculosis* DRN in Crohn's disease tissue. *Gut* 1992;33:390–896.

40. Wall S, Kunze ZM, Saboor S, et al. Identification of spheroplast-like agents isolated from tissues of patients with Crohn's disease and control tissues by polymerase chain reaction. *J Clin Microbiol* 1993;31:1241–1245.

41. Tompkins LS. Molecular methods in infectious disease epidemiology and virulence. *N Engl J Med* 1992;327:1290–1297.

42. Mathan VI, Mathan MM. Intestinal manifestations of invasive diarrheas and their diagnosis. *Rev Infect Dis* 1991;13: S311–S313.

43. Kelsall BL, Guerrant RL. Evaluation of diarrhea in the returning traveler. *Infect Dis Clin North Am* 1992;6:413–425.

44. Smith PD, Quinn TC, Strober W, Janoff EN, Masur H. 1992 Gastrointestinal infections in AIDS. *Ann Intern Med* 116: 63–77.

45. DeWitt TG. Acute diarrhea in children. *Pediatr Rev* 1989;11: 6–13.

46. Adkins HJ, Santiago LT. Increased recovery of enteric pathogens by use of both stool and rectal swab specimens. *J Clin Microbiol* 1987;25:158–159.

47. Wells JG, Morris GK. Evaluation of transport methods for isolating *Shigella* spp. *J Clin Microbiol* 1981;13:789–790.

48. Goossens H, Butzler JP. Isolation and identification of *Campylobacter* spp. In: Nachamkin I, Blaser MJ, Tompkins LS. Campylobacter jejuni: *current status and future trends,* Washington, DC: American Society for Microbiology; 1992:93–109.

49. Monfort JD, Stills Jr HF, Bech-Nielsen S. Effects of sample holding time, temperature, and atmosphere on the isolation of *Campylobacter jejuni* from dogs. *J Clin Microbiol* 1989;27: 1419–1420.

50. Luechtefeld NW, Wang WLL, Blaser MJ, Reller LB. Evaluation of transport and storage techniques for isolation of *Campylobacter fetus* supsp. *jejuni* from turkey fecal specimens. *J Clin Microbiol* 1981;13:438–443.

51. Wang WLL, Reller LB, Smallwood B, Luechtefeld NW, Blaser MJ. Evaluation of transport media for *Campylobacter jejuni* in human fecal specimens. *J Clin Microbiol* 1983;18:803–807.

52. Harris, JC, DuPont HL, and Hornick RB. Fecal leukocytes in diarrheal illness. *Ann Intern Med* 1972;76:697–703.

53. Pickering LK, DuPont HL, Olarte J, Conklin R, Ericsson C. Fecal leukocytes in enteric infections. *Am J Clin Pathol* 1976; 68:562–565.

54. Stoll BJ, Glass RI, Huq MI, Khan MU, Banu H, Holt J. Epidemiologic and clinical features of patients infected with Shigella who attended a diarrhea disease hospital in Bangladesh. *J Infect Dis* 1982;146:177–183.

55. Alvarado T. Faecal leucocytes in patients with infectious diarrhoea. *Trans R Soc Trop Med Hyg* 1983;77:316–320.

56. Hossain MA, Albert MJ. Effect of duration of diarrhoea and predictive values of stool leucocytes and red blood cells in the isolation of different serogroups or serogroups of *Shigella. Trans R Soc Trop Med Hyg* 1991;85:664–666.

57. Korzeniowski OM, Barada FA, Rouse JD, Guerrant RL. Value of examination for fecal leukocytes in the early diagnosis of shigellosis. *Am J Trop Med Hyg* 1979;28:1031–1035.

58. Guerrant RL, Araujo V, Soares E, et al. Measurement of fecal lactoferrin as a marker of fecal leukocytes. *J Clin Microbiol* 1992;30:1238–1242.

59. Thorson SM, Lohr JA, Dudley S, Guerrant RL. Value of methylene blue examination, dark-field microscopy, and carbolfuchsin Gram stain in the detection of *Campylobacter* enteritis. *J Pediatrics* 1985;106:941–943.

60. Paisley JW, Mirrett S, Lauer BA, Roe M, Reller LB. Darkfield microscopy of human feces for presumptive diagnosis of *Campylobacter fetus* subsp. *jejuni* enteritis. *J Clin Microbiol* 1982;15:61–63.

61. Kelly MT, Hickman-Brenner FW, Farmer JJ III. *Vibrio.* In: Balows, A, Hausler WJ, Jr, Herrmann KL, Isenberg HD, Shadomy HJ, eds. *Manual of clinical microbiology.* 5th ed. Washington, DC: American Society for Microbiology; 1991:384–395.

62. Tison DL. *Vibrio* infections. In: Wentworth BB, ed. *Diagnostic procedures for bacterial infections.* 7th ed. Washington, DC: American Public Health Association; 1987:599–611.

63. Ortega YR, Sterling CR, Gilman RH, Cama VA, Diaz F. Cyclospora species; a new protozoan pathogen of humans. *N Engl J Med* 1993;328:1308–1312.

64. Hoge CW, Shlim DR, Rajah R, et al. Epidemiology of diarrhoeal illness associated with coccidian-like organism among travellers and foreign residents in Nepal. *Lancet* 1993;341: 1175–1179.

65. Wurtz RM, Kocka FE, Peters CS, Weldon-Linne CM, Kuritza A, Yungbluth P. Clinical characteristics of seven cases of diarrhea associated with a novel acid-fast organism in the stool. *Clin Infect Dis* 1993;16:136–138.

66. Long EG, White EH, Carmichael WW, et al. Morphologic and staining characteristics of a cyanobacterium-like organism associated with diarrhea. *J Infect Dis* 1991;164:199–202.

67. Farmer JJ, Kelly MT. Enterobacteriaceae. In: Balows A, ed. *Manual of clinical microbiology.* 5th ed. Washington, DC: American Society for Microbiology; 1991:360–383.

68. Farmer JJ III, Wells JG, Griffin PM, Wachsmuth IK. Enterobacteriaceae infections. In: Wentworth BB, ed. *Diagnostic pro-*

cedures for bacterial infections. Washington, DC: American Public Health Association; 1987:233–296.

69. Echeverria P, Sethabutr O, Pitarangsi C. Microbiology and diagnosis of infections with *Shigella* and enteroinvasive *Escherichia coli*. *Rev Infect Dis* 1991;13:S220–S225.

70. Dusch H, Altwegg M. Comparison of Rambach Agar, SM-ID medium, and Hektoen enteric agar for primary isolation of nontyphi salmonellae from stool samples. *J Clin Microbiol* 1993; 31:410–412.

71. McGowan KL, Rubenstein MT. Use of a rapid latex agglutination test to detect *Salmonella* and *Shigella* antigens from gram-negative enrichment broth. *Am J Clin Pathol* 1989;92:679–682.

72. Rohner P, Dharan S, Auckenthaler R. Evaluation of the Well-colex Colour Salmonella test for detection of *Salmonella* spp. in enrichment broths. *J Clin Microbiol* 1992;30:3274–3276.

73. Fedorko DP, Lehman SM, Yu PKW, Germer JJ, Anhalt JP. Increased efficiency of stool culture for the detection of *Salmonella* and *Shigella*. *Diagn Microbiol Infect Dis* 1989;12: 463–466.

74. Taylor WI, Schelhart D. Isolation of shigellae. VI. Performance of media with stool specimens. *Appl Microbiol* 1971;16: 1387–1393.

75. Lue YA. Is enrichment broth necessary for stool cultures? *Clin Microbiol News* 1986;8:5–6.

76. Nordlander E, Phuphaisan S, Bodhidatta L, Arthur J, Echeverria P. Microscopic examination of stools and a latex slide agglutination test for the rapid identification of bacterial enteric infections in Khmer children. *Diag Microbiol Infect Dis* 1990;13: 273–276.

77. Ewing WH. *Edwards and Ewing's identification of Enterobacteriaceae*. 4th ed. New York: Elsevier; 1986.

78. Geers TA, Backes BA. Evaluation of two rapid methods to screen pathogens from stool specimens. *Am J Clin Pathol* 1989; 91:327–330.

79. Imperatrice CA, Nachamkin I. Evaluation of the Vitek EPS enteric pathogen screen card for detecting *Salmonella, Shigella,* and *Yersinia* spp. *J Clin Microbiol* 1993;31:433–435.

80. Ruiz J, Sempere MA, Varela MC, Gomez J. Modification of the methodology of stool culture for *Salmonella* detection. *J Clin Microbiol* 1992;30:525–526.

81. Ruiz J, Varela MC, Sempere MA, Lopez ML, Gomez J, Oliva J. Presumptive identification of *Salmonella enterica* using two rapid tests. *Eur J Clin Microbiol Infect Dis* 1991;10:649–651.

82. Farmer III JJ, Davis BR, Hickman-Brenner FW, et al. Biochemical identification of new species and biogroups of Enterobacteriaceae isolated from clinical specimens. *J Clin Microbiol* 1985;21:46–76.

83. Farmer JJ, McWorter AC, Brenner DJ, Morris GK. The *Salmonella–Arizona* group of Enterobacteriaceae: nomenclature, classification and reporting. *Clin Microbiol Newslett* 1984;6: 63–66.

84. Chagla AH, Borczyk AA, Aldom JE, Rosa SD, Cole DD. Evaluation of the L-pyrrolidonyl-β-naphthylamide hydrolysis test for the differentiation of members of the families Enterobacteriaceae and Vibrionaceae. *J Clin Microbiol* 1993;31:1946–1948.

85. Echeverria P, Taylor DN, Seriwatana J, Brown JE, Lexomboon U. Examination of colonies and stool blots for detection of enteropathogens by DNA hybridization with eight DNA probes. *J Clin Microbiol* 1989;27:331–334.

86. Begaud E, Jourand P, Morillon M, Mondet D, Germani Y. Detection of diarrheogenic *Escherichia coli* in children less than ten years old with and without diarrhea in New Caledonia using seven acetylaminofluorene-labeled DNA probes. *Am J Trop Med Hyg* 1993;48:26–34.

87. Malabi M, Venkatesan MM, Buysse JM, Kopecko DJ. Use of *Shigella flexneri ipaC* and *ipaH* gene sequences for the general identification of *Shigella* spp. and enteroinvasive *Escherichia coli*. *J Clin Microbiol* 1989;27:2687–2691.

88. Panda CS, Riley LW, Kumari SN, Khanna KK, Prakash K. Comparison of alkaline phosphatase-conjugated oligonucleotide DNA probe with the sereny test for identification of *Shigella* strains. *J Clin Microbiol* 1990;28:2122–2124.

89. Frankel G, Giron JA, Valmassoi J, Schoolnik GK. Multi-gene

90. Widjojoatmodjo MN, Fluit AC, Torensma R, Verdonk GPHT, Verhoef J. The magnetic immuno polymerase chain reaction assay for direct detection of salmonellae in fecal samples. *J Clin Microbiol* 1992;30:3195–3199.

91. Islam D, Lindberg AA. Detection of *Shigella dysenteriae* type 1 and *Shigella flexneri* in feces by immunomagnetic isolation and polymerase chain reaction. *J Clin Microbiol* 1992;30: 2801–2806.

92. Sethabutr O, Venkatesan M, Murphy GS, Eampokalap B, Hoge CW, Echeverria P. Detection of Shigellae and enteroinvasive *Escherichia coli* by amplification of the invasion plasmid antigen H DNA sequence in patients with dysentery. *J Infect Dis* 1993;167:458–461.

93. Lindberg AA, Cam PD, Chan N, Phu LK, Trach DD, Lindberg G, Karlsson K, Karnell A, Ekwall E. Shigellosis in Vietnam: seroepidemiologic studies with use of lipopolysaccharide antigens in enzyme immunoassays. *Rev Infect Dis* 1991;13: S231–S237.

94. Pàl T, Pàsca AS, Emódy L, Vörös S, Sélley E. Modified enzyme-linked immunosorbent assay for detecting enteroinvasive *Escherichia coli* and virulent shigella strains. *J Clin Microbiol* 1985;21:415–418.

95. Albert MJ, Ansaruzzaman M, Alim ARMA, Mitra AK. Fluorescent antibody staining test for rapid diagnosis of *Shigella dysenteriae* 1 Infection. *Diag Microbiol* 1992;15:359–361.

96. De Silva DGH, Candy DCA, Mendis LN, Chart H, Rowe B. Serological diagnosis of infection by *Shigella dysenteriae*-1 in patients with bacillary dysentery. *J Infect* 1992;25:273–278.

97. Blaser MJ, Reller LB. *Campylobacter enteritis*. *N Engl J Med* 1981;305:1444–1452.

98. Blaser MJ, Wang WLL. *Campylobacter* infections. In: Wentworth BB, ed. *Diagnostic procedures for bacterial infections*. 7th ed. Washington, DC: American Public Health Association; 1987:195–211.

99. Skirrow MB, Blaser MJ. Clinical and epidemiologic considerations. In: Nachamkin I, Blaser MJ, Tompkins LS. *Campylobacter jejuni: current status and future trends*. Washington, DC: American Society for Microbiology; 1992:3–8.

100. Penner JL. *Campylobacter, Helicobacter,* and related spiral bacteria. In: Balows A, Hausler WJ Jr, Herrmann KL, Isenberg HD, Shadomy HJ. *Manual of clinical microbiology*. 5th ed. Washington, DC: American Society for Microbiology; 1991: 402–409.

101. Penner JL. *The genus* Campylobacter: *a decade of progress*. *Clin Microbiol Rev* 1988;1:157–172.

102. Mishu B, Patton CM, Tauxe RV. Clinical and epidemiologic features of non-*jejuni*, non-*coli Campylobacter* species. In: Nachamkin I, Blaser MJ, Tompkins LS, eds. Campylobacter jejuni: *current status and future trends*. Washington, DC: American Society for Microbiology; 1992:31–41.

103. Simor AE, Wilcox L. Enteritis associated with *Campylobacter laridis*. *J Clin Microbiol* 1987;25:10–12.

104. Albert MJ, Tee W, Leach A, Asche V, Penner JL. Comparison of a blood-free medium and a filtration technique for the isolation of *Campylobacter* spp. from diarrhoel stools of hospitalised patients in central Australia. *J Med Microbiol* 1992;37: 176–179.

105. Guerrant RL, Lahita RG, Winn Jr WC, Roberts RB. Campylobacteriosis in man: pathogenic mechanisms and review of 91 bloodstream infections. *Am J Med* 1976;65:584–592.

106. Totten PA, Fennell CL, Tenover FC, et al. *Campylobacter cinaedi* (sp. nov.) and *Campylobacter fennelliae* (sp. nov.): two new *Campylobacter* species associated with enteric disease in homosexual men. *J Infect Dis* 1985;151:131–139.

107. Vandamme P, Falsen E, Pot B, Kersters K, De Ley J. Identification of *Campylobacter cinaedi* isolated from blood and feces of children and adult females. *J Clin Microbiol* 1990;28: 1016–1020.

108. Tee W, Anderson BN, Ross BC, Dwyer B. Atypical campylobacters associated with gastroenteritis. *J Clin Microbiol* 1987; 25:1248–1252.

109. Endtz HP, Ruijs GJHM, Zwinderman AH, van der Reijden T,

Biever M, Mouton RP. Comparison of six media, including a semisolid agar, for the isolation of various *Campylobacter* species from stool specimens. *J Clin Microbiol* 1991;29:1007–1010.

110. Karmali MA, Simor AE, Roscoe M, Flemming PC, Smith SS, Lane J. Evaluation of a blood-free, charcoal-based, selective medium for the isolation of *Campylobacter* organisms from feces. *J Clin Microbiol* 1986;23:456–459.

111. Ng LK, Stiles ME, Taylor DE. Inhibition of *Campylobacter jejuni* and *Campylobacter coli* by antibiotics used in selective growth media. *J Clin Microbiol* 1985;22:510–514.

112. Goossens H, Vlaes L, Galand I, Van den Borre C, Butzler J-P. Semisolid blood-free selective-motility medium for the isolation of campylobacters from stool specimens. *J Clin Microbiol* 1989;27:1077–1080.

113. Goossens H, and Butzler J-P. Isolation of *Campylobacter* spp. from stool specimens with a semisolid medium (letter). *J Clin Microbiol* 1991;29:2681–2682.

114. Endtz HP, Mouton RP. Isolation of *Campylobacter* spp from stool specimens with a semisolid medium (Letter). *J Clin Microbiol* 1991;29:2681–2682.

115. Bolton FJ, Hutchinson DN, Parker G. Reassessment of selective agars and filtration techniques for isolation of *Campylobacter* species from faeces. *Eur J Clin Microbiol Infect Dis* 1988;7:155–160.

116. Steele TW, Sangster N, Lanser JA. DNA relatedness and biochemical features of *Campylobacter* spp. isolated in central and south Australia. *J Clin Microbiol* 1985;22:71–74.

117. Altwegg M, Burnens A, Zollinger-Iten J, Penner JL. Problems in identification of *Campylobacter jejuni* associated with acquisition of resistance to nalidixic acid. *J Clin Microbiol* 1987;25:1807–1808.

118. Tenover FC, Baker C, Fennell CL, Ryan CA. Antimicrobial resistance in *Campylobacter* species. In: Nachamkin I, Blaser MJ, Tompkins LS, eds. Campylobacter jejuni: *current status and future trends*. Washington, DC: American Society for Microbiology; 1992:66–73.

119. Roop II RM, Smibert RM, Johnson JL, Krieg NR. Differential characteristics of catalase-positive campylobacters correlated with DNA homology groups. *Can J Microbiol* 1984;30:938–951.

120. Burnens AP, Nicolet J. Three supplementary diagnostic tests for *Campylobacter* species and related organisms. *J Clin Microbiol* 1993;31:708–710.

121. Popovic-Uroic T, Patton CM, Nicholson MA, Kiehlbauch JA. Evaluation of the indoxyl acetate hydrolysis test for rapid differentiation of *Campylobacter, Helicobacter,* and *Wolinella* species. *J Clin Microbiol* 1990;28:2335–2339.

122. Hodinka RL, Gilligan PH. Evaluation of the Campyslide agglutination test for confirmatory identification of selected *Campylobacter* species. *J Clin Microbiol* 1988;26:47–49.

123. Nachamkin I, Barbagallo S. Culture confirmation of *Campylobacter* spp. by latex agglutination. *J Clin Microbiol* 1990;28:817–818.

124. Tenover FC, Carlson L, Barbagello S, Nachamkin I. DNA probe culture confirmation assay for identification of thermophilic *Campylobacter* species. *J Clin Microbiol* 1990;28:1284–1287.

125. Oyofo BA, Thornton SA, Burr DH, Trust TJ, Pavlovskis OR, Guerry P. Specific detection of *Campylobacter jejuni* and *Campylobacter coli* by using polymerase chain reaction. *J Clin Microbiol* 1992;30:2613–2619.

126. Rautelin H, Renkonen OV, Kosunen TU. Emergence of fluoroquinolone resistance in *Campylobacter jejuni* and *Campylobacter coli* in subjects from Finland. *Antimicrob Agents Chemother* 1991;35:2065–2069.

127. Taylor DE, Ng LK, Lior H. Susceptibility of *Campylobacter* species to nalidixic acid, enoxacin, and other DNA gyrase inhibitors. *Antimicrob Agents Chemother* 1985;28:708–710.

128. Levine MM. *Escherichia coli* that cause diarrhea: enterotoxigenic, enteropathogenic, enteroinvasive, enterohemorrhagic, and enteroadherent. *J Infect Dis* 1987;155:377–389.

129. Taylor DN, Echeverria P, Sethabutr O, et al. Clinical and microbiologic features of *Shigella* and enteroinvasive *Escherichia coli* infections detected by DNA hybridization. *J Clin Microbiol* 1988;26:1362–1366.

130. Gordillo ME, Reeve GR, Pappas J, Mathewson JJ, DuPont HL, Murray BE. Molecular characterization of strains of enteroinvasive *Escherichia coli* O143, including isolates from a large outbreak in Houston, Texas. *J Clin Microbiol* 1992;30:889–893.

131. Toledo MRF, Trabulsi LR. Correlation between biochemical and serological characteristics of *Escherichia coli* and results of the Sereny test. *J Clin Microbiol* 1983;17:419–421.

132. Venkatesan M, Buysse JM, Vandendries EV, Kopecko DJ. Development and testing of invasion-associated DNA probes for the detection of *Shigella* spp. and enteroinvasive *Escherichia coli*. *J Clin Microbiol* 1988;26:261–266.

133. Cover TL, Aber RC. *Yersinia enterocolotica*. *N Engl J Med* 1989;321:16–24.

134. Simmonds SD, Noble MA, Freeman HJ. Gastrointestinal features of culture-positive *Yersinia enterocolitica* infection. *Gastroenterology* 1987;1:112–117.

135. Lee LA, Taylor J, Carter GP, Quinn B, Farmer III JJ, Tauxe RV, the *Yersinia enterocolitica* Collaborative Study Group. *Yersinia enterocolitica* O:3: an emerging cause of pediatric gastroenteritis in the United States. *J Infect Dis* 1990;163:660–663.

136. Van Noyen R, Selderslaghs R, Bekaert J, Wauters J, Vandepitte J. Causative role of *Yersinia* and other enteric pathogens in the appendicular syndrome. *Eur J Clin Microbiol Infect Dis* 1991;10:735–741.

137. Attwood SEA, Cafferkey MT, Kean BV. *Yersinia* infections in surgical practice. *Br J Surg* 1989;76:499–504.

138. Saebo A, Lassen J. A survey of acute and chronic disease associated with *Yersinia enterocolitica* infection. *Scand J Infect Dis* 1991;23:517–527.

139. Tak PP, Visser LG, Hoogkamp-Korstanje JAA. Unusual manifestations of *Yersinia enterocolitica* infections diagnosed using novel methods. *Clin Infect Dis* 1992;15:645–649.

140. Krogstad P, Mendelman PM, Miller VL, et al. Clinical and microbiologic characteristics of cutaneous infection with *Yersinia enterocolitica*. *J Infect Dis* 1992;165:740–743.

141. Tipple MA, Bland LA, Murphy JJ, et al. Sepsis associated with transfusion of red cells contaminated with *Yersinia enterocolitica*. *Transfusion* 1990;30:207–213.

142. Tsubokura M. Yersinioses other than plague. In: Balows A, Hausler WJ Jr, Ohashi M, Turano A, eds. *Laboratory diagnosis of infectious diseases: principles and practice: Bacterial, mycotic, and parasitic diseases*. I. New York: Springer-Verlag; 1988:540–549.

143. Morris Jr JG, Prado V, Ferreccio C, et al. *Yersinia enterocolitica* isolated from two cohorts of young children in Santiago, Chile: incidence of and lack of correlation between illness and proposed virulence factors. *J Clin Microbiol* 1991;29:2784–2788.

144. Cannon CG, Linnemann CC Jr. *Yersinia enterocolitica* infections in hospitalized patients: the problem of hospital-acquired infections. *Infect Control Hosp Epidemiol* 1992;13(3):139–143.

145. Bottone EJ, Sheehan DJ. *Yersinia enterocolitica*: guidelines for serologic diagnosis of human infections. *Rev Infect Dis* 1983;5:898–906.

146. Bissett ML, Powers C, Abbott SL, Janda JM. Epidemiologic investigations of *Yersinia enterocolitica* and related species: sources, frequency, and serogroup distribution. *J Clin Microbiol* 1990;28:910–912.

147. Blumberg HM, Kiehlbauch JA, Wachsmuth IK. Molecular epidemiology of *Yersinia enterocolitica* O:3 infections: use of chromosomal DNA restriction fragment length polymorphisms of rRNA genes. *J Clin Microbiol* 1991;29:2368–2374.

148. Agbonlahor DE. Characteristics of *Yersinia intermedia*–like bacteria isolated from patients with diarrhea in Nigeria. *J Clin Microbiol* 1986;23:891–893.

149. Hoogkamp-Korstanje JAA, de Koning J, Heesemann J. Persistence of *Yersinia enterocolitica* in man. *Infection* 1988;16:81–85.

150. Hoogkamp-Korstanje JAA, de Koning J, Heesemann J, Festen JJM, Houtman PM, van Oyen PLM. Influences of antibiotics on IgA and IgG response and persistence of *Yersinia enterocolitica* in patients with *Yersinia*-associated spondylarthropathy. *Infection* 1992;20:53–57.

151. Kachoris M, Ruoff KL, Welch K, Kallas W, Ferraro MJ. Rou-

tine culture of stool specimens for *Yersinia enterocolitica* is not a cost-effective procedure. *J Clin Microbiol* 1988;26:582–583.

152. Sharma NK, Doyle PW, Gerbasi SA, Jessop JH. Identification of *Yersinia* species by the API 20E. *J Clin Microbiol* 1990;28: 1443–1444.

153. Archer JR, Schell RF, Pennell DR, Wick PD. Identification of *Yersinia* spp. with the API 20E system. *J Clin Microbiol* 1987; 25:2398–2399.

154. Cornelis G, Laroche Y, Balligand G, Sory MP, Wauters G. *Yersinia enterocolitica,* a primary model for bacterial invasiveness. *Rev Infect Dis* 1987;9:64–87.

155. Miller VL, Farmer III JJ, Hill WE, Falkow S. The *ail* locus is found uniquely in *Yersinia enterocolitica* serotypes commonly associated with disease. *Infect Immun* 1989;57:122–131.

156. Miller VL, Falkow S. Evidence for two genetic loci in *Yersinia enterocolitica* that can promote invasion of epithelial cells. *Infect Immunol* 1988;56:1242–1248.

157. Pierson DE, Falkow S. Nonpathogenic isolated of *Yersinia enterocolitica* do not contain function *inv* homologous sequences. *J Bacteriol* 1990;172:1059–1064.

158. Kandolo K, Wauters G. Pyrazinamidase activity in *Yersinia enterocolitica* and related organisms. *J Clin Microbiol* 1985;21: 980–982.

159. Noble MA, Barteluk RL, Freeman HJ, Subramaniam R, Hudson JB. Clinical significance of virulence-related assay of *Yersinia* species. *J Clin Microbiol* 1987;25:802–807.

160. Delor I, Kaeckenbeeck A, Wauters G, Cornelis G. Nucleotide sequence of *yst,* the *Yersinia enterocolitica* gene encoding the heat-stable enterotoxin, and prevalence of the gene among pathogenic and nonpathogenic yersiniae. *Infect Immun* 1990; 58:2983–2988.

161. Nesbakken T, Kapperud G, Dommarsnes K, Skurnik M, Hornes E. Comparative study of a DNA hybridization method and two isolation procedures for detection of *Yersinia enterocolitica* O:3 in naturally contaminated pork products. *Appl Environ Microbiol* 1991;57:389–394.

162. Robins-Browne RM, Miliotis MD, Cianciosi S, Miller VL, Falkow S. Evaluation of DNA colony hybridization and other techniques for detection of virulence in *Yersinia* species. *J Clin Microbiol* 1989;27:644–650.

163. Ibrahim A, Liesack W, Stackebrandt E. Polymerase chain reaction-gene probe detection system specific for pathogenic strains of *Yersinia enterocolitica*. *J Clin Microbiol* 1992;30: 1942–1947.

164. Paerregaard A, Shand GH, Gaarslev K, Espersen F. Comparison of crossed immunoelectrophoresis, enzyme-lined immunosorbent assays, and tube agglutination for serodiagnosis of *Yersinia enterocolitica* serotype O:3 infection. *J Clin Microbiol* 1991;29:302–309.

165. Mäki-Ikola O, Heesemann J, Lahesmaa R, Toivanen A, Granfors K. Combined use of released proteins and lipopolysaccharide in enzyme-linked immunosorbent assay for serologic screening of *Yersinia* infections. *J Infect Dis* 1991;163:409–412.

166. Schoerner C, Wartenberg K, Röllinghoff M. Differentiation of serological responses to *Yersinia enterocolitica* serotype O9 and *Brucella* species by immunoblot or enzyme-linked immunosorbent assay using whole bacteria and *Yersinia* outer membrane proteins. *J Clin Microbiol* 1990;28:1570–1574.

167. Bartlett JG. *Clostridium difficile:* clinical considerations. *Rev Infect Dis* 1990;12:S243–S251.

168. Fekety R, Shah AB. Diagnosis and treatment of *Clostridium difficile* colitis. *JAMA* 1993;269:71–75.

169. Anand A. *Clostridium difficile* colitis: causes, cures (letter). *JAMA* 1993;269:2087.

170. McFarland LV, Surawicz CM, Stamm WE. Risk factors for *Clostridium difficile* carriage and *C. difficile*–associated diarrhea in a cohort of hospitalized patients. *J Infect Dis* 1990;162: 678–684.

171. Lyerly DM, Krivan HC, Wilkins TD. *Clostridium difficile:* its disease and toxins. *Clin Microbiol Rev* 1988;1:1–18.

172. Barbut F, Kajzer C, Planas N, Petit J-C. Comparison of three enzyme immunoassays, a cytotoxicity assay, and toxigenic culture for diagnosis of *Clostridium difficile*–associated diarrhea. *J Clin Microbiol* 1993;31:963–967.

173. Bennett RG, Laughon BE, Mundy LM, Bobo LD, Gaydos CA, Greenough III WB, Bartlett JG. Evaluation of a latex agglutination test for *Clostridium difficile* in two nursing home outbreaks. *J Clin Microbiol* 1989;27:889–893.

174. Peterson LR, Olson MM, Shanholtzer CJ, Gerding DN. Results of a prospective, 18-month clinical evaluation of culture, cytotoxin testing, and Culturette brand (CDT) latex testing in the diagnosis of *Clostridium difficile*–associated diarrhea. *Diag Microbiol Infect Dis* 1988;10:85–91.

175. Gerding DN. Disease associated with *Clostridium difficile* infection. *Ann Intern Med* 1989;110:255–257.

176. Doern GV, Coughlin RT, Wu L. Laboratory diagnosis of *Clostridum difficile*–associated gastrointestinal disease: comparison of a monoclonal antibody enzyme immunoassay for toxins A and B with a monoclonal antibody enzyme immunoassay for toxin A only and two cytotoxicity assays. *J Clin Microbiol* 1992;30:2042–2046.

177. DeGirolami PC, Hanff PA, Eichelberger K. Multicenter evaluation of a new enzyme immunoassay for detection of *Clostridium difficile* enterotoxin A. *J Clin Microbiol* 1992;30:1085–1088.

178. Chang TW, Lauermann M, Bartlett JG. Cytotoxicity assay in antibiotic-associated colitis. *J Infect Dis* 1979;140:765–777.

179. Bowman RA, Riley TV. Laboratory diagnosis of *Clostridium difficile*–associated diarrhoea. *Eur J Clin Microbiol Infect Dis* 1988;7:476–484.

180. Walpita P, Billman GF, Krous HF. Mammalian epithelial cell line kit for detection of *Clostridium difficile* toxin A. *J Clin Microbiol* 1993;31:315–319.

181. Tichota-Lee J, Jaqua-Stewart MJ, Benfield D, Simmons JL, Jaqua RA. Effect of age on the sensitivity of cell cultures to *Clostridium difficile* toxin. *Diag Microbiol Infect Dis* 1987;8: 203–214.

182. Maniar AC, Williams JW, Hammond GW. Detection of *Clostridium difficile* toxin in various tissue culture monolayers. *J Clin Microbiol* 1987;25:1999–2000.

183. Torres J, Camorlinga-Ponce M, Munoz O. Sensitivity in culture of epithelial cells from rhesus monkey kidney and human colon carcinoma to toxins A and B from *Clostridium difficile*. *Toxicon* 1992;30:419–426.

184. Allen SD, Baron EJ. *Clostridium*. In: Balows A, Hausler Jr WJ, Herrmann KL, Isenberg HD, Shadomy HJ, eds. *Manual of clinical microbiology*. 5th ed. Washington, DC: American Society for Microbiology; 1991:505–521.

185. Willey SH, Bartlett JG. Cultures for *Clostridium difficile* in stools containing a cytotoxin neutralized by *Clostridium sordellii* antitoxin. *J Clin Microbiol* 1979;10:880–884.

186. Lyerly DM, Barroso LA, Wilkins TD. Identification of the latex test-reactive protein of *Clostridium difficile* as glutamate dehydrogenase. *J Clin Microbiol* 1991;29:2639–2642.

187. George WL, Sutter VL, Citron D, Finegold SM. Selective and differential medium for isolation of *Clostridium difficile*. *J Clin Microbiol* 1979;9:214–219.

188. Marler LM, Siders JA, Wolters LC, Pettigrew Y, Skitt BL, Allen SD. Comparison of five cultural procedures for isolation of *Clostridium difficile* from stools. *J Clin Microbiol* 1992;30: 514–516.

189. Gumerlock PH, Tang YJ, Meyers FJ, Silva J Jr. Use of the polymerase chain reaction for the specific and direct detection of *Clostridium difficile* in human feces. *Rev Infect Dis* 1991; 13:1053–1060.

190. Centers for Disease Control. Update: cholera; western hemisphere. *MMWR* 1991;40:860.

191. Finelli L, Swerdlow D, Mertz K, Ragazzoni H, Spitalny K. Outbreak of cholera associated with crab brought from an area with epidemic disease. *J Infect Dis* 1992;166:1433–1435.

192. Morris Jr JG, Wilson R, Davis BR, et al. Non-O Group 1 *Vibrio cholerae* gastroenteritis in the United States. *Ann Intern Med* 1981;94:656–658.

193. Kelly MT, Peterson JW, Sarles HE Jr, Romanko M, Martin D, Hafkin B. Cholera on the Texas Gulf Coast. *JAMA* 1982; 247:1598–1599.

194. Morris Jr JG, Black RE. Cholera and other vibrioses in the United States. *N Engl J Med* 1985;312:343–350.

195. Joseph SW, Colwell RR, Kaper JB. Vibrio parahaemolyticus and Related halophilic vibrios. *CRC Critical Reviews in Microbiology* 1979;10:77–124.

196. Kelly MT, Stroh EMD. Urease-positive, Kanagawa-negative *Vibrio parahaemolyticus* from patients and the environment in the Pacific Northwest. *J Clin Microbiol* 1989;27:2820–2822.

197. Hoge CW, Watsky D, Peeler RN, Libonati JP, Israel E, Morris Jr JG. Epidemiology and spectrum of *Vibrio* infections in a Chesapeake Bay community. *J Infect Dis* 1989;160:985–992.

198. Lowry PW, McFarland LM, Peltier BH, et al. *Vibrio* gastroenteritis in Louisiana: a prospective study among attendees of a scientific congress in New Orleans. *J Infect Dis* 1989;160:978–984.

199. Hickman FW, Farmer JJ III, Hollis DG, et al. Identification of *Vibrio hollisae* sp. nov. from patients with diarrhea. *J Clin Microbiol* 1982;15:395–401.

200. Centers for Disease Control. *Vibrio vulnificus* infections associated with raw oyster consumption; Florida, 1981 to 1982. *MMWR* 1993;42:405–407.

201. Tacket CO, Hickman F, Pierce GV, Mendoza LF. Diarrhea associated with *Vibrio fluvialis* in the United States. *J Clin Microbiol* 1982;26:991–992.

202. Kelly MT, Hickman-Brenner FW, Farmer III JJ. *Vibrio*. In: Balows A, Hausler WJ Jr, Herrmann KL, Isenberg HD, Shadomy HJ, eds. *Manual of clinical microbiology.* 5th ed. Washington, DC: American Society for Microbiology; 1991:384–395.

203. Tison DL. *Vibrio* infections. In: Wentworth BB, ed. *Diagnostic procedures for bacterial infections.* 7th ed. Washington, DC: American Public Health Association; 1987:599–611.

204. Huq A, Alam M, Parveen S, Colwell RR. Occurrence of resistance to vibriostatic compound 0/129 in *Vibrio cholerae* 01 isolated from clinical and environmental samples in Bangladesh. *J Clin Microbiol* 1992;30:219–221.

205. MacDonell MT, Singleton FL, Hood MA. Diluent composition for use of API 20E in characterizing marine and estuarine bacteria. *Appl Environ Microbiol* 1982;44:423–427.

206. Colwell RR, Hasan JA, Huq A, et al. Development and evaluation of a rapid, simple, sensitive, monoclonal antibody-based co-agglutination test for direct detection of *Vibrio cholera* 01. *FEMS Microbiol Lett* 1992;76:215–219.

207. Almeida RJ, Hickman-Brenner FW, Sowers EG, Puhr ND, Farmer JJ III, Wachsmuth IK. Comparison of a latex agglutination assay and an enzyme-linked immunosorbent assay for detecting cholera toxin. *J Clin Microbiol* 1990;28:128–130.

208. Tabrizi S, Chen S, Fairley C, et al. Rapid detection of acute cholera in airline passengers by coagglutination assay. *J Infect Dis* 1993;168:797–799.

209. Ramamurthy T, Bhattacharya SK, Uesaka Y, et al. Evaluation of the bead enzyme-linked immunosorbent assay for detection of cholera toxin directly from stool specimens. *J Clin Microbiol* 1992;30:1783–1786.

210. Centers for Disease Control. Update: cholera; western hemisphere. *MMWR* 1991;40:562–565.

211. Chapman PA, Daly CM. Comparison of Y1 mouse adrenal cell and coagglutination assays for detection of *Escherichia coli* heat-lable enterotoxin. *J Clin Pathol* 1989;42:755–758.

212. Chapman PA, Daly CM. Evaluation of non-radioactive trivalent DNA probe (LT, ST1a, ST1b) for detecting enterotoxigenic *Escherichia coli*. *J Clin Pathol* 1993;46:309–312.

213. Scotland SM, Willshaw GA, Said B, Smith HR, Rowe B. Identification of *Escherichia coli* that produce heat stable enterotoxin ST by a commercially available enzyme-linked immunoassay and comparison of the assay with infant mouse and DNA probe tests. *J Clin Microbiol* 1989;27:1697–1699.

214. Faruque SM, Haider K, Albert MJ, et al. A comparative study of specific gene probes and standard bioassays to identify diarrhoeagenic *Escherichia coli* in paediatric patients with diarrhoea in Bangladesh. *J Med Microbiol* 1992;36:37–40.

215. Sommerfelt H, Grenwal HMS, Gaastra W, Svennerholm AM, Bhan VK. Use of nonradioactive DNA hybridization for identification of enterotoxigenic *Escherichia coli* harboring genes for colonization factor antigen i, coli surface antigen 4, or putative colonization factor 0166. *J Clin Microbiol* 1992;30:1823–1828.

216. Strockbine NA, Faruque SM, Kay BA, et al. DNA probe analysis of diarrhoeagenic *Escherichia coli*: detection of EAF-posi-

tive isolates of traditional enteropathogenic *E. coli* serotypes among Bangladeshi paediatric diarrhoea patients. *Mol Cell Probes* 1992;6:93–99.

217. Janda JM, Duffey PS. Mesophilic aeromonads in human disease: current taxonomy, laboratory identification, and infectious disease spectrum. *Rev Infect Dis* 1988;10:980–997.

218. Altwegg M, Geiss HK. Aeromonas as a human pathogen. *CRC Critical Rev Microbiol* 1989;16:253–286.

219. Pazzaglia G, Escalante JR, Sack RB, Rocca C, Benavides V. Transient intestinal colonization by multiple phenotypes of *Aeromonas* species during the first week of life. *J Clin Microbiol* 1990;28:1842–1846.

220. Pazzaglia G, Sack RB, Salazar E, et al. High frequency of coinfecting enteropathogens in *Aeromonas*-associated diarrhea of hospitalized Peruvian infants. *J Clin Microbiol* 1991;29:1151–1156.

221. Namdari H, Bottone EJ. Microbiologic and clinical evidence supporting the role of *Aeromonas caviae* as a pediatric enteric pathogen. *J Clin Microbiol* 1990;28:837–840.

222. Namdari H, Bottone EJ. Cytotoxin and enterotoxin production as factors delineating enteropathogenicity of *Aeromonas caviae*. *J Clin Microbiol* 1990;28:1796–1798.

223. Qadri SMH, Zafar M, Lee GC. Can isolation of *Aeromonas hydrophila* from human feces have any clinical significance? *Clin Gastroenterol* 1991;13:537–540.

224. Scott D Holmberg, Farmer III JJ. *Aeromonas hydrophila* and *Plesiomonas shigelloids* as causes of intestinal infections. *Rev Infect Dis* 1984;6:633–639.

225. Holmberg SD, Wachsmuth IK, Hickman-Brenner FW, Blake PA, Farmer JJ III. *Plesiomonas* enteric infections in the United States. *Ann Intern Med* 1986;105:690–694.

226. Brenden RA, Miller MA, Janda JM. Clinical disease spectrum and pathogenic factors associated with *Plesiomonas shigelloides* infections in humans. *Rev Infect Dis* 1988;10:303–316.

227. Kain KC, Kelly MT. Clinical features, epidemiology, and treatment of *Plesiomonas shigelloides* diarrhea. *J Clin Microbiol* 1989;27:1098–1001.

228. Olsvik O, Wachsmuth K, Kay B, Birkness KA, Yi A, Sack B. Laboratory observations on *Plesiomonas shigelloides* strains isolated from children with diarrhea in Peru. *J Clin Microbiol* 1990;28:886–889.

229. Processing and interpretations of bacterial fecal cultures. In: Isenberg HD, ed. *Clinical microbiology procedures handbook.* II. Washington, DC: American Society for Microbiology; 1992:1.10.1–1.10.25.

230. Pedler SJ, Orr KE. Examination of faeces for bacterial pathogens, Broadsheet 124. *Assoc Clin Pathol* 1990;43:410–415.

231. von Graevenitz A, Altwegg M. *Aeromonas* and *Plesiomonas*. In: Balows A, Hausler WJ Jr, Herrmann KL, Isenberg HD, Shadomy HJ, eds. *Manual of clinical microbiology.* 5th ed. Washington, DC: American Society for Microbiology; 1991:396–401.

232. Janda JM. *Aeromonas* and *Plesiomonas* infections. In: Wentworth BB, ed. *Diagnostic procedures for bacterial infections.* 7th ed. Washington, DC: American Public Health Association; 1987:37–44.

233. Altorfer R, Altwegg M, Zollinger-Iten J, von Graevenitz A. Growth of *Aeromonas* spp. on cefsulodin-irgasan-novobiocin agar selective for *Yersinia enterocolitica*. *J Clin Microbiol* 1985;22:478–480.

234. Carnahan AM, Behram S, Joseph SW. Aerokey II: a flexible key for identifying clinical *Aeromonas* species. *J Clin Microbiol* 1991;29:2843–2849.

235. Kuijper EJ, Steigerwalt AG, Schoenmakers BSCIM, Peeters MF, Zanen HC, Brenner DJ. Phenotypic characterization and DNA relatedness in human fecal isolates of *Aeromonas* spp. *J Clin Microbiol* 1989;27:132–138.

236. Schadow KH, Giger DK, Sanders CC. The Vitek system fails to detect β-lactam resistance in *Aeromonas*. Abstr 171. *Abstr Program 31st Intersci Conf Antimicrob Agents Chemother* Washington, DC: 1991:127.

237. Riley LW, Remis RS, Helgerson SD, et al. Hemorrhagic colitis associated with a rare *Escherichia coli* serotype. *N Engl J Med* 1983;308:681–685.

238. Wells JG, Davis BR, Wachsmuth IK, et al. Laboratory investigation of hemorrhagic colitis outbreaks associated with a rare *Escherichia coli* serotype. *J Clin Microbiol* 1983;18:512–520.

239. Cohen MB, Giannella RA. Hemorrhagic colitis associated with *Escherichia coli* O157:H7. *Adv Intern Med* 1991;37:173–195.

240. Cleary TG. *Escherichia coli* that cause hemolytic uremic syndrome. *Pediatr Infect* 1992;6:163–176.

241. Tarr PI, Neill MS, Clausen CR, Watkins SL, Christie DL, Hickman RO. *Escherichia coli* O157:H7 and the hemolytic uremic syndrome: importance of early cultures in establishing the etiology. *J Infect Dis* 1990;162:553–556.

242. Cordovéz A, Prado V, Maggi L, et al. Enterohemorrhagic *Escherichia coli* associated with hemolytic-uremic syndrome in Chilean children. *J Clin Microbiol* 1992;30:2153–2157.

243. Spika JS, Parsons JE, Nordenberg D, Wells JG, Gunn RA, Blake PA. Hemolytic uremic syndrome and diarrhea associated with *Escherichia coli* O157:H7 in a day care center. *J Pediatrics* 1986;109:287–291.

244. Carter AO, Borczyk AA, Carlson JAK, et al. A severe outbreak of *Escherichia coli* O157:H7 associated hemorrhagic colitis in a nursing home. *N Engl J Med* 1987;317:1496–1500.

245. Ritchie M, Partington S, Jessop J, Kelly MT. Comparison of a direct fecal Shiga-like toxin assay and sorbitol-MacConkey agar culture for laboratory diagnosis of enterohemorrhagic *Escherichia coli* infection. *J Clin Microbiol* 1992;30:461–464.

246. Karmali MA. Infection by verocytotoxin-producing *Escherichia coli*. *Clin Microbiol* 1989;2:15–38.

247. Pai CH, Gordon R, Sims HV, et al. Sporadic cases of hemorrhagic colitis associated with *Escherichia coli* O157:H7. *Ann Intern Med* 1984;101:738–742.

248. Griffin PM, Ostroff SM, Tauxe RV, et al. Illnesses associated with *Escherichia coli* O157:H7 infections; a broad clinical spectrum. *Ann Intern Med* 1988;109:705–712.

249. Ostroff SM, Kobayashi JM, Lewis JH. Infections with *Escherichia coli* O157:H7 in Washington state; the first year of statewide surveillance. *J Infect Dis* 1989;151:775–782.

250. Gunzer F, Bohm H, Russmann H, Bitzan M, Aleksic S, Karch H. Molecular detection of sorbitol-fermenting *Escherichia coli* O157 in patients with hemolytic-uremic syndrome. *J Clin Microbiol* 1992;30:1807–1810.

251. Ratnam S, March SB, Ahmed R, Bezanson GS, Kasatiya S. Characterization of *Escherichia coli* serotype O157:H7. *J Clin Microbiol* 1988;26:2006–2012.

252. Haldane DJM, Damm MAS, Anderson JD. Improved biochemical screening procedure for small clinical laboratories for vero (Shiga-like)-toxin-producing strains of *Escherichia coli* O157:H7. *J Clin Microbiol* 1986;24:652–653.

253. Farmer III JJ, Davis BR. H7 Antiserum-Sorbitol fermentation medium: a single tube screening medium for detecting *Escherichia coli* O157:H7 associated with hemorrhagic colitis. *J Clin Microbiol* 1985;22:620–625.

254. March SB, Ratnam S. Sorbitol-MacConkey medium for detection of *Escherichia coli* O157:H7 associated with hemorrhagic colitis. *J Clin Microbiol* 1986;23:869–872.

255. Karch H, Meyer T, Rüssmann H, Heesemann J. Frequent loss of Shiga-like toxin genes in clinical isolates of *Escherichia coli* upon subcultivation. *Infect Immun* 1992;60:3464–3467.

256. Karmali MA, Petric M, Lim C, et al. Sensitive method for detecting low numbers of verotoxin-producing *Escherichia coli* in mixed cultures by use of colony sweeps and polymyxin extraction of verotoxin. *J Clin Microbiol* 1985;22:614–619.

257. Karmali MA. Laboratory diagnosis of vertotoxin-producing *Escherichia coli* infections. *Clin Microbiol Newslett* 1987;9:65–70.

258. Scotland SM, Rowe B, Smith HR, Willsahw GA, Gross RJ. Verocytotoxin-producing strains of *Escherichia coli* from children with haemolytic uraemic syndrome and their detection by specific DNA probes. *J Med Microbiol* 1988;25:237–243.

259. Brian MJ, Frosolono M, Murray BE, Miranda A, Lopez EL, Gomez HF, Cleary TG. Polymerase chain reaction for diagnosis of enterohemorrhagic *Escherichia coli* infection and hemolytic-uremic syndrome. *J Clin Microbiol* 1992;30:801–1806.

260. Speirs JI, Akhtar M. Detection of *Escherichia coli* cytotoxins by enzyme-linked immunosorbent assays. *Can J Microbiol* 1991;37:650–652.

261. Toth I, Barrett TJ, Cohen ML, Rumschlag HS, Green JH, Wachsmuth IK. Enzyme-linked immunosorbent assay for products of the 60-megadalton plasmid of *Escherichia coli* serotype O157:H7. *J Clin Microbiol* 1991;29:1016–1019.

262. Law D, Ganguli LA, Donohue-Rolfe A, Acheson DWK. Detection by ELISA of low numbers of Shiga-like toxin-producing *Escherichia coli* in mixed cultures after growth in the presence of mitomycin. *J Med Microbiol* 1992;36:198–202.

263. Bitzan M, Karch H. Indirect hemagglutination assay for diagnosis of *Escherichia coli* O157 infection in patients with hemolytic-uremic syndrome. *J Clin Microbiol* 1992;30:1174–1178.

264. Kishore K, Rattan A, Bagga A, Srivastava RN, Nath N, Shiriniwas. Serum antibodies to Verotoxin-producing *Escherichia coli* (VTEC) strains in patients with haemolytic uraemic syndrome. *J Med Microbiol* 1992;37:364–367.

265. Robins-Browne RM, Yam WC, O'Gorman LE, Bettelheim KA. Examination of archetypal strains of enteropathogenic *Escherichia coli* for properties associated with bacterial virulence. *J Med Microbiol* 1993;38:222–226.

266. Levine MM, Edelman R. Enteropathogenic *Escherichia coli* of classical serotypes associated with infant diarrhea: epidemiology and pathogenesis. *Epidemiol Rev* 1984;6:31–51.

267. Nataro JP, Kaper JB, Robins-Browne R, Prado V, Vial P, Levine MM. Patterns of adherence of diarrheagenic *Escherichia coli* to HEp-2 cells. *Pædiatr Infect Dis* 1987;6:829–831.

268. Gomes TAT, Vieira MAM, Wachsmuth IK, Blake PA, Trabulsi LR. Serotype-specific prevalence of *Escherichia coli* strains with EPEC adherence factor genes in infants with and without diarrhea in Sao Paulo, Brazil. *J Infect Dis* 1989;160:131–135.

269. Cravioto AA, Tello A, Navarro A, et al. Association of *Escherichia coli* HEp-2 adherence patterns with type and duration of diarrhea. *Lancet* 1991;337:262–264.

270. Echeverria P, Orskov F, Orskov I, et al. Attaching and effacing enteropathogenic *Escherichia coli* as a cause of infantile diarrhea in Bangkok. *J Infect Dis* 1991;164:550–554.

271. Echeverria P, Serichantalerg O, Changchawalit S, et al. Tissue culture–adherent *Escherichia coli* in infantile diarrhea. *J Infect Dis* 1992;165:141–143.

272. Yamamoto T, Koyama Y, Matsumoto M, et al. Localized, aggregative, and diffuse adherence to HeLa cells, plastic, and human small intestines by *Escherichia coli* isolated from patients with diarrhea. *J Infect Dis* 1992;166:1295–1310.

273. Hill SM, Phillips AD, Walker-Smith JA. Enteropathogenic *Escherichia coli* and life threatening chronic diarrhoea. *Gut* 1991;32:154–158.

274. Pedroso MZ, Freymüller E, Trabulsi LR, Gomes TAT. Attaching-effacing lesions and intracellular penetration in HeLa cells and human duodenal mucosa by two *Escherichia coli* strains not belonging to the classical enteropathogenic *E. coli* serogroups. *Infect Immun* 1992;61:1152–1156.

275. Morris KJ, Rao GG. Conventional screening for enteropathogenic *Escherichia coli* in the UK. Is it appropriate or necessary? *J Hosp Infect* 1992;21:163–167.

276. Gangarosa EJ, Merson MH. Epidemiologic assessment of the relevance of the so-called enteropathogenic serogroups of *Escherichia coli* in diarrhea. *N Engl J Med* 1977;296:1210–1213.

277. Knutton S, Phillips AD, Smith HR, Gross RJ, Shaw R, Watson P, Price E. Screening for enteropathogenic *Escherichia coli* in infants with diarrhea by the fluorescent-actin staining test. *Infect Immun* 1991;59:365–371.

278. Farmer JJ III, Davis BR, Cherry WB, Brenner DJ, Dowell VR Jr, Balows A. "Enteropathogenic serotypes" of *Escherichia coli* which really are not. *J Pediatrics* 1977;90:1047–1049.

279. Orskov I, Orskov F, Jann B. Serology, chemistry and genetics of O and K antigens of *Escherichia coli*. *Bacteriol Rev* 1977;41:667–710.

280. Matthewson JJ, Carvioto A. HEp-2 cell adherence as an assay for virulence among diarrheagenic *Escherichia coli*. *J Infect Dis* 1989;159:1057–1060.

281. Vial P, Mathewson JJ, DuPont HL, Guers L, Levine MM. Comparison of two assay methods for patterns of adherence

to HEp-2 cells of *Escherichia coli* from patients with diarrhea. *J Clin Microbiol* 1990;28:882–885.

282. Shariff M, Bhan MK, Knutton S, Das BK, Saini S, Kimar R. Evaluation of the fluorescence actin staining test for detection of enteropathogenic *Escherichia coli*. *J Clin Microbiol* 1993; 31:386–389.

283. Nataro JP, Scaletsky ICA, Kaper JB, Levine MM, Trabulsi LR. Plasmid-mediated factors conferring diffuse and localized adherence of enteropathogenic *Escherichia coli*. *Infect Immun* 1985;48:378–383.

284. Donnenberg MS, Giron JA, Nataro JP, Kaper JP. A plasmid-encoded type IV fimbrial gene of enteropathogenic *Escherichia coli* associated with localized adherence. *Mol Microbiol* 1992; 6:3427–3437.

285. Girón JA, Ho ASY, Schoolnik GK. An inducible bundle-forming pilus of enteropathogenic *Escherichia coli*. *Science* 1991; 254:710–713.

286. Albert MJ, Ansaruzzaman M, Faruque SM, Neogi PKB, Haider K, Tzipori S. An ELISA for the detection of localized adherent classic enteropathogenic *Escherichia coli* serogroups. *J Infect Dis* 1991;164:986–989.

287. Jerse AE, Gicquelais KG, Kaper JB. Plasmid and chromosomal elements involved in the pathogenesis of attaching and effacing *Escherichia coli*. *Infect Immun* 1991;59:3869–3875.

288. Francis CL, Jerse AE, Kaper JB, Falkow S. Characterization of interactions of enteropathogenic *Escherichia coli* O127:H6 with mammalian cells in vitro. *J Infect Dis* 1991;164:693–703.

289. Girón JA, Jones T, Millán-Velasco F, Castro-Muñoz E, et al. Diffuse-adhering *Escherichia coli* (DAEC) as a putative cause of diarrhea in Mayan children in Mexico. *J Infect Dis* 1991; 163:507–513.

290. Ben I, Schmidt MA. AIDA-I, the adhesin involved in diffuse adherence of the diarrhoeagenic *Escherichia coli* strain 2787 (O126:H27), is synthesized via a precursor molecule. *Mol Microbiol* 1992;6:1539–1546.

291. Gunzburg ST, Chang BJ, Elliott SJ, Burke V, Gracey M. Diffuse and enteroaggregative patterns of adherence of enteric *Escherichia coli* isolated from aboriginal children from the Kimberley region of western Australia. *J Infect Dis* 1993;167: 755–758.

292. Bhan MK, Raj P, Levine MM, et al. Enteroaggregative *Escherichia coli* associated with persistent diarrhea in a cohort of rual children in India. *J Infect Dis* 1989;159:1061–1064.

293. Nataro JP, Deng Y, Maneval DR, German AL, Martin WC, Levine MM. Aggregative adherence fimbriae I of enteroaggregative *Escherichia coli* mediate adherence to HEp-2 cells and hemagglutination of human erythrocytes. *Infect Immun* 1992; 60:2297–2304.

294. Savarino SJ, Fasano A, Watson J, et al. Enteroaggregative *Escherichia coli* heat-stable enterotoxin 1 represents another subfamily of *E. coli* heat-stable toxin. *Proc Natl Acad Sci USA* 1993;90:3093–3097.

295. Baudry B, Savarino SA, Vial P, Kaper JP, Levine MM. A sensitive and specific DNA probe to identify enteroaggregative *Escherichia coli*, a recently discovered diarrheal pathogen. *J Infect Dis* 1990;161:1249–1251.

296. Albert MJ, Qadri F, Haque A, Bhuiyan NA. Bacterial clump formation at the surface of liquid culture as a rapid test for identification of enteroaggregative *Escherichia coli*. *J Clin Microbiol* 1993;31:1397–1399.

297. Dallabetta GA, Miotti PG. Chronic diarrhoea in AIDS patients in the tropics: a review. *Trop Doctor* 1992;January:3–9.

298. Bartlett JG, Belitsos PC, Sears CL. AIDS enteropathy. *Clin Infect Dis* 1992;15:726–735.

299. Greenson JK, Belitsos PC, Yardley JH, Bartlett JG. AIDS enteropathy: occult enteric infections and duodenal mucosal alterations in chronic diarrhea. *Ann Intern Med* 1991;114: 366–372.

300. Johanson JF, Sonnenberg A. Efficient management of diarrhea in the acquired immunodeficiency syndrome (AIDS). *Ann Intern Med* 1990;112:942–948.

301. Rabeneck L. Diagnostic workup strategies for patients with HIV-related chronic diarrhea. *J Clin Gastroenterol* 1992;16: 245–250.

302. Quinn TC, Goodell SE, Fenneili C, Wang SP, Schuffler MD, Holmes KK, Stamm WE. Infections with *Campylobacter jejuni* and *Campylobacter*-like organisms in homosexual men. *Ann Intern Med* 1984;101:187–192.

303. Laughon BE, Druckman DA, Vernon A, et al. Prevalence of enteric pathogens in homosexual men with and without acquired immunodeficiency syndrome. *Gastroenterology* 1988; 94:984–993.

304. Kiehn TE, Edwards FF, Brannon P, et al. Infections caused by *Mycobacterium avium* complex in immunocompromised patients: diagnosis by blood culture and fecal examination, antimicrobial susceptibility tests, and morphological and seroagglutination characteristics. *J Clin Microbiol* 1985;21:168–173.

305. Morris A, Reller LB, Salfinger M, Jackson K, Sievers A, Dwyer B. Mycobacteria in stool specimens: the nonvalue of smears for predicting culture results. *J Clin Microbiol* 1993;31: 1385–1387.

306. Hawkins CC, Gold JWM, Whimbey E, et al. *Mycobacterium avium* complex infections in patients with the acquired immunodeficiency syndrome. *Ann Intern Med* 1986;105:184–188.

307. Jacobson MA, Hopewell PC, Yajko DM, et al. Natural history of disseminated *Mycobacterium avium* complex infection in AIDS. *J Infect Dis* 1991;164:994–998.

308. Yajko DM, Nassos PS, Sanders CA, et al. Comparison of four decontamination methods for recovery of *Mycobacterium avium* complex from stools. *J Clin Microbiol* 1993;31:302–306.

309. Rolfe RD. Role of Anaerobic bacteria in other bowel pathology. In: Finegold SM, George WL, eds. *Anaerobic infections in humans*. New York: Academic Press; 1989:679–690.

310. Gracey M. The contaminated small bowel syndrome. In: Hentges DJ, ed. *Human intestinal microflora in health and disease*. New York: Academic Press; 1983:495–515.

311. Guerrant RL. Nausea, vomiting, and noninflammatory diarrhea. In: Mandell GL, Douglas RG, Bennett JE, eds. *Principles and practice of infectious diseases*. 2nd ed. New York: John Wiley and Sons; 1985:851–862.

312. Simon GI, Gorbach SL. Intestinal flora in health and disease. *Gastroenterology* 1984;86:174–193.

313. Bardhan PK, Gyr K, Belinger C, Vögtlin J, Frey R, Vischer W. Diagnosis of bacterial overgrowth after culturing proximal small-bowel aspirate obtained during routine upper gastrointestinal endoscopy. *Scand J Gastroenterol* 1992;27:253–356.

314. Craven DE, Steger KA. Nosocomial pneumonia in the intubated patient; new concepts on pathogenesis and prevention. *Infect Dis Clin North Am* 1989;3/4:843–866.

315. Penny ME. The role of the duodenal microflora as a determinant of persistent diarrhoea. *Acta Pædiatr* 1992;381: S114–S120.

316. Giuliano M, Barza M, Jacobus NV, Gorbach SL. Effect of broad-spectrum parenteral antibiotics on composition of intestinal microflora of humans. *Antimicrob Agents Chemother* 1987;31:202–206.

317. Chretien JH, Garagusi VF. Current management of fungal enteritis. *Med Clin North Am* 1982;66:675–684.

318. Gupta TP, Ehrinpreis MN. Diarrhea in hospitalized patients. *Gastroenterology* 1990;98:780–785.

319. Danna PL, Ruban C, Bellin E, Rahal JJ. Role of candida in pathogenesis of antibiotic-associated diarrhoea in elderly inpatients. *Lancet* 1991;337:511–514.

320. Hughes JM, Tauxe RV. Food-borne disease. In: Mandell GL, Douglas RG, Bennett JE, eds. *Principles and practice of infectious diseases*. 2nd ed. New York: John Wiley and Sons; 1985: 893–904.

321. Snydman DR. Food poisoning. In: Gorbach SL, Bartlett JG, Blacklow NR, eds. *Infectious diseases*. Philadelphia: WB Saunders; 1992:628–637.

322. Gradus MS. Public health criteria for the diagnosis of food-borne illness. *Clin Microbiol Newslett* 1986;8:85–92.

323. Bennett RW, Harmon SM. *Bacillus cereus* food poisoning. In: Balows A, Hausler WJ Jr, Ohashi M, Turano A, eds. *Laboratory diagnosis of infectious diseases: principles and practice: Bacterial, mycotic, and parasitic diseases*. I. New York: Springer-Verlag; 1988:83–93.

324. American Public Health Association. *Compendium of methods*

for the microbiological examination of foods. 2nd ed. Washington, DC: American Public Health Association; 1984.

325. Association of Official Analytical Chemists. *1980 Official methods of analysis.* 13th ed. Washington, DC: Association of Official Analytical Chemists; 1980.

326. Committee on Communicable Diseases Affecting Man, International Association of Milk, Food and Environmental Sanitarians, Inc. *1981 Procedures to investigate foodborne illness.* Ames, IA: International Association of Milk, Food and Environmental Sanitarians; 1981.

327. Woodruff BA, Griffin PM, McCroskey LM, et al. Clinical and laboratory comparison of botulism from toxin types A, B, and E in the United States, 1975–1988. *J Infect Dis* 1992;166: 1281–1286.

328. Solnick JV, Tompkins LS. *Helicobacter pylori* and gastroduodenal disease: pathogenesis and host-parasite interaction. *Infect Agents Dis* 1993;I:294–309.

329. Moss S, Calam J. *Helicobacter pylori* and peptic ulcers: the present position. *Gut* 1992;33:289–292.

330. Brown KE, Peura DA. Diagnosis of *Helicobacter pylori* infection. *Gastroenterol Clin North Am* 1993;22:105–115.

331. European Study Group on Antibiotic Susceptibility of *Helicobacter pylori*. Results of a multicentre European survey in 1991 of metronidazole resistance in *Helicobacter pylori*. *Eur J Clin Microbiol Infect Dis* 1992;11:777–781.

332. Rautelin H, Seppälä K, Renkonen OV, Vainio U, Kosunen TU. Role of metronidazole resistance in therapy of *Helicobacter pylori* infections. *Antimicrob Agents Chemother* 1992; 36:163–166.

333. Westblom TU, Unge P. Drug resistance of *helicobacter pylori:* memorandum from a meeting at the sixth international workshop on *Campylobacter, Helicobacter,* and related organisms. *J Infect Dis* 1992;165:974–975.

334. Bell GD, Powell K, Burridge SM, et al. Experience with "triple" anti-*Helicobacter pylori* eradication therapy: side effects and the importance of testing the pre-treatment bacterial isolate for metronidazole resistance. *Aliment Pharmacol Ther* 1992;6: 427–435.

335. Goodwin FRC, Path CS, Worsley BW. Microbiology of *Helicobacter pylori*. *Gastroenterol Clin North Am* 1993;22:5–19.

336. Westblom TU, Madan E, Midkiff BR. Egg yolk emulsion agar, a new medium for the cultivation of *Helicobacter pylori*. *J Clin Microbiol* 1991;29:819–821.

337. Owen RJ, Bell GD, Desai M, Moreno M, Gant PW, Jones PH, Linton D. Biotype and molecular fingerprints of metronidazole-resistant strains of *Helicobacter pylori* from antral gastric mucosa. *J Med Microbiol* 1993;38:6–12.

338. Millar MR, Pike J. Bactericidal activity of antimicrobial agents against slowly growing *Helicobacter pylori*. *Antimicrob Agents Chemother* 1992;36:185–187.

339. Loo VG, Sherman P, Matlow AG. *Helicobacter pylori* infection in a pediatric population: in vitro susceptibilities to omeprazole and eight antimicrobial agents. *Antimicrob Agents Chemother* 1992;36:1133–1135.

340. Glupczynski Y, Labbé M, Hansen W, Crokaert F, Yourassowsky E. Evaluation of the E test for quantitative antimicrobial susceptibility testing of *Helicobacter pylori*. *J Clin Microbiol* 1991;29:2072–2075.

341. Westblom TU, Madan E, Gudipati S, Midkiff BR, Czinn SJ. Diagnosis of *Helicobacter pylori* infection in adult and pediatric patients by using Pyloriset, a rapid latex agglutination test. *J Clin Microbiol* 1992;30:96–98.

342. Blecker U, Lanciers S, Hauser B, Vandenplas Y. Diagnosis of *Helicobacter pylori* infection in adults and children by using the Malakit *Helicobacter pylori*, a commercially available enzyme-linked immunosorbent assay. *J Clin Microbiol* 1993;31: 1770–1773.

343. Blecker U, Vandenplas Y. *Helicobacter pylori* serology (Letter). *J Clin Microbiol* 1993;31:173.

344. Westblom TU, Czinn SJ. *Helicobacter pylori* serology (letter). *J Clin Microbiol* 1993;31:173.

345. Czinn SJ, Carr HS, Speck WT. Diagnosis of gastritis caused by *Helicobacter pylori* in children by means of an ELISA. *Rev Infect Dis* 1991;13:S700–703.

346. Hirschl AM, Brandstätter G, Dragosics B, et al. Kinetics of specific IgG antibodies for monitoring the effects of anti-*Helicobacter pylori* chemotherapy. *J Infect Dis* 1993;168:763–766.

347. Van Zwet AA, Thijs JC, Kooistra-Smid AMD, Schirm J, Snijder JAM. Sensitivity of culture compared with that of polymerase chain reaction for detection of *Helicobacter pylori* from antral biopsy samples. *J Clin Microbiol* 1993;31: 1918–1920.

348. Westblom TU, Phadnis S, Yang P, Czinn SJ. Diagnosis of *Helicobacter pylori* infection by means of a polymerase chain reaction assay for gastric juice aspirates. *Clin Infect Dis* 1993;16: 367–371.

349. Wilson KH, Blitchington R, Frothingham R, Wilson JA. Phylogeny of the Whipple's-disease-associated bacterium. *Lancet* 1991;338:474–475.

350. MacDonald TT. Aetiology of Crohn's disease. *Arch Dis Child* 1993;68:623–625.

351. Stainsby KJ, Lowes JR, Allan RN, Ibbotson JP. Antibodies to *Mycobacterium paratuberculosis* and nine species of environmental mycobacteria in Crohn's disease and control subjects. *Gut* 1993;34:371–374.

352. Quinn TC, Stamm WE. Proctitis, proctocolitis, enteritis, and esophagitis in homosexual men. In: Holmes KK, Mårdh P-A, Sparling PF, Wiesner PJ, Cates W Jr, Lemon SM, Stamm WE, eds. *Sexually transmitted diseases.* 2nd ed. New York: McGraw-Hill; 1990;663–683.

353. Mårdh, P-A, Danielsson D. *Neisseria gonorrhoeae.* In: Holmes KK, Mårdh P-A, Sparling PF, Wiesner PJ, Cates W Jr, Lemon SM, Stamm WE, eds. *Sexually transmitted diseases.* 2nd ed. New York: McGraw-Hill; 1990:903–915.

354. Lewis JS, Kranig-Brown D, Trainor DA. DNA probe confirmatory test for *Neisseria gonorrhoeae. J Clin Microbiol* 1990;20: 40–50.

355. Schwarcz SK, Zenilman JM, Schnell D, et al. National surveillance of antimicrobial resistance in *Neisseria gonorrhoeae. JAMA* 1990;264:1413–1418.

356. Centers for Disease Control. Sexually transmitted disease treatment guidelines. *MMWR* 1989;38:S21–S23.

357. Stamm WE, Mårdh P-A. *Chlamydia trachomatis.* In: Holmes KK, Mårdh P-A, Sparling PF, Wiesner PJ, Cates W Jr, Lemon SM, Stamm WE, eds. *Sexually transmitted diseases.* 2nd ed. New York: McGraw-Hill; 1990:917–925.

358. Barnes RC. Laboratory diagnosis of human chlamydial infections. *Clin Microbiol Rev* 1989;2:119–136.

359. Larsen SA, Hunter EF, Creighton ET. Syphilis. In: Holmes KK, Mårdh P-A, Sparling PF, Wiesner PJ, Cates W Jr, Lemon SM, Stamm WE, eds. *Sexually transmitted diseases.* 2nd ed. New York: McGraw-Hill; 1990:927–933.

360. Larsen SA, Hunter EF, McGrew BE. Syphilis. In: Wentworth BB, Judson FN, eds. *Laboratory methods for the diagnosis of sexually transmitted diseases.* Washington, DC: American Public Health Association; 1987:1–42.

361. Jaffe HW, Musher DM. Management of the reactive syphilis serology. In: Holmes KK, Mårdh P-A, Sparling PF, Wiesner PJ, Cates W Jr, Lemon SM, Stamm WE, eds. *Sexually transmitted diseases.* 2nd ed. New York: McGraw-Hill; 1990: 935–939.

362. Finegold SM, Baron EJ, Wexler HM. *A clinical guide to anaerobic infections.* Belmont, CA: Star; 1992.

363. Hentges DJ. The anaerobic microflora of the human body. *Clin Infect Dis* 1993;16:S175–S180.

364. Nichols RL, Smith JW. Wound and intraabdominal infections: microbiological considerations and approaches to treatment. *Clin Infect Dis* 1993;16:S266–S272.

365. Citron DM, Appelbaum PC. How far should a clinical laboratory go in identifying anaerobic isolates, and who should pay? *Clin Infect Dis* 1993;16:S435–S438.

366. Mangels J, Edvalson I, Cox M. Rapid presumptive identification of *Bacteroides fragilis* group organisms with use of 4-methylumbelliferone-derivative substrates. *Clin Infect Dis* 16: S319–S321.

367. National Committee for Clinical Laboratory Standards. *Methods for dilution antimicrobial susceptibility tests for bacteria that grow aerobically.* Approved standard M7-A2. 2nd ed. Villanova, PA: NCCLS; 1990.

368. Finegold SM. Susceptibility testing of anaerobic bacteria. *J Clin Microbiol* 1988;26:1253–1256.
369. Wexler HM. Susceptibility testing of anaerobic bacteria; the state of the art. *Clin Infect Dis* 1993;16:S328–333.
370. Rosenblatt JE, Brook I. Clinical relevance of susceptibility testing of anaerobic bacteria. *Clin Infect Dis* 1993;16:S446–448.
371. Cuchural Jr GJ, Tally FP, Jacobus NV, et al. Susceptibility of the *Bacteroides fragilis* group in the United States: analysis by site of isolation. *Antimicrob Agents Chemother* 1988;32:717–722.
372. Appelbaum PC. Patterns of resistance and resistance mechanism in anaerobes. *Clin Microbiol News* 1992;14:49–56.
373. Bolmström A. Susceptibility testing of anaerobes with E test. *Clin Infect Dis* 1993;16:S367–370.
374. Citron DM, Ostovari MI, Karlsson A, Goldstein JC. Evaluation of the E test for susceptibility testing of anaerobic bacteria. *J Clin Microbiol* 1991;29:2197–2203.
375. Levison ME, Bush LM. Peritonitis and other intra-abdominal infection. In: Mandell GL, Douglas RG, Bennett JE, eds. *Principles and practices of infectious diseases.* 2nd ed. New York: John Wiley and Sons; 1985:636–670.
376. Weinstein MP, Reller LB, Murphy JB, Lichtenstein KA. The clinical significance of positive blood cultures; a comprehensive analysis of 500 episodes of bacteremia and fungemia in adults. I. Laboratory and epidemiologic observations. *Rev Infect Dis* 1983;5:35–53.
377. Aaronson MD, Bor DH. Blood cultures. *Ann Intern Med* 1987;106:246–253.
378. Roberts FJ. The value of the second blood culture. *J Infect Dis* 1993;168:795–796.
379. Ruoff KL, Miller SI, Garner CV, Ferraro MJ, Calderwood SB. Bacteremia with *Streptococcus bovis* and *Streptococcus salivarius:* clinical correlates of more accurate identification of isolates. *J Clin Microbiol* 1989;27:305–308.
380. Kornbluth AA, Danzig JB, Bernstein LH. *Clostridium septicum* infection and associated malignancy: report of two cases and review of the literature. *Medicine* 1989;68:30–37.
381. Gossling J. Occurrence and pathogenicity of the *Streptococcus milleri* group. *Rev Infect Dis* 1988;10:257–285.
382. Ruoff KL. *Streptococcus anginosus* ("*Streptococcus milleri*"): the unrecognized pathogen. *Clin Microbiol Rev* 1988;1:102–108.
383. Dorsher C, Rosenblatt J, Wilson W, et al. Anaerobic bacteremia: decreasing rate over a 15-year period. *Rev Infect Dis* 1991;13:633–636.
384. Murray P, Traynor P, Hopson D. Critical assessment of blood culture techniques: analysis of recovery of obligate and facultative anaerobes, strict aerobic bacteria, and fungi in aerobic and anaerobic blood culture bottles. *J Clin Microbiol* 1992;30:1462–1468.
385. Kelly MT, Roberts FJ, Henry D, Geere I, Smith JA. Clinical comparison of isoloator and BACTEC 660 resin media for blood culture. *J Clin Microbiol* 1990;28:1925–1927.
386. Tarrand JJ, Guillot C, Wenglar M, et al. Clinical comparison of the resin-containing BACTEC 26 Plus and the Isolator 10 blood culturing systems. *J Clin Microbiol* 1991;29:2245–2249.
387. Wilson ML, Davis TE, Mirrett S, et al. Controlled comparison of the BACTEC high-blood-volume fungal medium, BACTEC Plus 26 aerobic blood culture bottle, and 10-milliliter isolator blood culture system for detection of fungemia and bacteremia. *J Clin Microbiol* 1993;31:865–871.
388. Kiehn T, Cammarata R. Comparative recoveries of avium-intracellulare from Isolator lysis-centrifugation and BACTEC 13A blood culture systems. *J Clin Microbiol* 1988;26:760–761.
389. Runyon BA, Antillon MR, Akriviadis EA, McHutchison JG. Bedside inoculation of blood culture bottles with ascitic fluid is superior to delayed inoculation in the detection of spontaneous bacterial peritonitis. *J Clin Microbiol* 1990;28:2811–2812.
390. Ryan S, Fessia S. Improved method for recovery of peritonitis-causing microorganisms from peritoneal dialysate. *J Clin Microbiol* 1987;25:383–384.
391. Elston HR, Wang M, Philip A. Evaluation of isolator system and large-volume centrifugation method for culturing body fluids. *J Clin Microbiol* 1990;28:124–125.
392. Males BM, Walshe JJ, Garringer L, Koscinski D, Amsterdam D. AddiChek filtration, BACTEC, and 10-ml culture methods for recovery of microorganisms from dialysis effluent during episodes of peritonitis. *J Clin Microbiol* 1986;23:350–353.
393. Peterson PK, Matzke G, Keane WF. Current concepts in the management of peritonitis in patients undergoing continuous ambulatory peritoneal dialysis. *Rev Infect Dis* 1987;9:604–612.
394. Hakim A, Hisam N, Reuman PD. Environmental mycobacterial peritonitis complicating peritoneal dialysis: three cases and review. *Clin Infect Dis* 1993;16:426–431.
395. Ludlam HA, Price TN, Berry AJ, Phillips I. Laboratory diagnosis of peritonitis in patients on continuous ambulatory peritoneal dialysis. *J Clin Microbiol* 1988;9:1757–1762.
396. Koehler JE, Quinn FD, Berger TG, LeBoit PE, Tappero JW. Isolation of *Rochalimaea* species from cutaneous and osseous lesions of bacillary angiomatosis. *N Engl J Med* 1992;325:1625–1631.
397. Tappero JW, Mohle-Boetani J, Koehler JE, et al. The epidemiology of bacillary angiomatosis and bacillary peliosis. *JAMA* 1993;269:770–775.
398. Zangwill KM, Hamilton DH, Perkins BA, et al. Cat scratch disease in Connecticut; epidemiology, risk factors, and evaluation of a new diagnostic test. *N Engl J Med* 1993;329:8–20.
399. Relman DA. Isolation of rochalimaea species (letter). *N Engl J Med* 1993;328:1422–1423.
400. Koehler JE, Brenner DJ. Isolation of rochalimaea species (letter). *N Engl J Med* 1993;328:1422–1423.
401. Welch DF, Hensel DM, Pickett DA, San Joaquin VH, Robinson A, Slater LN. Bacteremia due to *Rochalimaea henselae* in a child: practical identification of isolates in the clinical laboratory. *J Clin Microbiol* 1993;31:2381–2386.
402. Regnery RL, Anderson BE, Clarridge III JE, Rodriguez-Barradas MC, Jones DC, Carr JH. Characterization of a novel *Rochalimaea* species, *R henselae* sp nov, isolated from blood of a febrile, human immunodeficiency virus-positive patient. *J Clin Microbiol* 1992;30:265–274.
403. Welch DF, Pickett DA, Slater LN, Steigerwalt AG, Brenner DJ. *Rochalimaea henselae* sp nov, a cause of septicemia, bacillary angiomatosis, and parenchymal bacillary peliosis.403.22 *J Clin Microbiol* 1992;30:275–280.
404. Dolan MJ, Wong MT, Regnery RL, et al. Syndrome of *Rochalimaea henselae* adenitis suggesting cat scratch disease. *Ann Intern Med* 1993;118:331–336.
405. Daly JS, Worthington MG, Brenner DJ, et al. *Rochalimaea elizabethae* sp nov isolated from a patient with endocarditis. *J Clin Microbiol* 1993;31:872–881.
406. Slater LN, Coody DW, Woolridge LK, Welch DF. Murine antibody responses distinguish *Rochalimaea henselae* from *Rochalimaea quintana*. *J Clin Microbiol* 1992;30:1722–1727.
407. Regnery RL, Olson JG, Perkins BA, Bibb W. Serological response to "*Rochalimaea henselae*" antigen in suspected cat-scratch disease. *Lancet* 1992;339:1443–1445.
408. Gilman RH, Terminel M, Hernandez-Mendoza P, Hornick RB. Relative efficiency of blood, urine, rectal swab, bone-marrow and rose-spot cultures for recovery of *Salmonella typhi* in typhoid fever. *Lancet* 1975;1:1211–1213.
409. Rubin FA, McWhirter PD, Burr D, et al. Rapid diagnosis of typhoid fever through identification of *Salmonella typhi* within 18 hours of specimen acquisition by culture of the mononuclear cell-platelet fraction of blood. *J Clin Microbiol* 1990;28:825–827.
410. Song JH, Cho H, Park MY, Na DS, Moon HB, Pai CH. Detection of *Salmonella typhi* in the blood of patients with typhoid fever by polymerase chain reaction. *J Clin Microbiol* 1993;31:1439–1443.
411. Heiba I, Girgis NI, Farid Z. Enzyme-linked immunosorbent assays (ELISA) for the diagnosis of enteric fever. *Trop Georg Med* 1989;41:213–217.
412. Quiroga T, Goycoolea M, Tagle R, Gonzalez F, Rodriguez L, Villarroel L. Diagnosis of typhoid fever by two serologic methods. *Diagn Microbiol Infect Dis* 1992;15:651–656.
413. Nardiello S, Pizzella T, Russo M, Galini B. Serodiagnosis of typhoid fever by enzyme-linked immunosorbent assay determi-

nation of anti–*Salmonella typhi* lipopolysaccharide antibodies. *J Clin Microbiol* 1984;20:718–721.

414. Sippel J, Bukhtiari N, Awan MB, et al. Indirect immunoglobulin G (IgG) and IgM enzyme-linked immunosorbent assays (ELISAs) and IgM capture ELISA for detection of antibodies to lipopolysaccharide in adult typhoid fever patients in Pakistan. *J Clin Microbiol* Vol 27:1298–1302.

415. Duthie R, French GL. Comparison of methods for the diagnosis of typhoid fever. *J Clin Pathol* 1990;43:863–865.

416. Ong LY, Pang T, Lim SH, Tan EL, Puthucheary SD. A simple adherence test for detection of IgM antibodies in typhoid. *J Med Microbiol* 1989;29:195–198.

417. Koeleman JGM, Regensburg DF, van Katwijk F, MacLaren DM. Retrospective study to determine the diagnostic value of the Widal test in a non-endemic country. *Eur J Clin Microbiol Infect Dis* 1992;11:167–170.

418. Kang G, Sridharan G, Jesudason MV, John TJ. Evaluation of modified passive hemagglutination assay for Vi antibody estimation in *Salmonella typhi* infections. *J Clin Pathol* 1992;45:740–741.

419. Rai GP, Zachariah K, Shrivastava S. Comparative efficacy of indirect hemagglutination test, indirect fluorescent antibody test and enzyme linked immunosorbent assay in serodiagnosis of typhoid fever. *J Tropical Med Hygi* 1989;92:431–434.

420. Wade DS, Nava HR, Douglass HO Jr. Neutropenic enterocolitis: clinical diagnosis and treatment. *Cancer* 1992;69:17–23.

421. Kleinhaus S, Weinberg G, Gregor MB. Necrotizing enterocolitis in infancy. *Surg Clin North Am* 1992;72:261–276.

422. Millar MR, MacKay P, Levene M, Langdale V, Martin C. Enterobacteriaceae and neonatal necrotising enterocolitis. *Arch Dis Child* 1992;67:53–56.

423. McKeown RE, Marsh TD, Amarnath U, et al. Role of delayed feeding and of feeding increments in necrotizing enterocolitis. *J Pediatrics* 1992;121:764–770.

424. Beeby PJ, Jeffery H. Risk factors for necrotising enterocolitis: the influence of gestational age. *Arch Dis Child* 1992;67:432–435.

425. Huppertz HI, Frauendienst G, Doerck M, von Stockhausen HB. Necrotising enterocolitis—a community-acquired infectious disease? *Lancet* 1992;339:241.

Infections of the Gastrointestinal Tract,
edited by M. J. Blaser, P. D. Smith, J. I. Ravdin,
H. B. Greenberg, and R. L. Guerrant
Raven Press, Ltd., New York © 1995.

CHAPTER 82

Laboratory Diagnosis of Infectious Gastroenteritis

Robert H. Yolken

The availability of laboratory methods for the detection and characterization of viral gastroenteritis represents an important advance in the study of this disease. The accurate diagnosis of an infected patient can establish the etiology of the diarrheal disease and can thus obviate the need for unnecessary medications or additional diagnostic assays. In addition, the identification of infected individuals in inpatient environments can result in the institution of infection control practices and the prevention of disease transmission to high-risk individuals (1,2). Also, the availability of accurate diagnostic assays has resulted in an improved understanding of disease epidemiology and in the identification of individuals at high risk for infection. Assays that can accurately detect gastrointestinal viruses in large numbers of clinical samples have been instrumental in the evaluation of the efficacy of immunization and other regimens directed at the prevention and treatment of gastroenteritis in humans (3–5).

The etiological agents of viral gastroenteritis are somewhat fastidious in terms of cultivation in tissue culture systems that are commonly employed in clinical laboratories. While the group A rotaviruses can be cultivated in a number of cell lines, protease activation is required for efficient replication (6). Enteric strains of adenoviruses and astroviruses can also be cultivated but require specialized cell lines and reaction conditions that are not generally available in clinical laboratories (7,8). Human enteric caliciviruses, and putative pathogens such as enteric coronaviruses and toroviruses, generally cannot be cultivated in available cell lines (9–13). Furthermore, the identification of enteric viruses in fecal samples following *in vitro* cultivation is impeded by the frequent occurrence of cytotoxicity due to bacterial toxins and other cytolytic materials commonly present in fecal samples (14). While cytotoxicity can be distinguished from viral replication by repeated passage of the sample, the need for such passage

increases the time and expense required for the attainment of an accurate diagnosis. Thus, while *in vitro* cultivation is an important research tool in terms of the study of prototype viruses and the analysis of viral replication, cultivation is not generally employed in clinical laboratories for the primary diagnosis of infections with enteric viruses.

In light of the limitations of cultivation assays for the detection of enteric viruses, a number of methods have been devised for the direct detection of viral particles, antigens, and nucleic acids in fecal and intestinal fluid samples. In fact, the need for the accurate detection of gastrointestinal viruses has provided a strong impetus for the development of assays for the direct detection of microorganisms in body fluids, a technology that has found applications in many other disease states (15). This chapter will review the principles of assays that are employed for the detection of pathogenic enteric viruses and will discuss some of the applications of these techniques. Most of the discussion will be directed at the detection and characterization of human rotaviruses since the assays for this agent have attained the most widespread usage and a great deal is known of their advantages and limitations. However, the principles discussed regarding rotaviruses may be applied to the detection and characterization of a wide range of viruses and other pathogens that infect the human gastrointestinal tract.

There are a large number of different assays that have been applied to the detection and characterization of intestinal viruses. These assays fall into three general categories: direct visualization, immunoassays, and nucleic acid detection assays.

DIRECT VISUALIZATION

Most of the viruses now recognized as etiological agents of diarrheal disease were originally detected by direct vis-

R. H. Yolken: Department of Pediatric Infectious Disease, Johns Hopkins Medical Center, Baltimore, Maryland 21205.

ualization utilizing electron microscopic techniques. The human rotaviruses as well as enteric strains of caliciviruses, coronaviruses, astroviruses, adenoviruses, and toroviruses were initially observed in human fecal or intestinal tissues by electron microscopy. In addition, electron microscopic techniques were instrumental in early studies that established these agents as human pathogens and that defined some of the their epidemiological characteristics (16–20). Electron microscopic techniques have the advantage of allowing for the detection of a wide range of recognized viral particles in a single observation of the fecal sample. In addition, such techniques are unique in that they allow for the detection and identification of novel viral agents of gastroenteritis. Furthermore, electron microscopic techniques play a central role in the purification of viruses necessary for the immunological and genetic characterization of newly discovered viruses (21,22). Electron microscopic techniques have thus played a central role in the development of the immunoassays and nucleic acid detection assays discussed below.

However, there are a number of limitations of electron microscopic assays in terms of their application to clinical diagnosis and large-scale studies. The first is that samples must be examined individually, thus limiting throughput and making it difficult to perform large-scale studies. Second, the performance of electron microscopic examinations requires access to specialized equipment and personnel trained in its use, resources that are unavailable in many clinical laboratory settings. Finally, the cost of electron microscopic procedures makes them difficult to apply on a general basis. For these reasons, the other direct detection assays have replaced electron microscopic examinations in most diagnostic situations (23). However, electron microscopy has potential utility in situations in which small numbers of samples need to be examined for large numbers of potentially infecting viruses. This might occur in the examination of samples from individuals at very high risk for infection, such as individuals who are immunocompromised or who are undergoing bone marrow transplantation. In addition, electron microscopy would be of use in the case of outbreaks of gastroenteritis in which common etiological agents have been excluded on the basis of other direct assay systems.

IMMUNOASSAYS

The identification and characterization of the agents of gastroenteritis has led to the development of immunoreagents capable of specific interaction with viral antigens. These immunoreagents have been applied to the detection of these agents in fecal and intestinal fluid samples. Immunoassays that have been applied to the direct detection of viral antigens in fecal samples have employed a number of formats including ones that utilize reagents labeled with radioactive, fluorescent, chemiluminescent, microparticulate, and enzymatic markers.

All of the these immunoassay formats are based on the interaction of antigens with labeled immunoglobulins and the measurement of the subsequent antigen–antibody in-

teractions. The sensitivity, specificity, and performance characteristics of the different immunoassays are thus dependent to a great extent on the affinity and reaction parameters of the immunoreagents employed (24,25). Since enteric viruses are generally assayed in the highly heterogeneous milieu of the human gastrointestinal tract, it is crucial that the immune agents be capable of reacting with antigens under a range of reaction conditions. In order to attain assay specificity, it is also crucial that the labeled immunoreagents not display cross-reactivities with antigens derived from dietary proteins, bacteria, intestinal epithelial, or other antigenic materials likely to be found in fecal and intestinal fluids. Fortunately, the development of techniques for the purification of viral particles has led to the availability of immunoreagents with acceptable levels of specificity. The specificity of the immunoassays can be further improved by the use of monoclonal antibodies and by the use of antibodies directed at viral proteins generated by molecular cloning and expression technologies (26).

Due to the heterogeneous nature of the reaction milieu inherent in the analyses of fecal samples, assays for the detection of enteric viruses generally employ a solid phase system to immunologically separate antigens from fecal samples prior to the performance of subsequent immunodetection reactions (Fig. 1). The use of a solid phase allows for the removal of antigens from potentially interfering substances in the sample and for the performance of subsequent immunological and enzymatic reactions in a defined environment. A number of different solid phase devices can be employed for these separations. Solid phase formats have been devised from plastic, paper, nitrocellulose, glass, or other potentially absorbent material. Immunoglobulins will absorb to these surfaces by means of hydrophobic attachment, allowing for the binding of immunoglobulins using simple reaction protocols (27,28). However, the use of covalent linkages allows for the binding of higher concentrations of immunoreactants and can result in improved reaction kinetics and assay performance (29).

Most currently available immunoassays employ a solid phase in the form of a macroscopic bead or a well of a microtitration plate. Although convenient in terms of the processing of large numbers of samples, such surfaces have relatively low capacities for immunoreagents. Immunoassays that employ such surfaces have relatively slow reaction kinetics and the performance of assays using such surfaces requires more than 4 hr of incubations at 37°C for the attainment of maximum assay sensitivity. The recent development of high-capacity solid phase surfaces consisting of microparticles or membranes can allow for the input of larger concentrations of immunoreagents and can result in improved reaction kinetics. For example, the use of nylon membranes allows for the detection of rotavirus antigens in fecal samples in less than 10 min, with a sensitivity equivalent to that of microplate assays that employ 4 hr of incubations (29).

Most of the immunoassays that are employed in diagnostic laboratories are directed at the detection of the target microorganism rather than at its antigenic characterization. Thus the immunoreagents that are employed are

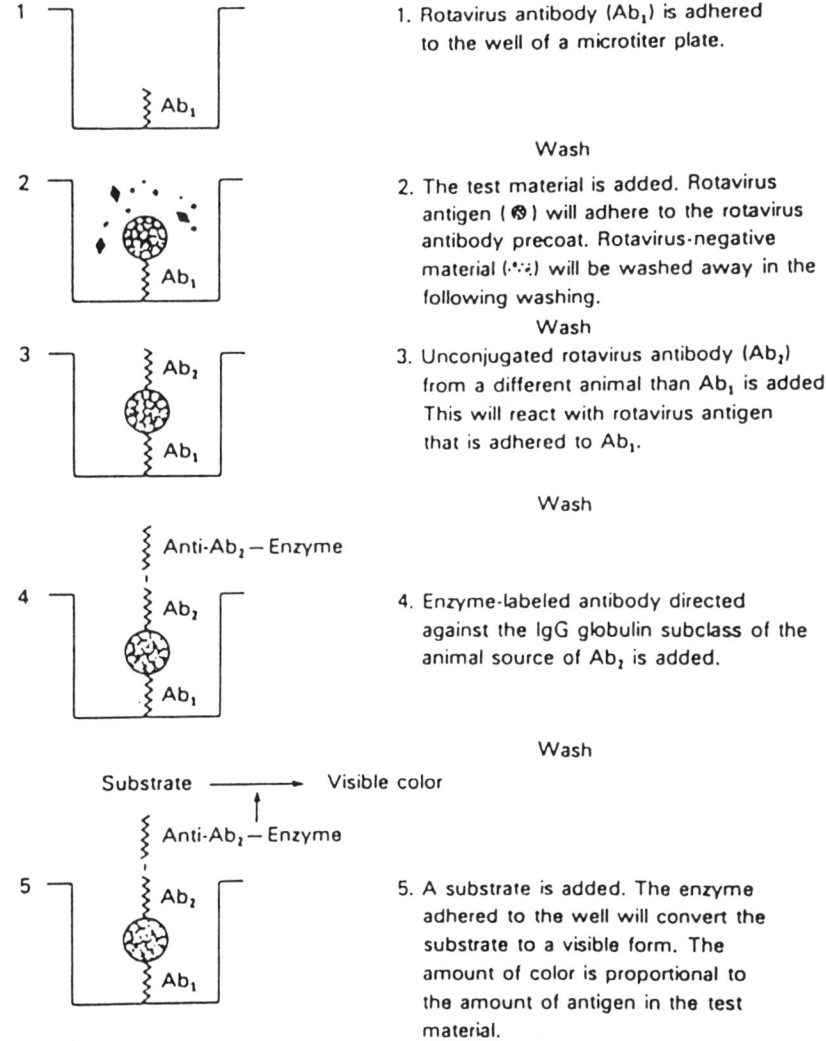

1. Rotavirus antibody (Ab_1) is adhered to the well of a microtiter plate.

Wash

2. The test material is added. Rotavirus antigen (⊗) will adhere to the rotavirus antibody precoat. Rotavirus-negative material (∷) will be washed away in the following washing.

Wash

3. Unconjugated rotavirus antibody (Ab_2) from a different animal than Ab_1 is added. This will react with rotavirus antigen that is adhered to Ab_1.

Wash

4. Enzyme-labeled antibody directed against the IgG globulin subclass of the animal source of Ab_2 is added.

Wash

5. A substrate is added. The enzyme adhered to the well will convert the substrate to a visible form. The amount of color is proportional to the amount of antigen in the test material.

FIG. 1. Indirect ELISA for rotavirus antigen measurement. From ref. 73, with permission.

generally directed at antigens present in all members of the target virus. However, the use of antibodies with more restricted reactivities can result in an immunoassay capable of more specific antigenic characterizations. Thus immunoassays for the detection of rotaviruses generally employ antibodies directed at the group reactive epitopes localized to the VP6 core protein. However, immunoassays have also been devised that employ monospecific or monoclonal reagents directed at epitopes located in the VP4 or VP7 proteins of the virus that define specific antigens of the infecting virus (26,30,31).

Immunoassays can employ a wide variety of labels to quantify the interaction of immunoreagents with target antigens. Labels that can be employed include ones that generate radioactive, fluorescent, chemiluminescent, or enzymatic markers. Many of the assays that have been employed for the detection of enteric viruses have made use of enzyme–substrate reactions as markers for immunoreactivity. Enzyme immunoassays (EIAs; also known as enzyme-linked immunosorbent assays, or ELISA) have the advantages of offering a high degree of magnifi-

cation due to the amplifying nature of enzyme–substrate reactivity. In addition, enzymes are relatively stable and a wide variety of suitable enzymatic markers and substrates are available at low cost. Since many enzyme–substrate reactions generate products that absorb light in the visible range of the spectrum, assays that employ such reactions are applicable to semiquantitative determinations by visual scoring or accurate quantitation by means of spectophotometric instrumentation (32). On the other hand, higher energy substrates, such as ones that generate fluorescent or chemiluminescent products, can be employed to decrease the time required for the performance of the assay and can in some circumstances increase assay reactivity (33–35).

The careful selection of immunoreagents can minimize the occurrence of false-positive reactions due to the immune recognition of extraneous antigens. However, nonspecific reactions can still occur in some fecal samples due to the binding to the Fc portion of the labeled immunoglobulins with bacterial proteins and other Fc-binding fecal materials (36,37). Control reactions are thus required in order to attain maximum assay specificity. Such reactions can be performed by reacting the sample with solid phase surfaces coated with control immunoreactants. Such immunoreactants can take the form of monoclonal antibodies of the same immunoglobulin subclass directed at irrelevant antigens or polyclonal antibodies obtained following immunization with irrelevant proteins (36). Alternately, specificity can be documented by the blocking of immunoreactivity by means of an independent source of antiviral antibodies (38). While this method of confirmation requires an extra reaction step, it offers the advantage of not requiring a different solid phase, and can thus be performed with any available immunoassay system provided that an additional source of antibodies is available.

Microparticles made of latex or other material can be employed as both the solid phase media and the detector. Such "agglutination" assays have the advantage of being rapid, due to the high concentration of immunoreagents, and relatively simple, since they can make use of visual scoring of the agglutination assay (38–40). However, such assays generally do not employ a separation procedure in which potential cross-reactive contaminants are removed prior to the completion of the assay. Agglutination formats are thus subject to false-positive reactions due to nonspecific agglutination and false-negative reactions due to the presence of materials in the stool that interfere with the immune reactions. In addition, since the assays are generally scored by visual inspection, they are subject to errors of assay interpretation. The availability of practical methods for the separation of microparticles from interfering reactants and for the quantitation of microparticles offers the future promise of accurate microparticle assays for the detection of enteric viruses (41).

There are a number of advantages of immunoassays for the detection of rotaviruses and selected other agents of viral gastroenteritis such as enteric adenoviruses and astroviruses in human clinical samples. The availability of formats for the large-scale manipulation of the solid phase and measurement of enzymatic reactions allows for the performance of a large number of assays in a single test run. Such formats allow for the detection of antigens in a practical and economical manner. In addition, the availability of rapid formats utilizing microparticles and other high-capacity solid phases allows for detection of viral antigens in a short time and for the immediate institution of appropriate interventions. Furthermore, the performance of immunoassays requires little in the way of sample preparation. For example, rectal swabs can be eluted in sample saline solutions and applied directly to the solid phase system. For this reason, immunoassays have been widely employed for the study of rotaviruses and remain the assay in most widespread usage in many areas of the world (42).

However, there are also a number of limitations of immunoassays in terms of the direct detection of microorganisms in fecal specimens. The most important limitation concerns assay sensitivity. While the actual sensitivity depends on the affinity characteristics of the immunoreagents, these affinity characteristics limit detection to the equivalent of approximately 10^4–10^5 viral particles. An additional limitation of immunoassays is that antigens can be complexed with endogenously produced antibodies and other materials present in the intestinal milieu that can bind viral antigens prior to the performance of the immunoassay. While these endogenously generated immune complexes can be dissociated by a number of chemical methods, it is difficult to employ such methods without destroying some of the antigens and thus lowering assay sensitivity. Finally, immunoassays are difficult to perform in situations in which the viral antigen has not been well characterized. Thus, while immunoassays have been widely employed for the detection of rotaviruses and adenoviruses, they are less widely used in the case of the newer viral agents.

NUCLEIC ACID DETECTION

Due to limitations inherent in the use of immunoassays, methods have been devised for the direct detection of viral nucleic acids in fecal and intestinal fluid specimens. Nucleic acid detection methods offer a number of advantages for the identification of viral pathogens in fecal samples (43,44). First of all, such assays require only that the nucleic acid sequence be identified; knowledge of the antigens present in the stool is not required for the assay. This constitutes a major advantage in the detection of newly discovered viral agents since unique nucleotide sequences are generally elucidated prior to the determination of whether they encode proteins that are shed into body fluids. Second, nucleic acids can be extracted from endogenous immune complexes, cellular membranes, and other physical states that might interfere with binding to labeled reagents. Nucleic acid binding techniques can thus detect viral infection in situations in which antigens are not accessible to labeled immunoreagents. Finally, numerous methods have been devised for the amplification of microbial nucleic acids from human body fluid samples. These techniques, which include the polymerase chain reaction (PCR) and related methodologies, allow for the detection of viruses at concentrations far below the levels determined by the equilibrium conditions of antigen–antibody reactions (45). For some viral enteric pathogens, such as Norwalk and related agents, the enhanced sensitivity of nucleic acid based assays is likely to improve on available immunoassays substantially. While nucleic acids can also be detected by hybridization protocols that do not employ amplification, the potential sensitivity of the amplification methods has made these techniques the most widely used in both research and clinical laboratories. Principles of these techniques related to the amplification of microbial nucleic acids from fecal, intestinal, and environmental samples are discussed below.

NUCLEIC ACID AMPLIFICATION TECHNIQUES IN FECAL SAMPLES

There are a number of considerations that are crucial to the successful amplification of microbial nucleic acids from fecal samples. Nucleic acid amplification involves a series of reactions consisting of the binding of oligonucleotides to complementary regions of target and the polymerase-catalyzed generation of copies of target sequences. It is thus necessary that the reaction milieu be suitable for the performance of these reactions. Since intestinal fluids in fecal samples contain a wide range of materials that can inhibit enzymatic reactions, it is important that the nucleic acid be separated from substances that might inhibit catalysis and amplification. In addition, intestinal fluids and fecal samples often contain nucleases that can break down nucleic acids prior to the performance of the enzymatic amplifications. The effect of enzymatic inhibitors and nucleases is particularly problematic in the analysis of samples for the presence of RNA genomes such as those present in rotaviruses, astroviruses, and caliciviruses. This difficulty is due to the fact that the thermostable DNA polymerases do not efficiently amplify RNA targets (46). It is thus necessary to convert RNA to DNA by reaction with reverse transcriptase prior to the performance of the cyclical amplification reactions. Since thermostable forms of reverse transcriptase are not generally available, this reaction needs to be performed at relatively low temperatures (37–40°C). In addition to decreasing the stringency of the reaction, the use of lower temperatures may augment the effect of the inhibitory materials. In addition, it is at these temperatures that ribonucleases and other nucleases display high levels of activity.

Many protocols for the performance of nucleic acid amplification utilize chemical denaturation with compounds such as phenol or guanidium followed by precipitation with ethanol or other alcohols in order to isolate nucleic acids (47). The performance of such reactions is adequate to separate DNA from compounds that inhibit DNA amplification. However, we have found that simple precipitation reactions are generally inadequate for the removal of materials that inhibit reverse transcription. While the exact nature of these materials has not been totally elucidated, they are likely to consist of heavy metals and other low molecular weight enzymatic inhibitors (48). While it might be suspected that such molecules could be removed by precipitation and similar techniques, the cationic nature of the substances can cause them to coprecipitate with nucleic acids and can make them difficult to remove by simple separation methodologies.

For these reasons a number of methods have been devised for the separation of RNA from inhibitory substances. These methods generally involve the isolation of nucleic acids by chemical denaturation followed by the physical separation of the nucleic acids from potentially contaminating materials. These separations can be accomplished by means of ion exchange chromatography, gel fractionation, detergent treatment, or differential polymers derived from silica and related materials (48–52). It should be noted in terms of the polymers that many synthetic materials that efficiently bind and separate DNA do not efficiently bind and elute RNA under the same reaction conditions (47). It is thus important that conditions specific for RNA binding and separation be devised for each reaction medium. In addition, the binding of double-stranded RNA, as would be found in rotaviruses and other reoviridae, often occur under conditions somewhat

different from those of the binding of single-stranded RNA as might be found in the caliciviradae. One general approach to the isolation of nucleic acids involves the use of oligonucleotide hybrids to capture target nucleotides on a solid phase surface prior to subsequent amplification. This principle, which is similar to that employed for the solid phase immunoassays, is outlined in Fig. 2 (53).

It should be noted that the titers of inhibitory substances found in fecal samples generally range from 1:2 to 1:100. Thus the dilution of fecal samples occurring beyond 1:100 generally results in the avoidance of inhibitory substances. In fact, many protocols for the detection of RNA in fecal samples employ the use of samples at such dilutions and thus avoid other problem inhibitors. However, it should be noted that the use of such samples alters the potential sensitivity of the assays since a minimum of 100 target molecules would be required for detection.

Another important consideration for the accurate detection of viral nucleic acids in fecal samples is the avoidance of false-positive reactions due to sample contamination. The manipulations required for the isolation of nucleic acids from fecal samples, as discussed above, can increase the likelihood of the inadvertent inoculation of contaminants into the reaction mixture. Of particular concern in this regard is the possibility of contamination with fragments of DNA amplified from other samples. Since these amplicons serve as templates for additional reactions, the presence of even small amounts of contaminating amplicons can result in a significant level of signal generation. It is thus extremely important that fecal samples be analyzed in such a way that contamination does not occur. Important steps in this regard are the use of dedicated tubes and transfer devices as well as the physical separation of areas in which samples are processed and the areas in which reaction tubes are opened following amplification. In addition, it is important that negative controls be included in each reaction and that assay results only be considered valid in situations in which all of the negative controls are devoid of amplification (54). In the case of RNA genomes, an additional control can be performed in which the sample is amplified without the prior conversion of RNA to cDNA by reaction with reverse transcriptase. The amplification of DNA without a reverse transcription reaction indicates that the started material contained amplifiable DNA and thus may have been contaminated from a previous reaction run.

The effect of amplicon carryover can be decreased by the use of modified nucleotides that can be selectively cleaved following the amplification reaction. For example, the nucleotide deoxyuracil can be substituted for deoxycytidine in the amplification mix. Nucleic acids that contain this nucleotide can be selectively cleaved by the enzyme deoxyuracil-N-glycanase (UNG). Since native nucleic acids do not contain this nucleotide, cleavage will be selective for nucleic acids generated by PCRs performed with this nucleotide. Such reactions thus result in a selective decrease of contaminating DNA as opposed to original target (55). However, it should be noted that such selective enzymatic reactions may not totally eliminate contaminating DNA when large amounts are present

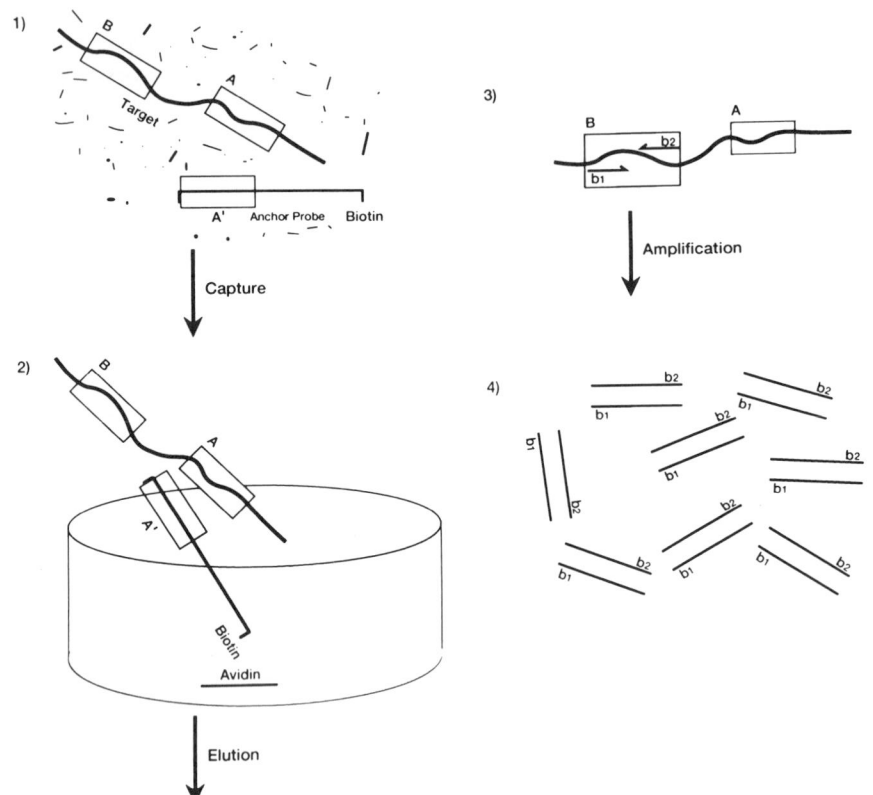

FIG. 2. Solid phase capture method for specific DNA amplification. The procedures used for solid phase capture and amplification are (*1*) Target nucleic acid is hybridized in liquid phase to a biotin labelled, single stranded RNA probe which is complementary to sequences located at one end of the target (region A). (*2*) The hybrid is bound to a solid phase coated with streptavidin. Contaminating materials such as enzyme inhibitors and amplified duplexes generated by extraneous reactions are removed by washing of the solid phase. (*3*) Following washing, target molecules are eluted from the solid phase by heating. (*4*) Region B of the target is amplified by repeated reactions with primers b_1 and b_2 and Taq polymerase using standard PCR protocol. (From ref. 53, with permission.)

in the reaction. In addition, the use of modified nucleotides can result in somewhat decreased assay sensitivity due to decreased incorporation of modified bases into the reaction products (56). Finally, none of these techniques will prevent contamination from genuine target nucleic acids introduced when the sample was collected or processed prior to extraction. Thus careful laboratory techniques must be continued throughout the collection, extraction, amplification, and detection processes. The use of solid phase capture systems, such as those depicted in Fig. 2, can also serve to decrease the rate of false-positive reactions due to sample contamination.

It should be noted that RNA can be converted to cDNA either by reaction with specific oligonucleotide primers or by the use of random oligonucleotides. Specific primers can be slightly more sensitive for amplification of small quantities of RNA in heterogeneous solutions. However, the use of random oligonucleotide primers (generally in the form of hexamers) has the advantage that a single reverse transcriptase reaction can be utilized to generate cDNA for the detection of a number of different viruses mediated by the use of oligonucleotide primers during the DNA amplification reaction. In light of the importance of the RNA extraction and conversion steps, as well as of the possible occurrences of sample inhibition and contamination, the use of random hexamers offers a number of advantages for the diagnostic application of nucleic acid amplification, especially in situations in which multiple nucleic acid targets will be amplified from the same clinical specimen.

Another consideration in the performance of nucleic

acid amplification reactions is the method employed for the detection of the amplified nucleic acids. In many research applications, the nucleic acid is simply visualized following reaction with ethidium bromide or another dye that selectively stains nucleic acids (57). Such methods have the advantage of being simple, rapid, and generally applicable to any target nucleic acid. However, the amplification of complex body fluids such as fecal material can lead to the generation of extraneous bands visible on gels due to base pairing between oligonucleotide primers and partially homologous nucleic acids extracted from the fecal milieu. Extraneous amplification is particularly problematic in the analysis of target RNA since the reverse transcriptase–mediated conversion of RNA to cDNA is generally performed at relatively low temperatures. It is thus not possible to increase the stringency of this reaction by the maintenance of the reactants at higher temperatures ("hot start") (58). The generation of extraneous bands can be modulated to some extent by the use of a second amplification reaction that employs oligonucleotide primers located internally to the ones used for the initial amplification (nested PCR). However, the performance of such protocols requires opening of the reaction tube prior to the completion of the reaction and thus increases the possibilities for contamination. In addition, multiple bands can still be visible due to the continued presence of the original oligonucleotide primers in the reaction milieu.

It is thus advisable that nucleic acid amplification reactions for the detection of microbial nucleic acids and fecal samples employ a specific hybridization technique to specifically identify the target nucleic acids. In addition, the use of such hybridization techniques can increase the functional sensitivity of the assay by identifying concentrations of amplified nucleic acids below that detectable by the use of simple standing techniques. Hybridization utilizing electrophoretic separation and transfer to nitrocellulose or other binding membranes (southern blot) is the standard method for accomplishing such identification. However, nucleic acids can also be identified by hybridization without the performance of the electrophoretic separation. This can be accomplished by liquid phase hybridization protocols in which hybridization is identified by precipitation, modulation of chemiluminescence, or the binding of antibodies that recognize nucleotide hybrids (59–64). The availability of practical methods for the accurate detection of amplified nucleic acids will play an important role in the development of practical methods for the detection of nucleic acids in fecal samples and for the increased availability of such assays in clinical laboratory environments.

CLINICAL INTERPRETATION OF RESULTS

As discussed above, the use of nucleic acid amplification results in assays with the capabilities of detecting viral nucleic acids at concentrations substantially below those that can be detected by other techniques such as immunoassay or electron neuron microscopy. This increased sensitivity allows for the potential amplification of microbial pathogens not detectable by other methods. For example, the shedding of rotavirus RNA can be detected by PCR techniques both before and after fecal antigen can be identified by immunoassay methods (Fig. 3)

(65). Nucleic acid amplification techniques thus can allow for the detection of microbial infection in patients for longer periods than that which could be accomplished by previously available diagnostic methodologies. Furthermore, nucleic acid amplification techniques have been developed for the detection of Norwalk virus, astroviruses, and enteric adenoviruses (65–68). As in the case of the assays for rotavirus, these assays can allow for the detection of virus in samples that do not contain virus detectable by other methodologies. Nucleic acid amplification techniques thus have the potential for improved detection of outbreaks and the better diagnosis of infected patients.

The availability of more sensitive diagnostic techniques raises the question as to whether the low levels of microbial nucleic acids that are detected by such methods are always indicative of a causal association between infection and illness. The question may also be raised as to whether low levels of viral nucleic acids that are detected during the course of an outbreak or in environmental sampling represent an infectious risk for other individuals. Such questions represents some of the potential benefits and potential pitfalls of sensitive diagnostic methodologies and can only be addressed by carefully performed prospective studies.

DETECTION OF VIRUS IN THE ENVIRONMENT

An important aspect of diagnostic methodologies for enteric pathogens concerns the identification of virus in the environment. While immunoassays and electron microscopy have been employed for this purpose, they generally lack the sensitivity for detailed studies. On the other hand, nucleic acid amplification procedures can be em-

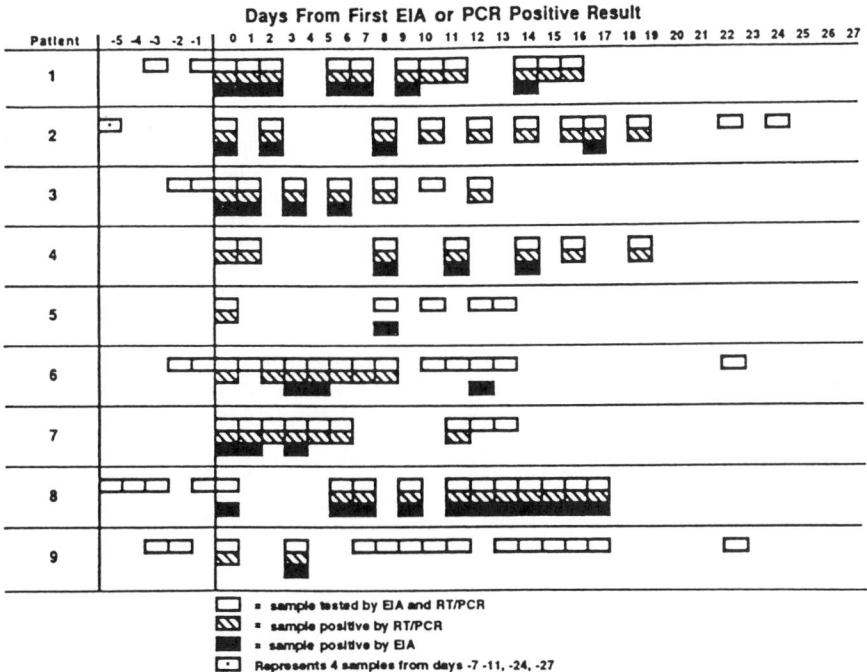

FIG. 3. Enzyme immunoassay (EIA) vs. polymerase chain reaction (PCR) for detection of group A rotavirus in serial fecal specimens. From ref. 65, with permission.

TABLE 1. *Detection of rotavirus in day care environment*

	Outbreak centers	Nonoutbreak centers	p^a
Toy balls	7/18 (39)	1/21 (5)	.012
Environment	8/39 (21)	1/44 (2)	.009
Floor	3/19 (16)	0/9	
Child area[b]	5/20 (25)	1/35 (3)	
Total	15/57	2/65 (3)	.001

From ref. 69, with permission.

Note: Data are no. positive/no. tested (%).

[a] Fisher's exact test, compared to incidence in outbreak center.

[b] Includes diaper change pads, diaper pail handles, and high chair seats.

ployed for the detection of low levels of virus in environmental samples. For example, we have utilized PCR for the detection of rotavirus in toys handled by infected children and in environmental samples obtained from the day care environment. Interestingly, the detection level of virus in the day care environment correlated to some extent with the occurrence of outbreaks of rotavirus diarrhea in the children attending the day care center (Table 1). In addition, rotavirus is found in samples, such as telephone headsets, that were not handled by the children thus indicating that rotavirus could be spread in the environment by adults (69,70). Similar assay have been employed for the detection of enteric viruses in water, shellfish, and other environmental sources (71,72). As in the case of the use of sensitive techniques for the detection of virus in stool, the potential infectivity of low levels of virus needs to be evaluated in further studies. The availability of assays for the accurate detection of enteric pathogens in water, food, and other environmental sources would represent a major contribution in terms of public health and disease prevention in a number of different populations.

ACKNOWLEDGMENT

This work was supported by NIH Cooperative Agreement 5U01AI30420.

REFERENCES

1. Grehn M, Kunz J, Sigg P, Slongo R, Zbinden R. Nosocomial rotavirus infections in neonates: means of prevention and control. *J Perinatal Med* 1990;18(5):369–374.
2. Brady MT, Pacini DL, Budde CT, Connell MJ. Diagnostic studies of nosocomial diarrhea in children: assessing their use and value. *Am J Infect Control* 1989;17(2):77–82.
3. Vesikari T, Ruuska T, Green KY, Flores J, Kapikian AZ. Protective efficacy against serotype 1 rotavirus diarrhea by live oral rhesus-human reassortant rotavirus vaccines with human rotavirus VP7 serotype 1 or 2 specificity. *Pediatr Infect Dis J* 1991;11(7):535–542.
4. Madore HP, Christy C, Pichichero M, et al. Field trial of rhesus rotavirus or human-rhesus rotavirus reassortant vaccine of VP7 serotype 3 or 1 specificity in infants. *J Infect Dis* 1991;166(2):235–243.
5. Clark HF, Borian FE, Plotkin SA. Immune protection of infants against rotavirus gastroenteritis by a serotype 1 reassortment of bovine rotavirus WC3. *J Infect Dis* 1990;161(6):1099–1104.
6. Bingnan F, Unicomb LE, Tu GL, et al. Cultivation and characterization of novel human group A rotaviruses with long RNA electropherotypes, subgroup II specificities, and serotype 2 VP7 genes. *J Clin Microbiol* 1991;29(10):2224–2227.
7. Brown M, Wilson-Friesen HL, Doane F. A block in release of progeny virus and a high particle-to-infectious unit ratio contribute to poor growth of enteric adenovirus types 40 and 41 in cell culture. *J Virol* 1992;66(5):3198–3205.
8. Mautner V, Mackay N, Morris K. Enteric adenovirus type 40: expression of E1B mRNA and proteins in permissive and non-permissive cells. *Virology* 1990;179(1):129–138.
9. Moe CL, Allen JR, Monroe SS, et al. Detection of astrovirus in pediatric stool samples by immunoassay and RNA probe. *J Clin Microbiol* 1991;29(11):2390–2395.
10. Yolken RH, Eiden JJ. Rotavirus, enteric adenoviruses, Norwalk viruses, caliciviruses, astroviruses, and other viruses causing gastroenteritis. In: Belshe RB, ed. *Textbook of human virology.* 2nd ed. St. Louis: Mosby Year Book; 1991:804–821.
11. Herrmann JE, Cubitt WD, Hudson RW, Perron-Henry DM, Oshiro LS, Blacklow NR. Immunological characterization of the Marin County strain of astrovirus. *Arch Virol* 1990;110(3–4):213–220.
12. Snijder EJ, den Boon JA, Horzinek MC, Spaan WJ. Comparison of the genome organization of toro- and cornonaviruses: evidence for two nonhomologous RNA recombination events during Berne virus evolution. *Virology* 1991;180(1):448–452.
13. Cubit WD. Human, small round structured viruses, caliciviruses and astroviruses (review). *Baillieres Clin Gastroenterol* 1990;4(3):643–656.
14. Kennedy E, Burke V, Pearman J, Robinson J, Gracey M. Cytotoxic effects of children's faeces: relation to diarrhoea due to Clostridium difficile and other enteric pathogens. *Ann Trop Paediatrics* 1991;11(2):107–112.
15. Yolken RH, Miotti P, Viscidi R. Immunoassays for the diagnosis and study of viral gastroenteritis. *Pediatr Infect Dis* 1986;5(1):46–52.
16. Bishop RF, Davidson GP, Holmes IH, et al. Virus particles in epithelial cells of duodenal mucosa from children with acute gastroenteritis. *Lancet* 1974;2:1281.
17. Thornhill TS, Wyatt RG, Kalica AR, et al. Detection by immune electron microscopy of 26–27 nm virus-like particles associated with two family outbreaks of gastroenteritis. *J Infect Dis* 1977;138:20.
18. Woode GN, Bridger JC, Jones JM, et al. Morphological and antigenic relationships between viruses (rotaviruses) from acute gastroenteritis of children, calves, piglets, mice and foals. *Infect Immun* 1976;14:804–810.
19. Cubit WD, McSwiggan DA. Calicivirus gastroenteritis in northwest London. *Lancet* 1981;1:975–977.
20. Madeley CR. Comparison of the features of astroviruses and caliciviruses seen in samples of feces by electron microscopy. *J Infect Dis* 1979;139:519–523.
21. Davies HA. Electron-microscopy and immune electron microscopy for detection of gastroenteritis viruses. In: Tyrrell DAJ, Kapikian AZ, eds. *Virus infections of the gastrointestinal tract.* New York: Marcel Dekker; 1982:37–49.
22. Christensen ML, Howard C. Viruses causing gastroenteritis. In: Balows A, Hausler WJ Jr, Herrmann KL, Isenberg HD, Shadomy HJ, eds. *Manual of clinical microbiology.* 5th ed. Washington, DC: American Society for Microbiology; 1991:950–958.
23. Dennehy PH, Gauntlett DR, Spangenberger SE. Choice of reference assay for the detection of rotavirus in fecal specimens: electron microscopy versus enzyme immunoassay. *J Clin Microbiol* 1990;28(6):1280–1283.
24. Yolken RH. Enzyme immunoassays for the detection of infectious antigens in body fluids: current limitations and future prospects. *Rev Infect Dis* 1982;4(1):35–68.
25. Yolken RH. Solid phase immunoassays for the detection of viral diseases. In: van Regenmortel MHV, Neurath AR eds. *Immuno-*

chemistry of viruses: the basis of serodiagnosis and vaccines. Amsterdam: Elsevier; 1985.

26. Midthun K, Valdesuso J, Kapikian AZ, Hoshino Y, Green KY. Identification of serotype 9 human rotavirus by enzyme-linked immunosorbent assay with monoclonal antibodies. *J Clin Microbiol* 1989;27(9):2112–2114.

27. Shekarchi IC, Sever JL, Lee YJ, Castellano G, Madden DL. Evaluation of various plastic microtiter plates with measles, toxoplasma, and gamma globulin antigens in enzyme-linked immunosorbent assays. *J Clin Microbiol* 1984;19:89–96.

28. Tijssen P. *Practice and theory of enzyme immunoassays.* Amsterdam: Elsevier; 1985.

29. Yolken RH, Eiden J, Leister F. Self contained enzymatic membrane immunoassay for detection of rotavirus antigen in clinical samples. *Lancet* 1986;2:1305–1307.

30. Coulson BS. Typing of human rotavirus VP4 by an enzyme immunoassay using monoclonal antibodies. *J Clin Microbiol* 1993; 31(1):1–8.

31. Woods PA, Gentsch J, Gouvea V, et al. Distribution of serotypes of human rotavirus in different populations. *J Clin Microbiol* 1992;30(4):781–785.

32. Yolken RH. Enzyme immunoassays for the detection of microbial antigens and prospects for improved assays. *Yale J Biol Med* 1986;59(1):25–31.

33. Hornsleth A, Aaen K, Gundestrup M. Detection of respiratory syncytial virus and rotavirus by enhanced chemiluminescence enzyme-linked immunosorbent assay. *J Clin Microbiol* 1988; 26(4):630–635.

34. Yolken RH, Leister FJ. Comparison of fluorescent and colorigenic substrates for enzyme immunoassays. *J Clin Microbiol* 1982;15(5):757–760.

35. Coutlee F, Viscidi RP, Yolken RH. Comparison of colorimetric, enzyme immunoassay for detection of DNA-RNA hybrids. *J Clin Microbiol* 1989;27(5):1002–1007.

36. Yolken RH, Stopa PJ. Analysis of non-specific reactions in enzyme-linked immunosorbent assay testing for human rotavirus. *J Clin Microbiol* 1979;10:703–710.

37. Lipson SM, Leonardi GP, Salo RJ, Schutzbank TE, Kaplan MH. Occurrence of nonspecific reactions among stool specimens tested by the Abbott TestPack rotavirus enzyme immunoassay. *J Clin Microbiol* 1990;28(6):1132–1134.

38. Kok TW, Burrell CJ. Comparison of five enzyme immunoassays, electron microscopy, and latex agglutination for detection of rotavirus in fecal specimens. *J Clin Microbiol* 1989;27(20): 364–366.

39. Kohli E, Pothier P, Denis F, Freymuth F, Goudeau A. Multicentre evaluation of a new commercial latex agglutination test using a monoclonal antibody for rotavirus detection. *Eur J Clin Microbiol Infect Dis* 1989;8(3):251–253.

40. Miotti PG, Eiden J, Yolken RH. Comparative efficiency of commercial immunoassays for the diagnosis of rotavirus gastroenteritis during the course of infection. *J Clin Microbiol* 1985;22(5): 693–698.

41. Miotti PG, Viscidi RP, Eiden J, Cerny E, Yolken RH. Centrifugation augmented solid-phase immunoassay (CASPIA) for the rapid diagnosis of infectious diseases. *J Infect Dis* 1986;154: 301–308.

42. Flewett TH, Arias CF, Avendano LF, et al. Comparative evaluation of the WHO and DAKOPATTS enzyme-linked immunoassay kits for rotavirus detection. *Bull WHO* 1989;67(4):369–374.

43. Viscidi RP, Yolken RH. Molecular diagnosis of infectious diseases by nucleic acid hybridization. *Mol Cell Probes* 1987;1: 3–14.

44. Yolken RH. Nucleic acids or immunologloglobulins: which are the molecular probes of the future? *Mol Cell Probes* 1988;2(2): 87–96.

45. Persing DH. Target selection and optimization of amplification reactions. In: Pershing DH, Smith TF, Tenover FC, White TJ, eds. *Diagnostic molecular microbiology: principles and applications.* Washington, DC: American Society for Microbiology; 1993:88–104.

46. Kawasaki ES. Amplification of RNA. In: Innis MA, Gelfand DH, Sninsky JJ, White TJ, eds. *PCR protocols: a guide to methods and applications.* San Diego: Academic Press; 1990:21–27.

47. Greenfield L, White TJ. Sample preparation methods. In: Pershing DH, Smith TF, Tenover FC, White TJ, eds. *Diagnostic molecular microbiology: principles and applications.* Washington, DC: American Society for Microbiology; 1993:122–137.

48. Wilde J, Eiden J, Yolken R. Removal of inhibitory substances from human fecal specimens for detection of group A rotaviruses by reverse transcriptase and polymerase chain reactions. *J Clin Microbiol* 1990;28:1300–1307.

49. Boom R, Sol CJA, Salimans, Jansen CL, Wertheim-van Dillen. Rapid and simple method for purification of nucleic acids. *J Clin Microbiol* 1990;28:495–503.

50. Chirgwin JM, Przybyla AE, MacDonald RJ, Rutter WJ. Isolation of biologically active ribonucleic acid from sources enriched in ribonuclease. *Biochemistry* 1979;5284–5299.

51. Buffone GJ, Demmler GJ, Schimbor CM, Greer J. Improved amplification of cytomegalovirus DNA from urine after purification of DNA with glass beads. *Clin Chem* 1991;1945–1949.

52. Lund A, Wasteson Y, Olsvik O. Immunomagnetic separation and DNA hybridization for detection of enterotoxigenic *Escherichia coli* in a piglet model. *J Clin Microbiol* 1991;29:2259–2262.

53. Yolken RH, Sierra-Honigmann AM, Viscidi RP. Solid phase capture method for the specific amplification of microbial nucleic acids—avoidance of false-positive and false-negative reactions. *Mol Cell Probes* 1991;5:151–156.

54. Persing DH. Polymerase chain reaction: trenches to benches. *J Clin Microbiol* 1990;29:1281–1285.

55. Longo MC, Berninger MS, Harley JL. Use of uracil DNA glycosylase to control carry-over contamination in polymerase chain reactions. *Gene* 1990;93:125–128.

56. Pang J, Modlin J, Yolken R. Use of modified nucleotides and uracil-DNA glycosylase (UNG) for the control of contamination in the PCR-based amplification of RNA. *Mol Cell Probes* 1992; 6:251–256.

57. Higuchi R, Dollinger G, Walsh PS, Griffith R. Simultaneous amplification and detection of specific DNA sequences. *Biotechnology* 1992;10:413–417.

58. Chou Q, Russell M, Birch DE, Raymond J, Bloch W. Prevention of pre-PCR mis-priming and priming dimerization improves low-copy-number amplifications. *Nucleic Acids Res* 1992;20: 1717–1723.

59. Bugawan D, Saiki RK, Levenson CH, Watson RM, Erlich HA. The use of non-radioactive oligonucleotide probes to analyze enzymatically amplified DNA for prenatal diagnosis and forensic HLA typing. *Biotechnology* 1988;6:943–947.

60. Ou C-Y, McDonough SH, Cabanas D, et al. Rapid and quantitative detection of enzymatically amplified HIV-1 DNA using chemiluminescent oligonucleotide probes. *AIDS Res Hum Retroviruses* 1990;6:1323–1329.

61. Nickerson DA, Kaiser R, Lappin S, Stewart J, Hood L, Landgren U. Automated DNA diagnostics usina an ELISA-based oligonucleotide ligation assay. *Proc Natl Acad Sci USA* 1990;87: 8923–8929.

62. Wahlberg J, Lundeberg J, Hultman T, Uhlen M. General colorimetric method for DNA diagnostics allowing direct solid-phase genomic sequencing of the positive samples. *Proc Natl Acad Sci USA* 1990;87:6569–6573.

63. Coutlee F, Yang B, Bobo L, Mayur K, Yolken R, Viscidi R. Enzyme immunoassay for detection of hybrids between PCR-amplified HIV-1 DNA and a RNA probe:PCR-EIA. *AIDS Res Hum Retroviruses* 1990;6(6):775–784.

64. Yolken RH. New methods for the quantitation of microbial nucleic acids. *Pure Appl Chem* 1991;63(8):1127–1130.

65. Wilde J, Yolken R, Willoughby R, Eiden J. Improved detection of rotavirus shedding by polymerase chain reaction. *Lancet* 1991;337:323–326.

66. Allard A, Albinsson B, Wadell G. Detection of adenoviruses in stools from healthy persons and patients with diarrhea by two-step polymerase chain reaction. *J Med Virol* 1992;37(2):149–157.

67. DeLeon R, Matsui SM, Baric RS, et al. Detection of Norwalk virus in stool specimens by reverse transcriptase–polymerase chain reaction and nonradioactive oligoprobes. *J Clin Microbiol* 1992;20(12):3151–3157.

68. Jiang X, Wang J, Graham DY, Estes MK. Detection of Norwalk virus in stool by polymerase chain reaction. *J Clin Microbiol* 1992;30(10):2529–2534.

69. Wilde J, Van R, Pickering L, Eiden J, Yolken R. Detection of rotaviruses in the day care environment by reverse transcriptase polymerase chain reaction. *J Infect Dis* 1992;166:507–511.

70. Butz AM, Fosarelli P, Dick J, Cusack T, Yolken R. Prevalence of rotavirus on high-risk fomites in day-care facilities. *Pediatrics* 1993;92(2):202–205.

71. Atmar RL, Metcalf TG, Neill FH, Estes MK. Detection of en- teric viruses in oysters by using the polymerase chain reaction. *Appl Environ Microbiol* 1993;59(2):631–635.

72. Yang F, Xu X. A new method of RNA preparation for detection of hepatitis A virus in environmental samples by the polymerase chain reaction. *J Virol Meth* 1993;43(1):77–84.

73. Kapikian AZ, Yolken RH, Greenberg HB, et al. Gastroenteritis viruses. In: Lennette EH, Schmidt NJ, eds. *Diagnostic proce- dures for viral, rickettsial and chlamydial infections.* 5th ed. Washington, DC: American Public Health Association; 1979: 927–995.

Infections of the Gastrointestinal Tract,
edited by M. J. Blaser, P. D. Smith, J. I. Ravdin,
H. B. Greenberg, and R. L. Guerrant
Raven Press, Ltd., New York © 1995.

CHAPTER 83

Use of the Parasitology Laboratory in the Diagnosis of Gastrointestinal Infections

Richard A. Oberhelman and Donald J. Krogstad

Parasitic infections of the gastrointestinal (GI) tract are a major cause of morbidity in developing countries and are increasingly important in certain populations from developed countries, particularly in patients with the acquired immunodeficiency syndrome (AIDS) (1). In contrast to bacterial and viral infections, parasitic infections of the GI tract may be diagnosed rapidly by direct microscopic examination of clinical specimens. However, the diagnosis of parasitic infections still presents at least four challenges for the clinician and the laboratory technician. First, excretion of parasitic pathogens in stool may be intermittent, requiring examination of several specimens collected at different times (2). Second, identification of various morphological stages of parasites and differentiation between potential pathogens and commensal parasites requires expertise, which may be insufficient in laboratories that handle small numbers of specimens. Third, the presence of multiple parasites in a single specimen may make it difficult to determine whether disease is caused by one or more than one pathogen. Finally, the correlation between the presence of parasitic pathogens in stool and clinical disease is not always straightforward, particularly in persons from developing countries who may harbor potential pathogens asymptomatically for prolonged periods.

COMMON CLINICAL SYNDROMES CAUSED BY PARASITIC PATHOGENS OF THE GI TRACT

Diarrhea is the most common clinical syndrome associated with parasitic infections of the GI tract. Common parasitic pathogens associated with diarrhea and other GI tract syndromes are shown in Table 1. Although the distinction between bloody diarrhea ("dysentery") and wa-

tery diarrhea is often useful because these clinical syndromes are associated with different parasitic pathogens, many parasites that cause dysentery by disruption or invasion of the enteric mucosa may also cause watery diarrhea. Thus, the differential diagnosis of diarrhea due to parasitic infection of the GI tract also depends on epidemiological factors such as geographic location, age of the patient, and whether the patient is native to the region, an expatriate resident, or a traveler (3). A thoughtful assessment of the differential diagnosis should be the first step in laboratory evaluation because many potential pathogens can be ruled out on clinical and epidemiological grounds, allowing the laboratory to focus on the techniques most likely to yield positive results.

Other clinical syndromes associated with parasitic infections of the GI tract are abdominal pain, failure to thrive, and GI blood loss/anemia. Abdominal pain is a frequent symptom in patients with diarrhea, but it may also be a presenting symptom of parasitic infection of the GI tract in the absence of diarrhea. "Failure to thrive" is the euphemism for malnutrition commonly used in the United States. Malnutrition due to chronic diarrhea, malabsorption, or both may result from parasitic infections of the GI tract, and both wasting (weight-for-height deficit) and stunting (height-for-age deficit) have been associated with parasitic infections (particularly helminthic infections) among children in developing countries (4–6). The relationship between parasitic infections of the GI tract and malnutrition is multifactorial, and parasitic infection of the GI tract in a child with malnutrition does not necessarily indicate a cause-and-effect relationship. Fecal blood loss may produce anemia from chronic dysentery due to parasitic infection, although severe anemia from parasitic infection is usually due to hookworm infection.

DIAGNOSTIC TECHNIQUES FOR PARASITIC INFECTIONS OF THE GI TRACT

The decision to obtain laboratory studies for parasitic pathogens in patients with the syndromes described above

---

R. A. Oberhelman and D. J. Krogstad: Department of Tropical Medicine, Tulane School of Public Health and Tropical Medicine, New Orleans, Louisiana 70112.

TABLE 1. *Common clinical syndromes caused by parasitic infections in the GI tract*

A. Diarrhea
  1. Bloody diarrhea ("dysentery")
     Entamoeba histolytica
     Balantidium coli
     Trichuris trichiura
     Schistosoma sp.
     Strongyloides stercoralis
  2. Watery diarrhea
     Giardia lamblia
     Cryptosporidium parvum
     Cyclospora spp. ("Cyanobacterium-like bodies")
     Isospora belli
     Microsporidium sp.
B. Abdominal pain (often not associated with diarrhea)
     Ascaris lumbricoides
     Strongyloides stercoralis
     Hookworm
     Schistosoma sp.
     Taeniasis
C. Failure to thrive (weight-for-height deficit)
  1. Parasitic infections frequently associated with diarrhea
     Giardia lamblia
     Trichuris trichiura
     Entamoeba histolytica
     Cryptosporidium parvum
     Isospora belli
  2. Parasitic infections *infrequently* associated with diarrhea
     Ascaris lumbricoides
     Strongyloides stercoralis
     Hookworm
     Taeniasis
D. GI blood loss/anemia
     Hookworm (*Necator* sp., *Ancylostoma* sp.)

should be based in part on clinical and epidemiological features. For example, a child from an urban area in the United States with watery diarrhea presenting during the same week as other children with confirmed rotaviral infection should not ordinarily be evaluated for parasitic infection of the GI tract. Factors that would suggest a parasitic etiology of diarrhea include illness of more than 10 days duration, contact with known cases of parasitic infection (such as outbreaks of giardiasis in a day care center), impaired host immunity (especially patients with HIV/AIDS), and recent travel to developing countries (3). When parasitic infection of the GI tract is a logical consideration, the most reasonable approach is to start with direct microscopy because of its low cost and potentially high yield. If direct microscopy does not provide a diagnosis, other tests that should be considered based on the clinical history include concentration techniques, special stains, antigen detection tests, and serological techniques.

Specimen Collection

Stool Specimens

Examination of stool specimens allows for the diagnosis of 35 species of pathogenic parasites (7) and is the initial method of choice for detection of parasitic pathogens in patients with all of the clinical syndromes listed above. If the initial stool specimen does not reveal a diagnosis, it is useful to collect an additional two or three specimens over a 7- to 10-day period due to intermittent passage of organisms and fluctuating numbers of parasites. Stool specimens should be collected in clean, labeled containers free of water and urine that could lyse trophozoite forms of protozoan parasites (7). Specimens collected from toilet bowls or from soil or grass should not be used because they may contain contaminating parasites. Stools with a mushy, liquid consistency are most likely to contain short-lived trophozoite forms, and these should optimally be examined within 30 min of collection. With refrigeration, protozoal cysts remain intact for several days and helminth eggs can be identified for at least a week after specimen collection. However, stool specimens for parasites should never be frozen as cysts and eggs are often destroyed at temperatures below 0°C. Mineral oil and bismuth preparations should be avoided prior to stool collection because they interfere with the detection and identification of parasites (2). Barium contrast material also interferes with stool examination and should not be administered for 2 weeks prior to stool collection. Certain antibiotics such as tetracycline may also eliminate or reduce the numbers of some parasites in the stool for weeks.

Stool preservatives are useful for stool specimens that cannot be examined immediately. The choice of preservative will vary in different clinical settings because all solutions present certain benefits and limitations. Most stool preservatives are poisonous to humans if ingested and should therefore be stored in places where they are inaccessible to children and animals. *Ten percent formalin (4% formaldehyde) in saline* is the least expensive preservative available, but it is not suitable for trophozoites (8). Preservation is accomplished by emulsifying 1–2 g of stool in 5 mL of 10% formalin. Protozoal cysts are well preserved in 10% formalin for many months. A *sodium acetate, acetic acid,* and *formalin solution (SAF fixative)* offers many of the benefits of 10% formalin as well as preserving trophozoites, although the quality of the smears can be inconsistent. *Merthiolate iodine formalin fixative (MIF)* is a more complex formalin mixture that preserves trophozoites as well as cysts, eggs, and larvae for several weeks. MIF is a convenient preservative for processing large numbers of specimens in the field, and the iodine in MIF allows for easy interpretation of temporary smears without further staining. However, the instability of the Lugol's iodine solution in MIF results in a short shelf life for this preparation (good for several weeks if stored in a dark, well-stoppered bottle). Concentration of specimens in 10% formalin and MIF can be performed by sedimentation, but not by routine flotation procedures. *Polyvinyl alcohol fixative (PVA)* is the best preservative for trophozoites and is stable for 6–12 months (8). Preservation is accomplished by mixing 1 part stool with 9 parts PVA. The resin in PVA provides additional stability and prevents collapse of fragile protozoal forms. Unlike MIF, PVA-preserved specimens require staining for microscopy and cannot be easily screened in the field. *Schaudinn's fixative* is also excellent for preservation of all stages of protozoa and helminths, and like PVA it can be used to prepare permanent smears (8). Unlike PVA, it does not contain resin to promote adhesiveness for mucoid specimens. Both PVA and Schaudinn's fixative contain mercuric chloride, an especially poisonous and environmentally hazardous solution. Mercuric chloride must be "washed out" of the preserved specimen by immersing fixed slides in 70% ethanol-iodine solution for 3–5 min in order to prevent crystalline precipitation; longer washout periods may adversely affect staining of organisms (9). Fixatives and solutions containing mercuric chloride should be handled as hazardous waste and should be disposed of in well-sealed containers according to Occupational Safety and Health Administration (OSHA) regulations.

Duodenal Contents

Examination of duodenal contents may be useful in some patients with suspected *Giardia* or *Strongyloides* infection when stool specimens are unrevealing. Fresh specimens can be obtained by duodenal intubation with a weighted flexible feeding tube, and parasites may be observed directly by wet mount. An alternative method for obtaining duodenal fluid is with an Enterotest capsule or a locally constructed string capsule device (Fig. 1) (2). The Enterotest capsule is a gelatin capsule with a weight on one end and nylon thread wrapped inside. The nylon yarn protruding from one end of the string is taped to the

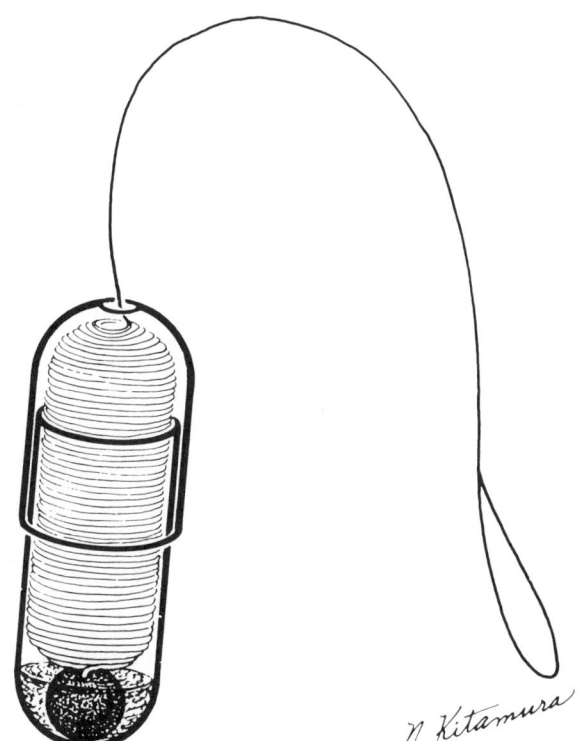

FIG. 1. The Enterotest capsule, for collection of duodenal secretions. (Illustration by Nobuko Kitamura. Photograph courtesy of L. Garcia and D. Bruckner.)

patient's cheek, and the capsule is swallowed. After 3–4 hr, when the end of the string has reached the duodenum, the string is removed. The presence of green, bile-stained fluid with pH >7 by test paper confirms the presence of duodenal fluid, which can then be examined by wet mount. *Duodenal biopsies* may be useful in some patients with chronic diarrhea when extensive evaluations are unrevealing, although this procedure requires more extensive technical expertise and should not be included in an initial evaluation. Biopsy specimens may reveal organisms such as *Isospora belli, Cryptosporidium parvum, Giardia lamblia,* and *Strongyloides stercoralis.*

Serum Specimens

Serological evaluation of patients with diarrheal diseases is of limited benefit because antibody tests do not distinguish between recent and old infections. Utility is greatest in nonendemic areas, in which the positive predictive value is greater. Blood for antibody detection should be collected in a sterile container in order to obtain serum for antibody testing. Sera are usually stored at −20°C or −70°C, and may be kept at 4°C for shorter times (days to 1–2 weeks). Repeated freezing and thawing should be avoided to prevent degradation of antibodies.

Macroscopic Examination of Stool and Perianal Secretions

Ascaris lumbricoides can often be observed directly in the stool of infected children, and they are easily identified by size (15–40 cm) and shape. *Enterobius vermicularis* eggs (50–60 × 20–30 μm) and adults (3–5 cm) are rarely visualized in the stool, but can be detected on the perianal area using the scotch tape test (see chapter by Gopinath and Keystone).

Biochemical and Microscopic Examination of Stool and Duodenal Secretions

Cytological and biochemical analysis of stool specimens may provide additional information to support the diagnosis of particular parasitic infections. The presence of *gross or occult blood* in the stool should be determined in most patients with symptoms that are possibly related to parasitic infections of the GI tract. Blood in the stool may indicate disruption of the mucus membrane or frank dysentery produced by pathogens that either invade or erode the intestinal mucosa. Lower GI tract bleeding may produce gross blood in the stool, although occult GI bleeding is more common and can only be detected biochemically. Parasites associated with bloody diarrhea include *E. histolytica, Trichuris trichiura,* and *Balantidium coli;* less common causes include *Strongyloides stercoralis* and *Schistosoma* spp. (Katayama fever). Other causes of blood in the stool should also be considered, including bacterial causes of dysentery and noninfectious causes of bleeding (e.g., diverticulitis, colonic polyps and cancers, hemorrhoids). Occult blood can be detected by reaction with guaiac solution, either as liquid suspension or by commercial test kits (e.g., Hemoccult cards). Tests for occult blood are very sensitive but, especially in the case of liquid guaiac reagent, they lack specificity. Tests for occult blood in stool may produce false-positive results from myoglobin in ingested meats (1).

Detection of microscopic *fecal fat* (steatorrhea) is an indication of fat malabsorption. Parasitic infections that are commonly associated with steatorrhea include giardiasis and strongyloidiasis. Excessive fecal fat produces a frothy appearance on gross examination and clear liquid fat droplets that may be observed on microscopic examination without special stains. Sudan stain may reveal needle-like crystals of fatty acids that are normal or large 10- to 75-μm orange globules suggestive of malabsorption (10). *Fecal leukocytes* indicate an inflammatory process in the GI tract and are commonly observed in bloody stool specimens from patients with dysentery. While the significance of scant numbers of fecal leukocytes may be questionable, the presence of large numbers (conventionally >20/high power field [HPF]) is suggestive of dysentery produced by parasites such as *E. histolytica, T. trichiura,* or *Balantidium coli* or by bacterial pathogens such as *Shigella* spp. One study demonstrated that fecal leukocytes were less numerous in the stools of patients with amebic dysentery (average 39 ± 6/HPF) than in specimens from patients with bacillary dysentery (average 81 ± 6), reflecting the greater extent of mucosal disease seen histologically in patents with shigellosis (11). *Charcot–Leyden crystals* (Fig. 2) are breakdown products of eosinophils seen in the stool of patients with amebiasis, *Isospora* infections, and helminthic infections (*Trichuris*, hookworm) (12). These crystals are needle-like and variable in size, and appear red–purple with trichrome stain. Charcot–Leyden crystals may be seen in stool specimens of patients with *Trichuris* infection even before worms or eggs appear in the stool (10). In cases of heavy infection with hookworms, these crystals may persist in the stool for several weeks after treatment.

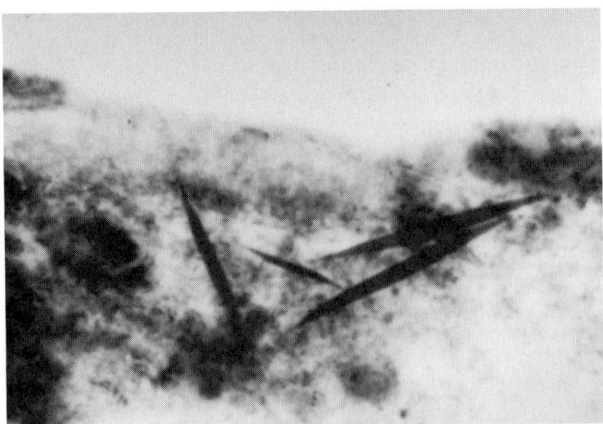

FIG. 2. Charcot–Leyden crystals (trichrome stain, oil immersion). Note the characteristic shape; various sizes will be present in a single specimen. The presence of these crystals indicates the presence of eosinophils in the contents of the intestinal lumen. (Courtesy of L. Garcia and D. Bruckner.) (See Plate 29.)

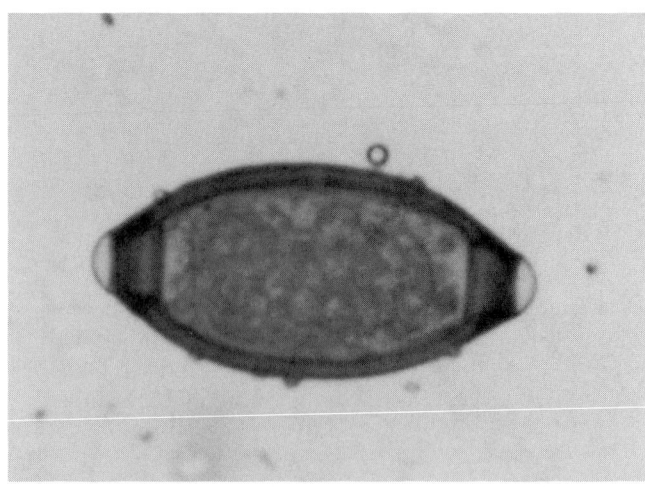

FIG. 3. *Trichuris trichiura* egg; iodine stain, wet mount. (Courtesy of L. Garcia and D. Bruckner.) (See Plate 30.)

Direct Microscopic Examination of Stool and Duodenal Secretions

Direct visualization of parasites in stool is the easiest and most definitive way to diagnose parasitic infections of the GI tract. The simplest and most inexpensive technique is a *saline preparation,* which is the method of choice for detection of motile trophozoites and flagellates (8). Helminth eggs may also be seen by this technique in patients with moderate to heavy infections. Saline preparations are performed by mixing a small amount of stool with a drop of physiological saline, and covering with a coverslip. Lugol's solution or D'Antoni's iodine may be added to enhance the distinctive morphology of parasites (Fig. 3). However, iodine kills organisms and eradicates motility; therefore, the slide should first be examined without staining. Proper technique requires an emulsion thin enough to be able to read newsprint through the slide; thicker solutions interfere with the ability to detect organisms. The *thick smear* or *Kato preparation* is especially useful for detection of small numbers of helminth eggs, especially for patients with suspected schistosomiasis (8). Thick smears do not permit detection of helminth larvae or protozoa. The advantage of this technique is that large amounts of stool (40–50 g) can be examined without concentration. Thick smears are performed by covering the fecal mass on a slide with a wettable cellophane strip that has been immersed in aqueous solution of glycerin (50%) with malachite green. After incubation for 1 hr the glycerin solution clears the fecal material, allowing for easy detection of helminth eggs. The disadvantage of the thick smear is that it requires a fresh specimen or a specimen that has been preserved soon after collection with sodium azide (3 mg/g of stool).

Stains of fecal smears may enhance detection of parasitic pathogens in certain cases. Although many laboratories in developed countries use stains routinely for all specimens, this technique is not cost effective for developing countries (13). Stains are most useful for detection

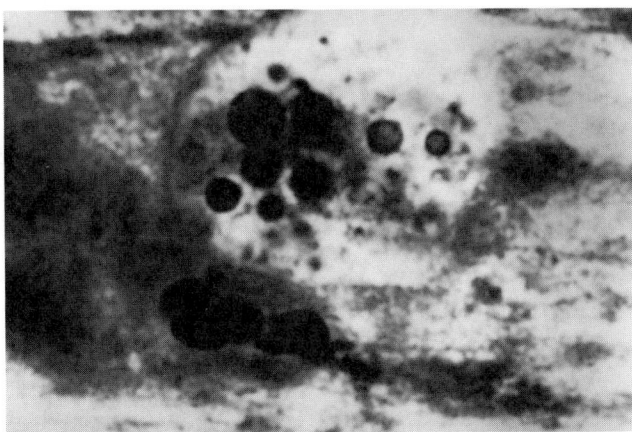

FIG. 4. *Entamoeba histolytica* trophozoite; trichrome stain. Note the presence of ingested red blood cells in the cytoplasm, which stain red with trichrome stain. (Courtesy of L. Garcia and D. Bruckner.) (See Plate 31.)

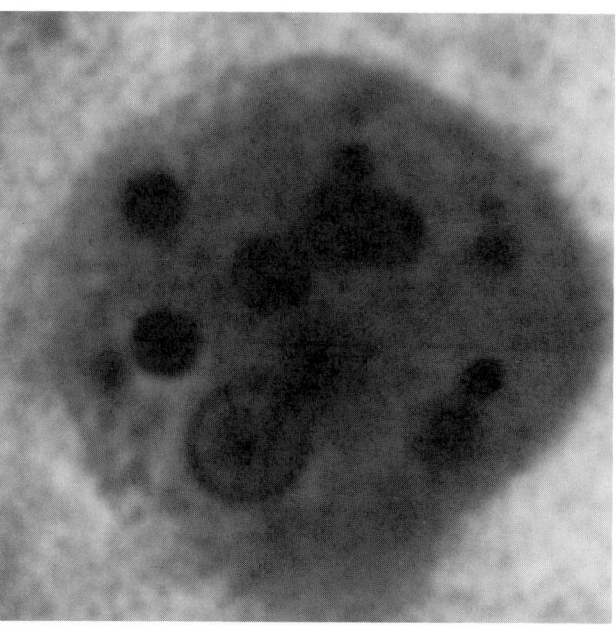

FIG. 5. *Entamoeba histolytica* trophozoite; iron and hematoxylin stain. In contrast to the example shown in Fig. 4, ingested red blood cells stain dark blue or black with iron and hematoxylin stain. (Courtesy of L. Garcia and D. Bruckner.)

of fragile trophozoite stages, for examination of specimens from patients with diarrhea, or to clarify parasite morphology when mixed infections are suspected. *Dientamoeba fragilis* is most easily detected in stained smears because it does not exist in a cyst stage. Trichrome stain (Fig. 4) is the most widely used technique because it is simple and sensitive. Although traditional methods required prolonged incubation periods for staining, new trichome staining techniques can be completed in 8–12 min (8). Nuclei of protozoa stain red to pink with trichome stain, with the exception of *Entamoeba coli* (purple staining). The *iron-hematoxylin stain* (Figs. 5 and 6) permits visualization of more detail, but it is also more complex and time consuming than the trichrome stain. Organisms stain darker and with greater contrast than with trichrome, allowing for easy detection of parasites while scanning at 40× magnification. The combination of preservation with PVA and iron-hematoxylin staining is probably the best technique for detection of *E. histolytica* trophozoites, as demonstrated in studies comparing this technique with other staining and concentration procedures (13). When looking for trophozoites stained unconcentrated specimens should always be evaluated since concentration techniques often destroy these fragile organisms. Proper procedures must be followed to wash out PVA when specimens are stained with iron-hematoxylin in order to prevent the dissolution of PVA in aqueous solution, causing the release of the stool specimen from the slide.

Quantitation of Parasitic Infections by Egg Counts

In some cases, quantitation of helminth eggs may provide clinically useful information. These techniques are most applicable for cases of schistosomiasis or infections with soil-transmitted nematodes (e.g., *Ascaris*, *Trichuris*, hookworm). Egg counts provide a rough estimate of worm burdens in population surveys conducted before and after

interventions (such as drug therapy), and they may aid the clinician managing an individual patient. Quantitation techniques have been standardized only for helminth eggs; assessment of parasite burdens for other GI tract organisms is less useful. Egg counts are always suspect due to the nature of the test. Results may be affected by characteristics of the specimen (e.g., consistency), parasite factors (e.g., duration of infection, presence of multiple parasites), and host factors (e.g., intermittent excretion, immunological responses).

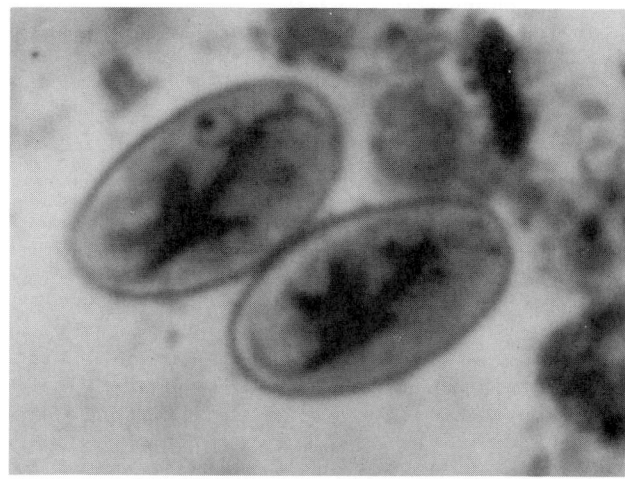

FIG. 6. *Giardia lamblia* cysts; iron and hematoxylin stain. (Courtesy of L. Garcia and D. Bruckner.) (See Plate 32.)

The *Stoll egg count* is the most widely used technique in reference laboratories (8). Although this method is relatively precise, it is of limited use in developing countries because it requires a special apparatus (Stoll flask, A. H. Thomas Co., Philadelphia, or another stoppered, calibrated flask). In brief, 4 mL of stool is added to 56 mL of 0.1 N sodium hydroxide solution in a stoppered flask containing small beads (about 5 mm diameter). After the flask has been allowed to stand 12–24 hr with intermittent agitation, a-0.075 mL (75-μL) sample is removed and placed on a microscope slide for examination. Eggs counted on the slide are multiplied by 200 to determine the number of eggs per gram of stool. The *direct smear egg count* is less precise but more adaptable to laboratories with limited resources. This technique is based on the preparation of standardized smears containing 1 or 2 mg of stool and counting all eggs on the smear in a standardized fashion. Since most laboratories are not able to make standard smears, many technicians estimate a 2-mg specimen for quantitation. This technique provides a rough estimate of worm burden when performed by experienced technicians, although practical limitations prevent reading smears made with excessively large amounts of stool (a 3-mg specimen will make the smear too thick to read). Egg counts per gram of stool are estimated by using the appropriate mathematical conversion factor, e.g., number of eggs in direct smear ($\approx$2 mg) $\times$ 500 = eggs/g.

Interpretation of egg counts depends on the infecting organism. An adult female *Ascaris* produces an average of 2000 eggs per gram of stool, and adult female hookworm and *Trichuris* produce about 50 eggs/g (8). "Light" infections with *Ascaris* are generally those with egg counts less than 20,000/g, "moderate" infections are those with egg counts between 20,000 and 100,000/g, and "heavy" infections are those with >100,000 eggs/g of stool. However, these counts must be interpreted with caution because any *Ascaris* infection can produce serious disease due to the potential effects of adult worms. Light infections with hookworm and *Trichuris* have egg counts less than 5000/g, "moderate" infections are those between 5000 and 25,000/g, and "heavy" infections are those exceeding 25,000/g. Hookworm infections may produce symptoms with relatively low egg counts (above 2500/g), while *Trichuris* rarely produces symptoms when egg counts are below 20,000/g.

Concentration Techniques for Diagnosis of Parasitic Infections

Concentration techniques are useful for detecting small numbers of parasites that may not be seen on direct smears, although trophozoites are destroyed by most concentration procedures (8). Concentration is based on the separation of other elements of stool that differ from parasites by size or density, and it is achieved either by sedimentation (removal of lighter elements in the supernatant) or by flotation (lifting of parasites out of a mass of denser objects). *Formalin-ether* and *formalin–ethyl acetate sedimentation* are common techniques performed in very similar ways. Ethyl acetate has been used more frequently

than ether in recent years because it is less explosive (8). The ethyl acetate technique is better than ether for visualization of *Giardia* cysts or *Taenia* eggs, although ethyl acetate is less effective than ether for dissolution of fat and mucus in stool specimens. Formalin–ethyl acetate sedimentation is performed by mixing stool with 10% formalin and normal saline and centrifugation, after which this procedure is repeated with addition of ethyl acetate to the formalin solution. Variations of this technique are described for stool specimens preserved in PVA, MIF, and other solutions. *Gravity sedimentation* is the simplest concentration technique, allowing for concentration of eggs, cysts, and larvae without a centrifuge or expensive equipment. The disadvantage of this technique is that parasites may be difficult to visualize because it also concentrates fecal debris. Gravity sedimentation is performed by mixing 10 g stool in 50–100 mL water, straining through gauze, and decanting the supernatant after allowing fecal material to settle in solution. This procedure is repeated until the supernatant is clear. Sedimentation can be enhanced by adding glycerin to the water (0.5% solution), and a 0.85% saline solution should be used instead of water if *Schistosoma* infection is suspected (schistosome eggs will hatch in water). The *Baermann larval extraction procedure* (Fig. 7) is another procedure used for concentration of nematode larvae, especially *Strongy-*

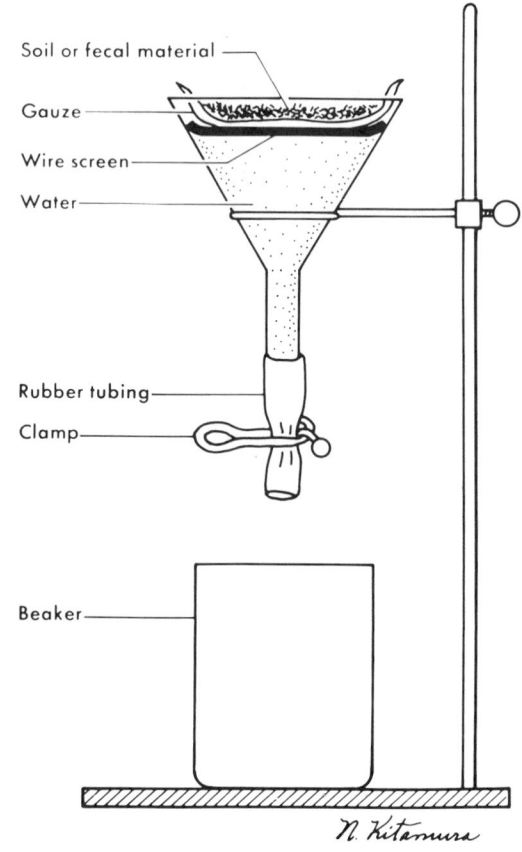

FIG. 7. The Baermann larval extraction apparatus. (Illustration by Nobuko Kitamura. Photograph courtesy of L. Garcia and D. Bruckner.)

loides (14). A wire mesh covered with a piece of gauze is placed over a closed funnel filled with water, and the stool specimen to be tested is placed on a filter paper and inverted specimen side down on the gauze. Larvae migrate from the stool and are concentrated at the bottom of the funnel. This technique can also be used to recover larvae from soil and tissue samples.

Flotation techniques provide cleaner specimens than sedimentation procedures, although they have the disadvantage of distorting some organisms in dense solutions. The *zinc sulfate flotation technique* is widely used to concentrate protozoal cysts and helminth eggs, but it is not suitable for concentrating fatty stool specimens or for detecting the eggs of trematodes (e.g., schistosomes) or most cestodes (e.g., tapeworms). Stool specimens to be examined are mixed in water and zinc sulfate solution, and following centrifugation the center of the surface film is stained and examined microscopically. *Sheather's sugar flotation technique* is especially suited for the detection of *Cryptosporidium* sp. in fresh or formalin-preserved specimens, although these can also be seen in zinc sulfate preparations. Some investigators report that *Cryptosporidium* oocysts are more refractile and easier to visualize by sugar flotation than by zinc sulfate flotation (8).

Special Staining Techniques for Parasite Identification

Certain parasitic infections of the GI tract require special staining procedures for diagnosis. *Cryptosporidium parvum,* unlike other coccidian parasites such as *Isospora belli,* does not stain by trichrome or iron-hematoxylin techniques. *Cryptosporidia* are generally diagnosed by a modified *Ziehl–Neelsen acid-fast stain* (Fig. 8). Several modifications of the Ziehl–Neelsen staining techniques that can be used to stain either fresh specimens or formalin-fixed specimens include the modified acid-fast stain (requires heat) and the Kinyoun carbol-fuschin stain, while the dimethylsulfoxide (DMSO)–modified acid-fast stain can only be performed on fresh specimens (8). Acid-fast stains have also been used to detect *Cyclospora* sp. ("*Cyanobacterium*-like bodies"), a parasite that has recently been associated with diarrheal disease in humans (15). *Cryptosporidium* oocysts stain an intense red color with black granules inside, whereas *Isospora* sp. generally demonstrate a red inner germinal mass (sporoblast) with only an outline of red around the cyst wall. *Auramine-rhodamine fluorescent staining* is also useful for detection of acid-fast organisms, but is limited by the need for a fluorescent microscope (16).

Microsporidia species, in particular *Enterocytozoon bieneusi,* are an increasingly important cause of diarrheal diseases in persons infected with HIV (17). These small organisms are very difficult to visualize in stool specimens, although recent studies have reported detection of these organisms in stool and duodenal secretions using a modified trichrome stain with a high concentration of chromotrope 2R (18). Microsporidia are usually seen on small intestine biopsy specimens using Giemsa stain. Intestinal biopsies stained with Giemsa may also reveal other parasitic pathogens, such as *Giardia lamblia.* Microsporidia have also been detected in stool by a modified Giemsa stain procedure, although technical requirements and unknown sensitivity will limit the usefulness of this technique (19).

Antibody Detection (Serological Techniques)

Serological tests are available for many enteric parasitic pathogens, although the usefulness of these tests is limited. The major problems of serological diagnosis are that serum antibodies may not reach high levels when infections are limited to the GI tract, and that it is often difficult to distinguish between recent and past infections. Serum antibody responses are produced in many cases of *giardiasis,* and *Giardia* IgM assays available in some research laboratories may be useful to detect recent infection. Commercial kits for detection of *Giardia*-specific antibodies are not available. Serological tests for *amebiasis* are most useful for the detection of invasive disease, particularly for cases of liver abscess, e.g., indirect hemagglutination titers (IHA) exceed 1:128 in 95% of liver abscess cases, 85% of dysentery cases (20). The IHA assay has greater sensitivity and specificity than other assays, such as counterimmune electrophoresis (CIE) and enzyme immunoassay (EIA), although titers do not correlate with severity of disease. Antibodies to *Cryptosporidium* may be detected by EIA for parasite-specific IgG and IgM, and these assays have been used as diagnostic tools for outbreaks (16). However, experience with these assays is limited and they are only available through research laboratories.

Antigen Detection Tests

Antigen detection tests for stool testing are available commercially for *Giardia* and *Cryptosporidium.* Several CIE and EIA kits can be used to detect *Giardia* from both fresh and formalin-preserved specimens, with sensitivities ranging from 90% to 98% and specificities from 87%

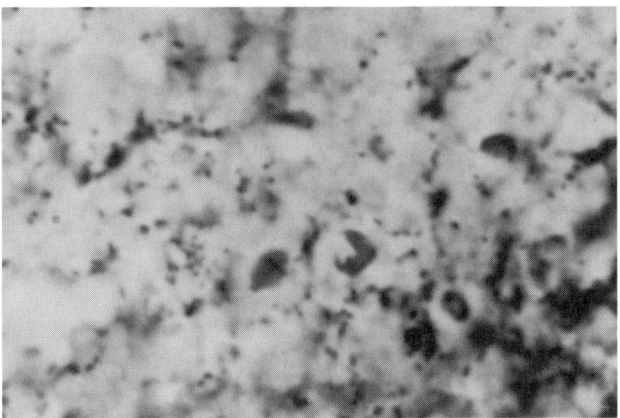

FIG. 8. *Cryptosporidium parvum* oocyts, modified acid-fast stain. (Courtesy of L. Garcia and D. Bruckner.) (See Plate 33.)

to 100% (21). Some CIE and EIA assays cannot be performed on specimens in stool preservatives. Immunofluorescent antibody (IFA) assays have also been used to detect *Giardia* cysts in frozen stool specimens, where cyst integrity may be distorted by freezing and thawing (21). One product is a combined IFA with monoclonal antibodies for *Giardia* cysts and *Cryptosporidium* oocysts for water testing purposes and testing of high-risk populations. Antigen detection tests have also been described for *E. histolytica* in stool by EIA, but these are used mostly as research tools.

Molecular Biological Approaches

The use of molecular technology has revolutionized the diagnosis of infectious diseases, and some DNA probes and polymerase chain reaction (PCR) assays have been developed for parasitic pathogens in the GI tract. *Cryptosporidium parvum* has been diagnosed by PCR in fixed, paraffin-embedded tissues, but this technique has not been reported for diagnosis of *Cryptosporidium* in stool (22). The presence of abundant genetic material from the fecal bacterial flora in stool requires the use of highly specific PCR assays in order to prevent false-positive reactions. DNA probes have been developed for *E. histolytica,* and some studies have shown close to 100% sensitivity of detection in stool with small numbers of samples (13). DNA probes (with or without PCR) provide the added advantage of specific antigen (gene) detection, a feature that has been applied to the differentiation of pathogenic and nonpathogenic *E. histolytica* at the molecular level (23). The advantages of DNA probes and PCR are that they can be used to process large numbers of specimens rapidly, results can be provided quickly, and with refinement they may be very cost-effective (13). Limitations of molecular technique include their restricted availability and the lack of sensitivity of some DNA probe tests. Further refinement will be necessary for these tests to become widely available and useful for the majority of clinicians.

Culture Techniques

Culture of parasitic pathogens of the GI tract is labor-intensive and rarely if ever indicated in medical practice. Culture techniques are best described for *E. histolytica* (24). Since these techniques require a very fresh specimen, they are not useful for processing specimens received in the mail. Several culture media for *E. histolytica* have been developed, e.g., Cleveland and Collier's Liver Extract as well as Modified Boeck and Drbohlov's LES. Specimens are incubated in culture media at 37°C, and fluid from the bottom of the flask is examined microscopically at 24–48 hr. Maintenance of viable cultures requires the inoculation of fresh media every 2–3 days, and aseptic technique is critical because bacterial contamination will kill the parasites. Culture methods have also been used to distinguish between pathogenic and nonpathogenic *E. histolytica* by enzymatic assays. The morphology of *E. histolytica* trophozoites in culture is essentially identical

to those seen in stool; cyst forms do not develop in liquid culture. Techniques for axenic cultivation of *Giardia* have also been described, although this procedure is rarely useful for diagnostic purposes.

SUMMARY AND OVERALL APPROACH TO THE PATIENT WHO MAY HAVE A PARASITIC INFECTION OF THE GI TRACT

The initial diagnostic evaluation must be guided by several factors, including the medical history, severity of disease, extent of medical evaluation for nonparasitic diseases, and cost effectiveness of the tests. Model algorithms for the evaluation of patients with diarrhea and other GI tract symptoms are shown in Tables 2 and 3. In general, the evaluation of the patient with diarrhea should follow a directed approach using diagnostic tools that are simple, inexpensive, and potentially useful for diagnosis of a variety of pathogens. These would include the biochemical and cytological tests described in this chapter and direct microscopic examination for parasites, along with selected tests for bacterial and viral pathogens (e.g., stool culture, rotaviral EIA). Some ''special stains'' are often included in the initial battery of tests, such as an acid-fast stain for the detection of *Cryptosporidium*.

For patients with prolonged diarrhea or other risk factors for parasitic infection whose initial evaluation is nonproductive, a second order of diagnostic tests may be useful. These tests should be selected based on the likely presence of particular parasites, since many tests are organism-specific or are limited in diagnostic scope. Second-order tests include thick fecal smears, concentration techniques (e.g., sucrose or zinc sulfate flotation for *Cryptosporidium*, Baermann extraction for *Strongyloides*), special stains (e.g., acid-fast stain for *Cryptosporidium*), and antigen detection tests (e.g., CIE or EIA for *Giardia*). The decision regarding which second-order tests to perform also depends on available laboratory resources, cost, and clinical usefulness of the information (e.g., can the infection that would be diagnosed be treated?). Although thick smears, concentration techniques, and special stains are usually not expensive tests, the limited experience of many diagnostic laboratories with these techniques may reduce the yield. When the receiving laboratory is inexperienced with techniques requested, these assays should be performed in a reference laboratory. Antigen detection tests may be more costly than other second-order tests, and their use should generally be limited to more complicated cases where the results will affect therapeutic decisions.

A third order of tests may be indicated for a few patients with severe disease or when unusual presentations of parasitic diseases are a diagnostic consideration. These tests would include antibody detection, molecular approaches, and culture techniques. In addition to the considerations mentioned for second-order tests, one must also consider lag time from test submission to results, especially for tests sent to reference laboratories that may perform such tests infrequently. In addition, in the case of serological tests one must consider whether the test result will distin-

TABLE 2. *Approach to the diagnosis of parasitic pathogens in the patient with diarrhea*[a]

Clinical features suggestive of a parasitic etiology:
  a. Duration of illness >10 days
  b. Recent travel to developing countries
  c. Consistent epidemiological pattern (e.g., outbreaks in day care centers)
  d. Altered host immunity (esp. HIV-positive)

Specimen collection:
  a. Unpreserved stool—for saline smear, egg counts, Baermann concentration, some antigen detection tests
  b. Preserved stool—
    For cysts and eggs: 10% formalin
    For cysts, eggs, and trophozoites: PVA, MIF Schaudinn's (SAF)[b]

First-Order Evaluation
Biochemical/cytological evaluation:
  a. Occult blood—Hemetest
  b. Fecal leukocytes—methylene blue stain
  c. Charcot–Leyden crystals
  d. Fecal fat—Sudan stain

Dysenteric (Bloody)
    Small volume, abundant mucus
    Soft consistency
    + Fecal leukocytes
    + Occult blood
    ± Fecal fat
    ± Charcot–Leyden[c]

Frequent etiologies shown in Table 1

Nondysenteric (watery)
    Large volume scant mucus
    Liquid consistency
    − Fecal leukocytes
    − Occult blood
    ± Fecal fat
    ± Charcot–Leyden[d]

Frequent etiologies shown in Table 1

Direct microscopy
    Saline smear for motile trophozoites
    Stained smear: trichrome or iron/hematoxylin

Direct microscopy
    Saline smear for motile trophozoites
    Stained smear: trichrome or iron/hematoxylin

Second-Order Evaluation
Thick smear if suspect helminth infection (especially *Schistosoma*):

Concentration techniques
    Formalin–ethyl acetate: for most cysts and eggs
    Zinc sulfate flotation: for most cysts and eggs (except *Strongyloides* and tapeworms)
    Baermann extraction: if *Strongyloides* is suspected

Concentration techniques
    Formalin–ethyl acetate: for most cysts and eggs
    Zinc sulfate flotation: for most cysts and eggs
    Sheather's sugar flotation: if suspect *Cryptosporidia*

Special Stains
    Acid-fast or rhodamine-auramine stain: if suspect *Cryptosporidia*, *Isospora*, or *Cyclospora*
    Giemsa stain: if suspect *Microsporidia*

Antigen Detection Tests
    for *Giardia*: EIA, CIE, IFA
    for *Cryptosporidium*: IFA
    (for *E. histolytica*: EIA)[b]

Third-Order Evaluation
Serological evaluation[b]
    Potentially useful serologies: for *E. histolytica*: IHA, (CIE, EIA)

Serological evaluation[b]
    Potentially useful serologies:
    for *Giardia*: (EIA)
    for *Cryptosporidium*: (EIA)

Culture techniques

Culture techniques

Molecular techniques

Molecular techniques

[a] Flow charts indicate the usual sequence for obtaining specific tests, based on the progression from the initial first-order evaluation to more sophisticated and directed studies. Differences in common diagnostic techniques for dysentery and watery diarrhea are shown. Most diagnostic evaluations do not require that all tests listed be performed; the extent of the diagnostic workup will depend on the results of preliminary diagnostic tests, the clinical picture, and the need for a definitive diagnosis.
[b] Choices shown in parentheses are generally less optimal than other choices.
[c] Charcot–Leyden crystals are characteristically seen in cases of dysentery due to *E. histolytica* and *Trichuris trichiura*.
[d] Charcot–Leyden crystals seen in cases of watery diarrhea are often associated with *Isospora belli* infection.

TABLE 3. *Approach to the diagnosis of parasitic pathogens in the patient with abdominal pain or failure to thrive[a]*

Clinical features suggestive of a parasitic etiology:
  Altered host immunity (esp. HIV-positive)
  Recent travel to developing country
Frequent etiologies shown in Table 1
Specimen collection:
  a. Unpreserved stool—for saline smear, egg counts, Baermann concentration, some antigen detection tests
  b. Preserved stool—
     For cysts and eggs: 10% formalin
     For cysts, eggs, and trophozoites: PVA, MIF Schaudinn's (SAF)[b]

First-Order Evaluation

Biochemical/cytological evaluation:
  a. Occult blood—Hemetest
  b. Fecal leukocytes—methylene blue stain
  c. Charcot–Leyden Crystals
  d. Fecal fat—Sudan Stain
Direct microscopy
  Saline smear for motile trophozoites
  Stained smear: trichrome or iron-hematoxylin

Second-Order Evaluation

Thick smear: if suspect helminth infection (especially *Schistosoma*)
Concentration techniques
  Formalin–ethyl acetate: for most cysts and eggs
  Zinc sulfate flotation: for most cysts and eggs (except *Strongyloides* and tapeworms)
  Baermann extraction: if *Strongyloides* is suspected
  Sheather's sugar flotation: if suspect *Cryptosporidia*
Special stains
  Acid-fast or rhodamine-auramine stain: if suspect *Cryptosporidia*, *Isospora*, or *Cyclospora*
Antigen detection tests
  for *Giardia*: EI, CIE, IFA
  for *Cryptosporidium*: IFA
  (for *E. histolytica*: EIA)[b]

Third-order Evaluation

Serological evaluation[b]
Potentially useful serologies:
  for *E. histolytica*: IHA, (CIE, EIA)
  for *Giardia*: (EIA)
  for *Cryptosporidium*: (EIA)

Culture techniques
Molecular techniques

─────────────────

[a] Flow charts indicate the usual sequence for obtaining specific tests, based on the progression from the initial first-order evaluation to more sophisticated and directed studies. Differences in common diagnostic techniques for dysentery and watery diarrhea are shown. Most diagnostic evaluations do not require that all tests listed be performed; the extent of the diagnostic workup will depend on the results of preliminary diagnostic tests, the clinical picture, and the need for a definitive diagnosis.

[b] Choices shown in parentheses are generally less optimal than other choices.

guish between past and recent infection and the degree of test standardization. The cost of most third-order tests is justified only in a limited number of patients.

ACKNOWLEDGMENT

The authors thank Dr. M. D. Little and Dr. Antonio D'Alessandro for their valuable help in the preparation of this manuscript.

REFERENCES

1. Guerrant RL, Bobak DA. Bacterial and protozoal gastroenteritis. *N Engl J Med* 1991;325:327–340.
2. Carroll MJ. Routine procedures for examination of stool and blood for parasites. *Pediatr Clin North Am* 1985;32:1041–1046.
3. Guerrant RL, Hughes JM, Lima NL, Crane J. Diarrhea in developed and developing countries: magnitude, special settings, and etiologies. *Rev Infect Dis* 1990;12(Suppl. 1):S41–S50.
4. Thein-Hliang, Thane-Toe, Than-Saw, Myat-Lay-Kyin, Myint-Lwin. A controlled chemotherapeutic intervention trial on the relationship between *Ascaris lumbricoides* infection and malnutrition in children. *Trans R Soc Trop Med Hyg* 1991;85:523–528.
5. Stephenson L, Latham MC, Kurz KM, Kinoti SN, Brigham H. Treatment with a single dose of albendazole improves growth of Kenyan schoolchildren with hookworm, *Trichuris trichiura*, and *Ascaris lumbricoides* infections. *Am J Trop Med Hyg* 1989; 41:78–87.
6. Stephenson LS, Crompton DWT, Latham MC, Schulpen TWJ, Nesheim MC, Jansen AAJ. Relationships between *Ascaris* infection and growth of malnourished preschool children in Kenya. *Am J Clin Nutr* 1980;33:1165—1172.
7. Desowitz RS. Fecal, blood, and urine examinations in parasitology. In: Goldsmith R, Heyneman D, eds. *Tropical medicine and parasitology.* Norwalk, CT: Appleton and Lange; 1989:866–875.
8. Ash LR, Orihel TC. *Parasites: a guide to laboratory procedures and identification.* Chicago: American Society of Clinical Pathologists Press; 1987.
9. Garcia LS, Bruckner DA. Macroscopic and microscopic examination of fecal specimens. In: *Diagnostic medical parasitology.* 2nd ed. Washington, DC: American Society for Microbiology; 1993:chap. 26.
10. Guerrant RL. Principles and syndromes of enteric infection. In: Mandell GL, Douglas RG Jr, Bennett JE, eds. *Principles and practice of infectious diseases.* New York: Churchill Livingstone; 1990.
11. Speelman P, McGaughlin R, Kabir I, Butler T. Differential clinical features and stool findings in shigellosis and amoebic dysentery. *Trans R Soc Trop Med Hyg* 1987;81:549–551.
12. Beaver PC, Jung RC, Cupp EW. Examination of specimens for parasites. In: *Clinical parasitology.* 9th ed. Philadelphia: Lea and Febiger; 1984;733–758.
13. Proctor EM. Laboratory diagnosis of amebiasis. *Clin Lab Med* 1991;11:829–859.
14. Garcia LS. Special laboratory examinations for parasitic infections. *Pediatr Clin North Am* 1985;32:1047–1061.
15. Ortega YR, Sterling CR, Gilman RH, Cama VA, Diaz F. *Cyclospora* species—a new protozoan pathogen of humans. *N Engl J Med* 1993;328:1308–1312.
16. Current WL, Garcia LS. Cryptosporidiosis. *Clin Microbiol Rev* 1991;4:325–358.
17. Schattenkerk J, Van Gool T, Van Ketel R, et al. Clinical significance of small intestinal microsporidiosis in HIV-1 infected individuals. *Lancet* 1991;337:895–898.
18. Weber R, Bryan RT, Owen RL, et al. Improved light-microscopical detection of *Microsporidia* spores in stool and duodenal aspirates. *N Engl J Med* 1992;326:161–166.
19. Orenstein JM, Chiang J, Steinberg W, Smith PD, Rotterdam H, Kotler DP. Intestinal microsporidiosis as a cause of diarrhea in

human immunodeficiency virus–infected patients: a report of 20 cases. *Hum Pathol* 1990;21:475–481.

20. Botero D. Amebiasis. In: Goldsmith R, Heyneman D, eds. *Tropical medicine and parasitology*. Norwalk, CT: Appleton and Lange; 1989:224–228.
21. Wolfe MS. Giardiasis. *Clin Microbiol Rev* 1992;5:93–100.
22. Laxer MA, D'Nicuola ME, Patel RJ. Detection of *Cryptosporidium parvum* DNA in fixed, paraffin-embedded tissue by the polymerase chain reaction. *Am J Trop Med Hyg* 1992;47:450–455.
23. Ambroise-Thomas P. Les sondes moléculaires dans l'étude et le diagnostique des maladies parasitaires. *Ann Parasitol Hum Comp* 1990;65(Suppl. 1):83–88.
24. Beaver PC, Jung RC, Cupp EW. Culture methods. In: *Clinical parasitology*. 9th ed. Philadelphia: Lea and Febiger; 1984:759–775.

Infections of the Gastrointestinal Tract,
edited by M. J. Blaser, P. D. Smith, J. I. Ravdin,
H. B. Greenberg, and R. L. Guerrant
Raven Press, Ltd., New York © 1995.

CHAPTER 84

Role of Endoscopy in the Evaluation of Gastrointestinal Infections

Harvey Young, Kathryn Swanson, Edward Slosberg, and John Cello

The advent of flexible endoscopy has dramatically changed the way in which we evaluate gastrointestinal (GI) pathology. This technology also plays a major role in the management of GI tract infections. The plethora of opportunistic GI infections seen in immunosuppressed patients has further expanded the utility of endoscopy. This chapter addresses the impact of endoscopy in the management of infections affecting the GI tract, the pancreas, and the biliary system. As the clinical syndromes of these infections have already been covered in detail elsewhere in this book, this chapter will concentrate on the endoscopic findings associated with these pathogens. The diagnostic efficacy of endoscopy in these infections will be compared to other diagnostic modalities. The specific therapeutic capabilities of endoscopy on some of these infections will be emphasized. Nosocomial infections induced by endoscopy and methods to prevent these infections will also be discussed.

ROLE OF ESOPHAGOGASTRODUODENOSCOPY IN INFECTIONS OF THE ESOPHAGUS, STOMACH, AND DUODENUM

Esophagogastroduodenoscopy provides a simple, safe, and direct examination of the mucosa from the esophagus to the duodenum. This procedure serves as a convenient method for tissue sampling in order to identify the specific pathogen involved in infections of this anatomic region.

H. Young, K. Swanson, and E. Slosberg: Department of Medicine, Stanford University School of Medicine, Stanford, California 94305.
J. Cello: Department of Medicine, San Francisco General Hospital, and University of California, San Francisco, California 94110.

Bacterial Infections

Helicobacter pylori *Gastritis*

H. pylori has gained widespread attention in the past decade. Its role in the pathogenesis of gastritis, gastric and duodenal ulceration has been well established. Its association with gastric carcinoma and lymphoma has been strongly suggested (1–4).

The endoscopic appearance of *H. pylori* infection is variable. Most commonly, patients have chronic gastritis, with mucosal erythema and sometimes gastroduodenal erosions (1,5,6). The mucosal erythema may be diffuse, focal, or in linear streaks. These changes are usually most prominent in the antrum. *H. pylori* can be found in 90–100% of duodenal ulcers and in 70% of gastric ulcers (2,5). However, the gastric mucosa may also appear entirely normal and still harbor the bacteria in biopsy specimens (5). These endoscopic changes are also frequently seen in gastritis induced by nonsteroidal antiinflammatory agents. Therefore, the endoscopic appearance alone cannot predict the presence or absence of *H. pylori*.

The normal esophagus does not appear to be affected by *H. pylori*. However, *H. pylori* organisms can be found in up to 62% of patients with Barrett's metaplasia in which the esophagus contains columnar-lined epithelium of the gastric type. The presence of the bacteria in these patients is not associated with esophagitis (6). *H. pylori* has also been found in dental plaque (7) and in heterotopic gastric mucosa (8).

During endoscopy, biopsies or rapid urease testing are necessary to confirm the presence of *H. pylori*. Biopsy specimens should be taken from both the antrum and the fundus. The organism is commonly found at both sites, but can be found in the fundus alone or in the antrum alone (1,5,9). Based on small studies, the taking of biopsies from either the antrum or fundus alone will yield positive results in 80–90% of cases, but the taking of biopsies from both sites will increase the yield to nearly 100%. Since the presence of *H. pylori* may be patchy, two biopsies should be taken in each area (10). The rapid urease tests have the advantage of providing immediate information, and have a sensitivity of 91–98% with a specificity of 100% compared to histological testing (2,11). They are also inexpensive. Histology adds the benefit of assessing microscopic evidence of inflammation. Culture of biopsy specimens is not routinely performed since it is relatively insensitive (1,2,5,9–11).

At present, endoscopic biopsy with either the rapid urease testing or histological examination is perhaps the most common method used to establish the diagnosis of active *H. pylori* infection. In the near future, newer noninvasive methods such as serology and breath tests probably will replace endoscopy in this function (see chapter by Holtmann and Talley).

Whipple's Disease

This is a rare disease that may affect many organ systems. It is caused by a gram-positive bacillus that has been identified using molecular genetic techniques, but has not yet been cultured *in vitro* (12; see chapter by Relman).

The symptoms are protean, and may include diarrhea, weight loss, fever, migratory arthritis, and central nervous system symptoms.

The small bowel is involved during the course of the illness in most patients, and the diagnosis is most commonly established after examination and biopsy of the postbulbar duodenal mucosa. The characteristic duodenal abnormality is a pale, yellow, shaggy mucosa alternating with erythematous, erosive, or friable mucosa (13,14) (Fig. 1). Alternatively, only yellow–white plaques or ero-

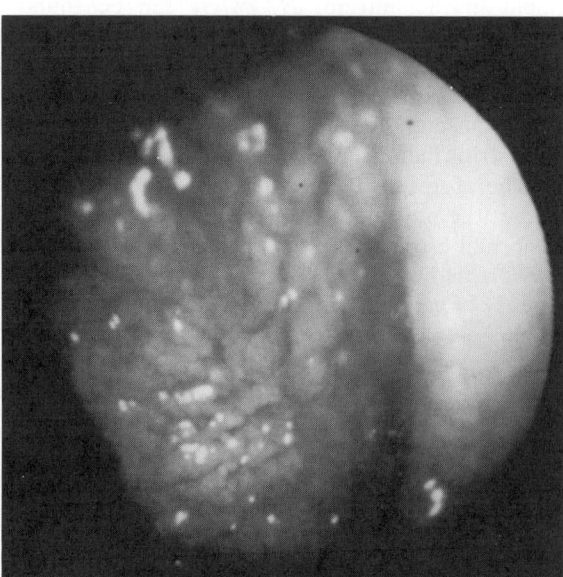

FIG. 1. Whipple's disease. Note characteristic coarsening of the villous pattern and pale, yellow, shaggy mucosa. (From ref. 14a, with permission.) (See Color Plate 34.)

sions may be seen. However, the affected mucosa may also appear normal. These endoscopic findings cannot be easily distinguished from infection of the small bowel by *Mycobacterium avium-intracellulare*. The endoscopic lesions correspond to the histological finding of period acid–Schiff (PAS)–positive macrophages distending the villi. The stomach may occasionally show endoscopic abnormalities, typically erosive or atrophic gastritis (14).

The diagnosis is suggested when duodenal biopsies show blunted villi packed with PAS-positive macrophages. These histological findings also occur in patients with *M. avium-intracellulare*. Special stains for mycobacteria should therefore be performed. When mucosal abnormalities are noted in the stomach, gastric biopsies may also show PAS-positive macrophages. Granulomas are also seen in histological specimens in 10% of patients (15).

The mucosal abnormalities regress with treatment, although biopsies may still show the presence of macrophages. With clinical relapse of the disease, the endoscopic lesions usually return.

Whipple's disease is often diagnosed late in its course, since it is rare and often produces a confusing clinical picture. When the diagnosis is being considered, early endoscopy with duodenal biopsies should be performed.

Bacterial Esophagitis

Bacterial esophagitis is an unusual cause of infectious esophagitis that occurs almost exclusively in immunocompromised patients (16–18). In the past it was mistakenly believed that bacteria simply colonize an esophagus already damaged by other factors, but it is now clear that bacterial invasion of the esophagus can occur without underlying esophageal damage. Bacterial esophagitis may occur in up to 12–16% of immunocompromised patients undergoing endoscopy for dysphagia (16,17). The most common organisms implicated are orally derived gram-positive cocci or gram-positive bacilli (16,17,19,20). Gram-negative bacilli are less commonly seen.

The endoscopic appearance ranges from mucosal erythema to frank circular or linear ulcerations with exudate to pseudomembrane formation. It appears that pseudomembranes, which indicate extensive epithelial destruction, are most commonly seen in severe cases, and these patients have an increased likelihood of associated bacteremia (16). The type of organism involved, however, cannot be predicted by the endoscopic appearance. Indeed, the endoscopic appearance of bacterial esophagitis can easily be mistaken for *Candida* or herpes esophagitis. However, bacterial colonization of herpetic and candidal ulcers should not be equated with true bacterial esophagitis (21). Bacterial invasion should be seen within the mucosa or deeper layers of the esophageal wall when biopsy specimens are examined, and no concomitant viral or fungal infections of the esophagus should be present (16). Therefore, endoscopy with biopsy is crucial in establishing the diagnosis of bacterial esophagitis.

Phlegmonous Gastritis

Phlegmonous gastritis is a rare bacterial infection of the gastric wall. Gram-positive organisms are most commonly implicated in the disease, with β-hemolytic *Streptococcus* found in 70% of cases (22). *E. coli, Proteus* sp. *Enterobacter, Staphylococcus* sp., and *Clostridium* sp. are other organisms that have been isolated (22,23). The infection extends from the submucosa to the serosa of the gastric wall, sparing the mucosa (22,24).

The endoscopic appearance of phlegmonous gastritis has not been well reported since most patients present with an acute abdomen and undergo exploratory laparotomy for diagnosis. Surgical findings include edematous gastric mucosa and thickened, rigid gastric folds. The gastric lumen may be narrowed suggesting the presence of a submucosal mass (25,26). Sometimes pus can be seen. The antrum is most commonly involved, but the whole stomach may be affected. The infection does not usually extend beyond the pylorus or proximal to the esophagogastric junction (22).

Other studies that are helpful in establishing the diagnosis of phlegmonous gastritis preoperatively include the demonstration of air in the gastric wall or edematous gastric folds by plain abdominal films (26,27), and upper GI barium study or abdominal computed tomography (CT) scan which will show thickened gastric folds (23,26,27).

These surgical and radiological changes should be evident during an endoscopic examination. However, the role of endoscopy in phlegmonous gastritis has not been defined due to the rarity of the disease and the acuity of the presentation. As early surgical intervention is indicated for both diagnosis and definitive treatment, endoscopic examination may not be important. However, if the diagnosis is unclear, demonstration of bacteria in endoscopic biopsies should help to confirm the diagnosis (26).

Viral Infections

Herpes Simplex

Herpes simplex virus (HSV) infection of the GI tract is typically seen in immunocompromised patients, but has also been described in healthy subjects (17,21,28–31). In the upper GI tract, the esophagus is the most commonly involved site and the stomach is affected infrequently.

The natural evolution of HSV involvement of the esophagus has not been well documented, but it is generally believed that the infection advances through several stages (32). Early in its course, endoscopy will reveal discrete vesicular lesions, but these short-lived vesicles are quickly replaced by ulcerations (21,33,34). By the time endoscopy is usually performed, the appearance will be that of single or multiple discrete punched-out ulcerations with normal intervening mucosa (21,29,51) (Fig. 2). The ulcerations are often less than 5 mm, but can be up to 1.5–2.0 cm in size. In later stages of the illness, they can become confluent. The ulcers may have the characteristic

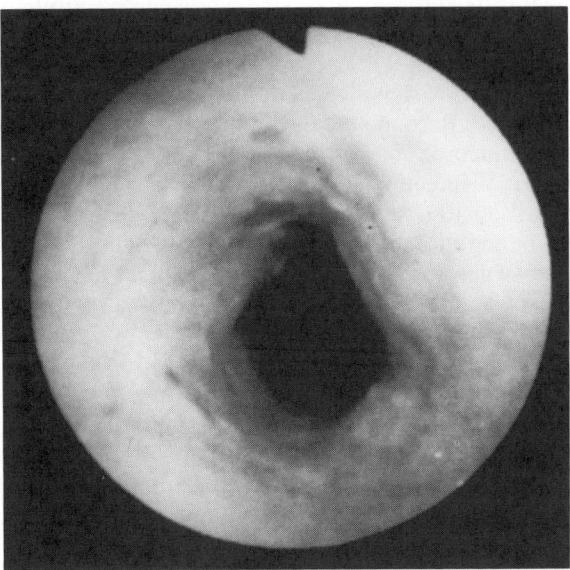

FIG. 2. HSV esophageal ulcer, early. Discrete punched-out ulcerations with normal intervening mucosa. (From ref. 14a, with permission.) (See Color Plate 35.)

raised yellow rims of exudate, the so-called volcano ulcers (21,35,50). In later stages, herpes esophagitis may be indistinguishable from *Candida* esophagitis with nonspecific diffuse exudative erosions and ulcerations (28,35) (Fig. 3).

Endoscopy with tissue sampling is the only way to confirm the diagnosis (21). As HSV infects epithelial cells, biopsy specimens must be taken from the ulcer margins in order to display the typical cell changes under microscopic examination (34). Biopsies taken from the ulcer center will usually yield only inflammatory changes. Cultures of specimens should also be sent. The sensitivity of a viral culture alone is approximately 76–89%, whereas histology alone is sensitive in 70–75% of cases. Frequently, only one of the two techniques may yield a positive result (32,33,36). Performing both tests increases the diagnostic yield substantially. Endoscopic brushing specimens have been shown in one limited retrospective study to be as accurate as biopsies for microscopic examination, but have a less diagnostic yield than biopsies when the

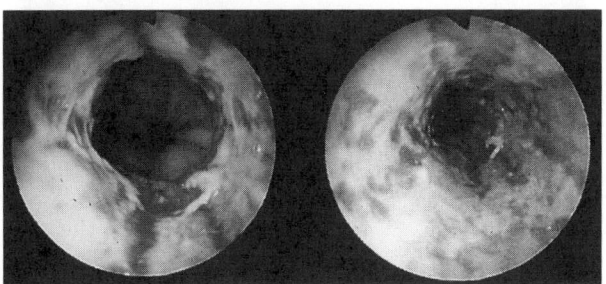

FIG. 3. HSV esophageal ulcer, late. Confluent, nonspecific, diffuse exudative ulcerations and erosions, which may be indistinguishable from *Candida* esophagitis.

material is used for culture (32). A prospective study designed to compare the efficacy of these two endoscopic sampling techniques is needed.

Other less invasive diagnostic tests for HSV infections are available. Barium studies of the esophagus may show variable mucosal abnormalities but cannot delineate between HSV infection and other mucosal abnormalities (35,51). A positive serological test for HSV does not imply active infection and is of no diagnostic value (51). The absence of active or past HSV stomatitis does not exclude HSV esophagitis. In fact, up to 80% of patients with well-documented HSV esophagitis will not even give a history of previous HSV stomatitis (32,33). It is logical to presume a diagnosis of HSV esophagitis in a patient with active HSV stomatitis and esophageal symptoms, but data validating this presumption are not available. Endoscopy with tissue sampling is the preferred method of establishing the diagnosis of HSV infection in the upper GI tract.

Cytomegalovirus

Gastrointestinal cytomegalovirus (CMV) disease is another opportunistic infection frequently seen in immunocompromised patients (36). CMV can occur anywhere in the GI tract (37,38). The endoscopic appearance is often characterized by ulcerations with sharp borders, which may be very deep and large (39). The ulcerations are rarely heaped up at the borders (40) and in general have little or no ulcer membrane or plaque. The intervening mucosa is typically normal (17) (Fig. 4). However, ulcerations are not a universal finding in GI CMV and the endoscopic appearance can be quite varied. Other endoscopic findings include gastric erythema with erosions, gastric nodules or polyps, and duodenal erythema (37,41,42) (Fig.

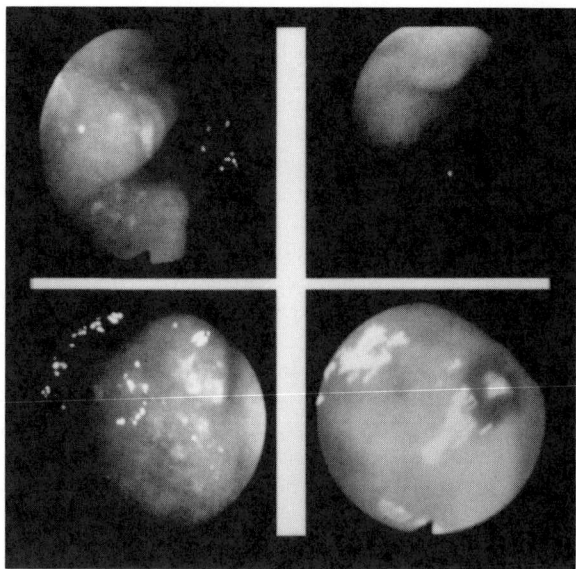

FIG. 5. Varied endoscopic appearance of CMV gastric lesions. Top left: Nodular gastritis with erosions. Top right: Nodular gastritis with minimal inflammation. Bottom left: Erosive gastritis. Bottom right: Gastric ulcerations. (From ref. 37, with permission.) (See Color Plate 36.)

5). In the upper GI tract, the distal esophagus, stomach, and duodenum are often affected. It is important to note that the ulcerations induced by CMV cannot be reliably distinguished from peptic ulcers, nor can they be positively differentiated from other infectious ulcerations based on endoscopic appearance (17).

Endoscopic biopsies early in the course of suspected infection should be performed to confirm the presence of CMV (40). Unlike HSV, CMV infects the stromal cells. CMV inclusion bodies are found in the granulation tissue of the ulcer base rather than in the tissue adjacent to the ulcer (40). Biopsies should therefore be taken from the ulcer bed and not near the ulcer borders. Biopsies from the edge of the ulceration are likely to show only inflammation (43). Similarly, if nonulcerated tissue is biopsied in the upper GI tract, it is unlikely that superficial biopsies will establish a diagnosis. Sampling of deeper lamina propria tissue is necessary (40). However, as ulcers caused by CMV may not be easily distinguishable from those induced by HSV, biopsies should be obtained from both the edge and the center of the ulcer crater. Some investigators have found that examination of biopsy specimens for inclusion bodies is the most sensitive and specific technique for diagnosing CMV infection (40). Others feel that cultures of brushing or biopsy specimens are more sensitive (36,39), though cultures often take weeks to become positive. The sensitivities of the two techniques vary widely in different studies. Biopsies for histological examination and cultures of biopsy specimens should be considered complementary, and both should be sent.

Brushings for cytological examination have yielded poor results in gastrointestinal CMV infection (17,36). In one study of AIDS patients with CMV esophagitis, brush-

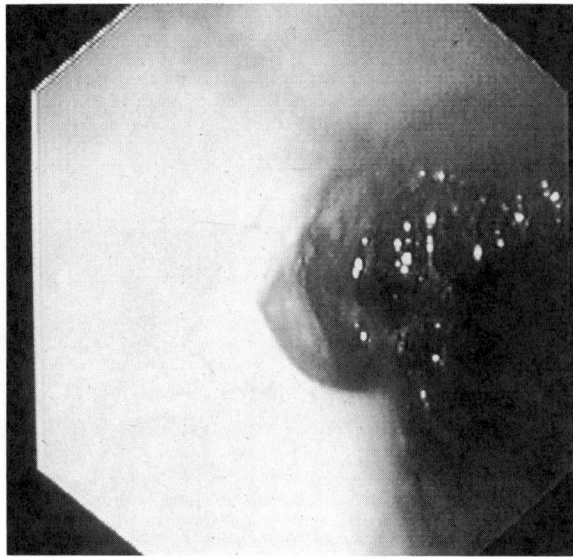

FIG. 4. CMV esophageal ulcer.

ings for cytology were positive in only 3% of cases (39). Similarly, serological tests are unreliable since they are often positive in the absence of clinical disease.

After a course of ganciclovir treatment for GI CMV, endoscopy with biopsies should be repeated to document the healing of the CMV-associated lesions. If CMV is still present in biopsy specimens, treatment may need to be continued (37).

Other Viral Infections

Varicella zoster can cause infection of the upper GI tract, often in patients with associated cutaneous herpes zoster lesions (44–46). Endoscopic findings are similar to those seen with herpes simplex virus, with vesicles, erosions, and ulcerations involving the esophagus or stomach. The GI lesions seem to improve with the skin lesions.

Esophageal ulcerations occurring with HIV seroconversion have been described (47,48). Endoscopy reveals multiple discrete shallow ulcerations that may be distributed over the length of the esophagus. The intervening mucosa is normal. Light microscopy and cultures of biopsy specimens are unrevealing, but electron microscopy of biopsy specimens shows retrovirus particles.

Epstein–Barr virus has also been reported to be a cause of esophageal ulceration in immunosuppressed patients (49).

Fungal Infections

Candida

Candida esophagitis is one of the most common causes of dysphagia or odynophagia in immunocompromised patients. It can also occur in patients without other predisposing illnesses (21,52,53). Although it most commonly affects the esophagus, all regions of the upper GI tract can be involved. Infection of both the stomach and small bowel has been described.

The classic endoscopic appearance of esophageal candidiasis is that of multiple raised white plaques, usually less than 1 cm in size (21,53,54). The surrounding mucosa is erythematous and friable (50,52). The plaques can become confluent and nodular, and can be associated with ulcerations (Figs. 6, 7). They are adherent to the mucosa and cannot easily be washed off. Although the presence of plaques is characteristic of candidiasis, the endoscopic appearance can be mistaken for other diseases, including reflux esophagitis and other infectious diseases. Therefore, specimens should be taken to confirm the presence of *Candida* (50). Gastric candidiasis may appear as erythematous mucosa with overlying patchy white exudate. It may also take on a nodular form, with small nodular projections against an inflamed mucosa, or an ulcerative form, with multiple gastric ulcerations (52,55) (Fig. 8). Similar findings can occur in the duodenum.

Endoscopic brushing smears or biopsies is the preferred method to confirm the diagnosis of *Candida* esophagitis

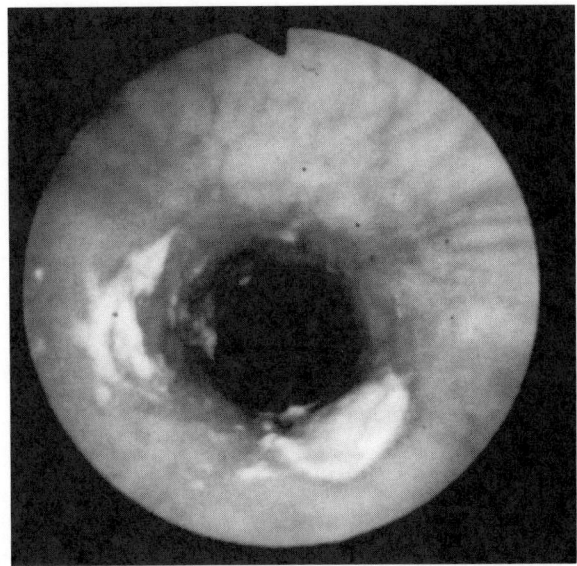

FIG. 6. *Candida* esophagitis. Discrete ulcer with white exudate and normal surrounding mucosa. (From ref. 14a, with permission.) (See Color Plate 37.)

(21,50,56). The cytology brush with its overlying protective sheath is placed through the biopsy channel of the endoscope, and brushing is carried out under endoscopic visualization. The brush is extended from the sheath and the brush is moved back and forth over the mucosa. The brush is then withdrawn into the sheath, and the two are pulled out together through the channel of the endoscope. The specimen should then be immediately smeared onto the slide for fixation. Brushing of the lesions has been shown in a number of studies to be superior to biopsy in

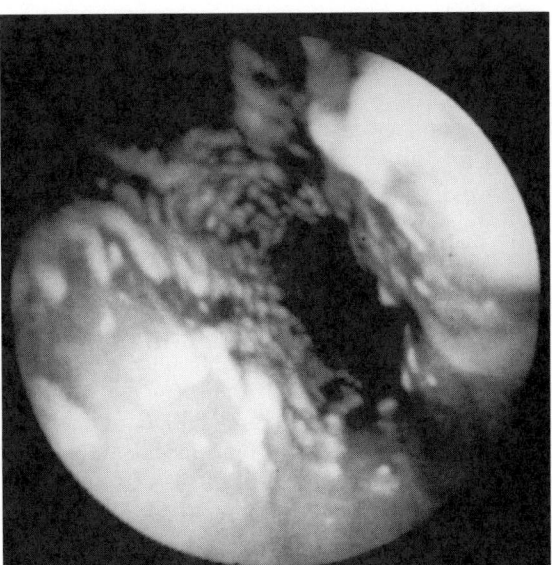

FIG. 7. *Candida* esophagitis. Severe, with extensive exudate and erythema. (From ref. 14a, with permission.) (See Color Plate 38.)

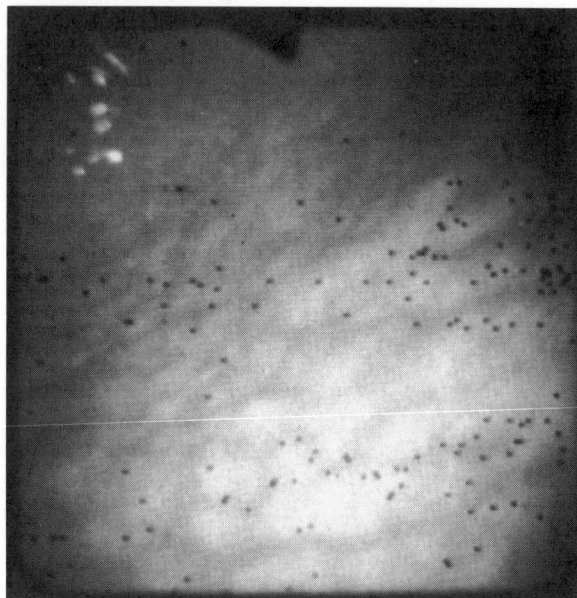

FIG. 8. *Candida* gastritis. Nodules in antrum. (From ref. 55, with permission.)

the diagnosis of esophageal candidiasis (50,56–58). Brushing allows sampling of a larger surface area than does biopsy alone, and it is thought that the fixation process may destroy or wash away some of the superficial hyphae in biopsy specimens (28). Cytological examination of esophageal brushing smears has a sensitivity of up to 100%, whereas histological examination of biopsy specimens is sensitive in only 10–75% of cases (53,56,58,59).

Blind brushing of the esophagus to establish the diagnosis of esophageal candidiasis has been studied in AIDS patients (57). This is performed by placing a sterile brush through an orally placed nasogastric tube. The sensitivity and specificity of blind brushing techniques are 87–96% and 87–100%, respectively, with false positives thought due to contamination of the nasogastric tube by oral thrush (57,60,61).

Barium esophagrams may be sensitive in up to 88% of cases, but the specificity is relatively low (62). The radiographs may show a shaggy, irregular mucosa or ulcerations, but the abnormalities do not distinguish between candidiasis and other types of infections (17,50–52,54).

Oral thrush is not a reliable predictor of *Candida* esophagitis. Approximately 70–80% of patients with symptomatic *Candida* esophagitis also have oral thrush (57). However, 20% of patients with oral thrush will not have *Candida* as a cause of their esophagitis (56,57,60).

Early endoscopy with brushing is currently the preferred method to confirm the diagnosis of *Candida* infection in the upper GI tract. Although the blind brushing technique appears to be an accurate tool for the diagnosis of *Candida* esophagitis in AIDS patients, its ability to exclude other concomitant infection has not been established. In some centers with a large population of AIDS patients, an empirical trial of antifungal therapy is often

given to these patients with mild symptoms of dysphagia without performing endoscopy (51,56). If the patient's symptoms do not improve after 7–10 days of therapy, endoscopy is performed. This approach is often taken even if oropharyngeal candidiasis is not seen, and its justification is based on the fact that esophageal candidiasis is the most common esophageal disease in these patients (51). In other immunosuppressed patients, such as transplant recipients, or in normal hosts in whom the diagnosis of candidiasis is being entertained, early endoscopy to confirm the *Candida* infection and exclude the presence of other serious infections is still the standard of care.

Other Fungal Infections

Histoplasmosis is well recognized as a pathogen of the esophagus, stomach, and small bowel, with endoscopic findings ranging from ulcerations to multiple small submucosal nodules to mass lesions (64) (Fig. 9). *Aspergillus* species can affect the GI tract and can cause ulcerations of variable configurations and mass lesions (63). The lesions may be segmental. Transmural infarction of the small bowel can occur due to vascular occlusion by Aspergillus organisms. Torulopsis glabrata has been described as causing focal esophageal ulcerations in immunocompromised patients (65).

In these and other fungal infections, it is important to recognize that the endoscopic features are not diagnostic, and biopsies and brushings should be performed.

Parasitic Infections

Anisakiasis

Anisakiasis is caused by the ingestion of *Anisakis* larvae in undercooked contaminated fish. The worm burrows

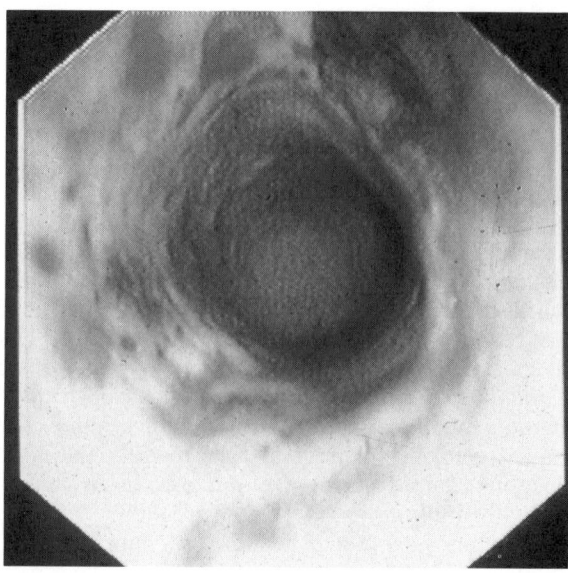

FIG. 9. Histplasmosis esophagitis.

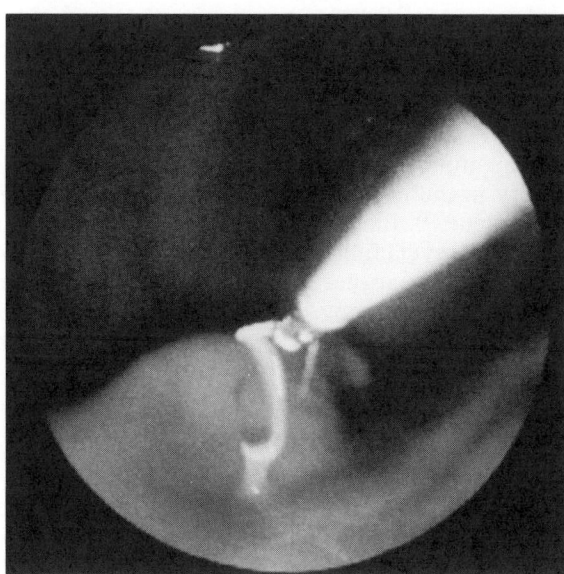

FIG. 10. Gastric anisakiasis. Anisakis larva being removed from the top of the inflammatory nodule. (From ref. 66, with permission.) (See Color Plate 39.)

into the gastric or intestinal mucosa causing severe abdominal symptoms. The stomach is affected in 75% of cases and the small or large bowel in 25% (66,67). A worm penetrating the gastric mucosa may be found by endoscopy (Fig. 10). The worm is surrounded by mucosal edema in 86% of cases, and a surrounding mass is seen in 43% of cases (66,67). In the stomach, the worm can be found in any area, but is most commonly located in the fundus.

Endoscopy is the main tool used for the diagnosis and treatment of anisakiasis. The disease is confirmed by locating the worm during endoscopy. Immunological assays for *Anisakis* antigens may be helpful when the worm cannot be recovered easily, but these assays are not available in routine clinical laboratories at present (68,69). Early endoscopic removal of the worm with biopsy forceps abates the symptoms and prevents the characteristic eosinophilic tissue reaction to the degenerating larvae, and is the definitive treatment (66–68). Therefore, early endoscopy is indicated in patients suspected to have anisakiasis.

Giardia lamblia

Giardia lamblia is the most common parasite implicated in gastrointestinal illness in the world (70–72). *Giardia* cysts are ingested and passed into the duodenum where they produce trophozoites which in turn colonize the upper intestine (71). The host may be asymptomatic during the course of the infection, or may develop either acute or chronic intestinal symptoms.

Endoscopy is not the first avenue of investigation for the diagnosis of giardiasis. Endoscopic findings are nonspecific. Inflammation, erosion, or nodularity of the duo-

denal mucosa may be seen (73). However, the mucosa may also appear entirely normal and still harbor the parasite. Cysts have also been found in gastric biopsy specimens, but only in the presence of chronic atrophic gastritis (74). It is thought that decreased gastric acidity may be necessary for colonization of the parasite in the stomach.

There is no gold standard for the diagnosis of *Giardia* infection. The most widely used method of diagnosis is the microscopic detection of cysts or trophozoites in multiple concentrated stool specimens (70). However, the sensitivity of this method is only 50–70% (71,75). There are now a number of antigen detection assays, such as enzyme-linked immunosorbent assay (ELISA), to detect *Giardia* antigen in fecal material (71,75,77–79). They use sera from animals immunized with *Giardia* trophozoites in order to detect *Giardia* antigen in stool specimens and appear to be quite accurate (75). The sensitivity and specificity of these systems are each approximately 90–99% in cases of giardiasis proven by microscopic examination of stool specimens (77–79).

If stool testing is negative and clinical suspicion for *Giardia* infection is high, endoscopy with small bowel biopsy or aspiration of duodenal fluid can be considered (80). Biopsies of the small bowel for microscopic examination yield positive results in 66% of cases (83). Endoscopic biopsy is as effective as the older peroral suction biopsy technique and is better tolerated (76,81). Although animal studies suggest that the midjejunum may be more heavily colonized with the organism than the duodenum (72), duodenal biopsies are adequate (81). Aspiration of duodenal fluid is sensitive in detecting the protozoan in up to 80% of cases. Duodenal aspirates can be obtained by instilling 10–20 mL of normal saline into the duodenum through the endoscope, then aspirating into a sterile trap. Normal saline should be used since the trophozoites undergo lysis in tap water (82). Passing a nasogastric tube into the duodenum to obtain an aspirate is often unsuccessful and is uncomfortable. Similarly, the Enterotest duodenal capsule (string test) is as sensitive as duodenal aspiration (83), but is often unsuccessful in reaching the duodenum (76). Endoscopic brush cytology has also yielded good results in two small studies (76,84). These patients had negative small bowel biopsies and stool studies for *Giardia,* but brush cytology of the duodenum showed the organism.

It should be emphasized that there are no studies directly comparing the sensitivities of antigen detection assays on fecal samples and small bowel biopsy or aspiration in diagnosing *Giardia* infection. It may be true that the detection of *Giardia* antigen in fecal samples may become the new gold standard, since the sensitivity and specificity of this technique appear to be quite high. It is unlikely that endoscopy will reveal many cases of giardiasis missed by antigen studies, and it should be considered a second-line investigative technique in the diagnosis of giardiasis. The major role of endoscopy may be in excluding other diseases that mimic *Giardia* infection.

Cryptosporidium *and* Isospora belli

Coccidian parasites such as *Cryptosporidium parvum* and *Isospora belli* are now commonly seen in patients with AIDS. Both can cause a debilitating GI syndrome characterized by diarrhea, abdominal pain, and weight loss. Although the parasites typically affect the small bowel, they can be found anywhere in the GI tract, from the pharynx to the rectum (85).

There are no gross endoscopic features thought to be specific for these protozoa (86). Biopsies of infected tissue may show nonspecific changes, such as atrophic mucosa and shortened villi in the small bowel (85). *Cryptosporidium* parasites may be seen along the intestinal epithelial surface.

Stool analysis is the main avenue of investigation for the diagnosis of *Cryptosporidium* and *Isospora* (86–89). In one study of 28 patients with *Cryptosporidium* infection, stool studies were positive in 71% of cases, with endoscopic biopsies positive in 29% (86). In another study, of 9 patients with *Cryptosporidium* detected in stool samples, only 3 had positive biopsies (89).

The role of endoscopy in the evaluation of these infections is primarily to exclude other possible infections affecting immunosuppressed patients. Endoscopy with biopsy has been shown to be of benefit in detecting CMV, *Mycobacterium avium-intracellulare,* and other infections in AIDS patients (86,89,90), that may present with similar symptoms of diarrhea, weight loss, and abdominal pain. It is also important to remember that a pathogen isolated in the stool is not necessarily the principle cause of the patient's illness, and other pathogens may be coexistent (86,90,91).

Other Parasitic Infections

Parasites occasionally discovered by upper endoscopy include hookworms, tapeworms, and ascaris (92–96) (Fig. 11). Schistosomal infection of the stomach and small bowel can occur, although the colon is more often involved (97,98). With schistosomal infection, endoscopy may show nonspecific inflammation and microulcerations of the mucosa, and biopsies will show live or degenerating ova (73,97).

Examination of stool samples is the main diagnostic modality in the evaluation of most parasitic diseases of the GI tract (99). Barium radiographs have also been useful and may reveal filling defects or barium in the worm's alimentary tract, suggesting the diagnosis of parasitic infection (73). Endoscopy is mainly performed to exclude other causes of abdominal symptoms when stool studies for parasites have been unrevealing.

Mycobacterium Infections

Mycobacterium tuberculosis

GI tuberculosis is rare, especially in the absence of pulmonary tuberculosis. Its diagnosis is therefore often delayed. The mycobacteria can affect the entire GI tract from the esophagus to the anus, but the most common site of involvement is the ileocecal region (100,101). The esophagus, stomach, and proximal small bowel are less commonly involved. The duodenum, for example, is infected 30 times less than the ileocecal region (102,103). Involvement of the stomach occurs in only 0.5–3% of tuberculous GI infections (104). However, if preexisting lesions exist in the upper GI tract, such as esophagitis, ulceration, or carcinoma, implantation of acid-fast bacilli in these areas occurs more easily (108,109).

Esophageal tuberculosis is most often a consequence of spread from adjacent lymph nodes (110). The most common site affected is therefore the midesophagus just above the carina, where the mediastinal lymph nodes are located (106,108,110) (Fig. 12). In the stomach, the pylo-

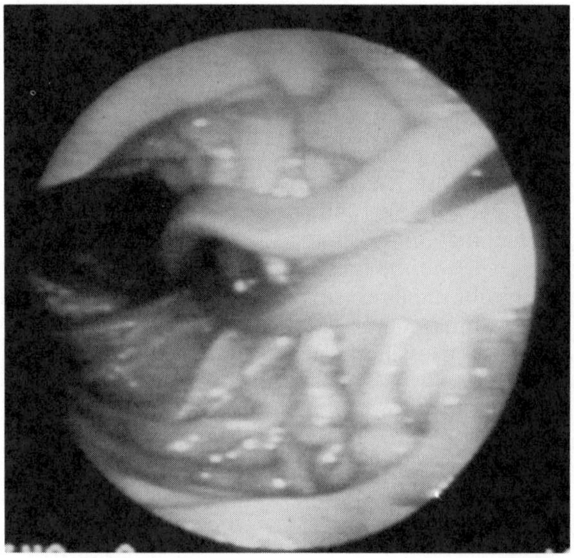

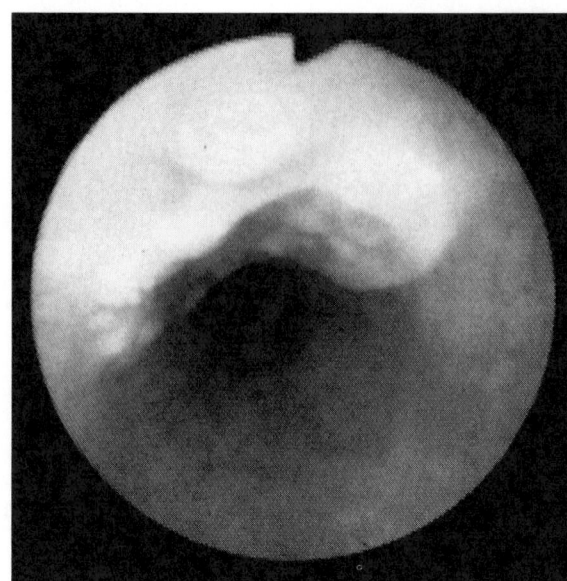

FIG. 11. *Ascaris* in duodenum. (Courtesy Dr. C. Michael Knauer.) (See Color Plate 40.)

FIG. 12. Esophageal tuberculosis. Presented as an ulcerated mass in mid-esophagus. (From ref. 110a, with permission.)

rus and lesser curvature of the antrum are most commonly involved, often leading to gastric outlet obstruction (105,107,111). The small bowel is often segmentally involved, which may lead to the mistaken diagnosis of Crohn's disease. Small bowel involvement commonly presents as intestinal obstruction secondary to stricture or mass formation (102,103,111–114). In one study, 75% of patients with duodenal tuberculosis presented with gastric outlet or intestinal obstruction (102).

The endoscopic appearance of upper GI tuberculosis is variable, but usually takes one of three forms: ulcerative, hypertrophic, or granular (106,108,110). The ulcerative form is the most common (107). The ulcers may be single or multiple, and often have irregular borders with a gray shallow base (100,108,113). The adjacent mucosa may be normal or may be erythematous (106). The hypertrophic form is caused by a fibrotic reaction of the mycobacteria and can mistakenly lead to a diagnosis of carcinoma (110). This form can cause obstruction and narrowing of the lumen. Finally, the least common type is the granular form. These are small, miliary tubercles on the mucosa. Strictures, fistulae, and sinuses may occur, and probing of hypertrophic masses or ulcers may uncover deep tracts to adjacent structures (106,109).

The endoscopic appearance is not diagnostic, and biopsies must be taken. Since the acid-fast bacilli are mostly submucosal, superficial biopsies may only show inflammation (101,103,104,106,107,112). Even with deeper biopsies, acid-fast bacilli and granulomas may not be identified on direct smear, but the yield is increased with deeper biopsies (101). At best, acid-fast bacilli can be identified only in about 50% of biopsy specimens, which is similar to the yield of gastric aspirates (102,110). Tissue should always be sent for mycobacterial culture.

Radiological studies are not pathognomonic in diagnosing GI tuberculosis. The findings of ulcers, strictures, pseudotumor masses, or even fistulae are nonspecific, and may be confused with Crohn's disease, tumor, or acid peptic disease (5,108,109).

Although endoscopy with biopsy is the procedure of choice (109), the limitations of endoscopy in the diagnosis of GI tuberculosis must be emphasized (112). Entertaining the diagnosis even in the absence of clear exposure to tuberculosis is critical. Biopsy specimens should be sent for histology, acid-fast bacilli staining, and culture. Surgical exploration is often performed because of the diagnosis of tuberculosis was not made preoperatively (111).

Mycobacterium avium-intracellulare

GI infection with *Mycobacterium avium-intracellulare* (MAI) is seen in the context of systemic infection in immunocompromised hosts (115,116). It may affect the entire GI tract, but commonly affects the duodenum. Endoscopic findings in the duodenum include the presence of fine white nodules thought to be characteristic of this infection (116) (Fig. 13). However, the endoscopic appearance can be easily mistaken as Whipple's disease. Ulcerations and fistulae have also been described (115,116).

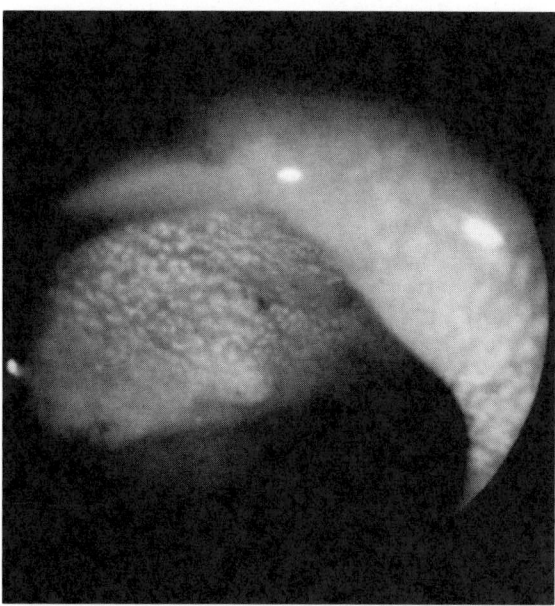

FIG. 13. MAI of the duodenum. Coarse, pale whitish-yellow, granular mucosa resembling Whipple's disease. (From ref. 116a, with permission.) (See Color Plate 41.)

Even with normal-appearing mucosa, MAI can be found in biopsy specimens.

In one study of 35 AIDS patients, biopsies were positive for acid-fast bacilli smear in up to 65% of patients with gastrointestinal MAI infection, and cultures of biopsy specimens were positive in up to 85% (116). Biopsies for histology, acid-fast bacilli smear, and culture should be submitted in patients with suspected MAI infection.

ROLE OF ENTEROSCOPY IN SMALL INTESTINE INFECTIONS

Currently, two types of endoscopes are available for examination of the small intestine. The Sonde-type enteroscopy involves the passage of a thin and long endoscope transnasally into the patient's duodenum. Peristalsis will then carry the endoscope to the terminal ileum in about 80% of the cases (117). This phase of the procedure takes about 6–8 hours. The small intestine is then examined upon withdrawal of the endoscope. However, this instrument lacks the ability to obtain tissue specimen or aspirates. The push-type enteroscopy is similar to routine upper endoscopy, but a special 240-cm-long endoscope is used (118). This instrument can be advanced to the midjejunum and is capable of tissue sampling. The procedure can be performed in 1–2 hr.

Although a large number of common bacterial, viral, and parasitic infections affect the small intestine and typically result in diarrhea, enteroscopy is seldom needed to make the diagnosis. Stool studies, clinical characteristics, and epidemiological considerations are generally more valuable in establishing the diagnosis of these infections.

Opportunistic infections of the small intestine in immunocompromised patients can often be detected by examination of the duodenum by routine upper endoscopy. The role of enteroscopy in these patients is yet to defined, but it is likely of minor importance.

ROLE OF FLEXIBLE SIGMOIDOSCOPY AND COLONOSCOPY IN INFECTIONS OF THE COLON AND TERMINAL ILEUM

Endoscopic examinations of the entire colon by colonoscopy, or to a limited extent by flexible sigmoidoscopy, are well tolerated. Intubation of the terminal ileum through the ileocecal valve is a routine maneuver during colonoscopy and has a success rate of over 80%. Endoscopic tissue sampling again plays an important role in the management of infectious process affecting these regions.

Bacterial Infections

Acute Bacterial Colitis

Common pathogens isolated from stool cultures in patients with acute bacterial colitis include *Campylobacter, Salmonella, Shigella,* toxigenic *E. coli* O157:H7, and *Clostridium difficile.* These organisms can cause a spectrum of clinical illness, ranging from an asymptomatic carrier state to acute hemorrhagic colitis. *C. difficile* causes pseudomembranous colitis and will be discussed separately.

There is a wide range of endoscopic findings in infectious colitis. Findings include edematous mucosa with loss of the normal vascular pattern, erythema, friability, ulcerations, and the presence of luminal exudate (119–121) (Fig. 14). Ulcerations may be small or several centimeters in size, and are of variable configuration (119,122). Pseudomembranes may also be found in a minority of cases associated with *E. coli* O157:H7 (127).

The endoscopic findings are variable depending on when endoscopy is performed in the course of the illness. The evolution of endoscopic findings was studied in a group of patients with acute shigellosis (122). During the

first week after presentation, edema was the dominant finding on colonoscopy. In the second and third weeks, slightly raised mucosal hemorrhages appearing as punctate spots, ulcerations, and friability were prominent. The punctate spots persisted after the other endoscopic abnormalities and clinical symptoms improved. Erythema was also present through the course of the disease, with diffuse involvement in early weeks and patchy involvement in later weeks. Luminal pus, mucus, and blood were maximal in the first 3 weeks. The endoscopic abnormalities lasted an average of 39 days, while the clinical symptoms lasted 23 days. Of importance, all patients eventually developed normal-appearing mucosa. Although this study was performed in patients with shigellosis, similar endoscopic changes are probably seen in acute colitis caused by other common pathogens (119,122,123). It is not possible to predict the bacterial organism involved on the basis of endoscopic examination.

The mucosal abnormalities may be segmental or continuous (119,123). Normal-appearing rectal mucosa on proctoscopy does not exclude an infectious colitis, and indeed normal proctoscopies were noted in 10 of 19 patients with *Campylobacter* isolated from stool samples in one study (124). The endoscopic findings of *E. coli* O157:H7–associated colitis are especially prominent in the right colon, although the whole large bowel can be involved (127–129,131). Either the cecum or the ascending colon will reveal endoscopic abnormalities in most cases, whereas the sigmoid colon will be abnormal less than half of the time, and the rectum less than one third of the time (130). There appears to be a gradation of endoscopic abnormalities from the cecum to the rectum, with the rectosigmoid often being normal or showing only moderate hyperemia (127,130).

One of the major concerns in a patient presenting with bloody diarrhea is differentiating an acute, self-limited, and presumably infectious colitis from idiopathic inflammatory bowel disease. Clinically, the symptoms may be identical. The endoscopic appearance is also generally not helpful (123–125). The presence of mucosal granularity has been suggested to be indicative of inflammatory bowel disease (122), but it can be seen in infectious colitis as well (119,120,123,125).

Biopsy specimens for histological examination may be helpful in differentiating between acute infectious colitis and inflammatory bowel disease. Although many histological features are seen in both illnesses, some features seem to be more specific for inflammatory bowel disease. One retrospective evaluation of rectal biopsy specimens from patients with either acute self-limited colitis or inflammatory bowel disease revealed that seven features were seen commonly in inflammatory bowel disease, but rarely in acute self-limited colitis (126). These features included distorted crypt architecture, increased number of round cells and neutrophils in the lamina propria, a villous surface, epithelioid granulomas, crypt atrophy, basal lymphoid aggregates, and basally located giant cells. The predictive probability of each of these features in diagnosing inflammatory bowel disease ranges from 79% to 100%.

In another study of colorectal biopsy specimens taken

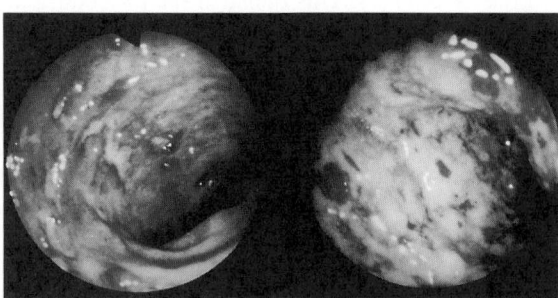

FIG. 14. Left: Severe *Shigalla flexineri* colitis with extensive coalescent superficial ulceration involving nearly the entire bowel circumference. Right: Improved appearance after two weeks of antibiotic therapy. (From ref. 14a, with permission.) (See Color Plate 42.)

from patients with bloody diarrhea within 4 days of presentation, the presence of crypt distortion and plasmacytosis in the lamina propria were diagnostic of ulcerative colitis, while edema, neutrophilic infiltration in the lamina propria, and crypts were diagnostic of acute self-limited colitis (125). The histological features in patients with acute self-limited colitis did not differ with the type of bacterial organisms isolated from the stool. However, as the histological changes in acute self-limited colitis rapidly evolve, biopsies taken later than 4 days after the onset of bloody diarrhea were not diagnostic.

Stool cultures should be the first tests performed in the evaluation of what is presumed to be an acute infectious diarrhea. In only 42–58% of patients with acute self-limited colitis, however, will stool studies be positive (125). When patients present with severe symptoms of colitis and rapid institution of treatment is necessary, sigmoidoscopy with biopsy should be performed to help differentiate between idiopathic inflammatory bowel disease and an infectious colitis. If the sigmoidoscopy is nondiagnostic, a colonoscopy should be considered, with concomitant examination of the terminal ileum.

Clostridium difficile–*Associated Colitis*

Clostridium difficile is the most common cause of pseudomembranous colitis. Although the name implies the presence of pseudomembranes, the endoscopic appearance of *C. difficile* colitis takes on many forms, and pseudomembranes, may not be seen in mild cases (132,133). The mucosa may appear only mildly granular, friable, or erythematous (133) before the appearance of pseudomembranes. The endoscopic appearance, as well as the pseudomembranes, seem to go through stages as the disease evolves (Fig. 15). Within the first few days after diarrheal symptoms begin, small 1- to 2-mm round yellowish spots dotting the colonic mucosa have been described (134). They appear as tiny lesions with erythematous bases and central yellow plaques, and may be confused with aphthous ulcerations or even mucus. Biopsies of these lesions confirm the presence of early pseudomembranes. The pseudomembranes later appear as elevated adherent yellow, white, or gray plaques. They are usually 2–5 mm in size at this stage, but can become confluent and extend several centimeters (135). The intervening mucosa may be normal, but can also be edematous and hyperemic.

Endoscopy often quickly establishes the diagnosis of *C. difficile* colitis. Proctoscopy alone is insufficient and will miss 23–70% of cases (136–139), since rectal sparing is common. Although flexible sigmoidoscopy will reveal abnormalities in most cases, up to 10% may be missed with sigmoidoscopy alone (137). In a prospective study of 22 patients with pseudomembranous colitis, 91% of patients could be diagnosed with sigmoidoscopy to 60 cm from the anus (137) with the remaining 9% having localized proximal colonic disease. The disease is limited to the colon, and even if there is proximal colonic involvement, there is usually an abrupt termination of the disease at the ileocecal valve (135).

It has been suggested that colonic biopsies are not en-

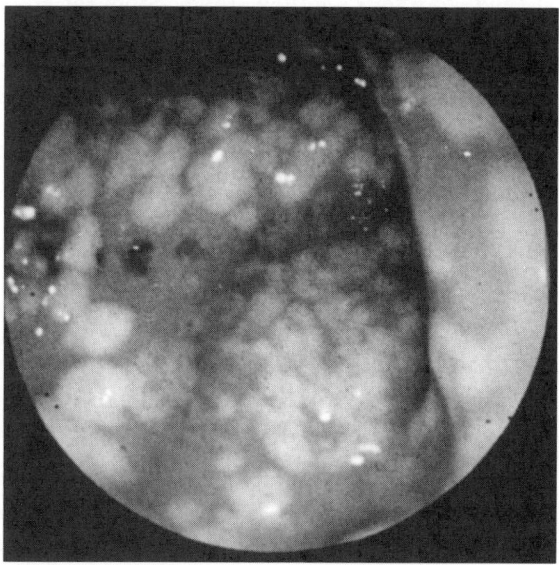

FIG. 15. Pseudomembranous colitis. Confluent colonic inflammation with pseudomembrane formation. This colonoscopic view illustrates the greenish pseudomembrane overlying the inflamed mucosal surface. (From ref. 133a, with permission.) (See Color Plate 43.)

tirely necessary if pseudomembranes are seen, since the diagnosis of pseudomembranous colitis can be established on visual grounds by an experienced observer. However, it is important to remember that other endoscopic abnormalities can be mistaken for pseudomembranes, and confirmation of pseudomembranes by histological examination is useful. In addition, even if pseudomembranes are not seen, biopsies of inflamed or granular mucosa may show the classic pseudomembranes microscopically (127,133,140). Biopsies should be performed routinely if pseudomembranous colitis is being considered.

The colitis is a result of two potent toxins elaborated by the organism (133). These toxins are the basis of diagnostic tests used in the evaluation of pseudomembranous colitis. The toxins are detected in stool samples. Although specific, the sensitivity of these tests is quite variable (133,141). Rapid ELISAs that detect the toxin are now in clinical use and appear to have a sensitivity of 80–90% (133,142). Recently, the polymerase chain reaction (PCR) technique has been used to identify the toxigenic *C. difficile* in stool specimens (143,144). This technique appears to be quite sensitive but is not in widespread clinical use.

C. difficile can be cultured from stool specimens in up to 97% of patients who meet clinical criteria for *C. difficile*–associated colitis (141). However, as many as 20% of hospitalized asymptomatic patients will harbor *C. difficile* in their stools without having colitis (133,145). In one study, only 11% of hospitalized patients with diarrhea who were culture-positive and cytotoxin-negative had pseudomembranes on sigmoidoscopy (145). Therefore clinical correlation and possibly endoscopic confirmation is important when a positive culture is obtained in patients with negative *C. dillicile* toxins (142).

The approach to a patient with suspected *C. difficile* is

to first send stool for *C. difficile* toxin. Stool for culture may also be sent. If patients are severely ill requiring a rapid diagnosis or if clinical suspicion is high when toxin and culture results are negative, endoscopy should be performed. Sigmoidoscopy will identify most cases, but colonoscopy will be necessary in the 10% of cases in which the disease is limited to the proximal colon.

Viral Infections

Cytomegalovirus Colitis

There has been a steady increase in the number of cases of CMV colitis with the increased population of transplant patients and patients with the acquired immunodeficiency syndrome (146,147). It is estimated that 20% of AIDS patients will at some time develop CMV GI disease (148).

As with upper GI CMV infection (see above), the endoscopic appearance of CMV colitis is one of mucosal ulcerations (146,149) (Fig. 16). The ulcers are discrete and can be quite large. Focal ulcerations occur, but in severe cases ulcers may be found throughout the colon. The surrounding mucosal may be edematous, erythematous, granular, and friable, and the changes may be continuous or discontinuous (149). In early stages, the mucosa may show only punctate superficial ulcerations. It is also noteworthy that the colonic mucosa may appear entirely normal and still harbor CMV inclusion bodies in biopsy specimens (147). In one study, 25% of AIDS patients with CMV infection of the colon had normal-appearing colonic mucosa with biopsies showing CMV inclusion bodies (147).

Localized CMV colitis has been described to be more common in the right colon (147,150), with a tendency toward sparing of the transverse and left colon. However, it has been noted that the rectosigmoid region is commonly involved in AIDS patients (147). Distal small bowel involvement is rare, composing only 1.4% of all cases of GI

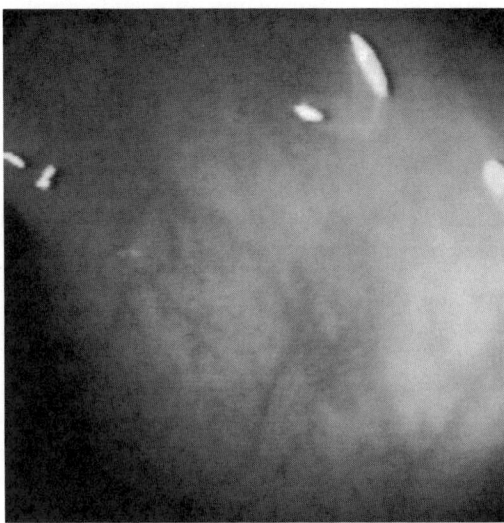

FIG. 16. CMV colitis, early. Punctate superficial ulcerations.

CMV infection (150). Even with diffuse colitis the disease often stops abruptly at the ileocecal valve, although isolated ileal CMV has also been reported (150). If colonoscopy is negative, passage of the colonoscope into the terminal ileum should be attempted.

Since the endoscopic changes are not specific for CMV, biopsies must be taken to establish the diagnosis. If ulcers are present, biopsies should be taken from the base of the ulcer (40). Even if the mucosa is normal, however, random biopsies should be taken if CMV colitis is being considered, such as in AIDS patients with diarrhea. The biopsies are more likely to show inclusion bodies if they are taken from the right colon rather than the left (38). It also appears that examination of colonic biopsies for inclusion bodies is more likely to yield a positive diagnosis than examination of biopsies of the upper GI tract, since the highest number of inclusion bodies is found in colonic biopsy specimens (38). It has been recommended that three random biopsies be taken from the cecum, transverse colon, and rectosigmoid colon in a patient suspected of having CMV colitis (147).

Viral cultures of biopsy specimens may take weeks to become positive, so that histological examination remains the mainstay of diagnosis. Stool cultures for CMV are unlikely to show CMV and are of no diagnostic value (147).

In patients with suspected CMV colitis, early endoscopy is warranted. Flexible sigmoidoscopy with biopsies should be performed as the initial study. If the examination is unrevealing, a colonoscopy is indicated as the disease is often localized in the proximal colon. Even with normal-appearing mucosa, random biopsies should be taken to exclude the presence of inclusion bodies.

Herpes Simplex Colitis

Herpes simplex infection of the proximal colon is very rare, although it is a common cause of proctitis in gay males. It is usually seen in immunocompromised patients but can occur in immunocompetent hosts as well (151). Colonoscopic findings include erythematous, friable mucosa, aphthous ulcerations, and multiple necrotic ulcers (151,152) (Fig. 17). Rectal ulcers caused by HSV are exquisitely tender; endoscopic examination of the infected anorectal area may require general anesthesia. It is probable that the evolution of mucosal changes is similar to that theorized in upper GI tract infection, with short-lived vesicles quickly evolving to form ulcerations. The entire colon may be involved with HSV colitis. As with HSV infection of the upper GI tract, biopsies should be taken from the margin of the ulcers and sent for both histological examination and culture.

Fungal Infections

Candida

GI candidiasis usually affects the upper GI tract, most notably the esophagus and stomach (see above). In an

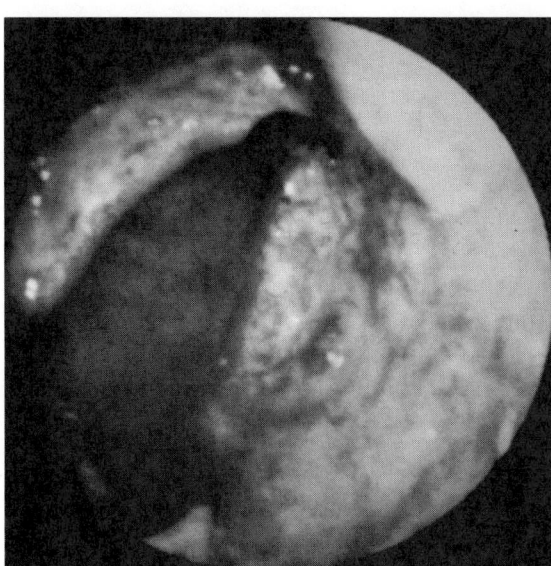

FIG. 17. HSV proctitis. Confluent, nearly circumferential ulceration of the anal canal and distal rectum. (From ref. 14a, with permission.) (See Color Plate 44.)

autopsy series of patients with GI *Candida* infection, the colon was involved in less than 4% of cases (154). Even with the prolonged survival of immunosuppressed patients and the high prevalence of *Candida* esophagitis in these patients, there does not seem to be an increase in invasive *Candida* infections of the lower GI tract (90,153). When the lower GI tract is involved, findings include small erosions and ulcerations, sometimes with overlying plaque (153).

Candida has been isolated from the stool in normal hosts and is thought to be nonpathogenic in these individuals. In hospitalized, debilitated patients with diarrhea, GI candidiasis has been implicated as but not conclusively proven to be a cause of the symptoms. Gupta reported on 10 ill patients with diarrhea who had positive stool cultures for *Candida* species and who responded to treatment with oral nystatin (153). Colonoscopies with biopsy in these patients were normal, suggesting a possible noninvasive role of *Candida* in the diarrheal illness. Based on this limited study, colonoscopy does not appear to play a significant role in patients with diarrhea and *Candida* isolated from stool cultures.

Parasitic Infections

Entamoeba histolytica

The clinical symptoms of amebic colitis can mimic other causes of diarrhea, and it should be considered in the differential diagnosis of any patient with symptoms suggestive of inflammatory bowel disease or bacterial colitis. Like inflammatory bowel disease, the symptoms may occur intermittently over years (155). It is important to recognize that the disease may be present in people with-

out obvious risk factors, such as recent travel to endemic areas (156,157). Ten percent of the world population (158) and 5% of the U.S. population (157) harbor *E. histolytica*, though up to 90% of these individuals are asymptomatic.

Endoscopic findings are nonspecific, and the colonic abnormalities are easily mistaken for acute idiopathic inflammatory bowel disease (155–157,159) (Fig. 18). Diffuse inflammatory changes and multiple ulcerations can be seen (157,160). The ulcers are typically shallow, discrete, and round, with surrounding mucosal elevation (155,159). They are of variable size, from a few mm to 2 cms and are usually covered by a white or yellow exudate. The intervening mucosa can be normal or inflamed and granular. Aphthous ulcers can also commonly be seen (155). The rectum is involved in most cases, although the entire colon can be involved. The right colon can show isolated abnormalities in about 10% of cases (155,161). Endoscopic ulcerations may persist for several weeks to months after clinical symptoms have resolved (156). Amebomas, presenting as mass polypoid mass lesions have also been described (162). These uncommon lesions occur mainly in the cecum and represent areas of the bowel in which the amebae have infiltrated the wall causing the inflamed mucosa to bulge into the lumen. In asymptomatic carriers of *E. histolytica*, the colonic mucosa appears grossly normal (158).

A definitive diagnosis of amebiasis is made by identifying amebic trophozoites and flask-shaped ulcers in colonic biopsy specimens (159). To increase the yield of finding the ameba, biopsies should be taken from the ulcer margins at the interface between the normal and ulcerated tissue. Even with adequate biopsy specimens, however, the ameba may easily be missed or may not be present in the specimen due to sampling error (160). One study suggests that as many as two thirds of biopsy specimens

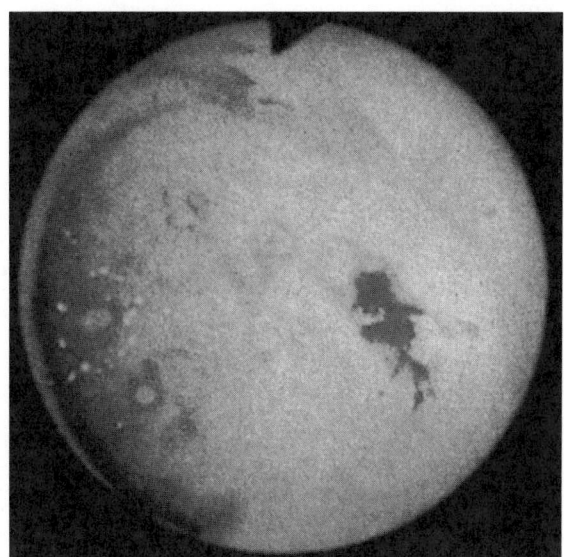

FIG. 18. Amebiasis of the colon. Small superficial ulcerations surrounded by an erythematous rim. Mucosa adjacent to the ulcers is unremarkable. (From ref. 14a, with permission.)

will be nondiagnostic in detecting ameba (159). In spite of this, histological examination of biopsy specimens is more sensitive than examination of fecal specimens (155,159). It is important to note that cathartics and enemas given before endoscopic evaluation may decrease the sensitivity of histological examination, since they can wash away and lyse the trophozoites (159). Because of this, some have recommended that no colonic preparation be given before endoscopic examination. Immediate microscopic examination of material aspirated or scraped from rectal lesions seen on proctoscopy has also been used to identify the parasite.

Stool studies for detection of amebic cysts have a high false-negative rate (157,161). The sensitivity of stool studies ranges from 50% to 60% (155,157,161). However, stool studies should be a routine test performed in patients being evaluated for possible infectious diarrhea. A stool ELISA test has been developed to detect *E. histolytica* infection and appears to differentiate between pathogenic and nonpathogenic forms (163). In a small study, the sensitivity and specificity of identifying pathogenic *E. histolytica* were 97% and 100%, respectively (163). This test is not yet available clinically.

Serological tests are positive in 85–95% of patients with invasive amebiasis (159,161), and asymptomatic cyst carriers usually have a negative serology (157). However, serological tests do not differentiate between past and present disease (158,161). The indirect hemagglutination (IHA) test, for instance, may remain elevated for as long as 20 years after the disease is cured (157,159). Serological testing should be correlated with clinical and endoscopic findings. Acute and convalescent serological titers should be sent 2–4 weeks apart, since false-negative tests can occur due to delayed seroconversion (157).

Stool studies and serological tests should be sent in any patient with new clinical symptoms suggestive of amebic colitis. Given the limitations of these tests, endoscopic examination of the colonic mucosa with biopsy sampling is an important part of the evaluation.

Schistosomiasis

Colonic involvement of schistosomiasis often presents with bleeding and diarrhea, but can also present with an abdominal mass (164). Colonoscopic findings include scattered mucosal erosions, edema, and erythema (165,166) (Fig. 19). Mucosal nodularity and polyps can also occur (164,166–168) (Fig. 20). Mucosal vascular alterations thought to be highly suggestive of this disease include loss of the reticular structure of blood vessels, vessel interruption, corkscrew vessels, and petechiae (166,169). Hypertrophy and fibrosis of the mucosa due to an inflammatory reaction to the submucosal schistosomal ova can cause formation of large masses simulating tumor (164). However, in 35–50% of patients, the mucosa appears normal, while biopsies demonstrate the presence of *Schistosoma* ova (165,167).

Biopsy specimens show granulomas containing *Schistosoma* ova (164) and are superior to stool examination. Biopsies should be taken from abnormal mucosal

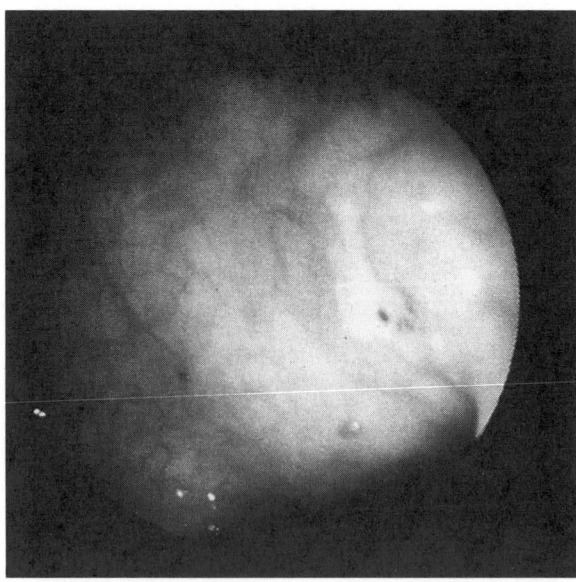

FIG. 19. Schistosomiasis of the colon. Scattered mucosal erosions, edema, and erythema. (From ref. 14a, with permission.)

lesions for the best yield, but random biopsies may still show the ova.

Stool examinations for ova and parasites were positive in only 11% of cases in which colonoscopic biopsies were positive for *Schistosoma mansoni* (165,167). Serological tests were positive in 53%, but the use of serology is limited since it does not distinguish between active and past infection. Therefore, colonoscopy with biopsy is a superior method for diagnosing intestinal schistosomiasis.

Mycobacterium Infections

Colonic Tuberculosis

Intestinal tuberculosis continues to present a diagnostic challenge, especially in the United States, where it is rela-

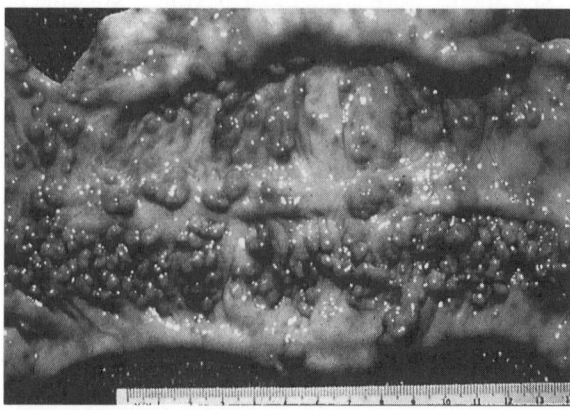

FIG. 20. Schistosomiasis of the colon. Gross specimen demonstrating mucosal nodularity and polyps. Histological examination of these polyps will demonstrate the ova. (From ref. 133a, with permission.)

tively uncommon. Although endoscopic and radiological findings have been well described, none are pathognomonic, and the diagnosis is still established by surgical intervention in many cases.

The ileocecal area is the most common site of infection with GI tuberculosis (100,103,170). In patients with colonic TB, the cecum is involved in up to 90% of cases, with the rectum involved the least often (171). However, segmental involvement of the colon without cecal lesions is being described more frequently (172). Typically, 4- to 8-cm segments of disease are seen with segmental tuberculosis, (173,174) and in approximately 30% of patients, two or more segments of the colon will be involved (174).

The colonic abnormalities usually take on an ulcerative form, a nodular hypertrophic form, or both (170–173, 175,176). Ulcers appear as multiple linear or round lesions with granular necrotic bases and edematous, elevated borders (170,175,176) (Fig. 21). Ulcers may be only a few millimeters, but can be several centimeters in dimension (174). Nodules and hypertrophic mucosa are also commonly seen. The nodules are typically 2–6 mm and can be densely packed (174). Ulcers are often interspersed among the nodules. Stricture formation is common. The ileocecal valve is characteristically deformed and edematous, and is associated with nodular mucosa and ulcerations in the majority of cases (170,171). Early colonoscopic abnormalities were described in 11 patients with pulmonary TB and normal barium enemas (171). Findings included small nodules resembling polyps in 70% of patients, and multiple small superficial ulcers in 30%. Biopsies were positive for acid-fast bacilli in all 11 patients. The cecum was also involved without ileal involvement in 4 cases, suggesting that cecal infection begins first, followed by ileal infection as the disease progresses.

Diagnosis requires histopathological demonstration of acid-fast bacilli or granulomas, or culture of *Mycobacte-*

rium from tissue specimens. Unfortunately, histological examination of endoscopic biopsy specimens has a poor diagnostic yield, partly due to the submucosal location of the *Mycobacterium* (170). Even with multiple biopsies taken from the same site to allow deeper sampling, histology is unrevealing in 20–60% of cases (170,172,174,175). Biopsy specimens are more frequently diagnostic if taken from an ulcerated lesion rather than a nodular lesion (48% vs. 25% in one series) (174). Kochhar reported two cases of intestinal tuberculosis diagnosed not by histology of biopsy specimens but by obtaining endoscopic fine-needle aspiration cytology samples from ileocecal nodules. The smears showed acid-fast bacilli in both patients, and may have had an increased yield because submucosal tissue was obtained. In another study of nine consecutive patients suspected of having intestinal TB, only two of nine biopsy samples showed acid-fast bacilli, whereas eight of nine brushing specimens showed acid-fast bacilli (177). The brushings were taken from a deep well created by first biopsying multiple times at the same site.

Culture of biopsy material is helpful, though it may take many weeks to become positive. Culture is positive in only about 40% of cases. However, the combination of histological examination and culture of biopsy specimens will yield a positive diagnosis in about 60% of cases (174).

Radiological studies may suggest the diagnosis, but the findings are nonspecific (170,173,174). The role of colonoscopy in the diagnosis of colonic tuberculosis is well established and should be performed in any patient suspected of having the disease. However, emphasis is placed on the difficulty in ascertaining the diagnosis in spite of extensive biopsy sampling.

ROLE OF ENDOSCOPIC RETROGRADE CHOLANGIOPANCREATOGRAPHY IN INFECTIONS OF THE PANCREATOBILIARY SYSTEM

Endoscopic retrograde cholangiopancreatography (ERCP) is currently the most definitive imaging technique in examining the biliary and pancreatic ducts. Although technically challenging, successful examination of the pancreatobiliary system by this method exceeds 90% of the cases in experienced hands. In addition to the ability of tissue sampling, ERCP with sphincterotomy or stent placement plays an important role in infections of the pancreatobiliary system by providing drainage of obstructed ducts.

Bacterial Infection

Bacterial Cholangitis

The most common cause of acute bacterial cholangitis is bile duct obstruction due to choledocholithiasis. Malignant or benign biliary strictures are important but less frequent causes of cholangitis. The patient's clinical presentation, laboratory data, and abdominal ultrasound or

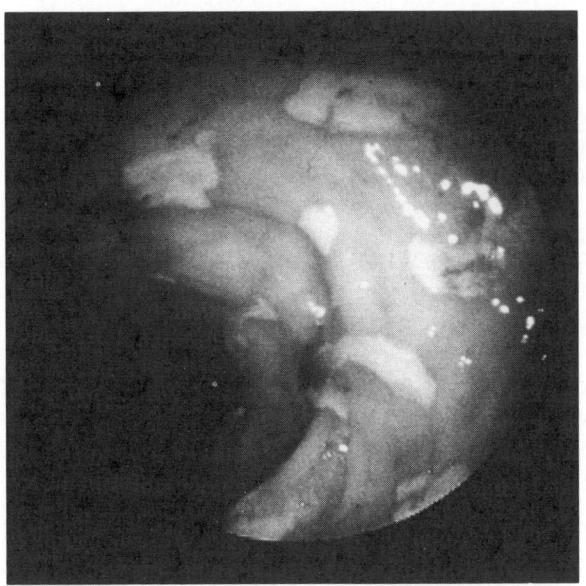

FIG. 21. Tuberculosis of the colon. Multiple round ulcers of the cecum. (From ref. 14a, with permission.)

CT provide adequate information to establish the proper diagnosis in the majority of cases. ERCP is seldom needed for diagnostic purposes in these patients.

However, in about 30% of patients with acute cholangitis, treatment with antibiotics alone is not adequate. Urgent decompression of the biliary tract is warranted (178). In experienced hands, ERCP can delineate the cause of bile duct obstruction in over 90% of cases (178,179). In addition, decompression of the bile duct by endoscopic sphincterotomy with stone extraction or by stent placement through a stricture has a success rate of over 85%. In a prospective study of patients with severe acute cholangitis due to choledocholithiasis, the mortality of patients who underwent emergency endoscopic drainage was 10% (180). This was significantly lower than the 32% observed in the group who underwent emergency surgical decompression. Endoscopic biliary drainage is also probably more preferable to percutaneous transhepatic biliary drainage. Prospective comparison of these two techniques in relieving malignant biliary obstruction suggested that the transhepatic approach was associated with higher complication rate due to intraperitoneal bile leak and hepatic bleed (181). However, direct comparison of these two drainage techniques in acute cholangitis has not been studied.

Viral Infections

HIV

AIDS cholangiopathy is now a well-recognized entity. Endoscopic cholangiogram will demonstrate biliary ductal abnormalities including strictures, dilation, sclerosis, and papillary stenosis. Although opportunistic infections such as CMV, cryptosporidiosis, and microsporidiosis are often implicated as the etiological factors of hepatobiliary pathology in these patients, 30–55% of cases fail to have any pathogen identified (182,183). This has been called AIDS cholangiopathy and considered to be directly related to local HIV infection. Some studies suggest that intrahepatic ductal irregularity is more indicative of concomitant infection with CMV or *Cryptosporidium* (184). Endoscopic sphincterotomy has been reported to provide long-term pain relief in these patients (184–186).

CMV

As much as 28% AIDS-related cholangitis has been documented to be secondary to CMV infection (187). The predominant clinical complaint at presentation is abdominal pain. Diagnosis of CMV infection is usually made in other regions of the body and is associated with disseminated infection. Endoscopic sphincterotomy relieves pain in more than 85% of these patients (187).

Fungal Infections

Pancreatobiliary infection due to fungal organisms has been infrequently reported. *Candida albicans* is the pre-

dominant organism noted (188,189). ERCP has been helpful in establishing the diagnosis in some cases by demonstrating ductal filling defects (188–190). Surgery has been the treatment of choice to date (190–192). The role of endoscopic management of these patients has yet to be defined.

Parasitic Infections

Cryptosporidia and Microsporidia

These organisms are the other common pathogens associated with cholangiopathy in AIDS patients (183, 193,194). The cholangiographic abnormalities cannot be differentiated from those induced by CMV (184). Endoscopic sphincterotomy also provides pain relief.

Ascaris

Ascaris lumbricoides is a major cause of acute obstructive cholangitis and pancreatitis throughout the world. In one region of India, ascariasis was considered to be an etiological factor in 23% of patients presenting with acute pancreatitis (195). ERCP is effective in identifying and extracting worms from both the biliary and pancreatic ducts with rapid relief of symptoms (196,197). Concomitant treatment with oral antihelminthic therapy is indicated for successful eradication of the parasite (195).

Echinococcus

Hydatid cysts of the liver are usually diagnosed after obtaining a clinical history, serology, and radiology findings including plain film of the abdomen, ultrasound, and CT scan. Surgical resection of the cyst with concomitant antihelminthic therapy with either mebendazole or albendazole has been the standard of treatment. Percutaneous drainage with hypertonic saline lavage of the cavity has also been advocated and offers a promising alternative to surgery (198). Intrabiliary rupture of a hepatic hydatid cyst occurs in 8–17% of cases and can lead to bile duct obstruction (199–202). ERCP is an effective diagnostic tool in this situation (203–205). Cholangiogram will often demonstrate irregularly shaped mobile filling defects, displacement and distortion of intrahepatic bile ducts by the hepatic cysts, and dilation of the pancreatic duct (206). Treatment options include sphincterotomy to facilitate drainage of cyst material, as well as lavage of the bile ducts and cysts with hypo- or hypertonic saline via a nasobiliary tube (204,207). Effective lavage of the cyst cavity requires continued communication with the biliary tree. These techniques have obviated the need for surgery in some cases, and long-term follow-up from 6 months to a year has demonstrated excellent results in most of these cases (206,208,209).

Liver Flukes

Clonorchis sinensis, Opisthorchis viverrini, and *Fasciola hepatica* follow similar patterns of existence within the bile ducts of a human host. Diagnosis, treatment, and management can be accomplished without the use of ERCP. The latter modality is employed when such complications as stricture or bacterial superinfection arise.

Mycobacterial Infections

Mycobacterium tuberculosis and *Mycobacterium avium-intracellulare* infections of the pancreatobiliary system are extremely rare. Frequently, tuberculosis of the pancreas is diagnosed postmortem (210). Since symptoms of these infections are predominantly related to other organs or organ systems, ERCP usually does not afford any earlier or greater diagnostic accuracy. Stenosis of the pancreatic duct secondary to tuberculosis diagnosed by ERCP in the setting of generalized *M. tuberculosis* infection has been reported (211).

ROLE OF ENDOSCOPY IN NOSOCOMIAL INFECTIONS

Nosocomial infections associated with endoscopy can be divided into three categories. The first group is the transmission of exogenous microorganisms to the patient by contaminated equipment. The second group is infection caused by the patient's endogenous enteric microorganisms that are introduced during endoscopy. The third group is transmission of infection from an infected patient to endoscopy personnel. The incidences of these events, the sources and types of microorganisms involved, and methods for preventing these infections are discussed in this section. This topic has been reviewed extensively in several recent reports (212,213).

Transmission of Infection by Contaminated Equipment

Incidence

The true incidence of transmission of pathogens by endoscopy is unknown. The number of reported cases of this event is remarkably small. Earlier reports on the incidence of patient infections due to endoscopy found rates for upper endoscopy, ERCP, colonoscopy, and colonoscopy plus polypectomy to be 0.008%, 0%, 0.01%, and 0.06%, respectively (214). From 1966 to 1987, 253 cases of infection transmitted by endoscopy were reported (213). The number of reported cases decreased to 28 in the period from 1988 to 1992. As approximately 40 million endoscopies were performed in this 4-year period, a crude and likely underestimate of incidence of infection transmitted by any endoscopy is therefore 1:1.8 million, or 0.000055% (212).

Types of Pathogens

Transmission of various species of *Salmonella* by either upper and lower endoscopy has been implicated in 84 patients (215–221). Forty-five cases of *Pseudomonas aeruginosa* transmission were reported (222–232). Most of these cases were associated with ERCP. Other bacterial organisms reported include *E. coli, Enterobacter cloacae* and *E. aerogenes* (231,233). *Staphylococcus epidermidis, Klebsiella* (234), *Serratia marcescens* (235), and *Helicobacter pylori* (236).

There is only one reported case of endoscopic transmission of hepatitis B (237). Several studies have demonstrated no transmission of hepatitis B in endemic areas where seronegative patients underwent endoscopies with equipment that had been used on hepatitis B surface and e-antigen–positive patients (238–240). As of June 1994, transmission of hepatitis C, HIV, CMV, and HSV by endoscopy has not been reported.

Two cases of endoscopic transmission of fungus (241,242) and one case of *Strongyloides stercoralis* transmission (243) have also been reported. So far transmission of *Mycobacterium* by GI endoscopy has not been documented.

Sources of Pathogens

Pathogens transmitted by endoscopy by and large can be traced back to inadequately cleaned endoscopic equipment. These organisms have been isolated from the endoscope's biopsy channels (215,226,227,229,230,244,245), biopsy forceps (218,246), water bottles (229), accessory suction equipment (215), and damaged endoscopes (247).

Contamination of equipment may be secondary to inadequate removal of debris prior to disinfection, ineffective cleaning or disinfecting agents (221,222,248,249), incomplete drying of equipment prior to storage (226), improper use of or poor design of automated cleaning machines (222,250,251), rinsing of equipment with tap water after disinfection (252), or handling of equipment by personnel before use.

Method of Prevention

The critical measure to prevent transmission of pathogens by endoscopy is proper cleaning of equipment. Sterilization of all endoscopes and accessories is not practical. Gas sterilization with ethylene oxide is too time consuming, and autoclaving damages the endoscope. High-level disinfection is the current standard of practice. This can be achieved by thorough manual cleaning of the equipment followed by soaking of the equipment in liquid chemical disinfectants. The recommended and most commonly used liquid disinfectant is 2% activated alkaline glutaraldehyde. Immersion of endoscopes in this solution for 5–10 min will eliminate all viral, fungal, and bacterial pathogens such as HBV, HIV, HSV, *Candida, Salmonella,* and *Pseudomonas.* Longer immersion time is needed to kill mycobacterial organisms. Bacterial spores are especially resistant to glutaraldehyde, but transmission of these organisms by endoscopy has not been reported. At present, the optimal immersion time in glutaraldehyde for complete disinfection is still controversial. A 20-min immersion is recommended by the Association for Practitioners in Infection Control.

Several organizations have published detailed guidelines for cleaning endoscopic equipment (253–255). Consensus of these recommendations includes:

1. Thorough manual cleaning of the endoscope immediately after use. This includes wiping of the instrument with detergent to remove debris and biofilm. Brushing of channels and removable parts of the endoscope is essential.
2. Immersion of instrument in 2% glutaraldehyde solution for at least 5 min. Ten to 20 minutes has also been recommended.
3. The disinfected endoscope must be dried with 70% alcohol and compressed air prior to storage in a hanging position.
4. Use of automated washers must be preceded by manual cleaning of the endoscope, and close monitoring of the washer for evidence of contamination must be performed.
5. Reusable accessories should be manually cleaned and then autoclaved.

Another approach to minimize transmission of pathogens by endoscopy is to use disposable equipment. Disposable accessories such as biopsy forceps and cannulas have enjoyed widespread use in recent years, and disposable endoscopes are being developed (213). However, consensus on the exclusive use of disposable equipment in endoscopy has not yet been established. Few objective data comparing the efficacy and safety of disposable equipment to reusable devices are available. The potential benefit of further reducing the small risk of infection transmission and the elimination of the cost of reprocessing equipment must be balanced against the expenses associated with equipment disposal and environmental impacts.

At present, strict adherence to equipment disinfection protocols is the best safeguard against transmission of infection by endoscopy. Adaptation of these disinfection guidelines may have contributed to the apparent decrease in reported transmission of infection by endoscopy since 1988. However, recent surveys suggested a 30–70% rate of noncompliance to recommended cleaning protocols by health care personnel (213). Further improvements in compliance with these guidelines by health care providers are needed.

Infections Due to Endogenous GI Flora

Transient bacteremia occurs with routine daily activity such as chewing hard candy (17%) and brushing one's teeth (25%), and does not lead to systemic infection (256). It is important to keep this in mind when examining data regarding procedure-induced bacteremia since only infrequently does systemic infection occur.

A wide range of endoscopy-induced bacteremia rates have been reported. Colonoscopy, sigmoidoscopy, and upper endoscopy are associated with lower rates of bacteremia, ranging from 0% to 19% (257–262). Biopsy during the procedure does not increase the incidence of bacteremia. More invasive procedures such as dilation of esophageal strictures, endoscopic laser therapy, injection sclerotherapy, and therapeutic ERCP may have bacteremia rates as high as 30–45% (262–264). However, much lower rates of bacteremia associated with these procedures have also been reported. Oropharyngeal flora such as *Streptococcus* and *Staphylococcus* species are the most common organisms isolated (256,258,259,262).

Despite the apparently high rate of bacteremia induced by various endoscopic procedures, the incidence of clinically significant infections as a result of these procedures is extremely low. Only a few cases of endocarditis, perinephric and brain abscesses have been reported (253,265–267). The risk of infectious complication in immunocompromised patients undergoing endoscopy is also not significantly different from that of patients with normal immune systems (268,269).

Use of prophylactic antibiotics prior to endoscopic procedures is a logical method to prevent serious infectious complications. However, there are no firm data demonstrating the benefit of prophylactic antibiotics in preventing endocarditis even in patients with prosthetic heart valves or in immunocompromised patients. As the true incidence of infection is probably very low in these patients, only very large randomized trials can demonstrate the efficacy of prophylactic antibiotics. These studies have not been and probably will never be conducted. Due to the serious consequences of endocarditis, prophylactic antibiotics prior to endoscopy are recommended in patients with prosthetic heart valves or surgically created systemic-pulmonary shunts, and in patients with a history of endocarditis (253). For other situations, including that of immunocompromised patients, the decision to use prophylactic antibiotics must be individualized. This will be influenced primarily by an individual physician's interpretation of the limited and often conflicting data available, and by the patient's condition and choice. Understandably, differences in opinion regarding these recommendations exist (253,270).

Transmission of Infections from Infected Patient to Endoscopy Personnel

Endoscopy personnel are at risk of acquiring infections transmitted directly from the patient or from contaminated equipment. The incidence of these events is unknown. The endoscopist may have a small risk of acquiring HBV when performing procedures in infected patients (271). Transmission of *H. pylori* during endoscopy has been implicated by the observation that the incidence of *H. pylori* infection in gastroenterologists (52%) appears to be higher than that in other endoscopy personnel, general practitioners, and age-matched controls (21%) (272).

Endoscopy personnel must exercise universal precautions in terms of protecting themselves against infections as patients' infection status may be unknown at the time of endoscopy. Use of protective measures such as gloves, gowns, masks, and eye coverings are recommended, especially when extensive contact with blood or other bodily fluid is anticipated. Handwashing must be done after each procedure even when gloves have been worn. Infection prevention guidelines during endoscopic procedures and endoscopy cleaning must be followed to maximize safety (273). In addition, vaccination against HBV in endoscopy personnel is appropriate.

Summary

Nosocomial infections caused by GI endoscopy are exceedingly rare, even allowing for possible underreporting of these events. The majority of the cases of infection transmission by endoscopy can be attributed to either inadequate disinfection protocols or noncompliance to these protocols. When proper adjustments in protocol are made, infection outbreaks are effectively terminated. Current standards of cleaning and disinfection therefore make gastrointestinal endoscopy a safe diagnostic and therapeutic tool in the management of GI disease.

REFERENCES

1. Dooley CP, Cohen H, Fitzgibbons PL, et al. Prevalence of *Helicobacter pylori* infection and histologic gastritis in asymptomatic persons. *N Engl J Med* 1989;321:1562–1566.
2. Dooley CP, Cohen J. The clinical significance of *Campylobacter pylori*. *Ann Intern Med* 1988;108:70–79.
3. Parsonnet J. *Helicobacter pylori* and gastric cancer. *Gastroenterol Clin North Am* 1993;22(1):89–104.
4. Parsonnett J, Hansen S, Rodriquez L, et al. *Helicobacter pylori* infection and gastric lymphoma. *N Engl J Med* 1994;330:1267–1271.
5. Strauss RM, Wang TC, Kelsey PB, et al. Association of *Helicobacter pylori* infection with dyspeptic symptoms in patients undergoing gastroduodenoscopy. *Am J Med* 1990;89:464–469.
6. Loffeld RJLF, Ten Tije BJ, Arends JW. Prevalence and significance of *Helicobacter pylori* in patients with Barrett's esophagus. *Am J Gastroenterol* 1992;87:1598–1600.
7. Nguyen AH, Engstrand L, Genta RM, Graham DY, El-Zaatari FAK. Detection of *Helicobacter pylori* in dental plaque by reverse transcription–polymerase chain reaction. *J Clin Microbiol* 1993;31:783–787.
8. Borhan-Manesh F, Farnum JB. Study of *Helicobacter pylori* colonization of patches of heterotopic gastric mucosa (HGM) at the upper esophagus. *Dig Dis Sci* 1993;38:142–146.
9. Hazell SL, Hennessy WR, Borody TJ, et al. *Campylobacter pyloridis* gastritis II: distribution of bacteria and associated inflammation in the gastroduodenal environment. *Am J Gastroenterol* 1987;82:297–301.
10. Goodwin CS, Worsley BW. Microbiology of *Helicobacter pylori Gastroenterol Clin North Am* 1993;22:5–19.
11. Brown KE, Peura DA. Diagnosis of *Helicobacter pylori* infection. *Gastroenterol Clin North Am* 1993;22:105–115.
12. Relman DA, Schmidt TM, MacDermott RP, Falkow S. Identification of the uncultured bacillus of Whipple's disease. *N Engl J Med* 1992;327:293–301.
13. Crane S, Schlippert W. Duodenoscopic findings in Whipple's disease. *Gastrointest Endosc* 1978;24:248–249.
14. Geboes K, Ectors N, Heidbuchel H, Rutgeerts P, Desmet V, Vantrappen G. Whipple's disease: endoscopic aspects before and after therapy. *Gastrointest Endosc* 1990;36:247–252.

14a.Silverstein FE, Tytgat, GNJ. *Atlas of gastrointestinal endoscopy*. Philadelphia: W.B. Saunders; 1987.
15. Ectors N, Geboes K, Wynants P, Desmet V. Granulomatous gastritis and Whipple's disease. *Am J Gastroenterol* 1992;87:509–513.
16. Walsh TJ, Bekutsis NJ, Hamilton SR. Bacterial esophagitis in immunocompromised patients. *Arch Intern Med* 1986;146:1345–1348.
17. Mcdonald GB, Sharma P, Hackman RC, et al. Esophageal infections in immunosuppressed patients after marrow transplantation. *Gastroenterol* 1985;88:1111–1117.
18. Ezzell JH, Bremer J, Adamec TA. Bacterial esophagitis: an often forgotten cause of odynophagia. *Am J Gastroenterol* 1990;85:296–298.
19. Mcmanus JPA, Webb JN. A yeast-like infection of the esophagus caused by *Lactobacillus acidophilus*. *Gastroenterol* 1975;68:583–586.
20. Howlett SA. Acute streptococcal esophagitis. *Gastrointest Endosc* 1979;25:150–151.
21. Goff JS. Infectious causes of esophagitis. *Annu Rev Med* 1988;39:163–169.
22. Nicholson BW, Maull KI, Scher LA. Phlegmonous gastritis: clinical presentation and surgical management. *South Med J* 1980;73:875–877.
23. Turner MA, Beachley MC, Stanley D. Phlegmonous gastritis. *AJR* 1979;133:527–528.
24. Lifton LJ, Schlossberg D. Phlegmonous gastritis after endoscopic polypectomy. *Ann Intern Med* 1982;97:373–374.
25. Stein LB, Greenberg RE, Ilardi CR, Kurtz L, Bank S. Acute necrotizing gastritis in a patient with peptic ulcer disease. *Am J Gastroenterology* 1989;84:1552–1554.
26. Miller AI, Smith B, Rogers AI. Phlegmonous gastritis. *Gastroenterology* 1975;68:231–238.
27. Cruz FO, Soffia PS, Del Rio PM, Fava MP, Duarte IF. Acute phlegmonous gastritis with mural abscess: CT diagnosis. *AJR* 1992;159:767–768.
28. Cardillo MR, Forte F. Brush cytology in the diagnosis of herpetic esophagitis. A case report. *Endoscopy* 1988;20:156–157.
29. Solammadevi SV, Patwardhan R. Herpes esophagitis. *Am J Gastroenterol* 1982;77:48–50.
30. McDonald GB, Shulman HM, Sullivan KM, Spencer GD. Intestinal and hepatic complications of human bone marrow transplantation. Part I. *Gastroenterology* 1986;90(2):460–477.
31. McDonald GB, Shulman HM, Sullivan KM, Spencer GD. Intestinal and hepatic complications of human bone marrow transplantation. Part II. *Gastroenterology* 1986;90(3):770–784.
32. McBane RD, Gross JB. Herpes esophagitis: clinical syndrome, endoscopic appearance, and diagnosis in 23 patients. *Gastrointest Endosc* 1991;37:600–603.
33. McBane RD, Gross JB. Herpes esophagitis: review of the clinical syndrome, endoscopic appearance, and diagnosis in 21 patients. *Gastrointest Endosc* 1990;36:192–193.
34. Agha FP, Lee HH, Nostrant TT. Herpetic esophagitis: a diagnostic challenge in immunocompromised patients. *Am J Gastroenterol* 1986;81:246–253.
35. Brady CE, Hover AR. Esophagitis in immunocompromised patients: a diagnostic challenge. *South Med J* 1983;76:1538–1541.
36. Alexander JA, Brouillette DE, Chien M-C, et al. Infectious esophagitis following liver and renal transplantation. *Dig Dis Sci* 1988;33:1121–1126.
37. Kaplan CS, Petersen EA, Icenogle TB, et al. Gastrointestinal cytomegalovirus infection in heart and heart–lung transplant recipients. *Arch Intern Med* 1989;149:2095–2100.
38. Hinnant KL, Rotterdam HZ, Bell ET, Tapper ML. Cytomegalovirus infection of the alimentary tract: a clinicopathological correlation. *Am J Gastroenterol* 1986;81:944–950.
39. Bonacini M, Young T, Laine L. The causes of esophageal symptoms in human immunodeficiency virus infection. *Arch Intern Med* 1991;151:1567–1572.
40. Culpepper-Morgan JA, Kotler DP, Scholes JV, Tierney AR. Evaluation of diagnostic criteria for mucosal cytomegalic inclusion disease in the acquired immune deficiency syndrome. *Am J Gastroenterol* 1987;82:1264–1270.
41. Jacobson MA, Mills J. Serious cytomegalovirus disease in the

acquired immunodeficiency syndrome (AIDS). *Ann Intern Med* 1988;108:585–594.

42. Freedman PG, Weiner BC, Balthazar EJ. Cytomegalovirus esophagogastritis in a patient with acquired immunodeficiency syndrome. *Am J Gastroenterol* 1985;80:434–437.

43. Theise ND, Rotterdam H, Dieterich D. Cytomegalovirus esophagitis in AIDS: diagnosis by endoscopic biopsy. *Am J Gastroenterol* 1991;86:1123–1126.

44. Gill RA, Gebhard RL, Dozeman RL, Sumner HW. Shingles esophagitis: endoscopic diagnosis in two patients. *Gastrointest Endosc* 1984;30:26–27.

45. Wisloff F, Bull-Berg J, Myron J. Herpes zoster of the stomach. *Lancet* 1979;2:953.

46. Artigas JMG, Saumell CB, Faure RA, Llebaria C. Herpes zoster of upper gastrointestinal tract. *Lancet* 1980;2:43.

47. Bartelsman JFWM, Lange JMA, Van Leeuwen R, Van den Tweel JG, Tytgat GNJ. Acute primary HIV-esophagitis. *Endoscopy* 1990;22:184–185.

48. Rabeneck L, Popovic M, Gartner S, et al. Acute HIV infection presenting with painful swallowing and esophageal ulcers. *JAMA* 1990;17:2318–2322.

49. Kitchen VS, Helbert M, Francis ND, et al. Epstein–Barr virus associated oesophageal ulcers in AIDS. *Gut* 1990;31:1223–1225.

50. Wheller RR, Peacock JE, Cruz JM, Richter JE. Esophagitis in the immunocompromised host: role of esophagoscopy in diagnosis. *Rev Infect Dis* 1987;9:88–96.

51. Wilcox CM. Esophageal disease in the acquired immunodeficiency syndrome: etiology, diagnosis, and management. *Am J Med* 1992;92:412–421.

52. Trier JS, Bjorkman DJ. Esophageal, gastric and intestinal candidiasis. *Am J Med* 1984;76:39–43.

53. Kodsi BE, Wickremesinghe PC, Kozinn PF, Iswara K, Goldberg PK. *Candida* esophagitis. A prospective study of 27 cases. *Gastroenterology* 1976;71:715–719.

54. Mathieson R, Dutta SK. *Candida* esophagitis. *Dig Dis Sci* 1983;28:365–370.

55. Minoli G, Terruzzi V, Butti G, Frigerio G, Rossini A. Gastric candidiasis: an endoscopic and histological study in 26 patients. *Gastrointest Endosc* 1982;28:59–61.

56. Porro GB, Parente F, Cernuschi M. The diagnosis of esophageal candidiasis in patients with acquired immune deficiency syndrome: is endoscopy always necessary? *Am J Gastroenterol* 1989;84:143–146.

57. Bonacini M, Laine L, Gal AA, Lee MH, Martin SE, Strigle S. Prospective evaluation of blind brushing of the esophagus for *Candida* esophagitis in patients with human immunodeficiency virus infection. *Am J Gastroenterol* 1990;85:385–389.

58. Young JA, Elias E. Gastro-oesophageal candidiasis: diagnosis by brush cytology. *J Clin Pathol* 1985;38:293–296.

59. Debongnie JC, Beyaert C, Legros G. Touch cytology, a useful diagnostic method for diagnosis of upper gastrointestinal tract infections. *Dig Dis Sci* 1989;34:1025–1027.

60. Rosario Mt, Raso Cl, Comer GM, Clain DJ. Transnasal brush cytology for the diagnosis of *Candida* esophagitis in the acquired immunodeficiency syndrome. *Gastrointest Endosc* 1989;35:102–103.

61. Korlipara AP, Shrinpreis MN, Luk GD, Peleman RR. Blind cytology brushing as a method of diagnosis of esophageal candidiasis. *Gastrointest Endosc* 1988;34:205.

62. Levine MS, Macones AJ Jr, Laufer I. *Candida* esophagitis: accuracy of radiographic diagnosis. *Radiology* 1985;154:581–587.

63. Prescott RJ, Harris M, Banerjee SS. Fungal infections of the small and large intestine. *J Clin Pathol* 1992;45:806–811.

64. Forsmark CE, Wilcox CM, Darragh TM, Cello JP. Disseminated histoplasmosis in AIDS: an unusual case of esophageal involvement and gastrointestinal bleeding. *Gastrointest Endosc* 1990;36:604–605.

65. Tom W, Aaron JS. Esophageal ulcers caused by *Torulopsis glabrata* in a patient with acquired immune deficiency syndrome. *Am J Gastroenterol* 1987;82:766–768.

66. Ikeda K, Kumashiro R, Kifune T. Nine cases of acute gastric anisakiasis. *Gastrointest Endosc* 1989;35:304–308.

67. Sugimachi K, Inokuchi K, Ooiwa T, Fujino T, Ishii Y. Acute gastric anisakiasis. Analysis of 178 cases. *JAMA* 1985;253:1012–1013.

68. Sakanari JA, Loinaz M, Deardorff TL, Raybourne RB, McKerrow JH, Frierson JG. Intestinal anisakiasis. A case diagnosed by morphologic and immunologic methods. *Am J Clin Pathol* 1988;90:107–113.

69. Sakanari JA, McKerrow JH. Anisakiasis. *Clin Microbiol Rev* 1989;2:278–284.

70. McHenry R, Bartlett MS, Lehman GA, O'Connor KW. The yield of routine duodenal aspiration for *Giardia lamblia* during esophagogastroduodenoscopy. *Gastrointest Endosc* 1987;33:425–426.

71. Flanagan PA. *Giardia*—diagnosis, clinical course and epidemiology. A review. *Epidemiol Infect* 1992;109:1–22.

72. Oberhuber G, Stolte M. Giardiasis: analysis of histological changes in biopsy specimens of 80 patients. *J Clin Pathol* 1990;43:641–643.

73. El Sheikh Mohemed AR, Al Karawi MA, Yasawy MI. Modern techniques in the diagnosis and treatment of gastrointestinal and biliary tree parasites. *Hepatogastroenterology* 1991;38:180–188.

74. Doglioni C, De Boni M, Ciclo R, et al. Gastric giardiasis. *J Clin Pathol* 1992;45:964–967.

75. Knisley CV, Engelkirk PG, Pickering LK, West MS, Janoff EN. Rapid detection of *Giardia* antigen in stool with the use of enzyme immunoassays. *Am J Clin Pathol* 1989;91:704–708.

76. Bendig DW. Diagnosis of giardiasis in infants and children by endoscopic brush cytology. *J Ped Gastroenterol Nutr* 1989;8:204–206.

77. Green EL, Miles MA, Warhurst DC. Immunodiagnostic detection of *Giardia* antigen in faeces by a rapid visual enzyme-linked immunosorbent assay. *Lancet* 1985;2:691–693.

78. Ungar BLP, Yolken RH, Nash TE, Quinn TC. Enzyme-linked immunosorbent assay for the detection of *Giardia lamblia* in fecal specimens. *J Infect Dis* 1984;149:90–97.

79. Janoff EN, Craft JC, Pickering LK, et al. Diagnosis of *Giardia lamblia* infections by detection of parasite-specific antigens. *J Clin Microbiol* 1989;27:431–435.

80. Kamath KR, Murugasu R. A comparative study of four methods for detecting *Giardia lamblia* in children with diarrheal disease and malabsorption. *Gastroenterol* 1974;66:16–21.

81. Achkar E, Carey WD, Petras R, Sivak MV, Revta R. Comparison of suction capsule and endoscopic biopsy of small bowel mucosa. *Gastrointest Endosc* 1986;32:278–281.

82. Korman SH. Endoscopic duodenal aspiration for diagnosis of giardiasis. *Gastrointest Endosc* 1989;35:354–355.

83. Rosenthal P, Liebman WM. Comparative study of stool examinations, duodenal aspiration, and pediatric Entero-Test for giardiasis in children. *J Pediatr* 1980;96:278–279.

84. Marshall JB, Kelley DH, Vogele KA. Giardiasis: diagnosis by endoscopic brush cytology of the duodenum. *Am J Gastroenterol* 1984;79:517–519.

85. Gellin BG, Soave R. Coccidian infections in AIDS. Toxoplasmosis, cryptosporidiosis and isosporiasis. *Med Clin North Am* 1992;76:205–234.

86. Rene E, Marche C, Regnier B, et al. Intestinal infections in patients with acquired immunodeficiency syndrome. A prospective study in 132 patients. *Dig Dis Sci* 1989;34:773–780.

87. Edwards P, Wodak A, Cooper DA, Thompson IL, Penny R. The gastrointestinal manifestations of AIDS. *Aust NZ J Med* 1990;20:141–148.

88. Angus KW. Cryptosporidiosis and AIDS. *Bailliere Clin Gastroenterol* 1990;4:425–441.

89. Connolly GM, Forbes A, Gleeson JA, Gazzard BG. The value of barium enema and colonoscopy in patients infected with HIV. *AIDS* 1990;4:687–689.

90. Ullrich R, Heise W, Bergs C, L'age M, Riecken EO, Zeitz M. Gastrointestinal symptoms in patients infected with human immunodeficiency virus: relevance of infective agents isolated from gastrointestinal tract. *Gut* 1992;33:1080–1084.

91. Cello JP. Evaluation of AIDS-related diarrhea. *Hosp Prac* 1993;28:95–102.

92. Dumont A, Seferian V, Barbier P. Endoscopic discovery and

capture of *Necator americanus* in the stomach. *Endoscopy* 1983;15:65–66.

93. Genta RM, Woods KL. Endoscopic diagnosis of hookworm infection. *Gastrointest Endosc* 1991;37:476–478.
94. Descombes P, Dupas JL, Capron JP. Endoscopic discovery and capture of *Taenia saginata*. *Endoscopy* 1981;13:44–45.
95. Jacob GS, Nakib A, Ruwaih AA. Ascariasis producing upper gastrointestinal hemorrhage. *Endoscopy* 1983;15:67.
96. Hamed AD, Akinola O. Intestinal ascariasis in the differential diagnosis of peptic ulcer disease. *Trop Geogr Med* 1990;42:37–40.
97. Contractor QQ, Benson L, Schulz TB, Contractor TQ, Kasturi N. Duodenal involvement in *Schistosoma mansoni* infection. *Gut* 1988;29:1011–1012.
98. Webbe G. Schistosomiasis: some advances. *Br Med J* 1981;283:1104–1106.
99. Salas SD, Heifetz R, Barrett-Connor E. Intestinal parasites in Central American immigrants in the United States. *Arch Intern Med* 1990;150:1514–1516.
100. Weissman D, Gumaste VV, Dave PB, Keh W. Bleeding from a tuberculous gastric ulcer. *Am J Gastrolenterol* 1990;85:742–744.
101. Abel ME, Chiu YS, Russell TR, Volpe P. Gastrointestinal tuberculosis. Report of four cases. *Dis Col Rect* 1990;33:886–889.
102. Vijayraghavan M, Arunabh, Sarda AK, Sharma AK, Chatterjee TK. Duodenal tuberculosis: a review of the clinicopathologic features and management of twelve cases. *Jpn J Surg* 1990;20:526–529.
103. Nair KV, Pai CG, Rajagopal KP, Ghat VN, Thomas M. Unusual presentations of duodenal tuberculosis. *Am J Gastroenterol* 1991;86:756–760.
104. Salpeter SR, Shapiro RM, Gasman JD. Gastric tuberculosis presenting as fever of unknown origin. *West J Med* 1991;155:412–413.
105. Gupta B, Mathew S, Bhalla S. Pyloric obstruction due to gastric tuberculosis and endoscopic diagnosis. *Postgrad Med J* 1990;66:63–65.
106. Gordon AH, Marshal JB. Esophageal tuberculosis: definitive diagnosis by endoscopy. *Am J Gastroenterol* 1990;85:174–177.
107. Tromba JL, Inglese R, Rieders B, Todaro R. Primary gastric tuberculosis presenting as pyloric outlet obstruction. *Am J Gastroenterol* 1991;86:1820–1822.
108. Eng J, Sabanathan S. Tuberculosis of the esophagus. *Dig Dis Sci* 1991;36:536–540.
109. Rosario MT, Raso CL, Comer GM. Esophageal tuberculosis. *Dig Dis Sci* 1989;34:1281–1284.
110. Tornieporth N, Lorenzo R, Gain T, Rosch T, Classen M. An unusual case of active tuberculosis of the oesophagus in an adult. *Endoscopy* 1991;23:294–296.
110a. Tornieporth N, Lorenz R, Gain T, et al. An unusual case of active tuberculosis of the oesophagus in an adult. *Endo* 1991;23:294–296.
111. Subei I, Attar B, Schmitt G, Levendoglu H. Primary gastric tuberculosis: a case report and literature review. *Am J Gastroenterol* 1987;82:769–772.
112. Regan F, Tran T. Duodenal tuberculosis—a continuing diagnostic challenge. *Postgrad Med J* 1990;66:787–791.
113. Sivasubramanian S, Senapaati MK. Tuberculosis of the stomach. *Trop Doctor* 1992;22:132–133.
114. Fukuya T, Yoshimitsu K, Kitagawa S, Masuda K, Ueyama T, Haraguchi Y. Single tuberculous stricture in the jejunum: report of 2 cases. *Gastrointest Radiol* 1989;14:300–304.
114a. Rosario Mt, Raso CL, Comer GM. Esophageal tuberculosis. *Dig Dis Sci* 1989;34:1281–1284.
115. De Silva R, Stoopack PM, Raufman J-P. Esophageal fistulas associated with mycobacterial infection in patients at risk for AIDS. *Radiology* 1990;175:449–453.
116. Gray JR, Rabeneck L. Atypical mycobacterial infection of the gastrointestinal tract in AIDS patients. *Am J Gastroenterol* 1989;84:1521–1524.
116a. Cotton PB, Tytgat GNJ, Williams CB. *Slide atlas of gastrointestinal endoscopy*. London: Current Science; 1992.
117. Lewis BS, Kornbluth A, Waye JD. Small bowel tumours: yield of enteroscopy. *Gut* 1991;32:763–765.

118. Barkin JS, Lewis BS, Reiner DK, et al. Diagnostic and therapeutic jejunoscopy with a new, longer enteroscope. *Gastrointest Endosc* 1992;38:55–58.
119. Loss RW, Mangla JC, Pereira M. *Campylobacter* colitis presenting as inflammatory bowel disease with segmental colonic ulcerations. *Gastroenterology* 1980;79:138–140.
120. Lambert ME, Schofield PF, Ironside AG, Mandal BK. *Campylobacter* colitis. *Br Med J* 1979;1:857–859.
121. Blaser MJ, Parsons RB, Wang W-LL. Acute colitis caused by *Campylobacter fetus* ss. *jejuni*. *Gastroenterology* 1980;78:448–453.
122. Khuro MS, Mahajan R, Zargar SA, et al. The colon in shigellosis: serial colonoscopic appearances in *Shigella dysenteriae* I. *Endoscopy* 1990;22:35–38.
123. Fry RD. Infectious enteritis. A collective review. *Dis Col Rect* 1990;33:520–527.
124. Drake AA, Gilchrist MJR, Washington JA, Huizenga KA, Van Scoy RE. Diarrhea due to *Campylobacter fetus* subspecies *jejuni*. A clinical review of 63 cases. *Mayo Clin Proc* 1981;56:414–423.
125. Nastrant TT, Kumar NB, Appelman HD. Histopathology differentiates acute self-limited colitis from ulcerative colitis. *Gastroenterology* 1987;92:318–328.
126. Surawicz CM, Belic L. Rectal biopsy helps to distinguish acute self-limited colitis from idiopathic inflammatory bowel disease. *Gastroenterology* 1984;86:104–113.
127. Kelly J, Oryshak A, Wenetsek M, Grabiec J, Handy S. The colonic pathology of *Escherichia coli* O157:H7 infection. *Am J Surg Pathol* 1990;14:87–92.
128. Griffin PM, Ostroff SM, Tauxe RV, et al. Illnesses associated with *Escherichia coli* O157:H7 infections. A broad clinical spectrum. *Ann Intern Med* 1988;109:705–712.
129. Shortsleeve MJ, Wilson ME. Finklestein M, Gardner RC. Radiologic findings in hemorrhagic colitis due to *Escherichia coli* O157:H7. *Gastrointest Radiol* 1989;14:341–344.
130. Griffin PM, Olmsteasd LC, Petras RE. *Escherichia coli* O157:H7–associated colitis. A clinical and histological study of 11 cases. *Gastroenterology* 1990;90:142–149.
131. Remis RS, MacDonald KL, Riley LW, et al. Sporadic cases of hemorrhagic colitis associated with *Escherichia coli* O157:H7. *Ann Intern Med* 1984;101:624–626.
132. Gerding DN. Disease associated with *Clostridium difficile* infection. *Ann Intern Med* 1989;110:255–257.
133. Fekety R, Shah AB. Diagnosis and treatment of *Clostridium difficile* colitis. *JAMA* 1993;269:71–75.
133a. Pounder RE, Allison MC, Dhillon AP. *Colour atlas of the digestive system*. London: Wolfe Publishing; 1989.
134. Gebhard RL, Gerding DN, Olson MM, et al. Clinical and endoscopic findings in patients early in the course of *Clostridium difficile*–associated pseudomembranous colitis. *Am J Med* 1985;78:45–48.
135. Tedesco FJ. Pseudomembranous colitis: pathogenesis and therapy. *Med Clin North Am* 1982;66:655–663.
136. Talbot RW, Walker RC, Beart RW Jr. Changing epidemiology, diagnosis, and treatment of *Clostridium difficile* toxin–associated colitis. *Br J Surg* 1986;73:457–460.
137. Tedesco FJ, Corless JK, Brownstein RE. Rectal sparing in antibiotic-associated pseudomembranous colitis: a prospective study. *Gastroenterology* 1982;83:1259–1260.
138. Seppala K, Hjelt L, Sipponen P. Colonoscopy in the diagnosis of antibiotic-associated colitis. A prospective study. *Scand J Gastroenterol* 1981;16:465–468.
139. Tedesco FJ. Antibiotic associated pseudomembranous colitis with negative proctosigmoidoscopy examination. *Gastroenterology* 1979;77:295–297.
140. Price AB, Davies DR. Pseudomembranous colitis. *J Clin Pathol* 1977;30:1–12.
141. Peterson LR, Olson MM, Shanholtzer CH, Gerding DN. Results of a prospective, 18-month clinical evaluation of culture, cytotoxin testing, and culturette brand (CDT) latex testing in the diagnosis of *Clostridium difficile*–associated diarrhea. *Diag Microbiol Infect Dis* 1988;10:85–91.
142. Lashner BA, Todorczuk J, Sahm DF, Hanauer SB. *Clostridium*

difficile culture-positive toxin-negative diarrhea. *Am J Gastroenterol* 1986;81:940–943.

143. Gumerlock PH, Tang YJ, Weiss JB, Silva J Jr. Specific detection of toxigenic strains of *clostridium difficile* in stool specimens. *J Clin Microbiol* 1993;31:507–511.

144. Kato N, Ou C-Y, Kato H, et al. Detection of toxigenic *Clostridium difficile* in stool specimens by the polymerase chain reaction. *J Infect Dis* 1993;167:455–458.

145. Gerding DN, Olson MM, Peterson LR, et al. *Clostridium difficile*–associated diarrhea and colitis in adults. A prospective case-controlled epidemiologic study. *Arch Intern Med* 1986;146:95–100.

146. Foucar E, Mukai K, Foucar K, Sutherland DER, Van Buren CT. Colonic ulceration in lethal cytomegalovirus infection. *Am J Clin Pathol* 1981;76:788–801.

147. Dieterich DT, Rahmin M. Cytomegalovirus colitis in AIDS: presentation of 44 patients and a review of the literature. *J AIDS* 1991;4(Suppl 1):S29–S35.

148. Dieterich DT, Kotler DP, Busch DF, et al. Gangiclovir treatment of cytomegalovirus colitis in AIDS: a randomized, double-blind, placebo-controlled multicenter study. *J Infect Dis* 1993;167:278–282.

149. Rene E, Marche C, Chevalier T, et al. Cytomegalovirus colitis in patients with acquired immunodeficiency syndrome. *Dig Dis Sci* 1988;33:741–750.

150. Weber FH, Frierson JF, Myers BM. Cytomegalovirus as a cause of isolated severe ileal bleeding. *J Clin Gastroenterol* 1992;14:52–55.

151. Colemont LJ, Pen JH, Peickmans PA, Degryse HR, Pattyn SR, Van Maercke YM. Herpes simplex virus type 1 colitis: an unusual cause of diarrhea. *Am J Gastroenterol* 1990;85:1182–1185.

152. Kinnaert R, Vereerstraeten P, Toussaint C. Diffuse herpes simplex virus colitis in a kidney transplant recipient successfully treated with acyclovir. *Transplantation* 1987;43:919–921.

153. Gupta TP, Ehrinpreis MN. *Candida*-associated diarrhea in hospitalized patients. *Gastroenterology* 1990;98:780–785.

154. Eras P, Goldstein MJ, Sherlock P. *Candida* infection of the gastrointestinal tract. *Medicine* 1972;51:367–379.

155. Matsui T, Iida M, Tada S, et al. The value of double-contrast barium enema in amebic colitis. *Gastrointest Radiol* 1989;14:73–78.

156. Sanderson IR, Walker-Smith JA. Indigenous amoebiasis: an important differential diagnosis of chronic inflammatory bowel disease. *Br Med J* 1984;289:823.

157. Patel AS, DeRidder PH. Amebic colitis masquerading as acute inflammatory bowel disease: the role of serology in its diagnosis. *J Clin Gastroenterol* 1989;11:407–410.

158. Variyam EP, Gogate P, Hassan M, et al. Nondysenteric intestinal amebiasis. Colonic morphology and search for *Entamoeba histolytica* adherence and invasion. *Dig Dis Sci* 1989;34:732–740.

159. Blumencranz H, Kasen L, Romeu J, Waye JD, LeLeiko NS. The role of endoscopy in suspected amebiasis. *Am J Gastroenterol* 1983;78:15–18.

160. Rozen P, Baratz M, Rattan J. Rectal bleeding due to amebic colitis diagnosed by multiple endoscopic biopsies: report of two cases. *Dis Col Rect* 1981;24:127–129.

161. Patterson M, Healy GR, Shabot JM. Serologic testing for amoebiasis. *Gastroenterology* 1980;78:1236–141.

162. Luterman L, Alsumait AR, Daly DS, Goresky CA. Colonoscopic features of cecal amebomas. *Gastrointest Endosc* 1985;31:204–206.

163. Haque R, Kress K, Wood S, et al. Diagnosis of pathogenic *Entamoeba histolytica* infection using a stool ELISA based on monoclonal antibodies to the galactose-specific adhesin. *J Infect Dis* 1993;167:247–249.

164. Zimbalist E, Gettenberg G, Brejt H. Ileocolonic schistosomiasis presenting as lymphoma. *Am J Gastroenerol* 1987;82:476–478.

165. Yasawy MI, El Shiekh Mohamed AR, Al Karawi MA. Comparison between stool examination, serology and large bowel biopsy in diagnosing *Schistosoma mansoni*. *Trop Doctor* 1989;19:132–134.

166. Raddawi JM, Nazer H, IIahi F. Unusual patterns of schistosomal disease of the colon. *Gastrointest Endosc* 1989;35:256–258.

167. El-Shiek Mohamad AR, Al Karawi MA, Yasawy MI. Schistosomal colonic disease. *Gut* 1990;31:439–442.

168. Radhakrishnan S, Al Nakib B, Shaikh H, Menon NK. The value of colonoscopy in schistosomal, tuberculous and amebic colitis. Two-year experience. *Dis Col Rect* 1986;29:891–895.

169. Sanguino J, Peixe R, Guerra J, Rocha C, Quina M. Schistosomiasis and vascular alterations of the colonic mucosa. *Hepatogastroenterology* 1993;40:184–187.

170. Kochhar R, Rajwanshi A, Goenka MK, et al. Colonoscopic fine needle aspiration cytology in the diagnosis of ileocecal tubercolosis. *Am J Gastroenterol* 1991;86:102–104.

171. Pettengell KE, Pirie D, Simjee AE. Colonoscopic features of early intestinal tuberculosis. Report of 11 cases. *South Afr Med J* 1990;79:279–280.

172. Shah S, Thomas V, Mathan M, et al. Colonoscopic study of 50 patients with colonic tuberculosis. *Gut* 1992;33:347–351.

173. Medina E, Orti E, Tome A, Quiles F, Canelles P, Mertinez A. Segmental tuberculosis of the colon diagnosed by colonoscopy. *Endoscopy* 1990;22:188–190.

174. Bhargava DK, Kushwaha AKS, Dasarathy S, Shriniwas DM, Chopra P. Endoscopic diagnosis of segmental colonic tuberculosis. *Gastrointest Endosc* 1992;38:571–574.

175. Morgante PE, Gandara MA, Sterle E. The endoscopic diagnosis of colonic tuberculosis. *Gastrointest Endosc* 1989;35:115–118.

176. Breiter JR, Hajjar J-J. Segmental tuberculosis of the colon diagnosed by colonoscopy *Am J Gastroenterol* 1981;76:369–373.

177. Bhasin DK, Roy P, Sharma M, Singh K, Malik AK, Panigrahi D. Acid-fast bacilli in colonoscopic brushings. *Lancet* 1991;338:184–185.

178. Leung JWC, Chung SCS, Sung JJY, et al. Urgent endoscopic drainage for acute supprative cholangitis. *Lancet* 1989;1:1307.

179. Ott DJ, Gilliam JH III, Zagoria RJ, Young GP: Interventional endoscopy of the biliary and pancreatic ducts: current indications and methods. *AJR* 1992;158:243–250.

180. Lai EC, Mok FP, Tan ES et al: Endoscopic biliary drainage for severe acute cholangitis. *N Engl J Med* 1992;326:1626–1628.

181. Speer AG, Russell RC, Hatfield ARW, et al. Randomised trial of endoscopic versus percutaneous stent insertion in malignant obstructive jaundice. *Lancet* 1987;2:57.

182. Cello JP. Acquired immunodeficiency syndrome cholangiopathy: spectrum of disease. *Am J Med* 1989;86:539–546.

183. Pol S, Romana CA, Richard S, et al. Microsporidia infection in patients with the human immunodeficiency virus and unexplained cholangitis. *N Engl J Med* 1993;328:95–99.

184. Benhamou Y, Caumes E, et al. AIDS-related cholangiopathy. Critical analysis of a prospective series of 26 patients. *Dig Dis Sci* 1993;38:1113–1118.

185. Dowsett JF, Miller R, et al. Sclerosing cholangitis in acquired immunodeficiency syndrome. Case reports and review of the literature. *Scand J Gastroenterol* 1988;23:1267–1274.

186. Schneiderman DJ, Cello JP, Laing FC. Papillary stenosis and sclerosing cholangitis in the acquired immunodeficiency syndrome. *Ann Intern Med* 1987;106:546–549.

187. Bouche H, Housset C, et al. AIDS-related cholangitis: diagnostic features and course in 15 patients. *J Hepatol* 1993;17:34–39.

188. Chung RT, Schapiro RH, Warshaw AL. Intraluminal pancreatic candidiasis presenting as recurrent pancreatitis. *Gastroenterology* 1993;104:1532–1543.

189. Ryan ME, Kirchner JP, Sell T, et al. Cholangitis due to Blastomyces dermatitidis. *Gastroenterology* 1989;96:1346–1349.

190. Ho F, Snape WJ Jr, Venegas R, et al. Choledochal fungal ball. An unusual cause of biliary obstruction. *Dig Dis Sci* 1988;33:1030–1034.

191. Magnussen CR, Olson JP, Ona FV, et al. *Candida* fungus balls in the common bile duct. Unusual manifestation of disseminated candidiasis. *Arch Intern Med* 1979;139:821–822.

192. Carstensen H, Nilsson KO, Nettelblad SC, et al. Common bile duct obstruction due to an intraluminal mass of candidiasis in a previously healthy child. *Pediatrics* 1986;77:858–861.

193. Pol S, Romana C, Richard S, et al. Enterocytozoon bieneusi

infection in acquired immunodeficiency syndrome-related sclerosing cholangitis. *Gastroenterology* 1992;102:1778–1781.

194. Girard PM, Rozenbaum W, et al. Cholangiopathy associated with microsporidia infection of the common bile duct mucosa in a patient with HIV infection. *Ann Intern Med* 1992;117:401–402.

195. Khuroo MS, Zargar SA, et al. Ascaris-induced acute pancreatitis. *Br J Surg* 1992;79:1335–1338.

196. el Sheikh Mohamed AR, al Karawi MA, et al. Modern techniques in the diagnosis and treatment of gastrointestinal and biliary tree parasites. *Hepatogastroenterology* 1991;38:180–188.

197. Krige JE, Lewis G, Bornman PC. Recurrent pancreatitis caused by a calcified ascaris in the duct of Wirsung. *Am J Gastroenterol* 1987;82:256–257.

198. Acunas B, Rozanes I, et al. Purely cystic hydatid disease of the liver: treatment with percutaneous aspiration and injection of hypertonic saline. *Radiology* 1992;182:541–543.

199. Xu MQ. Diagnosis and management of hepatic hydatidosis complicated with biliary fistula. *Chin Med J* 1992;105:69–72.

200. Aktan AO, Yalin R, et al. Surgical treatment of hepatic hydatid cysts. *Acta Chir Belg* 1993;93:151–153.

201. Ozmen V, Igci A, et al. Surgical treatment of hepatic hydatid disease. *Can J Surg* 1992;34:423–427.

202. Bilge A, Sozuer EM. Diagnosis and surgical treatment of hepatic hydatid disease. *HPB Surg* 1992;6:57–64.

203. Radin DR, Johnson MB. *Candida* cholangitis in a diabetic woman. *AJR* 1992;158:1029–1030.

204. al Karawi MA, Yasawy MI, el Shiekh Mohamed AR. Endoscopic management of biliary hydatid disease: report on six cases. *Endoscopy* 1991;23:278–281.

205. al Karawi MA, el Shiekh Mohamed AR, Yasawy MI. Advances in diagnosis and management of hydatid disease. *Hepatogastroenterology* 1990;37:327–331.

206. Van Steenbergen W, Fevery J, et al. Hepatic echinococcosis ruptured into the biliary tract. Clinical, radiological and therapeutic features during five episodes of spontaneous biliary rupture in three patients with hepatic hydatidosis. *J Hepatol* 1987;4:133–139.

207. al Karawi MA, Mohamed AR, et al. Non-surgical endoscopic trans-papillary treatment of ruptured echinococcus liver cyst obstructing the biliary tree. *Endoscopy* 1987;19:81–83.

208. Magistrelli P, Masetti R, et al. Value of ERCP in the diagnosis and management of pre- and postoperative biliary complications in hydatid disease of the liver. *Gastrointest Radiol* 1989;14:315–320.

209. Vignote ML, Mino G, et al. Endoscopic sphincterotomy in hepatic hydatid disease open to the biliary tree. *Br J Surg* 1990;77:30–31.

210. Ezratty A, Gumaste V, et al. Pancreatic tuberculosis: a frequently fatal but potentially curable disease. *J Clin Gastroenterol* 1990;12:74–77.

211. Stock KP, Riemann W, et al. Tuberculosis of the pancreas. *Endoscopy* 1981;13:178–80.

212. Transmission of infection by gastrointestinal endoscopy, ASGE Technology Assessment Position Paper, April 1993.

213. Spach DH, Silverstein FE, Stamm WE. Transmission of infection by gastrointestinal endoscopy and bronchoscopy. *Ann Intern Med* 1993;118:117–128.

214. Silvis SE, Nebel O, et al. Endoscopic complications. Results of the 1974 American Society for Gastrointestinal Endoscopy Survey. *JAMA* 1976;235:928–930.

215. Beecham HJ, Cohen ML, Parking WE: *Salmonella typhimurium:* transmission by fiberoptic upper gastrointestinal endoscopy. *JAMA* 1979; 241:1013–1015.

216. Chmel H, Armstron D. *Salmonella oslo:* a focal outbreak in a hospital. *Am J Med* 1976;60:203–208.

217. Dean AG. Transmission of *Salmonella typhi* by fiberoptic endoscopy. *Lancet* 1977;2:134.

218. Dwyer DM, Klein EG, et al. *Salmonella newport* infections transmitted by fiberoptic colonoscopy. *Gastrointest Endosc* 1987;33:84–87.

219. Holmberg SD, Osterholm MT, et al. Drug-resistant *Salmonella* from animals fed antimicrobials. *N Engl J Med* 1984;311:617–622.

220. Schliessler KH, Rozendaal B, et al. Outbreak of *Salmonella agona* infection after upper intestinal fiberoptic endoscopy. *Lancet* 1980;2:1246.

221. Tuffnell PG. *Salmonella* infections transmitted by a gastroscope. *Can J Public Health* 1976;67:141–142.

222. Struelens MJ, Rost F, et al. *Pseudomonas aeruginosa* and Enterobacteriaceace bacteremia after biliary endoscopy: an outbreak investigation using DNA macrorestriction analysis. *Am J Med* 1993;95:489–498.

223. Deviere J, Motte S, et al. Septicemia after endoscopic retrograde cholangiopancreatography. *Endoscopy* 1990;22:72–75.

224. Siegman-Igra Y, Isakov A, et al. *Pseudomonas aeruginosa* septicemia following endoscopic retrograde cholangiopancreatography, with a contaminated endoscope. *Scand J Infect Dis* 1987;19:527–530.

225. Davion T, Braillon A, et al. *Pseudomonas aeruginosa* liver abscesses following endoscopic retrograde cholangiopancreatography. Report of a case without biliary tract disease. *Dig Dis Sci* 1987;32:1044–1046.

226. Allen JI, Allen MO, et al. *Pseudomonas* infection of the biliary system resulting from use of a contaminated endoscope. *Gastroenterology* 1987;92:759–763.

227. Cryan EM, Falkiner FR, et al. *Pseudomonas aeruginosa* cross-infection following endoscopic retrograde cholangiopancreatography. *J Hosp Infect* 1984;5:371–376.

228. Schousboe M, Carte A, Sheppard PS. Endoscopic retrograde cholangiopancreatography: related nosocomial infections. *N Z Med J* 1980;92:275–277.

229. Doherty DE, Falko JM, et al. *Pseudomonas aeruginosa* sepsis following retrograde cholangiopancreatography (ERCP). *Dig Dis Sci* 1982;27:169–170.

230. Earnshaw JJ, Clark AW, et al. Outbreak of *Pseudomonas aeruginosa* following endoscopic retrograde cholangiopancreatography. *J Hosp Infect* 1985;6:95–97.

231. Elson CO, Hattori K, Balckstone MO. Polymicrobial sepsis following endoscopic retrograde cholangiopancreatography. *Gastroenterology* 1975;69:507–510.

232. Schoutens-Serruys E, Rost F, et al. The significance of bacterial contamination of fiberoptic endoscopes. *J Hosp Infect* 1981;2:392–394.

233. Noy MF, Harrison L, et al. The significance of bacterial contamination of fiberoptic endoscopes. *J Hosp Infect* 1980;1:53–61.

234. Parker HW, Geenen JE, et al. A prospective analysis of fever and bacteremia following ERCP. *Gastrointest Endosc* 1979;25:102–103.

235. Godiwala T, Andry M, et al. Consecutive *Serratia marcescens* infections following endoscopic retrograde cholangiopancreatography. *Gastrointest Endosc* 1988;34:345–347.

236. Langenberg W, Rauws EA, et al. Patient-to-patient transmission of *Campylobacter pylori* infection by fiberoptic gastroduodenoscopy and biopsy. *J Infect Dis* 1990;161:507–511.

237. Birnie GG, Quigley Em, et al. Endoscopic transmission of hepatitis B virus. *Gut* 1983;24:171–174.

238. Chiaramonte M, Farini R, et al. Risk of hepatitis B virus infection following upper gastrointestinal endoscopy: a prospective study in an endemic area. *Hepatogastroenterology* 1983;30:189–191.

239. Hoofnagle JH, Blake J, et al. Lack of transmission of type B hepatitis by fiberoptic upper endoscopy. *J Clin Gastroenterol* 1980;2:65–69.

240. Ayoola EA: The risk of type B hepatitis infection in flexible fiberoptic endoscopy. *Gastrointest Endosc* 1981;27:60–62.

241. Stuart D, Orelowitz J, et al. Fungemia with *Torulopsis glabrata* after endoscopic biliary stent replacement. *Am J Gastroenterol* 1992;87:883–885.

242. Ito M, Kato T, et al. Disseminated *Candida tropicalis* infection following endoscopic retrograde cholangiopancreatography. *J Infect* 1991;23:77–80.

243. Mandelstram P, Sugawa C, et al. Complications associated with esophagogastroduodenoscopy and with esophageal dilation. *Gastrointest Endosc* 1976;23:16–19.

244. Singh S, Singh N, et al. Contamination of an endoscope due to *Trichosporon beigelli*. *J Hosp Infect* 1989;14:49–53.

245. Tolon M, Thofern E, Miederer SE. Disinfection procedures of fiberscopes in endoscopic departments. *Endoscopy* 1976;8:24–29.

246. Karim QN, Rao GG, et al. Routine cleaning and the elimination of *Campylobacter pylori* from endoscopic biopsy forceps. *J Hosp Infect* 1989;13:87–90.

247. Hanson PJ. AIDS: practicing safe endoscopy. *Baillieres Clin Gastroenterol* 1990;4:477–494.

248. Axon AT, Phillips I, et al. Disinfection of gastrointestinal fiber endoscopes. *Lancet* 1974;1:656–658.

249. Hanson PJV, Gor D, et al. Contamination of endoscopes used in AIDS patients. *Lancet* 1989;2:86–88.

250. Struelens MJ, Rost F, et al. Septicemia after ERCP: outbreak linked to an automatic endoscopic disinfecting machine. 3rd International Conference on Nosocomial Infections, Atlanta, GA; 1990:32.

251. Alvarado CJ, Stoltz SM, Maki DG. Nosocomial infections from contaminated endoscopes: a flawed automatic endoscope washer. An investigation using molecular epidemiology. *Am J Med* 1991;91(3B Suppl):272s–280s.

252. Low DE, Micflikier AB, et al. Infectious complications of endoscopic retrograde cholangiopancreatography. *Arch Intern Med* 1980;140:1076–1077.

253. Infection control during gastrointestinal endoscopy. Guidelines for Clinical Application, ASGE Publication No. 1018. *Gastrointest Endosc* (Suppl)1988;34:37s–40s.

254. Axon AT, Bond W, et al. Endoscopic disinfection. In: *Working party reports of the World Congresses of Gastroenterology*, Sydney, Australia; August 1990:46–50.

255. Society of Gastroenterology Nurses and Associates, Inc. Recommended guidelines for infection control in gastrointestinal endoscopy settings, Monograph Series-1, 1990.

256. Kullman E, Borch K, Lindstrom E, Ansehn S, Ihse I, Anderberg B, Bacteremia following diagnostic and therapeutic ERCP. *Gastrointest Endosc* 1992;38:444–449.

257. LeFrock J, Ellis C, Turchik J, Weinstein L. Transient bacteremia associated with sigmoidoscopy *N Engl J Med* 1973;289:102–104.

258. Baltch A, Buhac I, Agrawal A, O'Connor P, Bram M, Malatino E. Bacteremia after upper gastrointestinal endoscopy. *Arch Intern Med* 1977;137:594–597.

259. Mellow M, Lewis R. Endoscopy-related bacteremia. *Arch Intern Med* 1976;136:667–669.

260. Norfleet R, Mulholland D, Mitchell P, Philo J, Walters E. Does bacteremia follow colonoscopy? *Gastroenterology* 1976;70:20–21.

261. Norfleet R, Mitchell P, Mulholland D, Philo J. Does bacteremia follow upper gastrointestinal endoscopy? *Am J Gastroenterology* 1981;76:420–422.

262. Schembre D, Bjorkman D. Review article: endoscopy related infections. *Aliment Pharmacol Ther* 1993;7:347–355.

263. Botoman V, Surawics C, Bacteremia with gastrointestinal endoscopic procedures. *Gastrointest Endosc* 1986;32:342–346.

264. Yin T, Ellis R, Dellipiani A. The incidence of bacteremia after outpatient Hurst bougienage in the management of benign esophageal stricture. *Endoscopy* 1983;15:289–290.

265. Wang WM, Chen CY, et al. Central nervous system infection after endoscopic injection sclerotherapy. *Am J Gastroenterol* 1990;85:865–867.

266. Tai DI, Lan CK, Hen HJ. Brain abscess following endoscopic injection sclerotherapy: report of a case. *J Formos Med Assoc* 1991;90:857–859.

267. Ritchie MT, Lightdale CJ, Botet JF. Bilateral perinephric abscesses: a complication of endoscopic injection sclerotherapy. *Am J Gastroenterol* 1987;82:670–673.

268. Kaw M, Przepiorka D, Sekas G. Infectious complications of endoscopic procedures in bone marrow transplant recipients. *Dig Dis Sci* 1993;38:71–74.

269. Bianco J, Sullivan P, Higano C, Appelbaum F, McDonald G, Singer J. Prevalence of clinically relevant bacteremia after upper gastrointestinal endoscopy in bone marrow transplant recipients. *Am J Med* 1990;89:134–136.

270. Dajani AS, Bisno AL, et al. Prevention of bacterial endocarditis. Recommendations by the American Heart Association. *JAMA* 1990;264:2919–2922.

271. Koretz RL, Chin K, Gitnick G. The endoscopists' risks from endoscopic transmission of hepatitis. *Gastroenterology* 1985;88:1454.

272. Mitchell H, Lee A, Carrick J. Increased incidence of *Campylobacter pylori* infection in gastroenterologists: further evidence to support person-to-person transmission of *C. pylori*. *Scand J Gastroenterology* 1989;24:396–400.

273. Martin MA, Reichelderfer M. APIC guidelines for infection prevention and control in flexible endoscopy. Association for Professionals in Infection Control and Epidemiology, Inc. 1991, 1992, and 1993 APIC Guidelines Committee. *Am J Inf Control* 1994;22:19–38.

Infections of the Gastrointestinal Tract,
edited by M. J. Blaser, P. D. Smith, J. I. Ravdin,
H. B. Greenberg, and R. L. Guerrant
Raven Press, Ltd., New York © 1995.

CHAPTER 85

Role of Radiological Procedures in the Diagnosis of Gastrointestinal Infections

Desiree E. Morgan and Robert E. Koehler

Radiology plays an important role in the detection and assessment of many gastrointestinal infections. Barium studies have for years been the most effective primary method, but computed tomography (CT) and ultrasonography are proving increasingly useful, particularly in colonic infections.

The double-contrast esophagram plays a major role in the detection and characterization of infectious esophagitis. The pattern of radiological abnormalities differs predictably from one infectious agent to another and can often suggest a specific etiology. Even small, superficial erosions can be detected in most patients when good double-contrast technique is employed.

In infections of the stomach, duodenum, and small intestine, there is a lesser role for radiological assessment. The gastric infections that cause gross morphological alterations of the stomach, principally tuberculosis, syphilis, and histoplasmosis, are rare. Most infectious enteritis is brief and self-limited, leaving little role for radiological studies. Infections of the small bowel in immunocompromised individuals do have radiological manifestations, but they are often nonspecific and fail to indicate the etiological agent.

Radiological methods have more to contribute in colitis. Single- and double-contrast barium enema findings are diagnostic in several of these conditions. Computed tomography is now the mainstay in the radiological assessment of suspected colonic diverticulitis. In patients with diverticulitis, CT provides not only confirmation of the disease, but also information regarding the presence of associated abscess or fistula. In complex and confusing cases of appendicitis, when radiological corroboration is needed to support equivocal clinical findings, CT is also very useful.

D. E. Morgan and R. E. Koehler: Department of Radiology, University of Alabama School of Medicine, Birmingham, Alabama 35233.

ESOPHAGUS

Infections of the esophagus are rare in otherwise healthy individuals. They occur most commonly in patients immunocompromised by hematological malignancy, AIDS, or pharmacological immunosuppression to prevent organ transplant rejection. To a lesser extent they also occur in patients with esophageal stasis. On occasion, monilial and herpetic esophagitis can be seen in otherwise healthy individuals. Compared to the conventional, single-contrast barium esophagram, the double-contrast barium esophagram has enabled better radiological recognition of the superficial mucosal abnormalities that occur in these diseases. In esophagitis due to *Candida* infection, for instance, the sensitivity of the double-contrast esophagram is approximately 90% (1). Typical radiological features support a decision to treat prior to or without endoscopic biopsy confirmation.

Candida

Candida esophagitis has a spectrum of radiographic findings. In mild disease there are widespread discrete, irregular mucosal plaques (2) (Fig. 1). This particular pattern is seen most often in patients immunocompromised by diseases other than AIDS (3). In patients with moderate disease, the plaques coalesce. Combined with the debris of necrotic epithelium, the plaques develop a more irregular mucosal outline. In its most severe stage, *Candida* esophagitis causes the esophageal mucosa to look shaggy with marked irregularity due to plaques, ulcers, and pseudomembranes (4) (Fig. 2). This fulminant form of *Candida* esophagitis is the form most often seen in AIDS patients (3).

Uncommon radiological presentations of *Candida* esophagitis include focal disease (5), stricture, complete obstruction with or without fungus ball, and perforation. Dramatic regression of the radiographic features of *Can-*

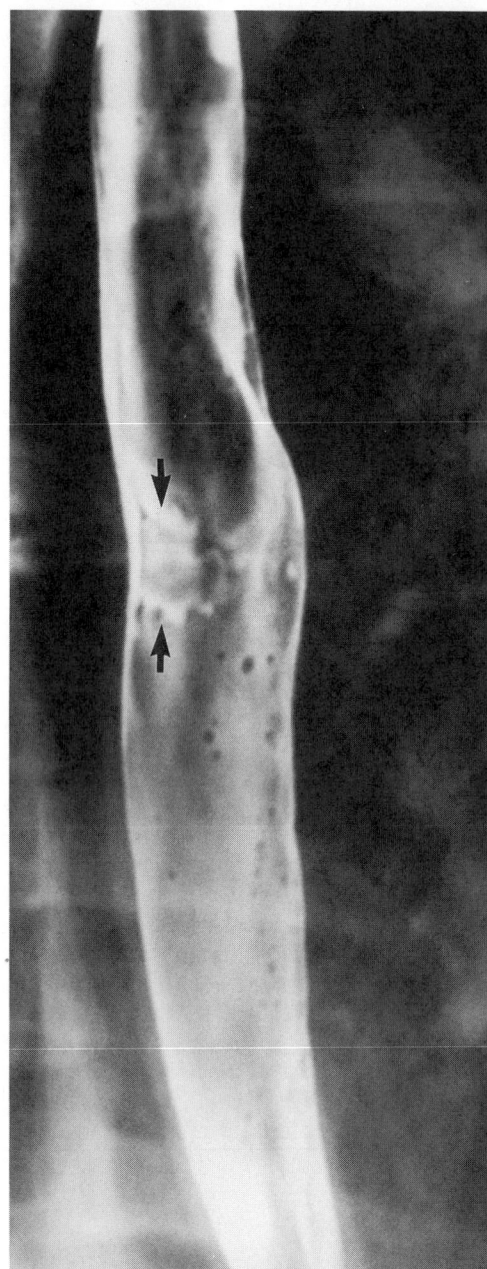

FIG. 1. Early esophageal moniliasis in a young patient receiving chemotherapy for lymphoma. Double-contrast esophagram shows a focal plaque-like area (*arrows*) in the midesophagus with an ulcerated plaque on the opposite wall.

dida esophagitis often occurs after treatment, but disappearance of the radiographic abnormalities may lag behind the clinical recovery. Because the infection may lead to permanent stricture or scarring, follow-up double-contrast esophagram is recommended (6).

Herpes Simplex

Esophagitis caused by herpes simplex virus (HSV) (Fig. 3) typically presents as small, discrete, punctate, linear

or stellate ulcers clustered in the midesophagus (6) or as multiple small, often diamond-shaped ulcers scattered throughout the esophagus. These develop on a background of otherwise normal mucosa (3). Because the radiographic appearance is not as specific as that of infection by *Candida,* and, because treatment carries more risk, biopsy confirmation of the radiological findings is warranted (4). An acute transient form of herpes esophagitis infrequently occurs in otherwise healthy individuals and has been reported to show numerous, tiny ulcers on

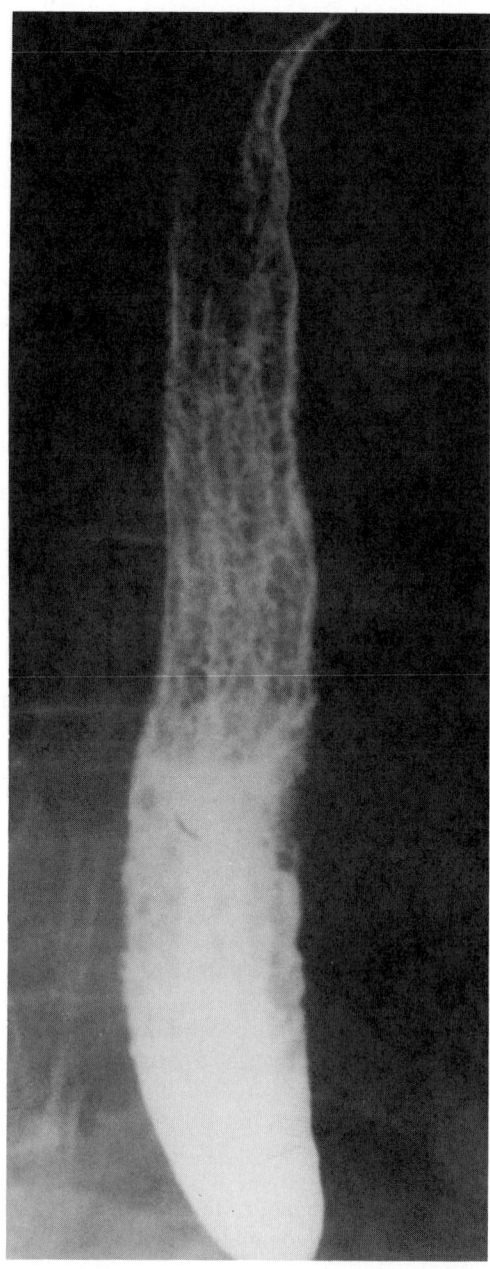

FIG. 2. Severe *Candida* esophagitis in an elderly man receiving steroids for chronic obstructive pulmonary disease. The diffuse shaggy irregularity of the mucosa in this double-contrast esophagram is typical for monilial infection.

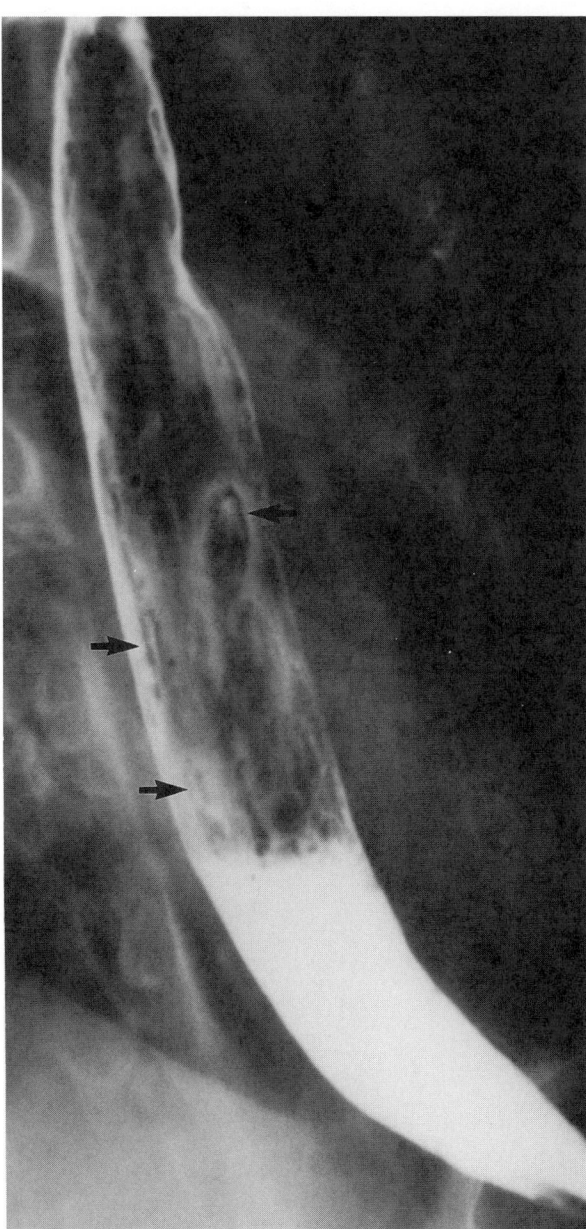

FIG. 3. Herpes simplex virus infection in an HIV-positive man with odynphagia. Numerous linear and punctate ulcers (*arrows*) appear as white barium collections surrounded by a darker halo of edematous tissue.

double-contrast esophagography. These ulcers typically occur in the midesophagus near the level of the left main bronchus (7). Advanced herpes esophagitis may also give rise to a diffusely "shaggy" esophagus, but concomitant *Candida* infection is usually present.

Cytomegalovirus

Cytomegalovirus (CMV) esophagitis occurs most often in patients with AIDS. It is characterized by one or more large (up to 2 cm), flat ulcers in the distal esophagus (Figs.

4 and 5). The surrounding mucosa usually appears normal. The radiographic features depend on the severity of the disease. Milder CMV infection presents as segmental areas of granular mucosa with superficial erosions and shallow, poorly defined ulcers (8,9).

Other Esophageal Infections

The human immunodeficiency virus itself has also been associated with esophagitis, usually occurring within

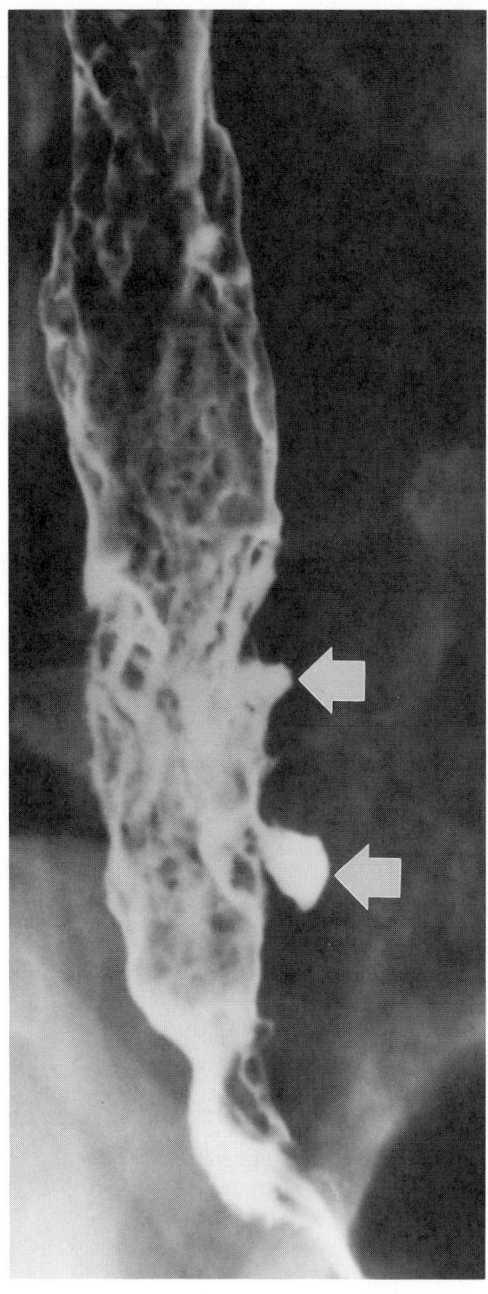

FIG. 4. Cytomegalovirus (CMV) esophageal ulcers in an HIV-positive man with nausea and vomiting. Esophagram shows two deep, discrete ulcers (*arrows*) typical of CMV infection. Note proximal and adjacent diffuse mucosal plaques due to monilial infection.

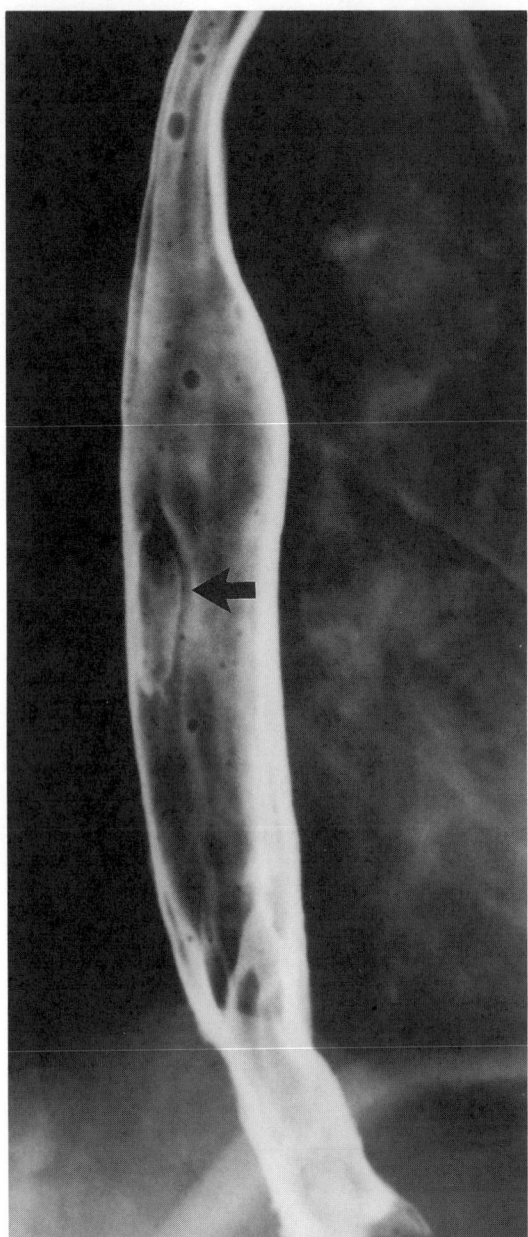

FIG. 5. A large CMV esophageal ulcer in a young male patient with AIDS. CMV may also cause shallow, longitudinally oriented, ovoid ulcers (*arrow*).

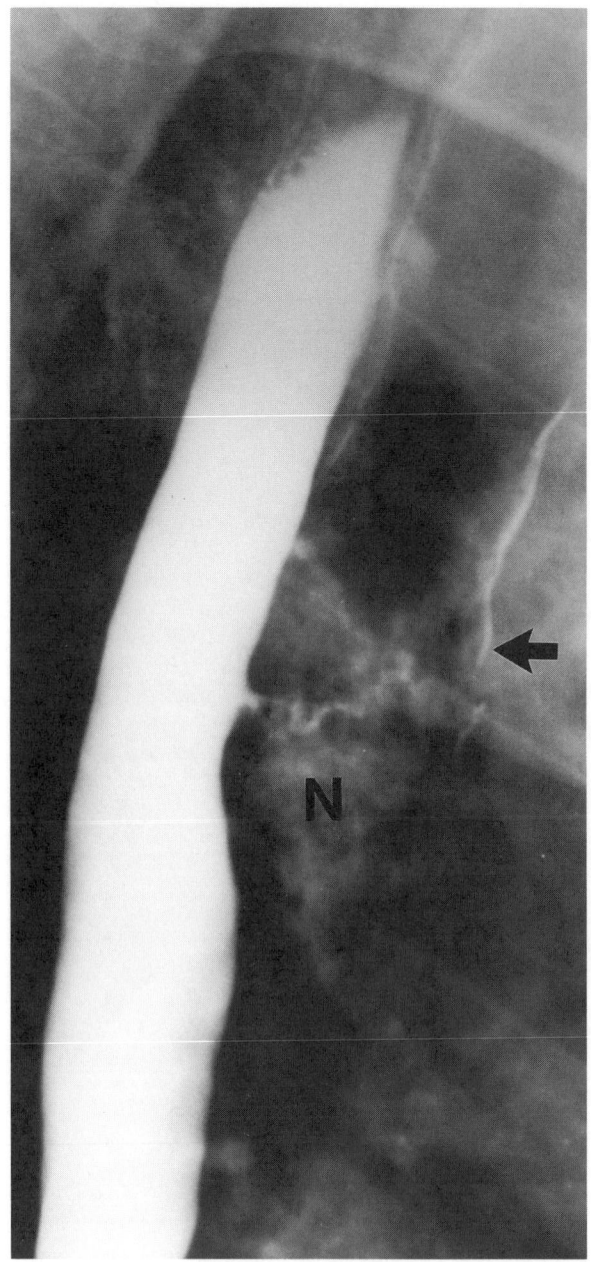

FIG. 6. Tracheoesophageal fistula due to histoplasmosis. This 54-year-old man noted a sensation of air passing from one portion of his chest to another when he lay on his left side. A single-contrast esophagram shows a pinpoint fistula filled with barium extending from the esophageal lumen through an enlarged, mediastinal, calcified lymph node (N) into the trachea (*arrow*).

weeks of seroconversion. Typically, transient, large, shallow, isolated (or less commonly multifocal) ulcers are seen in the distal esophagus (10). The appearance may be radiographically indistinguishable from that of CMV disease. This diagnosis is based on exclusion of another pathogen by biopsy.

Uncommon infectious causes of esophagitis include *Mycobacterium avium* complex, (MAC) which causes discrete ulceration of the esophagus, and *Mycobacterium tuberculosis,* which usually arises from contiguous, infected, necrotic, mediastinal lymph nodes and causes transmural inflammation that may lead to deep ulceration, intramural dissection, and bronchial fistula (11). Other

granulomatous infections may show similar findings. A small esophagobronchial fistula that passes through a calcified mediastinal lymph node is typical of infection with *Histoplasma capsulatum* (Fig. 6).

STOMACH

The radiographic differentiation of infectious diseases of the stomach is not often accurate due to the nonspecif-

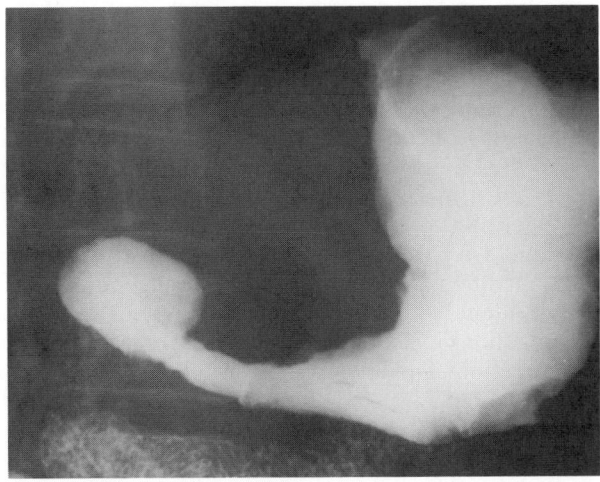

FIG. 7. Linitis plastica due to gastric syphilis is an 82-year-old Haitian male with a positive VDRL and 15-pound weight loss over one year. (Courtesy of Dr. Jack Farman.)

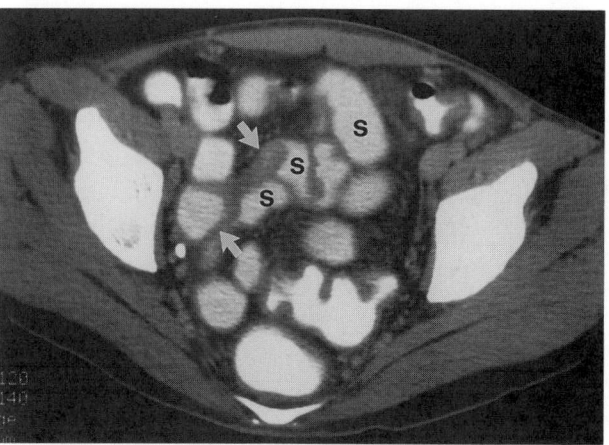

FIG. 8. Cryptosporidiosis in a 28-year-old man with AIDS and diarrhea. CT scan at the level of the pelvis shows focal thickening (*arrows*) of the wall of the small intestine (S).

icity and variability of findings on double-contrast radiographic examination. Recent reports describe aphthous ulcers or superficial erosions in the stomach due to fungal and viral infection (12), antral narrowing due to *Toxoplasma gondii* (13), and thickened rugal folds due to CMV, *Cryptosporidium,* and *T. gondii* in AIDS patients (12). The protean radiological features of CMV gastritis have also recently been described and range from fold thickening to aphthous ulceration to deep ulceration and fistula formation (14). The variety of findings in tuberculous infection of the stomach include an ulcerative form characterized by large, deep, chronic ulcers in the body of the stomach, and a hyperplastic form that produces thickening of the antrum and pylorus. Gastric syphilis (Fig. 7), most often due to the tertiary stage of syphilis, typically presents radiographically as diffuse thickening of the gastric wall with an intact mucosa, leading to funnel-shaped narrowing of the antrum, fold effacement, and decreased peristalsis (15). Endoscopic biopsy is required in the immunocompromised or other high-risk patient to determine the etiology of radiologically detected gastric infections (12).

SMALL INTESTINE

The role of radiographic studies in the evaluation of suspected small bowel infection involves identifying patients with mucosal abnormalities, characterizing the abnormalities as they relate to specific pathogens, and defining the location and extent of disease for biopsy planning. The barium small bowel follow through is often used in screening patients at risk for small bowel infections, with enteroclysis (small bowel enema) reserved for more difficult cases.

AIDS-Associated Infections

In patients with AIDS or other immunocompromising conditions, one of the most common small bowel infec-

tions is cryptosporidiosis (Fig. 8). This parasitic infection manifests itself radiographically as pronounced fold thickening, mostly in the duodenum and jejunum, with accompanying increase in the fluid content of the bowel (16). With longstanding disease, ileal and even colonic involvement can occur (17).

MAC infection may give rise to a variety of findings on barium studies of the small bowel, including irregular fold thickening and mild dilatation of the distal jejunum and ileum in a pattern similar to that of Whipple's disease (18). Enlarged lymph nodes may separate small bowel segments as seen on barium studies or the nodes may be seen directly on CT. Lymphadenopathy due to MAC infection is usually more extensive in the mesentery than in the retroperitoneum (4,19) and is accompanied by hepatosplenomegaly on CT (20). Abnormal lymph nodes range from small (1.0–1.5 cm) to large, bulky masses (17,20).

CMV infection of the small bowel (Fig. 9) may cause diffuse ulcers that can perforate or bleed (16). Multifocal disease of the bowel, especially when the duodenum is involved, should suggest AIDS (Fig. 10) even in patients thought not to be at high risk for the disease (21).

Bacterial Enteritides

Bacterial small bowel infections are seen predominantly in immunocompetent patients. Ileocecal tuberculosis resembles Crohn's disease radiologically, but tuberculosis should be suspected in patients with greater involvement of the cecum than terminal ileum, straightening of the ileocecal junction due to retraction of the cecum superiorly, abrupt transition from normal to diseased bowel, mesenteric adenopathy, and high-density ascites. Tuberculosis should also be in the differential diagnosis when there are transaxial, oval ulcers rather than the linear, longitudinal ulcers more typical of Crohn's disease (16). Tuberculous infection of the duodenum, which occurs most often in conjunction with gastric tuberculosis,

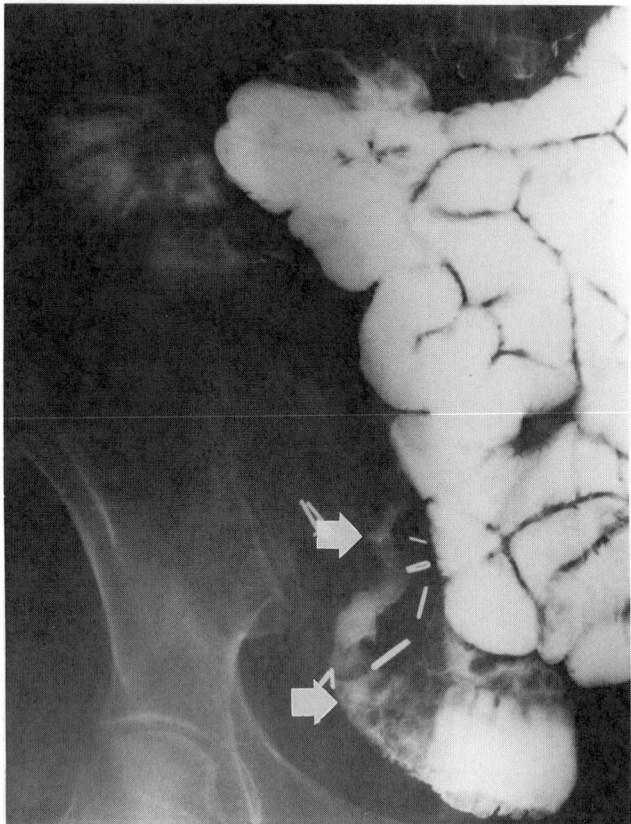

FIG. 9. CMV ileitis in a renal transplant recipient with small bowel obstruction. A barium study of the small intestine shows partial obstruction of the distal ileum (*arrows*) with irregularity of the lumen and thickening of the adjacent wall. Preoperatively, the findings were thought to be most consistent with lymphoma.

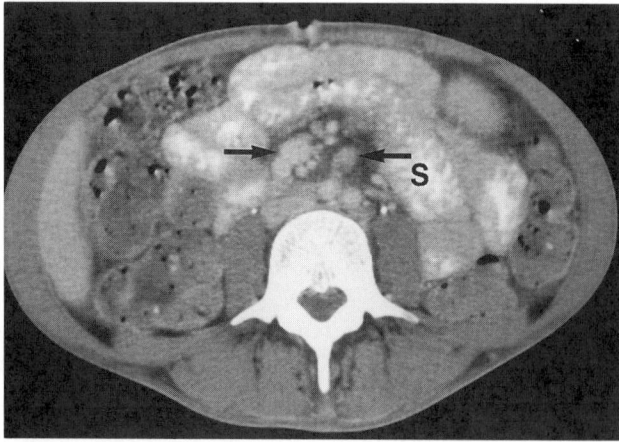

FIG. 10. Infectious enteritis due to CMV, *Mycobacterium avium* complex (MAC), and *Cryptosporidium* in a 37-year-old HIV-positive male with abdominal pain. CT scan through the midabdomen shows enlarged mesenteric lymph nodes (*arrows*) and diffuse thickening of the valvulae conniventes and the wall of the small intestine (S). The enlarged mesenteric nodes are consistent with MAC infection, and the small intestinal thickening is likely related to the cryptosporidiosis and/or CMV infection.

and the jejunum may also give rise to nodular mucosal thickening and lead to small bowel obstruction. The presence of enteroliths should also suggest tuberculosis (15).

Yersinia enterocolitica infection affects the terminal ileum, showing ulcers in the acute stage followed by thickening of the bowel wall and nodular fold thickening. *Salmonella* infection is manifested radiographically as gaseous distension of the small bowel without fluid levels on plain films. On barium studies there can be dilatation and fold thickening in the jejunum and fine ulceration of the terminal ileum. Intestinal transit is usually delayed. *Shigella* infection is also characterized by mucosal edema, hypersecretion, and hypermotility with rapid intestinal transit. Radiological studies may have a role in demonstrating complications such as perforation of the terminal ileum in typhoid fever, a situation in which the use of water-soluble contrast medium would be judicious.

Parasitic Infections

Parasitic infestations of the small bowel produce interesting and often characteristic radiographic findings. Giardiasis can cause thickening, blunting, and distortion of valvulae conniventes predominantly in the duodenum and proximal jejunum. Accompanying spasm and irritability, rapid bowel transit, and increased secretions may also be seen (15).

Because of the growing popularity of eating raw fish, the radiological manifestations of anisakiasis have come

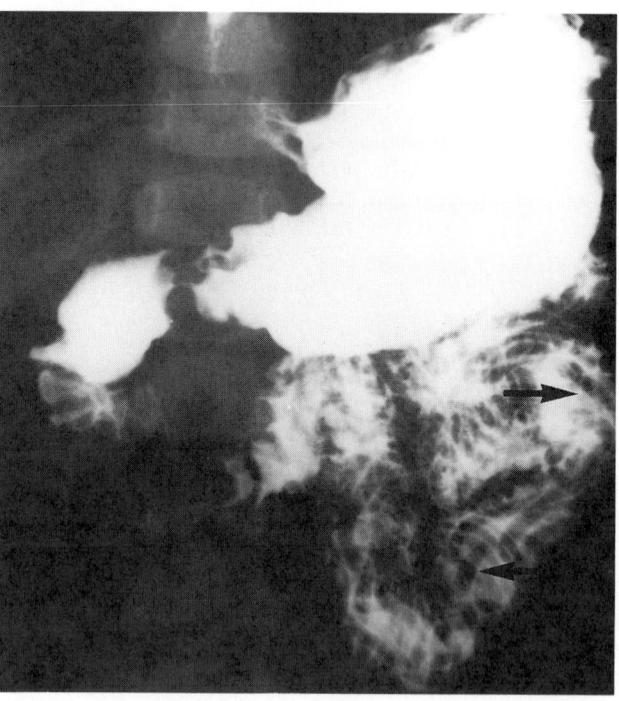

FIG. 11. Ascariasis in a 10-year-old child with recurrent asthmatic attacks. Numerous worms appear as linear filling defects (*arrows*) in the proximal jejunum in this small bowel barium follow-through study. Courtesy of the Department of Radiology, Children's Hospital of Alabama.

to attention. The findings on conventional small bowel follow-through are similar to those of Crohn's disease. Ultrasonographic features of anisakiasis include marked thickening of bowel loops and mucosal fold edema with decreased peristalsis. There may also be small amounts of ascites adjacent to the affected loops (22).

In helminthic infections, worms may be identified by barium radiography. In ascariasis, the worms appear as linear filling defects (Fig. 11) and may show ingested barium outlining their own gastrointestinal tracts. Also of importance is strongyloidiasis, especially in the immunocompromised patient. The radiological findings, similar to those of giardiasis, include prominent mucosal folds in the duodenum with excess mucous secretion and such rapid transit time that the proximal small bowel is sometimes difficult to evaluate. More extensive strongyloidiasis affects larger portions of the small bowel with dilatation and slower transit due to paralytic ileus (15).

COLON

A wide range of colonic infections may be seen radiologically. These infections are due to pathogens acquired locally, those acquired during international travel, and those commonly present in the immunocompromised patient. The standard radiographic method for evaluation of colitis is the double-contrast barium enema. Contraindications to barium enema include suspected perforation, toxic megacolon, and severe or fulminant colitis. In these situations it is safer to rely on a diagnostic enema per-

formed with water-soluble contrast material (25% solution of sodium diatrizoate) or to treat the patient based on nonradiological findings and consider barium enema at a later time if still needed. In immunocompromised patients, abdominal CT may be more useful as the initial radiological test because of its ability to demonstrate solid visceral disease and adenopathy as well as bowel abnormalities. Pericolonic inflammatory changes related to diverticulitis and appendicitis are also better evaluated by CT.

Common Protozoal and Bacterial Infections of the Colon

Amebiasis may present as haustral fold thickening due to mucosal edema (Fig. 12). Also seen are ulceration in the cecum and ascending colon with rigidity and bowel wall thickening. This can progress to the characteristic flask-shaped, undermined ulceration or fulminating colitis (toxic megacolon with deep ulcerations and perforation). Amebomas are tumor-like lesions within or adjacent to the colon wall, which are caused by direct transmural extension of amebic infection and accompanying bacterial infection (Fig. 13). They produce irregular, long, tapering strictures in the cecum and flexure regions. Tuberculous infection most commonly involves the ileocecal region, but may give rise to multifocal colitis and strictures with partial obstruction (15). A localized tuberculoma can mimic an annular carcinoma of the colon. *Yersinia, Campylobacter, Salmonella,* and *Shigella* (Fig. 14) may

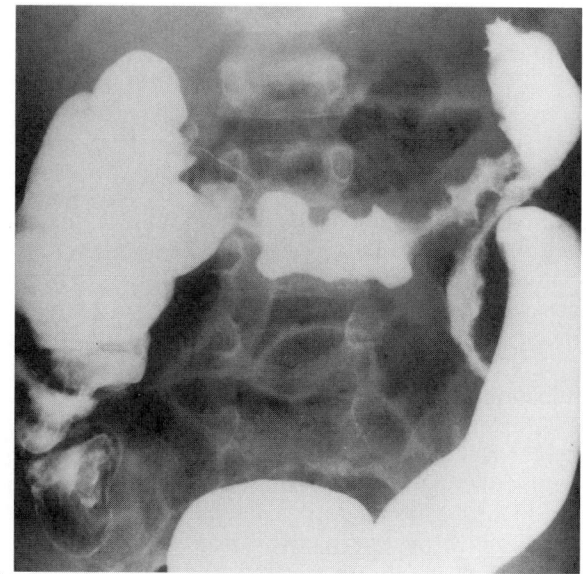

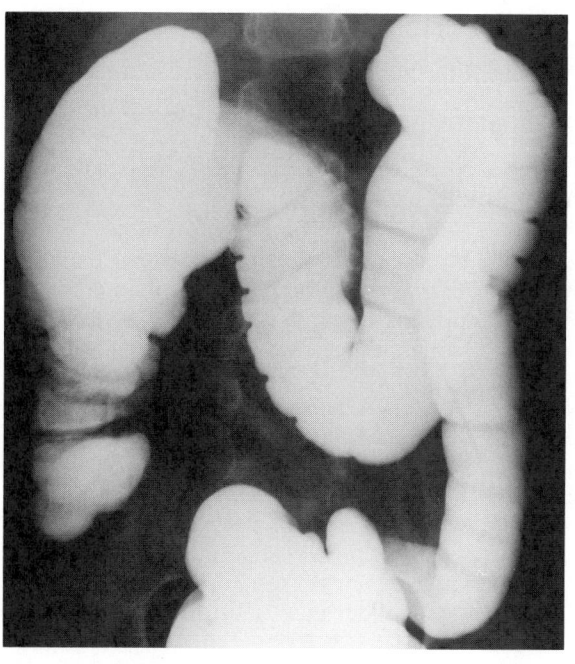

A

B

FIG. 12. A 10-year-old boy with crampy abdominal pain and diarrhea of 5 days duration and stool specimens positive for *E. histolytica* and *Salmonella* sp. **A:** Single-column barium enema performed in the acute phase shows marked edema and spasm in the region of the splenic flexure. **B:** The barium enema one month after therapy was normal. (Courtesy of the Department of Radiology, The Children's Hospital of Alabama.)

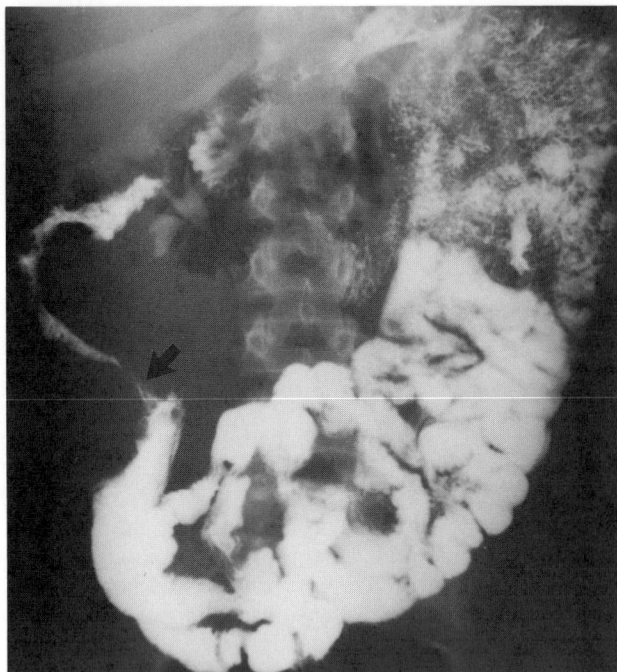

FIG. 13. Marked narrowing of the ascending colon (*arrow*) in a patient with amebic colitis. The displacement of the small intestine from the right midabdomen is due to the large inflammatory mass (ameboma) surrounding the affected right colon.

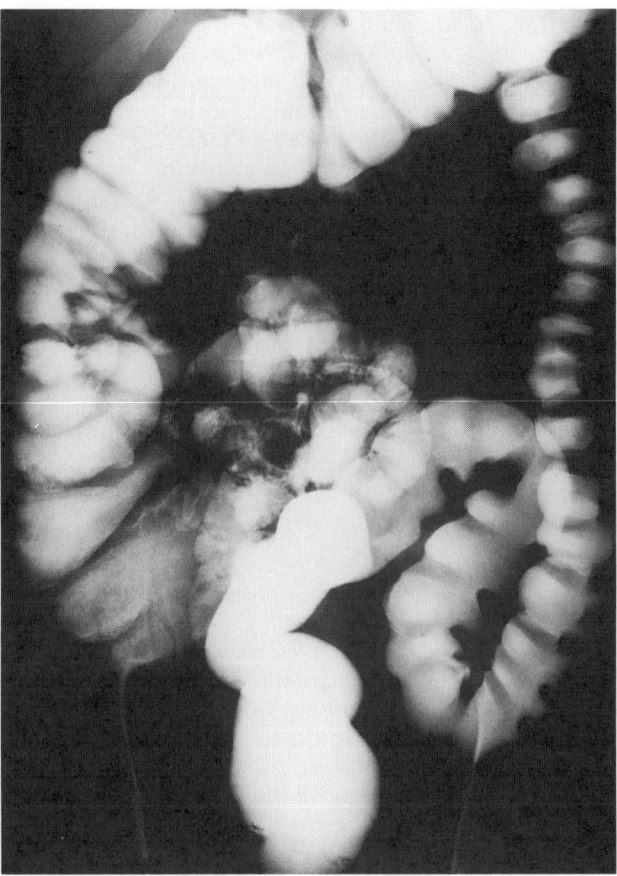

FIG. 14. Acute shigellosis. Barium enema shows the intrahaustral folds in the left colon are diffusely thickened by colonic edema, but no ulceration or other mucosal irregularities are seen.

all cause diffuse colitis with granular mucosal texture due to mucosal edema, or with fine ulcerations. The same findings may be demonstrated radiographically by pathogenic *Escherichia coli* infection, although diffuse colonic wall thickening with thumbprinting and spasm have also been noted.

Pseudomembranous Colitis

Therapy with broad-spectrum antibiotics can lead to overgrowth of *Clostridium difficile* and pseudomembranous colitis, manifesting on plain radiographs as diffuse dilation of the small and large bowel with characteristic transverse banding of the colon (Fig. 15). The transverse bands represent thickened haustral folds, which appear radiographically as broad bands of soft tissue traversing the air-filled lumen of the colon (23,24). On barium enema, mucosal edema and plaque-like lesions (the pseudomembranes) may be seen (4) (Fig. 16). Occasionally, rectal sparing or focal involvement will be noted (25). Sonography can also be used to demonstrate a thickened and echogenic colonic wall with effacement of the lumen (26). The CT findings are often the most helpful in identifying this disease (27,28). Characteristic features include circumferential, irregular, diffuse bowel wall thickening with eccentric polypoid fold thickening and the relative absence of pericolonic inflammatory changes (28) (Fig. 17). These CT findings are relatively specific, and in the proper clinical setting the diagnosis of pseudomembranous colitis can be confidently suggested.

Typhlitis

Typhlitis or neutropenic colitis is an inflammatory process affecting the cecum and sometimes the terminal ileum or appendix that was first described as a complication in patients with leukopathic conditions (29). The process presents on plain abdominal films as a right lower quadrant soft tissue mass with a dilated, fluid-filled cecum (16). CT may allow differentiation of typhlitis from pseudomembranous colitis. Typhlitis is limited to the cecum and right colon, and characteristically shows extensive mucosal edema and wall thickening in addition to pericolonic inflammatory fluid and thickening of fascial planes (4) (Fig. 18). Pneumatosis and subtle perforation may also be readily demonstrated by CT.

CMV Colitis

Cytomegalovirus (CMV) colitis occurs most often in patients with AIDS. On CT it shows a marked, diffuse,

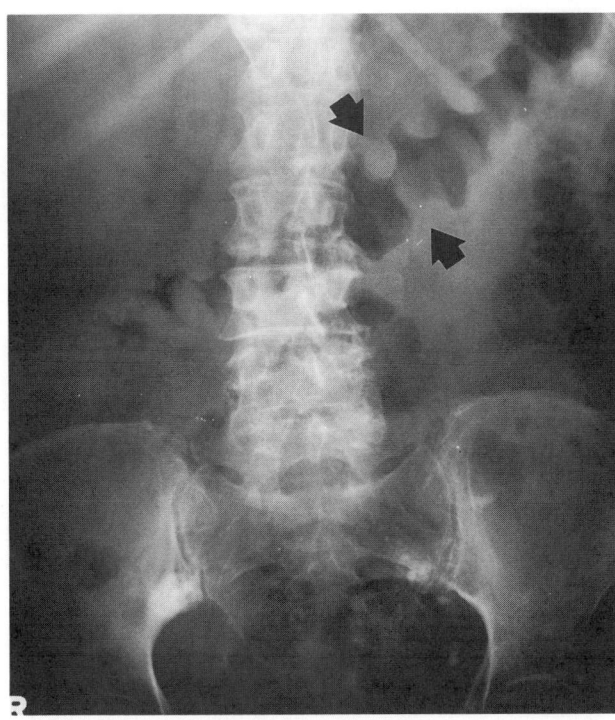

FIG. 15. An abdominal radiograph without contrast in a patient with severe pseudomembranous colitis. Pronounced thickening of the intrahaustral folds (*arrows*) is seen in the transverse colon.

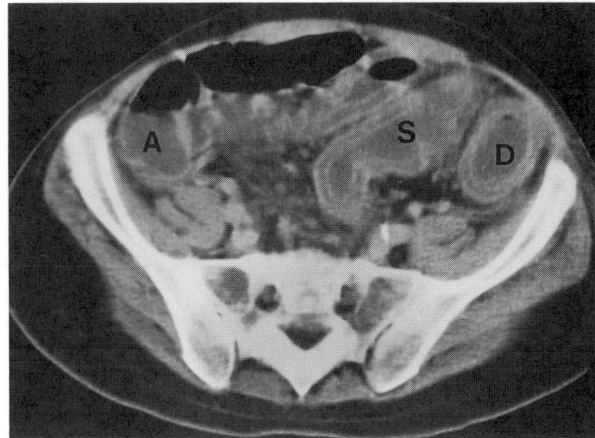

FIG. 17. Pseudomembranous colitis in a 33-year-old quadriplegic patient receiving multiple antibiotics. CT scan shows the thickened sigmoid (S) and descending (D) colonic wall, but a normal ascending colon (A).

or, less commonly, segmental bowel wall thickening (Fig. 19). The colon wall often is low in attenuation due to its edematous nature (30). The distinction between CMV colitis and pseudomembranous colitis on CT is sometimes difficult to make. With barium examination, fine mucosal nodularity in a pattern suggestive of lymphoid nodular hyperplasia may be seen in early CMV infection (4). This may progress to diffuse aphthous ulceration on a background of normal mucosa (Fig. 20). Deep ulceration develops in the severe stage of this disease. CMV colitis may be confined to the cecum (4). In this case differentiation from typhlitis is suggested by the absence of pericolonic changes.

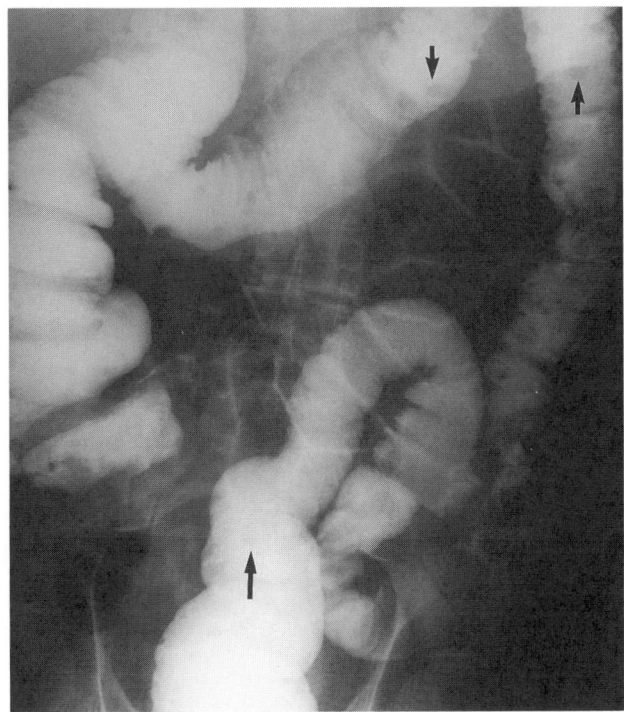

FIG. 16. Pseudomembranous colitis of moderate severity. Numerous plaque-like polypoid filling defects (*arrows*) due to pseudomembranes are distributed throughout the rectum and colon.

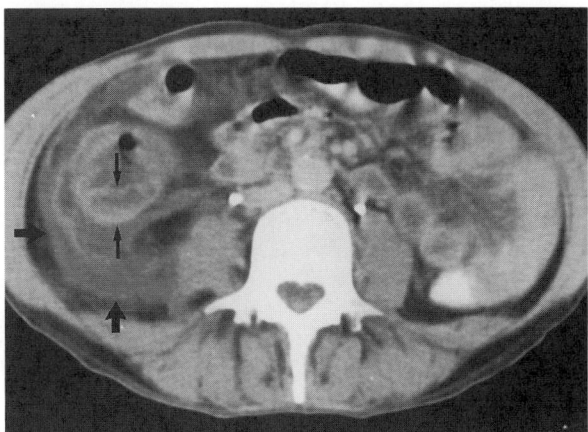

FIG. 18. Typhlitis in a 56-year-old man receiving chemotherapy for acute myelogenous leukemia. The patient presented with right lower quadrant abdominal pain and neutropenia. CT shows striking thickening of the wall (*small arrows*) of the ascending colon with markedly edematous pericolic fat (*arrows*).

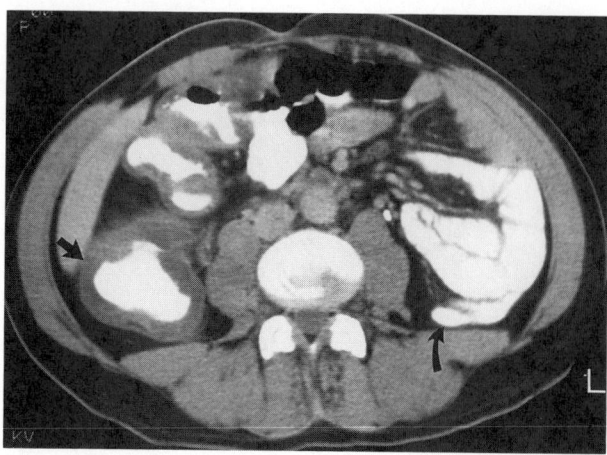

FIG. 19. Severe CMV colitis in a 38-year-old man with AIDS and diarrhea. Note thickening of the wall of the ascending colon (*straight arrow*) and a normal descending colon (*curved arrow*) in this CT scan with contrast.

Proctitis

Infectious proctitis is often seen in, but is not limited to, homosexual males, and is most commonly due to infection with *Neisseria gonococcus* and herpes simplex viruses (HSV) (Fig. 21). In mild cases of gonococcal proctitis the barium enema is normal. With more severe infection, diffuse ulceration, spasm, loss of distensibility, and widening

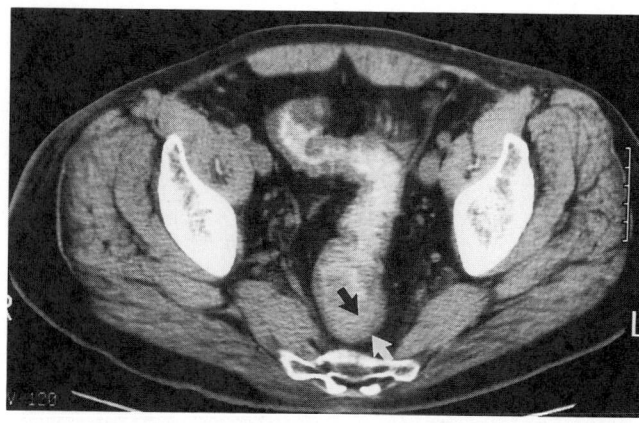

FIG. 21. Proctocolitis due to herpes simplex virus infection in a 40-year-old HIV-negative male with diabetic ketoacidosis and *Candida* sepsis. CT shows severe thickening (*arrows*) of the rectosigmoid colon where friable mucosa with punctate ulcers and mucosal edema was observed at colonoscopy.

of the presacral space are demonstrated on barium enema. Herpetic proctitis may show identical features, but it is often limited to the lower 10 cm of the rectum.

The radiographic feature of acute lymphogranuloma venereum (LGV) is primarily diffuse ulceration (Fig. 22). This may progress to loss of haustration, narrowing, spasm, fistula formation, and long strictures (Fig. 23) in severe, persistent disease (15,31). LGV, as well as gonococcal and HSV infections, may produce nonspecific CT

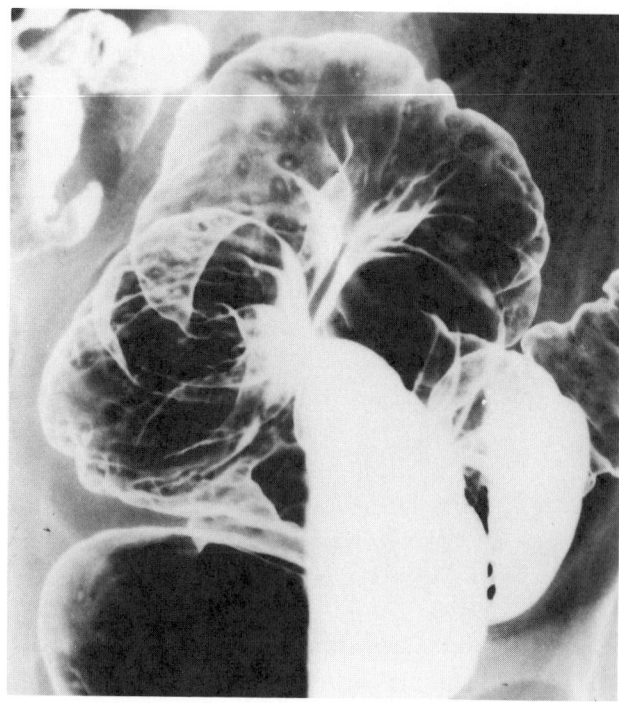

FIG. 20. CMV colitis. Air contrast study of the rectosigmoid region shows numerous discrete, punctate ulcers each of which is surrounded by a halo of edema. Courtesy of Dr. Emil Balthazar.

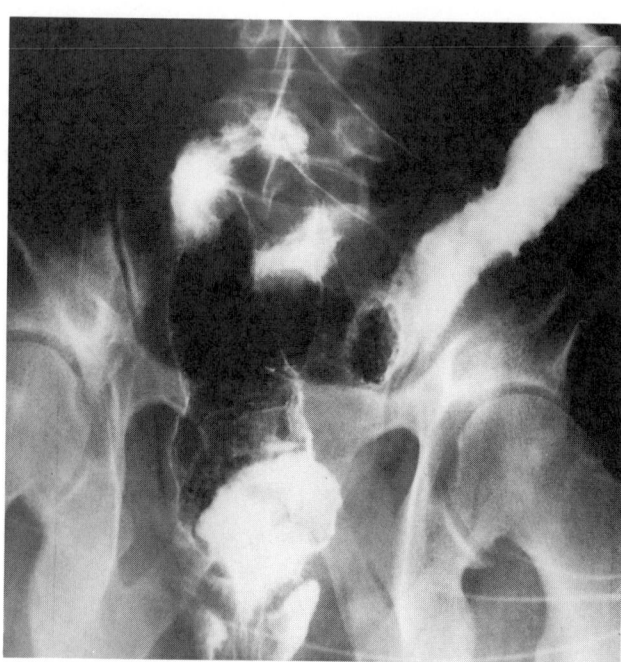

FIG. 22. Severe proctosigmoiditis due to lymphogranuloma venereum infection in a patient with AIDS. Barium enema shows diffuse shaggy irregularity of the ulcerated colonic mucosa and complete lack of normal haustration.

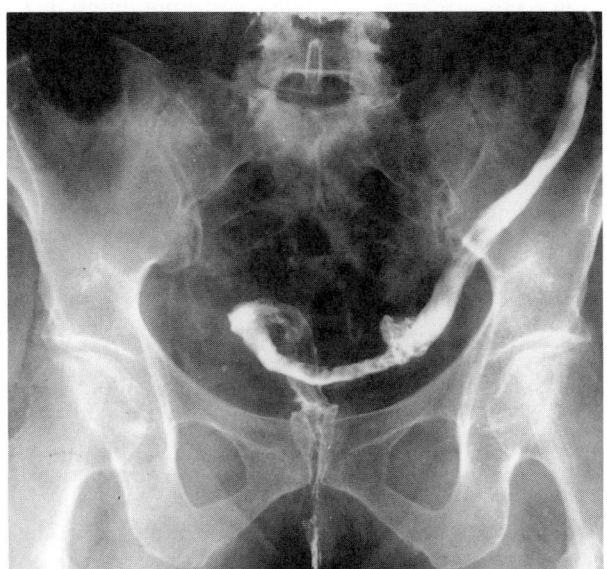

FIG. 23. Lymphogranuloma venereum infection of the rectum and sigmoid colon. The long stricture shown in this barium enema is typical of the late stages of this disease.

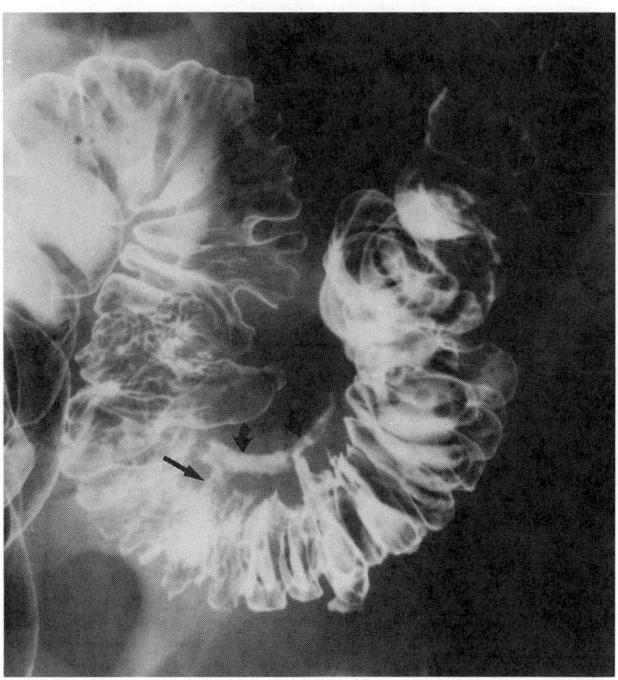

FIG. 24. Spot radiograph from an air contrast barium enema reveals sigmoid diverticula. A perforated diverticulum (*straight arrow*) is seen in continuity with an intramural sinus tract (*curved arrows*). Two other diverticula in the more proximal sigmoid colon also communicate with the intramural sinus tract.

signs of focal thickening of the rectal wall with abnormal soft tissue infiltration of the perirectal space.

The rarely occurring amebic and *Shigella* proctitis may extend to the sigmoid and descending colon, respectively, and show scattered areas of superficial and, later, deep collar button ulceration on barium enema examination (15).

Diverticulitis

The radiological evaluation of suspected diverticulitis should begin with an intravenous contrast–enhanced abdominal CT using oral and rectal contrast (3% meglumine diatrizoate solution). While the barium enema was the main radiological test used in the past to document diverticulitis (Fig. 24), CT has been shown not only to be more sensitive but to better demonstrate the extent and complications of diverticular inflammation (32). In patients with suspected diverticulitis, CT more often shows an alternative etiology for the signs and symptoms when diverticulitis is not present. Although sonographic identification of gut wall thickening, diverticula, pericolic and intramural fluid collections, and edema of the pericolic fat have been described (33,34), the value of sonography in the workup of suspected diverticulitis is not yet established.

The CT criteria for diverticulitis include the presence of colonic diverticula, localized inflammatory infiltration of the pericolic fat, focally thickened colon wall, intramural sinus tract, pelvic or abdominal abscess associated with an inflamed segment of colon, and fistula formation (especially sigmoid-vesical fistula) (35).

Radiographic stages of diverticulitis have been defined to correlate with optimal treatment planning. Stage 0 refers to the most common form of diverticulitis, which oc-

curs when diverticular inflammation is contained with the serosa (Fig. 25). This produces only thickening of the colon wall on CT and is usually responsive to antibiotic therapy alone. Stage I diverticulitis is defined by the presence of small (up to 3 cm) abscesses or phlegmon confined

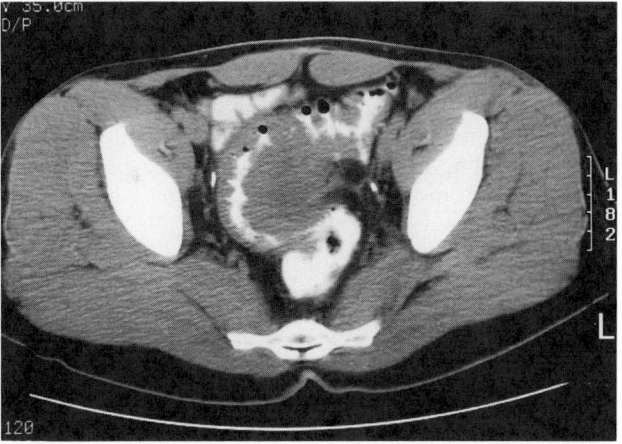

FIG. 25. Diverticulitis in a 30-year-old man with testicular carcinoma and acute onset of pelvic pain. CT scan using oral, rectal, and intravenous contrast at the level of the acetabular roofs demonstrates marked eccentric thickening of the wall of the sigmoid colon with narrowing of the lumen and effacement of the folds. Scattered, air-containing diverticula are also noted.

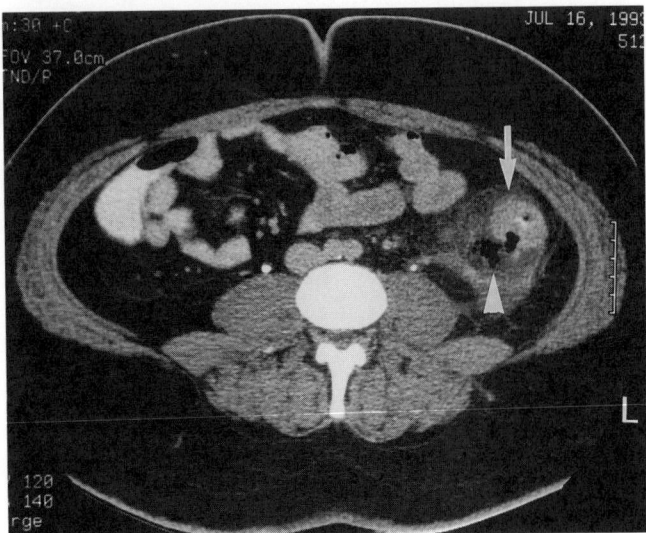

FIG. 26. Diverticulitis of the descending colon in a 37-year-old man who presented with left lower abdominal pain. CT shows marked thickening of the wall of the descending colon (*arrow*) and extraluminal gas (*arrowhead*) in the inflamed paracolic soft tissues, consistent with contained perforation.

to the mesentery (Fig. 26). It is also usually responsive to antibiotic therapy alone. In stage II diverticulitis an abscess spreads beyond the mesentery to become walled off by pelvic structures such as the small bowel or omentum. Such abscesses are often well suited for percutaneous CT-guided drainage. Stage III is marked by the spread of disease to other parts of the peritoneal cavity or retroperitoneum. Percutaneous drainage may allow surgery to be delayed until the patient's status improves (36). Stage IV is indistinguishable on CT from stage III but is accompanied by a clinical picture of acute peritonitis and life-threatening sepsis (35).

In cases in which the CT findings are unclear, barium enema examination is warranted for clarification. Patients with perforated colon carcinoma occasionally present with clinical and radiographic findings similar to those of diverticulitis, so it is prudent to perform a follow-up barium examination or colonoscopy 4–6 weeks after resolution of symptoms to evaluate the colonic mucosa for tumor.

Appendicitis

In prior years, patients with signs and symptoms of acute appendicitis often underwent operation without a preoperative radiological workup. Presently, patients with typical as well as atypical presentations are commonly evaluated prior to determination of therapy. CT and ultrasound recently replaced the barium enema as the most useful radiological examinations. In children, sonography of the right lower quadrant with graded compression is often the only preoperative imaging study performed. While sonography is also useful in adults (37–39),

operator performance variability and limitations due to body habitus and abdominal guarding have thus far limited the widespread application of this noninvasive method.

As with diverticulitis, CT has greater sensitivity and specificity for determining the extent and complications of appendicitis than does the barium enema, which has an accuracy ranging of 50% to 84% depending on demonstration of nonfilling of the appendix and an extrinsic mass effect on the cecum, terminal ileum, or ascending colon (40). The sensitivity and specificity of CT have been reported as 94% and 79%, respectively (38,41).

Uncomplicated appendicitis is characterized by the CT findings of appendiceal wall thickening and periappendiceal edema and inflammation (41,42). The abnormal appendix (Fig. 27) is seen in 13% to 60% of cases (43). Conversely, the normal appendix is visible in most unaffected patients and a confident diagnosis of no appendicitis can usually be made in this group. Focal indentation or eccentric thickening of the posteromedial cecum; thickening of the distal small bowel; thickening of the anterior renal fascia, lateroconal fascia, and abdominal wall muscles; and enlargement and blurring of the right psoas muscle also may be noted in patients with appendicitis. CT can often demonstrate appendicoliths not visible on plain abdominal radiographs (Fig. 28). This is important as appendicoliths are present in a higher percentage of patients with complicated (rather than uncomplicated) appendicitis (44).

Periappendiceal phlegmon or abscess can be located in the right lower quadrant, medial to the cecum, in the right anterior pararenal space, posterior to the right colon, or elsewhere in the abdomen, and can be accurately depicted by CT. Complications such as hepatic abscess or pylephlebitis are also well shown (41,45). Although right colonic diverticulitis, perforated right colonic neoplasm, and mucocele of the appendix occasionally mimic appendicitis on CT, it is usually possible to at least identify those patients with an inflammatory or neoplastic process severe

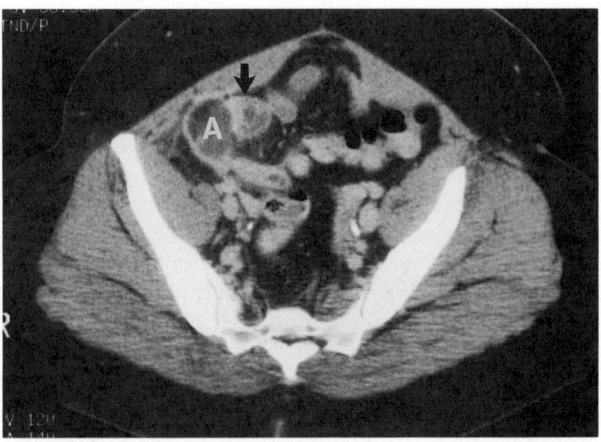

FIG. 27. A 34-year-old woman with acute appendicitis. CT obtained on the night of admission shows thickening of the appendiceal wall (*arrow*), which is seen in cross-section. Lateral to the inflamed appendix lies a 2-cm abscess (A).

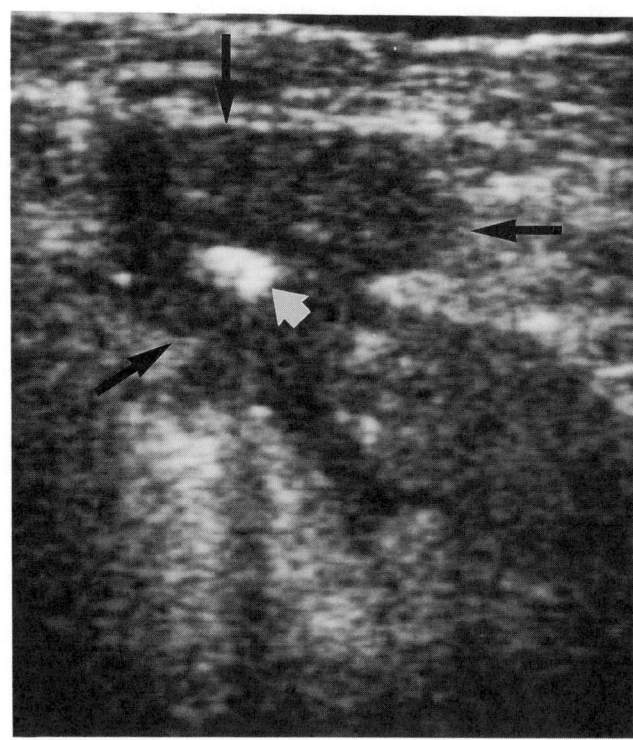

A

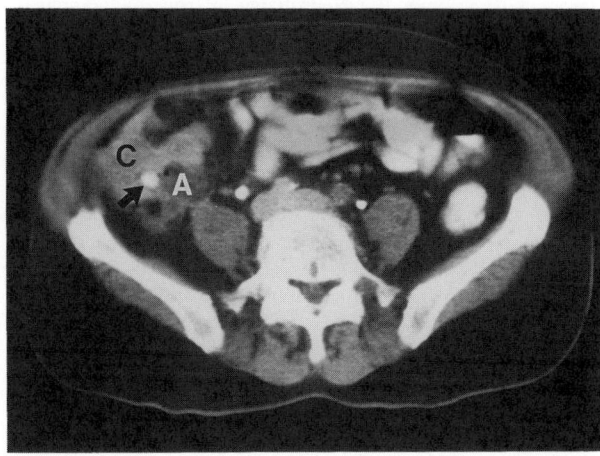

B

FIG. 28. A 64-year-old man with acute appendicitis. **A:** Ultrasonogram shows a right lower quadrant fluid collection (*arrows*) containing a calcified appendicolith (*arrowhead*). **B:** CT scan shows thickened cecal wall (**C**) and the appendicolith (*arrow*), which was not visible on the barium enema scout radiograph. An adjacent periappendiceal abscess (**A**) contains fluid and a single bubble of gas.

enough to warrant surgical intervention, even when an accurate preoperative diagnosis is not made.

REFERENCES

1. Levine MS, Macones AJ, Laufer I. *Candida* esophagitis: accuracy of radiographic diagnosis. *Radiology* 1986;158:597–603.
2. Levine MS. Radiology of esophagitis: a pattern approach. *Radiology* 1991;179:1–7.
3. Levine MS, Woldenbrg R, Herlinger H, Laufer I. Opportunistic esophagitis in AIDS: radiographic diagnosis. *Radiology* 1987; 165:815–820.
4. Jones B, Wall SD. Gastrointestinal disease in the immunocompromised host. In: Federle MP, ed. *Radiology of the immunocompromised host. Radiol Clin North Am.* Philadelphia: WB Saunders; 1992;30(3):555–577.
5. Farman J, Taavitian A, Rosenthan LE, Schwartz GE, Raufman J. Focal esophageal candidiasis in acquired immunodeficiency syndrome (AIDS). *Gastrointest Radiol* 1986;11:213–217.
6. Levine MS. *Radiology of the esophagus.* Philadelphia: WB Saunders; 1989.
7. Shortsleeve MJ, Levine MS. Herpes esophagitis in otherwise healthy patients: clinical and radiographic findings. *Radiology* 1992;182:859–861.
8. Balthazar EJ, Megibow AJ, Hulnick D, Cho KC, Beeranbaum E. Cytomegalovirus esophagitis in AIDS: radiographic features in 16 patients. *AJR* 1987;149:919–923.
9. Balthazar EJ, Megibow AJ, Hulnick DH. Cytomegalovirus esophagitis and gastritis in AIDS. *AJR* 1985;144:1201–1204.
10. Levine MS, Loercher G, Katzka DA, Herlinger H, Rubesin SE, Laufer I. Giant, human immunodeficiency virus–related ulcers in the esophagus. *Radiology* 1991;180:323–326.
11. de Silva R, Stoopack PM, Raufman J. Esophageal fistulas associated with mycobacterial infection in patients at risk for AIDS. *Radiology* 1990;175:449–453.
12. Falcone S, Murphy J, Weinfeld A. Gastric manifestations of AIDS: radiographic findings on upper gastrointestinal examination. *Gastrointest Radiol* 1991;16:95–98.
13. Smart PE, Weinfeld A, Thompson NE, Defortuna SM. Toxoplasmosis of the stomach: a cause of antral narrowing. *Radiology* 1990;174:369–370.
14. Farman J, Lerner ME, Ng C, et al. Cytomegalovirus gastritis: protean radiologic features. *Gastrointest Radiol* 1992;17:202–206.
15. Margulis AR, Burhenne HJ, eds. *Alimentary tract radiology.* 4th ed. St. Louis: CV Mosby; 1989.
16. Laufer I, Levine MS. *Double contrast gastrointestinal radiology.* 2nd ed. Philadelphia: WB Saunders; 1992.
17. Wall SD, Jones B. Gastrointestinal tract in the immunocompromised host: opportunistic infections and other complications. *Radiology* 1992;185:327–335.
18. Vincent ME, Robbins AH. *Mycobacterium avium-intracellulare* complex enteritis: pseudo-Whipple's disease in AIDS. *AJR* 1985;144:921–927.
19. Radin DR. Intraabdominal *Mycobacterium* tuberculosis vs *Mycobacterium avium-intracellulare* infections in patients with AIDS: distinction based on CT findings. *AJR* 1991;156:487–491.
20. Jeffrey RB Jr, Nyberg DA, Bottles K, et al. Abdominal CT in acquired immunodeficiency syndrome. *AJR* 1986;146:7–13.
21. Wall SD, Ominsky S, Altman DF, et al. Multifocal abnormalities of the gastrointestinal tract in AIDS. *AJR* 1986;146:1–5.
22. Shirahama M, Koga T, Ishibashi H, Uchida S, Ohta Y, Shimoda Y. Intestinal anisakiasis: US in diagnosis. *Radiology* 1992;185:789–793.
23. Stanley RJ, Melson GL, Tedesco FJ. The spectrum of radiographic findings in antibiotic-related pseudomembranous colitis. *Radiology* 1974;111:519–524.
24. Stanley RJ, Melson GL, Tedesco FJ. Plain-film findings in severe pseudomembranous colitis. *Radiology* 1976;118:7–11.
25. Rubesin SE, Levine MS, Glick SN. Pseudomembranous colitis with rectosigmoid sparing on barium studies. *Radiology* 1989; 170:811–815.
26. Downey DB, Wilson S. Pseudomembranous colitis: sonographic features. *Radiology* 1991;180:61–64.
27. Fishman EK, Kavuru M, Jones B, et al. Pseudomembranous colitis: CT evaluation of 26 cases. *Radiology* 1991;180:57–60.
28. Merine D, Fishman EK, Jones B. Pseudomembranous colitis: CT evaluation. *J Comput Assist Tomogr* 1987;11(6):1017–1020.

29. Amronin GD, Solomon RD. Necrotizing enteropathy: complications of treated leukemia or lymphoma patients. *JAMA* 1961; 192:23–27.

30. Balthazar EJ, Megibow AJ, Fazzini E, Opulencia JF, Engel I. Cytomegalovirus colitis in AIDS: radiographic findings in 11 patients. *Radiology* 1985;155:585–589.

31. Sider L, Mintzer RA, Mendelson EB, Rogers LF, Degesys GE. Radiographic findings of infectious proctitis in homosexual men. *AJR* 1982;139:667–671.

32. Cho KC, Morehouse HT, Alterman DD, Thornhill BA. Sigmoid diverticulitis: diagnostic role of CT—comparison with barium enema studies. *Radiology* 1990;176:111–115.

33. Wilson SR, Toi A. The value of sonography in the diagnosis of acute diverticulitis of the colon. *AJR* 1990;154:1199–1202.

34. Wada M, Kikuchi Y, Doy M. Uncomplicated acute diverticulitis of the cecum and ascending colon: sonographic findings in 18 patients. *AJR* 1990;155:283–287.

35. Neff CC, van Sonnenberg E. CT of diverticulitis. In: Gore RM, ed. *CT of the gastrointestinal tract*. *Radiol Clin North Am*. Philadelphia: WB Saunders; 1989;27:743–752.

36. Neff CC, van Sonnenberg E, Casola G, et al. Diverticular abscesses: percutaneous drainage. *Radiology* 1987;163:15–18.

37. Puylaert JBCM. Acute appendicitis: US evaluation using graded compression. *Radiology* 1986;158:355–360.

38. Abu-Yousef MM, Bleicher JJ, Maher JW, Urdaneta LF, Franken EA Jr, Metcalf AM. High-resolution sonography of acute appendicitis. *AJR* 1987;149:53–58.

39. Jeffrey RB, Laing FC, Lewis FR. Acute appendicitis: high-resolution real-time US findings. *Radiology* 1987;163:11–14.

40. Fedyshin P, Kelvin FM, Rice RP. Nonspecificity of barium enema findings in acute appendicitis. *AJR* 1984;143:99–102.

41. Balthazar EJ, Megibow AJ, Hulnick D, Gordon RB, Naidich DP, Beranbaum ER. CT of appendicitis. *AJR* 1986;147:705–710.

42. Fisher JK, Findly T. Diagnosing appendicitis by computed tomography. *Mo Med* 1988;85:15–20.

43. Balthazar EJ, Megibow AJ, Gordon RB, Whelan CA, Hulnick D. Computed tomography of the abnormal appendix. *J Comput Assist Tomogr* 1988;12(4):595–601.

44. Gale ME, Birnbaum S, Gerzof SG. CT of appendicitis and its local complications. *J Comput Assist Tomogr* 1985;9:34–37.

45. Feldberg MAM, Hendriks MJ, van Waes PFGM. Computed tomography in complicated acute appendicitis. *Gastrointest Radiol* 1985;10:289–295.

Infections of the Gastrointestinal Tract,
edited by M. J. Blaser, P. D. Smith, J. I. Ravdin,
H. B. Greenberg, and R. L. Guerrant
Published by Raven Press, Ltd., New York, 1995.

CHAPTER 86

Prophylaxis for Gastrointestinal Surgery

Douglas S. Kernodle and Allen B. Kaiser

Advances in anesthesia and antisepsis during the late 1800s ushered in the modern era of surgery. Abdominal surgery, in particular, underwent dramatic changes with the development of procedures to treat common acute and oftentimes fatal illnesses such as appendicitis. Also, surgical procedures became important in the management of chronic illnesses for which medical therapy alone had proved to be ineffective. So swift were the changes in general surgery that most of today's basic surgical procedures involving the gastrointestinal tract had been developed by World War I (1), predating the discovery and clinical use of antibiotics.

The surgical advances during that earlier era are even the more remarkable considering that many of these procedures involve portions of the gastrointestinal tract that are heavily colonized with bacteria. In 1920, Lord Moynihan wrote that "every operation in surgery is an experiment in bacteriology" (2). Nowhere is this statement more relevant than in surgery involving the gastrointestinal tract. For example, in the descending colon as many as 10^{12} bacteria are present per gram of stool (3,4). Before antibiotic prophylaxis became an accepted part of surgical management, procedures involving the colon were associated with infection rates of 30% to 60% (5). The infecting bacteria, usually *Escherichia coli* and *Bacteroides* species, generally were derived from the patient's endogenous flora.

The high incidence of wound infections in the preantibiotic era would be considered unacceptable by today's standards. Despite the relatively late acceptance of antibiotic prophylaxis as the standard of care in surgical practice (6), it is difficult to imagine modern gastrointestinal surgery without it. And in spite of its routine use, postoperative infections are still a major cause of surgical morbidity.

PATHOGENESIS OF SURGICAL WOUND INFECTIONS AND THE RATIONALE FOR ANTIBIOTIC PROPHYLAXIS

General Concepts

Based on the risk of bacterial contamination of the operative site, surgical wounds have been divided into several categories (7,8). Clean wounds are nontraumatic wounds in which no inflammation is encountered, no break in aseptic technique occurs, and the alimentary, respiratory, and urinary tracts are not entered. Clean-contaminated wounds are nontraumatic wounds in which a minor break in technique occurs or in which the gastrointestinal, respiratory, or urinary tracts are entered without significant spillage. This category includes cholecystectomy and appendectomy "in passing" in the absence of acute inflammation. Contaminated wounds are associated with procedures in which acute inflammation is encountered or there is visible spillage of material from a hollow viscus. Included in this category are procedures involving the biliary system in the presence of infected bile as well as surgery involving trauma, fecal contamination, a devitalized viscus, or pus from any source. Dirty wounds refer to surgery performed under conditions in which there is preexisting infection, for example, drainage of an abscess and surgical creation of a diverting colostomy following perforation of the colon. The use of antibiotics in this clinical setting is considered "therapeutic" rather than "prophylactic" (6,9). Several studies have demonstrated a correlation between the density of bacteria at the operative site with the subsequent risk of infection (10–12).

Whereas these categories historically have been useful in defining the epidemiology and risk of infectious complications, there is enough variance in the infection rates associated with different procedures within the same category as to make procedure-specific infection rates a superior indicator for hospital surveillance (13,14). Also, newer algorithms based on both patient and procedure-related risk factors appear to have better predictive value (15,16).

D. S. Kernodle: Infectious Diseases Section, Department of Veterans Affairs Medical Center, Nashville, Tennessee; and Department of Medicine, Vanderbilt University School of Medicine, Nashville, Tennessee 37232-2358.

A. B. Kaiser: Department of Medicine, Vanderbilt University School of Medicine, Nashville, Tennessee 37232-2358.

TABLE 1. *Host risk factors for wound infection following gastrointestinal surgery*

Extremes of age (i.e., very old or very young)
Diabetes
Prior irradiation of the operative site
Steroids and other immunosuppressive therapy
Severe obesity
Malnutrition
Cutaneous anergy
Low expression of HLA-DR (human leukocyte antigen-DR) on monocytes
Remote infection at the time of surgery (e.g., urinary tract infection)
Long duration of hospitalization prior to surgery
Gastric achlorhydria (gastroduodenal surgery)
Obstruction or perforation of viscus
Preoperative assessment score of 3, 4, or 5 (American Society of Anesthesiologists)

Risk Factors for Infection

A variety of host and technique-related variables have been identified as risk factors for the development of a surgical wound infection (Tables 1 and 2). Host factors include the extremes of age (i.e., the elderly and the very young), diabetes, severe obesity, concomitant steroid therapy, malnutrition, cutaneous anergy, the presence of remote infection at the time of surgery, and a long duration of time in the hospital prior to the operation (9,17–23).

Surgical Technique

The maintainance of adequate tissue perfusion in the postoperative period is of critical importance and in part reflects the care with which the surgeon handles body tissues and achieves hemostasis during the procedure. Tissue devitalization at a gross or microscopic level provides a niche wherein inoculated bacteria may grow in relative isolation from host defense mechanisms. Good surgical technique is one of the most important determinants of whether a wound becomes infected or not and

TABLE 2. *Operative risk factors for wound infection following gastrointestinal surgery*

No preoperative shower or inadequate preparation of skin with antiseptics
Shaving the operative site on the day prior to surgery
Prolonged length of procedure
Intraoperative contamination
Homologous blood transfusion
Excessive use of an electrosurgical knife
Poor hemostasis
Use of foreign material
Use of prophylactic abdominal drains
Injection of epinephrine into the wound
Appendectomy in passing added to elective cholecystectomy
Inadequate preparation of the colon (colorectal surgery)

is reflected in the "traditional surgical view that untidy operative techniques predispose to infection" (24). Other technical factors, including the method of preoperative hair removal (i.e., clipping or shaving), topical antisepsis, the choice of suture material, the use of electrocautery, whether or not a drain(s) is placed during surgery and if so its position (i.e., exiting via the incision versus a separate site and distance from an intestinal anastomotic site), and the use of intraoperative irrigation also have been correlated with the risk of wound infection (23,25–34).

Unique Risk Factors Among Gastrointestinal Procedures

Some gastrointestinal procedures have unique risks not shared by other surgical procedures. An "appendectomy in passing" added to elective cholecystectomy increases the infection rate from 1.4% to 4.5% (35). Gastric achlorhydria or the use of histamine (H_2) blocking agents have been associated with an increased risk of infection following gastric procedures (36,37). This is believed to be related to an increased number of bacteria in the stomach at the time of surgery stemming from the loss of the normal antibacterial effect of low gastric pH. In a canine model, vagotomy is associated with hypochlorhydria and a marked increase in the coliform population of the stomach (38). Obstruction or perforation of a viscus is a strong predictor of subsequent infection. Inadequate preparation of the colon with the retention of intestinal fluid and feces at the time of surgery is a strong risk factor for several types of septic complications, including dehiscence of the anastomotic site (39,40). Abdominal–perineal rectal resections have a greater risk of infection than intraperitoneal resections (41,42).

Blood Transfusion

The transfusion of homologous blood is an independent risk factor for infection in patients undergoing elective intra-abdominal surgery, with the majority of the infections occurring at sites other than the surgical wound (43,44). Homologous blood transfusions suppress cellular immunity in humans (45,46) and are associated with a reduced risk of rejection following renal allograft transplantation (47,48). In contrast, autologous blood transfusion does not appear to increase the risk of infection following surgery (49,50) and may even be immunostimulatory (50,51). The odds ratios for risk of infection among patients receiving homologous versus autologous blood transfusion in one randomized, prospective study was 2.84 (50).

Interrelationship of Risk Factors

Some risk factors for infection are interrelated, with a patient exhibiting one factor also being likely to have others. Haley et al. (15) have described an index to ascertain the risk of postoperative infection that involves combining a traditional assessment of the wound category (i.e., clean, clean-contaminated, or contaminated) with three patient and procedure-related factors. These include an operation involving the abdomen, a procedure lasting longer than 2 hr, and the presence of three or more underlying diagnoses (as a surrogate for identifying the complicated patient). Subsequently, this model for identifying patients at risk for infection has been further simplified: (a) a patient with an American Society of Anesthesiologists preoperative assessment score of 3, 4, or 5; (b) an operation classified as contaminated or dirty-infected; and (c) an operation lasting longer than T hours, where T depends on the procedure (16). In clean surgery, the importance of the duration of the operation appears diminished in studies in which antibiotic prophylaxis is readministered intraoperatively during long procedures (52,53). These observations suggest that the duration-related risk may be due to the lack of adequate antibiotic concentrations in the blood and tissues with longer surgical procedures, and that the risk of wound infection may be reduced by more aggressive prophylaxis.

The "Decisive Interval"

Whether or not a wound becomes infected is largely determined at the time of surgery. In experimental models, maneuvers initiated several hours following the inoculation of bacteria into the wound do not influence whether or not infection occurs (54–58). The demonstration that the efficacy of antibiotics in preventing wound infection is limited to only a few hours following the moment of bacterial inoculation implies that the wound microenvironment is not static. However, the changes that occur during this "decisive interval" are poorly understood. It is unclear whether the decisive interval is attributable to microbial factors (e.g., a shift from exponential to stationary phase growth with an accompanying decrease in bacterial susceptibility to antibiotics and possibly the expression of different microbial virulence factors) or to wound-related factors (e.g., gradually diminishing tissue perfusion and antibiotic delivery related to increased tissue oncotic pressure brought about by the effect of inflammatory mediators on vascular permeability). Both or neither of these examples may be important. It is likely, however, that the elucidation of the pathophysiology of the decisive interval will have a profound effect on developing strategies for preventing infection. The clinical relevance of the decisive interval in the prophylaxis of surgery has been established in clinical trials, in which the risk of infection is higher for patients who have prophylaxis initiated in the late intraoperative or postoperative period than in the immediate preoperative period (59,60).

Host Defenses and the Wound Microenvironment

Because of the large serosal surface of the peritoneum and the relative ease with which infection at the incisional site of a viscus may track to other parts of the abdomen and pelvis, it is important to consider the peritoneal defense systems in addition to the defenses of the skin and soft tissues through which the surgical incision was made. Three forms of peritoneal response to bacterial challenge have been described: (a) direct absorption of bacteria into the lymphatic stomata under the diaphragm, (b) the destruction of bacteria by phagocytosis, and (c) the localization of bacteria within an abscess (4,61).

Cellular and humoral factors contribute to the bacterial eradication from the peritoneum and the surgical wound site. In animal models, the initial clearing of a bacterial challenge to the peritoneum is mediated by macrophages, followed by the mobilization of neutrophils (62,63). Failure of peripheral monocytes to express the class II antigen HLA-DR, which is critical for the recognition of foreign antigens and the T lymphocyte proliferative response, has been associated with an increased incidence of infection and death among surgical and trauma patients (64,65). Whereas neutrophils can kill *Bacteroides fragilis* in the presence of serum, serum alone is not bactericidal (66). Immunoglobulins and the alternative complement pathways facilitate the opsonophagocytosis of *B. fragilis* (67). An anaerobic environment does not appear to adversely affect the microbicidal activity of neutrophils (68,69).

Cytokines also have a protective effect against disseminated and local infection in animal models. Systemic prophylaxis of mice with recombinant human tumor necrosis factor (TNF) inhibited local and bloodstream recovery of *Klebsiella pneumoniae* following insertion of a bacteria-laden thigh suture (70). TNF stimulates neutrophils to produce oxygen free radicals and promotes bacterial killing (71). Studies of the benefit of direct application of TNF into incisional wounds in animal models have yielded mixed results, however, and this practice has been associated with reduced tensile strength of the healing wound (72,73).

Microbial attachment to the wound tissues is believed to be important in the pathogenesis of wound infection. Coliforms and *B. fragilis* adhere to the peritoneal serosal mesothelium (74). The use of fibrinolytic agents inhibits abscess formation in investigational models (75,76), which is consistent with the hypothesis that the adherence of bacteria to fibrinous exudates is an essential step in wound infection pathogenesis.

Surgery and trauma induce systemic and local changes in the immune defense mechanisms of the host. Operative procedures impair neutrophil function and serum opsonizing capacity. The microbicidal activity of neutrophils obtained postoperatively from patients undergoing abdominal hysterectomy is reduced compared to neutrophils harvested from the same patients preoperatively, and it takes 9 days to return to normal (77). Neutrophils from an unfavorable wound environment can be stimulated to premature activation and degranulation in the absence of a bacterial stimulus more readily than can neutrophils from a well-perfused wound (78). Furthermore, the percentage of monocytes and neutrophils expressing complement receptors is reduced within pus compared to peripheral blood (79). The depletion of opsonizing factors within the milieu of an abscess also may contribute to decreased neutrophil bactericidal function (80,81).

The use of electrocautery alters the wound microenvironment. In an *in vitro* system, thermally killed fibroblasts activate the alternative complement pathway and deplete complement components that normally contribute to opsonophagocytosis of bacteria, leading ultimately to impaired neutrophil activity (82).

The formation of an abscess following intra-abdominal surgery is a complex process that appears to require lymphocytes. Renal transplant patients with lymphopenia who undergo appendectomy have a high incidence of bacteremia with *B. fragilis* without abscess formation (83). The capsule of *B. fragilis* promotes abscess formation, even when the bacteria are not viable (84). Following experimental inoculation of *B. fragilis*, antibiotics with good activity fail to prevent abscesses from developing but the combination of antibiotics with cell-free splenic extracts of animals previously challenged with *B. fragilis* prevents abscess formation (85). Furthermore, immunization against capsular polysaccharide protects by a T cell-dependent mechanism against abscess formation following *B. fragilis* inoculation (86,87). However, this protection can be reduced by the presence of foreign material.

Fecal roughage has a strong adjuvant effect on the ability of intestinal bacteria to induce abscess formation. The mechanism is believed to involve complement activation by the roughage and the depletion of complement-derived opsonins, with reduced opsonization of abscess-inducing bacteria (88). Roughage may also provide a niche wherein bacteria grow in relative isolation from the host defense mechanisms in much the same manner as described earlier for devitalized tissue.

Bacterial infection has an adverse effect on the tensile strength of intestinal anastomoses and the site of incisional healing (89,90). In a dog model, peroral antibiotics improve tensile strength of intestinal anastomoses and lessen the risk of dehiscence (40,90).

Major Wound Pathogens

Normal Flora and Wound Pathogens of the Gastrointestinal Tract

For most gastrointestinal procedures, the major wound pathogens come from the viscus entered during surgery, and an understanding of the gastrointestinal flora during health and disease is fundamental to effective surgical prophylaxis. This topic is covered in more detail in the chapter by Simon and Gorbach.

The flora of the esophagus and stomach reflect what is swallowed from the mouth; however, gastric acid has a potent antibacterial effect and renders the stomach nearly sterile under normal conditions (91). *Helicobacter pylori* and related organisms, the only known bacterial species adapted for living in the human stomach, are discussed elsewhere (see chapters by Riegg et al., Taylor and Parsonnet, and Holtman and Talley) and these fastidious organisms do not appear to be wound pathogens.

During the postprandial period, persons with a full stomach and relatively high gastric pH have counts of oral bacteria up to 10^5 CFU/mL (92). The quantitative gastric flora also increase under circumstances of hypochlorhydria and obstruction (36). The predominant species include streptococci, staphylococci, and lactobacilli (4); however, *B. fragilis* can be recovered from patients with achlorhydria or gastric carcinoma (4).

The biliary tract is normally sterile, and even in the setting of surgery for cholelithiasis the majority of patients have sterile bile (93). Infected bile from patients with acute cholecystitis and other biliary tract diseases from different institutions, geographic locations, and comprising different demographic populations shows marked variability in the aerobic and anaerobic organisms isolated (94–99). In general, aerobes are more common than anaerobes. Anaerobic cocci or *clostridium perfringens* are the most frequently recovered anaerobes. *Bacteroides fragilis* usually is not isolated; in one study it was recovered from 29% of elderly patients, however (100). Human bile acids normally inhibit the growth of *B. fragilis,* but among patients with gallstones, the inhibitory properties of the bile are diminished (101,102). In septicemia following cholecystectomy, the most common pathogens include *E. coli, Klebsiella* species, *Proteus* species, streptococci, and enterococci (103).

Although studies based on culturing fluid from the small intestine at autopsy or via peroral tubes suggest a complex microbial flora (4,104,105), aspirates obtained from living patients at the time of surgery show that the duodenum and jejunum are usually sterile or contain small numbers of ingested bacteria that are passing through (3,106). Heavier colonization occurs under conditions of gastric hypochlorhydria, intestinal stasis, cholelithiasis, and deficiencies in the secretion of pancreatic enzymes or bile acids (4,107–109).

The microflora of the colon include hundreds of different bacterial species but only a few have the propensity to cause infection (3,9,23). In the descending colon, bacterial counts are as high as 10^{12} CFU/g and bacteria account for 40% of the volume of stool (3,4). In the colon, 99.9% of the flora are anaerobic (3).

The patient's endogenous gastrointestinal flora are the major reservoir of pathogens causing postoperative infection. Polymicrobial infections are common, especially among procedures involving the appendix or colon. For example, patients undergoing surgery for perforated or gangrenous appendicitis have an average of eleven bacterial species, three aerobic and eight anaerobic, isolated from the operative specimen (110). *Escherichia coli* and *B. fragilis* are the most common aerobic and anaerobic pathogens, respectively. Despite the predominance of the intestinal flora, *Staphylococcus aureus*, the prototypic clean wound pathogen, is also commonly recovered from wound infections complicating colorectal surgery when the prophylactic regimen does not have activity against gram-positive pathogens (111). Presumably, they are derived either from the patient's endogenous skin or stool flora or exogenously from personnel involved in the procedure (112,113). Also, *S. aureus* has been recovered from 6% of wound infections and 12% of gastric secretions of patients undergoing gastric operations, demonstrating its pathogenic potential in surgery of the upper gastrointestinal tract (114). Staphylococci also have been problematic in studies when no prophylaxis was used in low-risk cholecystectomy patients (115,116) and are believed to come from the skin rather than the bile.

Virulence Determinants of E. coli *and* B. fragilis *in Wound Infection*

The most deleterious effects of wound sepsis or bacter-emia with *E. coli* are mediated by endotoxin (117). Endo-toxin induces the production of inflammatory mediators including TNF, interleukins, and prostaglandins by macrophages and other cells. These inflammatory media-tors produce local and systemic capillary damage and leakiness and, in severe cases, result in shock and multiorgan failure. Some strains of *E. coli* produce a hemolysin, which exhibits pore-forming capabilities and activity against a wide variety of cell types, including neutrophils (118). The hemolysin stimulates neutrophil degranulation and induces leukotriene generation. Hemoglobin and fer-ric iron augment *E. coli* virulence and lethality in *in vivo* peritonitis models (119–121).

In guinea pig models of intra-abdominal and cutaneous infections, *B. fragilis* is about 15 times more virulent than non-*B. fragilis* species including *B. thetaiotaomicron, B. ovatus, B. vulgatus*, and *B. distasonis* (122). The capsular polysaccharide of *B. fragilis* promotes abscess formation and reduces opsonophagocytosis (123,124). *Bacteroides fragilis* produces a variety of tissue-damaging enzymes including fibrinolysin, chondroitin sulfatase, collagenase, neuraminidase, heparinase, and hyaluronidase (125). The inducible production of superoxide dismutase in the pres-ence of oxygen facilitates aerotolerance (126). Production of succinic acid by *B. fragilis* and other anaerobes inhibits the respiratory burst and phagocytic killing capability of neutrophils by reducing the intraneutrophilic pH (127,128). This phenomenon also may help to protect aer-obic bacteria, including coliforms, in the wound from phagocytic killing (129,130). Although the lipopolysaccha-ride of *B. fragilis* contains endotoxin, it has low biological activity (3).

Microbial Synergism

By use of animal models, the peritonitis and abscess-formation stages of intra-abdominal infection have been correlated primarily with coliform and anaerobic flora, respectively (131,132). Despite the usefulness of this bi-phasic model in understanding infection pathogenesis, there also appear to be interactions between bacteria that are additive or synergistic in promoting infection. For ex-ample, the growth of some *Bacteroides* species is depen-dent on obtaining vitamin K produced by coliform copa-thogens (4,133,134). *Fusobacterium necrophorum* pro-duces a lipopolysaccharide that stimulates the growth of *B. intermedius* (135). The killing of *E. coli* by neutrophils is impaired in the presence of *B. fragilis* (136), and, as noted earlier, the production of succinic acid by anaer-obes may protect aerobes from neutrophils.

Concepts of Effective Prophylaxis

Spectrum of Activity

It is a basic tenet of antimicrobial prophylaxis that the regimen should be active against the major pathogens, and it is not necessary to cover those species among the normal flora that have little pathogenic potential. For po-tentially contaminated procedures involving the appen-dix, colon, or rectum, prophylaxis should be directed pri-marily against *B. fragilis* and the Enterobacteriaceae, in particular, *E. coli*. Anaerobic coverage appears to be less important for gastroduodenal and biliary tract proce-dures. Activity against *S. aureus*, which presumably is inoculated into the wound from the patient's endogenous skin flora or exogenously from operating room personnel, also has been recommended (23,111).

Whether or not resistant gram-negative pathogens such as *Pseudomonas aeruginosa* should be covered in the pro-phylactic regimen is controversial (137,138). Similarly, al-though enterococcal species including *E. faecalis* and *E. faecium* are commonly recovered from abdominal wound infections, the importance of providing coverage in the prophylactic regimen remains controversial. Animal model studies and clinical experience showing that poly-microbial infections, which include enterococci, can be eradicated successfully by using antibiotics that have poor activity against enterococci argue against the need for in-cluding a specific antienterococcal agent in the prophylac-tic regimen (4,139,140). On the other hand, enterococci increase the size of abscesses caused by other bacteria and can independently establish abscesses in animal models (4,141). In one study, postoperative enterococcal bacteremia was associated with increased patient morbid-ity (142). Among patients with prosthetic heart valves or with other risk factors for endocarditis, antienterococcal coverage with gentamicin plus either ampicillin or vanco-mycin should be given (143). Routine prophylaxis for pre-venting wound infection does not protect against endocar-ditis.

There are several recent changes in the antibiotic sus-ceptibility patterns of wound pathogens that may affect the efficacy of current routine prophylactic regimens. Iso-lates of *E. coli* and *Klebsiella* species that are resistant to the third-generation cephalosporins, including cefotaxime and ceftizoxime, have recently been described (144,145). This resistance is mediated via the substitution of several amino acids in positions close to the active site of the β-lactamases normally produced by these species. Failure of the third-generation cephalosporins to treat experimen-tal intra-abdominal abscesses caused by such strains has been reported (146). These mutant β-lactamases generally are susceptible to inhibition by β-lactamase inhibitors in-cluding clavulanic acid, sulbactam, and tazobactam (146,147). Also, the β-lactamases cannot hydrolyze the antianaerobic second-generation cephalosporins includ-ing cefoxitin, cefotetan, and cefmetazole; such agents maintain activity against these *E. coli* and *Klebsiella* strains. The emergence of vancomycin-resistant isolates of *E. faecium* as well as the widespread dissemination of methicillin-resistant strains of *S. aureus* (145) also may have implications for surgical prophylaxis.

Route of Administration

The principle on which most systemic antibiotic prophylaxis is based is the belief that antibiotics in the host tissues can augment natural immune defense mechanisms and help to kill bacteria that are inoculated into the wound. In some studies, topical and incisional administration of the antibiotic also have yielded good results (148–150).

The rationale for the administration of oral antibiotics before colonic surgery differs in that although some agents are absorbed systemically (e.g., erythromycin and metronidazole, but not neomycin), the primary goal is to reduce the potential pathogens among the normal gut flora at the time of surgery. Oral sulfanilamide was the first perioperative prophylactic antibiotic, being used for colorectal surgery in 1939 (151) and gastroduodenal surgery in 1941 (152). Oral prophylaxis is generally combined with mechanical preparation of the bowel to reduce colonic flora, including cathartics and/or isotonic lavage solutions (153,154).

Timing and Duration of Prophylaxis

For systemic prophylaxis, every effort should be made to ensure that free antibiotic levels are maintained above the minimal inhibitory concentration of common wound pathogens throughout the duration of the surgical procedure (23,155). Initiation of intravenous antibiotics in the operating room just before the induction of anesthesia provides time for the agent to distribute to body tissues prior to incision and avoids the premature administration associated with "on call" dosing. To prevent the serum and tissue concentrations of antibiotic from falling too low during long procedures, agents with a short half-life need to be redosed intraoperatively. Although a number of studies in the past have indicated that prolonged surgical procedures are associated with a higher infection rate (41,156), it is unclear whether a long procedure is truly a risk factor for infection or whether this association reflects inadequate intraoperative redosing.

For nonemergent colorectal procedures, an oral antibiotic regimen should be started on the afternoon prior to surgery in conjunction with isotonic lavage. Supplemental prophylaxis with a parenteral agent should be given when the duration of the procedure exceeds 3½ hr (41,156,157). Also, the timing of the administration of oral regimens is critical, and delays in the start of surgery from the originally scheduled time may diminish the efficacy of the oral regimen: under such circumstances, a systemic agent should be added.

In the setting of emergency surgery following abdominal trauma, parenteral prophylaxis should begin preoperatively and the duration of postsurgical antibiotic therapy should be based on the findings at the time of surgery. Thadepalli and Mandal (4) have recommended discontin-

uation of antibiotics if there is no hollow viscus injury; 48- to 72-hr coverage if the stomach, duodenum, or jejunum have been injured; and 7 days of therapy for colonic injuries.

Antibiotic Penetration

Under normal circumstances, the biliary concentrations of various antibiotics in the bile are markedly different (158–164). In the presence of cystic or common bile duct obstruction, however, the biliary concentration of most antibiotics falls dramatically (164–167). In general, antibiotic concentration in the bile does not correlate with prophylactic efficacy (168). Gentamicin, for example, is an effective prophylactic agent for biliary surgery even though minimal inhibitory concentrations are rarely achieved in the bile (169,170). Other antibiotics, including erythromycin, chloramphenicol, metronidazole, and clindamycin, are primarily excreted or detoxified in the liver (164,171). Caution should be exercised in the administration of these agents to patients with hepatic dysfunction.

Most antibiotics exhibit poor penetration into pancreatic secretions (164,172). An exception is chloramphenicol, which exhibits about 50% of its serum concentration in pancreatic juice. The "blood–pancreatic barrier" is reduced for some agents in the setting of acute pancreatitis (4,164,172–174).

Some of the common mistakes associated with antibiotic prophylaxis of gastrointestinal procedures are summarized in Table 3.

Adverse Effects

Complications of perioperative prophylaxis for the patient include pseudomembranous colitis from overgrowth of *Clostridium difficile,* allergic reactions, and bleeding problems induced by the methylthiotetrazole side chain of some of the cephalosporin antibiotics (164,175). The routine use of prophylaxis also has implications for the entire hospital and appears to correlate with development of increased resistance among common nosocomial pathogens. Not surprisingly, antibiotic prophylaxis increases the prevalence and quantity of antibiotic-resistant bacteria among the patient's skin and gastrointestinal flora (176–178).

TABLE 3. *Common errors in the administration of systemic perioperative prophylaxis*

Selection of an antibiotic that is not active against the important pathogens
Administering the initial dose too early ("on call") or too late
Failure to administer additional intraoperative doses during long operations
Continuing prophylaxis for longer than necessary

ANIMAL MODEL STUDIES OF PROPHYLAXIS AND EARLY THERAPY

The role of coliforms and anaerobes in abdominal sepsis has been elucidated in a rat model that simulates sepsis following colonic perforation and involves an intraperitoneal challenge with pooled cecal contents in a gelatin capsule placed via a midline abdominal incision (131,132,179). Without treatment, acute peritonitis and septicemia from coliforms caused rapid death in 35% to 45% of the animals, and all survivors develop abscesses with anaerobes as the predominant organisms. Different antibiotics, started 4 hr after inoculation and continued for 10 days, vary markedly in the ability to prevent early peritonitis/mortality versus abscess formation. In general, agents active against *E. coli* and other coliforms prevent early peritonitis and death, whereas drugs active against *B. fragilis* reduce abscess formation. Optimal results have been observed with regimens active against both coliforms and *B. fragilis*. Antibiotic efficacy as determined in this model appears to correlate well with the results of antibiotic prophylaxis in clinical trials of complicated appendectomy and colorectal surgery. The efficacy of prophylactically administered antibiotics has been established in an incisional model in which *E. coli* and *B. fragilis* are inoculated at the surgical site following the systemic administration of antibiotics (180).

SUMMARY OF CLINICAL TRIALS AND RECOMMENDATIONS

Gastroduodenal Surgery

Pathogens including *E. coli, Klebsiella* species, enterococci, *S. aureus*, and anaerobes frequently can be isolated from the gastric lumen of patients at the time of gastric surgery. In one study, 90% of patients with gastric carcinoma or gastric ulcers were colonized, compared to only 17% of patients undergoing surgery for duodenal ulcers (114). In general, the greatest risk factor for wound infection following gastroduodenal surgery is a breakdown in normal gastric acid secretion and prophylaxis is routinely recommended for patients with clinical conditions associated with decreased gastric acidity and/or abnormal motility (181). Patients undergoing gastric bypass surgery for morbid obesity also have high wound infection rates, which can be reduced with cefazolin prophylaxis (182). The prophylactic regimen should be directed primarily against coliforms; however, activity against gram-positive anaerobes and aerobes, including *S. aureus*, has been emphasized (41,181,183). Cefazolin, cefamandole, and cefuroxime appear to be as effective as antibiotics with activity against *B. fragilis* (184,185) (Table 4).

Biliary Tract Surgery

Although bile usually is sterile, 17% to 48% of patients undergoing biliary tract surgery have bacteria isolated from intraoperative cultures (103,168,186,187), and 90% of all wound infections occur in patients with infected bile (188). The major pathogens are aerobic, including *E. coli, Klebsiella* species, *Proteus* species, streptococci, and enterococci. Anaerobes are isolated infrequently, although *C. perfringens* is occasionally found. There is a strong correlation between the bacterial species isolated from preoperative bile cultures and blood cultures among patients with postcholecystectomy septicemia (168).

Historically, the decision whether or not to administer prophylactic antibiotics in biliary surgery has been based on risk stratification for the likelihood of positive bile cultures (23). Patients are at higher risk of infection at age greater than 60 years or with previous biliary tract surgery, common duct stones, and acute symptoms or laboratory abnormalities (i.e., elevated serum bilirubin or white blood cell count) (189–191). In this setting, the preoperative administration of an antibiotic with activity against aerobic flora, such as cefazolin, reduces the risk of infection (168,189,192,193). The risk of infection without antibiotic prophylaxis among uncomplicated patients undergoing elective cholecystectomy is small and routine prophylaxis has not been shown to be beneficial (95,189,194); however, many surgeons now routinely ad-

TABLE 4. *Recommendations for prophylactic antibiotics in gastrointestinal surgery*

Operative site	Indication	Antibiotic	Dose, route, and duration[a]
Gastroduodenal	High-risk patient[b]	Cefazolin	1–2 g preinduction of anesthesia
Biliary	High-risk patient[c]	Cefazolin	1–2 g preinduction of anesthesia
Appendectomy	All patients	Cefoxitin, cefotetan, or cefmetazole	1–2 g preinduction of anesthesia
Colorectal	Elective	Neomycin and erythromycin base	1 g of each at 1, 2, and 11 p.m. on the day prior to surgery
	Emergency, trauma, or for patients unable to take by mouth	Cefoxitin, cefotetan, or cefmetazole	1–2 g initially, postoperative doses may be given if surgical findings suggest infection

[a] Intraoperative doses of parenteral agents should be administered during long procedures.
[b] Includes patients with abnormalities in gastrointestinal motility or gastric acidity, including gastric carcinoma or ulcer, obstruction, bleeding, achlorhydria, or hypochlorhydria.
[c] Includes patients over the age of 60 years or with acute cholecystitis, obstructive jaundice, or common duct stones.

minister antibiotics to all patients undergoing biliary tract surgery regardless of risk (23).

Although the studies are not completely consistent, expanding the spectrum of coverage to include anaerobic bacteria or enterococci does not appear to reduce the risk of infection further. Most studies comparing cefazolin, cephalothin, or cefamandole to cefoxitin, cefotetan, or newer agents with broad antibacterial activity have demonstrated equivalent efficacy (184,192,195–198). The efficacy of single- and multiple-dose regimens are equivalent in most studies (192,199,200). Gentamicin is also effective and may be administered to patients who are allergic to β-lactams (169).

Whether antibiotic prophylaxis is needed during the postoperative manipulation of T tubes remaining in the biliary tract has not been evaluated prospectively. The bile is usually colonized with *E. coli, K. pneumoniae,* or enterococci in this clinical setting, however, and septicemia with the same species occurs in up to 9% of patients undergoing postoperative T-tube cholangiography (201,202). Culturing the bile prior to cholangiography and tailoring the prophylaxis to cover the bacterial strains that are isolated appear to be prudent precautions in this setting.

In recent years, laparoscopic cholecystectomy has been increasingly performed. Although controlled studies have not been done, a retrospective analysis of 77,604 procedures identified damage to the bile ducts as the major complication and infection appears to be uncommon (203). The role of antibiotic prophylaxis has not been established.

Appendectomy

Antibiotics are clearly efficacious in patients undergoing surgery for appendicitis with perforation; in this setting the patient already has established infection and the antibiotic course should be regarded as therapeutic rather than prophylactic (204,205). Whereas the benefits to the patient of perioperative antibiotics for appendicitis without perforation are less clear (206–214), such controversy is rendered academic by the imprecision of clinical discrimination prior to surgery between disease with or without perforation (204,215). The current standard of care is to provide prophylaxis for all patients undergoing surgery for possible appendicitis. Since such surgery usually is performed under emergent conditions, peroral prophylaxis is not feasible and parenteral agents should be used. The antibiotic regimen should have activity against both aerobic and anaerobic bacteria, and a variety of regimens have been shown to be efficacious (204,216–224). A regimen of one to three doses is appropriate unless there is evidence of gangrenous appendicitis or abscess formation at surgery, in which case a therapeutic course of antibiotics to treat active infection should be continued for at least 3 to 5 days.

Colorectal Surgery

Whereas colorectal surgery without antibiotic prophylaxis or with inappropriate agents is associated with infec-

tion rates up to 30% to 60%, less than 10% of patients receiving appropriate prophylaxis develop infection (5,204,225). Three basic approaches to prophylaxis are accepted for routine use: oral agents in combination with mechanical cleansing, parenteral prophylaxis, or a combination of both. The regimen should have activity against both aerobic and anaerobic bacteria (204,226).

Mechanical preparation of the colon and the use of oral antibiotics together with mechanical cleansing have been in practice longer than the routine use of systemic perioperative prophylaxis. Sulfanilamide was employed in colonic surgery by the late 1930s (151), at least 20 years prior to the pioneering work of Miles and Burke that led to the widespread acceptance of systemic antibiotic prophylaxis in surgery (56,58). Effective preparation of the colon is essential to the success of the oral prophylactic regimens; however, mechanical preparation without antibiotics reduces fecal bulk without altering the concentration of bacteria in the colon (227). Older procedures included the use of liquid diets, cathartics, and enema for up to 3 days; however, the more recent use of isotonic lavage appears comparable in its ability to remove feces and fluid (153,154).

A recent evaluation of the studies that employed a randomized, prospective design and included a sufficient number of patients to achieve statistical validity concluded that the lowest infection rates, from 3% to 9%, were observed among the trials that included an oral regimen, with or without systemic prophylaxis (204). The oral regimens are appropriate only for nonemergent procedures in which antibiotics can be administered on the afternoon and evening before surgery and for which sufficient time is available for mechanical cleansing of the colon by cathartics, enemas, or isotonic lavage. Although the combination of erythromycin and neomycin (1 g of each component at 1 P.M., 2 P.M., and 11 P.M. of the day before surgery) is the most carefully evaluated regimen in the United States (225,228,229), kanamycin has been substituted for neomycin and metronidazole for erythromycin with apparently similar efficacy (230–232). The addition of a systemic cephalosporin to oral erythromycin/neomycin is especially indicated in certain clinical settings (Table 5) (204). Several parenteral regimens have been shown to be efficacious including cefoxitin, cefotetan, and cefmetazole (53,233–237). Single-dose systemic prophylaxis appears to be just as efficacious as multiple-dose

TABLE 5. *Conditions for which systemic antibiotics should be added to oral prophylaxis in colorectal surgery*

The mechanical preparation is incomplete
Surgery lasting longer than 3½ hr
Surgery has been delayed substantially
Procedures involving rectal resection
Intestinal contents spill during the procedure
Surgery involving a site distal to an established colostomy[a]

---

[a] Oral antibiotics do not reach high intraluminal concentrations at sites distal to the colostomy.

regimens except among patients with inflammatory bowel disease (238–241).

Prophylaxis for Other Gastrointestinal Surgery and Procedures

Laparotomy

Data are not available to recommend prophylaxis for laparotomy, the division of adhesions, and other abdominal surgery in which a hollow viscus is not opened.

Small Bowel Surgery

Whereas the duodenum, jejunum, and upper ileum are normally sterile, fecal organisms can be found in large numbers in the setting of obstruction. Although randomized, prospective studies to establish the efficacy of prophylaxis in this clinical setting have not been performed, it appears prudent to administer systemic antibiotics that cover for both aerobic and anaerobic bacteria (242).

Percutaneous Endoscopic Gastrostomy

Cefazolin appears to be superior to placebo in preventing peristomal wound infections after percutaneous endoscopic gastrostomy (243). Single-dose prophylaxis is sufficient (244).

Liver Transplantation

During the first few weeks following liver transplantation, patients are at high risk for the development of infections caused by aerobic gram-negative bacilli and *Candida* species (245,246). In an effort to reduce the incidence of infection below that achieved with perioperative systemic prophylaxis alone, selective decontamination of the gastrointestinal flora with nonabsorbable oral antibiotics such as gentamicin, polymyxin, and nystatin has been advocated (247–249). However, no controlled trials have been done to study the efficacy of such regimens in preventing infection in patients undergoing liver transplantation. Because it may take days to weeks to achieve selective bowel decontamination and because of the impairment of gut peristalsis by surgery, it appears prudent to begin administering the oral regimen several days before the transplant liver is obtained (247). Perioperative systemic prophylaxis should have broad activity against coliforms. Cefotaxime, 2 g intravenously starting immediately before surgery and repeated every 6 hr during and every 8 hr after surgery for 48 hr, is an acceptable regimen (247).

EMERGING CONCEPTS AND OTHER CONSIDERATIONS

Prophylaxis with Biologics in Surgery

Among surgical patients at high risk for infection, the postoperative administration of intravenous immunoglobulins reduces the risk of infectious complications, usually at nonwound sites (250,251). No clear benefit has been observed following the administration of anti-endotoxin antibodies (251,252).

Bacterial Translocation in Surgery

The movement of gut bacteria across the intestinal mucosa to the mesenteric lymph nodes, lymphatics, and ultimately the systemic circulation is referred to as bacterial translocation. Under some circumstances, enteric flora appear to enter the systemic circulation directly via the portal venous system (253). In mice, translocation is dependent on the integrity of the intestinal mucosa and host immunity as well as the microflora (254,255). In some rodent models, the anaerobic flora appear to protect the animal from overgrowth and septicemia by aerobic species. A single dose of a β-lactam subcutaneously or bacitracin orally in guinea pigs leads to overgrowth by coliforms or *P. aeruginosa,* with a mortality rate approaching 50% (256,257). In mice, treatment with metronidazole facilitates translocation of *E. coli* (258). Furthermore, if the mice are immunosuppressed with steroids and cyclophosphamide prior to reducing anaerobic flora with clindamycin, *E. coli* septicemia and death will result (259). The manipulation of the intestines during surgery promotes translocation in animal models, primarily by *E. coli* and other coliforms (260). Selective decontamination of gram-negative colonization with nonabsorbable antibiotics that obtain high topical levels in the oropharynx and gut may substantially decrease nosocomial infection rates (50% to 80%) (261).

Cost Considerations

The primary reason for administering prophylactic antibiotics in surgery is the prevention of wound infection. Aside from this obvious benefit to the patient, however, the routine employment of prophylaxis has important cost implications for the institution.

Any assessment of the economic impact of surgical prophylaxis must balance the costs involved in purchasing and administering antibiotics with the costs of managing the infections that would have occurred if prophylaxis had not been given (262,263). The cost of antibiotic prophylaxis is considerable—it is estimated that one-third of all inpatient antibiotic use is for surgical prophylaxis (264,265).

In addition, surgical infections are costly. Surgical wound infections account for about 25% of all nosocomial infections, yet are responsible for 50% of infection-related costs (262). As many as 71% of all nosocomial infections occur in surgical patients (261). Infections at the operative site account for 40% of these, with the urinary tract (42%), respiratory tract (14%), and bloodstream (4%) as other major foci. Direct costs of postoperative infection include the costs of additional hospital stay as well as the costs of added medical studies and therapy to deal with the infection. The development of a postoperative wound infection approximately doubles the duration of the postoperative hospitalization (266). For patients undergoing uncomplicated gastrointestinal surgery, the extra expenses attributable to the management of nosocomial infection represent 6.8% of all patient-related costs (267).

Among the common types of nosocomial infection, surgical wound infection is the only one for which the rates have dropped consistently over the past decade (268,269). There is a general consensus that the benefits of perioperative prophylaxis in the selected operations where it is efficacious far outweigh the costs and consequences of this practice (262,270).

REFERENCES

1. Lyons AS, Petrucelli RJ II. *Medicine: an illustrated history.* New York: Abradale Press, Harry N Abrams, Inc, Publishers, 1987.
2. Bucknall TE. Factors affecting the development of surgical wound infections: a surgeon's view. *J Hosp Infect* 1985;6:1–8.
3. Bartlett JG. Anaerobic bacteria: general concepts. In: Mandell GL, Douglas RG, Bennett JE, eds. *Principles and practice of infectious diseases,* 3rd ed. New York: Churchill Livingstone, 1990;1828–1842.
4. Thadepalli H, Mandal AK. *Antimicrobial therapy in abdominal surgery: precepts and practices.* Boca Raton, FL: CRC Press, 1991.
5. Baum ML, Anish DS, Chalmers TC, et al. A survey of clinical trials of antibiotic prophylaxis in colon surgery: evidence against further use of no-treatment controls. *N Engl J Med* 1981;305:795–799.
6. Kaiser AB. Antimicrobial prophylaxis in surgery. *N Engl J Med* 1986;315:1129–1138.
7. Altemeier WA, Burke JF, Pluitt BA Jr, et al. *Manual on control of infection in surgical patients.* Philadelphia: Lippincott, 1976.
8. Simmons BP. CDC guidelines on infection control. *Infect Control* 1982;3:187–196.
9. The Medical Letter. Antimicrobial prophylaxis in surgery. *Med Lett* 1992;34:5–8.
10. Raahave D, Friis-Moller A, Bjerre-Jepsen K, Thiis-Knudsen J, Rasmussen LB. The infective dose of aerobic and anaerobic bacteria in postoperative wound sepsis. *Arch Surg* 1986;121:924–929.
11. Claesson B, Brandberg A, Nilsson LO, Kock NG. Quantitative recovery of contaminating bacteria at operation and the relation to postoperative infection in intestinal surgery. *Acta Chir Scand* 1981;147:285–288.
12. Houang ET, Ahmet Z. Intraoperative wound contamination during abdominal hysterectomy. *J Hosp Infect* 1991;19:181–189.
13. Davidson AIG, Clark C, Smith G. Postoperative wound infection: a computer analysis. *Br J Surg* 1971;58:333–337.
14. Garibaldi RA, Cushing D, Lerer T. Risk factors for postoperative infection. *Am J Med* 1991;91(Suppl 3B):158S–163S.
15. Haley RW, Culver DH, Morgan WM, et al. Identifying patients at high risk of surgical wound infection: a simple multivariate index of patient susceptibility and wound contamination. *Am J Epidemiol* 1985;121:206–215.
16. Culver DH, Horan TC, Gaynes RP, et al. Surgical wound infection rates by wound class, operative procedure, and patient risk index. *Am J Med* 1991;91(Suppl 3B):152S–157S.
17. Richet HM, Chidiac C, Prat A, et al. Analysis of risk factors for surgical wound infections following vascular surgery. *Am J Med* 1991;91(Suppl B):170S–172S.
18. Mead PB, Pories SE, Hall P, Vacek PM, Davis JH Jr, Gamelli RL. Decreasing the incidence of surgical wound infections. Validification of a surveillance-notification program. *Arch Surg* 1986;121:458–461.
19. Meakins JL, Pietsch JB, Bubenick O, et al. Delayed hypersensitivity: indicator of acquired failure of host defenses in sepsis and trauma. *Ann Surg* 1977;186:241–250.
20. Moesgaard F, Lykkegaard-Nielsen M. Preoperative cell-mediated immunity and duration of antibiotic prophylaxis in relation to postoperative infectious complications. A controlled trial in biliary, gastroduodenal and colorectal surgery. *Acta Chir Scand* 1989;155:281–286.
21. Griffith CDM, McLean Ross AH. Delayed hypersensitivity skin testing in elective colorectal surgery and relationship to postoperative sepsis. *J Parenter Enteral Nutr* 1984;8:279–280.
22. Siegman-Igra Y, Rozin R, Simchen E. Determinants of wound infections in gastrointestinal operations: the Israeli study of surgical infections. *J Clin Epidemiol* 1993;46:133–140.
23. Page CP, Bohnen JMA, Fletcher JR, et al. Antimicrobial prophylaxis for surgical wounds: guidelines for clinical care. *Arch Surg* 1993;128:79–88.
24. Elek SD, Conen PE. The virulence of *Staphylococcus pyogenes* for man. A study of the problems of wound infection. *Br J Exp Pathol* 1958;38:573–586.
25. Sharp WV, Belden TA, King PH, Teague PC. Suture resistance to infection. *Surgery* 1982;91:61–63.
26. McGeehan D, Hunt D, Chaudhuri A, Rutter P. An experimental study of the relationship between synergistic wound sepsis and suture materials. *Br J Surg* 1980;67:636–638.
27. Edlich RF, Tsung MS, Rogers W, Rogers P, Wangensteen OH. Studies in management of the contaminated wound: technique of closure of such wounds together with a note on a reproducible experimental model. *J Surg Res* 1968;8:585–592.
28. Kumagai SG, Rosales RF, Hunter GC, et al. Effects of electrocautery on midline laparotomy wound infection. *Am J Surg* 1991;162:620–623.
29. Budd DC, Cochram RC, Fouty WJ. Cholecystectomy with and without drainage: a randomized, prospective study of 300 patients. *Am J Surg* 1982;143:307–309.
30. Manz CW, Tendress CL, Osaka Y. The detrimental effects of drains on colonic anastomosis. *Dis Colon Rectum* 1970;13:17–25.
31. Raves JJ, Slifkin M, Diamond DL. A bacteriologic study comparing closed suction and simple conduit drainage. *Am J Surg* 1984;148:618–620.
32. Laufman H. Current use of skin and wound cleansers and antiseptics. *Am J Surg* 1989;157:359–365.
33. Schein M, Gecelter G, Freinkel W, Gerding H, Becker PJ. Peritoneal lavage in abdominal sepsis: a controlled clinical study. *Arch Surg* 1990;125:1132–1135.
34. Monson JRT, Guillou PJ, Keane FBV, Tanner WA, Brennan TG. Cholecystectomy is safer without drainage: the results of a prospective, randomized clinical trial. *Surgery* 1991;109:740–746.
35. Cruse PJE, Foord R. The epidemiology of wound infection: a ten-year prospective study of 63,939 wounds. *Surg Clin North Am* 1980;60:187–196.
36. Nichols RL, Smith JW. Intragastric microbial colonization in common disease states of the stomach and duodenum. *Ann Surg* 1975;182:557–561.
37. Gatehouse D, Dimock F, Burdon DW, Alexander-Williams J, Keighley MRB. Prediction of wound sepsis following gastric operations. *Br J Surg* 1978;65:551–554.
38. Broido PW, Gorbach SL, Condon RE, Nyhus LM. Upper intestinal microflora control, effects of gastric acid and vagal denervation on bacterial concentrations. *Arch Surg* 1973;106:90–93.
39. Irvin TT, Goligher JC. Aetiology of disruption of intestinal anastomosis. *Br J Surg* 1973;60:461–464.

40. Cohen SR, Cornell CN, Collins MH, et al. Healing of ischemic colonic anastomoses in the rat: role of antibiotic preparation. *Surgery* 1985;4:443–447.

41. Coppa GF, Eng K, Gough TH, Ranson JH, Lacalio SA. Parenteral and oral antibiotics in elective and rectal surgery. A prospective, randomized trial. *Am J Surg* 1983;145:62–65.

42. Tartter PI. Determinants of postoperative stay in patients with colorectal cancer. Implications for diagnostic-related groups. *Dis Colon Rectum* 1988;31:694–698.

43. Pinto V, Baldonedo R, Nicolas C, et al. Relationship of transfusion and infectious complications after gastric carcinoma operations. *Transfusion* 1991;31:114–118.

44. Wobbes TH, Bemelmans BLH, Kuypers JHC, Beerthuizen GIJM, Theewes AGM. Risk of postoperative septic complications after abdominal surgical treatment in relation to perioperative blood transfusion. *Surgery* 1990;171:59–62.

45. Fischer E, Lenhard V, Siefert P, Kluge A, Johannsen R. Blood transfusion induced suppression of cellular immunity in man. *Hum Immunol* 1980;3:187–194.

46. George CD, Morello PJ. Immunological effects of blood transfusion upon renal transplantation, tumor operations and bacterial infections. *Am J Surg* 1986;152:329–337.

47. Opelz G, Sengar DPS, Mickey MR, Terasaki PI. Effect of blood transfusion on subsequent kidney transplants. *Transplant Proc* 1973;5:253–259.

48. Keown PA, Descamps B. Improved renal allograft survival after blood transfusion; a non-specific, erythrocyte-mediated immunoregulatory process? *Lancet* 1979;1:20–22.

49. Mezrow CK, Bergstein I, Tartter PI. Postoperative infection following autologous and homologous blood transfusions. *Transfusion* 1992;32:27–30.

50. Heiss MM, Mempel W, Jauch K-W, et al. Beneficial effect of autologous blood transfusion on infectious complications after colorectal cancer surgery. *Lancet* 1993;342:1328–1333.

51. Alexander JW. Transfusion induced immunomodulation and infection. *Transfusion* 1991;31:195–196.

52. Nagachinta T, Stephens M, Reitz B. Risk factors for surgical-wound infection following cardiac surgery. *J Infect Dis* 1987; 156:967–973.

53. Kaiser AB, Petracek MR, Lea JW IV, et al. Efficacy of cefazolin, cefamandole, and gentamicin as prophylactic agents in cardiac surgery. *Ann Surg* 1987;206:791–797.

54. Howes EL. Prevention of wound infection by the injection of nontoxic antibacterial substances. *Ann Surg* 1946;124:268–276.

55. Miles AA, Niven JSF. The enhancement of infection during shock produced by bacterial toxins and other agents. *Br J Exp Pathol* 1950;31:73.

56. Miles AA, Miles EM, Burke J. The value and duration of defense mechanisms to the primary lodgement of bacteria. *Br J Exp Pathol* 1957;38:79–86.

57. Burke JF, Miles AA. The significance of vascular events in early infective inflammation. *J Pathol Bacteriol* 1958;76:1–19.

58. Burke JF. The effective period of preventive antibiotic action in experimental incisions and dermal lesions. *Surgery* 1961;50: 161–168.

59. Stone HH, Hooper CA, Kolb LD, et al. Antibiotic prophylaxis in gastric, biliary and colonic surgery. *Ann Surg* 1976;184: 443–452.

60. Classen DCM, Evans RS, Pestotnik SL, et al. The timing of prophylactic administration of antibiotics and the risk of surgical-wound infection. *N Engl J Med* 1992;326:281–286.

61. Hau T. Bacteria, toxins and the peritoneum. *World J Surg* 1990; 14:167–175.

62. Skau T, Nystrom PO, Ohman L, Stendahl O. The kinetics of peritoneal clearance of *Escherichia coli* and *Bacteroides fragilis* and participating defense mechanisms. *Arch Surg* 1986;121: 1033–1039.

63. Dunn DL, Berke RA, Ewald DC, Simmons RL. Macrophages and translymphatic absorption represent the first line of host defense of the peritoneal cavity. *Arch Surg* 1987;122:105–110.

64. Hershman MJ, Cheadle WG, Kuftinec D, Polk HC Jr, George CD. An outcome predictive score for sepsis and death following trauma. *Injury* 1988;19:263–266.

65. Cheadle WG, Hershman MJ, Wellhausen SR, Polk HC Jr.

66. HLA-DR antigen expression on peripheral blood monocytes correlates with surgical infection. *Am J Surg* 1991;161:639–645.

66. Bjornson AB, Altemeier WA, Bjornson SH. Comparison of the in vitro bactericidal activity of human serum and leukocytes against *Bacteroides fragilis* and *Fusobacterium mortiferum* in aerobic and anaerobic environments. *Infect Immun* 1976;14: 843–847.

67. Bjornson AB, Bjornson HS. Participation of immunoglobulin and the alternative complement pathway in opsonization of *Bacteroides fragilis* and *Bacteroides thetaiotaomicron*. *J Infect Dis* 1978;138:351–358.

68. Mandell GL. Bactericidal activity of aerobic and anaerobic polymorphonuclear neutrophils. *Infect Immun* 1974;9:337–341.

69. Wetherall BL, Pruull H, McDonald PJ. Oxygen-independent killing of *Bacteroides fragilis* by granule extracts from human polymorphonuclear leukocytes. *Infect Immun* 1984;43: 1080–1084.

70. Hershman MJ, Pietsch JD, Trachtenberg L, et al. Protective effects of recombinant human tumour necrosis factor α and interferon gamma against surgically simulated wound infection in mice. *Br J Surg* 1989;76:1282–1286.

71. Shalby MR, Aggarwal BB, Rinderknecht E, et al. Activations of human neutrophil functions by interferon and tumor necrosis factor. *J Immunol* 1985;135:2069–2073.

72. Mooney DP, Gamelli RL, O'Reilly M. Improved wound healing through the local delivery of tumour necrosis factor. *Surg Forum* 1988;39:77–79.

73. Steenfos HH, Hunt TK, Scheuenstuhl H, Goodson WH. Selective effects of tumor necrosis factor-alpha on wound healing in rats. *Surgery* 1988;106:171–176.

74. Edmiston CE, Gohen MP, Kornhall S, Jones FE, Condon RE. Fecal peritonitis: microbial adherence to serosal mesothelium and resistance to peritoneal lavage. *World J Surg* 1990;14: 176–183.

75. Rotstein OD, Kao J. Prevention of intra-abdominal abscesses by fibrinolysis using recombinant tissue plasminogen activator. *J Infect Dis* 1988;158:766–772.

76. Houston KA, McRitchie DI, Rotstein OD. Tissue plasminogen activator reverses the deleterious effect of infection on colonic wound healing. *Ann Surg* 1990;211:130–135.

77. El-Maallem H, Fletcher J. Effects of surgery on neutrophil granulocyte function. *Infect Immun* 1981;32:38–41.

78. Moelleken BRW, Mathes SJ, Amerhauser A, Scheuenstuhl H, Hunt TK. An adverse wound environment activates leukocytes prematurely. *Arch Surg* 1991;126:225–230.

79. Galandiuk S, Appel SH, Polk HC Jr. A biologic basis for altered host defenses in surgically infected abscesses. *Ann Surg* 1993; 217:624–633.

80. Zimmerli W, Lew PD, Waldvogel FA. Pathogenesis of foreign body infection. Evidence for a local granulocyte defect. *J Clin Invest* 1984;73:1191–2000.

81. Bamberger DM, Herndon BL. Bactericidal capacity of neutrophils in rabbits with experimental acute and chronic abscesses. *J Infect Dis* 1990;162:186–192.

82. Yamada Y, Hefter K, Burke JE, Gelfand JA. An in vitro model of the wound microenvironment: local phagocytic cell abnormalities associated with in situ complement activation. *J Infect Dis* 1987;155:998–1004.

83. Fisher MC, Balurate HJ, Long SS. Bacteremia due to *Bacteroides fragilis* after elective appendectomy in renal transplant recipients. *J Infect Dis* 1981;143:635–638.

84. McConville JH, Snyder MJ, Calia FM, Hornick RB. Model of intraabdominal abscess in mice. *Infect Immun* 1981;31: 507–509.

85. Gollapudi SV, Gupta A, Thadepalli H, Perez A. Use of lymphokines in treatment of experimental intra-abdominal abscess caused by *Bacteroides fragilis*. *Infect Immun* 1988;56: 2369–2372.

86. Onderdonk AB, Markham RB, Zaleznik DF, et al. Evidence of T cell-dependent immunity to *Bacteroides fragilis* in an intra-abdominal abscess model. *J Clin Invest* 1982;69:9–16.

87. Zaleznik DF, Finberg RW, Shapiro ME, Onderdonk AB, Kasper DL. A soluble suppressor T cell factor protects against

experimental intraabdominal abscesses. *J Clin Invest* 1985;75: 1023–1027.

88. Finlay-Jones JJ, Kenney PA, Nulsen MF, et al. Pathogenesis of intraabdominal abscess formation: abscess-potentiating agents and inhibition of complement-dependent opsonization of abscess-inducing bacteria. *J Infect Dis* 1991;164:1173–1179.

89. Raju DR, Jindrak K, Weiner M, Enquist IF. A study of the critical bacterial inoculum to cause a stimulus to wound healing. *Surg Gynecol Obstet* 1977;144:347–350.

90. LeVeen HH, Wapnick S, Falk G, et al. Effects of prophylactic antibiotics on colonic healing. *Am J Surg* 1976;131:47–53.

91. Giannella RP, Broitman SA, Zamcheck N. Gastric acid barrier to ingested microorganisms in man: studies in vivo and in vitro. *Gut* 1972;13:251–256.

92. Drasar BS, Hill MJ. *Human intestinal flora.* London: Academic Press, 1974.

93. Lou MA, Mandal AK, Alexander JL, Thadepalli H. Bacteriology of the human biliary tract and the duodenum. *Arch Surg* 1977;112:965–967.

94. England DM, Rosenblatt JE. Anaerobes in the human biliary tracts. *J Clin Microbiol* 1977;6:494–498.

95. Farnell MB, van Heerden JA, Beart RW Jr. Elective cholecystectomy. The role of biliary bacteriology and administration of antibiotics. *Arch Surg* 1981;116:537–540.

96. Fukunaga FH. Gallbladder bacteriology, histology and gallstones. Study of unselected cholecystectomy specimens in Honolulu. *Arch Surg* 1973;106:169–171.

97. Marne C, Pallares R, Martin R, Sitges-Serra A. Gangrenous cholecystitis and acute cholangitis associated with anaerobic bacteria in bile. *Eur J Clin Microbiol* 1986;5:35–39.

98. Goswitz JT. Bacteria and biliary tract disease. *Am J Surg* 1974; 128:644–646.

99. Claesson BE, Holmlund DEW, Matzsch TW. Microflora of the gallbladder related to duration of acute cholecystitis. *Surg Gynecol Obstet* 1986;162:531–535.

100. Shimada K, Inamatsu T, Yamashiro M. Anaerobic bacteria in biliary disease in elderly patients. *J Infect Dis* 1977;135: 850–854.

101. Floch MH, Binder HJ, Filburn B, Gershengoren W. The effect of bile acids on intestinal microflora. *Am J Clin Nutr* 1972;25: 1418–1426.

102. Thadepalli H, Chuah SK, Bansal MB, Lou MA. The effect of human bile on *Bacteroides fragilis* in human and disease. *Microbios* 1988;55:17–24.

103. Willis RG, Lawson WC, Hoare EM, Kingston RD, Sykes PA. Are bile bacteria relevant to septic complications following biliary surgery? *Br J Surg* 1984;71:845–849.

104. Gorbach SL, Plaut AG, Nahas L, et al. Studies of intestinal microflora. II. Microorganisms of the small intestine and their relations to oral and fecal flora. *Gastroenterology* 1967;53: 856–867.

105. Moore WEC, Cato EP, Holdeman LV. Anaerobic bacteria of the gastrointestinal flora and their occurrence in clinical infections. *J Infect Dis* 1969;119:641–649.

106. Thadepalli H, Lou MA, Bach VT, Matsui TK, Mandal AK. Microflora of the human small intestine. *Am J Surg* 1979;138: 845–850.

107. Cregan J, Hayward NJ. The bacterial content of the healthy human small intestine. *Br Med J* 1953;1:1356–1359.

108. Gorbach SL. Intestinal microflora. *Gastroenterology* 1971;60: 1110–1129.

109. Sykes PA, Boulter KH, Schofield PF. Alterations in small-bowel microflora in acute intestinal obstruction. *J Med Microbiol* 1976;9:13–22.

110. Bennion RS, Thompson JE, Baron EJ, Finegold SM. Gangrenous and perforated appendicitis with peritonitis: treatment and bacteriology. *Clin Ther* 1990;12(Suppl C):31–44.

111. Morris DL, Rodgers Wilson S, Pain J, et al. A comparison of aztreonam/metronidazole and cefotaxime/metronidazole in elective colorectal surgery: antimicrobial prophylaxis must include gram-positive cover. *J Antimicrob Chemother* 1990;25: 673–678.

112. Calia FM, Wolinsky E, Mortimer EA Jr, Abrams JS, Rammelkamp CH Jr. Importance of the carrier state as a source of

113. Weinstein HJ. The relation between the nasal-staphylococcal-carrier state and the incidence of postoperative complications. *N Engl J Med* 1959;260:1303–1307.

114. Stone HH. Gastric surgery. *South Med J* 1977;70:35–37.

115. Morran C, McNaught W, McArdle CS. Prophylactic cotrimoixazole in biliary surgery. *Br Med J* 1978;2:462–464.

116. Lewis RT, Allan CM, Goodall RG, et al. Cefamandole in gastroduodenal surgery: a controlled, prospective, randomized, double-blind study. *Can J Surg* 1982;25:561–563.

117. Bone RC. The pathogenesis of sepsis. *Ann Intern Med* 1991; 115:457–469.

118. Grimminger F, Sibelius U, Bhakdi S, Suttorp N, Seeger W. *Escherichia coli* hemolysin is a potent inductor of phosphoinositide hydrolysis and related metabolic responses in human neutrophils. *J Clin Invest* 1991;88:1531–1539.

119. Polk HC Jr, Miles AA. Enhancement of bacterial infection by ferric iron: kinetics, mechanisms, and surgical significance. *Surgery* 1971;70:71–77.

120. Kochan I, Kvach JT, Wiles TI. Virulence-associated acquisition of iron in mammalian serum by *Escherichia coli. J Infect Dis* 1977;135:623–632.

121. Dunn DL, Nelson RD, Condie RM, Simmons RL. Mechanisms of the adjuvant effect of hemoglobin in experimental peritonitis. VI. Effects of stroma-free hemoglobin and red blood cell stroma on mortality and neutrophil function. *Surgery* 1983;93: 653–659.

122. Maskell JP. The pathogenicity of *Bacteroides fragilis* and related species estimated by intra-abdominal-cutaneous infection in the guinea pig. *J Med Microbiol* 1981;14:131–140.

123. Onderdonk AB, Kasper DL, Cisneros RL, Bartlett JG. The capsular polysaccharide of *Bacteroides fragilis* as a virulence factor: comparison of the pathogenic potential of encapsulated and unencapsulated strains. *J Infect Dis* 1977;136:82–89.

124. Simon GL, Klempner MS, Kasper DL, Gorbach SL. Alterations in opsonophagocytic killing by neutrophils of *Bacteroides fragilis* associated with animal and laboratory passage: effect of capsular polysaccharide. *J Infect Dis* 1982;145:72–77.

125. Hofstad T. Pathogenicity of anaerobic gram-negative rods: possible mechanisms. *Rev Infect Dis* 1984;6:189–199.

126. Tally FO, Goldin BR, Jacobus NV, Gorbach SL. Superoxide dismutase in anaerobic bacteria of clinical significance. *Infect Immun* 1977;16:20–25.

127. Rotstein OD, Pruett TL, Fiegel VD, Nelson RD, Simmons RL. Succinic acid, a metabolic by-product of *Bacteroides* species, inhibits polymorphonuclear leukocyte function. *Infect Immun* 1985;48:402–408.

128. Rotstein OD, Nasmith PE, Grinstein S. The *Bacteroides* byproduct succinic acid inhibits neutrophil respiratory burst by reducing intracellular pH. *Infect Immun* 1987;55:864–870.

129. Ingham HR, Sisson PR, Tharagonnet D, Selkon JB, Codd AA. Inhibition of phagocytosis in vitro by obligate anaerobes. *Lancet* 1977;2:1252–1254.

130. Ingham HR, Sisson PR, Middleton RL, et al. Phagocytosis and killing of bacteria in aerobic and anaerobic conditions. *J Med Microbiol* 1981;14:391–399.

131. Weinstein WM, Onderdonk AB, Bartlett JG, Gorbach SL. Experimental intra-abdominal abscesses in rats: development of an experimental model. *Infect Immun* 1974;10:1250–1255.

132. Onderdonk AB, Bartlett JG, Louie T, Sullivan-Seigler N, Gorbach SL. Microbial synergy in experimental abscess. *Infect Immun* 1976;13:22–26.

133. Gibbons RJ, MacDonald JB. Hemin and vitamin K compounds as required factors for the cultivation of certain strains of *Bacteroides melaninogenicus. J Bacteriol* 1960;80:164.

134. Mayrand D, McBride BC. Ecological relationships of bacteria involved in a simple mixed anaerobic infection. *Infect Immun* 1980;27:44–50.

135. Price SB, McCallum RE. Studies on bacterial synergism in mice infected with *Bacteroides intermedius* and *Fusobacterium necrophorum. J Basic Microbiol* 1987;7:377–386.

136. Vel WA, Namavar WF, Verweij-van Vught AV, Pubben A, MacLaren DM. Killing of *Escherichia coli* by human polymor-

Staphylococcus aureus in wound sepsis. *J Hyg (London)* 1969; 67:49–57.

phonuclear leucocytes in the presence of *Bacteroides fragilis*. *J Clin Pathol* 1985;38:86–91.

137. Malangoni MA, Condon RE, Spiegel CA. Treatment of intra-abdominal infections is appropriate with single-agent or combination antibiotic therapy. *Surgery* 1985;98:648–655.

138. Yellin AE, Heseltine PN, Berne TV, et al. The role of *Pseudomonas* species in patients treated with ampicillin and sulbactam for gangrenous and perforated appendicitis. *Surg Gynecol Obstet* 1985;161:303–307.

139. Willey SH, Hindes RG, Eliopoulos GM, Moellering RC Jr. Effects of clindamycin and gentamicin and other antimicrobial combinations against enterococci in an experimental model of intra-abdominal abscess. *Surg Gynecol Obstet* 1989;169:199–202.

140. Gorbach SL, Thadepalli H. Clindamycin in pure and mixed anaerobic infections. *Arch Intern Med* 1974;134:87–92.

141. Matlow AG, Bohnen JMA, Nohr C, Christou N, Meakins J. Pathogenicity of enterococci in a rat model of fecal peritonitis. *J Infect Dis* 1989;160:142–145.

142. Garrison RN, Fry DE, Berberich S, Polk HC Jr. Enterococcal bacteremia: clinical implications and determinants of death. *Ann Surg* 1983;196:43–47.

143. Dajani AS, Bisno AL, Chung KJ, et al. Prevention of bacterial endocarditis. Recommendations by the American Heart Association. *JAMA* 1990;264:2919–2922.

144. Sirot D, Sirot J, Labia R, et al. Transferable resistance to third-generation cephalosporins in clinical isolates of *Klebsiella pneumoniae*: identification of CTX-1, a novel β-lactamase. *J Antimicrob Chemother* 1987;20:323–334.

145. Tenover FC. Novel and emerging mechanisms of antimicrobial resistance in nosocomial pathogens. *Am J Med* 1991;91(Suppl 3B):76S–81S.

146. Rice LB, Yao JDC, Klimm K, Eliopoulos GM, Moellering RC Jr. Efficacy of different β-lactams against an extended-spectrum β-lactamase-producing *Klebsiella pneumoniae* strain in the rat intra-abdominal abscess model. *Antimicrob Agents Chemother* 1991;35:1243–1244.

147. Fantin B, Pangon B, Potel G, et al. Activity of sulbactam in combination with ceftriaxone in vitro and in experimental endocarditis caused by an *Escherichia coli* producing SHV-like β-lactamase. *Antimicrob Agents Chemother* 1990;34:581–586.

148. Pitt HA, Postier RG, Gadacz TR, Cameron JL. The role of topical antibiotics in "high-risk" biliary surgery. *Surgery* 1982;91:518–524.

149. Dixon JM, Arnstrong CP, Duffy SW, Chetty U, Davies GC. A randomized prospective trial comparing the value of intravenous and preincisional cefamandole in reducing postoperative sepsis after operations upon the gastrointestinal tract. *Surg Gynecol Obstet* 1984;158:303–307.

150. Freischlag J, McGrattan M, Busuttil RW. Topical versus systemic cephalosporin administration in elective biliary operations. *Surgery* 1984;96:686–693.

151. Garlock JH, Seley GP. The use of sulfanilamide in surgery of the colon and rectum. Preliminary report. *Surgery* 1939;5:787–790.

152. Seley GP, Colp R. The bacteriology of peptic ulcers and gastric malignancies: possible bearing on complications following gastric surgery. *Surgery* 1941;10:369–380.

153. Soballe PW, Greif JM. Preoperative whole-gut lavage vs. traditional three-day bowel preparation in left colon surgery. *Mil Med* 1989;154:198–201.

154. Fleites RA, Marshall JB, Eckhauser ML, et al. The efficacy of polyethylene glycol-electrolyte lavage solution versus traditional mechanical bowel preparation for elective colonic surgery: a randomized, prospective, blinded clinical trial. *Surgery* 1985;98:708–717.

155. Redington J, Ebert SC, Craig WA. Role of antimicrobial pharmacokinetics and pharmacodynamics in surgical prophylaxis. *Rev Infect Dis* 1991;13(Suppl 10):S790–S799.

156. Kaiser AB, Herrington JL Jr, Jacobs JK, et al. Cefoxitin versus erythromycin, neomycin, and cefazolin in colorectal operations: importance of the duration of the surgical procedure. *Ann Surg* 1983;198:525–530.

157. Ehrenkranz NJ. Antimicrobial prophylaxis in surgery: mecha-

158. Brogard JM, Dorner M, Pinget M, Adloff M, Lavillaureix J. The biliary excretion of cefazolin. *J Infect Dis* 1975;131:625–633.

159. Ram MD, Watanatittan S. Levels of cefazolin in human bile. *J Infect Dis* 1973;128(Suppl):S361–S363.

160. Mendelson J, Portnoy J, Sigman H. Pharmacology of gentamicin in the biliary tract of humans. *Antimicrob Agents Chemother* 1973;4:538–541.

161. Pitt HA, Roberts RB, Johnson WD Jr. Gentamicin levels in the human biliary tract. *J Infect Dis* 1979;127:299–302.

162. Pulaski EJ, Fusillo MH. Gallbladder bile concentration of the major antibiotics following intravenous administration. *Surg Gynecol Obstet* 1955;100:571.

163. Hansbrough JF, Clark JE. Concentrations of cefoxitin in gallbladder bile of cholecystectomy patients. *Antimicrob Agents Chemother* 1982;22:709–710.

164. Kucers A, Bennett NMcK. *The use of antibiotics: a comprehensive review with clinical emphasis*, 4th ed. Philadelphia: Lippincott, 1987.

165. McLeish AR, Strachan CJL, Powis SJA, Wise R, Bevan PG. The influence of biliary disease on the excretion of cefazolin in human bile. *Surgery* 1977;81:426–430.

166. Brown RB, Martyak SN, Barza M, Curtis L, Weinstein L. Penetration of clindamycin phosphate into the abnormal human biliary tract. *Ann Intern Med* 1976;84:168–170.

167. Mortimer PR, Mackie DB, Haynes S. Ampicillin levels in human bile in the presence of biliary tract disease. *Br Med J* 1969;3:88–89.

168. Kanter MA, Geelhoed GW. Biliary antibiotics; clinical utility in biliary surgery. *South Med J* 1987;80:1007–1015.

169. Keighley MRB, Baddeley RM, Burden DW, et al. A controlled trial of parenteral prophylactic gentamicin therapy in biliary surgery. *Br J Surg* 1975;62:275–279.

170. Kaufman Z, Engelberg M, Eliashiv A, et al. Systemic prophylactic antibiotics in elective biliary surgery. *Arch Surg* 1984;119:1002–1004.

171. Davey PG. Pharmacokinetics in liver disease. *J Antimicrob Chemother* 1988;21:1–5.

172. Burns GP, Stein TA, Cohen M. Biliary and pancreatic excretion of cefamandole. *Antimicrob Agents Chemother* 1989;33:977–979.

173. Burns GP, Stein TA, Kabnick LS. Blood–pancreatic juice barrier to antibiotic excretion. *Am J Surg* 1986;151:205–208.

174. Trudel JL, Mutch DO, Brown PR, Richard GK, Brown RA. Antibiotic therapy for pancreatic sepsis: differences in bioactive blood and tissue levels. *Surg Forum* 1982;33:26.

175. Block BS, Mercer LJ, Ismail MA, et al. *Clostridium difficile*-associated diarrhea follows perioperative prophylaxis with cefoxitin. *Am J Obstet Gynecol* 1986;153:835–838.

176. Roberts NJ Jr, Douglas RG Jr. Gentamicin use and *Pseudomonas* and *Serratia* resistance: effect of a surgical prophylaxis regimen. *Antimicrob Agents Chemother* 1978;13:214–220.

177. Archer GL, Armstrong BC. Alteration of staphylococcal flora in cardiac surgery patients receiving antibiotic prophylaxis. *J Infect Dis* 1983;147:642–649.

178. Kernodle DS, Barg NL, Kaiser AB. Low-level colonization of hospitalized patients with methicillin-resistant coagulase-negative staphylococci and emergence of the organisms during surgical antibiotic prophylaxis. *Antimicrob Agents Chemother* 1988;32:202–208.

179. Bartlett JG, Louie TJ, Gorbach SL, Onderdonk AB. Therapeutic efficacy of 29 antimicrobial regimens in experimental intra-abdominal sepsis. *Rev Infect Dis* 1981;3:535–542.

180. Moesgaard F, Lykkegaard Nielsen MC, Justesen T. Wound infection rates after intraincisional plus systemic antibiotic prophylaxis in an animal model. *Eur J Clin Microbiol* 1984;3:538–541.

181. Nichols RL, Webb WR, Jones JW, Smith JW, LoCicero J. Efficacy of antibiotic prophylaxis in high risk gastroduodenal operations. *Am J Surg* 1982;143:94–98.

182. Pories WL, van Rij AM, Burlingham BT, Fulghum RS, Meel-

heim D. Prophylactic cefazolin in gastric bypass surgery. *Surgery* 1981;90:426–432.

183. Lewis RT, Allan CM, Goodall RG, et al. Discriminate use of antibiotic prophylaxis in gastroduodenal surgery. *Am J Surg* 1979;138:640–643.

184. Leaper DJ, Cooper MJ, Turner A. A comparative trial between cefotetan and cephazolin for wound sepsis prophylaxis during penetration into the obstructed biliary tree. *J Hosp Infect* 1986; 7:269–276.

185. Morris DL, Young D, Burdon DW, Keighley MRB. Prospective randomized trial of single dose cefuroxime against mezlocillin in elective gastric surgery. *J Hosp Infect* 1984;5:200–204.

186. Mason GR. Bacteriology and antibiotic selection in biliary tract surgery. *Arch Surg* 1968;97:533–537.

187. Pyrtek LJ, Bartus SA. An evaluation of antibiotics in biliary tract surgery. *Surg Gynecol Obstet* 1967;125:101–105.

188. Nielsen ML, Moesgaard F, Justesen T, Scheibel JH, Lindenberg S. Wound sepsis after elective cholecystectomy: restriction of prophylactic antibiotics to risk groups. *Scand J Gastroenterol* 1981;16:937–940.

189. Elliott DW. Biliary tract surgery. *South Med J* 1977;70:31–35.

190. Thompson JE Jr, Bennion RS, Doty JE, Muller EL, Pitt HA. Predictive factors for bactibilia in acute cholecystitis. *Arch Surg* 1990;125:261–264.

191. Lewis RT, Goodall RG, Marien B, Park M, Lloyd-Smith W, Wiegand FM. Biliary bacteria, antibiotic use, and wound infection in surgery of the gallbladder and common bile duct. *Arch Surg* 1987;122:44–47.

192. Meijer WS, Schmitz PIM, Jeekel J. Meta-analysis of randomized, controlled clinical trials of antibiotic prophylaxis in biliary tract surgery. *Br J Surg* 1990;77:283–290.

193. Lewis RT, Allan CM, Goodall RG, et al. A single preoperative dose of cefazolin prevents postoperative sepsis in high-risk biliary surgery. *Can J Surg* 1984;27:44–47.

194. Chetlin SH, Elliot DW. Preoperative antibiotics in biliary surgery. *Arch Surg* 1973;107:319–323.

195. Drumm J, Donovan IA, Wise R. A comparison of cefotetan and cephazolin for prophylaxis against wound infection after elective cholecystectomy. *J Hosp Infect* 1985;6:277–280.

196. Muller EL, Pitt HA, Thompson JE Jr, Doty JE, Mann LL, Manchester B. Antibiotics in infections of the biliary tract. *Surg Gynecol Obstet* 1987;165:285–292.

197. Baker RJ, Donahue PE, Finegold SM, et al. A prospective double-blind comparison of piperacillin, cephalothin and cefoxitin in the prevention of postoperative infections in patients undergoing intra-abdominal operations. *Surg Gynecol Obstet* 1985;161:409–415.

198. Dougherty SH, Saltzstein EC, Peacock JB, Mercer LC. Cefamandole versus cefoxitin prophylaxis in patients undergoing cholecystectomy. *Am Surg* 1988;54:495–499.

199. Kellum JM, Duma RJ, Gorbach SL, et al. Single-dose antibiotic prophylaxis for biliary surgery: cefazolin vs moxalactam. *Arch Surg* 1987;122:918–922.

200. Strachan CJL, Black J, Powis SJA, et al. Prophylactic use of cefazolin against wound infection after cholecystectomy. *Br Med J* 1976;1:1254–1256.

201. Keighley MRB, Lister DM, Jacobs SI, et al. Hazards of surgical treatment due to microorganisms in the bile. *Surgery* 1974;75: 578–583.

202. Pitt HA, Postier RG, Cameron JL. Postoperative T-tube cholangiography: is antibiotic coverage necessary? *Ann Surg* 1980; 191:30–34.

203. Deziel DJ, Millikan KW, Economou SG, et al. Complications of laparoscopic cholecystectomy: a national survey of 4,292 hospitals and an analysis of 77, 604 cases. *Am J Surg* 1993;165: 9–14.

204. Gorbach SL. Antimicrobial prophylaxis for appendectomy and colorectal surgery. *Rev Infect Dis* 1991;13(Suppl 10):S815–S820.

205. Krukowski ZH. Preventing wound infection after appendicectomy: a review. *Br J Surg* 1988;75:1023–1033.

206. Lewis FR, Holcroft JW, Boey J, Dunphy JE. Appendicitis—a critical review of diagnosis and treatment in 1000 cases. *Arch Surg* 1975;110:677.

207. Fine M, Busuttil RW. Acute appendicitis: efficacy of prophylactic pre-operative antibiotics in the reduction of septic morbidity. *Am J Surg* 1978;135:210–212.

208. Coleman RJ, Blackwood JM, Swan KG. Role of antibiotic prophylaxis in surgery for nonperforated appendicitis. *Am Surg* 1987;53:584–586.

209. Giacomantonio M, Bortolussi R, Gillis DA. Should prophylactic antibiotics be given perioperatively in acute appendicitis without perforation? *Can J Surg* 1982;25:555–556.

210. Foster PD, O'Toole RD. Primary appendectomy—the effect of prophylactic cephaloridine on post-operative wound infections. *JAMA* 1978;239:1411–1412.

211. Bauer T, Vennitis B, Holm B, et al. Antibiotic prophylaxis in acute nonperforated appendicitis. The Danish multicenter study group III. *Ann Surg* 1989;209:307–311.

212. Busuttil RW, Davidson RK, Fine M, Tompkins RK. Effect of prophylactic antibiotics in acute non-perforated appendicitis—a prospective, randomized, double-blind clinical study. *Ann Surg* 1981;194:502–509.

213. el-Sefi TA, el-Awadi HM, Shehata MI, Al-Hindi MD. The place of antibiotics in the prevention of post-appendicectomy sepsis: a prospective study of 400 cases. *Int J Surg* 1986;71:18–21.

214. Winslow RE, Dean RE, Harley JW. Acute nonperforating appendicitis. *Arch Surg* 1983;118:651–655.

215. Browder W, Smith JW, Vivoda LM, Nichols RL. Nonperforative appendicitis: a continuing surgical dilemma. *J Infect Dis* 1989;159:1088–1094.

216. Berne TV, Yellin AE, Appleman MD, Heseltine PNR. Antibiotic management of surgically treated gangrenous or perforated appendicitis. Comparison of gentamicin and clindamycin versus cefamandole versus cefoperazone. *Am J Surg* 1982;144: 8–13.

217. Berne TV, Appleman MD, Chenella FC, et al. Surgically treated gangrenous or perforated appendicitis. A comparison of aztreonam and clindamycin versus gentamicin and clindamycin. *Ann Surg* 1987;205:133–137.

218. Heseltine PNR, Yellin AE, Appleman MD, et al. Imipenem therapy for perforated and gangrenous appendicitis. *Surg Gynecol Obstet* 1986;162:43–48.

219. Saario I, Arvilommi H, Silvola H. Comparison of cefuroxime and gentamicin in combination with metronidazole in the treatment of peritonitis due to perforation of the appendix. *Acta Chir Scand* 1983;149:423–426.

220. Flannigan GM, Clifford RP, Carver RA, Yule AG, Madden NP. Antibiotic prophylaxis in acute appendicitis. *Surg Gynecol Obstet* 1983;156:209–211.

221. Morris WT, Innes DB, Richardson RA, et al. Prevention of post-appendicectomy sepsis by metronidazole and cefazolin: a controlled double blind trial. *Aust N Z J Surg* 1980;50:429–433.

222. Lau WY, Fan ST, Yui TF, et al. Prophylaxis of postappendicectomy sepsis by metronidazole and cefotaxime: a randomized, prospective and double blind trial. *Br J Surg* 1983;70: 670–672.

223. Foster MC, Kapila L, Morris DL, Slack RCB. A randomized comparative study of sulbactam plus ampicillin vs. metronidazole plus cefotaxime in the management of acute appendicitis in children. *Rev Infect Dis* 1986;8(Suppl 5):S634–S638.

224. O'Rourke MGE, Wynne JM, Morahan RJ, Green AJ, Walker RM, Wilson ME. Prophylactic antibiotics in appendicectomy: a prospective double blind randomized study. *Aust N Z J Surg* 1984;54:535–541.

225. Clarke JS, Condon RE, Bartlett JG, et al. Preoperative oral antibiotics reduce septic complications of colon operations: results of a prospective randomized, double-blind clinical study. *Ann Surg* 1977;186:251–259.

226. The Norwegian Study Group for Colorectal Surgery. Should antimicrobial prophylaxis in colorectal surgery include agents effective against both anaerobic and aerobic microorganisms? A double-blind, multi-center study. *Surgery* 1985;97:402–407.

227. Nichols RL, Broido P, Condon RE, Gorbach SL, Nyhus LM. Effect of preoperative neomycin–erythromycin intestinal preparation on the incidence of infection complications following colon surgery. *Ann Surg* 1973;178:453–462.

228. Bartlett JG, Condon RE, Gorbach SL, Clarke JS, Nichols RL,

Ochi S. Veterans Administration Cooperative Study on bowel preparation for elective colorectal operations: impact of oral antibiotic regimen on colonic flora, wound irrigation cultures and bacteriology of septic complications. *Ann Surg* 1978;188: 249–254.

229. Condon RE, Bartlett JG, Greenlee H, et al. Efficacy of oral and systemic antibiotic prophylaxis in colorectal operations. *Arch Surg* 1983;118:496–502.

230. Wapnick S, Guinto R, Reizis I, LeVeen HH. Reduction of postoperative infection in elective colon surgery with preoperative administration of kanamycin and erythromycin. *Surgery* 1979; 85:317–321.

231. Vergnes D, Moatti N. Pre-operative colonic preparation using kanamycin and metronidazole: qualitative and quantitative effects on the bacterial flora of the intestine. *J Antimicrob Chemother* 1980;6:709–716.

232. Washington JA II, Dearing WH, Jedd ES, Elveback LA. Effect of preoperative antibiotic regimen on development of infection after intestinal surgery. Prospective, randomized, double-blind study. *Ann Surg* 1974;4:567–572.

233. McDonald PJ, Karran SJ. A comparison of intravenous cefoxitin and a combination of gentamicin and metronidazole as prophylaxis in colorectal surgery. *Dis Colon Rectum* 1983;26: 661–664.

234. Hoffman CEJ, McDonald PJ, Watts JM. Use of preoperative cefoxitin to prevent infection after colonic and rectal surgery. *Ann Surg* 1981;193:353–356.

235. Periti P, Mazzei T, Tonelli F. Single-dose cefotetan vs. multiple-dose cefoxitin—antimicrobial prophylaxis in colorectal surgery. Results of a prospective, multicenter, randomized study. *Dis Colon Rectum* 1989;32:121–127.

236. Jagelman DG, Fabian TC, Nichols RL, Stone HH, Wilson SE, Zellner SR. Single dose cefotetan versus multiple-dose cefoxitin as prophylaxis in colorectal surgery. *Am J Surg* 1988;155: 71–76.

237. Griffith DL, Novak E, Greenwald CA, Metzler CM, Paxton LM. Clinical experience with cefmetazole sodium in the United States: an overview. *J Antimicrob Chemother* 1989;23(Suppl D):21–33.

238. Oostvogel HJM, van Vroonhoven TJMV, van der Werken C, Lenderink AW. Single-dose v. short-term antibiotic therapy for prevention of wound infection in general surgery. *Acta Chir Scand* 1987;153:571–575.

239. Juul P, Klaaborg KE, Kronberg O. Single or multiple doses of metronidazole and ampicillin in elective colorectal surgery. A randomized trial. *Dis Colon Rectum* 1987;30:526–528.

240. Higgins C, Allan RN, Keighley MRB, et al. Sepsis following surgery for inflammatory bowel disease. *Dis Colon Rectum* 1980;23:102–105.

241. Hares MM, Bentley S, Allan RN, Burdon DW, Keighley MRB. Clinical trials of the efficacy and duration of antibacterial cover for elective resection in inflammatory bowel disease. *Br J Surg* 1982;69:215–217.

242. Condon RE. Rational use of prophylactic antibiotics in gastrointestinal surgery. *Surg Clin North Am* 1975;55:1309–1318.

243. Jain NK, Larson DE, Schroeder KW, et al. Antibiotic prophylaxis for percutaneous endoscopic gastrostomy: a prospective, randomized, double-blind clinical study. *Ann Intern Med* 1987; 107:824–828.

244. Hollands MJ, Fletcher JP, Young J. Percutaneous feeding gastrostomy. *Med J Aust* 1989;151:328–331.

245. Colonna JO II, Winston DH, Brill JE, et al. Infectious complications in liver transplantation. *Arch Surg* 1988;123:360–364.

246. Kusne SJ, Dummer JS, Singh N, et al. Infections after liver transplantation: an analysis of 101 consecutive cases. *Medicine* (*Baltimore*) 1988;67:132–143.

247. Arnow PM, Furmaga K, Flaherty JP, George D. Microbiological efficacy and pharmacokinetics of prophylactic antibiotics in liver transplant patients. *Antimicrob Agents Chemother* 1992;36:2125–2130.

248. van Zeijl JH, Kroes ACM, Metselaar HJ, et al. Infections after auxiliary partial liver transplantation. Experiences in the first ten patients. *Infection* 1990;18:146–151.

249. Wiesner RH, Hermans PE, Rakela J, et al. Selective bowel decontamination to decrease gram-negative aerobic bacterial and *Candida* colonization and prevent infection after orthotopic liver transplantation. *Transplantation* 1988;45: 570–574.

250. Cafiero F, Gipponi M, Bonalumi U, et al. Prophylaxis of infection with intravenous immunoglobulins plus antibiotic for patients at risk for sepsis undergoing surgery for colorectal cancer: results of a randomized, multicenter clinical trial. *Surgery* 1992;112:24–31.

251. The Intravenous Immunoglobulin Collaborative Study Group. Prophylactic intravenous administration of standard immune globulin as compared with core-lipopolysaccharide immune globulin in patients at high-risk of postsurgical infection. *N Engl J Med* 1992;327:234–240.

252. Baumgartner J-D, Glauser MP, MuCutchan JA, et al. Prevention of gram-negative bacteremia shock and death in surgical patients by antibody to endotoxin core glycolipid. *Lancet* 1985; 2:59–63.

253. Mainous MR, Tso P, Berg RD, Deitch EA. Studies of the route, magnitude, and time course of bacterial translocation in a model of systemic inflammation. *Arch Surg* 1992;126:33–37.

254. Deitch EA, Bridges WM, Ma WJ, et al. Obstructed intestine as a reservoir for systemic infection. *Am J Surg* 1990;159: 394–401.

255. Deitch EA, Berg R. Bacterial translocation from the gut: a mechanism of infection. *J Burn Care Rehabil* 1987;8:475–482.

256. Farrar EW, Kent TH. Enteritis and coliform bacteremia in guinea pigs given penicillin. *Am J Pathol* 1965;47:629–642.

257. Kaiser AB, Kernodle DS, Parker RA. A low inoculum model of surgical wound infection. *J Infect Dis* 1992;166:393–399.

258. Wells CL, Maddaus MA, Jechorek RP, Simmons RL. Ability of intestinal *Escherichia coli* to survive within mesenteric lymph nodes. *Infect Immun* 1987;55:2834–2837.

259. Berg RD, Wommack E, Deitch EA. Immunosuppression and intestinal bacterial overgrowth synergistically promote bacterial translocation. *Arch Surg* 1988;123:1359–1364.

260. Salman FT, Buyruk MN, Gürler N, Çelik A. The effect of surgical trauma on the bacterial translocation from the gut. *J Pediatr Surg* 1992;27:802–804.

261. Tetteroo GWM, Wagenvoort JHT, Bruining HA. Role of selective decontamination in surgery. *Br J Surg* 1992;79:300–304.

262. McGowan JE Jr. Cost and benefit of perioperative antimicrobial prophylaxis: methods for economic analysis. *Rev Infect Dis* 1991;13(Suppl 10):S879–S889.

263. Roach AL, Kernodle DS, Kaiser AB. Selecting cost-effective antimicrobial prophylaxis in surgery: are we getting what we pay for? *Ann Pharmacother* 1990;24:183–185.

264. Shapiro M, Townsend TR, Rosner B, Kass EH. Use of antimicrobial drugs in general hospitals: patterns of prophylaxis. *N Engl J Med* 1979;301:351–355.

265. Kaiser AB. Overview of cephalosporin prophylaxis. *Am J Surg* 1988;155(Suppl 5A):52–55.

266. Green JW, Wenzel RP. Postoperative wound infection: a controlled study of the increased duration of hospital stay and direct cost of hospitalization. *Ann Surg* 1977;185:264–268.

267. Fabry J, Meynet R, Joron MT, et al. Cost of nosocomial infections: analysis of 512 digestive surgery patients. *World J Surg* 1982;6:362–365.

268. Horan TC, White JW, Jarvis WR, et al. Nosocomial infection surveillance, 1984. *MMWR Morb Mortal Wkly Rep* 1986; 35(1SS):17SS–34SS.

269. Olson M, O'Connor M, Schwartz ML. Surgical wound infections: a 5-year prospective study of 20,193 wounds at the Minneapolis VA Medical Center. *Ann Surg* 1984;199:253–259.

270. Liss RH, Batchelor FR. Economic evaluations of antibiotic use and resistance—a perspective: report of Task Force 6. *Rev Infect Dis* 1987;9(Suppl 3):S297–S312.

Infections of the Gastrointestinal Tract,
edited by M. J. Blaser, P. D. Smith, J. I. Ravdin,
H. B. Greenberg, and R. L. Guerrant
Raven Press, Ltd., New York © 1995.

CHAPTER 87

Pharmacology of Antimicrobial Agents Used in the Therapy of Gastrointestinal Infections

Jason D. Morrow and Kathleen M. Neuzil

Because an enormous number of pathogens are capable of infecting the gastrointestinal tract, many antimicrobial agents are available to treat these infections. For purposes of organization, this chapter is divided into sections dealing with antimicrobial drugs primarily used in the therapy of either bacterial, viral, mycobacterial, fungal, or parasitic infections. It should be recognized, however, that this division may be arbitrary since drugs like metronidazole, trimethoprim/sulfamethoxazole, or furazolidine may be useful against more than one class of organisms.

Despite the marked differences in the types of pathogens causing gastrointestinal infections, certain general statements can be made. First, the organism to be treated should be sensitive to the particular agent employed. Unfortunately, resistance represents an increasing impediment to the therapy of gastrointestinal pathogens. This is not only true for gram-negative bacilli such as *Salmonella* and *Shigella* but resistance is a significant problem in mycobacteria and has been documented in fungi, viruses, and, to some degree, parasites. Second, the antimicrobial agent that is administered must be able to reach the site of infection in concentrations adequate to kill or inhibit the growth of the organism. Thus intravenous therapy with an agent may be favored over oral therapy to ensure higher drug levels at the site of the infection. On the other hand, as is the case with vancomycin therapy of pseudomembranous colitis, for example, oral administration is favored over parenteral because of the much higher levels of the drug found in the intestinal lumen after oral therapy. Third, for many infections, more than one agent may be effective against a particular pathogen. Thus the use of one antimicrobial over another may be guided by issues such as relative cost, dosing frequency, adverse effect profile, or interpatient variables such as hypersensitivity to a particular agent.

Although antimicrobial therapy is often indicated for infections involving the gastrointestinal tract, antimicrobial agents themselves can predispose to infection. This is believed to occur as a result of alterations in normal gut flora by antimicrobials resulting in overgrowth of pathogenic organisms. An example of this is antibiotic-associated colitis due to *Clostridium difficile*.

It is the goal of this chapter to summarize the salient features of the antimicrobial agents used in the treatment of gastrointestinal infections; the emphasis is on pharmacokinetic and pharmacodynamic aspects of these agents as they relate to the gastrointestinal tract. In addition, adverse reactions and drug interactions are dealt with in detail. Throughout the chapter mention may be made of whether particular agents are considered by the authors to be drugs of first choice, alternative choice, or are of use in particular infections.

ANTIBACTERIAL AGENTS

Bacterial infections of the gastrointestinal tract range from pyogenic processes such as cholangitis and intra-abdominal abscess to enteric infections that include acute enterocolitis, enteric fever, and bacteremia. The number of individual pathogens capable of causing infection in the gastrointestinal tract is similarly large. For example, pyogenic infections are often associated with a mixture of many bacteria including gram-negative aerobic bacilli, gram-positive aerobic bacteria, and anaerobic organisms. Furthermore, a relatively large number of organisms including *Shigella, Salmonella,* and *Campylobacter* may cause enteric infections. Many agents exist to treat these infections and those more commonly used are discussed in this section.

J. D. Morrow and K. M. Neuzil: Divisions of Clinical Pharmacology and Infectious Diseases, Departments of Medicine and Pharmacology, Vanderbilt University School of Medicine, Nashville, Tennessee 37232-6602.

The Penicillins

Penicillins useful in the therapy of gastrointestinal infection include the natural penicillins (penicillin G and penicillin V), the aminopenicillins (ampicillin and amoxicillin), and the extended spectrum penicillins (ticarcillin, mezlocillin, and piperacillin).

Mechanism of Action. The penicillins are bactericidal. The exact mechanisms by which penicillins act are unknown but they reversibly bind and inhibit bacterial membrane enzymes such as carboxypeptidases, endopeptidases, and transpeptidases, which are termed penicillin binding proteins (PBPs) and are involved in bacterial cell wall synthesis and cell division (1–3). The most important mechanism of bacterial resistance to penicillins is by the production of β-lactamase. Another mechanism of penicillin resistance frequently occurring in gram-negative aerobic bacteria can involve inhibition of entry of the drug into the cell. Decreased affinity for PBPs or the development of tolerance that appears related to decreased autolytic activity in particular bacteria are other resistance mechanisms (4,5).

Adverse Effects. Although reasonably safe agents, adverse reactions to the penicillins are not infrequent and may be life-threatening (Table 1). Hypersensitivity reactions are relatively common, the most acutely life-threatening being anaphylaxis. Anaphylaxis occurs in 0.004% to 0.015% of penicillin treatment courses (6,7) and manifests clinically as laryngeal edema, bronchospasm, urticaria, gastrointestinal disturbances, and shock. The risk of a reaction of this type is best assessed with skin testing. Persons sensitive to penicillins also may have cross-reactions to other β-lactams, including cephalosporins and imipenem, but do not cross-react to aztreonam (8). One of the most common adverse reactions to penicillins is poorly characterized skin rashes, usually maculopapular, which probably have no immunological basis and are thus best termed "idiopathic." They most commonly occur with aminopenicillin administration, particularly in association with viral infections (9).

Both oral and parenteral administration of the penicillins may induce gastrointestinal disorders, although these side effects are more frequently observed with oral dosing (Table 1). They appear dose related and occur most frequently with oral administration of ampicillin. In adults, diarrhea occurs in between 5% and 20% of ampicillin-treated patients and is more common in the elderly, although it is usually not severe (10,11). Its cause is unclear but may be the result of direct local irritation by the penicillins or alterations in intestinal microflora. Antibiotic-associated pseudomembranous colitis occurs in 0.3% to 0.5% of persons treated with ampicillin, but it may occur with other penicillins (10). In addition, acute enterocolitis with abdominal pain and bloody diarrhea has been reported in several patients receiving oral penicillins (12). Other gastrointestinal side effects of the penicillins may include nausea, gastrointestinal moniliasis, anorexia, epigastric pain, and glossitis. Rarely, hepatic dysfunction occurs. Penicillins are associated with a number of other adverse effects (Table 1) (13–17).

Precautions. The penicillins should be used with caution in individuals with a prior history of an allergic type reaction or skin rash to β-lactam antibiotics. In these cases, skin testing is indicated prior to their administration. Safety of the penicillins has not been established conclusively in pregnancy although these agents are frequently used to treat infections in pregnant women because there is little evidence of adverse effects on the fetus (18). Nonetheless, these agents should be used in pregnancy only when clearly needed. Furthermore, the penicillins are distributed into breast milk and should be used with caution in nursing women. As a general rule, since the penicillins are cleared primarily by the kidney, dosage adjustment is indicated in renal failure.

Drug Interactions. The interactions of the penicillins with other agents may be either beneficial or, in most cases, adverse. The penicillins act synergistically with the aminoglycosides *in vitro* and *in vivo* against organisms including the enterococci, viridans streptococci, and many aerobic gram-negative rods (19). On the other hand, the action of the penicillins may be antagonized by bacteriostatic antibiotics including chloramphenicol and the tetracyclines, although clinical data supporting this are fairly scant (20). Probenecid administered shortly before penicillin increases serum levels and prolongs the serum half-life of penicillin by inhibiting renal tubular secretion and this may be of therapeutic benefit. Nonsteroidal anti-inflammatory agents also may increase the serum half-life of penicillin G. Of particular importance to women of childbearing age is that oral contraceptive efficacy may be decreased with ampicillin coadministration although some studies have contradicted this (21). Finally, the risk of rash with ampicillin administration appears increased with coadministration of allopurinol (22).

Penicillins Useful in the Treatment of Gastrointestinal Infections

The Natural Penicillins

Therapeutic Uses. Two members of this class, penicillin G (benzylpenicillin) and penicillin V (phenoxymethylpenicillin), are of use in gastrointestinal infection. Because of their limited spectrum, however, the natural penicillins are recommended for only a few gastrointestinal infections. These include abdominal actinomycosis, Whipple's disease, and illnesses in which particular clostridia, but not *C. difficile,* may play a role (23–25).

In Vitro Antimicrobial Activity. The natural penicillins are highly active *in vitro* against many β-hemolytic streptococci except group D streptococci. Against viridans streptococci, sensitivities vary. Anaerobic streptococci are usually highly susceptible as are most strains of anaerobic gram-positive sporing bacilli. Species of *Actinomyces* and *Arachnia* are also highly sensitive. Anaerobic gram-negative bacilli, in particular *Bacteroides,* vary in their sensitivity. Members of the *B. fragilis* group are often resistant. As a general rule, gram-negative aerobic bacteria are resistant.

TABLE 1. *Relative frequency of adverse reactions to the β-lactams used in gastrointestinal infection*

Reactions	Penicillins	Cephalosporins	Imipenem	Aztreonam
Hypersensitivity	+ + +	+ +	+ +	+
Skin rash (idiopathic)	+ + +	+ +	+	+
Gastrointestinal (GI)				
GI upset	+ + +	+ +	+ +	+
Diarrhea	+ + +	+ +	+	+
Antibiotic-associated colitis	+ + +	+ +	+	+
Hepatic dysfunction	+	+ +	+ +	+
Hematologic				
Blood dyscrasias	+ +	+ + +	+	+
Coagulation abnormalities	+	+ +	+	+
Renal dysfunction	+	+ +	+	+
Electrolyte abnormalities	+	+	+	Not reported
Central nervous system dysfunction	+	+	+ +	+
Cross-reaction to other β-lactams	+ + +	+ + +	+ + +	Not reported

+, Infrequent; + + +, frequent.

Clinical Pharmacology. Table 2 summarizes certain aspects of the clinical pharmacology of the penicillins used in gastrointestinal infection. Although most absorption of the oral penicillins occurs in the duodenum and upper jejunum, some may occur in the stomach and colon. Absorption of penicillin V tends to be increased in persons with achlorhydria and the elderly, probably due to decreased gastric inactivation. It is unclear whether food intake significantly affects the absorption of penicillin V but it is generally recommended that it not be administered at meal time. Absorption of penicillin V may be decreased in malabsorptive and prolonged diarrheal states (26,27).

The natural penicillins are widely distributed to tissues with the highest concentrations in the kidney and somewhat lower concentrations in the liver and gastrointestinal tract. The drugs readily distribute into peritoneal fluid and are found in therapeutic concentrations in bile (28); distribution into abscesses is poor. They readily enter hemato-mas and cross the placenta (29). The primary route of excretion of the natural penicillins is urine although penicillin G is also actively secreted in bile with up to 4.5% of the administered dose removed by this mechanism. Biliary excretion, in addition to urinary excretion, may be decreased by probenicid although the clinical significance of this is unknown. Little orally administered penicillin is excreted as active drug in the feces; that which is not absorbed is inactivated by colonic bacteria.

The Aminopenicillins

Therapeutic Uses. The two most important agents are ampicillin and amoxicillin and their indications include *Shigella* infections, typhoid and paratyphoid fevers, and certain other syndromes due to *S. typhi* and non-*typhi* *Salmonella*. However, the usefulness of the aminopenicillins is limited by the high rates of resistance among these

TABLE 2. *Selected pharmacokinetic data for the penicillins used in gastrointestinal infection*

Drug	Usual route of administration	Oral absorption (%)	Metabolized (%)	Urine recovery (%)	Biliary excretion[a]	Half-life (hr)
Natural penicillins						
Penicillin G	Intravenous	—	20	60–90	+	0.5
Penicillin V	Oral	60	55	29–37	+	0.5–1
Aminopenicillins						
Ampicillin	Intravenous	—	10	90	+	1
	Oral	40		40–45		
Amoxicillin	Oral	75–90	10	50–70	+	1
Extended generation penicillins						
Ticarcillin	Intravenous	—	10–15	75–85	+	1.2
Piperacillin	Intravenous	—	—	60–80	+ + + (up to 25%)	0.6–1.3
Mezlocillin	Intravenous	—	<10	45–70	+ + + (up to 25%)	0.8–1.2

With permission from ref. 5; and Division of Drugs and Toxicology, *Drug evaluations,* Summer 1992 Supplement. Chicago: American Medical Association, 1992.

[a] +, Biliary excretion is a minor route of elimination; + + +, significant biliary excretion.

enteric pathogens because of plasmid mediated β-lactamase production. The aminopenicillins are also effective in *Helicobacter pylori* infection in combination with other agents (30,31). In addition, they are frequently used in combination with other antibacterials for biliary tract infections and other intra-abdominal pyogenic processes. In combination with the aminoglycosides, the aminopenicillins are also useful for prophylaxis when gastrointestinal procedures are performed in patients at risk for endocarditis (32).

In Vitro Antimicrobial Activity. The spectrum of activity of the aminopenicillins includes essentially all organisms sensitive to penicillin G, as well as certain aerobic gram-negative bacteria including *Escherichia coli, Proteus mirabilis, Salmonella* species, *Shigella* species, and *H. pylori.* Of note, however, a significant percentage of non-*typhi Salmonella* and *Shigella* are resistant to the aminopenicillins. Ampicillin is more effective clinically against *Shigella* than is amoxicillin, which may be related to differences in the intrinsic antibiotic activity of the agents against *Shigella* rather than differences in luminal or serum concentrations of the drugs (33).

Clinical Pharmacology. Like the other penicillins, the aminopenicillins are absorbed from the duodenum and upper jejunum. Amoxicillin is more completely absorbed than ampicillin (Table 2) (34). Food in the gastrointestinal tract may affect absorption of the aminopenicillins with a greater effect on ampicillin than amoxicillin. Diarrhea does not appear to significantly affect aminopenicillin absorption (27). The aminopenicillins are widely distributed although levels in most tissues other than liver are often lower than serum levels (35). Therapeutic concentrations are achieved in infected and uninfected ascitic fluid (28). Biliary excretion results in high (up to 30 times serum) levels of aminopenicillins if biliary obstruction is not present. The drugs readily cross the placenta. The aminopenicillins are primarily excreted unchanged in the urine with relatively small amounts removed in the bile despite the high biliary levels noted. That portion of ampicillin or amoxicillin that is not absorbed is excreted in the feces.

The Extended Generation Penicillins

Therapeutic Uses. Three compounds—ticarcillin, mezlocillin, and piperacillin—are included in this category for the treatment of gastrointestinal infection. The primary use of these agents is for the treatment of serious intra-abdominal pyogenic infections such as abscess or perforation in which gram-negative organisms play a role (36–39).

In Vitro Antibacterial Activity. Extended generation penicillins are active against many gram-positive aerobic cocci like the other penicillins discussed but are more active against Enterobacteriaceae and *Pseudomonas aeruginosa.*

Clinical Pharmacology. For serious intra-abdominal infection, these agents are given intravenously although they can be administered intramuscularly but there is little oral absorption (Table 2) (39,40). After parenteral administration, they readily penetrate into ascitic, peritoneal, and wound fluids but not into abscess cavities (41). The drugs also pass into most tissues such as the gallbladder and intestinal mucosa, where they may attain therapeutic concentrations. For example, levels of piperacillin in the intestinal mucosa are about half those attained in serum (42). In the absense of biliary obstruction, biliary levels of ticarcillin are several times greater than serum and levels of piperacillin and mezlocillin are 5 to 300 times greater (22,43). The extended generation agents are primarily excreted via the kidney with significant biliary excretion occurring for mezlocillin and piperacillin.

The Cephalosporins

For ease of discussion, the large number of cephalosporin antibiotics can be divided into three major groups, or generations, based on increasing gram-negative antibacterial activity (Table 3).

Mechanism of Action. The mechanism of action of cephalosporins is incompletely understood but like penicillin appears to involve inhibition of enzymes critical to cell wall synthesis in susceptible bacteria (1,2). Mechanisms of resistance by bacteria to cephalosporins are the same as for the penicillins.

Adverse Effects. As a group, the cephalosporins are quite safe. Nonetheless, many adverse effects have been reported for these agents (Table 1). As with the penicillins, the most serious reactions are hypersensitivity reactions, which occur in 5% or less of patients (44,45). Hypersensitivity reactions are more common in persons with a history of sensitivity to penicillin, although the issue of a penicillin-allergic patient receiving a cephalosporin is controversial. As a general rule, however, cephalosporins should not be given to persons with a positive penicillin skin test or with a history of a severe reaction to a penicillin (6). In patients with less severe reactions to penicillin, the decision to administer a cephalosporin should be guided by clinical judgment.

Cephalosporin treatment can also lead to the development of a positive Coombs reaction and other blood dyscrasias (46). Prolonged coagulation parameters or hypoprothrombinemia has been reported in some patients receiving cephalosporins (47). Hypoprothrombinemia has been reported most commonly with drugs containing the tetrazolethiomethyl side chain including cefotetan, cefmetazole, and cefoperazone and appears to involve alterations in the production of vitamin K-dependent clotting factors. Cephalosporins, in general, also may act to disrupt vitamin K synthesis by inhibition of gut flora (48).

Gastrointestinal side effects occur more frequently with the oral cephalosporins than with the parenterally administered agents. Nonetheless, although adverse effects such as diarrhea occur, the incidence is relatively low. Cefoperazone may cause more diarrhea than other cephalosporins, potentially because of its high biliary excretion (49). The mechanism may relate to alterations in gut flora induced by these agents. Colitis due to *Clostridium difficile* may occur (50). In addition, treatment with ceftriaxone has been associated with sludge in the gallbladder, which has clinically manifested as cholecystitis (51,52).

TABLE 3. *Selected pharmacokinetic data for the cephalosporins and other β-lactams used in gastrointestinal infection*

Drug	Route of administration	Metabolized (%)	Urine recovery (%)	Biliary excretion[a]	Half-life (hr)
First generation					
Cephalothin	Intravenous	20–30	70–80	+	0.5–0.9
Cefazolin	Intravenous	—	95	+	1.8
Cephapirin	Intravenous	40	90	+	0.6–0.8
Cephradine	Intravenous	—	90	+	0.8
Second generation					
Cefoxitin	Intravenous	<2	80–95	+	0.7–1
Cefotetan	Intravenous	—	60–80	+	3–4.6
Cefmetazole	Intravenous	—	85	+	1.2
Third generation					
Cefotaxime	Intravenous	30–50 (metabolite activity)	85	+	1–1.1
Ceftizoxime	Intravenous	—	80–90	+	1.4–1.8
Ceftriaxone	Intravenous and intramuscular	—	40–65	+ + + (40% of dose)	6–9
Ceftazidime	Intravenous	—	80–90	+	1.9
Cefoperazone	Intravenous and intramuscular	—	25	+ + + (70% of dose)	1.9–2.1
Imipenem/ Cilastatin	Intravenous	25	95–99	+ (minimal)	1
Aztreonam	Intravenous	7	60–80	+	1.6–2.1

With permission from ref. 67; and Division of Drugs and Toxicology, *Drug evaluations,* Summer 1990 Supplement. Chicago: American Medical Association, 1990.

[a] +, Biliary excretion occurs but is a minor route of elimination; + + +, significant biliary excretion.

Precautions. As noted earlier, the decision to use cephalosporins in penicillin-allergic patients should be based on the type of penicillin reaction encountered, the results of skin testing if performed, and clinical judgment. The cephalosporins should be used only when clearly needed in pregnancy as their safety is not conclusively established. Nonetheless, no adverse effects in children born to women who received the drugs during pregnancy have been reported. The cephalosporins pass into breast milk (53). In general, dose adjustment of the cephalosporins is indicated in persons with renal dysfunction.

Drug Interactions. The cephalosporins may have enhanced nephrotoxicity when administered with other nephrotoxic agents such as aminoglycosides (54). Diuretics may worsen renal insufficiency when combined with cephalosporins. Cephalosporins containing the tetrazolethiomethyl side chain can induce a disulfiram-like reaction in patients ingesting alcohol (55).

Particular Agents Useful in the Treatment of Gastrointestinal Infection

First-Generation Cephalosporins

Therapeutic Uses. Four first-generation cephalosporins are available—cephalothin, cefazolin, cephradine, and cephapirin—for the treatment of gastrointestinal infections; however, their use is limited, largely because of their spectra of activity. Nonetheless, they are used extensively for surgical prophylaxis. In addition, they may also be of use in selected situations, often in combination with other agents, for the treatment of intra-abdominal pyogenic infections such as in biliary tract infections (56).

In Vitro Antimicrobial Activity. First-generation cephalosporins display a high degree of activity against gram-positive cocci with the exception of enterococci. They possess reasonable activity against *E. coli, Klebsiella pneumoniae,* and indole (−) *Proteus.* They are inactive against *B. fragilis* but often active against other *Bacteroides* species and other gram-negative anaerobes. They are also active against some *Clostridium* species.

Clinical Pharmacology. The first-generation agents are well distributed to many tissues including the gallbladder, stomach, and liver. Body fluids, including inflammatory exudates, ascitic fluid, and interstitial fluids, contain significant levels of cefazolin and presumably the other first-generation cephalosporins after parenteral administration (57,58). Abscess penetration is poor (59). In addition, although biliary excretion is low, therapeutic concentrations of cefazolin exist in the bile if obstruction is not present. The agents are variably metabolized and excreted in the urine (Table 3).

Second-Generation Cephalosporins

Therapeutic Uses. The second-generation cephalosporins of use in the treatment of gastrointestinal tract infections include cefoxitin, cefotetan, and cefmetazole. They are indicated in a wide variety of mixed organism pyogenic gastrointestinal infections, such as intestinal perforation and abscess (60,61), and should be administered intravenously for this indication.

In Vitro *Antimicrobial Activity*. As a class, these agents tend to be more active against gram-negative aerobic organisms than the first-generation agents and they are active against anaerobic organisms, in particular, *B. fragilis*.

Clinical Pharmacology. After intravenous administration, the second-generation cephalosporins are widely distributed to tissues and attain therapeutic levels in bile. Cefoxitin distributes well to peritoneal and interstitial fluid, where concentrations are similar to simultaneous serum levels (62). Abscess penetration is poor (59). Excretion of these compounds is primarily via the kidney as the unchanged drugs (Table 3).

Third-Generation Cephalosporins

Therapeutic Uses. The third-generation cephalosporins useful in the treatment of gastrointestinal infection are cefotaxime, ceftriaxone, ceftizoxime, cefoperazone, and ceftazidime. Since these agents possess enhanced gram-negative activity over first- and second-generation agents, they are useful, often in combination with other antibiotics, for the treatment of serious intra-abdominal pyogenic infections (63,64). Several agents including cefoperazone, ceftriaxone, and cefotaxime have clinical benefit in salmonellosis and typhoid fever (65,66).

In Vitro *Antimicrobial Activity*. Among different agents in this class, antimicrobial activity varies somewhat. As a general rule, cefotaxime, ceftizoxime, and ceftriaxone have excellent activity against group A and B streptococci, but ceftazidime and cefoperazone are less active. Enterococci are resistant to all third-generation agents. All third-generation cephalosporins generally possess good activity against most Enterobacteriaceae and specifically *Salmonella*, although cefoperazone is the least active. Against *P. aeruginosa*, ceftazidime has high activity, cefoperazone moderate, and the other agents are far less active. These agents are active against anaerobic gram-positive bacteria and *Bacteroides* species, but other agents are preferable.

Clinical Pharmacology. As a rule, these drugs distribute widely with therapeutic concentrations in peritoneal fluid and tissue fluids and in many tissues including the liver. Biliary concentrations are therapeutic and the highest levels are associated with cefoperazone and ceftriaxone. Passage into abscesses is poor (41). Metabolism and excretion of these agents are variable (Table 3)(67).

Other β-Lactam Antibiotics

Imipenem/Cilastatin

Imipenem is a carbapenem antibiotic useful in the treatment of serious mixed pyogenic bacterial infections such as perforation and abscess (68) and is an agent of choice for serious infections due to *Campylobacter fetus* (69). Imipenem is combined with cilastatin, a renal dehydropeptidase inhibitor, which limits its breakdown in the kidney (70).

As with other β-lactams, imipenem inhibits bacterial cell wall synthesis in susceptible organisms. It has particular affinity for PBP-2 in gram-negative bacteria (71) and resistance to imipenem generally results from altered PBPs. Although imipenem is resistant to many β-lactamases, it is hydrolyzed by *B. fragilis* β-lactamase (72).

The antibacterial spectrum of imipenem is extremely broad. It is highly active against most gram-positive cocci including, to some degree, enterococci. The spectrum of activity of imipenem also includes most Enterobacteriaceae, *P. aeruginosa*, and most clinically important anaerobes except *C. difficile* (72).

Oral absorption of imipenem does not occur due to instability of the compound in gastric acid and it is thus administered parenterally. The drug distributes widely in the body and, in particular, passes into the intestine, interstitial fluid, peritoneal fluid, and wound fluid, where therapeutic levels may be achieved (73). Nonetheless, levels appear low in duodenal and ileal fluid (74). In addition, the drug exists in moderately low levels in biliary fluid. This observation may explain its lack of marked association with diarrhea and lack of a major effect on bowel flora (75). Imipenem is predominantly excreted via the kidney with less than 1% excreted in feces (Table 3)(76,77).

Although imipenem is a fairly safe agent, adverse effects occur (Table 1). Allergic reactions consisting of rash and drug fever have been reported in 2.4% of patients and anaphylaxis has also occurred (78). In addition, apparent cross-reactions to imipenem in penicillin-allergic patients have been reported (79). Adverse central nervous system effects may be serious. Approximately 1% of patients develop seizures, which can be attributed directly to imipenem in a fraction of these patients (78). Risk factors appear to include other central nervous system disease, old age, renal insufficiency, and overdosage of imipenem. Persons with a history of a severe reaction to penicillin should not receive imipenem/cilastatin. In persons with central nervous system disorders, imipenem/cilastatin should be used with caution because of the risk of precipitating seizures. Dose adjustments should be made in persons with renal insufficiency. Use in pregnancy has not been studied carefully and thus this agent should be used with caution. Imipenem/cilastatin passes into breast milk. Few adverse drug interactions have been documented, although adverse central nervous system events have been reported in several individuals receiving ganciclovir or cyclosporine in combination with imipenem (80).

Aztreonam

Aztreonam is a monocyclic β-lactam antibiotic with a narrow spectrum of activity (81,82). Its use in gastrointestinal infections is for the treatment of serious intra-abdominal processes such as perforation and abscess in which aerobic gram-negative bacilli play a role (83). Parenterally administered aztreonam is effective in the treatment of enteric fever due to *Salmonella* species and it is effective orally for the treatment of traveler's diarrhea (84,85).

Like other β-lactams, aztreonam inhibits bacterial cell wall formation, possessing a high affinity for PBP-3 in aerobic gram-negative bacteria (81). Resistance to aztreonam appears related to alterations in permeability of the drug into organisms and possibly to inability to bind PBPs. Aztreonam is active against many gram-negative aerobic bacteria including Enterobacteriaceae, *P. aeruginosa, Salmonella, Shigella, Aeromonas,* and *Plesiomonas* species. Aztreonam is generally inactive against gram-positive aerobes and gram-positive and gram-negative anaerobic organisms (86). It does not significantly affect intestinal microflora.

Aztreonam is not absorbed orally (Table 3). Following parenteral administration, the drug distributes widely in the body and is detectable in tissues of the gallbladder, liver, and intestines with levels in the therapeutic range. Concentrations in bile are moderately high in the absence of biliary obstruction (87). In addition, it penetrates into peritoneal fluid with levels similar to those in serum. The primary route of excretion is the kidney. Only 1% of a parenterally administered dose appears in feces (88).

Overall aztreonam appears very safe and adverse reactions are uncommon (Table 1)(89). Cross-reactivity of aztreonam with penicillin does not appear to occur. Rashes and other hypersensitivity reactions are rare (90). Dosage adjustment is necessary in renal insufficiency. Aztreonam has not been carefully studied in pregnancy and thus should be used cautiously in this situation. It is present in breast milk in low concentrations. No adverse interactions with other drugs have been reported.

β-Lactamase Inhibitors

Three inhibitors of β-lactamase that do not possess significant intrinsic antibacterial activity of their own are available for use in combination with antimicrobial agents. These compounds are clavulanic acid, sulbactam, and tazobactam.

Clavulanic acid is an inhibitor of β-lactamase that is active against β-lactamases from a wide variety of gram-positive and gram-negative organisms (91). When administered orally, it is well absorbed and adequate levels appear in peritoneal fluid and in infected tissues of animals (92). Clavulanic acid is generally free of significant side effects although nausea and diarrhea have been reported to occur. Clavulanic acid is combined for use with either amoxicillin or ticarcillin. Amoxicillin/clavulanic acid is available as an oral preparation in a fixed ratio of 1:1. Its primary advantage over amoxicillin alone is enhanced activity against a wide range of β-lactamase-producing organisms including many gram-negative aerobes normally resistant to amoxicillin and *B. fragilis.* Clavulanic acid is also combined with ticarcillin in a fixed ratio of 30:1 (ticarcillin:clavulanic acid) and extends the spectrum of activity of ticarcillin to include additional Enterobacteriaceae.

Sulbactam is also a inhibitor of β-lactamase (93). It is available for parenteral use combined with ampicillin in a fixed ratio of 2:1 (ampicillin:sulbactam) and extends the spectrum of activity of ampicillin in a manner similar to clavulanic acid. Sulbactam penetrates well into body fluids and tissues. A small amount of the drug is eliminated via the bile and appears in the feces. Sulbactam has few, if any, adverse reactions (94).

A third, recently introduced, β-lactamase inhibitor is tazobactam. Tazobactam is combined with piperacillin and extends the spectrum of piperacillin against a number of β-lactamase-producing organisms.

The Aminoglycosides

Therapeutic Uses. The aminoglycosides comprise a large group of antibiotics possessing similar structures and spectra of activity. At present, eight aminoglycoside antibiotics are used for the treatment of gastrointestinal infections. For the purpose of treating serious intra-abdominal pyogenic infections due to gram-negative bacilli, gentamicin, tobramycin, netilmicin, and amikacin are used most commonly while kanamycin is infrequently employed. Streptomycin has antibacterial activity and is useful in the therapy of Whipple's disease but is more commonly employed for the treatment of tuberculosis (24). Neomycin is used primarily for the preparation of the bowel for surgery and, unlike the previously mentioned agents, is administered orally (95). Paromomycin is another orally administered aminoglycoside primarily used for the treatment of parasitic infections and will be discussed in that section.

Mechanism of Action. The aminoglycosides are bactericidal but the exact mechanism of their activity is unknown; inhibition of protein synthesis by interaction with either the 30S or 50S ribosomal subunit may be important but another, unknown, mechanism probably also is involved (96–99). Resistance to the aminoglycosides is not infrequent. Three mechanisms appear to play a role. The first is enzymatic inactivation of drug by three types of enzymes—acetyltransferases, phosphotransferases, and adenyltransferases. These enzymes are carried on plasmids and inactivate aminoglycosides by addition of acetyl, phosphate, or adenyl moieties to the drugs, respectively (100,101). This mechanism of inactivation is the one most commonly encountered in gram-negative bacteria. Two other mechanisms of resistance include ribosome binding site alteration and decreased uptake of antibiotic by resistant bacteria.

In Vitro *Antimicrobial Activity.* The spectrum of aminoglycoside activity generally includes aerobic and facultative gram-negative bacteria and staphylococci. With the exception of streptomycin, kanamycin, and neomycin, the aminoglycosides are active against *P. aeruginosa.*

Clinical Pharmacology. The aminoglycosides are poorly absorbed from the gastrointestinal tract. Thus the agents used to treat serious pyogenic infection—gentamicin, tobramycin, netilmicin, amikacin, and kanamycin—must be administered parenterally, preferably by the intravenous route. Streptomycin is usually administered intramuscularly. After administration, the aminoglycosides distribute primarily to extracellular fluids. Levels in body fluids and tissues are similar to or lower than serum levels (102,103). For example, levels of gentamicin in ascitic fluid are about one-half of serum levels but may increase in peritonitis, while levels of the other aminoglycosides in peritoneal fluid are 25% to 50% those in serum (28,104). These agents cross the placenta. The mean serum half-life is 2 to 3 hr but wide interperson variations exist. The aminoglycosides are primarily excreted via the kidney but small amounts are excreted in bile. The mean biliary concentration of gentamicin is 30% to 40% of plasma (105).

Adverse Effects. Because of the narrow toxic/therapeutic ratio of the aminoglycosides, adverse effects are not infrequently encountered. All aminoglycosides may cause ototoxicity, and both hearing and vestibular function can be affected. Ototoxicity is more likely to occur with prolonged and repeated dosing of aminoglycosides and its incidence may be as high as 25% (106). Risk factors for ototoxicity include the presence of bacteremia, fever, liver dysfunction, hypovolemia, and concomitant use of ethacrynic acid (106–108). The ototoxicity of aminoglycosides can be reversible or irreversible.

A second major adverse effect of aminoglycosides is nephrotoxicity. Between 8% and 26% of persons receiving aminoglycosides for several days develop reversible renal impairment (109,110) probably due to the fact that aminoglycosides are concentrated in the kidney. Risk factors for renal dysfunction include older age, female sex, liver disease, hypotension, and administration of other nephrotoxic agents. (111,112).

Rarely, the aminoglycosides produce neuromuscular paralysis (113), hypersensitivity reactions, liver dysfunction, and blood dyscrasias. Pseudomembranous colitis has been reported with oral but not with the parenteral use of aminoglycosides (114,115).

Precautions. Patients receiving parenteral aminoglycosides should have serum levels of the drugs monitored during therapy to avoid adversities. Dose adjustment is necessary in renal failure. These agents should be used with caution in persons with neuromuscular diseases. Aminoglycosides cross the placenta and streptomycin has been associated with deafness in children whose mothers received the agent while pregnant (116). This has not been demonstrated with other aminoglycosides but use of these agents in pregnancy is justified only for serious infections where the benefits outweigh the risks. Small amounts of aminoglycosides pass into breast milk (117).

Drug Interactions. Concurrent use of agents known to be ototoxic or nephrotoxic with aminoglycosides may worsen toxicity. In addition, concurrent use of general anesthetics and neuromuscular blockers may worsen neuromuscular blockade.

Neomycin

Neomycin is available for use orally to prepare the bowel for surgery. For this indication, it is often used in combination with erythromycin (95). Neomycin is poorly absorbed from the gastrointestinal tract with 97% of a dose eliminated via the feces (107). Nonetheless, measurable levels of the drug may exist in serum after oral dosing and thus systemic toxicity can occur, especially in persons with renal insufficiency. Side effects associated with neomycin therapy include intestinal malabsorption and superinfection.

The Quinolones

Therapeutic Uses. The quinolone antibiotics represent an important advance in the treatment of infections involving the gastrointestinal tract. Five agents are currently available for use in the United States. They are ciprofloxacin, ofloxacin, norfloxacin, lomefloxacin, and enoxacin. The most clinical information on treating gastrointestinal tract infections has been reported with ciprofloxcin, ofloxacin, and norfloxacin and thus those are the ones discussed.

The quinolones are usually administered orally. Ciprofloxacin is effective for treatment of enterocolitis due to enterotoxigenic *E. coli, Shigella, Salmonella,* and *Campylobacter* (118,119). Furthermore, norfloxacin has been efficacious in the treatment of severe bacterial diarrhea (120,121), while ofloxacin is effective for enteritis due to *Shigella* and other pathogens (122). Ciprofloxacin and ofloxacin also have been effective in the treatment of typhoid fever and in the eradication of the chronic *S. typhi* carrier state (123–125). The quinolones have been used in the treatment of *H. pylori* infections although they may frequently be ineffective due to development of resistance (126). The quinolones also are effective in the treatment of infections due to *Yersinia enterocolitica* and *Aeromonas hydrophila.* In addition, ciprofloxacin and ofloxacin, when administered intravenously, may be useful as an alternative therapy in serious intra-abdominal pyogenic infections in which gram-negative aerobic bacteria play a role.

Mechanism of Action. The quinolones are bactericidal agents although the mechanisms by which this occurs have not been fully elucidated; they inhibit the A subunit of deoxyribonucleic acid (DNA) topoisomerase (DNA gyrase) in susceptible organisms (127–129). Resistance to the quinolones is due to chromosomal mutations probably involving alterations in either DNA gyrase or changes in the permeability of the bacterial membrane to the drug (130). All quinolones exhibit cross-resistance to each other *in vitro.*

In Vitro *Antimicrobial Activity.* The quinolones all have similar activity that includes many aerobic gram-negative and some gram-positive bacteria. Many strains of bacteria resistant to the aminoglycosides and β-lactams are susceptible to the quinolones. These agents are highly active against most enteric pathogens including *Salmonella, Shigella, E. coli, Y. enterocolitica, Vibrio* species, *Campylobacter jejuni,* and *P. aeruginosa.* The quinolones are also active versus *H. pylori.* Most anaerobic bacteria including *C. difficile* and *B. fragilis* are resistant (131,132). In humans, ciprofloxacin and ofloxacin alter aerobic but

TABLE 4. *Pharmacokinetic data for the fluoroquinolones*

Drug	Oral bioavailability (%)	Excretion (%)				Half-life (hr)
		Parent compound	Metabolites	Renal	Bile/feces	
Norfloxacin	30–40	26–32	5–8	27	30	3.3
Ciprofloxacin	60–70	30–45	~15	29	30	3.3
Ofloxacin	95	70–90	~5	73	4–8	5–7

With permission from ref. 139; and Division of Drugs and Toxicology, *Drug evaluations*, Spring 1993 Supplement. Chicago: American Medical Association, 1993.

not anaerobic fecal flora (133). Ciprofloxacin and ofloxacin also have antimycobacterial activity.

Clinical Pharmacology. The quinolones are variably absorbed from the gastrointestinal tract and food generally delays their absorption (Table 4)(134–136). The agents distribute widely throughout the body and the highest levels of ciprofloxacin can be found in bile, intestinal fluid, liver, and gallbladder. For both ofloxacin and ciprofloxacin, these tissue and fluid levels exceed serum concentrations. The distribution of norfloxacin is more limited but it can be detected in the tissues and fluids mentioned above. The agents cross the placenta. Although quinolones exist in high levels in bile, this is a relatively minor route of elimination. Significant amounts of norfloxacin and ciprofloxacin are present in feces (Table 3), probably due, in large part, to incomplete absorption or gastrointestinal secretion; levels of ciprofloxacin after a 500-mg oral dose are about 900 μg/g feces. Intravenous administration of ciprofloxacin results in about 15% of the dose appearing in the feces. Four percent to 8% of orally administered ofloxacin appears in the feces.

Adverse Effects. Although the quinolones are quite safe, adverse reactions have been reported. Gastrointestinal side effects are most common (1% to 7%) and include nausea, vomiting, diarrhea, and anorexia. Antibiotic-associated colitis occurs infrequently (137,138). Central nervous system reactions occur in about 1% to 2% of patients and most commonly include drowsiness, insomnia, malaise, restlessness, and agitation. More severe reactions such as psychosis and seizures also have been reported. Skin and allergic reactions have been reported in 0.6% to 2.4% of patients and include skin rash, interstitial nephritis, vasculitis and joint swelling, and eosinophilia. Increases in hepatic transaminases and serum creatinine have also been documented (139).

Precautions. Use of the quinolones in pregnant women or in children is contraindicated based on animal studies showing cartilage erosion in weight-bearing joints of immature animals administered these agents (138). The dosage of these drugs should be adjusted in persons with renal insufficiency.

Drug Interactions. Antacids and sucralfate significantly lower the absorption of the quinolones from the gut as do iron preparations. In addition, ciprofloxacin and, to a lesser extent, ofloxacin increase plasma theophylline levels by inhibiting metabolism of this agent. Ciprofloxacin also prolongs the half-life of caffeine (140).

Clindamycin

Therapeutic Uses. Clindamycin is a lincosamide antibiotic used frequently in the management of serious intraabdominal pyogenic infection such as perforation and abscess (141). It is also active against *Actinomyces* species and may be an alternative to penicillin for infections caused by these organisms.

Mechanism of Action. Clindamycin is bacteriostatic and exerts its activity by binding to the 50S ribosomal subunit in susceptible bacteria. The result of this interaction is inhibition of peptide bond formation and protein synthesis (142). The mechanism whereby bacteria acquire resistance appears to involve alterations in the 50S ribosomal subunit binding site or the 23S ribonucleic acid (RNA) component of the 50S subunit (143).

In Vitro Antimicrobial Activity. Clindamycin has a broad antimicrobial spectrum of activity that includes many gram-positive aerobic organisms although enterococci are resistant. The compound exhibits potent *in vitro* activity against a wide range of microaerophilic and anaerobic bacteria including *Actinomyces* species, *Bacteroides* species including *B. fragilis,* microaerophilic streptococci, peptococci, peptostreptococci, and some clostridia. Aerobic gram-negative bacilli are resistant.

Clinical Pharmacology. Clindamycin can be administered orally, intramuscularly, or intravenously. Ninety percent of an oral dose is absorbed from the gastrointestinal tract and is increased even further in persons with celiac disease, jejunal diverticulosis, or Crohn's disease (144). Absorption does not appear significantly affected by food (145). After administration, clindamycin distributes widely to many body sites. It penetrates well into peritoneal fluid, liver, gallbladder, and the appendix and into ascitic fluid of individuals with bacterial peritonitis (28). Clindamycin penetrates well into abscesses and is present at therapeutic levels (146). It crosses the placenta and is found in human breast milk. The mean half-life is 2.4 to 3 hr. Biliary excretion also occurs and biliary levels of the drug are high in the absence of biliary obstruction (two to four times serum), although it is primarily metabolized in the liver and excreted in the urine (147). Some of the active drug is excreted in the feces (5% or less) (144). Both the liver and kidney are involved in the elimination of active drug; dosage reduction is indicated in severe hepatic and possibly renal disease.

Adverse Effects. By far the major adverse reactions associated with clindamycin therapy are antibiotic-associated diarrhea and pseudomembranous colitis due to *C. difficile* (148–150). These side effects are covered in detail in the chapter by Bartlett, which deals with antibiotic-associated colitis. Other adverse effects associated with clindamycin therapy include rash (in up to 10% of patients), neutropenia, drug fever, eosinophilia, and increases in liver function tests. Cardiopulmonary arrest has occurred with rapid intravenous infusion of this agent.

Precautions. As a general rule, development of diarrhea during clindamycin therapy warrants a search for *C. difficile* overgrowth and often drug cessation. The safety of this drug in pregnancy has not been established but there is no evidence that it is harmful.

Drug Interactions. Clindamycin has neuromuscular blocking effects and should be used cautiously with other drugs possessing this activity (151).

Metronidazole

Metronidazole is an important antimicrobial agent in the treatment of gastrointestinal infection. In addition to having excellent activity against many anaerobic bacteria, it also is active against the parasites *Giardia lamblia* and *Entamoeba histolytica* (152,153). Metronidazole is particularly useful in the treatment of intra-abdominal pyogenic infections in which anaerobes play a role (154). It also is effective in the treatment of antibiotic-associated colitis and *H. pylori* infection (31). Furthermore, it has been used to treat bowel overgrowth syndromes and Crohn's disease. Finally, it may be useful as perioperative prophylaxis in colon surgery (155,156).

Mechanism of Action. The selective antibacterial activity of metronidazole relates to reduction of the 5' nitro group on the molecule by electron transport proteins in susceptible organisms. The reduction products are reactive intermediates and are believed to be cytotoxic due to interactions with DNA or other macromolecules inside the cell (157). Resistance of anaerobic bacteria to metronidazole is unusual. Occasional resistant strains of *Bacteroides* species including *B. fragilis* have been studied. In one case, it appeared as though resistance was related to slow uptake of drug combined with decreased reduction to reactive intermediates (158,159).

In Vitro Antimicrobial Activity. Anaerobic organisms usually susceptible to metronidazole include *Bacteroides* species, *Fusobacterium*, *Clostridium*, *Veillonella*, *Peptococcus*, and *Peptostreptococcus*. In particular, *B. fragilis* is usually susceptible. Metronidazole is moderately active against *C. fetus* and against many *H. pylori* strains although resistance may develop in *H. pylori* in the course of therapy (160–162). Other aerobic organisms are generally considered resistant.

Clinical Pharmacology. Metronidazole is administered intravenously for serious intra-abdominal pyogenic infection and intravenously or orally for antibiotic-associated colitis due to *C. difficile*. The drug has been administered rectally and is moderately well absorbed from this site (157). When given orally, metronidazole is essentially completely absorbed from the gut and absorption is not affected by food. The drug distributes widely. Therapeu-

tic levels are found in bile. The drug distributes to abscess cavities including those in the liver where therapeutic concentrations are achieved. It penetrates well into the appendix and colonic wall (163). It readily crosses the placenta and passes into breast milk. The half-life is about 8 hr. Metronidazole is extensively metabolized and is primarily excreted in the kidney. Six percent to 15% is excreted in the feces, some of which is probably secreted across the colonic wall (164). Both oral and intravenous administration of metronidazole achieves therapeutic levels in feces in patients with *C. difficile* colitis (165).

Adverse Effects. The most common adverse reactions to metronidazole are usually gastrointestinal and include bad taste, nausea, epigastric distress, and anorexia. Interestingly, *C. difficile*-associated colitis has been reported with metronidazole use but is unusual, perhaps because metronidazole kills *C. difficile* (166). Rash, fever, and mental status changes have also been reported. Metronidazole has also been associated with seizures, encephalopathy, peripheral neuropathy, gynecomastia, pancreatitis, and reversible neutropenia (167).

Precautions. Patients should be monitored for neurologic dysfunction during therapy. The use of metronidazole in pregnancy is unsettled because of studies showing it to be a bacterial mutagen and to cause tumors in rodents given large doses (168). However, no evidence suggests that metronidazole is carcinogenic in humans. In addition, there is no evidence that metronidazole is teratogenic, in that congenital defects in infants are not increased if their mothers received metronidazole during pregnancy (157). Nonetheless, the benefits and risks should be weighed carefully when the drug is considered for use in the pregnant patient. In general, however, it is not recommended for use in women in the first trimester of pregnancy. Metronidazole passes into breast milk.

Drug Interactions. Metronidazole inhibits the metabolism of warfarin, and therefore prothrombin times should be monitored in individuals receiving both agents. Also importantly, metronidazole produces a disulfiram-like reaction in combination with alcohol ingestion. Furthermore, the combination of disulfiram and metronidazole has produced acute psychosis. Cimetidine may increase the serum half-life of metronidazole while phenobarbital shortens it. Metronidazole may also increase serum lithium levels.

Chloramphenicol

Therapeutic Uses. Chloramphenicol is an agent with a broad spectrum of activity, which is of use in the treatment of several gastrointestinal infections. It is considered one of the agents of choice for the treatment of invasive salmonellosis and typhoid fever although resistance among *Salmonella* species is increasing (169). Chloramphenicol also is an alternative agent, usually in combination with other drugs, for the treatment of serious intra-abdominal mixed pyogenic infection such as perforation or abscess (170).

Mechanism of Action. Chloramphenicol is bacteriostatic against most bacteria and appears to act by inhibition of bacterial protein synthesis by binding the 50S ribosomal subunit in susceptible bacteria (171,172). Bacterial resistance to chloramphenicol can be both natural and acquired. Resistance mechanisms in bacteria include (a) impermeability to the drug or (b) production of an enzyme, acetyltransferase, that acetylates the antibiotic to an inactive derivative (173). This latter mechanism is plasmid mediated and occurs in enteric bacteria (174–176).

In Vitro *Antimicrobial Activity.* Chloramphenicol is active *in vitro* against many gram-positive bacteria. Many gram-negative aerobes also are susceptible including *Salmonella* and *Shigella* species unless plasmid-mediated resistance has been acquired. *Enterobacter* and *P. aeruginosa* are usually resistant. Chloramphenicol is highly active against many anaerobes including *B. fragilis*.

Clinical Pharmacology. Chloramphenicol can be administered orally, intramuscularly, or intravenously for the treatment of gastrointestinal infection. For salmonellosis and typhoid fever, either of the three routes of administration can be beneficial although the oral route is most commonly used (177). Chloramphenicol is about 80% absorbed when administered orally and because of a high degree of lipid solubility it is distributed to many tissues where therapeutic levels can be obtained (178). It readily penetrates into ascitic fluid and in patients with peritonitis, peritoneal levels are half those of serum. The drug is present at high concentrations in the liver and spleen. Levels in abscesses are 10% to 20% of serum levels (41). The half-life is 1.5 to 4 hr. Chloramphenicol crosses the placenta and can be found in breast milk. Most of the drug is excreted in the urine as the glucuronide conjugate. Only small amounts (2% to 3%) of chloramphenicol are excreted in the bile and biliary concentrations are lower than serum. One percent is excreted in feces.

Adverse Effects. One of the most serious adverse effects of chloramphenicol administration is bone marrow suppression, of which two types exist (179). The first is reversible and dose related. It manifests as anemia (with a decrease of other cell lines), reticulocytopenia, and increased serum iron (180). The second type is idiosyncratic and characterized by aplastic anemia, which is unrelated to dose and usually occurs weeks to months after therapy. It is characterized by peripheral pancytopenia and a hypoplastic or aplastic marrow. The incidence is 1/25,000 to 1/40,000 courses of therapy and carries a poor prognosis. Chloramphenicol has also been implicated in induction of childhood leukemia (181) and hemolytic anemia associated with the Mediterranean form of glucose-6-phosphate dehydrogenase deficiency.

The drug has been associated with a disorder in neonates termed the "gray baby syndrome" characterized by abdominal distension, vomiting, flaccidity, cyanosis, and death. It is believed due to a decreased ability to conjugate and excrete chloramphenicol, leading to toxic levels of the drug. It also has been observed in adults when very large doses of the agent are given (182,183). Other reported toxicities have included optic neuritis, delirium, peripheral neuritis, and depression. Pseudomembranous colitis has been reported but is uncommon. Nausea, vomiting, diarrhea, and stomatitis also occur but are not common.

Precautions. Monitoring of patients' blood counts during therapy is important. Some authorities also measure blood levels of chloramphenicol. Dosage reduction of chloramphenicol may be necessary in renal and hepatic disease. Use in pregnancy has not been established but is probably contraindicated in near-term or breast-feeding women because of a concern about the decreased ability of neonates to conjugate the drug.

Drug Interactions. Chloramphenicol prolongs half-lives and increases serum concentrations of many drugs including the oral hypoglycemics, dicumarol, cyclophosphamide, and phenytoin, possibly by inhibiting their hepatic metabolism. Phenobarbital, phenytoin, and rifampin decrease serum concentrations of chloramphenicol. Furthermore, chloramphenicol may delay the response of anemia to therapy with iron, vitamin B_{12}, or folate. Whether or not it antagonizes the bactericidal effects of penicillin is unclear.

The Tetracyclines

Therapeutic Uses. Five different tetracycline antibiotics are available in the United States and can be divided based on their pharmacological properties (Table 5), although their antimicrobial activity is similar. The tetracyclines are one of the agents of choice for the treatment of infections due to *Vibrio cholerae* and other pathogenic vibrios (184). In addition, they are quite acceptable alternatives in the treatment of actinomycosis, gastroenteritis due to *Y. enterocolitica* and *C. jejuni*, Whipple's disease, and tropical sprue and are of use in the therapy of *H. pylori* infection in combination with other agents (24,185). Doxycycline has also been used to treat traveler's diarrhea but because of resistance among *E. coli* and other enteric pathogens, it is less effective than other agents (85). These agents are also useful for bowel overgrowth syndromes and for preoperative bowel sterilization (186). The tetracyclines can also be used to treat parasitic infections such as invasive intestinal amebiasis (187,188) and are useful in infections caused by *Balantidium coli* and *Dientamoeba fragilis*.

TABLE 5. *Selected pharmacokinetic features of the tetracyclines*

Drug	GI absorption (%)	Half-life (hr)	Urine recovery (%)
Short acting			
Oxytetracycline	58	6	70
Tetracycline	77	9	60
Intermediate acting			
Demeclocycline	66	12	39
Long acting			
Doxycycline	93	18	42
Minocycline	95	16	6

From ref. 178, with permission.

Mechanism of Action. The tetracyclines are actively taken up by bacteria where they reversibly bind to the 30S ribosomal subunit of susceptible bacteria to inhibit protein synthesis (189). Resistance to the tetracyclines primarily involves inhibition of accumulation of these agents intracellularly and is plasmid mediated (190). Resistance to one tetracycline implies resistance to the entire group.

In Vitro *Antibacterial Activity.* The spectrum of activity of the tetracyclines *in vitro* is very broad. These agents exhibit good activity against many gram-positive aerobic cocci including many strains of *Streptococcus pyogenes* and *S. agalactiae* and viridans and anaerobic streptococci. Enterococci are resistant. They are also active against many gram-positive bacilli including *C. tetani* and *Actinomyces israelii.* In addition, they are active against many gram-negative bacilli including *V. cholerae, C. jejuni, V. parahaemolyticus, V. vulnificus, H. pylori,* and *E. corrodens.* While the tetracyclines are active against some strains of *E. coli,* many Enterobacteriaceae are resistant including *Klebsiella, Enterobacter, Proteus, Serratia,* and *Shigella* species. *Pseudomonas aeruginosa* is usually resistant. Among gram-negative anaerobes, some *Bacteroides* strains are sensitive but many *B. fragilis* strains are resistant.

Clinical Pharmacology. All tetracyclines are absorbed from the proximal small intestine (Table 5). Food decreases absorption of the short and intermediate acting agents more than the longer acting ones. Achlorhydria does not significantly affect absorption (191). The tetracyclines penetrate fairly well into tissues and body fluids, but doxycycline and minocycline are more lipid soluble and are thus better able to penetrate tissues. In particular, these agents pass well into the intestinal epithelium (185). Furthermore, peritoneal fluid levels of doxycycline are about 75% of simultaneous serum levels. With minocycline, highest concentrations can be found in the intestinal tract, liver, gallbladder, and bile (192). The tetracyclines cross the placenta and are present in breast milk.

The tetracyclines are excreted in bile and levels 10 to 25 times serum concentrations occur. Overall, however, biliary excretion accounts for a small percentage of the administered dose of these agents. Tetracyclines excreted in the bile are partially reabsorbed in the intestines. With the exception of doxycycline and minocycline, the tetracyclines are incompletely absorbed from the gastrointestinal tract and concentrations may reach 1 mg/g feces after oral administration. Interestingly, although doxycycline is well absorbed, diffusion of this agent from the blood across the small bowel wall into the lumen of the bowel occurs and increases in renal failure (193).

Adverse Effects. Gastrointestinal side effects are fairly common adverse effects (Table 6). In patients receiving 2 g of tetracycline or its equivalent per day, the overall incidence is 10%. Fecal flora are greatly altered by the administration of the tetracyclines and this probably contributes significantly to the incidence of diarrhea. Furthermore, diarrhea tends to occur more commonly with poorly absorbed agents and may be due, in part, to direct chemical irritation of the bowel. Pseudomembranous colitis associated with *C. difficile* also occurs (186). Tetracy-

TABLE 6. *Adverse effects of the tetracyclines*

Effects	Relative frequency
Gastrointestinal	
Anorexia	+ + +
Nausea	+ + +
Vomiting	+ + +
Diarrhea	+ + +
Pseudomembranous colitis	+
Esophageal ulceration	+
Candidal overgrowth	+ +
Renal	
Elevated blood urea nitrogen and creatinine	+
Nephrogenic diabetes insipidus	+
Hepatic	
Hepatitis and hepatic dysfunction	+
Pancreatitis	+
Bones and teeth	
Discoloration of teeth	+ + (if given to children)
Bone growth depression	+ +
Nervous system	
Vestibular toxicity (minocycline)	+ + +
Pseudotumor cerebri	+
Other (drowsiness, lightheadedness)	+
Photosensitivity	+ +
Hypersensitivity reactions	+
Miscellaneous	
Thrombophlebitis (iv administration)	+ + +
Vaginitis (candidal)	+ +
Pigmentation of skin and nails	+
Jarisch–Herxheimer reaction	+
Blood dyscrasias	+

+, Infrequent; + + +, frequent.

clines are acidic agents (doxycycline has a pH of 3 in solution) and esophageal ulceration has been reported (194). Deposition of the tetracyclines in growing teeth and bones can result in serious cosmetic and medical problems for young children and the tetracyclines should thus be avoided in women in the last half of pregnancy or in children under 8 years old, unless there are strong reasons to administer these agents (186,191,195). In addition, minocycline is associated with a high incidence of vestibular dysfunction, which limits its utility (196).

Precautions. Use of tetracyclines in young children and in pregnant women is generally contraindicated. The drugs should be used with caution in renal and hepatic disease.

Drug Interactions. The tetracyclines chelate divalent and trivalent cations including Mg^{3+}, Fe^{2+}, Zn^{2+}, Al^{3+}, and Ca^{2+} and thus should generally not be administered concurrently with antacids, milk or milk products, vitamin and mineral preparations, or cathartics. Coingestion with subsalicylate bismuth significantly lowers the bioavailability of doxycycline (197) and the two agents should not be administered simultaneously. In addition, coadministration of doxycycline with carbamazepine, phenytoin, or barbiturates decreases the half-life of doxycycline. Tetracycline HCl may increase the anticoagulant effect of coumarin and may decrease digoxin metabolism, leading to markedly increased serum digoxin levels (195).

Vancomycin

Therapeutic Uses. Vancomycin is a glycopeptide antibiotic useful primarily in the therapy of infections due to gram-positive organisms. It is employed for two purposes related to gastrointestinal infection. First, when administered orally, it is one of the agents of choice for the treatment of antibiotic-associated pseudomembranous colitis caused by *C. difficile* (150). Second, administered intravenously it may be useful as an agent for the treatment of serious intra-abdominal pyogenic infection in which gram-positive organisms play a role (198).

A related agent, teicoplanin, is not currently available in the United States. It appears, however, to also be effective orally in the therapy of pseudomembranous colitis and has fewer side effects than vancomycin (199,200).

Mechanism of Action. Vancomycin is believed to exert its bactericidal activity by inhibition of assembly of the second stage of cell wall peptidoglycan polymers by complexing with the D-calanyl–D-alanine precursor. It also injures protoplasts by altering the cytoplasmic membrane and it impairs RNA synthesis (201,202). Resistance is unusual but has been reported in some enterococcal isolates. The mechanism of resistance is plasmid mediated and involves alteration in bacterial D-alanine:D-alanine ligase such that vancomycin is not recognized by the enzyme (203–205).

In Vitro *Antimicrobial Activity.* Vancomycin is active primarily against gram-positive bacteria. It is the agent of choice against methicillin-resistant *S. aureus* and is active against nearly all *Staphylococcus* strains. It is highly active against all Lancefield group streptococci except enterococci, which are killed only by very high concentrations of the drug. Viridans streptococci are also sensitive as are anaerobic and microaerophilic streptococci. In most cases *Clostridium* species, including *C. difficile,* are sensitive [minimal inhibitory concentration (MIC) < 8 µg/mL] (206).

Clinical Pharmacology. When administered intravenously, vancomycin distributes well into ascitic fluid, liver tissue, and abscesses (207). It readily crosses the placenta. After intravenous administration, little vancomycin appears in the feces and bile of most normal persons, although levels up to 100 µg/mL have been reported in the stool of some patients (208,209); primary excretion is in the urine. Oral administration of vancomycin is recommended for colitis due to *C. difficile*. Although not usually absorbed, clinically significant serum concentrations may occur in patients with pseudomembranous colitis and impaired renal function (210). Ingestion of a standard dose of 125 mg of vancomycin gives stool concentrations in the range of 100 to 800 µg/mL while 500 mg administered orally every 6 hr gives levels of 1000 to 9000 µg/mL (202,211).

Adverse Effects. Parenteral administration of vancomycin is associated with several adverse effects, most commonly including phlebitis at the site of injection,

fever, and chills. In addition, a syndrome associated with large or rapid infusions termed the "redman syndrome" is characterized by flushing of the upper body and face (212). Hypersensitivity reactions, leukopenia, and eosinophilia also have been reported. At least one case of *C. difficile* colitis associated with intravenous vancomycin therapy has also been reported (213). Neurotoxicity is another potential adversity associated with parenteral vancomycin therapy and manifests as hearing loss and auditory nerve damage (214). The hearing loss is often irreversible. Nephrotoxicity may be associated with vancomycin but is not common.

Precautions. Serum levels of vancomycin should be monitored during parenteral therapy and the dose adjusted in renal failure. Vancomycin should be used in pregnancy only when clearly needed. It is unknown whether vancomycin passes to breast milk.

Drug Interactions. The nephrotoxicity and/or ototoxicity of agents such as aminoglycosides, amphotericin B, cisplatin, and other agents may be worsened with concurrent vancomycin administration. Vancomycin should not be administered orally with cholestyramine as it complexes with this bile resin.

Erythromycin and the Newer Macrolides: Azithromycin and Clarithromycin

Erythromycin

Therapeutic Uses. Erythromycin is a broad spectrum antimicrobial agent useful in the treatment of enterocolitis caused by *Campylobacter jejuni* (215). In addition, erythromycin is frequently used in the preparation of the patient for bowel surgery and has been used in the therapy of invasive intestinal amebiasis (216,217).

Mechanism of Action. Erythromycin inhibits protein synthesis in susceptible organisms at the step of elongation by binding to the 50S ribosomal subunit (218). Resistance to erythromycin may occur by decreased permeability of the bacterial cell envelope to the drug, alteration in the 50S ribosomal protein binding site, alteration by methylation of adenine in the 23S ribosomal RNA, or inactivation of erythromycin by enzymatic hydrolysis (143).

In Vitro *Antimicrobial Activity.* The spectrum of activity of this agent is broad and includes most group A, viridans, and anaerobic streptococci, *A. israelii,* and most strains of *C. jejuni* and other *Campylobacter* species. *Clostridium perfringens* is modestly susceptible. Many *Bacteroides* species are sensitive (more than 90%) but most strains of *B. fragilis* are resistant.

Clinical Pharmacology. Erythromycin is usually administered orally. Since the active form, the free base, is inactivated by gastric acid, many formulations have been prepared to attempt to overcome this problem. These include enterically coated preparations of erythromycin base or derivatives such as salts and ester salts of the base (219). An important point is that despite the many preparations available, no one type appears to offer significant therapeutic advantages over another.

Erythromycin is absorbed from the small bowel and

food usually lowers this absorption. Dissociation or hydrolysis of the free base from its salt or ester occurs either in the intestine or plasma. Once absorbed, erythromycin distributes widely; it concentrates in the liver and spleen and persists in tissues longer than plasma. Good levels occur in ascitic fluid (40% of serum) (220,221). The drug crosses the placenta and is found in breast milk (222). The serum half-life is 1.5 to 2 hr. A large portion is excreted as active drug in the bile where levels may be 28 times that of serum. Some erythromycin excreted in bile is reabsorbed in the intestine. Fecal concentrations of erythromycin are often high owing probably to incomplete absorption. For example, fecal levels of 480 μg/mL have been reported after oral administration (219).

Adverse Effects. Erythromycin is an extremely safe agent but adverse effects occur. The most common are gastrointestinal, perhaps due to the fact that erythromycin stimulates gastrointestinal motility (223). Clinically, these effects manifest as dose-related cramps, vomiting, and diarrhea. Erythromycin can alter fecal flora to a large extent. Cholestatic hepatitis has been reported to occur chiefly in adults receiving the estolate preparation (224) and may be more common in pregnant women. Hepatic dysfunction also has been reported with other erythromycin preparations. Less common adverse effects include transient hearing loss and pseudomembranous colitis associated with *C. difficile* (225).

Precautions. Erythromycin estolate should not be used in persons with hepatic disease or in pregnancy. Other erythromycin preparations are frequently used to treat infections in pregnant women and have not been associated with an increased incidence of fetal defects (18). Nonetheless, use of erythromycin in pregnancy is indicated only when clearly needed.

Drug Interactions. Erythromycin interacts with many drugs metabolized by the hepatic cytochrome P450 system. Concomitant use of erythromycin and carbamazepine in adults has resulted in carbamazepine toxicity. Similar increases in serum levels and toxicity also occur with either cyclosporine or theophylline when they are coadministered with erythromycin. Erythromycin interacts with the antihistamine terfenadine and may lead to potentially serious cardiac arrhythmias. Thus the use of this agent and a related antihistamine, astemizole, with erythromycin is contraindicated (226). Erythromycin may also increase the bioavailability of digoxin and the anticoagulant effect of warfarin due to effects on fecal flora (222).

Azithromycin

Azithromycin is a new macrolide antibiotic related to erythromycin but with enhanced activity against gram-negative bacteria. In particular, the MIC of azithromycin against *C. jejuni* is in the range of 0.24 μg/mL compared with an MIC of 1 μg/mL for erythromycin (227,228). Azithromycin is better absorbed from the gastrointestinal tract than erythromycin but food also inhibits its absorption. Azithromycin concentrations in plasma are low but tissue concentrations are persistent and may be many

times those of serum. The highest concentrations are in the spleen, liver, and peritoneal fluid. Lower but still therapeutic levels exist in gastrointestinal tract mucosa (227,229). Azithromycin is taken up readily by macrophages. The plasma half-life is 11 to 14 hr. Azithromycin is primarily eliminated unchanged in the feces (66%). Transintestinal excretion may be a major route of elimination of the drug into the feces, in addition to the significant biliary excretion (230).

Side effects of the agent are most commonly gastrointestinal (12%) and include diarrhea, nausea, and abdominal pain. Headache and dizziness are uncommon. Interestingly, azithromycin does not appear to induce or inhibit cytochrome P450 enzymes and thus does not alter the pharmacokinetics of theophylline, warfarin, cimetidine, or other agents as does erythromycin, but until more data become available, concomitant use of azithromycin with these agents should be approached with caution (231). Furthermore, it is recommended that azithromycin not be used concurrently with astemizole or terfenadine.

Clarithromycin

Clarithromycin is closely related to erythromycin, differing only by methylation of the hydroxyl group at the sixth position of the lactone ring, which decreases acid catalyzed degradation. The spectrum of activity of clarithromycin is similar to erythromycin but in some cases is greater. In particular, the agent has marked *in vitro* activity against *H. pylori* with a mean MIC = 0.03 μg/mL compared to 0.25 μg/mL for erythromycin (232). It is also active against *Mycobacterium avium* complex. The drug is well absorbed from the gastrointestinal tract. Absorption is little affected by food. High levels of the drug can be found in the gastrointestinal tract, liver, and spleen (233,234). The half-life is 2.5 to 4.4 hr. A portion of the drug is excreted in the feces. The most common adverse effects include diarrhea, nausea, abnormal taste, and abdominal discomfort. Adverse effects, however, are fewer with clarithromycin than with erythromycin (232,235). Clarithromycin may increase carbamazepine levels due to cytochrome P450 inhibition.

Trimethoprim/Sulfamethoxazole

Therapeutic Uses. Trimethoprim/sulfamethoxazole (TMP/SMX) is a combination of the dihydrofolate reductase inhibitor trimethoprim and a sulfonamide. This agent is extremely useful in the treatment of a number of infections due to enteric pathogens including the common causes of traveler's diarrhea (*E. coli* and *Shigella*), *Salmonella* infections, and cholera, among others (85,236,237). In addition, TMP/SMX is effective against the protozoon *Isospora belli* (238). Despite the efficacy of TMP/SMX in treating enteric bacterial infections, resistance to this agent is increasing and in certain parts of the world, including the Americas, is frequently encountered (239–241).

Mechanism of Action. In susceptible bacteria, TMP/SMX inhibits sequential steps in the synthesis of tetrahydrofolate from para-aminobenzoic acid, which is required for synthesis of methionine, purines, glycine, and, most importantly, thymidine (242). The most important mechanism of resistance to TMP involves the production of plasmid-mediated dihydrofolate reductases resistant to TMP (243). Resistance to SMX can be chromosomally or plasmid mediated and can involve (a) overproduction of para-aminobenzoic acid, (b) decreased enzyme affinity for SMX, (c) decreased cell wall permeability to SMX, or (d) increased SMX inactivation (244).

In Vitro *Antimicrobial Activity.* TMP/SMX has a very wide spectrum of activity including *E. coli, Salmonella typhi* and other *Salmonella* species, and *Shigella* species. TMP/SMX also is active against *V. cholerae, Proteus mirabilis, Citrobacter, Y. enterocolitica,* and *A. hydrophila.* Other Enterobacteriaceae are moderately susceptible. Most gram-positive bacteria are susceptible *in vitro.* Anaerobic organisms are resistant.

Clinical Pharmacology. TMP/SMX is usually administered orally for enteric infections. TMP and SMX have similar pharmacological characteristics and thus will be discussed together. Each agent is well absorbed from the gastrointestinal tract primarily from the small intestine although SMX is also absorbed from the stomach. Oral absorption remains efficient in persons with acute gastroenteritis (245). TMP is more lipophilic than SMX and thus tissue levels of TMP are greater especially in the liver. Of note, SMX and TMP levels in the intestinal wall are one-tenth and two times simultaneous serum levels, respectively (246). TMP also penetrates well into most body fluids and bile and serum levels are similar. SMX is also widely distributed in the body, particularly to extracellular fluids (247,248). SMX can be detected in intestinal fluid and to a lesser degree in gastric juice. The half-lives of TMP and SMX are about 10 to 12 hr each. Only small amounts of the drug are excreted in the bile and ultimately in the feces with the major route of excretion via the kidney.

Adverse Effects. TMP/SMX usually is well tolerated but adverse reactions are not infrequent. Most reactions are skin rashes, which are usually mild although serious reactions such as toxic epidermal necrolysis have been reported. Sulfonamides cause a number of blood dyscrasias including leukopenia, thrombocytopenia, eosinophilia, and bone marrow aplasia. Hemolytic anemia may be related to both hypersensitivity and glucose-6-phosphate dehydrogenase deficiency. Other side effects can include drug fever, anaphylaxis, a lupus-like syndrome, renal and liver dysfunction, and gastrointestinal irritation including anorexia, nausea, and diarrhea. Pseudomembranous colitis is rare, perhaps because of a lack of activity toward anaerobic bacteria. Up to 80% of individuals with AIDS receiving this drug have adverse reactions including rash, fever, blood dyscrasias, and liver dysfunction (245,249–252).

Precautions. Use of TMP/SMX in pregnancy is only justified if the benefits of therapy outweigh the risks. TMP/SMX is generally contraindicated in the last trimester of pregnancy because sulfonamides may induce kernicterus in neonates since this agent displaces bilirubin from albumin binding sites. Although TMP has been shown to be teratogenic in animals, human studies have not shown an increase in congenital malformations in infants whose mothers took the drug during pregnancy.

Drug Interactions. Enhanced warfarin-induced anticoagulation can occur with TMP/SMX administration. TMP/SMX potentiates the hypoglycemic effects of oral hypoglycemics and also the bone marrow depression of methotrexate (245).

ANTIVIRAL AGENTS

A limited number of drugs exist for the treatment of viral infections involving the gastrointestinal tract. Of these, most have been developed for the therapy of herpesvirus infections and three agents are discussed in this section: acyclovir, ganciclovir, and foscarnet.

Acyclovir

Therapeutic Uses. Acyclovir, a nucleoside antiviral drug, is used for treatment and prophylaxis of herpes simplex and varicella zoster infections.

Mechanism of Action. The mechanism of action of acyclovir, a virustatic agent, involves selective inhibition of herpesvirus DNA synthesis. After uptake into infected cells, acyclovir is phosphorylated by virus-encoded thymidine kinase to acyclovir triphosphate, the active metabolite, which functions as a substrate for, and preferential inhibitor of, viral DNA polymerase (253). Viruses acquire resistance through selection of thymidine kinase deficient mutants, or alterations in viral thymidine kinases or DNA polymerases (254). Acyclovir is most active against herpes simplex virus type 1, followed by herpes simplex virus type 2 and varicella zoster virus. Epstein–Barr virus and cytomegalovirus (CMV) are much less sensitive (255).

Clinical Pharmacology. Acyclovir can be administered orally or intravenously. Oral absorption is variable and incomplete, with a bioavailability of 15% to 30%; serum levels are the same whether or not the drug is taken with food (256,257). After administration, acyclovir is widely distributed and tissue levels, including liver, are equivalent to or slightly greater than corresponding plasma levels (258). Acyclovir crosses the placenta and is found in high concentrations in human breast milk. Its half-life is 2.5 to 3 hr in patients with normal renal function and renal excretion is the major route of elimination (259).

Adverse Effects. Both oral and intravenous acyclovir are well tolerated. The major adverse effects of the intravenous preparation are nephrotoxicity, neurologic disturbances, and local phlebitis. Both oral and parenteral acyclovir are associated with rash, headache, nausea, and vomiting (255).

Precautions. Acyclovir is not teratogenic in animals at usual doses but has caused chromosomal damage at high dosages. It should therefore be used in pregnancy only when the potential risks are justified (260). Dose reduction is required with renal insufficiency.

Drug Interactions. Acyclovir decreases the renal clearance of methotrexate, and its own half-life may be prolonged by coadministration with probenecid.

Ganciclovir

Therapeutic Uses. Ganciclovir, an acyclic nucleoside analog of guanine, is used in immunocompromised patients for the treatment of CMV infections involving the gastrointestinal tract and is also for prophylaxis of CMV infections in bone marrow transplant recipients.

Mechanism of Action. Ganciclovir is virustatic. Upon entry into cells, ganciclovir undergoes phosphorylation to ganciclovir triphosphate, which inhibits viral DNA polymerase and causes premature termination of chain elongation by its incorporation as a false nucleotide. Resistance to ganciclovir can result from either reduced intracellular phosphorylation or alterations in DNA polymerase (261,262). Ganciclovir has antiviral activity against all human herpesviruses and is much more active than acyclovir against CMV (263).

Clinical Pharmacology. Because of poor oral absorption, ganciclovir is administered intravenously. In animal studies, ganciclovir is distributed widely, achieving levels similar to serum in liver, spleen, stomach, and the intestines. Its half-life is approximately 3 hr and 70% to 90% of the drug is eliminated unchanged by the kidney (264).

Adverse Effects. The most common adverse reaction associated with ganciclovir is bone marrow suppression—predominantly granulocytopenia and thrombocytopenia. Other reported adverse reactions are infrequent and include seizures, phlebitis, rash, nausea, diarrhea, liver function abnormalities, and eosinophilia (265,266).

Precautions. Ganciclovir has been shown to be carcinogenic and mutagenic in animal studies. Pregnancy should be avoided during and for several months after treatment with the agent (267). Ganciclovir passes into the breast milk of animals but it is unknown whether this occurs in humans. Dose adjustment is indicated in patients with renal impairment.

Drug Interactions. Ganciclovir should be used cautiously with other drugs possessing myelosuppressive effects. Generalized seizures have occurred in patients receiving ganciclovir and imipenem, but it is uncertain whether this incidence is greater than with either drug alone (268).

Foscarnet

Foscarnet is the synthetic, trisodium salt of phosphonoformic acid. It is useful in the treatment of CMV infection complicating immunodeficiency states and mucocutaneous lesions secondary to acyclovir-resistant herpes simplex virus.

Foscarnet is virustatic and it prevents replication of human herpesviruses by inhibiting viral DNA polymerases at a different site from nucleoside analogs such as ganciclovir and acyclovir. Clinical isolates of CMV resistant to ganciclovir and of herpes simplex virus resistant to acyclovir have generally been susceptible to foscarnet (269). Changes in viral DNA polymerases confer resistance to foscarnet in herpes simplex virus but resistance to foscarnet has not been reported in CMV (270). *In vitro*, foscarnet has antiviral activity against CMV, herpes simplex viruses 1 and 2, and varicella zoster and also inhibits the human immunodeficiency virus (HIV) (269). Because of poor oral absorption, foscarnet is administered intravenously. It is not metabolized to any significant extent and is eliminated principally by the kidney. Its half-life is 3 hr in patients with normal renal function (271).

The major adverse reaction associated with foscarnet therapy is nephrotoxicity, which may be lessened with saline hyperhydration (272,273). Metabolic derangements, including hypercalcemia, hypocalcemia, hypomagnesemia, hypokalemia, and hyperphosphatemia, are common. Other adverse reactions include penile ulceration, nausea and vomiting, seizures, transient neurological disturbances, and oral and esophageal ulcerations (274,275). There are no adequate human studies of foscarnet in pregnancy, and it should therefore be used only when clearly necessary. Pentamadine may potentiate the hypocalcemic effects of foscarnet. Dosage reduction is necessary in renal disease and foscarnet should be used cautiously with any nephrotoxic agent.

ANTIMYCOBACTERIAL AGENTS

This section focuses on agents used to treat the two most common mycobacterial diseases involving the gastrointestinal tract—disseminated tuberculosis and disseminated *Mycobacterium avium* complex (MAC) disease. Treatment recommendations for these infections have changed over the past several years because of emergence of multidrug-resistant tuberculosis and the increased incidence of atypical mycobacterial disease associated with the AIDS epidemic. Many older drugs have resurfaced, and several newer agents, such as clarithromycin and ciprofloxacin, now have a role in prophylaxis and therapy of mycobacterial disease (Table 7). Although

TABLE 7. *Therapy of mycobacterial infections involving the gastrointestinal tract*

Drug	M. tuberculosis First line	M. tuberculosis Second line	M. avium complex
Amikacin		X	X
Clarithromycin			X
Ciprofloxacin		X	X
Clofazimine			X
Cycloserine		X	X
Ethambutol	X		X
Ethionamide		X	
Isoniazid	X		
Para-aminosalicyclic acid		X	
Pyrazinamide	X		
Rifabutin			X
Rifampin	X		X
Streptomycin	X		X

each agent is discussed separately, the therapy of myco-bacterial infections involves the concurrent use of multiple drugs. Agents that possess both antimycobacterial and antibacterial activity, streptomycin, amikacin, clarithromycin, and ciprofloxacin, have been discussed in the antibacterial section of the chapter.

Isoniazid (INH)

Therapeutic Uses. Isoniazid (isonicotinic acid hydrazide, INH) is useful for the treatment of all forms of tuberculosis.

Mechanism of Action. INH inhibits the synthesis of mycolic acid, an important component of the cell wall of *Mycobacterium tuberculosis,* but it is unclear if this is its primary mechanism of action (276). The compound is bactericidal against growing *M. tuberculosis in vitro* and bacteriostatic against resting organisms (277). Resistance may be intrinsic or develop during therapy as a result of selection of drug-resistant mutants.

Clinical Pharmacology. INH can be administered orally or intramuscularly. The oral preparation is well absorbed from the gastrointestinal tract, although absorption is decreased by the presence of antacids (278). It is widely distributed in body fluids and tissues at concentrations similar to serum levels, with the highest concentrations in liver and bile (279,280). INH crosses the placenta and is excreted in breast milk. It is extensively metabolized to inactive products in the liver by N-acetylation, hydrolysis, and hydrazone formation. The amount of *N*-acetylisoniazid, the major metabolite formed, is determined genetically, as fast acetylators form more of this metabolite than slow acetylators (281). The clinical relevance of this is uncertain, although peripheral neuropathy is more common in slow acetylators (282). The half-life of INH varies from 1 to 4 hr, being shorter in fast acetylators. INH and its metabolites are primarily excreted in the urine.

Adverse Effects. Isoniazid causes mild hepatic dysfunction as manifested by increased liver enzymes in 10% to 20% of patients taking the drug (283). Liver function abnormalities may occur at any time during therapy but are most common in the first 3 months. Occasionally, continuation of INH will lead to progressive liver damage, which is age-related (284). Isoniazid is also neurotoxic as a result of enhancement of vitamin B$_6$ (pyridoxine) excretion, and its administration can lead to peripheral neuropathy. Patients at risk for nutritional deficiencies should be supplemented with pyridoxine while taking INH (285). Other less common side effects include gastrointestinal disturbances, rash, and seizures.

Precautions. Liver functions tests should be monitored during INH therapy. INH is a component of the multidrug regimen (along with rifampin and ethambutol) considered safe for use during pregnancy (286,287).

Drug Interactions. Isoniazid potentiates phenytoin, carbamazepine, and possibly acetaminophen toxicity (288). Coadministration with para-aminosalicylic acid increases levels of INH.

Rifampin

Therapeutic Uses. Rifampin, in combination with other drugs, is useful in the treatment of all forms of tuberculosis. It is also a component of combination therapy for MAC.

Mechanism of Action. Rifampin inhibits mycobacterial DNA-dependent RNA polymerase, and is bactericidal against *M. tuberculosis.* Resistance to rifampin develops rapidly if the drug is used alone; it is most likely due to a conformation change in the mycobacterial polymerase based on a point mutation (289).

Clinical Pharmacology. Rifampin is administered orally and is well absorbed from the gastrointestinal tract (290). It is widely distributed in body fluids and tissues, including the liver, bile, ascites, and pancreatic fluid, and it diffuses well into abscesses (291,292). It is metabolized in the liver to its active form and undergoes enterohepatic recirculation. The half-life of the drug is 3 hr and excretion is primarily via the bile. Rifampin crosses the placenta and is excreted in human breast milk (293).

Adverse Effects. Rifampin is associated with mild and transient disturbances in liver function especially during the first several weeks of its administration; however, this effect is self-limited in patients with no history of liver disease. There is little evidence that rifampin causes severe liver damage (294). Hypersensitivity reactions, manifested by flushing and pruritis, gastrointestinal disturbances, and an influenza-like syndrome are the most frequent clinical side effects. Hemolytic anemia, thrombocytopenia, acute renal failure, and respiratory insufficiency occur rarely (293). Rifampin turns body fluids orange and may permanently stain soft contact lenses.

Precautions. Rifampin is a component of a multidrug regimen (along with INH and ethambutol) considered safe for use during pregnancy (286). Liver function tests should be monitored during rifampin therapy.

Drug Interactions. Rifampin is a potent inducer of the hepatic cytochrome P450 enzyme system in humans. Clinically important interactions have been documented between rifampin and numerous other drugs, including oral anticoagulants, oral contraceptives, cyclosporine, ketoconazole, phenytoin, sulfonylureas, theophylline, and verapamil (295,296).

Ethambutol

Ethambutol is useful in the treatment of all forms of *M. tuberculosis* infection and disseminated MAC infection. Its precise mechanism of action is unknown but may involve inhibition of mycolic acid or RNA synthesis in mycobacteria (297). Ethambutol is administered orally and is well absorbed from the gastrointestinal tract. The drug is widely distributed, reaching high concentrations in intestinal tissues (298). Ascitic fluid concentrations are lower than corresponding serum concentrations. Ethambutol crosses the placenta and is excreted in human breast milk. It is eliminated primarily in the urine, and its half-life is 3.3 hr in patients with normal renal function (299).

The most important adverse effect of ethambutol is retrobulbar neuritis, which can lead to blurred vision, red–green color blindness, and decreased visual acuity. These ocular complications are infrequent and usually reversible but are more common if high dosages of the drug are administered for long periods of time (284). Visual acuity and red–green color discrimination should be monitored during ethambutol therapy. The majority of patients taking ethambutol develop hyperuricemia, which may cause gout. Other adverse effects include skin rash, peripheral neuropathy, gastrointestinal disturbances, and hypersensitivity reactions. Ethambutol is one of the drugs recommended for treatment of tuberculosis during pregnancy, although its adverse effects on the fetus are not entirely known since ocular toxicity is difficult to monitor in young children (286,288,300).

Pyrazinamide (PZA)

Pyrazinamide (PZA), in combination with other agents, is a first line drug for the treatment of tuberculosis. PZA is highly effective against phagocytized, tubercle bacilli, but its mechanism of action is unknown (301). Mycobacteria that lack the enzyme that hydrolyzes pyrazinamide to pyrazinoic acid are resistant to pyrazinamide (302).

PZA is administered orally and absorption is rapid and virtually complete (303,304). PZA is widely distributed throughout the body and accumulates in the liver; its half-life is 9 to 10 hr. PZA is metabolized by the hepatic microsomal enzyme system, and its metabolites are primarily excreted in the urine. It is also excreted in the bile, but levels are not therapeutic (301). The drug is excreted in human milk.

Hepatotoxicity is the most important adverse effect of PZA, being more common when larger doses are administered for longer durations (305). The most frequent adverse effect of PZA is a nongouty polyarthralgia associated with increased serum uric acid (303). Other adverse reactions include gastrointestinal intolerance and flushing. Liver function tests should be monitored during therapy with PZA. Routine use of PZA during pregnancy is not recommended because of the risk of teratogenicity (286). PZA has been reported to lower cyclosporine levels (306).

Clofazimine

Clofazimine is useful in the treatment of disseminated MAC infections in patients with AIDS. Its mechanism of action is unknown but may relate to iron chelation and free radical formation (307). The drug is administered orally and absorption is variable but increased with food (308). Clofazimine distributes widely to many body sites, particularly reticuloendothelial tissues, and it penetrates well into liver, spleen, lymph nodes, gallbladder, and distal small bowel, reaching concentrations higher than those in serum. Clofazimine tends to remain in tissues for up to several months. The compound crosses the placenta and is found in human breast milk. The serum half-life is

8 days and clofazimine is primarily excreted unchanged in the feces (308,309).

The most prominent adverse effect of clofazimine is a dose-related red–brown skin discoloration that is caused by the accumulation of the drug itself. Discoloration of sweat, hair, sputum, urine, and feces has also been observed as have gastrointestinal side effects, which include anorexia, nausea, vomiting, diarrhea, and crampy abdominal pain. The safety of clofazimine in pregnancy has not been well established. Infants born to mothers who received the drug during pregnancy may have darker skin color than expected, and this hyperpigmentation fades in the children who were not breast-fed (310). Breast-fed children of mothers receiving clofazimine may also develop skin discoloration. Clofazimine reduces rifampin absorption in patients with leprosy. The significance of this drug interaction in other patient populations is not known. Clofazimine is synergistic with clarithromycin against MAC *in vitro* (311).

Rifabutin

Rifabutin has recently been approved for the prophylaxis of MAC infections in patients with AIDS. The mechanism of action in mycobacterial infections is unknown but it inhibits DNA-dependent RNA polymerase in susceptible bacteria. Cross-resistance between rifabutin and rifampin occurs in MAC. Rifabutin is administered orally and is rapidly but incompletely absorbed from the gastrointestinal tract; its absorption is unaffected by food. The bioavailability is unpredictable, ranging from 85% in healthy adult volunteers to as low as 20% in patients infected with HIV (312,313). Rifabutin is highly lipophilic, with a propensity for intracellular tissue uptake. Its plasma half-life is 45 hr and it is extensively metabolized in the liver; it is excreted in feces, bile, and urine.

The most common adverse reactions associated with rifabutin therapy are rash, gastrointestinal intolerance, and neutropenia. Rifabutin recently has been associated with uveitis in HIV-infected patients. Body fluids may be colored brown–orange with rifabutin administration, and soft contact lenses may be permanently stained. Rifabutin induces hepatic cytochrome P450 enzymes and may enhance the clearance of some types of drugs, but to a lesser extent than rifampin. Rifabutin decreases plasma concentrations of zidovudine in HIV-positive patients (314).

Ethionamide

Ethionamide, a derivative of isonicotinic acid, is a second line agent for the treatment of tuberculosis. It exerts its antimycobacterial activity by inhibiting mycolic acid synthesis (315). Ethionamide is usually administered orally and is well absorbed (316). It can also be administered per rectum, but absorption is unpredictable (317). The compound is widely distributed to body sites and crosses the placenta. It has a half-life of 3 hr, is extensively metabolized, and is eliminated in the urine.

Gastrointestinal disturbances, including nausea, vomiting, anorexia, diarrhea, crampy abdominal pain, and metallic taste, are the most common adverse reactions to ethionamide and often limit its clinical use (318). Less common side effects include peripheral neuropathy, personality disturbances, rash, and hepatotoxicity. Ethionamide is teratogenic at high doses and should be avoided during pregnancy. It interferes with INH acetylation and hepatotoxicity may be worsened when administered with rifampin (319).

Para-aminosalicylic acid (PAS)

Para-aminosalicylic acid (PAS) is a second line antituberculous agent. PAS is administered orally and is rapidly absorbed from the gastrointestinal tract (320). It is well distributed to body sites; in animal studies it reaches high concentrations in the liver. Peritoneal fluid concentrations are equal to serum concentrations. The half-life of the drug is 1 hr and it is excreted primarily via the kidney with low concentrations in the bile. It is also excreted in human breast milk (321). Adverse effects are frequent and limit its use. Gastrointestinal disturbances, including nausea, vomiting, anorexia, cramping, and diarrhea, are almost universal. Hypersensitivity reactions occur in up to 5% of patients, manifested by fever, rash, pruritis, and eosinophilia (322). Less common adverse effects include hepatotoxicity, neutropenia, acute hemolytic anemia in patients with glucose-6-phosphate dehydrogenase deficiency, prolongation of the prothrombin time, and goiter (319,320). The safety of this drug in pregnancy is controversial because it may increase the risk of fetal malformation. PAS interferes with the absorption of rifampin and increases the serum levels and hepatotoxicity of INH (319).

Cycloserine

Cycloserine is useful as a second line agent against *M. tuberculosis* infection and as part of a combination regimen for disseminated MAC disease. It is well absorbed orally and distributes into bile, lymphatic tissue, and ascitic fluid. The half-life of cycloserine is 10 hr and it is excreted by glomerular filtration. It crosses the placenta and is present in human breast milk (323).

Adverse effects to cycloserine include central nervous system dysfunction and peripheral neuropathy, which may be aggravated by ethanol ingestion. Hepatotoxicity, fever, rash, and arrhythmia are rare side effects. Cycloserine should be used in pregnancy only when clearly indicated.

ANTIFUNGAL AGENTS

Fungal infections involving the gastrointestinal tract are most commonly due to *Candida* species, although other fungi may disseminate to involve the gastrointestinal tract. Agents most frequently used to treat these infections include amphotericin B and the azole group of drugs.

Amphotericin B

Therapeutic Uses. Amphotericin B, the first commercially available systemic antifungal drug, is used frequently in the treatment of deeply invasive fungal infections involving the gastrointestinal tract and for the prevention of invasive fungal disease in high-risk populations such as organ transplant recipients.

Mechanism of Action. Amphotericin B binds to sterols present in the cell membranes of susceptible fungi, resulting in altered membrane permeability (324). Oxidative damage and immunomodulation may also contribute to its antifungal properties. Resistance to amphotericin B is rare but may be acquired during therapy and is associated with alterations in membrane sterol composition (325,326).

Amphotericin has a broad spectrum of activity that includes most of the major fungal pathogens in humans such as *Candida albicans* and other *Candida* species, *Cryptococcus neoformans*, *Blastomyces dermatitidis*, *Paracoccidioides brasiliensis*, *Histoplasma capsulatum*, *Coccidioides immitis*, *Aspergillus* species, and most zygomycetes.

Clinical Pharmacology. Amphotericin B is poorly absorbed orally and is thus administered intravenously for treatment of systemic fungal infections. After intravenous infusion, concentrations of amphotericin B in body fluids are low compared with serum levels. In peritoneal fluid, for example, levels less than 50% of comparable serum concentrations are achieved. However, for localized fungal pertionitis, treatment with intraperitoneal amphotericin B has been successful (327). The agent is excreted in bile, where it reaches high concentrations. The highest tissue concentrations of amphotericin B are observed in reticuloendothelial tissues such as liver and spleen (328). Elimination of amphotericin B from serum follows a biphasic pattern, with an initial half-life of 24 to 48 hr, followed by a long elimination half-life of up to 15 days, which probably is due to the extremely slow release of the drug from peripheral tissues. Five percent to 10% of amphotericin B is excreted in urine and bile (329).

Adverse Effects. Infusion-related acute toxicities are common during amphotericin B administration and include rigors, fever, nausea, vomiting, headache, and local phlebitis. Less common but more severe acute reactions are hypotension, hypertension, and hyperkalemia in patients with renal failure. The most important long-term side effect is nephrotoxicity, with a permanent dose-related reduction in glomerular filtration rate in almost all patients treated. Renal tubular acidosis is common with large doses of amphotericin B. Other adverse reactions include headache, electrolyte disturbances, and hematologic side effects (329,330).

Precautions. Amphotericin B crosses the placenta and its safety during the first trimester of pregnancy has not been determined conclusively. A review of the limited experience on the use of amphotericin B during pregnancy, however, revealed no teratogenesis or permanent side effects in the infants of treated mothers (331).

Drug Interactions. Rifampin, tetracycline, and flucytosine may enhance the antifungal effects of amphotericin

TABLE 8. *Pharmacokinetic properties of azole antifungal agents*

Property	Ketoconazole	Fluconazole	Itraconazole
Route of administration	Oral	Oral, iv	Oral
Absorption favored at	Low pH	No pH effect	Low pH
Bioavailability	75%	85–90%	99%
Half-life	2–8 hr	~30 hr	15–20 hr
Effect of food on absorption	Both enhancement and reduction reported	None	Enhances
Effect of GI drugs on absorption	Antacids, anticholinergics, H_2 blockers ↓ absorption	No effect	Antacids ↓ absorption
Metabolism	Extensive (liver)	None	Extensive (liver)
Excretion	Feces/bile	Urine	Feces/urine
Dose adjustment in renal failure	None	Decrease	None

B. Studies of the interaction of amphotericin B with azole antifungal agents have yielded both antagonistic and synergistic effects on various fungi (332,333).

Azole Antifungal Agents

Therapeutic Uses. Ketoconazole, fluconazole, and itraconazole are useful in prophylaxis and therapy of mucosal candidiasis and invasive fungal infections and possess less toxicity than amphotericin B.

Mechanism of Action. The azole compounds inhibit a fungal cytochrome P450-dependent enzyme that is involved in the synthesis of ergosterol, a major component of the fungal cell membrane (334). Acquired resistance to the azoles is rare but when it has occurred, the fungi have been cross-resistant to other azole compounds (335). The azole antifungal agents exhibit a broad range of activity. The compounds demonstrate *in vitro* activity against *Candida albicans, Cryptococcus neoformans, Histoplasma capsulatum,* and *Coccidioides immitis.* Ketoconazole and itraconazole are effective against *Blastomyces dermatitidis.* Only itraconazole has any substantial activity against *Aspergillus* species (336).

Clinical Pharmacology. The pharmacokinetic properties of the azole antifungal agents differ substantially (Table 8). Fluconazole is the only azole available as either an intravenous or oral preparation. After administration, it distributes widely with high tissue levels, especially in the liver and spleen (337). Peritoneal fluid levels of fluconazole are roughly equivalent to plasma levels, and biliary levels are high. Itraconazole levels in liver and spleen also are high, being 3.5 and 1.9 times corresponding serum levels, respectively, and it penetrates well into abscess cavities (338,339). Ketoconazole diffuses rapidly into many body fluids including peritoneal fluid. Only its inactive metabolites are excreted in bile (340). All of the azole compounds are excreted in breast milk.

Adverse Effects. The azole antifungal agents are well tolerated and have excellent safety profiles (Table 9). The major side effects are nausea, vomiting, and hepatotoxicity. Ketoconazole has rarely been associated with severe hepatic toxicity, including some fatalities. Ketoconazole also inhibits mammalian steroid metabolism to a greater extent than the other azoles (341).

Drug Interactions and Precautions. The azole compounds inhibit the cytochrome P450 enzyme system not only in fungi but also in humans and thus alter the metabo-

TABLE 9. *Adverse effects and drug interaction profile of azole antifungal agents*

Drug	Adverse effect	Drug interactions	
		Drug effect potentiated by azoles	Plasma azole concentrations lowered by
Ketoconazole	GI disturbance Hepatotoxicity Antiandrogen effects Decreased cortisol response Hypersensitivity reactions	Warfarin, cyclosporine, phenytoin, oral hypoglycemics, terfenadine, astemizole	INH, rifampin
Fluconazole	GI disturbance Hepatotoxicity Stevens–Johnson syndrome	Warfarin, cyclosporine, phenytoin, oral hypoglycemics	Rifampin
Itraconazole	GI disturbance Hepatotoxicity Doses ≥ 600 mg/day: hypertension, severe hypokalemia, adrenal insufficiency, rhabdomyolysis	Warfarin, cyclosporine, phenytoin, oral hypoglycemics, terfenadine, astemizole, digoxin	INH, rifampin, phenobarbital, carbamazepine, phenytoin

TABLE 10. *Antiprotozoal agents useful for gastrointestinal infections*

Drug	Preferred therapy for infection	Alternative therapy for infection
Iodoquinol	*Entamoeba histolytica* (asymptomatic) *Dientamoeba fragilis*	*Balantidium coli* *Blastocystis hominis*[a]
Paromomycin	*Entamoeba histolytica* (asymptomatic) *Dientamoeba fragilis*	*Cryptosporidium*[a]
Diloxanide furoate[b]	*Entamoeba histolytica* (asymptomatic)	
Metronidazole (and other nitroimidazoles)	*Entamoeba histolytica* (invasive intestinal and extraintestinal) *Entamoeba polecki* *Giardia lamblia*	*Balantidium coli* *Blastocystis hominis*[a]
Emetine,[c] dehydroemetine[b]		*Entamoeba histolytica* (invasive intestinal and extraintestinal)
Chloroquine		*Entamoeba histolytica* (extraintestinal)
Tetracyclines	*Balantidium coli*	*Entamoeba histolytica* (invasive intestinal)
Erythromycins		*Entamoeba histolytica* (invasive intestinal)
Quinacrine	*Giardia lamblia*	
Furazolidine	*Giardia lamblia*	
Trimethoprim/ sulfamethoxazole	*Isospora belli*	

[a] Small numbers of patients have responded to this agent. No large trials have been reported.
[b] Available in the United States from Centers for Disease Control and Prevention.
[c] Not available in the United States.

lism of many drugs (Table 9). Ventricular arrhythmias have occurred in patients receiving ketoconazole or itraconazole and terfenadine, and the use of these azoles with terfenadine and a related antihistamine, astemizole, is contraindicated (342). Because of their potential for hepatotoxicity, liver function tests should be monitored prior to, and during, therapy with the azoles. The systemic azole antifungal agents have been shown to be teratogenic in animals at high doses, but no studies exist in humans. Their use in pregnancy should therefore be limited to situations in which the benefit outweighs this potentially serious side effect.

THE ANTIPARASITIC AGENTS

Agents to treat parasitic infections can be divided into two broad categories: those primarily used against protozoa (Table 10) and those active against helminths, either nematodes (Table 11), trematodes, or cestodes. For several agents, this division is artificial. For example, quinacrine and paromomycin are active against both protozoa and helminths. Furthermore, praziquantel, a very broad spectrum anthelmintic drug, is active against trematodes and cestodes.

As with other pathogens, resistance to new and old antiparasitic agents is of concern although with protozoa its clinical significance is unclear. The ability to induce resistance *in vitro* to commonly used antiprotozoal agents in pathogens such as *Entamoeba histolytica* or *Giardia lamblia* gives one pause for concern (343,344). Resistance also has been reported in helminths to all commonly used anti-infective agents. This is particularly true for parasitic infections in animals where widespread use of drugs such as the benzimidazoles, ivermectin, and levamisole has led

to a high frequency of resistance (345). At this time, the issue of resistance in helminths infecting humans is unclear. The possibility, however, that parasitic resistance will become a problem in human infections dictates the need for further understanding of factors affecting resistance, support for the development of new agents, and the judicious use of antiparasitic drugs already available to avoid the problem of selecting resistance through their indiscriminate use.

Agents Useful in the Treatment of Protozoal Infections

Iodoquinol (Diiodohydroxyquin)

Therapeutic Uses. Iodoquinol, a halogenated quinoline derivative used in the therapy of amebiasis, is considered to be an agent of choice in the treatment of asymptomatic cyst passage with cure rates greater than 80% (346,347). The drug also is useful in eradicating organisms from the bowel lumen of individuals with invasive intestinal or extraintestinal amebiasis after treatment with agents such as nitroimidazoles. It is not to be used, however, as sole therapy of invasive disease because treatment failures are common. Iodoquinol is also an agent of choice for the therapy of infection due to *Dientamoeba fragilis* and an alternative therapy of *Balantidium coli* infection (347). It has been employed in the treatment of *Blastocystis hominis,* although it is uncertain how often this organism is a human pathogen (348,349).

Mechanism of Action. The mechanism of action of iodoquinol is unknown although it has been hypothesized that the agent may chelate ferrous iron essential for metabolism in sensitive protozoa (187). Nonetheless, iodo-

TABLE 11. *Agents useful for nematode infections*

Drug	Preferred therapy	Alternative therapy
Mebendazole	*Capillaria philippinensis*	
	Ascaris lumbricoides	
	Enterobius vermicularis	
	Trichuris trichiura	
	Trichinella spiralis	
	Trichostrongylus	
	Hookworm	
	Angiostrongylus cantonensis	
Albendazole[a]	Hookworm	*Capillaria philippinensis*
	Ascaris lumbricoides	*Strongyloides stercoralis*
	Enterobius vermicularis	
	Trichuris trichiura	
	Echinococcus granulosus	
	Cysticercus cellulosae	
Thiabendazole	*Strongyloides stercoralis*	
	Trichinella spiralis	
Pyrantel pamoate	*Enterobius vermicularis*	
	Ascaris lumbricoides	
	Hookworm	
	Trichostrongylus	
Ivermectin[b]		*Strongyloides stercoralis*
Levamisole		*Ascaris lumbricoides*
Piperazine citrate		*Ascaris lumbricoides*
		Enterobius vermicularis

[a] Available in the United States from the manufacturer.
[b] Available in the United States from Centers for Disease Control and Prevention.

quinol is directly amebicidal and is active against both trophozoite and cyst forms of *E. histolytica* (350).

Clinical Pharmacology. Iodoquinol is administered orally. Approximately 5% of the drug is absorbed from the intestine and is excreted in the urine as sulfate and glucuronide conjugates (351). The bulk of iodoquinol is excreted in the feces and this is probably responsible for its antiamebic activity.

Adverse Effects. The most serious adverse effect caused by iodoquinol is neurotoxicity, which is related to dose and duration of therapy. The drug has been associated with optic and peripheral neuropathy. Administration of iodoquinol to children with chronic diarrhea has been associated with optic atrophy and vision loss (352,353). Dysesthesias and weakness also have been reported in adults as have agitation and confusion. Administration of large doses of halogenated quinolines for long periods of time has resulted in a syndrome of subacute myelo-opticoneuropathy (SMON) manifested by muscle pain, weakness, optic atrophy, and ataxia. This disorder was first described in Japan with the use of a related quinoline, iodochlorohydroxyquin (clioquinol) (354). The disorder reached epidemic proportions in the 1960s involving thousands of people. The agent was banned in Japan in 1970 and this led to an immediate and dramatic reduction in the incidence of SMON (355). Iodochloroxhydroxyquin is not available in the United States but is available in Mexico and other developing countries; travelers should be specifically warned against using this agent. Other side effects of iodoquinol may include gastrointestinal disorders such as nausea, vomiting, diarrhea, and constipation.

Absorption of iodoquinol may result in iodine toxicity

manifested clinically by generalized furunculosis (iodine toxicoderma) and other skin reactions. It also may cause thyroid enlargement and interfere with thyroid function studies.

Precautions. Iodoquinol should be administered with caution to patients with thyroid disease and is contraindicated in persons with renal or hepatic disease, optic neuropathy, or iodine hypersensitivity. Use in pregnancy or during lactation has not been established.

Paromomycin

Therapeutic Uses. Paromomycin, an aminoglycoside antibiotic used in the therapy of *E. histolytica* infection, is an agent of choice for the treatment of asymptomatic cyst passage with cure rates of at least 80% (356). It also has been used to treat mild to moderate intestinal disease with a high efficacy rate (357,358), although it may not be first line therapy for symptomatic disease since metronidazole is so effective (359). However, paromomycin is indicated for use in eradicating organisms from the bowel lumen of persons with invasive intestinal or extraintestinal disease once they have been treated with an agent such as a nitroimidazole. It should not be used as sole therapy for extraintestinal disease. Paromomycin also is effective in the therapy of gastrointestinal infection due to *Dientamoeba fragilis*. Furthermore, recent reports have suggested some efficacy in the treatment of *Cryptosporidium* infections in patients with AIDS (360–362). Paromomycin also has use in the treatment of cestodiasis due to *Taenia saginata, T. solium, Hymenolepis nana, Diphyllo-*

bothrium latum, and *Dipylidium caninum* with cure rates in excess of 90% in some studies, although other agents such as niclosamide or praziquantel are more commonly used (363).

Mechanism of Action. Paromomycin is directly amebicidal and has high *in vitro* activity against *Cryptosporidium parvum,* although the mechanism of action is not known (364). Paromomycin also markedly alters gut flora, which may have a detrimental effect on protozoa (187). Its mechanism of action against cestodes also is poorly understood, but when administered to humans, paromomycin causes destruction of cestode segments. This is of theoretical concern in the therapy of *T. solium* infection since humans are the intermediate host and the release of a large number of viable eggs could result in dissemination of larval forms to tissues.

Clinical Pharmacology. Paromomycin is poorly absorbed from the gastrointestinal tract with nearly 100% remaining in the intestinal lumen and is subsequently excreted in the feces. Thus levels in the bowel lumen are extremely high. Although the small portion that is absorbed is subsequently excreted in the urine, impaired gastrointestinal motility or intestinal ulcerations may enhance absorption and potentially result in adverse effects such as renal dysfunction (95).

Adverse Effects. Side effects of paromomycin therapy are mainly limited to the gastrointestinal tract and include anorexia, nausea, vomiting, diarrhea, and, rarely, rash and eosinophilia. Paromomycin has been reported to cause malabsorption of sugar and fats. Gastrointestinal overgrowth due to nonsusceptible organisms also may occur. Parenteral administration of paromomycin to animals results in severe renal damage.

Precautions. Paromomycin should not be used in persons with impaired renal function or with intestinal obstruction. Because it is poorly absorbed, it may be used during pregnancy if the benefits outweigh the risks (365).

Diloxanide Furoate

Therapeutic Uses. Diloxanide furoate is a luminally active agent used in the treatment of asymptomatic *E. histolytica* infection. The drug may also be useful in eradicating organisms from the bowel of persons with invasive intestinal disease or extraintestinal infection after treatment with agents such as nitroimidazoles. Diloxanide furoate is not recommended as the sole therapy for invasive intestinal or extraintestinal amebiasis due to low cure rates (358,366). Because diloxanide furoate is relatively inexpensive, effective (90% to 95% eradication), and well tolerated, it is an agent of choice for asymptomatic amebiasis (367). Diloxanide furoate (Furamide) is available in the United States only from the Centers for Disease Control and Prevention, Drug and Immunobiologics Service, 1600 Clifton Road, Bldg. 1 Room 1259, Atlanta, GA 30333; telephone 404/639-3670 days, 404/639-2888 nights and weekends.

Mechanism of Action. The mechanism of action of diloxanide is unknown but the compound is amebicidal *in vitro* against *E. histolytica.*

Clinical Pharmacology. After administration of diloxanide furoate orally to rats, most of the drug is hydrolyzed to free diloxanide by intestinal esterases. Diloxanide is then absorbed to a large extent and 60% to 90% of an administered dose is excreted in the urine after 48 hr, primarily in the form of a glucuronide conjugate. Four percent to 9% of the dose is excreted in the feces and this fraction is believed to be largely responsible for antiamebic activity of the drug. Delayed or reduced absorption of diloxanide furoate is believed to improve the luminal effect due to higher concentrations of the agent in the large bowel (368,369).

Adverse Effects. Diloxanide furoate is a safe agent. Side effects have generally been mild and include excessive flatulence, which is observed in a large percentage of patients (366,370). Occasionally, nausea, anorexia, diarrhea, or abdominal cramps occur.

Precautions. The safety of diloxanide in pregnancy has not been established and it is not recommended for use in this situation. It is unknown if it passes into human breast milk.

Metronidazole and Other Nitroimidazoles

Metronidazole

Metronidazole has revolutionized the therapy of many parasitic diseases. Not only is this agent extremely effective in the treatment of infection due to a number of organisms, but it also is associated with a relatively low incidence of side effects and is fairly inexpensive. Since much of the pharmacology of metronidazole has been discussed (in the section on Antibacterial Agents), this section briefly reviews aspects of the drug pertinent to antiprotozoal therapy. Metronidazole has a broad spectrum of activity and is considered the therapy of choice for both invasive intestinal and extraintestinal amebiasis (347,371). Because of its limited activity against cysts, however, metronidazole is often combined with a luminal agent, such as diloxanide (367). Metronidazole is also the therapy of choice for *Entamoeba polecki* infection and is very useful in the treatment of giardiasis and *Balantidium coli* infection (152). The mechanism of action of metronidazole against protozoa is believed to be the same as that against anaerobic bacteria (157,372). Clinically significant resistance to metronidazole has been reported infrequently and is poorly documented for both *E. histolytica* and *G. lamblia* but has been induced in *Giardia in vitro* (344).

Tinidazole

Tinidazole is a nitroimidazole closely related to metronidazole. Although not available in the United States, its indications for use are essentially the same as for metronidazole. It is an agent of choice in the therapy of invasive intestinal and extraintestinal amebiasis (347,367) and it is effective in the therapy of giardiasis (347,373). Tinidazole, like metronidazole, also is effective against anaerobic bacteria and may be of use in *Helicobacter pylori* infections (374,375). The mechanism of antimicrobial activity for tinidazole is believed to be the same as metronidazole. Tinidazole is usually administered as an oral preparation but has also been administered parenterally and per rectum. The drug is well absorbed from the gastrointestinal tract after oral administration (376); the serum half-life is 12 to 14 hr (377). Tinidazole is widely distributed in the body and the drug penetrates well into the bowel. Levels of tinidazole in the small intestine and colonic wall of rats are about one-half and two to four times simultaneous serum levels, respectively (378). The drug can be detected in these tissues in humans also. The agent is more lipid soluble than metronidazole and thus may penetrate tissues better. Levels in bile are similar to serum. Tinidazole is cleared mainly by metabolism (377,379). Urinary excretion accounts for 50% to 70% of the total dose. In the rat and dog, a significant percentage (15% to 20%) of an administered dose is excreted in the feces but only 2% to 3% is as unchanged drug (380).

The adverse effects of tinidazole are similar to metronidazole and are usually mild and infrequent. Nausea, vomiting, anorexia, and a metallic taste are most common. Tinidazole may cause neutropenia. As with metronidazole, it may produce a disulfiram-like reaction when administered with alcohol. Overall, adverse effects occur less frequently with tinidazole than metronidazole (347).

Ornidazole and Other Nitroimidazoles

Ornidazole is another nitroimidazole used in the therapy of protozoal infections in various parts of the world but is not available in the United States. It is effective in the therapy of amebic colitis, amebic liver abscess, and giardiasis (381,382). Its mechanism of action is believed to be the same as metronidazole and tinidazole. The agent is usually administered orally and is rapidly absorbed (383,384); its serum half-life is between 10 and 14 hr (164). Although it is primarily excreted in the urine as metabolized drug, about 22% is excreted in the feces. Adverse effects are similar to other nitroimidazoles although they may occur more frequently with ornidazole. In particular, dizziness is a frequent complaint.

Nimorazol, which is not available in the United States, is effective for giardiasis and amebiasis (373,385).

Emetine and Dehydroemetine

Therapeutic Uses. Previously, emetine and dehydroemetine were the agents of choice for the therapy of invasive intestinal and extraintestinal amebiasis. With the development of the nitroimidazoles, however, these agents are now considered alternative agents, to be used only when the nitroimidazoles are ineffective or contraindicated. Emetine and dehydroemetine are not indicated for the therapy of luminal disease since luminal concentrations of drug may be low (350). Thus, for the therapy of invasive intestinal amebiasis or extraintestinal disease, the emetines should be combined with a luminal agent.

Furthermore, for hepatic disease, the combination of chloroquine and an emetine yields a higher cure rate than either drug alone (386,387). Both emetine and dehydroemetine are toxic, which accounts, to a large extent, for their decreased use. Since dehydroemetine may be less toxic, there is no reason to use emetine over dehydroemetine and the former is no longer available in the United States (187). Dehydroemetine can only be obtained from the Centers for Disease Control and Prevention, Drug and Immunobiologics Service, 1600 Clifton Road, Bldg. 1 Room 1259, Atlanta GA 30333; telephone 404/639-3670 days, 404/639-2888 nights and weekends.

Mechanism of Action. Emetine and dehydroemetine are directly amebicidal, the former being somewhat more potent. Both agents are much more effective against amebic trophozoites than cysts. The mechanism of action appears to be inhibition of protein synthesis at the step of polypeptide elongation (372,388). Resistance to emetine can be induced in *E. histolytica in vitro* through induction of a protein produced by a multidrug resistance-like gene, which acts as a pump to remove emetine and other antiamebic agents from within the protozoa (343). The clinical relevance of this is unclear.

Clinical Pharmacology. The emetines are administered by the deep subcutaneous or intramuscular routes. Intravenous administration of these agents is contraindicated because of cardiac toxicity. Oral preparations of the emetines have been used for luminal disease with variable success but are not of use in invasive or extraintestinal infection (187). After administration, the emetines are absorbed from parenterally administered sites and excreted or metabolized slowly, although their disposition is poorly understood. The highest concentration of these agents is in the liver, which may account for their efficacy in hepatic amebiasis (350,389). The kidney is possibly the major route of excretion for the emetines although animal studies point to the gut as an important route of excretion (187,390).

Adverse Effects. Adverse reactions associated with the emetines are common (350). Both agents accumulate in the body and side effects are more common with prolonged administration. The most serious adverse reactions are cardiovascular and include hypotension, tachycardia, chest pain, dyspnea, and EKG changes. EKG changes occur in 25% to more than 50% of patients receiving emetine. They generally include QRS, T wave, and ST segment changes rather than arrhythmias. In general, cardiovascular side effects may be less frequent, severe, and persistent with dehydroemetine than with emetine although this is not conclusive (350,391,392).

Other adverse effects associated with the emetines include damage to the liver, kidney, gastrointestinal tract, and skeletal muscles. Gastrointestinal effects include diarrhea, nausea, and vomiting. Emetine-induced diarrhea occurs in up to 50% of patients (393). Other side effects can include headache, skeletal muscle weakness, local injection site pain, and rashes.

Precautions. These agents are contraindicated in pregnancy and in persons with kidney and heart disease. Retreatment of individuals not responding to therapy should be delayed 6 to 8 weeks to avoid toxicity. Persons receiving these agents should generally be hospitalized and cardiac status monitored.

Chloroquine

The primary use of chloroquine is for the prophylaxis and therapy of malaria. In addition, although it is effective in the therapy of extraintestinal amebiasis, the use of chloroquine is limited to those few patients who do not respond to nitroimidazole therapy. Chloroquine is quite useful in the therapy of hepatic amebiasis, probably because it achieves very high levels in hepatic tissue (394). Combination therapy with dehydroemetine or emetine improves cure rates (386,387). In some cases of severe infection, it also has been administered with nitroimidazoles. Chloroquine is not useful in invasive intestinal or asymptomatic infections (187,347).

Chloroquine is generally administered orally and is well absorbed (90%) (395). It has a very large volume of distribution and is extensively distributed to many tissues, most notably the liver (396). Levels in the bowel are much lower. Regarding its efficacy in treating hepatic amebiasis, chloroquine concentrates up to 700-fold in liver compared to serum. Chloroquine crosses the placenta (397).

The adverse reactions associated with chloroquine therapy are generally mild, are usually dose related, and include gastrointestinal discomfort consisting of nausea and diarrhea. Rash, headache, central nervous system stimulation, visual disturbances, and blood dyscrasias also occur. Acute hemolysis in persons with glucose-6-phosphate dehydrogenase deficiency has been reported occasionally. Long-term treatment with chloroquine has been associated with retinopathy. Patients receiving prolonged therapy should have visual examinations. Chloroquine should be used with caution in persons with liver disease and may be used during pregnancy if necessary. Chloroquine passes into human breast milk but the drug level is not thought harmful to a nursing infant. Concomitant administration of chloroquine and rabies vaccine intradermally may interfere with the antibody response to the vaccine. Cimetidine may inhibit metabolism of chloroquine and increase plasma levels of the drug.

Quinacrine

Quinacrine is an acridine derivative considered by many to be an agent of choice for the treatment of giardiasis because of cure rates of 90% to 95% (347,398). The cure rate, however, may be lower in children. Quinacrine also has been used for the treatment of tapeworm infestations but has been replaced, to some degree, by agents such as niclosamide. Quinacrine is active, however, against a wide range of cestodes including *Diphyllobothrium latum*, *Dipylidium caninum*, *Hymenolepis diminuta*, *H. nana*, *Taenia saginata*, and *T. solium*. Quinacrine is an attractive therapy for parasitic infections because it is effective and inexpensive, but it is associated with many adverse effects.

Mechanism of Action. Although quinacrine binds to DNA and inhibits nucleic acid synthesis, the mechanism of its activity is unknown (399). Quinacrine does not kill susceptible cestodes but causes the scolex of the cestode to dislodge from the intestinal wall. The worm is then passed with normal fecal flow. Interestingly, worms that are passed are often stained bright yellow.

Clinical Pharmacology. Quinacrine is administered orally and is well absorbed even in the presence of severe diarrhea. It distributes widely to tissues especially the pancreas, spleen, and liver, where it is tightly bound, and it crosses the placenta. Extremely high concentrations occur in liver after prolonged administration (396). Quinacrine is slowly eliminated from tissues and its metabolism is poorly understood although it is believed to be primarily excreted in the urine (350); trivial amounts are excreted in the bile.

Adverse Effects. The administration of quinacrine is associated with a number of side effects (400,401), commonly including nausea, vomiting, headaches, dizziness, diarrhea, and bright yellow coloring of the urine. Rashes and fever also may occur. Other rare adversities include dizziness, exfoliative dermatitis, reversible acute psychosis, and liver dysfunction (402). High doses of quinacrine can turn the skin yellow (403).

Precautions. Quinacrine should be used with caution in patients with psoriasis as it may exacerbate this condition. Quinacrine should only be used in pregnancy if the benefits justify the risk as the agent crosses the placenta. It is teratogenic in animals at high dosages and it should be used with caution in patients with renal and hepatic disease.

Drug Interactions. Quinacrine should not be used in combination with primaquine because it competes with primaquine for tissue binding sites and may markedly elevate plasma primaquine levels. If taken with alcohol, it may induce a disulfiram-like reaction.

Furazolidine

Therapeutic Uses. Furazolidine, a nitrofurantoin derivative, is an agent of choice for the therapy of giardiasis; cure rates are in the range of 75% to 90% (398). Although it is especially useful in children because it is available in liquid form, in the United States it is less commonly used than quinacrine or metronidazole. Furazolidine also is active against a number of enteric bacteria including *Salmonella*, *Shigella*, *Campylobacter*, *H. pylori*, *Vibrio cholerae*, *E. coli*, *Klebsiella*, *Enterobacter*, and *Bacteroides*. It is useful for the treatment of bacterial enterocolitis and traveler's diarrhea and for cholera (85,404,405).

Mechanism of Action. The antimicrobial activity of nitrofurans appears to involve reductive activation to compounds that damage DNA. The selective toxicity of furazolidine against *Giardia* may be due to its limited gut absorption and selective activation by reductases in the parasite (372).

Clinical Pharmacology. Following oral administration, furazolidine is very poorly absorbed from the gastrointestinal tract. About 5% or less of the oral dose is excreted in the urine as unchanged drug and metabolites although studies have been limited. Drug remaining in the intestine is inactivated to a large extent (406).

Adverse Effects. The most common adverse effects are nausea and vomiting with abdominal pain and diarrhea less frequent. Hypersensitivity reactions, fever, headache, and malaise also occur. Hemolysis may occur in persons with glucose-6-phosphate dehydrogenase deficiency. Furazolidine is mutagenic in bacteria and produces urinary tumors in mice (407). Rarely, a disulfiram-like reaction may occur with ethanol ingestion (372).

Precautions. Use in pregnancy has not been established but no adverse effects to the fetus have been noted. It is unknown if it passes into breast milk. Furazolidine may act as a monoamine oxidase inhibitor and thus should be given cautiously to individuals receiving indirectly acting sympathomimetic amines.

Agents Useful in the Treatment of Helminthic Infections and Intestinal Nematode Infections

Mebendazole

Therapeutic Uses. Mebendazole is a very useful broad spectrum anthelmintic benzimidazole (Table 11) (408,409). It is the agent of choice for infections due to *Capillaria philippinensis* (cure rates up to 100%), hookworm infections (cure rates higher than 90%), *A. lumbricoides*, pinworm (cure rate higher than 90%), *Trichuris trichiura* (high cure rates and 95% egg reduction), *Trichostrongylus, Angiostrongylus cantonensis,* and *Trichinella spiralis* (410–419). Administered at high doses, mebendazole may kill encysted larvae of *T. spiralis,* unlike thiabendazole. Mebendazole also has been used successfully in tapeworm infections due to *Taenia saginata* and *T. solium* (420), but other agents such as niclosamide are preferrable. The drug has also been useful in inoperable cystic hydatid disease caused by *E. granulosus* but albendazole is preferred (421).

Mechanism of Action. Mebendazole acts by inhibiting microtubule assembly and irreversibly blocking glucose uptake, thereby inhibiting glycogen stores and decreasing ATP formation in susceptible helminths. Parasite immobilization and death ensue. The agent is effective on adult worms, nematode larvae, and eggs (422). Resistance among animal parasites to mebendazole appears to involve alterations in the ability of the drug to bind parasite tubulin (345).

Clinical Pharmacology. After oral administration, only 5% to 10% of a dose is absorbed, which probably accounts for the marked activity of this agent against intraluminal organisms. Absorption is increased with fat intake (423). In individuals with hydatid disease, levels in cyst fluid are low (424). The half-life of mebendazole in plasma is 1.4 to 5.5 hr. Absorbed mebendazole is metabolized by the liver with excretion of the metabolites in urine and bile (425).

Adverse Effects. Mebendazole is relatively free of side effects when used at low doses to treat intestinal parasites. Transient abdominal pain and diarrhea occur with large parasite burdens. In addition, after administration of the agent for the treatment of ascariasis, worms may crawl through the mouth and nose of patients. Persons receiving large doses of the drug for hydatid disease may experience fever early in the course of treatment. Alopecia, reversible leukopenia and thrombocytopenia also have been reported as have pruritis and skin rashes (426). Mebendazole produces embryotoxicity and teratogenicity in pregnant rats and is thus contraindicated in pregnancy. It is unknown whether the agent passes into breast milk.

Drug Interactions. Mebendazole may increase the secretion of insulin and thus potentiate the effect of exogenously administered insulin and oral hypoglycemics. Carbamazepine and phenytoin decrease the serum concentration of mebendazole while cimetidine increases levels of mebendazole by inhibiting its metabolism (427).

Albendazole (and Flubendazole)

Therapeutic Uses. Albendazole, a benzimidazole compound related to mebendazole, possesses broad spectrum anthelmintic activity; its spectrum of activity is similar to mebendazole. Since albendazole is only available in the United States directly from the manufacturer, mebendazole is usually the preferred agent in this country. An exception is the therapy of hydatid disease because albendazole is more effective than mebendazole. Albendazole has been shown to be highly effective in the therapy of *A. duodenale* (90% cure and higher), *N. americanus* (80% cure and higher), *A. lumbricoides* (90% cure and higher), and pinworm infections (428–431). Approximately 65% to 75% of whipworm infections are cured by one dose of albendazole and egg counts decrease significantly (432); additional doses may improve results (428). The drug also is effective in capillariasis, strongyloidiasis, and *Trichostrongylus* infections. It also has been successful in the treatment of tapeworm and *Opisthorchis viverrini* infections but is generally not used (433,434). Finally, albendazole is an agent of choice for use as perioperative treatment or as an alternative to surgery in hydatid disease due to *E. granulosus* (435) and it is an agent of choice in cysticercosis (436).

Flubendazole is a fluorine analog of mebendazole, which has similar efficacy as mebendazole in a variety of helminthic infections (437). It is unavailable in the United States but is widely used in other parts of the world (408).

Mechanism of Action. Albendazole is effective against adult, larval, and, in some cases, egg forms of many nematodes and cestodes. Its mechanism of action is the same as mebendazole (345,438).

Clinical Pharmacology. After oral administration, absorption of albendazole from the gastrointestinal tract is low and unchanged drug cannot be detected in plasma. Fat increases intestinal absorption. Absorbed drug is rapidly converted to albendazole sulfoxide, an active metabolite. Therapeutic concentrations of this metabolite are detectable in plasma 4 hr after drug administration and significant quantities are present in hydatid cyst fluid (439,440). The half-life of the metabolite is about 8.5 hr. The primary route of excretion of absorbed albendazole is in the urine as the sulfoxide metabolite. The metabolite also is present in bile. The great majority of ingested albendazole is excreted in the feces.

Adverse Effects. When given in dosages to treat intestinal helminthiasis, albendazole is well tolerated. Constipation, diarrhea, abdominal pain, and dizziness are infrequent. Alopecia may be associated with prolonged therapy. Hematological and biochemical parameters remain unaltered following short-term therapy with albendazole, but rises in transaminases may occur with long-term dosing (441). Albendazole is contraindicated in pregnancy and it is unknown if it passes into breast milk.

Drug Interactions. With prolonged dosing, albendazole enhances its own metabolism by inducing hepatic microsomal enzymes (442). Thus it may interact with other microsomally metabolized drugs.

Thiabendazole

Therapeutic Uses. Thiabendazole is a benzimidazole anthelmintic, which is a drug of choice for the treatment of *Strongyloides stercoralis* and *Trichinella spiralis* infections. In trichinellosis, the agent is active against intestinal organisms and reduces the number of developing and migrating larvae but is ineffective against encysted larvae. In strongyloidiasis, cure rates are about 75% to 90% (443,444). It is active against adult worms and also prevents development of nematode eggs and larvae (445). In addition, thiabendazole is active against many other intestinal nematodes including *A. lumbricoides*, *E. vermicularis*, and *T. trichiura* but other more safe and effective agents are available.

Mechanism of Action. It had been believed that the primary mechanism of action of thiabendazole was to inhibit the mitochondrial fumarate reductase system in susceptible helminths (446); however, as with other benzimidazoles, thiabendazole also may act to inhibit microtubule assembly (447).

Clinical Pharmacology. Thiabendazole is rapidly and extensively absorbed (over 90%) after oral ingestion; its plasma half-life is about 1.2 hr. Thiabendazole is extensively metabolized and primarily excreted in the urine; 5% of an administered dose is recovered in the feces and 90% in the urine, of which less than 1% is unchanged (448–450).

Adverse Effects. Thiabendazole causes side effects in a high percentage (over 50%) of patients. Most commonly these include nausea, dizziness, malodorous urine and sweat, malaise, and neuropsychiatric disorders (426,444). Other less common adversities include anorexia, vomiting, abdominal pain, headache, flushing, and rashes. Administration of thiabendazole with meals may limit side effects. The agent should not be used during pregnancy as it has been reported to be teratogenic in mice. It is unknown whether it passes into breast milk. The drug should be used with caution in renal and hepatic disease.

Drug Interactions. Thiabendazole may compete with drugs metabolized by the liver and increase serum concentrations of drugs, such as xanthine derivatives including theophylline.

Pyrantel Pamoate

Pyrantel pamoate is an anthelmintic agent of choice in the treatment of enterobiasis, ascariasis, and hookworm infestations (347,451–454). This agent is also the drug of choice against *Trichostrongylus* species but is less active against trichuriasis. It acts as a depolarizing neuromuscular blocker, causing contracture of the worm and paralysis (426,455). The worm then is passed out with normal fecal flow.

Little is known of the pharmacokinetics of pyrantel because no simple analytical method exists to measure the drug in plasma. Nonetheless, absorption from the gastrointestinal tract is very low. Less than 4% of a dose is recovered in the urine during the 2 to 3 days after administration. The vast majority of the drug is excreted unchanged in feces, which accounts to a large degree for its efficacy (451,456).

The principal adverse effects of pyrantel are uncommon (5%) and include nausea, vomiting, cramps, and diarrhea. Headache may also occur (426,451,453). Transient increases in serum glutamic-oxaloacetic transaminase (SGOT) also have been reported. Use of pyrantel pamoate in pregnant women has not been reported and thus the use of this agent in pregnancy is justified only if the benefits outweigh the risk. It is unknown whether pyrantel passes into breast milk. Pyrantel and piperazine appear mutually antagonistic and should not be used together.

Ivermectin

Ivermectin is primarily of use in humans for the treatment of onchocerciasis, particularly when ocular involvement is present. It also is effective in humans for intestinal nematode infestations due to *Strongyloides stercoralis* with cure rates of about 90% to 100% in small studies and it is considered an alternative agent for infections due to this organism (457,458). Ivermectin is available in the United States only from the Centers for Disease Control and Prevention, Drug and Immunobiologics Service, 1600 Clifton Road, Bldg. 1 Room 1259, Atlanta, GA 30333; telephone 404/639-3670 days, 404/639-2888 nights and weekends.

The mechanism of action of ivermectin appears related to inhibition of neural transmission in nematodes by gamma-aminobutyric acid-dependent and -independent pathways (345,459). Resistance to ivermectin has been reported in animal helminths, but its mechanism is unknown. Pharmacokinetic studies of ivermectin in humans are limited (460). Nonetheless, the drug is readily absorbed from the gastrointestinal tract after oral administration. The mean plasma half-life is 12 hr. The drug is widely distributed and extensively metabolized in humans. Less than 1% is excreted in the urine with the major route of elimination of the parent drug and metabolites being the feces. The agent can be found in breast milk (461).

In general, ivermectin is a safe agent when administered to persons with intestinal nematode infections. Mild constipation has been reported most frequently. Transient liver and renal abnormalities have been observed in patients receiving the agent but it is unclear whether this was due to ivermectin. Ivermectin is not recommended in pregnancy as animal studies have associated the agent with congenital defects and maternal mortality (460).

Levamisole

Levamisole is an immunomodulating drug currently used in the United States primarily for the therapy of colon carcinoma. It possesses activity, however, against a broad range of intestinal nematodes and has been used extensively as an antiparasitic agent in animals (462). Levamisole can be used in treatment of *Ascaris* infections in humans with a cure rate over 90%, although it is considered an alternative agent for this indication (463–465). Levamisole also has activity against *S. stercoralis* and hookworm (454).

Levamisole acts as a cholinergic agonist in nematodes to induce sodium outflow, depolarization of muscle bag membranes, and muscle contraction, leading to paralysis and subsequent elimination of the worm (465,466). Resistance to levamisole among animal nematodes has been reported and may involve reduction in the sensitivity or number of cholinergic receptors to levamisole (345). Resistance in human parasites has not been well-documented.

Levamisole is rapidly absorbed from the gastrointestinal tract after oral administration. The elimination half-life is 3 to 4 hr. The drug is extensively metabolized by the liver in humans and excreted primarily in the kidney (70%); 5% of the drug (of which less than 0.2% is unchanged) is excreted in the feces (467). The overall incidence of adverse events is about 10%. The most common are gastrointestinal toxicities including nausea, vomiting, and diarrhea. Rash, a flu-like syndrome, dizziness, and ataxia also may occur. Agranulocytosis also has been reported (462,467). Levamisole should not be used in pregnancy unless the benefits justify the risks. In animals, extremely high doses are embryotoxic. It is unknown whether the agent passes into human breast milk but it passes into cow milk.

Piperazine Citrate

Piperazine citrate is an inexpensive second line anthelmintic agent useful in the therapy of ascariasis and enterobiasis. In the treatment of *A. lumbricoides,* cure rates range from 76% to 94% while it is more than 95% effective in the therapy of enterobiasis (468,469). The predominant effect of piperazine in helminths is to cause flaccid paralysis of the worm, resulting in helminth expulsion from the gut by normal fecal flow (426,470); this may occur by disruption of cellular ion channels in sensitive helminths.

Piperazine is rapidly but variably absorbed from the small intestine after oral administration. No data exist with regard to its pharmacokinetics. Some of the drug is metabolized, probably in the liver, and excreted in the urine. Interindividual variation in the rate of drug excre-

tion appears to exist (471,472). Piperazine is relatively safe. Infrequently, nausea, vomiting, diarrhea, and allergic reactions may develop (426). The drug accumulates in renal dysfunction. Large dosages can result in muscular incoordination, weakness, and confusion. It may induce or exacerbate seizures. Hepatitis and blood dyscrasias have been reported rarely. Piperazine is contraindicated in persons with seizures or renal disease. No harmful effects on the fetus have resulted from the administration of this agent to pregnant women. It is unknown whether it crosses into human breast milk. Concomitant administration of chlorpromazine and piperazine may induce seizures; thus use of these agents together should be approached with caution (473). Furthermore, piperazine and pyrantel pamoate have antagonistic modes of action and should not be administered concomitantly.

Agents Useful Against Trematode and Cestode Infections Involving the Gastrointestinal Tract

Praziquantel

Therapeutic Uses. Praziquantel represents a major advance in the therapy of helminthic infections (474,475). It has a very broad spectrum of activity, is safe, requires a relatively short course of therapy, and penetrates both tissues and infecting parasites well. Its major drawback is that it is relatively expensive compared to other anthelmintic agents.

The spectrum of activity of praziquantel (Table 12) includes all stages of infections due to pathogenic *Schistosoma* in humans including those caused by *Schistosoma mansoni, S. haematobium, S. japonicum, S. mekongii,* and *S. intercalatum* (476). For these pathogens, praziquantel is clearly the agent of choice. Cure rates for infections caused by these organisms vary between 75% and 100%; and no evidence of schistosomal resistance has been detected to date. In addition, praziquantel is the drug of choice in the treatment of other fluke infections (Table 12) (347,477–480). Praziquantel is also as effective as niclosamide in treating intestinal infections due to cestodes and is effective in the treatment of cysticercosis caused by *T. solium* larvae and is an agent of choice along with albendazole for this indication (436).

Mechanism of Action. Praziquantel is rapidly taken up by susceptible helminths. Praziquantel has two mechanisms of action against these organisms. First, at low concentrations, it increases muscular activity followed by contraction and spastic paralysis of the worm probably by making the membrane permeable to cations such as calcium and sodium (481). Second, praziquantel causes vacuolation and vesiculation of the tegument of the parasite, increasing its susceptibility to host defenses (482).

Clinical Pharmacology. Praziquantel is nearly completely absorbed (more than 90%) from the gastrointestinal tract after oral administration (483). The distribution of praziquantel occurs rapidly and is extensive with significant accumulation in liver and kidneys, which may explain its rapid elimination in urine and bile. Its plasma half-life is 3 to 8 hr. Most of the drug is metabolized and

TABLE 12. *Helminthic infections for which praziquantel is an effective therapy*

Organism	Therapy of choice	Alternate therapy
Trematodes		
All *Schistosoma* species	X	
Paragonimus westermani	X	
Clonorchis sinensis	X	
Opisthorchis viverrini	X	
Fasciolopsis buski	X	
Heterophyes heterophyes	X	
Fasciola hepatica		X
Cestodes (adult stage)		
Diphyllobothrium latum	X	
Taenia saginata	X	
Taenia solium	X	
Dipylidium caninum	X	
Hymenolepis nana	X	
Cestodes (larval stage)		
Cysticercus cellulosae (cysticercosis)	X	

80% to 85% of an administered dose of praziquantel is excreted in the urine in 4 days (484,485). Praziquantel crosses the blood–brain barrier and is effective in neurocysticercosis.

Adverse Effects. Praziquantel is generally well tolerated, but patients may have nausea, abdominal pain, fullness, dizziness, headache, or malaise. Many of these symptoms begin 30 min after administration of the drug and subside within several hours. Other infrequent side effects include diarrhea, urticaria, fever, rash, and liver dysfunction. Symptoms appear dose related (486). The incidence of side effects varies but can be as high as 40% to 50%. Patients with neurocysticercosis may develop a syndrome of headache, hyperthermia, seizures, and other central nervous system signs when treated with praziquantel. This is believed related to an inflammatory response to dying organisms in tissues and can be avoided by prior corticosteroid therapy.

No harmful effects resulting from the use of this agent in pregnant or lactating women have been reported but the manufacturer cautions against the use of the agent in this situation. It is unknown whether praziquantel crosses the placenta, but it passes into breast milk. No serious adverse drug interactions have been reported.

Oxamniquine

Since the introduction of praziquantel, oxamniquine has become an alternative agent for the therapy of *Schistosoma mansoni* infections. Despite being an alternative agent, millions of people have received oxamniquine and cure rates are over 80% (487,488). It is useful in all stages of *S. mansoni* infection, but its mechanism of action is unknown. Oxamniquine, however, induces a shift of worms from mesenteric vessels to the liver within a few days of administration, possibly because it causes muscular paralysis that impairs the adult worm suckers.

Male worms are retained in the liver and die. Females return to the mesenteric veins but are unable to lay eggs and subsequently die (489). Resistance to oxamniquine has been reported in several strains of *S. mansoni*, one obtained from a patient unresponsive to treatment (490). More commonly, however, there appear to be geographic variations in schistosome sensitivity to oxamniquine that is independent of acquired resistance.

Oxamniquine can be administered orally or intramuscularly although the former route is preferred. After oral administration, oxamniquine is well absorbed, but food in the small bowel may delay absorption. Little else is known about the pharmacology of oxamniquine other than that the half-life is 1 to 1.25 hr. The drug is extensively metabolized in the liver and only about 1% is excreted in urine as unchanged drug (491).

Dizziness and somnolence are the most common side effects (492). Other side effects include headache, nausea, abdominal pain, diarrhea, increases in liver transaminases, fever, and a Loeffler-like syndrome (426,493). Seizures have been reported rarely. Orange discoloration of the urine may occur. Oxamniquine should not be given to pregnant women as related compounds are teratogenic and carcinogenic although there is no evidence that this is true of oxamniquine. The drug also should be avoided in persons with a seizure disorder. It is unknown whether the drug passes into breast milk.

Bithionol

Bithionol is an anthelmintic that is the therapy of choice for the treatment of *F. hepatica* infection and is an alternative agent to praziquantel for paragonimasis (494,495). The cure rate is >90% in pulmonary paragonimiasis and is very high in *F. hepatica* infections. The anthelmintic activity of this agent may be related to interference in adenosine triphosphate (ATP) production in parasites through uncoupling of oxidative phosphorylation and in this regard its mechanism of action may be similar to niclosamide (496). Bithionol is administered orally but little is known of its pharmacology. Side effects occur frequently and include epigastric pain, nausea, vomiting, diarrhea, and photosensitization reactions. Cardiotoxicity also has been reported. The agent is available in the United States only from the Centers for Disease Control and Prevention, Drugs and Immunobiologics Service, 1600 Clifton Road, Bldg. 1 Room 1259, Atlanta, GA 30333; telephone 404/639-3670 days, 404/639-2888 nights and weekends.

Tetrachloroethylene

Tetrachloroethylene is a colorless, volatile liquid used as a second line agent in the therapy of intestinal fluke infections and also in hookworm infestations due to *N. americanus*. The cure rate of tetrachloroethylene in *F. buski* infections is higher than 80% and is similar in *N. americanus* infestations (497,498). Interestingly, the cure rate is far lower for *A. duodenale*. The mechanism of action of tetrachloroethylene is unknown. The agent is administered orally and its absorption is minimal in the absence of fatty food or alcohol. Tetrachloroethylene is a reasonably safe agent but can cause dizziness, nausea, vomiting, or a loss of consciousness. The drug is infrequently employed in the United States but is available for use as a veterinary preparation (426).

Niclosamide

Therapeutic Uses. Niclosamide is an important agent for the treatment of cestode infections. It is a drug of choice for *Taenia saginata, Diphyllobothrium latum,* and *Dipylidium caninum* (499,500). It is also an alternative agent of choice for *Hymenolepis nana.* It is not effective in cysticercosis or echinococcosis caused by tapeworm larvae infecting extraintestinal tissues (501). The drug is also a therapy of choice for *T. solium* infection although many authorities prefer quinacrine or praziquantel because niclosamide destroys *T. solium* segments during therapy, releasing eggs that could theoretically result in cysticercosis, although this has not been reported. Niclosamide also is an alternative therapy for *F. buski* infections.

Mechanism of Action. Niclosamide is believed to act by inhibition of oxidative phosphorylation in the mitochondria of cestodes resulting in scoleceal detachment and worm disintegration (500,502).

Clinical Pharmacology. Up to 15% to 20% of niclosamide is absorbed from the gut after oral administration. The absorbed portion is metabolized to the amino derivative. Little else is known about the pharmacology of this agent other than the material that remains in the gut is believed to exert the primary anthelmintic effect. Niclosamide is primarily excreted in the feces and may be metabolized to some extent in the gut.

Adverse Effects. In about 10% of patients, malaise, abdominal pain, and nausea occur on the day the drug is administered. Niclosamide has been used without adverse effects in pregnant women; nonetheless, its use in pregnancy is generally not recommended as cestode infections are usually not life-threatening. Alcohol may enhance gut absorption of niclosamide.

ACKNOWLEDGMENTS

This work was supported in part by NIH Grants GM42056 and GM15431. J. D. Morrow is a Howard Hughes Medical Institute Physician Research Fellow and the recipient of a Career Development Award from the International Life Sciences Institute. K. M. Neuzil was supported by NIH Training Grant GM07569. The secretarial assistance of Kathy Cunningham and Barbara Weaver was greatly appreciated.

REFERENCES

1. Blumberg PM, Strominger JL. Interaction of penicillin with the bacterial cell: penicillin-binding proteins and penicillin sensitive enzymes. *Bacteriol Rev* 1974;38:291–335.
2. Tomasz A. The mechanism of irreversible antimicrobial effects of penicillins: how the β-lactam antibiotics kill and lyse bacteria. *Annu Rev Microbiol* 1979;33:113–137.
3. Strominger JL. How penicillin kills bacteria: a short history. In: Schlessinger D, ed. *Microbiology—1977.* Washington, DC: ASM Publications, 1977;177–181.
4. Neu HE. Penicillins. In: Mandell GL, Douglas RG, Bennett JE, eds. *Principles and practice of infectious diseases,* 3rd ed. New York: Churchill Livingstone, 1990;230–246.
5. Penicillins. In: *Drug evaluations annual 1993.* Chicago: American Medical Association, 1993;1309–1343.
6. Weiss ME, Adkinson NF. β-lactam allergy. In: Mandell GL, Douglas RG, Bennett JE, eds. *Principles and practice of infectious diseases,* 3rd ed. New York: Churchill Livingstone, 1990; 264–269.
7. Idsoe O, Guthe T, Willcox RR, DeWeek AL. Nature and extent of penicillin side reactions, with particular reference to fatalities from anaphylactic shock. *Bull World Health Organ* 1968; 38:159–188.
8. Kaplan MS. Penicillin allergy. In: Lichtenstein LM, Fauci AS, eds. *Current therapy in allergy, immunology and rheumatology,* 4th ed. St Louis: BC Decker, 1992;126–131.
9. Arndt KA, Jick H. Rates of cutaneous reactions to drugs. *JAMA* 1976;235:918–923.
10. Gurwith MJ, Rabin HR, Love K, Co-Operative Antibiotic Diarrhea Study Group. Diarrhea associated with clindamycin and ampicillin therapy: preliminary results of a co-operative study. *J Infect Dis* 1977;135(Suppl):104–110.
11. Lusk RH, Fekety FR, Silva J, et al. Gastrointestinal side effects of clindamycin and penicillin therapy. *J Infect Dis* 1977; 135(Suppl):111–119.
12. Toffler RB. Acute colitis related to penicillin and penicillin derivatives. *Lancet* 1978;2:707–709.
13. Andrassy K, Weischedel E, Ritz E, Andrassy T. Bleeding in uremic patients after carbenicillin. *Thromb Haemost* 1976;36: 115–126.
14. Brunner FP, Frick PG. Hypokalemia, metabolic alkalosis and hypernatremia due to "massive" sodium penicillin therapy. *Br Med J* 1968;4:550–552.
15. Ruley EJ, Lisi LM. Interstitial nephritis and renal failure due to ampicillin. *J Pediatr* 1974;84:878–881.
16. Nichols PJ. Lead article. Neurotoxicity of penicillin. *J Antimicrob Chemother* 1980;6:161–165.
17. Wright AJ, Wilkowski CJ. The penicillins. *Mayo Clin Proc* 1987;62:806–820.
18. Brigg GG, Freeman RK, Yaffe SJ. *Drugs in pregnancy and lactation,* 3rd ed. Baltimore: Williams & Wilkins, 1990.
19. Colandra T, Cometta A. Antibiotic therapy for gram-negative bacteremia. *Infect Dis Clin North Am* 1991;5:817–834.
20. Lepper MH, Dowling HF. Treatment of pneumococcic meningitis with penicillin compared with penicillin plus aureomycin: studies including observations on apparent antagonism between penicillin and aureomycin. *Arch Intern Med* 1951;88: 489–494.
21. Back DJ, Breckenridge AM, Maciver M, et al. The effects of ampicillin on oral contraceptive steroids in women. *Br J Clin Pharmacol* 1982;13:280p–281p.
22. Penicillins. In: McEvoy GK, ed. *AHFS drug information 93—American Hospital Formulary Service.* Bethesda: American Society of Hospital Pharmacists, 1993;207–309.
23. Peabody JN, Seabury JH. Actinomycosis and nocardiosis. *Am J Med* 1960;28:99–115.
24. Keinath RD, Merrell DE, Vliestra R, Dobbins WO. Antibiotic treatment and relapse in Whipple's disease. Long term follow-up of 88 patients. *Gastroenterology* 1985;88:1867–1873.
25. Kucers A, Bennett NMcK. Penicillin G. In: *The use of antibiotics,* 4th ed. Philadelphia: Lippincott, 1987;3–81.
26. Bolme P, Erickson M. Absorption of phenoxymethylpenicillin in children. The influence of age, state of disease and pharmaceutical preparation. *Scand J Infect Dis* 1978;10:223–227.
27. Bolme P, Erickson M. Influence of diarrhea on the oral absorption of penicillin and ampicillin in children. *Scand J Infect Dis* 1975;7:141–145.
28. Gerding DN, Hall WH, Schierl EA. Antibiotic concentrations

in ascitic fluid of patients with ascites and bacterial peritonitis. *Ann Intern Med* 1977;86:708–713.

29. Bergman BR. Concentrations of dicloxacillin and benzylpenicillin in fracture hematoma. *Scand J Infect Dis* 1979;11:225–228.

30. Labenz J, Gyenes E, Ruhl GH, Borsch G. Efficacy of omeprazole and amoxicillin to eradicate HP. *Am J Gastroenterol* 1992;87:1271(abst).

31. Hentschel E, Brandstatter G, Dragosics B, et al. Effects of ranitidine and amoxicillin plus metronidazole on the eradication of *Helicobacter pylori* and the recurrence of duodenal ulcer. *N Engl J Med* 1993;328:308–312.

32. Prevention of bacterial endocarditis. *Med Lett* 1989;31:112.

33. Berant M, Wagner Y. Antibiotic treatment of shigellosis. *J Pediatr* 1979;95:334.

34. Sutherland R, Croydon EAP, Rolinson GN. Amoxycillin: a new semisynthetic penicillin. *Br Med J* 1972;3:13–16.

35. Stewart GT. *The penicillin group of drugs.* Amsterdam: Elseiver, 1965.

36. Ramirez-Ronda CH, Gutierrez J, Bermudez RH. Comparative effectiveness, safety and tolerance of mezlocillin and ticarcillin, a prospective, randomized trial. *J Antimicrob Chemother* 1982;9(Suppl A):125–129.

37. Pancoast SJ, Jahre JA, Neu HC. Mezlocillin in the therapy of serious infections. *Am J Med* 1979;67:747–752.

38. Winston DJ, Murphy W, Young LS, et al. Piperacillin therapy of serious bacterial infections. *Am J Med* 1980;69:255–261.

39. Brogden RN, Heel RC, Speight TM, Avery GS. Ticarcillin: a review of its pharmacologic properties and therapeutic efficacy. *Drugs* 1980;20:325–352.

40. Kucers A, Bennett NMcK. The newer antipseudomonal penicillins. In: *The use of antibiotics,* 4th ed. Philadelphia: Lippincott, 1987;225–253.

41. Joiner KA, Lowe BR, Dzink JL, Bartlett JG. Antibiotic levels in infected and sterile subcutaneous abscesses in mice. *J Infect Dis* 1981;143:487–494.

42. Holmes B, Richards DM, Brogden RN, Heel RC. Piperacillin: a review of its antibacterial activity, pharmacokinetic properties and therapeutic use. *Drugs* 1984;28:375–425.

43. Russo J, Thompson MIB, Russo ME, Saxon BA, Matsen JM, Moody FG, Rikkers LF. Piperacillin distribution into bile, gallbladder wall, abdominal skeletal muscle and adipose tissue in surgical patients. *Antimicrob Agents Chemother* 1982;22:488–492.

44. Thompson RL. Cephalosporin, carbapenem and monobactam antibiotics. *Mayo Clin Proc* 1987;62:821–834.

45. Donowitz GR, Mandell GL. Cephalosporins. In: Mandell GL, Douglas RG, Bennett JE, eds. *Principles and practice of infectious diseases,* 3rd ed. New York: Churchill Livingstone, 1990;246–257.

46. Bank NU, Kammer RB. Hematological complications associated with β-lactam antibiotics. *Rev Infect Dis* 1983;5(Suppl):380–393.

47. Nichols RL, Wikler MA, McDevitt JT, Lentnek AL, Hosutt JA. Coagulopathy associated with extended spectrum cephalosporins in patients with serious infections. *Antimicrob Agents Chemother* 1987;31:281–285.

48. Bang NU, Kammer RB. Hematologic complications associated with β-lactam antibiotics. *Rev Infect Dis* 1983;5(Suppl):380–393.

49. Carlberg H, Alestig K, Nord CE, Trollfors B. Intestinal side effects of cefoperazone. *J Antimicrob Chemother* 1982;10:483–487.

50. Bartlett JG, Willey SH, Chang TW, Lowe B. Cephalosporin associated pseudomembranous colitis due to *C. difficile. JAMA* 1979;242:2683–2685.

51. Jacobs RF. Ceftriaxone-associated cholecystitis. *Pediatr Infect Dis J* 1988;7:434–436.

52. Pigrau C, Pahissa A, Gropper S, Sureda D, Martinez-Vasques JM. Ceftriaxone-associated biliary pseudolithiasis in adults. *Lancet* 1989;2:165.

53. Cephalosporins and miscellaneous β-lactam antibiotics. In: McEvoy GK, ed. *AHFS drug information 93—American Hospital Formulary Service.* Bethesda: American Society of Hospital Pharmacists, 1993;92–186.

54. Wade JC, Petty BG, Conrad GS, et al. Cephalothin plus an aminoglycoside is more nephrotoxic than methicillin plus an aminoglycoside. *Lancet* 1978;2:604–606.

55. Reeves DS, Davies AJ. Antabuse effect with cephalosporins. *Lancet* 1980;2:540.

56. Kucers A, Bennett NMcK. Cephazolin, cephacetrile, and cephapirin. In: *The use of antibiotics,* 4th ed. Philadelphia: Lippincott, 1987;381–397.

57. Ellis BW, Standbridge R Del, Sikorski JM, Dudley HAF. Penetration into inflammatory exudate and wounds of 2 cephalosporins for the prevention of surgical infections. *J Antimicrob Chemother* 1975;1:291–296.

58. Ishiyama S, Nakayama I, Iwamoto H, Iwai S, Okui M, Matsubara T. Absorption, tissue concentration, and organ distribution of cefazolin. *Antimicrob Agents Chemother* 1970:476–480.

59. O'Keefe JP, Tally FP, Barza M, Gorbach SL. Penetration of cephalothin and cefoxitin into experimental infections with *Bacteroides fragilis. Rev Infect Dis* 1979;1:106–117.

60. Lau WY, Fan ST, Chu KW, et al. Cefoxitin versus gentamicin and metronidazole in prevention of post appendectomy sepsis: a randomized prospective trial. *J Antimicrob Chemother* 1986;18:613–619.

61. Wilson SE, Boswick JA, Duma RJ, et al. Cephalosporin therapy in intra-abdominal infections—a multi-center randomized comparative study of cefotetan, moxalactam, and cefoxitin. *Am J Surg* 1986;155:61–66.

62. Gillett AP, Wise R. Penetration of 4 cephalosporins into tissue fluid in man. *Lancet* 1978;1:962–964.

63. Eron LJ, Goldenberg RI, Park CH, Paretz DM. Ceftazidime therapy of serious bacterial infections. *Antimicrob Agents Chemother* 1983;23:236–241.

64. Stone HH, Geheber CE, Kolb CD, Dunlop WE. Clinical comparison of cefotaxime versus the combination of gentamicin plus clindamycin in the treatment of peritonitis and similar polymicrobial soft-tissue surgical infections. *Clin Ther* 1981;4(Suppl A):67–80.

65. Soe GB, Overturf GD. Treatment of typhoid fever and other systemic salmonelloses with cefotaxime, ceftriaxone, cefoperazone and other newer cephalosporins. *Rev Infect Dis* 1987;9:719–736.

66. The choice of antibacterial drugs. *Med Lett* 1992;34:49–56.

67. Cephalosporins and related agents. In: *Drug evaluations annual 1993.* Chicago: American Medical Association, 1993;1345–1402.

68. Kager L, Nord CE. Imipenem/cilastatin in the treatment of intraabdominal infections: a review of worldwide experience. *Rev Infect Dis* 1985;7(Suppl):518–521.

69. Sanford JP. *Guide to antimicrobial therapy 1992.* Dallas: Antimicrobial Therapy Inc, 1992.

70. Birnbaum J, Kahan FM, Kropp H, MacDonald JS. Carbapenems, a new class of β-lactam antibiotics: discovery and development of imipenem/cilastatin. *Am J Med* 1985;78(Suppl 6A):3–21.

71. Neu HC. Carbapenems: special properties contributing to their activity. *Am J Med* 1985;78(Suppl 6A):33–40.

72. Kropp H, Gerckens L, Sundelof JG, Kahan FM. Antibacterial activity of imipenem: first thienamycin antibiotic. *Rev Infect Dis* 1985;7(Suppl):389–410.

73. Clissold SP, Todd PA, Campoli-Richards DM. Imipenem/cilastatin—a review of its antibacterial activity, pharmacokinetic properties and therapeutic efficacy. *Drugs* 1987;33:183–241.

74. MacGregor RR, Gibson GA, Bland JA. Imipenem pharmacokinetics and body fluid levels in high dose patient treatment. In: *Proceedings 24th ICAAC ASM,* Washington, DC, 1984;abstract 597.

75. Wexler HM, Finegold SM. Impact of imipenem/cilastatin therapy on normal fecal flora. *Am J Med* 1985;78(Suppl 6A):41–46.

76. Rogers JD, Meisinger AP, Ferber F, Calandra GB, Demetriades VL, Bland JA. Pharmacokinetics of imipenem and cilastatin in volunteers. *Rev Infect Dis* 1985;7(Suppl):435–446.

77. Drusano GL, Standiford HC. Pharmacokinetic profile of imi-

penem/cilastatin in normal volunteers. *Am J Med* 1985; 78(Suppl 6A):47–53.

78. Wang C, Calandra GB, Aziz MA, Brown KR. Efficacy and safety of imipenem cilastatin: a review of worldwide clinical experience. *Rev Infect Dis* 1985;7(Suppl):528–536.

79. Calandra CB, Brown CR, Grad LC. Review of adverse experiences and tolerability in the first 2516 patients treated with imipenem/cilastatin. *Am J Med* 1985;78(Suppl 6A):73–78.

80. Zazgornick J, Schein W, Heimberger K, Shaheen FAM, Stockenhuber F. Potentiation of neurotoxic side effects by coadministration of imipenem to cyclosporine therapy in a kidney transplant recipient: synergism of side effects or drug interaction? *Clin Nephrol* 1986;26:265–266.

81. Brogden RN, Heel RC. Aztreonam—a review of its antibacterial activity, pharmacokinetic properties and therapeutic use. *Drugs* 1986;31:96–130.

82. Tunkel AR, Scheld WM. Aztreonam. *Infect Control Hosp Epidemiol* 1990;11:486–494.

83. Henry SA, Bendush CB. Aztreonam: worldwide overview of the treatment of patients with gram-negative infections. *Am J Med* 1985;78(Suppl 2A):57–64.

84. Girgis NL, Farid Z, Kilpatrick ME, Podgare JK, Sultan Y. Aztreonam compared to chloramphenicol in the treatment of enteric fevers. *Drugs Exp Clin Res* 1992;18:197–199.

85. Ericsson CD, DuPont HL. Travelers' diarrhea: approaches to prevention and treatment. *Clin Infect Dis* 1993;16:616–626.

86. Neu HC. Aztreonam activity, pharmacology and clinical uses. *Am J Med* 1990;88(Suppl 3C):2–6.

87. Martinez OV, Levi JU, Devlin RG. Biliary excretion of aztreonam in patients with biliary tract disease. *Antimicrob Agents Chemother* 1984;25:358–361.

88. Swabb EA. Review of the clinical pharmacology of monobactam antibiotic aztreonam. *Am J Med* 1985;78(Suppl 2A):11–18.

89. Newman TJ, Dreslinski GR, Tadros SS. Safety profile of aztreonam in clinical trials. *Rev Infect Dis* 1985;7:648–655.

90. Giamarellou H, Galanakis N, Douzinas E, et al. Evaluation of aztreonam in difficult to treat infections with prolonged post treatment follow-up. *Antimicrob Agents Chemother* 1984;26:245–250.

91. Neu HC, Fu CP. Clavulanic acid, a novel inhibitor of β lactamases. *Antimicrob Agents Chemother* 1978;14:650–655.

92. Boon RJ, Beale AS, Comber KR. Distribution of amoxicillin and clavulanic acid in infected animals and efficacy against experimental infections. *Antimicrob Agents Chemother* 1982;22:369–375.

93. Kerins DM. Ampicillin/sulbactam: a combination of an old and new agent in the treatment of infection. *Am J Med Sci* 1991;301:406–411.

94. Campoli-Richards DM, Brogden RN. Ampicillin/sulbactam: review of its antibacterial activity, pharmacokinetic properties and therapeutic uses. *Drugs* 1987;33:577–609.

95. Kucers A, Bennett NMcK. Neomycin, framycetin and paromomycin. In: *The use of antibiotics*, 4th ed. Philadelphia: Lippincott, 1987;739–753.

96. Tanaka N. Mechanism of action of aminoglycoside antibiotics. In: Umezawa H, Hooper IR, eds. *Handbook of experimental pharmacology*, vol 62. New York: Springer-Verlag 1982; 221–266.

97. Moellering RC. In vitro antibiotic activity of aminoglycoside antibiotics. *Rev Infect Dis* 1983;5(Suppl):212–232.

98. Pratt WB, Fekety R. Bactericidal inhibitors of protein synthesis. In: *The antimicrobial drugs*. New York: Oxford Press, 1986;153–183.

99. Philips I. The aminoglycosides. *Lancet* 1982;2:311–314.

100. Dickie P, Bryan LE, Pickard MA. Effect of enzyme adenylation on dihydrostreptomycin accumulation in *E. coli* carrying a R factor: model explaining aminoglycoside resistance by inactivating mechanisms. *Antimicrob Agents Chemother* 1978;14:569–580.

101. Davies JE. Resistance to aminoglycosides. Mechanisms and frequency. *Rev Infect Dis* 1983;5(Suppl):261–267.

102. Carbon C, Cantiepois A, Lamotte-Banillon S. Comparative distribution of gentamicin, tobramycin, sisomicin, netilmicin, and

103. Dan M, Halkin H, Rubenstein E. Interstitial fluid concentrations of aminoglycosides. *J Antimicrob Chemother* 1981;7:551–558.

104. Riff LJ, Jackson GG. Pharmacology of gentamicin in man. *J Infect Dis* 1971;124(Suppl):98–105.

105. Pitt HA, Roberts RB, Johnson WD. Gentamicin levels in the human biliary tract. *J Infect Dis* 1973;127:299–302.

106. Moore RD, Smith CR, Lietman PS. Risk factors for the development of auditory toxicity in patients receiving aminoglycosides. *J Infect Dis* 1984;149:23–30.

107. Sande MA, Mandell GL. The aminoglycosides. In: Gilman AG, Rall TW, Nies AS, Taylor P, eds. *Pharmacologic basis of therapeutics*, 8th ed. New York: Pergamon Press, 1990;1098–1116.

108. Mathog RH, Klein WJ. Ototoxicity of ethacrynic acid and aminoglycoside antibiotics in uremia. *N Engl J Med* 1967;280:1223–1224.

109. Smith CR, Baughman KL, Edwards CO, Rogers JF, Leitman PS. Controlled comparison of amikacin and gentamicin. *N Engl J Med* 1977;296:349–353.

110. Smith CR, Lipsky JJ, Laskin OL, Hellman DB, Mellits ED, Longstreth J, Lietman PS. Double-blind comparison of the nephrotoxicity and auditory toxicity of gentamicin and tobramycin. *N Engl J Med* 1980;302:1106–1109.

111. Moore RD, Smith CR, Lipsky JJ, Mellits ED, Lietman PS. Risk factors for renal dysfunction in patients treated with aminoglycosides. *Ann Intern Med* 1984;100:352–357.

112. Moore RD, Smith CR, Lietman PS. Increased risk of renal dysfunction due to interaction of liver disease and aminoglycosides. *Am J Med* 1986;80:1093–1097.

113. Pittinger CB, Eryasa Y, Adamson R. Antibiotic-induced paralysis. *Anesth Analg* 1970;49:487–501.

114. Bartlett JG. Antibiotic associated pseudomembranous colitis. *Rev Infect Dis* 1979;1:530–539.

115. Kappos A, Shinagawa N, Arabi Y, et al. Diagnosis of pseudomembranous colitis. *Br Med J* 1978;1:675–678.

116. Donald PR, Sellars SL. Streptomycin ototoxicity in the unborn child. *S Afr Med J* 1981;60:316–318.

117. The aminoglycosides. In: *Drug evaluations annual 1993*. Chicago: American Medical Association, 1993;1453–1478.

118. Dupont HL, Ericsson CD, Robinson A, Johnson PC. Current problems in antimicrobial therapy for bacterial enteric infection. *Am J Med* 1987;82(Suppl 4A):324–228.

119. Pichler HET, Diridl G, Stickler K, Wolf D. Clinical efficacy of ciprofloxacin compared with placebo in bacterial diarrhea. *Am J Med* 1987;82(Suppl 4A):329–332.

120. Lolekha S, Patanacharoen S. Clinical and microbiological efficacy of norfloxacin for the treatment of acute diarrhea. *Rev Infect Dis* 1988;10(Suppl):210–211.

121. DuPont HL, Corrado ML, Sabbaj J. Use of norfloxacin in the treatment of acute diarrheal disease. *Am J Med* 1987;82(Suppl):79–83.

122. Akalin HE, Firat M, Unal S, Serin A, Baykal M. Clinical efficacy of single dose or 1 day treatment with ofloxacin in shigellosis. *Rev Infect Dis* 1989;11(Suppl):1152–1153.

123. Ramirez CA, Bran JL, Mejia CR, Garcia JF. Open prospective study of the clinical efficacy of ciprofloxacin. *Antimicrob Agents Chemother* 1985;28:128–132.

124. Andriole VT. Clinical overview of the newer 4-quinolone antibacterial agents. In: Andriole VT, ed. *The quinolones*. London: Academic Press, 1988;155–200.

125. Diridl G, Pichler H, Wolf D. Four weeks treatment of adult chronic salmonella carriers with ciprofloxacin and its influence on fecal flora. In: *Proceedings of the 1st International Ciprofloxacin Workshop*. Amsterdam: Exerpta Medica, 1986; 370–372.

126. Forsmark CE, Wilcox CM, Cello JP, et al. Ciprofloxacin in the treatment of *H. pylori* in patients with gastritis and peptic ulcer. *J Infect Dis* 1990;162:998–999.

127. Wolfson JS, Hooper DC. Fluoroquinolones: structures, mechanisms of action and resistance and spectra of activity in vitro. *Antimicrob Agents Chemother* 1985;28:581–586.

128. Sato K, Hoshino K, Mitsuhashi Y. Mode of action of new quin-

olones: the inhibitory activity on DNA gyrase. *Prog Drug Res* 1992;38:121–132.

129. Hooper DC, Wolfson JS. Mode of action of the quinolone antimicrobial agents. *Rev Infect Dis* 1988;10(Suppl):14–21.

130. Hooper DC, Wolfson JS, Ng EY, Swartz MN. Mechanisms of action and resistance to ciprofloxacin. *Am J Med* 1987;82(Suppl 4A):12–20.

131. Sanders CS, Sanders WE, Goering RV. Overview of preclinical studies with ciprofloxacin. *Am J Med* 1987;82(Suppl 4A):2–12.

132. Sanders CC. Ciprofloxacin: in vitro activity, mechanism of action and resistance. *Rev Infect Dis* 1988;10:516–527.

133. Shah PM, Enzenberger R, Glogau O, Knothe H. Influence of oral ciprofloxacin or ofloxacin on the fecal flora of healthy volunteers. *Am J Med* 1987;82(Suppl 4A):333–335.

134. Hoffken G. Pharmacokinetics of ciprofloxacin after oral and parenteral administration. *Antimicrob Agents Chemother* 1985;27:375–379.

135. Monk JP, Campoli-Richards DM. Ofloxacin: a review of its antibacterial activity, pharmacokinetic properties and therapeutic use. *Drugs* 1987;33:346–391.

136. Holmes B. Norfloxacin: review of its antibacterial activity, pharmacokinetic properties and therapeutic use. *Drugs* 1985;30:482–513.

137. Stahlman R, Lode H. Safety overview: toxicity, adverse effects and drug interactions. In: Andriole VT, ed. *The quinolones.* London: Academic Press, 1988;201–233.

138. Christ W, Cehnert T, Vlbrich B. Specific toxicologic aspects of the quinolones. *Rev Infect Dis* 1988;10(Suppl):141–146.

139. Miscellaneous antibacterial drugs. In: *Drug evaluations annual 1993.* Chicago: American Medical Association, 1993;1523.

140. Brouwers JRBJ. Drug interactions with quinolone antibiotics. *Drug Safety* 1992;7:268–281.

141. Stone HH, Morris ES, Geheber CE, Kolb CE, Dunlop WE. Clinical comparison of cefotaxime with gentamicin plus clindamycin in the treatment of peritonitis and other soft tissue infections. *Rev Infect Dis* 1983;4(Suppl):439–443.

142. Davis BD. Chemotherapy. In: Davis BD, Dulbecco R, Eisen HN, Ginsberg HS, eds. *Microbiology,* 4th ed. Philadelphia: Lippincott, 1990;201–228.

143. Steigbigel NH. Erythromycin, lincomycin and clindamycin. In: Mandell GL, Douglas RG, Bennett JE, eds. *Principles and practice of infectious diseases,* 3rd ed. New York: Churchill Livingstone, 1990;308–317.

144. Keusch GT, Present DH. Summary of a workshop on clindamycin colitis. *J Infect Dis* 1976;133:578–587.

145. McGehee RF, Smith CB, Wilcox C, Finland M. Comparative studies of antibacterial activity in vitro and absorption and excretion of lincomycin and clindamycin. *Am J Med Sci* 1968;256:279–292.

146. LeFrock JL, Molavi A, Prince RA. Clindamycin. *Med Clin North Am* 1982;66:103–120.

147. Brown RB, Martyak SM, Barza M, Curtis L, Weinstein L. Penetration of clindamycin phosphate into the abnormal human biliary tract. *Ann Intern Med* 1976;84:168–170.

148. Kucers A, Bennett NMcK. Lincomycin and clindamycin. In: *The use of antibiotics,* 4th ed. Philadelphia: Lippincott, 1987;819–850.

149. Tedesco FJ, Barton RW, Alpers DH. Clindamycin associated colitis: a prospective study. *Ann Intern Med* 1974;81:429–433.

150. Fekety R, Shah AB. Diagnosis and treatment of *Clostridium difficile* colitis. *JAMA* 1993;29:71–75.

151. Fogdall RP, Miller RD. Prolongation of a pancuronium induced neuromuscular blockade by clindamycin. *Anesthesiology* 1974;41:407–408.

152. Wright SG, Tomkins AM, Ridley DS. Giardiasis: clinical and therapeutic aspects. *Gut* 1977;18:343–350.

153. Adams EB, MacLeod IN. Invasive amebiasis. I. Amebic dysentery and its complications. II Amebic liver abscess and its complications. *Medicine (Baltimore)* 1977;56:315–334.

154. Canadian Metronidazole–Clindamycin Study Group. Prospective randomized comparison of metronidazole and clindamycin, each with gentamicin, for the treatment of serious intraabdominal infection. *Surgery* 1983;93:221–229.

155. Taylor SA, Cowdery AM. The use of metronidazole in the preparation of the bowel for surgery. *Proc R Soc Med* 1977;70:481–482.

156. Brogden RN, Heel RC, Speight TM, Avery GS. Metronidazole in anaerobic infections: a review of its activity, pharmacokinetics, and therapeutic use. *Drugs* 1978;16:387–417.

157. Molavi A, Lefrock JL, Prince RA. Metronidazole. *Med Clin North Am* 1982;66:121–133.

158. Finegold SM, Mathisen GE. Metronidazole. In: Mandell GL, Douglas RG, Bennett JE, eds. *Principles and practice of infectious disease,* 3rd ed. New York: Churchill Livingstone, 1990;303–309.

159. Rasmussen BA, Bush K, Tally FP. Antimicrobial resistance in bacteroides. *Clin Infect Dis* 1993;16(Suppl 4):1390–1400.

160. McNulty CAM, Dent J, Wise R. Susceptibility of clinical isolates of *Campylobacter pyloridis* to antimicrobial agents. *Antimicrob Agents Chemother* 1985;28:837–840.

161. Glupcznski Y, Burette A, DeKoster E, et al. Metronidazole resistance in *Helicobacter pylori. Lancet* 1990;335:976–977.

162. Becx MCJM, Janssen AJHM, Claesner HOL, De Koning RW. Metronidazole-resistant *Helicobacter pylori. Lancet* 1990;335:539–540.

163. Kucers A, Bennett NMcK. Metronidazole. In: *The use of antibiotics,* 4th ed. Philadelphia: Lippincott, 1987;1290–1329.

164. Schwartz DE, Jeunet F. Comparative pharmacokinetic studies of ornidazole and metronidazole in man. *Chemotherapy* 1976;22:19–29.

165. Bolton RP, Culshaw MA. Fecal metronidazole concentrations during oral and intravenous therapy for antibiotic associated colitis due to *Clostridium difficile. Gut* 1986;27:1169–1172.

166. Saginau R, Hawley CR, Bartlett JG. Colitis associated with metronidazole therapy. *J Infect Dis* 1980;141:772–774.

167. Tally FP, Sutter VL, Finegold SM. Treatment of anaerobic infections with metronidazole. *Antimicrob Agents Chemother* 1975;7:672–675.

168. Rustia M, Shubik P. Induction of lung tumors and malignant lymphomas in mice by metronidazole. *J Natl Cancer Inst* 1972;48:721–729.

169. Chin TDY. Therapy of salmonellosis. *Ration Drug Ther* 1976;10:1.

170. Harding GKM, Buckwold FJ, Ronald AR, et al. Prospective, randomized comparative study of clindamycin, chloramphenicol, and ticarcillin, each in combination with gentamicin, in therapy for intraabdominal and female genital tract sepsis. *J Infect Dis* 1980;142:384–393.

171. Weissberger AS. Inhibition of protein synthesis by chloramphenicol. *Annu Rev Med* 1967;18:483–494.

172. Pratt WB, Fekety R. Bacteriostatic inhibitors of protein synthesis. In: *The antimicrobial drugs.* New York: Oxford University Press, 1986;184–228.

173. Okamoto S, Suzuki Y. Chloramphenicol, dihydrostreptamycin and kanamycin inactivating enzymes from multiple drug resistant *E. coli* carrying episome "R." *Nature* 1965;208:1301–1303.

174. Anderson ES, Smith HR. Chloramphenicol resistance in the typhoid bacillus. *Br Med J* 1972;3:329–331.

175. Anderson ES. Chloramphenicol resistant *S. typhi. Lancet* 1973;2:1494–1496.

176. Spika JS, Waterman SA, Shoo Hoo GW, et al. Chloramphenicol resistant *S. newport* traced through hamburger to dairy farms. *N Engl J Med* 1987;316:565–570.

177. Dupont HL, Hornick RB, Weiss CF, Snyder MJ, Woodward TE. Evaluation of chloramphenicol acid succinate therapy of induced typhoid fever and Rocky Mountain spotted fever. *N Engl J Med* 1970;282:53–57.

178. Standiford HC. Tetracyclines and chloramphenicol. In: Mandell GL, Douglas RG, Bennett JE, eds. *Principles and practice of infectious diseases,* 3rd ed. New York: Churchill Livingstone, 1990;284–295.

179. Yunis AA. Chloramphenicol-induced bone marrow suppression. *Semin Hematol* 1973;10:225–234.

180. Scott JL, Finegold SM, Belkin GA, Lawrence JS. A controlled double-blinded study of the hematologic toxicity of chloramphenicol. *N Engl J Med* 1965;272:1137–1142.

181. Shu XO, Linet MS, Gao RN, Gao YT, Bunton LA, Jin F,

Fraumeni JF. Chloramphenicol use and childhood leukemia in Shanghai. *Lancet* 1987;2:934–937.

182. Bartlett JC. Chloramphenicol. *Med Clin North Am* 1982;66: 91–102.

183. Burns LE, Hodgman JE, Cass AB. Fatal circulatory collapse in premature infants receiving chloramphenicol. *N Engl J Med* 1959;261:1318–1321.

184. Lead article. Antibiotics in cholera. *Lancet* 1966;1:801–802.

185. Kucers A, Bennett NMcK. Tetracyclines. In: *The use of antibiotics*, 4th ed. Philadelphia: Lippincott, 1987;979–1044.

186. Francke E, Neu HC. Chloramphenicol and tetracyclines. *Med Clin North Am* 1987;71:1155–1168.

187. Knight R. The chemotherapy of amoebiasis. *J Antimicrob Chemother* 1980;6:577–593.

188. Wilmot AJ. *Clinical amoebiasis*. Cambridge: Blackwell Scientific, 1962.

189. Craven GR, Gavin R, Fanning T. The transfer RNA binding site of the 30S ribosome and the site of tetracycline inhibition. *Symp Quant Biol* 1969;34:129–137.

190. Benveniste R, Davies J. Mechanisms of antibiotic resistance in bacteria. *Annu Rev Biochem* 1973;42:471–506.

191. Cunha BA, Comer JB, Jonas M. The tetracyclines. *Med Clin North Am* 1982;66:293–302.

192. MacDonald H, Kelly RG, Allen ES, Noble JF, Kanegis LA. Pharmacokinetic studies on minocycline in man. *Clin Pharmacol Ther* 1973;14:852–861.

193. Whelton A, Von Wittenau MS, Twomey TM, Walker WG, Bianchine JR. Doxycycline pharmacokinetics in the absence of renal function. *Kidney Int* 1974;5:365–371.

194. Bokey L, Hugh TB. Oesophageal ulceration associated with doxycycline therapy. *Med J Aust* 1975;1:236–237.

195. Tetracyclines and chloramphenicol. In: *Drug evaluations annual 1993*. Chicago: American Medical Association, 1993; 1435–1452.

196. Fanning WL, Guemp DW, Sofferman RA. Side effects of minocycline: a double-blind study. *Antimicrob Agents Chemother* 1977;11:712–717.

197. Feldman S, Pickering LK, Gleary TG, Ericsson CD. Influence of subsalicylate bismuth and absorption of doxycycline. *JAMA* 1982;247:2266–2267.

198. Geraci JE. Vancomycin. *Mayo Clin Proc* 1977;52:631–634.

199. Pantosti A, Luzzi I, Cardines R, Gianfrilli P. Comparison of the *in vitro* activities of teicoplanin and vancomycin against *Clostridium difficile* and their interactions with cholestyramine. *Antimicrob Agents Chemother* 1985;28:847–848.

200. deLalla F, Nicolin R, Rinaldi E, Scarpellini P, Rigoli R, Manfrin V, Tramarin A. Prospective study of oral teicoplanin versus oral vancomycin for therapy of pseudomembranous colitis and *Clostridium difficile*-associated diarrhea. *Antimicrob Agents Chemother* 1992;36:2192–2196.

201. Pratt WB, Fekety R. The inhibitors of cell wall synthesis I. In: *The antimicrobial drugs*. New York: Oxford University Press, 1986;85–112.

202. Fekety R. Vancomycin and teichoplanin. In: Mandell GL, Douglas RG, Bennett JE, eds. *Principles and practice of infectious diseases*, 3rd ed. New York: Churchill Livingstone, 1990; 317–322.

203. Leclerq R, Derlot E, Duval J, Courvalin P. Plasmid mediated resistance to vancomycin and teichoplanin in *Enterococcus faecium*. *N Engl J Med* 1988;319:157–161.

204. Goldmann DA. Vancomycin resistant *Enterococcus faecium*: headline news. *Infect Control Hosp Epidemiol* 1992;13: 695–699.

205. Bugg TDH, Dutka-Malen S, Arthur M, Courvalin P, Walsh CT. Identification of vancomycin resistance protein Van A as a D-alanine: D-alanine ligase of altered substrate specificity. *Biochemistry* 1991;30:2017–2021.

206. Watanakunakarn C. Mode of action and *in vitro* activity of vancomycin. *J Antimicrob Chemother* 1984;16(Suppl D):7–18.

207. Torres R, Sanders CV, Lewis AC. Vancomycin concentrations in human tissues—preliminary report. *J Antimicrob Chemother* 1979;5:475–477.

208. Geraci JE, Heilman FR, Nichols DR, Wellman WE, Ross GT. Some laboratory and clinical experiences with a new antibiotic, vancomycin. *Proc Staff Meet Mayo Clin* 1956;31:564–582.

209. Schaad UB, McCracken GH, Nelson JD. Clinical pharmacology and efficacy of vancomycin in pediatric patients. *J Pediatr* 1980;96:119–126.

210. Spitzer PC, Eliopoulas GM. Systemic absorption of enteral vancomycin in a patient with pseudomembranous colitis. *Ann Intern Med* 1984;100:533–534.

211. Tedesco F, Gurwith M, Markham R, Christie D, Bartlett JG. Oral vancomycin for antibiotic associated pseudomembranous colitis. *Lancet* 1978;2:226–228.

212. Polk RE, Healy DP, Schwartz LB, Rock DT, Garson ML, Roller K. Vancomycin and the red-man syndrome: pharmacodynamics of histamine release. *J Infect Dis* 1988;157:502–507.

213. Miller SN, Ringler RP. Vancomycin-induced pseudomembranous colitis. *J Clin Gastroenterol* 1987;9:114–115.

214. Levine JF. Vancomycin: a review. *Med Clin North Am* 1987; 71:1135–1145.

215. Salazar-Lindo E, Sack RB, Chea Woo E, Kay BA, Piscoya ZA, Leon-Barua R, Yi A. Early treatment with erythromycin of *Campylobacter jejuni*-associated dysentery in children. *J Pediatr* 1986;109:355–360.

216. Shafei AZ. Efficiency of a controlled release preparation of erythromycin stearate in the treatment of intestinal amebiasis. *Clin Med* 1969;76:38–44.

217. Powell SJ, Wilmot AJ, Elsdon-Dew R. A comparison of erythromycin, spiramycin and novobiocin in the treatment of acute amoebic dysentery. *J Trop Med Hyg* 1958;61:67–70.

218. Oleinick NC. The erythromycins. In: Corcoran JW, Hahn FE, eds. *Mechanisms of action of antimicrobial & antitumor agents*. New York: Springer-Verlag, 1975;396–419.

219. Gribble MJ, Chow AW. Erythromycin. *Med Clin North Am* 1982;66:79–89.

220. Kucers A, Bennett NMcK. Erythromycin. In: *The use of antibiotics*, 3rd ed. Philadelphia: Lippincott, 1987;851–882.

221. Macrolides and lincosamides. In: *Drug evaluations annual 1993*. Chicago: American Medical Association, 1993; 1419–1434.

222. Brittain DC. Erythromycin. *Med Clin North Am* 1987;71: 1147–1154.

223. Itoh Z, Suzuki T, Nakaya M, Inoue M, Mitsuhashi S. Gastrointestinal motor-stimulating activity of macrolide antibiotics and analysis of their side effects on the canine gut. *Antimicrob Agents Chemother* 1984;26:863–869.

224. Braun P. Hepatotoxicty of erythromycin. *J Infect Dis* 1969; 119:300–306.

225. Gantz NM, Zawacki JK, Dickerson J, Bartlett JG. Pseudomembranous colitis associated with erythromycin. *Ann Intern Med* 1979;91:866–867.

226. Safety of terfenadine and astemizole. *Med Lett* 1992;34:9–10.

227. Peters DH, Friedel HA, McTavish D. Azithromycin: a review of its antimicrobial activity, pharmacokinetic properties and clinical efficacy. *Drugs* 1992;44:750–799.

228. Ballow CH, Amsden GW. Azithromycin: the first azalide antibiotic. *Ann Pharmacother* 1992;26:1253–1261.

229. Foulds G, Shepard RM, Johnson RB. The pharmacokinetics of azithromycin in human serum and tissues. *J Antimicrob Chemother* 1990;25(Suppl A):73–82.

230. Schentag JJ, Ballow CH. Tissue directed pharmacokinetics. *Am J Med* 1991;91(Suppl 3A):5–11.

231. Hopkins S. Clinical toleration and safety of azithromycin. *Am J Med* 1991;91(Suppl 3A):40–45.

232. Peters DH, Clissold SP. Clarithromycin: a review of its antimicrobial activity, pharmacokinetic properties and therapeutic potential. *Drugs* 1992;44:117–164.

233. Sturgill MG, Rapp RP. Clarithromycin: review of a new macrolide antibiotic with improved microbiologic spectrum and favorable pharmacokinetic and adverse effect profiles. *Ann Pharmacother* 1992;26:1099–1108.

234. Kohno Y, Ohta K, Suwa T, Suga T. Autobacteriographic studies of clarithromycin and erythromycin in mice. *Antimicrob Agents Chemother* 1990;34:562–567.

235. Pichotta P, Gupta S, Prokocimer P, Pernet A. The overall safety of oral clarithromycin in comparative clinical studies.

30th Annual Interscience Conference on Antimicrobial Agents and Chemotherapy, Atlanta, GA, October 1990.

236. Kucers A, Bennet NMcK. Trimethoprim, co-trimoxazole. In: *The use of antibiotics*, 4th ed. Philadelphia: Lippincott, 1987; 1118–1202.

237. Cash RA, Northrup RS, Rahman ASMM. Trimethoprim and sulfamethoxazole in clinical cholera: comparison with tetracycline. *J Infect Dis* 1973;128(Suppl):749.

238. Pope JW, Verdier R, Joshus WD. Treatment and prophylaxis of *Isospora belli* infection in patients with the acquired immunodeficiency syndrome. *N Engl J Med* 1989;320:1044–1047.

239. Ryder RW, Blake PA, Murlin AC, et al. Increase in antibiotic resistance among isolates of *Salmonella* in the United States, 1967–1975. *J Infect Dis* 1980;142:485–491.

240. Dar L, Gupta BL, Rattan A. Multidrug resistant *Salmonella typhi* in Delhi. *Indian J Pediatr* 1992;59:221–224.

241. Mukherjee P, Mukherjee S, Dalal BK, Halden KK, Ghosh E, Palt K. Some prospective observations on recent outbreaks of typhoid fever in West Bengal. *J Assoc Physicians India* 1991; 39:445–448.

242. Pratt WB, Fekety R. The antimetabolites. In: *The antimicrobial drugs*. New York: Oxford University Press, 1986;229–251.

243. Richards N, Sojkaw J, Datta N, Wray C. Trimethoprim resistance plasmids and transposons in *Salmonella*. *Lancet* 1978;2: 1194–1195.

244. Then RL. Mechanisms of resistance to trimethoprim, the sulfonamides and trimethoprim-sulfamethoxazole. *Rev Infect Dis* 1982;4:261–269.

245. Foltzer MA, Reese RE. Trimethoprim–sulfamethoxazole and other sulfonamides. *Med Clin North Am* 1987;71:1177–1194.

246. Craig WA, Kunin CM. Distribution of TMP-SMX in tissues of rhesus monkeys. *J Infect Dis* 1973;128(Suppl):575–579.

247. Wilkinson PJ, Reeves DS. Tissue penetration of trimethoprim and sulphonamides. *J Antimicrob Chemother* 1979;5(Suppl B): 159–168.

248. Pater RB, Welling PO. Clinical pharmacokinetics of cotrimoxazole. *Clin Pharmacokinet* 1980;5:405–423.

249. Whartan JM, Coleman DL, Wofsy CB. Trimethoprim–sulfamethoxazole or pentamidine for *Pneumocystis carinij* pneumonia in the acquired immunodeficiency syndrome. *Ann Intern Med* 1986;105:37–44.

250. Lawson DH, Paice BJ. Adverse reactions to TMP-SMX. *Rev Infect Dis* 1985;4:429–433.

251. Sande MA, Volberding P. *The medical management of AIDS*, 2nd ed. Philadelphia: Saunders, 1990;224–227.

252. Sulfonamides and trimethoprim. In: *Drug evaluations annual 1993*. Chicago: American Medical Association, 1993; 1479–1497.

253. Elion GB. Selectivity of action of an antiherpetic agent, 9-(2-hydroxyethoxymethyl)guanine. *Proc Natl Acad Sci USA* 1977; 74:5716–20.

254. Palu G, Gerna G, Bevilacqua F, Marcello A. A point mutation in the thymidine kinase gene is responsible for acyclovir-resistance in herpes simplex virus type 2 sequential isolates. *Virus Res* 1992;25:133–144.

255. Dorsky DI, Crumpacker CS. Drugs five years later: acyclovir. *Ann Intern Med* 1987;107:859–874.

256. deMiranda P, Blum MR. Pharmacokinetics of acyclovir after intravenous and oral administration. *J Antimicrob Chemother* 1983;12(Suppl B):29–37.

257. O Brien JJ, Campoli-Richards DM. Acyclovir. An updated review of its antiviral activity, pharmacokinetic properties and therapeutic efficacy. *Drugs* 1989;37:233–309.

258. Wade JC, Hintz M, McGuffin RW, et al. Treatment of cytomegalovirus pneumonia with high dose acyclovir. *Am J Med* 1982; 73:249–255.

259. Acyclovir. In: McEvoy GK, ed. *AHFS drug information 93—American Hospital Formulary Service*. Bethesda: American Society of Hospital Pharmacists, 1993;366–369.

260. Acyclovir. In: Brigg GG, Freeman RK, Yaffe SJ, eds. *Drugs in pregnancy and lactation*, 3rd ed. Baltimore: Williams & Wilkins, 1990;99–100.

261. Biron KK, Fyfe JA, Stanat SC, Leslie LK, et al. A human cytomegalovirus mutant resistant to the nucleoside analog

9-{[2-hydroxy-1-(hydroxymethyl)ethoxy]methyl}guanine (BW B759U) induces reduced levels of BW B769U triphosphate. *Proc Natl Acad Sci USA* 1986;83:8769–8773.

262. Lurain NS, Thompson KD, Holmes EW, Read GS. Point mutations in the DNA polymerase gene of human cytomegalovirus that result in resistance to antiviral agents. *J Virol* 1992;66: 7146–7152.

263. Smee DF, Martin JC, Verheyden JP, Matthews TR. Anti-herpesvirus activity of the acyclic nucleoside 9-(1,3-dihydroxy-2-propoxymethyl)guanine. *Antimicrob Agents Chemother* 1983; 23:676–682.

264. Ganciclovir. In: McEvoy GK, ed. *AHFS drug information 93—American Hospital Formulary Service*. Bethesda: American Society of Hospital Pharmacists, 1993;386–390.

265. Paul S, Dummer S. Topics in clinical pharmacology: ganciclovir. *Am J Med Sci* 1992;304:272–277.

266. Dieterich DT, Kotler DP, Busch DF, et al. Ganciclovir treatment of cytomegalovirus colitis in AIDS; a randomized, double-blind, placebo-controlled multicenter study. *J Infect Dis* 1993;167:278–282.

267. Hayden FG, Douglas RD. Antiviral agents. In: Mandell GL, Douglas RG, Bennett JE, eds. *Principles and practice of infectious diseases*, 3rd ed. New York: Churchill Livingstone, 1990; 370–393.

268. Barton TL, Roush MK, Dever LL. Seizures associated with ganciclovir therapy. *Pharmacotherapy* 1992;12:413–415.

269. Crisp P, Clissold SP. Foscarnet. A review of its antiviral activity, pharmacokinetic properties and therapeutic use in immunocompromised patients with cytomegalovirus retinitis. *Drugs* 1991;41:104–129.

270. Derse D, Bastow KF, Cheng Y-C. Characterization of the DNA polymerases induced by a group of herpes simplex virus type I variants selected for growth in the presence of phosphonoformic acid. *J Biol Chem* 1982;257:10251–10260.

271. Aweek F, Gambertoglio J, Mills J, Jacobson MA. Pharmacokinetics of intermittently administered intravenous foscarnet in the treatment of acquired immunodeficiency syndrome patients with serious cytomegalovirus retinitis. *Antimicrob Agents Chemother* 1989;33:742–745.

272. Taburet AM, Katlama C, Blanshard C, et al. Pharmacokinetics of foscarnet after twice daily administrations for treatment of cytomegalovirus disease in AIDS patients. *Antimicrob Agents Chemother* 1992;36:1821–1824.

273. Blanshard C. Treatment of HIV-related cytomegalovirus disease of the gastrointestinal tract with foscarnet. *J Acquir Immune Defic Syndr* 1992;5(Suppl 1):S25–S28.

274. Ringden O, Lonnqvist B, Paulin T, et al. Pharmacokinetics, safety and preliminary clinical experiences using foscarnet in the treatment of cytomegalovirus infections in bone marrow and renal transplant recipients. *J Antimicrob Chemother* 1986; 17:373–387.

275. Saint-Marc T, Fournier F, Touraine JL, Marneff E. Uvula and oesophageal ulcerations with foscarnet. *Lancet* 1992;340:1443.

276. Wang L, Takayama K. Relationship between the uptake of isoniazid and its action on in vivo mycolic acid synthesis in *Mycobacterium tuberculosis*. *Antimicrob Agents Chemother* 1972; 2:438–441.

277. Jindani A, Aber VR, Edwards EA, Mitchison DA. Early bactericidal activity of drugs in patients with pulmonary TB. *Am Rev Respir Dis* 1980;121:939–947.

278. Hurwitz A, Schlozman DL. Effects of antacids on gastrointestinal absorption of isoniazid in rat and man. *Am Rev Respir Dis* 1974;109:41–47.

279. Kucers A, Bennett NMcK. Isoniazid. In: *The use of antibiotics*, 4th ed. Philadelphia: Lippincott, 1987;1351–1393.

280. LoDico CP, Levine BS, Goldberger BA, Caplan YH. Distribution of isoniazid in an overdose death. *J Anal Toxicol* 1992;16: 57–59.

281. Evans DA, Manley KA, McKusick VA. Genetic control of isoniazid metabolism in man. *Br Med J* 1960;2:485–491.

282. Alford RS. Antimycobacterial agents. In: Mandell GL, Douglas RG, Bennett JE, eds. *Principles and practice of infectious diseases*, 3rd ed. New York: Churchill Livingstone, 1990;350–352.

283. Mitchell JR. Isoniazid liver injury: clinical spectrum, pathology and probably pathogenesis. *Ann Intern Med* 1976;84:181–192.

284. American Thoracic Society. Preventive therapy of tuberculosis infection. *Am Rev Respir Dis* 1974;110:371.
285. American Thoracic Society. Treatment of tuberculosis and other mycobacterial diseases. *Am Rev Respir Dis* 1983;127:790–791.
286. CDC. Initial therapy for tuberculosis in the era of multidrug resistance. Recommendations of the advisory council for the elimination of tuberculosis. *MMWR Morb Mortal Wkly Rep* 1993;42:1–8.
287. Scheinhorn DJ, Angelillo VA. Antituberculous therapy in pregnancy. *West J Med* 1977;127:195–198.
288. Murphy R, Swartz R, Watkins PB. Severe acetaminophen toxicity in a patient receiving isoniazid. *Ann Intern Med* 1990;113:799–800.
289. Konno K, Oizumi K, Ariji F, Yamaguchi J, Oka S. Mode of action of rifampin on mycobacteria. *Am Rev Respir Dis* 1973;107:1002–1005.
290. Israili ZH, Rogers CM, El-Attar H. Pharmacokinetics of antituberculosis drugs in patients. *J Clin Pharmacol* 1987;27:78–83.
291. Pederzoli P. Rifampicin concentrations in pancreatic juice. *J Antimicrob Chemother* 1985;16:129–130.
292. Suter F. Rifampicin in collections of pus—a kinetic study in human abscesses. *J Antimicrob Chemother* 1984;13(Suppl C):43–47.
293. Frank LA. Clinical pharmacology of rifampin. *J Am Vet Med Assoc* 1990;197:114–117.
294. Grosset J, Leventis S. Adverse effects of rifampin. *Rev Infect Dis* 1983;5(Suppl 3):S440–S446.
295. Borcherding SM, Baciewicz AM, Self TH. Update on rifampin drug interactions II. *Arch Intern Med* 1992;152:711–716.
296. Venkatesan K. Pharmacokinetic drug interactions with rifampicin. *Clin Pharmacokinet* 1992;22:47–65.
297. Ethambutol. In: McEvoy GK, ed. *AHFS drug information 93—American Hospital Formulary Service.* Bethesda: American Society of Hospital Pharmacists, 1993;352–353.
298. Liss RW, Letourneau RJ, Schepis JD. Distribution of ethambutol in primate tissues and cells. *Am Rev Respir Dis* 1981;123:529–534.
299. Peets EA, Sweeney WM, Place VA, Byske DA. Absorption, excretion and metabolic fate of ethambutol in man. *Am Rev Respir Dis* 1965;91:51–56.
300. Wall MA. Treatment of tuberculosis during pregnancy. *Am Rev Respir Dis* 1980;122:989–993.
301. Stottmeier KD, Beam RE, Kubica GP. The absorption and excretion of pyrazinamide. Preliminary study in laboratory animals and in man. *Am Rev Respir Dis* 1972;98:70–74.
302. Butler WR, Kilburn JO. Susceptibility of *Mycobacterium tuberculosis* to pyrazinamide and its relationship to pyrazinamidase activity. *Antimicrob Agents Chemother* 1983;24:600–601.
303. Steele MA, DesPrez RM. The role of pyrazinamide in tuberculosis chemotherapy. *Chest* 1988;94:845–850.
304. Ellard EA. Bioavailability of isoniazid, rifampin, pyrazinamide in two commercially available combined formulas designed for use in short-course treatment of tuberculosis. *Am Rev Respir Dis* 1986;133:1076–1080.
305. Pilheu JA, DeSalvo MC, Koch O. Liver alterations in antituberculous regimens containing pyrazinamide. *Chest* 1981;80:720–722.
306. del Cerro LA, Hernandez FR. Effect of pyrazinamide on cyclosporin levels. *Nephron* 1992;62:113.
307. Alford RH. Antimycobacterial agents. In: Mandell GL, Douglas RG, Bennett JE, eds. *Principles and practice of infectious diseases,* 3rd ed. New York: Churchill Livingstone, 1990;358–359.
308. Holdiness MR. Clinical pharmacokinetics of clofazimine. *Clin Pharmacokinet* 1989;16:74–85.
309. Hastings RC, Franzblau SG. Chemotherapy of leprosy. *Annu Rev Pharmacol Toxicol* 1988;28:231–245.
310. Farb J, West DP, Pedvis-Leftick A. Clofazimine in pregnancy complicated by leprosy. *Obstet Gynecol* 1982;59:122–123.
311. Chaisson R, McCutchan A, Nightingale S, Young L. Managing *Mycobacterium avium* complex infection. *AIDS Clin Care* 1993;5:1–8.
312. Narang PK, Lewis RC, Bianchine JR. Rifabutin absorption in humans: relative bioavailability and food effect. *Clin Pharmacol Ther* 1992;52:335–341.
313. Skinner MH, Hsieh M, Torseth J, et al. Pharmacokinetics of rifabutin. *Antimicrob Agents Chemother* 1989;33:1237–1241.
314. Rifabutin. *Med Lett* 1993;35:36–38.
315. Kucers A, Bennett NMcK. Ethionamide. In: *The use of antibiotics,* 4th ed. Philadelphia: Lippincott, 1987;1426–1431.
316. Jenner PJ, Ellard GA, Gruer PK, Aber VR. A comparison of the blood levels and urinary excretion of ethionamide and prothionamide in man. *J Antimicrob Chemother* 1984;13:267–277.
317. Peloquin CA, James GT, McCarthy E, Goble M. Pharmacokinetic evaluation of ethionamide suppositories. *Pharmacotherapy* 1991;11:359–363.
318. Weinstein MJ, Hallett WY. Absorption and toxicity of ethionamide. *Am Rev Respir Dis* 1962;85:407–411.
319. Roussouw JS, Saunders SJ. Hepatic complications of antituberculous therapy. *Q J Med* 1975;44:1–22.
320. Robson JM, Sullivan FM. Antituberculous drugs. *Pharmacol Rev* 1963;15:169–221.
321. Aminosalicylic acid. In: McEvoy GK, ed. *AHFS drug information 93—American Hospital Formulary Service.* Bethesda: American Society of Hospital Pharmacists, 1993;347–348.
322. Lead article. Antituberculous drugs and the liver. *Br Med J* 1975;2:522–526.
323. Kucers A, Bennett NMcK. Cycloserine. In: *The use of antibiotics,* 4th ed. Philadelphia: Lippincott, 1987;1418–1421.
324. Palacios J, Serrano R. Proton permeability induced by polyene antibiotics. A plausible mechanism for their inhibition of maltose fermentation in yeast. *Fed Eur Biochem Soc Lett* 1978;91:198–201.
325. Merz WG, Sandford GR. Isolation and characterization of a polyene-resistant variant of *Candida tropicalis. J Clin Microbiol* 1979;9:677–680.
326. Powderly WG, Kobayashi GS, Herzig GP, Medoff G. Amphotericin B-resistant yeast infection in severely immunocompromised patients. *Am J Med* 1988;84:826–831.
327. Rahko PS, Davey WP, Wheat JL, Bartlett M. Treatment of *Torulopsis glabrata* peritonitis with intraperitoneal amphotericin B. *JAMA* 1983;249:1187–1188.
328. Collette N, van der Auwera P, Pascual Lopez A, Heymans C, Meunier F. Tissue concentrations and bioactivity of amphotericin B in cancer patients treated with amphotericin B-deoxycholate. *Antimicrob Agents Chemother* 1989;33:362–368.
329. Lyman CA, Walsh TJ. Systemically administered antifungal agents. *Drugs* 1992;44:9–35.
330. Barriere SL. Pharmacology and pharmacokinetics of traditional systemic antifungal agents. *Pharmacotherapy* 1990;10(Suppl):134S–140S.
331. Ismail MA, Lerner SA. Disseminated blastomycosis in a pregnant woman. Review of amphotericin B usage during pregnancy. *Am Rev Respir Dis* 1982;126:350–353.
332. Sud IJ, Feingold DS. Effect of ketoconazole on the fungicidal action of amphotericin B in *Candida albicans. Antimicrob Agents Chemother* 1983;23:185–192.
333. Graybill JR, Williams DM, Cutsem EV, et al. Combination therapy of experimental histoplasmosis and cryptococcosis with amphotericin B and ketoconazole. *Rev Infect Dis* 1980;2:551–554.
334. Vanden Bossche H, Bellens D, Colls W, et al. Cytochrome p-450: target for itraconazole. *Drug Dev Res* 1986;8:287–298.
335. Warnock DW, Burke J, Cope NJ, Johnson EM, von Fraunhofer NA, Williams EW. Fluconazole resistance in *Candida glabrata. Lancet* 1988;2:1310.
336. Denning DW, Tucker RM, Hanson LH, Stevens DA. Treatment of invasive aspergillosis with itraconazole. *Am J Med* 1989;86:791–800.
337. Bozzette SA, Gordon RL, Yen A, Rinaldi M, Ito MK, Fierer J. Biliary concentrations of fluconazole in a patient with candidal cholecystitis: case report. *Clin Infect Dis* 1992;15:701–703.
338. Grant SM, Clissold SP. Itraconazole. A review of its pharmacodynamic and pharmacokinetic properties, and therapeutic use in superficial and systemic mycoses. *Drugs* 1989;37:310–344.
339. Durand F, Bernuau J, Dupont B, et al. *Aspergillus* intraabdomi-

nal abscess after liver transplantation successfully treated with itraconazole. *Transplantation* 1992;54:734–735.

340. Brass C, Galgiani JN, Blaschke TF, Defelice R, O'Reilly RA, Stevens DA. Disposition of ketoconazole, an oral antifungal, in humans. *Antimicrob Agents Chemother* 1982;21:151–158.

341. Bodey GP. Azole antifungal agents. *Clin Infect Dis* 1992; 14(Suppl 1):S161–S169.

342. Safety of terfenadine and astemizole. *Med Lett* 1992;34:9–10.

343. Samuelson JC, Burke A, Courval JM. Susceptibility of an emetine-resistant mutant of *Entamoeba histolytica* to multiple drugs and to channel blockers. *Antimicrob Agents Chemother* 1992;36:2392–2397.

344. Townson SM, Laqua H, Upcroft P, Boreham PFL, Upcroft JA. Induction of metronidazole and furazolidine resistance in *Giardia*. *Trans R Soc Trop Med Hyg* 1992;86:521–522.

345. Prichard RK. Antihelminthic resistance in nematodes: extent, recent understanding and future directions for control and research. *Int J Parasitol* 1990;20:515–523.

346. Most H. Treatment of common parasitic infections of man encountered in the United States (second of 2 parts). *N Engl J Med* 1972;298:698–702.

347. Drugs for parasitic infections. *Med Lett* 1993;35:111–122.

348. Miller RA, Minshew BH. *Blastocystis hominis*, an organism in search of a disease. *Rev Infect Dis* 1988;10:930–938.

349. Doyle PW, Helgason MM, Mathias RG, Proctor EM. Epidemiology and pathogenicity of *Blastocystis hominis*. *J Clin Microbiol* 1990;28:116–121.

350. Rollo IM. Drugs used in the chemotherapy of amebiasis. In: Goodman LS, Gilman A, eds. *The pharmacological basis of therapeutics*, 5th ed. New York: Macmillan, 1975;1069–1080.

351. Berggren L, Hansson O. Absorption of intestinal antiseptics derived from 8-hydroxyquinolines. *Clin Pharmacol Ther* 1968; 9:67–70.

352. Fleisher DI, Hepler RS, Landau JW. Blindness during diiodohydroxyquin (Diodoquin) therapy: a case report. *Pediatrics* 1974;54:106.

353. Warning on diiodohydroxyquin. *Med Lett* 1974;16:71–72.

354. Clifford RF, Gawel M. Clioquinol neurotoxicity: an overview. *Acta Neurol Scand* 1984;100(Suppl):137–145.

355. Oakley GP. The neurotoxicity of the halogenated hydroxyquinolines. *JAMA* 1973;225:395–397.

356. Soderman WA. Amebiasis. *Am J Dig Dis* 1971;16:51–60.

357. Courtney KD, Thompson PE, Hodgkinson R, Fitzsimmons JR. Paromomycin as a therapeutic substance for intestinal amebiasis and bacterial enteritis. In: *Antibiotics annual 1959–1960*. New York: Antibiotica, 1960;304–309.

358. McAuley JB, Juranek DD. Luminal agents in the treatment of amebiasis. *Clin Infect Dis* 1992;14:1161–1162.

359. Reed SL. Reply. *Clin Infect Dis* 1992;14:1162.

360. Klezy K, Gold J, Blaze J, Jakes P. Paromomycin for the treatment of cryptosporidial diarrhea in AIDS patients. *AIDS* 1991; 5:1146–1147.

361. Fichtenbaum CJ, Ritchie DJ, Powderly WG. Use of paromomycin for treatment of cryptosporidiosis in patients with AIDS. *Clin Infect Dis* 1993;16:298–300.

362. Armitage K, Flanigan T, Carey J, et al. Treatment of cryptosporidiosis with paromomycin. A report of 5 cases. *Arch Intern Med* 1992;152:2497–2499.

363. Botero D. Paromomycin as effective treatment of *Taenia* infections. *Am J Trop Med Hyg* 1970;19:234–237.

364. Marshall RJ, Flanigan TP. Paromomycin inhibits *Cryptosporidium* infection of a human enterocyte cell line. *J Infect Dis* 1992;165:772–774.

365. D'Alauro F, Lee RV, Pao-In K, Khairalleh M. Intestinal parasites and pregnancy. *Obstet Gynecol* 1985;66:639–643.

366. Botero DR. Treatment of acute and chronic intestinal amoebiasis with entamide furoate. *Trans R Soc Trop Med Hyg* 1964; 58:419–421.

367. Reed SL. Amebiasis: an update. *Clin Infect Dis* 1992;14: 385–391.

368. Webster LT. Drugs used in the chemotherapy of protozoal infections. In: Gilman AG, Rall TW, Nies AS, Taylor P, eds. *The pharmacological basis of therapeutics*, 8th ed. New York: Pergamon Press, 1990;999–1007.

369. Wilmshurst EC, Cliffe EE. Absorption and distribution of amoebicides. In: Binns TB, ed. *Absorption and distribution of drugs*. Baltimore: Williams & Wilkins, 1964;191–198.

370. Wolfe MS. Non-dysenteric intestinal amoebiasis: treatment with diloxanide furoate. *JAMA* 1973;224:389–395.

371. Powell SJ, MacLeod I, Wilmot AJ, Elsdon-Dew R. Metronidazole in amoebic dysentery and amoebic liver abscess. *Lancet* 1966;2:1329–1331.

372. Pratt WB, Fekety R. Treatment of parasitic disease. In: *The antimicrobial drugs*. New York: Oxford University Press, 1986;385–413.

373. Levi GC, DeAvila CA, Neto VA. Efficacy of various drugs for the treatment of giardiasis. A comparative study. *Am J Trop Med Hyg* 1977;26:564–565.

374. Glupczynski Y, Burette A. Drug therapy for *Helicobacter pylori* infection: problems and pitfalls. *Am J Gastroenterol* 1990; 85:1545–1551.

375. Oderda G, Vaira D, Ainley C, et al. Eighteen month follow-up of *Helicobacter pylori* positive children treated with amoxicillin and tinidazole. *Gut* 1992;33:1328–1330.

376. Sawyer PR, Brogden RN, Pinder RM, Speight TM, Avery GS. Tinidazole: a review of its antiprotozoal activity and therapeutic efficacy. *Drugs* 1976;11:423–440.

377. Taylor JA, Migliardi JR, Von Wittenau MS. Tinidazole and metronidazole pharmacokinetics in man and mouse. *Antimicrob Agents Chemother 1970* 1971;267–270.

378. Wood BA, Faulkner JK, Monro AM. The pharmacokinetics, metabolism and tissue distribution of tinidazole. *J Antimicrob Chemother* 1982;10(Suppl A):43–57.

379. Kucers A, Bennett NMcK. Tinidazole. In: *The use of antibiotics*, 4th ed. Philadelphia: Lippincott, 1987;1330–1339.

380. Wood BA, Rycroft D, Monro AM. The metabolism of tinidazole in the rat and dog. *Xenobiotica* 1973;3:801–812.

381. Sankale M, Coly D, Thomas J, et al. Injectable ornidazole in severe amoebiasis. In: Siegnethaler W, Luthy R, eds. *Current chemotherapy. Proceedings of the 10th International Congress of Chemotherapy*, Zurich, Switzerland. Washington, DC: American Society for Microbiology, 1978;140–142.

382. Jokippi L, Kokippi AMM. Treatment of giardiasis: comparative evaluation of ornidazole and tinidazole as a single oral dose. *Gastroenterology* 1983;83:399–404.

383. Matheson I, Hernborg-Johannesson K, Bjorkvall B. Plasma levels after a single oral dose of 1.5 g ornidazole. *Br J Vener Dis* 1977;53:236–239.

384. Kucers A, Bennett NMcK. Nimorazole, ornidazole, carnidazole, secnidazole. In: *The use of antibiotics*, 4th ed. Philadelphia: Lippincott, 1987;1340–1343.

385. Pambo HO, Estambale BB, Chung CN, Donno L. Comparative study of aminosidine, etophamide and nimorazole, alone or in combination, in the treatment of intestinal amoebiasis in Kenya. *Eur J Clin Pharmacol* 1990;39:353–357.

386. Wilmot AJ, Powell SJ, Adams EB. Chloroquine compared with chloroquine and emetine combined in amebic liver abscess. *Am J Trop Med Hyg* 1959;8:623–632.

387. Scragg JN, Powell SJ. Emetine hydrochloride and dehydroemetine combined with chloroquine in the treatment of children with amoebic liver abscess. *Arch Dis Child* 1968;43: 121–123.

388. Huang T, Grollman AP. Novel inhibitors of protein synthesis in animal cells. *Fed Proc* 1970;29:209.

389. Gimble AI, Davison C, Smith PK. Studies on the toxicity, distribution, and excretion of emetine. *J Pharmacol Exp Ther* 1948;94:431–438.

390. Schwartz DE, Herrero J. Comparative pharmacokinetic studies of dehydroemetine and emetine in guinea pigs using spectrofluorometric and radiometric methods. *Am J Trop Med Hyg* 1965;14:78–83.

391. Powell SJ. The cardiotoxicity of systemic amebicides: a comparative electrocardiographic study. *Am J Trop Med Hyg* 1967; 16:447–450.

392. Yang WCT, Dubic M. Mechanism of emetine cardiotoxicity. *Pharmacol Ther* 1980;10:15–26.

393. Klatskin G, Friedman H. Emetine toxicity in man: studies on the nature of early toxic manifestations, their relation to the

dose level and their significance in determining safe dosage. *Ann Intern Med* 1948;28:892–914.

394. Sodeman WA, Doerner AA, Gordon EM, Gillikin CM. Chloroquine in hepatic amebiasis. *Ann Intern Med* 1951;35:331–341.

395. Walker O, Salako LA, Alvan G, Ericsson O, Sjoqvist F. The disposition of chloroquine in healthy Nigerians after single intravenous and oral dosages. *Br J Clin Pharmacol* 1987;23: 295–301.

396. Berliner RW, Earle DP, Taggart JV, et al. Studies on the chemotherapy of human malarias. VI. The physiological disposition, antimalarial activity and toxicity of several derivatives of 4-aminoquinolines. *J Clin Invest* 1948;27(Suppl):98–107.

397. Chloroquine. In: Dollery C, ed. *Therapeutic drugs.* Edinburgh: Churchill Livingstone, 1991;C188–C193.

398. Wolfe MS. Giardiasis. *Clin Microbiol Rev* 1992;5:93–100.

399. O'Brien RL, Olenick JG, Hahn FE. Reactions of quinine, chloroquine, and quinacrine with DNA and their effects on the DNA and RNA polymerase reactions. *Proc Natl Acad Sci USA* 1966;55:1511–1517.

400. Findlay GM. *Recent advances in chemotherapy,* vol II. London: J and A Churchill Ltd, 1951.

401. Smith JW, Wolfe MS. Giardiasis. *Annu Rev Med* 1980;31: 373–383.

402. Lindenmayer JP, Vargas P. Toxic psychosis following use of quinacrine. *J Clin Psychiatry* 1981;42:162–164.

403. Sokol RJ, Lichtenstein PK, Farrell MK. Quinacrine hydrochloride induced yellow discoloration of the skin in children. *Pediatrics* 1982;69:232–233.

404. Dupont HL, Ericsson CD, Galindo E, et al. Furazolidine versus ampicillin in the treatment of traveler's diarrhea. *Antimicrob Agents Chemother* 1984;26:160–163.

405. Chaudhuri RN, Sanyal SN, Neogy KN, Barua D, Manji P. Furazolidine in cholera. *Lancet* 1965;2:909.

406. Chamberlain RE. Chemotherapeutic properties of prominent nitrofurantoins. *J Antimicrob Chemother* 1976;2:325–336.

407. Treatment of giardiasis. *Med Lett* 1976;18:39–40.

408. Van den Bossche H, Rochette F, Horig C. Mebendazole and related antihelminthics. *Adv Pharmacol Chemother* 1982;19: 67–128.

409. Keystone JS, Murdock JK. Mebendazole. *Ann Intern Med* 1979;91:582–586.

410. Singson CN, Banzon TC, Cross JH. Mebendazole in the treatment of intestinal capillariasis. *Am J Trop Med Hyg* 1975;24: 932–934.

411. Banerjee D, Prakash O, Kaliyugaperunal V. A clinical trial of mebendazole (R17635) in cases of hookworm infection. *Indian J Med Res* 1972;60:562–536.

412. Vakil BJ, Dalal NJ. Comparative efficacy of new antihelminthics. *Prog Drug Res* 1975;19:166–175.

413. Wolfe MS, Wershing JM. Mebendazole: treatment of trichuriasis and ascariasis in Bahamian children. *JAMA* 1974;230: 1408–1411.

414. Miller MJ, Krupp IM, Little MD, Santos C. Mebendazole: an effective antihelminthic for trichuriasis in children. *Am J Trop Med Hyg* 1977;26:198–203.

415. Scrugg JN, Proctor EM. Mebendazole in the treatment of severe symptomatic trichuriasis in children. *Am J Trop Med Hyg* 1977;26:198–203.

416. Brugmans JP, Thienpant DC, Van Wigngaarden I, Vanparijs OF, Shuermans VL, Lauwers HL. Mebendazole in enterobiasis—radiochemical and pilot clinical study in 1278 subjects. *JAMA* 1971;217:313–316.

417. Fernando SSE, Denham DA. The effects of mebendazole on *Trichinella spiralis* in mice. *J Parasitol* 1976;62:874–876.

418. Levin ML. Treatment of trichinosis with mebendazole. *Am J Trop Med Hyg* 1983;32:980–983.

419. Ivanov KSS, Antonov VS, Knysch GG, et al. The clinical characteristics of 2 outbreaks of trichinellosis. *Med Parazitol (Mosb)* 1990;July/Aug:41–42.

420. Chavarria AP, Villarejas VM, Zeledan R. Mebendazole in the treatment of *Taenia solium* and *Taenia saginata*. *Am J Trop Med Hyg* 1977;26:118–120.

421. Beard TC, Rickard MD, Goodman HT. Medical treatment for hydatids. *Med J Aust* 1978;1:633–635.

422. Wagner ED, Chavarria AP. In vivo effects of a new antihelminthic, mebendazole (R-17635) on the eggs of *Trichuris trichiura* and hookworm. *Am J Trop Med Hyg* 1974;23:151–153.

423. Munst GJ, Karlaganis G, Bircher J. Plasma concentrations of mebendazole during treatment of echinococcosis. *Eur J Clin Pharmacol* 1980;17:375–378.

424. Morris DL, Gould SE. Serum and cyst concentration of mebendazole and flubendazole in hydatid disease. *Br Med J* 1982;285: 175.

425. Dawson M, Braithwaite PA, Roberts MA, Watson TR. The pharmacokinetics and bioavailability of a tracer dose of [^{3}H]-mebendazole in man. *Br J Clin Pharmacol* 1985;19:79–86.

426. Pratt WB, Fekety R. Chemotherapy of helminthic disease. In: *The antimicrobial drugs.* New York: Oxford University Press, 1986;414–446.

427. Bechkti A, Pirotte J. Cimetidine increases serum mebendazole concentrations: implications for treatment of hepatic hydatid cysts. *Br J Clin Pharmacol* 1987;24:390–392.

428. Rossignol JF, Maisonneuve H. Albendazole: placebo controlled study in 870 patients with intestinal helminthiasis. *Trans R Soc Trop Med Hyg* 1983;77:707–711.

429. Misra RC, Dewan R, Sachdev S, Sachdev K, Agarwal SK, Gupta PS. Albendazole: a new drug in the treatment of intestinal helminthiasis (nematodes and cestodes). *Curr Ther Res* 1983;33:758–761.

430. Ramalingam S, Sinniah B, Kirshnan U. Albendazole, an effective single dose broad spectrum antihelminthic drug. *Am J Trop Med Hyg* 1983;32:984–989.

431. Bassily S, El-Masry NA, Trabolsi B, Farid Z. Treatment of ancylostomiasis and ascariasis with albendazole. *Ann Trop Med Parasitol* 1984;78:81–82.

432. Coulaud JP, Rossignol JF. Albendazole: a new single dose antihelminthic study in 1455 patients. *Ann Trop Med Parasitol* 1984;78:81–82.

433. Albendazole. In: Dollery C, ed. *Therapeutic drugs.* Edinburgh: Churchill Livingstone, 1991;A31–A34.

434. Jagota SC. Albendazole, a broad spectrum antihelminthic, in the treatment of intestinal nematode and cestode infection: a multicenter study in 480 patients. *Clin Ther* 1986;8:226–231.

435. Morris DL, Dykes PW, Marriner S, et al. Albendazole: objective evidence of response in human hydatid disease. *JAMA* 1985;253:2053–2057.

436. Cruz M, Cruz I, Horton J. Albendazole versus praziquantel in the treatment of cerebral cysticercosis: clinical evaluation. *Tran R Soc Trop Med Hyg* 1991;85:244–247.

437. Kan SP. The antihelminthic effects of flubendazole on *Trichuris trichiura* and *A. lumbricoides*. *Trans R Soc Trop Med Hyg* 1982;77:668–670.

438. Barrowman MM, Marriner SE, Bogan JA. The binding and subsequent inhibition of tubulin polymerization in *Ascaris suum* in vitro by benzimidazole antihelminthics. *Biochem Pharmacol* 1984;33:3037–3040.

439. Wilson JF, Rausch RL, McMahon BJ, Schantz PM, Trujillo DE, O'Gorman MA, Wilson JF. Albendazole therapy in alveolar hydatid disease. A report of favorable results in 2 patients after short-term therapy. *Am J Trop Med Hyg* 1987;37:162–168.

440. Saimot AG. Albendazole as potential treatment for human hydatidosis. *Lancet* 1983;2:652–656.

441. Horton RJ. Chemotherapy of echinococcus infection in man. *Trans R Soc Trop Med Hyg* 1989;83:97–102.

442. Steiger U, Cotting J, Reichen J. Albendazole treatment of echinococcus in humans: effects on microsomal metabolism and drug tolerance. *Clin Pharmacol Ther* 1990;47:347–353.

443. Most H, Yoeli M, Campbell WC, Cuckler AC. The treatment of *Strongyloides* and *Enterobius* infections with thiabendazole. *Am J Trop Med Hyg* 1965;14:379–382.

444. Grove DI. Treatment of strongyloidiasis with thiabendazole: an analysis of toxicity and effectiveness. *Trans R Soc Trop Med Hyg* 1982;76:114–118.

445. Brown HD, Matzuk AR, Ilves IR, et al. Antiparasitic drugs. IV. 2-(4'thiazoyl)-benzimidazole, a new anthelminthic. *J Am Chem Soc* 1961;83:1764–1765.

446. Kohler P, Bachmann R. The effects of the antiparasitic drugs levamisole, thiabendazole, praziquantel and chloroquine on mi-

tochondrial electron transport in muscle tissue from *Ascaris suum. Mol Pharmacol* 1978;14:155–158.

447. Watts SDM, Rapson EB, Atkins AM, Lee DL. Inhibition of acetylcholinesterase secretion from *Nippostrongylus brasiliensis* by benzimidazole anthelmintics. *Biochem Pharmacol* 1982;31:3035–3040.

448. Stone OJ, Stone CT, Mullins JF. Thiabendazole: probable cure for trichinosis. *JAMA* 1964;187:536–538.

449. Bauer LA, Raisys VA, Watts MT, Ballinger J. The pharmacokinetics of thiabendazole and its metabolites in an anephric patient undergoing hemodialysis and hemoperfusion. *J Clin Pharmacol* 1982;22:276–280.

450. Tocco DJ, Rosenblum C, Martin CM, Robinson HJ. Absorption, metabolism, and excretion of thiabendazole in man and laboratory animals. *Toxicol Appl Pharmacol* 1966;9:31–39.

451. Pitts NE, Migliardi JR. Antiminth (pyrantel pamoate): the clinical evaluation of a new broad spectrum antihelminthic. *Clin Pediatr* 1974;13:87–94.

452. Bell WJ, Nassif S. Comparison of pyrantel pamoate and piperazine phosphate in the treatment of ascariasis. *Am J Trop Med Hyg* 1971;20:584–588.

453. Botero D, Castano A. Comparative study of pyrantel pamoate, bephenium hydroxynaphthoate and tetrachloroethylene in the treatment of *Necator americanus* infections. *Am J Trop Med Hyg* 1973;22:45–52.

454. Farahmandian I, Arfaa F, Reza M. Comparative studies on the evaluation of the effects of new antihelminthics on various intestinal nematodes in Iran. *Chemotherapy* 1977;23:98–105.

455. Aubry ML, Cowell P, Davey MJ, Shevde S. Aspects of the pharmacology of a new anthelmintic: pyrantel. *Br J Pharmacol* 1970;38:332–344.

456. Kimura Y, Kume M. Absorption, distribution, excretion and metabolism of pyrantel pamoate. *Pharmacometrics* 1971;5:347–358.

457. Freedman DO, Aierdt WS, Lujan A, Nutman TB. The efficacy of ivermectin in the chemotherapy of gastrointestinal helminthiasis in humans. *J Infect Dis* 1989;159:1151–1153.

458. Naquira C, Jimenez G, Guerra JG, et al. Ivermectin for human strongyloidiasis and other intestinal helminths. *Am J Trop Med Hyg* 1989;40:304–309.

459. Campbell WC, Fisher MH, Stapley ED, Albers-Schonberg G, Jacob TA. Ivermectin: a potent new antiparasitic agent. *Science* 1983;221:823–828.

460. Ette EI, Thomas WOA, Achumba JI. Ivermectin: a long acting microfilaricidal agent. *DICP* 1990;24:426–433.

461. Campbell WC, ed. *Ivermectin & abamectin.* New York: Springer-Verlag, 1989.

462. Campbell WC, Rew RS. *Chemotherapy of parasitic diseases.* New York: Plenum Press, 1986;272–273.

463. Guerrant RL, Schwartzmann JD, Pearson RD. Intestinal nematode infections. In: Strickland GT, ed. *Hunter's tropical medicine,* 7th ed. Philadelphia: Saunders, 1991;684–689.

464. Thienpont D, Brugmans J, Abadi K, Tanamal S. Tetramisole in the treatment of nematode infections of man. *Am J Trop Med Hyg* 1969;18:520–525.

465. Moens M, Dom J, Burke WE, Schlossberg S, Schermans V. Levamisole in ascariasis. A multicenter controlled evaluation. *Am J Trop Med Hyg* 1978;27:897–904.

466. Harrow ID, Gration KAF. Mode of action of the antihelminthics morantel, pyrantel and levamisole on muscle cell membrane of the nematode *Ascaris suum. Pesticide Sci* 1985;16:662–672.

467. *Physicians desk reference,* 47th ed. Montvale, NJ: Medical Economics Publishing, 1993;1164–1165.

468. Goodwin LG, Standen OD. Treatment of ascariasis with various salts of piperazine. *Br Med J* 1958;1:131–133.

469. Brown HW, Chan KF, Hussey KL. Treatment of enterobiasis and ascariasis with piperazine. *JAMA* 1956;161:515–520.

470. Saz HJ, Bueding E. Relationship between antihelminthic effects and biochemical and physiological mechanisms. *Pharmacol Rev* 1966;18:871–984.

471. Hana S, Tang A. Human urinary excretion of piperazine citrate from syrup formulation. *J Pharmaceut Sci* 1973;62:2024–2025.

472. Bellander T, Osterdahl BG, Hagmar L. Formation of *N*-mo-

nitrosopiperazine in the stomach and its excretion in the urine after oral intake of piperazine. *Toxicol Appl Pharmacol* 1985;80:193–198.

473. Boulos BM, Davis LE. Hazard of simultaneous administration of phenothiazine and piperazine. *N Engl J Med* 1969;280:1245–1246.

474. Andrews P, Thomas H, Pohlke R, Seubert J. Praziquantel. *Med Res Rev* 1983;3:147–200.

475. Pearson RD, Guerrant RL. Praziquantel: a major advance in antihelminthic therapy. *Ann Intern Med* 1983;99:195–198.

476. King CH, Mahmoud AAF. Drugs five years later: praziquantel. *Ann Intern Med* 1989;110:290–296.

477. Okeefe P, Edgett H. Efficacy and safety of praziquantel in treatment of *Clonorchis sinensis/Opisthorchis* viverrini: results of double blind placebo controlled trial in Southeast Asian refugees. *Curr Ther Res* 1986;40:411–417.

478. Knobloch J, Paz G, Feldmeier H, Wegner D, Voelker J. Serum antibody levels in human paragonimiasis before and after therapy with praziquantel. *Trans R Soc Trop Med Hyg* 1984;78:835–836.

479. Pachucki CT, Levandowski RA, Brown VA, Sonnenkalb BH, Vruno MJ. American parogonimiasis treated with praziquantel. *N Engl J Med* 1984;311:582–583.

480. Schiappacasse RH, Mohammadi D, Christie AJ. Successful treatment of severe infection with *Fasciola hepatica* with praziquantel. *J Infect Dis* 1985;152:1339–1340.

481. Pax R, Bennett JL, Fetterer R. A benzodiazepine derivative and praziquantel: effects on musculature of *Schistosoma mansoni* and *Schistosoma japonicum. Naunyn Schmiedebergs Arch Pharmacol* 1978;304:309–315.

482. Mehlhorn H, Becker B, Andrews P, Thomas H, Frenkel KJ. In vivo and in vitro experiments on the effects of praziquantel on *Schistosoma mansoni. Arz Drug Res* 1981;31(3a):544–554.

483. Leopold G, Ungethum W, Groll EJ, Diekmann HW, Nowak H, Wegner DHG. Clinical pharmacology in normal volunteers of praziquantel, a new drug against schistosomes and cestodes. *Eur J Clin Pharmacol* 1978;14:281–291.

484. Buhring KU, Diekmann HW, Muller H, Garbe A, Nowak H. Metabolism of praziquantel in man. *Eur J Drug Metab Pharmacokinet* 1978;3:179–190.

485. Praziquantel. In: Dollery C, ed. *Therapeutic drugs.* Edinburgh: Churchill Livingstone, 1991;189–195.

486. Ishizaki T, Kamo E, Boehme K. Double-blind studies of tolerance to praziquantel in Japanese patients with *Schistosoma japonicum* infections. *Bull World Health Organ* 1979;57:787–791.

487. Sleigh AC, Mott KE, Hoff R, Maguire JH, Da Franca Silva JT. Manson's schistosomiasis in Brazil: 11 year evaluation of successful disease control with oxamniquine. *Lancet* 1986;1:635–637.

488. Foster R. A review of clinical experience with oxamniquine. *Trans R Soc Trop Med Hyg* 1987;81:55–59.

489. Foster R, Cheetham BL. Studies with the schistosomicide oxamniquine (UK4271) I. Activity in rodents and in vitro. *Trans R Soc Trop Med Hyg* 1973;67:674–684.

490. Yeang FSW, Marshall I, Huggins M. Oxamniquine resistance in *S. mansoni:* fact or fiction. *Ann Trop Med Parasitol* 1987;81:337–339.

491. Kaye B, Woolhouse NM. The metabolism of oxamniquine, a new schistosomicide. *Ann Trop Med Parasitol* 1976;70:323–328.

492. Omer AHS. Oxamniquine for treating *Schistosoma mansoni* infection in Sudan. *Br Med J* 1978;2:163–165.

493. Katz N, Zicker F, Pereira JP. Field trials with oxamniquine in a *Schistosomiasis mansoni*-endemic area. *Am J Trop Med Hyg* 1977;26:234–244.

494. Kim JS. Treatment of *Paragonimus westermani* infections with bithionol. *Am J Trop Med Hyg* 1970;19:940–942.

495. Ashton WIG, Boardman DL, D'Sa JC, Everall PH, Houghton AWJ. Human fasciliasis in Shropshire. *Br Med J* 1970;3:500–502.

496. James DM, Gilles HM. *Antiparasitic drugs: pharmacology and usage.* Chichester: Wiley, 1985.

497. Plaut AG, Sanyakarn CK, Manning GS. A clinical study of

Fasciolopsis buski infection in Thailand. *Trans R Soc Trop Med Hyg* 1969;63:470–478.

498. Jung RC, McCroan JE. Efficacy of bephenium and tetrachloro-ethylene in mass treatment of hookworm infection. *Am J Trop Med Hyg* 1960;9:492–495.

499. Pearson RD, Hewlett EL. Niclosamide therapy for tapeworm infections. *Ann Intern Med* 1985;102:550–551.

500. Brown HW. Antihelminthics, new and old. *Clin Pharmacol Ther* 1968;10:5–21.

501. Keeling JED. The chemotherapy of cestode infections. *Adv Chemother* 1968;3:109–152.

502. Schiebel LW, Saz HJ, Bueding E. The anaerobic incorporation of ^{32}P into adenosinetriphosphate by *Hymenolepis diminuta*. *J Biol Chem* 1968;243:2229–2235.

Infections of the Gastrointestinal Tract,
edited by M. J. Blaser, P. D. Smith, J. I. Ravdin,
H. B. Greenberg, and R. L. Guerrant
Raven Press, Ltd., New York © 1995.

CHAPTER 88

Pharmacology of Agents Other than Antibiotics Used in Gastrointestinal Infections

David G. Binion and John G. Banwell

The four organs of the luminal gastrointestinal tract—esophagus, stomach, small intestine, and large intestine—are all susceptible to enteric infection. Symptoms of gastrointestinal infection are protean and can be grouped into four broad categories, based largely on the anatomic involvement of the disease process. Odynophagia and dysphagia, painful and difficult swallowing associated with pyrosis and regurgitation, are the classic symptoms of esophageal infection. Gastric infection may be associated with subsequent alterations in gastric function, including epigastric pain, nausea, vomiting, and gastric retention. Enteric infection of the small bowel results in diarrheal illnesses, associated with weight loss, abdominal cramping, and nutrient malabsorption. Colonic infections are also characterized by colicky abdominal pain, distension and ileus, diarrhea, rectal bleeding, and tenesmus. Anorectal pain is an additional common symptom complex that is often the result of primary infection, or the secondary sequela of some diarrheal illness. As a general principle, it is important to direct therapy at the offending pathogen. However, there is an important role for adjuvant treatment strategies to alleviate these symptom complexes of patient discomfort. An extensive pharmacopeia is available, which broadly includes: (a) *specific therapy,* consisting of agents that have defined modes of action that are generally understood and include antiemetics, anti-acid agents, antacids, prokinetic agents, analgesics, anti-inflammatory agents, and antidiarrheal compounds, which have defined pharmacologic actions; and (b) *nonspecific therapy,* which includes stool softeners, rectal suppositories, and retention enemas. Nonspecific therapy oftentimes represents treatment options available to patients over-the-

counter (OTC), where pharmacological action is poorly understood. Dietary constituents may also be important in allaying or exacerbating symptoms in the acute and recovering phases of disease. Therapy may be used to achieve cure of symptoms as well as for prophylaxis in some instances.

Understanding the pathophysiology of these four symptom complexes provides the best strategy for choice of appropriate pharmacotherapy. Symptomatic therapy for gastrointestinal infections should be considered adjunctive therapy: primary medical intervention will always be the use of appropriate antimicrobials, where this is available and curative.

PATHOPHYSIOLOGY OF GASTROINTESTINAL SYMPTOMS

Systemic Symptoms

The gastrointestinal tract has multiple functions, but primary are its role as portal of entry for liquids and nutrients and as an efficient recovery system for the 6 to 10 L of fluid and secretions that pass through the gastrointestinal system daily. Systemic symptoms related to gastrointestinal infection will typically contribute to an imbalance in these regulatory mechanisms for maintaining adequate fluid balance—either through inadequate intake, the sequela of anorexia, malaise, fever, myalgias, and nausea and vomiting, or through excess losses, a frequent result of acute diarrhea (1). Symptoms of dehydration and volume depletion are categorized as mild, moderate, or severe. In mild dehydration symptoms include thirst and restlessness, with unremarkable physical findings including moist mucous membranes and normal pulse. The fluid deficit in this setting is less than 50 mL/

D. G. Binion and J. G. Banwell: Case Western Reserve University School of Medicine, and Department of Medicine, Division of Gastroenterology, University Hospitals of Cleveland, Cleveland, Ohio 44106-5000.

kg of body weight. Moderate dehydration produces thirst and lethargy. Signs include sunken eyes and fontanelles in children, dry mucous membranes, skin turgor that retracts slowly to pinch, deep often rapid respiration, reduced urine that is dark in color, and rapid, weak pulse. Fluid deficit lies between 50 and 80 mL/kg of body weight. Severe dehydration is characterized by a drowsy patient, often cold and sweaty, with cyanotic extremities. Eyes are deeply sunken as are fontanelles. Skin is very dry, and turgor is poor with slow retraction to pinch. Respiration is deep and rapid, and urine output is nonexistent. Pulse is rapid, weak, and often not palpable. Fluid deficit in severe dehydration is often greater than 80 mL/kg of body weight (2).

The most important therapeutic response to volume depletion is restoration of fluid balance. It is most advantageous to utilize the gastrointestinal tract whenever possible to maintain fluid homeostasis, and oral rehydration solutions have been developed to facilitate this purpose. In the event that the gastrointestinal tract cannot tolerate nutrition and liquids or when a patient demonstrates findings of shock, intravenous fluid replacement is mandatory.

Nausea and Vomiting

Nausea and vomiting are frequent symptoms associated with gastrointestinal infections. These symptoms are the result of many varied stimuli that act on the sensory nervous system either directly in the gut or via circulatory and neuronal stimuli in the central nervous system (CNS). In the setting of enteric infection, nausea and vomiting usually are the result of one of two pathophysiologic mechanisms: local gastric mucosal irritation from ingested toxin and inflammatory products and functional or mechanical blockage of the gastroduodenal outlet (3).

Understanding of the emetic response evolved from neurological studies that demonstrated two distinct sites in the brainstem critical for control of emesis. The "vomiting center" located in the medulla coordinates and controls the final common motor mechanisms of vomiting, which reside in the lateral reticular formation. In addition, the "chemoreceptor trigger zone" (CTZ), an area rich in chemoreceptors that sample both blood and cerebrospinal fluid, lies adjacent to the area postrema. Both neuronal input as well as chemical and hormonal agents carried via the circulatory system can initiate vomiting but only through the vomiting center. In addition, other afferent input to the vomiting center arises from the vestibular system, central cortical areas, and the oropharynx and gastrointestinal tract (3).

Development of vomiting has been characterized by three physiologic steps. First, a preejection phase is characterized by gastric relaxation and retroperistalsis. Salivation, behavioral changes, and subjective nausea also characterize this phase whose duration is extremely variable, lasting from minutes to potentially days. The second, or ejection, phase is characterized by retching—the result of coordinated contraction of the abdominal muscles against a closed glottis. Retching allows for free retrograde flow of gastric contents into the esophagus, but the closed glottis prevents expulsion of these contents. The ejection phase culminates with vomiting, as the upper esophageal sphincter relaxes and intragastric contents are expelled via strong contraction of the abdominal musculature. The final postejection phase incorporates various systemic symptoms such as shivering, muscle weakness, and lethargy (4).

Treatment of nausea and vomiting relies on agents that act centrally or at the level of the gastrointestinal tract (4). The neurochemical mechanisms underlying emesis are continuing to be elucidated. Dopamine (D_2) receptors are implicated in the process of chemotherapy-induced emesis in the CNS. Specific D_2 receptor antagonists such as domperidone and phenothiazines, which block dopaminergic transmission, abolish emetic responses. Another group of centrally acting agents employed in the relief of nausea and vomiting are antagonists of histamine and acetylcholine and muscarinic receptor antagonists on the nucleus tractus solitarius. Much recent interest has focused on type D_3 serotonin receptors, which have been identified on vagal afferent fibers in the gastrointestinal tract and also centrally in the medulla. Increased urinary 5-hydroxy indoleacetic acid excretion, a major metabolite of serotonin, characterizes severe chemical-induced emesis. Prokinetic agents, such as metoclopramide, which act to increase gastric emptying, are also associated with a central antiemetic effect from antidopaminergic activity in the CTZ. Indeed, even nonspecific therapy, such as bismuth subsalicylate, has been demonstrated to have antiemetic, antinausea activity in volunteers challenged with ingested Norwalk agent. The mechanism of this action remains unclear but presumably depends on its effect within the gastrointestinal tract (5).

Many enteric infections produce nausea and vomiting, but typically they are acute and self-limited; symptomatic therapy may not be warranted in short-lived disease. However, patients with severe symptoms benefit from symptomatic use of centrally acting agents, which can prevent dehydration and need for hospitalization.

Upper Gastrointestinal Infections: Dysphagia/ Odynophagia/Pyrosis

Infections of the esophagus and stomach frequently manifest as difficulty and pain with swallowing (dysphagia and odynophagia) and with regurgitation. Infection of the gastric mucosa may also present with esophageal symptoms, the result of altered gastric motility, gastric retention, and gastroesophageal reflux or heartburn (6).

Dysphagia is an important and specific marker of esophageal pathology. Normally, swallowing once initiated voluntarily is followed by a peristaltic reflex. Patients with dysphagia are aware of difficulty in this process and typically complain of food "sticking" or "not going down right." Symptoms usually arise from two distinct mechanisms—mechanical obstruction of the esophagus or disordered esophageal propulsive function. Gastroesophageal infection produces dysphagia from a mechanism associated with ulceration of the mucosa to transmural inflammation of the esophagus.

Odynophagia, painful swallowing, often accompanies dysphagia. Invasion of enteric pathogens into and through the squamous epithelial layer of the esophagus results in mucosal inflammation and destruction and ulceration, with associated pain on ingestion of either a solid or liquid bolus. Pain may be so severe that it may preclude swallowing of even salivary secretions (7). Esophagitis may incorporate peptic components when associated with gastric reflux into the lower esophagus.

Pyrosis, or heartburn, is a common gastrointestinal complaint and is typically associated with reflux. The discomfort is usually described as "burning," and relief typically follows the ingestion of antacids. Enteric infection can be associated with heartburn in patients with cytomegalovirus (CMV) infection of the gastric mucosa, a common sequela of immunosuppression in organ transplantation. Altered gastric motility results in gastric stasis and a reservoir of acid stomach contents that readily refluxes into the esophagus, producing symptoms (23).

Odynophagia and dysphagia may be secondary complications of enteric infection when common medications cause caustic injury to the esophageal mucosa. Pill-induced esophagitis is a common, frequently underdiagnosed complication of oral medications. Many medications are responsible, with the antibiotics tetracycline and doxycycline, the antiviral azidothymidine (AZT), potassium supplements, and nonsteroidal anti-inflammatory pain relievers prominent on the list. Ingestion of medication in a recumbent position or with inadequate liquid to facilitate transit into the stomach results in pills partially dissolving within the esophagus and producing a caustic "burn" injury to the mucosal lining. The temporal relationship to the initiation of a prescription and careful history regarding the exact manner in which the patient consumes medications are important for making a correct diagnosis (8,9).

Symptomatic relief of severe odynophagia can be achieved through the use of antacids, along with topical analgesics (i.e., viscous lidocaine) frequently employed by radiation oncologists to relieve treatment-induced symptoms. Secondary acid-peptic injury can be relieved with the use of frequent antacids and antireflux measures, including head of bed elevation, frequent small meals, and postponing sleep for 4 hr following ingestion of the evening meal, to facilitate gastric emptying. The use of gastric antisecretory medications, such as histamine receptor antagonists, and proton pump inhibitors, such as omeprazol, is empiric. Deep penetrating ulcers of the esophagus associated with acquired immunodeficiency syndrome (AIDS) have been responsive to the use of frequent sucralfate slurries (7).

Small Bowel and Lower Gastrointestinal Infections: Diarrhea

Diarrhea, the passage of "too frequent, too loose stools," is a common sequela of gastrointestinal infection. The small and large intestines are highly specialized ab-

sorptive and secretory organs that function in tandem to recover 98% of the daily fluid volume that passes through the gastrointestinal tract. The efficiency of the intestines' ability to absorb nearly all of this 9-L daily volume of liquid—2 L from dietary consumption and approximately 7 L from various luminal secretions—is readily disturbed by gastrointestinal infection, with the resultant passage of diarrhea (10,11).

The pathophysiologic basis for diarrhea is twofold. Enteric pathogens, either directly or through inflammatory mediators, alter the normal mucosal electrolyte transport mechanisms. The classic sequela of enteric infection is secretory diarrhea, with the cholera toxin providing the example of an enterotoxigenic infection. It is now apparent that secretory diarrhea can also be induced through the release of inflammatory mediators associated with both enteroadhesive and enteroinvasive infections.

The basis of therapy in the treatment of infectious diarrhea is threefold (12). Antibacterial therapy directed at the responsible pathogen is often possible, but this is not always effective or immediate (13). Nonspecific nonantibiotic therapy often overshadows the role of antimicrobial therapy. Foremost is the requirement to restore fluid and electrolyte balance, which can be achieved with either intravenous or enteral rehydration solutions. These modalities of therapy are discussed in detail in the chapter by Snyder. In addition to restoring fluid balance, symptomatic pharmacotherapy with antidiarrheal agents may have a supportive role in restoring normal electrolyte and water transport.

Antidiarrheal agents fall into three categories. Binding agents that function intraluminally absorb liquid, toxins, or prosecretory factors within the gastrointestinal tract. Antimotility agents function by slowing the normal propulsive action of the gastrointestinal smooth muscle, thereby increasing the contact time between intraluminal liquid and the mucosa, enhancing the chance for absorption. A new category of antisecretory medications makes use of enteric hormonal control mechanisms to restore gastrointestinal homeostasis (14).

Anorectal Disorders

The anorectal region represents a transition from somatic cutaneous sensation to the visceral sensory pathways that subserve the colon and rectum. Perianal cutaneous sensation has the same modalities as the skin and traverses the pudendal nerve to spinal centers. Visceral afferent pathways originate in the rectum and adjacent structures such as the levator ani muscle. Non-noxious and noxious information is conveyed to the brain via small unmyelinated parasympathetic and sympathetic nerve fibers in which dorsal pathways transmit sensation of rectal fullness and the spinothalamic tract transmits pain to cortical levels.

Infections of the gastrointestinal tract often produce diarrhea, and the sequelae of increased defecatory frequency may include severe tenesmus, rectal pain, perianal excoriation, and discomfort. Sexually transmitted diseases of the lower bowel are associated with anal pain, tenesmus, and bleeding aggravated by defecation. Perianal condylomata are often painful with abrasion and minor trauma. Herpetic lesions of the sacral dermatomes may be associated with vesicles and pain in this site and frequently accompany impaired control of bladder and bowels due to associated pudendal and perianal nerve neuropathy.

PHARMACOLOGY AND PRINCIPLES OF USE OF SPECIFIC THERAPY

Antiemetic Drugs

Understanding the physiological mechanisms of emesis along with the evolution of a number of receptor antagonists have produced several agents that separately or in combination suppress emesis. Phenothiazine compounds (Table 1) are frequently used to alleviate mild to moderate nausea and vomiting caused by various factors, including gastrointestinal infection. The antiemetic effect may be increased by increasing dosage. Chlorpromazine, thiethylperazine, and prochlorperazine are three medications in this class with antiemetic efficacy (4).

In addition to their role as antipsychotics and sedatives, phenothiazine compounds have significant antiemetic properties due to their ability to block dopamine D_2 receptors in the CTZ. Prochlorperazine, the prototypical compound in the phenothiazine antiemetic class, has demonstrated significantly better efficacy than placebo in relieving emesis but is not as effective as tetrahydrocannabinol, the active ingredient of marijuana, or high-dose metoclopramide when compared in trials assessing relief of chemotherapy-induced emesis.

Prochlorperazine is available in parenteral, oral, or rectal suppository preparations. Recommended dosing is at 8-hr intervals. The side effect profile is significant. Autonomic side effects may include significant hypotension; hypersensitivity reactions in susceptible individuals may result in cholestatic jaundice. Prolactin release and secondary galactorrhea are also described. Antidopaminergic side effects include acute dystonic reactions and potentially chronic tardive dyskinesia, which prevent administration of high doses of these drugs.

Benzodiazepines

Benzodiazepines, particularly lorazepam and alprazolam, are used as antiemetics for mild emetic tendency. Their potency is low, however, and their most useful effect is for reducing anxiety and anticipatory vomiting.

Substituted Benzamides

Metoclopramide, originally developed as a prokinetic agent for treatment of gastroparesis, has mild antiemetic activity. Antiemetic activity is increased at higher doses but extrapyramidal reactions, anxiety, and depression, due to antidopaminergic side effects, often preclude its use.

Serotonin Antagonists

These recently developed agents, including Ondansetron, are free of antidopaminergic side effects and are very effective agents against severe chemotherapy-induced emesis. They are available in intravenous and oral formulations (15–17).

Butyrophenones, Corticosteroids, and Cannabinoids

These agents have useful antiemetic action but are rarely used or needed for relief of vomiting in gastrointestinal infections.

Anticholinergic Agents

These agents are used for motion-sickness-induced emesis.

TABLE 1. Antiemetic therapy

Drug	Antiemetic regimen	Initial dose
Phenothiazine	Prochlorperazine (Compazine) Chlorpromazine (Thorazine)	5–10 mg po or 25 mg by rectal suppository
Anticholinergic	Scopolamine (Transducer-Scop)	Patch application
Benzodiazepine	Lorezapam (Ativan) Alprazolam (Xanax)	0.1 mg po qid or 1–2 mg I.V.
Substituted benzamide	Metochlorpramide (Reglan)	10 mg po tid or 3 mg/kg IV q 2 hr × 2
Antihistamine	Diphenlhydramine (Benadryl)	25 mg IV q 2 hr ×2 or 25 mg po bid
Serotonin antagonists	Ondansetron (Zofran)	32 mg IV in divided dose 4–8 mg tid po

	Use in combination permits increase in efficacy and/or decrease in toxicity	
Effect	Primary antiemetic drug	Secondary drug
Improved efficacy	Serotonin antagonist Substituted benzamide	Phenothiazine Corticosteroid
Decrease in toxicity	Phenothiazine Substituted benzamide	Antihistamine Benzodiazepine

Combination of Antiemetic Drugs

Antiemetic drugs may be combined with the result of achieving a decrease in toxicity of the primary drug or increase in the efficacy of it. Table 1 provides uses for such agents.

Anti-acid and Antacid Agents

Antacids

Often considered the first pharmacologic step in the treatment of esophageal discomfort, antacids may play a role in the symptomatic relief of patients suffering from esophageal infection. Their efficacy stems from antacids' ability to raise esophageal pH by means of decreasing hydrogen ion concentration and thus prevent secondary injury to esophageal mucosa. There are a wide variety of preparations currently marketed, with a variety of active ingredients, including aluminum hydroxide, magnesium hydroxide, calcium carbonate, and aluminum phosphate (18).

Antacids are a safe, low-cost strategy in the treatment of esophagitis, gastritis, and upper gastrointestinal ulceration associated with injury by increased hydrogen ion and pepsin. Optimal efficacy may require frequent dosing to neutralize gastric pH; mild odynophagia/pyrosis symptoms can be relieved with four to six dosages per day. Antacids are best administered in a liquid form. Contraindications for the use of antacids are few. Aluminum-containing compounds classically produce a constipating side effect, while magnesium-based antacids can be diarrheagenic. It is important to avoid the use of magnesium-containing preparations in patients with chronic renal failure, as excess magnesium absorption can result in CNS depression, skin irritation, and, rarely, muscle paralysis and respiratory failure. A final consideration concerns the luminal action of antacid preparations. Concomitant ingestion of antacids with other medications can decrease oral availability. Tetracycline should not be taken with calcium-containing antacids, as it is readily bound within the lumen. Calcium-containing antacids are not recommended because they lead to acid rebound due to stimulation of endogenous gastrin release.

H₂ Antagonists

Severe symptoms may warrant acid-suppressive therapy with histamine receptor antagonists or proton pump inhibitors. Histamine type 2 receptor (H_2) antagonists represent structural analogs of histamine and compete for binding at the histamine receptor on the basolateral membrane of the gastric parietal cells (19), thereby blocking stimulus for acid secretion, although alternative mechanisms of action have been suggested. Basal acid output is reduced by up to 90% and nocturnal acid output by up to 67% with routine dosage. Intragastric and esophageal pH is raised, which also decreases activity of pepsin and thus promotes healing of mucosal lesions (20).

In the setting of esophageal or gastric infections, the use of H_2 receptor antagonists must be considered empiric, as no clinical trials assessing efficacy in this population have been conducted. However, many clinical observations support their use.

Omeprazol

The most potent inhibitor of parietal cell acid secretion, omeprazol, is a substituted benzimidazole that noncompetitively inhibits H^+/K^+ ATPase proton pump activity. Because omeprazol disables the proton pumps when it binds to the secretory membranes of parietal cells, its effect is long lasting, and in vivo half-life is estimated at 18 to 24 hr, and with steady-state conditions, acid inhibition may reach close to 100%. A single morning dose of omeprazol may decrease nocturnal acid secretion and meal-stimulated acid secretion by up to 50% (21).

Omeprazol's powerful acid inhibitory capabilities have made it the drug of choice for treatment of hypersecretion of gastric acid, refractory duodenal ulcer disease, and for poorly healing conditions such as errosive esophagitis and gastropathy. There are no trials assessing the use of omeprazol in the treatment of secondary acid/peptic related complications of enteric infection. Use of this compound may enhance healing of mucosal ulceration that is complicated by acid-related disease (19).

Prokinetic Agents

Prokinetic agents are drugs that increase contractile force and accelerate luminal transit. Effective agents often have antiemetic effects as well, particularly those with central antidopaminergic action (22). Prokinetic agents may have a useful role in patients with esophageal, gastroduodenal, and pseudo-obstructive dysmotility accompanying intestinal infections (23). Controlled studies have been limited and use has been recommended on an individual basis (24).

Bethanecol

Cholinergic activity of bethanecol is exerted via muscarinic receptors. Bethanecol has been used in a wide range of disorders with variable efficacy. It usually increases esophageal emptying and lower esophageal sphincter pressure but fails to improve gastric emptying. There have been few controlled studies (22). Adverse effects of abdominal cramps, skin flushing, and sweating and its lack of central antiemetic effects have led to it being superseded by more useful agents.

Erythromycin and Macrolides

It is well established that the antibiotic erythromycin has effects on human gastrointestinal motility with induction of the migratory motor complex and acceleration of gastric emptying. It mimics the action of the natural hormone motilin, but whether its sole action is exerted via motilin receptors remains uncertain (22). Study with other synthetic macrolides has revealed that the prokinetic effect can be distinguished from its antibiotic action. It has proved to have a useful therapeutic role in treatment of diabetic gastroparesis. Control studies in infectious disorders are not available. It is more effective when administered systemically and is an effective prokinetic agent at much lower doses than those used to achieve antibiotic therapy (22).

Cisapride

Cisapride is a benzamide derivative that is an effective promotility agent without antidopaminergic action or significant side effects. The primary mode of action is believed to be facilitation of acetylcholine release involving nerve endings at the myenteric plexus. Muscarinic cholinergic nerve receptors are not directly activated by cisapride. The functional effect of cisapride is to increase contraction in gastrointestinal smooth muscle, and the therapeutic benefit is best seen in patients with gastroesophageal reflux disease and gastric stasis. Cisapride increases the amplitude of contraction of lower esophageal sphincter pressure, thus helping to improve the anatomic barrier function of the lower esophageal sphincter. In the stomach, gastric emptying is facilitated by stimulation of digestive and interdigestive antroduodenal motility. As cisapride lacks antidopaminergic activity, it does not have the antiemetic effect associated with metoclopramide.

Cisapride dosing is recommended at 10 to 20 mg two to four times per day. Cisapride is currently approved for use in the treatment of gastroesophageal reflux disease. Prokinetic action that might benefit patients with secondary motility alterations, as in CMV gastritis, have not been assessed. At this time, use of cisapride in the patient with enteric infection must be considered empiric.

Metoclopramide

Metoclopramide is approved for clinical use in the United States for treatment of diabetic gastroparesis. Promotility effect stems from cholinomimetic effect on the gastrointestinal tract. The functional effect of metoclopramide is antegrade propulsion of gastric contents, increased lower esophageal sphincter pressure, and increased antral peristaltic function (25). The major drawback for use of metoclopramide stems from its central mechanism of action. Drowsiness and CNS depression are common complaints associated with use. The side effect profile includes other complaints associated with neuroleptic use, such as dystonic reactions. Excretion is almost entirely through the kidney, and dosage must be adjusted in patients with renal impairment. Dosage is typically 10 to 20 mg three times per day, although many patients cannot tolerate even lower dosages secondary to these side effects.

Use of metoclopramide in the treatment of enteric infection associated with gastric retention is anecdotal. No controlled studies have evaluated its benefit in patients with infectious motility disturbances of the gastrointestinal tract. Domperidone, an analogous antidopaminergic agent, is available for use in Europe. It has limited ability to cross the blood–brain barrier and primary action on the gastrointestinal tract.

Opiates and Their Synthetic Analogs

Opioid agonists are currently the most clinically effective of available antidiarrheal medications (Table 2). Opium, the parent compound, was known to have antidiarrheal medicinal properties as early as 3000 BC and was used by Sumerian physicians. Tincture of opium and the camphorated opium preparation paregoric were used in Europe in the 15th century, and both of these compounds are currently in use today, although undesirable for antidiarrheal therapy (26). Therapeutic efficacy of opioid compounds stems from their content of morphine, the major naturally occurring opioid compound. Morphine and codeine, the synthetic derivative of morphine, both have valuable antidiarrheal action but have been hindered in clinical application because of significant side effects including CNS narcotic effect, decreased respiration, release of prolactin, and potential dependence. Synthetic compounds that possess antidiarrheal activity, but not the side effect profile of morphine/codeine, have been developed. Diphenoxylate, a peripherally acting antidiarrheal with minimal central effects, is used in a preparation that is combined with subtherapeutic amounts of atropine, to provoke side effects if it is abused. Loperamide, an even more selective peripherally acting opioid antidiarrheal compound, has less ability to cross the blood–brain barrier and has no described narcotic abuse potential. It is free of prescribing restrictions for this reason (27). Diphenoxylate (Lomotil) and loperamide (Imodium) represent the most effective and most commonly used antidiarrheal medications available today (28–30).

Antidiarrheal efficacy stems from ability of the opioid antidiarrheal preparations to bind mu opiate receptors and to a lesser extent delta opiate receptors in the CNS, spinal cord, and enteric nervous system. Their mechanism of action is not entirely clear but appears to involve antisecretory, proabsorptive, as well as antimotility mechanisms. Antisecretory effect stems from the ability of opiates to block prosecretory neurotransmitters such as acetylcholine. Opiates promote release of the proabsorptive neurotransmitter norepinephrine. The most important pharmacologic activity in producing antidiarrheal effect stems from the ability of opiates to slow intestinal transit (31). Synthetic agents (codeine) may act preferentially on the small bowel in diarrheal states, whereas loperamide and morphine preferentially decrease colonic motility. The antimotility effect causes both delayed transit as well as dilatation of the bowel and increased capacitance to hold liquid. The net effect is to increase the time of liquid contacting the intestinal epithelium, allowing for more extensive absorption. An additional bene-

TABLE 2. *Antidiarrheal agents*

Drugs	Mechanism of action	Side effects	Therapeutic agents/ dosage

Opiates
  Natural extracts
    Paragoric tincture
    of opium
  Synthetic
    Codeine
    Diphenoxylate[a]
    Loperamide
	Act via mu receptors in CNS and enteric nervous system. Increases intestinal transit time. Effect on small bowel and colon. May cause dilatation, increased contraction of transverse musculature. Increases sphincter tone. Loperamide has its action on the enteric nervous system. Preferential efficacy and binding to enteric nerves. It is not a controlled substance under federal government schedules.	Natural extracts of variable content provide less advantage then synthetics. Toxic megacolon, enhanced bacterial invasion of invasive enteric organisms. CNS and respiratory depression. Potential for addiction.	1 dose qds for diarrhea for 48 hours as necessary. The opiate most preferred for antidiarrheal therapy. Not to be used for patients with fever or dysentery. Loperamide: 4 mg initially; 2 mg after each unformed stool to maximum of 8 mg/day.

Intraluminal agents
  Bulking agents
    Methylcellulose
    Psyllium
    Pectin
    Silicates
	Variably degraded in bowel lumen. Little water-holding capacity. As psyllium is increased in the diet, stool consistency is increased with an increase in sodium and potassium fecal losses and increase in viscosity. Clay suspensions are absorbents. Attapulgite (magnesium aluminum silicate) has greater holding power than kaolin. They may be useful in treatment in mild diarrheal disease.	Bloating, abdominal discomfort, nausea and vomiting, possible fecal impaction.	Konsyl, Donnagel; 2 tablespoons (Tbs), repeated after unformed stools not to exceed 14 Tbs.

Anticholinergic agents	Antisecretory activity via action on muscarinic receptor or enteric nerves and on epithelial cell ($M_2 > M_1$). Similar distribution on smooth muscle and CNS would account for antimotility effects.	Ileus and abdominal distal, peripheral vasodilatation, reduction in sweating, tachycardia, hyperpyrexia, hallucinations, coma, dry mucosa.	No anticholinergic agents are recommended for treatment of acute infectious diarrhea.
L-Adrenergic agonists	Receptors on CNS, enteric nerves, and the enterocyte. Major effects clinically are secondary to bowel motility changes. Antisecretory effect (proabsorption) mainly useful for diabetic diarrhea.	Centrally mediated postural hypotension, sedation, depression. Other agents may prove to be more therapeutically useful.	Clonidine
Phenothiazines	Phenothiazines inhibit calcium–calmodulin intracellular complex. In experimental studies, they inhibit intestinal secretion. Efficacy in human diarrheal studies has been demonstrated.	Sedation and postural hypotension may compromise patient cooperation with oral fluid replacement therapy. Chlorpromazine and trifluoperazine cause bradycardia, CNS depression, and gastric retention.	Chlorpromazine Trifluoperazine
Histamine receptor antagonists	H_1-H_3 histamine-mediated secretion may be reduced by specific receptor antagonist. H_1 and H_3 antagonists may have a useful role in reducing response to histamine release during acute, anaphylactic/allergic reactions and in association with release from mast cells during their activation. Histamine receptors are present on enteric nerves.	Sedation, nausea, and vomiting.	Terfenadine Aztenizole

Anti-inflammatory agents
  Eicosanoids
  Bismuth compounds
  Berberine
	May be useful in AIDS enteropathy. Inhibit prostaglandins; synthesis stimulates fluid absorption. Bacteriocidal, antitoxin action useful. Well tolerated in travelers with mild diarrhea. Berberine plant alkyloid with antidiarrheal properties attributed to antimotility, secretory, and antimicrobial effects.	Gastrointestinal ulceration, nausea, vomiting, and abdominal pain. Bismuth toxicity with very long-term use. Salicylate toxicity. Black feces. Mild nausea and vomiting. Well tolerated.	Bismuth subsalicylate (2 Tbs) each 30 mm for 8 doses.

Octreotide	Synthetic sandostatin with greater duration of action. Suppresses neuroendocrine cell secretion, intestinal fluid secretions, and motility (decreased peristalsis).	Painful when administered subcutaneously.	

table continues

TABLE 2. *Continued*

Drugs	Mechanism of action	Side effects	Therapeutic agents/dosage
Ketotifen Cromolyn sodium	Ketotifen has vesicle stabilizing action similar to cromolyn. May be of value in allergic eosinophilic gastroenteritis. Cromolyn sodium acts as a stabilizer of cell membranes. Reduces GI symptoms due to histamine release in systemic mastocytosis.		Gastrocrom, 2 capsules qid before meals
Dietary Starch Polysaccharides Glucose	Sustaining food intake and breast-feeding will reduce the duration of diarrhea in acute enteric infections. Glucose and starch serve as important constituents of WHO-ORS[b] and cereal-based ORS. Since diarrheal episodes result in attendant increased catabolism, ensuring food intake during illness may reduce weight loss in third world countries. Avoidance of poorly absorbed agents such as lactose, fructose, and sorbitol Avoidance of high dietary fiber foods (fruits and vegetables). Breast milk provides source of antibacterial/antiviral antibodies for passive immunization.		Pedialyte Ricelyte
Cholestyramine	Chloride salt of an anion exchange resin is hydrophilic but insoluble in water. The resin is not absorbed from the GI tract but will bind bacterial enteral toxins; especially useful in *C. difficile*-associated antibiotic colitis.	Constipation, hypoprothrombinemia, vitamin D and A deficiency, abdominal discomfort.	Questran
Serotonin antagonists	Main utility in reducing nausea and vomiting. Valuable in carcinoid syndrome, may have an antisecretory role in idiopathic atypical diarrheal disorders.	Tardive dyskinesia; mood change uncommon.	Methysergide Ketaserin Cyproheptadine
Glucocorticoids	Anti-inflammatory. Stimulate fluid absorption.	Steroid side effects; Cushing's syndrome.	Prednisone Hydrocortisone

[a] Contains atropine, which may cause toxic effects with an overdose.
[b] WHO-ORS, World Health Organization oral rehydration solution.

ficial pharmacologic action of loperamide is its ability to increase anal sphincter tone, which may aid in prevention of fecal incontinence.

Deleterious side effects of opiate antidiarrheal medications stem from their narcotic effect—producing CNS depression and potential addiction. Complications secondary to the desired therapeutic action—namely, ileus—and gut stasis leading to worsening of the enteric infection need also to be considered. Diarrhea represents the cathartic attempt of the body to rid itself of pathogens, and the antimotility effects of opioid medications can prolong the carrier state of an enteric infection, as well as precipitate the worsening of infection through microinvasion of the intestinal wall. For this reason opioid antidiarrheals are contraindicated in dysentery and colitis associated with invasive pathogens. In a worst case scenario, antimotility agents may facilitate the development of toxic megacolon in invasive bacterial infection. Use in the elderly has been associated with development of acute colonic pseudo-obstruction (Ogilvie's syndrome). However,

multiple studies have documented the safety of loperamide/diphenoxylate in patients with nonbloody diarrheas not accompanied by fever.

Dosing for loperamide and diphenoxylate is typically two 2-mg tablets following each liquid bowel movement with a recommended maximum of 8 tablets/day (32). In chronic nondysenteric diarrheal illness associated with human immunodeficiency virus (HIV) disease such as cryptosporidiosis and HIV enteropathy, the recommended maximum of 8 tablets/day can be cautiously exceeded. Regimens using twice the recommended dosage of loperamide have been advocated in patients with debilitating diarrheal symptoms (33). It is recommended that the use of high-dose loperamide be monitored carefully in these individual cases, as the likelihood of potential side effects is increased. It is likely that variable efficiency of opiates for diarrheal control is further confounded by irregular absorption from the bowel. Loperamide is actively metabolized by intestinal and hepatic P450 mixed function oxidases (34): its bioavailability may be altered by the rate of degradation in the bowel wall after absorption. Loperamide has limited absorption in short bowel syndromes.

Antisecretory Preparations

Adrenergic Agonists

The α_2-adrenergic receptor agonists have been found to stimulate NaCl and water absorption and inhibit stimulated chloride and water secretion. Clonidine, a centrally acting antihypertensive agent that has demonstrated some success in the treatment of secretory diarrhea states, particularly diabetic diarrhea, is the prototypical agent currently available in this class (35–37).

α_2-Receptors are found in the CNS and on enterocyte basolateral membranes, and it is postulated that any of these sites may be responsible for the antidiarrheal effect of α-adrenergic agonists. In addition to their antisecretory properties, α-adrenergic agents have an effect on small bowel motility. Similar to opiate medications, α_2-adrenergic agents increase luminal gut capacity and thus slow transit of fluid. Studies attempting to discern the major therapeutic effect have demonstrated a 15% change in intestinal secretion. Thus alteration in gut motility may represent the beneficial effect (38).

The practical use of α_2-adrenergic agonists is limited, as centrally mediated postural hypotension, sedation, and depression are common side effects. Methoxytolazine, an experimental agent in this class of medication, limits the CNS side effect profile associated with clonidine and holds promise for future directions in antidiarrheal pharmacotherapy.

Gastrointestinal Peptides

Somatostatin Analogs (Octreotide)

Increasing understanding of the normal role of gut peptides in gastrointestinal physiology has led to the recent development of synthetic compounds for clinical use. A synthetic analog of somatostatin—octreotide—represents the best available agent for clinical use to date (39,40).

Octreotide has numerous effects on gut physiology. Secretion is inhibited in the stomach, pancreas, and intestine. Gastrointestinal motility is inhibited in both the gallbladder and the stomach with decreased generation of migrating motor complexes, but intestinal migrating motor complexes are increased (41). Somatostatin acts as a general antagonist in the gut, inhibiting plasma concentrations of many gut hormones including gastrin, cholecystokinin, secretin, vasoactive intestinal peptide (VIP), glucagon, and motilin. Somatostatin also is known to decrease intestinal splanchnic blood flow and portal venous blood flow, modulate tissue proliferation, and inhibit intestinal absorption of calcium and sugars. Somatostatin, like most enteric hormones, has a short half-life, on the

order of 2 to 3 min. The development of the synthetic analog octreotide has overcome this pharmacologic handicap by stabilizing biologic activity and raising the half-life to 100 min (42,43).

The successful use of somatostatin to control secretory diarrhea secondary to the pancreatic tumor—VIPoma—and the carcinoid syndrome led clinical investigators to pioneer several trials of somatostatin injection therapy in the treatment of severe chronic diarrheal illness associated with HIV infection (42). Efficacy was demonstrated in an open label trial in 1989 that assessed increasing dosages of octreotide administered subcutaneously in 51 AIDS patients who were suffering from chronic diarrhea associated with cryptosporidiosis, *Mycobacterium avium intracellularis* (MAI), Microsporidia, and HIV enteropathy. Dosage of medication was initiated at 50 µg and was increased to a maximum of 500 µg three times per day. At the higher dosages of octreotide, 41% of patients responded with a decrease in stool volume by one-half. Two additional open label trials have corroborated octreotide's efficacy in the treatment of chronic HIV-related diarrhea. These trials were able to show patient improvement in symptoms at substantially lower dosages (50–100 micrograms administered subcutaneously three times per day) (34,45–47).

There are no absolute contraindications for the use of somatostatin or octreotide. Allergy has not been reported. Side effects associated with octreotide most commonly include local skin irritation and erythema at the injection site. These symptoms can be lessened by warming the loaded syringe between the palms prior to injection, and by injecting at a slow rate. Gastrointestinal side effects include nausea, abdominal cramping, and bloating. The most serious potential side effect, acute cholecystitis, the sequelae of gallstone formation from suppressed biliary motility, has not been reported in the use of octreotide in HIV-infected patients. Suppression of endocrine function (pituitary and thyroid) may accompany long term use. An additional concern regarding the use of octreotide injection therapy is cost. At our outpatient pharmacy, single dosages of octreotide injection varied from $8.00 to $24.00, making prolonged courses of therapy extremely costly. We recommend that octreotide therapy be used only following appropriate diagnostic strategies and adequate trials of conventional opiate antidiarrheal medications.

Anticholinergic Drugs

Atropine, hyocyamine, scopolomine, and synthetic agents such as dicyclomine and propantheline are the antimuscarinic drugs presently available. Experimental studies have demonstrated inhibitory effects on enteric nerves and epithelial and muscle cells through action on both M_1 and M_2 receptors and marked effects through parasympathetic nerve supply. However, in clinical practice, side effects associated with antimotility action (gastric retention and bowel dilatation, ileus, megacolon) preclude use of these agents in treatment of acute infectious diarrhea. Atropine is included with diphenoxylate as a means of discouraging overdose rather than for its antimuscarinic effects. It is believed that onset of tachycardia, a lack of sweating, urinary retention, and other side effects with overuse would dissuade the patient from overusing Lomotil.

Anti-inflammatory Drugs

Eicosanoids or 20 carbon unsaturated fatty acid derivatives of arachidonic acid include prostanoids, thromboxanes, leukotrienes, and lipoxins. Different eicosanoids, depending on the cell type of origin, are released by neural stimulation, mediators of inflammation such as bradykinin and cytokines, enteropathogens, laxatives, and irradiation. They may act as mediators of intestinal fluid secretion and, when derived from leukocytes, are more likely involved in inflammation of the bowel (47). Interaction between many inflammatory agents and the enteric nervous system is well demonstrated in experimental situations. However, evidence that eicosanoid synthesis inhibitors and/or receptor antagonists may inhibit intestinal secretion in humans remains conjectural at this time. Anti-inflammatory drugs do not fulfill a useful therapeutic role in gastrointestinal infections but have been used for pain relief associated with inflammatory states of the bowel.

Cyclooxygenase Inhibitors

Cyclooxygenase inhibitors such as indomethacin reduced fluid secretion in experimental amebiasis, cholera, cryptosporidiosis, and salmonellosis (48). Human cholera diarrhea was not ameliorated by aspirin or indomethacin. Other sites in the arachidonic acid cascade may also be susceptible to inhibition by specific inhibitors. Cellular release of histamine and other kinins from mast cells may be blocked by histamine antagonists and Ketotifen (49). Other inflammatory cells may be stabilized by steroids and may be susceptible to lipoxygenase inhibitory agents. Although potential for new developments in research are likely, no specific nonsteroidal anti-inflammatory drug (NSAID) could be recognized or recommended for use in this capacity in clinical medicine at this time. Their risk of causing significant gastrointestinal side effects and of exacerbating other inflammatory bowel disease provides no certainty of a strong benefit to risk ratio in their use in clinical management.

Bismuth Salts

Bismuth is one of the oldest preparations known in the treatment of gastrointestinal maladies, dating back to the late 18th century. Interest in the use of bismuth has undergone a resurgence with the increased understanding of the biology of *Helicobacter pylori* and in its etiologic role in peptic ulcer disease. In addition to its role in the treatment of *H. pylori*, bismuth has a well-established history in the nonspecific treatment of various upper and lower gastro-intestinal tract symptoms, including nausea and vomiting, abdominal cramping, and diarrhea (50,51).

Bismuth is the heaviest nonradioactive element. Therapeutic preparations are composed of bismuth salts. Two preparations are currently available—bismuth subsalicylate, marketed as Pepto-Bismol, and bismuth subcitrate, available in Europe as DeNol. Bismuth is largely insoluble in water, and very little of the two preparations, bismuth subsalicylate and bismuth subcitrate, are absorbed. Cases of fatal bismuth toxicity occurred in the 1970s, primarily in France and Australia, where preparations of bismuth subgallate were ingested chronically for the disparate purposes of deodorizing ostomy waste and as a health fad (51). Subgallate preparations contain higher bismuth concentrations in a more readily absorbable form. Manifestations of bismuth toxicity are primarily neurologic and include encephalopathy and coma. For these reasons, bismuth subgallate is no longer produced and the likelihood of toxicity with the available preparations is extremely low (52).

Potential toxicity that may result from the use of current bismuth preparations is salicylate toxicity. Bismuth subsalicylate (Pepto-Bismol) dissociates in the stomach, allowing ready absorption of the salicylate moiety. Salicylate is nearly completely absorbed from the proximal small bowel, and salicylate toxicity is a likely complication, particularly in patients using other forms of absorbable salicylate, namely, aspirin. Classic otologic, renal, and neurologic symptoms of aspirin toxicity will ensue.

Successful treatment of diarrhea with bismuth subsalicylate has been well documented (53). The exact mechanism of *in vivo* action has not been elucidated, but it is known that bismuth subsalicylate exhibits *in vitro* bactericidal activity against enterotoxigenic *Escherichia coli*. Ericsson and co-workers demonstrated that bismuth subsalicylate also reduced the fluid secretory activity of *E. coli* and cholera toxins. In addition, bismuth subsalicylate has been shown to bind cholera toxin *in vitro*.

It is not yet known whether bismuth represents the sole therapeutic moiety of the bismuth subsalicylate molecule. Salicylates antagonize toxin-induced intestinal secretion. Anti-inflammatory properties of salicylates have been well documented in the treatment of idiopathic inflammatory bowel disease, and the therapeutic role of salicylate in treating an inflammatory component of infectious diarrhea is foreseeable. It should be noted that the anti-inflammatory mechanism of action of salicylates is not completely understood but may involve scavenging of free radicals and prevention of proinflammatory prostaglandin formation (54). Gorbach and co-workers (55) demonstrated no significant fecal bactericidal action for bismuth subsalicylate.

In addition to its ability to ameliorate diarrhea, bismuth has demonstrated therapeutic efficacy in the treatment of upper gastrointestinal symptoms as well. In a study of volunteers infected with the Norwalk agent, bismuth was able to diminish nausea and vomiting associated with this viral infection. The mechanism for the antiemetic action is not understood (5).

Sucralfate

Sucralfate (Carafate) is a unique compound that has been used successfully in the treatment of peptic ulcers. Sucralfate consists of a sucrose molecular skeleton with sulfated hydroxyl residues, which is complexed with poly-aluminum hydroxide. It is insoluble in water and is poorly absorbed. The mechanism of action of sucralfate is believed to be multifactorial. The medication binds to all mucosal surfaces including ulcers and erosions. Forming a physical barrier to acid, pepsin, and bile salts is one of the proposed mechanisms of action. Additional mechanisms include cytoprotective effects, including bicarbonate secretion and promotion of prostaglandin-dependent mechanisms of mucosal healing.

The pill can form a slurry in water and has been used successfully for the treatment of esophageal ulcerations. This local therapy, taken two to four times daily, has been applied successfully to achieve healing of giant HIV-associated ulcers of the esophagus. Medication is well tolerated, and side effects are minimal.

NONSPECIFIC THERAPY

Dietary Considerations

An important adjunct for treatment of patients with gastrointestinal infections is dietary modifications. With diarrhea, avoidance of milk and milk products is an effective strategy both during diarrheal illness and for approximately 1 week following resolution of symptoms. Mild lactose intolerance often accompanies diarrheal illness, particularly rheovirus and parvovirus infections, and a secondary diarrheal illness can be avoided with simple dietary restriction (56). Initial foods that are recommended early in the course of enteric infection are broth-based soups, tea, dry toast, crackers, and gelatin. If this bland diet is tolerated for 24 hr, it is usually possible to advance the diet to include other easily tolerated foods, including high-carbohydrate, low-fat items such as rice, bananas, applesauce, and potatoes. An additional emphasis should also be placed on maintenance of hydration, with adequate intake of liquids. Avoidance of osmotically active agents such as sorbitol and fructose contained in many foods, fruits, and beverages should be advised to prevent a secondary osmotic-induced diarrhea (57).

Intraluminal Antidiarrheal Therapy

Dietary Fiber and Water-Holding Agents (Bulk-Forming Agents)

Dietary fiber, noncellulose polysaccharides that comprise the indigestible portion of the plant cell wall, is an agent that increases fecal bulk and helps promote normal bowel function. Fiber is usually regarded as a dietary component to prevent and treat constipation and maintain regular colonic function. Paradoxically, the mechanism of water absorption that promotes bowel regularity also functions to absorb excess water in the bowel lumen, thus symptomatically improving diarrhea.

Dietary fiber is composed of polysaccharides and lignins, the most common being cellulose, hemicellulose, pectin, mucilage, and gums (58). These carbohydrates are partially digested during passage through the colon by fecal bacteria. Degradation by bacterial action augments fecal bacterial mass, which additionally alters fecal consistency. In the diet they function to hold on to water at specific "hydrophilic sites" located on their molecules, increasing fecal bacterial cell mass and fecal water. They lead to generation of H_2, CO_2, and CH_4 gases (59).

The specific ability of dietary fiber to help alleviate symptoms of diarrhea has been formally evaluated. In a reproducible model of secretory diarrhea induced by the laxative phenolphthalein, six human volunteers showed linear improvement in stool consistency as dietary fiber (psyllium) was increased from 9 to 30 g/day. This same study failed to demonstrate improvement in symptoms with two other forms of dietary fiber—calcium polycarbophil and wheat bran (60).

An average dose of supplemental dietary fiber compounds provides an additional 2 to 4 g of fiber. Recommendations usually suggest a morning and an evening dose that is taken with a sufficient amount of water to prevent inadequate solubilization of the fiber and possible bezoar formation. A rare allergy to psyllium has been described, but this is associated most frequently with factory workers who are exposed to aerosolized psyllium and subsequently develop hypersensitivity. Fiber supplements normally have no side effects but may reduce the intake of nutrients due to satiety.

Dietary fiber supplementation represents a safe and reasonable starting point for nonspecific therapy of mild diarrheal disease although the quantities required to ameliorate diarrhea may augment satiety of ill patients.

Clay suspensions are compounds of aluminum and magnesium silica and have a time-honored place in acute diarrheal therapy. However, few studies are available to support claims that they are therapeutically useful. Magnesium aluminum silicate—attapulgite (Diasorb)—is 33 times more effective and absorbent than kaolin. It has been shown to be less effective than loperamide in symptomatic control of acute diarrhea. These agents are readily available to the public OTC, are free of side effects, and may be useful for treatment of mild diarrheal disease. They may have additional effects on enterotoxin binding and bacterial colonization in the bowel lumen.

Saccharomyces bouladii

Use of the nonpathogenic yeast *Saccharomyces bouladii* for the treatment of acute diarrheal disorders has been documented in recent controlled studies (61). Its main use has been in the treatment of antibiotic-associated diarrhea. Although its mode of action is uncertain, it is known to have an antagonistic action against the growth of various bacterial pathogens *in vivo* and *in vitro* with additional effects on mucosal disaccharidase activity and

Clostridium difficile toxin A binding. The *S. bouladii* needs to be in the growing state to provide its antagonistic effects. Stool culture after 3 days of oral therapy (250 mg bid) demonstrated concentrations of 10^8 organisms/mL of stool. Its major therapeutic role is for the prevention of recurrent relapse in *C. difficile* colitis diarrhea and in relapse of patients after treatment with vancomycin and metronidazole (61).

Cholestyramine

Cholestyramine (Questran) is a high molecular weight anion exchange resin that binds bile salts intraluminally. Bile salt binding resins are used most commonly for the treatment of bile salt-induced diarrhea, cholestatic liver disease, and as cholesterol-lowering agents. The sequestration of bile produces constipation in most individuals, and this phenomenon prompted trials of cholestyramine in the setting of enteric infection. Cholestyramine has demonstrated *in vitro* ability to bind *C. difficile* toxin and has demonstrated clinical efficacy in cases of mild pseudomembranous colitis. Moderate to severe colitis caused by *C. difficile* should always be treated with appropriate antibiotic therapy. A starting dosage of cholestyramine is 4 g mixed with liquid, taken before meals. It is important to note that bile salt-binding resins will bind other medications, so that time of administration of other medications should be 1 hr prior to or 4 hr after each dosage of cholestyramine (62).

Mucositis Treatment

Mucositis is a frequent complication of cancer chemotherapy regimens and radiation treatment to the thorax. Patients present with severe odynophagia and xerostomia, and the condition is often associated with superimposed enteric infection. Systemic analgesia and topical anesthetic agents can be used to provide pain relief. This treatment strategy carries inherent risks and should only be implemented in hospitalized patients under careful supervision, as analgesics may mask symptoms of clinical deterioration and carry risk of severe toxicity (63).

Patients with mucositis and superimposed viral or fungal esophageal infection may require analgesia with intravenous narcotic infusion. Local anesthetic agents are useful in patients with xerostomia. In the past, topical therapy consisted of cocktails of antacids combined with diphenhydramine and viscous lidocaine (64,65). Newer efforts to provide relief have utilized a "swish and spit" regimen of 2% lidocaine injectible solution. Patients typically tolerate the liquid form of lidocaine better than viscous gel. The major difficulty with this regimen is lidocaine toxicity that may lead to seizure, as lidocaine is readily absorbed from mucous membranes. It is imperative that patients are monitored and instructed not to ingest excess amounts of topical anesthetic.

Care of Anorectal Disorders

Perineal Care

Frequent bowel movements and attempts to clean the perineum with wiping will result in local tissue abrasion and irritation. Symptoms will typically resolve with the normalization of bowel habits, but much can be done to alleviate patient discomfort in the intervening time period. Perianal hygiene is emphasized, and this can be accomplished through the use of warm water baths to the perineum and perianal region for 10-min periods two to three times per day. It is important to emphasize not to use soap as part of the bathing regimen. Drying the perineum following baths should be done with absorbent cotton, and a similar protocol of warm water and cotton should be recommended for self-cleaning following bowel movements. Toilet paper and paper towels are avoided because of their abrasive nature (66).

With severe perianal inflammation, a short course of topical hydrocortisone creme can be applied to the perianal area. Relief from more severe discomfort has been described with the use of witchhazel applied via cotton pads. Desitin ointment (40% zinc oxide in a hydrophobic petroleum jelly base), used for the treatment of diaper rash, may also provide relief. Topical anesthetics are not recommended for the relief of perianal discomfort. The overall plan should recommend hygiene and avoidance of abrasive agents. Topical creams provide best results applied on a short-term basis but may lead to secondary skin sensitization and maceration if used chronically (67).

Stool Softeners

Stool softeners containing dioctyl sodium sulfosuccinate are anionic surfactants that lower the surface tension of stool, which theoretically might permit easier defecation. These agents also stimulate electrolyte secretion *in vitro*. However, placebo-controlled studies have failed to demonstrate changes in water content and stool weight or frequency of defecation when given in current recommended doses (68).

Rectal Suppositories

Rectal suppositories may provide a useful milieu to introduce medications such as antiemetics and anti-inflammatory agents (aminosalicylic acid) so as to act locally on the rectal mucosa. These agents are rarely of use in acute diarrheal disease when specific antibiotic therapy is often more useful. However, when patients have major involvement of the rectum in chronic disorders such as herpes simplex, cytomegalovirus, and chlamydia, topical therapy may play an adjunctive role.

Glycerine Suppositories

Glycerine suppositories generate increased intrarectal pressure when solubilized and may facilitate bowel evacuation in the constipated patient. Some other anti-inflammatory agents (bismuth subgallate) are either contraindicated or unresponsive in anorectal disease. Severe discomfort associated with tenesmus or urgency during evacuation may be ameliorated by use of antispasmodics and/or synthetic opiates.

Restoration of Fluid Balance

Oral Rehydration Solution

The most devastating sequelae of gastrointestinal infection are severe dehydration and death, which can accompany massive lower gastrointestinal fluid losses most typically from secretory diarrhea. The development of specifically designed orally administered solutions that augment normal fluid absorptive mechanisms has helped dramatically reduce morbidity and mortality associated with infectious diarrhea (69,70). Oral rehydration solutions are dependent on the ability of glucose in the intestinal lumen to stimulate water and electrolyte absorption. Originally, it was felt that movement of Na^+ and H_2O was coupled to active glucose absorption, and this mechanism alone explained the beneficial effect of oral rehydration solution. This mechanism does occur in the upper small intestine, but Fordtran and co-workers were able to demonstrate that 60% to 100% of the net absorption of Na^+ may in fact be a passive result of solvent drag that corresponds to the movement of glucose down a concentration gradient into the cell. Cl^- and bicarbonate are both effective stimuli for Na^+ absorption into the cell (70a).

The oral rehydration solution that has been recommended by the World Health Organization is an inexpensive, easily prepared liquid that incorporates table salt, baking soda, KCl, glucose, and water (2,71). This standard solution can be used by all ages. In milder forms of diarrhea, such as traveler's diarrhea, fluid replacement is typically in the range of 3 to 4 L in the adult and rarely exceeds 7 L. This amount of fluid replacement is readily achieved through the use of oral rehydration. Sugars other than glucose appear to be less effective in promoting absorption, but starches and other dietary polysaccharides are also effectively digested by hydrolytic enzymes to monosaccharide and short-chain polymers in the lumen (72). Detailed discussion of these issues are available in the chapter by Snyder.

CLINICAL USE AND PROPHYLAXIS

Prophylaxis of enteric infections, specifically traveler's diarrhea, can be accomplished through the use of antibiotic therapy. Two alternative regimens for prophylaxis that have proven efficacy include the use of lactobacillus preparations and bismuth subsalicylate (73). Lactobacilli inhibit the proliferation of enteropathogens by lowering the intraluminal pH, through their ability to metabolize carbohydrate to lactic acid and other organic acids (74). Bismuth has a short-term antimicrobial action, but its mechanism of action for preventing infection is not completely understood (75). Prophylaxis requires dosage with two 262-mg tablets taken four times daily. It is advisable that bismuth is taken at mealtime, as contaminated food represents an important vector for acquiring enteropathogenic infection. Although bismuth is not as effective as antimicrobials in preventing traveler's diarrhea, the protection rate utilizing four daily dosages is estimated at 65%. An equal amount of bismuth given only twice daily afforded only 40% protection, emphasizing the need to combine bismuth with meals (2,76–78).

FUTURE DIRECTIONS

Cytokines and Immune Modulators

Advances in understanding the immunologic control of mucosal inflammation have opened new avenues for therapeutic intervention (1). Although incompletely understood, this complex process appears to be mediated through activation of immune, mesenchymal, and epithelial cells in the mucosa, with additional immune cells recruited from the circulation. Inflammatory cells are controlled by the release of protein "signals" called cytokines. Cytokines have autocrine, paracrine, and endocrine effects that produce activation, proliferation, or differentiation of cells in the local environment or systemically. Cytokines mediate many symptoms associated with enteric infection, including diarrhea.

Advances in research of inflammatory bowel disease have highlighted new therapies that are specifically directed at the immunoregulatory role of cytokines. Interleukin-1 (IL-1), a cytokine with potent proinflammatory activity released by activated monocytes and macrophages, is elevated in inflammatory disease states of the bowel (79). This molecule can specifically be inhibited by the action of an endogenous protein that is found normally in the body, the IL-1 receptor antagonist, which competes for the IL-1 binding site (80). The genetic code for the IL-1 receptor antagonist has been defined, and this protein has been manufactured with recombinant DNA technology. Clinical trials of this specific cytokine blocker have been initiated in patients with colonic inflammation from ulcerative colitis, with promising results. It is exciting to hypothesize a similar role for other specific anti-inflammatory therapy in enteric infection, although this reality remains for the future.

Gastrointestinal Hormones

At the present time, one gastrointestinal peptide analog acting as a receptor agonist is available (the modified somatostatin molecule octreotide) (39). In the future, it is likely there will be an explosion of knowledge concerning gastrointestinal peptides with the development of peptide analogs and nonpeptide agonists and antagonists that will provide specific agents to deal with specific symptoms. For instance, VIP antagonists may be developed to counteract reflux esophagitis, neuropeptide Y antagonists to counteract vasoconstriction, and substance P antagonists to prevent inflammation. These possibilities are speculative and future knowledge will determine the outcome of useful therapeutic compounds (14).

Calmodulin Inhibitors

Development of antisecretory medication that may be able to decrease diarrheal volume by mechanisms directed at intestinal epithelial cell pathophysiology, without side effects, has long been a goal in gastrointestinal pharmacology. Enterotoxigenic *E. coli* produces secretory diarrhea through inappropriate activation of adenylate cyclase-mediated intestinal secretion in the epithelial cell. The biochemical pathways that activate adenylate cyclase rely on calcium and the protein calmodulin. Calmodulin complexes with calcium in the epithelial cell and ultimately stimulates adenylate cyclase, thus promoting intestinal secretion (81). Zaldaride maleate, a pyrolobenzoxazepine derivative, is a potent inhibitor of calmodulin activity and has demonstrated gastrointestinal antisecretory properties. Zaldaride maleate has been tested in a placebo-controlled trial of human subjects with enterotoxigenic *E. coli* and traveler's diarrhea (81). A dosage of 20 mg four times a day has been found to decrease frequency of diarrhea by 54% within 24 hr of initiating therapy. Control of symptoms of diarrhea without CNS side effects and aggravation of invasive bacterial enteritis is clearly a goal for future therapy.

Chloride-Channel Blockers

A therapeutic goal for antidiarrheal therapy would be to identify and use agents that would inhibit the chloride protein channel in the apical membrane of the intestinal epithelial cell, which is under the influence of intracellular messengers cyclic adenosine monophosphate (cAMP), cyclic guanosine monophosphate (cGMP), and ionized calcium (11). During the diarrheal state, translocation of chloride is the driving force for intestinal secretion of fluid. Recently, several compounds that are capable of blocking chloride channels have been developed. None, at present, are suitable for clinical use nor has their specificity been clearly established for particular chloride channels (there are several different chloride channels of different conductance in the epithelial cell). Moreover, some chloride-channel antagonists have had agonist effects *in vitro*. Exploration of this range of compounds has great promise for improving antidiarrheal therapy in the future (14).

REFERENCES

1. Sartor R. Cytokines in intestinal inflammation: pathophysiological and clinical considerations. *Gastroenterology* 1994;106: 533–539.
2. Banwell J. Treatment of traveler's diarrhea: fluid and dietary management. *Rev Infect Dis* 1986;8(Suppl 2):s182–s187.
3. Feldman M. Nausea and vomiting. In: Sleisenger MH, Fordtran JS, eds. *Gastrointestinal disease,* 4th ed. Philadelphia: Saunders, 1989;222–237.
4. Allan S. Antiemetics. *Gastroenterol Clin North Am* 1992;21(3): 597–611.
5. Steinhof M, Douglas RJ, Greenberg H, Callahan D. Bismuth subsalicylate therapy of viral gastroenteritis. *Gastroenterology* 1980;78:1495–1499.
6. Pope C. Heartburn, dysphagia, and other esophageal symptoms. In: Sleisenger MH, Fordtran JS, eds. *Gastrointestinal disease,* 4th ed. Philadelphia: Saunders, 1989;200–203.
7. Baehr P, McDonald G. Esophageal infections: risk factors, presentation, diagnosis, and treatment. *Gastroenterology* 1994;106: 509–532.
8. McCord G, Clouse R. Pill-induced esophageal strictures: clinical features and risk factors for development. *Am J Med* 1990;88: 512–518.
9. Kilkendall J. Pill-induced esophageal injury. *Gastroenterol Clin North Am* 1991;20(4):835–846.
10. Cooper B. Diarrhoea as a symptom. *Clin Gastroenterol* 1985; 14(3):599–613.
11. Fine K, Krejs G, Fordtran J. Diarrhea. In: Sleisenger M, Fordtran J, eds. *Gastrointestinal disease,* 4th ed. Philadelphia: Saunders, 1989;290–316.
12. Dukes G. Over-the-counter antidiarrheal medications used for the self-treatment of acute nonspecific diarrhea. *Am J Med* 1990; 88(Suppl 6A):24S–26S.
13. Brownlee HJ. Family practitioner's guide to patient self-treatment of acute diarrhea. *Am J Med* 1990;88(Suppl 6A):27S–29S.
14. Powell D, Szauter K. Nonantibiotic therapy and pharmacotherapy of acute infectious diarrhea. *Gastroenterol Clin North Am* 1993;22(3):683–707.
15. Talley N. Review article: 5-hydroxytryptamine agonists and antagonists in the modulation of gastrointestinal motility and sensation: clinical implications. *Aliment Pharmacol Ther* 1992;6: 273–289.
16. Grunberg S, Hesketh P. Control of chemotherapy-induced emesis. *N Engl J Med* 1993;329(24):1790–1796.
17. Herrstedt J, Sigsgaard T, Boesgaard M, Jensen T, Dombernowsky P. Ondansetron plus Metopimazine compared with Ondansetron alone in patients receiving moderately emetogenic chemotherapy. *N Engl J Med* 1993;328(15):1076–1084.
18. Van Ness M. Antacids. In: Van Ness MM, Gurney MS, eds. *Handbook of gastrointestinal drug therapy.* Boston: Little, Brown, 1989;7–12.
19. Andrea M, Van Ness M. H2-antagonists. In: Van Ness MM, Gurney MS, eds. *Handbook of gastrointestinal drug therapy.* Boston: Little, Brown, 1989;13–58.
20. Shamburek R, Schubert M. Control of gastric acid secretion: histamine H2-receptor antagonists and H+K+-ATPase inhibitors. *Gastroenterol Clin North Am* 1992;21(3):527–550.
21. Carboni M. Omeprazole. In: Van Ness MM, Gurney MS, eds. *Handbook of gastrointestinal drug therapy.* Boston: Little, Brown, 1989;83–89.
22. Reynolds J, Putnam P. Prokinetic agents. *Gastroenterol Clin North Am* 1992;21(3):567–596.
23. Van Thiel D, Gavaler J, Schade R, Chien M, Starzl T. Cytomegalovirus infection and gastric emptying. *Transplantation* 1992; 54(1):70–73.
24. Ramirez B, Richter J. Review article: promotility drugs in the treatment of gastro-oesophageal reflux disease. *Aliment Pharmacol Ther* 1993;7:5–20.
25. Litaker D. Metoclopramide. In: Van Ness MM, Gurney MS, eds. *Handbook of gastrointestinal drug therapy.* Boston: Little, Brown, 1989;77–82.
26. Miller R, Brown D. Opiates and the gut. *Viewpoints Dig Dis* 1984;16(2):5–8.
27. Ericsson C, Johnson P. Safety and efficacy of loperamide. *Am J Med* 1990;88(Suppl 6A):10S–14S.
28. DuPont H, Ericsson C, DuPont M, Cruz Luna A, Mathewson J. A randomized, open-label comparison of nonprescription loperamide and attapulgite in the symptomatic treatment of acute diarrhea. *Am J Med* 1990;88(Suppl 6A):20S–23S.
29. Burks T. Mechanisms of opioid antidiarrheal therapy. In: Leben-

thal E, Duffey M, eds. *Textbook of secretory diarrhea.* New York: Raven Press, 1990;409–419.

30. Awouters A, Megens A, Verlinden M, Schuurkes J, Niemegeers C, Janssen P. Loperamide: survey of studies on mechanism of its antidiarrheal activity. *Dig Dis Sci* 1993;38(6):977–995.

31. Awouters F, Niemegeers C, Janssen P. Pharmacology of antidiarrheal drugs. *Annu Rev Pharmacol Toxicol* 1983;23:279–301.

32. DuPont H, Flores Sanchez J, Ericsson C, et al. Comparative efficacy of loperamide hydrochloride and bismuth subsalicylate in the management of acute diarrhea. *Am J Med* 1990;88(Suppl 6A):15S–19S.

33. Simon A, Weiss L, Brandt L. Treatment options for AIDS-related esophageal and diarrheal disorders. *Am J Gastroenterol* 1992;87(3):274–281.

34. Watkins P. Drug metabolism by cytochrome P450 in the liver and small bowel. *Gastroenterol Clin North Am* 1992;21(3):511–526.

35. Dharmsathaphorn K. α2-Adrenergic agonists: a newer class of antidiarrheal drug. *Gastroenterology* 1986;91:769–775.

36. Pamukcu R, Chang E. Alpha-2-adrenergic agonists as antidiarrheal agents. In: Lebenthal E, Duffey M, eds. *Textbook of secretory diarrhea.* New York: Raven Press, 1990;383–393.

37. Chang E, Fedorak R, Field M. Experimental diabetic diarrhea in rats: intestinal mucosal denervation hypersensitivity and treatment with clonidine. *Gastroenterology* 1986;91:564–569.

38. Rabbani G, Butler T, Patte D, Abud R. Clinical trial of clonidine hydrochloride as an antisecretory agent in cholera. *Gastroenterology* 1989;97:321–325.

39. Maton P, Jensen R. Use of gut peptide receptor agonists and antagonists in gastrointestinal diseases. *Gastroenterol Clin North Am* 1992;21(3):551–566.

40. Redfern J, Mekhjian H, O'Dorisio T. Use of somatostatin-like peptides in the treatment of diarrhea. In: Lebenthal E, Duffey M, eds. *Textbook of secretory diarrhea.* New York: Raven Press, 1990;421–428.

41. Soudah H, Hasler W, Owyang C. Effect of octreotide on intestinal motility and bacterial overgrowth in scleroderma. *N Engl J Med* 1991;325:1461–1467.

42. Burroughs A, McCormick P. Somatostatin and octreotide in gastroenterology. *Aliment Pharmacol Ther* 1991;5:331–341.

43. Katz M, Erstad B. Octreotide, a new somatostatin analogue. *Clin Pharmacol* 1989;8:255–273.

44. Johanson J, Sonnenberg A. Efficient management of diarrhea in the acquired immunodeficiency syndrome (AIDS). *Ann Intern Med* 1990;112:942–948.

45. Cello J, Grendell J, Basuk P, et al. Effect of octreotide on refractory AIDS-associated diarrhea. *Ann Intern Med* 1991;115:705–710.

46. Cook D, Kelton J, Stanisz A, Collins S. Somatostatin treatment for cryptosporidial diarrhea in a patient with the acquired immunodeficiency syndrome (AIDS). *Ann Intern Med* 1988;108(5):708–709.

47. Rampton D, Collins C. Review article: thromboxanes in inflammatory bowel disease—pathogenic and therapeutic implications. *Aliment Pharmacol Ther* 1993;7:357–367.

48. Smith P, Blumberg J, Stoff J, Field M. Antisecretory effects of indomethacin on rabbit ileal mucosa in vitro. *Gastroenterology* 1981;80:356–365.

49. Podleski W, Panaszek B, Schmidt J, Burns R. Inhibition of eosinophils' degranulation by Ketotifen in a patient with milk allergy, manifested as bronchial asthma—an electron microscopic study. *Agents Actions* 1984;15:177.

50. Hailey F, Newsom J. Evaluation of bismuth subsalicylate in relieving symptoms of indigestion. *Arch Intern Med* 1984;144:269–272.

51. Marshall B. The use of bismuth in gastroenterology. *Am J Gastroenterol* 1991;86(1):16–25.

52. Bierer D. Bismuth subsalicylate: history, chemistry, and safety. *Rev Infect Dis* 1990;12(Suppl 1):s3–s8.

53. Figueroa-Quintanilla D, Salazar-Lindo E, Sack R, et al. A controlled trial of bismuth subsalicylate in infants with acute watery diarrheal disease. *N Engl J Med* 1993;328(23):1653–1658.

54. Goldenberg M, Honkomp L, Castellion A. The antidiarrheal action of bismuth subsalicylate in the mouse and rat. *Dig Dis* 1975;20(10):955–960.

55. Gorbach S, Cornick N, Silva M. Effect of bismuth subsalicylate on fecal microflora. *Rev Infect Dis* 1990;12(Suppl 1):s21–s23.

56. Martini M, Kukielka D, Savaiano D. Lactose digestion from yogurt: influence of a meal and additional lactose. *Am J Clin Nutr* 1991;53:1253–1258.

57. Johnson P, Ericsson C. Acute diarrhea in developed countries: a rationale for self-treatment. *Am J Med* 1990;88(Suppl 6A):5S–9S.

58. Cummings J. Cellulose and the human gut. *Gut* 1984;25:805–810.

59. Cummings J. Dietary fibre. *Br Med Bull* 1981;37(1):65–70.

60. Eherer A, Santa Ana C, Porter J, Fordtran J. Effect of psyllium, calcium polycarbophil, and wheat bran on secretory diarrhea induced by phenolphthalein. *Gastroenterology* 1993;104:1007–1012.

61. Pothoulakis C, Kelly C, Joshi M, et al. *Saccharomyces boulardii* inhibits *Clostridium difficile* toxin A binding and enterotoxicity in rat ileum. *Gastroenterology* 1993;104:1108–1115.

62. Gurney M. Bile salt binders. In: Van Ness MM, Gurney MS, eds. *Handbook of gastrointestinal drug therapy.* Boston: Little, Brown, 1989;298–302.

63. Strichnarz G, Govino B. Topical anesthesia. In: Miller RD, ed. *Anesthesia,* 3rd ed. New York: Churchill Livingstone, 1990;437–490.

64. DiPiro J, Talbert R, Hayes P, Yee G, Matzke G, Posey L, eds. *Pharmacotherapy: a pathophysiologic approach.* Norwalk, CT: Appleton & Lange, 1993;1879–1929.

65. Kinzie B. Treatment of stomatitis associated with antineoplastic-drug therapy. *Clin Pharmacol* 1988;7:14–17.

66. Lieberman D. Common anorectal disorders. *Ann Intern Med* 1984;101:837–846.

67. Cheskin L. Constipation and diarrhea. In: Barker LR, Burton JR, Zieve PD, eds. *Principles of ambulatory medicine,* 3rd ed. Baltimore: Williams & Wilkins, 1991;443–457.

68. Chapman R, Sillery J, Fontana D. Effect of oral dioctyl sodium sulfosuccinate on intake–output studies of human small and large intestine. *Gastroenterology* 1985;89:489.

69. Beaugerie L, Cosnes J, Verwaerde F, et al. Isotonic high-sodium oral rehydration solution for increasing sodium absorption in patients with short-bowel syndrome. *Am J Clin Nutr* 1991;53:769–772.

70. DiJohn D, Levine M. Treatment of diarrhea. *Infect Dis Clin North Am* 1988;2(3):719–745.

70a. Fordtran JS, Rector FC, Carter AW. The mechanics of sodium absorption in the human small intestine. *J Clin Invest* 1968;47:884–900.

71. Avery M, Snyder J. Oral therapy for acute diarrhea. *N Engl J Med* 1990;323(13):891–894.

72. Pizarro D, Posada G, Sandi L, Moran J. Rice-based oral electrolyte solutions for the management of infantile diarrhea. *N Engl J Med* 1991;324:517–521.

73. Kelsall B, Guerrant R. Evaluation of diarrhea in the returning traveler. *Infect Dis Clin North Am* 1992;6(2):413–425.

74. de dios Pozo-Olano J, Warram JJ, Gomez R, Cavazos M. Effect of a lactobacilli preparation on traveler's diarrhea: a randomized, double blind clinical trial. *Gastroenterology* 1978;74:829–830.

75. Dupont H, Ericsson C. Prevention and treatment of traveler's diarrhea. *N Engl J Med* 1993;328:1821–1827.

76. Steffen R. Worldwide efficacy of bismuth subsalicylate in the treatment of traveler's diarrhea. *Rev Infect Dis* 1990;12(Suppl 1):s80–s86.

77. Farthing M. Review article: prevention and treatment of traveller's diarrhoea. *Aliment Pharmacol Ther* 1991;5:15–30.

78. Tellier R, Keystone J. Prevention of traveler's diarrhea. *Infect Dis Clin North Am* 1992;6(2):333–354.

79. Youngman K, Simon P, West G, Cominelli F, Rachmilewitz D, Fiocchi C. Localization of intestinal interleukin-1 activity and protein and gene expression to lamina propria cells. *Gastroenterology* 1993;104:749–758.

80. Cominelli F, Nast C, Duchini A, Lee M. Recombinant interleukin-1 receptor antagonist blocks the proinflammatory activity of endogenous interleukin-1 in rabbit immune colitis. *Gastroenterology* 1992;103:365–371.

81. DuPont H, Ericsson C, Mathewson J, Marani S, Knellwolf-Cousin A, Martinez-Sandoval F. Zaldaride maleate, an intestinal calmodulin inhibitor, in the therapy of travelers' diarrhea. *Gastroenterology* 1993;104:709–715.

Infections of the Gastrointestinal Tract,
edited by M. J. Blaser, P. D. Smith, J. I. Ravdin,
H. B. Greenberg, and R. L. Guerrant
Raven Press, Ltd., New York © 1995.

CHAPTER 89

Therapy for Diarrheal Illness in Children

Larry K. Pickering and David O. Matson

Enteric infections generally are self-limited conditions that require fluid and electrolyte therapy (1). In some instances, specific antimicrobial therapy may eradicate fecal shedding of the causative organism, prevent transmission of the enteropathogen, abbreviate clinical symptoms, or prevent future complications. The number of enteropathogens capable of producing gastroenteritis is large, and the response of each to therapy varies. Organisms that commonly cause dehydration are the enteric viruses, *Vibrio cholerae,* and enterotoxigenic *Escherichia coli.* Invasive bacterial enteropathogens, including *Campylobacter jejuni, Shigella* species, *Salmonella* species, *E. coli* O157:H7, and *Yersinia enterocolitica,* may produce complications other than dehydration.

The major therapeutic considerations for children with gastroenteritis include (a) fluid and electrolyte replacement, (b) dietary intake, (c) nonspecific therapy with antidiarrheal compounds, and (d) specific therapy with antimicrobial agents. This chapter focuses on the latter two categories.

PRINCIPLES OF TREATING CHILDREN

Several basic principles underlie the treatment of children with acute infectious gastroenteritis.

1. Many bacterial, viral, and parasitic enteropathogens are capable of causing gastroenteritis. These organisms have varying degrees of response to antimicrobial agents (Table 1).
2. Diagnostic assays for several enteropathogens are cumbersome, costly, and/or available only in research or reference laboratories; their use may delay administration of appropriate antimicrobial therapy.
3. Enteropathogens are acquired through the fecal–oral route by contaminated food or water or are spread from person-to-person. In certain instances, antimi-

crobial therapy will reduce the potential of person-to-person transmission.
4. Infections in patients with defects in their host defense mechanisms, such as persons infected with the human immunodeficiency virus (HIV), are often severe, commonly disseminate, require prolonged therapy, and frequently relapse when therapy is stopped.
5. Development of resistance to antimicrobial agents by bacterial enteropathogens is an increasing problem.
6. *In vitro* drug susceptibility results do not always predict *in vivo* clinical response.
7. Safety factors and side effects preclude the use in children of certain antimicrobial agents (e.g., the fluoroquinolones) that are approved for administration to adults.

TABLE 1. *Potential benefit of antimicrobial therapy for enteropathogens or diseases produced by enteropathogens*

Potential benefit	Enteropathogen or disease
Established benefit	Amebiasis
	Antimicrobial associated colitis (*C. difficile*)
	Cholera
	Enterotoxigenic *E. coli*
	Giardiasis
	Invasive *E. coli*
	Isosporiasis
	Shigella
	Strongyloidiasis
	Any bacterium that produces bacteremia (e.g., *Salmonella typhi*)
Questionable or unknown	*Blastocystis hominis*
	Campylobacter jejuni
	Cryptosporidiosis
	Cyclospora
	Intestinal salmonellosis
	Enterohemorrhagic *E. coli*
	Yersinia enterocolitica
Therapy not available	Enteric viruses
	Enterocytozoon bieneusi

L. K. Pickering and D. O. Matson: Center for Pediatric Research, Children's Hospital of The King's Daughters, Eastern Virginia Medical School, Norfolk, Virginia 23510.

The recent rise in the number of persons who are immunodeficient has led to recognition of previously uncommonly encountered organisms, such as *Isospora, Enterocytozoon bieneusi,* and enteric viruses, as causes of diarrhea (2,3). These agents have expanded the list of potential causes of diarrhea in immunodeficient patients and treatment for these patients may be difficult because their course of illness often is severe, prolonged, or recurrent (4).

ANTIDIARRHEAL COMPOUNDS

Table 2 lists nonprescription and prescription compounds available for relief of symptoms of diarrhea (5–27); most are not approved for children younger than 2 or 3 years of age. These compounds may be classified by their mechanisms of action, which include alteration of intestinal motility, adsorption of fluid or toxins, alteration of intestinal microflora, and alteration of fluid and electrolyte secretion.

Many persons with diarrhea medicate themselves or their children before they seek medical care. Although self-medication usually results in no harm, several problems may occur. First, adverse effects may develop, including worsening of diarrhea because of slowing of intestinal motility by agents that alter their function (6–8), salicylate absorption from bismuth subsalicylate preparations (15–17), or prevention of absorption of medicines or nutrients in the gastrointestinal tract when they come in contact with adsorbents (18). Second, these compounds may interfere with identification of enteropathogens by microscopy, enzyme immunoassay (EIA), culture, or other diagnostic assays. Third, patients may have a false sense of security following use of a compound with no therapeutic benefit.

Drugs that alter intestinal motility usually have a rapid onset of action by producing segmental contractions of the intestine (23–25), which serves to retard movement of intestinal contents responsible for diarrhea and to restrict the intestinal distension responsible for pain. These agents also may inhibit intestinal secretion (5). Side effects include dizziness, dry mouth, drowsiness, tachycardia, constipation, and vomiting. These drugs should be avoided in patients with fever, toxemia, or bloody stools. They can worsen the clinical course of shigellosis (6), *Clostridium difficile* (19), and *E. coli* O157:H7 (28,29). Because of concern about safety of these compounds in children, including the potential for overdose, use of these compounds is not recommended in children (7,8,24).

Several antidiarrheal compounds are used as adsorbents (9,10) and are reported to work by adsorbing bacterial toxins and water to improve symptoms of diarrhea. All currently available compounds in this category contain activated attapulgite, which is a clay that acts as an adsorbent. It relieves diarrhea by reducing the number of bowel movements and improving stool consistency. Although attapulgite has been shown to be effective in animals (20,21), controlled studies showing the effectiveness of adsorbents in reducing the duration of diarrhea or the

TABLE 2. *Nonspecific diarrheal medications for patients with acute diarrhea*

Class	Generic name	Trade name	Earliest recommended age (year)	Comments
Alteration of intestinal motility	Loperamide hydrochloride	Imodium A-D	2	Side effects include drowsiness, dry mouth, dizziness, hypersensitivity, constipation, and emesis
		Pepto diarrheal control	2	
	Diphenoxylate-atropine	Lomotil[a]	2	Side effects include drowsiness, dizziness, dry mouth, flushing, urinary retention, respiratory depression, and coma
	Difenoxin HCl with atrophine sulfate	Motofen[a]	12	Side effects include drowsiness, dizziness, dry mouth, flushing, urinary retention, respiratory depression, and coma
Adsorbents	Activated attapulgite	Diasorb	3	Adsorbs nutrients and drugs
		Donnagel	3	Adsorbs nutrients and drugs
		Kaopectate	3	Adsorbs nutrients and drugs
		Rheaban	6	Adsorbs nutrients and drugs
Alteration of intestinal microflora	Lactobacillus-containing compounds	Lactinex	—	Contraindicated in patients with lactose intolerance; may cause gastric irritability and emesis
Alteration of secretion	Bismuth subsalicylate	Pepto-Bismol	3	Category III; contains salicylates and bismuth
	Octreotide	Sandostatin[a]	—	Used for relief of diarrhea caused by *Cryptosporidium* and *Enterocytozoon bieneusi*; not FDA approved for this indication

[a] Requires prescription.

loss of fluid and electrolytes in humans need to be conducted. Potential disadvantages include adsorption of nutrients, enzymes, and antibiotics in the intestine (18), particularly with prolonged use.

Lactobacillus preparations are given to recolonize the intestine with saccharolytic flora and to alter the intestinal pH to deter potential pathogens. Lactobacillus compounds are variable in content and no evidence exists that lactobacillus compounds are effective in the symptomatic treatment of diarrhea (11–13,30).

Bismuth subsalicylate, bismuth subnitrate, and bismuth subgallate are used as adjunctive therapy for acute diarrhea. The mechanism of action of these compounds is uncertain, although laboratory studies have shown that bismuth subsalicylate inhibits intestinal secretion caused by E. coli and cholera toxins (14). Bismuth subsalicylate in both liquid and tablet forms has been shown to be effective in prevention and treatment of acute diarrhea among adult students in Mexico (31,32). Controlled trials of bismuth subsalicylate demonstrated reduced frequency of unformed stools and increased stool consistency among adult volunteers receiving the Norwalk virus, as well as a decreased duration of diarrhea among children (26,33). Salicylate absorption has been reported following ingestion of bismuth subsalicylate (15,16). Bismuth-associated encephalopathy and other toxicities have been reported from the chronic administration of high doses of bismuth-containing compounds (17).

Octreotide acetate (Sandostatin) is a long-acting octapeptide that mimics the natural hormone somatostatin by inhibiting secretion of a variety of endocrine and exocrine hormones, including growth hormone, thyroid stimulating hormone, adrenocorticotropic hormone, insulin, glucagon, gastrin, secretin, pancreozymin, and pepsin. Octreotide is approved by the U.S. Food and Drug Administration (FDA) for symptomatic treatment of patients with metastatic carcinoid tumors because it suppresses or inhibits the severe diarrhea and flushing episodes associated with this disease. Octreotide also reduces the profuse, watery diarrhea associated with vasoactive intestinal peptide-secreting tumors. It has been used in patients with Cryptosporidium (22), but it has not been approved by the FDA for this purpose.

ANTIMICROBIAL THERAPY

Most children with acute infectious diarrhea will not benefit from therapy with an antimicrobial agent. To date, antimicrobial agents are not effective for treatment of gastroenteritis caused by viral enteropathogens that include rotavirus, enteric adenovirus, calicivirus, including the Norwalk virus, astrovirus, and unclassified viruses or by Enterocytozoon bieneusi. Patients with diarrhea associated with certain bacterial and protozoal agents may benefit from therapy (Table 1). Because resistance among enteric bacteria follows widespread use of antimicrobial agents and because resistant organisms can spread rapidly due to mobility of the world population, constant monitoring of susceptibility of bacterial isolates is critical for selection of appropriate antimicrobial agents for therapy (34).

BACTERIA

Antimicrobial-Associated Colitis

The specific cause of antimicrobial associated colitis (AAC) is a toxin produced by C. difficile. In patients with AAC, the most important aspects of therapy are discontinuation of the antimicrobial or antineoplastic agent and replacement of fluid and electrolytes. Approximately 25% of patients with mild disease may respond to these measures (35). If symptoms persist or worsen, or if the disease is severe, specific therapy with vancomycin (35–37), metronidazole (35,38), or bacitracin (39–41) should be administered (Table 3). All strains of C. difficile are susceptible to vancomycin, whereas resistance to metronidazole and bacitracin has been reported (42).

Oral vancomycin has been widely used for patients with severe AAC. Expense and bitter taste are major disadvantages, as is the potential for selecting vancomycin-resistant enterococcal flora. The oral preparation of metronidazole is a less expensive alternative for treating patients with mild-to-moderate disease (35), but it is not approved by the FDA for treatment of patients with this condition. Bacitracin, although a useful alternative to metronidazole and vancomycin, has a slower and less certain response rate than vancomycin (40,41) and is not approved by the FDA for this condition. Bacitracin can be toxic if absorbed from an inflamed intestine. Patients unable to take vancomycin orally should be treated with both metronidazole and vancomycin administered intravenously and with vancomycin administered by nasogastric tube, ostomy, enema, or rectal or colonic lavage (43,44), because parenteral therapy with vancomycin or metronidazole is not as effective as oral therapy. Relapses occur in 10% to 20% of patients treated with vancomycin, metronidazole, or bacitracin (35,37,41), generally 1 to 4 weeks after treatment is stopped. Recurrences are due to either germination of C. difficile spores that persist despite treatment or reinfection with C. difficile acquired from human or environmental exposure. Relapses generally respond to metronidazole or vancomycin.

Teicoplanin, a glycopeptide antibiotic, has been used successfully to treat patients with AAC (45), but additional studies are needed. Cholestyramine and other anion exchange resins were used in the past for treatment of patients with AAC when the cause was less clear and when bile acids were considered to be causative (46). Cholestyramine binds C. difficile toxin and may bind vancomycin. Because cholestyramine is not as effective as antimicrobial agents in severe disease, it generally is not used. Cholestyramine should not be used with orally administered vancomycin because of the potential of binding.

Salmonella

The syndrome produced by Salmonella dictates the selection and duration of antimicrobial therapy (Table 4).

TABLE 3. *Antimicrobial therapy for gastroenteritis caused by bacterial pathogens*

Organism	Antimicrobial agent	Each dose, mg/kg (maximum)	Hours between doses	Days of therapy
C. difficile	Vancomycin	5 (max 125–500)	6	7
	or			
	Metronidazole	7 (max 500)	8	7
C. jejuni	None or erythromycin	10 (max 250)	6	5–7
	or			
	Ciprofloxacin[a]	500 (max 1000)	12	5
V. cholerae O1	Tetracycline	10 (max 250)	6	3
	or			
	Doxycycline	6 (max 300)	Single dose	1
	or			
	TMP/SMX	5/25 (max 160/800)	12	3
V. cholerae O139[b]	Tetracycline	10 (max 250)	6	3
	or			
	Doxycycline	6 (max 300)	Single dose	1
Y. enterocolitica	None			
V. parahaemolyticus	None			
Enterotoxigenic E. coli	TMP/SMX	5/25 (max 160/800)	12	3–5
	or			
	Ciprofloxacin[a]	500 (max 1000)	12	3–5
Enteroinvasive E. coli	See Table 5	Same as for shigellosis		
Aeromonas species	See Table 5	Same as for shigellosis		
Plesiomonas shigelloides	TMP/SMX	5/25 (max 160/800)	12	3–5
	or			
	Ciprofloxacin[a]	500 (max 1000)	12	3–5

[a] Not FDA approved for individuals under 17 years of age.
[b] See text for alternatives.

Many practitioners do not recognize that antibiotics are likely to prolong symptoms or increase the risk of complications among persons who are nontyphoid *Salmonella* carriers or in patients who have mild gastroenteritis. Several randomized studies, including studies of newer antimicrobial agents, have demonstrated no difference between treated and untreated patients (47). Antimicrobial therapy may convert intestinal carriage to systemic disease with bacteremia (48), produce a bacteriologic and symptomatic relapse (49–51), encourage development or

selection of resistant strains, or prolong fecal excretion (49,51,52).

Antibiotic treatment of patients with *Salmonella* infection generally is restricted to those with (a) typhoid fever, including patients with clinical illness and carriers; (b) bacteremia from nontyphoidal strains, and (c) dissemination with localized suppuration. Antimicrobial therapy also should be considered in newborn infants and in patients with enterocolitis who have an underlying condition or disease that impairs host resistance, such as those with

TABLE 4. *Antimicrobial therapy for* Salmonella *infections in children*

Clinical manifestation	Antimicrobial agent	Each dose, mg/kg (maximum)	Hours between doses	Days of therapy
Carrier state with S. typhi	Amoxicillin with probenicid	15	8	42
Acute gastroenteritis	Probably none	See text for exceptions		
Bacteremia or enteric fever or both	Ampicillin	35 (max 1 g)	4	14
	or			
	Chloramphenicol	20 (max 1 g)	6	14
	or			
	TMP/SMX	5/25 (max 160/800)	12	14
	or			
	Ceftriaxone	75 (max 2 g)	12	14
	or			
	Cefotaxime	50 (max 3 g)	6	14
Dissemination with localized suppuration (osteomyelitis)	Same as above for bacteremia	—	—	4–6 weeks

acquired immunodeficiency syndrome (AIDS), a hemoglobinopathy including sickle cell anemia, lymphoma, leukemia, immunosuppression, or congenital heart disease or disorders of cardiac valves. Recommended antimicrobial agents include ampicillin, chloramphenicol administered intravenously or orally, and trimethoprim/sulfamethoxazole (TMP/SMX) (53,54). In the United States, attention has focused on resistance of nontyphoidal *Salmonella* strains, which have their major reservoir in animals. Several outbreaks of multiresistant *Salmonella* infection have been traced to animal sources in the United States and are a major problem in various parts of the world (55,56). All human isolates of *Salmonella* should have susceptibility testing performed.

In the United States, antimicrobial resistance of *S. typhi* has been a minor problem; only 2% to 3% of *S. typhi* strains are resistant to ampicillin and chloramphenicol (57). However, because of international travel, the potential exists for importation of resistant strains (52,57). From 1975 to 1984, 62% of the cases of acute typhoid fever in the United States were acquired in other countries, with Mexico (39%) and India (14%) being the major sources (57). California, Texas, and New York reported the greatest number of cases. In general, *S. typhi* has remained susceptible in comparison with the nontyphoidal *Salmonella* strains. Drugs that have been used successfully in the treatment of typhoid fever include chloramphenicol, ampicillin, and TMP/SMX. Cefotaxime, ceftriaxone, and cefoperazone are effective against *S. typhi* and nontyphoidal *Salmonella* strains that are resistant to ampicillin, chloramphenicol, and TMP/SMX (58–60). In prospective, randomized studies of children and adults with confirmed typhoid fever (60,61), ceftriaxone administered for 5 days was as effective and safe as a 2- to 3-week course of chloramphenicol. First- and second-generation cephalosporin antibiotics have been less effective than third-generation antibiotics and should not be used.

Ciprofloxacin is active *in vitro* against *Salmonella*, including *S. typhi*, and has been used clinically with success (62–64). Many other antibiotics are active *in vitro* against *Salmonella* strains, including *S. typhi*, but susceptibility correlates poorly with *in vivo* response (65). Corticosteroids can be beneficial in patients with typhoid fever in whom prompt relief of manifestations of toxemia might be lifesaving (66), but they may increase the relapse rate (67).

Antibiotics listed in Table 4 can be used for treatment of *Salmonella;* chloramphenicol should not be used if infection has disseminated to localized sites. Patients with defective host defense mechanisms, such as individuals with AIDS, should be treated with ampicillin or a third-generation cephalosporin (68–70). Ciprofloxacin has been reported to be effective in treatment of acute diarrhea due to *Salmonella* (71–73), recurrent *Salmonella* sepsis (74), and brain abscesses in a neonate (75). Duration of therapy is influenced by the site of infection and by the host. In a murine model, ciprofloxacin incorporated into liposomes was more effective than aqueous ciprofloxacin (76). Patients with bacteremia without a localized infection should be treated for 14 days, whereas those with localized infection, such as osteomyelitis or endocarditis, or patients

with AIDS and bacteremia should receive at least 4 to 6 weeks of therapy. In the majority of cases, chronic carriage of *S. typhi* is associated with gallbladder disease. The presence of cholelithiasis may significantly impact on the efficacy of therapy. When gallbladder disease was present, the failure rate of ampicillin was about 75% (77). In patients without gallbladder disease, ampicillin with probenecid or amoxicillin administered for 6 weeks is the treatment of choice for chronic enteric carriers (78,79). Norfloxacin (80) and ciprofloxacin (81) also have been reported to be successful in eradicating *S. typhi* in chronic carriers. Resistance of clinical isolates to and failure of treatment with ciprofloxacin have been noted in patients infected with *S. typhimurium* (82).

Shigella

In the United States, 60% of reported cases of diarrhea associated with *Shigella* are due to *S. sonnei; S. flexneri* serotypes account for the majority of the remaining cases. *Shigella dysenteriae* is an uncommon cause of diarrhea in the United States. Table 5 outlines suggested antimicrobial therapy for children who have presumed shigellosis or in whom *Shigella* has been isolated from stool. The treatment of choice for shigellosis is TMP/SMX for susceptible strains (83–92). *Shigella* strains have become progressively resistant to multiple antimicrobial agents, initially to sulfonamides, shortly after they became commercially available, then to tetracycline, chloramphenicol, and streptomycin less than 10 years after each was introduced, and subsequently to ampicillin, kanamycin, and TMP/SMX (93). In the United States, *S. flexneri* strains have remained relatively susceptible to ampicillin, whereas over half of the *S. sonnei* strains are resistant (86), except in certain native American populations where TMP/SMX resistance is common in *S. flexneri* and *S. sonnei* (86). In children with ampicillin-susceptible strains, ampicillin is an accepted treatment and can be given orally or intravenously. Amoxicillin is not as effective as ampicillin and should not be used (94). Single-dose tetracycline therapy is effective in the treatment of *Shigella* infection in adults regardless of clinical expression of illness and may be useful in treatment of disease from tetracycline-resistant strains (87). Treatment with tetracycline must be limited to adults because of tooth discoloration and bone deposition, which occur in children younger than 9 years of age. Furazolidone has been shown to be effective in children infected with susceptible strains (95,96). Patients who are transient, symptom-free carriers may be managed without antimicrobial therapy if they employ excellent standards of personal and public hygiene. Treatment of these patients, however, will reduce fecal shedding of the organism and may prevent spread of infection (88,89).

Parenterally and orally administered third-generation cephalosporins have been used successfully in the treatment of children with shigellosis (97–99). Two-day (98) and 5-day (99) courses of ceftriaxone were effective in eradication of *Shigella* from stool and reduction of the duration of diarrhea. In one study, a single parenteral dose of ceftriaxone produced a moderate reduction in diarrhea

TABLE 5. *Antimicrobial therapy for shigellosis*

Antimicrobial agent	Each dose, mg/kg (maximum)	Hours between doses	Days of therapy	Comment
TMP/SMX	5/25 (max 160/800)	12	5	Antimicrobial drug of choice; some strains are resistant
Ampicillin	20 (max 500)	6	5	Only for ampicillin-susceptible strains
Nalidixic acid	15 (max 1 g)	6	5	Use for TMP/SMX- and ampicillin-resistant strains; not FDA approved for this purpose
Ciprofloxacin	500 (max 1 g)	12	3–5	Resistant strains; not approved for persons under 17 years of age
Ceftriaxone	500 (max 1.5 g)	Single dose	3	Resistant strains; not FDA approved for this purpose
Cefixime	4 (max 200)	12	5	Resistant strains; not FDA approved for this purpose

but failed to eradicate *Shigella* strains from stools (100). Previous studies of first- and second-generation cephalosporins for treatment of shigellosis have demonstrated them to be ineffective (101–103). Cefixime administered orally has been shown to be therapeutic for children and adolescents whose isolates were resistant to TMP/SMX (97), although it is not approved by the FDA for this condition. Ceftibutin, an orally administered, third-generation cephalosporin, has shown good *in vitro* activity against various enteric pathogens and promising clinical efficacy in patients with shigellosis (104).

Ciprofloxacin, norfloxacin, and enoxacin have been used successfully to treat adults with shigellosis, even those infected with resistant strains (73,105–109). In a study evaluating dosing of ciprofloxacin in adults, ten 1-g doses (5 days) were an effective therapy for patients infected with *S. dysenteriae* type 1. For other *Shigella* species, a single, 1-g dose was sufficient (107). Ciprofloxacin is FDA approved for treatment of gastrointestinal tract infections caused by *S. sonnei* and *S. flexneri*. The fluoroquinolones, such as ofloxacin and ciprofloxacin, have greater activity against gram-negative bacteria than do the older deoxyribonucleic acid (DNA) gyrase inhibitors such as nalidixic acid. However, reduced susceptibility to ciprofloxacin and ofloxacin, probably due to mutation in the DNA gyrase subunit A gene, has been noted in *S. sonnei* strains isolated from patients with dysentery (110). Nalidixic acid can be used as an alternative drug (105,108,111), although resistance has been described (93,112,113).

Campylobacter

Campylobacter jejuni strains generally are susceptible to a wide variety of antimicrobial agents, including erythromycin, furazolidone, quinolones, aminoglycosides, tetracycline, chloramphenicol, imipenem, and clindamycin; by contrast, penicillin, ampicillin, and the cephalosporins are relatively inactive (114–117). Isolation of *Campylobacter* from stool does not mandate antibiotic therapy; the decision to institute therapy should be made on clinical grounds. In patients with *Campylobacter* enteritis, erythromycin represents the agent of choice. Ciprofloxacin has been approved by the FDA for treatment of *C. jejuni* enteritis in persons older than 17 years of age. In double-blind, placebo-controlled trials of treatment of patients with *Campylobacter* enteritis, erythromycin promptly eradicated *Campylobacter* from feces but did not alter the natural course of enteritis when administered 4 days or longer after the onset of symptoms. Studies in which therapy was initiated early in the course of illness gave conflicting results with regard to clinical resolution, although *C. jejuni* was eliminated from stools significantly faster in the treatment groups of both studies (118,119). Clindamycin or amoxicillin plus clavulanate are alternative choices in children, but studies supporting their effectiveness are limited. The treatment of choice for patients with septicemia appears to be parenterally administered gentamicin or ciprofloxacin in adults, although chloramphenicol, tetracycline, and erythromycin are alternate choices (120).

The frequency of isolation of erythromycin-resistant *Campylobacter* strains ranges from less than 1% in Canada and the United Kingdom (116,121–123) to 8% in Belgium and 10% in Sweden (124,125). In one study from the United States, 3% of *Campylobacter* strains from human sources were resistant to erythromycin (126). In the same study, a higher frequency of erythromycin resistance was noted in hog isolates, most of which were *C. coli* (126). Other studies have reported that the frequency of resistance in *C. coli* is much higher than in *C. jejuni* (114,126–128). This resistance may be due to production of ribonucleic acid (RNA) methylase or a mutational change of a ribosomal protein gene (121). Strains of *C. jejuni* and *C. coli* that show high-level resistance to erythromycin also appear to be resistant to clarithromycin and azithromycin (129). Development of resistance to ciprofloxacin in *Campylobacter* species has been reported in several studies (130–134). Resistance by *C. jejuni* to ciprofloxacin developed in two individuals during therapy with ciprofloxacin (135). These individuals failed microbiologically and one failed clinically.

Escherichia coli O157:H7

The role of antimicrobial therapy in patients with hemorrhagic colitis caused by *E. coli* O157:H7 or other Shiga-like toxin (SLT) producing *E. coli* is uncertain. In general, these *E. coli* strains have been susceptible to antimicrobial agents usually used for *E. coli*. Medications, including antibiotic therapy, do not appear to influence the duration of symptoms nor do they appear to alter the risk of progression to hemolytic-uremic syndrome (HUS) or thrombotic thrombocytopenic purpura (TTP) (136–138). That treatment of patients infected with *E. coli* O157:H7 may be harmful is raised by the following observations. (a) When *E. coli* O157:H7 was cultured with subinhibitory concentrations of certain antibiotics, including TMP/SMX, the intracellular and extracellular concentrations of SLT increase (139,140). (b) Because HUS and TTP are thought to be mediated by SLT, certain antibiotics may increase the amount of toxin released in the intestine resulting in an increased risk of systemic sequelae. (c) In nonrandomized studies of residents in an institution for the mentally retarded, five of eight individuals with HUS had received TMP/SMX compared with none of seven who had no subsequent complications (141). In another study, nursing home patients with *E. coli* O157:H7 infections who were treated with antimicrobial agents had an increased risk of death (142). The problem with these two clinical reports of antimicrobial use in patients with diarrhea due to *E. coli* O157:H7 is that antimicrobial agents were not administered in a randomized fashion and patients who had more severe illness were likely to have received medication (28,143). Therefore the outcome of treatment was more likely to be associated with poor outcome because the prognosis was worse at the onset of therapy (141). In contrast to the above observations, in one prospective, controlled trial, which evaluated the effect of TMP/SMX in children with proven *E. coli* O157:H7 enteritis, treatment had no effect on the progression of symptoms, fecal pathogen excretion, or incidence of HUS (144). Additional studies are needed to clarify the role of antimicrobial therapy for patients with infection due to SLT-producing *E. coli*.

Vibrio cholerae

Diarrhea caused by infection with *V. cholerae* O1 is uncommon in the United States, although the organism is endemic along the Gulf Coast (145). In addition, since appearing in Peru in 1991, *V. cholerae* has spread to most countries in South and North America. Oral fluid and electrolyte therapy is essential. Antimicrobial therapy for gastroenteritis from cholera will shorten the duration of diarrhea and reduce fluid losses. For most patients, either tetracycline or doxycycline are the drugs of choice (Table 3) (146–148). Other effective antimicrobial agents are TMP/SMX, furazolidone, and erythromycin (149–151).

The use of tetracycline or doxycycline is not recommended for children younger than 9 years of age; however, in severe cholera infections, benefits may offset the risk of tooth staining. Ciprofloxacin and ofloxacin are effective but are not approved for use in individuals under 17 years of age. *Vibrio cholerae* has remained relatively susceptible to antibiotics, most likely because only a few plasmid types are stable in these organisms. Nevertheless, resistance to tetracycline, streptomycin, chloramphenicol, sulfonamides, ampicillin, kanamycin, and TMP/SMX has been reported (93).

Vibrio cholerae O139 has been associated with a large outbreak of cholera-like disease in Bangladesh (152). This organism has been shown to be susceptible to tetracycline, ampicillin, chloramphenicol, erythromycin, and ciprofloxacin, but not to TMP/SMX and furazolidone, two agents often used to treat cholera in children (152).

Other Bacteria

Other bacteria that infrequently produce diarrhea in children in the United States are *E. coli* other than *E. coli* O157:H7, *Y. enterocolitica*, and *V. parahaemolyticus*. *Yersinia enterocolitica* appears to be a common cause of diarrhea among children in Europe and Canada (153), although it occurs infrequently in the United States (154). It usually is susceptible *in vitro* to aminoglycosides, chloramphenicol, tetracycline, TMP/SMX, third-generation cephalosporins, and quinolones (154,155). Strains are often resistant to penicillin, ampicillin, and first-generation cephalosporins. There are no data to support the use of antimicrobial agents in diarrhea caused by this organism. *Vibrio parahaemolyticus* gastrointestinal tract infection is self-limited, and antimicrobial therapy shortens neither the clinical course nor the duration of fecal excretion of the organism. Patients with *Y. enterocolitica*-induced septicemia should be treated with either gentamicin, chloramphenicol, or third-generation cephalosporin antibiotics. Good responses have been reported in treatment of *Y. enterocolitica* septicemia with third-generation cephalosporins and ciprofloxacin (156). Despite treatment, the mortality rate for this condition approaches 50%.

Diarrhea caused by enterotoxigenic *E. coli* usually is self-limited, but studies have shown that antimicrobial agents such as TMP/SMX or ciprofloxacin are effective (73,91,92,96,106). Ciprofloxacin is FDA approved for treatment of persons with diarrhea due to enterotoxigenic *E. coli*. Little is known about the treatment of enteroinvasive *E. coli* infection because it usually is not diagnosed. Antimicrobial therapy should be similar to that administered to patients with shigellosis. Susceptibility studies should be performed if the organism is isolated.

In vitro studies have shown that over 90% of 131 strains of *Aeromonas* species were susceptible to aminoglycosides, ureidopenicillins, third-generation cephalosporin antibiotics, aztreonam, quinolones, tetracycline, and chloramphenicol; over 75% were susceptible to TMP/SMX; and all strains were resistant to ampicillin (157). Differences in susceptibility patterns may exist among geographic areas and within species of *Aeromonas*. Invasive strains generally are treated with aminoglycosides, third-generation cephalosporins, or imipenem (158). Infections of the gastrointestinal tract may respond to TMP/SMX or ciprofloxacin, which is approved only for patients over 17 years of age.

Plesiomonas shigelloides has been identified as a cause of endemic and traveler's diarrhea. These organisms are susceptible to TMP/SMX, ciprofloxacin, cephalosporins, and imipenem (159). Many strains are resistant to aminoglycosides.

PROTOZOAL AGENTS

Because patients with AIDS frequently develop persistent diarrhea, there has been a renewed interest in parasitic infections involving the gastrointestinal tract. In patients with normal immune systems, infections with these organisms are generally of short duration and respond to therapy when available; however, the clinical course may be protracted in children with AIDS (3). Parasitic diseases of the gastrointestinal tract that fulfill the Centers for Disease Control and Prevention surveillance definition for AIDS are those caused by *Cryptosporidium* and *Isospora* (160). Tables 6, 7, and 8 show the recommended therapy for infection with enteric parasitic organisms (161). Several of these compounds have severe adverse effects that should be considered against the potential benefit of therapy.

Giardia lamblia

Quinacrine hydrochloride, metronidazole, and furazolidone are effective in treating patients with infection caused by *G. lamblia* (162). Metronidazole may be better tolerated than quinacrine, but it is more expensive and may be slightly less effective. In addition, metronidazole is carcinogenic in rodents and mutagenic in bacteria and is considered an investigational drug for this condition by the FDA. Quinacrine hydrochloride may produce a yellow discoloration of the skin that disappears after the drug

is stopped (163). Furazolidone is the only one of these three compounds available in liquid form; like quinacrine, it is less expensive than metronidazole. Furazolidone can be used in children (164) if compliance is a problem with quinacrine and metronidazole, both of which have an objectionable taste. The dosage schedule for children and adults is given in Table 6. Outside the United States tinidazole and ornidazole also are used to treat giardiasis. Tinidazole and ornidazole are nitroimidazoles similar to metronidazole and appear to be as effective as metronidazole and better tolerated.

Entamoeba histolytica

Iodoquinol is the recommended drug to eradicate both cysts and trophozoites of *E. histolytica* in the lumen of the gastrointestinal tract (Table 7). Invasive amebiasis of the intestine, liver, or other organs necessitates additional use of tissue amebicides such as metronidazole. Table 7 shows the recommended drugs for treatment of children with various forms of amebiasis (161).

Cryptosporidium

Infection with *Cryptosporidium* is self-limited in immunocompetent individuals; however, patients with AIDS may have large volume, intractable diarrhea. Specific antimicrobial therapy for *Cryptosporidium* is not available. Spiramycin has been used but generally is thought to be ineffective (165). Limited studies indicate paromomycin may be effective in rapid resolution of chronic diarrhea in most patients (166–168). Paromomycin has also been shown to inhibit *Cryptosporidium* infection of a human enterocyte cell line (169). In dexamethasone-immunosuppressed rats, azithromycin consistently prevented ileal infection with *Cryptosporidium parvum* in a dose-related manner (170). Azithromycin has been shown to be effective in treatment of two children with cancer who had severe diarrhea due to *Cryptosporidium* (171). Orally administered bovine transfer factor, hyperimmune colostrum, monoclonal antibody, cow milk immunoglobulin,

TABLE 6. *Antimicrobial therapy for giardiasis*

Antimicrobial agent	Each dose, mg/kg (maximum)	Hours between doses (route)	Days of therapy	Common side effects	Comment
Quinacrine HCl (Atabrine)	2 (max 100)	8	7	Dizziness, headache, vomiting, diarrhea	FDA approved for this purpose
Metronidazole (Flagyl)	5 (max 250)	8	7	Nausea, headache, dry mouth, metallic taste	Not FDA approved for this purpose
Furazolidone (Furoxone)	1.5 (max 100)	6	7	Nausea, vomiting	Available in liquid form
Paramomycin (Humatin)	10	8	7	Gastrointestinal tract disturbance	Not absorbed and not very effective; may be useful for treatment of giardiasis in pregnancy

TABLE 7. *Antimicrobial therapy for amebiasis*

Clinical manifestations	Antimicrobial agent	Each dose, mg/kg (maximum)	Hours between doses (route)	Days of therapy	Comment
Asymptomatic cyst excretor	Iodoquinol (Yodoxin)	10 (max 700)	8	20	Do not exceed maximum dose, because of possibility of optic neuritis
	or				
	Paromomycin (Humatin)	10	8	7	
	or				
	Diloxanide furoate (Furamide)[a]	7 (max 500)	8	10	Available from Centers for Disease Control and Prevention Drug Service[a]
Mild-to-moderate intestinal disease	Metronidazole (Flagyl) first	15 (max 750)	8	10	Not recommended for pregnant women, especially in first trimester
	Followed by iodoquinol or paromomycin	Same as above			
Severe intestinal disease	Metronidazole first	Same as above			
	Followed next by iodoquinol or dehydroemetine[a]	Same as above 0.5 to 0.75 im (max 45)	12	Up to 5	Available from CDC Drug Service
	Followed finally by iodoquinol	Same as above			
Liver abscess or extraintestinal amebic disease	Metronidazole	Same as above			Given with iodoquinol in two-stage treatment plan
	Iodoquinol	Same as above			After metronidazole
	or				
	Dehydroemetine[a]	Same as above			
	Chloroquine	10 mg base/kg/day (max 300 base/day)	Once	14–21	Given with chloroquine and iodoquinol in a two-stage treatment plan
	Plus iodoquinol	Same as above			

[a] Telephone number (404) 639-3670 or 639-2888.

and human serum immune globulin are all being evaluated (172–177). Octreotide (Sandostatin) may control the severe diarrhea that occurs in patients with AIDS as it has in patients with scleroderma (178), although it has no effect on the infection (22,178,179).

Isospora

Unlike *Cryptosporidium, Isospora* organisms respond to treatment with TMP/SMX (Table 8) (180). However, symptomatic disease recurs in 50% of patients (181). Recurrent disease may be prevented by prophylaxis with TMP/SMX or weekly doses of pyrimethamine-sulfadoxine (Fansidar). Both of these compounds are considered investigational by the FDA for isosporiasis. In sulfonamide-sensitive patients, such as those with AIDS, pyrimethamine has been effective in adults (182). In immunocompromised patients, therapy may need to be continued indefinitely. Patients who receive TMP/SMX or pyrimethamine-sulfadoxine should be monitored carefully for bone

marrow suppression, skin reactions, and allergic manifestations.

Strongyloides stercoralis

Persons infected with *S. stercoralis* should be treated with thiabendazole. In disseminated strongyloidiasis, thiabendazole therapy should be continued for at least 5 days. In immunocompromised patients with *Strongyloides* hyperinfection, it may be necessary to continue therapy longer (183); however, the mortality rate is high despite therapy. A thorough examination should be performed before immunosuppressive therapy is given to a patient with a history of infection with *S. stercoralis*. Treatment with albendazole or ivermectin also has been effective (184,185).

Enterocytozoon bieneusi

There is no established therapy for Microsporidia that infect the gastrointestinal tract, including *E. bieneusi* and

TABLE 8. *Antimicrobial therapy for enteric parasites in children*

Organism	Antimicrobial agent	Each dose, mg/kg (maximum)	Hours between doses	Days of therapy	Side effects
Cryptosporidium	None available; see text				Octreotide (Sandostatin) has provided symptomatic relief
Isospora belli	TMP/SMX	5/25 (max 160/800)	6	10 then every 12 hr for 3 weeks	Considered an investigational drug for this condition by FDA; studies lacking in children
Enterocytozoon bieneusi	None available				Octreotide (Sandostatin) has provided symptomatic relief
Strongyloides	Thiabendazole	25 (max 1.5 g)	12	2	In disseminated disease, continue for 5 days; dose may be toxic and require decrease; considered investigational drug for this condition by FDA
	or Ivermectin	200	Single dose	1–2	No studies in children
Blastocystis hominis	Metronidazole or	Same as for amebiasis (see Table 7)			Controlled studies not available
	Iodoquiniol	Same as for amebiasis (see Table 7)			
Cyclospora	TMP/SMX	5/25 (max 160/800)	12	3	No studies in children

For *Giardia lamblia,* see Table 6; for *Entamoeba histolytica,* see Table 7.

Septata intestinalis (186–190). Therapy with antiparasitic drugs, diet alteration, and antidiarrheal medications often fail to relieve diarrhea and malabsorption associated with microsporidiosis, although octreotide may provide symptomatic relief (179). In uncontrolled studies, albendazole has been reported to stop diarrhea and weight loss, as well as promote weight gain, in persons infected with *E. bieneusi* (187) and has been shown to cure *Septata intestinalis* infection (189,190), although improvement has not been uniform (187). Double-blind, placebo-controlled trials are needed to confirm the efficacy of albendazole in treating patients with intestinal microsporidiosis.

Blastocystis hominis

The clinical significance of *B. hominis* remains unclear, but use of metronidazole or iodoquinol in the same dose as used for mild-to-moderate intestinal disease from *E. histolytica* (Table 7) has been reported to be effective in uncontrolled studies (191,192).

Cyclospora

Cyclospora cayetanensis, a recently described coccidian parasite previously referred to as a cyanobacteria-like or coccidia-like body, causes moderate-to-severe self-limited diarrhea by injuring the small bowel (193). Although the majority of cases of diarrhea due to this organism have been among immunocompromised hosts, it may be a cause of protracted diarrhea in an immunocompetent host (194). A 3-day course of TMP/SMX may be beneficial (195), but additional studies are needed to determine the efficacy of TMP/SMX in treating individuals infected with *Cyclospora.*

PROTRACTED VIRAL INFECTIONS IN THE IMMUNOCOMPROMISED CHILD

Occasionally, a clinician will face the challenge of treating an immunocompromised child with protracted diarrhea associated with continual excretion of rotavirus, calicivirus, astrovirus, or other enteric viruses. The diarrhea in these children may be unremitting and fatal. Factors important for clearing viral infection in these individuals include an intact cellular immune system and the presence of specific neutralizing antibody. In these special situations, the administration of immunoglobulins enterically, as milk, colostrum, or specific immunoglobulin preparations, may reduce the burden of illness (196,197). These preparations usually are not standardized for level of antibody to any enteric virus and multiple agents frequently infect the child simultaneously. Therefore choice and dose of therapy frequently are empiric. However, in a tertiary care facility, immune electron microscopy, enzyme immunoassays, or neutralization tests may be available to evaluate the potency of antibody preparations and the virologic response to therapy.

NONSPECIFIC INTERVENTIONS FOR THE CHILD WITH ACUTE INFECTIOUS GASTROENTERITIS

A few measures are likely to limit the spread of infection from the affected children to potential contacts. Diaper changing areas should be separate from food preparation areas. Diapers should be disposed of directly in the changing area and bagged before moving outside the home or facility. A wipe-down fluid for the changing area should be used; a reasonable choice is a 1:100 dilution of household bleach or 70% alcohol for rotaviruses, made up fresh daily in a spray bottle. Handwashing facilities should be adjacent to diapering tables and should be employed frequently.

SUMMARY

Many organisms in multiple microbiologic classes cause acute infectious gastroenteritis among children. The diversity of etiologic agents is associated with differences in response to therapy, complexity in the diagnosis of specific causes of infection, and complexity of treatment options, especially because of the increasing prevalence of strains resistant to currently available antimicrobial agents. With a few exceptions, the constellation of symptoms associated with diarrhea is remarkably uniform. Because these agents usually are spread by the fecal–oral route, the potential for polymicrobial infection is high. Multiple agents should be suspected especially in the immunocompromised host and when the response to specific therapy for a detected pathogen is delayed. The recent discovery of a large number of enteric pathogens will provide opportunities for fruitful and careful investigations of treatment over the next several years.

REFERENCES

1. Duggan C, Santosham M, Glass RI. The management of acute diarrhea in children: oral rehydration, maintenance, and nutritional therapy. *Morb Mortal Wkly Rep* 1992;41(RR-16):1–19.
2. Grohmann GS, Glass RI, Pereira HG, et al. Enteric viruses and diarrhea in HIV-infected patients. *N Engl J Med* 1993;329:14–20.
3. Pickering LK. Infections of the gastrointestinal tract. In: Pizzo PA, Wilfert CM, eds. *Pediatric AIDS: the challenge of HIV infection in infants, children and adolescents,* 2nd ed. Baltimore: Williams & Wilkins, 1994.
4. Arbo A, Santos JI. Diarrheal disease in the immunocompromised host. *Pediatr Infect Dis J* 1987;6:894–906.
5. Higgins JA, Code CF, Orvis AL. The influence of motility on the rate of absorption of sodium and water from the small intestine of healthy persons. *Gastroenterology* 1956;31:708–716.
6. DuPont HL, Hornick RB. Adverse effect on Lomotil therapy in shigellosis. *JAMA* 1973;226:1525–1528.
7. Ginsburg CM. Lomotil (diphenoxylate and atropine) intoxication. *Am J Dis Child* 1973;125:241–242.
8. Rumack BH, Temple AR. Lomotil poisoning. *Pediatrics* 1974;53:495–500.
9. McClung HJ, Beck RD, Powers P. The effect of kaolin-pectin adsorbent on stool losses of sodium, potassium, and fat during a lactose-intolerance diarrhea in rats. *J Pediatr* 1980;96:769–771.
10. Portnoy BL, DuPont HL, Pruitt D, Abdo JA, Rodriguez JT. Antidiarrheal agents in the treatment of acute diarrhea in children. *JAMA* 1976;236:844–846.
11. Clements ML, Levine MM, Black RE, et al. Lactobacillus prophylaxis for diarrhea due to enterotoxigenic *Escherichia coli*. *Antimicrob Agents Chemother* 1981;20:104–108.
12. Levine MM, Hornick RB. Lactulose therapy in *Shigella* carrier state and dysentery. *Antimicrob Agents Chemother* 1975;8:581–584.
13. Pearce JL, Hamilton JR. Controlled trial of orally administered lactobacilli in acute infantile diarrhea. *J Pediatr* 1974;84:261–262.
14. Ericsson CD, DuPont HL, Evans DG, Evans DJ Jr, Pickering LK. Bismuth subsalicylate inhibits activity of crude toxins of *Escherichia coli* and *Vibrio cholerae. J Infect Dis* 1977;136:693–696.
15. Feldman S, Chen SL, Pickering LK, Cleary TG, Ericsson CD, Hulse M. Salicylate absorption from a bismuth subsalicylate antidiarrheal preparation (Pepto-Bismol). *Clin Pharmacol Ther* 1981;29:788–792.
16. Pickering LK, Feldman S, Ericsson CD, Cleary TG. Absorption of salicylate and bismuth from a bismuth subsalicylate containing compound (Pepto-Bismol). *J Pediatr* 1981;99:654–656.
17. Mendelowitz PC, Hoffman RS, Weber S. Bismuth absorption and myoclonic encephalopathy during bismuth subsalicylate therapy. *Ann Intern Med* 1990;112:140–141.
18. Parpia SH, Nix DE, Hejmanowski LG, Goldstein HR, Wilton JH, Schentag JJ. Sucralfate reduces the gastrointestinal absorption of norfloxacin. *Antimicrob Agents Chemother* 1989;33:99–102.
19. Novak E, Lee JG, Seckman CE, Phillips JP, DiSanto AR. Unfavorable effect of atropine–diphenoxylate (Lomotil) therapy in lincomycin-caused diarrhea. *JAMA* 1976;235:1451–1454.
20. Rateau JG, Morgant G, Droy-Priot MT, Parier JL. A histological, enzymatic and water–electrolyte study of the action of smectite, a mucoprotective clay, on experimental infectious diarrhoea in the rabbit. *Curr Med Res Opin* 1982;8:233–241.
21. Fioramonti J, Droy-Lefaix MT, Bueno L. Changes in gastrointestinal motility induced by cholera toxin and experimental osmotic diarrhoea in dogs: effects of treatment with an argillaceous compound. *Digestion* 1987;36:230–237.
22. Cook DJ, Kelton JG, Stanisz AM, Collins SM. Somatostatin treatment for cryptosporidial diarrhea in a patient with the acquired immunodeficiency syndrome (AIDS). *Ann Intern Med* 1988;108:708–709.
23. Diarrhoeal Diseases Study Group (UK). Loperamide in acute diarrhoea in childhood: results of a double-blind, placebo-controlled multicentre clinical trial. *Br Med J* 1984;289:1263–1267.
24. Vesikari T, Isolauri E. A comparative trial of cholestyramine and loperamide for acute diarrhoea in infants treated as outpatients. *Acta Paediatr Scand* 1985;74:650–654.
25. Bergström T, Alestig K, Thorén K, Trollfors B. Symptomatic treatment of acute infectious diarrhoea: loperamide versus placebo in a double-blind trial. *J Infect Dis* 1986;12:35–38.
26. Soriano-Brucher HE, Avendaño P, O'Ryan M, Soriano HA. Use of bismuth subsalicylate in acute diarrhea in children. *Rev Infect Dis* 1990;12:S51–S56.
27. Ericsson CD, DuPont HL, Mathewson JJ, West MS, Johnson PC, Bitsura JAM. Treatment of travelers' diarrhea with sulfamethoxazole and trimethoprim and loperamide. *JAMA* 1990;263:257–261.
28. Cimolai N, Carter JE, Morrison BJ, Anderson JD. Risk factors for the progression of *Escherichia coli* O157:H7 enteritis to hemolytic-uremic syndrome. *J Pediatr* 1990;116:589–592.
29. Cimolai N, Carter JE, Morrison BJ, Anderson JD. The progression of *Escherichia coli* O157:H7 enteritis to hemolytic uremic syndrome: anti-diarrheal agent use and age as risk factors? *Clin Invest Med* 1988;11(Suppl):C71.
30. Reuman PD, Duckworth DH, Smith KL, Kagan R, Bucciarelli RL, Ayoub EM. Lack of effect of *Lactobacillus* on gastrointestinal bacterial colonization in premature infants. *Pediatr Infect Dis* 1986;5:663–668.
31. DuPont HL, Ericsson CD, Johnson PC, Bitsura JAM, Dupont MW, de la Cabada FJ. Prevention of travelers' diarrhea by

the table formulation of bismuth subsalicylate. *JAMA* 1987;257: 1347–1350.

32. DuPont HL, Sullivan P, Pickering LK, Haynes G, Ackerman PB. Symptomatic treatment of diarrhea with bismuth subsalicylate among students attending a Mexican university. *Gastroenterology* 1977;73:715–718.

33. Figueroa-Quintanilla D, Salazar-Lindo E, Sack RB, et al. A controlled trial of bismuth subsalicylate in infants with acute watery diarrheal disease. *N Engl J Med* 1993;328:1653–1658.

34. Kunin CM. Resistance to antimicrobial drugs—a worldwide calamity. *Ann Intern Med* 1993;118:557–561.

35. Teasley PG, Gerding DN, Olson MM, et al. Prospective randomized trial of metronidazole versus vancomycin for *Clostridium difficile*-associated diarrhea and colitis. *Lancet* 1983;2: 1043–1046.

36. Batts DH, Martin D, Holmes R, Silva J, Fekety FR. Treatment of antibiotic-associated *Clostridium difficile* diarrhea with oral vancomycin. *J Pediatr* 1980;97:151–153.

37. Fekety R, Silva J, Kauffman C, Buggy B, Deery HG. Treatment of *Clostridium difficile* antibiotic-associated colitis with oral vancomycin. Comparison of two dosage regimens. *Am J Med* 1989;86:15–19.

38. Cherry RD, Portnoy D, Jabbari M, Daly DS, Kinnear DG, Goresky CA. Metronidazole: an alternate therapy for antibiotic associated colitis. *Gastroenterology* 1982;82:849–851.

39. Tedesco FJ. Bacitracin therapy in antibiotic associated pseudomembranous colitis. *Dig Dis Sci* 1980;25:783.

40. Young GP, Ward PB, Bayley N, et al. Antibiotic associated colitis due to *Clostridium difficile:* double-blind comparison of vancomycin with bacitracin. *Gastroenterology* 1985;89: 1038–1045.

41. Dudley MN, McLaughlin JC, Carrington G, Frick J, Nightingale CH, Quintiliani R. Oral bacitracin vs. vancomycin therapy for *Clostridium difficile*-induced diarrhea. A randomized double-blind trial. *Arch Intern Med* 1986;146:1101–1104.

42. Fekety R, Silva J, Toshniwal R, et al. Antibiotic-associated colitis: effects of antibiotics on the disease in hamsters. *Rev Infect Dis* 1979;1:386–396.

43. Bagwell CE, Langham MR Jr, Mahaffey SM, Talbert JL, Shandling B. Pseudomembranous colitis following resection for Hirschsprung's disease. *J Pediatr Surg* 1992;27:1261–1264.

44. Pasic M, Jost R, Carrel T, Segesser LV, Turina M. Intracolonic vancomycin for pseudomembranous colitis. *N Engl J Med* 1993;329:583.

45. deLalla F, Privitera G, Rinaldi E, Ortisi G, Santoro D, Rizzardini G. Treatment of *Clostridium difficile* associated disease with teicoplanin. *Antimicrob Agents Chemother* 1989;33: 1125–1127.

46. Burbige BJ, Milligan FD. Pseudomembranous colitis: association with antibiotics and therapy with cholesytramine. *JAMA* 1975;231:1157–1158.

47. Sanchez C, Garcia-Restoy E, Garau J, et al. Ciprofloxacin and trimethoprim/sulfamethoxazole versus placebo in acute uncomplicated *Salmonella* enteritis: a double-blind trial. *J Infect Dis* 1993;168:1304–1307.

48. Rosenthal SL. Exacerbation of *Salmonella* enteritis due to ampicillin. *N Engl J Med* 1969;280:147–148.

49. Aserkoff B, Bennett JV. Effect of antibiotic therapy in acute salmonellosis on the fecal excretion of salmonellae. *N Engl J Med* 1969;281:636–640.

50. Nelson JD, Kusmiesz H, Jackson LH, Woodman E. Treatment of *Salmonella* gastroenteritis with ampicillin, amoxicillin, or placebo. *Pediatrics* 1980;65:1125–1130.

51. Neill MA, Opal SM, Heelan J, et al. Failure of ciprofloxacin to eradicate convalescent fecal excretion after acute salmonellosis: experience during an outbreak in health care workers. *Ann Intern Med* 1991;114:195–199.

52. Mourad AS, Metwally M, El Deen A, et al. Multiple-drug-resistant *Salmonella typhi*. *Clin Infect Dis* 1993;17:135–136.

53. Pillay N, Adams EB, Coombes DN. Comparative trial of amoxicillin and chloramphenicol in treatment of typhoid fever in adults. *Lancet* 1975;2:333–334.

54. Robertson RP, Wahab MFA, Raasch FO. Evaluation of chloramphenicol and ampicillin in *Salmonella* enteric fever. *N Engl J Med* 1968;278:171–176.

55. Munoz P, Diaz MD, Rodriguez-Creixems M, Cercenado E, Pelaez T, Bouza E. Antimicrobial resistance of *Salmonella* isolates in a Spanish hospital. *Antimicrob Agents Chemother* 1993;37: 1200–1202.

56. Maioroni E, Lopez EL, Morrow AL, et al. Multiply resistant nontyphoidal *Salmonella* gastroenteritis in children. *Pediatr Infect Dis J* 1993;12:139–144.

57. Ryan CA, Hargrett-Bean NT, Blake PA. *Salmonella typhi* infections in the United States, 1975–1984: increasing role of foreign travel. *J Infect Dis* 1989;11:1–8.

58. Bryan JP, Rocha H, Scheld WM. Problems in salmonellosis: rationale for clinical trials with newer β-lactam agents and quinolones. *Rev Infect Dis* 1986;8:189–207.

59. Soe GB, Overturf GD. Treatment of typhoid fever and other systemic salmonelloses with cefotaxime, ceftriaxone, cefoperazone, and other newer cephalosporins. *Rev Infect Dis* 1987;9: 719–736.

60. Moosa A, Rubidge CJ. Once daily ceftriaxone vs. chloramphenicol for treatment of typhoid fever in children. *Pediatr Infect Dis J* 1989;8:696–699.

61. Islam A, Butler T, Kabir I, Alam NH. Treatment of typhoid fever with ceftriazone for 5 days or chloramphenicol for 14 days: a randomized clinical trial. *Antimicrob Agents Chemother* 1993;37:1572–1575.

62. Dutta P, Rasaily R, Saha MR, et al. Ciprofloxacin for treatment of severe typhoid fever in children. *Antimicrob Agents Chemother* 1993;37:1197–1199.

63. Ramirez CA, Bran JL, Mejia CR, Garcia J. Open, prospective study of the clinical efficacy of ciprofloxacin. *Antimicrob Agents Chemother* 1985;28:128–132.

64. Limson BM, Littana RT. Ciprofloxacin vs. co-trimoxazole in *Salmonella* enteric fever. *Infection* 1989;17:105–106.

65. Kaye D, Marselis JG, Hook EW. Susceptibility of *Salmonella* species to four antibiotics. *N Engl J Med* 1963;269:1084–1086.

66. Cooles P. Adjuvant steroids and relapse of typhoid fever. *J Trop Med Hyg* 1986;89:229–231.

67. Hoffman SL, Punjabi NH, Kumala S, et al. Reduction of mortality in chloramphenicol-treated severe typhoid fever by high dose dexamethasone. *N Engl J Med* 1984;310:82–88.

68. Jacobs JL, Gold JWM, Murray HW, Roberts RB, Armstrong D. *Salmonella* infections in patients with the acquired immunodeficiency syndrome. *Ann Intern Med* 1985;102:186–188.

69. Galser JB, Morton-Kute L, Berger SR, et al. Recurrent *Salmonella typhimurium* bacteremia associated with the acquired immunodeficiency syndrome. *Ann Intern Med* 1985;102:189–193.

70. Smith PD, Macher AM, Bookman AM, et al. *Salmonella typhimurium* enteritis and bacteremia in the acquired immunodeficiency syndrome. *Ann Intern Med* 1985;102:207–209.

71. Pichler H, Divide G, Wolf D. Ciprofloxacin in the treatment of acute bacterial diarrhea: a double-blind study. *Eur J Clin Microbiol* 1986;5:241–243.

72. Pichler HET, Divide G, Stickler K, Wolf D. Clinical efficacy of ciprofloxacin compared with placebo in bacterial diarrhea. *Am J Med* 1987;82(Suppl 4a):329–332.

73. Ericsson CD, Johnson PC, DuPont HL, Morgan DR, Bitsura JAM, de la Cabada J. Ciprofloxacin or trimethoprim/sulfamethoxazole as initial therapy for travelers' diarrhea. *Ann Intern Med* 1987;106:216–220.

74. Connolly MJ, Snow MH, Ingham HR. Ciprofloxacin treatment of recurrent *Salmonella* septicaemia in a patient with acquired immune deficiency syndrome. *J Antimicrob Chemother* 1986; 18:647–648.

75. Wessalowski R, Thomas L, Kivit J, Voit T. Multiple brain abscesses caused by *Salmonella enteritis* in a neonate: successful treatment with ciprofloxacin. *Pediatr Infect Dis J* 1993;12: 683–688.

76. Magallanes M, Dijkstra J, Fierer J. Liposome-incorporated ciprofloxacin in treatment of murine salmonellosis. *Antimicrob Agents Chemother* 1993;37:2293–2297.

77. Johnson WD Jr, Hook EW, Lindsey E, Kaye D. Treatment of chronic typhoid carriers with ampicillin. *Antimicrob Agents Chemother* 1973;3:439–440.

78. Phillips WE. Treatment of chronic typhoid carriers with ampicillin. *JAMA* 1971;217:913.

79. Nolan CM, White PC Jr. Treatment of typhoid carriers with amoxicillin. *JAMA* 1978;239:2352–2354.

80. Gotuzzo E, Guerra JG, Benavente L, et al. Use of norfloxacin to treat chronic typhoid carriers. *J Infect Dis* 1988;157:1221–1225.

81. Ferreccio C, Morriss G, Valdivieso C, et al. Efficacy of ciprofloxacin in the treatment of chronic typhoid carriers. *J Infect Dis* 1988;157:1235–1239.

82. Piddock LJV, Griggs DJ, Hall MC, Jin YF. Ciprofloxacin resistance in clinical isolates of *Salmonella typhimurium* obtained from two patients. *Antimicrob Agents Chemother* 1993;37:662–666.

83. Haltalin KC, Nelson JD, Kusmiesz HT. Comparative efficacy of nalidixic acid and ampicillin for severe shigellosis. *Arch Dis Child* 1973;48:305–312.

84. Nelson JD, Kusmiesz H, Jackson LH. Comparison of trimethoprim/sulfamethoxazole and ampicillin therapy for shigellosis in ambulatory patients. *J Pediatr* 1976;89:491–493.

85. Nelson JD, Kusmiesz H, Jackson LH, Woodman E. Trimethoprim/sulfamethoxazole therapy for shigellosis. *JAMA* 1976;235:1239–1244.

86. Griffin PM, Tauxe R, Redd SC, Puhr ND, Hargrett-Bean N, Blake PA. Emergence of highly trimethoprim/sulfamethoxazole-resistant *Shigella* in a native American population: an epidemiologic study. *Am J Epidemiol* 1989;129:1042–1051.

87. Pickering LK, DuPont HL, Olarte J. Single dose tetracycline therapy for shigellosis in adults. *JAMA* 1978;239:853–854.

88. Cheever FS. Treatment of shigellosis with antibiotics. *Ann NY Acad Sci* 1952;55:1063–1069.

89. Weissman JB, Gangarosa EJ, DuPont HL, Nelson JD, Haltalin KC. Shigellosis: to treat or not to treat? *JAMA* 1974;229:1215–1216.

90. Barada FA Jr, Guerrant RL. Sulfamethoxazole/trimethoprim versus ampicillin in treatment of acute invasive diarrhea in adults. *Antimicrob Agents Chemother* 1980;17:961–964.

91. DuPont HL, Reves RR, Galindo E, Sullivan PS, Wood LV, Mendiola JG. Treatment of travelers' diarrhea with trimethoprim/sulfamethoxazole and with trimethoprim alone. *N Engl J Med* 1982;307:841–844.

92. Oberhelman RA, de la Cabada FJ, Garibay EV, Bitsura JAM, DuPont HL. Efficacy of trimethoprim/sulfamethoxazole in treatment of acute diarrhea in a Mexican pediatric population. *J Pediatr* 1987;110:960–965.

93. Murray BE. Problems and mechanisms of antimicrobial resistance. *Infect Dis Clin North Am* 1990;3:423–439.

94. Nelson JD, Haltalin KC. Amoxicillin less effective than ampicillin against *Shigella in vitro* and *in vivo:* relationship of efficacy to activity in serum. *J Infect Dis* 1974;129:S222–S227.

95. Lexomboon U, Mansuwan P, Duangmani C, et al. Clinical evaluation of co-trimoxazole and furazolidone in treatment of shigellosis in children. *Br Med J* 1972;3:23–26.

96. DuPont HL, Ericsson CD, Galindo E, et al. Furazolidone versus ampicillin in the treatment of travelers' diarrhea. *Antimicrob Agents Chemother* 1984;26:160–163.

97. Ashkenazi S, Amir J, Waisman Y, et al. A randomized, double-blind study comparing cefixime and trimethoprim/sulfamethoxazole in the treatment of childhood shigellosis. *J Pediatr* 1993;123:817–821.

98. Eidlitz-Marcus T, Cohen YH, Nussinovitch M, Elian I, Varsano I. Comparative efficacy of two- and five-day courses of ceftriaxone for treatment of severe shigellosis in children. *J Pediatr* 1993;123:822–824.

99. Varsano I, Eidlitz-Marcus T, Nussinovitch M, Elian I. Comparative efficacy of ceftriazone and ampicillin for treatment of severe shigellosis in children. *J Pediatr* 1991;118:627–632.

100. Kabir I, Butler T, Khanam A. Comparative efficacies of single intravenous doses of ceftriazone and ampicillin for shigellosis in a placebo-controlled trial. *Antimicrob Agents Chemother* 1986;29:645–648.

101. Ostrower VG. Comparison of cefaclor and ampicillin in the treatment of shigellosis. *Postgrad Med J* 1979;55:82–84.

102. Orenstein WA, Ross L, Overturf GD, et al. Antibiotic treatment of acute shigellosis: failure of cefamandole compared to trimethoprim/sulfamethoxazole and ampicillin. *Am J Med Sci* 1981;282:27–33.

103. Nelson JD, Haltalin KC. Comparative efficacy of cephalexin and ampicillin for shigellosis and other types of acute diarrhea in infants and children. *Antimicrob Agents Chemother* 1975;7:415–420.

104. Prado D, Lopez E, Liu H, et al. Ceftibuten and trimethoprim/sulfamethoxazole for treatment of *Shigella* and enteroinvasive *Escherichia coli* disease. *Pediatr Infect Dis J* 1992;11:644–647.

105. Rogerie F, Ott D, Vandepitte J, Verbist L, Lemmens P, Habiyaremye I. Comparison of norfloxacin and nalidixic acid for treatment of dysentery caused by *Shigella dysenteriae* type 1 in adults. *Antimicrob Agents Chemother* 1986;29:883–886.

106. DuPont HL, Corrado ML, Sabbaj J. Use of norfloxacin in the treatment of acute diarrheal disease. *Am J Med* 1987;82(Suppl 6b):79–83.

107. Bennish ML, Salam MA, Khan WA, Khan AM. Treatment of shigellosis: III. Comparison of one- or two-dose ciprofloxacin with standard 5-day therapy. *Ann Intern Med* 1992;117:727–734.

108. De Mol P, Mets T, Lagasse R, Vandepitte J, Mutwewingabo A, Butzler JP. Treatment of bacillary dysentery: a comparison between enoxacin and nalidixic acid. *J Antimicrob Chemother* 1987;19:695–698.

109. Gotuzzo E, Oberhelman RA, Maguiña C, et al. Comparison of single-dose treatment with norfloxacin with standard 5 day treatment with trimethoprim/sulfamethoxazole for acute shigellosis in adults. *Antimicrob Agents Chemother* 1989;33:1101–1104.

110. Horiuchi S, Inagaki Y, Yamamoto N, Okamura N, Imagawa Y, Nakaya R. Reduced susceptibilities of *Shigella sonnei* strains isolated from patients with dysentery to fluoroquinolones. *Antimicrob Agents Chemother* 1993;37:2486–2489.

111. Salam MA, Bennish ML. Therapy for shigellosis. I. Randomized, double-blind trial of nalidixic acid in childhood shigellosis. *J Pediatr* 1988;113:901–907.

112. Bennish ML, Salam MA, Hossain MA, et al. Antimicrobial resistance of *Shigella* isolates in Bangladesh, 1983–1990: increasing frequency of strains multiply resistant to ampicillin, trimethoprim/sulfamethoxazole, and nalidixic acid. *Clin Infect Dis* 1992;14:1055–1060.

113. Burstein S, Regalli G. *In vitro* susceptibility of *Shigella* strains isolated from stool cultures of dysenteric patients. *Scand J Gastroenterol* 1989;24(Suppl):34–38.

114. LaChance N, Gaudreau C, Lamothe F, Turgeon F. Susceptibilities of β-lactamase-positive and -negative strains of *Campylobacter coli* to β-lactam agents. *Antimicrob Agents Chemother* 1993;37:1174–1176.

115. Chow AW, Pattern V, Bednorz D. Susceptibility of *Campylobacter fetus* to twenty-two antimicrobial agents. *Antimicrob Agents Chemother* 1978;13:416–418.

116. Karmali MA, DeGrandis S, Fleming PC. Antimicrobial susceptibility of *Campylobacter jejuni* with special reference to resistance patterns of Canadian isolates. *Antimicrob Agents Chemother* 1981;19:593–597.

117. Taylor DE, Courvalin P. Mechanisms of antibiotic resistance in *Campylobacter* species. *Antimicrob Agents Chemother* 1988;32:1107–1112.

118. Salazar-Lindo E, Sack B, Chea-Woo E, et al. Early treatment with erythromycin of *Campylobacter jejuni*-associated dysentery in children. *J Pediatr* 1986;109:355–360.

119. Williams D, Schorling J, Barrett LJ, et al. Early treatment of *Campylobacter jejuni* enteritis. *Antimicrob Agents Chemother* 1989;33:248–250.

120. The choice of anti-bacterial drugs. *Med Lett* 1992;34:49–56.

121. Yan W, Taylor DE. Characterization of erythromycin resistance in *Campylobacter jejuni* and *Campylobacter coli*. *Antimicrob Agents Chemother* 1991;35:1989–1996.

122. Brunton WAT, Wilson AAM, Macrae RM. Erythromycin-resistant campylobacters. *Lancet* 1978;2:1385.

123. Taylor DE, Chang N, Garner RS, Sherburne R, Mueller L. Incidence of antibiotic resistance and characterization of

plasmids in *Campylobacter jejuni* strains isolated from clinical sources in Alberta, Canada. *Can J Microbiol* 1986;32:28–32.

124. Vanhoof R, Vanderlinden MP, Dierickx R, Lauwers S, Yourassowsky E, Butzler JP. Susceptibility of *Campylobacter fetus* subsp. *jejuni* to twenty-nine antimicrobial agents. *Antimicrob Agents Chemother* 1978;14:553–556.

125. Walder M, Forgren A. Erythromycin-resistant campylobacters. *Lancet* 1978;2:1201.

126. Wang WLL, Reller LB, Blaser MJ. Comparison of antimicrobial susceptibility patterns of *Campylobacter jejuni* and *Campylobacter coli*. *Antimicrob Agents Chemother* 1984;26:351–353.

127. Taylor DN, Blaser MJ, Echeverria PE, Pitarangsi C, Bodhidatta L, Wang WLL. Erythromycin-resistant *Campylobacter* infections in Thailand. *Antimicrob Agents Chemother* 1987;31:438–442.

128. Sagara H, Mochizuki A, Okamura N, Nakaya R. Antimicrobial resistance of *Campylobacter jejuni* and *Campylobacter coli* with special reference to plasmid profiles of Japanese clinical isolates. *Antimicrob Agents Chemother* 1987;31:713–719.

129. Taylor DE, Chang N. *In vitro* susceptibilities of *Campylobacter jejuni* and *Campylobacter coli* to azithromycin and erythromycin. *Antimicrob Agents Chemother* 1991;35:1917–1918.

130. Reina J, Alomar P. Fluoroquinolone-resistance in thermophilic *Campylobacter* spp. isolated from stools of Spanish patients. *Lancet* 1990;336:186.

131. Rautelin H, Renkonen O-V, Kosunen TU. Emergence of fluoroquinolone resistance in *Campylobacter jejuni* and *Campylobacter coli* in subjects from Finland. *Antimicrob Agents Chemother* 1991;35:2065–2069.

132. Endtz HP, Mouton RP, van der Reyden T, Ruijs GJ, Biever M, van Klingeren B. Fluoroquinolone resistance in *Campylobacter* spp isolated from human stools and poultry products. *Lancet* 1990;335:787.

133. Sanchez R, Fernández-Baca V, Diaz MD, Muñoz P, Rodriguez-Créixems M, Bouza E. Evolution of susceptibilities of *Campylobacter* spp. to quinolones and macrolides. *Antimicrob Agents Chemother* 1994;38:1879–1882.

134. Navarro F, Miro E, Fuentes I, Mirelis B. *Campylobacter* species: identification and resistance to quinolones. *Clin Infect Dis* 1993;17:815–816.

135. Segreti J, Gootz TD, Goodman LJ, et al. High-level quinolone resistance in clinical isolates of *Campylobacter jejuni*. *J Infect Dis* 1992;165:667–670.

136. Ostroff SM, Kobayashi JM, Lewis JH. Infections with *Escherichia coli* O157:H7 in Washington State. *JAMA* 1989;262:355–359.

137. Riley LW, Remis RS, Helgerson SD, et al. Hemorrhagic colitis associated with a rare *Escherichia coli* serotype. *N Engl J Med* 1983;308:681–685.

138. Ryan C, Tauxe R, Hosek G, et al. *Escherichia coli* O157:H7 diarrhea in a nursing home: clinical, epidemiological, and pathological findings. *J Infect Dis* 1986;154:631–637.

139. Karch H. Growth of *Escherichia coli* in the presence of trimethoprim/sulfamethoxazole facilitates detection of Shiga-like toxin producing strains by colony blot assay. *FEMS Microbiol Lett* 1986;35:141–145.

140. Walterspiel JN, Ashkenazi S, Morrow AL, Cleary TG. Effect of subinhibitory concentrations of antibiotics on the release of Shiga-like toxin I. *Infection* 1992;20:25–29.

141. Pavia AT, Nichols CR, Green DP, et al. Hemolytic-uremic syndrome during an outbreak of *Escherichia coli* O157:H7 infections in institutions for mentally retarded persons: clinical and epidemiologic observations. *J Pediatr* 1990;116:544–551.

142. Carter AO, Borczyk AA, Carlson JAK, et al. A severe outbreak of *Escherichia coli* O157:H7-associated hemorrhagic colitis in a nursing home. *N Engl J Med* 1987;317:1496–1500.

143. Butler T, Islam MR, Azad MAK, Jones PK. Risk factors for development of hemolytic uremic syndrome during shigellosis. *J Pediatr* 1987;110:894–897.

144. Prouix F, Turgeon JP, Delage G, Lafleur L, Chicoine L. Randomized, controlled trial of antibiotic therapy for *Escherichia coli* O157:H7 enteritis. *J Pediatr* 1992;121:299–303.

145. Blake PA, Allegra DT, Snyder JD, et al. Cholera—a possible endemic focus in the United States. *N Engl J Med* 1980;302:305–309.

146. Kobari K, Uylangco C, Vasco J, Takahira Y, Shimizu N. Observations on cholera treated orally and intravenously with antibiotics: with particular reference to the number of vibrios excreted in the stool. *Bull World Health Organ* 1967;37:751–762.

147. Lindenbaum J, Greenough WB III, Islam MR. Antibiotic therapy of cholera. *Bull World Health Organ* 1967;36:871–883.

148. Wallace CK, Anderson PN, Brown TC, et al. Optimal antibiotic therapy in cholera. *Bull World Health Organ* 1968;39:239–245.

149. Swerdlow DL, Ries AA. Cholera in the Americas: guidelines for the clinician. *JAMA* 1992;267:1495–1499.

150. Rahaman MM, Majid MA, Alam AKM, Islam R. Effects of doxycycline in actively purging cholera patients. A double-blind clinical trial. *Antimicrob Agents Chemother* 1976;10:610–612.

151. Sack DA, Islam S, Rabbani H, Islam A. Single-dose doxycycline for cholera. *Antimicrob Agents Chemother* 1978;14:462–464.

152. Cholera Working Group. Large epidemic of cholera-like disease in Bangladesh caused by *Vibrio cholerae* O139 synonym Bengal. *Lancet* 1993;342:387–390.

153. Marks MI, Pai CH, Lafleur L, Lackman L, Hammerberg O. *Yersinia enterocolitica* gastroenteritis: a prospective study of clinical bacteriologic and epidemiologic features. *J Pediatr* 1980;96:26–31.

154. Kohl S. *Yersinia enterocolitica* infection. *Pediatr Clin North Am* 1979;26:433–443.

155. Hoogkamp-Korstanje JAA. Antibiotics in *Yersinia enterocolitica* infections. *J Antimicrob Chemother* 1987;20:123–131.

156. Gayraud M, Scavizzi MR, Mollaret HH, Guillevin L, Hornstein MJ. Antibiotic treatment of *Yersinia enterocolitica* septicemia: a retrospective review of 43 cases. *Clin Infect Dis* 1993;17:405–410.

157. Koehler JM, Ashdown LR. *In vitro* susceptibilities of tropical strains of *Aeromonas* species from Queensland, Australia, to 22 antimicrobial agents. *Antimicrob Agents Chemother* 1993;37:905–907.

158. Parras F, Diaz MD, Reina J, Moreno S, Guerrero C. Meningitis due to *Aeromonas* species: case report and review. *Clin Infect Dis* 1993;17:1058–1060.

159. Kain KC, Kelly MT. Clinical features, epidemiology, and treatment of *Plesiomonas shigelloides* diarrhea. *J Clin Microbiol* 1989;27:998–1001.

160. Castro KG, Ward JW, Slutsker L, et al. 1993 revised classification system for HIV infection and expanded surveillance case definition for AIDS among adolescents and adults. *Clin Infect Dis* 1993;17:802–810.

161. Drugs for parasitic infections. *Med Lett* 1993;35:111–122.

162. Pickering LK, Engelkirk PG. *Giardia lamblia*. *Pediatr Clin North Am* 1988;35:565–577.

163. Sokol RJ, Lichtenstein PK, Farrell MK. Quinacrine hydrochloride-induced yellow discoloration of the skin in children. *Pediatrics* 1982;69:232–233.

164. Craft JC, Murphy T, Nelson JD. Furazolidone and quinacrine: comparative study of therapy for giardiasis in children. *Am J Dis Child* 1981;135:164–166.

165. Pilla AM, Rybak MJ, Chandrasekar PH. Spiramycin in the treatment of cryptosporidiosis. *Pharmacotherapy* 1987;7:188–190.

166. Armitage K, Flanigan T, Carey J, et al. Treatment of cryptosporidiosis with paromomycin. *Arch Intern Med* 1992;152:2497–2499.

167. Fichtenbaum CJ, Ritchie DJ, Powderly WG. Use of paromomycin for treatment of cryptosporidiosis in patients with AIDS. *Clin Infect Dis* 1993;16:298–300.

168. Wallace MR, Nguyen M-T, Newton JA Jr. Use of paromomycin for the treatment of cryptosporidiosis in patients with AIDS. *Clin Infect Dis* 1993;17:1070–1071.

169. Marshall RJ, Flanigan TP. Paromomycin inhibits *Cryptosporidium* infection of a human enterocyte cell line. *J Infect Dis* 1992;165:772–774.

170. Rehg JE. Activity of azithromycin against cryptosporidia in immunosuppressed rats. *J Infect Dis* 1991;163:1293–1296.

171. Vargas SL, Shenep JL, Flynn PM, Pui C-H, Santana VM, Hughes WT. Azithromycin for treatment of severe *Cryptosporidium* diarrhea in two children with cancer. *J Pediatr* 1993;123: 154–156.

172. Perryman LE, Riggs MW, Mason PH, Fayer R. Kinetics of *Cryptosporidium parvum* sporozoite neutralization by monoclonal antibodies, immune bovine serum, and immune bovine colostrum. *Infect Immun* 1990;58:257–259.

173. Borowitz SM, Saulsbury FT. Treatment of chronic cryptosporidial infection with orally administered human serum immune globulin. *J Pediatr* 1991;119:593–595.

174. Bjorneby JM, Hunsaker BD, Riggs MW, Perryman LE. Monoclonal antibody immunotherapy in nude mice persistently infected with *Cryptosporidium parvum*. *Infect Immun* 1991;59: 1172–1176.

175. Louie E, Borkowsky W, Klesius PH, et al. Treatment of cryptosporidiosis with oral bovine transfer factor. *J Clin Immunol Pathol* 1987;44:329–334.

176. Tzipori S, Robertson D, Chapman C. Remission of diarrhea due to cryptosporidiosis in an immunodeficient child treated with hyperimmune bovine colostrum. *Br Med J* 1986;293:1276.

177. Perryman LE, Kegerreis KA, Mason PH. Effect of orally administered monoclonal antibody on persistent *Cryptosporidium parvum* infection in scid mice. *Infect Immun* 1993;61: 4906–4908.

178. Soudah HC, Hasler WL, Owyang C. Effect of octreotide on intestinal motility and bacterial overgrowth in scleroderma. *N Engl J Med* 1991;325:1461–1467.

179. Cello JP, Grendell JH, Basuk P, et al. Effect of octreotide on refractory AIDS-associated diarrhea: a prospective multicenter clinical trial. *Ann Intern Med* 1991;115:705–710.

180. Pape JW, Verdier R-I, Johnson WD Jr. Treatment and prophylaxis of *Isospora belli* infection in patients with the acquired immunodeficiency syndrome. *N Engl J Med* 1989;320: 1044–1047.

181. DeHovitz JA, Page JW, Boney M, Johnson WD. Clinical manifestations and therapy of *Isospora belli* infection in patients with the acquired immunodeficiency syndrome. *N Engl J Med* 1986;315:87–90.

182. Weiss LM, Perlman DC, Sherman J, Tanowitz H, Wittner M. *Isospora belli* infection: treatment with pyrimethamine. *Ann Intern Med* 1988;109:474–475.

183. Lessnau KD, Can S, Talavera W. Disseminated *Strongyloides stercoralis* in human immunodeficiency virus-infected patients: treatment failure and a review of the literature. *Chest* 1993;104: 119–122.

184. Lyagoubi M, Datry A, Mayorga R, et al. Chronic persistent strongyloidiasis cured by ivermectin. *Trans R Soc Trop Med Hyg* 1992;86:541.

185. Naguira C, Jiminez G, Guerra JG, et al. Ivermectin for human strongyloidiasis and other intestinal helminths. *Am J Trop Med Hyg* 1989;40:304–309.

186. Rijpstra AC, Canning EU, Van-Ketel RJ, Ettinck-Schattenkerk JK, Laarman JJ. Use of light microscopy to diagnose small intestinal microsporidiosis in patients with AIDS. *J Infect Dis* 1988;157:827–831.

187. Dieterich DT, Lew EA, Kotler DP, Poles MA, Orenstein JM. Treatment with albendazole for intestinal disease due to *Enterocytozoon bieneusi* in patients with AIDS. *J Infect Dis* 1994; 169:178–183.

188. Molina JM, Sarfati C, Beauvais B, et al. Intestinal microsporidiosis in human immunodeficiency virus-infected patients with chronic unexplained diarrhea: prevalence and clinical biologic features. *J Infect Dis* 1993;167:217–221.

189. Cali A, Kotler DP, Orenstein JM. *Septata intestinalis* n.g., n.sp., an intestinal microsporidian associated with chronic diarrhea and dissemination in AIDS patients. *J Eukaryot Microbiol* 1993;40:101–112.

190. Blanshard C, Ellis DS, Tovey DG, Dowell S, Gazzard BG. Treatment of intestinal microsporidiosis with albendazole in patients with AIDS. *AIDS* 1992;6:311–313.

191. Grossman I, Weiss LM, Simon D, Tanowitz HB, Wittner M. *Blastomycosis hominis* in hospital employees. *Am J Gastroenterol* 1992;87:729–732.

192. Boreham PF, Stenzel D. *Blastocystis* in humans and animals: morphology, biology, and epizootiology. *Adv Parasitol* 1993; 32:1–70.

193. Connor BA, Shlim DR, Scholes JV, Rayburn JL, Reidy J, Rajaj R. Pathologic changes in the small bowel in nine patients with diarrhea associated with a coccidia-like body. *Ann Intern Med* 1993;119:377–382.

194. Hale D, Aldeen W, Carroll K. Diarrhea associated with cyanobacterialike bodies in an immunocompetent host. *JAMA* 1994; 271:144–145.

195. Madico G, Gilman RH, Miranda E, Cabrera L, Sterling CR. Treatment of *Cyclospora* infections with co-trimoxazole. *Lancet* 1993;342:122–123.

196. Yolken R, Kinney J, Wilde J, Willoughby R, Eiden J. Immunoglobulins and other modalities for the prevention and treatment of enteric viral infections. *J Clin Immunol* 1990;10:80S–87S.

197. Losonsky GA, Johnson JP, Winkelstein JA, Yolken RH. Oral administration of human serum immunoglobulin in immunodeficient patients with viral gastroenteritis. *J Clin Invest* 1985;76: 2362–2367.

Infections of the Gastrointestinal Tract,
edited by M. J. Blaser, P. D. Smith, J. I. Ravdin,
H. B. Greenberg, and R. L. Guerrant
Raven Press, Ltd., New York © 1995.

CHAPTER 90

Oral Therapy for Diarrhea

John D. Snyder

Diarrhea continues to be a major problem in developing and developed countries. The greatest impact from diarrhea is in developing countries where approximately 1.5 billion diarrheal episodes and 4 million deaths occur each year in children less than 5 years old (1). The impact of diarrheal illness is not so overwhelming in the United States, but it is still a major problem. Outpatient visits for diarrhea account for as many as 20% of acute care visits by young children at large urban hospitals (2) and the incidence of hospital admissions due to diarrhea was reported to be 7.9 per 1000 infants in 1984 (3). Diarrhea accounts for approximately 400 infant deaths in the United States each year, which is about 10% of the potentially preventable deaths in this age group (4). The magnitude of the problem in developing countries approximates that seen in the United States at the turn of the 20th century (5). A substantial decrease in the incidence of diarrhea in developing countries will likely not occur until improvements in sanitation, hygiene, and the general standard of living occur.

The critical element of effective therapy for acute diarrhea is the replacement of fluid in electrolyte losses. For over 50 years intravenous (iv) therapy has been a successful method of administration of the fluid and electrolytes lost during diarrhea. Efforts to find a less expensive and more easily administered therapy have led to the development of effective oral therapy for acute diarrhea (6). This therapy, which has evolved over the past 25 years to include oral rehydration therapy (ORT) of fluid and electrolytes and appropriate early feeding, will be the major focus of this chapter.

HISTORY OF ORAL THERAPY

ORT

The first studies of the optimal method to replace fluid and electrolyte losses from diarrhea began about 150 years

ago (7). Despite these initial efforts, cholera epidemics continued to be associated with high mortality rates until investigators eventually documented that stool losses of water, sodium, potassium, chloride, and base must be restored to ensure the most effective rehydration (8). Early attempts at parenteral administration of therapy were largely failures because of inadequate aseptic technique, primitive equipment, and limited understanding of mechanisms of maintaining intravascular volume (9). Approximately 50 years ago, iv therapy became the first successful method of administration of fluid and electrolytes and was widely accepted as the standard for rehydration therapy (10). The success of iv therapy increased with the realization of the importance of correcting acidosis with administration of base and subsequently with the appreciation of the importance of replacing potassium losses (11). However, several important limitations of iv therapy stimulated the search for simpler, less expensive methods to rehydrate patients with diarrhea and dehydration. These limitations, which are especially important in developing countries where the burden of diarrhea is greatest, include the expenses for sterile solutions, needles, and tubing; the need for administration by skilled health workers; and the requirement for specialized facilities (6).

The initial efforts to develop effective orally administered fluid and electrolyte solutions were begun by Harrison at Johns Hopkins and Darrow at Yale in the early 1950s (12). Harrison and his colleagues included sodium (60 mmol/L), potassium (20 mmol/L), chloride (54 mmol/L), and lactate (33 mmol/L) and added 3.3 g/L of glucose for protein-sparing purposes (13). The first commercial oral glucose–electrolyte solution (Lytren) was introduced shortly thereafter, but this solution had a much higher carbohydrate content and osmolality than Harrison's solution. An important setback to the development of oral therapy for diarrhea then occurred when an outbreak of hypernatremic dehydration coincided with the introduction of hyperosmolar Lytren (14). Several other factors contributed in large part to this epidemic including the incorrect mixing of home-prepared sugar and salt preparations, inappropriate administration of the early forms of

J. D. Snyder: GI/Nutrition Division, Department of Pediatrics, University of California Medical Center, San Francisco, California 94143.

iv solutions, and the recommended use of boiled skim milk, a very hypertonic solution (14). At the time, the epidemic was incorrectly attributed to the sodium content of the solutions rather than to their excessive carbohydrate concentrations and osmolality (14). These misconceptions influenced a generation of pediatricians and slowed the acceptance of the physiologically based oral rehydration solutions that followed.

Physiologic Principles

The discovery of the coupled transport of sodium and glucose or other small organic molecules in the early 1960s is the foundation on which effective ORT was developed (15). Coupled transport causes enhanced absorption of salt and water from the intestinal lumen across the epithelium and is effective even during intestinal inflammation caused by enteritis (8,15).

A large number of controlled clinical trials in adults and children began just after the discovery of coupled transport and have demonstrated the safety and efficacy of oral rehydration solutions for all types of diarrhea (1,6,16–19). Several formulations have been studied and used but by far the most widely and successfully used of these ORT solutions has been the World Health Organization (WHO)/UNICEF oral rehydration salts. This solution contains glucose (20 g/L) and three salts: sodium chloride (3.5 g/L), potassium chloride (1.5 g/L), and either trisodium citrate (2.9 g/L) or sodium bicarbonate (2.5 g/L) (Table 1). For maximum cotransport of electrolytes, glucose, and water, the ratio of carbohydrate to sodium should not exceed 2:1, because excess carbohydrate can produce osmotic retention of water in the intestine (20). Clinical trials of ORT in health facilities and communities have consistently demonstrated its ability to successfully rehydrate 90% or more of patients with dehydration from all causes of acute diarrhea (1), to reduce significantly case/fatality ratios (1,21), to be substantially less expensive than iv therapy (22), and to be administered safely and effectively by family members, even with little or no formal education (21). ORT solutions are usually packaged in aluminum foil packets, which give it a long shelf-life even in hot, humid conditions.

Feeding

Interest in the role of feeding during diarrhea has been present for many years. Some of the earliest studies of

the potential feeding component of oral therapy were carried out by Chung and Viscerova in the late 1940s (23,24). Using careful nutrient balance experiments, they demonstrated that effective intestinal absorption occurs during diarrhea and that absorption is roughly proportional to intake (23,24). However, these observations had little effect on the traditional practice of withholding feedings until the diarrhea stopped (25). This practice was recommended primarily because of the concern for the development of malabsorption, which could worsen the diarrhea (25).

Only in the past decade have investigators begun to reevaluate the findings of Chung and Viscerova and to explore the possibility of using feeding as a central component of oral therapy. The inclusion of effective feeding is of obvious importance, especially in developing countries where diarrhea and malnutrition are so closely linked (1,6).

Physiologic Principles

Studies of the effect of diarrhea on nutrient uptake have demonstrated that the luminal and mucosal phases of digestion and absorption can be preserved to a substantial degree (26). The luminal phase is fairly well preserved, especially with regard to carbohydrate and protein digestion and absorption. This is because pancreatic enzymes play such a major role in luminal digestion and pancreatic function appears to be normal or nearly normal during diarrhea (27,28). In addition, salivary and breast milk amylase, which are important in carbohydrate digestion, also appear to be relatively unaffected by diarrhea (26). Fat digestion, which is a complex process involving multiple factors including bile salts, fatty acid binding protein, and apolipoprotein, as well as pancreatic lipase, is affected the most of the macronutrients in the luminal phase. The coefficient of absorption of fat is about 50% to 60% in most studies (23,29).

The negative effect of diarrhea is greater on the mucosal phase of digestion and absorption (27,30). This is especially true when diarrhea is associated with an altered absorptive surface due to damaged enterocytes.

Carbohydrate digestion can be affected because of the decreased levels of brush border disaccharidases. Lactase levels are decreased most during diarrhea, followed by sucrase, while the effect is least on glucoamylase (31). The relative preservation of glucoamylase levels provides

TABLE 1. *Composition of representative glucose electrolyte solution (GES)*

GES	Concentration (mmol/L)					
	CHO	Na	CHO:Na	K	Base	Osmolality
Naturalyte (Unlimited Beverages)	140	45	3.1	20	48	265
Pediatric Electrolyte (NutraMax)	140	45	3.1	20	30	250
Pedialyte (Ross)	140	45	3.1	20	30	250
Infalyte (Mead Johnson)	70	50	1.4	25	30	200
Rehydralyte (Ross)	140	75	1.9	20	30	310
WHO/UNICEF ORS	111	90	1.2	20	30	310

CHO, carbohydrate; ORS, oral rehydration salts.

an important reason why starches have proved to be so successful in ORT and appropriate early feeding (32).

Although lactase enzyme levels are often decreased in diarrhea, clinically important lactose intolerance is uncommon, indicating that substantial quantities of lactose can be digested (33,34). The effect of diarrhea on monosaccharide absorption depends on the extent of injury, but even in severe cases, this mechanism is often very effective (35). The coefficient of absorption for carbohydrate using a variety of mixed diets is about 85% to 90% during diarrhea (23,29).

The brush border peptidase enzymes are also decreased during diarrhea, especially when extensive mucosal damage occurs (27). The combined effect of diarrhea on luminal and mucosal digestion results in a coefficient of absorption of protein similar to that for fat—about 60% (23,29).

The impact of diarrhea on the mucosal phase of fat digestion also depends on the amount of mucosal damage (26). When severe injury has occurred, fewer enterocytes are available for triglyceride resynthesis and chylomicron formation.

CURRENT PRACTICES OF OPTIMAL ORAL THERAPY: ORT AND APPROPRIATE EARLY FEEDING

ORT

Based on the data from the large number of controlled clinical trials conducted in the first decade after the introduction of glucose–electrolyte ORT, the WHO and UNICEF incorporated ORT as the cornerstone of their child survival efforts beginning in 1978 (36). Further trials confirming the safety and efficacy of ORT, most often using the WHO/UNICEF formulation, have now been carried out in nearly every country in the world (1). In the United States, several commercial solutions similar to the WHO/UNICEF solution are widely available (Table 1). In controlled trials in this country, solutions with sodium concentrations of 50 to 90 mEq/L have proved to be effective in the treatment of well-nourished children with mild to severe dehydration (22,37–39).

Glucose–electrolyte solutions formulated on physiologic principles must be distinguished from other popular liquids, which have been used inappropriately to treat diarrhea (Table 2). Unfortunately, the use of these nonphysiologic solutions is still widespread (40).

Enhanced ORT

Although ORT has been hailed as "potentially the most important medical advance this century" (41) and is credited with saving an estimated one million lives each year (1), it has limitations. Perhaps the most important is that, although it is extremely effective at replacing fluid and electrolyte losses, glucose–electrolyte ORT has no beneficial effect on the volume or duration of diarrhea.

To improve the absorption of ORT, additional cotransport molecules must be added without substantially adding to the osmotic load of the solution (32). Initially, amino acids were added to ORT as a means of increasing the number of cotransport molecules (32). However, results in children have shown little or no benefit over standard ORT, and important limitations such as increased urine output and azotemia have been reported (42,43).

Polymers of glucose and amino acids were promising because of their effective cotransport properties and lower osmolality (44) but in their purified form are very expensive. However, naturally occurring foods, especially grains, contain polymers of starch and simple proteins that can provide glucose, amino acids, and oligopeptides to the transporting villi without exacting an osmotic penalty (32). The most success with enhanced ORT formulations has been with cereal-based solutions in less developed countries (6). By far the most experience has been with rice-based solutions (32,45,46), but successful use of maize, wheat, and sorghum also has been reported (47,48). Cereal-based solutions can reduce stool volume by more than 30% in children with toxigenic diarrhea and by close to 20% in those with nontoxigenic diarrhea when compared to standard WHO oral rehydration salts (49). These solutions can easily be made at home, and the use of starch greatly reduces the chance of producing an osmotic diarrhea. However, they have several potential disadvantages in developing countries. They require fuel and time to prepare, and they can become contaminated if kept unrefrigerated.

Further development of cereal-based ORT may not occur because of the success of early, aggressive nutritional therapy. Initial studies have indicated that glucose–electrolyte ORT plus early appropriate feeding is as effective as the use of cereal-based ORT and provides obvious nutritional advantages (50,51).

Hypo-osmolar solutions using refined glucose polymers also have been evaluated (e.g., Infalyte, Table 1). They are more costly to produce than the cereal-based solutions and have no greater impact on stool volume and duration

TABLE 2. *Composition of representative clear liquids*

| Liquid | Concentration (mmol/L) | | | | | |
	CHO	Na	CHO:Na	K	Base	Osmolality
Cola	700 (fructose, glucose)	2	350	0	13	750
Apple juice	690 (fructose, glucose, sucrose)	3	230	32	0	730
Chicken broth	0	250	—	8	0	500
Gatorade	255 (sucrose, glucose)	20	13	3	3	330

CHO, carbohydrate.

of diarrhea compared to standard glucose–electrolyte ORT (52).

Indications for Use

The WHO and American Academy of Pediatrics (AAP) recommend the use of ORT to treat all degrees of dehydration and to provide maintenance fluid and electrolytes for all cases of diarrhea and dehydration (1,20). In cases of severe dehydration (10% or greater fluid deficit, shock or near shock) iv (or intraosseous) rehydration should be started immediately if available. In patients who can tolerate enteral solutions, ORT can be used to treat severe dehydration if parenteral therapy is not available (1,33). ORT is effective in treating all types of diarrhea including those caused by invasive, adherent, or toxin-producing organisms (6,33).

Contraindications to Use

ORT can be used for nearly all cases of diarrhea but several important limitations to its use must be remembered. ORT should not be used in unconscious persons or those with ileus (33). Monosaccharide malabsorption occurs in only about 1% of acute diarrhea cases but, when present, is a contraindication to the use of ORT (33). Patients suspected of glucose malabsorption, based on poor response to ORT, should be treated with iv therapy.

ORT can be used effectively in cases of dysentery to replace fluid and electrolyte losses but antimicrobial therapy should also be used (53).

Vomiting commonly accompanies diarrhea and more than 90% of patients with diarrhea and vomiting can be treated with ORT if it is given frequently in small volumes (33). Severe, intractable vomiting occurs rarely but may require parenteral therapy.

Efforts to Increase Utilization

ORT is estimated to be used in about 25% to 30% of the patients who could benefit from its use in the United States and in developing countries (1,12). The reasons for this relative underutilization include the logistic and economic difficulties in producing and supplying prepackaged ORT to families in the developing world, the need for labor-intensive administration, and the difficulty in overcoming the reliance on the long-time successful practice of iv therapy (12).

The substantial impact of ORT on the morbidity and mortality of diarrhea may increase with the growing awareness of the effectiveness of ORT and continued success of the promotional activities of organizations like the WHO and UNICEF (1,6). The further evolution of oral therapy to include more effective treatment, which can reduce stool volume and diarrhea duration, also will likely have a major impact on its use. As the experience with the use of locally available, culturally acceptable ingredients to make effective oral therapy increases, further barriers to its use may fall.

Applications Beyond Diarrhea

In addition to diarrhea, ORT can be used in other conditions associated with fluid and electrolyte losses, such as burns (12). Since the gastrointestinal tract is usually intact in burn patients, ORT can have an important role, especially in patients in whom iv access is difficult. The use of the oral rather than the iv route helps to reduce the risk of infection in these patients who have a skin barrier.

The efforts to improve oral therapy to include effective feeding regimens may be very beneficial in diseases with an important component of malnutrition. For example, these regimens may prove to be helpful in acquired immunodeficiency syndrome (AIDS) patients who often have some element of altered intestinal function and malnutrition (54).

Appropriate Early Feeding

The recommendation to include feeding along with ORT as an important component of oral therapy for diarrhea is a more recent development in the evolution of optimal therapy. The common practice previously used in this and many countries was to withhold feedings during diarrhea; however, the validity of this practice has been rigorously questioned (25). The rationale for withholding food during diarrhea was based primarily on the concern for malabsorption, which can occur because of an altered intestinal mucosa, decreased brush border enzymes, and more rapid intestinal transit time (25). The theoretical risk of increased macromolecular uptake across the damaged mucosa leading to intestinal allergy has been postulated but has never been shown to be of practical importance in diarrhea (55).

An increasing series of studies indicates that feeding can have a direct beneficial effect on the outcome of acute diarrhea (56–68). The most important benefit of feeding is to offer nutritional rehabilitation to the patient with diarrhea, especially in developing countries. In addition, intestinal nutrient uptake has long been known to be an important factor involved in repair following injury (69,70). Factors that influence the success of feeding include the age of the child, the etiology of the diarrhea, the severity of the stooling, and, especially, the composition and complexity of the diet (25).

As discussed earlier, some element of malabsorption is often associated with diarrhea, but it is rarely complete, and substantial percentages of dietary carbohydrate, fats, and protein are absorbed (23,29). A variety of early feeding regimens have been studied including breast milk (56–59), dilute or full-strength animal milk or animal milk formulas (56,57,59,60), dilute and full-strength lactose-free formulas (57,62,63), and staple food diets with milk (66–69). These studies have demonstrated that an unrestricted diet does not affect the course or symptoms in children with mild diarrhea (59–61). In fact, appropriate early feeding can help reduce stool output (29,56,62,66,68) and duration of diarrhea (57,62,64,65,68,69), compared to the use of ORT or iv therapy alone. Perhaps most importantly, early feeding can also result in improved initial nutritional outcome (64,65).

Cereal-based diets appear to be especially effective during diarrhea (68–70), but if cereals or legumes are the sole source of protein, an incomplete amino acid profile, deficient in essential amino acids, is likely to result (71). Also, a greater proportion of protein may be required in cereal- or legume-based diets because of their digestibility (71). A potential solution to this problem is to include milk, a more complete protein source, with cereals to improve the amino acid profile and digestibility.

The amount of lactose that can be tolerated by children with diarrhea is still subject to controversy, but several principles have become clear (34). Breast-fed infants who receive a higher concentration of lactose than children receiving cow's milk or cow's milk formula can be fed safely through diarrhea (25). Full-strength animal milk or animal milk formula is usually well tolerated by children who have mild, self-limited diarrhea, which is very common in the United States (59). A recent meta-analysis on the use of lactose in children with acute diarrhea found that most can safely tolerate full-strength animal milk (34). As long as children are carefully monitored to identify the few who will develop signs of intolerance (increased stool volume and frequency, bloating, and cramps), full-strength milk should be used as part of appropriate early feeding (34).

Combining milk with staple foods like cereals is well tolerated by children who normally take solid foods (60,62,66–69). These mixed diets are better tolerated than milk alone (69) and are thought to be successful in part because of the smaller total lactose load and because solid foods help delay gastric emptying and thus slow transit time (72).

Recent studies of diets such as chicken and cereal (29), cereal and milk (68), and cereal and legumes (69) have confirmed that a substantial proportion of nutrients can be absorbed from mixed diets by young children and infants with acute diarrhea. These studies indicate that diets of naturally occurring, culturally acceptable, inexpensive foods can be effective in diarrhea. The implications of these findings are significant from a health policy standpoint because they provide hope that the important ingredients of successful feeding therapy are already present, even in developing countries.

THERAPEUTIC GUIDELINES

The specific guidelines for oral therapy of children with diarrhea are related to the degree of dehydration. The clinical assessment of dehydration is critical to effective oral therapy.

Evaluation

A careful history is essential to guiding and focusing the evaluation process. The history should seek information of an associated illness including meningitis, sepsis, pneumonia, otitis media, or urinary tract infection, which can cause similar symptoms. The history also should evaluate possible risk factors for a causative agent such as travel to lesser developed countries, use of untreated water, exposure to animals, involvement in a day care setting, or recent use of antibiotics. The dietary history also is important, as food allergies and excessive intake of juice can cause diarrhea in infants and young children (73).

The physical examination must include an accurate body weight as part of the assessment of hydration. The assessment of hydration also includes evaluation of the skin turgor, moisture of the mucous membranes, firmness of the orbits, mental status, and presence or absence of postural changes in the heart rate or blood pressure (Table 3). The fullness of the anterior fontanelle should also be assessed in young infants. Recent studies have indicated that tenting of the skin, rapid and deep breathing (evidence of acidosis), and delayed capillary refill time can be especially helpful in determining the severity of dehydration (74,75). The physical examination also can be helpful in detecting electrolyte abnormalities. Altered sensorium should raise the possibility of hypernatremia and abnormal neuromuscular states can be seen with hypokalemia. Hyperkalemia can cause cardiac arrhythmias. In general, the other portions of the physical examination are not helpful in evaluating the severity or etiology of the diarrheal illness.

The laboratory evaluation is only rarely required in the immunocompetent child with acute diarrhea. Serum chemistries are usually not helpful, although electrolytes should be obtained when clinical signs and symptoms of sodium or potassium abnormalities are present (33). A microscopic stool evaluation using either a Wright's stain or Gram stain identifies the presence of red or white blood cells in the stool. Stool cultures have a very low yield of enteric pathogens when red and white blood cells are not present (76).

Therapeutic Recommendations

No Detectable Dehydration

ORT is recommended to replace the ongoing stool and emesis losses (20,33). Stool losses are replaced with 10 mL/kg for each stool and emesis losses are replaced using ½-cup increments (33). However, children with no dehydration are the least likely to take ORT, in part because of the slightly salty taste of the solutions. Fortunately, if the stool output remains modest, ORT may not be required. If no dehydration develops, which is the case in the great majority of diarrhea cases in the United States, continued age-appropriate feeding is the only therapy required. Nonweaned infants should receive breast milk or continued use of the regular formula. The formula does not require dilution if the diarrhea remains mild. If a diluted formula is used, the concentration should be increased rapidly if the diarrhea does not worsen. Weaned infants and children should have their regular diet contin-

TABLE 3. *Assessment of dehydration*

Evaluators	Mild (<5%)	Moderate (5–9%)	Severe (≤10%)
Blood pressure	Normal	↓ ↓	↓ ↓ ↓
Heart rate	Normal	Normal to increased	Tachycardia
Skin	Normal	Decreased turgor	Decreased turgor
Fontanelle	Normal	Sunken	Sunken
Mucous membranes	Slightly dry	Dry	Dry
Eyes	Normal	Sunken orbits	Sunken orbits
Extremities	Perfused	Delayed capillary refill	Cool, mottled
Mental status	Normal	Lethargy	Lethargy, coma
Urine output	Slightly decreased	Decreased	Absent
Thirst	↑	↑ ↑	↑ ↑ ↑

Adapted from ref. 33.

ued, emphasizing complex carbohydrates (such as rice, wheat, and potatoes), meats (especially chicken), and the child's regular milk or formula. Foods high in simple sugars and fats should be avoided (33).

Mild Dehydration (Less than 5%)

Dehydration should be corrected by giving 50 mL/kg of ORT over 4 to 6 hr (33). Rapid restoration of the circulating blood volume helps to correct acidosis and improves tissue perfusion, which aids the early refeeding process. Replacement of continuing stool and emesis losses is accomplished as outlined earlier. As soon as the dehydration is corrected, feeding should begin following the guidelines given earlier.

Moderate Dehydration (5% to 9%)

Dehydration is corrected by giving 100 mL/kg of ORT over 4 to 6 hr. At the end of each hour of rehydration, continuing stool losses and emesis volume should be calculated and the total added to the amount remaining to be given.

When rehydration is complete, feeding is continued following the guidelines given earlier.

Severe Dehydration (More than 10%)

By definition, severe dehydration designates shock or a near shock-like condition (33), and should be treated as a true medical emergency. A large bore catheter should be used for the infusion of Ringer's lactate, normal saline, or similar solution and boluses of 20 to 40 mL/kg should be administered until signs of shock resolve. Fluid and electrolyte resuscitation may require more than one intravenous site and the use of alternate access sites including venous cutdown, femoral vein, or interosseous locations may be needed (33). As the level of consciousness improves, ORT can be instituted. The hydration status must be frequently reassessed to monitor the effectiveness of the therapy.

When rehydration is complete, feeding is continued as described earlier.

REFERENCES

1. Cleason M, Merson MH. Global progress in the control of diarrheal diseases. *Pediatr Infect Dis J* 1990;9:345–355.
2. Koloff KL, Wasserman SS, Steciak JY, et al. Acute diarrhea in Baltimore children attending an outpatient clinic. *Pediatr Infect Dis J* 1988;7:753–759.
3. Hospital use by children in the United States and Canada. *Comp Int Vital Health Statistics Rep* 1984;5:1.
4. Ho MS, Glass RI, Pinsky PF. Diarrheal deaths in American children: are they preventable? *JAMA* 1988;260:3281–3285.
5. Levine MM, Edelman R. Acute diarrheal infections in infants. I. Epidemiology, treatment and prospects for immunoprophylaxis. *Hosp Pract* 1979;14:89–100.
6. Hirschhorn N, Greenough WB III. Progress in oral rehydration therapy. *Sci Am* 1991;264:50–56.
7. O'Shaughnessy WB. Proposal for a new method of treating the blue epidemic cholera. *Lancet* 1830;1:366.
8. Phillip RA. Water and electrolyte losses in cholera. *Fed Proc* 1964;23:705–712.
9. Cosnett JE. The origins of intravenous fluid therapy. *Lancet* 1989;1:768–771.
10. Watten RH, Morgan FM, Songkhla VN, et al. Water and electrolyte studies in cholera. *J Clin Invest* 1959;38:1879–1889.
11. Finberg L. The role of oral electrolyte–glucose solutions in hydration for children: international and domestic aspects. *J Pediatr* 1980;96:51–54.
12. Avery ME, Snyder JD. Oral therapy for acute diarrhea: the underused simple solution. *N Engl J Med* 1990;323:891–894.
13. Harrison HE. The treatment of diarrhea in infancy. *Pediatr Clin North Am* 1954;1:335–348.
14. Paneth N. Hypernatremic dehydration in infancy: an epidemiologic review. *Am J Dis Child* 1980;134:785–791.
15. Curran PF. NaCl and water transport by rat ileum in vitro. *J Gen Physiol* 1960;43:1137–1148.
16. Carpenter CC, Mitra PP, Sack RB. Clinical studies in Asiatic cholera. 1. Preliminary observations, November, 1962–March, 1963. *Bull Johns Hopkins Hosp* 1966;118:165–173.
17. Hirschhorn NB, Kinzie JL, Sachar DB, et al. Decrease in net stool output in cholera during intestinal perfusion with glucose-containing solutions. *N Engl J Med* 1968;279:174–181.
18. Gutman RA, Drutz DL, Whalen BE Jr. Double blind fluid therapy evaluation in pediatric cholera. *Pediatrics* 1969;44:922–931.
19. Nalin DR, Cash RA. Oral or nasogastric maintenance therapy in pediatric cholera patients. *J Pediatr* 1971;78:355–358.
20. AAP Committee on Nutrition. Use of oral fluid therapy and post-treatment feeding following enteritis in children in a developed country. *Pediatrics* 1985;75:358–361.
21. Mahalanalis D, Choudri AB, Bagchi NG, et al. Oral fluid therapy

of cholera among Bangladesh refugees. *Johns Hopkins Med J* 1973;132:197–205.

22. Listernik R, Zieseri E, Davis AT. Outpatient oral rehydration in the United States. *Am J Dis Child* 1986;140:211–215.

23. Chung AW. The effect of oral feeding at different levels on the absorption of foodstuffs in infantile diarrhea. *J Pediatr* 1948;33:14–22.

24. Chung AW, Viscerova B. The effect of early oral feeding versus early oral starvation on the course of infantile diarrhea. *J Pediatr* 1948;33:14–22.

25. Brown KH, MacLean WL Jr. Nutritional management of acute diarrhea; an appraisal of the alternatives. *Pediatrics* 1984;73:119–128.

26. Thobani S, Molla AM, Snyder JD. Nutritional therapy for persistent diarrhea. In: Baker S, Baker R, Davis A, eds. *Pediatric enteral nutrition*. New York: Rhineholt Publishers, 1994.

27. Auricchio S. Peptide digestion and absorption in the small intestinal mucosa during acute and chronic diarrhea. In: Lebenthal E, ed. *Chronic diarrhea in children*. New York: Nestle, Vevey/Raven Press, 1984.

28. Fine KD, Kreijs GJ, Fordtran JS. Diarrhea. In: Sleisenger MH, Fordtran JS, eds. *Gastrointestinal disease: pathophysiology, diagnosis and management*. Philadelphia: Saunders, 1989.

29. Molla A, Molla AM, Sarker S, et al. Absorption of nutrients during diarrhea due to V. *cholerae*, E. *coli*, rotavirus and shigella. In: Chen LC, Scrimshaw HA, eds. *Diarrhea and malnutrition: interactions, mechanisms and interventions*. New York: Plenum Press, 1981;114–123.

30. Molla A, Molla AM, Sarker S, Khatun M, Rahaman MM. Effects of acute diarrhea on absorption of macronutrients during disease and after recovery. *Scand J Gastroenterol* 1983;18:537–543.

31. Barnes GL, Townley RW. Duodenal mucosal damage in 31 infants with gastroenteritis. *Arch Dis Child* 1973;48:343–349.

32. Carpenter CCJ, Greenough WB, Pierce NF. Oral rehydration therapy—the role of polymeric substrates. *N Engl J Med* 1988;319:1346–1348.

33. Duggan C, Santosham M, Glass R. The management of acute diarrhea in children: oral rehydration, maintenance and nutritional therapy. *MMWR Morb Mortal Wkly Rep* 1992;41:1–20.

34. Brown KH, Peerson JM, Fontaine O. Use of non-human milks in the dietary management of young children with acute diarrhea: a meta-analysis of clinical trials. *Pediatrics* 1994;93:17–27.

35. Hirschhorn N. The treatment of acute diarrhea in children: an historical and physiological perspective. *Am J Clin Nutr* 1980;33:637–663.

36. *The state of the world's children 1993*. Oxford: Oxford University Press for UNICEF, 1993.

37. Santosham M, Daum RS, Dillman L, et al. Oral rehydration therapy of infantile diarrhea: a controlled study of well-nourished children hospitalized in the United States and Panama. *N Engl J Med* 1982;306:1070–1076.

38. Tamer AM, Friedman LB, Maxwell SRW, et al. Oral rehydration of infants in a large urban U.S. medical center. *J Pediatr* 1986;107:14–19.

39. Santosham M, Burns B, Nadkarni V, et al. Oral rehydration therapy for acute diarrhea in ambulatory children in the United States: a double-blind comparison of four different solutions. *Pediatrics* 1985;76:159–166.

40. Snyder JD. Use and misuse of oral therapy for diarrhea: comparison of U.S. practices with American Academy of Pediatrics recommendations. *Pediatrics* 1991;87:28–33.

41. Editorial. Oral glucose/electrolyte therapy for acute diarrhea. *Lancet* 1975;1:79–80.

42. Santosham M, Burns BA, Reid R, et al. Glycine-based oral rehydration solution: reassessment of safety and efficacy. *J Pediatr* 1986;109:795–801.

43. Ribeiro HD Jr, Lifshitz F. Alanine-based oral rehydration therapy for infants with acute diarrhea. *J Pediatr* 1991;118:S86–S90.

44. Field M. New strategies for treating watery diarrhea. *N Engl J Med* 1977;297:1121–1122.

45. Molla AM, Hossain M, Sarker SA, et al. Rice-powder electrolyte solution as oral therapy in diarrhoea due to *Vibrio cholerae* and *Escherichia coli*. *Lancet* 1982;1:1317–1319.

46. Patra FC, Mahalanabis D, Jalan KN, et al. Is oral rice electrolyte

47. Molla AM, Molla A, Nath SK, et al. Food-based oral rehydration salt solution for acute childhood diarrhea. *Lancet* 1989;2:429–431.

48. Alam AN, Sarker SA, Molla AM, et al. Hydrolyzed wheat based oral rehydration solution for acute diarrhea. *Arch Dis Child* 1987;62:440–442.

49. Gore SM, Fontaine O, Pierce NF. Impact of rice based oral rehydration solution on stool output and duration of diarrhoea: meta-analysis of 13 clinical trials. *Br Med J* 1992;304:287–291.

50. Santosham M, Fayad I, Hashem M, et al. A comparison of rice-based oral rehydration solution and "early feeding" for the treatment of acute diarrhea in infants. *J Pediatr* 1990;116:868–875.

51. Fayad IM, Hashem M, Duggan C, et al. Comparative efficacy of rice-based oral rehydration salts versus early reintroduction of food. *Lancet* 1993;342:772–775.

52. Pizarro D, Posada G, Sandi L, Moran JR. Rice-based oral electrolyte solutions for the management of infantile diarrhea. *N Engl J Med* 1991;324:517–521.

53. *The rational use of drugs in the management of acute diarrhoea in children*. Geneva: World Health Organization, 1990.

54. Greenson JK, Belitsos PC, Yardly JH, Bartlett JG. AIDS enteropathy: occult enteric infections and duodenal mucosal alterations in chronic diarrhea. *Ann Intern Med* 1991;114:366–372.

55. Snyder JD. Dietary protein sensitivity: is it an important risk factor for persistent diarrhea? *Acta Paediatr* 1992;81(S381):78–81.

56. Vanderhoof JA. Short bowel syndrome. In: Lebenthal E, ed. *Textbook of gastroenterology and nutrition in infancy*, 2nd ed. New York: Raven Press, 1989;794.

57. Isolauri E, Juntunen M, Wiren S, et al. Intestinal permeability changes in acute gastroenteritis: effects of clinical factors and nutritional management. *J Pediatr Gastroenterol Nutr* 1989;8:466–473.

58. Khin Maung U, Nyunt-Nyunt Wai, Myo Khon, et al. Effect of clinical outcome of breast feeding during acute diarrhoea. *Br Med J* 1985;290:587–589.

59. Margolis PA, Litteer T. Effects of unrestricted diet on mild infantile diarrhea. *Am J Dis Child* 1990;144:162–164.

60. Gozala E, Weitzman S, Weitzman Z, et al. Early versus late refeeding in acute infantile diarrhoea. *Isr J Med Sci* 1988;24:175–179.

61. Fox R, Leen CLS. Acute gastroenteritis in infants under 6 months old. *Arch Dis Child* 1990;65:936–938.

62. Rees L, Brooke CGD. Gradual reintroduction of full-strength milk after acute gastroenteritis in children. *Lancet* 1979;1:770–771.

63. Placzek M, Walker-Smith JA. Comparison of two feeding regimens following acute gastroenteritis in infancy. *J Pediatr Gastroenterol Nutr* 1984;3:245–248.

64. Santosham M, Foster S, Reid R, et al. Role of soy-based, lactose-free formula during treatment of acute diarrhea. *Pediatrics* 1985;76:292–298.

65. Brown KH, Gastanaduy AS, Saaverdra JM, et al. Effect of continued oral feeding on clinical and nutritional outcomes of acute diarrhea in children. *J Pediatr* 1988;112:191–200.

66. Hjelt K, Paerregard A, Petersen W, et al. Rapid versus gradual refeeding in acute gastroenteritis in childhood: energy intake and weight gain. *J Pediatr Gastroenterol Nutr* 1989;8:75–80.

67. Isolauri E, Vesakari T. Oral rehydration, rapid refeeding and cholestyramine for treatment of acute diarrhoea. *J Pediatr Gastroenterol Nutr* 1985;4:366–374.

68. Brown KH, Perez F, Gastanaduy AS. Clinical trial of modified whole milk, lactose-hydrolyzed whole milk, or cereal–milk mixtures for the dietary management of acute childhood diarrhea. *J Pediatr Gastroenterol Nutr* 1991;12:340–350.

69. Alarcon P, Montoya R, Perez F, et al. Clinical trial of home available, mixed diets versus a lactose-free, soy-protein formula for the dietary management of acute childhood diarrhea. *J Pediatr Gastroenterol Nutr* 1991;12:224–232.

70. Molla AM, Molla A, Rhode J, Greenough WB III. Turning off the diarrhea: the role of food and ORS. *J Pediatr Gastroenterol Nutr* 1989;8:81–84.

71. Brown KH. Appropriate diets for the rehabilitation of malnour-

ished children in the community setting. *Acta Paediatr Scand Suppl* 1991;374:151–159.

72. Martini MC, Savaiano DA. Reduced intolerance symptoms from lactose consumed during a meal. *Am J Clin Nutr* 1988;47:57–60.

73. Hyams JS, Leichner AM. Apple juice: an unappreciated cause of chronic diarrhea. *Am J Dis Child* 1985;139:503–505.

74. Saavedra JM, Harris GD, Li S, Finberg L. Capillary refilling (skin turgor) in the assessment of dehydration. *Am J Dis Child* 1991;145:296–298.

75. Schriger DL, Baraff L. Defining normal capillary refill: variation with age, sex and temperature. *Ann Emerg Med* 1988;17:932–935.

76. Guerrant RL, Bobak DA. Bacterial and protozoal gastroenteritis. *N Engl J Med* 1991;325:327–340.

Infections of the Gastrointestinal Tract,
edited by M. J. Blaser, P. D. Smith, J. I. Ravdin,
H. B. Greenberg, and R. L. Guerrant
Raven Press, Ltd., New York © 1995.

CHAPTER 91

Current Vaccines to Prevent Enteric Infections

Daniel J. Skiest and David R. Hill

The prevention of bacterial enteric infections involves two strategies. The first is care in the ingestion of potentially contaminated food and water; the second is immunization. There are currently vaccines against only two enteric bacteria: *Salmonella typhi* and *Vibrio cholerae*. While vaccines are being developed against agents such as toxigenic *Escherichia coli,* they are not currently available (see the chapter by Levine). Neither the vaccines against typhoid or cholera provide complete protection against infection, and therefore they should be given in the context of counseling about food and liquid hygiene. Outside the immunization of military personnel and some laboratory workers, these vaccines have been used primarily in the international traveler, for whom they are usually administered with other immunizations and in the setting of general advice about health and travel (1,2).

The discipline of travel medicine—the prevention and management of illness in travelers—has seen dramatic growth in recent years as a subspecialty of clinical tropical medicine and infectious diseases (3,4). Careful epidemiologic studies on the risk of illness such as traveler's diarrhea and malaria have been carried out as well as the use of various prevention strategies. The most common illness is traveler's diarrhea, occurring in 20% to 50% of persons going to the developing world (see the chapter by DuPont) (5). One of the most serious illnesses is malaria, which can occur in 0.2% to 2.5% of travelers to Africa depending on their itinerary and whether they are compliant with antimalarials (6–10). While for most people traveler's diarrhea is a mild, self-limited illness, other people can be incapacitated and bedridden, losing a few days

of a long sought-after holiday or important business trip. In addition to traveler's diarrhea, other more serious enteric illnesses can occur: two of these are typhoid fever and cholera. The incidence of typhoid fever varies from 3.5 cases/1,000,000 travelers to Eastern Europe to 1.2 cases/10,000 travelers to the Indian subcontinent (11). While cholera had been a rare illness in travelers, the recent epidemic in Latin America, which began in January 1991, has increased the risk, such that in the United States there are one to two cases in returned travelers per week, with some of the cases being severe (12,13). In addition, the recognition of a new serogroup of *Vibrio cholerae* (O139) causing cholera-like illness in Asia will make the control of cholera by preventive measures and vaccination all the more difficult (14).

As mentioned, the most effective strategy against the prevention of enteric illness is to avoid contaminated food and liquids. This can be done by not drinking tap water, by not placing ice cubes in drinks, and by avoiding ground-grown, leafy vegetables. Cooked foods, bottled and carbonated beverages, and heated liquids are generally safe. Meats, and especially seafood, should be well cooked. To increase the level of protection, one can be immunized against several of the enteric diseases, as well as against other infections that are a potential risk for the traveler, such as tetanus, diphtheria, measles, and meningococcal disease. Immunization schedules are listed in Table 1.

This chapter discusses only the existing vaccines for enteric bacterial infections—those against typhoid fever and cholera. The chapter by Levine discusses vaccines in development.

D. J. Skiest: Division of Infectious Diseases, University of Texas, Southwestern Medical School, Dallas, Texas 75235-9113.

D. R. Hill: Department of Medicine, International Traveler's Medical Service; and Division of Infectious Diseases, University of Connecticut School of Medicine, Farmington, Connecticut 06030-3212.

SALMONELLA TYPHI

Enteric fever caused by *Salmonella typhi* as well as other *Salmonella* species remains a significant problem in underdeveloped countries for both the natives of and travelers to these regions. Although the incidence of ty-

TABLE 1. *Immunizations and*

Vaccine	Type	Schedule[a]
Toxoid vaccine		

Tetanus-diphtheria (Td)	Adsorbed toxoids	Primary:
		    2 doses (0.5 mL) im, 4–8 wk apart; 3rd dose 6–12 mo later
		Booster:
		    Every 10 yr

Inactivated bacterial vaccines		

Cholera	Phenol-killed *Vibrio cholerae* (4×10^9/mL)	Primary:
		    0.5 mL im or sc, or 0.2 mL id; give 2 doses 1 wk to 1 mo apart at least 6 d before travel
		Booster:
		    0.5 mL im or sc
		          —or—
		    0.2 mL id given every 6 mo

Streptococcus pneumoniae	Polysaccharide containing 23 serotypes	Primary:
		    1 dose (0.5 mL) sc or im
		Booster:
		    Recommended for some patients at high risk

Neisseria meningitidis	Polysaccharide containing four serotypes (A, C, Y, W135)	Primary:
		    1 dose (0.5 mL) sc
		Booster:
		    Not officially recommended, may be given after 5 yr

Typhoid	Heat–phenol-inactivated *Salmonella typhi* (10^9/mL)	Primary:
		    2 doses (0.5 mL) sc, given 4 wk or more apart
		Booster:
		    0.5 mL sc or 0.1 mL id, every 3 yr

Typhoid	Vi polysaccharide	Primary:
		    1 dose (0.5 mL) sc or im
		Booster:
		    Not officially recommended, may be given after 3 yr

Attenuated live bacterial vaccine		

Typhoid	Attenuated Ty21a strain of *Salmonella typhi*	Primary:
		    1 capsule po given on alternate days for 4 doses
		Booster:
		    Every 5 yr

Attenuated live virus vaccines		

Measles	Attenuated live virus (available in monovalent form or combined with rubella [MR] ± mumps [MMR])	Primary:
		    2 doses (0.5 mL) sc; see text for interval between doses
		Booster:
		    None

Mumps	Attenuated live virus	Primary:
		    1 dose (0.5 mL) sc (usually given as part of MMR vaccine)
		Booster:
		    None

Poliomyelitis	Attenuated live virus, trivalent	Primary:
		    3 doses po, the first 2 given at a 6- to 8-wk interval, the 3rd 8–12 mo later
		Booster:
		    1 dose po

prophyaxis for foreign travel

Indications	Precautions and contraindications[b]	Side effects[b]
All adults	First trimester of pregnancy Hypersensitivity or neurologic reaction to previous doses Severe local reaction	Local reactions Occasional fever, systemic symptoms Arthus-like reactions in persons with multiple previous boosters Rare systemic allergy
No longer required by individual countries May be considered for individuals with compromised gastrointestinal function and high-risk travel (see text)	Safety in pregnancy is unknown Previous severe local or systemic reaction	Local reaction of pain, erythema, and induration lasting 1–2 d Occasional fever, malaise
Persons ≥2 yr at increased risk of pneumococcal disease and its complications Healthy adults 65 yr or older Travelers to areas with epidemic meningococcal disease Asplenia or certain complement-deficiency states	Safety in pregnancy is unknown Previous pneumococcal vaccination Safety in pregnancy is unknown	Approximately 50% of patients have mild erythema and pain at injection site Systemic reaction in <1% of patients Arthus-like reaction with booster doses Infrequent, mild local reactions
Risk for exposure to typhoid fever (see text)	Previous severe local or systemic reaction Acetone-killed vaccines should not be given id	Frequent local reaction of pain, swelling, and induration Occasional systemic reaction
Risk for exposure to typhoid fever (see text)	Safety in pregnancy is unknown Hypersensitivity to vaccine components	Local pain and induration in 10%–20% Systemic reaction in <5%
Risk for exposure to typhoid fever (see text)	Safety in pregnancy is unknown Immunocompromised host[c] Children <6 yr Persons with an acute febrile or gastrointestinal illness Persons taking antibiotics Capsules must be refrigerated	Infrequent gastrointestinal upset, rash
Persons born after 1956 who have not had documented measles infection or received 2 doses of live measles vaccine	Pregnancy Immunocompromised host[c] (HIV-infected persons can be considered for vaccination) History of anaphylaxis to eggs or neomycin	Temperature of ≥39.4°C, 5–21 d after vaccination, in 5%–15% Transient rash in 5% Of persons previously immunized with killed vaccine (1963–1967), 4%–55% have a local reaction
Persons born after 1956 who have not had documented mumps	Pregnancy Immunocompromised host[c] History of anaphylaxis to eggs or neomycin	Mild allergic reactions uncommon Rare parotitis
Children and adolescents <18 yr of age	Immunocompromised host[c] or immunocompromised contacts of recipients	Rare paralysis (see text)
Boost previously immunized persons; complete series in partially immunized adults; alternative to inactivated poliomyelitis vaccine in previously unimmunized adults when there is <1 mo before travel	Not used for primary immunization in persons >18 yr	

TABLE 1.

Vaccine	Type	Schedule[a]
Rubella	Attenuated live virus	Primary: 1 dose (0.5 mL) sc (usually given as part of MR or MMR) Booster: None
Yellow fever	Attenuated live virus	Primary: 1 dose (0.5 mL) sc, 10 d to 10 yr before travel Booster: Every 10 yr
Inactivated virus vaccines Hepatitis B	Yeast-derived recombinant hepatitis B surface antigen	Primary:[d] 3 doses (1.0 mL); im in deltoid, at 0, 1, and 6 mo Booster: Not routinely recommended
Poliomyelitis	Killed poliomyelitis virus, trivalent; enhanced potency	Primary: 2 doses (0.5 mL) sc at a 4–8 wk interval 3rd dose 6–12 mo after 2nd dose Booster: 1 lifetime dose (0.5 mL) sc
Influenza	Inactivated whole and split influenza A and B virus	Annual vaccination with current vaccine
Japanese B encephalitis	Inactivated virus	Primary: 3 doses (1.0 mL) sc at 0, 7, and 30 d Booster: 1 dose at 2 yr
Rabies	Inactivated virus grown in human diploid cells	Preexposure: 1 mL im in deltoid or 0.1 mL id on days 0, 7, and 21 or 28 Booster: Depends on risk category and is based on serologic testing. Dose is 1.0 mL im or 0.1 mL id
Passive prophylaxis Immune globulin	Fractionated immunoglobulins (primary IgG)	Travel of <3 mo duration: 0.02 mL/kg Travel >3 mo: 0.06 mL/kg every 4–6 mo

Adapted from ref. 2.

[a] Manufacturer's full prescribing information should be consulted. Doses are for adults. Children's doses may vary and text or manufacturer's information should be consulted.

[b] Only major precautions, contraindications, and side effects listed.

Continued.

Indications	Precautions and contraindications[b]	Side effects[b]
All persons, particularly women of childbearing age, without documented illness or live vaccine on or after 1st birthday	Pregnancy Immunocompromised host[c] History of anaphylaxis to neomycin	Up to 40% postpubertal females have joint pains, transient arthritis, beginning 3–25 d after vaccination, persisting 1–11 d Frank arthritis in <2%
As required by individual countries	Avoid in pregnant women, unless high-risk travel Prudent to avoid vaccinating infants <9 mo Immunocompromised host[c] Hypersensitivity to eggs	2%–5% have mild headache, myalgia, fever, 5–10 d after vaccination Rare immediate hypersensitivity
Health-care workers in contact with blood Persons residing for >6 mo in areas of high endemicity for hepatitis B surface antigen Others at risk for contact with blood, body fluids, or potentially contaminated medical or dental instruments	Although safety to fetus is not known, pregnancy is not a contraindication in high-risk persons	Mild local reactions in 10%–20%
Preferred for persons 18 yr and older and for immunocompromised hosts[c]	Safety in pregnancy is unknown Anaphylactic reactions to streptomycin or neomycin	Mild local reaction
Persons ≥6 mo of age at increased risk of complications from influenza Healthy adults >65 yr old Medical personnel	First trimester of pregnancy is a relative contraindication Anaphylaxis to eggs	Mild local reactions in < one-third Occasional systemic reaction of malaise, myalgia, beginning 6–12 hr after vaccination and lasting 1–2 d Rare allergic reaction
Travelers to areas of risk with rural exposure or prolonged residence	Safety in pregnancy is unknown; administer only if high risk Allergy to mice or rodents Previous severe reaction Vaccinees should not depart for travel within 10 d of immunization so they can be observed for adverse reactions	Local mild reactions lasting 1–3 d Occasional malaise, myalgias, and fever Unusual (0.2–5/1000) severe systemic hypersensitivity reaction
Travel to areas for >1 mo where rabies is a constant threat	Allergy to previous doses May be given in pregnancy if indicated The id route should be completed ≥30 d before travel The id route should not be used with concurrent chloroquine or mefloquine administration	Approximately 30% have local reactions Approximately 20% have mild systemic reactions of headache, nausea, aches, and dizziness Rare neurologic illness Occasional (6%) immune-complex reactions with booster doses occurring 2–21 d after vaccination
For prevention of hepatitis A Some travelers may benefit from pretravel hepatitis A antibody testing		Transient local discomfort Rare systemic reaction

[c] Persons immunocompromised because of immunodeficiency diseases, leukemia, lymphoma, generalized malignancy, or acquired immunodeficiency syndrome (AIDS), or immunosuppressed from therapy with corticosteroids, alkylating agents, antimetabolites, or radiation.

[d] One vaccine (Engerix-B) can be given in an alternative four-dose schedule of 0, 1, 2, and 12 months.

im, Intramuscularly; sc, subcutaneously; id, intradermally; po, orally.

phoid fever in the United States steadily decreased from the beginning of the century until the mid-1960s, since then it has remained fairly stable with approximately 500 cases/year (11). However, the proportion of cases associated with foreign travel has increased. International travelers now account for greater than two-thirds of reported cases in the United States (11). The choices for vaccination against typhoid fever have recently been expanded by the availability of two new vaccines. These supplement the parenteral, killed, whole-cell vaccine, which has been available for many years. The new vaccines, while more costly, are seen as advances because of their engineering, their ease of administration (one oral and the other a single parenteral dose), and their decreased side effects compared with the killed, whole-cell vaccine.

Typhoid Vaccine Development

Killed, Whole-Cell Vaccine

A parenteral, heat-killed and phenol-preserved whole-cell typhoid vaccine was first used in 1896. An alcohol-inactivated whole-cell vaccine, which was developed in the 1940s, was compared to the phenol-preserved vaccine in the 1950s and was found to be less efficacious (15). In the 1960s and 1970s, controlled trials, which were conducted in persons residing in endemic areas, demonstrated efficacy rates of 51% to 77% for the heat, phenolized vaccine and 56% to 90% for an acetone-inactivated vaccine (16–21). This protection was maintained for at least 3 years and in some studies for as long as 7 years (17,22,23). Although the acetone-inactivated vaccine often demonstrated slightly higher levels of protection in these initial studies, it is more costly to produce and may be associated with a higher incidence of side effects. For example, if it is given intradermally it is poorly tolerated (24). Thus the heat-killed, phenol-inactivated vaccine is used primarily. In the United States, the acetone vaccine is only available within the Armed Services.

In nonimmune travelers to areas endemic for typhoid fever, there is some evidence for a protective effect of the heat-killed, phenol-inactivated vaccine (25). While a moderate degree of protection can be afforded by these killed vaccines, they are associated with a significant degree of both local and systemic adverse effects. The killed vaccine had been combined with one against paratyphoid A and B. However, the efficacy of this vaccine was never established and the combined antigens contributed to increased side effects; thus the vaccine is no longer manufactured in the United States (26). It is not clear if the whole-cell, killed vaccine offers any protection against the other agents of salmonella enteric fever.

Oral, Killed Vaccines

Oral, killed, whole-cell vaccines have been studied and although they were well-tolerated they have not been protective in clinical trials even with multiple doses of high numbers of bacteria (23,27,28). This lack of efficacy is likely related to the inadequate immune response evoked by the killed vaccine (29).

Live Oral Vaccines

The first efforts to produce an attenuated oral vaccine centered on streptomycin-dependent derivatives (30). While these were immunogenic when administered fresh, they lost efficacy following lyophilization. Thus they were not felt to be practical and were not pursued further as vaccine candidates. In the early 1970s a mutant strain of S. typhi, known as Ty21a, was described, which had a mutation of the galE gene, which encodes for the enzyme uridine diphosphate (UDP)-galactose-4-epimerase (31,32). This enzyme catalyzes the reversible isomerization of UDP-glucose to UDP-galactose. UDP-galactose is an essential precursor for lipopolysaccharide (LPS) synthesis (Fig. 1). The presence of intact LPS is required for the development of immunity (32,33). In the absence of this enzyme the bacteria must use exogenous galactose to form UDP-galactose. However, in this process toxic amounts of galactose-1-phosphate and UDP-galactose accumulate in the bacterial cell and result in cell lysis. The Ty21a mutant has moderate resistance to these galactose intermediates by having decreased levels of galactokinase and Gal-1-P-uridyltransferase compared with the parental strain (31,32). It remains capable of producing sufficient LPS to be immunogenic but does not undergo sustained replication and therefore is avirulent and incapable of producing typhoid fever (31,34). In addition to this important mutation, Ty21a has several other mutations that make it well tolerated, including the lack of Vi polysaccharide, which is a well-described virulence factor for S. typhi.

The Ty21a strain was first shown to protect mice when challenged with S. typhi, and in subsequent human studies, five to eight doses (3×10^{10} to 10×10^{10} fresh bacteria/dose) provided 87% protection for volunteers challenged with 10^5 S. typhi organisms (35). In the human trials the vaccine was well tolerated without serious adverse effects.

The human challenge studies led to large field trials conducted in Egypt, Chile, and Indonesia. These have demonstrated variable efficacy (42% to 96%) (36–41). The initial field trial conducted by Wahdan et al. (36,37) in Egypt from 1978 to 1981 included nearly 32,500 children aged 6 to 7 years. The children were randomized to receive three doses of a liquid suspension of lyophilized vaccine (containing 1×10^9 to 8×10^9 organisms) or placebo on alternate days, after ingesting chewable $NaHCO_3$ (to neutralize gastric acid). The vaccine was well tolerated and no serious adverse effects were noted. Mild side effects were infrequent and included nausea, vomiting, and mild abdominal pain. The overall efficacy rate at 3 years was 96%.

Following this field trial a gelatin capsule formulation of Ty21a, which differed from the liquid formulation utilized in the Egyptian study, was licensed in Switzerland. A retrospective study of Swiss travelers who received this formulation indicated that this vaccine was ineffective in

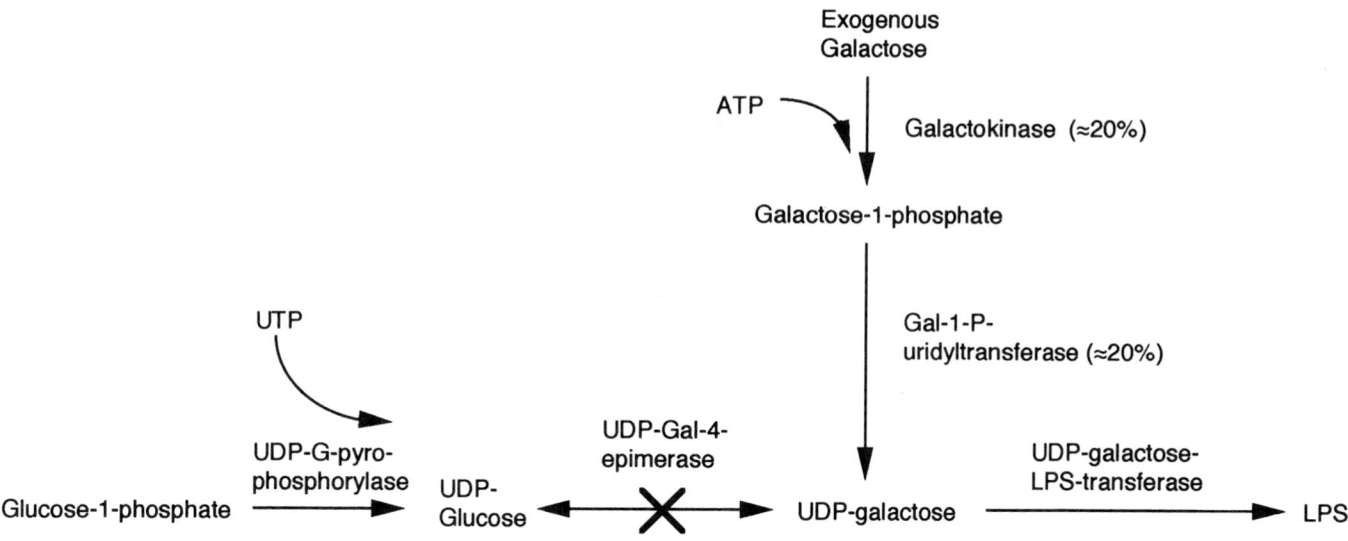

FIG. 1. Schematic of the incorporation of glucose and galactose into the lipopolysaccharide (LPS) of *Salmonella typhi* gal E mutants. The Ty21a strain entirely lacks UDP-galactose-4-epimerase (X) and therefore utilizes exogenous galactose. The enzymes galactokinase and Gal-1-P-uridyltransferase are at levels approximately 20% of the parental strains. This confers partial resistance to galactose-induced bacterial lysis. UTP, uridine triphosphate; UDP, uridine diphosphate; G, glucose; gal, galactose; ATP, adenosine triphosphate. (Adapted from ref. 32.)

this population (42). The authors of this report suggested the low efficacy rate may have been secondary to the use of a formulation that contained fewer organisms per dose, inconsistent refrigeration of vaccine, and, in some cases, possible ingestion of antibiotics. Compliance was not ascertained.

Subsequently, field trials of Ty21a were conducted in Santiago, Chile, an area highly endemic for typhoid fever (38–40). Overall, these studies demonstrated a 67% efficacy rate at 5 years. In the largest study, 109,000 children aged 6 to 21 years were divided into three groups; each group was given three doses of placebo, lyophilized Ty21a (1×10^9 to 3×10^9 organisms/dose) in enteric-coated capsules or Ty21a in gelatin capsules with $NaHCO_3$. Short-interval dosing (2 days) was also compared with long-interval dosing (21 days) for the group that received the actual vaccine. The highest efficacy of 67% at 3 years was obtained in children given enteric-coated capsules in the short-interval dosing (38). Of note, the older a child was, the better the efficacy. Children aged 6 to 9 years had 59% efficacy, whereas children aged 15 years and older had 85% efficacy, suggesting a possible booster effect of vaccination in individuals with a high likelihood of environmental exposure because of increasing age. Follow-up at 5 years indicated continued protective efficacy of 66% in this cohort (23). In order to determine the most effective dosing regimen, 190,000 Chilean school children were enrolled in a study that compared two, three, or four doses of the enteric-coated Ty21a given on alternate days (39). The four-dose regimen was superior to the other two regimens, achieving a 40% lower incidence of typhoid fever compared with the three-dose regimen.

The marked difference in protective efficacy noted in the Egyptian versus the Chilean trials raised important

questions. Possible explanations for the differences included rates of exposure to *S. typhi* for each population, different vaccine formulations, and genetic differences in susceptibility. In Chile there was a twofold to threefold higher incidence of typhoid fever compared with Egypt. It is known that larger inocula can overwhelm the protective effect of vaccination (43). The Egyptian trials used a liquid formulation, whereas the Chilean trials used an enteric-coated preparation. The variable of vaccine formulation was directly studied in Chile (44). This trial of nearly 82,000 children aged 5 to 19 confirmed the superiority of a liquid preparation compared to enteric-coated capsules. Possible reasons for this superiority included the ability of organisms in the liquid vaccine to contact the tonsils, which may provide an enhanced immunologic response. Also, lyophilized organisms in the liquid vaccine may have been more viable because of reconstitution immediately prior to administration (15,44).

The final field trial of Ty21a was in Indonesia and enrolled 20,500 children and adults aged 3 to 44 years (41). Three weekly doses of liquid vaccine or enteric-coated formulations (approximately 4×10^9 bacteria/capsule) were compared against placebo. The liquid formulation was consistently more efficacious than enteric-coated capsules, 53% versus 42% efficacy at 30 months; however, this difference did not reach statistical significance.

The overall lower efficacy compared with previous trials was again an area of concern. Unfortunately, in Indonesia only three doses of vaccine were given and at weekly intervals, both of which have previously been shown to be less effective than four doses at shorter intervals (36,38,39). Also the higher incidence of typhoid in Indonesia and differences in population susceptibilities could have been important variables.

TABLE 2. *Currently available*

Vaccine	Type	Route	Refrigeration required?	Number of doses
Whole cell	Heat- and phenol-inactivated	Subcutaneous	No	Two at 4-wk interval
Ty21a	Live, attenuated	Oral	Yes	Four at 2-d interval
Vi	Capsular polysaccharide	Intramuscular	No	One

a Duration of protective efficacy according to either field studies or the manufacturer's recomendations. The manufacturer's duration is taken from the interval at which boosting is recommended.

The currently available Ty21a vaccine is formulated as enteric-coated capsules, in a four-dose schedule, using 2×10^9 to 6×10^9 organisms/capsule (45). While this can be expected to provide about 60% to 70% protection in persons who reside in the developing world, it is not clear that this level of protection can be achieved in nonimmune travelers. The initial volunteer studies demonstrated excellent protection, but more doses with higher numbers of bacteria were used (35). Additionally, the capsule formulation in the second Chilean study only gave 17% protection to children 5 to 6 years of age, a group who may resemble travelers because of low levels of endemic exposure to typhoid (44). Thus, while the liquid preparation may afford the best protection, it has not been manufactured for commercial use.

One study has indirectly addressed this issue of protection of the nonimmune traveler, by retrospectively reviewing cases of typhoid in travelers in Nepal (25). There was a suggestion of decreased efficacy of the Ty21a vaccine compared with parenteral preparations, but again, the persons who had received oral vaccine may have had an earlier, less effective preparation (42). Because the incidence of typhoid in travelers is so low it is unlikely that a prospective study in this population will be able to be carried out. Given this uncertainty, recipients of vaccine should be told of the persistent risk of typhoid and counseled about food and liquid hygiene. It is not clear if the oral vaccine will provide protection against paratyphoid A or B, but if there is any cross-protection it is likely to be minimal (25,41).

Vi Antigen Vaccine

The Vi antigen (virulence antigen) is the capsular polysaccharide of *S. typhi* and is composed of highly polymerized *O*-acetyl and *N*-acetyl-D-galacturonic acid. Vi antigen enhances resistance to phagocytosis and the action of complement, making Vi$^+$ strains more virulent than Vi$^-$ strains (46,47). Strains of *S. typhi* isolated from cases of typhoid fever almost always have Vi capsular antigen on their surface. Antibodies to Vi antigen are seen in infection, correlate with chronic, asymptomatic carriage of *S. typhi*, and may play a partially protective role in typhoid fever (46–49). Because of the important role of the Vi antigen in pathogenesis of typhoid fever, it was considered to be a good vaccine candidate. Studies in the 1950s of a parenteral Vi antigen vaccine performed by Landy et al. (47,50) did not demonstrate a protective effect in

either chimpanzees or humans. This was attributed to the fact that during vaccine preparation the Vi antigen was denatured (15,23,43,47,51). When prepared by detergent extraction and subsequent purification, the antigenic characteristics are maintained and the parenteral Vi antigen vaccine has been well tolerated, immunogenic, and moderately effective (47,52,53). Immunogenicity was first shown by Tacket and colleagues (52) in a phase I trial. High titers of anti-Vi antibodies were demonstrated in recipients of a single dose of parenteral vaccine and were maintained at 3 years (52,54). Lots that were highly purified to decrease the amount of contaminating LPS were tolerated the best.

Two field trials have been conducted to assess the efficacy of a single, intramuscular dose of 25 µg of Vi antigen (55,56). In a double-blind, randomized controlled trial in Nepal of 6900 children and adults over the age of 4 years, the vaccine had a 72% protective rate for at least 17 months. Efficacy correlated with the development of anti-Vi polysaccharide antibodies. Side effects were minor and consisted of local reactions and low-grade fever. In a double-blind, randomized controlled trial in South Africa involving over 11,300 children aged 5 to 16 years, a 64% efficacy rate at 21 months was seen. A significant increase in anti-Vi antibodies was also seen at 6 and 12 months.

Recommendations for Vaccine Use

There are currently three vaccines for the prevention of infection secondary to *S. typhi:* the parenteral, whole-cell, heat-killed, phenol-inactivated vaccine (Typhoid Vaccine, Wyeth Laboratories Inc., Philadelphia, PA, USA); the oral live-attenuated Ty21a strain of *S. typhi* (Vivotif Berna Vaccine, Swiss Serum and Vaccine Institute, Berne, Switzerland); and the parenteral Vi antigen polysaccharide vaccine (TYPHIM Vi, Pasteur Mérieux, Lyon, France) (Table 2). The killed whole-cell and the Ty21a vaccines are licensed throughout the world, whereas the Vi antigen vaccine is not yet available in North America. Each has been shown to be moderately effective in preventing typhoid in persons living in endemic countries. There have been no direct comparisons of protective efficacy for any of these vaccines. No trials of vaccine efficacy have been performed in nonimmune individuals, and therefore vaccine efficacy may be lower in these persons.

In the United States the following groups are generally recommended for vaccination (1,21,26). First, travelers to areas where there is a recognized risk of exposure to

Salmonella typhi *vaccines*

Cost	Side effects	Field efficacy	Immunogenic in children ≤5 yr	Protective duration[a]	
				Field	Manufacturer
Low	Moderate, occasionally severe	50%–77%	Yes	3–7 yr	3 yr
High	Mild	42%–96% (70%)	Yes in 4- and 5-yr olds	5 yr	5 yr
High	Mild to moderate	64%–72%	Unknown	17–21 mo	3 yr

food and/or water contaminated with *S. typhi*. These areas include many countries of the developing world in Asia, Africa, and Latin America, particularly when the traveler visits areas of poor sanitation such as may occur in small villages and rural sites. Second, microbiology laboratory workers with exposure to *S. typhi*. And third, household contacts of known carriers of *S. typhi*. In contrast, the following groups are not at sufficient risk to contract *S. typhi* and should not be vaccinated: sewer workers not working in an endemic area, persons attending summer camps in rural sites, and persons residing in areas where flooding has occurred. In addition, vaccination has no role in controlling a common source outbreak. At the time of administration it should be emphasized that no vaccine, irrespective of the formulation or route of administration, is 100% effective, and that precautions about food and water sanitation need to be adhered to.

With three vaccines available throughout much of the world, the question arises as to which vaccine is preferable for the major consumers of vaccine, travelers, and the major group at risk, school-aged children residing in endemic areas. For each vaccine, issues of ease of administration, cost, side effects, immunogenicity, efficacy, and duration of protection need to be considered (Table 2). For persons traveling from the developed world, the Ty21a or Vi antigen vaccine is often preferred because of ease of administration, lower side effect profile compared with the whole-cell, killed vaccine, and potentially longer duration of activity. In addition, the shorter vaccination schedule of 6 days with the Ty21a vaccine and one dose with Vi antigen vaccine allows completion within a week compared with a month for the killed vaccine. This may be particularly useful for travelers who need to be protected within a short period prior to travel. An advantage of the Vi antigen vaccine is that compliance is assured since only one dose of vaccine is required. When cost is considered, the killed whole-cell vaccine is less expensive than either of the other two, but for most international travelers vaccine costs are a small expense compared to the overall cost of their journey. Ultimately, the recipient must decide based on the timing of the trip, one's tolerance of side effects, and one's ability to pay for vaccination.

When considering vaccination of children in the developing world, issues of cost, efficacy, and ease of administration are foremost (23,57). The costs of Ty21a and Vi antigen vaccines are high and would need to be decreased prior to their inclusion in mass vaccination. In addition, the Ty21a and Vi antigen vaccines have not been adequately studied in children less than 5 years of age. Data

from other polysaccharide vaccines would suggest that the response to Vi polysaccharide would be low unless it was complexed to an adjuvant (58). While Ty21a vaccine is well tolerated in children aged 6 months to 6 years, it is poorly immunogenic as currently formulated in children less than 3½ years of age (59,60). Therefore, if these newer vaccines were used, they would need to be targeted toward school-aged children, an appropriate group since they have a high incidence of disease. The Ty21a vaccine requires refrigeration, and although it can be administered by unskilled personnel, it requires compliance with four doses (39). Vi antigen vaccine does not require refrigeration, may be given in one dose, but does require a health care provider for administration.

Side effects and the need for two doses at a 1-month interval are important factors with the whole-cell, killed vaccine since cost is less of a concern. This vaccine has been used in a large campaign of annual vaccination of school children aged 7 to 12 years in Thailand (61). It was effective in decreasing the incidence of typhoid fever; however, it was associated with a high incidence of side effects and was costly to run on an annual basis. In considering duration of protective efficacy, the Vi antigen vaccine has formally been studied only to 21 months, but in volunteers antibody titers persisted for 3 years (54). Ty21a vaccine has been shown to be protective for at least 5 years and that remains as the appropriate booster interval at present (21,23,45). The true duration of protection of both of these vaccines needs to be determined. Thus two goals to be achieved, before either of the new vaccines is included in the routine immunization of children in the developing world, are to lower costs and improve efficacy.

Vaccine Administration

Whole-Cell, Killed Vaccine

Primary immunization of adults and children 10 years of age and older consists of two doses of vaccine given at least 4 weeks apart (Table 1) (26,62). For children under 10 years of age, the dose is decreased to 0.25 mL. The vaccine should not be given to children less than 6 months of age (1,57). If less than 4 weeks are available, three doses may be administered at weekly intervals, although the efficacy of this schedule is not known. Booster doses for individuals at repeated or continuous exposure to *S. typhi* are given at 3-year intervals and may be given either subcutaneously or, in a lower dose of 0.1 mL, intradermally. Acetone-inactivated vaccine must not be given intradermally because of severe local reactions. Boosters in children 6 months to 10 years of age can also be given subcutaneously (0.25 mL) or intradermally (0.1 mL).

Side effects associated with this vaccine usually occur in the first 24 hr and dissipate by 48 to 72 hr. They include fever (14% to 29% of recipients), headache (9% to 30%), severe local pain and/or swelling (6% to 40%), work or school absenteeism (15% to 26%), and rare reports of hypotension, chest pain, anaphylaxis, liver damage, neurologic problems, and reactive arthropathy (19,22,26,63,64). There are no specific contraindications to this vaccine except for a history of a severe reaction following administration of a previous dose. Vaccination should be postponed if the recipient has a febrile illness. There are no data on the use of this vaccine in pregnancy, but because of the potential for febrile reactions it is prudent not to vaccinate during pregnancy (65,66). In immunocompromised patients such as those with human immunodeficiency virus (HIV) infection, the inactivated vaccine is theoretically preferable to the live attenuated vaccine; however, there are no specific data on its use or efficacy in such circumstances (66–68).

Live, Attenuated, oral Ty21a Vaccine

For adults and children 6 years of age or older in the United States the dose is one enteric-coated capsule every other day for a total of four doses. Capsules should be given with a cool or warm liquid (less than 37°C), approximately 1 hr prior to a meal. Patients should be instructed to refrigerate the vaccine and to take each of the doses in the prescribed manner in order to obtain maximum efficacy. One study showed that with careful instructions, 82% of patients can be completely compliant (69). Although the package insert states that the vaccine should not be given to children less than 6 years of age, studies have shown a low incidence of adverse reactions in young children, and efficacy has been demonstrated in children as young as 4 years of age (38,41,59). It is likely that the manufacturer will release a pediatric formulation in the near future for children 4 years and older.

The optimal interval for boosting has not been determined. The manufacturer recommends revaccination with the complete four doses at a 5-year interval; however, these recommendations could change as data on duration of protection become available (21,26,45). It appears that giving a second, booster course of the oral vaccine will result in a brisk response, which would be helpful with protecting against S. typhi itself as well as using the Ty21a strain as a carrier for other antigens (70). Another study addressed the question of the immunologic response to being initially vaccinated (primed) with oral or parenteral vaccine and then boosted with the converse vaccine (71). In this study there was neither enhancement nor suppression of a response in individuals primed parenterally and boosted orally. For those who had been primed orally and boosted parenterally there was an enhanced response. These studies show that there is no adverse interaction

between heat-killed, whole-cell vaccine and the Ty21a strain vaccine. Finally, information from vaccine trials, which showed increased levels of efficacy in older recipients of vaccine, suggests that the oral vaccine may be acting as a booster following previous natural exposure to S. typhi (38).

Mild side effects with Ty21a vaccine are infrequent and have included nausea, vomiting, abdominal discomfort, rash, and urticaria (21,45). In the Chilean field trials, these side effects did not appear to be significantly higher in vaccine recipients compared with recipients of placebo (21,23). Postmarketing surveillance by the manufacturer indicates that there is a very low rate of adverse reactions (21,72). The only contraindication to receipt of vaccine is known hypersensitivity to a previous dose. Administration should be delayed in individuals with a febrile or gastrointestinal illness, and it should not be given concomitantly with sulfonamide-type drugs or antibiotics, since they may inhibit bacterial replication in the gastrointestinal tract, which is required for the development of immunity. A history of severe adverse reaction to the parenteral vaccine is not a contraindication to receipt of the oral vaccine. There are no human data on the Ty21a vaccine in pregnancy and in the United States it is considered a category C agent. It should probably not be used unless there is a high risk of exposure (26,45,66). Ty21a vaccine, because it is a live vaccine, should not be given to immunodeficient individuals, including patients with HIV infection, although there have been no reports of adverse outcomes following administration (66–68). Limited data have demonstrated that mefloquine, an antimalarial agent, has in vitro activity against the Ty21a strain and probably should not be given simultaneously with the vaccine. The manufacturer recommends that mefloquine be taken at least 8 hr before receiving Ty21a, although others have suggested a longer interval (72–75). There is no evidence that simultaneous administration of oral polio vaccine and Ty21a diminishes the immune response to either vaccine (72,75).

Vi Antigen Vaccine

A single intramuscular dose of 25 μg of Vi antigen preserved in phenol may be given to adults and children age 2 years and older. However, the manufacturer indicates that the immune response to vaccination in children between 2 and 5 years of age has not been studied specifically (76). No formal recommendations have been made concerning booster doses, but persons may be revaccinated after 3 years. Since the polysaccharide is a T-cell-independent antigen, second injections have not been shown to boost titers (47,77). Because of this, efforts have focused on conjugating the Vi antigen to enhance the booster response (23,78).

The vaccine is generally well tolerated with the few side effects limited to local pain and induration in about 10% to 20% of vaccine recipients. Less than 5% of recipients develop fever and systemic reactions (56,76,79). Contraindications include hypersensitivity to vaccine components. The vaccine has not been studied in pregnant women and should be avoided unless there is a high-risk situation.

VIBRIO CHOLERAE

Cholera remains a major cause of morbidity and mortality particularly for children of the developing world in spite of efforts to both control its spread and treat its victims (80). While oral rehydration formulas have been critically important in the treatment of diarrheal disease worldwide, vaccination against cholera has not played a substantial role (81–83). That is likely because of the limited efficacy of the currently available parenteral vaccine. The problem of cholera has recently been emphasized in the Western hemisphere because of the ongoing cholera epidemic that began in January 1991. In Mexico, Central America, and South America it has affected over 1 million persons, with a case fatality ratio of 0.9%, and has accounted for a steady number of cases in the United States (12,13). It is clear that until sewage can be disposed of properly and water supplies made potable, cholera will not be controlled and there remains the need for a low-cost, effective, and well-tolerated vaccine.

Despite extensive work by several investigators over many years, only one vaccine against cholera is currently licensed in the United States (84,85). This parenteral, whole-cell vaccine is considered to have little clinical utility, because of its limited effectiveness and short duration of activity (86). It is also least effective in young children, who are at greatest risk for both infection as well as the morbidity and mortality from cholera (87–89). Because of the disappointing results obtained with parenteral vaccines, researchers have shifted their focus to oral vaccines, which simulate natural infection and stimulate intestinal immunity, thereby theoretically providing better protection (77,90–93). One of these vaccines, CVD 103-HgR is soon to be licensed in Europe and is reviewed in the chapter by Levine.

Parenteral Vaccine Studies

The immunology of natural infection with *Vibrio cholerae* is discussed in the chapter by Levine; however, a few salient points with respect to immunization are reviewed here. Both experimental and natural infections with *V. cholerae* are associated with the development of long-lasting, effective immunity against the homologous biotype (93–98). Thus in endemic areas where exposure to *V. cholerae* occurs early in life and often, adults have much lower disease rates than children and recurrent infection with *V. cholerae* is rare (94,99–103). Studies in volunteers conducted by Cash and subsequently by Levine demonstrated that infection with *V. cholerae* can provide protection of up to 3 years (the longest period tested) in 90% to 100% of volunteers (94,96,98,104,105). Glass et al. (103) showed that in an endemic area (Bangladesh) an initial clinical infection reduced the risk of a second clinically apparent infection by approximately 90%.

There are two levels at which the host develops immunity—systemic and intestinal. Most studies have shown a correlation between systemic vibriocidal antibodies and a decreased risk of subsequent infection with *V. cholerae*

(99,100,106–108). However, despite this correlation vibriocidal titers may merely be a marker of previous infection and may not in themselves be protective, and other antibodies, such as local intestinal immunoglobulin A (IgA), or other factors may play a role (94,100,109,110). Another major component of the systemic immune response is the development of antitoxin antibodies; however, they do not appear to be the major determinant of long-term protective immunity (93,95,97,111).

Intestinal immunity is likely to play the major role in protection against this noninvasive infection. Studies have shown that breast-fed infants of mothers with high levels of IgA antibodies to cholera toxin and LPS in breast milk are protected against disease, although they are not protected against colonization (112). In challenge experiments of volunteers previously infected with cholera, a brisk secretory response can be elicited nearly 3 years after original infection (96). Unfortunately, parenteral, whole-cell, killed vaccines do not sufficiently induce this intestinal secretory antibody response compared with oral vaccines or natural infection, thus helping to explain their limited efficacy and the recent focus on oral vaccines (93,94,113).

The major classes of vaccines that have been studied include parenteral, whole-cell vaccines; cell-free vaccines directed against either toxin or bacterial antigens; oral, killed vaccines; and oral, live-attenuated vaccines. This chapter focuses on the parenteral vaccines, since oral vaccines are not currently licensed. New killed and live oral vaccines are reviewed in the chapter by Levine. Shortly after the discovery of the etiologic agent of cholera by Koch in 1883, the first cholera vaccine was tested by Ferran in 1884 (114). This parenteral vaccine, which consisted of live attenuated vibrio organisms was associated with significant adverse reactions and had little demonstrable efficacy. Another parenteral vaccine, which consisted of two attenuated strains of *Vibrio cholerae* administered separately, was developed and tested by Haffkine in the 1890s (115). This vaccine also had significant side effects but was partially effective. During the 1920s and 1930s a killed oral *V. cholerae* vaccine, known as the bilivaccine vaccine, was tested. Although this vaccine had some efficacy, it was associated with limiting gastrointestinal side effects because it was combined with bile (94). It was not until the early 1960s that large randomized, controlled trials were conducted of parenteral vaccines. These were conducted mainly in Bangladesh, the Philippines, and India. The trials demonstrated only a moderate degree of efficacy for the vaccines with a short duration of protection. Several chemicals (phenol, formalin, organic mercurials) and heat were used to inactivate the vibrios. The current vaccine in the United States uses a combination of heat and phenol inactivation (85).

The data from these field trials conducted in the 1960s and 1970s can be summarized as follows (previously summarized by Jóo in ref. 86) (87,88,108,109,116–123). In most studies the overall efficacy was approximately 50% to 65%, although a few studies reported higher efficacy rates. Two of the most important variables affecting efficacy were the interval since vaccination and the age at vaccination. Duration of protection was limited, averaging 3 to 6 months, and, depending on the group vaccinated, declined sharply thereafter. The vaccine was more effective in older age groups and generally ineffective in children under 4 years of age. Vaccination did not protect against the development of a carrier state following infection nor did it prevent asymptomatic infection. Widespread use of the vaccine in an endemic area would shorten an outbreak of cholera if given early in the outbreak; however, there was no limitation of the spread of infection and establishment of the carrier state or amelioration of the symptoms of cholera (86,124). Vaccination of family contacts was not useful (125). Vaccination with either classical or El Tor biotype protected against disease with El Tor biotype. Inaba serotype vaccine protected against infection with either Inaba or Ogawa serotypes; however, vaccination with Ogawa did not protect against Inaba (86,89,94,110,120,122). The use of adjuvants (including oil, aluminum hydroxide, and aluminum phosphate) with the whole-cell vaccine generally increased efficacy and extended the duration of protection; however, they caused serious local reactions that precluded their use (86,94,122,126).

When healthy volunteers from nonendemic areas were compared to volunteers from endemic areas, the former had significantly weaker immune responses to parenteral cholera vaccination. This is probably due to the lack of a booster effect, which natural (subclinical) infection confers on older children and adults in endemic areas (86,88,89,109,127). This would also apply to vaccination of nonimmune travelers and suggests that efficacy would be lower in them, a possibility that is similar to that seen with immunization against typhoid fever. In summary, these clinical and experimental trials demonstrated that the whole-cell parenteral vaccine had limited efficacy in any setting and led researchers to explore other approaches for vaccination.

Another approach for parenteral vaccines was to use cell-free preparations—toxoids (formaldehyde, formalin and glycine, or glutaraldehyde-treated toxin), procholeragenoid, and B subunit vaccines (94). In addition, there were studies using bacterial antigens consisting of purified Ogawa or Inaba lipopolysaccharide. Finally, vaccines were tested that consisted of a combination of killed whole cells and toxoids. In general, the toxoid vaccines were associated with either a high incidence of side effects or were not efficacious in clinical trials. A few (a formaldehyde treated toxoid, purified B subunit, and a procholeragenoid toxoid) showed some initial potential but were never tested in clinical trials (94,95). The purified lipopolysaccharide antigens showed some efficacy but, like the whole-cell vaccine, protection was limited (43% to 90%), of short duration, and was least effective in children less than 5 years of age (110,118,120). Further research on the purified antigen vaccines was not conducted.

Recommendations for Vaccine Use

In general, parenteral cholera vaccine should not be used for citizens of the United States or other developed countries traveling abroad, for several reasons (12,83,84).

First, despite a recent increase in the number of cholera infections in U.S. travelers, the risk of acquiring cholera by traveling abroad still remains very low. Many of the cases acquired from Latin America were associated with an error in food choice or preparation and therefore could have been avoided with proper precautions. Before the current Latin American outbreak, the risk was estimated at 1 case per 500,000 travelers (128). This was based on only 51 reported cases of cholera imported to Europe, the United States, and Canada by native citizens who had traveled abroad from 1975 through 1981; there were only ten cases of cholera reported in U.S. travelers from 1961 to 1982 (128,129). Second, as discussed, the parenteral killed vaccines have limited efficacy. Third, in 1970 the U.S. Public Health Service eliminated the requirement for vaccination for persons arriving in the United States from cholera-infected areas. Finally, in 1973 the World Health Organization eliminated from their International Health Regulations the requirement for cholera vaccination for travel between countries, and currently no country requires a certificate of vaccination against cholera (1,84,130). A recent decision analysis from Canada recommended against vaccination of North American travelers (131). Using an attack rate of one case of cholera per million journeys (probably an underestimate currently), they calculated a cost of $28.7 million to prevent one case of cholera. Until more efficacious vaccines become available, the best way for travelers to avoid cholera is to avoid potentially contaminated food and water (83,84,132).

Although these international regulations are formally in effect, some local authorities may still require evidence of cholera immunization. For travelers to these areas, a letter of medical contraindication can be included with their International Certificate of Vaccination, or a single dose of vaccine may be administered and, if properly recorded, will satisfy international health regulations for a period of 6 days to 6 months following the date of immunization. For those short-term travelers who are at high risk for enteric infection by virtue of decreased gastric acidity, or for whom a diarrheal illness may be particularly debilitating, such as those with inflammatory bowel disease or a colostomy, vaccination can be considered.

In areas of the world where cholera is currently endemic or epidemic, the vaccine is not recommended as an adjunctive control measure (83,124). This is because of the reasons previously presented, but also because the vaccine has poor and short duration efficacy in young children for whom the consequences of cholera are most severe.

Vaccine Administration

The only available cholera vaccine in the United States is a whole-cell parenteral vaccine made from a combination of phenol-inactivated suspensions of classic Inaba and Ogawa serotypes. Primary immunization consists of two doses of vaccine (approximately 4×10^9 bacteria/dose) given 1 week to 1 month apart (Table 1) (1,84,85). The vaccine can be given via the subcutaneous, intramuscular, or intradermal route, although the latter route should not be used for patients less than 5 years of age. The vaccine is not recommended for infants less than 6 months of age. A single booster dose of vaccine can be given by the same routes at 6-month intervals.

Serious adverse reactions secondary to the parenteral vaccine are very uncommon; however, minor side effects are frequent, including pain, erythema, and induration at the injection site, which is sometimes accompanied by systemic symptoms of malaise, headache, and fever (84–86). There has been one report of possible transmission of hepatitis B, when the vaccine was given in a setting where needles and syringes were reused and inadequately sterilized (133). Cholera vaccine and yellow fever vaccine should preferably be given at least 3 weeks apart because of the decreased immune response to both vaccines when given simultaneously or within 3 weeks of each other (134). There are no data on usage of the vaccine in pregnancy (category C), but, as with typhoid vaccine, it is prudent to avoid it because of the potential for a febrile reaction and the minimal benefit (65,66,84).

The progress made in the past few years in vaccination against typhoid fever is exciting and has increased the options for protecting both international travelers and inhabitants of endemic areas. It is likely that the information obtained from studies of the Ty21a strain of *S. typhi* will lead to the development of new genetic mutants, which can deliver multiple antigens to the gut. Research on oral cholera vaccines, specifically attenuated live vaccines, also holds the greatest promise for a successful vaccine, although the emergence of a new cholera strain, *V. cholerae* (O139), will continue to challenge efforts to control this disease. Further progress is needed to develop even more efficacious and safe vaccines.

REFERENCES

1. *Health information for international travel, 1994.* Atlanta, GA: US Department of Health and Human Services, Public Health Service, 1994. (HHS publication no [CDC]93-8280).
2. Hill DR, Pearson RD. Health advice for international travel. *Ann Intern Med* 1988;108:839–852.
3. Kozarsky PE, Lobel HO, Steffen R. Travel medicine 1991: new frontiers. *Ann Intern Med* 1991;115:574–575.
4. Gardner P, ed. Health issues of international travel. *Infect Dis Clin North Am* 1992;6:275–502.
5. Dupont HL, Ericsson CD. Prevention and treatment of traveler's diarrhea. *N Engl J Med* 1993;328:1821–1827.
6. Lackritz EM, Lobel HO, Howell BJ, Bloland P, Campbell CC. Imported *Plasmodium falciparum* malaria in American travelers to Africa. Implications for prevention strategies. *JAMA* 1991;265:383–385.
7. Lobel HO, Phillips-Howard PA, Brandling-Bennett AD, et al. Malaria incidence and prevention among European and North American travelers to Kenya. *Bull World Health Organ* 1990; 68:209–215.
8. Steffen R, Heusser R, Machler R, et al. Malaria chemoprophylaxis among European tourists in tropical Africa: use, adverse reactions, and efficacy. *Bull World Health Organ* 1990;68: 313–322.
9. Phillips-Howard P, Radalowicz A, Mitchell J, Bradley DJ. Risk of malaria in British residents returning from malarious areas. *Br Med J* 1990;300:499–503.
10. Wyler D. Malaria chemoprophylaxis for the traveler. *N Engl J Med* 1993;329:31–37.
11. Ryan CA, Hargrett-Bean NT, Blake PA. *Salmonella typhi* in-

fections in the United States, 1975–1984: increasing role of foreign travel. *Rev Infect Dis* 1989;11:1–8.
12. Centers for Disease Control. Cholera associated with international travel, 1992. *MMWR Morb Mortal Wkly Rep* 1992;41: 664–667.
13. Centers for Disease Control. Update: cholera—Western hemisphere, 1992. *MMWR Morb Mortal Wkly Rep* 1993;42:89–91.
14. Cholera Working Group, International Centre for Diarrheal Diseases Research, Bangladesh. Large epidemic of cholera-like disease in Bangladesh caused by *Vibrio cholerae* O139 synonym Bengal. *Lancet* 1993;342:387–390.
15. Levine MM, Hone DM. Typhoid fever. In: Cryz S, ed. *Vaccines and immunotherapy.* New York: Pergamon Press, 1991; 59–72.
16. Ashcroft MT, Ritchie JM, Nicholson CC. Controlled field trial in British Guiana school children of heat-killed-phenolized and acetone-killed lyophilized typhoid vaccines. *Am J Hyg* 1964; 79:196–206.
17. Ashcroft MT, Singh B, Nicholson CC, Ritchie JM, Sobryan, Williams F. A seven-year field trial of two typhoid vaccines in Guyana. *Lancet* 1967;2:1056–1059.
18. Yugoslav Typhoid Commission. A controlled field trial of the effectiveness of acetone-dried and inactivated and heat-phenol-inactivated typhoid vaccines in Yugoslavia. *Bull World Health Organ* 1964;30:623–630.
19. Hejfec LB, Salmin LV, Lejtman MZ, et al. A controlled field trial and laboratory study of five typhoid vaccines in the USSR. *Bull World Health Organ* 1966;34:321–339.
20. Polish Typhoid Committee. Controlled field trials and laboratory studies on the effectiveness of typhoid vaccines in Poland, 1961–64. Final report. *Bull World Health Organ* 1966;34: 211–222.
21. Woodruff BA, Pavia AT, Blake PA. A new look at typhoid vaccination. Information for the practicing physician. *JAMA* 1991;265:756–759.
22. Tapa S, Cvjetanovic B. Controlled field trial on the effectiveness of one and two doses of acetone-inactivated and dried typhoid vaccine. *Bull World Health Organ* 1975;52:75–80.
23. Levine MM, Taylor DN, Ferreccio C. Typhoid vaccines come of age. *Pediatr Infect Dis J* 1989;8:374–381.
24. Edwards EA, Johnson JP, Pierce WE, Peckinpaugh RO. Reactions and serologic response to monovalent acetone-inactivated typhoid vaccine and heat-killed TAB vaccine when given by jet-injection. *Bull World Health Organ* 1974;51:501–505.
25. Schwartz E, Shlim DR, Eaton M, Jenks N, Houston R. The effect of oral and parenteral typhoid vaccination on the rate of infection with *Salmonella typhi* and *Salmonella paratyphi* A among foreigners in Nepal. *Arch Intern Med* 1990;150:349–351.
26. Immunizations Practices Advisory Committee (ACIP): typhoid immunization. *MMWR Morb Mortal Wkly Rep* 1990;39(RR-10):1–5.
27. Chuttani CS, Prakash K, Gupta P, Grover V, Kumar A. Controlled field trial of a high-dose oral killed typhoid vaccine in India. *Bull World Health Organ* 1977;55:643–644.
28. Borgono JM, Corey G, Englehardt H. Field trials with killed oral typhoid vaccines. *Dev Biol Stand* 1976;33:80–84.
29. Kantele A, Arvilommi H, Kantele JM, Rintala L, Makela PH. Comparison of the immune response to live oral, killed oral or killed parenteral *Salmonella typhi* Ty21a vaccines. *Microbial Pathog* 1991;10:117–126.
30. Levine MM, Dupont HL, Hornick RB, et al. Attenuated, streptomycin-dependent *Salmonella typhi* oral vaccine: potential deleterious effects of lyophilization. *J Infect Dis* 1976;133: 424–429.
31. Germanier R, Fürer E. Isolation and characterization of gal E mutant Ty21a of *Salmonella typhi*: a candidate for a live, oral typhoid vaccine. *J Infect Dis* 1975;131:553–558.
32. Germanier R, Fürer E. Immunity in experimental salmonellosis. II. Basis for the avirulence and protective capacity of gal E mutants of *Salmonella typhimurium*. *Infect Immun* 1971; 4:663–673.
33. Germanier R. Immunity in experimental salmonellosis. I. Protection induced by rough mutants of *Salmonella typhimurium*. *Infect Immun* 1970;2:309–315.

34. Germanier R. Typhoid fever. In: R. Germanier, ed. *Bacterial vaccines*. Orlando, FL: Academic Press, 1984;137–165.

35. Gilman RH, Hornick RB, Woodward WE, et al. Evaluation of a UDP-glucose-4-epimeraseless mutant of *Salmonella typhi* as a live oral vaccine. *J Infect Dis* 1977;136:717–723.

36. Wahdan MH, Série C, Germanier R. A controlled field trial of live oral typhoid vaccine Ty21a. *Bull World Health Organ* 1980; 58:469–474.

37. Wahdan MH, Série C, Cerisier Y, Sallam S, Germanier R. A controlled field trial of live *Salmonella typhi* strain Ty21a oral vaccine against typhoid: three-year results. *J Infect Dis* 1982; 145:292–295.

38. Levine MM, Ferreccio C, Black RE, et al. Large-scale field trial of Ty21a live oral typhoid vaccine in enteric-coated capsule formulation. *Lancet* 1987;1:1049–1052.

39. Ferreccio C, Levine MM, Rodriguez H, Contreras R, Chilean Typhoid Committee. Comparative efficacy of two, three, or four doses of Ty21a live oral typhoid vaccine in enteric-coated capsules: a field trial in an endemic area. *J Infect Dis* 1989;159: 766–769.

40. Black RE, Levine MM, Ferreccio C, et al. Efficacy of one or two doses of Ty21a *Salmonella typhi* vaccine in enteric coated capsules in a controlled field trial. *Vaccine* 1990;8:81–84.

41. Simanjuntak CH, Paleologo FP, Punjabi NH, et al. Oral immunization against typhoid fever in Indonesia with Ty21a vaccine. *Lancet* 1991;338:1055–1059.

42. Hirschel B, Wuthrich R, Somaini B, et al. Inefficacy of the commercial live oral Ty21a vaccine in the prevention of typhoid fever. *Eur J Clin Microbiol* 1985;4:295–298.

43. Hornick RB, Griesman SE, Woodward TE, et al. Typhoid fever: pathogenesis and immunologic control. *N Engl J Med* 1970;283:686–691.

44. Levine MM, Ferreccio C, Cryz S, Ortiz E. Comparison of enteric-coated capsules and liquid formulation of Ty21a typhoid vaccine in randomised controlled field trial. *Lancet* 1990;336: 891–894.

45. Product information. Vivotif Berna Vaccine. Swiss Serum and Vaccine Institute, Switzerland, 1991.

46. Hook EW. *Salmonella* species (including typhoid fever). In: Mandell GL, Douglas RG, Bennett JE, eds. *Principles and practice of infectious diseases*, 3rd ed. New York: Churchill Livingstone, 1990;1700–1716.

47. Robbins JD, Robbins JB. Reexamination of the protective role of the capsular polysaccharide (Vi antigen) of *Salmonella typhi*. *J Infect Dis* 1984;150:436–449.

48. Lanata C, Levine MM, Ristori C, et al. Vi serology in detection of chronic *Salmonella typhi* carriers in an endemic area. *Lancet* 1983;2:411–413.

49. Landy M. Studies on Vi antigen. VII. Characteristics of the immune response in the mouse. *Am J Hyg* 1957;65:81–93.

50. Landy M. Studies on Vi antigen. VI. Immunization of human beings with purified Vi antigen. *Am J Hyg* 1954;60:52–62.

51. Gaines S, Landy M, Edsall G, et al. Studies on infection and immunity in experimental typhoid fever. III. Effect of prophylactic immunization. *J Exp Med* 1961;114:327–342.

52. Tacket CO, Ferreccio C, Robbins JB, et al. Safety and immunogenicity of two *Salmonella typhi* Vi capsular polysaccharide vaccine candidates. *J Infect Dis* 1986;154:342–345.

53. Levin DM, Wong KH, Reynolds HY, Sutton A, Northrup RS. Vi antigen from *Salmonella typhosa* and immunity against typhoid fever. II. Safety and antigenicity in humans. *Infect Immun* 1975;12:1290–1294.

54. Tacket CO, Levine MM, Robbins JB. Persistence of Vi antibody titers three years after vaccination with Vi polysaccharide against typhoid fever. *Vaccine* 1988;6:307–308.

55. Archarya VL, Shrestha MB, Cadoz M, et al. Prevention of typhoid fever in Nepal with the Vi capsular polysaccharide of *Salmonella typhi:* a preliminary report. *N Engl J Med* 1987; 371:1101–1104.

56. Klugman KP, Gilbertson IT, Koornhof HJ, et al. Protective effect of Vi capsular polysaccharide vaccine against typhoid fever. *Lancet* 1987;2:1165–1169.

57. Preblud SR, Tsai TF, Brink EW, Nahlen BL, Parsonnet J. International travel and the child younger than two years: I. Rec-

ommendations for immunization. *Pediatr Infect Dis J* 1989;8: 416–425.

58. Eskola J, Käyhty H, Takala AK, et al. A randomized, prospective field trial of a conjugate vaccine in the protection of infants and young children against invasive *Haemophilus influenzae* type b disease. *N Engl J Med* 1990;323:1381–1387.

59. Olanratmanee T, Levine M, Losonsky G, Thisyakorn U, Cryz SJ. Safety and immunogenicity of *Salmonella typhi* Ty21a liquid formulation vaccine in 4- to 6-year-old Thai children. *J Infect Dis* 1992;166:451–452.

60. Murphy JR, Grez L, Schlesinger L, et al. Immunogenicity of *S. typhi* Ty21a for young children. *Infect Immun* 1991;59: 4291–4293.

61. Bodhidatta L, Taylor DN, Thisyakorn U, Echeverria P. Control of typhoid fever in Bangkok, Thailand, by annual immunization of schoolchildren with parenteral typhoid vaccine. *Rev Infect Dis* 1987;9:841–845.

62. Product information. Typhoid vaccine. Wyeth Laboratories Inc., Philadelphia, PA, United States, 1982.

63. Rone JK. Severe systemic reactions to typhoid vaccination: two cases and a review of the literature. *Mil Med* 1990;155: 272–274.

64. Kelleher PC, Kelley LR, Rickman LS. Anaphylactoid reaction after typhoid vaccine [Letter]. *Am J Med* 1990;89:822–824.

65. Barry M, Bia F. Pregnancy and travel. *JAMA* 1989;261: 728–731.

66. Hill DR. Immunizations for foreign travel. *Yale J Biol Med* 1992;65:293–315.

67. Wilson ME, von Reyn CF, Fineberg HV. Infections in HIV-infected travelers: risks and prevention. *Ann Intern Med* 1991; 114:582–592.

68. Centers for Disease Control and Prevention. Recommendations of the Advisory Committee on Immunizations Practices (ACIP): use of vaccines and immune globulins in persons with altered immunocompetence. *Morb Mortal Wkly Rep* 1993; 42(RR-5):1–18.

69. Kaplan DT, Hill DR. Compliance with live, oral Ty21a typhoid vaccine [Letter]. *JAMA* 1992;267:1074.

70. Kantele A, Makela PH. Different profiles of the human immune response to primary and secondary immunization with an oral *Salmonella typhi* Ty21a vaccine. *Vaccine* 1991;9:423–427.

71. Forrest BD, Labrooy JT, Dearlove CE, Shearman DJC. Effect of parenteral immunization on the intestinal immune response to *Salmonella typhi* Ty21a. *Infect Immun* 1992;60:465–471.

72. Cryz SJ. Postmarketing surveillance experience with live oral Ty21a vaccine [Letter]. *Lancet* 1993;341:49–50.

73. Horowitz H, Carbonaro CA. Inhibition of the *Salmonella typhi* oral vaccine strain, Ty21a, by mefloquine and chloroquine [Letter]. *J Infect Dis* 1992;166:1462–1464.

74. Brachman PS, Metchock B, Kozarsky PE. Effects of antimalarial chemoprophylactic agents on the viability of the Ty21a typhoid vaccine strain [Letter]. *Clin Infect Dis* 1992;15: 1057–1058.

75. Wolfe MS. Precautions with oral live typhoid (Ty21a) vaccine [Letter]. *Lancet* 1990;336:631–632.

76. Product information. TYPHIM Vi. Pasteur Mérieux, Lyon, France, 1993.

77. Levine MM. Enteric vaccines. *Lancet* 1990;335:958–961.

78. Szu SC, Stone AL, Robbins JD, et al. Preparation and characterization of conjugates of the Vi capsular polysaccharide and carrier proteins. *J Exp Med* 1987;166:1510–1524.

79. Cumberland NS, Roberts J, Arnold WSG, Patel RK, Bowker CH. Typhoid Vi: a less reactogenic vaccine. *J Int Med Res* 1992;20:247–253.

80. Guerrant RL, Guerrant DI. The history of cholera and update on gastrointestinal infections. *Curr Opin Infect Dis* 1993;6: 37–40.

81. Avery ME, Snyder JD. Oral therapy for acute diarrhea. The underused simple solution. *N Engl J Med* 1990;323:891–894.

82. Guerrant RL, Bobak DA. Bacterial and protozoal gastroenteritis. *N Engl J Med* 1991;325:327–340.

83. Swerdlow DL, Ries AA. Cholera in the Americas. Guidelines for the clinician. *JAMA* 1992;267:1495–1499.

84. Centers for Disease Control. Cholera vaccine. Recommenda-

tions of the Immunization Practices Advisory Committee. *MMWR Morb Mortal Wkly Rep* 1988;37:617–624.

85. Product information. Cholera vaccine. Wyeth Laboratories Inc., Philadelphia, PA, United States, 1984.

86. Jóo I. Cholera vaccines. In: Barua D, Burrows W, eds. *Cholera*. Philadelphia: Saunders, 1974;333–355.

87. Philippines Cholera Committee. A controlled field trial of the effectiveness of various doses of cholera vaccine in the Philippines. *Bull World Health Organ* 1968;38:917–923.

88. Mosley WH, McCormack WM, Fahimuddin M, et al. Report of the 1966–67 cholera vaccine field trial in rural East Pakistan. 1. Study design and results of the first year of observation. *Bull World Health Organ* 1969;40:177–185.

89. Philippines Cholera Committee. A controlled field trial of the effectiveness of monovalent classical and El Tor cholera vaccines in the Philippines. *Bull World Health Organ* 1973;49:13–19.

90. Clemens JD, Sack DA, Harris JR, et al. Field trials of oral cholera vaccines in Bangladesh: results from three-year follow-up. *Lancet* 1990;335:270–273.

91. Clemens JD, Sack DA, Rao MR, et al. Evidence that inactivated oral cholera vaccines both prevent and mitigate *Vibrio cholerae* O1 infections in a cholera-endemic area. *J Infect Dis* 1992;166:1029–1034.

92. Tacket CO, Losonsky G, Nataro JP, et al. Onset and duration of protective immunity in challenged volunteers after vaccination with live oral cholera vaccine CVD 103-HgR. *J Infect Dis* 1992;166:837–841.

93. Levine MM, Kaper JB. Live oral vaccines against cholera: an update. *Vaccine* 1993;11:107–212.

94. Levine MM, Pierce NF. Immunity and vaccine development. In: Barua D, Greenough WB, eds. *Cholera*. New York: Plenum Medical Book Company, 1992;285–327.

95. Greenough WB. *Vibrio cholerae*. In: Mandell GL, Douglas RG, Bennett JE, eds. *Principles and practice of infectious diseases*, 3rd ed. New York: Churchill Livingstone, 1990;1636–1646.

96. Levine MM, Black RE, Clements ML, Cisneros L, Nalin DR, Young CR. Duration of infection-derived immunity to cholera. *J Infect Dis* 1981;143:818–820.

97. Levine MM, Nalin DR, Craig JP, et al. Immunity to cholera in man: relative role of antibacterial versus antitoxic immunity. *Trans R Soc Trop Med Hyg* 1979;73:3–9.

98. Levine MM, Black RE, Clements ML, Nalin DR, Cisneros L, Finklestein RA. Volunteer studies in development of vaccines against cholera and enterotoxigenic *Escherichia coli:* a review. In: Holme T, Holmgren J, eds. *Acute enteric infections in children: new prospects for treatment and prevention*. Amsterdam: Elsevier, 1981;443–459.

99. Mosley WH, Benenson AS, Barui R. A serological survey for cholera antibodies in rural East Pakistan. 1. The distribution of antibody in the control population of a cholera-vaccine field-trial area and the relation of antibody titre to the pattern of endemic cholera. *Bull World Health Organ* 1968;38:327–334.

100. Mosley WH. The role of immunity in cholera. A review of epidemiological and serological studies. *Tex Rep Biol Med* 1969;27(Suppl 1):227–241.

101. Woodward WE. Cholera reinfection in man. *J Infect Dis* 1971;123:61–66.

102. Gangarosa EJ, Mosley WH. Epidemiology and surveillance of cholera. In: Barua D, Burrows W, eds. *Cholera*. Philadelphia: Saunders, 1974;381–403.

103. Glass RI, Becker S, Huq MI, et al. Endemic cholera in rural Bangladesh, 1966–1980. *Am J Epidemiol* 1982;116:959–970.

104. Cash RA, Music SI, Libonati JP, et al. Response of man to infection with *Vibrio cholerae*. Protection from illness afforded by previous disease and vaccine. *J Infect Dis* 1974;130:325–333.

105. Clements ML, Levine MM, Young CR, et al. Magnitude, kinetics, and duration of vibriocidal antibody responses in North Americans after ingestion of *Vibrio cholerae*. *J Infect Dis* 1982;145:465–473.

106. Sack RB, Barua D, Saxena R, Carpenter CCJ. Vibriocidal and agglutinating antibody pattern in cholera patients. *J Infect Dis* 1966;116:630–640.

107. McCormack WM, Chakraborty J, Rahman ASMM, Mosley WH. Vibriocidal antibody in clinical cholera. *J Infect Dis* 1969;120:192–201.

108. Glass RI, Svennerholm AM, Khan MR, Huda S, Huq MI, Holmgren J. Seroepidemiological studies of El Tor cholera in Bangladesh: association of serum antibody levels with protection. *J Infect Dis* 1985;151:236–242.

109. Mosley WH, Aziz KMA, Rahman ASMM, Chowdhury AKMA, Ahmed A, Fahimuddin M. Report of the 1966–67 cholera vaccine trial in rural East Pakistan. 4. Five years of observation with a practical assessment of the role of a cholera vaccine in cholera control programmes. *Bull World Health Organ* 1972;47:229–238.

110. Mosley WH, Aziz KMA, Rahman ASMM, Chowdhury AKMA, Ahmed A. Field trials of monovalent Ogawa and Inaba cholera vaccines in rural Bangladesh—three years of observation. *Bull World Health Organ* 1973;49:381–387.

111. Pierce NF, Kaniecki K, Northrup RS. Protection against experimental cholera by antitoxin. *J Infect Dis* 1972;126:606–616.

112. Glass RI, Svennerholm AM, Stoll BJ, et al. Protection against cholera in breast-fed children by antibodies in breast milk. *N Engl J Med* 1983;308:1389–1392.

113. Ganguly R, Clem LW, Bencic Z, Sinha R, Sakazaki R, Waldman RH. Antibody response in the intestinal secretions of volunteers immunized with various cholera vaccines. *Bull World Health Organ* 1975;52:323–330.

114. Ferran J. Nota sobre la profilixas del cholera por medio de inyecciones hipodermicas de cultivo puro del bacilo virgula. *Siglo Med* 1885;32:480.

115. Haffkine WM. Les vaccinations anticholeriques aux Indes. *Bull Inst Pasteur* 1906;4:690–705,737–747.

116. Oseasohn RO, Benenson AS, Fahimuddin M. Field trial of cholera vaccine in rural East Pakistan. *Lancet* 1965;1:450–453.

117. Benenson AS, Joseph PR, Oseasohn RO. Cholera vaccine trials in East Pakistan. 1. Reaction and antigenicity studies. *Bull World Health Organ* 1968;38:347–357.

118. Benenson AS, Mosley WH, Fahimuddin M, Oseasohn RO. Cholera vaccine field trials in East Pakistan. 2. Effectiveness in the field. *Bull World Health Organ* 1968;38:359–372.

119. Mosley WH, McCormack WM, Ahmed A, Chowdhury AKMA, Barui RK. Report of the 1966–67 cholera vaccine field trial in rural East Pakistan. 2. Results of the serological surveys in the study population—the relationship of case rate to antibody titre and an estimate of the inapparent infection rate with *Vibrio cholerae*. *Bull World Health Organ* 1969;40:187–197.

120. Mosley WH, Woodward WE, Aziz KMA, et al. The 1968–1969 cholera vaccine trial in rural East Pakistan. Effectiveness of monovalent Ogawa and Inaba vaccines and a purified Inaba antigen, with comparative results of serological and animal protection tests. *J Infect Dis* 1970;121(Suppl):S1–S9.

121. Das Gupta A, Sinha R, Shrivastava DL, Taneja BL, Rao MS, Abou-Gareeb AH. Controlled field trial of the effectiveness of the cholera and cholera El Tor vaccines in Calcutta. *Bull World Health Organ* 1967;37:371–385.

122. Azurin JC, Cruz A, Pesigan TP, et al. A controlled field trial of the effectiveness of cholera and cholera El Tor vaccines in the Philippines. *Bull World Health Organ* 1967;37:703–727.

123. Philippines Cholera Committee. A controlled field trial of the effectiveness of monovalent classical and El Tor cholera vaccines in the Philippines. *Bull World Health Organ* 1973;49:13–19.

124. Sommer A, Mosley WH. Ineffectiveness of cholera vaccination as an epidemic control measure. *Lancet* 1973;1:1232–1234.

125. Sommer A, Khan M, Mosley WH. Efficacy of vaccination of family contacts of cholera cases. *Lancet* 1973;1:1230–1232.

126. Pal SC, Deb BC, Sen Gupta PG, et al. A controlled field trial of an aluminum phosphate-adsorbed cholera vaccine in Calcutta. *Bull World Health Organ* 1980;58:741–745.

127. Svennerholm A-M, Hanson LA, Holmgren J, et al. Different secretory immunoglobulin A antibody responses to cholera vaccination in Swedish and Pakistani women. *Infect Immun* 1980;30:427–430.

128. Snyder JD, Blake PA. Is cholera a problem for US travelers? *JAMA* 1982;247:2268–2269.
129. Morger H, Steffen R, Schär M. Epidemiology of cholera in travellers, and conclusions for vaccination recommendations. *Br Med J* 1983;286:184–186.
130. World Health Organization. *International travel and health. Vaccination requirements and health advice.* Geneva: World Health Organization, 1994.
131. MacPherson DW, Tonkin M. Cholera vaccine: a decision analysis. *Can Med Assoc J* 1992;146:1947–1955.
132. Prevention and treatment of cholera. *Med Lett Drug Ther* 1991;33:107–108.
133. Gellert G, Wagner G, Ehling LR. Risks of cholera immunisation at port of entry [Letter]. *Lancet* 1991;337:552.
134. Felsenfeld O, Wolf RH, Gyr K, et al. Simultaneous vaccination against cholera and yellow fever. *Lancet* 1973;1:457–458.

Infections of the Gastrointestinal Tract,
edited by M. J. Blaser, P. D. Smith, J. I. Ravdin,
H. B. Greenberg, and R. L. Guerrant
Raven Press, Ltd., New York © 1995.

CHAPTER 92

Development of Bacterial Vaccines

Myron M. Levine

PRIORITIZATION OF THE VACCINES NEEDED

Infections of the gastrointestinal tract, including diarrheal diseases, dysenteries, and enteric fevers, constitute an important public health problem worldwide. The populations at greatest risk include infants and young children in less developed countries (1–5) and travelers from industrialized countries who visit less developed areas of the world (6–8). Within industrialized countries, infants and the elderly suffer much higher incidence rates of diarrheal disease than other segments of the population. In North America, endemic diarrhea is also a recognized problem among children attending day care centers (9–11), patients in custodial institutions for the mentally retarded and psychotic (12,13), and native Americans on tribal reservations (14,15).

Prior to 1973, a specific etiologic agent could not be ascribed to most cases of infectious diarrhea. Without knowledge of the infectious agents responsible for gastrointestinal infections in high-risk populations, it was not possible to undertake the development of vaccines. Nor in that era was there reason to predict that immunoprophylaxis might one day represent a feasible and rational approach to the control of diarrheal disease. However, since the early 1970s a plethora of viral, bacterial, and protozoal agents have been identified as causes of diarrhea. Indeed, the list of diarrheal pathogens has lengthened so markedly in the past 20 years that, at first glance, one might wonder whether a score of distinct vaccines might be necessary to prevent and control gastrointestinal infections. Fortunately, this is not the case since only a relative handful of etiologic agents account for the vast majority of infections of clinical and epidemiologic importance. The relative importance of the various diarrheal agents can be quantitated from several different perspectives, including (a) association with severe and dehydrating diarrhea that requires treatment at health centers or

hospitals (4,16–20), (b) association with high incidence mild diarrhea (1,2,4,5,21), (c) propensity to cause explosive epidemics and pandemics of severe disease (22–26), (d) correlation with adverse nutritional consequences (27), and (e) frequency as agents of traveler's diarrhea (6–8). By this analysis, a small number of bacterial agents, including enterotoxigenic *Escherichia coli* (ETEC), enteropathogenic *E. coli*, *Shigella*, and *Vibrio cholerae* (O1 and O139), and one virus, rotavirus, combine to cause a major proportion of the diarrheal illness of public health importance. Similarly, *Salmonella typhi* is by far the leading cause of enteric fever. Consequently, if safe, practical, and effective vaccines existed against just these few pathogens, much of the morbidity and mortality due to enteric infections could be eliminated (28). Accordingly, these are the enteropathogens targeted by the World Health Organization as those for which new or improved vaccines should be developed (5,28,29). The status of newly developed vaccines against the above-mentioned bacterial pathogens will be reviewed in this chapter, emphasizing those vaccines that have reached the stage of licensure, controlled field trials of efficacy, or clinical trials in volunteers.

VACCINES AGAINST TYPHOID FEVER

Recently Licensed Vaccines Against Typhoid Fever

The parenteral heat-inactivated phenol-preserved whole-cell typhoid vaccine that was developed at the end of the 19th century was shown in randomized, placebo-controlled field trials sponsored by the World Health Organization in the 1960s to confer a moderate level of protection (60% to 67% vaccine efficacy) that endures for at least 7 years (30,31). However, this vaccine was never an acceptable public health tool because it elicits severe adverse reactions so frequently. Approximately 25% of recipients of inactivated whole-cell vaccine develop high fever and malaise, leading to absenteeism from school or work in approximately 15% of vaccinees (32–34). The

M. Levine: Center for Vaccine Development, University of Maryland School of Medicine, Baltimore, Maryland 21201.

TABLE 1. *Comparison of the characteristics of live oral vaccine Ty21a and parenteral Vi polysaccharide vaccine*

Characteristic	Ty21a	Vi	Killed WCV[a]
Type of vaccine	Live	Subunit	Whole cell
Route of administration	Oral	Parenteral	Parenteral
Immunization schedule	3 or 4 doses (given every other day)	1 dose	2 doses (monthly)
Strict cold chain required	Yes	No	No
Well tolerated	Yes	Yes	No
Efficacy	60%–96%	64%–72%	51%–67%
Duration of efficacy	7 yr	3 yr	3–7 yr
Evidence of a herd immunity effect	Yes	?	?
Interferes with use of serum Vi antibody as a screening test to detect chronic typhoid carriers	No	Yes	Unlikely

[a] Heat-inactivated, phenol-preserved, whole-cell vaccine.

1980s saw the advent of two new vaccines to prevent typhoid fever that confer at least the same level of protection as the parenteral whole-cell vaccine but are well tolerated (35). These vaccines, attenuated strain Ty21a used as a live oral vaccine and purified Vi polysaccharide administered as a parenteral vaccine, have been licensed in many countries worldwide. The development of these vaccines and the clinical and epidemiologic data that support their safety and efficacy have previously been reviewed in depth (30,31,35,36). Salient features of the Ty21a, Vi polysaccharide, and the heat-inactivated phenol-preserved whole-cell vaccines are summarized in Table 1.

While the Ty21a and purified Vi vaccines constitute notable advances over earlier typhoid vaccines, nonetheless each suffers from certain drawbacks. Consequently, various investigators have undertaken to develop newer typhoid vaccine candidates that will overcome the drawbacks of Ty21a and Vi polysaccharide.

Live Oral Typhoid Vaccines

Characteristics of an Ideal Live Oral Typhoid Vaccine

To serve as an ideal oral typhoid vaccine, an attenuated strain of *S. typhi* would have the following characteristics:

1. Attenuation would be achieved by precise deletion mutations in two separate genetic loci, each independently leading to attenuation.
2. The vaccine strain would contain a marker to readily differentiate it from wild type *S. typhi* strains.
3. The vaccine strain would be hardy, allowing a high yield upon large-scale fermentation and lyophilization.
4. The vaccine would be well tolerated, causing no notable adverse reactions.
5. The vaccine strain would be highly immunogenic, eliciting significant protection following administration of a single oral dose.
6. The vaccine would be only minimally excreted.

Modern Strategies to Attenuate S. typhi

Two broad strategies are being followed to develop new attenuated *S. typhi* vaccine candidates: (a) inactivation of "housekeeping genes" or (b) inactivation of genes encoding specific virulence properties. Specific examples of these two approaches are given below.

Single aro Mutants

In the 1950s, Bacon (37) first demonstrated that mutants of *Salmonella* that were auxotrophic for aromatic compounds were attenuated in a mouse model. *Salmonella* organisms contain genetic information that encodes a series of enzymes leading to the synthesis of chorismic acid (38), a critical intermediate in the aromatic amino acid biosynthesis pathway. From chorismic acid, *Salmonella* can synthesize the aromatic amino acids tryptophane, tyrosine, and phenylalanine, as well as para-aminobenzoic acid (PABA, a precursor of folic acid) and 2,3-dihydroxybenzoate (DHB, precursor of an iron-binding protein).

Inactivation of the genes *aroA*, *aroC*, or *aroD* that encode enzymes in this biosynthesis pathway interrupts the synthesis of chorismic acid, disrupting the pathway. *Salmonella typhimurium* organisms harboring mutations in *aroA*, *aroC*, or *aroD* are highly attenuated when inoculated orally into mice (39,40). After they have invaded mice to gain their intracellular niche, these mutants can acquire the aromatic amino acids tryptophane, tyrosine, and phenylalanine but are unable to scavenge PABA and DHB since these are not present in adequate concentrations in mammalian tissues. As a consequence, the *aro* mutants cannot sustain proliferation and are attenuated. Nevertheless, they remain viable in tissue long enough to be able to stimulate cell-mediated immune responses, as well as mucosal and serum antibodies, and to confer a high level of protection (41–46).

Stocker (38) first proposed that *aro* mutants of *S. typhi* might be sufficiently attenuated to be used as live oral vaccines. Edwards and Stocker (47) constructed a prototype vaccine strain, 541Ty, harboring a mutation in *aroA*. The mutation was derived by Tn10 inactivation of *aroA* in *S. typhimurium* followed by illegitimate excision of the transposon, leading to a deletion in *aroA*. Using P22 transduction, this mutation was moved into a wild type *S. typhi* strain (CDC 1080) of phage type A. Edwards and Stocker added an independently attenuating mutation in *purA* (which creates a dependency on adenine) as an additional safeguard. A further derivative, strain 543Ty, was created by selecting a mutant of 541Ty that was unable to express Vi capsular polysaccharide.

Levine et al. (48) extensively studied the safety and immunogenicity of strains 541Ty and 543Ty in Phase 1 clinical trials in volunteers. Both strains were well tolerated in oral doses as high as 10^{10} colony forming units (CFU) administered with buffer. Excretion of these mutants was short-lived, usually lasting only 2 days. By stimulating peripheral blood mononuclear cells collected before and at several time points after vaccination with various *S. typhi* antigens, Levine et al. (48) showed that most vaccinees manifested a cell-mediated immune response to the vaccine strains. Similarly, all vaccinees exhibited antibody-dependent mononuclear cell-mediated inactivation of *S. typhi* following immunization with these vaccines. In contrast to these cell-mediated immune responses, the serological response was quite disappointing: only 10% of the vaccinees developed significant rises in serum antibodies or in surface immunoglobulin A (SIgA) intestinal antibodies against *S. typhi* antigens.

The overall conclusion upon completion of the clinical trials with strains 541Ty and 543Ty was that these vaccine candidates were overly attenuated, probably because of the mutation in *purA*. Subsequently, O'Callaghan et al. (49), as well as Stocker's group themselves (50), showed that mutations in *purA* can hyperattenuate *S. typhimurium* for mice.

Double aro *Mutants*

Following on the pioneering work of Edwards and Stocker (47), Hone et al. (51,178) utilized recombinant deoxyribonucleic acid (DNA) techniques to construct mutants harboring precise deletion mutations in two separate *aro* genes, *aroC* and *aroD*. Since these two genes are far apart on the *S. typhi* chromosome and each is independently attenuating, the combination serves as a safety factor against the unlikely event of a single recombinational event that might theoretically restore one of the wild type *aro* genes. While the probability of even a single such recombinational event is exceedingly small, the chance of two such events occurring is infinitesimal.

Hone et al. (51,178) constructed strain CVD 906 by introducing deletion mutations in *aroC* and *aroD* into wild type strain ISP 1820, isolated from the blood of a Chilean schoolchild with uncomplicated acute typhoid fever in the 1980s. Strain CVD 908 was prepared by introducing the identical deletions in *aroC* and *aroD* in wild type strain Ty2, the parent from which vaccine strain Ty21a was derived. In Phase 1 clinical trials, both CVD 906 and CVD 908 were clearly attenuated compared to what would be expected if their wild type parent strains were to be administered in comparable dosages with buffer. Nevertheless, there was a clear-cut difference in the clinical behav-

ior between the two vaccine candidate strains. At the highest dosage level administered, 10^7 CFU, CVD 906 was insufficiently attenuated, causing febrile adverse reactions in a proportion of vaccinated subjects (51,52). In contrast, in these Phase 1 studies CVD 908 was well tolerated and did not cause febrile responses, malaise, or other adverse reactions (52,53). Both CVD 906 and CVD 908 were impressively immunogenic, eliciting serum antibody and mucosal immune responses, as well as cell-mediated immune responses following administration of a single oral dose (51–53). Two assays, in particular, were helpful in monitoring the immune response because they correlated with the protection observed in field trials of attenuated strain Ty21a that were carried out in Santiago, Chile. These include serum IgG O antibody measured by enzyme-linked immunoadsorbent assay (ELISA) (30) and enumeration of gut-derived IgA O antibody secreting cells (ASCs) detected in peripheral blood (54). Although these immune responses are not deemed to be mediators of protection *per se,* they serve as helpful correlates. Viewed from this perspective, the serum IgG O antibody and the ASC responses elicited by a single well-tolerated dose of CVD 908 are quite remarkable (Table 2). These prominent responses are compared in Table 2 with the 10% to 17% rates of seroconversion encountered following administration of a single dose of Ty21a, Vi + Ty21a, 541Ty, or 543Ty (48,55).

It has been well recognized from studies with attenuated *aro* mutants of *S. typhimurium* in mice and in calves that these vaccine organisms disseminate via the lymph drainage, thoracic duct, and bloodstream to reach all organs of the reticuloendothelial system including the spleen, liver, bone marrow, and lymph nodes (40,41). They survive for approximately 1 to 2 weeks within the fixed macrophages of the reticuloendothelial system, during which time they elicit potent immune responses (42–45). It was proposed that *aro* mutants of *S. typhi* would behave similarly in humans. By systematic repetitive culturing of the blood of vaccinees beginning within hours after vaccination and continuing through 12 days, it has been possible to detect vaccine organisms. The vaccinemias are detected in a proportion of vaccinated individuals on days 4 to 8, but never before or thereafter (52,53). Phase 2 studies with CVD 908 involving larger numbers of subjects are planned to explore further the safety and immunogenicity of this vaccine strain.

cya,crp *and* cya,crp,cdt *Mutants*

In *Salmonella,* the products encoded by *cya* (adenylate cyclase) and *crp* [the cyclic adenosine monophosphate (AMP) receptor protein] comprise a global regulatory system that regulates the transcription of multiple genes and operons. These include genes concerned with the transport and breakdown of catabolites, expression of fimbriae, flagella, and one outer membrane protein, and transport systems for carbon sources. Curtiss and Kelly (56) prepared deletion mutations in *cya* and *crp* in *S. typhimurium* by illegitimate excision of a transposon that had been inserted into each of these genes. The Δ*cya* and Δ*crp*

TABLE 2. *Immunogenicity of a single dose of attenuated* S. typhi *oral vaccine strain CVD 908 compared with earlier well-tolerated live oral typhoid vaccines administered as a single dose*

Vaccine	CFU/dose	Serum IgG O antibody seroconversion	IgA O antibody secreting cells	
			Responders	Mean number of cells[a]
Ty21a [galE, Vi-]	10^9	5/36 (14%)	20/20	45
Vi + Ty21a	10^9	1/6 (17%)	—	—
541Ty [aroA, purA]	$10^9, 10^{10}$	2/18 (11%)	—	—
CVD 908 [aroC, aroD]	10^8	6/6 (100%)	6/6	1062
CVD 908 [aroC, aroD]	10^7	11/12 (92%)	11/12	352
CVD 908 [aroC, aroD]	10^5	2/5 (40%)	3/5	54
CVD 908 [aroC, aroD]	10^4	4/7 (57%)	5/6	17

[a] IgA O antibody secreting cells (ASCs) per 10^6 peripheral blood mononuclear cells.

of *S. typhimurium* were then moved into wild type *S. typhi* strain Ty2 by transduction with phage P22. The resultant *S. typhi* vaccine strain was designated X3927. When Phase 1 clinical trials were undertaken with low doses of X3927 (10^4 and 10^5 CFU), febrile and other notable adverse reactions were encountered in a few vaccinees (52).

Curtiss and Kelly proceeded to introduce an additional putatively attenuating mutation into X3927 to achieve a greater level of clinical safety. To accomplish this, they selected a mutation in *cdt*, a gene that affects the propensity of *Salmonella* to invade beyond the gut-associated lymphoid tissues to reach the deep organs of the reticuloendothelial system. The further modified strain, designated X4073, was well tolerated and moderately immunogenic when administered to volunteers in doses of 10^4 to 10^6 CFU in Phase 1 clinical trials. Some volunteers given doses containing 10^8 CFU of this vaccine strain, with or without a plasmid carrying a gene encoding hepatitis B pre-S1 and pre-S2 protein, developed febrile or mild diarrheal adverse reactions (C. Tacket et al., *unpublished observations*).

Mutants with Inactivation of phoP or ompR Regulatory Genes

The pathogenesis of *S. typhimurium* infection in mice bears a number of similarities to that of *S. typhi* infection in humans. Therefore the degree of attenuation of certain mutations on *S. typhimurium* in mice is often the basis for introducing homologous mutations in *S. typhi* in the hope of achieving a similar level of attenuation of that human host-restricted pathogen. Although overall this approach has proved to be valuable, mutations that attenuate *S. typhimurium* for mice do not always achieve a comparable level of attenuation of *S. typhi* for humans (51, 52,57).

Salmonella typhimurium and *S. typhi* must have the ability to adapt to two quite different environments. Upon excretion by their mammalian hosts, *Salmonella* must survive in the external environment until they are once again ingested by a susceptible host. At that point, they must re-adapt to existence within phagolysosomes of fixed macrophages. *Salmonella* organisms have at least two systems of regulatory genes encoding proteins that

sense the environment. Certain environmental conditions lead to signal transductions that set into motion activation or repression of various genes. One such regulatory system is the two-gene operon of *envZ* and *ompR*, which regulate the relative expression of outer membrane porins OmpC and OmpF (58). Under conditions of low osmolarity, such as might be encountered in the external environment, expression of *ompF* is favored. In contrast, under the higher osmolar conditions found in the intestine of mammals, *ompC* expression is enhanced. Inactivation of *ompR* results in demonstrable attenuation of *S. typhimurium* for mice (58). The degree of attenuation is more than can be accounted for merely by the inactivation of *ompC*, *ompF*, or both. Undoubtedly, *ompR* serves as a regulator of additional, as yet unrecognized, genes involved in the virulence of *Salmonella*. Based on the attenuating effect observed when *ompR* is inactivated in *S. typhimurium*, mutation of *ompR* has been proposed as a possible attenuating lesion to be introduced in construction of an acceptably attenuated *S. typhi* oral vaccine strain (58). However, so far no clinical trials have been reported with *S. typhi* bearing mutations in *ompR*.

phoP/phoQ constitutes another two-component regulatory system that allows *Salmonella* to adapt to the stressful conditions present within phagolysosomes of macrophages (59,60). *phoP* leads to activation of certain genes (*pag*, phoP-activated genes) and repression of others (*prg*, phoP-repressed genes). Inactivation of *phoP* results in measurable attenuation of *S. typhimurium* for mice (59–61). Mutations in *phoP* have also been proposed as possible attenuating lesions to be introduced into *S. typhi* to prepare new candidate live oral vaccine strains.

pagC Mutants

One of the genes activated by the *phoP/phoQ* regulatory system is *pagC*, which encodes a protein believed to confer upon *Salmonella* the ability to survive within the low pH hostile environment of the phagosome within macrophages (59,61). Mutations of *pagC* have been proposed as potential attenuating mutations to be used in concert with other attenuating mutations in constructing an improved live oral typhoid vaccine strain.

Combinations of Putative Attenuating Mutations

Clinical trials in humans with candidate attenuated *S. typhi* vaccine strains have revealed a number of surprises. Some mutations that were expected to be sufficiently attenuating, based on the effects of such mutations on *S. typhimurium* in mice, have proved ineffective or insufficient when *S. typhi* organisms bearing the same mutations were administered to humans (51,52,57). Examples include a *galE* mutant (57) and a *cya,crp* mutant (52). Moreover, the identical mutations (e.g., *aroC* and *aroD*) that acceptably attenuate one wild type strain (Ty2) may not adequately attenuate another wild type strain (ISP 1820) (51–53). These surprises and inconsistencies have rendered the development of new live oral typhoid vaccines more difficult and more capricious than was anticipated a few years ago. In other words, the recombinant DNA technology to construct defined mutants of *S. typhi* has outpaced our knowledge of the pathogenesis of *S. typhi* infection and therefore our ability to predict accurately the phenotypic effect of specific mutations.

Nevertheless, results of clinical trials performed in recent years have provided a wealth of information, which can now be used to "mix and match" mutations that by themselves are otherwise insufficiently attenuating. From combinations of these mutations in selected wild type strains there may arise vaccine candidates with a better profile of safety and immunogenicity. Moreover, yet other putative attenuating mutations have been proposed (62,63) that could be combined with earlier mutations that have achieved only partial attenuation.

Attenuated S. typhi *Mutants as Live Vector Vaccines*

One of the most exciting emerging strategies in modern vaccinology is the use of live vector vaccines to express antigens of other microorganisms and deliver them to the immune system. This approach is also referred to as the use of "live carrier vaccines" or live "antigen delivery systems" (64,65). Attenuated *S. typhi* is a particularly promising live vector for use in humans because (a) the hybrid vaccine can be administered orally, (b) *Salmonella* organisms stimulate a broad immune response (including serum antibodies, SIgA mucosal antibodies, and a variety of cell-mediated immune responses), and (c) there exists extensive experience in the genetic manipulation of *Salmonella*.

Early attempts at live vector vaccines utilized attenuated *S. typhi* Ty21a, which was modified to express the O antigen of *Shigella sonnei* (by introduction of the 120 MDa plasmid of *S. sonnei*) (66) and the O antigen of *Vibrio cholerae* O1 serotype Inaba (by introduction of the *rfa* region of *Escherichia coli* and the *rfb* region of *V. cholerae* O1 Inaba) (67). Administered as three spaced doses each containing 10^{10} CFU, each of these vaccines stimulated modest to moderate immune responses to the foreign antigen and demonstrated some degree of protection in experimental challenge studies (68,69), although results were not always consistent (70).

The new generation of attenuated *S. typhi* vaccine strains such as CVD 908 are also being modified to serve as live vectors. In a prototype experiment, a gene encoding the circumsporozoite protein (CSP) of *Plasmodium falciparum* was integrated into the chromosome of CVD 908 in the Δ*aroC* locus (71). When two 10^7 CFU doses of this live vector vaccine were fed to ten volunteers, 1 week apart, two volunteers made serological responses and a third developed CD8 + cytotoxic lymphocytes that recognized target cells expressing CSP (71). Thus there exists great expectation that attenuated *S. typhi* strains may play a role far beyond their ability to protect against typhoid fever if they prove to be competent live vectors that can deliver foreign antigens to the human immune system.

Parenteral Vi Polysaccharide–Carrier Protein Conjugate Vaccines

Purified Vi polysaccharide behaves like a T-lymphocyte-independent antigen (36). The serum antibody response is not boosted by administration of additional doses of Vi vaccine. Moreover, the immunogenicity of Vi in infants is somewhat less than in older children. However, when Vi is conjugated to carrier proteins, such as tetanus or diphtheria toxoids, cholera toxin or cholera toxin B subunit, B subunit of LT, or *Pseudomonas aeruginosa* exotoxin A, it behaves as a T-lymphocyte-dependent antigen (72,73). In studies in animal models, subsequent inoculations with Vi conjugate clearly boost the serum Vi antibody titer. The molecular weight of the Vi polysaccharide that is conjugated to the carrier protein influences the extent of the serological response. Native Vi was superior to a lower molecular weight derivative (73). Clinical studies in humans with Vi conjugate vaccines are underway.

If the Vi conjugate vaccine meets its expectations in clinical trials in humans, the anticipated advantages that it should show over the purified Vi polysaccharide would include (a) elicitation of higher antibody levels following the initial dose of vaccine, (b) induction of memory so that a boost in Vi antibody titer will follow a second immunization, and (c) stimulation of a higher level of protection than the 65% efficacy stimulated by purified Vi. On the other hand, expected drawbacks to the conjugate vaccine include greater expense, a multiple dose immunization schedule and the need for a cold chain.

NEW VACCINES AGAINST CHOLERA

Until late 1992, dogma taught that epidemic and pandemic cholera was always caused by strains expressing serogroup O1 antigen. The occurrence of epidemic cholera in the Indian subcontinent in 1992 and 1993 caused by a *V. cholerae* strain that does not express O1 antigen and its spread to multiple neighboring countries have led to a reconsideration of this position. The new epidemic strain has tentatively been designated *V. cholerae* O139 (26,74). Understandably, cholera vaccine development activities during the past century have focused on vaccines against *V. cholerae* O1, as will most of the discussion in this chapter. Nevertheless, recent work on the development of vaccines against O139 cholera will also be reviewed.

Improved Oral, Inactivated, Whole-Cell Vaccine

Two oral, inactivated, antigen vaccines were evaluated for efficacy in a large-scale, randomized, placebo-controlled field trial carried out in Bangladesh in the 1980s (75–77). A three-dose immunization regimen was used with an interval of 6 weeks between doses (75). One vaccine consisted of inactivated *V. cholerae* O1 (10^{11} organisms/dose) plus B subunit of cholera toxin (1 mg/dose), while the other vaccine contained only the inactivated vibrios. Each dose of the inactivated *V. cholerae* component included a mixture of both biotypes, classical and El Tor, and both serotypes, Inaba and Ogawa, and included both heat-inactivated and formalin-inactivated bacteria (75). Over 3 years of follow-up, the combination vaccine conferred 50% and the whole-cell only vaccine provided 53% protection against cholera (77). More detailed analysis revealed that notably lower levels of protection were conferred on children less than 6 years of age, subjects of blood group O (an important risk factor for the development of cholera gravis) and against El Tor rather than classical biotype cholera (77,78).

The developers of the oral, inactivated combination vaccine (J. Holmgren et al., Göteborg, Sweden) have modified it in an attempt to improve protection and diminish cost. The modifications include (a) utilizing B subunit prepared from a recombinant organism, which decreases production costs because of the increased yield of antigen; (b) increasing the proportion of inactivated vibrios that are of the El Tor biotype; and (c) modifying the conditions under which the bacteria are cultivated so that the El Tor vibrios enhance their expression of mannose-sensitive hemagglutination pili (79) and classical vibrios express toxin coregulated pili (80), antigens believed to be important in stimulating protective immune responses (79,81). A large-scale field trial is expected to be initiated in Latin America in 1994 to assess the efficacy of this modified version of the oral, inactivated combination vaccine.

Attenuated *V. cholerae* O1 Strains as Live Oral Cholera Vaccines

Attributes of an Ideal Cholera Vaccine

An ideal cholera vaccine would provide a high level of long-term protection following administration of just a single dose and the onset of protection would commence within a few days of vaccination. Such a vaccine would be given orally for practicality and to stimulate optimally the mucosal immune system of the intestine. An ideal cholera vaccine would satisfactorily protect groups such as young children and individuals of blood group O that have not been well-protected by earlier cholera vaccines such as the parenteral or oral inactivated vaccines (77,78,82). Lastly, an ideal cholera vaccine would be packaged in a practical formulation that would facilitate mass vaccination, including young children, and would be inexpensive. During the past decade considerable progress has been made in constructing recombinant bacteria and adapting them for use as live oral cholera vaccines. In extensive clinical studies carried out so far, one such recombinant strain, CVD 103-HgR, exhibits many of the features of an ideal cholera vaccine (83). Recent developments and progress in the use of recombinant bacteria as live oral cholera vaccines will be reviewed in this chapter.

Rationale for Live Cholera Vaccines

A series of observations form the rationale for the use of attenuated *V. cholerae* O1 prepared by recombinant DNA methods as live oral cholera vaccines.

1. A single clinical infection due to wild type *V. cholerae* O1 confers significant protection against cholera upon subsequent exposure to wild type *V. cholerae* O1 (82–89).
2. Whereas many virulence properties contribute to the pathogenesis of cholera, the *in vivo* expression of cholera enterotoxin is an absolute necessity for the profuse purging of voluminous rice water stools that is characteristic of cholera gravis (88).
3. The fundamental protective immunity to cholera is antibacterial rather than antitoxic in nature (82,89), although in the short term antitoxic immunity may synergistically enhance antibacterial immunity (75, 88).
4. The degree of stimulation of serum vibriocidal antibody following ingestion of a live oral cholera vaccine or following infection with wild type *V. cholerae* O1 constitutes the best correlate for the elicitation of antibacterial immunity in the intestine (82,83,90–93).
5. Whereas many antigens on the surface of *V. cholerae* O1 have been identified, recognition of precisely which antigens or combination of antigens constitute the protective repertoire is still the subject of study and debate (79,94–104).

Infection-Derived Immunity

Information on the extent to which a prior clinical infection with wild type enterotoxigenic *V. cholerae* O1 stimulates protection against cholera in the face of subsequent challenge with wild type *V. cholerae* O1 comes from two sources: volunteer studies and epidemiologic studies in endemic areas. The results of rechallenge studies in volunteers shown in Table 3 vividly demonstrate that an initial clinical infection with either classical biotype or El Tor biotype *V. cholerae* O1 confers 90% (El Tor) to 100% (classical) protection against clinical illness when the volunteers are rechallenged with *V. cholerae* O1 of the same biotype (83,87,88). Protection is equal against rechallenge with either the homologous or heterologous serotype (i.e., either Inaba or Ogawa) within the same biotype. In studies with classical biotype vibrios, protection was seen to per-

TABLE 3. *Protective efficacy in volunteers against biotype homologous challenge conferred by prior clinical infection with pathogenic* Vibrio cholerae *O1 of classical or El Tor biotype*

Immunizing V. cholerae biotype	Attack rate for diarrhea[a]		Protective efficacy	Isolation of V. cholerae from direct coprocultures	
	Controls	Veterans[b]		Controls	Veterans
Classical	24/27 (89%)	0/16 (0%)	100%	26/27 (96%) p = 0.012	0/16 (0%)
El Tor	32/37 (86%)	2/22 (9%)	90%	34/37 (92%)	8/22 (36%)

[a] Challenge with 10^6 pathogenic *V. cholerae* O1 given with $NaHCO_3$.

[b] Includes both serotype-homologous and serotype-heterologous challenges. Volunteers who developed diarrhea following ingestion of *V. cholerae* O1 on initial challenge were rechallenged 4 to 6 weeks later with *V. cholerae* O1 of either the same or the heterologous serotype within the identical biotype.

sist as long as 3 years, the longest interval tested (86). Unfortunately, no data are available from cross-biotype rechallenge studies in volunteers with wild type vibrios to ascertain the degree of cross-biotype immunity evident in this model. One notable difference observed in relation to biotype was the extent of excretion of *V. cholerae* O1 (Table 3). The level of excretion of *V. cholerae* O1 was so low in volunteers rechallenged with classical biotype vibrios that direct cultures of stool onto thiosulfate–citrate–bile salts–sucrose (TCBS) medium were all negative. In contrast, *V. cholerae* O1 biotype El Tor could be recovered on direct coprocultures from approximately 30% of individuals who were rechallenged with that biotype. The data from these volunteer studies suggest that in some manner classical biotype vibrios appear to stimulate a more potent immunity than El Tor vibrios.

Natural infection-derived immunity has been studied among persons living in Matlab Bazaar, Bangladesh, an area where cholera is highly endemic. Woodward (105) described repeat infections in 14 subjects, of which six represent individuals who experienced clinical cholera infections both times. In five of these instances, the initial clinical infection occurred in a child 5 years of age or less. One or the other infection was asymptomatic in the other eight cases. Woodward concluded that cholera is not a highly immunizing disease but a lack of precise denominators prevented him from adequately comparing the risk of the general population and persons who experienced an earlier episode of cholera.

A decade later, Glass et al. (85) again reviewed data from Matlab Bazaar and concluded that an initial clinical infection diminishes by approximately 90% the risk of experiencing a subsequent episode of clinical cholera (Table 4). The data of Glass et al. (85) were mainly with classical biotype infections. Based on life table analysis, 29 clinical cholera infections were expected but only three were observed in persons who had an initial clinical cholera infection. Two represented El Tor/El Tor recurrences and one was a classical/classical recurrence. All three individuals who experienced these recurrent episodes of cholera had their first illness when they were young children 5 years of age or less.

Lastly, Clemens et al. (84) reviewed the frequency of repeat clinical cholera infections in Matlab. These investigators observed that an initial clinical infection due to *V. cholerae* O1 of classical biotype conferred 100% protection against subsequent cholera due to either biotype. In contrast, an initial infection with El Tor biotype was seen to be unprotective against subsequent cholera due to the heterologous classical biotype and to be poorly protective (29% efficacy) even against subsequent cholera due to the homologous El Tor biotype (Table 4).

The volunteer model and the field studies concur in demonstrating the superior protective immunity that follows an initial clinical infection with classical biotype *V. cholerae* O1. The discrepancy over the degree of immunity following clinical infection due to biotype El Tor may be explained by the duration of follow-up. The high level of protection attributed to El Tor cholera infection in volunteers was tested only after 2 months. It is conceivable that the protective immunity conferred by El Tor vibrios wanes over time. In the epidemiologic studies in Bangladesh, the El Tor infection-derived immunity was examined over years rather than several months. Under any circumstances, after reviewing the above data, one might conclude that if the intention is to utilize recombinant *V. cholerae* O1 strains as live oral vaccines, it would be wise to include strains of classical biotype; arguably, attenuated classical strains alone might suffice.

Cholera Enterotoxin Is a Prerequisite for Cholera Gravis

The well-studied molecular pathogenesis of cholera infection is characterized by cascades of coordinately regu-

TABLE 4. *Infection-derived immunity conferred by clinical infection with different biotypes of* Vibrio cholerae *O1: observations from field studies in a cholera-endemic area of Bangladesh*

Study (reference)	Biotype of initial infection	Biotype of subsequent infection	Protective efficacy
Glass et al. (85)	Mostly classical	Mostly classical	90%
Clemens et al. (84)	Classical	Classical	100%
	Classical	El Tor	100%
	El Tor	El Tor	29%
	El Tor	Classical	0%

lated virulence properties as *V. cholerae* O1 converts itself from an environmental niche in brackish water to adapt to survival in the human small intestine (106). Of the many recognized virulence properties of *V. cholerae* O1 (88), one that *must* be expressed for the syndrome of cholera gravis to ensue is the elaboration *in vivo* of cholera enterotoxin. Direct experimental evidence supports this claim. Administration of minute quantities of purified cholera enterotoxin to healthy adult North American volunteers results in severe purging and a syndrome resembling cholera gravis (88). Ingestion of as little as 5.0 μg of purified cholera enterotoxin resulted in diarrhea in four of five volunteers, one of whom passed a total diarrheal stool volume of more than 5.0 L. (Note: A total purge of 5.0 L or more is the criterion that defines severe cholera in the volunteer model). Two volunteers who ingested a mere 25.0 μg of purified cholera enterotoxin each purged more than 20 L (88).

These data emphasize the fundamental importance of inactivating the ability of candidate live vaccine strains to express cholera holotoxin. Whatever residual diarrhea may be elicited by such strains, they would be incapable of causing cholera gravis.

Critical Role of Antibacterial Immunity

A wealth of evidence supports the contention that the main mechanism of protection against *V. cholerae* O1 involves antibacterial rather than antitoxic immunity:

1. Parenteral, whole-cell, inactivated vaccines that elicit serum vibriocidal antibody but not antitoxin confer significant protection, albeit for only short periods (several months) (82).
2. Parenteral toxoids that stimulate high levels of serum antitoxin do not confer credible protection, even short-term (107,108).
3. Over 3 years of surveillance in a controlled field trial in Bangladesh, three spaced doses (6 weeks apart) of an oral vaccine consisting of only inactivated *V. cholerae* O1 conferred virtually identical protection (52% efficacy) as three doses of the same inactivated *V. cholerae* O1 vaccine given in combination with B subunit (50% efficacy) (77). Although the large doses of B subunit stimulated strong antitoxic serologic responses in the intestine and in serum, this was not accompanied by any long-term enhancement of the protection conferred by the inactivated bacteria alone (77).
4. A single oral dose of a recombinant A⁻B⁻ *V. cholerae* O1 El Tor candidate vaccine strain (JBK 70) conferred on volunteers 89% protection against experimental challenge with wild type *V. cholerae* El Tor (109). Whatever mechanisms were operative in conferring the high level of protection, antitoxin was not among them since this strain elaborated neither the A nor the B subunit of cholera toxin and did not stimulate an antitoxic immune response.

Serum Vibriocidal Antibody as a Correlate of Protection

Vibriocidal antibody is measured by bacterial lysis when serial dilutions of serum are incubated with a large standardized inoculum of *V. cholerae* O1 in the presence of guinea pig complement (110). Following natural or experimental infection of humans, one observes many-fold rises in the titer of serum vibriocidal antibody. In cholera endemic areas, the repeated ingestion of *V. cholerae* O1 gives rise to long-lived elevated titers of IgG vibriocidal antibody; indeed, in endemic areas the prevalence and geometric mean titer of vibriocidal antibody increase with age (90–93). Such elevated titers are correlated with protection (90–93). Vibriocidal responses following experimental challenge of adult volunteers tend to be mainly IgM and are short-lived, typically falling to a level twofold over baseline within 6 to 12 months. Nevertheless, the initial short-lived serum vibriocidal response is a marker for the elicitation of long-lived intestinal immunity since such volunteers are protected as long as 3 years after initial challenge, despite the fact that they no longer have elevated vibriocidal titers (86). Thus the potent serum vibriocidal antibody response that appears following the ingestion of live oral antigens, be they wild type or attenuated vibrios, serves as a marker for the stimulation of a potent intestinal immunity that endures long after the serum vibriocidal antibody titers have returned toward baseline levels (83,86,111).

For the above reasons, serum vibriocidal antibody is monitored as the proxy for elicitation of a protective intestinal immune response following the administration of candidate live oral vaccines (83). In general, the more potent the serum vibriocidal immune response following oral vaccination, the greater the protective immunity induced.

Protective Surface Antigens of V. cholerae O1

Many surface antigens have been proposed to play a role as protective antigens (88,94,95,97–103). These include lipopolysaccharide (LPS) O antigen, pili (fimbriae), outer membrane proteins, and certain hemagglutinins. However, the relative importance of the various recognized antigens is disputed. To further complicate the issue, there exist antigens that are expressed *in vivo* but are not readily observed when *V. cholerae* O1 are cultured *in vitro*, despite attempts to mimic *in vivo* conditions (112,113).

Approximately 85% to 90% of the vibriocidal antibodies stimulated by wild type infection are directed against the LPS O antigen (88,94,101). However, important protective antibodies are believed to reside among the vibriocidal antibodies that are directed against antigens other than LPS (88,94,101). Toxin coregulated pili must be expressed for classical biotype *V. cholerae* O1 to elicit strong vibriocidal responses (81). Yet the immune response to the pili themselves is minimal (95).

Early Generations of Attenuated V. cholerae O1 Recombinant Vaccine Candidates

The main approach followed in developing live recombinant vaccines against cholera has been to disarm known pathogenic strains of certain specific virulence properties, thereby presumably rendering them incapable of causing cholera yet leaving intact the various surface antigens (known and unknown) involved in protection. This approach has been pioneered by research groups at the Center for Vaccine Development of the University of Maryland School of Medicine (83,114–117) and at Harvard Medical School (118,119).

A radically different approach has been taken by investigators in Australia, who have utilized an attenuated *S. typhi* vaccine strain to express a putative protective antigen of *V. cholerae* O1 and to deliver that vibrio antigen to the human intestinal immune system (67). Each of these approaches is discussed below.

First- and Second-Generation Attenuated V. cholerae O1 Recombinant Vaccine Candidates

A series of early vaccine candidates was constructed from wild type *V. cholerae* strains known to be pathogenic for volunteers by introducing deletions in the chromosomal genes encoding the A (ADP ribosylating "toxic") subunit (115,118) or both the A and B (nontoxic binding) subunits (116) of cholera enterotoxin. It was observed that these first-generation vaccine strains, such as JBK 70, CVD 101, and 395N1, were markedly attenuated compared to their wild type parents (109). These strains were clearly incapable of causing severe diarrhea (109). Nevertheless, residual reactogenicity remained (109). Approximately one-half of the volunteers suffered adverse reactions such as combinations of malaise, nausea, vomiting, abdominal cramps, low-grade fever, headache, and mild diarrhea. Although these first-generation strains were unacceptably reactogenic, a single oral dose of these vaccine strains containing as few as 10^3 CFU, given with sodium bicarbonate buffer, elicited potent vibriocidal responses. The objective of subsequent research was to diminish reactogenicity, while retaining immunogenicity with a single oral dose. Among the second generation of attenuated candidates were strains with deletions in *hlyA*, which encodes the El Tor hemolysin. In animal models the El Tor hemolysin exhibits enterotoxic activity (120). The resultant strains, CVD 104 and 105, representing further derivatives of JBK 70 and CVD 101, respectively, appeared somewhat further attenuated but were still unacceptably reactogenic (109).

Another second-generation vaccine candidate, CVD 102, a thymine-dependent auxotroph derived from CVD 101 (109), was unable to proliferate in the human intestine. CVD 102 did not cause adverse reactions when fed to volunteers in a dose of 10^7 CFU but the vibriocidal responses were so diminished compared to CVD 101 that this strain was not considered capable of immunizing with a single dose vaccine and so further clinical studies were abandoned.

TABLE 5. *Effect of inactivation of toxR (gene that coordinates the regulation of multiple virulence properties) or tcpA (encodes the structural subunit of toxin coregulated pili [TCP]) on the degree of stimulation of serum vibriocidal antibodies by adult vaccinees*

Vaccine strain	Seroconversion	Peak postvaccination GMT of vibriocidal antibody
395N1[a]	7/8	2153
JJM43[b]	2/7	230
TCP2[c]	0/8	52

[a] A⁻B⁺ derivative of wild type strain classical Ogawa 395 in which a deletion has been made in *ctxA*.
[b] Further derivative of 395N1 in which *toxR* has been inactivated.
[c] Further derivative of 395N1 in which *tcpA*, which encodes the structural subunit of the TCP colonization factor, has been inactivated.

Two additional second-generation vaccine strains provided invaluable information in directing further live cholera vaccine development (81). JJM43 is a further derivative of strain 395N1 (*ctxA* mutant of Ogawa 395) in which the regulatory gene *toxR* is inactivated, making the vaccine candidate unable to respond to environmental signals and unable to coordinate the regulation of virulence gene expression (106). TCP2 is another derivative of 395N1 in which *tcpA*, the gene encoding the structural subunit of cholera toxin coregulated pilus, has been inactivated (121). Each of these strains exhibited greatly diminished ability to colonize the intestine of volunteers and to elicit vibriocidal antibody responses (Table 5) (81). Results of these studies emphasize the importance of retaining intact the fimbrial colonization factors and the master regulatory gene (*toxR*) of *V. cholerae* O1 in attenuated *V. cholerae* candidate live vaccines.

Construction of Attenuated V. cholerae O1 Vaccine Strain CVD 103

It was not clear whether or not the residual reactogenicity of the first generation of recombinant *V. cholerae* O1 vaccine candidate strains was due to the expression of as yet uncharacterized enterotoxins or whether the very act of adherence of vibrios to enterocytes somehow results in secretion or diminished absorption by the enterocytes (109). In the mid-1980s, O'Brien et al. (122) reported that most wild type strains of *V. cholerae* O1 elaborate minute quantities of a Shiga-like toxin that is cytotoxic for HeLa cells in tissue culture and that is neutralized, at least partially, by Shiga antitoxin. One wild type strain known to be pathogenic for volunteers but that was negative for this putative Shiga-like toxin was classical Inaba strain 569B (123). It was not known whether or not this Shiga-like toxin might play a role in the residual reactogenicity encountered in volunteers fed vaccine candidates CVD 101, CVD 104, CVD 105, JBK 70, and 395N1, all of which were derived from wild type parent strains that elaborated the Shiga-like toxin. Accordingly, there was interest in testing vaccine candidate CVD 103, an A⁻B⁺ derivative of classical 569B. Whatever the underlying explanation, the clinical studies of CVD 103 constituted a breakthrough; this vaccine strain was well tolerated yet highly immunogenic and protective (109,123). A single dose of CVD 103 vaccine elicited seroconversions of vibriocidal antibody in 90% of vaccinees and of antitoxin in more than 80% and conferred on volunteers significant protection against challenge with pathogenic *V. cholerae* O1 of either serotype or biotype (109,123).

An Ad Hoc Advisory Committee that included representation from the National Institute of Allergy and Infectious Diseases, the Food and Drug Administration, the U.S. Agency for International Development, and the World Health Organization recommended that a unique marker be introduced into CVD 103 before undertaking clinical studies outside physical containment in less developed countries. The purpose of such a marker would be to allow the vaccine strain to be readily differentiated from wild type strains. Accordingly, Ketley et al. (114,117,123) introduced a gene encoding resistance to Hg⁺⁺ (*mer*) or encoding the production of urease into the *hylA* locus of the chromosome of CVD 103. The derivative encoding resistance to Hg⁺⁺ was designated CVD 103-HgR (114,117,123). CVD 103-HgR is phenotypically resistant to Hg⁺⁺, a property not found in wild type *V. cholerae* O1 strains recovered in nature.

Clinical and Field Studies with CVD 103-HgR

Overview

To date, approximately 6000 subjects ranging in age from 24 months to 50 years have participated in placebo-controlled clinical trials establishing the safety and immunogenicity of CVD 103-HgR. These trials have been carried out in industrialized countries (United States, Switzerland, Italy) (83,123–127) and in developing countries with endemic cholera (Indonesia, Thailand) (128–130), epidemic cholera (Peru, Colombia) (131), or little or no cholera (Chile, Costa Rica) (132). For these studies, a practical formulation of the vaccine was used, consisting of two aluminum foil sachets, one containing lyophilized vaccine (and aspartame as sweetener) and the other containing buffer (to protect the vaccine strain from gastric acid). The two sachets are mixed in a cup containing 100 mL of water and the resultant suspension is ingested by the subject. In 1993, a large-scale field trial was initiated in approximately 67,000 subjects in North Jakarta, Indonesia, to assess the efficacy of a single dose of CVD 103-HgR in preventing cholera under natural conditions of challenge.

Safety of CVD 103-HgR

Table 6 summarizes the results of clinical studies that have assessed the safety of CVD 103-HgR. Initial studies in adult U.S. volunteers did not include placebo control groups. However, subsequently, multiple studies in adults, school-age children, and preschool children were of randomized, double-blind, and placebo-controlled design (124–130). Since CVD 103-HgR was derived from a pathogenic parent strain (classical 569B) that is known to be capable of causing cholera gravis in volunteers, considerable attention has been directed to ascertaining whether CVD 103-HgR causes diarrhea. As summarized in Table 6, a large clinical experience now attests to the safety of this vaccine strain in all age groups. Diarrheal adverse reactions have not been observed more often in vaccinees than in placebo recipients in controlled trials. Placebo-controlled studies in infants and toddlers 7 to 23 months of age are planned to begin shortly.

Immunogenicity of CVD 103-HgR

Since vibriocidal antibody is currently considered to be the best correlate of protection and the best measure of the successful stimulation of antibacterial immunity, the serum vibriocidal antibody response has been used to assess the immunogenicity of CVD 103-HgR (83,111, 123–132); fourfold or greater rise is considered significant (i.e., seroconversion).

Immunogenicity in Populations in Industrialized Countries

In clinical studies in North Americans, Swiss, and Italian volunteers, a single 5 × 10⁸ CFU dose of CVD 103-HgR has elicited fourfold or greater rises in vibriocidal antibody in approximately 90% of vaccinees. Table 7 summarizes the serum vibriocidal antibody responses in the first 156 Maryland adult volunteers who received CVD 103-HgR; these data comprise results from the vaccination of multiple groups who received different lots of vaccine. Ninety-two percent of individuals who ingested a single dose containing 5 × 10⁸ CFU of CVD 103-HgR seroconverted, with 50% attaining reciprocal titers ≥2560 (arbitrarily considered a high titer based on earlier studies with other cholera vaccines). In Table 7 are also shown the serological responses from a cohort of 94 young adults who were immunized with a single 5 × 10⁸ CFU dose of CVD 103-HgR from a single representative lot. Once again, a high rate of seroconversion (97%) and a high geometric mean (antibody) titer (GMT) are observed.

Two explanations have been advanced to account for the vigorous immunogenicity of this live oral vaccine. The first relates to the fact that initiation of the intestinal immune response begins with uptake of antigen by the dome-like epithelial cells (so-called M cells) that cover the Peyer's patches and other organized lymphoid tissue of the gut (133). Owen et al. (134) have shown that in rabbit ileal loops containing a Peyer's patch, live *V. cholerae* O1 are taken up more readily by the M cells than inactivated bacteria. The second is based on the observation that *V. cholerae* O1 infection requires coordinate regulation of multiple tightly controlled virulence properties that are

TABLE 6. *Rate of diarrheal adverse reactions in recipients of CVD 103-HgR live oral cholera vaccine versus placebo recipients in randomized, double-blind trials in adults and children*

Age group and site	Vaccine dose (in CFU)	Rate of diarrhea Vaccinees	Controls	p	Reference
Adults					
United States	5×10^8	1/200 (0.5%)	—		83
United States	5×10^8	1/94 (1.1%)	0/94 (0%)	NS	126
Switzerland	5×10^8	1/25 (4%)	2/25 (8%)	NS	124
Thailand	5×10^8	0/12 (0%)	0/12 (0%)	NS	128
Thailand	5×10^8	11/102 (11%)	13/104 (13%)	NS	129
Thailand	5×10^8	0/103 (0%)	—		129
Thailand	5×10^9	5/119 (4%)	2/89 (2%)	NS	129
Peru	5×10^8	2/41 (4.9%)	3/40 (7.5%)	NS	131
	5×10^9	5/41 (12.2%)	3/40 (7.5%)	NS	131
Chile	5×10^9	0/40 (0%)	1/41 (2.4%)	NS	132
5–9 year olds					
Indonesia	$5 \times (10^6–10^8)$	10/209 (4.8%)	4/65 (6.2%)	NS	130
	$5 \times (10^9–10^{10})$	4/124 (3.2%)	4/32 (12.5%)	NS	
Chile	5×10^9	2/178 (1.1%)	1/171 (0.6%)	NS	
Costa Rica	5×10^9	2/196 (1.0%)	4/193 (2.1%)	NS	
Peru	5×10^8	1/40 (2.5%)	1/40 (2.5%)	NS	
	5×10^9	1/40 (2.5%)	1/40 (2.5%)	NS	
24–59 month olds					
Indonesia	5×10^9	18/155 (11.6%)	12/148 (8.1%)	NS	135
Costa Rica	5×10^9	2/118 (1.7%)	2/118 (1.7%)	NS	
Chile	5×10^9	4/100 (4.0%)	4/100 (4.0%)	NS	

activated or depressed by regulatory genes that respond to environmental signals (106). For example, ToxR, the product of the *toxR* regulatory gene, directly or indirectly (through *toxT*) regulates 18 other genes including cholera toxin and the toxin coregulated pilus colonization factor (106). With inactivated vaccine, the surface antigens present during growth in the fermentor are the surface antigens that will be exposed to the intestinal immune system; the inactivated vibrios cannot change in response to envi-ronmental stimuli in the intestine. In contrast, in CVD 103-HgR *toxR* is intact and this live vaccine organism can modify and express the new proteins that are required to survive in and colonize the intestine. Some of these *in vivo*-activated gene products are immunogenic and may play a role in protection. A clear-cut demonstration of the effect of the *toxR* regulation of virulence properties on the degree of stimulation of vibriocidal antibodies was reported by Herrington et al. (81) summarized in Table 5.

TABLE 7. *Serum vibriocidal antibody response of U.S. adults immunized with a single 5×10^8 CFU oral dose of CVD 103-HgR or adult and pediatric populations in several developing countries immunized with a single 5×10^9 CFU dose*

Site of study	Seroconversion rate	Prevaccination GMT	Peak postvaccination GMT	Reference
United States (adults)				
Multiple lots	143/155 (92%)	16	1699	83
Single lot	91/94 (97%)	20	2656	126
Thailand				
Adults	39/48 (48%)[a]	82	368	129
Chile				
Adults	34/40 (85%)	15	222	
5–9 year olds	127/171 (74%)	20	328	132
Peru				
Adults (high SEL)[b]	31/40 (78%)	14	374	131
Adults (low SEL)	28/39 (72%)	16	202	131
Indonesia				
5–9 year olds (lot C)	27/31 (87%)	43	800	130
5–9 year olds (lot F)	21/28 (75%)	51	453	130
2–4 year olds	94/125 (75%)	24	243	135

[a] Number who seroconvert/number vaccinated (%).
[b] SEL, socioeconomic level.

Herrington et al. (81) fed to volunteers a series of isogenic vaccine strains constructed by Mekalanos and co-workers (119,121) that included 395N1, JJM43, and TCP2. Strain 395N1 is an A^-B^+ derivative of wild type classical Ogawa 395; JJM43 is a further mutant of 395N1 in which *toxR* is inactivated, whereas TCP2 is a derivative of 395N1 in which *tcpA* (gene encoding the structural subunit of TCP) is inactivated. When adult Maryland volunteers were immunized orally with these three strains the vibriocidal responses were markedly diminished in recipients of the derivatives harboring mutations in *toxR* or *tcpA* (Table 5).

Immunogenicity in Populations in Less Developed Countries

When community studies of adults and children began in less developed countries where cholera was endemic or epidemic, it was found that the 5×10^8 CFU dosage level, which is highly immunogenic in subjects in industrialized countries (>90% seroconversion), elicited seroconversions of vibriocidal antibody in only about 25% of Thai soldiers (129) and in only 16% of Indonesian children (130). It was subsequently found that many individuals in endemic areas already have elevated vibriocidal titers and are presumably at least partially immune (129,130). In several studies the baseline vibriocidal GMT in subjects who did not seroconvert (i.e., at least a fourfold rise in titer) was significantly higher than the baseline GMT of individuals who did seroconvert (129,130). In such persons with elevated baseline titers, a further rise in serum vibriocidal antibody is not a good measure of vaccine "take" or boosting. It was found that in these populations administering a single dose of vaccine containing one log higher number of vaccine organisms (i.e., 5×10^9 CFU) markedly increases the vibriocidal seroconversion. With a single 5×10^9 CFU dose of vaccine, high rates of seroconversion of vibriocidal antibody (usually 75% to 85%) have been achieved in the less developed country populations studied so far (129–132,135). Table 7 shows vibriocidal antibody responses in adult populations in Thailand, Peru, and Chile and pediatric populations in Indonesia and Chile.

Efficacy

Experimental Challenge Studies to Assess Vaccine Efficacy

A series of challenge studies have been carried out in the volunteer model of experimental cholera. A total of ten such challenges have been performed, three with volunteers who received CVD 103 and seven with volunteers who received CVD 103-HgR (83,123,127). In all but one study only a single dose of vaccine was administered; in one study (El Tor Ogawa challenge) the volunteers ingested two doses of vaccine 1 week apart. Subsequent immunogenicity studies have detected no difference in the

TABLE 8. *Efficacy of CVD 103 and CVD 103-HgR live oral cholera vaccines evaluated in experimental challenge studies in volunteers[a]*

Vaccine	Interval between vaccination and challenge[b]	Protective efficacy
CVD 103		
Classical Inaba	4 wk	87%
Classical Ogawa	4 wk	82%
El Tor Inaba	4 wk	67%
CVD 103-HgR		
Classical Inaba	4 wk	100%
Classical Inaba	24 wk	100%
Classical Inaba	1 wk	100%
El Tor Inaba	4 wk	62%
El Tor Ogawa	4 wk	64%
El Tor Ogawa	4 wk	49%
El Tor Ogawa	1 wk	54%

[a] This summary includes data from Levine et al. (83,123), Tacket et al. (127), and unpublished data.
[b] In all but one study subjects received a single dose of vaccine; before challenge with El Tor Ogawa vaccinees received two doses, 1 week apart.

vibriocidal antibody response between groups of subjects who receive a single dose of CVD 103-HgR versus those who get two doses 1 week apart (129).

In each of these ten challenge studies (Table 8), CVD 103-HgR (or its parent CVD 103) conferred significant protection against challenge with fully enterotoxigenic wild type *V. cholerae* O1 (strains that caused cholera diarrhea in 78% to 100% of unimmunized control volunteers). The overall protection was quite high against challenge with classical biotype (82% to 100%, irrespective of serotype) and moderate with El Tor biotype (49% to 67%, irrespective of serotype). However, a more relevant way to consider the challenge data is from the perspective of prevention of severe and moderate diarrhea, since it is the syndrome of cholera gravis that establishes cholera as a public health problem. Table 9 summarizes the eight challenge studies with respect to protection against diarrhea of different severity determined by total diarrheal stool volume. CVD 103 and CVD 103-HgR provide complete protection against severe (≥ 5.0 L total purge) and moderate (≥ 3.0 L total purge) volume diarrhea. In fact,

TABLE 9. *Efficacy of CVD 103 and CVD 103-HgR live oral cholera vaccines against experimental challenge with wild type* V. cholerae *O1*

Severity of diarrhea[a]	Controls	Vaccinees	Efficacy	p value
≥ 5.0 L	9/88	0/101	100%	<0.001
≥ 3.0 L	19/88	0/101	100%	<0.0001
> 2.0 L	28/88	2/101	94%	<0.0001
≥ 1.0 L	42/88	7/101	86%	<0.0001
Any diarrhea	70/88	19/101	76%	<0.0001

[a] Total diarrheal stool volume in liters during episode of experimental cholera.

of the 19 vaccinees who manifested diarrhea following challenge with wild type *V. cholerae* O1, only two subjects purged a total diarrheal stool volume of 2.0 L or more. Thus CVD 103-HgR is highly protective against severe and moderate cholera of the type that would lead to dehydration.

A single dose of CVD 103-HgR provided 100% protection in volunteers who were challenged with wild type *V. cholerae* O1 (classical Inaba) 6 months after immunization (the longest interval so far tested) (127). Moreover, when a group of volunteers were challenged with classical Inaba a mere 8 days after ingesting a single dose of CVD 103-HgR, they were also 100% protected against cholera (127). A challenge organism of the homologous biotype and serotype was used in these studies to maximize the chance of finding a beneficial effect because these are the shortest and longest intervals between vaccine and challenge that have ever been tested for any candidate vaccine in the volunteer model.

Field Trials of Efficacy in Endemic Areas

In 1993, a large-scale, randomized, placebo-controlled field trial was initiated in about 67,000 subjects 2 to 42 years of age in North Jakarta to assess the efficacy of a single oral dose of CVD 103-HgR in protecting against cholera in a population exposed to natural challenge in an endemic area. The aims of this study include measuring vaccine efficacy in persons less than 6 years of age (an age group not well protected by earlier vaccines) and comparing efficacy in persons of blood group O versus other blood groups. Surveillance will be maintained for at least 3 years before data are analyzed.

Newer Attenuated *V. cholerae* O1 Vaccine Strains

New Virulence Properties Encoded Within the Virulence Cassette

Investigators at the Center for Vaccine Development of the University of Maryland have identified two new toxins that are elaborated by virulent *V. cholerae* O1, in addition to cholera toxin. The genes that encode these two toxins, *Zonula occludens* toxin (ZOT) (136,137) and accessory cholera toxin (ACE) (138), are located on the "cholera toxin element" or "virulence cassette" of the cholera chromosome contiguous to *ctxAB* that encodes cholera toxin. Also located on this region of the chromosome is the gene *cep*, which encodes core encoded pili, an accessory colonization factor (139).

Construction of CVD 110

The virulence cassette region of the chromosome in El Tor strains is found between two insertion-like sequences, RS, that make this transposon-like region of the chromosome unstable and subject to duplication or deletion (140).

Accordingly, it has been possible to construct new vaccine candidate strains from wild type El Tor parent strains by deleting the entire cholera toxin virulence cassette that falls between the two RS elements (141). Thus these new candidates lack ZOT and ACE, as well as cholera toxin and the accessory colonization factor. Michalski et al. (141) then introduced the gene encoding B subunit under control of its native promoter into another chromosomal locus, *hlyA*, along with a gene encoding resistance to Hg^{++}.

Construction of Bahr-3, Bang-3, Peru-3, Peru-5, and Peru-14

The research team directed by Mekalanos (142) have also prepared a series of interesting El Tor vaccine candidates generated from wild type El Tor strains, as summarized in Table 10. The virulence of wild type parent strains El Tor Inaba P27459 from Bangladesh and El Tor Ogawa E7946 from Bahrain have been established in volunteer studies (87,143). The various vaccine constructs have in common a deletion of the virulence cassette that contains *ctxAB*, *zot*, *ace*, and *cep*, as well as factors RS1 and attRS1, which are involved in site-specific and homologous recombination. All these live El Tor vaccine candidates except Peru-5 have an inactivation of *recA* as a consequence of the insertion into that gene of *ctxB* fused to a promoter from the heat shock gene *htpG*. In the Peru-5 strain, *ctxB* under its native promoter is inserted into *lacZ*. All five of these vaccine candidates have been evaluated in Phase 1 clinical trials.

Clinical Trials with CVD 110, Bahr-3, Bang-3, Peru-3, Peru-5, and Peru-14

Quite surprising and rather disappointing results were obtained when Phase 1 clinical trials were carried out with the new generation of El Tor candidate strains, particularly CVD 110 (141) and Bahr-3 (142). Candidate vaccine strains CVD 110 and Bahr-3, which were both derived from volunteer-tested wild type strain El Tor Ogawa E7946 (isolated from an epidemic in Bahrain), each caused mild to moderate diarrhea in most of the vaccinees, accompanied by headache, malaise, abdominal cramps, or low-grade fever (144–146). These are important findings because they demonstrate that *V. cholerae* O1 candidate vaccine strains that are derived from known virulent strains by deleting the capacity to express cholera toxin, ZOT, ACE, El Tor hemolysin, and CEP still retain the propensity to cause definite diarrheal illness. The pathophysiologic explanation for the residual diarrheogenic potential of these strains has yet to be elucidated. One possibility is that additional, so far unidentified, enterotoxins are elaborated *in vivo*. An alternative plausible explanation is that the act of adherence of vaccine strains to enterocytes in the proximal small intestine *per se* results in net secretion.

TABLE 10. *Attenuated El Tor vaccine candidates evaluated in Phase 1 and 2 clinical trials for safety and immunogenicity*

Vaccine strain	Wild type parent	Characteristics of strain	Dose (CFU)	Attack rate[a]	Mean total stool volume	Other adverse reactions[b]	Vibriocidal antibody sero-conversions[c]
CVD 104	In N16961	ΔctxAB, ΔhlyA	10^7	2/6	0.7 L		6/6
CVD 110	Og E7946	Deletion of *ctx* virulence cassette,[d] Δ*hlyA*::*mer*, *ctxB*	10^8	7/10	0.86 L	8/10	10/10
Bahr-3	Og E7946	Deletion of *ctx* virulence cassette,[d] Δ*recA*::$_{htp}$P-*ctxB*	2×10^6	2/3	3.1 L	3/3	3/3
Bang-3	In P27459	Deletion of *ctx* virulence cassette,[d] Δ*recA*::$_{htp}$P-*ctxB*	4×10^6	1/3	0.3 L	3/3	3/3
Peru-3	In C6709	Deletion of *ctx* virulence cassette,[d] Δ*recA*::$_{htp}$P-*ctxB*	4×10^6, 1×10^8	2/6	0.4 L	0/6	5/6
Peru-5	In C6709	Deletion of *ctx* virulence cassette,[d] *lacZ*::$_{ctx}$P-*ctxB*	4×10^6	1/3	0.5 L	2/3	3/3
Peru-14	In C6709	Motility-deficient mutant of Peru-3	2×10^6, 9×10^8	1/12	0.3 L	0/12	12/12

[a] Number with diarrhea/number of subjects vaccinated.
[b] Any combination of abdominal cramps, nausea, vomiting, or fever.
[c] Fourfold or greater rises in titer.
[d] This results in deletion of the region of the chromosome that contains *ctxAB*, *zot*, *ace*, *cep*, and *orfU*.

As summarized in Table 10, mild diarrhea, usually accompanied by other gastrointestinal adverse reactions, was also observed in volunteers who ingested a single dose of the Bang-3, Peru-3, and Peru-5 strains. The attack rate for such adverse reactions and the total diarrheal stool volumes (about 300–500 mL) were similar to what was observed with earlier generation vaccine candidate strain CVD 104 (109). Although dealing with small numbers of subjects, Taylor et al. noted that while two of six recipients of the Peru-3 strain developed mild diarrhea (400 mL stool volumes), they did not manifest the accompanying adverse reactions (such as abdominal cramps, malaise, nausea, or vomiting) that can thwart the acceptability of a vaccine. Mekalanos and colleagues thereupon selected a motility-deficient mutant of Peru-3, designated Peru-14, for further clinical evaluation. Of 12 volunteers given a dose of 2×10^6 or 9×10^8 CFU of Peru-14 with buffer, only one subject developed diarrhea and this was not accompanied by accessory gastrointestinal adverse reactions. Further studies with the Peru-14 strain are planned.

Four months after the Phase 1 clinical trial that assessed the safety and immunogenicity of the candidate vaccine strains, Taylor et al. (145,146) challenged eight volunteers who had received a dose of Peru-3 or Peru-5 with 1.8 $\times$ 10^6 CFU of wild type El Tor Inaba N16961. Three unimmunized volunteers served as controls. While diarrhea occurred in all three controls, seven of the eight vaccinees were protected (vaccine efficacy = 87%). The vaccinee who developed diarrhea had not developed a vibriocidal antibody response nor did that subject excrete the vaccine strain.

Vaccines to Prevent Cholera Caused by *V. cholerae* O139

Beginning in late 1992 and in early 1993 in India and Bangladesh, there appeared epidemic cholera caused by a *V. cholerae* strain of a serogroup other than O1. This new epidemic strain has been given the designation O139 (26,147). *Vibrio cholerae* O139 appears to have pandemic potential as cases of O139 cholera have been documented in Thailand, China, Malaysia, Pakistan, and Kazakhstan. Travel-associated cases have been observed in California and the United Kingdom. In cholera-endemic areas of Bangladesh, attack rates for O1 cholera are highest in young children and decrease in older age groups, indicative of acquisition of immunity from repeated antigenic contact. In contrast, attack rates for O139 cholera have been high in adults compared with children, suggesting that antibacterial and antitoxic immunity elicited by *V. cholerae* O1 does not provide cross-protection against *V. cholerae* O139. Recognizing that the early epidemiologic behavior of *V. cholerae* O139 may constitute the harbinger of an eighth pandemic of cholera (148), the World Health Organization, the U.S. National Institutes of Health, and other agencies have encouraged the accelerated development of vaccines against O139 cholera as a high priority.

Investigators at the University of Maryland documented the virulence of a prototype wild type O139 strain, AI1837, by means of experimental challenge studies in volunteers (149). The attack rates and severity of diarrhea following ingestion of *V. cholerae* O139 strain AI1837 with buffer resemble those observed in volunteers challenged with *V. cholerae* O1 of the El Tor biotype. Seven volunteers who experienced O139 cholera were rechallenged 2 months later, along with 13 naive control subjects. Eleven of 13 controls developed O139 cholera versus only one of seven "veterans" (14%) (who manifested only mild diarrhea) ($p = 0.004$) (149). Thus, in the volunteer model, an initial clinical infection caused by wild type *V. cholerae* O139 elicits immune responses that confer 83% protection against a challenge inoculum capable of causing a high attack rate in naive volunteers. These observations encourage the expectation that moderate levels of protective immunity may also be achieved by means of O139 vaccine candidates.

The scientific approaches being pursued to develop O139 vaccines follow the same strategies for developing vaccines against O1 cholera. Holmgren and associates at the University of Göteborg have prepared an oral nonliving antigen vaccine consisting of inactivated *V. cholerae* O139 in combination with B subunit of cholera toxin (150). In contrast, investigators at the Center for Vaccine Development of the University of Maryland and at Harvard University have constructed live oral vaccine candidates, as described in more detail below.

Live Oral Vaccines against O139 Cholera

Molecular biologists at the Center for Vaccine Development (151) engineered an attenuated *V. cholerae* O139 vaccine candidate by deleting from volunteer-tested wild type strain Al1837 the entire "virulence cassette" region of the chromosome that includes the genes encoding cholera toxin, ZOT, ACE, and the core encoded pili. A gene encoding resistance to Hg^{++} and the gene encoding B subunit under control of its native promoter were introduced into the chromosome in the *hlyA* locus, thereby inactivating that hemolysin/cytotoxin/enterotoxin as well. The resultant vaccine candidate is designated CVD 112. A further derivative, CVD 112-RM, harbors a deletion mutation in *recA*, thereby diminishing the ability of the vibrio to recombine foreign DNA into its chromosome. The *recA* mutation serves to diminish even further the already unlikely possibility of reacquisition of the virulence cassette by a recombinational event with wild type *V. cholerae* O1 or O139 (152). These O139 vaccine candidates, CVD 112 and CVD 112-RM, are entering Phase 1 clinical trials to assess their safety and immunogenicity.

Waldor and Mekalanos (153) have also constructed attenuated vaccine candidates, starting from wild type strain M010. An attenuated derivative designated Bengal-2 has deletion of the virulence cassette that contains *ctxAB, zot, ace,* and *cep* as well as RS1 and attRS1 (factors that are involved in virulence cassette site-specific and homologous recombination). A recombinant gene encoding B subunit under control of the promoter from heat shock gene *htpG* ($_{htpG}$P) was then inserted into *recA*, resulting in inactivation of that gene. The resultant strain has been designated Bengal-3. Waldor and Mekalanos (153) report that *in vitro* Bengal-3 elaborates 25-fold more B subunit than its wild type parent, MO10. Phase 1 clinical trials to assess the safety and immunogenicity of Bengal-3 are underway.

NEW VACCINES AGAINST SHIGELLA

Early Generations of *Shigella* Vaccines

Killed *Shigella* organisms inoculated parenterally stimulate high levels of circulating antibody but have failed to protect monkeys or humans from experimental or natural challenge (154–156). In contrast, attenuated strains of *Shigella* have been used successfully as live oral vaccines since the 1960s (157–165). Vaccine strains developed in the 1960s, including the streptomycin-dependent mutants of Mel et al. (157–163) and the T_{32} mutant of Istrati et al. (164,165), were shown to be safe and protective. The streptomycin-dependent *S. sonnei* and *S. flexneri* 2a were evaluated by the U.S. Public Health Service as possible interventions to assist in the control of endemic shigellosis in custodial institutions with encouraging results in one of two venues (161,162,166). Nevertheless, those vaccines suffer from certain drawbacks that limited their use and encouraged further research to develop improved vaccines. The drawbacks include the requirement for multiple doses, the large number of vaccine organisms required per dose (which affected production cost), the necessity to administer an annual booster to maintain protection (160), genetic reversions (167), lack of knowledge of the molecular basis of attenuation, and dose-related vomiting in a few percent of recipients of vaccine (usually after the first dose) (157–160,162,163). Extraordinary advances have been made in our knowledge of the molecular pathogenesis of *Shigella* infections, which have been applied to prepare several generations of new vaccine candidates. However, in practical terms, little progress has been made since the mid-1960s with respect to providing a well-tolerated multivalent *Shigella* vaccine that can confer protection long-term after administration of only one or two doses. Experience with a number of the most notable vaccine candidates will be summarized below.

Noninvasive *E. coli* Expressing *S. flexneri* 2a O Antigens

It can be fairly stated that the era of live vector bacterial vaccines was ushered in when Formal and co-workers (168) prepared a prototype *Shigella* vaccine by introducing the *his*$^+$ and *met*$^+$ loci of *S. flexneri* 2a into an *E. coli* strain by conjugal transfer; the former locus being closely linked with *S. flexneri* group 3,4 antigens and the latter closely linked with the type II serotype-specific antigen (168). The resultant "hybrid," strain PGAI 42-I-15, consisted of *E. coli* expressing smooth *S. flexneri* 2a group- and type-specific antigens (169).

When fed to adult volunteers in doses containing 3×10^{10} CFU, strain PGAI 42-I-15 was well tolerated, thereby meeting expectations of safety. Judged by seroconversion of O antibodies measured by hemagglutination (169), this live oral vaccine was notably less immunogenic than the streptomycin-dependent and mutant hybrid vaccines tested several years earlier (162,170). Most importantly, the hybrid vaccine failed to protect volunteers against experimental shigellosis in two separate challenge studies with wild type *S. flexneri* 2a (169). Results of these clinical studies led to the concept that live oral *Shigella* vaccines may have to exhibit some degree of epithelial cell invasiveness in order to elicit protective immunity, particularly if the immunization schedule were to involve only one or two doses.

Ty21a–*S. sonnei* Bivalent Hybrid Vaccine Strain 5076-1C

Considerable progress in the live vector vaccine concept was made when Formal et al. (66) prepared a candidate *Shigella sonnei* vaccine by inserting into attenuated *S. typhi* strain Ty21a the 120-MDa plasmid of *S. sonnei* that contains the genes encoding the *S. sonnei* O antigen. The resultant hybrid strain, 5076-1C, which expresses both the *S. typhi* and *S. sonnei* O antigens, was well tolerated and surprisingly immunogenic (68,171), and several lots of this vaccine conferred significant protection in experimental challenge studies in adult volunteers (68). Protection was particularly strong against more severe forms of shigellosis characterized by fever and dysentery. Disappointingly, because of lot-to-lot variation in protective efficacy, controlled field trials were not undertaken (70).

E. coli K-12 with the 140-MDa *S. flexneri* Invasiveness Plasmid, Chromosomal Genes for Expression of the Group- and Type-Specific Antigens of *S. flexneri* 2a, and a Mutation in *aroD*

Another intriguing approach taken by Formal et al. (172) to develop new *Shigella* vaccines was to introduce the chromosomal genes that code for the group- and type-specific O antigens of *S. flexneri* 2a into rough *E. coli* K-12, along with the 140-MDa plasmid of *S. flexneri* associated with epithelial cell invasiveness. This resulted in a modified *E. coli* K-12 that elaborates smooth *S. flexneri* 2a lipopolysaccharide O antigens and invades epithelial cells yet does not cause keratoconjunctivitis in the guinea pig eye test (a test of the strain's ability to invade epithelial cells and invoke an inflammatory process) and is safe for monkeys (172). In initial clinical trials in humans, however, a prototype vaccine (strain ECSf2a-1) was well tolerated at low dosage levels (10^7 and 10^7 CFU) but caused adverse reactions in 4 of 13 subjects who ingested vaccine doses containing 10^9 CFU; the untoward reactions included diarrhea, fever, and dysentery (173). Based on this experience, Newland et al. (174) further modified the construct by introducing a mutation in *aroD* rendering the strain (ECSf2a-2) auxotrophic for para-aminobenzoic acid, a substrate not available in sufficient quantity in

human tissues. It was anticipated that the *aroD* mutation would increase the degree of attenuation.

Extensive Phase 2 clinical trials have been carried out with ECSf2a-2 in several different healthy adult populations in the United States and in Israel to assess the safety and immunogenicity of ECSf2a-2. In healthy young adult civilians immunologically naive to *S. flexneri* 2a, vaccine doses containing 5.0×10^6 to 2.1×10^9 CFU were well tolerated. However, adverse reactions that included fever (as high as 39.1°C), mild diarrhea, or dysentery (scanty stools containing blood and mucus) occurred in two of four individuals who received a single 1.8×10^{10} CFU dose and in 4 of 23 individuals who were fed three doses of vaccine each containing 2.5×10^9 CFU (173). Gut-derived antibody secreting cells that elaborate IgA specific for *S. flexneri* 2a O antigen were detected in the peripheral blood of all 30 vaccinees who were tested and rises in serum O antibody (IgG or IgA) were recorded in 60% of the 38 vaccinees. Two experimental challenge studies were carried out in which vaccinees and a control group of unvaccinated volunteers were given wild type *S. flexneri* 2a to assess vaccine efficacy (173). Overall, 48% vaccine efficacy was observed in the first challenge study and 36% in the second.

ECSf2a-2 was evaluated in a large Phase 2 study in Israeli soldiers in a collaboration between the Walter Reed Army Institute of Research and the Department of Preventive Medicine of the Israel Defense Forces. Overall, the vaccine was well tolerated. However, following the first dose of vaccine, there was a significantly increased occurrence of mild adverse gastrointestinal reactions in recipients of vaccine versus those who got placebo. The protective efficacy of a three-dose regimen of ECSf2a-2 is currently being evaluated in a randomized, placebo-controlled field trial in a military population in Israel.

Mutants of *Shigella* Auxotrophic for Aromatic Amino Acids

The cardinal virulence properties of *Shigella* are its ability to invade epithelial cells of the distal ileum and colon and to multiply within the cytoplasm of those cells leading to cell death (175,176). Much of the pathology of shigellosis is consequent to this epithelial damage. In order to be able to proliferate within enterocytes and colonocytes, *Shigella* organisms possess a biosynthesis system for aromatic compounds, which allows them to synthesize para-aminobenzoic acid (PABA), as well as tryptophane, phenylalanine, and tyrosine, from chorismic acid, the end product of the biosynthesis pathway. PABA, which is necessary for growth, is not available in sufficient quantity in human tissues.

Recognizing that some strains of *S. typhimurium* (41,46), *S. dublin* (177), and *S. typhi* (53,178) have been successfully attenuated by means of mutations in the aromatic pathway, Lindberg et al. (179–182) prepared analogous auxotrophic strains of *Shigella* for evaluation as potential live oral vaccines. A prototype strain of serotype *S. flexneri* Y was produced by transducing into *Shigella* a Tn10-inactivated *aroD* from *E. coli*, resulting in strain

Sfl114 (179,180); the tetracycline resistance gene encoded by Tn10 renders Sfl114 resistant. Although this candidate vaccine strain invaded monolayers of HEp-2 cells in tissue culture, it exhibited a greatly diminished plaque formation. More importantly, Sfl114 did not cause keratoconjunctivitis when inoculated into the conjunctival sac of guinea pigs and the vaccine strain was safe and protective in monkeys challenged experimentally (182). Mild intestinal discomfort was reported in 3 of 25 Vietnamese subjects given 10^9 CFU and in 13 of 24 (54%) fed 10^{10} CFU of Sfl114 vaccine. These clinical data are difficult to interpret because the adult subjects come from an area where *S. flexneri* is endemic and they had serological evidence of prior exposure.

Karnell et al. (183) developed a further derivative, Sfl124, by selecting a tetracycline-sensitive mutant that lost the Tn10. Moreover, illegitimate excision of the transposon resulted in a large deletion in *aroD*. Sfl124 exhibited the same properties of attenuation as its parent in tissue culture and in the guinea pig eye test. Colonoscopy of monkeys following ingestion of an initial high dose of Sfl124 revealed evidence of mild (but definite) inflammation of the intestinal mucosa. Two of 21 Swedish volunteers who ingested one or three doses of vaccine containing 2×10^9 CFU developed mild diarrhea (184). It became increasingly difficult to interpret clinical results with Sfl124 and Sfl114 when it became apparent from clinical studies carried out at the Center for Vaccine Development that the putative wild type *S. flexneri* Y parent strain from which the vaccine strains were derived was only minimally pathogenic in volunteers.

In order to assess clearly the effect of *aro* mutations on a *Shigella* strain of well-established virulence, Verma et al. (181) introduced *aroD* and *aroA* deletion mutations into *S. flexneri* 2a strain 2457T. This wild type strain is the standard challenge strain used to induce experimental shigellosis in monkeys and in volunteers (173,185). Mutants harboring single deletions in *aroA* (this strain also had a mutation in *serC*) or *aroD* and an *aroA,aroD* double mutant (strain 1092) were all attenuated compared to the wild type parent, as demonstrated in tissue culture assays and guinea pig eye tests. The *aroD* mutant was protective in orally immunized monkeys (186). The *aroA* mutant and the *aroA,aroD* double mutant provided orally immunized guinea pigs little protection against conjunctival challenge with 10^8 CFU of the wild type *S. flexneri* parent strain 2457T (186). However, the single *aroD* mutant strain conferred upon guinea pigs a moderate level of protection against a similar challenge (186).

In adult Swedish volunteers, doses of 10^8 CFU of the *aroD S. flexneri* 2a mutant were well tolerated. However, when volunteers were given a 10^9 CFU dose, four of nine developed mild diarrhea and fever (187). The basis of these adverse reactions is not entirely clear. The fever and diarrhea may be the consequence of cytokines released following invasion of the intestinal mucosa (188); alternatively, the mild diarrhea may be caused by secretagogues elaborated by the polymorphonuclear neutrophilic leukocytes (189,190) that accompany the mild inflammatory response elicited by this epithelial cell invasive vaccine or by recently discovered enterotoxins (191).

iuc,icsA Mutants

In the 1960s, it was recognized that the xylose rhamnose region of the *S. flexneri* chromosome played a role in virulence. Formal et al. (192) were able to attenuate the intracellular growth of *S. flexneri* 2a by conjugal transfer into *Shigella* of the xylose rhamnose region of *E. coli*. In later years it was shown that this chromosomal region of *Shigella* contained the *iucABCD* operon responsible for production of the hydroxamate siderophore aerobactin (175) and *iutA*, which encodes the 76-kDa receptor protein located on the bacterial outer membrane (193). *iuc* Mutants of *S. flexneri* remain invasive for epithelial cells and their growth within such cells resembles wild type *Shigella* (194). In contrast, Nassif et al. (194) obtained evidence that *iuc* mutants are attenuated in their capacity to cause keratoconjunctivitis in guinea pigs and to cause fluid accumulation after inoculation into the lumen of rabbit ileal loops; the attenuation observed was dose dependent. It thus appears that *iuc* mutants are demonstrably limited in their capacity to grow in extracellular environments but once they attain an intracellular niche they appear able to scavenge sufficient iron to maintain normal bacterial growth.

Located on the large invasiveness plasmid of *Shigella* is *virG* (also known as *icsA*), a gene that encodes a 120-kDa protein (so-called VirG or IcsA) involved in intracellular spread of the bacteria as well as cell to cell spread (195–199). This protein is secreted as a 95-kDa protein in the outer membrane, following a carboxy terminal cleavage of the 120-kDa moiety.

Sansonetti and co-investigators (200,201) have engineered candidate *S. flexneri* vaccine candidate strains by introducing mutations in *iuc*, *iut*, and *icsA*. A prototype *iuc,icsA* double mutant of this variety, *S. flexneri* 5 strain SC5700, did not cause diarrhea when fed to monkeys in does of 5×10^{10} CFU (200,201). Candidates of this variety are currently entering preliminary clinical trials to assess their safety and immunogenicity. These investigators are also exploring the use of other putatively attenuating mutations, such as one (*ompB*) that interferes with the bacteria's ability to perform osmoregulation, in conjunction with mutations in *icsA* in order to achieve vaccine candidates with the proper balance of safety and immunogenicity (202). In rhesus monkeys an *icsA,ompB* double mutant strain was well tolerated without inflammatory changes (202).

Since recombinant mutations in *virG* (*icsA*) are being discussed in the context of development of vaccine strains, it is worth noting that Venkatesan et al. (203) recently used molecular techniques to characterize the T_{32} strain of *S. flexneri* 2a, which was developed by Istrati et al. (164) in the 1960s and was used extensively in Rumania as a live oral vaccine. Venkatesan et al. (203) show that the large plasmid present in noninvasive strain T_{32} has undergone a spontaneous deletion of *virG*, *ipaBCDA*, and *invA*.

Double Mutant Vaccine Strains with Inactivations in *aroA* and *virG*

Noriega et al. (204) have constructed a double mutant of wild type *S. flexneri* 2a strain 2457T with precise deletion mutations in chromosomal gene *aroA* and in plasmid gene *virG*. This double mutant strain is attenuated in guinea pigs. Moreover, by inoculating very high doses into the conjunctival sac of guinea pigs they were able to show that the *aroA,virG* double mutant is significantly more attenuated in that animal model than an *aroA* strain (representing an intermediate in construction of the double mutant). Two oral immunizations with the *aroA,virG* double mutant conferred on guinea pigs significant protection against keratoconjunctivitis when they were challenged in the conjunctival sac with a dose of wild type *S. flexneri* 2a that caused 100% purulent keratoconjunctivitis in the control animals. Clinical trials with vaccine candidate are commencing in 1994.

Vaccines Against Shiga Dysentery

Because of the severe clinical syndrome caused by *S. dysenteriae* 1 (Shiga's bacillus), its propensity for pandemic spread, and its resistance to most clinically relevant antibiotics, a vaccine to prevent Shiga dysentery is a high priority. Several vaccine candidates are in preparation, including live oral vaccines. Attenuated *S. dysenteriae* 1 strains under development have deletions in *stxA,* which encodes the A subunit of Shiga toxin; in addition to other attenuating mutations such as deletions in *aro* and *virG* (201), such mutants continue to express the nontoxic B subunit. The elucidation of the intricacies of *S. dysenteriae* 1 O antigen expression and cloning of the genes necessary for O antigen and for the B subunit of Shiga toxin also make it possible to construct Shiga vaccines using the live vector approach (205–209).

Modern Parenteral Vaccines

O Polysaccharide–Carrier Protein Conjugate Vaccines

Robbins and co-investigators (210,211) have developed candidate parenteral *Shigella* vaccines consisting of the O polysaccharide conjugated to carrier proteins such as tetanus toxoid. They hypothesize that the reason that parenteral, killed, whole-cell *Shigella* vaccines were not protective is that they likely stimulated IgM O antibodies (154–156), whereas the conjugate vaccines elicit IgG O antibodies. Robbins contends that IgG but not IgM antibodies are protective. Clinical trials to assess the safety and immunogenicity of *S. flexneri* 2a and *S. sonnei* conjugate vaccines are in progress.

Ribosomal Vaccines

Levenson et al. (212–214) have prepared purified ribosomal vaccines against *S. sonnei* that are administered by subcutaneous inoculation. In monkeys one or two inoculations of the ribosomal vaccines containing low (600 μg) or high (3000–5000 μg) dosages were generally well tolerated although some local reactions at the site of inoculation were observed in monkeys that received the high dosages. In challenge studies with wild type *S. sonnei* carried out 4 to 22 weeks after immunization, a high level of protection was recorded. Overall, 89% protective efficacy was observed with the ribosomal vaccines in monkey studies.

In guinea pig challenge studies with *S. sonnei* and *S. flexneri* ribosomal vaccines, the vaccine protected only against wild type challenge with the homologous serotype. Such serogroup and serotype specificity is the same as has been observed with various live oral vaccines (158–161), as well as with immunity elicited by wild type infection (185,215). Levenson et al. believe that their vaccine consists of the O polysaccharide complexed to ribosomal protein, thereby having certain similarities to the O-polysaccharide–protein conjugate vaccines being developed by Robbins and associates. Heretofore, only one clinical trial in humans has been carried out with the ribosomal vaccine wherein subcutaneous doses of 100 or 200 μg were well tolerated by all subjects.

VACCINES AGAINST ENTEROTOXIGENIC *E. COLI*

Antigenic Diversity Among Human ETEC Pathogens

Analysis of the antigenic structure of enterotoxigenic *E. coli* (ETEC) strains from an endemic area shows many different O:H serotypes, at least ten distinct antigenic types of fimbrial colonization factors (CFA/I, CS1 to CS7, CS17, PCF O20, PCF O159:H4, and PCF O166 fimbriae), and three different toxin phenotypes (LT, ST, and LT/ST) (1,2,4,216–219). Most authorities agree that in order to provide broad spectrum protection against ETEC infections for humans, a vaccine will have to contain fimbrial antigens representative of the most prevalent ETEC pathogens (216–219). The most common fimbrial colonization factors of human ETEC are colonization factor antigen I (CFA/I), the CFA/II family, and the CFA/IV family of antigens. CFA/I is a single antigenic moiety. Coli surface antigens 1 (CS1), 2 (CS2), and 3 (CS3) constitute the CFA/II family of antigens (220–222). All CFA/II strains express CS3, either alone or in conjunction with CS1 or CS2. CS4, CS5, and CS6 comprise the CFA/IV family of antigens (223). All CFA/IV strains express CS6, either alone or in conjunction with CS4 or CS5. Other fimbrial colonization factors such as PCF O159, PCF O166, PCF O20, CS7, and CS17 are much less frequent (224–227). Carriage of the genes to express a particular fimbrial colonization factor is closely correlated with O:H serotype and with toxin phenotype (219).

Analysis of ETEC isolates from diverse geographic areas shows that CFA/I and CS1-6 are found on the majority of isolates (Table 11). About 90% of isolates that elaborate both heat-labile and heat-stable enterotoxins (LT and ST, respectively) express these CFAs, while they are

TABLE 11. *Prevalence of major fimbrial colonization factor antigens among enterotoxigenic* E. coli *isolates from adults with traveler's diarrhea and from children with diarrhea in less developed countries*

Report	Geographic source	Enterotoxin profile	Number of isolates	Percentage of isolates expressing fimbrial antigens		
				CFA/I	CFA/II	CFA/IV
Traveler's diarrhea						
Levine et al., 1983	Morocco, Honduras, Kenya, Zaire	All	36	11.1	13.9	NT
		LT/ST	10	30.0	40.0	NT
		ST	12	8.3	0.0	NT
		LT	14	0.0	0.0	NT
Wolf et al., 1993	Saudi Arabia, Egypt	All	189	11.6	33.9	30.7
		LT/ST	84	15.5	64.3	4.8
		ST	73	12.3	8.2	43.8
		LT	32	0.0	6.3	21.9
Pediatric diarrhea						
Gothefors et al., 1985	Bangladesh	All	67	56.7	17.9	NT
		LT/ST	43	67.4	25.6	NT
		ST	18	50.0	5.6	NT
		LT	6	0.0	0.0	NT
Binsztein et al., 1991	Argentina	All	109	44.4	11.9	17.4
		LT/ST	15	0.0	80.0	0.0
		ST	71	35.2	1.4	26.8
		LT	23	0.0	0.0	0.0
Levine et al., 1993	Chile	All	93	11.8	26.9	5.4
		LT/ST	19	0.0	100	0.0
		ST	28	39.3	0.0	17.9
		LT	46	0.0	13.0	0.0

NT, not tested.

found on about 60% of ST-only strains. Generally, less than 10% of LT-only strains bear these CFAs. Thus, if a multivalent ETEC vaccine contained just CFA/I and CS1-6, it could theoretically provide protection against approximately 50% to 80% of ETEC strains in most geographic areas (Table 11). If an LT toxoid (such as B subunit of LT) were included, and if such a vaccine were well tolerated and efficacious, the multivalent vaccine might provide relatively broad protection against about 80% to 90% of ETEC strains worldwide. Inclusion of the less frequent fimbrial antigens (e.g., PCF O159, PCF O166, CS17) in the multivalent vaccine (that would also include LT B) might expand the potential spectrum of coverage to greater than 90% of ETEC strains.

Infection-Derived Immunity

Despite the antigenic heterogeneity of ETEC, evidence from both volunteer studies and from epidemiological surveys shows that prior infection with enterotoxigenic *E. coli* confers immunity (228–231). A review of these studies leads to the conclusion that in endemic areas multiple infections with distinct strains bearing different fimbrial colonization factor antigens and of different toxin phenotypes must occur in order for broad spectrum immunity to be elicited.

Volunteer Studies

Studies in a volunteer model of ETEC clearly show that an initial clinical infection elicits significant protection

against homologous rechallenge but not against challenge with an ETEC strain expressing heterologous surface antigens (229,232).

Epidemiologic Studies

In less developed countries, infants and young children experience up to three separate clinical ETEC infections per year during the first 3 years of life (1,2,4,21), after which the incidence of ETEC diarrhea drastically falls (230). It is obvious that this lower incidence in older individuals is due to acquired immunity rather than to other age-related host factors, since adult travelers from industrialized countries who visit less developed countries where ETEC pediatric diarrhea is endemic suffer high attack rates of ETEC travelers' diarrhea (6–8). Analysis of the antigenic make-up of the strains that cause endemic pediatric diarrhea and those that cause traveler's diarrhea, including O:H serotypes and fimbrial antigenic types reveals that they are the same (4,219,233–236). Travelers from industrialized countries who remain in less developed countries for at least a year and travelers who arrive from other less developed countries suffer significantly lower incidence rates of ETEC diarrhea than newly arrived travelers from industrialized countries (231). These data provide further support for the concept of acquired immunity.

A few prospective epidemiologic field studies provide direct evidence that acquired immunity is largely directed at fimbrial colonization factors of ETEC (21). However, most epidemiologic data provide only indirect evidence (237).

Rabbit Model of Human ETEC Infection

In a rabbit model of ETEC infection followed by experimental challenge by the reversible intestinal tie adult rabbit diarrhea (RITARD) method that is used to study immunity (238), it is apparent that the protective immunity of prior infection is directed at fimbrial CFAs (239,240).

Immune Responses Observed

Protection derived from wild type infections is believed to be mediated by SIgA antibody directed primarily against fimbrial colonization factors and to a lesser extent against LT; ST, which is a small peptide, does not stimulate neutralizing ST antitoxin following natural infection. In the course of natural infection (241,242), as well as in experimental challenge of volunteers (220,228,243), humans mount intestinal SIgA and serum IgG antibody responses to the CFAs expressed by the ETEC strain responsible for diarrhea.

Multiple Strategies to Develop ETEC Vaccines

Various investigators have taken distinct approaches in attempting to develop ETEC vaccines that will give broad spectrum immunity. The vaccine candidates can be divided into nonliving antigen categories and live oral vaccines. The various approaches will be summarized below.

Passive Protection with Oral Immunoglobulin

Tacket et al. (243) immunized cows with ETEC strains expressing different fimbrial antigens including CFA/I. A bovine immunoglobulin concentrate was prepared from the milk of the cows. In a randomized, placebo-controlled, double-blind clinical trial in volunteers, all ten subjects who received the ETEC milk immunoglobulin concentrate were completely protected against challenge with a wild type ETEC strain that expresses CFA/I, LT, and ST and that caused diarrhea in 90% of the ten volunteers that got the control preparation. Although passive protection is neither practical nor economical for long-term immunoprophylaxis, the results reported by Tacket et al. (243) generate optimism for the concept of prevention of ETEC diarrhea. If active immunization with oral vaccines can succeed in eliciting high titers of intestinal antibody, it may be possible to confer protection that will be more enduring.

Nonliving Antigen Vaccines

LT/ST Toxoids

Klipstein et al. (244) evaluated an oral toxoid vaccine consisting of synthetic ST cross-linked to a synthetic pep-

tide containing the immunodominant epitope of human LT (LTh). Three spaced doses of this oral toxoid were well tolerated by volunteers and stimulated anti-ST and anti-LT in serum and intestinal fluid. The efficacy of this or other synthetic peptide toxoid vaccines has not yet been determined in experimental challenges or in field trials.

The killed whole vibrio/B subunit combination oral vaccine against cholera recently field-tested in Bangladesh provided significant protection against diarrhea due to LT-producing *E. coli,* including both LT and LT/ST strains, in the initial 3 months following vaccination (245). This short-lived protection was apparently based on the strong antigenic similarity between LT and cholera toxin. Short-term protection against traveler's diarrhea caused by LT-producing ETEC was also observed in a randomized, placebo-controlled, double-blind trial carried out among Finnish travelers to Morocco, who were immunized with the combination whole vibrio/B subunit vaccine (246).

Purified Colonization Factor Fimbriae as Vaccines

De la Cabada et al. (247) immunized rabbits orally with multiple doses of purified CFA/I fimbriae. Significant protection was observed when the rabbits were then challenged by the modified RITARD model (238).

Two groups of investigators have explored the immunogenicity and efficacy in humans of ETEC vaccines based on purified fimbriae to elicit anti-colonization immunity. Evans et al. (248) administered a combination of purified CFA/I and CFA/II (the precise CS antigens that they used were not identified) fimbriae to volunteers. Four doses, each containing 1 mg of CFA/I and 1 mg of CFA/II, were given by mouth in a glass of milk on consecutive days; on the 11th and 17th day after primary immunization a booster dose containing 2 mg of CFA/I and 2 mg of CFA/II fimbriae was administered. Two of 11 vaccinees manifested significant rises in CFA/I antibody in serum and two others had rises in serum antibody to CFA/II fimbriae. None manifested rises in SIgA anti-fimbrial antibody in saliva (measured as a convenient proxy in place of intestinal antibody). Some of these vaccinees were challenged with pathogenic ETEC expressing CFA/I and others with ETEC bearing CFA/II; in neither instance were the vaccinees significantly protected. An additional group of eight volunteers with no detectable anti-CFA/I antibody prevaccination were given a single 50-μg subcutaneous dose of fimbriae followed by two 0.5-mg oral boosters given 1 week apart. Using this regimen of immunization, Evans et al. (248) detected significant rises in intestinal IgA anti-CFA/I in four vaccinees (50%). These investigators noted that CFA fimbriae were destroyed by human gastric contents containing pepsin.

Levine et al. (249) showed that application of multiple 2.0-mg doses of a CFA/II (CS1 and CS3) purified fimbriae vaccine to the mucosal surface of an exteriorized Thirty-Vella intestinal loop of a rabbit elicited impressive titers of SIgA anti-fimbrial antibody in intestinal washes. They then immunized intact adult rabbits orally with multiple doses of the purified CS1/CS3 fimbriae vaccine given with NaHCO₃. When these rabbits were challenged by the RITARD method, significant protection was not observed (249).

Subsequently, Levine et al. (249,250) immunized healthy adult volunteers with multiple oral doses of the purified CS1/CS3 fimbriae vaccine. Despite pretreatment with cimetidine to diminish gastric acid secretion and administration of the vaccine with 2.0 g of NaHCO₃ to neutralize gastric acid, serum and intestinal SIgA antibodies were detected in only two of ten vaccinees (249,250). Shortly thereafter, Schmidt et al. (251) demonstrated that gastric juice, even when neutralized to pH 7.0, adversely affected the antigenicity of this fimbrial vaccine. Based on this observation, Levine et al. (250) investigated the immunogenicity of the purified CS1/CS3 fimbriae vaccine when it was administered by direct instillation into the small intestine (via an intestinal tube), thereby bypassing the stomach. Using this regimen, significant rises in SIgA intestinal anti-fimbrial antibody were recorded in four of five vaccinees; this represents a significantly higher seroconversion rate than occurred in the group that was vaccinated orally (of whom only two of ten seroconverted) (p = 0.05, single tail Fisher's exact test).

Polylactide–Polyglycolide Microspheres and Other Antigen Delivery Systems

Based on the above studies, it became apparent that more effective and innovative ways would have to be devised to deliver soluble protein antigens that are sensitive to gastric juice into the small intestine without them suffering the ravages of the gastric contents. The use of various microspheres and biodegradable polymers is being explored as a possible solution to this problem (252,253). Edelman et al. (253) incorporated purified CFA/I fimbriae into biodegradable polymer microspheres composed of poly (D,L-lactide–coglycolide). Rabbits were immunized orally with these microspheres or with native purified CFA/I. Only rabbits immunized with the CFA/I delivered in microspheres exhibited high titers of serum CFA/I antibody, suggesting that the microspheres protected the fimbriae from the deleterious effects of gastric juice.

Reid et al. (252) incorporated the CFA/II (CS1/CS3) fimbrial vaccine used by Levine et al. (220,250) into poly (D,L-lactide–coglycolide) microspheres. Preliminary clinical trials are underway to investigate the utility of this antigen delivery system in humans. A feasibility clinical trial was carried out in volunteers by Tacket et al. (254), who administered CS1/CS3 purified fimbriae vaccine in microspheres directly via intestinal tube. The vaccine was well tolerated by ten subjects. Gut-derived trafficking IgA antibody secreting cells that make specific antibody when stimulated by CS1/CS3 antigen were detected in peripheral blood in five volunteers and five developed significant rises in jejunal fluid SIgA antibody to CS1/CS3 fimbrial antigen.

Formalin-Inactivated Whole-Cell Vaccine

To explore the safety, immunogenicity, and efficacy of a simple-to-prepare, killed, whole-cell vaccine, Tacket et al. (unpublished data) administered formalin-inactivated fimbriated ETEC to volunteers. The vaccine was prepared from E. coli strain E1392-75-2A, an O6:H16 biotype A strain that expresses CS1 and CS3 fimbriae but does not elaborate LT or ST (249,250,255). When used previously as a live oral vaccine (vide infra) (249,250,255), a single dose of E1392-75-2A provided significant protection to volunteers against experimental challenge with an LT/ST ETEC strain of serotype O139:H28 that expresses CS1 and CS3. E1392-75-2A bacteria were formalin-inactivated by collaborating investigators at the U.S. Army Vaccine Production Facility of the Walter Reed Army Institute of Research at Forest Glen, Maryland. Electron microscopy documented that the E1392-75-2A bacteria in the vaccine suspension were fimbriated (217). In an initial study, three doses of vaccine (each containing 5×10^{10} inactivated bacteria) with NaHCO₃ were given at 2-week intervals to nine volunteers. Significant rises in CFA antibody were detected in serum in two of nine vaccinees, while four of nine had rises in intestinal SIgA anti-fimbrial antibody. A small challenge study was carried out in which four vaccinees and ten controls were challenged with pathogenic ETEC strain E24377A (O139:H28, CS1, CS3, LT/ST). No evidence of protection was detected in this small preliminary study; diarrhea occurred in two of four vaccinees and in six of ten controls.

Oral Whole-Cell Vaccine Inactivated by Treatment with Colicin

Evans et al. (256,257) discovered that inactivation of ETEC strain H10407 (O78:H11, CFA/I, LT⁺/ST⁺) by treatment of cultures with colicin E2 (derived from E. coli strain E-279) results in loss of viability of the bacterial cells by in situ digestion of DNA without damage to the surface antigens such as fimbrial colonization factors. These investigators have shown that immunization of volunteers with several oral doses of the colicin-inactivated bacteria significantly protected the vaccinees against challenge with viable ETEC. Groups of volunteers were given, with NaHCO₃ buffer, a priming dose containing 3×10^{10} colicin-inactivated H10407 bacteria. One month later an identical booster dose was given. The colicin-inactivated vaccine was well tolerated and the majority of vaccinees manifested significant rises in intestinal SIgA antibody to both CFA/I and to LT. A vaccine efficacy level of 75% was observed when the vaccinees and controls were challenged with viable, pathogenic ETEC of the homologous strain (H10407, O78:H11, LT⁺/ST⁺, CFA/I) or a heterologous serotype expressing CFA/I (O63:H⁻, CFA/I, LT⁺/ST⁺).

Inactivated Whole Bacterial Cells Plus Toxoid

Based on their experiences with a combination nonliving oral cholera vaccine consisting of the B subunit of cholera toxin given along with inactivated *V. cholerae* O1 of different serotypes and biotypes, Svennerholm et al. (218,258) are developing an analogous vaccine to prevent ETEC diarrhea. Studies by these investigators in a rabbit model have shown that a combination vaccine that stimulates both antibacterial and antitoxic immunity confers greater protection against ETEC than vaccines that stimulate only one or the other type of immunity (240).

In the combination vaccine proposed by these investigators, formalin-inactivated bacteria are used to stimulate antibacterial immunity, while the B subunit of LT elicits anti-LT immunity. If a highly immunogenic ST toxoid were to be developed, it might also be included (259). To achieve broad spectrum protection, the bacterial organisms used in the vaccine include strains of different O:H serotypes expressing the most important fimbrial colonization factor antigens. Studies of the safety and immunogenicity of this vaccine candidate are ongoing.

Live Oral Vaccines

Attenuated E. coli *as Live Oral Vaccines Against ETEC*

The *E. coli* E1392-75-2A is a CFA/II-positive mutant that was derived in the Central Public Health Laboratory, Colindale, wherein the genes encoding LT and ST spontaneously deleted from the CFA/II plasmid. Consequently, E1392-75-2A, which expresses CS1 and CS3 fimbrial antigens, is negative when tested with toxin assays and gene probes for LT and ST. Levine et al. (219,249,250,255) utilized strain E1392-75-2A to explore fundamental questions of anticolonization immunity in the absence of antitoxic immunity. All volunteers who were fed 1×10^{10} to 5×10^{10} CFU doses of strain E1392-75-2A developed significant rises in intestinal fluid SIgA antibody to CS1 and CS3 fimbriae. The GMT of anti-fimbrial CS1 and CS3 SIgA antibody in these volunteers was tenfold higher than the peak postvaccination GMT of volunteers who received enteral immunization with multiple doses of purified CS1 and CS3 fimbriae.

A group of vaccinees, who were immunized with a single 5×10^{10} CFU dose of E1392-75-2A with $NaHCO_3$ were challenged 1 month later, along with unimmunized control volunteers. The pathogenic ETEC challenge strain used, E24377A, was of heterologous serotype O139:H28, possessed CS1 and CS3, and elaborated LT and ST. The vaccinees were significantly protected ($p <$ 0.005, 75% vaccine efficacy) against ETEC diarrhea (219). By means of bacteriological studies, it was shown that anticolonization immunity was responsible for the protection. In the challenge study, all participants, both vaccinees and unimmunized controls, excreted the ETEC challenge strain and there was no difference between the groups in the mean number of ETEC per gram of stool. In contrast, a striking difference was found in duodenal cultures that monitored colonization of the proximal small intestine, the critical site of ETEC–host interaction. The challenge strain was recovered from duodenal cultures of five of six controls (mean 7×10^3 CFU/mL) versus only 1 of 12 vaccinees (10^1 CFU/mL) ($p < 0.004$). Levine et

al. (219) interpreted these results to mean that SIgA anti-CS1 and anti-CS3 fimbrial antibody in the proximal intestine stimulated by the live oral vaccine prevented challenge ETEC from colonizing the proximal small intestine. Since the immune response was not bactericidal, the ETEC organisms were carried by peristalsis to the large intestine, where they could colonize without causing diarrheal illness.

While the E1392-75-2A strain provided invaluable information when used as a prototype live oral vaccine, it caused mild diarrhea in approximately 15% of the recipients who ingested it, an unacceptable rate of adverse reactions. Therefore research is ongoing to prepare a live oral ETEC vaccine that will be acceptably immunogenic and efficacious without causing mild diarrhea or other adverse reactions. An approach being pursued by investigators at the Center for Vaccine Development of the University of Maryland involves a live oral vaccine containing a mixture of strains modified from the same background strain that collectively express all the important fimbrial colonization factors. In addition, this live vaccine will elaborate LT B.

Attenuated Salmonella *Strains Expressing ETEC Antigens*

Because of their intimate interaction with and prolonged residence within the gut-associated lymphoid tissue, attenuated *Salmonella* make extremely attractive live vectors to express foreign genes encoding protective antigens of other bacterial enteropathogens and to deliver those antigens to the human immune system (64,65). Hone et al. (260) showed that genes encoding the structural subunit of K88 colonization factor fimbriae of porcine ETEC could be integrated into the chromosome of a *galE S. typhimurium* mutant, leading to production of K88 fimbriae by the *Salmonella*. Yamamoto et al. (261) introduced a CFA/I-ST plasmid into attenuated *S. typhi* strain Ty21a and demonstrated that the *Salmonella* could express *E. coli* CFA/I fimbriae.

A new generation of attenuated *S. typhi* strains has appeared that is based on mutations in genes encoding enzymes critical for the aromatic amino acid biosynthesis pathway (38,40,178). CVD 908 is an Δ*aroC*, Δ*aroD* attenuated *S. typhi* recombinant vaccine strain that has proved to be well tolerated and highly immunogenic using a single-dose immunization schedule in Phase 1 clinical trials (53). Cassettes containing the multiple cloned genes necessary for expression of CFA/I fimbriae have been introduced into CVD 908 on plasmids as well as integrated into the chromosome (262,263). In both instances, CVD 908 has expressed CFA/I fimbriae. Similarly, the CS3 operon has been introduced into CVD 908 both integrated into the *aroC* locus of the chromosome and on a plasmid. Lastly, Giron et al. (263) succeeded in simultaneously expressing both CS3 and CFA/I in the same CVD 908 strain. Thus, by means of recombinant DNA technology, it has been possible to construct a multivalent fimbrial vaccine strain expressing two fimbrial antigens that are never found together in the same bacterial strain in nature.

Considerable progress is being made toward development of a *Salmonella*-based live vector vaccine in which the important fimbrial colonization factor antigens are expressed along with B subunit of LT (216,217). Other non-invasive attenuated bacterial strains are also attractive as potential live vectors to express fimbriae, including attenuated *V. cholerae* strain CVD 103-HgR (83,264).

Attenuated Shigella Strains Expressing ETEC Antigens

In another variation of the live vector vaccine concept, Noriega et al. have introduced plasmids encoding CFA/I fimbriae and CS3 fibrillae (the common antigen of the CFA/II family) into an attenuated *aroA,virG* double mutant strain of *S. flexneri* 2a (204a). These investigators achieved simultaneous coexpression of the two fimbrial antigens in the attenuated *Shigella* strain, raising the prospect of eventually attaining a combined multivalent vaccine against *Shigella* and ETEC.

VACCINES AGAINST ENTEROPATHOGENIC E. COLI

Enteropathogenic *E. coli* (EPEC) was the first category of *E. coli* to be incriminated as a cause of diarrhea, beginning in the 1940s (265). Originally, they were defined only by their O:H serotypes, and somewhat later by serotype and lack of LT and ST production and absence of *Shigella*-like invasiveness properties (265). Even without knowing the virulence properties involved in pathogenesis of EPEC infections or of the immune responses that might be protective, during the late 1960s and early 1970s investigators in Germany and Hungary prepared candidate vaccines. During this period, nosocomial infection was a serious problem for very young infants admitted to hospital, with strains of serogroups O55 and O111 being the predominant pathogens. The oral vaccines clinically tested in Eastern Europe and shown to be well tolerated include a sodium deoxycholate Boivin extract prepared from O55 and O111 strains (266); a deoxycholate Boivin preparation from O111, O55, and O86 strains (267,268); formalin-inactivated O111, O55, and O86 whole bacteria (267); and attenuated streptomycin-dependent O111 organisms (269).

The efficacy of the formalin-inactivated and streptomycin-dependent vaccines was not evaluated in controlled field trials. The Boivin extract vaccines had some investigation of their efficacy, which demonstrated variable success. Further studies with these vaccines were abandoned.

In recent years the virulence properties of EPEC have been elucidated in studies of molecular pathogenesis (219,270). They possess a chromosomal gene, *eaeA*, that encodes a 94-kDa protein, intimin, that is associated with intimate adherence to the cell membranes of enterocytes (271). EPEC organisms harbor a 55- to 65-MDa virulence plasmid (the EPEC adherence factor plasmid) that encodes a gene that regulates expression of the 94-kDa protein (219,270,271). This plasmid also encodes the genes

necessary for expression of bundle forming pili (BFP), which constitute a preliminary adherence factor of EPEC that functions prior to the intimate adherence step mediated by the 94-kDa protein intimin (272). The BFP of EPEC are type IV pili and are attractive as potential immunogens. It is hypothesized that stimulation of intestinal SIgA antibodies to BFP by an immunogenic vaccine might impede the characteristic localized attachment of EPEC, thereby preventing clinical illness.

There exist *E. coli* organisms analogous to EPEC that constitute natural diarrheal pathogens of juvenile rabbits (273,274). Study of the prototype EPEC-like pathogen of rabbits, strain RDEC-1, has yielded insights on the pathogenesis of and immunity to human EPEC (273,274). RDEC-1 results in intimate attachment and effacement of enterocyte membranes identical to the lesions of EPEC. RDEC-1 also harbors a plasmid that encodes a fimbrial colonization factor, AF/R1 pili (275). McQueen et al. (276) incorporated the AF/R1 pilus adhesin of strain RDEC-1 into poly (D,L-lactide–coglycolide) microspheres and immunized rabbits with the microspheres. Following challenge with wild type *E. coli* RDEC-1, vaccinated rabbits were significantly protected from illness and weight loss, compared with unimmunized control rabbits (276). By analogy, these animal data support the concept of a BFP-based vaccine to prevent EPEC diarrhea in humans.

Another approach to develop a vaccine against EPEC might rely on strains of EPEC attenuated by inactivation of the genes involved with intimate attachment to enterocytes and effacement of the microvilli, accompanied by appropriate modifications of the bacteria (e.g., mutations in *recA*) to minimize the chance of reacquisition of the wild type genes by recombination.

Whatever EPEC vaccine candidates become available in the future for clinical trials, since EPEC gastroenteritis is a diarrheal illness that is largely confined to the first 6 months of life, active immunization would require that a vaccine be highly safe so that ultimately it could be administered in the neonatal period. It would be preferable if the vaccine were effective following administration of just a single dose, in order to elicit a very rapid onset of protection. Considerable epidemiologic evidence demonstrates that breast-fed infants are at low risk of EPEC diarrhea (265). It is believed that such protection has an immunologic basis by means of maternal SIgA antibodies in breast milk (277).

REFERENCES

1. Black RE, Brown KH, Becker S, et al. Longitudinal studies of infectious diseases and physical growth in rural Bangladesh. II. Incidence of diarrhea and association with known pathogens. *Am J Epidemiol* 1982;115:315–324.
2. Guerrant RL, Kirchhoff LV, Shields DS, et al. Prospective study of diarrheal illness in northeastern Brazil: patterns of disease, nutritional impact, etiologies, and risk factors. *J Infect Dis* 1983;148:986–997.
3. Snyder JD, Merson MH. The magnitude of the global problem of acute diarrhoeal disease: a review of active surveillance data. *Bull World Health Organ* 1982;60:605–613.
4. Levine MM, Ferreccio C, Prado V, et al. Epidemiologic studies of *Escherichia coli* infections in a low socioeconomic level peri-

urban community in Santiago, Chile. *Am J Epidemiol* 1993;138: 849–869.

5. Levine MM, Losonsky G, Herrington D, et al. Pediatric diarrhea: the challenge of prevention. *Pediatr Infect Dis* 1986;5: S29–S43.

6. Merson MH, Morris GK, Sack DA, et al. Travelers' diarrhea in Mexico. A prospective study of physicians and family members attending a congress. *N Engl J Med* 1976;294:1299–1305.

7. Black RE. Pathogens that cause travelers' diarrhea in Latin America and Africa. *Rev Infect Dis* 1986;8S:S131–S141.

8. Taylor DN, Echeverria P. Etiology and epidemiology of travelers' diarrhea in Asia. *Rev Infect Dis* 1986;8S:S136–S141.

9. Weissman JB, Gangarosa EJ, Schmerler A, et al. Shigellosis in daycare centers. *Lancet* 1975;1:88–90.

10. Pickering LK, Evans DG, DuPont HL, et al. Diarrhea caused by *Shigella*, rotavirus, and *Giardia* in daycare centers: prospective study. *J Pediatr* 1981;99:51–56.

11. Pickering LK, Bartlett AV, Woodward WE. Acute infectious diarrhea among children in daycare: epidemiology and control. *Rev Infect Dis* 1986;8:539–547.

12. DuPont HL, Gangarosa EJ, Reller LB, et al. Shigellosis in custodial institutions. *Am J Epidemiol* 1970;92:172–179.

13. Levine MM, Rice PA, Gangarosa EJ, et al. An outbreak of sonnei shigellosis in a population receiving oral attenuated *Shigella* vaccines. *Am J Epidemiol* 1974;99:30–36.

14. Blaser MJ, Pollard RA, Feldman RA. Shigella infections in the United States, 1974–1980. *J Infect Dis* 1983;147:771–775.

15. Griffin PM, Tauxe RV, Redd SC, et al. Emergence of highly trimethoprim-sulfamethoxazole-resistant *Shigella* in a native American population: an epidemiological study. *Am J Epidemiol* 1989;129:1042–1051.

16. Black RE, Merson MH, Huq I, et al. Incidence and severity of rotavirus and *Escherichia coli* diarrhoea in rural Bangladesh. *Lancet* 1981;1:141–143.

17. Kotloff KL, Wasserman SS, Steciak JY, et al. Acute diarrhea in Baltimore children attending an outpatient clinic. *Pediatr Infect Dis J* 1988;7:753–759.

18. Mata LJ, Simhon A, Padilla R. Diarrhea associated with rotaviruses, enterotoxigenic *Escherichia coli*, *Campylobacter*, and other agents in Costa Rican children, 1976–1981. *Am J Epidemiol* 1983;32:146–153.

19. Levine MM, Prado V, Robins-Browne R, et al. Use of DNA probes and HEp-2 cell adherence assay to detect diarrheagenic *Escherichia coli*. *J Infect Dis* 1988;158:224–228.

20. Stoll BJ, Glass RI, Huq MI, et al. Surveillance of patients attending a diarrhoeal disease hospital in Bangladesh. *Br Med J* 1982;285:1185–1188.

21. Cravioto A, Reyes RE, Ortega R, et al. Prospective study of diarrhoeal disease in a cohort of rural Mexican children: incidence and isolated pathogens during the first two years of life. *Epidemiol Infect* 1988;101:123–134.

22. Gangarosa EJ, Perera DR, Mata LJ, et al. Epidemic Shiga bacillus dysentery in Central America. II. Epidemiologic studies in 1969. *J Infect Dis* 1970;122:181–190.

23. Rahaman MM, Khan MM, Aziz KMS, et al. An outbreak of dysentery caused by *Shigella dysenteriae* type 1 on a Coral Island in the Bay of Bengal. *J Infect Dis* 1975;132:15–19.

24. Goodgame RW, Greenough WB. Cholera in Africa: a message for the West. *Ann Intern Med* 1975;82:101–106.

25. Mhalu F, Mmari PW, Ijumba J. Rapid emergence of El Tor *Vibrio cholerae* resistant to antimicrobial agents during the first six months of fourth cholera epidemic in Tanzania. *Lancet* 1979;1:345–347.

26. Cholera Working Group, International Centre for Diarrhoeal Diseases Research, Bangladesh. Large epidemic of cholera-like disease in Bangladesh caused by *Vibrio cholerae* O139 synonym Bengal. *Lancet* 1993;342:387–390.

27. Black RE, Brown KH, Becker S. Effects of diarrhea associated with specific enteropathogens on the growth of children in rural Bangladesh. *Pediatrics* 1984;73:799–805.

28. Levine MM. Modern vaccines. Enteric infections. *Lancet* 1990;335:958–961.

29. Diarrhoeal Diseases Control Programme World Health Organization. *Biomedical and epidemiological research priorities of global scientific working groups.* WHO/CDD/86.8 Rev 1. Geneva: World Health Organization 1987.

30. Levine MM, Ferreccio C, Black RE, et al. Progress in vaccines against typhoid fever. *Rev Infect Dis* 1989;11(Suppl 3): S552–S567.

31. Levine MM. Typhoid fever vaccines. In: Plotkin SA, Mortimer A Jr, eds. *Vaccines*. Philadelphia: Saunders, 1988;333–361.

32. Ashcroft MT, Morrison-Ritchie J, Nicholson CC. Controlled field trial in British Guyana schoolchildren of heat-killed-phenolized and acetone-killed lyophilized typhoid vaccines. *Am J Hyg* 1964;79:196–206.

33. Yugoslav Typhoid Commission. A controlled field trial of the effectiveness of acetone-dried and inactivated and heat-phenol-inactivated typhoid vaccines in Yugoslavia. *Bull World Health Organ* 1964;30:623–630.

34. Hejfec LB, Salmin LV, Lejtman MZ, et al. A controlled field trial and laboratory study of five typhoid vaccines in the USSR. *Bull World Health Organ* 1966;34:321–339.

35. Levine MM, Taylor DN, Ferreccio C. Typhoid vaccines come of age. *Pediatr Infect Dis J* 1989;8:374–381.

36. Robbins JD, Robbins JB. Reexamination of the protective role of the capsular polysaccharide Vi antigen of *Salmonella typhi*. *J Infect Dis* 1984;150:436–449.

37. Bacon GA, Burrows TW, Yates M. The effects of biochemical mutation on the virulence of *Bacterium typhosum*: the loss of virulence of certain mutants. *Br J Exp Pathol* 1951;32:85–96.

38. Stocker BAD. Auxotrophic *Salmonella typhi* as live vaccine. *Vaccine* 1988;6:141–145.

39. Hoiseth S, Stocker BAD. Aromatic-dependent *Salmonella typhimurium* are non-virulent and effective as live vaccines. *Nature* 1981;292:238–239.

40. Dougan G, Chatfield S, Pickard D, et al. Construction and characterization of vaccine strains of *Salmonella* harbouring mutations in two different *aro* genes. *J Infect Dis* 1988;158:1329–1335.

41. Robertson JA, Lindberg AA, Hoiseth S, et al. *Salmonella typhimurium* infection in calves: protection and survival of virulent challenge bacteria after immunization with live or inactivated vaccines. *Infect Immun* 1983;41:742–750.

42. Lindberg AA, Robertsson JA. *Salmonella typhimurium* infection in calves: cell-mediated and humoral immune reactions before and after challenge with live virulent bacteria in calves give live or inactivated vaccines. *Infect Immun* 1983;41: 751–757.

43. Eisenstein TK, Killar LM, Stocker BAD, et al. Cellular immunity induced by avirulent *Salmonella* in LPS-defective C3H/HeJ mice. *J Immunol* 1984;133:958–961.

44. Killar LM, Eisenstein TK. Immunity to *Salmonella typhimurium* infection in C3H/HeJ and C3H/HeNCrlBR mice: studies with an aromatic-dependent live *S. typhimurium* strain as a vaccine. *Infect Immun* 1985;47:605–612.

45. Killar LM, Eisenstein TK. Cellular immunity induced by avirulent *Salmonella* in LPS-defective C3H/HeJ mice. *J Immunol* 1984;133:3991–3995.

46. Jones PW, Dougan G, Hayward C, et al. Oral vaccination of calves against experimental salmonellosis using a double *aro* mutant of *Salmonella typhimurium*. *Vaccine* 1991;9:29–34.

47. Edwards MF, Stocker BAD. Construction of *aroA his pur* strains of *Salmonella typhi*. *J Bacteriol* 1984;170:3991–3995.

48. Levine MM, Herrington D, Murphy JR, et al. Safety, infectivity, immunogenicity, and in vivo stability of two attenuated auxotrophic mutant strains of *Salmonella typhi*, 541Ty and 543Ty, as live oral vaccines in humans. *J Clin Invest* 1987;79: 888–902.

49. O'Callaghan D, Maskell D, Liew F, et al. Characterization of aromatic- and purine-dependent *Salmonella typhimurium*: attenuation, persistence, and ability to induce protective immunity in BALB/c mice. *Infect Immun* 1988;56:419–423.

50. Sigwart DF, Stocker BAD, Clements JD. Effect of a *purA* mutation on efficacy of *Salmonella* live-vaccine vectors. *Infect Immun* 1989;57:1858–1861.

51. Hone DM, Tacket C, Harris A, et al. Evaluation in volunteers of a candidate live oral attenuated *S. typhi* vector vaccine. *J Clin Invest* 1992;90:1–9.

52. Tacket CO, Hone DM, Curtiss R III, et al. Comparison of the safety and immunogenicity of ΔaroC ΔaroD and Δcya Δcrp Salmonella typhi strains in adult volunteers. Infect Immun 1992;60:536–541.

53. Tacket CO, Hone DM, Losonsky GA, et al. Clinical acceptability and immunogenicity of CVD 908 Salmonella typhi vaccine strain. Vaccine 1992;10:443–446.

54. Kantele A. Antibody-secreting cells in the evaluation of the immunogenicity of an oral vaccine. Vaccine 1990;8:321–326.

55. Tacket CO, Losonsky G, Taylor DN, et al. Lack of immune response to the Vi component of a Vi-positive ee variant of the Salmonella typhi live oral vaccine strain Ty21a in human studies. J Infect Dis 1991;163:901–904.

56. Curtiss R III, Kelly SM. Salmonella typhimurium deletion mutants lacking adenylate cyclase and cyclic AMP receptor protein are avirulent and immunogenic. Infect Immun 1987;55:3035–3043.

57. Hone DM, Attridge SR, Forrest B, et al. A galE via (Vi antigen-negative) mutant of Salmonella typhi Ty2 retains virulence in humans. Infect Immun 1988;56:1326–1333.

58. Dorman CJ, Chatfield S, Higgins CF, et al. Characterization of porin and ompR mutants of a virulent strain of Salmonella typhimurium: ompR mutants are attenuated in vivo. Infect Immun 1989;57:2136–2140.

59. Miller SI, Kukral AM, Mekalanos JJ. A two-component regulatory system (phoP phoQ) controls Salmonella typhimurium virulence. Proc Natl Acad Sci USA 1989;86:5054–5058.

60. Galan J, Curtiss R III. Virulence and vaccine potential of phoP mutants of Salmonella typhimurium. Microb Pathog 1989;6:433–443.

61. Alpuche Aranda CM, Swanson JA, Loomis WP, et al. Salmonella typhimurium activates virulence gene transcription within acidified macrophage phagosomes. Proc Natl Acad Sci USA 1992;89:10079–10083(abst)

62. Johnson K, Charles I, Dougan G, et al. The role of a stress-response protein in Salmonella-typhimurium virulence. Mol Microbiol 1991;5:401–407.

63. Benjamin WH Jr, Hall P, Briles DE. A hemA mutation renders Salmonella typhimurium avirulent in mice, yet capable of eliciting protection against infection with S. typhimurium. Microb Pathog 1991;11:289–295.

64. Levine MM, Hone D, Heppner DG, et al. Attenuated Salmonella as carriers for the expression of foreign antigens. Microecol Ther 1990;19:23–32.

65. Dougan G, Hormaeche CE, Maskell DJ. Live oral Salmonella vaccines: potential use of attenuated strains as carriers of heterologous antigens to the immune system. Parasite Immunol 1987;9:151–160.

66. Formal SB, Baron LS, Kopecko DJ, et al. Construction of a potential bivalent vaccine strain: introduction of Shigella sonnei form I antigen genes into the galE Salmonella typhi Ty21a typhoid vaccine strain. Infect Immun 1981;34:746–750.

67. Forrest B, LaBrooy JT, Attridge SR, et al. A candidate live oral typhoid/cholera hybrid vaccine is immunogenic in man. J Infect Dis 1989;159:145–146.

68. Black RE, Levine MM, Clements ML, et al. Prevention of shigellosis by a Salmonella typhi–Shigella sonnei bivalent vaccine. J Infect Dis 1987;155:1260–1265.

69. Tacket CO, Forrest B, Morona R, et al. Safety, immunogenicity, and efficacy against cholera challenge in humans of a typhoid–cholera hybrid vaccine derived from Salmonella typhi Ty21a. Infect Immun 1990;58:1620–1627.

70. Herrington DA, Van de Verg L, Formal SB, et al. Studies in volunteers to evaluate candidate Shigella vaccines: further experience with a bivalent Salmonella typhi–Shigella sonnei vaccine and protection conferred by previous Shigella sonnei disease. Vaccine 1990;8:353–357.

71. Gonzalez C, Hone D, Noriega F, et al. Salmonella typhi strain CVD 908 expressing the circumsporozoite protein of Plasmodium falciparum: strain construction, safety, and immunogenicity. J Infect Dis 1994;169:927–931.

72. Szu SC, Stone AL, Robbins JD, et al. Vi capsular polysaccharide–protein conjugates for prevention of typhoid fever. Prepa-

ration, characterization, and immunogenicity in laboratory animals. J Exp Med 1987;166:1510–1524.

73. Szu SC, Li X, Schneerson R, et al. Comparative immunogenicities of Vi polysaccharide–protein conjugates composed of cholera toxin or its B subunit as a carrier bound to high- or low-molecular weight-Vi. Infect Immun 1989;57:3823–3827.

74. Rabbani GH, Mahalanabis D. New strains of Vibrio cholerae O139 in India and Bangladesh: lessons from the recent epidemics. J Diarrhoeal Dis Res 1993;11:63–66.

75. Clemens JD, Sack DA, Harris JR, et al. Field trial of oral cholera vaccines in Bangladesh. Lancet 1986;2:124–127.

76. Clemens J, Harris J, Sack D, et al. Field trial of oral cholera vaccines in Bangladesh: results of one year of follow-up. J Infect Dis 1988;158:60–69.

77. Clemens JD, Sack DA, Harris JR, et al. Field trial of cholera vaccines in Bangladesh: results from three year follow-up. Lancet 1990;335:270–273.

78. Clemens JD, Sack DA, Harris JR, et al. ABO blood groups and cholera: new observations on specificity of risk and modifications of vaccine efficacy. J Infect Dis 1989;159:770–773.

79. Osek J, Svennerholm A-M, Holmgren J. Protection against Vibrio cholerae El Tor infection by specific antibodies against mannose-binding hemagglutinin pili. Infect Immun 1992;60:4961–4964.

80. Taylor RK, Miller VL, Furlong DB, et al. Use of phoA gene fusions to identify a pilus colonization factor coordinately regulated with cholera toxin. Proc Natl Acad Sci USA 1987;84:2833.

81. Herrington DA, Hall RH, Losonsky G, et al. Toxin, toxin-coregulated pili, and the toxR regulon are essential for Vibrio cholerae pathogenesis in humans. J Exp Med 1988;168:1487–1492.

82. Levine MM, Pierce NF. Immunity and vaccine development. In: Barua D, Greenough WB III, eds. Cholera. New York: Plenum Medical 1992;285–327.

83. Levine MM, Kaper JB. Live oral vaccines against cholera: an update. Vaccine 1993;11:207–212.

84. Clemens JD, van Loon F, Sack DA, et al. Biotype as determinant of natural immunising effect of cholera. Lancet 1991;337:883–884.

85. Glass RI, Becker S, Huq I, et al. Endemic cholera in rural Bangladesh, 1966–1980. Am J Epidemiol 1982;116:959–970.

86. Levine MM, Black RE, Clements ML, et al. Duration of infection-derived immunity to cholera. J Infect Dis 1981;143:818–820.

87. Levine MM, Black RE, Clements ML, et al. Volunteer studies in development of vaccines against cholera and enterotoxigenic Escherichia coli: a review. In: Holme T, Holmgren J, Merson MH, Mollby R, eds. Acute enteric infections in children. New prospects for treatment and prevention. Amsterdam: Elsevier/North-Holland Biomedical Press, 1981;443–459.

88. Levine MM, Kaper JB, Black RE, et al. New knowledge on pathogenesis of bacterial enteric infections as applied to vaccine development. Microbiol Rev 1983;47:510–550.

89. Levine MM, Nalin DR, Craig JP, et al. Immunity of cholera in man: relative role of antibacterial versus antitoxic immunity. Trans R Soc Trop Med Hyg 1979;73:3–9.

90. Mosley WH, Ahmad S, Benenson AS, et al. The relationship of vibriocidal antibody titre to susceptibility to cholera in family contacts of cholera patients. Bull World Health Organ 1968;38:777–785.

91. Mosley WH, Benenson AS, Barui R. A serological survey for cholera antibodies in rural east Pakistan. I. The distribution of antibody in the control population of a cholera vaccine field-trial area and the relation of antibody titer to the pattern of endemic cholera. Bull World Health Organ 1968;38:327–334.

92. Glass RI, Svennerholm AM, Khan MR, et al. Seroepidemiological studies of El Tor cholera in Bangladesh: association of serum antibody levels with protection. J Infect Dis 1985;151:236–242.

93. Clemens JD, van Loon F, Sack DA, et al. Field trial of oral cholera vaccines in Bangladesh: serum vibriocidal and antitoxic antibodies as markers of the risk of cholera. J Infect Dis 1991;163:1235–1242.

94. Chongsa-Nguan M, Chaicumpa W, Kalambaheti T, et al. Vibriocidal antibody and antibodies to *Vibrio cholerae* lipopolysaccharide, cell-bound haemagglutinin and toxin in Thai population. *Southeast Asian J Trop Med Public Health* 1986;17:558–566.

95. Hall RH, Losonsky G, Silveira AP, et al. Immunogenicity of *Vibrio cholerae* O1 toxin-coregulated pili in experimental and clinical cholera. *Infect Immun* 1991;59:2508–2512.

96. Jonson G, Holmgren J, Svennerholm AM. Epitope differences in toxin-coregulated pili produced by classical and El Tor *Vibrio cholerae*-O1. *Microb Pathog* 1991;11:179–188.

97. Neoh SH, Rowley D. The antigens of *Vibrio cholerae* involved in the vibriocidal action of antibody and complement. *J Infect Dis* 1970;121:505–513.

98. Parsot C, Taxman E, Mekalanos JJ. ToxR regulates the production of lipoproteins and the expression of serum resistance in *Vibrio cholerae*. *Proc Natl Acad Sci USA* 1991;88:1641–1645.

99. Richardson K, Kaper JB, Levine MM. Human immune response to *Vibrio cholerae* O1 whole cells and isolated outer membrane antigens. *Infect Immun* 1989;57:495–501.

100. Sciortino CV. Protection against infection with *Vibrio cholerae* by passive transfer of monoclonal antibodies to outer membrane antigens. *J Infect Dis* 1989;160:248–252.

101. Sharma DP, Attridge S, Hackett J, et al. Nonlipopolysaccharide protective antigens shared by classical and El Tor biotypes of *Vibrio cholerae*. *J Infect Dis* 1987;155:716–723.

102. Sharma DP, Thomas C, Hall RH, et al. Significance of toxin-coregulated pili as protective antigens of *Vibrio cholerae* in the infant mouse model. *Vaccine* 1989;7:451–456.

103. Sun D, Tillman DJ, Marion TN, et al. Production and characterization of monoclonal antibodies to the toxin coregulated pilus (TCP) of *Vibrio cholerae* that protect against experimental cholera in infant mice. *Serodiag Immunother Infect Dis* 1990;4:73–81.

104. Svennerholm AM, Levine MM, Holmgren J. Weak serum and intestinal antibody responses to *Vibrio cholerae* soluble hemagglutinin in cholera patients. *Infect Immun* 1984;45:792–794.

105. Woodward WE. Cholera reinfection in man. *J Infect Dis* 1971;123:61–66.

106. DiRita VJ, Parsot C, Jander G, et al. Regulatory cascade controls virulence in *Vibrio cholerae*. *Proc Natl Acad Sci USA* 1991;88:5403–5407.

107. Curlin G, Levine R, Aziz KMA, et al. Field trial of cholera toxoid. In: *Proceedings of the 11th Joint Conference on Cholera, US–Japan Cooperative Medical Science Program*. Washington, DC: US HEW, 1974;314–329.

108. Noriki H. Evaluation of toxoid field trial in the Phillipines. In: *Proceedings of the 12th Joint Conference on Cholera, US–Japan Cooperative Medical Science Program*. Tokyo: Fuji, 1976;302–310.

109. Levine MM, Kaper JB, Herrington D, et al. Volunteer studies of deletion mutants of *Vibrio cholerae* O1 prepared by recombinant techniques. *Infect Immun* 1988;56:161–167.

110. Benenson AS, Saad A, Mosley WH, et al. Serological studies in cholera. 3. Serum toxin neutralization—rise in titre in response to infection with *Vibrio cholerae*, and the level in the "normal" population in East Pakistan. *Bull World Health Organ* 1968;38:287–295.

111. Losonsky GA, Tacket CO, Wasserman SS, et al. Secondary *Vibrio cholerae*-specific cellular antibody responses following wild-type homologous challenge in people vaccinated with CVD 103-HgR live oral cholera vaccine: changes with time and lack of correlation with protection. *Infect Immun* 1993;61:729–733.

112. Jonson G, Svennerholm AM, Holmgren J. *Vibrio cholerae* expresses cell surface antigens during intestinal infection which are not expressed during in vitro culture. *Infect Immun* 1989;57:1809–1815.

113. Sigel SP, Payne SM. Effect of iron regulation on growth, siderophore production, and expression of outer membrane proteins of *Vibrio cholerae*. *J Bacteriol* 1982;150:148–155.

114. Kaper JB, Levine MM. Recombinant attenuated *Vibrio cholerae* strains used as live oral vaccines. *Res Microbiol* 1990;141:901–906.

115. Kaper JB, Lockman H, Baldini MM, et al. A recombinant live oral cholera vaccine. *Bio/Technology* 1984;2:345–349.

116. Kaper JB, Lockman H, Baldini MM, et al. Recombinant nontoxinogenic *Vibrio cholerae* strains as attenuated cholera vaccine candidates. *Nature* 1984;308:655–658.

117. Ketley JM, Michalski J, Galen J, et al. Construction of genetically marked *Vibrio cholerae* O1 vaccine strains. *FEMS Microbiol Lett* 1993;111:15–21.

118. Mekalanos JJ, Swartz DJ, Pearson GD, et al. Cholera toxin genes: nucleotide sequence, deletion analysis and vaccine development. *Nature* 1983;306:551–557.

119. Pearson GD, DiRita VJ, Goldberg MB, et al. New attenuated derivatives of *Vibrio cholerae*. *Res Microbiol* 1990;141:893–899.

120. Madden JM, McCardell BA, Shah DB. Cytotoxin production by members of genus *Vibrio*. *Lancet* 1984;1:1217–1218.

121. Taylor RK, Shaw C, Peterson K, et al. Safe, live *Vibrio cholerae* vaccines. *Vaccine* 1984;6:151–154.

122. O'Brien AD, Chen ME, Holmes RK, et al. Environmental and human isolates of *Vibrio cholerae* and *Vibrio parahaemolyticus* produce a *Shigella dysenteriae* 1 (Shiga)-like cytotoxin. *Lancet* 1984;1:77.

123. Levine MM, Kaper JB, Herrington D, et al. Safety, immunogenicity, and efficacy of recombinant live oral cholera vaccines, CVD 103 and CVD 103-HgR. *Lancet* 1988;2:467–470.

124. Cryz SJ, Levine MM, Kaper JB, et al. Randomized double-blind placebo controlled trial to evaluate the safety and immunogenicity of the live oral cholera vaccine strain CVD 103-HgR in Swiss adults. *Vaccine* 1990;8:577–580.

125. Cryz SJ Jr, Levine MM, Losonsky G, et al. Safety and immunogenicity of a booster dose of *Vibrio cholerae* CVD 103-HgR live oral cholera vaccine in Swiss adults. *Infect Immun* 1992;60:3916–3917.

126. Kotloff KL, Wasserman SS, ODonnell S, et al. Safety and immunogenicity in North Americans of a single dose of live oral cholera vaccine CVD 103-HgR: results of a randomized, placebo-controlled, double-blind crossover trial. *Infect Immun* 1992;60:4430–4432.

127. Tacket CO, Losonsky G, Nataro JP, et al. Onset and duration of protective immunity in challenged volunteers after vaccination with live oral cholera vaccine CVD 103-HgR. *J Infect Dis* 1992;166:837–841.

128. Migasena S, Pitisuttitham P, Prayurahong P, et al. Preliminary assessment of the safety and immunogenicity of live oral cholera vaccine strain CVD 103-HgR in healthy Thai adults. *Infect Immun* 1989;57:3261–3264.

129. Su-Arehawatana P, Singharaj P, Taylor DN, et al. Safety and immunogenicity of different immunization regimens of CVD 103-HgR live oral cholera vaccine in soldiers and civilians in Thailand. *J Infect Dis* 1992;165:1042–1048.

130. Suharyono, Simanjuntak C, Witham N, et al. Safety and immunogenicity of single-dose live oral cholera vaccine CVD 103-HgR in 5–9-year-old Indonesian children. *Lancet* 1992;340:689–694.

131. Gotuzzo E, Butron B, Seas C, et al. Safety, immunogenicity, and excretion pattern of single-dose live oral cholera vaccine CVD 103-HgR in Peruvian adults of high and low socioeconomic levels. *Infect Immun* 1993;61:3994–3997.

132. Lagos R, Avendano A, Horwitz I, et al. Tolerancia e immunogenicidad de ina dosis oral de la cepa de *Vibrio cholerae* O1, viva-atenuada, CVD 103-HgR: estudio de doble ciego en adultos Chilenos. *Rev Med Chile* 1993;121:857–863.

133. McGhee JR, Mestecky J, Dertzbaugh MT, et al. The mucosal immune system: from fundamental concepts to vaccine development. *Vaccine* 1992;10:75–88.

134. Owen RL, Pierce NF, Apple RT, et al. M cell transport of *Vibrio cholerae* from the intestinal lumen into Peyer's patches: a mechanism for antigen sampling and for microbial transepithelial migration. *J Infect Dis* 1986;153:1108–1118.

135. Simanjuntak CH, O'Hanley P, Punjabi NH, et al. The safety, immunogenicity, and transmissibility of single-dose live oral cholera vaccine CVD 103-HgR in 24 to 59 month old Indonesian children. *J Infect Dis* 1993;168:1169–1176.

136. Fasano A, Baudry B, Pumplin DW, et al. *Vibrio cholerae* pro-

duces a second enterotoxin, which affects intestinal tight junctions. *Proc Natl Acad Sci USA* 1991;88:5242–5246.

137. Baudry B, Fasano A, Ketley J, et al. Cloning of a gene (*zot*) encoding a new toxin produced by *Vibrio cholerae*. *Infect Immun* 1992;60:428–434.

138. Trucksis M, Galen JE, Michalski J, et al. Accessory cholera enterotoxin (Ace), the third member of a *Vibrio cholerae* virulence cassette. *Proc Natl Acad Sci USA* 1993;90:5267–5271.

139. Pearson GD, Woods A, Chiang SL, et al. CTX genetic element encodes a site-specific recombination system and an intestinal colonization factor. *Proc Natl Acad Sci USA* 1993;90:3750–3754.

140. Goldberg I, Mekalanos JJ. Effect of a recA mutation on cholera toxin gene amplification and deletion events. *J Bacteriol* 1986;165:723–731.

141. Michalski J, Galen JE, Fasano A, et al. *Vibrio cholerae* CVD110: a live oral attenuated El Tor vaccine strain. *Infect Immun* 1993;61:4462–4468.

142. Roberts A, Pearson G, Mekalanos J. Cholera vaccine strains derived from a 1991 Peruvian isolate of *Vibrio cholerae* and other El Tor strains. *Abstr 28th Joint US–Japan Cooperative Medical Science Program, Cholera Panel* 1992;28:43–47(abst).

143. Levine MM, Black RE, Clements ML, et al. The pathogenicity of nonenterotoxigenic *Vibrio cholerae* serogroup O1 biotype El Tor isolated from sewage water in Brazil. *J Infect Dis* 1982;145:296–299.

144. Tacket CO, Losonsky G, Nataro JP, et al. Safety and immunogenicity of live oral cholera vaccine candidate CVD 110, a ΔctxA Δzot Δace derivative of El Tor Ogawa *Vibrio cholerae*. *J Infect Dis* 1993;168:1536–1540.

145. Taylor DN, Hack DC, Killeen KP, et al. Safety, immunogenicity, and efficacy of live, attenuated *Vibrio cholerae* El Tor cholera vaccine candidates in humans. *IDSA* 1993;199:35-A(abst).

146. Taylor DN, Hack DC, Killeen KP, et al. Development of a live, oral, attenuated vaccine against El Tor cholera. *29th Joint Conference on Cholera and Related Diseases* 1993;189–193(abst).

147. Ramamurthy T, Garg S, Sharma R, et al. Emergence of a novel strain of *Vibrio cholerae* with epidemic potential in southern and eastern India. *Lancet* 1993;341:703–704.

148. Swerdlow DL, Mintz ED, Rodriguez M, et al. Waterborne transmission of epidemic cholera in Trujillo, Peru: lessons for a continent at risk. *Lancet* 1992;340:28–32.

149. Johnson JA, Salles CA, Panigrahi P, et al. *Vibrio cholerae* O139 synonym Bengal is closely related to *Vibrio cholerae* El Tor, but has important differences. *Infect Immun* 1994;62:2108–2110.

150. Sack RB, Albert MJ. Summary of a meeting on cholera vaccines. *J Diarr Dis Res* (in press).

151. Johnson JA, Albert MJ, Panigrahi P, et al. Non-O1 *Vibrio cholerae* (O139 synonym Bengal) from the India/Bangladesh epidemic are encapsulated. *29th Joint Conference on Cholera and Related Diseases* 1993;35–38(abst).

152. Kaper JB, Michalski J, Ketley J, et al. Potential for reacquisition of cholera enterotoxin genes by attenuated *Vibrio cholerae* vaccine strain CVD 103-HgR. *Infect Immun* 1994;62:1480–1483.

153. Waldor MK, Mekalanos JJ. Emergence of a new cholera pandemic: molecular analysis of virulence determinants in *Vibrio cholerae* O139 and development of a live vaccine prototype. *J Infect Dis* 1994;170:278–283.

154. Formal SB, Maenza RM, Austin S, et al. Failure of parenteral vaccines to protect monkeys against experimental shigellosis. *Proc Soc Exp Biol (NY)* 1967;125:347–349.

155. Shaughnessy H, Olsson R, Bass K, et al. Experimental human bacillary dysentery. *JAMA* 1946;132:362–368.

156. Higgins AR, Floyd TM, Kader MA. Studies in shigellosis. III. A controlled evaluation of a monovalent *Shigella* vaccine in a highly endemic environment. *Am J Trop Med Hyg* 1955;4:281–288.

157. Mel DM, Terzin AL, Vuksic L. Studies on vaccination against bacillary dysentery. 3. Effective oral immunization against *Shigella flexneri* 2a in a field trial. *Bull World Health Organ* 1965;32:647–655.

158. Mel DM, Arsic BL, Nikolic BD, et al. Studies on vaccination against bacillary dysentery. 4. Oral immunization with live monotypic and combined vaccines. *Bull World Health Organ* 1968;39:375–380.

159. Mel DM, Gangarosa EJ, Radovanovic ML, et al. Studies on vaccination against bacillary dysentery. 6. Protection of children by oral immunization with streptomycin-dependent *Shigella* strains. *Bull World Health Organ* 1971;45:457–464.

160. Mel DM, Arsic BL, Radovanovic ML, et al. Live oral *Shigella* vaccine: vaccination schedule and the effect of booster dose. *Acta Microbiol Acad Sci Hung* 1974;21:109–114.

161. Levine MM, Gangarosa EJ, Barrow WB, et al. Shigellosis in custodial institutions. *Am J Epidemiol* 1976;133:424–429.

162. Levine MM, DuPont HL, Gangarosa EJ, et al. Shigellosis in custodial institutions. II. Clinical, immunologic and bacteriologic response of institutionalized children to oral attenuated shigella vaccines. *Am J Epidemiol* 1972;96:40–49.

163. DuPont HL, Hornick RB, Snyder MJ, et al. Immunity in shigellosis. II. Protection induced by oral live vaccine or primary infection. *J Infect Dis* 1972;125:12–16.

164. Istrati G, Meitert T, Ciufecu C. Recherches sur l'immunite active de l'homme dans la dysenterie bacillaire. *Arch Roumaines Pathol Exp Microbiol* 1965;24:677–686.

165. Cooperation Group of Dysentery Vaccine, Bing Rui W. Study on the effect of oral immunization of T₃₂Istrati strain against bacillary dysentery in field trials. *Arch Roumaines Pathol Exp Microbiol* 1984;43:285–289.

166. Levine MM, Gangarosa EJ, Werner M, et al. Shigellosis in custodial institutions. III. Prospective clinical and bacteriologic surveillance of children vaccinated with oral attenuated *Shigella* vaccine. *J Pediatr* 1974;84:803–806.

167. Levine MM, Gangarosa EJ, Barrow WB, et al. Shigellosis in custodial institutions. IV. In vivo stability and transmissibility of oral attenuated streptomycin-dependent *Shigella* vaccines. *J Infect Dis* 1975;131:704–707.

168. Formal SB, Gemski P Jr, Baron LS, et al. Genetic transfer of *Shigella flexneri* antigens to *E. coli* K-12. *Infect Immun* 1970;1:279–287.

169. Levine MM, Woodward WE, Formal SB, et al. Studies with a new generation of oral attenuated shigella vaccine: *Escherichia coli* bearing surface antigens of *Shigella flexneri*. *J Infect Dis* 1977;136:577–582.

170. DuPont HL, Hornick RB, Snyder MJ, et al. Immunity in shigellosis. I. Response of man to attenuated strains of *Shigella*. *J Infect Dis* 1972;125:5–11.

171. Van de Verg L, Herrington DA, Murphy JR, et al. Specific immunoglobulin A-secreting cells in peripheral blood of humans following oral immunization with a bivalent *Salmonella typhi–Shigella sonnei* vaccine or infection by pathogenic sonnei. *Infect Immun* 1990;58:2002–2004.

172. Formal SB, Hale TL, Kapfer C, et al. Oral vaccination of monkeys with an invasive *Escherichia coli* K-12 hybrid expressing *Shigella flexneri* 2a somatic antigen. *Infect Immun* 1984;46:465–469.

173. Kotloff KL, Herrington DA, Hale TL, et al. Safety, immunogenicity, and efficacy in monkeys and humans of invasive *Escherichia coli* K-12 hybrid vaccine candidates expressing *Shigella flexneri* 2a somatic antigen. *Infect Immun* 1992;60:2218–2224.

174. Newland JW, Hale TL, Formal SB. Genotypic and phenotypic characterization of an *aroD* deletion-attenuated *Escherichia coli* K12-*Shigella flexneri* hybrid vaccine expressing *S. flexneri* 2a somatic antigen. *Vaccine* 1992;10:766–776.

175. Hale TL. Genetic basis of virulence in *Shigella* species. *Microbiol Rev* 1991;55:206–224.

176. Sansonetti PJ. Molecular and cellular biology of *Shigella flexneri* invasiveness: from cell assay systems to shigellosis. *Curr Top Microbiol Immunol* 1992;180:1–19.

177. Smith BP, Reina-Guerra M, Stocker BAD, et al. Aromatic-dependent *Salmonella dublin* as a parenteral modified live vaccine for calves. *Am J Vet Res* 1984;45:2231–2235.

178. Hone DM, Harris AM, Chatfield S, et al. Construction of genetically-defined double *aro* mutants of *Salmonella typhi*. *Vaccine* 1991;9:810–816.

179. Lindberg AA, Karnell A, Pal T, et al. Construction of an auxo-

trophic *Shigella flexneri* strain for use as a live vaccine. *Microb Pathog* 1990;8:433–440.

180. Lindberg AA, Karnell A, Stocker BA, et al. Development of an auxotrophic oral live *Shigella flexneri* vaccine. *Vaccine* 1988;6: 146–150.

181. Verma NK, Lindberg AA. Construction of aromatic dependent *Shigella flexneri* 2a live vaccine candidate strains: deletion mutations in the *aroA* and the *aroD* genes. *Vaccine* 1991;9:6–9.

182. Karnell A, Stocker BA, Katakura S, et al. An auxotrophic live oral *Shigella flexneri* vaccine: development and testing. *Rev Infect Dis* 1991;13(Suppl 4):S357–S361.

183. Karnell A, Stocker BA, Katakura S, et al. Live oral auxotrophic *Shigella flexneri* SFL124 vaccine with a deleted *aroD* gene: characterization and monkey protection studies. *Vaccine* 1992;10:389–394.

184. Li A, Pal T, Forsum U, et al. Safety and immunogenicity of the live oral auxotrophic *Shigella flexneri* SFL124 in volunteers. *Vaccine* 1992;10:395–404.

185. Formal SB, Oaks EV, Olsen RE, et al. Effect of prior infection with virulent *Shigella flexneri* 2a on the resistance of monkeys to subsequent infection with *Shigella sonnei*. *J Infect Dis* 1991; 164:533–537.

186. Karnell A, Cam PC, Verma N, et al. AroD deletion attenuates *Shigella flexneri* strain 2457T and makes it a safe and efficacious oral vaccine in monkeys. *Vaccine* 1993;11:830–836.

187. Karnell A, Li A, Zhao CR, et al. Safety and immunogenicity study of the auxotrophic *Shigella flexneri* 2a vaccine SFL1070 with a deleted *aro* gene in adult Swedish volunteers. *Vaccine* (in press).

188. Lanfranchi GA, Tragnone A. Serum and faecal tumour necrosis factor as marker of intestinal inflammation. *Lancet* 1992;339: 1053.

189. Madara JL, Parkos C, Colgan S, et al. Cl⁻ secretion in a model intestinal epithelium induced by a neutrophil-derived secretagogue. *J Clin Invest* 1992;89:1934–1944.

190. Madara JL, Patapoff TW, Gillece-Castro B, et al. 5'-Adenosine monophosphate is the neutrophil-derived paracrine factor that elicits chloride secretion from T84 intestinal epithelial cell monolayers. *J Clin Invest* 1993;91:2320–2325.

191. Fasano A, Maneval DR Jr, Noriega F, et al. Enterotoxic factors elaborated by *Shigella flexneri* 2a. *29th Joint Conference on Cholera and Related Diseases* 1993;158–163(abst).

192. Formal SB, LaBrec EH, Palmer A, et al. Abortive intestinal infection with *Escherichia coli–Shigella flexneri* hybrid strain. *J Bacteriol* 1965;89:1374–1382.

193. Griffiths E, Stevenson P, Hale TL, et al. Synthesis of aerobactin and a 76,000-dalton iron-regulated outer membrane protein by *Escherichia coli* K-12–*Shigella flexneri* hybrids and by enteroinvasive strains of *Escherichia coli*. *Infect Immun* 1985;49: 67–71.

194. Nassif X, Mazert MC, Mounier J, et al. Evaluation with an iuc::Tn10 mutant of the role of aerobactin production in the virulence of *Shigella flexneri*. *Infect Immun* 1987;55: 1963–1969.

195. Makino S, Sasakawa C, Kamata K, et al. A genetic determinant required for continuous reinfection of adjacent cells on large plasmid in *S. flexneri* 2a. *Cell* 1986;46:551–555.

196. Bernardini ML, Mounier J, D'Hauteville H, et al. Identification of icsA, a plasmid locus of *Shigella flexneri* that governs bacterial intra- and intercellular spread through interaction with F-actin. *Proc Natl Acad Sci USA* 1989;86:3867–3871.

197. Lett M, Sasakawa C, Okada N, et al. *virG*, a plasmid-coded virulence gene of *Shigella flexneri*: identification of the *virG* protein and determination of the complete coding sequence. *J Bacteriol* 1989;171:353–359.

198. Vasselon T, Mounier J, Hellio R, et al. Movement along actin filaments of the perijunctional area and de novo polymerization of cellular actin are required for *Shigella flexneri* colonization of epithelial Caco-2 cell monolayers. *Infect Immun* 1992;60: 1031–1040.

199. Goldberg MB, Sansonetti PJ. *Shigella* subversion of the cellular cytoskeleton: a strategy for epithelial colonization. *Infect Immun* 1993;61:4941–4946.

200. Sansonetti PJ, Arondel J. Construction and evaluation of a double mutant of *Shigella flexneri* as a candidate for oral vaccination against shigellosis. *Vaccine* 1989;7:443–450.

201. Fontaine A, Arondel J, Sansonetti PJ. Construction and evaluation of live attenuated vaccine strains of *Shigella flexneri* and *Shigella dysenteriae* 1. *Res Microbiol* 1990;141:907–912.

202. Sansonetti PJ, Arondel J, Fontaine A, et al. OmpB (osmo-regulation) and icsA (cell-to-cell spread) mutants of *Shigella flexneri*: vaccine candidates and probes to study the pathogenesis of shigellosis. *Vaccine* 1991;9:416–422.

203. Venkatesan M, Fernandez Prada C, Buysse JM, et al. Virulence phenotype and genetic characteristics of the T32-IS-TRATI *Shigella flexneri* 2a vaccine strain. *Vaccine* 1991;9: 358–363.

204. Noriega FR, Wang JY, Losonsky G, et al. Construction and characterization of attenuated ΔaroA ΔvirG *Shigella flexneri* strain CVD 1203, a prototype live oral vaccine. *Infect Immun* 1994;62:5168–5172.

204a.Noriega FR, Giron J, Xu JG, et al. Construction and characterization of oral attenuated *Shigella* vaccine candidates and their potential use as live vector-hybrid vaccines. *29th Joint Conference on Cholera and Related Diseases* 1993;166–168(abst).

205. Watanabe H, Timmis KN. A small plasmid in *Shigella dysenteriae* 1 specifies one or more functions essential for O antigen production and bacterial virulence. *Infect Immun* 1984;43: 391–396.

206. Sturm S, Timmis KN. Cloning of the rfb gene region of *Shigella dysenteriae* 1 and construction of an rfb-rfp gene cassette for the development of lipopolysaccharide-based live anti-dysentery vaccines. *Microb Pathog* 1986;1:289–297.

207. Sturm S, Jann B, Jann K, et al. Genetic and biochemical analysis of *Shigella dysenteriae* 1 O antigen polysaccharide biosynthesis in *Escherichia coli* K-12: 9 kb plasmid of *S. dysenteriae* 1 determines addition of a galactose residue to the lipopolysaccharide core. *Microb Pathog* 1986;1:299–306.

208. Su GF, Brahmbhatt HN, Wehland J, et al. Construction of stable LamB-Shiga toxin B subunit hybrids: analysis of expression in *Salmonella typhimurium aroA* strains and stimulation of B subunit-specific mucosal and serum antibody responses. *Infect Immun* 1992;60:3345–3359.

209. Su GF, Brahmbhatt HN, Wehland J, et al. Extracellular export of Shiga toxin B-subunit/haemolysin A (C-terminus) fusion protein expressed in *Salmonella typhimurium aroA*-mutant and stimulation of B-subunit specific antibody responses in mice. *Microb Pathog* 1992;13:465–476.

210. Robbins JB, Schneerson R. Polysaccharide–protein conjugates: a new generation of vaccines. *J Infect Dis* 1990;161: 821–832.

211. Polotsky YE, Robbins JB, Bryla D, et al. Comparison of conjugates composed of lipopolysaccharide from *Shigella flexneri* type 2a detoxified by two methods and bound to tetanus toxoid. *Infect Immun* 1994;62:210–214.

212. Levenson V, Chernokhvostova EV, Lyubinskaya MM, et al. Parenteral immunization with *Shigella* ribosomal vaccine elicits local IgA response and primes for mucosal memory. *Int Arch Allergy Appl Immunol* 1988;87:25–31.

213. Levenson VI, Egorova TP. Polysaccharide nature of O antigen in protective ribosomal preparations from Shigella: experimental evidence and implications for the ribosomal vaccine concept. *Res Microbiol* 1990;141:707–720.

214. Levenson V, Egorova TP, Belkin ZP, et al. Protective ribosomal preparation from *Shigella sonnei* as a parenteral candidate vaccine. *Infect Immun* 1991;59:3610–3618.

215. Ferreccio C, Prado V, Ojeda A, et al. Epidemiologic patterns of acute diarrhea and endemic *Shigella* infections in a poor periurban setting in Santiago, Chile. *Am J Epidemiol* 1991;134: 614–627.

216. Levine MM, Giron JA, Noriega F. Fimbrial vaccines. In: Klemm P, ed. *Fimbriae: adhesion, biogenics, genetics and vaccines*. Boca Raton, FL: CRC Press, 1994.

217. Levine MM. Vaccines against enterotoxigenic *Escherichia coli* infections. Vaccines based predominantly on antibacterial immunity. In: Woodrow GC, Levine MM, eds. *New generation vaccines: the molecular approach*. New York: Marcel Dekker, 1990;649–660.

218. Svennerholm AM, Holmgren J, Sack DA. Development of oral vaccines against enterotoxinogenic *Escherichia coli* diarrhoea. *Vaccine* 1989;7:196–198.
219. Levine MM. *Escherichia coli* that cause diarrhea: enterotoxigenic, enteropathogenic, enteroinvasive, enterohemorrhagic, and enteroadherent. *J Infect Dis* 1987;155:377–389.
220. Levine MM, Ristaino P, Marley G, et al. Coli surface antigens 1 and 3 of colonization factor antigen II-positive enterotoxigenic *Escherichia coli*: morphology, purification, and immune responses in humans. *Infect Immun* 1984;44:409–420.
221. Smyth CJ. Two mannose-resistant hemagglutinins on enterotoxigenic *Escherichia coli* of serotype O6:H16 or H-isolated from traveller's and infantile diarrhea. *J Gen Microbiol* 1982;128:2081–2096.
222. Cravioto A, Scotland SM, Rowe B. Hemagglutination activity and colonization factor antigens I and II in enterotoxigenic and non-enterotoxigenic strains of *Escherichia coli* isolated from humans. *Infect Immun* 1982;36:189–197.
223. Thomas LV, McConnell MM, Rowe B, et al. The possession of three novel coli surface antigens by enterotoxigenic *Escherichia coli* strains positive for the putative colonization factor PCF8775. *J Gen Microbiol* 1986;131:2319–2326.
224. Tacket CO, Maneval DR, Levine MM. Purification, morphology, and genetics of a new fimbrial putative colonization factor of enterotoxigenic *Escherichia coli* O159:H4. *Infect Immun* 1987;55:1063–1069.
225. McConnell MM, Chart H, Field AM, et al. Characterization of putative colonization factor (PCF0166) of enterotoxigenic *Escherichia coli* of serogroup O166. *J Gen Microbiol* 1989;135:1135–1144.
226. McConnell MM, Hibberd ML, Field AM, et al. Characterization of a new colonization factor (CS17) from a human enterotoxigenic *Escherichia coli* of serotype O114:H21 which produces only heat-labile enterotoxin. *J Infect Dis* 1990;161:343–347.
227. Viboud G, Binsztein N, Svennerholm AM. A new fimbrial putative colonization factor, PCF020, in human enterotoxigenic *Escherichia coli*. *Infect Immun* 1993;61:5190–5197.
228. Evans DG, Satterwhite TK, Evans DJ Jr, et al. Differences in serological responses and excretion patterns of volunteers challenged with enterotoxigenic *Escherichia coli* with and without the colonization factor antigen. *Infect Immun* 1978;19:883–888.
229. Levine MM, Nalin DR, Hoover DL, et al. Immunity to enterotoxigenic *Escherichia coli*. *Infect Immun* 1979;23:729–736.
230. Black RE, Merson MH, Rowe B, et al. Enterotoxigenic *Escherichia coli* diarrhoea: acquired immunity and transmission in an endemic area. *Bull World Health Organ* 1981;59:263–268.
231. DuPont HL, Olarte J, Evans DG, et al. Comparative susceptibility of Latin American and United States students to enteric pathogens. *N Engl J Med* 1976;285:1520–1521.
232. Levine MM, Rennels MB, Cisneros L, et al. Lack of person-to-person transmission of enterotoxigenic *Escherichia coli* despite close contact. *Am J Epidemiol* 1980;111:347–355.
233. Levine MM, Ristaino P, Sack RB, et al. Colonization factor antigens I and II and type 1 somatic pili in enterotoxigenic *Escherichia coli*: relation to enterotoxin type. *Infect Immun* 1983;39:889–897.
234. Wolf MK, Taylor DN, Boedeker E, et al. Characterization of enterotoxigenic *Escherichia coli* isolated from US troops deployed to the Middle East. *J Clin Microbiol* 1993;31:851–856.
235. Gothefors L, Ahren C, Stoll B, et al. Presence of colonization factor antigens on fresh isolates of fecal *Escherichia coli*: a prospective study. *J Infect Dis* 1985;152:1128–1133.
236. Binsztein N, Jouve M, Viboud G, et al. Colonization factors of enterotoxigenic *Escherichia coli* isolated from children with diarrhea in Argentina. *J Clin Microbiol* 1991;29:1893–1898.
237. Clemens JD, Svennerholm AM, Harris JR, et al. Seroepidemiologic evaluation of anti-toxic and anti-colonization factor immunity against infections by LT-producing *Escherichia coli* in rural Bangladesh. *J Infect Dis* 1990;162:448–453.
238. Spira WM, Sack RB, Froehlich JL. Simple adult rabbit model for *Vibrio cholerae* and enterotoxigenic *Escherichia coli* diarrhea. *Infect Immun* 1981;32:739–747.
239. Svennerholm AM, Vidal YL, Holmgren J, et al. Role of PCF8775 antigen and its coli surface subcomponents for colonization, disease, and protective immunogenicity of enterotoxigenic *Escherichia coli* in rabbits. *Infect Immun* 1988;56:523–528.
240. Ahren C, Svennerholm AM. Synergistic protective effect of antibodies against *Escherichia coli* enterotoxin and colonization factor antigens. *Infect Immun* 1982;38:74–79.
241. Stoll BJ, Svennerholm AM, Gothefors L, et al. Local and systemic antibody responses to naturally acquired enterotoxigenic *Escherichia coli* diarrhea in an endemic area. *J Infect Dis* 1986;153:527–534.
242. Deetz TR, Evans DJ Jr, Evans DG, et al. Serologic responses to somatic O and colonization factor antigens of enterotoxigenic *Escherichia coli*. *J Infect Dis* 1979;140:114–118.
243. Tacket CO, Losonsky G, Link H, et al. Protection by milk immunoglobulin concentrate against oral challenge with enterotoxigenic *Escherichia coli*. *N Engl J Med* 1988;318:1240–1243.
244. Klipstein FA, Engert RF, Houghten RA. Immunisation of volunteers with a synthetic peptide vaccine for enterotoxigenic *Escherichia coli*. *Lancet* 1986;1:471–473.
245. Clemens JD, Sack DA, Harris JR, et al. Cross-protection by B subunit–whole cell cholera vaccine against diarrhea associated with heat-labile toxin-producing enterotoxigenic *Escherichia coli*: results of a large-scale field trial. *J Infect Dis* 1988;158:372–377.
246. Peltola H, Siitonen A, Kyrönseppä H, et al. Prevention of travellers' diarrhoea by oral B-subunit/whole-cell cholera vaccine. *Lancet* 1991;338:1285–1289.
247. De la Cabada FJ, Evans DG, Evans DJ Jr. Immunoprotection against enterotoxigenic *Escherichia coli* diarrhea in rabbits by peroral administration of purified colonization factor antigen I (CFA/I). *FEMS Microbiol Lett* 1981;11:303–307.
248. Evans DG, Graham DY, Evans DJ Jr, et al. Administration of purified colonization factor antigens (CFA/I, CFA/II) of enterotoxigenic *Escherichia coli* to volunteers. *Gastroenterology* 1984;87:934–940.
249. Levine MM, Black RE, Clements ML, et al. Prevention of enterotoxigenic *Escherichia coli* diarrheal infection by vaccines that stimulate antiadhesion (antipili) immunity. In: Boedeker EC, ed. *Attachment of organisms to the gut mucosa*. Boca Raton, FL: CRC Press, 1984;223–244.
250. Levine MM, Morris JG, Losonsky G, et al. Fimbriae (pili) adhesins as vaccines. In: Lark DL, Normark S, Uhlin BE, Wolf-Watz H, eds. *Protein–carbohydrate interactions in biological systems. The molecular biology of microbial pathogenicity*. London: Academic Press, 1986;143–145.
251. Schmidt MA, Kelley EP, Tseng LY, et al. Towards an oral *E. coli* pilus vaccine for traveler's diarrhea: susceptibility to proteolytic digestion. *Gastroenterology* 1985;82:1575.
252. Reid RH, Boedeker EC, McQueen CE, et al. Preclinical evaluation of microencapsulated CFA/II oral vaccine against enterotoxigenic *E. coli*. *Vaccine* 1993;11:159–167.
253. Edelman R, Russel RG, Losonsky GA, et al. Immunization of rabbits with enterotoxigenic *E. coli* colonization factor antigen (CFA/I) encapsulated in biodegradable microspheres of poly-(lactide-co-glycolide). *Vaccine* 1993;11:155–158.
254. Tacket CO, Reid RH, Boedeker EC, et al. Enteral immunization and challenge of volunteers given enterotoxigenic *E. coli* CFA/II encapsulated in biodegradable microspheres. *Vaccine* 1994;12:1270–1274.
255. Levine MM. Travellers' diarrhoea: prospects for successful immunoprophylaxis. *Scand J Gastroenterol Suppl* 1983;84:121–134.
256. Evans DJ Jr, Evans DG, Opekun A, et al. Immunoprotective oral whole cell vaccine for enterotoxigenic *Escherichia coli* diarrhea prepared by in situ destruction of chromosomal and plasmid DNA with colicin E2. *FEMS Microbiol Lett* 1988;47:9–18.
257. Evans DG, Evans DJ Jr, Opekun A, et al. Non-replicating whole cell vaccine protective against enterotoxigenic *Escherichia coli* (ETEC) diarrhea: stimulation of anti-CFA (CFA/I) and anti-enterotoxin (anti-LT) intestinal IgA and protection

against challenge with ETEC belonging to heterologous serotypes. *FEMS Microbiol Lett* 1988;47:117–125.

258. Wenneras C, Svennerholm AM, Ahren C, et al. Antibody-secreting cells in human peripheral blood after oral immunization with an inactivated enterotoxigenic *Escherichia coli* vaccine. *Infect Immun* 1992;60:2605–2611.

259. Saarilahti HT, Palva ET, Holmgren J, et al. Fusion of genes encoding *Escherichia coli* heat-stable enterotoxin and outer membrane protein OmpC. *Infect Immun* 1989;57:3663–3665.

260. Hone D, Attridge S, van den Bosch L, et al. A chromosomal integration system for stabilization of heterologous genes in *Salmonella* based vaccine strains. *Microb Pathog* 1988;5:407–418.

261. Yamamoto T, Tamura Y, Yokota T. Enteroadhesion fimbriae and enterotoxin of *Escherichia coli*: genetic transfer to a streptomycin-resistant mutant of the *galE* oral route live-vaccine *Salmonella typhi* Ty21a. *Infect Immun* 1985;50:925–928.

262. Xu JG, Levine MM, Hone DM. Expression of CFA/I in candidate attenuated *Salmonella typhi* live oral vector vaccine strain CVD 908. *Proceedings of the 92nd Meeting of the American Society for Microbiology* 1993;84(abst).

263. Giron JA, Xu JG, Gonzalez CR, et al. Simultaneous constitutive expression of CFA/I and CS3 colonization factors of enterotoxigenic *Escherichia coli* in genetically defined double aro mutant *Salmonella typhi* strain CVD 908. [*Submitted*].

264. Viret J, Cryz SJ, Lang A, et al. Molecular cloning and characterization of the genetic determinants that express the complete *Shigella* serotype (*Shigella sonnei*) lipopolysaccharide in heterologous live attenuated vaccine strains. *Mol Microbiol* 1993;7:239–252.

265. Levine MM, Edelman R. Enteropathogenic *Escherichia coli* of classic serotypes associated with infant diarrhea: epidemiology and pathogenesis. *Epidemiol Rev* 1984;6:31–51.

266. Mochmann H, Ocklitz HW, Weh L, et al. Oral immunization with an extract of *Escherichia coli* enteritidis. *Acta Microbiol Acad Sci Hung* 1974;21:193–196.

267. Rauss K, Ketyi I, Matusovitis E, et al. Specific oral prevention of infantile enteritis. III. Experiments with corpuscular vaccine. *Acta Microbiol Acad Sci Hung* 1972;19:19–28.

268. Rauss K, Ketyi I, Szendrai L, et al. Immunization of infants against *Escherichia coli* enteritis. *Acta Microbiol Acad Sci Hung* 1974;21:181–185.

269. Linde K, Koch H. Untersuchungen zur oralen immunisierung gegen Colienteritis mit streptomycin-dependenten coli-keiman. *Zentralbl Bakteriol Parasitenkd Infektionskr Hyg Abt 1 Orig* 1969;211:476–485.

270. Donnenberg MS, Kaper JB. Enteropathogenic *Escherichia coli*. *Infect Immun* 1992;60:3953–3961.

271. Jerse AE, Kaper JB. The eae gene of enteropathogenic *Escherichia coli* encodes a 94 kDa membrane protein, the expression of which is influenced by the EAF plasmid. *Infect Immun* 1991;59:4302–4309.

272. Giron JA, Ho ASY, Schoolnik GK. An inducible bundle-forming pilus of enteropathogenic *Escherichia coli*. *Science* 1991;254:710–713.

273. Takeuchi A, Inman LR, O'Hanley O, et al. Scanning and transmission electron microscopic study of *Escherichia coli* O15 (RDEC-1) enteric infection in rabbits. *Infect Immun* 1978;19:686–694.

274. Boedeker EC, Cheney CP. *Escherichia coli* (strain RDEC-1) diarrhea in the rabbit: an animal model for enteropathogenic *E. coli* (EPEC) infection of human infants. In: Pfeiffer CJ, ed. *Animal models for intestinal disease*. Boca Raton, FL: CRC Press, 1985;27–40.

275. Wolf MK, Andrews GP, Fritz DL, et al. Characterization of the plasmid from *Escherichia coli* RDEC-1 that mediates expression of adhesin AF/R1 and evidence that AF/R1 pili promote but are not essential for enteropathogenic disease. *Infect Immun* 1988;56:1846–1857.

276. McQueen CE, Boedeker EC, Reid RH, et al. Pili in microspheres protect rabbits from diarrhoea induced by *E. coli* strain RDEC-1. *Vaccine* 1993;11:201–206.

277. Cravioto A, Tello A, Villafán H, et al. Inhibition of localized adhesion of enteropathogenic *Escherichia coli* to HEp-2 cells by immunoglobulin and oligosaccharide fractions of human colostrum and breast milk. *J Infect Dis* 1991;163:1247–1255.

278. Lagos R, Avendaño A, Prado V, et al. Attenuated live oral cholera vaccine strain CVD 103-HgR elicits significantly higher serum vibriocidal antibody titers in persons of blood group O. *Infect Immun* 1995;63: (*in press*).

Infections of the Gastrointestinal Tract,
edited by M. J. Blaser, P. D. Smith, J. I. Ravdin,
H. B. Greenberg, and R. L. Guerrant
Raven Press, Ltd., New York © 1995.

CHAPTER 93

Vaccines for Enteric Viral Pathogens

Paul A. Offit and H. Fred Clark

Several different viruses including rotavirus, adenovirus, small round viruses (e.g., Norwalk and Norwalk-like viruses), coronavirus, astrovirus, and calicivirus are important causes of acute gastroenteritis (1). The worldwide impact of these viral infections has excited interest in disease prevention by immunization. Viruses that infect the intestine replicate primarily in villous epithelial cells, which line the small intestine; neither viremia nor virus replication at sites distant from the intestine are important in viral pathogenesis. Therefore a successful vaccine will be one that induces an immune response active at the intestinal mucosal surface.

There are several features of the intestinal mucosal immune system that are unique (2). The intestine is a rich source of antigen-presenting cells, T cells, and immunoglobulin A (IgA)-bearing B cells. Antigen-presenting cells such as macrophages, follicular dendritic cells, and B cells in Peyer's patches present antigen to T helper cells and IgA-bearing precursor B cells. Indeed, an adult human will make approximately 5 g of IgA at the mucosal surface each day. In addition, T helper cells with the capacity to stimulate cytotoxic T cells via cytokines such as interleukin-2 (IL-2) and interferon-γ (IFN-γ) (Th1 cells) and B cells via cytokines such as IL-4, IL-5, IL-6, and IL-10 (Th2 cells) are present in large numbers in Peyer's patches, the intestinal lamina propria, and mesenteric lymph nodes (3).

Currently, a number of strategies including oral or parenteral immunization with live attenuated viruses, bacterial or viral vectors expressing individual viral proteins, purified viral proteins, as well as various antigen-delivery systems [e.g., liposomes, immune-stimulating complexes (ISCOMS), and microencapsulation] are being considered for human use. Development of successful vaccines will depend on a thorough understanding of the soluble and cellular components of the mucosal immune response,

which determine protection against disease. For example, protection against rotavirus infection in experimental animals has been shown to be dependent on both virus-specific neutralizing antibodies and virus-specific cytotoxic T cells (reviewed in ref. 4). If these animal model studies are predictive of events occurring in human infection, then both antibodies and cytotoxic T lymphocytes (CTLs) must be induced by rotavirus vaccination. Therefore an immunization strategy that induces Th2 cells at the expense of Th1 cells or vice versa may not be adequate to induce a protective response; induction of Th2 versus Th1 cells may be dependent on both the route of inoculation (i.e., oral versus parenteral) (5) and the nature of the virus antigen (i.e., replicating virus versus purified virus protein).

ROTAVIRUS

Immune Response After Natural Infection

The humoral immune response of infants and young children following rotavirus infection has been studied extensively (6–9). Within the first week of illness, rotavirus-specific IgM is detected in the duodenal fluid and serum. Within 4 months of infection, rotavirus-specific IgG and secretory immunoglobulin A (sIgA) are detected in duodenal fluid and rotavirus-specific IgG and monomeric IgA are detected in serum. One year after infection, rotavirus-specific IgG but not IgA is detected in serum, and neither IgG nor sIgA is detected at the mucosal surface. Because of its persistence in serum after natural infection, circulating rotavirus-specific IgG provides an excellent marker for previous exposure to rotavirus in older infants and children. In addition, fecal or duodenal IgA provides an excellent marker for recent infection (either primary infection or reinfection) because of the relatively rapid disappearance of this isotype from the intestinal mucosal surface (10). The humoral immune response to rotavirus infection in neonates is similar to that found in infants (11,12).

P. A. Offit and H. F. Clark: Division of Allergy, Immunology and Infectious Diseases, The Children's Hospital of Philadelphia, The University of Pennsylvania School of Medicine, and The Wistar Institute of Anatomy and Biology, Philadelphia, Pennsylvania 19104.

Rotavirus-specific T helper cells are detected in the circulation within several weeks of primary, symptomatic infection of infants (13). This finding is consistent with the observation that lymphocytes originating in the murine small intestine migrate to the circulation after entrance through the thoracic duct (14) and therefore, similar to circulating rotavirus-specific sIgA, circulating rotavirus-specific T cells probably are a specific indicator of intestinal T cell responses.

The capacity of one rotavirus serotype to evoke antibodies that cross-react with rotaviruses of different serotypes after primary infection remains unclear. Rotavirus serotype specificity is determined by two rotavirus surface proteins, VP4 (P type) and VP7 (G type) (15,16). Sera from animals parenterally inoculated with human rotaviruses have been used to define at least nine different human rotavirus G types (G types 1 to 4, 6, 8, 9, 10, and 12) (17–20). Comparative sequence analysis has been used to distinguish at least six human rotavirus P types (17,21,22). The P and G type specificities of the humoral immune response after natural infection have been difficult to determine. However, a preponderance of evidence supports the hypothesis that VP4 may be more important than VP7 in evoking virus-specific neutralizing antibodies in serum during natural infection (13,23–28). The capacity of the humoral immune response to distinguish different human rotavirus P types after natural infection has not been determined.

Protection Against Disease by Natural Infection

Natural infection with rotaviruses protects against clinically significant disease caused by reinfection. Neonates infected within the first 2 weeks of life are usually protected against moderate-to-severe disease but not reinfection (29,30). Similarly, infants and young children are protected against symptomatic disease after primary infection, independent of whether the primary infection was symptomatic or asymptomatic (11,31); protection lasted for at least 2 years. On the other hand, symptomatic reinfection 1 year following primary infection (even with the same serotype) is well described (29,32–43). Therefore, although the data are somewhat contradictory, protection against rotavirus disease induced by natural infection may in many cases be short-lived. It remains unclear whether serotype is important in protection against reinfection (35,44).

There remains no definitive immunologic correlate of protection against rotavirus disease. However, because replication of rotaviruses occurs exclusively among mature villous epithelial cells of the small intestine, protection is probably best predicted by the immunologic response occurring at the intestinal mucosal surface. High levels of fecal, rotavirus-specific IgA correlate with protection against disease (45,46). Of interest, high levels of rotavirus-specific IgG in serum also correlate with protection against relatively severe disease (33,47,48). Although the quantity of serotype-specific neutralizing antibodies in serum directed against the challenge virus has been found to correlate directly with protection against disease

(35), this has not been a consistent finding (44). Possibly, high levels of rotavirus-specific IgG in serum are predictive of persistence of rotavirus-specific sIgA at the intestinal mucosal surface. The short-lived sIgA response (in contrast with the relative persistence of circulating, rotavirus-specific IgG) is consistent with the often short-lived nature of protection against disease induced by natural infection and further supports the correlation between rotavirus-specific sIgA at the intestinal surface and protection against disease. There are no studies in humans examining the relationship between the presence of circulating rotavirus-specific T helper cells or cytotoxic T cells and protection against disease.

Protection Against Disease by Breast-feeding or Transplacental Transfer of Antibodies

Virtually all women, independent of socioeconomic background, have rotavirus-specific binding antibodies (primarily sIgA) and rotavirus-specific neutralizing antibodies in colostrum and milk (49–53). Levels of virus-specific binding and neutralizing antibodies appear to decline in milk during the first 6 months of life (49,53). The presence of virus-specific neutralizing antibodies in milk may in part be responsible for the decreased incidence of symptomatic rotavirus infection in early infancy (54,55).

It remains unclear whether breast-feeding protects against relatively severe rotavirus disease in infants (34,56–63). Higher levels of rotavirus-specific neutralizing antibodies in colostrum and milk are detected in mothers of uninfected as compared to infected neonates (58). However, a number of studies failed to demonstrate an association between breast-feeding and protection against rotavirus disease (59–63). Similar to passive protection studies performed in animals (63), the capacity of colostrum or milk to protect against disease may be dependent on the titer of serotype-specific neutralizing antibodies (64). Levels of neutralizing antibodies in milk, which are protective against challenge, may only occasionally be reached after natural infection. Therefore studies including low numbers of infants may give conflicting results.

It is unclear whether passive protection is afforded by transplacental transfer of maternal, rotavirus-specific IgG (65–67).

Protection Against Disease by Oral Administration of Antibodies

Prophylactic protection against rotavirus infection and clinically significant rotavirus disease can be afforded by oral administration of either serum immunoglobulins or bovine milk containing high titers of rotavirus-specific neutralizing antibodies (obtained after hyperimmunization of cattle) (68,69). However, amelioration of acute disease in infants is not afforded by passive administration of bovine milk containing high titers of rotavirus-neutralizing antibodies (70). Because rotavirus replication in the small intestine is limited to several days, administration of antibodies at the time of clinical disease is probably too late to alter the clinical course. However, in children with immunodeficiency disorders (where rotavirus replication may occur over many weeks or months), rotavirus-specific immunoglobulin preparations administered orally may ablate shedding and ameliorate disease (71).

Protection Against Disease by Immunization

Given the infant mortality associated with rotavirus gastroenteritis in the developing world, prevention of disease by universal immunization would be ideal. In developed countries, the prevalence of rotavirus morbidity, including hospitalizations, also indicates that an effective vaccine against rotavirus disease would be cost-effective. Attempts to develop a rotavirus vaccine for infants were initiated soon after the discovery of human rotavirus and continue to be actively pursued.

Vaccine development has not evolved based on any clear understanding of the critical immunoprotective antigenic components of rotavirus, nor from knowledge of the critical protective component(s) of the host immune response. Rather, development has largely been based on empirical thinking and, until recently, has largely been disappointing.

Animal-Origin Rotavirus Vaccines

The first veterinary vaccine actually also became the first human candidate vaccine. A bovine (G type 6) rotavirus isolated in bovine cell culture and passed 147 times (including 30 passages at a reduced incubation temperature of 30°C) was designated Nebraska calf diarrhea virus (NCDV) (72).

Use of NCDV as an oral vaccine administered to day-old calves was reported in 1972 (73). Protective efficacy was reported based on clinical studies that did not include double-blind controlled trials (73). In subsequent properly controlled trials, NCDV was found to be ineffective (74,75). Nevertheless, its clinical use in veterinary medicine continued.

The only known clinically successful programs of vaccination against rotavirus involve parenteral vaccination of cattle when pregnant to induce high titers of passively transferred rotavirus-specific antibodies in colostrum and milk (76,77). Although this approach is successfully applied in Europe and South America, it requires the administration parenterally of rotavirus with an oily adjuvant (78). This requirement currently precludes application for humans.

After adaptation to growth in primate cell culture, NCDV was renamed strain RIT 4237 and clinically evaluated as a human rotavirus vaccine candidate. This and all other experimental rotavirus vaccines that have been brought to clinical trials are live vaccines given orally to infants; an approach exclusively pursued despite the fact that no live oral rotavirus vaccine, veterinary or human, has yet proved to be consistently effective.

RIT 4237 vaccine was given in high dose (approximately $10^{8.0}$ TCID$_{50}$) to adults and subsequently to infants as young as 1 month of age with virtually no adverse clinical effects. Little virus was shed in feces; apparently replication in the infant intestinal tract was minimal (79–81).

Placebo-controlled efficacy studies in Finnish infants were characterized by protection rates of 50% to 58% against rotavirus diarrhea but higher (82% to 88%) protection rates against moderate-to-severe (i.e., clinically significant) rotavirus diarrhea (82). Subsequent efficacy trials in The Gambia and in Rwanda in Africa and on the White River Indian Reservation (83) in the United States revealed no protection induced by RIT 4237 against rotavirus disease (84,85). A trial comparing the protective effect of one, two, or three doses of RIT 4237 vaccine in Lima, Peru, represented an exception among rotavirus vaccine trials: efficacy was demonstrated in a developing world environment (86). It was not clear whether multiple doses were necessary for optimum effect. However, factors related to demonstrable efficacy were immunization of infants in the first year of life, natural challenge with G type 1 rotavirus, and disease in which rotavirus infection was not associated with other enteric pathogens. Up to 75% protection against severe rotavirus disease was reported. Nevertheless, because of inconsistent results, RIT 4237 has been withdrawn as a vaccine candidate.

Another bovine-origin rotavirus vaccine candidate (strain WC3) was evaluated in low (12th) cell culture passage, in hopes that a less extensively passaged virus would be more immunogenic. The WC3 strain virus is, like NCDV, G type 6 but has a P type distinct from NCDV. It is given orally as a live virus in high titer [usually $\geq 10^{7.0}$ plaque-forming units (PFU)].

WC3 rotavirus has been given to more than 700 infants (some as young as 1 month old) with no adverse effects noted (87–90). In an initial trial, fecal shedding of virus was observed in 30% of infants; in subsequent trials the incidence has been lower (88). Immune response rates measured by serum-neutralizing antibodies to WC3 rotavirus have ranged from 70% to 100% in trials performed in developed countries (67,87–90).

In immunologically naive infants, WC3 vaccine does not induce serum neutralizing antibodies to viruses of human serotypes. However, infants seropositive to human rotavirus may develop a broad heterotypic "booster" neutralizing antibody response including considerable activity directed to human serotypes (88).

An initial double-blind placebo-controlled efficacy trial of WC3 vaccine conducted in Philadelphia yielded a 76% vaccine-associated protection rate against all rotavirus disease and 100% protection against moderate-to-severe disease (87). However, in a subsequent trial performed in Cincinnati, WC3 induced only 17% protection against all disease episodes; a modest but significant degree of protection was seen against moderate-to-severe disease (67). In each of these studies the natural challenge virus was G type 1. In subsequent WC3 efficacy trials performed in the Central African Republic (90) and in China, protection rates obtained against all rotavirus disease were 0% and 50%, respectively. The WC3 vaccine is no longer being actively investigated.

The most extensively tested of the animal-origin rotavirus vaccines was rhesus rotavirus (RRV). RRV was isolated from a monkey with diarrhea (91). It is a G type 3 rotavirus but the VP7 is clearly distinguishable from human G type 3 on the basis of amino acid sequence and reactivity with monoclonal antibodies (92). RRV was clinically evaluated as vaccine at the 16th cell culture passage level propagated in monkey diploid cells (93). The dose tested was commonly $10^{4.0}$ or $10^{5.0}$ PFU per infant.

RRV is, in comparison to bovine-origin rotaviruses, both more immunogenic and more reactogenic (94,95). RRV shares with many G type 3 rotaviruses a capacity to cause gastroenteritis in newborn mice, a property that is lacking or much less efficient in bovine-origin (G type 6) or other serotype rotaviruses (96). RRV also shares with G type 3 strain HCR3a a particular capacity to cause hepatitis, extrahepatic biliary obstruction, and sometimes death in certain strains of inbred mice and in severe combined immunodeficient (SCID) mice (97,98). RRV is also shed in the feces of more than half of inoculated infants (95). Transient fever occurring 2 to 4 days after inoculation was observed in 20% to 40% of infants; in some trials a small number of inoculated infants also exhibited mild symptoms of gastroenteritis (95).

RRV differs from bovine-origin rotaviruses in its efficient immunogenicity in adults and in its demonstrated capacity to induce secretory intestinal antibody in immunized infants (99). Like the bovine-origin rotaviruses, RRV induces a neutralizing antibody response directed to human rotavirus serotypes only in previously seropositive infants.

The results of placebo-controlled efficacy trials of RRV in infants have varied from no protection to as much as 65% protection against all rotavirus disease (79,100,101). In some trials protection against moderate-to-severe disease exceeded that against all rotavirus disease (102). The most puzzling result was obtained in two efficacy trials conducted 2 years apart in Rochester, New York. Despite the fact that the wild-type virus was G type 1 in both test seasons, RRV provided no protection during the first year but 65% protection against all rotavirus disease the second trial season (100,101)!

Only in a single efficacy trial of RRV was the natural challenge virus of G type 3. In this trial RRV provided 70% protection against G type 3 rotavirus disease and 67% protection against non-G type 3 rotavirus disease (103). RRV is no longer a candidate vaccine.

In summary, each of the three animal-origin rotavirus vaccines has ultimately proved to be too inefficient to pursue for universal application. Nevertheless, a few generalizations may be derived from the numerous clinical trials. (a) These rotaviruses are generally well tolerated at any age including newborn. (b) The immune response is most efficient when maternally derived immunity has waned (age 4 to 6 months). (c) The serum neutralizing antibody response is homotypic only, except in infants with evidence of previous rotavirus infection. (d) The advantage of booster doses has not been demonstrated. (e) Gastric buffering by pretreatment with antacid increases immunogenic efficiency (104). (f) Nursing may decrease the immune response to RRV but probably not to bovine rotavirus. (g) When rotavirus is coadministered with oral polio vaccine, there is probably little interference with the

normal immune response to either virus (105). (h) Heterotypic protection against human rotavirus gastroenteritis is induced, but the mechanism is unknown. The importance of serotype has not been demonstrated.

Human × Animal Reassortant Rotavirus Vaccines

Some, but by no means all, rotavirus vaccine/challenge experiments in domestic animals indicated that protection was serotype specific (106–108). This fact, coupled with the unsatisfactory performance of heterotypic animal-origin rotaviruses in human infants, led investigators to develop a second generation of candidate vaccines bearing human rotavirus type-specific surface proteins. Such recombinants or "reassortants" were developed by mixed infection in cell culture of human and animal rotaviruses followed by selection of progeny virus bearing the gene coding for human virus G protein (VP7) and the remaining genome of animal rotavirus origin. The VP7 gene was selected because it is the most highly represented surface protein and, as the predominant immunogen in parenterally inoculated hyperimmunized animals, determines serotype (17).

Reassortants bearing human G type specificity have been prepared from both simian RRV and bovine WC3 rotaviruses (109,110). Reassortants exhibit a level of attenuation characteristic of the animal rotavirus parent. Such reassortants express an enhanced ability to induce neutralizing antibodies to the homotypic human rotavirus. However, reassortants also induce neutralizing antibodies to the animal rotavirus parent, based on the retained animal rotavirus surface protein VP4 (P). For reasons that are not clear, reassortants containing human rotavirus G type on either an RRV or WC3 virus genome induce neutralizing antibodies most efficiently to RRV or WC3 virus, respectively (111,112).

RRV reassortants were developed with VP7 of either human G type 1, 2, or 4 antigenic specificity. These were evaluated either individually or, most recently, as a quadrivalent vaccine containing type 1, 2, and 4 reassortants and RRV itself as the G type 3 component.

RRV reassortants efficiently induce neutralizing antibodies to RRV, but 50% or less of infants commonly develop neutralizing antibodies to human G1, G2, G3, or G4 (111,112). RRV reassortants induced transient fevers in a small percentage of infants in developed countries but not in an initial trial in Venezuela (112). Although a majority of the quadrivalent RRV reassortant trials were performed with vaccine containing each component reassortant at a dose of 1×10^4 or 1×10^5 PFU, a recent trial in Venezuela included evaluation of the effect of a maximum concentration of 1×10^6 PFU of each. Equal rates of induction of fever (23% to 26%) and equal levels of immunogenicity were detected with the highest dose and with the vaccine containing 1×10^5 PFU of each component (113).

Limited data on protection are available. In a trial in Rochester, New York, administration of RRV type 1 reassortant was associated with 77% protection against rotavirus disease (in this same trial RRV alone gave 65% protection) (101). In a Finnish efficacy trial, RRV G type 1 and G type 2 reassortants given separately provided infants with the same degree of protection (65% and 67%, respectively) against rotavirus disease caused by a natural G type 1 virus challenge (114).

In a large, multicenter trial, the protective efficacy in infants of three doses of quadrivalent RRV reassortant was compared with that of three doses of G type 1 reassortant RRV. The two different vaccine preparations gave an identical rate of protection (63% to 65%) in a season when the natural challenge was G type 1 (115). Additional trials of the quadrivalent RRV vaccine are in progress.

A WC3 reassortant with human G type 1 was innocuous in infants at doses to $10^{7.3}$ PFU and was shed only rarely in feces; this reassortant induced antibody to WC3 in nearly 100% of inoculated infants and antibody to G type 1 rotaviruses in up to 50% (116). In a small initial efficacy trial in suburban Philadelphia, Pennsylvania, infants given two doses of the WC3 type 1 reassortant were completely protected against rotavirus disease despite the fact that only 22% of vaccinees developed a G type 1-specific serum neutralizing antibody response (117). In two subsequent three-dose trials of this reassortant, protection rates against all rotavirus disease obtained in Rochester (237 infants) and in Philadelphia (88 infants) were 63% and 73%, respectively (J. Treanor and H. F. Clark, *personal communication*). Protection rates against moderate-to-severe rotavirus disease were 84% and 100%, respectively. In both cities, the natural challenge virus was predominantly G type 1.

Single gene reassortants in which the gene coding for human rotavirus P type 1 is added to a WC3 genome are now being investigated. In a pilot experiment exploring immunogenicity, infants given a mixture of two reassortant strains—one containing P type 1 and one containing G type 1—developed an immune response to P type 1 G type 1 rotavirus with much greater efficiency than did those given either (a) the G type 1 or P type 1 monovalent reassortant alone or (b) a double reassortant containing both human P1 and G1 (118). Reassortant rotavirus vaccines containing different human P and G types on a WC3 background are now being evaluated in clinical trials.

Human-Origin Rotavirus Vaccines

Although the immunogenicity in infants of many animal-origin rotaviruses and their reassortants has been disappointing, there is little reason to believe that human-origin rotaviruses will be more effective. The human-origin rotavirus that has received the most attention is a newborn "nursery" strain M37 (G type 1). M37 has been inefficient at inducing G type 1-specific antibodies in orally inoculated infants (119) and has not induced protection against rotavirus disease (120). Cold-adapted human-origin rotaviruses of G types 1 and 3 have been evaluated in infants; human rotavirus type-specific neutralizing antibody responses occurred irregularly and were low in titer (H. F. Clark and F. Borian, *unpublished data*).

Future Directions

It appears that the vaccine candidates that will first find widespread clinical application will be human × animal rotavirus reassortants. These will be multivalent with several G types and possibly P types. They will be based on either the RRV or WC3 genome background. Either or both of these products may be licensed before the end of this decade.

It is likely that no live attenuated orally administered rotavirus vaccine will be 100% efficient. An ideal protective immune response may require a greater antigenic stimulus than that provided by the limited replication in intestinal mucosal epithelium characteristic of the present vaccine candidates. Therefore we anticipate in the near future exploration of novel immunization strategies incorporating varied routes of antigen inoculation and innovative delivery systems for virion or subvirion rotavirus components.

OTHER ENTERIC VIRUSES

There are currently no candidate vaccines for enteric viruses other than rotaviruses, which have undergone clinical trials of safety or efficacy. Small round viruses, astroviruses, caliciviruses, enteric coronaviruses, and adenoviruses have been less adaptable to growth in tissue culture than rotaviruses. Therefore development of live, attenuated viruses for use in humans has been difficult. However, the cloning and expression of individual viral genes in other bacterial or other viral vectors (e.g., expression of Norwalk virus genes in a baculovirus vector) (121) offer an interesting approach for vaccine development in the future. Long-term immunity to Norwalk and Norwalk-like viruses has not been demonstrated after natural or experimental infection. In the absence of natural immunity, prospects for successful vaccination must be viewed with some caution.

REFERENCES

1. Christensen ML. Human viral gastroenteritis. *Clin Microbiol Rev* 1989;2:51–89.
2. McGhee JR, Kiyono H. New perspectives in vaccine development: mucosal immunity to infections. *Infect Agents Dis* 1993; 2:55–73.
3. Mossman RR, Coffman RL. Th1 and Th2 cells: different patterns of lymphokine secretion lead to different functional properties. *Annu Rev Immunol* 1989;7:145–173.
4. Offit PA. Rotaviruses: immunologic determinants of protection against infection and disease. *Adv Virus Res* 1994;44:161–202.
5. Xu-Amano J, Aicher WK, Taguchi T, Kiyono H, McGhee JR. Selective induction of Th2 cells in murine Peyer's patches by oral immunization. *Int Immunol* 1992;4:433–435.
6. Davidson G, Hogg R, Kirubakaran C. Serum and intestinal immune response to rotavirus enteritis in children. *Infect Immun* 1983;40:447–452.
7. Riepenhoff-Talty M, Bogger-Goren S, Li P, Carmody P, Barrett H, Ogra P. Development of serum and intestinal antibody response to rotavirus after naturally acquired rotavirus infection in man. *J Med Virol* 1981;8:215–222.
8. Grimwood K, Lund J, Coulson B, Hudson I, Bishop R, Barnes G. Comparison of serum and mucosal antibody responses fol-

lowing severe acute rotavirus gastroenteritis in young children. *J Clin Microbiol* 1988;26:732–738.

9. Aiyar J, Ban M, Bhandari N, Kumar R, Raj P, Sazawal S. Rotavirus-specific antibody response in saliva of infants with rotavirus diarrhea. *J Infect Dis* 1990;162:1383–1384.

10. Coulson B, Grimwood K, Masendycz P, Lund J, Mermelstein N, Bishop R, Barnes G. Comparison of rotavirus immunoglobulin A coproconversion with other indices of rotavirus infection in a longitudinal study in childhood. *J Clin Microbiol* 1990;28:1367–1374.

11. Bishop R, Lund J, Cipriani E, Unicomb L, Barnes G. Clinical, serological and intestinal immune responses to rotavirus infections in humans. In: de la Maza L, Peterson E, eds. *Medical virology*. New York: Plenum Press, 1990.

12. Losonsky G, Reymann M. The immune response in primary asymptomatic and symptomatic rotavirus infection in newborn infants. *J Infect Dis* 1990;161:330–332.

13. Offit P, Hoffenberg E, Santos N, Gouvea V. Rotavirus-specific humoral and cellular immune response after primary, symptomatic infection. *J Infect Dis* 1993;167:1436–1440.

14. Guy-Grand D, Griscelli C, Vassali P. The mouse gut T lymphocyte, a novel type of cell: nature, origin, and traffic in mice in normal and graft-versus-host conditions. *J Exp Med* 1978;148:1661–1677.

15. Hoshino Y, Sereno M, Midthun K, Flores J, Kapikian A, Chanock R. Independent segregation of two antigenic specificities (vp3 and vp7) involved in neutralization of rotavirus infectivity. *Proc Natl Acad Sci USA* 1985;82:8701–8704.

16. Offit P, Blavat G. Identification of the two rotavirus genes determining neutralization specificities. *J Virol* 1986;57:376–378.

17. Estes M, Cohen J. Rotavirus gene structure and function. *Microbiol Rev* 1989;53:410–449.

18. Browning G, Fitzgerald T, Chalmers R, et al. A novel group A rotavirus G serotype: serological and genomic characterization of equine isolate F123. *J Clin Microbiol* 1991;29:2043–2046.

19. Taniguchi K, Urasawa T, Kobayashi N, et al. Nucleotide sequence of vp4 and vp7 genes of human rotaviruses with subgroup I specificity and long RNA pattern: implication for new G serotype specificity. *J Virol* 1990;64:5640–5644.

20. Beards G, Xu L, Ballard A, et al. A serotype 10 human rotavirus. *J Clin Microbiol* 1992;30:1432–1435.

21. Gentsch J, Glass R, Woods P, et al. Identification of group A rotavirus gene 4 types by polymerase chain reaction. *J Clin Microbiol* 1992;30:1365–1373.

22. Gorziglia M, Larralde G, Kapikian A, Chanock R. Antigenic relationships among human rotaviruses as determined by outer capsid protein vp4. *Proc Natl Acad Sci USA* 1990;87:7155–7159.

23. Clark H, Dolan K, Horton-Slight P, Palmer J, Plotkin S. Diverse serologic response to rotavirus infection of infants in a single epidemic. *Pediatr Infect Dis J* 1985;4:626–631.

24. Puerto F, Padilla-Noriega L, Zamora-Chavez A, Briceno A, Puerto M, Arias C. Prevalent patterns of serotype-specific seroconversion in Mexican children infected with rotavirus. *J Clin Microbiol* 1987;25:960–963.

25. Brussow H, Offit P, Gerna G, Bruttin A, Sidoti J. Polypeptide specificity of antiviral serum antibodies in children naturally infected with human rotavirus. *J Virol* 1990;64:4130–4136.

26. Gerna G, Sarasini Z, Torsellini M, Torre D, Parea M, Battaglia M. Group- and type-specific serologic response in infants and children with primary rotavirus infections and gastroenteritis caused by a strain of known serotype. *J Infect Dis* 1990;161:1105–1111.

27. Ward R, Knowlton D, Schiff G, Hoshino Y, Greenberg H. Relative concentrations of serum neutralizing antibody to vp3 and vp7 proteins in adults infected with a human rotavirus. *J Virol* 1988;62:1543–1549.

28. Ward R, McNeal M, Sander D, Greenberg H, Bernstein D. Immunodominance of the vp4 neutralization protein of rotavirus in protective natural infections of young children. *J Virol* 1993;67:464–468.

29. Bishop R, Barnes G, Cipriani E, Lund J. Clinical immunity

30. Bhan MK, Lew JF, Sazawal S, Das BK, Gentch JR, Glass RI. Protection conferred by neonatal rotavirus infection against subsequent rotavirus diarrhea. *J Infect Dis* 1993;168:282–287.

31. Bernstein D, Sander D, Smith V, Schiff G, Ward R. Protection from rotavirus reinfection: 2-year prospective study. *J Infect Dis* 1990;164:277–283.

32. Yolken R, Wyatt R, Zissis G. Epidemiology of human rotavirus types 1 and 2 as studied by enzyme-linked immunosorbent assay. *N Engl J Med* 1978;299:1156–1161.

33. Black R, Greenberg H, Kapikian A, Brown K, Becker S. Acquisition of serum antibody to Norwalk virus and rotavirus in relation to diarrhea in a longitudinal study of young children in rural Bangladesh. *J Infect Dis* 1982;145:483–489.

34. Mata L, Simhon A, Urratia J, Kronmal R, Fernandez R, Garcia B. Epidemiology of rotaviruses in a cohort of 45 Guatemalan Mayan Indian children observed from birth to the age of three years. *J Infect Dis* 1983;148:452–461.

35. Chiba S, Nakata S, Urasawa T, et al. Protective effect of naturally acquired homotypic and heterotypic rotavirus antibodies. *Lancet* 1986;1:417–421.

36. Ward R, Bernstein D, Young E, Sherwood J, Knowlton D, Schiff G. Human rotavirus studies in volunteers: determination of infectious dose and serological response to infection. *J Infect Dis* 1986;154:871–880.

37. Linares A, Gabbay Y, Mascarenhas J, Freitas R, Flewett T, Beards G. Epidemiology of rotavirus subgroups and serotypes in Belem, Brazil: a three-year study. *Ann Inst Pasteur/Virol* 1988;139:89–99.

38. Georges-Courbot M, Monges J, Beraud-Cassel A, Gouandika I, Georges A. Prospective longitudinal study of rotavirus infections in children from birth to two years of age in Central Africa. *Ann Inst Pasteur/Virol* 1988;139:421–428.

39. Friedman M, Gaul A, Sarov B, et al. Two sequential outbreaks of rotavirus gastroenteritis: evidence for symptomatic and asymptomatic reinfection. *J Infect Dis* 1988;158:814–822.

40. Grinstein S, Gomez J, Bercovich J, Biscorn E. Epidemiology of rotavirus infection and gastroenteritis in prospectively monitored Argentine families with young children. *Am J Epidemiol* 1989;130:300–308.

41. Reves R, Hossain M, Midthun K, Kapikian A, Naguib T, Zaki A, Dupont H. An observational study of naturally-acquired immunity to rotavirus diarrhea in a cohort of 363 Egyptian children. *Am J Epidemiol* 1989;130:981–988.

42. O'Ryan M, Matson D, Estes M, Bartlett A, Pickering L. Molecular epidemiology of rotavirus in young children attending day care centers in Houston. *J Infect Dis* 1990;162:810–816.

43. De Champs C, Laveran H, Peigue-Lafeville H, Chambon M, Demeocq F, Gaulme J, Beytout D. Sequential rotavirus infections: characterization of serotypes and electropherotypes. *Res Virol* 1991;142:39–45.

44. Ward R, Clemens J, Knowlton D, et al. Evidence that protection against rotavirus diarrhea after natural infection is not dependent on serotype-specific neutralizing antibody. *J Infect Dis* 1992;166:1251–1257.

45. Coulson B, Grimwood K, Hudson I, Barnes G, Bishop R. Role of coproantibody in clinical protection of children during reinfection with rotavirus. *J Clin Microbiol* 1992;30:1678–1684.

46. Matson D, O'Ryan M, Herrera I, Pickering L, Estes M. Fecal antibody responses to symptomatic and asymptomatic rotavirus infections. *J Infect Dis* 1993;167:577–583.

47. Ryder R, Singh N, Reeves W, Kapikian A, Greenberg H, Sack R. Evidence of immunity induced by naturally acquired rotavirus and Norwalk virus infection on two remote Panamanian islands. *J Infect Dis* 1985;151:99–105.

48. Clemens J, Ward R, Rao M, et al. Seroepidemiologic evaluation of antibodies to rotavirus as correlates of the risk of clinically significant rotavirus diarrhea in rural Bangladesh. *J Infect Dis* 1992;165:161–165.

49. Yolken R, Wyatt R, Mata L, Urratia J, Garcia B, Chanock R, Kapikian A. Secretory antibody directed against rotavirus in human milk—measurement by means of enzyme-linked immunosorbent assay. *J Pediatr* 1978;93:916–921.

50. Cukor G, Blacklow N, Capozza F, Panjvani Z, Bednarek F. Persistence of antibodies to rotavirus in human milk. *J Clin Microbiol* 1979;9:93–96.

51. Otnaess A, Ostavik I. The effect of human milk fractions on rotavirus in relation to the secretory IgA content. *Acta Pathol Microbiol Scand* 1980;88:15–21.

52. Bell L, Clark H, Offit P, Slight P, Arbeter A, Plotkin S. Rotavirus serotype-specific neutralizing activity in human milk. *Am J Dis Child* 1988;142:275–278.

53. Ringenbergs M, Albert M, Davidson G, Goldsworthy W, Haslam R. Serotype-specific antibodies to rotavirus in human colostrum and breast milk and in maternal and cord blood. *J Infect Dis* 1988;158:477–480.

54. Perez-Schael I, Daoud G, White L, Urbina G, Daoud N, Perez M, Flores J. Rotavirus shedding by newborn children. *J Med Virol* 1984;14:127–136.

55. Chrystie I, Totterdell B, Banatvala J. Asymptomatic endemic rotavirus infections in the newborn. *Lancet* 1978;1:1176–1178.

56. Duffy L, Byers T, Riepenhoff-Talty M, La Scolea L, Zielezny M, Ogra P. The effects of infant feeding on rotavirus-induced gastroenteritis: a prospective study. *Am J Public Health* 1986; 76:259–263.

57. Duffy L, Riepenhoff-Talty M, Byers T, La Scolea L, Zielezny M, Dryja D, Ogra P. Modulation of rotavirus enteritis during breast-feeding. *Am J Dis Child* 1986;140:1164–1168.

58. Zheng B, Ma G, Tam J, et al. The effects of maternal antibodies on neonatal rotavirus infection. *Pediatr Infect Dis J* 1992;10: 865–868.

59. Cushing A, Anderson L. Diarrhea in breast-fed and non-breast-fed infants. *Pediatrics* 1982;70:921–925.

60. Totterdell B, Nicholson K, MacLeod J, Chrystie I, Banatvala J. Neonatal rotavirus infection: role of lacteal neutralising alpha₁-anti-trypsin and nonimmunoglobulin antiviral activity in protection. *J Med Virol* 1982;10:37–44.

61. Weinberg R, Tipton G, Klish W, Brown M. Effect of breast-feeding on morbidity in rotavirus gastroenteritis. *Pediatrics* 1984;74:250–253.

62. Glass R, Stoll B, Wyatt R, Hoshino Y, Banu H, Kapikian A. Observations questioning a protective role for breast-feeding in severe rotavirus diarrhea. *Acta Pediatr Scand* 1986;75: 713–718.

63. Blake P, Ramos S, MacDonald K, et al. Pathogen-specific risk factors and protective factors for acute diarrheal disease in urban Brazilian infants. *J Infect Dis* 1993;167:627–632.

64. Offit P, Clark H. Maternal antibody-mediated protection against gastroenteritis due to rotavirus in newborn mice is dependent on both serotype and titer of antibody. *J Infect Dis* 1985;152:1152–1158.

65. Totterdell B, Chrystie I, Banatvala J. Cord blood and breast-milk antibodies in neonatal rotavirus infection. *Br Med J* 1980; 2:828–830.

66. Jayashree S, Bhan M, Raj P, Kumar R, Svensson L, Stintzing G, Bhandari N. Neonatal rotavirus infection and its relation to cord blood antibodies. *Scand J Infect Dis* 1988;20:249–253.

67. Bernstein D, Smith V, Sander D, Pax K, Schiff G, Ward R. Evaluation of WC3 rotavirus vaccine and correlates of protection in healthy infants. *J Infect Dis* 1990;162:1055–1062.

68. Barnes G, Hewson P, McLellan J, Doyle L, Knoches A, Kitchen W, Bishop R. A randomized trial of oral gammaglobulin in low-birth-weight infants infected with rotavirus. *Lancet* 1982;1:1371–1373.

69. Davidson G, Daniels E, Nunan H, et al. Passive immunization of children with bovine colostrum containing antibodies to human rotavirus. *Lancet* 1989;1:709–712.

70. Hilpert H, Brussow H, Mietens C, Sidoti J, Lerner L, Werchau H. Use of bovine milk concentrate containing antibody to rotavirus to treat rotavirus gastroenteritis in infants. *J Infect Dis* 1987;156:158–165.

71. Guarino A, Guandalini S, Albano F, Mascia A, Ritis G, Rubino A. Enteral immunoglobulins for treatment of protracted rotaviral diarrhea. *Pediatr Infect Dis J* 1991;10:612–614.

72. Mebus CA, White RG, Bass EP, et al. Immunity to neonatal calf diarrhea virus. *J Am Vet Med Assoc* 1973;163:880–883.

73. Mebus CA, White RG, Stair FL, et al. Neonatal calf diarrhea: results of a field trial using a reo-like virus vaccine. *Vet Med Am Clin* 1972;67:173–174.

74. Thurber ET, Bass EP, Beckenhauer WH. Field trial evaluation of a reocoronavirus calf diarrhea vaccine. *Can J Comp Med* 1977;41:131–136.

75. Acres SD, Radostits OM. The efficacy of a modified live reo-like virus vaccine and an *E. coli* bacteria for prevention of acute neonatal diarrhea of beef calves. *Can Vet J* 1976;17:197–212.

76. Bachmann PA. Immunity and immunization against rotavirus in animals—a synopsis. In: Holmgren J, Lindberg A, Mollby R, eds. *Development of vaccines and drugs against diarrhea.* Lund, Sweden: Studentlitteratur, 1985:215–220.

77. Saif LJ, Smith KL, Landmeier BJ, Bohl EH, Theil KW. Immune response of pregnant cows to bovine rotavirus immunization. *Am J Vet Res* 1983;45:49–58.

78. Bellinzoni RC, Blackhall J, Baro N, et al. Efficacy of an inactivated oil-adjuvanted rotavirus vaccine in the control of calf diarrhoea in beef herds in Argentina. *Vaccine* 1989;7:263–268.

79. Vesikari T, Ruuska T, Delem A, Andre FE. Neonatal rotavirus vaccination with RIT 4237 bovine rotavirus vaccine: a preliminary report. *Pediatr Infect Dis J* 1987;6:164–169.

80. Vesikari T, Isolauri E, Delem A, et al. Immunogenicity and safety of live oral attenuated bovine rotavirus vaccine strain RIT 4237 in adults and young children. *Lancet* 1983;2:807–811.

81. Vesikari T, Isolauri E, D'Hondt E, et al. Protection of infants against rotavirus diarrhoea by RIT 4237 attenuated bovine rotavirus strain vaccine. *Lancet* 1984;1:977–980.

82. Vesikari T, Isolauri E, Delem A, et al. Clinical efficacy of the RIT 4237 live attenuated bovine rotavirus vaccine in infants vaccinated before a rotavirus epidemic. *J Pediatr* 1985;107: 189–194.

83. Santosham M, Letson GW, Wolff M, et al. A field study of the safety and efficacy of two candidate rotavirus vaccines in a native American population. *J Infect Dis* 1991;163:483–487.

84. Hanlon P, Hanlon K, Marsh V, et al. Trial of an attenuated bovine rotavirus vaccine (RIT 4237) in Gambian infants. *Lancet* 1987;1:1342–1345.

85. DeMol P, Zissis G, Butzler JP, et al. Failure of live, attenuated oral rotavirus vaccine. *Lancet* 1986;2:108.

86. Lanata CF, Black RE, deAguila R, et al. Protection of Peruvian children against rotavirus diarrhea of specific serotypes by one, two or three doses of the RIT 4237 attenuated bovine rotavirus vaccine. *J Infect Dis* 1989;159:452–459.

87. Clark HF, Borian FE, Bell LM, Modesto K, Gouvea V, Plotkin SA. Protective effect of WC3 vaccine against rotavirus diarrhea in infants during a predominantly serotype 1 rotavirus season. *J Infect Dis* 1988;158:570–587.

88. Clark HF, Furukawa T, Bell LM, et al. Immune response of infants and children to low passage bovine rotavirus (strain WC3). *Am J Dis Child* 1986;140:350–356.

89. Garbag-Chenon A, Fontaine J-L, Lasfargues G, et al. Reactogenicity and immunogenicity of rotavirus WC3 vaccine in 5–12-month old infants. *Ann Inst Pasteur* 1989;140:207–217.

90. Georges-Courbot MC, Monges J, Siopathis MR, et al. Evaluation of the efficacy of a low passage bovine rotavirus vaccine (strain WC3) in children in Central Africa. *Res Virol* 1991;142: 405–411.

91. Stuker G, Oshiro LS, Schmidt NJ. Antigenic comparisons of two new rotaviruses from rhesus monkeys. *J Clin Microbiol* 1980;11:202–203.

92. Nishikawa K, Hoshino Y, Taniguchi K, et al. Rotavirus vp7 neutralization epitopes of serotype 3 strains. *Virology* 1989; 171:503–515.

93. Kapikian AZ, Midthun K, Hoshino Y, et al. Rhesus rotavirus: a candidate vaccine for prevention of human rotavirus disease. In: Lerner RA, Chanock RM, Brown F, eds. *Molecular and chemical basis of resistance to parasitic, bacterial, and viral diseases.* Cold Spring Harbor, NY: Cold Spring Harbor Laboratory, 1985.

94. Vesikari T, Kapikian AZ, Delem A, et al. A comparative trial of rhesus monkey (RRV-1) and bovine (RIT 4237) oral rotavirus vaccines in young children. *J Infect Dis* 1986;153:832–839.

95. Losonsky GA, Rennels MB, Kapikian AZ, et al. Safety, infec-

tivity, transmissibility and immunogenicity of rhesus rotavirus vaccine (MMU18006) in infants. *Pediatr Infect Dis J* 1986;5: 25–29.

96. Bell LM, Clark HF, O'Brien EA, Kornstein MJ, Plotkin SA, Offit PA. Gastroenteritis caused by human rotaviruses (serotype 3) in a suckling mouse model. *Proc Soc Exp Biol Med* 1987;184:127–132.

97. Uhnoo I, Riepenhoff-Talty M, Dharakul T, Chegas P, Fisher J, Greenberg H, Ogra P. Extramucosal spread and development of hepatitis in immunodeficient and normal mice infected with rhesus rotavirus. *J Virol* 1990;64:361–368.

98. Riepenhoff-Talty M, Schaekel K, Clark HF, et al. Group A rotaviruses produce extrahepatic biliary obstruction in orally inoculated newborn mice. *Pediatr Res* 1993;33:394–399.

99. Wright PF, Tajima T, Thompson J, et al. Candidate rotavirus vaccine (rhesus rotavirus strain) in children: an evaluation. *Pediatrics* 1987;80:473–480.

100. Christy C, Madore HP, Pichichero ME, et al. Field trial of rhesus rotavirus vaccine in infants. *Pediatr Infect Dis J* 1988; 7:647–650.

101. Madore H, Christy C, Pichichero M, et al. Field trial of rhesus rotavirus or human–rhesus rotavirus reassortant vaccine of vp7 serotype 3 or 1 specificity in infants. *J Infect Dis* 1992;166: 235–243.

102. Gothefors L, Wadell G, Juto P, et al. Prolonged efficacy of rhesus rotavirus vaccine in Swedish children. *J Infect Dis* 1989; 159:753–757.

103. Perez-Schael I, Garcia D, Gonzalez M, et al. A prospective study of diarrheal diseases in Venezuelan children to evaluate the efficacy of rhesus rotavirus vaccine. *J Med Virol* 1990;30: 219–229.

104. Pichichero M, Losonsky G, Rennels M, et al. Oral rhesus rotavirus vaccine-serotype 3 (RRV): effects of dose, formula buffering, and breast feeding. *Pediatr Res* 1989;25:187A.

105. Ho MS, Floyd RL, Glass RI, et al. Simultaneous administration of rhesus rotavirus vaccine and oral poliovirus vaccine: immunogenicity and reactogenicity. *Pediatr Infect Dis J* 1989;8: 692–696.

106. Woode GN, Kelso NE, Simpson TF, et al. Antigenic relationships among some bovine rotaviruses: serum neutralization and cross-protection in gnotobiotic calves. *J Clin Microbiol* 1983; 18:358–364.

107. Gaul SK, Simpson TF, Woode GN, et al. Antigenic relationships among some animal rotaviruses: virus neutralization in vitro and cross-protection in piglets. *J Clin Microbiol* 1982;16: 495–503.

108. Snodgrass DR, Ojeh CK, Campbell I, et al. Bovine rotavirus serotypes and their significance for immunization. *J Clin Microbiol* 1984;20:342–346.

109. Midthun K, Greenberg H, Hoshino Y, et al. Reassortant rotaviruses as potential live rotavirus vaccine candidates. *J Virol* 1985;53:949–954.

110. Clark HF, Borian FE, Modesto K, et al. Serotype 1 reassortant of bovine rotavirus WC3, strain WI79-9, induces a polytypic antibody response in infants. *Vaccine* 1990;8:327–332.

111. Perez-Schael I, Blanco M, Vilar M, et al. Clinical studies of a quadrivalent rotavirus in Venezuelan infants. *J Clin Microbiol* 1990;28:553–558.

112. Pichichero ME, Marsocci SM, Francis AB, et al. A comparative evaluation of the safety and immunogenicity of a single dose of unbuffered oral rhesus rotavirus serotype 3, rhesus/human reassortant serotypes 1, 2, and 4 and combined (tetravalent) vaccines in healthy infants. *Vaccine* 1993;11:747.

113. Flores J, Perez-Schael I, Blanco M, et al. Reactogenicity and immunogenicity of a high-titer rhesus rotavirus-based quadrivalent rotavirus vaccine. *J Clin Microbiol* 1993;31:2439–2445.

114. Vesikari T, Ruuska T, Green K, et al. Protective efficacy against serotype 1 rotavirus diarrhea by live oral rhesus–human reassortant rotavirus vaccines with human rotavirus vp7 serotype 1 or 2 specificity. *Pediatr Infect Dis J* 1992;11:535–542.

115. Sack D. Efficacy of rhesus rotavirus monovalent or tetravalent oral vaccines in US children. *ICAAC* 1992:344.

116. Borian FE, Clark HF, Plotkin SA. Immune response of infants to sequential dosing regimens of WC3 and WI79-9 oral rotavirus vaccines. *ICAAC* 1990;1226.

117. Clark HF, Borian F, Plotkin SA. Immune protection of infants against rotavirus gastroenteritis by a serotype 1 reassortant of bovine rotavirus WC3. *J Infect Dis* 1990;161:1099–1104.

118. Clark HF, Welsko D, Offit P. Infant responses to bovine rotavirus WC3 reassortants containing human rotavirus vp7, vp4, or vp7 + vp4. *ICAAC* 1992;1394.

119. Midthun K, Halsey NA, Jett-Goheen X, et al. Safety and immunogenicity of human rotavirus vaccine strain M37 in adults, children and infants. *J Infect Dis* 1991;164:792–796.

120. Vesikari T, Ruuska T, Koivu H-P, et al. Evaluation of the M37 human rotavirus vaccine in 2-to-6-month-old infants. *Pediatr Infect Dis J* 1991;10:912–917.

121. Jiang X, Wang M, Graham D, Estes MK. Expression, self-assembly, and antigenicity of the Norwalk virus capsid protein. *J Virol* 1992;66:6527–6532.

Infections of the Gastrointestinal Tract,
edited by M. J. Blaser, P. D. Smith, J. I. Ravdin,
H. B. Greenberg, and R. L. Guerrant
Raven Press, Ltd., New York © 1995.

CHAPTER 94

Vaccines to Prevent Infection by Gastrointestinal Parasites

Frederick P. Heinzel and Jonathan I. Ravdin

Billions of humans, perhaps up to one-third of the world's population, suffer intestinal infections with protozoan or helminthic parasites each year (1). Despite the substantial mortality and morbidity that result (Table 1), there is yet no vaccine available for human use that is effective against enteric parasites. This chapter specifically addresses practical and theoretical problems encountered in the development of vaccines active against enteric parasites. This includes the need to better characterize the nature of protective immunity against these diverse organisms and the importance of designing vaccines for the specific induction of mucosal immunity. In comparison to viral or bacterial agents of infection, parasites (here meaning the traditional and arbitrary grouping together of pathogenic protozoa and worms) are eukaryotes with complex life cycles. These organisms are also distinct in size, reproductive strategy, and tendency toward intra- or extracellular infection. Helminths are macroparasites (millimeters to centimeters in size), generally incapable of reproduction in a single host, rarely intracellular pathogens, and usually existing in multiple developmental stages during the course of infection. Protozoa are microparasites (micrometers in size), short lived, frequently intracellular invaders during at least one developmental stage, and able to reproduce asexually within a single host. Protozoan developmental cycles may be simple (*Giardia*) or complex (*Plasmodium*).

These factors have important effects on the nature of host immunity against infection. When multiple parasitic stages are present during infection, each may be antigenically distinct, susceptible to different types of host response, and may display shifting trophisms for different host tissues. If few antigens are conserved during maturation, immune responses developed against one stage may be ineffective or irrelevant against the succeeding devel-

opmental forms. The biology of schistosomiasis in mammalian hosts illustrates these features (see the chapter by King and Mahmoud). Infecting cercariae enter through the skin and metamorphose into schistosomula that migrate into the lung and liver. After several weeks, schistosomula mature into adult worms, take up permanent residence in the venous plexi of the gastrointestinal or urinary tract, and there lay eggs that migrate into the mucosa of these hollow viscera. Immune responses against any of these stages, including ova deposited into the intestinal tissues, exhibit incomplete cross-reactivity and can result in clinical syndromes that are stage and tissue specific. These might include an initial dermatitis at the site of entry, systemic manifestations of Katayama fever early in infection, or late-onset cirrhosis caused by fibrotic reactions to eggs deposited in the liver. As will be discussed later, protective immunity against larval or adult *Schistosoma* appears to require different types of humoral and/or cellular responses.

An additional impediment to vaccine development is that most parasites exhibit extreme antigenic heterogeneity within a species, complicating the task of identifying conserved immunodominant antigens that could protect against multiple strains endemic to the same area. High rates of mutation in genes encoding targets of host immunity may generate further antigenic variation within each strain of parasite. This rate has been estimated to be as high as 2% per generation in the case of malaria and is also apparent in intestinal protozoan agents (2); worms may be more genetically stable. Extreme forms of antigenic variation occur by gene switching, as exemplified by *Trypanosoma brucei* (3). Sporadic activation of each member of a large pool of structural genes encoding antigenically distinct surface proteins results in the outgrowth of new parasite clones. These can temporarily escape cytotoxic antibody responses directed against previous forms of the protein. When repeated, this process markedly extends the duration of infection.

The slow pace of antiparasite vaccine development also

F. P. Heinzel and J. I. Ravdin: Department of Medicine, Case Western Reserve University School of Medicine, and the Cleveland VA Medical Center, Cleveland, Ohio 44106.

TABLE 1. *Worldwide prevalence and mortality of gastrointestinal parasites in humans*

Parasite	Infections (millions)	Annual number of deaths	Average days of disability/case
Hookworm	900	60,000	100
Ascaris	1000	20,000	7–10
Trichuris	750	Unknown	7–10
Strongyloides	80	Unknown	Unknown
Schistosomiasis	200	500,000	600–1000
Entamoeba	500	100,000	7–10
Giardia	200	Unknown	5–7

Adapted from J. A. Walsh in ref. 1 and estimates from the World Health Organization and its special Programme for Research and Training.

reflects the inherent complexity of host–pathogen relationships that have probably coevolved over millions of years. Parasite transmission may be slow and inefficient if multiple intermediate hosts and/or arthropod vectors are required during the life cycle. This results in evolutionary pressure favoring chronicity of infection as one way to increase the probability of transmission. Consequently, many parasites have acquired intricate strategies for the evasion or subversion of host immunity. This may allow adult worms to survive in host tissues for up to 30 years, in the case of *Schistosoma,* or for a year or two in the case of intestinal parasites such as *Ascaris* (1). In addition to antigenic variation and switching, mechanisms of evasion include antigenic sequestration and camouflage, whereas other parasites achieve latency or chronicity when they preferentially elicit nonparasiticidal immune responses that antagonize nascent protective host responses. In this regard, infection may be maintained in a small number of humans who are genetically predisposed for chronic infection because they fail to generate sterilizing immunity (4,5). These intricate host–parasite interactions have recently been reviewed in depth (6–8). Finally, host responses elicited by chronic parasitic infection may damage host tissues due to bystander effect or to infection-related autoimmunity, as illustrated by the T cell- and cytokine-dependent pathology of schistosomal cirrhosis (9,10), and the autoantibody-mediated cardiomyopathy and neuropathy of American trypanosomiasis (Chagas' disease) (11). This raises concern over the possibility that some vaccines, rather than being protective, might prime the host for immunopathology. These current observations on host–parasite biology largely serve to highlight the fragmented nature of our understanding of which immune responses are protective, exacerbative, or merely irrelevant with regard to the expression of disease. Indeed, the usual models of "natural immunity" available for most bacterial or viral illness seem not to exist for important human helminth and protozoan pathogens. Specifically, protection against reinfection with *Schistosoma mansoni* or *Plasmodium falciparum* is, at best, incomplete even in highly endemic areas (1).

The belief that these infections are not sufficiently devastating to justify the cost and effort of discovery also may have limited the development of vaccines against intestinal parasites. Although symptoms of enteric parasitosis may not be evident by local criteria, abnormalities in the intestinal mucosa consistent with mild malabsorption are frequent in inhabitants of endemic areas (12) and suggest that broad physiologic consequences of persistent infection may be underappreciated. Recent data have demonstrated that "asymptomatic" infection with *Ascaris* and *Trichuris,* which yearly afflict over a billion humans worldwide, may be associated with delayed mental development and growth in children (13,14). This combination of high prevalence and insidious morbidity is a significant impediment to the well-being and economic productivity of a large portion of the world's population (15,16). Ironically, economic concern over lost agricultural productivity due to infection of cattle and sheep by intestinal parasites has led to the development and distribution of effective vaccines long before similar progress is evident against homologous human infections.

Although a variety of environmental or vector control solutions are available to limit the persistence or transmission of parasites, convincing data are lacking that these efforts alone will effectively or economically control local disease. On this basis, the production of reasonably inexpensive and effective vaccines against gastrointestinal parasites is a highly desired goal. The subsequent discussions will focus on the nature of protective immunity against certain types of intestinal parasites, the technology available for vaccine construction and the progress obtained to date in the development of vaccines effective against these organisms. Because many of these host–parasite responses occur within the intestinal tissues, a brief overview of mucosal immunity is provided.

HOST DEFENSES OF THE GASTROINTESTINAL MUCOSA

The intestinal tract is an organ with a surface area of nearly 400 m² that is constantly exposed to benign antigenic challenges from the residential flora and dietary biomolecules but is also the preferred portal of entry for pathogenic viruses, bacteria, and parasites. The mucosal immune system has evolved structural and functional specializations distinct from the peripheral immune system to deal with these disparate exposures.

Natural Immunity

The first line of defense in the gut is provided by natural tissue barriers (17). Although most microbial pathogens entering the gastrointestinal tract by oral uptake are inactivated by gastric acidity, parasite ova and cysts are resistant and may even require exposure to low pH to trigger excystation. Potentially expulsive intestinal peristalsis is ineffective against intestinal parasites that are usually selectively adherent to the epithelium or motile and able to resist the luminal flow. The mucous layer of the intestinal epithelium is thought to resist penetration by some microbes but is easily permeable to most parasitic worms and protozoa. Indeed, *Entamoeba histolytica* adherence lectin molecules attach to carbohydrate determinants within the mucous layer (18). Other potential barriers against infection are provided by the rapid turnover of intestinal epithelia, which may shed parasitized cells before infection spreads, and the normal flora of the gut, which may compete with invading parasites for mucosal attachment sites or may modify mucosal receptors for parasite adherence.

Polymorphonuclear cells and the proteins of the alternative complement system are rapidly recruited, and antigen-nonspecific defenses against invasive pathogens are capable of limiting infection until specific T and B cell responses can be generated. These early defenses may be effective against those gastrointestinal protozoa known to activate complement and be susceptible to lysis and/or opsonophagocytosis when incubated with serum. The serum sensitivity of *Giardia* may help to prevent ingress of infection from the intestinal mucosa (19). In contrast, most tissue-invasive protozoa, including *Trypanosoma cruzi*, *Toxoplasma gondii*, *Leishmania*, and *Entamoeba histolytica*, resist complement activation or complement-dependent lysis (20,21). Helminths are also targets for complement activation, although their thick, chitinous cuticle and shedding of surface components may defeat the cytocidal effects of the membrane attack complex (22). Whether neutrophils and complement are active within the intestinal lumen is less certain, although inflammation of the mucosa presumably leads to transmural release of polymorphonuclear cells and serum proteins.

The large size of gastrointestinal nematodes rules out killing by classical opsonophagocytosis, whereas ingestion and killing by phagocytic cells is central to the clearance of invasive protozoa (23). Nevertheless, helminths remain susceptible to killing by extracellular products of phagocyte activation and degranulation (24). Toxic compounds include oxidants, such as superoxide and nitric oxide, oxidative enzymes capable of converting superoxide into halous acids and other products, and toxic proteins, such as the major basic protein of eosinophils (25). Superoxide synthesis is triggered in neutrophils, eosinophils, and macrophages in response to the cross-linking of surface Fc receptors by immunoglobulin G- (IgG)-, IgA-, and/or IgE-coated parasites. Engagement of the phagocyte complement receptors by surface-bound products of complement activation may enhance these responses (26). Superoxide-generated free radicals, peroxides, and halide acids mediate their lethality by forming toxic lipid peroxides and carbonyls within the parasite cell membrane or by deactivating parasite enzymes (27). Nitric oxide generated by activated phagocytic, mesenchymal, endothelial, and epithelial cells can additionally damage parasite nucleic acids and proteins (28). To counter these oxidative threats, many parasites produce detoxifying enzymes, including catalases, glutathione reductase/transferases, and superoxide dismutase (27,29–31). Since these detoxifying enzymes may be critical for parasite survival in the host and may be inhibited by specific antibody responses, they are candidate antigens for use in vaccine design.

Antigen-Specific Immune Responses

Acquired resistance to many gastrointestinal parasites, when it is evident, is a function of cell-mediated immunity and antibody responses. However, the biology of T and B cells in the gut-associated lymphoid tissue (GALT) is distinct from that of the peripheral lymph nodes and spleen (the peripheral lymphoid system), as detailed elsewhere in this textbook. These differences will be explored here in relation to their importance in vaccine design. Briefly, the GALT is a functionally distinct lymphoid organ possessing its own population of memory and effector lymphocytes. The GALT is predisposed to specific pathways of T and B cell differentiation that are highly relevant in antiparasitic immunity (Fig. 1). Cells primed within the GALT preferentially recirculate within mucosal tissues; previous exposure to antigen within the intestine is more likely than peripheral immunization to induce long-lasting resistance against enteric infection (32,33).

Mucosal immune responses are generated within the Peyer's patches of the small intestine, submucosal lymphoid patches in the colon, and homologous tissues underlying the respiratory and oral mucosa. The transport of antigen from the intestinal lumen into the Peyer's patches is mediated by specialized epithelial M cells that ingest and convey particulate and soluble materials to the submucosal tissues (34). M cells are major histocompatibility complex II (MHC II) negative and presumably do not contribute to antigen presentation. Instead, antigen presenting cells in the Peyer's patches consist of macrophages and dendritic cells that process materials provided by M cell transport. The resulting antigenic peptides or linearized proteins present in the surface groove of the MHC II heterodimer are then capable of activating antigen-specific CD4+ T cells. B cells present in these tissues probably also contribute to CD4+ T cell activation during secondary responses, especially when low concentrations of antigen necessitate efficient uptake provided by antigen-specific Ig molecules on the surface of the B cell. CD8+ T cells are activated by exposure to short peptides present on MHC I following cytoplasmic infection or transcytosolic leakage of protein from the endosomal–lysosomal system (35). Activated T cells proliferate, transiently circulate within the systemic bloodstream and lymphatics, and eventually distribute throughout submucosal tissues. This tissue specificity is linked to an increased affinity for specific receptors on the endothelium of the mucosal tissues, including the recently described mucosal MadCAM molecule (36). Memory and effector T cells representative of prior mucosal antigenic challenges are widely distributed in the lamina propria of the gut and within the epithelial layer as intraepithelial lymphocytes (IELs).

Activated CD4+ T cells may become functionally specialized into phenotypically distinct T helper type 1 or type 2 (Th1 or Th2) cells. These subsets are defined by the synthesis of mutually exclusive sets of cytokines and by the expression of distinct effector functions (37). Specifically, Th1 cells generate interleukin-2 (IL-2), inter-

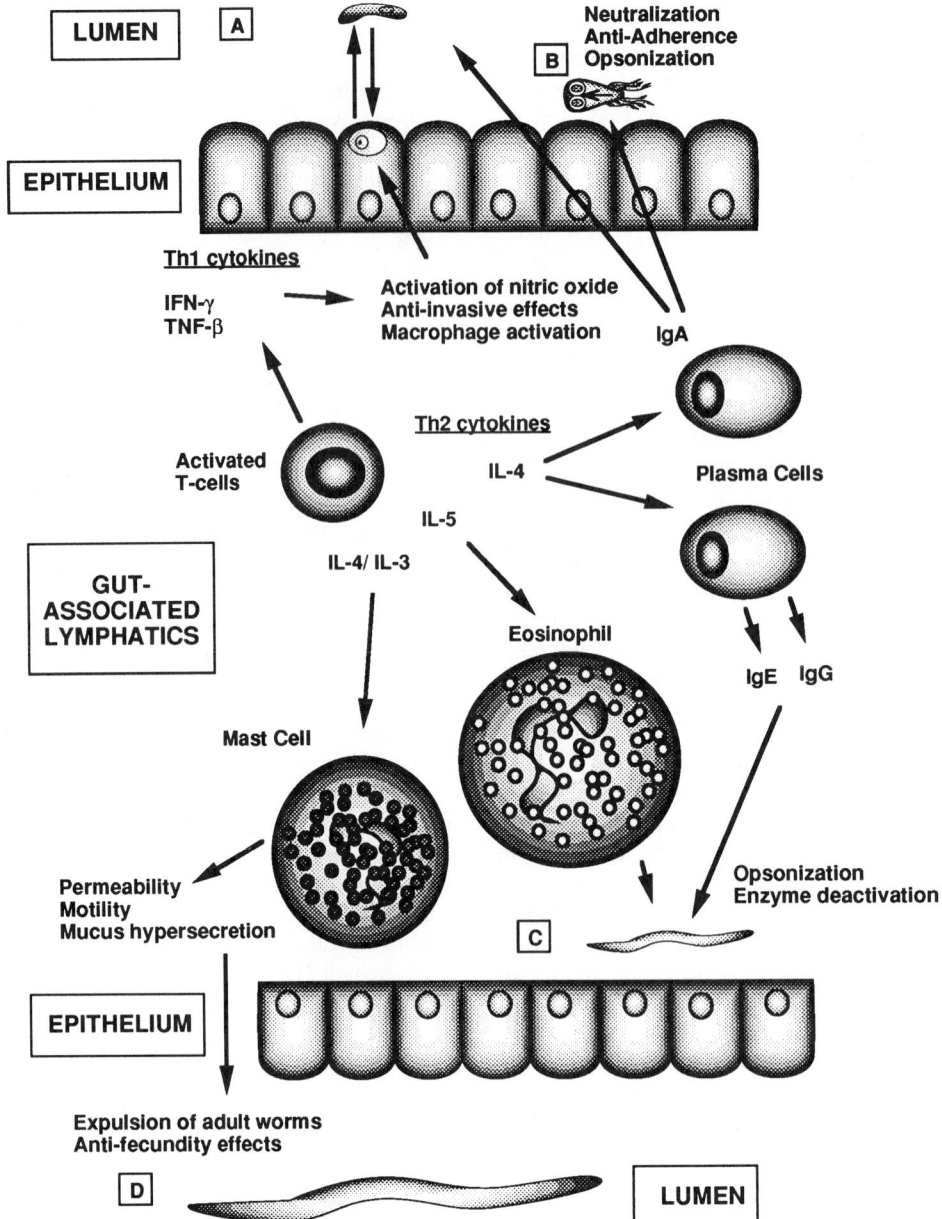

FIG. 1. Highly schematic illustration of the different forms of protective immunity generated by the mucosal immune system against parasites of the intestine. Following activation by parasite antigens, T cells within the GALT release proinflammatory cytokines that activate tissue macrophages and that stimulate nitric oxide synthesis in the epithelium, resulting in microbicidal responses directed against the intraepithelial stages of the protozoa, *Cryptosporidium parvum* (**A**). Under the influence of Th2-type cells, B lymphocytes are activated to become IgA-secreting plasma cells within the lamina propria. Dimeric IgA is transported across the epithelium into the gastrointestinal lumen, where it disrupts adherence to the mucosal surface by protozoa, such as *Giardia* trophozoites (**B**) and the extracellular merozoite stage of *Cryptosporidium*. IgA may also opsonize luminal parasites for killing by mucosal phagocytes (not shown). Tissue-dwelling helminths, such as *Schistosoma* (**C**), elicit Th2-type cell responses that result in eosinophil, mast cell, and IgE production. Opsonization of worms by IgE and IgG trigger the activation and degranulation of eosinophils and other phagocytes. Production of parasite-specific antibodies also inactivates detoxifying enzymes important for worm survival in the presence of phagocyte secretory products. Mast cells displaying cytophilic IgE are activated by exposure to parasite antigen and release factors promoting intestinal motility and hypersecretion of mucus. This facilitates the expulsion of adult worms, such as *Ascaris lumbricoides* (**D**), from the intestinal lumen.

feron-γ (IFN-γ), and tumor necrosis factor (TNF) upon antigenic stimulation. Because IFN-γ and TNF mediate proinflammatory and phagocyte-activating activities, Th1 cells are involved in the expression of delayed type hypersensitivity and are important constituents of cell-mediated immunity. In contrast, Th2 cells produce mostly B cell-stimulatory cytokines, including IL-4, IL-5, IL-6, and IL-13. Through the actions of IL-5 and IL-4 these T cells promote the increased production of eosinophils and IgE molecules. Both CD4+ T cell subsets possess ligands for B cell surface receptors, such as CD40, B7, and CD72, that transduce costimulatory signals during lymphocyte activation (38). However, Th2 cells are especially effective in promoting B cell proliferation, differentiation, and antibody synthesis and probably account for most of the "T helper" functions classically associated with CD4+ T lymphocytes. Th1 and Th2 cells possess mutually counterregulatory functions (39). IFN-γ produced by Th1 cells inhibits Th2 differentiation and function, whereas Th2-derived IL-4 and IL-10 block Th1 activation and antagonize the proinflammatory/macrophage-activating functions of IFN-γ. Because of these cross-regulatory networks, chronic parasitic infection with parasites tends to result in unbalanced expansions of Th1 and Th2 cells (7); the significance of this in specific parasitic infections and in vaccine design will be described in greater detail.

Compared to spleen and the peripheral lymph nodes, mucosal CD4+ T cells are especially predisposed toward Th2 cell development (40). This tendency may serve two functions important for normal immunologic homeostasis. First, because IL-10 and IL-4 counteract proinflammatory cellular responses, the presence of Th2 cells in the GALT may be important in suppressing deleterious inflammatory responses against constitutive antigenic exposures provided by the diet and the normal gut microbial flora. Indeed, the presence of large numbers of differentiated T cells in the mucosa with increased expression of activation markers is consistent with a state of constant physiologic activation in response to luminal antigens. Another endogenous anti-inflammatory factor, transforming growth factor-β (TGF-β), is also prevalent within many epithelial surfaces and has suppressive effects on the production and function of IFN-γ and TNF. That these cytokines mediate important homeostatic effects in suppressing inflammation is demonstrated by the appearance of severe autoimmune enteritis and colitis in mice containing homozygous inactivations in the TGF-β and IL-10 genes (41,42). A second consequence of increased Th2 cytokine production within the intestinal mucosa is that IL-4, IL-5, and TGF-β stimulate immunoglobulin class switching and synthesis of IgA (43–45), provided that activated T cells provide the surface ligand for B cell CD40 (46). Because IgA development requires both soluble and cognate T cell signals (T cell-dependent B cell activation), T cell-deficient hosts are incapable of antigen-specific IgA responses.

IFN-γ-producing Th1 cells are also prevalent in the lamina propria, although constitutive expression of proinflammatory function is apparently downregulated by the local cytokine milieu. Activated Th1 cells are adapted for the recruitment of cellular defenses against infectious agents, especially intracellular parasites. Th1 derived IFN-γ and TNF stimulate nitric oxide synthesis within endothelial, epithelial, and phagocytic cells and upregulate the production of superoxide and other oxidants by phagocytes (47). These highly reactive nitrogen and oxygen intermediates are critically involved in the killing of both helminths and protozoa. Phagocytosis and other microbicidal responses associated with granulocyte-mediated clearance of extracellular parasites are also enhanced following exposure to Th1 cytokines. CD8+ T cells can also generate IFN-γ and TNF, provided that the eliciting antigen is loaded onto MHC I in the cellular cytoplasm; a role for CD8+ T cells in resistance against intracytoplasmic protozoa has been well described (48). Natural killer (NK) cells nonspecifically stimulated by IL-12 and/or TNF released from macrophages can also be significant sources of IFN-γ during acute systemic infections and may affect indirectly the differentiation of antigen-specific T cells (49). Whether NK cells thereby protect against infection at mucosal sites is unknown.

Some CD4+ Th1 and CD8+ T cells are capable of cellular cytotoxicity against infected host cells containing intracellular microbes (7). Recently, partial human immunity against reinfection with *Plasmodium falciparum* in West Africa was linked to MHC I-restricted, CD8+ cytotoxic T cell responses against hepatic stage parasites (50). Although cytotoxic T cell effector cells are known to be present within the lamina propria and intraepithelial cell populations, the role of this response in resistance against gastrointestinal parasitism is not well defined. T cells bearing the alternative γδ T cell receptor are present within the mucosa; their functions in normal intestinal immunology and in protection against infection are also not well known (51).

Humoral responses within the GALT are dominated by synthesis of IgA and the transmucosal secretion of this antibody onto the luminal surface of the epithelium (52). Presumably because of the favorable Th2 cell environment (43), the lamina propria of the intestine and other mucosal tissues is essentially filled with IgA+ plasma cells. Polymeric IgA produced locally or systemically is transported onto the mucosal surface by the epithelial secretory component receptor (53,54). Secretory IgA is by far the most prevalent class of immunoglobulin on mucosal surfaces and has been well characterized for its ability to protect against enteral and respiratory infections (52,55). Naturally acquired immunity against several protozoan parasites has been linked to the production of specific IgA antibodies, notably against infection with *Cryptosporidium, Eimeria,* and *Giardia* (56). IgA may also neutralize microbial toxins and block microbial adherence to mucosal receptors. Although inactive as a trigger for the classic pathway of complement activation, IgA may stimulate opsonophagocytosis and lysosomal degranulation when it engages IgA-specific Fc receptors present on mucosal neutrophils and macrophages (57). Other functions of IgA unrelated to parasite immunity, such as cytosolic neutralization of viruses, immune exclusion of dietary antigens, and removal of submucosal antigens, are discussed elsewhere in this text.

IMMUNITY AGAINST SPECIFIC ENTERIC PARASITES

The pathobiology of each distinct parasite critically influences the character and efficacy of the elicited immune response. Important variables in this regard include the location of infection (extracellular, intracellular, or intraluminal), the size and complexity of the organism, the presence of molecular virulence factors (toxins, enzymes, or adhesion proteins), and the immune evasion strategies employed by the pathogen. Four general classes of parasitic infection involving the gastrointestinal tract can be identified and these categories provide a practical framework for discussion of mucosal immunity directed against these extremely diverse helminths and protozoa.

1. Infections caused by helminths. These include organisms that enter into visceral tissues during the larval stage and that subsequently localize to the gastrointestinal tract as adult worms (*Ascaris*, hookworm, *Strongyloides*), worms with purely luminal or mucosal lifestyles (pinworms, *Trichuris*, most tapeworms), worms that are primarily tissue-dwelling and that secondarily cause intestinal disease during egg-laying (*Schistosoma*), and worms for which humans are intermediate hosts and that manifest as visceral infection (*Trichinella, Taenia solium, Echinococcus*).
2. Infections caused by protozoa with at least one developmental stage that requires intracellular parasitization of the intestinal epithelium (*Cryptosporidium*, enterozoa, *Isospora*).
3. Infections caused by protozoa that are strictly intraluminal parasites (*Giardia*).
4. Protozoa that are extracellular gastrointestinal parasites with tissue-invasive proclivities (*Entamoeba, Balantidium coli*).

Helminthic Infections

Role of Th2 Responses in Immunity

Trematode and nematode parasites are among the commonest enteric infectious agents in the world. Although some cause relatively asymptomatic infections such as *Ascaris lumbricoides* and *Trichuris trichiura*, their extreme prevalence and cumulative low-grade morbidity assume epidemiologic importance. Before attaining their adult location in the intestinal lumen, invasion of visceral tissues may occur during migratory larval stages. These infections frequently manifest with a distinctive triad of eosinophilia, mastocytosis, and increased levels of circulating IgE (6). The similarity between these responses and the typical manifestations of allergic disorders has led to speculation that immediate type hypersensitivity responses are adaptations for control of helminthic infection. Indeed, prior infection with *Ascaris* or *Echinococcus* may sensitize individuals for atopic-like responses upon repeated contact with parasitic antigens (58,59). Rats infected with *Nippostrongylus brasiliensis* can also be in-duced to anaphylaxis when challenged with parasite antigen (60).

The mechanistic relationship between immediate hypersensitivity and protection against helminthic infection, or whether these responses are protective at all, remains widely debated. There is greater agreement that IgE, eosinophilia, and mastocytosis reflect the *in vivo* activation of Th2 CD4+ lymphocytes during helminthic infection (61). This is consistent with the known abilities of IL-4 to promote IgE synthesis and of IL-5 to act as a specific growth factor for eosinophils (62,63). IL-3 and IL-4 produced by Th2 cells may also contribute to the hyperplastic mast cell response present in the infected intestinal mucosa (64). The reason why Th2 responses are so frequently induced by worms has not been fully explained, although some have suggested an etiologic role for proteinases elaborated by helminths during morphologic differentiation and tissue penetration (65). In animal models of intestinal worm infection, such as *Trichinella spiralis*, both Th1 and Th2 cell development may be apparent, although these cell types are compartmentalized to the spleen and mesenteric lymph nodes, respectively (66). Finally, it is not entirely clear if the Th2 response is indiscriminantly elicited by all parasite antigens (usually consisting of dozens or hundreds of proteins) due to an "adjuvant" effect or reflects an especially strong response against a relatively small number of Th2-inducing molecules.

Does IgE protect against reinfection with helminthic parasites? In areas highly endemic for schistosomiasis, reinfection is least frequent in drug-cured individuals with the highest serum concentrations of IgE specific for *Schistosoma* (67,68). In contrast, increased amounts of schistosome-specific IgM or IgG4 antibodies capable of blocking IgE recognition of antigen predicted a higher reinfection rate (69). The mechanisms by which IgE might benefit the host during helminth infection are only partially understood. IgE-coated parasites have been shown to activate macrophages, eosinophils, and platelets bearing the low-affinity Fc receptor for IgE (FcεRII or CD23) (70). Engagement of this receptor activates cytotoxic responses capable of killing multicellular organisms *in vitro*, although *in vivo* correlates are lacking (71). IgE can also trigger immediate hypersensitivity responses by mast cells and basophils bearing cytophilic IgE antibody specific for parasite antigen. Cross-linking of cell-associated IgE on high-affinity Fc receptors (FcεRI) induces synthesis and release of eicosanoids and amines that stimulate intestinal peristalsis and mucus hypersecretion. These physiologic responses have postulated roles in parasite expulsion (72). Other products of mast cell activation recruit eosinophils that may contribute to antihelminthic immunity. *In vivo* data from selected animals models of parasitosis add support to a protective role for IgE, as demonstrated for intestinal infection with *Trichinella spiralis* in rats (73,74). However, ablation of circulating IgE by treatment with anti-IgE monoclonal antibody did not inhibit resistance against reinfection by *Heligosigmoides polygyrus* in another well-defined rodent model of intestinal parasitism (65).

Marked tissue and peripheral eosinophilia frequently

accompany helminth infection, reflecting the selective hematopoietic effects of IL-5 produced by antigen-specific Th2 cells (7). Eosinophils are antiparasite effector cells with well-defined cytotoxic effects directed against cultured adult and larval worms (23,71). Eosinophils from worm-infected humans appear to be activated for greater cytotoxicity (75) and express both the low-affinity FcεRII and high-affinity FcεRI receptors for IgE. These receptors trigger eosinophil degranulation when engaged by IgE-coated parasites (76). Fc receptors specific for IgG-coated parasites trigger similar responses. Some *in vivo* data support a role for these cells in recovery from acute illness. Eosinophil responses can be abrogated by treatment with anti-eosinophil antibodies or with anti-IL-5 antibodies prior to experimental infection. In a mouse model utilizing the gastrointestinal helminth *Strongyloides venezuelensis*, depletion of eosinophils by anti-IL-5 therapy inhibited parasite removal during the transient lung phase without any effect on the intensity of the subsequent adult intestinal phase (77). Similar experiments in a mouse model of schistosomiasis have provided conflicting results, depending on whether polyclonal anti-eosinophil antibodies or monoclonal anti-IL-5 antibodies were used (63,78).

Mast cell numbers are also increased in the gastrointestinal tract during worm infection (79) in response to Th2-related release of mast cell growth factors, such as IL-3 and IL-4 (64). An association between increased mast cell activity and expulsion of adult worms has been noted (80), presumably triggered by binding of cytophilic IgE on mast cells to parasites or their soluble antigens. Postulated mechanisms of mast cell-mediated protection include mucus production, epithelial shedding, release of motility-inducing leukotrienes, and transmural exudation of antibodies and complement (81). Activated mast cells also synthesize and release regulatory cytokines, suggesting a contributory role in the differentiation of local T cell responses (82).

Direct Effects of Th2 Cytokines on Host Resistance to Intestinal Parasitosis

Alternatively, since IgE and eosinophil production are indicative of Th2 CD4+ cell activity, it may be that critical protective responses are directly mediated by Th2-derived cytokines. In this regard, expulsion of *Heligosigmoides polygyrus* by infected mice was markedly suppressed by anti-IL-4 or anti-IL-4 receptor antibodies, but not by anti-IgE or anti-IL-5 antibodies (83), suggesting that IL-4-responsive effector cells in the gastrointestinal tract are responsible for expelling adult worms. Despite initial speculation that these were mast cells, mice genetically deficient in mast cells suffer no aberration in parasite clearance (82). Alternatively, IL-4 may be required only through its autocrine growth effect on Th2 cells (7,84,85) and it is the subsequent loss of other Th2 activities that counteract anthelminthic immunity in anti-IL-4-treated animals (65). This hypothesis is consistent with the observed attenuation of anthelminthic immunity by IFN-α and IFN-γ, which inhibit Th2 cell development and func-

tion (65). Recently, expulsion of the intestinal murine helminth, *Trichuris muris,* was found to be similarly dependent on IL-4 activity *in vivo* and to be inhibited by IFN-γ (86).

Th2 cell functions can contribute to immunopathology during infection. Th2 cell activity is important in the formation of granulomas in schistosomiasis, a response that can lead to hepatic fibrosis, portal hypertension, and intestinal dysfunction (87). Intense hypereosinophilia induced by Th2 cell cytokines is associated with pulmonary and cardiac pathology as a result of the cumulative toxic effect of major basic protein released from these cells (88,89).

Role of Other Immune Responses

Some non-IgE antibodies generated against secretory products of the tissue- and intestine-dwelling helminths may contribute to host protection by inactivating parasite-secreted detoxifying enzymes, such as catalase, superoxide dismutase, and glutathione peroxidase (27). Specific protective effects have been identified *in vivo* that are mediated by neutralizing antibodies directed against antioxidant enzymes, such as *Fasciola hepatica* and *Schistosoma mansoni* glutathione transferases (90,91). Cytotoxic antibodies directed against the worm intestine may inhibit growth and reproduction of adult worms that feed on blood obtained from submucosal vessels (typical of the hookworms and *Trichuris trichiura*). Serum IgG and IgM antibodies combined with ingested complement, presumably to mediate cytolytic reactions within the worm intestine. Alternatively, antibodies directed against parasite-derived anticoagulation factors may disable the efficient ingestion and digestion of blood when the intestine is blocked by clotted blood. In some instances a Th1 cell response can protect against reinfection with worms. The best studied example of this is the immobilization of schistosomula within the lung by inflammatory responses dependent on proinflammatory T cells producing IFN-γ (92). Eosinophilic responses in the lung were inversely correlated with protection. However, egg-laying behavior in adult schistosomes requires the presence of TNF, usually a Th1-dependent cytokine, and ovulation is absent in T cell-deficient mice (9).

In summary, the host response to helminths is complex and does not easily lend itself to *in vivo* mechanistic analyses. For a majority of the experimental systems studied, Th2 responses seem to convey protection against reinfection or facilitate early expulsion of adult worms from the intestine. It is not certain if Th2 or IgE responses directed to any specific antigen have critical importance during natural immunity. Instead, it may be the nature, rather than the specificity, of the immune response that provides the protective effect. Whether vaccine candidates should focus on identifying uniquely immunoprotective antigens or on inducing strong Th2 immune responses to mixtures of antigens will require further study.

Intracellular Parasitic Infections

A few protozoan pathogens with obligate intracellular developmental stages are important causes of human intestinal disease. The most significant of these are the species of *Cryptosporidium* that cause sporadic cases of self-limited diarrhea or, when agricultural waste enters community water supplies, city-wide epidemics (93,94). The life cycle of *Cryptosporidium* resembles that of other closely related *Apicomplexa* protozoa, including *Toxoplasma* and *Plasmodium,* and consists of alternating extracellular and intracellular developmental stages with separate asexual and sexual replicative cycles. Briefly, ingested oocysts excyst in the intestine, giving rise to four motile sporozoites that invade the cells of the columnar epithelium. Asexual reproduction within this intracellular site results in the formation and release of merozoites that then infect new enterocytes. Gametocytes are formed as part of a sexual stage leading to oocyst formation and subsequent release into the environment (93).

Naturally acquired immunity against these protozoa is evident in the self-limited nature of cryptosporidiosis in children and previously uninfected animals (95). However, immunodeficient patients, especially those with acquired immunodeficiency syndrome (AIDS), can develop severe chronic diarrhea, resulting in protein wasting enteropathy and malabsorption. Indeed, a strong correlation exists between persistence of disease and low CD4+ T cell counts; CD4+ counts above 200/mm³ were associated instead with self-limited illness (96). Consequently, a role for T lymphocytes in resolution of disease is a reasonable deduction that has been supported experimentally in animal studies (97). Antibodies may also be important in immunity, as patients with immunoglobulin deficiencies are predisposed to chronic infection (98,99). The development of *in vitro* cell invasion assays, using *Cryptosporidium* sporozoites and cultured epithelial cells, has further shown that uptake and intracellular development can be blocked by hyperimmune bovine colostrum antibodies (100). Several sporozoite surface antigens have been characterized that may contribute to cellular adhesion and entry and that are obvious candidates for vaccine development. Indeed, monospecific antibodies directed against these determinants inhibit the infection of mice when coadministered orally with *Cryptosporidium* (100).

Animal models of gastrointestinal infection with *Cryptosporidium* or with closely related *Eimeria* species have provided additional insights into the relative importance of antibody and cell-mediated immunity in protection against gastrointestinal protozoa. Resistance against reinfection was confirmed as partially T cell dependent. Depletion of CD4+ T cells following injection with anti-CD4 monoclonal antibodies exacerbated disease in mice infected with *Cryptosporidium,* as did treatment with anti-IFN-γ monoclonal antibodies (101). The protective effects of IFN-γ were multiple in these experimental systems. Specifically, IFN-γ-treated cells were resistant to invasion by sporozoites and better able to contain the growth of intracellular parasites (102). The activation of local macrophages by interferon may also promote para-

site removal through enhanced local production of superoxide, nitric oxide, and related oxidative reactants by these phagocytes. Epithelial cells may be similarly induced to kill intracellular parasites through the IFN-γ-mediated activation of nitric oxide synthease (28,103). These findings suggest that protective immunity depends on a combination of neutralizing antibodies to block parasite attachment and invasion of the epithelium, as well as antigen-specific CD4+ T cell responses capable of orchestrating microbicidal and counterinvasive responses within mucosal cells (103).

Intraluminal Protozoan Infections

Giardia lamblia is a common cause of infectious diarrhea throughout temperate climates (104). *Giardia* cysts are ingested by drinking contaminated water and these excyst within the duodenum or jejunum. The binucleate, motile trophozoite of *Giardia* subsequently replicates within the small intestine, where it feeds and generates new infective cysts. Tissue invasion is not thought to be significant; instead, the parasite adheres firmly to the mucosal surface using its ventral disc structure and apparently obtains nutrients from luminal contents and mucosal juices. As with *Cryptosporidium* infections, resistance to repeated infection is usually the rule, although some individuals can develop chronic infection that persists for years. Both parasite- and host-related factors may be responsible for the variable clinical expression of this infection (105). Giardiasis results in prompt seroconversion to the immunodominant surface antigens of the parasite. Since IgG and IgM are directly toxic to cultured trophozoites (106) and because hypogammaglobulinemic humans do not clear infection well, it is likely that the local mucosal antibody response contributes to recovery (56). Presumably, damaged or inflamed epithelium would permit local release of phagocytes and *Giardia*-specific IgG antibodies. IgM also can be transported via the polymeric secretory immunoglobulin receptor. Alternatively, opsonization from secretory antibodies might occur via IgA-specific receptors expressed on mucosal phagocytes. Despite the evident importance of mucosal adherence in the biology of *Giardia,* there is not yet any data supporting anti-adherence antibodies as determinants of acquired resistance.

T cell responses are also essential for eradication of giardiasis in animal models. Depletion of CD4+ T cells in mice by cytotoxic antibody therapy or due to inheritance of an athymic state results in persistent infection (107). Depletion of CD8+ T cells has no effect. As in humans, B cell-deficient mice are also highly susceptible to infection (108). However, since humans with AIDS do not have altered susceptibility to giardiasis, it is probable that the observed dependence on T cells in the naive mouse model reflects CD4+ helper activity required for B cell activation during primary exposures and does not indicate a critical direct role for cellular immunity.

Invasive Protozoan Infection

Specific immunity to *Entamoeba histolytica* relates only to the pathogenic form of the organism that causes symptomatic colitis and liver abscess and that comprises 10% to 40% of asymptomatic human infections. Epidemiologic, antigenic, and genomic deoxyribonucleic acid (DNA) studies indicate that there are distinct nonpathogenic (termed *E. dispar*) and pathogenic strains of *E. histolytica* (109–113). Nonpathogenic organisms are limited to intraluminal infections and do not elicit humoral antibody responses (114); other specific immune responses have not been studied. All infections with pathogenic *E. histolytica* strains apparently elicit secretory, humoral, and cell-mediated immune responses.

Entamoeba histolytica cysts are the infective form, resistant to desiccation and the acid pH of the stomach. As with *Giardia*, excystation occurs in the small bowel and trophozoites exclusively colonize the colon, where they feed on bacteria and other debris. The factors that induce encystation are unknown, but excretion of cysts (up to 15 million per day) completes the life cycle. Patent human infection can be induced by ingestion of a single cyst. It is debated whether subclinical invasion occurs during all intestinal infections with pathogenic organisms. Important parasite virulence factors include the basement membrane-degrading cysteine proteinases (115,116), a galactose-inhibitable adherence lectin that mediates attachment to colonic mucous and host cells (117–120), and a pore-forming protein that has a putative role in the amebic contact-dependent cytotoxicity that follows binding by the galactose-inhibitable lectin (121,122). A complete review of the pathogenic mechanisms of *E. histolytica* and all aspects of the host immune response are provided in the chapter by Reed and Ravdin.

There are no prospective, controlled studies that demonstrate natural immunity in humans to intraluminal infection or invasive amebiasis. Asymptomatic infection with nonpathogenic or pathogenic *E. histolytica* clears within 9 to 12 months without treatment (123,124). Susceptibility to reinfection in endemic areas has not been studied. However, subjects with serum anti-amebic antibodies have a lower point prevalence of *E. histolytica* intestinal infection (125). In addition, recurrence of amebic liver abscess is unusual (126), unless the concurrent intestinal infection was not eradicated (127). In experimental animal models of amebic liver abscess, pharmacologic cure resulted in resistance to subsequent intrahepatic parasitic challenge (128).

Invasive *E. histolytica* trophozoites are resistant to the lytic mechanisms of complement via cysteine proteinase-mediated degradation of the C3 complement component and by binding of the C8 and C9 components by the galactose-inhibitable adherence lectin, preventing formation of complete C5b–C9 membrane attack complexes (129,130). Invasive intestinal and hepatic amebiasis elicits a secretory IgA (sIgA) response to amebic antigens (131,132), and specifically the adherence lectin 170-kDa subunit (133). Anti-amebic sIgA has been found in colostrum and saliva (131–135) but has not been studied in local colonic secretions. The trophozoite possesses a potent defense against sIgA, degradation of IgA by extracellular cysteine proteinases (Fig. 2) (136). IgA degradation by *E. histolytica* is complete; specific cleavage at the hinge site as described for bacterial IgA proteinases was not found (136). Serum anti-amebic IgM and IgG antibody responses occur

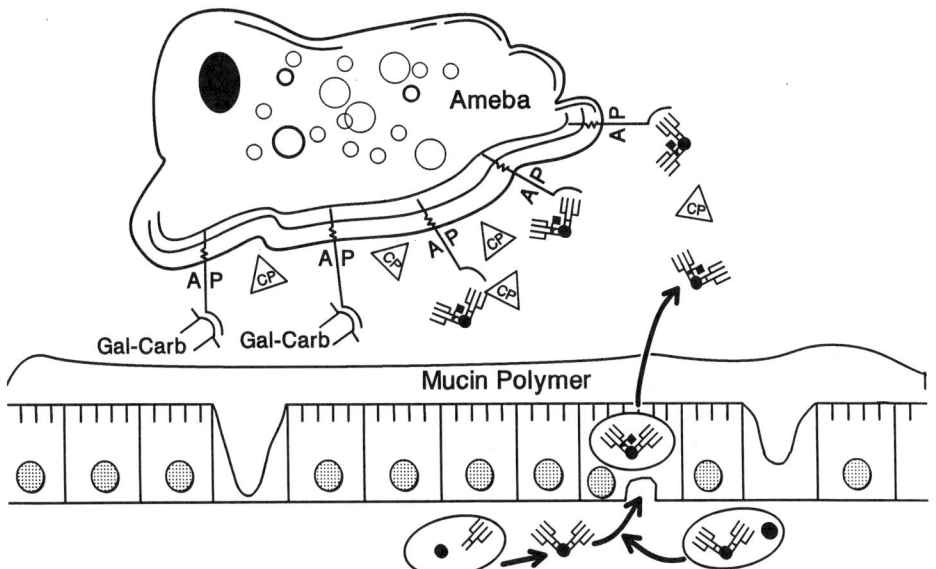

FIG. 2. Schematic illustration of the interactions between *Entamoeba histolytica* and secretory IgA. Ameba attaches to galactose-containing carbohydrate determinants on the intestinal mucins through interactions with the 170-kDa galactose-inhibitable lectin adherence protein (AP). IgA antibodies directed against the adherence protein are synthesized in the lamina propria, dimerized, and transported through the secretory component pathway. Luminal IgA binds and neutralizes the adherence protein. Cysteine proteinase (CP) is produced by the ameba in defense and this enzyme cleaves luminal IgA, thus compromising host immunity against invasion.

within the first 7 days of symptomatic invasive amebiasis (137,138). However, all asymptomatic individuals found to harbor pathogenic *E. histolytica* possess serum anti-amebic antibodies (114,138). The 170-kDa subunit of the galactose-inhibitable lectin is a highly conserved parasite antigen; over 95% of patients with amebic liver abscess have serum IgM or IgG antibody to this protein (114,138). Fortunately, significant antigenic variation or heterogeneity has not been found in *E. histolytica*.

It is unclear if serum anti-amebic antibody provides a neutralizing or protective response against *E. histolytica*. There is relentless progression of established invasive disease despite development of high titers of serum antibody, including neutralizing antibodies to the adherence lectin (114). *In vitro*, via capping, trophozoites repeatedly shed attached anti-amebic IgG antibodies without loss of viability (139). In addition, antibody-dependent cellular cytotoxicity has not been found to be operative against *E. histolytica*. In contrast, recent studies of passive immunization with polyclonal anti-lectin antibodies in immunocompetent gerbils (139,140) and with antisera raised to whole trophozoites in severe combined immunodeficient (SCID) mice (141) provided partial protection against amebic liver abscess, suggesting some role for serum antibody in host immunity.

Cell-mediated immunity clearly has an important role in combating the trophozoites that are residing in tissue. Peripheral blood lymphocytes from patients cured of invasive amebiasis proliferate and produce IFN-γ upon stimulation with amebic antigen (142,143). Supernates from stimulated lymphocytes activate human monocyte-derived macrophage amebicidal activity (via oxidative and nonoxidative mechanisms) (144). IFN-γ is sufficient to activate human macrophage amebicidal activity; however, neutralizing anti-IFN-γ monoclonal antibody only partially inhibits the activity of stimulated lymphocyte supernatants, indicating that other lymphokines are also contributory (143). In the murine system, TNF has been shown to activate macrophage and neutrophil amebicidal activity (145–147). Interestingly, CD8 lymphocytes from serum anti-amebic antibody positive subjects became directly amebicidal when stimulated with amebic antigen *in vitro*. This is an antigen-specific event; CD8 cell lines stimulated with nonrelated antigens (i.e., tuberculosis) are not cytotoxic for the parasite and are rapidly killed by trophozoites. Mice demonstrate natural immunity to intrahepatic injection of trophozoites; however, the T and B cell-deficient SCID mice do develop necrotic amebic liver abscesses (141).

STRATEGIES FOR VACCINE DEVELOPMENT

Overview of Vaccine Strategies Relative to Parasitic Disease

Successful vaccine design has usually been an empiric exercise, relying on the formulation of noninfectious antigenic preparations that provide measurable resistance against infection. Characterization of the mechanism of protective immunity thus engendered has often followed demonstration of efficacy. This approach has proved useful against viral and bacterial pathogens that are especially susceptible to the effects of neutralizing or opsonizing antibodies. However, similar methodology has not been as useful against metazoan or protozoan parasites, where the immunologic goals of vaccination are less well understood. The need to elicit mucosal immunity against intestinal parasites adds another dimension of complexity to consider in vaccine design against enteric infections. The following discussions will address different approaches to vaccine design that may be applicable to intestinal parasites, focusing on the different forms of antigen that might be used and on the contributions of vaccine formulation and adjuvant in optimizing mucosal responses.

Live, Attenuated Vaccines

The most desirable form of antigen for inducing prophylactic immunity is viable, but nonpathogenic, forms of the selected microorganism. This provides a broad range of protein and carbohydrate antigens produced in their native configuration. Furthermore, *in vivo* replication and persistence of the organism amplify the host response beyond that elicited by purely nonviable antigenic mixtures. In addition to provoking long-lived antibody responses, live challenge with attenuated organisms generates strong cell-mediated immunity (148). This is an important consideration when the targeted parasite is intracellular, and antigen-specific effector T cells are important determinants of resistance (149). Examples of this approach to vaccination include the use of vaccinia virus to prevent infection with the antigenically similar smallpox virus (150), and the use of attenuated mumps, measles, rubella, and yellow fever vaccines. Attenuated live bacterial vaccines with demonstrated efficacy include the Bacille bilié de Calmette-Guérin (BCG) strain of *Mycobacterium bovis* (151). Nonvirulent strains of *enteric* pathogens are especially useful because they reproduce and cause abortive infection of the *mucosal* immune system, leading to strong local IgA and T cell responses that would be less efficiently generated by peripheral vaccination. This avoids the problem of antigen delivery to the intestine and has proved clinically useful in the form of attenuated Sabin strain of poliovirus. Recently, the use of orally delivered avirulent Ty21a strain of *Salmonella typhi* and attenuated *Vibrio cholerae* strains have been subjected to clinical studies with some evidence of clinical efficacy in highly endemic areas (152,153).

This approach has been tried for some parasitic agents of disease. Gamma-irradiated canine hookworm and bovine lungworm larvae provided the first demonstrations of vaccine-induced immunity against helminthic parasites. Vaccination with gamma-irradiated sporozoites has long been used as a murine model of acquired resistance against *Plasmodium falciparum* (154). Although useful in defining protective vaccine immunity, this approach has practical limitations preventing successful scale-up for field use against a wider variety of parasitic targets. Many pathogenic protozoa and helminths cannot be grown in culture under economically feasible conditions and may not survive long in an antigenically useful form following irradiation. Although some protozoa can be propagated in culture as avirulent forms, the possibility of reversion to a pathogenic trait—due to the often complex and unpredictable molecular genetics of these organisms—gives pause to the idea of clinical trials with live, attenuated protozoa. As the molecular biology of these organisms becomes better known, it may be possible to engineer avirulent forms by inserting selected "suicide" genes into wild type protozoa (155). Indeed, transfection methodologies useful in studies of protozoa have allowed the bioengineering of recombinant strains of *Leishmania major* and *Toxoplasma gondii* (156,157). However, genetic transfection of pathogenic helminths has not been achieved.

Inactivated Whole Organisms

Alternatively, inactivated whole organisms (heat-killed or formalin-fixed) can be used as immunogens, maintaining the benefit of multicomponent antigenic structure without the risk of symptomatic infection. However, the intensity of the immune response suffers from the inability of these preparations to proliferate in the host tissues. Furthermore, the inactivation process may subtly alter the immune responses. For instance, the generation of cytotoxic or inflammatory CD8+ T cells against viral agents may be hindered if critical antigenic peptides are not loaded onto MHC I in the absence of cytoplasmic synthesis of viral proteins (35). Again, an economic source of large numbers of inactivated parasites, devoid of biohazardous materials, remains a major hurdle to further development.

Subunit Vaccines

Given the complexities of obtaining preparations of attenuated or inactivated parasites, can distinct antigens be found that give rise to long-lasting immunity? In contrast to the "shotgun" approach of whole-organism vaccination, the design of subunit parasite vaccines requires that we understand what constitutes protective, exacerbative, or irrelevant forms of immunity in parasite-infected humans and experimental animals. The designated antigen might be a target for cytotoxic responses, in which case it must be accessible to *in vivo* cellular and humoral immunity. Alternatively, candidate immunogens might represent functionally important molecules that are inactivated by humoral immune responses and that are necessary for the viability and/or virulence of the pathogen. Examples include antitoxin responses, analogous to that generated by tetanus and diphtheria toxoid, and anti-adherence antibodies similar to neutralizing humoral immunity against viruses. Neutralizing antibodies directed against the adhesion proteins of *Entamoeba histolytica*, *Giardia* species, and *Cryptosporidium* species may disrupt binding of the parasite to intestinal mucosa and thereby local colonization and reproduction. Any putative adherence protein should receive considerable scrutiny as a vaccine candidate. The galactose-inhibitable lectin of *Entamoeba histo-*

lytica is the best characterized example of a candidate vaccine antigen of this sort.

Subunit vaccines can effectively generate protective humoral immune responses, especially when the antigenic protein is aggregated by formalin treatment. However, significant cell-mediated immunity may be difficult to elicit without the use of potent adjuvants with clinically unacceptable side effects. Furthermore, T cell responses against a single protein may not be consistently obtained if a few key peptide epitopes are not effectively presented by MHC haplotypes prevalent in the local population (158). Nevertheless, this approach uses reasonably economical methodology to produce large quantities of recombinant antigen, without risk of contamination by virulent organisms, and available in a stable lyophilized form amenable to storage and transport. However, despite impressive advances in cataloging immunodominant antigens of the important parasites, few of these have progressed into clinical investigation as vaccine components (Table 2).

Curiously, some of the best examples of antibody-mediated resistance against intestinal parasitism were not predicted because the elicited response is directed against antigens normally not recognized during native infection (159). Examples of protective immunity against such "concealed" antigens are highlighted by vaccines introduced recently against cattle ticks and sheep intestinal nematodes. Antibodies elicited by a tick-specific gut antigen are ingested with complement during a blood meal, destroy the arthropod intestine, and thereby disrupt *Boophilus microplus* egg laying (160). Since many helminthic infections do not give rise to impressive "natural" immunity, these observations suggest that the search for "unnatural" types of immunity may be worth pursuing.

Peptide Vaccines

Assuming protective proteins can be found, it may be possible to identify uniquely immunogenic epitopes that are sufficiently conserved to justify the construction of oligopeptide vaccines. Peptides would be relatively easy and inexpensive to mass-produce; they also store well and bear absolutely no risk of accidental virulence. However, immunogenicity is poor, especially for the generation of long-lived cell-mediated immunity. New approaches in adjuvant and antigen delivery technology will be required to make oligopeptides clinically useful. As with subunit immunogens, some individuals possessing the wrong MHC or T cell receptor repertoire may be unresponsive to the small number of potential epitopes thus provided (158). However, a "cocktail" approach to peptide vaccination, using multiple peptide epitopes, circumvents this drawback. A recent advance in the formulation of oligopeptide vaccines has been the use of multiple antigenic peptide (MAP) constructs, containing four or more peptides linked to a branching lysine core (161). Although originally designed to induce antibodies *in vivo*, the use of combined T and B cell epitopes from parasite-derived triose phosphate isomerase in a MAP construct elicits

TABLE 2. *Candidate vaccines against parasites of the gastrointestinal tract*

Parasite	Amount of protection
Schistosoma mansoni (reviewed in ref. 181)	
Cercariae/worm extracts	40%–90% protective in rodent models
Glutathione-*S*-transferase	50%–70% Protective in rodent and primate models; antifecundity vaccine (182)
Triose phosphate isomerase	38% Protective in mouse model
Paramyosin	30%–40% Protective in mouse model
Fasciola hepatica	
Glutathione-*S*-transferase	50% Protection; directed against juvenile worms (90)
Taenia species	
Taenia ovis 45S protein (fusion with GST)	97% Protection in lambs (186,188)
Ascaris species	
Ascaris suum extracts	89% Protection in mice; liposomal carrier with levamisole as adjuvant (185)
Ancyclostoma species	
Irradiated larvae (dog)	60% Protection in dogs (184)
Other enteric helminths	
Haemonchus contortus (various antigens)	80% Protection in lambs
Giardia lamblia	
56–65 kDa cysteine-rich protein	80% Protection in mice against homologous strains of *Giardia* (192)
Cryptosporidium species	
Sporozoite/merozoite gp15, gp20, p23	Antibodies confer passive protection in mouse model (97,100)
Entamoeba histolytica	
260-kDa Galactose-inhibitable lectin	67% Protection against liver abscess in gerbil model (201)
29-kDa Surface protein	56% Protection against liver abscess in gerbil model (205)
Recombinant 47-kDa segment of lectin 170-kDa subunit	67% Protection against liver abscess in gerbil model (203)

both cellular and humoral immune responses in a mouse model of schistosomiasis (162).

The use of single-antigen vaccines, whether peptides or whole proteins, introduces the problem of eliciting immunity against multistage parasites when the immunogen is unique only to a single developmental stage. The effort to develop an antimalarial vaccine has had to address this issue, since naturally acquired immunity against infection seems to involve distinct and nonoverlapping host responses against circulating sporozoites, intracellular hepatic schizonts, blood-borne gametocytes, and extracellular and intracellular blood stage parasites (163). At each stage, protective immunity might variably consist of anti-adherence antibodies, cytotoxic antibodies, Th1 CD4+ or Th2 CD4+ T cell responses, or CD8+ cytotoxic T cell responses. It is now accepted dogma that a single-antigen vaccine will not be appropriate for clinical use against malaria, leading to the formulation of multistage-specific protein or peptide vaccines. Specifically, a MAP vaccine containing T and B cell epitopes for multiple stages of *Plasmodium falciparum* has already proved successful in preventing human malaria in endemic areas (164).

Finally, polysaccharide antigens may be important targets for neutralizing or opsonizing antibody responses against mucosal pathogens. In this regard, purified Vi antigen of *Salmonella typhi* has proved to be a highly protective immunogen in humans living in areas highly endemic for typhoid fever (165). The disadvantage to polysaccharide vaccines is that they only elicit humoral immune responses and rarely provoke IgG synthesis with long-term memory unless conjugated to protein carriers, a modification easily provided using current technology (166).

Induction of Mucosal Immunity Effective Against Intestinal Parasites

Vaccines effective against gastrointestinal parasite infection may need to be especially formulated to optimally induce mucosal immunity. Due to targeted recirculation of antigen-primed T cells and B cells, immunization at mucosal sites is clearly preferred for optimizing intestinal immune responses (32,33). Assuming that the techniques and science of oral immunization can be mastered, this approach has several advantages over parenteral vaccines. First, the quality control standards for biologics taken orally need not be as strict (or expensive) as for injectable preparations. Second, oral administration will minimize the need to have trained medical personnel available. Third, because of lymphocyte recirculation through the various mucosal lymphoid systems, oral immunization may also promote protective immunity within the bronchial and upper respiratory tract mucosa against the migratory larval forms of *Strongyloides* and *Ascaris*. Whatever the route of administration, vaccine design may need to be altered to induce specific types of immune response associated with protective antiparasite immunity. For protozoa that require mucosal adherence to permit multiplication or tissue invasion, this amounts to responses supporting synthesis of neutralizing IgA antibodies. For intracellular pathogens, such as *Cryptosporidium*, protection may also require that Th1 cell responses be generated. In contrast, helminths may require Th2 responses to mediate expulsion of adult worms.

Delivery of inactivated or recombinant antigen requires

some protection against the proteolytic functions of the upper gastrointestinal tract. Methods evolved to circumvent this problem include the use of lipsomes and biodegradable microspheres to deliver antigen distally within the gut. As of yet, this approach has not been specifically utilized against parasitic infections and the background of this technology is discussed in greater detail in the chapter by Skiest and Hill. Another approach, applicable to recombinant immunogens with demonstrated efficacy is to genetically engineer avirulent bacteria or viruses for expression of the desired protein following oral administration. Considerable experience with this approach has already been obtained using attenuated strains of *Salmonella* that invade and replicate directly within the mucosal lymphoid tissues (167). One such recombinant vector induced strong cell-mediated immune responses against antigens of *Plasmodium berghei* (168). Similarly, both cellular and antibody responses were observed following oral immunization with *Salmonella* expressing hepatitis B virus antigens (169). Other potential live vectors for the expression of parasite antigens include recombinant BCG, fowlpox virus, and vaccinia (170–173). Not all these systems would be amenable to oral administration, however. The use of intracellular vectors, such as *Salmonella* and recombinant viruses, also affords a means to deliver antigen for loading on MHC I. Indeed, these vectors have demonstrated success in eliciting antigen-specific CD8+ T cells that might prove effective in clearing intracellular parasitism (174).

Adjuvants

Protein or peptide antigens alone may not be sufficiently immunogenic to induce effective and durable levels of humoral or cellular immunity. A long list of substances that enhance immunogenicity by inducing inflammation are known and collectively referred to as adjuvants (175). However, many of these substances, such as Freund's adjuvant, are too proinflammatory to be acceptable for human use (176). The relatively weak adjuvant, aluminum hydroxide, has been used for a variety of human vaccines but may not be useful for the induction of strong mucosal immunity. Several candidate adjuvants are currently under study that may dramatically improve the effectiveness of oral immunization (177).

The best studied of these is the cholera toxin subunit B protein derived from *Vibrio cholerae*. This protein interacts with specific ganglioside receptors on intestinal epithelial cells and is known to be a potent mucosal immunogen that elicits strong IgA responses when given orally (178). Through unclear mechanisms, probably mediated by induction of Th2 cells or downregulation of "suppressor" T cells, cholera toxin markedly increases the immunogenicity of coadministered proteins, such as tetanus toxoid (179). Again, IgA responses are favored. For those parasitic infections contained by mucosal IgA responses, for example, anti-adherence antibodies directed against *Entamoeba*, *Giardia*, and *Cryptosporidium*, these data would suggest that recombinant parasite proteins might be incorporated into a mixture (or chemically fused) with cholera toxin to generate the appropriate protective response. This approach may also produce protective Th2 responses effective in the eradication of luminal worms, although the mechanism of this protection remains poorly defined as discussed earlier.

Alternatively, for peripheral vaccination, the use of cytokines has recently been explored as a means to both increase immunogenicity and to direct the nature of the subsequent immune response to an antigen. Indeed, most adjuvant effect may be due to locally elicited cytokines (176). Specifically, recombinant IL-12 has been shown to promote Th1 CD4+ T cell responses when coadministered with *Leishmania major* antigen, resulting in resistance against progressive infection in genetically susceptible mice (180). Again, this might be useful when Th1 cell-mediated cytotoxic or proinflammatory reactions would be desired for eradication of intracellular parasites. Because Th1 cells may antagonize the differentiation and synthetic abilities of IgA-producing B cells, rIL-12 would be an undesirable adjuvant for worm and protozoan infections requiring this mucosal response.

PROGRESS IN VACCINE DESIGN AND FUTURE DIRECTIONS

Vaccination Against Intestinal Helminths

To date there has been no trial of anthelminthic vaccination in humans. Data from animal models of intestinal parasitism suggest that live infection induces lasting immunity against rechallenge, although these effects are not consistent among different species of helminth. Some progress has been made against tissue-invasive helminths that secondarily involve the gut, such as the trematode *Schistosoma mansoni*, where several candidate antigens have been generated in recombinant form and characterized in animal models (10). Immunization of primates or rodents with glutathione-*S*-transferase (GST), triose phosphate isomerase, and paramyosin (or Sm97), among others, have provided rates of protection ranging from 40% to 80% upon challenge with measured inocula of infectious cercariae (181). These rates approach the protective efficacy provided using crude extracts of schistosomula or adult worm excretory proteins. In most cases, the target of protective immunity is the larval schistosomula, a feature in accord with epidemiologic observations showing that naturally acquired immunity is expressed as a decreased reinfection rate and does not correspond with eradication of adult worms from previous infections. Other vaccines may inhibit adult worm fecundity and act to block immunopathology rather than worm infestation (182). Although rates of vaccine protection are not as great as that seen for viral or bacterial vaccines, even small decreases in the eventual egg burden may have a clinically significant effect on the resulting immunopathology. Immunizations directed against antioxidant enzymes of other trematodes, such as the glutathione-*S*-transferase of *Fasciola hepatica*, have demonstrated efficacy in an experimental sheep model (27,90). Immunity in this case was directed against juvenile worms and was associated with a 50% reduction in adult worm burden, a degree of protection associated with marked improvements in anemia and liver function relative to unimmunized controls.

Greater success has been had in the immunization against intestinal nematode parasites of cattle (183). *Haemonchus contortus* is a stomach-dwelling parasite of sheep that is estimated to cause $500 million in damage to the Australian sheep industry. Empirically, it was determined that immunization with irradiated larvae was sufficient to achieve more than 80% protection of susceptible lambs. Recently, recombinant antigens have been found that are also highly effective when given by subcutaneous injection. Protection seems to result from ingestion of cytotoxic antibodies by these worms as they feed on submucosal blood, the apparent target being an intestinal protein called contortin that is effective when used as a recombinant vaccinogen. This may serve as a useful model for designing vaccines effective against homologous blood-feeding nematodes of humans, such as the hookworms *Necator americanus* and *Ancylostoma duodenale* and the whipworm *Trichuris trichiura*. An effective antihookworm vaccine, using inactivated larvae harvested from infected dog stool, has been characterized (184). Some cross-reactivity with other *Ancyclostoma* species was noted, suggesting that this model deserves further exploration for insights into protective immunogens. Relatively little research exists on candidate vaccines effective against human intestinal nematodes, such as *Ascaris lumbricoides,* although liposome-encapsulated extracts of *Ascaris suum* combined with levamisole as an adjuvant were 88.9% effective in preventing infection in mice (185).

Development of vaccines effective against cestodes has centered on providing immunoprotection against the larval stages of tapeworms within their intermediate hosts (186). This phase of the life cycle of *Echinococcus granulosus* and *Taenia solium* causes significant disease in humans and these and related parasites are major concerns in the raising of domestic animals (187). The economic benefit provided by eradication of tissue parasitism in domestic animals has already spurred development of an effective vaccine against the sheep tapeworm, *Taenia ovis* (188). Relying on the observation that irradiated oncospherules were effective in preventing tissue phase infection in lambs, *T. ovis* oncosphere cDNA libraries were screened by immunoblotting with sera from infected sheep. One recombinant protein thus identified (GST-45S) was expressed as a fusion protein with *S. japonicum* glutathione-*S*-transferase and provided an outstanding 97% efficacy against experimental infection. An exciting footnote to these studies has been the recognition of substantial cross-reactivity between the GST-45S antigen and proteins expressed by *Echinococcus granulosus,* which is a cause of considerable morbidity in human intermediate hosts. The nature of protective immunity is not precisely determined, although the ability of passive immunization to provide significant protection against larval infection suggests that a humoral response is important to long-lasting immunity. These veterinary vaccines not only provide a model for human vaccine development but might benefit humans living in agricultural areas by diminishing

the exposure to zoonotic *Taenia* and *Echinococcus* infections.

Vaccination Against Intracellular Intestinal Protozoa

The characterization of neutralizing antibody responses directed against sporozoite and merozoite antigens suggests that development of a *Cryptosporidium* vaccine may be feasible. However, it is still unknown if the protective epitopes involved will provide cross-protection against what are thought to be a large number of serologically distinct strains and species of this parasite. Much more progress has been made in developing vaccines effective against avian species of *Eimeria* that have had important economic consequences for the broiler industry (189,190). Specifically, highly conserved recombinant antigens from *Eimeria* species have been used to prophylactically immunize chicks (191). Live, attenuated strains of *Eimeria* have also been developed that are proven efficacious and marketed for widespread use.

Vaccination Against Intraluminal Protozoa

The major protective responses against giardiasis seem to be antibody mediated, although the frequent occurrence of chronic infection in seropositive individuals suggests that other immune or parasite-related factors influence the outcome of infection. In this regard, insights into the biologic diversity of *Giardia* are only now being explored that may identify important virulence factors. One potential protective immunogen, the 56- to 69-kDa cysteine-rich surface protein, has been characterized in a mouse model of protective vaccination against homologous strains of *Giardia* (192). However, these cell surface antigens of *Giardia* exhibit considerable strain heterogeneity. Furthermore, *in vivo* and *in vitro* antigen variations occur under the selective pressure of host immunity and these variants may be able to maintain infection (193–197). Consequently, the prospects for eventual development of an effective anti-*Giardia* vaccine are speculative until further research into the biology of the parasite reveals more conserved antigens that are potential targets of protective immunity.

Vaccination Against Enteroinvasive Protozoa

Research on development of an amebiasis vaccine has followed two pathways: the first builds on a knowledge of the mechanisms of disease pathogenesis and the second on use of the generalizable strategy of identifying highly conserved surface antigens to be targeted by humoral and T cell-mediated immune mechanisms. Currently, there are three promising antigens under study.

The most promising antigen is the 260-kDa galactose-inhibitable adherence lectin, which consists of a 170-kDa heavy subunit and a 35-kDa light subunit (117,118,141). Monoclonal antibodies to the lectin completely inhibit the galactose-specific binding of trophozoites to purified colonic mucins, suggesting that a blocking IgA response in the gut may be useful (120,198). In addition, the genes for the 170-kDa heavy subunit have been cloned and sequenced (199,200), providing opportunities for study of recombinant antigens. The native 260-kDa lectin was found to be protective in the gerbil model of amebic liver abscess, having 67% vaccine efficacy following intraperitoneal or subcutaneous immunization with Freund's adjuvant (201). By use of expression polymerase chain reaction (PCR), Wan and co-workers (202) produced small amounts of recombinant radiolabeled 170-kDa heavy subunit and found it possessed galactose-binding activity. Chu-Jing et al. (203) have reported that a recombinant 47-kDa portion of the 170-kDa subunit, amino acids 757 to 1132, was highly protective in the gerbil model of amebic liver abscess (Table 2). Current work is focused on development of animal models of intestinal amebiasis, such as in the baboon, to study the efficacy of oral immunization of recombinant lectin subunits with cholera toxin. In addition, use of passive immunization with anti-lectin IgA monoclonal antibodies may provide important information regarding the feasibility of eliciting a blocking S-IgA response.

Two other surface antigens of *E. histolytica* have exhibited some promise as vaccine candidates. The recombinant serine-rich surface protein identified by Stanley and co-workers is effective in a modified gerbil model of amebic liver abscess (presented at the Fogarty Conference on Amebiasis, September 1993). Rabbit antiserum raised to this surface antigen was protective in the SCID mice model of amebic liver abscess. Although antibody to the serine-rich protein partially inhibits parasite adherence, the protein itself has no binding activity and its function has not been characterized. The 29-kDa antigen first described by Soong and co-workers (204) and cloned in a number of laboratories appears to function as an adherence protein. This protein is somewhat specific as a liver-stage antigen as serum antibodies from patients with liver abscess but not with colitis recognize native or recombinant protein (205). The entire recombinant antigen is highly immunogenic and partially protective in the gerbil model of amebic liver abscess.

Development of an amebiasis subunit vaccine appears highly feasible given the number of well-characterized vaccine candidates, the lack of antigenic variation, and the high degree of antigenic relatedness among strains. The absence of any significant nonhuman reservoirs suggests that development of an adherence-inhibitory intestinal IgA response that succeeds in preventing human intestinal colonization could eradicate the parasite.

CONCLUSION

Development of immunizations active against gastrointestinal parasites is only slowly advancing toward clinical reality, despite considerable progress in the widespread use of vaccines effective against viral and bacterial agents of human disease. New insights into the molecular pathogenesis of parasitic infection, the complex host–parasite biology of these illnesses, and the basic immunology of

mucosal tissues strongly suggest that the rational design of antiparasite vaccines is possible. However, as detailed in this chapter, no single strategy is likely to be effective when the nature of protective immunity may be quite distinct for different protozoan and helminthic pathogens. The problem is even greater for those enteric parasitic infections not obviously associated with naturally acquired immunity. Nevertheless, several recombinant vaccines for use against human schistosomiasis are ready for clinical study and a recombinant vaccine against amebic dysentery may be suitable for human trials in the near future. Furthermore, recombinant vaccines against protozoan, tapeworm, and trematode (fluke) infections of domestic animals have been employed successfully and strongly suggest that similar approaches, perhaps using the same conserved vaccine antigens, may have utility against homologous human infections.

ACKNOWLEDGMENTS

This work was supported by NIH grants AI27461 (F.P.H.) and AI18841 (J.I.R.).

REFERENCES

1. Warren KS, Mahmoud AAF, eds. *Tropical and geographic medicine.* New York: McGraw-Hill, 1990.
2. Howard RJ. Asexual deviants take over. *Nature* 1992;357:647.
3. Donelson JE. Antigenic variation in African trypanosomes. *Contrib Microbiol Immunol* 1997;8:138.
4. Haswell EM, Elkins DB, Anderson RM. Evidence for predisposition in humans to infection with *Ascaris,* hookworm, *Enterobius* and *Trichuris* in a South Indian fishing community. *Parasitology* 1987;95:323.
5. Badaro R, Jones TC, Carvalho EM, et al. New perspectives on a subclinical form of visceral leishmaniasis. *J Infect Dis* 1986;154:1003.
6. Maizels RM, Bundy DAP, Selkirk ME, Smith DF, Anderson RM. Immunological modulation and evasion by helminth parasites in human populations. *Nature* 1993;365:797.
7. Sher A, Coffman RL. Regulation of immunity to parasites by T cells and T cell-derived cytokines. *Annu Rev Immunol* 1992;10:385.
8. David JR. Host–parasite interface: immune evasion. In: Warren KS, Mahmoud AAF, eds. *Tropical and geographic medicine.* New York: McGraw-Hill, 1990;117.
9. Amiri P, Locksley RM, Parslow TG, Sadick M, Rector E, Ritter D, McKerrow JH. Tumour necrosis factor α restores granulomas and induces parasite egg-laying in schistosome-infected SCID mice. *Nature* 1992;356:604.
10. Pearce EJ. Proselytizing with immunity. *Nature* 1993;363:19.
11. Van Voorhis WC, Schlekewy L, Trong HL. Molecular mimicry by *Trypanosoma cruzi:* The Fl-160 epitope that mimics mammalian nerve can be mapped to a 12-amino acid peptide. *Proc Natl Acad Sci USA* 1991;88:5993.
12. Lindenbaum J. Tropical enteropathy. *Gastroenterology* 1973;64:637.
13. Halloran M. Infectious disease and the UNESCO basic education initiative. *Parasitol Today* 1989;5:359.
14. Stephenson LS. *The impact of helminth infections on human nutrition: schistosomes and soil-transmitted helminths.* London: Taylor and Francis, 1987.
15. Guyatt HL, Evans D. Economic considerations for helminth control. *Parasitol Today* 1992;8:397.
16. Tanner M. Evaluation of public health impact of schistosomiasis. *Trop Med Parasitol* 1989;40:143.

17. Sarker SA, Gyr K. Non-immunological defence mechanisms of the gut. *Gut* 1992;33:987.
18. Ravdin JI. *Entamoeba histolytica:* pathogenic mechanisms, human immune response, and vaccine development. *Clin Res* 1990;38:215.
19. Hill DR, Rurge JJ, Pearson RD. Susceptibility of *Giardia lamblia* trophozoites to the lethal effect of human serum. *J Immunol* 1984;132:2046.
20. Hall BF, Joiner KA. Strategies of obligate intracellular parasites for evading host defences. *Parasitol Today* 1991;7:A22.
21. Caledron J, Tovar R. Loss of susceptibility to complement lysis in *Entamoeba histolytica* HM1 by treatment with human sera. *Immunology* 1986;58:467.
22. Blaxter M, Page A, Rudin W, Maizels R. Nematode surface coats: actively evading immunity. *Parasitol Today* 1992;8:243.
23. Mahmoud AAF. Eosinophilia. In: Warren KS, Mahmoud AAF, eds. *Tropical and geographic medicine.* New York: McGraw-Hill, 1990;65.
24. Butterworth AE. Cell mediated damage to helminths. *Adv Parasitol* 1984;23:143.
25. Gleich GJ, Adolphson CR. The eosinophilic leukocyte: structure and function. *Adv Immunol* 1986;39:177.
26. Horowitz MA. Phagocytosis of microorganisms. *Rev Infect Dis* 1982;4:104.
27. Brophy PM, Pritchard DI. Immunity to helminths: ready to tip the biochemical balance? *Parasitol Today* 1992;8:419.
28. Liew FY, Cox FEG. Nonspecific defence mechanism: the role of nitric oxide. *Parasitol Today* 1991;7:A17.
29. Leid RW, Suquet CM. A superoxide dismutase of metacestodes of *Taenia taeniaeformis. Mol Biochem Parasitol* 1986;18:301.
30. Leid RW, Suquet CM, Tanigoshi L. Parasite defense mechanisms for evasion of host attack: a review. *Vet Parasitol* 1987;25:147.
31. Leid RW, Suquet CM, Tanigoshi L. Oxygen detoxifying enzymes in parasites: a review. *Acta Leiden* 1989;57:107.
32. Holmgren J, Czerkinsky C, Lycke N, Svennerholm. Mucosal immunity: implications for vaccine development. *Immunobiology* 1992;184:157.
33. McGhee JR, Mestecky J. In defense of mucosal surfaces: development of novel vaccines for IgA responses protective at the portals of entry of microbial pathogens. *Infect Dis Clin North Am* 1990;4:315.
34. Keren DF. Antigen processing in the mucosal immune system. *Semin Immunol* 1992;4:217.
35. Brodsky FM, Guagliardi LE. The cell biology of antigen processing and presentation. *Annu Rev Immunol* 1991;9:707.
36. Briskin MJ, McEvoy LM, Butcher EC. MAdCAM-1 has homology to immunoglobulin and mucin-like adhesion receptors and to IgA1. *Nature* 1993;363:461.
37. Mosmann T, Coffman R. TH1 and TH2 cells: different patterns of lymphokine secretion lead to different functional properties. *Annu Rev Immunol* 1989;7:145.
38. Parker DC. T cell-dependent B cell activation. *Annu Rev Immunol* 1993;11:331.
39. Fitch FW, McKisic MD, Lancki DW, Gajewski TF. Differential regulation of murine T lymphocyte subsets. *Annu Rev Immunol* 1993;11:29.
40. Taguchi T, McGhee JR, Coffman RL, Beagley KW, Eldridge JH, Takatsu K, Kiyono H. Analysis of Th1 and Th2 cells in murine gut-associated tissues: frequencies of CD4+ and CD8+ T cells that secrete IFN-γ and IL-5. *J Immunol* 1990;145:68.
41. Kuhn R, Lohler J, Rennick D, Rajewsky K, Muller W. Interleukin-10-deficient mice develop chronic enterocolitis. *Cell* 1993;75:263.
42. Shull MM, Ormsby I, Kier A, et al. Targeted disruption of the mouse transforming growth factor-β1 gene results in multifocal inflammatory disease. *Nature* 1992;359:693.
43. Fujihashi K, McGhee JR, Lue C, et al. Human appendix B cells naturally express receptors for and respond to interleukin 6 with selective IgA1 and IgA2 synthesis. *J Clin Invest* 1991;88:248.
44. Murray PD, McKenzie DT, Swain SL, Kagnoff MF. Interleu-

kin 5 and interleukin 4 produced by Peyer's patch T cells selectively enhance immunoglobulin A expression. *J Immunol* 1987;139:2669.
45. Defrance T, Vanbervliet B, Briere F, Durand I, Rousset F, Banchereau J. Interleukin 10 and transforming growth factor β cooperate to induce anti-CD40 activated naive human B cells to secrete immunoglobulin A. *J Exp Med* 1992;175:671.
46. Banchereau J, Rousset F. Growing human B lymphocytes in the CD40 system. *Nature* 1991;353:678.
47. Farrar MA, Schreiber RD. The molecular cell biology of interferon-γ and its receptor. *Annu Rev Immunol* 1993;11:571.
48. Tarleton RL, Koller BH, Latour A, Postan M. Susceptibility of β2-microglobulin-deficient mice to *Trypanosoma cruzi* infection. *Nature* 1992;356:338.
49. Tripp CS, Wolf SF, Unanue ER. Interleukin-12 and tumor necrosis factor-α are costimulators of interferon-γ production by natural killer cells in severe combined immunodeficiency mice with listeriosis, and interleukin-10 is a physiologic antagonist. *Proc Natl Acad Sci USA* 1993;90:38.
50. Hill A, Elvin J, Willis A, et al. Molecular analysis of the association of HLA-B53 and resistance to severe malaria. *Nature* 1992;360:434.
51. Haas W, Pereira P, Tonegawa S. Gamma/delta cells. *Annu Rev Immunol* 1993;11:637.
52. Underdown B, Schiff M. Immunoglobulin A: strategic defense initiative at the mucosal surface. *Annu Rev Immunol* 1986;4:389.
53. Kaetzel CS, Robinson JK, Chintalacharuvu KR, Vaerman JP, Lamm ME. The polymeric immunoglobulin receptor (secretory component) mediates transport of immune complexes across epithelial cells: a local defense function for IgA. *Proc Natl Acad Sci USA* 1991;88:8796.
54. Lamm ME. Cellular aspects of immunoglobulin A. *Adv Immunol* 1976;22:223.
55. Childers NK, Bruce MG, McGhee JR. Molecular mechanisms of immunoglobulin A defense. *Annu Rev Microbiol* 1989;43:503.
56. Heyworth MF. Immunology of *Giardia* and *Cryptosporidium* infections. *J Infect Dis* 1992;166:465.
57. Hostoffer RW, Krukovets I, Berger M. Increased FcαR expression and IgA-mediated function on neutrophils induced by chemoattractants. *J Immunol* 1993;150:4532.
58. Ottesen EA, Neva FA, Paranjape RS, Tripathy SP, Thiruvengadam KV, Beaven MA. Specific allergic sensitisation to filarial antigens in tropical eosinophilia syndrome. *Lancet* 1979;1:1158.
59. Ottesen E. Parasite infections and allergic reaction—how each affects the other. In: *Bronchial asthma: mechanisms and therapeutics,* 2nd ed. New York: Little, Brown, 1985.
60. Moqbel R, King SJ, MacDonald A, Miller H, Cromwell O, Shaw RJ, Kay AB. Enteral and systemic release of leukotrienes during anaphylaxis of *Nippostrongylus brasiliensis*-primed rats. *J Immunol* 1986;137:296.
61. King CL, Nutman TB. Biological role of helper T-cell subsets in helminth infections. *Chem Immunol* 1992;54:136.
62. Coffman RL, Seymour BWP, Hudak S, Jackson J, Rennick D. Antibody to interleukin-5 inhibits helminth induced eosinophilia in mice. *Science* 1989;245:308.
63. Sher A, Coffman RL, Hieny S, Cheever AW. Ablation of eosinophil and IgE responses with anti-IL-5 or anti-IL-4 antibody fails to affect immunity against *Schistosoma mansoni* in the mouse. *J Immunol* 1990;145:3911.
64. Madden KB, Urban JF, Ziltener HJ, Schrader JW, Finkelman FD, Katona IM. Antibodies to IL-3 and IL-4 suppress helminth-induced intestinal mastocytosis. *J Immunol* 1991;147:1387.
65. Urban JF Jr, Madden KB, Svetic A, et al. The importance of Th2 cytokines in protective immunity to nematodes. *Immunol Rev* 1992;127:205.
66. Kelly EAB, Cruz ES, Hauda KM, Wassom DL. IFN-γ- and IL-5-producing cells compartmentalize to different lymphoid organs in *Trichinella spiralis*-infected mice. *J Immunol* 1991;147:306.
67. Butterworth AE, Capron M, Cordingley JS, et al. Immunity

after treatment of human schistosomiasis mansoni. II. Identification of resistant individuals, and analysis of their immune responses. *Trans R Soc Trop Med Hyg* 1985;79:393.

68. Hagan P, Blumenthal UJ, Dunn D, Simpson AJ, Wilkins HA. Human IgE, IgG4 and resistance to reinfection with *Schistosoma haematobium*. *Nature* 1991;349:243.

69. Butterworth AE, Bensted SR, Capron A, et al. Immunity in human schistosomiasis mansoni: prevention by blocking antibodies of the expression of immunity in young children. *Parasitology* 1987.

70. Conrad DH. FcεRII/CD23: The low affinity receptor for IgE. *Annu Rev Immunol* 1990;8:623.

71. Capron A, Dessaint JP, Capron M, Ouma JH, Butterworth AE. Immunity to schistosomes: progress toward vaccine. *Science* 1987;238:1065.

72. Metzger H, Alcaraz G, Hohman R, et al. The receptor with high affinity for immunoglobulin E. *Annu Rev Immunol* 1986; 4:419.

73. Dessein AJ, Parker WL, James SL, David JR. IgE antibody and resistance to infection I. Selective suppression of the IgE antibody response in rats diminishes the resistance and the eosinophil response to *Trichinella spiralis* infection. *J Exp Med* 1981;153:423.

74. Ahmad A, Wang CH, Bell RG. A role for IgE in intestinal immunity. Expression of rapid expulsion of *Trichinella spiralis* in rats transfused with IgE and thoracic duct lymphocytes. *J Immunol* 1991;146:3563.

75. David J, Vadas M, Butterworth A. Enhanced helminthotoxic capacity of eosinophils from patients with eosinophilia. *N Engl J Med* 1980;303:1147.

76. Gounni AS, Lamkhioued B, Ochiai K, et al. High-affinity IgE receptor on eosinophils is involved in defence against parasites. *Nature* 1994;367:183.

77. Korenaga M, Hitoshi Y, Yamaguchi N, Sato Y, Takatsu K, Tada I. The role of interleukin-5 in protective immunity to *Strongyloides venezuelensis* infection in mice. *Immunology* 1991;72:502.

78. Mahmoud AAF, Warren KS, Peters PA. A role for the eosinophil in acquired resistance to *Schistosoma mansoni* infection as determined by antieosinophil serum. *J Exp Med* 1975;142:805.

79. Befus AD, Bienenstock J. Immunologically mediated intestinal mastocytosis in *Nippostrongylus brasiliensis*-infected rats. *Immunology* 1979;38:95.

80. Woodbury RG, Miller HR, Huntley JF, Newlands G, Palliser AC, Wakelin D. Mucosal mast cells are functionally active during the spontaneous expulsion of primary intestinal nematode infections in the rat. *Nature* 1984;312:450.

81. Douch P, Harrison G, Buchanan L, Greer K. In vitro bioassay of sheep gastrointestinal mucus for nematode paralyzing activity mediated by a substance with properties characteristic of SRS-A. *Int J Parasitol* 1983;13:207.

82. Galli S. New concepts about the mast cell. *N Engl J Med* 1993; 328:257.

83. Urban JFJ, Katona IM, Paul WM, Finkelman RD. Interleukin 4 is important in protective immunity to a gastrointestinal nematode infection in mice. *Proc Natl Acad Sci USA* 1991;88:5513.

84. Coffman RL, Varkila K, Scott P, Chatelain R. Role of cytokines in the differentiation of CD4+ T-cell subsets in vivo. *Immunol Rev* 1991;123:189.

85. Heinzel FP, Sadick MD, Mutha S, Locksley RM. Production of interferon-γ, IL-2, IL-4 and IL-10 by CD4+ lymphocytes in vivo during healing and progressive murine leishmaniasis. *Proc Natl Acad Sci USA* 1991;88:7011.

86. Else KJ, Finkelman FD, Maliszewski CR, Grencis RK. Cytokine mediated regulation of chronic intestinal helminth infection. *J Exp Med* 1984;179:347.

87. Chensue S, Terebuh P, Warmington K, Hershey S, Evanoff H, Kunkel S, Higashi G. Role of IL-4 and IFN-γ in *Schistosoma mansoni* egg-induced hypersensitivity granuloma formation. Orchestration, relative contribution and relationship to macrophage function. *J Immunol* 1992;148:900.

88. Ive FA, Willis AJ, Ikeme AC, Brockington IF. Endomyocardial fibrosis and filariasis. *Q J Med* 1967;36:495.

89. Brockington IF, Olsen EG. Eosinophilia and endomyocardial fibrosis. *Postgrad Med J* 1972;48:740.

90. Sexton J, Milner A, Panaccio M, et al. Glutathione-S-transferase. Novel vaccine against *Fasciola hepatica* infection in sheep. *J Immunol* 1990;145:3905.

91. Mitchell GF. Animal models of human parasitic diseases and the testing of vaccines. *Parasitol Today* 1989;5:34.

92. Smythies L, Coulson P, Wilson RA. Monoclonal antibody to IFN-γ modifies pulmonary inflammatory responses and abrogates immunity to *Schistosoma mansoni* in mice vaccinated with attenuated cercariae. *J Immunol* 1992;149:3654.

93. Current WL, Garcia LS. Cryptosporidiosis. *Clin Microbiol Rev* 1991;4:25.

94. Hayes EB, Matte TD, O'Brien TR, et al. Large community outbreak of cryptosporidosis due to contamination of a filtered public water supply. *N Engl J Med* 1989;320:1372.

95. DuPont HL. Cryptosporidiosis and the healthy host. *N Engl J Med* 1985;312:1319.

96. Flanigan T, Whalen C, Turner J, Soave R, Toerner J, Havlir D, Kotler D. *Cryptosporidium* infection and CD4 counts. *Ann Intern Med* 1992;10:840.

97. Petersen C. Cryptosporidiosis in patients infected with the human immunodeficiency virus. *Clin Infect Dis* 1992;15:903.

98. Ochs HD, Ament ME, Davis SD. Giardiasis with malabsorption in X-linked agammaglobulinemia. *N Engl J Med* 1972;287:341.

99. Jacyna MR, Parkin J, Goldin R, Baron JH. Protracted enteric cryptosporidial infection in selective immunoglobulin A and saccharomyces opsonin deficiencies. *Gut* 1990;31:714.

100. Petersen C. Cellular biology of *Cryptosporidium parvum*. *Parasitol Today* 1993;9:87.

101. Ungar BLP, Kao T, Burris JA, Finkelman FD. *Cryptosporidium* infection in an adult mouse model. Independent roles for IFN-γ and CD4+ T lymphocytes in protective immunity. *J Immunol* 1991;147:1014.

102. Kogut MH, Lange C. Interferon-gamma-mediated inhibition of the development of *Eimeria tenella* in cultured cells. *J Parasitol* 1989;75:313.

103. Ovington KS, Smith NC. Cytokines, free radicals and resistance to *Eimeria*. *Parasitol Today* 1992;8:422.

104. Wolfe MS. Giardiasis. *N Engl J Med* 1978;298:319.

105. Farthing MJ. Giardia comes of age: progress in epidemiology, immunology and chemotherapy. *J Antimicrob Chemother* 1992;30:563.

106. Nash T, Aggarwal A. Cytotoxicity of monoclonal antibodies to a subset of *Giardia* isolates. *J Immunol* 1986;136:2628.

107. Heyworth MF, Carlson JR, Ermak TH. Clearance of *Giardia muris* infection requires helper/inducer T lymphocytes. *J Exp Med* 1987;165:1743.

108. Roberts-Thomson IC. Genetic studies of human and murine giardiasis. *Clin Infect Dis* 1993;16(Suppl 2):S98.

109. Sargeaunt P, Williams J, Grene J. The differentiation of invasive and non-invasive *Entamoeba histolytica* by isoenzyme electrophoresis. *Trans R Soc Trop Med Hyg* 1978;72:5.

110. Clark C, Diamond L. Ribosomal RNA genes of "pathogenic" *Entamoeba histolytica* are distinct. *Mol Biochem Parisitol* 1991;49:297.

111. Tannich E, Horstmann R, Knobloch J. Genomic DNA differences between pathogenic and nonpathogenic *Entamoeba histolytica*. *Proc Natl Acad Sci USA* 1989;86:5.

112. Diamond L, Clark C. A redescription of *Entamoeba histolytica* Schaudinn. 1903 (Emended Walker. 1911). Separating it from *Entamoeba dispar* Brumpt. 1925. *J Eukaryotic Microbiol* 1993; 40:340.

113. Petri WJ, Jackson T, Gathiram V. Pathogenic and nonpathogenic strains of *Entamoeba histolytica* can be differentiated by monoclonal antibodies to the galactose-specific adherence lectin. *Infect Immun* 1990;58:1802.

114. Ravdin JI, Jackson TFHG, Petri WA, et al. Association of serum antibodies to adherence lectin with invasive amebiasis and asymptomatic infection with *Entamoeba histolytica*. *J Infect Dis* 1990;162:768.

115. Reed S, Bouvier J, Pollack A. Cloning of a virulence factor of *Entamoeba histolytica*. *J Clin Invest* 1993;91:1532.

116. Keene W, Petitt M, Allen S. The major neutral proteinase of *Entamoeba histolytica*. *J Exp Med* 1986;163:536.

117. Petri WA, Smith RD, Schlesinger PH, Ravdin JI. Isolation of the galactose-binding lectin which mediates the in vitro adherence of *Entamoeba histolytica*. *J Clin Invest* 1987;80:1238.

118. Petri WA Jr, Chapman MD, Snodgrass T, Mann BJ, Broman J, Ravdin JI. Subunit structure of the galactose and *N*-acetyl-D-galactosamine-inhibitable adherence lectin of *Entamoeba histolytica*. *J Biol Chem* 1989;264:3007.

119. Ravdin J, Guerrant R. The role of adherence in cytopathogenic mechanisms of *Entamoeba histolytica*. Study with mammalian tissue culture cells and human erythrocytes. *J Clin Invest* 1981; 68:1305.

120. Chadee K, Petri WA, Innes DJ, Ravdin JI. Rat and human colonic mucins bind to and inhibit the adherence of lectin of *Entamoeba histolytica*. *J Clin Invest* 1987;80:1245.

121. Lynch E, Rosenberg I, Gitler C. An ion-channel forming protein produced by *Entamoeba histolytica*. *EMBO J* 1982;1:80.

122. Leippe M, Tannich E, Nicke IR, Vandergoot G, Horstmann R, Mullereberhard J. Primary and secondary structure of the pore-forming peptide of pathogenic *Entamoeba histolytica*. *EMBO J* 1992;11:3501.

123. Nanda R, Baveja U, Anand B. *Entamoeba histolytica* cyst passers: clinical features and outcome in untreated subjects. *Lancet* 1984;2:30.

124. Gathiram V, Jackson T. A longitudinal study of asymptomatic carriers of pathogenic zymodemes of *Entamoeba histolytica*. *S Afr Med J* 1987;72:669.

125. Choudhuri G, Prakash V, Kumar A. Protective immunity to *Entamoeba histolytica* infection in subjects with antiamoebic antibodies residing in a hyperendemic zone. *Scand J Infect Dis* 1991;23:77.

126. DeLeon A. Prognostico tardio en el absceso hepatico amibiano. *Arch Invest Med (Mex)* 1970;1(Suppl 1):205.

127. Irusen E, Jackson T, Simjee A. Asymptomatic intestinal colonization by pathogenic *Entamoeba histolytica* in amebic liver abscess: prevalence, response to therapy and pathogenic potential. *Clin Infect Dis* 1992;14:889.

128. Meerovitch E, Chadee K. In vivo models of immunity in amebiasis. In: *Amebiasis: human infection by Entamoeba histolytica*. New York: Churchill Livingstone, 1988;425.

129. Braga L, Ninomiya H, McCoy J, et al. Inhibition of the complement membrane attack complex by the galactose-specific adhesion of *Entamoeba histolytica*. *J Clin Invest* 1992;90:1131.

130. Reed S, Gigli I. Lysis of complement-sensitive *Entamoeba histolytica* by activated terminal complement components. *J Clin Invest* 1990;86:18.

131. Aceti A, Pennica A, Celestino D, et al. Salivary IgA antibody detection in invasive amebiasis and in asymptomatic infection. *J Infect Dis* 1961;164:6.

132. del Muro R, Acosta E, Merino E, Glender W, Ortiz-Ortiz L. Diagnosis of intestinal amebiasis using salivary IgA antibody detection. *J Infect Dis* 1990;162:1360.

133. Kelsall B, Jackson J, Pearson R, Ravdin J. The 260kD galactose-binding lectin of *Entamoeba histolytica* is a mucosal immunogen in both human and rats. *Clin Res* 1991;39:240.

134. Grundy M, Cartwright T, Lundin L, et al. Antibodies against *Entamoeba histolytica* in human milk and serum in Kenya. *J Clin Microbiol* 1993;17:753.

135. Islam A, Stoll B, Ljungstrom I, et al. The prevalence of *Entamoeba histolytica* in lactating women and in their infants in Bangladesh. *Trans R Soc Trop Med Hyg* 1988;82:99.

136. Kelsall B, Ravdin J. Proteolytic degradation of human IgA by *Entamoeba histolytica*. *J Infect Dis* 1993;168:1319.

137. Ravdin J. Animal models of vaccine development. Presented at the Fogarty Conference on Amebiasis. Washington, DC, 1993.

138. Abd-Alla M, El-Hawey A, Ravdin J. Use of an enzyme-linked immunosorbent assay to detect anti-adherence protein antibodies in sera of patients with invasive amebiasis in Cairo, Egypt. *Am J Trop Med Hyg* 1992;47:800.

139. Calderon J. The role of complement in host defense against *Entamoeba histolytica*. In: *Amebiasis: human infection by Entamoeba histolytica*. New York: Churchill Livingstone, 1988; 453.

140. Ravdin J, Westerdahl C. Protective immunity following vaccination with the galactose-specific adherence protein of *Entamoeba histolytica* is mediated, in part, by adherence-inhibitory serum antibodies. *Clin Res* 1992;40:174A.

141. Cieslak P, Virgin H, Stanley S. A severe combined immunodeficient (SCID) mouse model for infection with *Entamoeba histolytica*. *J Exp Med* 1992;176:1605.

142. Salata RA, Martinez-Palomo C, Murphy CF, et al. Patients treated for amebic liver abscess develop a cell-mediated immune response effective in vitro against *Entamoeba histolytica*. *J Immunol* 1986;136:2633.

143. Salata R, Murray H, Rubin B, et al. The role of gamma interferon in the generation of human macrophages and T lymphocytes cytotoxic for *Entamoeba histolytica*. *Am J Trop Med Hyg* 1987;37:72.

144. Salata R, Ravdin J. Review of human immune mechanisms directed against *Entamoeba histolytica*. *Infect Dis Dig* 1986;7: 16.

145. Denis M, Chadee K. Murine T-cell clones against *Entamoeba histolytica*: in vivo and in vitro characterization. *Immunology* 1989;66:76.

146. Denis M, Chadee K. Cytokine activation of murine macrophages for in vitro killing of *Entamoeba histolytica* trophozoites. *Infect Immun* 1989;57:1750.

147. Wang W, Keller L, Chadee K. Modulation of tumor necrosis factor production by macrophages in *Entamoeba histolytica* infection. *Infect Immun* 1992;60:3.

148. Ada GL. Vaccines and the challenge of parasitic infections. In: *Immunology and molecular biology of parasitic infections*. Boston, MA: Blackwell Scientific Publications, 1993;126.

149. James SL, Scott PA. Induction of cell-mediated immunity as a strategy for vaccine production against parasites. In: *The biology of parasitism: a molecular and immunologic approach*. New York: Alan R Liss, 1988;249.

150. Behbehani AM. The smallpox story: life and death of an old disease. *Microbiol Rev* 1983;47:455.

151. Luelmo F. BCG vaccination. *Am Rev Respir Dis* 1982;125:70.

152. Hone D, Tacket C, Harris A, Kay B, Losonsky G, Levine M. Evaluation in volunteers of a candidate live oral attenuated *Salmonella typhi* vector vaccine. *J Clin Invest* 1992;90:412.

153. Tacket C, Clemens J, Kaper JB. Cholera vaccines. *Biotechnology* 1992;20:53.

154. Hoffman S, Nussenzweig V, Sadoff J, Nussenzweig R. Progress toward malaria preerythrocytic vaccines. *Science* 1991;252:520.

155. Tobin JF, Reiner SL, Hatam F, Zheng S, Leptak CL, Wirth DF, Locksley RM. Transfected leishmania expressing biologically active IFN-γ. *J Immunol* 1993;150:5059.

156. Laban A, Wirth DF. Transfection of *Leishmania enriettii* and expression of chloramphenicol acetyltransferase gene. *Proc Natl Acad Sci USA* 1989;86:9119.

157. Kim K, Soldati D, Boothroyd JC. Gene replacement in *Toxoplasma gondii* with chloramphenicol acetyltransferase as selectable marker. *Science* 1993;262:911.

158. Good M, Kumar S, Miller LH. The real difficulties for malaria sporozoite vaccine development: non-responsiveness and antigenic variation. *Immunol Today* 1988;9:351.

159. Willadsen P, Eisemann CH, Tellam RL. "Concealed" antigens: expanding the range of immunological targets. *Parasitol Today* 1993;9:132.

160. Willadsen P. Immunologic control of a parasitic arthropod. Identification of a protective antigen from *Boophilus microplus*. *J Immunol* 1969;143:1346.

161. Posnett DN, McGrath H, Tam JP. A novel method for producing anti-peptide antibodies. Production of site-specific antibodies to the T cell antigen receptor β-chain. *J Biol Chem* 1988; 263:1719.

162. Reynolds SR, Dahl CE, Harn DA. T and B eptiope determination and analysis of multiple antigenic peptides for the *Schistosoma mansoni* experimental vaccine triose-phosphate isomerase. *J Immunol* 1994;152:193.

163. Nardin EH, Nussenzweig RS. T cell responses to pre-erythrocytic stages of malaria. *Annu Rev Immunol* 1993;11:687.

164. Valero MV, Amador L, Galindo C, et al. 3. Vaccination with

SPf66, a chemically synthesized vaccine, against *Plasmodium faciparum* malaria in Colombia. *Lancet* 1993;341:705.

165. Acharya I, Lowe C, Thapa R, et al. Prevention of typhoid fever in Nepal with Vi capsular polysaccharide of *Salmonella typhi*. A preliminary report. *N Engl J Med* 1987;317:1101.

166. Robbins JB, Scheerson R. Polysaccharide–protein conjugates: a new generation of vaccines. *J Infect Dis* 1990;161:821.

167. Cardenas L, Clements JD. Oral immunization using live attenuated *Salmonella* spp. as carriers of foreign antigens. *Clin Microbiol Rev* 1992;5:328.

168. Sadoff J, Ballou W, Baron L, et al. Oral *Salmonella typhimurium* vaccine expressing circumsporozoite protein protects against malaria. *Science* 1988;240:336.

169. Schodel F, Milich DR, Will H. Hepatitis B virus nucleocapsid/pre-S2 fusion proteins expressed in attenuated *Salmonella* for oral vaccination. *J Immunol* 1990;145:4317.

170. Moss B. Vaccinia virus: a tool for research and vaccine development. *Science* 1991;252:1662.

171. Stover K, de la Cruz V, Fuerst T, et al. New use of BCG for recombinant vaccines. *Nature* 1991;351:456.

172. Taylor J, Weinbverg R, Languet B, Desmettre P, Paoletti E. Recombinant fowlpox virus inducing protective immunity in non-avian species. *Vaccine* 1988;6:497.

173. Taylor J, Paoletti E. Fowlpox virus as a vector in non-avian species. *Vaccine* 1988;6:466.

174. Shen L, Chen ZW, Miller MD, Stallard V, Letvin N. Recombinant virus vaccine-induced SIV-specific CD8+ cytotoxic T lymphocytes. *Science* 1991;252:440.

175. Lussow AR, Aguado MT, Giudice G, Lambert PH. Towards vaccine optimisation. *Immunol Lett* 1990;25:255.

176. Warren HS, Vogel FR, Chedid L. Current status immunological adjuvants. *Annu Rev Immunol* 1986;4:369.

177. Del Giudice G. New carriers and adjuvants in the development of vaccines. *Curr Opin Immunol* 1992;4:454.

178. Elson CO, Ealding W. Generalized systemic and mucosal immunity in mice after mucosal stimulation with cholera toxin. *J Immunol* 1984;132:2736.

179. Xu-Amano J, Kiyono H, Jackson R, et al. Helper T cell subsets for immunoglobulin A responses: oral immunization with tetanus toxoid and cholera toxin as adjuvant selectively induces Th2 cells in mucosa associated tissues. *J Exp Med* 1993;178:1309.

180. Afonso LCC, Scharton TM, Vieira LQ, Wysocka M, Trinchieri G, Scott P. The adjuvant effect of interleukin-12 in a vaccine against *Leishmania major*. *Science* 1994;263:235.

181. Newport GR, Colley DG. Schistosomiasis. In: *Immunology and molecular biology of parasitic infections*. Boston, MA: Blackwell Scientific Publications, 1993;387.

182. Xu CB, Verwaerde C, Gras-Masse H, Fontaine J. *Schistosoma mansoni* 28-kDa glutathione *S*-transferase and immunity against parasite fecundity and egg viability. *J Immunol* 1993;150:940.

183. Emery DL, Wagland BM. Vaccines against gastrointestinal nematode parasites of ruminants. *Parasitol Today* 1991;7:347.

184. Miller TA. Industrial development and field use of the canine hookworm vaccine. *Adv Parasitol* 1978;16:333.

185. Lukes S. *Ascaris suum*—vaccination of mice with liposome encapsulated antigen. *Vet Parasitol* 1992;43:105.

186. Lightowlers MW, Mitchell GF, Rickard MD. Cestodes. In: *Immunology and molecular biology of parasitic infections*. Boston, MA: Blackwell Scientific Publications, 1993;438.

187. Mitchell GH. A vaccine for ovine cysticercosis. *Vaccine* 1989;7:379.

188. Johnson K, Harrison G, Lightowlers M, et al. Vaccination against ovine cysticercosis using a defined recombinant antigen. *Nature* 1989;338:585.

189. Smith N, Eckert J, Braun R. Coccidiosis research in Europe. *Parasitol Today* 1993;9:236.

190. Ellis J, Tomley F. Development of a genetically engineered vaccine against poultry coccidiosis. *Parasitol Today* 1991;7:344.

191. Bhogal BS, Miller GA, Anderson AC, Jessee EJ. Potential of a recombinant antigen as a prophylactic vaccine for day-old broiler chickens against *Eimeria acervulina* and *Eimeria tenella* infections. *Vet Immunol Immunopathol* 1992;31:323.

192. Vinayak VK, Kum K, Khanna R, Khuyller M. Systemic-oral immunization with 56 kDa molecule of *Giardia lamblia* affords protection in experimental mice. *Vaccine* 1992;10:21.

193. Nash T, Herrington D, Leveine M, Conrad J, Merritt J. Antigenic variation of *Giardia lamblia* in experimental human infections. *J Immunol* 1990;4:362.

194. Nash T. Surface antigen variability and variation in *Giardia lamblia*. *Parasitol Today* 1992;8:229.

195. Nash T, Mowatt MR. Characterization of a *Giardia lamblia* variant-specific surface protein (VSP) gene from isolate GS/M and estimation of the VSP gene repertoire size. *Mol Biochem Parasitol* 1992;51:219.

196. Aggarwal A, Nash T. Antigenic variation of *Giardia lamblia* in vivo. *Infect Immun* 1987;56:1420.

197. Gottstein B, Nash TE. Antigenic variation in *Giardia lamblia*: infection of congenitally athymic nude and scid mice. *Parasite Immunol* 1991;13:649.

198. Chadee K, Petri W, Johnson M, et al. Binding and internalization of purified rat colonic mucins by the Gal/GalNAc adherence lectin of *Entamoeba histolytica*. *J Infect Dis* 1988;158:398.

199. Mann B, Chung C, Dodson J, et al. Neutralizing monoclonal antibody epitopes of the *Entamoeba histolytica* galactose adhesion map to the cysteine-rich extracellular domain of the 170-kilodalton heavy subunit. *Infect Immun* 1993;61:1772.

200. Tannich E, Ebert F, Horstmann R. Primary structure of the 170-kDa surface lectin of pathogenic *Entamoeba histolytica*. *Proc Natl Acad Sci USA* 1991;88:1849.

201. Petri W Jr, Ravdin J. Protection of gerbils from amebic liver abscess by immunization with the galactose-specific adherence lectin of *Entamoeba histolytica*. *Infect Immun* 1991;59:97.

202. Wan PSK, Ravdin JI, Soong CJ, Kain KC. Galactose-specific binding of recombinant *Entamoeba histolytica* adhesion lectin 170kDa subunit maps to the cysteine-rich region. *Am J Trop Med Hyg Suppl* 1993;49:127.

203. Chu-Jing GS, Kain KC, Abd-Alla M, Jackson TFHG, Ravdin JI. A recombinant cysteine-rich section of the *Entamoeba histolytica* galactose-inhibitable adherence lectin is efficacious as a subunit vaccine in the gerbil (*Meriones unguiculatus*) model of amebic liver abscess. *J Infect Dis* (in press).

204. Soong G, Torian B, Abd-Alla M, Jackson T, Gatharim V, Ravdin J. Protection of gerbils from amebic liver abscess by immunization with recombinant *Entamoeba histolytica* 29-kDa antigen. *Infect Immun* (in press).

205. Torian B, Flores B, Stroeher V, et al. cDNA sequence analysis of a 29kDa cysteine-rich surface antigen of pathogenic *Entamoeba histolytica*. *Proc Natl Acad Sci USA* 1990;87:6358.

Infections of the Gastrointestinal Tract,
edited by M. J. Blaser, P. D. Smith, J. I. Ravdin,
H. B. Greenberg, and R. L. Guerrant
Raven Press, Ltd., New York © 1995.

CHAPTER 95

Antimicrobial Resistance of Enteric Pathogens

Michael L. Bennish and Stuart B. Levy

Resistance of enteric pathogens to antimicrobial agents is a problem of increasing clinical and public health concern, most particularly in developing countries, but also in the United States and other industrialized countries (1–5). Although multiply-resistant enteric pathogens have been a problem for over 40 years, the last decade has witnessed an alarming worldwide increase in resistance to commonly used antimicrobial agents (1,3,6–9). Although different definitions of multiply-resistant have been used in the literature, in this chapter the term multiply-resistant will be used to refer to bacterial strains resistant to two or more antimicrobial agents to which most strains of that bacterial species had previously been susceptible (10).

This rise in antimicrobial resistance has had a number of important effects. For patients, especially those in developing countries where both enteric infections and antimicrobial resistance are most common, the increase in multiply-resistant strains of enteric pathogens has resulted in an increase in both morbidity and mortality (11,12). For physicians, despite the rapid increase in the number of marketed antimicrobial agents, it has limited the available options for antimicrobial treatment of enteric infections (7,8,13). The increase in resistance among enteric pathogens is in part a reflection of the increase of multiply-resistant Enterobacteriaceae (14,15), because in the gut resistance genes are often transferred from this source to enteric pathogens, and vice versa (16–19). Thus an increase in resistance of enteric pathogens can affect the management of a broad range of infections resulting from bacteria resident in the gut. For public health authorities in developing countries, resistance to commonly used antimicrobial agents has meant that they must find additional funds in already overburdened health budgets for the supply of newer, more expensive antimicrobial agents to which enteric pathogens remain susceptible. In industrialized countries, increasing health care costs have forced insurers, both government and private, to reexamine expenditures for pharmaceuticals, often requiring patients to pay an increasing proportion of the costs of the expensive pharmaceutical agents needed for the treatment of multiply-resistant enteric infections.

This chapter reviews the prevalence of resistance among the major enteric bacterial pathogens, examines the mechanisms of bacterial resistance to antimicrobial agents, and discusses antimicrobial usage patterns that affect the development of resistance. The consequences of the recent increase in the prevalence of resistance and strategies for improving the rational use of antimicrobials in the treatment of enteric infections are also addressed.

MAGNITUDE OF THE PROBLEM

The majority of enteric infections do not require treatment with an antimicrobial agent (20) (see the chapter by Morrow and Neuzil for detailed discussions of the indications for antimicrobial therapy of enteric infections). Unfortunately, it is among the relatively few enteric pathogens—*Salmonella, Shigella,* and *Vibrio cholerae*—that often require antimicrobial treatment that the problem of antimicrobial resistance is greatest. This is not entirely surprising, as the widespread use of antimicrobial agents has resulted in the selection of strains resistant to commonly used antimicrobial agents.

It is, however, difficult to determine for most pathogens the precise extent of antimicrobial resistance (2,21). In the absence of effective surveillance systems in most countries, information on trends in antimicrobial resistance are usually derived from publications on resistance

M. L. Bennish: Departments of Pediatrics and of Medicine, Tufts University School of Medicine, and Floating Hospital for Children, New England Medical Center, Boston, Massachusetts 02111.
S. B. Levy: Departments of Molecular Biology/Microbiology and of Medicine, and Center for Adaptation Genetics and Drug Resistance, Tufts University School of Medicine, and New England Medical Center, Boston, Massachusetts 02111.

patterns at individual medical facilities. It is likely that many of these reports overestimate the prevalence of resistance in the community. Patients who fail initial therapy provided by community medical practitioners selectively come to tertiary medical facilities, where facilities for microbiologic diagnosis are available, and where there are investigators likely to collate and publish the results. In addition, in medicine (as in most other spheres of human life) "no news is good news," and it is probable that publications on antimicrobial resistance are biased in favor of reporting the development of bacterial strains with new resistance patterns.

On the other hand, there are a number of factors that serve to underestimate the prevalence of resistance. Resistant antimicrobial strains can arise in areas of developing countries where microbiologic facilities are not available, and outbreaks of multiply-resistant strains of enteric pathogens can continue for prolonged periods before they are first recognized. That this is so is reflected in the inordinate number of reports on antimicrobial resistance in developing countries that originate from visiting medical investigators from industrialized countries, rather than from local investigators. Given that most developing countries lack both foreign or local investigative capacity, the true extent of antimicrobial resistance in these countries remains unknown. Determination of bacterial susceptibility is itself susceptible to the vagaries of the methods used, and thus results obtained using different methods of susceptibility testing may not be directly comparable. In developing countries the too frequent use of reagents that are out-of-date, or inadequately stored, are another impediment to obtaining reliable information on bacterial resistance (22,23).

Resistance patterns are frequently changing (unfortunately often for the worse), making the prevalence of resistance a "moving target." With the notable exception of *Morbidity and Mortality Weekly Report* from the United States Centers for Disease Control and Prevention (and similar publications in a few other industrialized countries), the delay between the identification of a new resistant bacterial strain and its reporting in the medical literature can often be a year or more. Thus general knowledge of the progression of resistance often is delayed. Lastly, both in industrialized and developing countries there can be substantial variability in resistance patterns within countries, states, or cities. To paraphrase the ex-Speaker of the United States House of Representatives, "Tip" O'Neill, who said "all politics are local," all resistance is also local. Hospitals within the same community, or in adjacent communities, can be confronted by markedly different antimicrobial resistance patterns. Thus for all of the reasons noted above, discussions such as this one can at best indicate general trends in the patterns of resistance, with locally gathered surveillance data remaining the best guide to selection of treatment within individual communities. A summary of recent published information on resistance patterns of enteric pathogens follows.

Campylobacter

The efficacy of antimicrobial agents in treating most *Campylobacter* infections is problematic, and, as a consequence, the issue of resistance has less immediacy than it does for infections with enteric pathogens for which antimicrobial therapy is clearly indicated. Erythromycin is the drug that has historically been used, with modest or no effect, to treat *Campylobacter* infections (24–26a); many strains of *C. jejuni* and *C. coli* remain susceptible to this agent (27,28), though resistance rates among *C. coli* have tended to be higher than among *C. jejuni* (27,29). There are countries in which high rates of resistance to erythromycin have been reported, such as the 53% rate of resistance reported from orphanages in Bangladesh (26) and the 51% resistance rate reported from Singapore (30), but such high resistance rates remain exceptional. *Campylobacter* that are resistant to erythromycin are also resistant to the newer macrolide agents azithromycin and clarithromycin (31–33).

Because of the limited efficacy of erythromycin in the treatment of *Campylobacter* infections, there was considerable initial enthusiasm for the potential role of the newer quinolone agents, which had excellent *in vitro* activity against *Campylobacter* (34). Use of the new quinolone agents to treat *Campylobacter* infections and their widespread use for the treatment of other infections have resulted in the rapid emergence of resistant *Campylobacter* strains (35–38), primarily because of alteration in the drug target, bacterial deoxyribonucleic acid (DNA) gyrase (39–42), and possibly also because of decreased accumulation of the drug within the bacteria.

Diarrheogenic *Escherichia coli*

Information on antimicrobial resistance among the various types of diarrheogenic *E. coli* (enterotoxigenic, enteropathogenic, enteroinvasive, and enterohemorrhagic) is limited because, with the exception of enterohemorrhagic *E. coli*, most clinical microbiologic laboratories do not identify these organisms. Most studies suggest that the resistance pattern of diarrheogenic *E. coli* mimic the resistance pattern of the larger agglomeration of *E. coli* existing in the community (6). Exceptions to this generalization are a study analyzing *E. coli* from the United States, which found that antimicrobial resistance among strains of *E. coli* producing heat-labile toxin was lower than among strains producing heat-stable toxin, or strains that did not produce either toxin (43), and a report of a limited number of *E. coli* from Brazil, which found that resistance to trimethoprim–sulfamethoxazole (TMP-SMX) among enteropathogenic strains of *E. coli* (50%) was significantly higher than for enterotoxigenic *E. coli* (10%) or enteroinvasive *E. coli* (11%) (14). Resistance of toxigenic *E. coli* to commonly used antimicrobial agents has generally been high in developing countries, with resistance rates to ampicillin and trimethoprim–sulfamethoxazole of 48% and 39%, respectively, in isolates from American soldiers participating in the Gulf War (44), and trimethoprim resistance rates of 25% in children coming to a hospital in Bangkok in 1986 (45). Lower rates of resistance to trimethoprim–sulfamethoxazole have been reported in isolates from American students in Mexico (9% of isolates obtained from 1987 to 1989) (46) and in children in Bangladesh (4%) (47). In both of these studies, rates of resistance to ampicillin were higher than for trimethoprim–sulfamethoxazole, with ampicillin resistance being 26% in Mexico and 23% in Bangladesh (46,47).

A number of studies have found that the genes encoding antimicrobial resistance and toxin production in some strains of toxigenic *E. coli* are carried on the same plasmid (48–50) and that both of these traits can be transferred simultaneously during conjugation experiments (49). This finding raised the specter that increasing use of antimicrobial agents in the community would, by selecting for multiply-resistant strains, also increase the prevalence of toxigenic *E. coli*. To date, there has been no epidemiologic evidence to substantiate that this has occurred.

Helicobacter pylori

Although *H. pylori* infection results in ulcer disease rather than diarrhea, it is an enteric infection for which antimicrobial therapy is used, and in which antimicrobial resistance has been a substantial problem. There are at least three classes of drugs used to treat *H. pylori* infections, which frequently select for strains with chromosomally mediated resistance to the drug being used (51). These are the quinolones (including ciprofloxacin, norfloxacin, and ofloxacin), the macrolides (including erythromycin and the newer macrolide agents azithromycin and clarithromycin), and the imidazoles (metronidazole and tinidazole, the latter not currently marketed in the United States) (51,52). Metronidazole resistance appears to be common in developing countries, where resistance rates in patients newly diagnosed with *H. pylori*-induced ulcer disease have been reported as being 65% in Brazil (53) and 84% in Zaire (54), although a resistance rate of only 11% was reported from a small series of patients in Malaysia (55). Rates of resistance in industrialized countries have ranged from 7% in Spain (56) to 50% in Finland (57).

Reported resistance rates are dependent on how the study population has been selected, with resistance rates being substantially higher in patients who have previously been treated with metronidazole (58). In at least some reports from industrialized countries, higher resistance rates have been reported from women than from men (56,59,60). The higher rates of resistance among women and persons from developing countries have been attributed, without definitive proof, to more common use of metronidazole in these two groups—in developing countries for the treatment of parasitic infections, and in women for the treatment of gynecologic infections.

To reduce the rate at which resistance develops, and to increase the efficacy of treatment, triple drug regimens have been used (51,61,62), with one of the more popular regimens consisting of bismuth, tetracycline, and metronidazole (51,59,63). Such regimens produce rates of cure of 90% or more in patients infected with metronidazole-susceptible strains, but rates of only 19% to 75% in infections caused by metronidazole-resistant strains of *H. pylori* (51,59,62–65).

Non-typhi Salmonella

In the United States and in many other countries, the vast majority of non-typhi *Salmonella* infections are either never identified or are never reported to public health authorities (Table 1) (66). Thus determining the true prevalence of resistance among the many hundreds of serotypes of non-typhi *Salmonella* is especially problematic. Reports from existing surveillance systems, from hospitals, and from outbreak investigations, however, suggest that resistance among the non-typhi *Salmonella* is a continuing problem, especially in developing countries.

Although chloramphenicol and tetracycline had once been the drugs of choice for the treatment of non-typhi *Salmonella* infections, increasing resistance and concerns about toxicity in children had led, by the 1970s, to their being replaced by ampicillin or trimethoprim–sulfamethoxazole in those *Salmonella* infections that required treatment. High rates of resistance (50% to 100%) to either ampicillin or trimethoprim–sulfamethoxazole (or both) have, however, now been reported from medical facilities in Africa (Algeria, Central African Republic, Kenya, Rwanda) (67–70), Asia (Iran, Saudi Arabia) (71,72), and South America (Argentina, Brazil) (73,74). These reports are from hospital surveillance systems as well as from studies of outbreaks caused by multiply-resistant strains. Reports from medical facilities in other tropical countries (Hong Kong, Kuwait, Singapore, Sudan, Thailand) have found considerably lower rates of resistance (75–79). Not surprisingly, in developing countries (as in industrialized countries), resistance patterns of *Salmonella* can vary markedly between institutions, as is seen in reports from Thailand (79,80).

National surveillance in the United States and United Kingdom and provincial surveillance in Ontario, Canada, have found consistently low rates of resistance among *Salmonella*, with 12% or fewer (depending on the species tested) of all isolates being resistant to either ampicillin or trimethoprim–sulfamethoxazole (81–84). Hospital-based reporting from the United States has found slightly higher rates of resistance than did the national surveillance system of the Centers for Disease Control and Prevention—20% compared to 9%, respectively, for resistance to ampicillin, and 3% versus 1% for trimethoprim–sulfamethoxazole (82,85). Low (<2%) rates of resistance to trimethoprim–sulfamethoxazole have also been reported from hospitals in Spain (86,87). The lowest rates of resistance have perhaps been found in New Zealand, where, in 1987, 3% of *Salmonella* isolates reported to the national surveillance system were resistant to ampicillin and 1% to trimethoprim (88).

Many outbreaks due to multiply-resistant strains of *Salmonella* have been reported in the United States, with perhaps the most spectacular being an outbreak originating from a dairy in Illinois that was caused by a strain of *S. typhimurium* resistant to both ampicillin and tetracycline that resulted in at least 16,000 culture confirmed cases of salmonellosis (89). Resistance does not appear to be species specific, as multiply-resistant strains of a number of different species of *Salmonella* have been reported.

TABLE 1. *Non-typhi* Salmonella: *selected recent reports of antimicrobial resistance to commonly used agents*

Location (reference)	Year isolates were obtained	Origin of isolates	Number of isolates and species	Percentage of resistance to indicated antimicrobial agent		
				Amp	TMP-SMX	Other antimicrobial agents
Australia–Oceania						
New Zealand (88)	1987	National surveillance	1122 *Salmonella*	3	1[a]	No resistance to norfloxacin
Africa						
Nairobi, Kenya (69)	1985	Hospital	417 *S. typhimurium*	12	14	
Asia						
Taiwan (111)	1978–1987	Six hospitals	1430 *S. typhimurium*	92	48	
Tehran, Iran (71)	1983–1986	Children with diarrhea	508 *Salmonella*	85	74	
Hong Kong (75)	1985–1988	Hospital	720 *Salmonella*	17	6	No resistance to five newer fluoroquinolones or to cefotaxime
Singapore (77)	1985–1989	Hospital	487 *Salmonella*	5	14	
Bangkok, Thailand (79)	1986	Children's hospital	187 *Salmonella*	17	9	
Riyadh, Saudi Arabia (72)	1986–1987	Hospital	131 *Salmonella*	46	64	
Kuwait (76)	1989	Hospital	124 *Salmonella*	6	2	
Europe						
United Kingdom (83)	1988	Central Public Health Laboratory	6898 *S. enteritidis*	10	<1[a]	
			6444 *S. typhimurium*	12	2[a]	
			1120 *S. virchow*	6	11[a]	
			3952 Other *Salmonella* species	5	9[a]	
Madrid, Spain (86)	1988–1991	Hospital	961 *Salmonella*	32	2	
North America						
United States (85)	1984	National hospital monitoring	1293 *Salmonella*	20	3	
United States (82)	1984–1985	CDC national surveillance	485 *Salmonella*, 36% *S. typhimurium*	9	1	
South America						
Buenos Aires, Argentina (73)	1990	Children's hospital	75 Multiply-resistant *Salmonella* isolates (85% *S. typhimurium*)	100	93	96% Resistant to cefotaxime

[a] Tested to trimethoprim only.
Amp, ampicillin; TMP-SMX, trimethoprim–sulfamethoxazole.

The newer quinolone agents and extended spectrum (third-generation) cephalosporins have been used to treat *Salmonella* infections caused by strains resistant to both ampicillin and trimethoprim–sulfamethoxazole (90). There have now, however, been an increasing number of reports of strains of *Salmonella* that are either resistant, or have decreased susceptibility, to these newer agents (91–95).

Salmonella typhi

Although *S. typhi* infection produces a number of systemic manifestations for which it is best known, diarrhea does occur with *S. typhi* infection (Table 2) (96). Chloram-phenicol has been the agent of choice for the treatment of typhoid fever since the 1950s (97,98). Resistance to this agent had, until recently, been relatively uncommon (98,99). A major outbreak of chloramphenicol-resistant *S. typhi* occurred in Mexico in the early 1970s (100), and a similar outbreak occurred in Vietnam at about the same time (101,102). In part because the Mexican epidemic of chloramphenicol-resistant *S. typhi* arose shortly after the onset of a major epidemic of multiply-resistant (including chloramphenicol-resistant) *S. dysenteriae* type 1 in Latin America (103–105), and in part because the epidemic occurred in a country adjacent to the United States, it received considerable attention in the medical and lay communities in the United States (and in England) (106) and helped to heighten awareness of the problem of antimicrobial resistance (107).

TABLE 2. *Selected recent reports of multiply-resistant* Salmonella typhi *or* paratyphi

Location (reference)	Number of isolates	Years isolated	Chloramphenicol resistance rate	Resistance to other antimicrobial agents
Lima, Peru (109)	241	1981–1983	30%	All Chl-resistant strains also resistant to Tet and SMX; half of Chl-resistant strains also resistant to TMP
Karachi, Pakistan (113)	355	1986–1989	20%	All Chl-resistant strains also resistant to Amp and TMP-SMX
Dhaka, Bangladesh (114)	135	1990	12%	All Chl-resistant isolates also resistant to Amp and TMP-SMX
New Delhi, India (115)	158	1990	50%	Chl-resistant isolates also resistant to Amp and TMP-SMX but susceptible to third-generation cephalosporins and newer quinolones
Calcutta, India (117)	53	1990	100%	All strains also resistant to Amp and TMP-SMX but susceptible to newer quinolones
Karnataka, India (118)	134	1990–1991	78%	All Chl-resistant isolates also resistant to Amp and TMP-SMX but susceptible to newer quinolones
South Africa (119)	6	1991	100%	All six isolates resistant to Amp and TMP-SMX but susceptible to third-generation cephalosporins and newer quinolones

Amp, ampicillin; Chl, chloramphenicol; Tet, tetracycline, TMP-SMX, trimethoprim–sulfamethoxazole.

The incidence of infections with chloramphenicol-resistant *S. typhi* infections, however, declined in Mexico and in other countries of Latin America following this outbreak. Although occasional infections with chloramphenicol-resistant strains of *S. typhi* occurred in countries where the infection was endemic (6,69,72,75,78,108–111), such strains did not become highly prevalent in any typhoid endemic country until an epidemic of multiply-resistant *S. typhi* occurred in South Asia in the late 1980s (112). This epidemic strain (which now appears to have become endemic) is resistant to chloramphenicol, ampicillin, and trimethoprim–sulfamethoxazole. Reports from hospitals in India, Pakistan, and Bangladesh suggest that half or more of all *S. typhi* infections in those countries are now caused by this multiply-resistant strain (Table 2) (113–118). Strains of *S. typhi* resistant to chloramphenicol, ampicillin, and trimethoprim–sulfamethoxazole have also been identified in Africa (119,120) and South America (109) but epidemics on the scale of those reported from the Indian subcontinent have not (yet) been reported.

Shigella

Shigella has a dubious place of distinction in the annals of antimicrobial resistance, as it is in shigellae that transmissible antimicrobial resistance by plasmids (initially known as R, or resistance, factors) was first described (121). First identified in Japan in the late 1950s after endemic strains of *Shigella* simultaneously developed resistance to chloramphenicol, sulfonamides, streptomycin, and tetracycline, plasmid-mediated transfer of resistance determinants has been identified (as described in detail later) as one of the major mechanisms by which bacteria acquire antimicrobial resistance (122,123).

Since acquiring resistance in the 1940s and 1950s to the sulfonamides (121), the first antimicrobial agents used in the treatment of shigellosis, shigellae have ineluctably developed resistance to almost all other agents used for the treatment of this infection. Due to the rapid dissemination of resistance plasmids, by the 1970s shigellae were also commonly resistant to tetracycline and chloramphenicol (123,124). The introduction of ampicillin and trimethoprim–sulfamethoxazole in the late 1960s and early 1970s provided effective alternative agents for the treatment of this infection, but by the mid-1980s resistance to these two agents was widespread among all four species of *Shigella* (124). Currently, in most countries in Asia and Africa (both developed and less developed) and in some Latin American countries, half or more of all *Shigella* isolates are resistant to ampicillin and trimethoprim–sulfamethoxazole (Table 3) (7,8,125–145). Resistance is particularly common among strains of *S. dysenteriae* type 1 (Table 3) (8,125,126,129,131,134).

In the United States, recent surveillance reports have found that less than 10% of tested strains of either *S. flexneri* or *S. sonnei* (the two most common species of *Shigella* in the United States) are resistant to trimethoprim–sulfamethoxazole, though resistance to ampicillin among strains of these two species has increased to 19% and 40%, respectively (146). Outbreaks of *S. sonnei* resistant to both of these agents have been reported in the United States, however, (147), and multiply-resistant *S. flexneri* and *S. sonnei* are now endemic in Indian reservations in the American Southwest (12). Reports from a number of western European countries (where a substantial proportion of all *Shigella* infections are acquired during travel outside the country), Bulgaria, and Canada also indicate levels of resistance to ampicillin and trimetho-

TABLE 3. Shigella: *selected recent reports of antimicrobial resistance to commonly used agents*

Location (reference)	Year isolates were obtained	Origin of isolates	Number of isolates and species	Percentage of resistance to indicated antimicrobial agent			
				Amp	NA	TMP-SMX	Other antimicrobial resistance
Africa							
Lagos, Nigeria (137)	1988–1989	Hospital	100 *Shigella*	70	0	74	No isolates resistant to Cip
Djibouti (143)	1991–1992	Hospital	57 *S. flexneri*	89[a]	0	32	No isolates resistant to Cip
			59 *S. sonnei*	12[a]	0	83	
Asia							
Kaohsiung, Taiwan (141)	1982–1987	Hospital	53 *S. flexneri*	81	17	9	
			60 *S. sonnei*	27	33	13	
Manila, The Philippines (136)	1982–1988	Hospital	327 *S. flexneri*	65	—[b]	12	
			138 Other *Shigella*	19	—	8	
Dhaka, Bangladesh (8)	1983–1990[c]	Diarrhea treatment center	1348 *S. boydii*	18	1	18	
			4732 *S. dysenteriae* 1	54	33	85	
			471 *S. dysenteriae* 2–10	12	<1	11	
			8537 *S. flexneri*	46	2	23	
			736 *S. sonnei*	17	1	27	
Teheran, Iran (133)	1984–1985	Hospital	100 *Shigella*	76	0	67	
Singapore (139)	1986–1990	Hospital	305 *S. flexneri*	83	—	37	
			170 *S. sonnei*	22	—	17	
Bangkok, Thailand (140)	1988	Hospital	1280 *S. flexneri*	98	0	88	
			265 Other *Shigella*	36	1	73	
Saudi Arabia (44)	1990	American soldiers in the Gulf War	113 *Shigella*	21	—	85	No isolate resistant to Cip
Tel Aviv, Israel (145)	1991–1992	Hospital	132 *S. sonnei*	80	—	95	No isolate resistant to ofloxacin
Europe							
United Kingdom (148)	1983	Central Public Health Laboratory	286 Isolates of *Shigella* other than *S. sonnei*	48	—	17[d]	
The Netherlands (151)	1984–1989	National surveillance	1532 *S. flexneri*	47	—	18[d]	
			1549 *S. sonnei*	14	—	35[d]	
Nizhny Novgorod, Russia (153)	1986–1989	Hospital	322 *Shigella*	20	—	—	
Finland (150)	1988	Finnish travelers	207 *Shigella*	26	0	42[d]	No isolates resistant to Cip
North America							
United States (12)	1985	Indian Health Service Clinics	72–224 *S. flexneri*	40	—	20	
			69–102 *S. sonnei*	85	—	21	
United States (146)	1985–1986	CDC nationwide surveillance	88 *S. flexneri*	19	1	9	
			152 *S. sonnei*	40	0	7	
Guadalajara, Mexico (46)	1987–1989	Visiting American students	89 *Shigella*	23	—	8	No isolates resistant to Cip
Ontario, Canada (152)	1990	Provincial Public Health Laboratory	254 *S. flexneri*	67	—	30	
			290 *S. sonnei*	39	—	38	
South America							
Lima, Peru (135)	1986–1987	Private physicians' offices	115 *Shigella*	60	4	35	

[a] Tested to amoxicillin
[b] Dash indicates not tested against this antimicrobial agent.
[c] Resistance to nalidixic acid determined for the years 1986 through 1990.
[d] Tested to trimethoprim component only.
Amp, ampicillin; NA, nalidixic acid; TMP-SMX, trimethoprim–sulfamethoxazole; Cip, ciprofloxacin.

prim–sulfamethoxazole that preclude their use as empiric treatment for presumptive *Shigella* infections (148–152). Similar resistance patterns have been identified in the republics of the former Soviet Union (153).

In locations where resistance to ampicillin and trimethoprim–sulfamethoxazole is common, the older quinolone agent nalidixic acid has been used as a first-line agent for treating *Shigella* infections (154). Resistance to nalidixic acid has developed rapidly in areas where it has been introduced as a first-line agent (8,155,156), especially among *S. dysenteriae* type 1 strains. In Bangladesh, where *S. dysenteriae* type 1 is both endemic and periodically epidemic, more than half of all *S. dysenteriae* type 1 strains are currently resistant to nalidixic acid (8). Nalidixic acid-resistant strains of *Shigella* remain susceptible to the newer quinolones, albeit with reduced susceptibility (156–158). Resistance to the newer quinolone agents is not yet a common problem among *Shigella*, but the recent emergence of quinolone-resistant *E. coli* (159,160) suggests that this problem may not be long in coming.

Most multiply-resistant strains of *Shigella*, including ampicillin-resistant strains, remain susceptible to pivamdinocillin, a β-lactam agent that selectively binds to penicillin binding protein 2 (161), and to the third-generation cephalosporins. The former is now commonly used in the treatment of childhood shigellosis where multiply-resistant strains of *Shigella* are common; the latter are being evaluated in clinical trials.

Vibrio cholerae O1

Tetracycline, or its congener, doxycycline, has been the agent of choice for treating cholera since tetracycline was shown effective in the treatment of *V. cholerae* O1 infection in 1964 (162,163). During the 1960s and early 1970s sporadic resistance of *V. cholerae* O1 to tetracycline was reported in areas affected by the seventh cholera pandemic (164). The initially reported strains of tetracycline-resistant *V. cholerae* most often remained susceptible to ampicillin and trimethoprim–sulfamethoxazole, or to furazolidone, a nonabsorbable antimicrobial agent also used in the treatment of cholera (164–166). In the late 1970s and early 1980s, however, cholera outbreaks caused by strains of *V. cholerae* O1 with plasmid-mediated resistance to tetracycline, ampicillin, and trimethoprim-sulfamethoxazole (but most often susceptible to furazolidone) were reported from East Africa, Bangladesh, and Thailand (Table 4) (167–171). Similar strains have also been identified in South America, the continent most recently affected by the seventh cholera pandemic (172). A strain of *V. cholerae* O1 resistant to tetracycline, ampicillin, trimethoprim–sulfamethoxazole, and furazolidone has now become endemic in the Ganges Delta in Bangladesh and West Bengal, India (173), the historic home of *V. cholerae* O1. The newer quinolones have been the only available antimicrobial agents shown to be effective for treating this multiply-resistant strain (174). *Vibrio cholerae* O139, a recently identified serotype of *V. cholerae* that, like *V. cholerae* O1, is capable of causing epidemic cholera, remains (at least early in the epidemic) susceptible to tetracycline and other commonly used antimicrobial agents (175,176).

Traveler's Diarrhea

The bacterial enteric pathogens that infect travelers to developing countries are a selected sample of the enteric pathogens resident at the site of travel (6). Studies from a diverse array of developing countries have found that enterotoxigenic *E. coli* is the most common cause of traveler's diarrhea, with *Salmonella*, *Shigella*, and *Campylobacter* being other common bacterial causes of traveler's diarrhea (177–180). The pattern of antimicrobial resistance of the bacterial strains infecting travelers is a reflection of the resistance pattern in the country of travel (6,181). In most developing countries, the prevalence of multiply-resistant *E. coli* is considerably higher than it is in industrialized countries (14,15). Thus antimicrobial agents, such as trimethoprim–sulfamethoxazole or doxycycline, that might still be effective for treating *E. coli* infections in industrialized countries, or that might in the past have been effective for treating traveler's diarrhea due to *E. coli*, are unlikely to be currently effective for treating traveler's diarrhea (182,183). As with all organisms, there is considerable regional variation, and relatively recent reports suggest that trimethoprim–sulfamethoxazole may still be effective in treating or preventing diarrhea in students going to Guadalajara for their summer studies (184), though it may be ineffective for preventing diarrhea in those persons embarking on an exploration of the wonders of Thailand (183).

The use of antimicrobial agents for the prophylaxis of traveler's diarrhea has been the source of debate, not only because of the question of how efficacious a strategy it is for preventing traveler's diarrhea, but also because of concerns about the effect that prophylaxis has on enhancing colonization of the gut (and presumably other sites) with resistant bacteria. Travelers to Mexico who took trimethoprim alone, or trimethoprim combined with sulfamethoxazole, as prophylaxis for diarrhea were rapidly colonized with trimethoprim–resistant strains of *E. coli* (185). Almost all resistant strains of *E. coli* carried an identical plasmid coding for the same resistance determinant (186). Colonization with resistant strains of *E. coli* can occur in the majority of travelers, however, even in the absence of antimicrobial prophylaxis (187). The use of

TABLE 4. *Recent reports of tetracycline-resistant* V. cholerae *O1*

Country (reference)	Year	Number of isolates and biotype	Percentage of resistance to tetracycline	Resistance to other antimicrobial agents
Thailand (171)	1982	31 El Tor	100	All isolates also resistant to Amp, Chl, and TMP-SMX
Kenya (169)	1983	245 El Tor	96	75% Also resistant to Amp; all isolates susceptible to Chl and NA
India (173)	1989–1990	141 El Tor	63	96% Resistant to Fur and Amp, 83% to TMP-SMX, and 54% to Chl
Ecuador (172)	1992	12 El Tor	17	The two tetracycline-resistant strains also resistant to Amp, Chl, and TMP-SMX

Amp, ampicillin; Chl, chloramphenicol; Fur, furazolidone; NA, nalidixic acid; TMP-SMX, trimethoprim–sulfamethoxazole.

norfloxacin, rather than trimethoprim–sulfamethoxazole, as prophylaxis for diarrhea in students traveling to Mexico did not result in the development of gut colonization with resistant Enterobacteriaceae, largely because norfloxacin completely eradicated the gram-negative aerobic fecal flora, an accomplishment of dubious merit (188). However, as was found with other agents, the continued use of the quinolones can result in the development of quinolone-resistant enteric flora, as has now been reported for *E. coli* (159,160). As in the general population, the use of fluoroquinolone agents in travelers also results in the development of quinolone-resistant *Campylobacter* (189).

MECHANISMS OF RESISTANCE

Resistance has emerged to all of the currently available antimicrobial agents and in many different kinds of bacteria (1,2,190). While some resistance traits may be intrinsic—that is, part of the normal bacterial genome—most of those confronted now are acquired from other bacteria. Once transferred and expressed, the resistance traits essentially create a novel strain of the species—one that is resistant to antimicrobial agents to which it had been previously susceptible.

Antibiotic resistance is not new: it was observed among streptococci, gonococci, and meningococci soon after sulfonamides were introduced to treat these pathogens (191). When penicillin was introduced in the 1940s, resistance to penicillin unexpectedly emerged among the staphylococci. These organisms bore plasmids containing a gene for a β-lactamase that destroyed the penicillin. These resistant forms of staphylococcus were already present at some level in the environment (for reasons that are not clear) when penicillin was introduced. Under the selective pressure of penicillin, penicillin-resistant staphylococci increased in frequency in one London hospital from 14% in 1946 to 59% by 1950.

The resistance specified for sulfonamides and penicillin was to the single drug. A more difficult era of resistance became evident during the 1960s—that of multidrug resistance. At the end of the 1950s in Japan, multiresistant *S. dysenteriae* and *E. coli* were isolated from the feces of the same individual with diarrhea (192). The resistances (to tetracycline, chloramphenicol, sulfonamide, and streptomycin) were not individual mutations on the chromosome but were transferable on a self-replicating DNA element now known as a plasmid, then called an R factor (121). That plasmids could transfer between and among different genera of the Enterobacteriaceae was novel; the only plasmids known at the time, the F factors, had transferability limited to *E. coli*. This event forewarned an extensive transfer of resistance determinants among different bacteria, which we observe today.

Resistance Gene Transfer

There are three ways by which genes can be transferred among bacteria of the same and different species. Plasmid transfer occurs via a process called *conjugation,* by which a plasmid, bearing genes for resistance and other traits, moves from one organism to another (Fig. 1). This form of gene transfer is common among bacteria of the intestinal tract and involves plasmids of many different types, distinguished by their origins of replication and by their "incompatibility" trait, that is, the inability of the same type plasmids to remain stably in the same cell. Plasmids may be small, with as few as 1 kilobase, or large, with several hundred kilobases. In general, plasmids represent only a few percent of the DNA of the single chromosome in bacteria. Those plasmids that transfer by conjugation tend to be large because the transfer apparatus requires many genes. The F transfer system, for instance, needs more than 15 Kb of DNA (193). Conjugation takes place by the attachment of a pilus protein from the donor bacterium to a recipient bacterium, which leads to a joining of the two organisms. Before transfer of the plasmid into the recipient, the plasmid is duplicated in the donor. The original donor therefore never loses the plasmid and is able to donate plasmids to multiple organisms. Moreover, the recipient becomes a new donor. Thus there is a cascade of resistance gene transfer from one donor to new recipients and the creation of multiple new donors able to transfer to other recipients.

A second, less widespread mechanism of gene transfer is that of *transduction,* which relies on bacterial viruses called bacteriophages, which incorporate small pieces of the host bacterial chromosome or resident plasmid into their protein shell (194). Phages have specific cell wall receptor sites by which they attach and inject their DNA into the recipient cell. Therefore the extent of spread via phages is limited by the kinds of bacteria that have these receptors. Phages tend to be specific for particular genera. Still, this is a mechanism by which genes can spread among different, but related, species.

Finally, there is the method of *transformation,* which involves the uptake of released, free DNA into a new recipient organism (195). This process requires a specific uptake system in the recipient and often particular sequences in the DNA being taken up. However, it is a common mechanism for transfer of genetic information among some gram-positive organisms such as *Streptococcus pneumoniae,* and among some gram-negative bacteria, such as *Hemophilus influenzae.* It is not a common mechanism for transfer among gram-negative organisms in the gastrointestinal tract.

Allied to these three gene transfer processes is yet another genetic mechanism, which influences the transferability, maintenance, and stability of the resistance determinants. This genetic event, called *transposition,* comes into play inside the cell once the transfer event has occurred (196). It involves the movement of the resistance gene to DNA structures within the cell. Many resistance determinants lie on discrete pieces of DNA called *transposons,* which have the ability to move from one DNA vehicle (phage, plasmid, chromosome) to another. By integrating into the DNA, they become a part of that DNA molecule. In this way, resistance genes, which enter a cell on a plasmid that cannot exist in the cell, can "jump" from the entering plasmid onto the chromosome or onto a resident plasmid. The result is transfer of the resistance

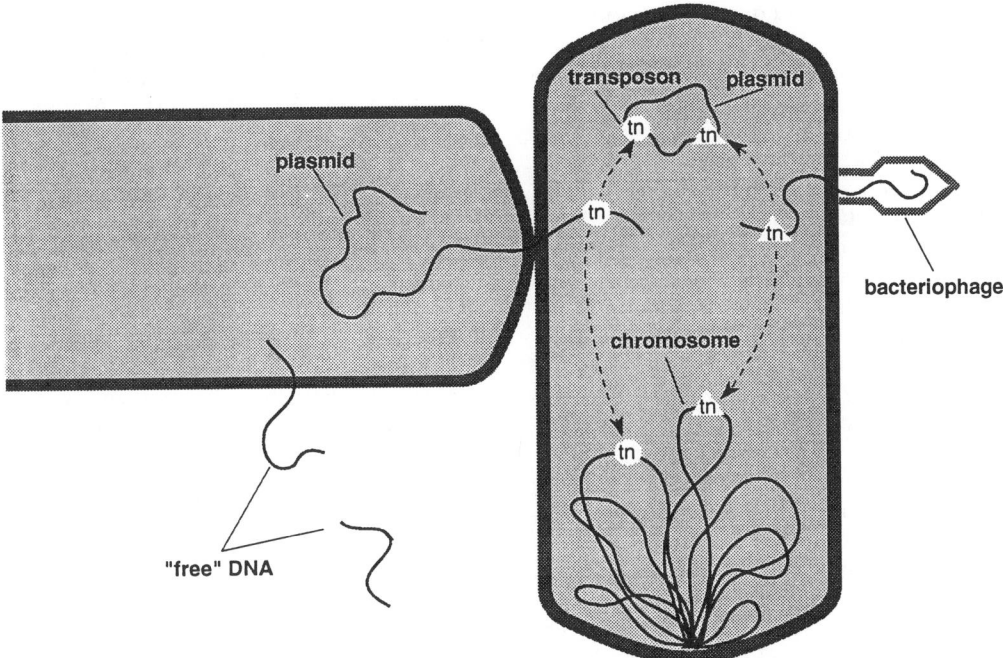

FIG. 1. Mechanisms for resistance gene transfer in bacteria. Transfer of resistance genes by conjugation (the transfer between two bacteria via pili), transduction (the transfer by viruses or bacteriophages), and transformation (uptake of free DNA) contribute to the high frequency of antimicrobial resistance. Movement of small DNA elements called transposons (*tn*), which contain antimicrobial resistance genes, occurs among various DNA molecules. (Adapted from ref. 2.)

gene, although the vehicle of transfer (i.e., the plasmid, the phage, or the free DNA) is lost. This is the likely method by which the β-lactamase gene on a transposon has moved from gram-negative intestinal organisms like *E. coli* into *H. influenzae* and *Neisseria gonorrheae,* as first noted in the mid-1970s.

Thus an intricate and sophisticated number of processes (conjugation, transduction, transformation, and transposition) (Fig. 1) alone or together, allow wide genetic exchange among bacteria of different types, including those that reside in the gastrointestinal tract. In fact, in an analysis of gene transfer among different genera, one could propose that the *Enterococcus* and the Enterobacteriaceae, both members of the intestinal flora, could act as major reservoirs of antibiotic resistance and other genes for their eventual transfer into many different genera (197).

Genetics and Mechanisms of Antimicrobial Resistance

Drug Inactivation

Antimicrobial resistance can be produced by a number of different mechanisms, each of which is generally specific for a particular antimicrobial agent (Table 5). Among the most common mechanisms are those that *degrade* or *modify* the antimicrobial agent.

Degradation is the chief mechanism by which penicillins and cephalosporins are inactivated in both gram-posi-

tive and gram-negative organisms. The initially recognized penicillinases and cephalosporinases were able to break the β-lactam ring of first-generation β-lactam antibiotics.

Penicillinase genes may be acquired on plasmids or be part of the cell's intrinsic genetic apparatus (198). The

TABLE 5. *Mechanisms of resistance to antimicrobial agents*

Mechanism	Drug
Degradation of the antibiotic	Penicillins, cephalosporins
Modification of the antimicrobial agent	Aminoglycosides, chloramphenicol
Active efflux	Tetracyclines, quinolones, chloramphenicol, macrolides
Reduced uptake	Tetracyclines, quinolones, chloramphenicol, β-lactams
Altered target	
Ribosome	Tetracycline, macrolides
Gyrase	Quinolones
RNA polymerase	Rifampin
Substitute target	
Enzymes in folic acid synthesis	Trimethoprim, sulfonamides
Membrane-associated proteins	Penicillins, cephalosporins, vancomycin

TEM-1 β-lactamase gene is found commonly among Enterobacteriaceae; it is generally located on a transposon. The plasmid and transposon location helps explain its current widespread distribution. Besides TEM-1, many different β-lactamase genes have been described among the intestinal bacteria (199). With the introduction of second- and third-generation β-lactam agents, resistance to these agents has also appeared. β-Lactamases have been identified that have an extended spectrum of activity. Of particular interest, these novel β-lactamases have evolved from the previously selected β-lactamase genes, namely, TEM-1 and SHV-1. By a small number of mutations, the older resistance genes have now enlarged their spectrum. First recognized among *Klebsiella* and *Enterobacter,* they are now found among *E. coli* and other members of the Enterobacteriaceae (200).

If intestinal bacteria, such as *E. coli* or *Klebsiella,* are resistant to β-lactam antibiotics, the mechanism will be a β-lactamase, of narrow or extended spectrum, generally carried on plasmids (198,199). Of particular interest, as well, are the inducible chromosomal β-lactamases in many of the enteric organisms (198). These enzymes are not normally expressed at high level but they can be induced by certain cephalosporins and, upon induction, have activity against other β-lactam drugs (198). Mutants that express the enzymes constitutively have been found among *E. coli* and other Enterobacteriaceae (198).

Another drug-inactivating mechanism of resistance leads to modification of the antimicrobial agent. This mechanism is illustrated in resistance to the aminoglycosides (e.g., gentamicin, tobramycin, and kanamycin) and to chloramphenicol. By an ever increasing number (more than two dozen) of enzymes that phosphorylate, adenylate, or acetylate the antibiotic, bacteria resist aminoglycosides of all types (201). The modified drugs are inactive, having difficulty being taken up into the cell and binding to the ribosome, which is their site of action. Chloramphenicol is also inactivated by an acetyl side chain, the result of an acetyltransferase (202).

Active Efflux

These aforementioned mechanisms are targeted at the antimicrobial agent: they represent drug-directed mechanisms. A different kind of drug-directed mechanism is that of active efflux. This resistance mechanism was initially described for the tetracyclines (203). More recently, efflux systems for the quinolones (204,205) and chloramphenicol (206) have been identified among gram-negative bacteria. Each of the efflux systems is unique and generally exports a single substrate family (e.g., tetracyclines). There are examples, however, of other efflux systems that appear to have multiple substrates (207). One example is the *Bacillus* multidrug resistance protein (Bmr) found in *Bacillus subtilis* (208).

Among the intestinal organisms, the major drug resistance mediated by active efflux is that to the tetracyclines. There are many different efflux-mediated tetracycline resistance determinants (209,210). At least seven are currently known, distinguished by DNA::DNA hybridiza-

tions, and show genetic organization and amino acid sequences that are highly homologous. The determinants have been classified by letters into classes (class A, class B, etc. or Tet(A), Tet(B), etc.). Among *E. coli,* the Tet(B) determinant, residing on transposon *10,* is the most common, followed by classes A and C (209,211). Among *Aeromonas,* at least in one study, class E was common (212). Other studies show different distributions of the determinants among different genera. The recently described class H determinant came from *Pasteurella* (213) and class G was found in *Vibrio* (214). All determinants specify a structural protein, TetA, and a repressor of its transcription (TetR). The efflux of tetracycline occurs as a cation (Mg^{2+}):tetracycline complex in exchange for a proton (215). Efflux is also one of the mechanisms for tetracycline resistance in *Clostridium perfringens.* The efflux determinant also involves an inner membrane protein, but it shows only limited likeness to the Tet efflux systems in gram-negative bacteria (216).

Efflux is also a mechanism for resistance to quinolones and chloramphenicol. The genetic determinants appear to be on the chromosome and their impact *vis-à-vis* resistance is enhanced by changes in drug influx. For instance, an endogenous efflux system for quinolones and one for chloramphenicol have been identified in *E. coli* (203,206). They are not clinically relevant unless their activity is augmented by a decrease in drug permeability (217).

One form of macrolide resistance by efflux has been described among the staphylococci, namely, *S. epidermidis.* Unlike the tetracycline and quinolone efflux system, it is not energized by proton motive force, but by adenosine triphosphate (ATP) (218). Whether this resistance determinant will enter into other species and organisms such as enterococcus is to be seen.

Decreased Uptake

Reduced penetration of the drug into the cell can occur by reducing the outer membrane porins through which many of the more hydrophilic antimicrobial agents, such as tetracyclines, quinolones, chloramphenicol, and the penicillins, enter into the cell. By loss of the porins, susceptibility to the drug may decrease two- to four-fold. If this mechanism of reduced penetration is added to those of a β-lactamase (219) or to an efflux system (217), there is an amplification of resistance. The combination of the two mechanisms provides higher levels of resistance. The decreased uptake is mediated by various chromosomal mutations in the cell, including one in the regulatory locus *mar,* which leads to increased resistance to multiple antibiotics and other toxic elements (217).

Changing the Target

Other mechanisms of resistance act by changing or altering the target of the antimicrobial agent. The ribosome, the target for tetracyclines and the macrolides, is altered by some resistance determinants to these drugs. For tetracyclines, the widely spread Tet(M) resistance determinant, found in enterococcus, *Neisseria, H. ducreyi,* streptococcus, staphylococcus, and many organisms of the genitourinary tract (220), and other related determinants, such as Tet(O) in *Campylobacter,* Tet(Q) in *Bacteroides,* Tet(S) in *Listeria,* or TetB(P) in *Clostridium perfringens,* encode an approximately 68,000 molecular weight cytoplasmic protein that loosely associates with the ribosome. By a mechanism yet unclear, the protein protects the ribosome from being inhibited by tetracyclines (221,222).

One kind of macrolide resistance, known as *erm,* is determined by highly related macrolide resistance determinants. The *erm* gene encodes a methylase that causes a methylation of the 23S ribosomal ribonucleic acid (RNA) (225). The *erm* determinants are common among the gram-positive organisms, where erythromycin is used more widely. However, they are also the basis of clindamycin resistance among *Bacteroides.* With the rise of extended spectrum macrolides, one may begin to see these and other mechanisms of macrolide resistance appear in gram-negative bacteria. One, an antibiotic degradation mechanism for erythromycin on a plasmid, was recently described in *E. coli* (224).

Another mechanism of resistance related to an altered target is that for the quinolones. In addition to active efflux and decreased penetration as mechanisms of resistance, a mutation in the target enzyme, DNA gyrase, provides the high-level resistance to this family of antimicrobials (225). Spontaneous mutations in the gene for the gyrase make the enzyme no longer susceptible to the quinolones. There is some evidence to suggest that the gyrase mutation may follow as a second step event in bacteria in which lower-level resistance via decreased uptake or increased efflux is present (217).

A mutation in the RNA polymerase, the target for rifampin and related drugs, is the basis for resistance to this drug.

Target Substitution

A second form of target modification is the addition of a drug-resistant target to the one that is susceptible to the antimicrobial. Early examples of this mechanism are those for resistance to sulfonamides and trimethoprim. These antimicrobials each inactivate an enzyme involved in folic acid biosynthesis. The resistance determinants, borne on transposons and plasmids, encode substitute enzymes, which are not sensitive to trimethoprim (dihydrofolate reductase) (226) or to sulfonamides (dehydropteonoate) (227). Thus high expression of the substitute enzyme allows the cells to grow despite contact with the antimicrobials, which inhibit the endogenous chromosomal enzymes.

Resistance to penicillins and other β-lactam antibiotics can be mediated by changes in the penicillin binding proteins (PBPs) in the cell wall of these organisms (228). This is a mechanism of resistance that is frequent among certain gram-positive bacteria, such as staphylococcus and pneumococcus, but may also appear among the gram-negative bacteria.

Another cell wall change leading to resistance is that

to vancomycin. This determinant has been identified on plasmids among the enterococcus. Vancomycin-resistant enterococci are now a major nosocomial problem. The substitution of D-ala-D-lac for D-ala-D-ala at the terminus of the cell peptidoglycan precursor makes this organism no longer susceptible to vancomycin (229).

Regulatory Locus Mutation

Mutations in a recently described reguatory locus for multiple antibiotic resistance (*mar*) leads to resistance to multiple antibiotics, oxidative stress compounds and response to weak acids in *E. coli* and other members of the *Enterobacteriaceae.* Constitutive expression of the normally repressed *mar* operon leads to activation of the other chromosomal genes, leading to the multidrug resistance phenotype, generally via changes in the uptake or efflux (217,229a).

EPIDEMIOLOGICAL FACTORS AFFECTING THE DEVELOPMENT OF RESISTANCE

Human Use of Antimicrobial Agents

Although some bacterial species are intrinsically resistant to particular antimicrobial agents, and plasmids with or without resistance determinants have been identified in bacterial strains saved from the preantibiotic era (230,231) (or isolated from communities not exposed to antimicrobial agents) (232), widespread resistance has only occurred since the introduction and intensive use of antimicrobial agents. The "why" of this increase in resistance is intuitively obvious: organisms that are resistant to antimicrobial agents have a survival advantage over those that are killed by these agents. The "how" is less evident: although many antimicrobial agents are in use, resistance develops in erratic, and not easily predictable, patterns. How does resistance develop in one genus and not another? How does resistance develop in one locality and not another? How do some resistant strains disseminate and not others? How do some persons in a community (or in a hospital) become infected with an antimicrobial-resistant strain of bacteria, while others in the same community become infected with an antimicrobial-susceptible strain of the same species of bacteria?

The answers to these questions lie in part with the ingenuity of bacteria (200,233). As discussed above, mechanisms conferring resistance may be shared among different bacterial species. But even after a bacterial strain acquires the apparatus for antimicrobial resistance, there still needs to be the selective pressure of antimicrobial use for that strain to become prevalent. The quantitative and qualitative components of that selective pressure, however, are not certain (234).

The empiric observation that antimicrobial resistance among bacterial enteric pathogens and among commensal Enterobacteriaceae is more common in developing countries than in industrialized countries suggests that there

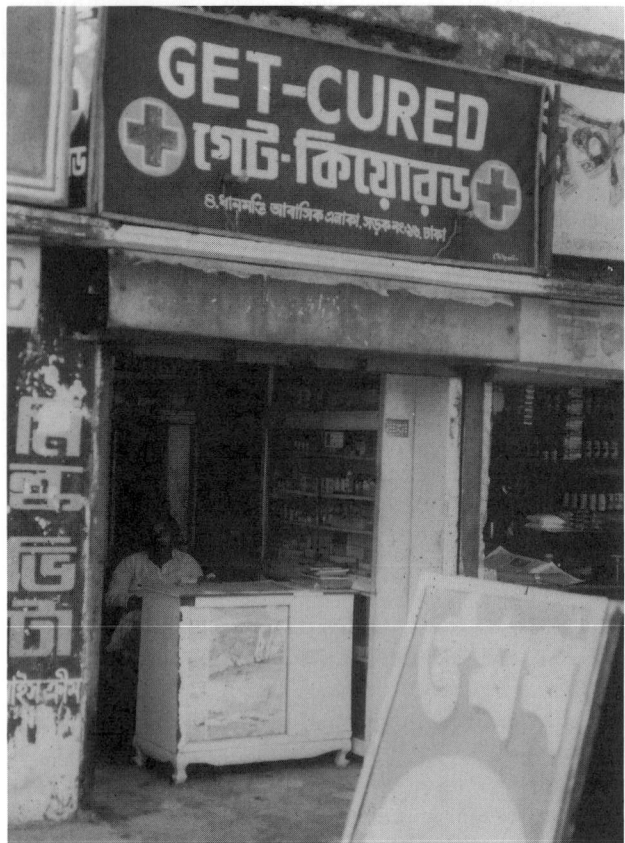

FIG. 2. A retail pharmacy in Bangladesh. Such pharmacies are usually owned and operated by persons with no formal medical training and who dispense pharmaceuticals without prescription. Pharmacies such as this are the most common source of pharmaceuticals (and a common source of primary medical care) in developing countries.

are practices in the former that facilitate the development of resistance. Indeed, antimicrobial use patterns clearly differ between developing and industrialized countries in a number of important ways (235,236). In most developing countries antimicrobial agents are available without prescription from pharmacies (237–244), and most pharmacies are staffed by personnel with no medical training (Fig. 2) (238,244). Treatment obtained from such pharmacies (and from medical practitioners, both trained and untrained) is often irrational (235,238,244–247) and is strongly driven by economic incentives, as the more drugs sold the greater the profit for the pharmacy. Irrational prescribing of antimicrobial agents is especially common, as these drugs are particularly sought by patients, and in some countries they have attained the status of indigenous, herbal remedies (248–249). In a number of studies from developing countries, 30% or more of patients with watery diarrhea, for which antimicrobial therapy is not routinely recommended, will receive treatment with an antimicrobial agent (250–252). Unfortunately, prescribing practices by physicians are often not any better than those of untrained medical practitioners. Many prescriptions from both physicians and other medical practitioners are

for multiple antimicrobial agents (Fig. 3), often for diseases for which at most one, and very often no, antimicrobial agent is indicated (253,254).

The irrational use of antimicrobial agents is compounded by the marketing in many developing countries of drugs combining several antimicrobial agents (255,256). Popular combinations of drugs for oral administration in developing countries have been chloramphenicol and streptomycin (sold as Chloro-Strep in many countries) (Fig. 4) and chloramphenicol and tetracycline (240). Such irrational combinations of drugs are likely to be particularly proficient in selecting multiply-resistant strains of bacteria, because genes coding for resistance are often closely linked, either on a plasmid or because a single chromosomal operon can control expression of different resistance mechanisms (257). In the past, many of these irrational combinations of drugs were marketed in developing countries by large multinational pharmaceutical companies despite their not being licensed for use in the industrialized country where the multinational firm is headquartered (258). Pressure from consumer groups has been effective in convincing many multinational companies to withdraw these products from the market, but such drugs are still often produced in developing countries by local companies (258a).

In an effort to reduce cost, inadequately short courses of antimicrobial therapy are often purchased by patients in developing countries (238). This pattern of dosing is also thought to increase the rate at which antimicrobial resistance develops, though this has been conclusively demonstrated only for *Mycobacterium tuberculosis* infections. It has been well demonstrated, however, that chronic administration of subtherapeutic doses of antimicrobial agents will lead to the development of resistance among Enterobacteriaceae (2).

There are a number of factors in addition to economic incentives that encourage the irrational use of drugs. One is that the information available on rational prescribing to physicians and other health workers in both industrialized and developing countries is limited (259,260). In comparison to industrialized countries, an even greater share of information on pharmaceuticals in developing countries is provided by company representatives or company advertising that is often either incomplete or incorrect (261,262). On an optimistic note, there has been some improvement reported in these practices in recent years (263), though in most developing countries the ratio of pharmaceutical company representatives to physicians (1:3, or 1:4) remains five to ten times what it is in developed countries (264).

Prescribing practices in developing countries are also affected by the very brief amount of time most health care workers spend with patients. Patient visits usually last at most a few minutes, and the provision of a pharmaceutical agent furnishes a convenient means of ending the encounter. From the health care worker's perspective (and similar to what has been witnessed in industrialized countries), rapidly concluding a patient visit by providing an antimicrobial agent is often a more expeditious use of time than attempting to explain (counter to the patient's expectations) why no pharmaceutical agent is needed.

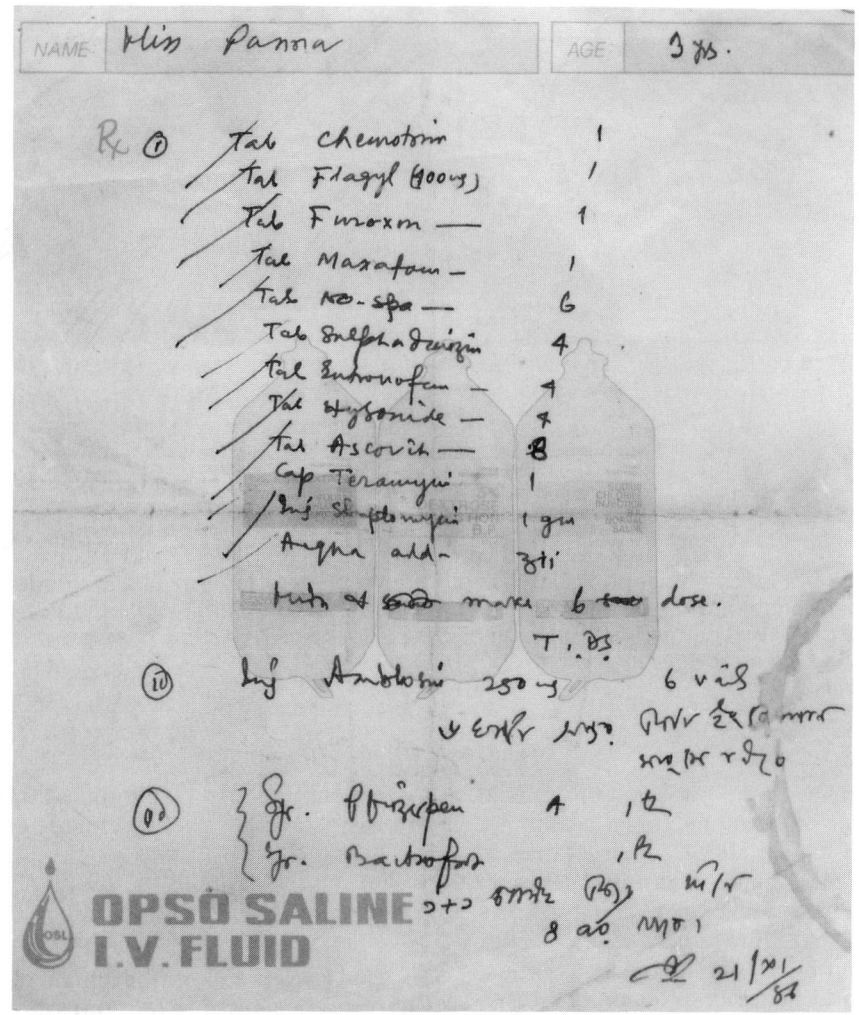

FIG. 3. Prescriptions for patients with shigellosis in Bangladesh. **A:** Example of a prescription for a 3-year-old girl with shigellosis. The prescription is for 16 different medications, including eight different antimicrobial agents. **B:** Example of a prescription for an 18-year-old with shigellosis. The diagnosis was correct, but four different antimicrobial agents were prescribed, including three (chloramphenicol, streptomycin, and metronidazole) that would not have been effective in the treatment of shigellosis at the time the prescription was written.

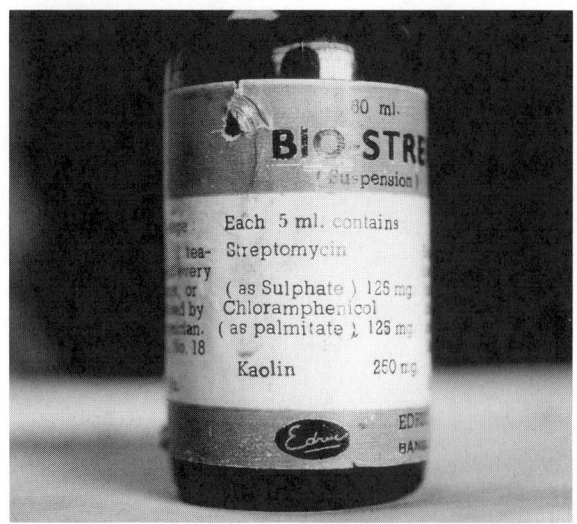 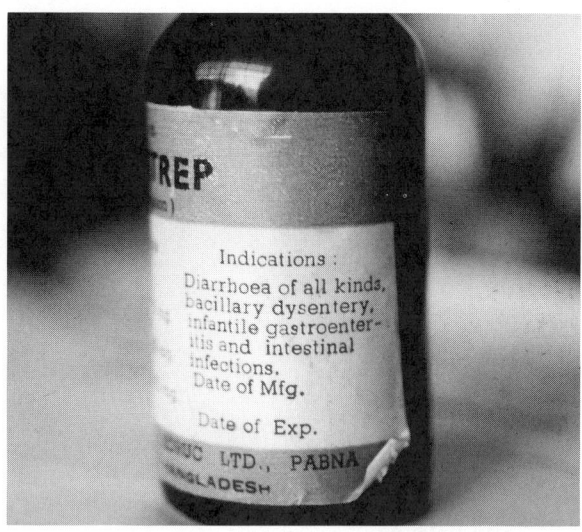

FIG. 4. Antimicrobial combinations, such as chloramphenicol–streptomycin, are frequently marketed in developing countries for the treatment of diarrhea. **A:** Listing of the ingredients of this combination drug. **B:** The manufacturer's indications for use. This drug has now been banned under the Bangladesh drug policy.

Despite these problems with the provision of drugs in developing countries, far more antimicrobial agents are consumed per capita in industrialized countries than in developing countries (265), and prescribing patterns, though perhaps better than in developing countries, are still far from ideal (266–268). Thus other factors besides the magnitude of inappropriate antimicrobial use must contribute to the high prevalence of antimicrobial resistance found in developing countries. Such factors may include the high rate of transmission of enteric pathogens that occurs because of poor hygiene and crowding, and the lack of surveillance systems to detect and control outbreaks of resistant bacteria.

The ingestion of antimicrobial agents for symptoms unrelated to diarrhea has also been shown in a number of studies to markedly increase the risk of developing symptomatic enteric infection with multiply-resistant organisms. This has been most conclusively demonstrated for *Salmonella* (269,270). This is thought to occur because gut flora that act to inhibit colonization or growth of *Salmonella* are suppressed by antimicrobial therapy, thus allowing the multiply-resistant strain of *Salmonella* to flourish. In one study, symptomatic infection with a multiply-resistant strain of *Salmonella* (as opposed to a susceptible strain of *Salmonella*) was 50 times more common in patients who had recently ingested an antimicrobial agent for an unrelated illness than in persons who had not taken an antimicrobial agent (269). In four outbreaks of multiply-resistant *Salmonella* studied in the United States, recent ingestion of an antimicrobial agent for an unrelated illness was estimated to have increased the total number of symptomatic cases from 16% to 64% in these four outbreaks (66). Prior antimicrobial use can also increase the risk of infection with an antimicrobial-susceptible strain of *Salmonella* (271). Treatment of symptomatic *Salmonella*

infections can also result in the acquisition of antimicrobial resistance by the infecting strain (272).

Veterinary Use of Antimicrobial Agents

The widespread use of antimicrobial agents in veterinary medicine also exerts pressure for the selection of resistant bacteria, although how important a contribution this makes to human enteric infections with resistant organisms has been a subject of debate (269,273,274). Antimicrobial agents are widely used in farm animals raised for human consumption. Recent estimates are that in the United States about half of the antimicrobial agents produced annually, by weight, are used in nonhuman animals, and that this constitutes 13% of the total value of antimicrobial agents consumed (273–275). Much of the antimicrobial use in animals is provided at subtherapeutic levels in feed for the purpose of growth promotion, or for prophylaxis in animals at high risk of infection, such as those being raised in densely inhabited, confined quarters, or animals being shipped to market (273).

At least three of the most important bacterial enteric pathogens, *Yersinia, Campylobacter,* and *Salmonella,* are zoonoses, with a major reservoir for all three pathogens being farm animals raised for human consumption. Human infections with multiply-resistant strains of nontyphoidal *Salmonella* have been traced to beef produced from animals fed tetracycline or chloramphenicol (11,269,270,277). Because beef from single slaughterhouses can be widely distributed (and difficult to trace), it is often hard to identify infections from animal-derived strains unless they have unusual characteristics, such as an uncommon serotype, resistance pattern, or plasmid (278). It is therefore likely that the extent of transmission of multiply-resistant strains of enteric pathogens from animal to human is considerably underestimated. One study of multiply-resistant *Salmonella* outbreaks in the United States did, however, estimate that 69% of such outbreaks were attributable to an animal source (11). Once multiply-resistant strains have spread from animal to human, they may then spread from human to human, thus increasing the impact that such multiply-resistant strains have in the human community but decreasing the likelihood that the original animal source of infection will be identified (278). The use of antimicrobial agents in animal feed has also resulted in the development of resistant strains of *Campylobacter* and *Yersinia*, although there is yet no conclusive evidence (as there is with *Salmonella*) that these strains have been transmitted to humans, although that event seems likely (279,280).

The use of antibiotics in animal feed can also increase the prevalence of resistant fecal bacteria in farm workers caring for these animals (281) and result in the direct spread of resistant enteric pathogens to farm workers. An example of the latter was an outbreak of multiply-resistant *Salmonella* that occurred in a nursery and that was traced to infected calves on a farm where one of the mothers of the newborns lived (282). In fairness to animals, it should also be pointed out that the traffic in antimicrobial-resistant bacteria is a two-way street: animals may also acquire multiply-resistant bacteria from humans, as has been shown in baboons feeding from refuse heaps near Kenyan tourist lodges (283).

Spread of Resistance

Antimicrobial resistance is cosmopolitan. There are a number of reasons for this. One is jetliners. More people travel, and travel faster and farther, than before commercial transportation by jet was available. In many industrialized countries a common (and in some cases the most common) origin of antimicrobial-resistant enteric infections is from travelers returning from developing countries or from emigrants from developing countries (99,146,148,150,151,158). Such strains may establish residence in the country to which they have been transported. Second, the food supply in most developed countries is no longer local in origin. Seafood, beef, and produce (or pet turtles) (284) may be imported into the United States or other industrialized countries from many locales, including countries where antimicrobial-resistant enteric infections are common. Third, resistance plasmids are inveterate travelers. The movement of plasmids is a much more efficient means of disseminating resistance than the independent development of resistance at different geographic sites. Resistance plasmids may travel to a new geographic locale in one genus of bacteria and quickly disseminate to other genera. Using molecular techniques to type plasmids, the intercontinental spread of a plasmid carrying resistance to gentamicin has been demonstrated (285). It is likely that resistance to other antimicrobial agents has also spread in this fashion.

IMPACT OF RESISTANCE ON THE THERAPY OF ENTERIC INFECTIONS

In areas where multiply-resistant strains of enteric pathogens are common, the impact of bacterial resistance on the treatment of diarrhea has been profound (7,13,156). The high prevalence of multiply-resistant strains of enteric bacterial pathogens in developing countries has required the use of agents that are often more expensive, more toxic, or less effective than the agents they replaced.

In developing countries the drugs of choice for the treatment of enteric infections in the early 1980s are now, for the most part, no longer useful because of the increase of multiply-resistant infections. Ampicillin and trimethoprim–sulfamethoxazole, which, because of their low cost, relative lack of toxicity, availability in oral and intravenous formulations, and good *in vitro* and *in vivo* activity, had been used for treating *Shigella*, *V. cholerae*, and *S. typhi* infections, are often no longer useful for the treatment of any of these infections. In Bangladesh more than half of the isolates of each of these three species are now resistant to these two drugs. Other agents that had also been in common use—chloramphenicol, nalidixic acid, and tetracycline—have also been rendered useless because of the increased prevalence of multiply-resistant strains.

Although the retail price of newer antimicrobial agents is usually less in developing countries than in industrialized countries, they remain markedly more expensive than older agents and in relation to income are more expensive than they are in industrialized countries. Table 6 lists the prices at pharmacies in Bangladesh and Boston of older antimicrobial agents used in the treatment of enteric infections, and the newer agents that have replaced them. Alternative agents have limitations in addition to cost. Some drugs, such as the β-lactam agent pivamdinocillin, which is used to treat multiply-resistant *Shigella* infections, are less widely available than older agents, especially in rural areas. Other agents, such as the newer quinolones, are not approved for use in children because of concerns about potential toxicity to developing bones and joints. And some agents, such as the third-generation cephalosporins that have been used in the treatment of typhoid fever, are administered parenterally. In desperation, some centers are now using older agents, such as furazolidone, that have been shown to be active *in vitro* against multiply-resistant strains of enteric pathogens such as *Shigella*, but whose activity *in vivo* is limited.

Although the problem of multiply-resistant enteric pathogens is particularly acute in Bangladesh, it is hardly confined to Bangladesh or to the Indian subcontinent, as can be seen from Tables 1 to 4. Epidemics of *Shigella* resistant to all locally available antimicrobial agents (ampicillin, trimethoprim–sulfamethoxazole, and nalidixic acid) have occurred in a number of African countries (156), and systemic *Salmonella* infections resistant to even third-generation cephalosporins have been reported from newborn nurseries (93).

The costs associated with infection with multiply-resistant organisms extend beyond simply the need to use a

TABLE 6. *Cost of 5 days of treatment with antimicrobial agents used for enteric infections*

Agent	Dose	Number of doses	Cost in United States[a]	Cost as percentage of daily income in United States[b]	Cost in Bangladesh[c]	Cost as percentage of daily income in Bangladesh[b]
Older agents						
Amoxicillin	500 mg	15	$6.60	8%	$2.25	281%
Ampicillin	500 mg	20	$5.39	6%	$2.00	250%
Erythromycin base	333 mg	15	$6.64	8%	$3.38	423%
Tetracycline	500 mg	20	$5.28	6%	$1.30	163%
Trimethoprim–sulfamethoxazole	Double-strength tablet	10	$5.00	6%	$0.70	88%
Newer agents						
Amoxicillin–clavulanic acid	500 mg amoxicillin	15	$54.37	62%	NM[d]	—
Cefixime	8 mg/kg/d	150-mL bottle (20 mg/mL)	$36.00	41%	NM[d]	—
Ciprofloxacin	500 mg	10	$44.00	50%	$3.75[e]	469%
Norfloxacin	400 mg	10	$36.20	42%	NM[d]	—

[a] Charge to the patient at the outpatient pharmacy of the New England Medical Center, January 1994.
[b] Calculated from per-capita annual income divided by 250 working days per year. (Values for per-capita income obtained from ref. 286: $21,790 for the United States and $200 for Bangladesh.)
[c] Retail price fixed by the Government of Bangladesh.
[d] NM, not marketed.
[e] Patent rights for newer drugs not recognized by the Government of Bangladesh.

newer, more expensive antimicrobial agent for treatment. Although enteric infections are often treated empirically (especially in developing countries), the prospect of infection with a resistant organism will often prompt a physician to obtain a culture of stool. In January 1994, the cost of a stool culture for the isolation of *Campylobacter, Shigella,* and *Salmonella* at the New England Medical Center in Boston was $43; isolation of *Yersinia* and enterohemorrhagic *E. coli* are each an additional $42 charge, and the cost of susceptibility testing if a pathogen is identified is $24. If all these tests are performed, the total cost is then $151. Although costs for such tests in developing countries are often less (if the test is available, which is often not the case), in comparison to income they remain expensive. Because the provision of effective therapy is often delayed in patients infected with multiply-resistant enteric pathogens, patients infected with such strains may also incur more morbidity, thereby increasing the cost of illness even further, and are more likely to transmit the infection to other persons. Added to the medical costs are the loss of wages caused by absence from work.

The high prevalence of multiply-resistant infections in developing countries plays havoc with the standard diarrhea treatment algorithms promulgated by the World Health Organization and other public health organizations. These diarrhea treatment algorithms are based on symptom complexes (287,288). Children with dysentery are presumed to be infected with *Shigella,* children and adults with profound watery diarrhea in cholera endemic (or epidemic) areas are assumed to be infected with *V. cholerae,* and patients with the classic features of enteric fever are presumed to be infected with *S. typhi* or *S. para-*

typhi. Antimicrobial treatment is initiated based on these symptoms. When resistance is uncommon, these algorithms work well: community health care workers need only carry one or two drugs (in addition to oral rehydration salts) for the treatment of diarrhea when visiting villages, and a relatively uniform treatment can be provided to patients. When multiply-resistant organisms are highly prevalent, the utility of such simple algorithms often breaks down, as initial empiric therapy is far less likely to be effective, and frequent follow-up visits are required. At what prevalence of resistance an antimicrobial agent ceases to be useful as a first-line drug for empiric therapy depends on a number of factors, but at the International Centre for Diarrhoeal Disease Research in Bangladesh a prevalence of resistance of 20% or more is the arbitrary level at which a drug is no longer used for initial empiric therapy.

EFFORTS TO CONTROL RESISTANCE

Regulatory Efforts

Efforts to regulate drug use patterns thought to enhance the development of antimicrobial resistance have been undertaken by both governments and hospitals. In developing countries the major focus of efforts to regulate and rationalize antimicrobial use has been essential drug programs supported by the World Health Organization and the United Nations Children Fund (UNICEF) (289,290). The World Health Organization has established a model list of essential drugs for use in developing countries (291).

The most recent list includes 13 antibacterial agents for routine use in developing countries and selected supplementary agents (newer fluoroquinolones, third-generation cephalosporins) that are to be used when resistance to the standard agents becomes common. This essential drugs list and similar policy statements emanating from expert commissions convened by the World Health Organization (292) serve as recommendations to governments in the developing world; the decision to implement these programs rests with the individual country. Although the essential drugs list has served as a model for drug use in government health programs (where drugs are often supplied by international donors such as UNICEF), in most developing countries the vast majority of drugs are obtained from nongovernment sources, including licensed and unlicensed drug dispensers and private medical practitioners (237,238,241–246,250,251). Studies conducted in Yemen and other developing countries suggest that when essential drug programs are introduced into the government health service they can effect a reduction in the use of unwarranted injections and the number of drugs supplied (293). This effect is largely a result of decreased availability of nonessential drugs, rather than because of improved knowledge on the part of medical practitioners (293).

With one notable exception (the Bangladesh National Drug Policy), the essential drugs programs that would control the drugs available in the private market have not been implemented by governments in developing countries with free-market economies. The Bangladesh policy, which was adopted in 1982, established an essential drugs list for use by both private and government facilities, banned the import of nonessential drugs, and established price controls on drugs (294,295). The implementation of this policy was strongly opposed by international pharmaceutical companies and by the United States Government at that time (294). The essential drugs program in Bangladesh has not, however, had an apparent effect on the development of resistance among enteric pathogens and has, because of continued pressure from the pharmaceutical industry, been much diluted by the addition of many nonessential antimicrobial agents to the list of approved drugs (295).

Few efforts to regulate prescribing behavior in developing countries have been undertaken (239). The paucity of physicians in developing countries (many developing countries have less than one physician per 5000 population, compared to a ratio of 1:500 or less in most industrialized countries) (264,294) makes limiting the availability of antimicrobial agents to a prescription-only basis difficult (239). Although one solution to the problem of irrational use of drugs would be to limit drug dispensing or prescribing to medical workers with some training (in developing countries the majority of trained medical practitioners are not physicians, but community health care workers or paramedics), in practice such a solution is difficult because of the political force of the licensed drug dispensers and pharmaceutical companies (296). In Bangladesh (population 120,000,000), for instance, there are 21,000 doctors, but 150 drug companies, 20,000 licensed pharmacies, and perhaps twice as many unlicensed pharmacies (295). Over half of all health expenditures are for the purchase of drugs (275,295). Even within the formal, physician-dominated segment of the medical system (hospitals, office practices), there has been little headway in implementing peer review or medical audit systems that would help to control the irrational use of antimicrobial agents. This is in part due to the major differences in perceptions and social class between those in authority (in national governments or international organizations) who would impose restraints, and the practitioners and patients who prescribe and use drugs (297). To overcome these obstacles to rational drug use, some experts have suggested using social marketing techniques rather than regulation (which is often unenforceable in developing countries) as the best way to improve drug prescribing and drug use habits (298). Such an approach, however, neglects the strong economic incentive for the continued overprescribing of antimicrobial agents.

In industrialized countries hospitals have had some success in limiting the use of newer antimicrobial agents by either not including them on the formulary or by requiring that they be approved for use by, or discussed with, an infectious disease consultant before the drug is provided (299–301). Efforts to control the outpatient use of antimicrobial agents have proved less successful. Indeed, factors influencing the use of antimicrobial agents in industrialized countries (especially among outpatients) are similar to those at work in developing countries—a disproportionate influence of pharmaceutical companies through advertising of often dubious merit (often provided under the guise of educational programs) (259,302) and the desire by physicians to prescribe the latest "antimicrobial–sedative" combination agent—"antimicrobial" for the patient and "sedative" for the physician, who is able to sleep well at night convinced that he/she has prescribed an agent that will be effective against all possible bacterial organisms and all possible infectious diseases. Perhaps the most effective restraint on prescribing will come through restrictions imposed by third-party payers—the insurance companies and government agencies that want to reduce their costs. The constraints on reimbursements and formulary selection imposed by third-party payers through capitation payments and managed care systems will inevitably result in a reduction in the use of newer, more expensive antimicrobial agents (303).

Regulatory efforts have also been imposed on the use of antimicrobial agents for veterinary use. The European Union has taken a stricter approach to the regulation of antimicrobial supplementation of animal feed than the United States, having banned the use of tetracycline and other antimicrobial agents used in humans as supplements to animal feed (274,304). The prohibition on the use of tetracycline in animal feed in The Netherlands in 1974 was associated with a decline in the number of tetracycline-resistant *Salmonella* isolated from animals and from humans (304). Although the issue of antimicrobial supplementation of animal feed has been the subject of a number of government-sponsored reviews in the United States (305), bans similar to those in Europe have not been put into effect (274).

Directly observed administration of antimicrobial

agents has been shown to lower the rate of acquired drug resistance in patients with tuberculosis in the United States (306). Such a system would be difficult to implement for enteric infections, which are many times more common than tuberculosis. One option for assuring compliance with therapy in enteric infections, however, would be to use single-dose therapy, which has been shown to be effective in the treatment of shigellosis (157,307) and cholera (166,308) and which could be administered directly at a physician's office or in an outpatient clinic.

Educational Efforts

Traditional continuing medical education efforts, which are often didactic in nature and require only the passive participation of medical practitioners, have had modest or no impact on the prescribing behavior of physicians in industrialized countries (303,309–313). One reason for this is succinctly summarized by Goldfinger: "an overemphasis on cognitive issues in education stems from the platonic fallacy that knowledge is a virtue and if only one knew the facts, his performance would be outstanding" (314). More innovative methods, including office visits by clinical pharmacists and physician counselors (the public health equivalent of the pharmaceutical company detail representative) (310,311) or the use of advertising methods similar to those employed by pharmaceutical companies (315), have had greater impact. These methods have been shown to reduce the unwarranted use of expensive antimicrobial agents and, in the end, to be cost-effective. These programs must be continued to have a sustained effect, however.

Much less attention has been paid to educating consumers in an effort to change their perceptions and reduce demand. Among the public, both in developing and industrialized countries, antimicrobial agents retain their cachet as miracle drugs that will potentially benefit most afflictions and that carry little or no risk (2). The concept that inappropriate use of antimicrobial agents by individuals contributes to the problem of antimicrobial resistance in the community is a difficult one to communicate, especially when the individual involved is ill and desirous of taking an antimicrobial agent. Physician and consumer movements that aim to change these perceptions and that provide information on the relative risks and benefits of antimicrobial therapy have appeared. These include the Alliance for the Prudent Use of Antibiotics (2), Health Action International (255,256), the International Organization of Consumers Union (295), and the International Network for Rational Use of Drugs (316). How effective these organizations are in altering perceptions remains to be seen, but as part of broader consumer and ecologic movements (e.g., the green parties in Europe), they are likely to result in changes in consumer attitudes over the long term. Changes in attitudes and behavior will also be required of academic physicians who, by conducting drug trials, publishing in the medical literature, and speaking at industry-sponsored symposia, strongly influence drug utilization (317).

CONCLUSION

Although antimicrobial resistance is a problem in the treatment of many diseases, the problem of antimicrobial resistance in enteric infections is particularly acute. In many areas, bacteria causing diarrhea—*Shigella, Salmonella,* and *Vibrio cholerae*—are largely resistant to the antimicrobial agents that until recently had commonly been used to treat these infections. This has necessitated the use of newer, more expensive agents (most commonly the newer quinolones) to which enteric pathogens remain susceptible. The optimist's assumption (based on previous experience) that new antimicrobial agents will inevitably be identified to treat multiply-resistant pathogens, especially now that structure-based design of antimicrobial agents is possible (318), is counterpoised to the pessimist's assumption (also based on previous experience) that resistance will inevitably develop to antimicrobial agents in common use (200,233). The recent occurrence of strains of enterococci (229) and *Mycobacterium tuberculosis* (319) resistant to all available antimicrobial agents suggests that the pessimist's view—that development of new antimicrobial agents will not keep pace with the development of resistance—may be the more realistic one.

The definitive answers to the question of how to prevent the further development of resistance are not yet clear. The complex ecology of enteric pathogens, involving humans, animals, and the environment, along with the difficulties in even imprecisely determining the extent and pattern of antimicrobial use, makes this a difficult question to answer. The current crisis in antimicrobial resistance among enteric pathogens and other bacteria, however, might not allow for interventions designed to control the emergence of bacterial resistance to be delayed until such definitive answers are available (320).

REFERENCES

1. Neu HC. The crisis in antibiotic resistance. *Science* 1992;257: 1064–1072.
2. Levy SB. *The antibiotic paradox. How miracle drugs are destroying the miracle.* New York: Plenum Publishing, 1992.
3. Tomasz A. Multiple-antibiotic-resistant pathogenic bacteria. A report on the Rockefeller University workshop. *N Engl J Med* 1994;330:1247–1251.
4. O'Brien TF, Members of Task Force 2. Resistance of bacteria to antibacterial agents: report of Task Force 2. *Rev Infect Dis* 1987;9(Suppl 3):S244–S260.
5. Farrar WE. Antibiotic resistance in developing countries. *J Infect Dis* 1985;152:1103–1106.
6. Murray BE. Resistance of *Shigella, Salmonella,* and other selected enteric pathogens to antimicrobial agents. *Rev Infect Dis* 1986;8:S172–S181.
7. Bennish ML, Salam MA. Rethinking options for the treatment of shigellosis. *J Antimicrob Chemother* 1992;30:243–247.
8. Bennish ML, Salam MA, Hossain MA, et al. Antimicrobial resistance of *Shigella* isolates in Bangladesh, 1983–1990: increasing frequency of strains multiply resistant to ampicillin, trimethoprim-sulfamethoxazole, and nalidixic acid. *Clin Infect Dis* 1992;14:1055–1066.
9. Kunin CM. Resistance to antimicrobial drugs—a worldwide calamity. *Ann Intern Med* 1993;118:557–561.
10. Weinstein RA, Kabins SA. Strategies for prevention and con-

trol of multiple drug-resistant nosocomial infection. *Am J Med* 1981;70:449–454.

11. Holmberg SD, Wells JG, Cohen ML. *Salmonella:* investigations of U.S. outbreaks, 1971–1983. *Science* 1984;225:833–835.

12. Griffin PM, Tauxe RV, Redd SC, Puhr ND, Hargrett-Bean N, Blake PA. Emergence of highly trimethoprim-sulfamethoxazole-resistant *Shigella* in a native American population: an epidemiologic study. *Am J Epidemiol* 1989;129:1042–1051.

13. Reid TMS. The treatment of non-typhi salmonellosis. *J Antimicrob Chemother* 1992;29:4–8.

14. Murray BE, Alvarado T, Kyung-Hee K, et al. Increasing resistance to trimethoprim-sulfamethoxazole among isolates of *Escherichia coli* in developing countries. *J Infect Dis* 1985;152:1107–1112.

15. Lester SC, Pla MDP, Wang F, Schael IP, Jiang H, O'Brien TF. The carriage of *Escherichia coli* resistant to antimicrobial agents by healthy children in Boston, in Caracas, Venezuela, and in Qin Pu, China. *N Engl J Med* 1990;323:286–289.

16. Tauxe RV, Cavanagh TR, Cohen ML. Interspecies gene transfer in vivo producing an outbreak of multiply resistant shigellosis. *J Infect Dis* 1989;160:1067–1070.

17. Archambaud M, Gerbaud G, Labau E, Marty N, Courvalin P. Possible in-vivo transfer of β-lactamase TEM-3 from *Klebsiella pneumoniae* to *Salmonella kedougou*. *J Antimicrob Chemother* 1991;27:427–436.

18. Schwalbe RS, Hoge CW, Morris JG, O'Hanlon PN, Crawford RA, Gilligan PH. In vivo selection for transmissible drug resistance in *Salmonella typhi* during antimicrobial therapy. *Antimicrob Agents Chemother* 1990;34:161–163.

19. Datta N, Richards H. *Salmonella typhi* in vivo acquires resistance to both chloramphenicol and co-trimoxazole. *Lancet* 1981;1:1181–1183.

20. WHO Diarrhoeal Diseases Control Programme. *The rational use of drugs in the management of acute diarrhoea in children.* Geneva: World Health Organization, 1990.

21. Cohen ML. Epidemiology of drug resistance: implications for a post-antimicrobial era. *Science* 1992;257:1050–1055.

22. Escamilla J, Kilpatrick ME, Florez Ugarte H. Spurious sulfamethoxazole-trimethoprim resistance of *Salmonella typhi*. *J Clin Microbiol* 1986;23:205–206.

23. Goldstein FW, Murray BE. Sulfonamide and trimethoprim resistance in *Salmonella typhi* [Letter]. *J Clin Microbiol* 1987;25:1344–1345.

24. Anders BJ, Lauer BA, Paisley JW, Reller LB. Double-blind placebo controlled trial of erythromycin for treatment of *Campylobacter enteritis*. *Lancet* 1982;1:131–132.

25. Salazar-Lindo E, Sack RB, Chea-Woo E, et al. Early treatment with erythromycin of *Campylobacter jejuni*-associated dysentery in children. *J Pediatr* 1986;109:355–360.

26. Taylor DN, Blaser MJ, Echeverria P, Pitarangsi C, Bodhidatta L, Wang WL. Erythromycin-resistant *Campylobacter* infections in Thailand. *Antimicrob Agents Chemother* 1987;31:438–442.

26a. Williams D, Schorling J, Barrett LJ, et al. Early treatment of *Campylobacter jejuni* enteritis. *Antimicrob Agents Chemother* 1989;33:248–250.

27. Sjögren E, Kaijser B, Werner M. Antimicrobial susceptibilities of *Campylobacter jejuni* and *Campylobacter coli* isolated in Sweden: a 10-year follow-up report. *Antimicrob Agents Chemother* 1992;36:2847–2849.

28. Van der Auwera P, Scorneaux B. *In vitro* susceptibility of *Campylobacter jejuni* to 27 antimicrobial agents and various combinations of β-lactams with clavulanic acid or sulbactam. *Antimicrob Agents Chemother* 1985;28:37–40.

29. Sagara H, Mochizuki A, Okamura N, Nakaya R. Antimicrobial resistance of *Campylobacter jejuni* and *Campylobacter coli* with special reference to plasmid profiles of Japanese clinical isolates. *Antimicrob Agents Chemother* 1987;31:713–719.

30. Lim YS, Tay L. A one-year study of enteric *Campylobacter* infections in Singapore. *J Trop Med Hyg* 1992;95:119–123.

31. Taylor DE, Chang N. In vitro susceptibilities of *Campylobacter jejuni* and *Campylobacter coli* to azithromycin and erythromycin. *Antimicrob Agents Chemother* 1991;35:1917–1918.

32. King A, Phillips I. A comparison of the in-vitro activity of clar-

ithromycin, a new macrolide antibiotic, with erythromycin and other oral agents. *J Hosp Infect* 1991;19(Suppl A):3–9.

33. Loza E, Beltrán JM, Baquero F, León A, Cantón R, Garijo B, Spanish Collaborative Group. Comparative in vitro activity of clarithromycin. *Eur J Clin Microbiol Infect Dis* 1992;11:856–866.

34. Hirschl AM, Wolf D, Berger J, Rotter ML. In vitro susceptibility of *Campylobacter jejuni* and *Campylobacter coli* isolated in Austria to erythromycin and ciprofloxacin. *Zentralbl Bakteriol* 1990;272:443–447.

35. Reina J, Borrell N, Serra A. Emergence of resistance to erythromycin and fluoroquinolones in thermotolerant *Campylobacter* strains isolated from feces 1987–1991. *Eur J Clin Microbiol Epidemiol* 1992;11:1163–1166.

36. Rautelin H, Renkonen O-V, Kosunen TU. Emergence of fluoroquinolone resistance in *Campylobacter jejuni* and *Campylobacter coli* in subjects from Finland. *Antimicrob Agents Chemother* 1991;35:2065–2069.

37. Wretlind B, Strömberg A, Östlund L, Sjögren, Kaijser B. Rapid emergence of quinolone resistance in *Campylobacter jejuni* in patients treated with norfloxacin. *Scand J Infect Dis* 1992;24:685–686.

38. Mirelis B, Miro E, Navarro F, Ogalla CA, Bonal J, Prats G. Increased resistance to quinolone in Catalonia, Spain. *Diagn Microbiol Infect Dis* 1993;16:137–139.

39. Wang Y, Huang WM, Taylor DE. Cloning and nucleotide sequence of the *Campylobacter jejuni* gyrA gene and characterization of quinolone resistance mutations. *Antimicrob Agents Chemother* 1993;37:457–463.

40. Gootz TD, Martin BA. Characterization of high-level quinolone resistance in *Campylobacter jejuni*. *Antimicrob Agents Chemother* 1991;35:840–845.

41. Segreti J, Gootz TD, Goodman LJ, et al. High-level quinolone resistance in clinical isolates of *Campylobacter jejuni*. *J Infect Dis* 1992;165:667–670.

42. Taylor DE, Courvalin P. Mechanisms of antibiotic resistance in *Campylobacter* species. *Antimicrob Agents Chemother* 1988;32:1107–1112.

43. DeBoy JM II, Wachsmuth IK, Davis BR. Antibiotic resistance in enterotoxigenic and non-enterotoxigenic *Escherichia coli*. *J Clin Microbiol* 1980;12:264–270.

44. Hyams KC, Bourgeois AL, Merrell BR, et al. Diarrheal disease during Operation Desert Shield. *N Engl J Med* 1991;325:1423–1428.

45. Chatkaeomorakot A, Echeverria P, Taylor DN, Seriwatana J, Leksomboon U. Trimethoprim-resistant *Shigella* and enterotoxigenic *Escherichia coli* strains in children in Thailand. *Pediatr Infect Dis J* 1987;6:735–739.

46. Bandres JC, Mathewson JJ, Ericsson CD, DuPont HL. Trimethoprim/sulfamethoxazole remains active against enterotoxigenic *Escherichia coli* and *Shigella* species in Guadalajara, Mexico. *Am J Med Sci* 1992;303:289–291.

47. Faruque SM, Rahman MM, Alim ARMA, Hoq MM, Albert MJ. Antibiotic resistance pattern of heat-labile enterotoxin (LT) producing *Escherichia coli* isolated from children with diarrhoea in Bangladesh: clonal relationships among isolates with different resistant phenotypes. *J Diarrhoeal Dis Res* 1993;11:143–147.

48. Echeverria P, Verhaert L, Ulyangco CV, et al. Antimicrobial resistance and enterotoxin production among isolates of *Escherichia coli* in the Far East. *Lancet* 1978;2:589–592.

49. Echeverria P, Murphy JR. Enterotoxigenic *Escherichia coli* carrying plasmids coding for antibiotic resistance and enterotoxin production. *J Infect Dis* 1980;142:273–278.

50. Silva MLM, Scaletsky ICA, Reis MHL, Affonso MHT, Trabulsi LR. Plasmid coding for drug resistance and production of heat-labile and heat-stable toxins harbored by an *Escherichia coli* strain of human origin. *Infect Immun* 1983;39:970–973.

51. Marshall BJ. Treatment strategies for *Helicobacter pylori* infection. *Gastroenterol Clin North Am* 1993;22:183–197.

52. Haas CE, Nix DE, Schentag JJ. In vitro selection of resistant *Helicobacter pylori*. *Antimicrob Agents Chemother* 1990;34:1637–1641.

53. Queiroz DMM, Coimbra RS, Mendes EN, et al. Metronida-

zole-resistant *Helicobacter pylori* in a developing country [Letter]. *Am J Gastroenterol* 1993;88:322–323.

54. Glupczynski Y, Burette A, De Koster E, et al. Metronidazole resistance in *Helicobacter pylori* [Letter]. *Lancet* 1990;1: 976–977.

55. Parasakthi N, Goh KL. Metronidazole resistance among *Helicobacter pylori* strains in Malaysia [Letter]. *Am J Gastroenterol* 1992;87:808.

56. European Study Group on Antibiotic Susceptibility of *Helicobacter pylori*. Results of a multicentre European survey in 1991 of metronidazole resistance in *Helicobacter pylori*. *Eur J Clin Microbiol Infect Dis* 1992;11:777–781.

57. Westblom TU, Unge P. Drug resistance of *Helicobacter pylori*: memorandum from a meeting at the Sixth International Workshop on *Campylobacter, Helicobacter,* and related organisms [Letter]. *J Infect Dis* 1992;165:974–975.

58. Xia HX, Daw MA, Beattie S, Keane CT, O'Morain CA. Prevalence of metronidazole-resistant *Helicobacter pylori* in dyspeptic patients. *Irish J Med Sci* 1993;162:91–94.

59. Rautelin H, Seppälä K, Renkonen O-V, Vainio U, Kosunen TU. Role of metronidazole resistance in therapy of *Helicobacter pylori* infections. *Antimicrob Agents Chemother* 1992; 36:163–166.

60. Tucci A, Varoli O, Corinaldesi R, et al. Evaluation of *Helicobacter pylori* sensitivity to amoxycillin and metronidazole in dyspeptic patients. *Ital J Gastroenterol* 1993;25:65–67.

61. Glupczynski Y, Burette A. Drug therapy for *Helicobacter pylori* infection: problems and pitfalls. *Am J Gastroenterol* 1990; 12:1545–1551.

62. Logan RPH, Gummett PA, Misiewicz JJ, Karim QN, Walker MM, Baron JH. One week eradication regimen for *Helicobacter pylori*. *Lancet* 1991;338:1249–1252.

63. Bell GD, Powell K, Burridge SM, et al. Experience with "triple" anti-*Helicobacter pylori* eradication therapy: side effects and the importance of testing the pretreatment bacterial isolate for metronidazole resistance. *Aliment Pharmacol Ther* 1992;6: 427–435.

64. Bell GD, Powell KU, Burridge SM, et al. *Helicobacter pylori* eradication: efficacy and side effect profile of a combination of omeprazole, amoxycillin and metronidazole compared with four alternative regimens. *Q J Med* 1993;86:743–750.

65. Logan RPH, Gummett PA, Misiewicz JJ, Karim QN, Walker MM, Baron JH. Two-week eradication regimen for metronidazole-resistant *Helicobacter pylori*. *Aliment Pharmacol Ther* 1993;7:149–153.

66. Cohen ML, Tauxe RV. Drug-resistant *Salmonella* in the United States: an epidemiologic perspective. *Science* 1986;234: 964–969.

67. Zoukh K. Résistance aux antibiotiques des *Salmonella*, autres que *typhi* et *paratyphi* isolées en Algérie de 1979 à 1985 (French). *Pathol Biol* (*Paris*) 1988;3:255–257.

68. Georges-Courbot MC, Wachsmuth IK, Bouquety JC, Siopathis MR, Cameron DN, Georges AJ. Cluster of antibiotic-resistant *Salmonella enteritidis* infections in the Central African Republic. *J Clin Microbiol* 1990;28:771–773.

69. Mirza NB, Wamola IA. *Salmonella typhimurium* outbreak at Kenyatta National Hospital (1985). *East Afr Med J* 1989;66: 453–457.

70. Lepage P, Bogaerts J, Van Goethem C, Hitimana DG, Nsengumuremyi F. Multiresistant *Salmonella typhimurium* systemic infection in Rwanda. Clinical features and treatment with cefotaxime. *J Antimicrob Chemother* 1990;26(Suppl A):53–57.

71. Farhoudi-Moghaddam AA, Katouli M, Jafari A, Bahavar MA, Parsi M, Malekzadeh F. Antimicrobial drug resistance and resistance factor transfer among clinical isolates of salmonellae in Iran. *Scand J Infect Dis* 1990;22:197–203.

72. Chowdhury MNH. Antibiotic sensitivity pattern: experience at University Hospital, Riyadh, Saudi Arabia. *J Hyg Epidemiol Microbiol Immunol* 1991;35:289–301.

73. Maiorini E, Lopez EL, Morrow AL, et al. Multiply resistant nontyphoidal *Salmonella* gastroenteritis in children. *Pediatr Infect Dis J* 1993;12:139–144.

74. Campos CL, Hofer E. Antimicrobial resistance among *Salmo-*

nella serovars isolated from different sources in Brazil during 1978–1983. *Antonie Van Leeuwenhoek* 1989;55:349–359.

75. Ling JM, Zhou G-M, Woo THS, French GL. Antimicrobial susceptibilities and β-lactamase production of Hong Kong isolates of gastroenteric salmonellae and *Salmonella typhi*. *J Antimicrob Chemother* 1991;28:877–885.

76. Dhar R, Marafi E. Antibiotic susceptibility patterns of selected bacterial isolates in a general hospital in Kuwait. *J Trop Med Hyg* 1991;94:111–115.

77. Kumarasinghe G, Lim YS, Chow C, Bassett DCJ. Prevalence of bacterial agents of diarrhoeal disease at the National University Hospital, Singapore and their resistance to antimicrobial agents. *Trop Geogr Med* 1992;44:229–232.

78. Hassan HS. Sensitivity of *Salmonella* and *Shigella* to antibiotics and chemotherapeutic agents in Sudan. *J Trop Med Hyg* 1985;88:243–247.

79. Rasrinaul L, Suthienkul O, Echeverria PD, et al. Foods as a source of enteropathogens causing childhood diarrhoea in Thailand. *Am J Trop Med Hyg* 1988;39:97–102.

80. Jayanetra P, Vorachit M, Pilantanapak A, Panbangred W, Bangtragulnonth A, Panurai R. *Salmonella krefeld* in Thailand: I. Epidemiology, infection and drug resistance. *Southeast Asian J Trop Med Public Health* 1990;21:354–360.

81. Rodrigue DC, Cameron DN, Puhr ND, et al. Comparison of plasmid profiles, phage types, and antimicrobial resistance patterns of *Salmonella enteritidis* isolates in the United States. *J Clin Microbiol* 1992;30:854–857.

82. MacDonald KL, Cohen ML, Hargrett-Bean NT, et al. Changes in antimicrobial resistance of *Salmonella* isolated from humans in the United States. *JAMA* 1987;258:1496–1499.

83. Ward LR, Threlfall EJ, Rowe B. Multiple drug resistance in salmonellae in England and Wales: a comparison between 1981 and 1988. *J Clin Pathol* 1990;43:563–566.

84. Antimicrobial resistance of *Salmonella* isolates from human and animal sources in Ontario. *Can Dis Wkly Rep* 1990;16-21: 99–102.

85. Lorian V. *Salmonella* susceptibility patterns in hospitals from 1975 through 1984. *J Clin Microbiol* 1986;23:826–827.

86. Muñoz P, Díaz MD, Rodríquez-Créixems M, Cercenado E, Peláez T, Bouza E. Antimicrobial resistance of *Salmonella* isolates in a Spanish hospital. *Antimicrob Agents Chemother* 1993; 37:1200–1202.

87. Rivera MJ, Rivera N, Castillo J, Rubio MC, Gómez-Lus R. Molecular and epidemiological study of *Salmonella* clinical isolates. *J Clin Microbiol* 1991;29:927–932.

88. Heffernan HM. Antibiotic resistance among salmonella from human and other sources in New Zealand. *Epidemiol Infect* 1991;106:17–23.

89. Ryan CA, Nickels MK, Hargrett-Bean NT, et al. Massive outbreak of antimicrobial resistant salmonellosis traced to pasteurized milk. *JAMA* 1987;258:3269–3274.

90. Barnass S, Franklin J, Tabaqchali S. The successful treatment of multiresistant nonenteric salmonellosis with seven day oral ciprofloxacin [Letter]. *J Antimicrob Chemother* 1990;25: 299–300.

91. Howard AJ, Joseph TD, Bloodworth LLO, Frost JA, Chart H, Rowe B. The emergence of ciprofloxacin resistance in *Salmonella typhimurium* [Letter]. *J Antimicrob Chemother* 1990;26: 296–298.

92. Gibb AP, Lewin CSJ, Garden OJ. Development of quinolone resistance and multiple antibiotic resistance in *Salmonella bovismorbificans* in a pancreatic abscess [Letter]. *J Antimicrob Chemother* 1991;28:318–321.

93. Hammami A, Arlet G, Ben Redjeb S, et al. Nosocomial outbreak of acute gastroenteritis in a neonatal intensive care unit in Tunisia caused by multiply drug resistant *Salmonella wien* producing SHV-2 beta-lactamase. *Eur J Clin Microbiol Infect Dis* 1991;10:641–646.

94. Bauernfeind A, Casellas JM, Goldberg M, et al. A new plasmidic cefotaximase from patients infected with *Salmonella typhimurium*. *Infection* 1992;20:158–163.

95. Piddock LJV, Griggs DJ, Hall MC, Jin YF. Ciprofloxacin resistance in clinical isolates of *Salmonella typhimurium* obtained

from two patients. *Antimicrob Agents Chemother* 1993;37: 662–666.

96. Roy SK, Speelman P, Butler T, Nath S, Rahman H, Stoll BJ. Diarrhea associated with typhoid fever. *J Infect Dis* 1985;151: 1138–1143.

97. Woodward TE, Smadel JE, Parker RT, Wisseman CL. Treatment of typhoid fever with antibiotics. *Ann NY Acad Sci* 1952; 55:1043–1055.

98. Rowe B, Threlfall EJ, Ward LR. Does chloramphenicol remain the drug of choice for typhoid? *Epidemiol Infect* 1987;98: 379–383.

99. Ryan CA, Hargrett-Bean NT, Blake PA. *Salmonella typhi* infections in the United States, 1975–1984: increasing role of foreign travel. *Rev Infect Dis* 1989;11:1–8.

100. Olarte J, Galindo E. *Salmonella typhi* resistant to chloramphenicol, ampicillin, and other antimicrobial agents: strains isolated during an extensive typhoid fever epidemic in Mexico. *Antimicrob Agents Chemother* 1973;4:597–601.

101. Butler T, Linh NN, Arnold K, Pollack M. Chloramphenicol-resistant typhoid fever in Vietnam associated with R factors. *Lancet* 1973;2:983–985.

102. Brown JD, Mo DH, Rhoades ER. Chloramphenicol-resistant *Salmonella typhi* in Saigon. *JAMA* 1975;231:162–166.

103. Olarte J, Filloy L, Galindo E. Resistance of *Shigella dysenteriae* type 1 to ampicillin and other antimicrobial agents: strains isolated during a dysentery outbreak in a hospital in Mexico City. *J Infect Dis* 1976;133:572–575.

104. Farrar WE Jr, Eidson M. R factors in strains of *Shigella dysenteriae* type 1 isolated in the Western Hemisphere during 1969–1970. *J Infect Dis* 1971;124:327–329.

105. Thorne GM, Farrar WE Jr. Genetic properties of R factors associated with epidemic strains of *Shigella dysenteriae* type 1 from Central America and *Salmonella typhi* from Mexico. *J Infect Dis* 1973;128:132–136.

106. Anderson ES, Smith HR. Chloramphenicol resistance in the typhoid bacillus. *Br Med J* 1972;3:329–331.

107. Gangarosa EJ, Bennett JV, Wyatt C, et al. An epidemic-associated episome? *J Infect Dis* 1972;126:215–218.

108. Zoukh K. Sensibilité aux antibiotiques des souches de *Salmonella* typho-paratyphoïdiques isolées en Algérie de 1979 à 1984. *Pathol Biol (Paris)* 1986;5:608–610.

109. Goldstein FW, Chumpitaz JC, Guevara JM, Papadopoulou B, Acar JF, Vieu JF. Plasmid-mediated resistance to multiple antibiotics in *Salmonella typhi*. *J Infect Dis* 1986;153:261–266.

110. Mikhail IA, Haberberger RL, Farid Z, Girgis NI, Woody JN. Antibiotic-multiresistant *Salmonella typhi* in Egypt. *Trans R Soc Trop Med Hyg* 1989;83:120.

111. Peng CF. Incidence and antimicrobial resistance of *Salmonella* serotypes in southern Taiwan from 1978 through 1987. *Kaohsiung J Med Sci* 1992;8:247–254.

112. Threlfall EJ, Ward LR, Rowe B, et al. Widespread occurrence of multiple drug-resistant *Salmonella typhi* in India. *Eur J Clin Microbiol Infect Dis* 1992;11:990–993.

113. Bhutta ZA, Naqvi SH, Razzaq RA, Farooqui BJ. Multidrug-resistant typhoid in children: presentation and clinical features. *Rev Infect Dis* 1991;13:832–836.

114. Albert MJ, Haider K, Nahar S, Kibriya AKMG, Hossain MA. Multiresistant *Salmonella typhi* in Bangladesh [Letter]. *J Antimicrob Chemother* 1991;27:554–555.

115. Dar L, Gupta BL, Rattan A, Bhujwala RA, Shriniwas. Multidrug resistant *Salmonella typhi* in Delhi. *Indian J Pediatr* 1992; 59:221–224.

116. Rao RS, Amarnath SK, Sujatha S. An outbreak of typhoid due to multidrug resistant *Salmonella typhi* in Pondicherry. *Trans R Soc Trop Med Hyg* 1992;86:204–205.

117. Saha MR, Dutta P, Bhattacharya SK, et al. Occurrence of multi-drug resistant *Salmonella typhi* in Calcutta. *Indian J Med Res [A]* 1992;95:179–180.

118. Rao PS, Rajashekar V, Varghese GK, Shivananda PG. Emergence of multidrug-resistant *Salmonella typhi* in rural southern India. *Am J Trop Med Hyg* 1993;48:108–111.

119. Coovadia YM, Gathiram V, Bhamjee A, et al. An outbreak of multiresistant *Salmonella typhi* in South Africa. *Q J Med* 1992; 82:91–100.

120. Gebre-Yohannes A, Tekle B, Limenih Y. Chloramphenicol-resistant *Salmonella typhi* from a patient in Addis Ababa. *Ethiop Med J* 1992;30:119–122.

121. Watanabe T. Infective heredity of multiple drug resistance in bacteria. *Bacteriol Rev* 1963;27:87–115.

122. Mitsuhashi S. Review: the R factors. *J Infect Dis* 1969;119: 89–100.

123. Farrar WE Jr, Eidson M. Antibiotic resistance in *Shigella* mediated by R factors. *J Infect Dis* 1971;123:477–484.

124. Salam MA, Bennish ML. Antimicrobial therapy for shigellosis. *Rev Infect Dis* 1991;13(Suppl 4):S332–S341.

125. Frost JA, Rowe B, Vandepitte J. Acquisition of trimethoprim resistance in epidemic strain of *Shigella dysenteriae* type 1 from Zaire. *Lancet* 1982;1:963.

126. Malengreau M, Molima-Kaba, Gillieaux M, De Feyter M, Kyele-Duibone, Mukolo-Ndjolo. Outbreak of Shigella dysentery in eastern Zaire, 1980–1982. *Ann Soc Belge Med Trop* 1983;63:59–67.

127. Chun D, Cho DT, Seol SY, Suh MH, Lee YC. R plasmids conferring multiple drug resistance from shigella isolated in Korea. *J Hyg (Camb)* 1984;92:153–160.

128. Jegathesan M. Serotype prevalence and antibiotic susceptibility of *Shigella* strains isolated in Malaysia during 1980 and 1981. *J Diarrhoeal Dis Res* 1984;2:102–104.

129. Ebright JR, Moore EC, Sanborn WR, Schaberg D, Kyle J, Ishida K. Epidemic Shiga bacillus dysentery in Central Africa. *Am J Trop Med Hyg* 1984;33:1192–1197.

129a. Tiemens KM, Shipley PL, Correia RA, Shields DS, Guerrant RL. Sulfamethoxazoletrimethoprim-resistant *Shigella flexneri* in northeastern Brazil. *Antimicrob Agents Chemother* 1984;25: 653–654.

130. Chugh TD, Suheir A, Mahboob AG, Neil L, El-Bishbishi E. Plasmid-mediated drug resistance of shigellae in Kuwait. *Antonie Van Leeuwenhoek* 1985;51:241–247.

131. Huppertz HI. An epidemic of bacillary dysentery in western Rwanda 1981–1982. *Cent Afr J Med* 1986;32:79–82.

132. Huq MI, Al Ghamdi MA, Haider K, Alim ARMA. Antimicrobial susceptibility pattern of the clinical isolates of *Shigella* sp. in the eastern province of Saudi Arabia. *Asian Med J* 1987;30: 228–234.

133. Nikkah J, Mehr-Movahead A. Antibiotic resistance among *Shigella* species isolated in Tehran, Iran. *Ann Trop Med Parasitol* 1988;82:481–483.

134. Taylor DN, Bodhidatta L, Brown JE, et al. Introduction and spread of multi-resistant *Shigella dysenteriae* I in Thailand. *Am J Trop Med Hyg* 1989;40:77–85.

135. Burstein S, Regalli G. In vitro susceptibility of *Shigella* strains isolated from stool cultures of dysenteric patients. *Scand J Gastroenterol* 1989;24(Suppl 169):34–38.

136. Leaño FT, Saniel MC, Monzon OT. Prevalent serogroups and antimicrobial susceptibility of *Shigella* strains in metro Manila, 1982–1988. *Southeast Asian J Trop Med Public Health* 1990; 21:207–213.

137. Olukoya DK, Oni O. Plasmid profile analysis and antimicrobial susceptibility patterns of shigella isolates from Nigeria. *Epidemiol Infect* 1990;105:59–64.

138. Smollan G, Block C. Development of antimicrobial drug resistance among shigellae isolated at an Israeli hospital from 1977 through 1990. *Public Health Rev* 1990/91;18:319–327.

139. Lim YS, Tay L. Serotype distribution and antimicrobial resistance of *Shigella* isolates in Singapore. *J Diarrhoeal Dis Res* 1991;9:328–331.

140. Lolekha S, Vibulbandhitkit S, Poonyarit P. Response to antimicrobial therapy for shigellosis in Thailand. *Rev Infect Dis* 1991; 13(Suppl 4):S342–S346.

141. Lin S-R, Chang S-F. Drug resistance and plasmid profile of shigellae in Taiwan. *Epidemiol Infect* 1992;108:87–97.

142. Thisyakorn USA, Rienprayoon S. Shigellosis in Thai children: epidemiologic, clinical and laboratory features. *Pediatr Infect Dis J* 1992;11:213–215.

143. Cavallo PJD, Bercion R, Baudet J-M, Samson T, France M, Meyran J. Étude de la sensibilité aux antibiotiques de 140 souches de Shigelles isolées à Djibouti (French). *Bull Soc Pathol Exot Filiales (Paris)* 1993;86:35–40.

144. Haider K, Malek MA, Albert MJ. Occurrence of drug resistance in *Shigella* species isolated from patients with diarrhoea in Bangladesh [Letter]. *J Antimicrob Chemother* 1993;32: 509–511.

145. Dan M. Marked decrease in susceptibility of *Shigella* to ampicillin and cotrimoxazole in Israel. *Eur J Clin Microbiol Infect Dis* 1993;12:143–144.

146. Tauxe RV, Puhr ND, Wells JG, Hargrett-Bean N, Blake PA. Antimicrobial resistance of *Shigella* isolates in the USA: the importance of international travelers. *J Infect Dis* 1990;162: 1107–1111.

147. Wharton M, Spiegel RA, Horan JM, et al. A large outbreak of antibiotic-resistant shigellosis at a mass gathering. *J Infect Dis* 1990;162:1324–1328.

148. Gross RJ, Threlfall EJ, Ward LR, Rowe B. Drug resistance in *Shigella dysenteriae, S. flexneri* and *S. boydii* in England and Wales: increasing incidence of resistance to trimethoprim. *Br Med J* 1984;288:784–786.

149. Bratoeva MP, John JF Jr. Dissemination of trimethoprim-resistant clones of *Shigella sonnei* in Bulgaria. *J Infect Dis* 1989; 159:648–653.

150. Heikkilä E, Siitonen A, Jahkola M, Fling M, Sundström L, Huovinen P. Increase of trimethoprim resistance among *Shigella* species, 1975–1988: analysis of resistance mechanisms. *J Infect Dis* 1990;161:1242–1248.

151. Voogd CE, Schot CS, van Leeuwen WJ, van Klingeren B. Monitoring of antibiotic resistance in shigellae isolated in The Netherlands 1984–1989. *Eur J Clin Microbiol Infect Dis* 1992; 11:164–167.

152. Harnett N. High level resistance to trimethoprim, cotrimoxazole and other antimicrobial agents among clinical isolates of *Shigella* species in Ontario, Canada—an update. *Epidemiol Infect* 1992;109:463–472.

153. Garanin BA. Antibiotic sensitivity of *Shigella* (Russian). *Antibiot Khimioter* 1992;37:19–20.

154. Salam MA, Bennish ML. Therapy for shigellosis. 1. Randomized, double-blind trial of nalidixic acid in childhood shigellosis. *J Pediatr* 1988;113:901–907.

155. Munshi MH, Sack DA, Haider K, Ahmed ZU, Rahaman MM, Morshed MG. Plasmid-mediated resistance to nalidixic acid in *Shigella dysenteriae* type 1. *Lancet* 1987;2:419–421.

156. Ries AA, Wells JG, Olivola D, et al. Epidemic *Shigella dysenteriae* type 1 in Burundi: pan-resistance and the implications for prevention. *J Infect Dis* 1994;169:1035–1041.

157. Bennish ML, Salam MA, Khan WA, Khan AM. Treatment of shigellosis: III. Comparison of one- or two-dose ciprofloxacin with standard 5-day therapy. A randomized, blinded trial. *Ann Intern Med* 1992;117:727–734.

158. Horiuchi S, Inagaki Y, Yamamoto N, Okamura N, Imagawa Y, Nakaya R. Reduced susceptibilities of *Shigella sonnei* strains isolated from patients with dysentery to fluoroquinolones. *Antimicrob Agents Chemother* 1993;37:2486–2489.

159. Cometta A, Calandra T, Bille J, Glauser MP. *Escherichia coli* resistant to fluoroquinolones in patients with cancer and neutropenia [Letter]. *N Engl J Med* 1994;330:1240.

160. Kern WV, Andriof E, Oethinger M, Kern P, Hacker J, Marre R. Emergence of fluoroquinolone-resistant *Escherichia coli* at a cancer center. *Antimicrob Agents Chemother* 1994;38:681–687.

161. Mitra AK, Kabir I, Hossain MA. Pivmecillinam-resistant *Shigella dysenteriae* type 1 infection in Bangladesh [Letter]. *Lancet* 1990;335:1461–1462.

162. Greenough WB III, Gordon RS Jr, Rosenberg IS, Davies BI, Benenson AS. Tetracycline in the treatment of cholera. *Lancet* 1964;1:355–357.

163. *Guidelines for cholera control. Programme for control of diarrhoeal disease.* WHO/CDD/SER/80.4 Rev 2. Geneva: World Health Organization, 1992.

164. Kobari K, Takakura I, Nakatomi M, Sogame S, Uylangco C. Antibiotic-resistant strains of El Tor *Vibrio* in the Philippines and the use of furalazine for chemotherapy. *Bull World Health Organ* 1970;43:365–371.

165. O'Grady F, Lewis MJ, Pearson NJ. Global surveillance of antibiotic sensitivity of *Vibrio cholerae. Bull World Health Organ* 1976;54:181–185.

166. Rabbani GH, Butler T, Shahrier M, Mazumdar R, Islam MR. Efficacy of a single dose of furazolidone for treatment of cholera in children. *Antimicrob Agents Chemother* 1991;35: 1864–1867.

167. Mhalu FS, Mmari PW, Ijumba J. Rapid emergence of El Tor *Vibrio cholerae* resistance to antimicrobial agents during first six months of fourth cholera epidemic in Tanzania. *Lancet* 1979;1:345–347.

168. Glass RI, Huq MI, Alim ARMA, Yunus M. Emergence of multiply antibiotic-resistant *Vibrio cholerae* in Bangladesh. *J Infect Dis* 1980;142:939–942.

169. Ichinose Y, Ehara M, Watanabe S, et al. The characterization of *Vibrio cholerae* isolated in Kenya in 1983. *J Trop Med Hyg* 1986;89:269–276.

170. Finch MJ, Morris JG, Kaviti J, Kagwanja W, Levine MM. Epidemiology of antimicrobial resistant cholera in Kenya and East Africa. *Am J Trop Med Hyg* 1988;39:484–490.

171. Tabtieng R, Wattanasri S, Echeverria P, et al. An epidemic of *Vibrio cholerae El Tor Inaba* resistant to several antibiotics with a conjugative group C plasmid coding for type II dihydrofolate reductase in Thailand. *Am J Trop Med Hyg* 1989;41: 680–686.

172. Threlfall EJ, Said B, Rowe B, Dávalos-Pérez A. Emergence of multiple drug resistance in *Vibrio cholerae* O1 El Tor from Ecuador [Letter]. *Lancet* 1993;342:1173.

173. Ramamurthy T, Pal A, Bhattacharya MK, et al. Serovar, biotype, phagetype, toxigenicity and antibiotic susceptibility patterns of *Vibrio cholerae* isolated during two consecutive cholera seasons (1989–1990) in Calcutta. *Indian J Med Res* [A] 1992;95:125–129.

174. Bhattacharya SK, Bhattacharya MK, Dutta P, et al. Double-blind, randomized, controlled clinical trial of norfloxacin for cholera. *Antimicrob Agents Chemother* 1990;34:939–940.

175. Cholera Working Group, International Centre for Diarrhoeal Disease Research, Bangladesh. Large epidemic of cholera-like disease in Bangladesh caused by *Vibrio cholerae* O139 synonym Bengal. *Lancet* 1993;342:387–390.

176. Nair GB, Ramamurthy T, Bhattacharya SK. Spread of *Vibrio cholerae* O139 Bengal in India. *J Infect Dis* 1994;169: 1029–1034.

177. Speelman P, Struelens MJ, Sanyal SC, Glass RI. Detection of *Campylobacter jejuni* and other potential pathogens in travellers' diarrhoea in Bangladesh. *Scand J Gastroenterol* 1983; 18(Suppl 84):19–23.

178. Black RE. Pathogens that cause travelers' diarrhea in Latin America and Africa. *Rev Infect Dis* 1986;8(Suppl 2):S131–S135.

179. Taylor DN, Echeverria P. Etiology and epidemiology of travelers' diarrhea in Asia. *Rev Infect Dis* 1986;8(Suppl 2):S136–S141.

180. DuPont HL, Ericsson CD. Prevention and treatment of travelers' diarrhea. *N Engl J Med* 1993;328:1821–1827.

181. Bhattacharya SK, Sen D, Nair GB, Bhattacharya MK, Datta P, Datta D. Multiply drug-resistant *Shigella dysenteriae* type 1 and travelers' diarrhea [Letter]. *J Infect Dis* 1986;154:729–730.

182. Sack RB, Santosham M, Froehlich JL, Medina C, Orskov F, Orskov I. Doxycycline prophylaxis of travelers' diarrhea in Honduras, an area where resistance to doxycycline is common among enterotoxigenic *Escherichia coli. Am J Trop Med Hyg* 1984;33:460–466.

183. Arthur JD, Echeverria P, Shanks GD, Karwacki J, Bodhidatta L, Brown JE. A comparative study of gastrointestinal infections in United States soldiers receiving doxycycline or mefloquine for malaria prophylaxis. *Am J Trop Med Hyg* 1990;43: 608–613.

184. Ericsson CD, Johnson PC, DuPont HL, Morgan DR, Bitsura JAM, de la Cabada FJ. Ciprofloxacin or trimethoprim-sulfamethoxazole as initial therapy for travelers' diarrhea. *Ann Intern Med* 1987;106:216–220.

185. Murray BE, Rensimer ER, DuPont HL. Emergence of high-level trimethoprim resistance in fecal *Escherichia coli* during oral administration of trimethoprim or trimethoprim-sulfamethoxazole. *N Engl J Med* 1982;306:130–135.

186. Rudy RP, Murray BE. Evidence for an epidemic trimethoprim-

resistance plasmid in fecal isolates of *Escherichia coli* from citizens of the United States studying in Mexico. *J Infect Dis* 1984;150:25–29.

187. Murray BE, Mathewson JJ, DuPont HL, Ericsson CD, Reves RR. Emergence of resistant fecal *Escherichia coli* in travelers not taking prophylactic antimicrobial agents. *Antimicrob Agents Chemother* 1990;34:515–518.

188. Johnson PC, Ericsson CD, Morgan DR, DuPont HL, Cabada FJ. Lack of emergence of resistant fecal flora during successful prophylaxis of traveler's diarrhea with norfloxacin. *Antimicrob Agents Chemother* 1986;30:671–674.

189. Petruccelli BP, Murphy GS, Sanchez JL, et al. Treatment of traveler's diarrhea with ciprofloxacin and loperamide. *J Infect Dis* 1992;165:557–560.

190. Levy SB, Marshall B, Schluederberg S, Rowse D, Davis J. High frequency of antimicrobial resistance in human fecal flora. *Antimicrob Agents Chemother* 1988;32:1801–1806.

191. Levy SB. Microbial resistance to antibiotics: an evolving and persistent problem. *Lancet* 1982;1:83–88.

192. Akiba T, Koyama L, Ishiki Y, Kimura S, Rukushima T. On the mechanism of the development of multiple drug resistant clones of *Shigella. Jpn J Microbiol* 1960;4:219–227.

193. Ippen-Ihler K. Bacterial conjugation. In: Levy SB, Miller RV, eds. *Gene transfer in the environment*. New York: McGraw-Hill, 1989;33–72.

194. Kokjohn TA. Transduction: mechanism and potential for gene transfer in the environment. In: Levy SB, Miller RV, eds. *Gene transfer in the environment*. New York: McGraw-Hill, 1989; 73–98.

195. Stewart GJ. The mechanism of natural transformation. In: Levy SB, Miller RV, eds. *Gene transfer in the environment*. New York: McGraw-Hill, 1989;139–164.

196. Berg DE. Transposable elements in prokaryotes. In: Levy SB, Miller RV, eds. *Gene transfer in the environment*. New York: McGraw-Hill, 1989;99–138.

197. DeFlaun MF, Levy SB. Genes and their varied hosts. In: Levy SB, Miller RV, eds. *Gene transfer in the environment*. New York: McGraw-Hill, 1989;1–32.

198. Sanders CC, Sanders WE Jr. β-Lactam resistance in gram-negative bacteria: global trends and clinical impact. *Clin Infect Dis* 1992;15:824–839.

199. Sanders CC. β-Lactamases of gram-negative bacteria: new challenges for new drugs. *Clin Infect Dis* 1992;14:1089–1099.

200. Jacoby GA, Medeiros AA. More extended-spectrum β-lactamases. *Antimicrob Agents Chemother* 1991;35:1697–1704.

201. Shaw KJ, Rather PN, Hare RS, Miller GH. Molecular genetics of aminoglycoside resistance genes and familial relationships of the aminoglycoside-modifying enzymes. *Microbiol Rev* 1993;57:138–163.

202. Leslie AGW, Moody PCE, Shaw WV. Structure of chloramphenicol acetyltransferase at 1.75-Å resolution. *Proc Natl Acad Sci USA* 1988;85:4133–4137.

203. McMurry LM, Petrucci R, Levy SB. Active efflux of tetracycline encoded by four genetically different tetracycline resistance determinants in *E. coli. Proc Natl Acad Sci USA* 1980; 77:3974–3977.

204. Cohen SP, Hooper DC, Wolfson JS, Souza KS, McMurry LM, Levy SB. Endogenous active efflux of norfloxacin in susceptible *Escherichia coli. Antimicrob Agents Chemother* 1988;32: 1187–1191.

205. Celesk RA, Robillard NJ. Factors influencing the accumulation of ciprofloxacin in *Pseudomonas aeruginosa. Antimicrob Agents Chemother* 1989;33:1921–1926.

206. McMurry LM, George AM, Levy SB. Active efflux of chloramphenicol in susceptible *Escherichia coli* and in multiple antibiotic resistant (Mar) mutants. *Antimicrob Agents Chemother* 1994;38:542–546.

207. Lewis K. Multidrug resistance pumps in bacteria: variations on a theme. *Trends Biochem Sci* 1994;19:119–123.

208. Neyfakh AA, Bidnenko VE, Chen LB. Efflux-mediated multidrug resistance in bacteria: similarities and dissimilarities with mammalian system. *Proc Natl Acad Sci USA* 1991;88: 4781–4785.

209. Levy SB. Evolution and spread of tetracycline resistance determinants. *J Antimicrob Chemother* 1989;24:1–3.

210. Levy SB. Active efflux mechanisms for antimicrobial resistance. *Antimicrob Agents Chemother* 1992;36:695–703.

211. Marshall B, Tachibana C, Levy SB. Frequency of tetracycline resistance determinant classes among lactose-fermenting coliforms. *Antimicrob Agents Chemother* 1983;24:835–840.

212. DePaola A, Flynn PA, McPhearson RM, Levy SB. Phenotypic and genotypic characterization of tetracycline and oxytetracycline resistant *Aeromonas* from cultured channel catfish (*Ictalurus punctatus*) and their environments. *Appl Environ Microbiol* 1988;54:1861–1863.

213. Hansen LM, McMurry LM, Levy SB, Hirsh DC. A new tetracycline resistance determinant (TetH) from *Pasteurella multocida* specifying active efflux of tetracycline. *Antimicrob Agents Chemother* 1993;37:2699–2705.

214. Zhao J, Aoki T. Nucleotide sequence analysis of the class G tetracycline resistance determinant from *Vibrio anguillarum. Microbiol Immunol* 1992;36:1051–1060.

215. Yamaguchi A, Udagawa T, Sawai T. Transport of divalent cations with tetracycline as mediated by the transposon Tn*10*-encoded tetracycline resistance protein. *J Biol Chem* 1990;265: 4809–4813.

216. Sloan J, McMurry LM, Lyras D, Levy SB, Rood JI. The *Clostridium perfringens* TetP determinant comprises two overlapping genes: *tetA*(P) which mediates active tetracycline efflux and *tetB*(P) which is related to the ribosomal protection family of tetracycline resistance determinants. *Mol Microbiol* 1993; 11:403–415.

217. Cohen SP, McMurry LM, Hooper DC, Wolfson JS, Levy SB. Cross-resistance to fluoroquinolones in multiple antibiotic resistant (Mar) *Escherichia coli* selected by tetracycline or chloramphenicol: decreased drug accumulation associated with membrane changes in addition to OmpF reduction. *Antimicrob Agents Chemother* 1989;33:1318–1325.

218. Ross JI, Eady EA, Cove JH, Cunliffe WJ, Baumberg S, Wostten JC. Inducible erythromycin resistance in staphylococcus is encoded by a member of the ATP-binding transport super-gene family. *Mol Microbiol* 1990;4:1207–1214.

219. Nikaido H. Outer membrane barrier as a mechanism of antimicrobial resistance. *Antimicrob Agents Chemother* 1989;33: 1831–1836.

220. Roberts MC. Gene transfer in the urogenital and respiratory tract. In: Levy SB, Miller RV, eds. *Gene transfer in the environment*. New York: McGraw-Hill, 1989;347–376.

221. Burdett V. Purification and characterization of Tet(M), a protein that renders ribosomes resistant to tetracycline. *J Biol Chem* 1991;26:2872–2877.

222. Manavothu EK, Fernandez CL, Cooperman BS, Taylor DE. Molecular studies on the mechanisms of tetracycline resistance mediated by Tet(O). *Antimicrob Agents Chemother* 1990;34: 71–77.

223. Weisblum B, Holder SB, Halling SM. Deoxyribonucleic acid sequence common to staphylococcal and streptococcal plasmids which specify erythromycin resistance. *J Bacteriol* 1979;138:990–998.

224. Arthur M, Autissier D, Courvalin P. Analysis of the nucleotide sequence of the *ereB* gene encoding the erythromycin esterase type II. *Nucleic Acids Res* 1986;14:4987–4999.

225. Yoshida H, Nakamura M, Bogaki M, Ito H, Kojima T, Hattori H, Nakamura S. Mechanism of action of quinolones against *Escherichia coli* DNA gyrase. *Antimicrob Agents Chemother* 1993;37:839–845.

226. Amyes SGB, Towner KJ. Trimethoprim resistance: epidemiology and molecular aspects. *J Med Microbiol* 1990;31:1–19.

227. Radstrom P, Swedberg G, Skold O. Genetic analyses of sulfonamide resistance and its dissemination in gram-negative bacteria illustrate new aspects of R plasmid evolution. *Antimicrob Agents Chemother* 1991;35:1840–1848.

228. Georgopapadakou NH. Penicillin-binding proteins and bacterial resistance to β-lactams. *Antimicrob Agents Chemother* 1993;37:2045–2053.

229. Bugg TD, Wright GD, Dutka-Malen S, Arthur M, Courvalin P. Molecular basis for vancomycin resistance in *Enterococcus*

faecium BM4147: biosynthesis of a depsipeptide peptidoglycan precursor by vancomycin resistance proteins VanH and VanA. *Biochemistry* 1991;30:10408–10415.

229a. Cohen SP, Hachler H, Levy SB. Genetic and functional analysis of multiple antibiotic resistance (*mar*) locus in *Escherichia coli*. *J Bacteriol* 1993;175:1484–1492.

230. Smith DH. R factor infection of *Escherichia coli* lyophilized in 1946. *J Bacteriol* 1967;94:2071–2072.

231. Hughes VM, Datta N. Conjugative plasmids in bacteria of the "pre-antibiotic" era. *Nature* 1983;302:725–726.

232. Davis CE, Anandan J. The evolution of R factor. A study of a "preantibiotic" community in Borneo. *N Engl J Med* 1970; 282:117–122.

233. Jacoby GA, Archer G. New mechanisms of bacterial resistance to antimicrobial agents. *N Engl J Med* 1991;324:601–612.

234. McGowan JE Jr. Antimicrobial resistance in hospital organisms and its relation to antibiotic use. *Rev Infect Dis* 1983;5: 1033–1048.

235. Lee D. Drug utilization in Panama. *J Clin Epidemiol* 1991; 44(Suppl II):31S–38S.

236. Silverman M, Lydecker M, Lee PR. *Bad medicine. The prescription drug industry in the third world.* Stanford, CA: Stanford University Press, 1992.

237. Amidi S, Ajamee G, Sadeghi HRM, Yourshalmi P, Gharehjeh AM. Dispensing drugs without prescription and treating patients by pharmacy attendants in Shiraz, Iran. *Am J Public Health* 1978;68:495–496.

238. Hossain MM, Glass RI, Khan MR. Antibiotic use in a rural community in Bangladesh. *Int J Epidemiol* 1982;11:402–405.

239. Simon HJ, Folb PI, Rocha H. Policies, laws, and regulations pertaining to antibiotics: report of Task Force 3. *Rev Infect Dis* 1987;9(Suppl 3):S261–S269.

240. Hardon AP. The use of modern pharmaceuticals in a Filipino village: doctors' prescription and self medication. *Soc Sci Med* 1987;25:277–292.

241. van der Geest S. Self-care and the informal sale of drugs in South Cameroon. *Soc Sci Med* 1987;25:293–305.

242. Greenhalgh T. Drug prescription and self-medication in India: an exploratory survey. *Soc Sci Med* 1987;25:307–318.

243. Wolffers I. Drug information and sale practices in some pharmacies of Colombo, Sri Lanka. *Soc Sci Med* 1987;25:319–321.

244. Ronsmans C, Bennish ML, Chakraborty J, Fauveau V. Current practices for treatment of dysentery in rural Bangladesh. *Rev Infect Dis* 1991;13(Suppl 4):S351–S356.

245. Thamlikitkul V. Antibiotic dispensing by drug store personnel in Bangkok, Thailand. *J Antimicrob Chemother* 1988;21:125–131.

246. Schorling JB, de Souza MA, Guerrant R. Patterns of antibiotic use among children in an urban Brazilian slum. *Int J Epidemiol* 1991;19:293–299.

247. Bennish M. The Bangladesh drug policy; the next step: using good drugs "goodly." *Bangladesh J Child Health* 1987;11: 63–72.

248. Haak H, Hardon AP. Indigenised pharmaceuticals in developing countries: widely used, widely neglected. *Lancet* 1988;2: 620–621.

249. Michel JM. Why do people like medicines? A perspective from Africa. *Lancet* 1985;1:210–211.

250. Lerman SJ, Shepard DS, Cash RA. Treatment of diarrhoea in Indonesian children: what it costs and who pays for it. *Lancet* 1985;2:651–654.

251. Tomson G, Sterky G. Self-prescribing by way of pharmacies in three Asian developing countries. *Lancet* 1986;2:620–621.

252. Bojalil R, Calva JJ. Antibiotic misuse in diarrhea. A household survey in a Mexican community. *J Clin Epidemiol* 1994;47: 147–156.

253. Aswapokee N, Vaithayapichet S, Heller RF. Pattern of antibiotic use in medical ward of a University Hospital, Bangkok, Thailand. *Rev Infect Dis* 1990;12:136–141.

254. Obaseiki-Ebor EE, Akerele JO, Ebea PO. A survey of antibiotic outpatient prescribing and antibiotic self-medication. *J Antimicrob Chemother* 1987;20:759–763.

255. Chetley A. *Antibiotics: the wrong drugs for diarrhoea.* The Hague: Health Action International, 1987.

256. Chetley A. *Antibiotics and diarrhoea: a dangerous combination.* Amsterdam: Health Action International, 1993:35–40.

257. Cohen SP, Yan W, Levy SB. A multidrug resistance regulatory chromosomal locus is widespread among enteric bacteria. *J Infect Dis* 1993;168:484–488.

258. Gustafsson LL, Wide K. Marketing of obsolete antibiotics in Central America. *Lancet* 1981;1:31–33.

258a. Anand MP. Marketing durgs in the third world [letter]. *Lancet* 1986;2:222.

259. Herxheimer A. Basic information that prescribers are not getting about drugs. *Lancet* 1987;1:31–32.

260. Lexchin J. Doctors and detailers: therapeutic education or pharmaceutical promotion? *Int J Health Serv* 1989;19:663–679.

261. Silverman M, Lee PR, Lydecker M. Drug promotion: the third world revisited. *Int J Health Serv* 1986;16:659–667.

262. Chetley A. *The antibiotic crisis.* Amsterdam: Health Action International, 1993:51–68.

263. Lee PR, Lurie P, Silverman MM, Lydecker M. Drug promotion and labeling in developing countries: an update. *J Clin Epidemiol* 1991;44(Suppl II):49S–55S.

264. Kunin CM, Lipton NI, Tupasi T, et al. Social, behavioral, and practical factors affecting antibiotic use worldwide: report of Task Force 4. *Rev Infect Dis* 1987;9(Suppl 3):S270–S285.

265. Liss RH, Batchelor FR. Economic evaluations of antibiotic use and resistance—a perspective: report of Task Force 6. *Rev Infect Dis* 1987;9(Suppl 3):S297–S312.

266. Swindell PJ, Reeves DS, Bullock DW, Davies AJ, Spence CE. Audits of antibiotic prescribing in a Bristol hospital. *Br Med J* 1983;286:118–122.

267. Goodburn E, Mattosinho S, Mongi P, Waterston T. Management of childhood diarrhoea by pharmacists and parents: is Britain lagging behind the third world? *Br Med J* 1991;302: 440–443.

268. Frieden TR, Mangi RJ. Inappropriate use of oral ciprofloxacin. *JAMA* 1990;264:1438–1440.

269. Holmberg SD, Osterholm MT, Senger KA, Cohen ML. Drug-resistant *Salmonella* from animals fed antimicrobials. *N Engl J Med* 1984;311:617–622.

270. Spika JS, Waterman SH, Soo Hoo GW, et al. Chloramphenicol-resistant *Salmonella newport* traced through hamburger to dairy farms. *N Engl J Med* 1987;316:565–570.

271. Pavia AT, Shipman LD, Wells JG, et al. Epidemiologic evidence that prior antimicrobial exposure decreases resistance to infection by antimicrobial-sensitive *Salmonella*. *J Infect Dis* 1990;161:255–260.

272. Aserkoff B, Bennett JV. Effect of antibiotic in acute salmonellosis on the fecal excretion of salmonellae. *N Engl J Med* 1969;281:636–640.

273. Levy SB. Playing antibiotic pool: time to tally the score [Editorial]. *N Engl J Med* 1984;311:663–665.

274. DuPont HL, Steele JH. Use of antimicrobial agents in animal feeds: implications for human health. *Rev Infect Dis* 1987;9: 447–460.

275. Col NF, O'Connor RW. Estimating worldwide current antibiotic usage: report of Task Force I. *Rev Infect Dis* 1987;9(Suppl 3):S232–S243.

276. Corrier DE, Purdy CW, DeLoach JR. Effects of marketing stress on fecal excretion of *Salmonella* spp in feeder calves. *Am J Vet Res* 1990;51:866–869.

277. Anderson ES. Drug resistance in *Salmonella typhimurium* and its implications. *Br Med J* 1968;3:333–339.

278. O'Brien TF, Hopkins JD, Gilleece ES, et al. Molecular epidemiology of antibiotic resistance in *Salmonella* from animals and human beings in the United States. *N Engl Med J* 1982;307: 1–6.

279. Trallero EP, Zigorraga C, Cilla G, Idigoras P, Lopategui CL, Solaun L. Animal origin of the antibiotic resistance of human pathogenic *Yersinia enterocolitica* [Letter]. *Scand J Infect Dis* 1988;20:573.

280. Endtz HP, Ruijs GJ, van Klingeren B, Jansen WH, van der Reyden T, Mouton RP. Quinolone resistance in *Campylobacter* isolated from man and poultry following the introduction of fluoroquinolones in veterinary medicine. *J Antimicrob Chemother* 1991;27:199–208.

281. Levy SB, FitzGerald GB, Macone AB. Changes in intestinal flora of farm personnel after introduction of a tetracycline-supplemented feed on a farm. *N Engl J Med* 1976;295:583–588.
282. Lyons RW, Samples CL, DeSilva HN, Ross KA, Julian EM, Checko PJ. An epidemic of resistant *Salmonella* in a nursery: animal-to-human spread. *JAMA* 1980;243:546–547.
283. Rolland RM, Hausfater G, Marshall B, Levy SB. Antibiotic-resistant bacteria in wild primates: increased prevalence in baboons feeding on human refuse. *Appl Environ Microbiol* 1985;49:791–794.
284. D'Aoust JY, Daley E, Crozier M, Sewell AM. Pet turtles: a continuing international threat to public health. *Am J Epidemiol* 1990;132:233–238.
285. O'Brien TF, Pla MDP, Mayer KH, et al. Intercontinental spread of a new antibiotic resistance gene on an epidemic plasmid. *Science* 1985;230:87–88.
286. Grant JP. *The state of the world's children, 1994.* Oxford: Oxford University Press, 1993.
287. Ronsmans C, Bennish ML, Wierzba T. Diagnosis and management of dysentery by community health workers. *Lancet* 1988;2:552–555.
288. *A manual for the treatment of diarrhoea.* WHO/CDD/SER/80.2 Rev 2. Geneva: World Health Organization, 1990.
289. Hogerzeil HV, Bimo, Ross-Degan D, et al. Field tests for rational drug use in twelve developing countries. *Lancet* 1993;342:1408–1410.
290. Munishi GK. The development of the essential drugs program and implications for self-reliance in Tanzania. *J Clin Epidemiol* 1991;44(Suppl II):7S–14S.
291. *The use of essential drugs. Model list of essential drugs* (seventh list). WHO Technical Report Series 825. Geneva: World Health Organization, 1992.
292. Control of antibiotic-resistant bacteria: memorandum from a WHO meeting. *Bull World Health Organ* 1983;61:423–433.
293. Hogerzeil HV, Walker GJA, Sallami AO, Fernando G. Impact of an essential drugs programme on availability and rational use of drugs. *Lancet* 1989;1:141–142.
294. Tiranti DJ. *Essential drugs. The Bangladesh example—four years from 1982–1986.* Oxford: International Organization of Consumers' Unions/New Internationalist Publications/War on Want, 1986.
295. Chetley A. *From policy to practice. The future of the Bangladesh National Drug Policy.* Penang, Malaysia: International Organization of Consumers Unions, 1992.
296. Kanji N, Hardon A, Harnmeijer JW, Mamdani M, Walt G. *Drug policy in developing countries.* London: Zed Books Ltd, 1992.
297. Sterky G, Tomson G, Diwan VK, Sachs L. Drug use and the role of patients and prescribers. *J Clin Epidemiol* 1991;44(Suppl II):67S–72S.
298. Higginbotham N, Streiner DL. The social science contribution to pharmacoepidemiology. *J Clin Epidemiol* 1991;44(Suppl II):73S–82S.
299. McGowan JE Jr, Finland M. Infection and antibiotic usage at Boston City Hospital: changes in prevalence during the decade 1964–1973. *J Infect Dis* 1974;129:421–428.
300. Recco RA, Gladstone JL, Friedman SA, Gerken EH. Antibiotic control in a municipal hospital. *JAMA* 1979;241:2283–2286.
301. Seligman SJ. Reduction in antibiotic costs by restricting use of an oral cephalosporin. *Am J Med* 1981;71:941–944.
302. Wade VA, Mansfield PR, McDonald PJ. Drug companies' evidence to justify advertising. *Lancet* 1989;2:1261–1264.
303. Avorn J, Harvey K, Soumerai SB, Herxheimer A, Plumridge R, Bardelay G. Information and education as determinants of antibiotic use: report of Task Force 5. *Rev Infect Dis* 1987;9(Suppl 3):S286–S296.
304. van Leeuwen WJ, van Embden J, Guinée P, et al. Decrease of drug resistance in *Salmonella* in The Netherlands. *Antimicrob Agents Chemother* 1979;16:237–239.
305. Committee on Human Health Risk Assessment of Using Subtherapeutic Antibiotics in Animal Feeds. *Human health risks with the subtherapeutic use of penicillin or tetracyclines in animal feed.* Washington, DC: National Academy Press, 1989.
306. Weis SE, Slocum PC, Blais FX, et al. The effect of directly observed therapy on the rates of drug resistance and relapse in tuberculosis. *N Engl J Med* 1994;330:1179–1184.
307. Gilman RH, Spira W, Rabbani H, Ahmed W, Islam A, Rahaman MM. Single-dose ampicillin therapy for severe shigellosis in Bangladesh. *J Infect Dis* 1981;143:164–169.
308. Alam AN, Alam NH, Ahmed T, Sack DA. Randomised double blind trial of single dose doxycycline for treating cholera in adults. *Br Med J* 1990;300:1619–1621.
309. Sibley JC, Sackett DL, Neufeld V, Gerrard B, Rudnick KV, Fraser W. A randomized trial of continuing medical education. *N Engl J Med* 1982;306:511–515.
310. Schaffner W, Ray WA, Federspiel CF, Miller WO. Improving antibiotic prescribing in office practice. A controlled trial of three educational methods. *JAMA* 1983;250:1728–1732.
311. Avorn J, Soumerai SB. Improving drug-therapy decisions through educational outreach. A randomized controlled trial of academically based "detailing." *N Engl J Med* 1983;308:1457–1463.
312. Schroeder SA, Myers LP, McPhee SJ, et al. The failure of physician education as a cost containment strategy. *JAMA* 1984;252:225–230.
313. Ray WA, Schaffner W, Federspiel CF. Persistence of improvement in antibiotic prescribing in office practice. *JAMA* 1985;253:1774–1776.
314. Goldfinger SE. Continuing education and general internal medicine. *Arch Intern Med* 1977;137:1311–1315.
315. Harvey KJ, Stewart R, Hemming M, Naismith N, Moulds RFW. Educational antibiotic advertising. *Med J Aust* 1986;145:28–32.
316. Quick JD, Laing RO, Ross-Degnan DG. Intervention research to promote clinically effective and economically efficient use of pharmaceuticals: the international network for rational use of drugs. *J Clin Epidemiol* 1991;44(Suppl II):57S–65S.
317. Kunin CM. The responsibility of the infectious disease community for the optimal use of antimicrobial agents. *J Infect Dis* 1985;151:388–398.
318. Kuntz ID. Structure-based strategies for drug design and discovery. *Science* 1992;257:1078–1082.
319. Bloom BR. Tuberculosis. Back to a frightening future. *Nature* 1992;358:538–539.
320. Levy SB. Confronting multidrug resistance. A role for each of us. *JAMA* 1993;269:1840–1842.

Infections of the Gastrointestinal Tract,
edited by M. J. Blaser, P. D. Smith, J. I. Ravdin,
H. B. Greenberg, and R. L. Guerrant
Raven Press, Ltd., New York © 1995.

CHAPTER 96

Prevention and Control of Nosocomial Enteric Infections

Anne M. Anglim, William Schaffner, and Barry M. Farr

Nosocomial gastrointestinal tract infections cause substantial additional morbidity, mortality, and hospital costs (1). A case definition has been formulated by the Centers for Disease Control and Prevention (CDC), enabling standardized surveillance and reporting of nosocomial infections (2). Use of this definition should allow comparison among studies and analysis of secular trends. The CDC definition of nosocomial gastroenteritis requires either of the following:

1. The acute onset of diarrhea in a hospitalized patient, characterized by liquid stool for more than 12 hr, with or without vomiting and/or fever (>38°C).

or

2. Two of the following symptoms with no other recognized cause: nausea, vomiting, abdominal pain, or headache. These symptoms must occur in conjunction with objective evidence of enteric infection, obtained by either stool culture, antigen or antibody assay of feces or blood, routine or electron microscopic examination of stool, or toxin assay.

The amount of time the patient has been hospitalized before the onset of symptoms and the incubation period of the particular etiology of gastroenteritis are used to differentiate community-acquired from nosocomial illness (Table 1). Three days after admission is a frequently used cutpoint for distinguishing nosocomial from community-acquired infections. It may, however, be deceptive for pathogens with longer or shorter average incubation periods. Moreover, the incubation period of a particular infection can be longer than expected; altered immunological function may also result in development of symptoms

from a previously inactive infection. Hospital spread of pathogens from the community can result from hospital employees working while ill. Visitors can also bring in pathogens from the community. Finally, the workup of nosocomial diarrhea in patients with acquired immunodeficiency syndrome (AIDS) or those in developing countries is especially difficult because of the high endemic rate of enteric disease in these populations and the wide variety of pathogens known to infect these patients.

The hospitalized patient who develops diarrhea should be evaluated for noninfectious conditions. Inflammatory bowel disease, endocrine disturbances, exocrine deficiencies, or mechanical processes such as fecal impaction can be detected by history, physical examination, and supplemental laboratory tests. Medications are another potential cause of diarrhea in the hospitalized patient with laxatives, cathartics, antacids, quinidine, and digoxin being frequently implicated. Cytotoxic chemotherapeutic drugs, antibiotics, and enteral nutritional formulas not only cause noninfectious diarrhea but also increase risk for infectious gastroenteritis.

IMPORTANCE OF NOSOCOMIAL GASTROENTERITIS

The CDC's National Nosocomial Infections Surveillance (NNIS) Program (3), a voluntary network of participating hospitals that report data on nosocomial infections, has provided much of the data regarding nosocomial gastroenteritis. The most current available surveillance data are from 1985 to 1991. During those years, the crude rate of gastroenteritis was 10.5/10,000 discharges, an apparent eightfold increase over rates from 1980 to 1984 (4). This increase could be due to a combination of improved surveillance and reporting techniques, advances in diagnostic technology, or a true increase in infection.

Modifications in case finding can substantially alter rates of nosocomial gastroenteritis. This is exemplified by

A. M. Anglim and B. M. Farr: University of Virginia Health Sciences Center, Charlottesville, Virginia 22908.

W. Schaffner: Vanderbilt University School of Medicine, Nashville, Tennessee 37232-0263.

TABLE 1. *Pathogens in nosocomial gastroenteritis*

Agent	Incubation period	Modes of transmission	Duration of illness[a]
Adenovirus	8–10 days	Unknown	8 days
Aeromonas species	Unknown	Food ingestion	1–7 days
Bascillus cereus	1–6 hr (short) 8–16 hr (long)	Food ingestion	<24 hr
Campylobacter jejuni	3–5 days	Food ingestion, direct contact	2–10 days
Clostridium botulinum	18–36 hr	Food ingestion	Weeks–months
C. difficile	Unknown	Direct/indirect contact	5 days–10 wk[b]
C. perfringens	8–16 hr	Food ingestion	24–72 hr
Cryptosporidium	2–14 days	Food/water ingestion, direct and indirect contact	Weeks–months
Entamoeba histolytica	7–14 days	Food/water ingestion, direct and indirect contact	Variable
Escherichia coli			
ETEC	16–72 hr	Food/water ingestion	3–5 days
EPEC	16–48 hr	Food/water ingestion, direct and indirect contact	5–15 days
EIEC	16–48 hr	?Food/water ingestion	2–7 days
EHEC	72–120 hr	Food ingestion, direct and indirect contact	2–12 days
Giardia lamblia	7–14 days	Food/water ingestion, direct and indirect contact	Weeks–months
Listeria monocytogenes	3–70 days	Food ingestion, ?direct or indirect contact	Variable
Norwalk agent(s)	24–48 hr	Food/water ingestion, direct and indirect contact, ?aerosol	24–48 hr
Rotavirus	24–72 hr	Direct and indirect contact, ?aerosol	4–6 days
Salmonellae	16–72 hr	Food ingestion, direct and indirect contact	2–7 days
Shigellae	16–72 hr	Food/water ingestion, direct and indirect contact	2–7 days
Staphylococcus aureus	1–6 hr	Food ingestion	<24 hr
Yersinia enterocolitica	3–7 days	Food ingestion, direct contact	1–3 wk

[a] Course of illness without antimicrobial therapy.
[b] After stopping antibiotics.

cases of nosocomial infectious diarrhea increasing 150- to 200-fold at the University of Virginia Hospital after the Clinical Microbiology Laboratory was requested to notify infection control personnel of all positive *Clostridium difficile* results (1). Stool ova and parasite exams and bacterial cultures for *Salmonella*, *Shigella*, and *Campylobacter* species yield so few diagnoses in the evaluation of sporadic nosocomial diarrhea that they are not recommended for routine use (5,6). *Clostridium difficile* and rotavirus have been the most frequent causes of nosocomial diarrhea (Table 2).

A study from a children's hospital found that infections of the gastrointestinal tract were exceeded only by those of the respiratory tract as causes of nosocomial infection (9); these infections were confirmed to be viral by stool electron microscopy. The study suggested that the availability and use of testing capabilities for viral pathogens may explain some of the increase in rates of nosocomial gastrointestinal tract infections that has been evident in the past decade.

Rates of nosocomial gastroenteritis several hundred times higher than the NNIS data have been found in surveillance studies conducted in several hospitals. A study observing an adult medical intensive care unit and two pediatric wards during 1985 and 1986 found a rate of nosocomial diarrhea of 2.6/100 admissions, with a pathogen identified in about 40% of cases (11). In these particular wards, nosocomial diarrhea was the most frequently identified nosocomial infection, occurring in 7.7 and 2.3 per 100 admissions in adults and children, respectively.

NNIS data suggest that most infections occur in the elderly, with 64% involving patients 60 years or older (4). Such a finding may reflect a relative lack of viral diagnostic capabilities in NNIS participating hospitals, or infrequent testing for viral pathogens in sporadic diarrhea in hospitals that do have facilities. Viral nosocomial diarrhea has been most frequently documented in children (6–8).

Although accounting for less than 1% of nosocomial infections reported from NNIS hospitals during the 1970s (17), gastroenteritis, primarily due to *Salmonella* species and enteropathogenic *Escherichia coli* made up 21% of nosocomial epidemics investigated by the CDC from 1956 to 1979 (18). In contrast, gastrointestinal disease made up only 7.4% of nosocomial epidemics investigated by the CDC between 1980 and 1991 (4), perhaps because there are fewer hospital epidemics due to gastroenteritis. Just as plausibly, hospitals and local health departments may be managing more outbreaks without requesting CDC assistance.

Recent studies have examined the mortality attributable to nosocomial gastroenteritis. Zaidi and associates (19) prospectively evaluated adult patients in a Mexico City referral hospital, finding an 18% mortality rate in patients with nosocomial diarrhea compared with 5% in matched controls. Also evident was a 7% complication rate from diarrhea, such as volume depletion, gastrointestinal bleeding, and candidemia. A study of bone marrow transplant recipients also found a significantly increased mortality in patients with nosocomial gastroenteritis (12). Those infected with viral pathogens or *C. difficile* had a 55% case-fatality rate over the 9-month study period, versus 13% in matched controls. Patients with gastrointesti-

TABLE 2. *Pathogens isolated in endemic nosocomial gastroenteritis*

Etiologic agent	Study (references)	Number of positive cultures	Total number tested	Relative frequency
Viral				
Rotavirus	6–14	343	919	0.37
Adenovirus	6,8,9,15	31	413	0.08
Calicivirus	8	13	80	0.16
Astrovirus	8	11	80	0.14
Minireovirus	8	10	80	0.13
Coxsackievirus	12	4	78	0.05
Coronavirus	9	2	65	0.03
Norwalk agent	8	2	80	0.03
Other viruses	9	11	65	0.17
Bacterial				
Clostridium difficile	6,10–12,15	94	324	0.29
Salmonellae	10,11,16	13	435	0.03
Shigellae	10,16	15	405	0.04
Fungal				
Candida species	10	19	45	0.42[a]

[a] Yeast was identified in the stool cultures of 55% of control patients.

nal infections also had an average duration of hospitalization of 66 days compared to 46 days for the controls.

Some have proposed that an increased risk for other nosocomial infections following nosocomial gastroenteritis may contribute to increased mortality. Lima and associates (20) found that nosocomial diarrhea was a significant risk factor for nosocomial urinary tract infections, which were ten times more common in patients with preceding diarrhea than in those without diarrhea. This may occur as a result of colonization of the urethral meatus with enteric flora during the diarrhea (21–24).

MECHANISMS OF SPREAD

The transmission of hospital-acquired gastrointestinal tract infections has been clarified by newly developed techniques in molecular epidemiology (25). Transmission can occur by any of the following:

1. Spread among patients by contaminated hands of hospital workers.
2. Direct patient-to-patient contact.
3. Dissemination by a vehicle such as contaminated medical equipment, food, or water.
4. Environmental contamination and subsequent direct or indirect spread.

Nosocomial gastroenteritis is usually spread by the hands of hospital personnel. Contamination of hands has been documented in 59% of health-care workers after routine contact with patients colonized with *C. difficile;* contamination was also demonstrable after handling patient charts (26). Another study showed a significant reduction of nosocomial transmission of *C. difficile* by the routine use of gloves (27). Accentuating the need for consistent use of barrier precautions is the finding that 21% of asymptomatic patients in one Veterans Administration Hospital study were colonized with *C. difficile* (28).

The use of molecular markers has proved useful in defining transmission patterns of *C. difficile.* Serogroup analysis of one outbreak found clusters of infection on hospital wards and provided a gauge of efficacy of infection control measures (29). The technique allowed discrimination of serotypes with tendencies for epidemic spread. Hospital-wide transmission has been documented with such procedures as restriction endonuclease analysis of chromosomal deoxyribonucleic acid (DNA), which in one instance was able to identify one clone as the cause of nosocomial diarrhea on several wards of a hospital (29).

Acquisition and transmission of sporadic *C. difficile* cases have been studied using immunoblot typing (26). On one ward, 22.7% of patients acquired *C. difficile,* with 37% of these developing diarrhea. Thus it was suggested that most hospitalized patients who develop *C. difficile* disease become infected with the organism in the hospital. This method also showed person-to-person spread, with spatial clustering of affected patients and caregivers. Positive cultures were still evident in 82% of infected patients at time of discharge.

McFarland and associates (26) have suggested that asymptomatic carriers are an important mechanism for the spread of *C. difficile* associated diarrhea (CDAD) (26). Of 92 initially culture-negative patients, 23 (25%) acquired *C. difficile* from exposure to a roommate with a positive culture. Asymptomatic roommates were the source of *C. difficile* colonization in 14 (61%) of these 23 patients. In another study, 42% of asymptomatic excretors shed nontoxigenic, nonpathogenic organisms (30). Symptomatic patients were more likely to harbor toxigenic strains and excrete greater organism loads, theoretically increasing possibility of transmission (29).

Contamination of the hospital environment has a potential role in the spread of nosocomial enteric disease (26,31,32). *Clostridium difficile* spores can remain viable for 5 months on inanimate surfaces (32). One study showed that 8% of cultures of surfaces such as bedrails, commodes, floors, call buttons, bedpans, and windowsills were positive in the rooms of uninfected patients; 29% were positive in the rooms of patients with asymptomatic carriage. Of those cultures taken from rooms of patients with CDAD, 49% were positive (26).

Nosocomial *Salmonella* gastroenteritis is characteristically associated with foodborne epidemics (33). In the developed world, point-source outbreaks due to contaminated food comprise most hospital-acquired *Salmonella* disease. After entry into the hospital, a sustained period of secondary person-to-person spread of *Salmonella* frequently results (34), often aided by employees who transmit organisms on their hands (35). Asymptomatic carriers may also be vectors of spread (36). Such patients or hospital workers may harbor enough of an infective burden to produce disease in those who are vulnerable to infection. Susceptibility to infection can be increased by achlorhydria, malignancy, human immunodeficiency virus (HIV) infection, hemoglobinopathies, or prior antibiotic treatment. As a result of these multiple routes of spread, an originally foodborne epidemic continued for 5 years (36), maintained by food handlers, medical personnel, or patients who were colonized and/or infected with the organism.

Foods most often associated with nosocomial salmonellosis have included eggs, poultry, meat, and protein supplements. Pharmacologic agents and blood products have also been found to cause outbreaks (37). Contaminated animal extracts of pancreas, thyroid, pituitary, or liver were documented to occur in the years before the breakthrough of recombinant technology (33). The contamination of such objects as a delivery room suction apparatus (33) and endoscopy equipment (38) have also been responsible for outbreaks. A recent report of a *S. hadar* outbreak in a nursing home demonstrated spread from patients to laundry workers handling linens soiled by incontinent infected patients (39).

In the developing world, nosocomial salmonellosis has illustrated the consequences of liberal antibiotic utilization. In many regions, hospitals have become abundant sources of multiply-resistant organisms (40). Multiply-resistant *Salmonella* species have been linked to several hospital outbreaks that have had considerable mortality rates (35). In a Tunisian special care nursery, an outbreak of *S. wien* that was marked by significant secondary spread had a 33% case–fatality rate (35). The development of a *Salmonella* species with plasmids carrying the extended-spectrum β-lactamase SHV-2 was likely fostered by extensive use of cefotaxime. Its subsequent spread was accelerated by casual adherence to the hospital's infection control policies.

Gastroenteritis of viral etiology frequently spreads within hospitals by contact with contaminated hands. There are anecdotal reports suggesting an additional route of spread by aerosol, possibly by movement of contaminated laundry (41,42). Efforts to prevent nosocomial viral gastroenteritis should consider the problem of hospital employees working while ill with gastrointestinal symptoms (43). Despite being an illness with a short duration and of minimal consequence to the employee, viral gastroenteritis can produce serious disease in many hospitalized patients. Assessment of the importance of both the aerosol route and of the health-care worker in transmission of viral gastroenteritis warrants further study.

Of epidemics investigated by the CDC during 1956 to 1975, 11% were false outbreaks. The gastrointestinal tract was involved in 20% of these pseudoepidemics, the second most common site involved (44). Specimen processing mistakes, misdiagnosis, and misinterpretation of surveillance findings produced false spatial and temporal relationships of alleged infections. A group of "infections" were due to *Salmonella saint-paul* contamination of a saline solution used for specimen processing in a hospital laboratory. Two other outbreaks were reported because of improper discrimination between community-acquired and nosocomial infection. A nursery outbreak, thought to be due to *S. aureus*, resulted from dependence on positive stool cultures in the absence of clinical evaluation. Judicious analysis of epidemiologic findings can prevent wasting resources on investigation of pseudoepidemics.

The indigenous flora of the intestinal tract may provide a source for the development and spread of bacteria resistant to antimicrobial agents. Studies have demonstrated increased fecal colonization in both hospitalized patients and those in community surveys, irrespective of whether antimicrobials were administered (45–47). Similarly, diapered children in day-care centers have been shown to harbor trimethoprim-resistant as well as multiresistant *E. coli* in their stools. Carriage in that setting was not correlated with recent antibiotic use (48). Extended courses of ampicillin for urinary tract infection have, however, been associated with the development of resistant *E. coli* (49). Studies in volunteers have shown an association between the administration of oral glycopeptides and the development of glycopeptide-resistant enterococci in fecal flora (50). The spread of vancomycin-resistant enterococci has produced the suggestion that the equally effective and considerably less expensive oral metronidazole should replace vancomycin as the treatment of choice for *C. difficile* colitis (51). The relationship between antimicrobials, indigenous gut flora, and the emergence of antimicrobial resistance merits further study.

ENVIRONMENTAL DETERMINANTS OF INFECTION

Risk for nosocomial gastrointestinal tract infection is the aggregate of an intricate relationship between host defenses and exposure to pathogens in the hospital environment. An understanding of the environmental factors that influence the development of nosocomial diarrhea provides the basis for measures that prevent acquisition of infection. Extrinsic factors predisposing to nosocomial gastrointestinal tract infections include nasogastric intubation, which allows introduction of bacteria into the gastrointestinal tract (52), and enteral feeding (19). Although bacterial contamination of nutritional formulas has occasionally been reported to produce a nosocomial gastrointestinal illness (53), diarrhea from enteral supplements is usually an osmotic process. Zaidi and associates (19), however, found that patients with nosocomial diarrhea were 67 times more likely to have received enteral feeding supplementation and identified pathogenic organisms in 59% of cases.

Transmission of nosocomial gastroenteritis can occur by cross-infection in crowded hospital environments. Ford-Jones and co-workers (8) found an association between nosocomial gastroenteritis and the number of patients in a room. Infection rates of 15.7 cases/1000 patient-days were found for rooms with one patient, 27.7 cases/1000 for rooms with two to three patients, and 45.2 cases/1000 for rooms with four or more patients. Diaper use was associated with a fivefold increased risk of nosocomial gastroenteritis.

Several studies of nosocomial gastroenteritis have linked prior antimicrobial use to an increased incidence of infection presumably by effects on the resident intestinal microflora (54). Thibault and associates (55) found that the risk of CDAD increased with the number of antibiotics administered to a patient. Risk was further magnified depending on the type of antibiotic used, with the highest odds ratio found with clindamycin usage. The anomalous finding of an increased risk associated with metronidazole use was likely due to its administration with other antibiotics.

INSTITUTIONAL FOODBORNE DISEASES

Patients in hospitals, nursing homes, and custodial facilities are predisposed to acquire and suffer serious effects of foodborne gastrointestinal disease. Thus institutional food services are challenged with procuring quality food at low cost, appropriately storing food items before consumption, adequately preparing and cooking for large numbers of patients, and serving it before spoilage occurs.

Of foodborne outbreaks documented by the CDC during a 12-year period, hospitals and nursing homes were the settings for 3.1% of the outbreaks and 5.1% of total cases. These locations contributed 24.1% of deaths due to epidemic foodborne disease (56). The grave consequences of these outbreaks are illustrated by a 35% mortality rate in one nursing home outbreak of E. coli O157:H7, linked to sandwiches (57). Most institutional epidemics, however, have less serious outcomes. Salmonellosis in nursing homes has historically been a major determinant of foodborne morbidity and mortality. Salmonella accounted for 52% of outbreaks and 81% of deaths in outbreaks of confirmed etiology in 1975 to 1987, resulting in a case–fatality rate of 3.8% (58).

In institutions, foodborne gastrointestinal illness typically follows a biphasic epidemic pattern, with a primary source, contaminated food, that infects a large number rapidly. Subsequent transmission generally follows (59), with a characteristically more sluggish course. Such transmission relies on cross-infection among patients, healthcare workers, or visitors.

Nosocomial foodborne epidemics most often are caused by Salmonella species, S. aureus, and C. perfringens (56). As clinical laboratories commonly lack the diagnostic testing abilities for such entities as Norwalk and related agents and many E. coli, their relative importance in institutional foodborne illness is not well defined.

Epidemics may be caused by many different food vehicles. Salmonella species are associated with poultry, meat loaf, and egg-based foods, such as eggnog and scrambled eggs. Recipes made with meat are frequent vehicles of C. perfringens gastroenteritis. Salads have been incriminated in many S. aureus outbreaks. Although bacterial contamination of feeding formulas appears to be a relatively rare phenomenon, enteral feeding supplements have occasionally been found to be responsible for disease due to agents such as Enterobacter sakazakii (53) and other Enterobacter species.

Numerous food preparation errors have produced outbreaks of gastroenteritis. Most often cited have been food storage problems, such as inadequate refrigeration. Other frequently reported difficulties have included substandard hygienic practices by food workers, equipment contamination, incomplete cooking, and use of food that was contaminated during the initial processing (56).

Spatial and temporal clustering of gastrointestinal illness should suggest a potential common source. The likely pathogen may reveal itself in characteristic presenting symptoms. Early verification of enteroinvasive infection is possible by fecal leukocyte analysis. The putative agent's incubation period may provide clues regarding the source of the outbreak. Thus an early differential diagnosis may facilitate evaluation. Timely implementation of practices to limit ongoing transmission may then be undertaken.

The prevention of foodborne nosocomial infection must concentrate on (a) proper food preparation, storage, and distribution; and (b) the health and hygiene of food service personnel. Regulations in these areas are provided by the Joint Commission on Accreditation of Healthcare Organizations (JCAHO). In addition, the Association for Practitioners in Infection Control (APIC) publishes guidelines for hospitals and nursing homes, each of which are usually supervised by an infection control committee. Pivotal considerations in the formulation of hygienic practices in food preparation are (a) use of proper temperatures for storage of food, (b) prevention of contact between cooked food and uncooked items or kitchen workers carrying pathogenic organisms, (c) proper maintenance of equipment, and (d) training of food service personnel. Food service personnel must be competent in proper equipment use and care and must use acceptable personal hygiene practices. Particularly important, but frequently overlooked, is the need for employees to be educated in the necessity for medical evaluation of diarrhea and of dermatologic conditions associated with staphylococcal carriage.

Foodborne nosocomial illness is a very preventable cause of hospital-acquired morbidity. Illnesses due to Salmonella species and enterohemorrhagic E. coli are capable of causing significant morbidity and mortality in seriously ill hospitalized patients and the nursing home population. However, with diligent regard given to simple infection control procedures, hygienic food preparation, and the involvement of employee health services, foodborne nosocomial illness need not be an ongoing problem in hospitals and other facilities.

COMMON PATHOGENS THAT CAUSE NOSOCOMIAL GASTROENTERITIS

Aerobic Gram-Negative Organisms

Escherichia coli

Escherichia coli is an important etiology of noninflammatory diarrhea in developing countries and the leading cause of traveler's diarrhea. In contrast, the incidence of nosocomial diarrhea due to the pathogenic *E. coli* is perceived to be low, although routine testing for such organisms is not possible in many clinical laboratories. Reference laboratories with such diagnostic capabilities are not often employed in the evaluation of endemic diarrhea, obscuring the true prevalence of sporadic nosocomial diarrhea caused by *E. coli*. Several noteworthy institutional epidemics nonetheless reveal this organism's relevance as a nosocomial pathogen.

Despite a perceived identity as an agent responsible for sporadic disease, enterohemorrhagic *E. coli* (EHEC) serotype O157:H7 is now recognized as the causative pathogen in a four-state outbreak that affected over 500 people. Linked to undercooked hamburger meat from a national chain of fast food restaurants, infection was often marked by hemorrhagic colitis. Forty cases were complicated by hemolytic–uremic syndrome (HUS), resulting in four deaths (60). Both citizens and public officials were explicitly shown the necessity for strict food hygiene standards to protect the nation's food supply (61).

Hospital epidemics due to EHEC have not been reported, although nursing home outbreaks have been noted (57,62). One reported an attack rate of 32.5% (55 of 169) among the patients (57). Twelve of the residents developed HUS, with 11 resultant deaths. Nineteen residents died, resulting in a case–fatality rate of 35%. The epidemic showed a biphasic pattern, with secondary person-to-person spread and moderately high attack rates among the nursing home staff. It is possible that indolent outbreaks, as well as sporadic cases of EHEC gastroenteritis, may be detected by the submission of stool cultures for patients with thrombotic thrombocytopenic purpura (TTP) or HUS (63).

Decades ago, enteropathogenic *E. coli* (EPEC) was associated with epidemic infantile diarrhea. Numerous outbreaks, both in the hospital and community, were ascribed to EPEC between 1940 and 1970 (64). Nosocomial infantile diarrhea was a frequent occurrence in nurseries, with outbreaks marked by high attack rates and case–fatality rates of 50%, usually from sepsis, shock, and acidosis (65). Children were usually afebrile, with poor feeding and watery diarrhea ensuing over 3 to 6 days (66). For reasons that have been ascribed to altered virulence of the organism, improved rehydration techniques, and antibiotic therapy, cases in recent years have been substantially milder. Volume depletion may still nonetheless require hospital care (67).

The index case of an outbreak of EPEC is characteristically an infant infected perinatally. Special care nurseries are therefore especially vulnerable to rapid spread of EPEC, due to the presence of source patients in an often crowded ward of vulnerable newborns. Transmission by asymptomatic carriers may be important in the nursery. In one epidemic, 5% of asymptomatic pediatric patients and about one-third of antepartum mothers had EPEC in their stool (68). Despite its departure from the United States and western Europe (69), institutional diarrhea caused by EPEC is an ongoing challenge in the developing nations of Africa, Asia, and South America (70).

Enterotoxigenic *E. coli* (ETEC) has been the cause of two documented nosocomial outbreaks (71,72). One 9-month-long outbreak, spread by contaminated enteral feedings, was linked to a strain elaborating a heat-stable enterotoxin. This serotype was seemingly unable to colonize adults despite its prevalence in the special care nursery (71). In addition, the responsible strain was unique in that a common plasmid carried resistance genes for multiple antibiotics as well as the enterotoxin gene (73).

Salmonella

Salmonella species remain prominent causes of nosocomial disease. Of U.S. cases of *Salmonella,* up to 35% are documented to originate from hospitals and extended care facilities (33). With only *S. aureus* as a greater cause of epidemic illness in the hospital (18), *Salmonella* accounts for 81% of deaths from foodborne disease in nursing homes (58). *Salmonella* is also an important cause of hospital-acquired morbidity among infants and children, with about 50% of all nosocomial salmonellosis occurring in neonatal and pediatric wards (74). Unlike infections in adults, which often stem from consumption of a food vehicle, cross-infection is the primary mode of spread of pediatric infection. Nursery outbreaks have followed admission of a parturient patient with diarrhea due to *Salmonella* (75).

Most nosocomial outbreaks due to *Salmonella* have been due to a common source (18). Vehicles that have been linked to these epidemics include diagnostic agents, blood products, medications, banked human milk, and enteral feeding supplements containing yeast or raw egg. Contaminated equipment such as endoscopes (76) and suction apparatuses have also been implicated (34). The food sources most often cited are dairy products, poultry, and eggs.

It is not certain whether those who asymptomatically excrete the organism are important sources of nosocomial transmission. Convalescent shedding of *Salmonella* is frequent, evident for a median of 5 weeks after overt disease. In patients younger than 5 years of age and in those infected with serotypes other than *S. typhimurium,* prolonged excretion can be seen (77). Carriage may continue for over 1 year in less than 1% of patients with nontyphoidal disease and in 1% to 3% of those with *S. typhi.* Prolonged excretion is most frequent in the older patients and those with gallbladder disease (78).

Despite a lack of data demonstrating nosocomial spread of *Salmonella* by asymptomatic carriers, apprehension continues to exist. Prevention of the dissemination of infection from such persistent excretors can practically be avoided by fastidious use of enteric isolation procedures. Although *Salmonella* organisms are present on the hands of carriers after defecation, they are removed by handwashing with soap and water (79).

Hospital employees recuperating from salmonellosis must nonetheless be considered a risk for nosocomial transmission and those with contact with patients or food should be confirmed to be culture-negative on two consecutive cultures before returning to such duties. *Salmonella* excretion can be intermittent, however, and positive stool cultures have been found after four to nine consecutive negative cultures in 17% of patients (77). Rectal swabs, which are unable to reliably detect fewer than 10^3 organisms/g of feces, are not recommended for use instead of stool cultures because of poor sensitivity (80).

Because of the problems in demonstrating clearance of *Salmonella* and the erratic ability of antibiotics to eliminate carriage, a reasonable and cost-effective strategy is advocating uniform handwashing by all employees in patient care and food service positions. Those who show evidence of ongoing *Salmonella* carriage must not have direct patient or food contact. A trial of ampicillin therapy can be considered in some employees. The administration of 4 to 5 g of ampicillin daily for 4 to 6 weeks has been able to eradicate *Salmonella* from chronic excretors. Another study demonstrated success in 70% of 17 carriers without cholelithiasis. In only 23% of patients with biliary stones, however, were negative cultures obtained (81). The use of ampicillin eliminated *Salmonella* in 13 (87%) of the long-term excretors who were observed for 7 to 54 months (82). The frequency of adverse drug effects in the study sample was remarkable: 53% of patients reported loose stools, 40% rash, and 20% eosinophilia.

Fluoroquinolones have been evaluated as alternatives to ampicillin and its accompanying difficulties of poor tolerance and potential resistance. One study documented that 10 of 12 (83%) patients who finished 4 weeks of ciprofloxacin had negative cultures after 1 year (83). The rather severe option of cholecystectomy can be contemplated for a *Salmonella* carrier, weighing the uncertainty of nosocomial transmission versus the risks of an operation. A foodborne outbreak of salmonellosis affecting 203 nurses showed no evidence of spread to patients in spite of 77 nurses working 120 shifts while symptomatic (84). It is difficult to extrapolate these findings to such susceptible patients as neonates and those who are immunosuppressed, since none of the infected nurses worked with these groups.

The use of antibiotics can prolong bacterial shedding (85) as well as foster the development of resistance to antimicrobial agents. Moreover, antibiotic therapy has also been shown to increase the risk of infection (86). Nonetheless, these concerns are outweighed by a risk of grave sequelae in such patients as newborns, immunosuppressed, or those with severe infection. These patients should therefore receive antibiotics for treatment of disease.

Nosocomial salmonellosis is more frequently seen in the developing world. In Africa, South America, and Asia, hospitals have been identified as wellsprings for evolution and spread of multiply-resistant *Salmonella* (40). Certain serotypes have acquired resistance to ampicillin. In addition, significant numbers have developed resistance to aminoglycosides, chloramphenicol, monobactams, trimethoprim–sulfamethoxazole, other penicillins, and extended-spectrum cephalosporins. A study from Argentina found that 70% of its *Salmonella* isolates were resistant to multiple antibiotics. In addition, 59% of these pathogens were hospital acquired. Illness caused by resistant strains was as severe as that caused by sensitive isolates, thus suggesting no diminution in virulence with the development of resistant phenotypes (87).

Shigella

Unlike *Salmonella*, *Shigella* species are an exceedingly uncommon cause of hospital-acquired diarrhea. Shigellosis was reported in only 1 of 3363 patients with nosocomial gastroenteritis recorded by the NNIS Program between 1986 and 1989, although *Shigella* has been regarded as one of the most infectious of bacterial agents with a dose of 100 organisms sufficient to produce disease (88).

The few occurrences of nosocomial shigellosis have primarily originated from direct contact. Scattered outbreaks have been reported in custodial care facilities (89) and nurseries (90). The likely mode of spread has been postulated to be the hands of employees with caregiving duties (91). The low incidence of hospital spread of *Shigella* was shown in a Kenyan study, where the organism is endemic and frequently present in newly admitted patients (16).

In contrast to *Salmonella*, all *Shigella* infections should be treated with antibiotics. An agent such as a fluoroquinolone or trimethoprim–sulfamethoxazole will abbreviate the course of clinical illness and reduce fecal shedding of the pathogen. Because of the low incidence of nosocomial shigellosis, an infection that develops in a hospitalized patient must be investigated.

Yersinia enterocolitica

The potential of *Y. enterocolitica* as a nosocomial pathogen has become more apparent in the last 10 years. Although less common than *C. jejuni*, *Y. enterocolitica* is a common cause of community-acquired gastroenteritis in industrialized nations, particularly in the countries of northern Europe. Of the 50 known serotypes, most illness in humans results from infection with O8, O9, O27, and especially O3 (92). Because of the prevalence of nonpathogenic serotypes, any *Y. enterocolitica* strain isolated from a clinical specimen should undergo serotyping. This will help to associate pathogen with illness as well as to establish any epidemiologic link between cases (93).

Community outbreaks have been traced to milk (94),

chitterlings (95), tofu packed in spring water (96), and bean sprouts packed in well water (97), with foods produced from pigs most often incriminated (97,98). Instances of nosocomial bloodstream infection, caused by transfusion of contaminated packed red blood cells producing a sepsis syndrome due to *Y. enterocolitica,* have received significant publicity in recent years. The ten reported cases in nine states had a case–fatality rate of 70%. Almost half of the donors of the implicated blood had gastrointestinal symptoms within 3 weeks before donation but were asymptomatic at the time of donation. All donors demonstrated evidence of recent *Yersinia* infection by serological testing (99,100).

A few clusters of nosocomial gastroenteritis due to *Yersinia* have been documented in the last 20 years (101,102). A study by Cannon and Linnemann (103) analyzed 4 years of surveillance. They determined that five patients had hospital-acquired *Yersinia* infection. They concluded that the infections usually originated from a patient with community-acquired yersiniosis and that nosocomial spread only would occur to one subsequent patient, suggesting that direct transmission of *Y. enterocolitica* seems to occur rarely.

Campylobacter jejuni

Campylobacter jejuni is increasingly recognized as an important cause of invasive gastroenteritis. More prevalent than *Salmonella* or *Shigella,* it is perhaps the most common cause of bacterial diarrhea in the developed world (104). Population studies have shown a bimodal distribution of age-specific incidence, with the first peak in children less than 1 year old and the second occurring in patients 15 to 29 years old (105,106).

Despite its importance as a community-acquired pathogen, nosocomial transmission of *C. jejuni* has been documented only rarely. Foodborne illness has been confirmed in nursing homes, with milk the reported vehicle (58). Reports of a case of bacteremia from a contaminated blood transfusion (107) and vertically transmitted cases of enteritis in neonates have been published (108). Asymptomatic excretors of *Campylobacter* do not seem to disseminate the disease (104).

Aeromonas Species and Other Gram-Negative Bacteria

In addition to EPEC, other Enterobacteriaceae are known to cause epidemic infantile diarrhea, particularly *Klebsiella* and *Citrobacter* species (109). One diarrheal outbreak was caused by multiple species using a common enterotoxin, likely disseminated by a plasmid or bacteriophage (110). Such noteworthy events are seldom detected using the facilities in most hospital laboratories.

Aeromonas species are controversial pathogens, which only recently have been found to cause gastrointestinal illness. They appear, however, unable to produce disease in healthy adults (111); in volunteer studies, even large bacterial loads did not cause symptoms (112). The mechanisms by which *Aeromonas* causes disease are not yet well defined but include a heat-labile cytotonic enterotoxin (113) and another enterotoxin that cross-reacts with cholera toxin (114) and has enteroinvasive traits (115).

Both seasonal and geographic associations have been reported with *Aeromonas* infections (116). *Aeromonas* species have been recovered from 52.8% of Peruvian infants hospitalized with diarrhea, versus 8.7% of controls (117). In Australia, only rotavirus is a more common cause of endemic diarrhea in pediatric populations (118). In contrast, a study evaluating diarrhea in Brazilian children did not isolate *Aeromonas* in a single culture (119).

Isolation of *Aeromonas* species from hospital water sources (120) implies a possibility for nosocomial epidemics. Actual reports, however, have been rare. One described respiratory colonization with resultant pneumonia or extrapulmonary infections (but not diarrhea) in 19 patients (121). Another apparent outbreak of *Aeromonas* occurred in a nursing home where 17 patients developed a brief illness of nonbloody diarrhea over a 3-day period (122). Of 11 cultures submitted, four grew *A. hydrophila.* In neither outbreak was a common source found, nor were cultures tested for the presence of a toxin.

Gram-Positive Aerobic Bacteria

Listeria monocytogenes

Listeria monocytogenes is a motile, nonspore-forming gram-positive rod that is ubiquitous in the environment and among animals (123). Approximately 20% of sporadic cases (124) and many large outbreaks have been traced to contaminated food. Common sources of major outbreaks have been pasteurized milk (125), cheese (126), coleslaw (127), and undercooked meats (124). It also has frequently been isolated from commercially prepared foods intended for instant use, with a number of products recalled or not released as a result (128).

The spectrum of clinical manifestations caused by *Listeria* ranges from transient, asymptomatic carriage (123) to sepsis and meningoencephalitis (129). One-third of patients with listeriosis in a large British survey were infected during pregnancy (130), most often as a nonspecific febrile illness. Transplacental transmission can be inconsequential (131) or catastrophic, with stillbirth, prematurity, neonatal sepsis/meningitis, and granulomatosis infantiseptica resulting (130). The reporting of gastrointestinal symptoms prior to the development of invasive listeriosis has roused speculation that the organism, or perhaps a coinfecting pathogen, may be damaging the intestinal mucosa and allowing the invasion of *Listeria* (132).

Only 10% to 30% of patients have no identifiable predisposition for infection (129). Invasive disease in the general population is rare, with a risk for adults of 0.5/100,000 population (128), despite point prevalence gut colonization rates of 0.6% to 16% in the general population and longitudinal studies showing transient carriage occurring in 70% of people (133).

Hospital-associated outbreaks of listeriosis have been described. One outbreak in 1979, traced to raw vegetables, affected 20 patients in eight Boston-area hospitals.

Ten of these patients were immunosuppressed (134). An unusual epidemic in a Costa Rican nursery documented cross-infection from an index case, an infant with neonatal listeriosis, via a contaminated bottle of mineral oil that was used on other infants (135). Although not associated with gastroenteritis, it should be emphasized that no other foodborne illness has a higher case–fatality rate; nonperinatal cases of listeriosis reported in a nationwide survey in 1986 had a case–fatality rate of 35% (128).

Listeria monocytogenes requires temperatures of at least 70°C to kill the organism (123). The agent can also grow at temperatures near the freezing point, which allows for "cold enrichment" techniques and facilitates its isolation in the microbiology laboratory (123). Person-to-person transmission of infection has not yet been firmly described, with a few reports of small outbreaks suggesting spread by fomites or hospital workers (136). Nosocomial outbreaks should be investigated with a technique, such as multilocus enzyme electrophoresis (137), that allows subtyping in addition to more routine serotyping.

Staphylococci

Staphylococcal foodborne disease is a common institutional occurrence. Foodborne *S. aureus* outbreaks made up 8% of hospital and 23% of nursing home outbreaks reported to the CDC during the years 1975 to 1987 (56). Although mortality is rare, with a 0.4% case–fatality rate in the CDC nursing home survey (58), morbidity can be considerable. Hospitalization rates have been reported to be about 8% (58), often required by the rapid volume depletion and electrolyte derangements that can be a result of the vomiting produced by this explosive illness.

The source of epidemic staphylococcal food poisoning is often a food handler with hands colonized with *S. aureus,* perhaps following a skin infection. Disease can ensue if food prepared by the carrier is stored at an improper temperature or not served promptly. Interruption of this chain of events can be accomplished by (a) conscientious employee hygiene with handwashing, the use of gloves, or the exclusion of food handlers with skin infections; (b) proper refrigeration of foods at temperatures below 4°C, especially after partial cooking (138); and (c) rapid serving of food kept at room temperature.

In the last decade methicillin-resistant *S. aureus* (MRSA) and coagulase-negative staphylococci have received widespread attention as increasingly important nosocomial pathogens. Despite a reputation as primarily a bloodstream and wound pathogen, a few reports have implicated MRSA as a cause of antibiotic-associated diarrhea (139).

Anaerobic Organisms

Clostridium difficile

A gram-positive, spore-forming, obligate anaerobe, *C. difficile* has been shown to be the predominant microbial etiology of nosocomial diarrhea. In early experiments, hamsters given antibiotics were noted to develop severe colitis (140), providing insight into the pathogenesis of antibiotic-associated pseudomembranous colitis. A cytotoxin neutralized by *C. sordelli* antitoxin was identified in the hamster feces (141). It was subsequently associated with *C. difficile* and is now known as toxin B (142). An enterotoxin (toxin A) is also elaborated by *C. difficile,* producing intestinal fluid secretion and hemorrhage in an animal model (143). Although toxin A is thought to express the clinical symptoms, most strains of *C. difficile* produce both toxins (144).

Until recently, tissue culture assay to detect cytopathic effects of toxin B had been considered the gold standard for diagnosis of antibiotic-associated colitis. Used independently, it was reported to have a sensitivity between 67% (145) and 100% (146) and a specificity of 99% (145,147). Disadvantages, however, exist with this test. It is technically difficult to perform, restricting availability (144). Crucial for accuracy of the assay is the proper care of cell lines, impractical for some laboratories. Diagnostic precision is also contingent on the selection of an appropriate dilution titer to define a positive result (148).

Recent studies have given cause for concern over the specificity of the cytotoxin assay. Zaidi and associates (19) found *C. difficile* toxin more often in asymptomatic patients than in those with diarrhea. Another study showed a 5% rate of asymptomatic toxin carriage in hospitalized adults (28).

Other rapid assays for *C. difficile* toxin have been developed that seek to remedy the technical problems with the cytotoxin assay. Several commercial enzyme immunoassay (EIA) tests are available that can detect toxin A, B, or both. Latex agglutination tests have also been developed. They are rapid and simple to perform, but sensitivities have ranged from 71% to 92% when compared with a cytotoxin assay (148). Many of these kits have either insufficient sensitivity or an excessive number of indeterminate results to allow use as a definitive test (10,146,149). Other diagnostic tests, such as a polymerase chain reaction that uses primers from both toxins A and B, have shown promise (150,151).

Techniques for culturing *C. difficile* commonly use a selective egg-yolk agar base medium with cycloserine, cefoxitin, and fructose (CCFA) (152). Because the rate of asymptomatic *C. difficile* carriage in hospitalized patients is about 16% (26), culture alone should not be used for the diagnosis of CDAD. To facilitate epidemiologic studies, 0.1% sodium taurocholate can be added to CCFA to increase recovery of *C. difficile* from environmental sources by increasing spore germination (153). Likewise, alcohol shock enrichment also seems to increase yield from cultures of suspected *C. difficile* carriers (154,155). Because of the high rate of asymptomatic carriage of *C. difficile* in hospitalized patients, the evaluation of antibiotic-associated colitis must use both clinical and laboratory criteria (28,145).

Follow-up cultures to document cure do not seem to be helpful in patients with CDAD. After treatment, high rates of asymptomatic colonization persist (156). Although transmission may occur from an asymptomatic excretor, eradication of *C. difficile* carriage has not been usually successful and is not advised. One recent study found that the use of metronidazole had no effect on excretion and vancomycin had only a temporary influence on excretion rates (157). Therefore the recommended measures to interrupt nosocomial outbreaks of CDAD are use of enteric precautions, glove and gown use, handwashing, and use of private rooms and cohorting if patient hygiene is poor. Contaminated electronic thermometers have been linked to an outbreak of CDAD. Discontinuation of their use was temporally associated with cessation of the outbreak (158). Some data suggest that handwashing with chlorhexidine is more effective in eradicating *C. difficile* than plain soap and water (26).

Clostridium perfringens

Nosocomial gastroenteritis due to *C. perfringens* is the third most common foodborne illness in hospitals and nursing homes (56). Following an incubation period of 6 to 24 hr, diarrhea and abdominal cramps develop, usually in the absence of systemic toxicity. The illness lasts up to 24 hr and resolves without therapy (159). Although typically benign, deaths due to *C. perfringens* food poisoning have been reported (58).

Toxigenic strains of *C. perfringens* are usually found in meats, stews, poultry, gravies, and meat pies (160) that became contaminated during prolonged cooling and storage at room temperature (161). Heat-stable spores are able to survive cooking and germinate with cooling. Optimal growth in meat occurs at a temperature of 43°C to 47°C (160). Thus it is the storage of food at inappropriate temperatures that will most likely favor the growth of *C. perfringens*. Cooked foods must therefore be promptly refrigerated at a temperature of no greater than 4°C and, if reheated, cooked to a temperature of at least 100°C, which will inactivate both the toxin and *C. perfringens* spores that might have germinated due to insufficient refrigeration (162).

Syndromes other than foodborne gastroenteritis have been associated with *C. perfringens*. Sporadic diarrhea has been reported and shown to be independent of contaminated food ingestion. This illness follows a protracted clinical course, akin to that of *Salmonella* or *Campylobacter* species (163). Cases of antibiotic-associated diarrhea have also been reported (164). *Clostridium perfringens* (165) and *C. butyricum* (166) have both been implicated in the pathogenesis of infant necrotizing enterocolitis (NEC). The discovery that *C. perfringens* type C was the etiologic agent in pigbel (167) (a syndrome of necrotizing enteritis described in highland natives of New Guinea, which classically occurs after ritual consumption of a large pork meal), suggested that NEC may be caused by a bacterial toxin.

Viral Pathogens

Rotavirus

Rotavirus is the major worldwide cause of childhood diarrhea, producing substantial mortality in the children

of developing nations (168). In the United States and western Europe, diarrheal mortality is rare, but 35% of wintertime pediatric hospital admissions for gastroenteritis are due to rotavirus (169). Children between 6 months and 2 years old experience the bulk of disease, with 62% of children having had at least one infection by 2 years of age (170). Hospitalization rates for children have been reported to be as high as 8.5 admissions/1000 children (171).

After an incubation period of 48 to 72 hr, there is the onset of fever and vomiting that generally lasts about 2 days. A watery diarrhea follows that is devoid of blood and leukocytes, subsiding within 8 days (4). Viral shedding in the feces is usual from the third to eighth days of illness. Although clinically inapparent infection can occur in any age group, it is most commonly seen in adults. In contrast, children aged 6 to 24 months most often have pronounced symptoms (172). Infected patients may excrete viral loads as high as 10^{12} organisms/g of feces (173).

Rotavirus has been found to exist on environmental surfaces for up to 10 days (174). A simian rotavirus can survive acid and alkaline exposures, freeze-thawing, ether, and chloroform (175), as well as chlorhexidine (176). The most effective disinfectant has been found to be 95% ethanol (177), with glutaraldehyde and povidone-iodine also useful (176).

The infectious nature of rotavirus has been shown in household studies that describe a 40% seroconversion rate among parents of children with rotavirus gastroenteritis (178). Thus it may not be surprising that an analysis of a children's hospital found that only *S. aureus* was more common as a nosocomial pathogen (5). The development of electron microscopy in the 1970s allowed diarrheal illness to be correlated with demonstration of the virus in stool specimens. The first outbreaks were reported from nurseries in England (179), Australia (180), and the United States (181). These accounts described high attack rates, but with only a fraction of infected infants having detectable symptoms.

Transmission is thought to be horizontal, supported by the detection of rotavirus in the handwashings of asymptomatic caregivers of patients with diarrhea (182). Emphasizing the practical importance of person-to-person spread, several institutions have ended outbreaks by cohorting infected patients and caregivers (181,183). In contrast, one study was unable to find efficacy by using early screening of symptomatic patients with ELISA testing and isolation. This very small study found no difference in transmission rates from cases identified during two separate 5-week surveillance periods, occurring before and after the introduction of rapid testing for rotavirus (13).

Although solid data are lacking, conjecture has been raised about the potential for aerosol spread (184,185). The frequent occurrence of simultaneous respiratory symptoms with rotavirus gastroenteritis implies a need for further investigation of this possible mode of transmission.

Nosocomial rotavirus gastroenteritis has been documented in adults, with multiple outbreaks reported among elderly patients (183,186). One outbreak affected 19 out of 34 patients, with six severe cases of gastroenteritis and two deaths (187). Yolken and colleagues (12) studied adult bone marrow transplant recipients and found that 9 of 31 patients with infectious diarrhea had disease due to rotavirus. Other studies have found this entity to be the etiologic agent in 1% to 4% of nosocomial gastroenteritis in adults (68).

In some populations, rotavirus infection may be more severe. Immunodeficient patients may experience chronic diarrhea and prolonged viral shedding (188). Potential for more serious illness with protracted infectivity likewise exists for elderly (187) and transplant patients (12,189).

The epidemiologic study of rotavirus has greatly been facilitated by improved diagnostic technologies. The use of enzyme-linked immunoadsorbent assay (ELISA) testing has made case-finding rapid, inexpensive, and simple. These commercially available kits can detect rotavirus inner capsid antigen in stools with a sensitivity early in the illness equivalent to that of virus isolation and visualization by electron microscopy (190). Latex agglutination tests, although less sensitive than ELISA (191), are also rapid and readily available. The use of polymerase chain reaction (PCR) can detect rotavirus antigen at concentrations 1000 times lower than electron microscopy or immunoassay methods (192).

Polyacrylamide gel electrophoresis (PAGE) has been used to differentiate rotavirus strains. Using variations in migration patterns of the RNA segments in the virus genome to define strains, PAGE (or "electropherotyping") is a powerful technique for epidemiologic analysis (193,194). Its ability to classify rotaviruses or analyze organisms over time or in widely separated outbreaks is limited by the fact that a given electropherotype does not always correlate with DNA hybridization patterns or serotype (195,196). Despite these shortcomings, electropherotyping is useful in the study of individual outbreaks. It has shown infant-to-infant transmission, with involvement of multiple strains in an outbreak (197). One outbreak with an initial predominance of one electropherotype had subsequent appearance of highly variable RNA segments by PAGE (198), suggesting that a rotavirus strain may evolve during an epidemic, either by genetic reassortment ("antigenic drift") or by introduction of other strains with multiple infections.

Efforts to prevent nosocomial rotavirus infection should concentrate on diagnosing patients newly admitted with diarrhea and early isolation using enteric precautions, those shown to be the most important sources of nosocomial rotavirus outbreaks (199). Other efforts should include strengthening of hygienic practices, particularly handwashing, among hospital staff, who have also been implicated in nosocomial spread of rotavirus (181). Vaccines are being produced, using both attenuated animal and reassortment vaccine types, with promising but somewhat erratic results being obtained in clinical trials. Finnish trials demonstrated efficacy of 0% to 67% against rotavirus diarrhea but vaccines provided protection in 44% to 100% of recipients in other studies (200).

Adenovirus

The role of adenoviruses in childhood enteric disease is now firmly established after their first identification by electron microscopy in the stools of infants with diarrhea in 1975 (201,202). Strains linked to gastroenteritis are called enteric adenoviruses and belong to serogroups 40 and 41 (203). These strains are often referred to as "uncultivable" adenoviruses because of fastidious growth requirements in cell culture.

For children under 2 years old, only rotavirus is a more common cause of community-acquired gastroenteritis (204,205). Serologic evidence of prior infection is present in 50% of children by age 4 (206). Unlike rotavirus, there is no seasonal variability in infection rates (205,207). Person-to person transmission is the probable route of spread (208) although spread to adults is uncommon (205,207). The prevalence of latent infection is illustrated by a prospective study that found that 46% of infected children were asymptomatic (204). Infection appears to confer long-term immunity.

Nosocomial acquisition of adenovirus was first reported by Flewett and co-workers (201). They described a diarrheal illness of 24- to 48-hr duration affecting 6 of 19 children and one nurse in a pediatric ward. Adenovirus-like particles were found on stool electron microscopy in four of six ill children and the nurse, but none of the well children (201). In another study, Yolken and associates (209) described adenovirus in the stools of 14 (52%) of 27 hospitalized infants with gastroenteritis, with 13/14 (93%) of these affected patients having concurrent respiratory symptoms. Nosocomial acquisition was suggested by the fact that 5 of the 14 children with gastroenteritis were not excreting adenovirus at the time of admission (209). Only one (1.3%) of 72 asymptomatic children had adenovirus detectable on stool examination. Another prospective study of hospitalized children under 2 years of age determined that adenovirus was the third most common cause of nosocomial diarrhea in this age group, causing 6.2% of cases (210). A study of bone marrow transplant recipients with a mean age of 21 years discovered that the incidence of gastroenteritis due to adenovirus was equal to that of *C. difficile* and is associated with a 45% mortality (12).

Small, Round Structured Viruses (Norwalk and Other Agents)

A syndrome of acute nausea and vomiting commonly occurs during the winters in temperate climates. This illness aggregates in families, usually affecting children 1 to 10 years old, but not sparing adults. Until recently, this illness was identified as "winter vomiting disease" (211), reflecting the lack of a known etiology.

Investigation of a large outbreak of winter vomiting disease in Norwalk, Ohio (212), revealed the first of a collection of small (20 to 35 nm), round structured viral agents that were subsequently linked to gastroenteritis (213). Of the outbreaks of acute nonbacterial gastroenteritis investigated by the CDC during 1976 to 1981, 42% were caused by the Norwalk and related entities (214).

These viruses are generally identified either by immune electron microscopy or by paired serology. Other methods have been developed, such as an ELISA (215) and PCR (216) for the Norwalk agent, and ELISA for both the calicivirus (217) and astrovirus (218), but routine use is limited by availability of reagents.

Most Norwalk-related outbreaks result from such contaminated vehicles as water (219), salad (220), or shellfish (214). Nursing homes have been the most common sites for institutional epidemics. In fact, it was the study of an outbreak in a California nursing home that initially recognized the Marin County agent (221). High attack rates have been reported; another nursing home epidemic affected 64% of its 120 residents as well as 29% of the staff (222). Nine (12%) of the residents required hospitalization, and two deaths occurred. Documentation of this outbreak was incomplete; stool electron microscopy was not performed nor was a vehicle for the outbreak found.

Person-to-person spread seems to perpetuate some outbreaks (223). Investigators in an emergency department found some ill patients and staff without any history of direct contact with other ill patients. It was theorized that movement of infectious laundry extended the area where virus could be spread (42). Despite conjecture regarding an aerosol route in this instance, as well as another nursing home outbreak (41), confirmation of this route for the spread of gastrointestinal illness remains forthcoming.

Testing for this class of viruses is not commonly done in clinical laboratories. Therefore, without prospective surveillance, recognition of early outbreaks as well as sporadic cases is unlikely. Also complicating investigations is the short duration of the illness. Stool and blood must be obtained in the presence of symptoms. Specimens must then be evaluated quickly for best results using immune electron microscopy or serology (208).

Other viruses have been associated with nosocomial gastroenteritis. They include coronaviruses, echoviruses, and coxsackieviruses. These agents have primarily been linked to outbreaks in infants.

Protozoa

Cryptosporidium

The initial correlation of infection with *Cryptosporidium* and human disease was first reported in 1976 by two investigators (224,225). This organism produces an illness in which both the severity and duration of illness are modified by the competence of the patient's immune system (226). An intractable, frequently fatal, diarrhea occurs in AIDS patients, with less severe disease in normal hosts (227). The illness can result from exposure to infected animals and humans, in addition to consumption of water (228). Nosocomial transmission between patients and from infected patients to hospital personnel has been reported (229–232). One outbreak affected all six patients in a bone marrow transplantation unit after a recently admitted patient shared a room with a patient with cryptosporidiosis on another unit (230). Convalescent shedding of organisms can persist after cessation of symptoms but will generally subside within 2 weeks (233).

Cryptosporidium oocysts are extremely difficult to inactivate. They survive the chlorination in public water supplies, as well as such common disinfectants as iodophors, hypochlorite, and 5% formaldehyde. Heat ($\geq 60°C$), formalin ($\geq 10\%$), and ammonia ($\geq 50\%$) appear to be effective in killing the organism (228,234–237). Even concentrated to 100%, hypochlorite alone appears to be only partially effective in eradicating oocysts.

Laboratory diagnosis is most often made by microscopic examination of stool using a Kinyoun acid-fast stain looking for oocysts (238,239). Since oocyst shedding is not always continuous, evaluation of multiple specimens may increase yield (233). Recently available is an EIA kit, shown in one study to have a sensitivity and specificity of 100% compared to a standard of immunofluorescence (240). Concentration methods (241) may assist in epidemic investigation by evaluating suspected nosocomial cases, detecting oocysts in water, other environmental samples, or in a specimen from a contact of a patient with cryptosporidiosis. Serologic methods, such as ELISA, may be more practical for larger scale studies that are evaluating prevalence. They have a 95% sensitivity when both immunoglobulin M (IgM) and IgG antibodies are used (242). As in other pathogens, efforts to control institutional spread must rely on aggressive identification of infected patients and strict enteric precautions. Because of the difficulty with effective environmental disinfection, the severity of illness in the immunocompromised, and only recent emergence of a potentially useful treatment, such preventive measures are even more crucial.

Entamoeba histolytica

Although it is a known cause of diarrhea in custodial institutions (243) and in AIDS patients (244), *E. histolytica* is a rare nosocomial pathogen. One noteworthy outbreak of amebiasis, however, was connected to an improperly maintained colonic irrigation machine in a chiropractor's office. Over 2½ years, 36 cases of the illness, including six deaths, were reported (245).

Although hospital-acquired amebiasis occurs in developing countries (19), it is generally felt to be a reactivation illness. Not only do affected patients appear to lack identifiable risk factors for recent acquisition of infection, but no geographical or spatial clustering of cases is evident. Most patients had received prior corticosteroids or chemotherapy, with resultant suppression of cell-mediated immunity permitting recrudescence of dormant infection. If there is ever a concern regarding possible nosocomial transmission of *E. histolytica*, methods such as DNA hybridization (246) and PCR (247) may be useful in elucidating modes of transmission.

Giardia lamblia (G. duodenalis)

Currently the most frequently identified intestinal parasite in the United States, *G. lamblia* has caused numerous large waterborne community outbreaks (248,249). *Giardia lamblia* also is a well-known etiology of diarrhea in both day-care centers (250) and custodial institutions (251). One outbreak in a nursing home has also been documented (252). The ingestion of water contaminated by cysts is a characteristic route of acquisition, with person-to-person spread next in frequency. Indirect transmission of *Giardia* cysts can occur, resulting from their survival on environmental surfaces (253) and resistance to many disinfectants (254).

Children in day-care centers may excrete cysts for as long as 6 months in the absence of overt symptoms (250). Up to 50% of children younger than 3 years of age demonstrate silent fecal shedding of cysts. Other studies have found that 25% of family members of children in day-care have evidence of *Giardia* infection (255). Handwashing is nonetheless effective in curtailing spread of this agent in the day-care center (256).

The organism is visible on either a saline wet-mount examination of a fresh stool specimen or a preserved sample that is stained with trichrome or hematoxylin. Some recommend use of a concentration method (257), sampling of duodenal contents by a string test (258), or endoscopy with brushings/biopsy (259) if initial stool microscopy is unproductive. The use of an ELISA that can detect *Giardia* in stool with a sensitivity and specificity of over 90% may assist epidemiologic study (260). The PCR could add power to such investigation by virtue of its ability to distinguish subgroups of *G. lamblia* (261).

Fungal Pathogens

Candida *Species*

The isolation of *Candida* from 65% of stool specimens from healthy persons (262) has confounded efforts to understand the potential of *Candida* to cause serious nosocomial disease. The organism's role beyond that of a saprophyte has nonetheless grown, largely as a result of the increasing use of immunosuppressive and cytotoxic agents, as well as the expansion of the AIDS epidemic. Gastrointestinal candidiasis may manifest as invasive enteritis in immunocompromised hosts, or a noninvasive overgrowth syndrome (263).

Case–control studies show that colonization with *Candida* is a risk factor for the development of candidemia (264,265), which carries a mortality rate as high as 38% (266). It has been demonstrated by restriction endonuclease digestion with fungal DNA that colonizing strains are identical to those that appear in the blood (267). It is postulated that fungal invasion of the gastrointestinal tract mucosa leads to the organism's subsequent hematogenous spread (268). A healthy human volunteer developed fever and rigors hours after swallowing a saline suspension containing 10^{12} *C. albicans* cells and was documented to have candidemia and candiduria (269).

Although its pathogenesis is unclear, an illness of watery diarrhea, with *Candida* overgrowth in the absence of mucosal invasion, has been documented (270). Some suggest a toxin-mediated process produces the disease (271). In contrast, deranged small intestinal brush border enzyme activity is felt by others to be the primary lesion (272). This syndrome has been described most commonly in neonates (273) and debilitated patients (270), with a uniformly positive response to oral nystatin (270,274).

Despite their use being almost exclusively in research centers, serotyping techniques have contributed to an understanding of the acquisition and transmission of *Candida* (275). Doebbling and co-workers (276) have utilized contour-clamped homogeneous electric field electrophoresis to demonstrate hand carriage of *Candida* in healthcare personnel, thus implying a potential for direct spread. DNA fingerprinting and biotyping have been used together, producing precise discrimination among clinical specimens (277). Unfortunately, early and reliable diagnosis of invasive candidiasis in the clinical setting is still difficult, generally necessitating blood culture and biopsy of appropriate anatomic sites. New rapid tests for *Candida* species, applying EIA to detect either cell wall (278) or cytoplasmic (279) antigens, have shown potential in selected samples but seem to be limited by poor specificity in patient groups at a lesser risk for candidiasis (280).

OUTBREAK DETECTION AND MANAGEMENT

Optimally, the hospital with sufficient resources and personnel should conduct regular ward-based surveillance of all units and review all microbiology data (281). Institutions with more limited facilities can effectively perform surveillance for nosocomial gastroenteritis by routine review of positive stool results, coupled with periodic observation of high-risk wards, such as the newborn and special-care nurseries, intensive care units, and oncology wards. This method incorporates aspects of laboratory surveillance and selective chart review (282,283). Such use of surveillance to detect sporadic cases of *C. difficile* diarrhea has been demonstrated to be useful in decreasing spread of that organism within the hospital (29). Rapid interpretation of positive stool assays for *C. difficile* can permit early institution of procedures to limit nosocomial spread, including glove use with patient contact, gowns if soiling is likely, and a private room if the patient hygiene is poor, in addition to routine handwashing. Chlorhexidine may be superior to nonantimicrobial soap in eliminating organisms such as *C. difficile* from the hands of hospital employees (26).

After confirmation of a nosocomial outbreak of gastroenteritis, epidemiologic investigation should begin, with initial isolation measures being undertaken concurrent with the gathering of preliminary data. If a large number of persons appear to be affected, cohorting of patients and caregivers should be considered. Prompt notification of the local or state health department is advisable, as nursing homes and small hospitals may not have the necessary facilities for an appropriate investigation. Larger hospitals may still benefit from the support of the state health department, which can perform serotyping or test for such organisms as pathogenic *E. coli* or Norwalk and related agents.

PREVENTION OF NOSOCOMIAL GASTROENTERITIS

Prevention of gastrointestinal infections in hospitalized patients lies with the awareness that these diseases are fundamentally spread by the fecal–oral route. Subsequently, transmission to others may occur by direct physical contact, or indirectly by the hands of caregivers or contact with inanimate surfaces. Gastrointestinal pathogens may also be acquired by a contaminated common vehicle such as food, water, medication, or equipment. Thus approaches to control these infections require incorporation of these concepts.

Of paramount importance is handwashing between patient and food contact, as well as the use of enteric precautions. Although originally enacted to prevent employee exposure to bloodborne viral agents, the use of universal precautions (284) reduces nosocomial transmission of agents such as *C. difficile*. In one medical center, the institution of an employee educational program that urged glove use for contact with any moist body substance resulted in an 80% decrease in the incidence of *C. difficile*-associated diarrhea (27). Handwashing after all patient contact (285) and changing gloves between patients should be urged (286). Strategies must improve handwashing compliance rates estimated to be 40% in one intensive care unit survey (287). Also requiring correction is the belief of many hospital employees that they are consistently observing handwashing protocols, in contrast to observed inadequate compliance with hygienic procedures (288).

Contamination of such equipment as endoscopy and respiratory therapy devices has been found to be associated with institutional spread of enteric diseases, notably *C. difficile, Salmonella* species, and *Helicobacter pylori* (31,32,38,76,289,290). Most implicated equipment is classified as "semicritical" (291), needing a minimum of high-level disinfection due their close proximity to nonintact skin or mucous membranes. One nationwide sample found a significant heterogeneity in protocols used for disinfection of endoscopic devices (292). In addition, manual cleaning, the first and essential step in proper disinfection, is complicated by the intricate design and fragility of endoscopes (293). An inadequate performance of this step makes prolonged chemical disinfection with high-potency germicides necessary. Such an alternative can include either a 20-min treatment in 2% glutaraldehyde or ethylene oxide sterilization as another option (294). Incomplete rinsing of devices after exposure to such agents has been documented to cause a dermatitis in employees and, in patients, a chemical colitis with an endoscopic appearance similar to pseudomembranous colitis (295). Automated washers do not totally eliminate potential for contamination of devices. Alvarado et al. (296) reported nosocomial *P. aeruginosa* infections originating from an endoscope washer that was contaminated with the same strain. The internal components were noted to be colonized with *Pseudomonas,* with positive cultures of rinse-cycle water seen over a 1-year period. The washer's self-operating decontamination procedure had failed to eliminate the organism. Colonization was successfully eradicated by the addition of a step after machine cleansing and disinfection: rinsing external surfaces and endoscope channels using 70% alcohol and subsequent drying with forced air. In situations where the source of contamination is unknown, sterilization with ethylene oxide can be used if infections seem to be occurring due to problems with high-level disinfection.

Clinical thermometers are also a semicritical item and should undergo high-level disinfection, most easily done with 70% to 90% isopropyl alcohol (294). Outbreaks of *C. difficile* have been associated with electronic rectal thermometers, with their successful cessation by substituting disposable thermometers (158). A crossover study comparing disposable thermometers to electronic thermometers demonstrated a 64% reduction in rates of *C. difficile* infection with use of the disposable device (297).

Disinfection of environmental surfaces is a relatively uncomplicated procedure. Any of a number of agents, such as 70% to 90% isopropyl alcohol, sodium hypochlorite, or detergents with phenol, iodophor, or ammonia (294), can be used for low-level disinfection of noncritical items (those coming in contact with intact skin) and surfaces.

Prevention should also center on patients. Established risk factors for nosocomial diarrhea should be minimized to lessen the chance of its development. These strategies can include reducing antimicrobial utilization, using sucralfate instead of antacids or H_2 blockers if ulcer prophylaxis is needed, limiting enema use, and reducing duration of nasogastric tube use. Some innovative approaches have been tried, with uneven results. The administration of nonpathogenic bacteria and yeasts has been attempted in an effort to prevent antibiotic-associated diarrhea. One study demonstrated a significant decrease in the incidence of antibiotic-associated diarrhea by using a saprophytic yeast *Saccharomyces boulardii.* The yeast, however, had no impact on the colonization of *C. difficile* as well as the toxin (298).

Hospital and food service employee education should emphasize relevant aspects of personal health. The Study on the Efficacy of Nosocomial Infection Control (SENIC) project addressed the attitudes of hospital employees toward their own illnesses (299). It was discovered that infection control nurses often had negligible authority to mandate suspension from patient contact for employees with communicable diseases. The study also reported that 68% of nurses believed that working with diarrheal symptoms was acceptable, in comparison to 4% in the presence of fever and sore throat. Outbreaks of gastroenteritis due to Norwalk and related agents have been traced to health-care providers working in the presence of gastrointestinal symptoms (43). The customarily brief course of gastroenteritis can permit an ill employee to spread the infection at work and experience subsequent cessation of symptoms, evading the notice of supervisors, employee health, or infection control personnel. To avert this type of scenario, the institution's employee health service, perhaps with infection control, must take on a more proactive approach. Illness should promptly be identified. Educational interventions must stress that patient contact must be avoided in the presence of illness, in spite of notions that a condition is minor. Finally, the success of such interventions rests on the certainty that employees will not receive financial penalty for time lost from duty due to illness (300).

Employees with gastroenteritis should be evaluated and

released from direct patient or food contact until symptoms subside. Most of these illnesses will only require supportive treatment. If there is concern over an invasive illness or a possible institutional outbreak, more thorough evaluation is indicated with stool samples submitted for bacterial culture and perhaps ova and parasite examination. In this way, a specific diagnosis can be made to not only guide treatment but also to estimate the risk for further dissemination (301). A significant concern is to consider those entities that are likely to be excreted for a prolonged interval after recovery from acute illness. For nontyphoidal *Salmonella* or *Shigella* infections, an asymptomatic employee should have at least two negative stool cultures before resuming duties (302). For the most valid results, stool specimens should be collected at least 24 hr apart and at least 48 hr after discontinuation of antibiotics. More than 50% of those having salmonellosis will have negative cultures within 5 weeks after the illness, with 90% by 9 weeks (77). A health-care worker with disease due to most agents may resume work after cessation of symptoms, with explicit advice to use universal precautions and handwashing.

Prevention of institutional foodborne disease must focus on maintaining hygienic food storage and preparation procedures. Kitchen surfaces as well as equipment should be kept fastidiously clean. Food should be sought from reliable sources, avoiding unpasteurized products. Appropriate temperatures, either above 60°C or below 7°C, must be used for storage of food. Thawing must be complete before cooking, optimally done while the food is refrigerated. Although modified ultraviolet lamps have been used to eradicate *Salmonella* species on culture plates (303), the technique is not currently applicable to food disinfection. Proper training of food service personnel cannot be overemphasized, as they are most able to prevent foodborne disease spread.

REFERENCES

1. Farr BM. Diarrhea: a neglected nosocomial hazard? [Editorial]. *Infect Control Hosp Epidemiol* 1991;12:343–344.
2. Garner JS, Jarvis WR, Emori TG, Horan TC, Hughes JM. CDC definitions for nosocomial infections. *Am J Infect Control* 1988; 16:128–140.
3. Emori TG, Culver DH, Horan TC, et al. National nosocomial infections surveillance system (NNIS): description of surveillance methods. *Am J Infect Control* 1991;19:19–35.
4. Hughes JM, Jarvis WR. Nosocomial gastrointestinal infections. In: R Wenzel, ed. *Prevention and control of nosocomial infections*. Baltimore: Williams & Wilkins, 1993;708–745.
5. Siegal DL, Edelstein PH, Nachamakin I. Inappropriate testing for diarrheal diseases in the hospital. *JAMA* 1990;263:979–982.
6. Brady MT, Pacini DL, Budde CT, Connell MJ. Diagnostic studies of nosocomial diarrhea in children: assessing their use and value. *Am J Infect Control* 1989;17:77–82.
7. Lam BCC, Tam J, Ng MH, Yeung CY. Nosocomial gastroenteritis in pediatric patients. *J Hosp Infect* 1989;14:351–355.
8. Ford-Jones EL, Mindorff CM, Gold R, Petrie M. The incidence of viral-associated diarrhea after admission to a pediatric hospital. *Am J Epidemiol* 1990;131:711–718.
9. Welliver RC, McLaughlin S. Unique epidemiology of nosocomial infection in a children's hospital. *Am J Dis Child* 1984; 138:131–135.
10. Lima NL, Farr BM, Lima MEF, et al. Etiologies of nosocomial

11. Guerrant RL, Hughes JM, Lima NL, Crane J. Diarrhea in developed and developing countries: magnitude, special settings, and etiologies. *Rev Infect Dis* 1990;12(Suppl):s41–s50.
12. Yolken RH, Bishop CA, Townsend TR, et al. Infectious gastroenteritis in bone marrow transplant recipients. *N Engl J Med* 1982;306:1009–1012.
13. Dennehy PH, Tenle WE, Fisher DJ, Beloudis BA, Peter G. Lack of impact of rapid identification of rotavirus-infected patients on nosocomial rotavirus infections. *Pediatr Infect Dis J* 1989;8:290–296.
14. Cone R, Mohan K, Thouless M, Corey L. Nosocomial transmission of rotavirus infection. *Pediatr Infect Dis J* 1988;7(2): 103–109.
15. Yannelli B, Qurevich I, Schoch PE, Cunha BA. Yield of stool cultures, ova and parasite tests, and *Clostridium difficile* determinations in nosocomial diarrheas. *Am J Infect Control* 1988; 16:246–249.
16. Paton S, Nicolle L, Mwongera M, et al. *Salmonella* and *Shigella* gastroenteritis at a public teaching hospital in Nairobi, Kenya. *Infect Control Hosp Epidemiol* 1991;12:710–717.
17. Hughes JM, Jarvis WR. Nosocomial gastrointestinal infections. In: R Wenzel, ed. *Prevention and control of nosocomial infections*. Baltimore: Williams & Wilkins, 1987;405–439.
18. Stamm WE, Weinstein RA, Dixon RE. Comparison of endemic and epidemic nosocomial infections. *Am J Med* 1981;70: 393–397.
19. Zaidi M, Ponce de Leon S, Ortiz RM, et al. Hospital-acquired diarrhea in adults: a prospective case-controlled study in Mexico. *Infect Control Hosp Epidemiol* 1991;12:349–355.
20. Lima NL, Guerrant RL, Kaiser DL, Germanson T, Farr BM. A retrospective cohort study of nosocomial diarrhea as a risk factor for nosocomial infection. *J Infect Dis* 1990;161:948–952.
21. Garibaldi RA, Burke J, Britt MR, Miller WA, Smith CB. Meatal colonization and catheter-associated bacteriuria. *N Engl J Med* 1980;303:316–318.
22. Schaeffer AJ, Chmiel J. Urethral meatal colonization in the pathogenesis of catheter-associated bacteriuria. *J Urol* 1983; 130:1096–1099.
23. Daifuku R, Stamm WE. Association of rectal and urethral colonization with urinary tract infection in patients with indwelling catheters. *JAMA* 1984;252:2028–2030.
24. Monti S, Opal SM, Palardy JE, Boyce JM. Nosocomial *C. difficile* diarrhea: risk factors, complications, and cost [Abstract]. Second Annual SHEA Meeting. Baltimore, MD, Apr 12–14, 1992.
25. Eisenstein BI. New molecular techniques for microbial epidemiology and the diagnosis of infectious diseases. *J Infect Dis* 1990;161:595–602.
26. McFarland LV, Mulligan ME, Kwok RYY, Stamm WE. Nosocomial acquisition of *Clostridium difficile* infection. *N Engl J Med* 1989;320:204–210.
27. Johnson S, Gerding DN, Olson MM, et al. Prospective controlled study of vinyl glove use to interrupt *Clostridium difficile* nosocomial transmission. *Am J Med* 1990;88:137–140.
28. Gerding DN, Olson MM, Peterson LR, et al. *Clostridium difficile* associated diarrhea and colitis in adults. A prospective case-controlled epidemiologic study. *Arch Intern Med* 1986; 146:95–100.
29. Struelens MJ, Maas A, Nonhoff C, et al. Control of nosocomial transmission of *Clostridium difficile* based on sporadic case surveillance. *Am J Med* 1991;91(Suppl 3B):138s–144s.
30. Gerding DN, Peterson LR, Johnson S. The silent sea of *C. difficile* [Abstract A80]. Third Decennial Internationl Conference of Nosocomial Infections. Atlanta, GA, July 31–Aug 3, 1990.
31. Kaatz GW, Gitlin SD, Schaberg DR, et al. Acquisition of *Clostridium difficile* from the hospital environment. *Am J Epidemiol* 1988;127:1289–1294.
32. Fekety R, Kim KH, Brown D, Batts DH, Cudmore M, Silva JJ. Epidemiology of antibiotic-associated colitis. Isolation of

diarrhea at a university hospital in northeastern Brazil (Abstract #1297). 33rd Interscience Conference on Antimicrobial Agents and Chemotherapy. New Orleans, LA, Oct 17–20, 1993.

Clostridium difficile from the hospital environment. *Am J Med* 1981;70:906–908.

33. Baine WB, Gangarosa EJ, Bennett JV, Barker WH Jr. Institutional salmonellosis. *J Infect Dis* 1973;128:357–360.

34. Rice PA, Craven PC, Wells JG. *Salmonella heidelberg* enteritis and bacteria: an epidemic on two pediatric wards. *Am J Med* 1976;60:509–516.

35. Hammami A, Arlet G, Ben Redjeb S, et al. Nosocomial outbreak of acute gastroenteritis in a neonatal intensive care unit in Tunisia caused by multiply drug resistant *Salmonella wien* producing SHV-2 beta-lactamase. *Eur J Clin Microbiol Infect Dis* 1991;10:641–646.

36. Linnemann CC Jr, Cannon CG, Staneck JL, McNeely BL. Prolonged epidemic of salmonellosis: use of trimethoprim–sulfamethoxazole for control. *Infect Control* 1985;6:221–225.

37. Haley CE, Guerrant RL. Institutional salmonellosis. *Asepsis* 1982;4:7–12.

38. Dwyer DW, Klein EG, Istre GR, Robinson MG, Neumann DA, McCoy GA. *Salmonella newport* infections transmitted by fiberoptic colonoscopy. *Gastrointest Endosc* 1987;33:84–87.

39. Standaert SM, Hutcheson RH, Schaffner W. Nosocomial transmission of salmonella gastroenteritis to laundry workers in a nursing home. *Infect Control Hosp Epidemiol* 1994;15:22–26.

40. Riley LW, Ceballos O, Tabuls LR, Fernandes de Toledo MR, Blake PA. The significance of hospitals as reservoirs for epidemic multiresistant *Salmonella typhimurium* causing infection in urban Brazilian children. *J Infect Dis* 1984;150:236–241.

41. Gellert GA, Waterman SH, Ewert D, et al. An outbreak of acute gastroenteritis caused by a small round structured virus in a geriatric convalescent facility. *Infect Control Hosp Epidemiol* 1990;11:459–464.

42. Sawyer LA, Murphy JJ, Kaplan JE, et al. 25- to 30-nm particle associated with a hospital outbreak of acute gastroenteritis with evidence for airborne transmission. *Am J Epidemiol* 1988;127:1261–1271.

43. Butcher I, Kudesia G, Gordon J, Miller J. Small round structured viruses and their spread [Letter]. *Lancet* 1989;1:443.

44. Weinstein RA, Stamm WE. Pseudoepidemics in hospital. *Lancet* 1977;2:862–864.

45. Datta N. Drug resistance and R factor in the bowel bacteria of London patients before and after admission to hospital. *Br Med J* 1969;2:407–411.

46. McGowan JE. Antimicrobial resistance in hospital organisms and its relation to antibiotic use. *Rev Infect Dis* 1983;5:1033–1048.

47. Isameel NA. Resistance of bacteria from human faecal flora to antimicrobial agents. *J Trop Med Hyg* 1993;96:51–55.

48. Reves RR, Fong M, Pickering LK, Bartlett AI, Alvarez M, Murray BE. Risk factors for fecal colonization with trimethoprim-resistant and multiresistant *E coli* among children in day-care centers in Houston, Texas. *Antimicrob Agent Chemother* 1990;34:1429–1434.

49. Datta N, Faiers MC, Reeves WS, Brumfitt W, Orskov F, Orskov I. R-factors in *Escherichia coli* in faeces after oral chemotherapy in general practice. *Lancet* 1971;1:321–315.

50. Van der Auwesa P, Defresne N, Grenier P, Meunier F. Emergence of resistant (R) *Enterococcus faecium* and coagulase negative staphylococci (CNS) in fecal flora of volunteers receiving teicoplanin [Abstract 258]. 30th Interscience Conference of Antimicrobial Agents and Chemotherapy. Atlanta, GA, 1990.

51. Spera RV Jr, Farber BF. Multiply-resistant *Enterococcus faecium*. The nosocomial pathogen of the 1990s. *JAMA* 1992;268(18):2563–2564.

52. Brown E, Talbot GH, Axelrod P, Provencher M, Hoegg C. Risk factors for *Clostridium difficile* toxin-associated diarrhea. *Infect Control Hosp Epidemiol* 1990;11:283–290.

53. Simmons BP, Gelfand MS, Haas M, Metts C, Ferguson J. *Enterobacter sakazakii* infections in neonates associated with intrinsic contamination of a powdered infant formula. *Infect Control Hosp Epidemiol* 1989;10:398–401.

54. Mentzing LO, Ringertz O. *Salmonella* infection in tourists. II. Prophylaxis against salmonellosis. *Acta Pathol Microbiol Scand* 1968;74:405–413.

55. Thibault A, Miller MA, Gaese C. Risk factors for the develop-

ment of *Clostridium difficile*-associated diarrhea during a hospital outbreak. *Infect Control Hosp Epidemiol* 1991;12:345–348.

56. Villarino ME, Vugia DJ, Bean NH, Jarvis WR, Hughes JM. Foodborne disease prevention in health care facilities. In: Brachman P, Bennett J, eds. *Hospital infections*. Boston: Little, Brown, 1992;345–358.

57. Carter AO, Borezyk AA, Carlson JAK, et al. A severe outbreak of *Escherichia coli* O157:H7-associated hemorrhagic colitis in a nursing home. *N Engl J Med* 1987;327:1496–1500.

58. Levine WC, Smart JF, Archer DL, Bean NH, Tauxe RV. Foodborne disease outbreaks in nursing homes, 1975 through 1987. *JAMA* 1991;266:2105–2109.

59. Steere AC, Craven PJ, Hall WJ III, et al. Person-to-person spread of *Salmonella typhimurium* after a hospital common-source outbreak. *Lancet* 1975;1:319–321.

60. Centers for Disease Control. Update: multistate outbreak of *Escherichia coli* O157:H7 infections from hamburgers—western United States, 1992–1993. *MMWR Morb Mortal Wkly Rep* 1993;42:258–263.

61. MacDonald KL, Osterholm MT. The emergence of *Escherichia coli* O157:H7 infection in the United States. The changing epidemiology of foodborne disease. *JAMA* 1993;269:2264–2266.

62. Ryan CA, Tauxe RV, Hosek GW, et al. *Escherichia coli* O157:H7 diarrhea in a nursing home: clinical, epidemiological, and pathological findings. *J Infect Dis* 1986;154:631–638.

63. Ostroff SM, Griffin PM, Tauxe RV, et al. A statewide outbreak of *Escherichia coli* O157:H7 infections in Washington State. *Am J Epidemiol* 1990;132:239–247.

64. Levine MM, Edelman R. Enteropathogenic *Escherichia coli* of classic subtypes associated with infant diarrhea: epidemiology and pathogenesis. *Epidemiol Rev* 1984;6:31–51.

65. Giles C, Sangster G, Smith J. Epidemic gastroenteritis of infants in Aberdeen during 1947. *Arch Dis Child* 1949;24:45–53.

66. Levine MM, Bergquist EJ, Nalin DR, et al. *Escherichia coli* strains that cause diarrhea but do not produce heat-labile or heat-stable enterotoxins and are non-invasive. *Lancet* 1978;1:1119–1122.

67. Bower JR, Congeni BL, Cleary TG, et al. *Escherichia coli* O114: nonmotile as a pathogen in an outbreak of severe diarrhea associated with a day care center. *J Infect Dis* 1989;160:243–247.

68. DuPont HL, Ribner BS. Infectious gastroenteritis. In: Bennett J, Brachman P, eds. *Hospital infections*. Boston: Little, Brown, 1992;641–657.

69. Morris KJ, Rao GG. Conventional screening for enteropathogenic *Escherichia coli* in the U.K. Is it appropriate or necessary? *J Hosp Infect* 1992;21:163–167.

70. Western KA, St John RK, Shearer LA. Hospital infection control—an international perspective [Editorial]. *Infect Control* 1982;3:453–455.

71. Ryder RW, Wachsmuth IK, Buxton AE, et al. Infantile diarrhea produced by heat-stable enterotoxigenic *E. coli*. *N Engl J Med* 1976;295:849–853.

72. Gross RJ, Rowe B, Henderson A, Byatt ME, MacLaurin JC. A new *Escherichia coli* O-group, O159, associated with outbreaks of enteritis in infants. *Scand J Infect Dis* 1976;8:195–198.

73. Wachsmuth IK, Falkow S, Ryder RW. Plasmid-mediated properties of a heat-stable enterotoxin-producing *Escherichia coli* associated with infantile diarrhea. *Infect Immun* 1976;14:403–407.

74. DuPont HL. Nosocomial salmonellosis and shigellosis. *Infect Control Hosp Epidemiol* 1991;12:707–709.

75. Lyons RW, Samples CL, DeSilva HN, Ross KA, Julian EM, Checko PJ. An epidemic of resistant *Salmonella* in a nursery. *JAMA* 1980;243:346–347.

76. Chmel H, Armstrong D. *Salmonella oslo*: a focal outbreak in a hospital. *Am J Med* 1976;60:203–208.

77. Buchwald DS, Blaser MJ. A review of human salmonellosis: II. Duration of excretion following infection with nontyphi *Salmonella*. *Rev Infect Dis* 1984;6:345–356.

78. Musher DM, Rubenstein AD. Permanent carriers of nontyphoidal salmonellae. *Arch Intern Med* 1973;132:869–872.

79. Pether JVS, Scott RHD. *Salmonella* carriers: are they danger-

ous? A study to identify finger contamination with salmonellae by convalescent carriers. *J Infect* 1982;5:81–88.

80. McCall CE, Martin WT, Boring JR. Efficiency of cultures of rectal swabs and fecal specimens in detecting *Salmonella* carriers: correlation with numbers of salmonellae excreted. *J Hyg (Lond)* 1966;64:261–269.

81. Perkins JC, Devetski RL, Dowling HF. Ampicillin in the treatment of *Salmonella* carriers. Report of six cases and summary of the literature. *Arch Intern Med* 1966;118:528–533.

82. Simon HJ, Miller RC. Ampicillin in the treatment of chronic typhoid carriers. Report of fifteen treated cases and a review of the literature. *N Engl J Med* 1966;274:807–815.

83. Ferreccio C, Morris JG Jr, Valdivieso C, et al. Efficacy of ciprofloxicin in the treatment of chronic typhoid carriers. *J Infect Dis* 1988;157:1235–1239.

84. Tauxe RV, Hassan FL, Findeisen KO, Sharrar RG, Blake PA. Salmonellosis in nurses: lack of transmission to patients. *J Infect Dis* 1988;157:370–373.

85. Askerkoff B, Bennett JV. Effect of antibiotic therapy in acute salmonellosis on the fecal excretion of salmonellae. *N Engl J Med* 1969;281:636–640.

86. Pavia AT, Shipman LD, Wells JG, et al. Epidemiologic evidence that prior antimicrobial exposure decreases resistance to infection by antimicrobial-sensitive *Salmonella*. *J Infect Dis* 1990;161:255–260.

87. Maiorini E, Lopez EL, Morrow AL, et al. Multiply resistant nontyphoidal *Salmonella* gastroenteritis in children. *Pediatr Infect Dis* 1993;12:139–143.

88. DuPont HL, Levine MM, Hornick RB, Formal SB. Inoculum size in shigellosis and implications for expected mode of transmission. *J Infect Dis* 1989;159:1126–1128.

89. DuPont HL, Gangarosa EJ, Reller LB, et al. Shigellosis in custodial institutions. *Am J Epidemiol* 1970;92:172–179.

90. Salzman TC, Scher CD, Moss R. Shigellae with transferable drug resistance: outbreak in a nursery for premature infants. *Pediatr Res* 1967;71:21–26.

91. Weissman JB, Hutcheson RH. Shigellosis transmitted by nurses. *South Med J* 1976;69:1341–1346.

92. Lee LA, Taylor J, Carter GP, et al. *Yersinia enterocolitica* O: 3: an emerging cause of pediatric gastroenteritis in the United States. *J Infect Dis* 1991;163:660–663.

93. Jarvis WR. *Yersinia enterocolitica:* a new or unrecognized nosocomial pathogen? [Editorial]. *Infect Control Hosp Epidemiol* 1992;13:137–138.

94. Shayegani M, Morse D, DeForge I, Root T, Parsons LM, Maupin PS. Microbiology of a major foodborne outbreak of gastroenteritis caused by *Yersinia enterocolitica* serogroup O:8. *J Clin Microbiol* 1983;17:35–40.

95. Lee LA, Gerber AR, Lonsway DR, et al. *Yersinia enterocolitica* O:3 infections in infants and children associated with household preparation of chitterlings. *N Engl J Med* 1990;322: 984–987.

96. Tacket CO, Ballard J, Harris N, et al. An outbreak of *Yersinia enterocolitica* infections caused by contaminated tofu (soybean curd). *Am J Epidemiol* 1985;121:705–711.

97. Aber RC, McCarthy MA, Berman R, DeMelfi T, Witte E. An outbreak of *Yersinia enterocolitica* gastrointestinal illness among members of a Brownie troop in Centre County, Pennyslvania [Abstract 860]. 22nd Interscience Conference on Antimicrobial Agents and Chemotherapy. Miami Beach, FL, Oct 4–6, 1982.

98. Tauxe RV, Vandepitte J, Wauters G, et al. *Yersinia enterocolitica* infections and pork: the missing link. *Lancet* 1987;1: 1129–1132.

99. Tipple MA, Bland LA, Murphy JJ, et al. Sepsis associated with transfusion of red cells contaminated with *Yersinia enterocolitica*. *Transfusion* 1990;30:207–213.

100. Centers for Disease Control. *Yersinia enterocolitica* bacteremia and endotoxin shock associated with red blood cell transfusions—United States, 1991. *MMWR Morb Mortal Wkly Rep* 1991;40:176–178.

101. Rutnam S, Mercer E, Picco B, Parsons S, Butler R. A nosocomial outbreak of diarrheal disease due to *Yersinia enterocolitica* serotype O:5; biotype 1. *J Infect Dis* 1982;145:242–247.

102. Toivanen P, Toivanen A, Olkkonen L, Aantaa S. Hospital outbreak of *Yersinia enterocolitica* infections. *Lancet* 1973;1: 801–803.

103. Cannon CG, Linnemann CC Jr. *Yersinia enterocolitica* infections in hospitalized patients: the problem of hospital-acquired infections. *Infect Control Hosp Epidemiol* 1992;13:139–143.

104. Blaser MJ, Wells JG, Feldman RA, Pollard RA, Aller JR, Group CDDS. *Campylobacter enteritis* in the United States: a multicenter study. *Ann Intern Med* 1983;98:360–365.

105. Riley LW, Finch MJ. Results of a first year of surveillance of *Campylobacter* infections in the United States. *J Infect Dis* 1985;151:956–959.

106. Tauxe RV, Deming MS, Blake PA. *Campylobacter jejuni* infections on college campuses: a national survey. *Am J Public Health* 1985;75:659–660.

107. Pepersack F, Prigogyne T, Butzler JP, Yourassowsky E. *Campylobacter jejuni* post-transfusional septicaemia [Letter]. *Lancet* 1979;2:911.

108. Karmali MA, Norrish B, Lior H, Heyes B, Monteath A, Montgomery H. *Campylobacter* enteritis in a neonatal nursery. *J Infect Dis* 1984;149:847–877.

109. Guarino A, Capano G, Malamisura B, Alessio M, Guandalini S, Rubin A. Production of *Escherichia coli* STa-like heat-stable enterotoxin by *Citrobacter freundii* isolated from humans. *J Med Microbiol* 1987;25:110–114.

110. Guerrant RL, Dickens MD, Wenzel RP, Kapikian AZ. Toxigenic bacterial diarrhea: nursery outbreak involving multiple bacterial strains. *J Pediatr* 1976;89:885–891.

111. Moyer NP. Clinical significance of *Aeromonas* species isolated from patients with diarrhea. *J Clin Microbiol* 1987;25: 2044–2048.

112. Morgan DR, Johnson PC, DuPont HL, Satterwhite TK, Wood LV. Lack of correlation between known virulence properties of *Aeromonas hydrophila* and enteropathogenicity for humans. *Infect Immun* 1985;50:62–65.

113. Chakraborty T, Montenegro MA, Sanyal SC, Helmuth R, Bulling E, Timmis KN. Cloning of the enterotoxin gene from *Aeromonas hydrophila* provides conclusive evidence of production of a cytotonic cytotoxin. *Infect Immun* 1984;46:435–441.

114. Shimada T, Sakazaki R, Horigome K, Uesaka Y, Niwano K. Production of cholera-like enterotoxin by *Aeromonas hydrophila*. *Jpn J Med Sci Biol* 1984;37:141–144.

115. Pazzaglia G, Sack RB, Bourgeois AL, Froelich J, Eckstein J. Diarrhea and intestinal invasiveness of *Aeromonas* strains in the removable intestinal tie rabbit model. *Infect Immun* 1990; 58:1924–1931.

116. Altwegg M, Geiss HK. *Aeromonas* as a human pathogen. *Crit Rev Microbiol* 1989;16:253–286.

117. Pazzaglia G, Sack RB, Salazar E, et al. High frequency of coinfecting enteropathogens in *Aeromonas*-associated diarrhea of hospitalized Peruvian infants. *J Clin Microbiol* 1991;29: 1151–1156.

118. Hazen TC, Fliermans CB, Hirsch RP, Esch GW. Prevalence and distribution of *Aeromonas hydrophila* in the United States. *Appl Environ Microbiol* 1978;36:731–738.

119. Schorling JB, Wanke CA, Schorling SK, McAuliffe JF, de Souza MA, Guerrant RL. A prospective study of persistent diarrhea among children in an urban Brazilian slum. *Am J Epidemiol* 1990;132:144–156.

120. Millership SE, Stephenson JR, Tabaqchalis S. Epidemiology of *Aeromonas* species in a hospital. *J Hosp Infect* 1988;11: 169–175.

121. Mellersh AR, Norman P, Smith GH. *Aeromonas hydrophila:* an outbreak of hospital infection. *J Hosp Infect* 1984;5: 425–430.

122. Bloom HG, Bottone EJ. *Aeromonas hydrophila* diarrhea in a long-term care setting. *J Am Geriatr Soc* 1990;38:804–806.

123. Farber JM, Peterkin PI. *Listeria monocytogenes:* a foodborne pathogen. *Microbiol Rev* 1991;55:476–511.

124. Schwartz B, Ciesielski CA, Broome CV, et al. Association of sporadic listeriosis with consumption of uncooked hot dogs and undercooked chicken. *Lancet* 1988;2:779–782.

125. Fleming DW, Cochi SL, MacDonald KL, et al. Pasteurized

milk as a vehicle of infection in an outbreak of listeriosis. *N Engl J Med* 1985;312:404–407.

126. Linnan MJ, Mascola L, Lou XD, et al. Epidemic listeriosis associated with Mexican-style cheese. *N Engl J Med* 1988;319: 823–829.

127. Schlech WF III, Lavigne PM, Bortolussi RA, et al. Epidemic listeriosis—evidence for transmission by food. *N Engl J Med* 1983;308:203–206.

128. Gellin BG, Broome CV, Bibb WF, Weaver RE, Gaventa S, Mascola L. The epidemiology of listeriosis in the United States—1986. *Am J Epidemiol* 1991;133:392–401.

129. Nieman RE, Lorber B. Listeriosis in adults: a changing pattern. Report of eight cases and review of the literature, 1968–1978. *Rev Infect Dis* 1980;2:207–227.

130. McLauchlin J. Human listeriosis in Britain 1967–1985: a summary of 772 cases. 1. Listeriosis during pregnancy and in the newborn. *Epidemiol Infect* 1990;104:181–189.

131. MacGowan AP, Cartlidge PH, MacLeod F, McLaughlin J. Maternal listeriosis in pregnancy without fetal or neonatal infection. *J Infect* 1991;22:55–57.

132. Schwartz B, Hexter D, Broome DV, et al. Investigation of an outbreak of listeriosis: a new hypothesis for the etiology of epidemic *Listeria monocytogenes* infections. *J Infect Dis* 1989; 159:680–685.

133. Lamont RJ, Postlethwaite R, MacGowan AP. *Listeria monocytogenes* and its role in human infection. *J Infect* 1988;17:7–28.

134. Ho JL, Shands KN, Friedland G, Eckind P, Fraser DW. An outbreak of type 4b *Listeria monocytogenes* infection involving patients from eight Boston hospitals. *Arch Intern Med* 1986; 146:520–524.

135. Schuchat A, Lizano C, Broome CV, Swaminathan B, Kim C, Winn K. Outbreak of neonatal listeriosis associated with mineral oil. *Pediatr Infect Dis J* 1991;10:183–189.

136. Nelson KE, Warren D, Tomasi AM, Raju TN, Vidyasagar D. Transmission of neonatal listeriosis in a delivery room. *Am J Dis Child* 1985;139:903–905.

137. Bibb WF, Schwartz B, Gellin BG, Plikaytis BD, Weaver RE. Analysis of *Listeria monocytogenes* by multilocus enzyme electrophoresis and application of the method to epidemiologic investigations. *Int J Food Microbiol* 1989;8:233–239.

138. Bryan FL. What the sanitarian should know about staphylococci and salmonellae in non-dairy products. 1. Staphylococci. *J Milk Food Technol* 1968;31:110–116.

139. Batts DH, Silva J, Fekety R. Staphylococcal enterocolitis. In: Nelson J, Grassi C, eds. *Current chemotherapy and infectious disease.* Washington, DC: American Society for Microbiology, 1980;944–945.

140. Lusk RH, Fekety R, Silva J, Browne RA, Ringler DH, Abrams GD. Clindamycin-induced enterocolitis in hamsters. *J Infect Dis* 1978;137:464–475.

141. Rifkin GD, Fekety FR, Silva J, Sack RB. Antibiotic-associated colitis: implication of a toxin neutralized by *Clostridium sordelli* antitoxin. *Lancet* 1977;2:1103–1106.

142. Bartlett JG. Antibiotic-associated pseudomembranous colitis. *Rev Infect Dis* 1979;1:530–539.

143. Lima AAM, Lyerly DM, Wilkins TD, Innes DJ, Guerrant RL. Effects of *Clostridium difficile* toxins A and B in rabbit small and large intestine in vivo and on cultured cells in vitro. *Infect Immun* 1988;56:582–588.

144. Bartlett JG. Antibiotic-associated diarrhea. *Clin Infect Dis* 1992;15:573–581.

145. Peterson LR, Olson MM, Shanholtzer CJ, Gerding DN. Results of a prospective, 18-month clinical evaluation of culture, cytotoxin testing, and culturette brand (CDT) latex testing in the diagnosis of *Clostridium difficile*-associated diarrhea. *Diagn Microbiol Infect Dis* 1988;10:85–91.

146. Shanholtzer CJ, Willard KE, Holter JJ, Olson MM, Gerding DN, Peterson LR. Comparison of VIDAS *C. difficile* toxin A immunoassay (CDA) with *C. difficile* culture, cytotoxin, and latex test. *J Clin Microbiol* 1992;30:1837–1840.

147. Barbut F, Kajzer C, Planas N, Petit JC. Comparison of three enzyme immunoassays, a cytotoxicity assay and toxigenic culture for the diagnosis of *Clostridium difficile*-associated diarrhea. *J Clin Microbiol* 1993;31:963–967.

148. Peterson LR, Kelly PJ. Role of the clinical microbiology laboratory in the management of *Clostridium difficile*-associated diarrhea. *Infect Dis Clin North Am* 1993;7:277–293.

149. Doern GV, Coughlin RT, Wu L. Laboratory diagnosis of *Clostridium difficile*-associated gastrointestinal disease: comparison of monoclonal antibody enzyme immunoassay for toxins A and B with a monoclonal antibody enzyme immunoassay for toxin A only and two cytotoxicity assays. *J Clin Microbiol* 1992;30:2042–2046.

150. Kato N, Ou C-Y, Kato H, et al. Identification of toxigenic *Clostridium difficile* in stool specimens by the polymerase chain reaction. *J Infect Dis* 1993;162:455–458.

151. Gumerlock PH, Tary YJ, Weiss JB, Silva J Jr. Specific detection of toxigenic strains of *Clostridium difficile* in stool specimens. *J Clin Microbiol* 1993;31:507–511.

152. George WL, Sutter VL, Citron D, Finegold SM. Selective and differential medium for isolation of *Clostridium difficile*. *J Clin Microbiol* 1979;9:214–219.

153. Wilson KH, Kennedy MJ, Fekety R. Use of sodium taurocholate to enhance spore recovery on a medium selective for *Clostridium difficile*. *J Clin Microbiol* 1982;15:443–446.

154. Clabots CR, Gerding SJ, Olson MM, Peterson LR, Gerding DN. Detection of asymptomatic *Clostridium difficile* carriage by an alcohol shock procedure. *J Clin Microbiol* 1989;27: 2386–2387.

155. Riley TV, Brazier JS, Hassan H, Williams K, Phillips KD. Comparison of alcohol shock enrichment and selective enrichment for the isolation of *Clostridium difficile*. *Epidemiol Infect* 1987;99:355–359.

156. Teasley DG, Gerding DN, Olson MM, et al. Prospective randomized trial of metronidazole versus vancomycin for *Clostridium difficile*-associated diarrhoea and colitis. *Lancet* 1983;2: 1043–1046.

157. Johnson S, Homann SR, Bettin KM, et al. Treatment of asymptomatic *Clostridium difficile* carriers (fecal excretors) with vancomycin or metronidazole. A randomized, placebo controlled trial. *Ann Intern Med* 1992;117:297–302.

158. Brooks SE, Veal RO, Kramer M, Dore L, Schupf N, Adachi M. Reduction in the incidence of *Clostridium difficile*-associated diarrhea in an acute care hospital and a skilled nursing facility following replacement of electronic thermometers with single-use disposables. *Infect Control Hosp Epidemiol* 1992;13: 98–103.

159. Shandera WX, Tacket CO, Blake PA. Food poisoning due to *Clostridium perfringens* in the United States. *J Infect Dis* 1983; 147:167–170.

160. Hall HE, Angelotti R. *Clostridium perfringens* in meat and meat products. *Appl Microbiol* 1965;13:352–357.

161. Peterson LR, Musher R, Cooper GH, Bruce AR, Hadler JL. A large *Clostridium perfringens* foodborne outbreak with an unusual attack rate pattern. *Am J Epidemiol* 1988;127:605–611.

162. Hobbs BC. *Clostridium perfringens* and *Bacillus cereus* infections. In: Riemann H, ed. *Foodborne infections and intoxications.* New York: Academic Press, 1969;131–173.

163. Larson HE, Borriello SP. Infectious diarrhea due to *Clostridium perfringens*. *J Infect Dis* 1988;157:390–391.

164. Schwartz JN, Hamilton JP, Fekety R, et al. Ampicillin-induced enterocolitis: implication of toxigenic *Clostridium perfringens* type C. *J Pediatr* 1980;97:661–663.

165. Kosloske AM, Ball WS Jr, Umland E, Skipper B. Clostridial necrotizing enterocolitis. *J Pediatr Surg* 1985;20:155–159.

166. Sturm R, Staneck JL, Stauffer LR, Neblett WW. Neonatal necrotizing enterocolitis associated with penicillin-resistant, toxigenic *Clostridium butyricum*. *Pediatrics* 1980;66:928–931.

167. Murrell TGC, Egerton JR, Rampling A, Samels J, Walker PD. The ecology and epidemiology of the pig-bel syndrome in man in New Guinea. *J Hyg (Lond)* 1966;64:375–396.

168. Guerrant RL, Kirchoff LV, Shields DS, et al. Prospective study of diarrheal diseases in northeastern Brazil: patterns of disease, nutritional impact, and risk factors. *J Infect Dis* 1983;148: 986–997.

169. Ho MS, Glass RI, Pinsky PF, Anderson LJ. Rotavirus as a cause of diarrheal morbidity and mortality in the United States. *J Infect Dis* 1988;158:1112–1116.

170. Gurwith M, Wenman W, Hinde D, Feltham S, Greenberg H. A prospective study of rotavirus infection in infants and young children. *J Infect Dis* 1981;144:218–224.

171. Matson DO, Estes MK. Impact of rotavirus at a large pediatric hospital. *J Infect Dis* 1990;162:598–604.

172. Wenman WM, Hinde D, Feltham S. Rotavirus in adults: results of a prospective family study. *N Engl J Med* 1979;301:303–306.

173. Flewett TH. Rotavirus in the home and hospital nursery. *Br Med J* 1983;287:568–569.

174. Sattar SA, Lloyd-Evans N, Springthorpe VA. Institutional outbreaks of rotavirus diarrhoea: potential role of fomites and environmental surfaces as vehicles for virus transmission. *J Hyg (Lond)* 1986;96:277–289.

175. Estes MK, Palmer EL, Obijeski JF. Rotaviruses: a review. *Curr Top Microbiol Immunol* 1983;105:123–184.

176. Sattar SA, Raphael RA, Lochnan H, Springthorpe VS. Rotavirus inactivation by chemical disinfectants and antiseptics used in hospitals. *Can J Microbiol* 1983;29:1464–1469.

177. Tan JA, Schnagel RD. Inactivation of a rotavirus by disinfectants. *Med J Aust* 1981;1:19–23.

178. Haug KW, Orstavik I, Kuelstad G. Rotavirus infections in families. *Scand J Infect Dis* 1978;10:265–269.

179. Chrystie IL, Totterdell BM, Banatvala JE. Asymptomatic endemic rotavirus infection in the newborn. *Lancet* 1978;1:1176–1178.

180. Bishop RI, Hewstone AS, Davidson GP, Townnley RRW, Holmes IH, Ruck BJ. An epidemic of diarrhoea in human neonates involving a reovirus-like agent and "enteropathogenic" serotypes of *E. coli*. *J Clin Pathol* 1976;29:46–49.

181. Rodriguez WJ, Kim HW, Brandt CD, Fletcher AB, Parrott RH. Rotavirus: a cause of nosocomial infection in the nursery. *J Pediatr* 1982;101:274–277.

182. Samadi AR, Huq MI, Ahmed OS. Detection of rotavirus in handwashings of attendants of children with diarrhoea. *Br Med J* 1983;286:188.

183. Cubitt WD, Holzel H. Outbreak of rotavirus infection in a long-stay ward of a geriatric hospital. *J Clin Pathol* 1980;33:306–308.

184. Stals F, Walther FJ, Bruggeman CA. Faecal and pharyngeal shedding of rotavirus and rotavirus IgA in children with diarrhea. *J Med Virol* 1984;14:333–339.

185. Santosham M, Yolken RN, Quiroz E, et al. Detection of rotavirus in respiratory secretions of children with pneumonia. *J Pediatr* 1983;103:583–585.

186. Holzel H, Cubitt DW, McSwiggen DA, Sanderson PJ, Church J. An outbreak of rotavirus infection among adults in a cardiology ward. *J Infect* 1980;2:33–37.

187. Marrie TJ, Lee SHS, Faulkner RS, Ethier J, Young CH. Rotavirus infection in a geriatric population. *Arch Intern Med* 1982;142:313–316.

188. Saulsbury FT, Winkelstein JA, Yolken RH. Chronic rotavirus infection in immunodeficiency. *J Pediatr* 1980;97:61–65.

189. Peigue-Lafeuille H, Henquell C, Chambon M, Gazuy N, DeChamps C, Cluzel R. Nosocomial rotavirus infections in adult renal transplant recipients. *J Hosp Infect* 1991;18:67–70.

190. Miotti PG, Eiden J, Yolken RH. Comparative efficacy of commercial immunoassays for the diagnosis of rotavirus gastroenteritis during the course of infection. *J Clin Microbiol* 1985;22:693–698.

191. Doern GV, Herrmann JE, Henderson P. Detection of rotavirus with a new polyclonal antibody enzyme immunoassay (Rotazyme II) and a commercial latex agglutination test (Rotalex): comparison with a monoclonal antibody enzyme immunoassay. *J Clin Microbiol* 1986;23:226–229.

192. Wilde J, Yolken RH, Willoughby R, Eiden J. Improved detection of rotavirus shedding by polymerase chain reaction. *Lancet* 1991;337:323–326.

193. Spencer E, Avendano LF, Araya M. Characteristics and analysis of electropherotypes of human rotavirus isolated in Chile. *J Infect Dis* 1983;148:41–48.

194. Steele HM, Garnham S, Beards GM, Brown DWG. Investigation of an outbreak of rotavirus infection in geriatric patients by serotyping and polyacrylamide gel electrophoresis (PAGE). *J Med Virol* 1992;37:132–136.

195. Chanock SJ, Wenske EA, Fields BN. Human rotaviruses and genomic RNA [Editorial]. *J Infect Dis* 1983;48:49–50.

196. Clark IN, McCrae MA. Structural analysis of electrophoretic variation in the genomic profiles of rotavirus field isolates. *Infect Immun* 1982;36:492–497.

197. Rodriguez WJ, Kim HW, Brandt CD, Gardner MK, Parrott RH. The use of electrophoresis of RNA from human rotavirus to establish identity of strains involved in outbreaks in a tertiary care nursery. *J Infect Dis* 1983;148:34–40.

198. Konno T, Sato T, Suzuki H, et al. Changing RNA patterns in rotavirus of human origin: demonstration of a single dominant pattern at the start of an epidemic and various patterns thereafter. *J Infect Dis* 1984;149:683–687.

199. Gaggero A, Avendano LF, Fernandex J, Spencer E. Nosocomial transmission of rotavirus from patients admitted with diarrhea. *J Clin Microbiol* 1992;30:3294–3297.

200. Vesikari T. Clinical trials of live oral rotavirus vaccines; the Finnish experience. *Vaccine* 1993;11:255–261.

201. Flewett TH, Bryden AS, Davies H, Morris CA. Epidemic viral enteritis in a long-stay children's ward. *Lancet* 1975;1:4–5.

202. Uhnoo I, Wadell G, Svensson L, Johansson ME. Importance of enteric adenoviruses 40 and 41 in acute gastroenteritis in infants and young children. *J Clin Microbiol* 1984;20:365–372.

203. Horwitz MS. Adenoviruses. In: Fields B, Knipe D, eds. *Virology*. New York: Raven Press, 1990;1723–1740.

204. Van R, Wun C-C, O'Ryan ML, Matson DO, Jackson L, Pickering LK. Outbreaks of human enteric adenovirus types 40 and 41 in Houston day care centers. *J Pediatr* 1992;120:516–521.

205. Brandt CD, Kim HW, Rodriguez WJ, et al. Adenovirus and pediatric gastroenteritis. *J Infect Dis* 1983;151:437–443.

206. Shinozak T, Araki K, Ushijima H, Fujii R. Antibody response to enteric adenovirus types 40 and 41 in sera of various age groups. *J Clin Microbiol* 1987;25:1679–1682.

207. Rodriguez WJ, Kim HW, Brandt CD, et al. Fecal adenoviruses from a longitudinal study of families in metropolitan Washington, DC: laboratory, clinical and epidemiologic observations. *J Pediatr* 1985;107:514–520.

208. Centers for Disease Control. Viral agents of gastroenteritis: public health importance and outbreak management. *MMWR Morb Mortal Wkly Rep* 1990;39(RR-5):1–24.

209. Yolken RH, Lawrence F, Leister F, Takiff HE, Strauss SE. Gastroenteritis with enteric type adenovirus in hospitalized infants. *J Pediatr* 1982;101:21–26.

210. Kotloff KL, Losonsky GA, Morris JG Jr, Wasserman SS, Singh-Naz N, Levine MM. Enteric adenovirus infection and childhood diarrhea: an epidemiologic study in three clinical settings. *Pediatrics* 1989;84:219–225.

211. Zahorsky J. Hyperemesis hiemis or the winter vomiting disease. *Arch Pediatr* 1929;46:391–395.

212. Adler JL, Zickl R. Winter vomiting disease. *J Infect Dis* 1969;119:668–673.

213. Kapikian AZ, Wyatt RG, Dolin R, Thornhill TS, Kalica AR, Chanock RM. Visualization by immune electron microscopy of a 27nm particle associated with acute infectious nonbacterial gastroenteritis. *J Virol* 1972;10:1075–1081.

214. Kaplan JE, Gary GW, Baron RC, Schonberger LB, Feldman R, Greenberger HB. Epidemiology of Norwalk gastroenteritis and the role of Norwalk virus in outbreaks of acute nonbacterial gastroenteritis. *Ann Intern Med* 1982;96:756–761.

215. Herrmann JE, Nowak NA, Blacklow NR. Detection of Norwalk virus in stools by enzyme immunoassay. *J Med Virol* 1985;17:127–133.

216. DeLeon R, Matsui SM, Barrie RS, et al. Detection of Norwalk virus in stool specimens by reverse transcriptase polymerase chain reaction and nonradioactive oligoprobes. *J Clin Microbiol* 1992;30:3151–3157.

217. Nakata S, Estes MK, Chiba S. Detection of human calicivirus antigen and antibody by enzyme-linked immunosorbent assays. *J Clin Microbiol* 1988;26:2001–2005.

218. Herrmann JE, Nowak NA, Perron-Henry DM, Hudson RW, Cubitt WD, Blacklow NR. Diagnosis of astrovirus gastroenteritis by antigen detection with monoclonal antibodies. *J Infect Dis* 1990;161:226–229.

219. Taylor JW, Gary GW Jr, Greenberg HB. Norwalk-related viral

gastroenteritis due to contaminated drinking water. *Am J Epidemiol* 1981;114:584–592.

220. Griffin MR, Surowiec JJ, McCloskey DI, et al. Foodborne Norwalk virus. *Am J Epidemiol* 1982;115:178–184.

221. Oshiro LS, Haley CE, Roberto RR, et al. A 27nm virus isolated during an outbreak of acute infectious nonbacterial gastroenteritis in a convalescent hospital: a possible new serotype. *J Infect Dis* 1981;143:791–795.

222. Pegues DA, Woernle CH. An outbreak of acute nonbacterial gastroenteritis in a nursing home. *Infect Control Hosp Epidemiol* 1993;14:87–94.

223. Kaplan J, Schonberger L, Varano G, Jackman N, Bled J, Gary GW. An outbreak of acute nonbacterial gastroenteritis in a nursing home. Demonstration of person-to-person transmission by temporal clustering of cases. *Am J Epidemiol* 1982;116:940–948.

224. Nime FA, Burek JD, Page DL, Holscher MA, Yardley JH. Acute enterocolitis in a human being infected with the protozoan *Cryptosporidium*. *Gastroenterology* 1976;70:592–598.

225. Meisel JL, Perea DR, Meligro C, Rubin CE. Overwhelming watery diarrhea associated with a *Cryptosporidium* in an immunosuppressed patient. *Gastroenterology* 1976;70:1156–1160.

226. Soave R, Armstrong D. *Cryptosporidium* and cryptosporidiosis. *Rev Infect Dis* 1986;8:1012–1023.

227. Current WL, Reese NC, Ernst JV, Bailey WS, Heyman MB, Weinstein WM. Human cryptosporidiosis in immunocompetent and immunodeficient persons: studies of an outbreak and experimental transmission. *N Engl J Med* 1983;308:1252–1257.

228. Fayer R, Ungar BLP. *Cryptosporidium* spp. and cryptosporidiosis. *Microbiol Rev* 1986;50:458–483.

229. Baxby D, Hart CA, Taylor C. Human cryptosporidiosis: a possible cause of hospital infection. *Br Med J* 1983;287:1760–1761.

230. Martino P, Gentile G, Caprioli A, et al. Hospital-acquired cryptosporidiosis in a bone marrow transplantation unit. *J Infect Dis* 1988;158:647–649.

231. Koch KL, Phillips DJ, Aber R, Current WL. Cryptosporidiosis in hospital personnel: evidence for person-to-person transmission. *Ann Intern Med* 1985;102:593–596.

232. Dryjanski J, Gold JW, Ritchie MT, Kurtz RC, Lim SL, Armstrong D. Cryptosporidiosis: case report in health team worker. *Am J Med* 1986;1986:751–752.

233. Jokipii L, Jokipii AMM. Timing of symptoms and oocyst excretion in human cryptosporidiosis. *N Engl J Med* 1986;315:1643–1647.

234. Tzipori S. *Cryptosporidium* in animals and humans. *Microbiol Rev* 1983;47:84–96.

235. Tzipori S. Cryptosporidiosis in humans and animals. *Microbiol Rev* 1983;47:84–86.

236. Sundermann CA, Lindsay DS, Blagburn BL. Evaluation of disinfectants for ability to kill avian *Cryptospordium* oocysts. *Companion Anim Pract* 1987;2:36–39.

237. Campbell I, Tzipori S, Hutchinson G, Angus KW. Effect of disinfectants on survival of cryptosporidal oocysts. *Vet Rec* 1982;111:414–415.

238. Henricksen SA, Pohlenz JFL. Staining of cryptosporidia by a modified Ziehl–Neelson technique. *Acta Vet Scand* 1981;22:594–596.

239. Ma P, Soave R. Three-step stool examination for cryptosporidiosis in 10 homosexual men with protracted watery diarrhea. *J Infect Dis* 1983;147:824–828.

240. Siddons CA, Chapman PS, Rush BA. Evaluation of an enzyme immunoassay kit for detecting *Cryptosporidium* in faeces and environmental samples. *J Clin Pathol* 1992;45:479–482.

241. Weber R, Bryan RT, Juranek DD. Improved stool concentration procedure for detection of cryptosporidium oocysts in fecal specimens. *J Clin Microbiol* 1992;30:2869–2873.

242. Ungar BL, Soave R, Fayer R, Nash TE. Enzyme immunoassay detection of immunoglobulin M and G antibodies to *Cryptosporidium* in immunocompetent and immunocompromised patients. *J Infect Dis* 1986;153:570–578.

243. Petri WA Jr, Ravdin JI. Amebiasis in institutionalized populations. In: Ravdin JI, ed. *Amebiasis*. New York: Wiley, 1988;576–581.

244. Smith PD, Lane HC, Gill VJ, et al. Intestinal infections in patients with the acquired immunodeficiency syndrome (AIDS). *Ann Intern Med* 1988;108:328–333.

245. Istre GR, Kreiss K, Hopkins RS, et al. An outbreak of amebiasis spread by colonic irrigation at a chiropractic clinic. *N Engl J Med* 1982;307:339–341.

246. Samuelson J, Acuna-Soto R, Reed S, Biagi F, Wirth D. DNA hybridization probe for clinical diagnosis of *Entamoeba histolytica*. *J Clin Microbiol* 1989;27:671–676.

247. Acuna-Soto R, Samuelson J, De Giralami P, et al. Application of polymerase chain reaction to the epidemiology of pathogenic and nonpathogenic *Entamoeba histolytica*. *Am J Trop Med Hyg* 1993;48:58–70.

248. Craun GF. Waterborne giardiasis in the United States 1965–1984. *Lancet* 1986;2:513–514.

249. Kent GP, Greenspan JR, Herndon JL, et al. Epidemic giardiasis caused by a contaminated public water supply. *Am J Public Health* 1988;78:139–143.

250. Pickering LK, Woodward WE, DuPont HL, Sullivan P. Occurrence of *Giardia lamblia* in children in day care centers. *J Pediatr* 1984;104:522–526.

251. Yoeli M, Most H, Hammond J, Scheinesson GP. Parasitic infection in a closed community: results of a 10 year survey in Willowbrook State Hospital. *Trans R Soc Trop Med Hyg* 1972;66:764–776.

252. White KE, Hedber CW, Edmonson LM, Jones DBW, Osterholm MT, MacDonald KL. An outbreak of giardiasis in a nursing home with evidence for multiple modes of transmission. *J Infect Dis* 1989;160:298–304.

253. Flanagan PA. Giardiasis—diagnosis, clinical course and epidemiology. A review. *Epidemiol Infect* 1992;109:1–22.

254. Hoff JC. Inactivation of microbial agents by chemical disinfectants. EPA-600/2-86-067. Cincinnati, OH: Water Engineering Research Laboratory, US Environmental Protection Agency, 1986.

255. Black RE, Dykes AC, Sinclair SP, Wells JG. Giardiasis in day-care centers: evidence of person-to-person transmission. *Pediatrics* 1977;60:486–491.

256. Black RE, Dykes AC, Anderson KE, et al. Handwashing to prevent diarrhea in day care centers. *Am J Epidemiol* 1982;113:445–451.

257. Paerregaard A, Kjelt K, Krasilnikoff PA. The diagnosis of childhood giardiasis. *J Pediatr Gastroenterol Nutr* 1990;10:275.

258. Bezjak B. Evaluation of a new technic for sampling duodenal contents in parasitologic diagnosis. *Am J Dig Dis* 1972;17:848–850.

259. Bendig DW. Diagnosis of giardiasis in infants and children by endoscopic brush cytology. *J Pediatr Gastroenterol Nutr* 1989;8:204–206.

260. Knisley CV, Engelkirk PG, Pickering LK, West MS, Janoff EN. Rapid detection of *Giardia* antigen in stool with the use of enzyme immunoassays. *Am J Clin Pathol* 1989;91:704–708.

261. Weiss JB, van Keulen H, Nash TE. Classification of subgroups of *Giardia lamblia* based on ribosomal DNA gene sequence using polymerase chain reaction. *Mol Biochem Parasitol* 1992;54:73–86.

262. Cohen R, Roth FJ, Delgado E, Ahearn DG, Kalser MH. Fungal flora of the normal human small and large intestine. *N Engl J Med* 1969;208:638–641.

263. Chretien JH, Garagusi VF. Current management of fungal enteritis. *Med Clin North Am* 1982;66:675–687.

264. Karabinis A, Hill C, Leclercq B, Tancrede C, Baume D, Andremont A. Risk factors for candidemia in cancer patients: a case–control study. *J Clin Microbiol* 1988;126:429–432.

265. Wey SB, Mori M, Pfaller MA, Woolson RF, Wenzel RP. Risk factors for hospital-acquired candidemia. A matched case–control study. *Arch Intern Med* 1989;149:2349–2353.

266. Wey SB, Mori M, Pfaller MA, Woolson RF, Wenzel RP. Hospital-acquired candidemia: the attributable mortality and excess length of stay. *Arch Intern Med* 1988;148:2642–2645.

267. Regan DR, Pfaller MA, Hollis RJ, Wenzel RP. Characterization of the sequence of colonization and nosocomial candidemia using DNA fingerprinting and a DNA probe. *J Clin Microbiol* 1990;28:2733–2738.

268. Stone HH, Kolb LD, Currie CA, Geheber CE, Cuzzell JZ.

Candida sepsis: pathogenesis and principles of treatment. *Ann Surg* 1974;179:697–711.

269. Krause W, Matheis H, Wulf K. Fungaemia and funguria after oral administration of *Candida albicans. Lancet* 1969;1: 598–599.

270. Gupta T, Ehrinpreis MN. *Candida*-associated diarrhea in hospitalized patients. *Gastroenterology* 1990;98:780–785.

271. Cutler JE, Friedman L, Milner KC. Biological and chemical characterization of toxic substances from *Candida albicans. Infect Immun* 1972;6:616–627.

272. Barnes GL, Bishop RF, Townley RRW. Microbial flora and disaccharidase depression in infantile gastroenteritis. *Acta Pediatr Scand* 1974;63:423–426.

273. Kozinn PJ, Taschdjian CL. Enteric candidiasis. *Pediatrics* 1962;30:71–85.

274. Margolis BD, Tsang T-K, Kuo D. Persistent diarrhea secondary to *Candida* overgrowth [Letter]. *Am J Gastroenterol* 1990; 85:329–330.

275. Pfaller MA. Epidemiological typing methods for mycoses. *Clin Infect Dis* 1992;14(Suppl)s4–s10.

276. Doebbling BN, Hollis RJ, Wenzel RP, Pfaller MA, Reagan DR. Method of *Candida* typing by contour-clamped homogeneous electric fields electrophoresis (CHEF) [Abstract]. Interscience Conference on Antimicrobial Agents and Chemotherapy. Anaheim, CA, Oct 11–14, 1992.

277. Pfaller MA, Cabezudo I, Hollis RJ, Huston B, Wenzel RP. The use of biotyping and DNA fingerprinting in typing *Candida albicans* from hospitalized patients. *Diagn Microbiol Infect Dis* 1990;13:481–489.

278. Pfaller MA, Cabezudo I, Buschelman B, et al. Value of the Hybritech ICON *Candida* assay in the diagnosis of invasive candidiasis in high-risk patients. *Diagn Microbiol Infect Dis* 1993;16:53–60.

279. Walsh TJ, Hathorn JW, Sobel JD, et al. Detection of circulating *Candida* enolase by immunoassay in patients with cancer and invasive candidiasis. *N Engl J Med* 1991;324:1026–1031.

280. Kealey GD, Heinle JA, Lewis RW II, Pfaller MA, Rosenquist MD. Value of *Candida* antigen assay in the diagnosis of systemic candidiasis in burn patients. *J Trauma* 1992;32:285–288.

281. Centers for Disease Control. Outline for surveillance and control of nosocomial infections. Feb. 1981.

282. Wenzel RP, Osterman CA, Hunting KJ, Gwaltney JM Jr. Hospital-acquired infections. I: Surveillance in a university hospital. *Am J Epidemiol* 1976;103:251–259.

283. Lima NL, Periera CRB, Souza IC, et al. Selective surveillance for nosocomial infections in a Brazilian hospital. *Infect Control Hosp Epidemiol* 1993;14:197–202.

284. Centers for Disease Control. Recommendations for precautions of HIV transmission in health care settings. *MMWR Morb Mortal Wkly Rep* 1987;36:s3–s18.

285. Conley JM, Hill S, Ross J, Lertzman J, Louie TJ. Handwashing practices in an intensive care unit: the effects of an educational program and its relationship to infection rates. *Am J Infect Control* 1989;17:303–339.

286. Doebbling BN, Pfaller MA, Houston AK, Wenzel RP. Removal of nosocomial pathogens from the contaminated glove: implica-

tions for glove reuse and handwashing. *Ann Intern Med* 1988; 109:394–398.

287. Doebbling BN, Stanley GL, Sheetz CT, et al. Comparative efficacy of alternative hand-washing agents in reducing nosocomial infections in intensive care units. *N Engl J Med* 1992;327: 88–93.

288. Simmons B, Bryant J, Neiman K, Spencer L, Arheart K. The role of handwashing in prevention of endemic intensive care unit infections. *Infect Control Hosp Epidemiol* 1990;11: 589–594.

289. Katoh M, Saito D, Noda T, et al. *Helicobacter pylori* may be transmitted through gastrofiberscope even after manual Hyamine washing. *Jpn J Cancer Res* 1993;84:117–119.

290. Langenberg W, Rauws EAJ, Oudbier JH, Tytgat GNJ. Patient-to-patient transmission of *Campylobacter pylori* infection by fiberscopic gastroduodenoscopy and biopsy. *J Infect Dis* 1990; 161:507–511.

291. Spaulding EH. Chemical disinfection of medical and surgical materials. In: Lawrence C, Block S, eds. *Disinfection, sterilization and preservation.* Philadelphia: Lea & Febiger, 1968; 517–531.

292. Gorse GJ, Messner RL. Infection control practices in gastrointestinal endoscopy in the United States. *Infect Control Hosp Epidemiol* 1991;12:289–296.

293. Favero MS. Strategies for disinfection and sterilization of endoscopes: the gap between basic principles and actual practice. *Infect Control Hosp Epidemiol* 1991;12:279–281.

294. Rutala WA. APIC guideline for selection and use of disinfectant. *Am J Infect Control* 1990;18:99–117.

295. Jonas G, Mahoney A, Murray J, Gertler S. Chemical colitis due to endoscope cleaning solutions: a mimic of pseudomembranous colitis. *Gastroenterology* 1988;95:1403–1408.

296. Alvarado CJ, Stolz SM, Maki DG. Nosocomial infections from contaminated endoscopes: a flawed automated endoscope washer: an investigation using molecular epidemiology. *Am J Med* 1991;91(Suppl 3B):272s–280s.

297. Jernigan JA, Giuliano K, Guerrant RL, Farr BM. Effect of disposable thermometer use on rates of nosocomial *Clostridium difficile* diarrhea and total nosocomial infections: a randomized controlled study [Abstract 62]. 33rd Interscience Conference on Antimicrobial Agents and Chemotherapy. New Orleans, LA, Oct 17–20, 1993.

298. Surawicz CM, Elmer GW, Speelman P, McFarland LV, Chinn J, van Belle G. Prevention of antibiotic associated diarrhea by *Saccharomyces boulardii:* a prospective study. *Gastroenterology* 1989;96:981–988.

299. Haley R, Emori T. The employee health service and infection control in U.S. hospitals, 1976–1977 II. *JAMA* 1981;246: 962–966.

300. Valenti WM. Employee work restrictions for infection control. *Infect Control* 1984;5:583–584.

301. Williams WW. Guideline for infection control in hospital personnel. *Infect Control* 1983;4:326–349.

302. Benenson AS. *Control of communicable diseases in man,* 15th ed. Washington, DC: American Public Health Association, 1990.

303. Bank HL, John JF, Atkins LM, Schmehl MK, Dratch RJ. Bactericidal action of modulated ultraviolet light on six groups of *Salmonella. Infect Control Hosp Epidemiol* 1991;12:486–489.

Infections of the Gastrointestinal Tract,
edited by M. J. Blaser, P. D. Smith, J. I. Ravdin,
H. B. Greenberg, and R. L. Guerrant
Raven Press, Ltd., New York © 1995.

CHAPTER 97

Responding to Changes in Host, Pathogen, and Environment

Roger A. Feldman

Many changes in the environment have impacted on enteric infections in humans. These include changes in the human host, with an increasing number of elderly persons whose immune responses are muted, and with increasing numbers of immunosuppressed persons following treatments for cancer, organ transplants, and human immunodeficiency virus (HIV) infection. There are changes in the ways foods are transported, delivered, and handled, so that some foods, which once came from many suppliers, may now come from only a few; foods that were locally produced may now be shipped half-way around the world; foods once only locally available may now be available worldwide; and foods once collected in local areas may now be collected throughout wide areas. There are, in addition, agents now associated with human infection that have in the past rarely been identified or were not known to be associated with human illness. All these changes have their effects on the frequency and character of human enteric infections, and many have been described in previous chapters. This chapter focuses on the effects of these changes in environment and comments on methods of control available to reduce associated risks.

MODIFIED RESERVOIRS

There have been changes in the reservoirs in which the infectious agents are located, and control methods that worked in the past are now ineffective or have yet to be developed. An example concerns *Vibrio cholerae* and its association with uncooked or partially cooked food, often seafood (1). For over 100 years, *V. cholerae* transmission has been associated with water, so that development and maintenance of a clean and protected water supply were appropriate ways to deal with control of *V. cholerae* infec-

tions (2). In some countries, further development of clean water supplies is limited by available finances (3), but aside from efforts at vaccination as a method of control (4), improving the clean water supply has been central to control activities. As described in the chapters by Bullerton and Calderwood and by Morris, which deal with *V. cholerae* infections, recent outbreaks of *V. cholerae* in Africa, Europe, South America, and North America have pointed to foods, often seafoods, as vehicles, with water as a reservoir (5). One control method is to effectively cook foods, particularly seafoods, but some of these foods lose their appeal when overcooked and remain a risk when partially cooked.

Another example has been the demonstration that chicken eggs with intact shells may serve as a reservoir for *Salmonella enteritidis* (6). Although it was well known that duck eggs could harbor salmonellae, intact-shell chicken eggs appeared to be an insignificant reservoir until quite recently (7–10). Whatever the explanation, and one possibility relates to the centralization of production of chickens, the world of commerce and the food preparation habits of the general public were not prepared to consider an intact chicken egg as a reservoir for an infectious agent. Mayonnaise, a variety of sauces, soft-boiled eggs, scrambled eggs, egg nogs, and other products utilizing raw eggs had been developed successfully when eggs were not a major reservoir for *Salmonella*. Present circumstances require either that the reservoir be eliminated or that food practices be changed. Neither of these is particularly easy to effect.

Hospital newborn and intensive care nurseries are places where both normal and seriously ill children can be treated safely. There were enteric disease outbreaks in newborn nurseries in developed countries in the 1940s (11), but surveillance and rigorous control measures reduced their frequency. However, some hospital newborn nurseries have become reservoirs for *Salmonella* infection. In Brazil (12), China (13), India (14), and elsewhere (15,16), contamination of a newborn nursery with *Salmonella* has produced a problem difficult to control.

R. A. Feldman: Department of Epidemiology and Medical Statistics, The London Hospital Medical College at QMW, London E1 4NS, England.

Modern microbiologic laboratories have occasionally played a role as a reservoir. To monitor the competence of a microbiologic laboratory, organisms were sent as unknowns from a central source to laboratories throughout the system. *Salmonella typhi,* multiresistant, often was chosen as one of these unknowns and was shipped to laboratories that rarely saw *S. typhi* from patients. One unexpected result was that laboratory technicians, and even their family members, became infected with the test strain (17).

Other reservoirs for enteric infections exist for which control measures are not yet easily developed. Spices and other dried condiments often become contaminated in the process of collection and drying, and this contamination may be maintained during bulking and subsequent shipment. Outbreaks associated with black pepper (18), dry coconut (19), chocolate (20,21), and many other condiments have been described. The most obvious method to control this reservoir is treatment of bulk materials before their distribution. A variety of methods, including radiation, have been tried (22), but none has been universally accepted.

These changes in enteric agent reservoirs pose new problems for control—either of the agent before it enters the reservoir, of control of the reservoir once contaminated, or of new ways of food preparation based on the knowledge that previously safe foods are no longer safe as once prepared.

MODIFIED HOST RESISTANCE

Although there are increasing uses of immunosuppressive therapy for cancer and organ transplants, and there is immunosuppression with HIV infection, the largest number of persons with modified host resistance are pregnant women, newborns, and the elderly. *Listeria* causes illness in all three of these latter groups and may be considered as a model foodborne organism, even though it does not typically cause clinical illness relating to the gastrointestinal tract. Although outbreaks are increasingly being reported, it is probable that reservoirs for *Listeria* are not now expanding. Control of *Listeria* in the environment has not been attempted, nor is there evidence of increased frequency of *Listeria* in the environment. The explanation of the *Listeria* outbreaks stems in part from the recent ability to identify the vehicles for *Listeria* infections. Following the outbreak of cabbage-associated listeriosis in Nova Scotia (23), a series of case–control studies, outbreak investigations, and laboratory studies identified a variety of foods associated with *Listeria* infections (24–27). Control of *Listeria* in soft cheese and in other vehicles identified as significant in foodborne listeriosis is difficult, since the sources of *Listeria* are multiple. Pasteurization is modestly effective, but changes in the habits of individuals concerning the foods they eat are more likely to be needed to control this infection in those persons with modified host resistance. When one looks at the number of infectious agents that could cause disease in the immunosuppressed, and the number of such persons, it is evident that a market exists for foods for this group. There are foods that are salt free or salt reduced, fat free or fat reduced, sugar free or sugar reduced, and there is a market potential for special foods for the immunosuppressed.

MODIFIED VEHICLES OF INFECTION

The use of ground beef for food is well known, long established, and has been a staple for many fast food manufacturers. Steak tartar is on many menus and there are many people in the world who feel that eating rare or partially cooked beef is the best way to utilize this particular product. When outbreaks of hemorrhagic colitis associated with *Escherichia coli* O157:H7 were traced to beef products (28,29), in particular to ground beef, new control methods were needed. Either hamburgers had to be well cooked, the organism eliminated from the ultimate reservoir (usually cattle), or ways found to prevent the entry of the organism into meat products following slaughter. The increase in hemorrhagic colitis and its complications (30–33), in association with recognized outbreaks, suggest that something new has occurred. Perhaps, in the past, the food processing industry was not as centralized as it is at present, so that contamination of food, at a low level, could not lead to disease occurrence in wide areas and in large numbers. The details are presented in the chapter by Griffin. It appears that this increasing problem is an example of a modified vehicle of infection.

Another potential new vehicle for enteric infection is direct use of human sewage or reused wastewater. Anxieties have arisen concerning the potential that there will be contamination of raw vegetables and fruits by reused wastewater. Wastewater, sometimes reused wastewater, is used in many parts of the world in association with foods shipped by air and then eaten raw in another part of the world. The potential for infectious agents to be spread by wastewater is great, and control of this practice is difficult. Outbreaks associated with picked fresh fruits (34–36) or vegetables (37–39) may be associated with contaminated water or impaired personal hygiene.

Distribution of vacuum-packed foods, not maintained under refrigeration, is an increasing practice. Anxieties concerning side effects of nitrates as a preservative have reduced its use. Potentially, this phenomenon allows sporulation of *Clostridium* and could increase the risk of foodborne botulism (40). When canning was the major form of food preservation, botulism was controlled by careful time–temperature regulations. Present use of alternative methods of food preservation has the potential to lead to problems associated with *Clostridium botulinum.*

MODIFIED PATHOGENS

With each of the major new enteric outbreaks that have occurred in the last two decades, two questions need to be answered. Is the agent new? Is it modified or has something else changed to allow disease occurrence? In the United Kingdom, a new disease, bovine spongiform encephalopathy (BSE), occurred following a change in regulations concerning rendering of animal waste (41). A less expensive process to produce tallow was introduced, and the residual material from animals, including sheep, was used for cattle food. The result, in this instance, may have been the transmission of a sheep prion disease to cattle. BSE developed in cattle presumably as a result of a transformation of the sheep prion agent to one that infected cattle. Almost immediately, the question arose as to whether such a transformed agent would have the same characteristics as its parent, which did not appear to be pathogenic for humans, or would, in its new host, have modified pathogenicity for humans.

MODIFIED METHODS OF CONTROL

With each of the preceding examples, there are questions about which control measures are available to deal with modified environments, modified host resistances, modified reservoirs, modified vehicles of infection, and modified pathogens. The cheapest method is to avoid foods with known risks. Although the least expensive, it is often also the least successful. Documenting the risks associated with eating of uncooked shellfish appears to have an imperceptible effect. A more successful method is to reduce the hazard in a food before it reaches the human host. More expensive and less effective control methods are those that are performed after contamination already has occurred. For example, elimination of *Salmonella enteritidis* infection from breeding poultry flocks would be the most effective way to reduce the potential for transmission by eggs, while instruction of consumers to better cook their eggs is likely to be incompletely successful. There are, in addition to such direct measures, others that can reduce the magnitude of contamination.

One method to reduce specific bacterial contamination of poultry is the oral introduction of anaerobic flora from the gastrointestinal tract of adult birds to newly hatched chicks, a method called "competitive exclusion." The commercial use of the competitive exclusion (CE) concept was developed in the early 1970s in Finland by Nurmi and others (42). Fifteen years after the introduction of CE treatment, over 70% of Finnish poultry producers use it routinely. The number of *Salmonella*-positive flocks is less than 5% and the incidence of *Salmonella*-contaminated broiler carcasses has been 5% to 11% in the 1990s. The average number of *Salmonella* cells on contaminated carcasses is generally less than 5 per carcass (43). CE treatment protects against all *Salmonella* serotypes capable of intestinal colonization. For example, it protected against oral challenge by *Salmonella enteritidis* PT4. The average number of salmonellae was less than 10 colony forming units (CFU)/g of cecal contents in the treated birds and more than 10×10^6 CFU/g in the untreated birds (44). Spray or "droplet" application and administration in the first drinking water gave similar protection, although the degree of protection obtained varied with the type of preparation and host origin (45). Although the CE product (Broilact) was effective against *Salmonella*, it was inactive against *Campylobacter* (46). Other products have

been developed for *Campylobacter* and could be developed for other infectious agents. If this method could be applied more widely in the commercial production of poultry, it might reduce the frequency of foodborne illness associated with poultry products.

Another method to reduce bacterial contamination of food is use of irradiation (47). Although there is much anxiety about radiation in foods (48), this stems in part from the confusion concerning irradiation of foods and contamination following accidents like that at Chernobyl, where there was exposure of food animals and farming areas to radioactive materials. The industrial applications of ionizing radiation, including sterilization of medical supplies, are well established all over the world, with the efficacy dependent on accurate dosimetry assuring both an effective result at the lowest cost and the safety of consumers (49). Food irradiation has been demonstrated to be safe, effective, and versatile as a process of food preservation, decontamination, or disinfection (50). There is increasing recognition and acceptance of food irradiation based on the Codex Standard for Irradiated Foods and its associated Code of Practice (51). Clear economic advantages and health benefits of sterilizing food in this manner exist. Toxicological and nutritional evaluations have repeatedly confirmed the safety of irradiated foods. Effects on nutritional quality are frequently comparable with heat treatment and sometimes more conservative, particularly if oxygen is excluded (52). Animal feeding studies, conducted during a 12-year program from the 1970s through the early 1980s, using doses of up to 10 kilogray (10 kGy) of irradiated wheat flour, potatoes, rice, iced ocean fish, mangoes, spices, dried dates, and cocoa powder in feeding experiments, demonstrated the safety of these foods when fed to a variety of animals over long periods of time (22).

One problem with public acceptance of food irradiation relates to the reliability of labeling concerning use of irradiation. Irradiated foods should be appropriately labeled. Tests for the use of radiation would help to enforce necessary controls. Various methods are available that reveal the previous use of irradiation treatment. The three most successful methods now in use are thermoluminescence, electron spin resonance (ESR) spectroscopy, and detection of volatiles (53). ESR spectroscopy can be used for the detection of irradiation of various groups of foodstuffs and has been used to develop an official method according to the German law section 35 LMBG (54). Calcified tissues in several foods give rise to characteristic ESR spectra on irradiation (55). The limits of detection of irradiation vary among the studied animal species.

Irradiation is highly effective against bacterial pathogens that are found on chickens (56). Both *Salmonella* and *L. monocytogenes* may be safely eliminated from broiler chicken carcasses (57). Irradiation is potentially an effective method to control *E. coli* O157:H7 foodborne contamination. No measurable verotoxin from *E. coli* O157:H7 was found in finely ground lean beef that had been heavily contaminated (10^5), then irradiated, and then subjected to temperature abuse at 35°C for 20 hr (58).

Liver fluke infection by *Opisthorchis viverrini* is the leading cause of foodborne parasitic disease in Thailand.

Approximately one-third of the population and 60% of the workforce in the northeastern region of the country are infected by this parasite. Irradiation of fish flesh infected by metacercariae of *O. viverrini* is an effective method of control. Economic analyses indicate that the public health benefit from preventing infection with this parasite could outweigh the investment cost of irradiation facilities (59).

Reduction of indigenous microflora in mechanically deboned chicken meat by irradiation may create better conditions for the growth of salmonellae and may thus increase the risk of salmonellosis when accidental contamination and temperature abuse occur after a radiation treatment (60). Gamma rays do not induce radioactivity in foods, but x-rays and fast electrons can induce short-lived radioactivity if sufficiently energetic. This consideration imposes limitations on the radiation energies that can be used, and the World Health Organization recommends doses of less than 10 kGy. With these doses, there is no problem with radiation in the food (61).

There remain questions about the routine use of irradiation as a method of decontamination of foods. Selective changes in the microflora, caused by nonsterilizing radiation doses, might make known pathogens more likely to occur or bring into prominence unfamiliar pathogens. Mutations might make pathogens more virulent or more difficult to recognize, and new pathogens might arise (62). Irradiation of food to control microbial load has been regarded by many with suspicion because current and some proposed labeling does not indicate that it has been used (63). Now that effective detection methods are available, this no longer need be a problem.

Irradiation produces chemical changes in foodstuffs, and some foods, such as dairy products, are unsuitable for irradiation (22). Some loss in nutritional quality can take place. At low doses (up to 1 kGy), the loss of nutrients is insignificant. With medium doses (1 to 10 kGy), vitamin losses may occur in foods exposed to air during irradiation or storage (22). Irradiation does not eliminate all risk from microbial contamination. As a result, irradiated foods must be stored and handled with the same regard for safety as that accorded nonirradiated or other unsterilized foods (22).

In order to cope with the many changes that are occurring in microbes, reservoirs, hosts, and economic realities, attitudes and methods must respond to the changes, and we must be prepared to try new approaches to reduce the magnitude and character of the burden of enteric disease that faces us.

REFERENCES

1. Taylor JL, Tuttle J, Pramukul T, et al. An outbreak of cholera in Maryland associated with imported commercial frozen fresh coconut milk. *J Infect Dis* 1993;167:1330–1335.
2. Glass RI, Black RE. The epidemiology of cholera. In: Barua D, Greenough WB III, eds. *Cholera.* New York: Plenum Medical Book, 1992;129–154.
3. Swerdlow DL, Mintz ED, Rodriguez M, et al. Waterborne transmission of epidemic cholera in Trujillo, Peru: lessons for a continent at risk. *Lancet* 1992;340:28–33.
4. Levine MM, Kaper JB. Live oral vaccines against cholera: an update. *Vaccine* 1993;11:207–212.
5. St Louis ME, Porter JD, Helal A, et al. Epidemic cholera in West Africa: the role of food handling and high-risk foods. *Am J Epidemiol* 1990;131:719–728.
6. Gast RK, Beard CW. Research to understand and control *Salmonella enteritidis* in chickens and eggs. *Poult Sci* 1993;72:1157–1163.
7. Binkin N, Scuderi G, Novaco F, et al. Egg-related *Salmonella enteritidis,* Italy, 1991. *Epidemiol Infect* 1993;110:227–237.
8. Poppe C, Johnson RP, Forsberg CM, Irwin RJ. *Salmonella enteritidis* and other *Salmonella* in laying hens and eggs, from flocks with *Salmonella* in their environment. *Can J Vet Res* 1992;56:226–232.
9. Altekruse S, Koehler J, Hickman-Brenner F, Tauxe RV, Ferris K. A comparison of *Salmonella enteritidis* phage types from egg-associated outbreaks and implicated laying flocks. *Epidemiol Infect* 1993;110:17–22.
10. Hedberg CW, David MJ, White KE, MacDonald KL, Osterholm MT. Role of egg consumption in sporadic *Salmonella enteritidis* and *Salmonella typhimurium* infections in Minnesota. *J Infect Dis* 1993;167:107–111.
11. Neter E. Epidemic and endemic diarrheal diseases of the infant. *Ann NY Acad Sci* 1956;66:3–230.
12. Riley LW, Ceballos BS, Trabulsi LR, Fernandes de Toledo MR, Blake PA. The significance of hospitals as reservoirs for endemic multiresistant *Salmonella typhimurium* causing infection in urban Brazilian children. *J Infect Dis* 1984;150:236–241.
13. Shi J. A survey of nosocomial infection by *Salmonella typhimurium. Chung Hua Liu Hsing Ping Hsueh Tsa Chih (Chinese J Epidemiol)* 1990;11:284–287.
14. Joseph AT, Rammurty DV, Srivastava L, Gupta R, Mohan M, Anand NK. *Salmonella senftenberg* outbreak in a neonatal unit. *Indian Pediatr* 1990;27:157–160.
15. Khan MA, Abdur-Rab M, Israr N, et al. Transmission of *Salmonella worthington* by oropharyngeal suction in hospital neonatal unit. *Pediatr Infect Dis J* 1991;10:668–672.
16. Hammami A, Arlet G, Ben Redjeb S, et al. Nosocomial outbreak of acute gastroenteritis in a neonatal intensive care unit in Tunisia caused by multiply drug resistant *Salmonella wien* producing SHV-2 beta-lactamase. *Eur J Clin Microbiol Infect Dis* 1991;10:641–646.
17. Blaser MJ, Hickman FW, Farmer JJ 3rd, Brenner DJ, Balows A, Feldman RA. *Salmonella typhi:* the laboratory as a reservoir of infection. *J Infect Dis* 1980;142:934–938.
18. Gustavsen S, Breen O. Investigation of an outbreak of *Salmonella oranienburg* infections in Norway, caused by contaminated black pepper. *Am J Epidemiol* 1984;119:806–812.
19. Schaffner CP, Mosbach K, Bibit VS, Watson CH. Coconut and *Salmonella* infection. *Appl Microbiol* 1967;15:471–475.
20. Craven PC, Mackel DC, Baine WB, Barker WH, Gangarosa EJ. International outbreak of *Salmonella eastbourne* infection traced to contaminated chocolate. *Lancet* 1975;1:788–792.
21. Gill ON, Sockett PN, Bartlett CL, et al. Outbreak of *Salmonella napoli* infection caused by contaminated chocolate bars. *Lancet* 1983;1:574–577.
22. World Health Organization. *Food irradiation: a technique for preserving and improving the safety of food.* Geneva: World Health Organization, 1988;39.
23. Schlech WF 3rd, Lavigne PM, Bortolussi RA, et al. Epidemic listeriosis—evidence for transmission by food. *N Engl J Med* 1983;308:203–206.
24. Schuchat A, Swaminathan B, Broome CV. Epidemiology of human listeriosis. *Clin Microbiol Rev* 1991;4:169–183.
25. Schuchat A, Deaver KA, Wenger JD, et al. Role of foods in sporadic listeriosis. I. Case–control study of dietary risk factors. The Listeria Study Group. *JAMA* 1992;267:2041–2045.
26. Pinner RW, Schuchat A, Swaminathan B, et al. Role of foods in sporadic listeriosis. II. Microbiologic and epidemiologic investigation. The Listeria Study Group. *JAMA* 1992;267:2046–2050.
27. Art D, Andre P. Clinical and epidemiological aspects of listeriosis in Belgium, 1985–1990. *Int J Med Microbiol* 1991;275:549–556.
28. Riley LW. The epidemiologic, clinical, and microbiologic fea-

tures of hemorrhagic colitis. *Annu Rev Microbiol* 1987;41:383–407.

29. Ostroff SM, Griffin PM, Tauxe RV, et al. A statewide outbreak of *Escherichia coli* O157:H7 infections in Washington State. *Am J Epidemiol* 1990;132:239–247.

30. Griffin PM, Tauxe RV. The epidemiology of infections caused by *Escherichia coli* O157:H7, other enterohemorrhagic *E. coli,* and the associated hemolytic uremic syndrome. *Epidemiol Rev* 1991;13:60–98.

31. Tarr PI, Hickman RO. Hemolytic uremic syndrome epidemiology: a population-based study in King County, Washington, 1971 to 1980. *Pediatrics* 1987;80:41–45.

32. Tarr PI, Neill MA, Allen J, Siccardi CJ, Watkins SL, Hickman RO. The increasing incidence of the hemolytic-uremic syndrome in King County, Washington: lack of evidence for ascertainment bias. *Am J Epidemiol* 1989;129:582–506.

33. Martin DL, MacDonald KL, White KE, Soler JT, Osterholm MT. The epidemiology and clinical aspects of the hemolytic uremic syndrome in Minnesota. *N Engl J Med* 1990;323:1161–1167.

34. Fredlund H, Back E, Sjoberg L, Tornquist E. Water-melon as a vehicle of transmission of shigellosis. *Scand J Infect Dis* 1987;19:219–221.

35. Niu MT, Polish LB, Robertson BH, et al. Multistate outbreak of hepatitis A associated with frozen strawberries. *J Infect Dis* 1992;166:518–524.

36. Anonymous. Multistate outbreak of *Salmonella poona* infections—United States and Canada, 1991. *MMWR Morb Mortal Wkly Rep* 1991;40:549–552.

37. Warner RD, Carr RW, McCleskey FK, Johnson PC, Elmer LM, Davison VE. A large nontypical outbreak of Norwalk virus. Gastroenteritis associated with exposing celery to nonpotable water and with *Citrobacter freundii*. *Arch Intern Med* 1991;151:2419–2424.

38. Rosenblum LS, Mirkin IR, Allen DT, Safford S, Hadler SC. A multifocal outbreak of hepatitis A traced to commercially distributed lettuce. *Am J Public Health* 1990;80:1075–1079.

39. Martin DL, Gustafson TL, Pelosi JW, Suarez L, Pierce GV. Contaminated produce—a common source for two outbreaks of *Shigella* gastroenteritis. *Am J Epidemiol* 1986;124:299–305.

40. Nurmi E, Hirn J. Integration of hygiene into food technology. In: Lindroth S, Ryynänen SSI, eds. *Food technology in the year 2000. Bibliotheca Nutritio et Dieta,* vol 47, Basel: Karger, 1990; 12–18.

41. Tyrrell DA. An overview of bovine spongiform encephalopathy (BSE) in Britain. *Dev Biol Stand* 1992;76:275–284.

42. Nurmi E, Nuotio L, Schneitz C. The competitive exclusion concept: development and future. *Int J Food Microbiol* 1992;15:237–240.

43. Hirn J, Nurmi E, Johansson T, Nuotio L. Long-term experience with competitive exclusion and salmonellas in Finland. *Int J Food Microbiol* 1992;15:281–285.

44. Schneitz C, Nuotio L, Mead G, Nurmi E. Competitive exclusion in the young bird: challenge models, administration and reciprocal protection. *Int J Food Microbiol* 1992;15:241–244.

45. Schneitz C, Hakkinen M, Nuotio L, Nurmi E, Mead G. Droplet application for protecting chicks against *Salmonella* colonisation by competitive exclusion. *Vet Rec* 1990;126:510.

46. Aho M, Nuotio L, Nurmi E, Kiiskinen T. Competitive exclusion of campylobacters from poultry with K-bacteria and Broilact. *Int J Food Microbiol* 1992;15:265–275.

47. World Health Organization. *Food irradiation: a technique for preserving and improving the safety of food.* Geneva: World Health Organization, 1988;1–84.

48. Murray DR. *Biology of food irradiation.* New York: Wiley, 1990.

49. Bartolotta A, Onori S, Pantaloni M. Comparative calibration of dosimetry methods used around industrial irradiation plants in Italy. *Ann Ist Super Sanita* 1989;25:319–326.

50. Olszyna-Marzys AE. Radioactivity and foods. *Bull Pan Am Health Organ* 1991;25:27–40.

51. Sigurbjornsson B, Loaharanu P. Irradiation and food processing. *Bibl Nutr Dieta* 1989;43:13–30.

52. Diehl JF. Food irradiation: is it an alternative to chemical preservatives? *Food Addit Contam* 1992;9:409–416.

53. Raffi J, Stevenson MH, Kent M, Thiery JM, Belliardo JJ. European intercomparison on electron spin resonance identification of irradiated foodstuffs. *Int J Food Sci Technol* 1992;27:111–124.

54. Helle N, Linke B, Mager M, Schreiber G, Bogl KW. Status of the development of electron spin resonance measurement for the detection of irradiated food. *Z Ernahrungswiss* 1992;31:205–218.

55. Dodd NJ, Lea JS, Swallow AJ. The ESR detection of irradiated food. *Int J Radiat Appl Instrum [A]* 1989;40:1211–1214.

56. Kohler B, Hubner H, Krautschick M. The use of ionizing radiation for the decontamination of salmonella-containing slaughtered broiler chickens and powdered eggs. *Z Gesamte Hyg* 1989;35:665–668.

57. Lewis SJ, Corry JE. Survey of the incidence of *Listeria monocytogenes* and other *Listeria* spp. in experimentally irradiated and in matched unirradiated raw chickens. *Int J Food Microbiol* 1991;12:257–262.

58. Thayer DW, Boyd G. Elimination of *Escherichia coli* O157:H7 in meats by gamma irradiation. *Appl Environ Microbiol* 1993;59:1030–1034.

59. Loaharanu P, Sornmani P. Preliminary estimates of economic impact of live fluke infection in Thailand and the feasibility of irradiation as a control measure. *Southeast Asian J Trop Med Public Health* 1991;22(Suppl):384–390.

60. Szczawinska ME, Thayer DW, Phillips JG. Fate of unirradiated *Salmonella* in irradiated mechanically deboned chicken meat. *Int J Food Microbiol* 1991;14:314–324.

61. Swallow AJ. Wholesomeness and safety of irradiated foods. *Adv Exp Med Biol* 1991;289:11–31.

62. Farkas J. Microbiological safety of irradiated foods. *Int J Food Microbiol* 1989;9:1–15.

63. Murray DR. *Biology of food irradiation.* New York: Wiley, 1990;183–187.

Subject Index